Zakim and Boyer's Hepatology

Zakim and Boyer's Hepatology

A Textbook of Liver Disease

SIXTH EDITION

THOMAS D. BOYER, MD
Chairman of Medicine
Robert and Irene Flinn Professor of Medicine
Director, Liver Research Institute
University of Arizona College of Medicine
Tucson, Arizona

MICHAEL P. MANNS, MD
Professor and Chairman
Department of Gastroenterology, Hepatology, and Endocrinology
Hannover Medical School
Hannover, Germany

ARUN J. SANYAL, MBBS, MD
Charles Caravati Professor of Medicine
Chairman, Division of Gastroenterology, Hepatology, and Internal Medicine
Virginia Commonwealth University School of Medicine
Richmond, Virginia

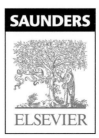

SAUNDERS

ELSEVIER

1600 John F. Kennedy Blvd.
Ste 1800
Philadelphia, PA 19103-2899

ZAKIM AND BOYER'S HEPATOLOGY   ISBN: 978-1-4377-0881-3

Previous editions copyrighted 1982, 1990, 1996, 2003, 2006

Library of Congress Cataloging-in-Publication Data

Zakim and Boyer's hepatology: a textbook of liver disease / [edited by] Thomas D. Boyer, Michael P. Manns, Arun J. Sanyal.—6th ed.
    p. ; cm.
    Hepatology
    Includes bibliographical references and index.
    ISBN 978-1-4377-0881-3 (hardcover : alk. paper)
    1. Liver—Diseases.   I. Boyer, Thomas D.   II. Manns, Michael P. (Michael Peter)   III. Sanyal, Arun
J.   IV. Zakim, David.   V. Title: Hepatology.
    [DNLM: 1. Liver Diseases.   WI 700]
    RC845.H46 2012
    616.3'62—dc23

                                                                        2011024933

Senior Acquisitions Editor: Kate Dimock
Senior Developmental Editor: Janice M. Gaillard
Editorial Assistant: Kate Crowley
Publishing Services Manager: Anne Altepeter
Senior Project Manager: Cheryl A. Abbott
Design Direction: Steven Stave
Marketing Manager: Abby Swartz

Printed in China

Last digit is the print number: 9 8 7 6 5 4 3 2 1

Contributors

Paul C. Adams, MD
Professor of Medicine
Department of Medicine
University Hospital
London, Ontario, Canada

Helmut Albrecht, MD
Heyward Gibbes Distinguished Professor
    of Medicine and Division Chief
Division of Infectious Diseases
School of Medicine
University of South Carolina
Columbia, South Carolina

Jasmohan Bajaj, MBBS, MD, MSc
Associate Professor of Medicine
Division of Gastroenterology, Hepatology,
    and Nutrition
Department of Medicine
Virginia Commonwealth University
    and McGuire Veterans Administration
    Medical Center
Richmond, Virginia

Soon Koo Baik, MD
Department of Medicine
Yonsei University Wonju College of Medicine
Wonju, Korea

Ulrich Beuers, MD
Professor of Gastroenterology and Hepatology
Department of Gastroenterology
    and Hepatology
Tytgat Institute for Liver and Intestinal Research
Academic Medical Center
University of Amsterdam
Amsterdam, Netherlands

Scott W. Biggins, MD, MAS
Assistant Professor, Section of Hepatology
    and Liver Transplantation
Division of Gastroenterology
Anschutz Medical Campus
University of Colorado, Denver
Aurora, Colorado

Henri Bismuth, MD
Centre Hepato Biliaire
Paris, France

Kirsten Muri Boberg, MD, PhD
Consulting Physician
Norwegian PSC Research Center
Clinic for Specialized Medicine and Surgery
Oslo University Hospital, Rikshospitalet
Oslo, Norway

Herbert L. Bonkovsky, MD
Vice President, Research
Director, The Liver, Digestive, and Metabolic
    Disorders Laboratory
Department of Medicine
Division of Education and Research
Carolinas Medical Center
Charlotte, North Carolina;
Professor, Medicine
University of Connecticut Health Center
Farmington, Connecticut;
Professor, Biology
University of North Carolina, Charlotte
Charlotte, North Carolina;
Clinical Professor, Medicine
University of North Carolina, Chapel Hill
Chapel Hill, North Carolina

Jaime Bosch, MD, PhD
Professor of Medicine
University of Barcelona
Liver Unit Hospital Clinic
Barcelona, Spain

Thomas D. Boyer, MD
Chairman of Medicine
Robert and Irene Flinn Professor of Medicine
Director, Liver Research Institute
University of Arizona College of Medicine
Tucson, Arizona

Elizabeth M. Brunt, MD
Professor, Pathology and Immunology
Washington University School of Medicine
St. Louis, Missouri

Martin Caselitz, MD
Assistant Professor of Medicine (Privatdozent)
Medical Clinic II, Klinikum Deggendorf
Deggendorf, Germany

Wolfgang H. Caselmann, MD, PhD
Professor of Medicine
Head of Division, Bavarian State Ministry
    of the Environment and Public Health
Munich, Germany

Matt Cave, MD
Assistant Professor
Department of Medicine
Division of Gastroenterology, Hepatology,
    and Nutrition
Department of Pharmacology and Toxicology
University of Louisville
Louisville, Kentucky

Henry Lik-Yuen Chan, MD, FRCP
Professor, Division of Gastroenterology
    and Hepatology
Director, Cheng Suen Man Shook Centre
    for Hepatitis Research
Director, Center for Liver Health
Department of Medicine and Therapeutics
The Chinese University of Hong Kong, Shatin
Hong Kong, China

Kyong-Mi Chang, MD
Associate Professor of Medicine
Department of Medicine
Philadelphia Veterans Administration Medical
    Center and University of Pennsylvania
Philadelphia, Pennsylvania

Alessia Ciancio, MD, PhD
University of Turin
AOU San Giovanni Battista di Torino
Dip Gastro-Hepatology
Torino, Italy

Massimo Colombo, MD
Professor, First Division of Gastroenterology
Fondazione IRCCS Ca'Granda Ospedale
    Maggiore Policlinico
Universita degli Studi di Milano
Milan, Italy

Hari S. Conjeevaram, MD, MS
Associate Professor, Department of Internal
    Medicine
Director, GI Fellowship Training Program
University of Michigan
Ann Arbor, Michigan

Diane W. Cox, PhD, CCMG, FRSC
Professor, Medical Genetics
University of Alberta, Edmonton
Alberta, Canada

Chris P. Day, FMedSci
Professor, Institute of Cellular Medicine
Newcastle University
Newcastle upon Tyne, United Kingdom

R. Brian Doctor, PhD
Associate Professor
Department of Medicine
University of Colorado, Denver
Denver, Colorado

Ronald P.J. Oude Elferink, PhD
Tytgat Institute for Liver and Intestinal Research
Academic Medical Center
University of Amsterdam
Amsterdam, Netherlands

Scott A. Elisofon, MD
Instructor in Pediatrics
Harvard Medical School;
Division of Pediatric Gastroenterology
Children's Hospital, Boston
Boston, Massachusetts

Hashem B. El-Serag, MD, MPH
Professor of Medicine
Chief, Gastroenterology and Hepatology
Michael E. DeBakey Veterans Administration
    Medical Center and Baylor College of Medicine
Houston, Texas

Gamal Esmat, MD
Professor of Tropical Medicine and Hepatology
Department of Tropical Medicine
Faculty of Medicine
Cairo University
Cairo, Egypt

Gregory T. Everson, MD
Professor of Medicine
School of Medicine
Director of Hepatology
Division of Gastroenterology and Hepatology
University of Colorado, Denver
Aurora, Colorado

Keith Cameron Falkner
Senior Research Associate
Department of Medicine
Division of Gastroenterology, Hepatology,
    and Nutrition
University of Louisville
Louisville, Kentucky

Michael B. Fallon, MD
Professor of Medicine
Division Director, Division of Gastroenterology,
    Hepatology, and Nutrition
University of Texas Health Science Center
    at Houston
Houston, Texas

Sandy Feng, MD, PhD
Associate Professor of Surgery
Director, Abdominal Transplant Surgery
    Fellowship
University of California, San Francisco
San Francisco, California

Hans-Peter Fischer, MD
Professor, Department of Pathology
Bonn University
Bonn, Germany

Brett E. Fortune, MD
Gastroenterology/Hepatology Fellow
Division of Gastroenterology and Hepatology
University of Colorado
Aurora, Colorado

Scott L. Friedman, MD
Fishberg Professor of Medicine
Division of Liver Diseases
Mount Sinai School of Medicine
New York, New York

J.C. García-Pagán, MD, PhD
Senior Consultant in Hepatology
Liver Unit, Hospital Clinic
Barcelona, Spain;
Senior Research, IDIBAPS and CIBERehd
Barcelona, Spain

Guadalupe Garcia-Tsao, MD
Professor of Medicine
Internal Medicine/Digestive Diseases
Yale University
New Haven, Connecticut;
Chief, Digestive Diseases
Veterans Administration Connecticut
    Healthcare System
West Haven, Connecticut

Fayez K. Ghishan, MD
Horace W. Steele Endowed Chair
    in Pediatric Research
Professor and Head
Director, Steele Children's Research
    Center, Pediatrics
University of Arizona
Tucson, Arizona

Gregory J. Gores, MD
Reuben R. Eisenberg Professor of Medicine
Division of Gastroenterology and Hepatology
College of Medicine
Mayo Clinic
Rochester, Minnesota

Rainer W. Gruessner, MD, FACS
Professor of Surgery and Immunology
Chairman, Department of Surgery
University of Arizona
Tucson, Arizona

Sanjeev Gupta, MBBS, MD, FRCP
The Eleazar and Feige Reicher Chair
    in Translational Medicine
Professor of Medicine (Gastroenterology
    and Liver Diseases) and Pathology
Albert Einstein College of Medicine
Bronx, New York

Ghassan M. Hammoud, MD, MPH
Assistant Professor of Clinical Medicine
Director, Section of Hepatology
    and Biliary Disease
Division of Gastroenterology and Hepatology
University of Missouri School of Medicine
Columbia, Missouri

**E.J. Heathcote, MBBS, MD, FRCP,
    FRCP(C)**
The Francis Family Chair
    in Hepatology Research
Professor of Medicine
University of Toronto;
Head, Patient-Based Clinical Research
Toronto Western Research Institute
Toronto Western Hospital
Toronto, Ontario, Canada

Steve M. Helmke, PhD
Research Instructor
Division of Gastroenterology and Hepatology
University of Colorado School of Medicine
Aurora, Colorado

**G.M. Hirschfield, MA, MB BChir,
    MRCP, PhD**
Staff Hepatologist/Assistant Professor
Liver Centre, Toronto Western Hospital
Department of Medicine
University of Toronto
Toronto, Ontario, Canada

Douglas Hunt, MD
Department of Medicine
Division of Gastroenterology and Hepatology
Scripps Green Hospital
La Jolla, California

Massimo Iavarone, MD, PhD
First Division of Gastroenterology
Fondazione IRCCS Ca' Granda
    Maggiore Hospital
Milan, Italy

Jamal A. Ibdah, MD, PhD, AGAF
Professor and Raymond E. and Vaona H. Peck
    Research Chair
Director, Digestive Health Center
Director, University of Missouri Columbia
    Institute for Clinical and Translational Science
Senior Associate Dean for Research
School of Medicine
University of Missouri, Columbia
Columbia, Missouri

Françoise Imbert-Bismut, PhD
APHP UPMC Liver Center
Biochemistry Unit
Paris, France

Peter L.M. Jansen, MD, PhD
Professor, Gastroenterology and Hepatology
Academic Medical Center
Amsterdam, Netherlands

Benjamin F. Johnson, MD
Assistant Physician
Department of Medicine
University of California, San Diego
San Diego, California

Maureen M.F. Jonas, MD
Associate Professor, Pediatrics
Harvard Medical School;
Senior Associate in Medicine
Division of Gastroenterology
Children's Hospital, Boston
Boston, Massachusetts

Dean P. Jones, PhD
Professor of Medicine
Director, Clinical Biomarkers Laboratory
Division of Pulmonary, Allergy, and Critical
    Care Medicine
Emory University
Atlanta, Georgia

Patrick S. Kamath, MD
Professor of Medicine
Division of Gastroenterology and Hepatology
Mayo Clinic College of Medicine
Rochester, Minnesota

Tom H. Karlsen, MD, PhD
Department of Organ Transplantation,
   Gastroenterology, and Nephrology
Oslo University Hospital Rikshospitalet
Oslo, Norway

**Deirdre Kelly, FRCPH, FRCP, FRCPI,
   MD, MB, BA**
Professor of Paediatric Hepatology
The Liver Unit
Birmingham Children's Hospital
Birmingham, West Midlands, United Kingdom

J. Kettelle, MD
Assistant Professor of Clinical Surgery
Surgery
University of Arizona
Tucson, Arizona

Khalid M. Khan, MB, ChB
Associate Professor
Surgery
University of Arizona
Tucson, Arizona

Percy Knolle, MD
Professor, Institutes of Molecular Medicine
   and Experimental Immunology
Friedrich-Wilhelms-Universität Bonn
Bonn, Germany

David J. Kramer, MD, FACP
Professor of Medicine, College of Medicine
Director, Transplant Critical Care Service
Mayo Clinic
Jacksonville, Florida

Manoj Kumar, MD, DM
Department of Gastroenterology
G.B. Pant Hospital
New Delhi, India

Navaneeth C. Kumar, MD, MBBS
Chennai, India

Jennifer C. Lai, MD
Fellow in Gastroenterology
University of California, San Francisco
San Francisco, California

Réal Lapointe, MD, FRCSC
Professor of Surgery
Head of Division of General Surgery
Department of Surgery
University of Montreal
Montreal, Quebec, Canada;
Head of Hepato-Pancreato-Biliary and Liver
   Transplant Service
Department of Surgery
Montreal University Medical Center
Montreal, Quebec, Canada

Konstantinos N. Lazaridis, MD
Associate Professor of Medicine
Department of Gastroenterology and Hepatology
The Mayo Clinic
Rochester, Minnesota

André Lechel, MD
Institute of Molecular Medicine
   and Max-Planck-Research Department
   for Stem Cell Aging
Ulm University
Ulm, Germany

Samuel S. Lee, MD, FRCPC
Professor of Medicine
University of Calgary
Calgary, Alberta, Canada

Riccardo Lencioni, MD
Director, Division of Diagnostic Imaging
   and Intervention
Pisa University Hospital;
Associate Professor of Radiology
University of Pisa
Pisa, Italy

Cynthia Levy, MD
Associate Professor of Medicine
Center for Liver Diseases
Division of Hepatology
University of Miami Miller School of Medicine
Miami, Florida

Keith D. Lindor, MD
Dean, Mayo Medical School
Professor of Medicine
Division of Gastroenterology and Hepatology
Mayo Clinic
Rochester, Minnesota

**Stephen Locarnini, MBBS, BSc(Hon),
   PhD, FRC(Path)**
Professor
Head, Research and Molecular Development
Victorian Infectious Diseases
   Reference Laboratory
North Melbourne, Victoria, Australia

Anna S.F. Lok, MD
Professor, Internal Medicine
University of Michigan
Ann Arbor, Michigan

Harmeet Malhi, MBBS
Assistant Professor of Medicine
Department of Medicine
Division of Gastroenterology and Hepatology
Mayo Clinic
Rochester, Minnesota

Michael P. Manns, MD
Professor and Chairman
Department of Gastroenterology, Hepatology,
   and Endocrinology
Hannover Medical School
Hannover, Germany

Jorge A. Marrero, MD, MS
Keith S. Henley, MD, Collegiate Professor
   of Gastroenterology
Director, Multidisciplinary Liver Tumor Clinic;
Department of Medicine
University of Michigan
Ann Arbor, Michigan

Craig McClain, MD
Professor, Departments of Medicine
   and Pharmacology and Toxicology
Distinguished University Scholar
Associate Vice President
   for Translational Research
University of Louisville
Louisville, Kentucky

Robert McCuskey, AB, PhD
Professor Emeritus of Cell Biology
   and Anatomy, Physiology, and Pediatrics
Department of Cell Biology and Anatomy
University of Arizona
Tucson, Arizona

Barbara H. McGovern, MD
Associate Professor
Tufts University School of Medicine
Boston, Massachusetts

John G. McHutchison, MD
Senior Vice President
Liver Diseases
Gilead Sciences, Inc.
Foster City, California

Darius Moradpour, MD
Professor and Chief
Division of Gastroenterology and Hepatology
Centre Hospitalier Universitaire Vaudois
University of Lausanne
Lausanne, Switzerland

Victor J. Navarro, MD
Professor of Medicine, Pharmacology,
   and Experimental Therapeutics
Thomas Jefferson University
Philadelphia, Pennsylvania

James Neuberger, DM, FRCP
Consultant Physician
Liver Unit
Queen Elizabeth Hospital
Birmingham, United Kingdom

Moises I. Nevah R., MD
Clinical Fellow
Division of Gastroenterology, Hepatology,
   and Nutrition
Department of Medicine
University of Texas Health Science
   Center, Houston
Houston, Texas

Yulia A. Nevzorova, PhD
Department of Medicine III
University Hospital Aachen
Aachen, Germany

Heather M. Patton, MD
Assistant Clinical Professor of Medicine
Division of Gastroenterology
University of California, San Diego
San Diego, California

François Penin, PhD
Intitut de Biologie et Chimie des Protéines
University of Lyon
Lyon, France

David Perlmutter, MD
Vira I. Heinz Professor and Chair, Pediatrics
Professor, Cell Biology and Physiology
University of Pittsburgh School of Medicine;
Physician-in-Chief and Scientific Director
Children's Hospital of Pittsburgh of UPMC
Pittsburgh, Pennsylvania

Aurélie Plessier, MD
Hepatology
Hopital Beaujon
Clichy, France

Thierry Poynard, MD, PhD
Professor of Hepatology
Department Head
UPMC APHP Liver Center
Groupe Hospitalier Pitié Salpêtrière
Paris, France

Puneet Puri, MBBS, MD
Assistant Professor of Medicine
Division of Gastroenterology, Hepatology,
    and Nutrition
Virginia Commonwealth University
    School of Medicine
Richmond, Virginia

Charles Rice, PhD
Maurice R. and Corinne P. Greenberg Professor
Head, Laboratory of Virology
    and Infectious Disease
Scientific and Executive Director
Center for the Study of Hepatitis C
The Rockefeller University
New York, New York;
New York–Presbyterian Hospital
Weill Medical College of Cornell University
Ithaca, New York

Mario Rizzetto, MD
Experimental Department of Gastroenterology
San Giovanni Battista Hospital
Turin, Italy

Eve A. Roberts, MD, MA, FRCPC
Adjunct Professor, Paediatrics
Medicine and Pharmacology
University of Toronto
Toronto, Ontario, Canada;
Adjunct Scientist
Genetics and Genome Biology
Hospital for Sick Children Research Institute
Toronto, Ontario, Canada

Don C. Rockey, MD
Dr. Carey G. King, Jr., and Dr. Henry M.
    Winans, Sr., Chair in Internal Medicine
Chief, Division of Digestive and Liver Diseases
University of Texas Southwestern
    Medical Center
Dallas, Texas

**Jayanta Roy-Chowdhury, MD, MRCP,
AGAF**
Professor, Department of Medicine
Division of Gastroenterology and Liver Diseases
Professor, Department of Genetics
Albert Einstein College of Medicine
Bronx, New York

Namita Roy-Chowdhury, PhD
Professor, Department of Medicine
Division of Gastroenterology and Liver Diseases
Professor, Department of Genetics
Albert Einstein College of Medicine
Bronx, New York

K. Lenhard Rudolph, MD
Director, Institute of Molecular Medicine
    and Max-Planck-Research Department
    on Stem Cell Aging
Ulm University
Ulm, Germany

Mark W. Russo, MD, MPH
Medical Director of Liver Transplantation
Department of Medicine
Carolinas Medical Center
Charlotte, North Carolina

Sammy Saab, MD, MPH, AGAF
Associate Professor
Medicine and Surgery
Head, Outcomes Research in Hepatology
David Geffen School of Medicine at University
    of California, Los Angeles
Los Angeles, California

Arun J. Sanyal, MBBS, MD
Charles Caravati Professor of Medicine
Chairman, Division of Gastroenterology,
    Hepatology, and Internal Medicine
Virginia Commonwealth University
    School of Medicine
Richmond, Virginia

S.K. Sarin, MD, DM, FNASc
Professor
Head of Hepatology
Director
Institute of Liver and Biliary Sciences (ILBS)
New Delhi, India

Erik Schrumpf, MD, PhD
Professor, Head of Section of Gastroenterology
    and Hepatology
Medical Department
Oslo University Hospital–Rikshospitalet
Oslo, Norway

Leonard B. Seeff, MD
Senior Scientific Officer
National Institute of Diabetes and Digestive
    and Kidney Disease
National Institutes of Health
Bethesda, Maryland

S. Seijo, MD
Hepatic Hemodynamic Laboratory
Liver Unit
Institut de Malalties Digestives I Metaboliques
IDIBAPS, Clinic Hospital
Barcelona, Spain

Vijay H. Shah, MD
Director, Office of Postdoctoral Affairs
Professor of Medicine and Research Chair
Division of Gastroenterology and Hepatology
Mayo Clinic
Rochester, Minnesota

Steven I. Shedlofsky, MD
Professor of Medicine
Internal Medicine
University of Kentucky College of Medicine
Lexington, Kentucky

Daniel Shouval, MD
Professor of Medicine
Director, Liver Unit
Hadassah-Hebrew University Hospital
Jerusalem, Israel

Claude B. Sirlin, MD
Associate Professor
University of California, San Diego
San Diego, California

Maxwell L. Smith, MD
Director of Liver and Transplant Pathology
Assistant Professor
University of Colorado Anschutz Medical
    Campus
Aurora, Colorado

Emmanuil Smorodinsky, MD
Liver Imaging Group
Department of Radiology
University of California, San Diego
San Diego, California

Ulrich Spengler, MD
Professor, Department of Internal Medicine 1
University of Bonn
Bonn, Germany

Richard K. Sterling, MD, MSc
Professor of Medicine
Associate Chair of Education and Training
Chief of Hepatology
Division of Gastroenterology, Hepatology,
    and Nutrition
Medical Director, HIV Liver Disease
Virginia Commonwealth University
    School of Medicine
Richmond, Virginia

Stephen F. Stewart, MD, PhD
Consultant Hepatologist
Liver Unit
Freeman Hospital
Newcastle upon Tyne, United Kingdom

Doris B. Strader, MD
Associate Professor of Medicine
Internal Medicine/Division of Gastroenterology
    and Hepatology
Fletcher Allen Health Care
Burlington, Vermont

Christian P. Strassburg, MD
Professor of Gastroenterology and Hepatology
Department of Gastroenterology, Hepatology,
    and Endocrinology
Hannover Medical School
Hannover, Germany

R. Todd Stravitz, MD
Professor of Medicine
Hume-Lee Transplant Center,
    Section of Hepatology
Virginia Commonwealth University
    School of Medicine
Richmond, Virginia

Priti Sud, MD
Gastroenterology Fellow
University of Arizona
Tucson, Arizona

Mark S. Sulkowski, MD
Associate Professor of Medicine
The Johns Hopkins University
Baltimore, Maryland

Jayant A. Talwalkar, MD, MPH
Associate Professor of Medicine
Division of Gastroenterology and Hepatology
Mayo Clinic
Rochester, Minnesota

Norah A. Terrault, MD, MPH
Professor of Medicine
University of California, San Francisco
San Francisco, California

Hans L. Tillmann, MD
Assistant Professor
Gastroenterology/Hepatology Research
Duke Clinical Research Institute
Durham, North Carolina

Christian Trautwein, MD
Professor of Medicine
Department of Internal Medicine
    (Gastroenterology, Hepatology,
    and Metabolic Diseases)
University Hospital, RWTH Aachen
Aachen, Germany

Parsia A. Vagefi, MD
Clinical Instructor in Surgery
University of California, San Francisco
San Francisco, California

Dominique Valla, MD
Professor of Hepatology
Universté Denis Diderot and INSERM U773
Paris, France;
Head, Liver Unit
INSERM U773
Hôpital Beaujon
Clichy, France

Siegfried Wagner, MD, AGAF
Klinikum Deggendorf
Medizinizche Klinik II
Deggendorf, Germany;
Department of Gastroenterology, Hepatology,
    and Endocrinology
Medical School of Hannover
Hannover, Germany

Nadia Warner, MD
Molecular Research and Development
Victorian Infectious Diseases Reference
    Laboratories
Melbourne, Victoria, Australia

Vincent Wai-Sun Wong, MD
Associate Professor
Department of Medicine and Therapeutics
The Chinese University of Hong Kong
Hong Kong, China

Naglaa Zayed, MD
Assistant Professor of Tropical Medicine
    and Hepatology
Faculty of Medicine, Cairo University
Cairo, Egypt

Preface

In 1982 the first edition of *Hepatology: A Textbook of Liver Disease* was published. The book was based on pathophysiologic principles in the belief that these "principles form the basis for interpreting concepts about disease and for evaluating the validity of research." The first 12 chapters focused on normal hepatic function. The next 10 chapters focused on alterations of normal function leading to clinical illnesses, such as hepatic encephalopathy, and the last 24 chapters focused on specific disease states. There were only two chapters on viral hepatitis: one on the biology of hepatitis viruses and the second on clinical features of viral hepatitis. A single chapter on liver transplantation was included in the first edition. Over the next almost 30 years, the book has changed dramatically, largely as a reflection of the tremendous progress that has been achieved in the field of hepatology. Because we now understand better the abnormal pathophysiology seen in the patient with liver disease, this new edition focuses more on the abnormal, rather than the normal, physiology. However, the current editors, Drs. Boyer, Manns, and Sanyal, believe that a basic understanding of both normal and abnormal physiology present in the patient with liver disease is critical to provide a high level of care for this difficult patient population, as well as to advance the field of hepatology. We hope that this sixth edition of *Zakim and Boyer's Hepatology: A Textbook of Liver Disease* will serve practicing hepatologists and gastroenterologists; general physicians, such as internists and general practitioners; and basic scientists who want to know more about the clinical spectrum, therapeutic approaches, and unmet needs of the diseases they investigate and treat.

Teresa Wright and Michael Manns were new editors for the fifth edition of *Zakim and Boyer's Hepatology: A Textbook of Liver Disease*. Dr. Wright moved into industry; therefore, Dr. Arun Sanyal joined Drs. Boyer and Manns as the third editor for the sixth edition. Each of the editors brings unique expertise to the book, and we believe this experience and knowledge is reflected in the sixth edition.

The sixth edition contains five new chapters. Three cover new topics on viral hepatitis. One discusses hepatitis B and C infection in the non-liver transplant population, and the second discusses HIV and HCV co-infection and drug toxicity. The third new viral hepatitis chapter covers pathogenesis of liver injury in HBV and HCV. The fourth new chapter on the pathogenesis of hepatocellular carcinoma and the fifth new chapter on imaging techniques for the diagnosis of liver disease complete the new additions. As in the past, we have changed the authors on approximately one third of the chapters to provide fresh perspectives on subjects that have appeared in previous editions.

To keep the book at a reasonable size and reduce cost, each chapter has only 100 of the most current references in the printed book. Additional cited references will be on the Elsevier Expert Consult website, which will keep the tradition of the book being well referenced without being too large. The style that was used for the previous edition, including placing the color photomicrographs and photos within each chapter, is used again in this edition. We believe the book is more readable using this format.

Hepatology, like medicine in general and infectious diseases in particular, does not respect any borders. Liver diseases are a significant global health burden. Over the past 40 to 50 years, the discipline of hepatology has provided examples of discoveries in basic science that are immediately transformed into novel diagnostic procedures, molecular-based therapies, antitoxins, and vaccines. The discovery of the five major hepatotropic viruses is an example of success for translational medicine. Effective treatment for acetaminophen overdose has been developed from basic studies of drug metabolism and toxicity. Liver transplantation has evolved into a routine, lifesaving procedure. We have seen the global success of hepatitis A and B vaccination programs, and we are now following the clinical development of new generations of direct-acting anti-HCV drugs that hopefully will provide more effective and less toxic anti-HCV therapies. Finally, hepatocellular carcinoma, which is one of the top killers globally and one of the most important complications of end-stage liver disease, has become an area for innovative molecularly targeted anti-cancer therapies. We will be very pleased if this sixth edition is regarded as an international textbook for a global readership helping to combat a global health burden.

Acknowledgments

The creation of a book of this size involves numerous individuals. We are grateful to all of the contributors for their timely delivery of the manuscripts and the excellence of the chapters that they have written. This book would never have been published without the professional staff at Elsevier. Druanne Martin and Kate Dimock were instrumental in the creation of this edition of *Zakim and Boyer's Hepatology: A Textbook of Liver Disease.* They were there to solve problems and encourage all of us to make the best book possible. Janice Gaillard and Cheryl Abbott have been of equal importance during the production of this edition. Their work has led to a book with a new and exciting appearance, from the cover by illustrator Richard Tibbitts, to the tables, to the high-quality full-color design by Steven Stave. We realize that there are numerous other people at Elsevier who have contributed to *Zakim and Boyer's Hepatology*, and we are grateful for their efforts as well.

Lastly, we would like to thank our families, who have supported us during the genesis of this book.

Contents

xiv　　Contents

Section I

Pathophysiology of the Liver

Anatomy of the Liver

Robert McCuskey

Introduction

Overview of the Structure and Function of the Liver

The liver is the largest organ in the human body. It is incompletely separated into lobes that are covered on their external surfaces by a thin connective tissue capsule. The liver is composed of several cell types that not only interact with each other but also are adapted to perform specific functions. The principal cell type is the hepatic parenchymal cell, generally referred to as the hepatocyte, which accounts for 60% of the total cell population and 80% of the volume of the organ. Hepatocytes are organized into plates or laminae that are interconnected to form a continuous three-dimensional lattice (**Fig. 1-1**). Between the plates of hepatocytes are spaces occupied by hepatic sinusoids—the large-bore fenestrated capillaries of the liver that nourish each parenchymal cell on several sides (see **Fig. 1-1**).

The sinusoidal space, and the non-parenchymal cells associated with sinusoids, comprises the majority of the remaining liver volume. The non-parenchymal cells include sinusoidal endothelial cells, perisinusoidal stellate cells (fat-storing cells of Ito), and intraluminal Kupffer cells. An interconnecting network of minute intercellular channels forms bile canaliculi, which course between adjacent hepatocytes (see **Fig. 1-1, A**) and receive bile secreted from hepatocytes. From the canaliculi the bile then drains through short bile ductules (cholangioles, which are partially lined by cuboidal epithelial cells) to bile ducts.

Hepatocytes execute most of the functions generally associated with the liver. They extract and process nutrients and other materials from the blood, and they produce both exocrine and endocrine secretions, as described in the following paragraphs.

Bile Synthesis and Secretion

Hepatocytes synthesize bile acids from cholesterol; bile acids act as fat emulsification agents in the lumen of the small intestine.

Bilirubin, a toxic metabolite generated from the metabolism of heme, is excreted by hepatocytes as follows. Insoluble, unconjugated bilirubin is produced as a by-product of red blood cell destruction in the spleen and usually circulates in the blood plasma as a complex with albumin. Hepatocytes absorb and convert unconjugated bilirubin to its conjugated, soluble form, which is then secreted into bile canaliculi.

Protein Synthesis

Hepatocytes synthesize proteins for hepatic and nonhepatic use. Proteins for hepatic use include a wide variety of liver-specific enzymes that perform the many synthetic and detoxifying functions of the liver. With the exception of immunoglobulins, which are synthesized by plasma cells, proteins secreted by hepatocytes include all of the major plasma proteins (e.g., albumin, transferrin, prothrombin, fibrinogen, lipoproteins, complement proteins).

Glucose Homeostasis

Hepatocytes help to maintain steady blood glucose levels. In response to pancreatic islet hormones, hepatocytes either synthesize glycogen from glucose or metabolize glycogen to produce glucose (glycogenolysis); hepatocytes can also

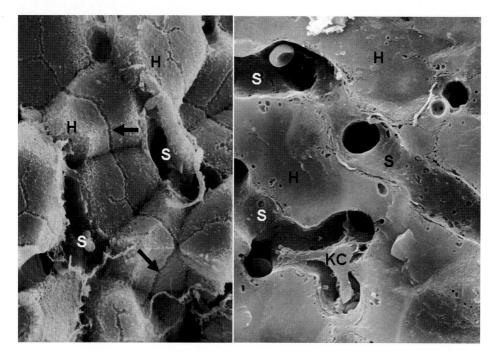

Fig. 1-1 Laminae of hepatic parenchymal cells *(H)* interconnected to form a three-dimensional lattice containing a labyrinth of spaces occupied by sinusoids *(S)*. KC, Kupffer cell. *(Modified from McCuskey RS. Functional morphology of the liver with emphasis on its microvasculature. In: Tavoloni N, Berk PD, editors. Hepatic transport and bile secretion. New York: Raven Press, 1993: 2, ©1993, with permission from Lippincott Williams & Wilkins [http://lww.com].)*

manufacture glucose from other carbohydrates (e.g., fructose) and from amino acids (gluconeogenesis).

Metabolism of Drugs and Toxins

Hepatocyte enzymes metabolize drugs and toxins delivered to the liver from the gut via the portal circulation.

The functions of the three types of hepatic non-parenchymal cells are listed in the following paragraphs.

Kupffer Cells

These large, irregularly shaped cells are attached to the luminal surface of the sinusoidal wall and are responsible for the following functions:

- Phagocytosis of blood-borne toxicants and particulates such as bacteria from the circulation
- Secretion of mediators (e.g., inflammatory mediators) that affect the function of adjacent cells and cells in distant sites
- Production of beneficial and toxic substances that contribute to host defense as well as liver injury

Sinusoidal Endothelial Cells

These cells form a leaky barrier between the parenchymal cells and the blood flowing in sinusoids. The fenestrated morphology of the endothelial cells acts as a sieve that both prevents red blood cells and other cellular components from interacting with hepatocytes and allows rapid access of hepatocytes to select substances in the blood.

Stellate Cells

Two of the functions of these star-shaped cells that are external to the sinusoidal endothelium are the following:

- Stellate cells store vitamin A and other fat-soluble vitamins.
- When stellate cells are activated they synthesize collagen; thus they are important in the development of cirrhosis.

The structure of the liver at the tissue, cellular, and molecular levels has evolved to serve the previously listed functions and is the subject of the remainder of this chapter.

Gross Anatomy

The mature liver lies mainly in the right hypochondriac and epigastric regions of the abdominal cavity, below the diaphragm. The liver is attached to the diaphragm and protected by the ribs. Its morphology has been extensively reviewed.[1,2] Briefly, in adults the healthy liver weighs approximately 1500 g and extends along the midclavicular line from the right fifth intercostal space to just inferior to the costal margin. The anterior border of the liver then extends medially and crosses the midline just inferior to the xiphoid process. A small portion of the organ projects across the midline and lies in the upper left abdominal quadrant.

The dual blood supply of the liver enters the organ at its hilus (porta hepatis) accompanied by the hepatic bile duct, lymphatics, and nerves. Approximately 80% of the blood entering the liver is poorly oxygenated and is supplied by the portal vein. This is the venous blood flowing from the intestines, pancreas, spleen, and gallbladder. The remaining 20% of the blood supply is well oxygenated and delivered by the hepatic artery.

Anatomically, the liver is divided into right and left lobes by the falciform ligament, which is a peritoneal fold connecting the liver to the anterior abdominal wall and the diaphragm (**Fig. 1-2**). The right lobe is further subdivided inferiorly and

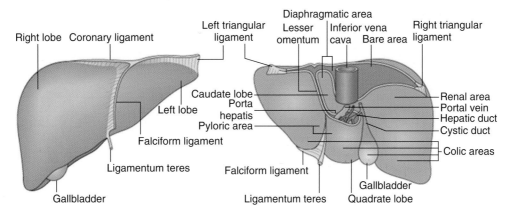

Fig. 1-2 **Lobes, surfaces, and ligaments of the liver viewed anteriorly** *(left)* **and from a posteroinferior perspective** *(right)*. *(Modified from Moore KL, Dalley AF. Clinically oriented anatomy, 4th ed. Philadelphia: Lippincott Williams & Wilkins, 1999: 264, ©1999, with permission from Lippincott Williams & Wilkins [http://lww.com].)*

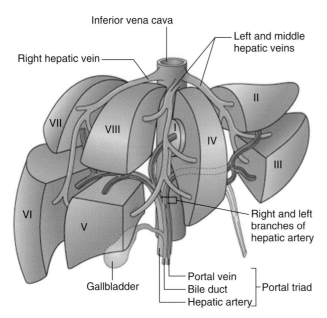

Fig. 1-3 **Segmentation of the liver based on principal divisions of the portal vein and hepatic artery.** *(Modified from Moore KL, Dalley AF. Clinically oriented anatomy, 4th ed. Philadelphia: Lippincott Williams & Wilkins, 1999: 268, ©1999, with permission from Lippincott Williams & Wilkins [http://lww.com].)*

posteriorly into two smaller lobes—the caudate and quadrate lobes. The functional division, however, is a plane that passes through the gallbladder and inferior vena cava and that defines the halves of the liver supplied by the right and left branches of the portal vein and hepatic artery, together with biliary drainage into the right and left hepatic ducts. As a result, the quadrate lobe and a large portion of the caudate lobe belong functionally to the left hemiliver. Further functional subdivision of the liver into eight segments having independent vascular and biliary supplies has been reported (**Fig. 1-3**) and is an important consideration when liver resection is required.[1-3]

The liver is encapsulated by a thin connective tissue layer (Glisson's capsule) consisting mostly of regularly arranged type I collagen fibers, scattered type III fibers, fibroblasts, mast cells, and small blood vessels. On the surfaces facing the abdominal cavity this connective tissue layer is covered by the simple squamous mesothelial cells of the peritoneal lining. At the site of attachment of the falciform ligament to the liver, the two leaves of the ligament separate to form an area devoid of peritoneum, the "bare area," on the superior surface of the liver. The right and left leaves of the falciform ligament then merge with reflections of the peritoneum extending from the diaphragm, respectively forming the triangular and coronary ligaments.

Development of the Liver

The development of the liver has been extensively described[1,2,4,5] and is illustrated in **Figure 1-4**. Briefly, the liver primordium appears in human embryos during the third week of gestation as an endodermal bud from the ventral foregut just cranial to the yolk sac. This bud becomes the hepatic diverticulum as it enlarges, elongates, and develops a cavity contiguous with the foregut. The hepatic diverticulum grows into the septum transversum—a plate of mesenchyme that incompletely separates the pericardial and peritoneal cavities—and consists of three portions: (1) the hepatic portion forms the hepatic parenchymal cells as well as the intrahepatic bile ducts, (2) the cystic portion forms the gallbladder, and (3) the ventral portion forms the head of the pancreas.

During the fourth week of development, buds of epithelial cells extend from the hepatic diverticulum into the mesenchyme of the septum transversum as thick, multicellular anastomosing cords. They become interspersed within the developing anastomotic network of capillaries arising from the vitelline veins, thus beginning to establish the close relationship of the hepatic parenchymal cells to the sinusoids. The anastomotic pattern of both multicellular cords of parenchymal cells and sinusoids persists until several years after birth, by which time cords consisting of two or more parenchymal cells bounded on several sides by sinusoids have become plates consisting of single parenchymal cells bounded on at least two sides by sinusoids, particularly in the centrilobular region. By 7 weeks the vitelline veins unite to form the portal vein. The hepatic artery is derived from the celiac axis and its ingrowth into the hepatic primordium closely follows that of the bile ducts.[6] Between the sixth week and birth the fetal liver serves as a hematopoietic organ and as the primary site for fetal blood formation until the third trimester, when most hematopoietic sites disappear as the bone marrow develops.

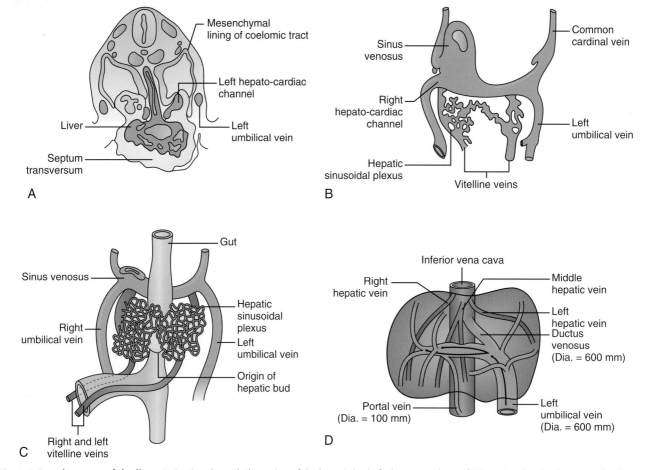

Fig. 1-4 Development of the liver. A, Section through the region of the hepatic bud of a human embryo of 25 somites (26 days). **B,** Vascular channels associated with the developing liver in a human embryo of 30 somites. **C,** Vascular channels at a later stage showing development of the sinusoidal network. **D,** Portal hepatic circulation in a human embryo of 17 mm (7 weeks). *(Reproduced from MacSween RNM, et al. Functional morphology of the liver with emphasis on its microvasculature. In: MacSween RNM, et al., editors. Pathology of the liver, 4th ed. London: Churchill Livingstone, 2002: 4, ©2002, with permission of Elsevier.)*

Microscopic Anatomy
Vasculature, Biliary System, Innervation

Vasculature

Both the hepatic portal vein and the hepatic artery, together with afferent nerves, enter the liver at the hilus. The hilus is also the site where efferent bile ducts as well as lymphatics and nerves exit the liver. Branches of the hepatic artery, hepatic portal vein, main bile duct, and main lymphatic vessel travel together in portal tracts through the liver parenchyma (**Fig. 1-5**). Portal tracts are sometimes referred to as portal triads, with each triad consisting of a branch of the hepatic artery, a branch of the portal vein, and a branch of the bile duct. Although portal tracts contain five elements, the lymphatic vessel is usually collapsed and inconspicuous as are the autonomic nerves, resulting in only three elements (i.e., triad) being visible in sections through portal tracts. After repeated bifurcation, terminal branches of the blood vessels (portal venules and hepatic arterioles) supply blood to the sinusoids (**Fig. 1-6**). Branches of hepatic arterioles also supply the peribiliary plexus of capillaries nourishing the bile ducts, and then drain into sinusoids (via arterio-sinus twigs) (**Fig. 1-7**) or occasionally into portal venules (arterio-portal anastomoses). Because all these vessels are independently contractile, the sinusoids receive a varying mixture of portal venous and hepatic arterial blood.[7,8] After flowing through the sinusoids, blood is collected in small branches of hepatic veins termed central venules (also referred to as terminal hepatic venules) (see **Fig. 1-6**). These veins course independently of the portal tracts and drain via hepatic veins, which emerge from the liver's dorsal surface and join the inferior vena cava.

Lymphatic vessels originate as blind-ending capillaries in the connective tissue spaces within the portal tracts.[9] The fluid contained in these lymphatics moves toward the hepatic hilus and eventually into the cisternae chyli and thoracic duct. Some scholars believe the perisinusoidal space of Disse functions as a lymphatic space that channels plasma to the true lymphatics coursing in the portal tract. However, anatomic connections between the space of Disse and the portal tract have not been identified.[9] Lymph also leaves the liver in small lymphatics associated with the larger hepatic veins, which empty into larger lymphatics along the wall of the inferior vena cava. Lymphatics in the hepatic capsule drain to vessels either at the hilum or around the hepatic veins and inferior vena cava.[1]

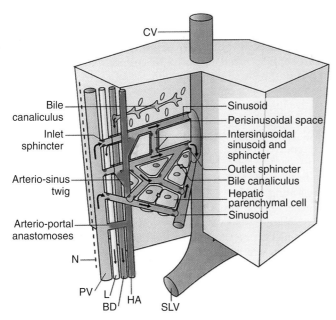

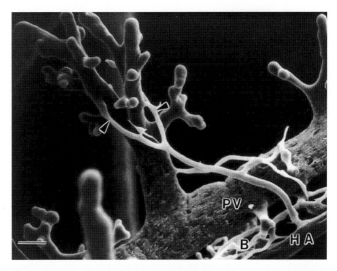

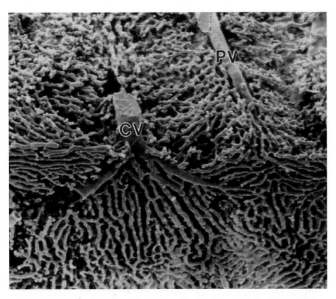

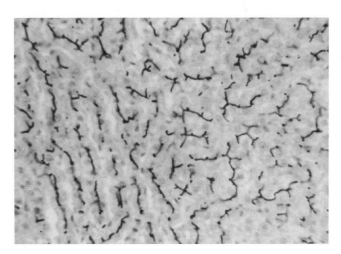

Fig. 1-5 Hepatic microvasculature as determined by in vivo microscopic studies. *BD,* bile ductule; *CV,* central venule; *HA,* hepatic arteriole; *L,* lymphatic; *N,* nerve; *PV,* portal venule; *SLV,* sublobular hepatic vein. *Arrows* indicate direction of flow. *(Modified from McCuskey RS. Functional morphology of the liver with emphasis on its microvasculature. In: Tavoloni N, Berk PD, editors. Hepatic transport and bile secretion. New York: Raven Press, 1993: 2, ©1993, with permission from Lippincott Williams & Wilkins [http://lww.com].)*

Fig. 1-7 Terminal branches *(arrowheads)* from hepatic arteriole *(HA)* frequently end in inlet venules or terminal portal venules where sinusoids originate. B, peribiliary plexus supplied by the adjacent hepatic arteriole; PV, portal venule. *(Modified from McCuskey RS. Functional morphology of the liver with emphasis on its microvasculature. In: Arias IM, et al., editors. The liver: biology and pathobiology, 3rd ed. New York: Raven Press, 1994: 1095, ©1994, with permission from Lippincott Williams & Wilkins [http://lww.com].)*

Fig. 1-6 Vascular cast of the hepatic microvasculature illustrating the tortuous anastomotic sinusoids adjacent to the portal venule *(PV)* and the more parallel and larger sinusoids near the central venule *(CV).* *(Modified from McCuskey RS. The hepatic microvascular system. In: Tavoloni N, Berk PD, editors. Hepatic transport and bile secretion. New York: Raven Press, 1993: 4, ©1993, with permission from Lippincott Williams & Wilkins [http://lww.com].)*

Fig. 1-8 Bile canalicular network filled with dye injected retrograde into the bile duct.

Biliary System

Bile canaliculi are spaces 1 to 2 μm wide formed between adjacent hepatocytes (see **Fig. 1-1, A**).[10,11] They are interconnected and form a network of minute intercellular channels (**Fig. 1-8**) that receive the bile secreted from hepatocytes.

These minute biliary channels are specialized regions of adjacent hepatic parenchymal cells and will be discussed in more detail together with the ultrastructure of these cells. The bile canaliculi drain through short bile ductules (cholangioles), partially lined by cuboidal epithelial cells, to bile ducts, lined with simple cuboidal epithelium, which course along with branches of the portal vein and hepatic artery in portal tracts. Bile ducts drain through larger left and right hepatic ducts, which exit the liver at the hilus to form the common bile duct. These ducts are lined with simple columnar epithelial cells. Branches of the hepatic artery supply an extensive peribiliary plexus of capillaries (see **Fig. 1-7**).

Innervation

Aminergic, peptidergic, and cholinergic nerves are contained in the portal tracts and affect both intrahepatic blood flow and hepatic metabolism.[12,13] The role of neural elements in regulating blood flow through the hepatic sinusoids, solute exchange, and parenchymal function is incompletely understood. This is due in part to limited investigation in only a few species, whose hepatic innervation may differ significantly from that of humans. For example, most experimental studies have used rats and mice, whose livers have little or no intralobular innervation. In contrast, most other mammals, including humans, have aminergic and peptidergic nerves extending from the perivascular plexus in the portal space into the lobule (**Fig. 1-9**), where they course in the space of Disse in close relationship to stellate cells and hepatic parenchymal cells (**Fig. 1-10**). Although these fibers extend throughout the lobule, they predominate in the periportal region. Cholinergic innervation, however, appears to be restricted to structures in the portal space and immediately adjacent hepatic parenchymal cells. Neuropeptides have been co-localized with neurotransmitters in both adrenergic and cholinergic nerves. Neuropeptide Y (NPY) has been co-localized in aminergic nerves supplying all segments of the hepatic portal venous and the hepatic arterial and biliary systems. Nerve fibers immunoreactive for substance P (SP) and somatostatin (SOM) follow a similar pattern of distribution. Intralobular distribution of all of these nerve fibers is species dependent and similar to that reported for aminergic fibers. Vasoactive intestinal peptide (VIP) and calcitonin gene-related peptide (CGRP) are reported to co-exist in cholinergic and sensory afferent nerves innervating portal veins and hepatic arteries and their branches, but not the other vascular segments or the bile ducts. Nitrergic nerves immunoreactive for neuronal nitric oxide (nNOS) are located in the portal tract, where nNOS co-localizes with both NPY- and CGRP-containing fibers.

Hepatic Functional Units

The organization of each liver lobe into structural or functional units related to function and/or disease has been the subject of considerable debate during the past century. Several models, none of which are mutually exclusive, have been proposed and are illustrated in **Figure 1-11**.

The classic hepatic lobule is a polygonal structure having as its central axis a central venule, with portal tracts distributed along its peripheral boundary.[14] The peripheral boundaries of these lobules are poorly defined in most species, including humans (**Fig. 1-12**). In some species (e.g., pigs, seals) there is considerably more connective tissue in the liver that is distributed along the peripheral boundary of classic lobules, thereby demarcating each lobule. Considerable sinusoidal anastomoses occur between adjacent lobules, and thus the blood collected by each central venule is supplied by several portal venules.

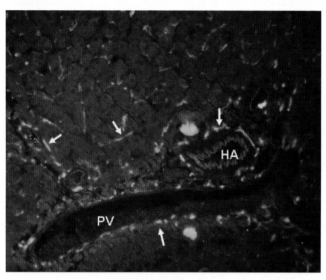

Fig. 1-9 Intrahepatic aminergic innervation in the dog. Brightly fluorescent nerve fibers are adjacent to the portal vein (PV), hepatic artery (HA), and bile duct (not visible in this section) and are also distributed intralobularly along the sinusoids (arrows).

The hepatic acinus[15] is a unit having no distinct morphologic boundaries. Its axis is a portal tract and its peripheral boundary is circumscribed by an imaginary line connecting the neighboring terminal hepatic venules (central hepatic venules of the classic lobule), which collect blood from sinusoids. Contained within the acinus are three zones, each having different levels of oxygenation and metabolic functions.

In yet another model of lobular organization, the lobule is defined by bile drainage. So-called "portal lobules"[16] have at their center a portal tract, with central veins present around the periphery of each lobule.

Currently the concept of subunits of the classic lobule forming functional units is the most consistent with existing evidence.[17-19] In this model, each "classic" lobule consists of several "primary lobules." Each primary lobule is cone-shaped, having its convex surface at the periphery of the classic lobule supplied by terminal branches of portal venules and hepatic arterioles, and its apex at the center of the classic lobule drained by a central (terminal hepatic) venule. These "primary lobules" were renamed hepatic microvascular subunits (HMS) and were demonstrated to consist of a group of sinusoids supplied by a single inlet venule and its associated termination of a branch of the hepatic arteriole from the adjacent portal space (see **Fig. 1-12**). Further confirmation of this HMS concept was obtained by studying their development

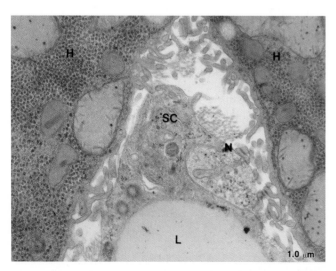

Fig. 1-10 Nerve fiber (N) closely associated with a stellate cell (SC) in the space of Disse of a dog. H, hepatic parenchymal cell; L, lipid droplet.

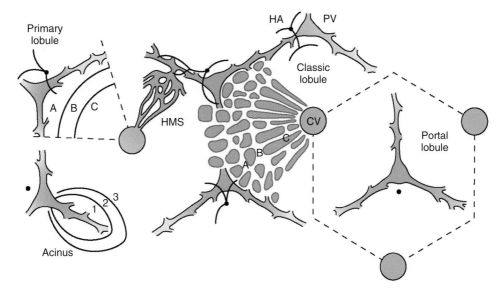

Fig. 1-11 Contiguous hepatic lobules illustrating the interconnecting network of sinusoids derived from two portal venules *(PV)*. Note that the sinusoids become more parallel as they course toward the central venule *(CV)*, which forms the axis of the classic lobule. Hepatic arterioles *(HA)* supply blood to sinusoids near the periphery of the lobule, usually by terminating in inlet venules or terminal portal venules. As a result, three zones *(1, 2, 3)* of differing oxygenation and metabolism have been postulated to comprise a hepatic acinus, with its axis being the portal tract *(lower left)*. Several acini would comprise the portal lobule *(lower right)*. Each classic lobule contains several cone-shaped subunits having convex surfaces supplied by portal and arterial blood at the periphery and its apex at the central venule *(upper left)*. A, B, and C represent hemodynamically equipotential lines in a "primary lobule." A recent modification further subdivides lobules into conical hepatic microcirculatory subunits *(HMS)*, each being supplied by a single inlet venule. *(Modified from McCuskey RS. Functional morphology of the liver with emphasis on its microvasculature. In: Tavoloni N, Berk PD, editors. Hepatic transport and bile secretion. New York: Raven Press, 1993: 4, ©1993, with permission from Lippincott Williams & Wilkins [http://lww.com].)*

in neonatal livers.[20] Accompanying the HMS are hepatic parenchymal cells and the associated cholangioles and canaliculi. Hepatocellular metabolic gradients also have been demonstrated to conform to this proposed functional-unit concept.[21]

Hepatic Parenchymal Cells

Hepatic parenchymal cells, commonly referred to as hepatocytes, are polyhedral cells approximately 20 to 30 μm in diameter; they have a volume of approximately 5000 μm^3 and are organized into anastomotic sheets (see **Fig. 1-1**).[22-24] They are epithelial cells, and like other polarized epithelial cells they have distinct apical, lateral, and basal surfaces. The basal surfaces of hepatocytes face the sinusoidal endothelium. Their plasma membranes have microvilli that extend into the space of Disse (the space between hepatocytes and endothelial cells), increasing the surface area available for the exchange of materials between hepatocytes and blood plasma. The apical surfaces of hepatocytes face adjacent hepatocytes and enclose the bile canaliculi, minute spaces forming a network of channels that carry the bile secretion (exocrine secretion) of hepatocytes (**Figs. 1-13 and 1-14**). The apical surfaces also form microvilli to increase the surface area available for secretion. This is also referred to as the canalicular domain of the plasma membrane. The lateral membranes of hepatocytes extend from the bile canaliculi to the space of Disse and form cell–cell junctions, including gap junctions that facilitate communication between hepatocytes and tight junctions that seal the bile

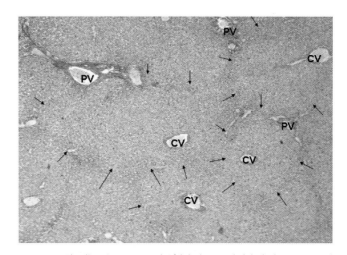

Fig. 1-12 The liver is composed of lobules; each lobule has a central venule *(CV)* as its axis and peripheral boundaries that are poorly defined *(arrows)* but contain branches of the portal vein *(PV)*, hepatic artery, and bile duct.

canalicular lumen from the interstitial space (see **Figs. 1-13 and 1-14**). These tight junctions are critical in that they prevent leakage of plasma into bile as well as backflow of bile from canaliculi into the blood. Functionally, the basal and lateral membranes are frequently considered a unit—the basolateral membrane.

Hepatocytes may have one nucleus but typically have two nuclei, and their cytoplasm contains numerous mitochondria as well as a prominent Golgi apparatus located between the nucleus and the bile canaliculi, rough endoplasmic reticulum,

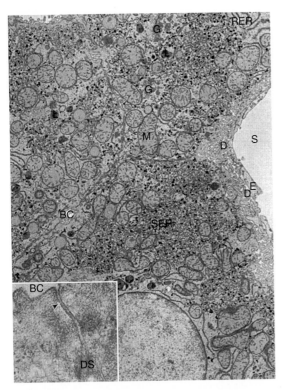

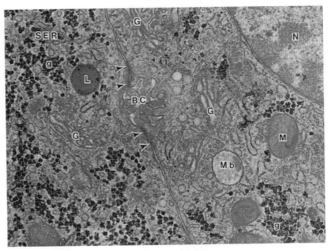

Fig. 1-14 **Two adjacent hepatic parenchymal cells and enclosed bile canaliculus (BC) and associated organelles.** G, Golgi; g, glycogen; L, lysosome; M, mitochondria; Mb, microbody (peroxisome); N, nucleus; SER, smooth endoplasmic reticulum. *Arrowheads*, tight junctions. *(Reproduced from Jones AL. Anatomy of the normal liver. In: Zakim D, Boyer TD, editors. Hepatology: a textbook of liver disease, 3rd ed. Philadelphia: WB Saunders, 1996: 22, ©1996, with permission of Elsevier.)*

Fig. 1-13 **Portions of three hepatic parenchymal cells having bile canaliculi (BC) located between adjacent cells.** D, space of Disse; E, endothelial cell; L, lysosome; M, mitochondria; RER, rough endoplasmic reticulum; S, sinusoid; SER, smooth endoplasmic reticulum. *Inset* is a higher magnification of a tight junction *(arrowhead)* between adjacent parenchymal cells. DS, Desmosome. *(Reproduced from Jones AL. Anatomy of the normal liver. In: Zakim D, Boyer TD, editors. Hepatology: a textbook of liver disease, 3rd ed. Philadelphia: WB Saunders, 1996: 22, ©1996, with permission of Elsevier.)*

and smooth endoplasmic reticulum, with associated rosettes of glycogen particles.[24] They also contain numerous endosomes, lysosomes, and peroxisomes. Fat droplets also may be present.

Plasma Membrane

The plasma membrane is a dynamic structure[24-26] that has a variety of regions having specific functions and characteristics. The basal plasma membrane of each hepatocyte faces one or more sinusoids, where its surface area is greatly increased by microvilli that extend into the space of Disse (see **Fig. 1-13**) to facilitate the uptake of blood-borne substances into hepatocytes and the secretion of constitutively produced substances into the blood. This exchange of products across the plasma membrane in the space of Disse is further facilitated by the absence of a typical epithelial basal lamina; the sinusoidal endothelium also has a greatly reduced or absent basal lamina. The apical surface of the plasma membrane is limited to the bile canaliculi, which are channels formed by tight junctions between adjacent hepatocytes (see **Figs. 1-13 and 1-14**). Microvilli extend into the bile canaliculi, expanding the surface area of the apical plasma membrane that is available for secretion of bile.

Communication between hepatocytes is provided by gap junctions, which are an assemblage of many connexons—membrane pores formed by the circular arrangement of six

transmembrane proteins called connexins. Connexons in opposing plasma membranes are directly aligned and form aqueous channels that allow the passage of ions and small molecules. Cellular metabolic products, as well as chemical and electrical signals, can pass between cells. Hepatocytes express specific genes for their unique connexin proteins. Desmosomes, as well as "knob and groove" or interdigitating undulations of adjacent plasma membranes, attach cells together in addition to the tight junctions forming bile canaliculi.

The molecular structure of the hepatocyte plasma membrane includes specializations such as membrane proteins that are receptors for hormones (e.g., insulin, glucagon) and receptors that bind other substances, such as circulating immunoglobulin A (IgA), and also contribute the secretory component required for IgA function. Assorted carrier and channel protein membrane components regulate/facilitate the great variety of substances that enter and exit hepatocytes by ways other than receptor-mediated transport, endocytosis, and exocytosis. Hepatocyte uptake and the release of glucose affect the blood glucose levels and also account for the variable intracellular glycogen deposits that have been characterized in a variety of physiologic conditions.

Nucleus

Hepatocytes have one or two spherical nuclei containing one or more prominent nucleoli (see **Figs. 1-13 and 1-14**).[1,2,5,24] Some of the nuclei are polyploid and their number increases as the cell ages. Polyploid nuclei are characterized by their greater size, which is directly proportional to their ploidy. Multinucleated hepatocytes and polyploidy are consistent with high cellular function and demands and are mechanisms by which both nuclear "machinery" and cytosomal "machinery" are increased to meet these functional demands. The high level of hepatocellular activity is also reflected in the high percentage of nuclei that are euchromatic, which indicates that transcription of most of the genome is occurring continuously; thus almost all of the deoxyribonucleic acid (DNA) is in the extended configuration, and little heterochromatin is observed. Hepatocytes engaged in the synthesis of many proteins have a large nucleolus (sometimes several) that can be recognized by light microscopy, and this characteristic is typical of hepatocytes. Electron microscopy reveals the nucleolus to consist of pale-staining areas of nucleolar organizer DNA, an electron-dense granular portion of ribonucleoprotein particles forming ribosomal subunits, and a fibrillar region of transcripts of rRNA. Heterochromatic nucleolar-associated chromatin is found at the nucleolus periphery. Nucleoli are the sites of translation of rRNA into protein-rich ribosomal subunits that exit the nucleus through pores in the double membrane nuclear envelope.

Endoplasmic Reticulum, Ribosomes, and Golgi Apparatus

Rough endoplasmic reticulum (RER), smooth endoplasmic reticulum (SER), and Golgi complex are abundant in mammalian hepatocytes (see **Figs. 1-13 and 1-14**).[1,2,24,27] Their functions are related mainly to the synthesis and conjugation of proteins, metabolism of lipids and steroids, detoxification and metabolism of drugs, and breakdown of glycogen. The endoplasmic reticulum forms a continuous three-dimensional network of tubules, vesicles, and lamellae. Almost 60% of the endoplasmic reticulum has ribosomes attached to its cytoplasmic surface and is known as the RER. The remaining 40% constitutes the SER, which lacks a coating of ribosomes. The membranes of the endoplasmic reticulum are 5 to 8 nm thick. The lumen of the RER is approximately 20 to 30 nm wide, whereas that of the SER is larger (30 to 60 nm). The morphologic characteristics and amount of the endoplasmic reticulum may vary in the different zones of the liver lobule.

RER is arranged in aggregates of flat cisternae that may be found throughout the cytoplasm. It is more frequently distributed in the perinuclear, pericanalicular, and vascular regions of hepatocytes, and it is more abundant in periportal cells than in centrilobular cells.[28] The numerous attached membrane-bound ribosomes consist of a large and a small subunit, with the large subunit attached to the RER. Free ribosomes and polyribosomes are also present within the hepatocyte cytoplasm. Ribosomes contain RNA and ribosomal proteins and play a key role in the synthesis of proteins.

SER is less common and has a more complex arrangement than RER.[24] It is usually much more abundant in centrilobular than in periportal hepatocytes.[28,29] The cytoplasm within the SER tubules is usually slightly more electron-dense than the surrounding cytoplasm. SER membranes are irregular in size and present a tortuous course. They may be tubular or vesicular in structure, with a width of 20 to 40 nm. SER is mainly distributed near the periphery of the cell. It is often in close relation to RER and Golgi membranes, as well as to glycogen inclusions.[24]

The ER is not the only site of protein synthesis in hepatocytes. Abundant free ribosomes in the cytoplasm participate in the synthesis of some proteins that will be secreted, but especially of all structural proteins for the hepatocyte. Messages encoding proteins that are to remain within the cytoplasm or are destined to enter the nucleus, peroxisomes, or mitochondria are completely synthesized by free ribosomes.

The Golgi complex is a three-dimensional structure in hepatocytes consisting of numerous membranes and vacuoles.[8,24,27] Multiple Golgi complexes exist in each hepatic parenchymal cell. Whether or not these complexes are interconnected (functionally forming a single large organelle) is uncertain. The Golgi generally is distributed near the bile canaliculus or nucleus. The Golgi apparatus presents a characteristic heterogeneity. It is usually formed by a stack of four to six parallel cisternae, often with dilated bulbous ends containing electron-dense material. The cisternae may be up to 1 μm in diameter with a lumen that is 30 nm wide. This structure shows a convex or proximal portion facing the nucleus and the endoplasmic reticulum (*cis* Golgi), where small vesicles transfer proteins from the endoplasmic reticulum, and a concave part (*trans* Golgi), where vesicles and vacuoles (secretory granules) originate to transport the contained secretory proteins to the plasma membrane for discharge into the space of Disse. Both *cis* and *trans* Golgi are connected by means of the medial Golgi. The latter is the intermediate station between endoplasmic reticulum and Golgi products, such as secretory granules or secondary lysosomes (GERL). This arrangement of Golgi stacks corresponds to its morphofunctional polarization related to the pathway of protein passage through this structure. Proteins in fact enter via the *cis* Golgi, pass through the medial Golgi, and leave this structure via the exit pole (*trans* Golgi). Two main types of secretory vesicle can be identified within the Golgi apparatus: smaller presecretory granules of 50-nm diameter and larger secretory granules 400 to 600 nm in diameter containing proteins such as very low-density lipoproteins.[30]

Mitochondria

Mitochondria are large organelles and are very numerous in hepatocytes (1 to 2000 per cell) (see **Figs. 1-13 and 1-14**), constituting approximately 18% to 20% of the cell volume.[31] They play a role in the oxidative phosphorylation and oxidation of fatty acids and in all metabolic processes of the hepatocyte.[24] Although the mitochondria are dispersed ubiquitously within hepatocytes, they are more concentrated near sites of adenosine triphosphate (ATP) utilization and are often associated with the RER. Such a relationship seems to be important during the formation of cytoplasmic membranes (SER) and cytochromes.

Mitochondria in hepatocytes may be round or elongated, with a width of 0.4 to 0.6 μm and a length of 0.7 to 1.0 μm. Longer (up to 4 μm) and larger (up to 1.5 μm in diameter) mitochondria are more numerous in periportal hepatocytes.[31] Mitochondria are bounded by an outer and an inner membrane, each 5 to 7 nm thick. The outer membrane possesses special pores that allow the passage of molecules smaller than approximately 2000 daltons (Da). The inner membrane's surface area is greatly increased by the presence of numerous cristae, which fold within the mitochondrial matrix. The space between inner and outer membranes presents a low-density matrix and ranges from about 7 to 10 nm in thickness. Mitochondria have a relatively low-density matrix in which lamellar or tubular cristae and a variable amount of small dense granules can be observed. The dense granules have a diameter of 20 to 50 nm. In addition, filaments of circular mitochondrial DNA about 3 to 5 nm in width and granules approximately 12 nm in diameter containing mitochondrial RNA are also present. The DNA codes for some of the mitochondrial proteins that are synthesized in ribosomes within the organelle, but most of the mitochondrial protein is encoded by nuclear DNA. Mitochondria are self-replicating and have a half-life of approximately 10 days.

Lysosomes

Lysosomes in hepatocytes (see **Figs. 1-13 and 1-14**) consist of a heterogeneous population of organelles containing hydrolytic enzymes that are morphologically and functionally interrelated.[24,32] These organelles form rounded single-membrane–bound dense bodies, autophagic vacuoles, multivesicular bodies, coated vesicles, and the GERL. The GERL are similar to a cytoplasmic pool of structures located proximal to the Golgi apparatus; however, they are not part of the Golgi apparatus. Instead, GERL consist of smooth-surfaced membranes (similar to a specialized area of smooth ER) with the same hydrolase activity of the lysosome (but without the typical morphology of spherical organelles) and probably have a major role in the formation of lysosomes and hepatocyte lipoprotein metabolism.

Several classes of lysosomes can be identified within the hepatocyte cytoplasm: (1) primary lysosomes, small in size, are considered from a functional point of view to be in a resting phase; (2) secondary lysosomes are functionally activated; (3) autophagic vacuoles contain parts of the degrading cytoplasmic organelles and are often delimited by a double membrane; and, finally, (4) residual bodies are larger than primary and secondary lysosomes and are usually more numerous in older organisms. The residual bodies contain the residues of nondigested material or pigments such as lipofuscins (which are considered undigestible permanent residues). Lipofuscin granules are the most numerous lysosomal bodies present in human hepatocytes.[28]

Lysosomes are frequently found near the plasma membrane proximal to the bile canaliculus, forming the so-called "peribiliary dense bodies" of early histologic descriptions. The lysosomes in periportal hepatocytes are often larger and more positive for acid phosphatase than those in centrilobular hepatocytes.[28,29]

Peroxisomes (Microbodies)

Peroxisomes are subcellular organelles that are usually rounded or slightly oval in shape, are surrounded by a single membrane (see **Fig. 1-14**), and participate mainly in oxidative processes.[24,33] Each hepatocyte may contain 300 to 600 peroxisomes. These organelles are characteristically more numerous and larger in hepatocytes than in other mammalian cells.[28] They contain a fine granular matrix and in some species (but not humans) a denser paracrystalline structure may be present. The peroxisome size ranges between 0.2 and 1.0 μm. They are often found grouped in clusters near the endoplasmic reticulum. However, the presence of direct connections (the so-called "tails") with endoplasmic reticulum or other peroxisomes (peroxisomal reticulum) is still under investigation. Peroxisomes may be more numerous in pericentral hepatocytes, but they are generally homogeneously distributed within the hepatic lobule.[28,29] Peroxisomes are believed to originate as a focal protrusion of the RER.

Cytoplasmic Inclusions

The hepatocyte is extremely rich in cytoplasmic inclusions. These are functionally related to the enhanced metabolic activity of the liver cells. The more frequently observed cytoplasmic inclusions are glycogen granules, lipid droplets, and pigments of various nature.[24]

Glycogen granules are the most abundant inclusions in normal hepatocytes (see **Figs. 1-13 and 1-14**).[24,28] At the electron microscopy level they are stained by lead salts, and may occur either in the monoparticulate form (β particles, 15 to 30 nm in size) or, more frequently, as aggregates of smaller particles arranged to form "rosettes" (α particles). Glycogen granules are dispersed in the cytoplasm, but are often associated with the SER. Glycogen is depleted during fasting, disappearing first from periportal hepatocytes and then from centrilobular cells. Upon refeeding, the sequence reverses.

Lipid inclusions appear as empty vacuoles or osmiophilic droplets and are usually not surrounded by membranes. Fat droplets may vary in size and quantity, and their levels correspond mainly to triglyceride levels in the hepatocyte.[29]

A variable amount of iron-containing granules are often present within the hepatocyte cytoplasm. These are related to the apoferritin-ferritin system (the so-called "hepatic iron buffer"). Liver iron metabolism occurs in hepatocytes; nevertheless, the pathway of iron transport from the blood to the hepatocytes has not yet been fully elucidated. In addition to hepatocytes, liver endothelial cells and Kupffer cells[34] also possess receptors for transferrin, a glycoprotein implicated in cellular iron uptake, thus suggesting that iron transport involves a transendothelial (transcytosis) mechanism. Hepatocytes contain iron in the form of ferritin particles. With an approximately spherical shape, the iron-containing protein ferritin consists of a protein shell (apoferritin) 11 nm in diameter and an iron-containing central core approximately 5 nm in diameter. Hepatocyte iron deposits may also occur as single membrane-bound lysosomal bodies (residual bodies) forming aggregates of iron-containing electron-dense particles (siderosomes-hemosiderin granules).

Cytoskeleton and Cytomatrix

The cytoskeleton is a structure that is considered to regulate the shape, subcellular organization, and movements of the cells. In the hepatocyte the cytoskeletal organization[30] is dependent on the arrangement of the three main components of this structure: the microfilaments, the intermediate filaments, and the microtubules. These filament types are regularly distributed in the cytoplasm and characterize the cytomatrix, which together with other finer filaments (microtrabeculae) is believed to contribute to the "gel" consistency of cytoplasm. Microfilaments, made of actin, and microtubules, consisting of tubulin, are both involved in intracellular motility. Microtubules are considered to be implicated in determining cell shape, completing mitosis, and regulating the intracellular transport of vesicles.[35] Especially in the liver, these structures assume a relevant role in the secretion of lipoproteins and albumin, and the release of lipids into bile. Microfilaments are more directly related to bile secretion. In fact, they are normally found around the bile canaliculi (pericanalicular web). Many experimental studies have shown that microfilaments play an active role in the dilatation and contraction of bile canaliculi.[36,37] Thus they may control the bile canalicular caliber and bile flow. Intermediate filaments show a more complex architecture. They correspond to the epithelial cell "tonofilaments" of the old nomenclature. In the liver they show a relationship with the Mallory bodies (the structural marker of human alcoholic liver disease). They are located around the nucleus, near the cell border, in the cytoplasmic network, and around the bile canaliculi.

There is very little information available about the presence of microtubules or microfilaments in differentiating hepatocytes. In mice these structures have been recognized as dense bundles occurring near the nucleus and the plasma membrane in late developmental stages.[38] Their presence could have some importance in bile canaliculus and desmosome differentiation.

Non-Parenchymal Cells

The hepatic sinusoid is a unique, dynamic microvascular structure that serves as the principal site of exchange between the blood and the perisinusoidal space (i.e., space of Disse), and projecting into the space of Disse are microvilli of the hepatic parenchymal cells that form the external lining of this space.[7] The sinusoid is composed of non-parenchymal cells, of which there are four recognized types (**Figs. 1-15 and 1-16**).[7,39] These are (1) fenestrated endothelial cells and (2)

phagocytic Kupffer cells, which form the sinusoid lining that is in contact with the blood; (3) extraluminal stellate cells, also referred to as fat-storing cells (of Ito), lipocytes, or perisinusoidal cells, which serve as specialized pericytes that extend processes throughout the space of Disse; and (4) pit cells, which are immunoreactive natural killer (NK) cells that are attached to the luminal surface of the sinusoid and are part of a population of liver-associated lymphocytes (LAL).[40] Additional cells and cell processes may be present in the perisinusoidal space (of Disse) of some species, most notably mast cells in the dog[41] and adrenergic and peptidergic nerves in most mammalian species, except mouse and rat.[12] The perisinusoidal space is considered by some scholars to function as a lymphatic space that channels plasma to the true lymphatics coursing in the portal tract. Although this hypothesis would help to explain the large efflux of lymph from the liver, it may not be valid because anatomic connections between the space of Disse and the lymphatics in the portal tract have not been identified. For a review of intrahepatic lymphatics, see Trutmann and Sasse.[9]

The majority of the non-parenchymal cells have been studied both in situ and in vitro. Together, sinusoidal cells represent approximately 6% of the total liver volume, but account for 30% to 35% of the total number of liver cells.[42,43] The purpose of this chapter is to present an overview of the structural and functional features of these sinusoidal cells, which together provide a physical and selective barrier between the blood and the parenchyma that is dynamic and responsive to a wide variety of physical and chemical stimuli. Whereas sinusoidal lining cells have the capacity to divide and proliferate, especially when stimulated by immune system modifiers,[44] sinusoidal macrophages and NK cells may also be increased in numbers by the respective recruitment and subsequent modification of monocytes and lymphocytes, principally of bone marrow origin.[45]

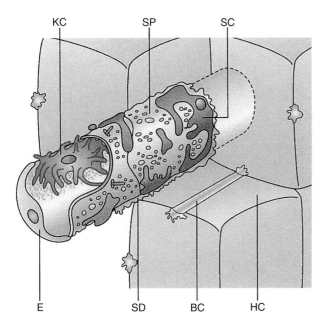

Fig. 1-15 **Sinusoid wall and contiguous hepatic parenchymal cells (HC).** BC, bile canaliculus; E, endothelium; KC, Kupffer cell; SC, stellate cell; SD, space of Disse; SP, sieve plate of fenestrae. *(Modified from McCuskey RS. In: Tavoloni N, Berk PD, editors. Hepatic transport and bile secretion. New York: Raven Press, 1993: 6, ©1993, with permission from Lippincott Williams & Wilkins [http://lww.com].)*

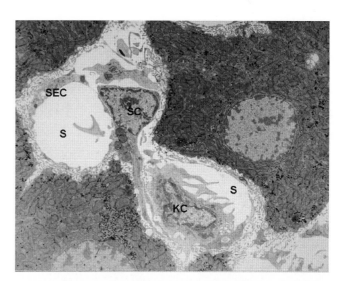

Fig. 1-16 **Sinusoid (S) lined by endothelial cells (SEC) having attenuated cytoplasm with a Kupffer cell (KC) attached to the luminal surface and a stellate cell (SC) lying externally in the space of Disse.** *(Modified from McCuskey RS. Functional morphology of the liver with emphasis on its microvasculature. In: Tavoloni N, Berk PD, editors. Hepatic transport and bile secretion. New York: Raven Press, 1993: 6, ©1993, with permission from Lippincott Williams & Wilkins [http://lww.com].)*

Sinusoidal Endothelial Cells

Similar to endothelial cells found in capillaries elsewhere throughout the body, contiguous sinusoidal endothelial cells in the liver form the basic tubular vessel for transvascular exchange between the blood and the surrounding tissue (see **Fig. 1-15**) and represent approximately 50% of the number and volume of sinusoidal cells.[42,43] The morphology of hepatic sinusoidal endothelial cells has been reviewed by several authors.[39,46] These cells are unique to the liver in that their extensive, attenuated cytoplasm contains numerous fenestrae, approximately 170 nm in diameter, that lack diaphrams and that are clustered in groups known as sieve plates[47] (see **Figs. 1-16 to 1-18**). In addition, this specialized endothelium generally lacks a basal lamina in healthy individuals; this allows solutes and small particles to have direct access to the perisinusoidal space–containing processes of fat-storing cells and the microvilli of hepatic parenchymal cells.

The endothelium of the sinusoids exhibits heterogeneity. The fenestrae are not uniform in size or distribution throughout the length of the sinusoid, from its origin at the portal venule to its termination in the central venule. At the periportal end of the sinusoid the fenestrae are somewhat larger than those located centrilobularly, but their numbers are fewer, which, when combined with the sinusoid having a smaller diameter at the periportal end than the centrilobular end, results in a higher centrilobular endothelial porosity.[47,48] The functional significance of these regional differences is unclear, but it is tempting to relate them to the functional metabolic heterogeneity that has been demonstrated for hepatocytes in different regions of the lobule,[21,49-51] as well as to the portal–central intralobular oxygen gradient.[52]

The fenestrae constitute only 6% to 8% of the surface area of the endothelial lining. They form a selective barrier between the blood and parenchyma that acts as a dynamic and discriminating sieve for particulates such as chylomicron remnants.[47] Transport of particulates somewhat larger than the size of the fenestrae is postulated to be accomplished by the "forced sieving" and "endothelial massage" concomitant with the passage of blood cells, particularly leukocytes, through the sinusoids and the resulting interaction of these cells with the endothelial wall.[47]

The endothelial fenestrae are dynamic structures whose diameters are affected by luminal blood pressure, vasoactive substances, drugs, and toxins.[47,53,54] The mechanism for active control of the diameters of these fenestrae appears to reside in actin-containing components of the cytoskeleton.[54-57] Additional cytoskeletal components form rings that delineate both the fenestrae and the sieve plates.[55,58] As a result, the fenestrae are thought to regulate the passage of large substances, such as chylomicron remnants, through the endothelium while allowing free exchange of plasma and large proteins between the blood and the space of Disse. The sinusoidal endothelial filter thereby influences the fat balance between the liver and other organs, the cholesterol level in the plasma, and the delivery of retinoids to parenchymal and fat-storing cells. The number of fenestrae present in the hepatic sinusoid decreases as the individual ages.[59]

The surfaces of the sinusoidal endothelial cells are relatively smooth compared with those of Kupffer cells and are generally lacking in filopodia or lamellipodia (see **Figs. 1-16 to 1-18**). The perikaryon contains mitochondria, some scattered components of both smooth and rough endoplasmic reticulum, and a well-developed Golgi apparatus. Throughout the cytoplasm are located numerous vacuoles and organelles associated with the uptake, transport, and degradation of material. These include bristle-coated pits (which are invaginations from the cell membrane), bristle-coated micropinocytotic

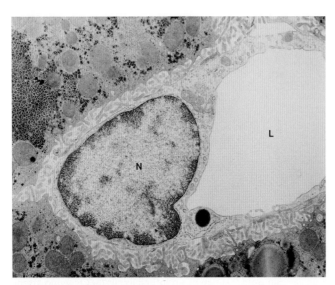

Fig. 1-17 **Sinusoidal endothelial cell with limited perinuclear cytoplasm that contains a few organelles, such as mitochondria, a lysosome, and a few cisternae of endoplasmic reticulum.** The endothelial cell rests on the microvilli filling the space of Disse. L, sinusoidal lumen; N, nucleus. *(Modified from Wisse E, et al. Structure and function of sinusoidal lining cells in the liver. Toxicol Pathol 1996;24:100–111, with permission.)*

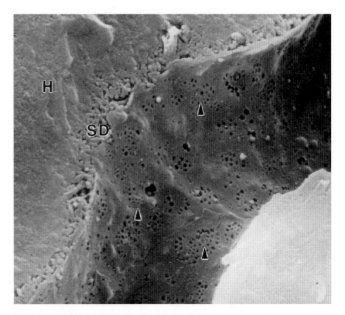

Fig. 1-18 **Sinusoid illustrating fenestrae organized in clusters as "sieve plates" *(arrowheads)*.** H, hepatic parenchymal cell; SD, space of Disse; *(Reproduced from McCuskey RS. Functional morphology of the liver with emphasis on its microvasculature. In: Tavoloni N, Berk PD, editors. Hepatic transport and bile secretion. New York: Raven Press, 1993: 7, ©1993, with permission from Lippincott Williams & Wilkins [http://lww.com].)*

vesicles, endosomes, transfer tubules, and lysosomes.[39,60] The fact that these endothelial cells contain 45% by volume of the pinocytotic vesicles in the liver as well as 14% of the lysosomes[42,43] indicates the high degree of endocytotic activity present in these cells.

The variety of substances known to be endocytosed by sinusoidal endothelial cells includes proteins, glycoproteins, lipoproteins, glycosaminoglycans,[61–63] and, under certain conditions, larger particulates, which are phagocytosed in the absence of functional Kupffer cells.[64] A number of receptors to accomplish this have been identified on the cell surface, including Fc receptors for immune complexes, transferrin (Tf) receptors, scavenger receptors, mannose, galactose, apo-E, and C-III receptors. Of these, the scavenger and apo-E receptors are particularly abundant on endothelial cells compared with Kupffer cells, as are mannose/N-acetylglucosamine receptors. This indicates the important role played by the sinusoidal endothelial cells in the processing and metabolism of lipoproteins. In addition, sinusoidal endothelial cells have been demonstrated to play a significant role in the removal of advanced glycation end products (AGE) molecules.[62]

The endothelial cells also are secretory and release interleukin-1 (IL-1), IL-6, and interferon.[39,62] In addition, these cells produce eicosanoids, particularly prostaglandins PGI_2 and PGE_2 and thromboxane A_2 (TXA_2), as well as endothelin and nitric oxide.[39] Thus, along with Kupffer cells, the endothelium participates in host defense mechanisms and regulation of sinusoidal blood flow in the liver. In addition, sinusoidal endothelial cells constitutively express the intercellular adhesion molecule ICAM-1, which along with vascular cell adhesion molecule-1 (VCAM-1) is up-regulated by inflammatory stimuli either in a direct manner or by mediators released from stimulated Kupffer cells, resulting in increased adhesion of leukocytes to the endothelial surfaces.[65] Finally, sinusoidal endothelial cells may participate in local immune responses in the liver by acting as antigen-presenting cells and resembling immature dendritic cells (see Chapter 9).[66,67]

Kupffer Cells

Kupffer cells constitute the largest population of fixed macrophages in most vertebrates. They are components of the walls of hepatic sinusoids and play a significant role in the removal by endocytosis of particulates and cells from the portal blood, as well as toxic, infective, and foreign substances, particularly those of intestinal origin.[63] Kupffer cells also are the source of a variety of beneficial, vasoactive, and toxic mediators that are involved in host defense mechanisms, as well as some disease processes in the liver.[63,68] Included among the substances released are eicosanoids, free radicals, cytokines, interferon, platelet-activating factor, and lysosomal enzymes.

The morphology of mammalian Kupffer cells, including those in humans, has been described and extensively reviewed.[63] Kupffer cells are macrophages that constitute one of the cellular components of hepatic sinusoids (see **Figs. 1-15, 1-16, 1-19, and 1-20**). At this site they are anchored to the luminal surface of the sinusoidal endothelium and thus are exposed to the bloodstream. Occasionally, Kupffer cells also are interdigitated between endothelial cells. However, Kupffer cells are unevenly distributed within hepatic lobules, with the majority being found in the periportal region, where they are

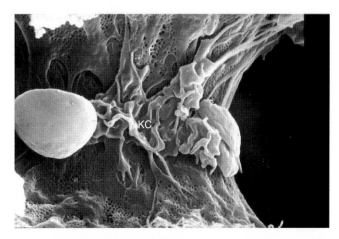

Fig. 1-19 **Kupffer cell (KC) attached to luminal surface of sinusoidal endothelium by processes that penetrate fenestrae.** (Modified from McCuskey RS. Functional morphology of the liver with emphasis on its microvasculature. In: Tavoloni N, Berk PD, editors. Hepatic transport and bile secretion. New York: Raven Press, 1993: 7, ©1993, with permission from Lippincott Williams & Wilkins [http://lww.com].)

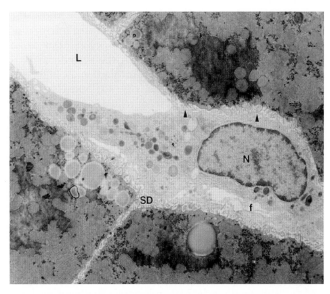

Fig. 1-20 **Kupffer cell containing lysosomes with varying density and diameter, vacuoles, and a nucleus (N).** Kupffer cells are sometimes seen in direct contact with the microvilli of the parenchymal cells (arrowhead). f, fenestrae; L, Sinusoidal lumen; SD, space of Disse. (Modified from Wisse E, et al. Structure and function of sinusoidal lining cells in the liver. Toxicol Pathol 1996;24:100–111, with permission.)

larger and have greater phagocytic activity than Kupffer cells located in the centrilobular region of the lobule.[44,69] In addition, Kupffer cells are often located at the junctions of sinusoids. As a result, the majority of Kupffer cells are strategically located to remove foreign materials as they enter the liver lobule.

Kupffer cells often present a large irregular surface, caused by numerous microvilli, filopodia, and lamellipodia extending from the cellular surface (see **Figs. 1-16 and 1-19**).[63] Attachment to the endothelium appears to be by cytoplasmic processes that often penetrate the endothelial fenestrae to enter the space of Disse, where they may contact stellate cells and, occasionally, parenchymal cells. Other processes frequently extend across the lumen to anchor in the opposite wall of the sinusoid. As a result, Kupffer cells often have a branched or "stellate" appearance. Although Kupffer cells frequently contact other sinusoidal cell types, no organized junctions have been visualized between Kupffer cells and these contiguous cells. The surface of Kupffer cells is covered with a fuzzy coat of unknown composition that normally is not preserved by perfusion fixation with glutaraldehyde.[70,71] It can, however, be seen coating the inner surface of the membranes of large pinocytotic vacuoles, and as a dense midline within membranous invaginations known as "worm-like" bodies or vermiform processes. These structures are believed to be unique to Kupffer cells, as are annulate lamellae.[72] The latter are sometimes found connected to the RER and are considered to represent a particular arrangement of the RER. These latter two structures, along with the nuclear membrane, stain positive for endogenous peroxidase. Although this is a specific marker for Kupffer cells in the rat liver[71,73] it is not as useful in other species, because of a similar positivity in large numbers of endothelial cells. More recently, monoclonal antibodies also have been used to identify macrophages and Kupffer cells.[74,75]

In addition to the previously mentioned structures, the cytoplasm of Kupffer cells contains bristle-coated micropinocytotic vesicles and a number of clear vacuoles and dense bodies (lysosomes), which, along with the vermiform processes and fuzzy-coated vacuoles, are involved in the high level of endocytotic and digestive activity attributed to these cells.[63,72] Additionally, the usual set of cellular organelles is also present in the cytoplasm, including mitochondria, RER, free ribosomes, Golgi apparatus, microtubules, microfilaments, intermediate filaments, centrioles, and a nucleolus.[63,72] However, fat droplets, autophagic vacuoles, multivesicular bodies, peroxisomes, and smooth endoplasmic reticulum have not been reported in Kupffer cells in situ.

The endocytotic mechanisms of Kupffer cells have been studied both in situ and, in greater detail, in isolated cultured cells. Four morphologically recognizable endocytotic mechanisms for Kupffer cells fixed in situ by perfusion have been described: bristle-coated micropinocytosis; pinocytosis veriformis; pinocytosis (fuzzy-coated vacuole); and phagocytosis.[63,72] Of these, the principal endocytotic mechanisms, both in vivo and in vitro, are thought to be phagocytosis and bristle-coated micropinocytosis. Phagocytosis of particulates larger than 0.3 to 0.5 µm (e.g., latex, bacteria) is performed by hyaloplasmic pseudopodia, which extend from the cell surface to engulf the particulate. Phagocytosis of particulates >0.5 µm (e.g., latex) has been used as a marker to distinguish Kupffer cells from other sinusoidal lining cells under normal conditions.[73] However, as noted previously the sinusoidal endothelium is also capable of phagocytosing latex particles if Kupffer cells are injured.[64] Bristle-coated micropinocytosis is believed to be responsible for both receptor-mediated and non–receptor-mediated fluid-phase endocytosis. Several receptors have been demonstrated on Kupffer cells, including Fc and C3 receptors, N-acetyl-D-galactosamine receptors, and N-acetylglucosamine/mannose receptors.

The origin and cell kinetics of Kupffer cells continue to be debated between scholars who are proponents of a monocytic origin and those favoring self-replication.[44,76] Taken together, the data seem to support both points of view. Healthy Kupffer cells have long residence times and slow rates of self-replication, augmented by some recruitment and transformation of monocytes. Monocyte recruitment becomes more important during stimulation of Kupffer cell function (e.g., after exposure to zymosan or bacille Calmette-Guérin [BCG]).[77–79]

Stellate Cells

External to the endothelium, perisinusoidal cells known as stellate cells (previously known as fat-storing cells, Ito cells, or lipocytes) are located in the space of Disse (see **Figs. 1-15, 1-16, and 1-21**), with a higher number present in the periportal area.[80,81] These cells contain fat droplets and are the major storage site of retinoids, including vitamin A, which emits a characteristic, rapidly quenched autofluorescence when excited with 328-nm ultraviolet light. Two types of fat droplets are recognized: those with and those without a limiting membrane.[80]

The nuclear area of the stellate cell is frequently located in recesses between hepatic parenchymal cells, whereas the thin, multiple cytoplasmic processes of these cells course through the perisinusoidal space and extensively embrace the abluminal surfaces of the endothelium that surrounds the sinusoid like a cylindrical basket. This close relationship of the processes of the stellate cell to the sinusoid wall, the presence of large numbers of cytoplasmic microtubules and microfilaments, the positive immunostaining of desmin and smooth muscle α-actin, and the close association of nerve fibers (see **Fig. 1-10**), coupled with the demonstration of contractile activity in these cells both in vivo and in vitro, strongly suggest that stellate cells play a role in the local regulation of blood flow through the hepatic sinusoids.[82,83]

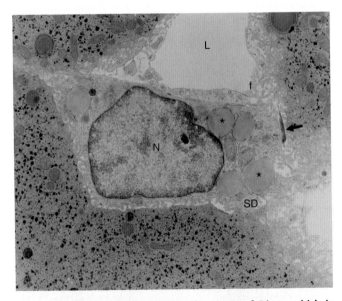

Fig. 1-21 Stellate cell lying within the space of Disse, which is covered by the endothelial lining. Fat droplets (*asterisks*) and cisternae of the endoplasmic reticulum are located in the cytoplasm. A small bundle of collagen fibers (*arrow*) is associated with the cell. f, fenestrae; L, sinusoidal lumen; N, nucleus; SD, space of Disse. (*Modified from Wisse E, et al. Structure and function of sinusoidal lining cells in the liver. Toxicol Pathol 1996;24:100–111, with permission.*)

Healthy individuals have little or no basal lamina and collagen associated with the sinusoidal endothelium. As a result, the sinusoid wall is a highly permeable structure that permits continuity of plasma between the blood and the hepatocyte. However, with certain types of liver injury (e.g., cirrhosis) basement membrane material and collagen fibrils accumulate in the perisinusoidal space, resulting in "capillarization" of the sinusoid and impaired transvascular exchange.[84] The perisinusoidal stellate cells are thought to be responsible for the synthesis of this material, following their transformation into myofibroblast-like cells having reduced numbers of fat droplets and vitamin A as well as an increased capacity to secrete extracellular matrix materials, including collagen types I and III to VI, fibronectin, laminin, tenascin, undulin, hyaluronic acid, biglycan, decorin, syndecan-containing chondroitin sulfate, heparan, and dermatan sulfate.[85]

Liver-Associated Lymphocytes

Pit cells are derived from circulating large granular lymphocytes (LGL)[86] that become attached to the sinusoidal wall (**Fig. 1-22**); LGL possess natural killer (NK) activity and are part of a population of liver-associated lymphocytes (LAL).[40,87] Pit cells contain azurophilic granules that stain for acid phosphatase, suggesting that they are lysosomal in nature.[88,89] In addition, the cytoplasm of these cells contains characteristic rod-cored vesicles as well as multivesicular bodies, a Golgi apparatus, and mitochondria, all of which exhibit polarity

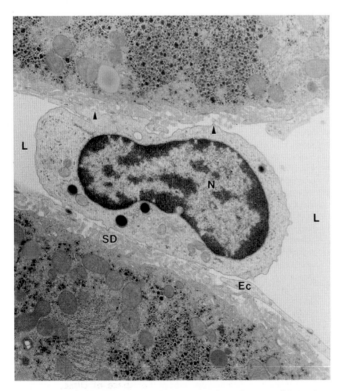

Fig. 1-22 **Pit cell with typical dense granules.** This pit cell is in close contact with the endothelial lining and is seen to contact microvilli of the parenchymal cells *(arrowhead)*. Ec, endothelial cell; f, fenestrae; L, sinusoidal lumen; N, nucleus; SD, space of Disse. *(Modified from Wisse E, et al. Structure and function of sinusoidal lining cells in the liver. Toxicol Pathol 1996;24:100–111, with permission.)*

toward one side of an eccentric, indented nucleus. Although the majority of attachments to the sinusoidal wall are to endothelial cells, adhesion to Kupffer cells is not uncommon.

Pit cells have been shown to spontaneously kill tumor cells as well as produce a cytolytic factor that is up-regulated by biologic response modifiers such as zymosan, as well as by IL-2.[87] These substances also induce proliferation of pit cells, as does partial hepatectomy, perhaps through the activation of Kupffer cells. Finally, two types of pit cell have been recognized: high density (HD) and low density (LD). The LD pit cells have a greater number of smaller granules, as compared with the granules found in HD cells; in addition, LD cells exhibit more cytotoxicity.[90]

Heterogeneity

Within the hepatic lobules, the parenchyma exhibits considerable heterogeneity along the portal venous–central venous axis, both ultrastructurally and in various enzyme activities. This results in an intralobular metabolic zonation, with different cellular functions represented in different zones within each lobule.[49,50] For example, the key enzymes involved in glucose uptake and release and in the formation of urea and glutamine are reciprocally located with glucogenic and urea cycle enzymes, principally in the periportal zone, and with glycolytic and glutaminogenic enzymes, in the centrilobular zone. Mixed-function oxidation and glucuronidation are mainly centrilobular functions, whereas sulfation is principally a periportal function. This zonation of enzymatic functions also is reflected ultrastructurally in differences in mitochondria and smooth endoplasmic reticulum among different zones. As a result of this zonation, as well as the portal-central oxygen gradient, most toxicologic and pathologic events in the liver show a considerable degree of zonal preference. An example of toxicants eliciting periportal injury is allyl alcohol; carbon tetrachloride and acetaminophen elicit centrilobular injury.

The sinusoids are composed of specialized non-parenchymal cells and also exhibit structural and functional heterogeneity.[7,8] Near their origins from portal venules and hepatic arterioles, sinusoids are slightly narrower as well as tortuous and anastomotic, forming interconnecting polygonal networks; farther away from the portal venules the sinusoids become organized as parallel vessels that terminate in central venules (terminal hepatic venules). Short intersinusoidal vessels connect adjacent parallel sinusoids. The volume of liver occupied by sinusoids in the periportal area is also greater than that surrounding central venules. However, because of the smaller size and the anastomotic nature of the periportal sinusoids, the surface area available for exchange in the periportal sinusoids (surface area/volume ratio) is greater than that found in centrilobular sinusoids. The size and pattern of distribution of endothelial fenestrae differ along the length of the sinusoid. At the portal end the fenestrae are larger but comprise less of the endothelial surface area than they do in the pericentral region. The functional significance of these regional differences is unclear but relates to the functional metabolic heterogeneity that has been demonstrated for hepatocytes in different regions of the lobule. This, in turn, may depend on the recognized portal-central intralobular oxygen gradient.

References

1. Saxena R, Zucker SD, Crawford JM. Anatomy and physiology of the liver. In: Zakim D, Boyer TD, editors. Hepatology: a textbook of liver disease. Philadelphia: WB Saunders, 2003: 3–30.

2. Wanless IR. Physioanatomic considerations. In: Schiff ER, Sorrell MF, Maddrey WC, editors. Schiff's diseases of the liver, 8th ed. Philadelphia: Lippincott-Raven, 1999: 3–37.

3. Blumgart LH, Hann LE. Surgical and radiologic anatomy of the liver and biliary tract. In: Blumgart LH, Fong Y, editors. Surgery of the liver and biliary tract. Vol. 1. London: Harcourt, 2000: 1–34.

4. Zaret KS. Embryonic development of the liver. In: Boyer JL, et al, editors. The liver: biology and pathobiology, 4th ed. Philadelphia: Lippincott Williams & Wilkins, 2001: Chapter 2.

5. MacSween RNM, Scothorne RJ. Developmental anatomy and normal structure. In: MacSween RNM, et al, editors. Pathology of the liver, 4th ed. London: Churchill Livingstone, 2002: 1–66.

6. Nakanuma Y, et al. Microstructure and development of the normal and pathologic biliary tract in humans, including blood supply. Microsc Res Tech 1997;38:552–570.

7. McCuskey RS. The hepatic microvascular system. In: Arias IM, et al, editors. The liver: biology and pathobiology, 3rd ed. New York: Raven Press, 1994: 1089–1106.

8. McCuskey RS. Morphologic mechanisms for regulating blood flow through hepatic sinusoids. Liver 2000;20:3–7.

9. Trutmann M, Sasse D. The lymphatics of the liver. Anat Embryol 1994;190: 201–209.

10. Ludwig J, et al. Anatomy of the human biliary system studied by quantitative computer-aided three-dimensional imaging techniques. Hepatology 1998;27: 893–899.

11. Motta PM. Scanning electron microscopy of the liver. Prog Liver Dis 1982;7: 1–16.

12. McCuskey RS. Distribution of intrahepatic nerves: an overview. In: Shimazu T, editor. Liver innervation. London: John Libbey, 1996: 17–22.

13. McCuskey RS. Anatomy of efferent hepatic nerves. Anat Rec 2004;280A:821–826.

14. Kiernan F. The anatomy and physiology of the liver. Trans Roy Soc Lond 1883;123:711–770.

15. Rappaport AM. The microcirculatory hepatic unit. Microvasc Res 1973;6: 218–228.

16. Mall FP. On the origin of the lymphatics in the liver. A study of the structural unit of the liver. Am J Anat 1906;5:227–308.

17. Matsumoto T, Kawakami M. The unit-concept of hepatic parenchyma—a reexamination based on angio architectural studies. Acta Pathol Jpn 1982;32:285–314.

18. Ekataksin W, Wake K. New concepts in biliary and vascular anatomy of the liver. In: Boyer JL, Ockner RK, editors. Progress in liver diseases. Vol. XV. Philadelphia: WB Saunders, 1997: 1–30.

19. Ekataksin W, et al. The hepatic microcirculatory subunits: An over-three-century-long search for the missing link between the exocrine unit and an endocrine unit in mammalian liver lobules. In: Motta PM, editor. Recent advances in microscopy of cells, tissues and organs. Rome: University of Rome "La Sapienza", 1997: 407–412.

20. McCuskey RS, et al. Hepatic microvascular development in relation to the morphogenesis of hepatocellular plates in neonatal rats. Anat Rec 2003;275A: 1019–1030.

21. Teutsch HF, Schuerfeld D, Groezinger E. Three-dimensional reconstruction of parenchymal units in the liver of the rat. Hepatology 1999;29:494–505.

22. Elias H, Sherrick JC. Morphology of the liver. New York: Academic Press, 1969.

23. Motta P, Muto M, Fujita T. The liver cell. Tokyo: Igaku-Shoin, 1978: 30–33.

24. Cardell EL, Cardell RR. Structure and function of hepatic parenchymal cells. In: McCuskey RS, Earnest DL, editors. Comprehensive toxicology. Vol. 9. Hepatic and gastrointestinal toxicology. Oxford: Elsevier Science, 1997: 11–34.

25. Schachter D. The hepatocyte plasma membrane: organization, differentiation, biogenesis, and turnover. In: Arias IM, et al, editors. The liver: biology and pathobiology, 4th ed. Philadelphia: Lippincott Williams & Wilkins, 2001: 77–81.

26. Doyle D, Bujanover Y, Petell JK. Plasma membrane: biogenesis and turnover. In: Arias IM, et al, editors. The liver: biology and pathobiology. New York: Raven Press, 1988: 61–69.

27. Lippincott-Schwarz J. The endoplasmic reticulum and Golgi complex in secretory membrane transport. In: Arias IM, et al, editors. The liver: biology and pathobiology, 4th ed. Philadelphia: Lippincott Williams & Wilkins, 2001: 119–131.

28. Tanikawa K. Ultrastructural aspects of the liver and its disorders, 2nd ed. New York: Igaku-Shoin, 1979.

29. Weibel ER, et al. Correlated morphometric and biochemical studies on the liver cell: i. morphometric model, stereologic methods, and normal morphometric data for rat liver. J Cell Biol 1969;42:68–91.

30. Phillips MJ. Biology and pathobiology of actin in the liver. In: Arias IM, et al, editors. The liver: biology and pathobiology, 3rd ed. New York: Raven Press, 1994: 19–32.

31. Hinkle PC. Mitochondria. In: Arias IM, et al, editors. The liver: biology and pathobiology. New York: Raven Press, 1994: 309–317.

32. Sahagian GG, Novikoff PM. Lysosomes. In: Arias IM, et al, editors. The liver: biology and pathobiology. New York: Raven Press, 1994: 275–291.

33. Lazarow PB. Peroxisomes. In: Arias IM, et al, editors. The liver: biology and pathobiology, 3rd ed. New York: Raven Press, 1994: 293–307.

34. Kishimoto T, Tavassoli M. Transendothelial transport (transcytosis) of iron-transferrin complex in the rat liver. Am J Anat 1987;178:241–249.

35. Crawford J. The role of vesicle-mediated transport pathways in hepatocellular bile secretion. Semin Liver Dis 1996;16:169–189.

36. Kawahara H, French SW. Role of cytoskeleton in canalicular contraction in cultured differentiated hepatocytes. Am J Pathol 1990;136:521–532.

37. Watanabe N, et al. Motility of bile canaliculi in the living animal: implications for bile flow. J Cell Biol 1991;113:1069–1080.

38. Sugisaki T, Sagakuchi T. Intracytoplasmic tonofilaments: a desmosome-like structure in the mouse fetal liver cell. J Ultrastruct Res 1977;59:178–184.

39. Wisse E, et al. Structure and function of sinusoidal lining cells in the liver. Toxicol Pathol 1996;24:100–111.

40. Winnock M, et al. Liver-associated lymphocytes: role in tumor defense. Semin Liver Dis 1993;13:81–92.

41. McCuskey PA. Electron and fluorescence microscopic study of mast cells and adrenergic innervation in Beagle dog liver. In: Wisse E, Knook DL, Decker K, editors. Cells of the hepatic sinusoids. Vol. 2. Leiden: Kupffer Cell Foundation, 1989: 260–265.

42. Blouin A. Morphometry of the liver sinusoidal cells. In: Wisse E, Knook DL, editors. Kupffer cells and other liver sinusoidal cells. Amsterdam: Elsevier Biomedical, 1977: 61–71.

43. Blouin A, Bolender RP, Weibel ER. Distribution of organelles and membranes between hepatocytes and non hepatocytes in the rat liver parenchyma. A stereological study. J Cell Biol 1977;72:441–455.

44. Bouwens L, et al. Quantitation, tissue distribution and proliferation kinetics of Kupffer cells in normal rat liver. Hepatology 1986;6:718–722.

45. Bouwens L, et al. Electron microscopic observations on the accumulation of large granular lymphocytes (pit cells) and Kupffer cells in the liver of rats treated with continuous infusion of interleukin-2. Hepatology 1990;12: 1365–1370.

46. Brouwer A, Knock DL, Wisse E. Sinusoidal endothelial cells and perisinusoidal fat-storing cells. In: Arias IM, et al, editors. Liver: biology and pathobiology. New York: Raven Press, 1988: 665–682.

47. Wisse E, et al. The liver sieve: consideration concerning the structure and function of endothelial fenestrae, the sinusoid wall and the space of Disse. Hepatology 1985;5:683–692.

48. Vidal-Vanaclocha F, Barbera-Guillem E. Fenestration patterns in endothelial cells of rat liver sinusoids. J Ultrastruct Res 1985;90:115–123.

49. Gumucio JJ, et al. The biology of the liver cell plate. In: Arias I, et al, editors. The liver: biology and pathobiology, 3rd ed. New York: Raven Press, 1994: 1143–1163.

50. Jungermann K. Metabolic zonation of liver parenchyma. Semin Liver Dis 1988;8:329–341.

51. Teutsch HF. Regionality of glucose-6-phosphate hydrolysis in the liver lobule of the rat: metabolic heterogeneity of "portal" and "septal" sinusoids. Hepatology 1988;8:311–317.

52. Lemasters JJ, Ji S, Thurman RG. Centrilobular injury following hypoxia in isolated, perfused rat liver. Science 1981;213:661–663.

53. Fraser R, Dobbs BR, Rogers GWT. Lipoproteins and the liver sieve: the role of the fenestrated sinusoidal endothelium in lipoprotein metabolism, atherosclerosis, and cirrhosis. Hepatology 1995;21:863–874.

54. Arias IM. The biology of hepatic endothelial fenestrae. In: Schaffner F, Popper H, editors. Progress in liver diseases. Vol. IX. Philadelphia: WB Saunders, 1990: 11–26.

55. Braet F, et al. Structure and dynamics of the fenestrae-associated cytoskeleton of rat sinusoidal endothelial cells. Hepatology 1995;21: 180–189.

56. Oda M, Han JY, Yokomori H. Local regulators of hepatic sinusoidal microcirculation: recent advances. Clin Hemorheol Microcirc 2000;23:85–94.

57. Oda M, et al. Hepatic sinusoidal endothelial fenestrae are a stationary type of fused and interconnected caveolae. In: Wisse E, et al, editors. Cells of the hepatic sinusoid. Vol. 8. Leiden: Kupffer Cell Foundation, 2001: 94–98.

58. Braet F, et al. A novel structure involved in the formation of liver endothelial cell fenestrae revealed by using the actin inhibitor misakinolide. Proc Natl Acad Sci USA 1998;95:13635–13640.
59. Le Couteur DG, et al. Old age and the hepatic sinusoid. Anat Rec (Hoboken) 2008;291:672–683.
60. Wisse E. An electron microscopic study of the fenestrated endothelial lining of rat liver sinusoids. J Ultrastruct Res 1970;31:125–150.
61. Smedsrod B, et al. Advanced glycation end products are eliminated by scavenger-receptor-mediated endocytosis in hepatic sinusoidal Kupffer and endothelial cells. Biochem J 1997;322:567–573.
62. Smedsrod B, et al. Cell biology of liver endothelial and Kupffer cells. Gut 1994;35:1509–1516.
63. Wisse E, et al. Structure and function of sinusoidal lining cells in the liver. Toxicol Pathol 1996;24:100–111.
64. Steffan A-M, et al. Phagocytosis, an unrecognized property of murine endothelial liver cells. Hepatology 1986;6:830–836.
65. VanOosten M, et al. Vascular adhesion molecule-1 and intercellular adhesion molecule-1 expression on rat liver cells after lipopolysaccharide administration in vivo. Hepatology 1995;22:1538–1546.
66. Knolle PA, Gerken G. Local control of the immune response in the liver. Immunol Rev 2000;174:21–34.
67. Knolle PA, Limmer A. Neighborhood politics: the immunoregulatory function of organ-resident liver endothelial cells. Trends Immunol 2001;22:432–437.
68. Decker K. Biologically active products of stimulated liver macrophages. Eur J Biochem 1990;192:245–261.
69. McCuskey RS, et al. Species differences in Kupffer cells and endotoxin sensitivity. Infect Immun 1984;45:278–280.
70. Emeis JJ. Morphologic and cytochemical heterogeneity of the cell coat of rat liver Kupffer cells. J Reticuloendothelial Soc 1976;20:31–50.
71. Wisse E. Observations on the fine structure and peroxidase cytochemistry of normal rat liver Kupffer cells. J Ultrastruct Res 1974;46:393–426.
72. Wisse E, Knook DL. The investigation of sinusoidal cells: a new approach to the study of liver function. In: Popper H, Schaffner F, editors. Progress in liver diseases. Vol. VI. New York: Grune & Stratton, 1979: 153–171.
73. Widmann JJ, Cotran RS, Fahimi HD. Mononuclear phagocytes (Kupffer cells) and endothelial cells. Identification of two functional cell types in rat liver sinusoids by endogenous peroxidase activity. J Cell Biol 1972;52:159–170.
74. Bodenheimer HC, et al. Characterization of a new monoclonal antibody to rat macrophages and Kupffer cells. Hepatology 1988;8:1667–1672.
75. Malorny U, Michels E, Sorg C. A monoclonal antibody against an antigen present on mouse macrophages and absent from monocytes. Cell Tissue Res 1986;243:421–428.
76. Bouwens L, Baekeland M, Wisse E. Cytokinetic analysis of the expanding Kupffer-cell population in rat liver. Cell Tissue Kinet 1986;19:217–226.
77. Bouwens L, Knook DL, Wisse E. Local proliferation and extrahepatic recruitment of liver macrophages (Kupffer cells) in partial-body irradiated rats. J Leukocyte Biol 1986;39:687–697.
78. Bouwens L, Wisse E. Proliferation, kinetics, and fate of monocytes in rat liver during a zymosan-induced inflammation. J Leukocyte Biol 1985;37:531–543.
79. Deimann W, Fahimi H. The appearance of transition forms between monocytes and Kupffer cells in the liver of rats treated with glucan. J Exp Med 1979;149:883.
80. Wake K. Development of vitamin A-rich lipid droplets in multivesicular bodies of rat liver stellate cells. J Cell Biol 1974;63:683–691.
81. Wake K. Perisinusoidal stellate cells (fat-storing cells, interstitial cells, lipocytes), their related structure in and around liver sinusoids, and vitamin A-storing cells in extrahepatic organs. Int Rev Cytol 1980;66:303–353.
82. Zhang JX, Pegoli W, Clemens MG. Endothelin-1 induces direct constriction of hepatic sinusoids. Am J Physiol 1994;266:G624–G632.
83. Rockey DC. Hepatic blood flow regulation by stellate cells in normal and injured liver. Semin Liver Dis 2001;21:337–349.
84. LeBail B, et al. Fine structure of hepatic sinusoids and sinusoidal cells in disease. J Electron Microsc Tech 1990;14:257–282.
85. Gressner AM. Perisinusoidal lipocytes and fibrogenesis. Gut 1994;35:1331–1333.
86. Vanderkerken K, et al. Origin and differentiation of hepatic natural killer cells (pit cells). Hepatology 1993;18:919–925.
87. Bouwens L, Wisse E. Pit cells in the liver. Liver 1992;12:3–9.
88. Bouwens L, et al. Large granular lymphocytes or pit cells from rat liver: Isolation, ultrastructural characterization and natural killer cell activity. Eur J Immunol 1987;17:37–42.
89. Kaneda K, Wake K. Distribution and morphological characteristics of the pit cells in the liver of the rat. Cell Tissue Res 1983;233:485–505.
90. Vanderkerken K, Bouwens L, Wisse E. Characterization of a phenotypically and functionally distinct subset of large granular lymphocytes (pit cells) in rat liver sinusoids. Hepatology 1990;12:70–75.

Chapter 2

Liver Regeneration

Yulia A. Nevzorova and Christian Trautwein

ABBREVIATIONS

Alb albumin	**Gab** growth factor receptor–bound protein	**RIP** receptor interacting protein
APG acute-phase gene	**GFP** green fluorescent protein	**S1P** spingosine 1-phospate
APR acute-phase response	**HGF** hepatocyt growth factor	**Shp2** SH2-domain-containing protein tyrosine phosphatase 2
Bcl B-cell lymphoma protein	**I/R** ischemia reperfusion	**Skp2** S-phase kinase-associated protein 2
c-met mesenchymal-epithelial transition factor	**IAP** inhibitor of apoptosis	**SOCS** suppressors of cytokine signaling
CCl₄ carbon tetrachloride	**IL** interleukin	**S-phase** synthesis phase
Cdc cell division control	**IRES** internal ribosome entry site	**STAT** signal transducer and activator of transcription
Cdk cyclin dependent kinase	**JAKs** Janus kinase	
Cip/Kip cyclin-dependent kinase inhibitor	**JNK** Jun terminal kinase	**TGF** transforming growth factor
E2F electro-acoustic 2 factor	**LPS** lipopolysaccharides	**TNF** tumor necrosis factor
Edg endothelial differentiation gene	**MAPK** mitogen-activated protein kinase	**TNFR** tumor necrosis factor receptor
EGF epidermal growth factor	**MCM** mini-chromosome maintenance	**TRADD** tumor necrosis factor receptor–associated death domain
EGFR epidermal growth factor receptor	**M-phase** mitosis phase	
Erk extracellular signal-regulated kinase	**NF-κB** nuclear factor-kB	**TRAF** tumor necrosis factor–associated factor
FADD fas-associated death domain	**PCNA** proliferating cell nuclear antigen	
G1-phase Gap 1 phase	**PH** partial hepatectomy	**uPaR** urikinase receptor
G2-phase Gap 2 phase	**Ras** rat sarcoma	
	Rb retinoblastoma protein	

Introduction

A striking property of the liver is its unique ability to regenerate and thereby restore its original mass after tissue loss. Major progress has been achieved during the last 50 years in understanding the mechanisms involved in controlling this process. However, this phenomenon has been discussed since Greek mythology: The Titan Prometheus stole the fire from Zeus and brought it to mankind. Zeus punished him by chaining Prometheus to a rock in the Caucasus Mountains. Every day an eagle came and ate from his liver, which regenerated overnight.

The liver has a large metabolic task to perform and normally hepatocyte proliferation in the liver is a rare event. However, liver regeneration is induced following different mechanisms of injury. Examples in humans are liver regeneration after acute liver damage from viral infection or following liver resection. Moreover, in recent years liver transplantation and especially split liver transplantation have become very important areas of research because of the shortage of donor livers. Therefore animal models to study liver regeneration are of direct relevance to better understand the physiologic mechanisms that occur in liver transplant patients. Additionally, the direct clinical application of split liver transplantation allows further proof of the concepts that have been gathered in animal models.

Different animal models to study liver regeneration have been established, mainly in rats and mice. More recently, mouse models have been favored because genetic manipulation in these species allows the researcher to directly address the function of specific genes involved in hepatocyte proliferation after injury (**Table 2-1**). The best studied model to investigate mechanisms relevant for liver regeneration is the one of partial hepatectomy (PH) (**Fig. 2-1**). Here, in mice or rats 70% of the liver is surgically removed and the impact on cell cycle progression of parenchymal and non-parenchymal liver cells can be investigated. In this classical model, the first wave of hepatocyte proliferation is found in rats after 24 hours and in mice after 40 hours. Non-parenchymal cells follow hepatocyte proliferation several hours later (**Fig. 2-2**).[1]

In this simple model of partial hepatectomy, basic mechanisms involved in controlling hepatocyte proliferation have become evident. The correct liver weight/body weight ratio can be restored quite rapidly and takes between 7 and 10 days in rodents. This ratio is relatively constant and reflects the balance between liver function and the body's demands for this function. After resection the removed liver lobes are not replaced; instead, hepatocytes in the remaining lobes

Table 2-1 Knock Out Animal Models Used to Study Liver Regeneration

DISRUPTED GENE	PHENOTYPE AFTER PARTIAL HEPATECTOMY	REFERENCES
Interleukin-6 (IL-6) (Constitutive knockout mice)	Impaired liver regeneration characterized by liver necrosis and failure	7
STAT3 (Liver specific conditional knockout mice)	Significant reduction of DNA synthesis, abnormalities in activation of immediate-early gene and cell cycle regulators	11
Gp130 (Liver specific conditional knockout mice)	Normal liver regeneration; impaired regeneration after LPS treatment	13
Gp130ΔSTAT (Liver specific conditional knockout mice) Gp130ΔRAS (Liver specific conditional knockout mice)	Block of acute-phase gene regulation Enhanced acute-phase response regulation; up-regulation of SOCS3 delay of hepatocyte proliferation	18
SOCS3 (Liver specific conditional knockout mice)	Hepatocytes acquire enhanced proliferation capacity	21
TNF-R1 (Constitutive knockout mice) TNF-R2 (Constitutive knockout mice)	Deficient DNA synthesis and massive lipid accumulation Liver regeneration not affected	24
IKK2 (Liver specific conditional knockout mice)	Earlier hepatocyte proliferation and more rapid cell cycle progression	50
JNK1–/– (Constitutive knockout mice) JNK2 (Constitutive knockout mice)	Impaired liver regeneration Liver regeneration not affected	176
Bax inhibitor-1 (Bi-1) (Constitutive knockout mice)	Accelerated liver regeneration	61
c-jun (Liver specific conditional knockout mice)	Impaired liver regeneration correlates with increased protein level of p21	73
c-Myc (Liver specific conditional knockout mice)	Compromised liver regeneration	77
c-met (Liver specific conditional knockout mice)	Regeneration of liver is impaired	84
EGFR (Liver specific conditional knockout mice)	Impaired liver regeneration	100
β-Catenin (Liver specific conditional knockout mice)	Suboptimal delay of proliferation	91
TGF-α (Constitutive knockout mice)	Liver regeneration proceeds normally	102
Notch interferon-inducible (Liver specific conditional knockout mice)	Slower restoration of liver mass with reduced proliferative response	111
E2F1 depletion (Liver specific conditional knockout mice)	No influence on regenerative capacity	130
Cyclin D (Constitutive knockout mice)	Insufficient delay in S phase	134
Cyclin E1 (Constitutive knockout mice)	Normal liver regeneration with slight delay of G1/S-phase transition; absent endoreplication in hepatocytes	138
Cyclin E2 (Constitutive knockout mice)	Accelerated liver regeneration	138
Cdk2 (Constitutive knockout mice)	Insufficient delay in S phase	139
Cdk2/Cdk4 (Conditional ablation of CDK2constitutive CDK4 knockout)	No detectable abnormalities	121
p21 (Constitutive knockout mice)	Increased hepatocyte proliferation	149
p27 (Constitutive knockout mice)	Accelerated liver regeneration	151
Skp2 (Constitutive knockout mice)	Restoration of individual cells achieved not by proliferation but by enlargement of cells	155

Continued

Table 2-1 **Knock Out Animal Models Used to Study Liver Regeneration—cont'd**		
DISRUPTED GENE	**PHENOTYPE AFTER PARTIAL HEPATECTOMY**	**REFERENCES**
p27/Skp2 (Constitutive knockout mice)	Normal regeneration	156
p18 (Constitutive knockout mice)	Normal regeneration	158
p18/p21 (Constitutive knockout mice)	Shortened G1 phase	158
p18/p27 (Constitutive knockout mice)	Increase of proliferation	158
TGF-β receptor II (Liver specific conditional knockout mice)	Earlier and increased DNA synthesis; increased liver weight after resection	167
Sphingosine 1-phosphate receptor 2–deficient mice (Constitutive knockout mice)	High proliferation and enhanced liver weight/body weight ratio	175

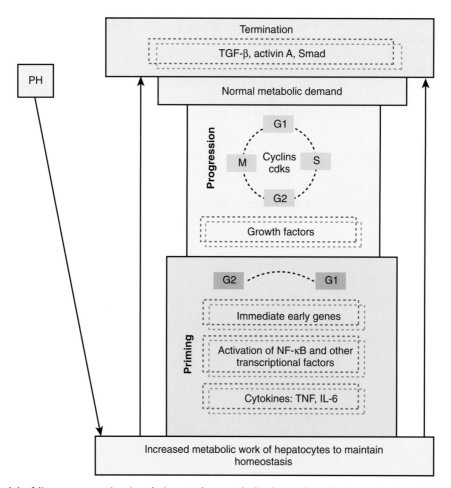

Fig. 2-1 Multistep model of liver regeneration in relation to the metabolic demands and mitogenic signals. The process can be divided into three phases: priming, progression, and termination. Priming is initiated by cytokines sensitizing the cells to growth factors. Growth factors and cyclins move cells through the cell cycle. Termination with a prominent role of the TGF-β family is essential to return the liver to the quiescent state.

proliferate. Therefore liver regeneration can also be described as compensatory hyperplasia. After liver mass is restored hepatocytes receive signals that lead to the cessation of proliferation. Thus liver regeneration is a tightly regulated process in which hepatocytes enter the cell cycle and then become quiescent again.

Besides the proliferative response after resection or injury, the liver also has the capacity to proliferate without loss of tissue, and this event is called direct hyperplasia. Different agents (e.g., nuclear receptors) have been characterized that trigger direct hyperplasia.[2] However, this chapter will focus on mechanism of liver regeneration (compensatory hyperplasia).

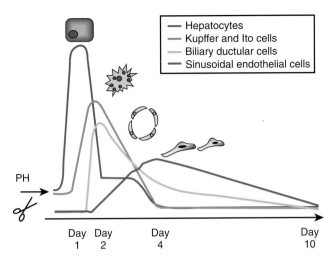

Fig. 2-2 Time kinetics of DNA synthesis in different liver cell types during liver regeneration after partial hepatectomy. The four major types of liver cells undergo DNA synthesis at different time points after PH. In rats hepatocyte DNA synthesis peaks at 24 hours, whereas the other cell types proliferate later. Regenerating hepatocytes produce growth factors that can function as mitogens for these cells. It has been suggested that hepatocytes are also involved in stimulating proliferation of the other cells by a paracrine mechanism. PH, Partial hepatectomy.

In the past 50 years different topics of liver regeneration have been proposed. In the beginning the model of partial hepatectomy was established and morphologic and metabolic changes during hepatocyte proliferation were studied. Subsequently, it became obvious that growth factors are involved in controlling the exact timing of cell cycle progression of hepatocytes. In further studies the intracellular events, especially in the nucleus, were investigated, which resulted in the analysis of changes in the expression and activity of transcription factors. Currently, because of the broad spectrum of capabilities offered by genetically manipulated mice, complex pathways interacting during liver regeneration have been investigated and it has become possible to dissect the essential mechanisms that are needed to restore liver mass after liver injury.

The events of liver regeneration can be divided into the following three phases (see **Fig. 2-1**):
1. Initiation/priming—induction of hepatocytes into a state of replicative competence
2. Progression—expansion of the entire hepatocyte population
3. Termination—suppression of cell proliferation

However, there are no distinct borders among these processes, because all phases are closely linked and share several mechanisms.[3,4]

Initiation Phase

The events occurring in the early period up to 5 hours after partial hepatectomy (PH) have been called "priming." During the initiation phase hepatocytes are primed for subsequent replication. Initiation factors include interleukin-6 (IL-6) and tumor necrosis factor-α (TNF).

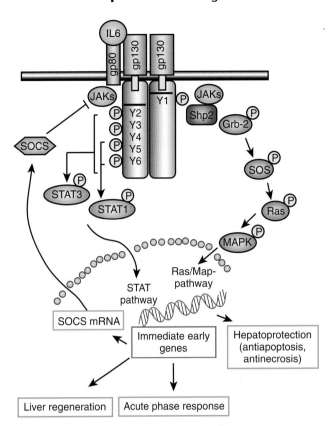

Fig. 2-3 Interleukin-6–dependent signaling. On the cell surface interleukin-6 (IL-6) first interacts with the IL-6 receptor (IL-6R)/gp80. This complex interacts with gp130 molecules and in turn triggers intracellular dimerization. Receptor-bound Janus kinases (JAKs: Jak1/2/Tyk2) become activated and phosphorylate tyrosines as the intracellular part of gp130. The phosphorylated tyrosines are essential to activate downstream pathways. Although phosphorylation of the second tyrosine is important to trigger the Ras/Map pathway via the SH₂ domain containing protein tyrosine phosphatase 2 (Shp2), the four distal tyrosines are essential to activate Stat transcription factors.

Interleukin-6

Interleukin 6 (IL-6) is known as a multifunctional cytokine that regulates hematopoiesis and inflammation. IL-6 first binds the IL-6 receptor (gp80) and then interacts with gp130. Subsequently, dimerization of two gp130 molecules activates Janus kinases (Jaks), which phosphorylate specific tyrosine residues of gp130 and thus activate the SHP2/Erk/Map pathways or the transcription factors STAT1 and STAT3 (**Fig. 2-3**).[5,6]

Studies in knockout mice indicated that normal liver regeneration after PH requires IL-6. The first experiments published by Taub's group demonstrated that IL-6−/− animals had a defect in hepatocyte proliferation after partial hepatectomy. Significantly more of the knockout mice died compared with the wild-type (wt) controls.[7] Livers show impaired regeneration characterized by necrosis and G1-phase abnormalities, including absence of STAT3 activation. Pretreatment of IL-6−/− mice with IL-6 rescues STAT3 binding, gene expression, and hepatocyte proliferation to almost normal level and prevents liver damage.[7]

The relevance of these findings was further emphasized by the finding that the defect in liver regeneration found in tumor necrosis factor-1 (TNFR-1–/–) mice could be reverted by IL-6 injection.[8] Through these two findings the hypothesis was raised that IL-6 is an essential factor involved in propelling the resting hepatocyte into the cell cycle. Further experiments aimed at better defining the pathways activated by IL-6 are essential for liver regeneration.

The most prominent factor activated by IL-6 in hepatocytes is STAT3. Treatment of IL-6–/– mice after partial hepatectomy with stem cell factor restored STAT3 activation and DNA synthesis.[9] Because STAT3 knockout mice are embryonal lethal[10] conditional knockout mice with a hepatocyte-specific knockout for STAT3 were used to study the role of IL-6/gp130-dependent STAT3 activation during liver regeneration. These animals also showed impairment in liver regeneration resembling the results of IL-6–/– animals.[11] Therefore these results suggested that especially the STAT3 pathway appears necessary for liver regeneration following partial hepatectomy. However, in these animals there was strong STAT1 activation, which is normally not found after partial hepatectomy. STAT1 is known to mediate effects opposite those of STAT3. Therefore this experimental setting has major limitations in solving the role of STAT3 during liver regeneration.

Blindenbacher and colleagues performed a careful study in IL-6–/– mice to better define the role of IL-6 during liver regeneration.[12] They tested whether IL-6 has a direct impact on hepatocyte proliferation or on body homeostasis. By using intravenous or subcutaneous IL-6 injection the authors determined that IL-6 is not directly involved in stimulating hepatocyte proliferation; instead, its primary purpose is to maintain body homeostasis in order to allow normal liver regeneration.

These results were further confirmed in conditional knockout animals for gp130. These mice showed normal liver regeneration compared with wild-type animals.[13] However, after lipopolysaccharide (LPS) injection—mimicking bacterial infection—more of the gp130–/– animals died, compared with controls, and showed impaired hepatocyte proliferation. Taken together, the work of these groups indicates that IL-6/gp130 is involved in contributing to liver regeneration through a mechanism that is not directly related to cell cycle control.

At present, the pathways that are relevant to mediate this effect are not completely understood. However, in recent years several reports demonstrate that IL-6 activates anti-apoptotic pathways also in hepatocytes. Earlier experiments by Kovalovich and colleagues demonstrated that IL-6 can activate Bcl-xL expression; in addition, it has also been suggested that IL-6 has a role in the activation of Akt.[14,15] Therefore these results indicate that IL-6/gp130 might be relevant to directly protect hepatocytes during cell cycle progression.

Additionally, IL-6 induces pathways involved in mediating immune-dependent mechanisms. IL-6 via STAT3 is the major cytokine that induces the acute-phase response (APR) in the liver. The APR is a first line of defense in the body but is also involved in the regulation of other pathophysiologic mechanisms (e.g., macrophage activation, interaction with the complement system).[16] Besides controlling APR expression, IL-6 contributes to the regulation of the TH1/TH2 response.[17] Therefore these IL-6–dependent tasks could also be relevant in contributing to body homeostasis after partial hepatectomy.

Two main pathways leading to Ras/Erk or STAT3 activation are essential (see **Fig. 2-3**). To dissect these two pathways

during hepatocyte proliferation, PH was performed in animals deficient for either hepatocyte-specific gp130-dependent Ras-Erk or STAT activation.

Deletion of gp130-dependent signaling had a major impact on acute-phase gene (APG) regulation after PH. APG regulation was blocked in gp130Δ STAT animals, whereas gp130Δ Ras mice showed an enhanced APG response and significantly stronger SOCS3 regulation. Unexpectedly, this response was associated with a delayed start of hepatocyte proliferation. A more detailed analysis of cell cycle parameters demonstrated that the G1/S-phase transition was also delayed in these animals.

Taken together these results indicate that gp130-dependent STAT signaling during liver regeneration in hepatocytes via SOCS3 controls the timing of the G1/S-phase transition, thereby providing protective signals that are important to allow hepatocyte proliferation during stress conditions.[18]

The suppressors of cytokine signaling (SOCS) constitute one important family of negative regulators that mediate

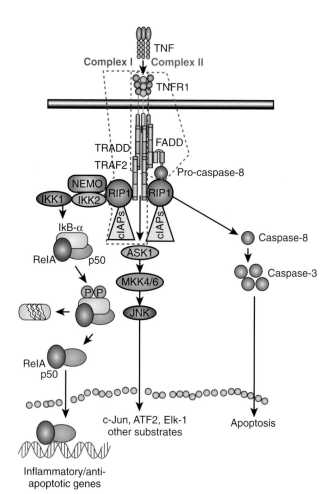

Fig. 2-4 TNF-dependent signal transduction. Binding of TNF to its cognate receptor TNFR1 results in the release of SODD and formation of a receptor-proximal complex containing the important adapter proteins TRADD, TRAF2, RIP, and FADD. These adapter proteins in turn recruit additional key pathway-specific enzymes (e.g., caspase 8, IKK2) to the TNFR1 complex, where they become activated and initiate downstream events leading to apoptosis via caspase 8, NF-κB activation involving the IKK-complex, and Jun kinase (JNK) activation.

immune responses. Most SOCS proteins are expressed following STAT activation and therefore function as classic negative regulators—they inhibit cytokine-mediated signal transduction.[19]

Mice deficient in SOCS3 die in utero because of placental defects.[20] Analyses of hepatocyte-specific Socs3−/− mice revealed that SOCS3 expression at early stages of liver regeneration is an essential element that coordinates the termination of the main cytokine response with the activation of growth factors that regulate cell cycle progression. In the absence of SOCS3, hepatocytes acquire an enhanced proliferation capacity, both in vivo and in cell culture.[21]

Tumor Necrosis Factor-α

Tumor necrosis factor is a multifunctional cytokine. In the liver it acts as a cytotoxic agent in many types of hepatic injury and is also an important mediator of hepatocyte proliferation.[22] It has been shown that TNF levels increased in the blood immediately after partial hepatectomy in normal animals and that administration of anti-TNF antibodies inhibited liver regeneration after surgery.[23]

TNF signals through two distinct receptors, TNFR1 and TNFR2, of which TNF-R1 initiates the majority of TNF's biologic activities in hepatocytes. After PH, TNFR1−/− show deficient DNA synthesis and massive lipid accumulation in hepatocytes. In contrast, TNFR2−/− mice have normal liver structure and similar levels of hepatocyte DNA replication compared to wild-type mice.[24]

Upon stimulation of tumor necrosis factor receptor 1 (TNFR1), TNF receptor–associated death domain (TRADD) provides a scaffold for the assembly of complex I at the plasma membrane by binding receptor interacting protein 1 (RIP1), TNF receptor–associated factor 2 (TRAF2) or TRAF5, and the inhibitor of apoptosis proteins (IAPs) cIAP1 and cIAP2. This complex is crucial for activating NF-κB and mitogen-activated protein kinase (MAPK) pathways, which ultimately activates c-Jun NH$_2$-terminal kinase (JNK) (**Fig. 2-4**).

After internalization of the TNFR1 receptor, secondary cytosolic complexes dependent on either TRADD (complex IIA) or RIP1 (complex IIB) are formed to initiate apoptosis. Complex IIA formation involves Fas-associated death domain (FADD) mediated recruitment and activation of caspase 8 for RIP1 and RIP3 cleavage. Complex IIB is formed in the presence of Smac mimetics and acts independently of TRADD through a RIP1-FADD scaffold to activate caspase 8 in a RIP1 kinase–dependent way.[25,26]

Activation of NF-κB by TNF requires a complex network of kinases. First the IKK complex interacts with TRAF2 and RIP. Upon activation, the IKK kinase phosphorylates I-κB, which results in its degradation, and as a consequence NF-κB is released to the nucleus where target gene transcription begins.

The signals transduced by the receptors converge on the I-κB kinase complex (IKK), consisting of the catalytic subunits IKK-α (IKK1) and IKK-β (IKK2) and the regulatory subunit NEMO (NF-κB essential modulator).[27–29]

In vitro IKK1 and IKK2 can form homodimers and heterodimers.[30] Both IKK1 and IKK2 are able to phosphorylate I-κB in vitro; however, compared with IKK1, IKK2 has a higher kinase activity in vitro.[31–33]

The IKK complex phosphorylates I-κBs at the N-terminal domain at two conserved serines (S32 and S36 in human I-κBα). After phosphorylation, the I-κBs undergo a second posttranslational modification: polyubiquitination by a cascade of enzymatic reactions, mediated by the β-TrCP-SCF complex (or the E3IkB-ubiquitin ligase complex). This process is followed by the degradation of I-κB proteins by the proteasome, thus releasing NF-κB from its inhibitory I-κB binding partner. This uncovers the nuclear translocation signal and thus NF-κB translocates to the nucleus and activates transcription of NF-κB–dependent target genes.[34,35] Because the enzymes that catalyze the ubiquitination of I-κB are constitutively active, the only regulated step in NF-κB activation appears to be in most cases the phosphorylation of I-κB molecules.

During embryogenesis, IKK2 and NEMO appear to be critical subunits for NF-κB activation and for protection of cells from proinflammatory cytokines such as TNF. Mice lacking IKK1 die shortly after birth and display a phenotype marked by thickening of skin and limb as well as skeletal defects.[36,37] In contrast, IKK2−/− mice die in utero approximately at embryonic day 12.5 as a result of massive apoptosis in the liver.[38–40] A similar phenotype was noted in mice lacking the regulatory subunit NEMO, which also die from massive apoptosis in the liver.[41,42] Interestingly, in adult mice hepatocyte-specific ablation of NEMO caused spontaneous development of hepatocellular carcinoma, preceded by chronic liver disease with hepatitis, steatohepatitis, and fibrosis.[43]

After PH, NF-κB in the liver is rapidly activated within 30 minutes.[44] Although the role of NF-κB during liver regeneration has been previously investigated using different models, it still remains controversial.

One important question is whether NF-κB is able to directly promote hepatocyte proliferation in this model. NF-κB has been shown to be able to directly stimulate the transcription of genes that encode G1-phase cyclins and a NF-κB binding site is present in the cyclin D1 promoter.[45,46] Initially, experiments were performed using an adenovirus expressing the nondegradable I-κBα super-repressor, which blocks NF-κB activation. These studies indicated that NF-κB activation after partial hepatectomy is required for liver regeneration. Animals treated with the virus showed a lack of hepatocyte proliferation and increased apoptosis.[47]

In contrast, Chaisson and colleagues used transgenic mice that expressed the nondegradable I-κBα super-repressor specifically in hepatocytes. However, only 60% of the hepatocytes expressed the transgene. These mice—in contrast to the adenovirus experiments—showed normal hepatocyte proliferation after PH.[48]

A recent study showed that PH in hepatocyte-specific IKK2 knockout mice triggered a more rapid and pronounced inflammatory response in non-parenchymal liver cells. This resulted in earlier hepatocyte proliferation and more rapid cell cycle progression. These results support previous findings that IKK2 hepatocyte-specific knockout mice provide an attenuated inflammatory response after ischemia reperfusion (I/R).[49] Taken together, these findings contribute essentially to the understanding of the role of IKK2 and consequently NF-κB signaling in injury-induced liver regeneration. The crosstalk between non-parenchymal cells and hepatocytes during this process is important to preserve the balance of NF-κB activity between the liver cell compartments in order to maintain liver homeostasis and efficiently counteract injury.[50]

TNF also triggers Jun kinase (JNK) activation.[51,52] JNK activity begins to increase within 5 minutes and reaches its peak of approximately 50-fold above basal levels within 1 hour after PH, returning to basal activity 3 hours post-PH.[53] Treatment with the JNK inhibitor SP600125 reduced hepatocyte proliferation.[54]

The JNK subgroup consist of three members—JNK1, JNK2, and JNK3—that are highly homologous.[55] JNK1 and JKN2 are ubiquitously expressed, while JNK3 expression is restricted to the brain, heart, and testis. Experiments with knockout mice revealed that in spite of significant structural homology between JNK1 and JNK2, both play different roles during liver regeneration. It was clearly demonstrated that JNK1 but not JNK2 is a positive regulator of hepatocyte proliferation.

Following two-thirds hepatectomy, JNK2–/– mice display hepatocyte proliferation rates similar to those of controls. In contrast, the hepatocyte proliferation ratio in JNK1–/– mice is reduced by 80%. Impaired liver regeneration in JNK1–/– correlates with increased p21 expression. Combined deletion of p21 and JNK1–/– restored hepatocyte proliferation, suggesting that decreased proliferation in JNK1–/– is linked to increased p21 levels during liver regeneration.[56]

Interestingly, c-Myc expression is also reduced in regenerating liver of JNK–/– mice. Hydrodynamic transfection of a c-Myc IRES CFP plasmid into JNK1–/– mice triggered significant stronger hepatocyte proliferation after PH. These data strongly indicate that JNK1 facilitates mouse liver cell proliferation controlling p21 and c-Myc expression. JNK1 activation and decreased p21 levels are important for cell proliferation during liver regeneration. p21 expression repressed by c-Myc attenuates proliferation of liver cells, probably via suppression of cyclin D1. This pathway is negatively regulated by p38-α and the NF-κB stress-signaling pathway and appears to be independent of c-jun.[56]

Via FADD, TNF can trigger apoptosis via caspase, 8 activation. This pathway can be activated by many of the TNF family members (e.g., FAS, TRAIL). However, in contrast to TNF, hepatocytes are more sensitive to Fas-induced apoptosis because after receptor binding the counter-balancing effect of NF-κB activation is missing.[57] During liver regeneration after partial hepatectomy, hepatocytes are less sensitive to Fas-induced apoptosis. Additionally, Fas stimulation enhances hepatocyte proliferation, indicating that the FADD/caspase 8 pathway during liver regeneration induces pro-proliferative effects.[58] In agreement with this hypothesis are results from transgenic mice overexpressing the anti-apoptotic protein Bcl-2 in hepatocytes, showing a delay in hepatocyte cell cycle progression during liver regeneration.[59,60] Deletion of anti-apoptotic protein Bax inhibitor-1 (Bi-1) accelerates liver regeneration after partial hepatectomy. Regenerated hepatocytes in Bi-1–/– mice quickly enter the cell cycle, and this is associated with an earlier increase of cyclins and cyclin-dependent kinases and a faster degradation of cell cycle inhibitors.[61]

Caspase 8 is an important initiator of the apoptotic cascade. After PH it is induced. However, it does not lead to apoptosis. There are several options to explain this observation after PH[62]:

1. The NF-κB and c-jun pathways inhibit apoptosis.[63,64]
2. IL-6 can protect hepatocytes from apoptosis.[65]
3. Anti-apoptotic proteins can be activated (e.g., Bcl-x Bxl2).

Therefore during the first hours after PH[66] caspase 8 seems to play a non-apoptotic role and very likely is involved in initiating hepatocyte proliferation during the initial stage of liver regeneration.[67]

Immediate Early Genes

Subsequent to priming/initiation, several immediate early-phase genes related to hepatocyte proliferation are induced within the 2 hours after PH.[4] The almost immediate activation of these genes is the first step in a cascade of events that leads to DNA synthesis (**Fig. 2-5**).

Detailed studies of the immediate early response genes revealed that more than 70 genes are activated during the first few hours after PH. The most important among these genes are c-fos, c-jun, and c-Myc.[68] Their activation follows the order fos-jun-myc. Increased expression is transient and returns to normal around 4 hours after surgery.[3]

Expression levels of both c-fos and c-jun almost increase in parallel during the first hour of liver regeneration. Although both c-fos and c-jun transcription levels are elevated shortly after partial hepatectomy, the increase in the c-fos and c-jun mRNA level is much higher than the transcriptional enhancement, implying that posttranscriptional mechanisms also play a role in the regulation of mRNA abundance.[68]

Null mutation in the c-fos proto-oncogene is not always lethal. Approximately 40% of the homozygous mutant animals live as long as their control littermates, showing that c-fos expression is not required for the growth of most cell types.[69,70] These mice can be used as a powerful model to clarify the role of the absence of c-fos expression during liver regeneration, particular because the expression of the other members of the fos family (fra1, fra2, and fra3) does not change after PH and thus is not expected to compensate for the absence of c-fos expression.[69]

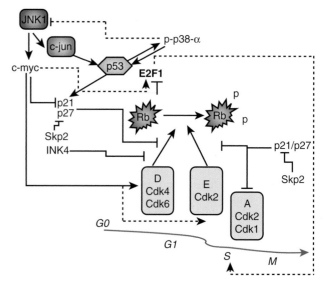

Fig. 2-5 Signaling network involving immediate early genes. Mechanistic link in the complex signaling network involving immediate early genes such as c-jun and c-myc and cell cycle regulators such p53/p21, p38-α, Rb, and E2F, which are essential for regulating the restoration of liver mass following stress responses after PH and liver injury.

Mice lacking *c-jun* die around embryonic day E13.0 and exhibit impaired hepatogenesis, altered fetal liver erythropoiesis, and generalized edema attributable to increased apoptosis in hepatoblasts and hematopoietic cells.[71,72] In contrast, mice with conditional deletion of *c-jun* in the liver are born with Mendelian frequencies. They do not develop any signs of impaired liver function and are phenotypically normal except for reduced body weight.

However, after partial hepatectomy, half of *c-jun* knockout mice die and liver regeneration is impaired. The failure to regenerate is accompanied by increased cell death and lipid accumulation in hepatocytes. At the molecular level, impaired hepatocyte proliferation correlates with increased protein level of p21, an inhibitor of cyclin-dependent kinases, resulting in inefficient G1/S-phase progression.[73]

The Wagner group showed that the increase in p21 protein level in *c-jun* deficient livers is p53 dependent and sufficient to block hepatocyte proliferation. They demonstrated that the defecting liver regeneration is completely rescued in p53 or p21 *c-jun* double knockout animals.

Interestingly, up-regulation of p21 protein in regenerating liver of *c-jun* mice correlates with increased phosphorylation of p38, a stress kinase known to stabilize p21. The conditional loss of both p38-α and *c-jun* in the liver abrogated elevated expression of p21 protein and rescued impaired hepatocyte proliferation. Taken together these data demonstrate a mechanistic link in the complex signaling network involving *c-jun*, p53/p21, and p38-α, which is essential for regulating the restoration of liver mass following stress responses such as PH and liver injury. During liver regeneration, p53 and p38 are kept at low basal activities by *c-jun*, preventing p21 protein accumulation and allowing hepatocyte proliferation. In the absence of *c-jun*, a p53-dependent and p21-mediated G1/S cell cycle block inhibits liver regeneration.[74] The transcriptional activity of *c-jun* is regulated by c-Jun N-terminal kinases (JNKs).

The *c-Myc* protein is a transcription factor implicated in the regulation of different biologic processes, such as apoptosis, cell growth, and proliferation. After PH the *c-myc* proto-oncogene reaches peak expression at 2 to 4 hours and begins to decline at 6 hours after surgery. The protein products of these nuclear proto-oncogenes are induced early in the transition from G0 to G1.[75]

c-myc knockout mice are embryonic lethal between 9.5 and 10.5 days of gestation. The embryos have multiple abnormalities; they are generally smaller and retarded in development compared with their littermates.[76]

Perinatal inactivation of *c-Myc* (*c-Mycfl/fl; cre+*, activated by pIpC) in liver causes disorganized organ architecture, decreased hepatocyte size, and cell ploidy. PH in these mice results in compromised liver regeneration and reduced PCNA expression. These data demonstrate that postnatal hepatocyte proliferation does not require *c-Myc*, although it is necessary for liver regeneration in adult mice.[77]

Progression Phase

Progression of primed hepatocytes through G1 and subsequent replicative cycling is dependent on hepatocyte growth factor (HGF), epidermal growth factor (EGF), and transforming growth factor-α (TGF-α) signaling, after which the proliferation process seems to proceed autonomously under the control of cyclins and cyclin-dependent kinases.[4]

HGF is the best characterized mitogenic growth factor involved in stimulating liver regeneration and was first isolated and purified from the serum of a patient with fulminant hepatic failure and from rats after partial hepatectomy.[78] Meanwhile it has become evident that HGF and the scatter factor are the same molecules[79] and thus the protein also has tasks in other organs besides the liver.

Activation of intracellular pathways via HGF occurs after binding to its receptor c-met (**Fig. 2-6**).[80] Crucial for the downstream activation of c-met–dependent pathways is the phosphorylation of two tyrosine residues at its intracellular domain. Tyrosine phosphorylation creates docking sites for substrates. The most relevant partner is Gab1. Through a specific Met binding site, Gab1 interacts with c-met and becomes phosphorylated. Phosphorylated Gab1 binds signal molecules such as the SH2-domain-containing protein tyrosine phosphatase 2 (Shp2), PI3K, phospholipase C, and Crk. One of the prominent downstream pathways, which becomes activated

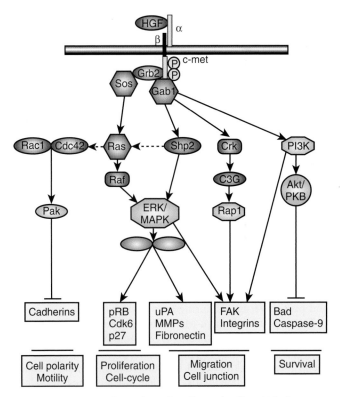

Fig. 2-6 **HGF/c-met–dependent signaling.** After ligand binding, tyrosines at the intracellular part of the c-met receptor become phosphorylated and serve as docking sites for different adapter molecules (e.g., Gab1, Grb2, phosphatidylinositol 3-kinase). As a consequence specific signaling molecules such as Ras, Shp2, and Crk become activated and trigger downstream pathways. These cascades are essential in stimulating gene expression and/or functions involved in proliferation, migration, or survival, for example. Some of the prominent pathways that are activated are the Ras/Raf/ERK/MAP kinase or PI3K/Akt/PKB pathways. *ERK/MAP KINASE,* extracellular signal-regulated kinase/mitogen-activated protein kinase; Gab1, growth factor receptor–bound protein-2 (Grb2) associated binder 1; Pak, p21-activated protein kinase; PI3K, phosphatidylinositol 3-kinase; PKB, protein kinase B; Shp2, SH2-domain-containing-protein tyrosine phosphatase 2; Sos, son-of-sevenless; met-α and -β receptor subunits. (Modified from Birchmeier C, et al. Met: metastasis, motility and more. Nat Rev Mol Cell Biol 2003;4:915–925[80]).

through c-met/Gab1/Shp2, is the ERK/MAPK pathway that triggers transcription factors such as ETS/AP1 and adhesion molecules. This mechanism is directly involved in mediating cell proliferation; however, PI3K via Akt/protein kinase B confers cell survival. Besides these main signaling pathways c-met also activates Jun terminal kinase (JNK), signal transducer and activator of transcription (Stat) 3, nuclear factor κB (NF-κB), and β-catenin (for a review, see Birchmeier et al.[80]).

c-met can also interact with other membrane receptors on the surface of the cell (e.g., E-cadherin, β4-integrin, Fas). This receptor crosstalk may also have a direct effect on the cellular response of the cell (for review, see Birchmeier et al.[80]). Therefore HGF/c-met can interact on different levels with cell cycle progression during liver regeneration.

Mice lacking HGF fail to complete embryonic development and die in utero. The mutation affects the embryonic liver, which is reduced in size and shows extensive loss of parenchymal cells. In addition, development of the placenta, particular of trophoblast cells, is impaired.[81]

It has been shown[82] that exogenous hepatocyte growth factor is a powerful mitogen for the intact murine liver. A 5-day infusion of human HGF into the portal vein resulted in an increase in relative liver mass and induction of hepatocyte proliferation.

After partial hepatectomy HGF plasma levels increase 10-fold to 20-fold. The phosphorylation of the HGF receptor c-met is observed as early as 1 to 15 minutes after PH with the largest increase at 60 minutes.[83]

The role of c-met for cell cycle progression during liver regeneration recently has been further clarified by two independent groups using conditional c-met knockout mice.[84,85] These experiments provided evidence that after partial hepatectomy, ERK activation is selectively mediated via the HGF/c-met system, which is associated with a reduction in DNA synthesis.[84] Also after carbon tetrachloride (CCl₄) injury, impaired regeneration was found and inflammatory changes in the liver of these animals were more prolonged. Additionally, the animals, which lack c-met expression, show higher sensitivity versus Fas-induced apoptosis.[84] Therefore conditional ablation of the c-met receptor in hepatocytes shows that the signaling pathway is essential for providing proliferative and protective signals during liver regeneration.

The role of HGF and c-Met in liver regeneration in rat after PH was also investigated using HGF and c-Met ShRNA. Interference with HGF has a measurable but moderate effect on the proliferation kinetics of hepatocytes. Indeed, interference with Met is associated with complete block of the cell cycle.[86]

Another important downstream effector of HGF/c-Met signal transduction is β-catenin. β-Catenin forms a complex with c-met on the hepatocyte membrane that dissociates upon stimulation with HGF. The dissociation is tyrosine phosphorylation dependent and results in β-catenin nuclear translocation and up-regulation of target genes such as *cyclin D*, *c-myc*, and *uPaR* (**Fig. 2-7**).[87]

Activation of the Wnt/β-catenin pathway has been observed during early liver development and during liver regeneration.

As early as 5 minutes after partial hepatectomy, an increase in β-catenin protein level and its translocation to the nucleus can be detected.[88]

HGF-mediated signaling pathways and β-catenin cooperate in activating hepatocyte proliferation, which is crucial for liver development and its regeneration.

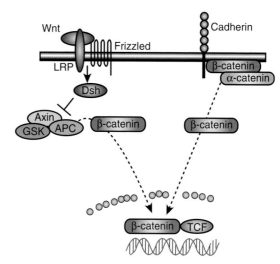

Fig. 2-7 **Schematic cartoon of β-catenin activation via Wnt and cadherin.** Binding of Wnt to its receptors Frizzled and LRP (lipoprotein receptor–related protein) results in activation of Dsh, accumulation of β-catenin, and interaction with TCF, which regulates target gene transcription. In unstimulated cells the level of β-catenin is kept low through degradation by the proteasome system involving Axin, adenomatous polyposis coli (APC), and glycogen synthase-3β (GSK). Dsh (dishevelled) uncouples β-catenin from this protein complex. Additionally, the cytoplasmic domains of type I cadherin bind β-catenin and thus link the protein via α-catenin to the actin cytoskeleton. The interaction of these molecules is controlled by phosphorylation. In general, activation of tyrosine kinases (e.g., by growth factors) results in loss of cadherin-mediated cell–cell adhesion and thus increases β-catenin expression and gene transcription. Both possibilities for activation of β-catenin result in the activation of processes involved in cell adhesion and cell migration that play a role during liver regeneration.

The delivery of the human HGF gene by a hydrodynamic tail vein injection of plasmid DNA leads to hepatomegaly via β-catenin activation in the liver. Additionally, β-catenin transgenic mice show a 15% to 20% increase in liver weight/body weight ratio.[89,90]

Liver-specific β-catenin knockout mice demonstrate significantly smaller livers, and HGF gene delivery failed to induce hepatomegaly in these mice.[90]

After PH conditional β-catenin knockout mice were sick and lethargic during the first 48 hours and proliferation was significantly decreased. However, all mice survived and an increase in hepatocyte proliferation was only detected at the third day.[91]

The following conclusions can be reached from consideration of all of these data:
1. HGF is a direct mitogen for hepatocytes.
2. HGF can induce most of the changes during liver regeneration after administration into intact mice and rats.
3. HGF's receptor (c-met) is activated very early after PH and elimination of c-met results in impaired liver regeneration.
4. β-Catenin is essential for normal liver growth and development. In the absence of β-catenin, liver regeneration is delayed.
5. Given its properties and action, HGF appears to be an essential growth factor to stimulate liver regeneration.[92]

Epidermal Growth Factor and Transforming Growth Factor-α

The epidermal growth factor receptor (EGFR/Erbb1) belongs to a family of structurally related tyrosine kinase receptors including Erbb2/neu, Erbb3, and Erbb4. Several growth factors such as epidermal growth factor (EGF), transforming growth factor-α (TGF-α), amphiregulin, heparin-binding EGF (HB-EGF), β-cellulin, and epiregulin can bind EGFR and induce receptor dimerization. Consecutive activation of the intrinsic tyrosine kinase induces complex downstream pathways (**Fig. 2-8**).[93–95]

In mice, EGF is produced mainly in salivary glands and is abundant in male animals. Mice lacking EGFR die between midgestation and postnatal day 20 depending on their genetic background, with defects in placenta, brain, bone, skin, and lung.[96]

Two possible EGFR activation loops have been suggested. Initially, activation of EGFR can occur through binding to circulating EGF. After PH plasma levels of EGF rise, which results in an increased EGF/EGFR ratio in the liver. This suggests that EGFR plays a mytogenic role in the initial phase of liver regeneration.[97]

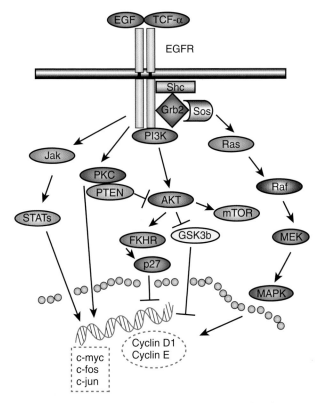

Fig. 2-8 Signaling via the epidermal growth factor (EGF) receptor. Binding of EGF or TGF-α to the EGF receptor (EGFR/Erbb1) or other members of the family (Erbb2/neu, Erbb3, and Erbb4) results in intracellular receptor homodimerization or heterodimerization. This event stimulates intrinsic tyrosine kinases and phosphorylation of the intracellular receptor domains. As a consequence, the Ras/Raf/MAP kinase cascade and other signaling pathways (e.g., PI3K, protein kinase C [PKC], Stat proteins) are activated, which translate the different EGF-dependent functions on the cellular level.

Good evidence for the important role of EGF during liver regeneration was obtained from experiments in sialoadenectomized mice and rats. In these animals DNA synthesis is reduced after 48 hours, but application of EGF can restore the phenotype.[98]

Recent experiments using transgenic mice that overexpress HB-EGF–like growth factors showed accelerated hepatocyte proliferation (five times higher in the liver of transgenic mice compared with wild type) and high liver weight/body weight ratio after PH. These data suggest that HB-EGF functions as a hepatotrophic factor in vivo.[99]

An interesting study has been performed using mice with a loxP-flanked EGFR allele.[100] Inducible Mx-cre deletion in the liver of adult mice results in impaired liver regeneration after PH. Analysis of cell cycle progression in EGF-deleted livers revealed reduction of cyclin D, Cdk2, and Cdk1 expression, which identifies EGFR as a critical growth factor receptor for hepatocyte proliferation by regulating efficient G1/S-phase transition in the initial phases after PH.

At later stages of liver regeneration, an increased expression of TGF-α is observed in hepatocytes. TGF-α binds to EGFR with lower affinity than EGF but is usually more potent in stimulating DNA synthesis in vivo and in culture.[22] It is produced by hepatocytes and acts on these cells through an autocrine mechanism.

TGF-α mRNA and protein levels in rat liver are developmentally regulated. A high expression is found during the last days of gestation and the first postnatal week.

During liver regeneration after PH in rats, TGF-α mRNA starts to increase 4 hours after PH and reaches a maximum before the peak of DNA synthesis. Protein levels are increased at 24 and 48 hours after surgery.[101] However, in mice carrying a homozygous deletion of the TGF-α gene, liver regeneration proceeded normally, indicating that TGF-α in physiologic doses is dispensable for liver regeneration.[102]

A model to study the effect of constitutive overexpression of TGF-α in the liver of adult mice was provided by a transgenic line that overexpressed human TGF-α. These results demonstrate that constitutive TGF-α overexpression causes increased hepatocyte proliferation and liver enlargement in young animals and is associated with a delay in the occurrence of hepatic polyploidy. These findings as well as the response of transgenic mice to partial hepatectomy show that constitutive overexpression of TGF-α initially caused increased but regulated hepatocyte proliferation that in older animals was compensated in part by faster cell turnover.[103]

The constitutive knockout mice for Erbb2, Erbb3, and Erbb4 die during midgestation.[104–106] However, until now no liver phenotype for all these mice has been reported.

The following conclusions can be reached from consideration of all of these data:
1. TGF-α and EGF are growth factors with important roles in hepatocyte proliferation.
2. EGF is an early signal that acts on G0 cells.
3. TGF-α acts on hepatocytes that have already entered the cell cycle and functions as a cell cycle progression agent.[103]

Notch/Jagged Signaling

The Notch/Jagged signaling pathway is relevant in different systems for cell growth and differentiation. Binding of Jagged to Notch results in a complex cascade reaction whereby the intracellular domain of NOTCH (NICD) is cleaved and migrates to the nucleus, where it functions as a transcriptional factor and mediates expression of several genes related to the cell cycle, including *Myc* and *cyclin D1*.[92]

The Notch/Jagged system seems to be directly involved in triggering cell proliferation during liver regeneration in the priming phase. After PH, nuclear translocation of the intracellular domain of Notch (NICD) increased and peaked within 15 minutes, indicating activation of Notch. Addition of recombinant Jagged-1 protein to a primary culture of hepatocytes stimulated hepatocyte DNA synthesis.

Jag1, Notch1, and Notch are essential for normal embryonic development, because mice with disruption of either gene die in midgestation.[107–109] Therefore other approaches have been used. Treatment with siRNA for Notch and Jagged-1 2 days before PH significantly suppressed proliferation of hepatocytes 2 to 4 days after surgery.[110]

Elimination of Notch using the interferon-inducible Cre/lox system soon after birth results in hepatic nodular hyperplasia. The increase of liver weight together with nodular deformation is the result of spontaneous proliferation in the absence of Notch1. Additionally, restoration of liver mass after PH is slower in Notch knockout mice compared with the control group, showing a reduced proliferative response as evidenced by BrdU incorporation.[111]

Cell Cycle Related Genes

Higher expression of immediate early genes and the activation of transcription factors are followed by the expression of cell cycle related genes. They include both inducers and inhibitors of the cycle. In mice, at the time between 30 and 36 hours post-PH, most of the hepatocytes cross the G1/S-phase boundary.[112] A peak of DNA synthesis is observed at 40 hours and mitosis occurs a few hours later. This process requires a tight coordination of several pathways.

Cyclins and their partners, the cyclin-dependent kinases (Cdks), represent the molecular basis of the cell cycle.[113] In mammals each phase (G1, S, G2, M) of the cell cycle machinery is characterized by its own set of Cdks and cyclins.[114] The most important mammalian cyclin-Cdk complexes currently known are the G1 cyclins D and E in complex with Cdk4/6 and Cdk2, respectively, and the mitotic cyclins A and B, which are associated with Cdk1 (**Fig. 2-9**).[115,116]

This model has been challenged by recent genetic evidence that mice can survive in the absence of individual interphase Cdks; studies have shown that Cdk4,[117] Cdk6,[118] and Cdk2[119] knockout mice are viable. Moreover, most mouse cell types proliferate in the absence of two or even three Cdks. Similar results have been reported after ablation of cyclins.

However, the group of Barbacid recently showed that Cdk1 activity alone can drive the mammalian cell cycle through cell division, as also shown for unicellular organisms such as yeast.[120] The embryos lacking all interphase Cdks (Cdk2, -3, -4, and -6) undergo organogenesis and develop to midgestation. In these embryos, Cdk1 binds to all cyclins, resulting in the phosphorylation of the retinoblastoma protein and the expression of genes that are regulated by E2F transcriptional factors.

The cell cycle starts from Cdk4 and Cdk6, which are activated by the D-type cyclins and have been implicated in the early phase.[121] They initiate phosphorylation of members of

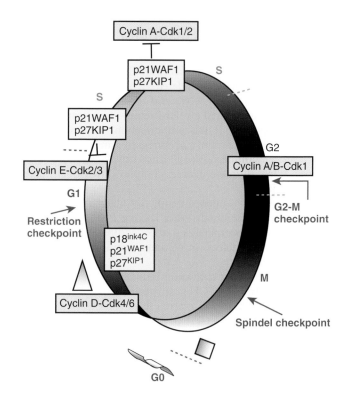

Fig. 2-9 Cell cycle progression. Cell cycle progression is dependent on the orchestrated expression and activation of specific catalytic enzymes (Cdks) with their regulatory units (cyclins). The resting hepatocyte (Go) is activated by different stimuli to enter the cell cycle. During the G1 phase, cyclin D-Cdk4/6 complexes become activated followed by cyclin E-Cdk2/3 complexes during the G1/S phase. During the S phase the cyclin A-Cdk1/2 complex is necessitate and during the G2/M phase cyclin A/B-Cdk1 is required. Additionally, cell cycle progression is controlled through a complex network of proteins where the cyclin-dependent kinase inhibitors (CKIs) play an important role. They interact with the specific cyclin/Cdk complexes and thus can manipulate their activity.

the retinoblastoma (Rb) protein family pRb—p107 and p130. The unphosphorylated Rb proteins repress gene transcription by binding and thereby inhibiting E2F transcription factors. Phosphorylation of Rb results in the release of E2F.[122] Consequently, activation of E2F in G1 allows the transcription of genes required for cell cycle progression and also relieves transcriptional repression (see **Fig. 2-5**).[123]

Inactivation of both *Rb* alleles in mice results in unscheduled cell proliferation, apoptosis, and widespread developmental defects, leading to embryonic death at day 14.5.[124] To investigate the action of pRb in liver, a model of tissue-specific inactivation of RB was developed. Rbf/f Alb Cre mice are born at the expected ratio and histologic analysis of neonatal liver reflected no gross changes in either the hepatic or the hematopoietic cells in the liver. However, liver-specific pRb loss results in E2F target gene deregulation and elevated cell cycle progression during postnatal growth. Therefore 21-day-old mice with liver-specific deletion of pRB demonstrate elevated levels of cyclin E, MCM7, PCNA, and p107 and an increased number of hepatocytes in the S phase, which was not reflective of a gross deregulation of proliferation. In adult livers (16-week-old mice) E2F targets are repressed and hepatocytes become quiescent independent of pRB, suggesting that other factors may compensate for the loss of pRb. It also has been shown that deletion of pRb in the liver results in development of pleomorphism associated with elevated ploidy.[125]

Numerous experiments have shown that E2F plays a critical role in cell cycle control. Inhibition or lack of E2F activity will block G1- to S-phase progression in mammalian cells, and ectopic expression of several E2F proteins is sufficient to induce S phase in quiescent cells. Various properties of individual E2F family members suggest a distinct functional role for these proteins: E2F1, E2F2, and E2F3 appear to play a positive role in cell cycle progression, while E2F4, E2F5, and E2F6 most likely contribute to repression of cell growth.[126–128]

Interestingly, transgenic mice expressing E2F1 under the control of the albumin promoter after PH demonstrate an overall proliferation rate comparable to wild-type controls.[129] These data argue that overexpression of E2F1 does not provide any growth advantage during compensatory regeneration after PH. Similar results were obtained[130] in E2F1−/− mice; thus in the liver E2F1 does not seem to influence its regenerative capacity.

Retinoblastoma proteins are activated by cyclin D/Cdk4-Cdk6.[131] D-type cyclins represent a very unique component of the cell cycle apparatus. Unlike other cyclins that are periodically induced during cell cycle progression, the level of D-cyclins is controlled by the extracellular mitogen environment. For this reason, D-type cyclins are believed to serve as "links" between the extracellular environment and core cell cycle machinery.[132]

Recent data indicate that cyclins D1 and D3 are regulated differently in the regenerating liver and also perform different biochemical functions. Cyclin D1 primarily forms complexes with Cdk4, which are markedly activated in the regeneration liver and readily sequester the cell cycle inhibitory proteins, such as p21 and p27. Cyclin D3 binds to both Cdk4 and Cdk6. Cyclin D3/Cdk6 activity is readily detectable in the quiescent liver and changes little after PH. This complex appears to play a minor role in sequestering p21 and p27.[133]

Treatment of D1−/− mice with the powerful hepatomitogen TCPOBOP showed that the lack of cyclin D1 expression transiently delays entry into the S phase but is not sufficient to inhibit the response of hepatocytes to mitogenic stimuli. It has also been suggested that cyclin E may functionally replace cyclin D1 during this process.[134]

In contrast to growth factor inducible D-type cyclins, the expression of E-type cyclins is controlled by an autonomous mechanism and peaks sharply at the G1/S border.[135] After passing the restriction point, the cell cycle becomes substantially less responsive to extracellular factors, which can delay entry into S phase or even arrest the cell cycle. The regulation of the cell cycle progression through the restriction point is believed to be the main function of E-type cyclins.

Two E-type cyclins—E1 and E2, which specifically bind to Cdk2—have been described. Active Cdk2-cyclin E complexes complete pRB phosphorylation.[136]

From previous work[137] it is known that E-type cyclins are critical for cell cycle reentry from quiescence and therefore play an essential role during the G0/G1-S phase transition, at least in murine embryonic fibroblasts. E1 and E2 knockout mice are viable and develop normally; however, E1/E2 double

knockout embryos die by E11.5 because of failure of endoreplication of trophoblast giant cells.[137]

In the partial hepatectomy model it was shown that cyclin E1 deletion results in normal liver regeneration with slight delay of the G1/S-phase transition but absent endoreplication in hepatocytes. In contrast, cyclin E2 knockout mice showed overexpression of cyclin E1 and prolonged Cdk2 kinase activity, leading to earlier and sustained DNA synthesis. Higher DNA synthesis in cyclin E2−/− mice is associated with higher polyploidy in the dividing hepatocytes as a result of endoreplication. Consistently, cyclin E2−/− mice showed a 45% higher liver weight/body weight ratio compared with wild-type animals after regeneration as a result of excessive polyploidization.[138]

Cdk2, a kinase previously believed to be essential for driving cells through the G1/S transition, is dispensable for normal embryonic development and adult homeostasis as Cdk2 knockout mice are viable. These animals do not have any abnormalities, except meiotic failure, which results in male and female sterility.[119]

The group of Kaldis[139] showed that the G1/S checkpoint transition in the regenerative liver is intact in the absence of Cdk2. Only a slight delay of S-phase onset was found in Cdk2 knockout mice. These observations suggested at least in part compensatory activities between Cdk2 and Cdk4. Interestingly, Cdk2/Cdk4 double knockout mice die during embryogenesis around E15 as results of heart defect.[140]

Additionally, conditional ablation of Cdk2 in adult Cdk4 knockout mice does not result in detectable abnormalities. Hepatocytes of double knockout mice 9 days after PH showed no obvious abnormalities and size differences when compared with control mice. Histologic characterization of liver sections revealed normal morphology. Taken together, these findings provide convincing evidence that adult mammalian cells proliferate normally in the absence of Cdk2 and Cdk4.[121]

Among the cyclin family, cyclin A is especially interesting because it can activate two different cyclin-dependent kinases (Cdk2 and Cdk1/Cdc2) and function in both S phase and mitosis.[141] Cyclin A starts to accumulate during S phase and is abruptly degraded before metaphase. The synthesis of cyclin A is mainly controlled at the transcription level, involving E2F and other transcription factors.[142]

Entry into mitosis in eukaryotic cells is controlled by activation of the serine/threonine kinase Cdc2, which interacts with one of several B-type cyclins. Once the activated cyclin B/Cdc2 complex moves into the nucleus, it can phosphorylate a variety of substrates, including histone H1, microtubule-associated proteins (MAPs), nuclear lamins, and centrosomal proteins. These nuclear phosphorylation events regulate the initiation and progression of mitosis.[143] Numerous reports have shown marked increases in cyclin A2 mRNA and protein expression concomitantly with DNA replication after PH.[144]

Cyclin B transcript levels are barely detectable in quiescent hepatocytes. When these cells are induced to proliferate after PH, the cyclin B transcriptional level is coordinately regulated, with maximal expression during S phase and G2.[145]

The functions of cyclins A and B during liver regeneration have to be fully studied and need to be better understood. These experiments are probably complex because constitutive disruption of cyclins A2 and B1 results in embryonic lethality.[146]

The activity of cyclin/Cdk complexes is negatively regulated by Cdk-inhibitory proteins, which can be classified into two families—the INK4 family (p15, p16, p18, and p19) inhibits Cdk4 and Cdk6; the Cip/Kip family inhibits numerous Cdks.[147]

p21 is detected in quiescent liver; it is markedly induced after PH during G1 phase and peaks during the postreplicative phase.[12] p21 knockout mice develop normally and demonstrate no developmental or phenotypic abnormalities.[148] However, p21−/− mice demonstrated evidence of markedly accelerated hepatocyte progression through G1 phase after PH. These results suggest that p21 modulates Cdk activity in regenerating liver and controls progression through the G1 phase of the cell cycle.[149]

p27 is also involved in growth regulation of hepatocytes during liver regeneration and acts as an inhibitor of Cdks activity in the pre- and postreplicative phases of the cell cycle.[149]

p27 knockout mice display increased body size and multiple organ hyperplasia.

The liver weight/body weight ratio in p27−/− mice, however, was similar to that in wild-type animals.[150]

After PH in p27-deficient mice, the timing of DNA synthesis is significantly accelerated. However, the timing of S-phase entry most strongly affects the cells around the pericentral region, without affecting the total cell population.[151]

Degradation of p27 is required for the cellular transition from the quiescent to the proliferative state. Skp2 is a rate-limiting component of the machinery that ubiquitinates and degrades phosphorylated p27. This process is mediated by complexes containing cyclin E/A and Cdk2.

In G0 or early G1 phase, p27 cannot be degraded, because of the low level of both Skp2 and cyclin E. Following mitogenic stimulation the amount of Skp2 and cyclin E increases and causes rapid p27 degradation. During the S and G2 phases, low levels of p27 are found, which are controlled by the high levels of Skp2 and cyclin A-Cdk2.[152,153]

Skp2−/− animals are viable; they have reduced body and organ size but increased mass of individual cells and polyploidy. Skp2−/− cells also exhibit increased accumulation of cyclin E and p27.[152,154]

Restoration of liver mass and function in the Skp2−/− mutant mice after PH is achieved not by cellular proliferation but by the enlargement of individual cells. Skp2−/− cells are able to enter S phase but not M phase, a characteristic of endoreplication. The enlargement and polyploidy of Skp2−/− hepatocytes are consistent with the repeated occurrence of S phase without completion of mitosis.[155]

Based on the hypothesis that p27 accumulation may contribute to some of the observed changes in Skp2−/− mice, an interesting study was performed in skp2/p27 double knockout mice. After PH loss of p27 in double knockout animals can rescue the cell size and ploidy phenotype. Double knockout mice also showed normal kinetics of cell cycle entry and progression. This observation makes p27 an essential target of skp2-dependent protein turnover.[156]

p18 (INK4c) belongs to the family of cyclin-dependent kinase inhibitory proteins. The constitutive p18 INK4c deficient mice develop gigantism and widespread organomegaly.[157] p18 expression is found in quiescent hepatocytes and it is slightly up-regulated after PH. Interestingly, no significant phenotype after PH in p18−/− animals was found. This finding very likely can be explained by functional redundancy of p18 with other cell cycle inhibitors.

This supported earlier findings in p21/p18 knockout animals: the G1 phase was shortened, as evidenced by an earlier onset of cyclin D and PCNA expression and Cdk2 activation after PH.[158]

Mice lacking both p18 and p27 initially develop normally, but later they appear visibly thin, ataxic, and dehydrated and then die from pituitary tumors at the age of 3.5 months.[157] After PH in double p18/p27 knockout mice the G1 phase was unchanged, but the amount of proliferating hepatocytes 48 hours after PH was elevated. This suggests that the two Cdk inhibitors collaborate in regulating the number of hepatocytes entering the S phase. These results indicate that the timing and strength of DNA synthesis in hepatocytes after PH are tightly regulated through the collaboration of different cell cycle inhibitors.

Termination Phase

Subsequent to the expansion phase, the growth response must finally be terminated. The most prominent factor in this process is transforming growth factor-β (TGF-β).

TGF-β is a multifunctional cytokine involved in different mechanisms (e.g., growth and development). Three forms of TGF-β (TGF-β 1-3) are known in mammals, which have 80% identity on the amino acid level. All TGF-β forms bind directly or via co-receptors to the TGF-β type II receptor. In turn they recruit, bind, and transphosphorylate type I receptors, thereby stimulating their protein kinase activity. The activated type I receptors phosphorylate Smad2 or Smad3, which then bind to Smad4. The resulting Smad complex translocates to the nucleus to interact in a cell-specific manner with various transcription factors to regulate target gene transcription (**Fig. 2-10**; for review, see Shi and Massague).[159]

In many cells TGF-β inhibits cell proliferation in G1 as it stimulates cyclin-dependent protein kinase inhibitor p15 and blocks the function or production of essential cell cycle regulators (e.g., cyclin-dependent protein kinases 2 and 4, cyclins D1 and D4).[160]

A role for TGF-β in hepatocytes was first detected in vitro, where it has strong antiproliferative activity.[161] After partial hepatectomy TGF-β mRNA increases immediately[162] and infusion of TGF-β after partial hepatectomy transiently delays the start of DNA synthesis.[163] Additionally, during liver regeneration hepatocytes acquire a transient resistance against TGF-β by down-regulation of TGF-β receptors[164] or by up-regulation of inhibitors of the TGF-β signaling pathway.[165] Therefore these results suggest that TGF-β-dependent signaling is directly involved in controlling liver regeneration at different stages. At the beginning the pathway is down-regulated in order to allow hepatocytes to enter the cell cycle; however, after DNA synthesis TGF-β sensitivity is restored in order to limit hepatocyte proliferation and terminate liver regeneration.[166]

The concept that TGF-β-dependent signaling is especially involved in the early phase of liver regeneration has been further confirmed in hepatocyte-specific knockout mice for TGF-β receptor 2 (TGFR2). These animals show an earlier and increased DNA synthesis. Additionally, liver weight in the regenerating liver is increased after partial hepatectomy.[167] However, there was no major difference in cessation of DNA synthesis between TGFR2−/− animals and controls, indicating that additional pathways are involved in blocking DNA synthesis after partial hepatectomy.[168]

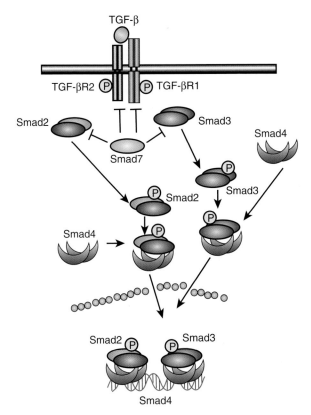

Fig. 2-10 TGF-β–dependent signaling. Binding of TGF-β induces phosphorylation and activation of the TGF-β-receptor 1 (TGF-βR1) by the TGF-β-receptor 2 (TGF-βR2). TGF-βR1 phosphorylates Smad2 and Smad3. Both factors interact with Smad4 in the cytoplasm or nucleus and regulate gene transcription in several ways. This includes by binding and interacting with other transcription factors, interacting with co-repressors, and binding to factors such as CBP and p300 involved in mediating gene transcription. Smad7 represses signaling by other Smads in order to down-regulate the cascades. Besides activating Smads, TGF-β also induces the ERK/MAP kinase cascade that is involved in modulating/inhibiting Smad proteins.

A second member of the TGF-β superfamily—activin A—has also been suggested to block hepatocyte proliferation in vitro and after partial hepatectomy.[169] Activin A induces intracellular Smad activation through its type II receptor, comparable to TGF-β. Therefore it has been suggested that activin A and TGF-β have similar roles in terminating liver regeneration. Kogure and co-workers infused follistatin—an activin A receptor antagonist—during liver regeneration and demonstrated that hepatocyte proliferation and increased liver weight are induced.[170] In the TGFR2−/− animals activin A expression was increased compared with controls. Additionally, after follistatin infusion in TGFR2−/− hepatocyte proliferation was increased after 120 hours, again indicating that the activin A–induced pathway is involved in terminating liver regeneration.[168] However, because activin A and TGF-β activate very similar intracellular pathways, there is a high probability that the two pathways are able to compensate for each other.

Smad family proteins Smad2 and Smad3 are activated by TGF-β activin/nodal receptors and mediate transcriptional regulation. Although Smad2 and Smad3 are highly similar and share regulation and overlapping function, several distinct differences determine their unique patterns of gene activation and signal transduction.

Smad2-deficient embryos die around day 7.5 of gestation because of failure of gastrulation.[171] In contrast, Smad3 null mice, although smaller than wild-type littermates, are viable and survive to adulthood.[172] Mice with hepatocyte-specific deletion of Smad2 or a double knockout of Smad2 and Smad3 are viable and develop a normal adult liver. However, after carbon tetrachloride injury hepatocyte proliferation is significantly increased in Smad2 knockout mice, and transplanted Smad2-deficient hepatocytes have a significant and persistently higher growth rate. Surprisingly, Smad2-deficient hepatocytes, stimulated by TGF-β in primary cell culture, are unable to maintain G1 arrest and apoptosis. Collectively, these results demonstrate that Smad2 suppresses hepatocyte growth and differentiation independent of TGF-β signaling.[173]

Besides TGF-β and activin A, alternative signaling cascades have been discussed that might be involved in terminating liver regeneration. An attractive candidate is sphingosine 1-phosphate (S1P) because interaction with the G-protein-coupled endothelial differentiation gene *Edg5* activates Rho activity in hepatocytes, which is growth-inhibitory. As shown for TGF-β *Edg5* also increases 24 to 72 hours after partial hepatectomy and administration of S1P during liver regeneration increases Rho activity and inhibits DNA synthesis.[174] Sphingosine 1-phosphate receptor 2–deficient mice (S1PR2) after partial hepatectomy demonstrate high proliferation and an enhanced liver weight/body weight ratio.[175]

Different pathways do exist that are involved in inhibiting hepatocyte proliferation. Further research in this area very likely will also help to develop new treatment options to limit uncontrolled growth of hepatocytes.

Key References

Apte U, et al. Activation of Wnt/beta-catenin pathway during hepatocyte growth factor-induced hepatomegaly in mice. Hepatology 2006;44(4):992–1002. (Ref.90)

Baena E, et al. c-Myc regulates cell size and ploidy but is not essential for postnatal proliferation in liver. Proc Natl Acad Sci USA 2005;102(20):7286–7291. (Ref.77)

Bailly-Maitre B, et al. Mice lacking bi-1 gene show accelerated liver regeneration. Cancer Res 2007;67(4):1442–1450. (Ref.61)

Barriere C, et al. Mice thrive without Cdk4 and Cdk2. Mol Oncol 2007;1(1):72–83. (Ref.121)

Behrens A, et al. Impaired postnatal hepatocyte proliferation and liver regeneration in mice lacking c-jun in the liver. EMBO J 2002;21(7):1782–1790. (Ref.73)

Ben Moshe T, et al. Role of caspase-8 in hepatocyte response to infection and injury in mice. Hepatology 2007;45(4):1014–1024. (Ref.67)

Berthet C, et al. Combined loss of Cdk2 and Cdk4 results in embryonic lethality and Rb hypophosphorylation. Dev Cell 2006;10(5):563–573. (Ref.140)

Birchmeier C, et al. Met, metastasis, motility and more. Nat Rev Mol Cell Biol 2003;4(12):915–925. (Ref.80)

Blindenbacher A, et al. Interleukin 6 is important for survival after partial hepatectomy in mice. Hepatology 2003;38(3):674–682. (Ref.12)

Boonstra J. Progression through the G1-phase of the on-going cell cycle. J Cell Biochem 2003;90(2):244–252. (Ref.113)

Borowiak M, et al. Met provides essential signals for liver regeneration. Proc Natl Acad Sci USA 2004;101(29):10608–10613. (Ref.84)

Chaisson ML, et al. Hepatocyte-specific inhibition of NF-kappaB leads to apoptosis after TNF treatment, but not after partial hepatectomy. J Clin Invest 2002;110(2):193–202. (Ref.48)

Conner EA, et al. Dual functions of E2F-1 in a transgenic mouse model of liver carcinogenesis. Oncogene 2000;19(44):5054–5062. (Ref.129)

Croquelois A, et al. Inducible inactivation of Notch1 causes nodular regenerative hyperplasia in mice. Hepatology 2005;41(3):487–496. (Ref.111)

Declercq W, Vanden Berghe T, Vandenabeele P. RIP kinases at the crossroads of cell death and survival. Cell 2009;138(2):229–232. (Ref.25)

Delhase M, et al. Positive and negative regulation of IkappaB kinase activity through IKKbeta subunit phosphorylation. Science 1999;284(5412):309–313. (Ref.31)

Desbarats J, Newell MK. Fas engagement accelerates liver regeneration after partial hepatectomy. Nat Med 2000;6(8):920–923. (Ref.58)

Dierssen U, et al. Molecular dissection of gp130-dependent pathways in hepatocytes during liver regeneration. J Biol Chem 2008;283(15):9886–9895. (Ref.18)

Eferl R, et al. Functions of c-Jun in liver and heart development. J Cell Biol 1999;145(5):1049–1061. (Ref.72)

Elliott J. SOCS3 in liver regeneration and hepatocarcinoma. Mol Interv 2008;8(1):19–21, 2. (Ref.19)

Fausto N. Liver regeneration. J Hepatol 2000;32(Suppl 1):19–31. (Ref.3)

Galluzzi L, Kepp O, Kroemer G. RIP kinases initiate programmed necrosis. J Mol Cell Biol 2009;1(1):8–10. (Ref.26)

Geng Y, et al. Cyclin E ablation in the mouse. Cell 2003;114(4):431–443. (Ref.137)

Giacinti C, Giordano A. RB and cell cycle progression. Oncogene 2006;25(38): 5220–5227. (Ref.122)

Guttridge DC, et al. NF-kappaB controls cell growth and differentiation through transcriptional regulation of cyclin D1. Mol Cell Biol 1999;19(8):5785–5799. (Ref.45)

Hayashi E, et al. Loss of p27(Kip1) accelerates DNA replication after partial hepatectomy in mice. J Surg Res 2003;111(2):196–202. (Ref.151)

Hinz M, et al. NF-kappaB function in growth control: regulation of cyclin D1 expression and G0/G1-to-S-phase transition. Mol Cell Biol 1999;19(4):2690–2698. (Ref.46)

Hu Y, et al. Abnormal morphogenesis but intact IKK activation in mice lacking the IKKalpha subunit of IkappaB kinase. Science 1999;284(5412):316–320. (Ref.36)

Huh CG, et al. Hepatocyte growth factor/c-met signaling pathway is required for efficient liver regeneration and repair. Proc Natl Acad Sci USA 2004;101(13):4477-4482. (Ref.85)

Hui L, et al. Proliferation of human HCC cells and chemically induced mouse liver cancers requires JNK1-dependent p21 downregulation. J Clin Invest 2008;118(12):3943–3953. (Ref.176)

Hui L, et al. Proliferation of human HCC cells and chemically induced mouse liver cancers requires JNK1-dependent p21 downregulation. J Clin Invest 2008;118(12):3943–3953. (Ref.56)

Ikeda H, et al. Antiproliferative property of sphingosine 1-phosphate in rat hepatocytes involves activation of Rho via Edg-5. Gastroenterology 2003;124(2):459–469. (Ref.174)

Ikeda H, et al. Sphingosine 1-phosphate regulates regeneration and fibrosis after liver injury via sphingosine 1-phosphate receptor 2. J Lipid Res 2009;50(3):556–564. (Ref.175)

Ju W, et al. Deletion of Smad2 in mouse liver reveals novel functions in hepatocyte growth and differentiation. Mol Cell Biol 2006;26(2):654–667. (Ref.173)

Kaldis P, Aleem E. Cell cycle sibling rivalry: Cdc2 vs. Cdk2. Cell Cycle 2005;4(11):1491–1494. (Ref.114)

Karin M. How NF-kappaB is activated: the role of the IkappaB kinase (IKK) complex. Oncogene 1999;18(49):6867–6874. (Ref.35)

Kiso S, et al. Liver regeneration in heparin-binding EGF-like growth factor transgenic mice after partial hepatectomy. Gastroenterology 2003;124(3):701–707. (Ref.99)

Kohler C, et al. Expression of Notch-1 and its ligand Jagged-1 in rat liver during liver regeneration. Hepatology 2004;39(4):1056–1065. (Ref.110)

Kossatz U, et al. Skp2-dependent degradation of p27kip1 is essential for cell cycle progression. Genes Dev 2004;18(21):2602–2607. (Ref.156)

Kovalovich K, et al. Interleukin-6 protects against Fas-mediated death by establishing a critical level of anti-apoptotic hepatic proteins FLIP, Bcl-2, and Bcl-xL. J Biol Chem 2001;276(28):26605–26613. (Ref.15)

Kozar K, Sicinski P. Cell cycle progression without cyclin D-CDK4 and cyclin D-CDK6 complexes. Cell Cycle 2005;4(3):388–391. (Ref.132)

Ledda-Columbano GM, et al. Loss of cyclin D1 does not inhibit the proliferative response of mouse liver to mitogenic stimuli. Hepatology 2002;36(5):1098–1105. (Ref.134)

Leone G, et al. Myc requires distinct E2F activities to induce S phase and apoptosis. Mol Cell 2001;8(1):105–113. (Ref.126)

Li Q, et al. Severe liver degeneration in mice lacking the IkappaB kinase 2 gene. Science 1999;284(5412):321–325. (Ref.38)

Li W, et al. STAT3 contributes to the mitogenic response of hepatocytes during liver regeneration. J Biol Chem 2002;277(32):28411–28417. (Ref.11)

Li ZW, et al. The IKKbeta subunit of IkappaB kinase (IKK) is essential for nuclear factor kappaB activation and prevention of apoptosis. J Exp Med 1999;189(11):1839–1845. (Ref.39)

Luedde T, et al. Deletion of IKK2 in hepatocytes does not sensitize these cells to TNF-induced apoptosis but protects from ischemia/reperfusion injury. J Clin Invest 2005;115(4):849–859. (Ref.49)

Luedde T, et al. Deletion of NEMO/IKKgamma in liver parenchymal cells causes steatohepatitis and hepatocellular carcinoma. Cancer Cell 2007;11(2):119–132. (Ref.43)

Luedde T, et al. p18(INK4c) collaborates with other CDK-inhibitory proteins in the regenerating liver. Hepatology 2003;37(4):833–841. (Ref.158)

Luedde T, Beraza N, Trautwein C. Evaluation of the role of nuclear factor-kappaB signaling in liver injury using genetic animal models. J Gastroenterol Hepatol 2006;21 Suppl 3:S43–S46. (Ref.42)

Macias-Silva M, et al. Up-regulated transcriptional repressors SnoN and Ski bind Smad proteins to antagonize transforming growth factor-beta signals during liver regeneration. J Biol Chem 2002;277(32):28483–28490. (Ref.165)

Malato Y, et al. Hepatocyte-specific inhibitor-of-kappaB-kinase deletion triggers the innate immune response and promotes earlier cell proliferation during liver regeneration. Hepatology 2008;47(6):2036–2050. (Ref.50)

Malumbres M, et al. Mammalian cells cycle without the D-type cyclin-dependent kinases Cdk4 and Cdk6. Cell 2004;118(4):493–504. (Ref.118)

Mayhew CN, et al. Liver-specific pRB loss results in ectopic cell cycle entry and aberrant ploidy. Cancer Res 2005;65(11):4568–4577. (Ref.125)

Michalopoulos GK. Liver regeneration. J Cell Physiol 2007;213(2):286–300. (Ref.92)

Minamishima YA, Nakayama K. Recovery of liver mass without proliferation of hepatocytes after partial hepatectomy in Skp2-deficient mice. Cancer Res 2002;62(4):995–999. (Ref.155)

Monga SP, et al. Changes in WNT/beta-catenin pathway during regulated growth in rat liver regeneration. Hepatology 2001;33(5):1098–1109. (Ref.88)

Monga SP, et al. Hepatocyte growth factor induces Wnt-independent nuclear translocation of beta-catenin after Met-beta-catenin dissociation in hepatocytes. Cancer Res 2002;62(7):2064–2071. (Ref.87)

Moroy T, Geisen C. Cyclin E. Int J Biochem Cell Biol 2004;36(8):1424–1439. (Ref.136)

Nakayama K, et al. Targeted disruption of Skp2 results in accumulation of cyclin E and p27(Kip1), polyploidy and centrosome overduplication. EMBO J 2000;19(9):2069–2081. (Ref.154)

Natarajan A, Wagner B, Sibilia M. The EGF receptor is required for efficient liver regeneration. Proc Natl Acad Sci USA 2007;104(43):17081–17086. (Ref.100)

Nevzorova YA, et al. Aberrant cell cycle progression and endoreplication in regenerating livers of mice that lack a single E-type cyclin. Gastroenterology 2009;137(2):691–703. (Ref.138)

Ni HM, et al. Differential roles of JNK in ConA/GalN and ConA-induced liver injury in mice. Am J Pathol 2008;173(4):962–972. (Ref.63)

Oe S, et al. Intact signaling by transforming growth factor beta is not required for termination of liver regeneration in mice. Hepatology 2004;40(5):1098–1105. (Ref.168)

Olayioye MA, et al. The ErbB signaling network: receptor heterodimerization in development and cancer. EMBO J 2000;19(13):3159–3167. (Ref.93)

Ortega S, et al. Cyclin-dependent kinase 2 is essential for meiosis but not for mitotic cell division in mice. Nat Genet 2003;35(1):25–31. (Ref.119)

Paranjpe S, et al. Cell cycle effects resulting from inhibition of hepatocyte growth factor and its receptor c-Met in regenerating rat livers by RNA interference. Hepatology 2007;45(6):1471–1477. (Ref.86)

Porter LA, Donoghue DJ. Cyclin B1 and CDK1: nuclear localization and upstream regulators. Prog Cell Cycle Res 2003;5:335–347. (Ref.143)

Ren X, et al. Stem cell factor restores hepatocyte proliferation in IL-6 knockout mice following 70% hepatectomy. J Clin Invest 2003;112(9):1407–1418. (Ref.9)

Rickheim DG, et al. Differential regulation of cyclins D1 and D3 in hepatocyte proliferation. Hepatology 2002;36(1):30–38. (Ref.133)

Riehle KJ, et al. Regulation of liver regeneration and hepatocarcinogenesis by suppressor of cytokine signaling 3. J Exp Med 2008;205(1):91–103. (Ref.21)

Roberts AW, et al. Placental defects and embryonic lethality in mice lacking suppressor of cytokine signaling 3. Proc Natl Acad Sci USA 2001;98(16):9324–9329. (Ref.20)

Romero-Gallo J, et al. Inactivation of TGF-beta signaling in hepatocytes results in an increased proliferative response after partial hepatectomy. Oncogene 2005;24(18):3028–3041. (Ref.167)

Rudolph D, et al. Severe liver degeneration and lack of NF-kappaB activation in NEMO/IKKgamma-deficient mice. Genes Dev 2000;14(7):854–862. (Ref.41)

Sabapathy K, Wagner EF. JNK2: a negative regulator of cellular proliferation. Cell Cycle 2004;3(12):1520–1523. (Ref.55)

Santamaria D, et al. Cdk1 is sufficient to drive the mammalian cell cycle. Nature 2007;448(7155):811–815. (Ref.120)

Satyanarayana A, et al. Gene expression profile at the G1/S transition of liver regeneration after partial hepatectomy in mice. Cell Cycle 2004;3(11):1405–1417. (Ref.112)

Satyanarayana A, Hilton MB, Kaldis P. p21 inhibits Cdk1 in the absence of Cdk2 to maintain the G1/S phase DNA damage checkpoint. Mol Biol Cell 2008;19(1):65–77. (Ref.139)

Schlessinger J. Cell signaling by receptor tyrosine kinases. Cell 2000;103(2):211–225. (Ref.94)

Schwabe RF, et al. c-Jun-N-terminal kinase drives cyclin D1 expression and proliferation during liver regeneration. Hepatology 2003;37(4):824–832. (Ref.54)

Shi Y, Massague J. Mechanisms of TGF-beta signaling from cell membrane to the nucleus. Cell 2003;113(6):685–700. (Ref.159)

Skarpen E, et al. Altered regulation of EGF receptor signaling following a partial hepatectomy. J Cell Physiol 2005;202(3):707–716. (Ref.97)

Skaug B, Jiang X, Chen ZJ. The role of ubiquitin in NF-kappaB regulatory pathways. Annu Rev Biochem 2009;78:769–796. (Ref.29)

Stepniak E, et al. c-Jun/AP-1 controls liver regeneration by repressing p53/p21 and p38 MAPK activity. Genes Dev 2006;20(16):2306–2314. (Ref.74)

Streetz KL, et al. Lack of gp130 expression in hepatocytes promotes liver injury. Gastroenterology 2003;125(2):532–543. (Ref.14)

Strey CW, et al. The proinflammatory mediators C3a and C5a are essential for liver regeneration. J Exp Med 2003;198(6):913–923. (Ref.16)

Takeda K, et al. Role of early continuous regional arterial infusion of protease inhibitor and antibiotic in nonsurgical treatment of acute necrotizing pancreatitis. Digestion 1999;60(Suppl 1):9–13. (Ref.37)

Tan X, et al. Conditional deletion of beta-catenin reveals its role in liver growth and regeneration. Gastroenterology 2006;131(5):1561–1572. (Ref.91)

Tan X, et al. Epidermal growth factor receptor: a novel target of the Wnt/beta-catenin pathway in liver. Gastroenterology 2005;129(1):285–302. (Ref.89)

Tanaka M, et al. Embryonic lethality, liver degeneration, and impaired NF-kappa B activation in IKK-beta-deficient mice. Immunity 1999;10(4):421–429. (Ref.40)

Vail ME, et al. Bcl-2 expression delays hepatocyte cell cycle progression during liver regeneration. Oncogene 2002;21(10):1548–1555. (Ref.60)

Vail ME, Pierce RH, Fausto N. Bcl-2 delays and alters hepatic carcinogenesis induced by transforming growth factor alpha. Cancer Res 2001;61(2):594–601. (Ref.59)

Volkmann X, et al. Caspase activation is associated with spontaneous recovery from acute liver failure. Hepatology 2008;47(5):1624–1633. (Ref.67)

Wuestefeld T, et al. Interleukin-6/glycoprotein 130-dependent pathways are protective during liver regeneration. J Biol Chem 2003;278(13):11281–11288. (Ref.13)

Wullaert A, et al. Hepatic tumor necrosis factor signaling and nuclear factor-kappaB: effects on liver homeostasis and beyond. Endocr Rev 2007;28(4):365–386. (Ref.64)

Yam CH, Fung TK, Poon RY. Cyclin A in cell cycle control and cancer. Cell Mol Life Sci 2002;59(8):1317–1326. (Ref.142)

Yamamoto Y, Gaynor RB. IkappaB kinases: key regulators of the NF-kappaB pathway. Trends Biochem Sci 2004;29(2):72–79. (Ref.34)

Yarden Y, Sliwkowski MX. Untangling the ErbB signalling network. Nat Rev Mol Cell Biol 2001;2(2):127–137. (Ref.95)

Zimmermann A. Regulation of liver regeneration. Nephrol Dial Transplant 2004;19(Suppl 4):6-10. (Ref.4)

Zorde-Khvalevsky E, et al. Toll-like receptor 3 signaling attenuates liver regeneration. Hepatology 2009;50(1):198–206. (Ref.62)

A complete list of references can be found at www.expertconsult.com.

Chapter 3

Mechanisms of Liver Cell Destruction

Harmeet Malhi

ABBREVIATIONS

ATF4 activating transcription factor 4
ATF6 activating transcription factor 6
CHOP C/EBP-homologous protein
eIF2-α eukaryotic translation initiation factor 2α
ER endoplasmic reticulum
FADD Fas-associated death domain
FasL Fas ligand
IRE1 inositol-requiring protein 1
JNK c-jun N-terminal kinase

NF-κB nuclear factor κB
NK natural killer
PERK PKR–like ER kinase
PKR double-stranded RNA-dependent protein kinase
TNF-α tumor necrosis factor-α
TNFR1 tumor necrosis factor receptor 1
TNFR2 tumor necrosis factor receptor 2
TRAF2 tumor necrosis factor receptor–associated factor 2

TRAIL tumor necrosis factor–related apoptosis-inducing ligand
TRAIL-R1 tumor necrosis factor–related apoptosis-inducing ligand receptor 1
TRAIL-R2 tumor necrosis factor–related apoptosis-inducing ligand receptor 2
XBP1 X-box binding protein 1

Introduction

The liver is a dynamic organ characterized by several unique properties, including self-renewal, that permit its daily exposure to ingested nutrients, gut-derived endobiotics, and xenobiotic metabolism without adverse consequences. The unique position of the liver also confers vulnerability to a wide variety of insults and injury. These are characterized by cell death, which can target any cell type in the liver. Hepatocytes, the most abundant cell type, are most commonly affected in both acute and chronic liver diseases.[1,2] Other cell types, such as endothelial cells and biliary epithelial cells, are affected in a disease-specific manner.[2] Hepatic inflammation facilitates, accelerates, and augments liver injury. Indeed, the innate immune system plays a key role in liver injury. Hepatocyte cell death is a unifying mechanistic theme throughout the temporal spectrum of liver injury (**Fig. 3-1**). Acute liver injury, defined arbitrarily on the basis of duration, can either resolve completely or progress into fulminant hepatic failure or chronic liver injury. In resolved acute injury, liver architecture and function are restored completely, without any enduring evidence of earlier cell death. However, chronic liver injury is characterized by ongoing cell death and, ultimately, the development of hepatic fibrosis. Progressive fibrosis results in cirrhosis of the liver and its well-known complications.

Hepatocyte cell death has been recognized histologically in many acute and chronic liver diseases, as well as in fulminant hepatic failure. Modes of cell death in the liver can be defined morphologically or mechanistically. Traditionally, cell death has been defined morphologically. In liver disease apoptotic cell death, necrotic cell death, and autophagic cell death have

been described. Mechanistically, the modes of cell death relevant to the liver are apoptosis, necrosis, necroptosis, and autophagy. These modes of cell death have been classified on the basis of their cellular and molecular pathways, in addition to their morphology. Although morphologic features continue to be distinct for these modes of cell death and aid in the histologic identification of each mode, increasingly the molecular mediators of these pathways are being elucidated. In the liver an injurious stimulus can result in both apoptotic and necrotic cell death, depending on the state of the cell.[3,4] Upon activation of apoptotic signaling by death receptors, in cells deficient in key mediators of apoptosis, cell death ensues by an alternative pathway, termed necroptosis.[5,6] Furthermore, even though a given cell dies by one mode of cell death, in a particular disease or in response to a death-inducing stimulus multiple pathways are activated in the context of the whole liver. Thus advances in understanding the processes of liver cell death are more important than labeling death on the basis of morphology alone. In this chapter, each morphologic mode of cell death and its known molecular mediators are presented in an integrated manner along with their relevance to liver injury. In some instances liver-specific information is lacking and paradigms are based on other model systems.

Apoptosis

Apoptotic hepatocytes can be identified in almost every etiology of liver injury. In patients with yellow fever, the pathologist William T. Councilman (1854-1933) described what are now recognized as apoptotic hepatocytes, eponymously known also as Councilman bodies. Apoptotic cells

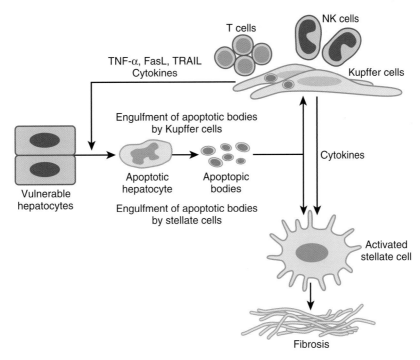

Fig. 3-1 Apoptosis, inflammation, and fibrosis in the liver. In disease states apoptosis of vulnerable hepatocytes triggers an inflammatory response. Kupffer cells are activated by engulfment of apoptotic bodies, the primary means of removal of apoptotic bodies. Kupffer cells and cells of the innate immune system secrete death ligands, which induce further apoptosis of vulnerable hepatocytes as well as inflammatory cytokines. Stellate cells are activated in chronic injury by a combination of engulfment of apoptotic bodies and cytokines, leading to hepatic fibrosis.

are characterized morphologically by cell shrinkage, chromatin condensation (pyknosis), nuclear fragmentation (karyorrhexis), and formation of membrane-bound apoptotic bodies and their elimination by phagocytosis. Since its earliest description, apoptosis has been recognized as programmed cell death (i.e., regulated either by a developmental program using intrinsic cellular mediators or by extrinsic factors). Physiologic apoptosis, such as developmental apoptosis or homeostatic removal of senescent cells, is not associated with an inflammatory response. However, pathologic apoptosis, as in acute or chronic liver disease, activates inflammatory pathways. Engulfment of apoptotic bodies by Kupffer cells leads to their activation and secretion of inflammatory cytokines, including tumor necrosis factor-α (TNF-α) and Fas ligand (FasL).[7] Apoptotic body engulfment also activates stellate cells and promotes hepatic fibrogenesis.[8] Indeed, in mouse models of liver injury inhibition of apoptosis attenuates both the inflammatory response and fibrosis, thus solidifying the importance of apoptosis in disease pathogenesis.[7,9,10] Apoptotic cell death of activated stellate cells, in turn, is a mechanism for fibrosis resolution and abrogation of the fibrotic response.[11]

Hepatocyte apoptosis can be initiated either by the extrinsic—or death receptor—pathway or by the intrinsic pathway (**Fig. 3-2**). The death receptors are cell surface receptors that are activated upon ligation with their cognate ligands. The receptors present on hepatocytes and their ligand pairs are Fas and Fas ligand (FasL); tumor necrosis factor receptors 1 and 2 (TNFR1 and TNFR2, respectively) and TNF-α ligand; and tumor necrosis factor–related apoptosis-inducing ligand receptors 1 and 2 (TRAIL-R1 and TRAIL-R2, respectively) and TRAIL ligand. The intrinsic (mitochondrial) pathway of apoptosis is activated by intracellular stress, such as oxidative stress or metabolic stress, and by organelle dysfunction, such as DNA damage, endoplasmic reticulum (ER) stress, and lysosomal permeabilization. In hepatocytes, both the intrinsic and extrinsic pathways of apoptosis converge on mitochondria, and mitochondrial permeabilization is an obligate step in the execution of apoptosis. Mitochondrial permeabilization results in the activation of effector caspases (cysteine proteases that cleave aspartate residues), which degrade intracellular targets and result in the characteristic apoptotic morphology.

The Extrinsic Apoptosis Pathway
Death Receptors

Death receptors belong to the tumor necrosis factor/nerve growth factor superfamily. They are type I transmembrane proteins with a conserved cytoplasmic death domain (DD). The DD facilitates homotypic interactions with adaptor proteins, via their death domain motifs. Death receptors are activated upon ligation with their cognate ligands (i.e., cytokines, which are type II transmembrane proteins) and can also be cleaved by metalloproteases into soluble circulating forms. Tumor necrosis factor-α (TNF-α), Fas ligand (FasL), and tumor necrosis factor–related apoptosis-inducing ligand (TRAIL) are ligands—that along with their receptors TNFR1, Fas, and TRAIL-R1 and TRAIL-R2, respectively—have well-recognized roles in liver injury. Receptor-ligand binding initiates a signaling cascade that starts with homooligomerization

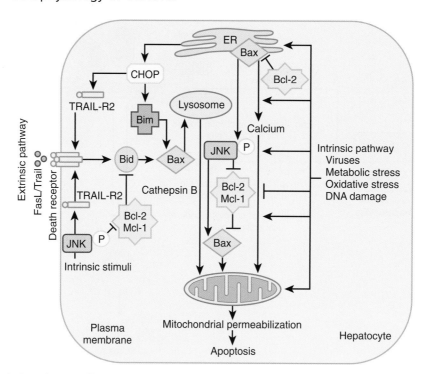

Fig. 3-2 Extrinsic and intrinsic pathways of hepatocyte apoptosis converge on mitochondria. Death receptor–ligand pairs mediate the extrinsic pathway of apoptosis. Upon receptor ligation the death-inducing signaling complex (DISC) is formed with subsequent caspase 8 activation, Bid cleavage, and eventual mitochondrial permeabilization. Bcl-2 proteins regulate this pathway as well as the intrinsic pathway. Intracellular stress capable of inducing apoptosis can activate the intrinsic pathway of cell death at many different levels. Lysosomal permeabilization, with release of cathepsin B, leads to mitochondrial permeabilization. Endoplasmic reticulum (ER) stress can lead to pro-apoptotic JNK activation or alter calcium homeostasis. Intracellular stressors can directly act on mitochondria, activate JNK, or alter expression of Bcl-2 family pro-apoptotic and anti-apoptotic proteins.

of the ligated receptor and recruitment of adaptor proteins followed by activation of initiator caspases 8 and 10. This signaling platform is designated the death-inducing signaling complex (DISC), for Fas- and TRAIL-initiated signals. TNF-α signaling is distinct from Fas and TRAIL, and activates inflammatory and prosurvival signals before the onset of apoptotic signals. One level of regulation of apoptotic signals that emanate from ligated death receptors is at the level of the DISC. Cellular caspase 8 (FLICE)–like regulatory proteins (cFLIP) function as dominant negative regulators of caspase 8 activation at the DISC. cFLIP isoforms share homology with caspase 8, preventing its homodimerization.[12] Overexpression of cFLIP$_L$ (one of several isoforms) in vitro can inhibit apoptotic signaling from Fas, TNFR1, TRAIL-R1, and TRAIL-R2. Cells can be sensitized to TNF-α–induced apoptosis by enhanced degradation of cFLIP$_L$ via c-jun N-terminal kinase (JNK) mediated ubiquitination and proteasomal degradation.[13]

Fas

Fas is ubiquitously expressed on various liver cell types and can induce apoptosis of hepatocytes, cholangiocytes, sinusoidal endothelial cells, stellate cells, and Kupffer cells.[2] Fas (CD95/APO-1) is activated naturally by binding to membrane-bound FasL (i.e., soluble FasL) or experimentally by exposure to agonistic antibodies. Cells of the innate immune system, Kupffer cells, and natural killer (NK) cells as well as cytotoxic T lymphocytes (CTL) are endogenous sources of FasL. Fas

DISC is formed upon ligation and oligomerization of Fas, which leads to recruitment of the adaptor molecule Fas-associated death domain (FADD) through its DD. FADD also possesses a death effector domain (DED), which recruits procaspase 8, again via a homotypic interaction. Procaspase 8 is activated by autoproteolytic cleavage to caspase 8. Downstream of caspase 8, cells dying via Fas-induced signals can be classified as either type I or type II.[14] In type I cells, such as lymphocytes, caspase 8 activated at the DISC is sufficient to activate the effector caspase, caspase 3. However, in type II cells, such as hepatocytes, caspase 8 cleaves Bid, a pro-apoptotic Bcl-2 family protein, thus activating the intrinsic apoptotic pathway. The cleaved fragment, tBid, activates the pro-apoptotic proteins Bax and Bak, leading to mitochondrial outer membrane permeabilization (MOMP) and eventual activation of caspase 3. In addition to Bid, another key determinant of the response to Fas-induced signals is X-chromosome linked inhibitor of apoptosis protein (XIAP). XIAP binds to and inhibits active caspase 3; therefore in cells deficient in XIAP, type I signaling predominates[15] (**Fig. 3-3**).

Sensitivity to Fas-induced cell death can be modulated in many ways. The availability of cell surface Fas is one such determinant. In healthy liver Fas is compartmentalized intracellularly mostly in the Golgi and *trans*-Golgi network, preventing spontaneous oligomerization and cell death. Translocation from the Golgi network to the cell surface (e.g., upon stimulation with bile salts) enhances Fas availability, without the need for translation of new protein.[16] Cell surface Fas is also bound to the hepatocyte growth factor (HGF)

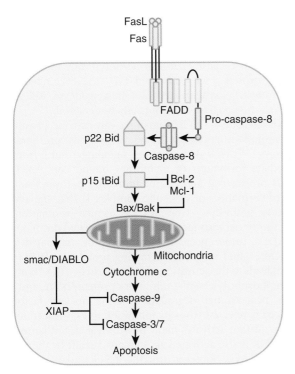

Fig. 3-3 Fas receptor signaling. The extrinsic apoptotic pathway of Fas ligand–induced cell death occurs upon receptor ligation. The adaptor protein Fas-associated death domain (FADD) binds to the intracellular death domain (DD) of the oligomerized receptor. Through homotypic interaction via its death effector domain (DED), FADD recruits procaspase 8, followed by autoproteolytic cleavage and homodimerization to form active caspase 8. Caspase 8 cleaves the pro-apoptotic protein Bid to tBid, which in turn activates Bax and Bak, resulting in mitochondrial outer membrane permeabilization and release of mitochondrial intermembrane space contents, with eventual activation of caspase 3/7. Hepatocytes are type II cells, with regard to Fas-induced cell death. Thus death signaling is sensitive to the anti-apoptotic Bcl-2 family proteins, as well as XIAP.

receptor Met, leading to its sequestration and diversion from cell death pathways.[17] Met competes with the cognate ligand, FasL, for Fas binding, and at low concentrations of FasL, receptor ligation is prevented. The binding of HGF to Met releases Fas from inhibition, and a higher concentration of FasL can also overcome the inhibition; both situations would favor apoptotic signaling. Fas receptor expression is also regulated transcriptionally. Enhanced expression, such as in fatty liver, confers sensitivity to Fas-induced apoptosis.[18] Following receptor ligation, sensitivity to apoptosis is further modulated by several pro-apoptotic and anti-apoptotic proteins. cFLIP inhibits caspase 8 activation at the level of the DISC (see preceding paragraph). Bcl-2 family proteins and XIAP determine a cell's response to Fas-induced death signals.

The liver develops normally in Fas-deficient mice even though they exhibit hepatic hyperplasia attributable to infiltration by lymphocytes and the accumulation of hepatocytes. Hepatocytes are exquisitely sensitive to Fas-induced cell death. In an experimental model using an agonistic antibody, Fas induced fulminant hepatic failure and lethality in mice.[4] The vital role of Bcl-2 family proteins in regulating sensitivity to Fas-induced apoptosis was also demonstrated in a similar experiment. Overexpression of the anti-apoptotic protein

Bcl-2 rescued animals from Fas-induced liver failure and death.[19] Mice lacking the pro-apoptotic Bcl-2 protein Bid fail to develop hepatocyte apoptosis and lethality upon exogenous administration of Fas.[20] As expected, overexpression of Met also protected mice from Fas-induced apoptosis.[21] Experimental strategies to minimize hepatocyte apoptosis and rescue lethality have also successfully used small interfering ribonucleic acid (siRNA) to silence Fas expression.[22]

In many experimental models of liver disease, Fas-induced hepatocyte apoptosis is a key pathogenic event. In a murine model of dietary fatty liver, Fas receptor expression is enhanced.[18] This is associated with sensitization to Fas-induced apoptosis. In cell culture systems, steatotic hepatocytes are sensitized to Fas-induced apoptosis.[23] Hydrophobic bile salts accumulate in the liver in cholestasis and are toxic. Glycochenodeoxycholate (GCDC), a toxic hydrophobic bile salt, induces hepatocyte apoptosis, which is partially Fas dependent. GCDC can sensitize cells to Fas-induced apoptosis, as well as spontaneous Fas oligomerization, by increasing translocation of Fas from the cytosol to the surface of the cell.[16,24] Bile salts can also sensitize cells to Fas-induced apoptosis by phosphorylation-induced activation of Fas via the Src family kinase Yes.[25] Furthermore, in the bile duct ligation mouse model of cholestatic liver injury, Fas-deficient mice (*lpr*) demonstrate abrogation of hepatocyte apoptosis and liver injury as well as hepatic fibrosis.[10]

In patients with acute liver failure, soluble Fas (sFas) levels are elevated, regardless of etiology.[26] Hepatic Fas expression correlates with apoptosis, suggesting a role for Fas-induced apoptosis in the pathogenesis of fulminant hepatic failure. This has been demonstrated in patients with drug-induced liver injury, acetaminophen-induced liver failure, and fulminant hepatitis B.[26-28] In chronic hepatitis C, infected hepatocytes demonstrate enhanced expression of Fas, and infiltrating, activated lymphocytes demonstrate enhanced expression of FasL.[29] Fas expression correlates with hepatocyte apoptosis as well as fibrosis.[30] However, not all infected hepatocytes are removed by apoptosis in spite of the activation of the Fas system, suggesting that viral factors may modulate apoptosis, permitting survival of infected cells to establish chronic infection. Patients with chronic hepatitis B and C have elevated circulating levels of soluble Fas (sFas), which correlate with treatment.[31] In liver biopsy samples from patients with chronic hepatitis B, Fas expression correlates with the activity of viral hepatitis, and Fas-positive cells are located in areas of immunologic activity.[32] Apoptosis and Fas expression are significantly increased in liver biopsy samples from patients with alcoholic hepatitis as well as nonalcoholic steatohepatitis (NASH).[1,33] Further sensitization to Fas in fatty liver is imparted by release from Met-induced inhibition.[34]

Trail

A systematic approach to identify proteins similar to TNF-α led to the identification of TRAIL; it was also found to have significant homology with FasL. TRAIL ligand binds to five known receptors, of which two, TRAIL receptor 1 (TRAIL-R1/death receptor [DR] 4) and TRAIL receptor 2 (TRAIL-R2/DR 5/Killer/TRICK2), can propagate apoptotic signals and are of relevance to liver injury.[35] TRAIL signaling shares many of the molecular mediators and regulators described previously for Fas. Upon receptor ligation, oligomerization, recruitment of

FADD, formation of the DISC, activation of procaspase 8, and cleavage of Bid occur in a similar manner. cFLIP$_L$ can inhibit TRAIL-induced apoptosis at the DISC.[12] Bcl-2 family proteins regulate sensitivity to TRAIL, because mitochondrial permeabilization is required for TRAIL-induced hepatocyte apoptosis. TRAIL receptor ligation also activates nuclear factor κB (NF-κB) and JNK via adaptor proteins. NFκB transcriptionally activates proinflammatory, prosurvival, and anti-apoptotic genes. JNK can have an anti-apoptotic effect or pro-apoptotic effect, depending on the stimulus and duration of JNK activation.

Normal human liver is resistant to the apoptotic effects of TRAIL.[36] However, TRAIL can induce apoptosis in hepatocytes that are diseased or stressed. This is an important consideration in patients receiving TRAIL agonistic antibodies for cancer chemotherapy, to minimize potential hepatotoxicity. Sensitization to TRAIL has been observed in experimental acute hepatitis and chronic viral hepatitis as well as in nonalcoholic fatty liver disease.[23,37,38] In mouse models of concanavalin A–mediated acute hepatitis and *Listeria monocytogenes* infection, TRAIL-deficient mice are resistant to liver injury.[37] Adoptive transfer of TRAIL-expressing liver mononuclear cells restored sensitivity to concanavalin A (ConA). Thus sensitivity to TRAIL can be regulated by the presence of TRAIL-expressing cells of the innate immune system or cell surface expression of TRAIL-R1 and TRAIL-R2. Enhanced expression of TRAIL-R2 (DR5) on hepatocytes with constitutive activation of NFκB also results in sensitization to TRAIL toxicity, suggesting that NFκB-mediated chronic inflammation sensitizes to TRAIL-induced apoptosis, consistent with previous observations.[39] The stress kinase JNK, as well as the transcription factor CHOP, can up-regulate TRAIL-R2 expression, thereby sensitizing stressed cells to apoptosis.[23,40] In cell culture systems, hepatitis C and hepatitis B viral proteins can modulate TRAIL receptor expression. This may be pro-apoptotic, with enhanced TRAIL receptor expression leading to removal of infected cells, or anti-apoptotic, with diminished TRAIL-R2 expression promoting survival of an infected cell and the establishment of chronic infection.

The expression of TRAIL-R1 and TRAIL-R2 is enhanced in liver biopsy samples from patients with chronic liver disease.[36] This has been observed in patients with nonalcoholic fatty liver disease (NAFLD), chronic hepatitis C, and chronic hepatitis B.[23,36,38] Utilizing explanted liver specimens from patients with NAFLD or hepatitis C, sensitization to TRAIL-induced apoptosis was demonstrated.[36] In patients with hepatitis B, TRAIL-expressing NK cells of the innate immune system are enriched in the liver, providing a mechanism to remove virus-infected cells; indeed, flares of inflammation correlate with NK cell expression of TRAIL.[38]

Tumor Necrosis Factor-α

Tumor necrosis factor-α was named for its ability to induce tumor cell death during the process of its discovery and characterization. Phenomenal research has established a role for this cytokine in a myriad of biologic processes.[41] In the liver TNF-α mediates injury, inflammation, regeneration, and cell death. It is produced by cells of the immune system but can also be expressed by hepatocytes, both in a membrane-bound form and in a soluble form. There are two distinct receptors on hepatocytes that can bind TNF-α— tumor necrosis factor receptor 1 (TNFR1) and tumor necrosis factor receptor 2 (TNFR2). Only TNFR1 possesses an intracellular DD and therefore the ability to activate the apoptotic program via activation of caspase 8. It also homotypically interacts with adaptor proteins, via conserved DD.[42] TNFR2 may play a cooperative or synergistic role in hepatocyte cell death; however, the mechanism is not fully understood.[43]

TNF-α–ligated TNFR1 signaling can activate prosurvival and proinflammatory pathways as well as pro-apoptotic pathways.[44-46] This dichotomous signaling results from the immediate formation of membrane-bound complex I that signals prosurvival and proinflammatory pathways and the delayed formation of cytosolic complex II that signals pro-apoptotic pathways.[45] Complex I is formed by adaptor proteins, tumor necrosis factor receptor–associated death domain (TRADD), tumor necrosis factor receptor–associated factor 2 (TRAF2), and receptor interacting protein 1 (RIP-1) (**Fig. 3-4**). It leads to the activation of the IκB kinase (IKK) complex, which phosphorylates the inhibitory protein, IκBα, and leads to its proteasomal degradation. Thus nuclear factor κB (NF-κB) is released from its inhibition. NFκB is a transcription factor that activates many prosurvival and inflammatory genes. JNK is also activated via a kinase cascade by the adaptor protein TRAF2. Subsequently, the TNFR1/adaptor complex undergoes a conformational change and recruits the adaptor protein FADD, forming complex II, which leads to activation of caspase 8, cleavage of Bid, and subsequent apoptotic signaling. TNF-α can also mediate non-apoptotic cell death via the adaptor protein RIP1 (as described earlier in this section). Thus complex and opposing signals emanate from ligated TNFR1.

In general, TNF-α signaling in vivo is inflammatory or promotes survival.[47] However, cell death can occur under specific conditions and in experimental models. Hepatocytes can be sensitized to TNF-α–induced apoptosis by inhibition of NFκB signaling, or by utilization of inhibitors of transcription or translation, thus preventing the formation of prosurvival factors and shifting the balance of TNF-α signaling toward cell death. Prolonged JNK activation can also promote TNF-α–induced cell death. Enhanced proteasomal degradation of cFLIP and also activation of Bim are two ways in which JNK can sensitize to TNF-α–induced cell death.[13,48] TNF-α is essential for liver regeneration after partial hepatectomy.[44] In mice with constitutive activation of TNF-α chronic hepatitis ensues.[49] In experimental orthotopic liver transplantation studies using mice deficient in TNFR1 (TNFR1 −/−) and wild type as donors and recipients, it was demonstrated that in the graft TNFR1 is protective and in the recipient TNFR1 promotes injury.[50] Ethanol-fed rats demonstrated elevated circulating levels of TNF-α.[51] In a murine model of alcoholic liver disease, TNFR1-deficient mice demonstrated decreased inflammation, apoptosis, and injury.[52] This effect was specific to TNFR1-deficient mice; TNFR2-deficient mice were not protected from ethanol toxicity.[53]

Evidence for activation of the TNF-α signaling pathway can be found in most acute and chronic hepatitides. In fulminant hepatitis, serum levels of TNF-α and its receptors are elevated and correlate with prognosis.[54,55] Circulating TNF-α levels are elevated in patients with chronic hepatitis B virus (HBV).[56] In liver biopsy samples, TNF-α expressing mononuclear cell infiltration correlates with markers of HBV replication and

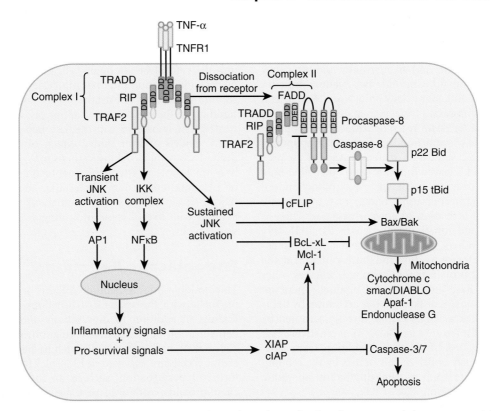

Fig. 3-4 Complex I and complex II of TNF-α signaling. Complex I is formed upon ligation of tumor necrosis factor receptor 1 (TNFR1) with TNF-α. Recruitment of adaptor proteins, TNF-R1–associated death domain protein (TRADD) and receptor-interacting protein (RIP), is via homotypic interaction between their respective death domains (DD), and of (TRAF2) via its kinase domain or an intermediate domain. These adaptors mediate the activation of nuclear factor κB (NF-κB), and the transient activation of c-jun N-terminal kinase (JNK), with subsequent up-regulation of anti-apoptotic genes and inflammatory genes. RIP also mediates sustained JNK activation. Complex II is formed upon receptor dissociation and the recruitment of FADD, which, via its death effector domain (DED), recruits and activates caspase-8 with subsequent mitochondrial permeabilization.

liver inflammation on histologic examination.[57] TNF-α receptor expression is observed in hepatocytes, sinusoidal endothelial cells, and mononuclear cells, and it also correlates with liver histology. In chronic hepatitis C, elevated receptor levels correlate with viral decay in response to therapy.[58] A TNF-α promoter genetic polymorphism that confers enhanced TNF-α expression is associated with steatohepatitis in patients with biopsy-proven alcoholic liver disease.[59] Serum levels of TNF-α receptors correlate with disease severity in patients with alcoholic hepatitis, and TNFR1 levels correlate with 3-month mortality.[60,61] Both experimental and clinical data point toward a key role for TNF-α in the pathogenesis of alcoholic hepatitis; however, this is not straightforward because blockade of TNF-α signaling with etanercept is associated with a higher mortality in patients with moderate to severe alcoholic hepatitis.[62]

The Intrinsic Apoptosis Pathway
Mitochondria

Mitochondria play a key role in hepatocyte cell death. Mitochondria are double-membraned organelles enclosing an intermembrane space that isolates and contains several mediators of apoptosis, including cytochrome *c*, AIF (apoptosis

inducing factor), SMAC/DIABLO (second mitochondrial activator of caspase/direct IAP binding protein with low p*I*), HtrA2/Omi, and endonuclease G.[63] Mitochondrial outer membrane permeabilization (MOMP), an essential step in apoptosis, results in release of these mediators into the cytosol. MOMP can occur either by selective permeabilization using the pro-apoptotic Bcl-2 family proteins Bax and Bak, or by following the mitochondrial permeability transition via the mitochondrial permeability transition pore. Bax- and Bak-dependent MOMP is regulated by the Bcl-2 protein family. Cytochrome *c* interacts with apoptotic peptidase activating factor-1 (APAF-1) to form the apoptosome, which recruits and activates procaspase 9. Caspase 9 recruits and activates the executioner caspases 3 and 7, which in turn cleave key substrates and result in the typical apoptotic morphology. The inhibitors of apoptosis (IAP) proteins inhibit terminal caspase activation, and are in turn inhibited by the mitochondrial protein SMAC, which promotes their polyubiquitination and degradation, thus favoring caspase activation.

Bcl-2 Protein Family

The intrinsic or mitochondrial pathway of apoptosis is regulated by the Bcl-2 (B-cell lymphoma-2) protein family.[64] The Bcl-2 protein family has classically been divided into three broad subfamilies based on four homologous domains, designated Bcl-2 homology (BH) domains. The anti-apoptotic members have multiple BH domains, and include Bcl-2, Mcl-1, Bcl-xL and A1, and Bcl-w. The pro-apoptotic multi-domain proteins include Bax, Bak, and Bok. The BH3-only proteins are pro-apoptotic, and as their name indicates they only share the BH3 domain with other Bcl-2 family proteins. This group includes Bid, Bim, Bad, Bmf, Noxa, Puma, and Bik. Bid plays an important role in hepatocyte apoptosis because the extrinsic or death receptor pathway of apoptosis requires the intrinsic or mitochondrial pathway of apoptosis, which it activates via caspase 8–mediated cleavage of the pro-apoptotic protein Bid. Cleaved Bid (tBid) and other BH3-only proteins then result in activation of Bak or Bax, mitochondrial outer membrane permeabilization, release of pro-apoptotic factor, and eventual activation of effector caspases. There is some redundancy and functional overlap in the BH3-only proteins; however, others function in a cell- and stimulus-specific manner. Furthermore, Bim and Puma can bind all the anti-apoptotic Bcl-2 protein family members, whereas other BH3-only proteins have more restricted binding. There are two proposed mechanisms of Bak and Bax activation by BH3-only proteins: (1) Bak and Bax can be directly activated by the BH-3 protein of interest (e.g., tBid); (2) alternatively, Bak or Bax can be activated by relief of inhibition from anti-apoptotic proteins such as Bcl-2. This occurs by the binding of the pro-apoptotic BH3-only protein with the anti-apoptotic family member, thus releasing Bak or Bax.

Bid is a key mediator of the apoptotic pathway in hepatocytes. Bid-deficient mice are protected from Fas-induced hepatocyte apoptosis and lethality.[20] In a murine model of cholestatic injury, interference with Bid expression by antisense oligonucleotide ameliorates hepatocyte apoptosis and liver injury.[65] Bid mediates not only mitochondrial permeabilization but also lysosomal permeabilization downstream of TNF-α–induced apoptosis. Bim and Puma are up-regulated by the toxic free fatty acid palmitate, which sensitizes hepatocytes to apoptosis.[66,67] Mice genetically deficient in Bcl-xL demonstrated enhanced spontaneous apoptosis, signifying a critical role for Bcl-xL in maintaining hepatic homeostasis.[68] On the other hand, overexpression of Bcl-2 ameliorated Fas-induced apoptosis in mice.[19] These mice also developed hepatic fibrosis, strengthening the link between hepatocyte apoptosis and hepatic fibrosis. In chronic viral hepatitis, expression of Bcl-2 protein family members can be regulated by viral proteins, promoting or inhibiting apoptosis of the infected hepatocytes.[69,70] Thus the Bcl-2 protein family determines the susceptibility of a given hepatocyte to extrinsic or intrinsic death stimuli.

Lysosomes

Lysosomes are membrane-bound organelles that can be involved in both the extrinsic and intrinsic pathways of apoptosis.[71] Within cells, lysosomes sequester hydrolytic enzymes, which are active at an acidic pH and maintain an intraluminal acidic milieu. These enzymes break down intracellular organelles and macromolecules delivered to the lysosomes for turnover. Permeabilization of the lysosomal membrane results in release of lysosomal enzymes into the cytosol, including cathepsin B, a lysosomal protease that is active at neutral pH. In hepatocyte apoptosis via the lysosomal pathway this event occurs upstream of mitochondrial permeabilization. Lysosomes can be permeabilized by death receptors or by

intracellular stressors (e.g., free fatty acids, sphingosine, reactive oxygen species).[72] Massive lysosomal permeabilization is a feature of necrotic cell death, with release of lytic enzymes into the cytosol of the dying cell. In the liver initial experiments with ischemic and toxic injury demonstrated lysosomal rupture in necrotic cell death.[73] With advances in the understanding of the regulation of apoptosis, it has been demonstrated that lysosomes can mediate hepatocyte apoptosis in many models of liver injury. Much of this information is derived from mice lacking cathepsin B. The absence of this lysosomal protease attenuates apoptosis and injury in models of ischemia-reperfusion, cholestasis, and TNF-α.[9,74,75] Furthermore, serum levels of lysosomal enzymes are elevated in patients with liver disease, indicating activation of the lysosomal pathway.[76]

Endoplasmic Reticulum

The endoplasmic reticulum (ER) is a membrane-bound organelle with the specialized function of oxidative protein folding, in addition to biosynthesis of lipids and steroids, detoxification of drugs, and regulation of cytosolic calcium concentration. Secretory cells such as hepatocytes and pancreatic β cells are enriched in ER. The ER is sensitive to many forms of perturbation, such as an increase in the load of client proteins, oxidative stress, metabolic stress, and calcium depletion (Fig. 3-5). ER stress is sensed by three transmembrane ER stress sensors—inositol-requiring protein 1α (IRE-1α), activating transcription factor 6 (ATF6), and PKR–like ER kinase (PERK)—that activate a series of signaling events known collectively as the unfolded protein response (UPR).[77] The three arms of the UPR act in concert to adapt to ER stress. IRE-1α uniquely splices transcription factor X-box binding protein 1 (XBP1) mRNA, activating UPR genes that encode for chaperones and components of the ER-associated protein degradation (ERAD) pathway. PERK-mediated phosphorylation of eIF-2α leads to translation attenuation and reduction in the client load in the ER. However, certain genes are selectively translated following phosphorylation of eIF-2α. These include activating transcription factor 4 (ATF4) and transcription of C/EBP-homologous protein (CHOP). ATF6 is cleaved in the Golgi compartment to a transcriptionally active form that translocates to the nucleus and activates UPR target genes. Unresolved or sustained ER stress is associated with failure of adaptation and results in cell death. The UPR and ER are linked to the cellular apoptotic machinery at many levels. IRE-1α can activate the stress kinase c-jun N-terminal kinase via the adaptor proteins TRAF2 and ASK1. CHOP can sensitize cells to apoptosis by regulating the expression of TRAIL-R2, the pro-apoptotic Bcl-2 family protein Bim, and the anti-apoptotic protein Bcl-2.[78-80] Perturbations in calcium homeostasis can affect cell death pathways. In experimental models of diabetes and diet-induced obesity, the UPR is activated in pancreatic β cells and the liver.[77,81] In obese patients undergoing bariatric surgery, UPR markers were activated in the liver and correlated with weight loss.[82] In a murine model of ethanol-induced liver injury, CHOP deletion abrogated hepatocyte apoptosis, though no differences were observed in ALT levels.[83] The hepatitis C viral protein nonstructural protein 4B and hepatitis B X protein can also activate the UPR.[84,85] Furthermore, disruption of any of the arms of the

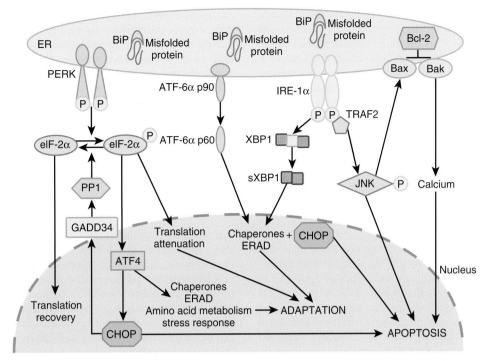

Fig. 3-5 The endoplasmic reticulum stress pathway. Endoplasmic reticulum stress is mediated via three transmembrane stress sensors: inositol-requiring protein 1α (IRE-1α), activating transcription factor 6α (ATF-6α), and PKR–like ER kinase (PERK). Upon the accumulation of misfolded proteins in the ER, the chaperone immunoglobulin binding protein of B cells (BiP/GRP78) binds to these client proteins, releasing the ER stress sensors from inhibitory BiP binding. ATF-6α is cleaved in the Golgi and translocates to the nucleus, activating UPR genes. IRE-1α has kinase activity as well as endoribonucleolytic activity; it is activated by autophosphorylation and splices the transcription factor X-box binding protein 1 (XBP1) to sXBP1, as well as by activation of JNK via TRAF2. Eukaryotic initiation factor 2α (eIF-2α) is phosphorylated by PERK, leading to attenuation of translation, thereby decreasing the client protein load in the ER. Activating transcription factor 4 (ATF4) and CHOP are selectively up-regulated following phosphorylation of eIF-2α. Failure of adaptation to ER stress results in apoptosis. The transcription factor CHOP can enhance the expression of the pro-apoptotic protein Bim, or the TRAIL receptor TRAIL-R2. Perturbations of calcium homeostasis as well as JNK activation can promote ER stress-induced apoptosis. The up-regulation of growth arrest and DNA damage protein 34 (GADD34) leads to dephosphorylation of eIF-2α via protein phosphatase 1 (PP1). This can lead to translational recovery or worsen ER stress by increasing the load of client proteins.

UPR led to microvesicular hepatic steatosis.[86] Thus the UPR is activated in the diseased liver, and further studies will elucidate its role in adaptation, cell death, inflammation, and injury in the liver.

C-jun N-Terminal Kinase

Members of the mitogen-activated protein kinase family, c-jun N-terminal kinases (JNK) are stress kinases activated by a number of intracellular or extracellular stressors (e.g., death ligands, ER stress, cytokines, ultraviolet irradiation, reactive oxygen species). Only two of the three known genes are expressed in the liver, encoding for JNK1 and JNK2 isoforms.[87] Sustained JNK activation can promote cell death by transcriptionally enhancing the expression of death receptors.[23] Phosphorylation can lead to inactivation of anti-apoptotic Bcl-2 family proteins or activation of pro-apoptotic proteins (e.g., Bim), resulting in mitochondrial permeabilization.[88,89] Both isoforms can mediate cell death via distinct pathways and in a stimulus-specific manner. In a toxin-induced liver injury model, caspase 8 activation, Bid cleavage, and mitochondrial permeabilization were JNK2 dependent.[90] Furthermore, JNK1 supported degradation of cFLIP, thereby promoting death receptor–induced cell death by TNF-R1, Fas, or TRAIL-R1/R2.[13] In murine models of dietary obesity, mice deficient in

JNK1 were protected from hepatocyte apoptosis and liver injury.[91] In a cellular model of steatotic hepatocyte apoptosis, JNK2 isoforms played a predominant role.[92] Mice deficient in JNK2 were protected from toxin-induced liver injury.[90] Although JNK2 was predominant, both isoforms mediated the toxicity of acetaminophen.[93]

Necrosis

Necrotic morphology is characterized by oncosis, an increase in cell volume, swelling of organelles, and rupture of the plasma membrane.[94] Necrosis was recognized in the liver in studies involving overwhelming acute metabolic insults (e.g., ischemia, toxins). In an experimental model of ischemic injury based on portal vein branch ligation, large portions of the affected hepatic parenchyma demonstrated necrotic morphology.[73] Interestingly, the presentation of a distinct morphology of cell death in the viable, periportal hepatocytes led to the description and establishment of apoptotic cell death in the liver. Necrotic cell death was considered unregulated; however, some of the molecular pathways involved in necrosis have been recently recognized and are discussed further under Necroptosis. Necrotic death is characterized by plasma membrane bleb formation, mitochondrial membrane permeability transition, and lysosomal rupture followed by plasma membrane bleb rupture.[2] Mitochondrial permeability transition (MPT) is regulated by the mitochondrial permeability transition pore (MPTP) on the inner mitochondrial membrane, which is formed by a voltage-dependent anion channel, adenosine nucleotide transporter, and cyclophilin D. Opening of the MPT leads to mitochondrial swelling, eventual rupture of the outer mitochondrial membrane, and release of the contents of the intermembrane space into the cytosol.[95] Experiments in genetic knockout mice have demonstrated that of these three proteins, cyclophilin D is essential for the MPT.[96] Mitochondria from mice deficient in cyclophilin D are resistant to MPT, and hepatocytes are protected from cell death induced by calcium overload or oxidative stress.

Necroptosis

Cell death initiated by classic apoptotic signals in cells that cannot execute apoptosis because of the deficiency of mediators or the use of pharmacologic inhibitors of apoptosis is referred to as necroptosis. It shares both mechanistic features of apoptosis, such as activation by death receptors, and the morphologic appearance of necrosis. Fas-induced cell death in a lymphocyte cell line deficient in caspase 8 occurred without caspase activation, and demonstrated necrotic morphology.[5] Necroptosis is mediated by the adaptor proteins RIP1 and RIP3.[97] Genome-wide screening has led to the identification of several genes that regulate necroptosis, including some that are shared between apoptosis and necroptosis.[6]

Autophagy

Autophagy is a cellular catabolic process that plays a role in many biologic functions, including cellular homeostasis (by removal of obsolete or expanded organelles), cell survival under conditions of nutrient deprivation, development, innate and adaptive immunity, neurodegeneration, tumor suppression, and cell death.[98,99] Macroautophagy (referred to as autophagy here) is one form of autophagy. It refers to the formation of cytosolic double membrane–bound autophagosomes that contain a cargo of cytoplasm and organelles destined to the lysosomes for degradation. Autophagosomes fuse with lysosomes to form autolysosomes or autophagic vacuoles. As with other modes of cell death, morphologic criteria are used to define autophagic cell death, also known as type II programmed cell death. The recognition of autophagic cell death is based on the massive accumulation of double-membraned autophagosomes in the cytoplasm of dying cells, in the absence of chromatin condensation.[94] The accumulation of autophagosomes can occur as a result of many perturbations, such as defects in the fusion of autophagosomes with lysosomes or defects in apoptotic cells, and does not imply that the cell is dying from autophagic mechanisms.[100] Furthermore, autophagy is regulated by nutrient availability via TOR (target of rapamycin)-mediated suppression and clearly promotes cellular survival under nutrient deprivation and growth factor withdrawal.[101,102] Although autophagic vacuoles have been observed in dying cells, only in very select conditions has it been demonstrated that cells are actually dying by autophagy. Screening strategies based on genetic mutants in yeast have led to the identification and elucidation of genes that regulate autophagy both in yeast and in mammals, and this has accelerated research in this field in recent years.

Autophagic processes have been observed in the liver under diverse stress conditions. Autophagy is prominent in the liver during nutrient and growth factor deprivation.[103] Autophagy leads to resorption of Mallory-Denk bodies in the liver.[104] The accumulation of aggregation-prone mutant α_1-antitrypsin within the endoplasmic reticulum in hepatocytes is also associated with the activation of autophagy.[105] In this disease autophagy plays an important role in the removal of aggregated protein. Mice deficient in constitutive autophagy develop liver injury.[106] Thus the activation of autophagy in the liver is most likely protective; however, whether it plays a role in liver cell death and injury is an area of active research.

Conclusion

Apoptosis is a prominent mechanism for hepatocyte cell death and a mechanistic link between insult and injury in the liver. Furthermore, hepatocyte apoptosis also incites activation of inflammatory pathways and fibrogenic processes. Other modes of cell death are also recognized in the liver, and are areas of active research. At a cellular level multiple apoptotic pathways can be activated by death-inducing stimuli; these can be cooperative or oppose each other, with eventual mitochondrial permeabilization and hepatocyte cell death occurring secondary to the predominant pathway. At an organismal level, multiple modes of cell death may be activated and detected in response to the same injurious stimulus. Manipulations to inhibit hepatocyte cell death are potential strategies for the development of novel therapies for acute and chronic liver diseases.

Key References

Aggarwal BB. Signalling pathways of the TNF superfamily: a double-edged sword. Nat Rev Immunol 2003;3:745–756. (Ref.41)

Akpolat N, et al. Relationship between serum cytokine levels and histopathological changes of liver in patients with hepatitis B. World J Gastroenterol 2005;11:3260–3263. (Ref.56)

Baines CP, et al. Loss of cyclophilin D reveals a critical role for mitochondrial permeability transition in cell death. Nature 2005;434:658–662. (Ref.96)

Barreyro FJ, et al. Transcriptional regulation of Bim by FoxO3A mediates hepatocyte lipoapoptosis. J Biol Chem 2007;282:27141–27154. (Ref.66)

Baskin-Bey ES, et al. Cathepsin B inactivation attenuates hepatocyte apoptosis and liver damage in steatotic livers after cold ischemia-warm reperfusion injury. Am J Physiol Gastrointest Liver Physiol 2005;288:G396–G402. (Ref.74)

Beraza N, et al. Hepatocyte-specific NEMO deletion promotes NK/NKT cell- and TRAIL-dependent liver damage. J Exp Med 2009;206:1727–1737. (Ref.39)

Blommaart EF, Luiken JJ, Meijer AJ. Autophagic proteolysis: control and specificity. Histochem J 1997;29:365–385. (Ref.103)

Boetticher NC, et al. A randomized, double-blinded, placebo-controlled multicenter trial of etanercept in the treatment of alcoholic hepatitis. Gastroenterology 2008;135:1953–1960. (Ref.62)

Boya P, et al. Inhibition of macroautophagy triggers apoptosis. Mol Cell Biol 2005;25:1025–1040. (Ref.100)

Boya P, Kroemer G. Lysosomal membrane permeabilization in cell death. Oncogene 2008;27:6434–6451. (Ref.72)

Budd RC, Yeh WC, Tschopp J. cFLIP regulation of lymphocyte activation and development. Nat Rev Immunol 2006;6:196–204. (Ref.12)

Canbay A, et al. Kupffer cell engulfment of apoptotic bodies stimulates death ligand and cytokine expression. Hepatology 2003;38:1188–1198. (Ref.7)

Canbay A, et al. Cathepsin B inactivation attenuates hepatic injury and fibrosis during cholestasis. J Clin Invest 2003;112:152–159. (Ref.9)

Canbay A, et al. Fas enhances fibrogenesis in the bile duct ligated mouse: a link between apoptosis and fibrosis. Gastroenterology 2002;123:1323–1330. (Ref.10)

Canbay A, et al. Apoptotic body engulfment by a human stellate cell line is profibrogenic. Lab Invest 2003;83:655–663. (Ref.8)

Cazanave SC, et al. JNK1-dependent PUMA expression contributes to hepatocyte lipoapoptosis. J Biol Chem 2009;284:26591–26602. (Ref.67)

Chang L, et al. The E3 ubiquitin ligase itch couples JNK activation to TNFalpha-induced cell death by inducing c-FLIP(L) turnover. Cell 2006;124:601–613. (Ref.13)

Conzelmann LO, et al. Graft tumor necrosis factor receptor-1 protects after mouse liver transplantation whereas host tumor necrosis factor receptor-1 promotes injury. Transplantation 2006;82:1214–1220. (Ref.50)

Corazza N, et al. TRAIL receptor-mediated JNK activation and Bim phosphorylation critically regulate Fas-mediated liver damage and lethality. J Clin Invest 2006;116:2493–2499. (Ref.89)

Costelli P, et al. Mice lacking TNFalpha receptors 1 and 2 are resistant to death and fulminant liver injury induced by agonistic anti-Fas antibody. Cell Death Differ 2003;10:997–1004. (Ref.46)

Czaja MJ. The future of GI and liver research: editorial perspectives. III. JNK/AP-1 regulation of hepatocyte death. Am J Physiol Gastrointest Liver Physiol 2003;284:G875–G879. (Ref.87)

Deng X, et al. Novel role for JNK as a stress-activated Bcl2 kinase. J Biol Chem 2001;276:23681–23688. (Ref.88)

Dunn C, et al. Cytokines induced during chronic hepatitis B virus infection promote a pathway for NK cell-mediated liver damage. J Exp Med 2007;204:667–680. (Ref.38)

Faubion WA, et al. Toxic bile salts induce rodent hepatocyte apoptosis via direct activation of Fas. J Clin Invest 1999;103:137–145. (Ref.24)

Feldstein AE, et al. Hepatocyte apoptosis and Fas expression are prominent features of human nonalcoholic steatohepatitis. Gastroenterology 2003;125:437–443. (Ref.1)

Feldstein AE, et al. Diet associated hepatic steatosis sensitizes to Fas mediated liver injury in mice. J Hepatol 2003;39:978–983. (Ref.18)

Green DR. Apoptotic pathways: ten minutes to dead. Cell 2005;121:671–674. (Ref.63)

Green DR, Kroemer G. The pathophysiology of mitochondrial cell death. Science 2004;305:626–629. (Ref.95)

Gregor MF, et al. Endoplasmic reticulum stress is reduced in tissues of obese subjects after weight loss. Diabetes 2009;58:693–700. (Ref.82)

Grove J, et al. Association of a tumor necrosis factor promoter polymorphism with susceptibility to alcoholic steatohepatitis. Hepatology 1997;26:143–146. (Ref.59)

Guicciardi ME, et al. Cathepsin B contributes to TNF-alpha-mediated hepatocyte apoptosis by promoting mitochondrial release of cytochrome c. J Clin Invest 2000;106:1127–1137. (Ref.75)

Guicciardi ME, Leist M, Gores GJ. Lysosomes in cell death. Oncogene 2004;23:2881–2890. (Ref.71)

Gunawan BK, et al. c-Jun N-terminal kinase plays a major role in murine acetaminophen hepatotoxicity. Gastroenterology 2006;131:165–178. (Ref.93)

Harada M, et al. Autophagy activation by rapamycin eliminates mouse Mallory-Denk bodies and blocks their proteasome inhibitor-mediated formation. Hepatology 2008;47:2026–2035. (Ref.104)

Hayashi N, Mita E. Involvement of Fas system-mediated apoptosis in pathogenesis of viral hepatitis. J Viral Hepat 1999;6:357–365. (Ref.29)

He Q, et al. Celecoxib and a novel COX-2 inhibitor ON09310 upregulate death receptor 5 expression via GADD153/CHOP. Oncogene 2007;27:2656–2660. (Ref.40)

Higuchi H, et al. Bid antisense attenuates bile acid-induced apoptosis and cholestatic liver injury. J Pharmacol Exp Ther 2001;299:866–873. (Ref.65)

Hitomi J, et al. Identification of a molecular signaling network that regulates a cellular necrotic cell death pathway. Cell 2008;135:1311–1323. (Ref.6)

Iredale JP, et al. Mechanisms of spontaneous resolution of rat liver fibrosis. Hepatic stellate cell apoptosis and reduced hepatic expression of metalloproteinase inhibitors. J Clin Invest 1998;102:538–549. (Ref.11)

Ji C, Deng Q, Kaplowitz N. Role of TNF-alpha in ethanol-induced hyperhomocysteinemia and murine alcoholic liver injury. Hepatology 2004;40:442–451. (Ref.52)

Ji C, et al. Role of CHOP in hepatic apoptosis in the murine model of intragastric ethanol feeding. Alcohol Clin Exp Res 2005;29:1496–1503. (Ref.83)

Jost PJ, et al. XIAP discriminates between type I and type II FAS-induced apoptosis. Nature 2009;460:1035–1039. (Ref.15)

Kaufmann T, et al. Fatal hepatitis mediated by tumor necrosis factor TNFalpha requires caspase-8 and involves the BH3-only proteins Bid and Bim. Immunity 2009;30:56–66. (Ref.48)

Kawahara A, et al. Caspase-independent cell killing by Fas-associated protein with death domain. J Cell Biol 1998;143:1353–1360. (Ref.5)

Kerr JF. History of the events leading to the formulation of the apoptosis concept. Toxicology 2002;181–182,471–474. (Ref.73)

Komatsu M, et al. Homeostatic levels of p62 control cytoplasmic inclusion body formation in autophagy-deficient mice. Cell 2007;131:1149–1163. (Ref.106)

Kroemer G, et al. Classification of cell death: recommendations of the Nomenclature Committee on Cell Death 2009. Cell Death Differ 2009;16:3–11. (Ref.94)

Lacronique V, et al. Bcl-2 protects from lethal hepatic apoptosis induced by an anti-Fas antibody in mice. Nat Med 1996;2:80–86. (Ref.19)

Lapinski TW, et al. Serum concentration of sFas and sFasL in healthy HBsAg carriers, chronic viral hepatitis B and C patients. World J Gastroenterol 2004;10:3650–3653. (Ref.31)

Li B, et al. Hepatitis B virus X protein (HBx) activates ATF6 and IRE1-XBP1 pathways of unfolded protein response. Virus Res 2007;124:44–49. (Ref.85)

Li S, et al. Hepatitis C virus NS4B induces unfolded protein response and endoplasmic reticulum overload response-dependent NF-kappaB activation. Virology 2009;391:257–264. (Ref.84)

Liang X, et al. Hepatitis B virus sensitizes hepatocytes to TRAIL-induced apoptosis through Bax. J Immunol 2007;178:503–510. (Ref.70)

Lin HZ, et al. Chronic ethanol consumption induces the production of tumor necrosis factor-alpha and related cytokines in liver and adipose tissue. Alcohol Clin Exp Res 1998;22:231S–237S. (Ref.51)

Lum JJ, et al. Growth factor regulation of autophagy and cell survival in the absence of apoptosis. Cell 2005;120:237–248. (Ref.102)

Lum JJ, DeBerardinis RJ, Thompson CB. Autophagy in metazoans: cell survival in the land of plenty. Nat Rev Mol Cell Biol 2005;6:439–448. (Ref.98)

Malhi H, et al. Free fatty acids sensitise hepatocytes to TRAIL mediated cytotoxicity. Gut 2007;56:1124–1131. (Ref.23)

Malhi H, et al. Free fatty acids induce JNK-dependent hepatocyte lipoapoptosis. J Biol Chem 2006;281:12093–12101. (Ref.92)

Malhi H, Gores GJ, Lemasters JJ. Apoptosis and necrosis in the liver: a tale of two deaths? Hepatology 2006;43:S31–S44. (Ref.2)

Matsumura H, et al. Necrotic death pathway in Fas receptor signaling. J Cell Biol 2000;151:1247–1256. (Ref.3)

McCullough KD, et al. Gadd153 sensitizes cells to endoplasmic reticulum stress by down-regulating Bcl2 and perturbing the cellular redox state. Mol Cell Biol 2001;21:1249–1259. (Ref.80)

Micheau O, Tschopp J. Induction of TNF receptor I-mediated apoptosis via two sequential signaling complexes. Cell 2003;114:181–190. (Ref.45)

Mochizuki K, et al. Fas antigen expression in liver tissues of patients with chronic hepatitis B. J Hepatol 1996;24:1–7. (Ref.32)

Mohammed FF, et al. Abnormal TNF activity in Timp3-/- mice leads to chronic hepatic inflammation and failure of liver regeneration. Nat Genet 2004;36:969–977. (Ref.49)

Natori S, et al. Hepatocyte apoptosis is a pathologic feature of human alcoholic hepatitis. J Hepatol 2001;34:248–253. (Ref.33)

Naveau S, et al. Plasma levels of soluble tumor necrosis factor receptors p55 and p75 in patients with alcoholic liver disease of increasing severity. J Hepatol 1998;28:778–784. (Ref.60)

Ozcan U, et al. Endoplasmic reticulum stress links obesity, insulin action, and type 2 diabetes. Science 2004;306:457–461. (Ref.81)

Perlmutter DH. Autophagic disposal of the aggregation-prone protein that causes liver inflammation and carcinogenesis in alpha-1-antitrypsin deficiency. Cell Death Differ 2009;16:39–45. (Ref.105)

Pianko S, et al. Fas-mediated hepatocyte apoptosis is increased by hepatitis C virus infection and alcohol consumption, and may be associated with hepatic fibrosis: mechanisms of liver cell injury in chronic hepatitis C virus infection. J Viral Hepat 2001;8:406–413. (Ref.30)

Puthalakath H, et al. ER stress triggers apoptosis by activating BH3-only protein Bim. Cell 2007;129:1337–1349. (Ref.79)

Reinehr R, et al. Involvement of the Src family kinase yes in bile salt-induced apoptosis. Gastroenterology 2004;127:1540–1557. (Ref.25)

Rivero M, et al. Apoptosis mediated by the Fas system in the fulminant hepatitis by hepatitis B virus. J Viral Hepat 2002;9:107–113. (Ref.28)

Rutherford AE, et al. Serum apoptosis markers in acute liver failure: a pilot study. Clin Gastroenterol Hepatol 2007;5:1477–1483. (Ref.26)

Rutkowski DT, et al. UPR pathways combine to prevent hepatic steatosis caused by ER stress-mediated suppression of transcriptional master regulators. Dev Cell 2008;15:829–840. (Ref.86)

Scaffidi C, et al. Two CD95 (APO-1/Fas) signaling pathways. Embo J 1998;17:1675–1687. (Ref.14)

Schattenberg JM, et al. JNK1 but not JNK2 promotes the development of steatohepatitis in mice. Hepatology 2006;43:163–172. (Ref.91)

Scheuner D, Kaufman RJ. The unfolded protein response: a pathway that links insulin demand with beta-cell failure and diabetes. Endocr Rev 2008;29:317–333. (Ref.77)

Schneider P, et al. TRAIL receptors 1 (DR4) and 2 (DR5) signal FADD-dependent apoptosis and activate NF-kappaB. Immunity 1997;7:831–836. (Ref.35)

Schumann J, et al. Parenchymal, but not leukocyte, TNF receptor 2 mediates T cell-dependent hepatitis in mice. J Immunol 2003;170:2129–2137. (Ref.43)

Sodeman T, et al. Bile salts mediate hepatocyte apoptosis by increasing cell surface trafficking of Fas. Am J Physiol Gastrointest Liver Physiol 2000;278:G992–G999. (Ref.16)

Song E, et al. RNA interference targeting Fas protects mice from fulminant hepatitis. Nat Med 2003;9:347–351. (Ref.22)

Spahr L, et al. Soluble TNF-R1, but not tumor necrosis factor alpha, predicts the 3-month mortality in patients with alcoholic hepatitis. J Hepatol 2004;41:229–234. (Ref.61)

Streetz K, et al. Tumor necrosis factor alpha in the pathogenesis of human and murine fulminant hepatic failure. Gastroenterology 2000;119:446–460. (Ref.54)

Suzuki H, et al. Hepatocyte growth factor protects against Fas-mediated liver apoptosis in transgenic mice. Liver Int 2009;29:1562–1568. (Ref.21)

Tagami A, Ohnishi H, Hughes RD. Increased serum soluble Fas in patients with acute liver failure due to paracetamol overdose. Hepatogastroenterology 2003;50:742–745. (Ref.27)

Takehara T, et al. Hepatocyte-specific disruption of Bcl-xL leads to continuous hepatocyte apoptosis and liver fibrotic responses. Gastroenterology 2004;127:1189–1197. (Ref.68)

Tokushige K, et al. Significance of soluble TNF receptor-I in acute-type fulminant hepatitis. Am J Gastroenterol 2000;95:2040–2046. (Ref.55)

Torre F, et al. Kinetics of soluble tumour necrosis factor (TNF)-alpha receptors and cytokines in the early phase of treatment for chronic hepatitis C: comparison between interferon (IFN)-alpha alone, IFN-alpha plus amantadine or plus ribavirin. Clin Exp Immunol 2004;136:507–512. (Ref.58)

Tsamandas AC, et al. Potential role of bcl-2 and bax mRNA and protein expression in chronic hepatitis type B and C: a clinicopathologic study. Mod Pathol 2003;16:1273–1288. (Ref.69)

Volkmann X, et al. Increased hepatotoxicity of tumor necrosis factor-related apoptosis-inducing ligand in diseased human liver. Hepatology 2007;46:1498–1508. (Ref.36)

Wang X, et al. A mechanism of cell survival: sequestration of Fas by the HGF receptor. Met Mol Cell 2002;9:411–421. (Ref.17)

Wang Y, et al. Tumor necrosis factor-induced toxic liver injury results from JNK2-dependent activation of caspase-8 and the mitochondrial death pathway. J Biol Chem 2006;281:15258–15267. (Ref.90)

Yamada Y, et al. Analysis of liver regeneration in mice lacking type 1 or type 2 tumor necrosis factor receptor: requirement for type 1 but not type 2 receptor. Hepatology 1998;28:959–970. (Ref.44)

Yamaguchi H, Wang HG. CHOP is involved in endoplasmic reticulum stress-induced apoptosis by enhancing DR5 expression in human carcinoma cells. J Biol Chem 2004;279:45495–45502. (Ref.78)

Yin M, et al. Essential role of tumor necrosis factor alpha in alcohol-induced liver injury in mice. Gastroenterology 1999;117:942–952. (Ref.53)

Yin XM, et al. Bid-deficient mice are resistant to Fas-induced hepatocellular apoptosis. Nature 1999;400:886–891. (Ref.20)

Youle RJ, Strasser A. The BCL-2 protein family: opposing activities that mediate cell death. Nat Rev Mol Cell Biol 2008;9:47–59. (Ref.64)

Yu L, et al. Regulation of an ATG7-beclin 1 program of autophagic cell death by caspase-8. Science 2004;304:1500–1502. (Ref.99)

Zhang DW, et al. RIP3, an energy metabolism regulator that switches TNF-induced cell death from apoptosis to necrosis. Science 2009;325:332–336. (Ref.97)

Zheng SJ, et al. Critical roles of TRAIL in hepatic cell death and hepatic inflammation. J Clin Invest 2004;113:58–64. (Ref.37)

Zou C, et al. Lack of Fas antagonism by Met in human fatty liver disease. Nat Med 2007;13:1078–1085. (Ref.34)

A complete list of references can be found at www.expertconsult.com.

Chapter 4

Mechanisms of Bile Secretion

Peter L.M. Jansen, Ulrich Beuers, and Ronald P.J. Oude Elferink

ABBREVIATIONS

AA amino acids
ABC ATP-binding cassette
ASBT apical sodium-dependent bile salt transporter
BSEP bile salt export pump
CAR constitutively activated receptor
C/EBP CCAAT-enhancer binding protein
CYP cytochrome P-450
CYP7A1 cholesterol 7α-hydroxylase
DR direct repeats
FGF19 fibroblast growth factor 19
FXR farnesoid X receptor
GSH reduced glutathione
GSSG oxidized GSH
HNF hepatocyte nuclear factor
I-BABP intestinal bile salt binding protein
IR inverted repeat

LXR liver X receptor
MDR1 multidrug resistance protein 1
Mdr2 rodent phosphatidylcholine transporter
MDR3 human phosphatidylcholine transporter
MRP multidrug resistance–associated protein and its homologues
NHR nuclear hormone receptor
NTCP human Na$^+$/taurocholate co-transport polypeptide
Ntcp rat Na$^+$/taurocholate co-transport polypeptide
OATP human organic anion–transporting protein
Oatp rat organic anion–transporting protein

OCT organic cation transporter
PC phosphatidylcholine
PPAR peroxisome proliferator activated receptor
PS phosphatidylserine
PXR pregnane X receptor
RAR 9-*cis*-retinoic acid receptor
RE responsive element
ROS reactive oxygen species
RXR retinoid X receptor
SHP1 small heterodimer partner 1
SLC solute carrier protein
SP1 stimulating protein 1
TM transmembrane α-helix
TNF-α tumor necrosis factor-α

Introduction

Generation of bile flow depends on the transepithelial movement of solutes and organic molecules. Bile is primarily produced in hepatocytes, and the composition of bile is modified in the bile ducts. Bile is formed by a process of osmotic filtration in response to osmotic gradients created within the lumen of the bile canaliculus. This osmotic gradient is established by ongoing active secretion of solutes across the canalicular membrane of hepatocytes into the canalicular lumen. Water follows passively through the leaky pores of tight junctions and via transcellular paths mediated by water channels or aquaporins. Bile secretion serves different important functions. First, it is one of the main mechanisms for the disposition of endogenous and exogenous amphipathic compounds, including drugs, toxins, and waste products. Second, it supplies bile salts to the intestine, which is of crucial importance for the emulsification and subsequent digestion and absorption of dietary lipids. Since it became evident that bile salts are ligands for nuclear hormone receptors in liver and gut, a third function can be assigned to bile—carrier of signaling molecules from liver to gut. The enterohepatic cycling of bile salts is a main determinant of bile flow; however, the secretion of bile salts, cholesterol, phospholipids, and glutathione contributes to the formation of bile.

Bile salts are the predominant organic solutes in bile, and their vectorial secretion from blood into bile represents the major driving force for hepatic bile formation. Although bile is isoosmotic in relation to plasma, bile salts are concentrated up to 1000-fold in bile, necessitating active transport by hepatocytes. After their secretion into the canaliculus, bile salts are prevented from regurgitation into the systemic circulation by hepatocyte tight junctions, the integrity of which is disturbed during bile duct obstruction. The total bile salt pool size in adult humans can reach 50 to 60 mmol/kg body weight, corresponding to 3 to 4 g, and is largely stored in the gallbladder during the fasting state. Rats lack this reservoir function because of the absence of a gallbladder. The human bile salt pool circulates 6 to 10 times per 24 hours, resulting in a daily bile salt secretion of 20 to 40 g. Despite a high degree of intestinal bile salt conservation, about 0.5 g of bile salt is lost each day by fecal excretion. This loss is compensated for by de novo hepatic bile salt synthesis. The intrinsic link between intestinal bile salt absorption and hepatic synthesis has been found to be a complex system involving specific bile salt binding nuclear receptors and a hormone called fibroblast growth factor 19 (FGF19). By this mechanism, bile salts can regulate their own enterohepatic circulation. Through interaction with the farnesoid X receptor (FXR) in the terminal ileum, the subsequent secretion of FGF19 into the portal blood, and the interaction between FGF19 and its receptor FGFR4 on the surface of hepatocytes, bile salts regulate their own biosynthesis, hepatic uptake, and secretion. FXR and FGF19 also regulate key steps in hepatic cholesterol, carbohydrate, and lipid metabolism and thus serve as a bridge between gut and liver and between bile salts and a range of metabolic reactions.

Uptake of bile salts from the sinusoidal blood and secretion across the canalicular membrane are the major determinants governing the rate of bile secretion. Disturbances of bile salt transport are important causes of acquired and genetic forms of cholestatic liver disease. In case of impaired bile salt secretion, the liver can generate a number of adaptations to detoxify or secrete bile salts via alternate pathways. When these fail or are overwhelmed, liver damage will ensue with consequent malnutrition secondary to reduced intestinal absorption of lipids and fat-soluble vitamins.

Bile Secretion

The liver is specialized in the processing of albumin-bound compounds and as such its function is complementary to that of the kidney. Anatomically the liver is well equipped for its function. Microscopically the liver resembles a sponge in which the holes permit passage of blood and the solid material consists of sinusoidal endothelium, macrophages, stellate cells, and hepatocytes. The hepatocytes are arranged in plates. Within these plates there is a network of bile canaliculi. Thus bile canaliculi have no specialized cell layer; they are surrounded by hepatocytes and the canalicular membranes of two adjacent hepatocytes form the boundary of a bile canaliculus.

On closer examination the sponge has an ordered structure with rows of hepatocytes in plates radiating from portal areas towards a terminal hepatic vein. This association between the portal triads and the terminal hepatic veins defines the smallest anatomic unit in the liver—the hepatic acinus.[1] In the human liver these acini are not isolated units, but are interconnected in the periportal area.[2] When the network of bile canaliculi exits the hepatic acinus at the level of the portal triad, the bile canaliculus acquires its own cell layer—the cholangiocytes.

The portal blood carries metabolites from the intestine directly to the liver. In the liver the portal blood flows through the sinusoids from the portal triads towards the terminal hepatic vein. The fenestrated sinusoidal endothelium lacks a basal membrane and thus allows easy passage of molecules as large as albumin from the blood to the surface of the hepatocytes. The hepatocytes and endothelium are separated by a 10- to 15-μm-wide space of Disse. In a three-dimensional view, single layers of hepatocytes form plates that are perfused on both sides by portal venous blood. A bile canalicular network is hidden within these plates. After immunohistochemical staining with antibodies directed against canalicular proteins, this network is revealed and appears similar to chicken wire. Because of its three-dimensional structure, the chicken wire structure, when seen in the plane of the microscope, seems incomplete. With antibodies against basolateral proteins one obtains a more regular honeycomb structure. Analogous to the honeycomb, each hole in the chicken wire is a hepatocyte, indicating that each individual hexagonal hepatocyte is surrounded by a canaliculus. Within the plates of hepatocytes, the canaliculi form a cul-de-sac in the pericentral region, thus ensuring a strict separation between blood and bile. Near the portal triads they are connected with the bile ducts via the canals of Hering. Many canaliculi drain into one canal of Hering.[3] Bile flows from the pericentral

to the portal zone, opposite to the direction of the flow of blood.

The fenestrated endothelium of the hepatic sinusoids allows passage of small molecules, proteins, and large particles such as chylomicrons. Blood cells cannot pass. Thus the sinusoidal endothelium acts as a dynamic biofilter.[4] The diameter of the fenestrae changes upon alterations in portal pressure—for instance, after a meal. In addition, agents such as alcohol, nicotine, and serotonin induce changes in the diameter of the fenestrae. In liver cirrhosis this regulation is disrupted; the sinusoids lose their fenestrations and acquire a basement membrane. This may contribute to liver dysfunction and portal hypertension.[5]

The space of Disse is continuous with the spaces between the hepatocytes. The diameter of white blood cells (WBCs) is larger than the diameter of the sinusoids. Therefore upon passage of WBCs the space of Disse is temporarily obliterated and the endothelium is pressed against the hepatocytes. During these periods the hepatocyte plasma membrane is directly in contact with the blood space. The space of Disse is continuous with the lymph vessels. Thus hepatic lymph is generated in the space of Disse.

Tight junctions form a barrier between these intercellular spaces and the bile canalicular lumen. Tight junctions between hepatocytes are permeable to water and electrolytes and have a limited permeability for organic cations.[6] They are impermeable for organic anions. Tight junctions are complex structures in which the transmembrane proteins occludins and claudins interact with similar proteins in neighboring cells and with the cytoplasmic tight junction proteins ZO-1 and ZO-2.[7] In cholestatic liver disease the tight junction permeability is changed, allowing passage of organic anions from bile to the interstitial space of Disse.[8]

The many agents for which the tight junctions form an impermeable barrier have to traverse the hepatocyte en route from blood to bile. Receptor-mediated endocytosis and pinocytosis play a role in the transcellular routing of proteins and macromolecules. For small charged molecules the exact mechanism of vectorial transcellular transport is still obscure. Single-pass perfusion experiments with isolated perfused rat liver preparations showed that 2 to 3 minutes were required for the paracellular permeation from blood to bile, whereas 5 to 20 minutes are needed for transcellular transport.[9] A relatively fast transcellular component is not inhibited by microtubule inhibitors, whereas a slower component is inhibited by these agents and therefore seems to be associated with intracellular vesicles or with so-called "lipid rafts."[10]

The canalicular domain is the hepatocyte plasma membrane section that surrounds the canaliculus. In fact, it surrounds half of the canaliculus because the domains of two adjacent hepatocytes, linked via tight junctions, form the complete surrounding membrane. A canalicular network in an entire liver plate is in contact with a large number of hepatocytes. Hepatocytes secrete bile salts, which are toxic detergents that have to be neutralized by cholesterol and phospholipids. Therefore hepatocytes must communicate with each other in order to tune the secretory activity of adjacent hepatocytes. If this communication did not exist, the bile salts secreted by one hepatocyte would damage the neighboring cell. This communication occurs via the gap junctions. Gap junctions allow passage of small signaling molecules, such as calcium and/or nucleotides, from one hepatocyte to the other.

Electron microscopy of the canalicular membrane shows microvilli, which contain a number of proteins with a specialized transport function (**Fig. 4-1**). These proteins predominantly belong to the large ABC-transporter superfamily.[11,12] In fact, almost all compounds destined for biliary secretion are handled by these proteins. The canalicular pumps are embedded within lipid microdomains of the canalicular membranes. The lipid composition of these microdomains is important for the function of the pumps and derangements of intracellular lipid trafficking may lead to dysfunction of the surface pumps. Progressive familial intrahepatic cholestasis type 1 (see below) may be an example of a disease attributable to dysfunction of a membrane transporter (ABCB11) caused by disturbance of the canalicular membrane lipid composition.

The canalicular membrane represents approximately 15% of the total surface area of hepatocytes. It contains transport proteins that are able to pump the cholephilic compounds into bile against a 100-fold concentration gradient. This active ATP-dependent transport can be considered the principal driving force of bile flow. In terms of energy, bile formation is a costly process: for example, the secretion of one molecule of unconjugated bilirubin requires four molecules of ATP

equivalents (i.e., two molecules of UDP-glucuronic acid for conjugation and two molecules of ATP for canalicular transport). However, bile formation has at least a dual function: it rids the body of metabolic waste and it is important for the intestinal digestion of energy-rich lipids. The inability to produce bile is associated with rapid weight loss. Therefore the energy required to produce bile seems well spent.

The portal blood is rich in metabolites. Many of these metabolites are absorbed from the blood in the first hepatocytes of the hepatic acinus. Studies with fluorescent or radiolabeled bile salts and fatty acids revealed a steep acinar gradient with a concentration that was high in the periportal hepatocytes and low in the pericentral hepatocytes. This indicates that bile salts and fatty acids are efficiently extracted in these first hepatocytes.[13,14] Depending on the bile salt species, up to 98% is removed by the liver during one passage.

Bile salts repress their own synthesis by inhibiting the first committed step of the classical neutral pathway, microsomal cholesterol 7α-hydroxylase or Cyp7A1, and the first step of the so-called acidic pathway, the mitochondrial sterol 27-hydroxylase Cyp8B1.[15] Thus the periportal hepatocytes are intensively involved in the enterohepatic cycling of bile salts,

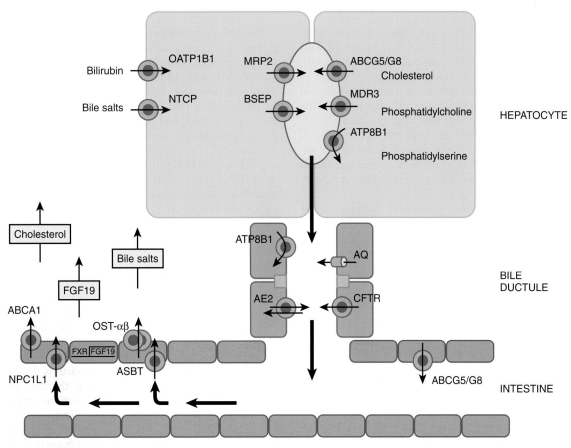

Fig. 4-1 **Human hepatic transporter proteins involved in bile formation.** Transporter proteins located in the basolateral membrane are responsible for the the uptake of bile salts (NTCP), bulky organic anions, uncharged compounds (OATPs), and cations (OATPs, OCT1). Transporter proteins located in the canalicular membrane are responsible for the biliary secretion of compounds such as bile salts, phosphatidylcholine, cholesterol, bilirubin conjugates, and oxidized and reduced glutathione. These transporter proteins comprise the bile salt transporter BSEP, the phosphatidylcholine translocator MDR3, the anionic conjugate transporter MRP2, and the multidrug transporter MDR1 (not shown). The organic anion transporters MRP3, MRP4, and OST-α/β are present at very low levels in normal hepatocytes but are up-regulated during cholestasis (see Fig. 4-2). ABCG5/G8 are two half-transporters (half the molecular mass of regular ABC transporters) and together act as cholesterol and plant sterol transporters. Fibroblast growth factor 19 (FGF19) is synthesized in the terminal ileum upon binding of bile salts to FXR. Niemann-Pick C1-Like 1 (NPC1L1) protein is the intestinal cholesterol transporter. Bile salts and cholesterol participate in an enterohepatic cycle.

whereas the hepatocytes in the pericentral zone are more active in de novo biosynthesis.[16]

When bile leaves the hepatic acinus it enters the bile ducts. These structures are visible on light microscopy as portal triads—a bile duct accompanied by one or two hepatic arteries and a branch of the portal vein. From the bile ducts, bile flows via the intrahepatic and extrahepatic ducts to the intestine. Although cholangiocytes or bile duct epithelial cells in total volume contribute no more than 3% to 5% to the total liver, bile ducts in normal human liver are estimated to be 1 km in length. Small and large cholangiocytes have distinct morphologic and functional features and differ in proliferative capacity.[17] Cholangiocytes have a collection of transporter proteins, electrolyte exchangers, and water channels on their apical and basolateral surfaces, indicating that the bile duct epithelium has both an absorptive and a secretory function. It is not surprising, therefore, that bile composition is considerably modified in the bile ducts. Here, bile becomes enriched in bicarbonate and chloride whereas glucose and glutamate are reabsorbed. Also, bile salts may to some extent be reabsorbed.[18] Indirect proof for bile salt reabsorption is the presence of the apical sodium-dependent bile salt transporter ASBT (SLC10A2) and the observed uptake of fluorescent bile salts in the bile duct epithelium.

Bile is rich in mucin, which is produced in the gallbladder. Therefore the substance that enters the duodenum after passing through the ampulla of Vater is a rather viscous, mucin-containing yellow fluid composed of phospholipids, cholesterol, and bile salts. The yellow color is attributable to bilirubin, which is present in millimolar quantities. Bile also contains amino acids, carnitine, and many other solutes. Bile entering the duodenum contains very little glutathione. This tripeptide is almost completely degraded and its components are largely reabsorbed in the bile ducts.[19] Some drugs are highly concentrated in bile. An example is ceftriaxone, which can even precipitate out of solution and form gallstones, particularly in children.[20]

Unconjugated bile salts are reabsorbed throughout the small intestine, and conjugated bile salts are reabsorbed in the ileum. ASBT mediates bile salt uptake into the ileal epithelium (**Table 4-1**). Human ASBT transports conjugated and unconjugated bile salts with a higher affinity for dihydroxy bile salts than trihydroxy bile salts. Some sodium-independent bile salt transport may be mediated by Oatp3 (Slc21a7), which is present in all small intestinal segments,[21] and the bulk of unconjugated bile salts may be reabsorbed by passive diffusion. After uptake the bile salt molecules move through the enterocyte to the basolateral domain. The 14-kilodalton ileal bile salt binding protein (I-BABP) may play a role in this passage. The organic solute transporters Ostα-Ostβ[22] in the basolateral membrane of the enterocyte mediate the secretion of bile salts from the enterocyte to the portal blood.

Reabsorption in the small bowel is very efficient because only about 10% of the total biliary bile salts that enter the duodenum escape reabsorption. These remaining bile salts enter the colon, where they become subject to bacterial metabolism that converts primary to secondary bile salts. Some of these bile salts, such as deoxycholate and lithocholate, become reabsorbed in the colon by as yet undefined transport mechanisms or perhaps by passive diffusion.

Phospholipids are hydrolyzed in the intestine and the monophosphate and diphosphate esters are subsequently reabsorbed. Phospholipids in the intestinal lumen are important for the formation of chylomicrons. Formation of these lipoproteins is disturbed in Abcb4 (Mdr2(−/−)) knockout mice, which lack phospholipids in bile.[23] Cholesterol reabsorption is 60% to 80%, depending on conditions and the expression of proteins, which may show species differences. Until recently cholesterol absorption in the intestine was considered to occur passively, only to some extent facilitated by proteins. However, in recent years it has become apparent that intestinal cholesterol absorption is a complex process involving separate counteracting transport systems.

In drug therapy one has to realize that drugs may also participate in the enterohepatic cycling. This adds considerably to their biologic half-life. Ceftriaxone is one example; because of its enterohepatic cycling it must be dosed only once per day. There is evidence that unconjugated bilirubin or bilirubin photoproducts also participate in the enterohepatic circulation.[24] Oral bilirubin trapping agents, such as fresh calcium phosphate, interrupt this cycling and lower serum bilirubin levels in patients with disturbed hepatic bilirubin glucuronidation (e.g., patients who have Crigler-Najjar syndrome). Agents that reduce the gastrointestinal transit time lower serum bilirubin levels in Gunn rats, the animal model of Crigler-Najjar syndrome, by reducing passive reabsorption of unconjugated bilirubin.[25]

Collectively, hepatocytes, bile ductuli, and ducts can be considered as a "hepatic secretory unit," with a certain analogy to the nephron. In both organs there is a primary solution that is produced by filtration, which in the liver occurs through the tight junctions, and active secretion by the hepatocytes. This "primary" bile is modified in the bile ducts through reabsorption of unconjugated and conjugated bile salts, glucose, glycine, and glutamate and by secretion of water, chloride, and bicarbonate. To support these functions cholangiocytes express the apical Na$^+$-dependent bile salt transporter (ASBT or NTCP2, gene symbol Slc10a2), the cystic fibrosis transmembrane conductance regulator (CFTR, ABCC7), a Cl$^-$/HCO$_3^-$ exchanger (AE2, SLC4A2), and an aquaporin (AQP1). Similar to the nephron this ductular secretion is under both hormonal and adrenergic and cholinergic neuronal control with an abundance of calcitonin gene-related peptide (CGRP), substance P, vasoactive intestinal peptide (VIP), and somatostatin-containing nerves around human bile ductules.[26] Hormones that influence the secretory function of bile ducts include secretin, cholecystokinin, bombesin, gastrin, and somatostatin. During cholestasis abundant proliferation of bile ductules is observed and this proliferation is under hormonal control with glucagon-like peptide 1, estrogens, and growth hormone playing a major role. The proliferative effect of estrogens protects the bile ducts against disappearance by apoptosis in primary biliary cirrhosis, a disease mainly affecting women.[27]

Hepatic Transport Proteins

To secrete bile and to excrete metabolites of toxic substances, hepatocytes must transport bile salts, phospholipids, and other solutes from blood to bile. Various basolateral transporters for organic solutes have been characterized. These transporters belong to the solute carrier superfamily and comprise the sodium-dependent transporter for the uptake of bile salts (NTCP; gene symbol SLC10A1), transporters for amphiphilic

Table 4-1 Human Hepatic Transporter Proteins

NAME	GENE	CHROMOSOME	LOCALIZATION*	TRANSPORT FUNCTION*	PHENOTYPE WHEN DEFECTIVE
NTCP	SLC10A1	14q24.1-24.2	H-BL	BS	
ASBT	SLC10A2	13q33	CH-A, E-A	BS	Bile salt diarrhea
OCT1	SLC22A1	6q26	H-BL, E-BL	OC	
OAT2	SLC22A7	6p21.2-21.1	H-BL	OA	
OATP	SLC21A3	12p12	H-BL	BS, OA, OC	
OATP2	SLC21A6	12p	H-BL	B, BS, OA, OC	
OATP8	SLC21A8	12p12	H-BL	BS, OA, OC	
OATP-B	SLC21A9	11q13	H-BL	OA	
	SLC1B1				
ABCA1	ABCA1	9q31	H-BL, E-BL	Phospholipid	High-density lipoprotein deficiency, Tangier type
MDR1	ABCB1	7q21	H-A, CH-A	Drugs, chemotherapeutics	
MDR3	ABCB4	7q21	H-A	PC	PFIC3, ICP, intrahepatic gallstones
BSEP	ABCB11	2q24	H-A	BS	PFIC2, BRIC2
MRP1	ABCC1	16p13.12-p13	H-BL, CH-BL	OA, OA conjugates	
MRP2	ABCC2	10q23-q24	H-A, E-A	OA, OA conjugates	Dubin-Johnson syndrome
MRP3	ABCC3	17q21.3	H-BL, CH-BL	OA conjugates	
MRP4	ABCC4	13q31	H-BL	BS sulfates	
MRP6	ABCC6	16p13.1	H-BL	Peptides, endothelin receptor antagonist BQ123	Pseudoxanthoma elasticum
CFTR	ABCC7	7q31.2	CH-A	Chloride	Cystic fibrosis
ABCG2	ABCG2	4q22-q23	H-A	Chemotherapeutics, chlorophyll metabolites, protoporphyrin	Photosensitivity (mice)
ABCG5	ABCG5	2p21	H-A, E-A	Plant sterols	Sitosterolemia
ABCG8	ABCG8	2p21	H-A, E-A	Plant sterols	Sitosterolemia
FIC1	ATP8B1	18q21-q22	H-A, CH-A, E-A	Aminophospholipid translocation	PFIC1, BRIC1, ICP
WND	ATP7B	13q14.3	H-INT	Copper	Wilson's disease
NPC1L1	NPC1L1	7p13	E-A, H-A	Cholesterol	Inhibited by ezetimibe

A, apical; B, bilirubin; BL, basolateral; BS, bile salts; CH, cholangiocytes; E, enterocytes; H, hepatocytes; ICP, intrahepatic cholestasis of pregnancy; INT, intracellular; MDR, multidrug resistance; OA, organic anions; OC, organic cations; PC, phosphatidylcholine; PFIC, progressive familial intrahepatic cholestasis

substrates such as members of the subfamilies of organic anion–transporting polypeptides (OATPs; gene family SLC21A), and organic cation transporters (OCTs; gene family SLC22A) (see **Table 4-1**).

Basolateral Transport Proteins

NTCP represents the major bile salt uptake system of hepatocytes, localized exclusively in the basolateral membrane of hepatocytes (see **Table 4-1 and Fig. 4-1**).[28] Ntcp preferentially mediates Na$^+$-dependent transport of conjugated bile salts such as taurocholate, and this transport comprises the predominant, if not exclusive, fraction in hepatic bile salt uptake.[29] Human liver NTCP transports conjugated bile salts and human NTCP has a higher affinity (K_M 6 μM) for taurocholate than rat Ntcp (K_M 25 μM).[30] Rat Ntcp has broad substrate

specificity. In addition to bile salts, sulfated steroids, bromo-sulfophthalein (BSP), and thyroid hormones have been shown to be transported by this protein.

Transcriptional regulators of the Slc10a gene include hepatocyte nuclear factor 1α (HNF1-α), HNF4-α, and the retinoid X receptor/retinoic acid receptor (RXR-α/RAR-α) dimer. A protein called short heterodimer partner (SHP) interferes with the transcription of Ntcp by RXR/RAR, particularly at high bile salt concentrations in which the farnesoid X receptor (FXR) is activated that drives SHP expression.[31] There is debate whether this type of regulation also holds true for human NTCP.[32] The human SLC10A gene is activated by glucocorticoid binding to the glucocorticoid receptor. At high bile salt concentrations SHP abrogates this activation by glucocorticoids.[33] Ntcp expression at the basolateral membrane is also regulated by posttranslational mechanisms. cAMP increases the basolateral expression of NTCP,[34,35] and cytokines decrease NTCP expression.[36] A phosphoinositide-3-kinase (PI3K)/phosphokinase B (PKB)-dependent activation of protein kinase C-ε, involved in the regulation of Mrp2 at the canalicular membrane, does not seem to be implicated in the regulation of Ntcp.[37]

An important feature of the Na$^+$-independent bile salt uptake pathway is its wide substrate preference, indicating that this is not mediated by NTCP but by the OATPs, transport carriers of drugs, bile salts, and bilirubin. OATP substrates include conjugated and unconjugated bile salts, cardiac glycosides, estrogens, neutral steroids, thyroid hormones, linear and cyclic peptides, selected organic cations, anti-HIV drugs, statins, and chemotherapeutics. OATPs are localized in the basolateral membrane of hepatocytes. In human liver the major organic anion carrier proteins are OATP1B1 (OATP2, OATP-C, gene symbol SLCO1B1) and OATP1B3 (OATP8, SLCO1B3). OATP1B1 transports a large number of organic anions, including drugs such as the statins and probably also bilirubin. OATP1B3 also transports bilirubin (albeit with less affinity than that demonstrated by OATP1B1), bilirubin monoglucuronide, paclitaxel, and digoxin.[38,39] Similar to NTCP, the expression of these proteins also is regulated on a transcriptional and a posttranscriptional level. For instance, HNF-1α activates the SLCO1B1 promoter and bile salts via their action on HNF-4α or via FXR/SHP suppress HNF-1α activity and thus reduce OATP1B1 expression.[40] This might explain the down-regulation of this protein observed in a variety of cholestatic liver diseases.[41-44] A genome-wide association study revealed polymorphisms of SLCO1B1 strongly associated with an increased risk of simvastatin-induced myopathy.[45] In another study irinotecan toxicity has been associated with SLCO1B1 polymorphisms.[46]

A variety of small organic cations, including drugs, choline, or monoamine neurotransmitters, are translocated by OCT1 (SLC22A1).[47] Of the five SLC22A family members only OCT1 is of relevance for the liver. Human OCT1[48] is 78% identical to rat Oct1 and has comparable substrate specificity.

Canalicular Transport Proteins

Most canalicular transport systems involved in bile formation belong to the 48 members of the ATP-binding cassette (ABC) transporter superfamily, which is one of the largest superfamilies of proteins in prokaryotes and eukaryotes.[49] With respect to bile formation, four subclusters of this superfamily are most important—the A, B, C, and D clusters (see **Table 4-1**).

The Bile Salt Export Pump BSEP (ABCB11)

The bile salt excretory pump (BSEP, ABCB11) is critical for ATP-dependent transport of bile salts across the hepatocyte canalicular membrane and for generation of bile salt–dependent bile secretion (**Fig. 4-2**).[50] Patients genetically lacking BSEP have a severe cholestatic liver disease characterized by high serum bile salt levels—progressive familial intrahepatic cholestasis type 2 (PFIC type 2).[51,52] Bsep(−/−) mice are cholestatic in the sense that taurocholate accumulates in their plasma because its secretion into bile is strongly impaired.[53] However, in contrast to human patients, the mice excrete substantial amounts of tauromuricholate into bile as well as tetrahydroxy bile salt metabolites. Apparently, Bsep is

not the only bile salt transporting system in the canalicular membrane because other systems, such as Mdr1a/1b in the mouse, are probably capable of excreting hydrophilic bile salts.[54] These transporters may serve as escape routes that prevent severe and progressive cholestasis. As a possible consequence the mice have very few histopathologic indications of liver injury. The possible role of MDR1 in humans in bile salt secretion has not yet been elucidated (see the following section: MDR1 P-Glycoprotein [ABCB1]).

The regulation of rat Bsep has been studied under conditions of endotoxin treatment, bile duct ligation, and ethinylestradiol-induced cholestasis.[55,56] In these cholestatic and stress response models, Bsep mRNA and protein expression levels only slightly decreased compared with levels of the basolateral bile salt carrier Ntcp[57] (i.e., Oatp1, Oatp2) or the canalicular transporter Mrp2.[56,58] Thus Bsep may continue to secrete bile salts, although at impaired rates. Remarkably, after partial hepatectomy the mRNA level of Bsep was only slightly decreased and the protein level of Bsep was unaffected in contrast to the bile salt uptake transporter Ntcp.[58,59] This may explain that after partial hepatectomy the remnant liver is not cholestatic and not damaged by excess bile salts. Also in human liver disease BSEP expression is usually unaffected.[60,61]

Expression of BSEP is sensitive to the flux of bile salts through the hepatocyte. The BSEP promoter contains an IR-1 element that serves as a binding site for the farnesoid X receptor, a nuclear receptor for bile salts.[62] FXR activity requires heterodimerization with RXRα, and when bound by bile salts the complex effectively regulates the transcription of several genes involved in bile salt homeostasis. By this mechanism bile salts transcriptionally regulate the activity of BSEP, preventing increased hepatocellular levels of potential toxic bile salts (see **Fig. 4-2**). In addition to BSEP, FXR has a large number of target genes, some quite unrelated to bile salt metabolism. Therefore the use of potent FXR ligands as drugs has to be considered with caution because these ligands could have unpredictable side effects.[63]

MDR1 P-Glycoprotein (ABCB1)

MDR1 in humans and Mdr1a and Mdr1b in rodents are encoded by the *ABCB1*, Abcb1a, and Abcb1b genes, respectively. Various physiologic functions of MDR1/Mdr1 have been demonstrated or postulated, such as transport of exogenous and endogenous metabolites or toxins,[64] steroid hormones,[65] hydrophobic peptides,[66] amphiphilic cationic drugs,[67] and bile salts.[54] To establish the physiologic function of Mdr1 and Mdr2, a set of gene knockout mice was generated.[68] These mutant mice did not express either functional Mdr1a (Abcb1a(−/−)),[69] Mdr1b (Abcb1b(−/−)),[68] or Mdr2 (Abcb2(−/−)).[70] Double-knockout mice were also produced (Abcb1a(−/−)/Abc1b(−/−)).[68] These mice were all fertile. The *Abcb1* knockout mice exhibited an almost normal phenotype under laboratory conditions.[68] From experiments with mice with Abcb1a/1b(−/−) gene knockout, no changes in bile composition became apparent.[71] Disruption of both genes in mice has no effect on the normal laboratory life of these mice, but renders them hypersensitive to drugs. MDR1 appears to be especially important in protecting the brain. In the gut, where MDR1 pumps from the enterocyte towards the lumen, MDR1 limits the uptake of hydrophobic drugs. In analogy,

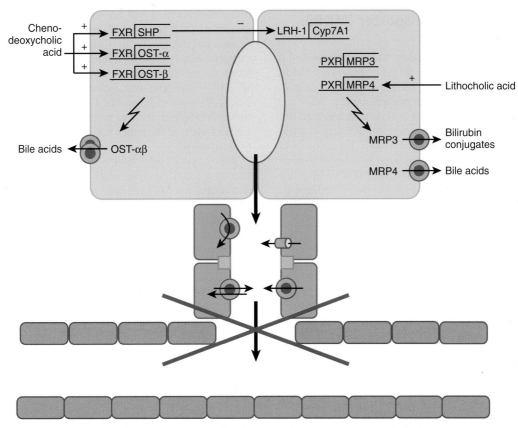

Fig. 4-2 Hepatic gene regulation by bile salts and role of members of the nuclear hormone superfamily. During cholestasis bile salts accumulate and chenodeoxycholic acid and lithocholic acid bind to FXR and PXR, respectively. These nuclear hormone receptors act as transcription factors for a number of genes, including SHP1, a gene that encodes a small protein that interacts with LRH1-mediated gene regulation of Cyp7A1, the gatekeeping enzyme of bile acid synthesis. Activation of FXR and PXR causes the induction of the basolateral ATP-dependent transporters MRP3, MRP4, and OST-α/β that act as escape routes in cholestatic conditions. Solutes that are transported back to the blood are eventually secreted by the kidneys.

MDR1 may protect the hepatocyte against hydrophobic toxic drugs by transporting them into the bile. MDR1 polymorphisms have been reported to be relevant in cancer chemotherapy, in immunosuppressive therapy, in organ transplant recipients, and for the natural clinical course of cancer patients.[72]

The regulation of MDR1 and its rodent homologues has been studied in detail. It is clear that ABCB1 promoter activation is part of a general stress response resulting in cellular resistance. p53 is involved in the basal regulation of human ABCB1 and rat Abcb1a and Abcb1b.[73] Although wild-type p53 represses Abcb1a expression, overexpression of mutant p53 resulted in markedly elevated levels of rat Abcb1a mRNA and protein. Similar regulation was reported for ABCB1. A functional p53 binding site has been identified in the rat Abcb1b promoter.[74] Wild-type p53 was shown to up-regulate Abcb1b promoter activity and mediates the endogenous expression of rat Abcb1b. These results and other studies indicate that the two rodent Abcb1 genes are differentially regulated. The expression of Abcb1a in rat liver is not affected by endotoxin treatment and increases only slightly after bile duct ligation or partial hepatectomy.[58] In contrast, Abcb1b expression is markedly enhanced during endotoxin-induced and bile duct ligation–induced cholestasis, and even more in the remnant liver after partial hepatectomy. Up-regulation

of *Abcb1b* during liver regeneration, after partial hepatectomy, or after endotoxin treatment is at least in part TNF-α dependent. In fact, activation of the rat Abcb1b gene by TNF-α is a result of NFκB signaling.[75] Abcb1b up-regulation, at least in part, may provide anti-apoptotic protection against oxidative stress-induced cell damage. Bsep(−/−) mice have a far less severe genotype than humans lacking BSEP expression. The rationale for this may be that in mice Abc1a/1b are able to compensate for the lack of Bsep expression. Thus triple-knockout mice (Bsep(−/−), Mdr1a(−/−), Mdr1b(−/−)) showed a significantly more severe cholestatic phenotype than single Bsep(−/−) or double Mdr1a(−/−), Mdr1b(−/−) knockout mice.[54] These findings indicate that although BSEP is a transporter for hydrophobic bile salts, MDR1 may be able to transport hydrophilic bile salts. This compensatory role of MDR1/Mdr1 is probably more effective in mice than in humans because mice are able to synthesize hydrophilic hydroxylated bile salts.

PXR is a nuclear hormone receptor that binds pregnenolone 16α-carbonitrile (PCN), rifampicin, and lithocholic acid. These ligands induce CYP3A4 expression as well as the expression of enzymes of the UDP-glucuronosyltransferase family (i.e., UGT1A1, UGT1A6), and thus protect the body from harmful chemical agents. PXR also regulates drug efflux by inducing the expression of MDR1.[76]

MDR3 Phospholipid Transporter (MDR3, mdr2; ABCB4, Abcb4)

In the liver, human MDR3 and rodent Mdr2 are expressed in canalicular membranes[77] (see **Fig. 4-1**). The function of Mdr2 became apparent after producing Abcb2(−/−) knockout mice, resulting in a complete absence of phospholipid in bile.[78]

From these and other studies it is now well accepted that Mdr2 as well as its human counterpart, MDR3, acts as a flippase, translocating phospholipids through the canalicular membrane.[79] The currently accepted hypothesis for the mechanism of phospholipid secretion is that MDR3/Mdr2 flips phosphatidylcholine from the inner to the outer leaflet of the lipid bilayer. These lipids are probably concentrated in microdomains in the exoplasmic hemileaflet of the canalicular membrane.[80] Bile salts solubilize PC from these microdomains either in the form of vesicles or as mixed bile salt/PC micelles.

Cholesterol secretion is strongly reduced but can be increased in Abcb4 knockout mice by enriching the bile with taurocholate.[81] In a physiologic sense, these mice are not cholestatic because the bile salt secretion is normal and bile flow is elevated.[78] However, when stressed with oral cholate feeding, serum bilirubin levels and serum alkaline phosphatase activity increase, showing that under these conditions these mice become cholestatic. Also there are histologic features similar to those observed in cholestasis, such as bile ductular proliferation and feathery degeneration of hepatocytes.[70] Biliary bile salt secretion in these mice is not accompanied by phospholipids. Therefore the bile they produce is cytotoxic. Older mice with the gene disruption develop liver tumors.[70] The human counterparts of the Mdr2 knockout mice are patients with progressive familial intrahepatic cholestasis (PFIC type 3) (see Genetic Defects of Bile Secretion). Expression of Mdr2 in rodent liver appears to be unaltered under most conditions of cellular stress.[82] Mdr2 expression was not affected after endotoxin treatment[55] and was only slightly enhanced after partial hepatectomy.[58] When mice received a diet that was supplemented with fibrates, this increased Mdr2 mRNA and protein levels and increased PC secretion, suggesting involvement of PPAR-α in Mdr2 gene expression.[83] In mice fed a diet supplemented with the hydrophobic bile salt cholate, Mdr2 mRNA levels were induced, which was functionally reflected in a concomitant increase of the maximal PC secretion capacity.[84] Administration of the (relatively) hydrophilic bile salt ursodeoxycholate did not influence the Mdr2 mRNA levels or the maximal PC output capacity.[84] Bile salt–mediated induction of Abcb4 at least partly involves activation of FXR.[85]

The Multidrug Resistance Protein MRP2 (ABCC2)

MRP2 is located in the canalicular membrane of hepatocytes as well as the apical membranes of enterocytes, and in renal tubular cells, the blood-brain barrier, and tubuli seminiferi (see **Fig. 4-1**). In the liver endogenous and xenobiotic lipophilic compounds are converted into more hydrophilic anionic conjugates with glutathione, glucuronate, or sulfate. These conjugates are transported across the canalicular membrane into bile by MRP2. MRP2 contributes to bile formation by transporting glutathione, a major driving force for bile salt–independent bile flow. In Dubin-Johnson syndrome MRP2 is genetically lacking.[86] These patients have a mild conjugated hyperbilirubinemia but are otherwise quite healthy. In fact, certain ABCC2 gene polymorphisms have a protective effect when receiving irinotecan (Camptothecin), a chemotherapeutic agent that in 25% of patients causes severe diarrhea. Irinotecan is metabolized by carboxylesterases, UGT1A1 and UGT1A7,[87] and the metabolites are secreted into bile via MRP2. Patients with the ABCC2*2 gene variant secrete less of these metabolites and are protected against diarrhea. This is particularly true for patients who have a normal glucuronidation capacity.[88]

Rats lacking Mrp2 have a normal life span and a normal breeding capacity. These rats have been invaluable for the demonstration of canalicular transporter function for the disposition of drugs and endogenous metabolites.[89] MRP2 gene expression is regulated by three nuclear receptors: PXR, FXR, and CAR.[90] Thus the PXR and CAR ligands, rifampicin and phenobarbital, respectively, induce MRP2 expression and thereby help in the elimination of organic anions such as bilirubin from the liver. The promoter regions of the human MRP2 genes and the rat Mrp2 genes have been isolated.[91] Interestingly, in cholestasis Mrp2 is up-regulated in the kidney.[92] This helps in eliminating organic anions, glucuronide, and glutathione conjugates when hepatobiliary function is impaired.

The Basolateral Anionic Conjugate and Bile Salt Transporters MRP3 and MRP4

MRP3 (ABCC3) is a transporter protein that supports the basolateral export of organic anions, including glutathione and glucuronide conjugates as well as bile salts from hepatocytes.[93] For bile salts its affinity is low and its expression in normal liver is also low.[94] Under control conditions MRP3 is expressed in the centrilobular hepatocytes, in bile duct epithelium, and in the gallbladder.[95] Basolateral MRP3 expression is up-regulated during cholestasis and in livers of patients with Dubin-Johnson syndrome.[61,96] Mrp3 is significantly up-regulated in Mrp2-deficient TR− rats and EHBR rats, in bilirubin-UDP-glucuronosyltransferase–deficient Gunn rats, and in bile duct–ligated rats.[93,97-99] These are models with conjugated hyperbilirubinemia, unconjugated hyperbilirubinemia, and cholestasis, respectively. MRP3 clearly is the inducible counterpart of MRP2. MRP3 transcription is regulated by the drug-activated nuclear hormone receptors CAR and PXR.[100] The identities of the natural agents that induce MRP3 are less clear. Feeding rats a docosahexanoic acid–enriched diet causes an increased lipid peroxidation in the liver; in Mrp2-deficient EHBR rats this is associated with a significant up-regulation of Mrp3.[98] This enables the urinary secretion of the metabolic products as mercapturic acid. Thus lipid peroxidation–induced cellular stress may induce Mrp3. MRP3 is the dominant glucuronide and glutathione conjugate overflow system.

MRP4 (ABCC4) is an inducible basolateral transporter that co-transports reduced glutathione and the taurine and glycine conjugates of cholic acid.[101] It is also a high-affinity transporter of sulfated bile salts and the sulfate conjugate of dihydroepiandrosterone.[102] The drug-activated receptor CAR activates transcription of the Abcc4 gene and the dihydroepiandrosterone sulfotransferase 2a1 gene. The latter is the main sulfa-conjugating enzyme in the liver and as such prepares substrates for Mrp4-mediated transport. MRP4 is the primary high-affinity bile salt overflow system and expression of Mrp4 represents a major adaptation of the liver to cholestasis. In Mrp4(−/−) (knockout) mice cholestasis induced by bile duct ligation causes significantly more liver damage than cholestasis induced in wild-type or Mrp3(−/−) mice.

ATP8B1

ATP8B1 is not an ABC transporter but a member of the type 4 subfamily of P-type ATPases (P4 ATPase). P4 ATPases are transmembrane proteins that mediate the translocation of phospholipids from the exoplasmic to the cytoplasmic leaflet of biologic membranes.[103] In most eukaryotic cells phosphatidylcholine and sphingolipids are concentrated in the exoplasmic leaflet, whereas the aminophospholipids phosphatidylserine (PS) and phosphatidylethanolamine (PE) are largely confined to the cytoplasmic leaflet of the plasma membrane.[104] This asymmetric distribution is actively maintained by proteins termed floppases and flippases.[105]

The canalicular membrane is a rigid, detergent-resistant membrane that is enriched in cholesterol and sphingomyelin (SM).[106] This allows tight packing of the membrane lipids into a so-called "liquid-ordered" state and makes the membrane extremely resistant to bile salt–mediated lipid extraction.[107] ATP8B1 is indispensable in maintaining this detergent-resistant state of the canalicular membrane.[108] Work from our lab demonstrated that ATP8B1-mediated PS translocation requires co-expression of a putative β-subunit termed CDC50A.[109] Only when ATP8B1 and CDC50A were co-expressed was ATP8B1 released from the endoplasmic reticulum and localized to the plasma membrane of CHO cells; this coincided with a significant increase in NBD-PS and natural PS internalization. Recently, Cai and colleagues demonstrated with rat hepatocyte sandwich cultures that Atp8b1 deficiency resulted in enhanced accumulation of NBD-PS in the canalicular lumen compared with control.[110]

Having established that ATP8B1 is an aminophospholipid translocase that helps in maintaining a detergent-resistant state of canalicular membranes, one may ask how this relates to cholestasis. We have recently demonstrated that canalicular membranes of bile salt–fed cholestatic Atp8b1-deficient mice have a dramatically reduced cholesterol/phospholipid ratio compared with those of bile salt–fed wild-type controls.[111] The cholesterol content of the membrane is an essential determinant of the activity of the major bile salt transporter BSEP and of the conjugated bilirubin transporter MRP2 (encoded by the *ABCC2* gene). In fact, there is a linear relationship between membrane cholesterol content and BSEP activity. In line with these observations, Cai and colleagues recently demonstrated that Bsep activity was reduced by 40% compared with control in Atp8b1-deficient rat hepatocytes.[110] ATP8B1 deficiency thus leads to loss of membrane cholesterol and the normal phospholipid asymmetry of the canalicular membrane. This impairs the activity of BSEP and, as a consequence, causes cholestasis. In benign recurrent intrahepatic cholestasis (BRIC) the cholestasis is intermittent and recurring. What triggers these cholestatic episodes that can last for weeks to months? Recent publications shed some new light on this intriguing phenomenon. van der Velden and colleagues show that a number of missense mutations are associated with a folding defect of the ATP8b1 protein. These folding defects are temperature sensitive: 30° C is a permissive temperature that enables the normal folding of the protein whereas at higher temperatures protein folding is significantly impaired.[112] The cholestatic attacks in BRIC patients are sometimes preceded by fever, and the temperature elevation may enhance the expression of the folding defect. An alternative explanation is offered by Folmer and colleagues.[113] These authors argue that in nonjaundiced BRIC patients, BSEP expression is just enough to maintain bile flow but there is not enough reserve to cope with a cytokine-induced impairment of BSEP expression during a viral or bacterial disease.[113] Because of the instability of the canalicular membrane in BRIC patients, cholestasis is self-perpetual. Membrane stability has to be restored to end the cholestatic episode.

ABCG5/ABCG8

Similar to all other members of the ABC G-subfamily, ABCG5 and ABCG8 consist of a single ATP-binding cassette in the amino terminal followed by six putative transmembrane helices; to become functionally active they must dimerize, and hence they are referred to as half-transporters. In contrast to the other G-family members, these two half-transporters represent a heterodimer and no evidence exists that homodimerization of either of the two results in active transport of a substrate across the plasma membrane of cells. The strongest evidence that ABCG5 and ABCG8 act as obligate heterodimers is obtained from genetic data: sitosterolemia, a disease resulting from a deficiency of functional sterol transport, is caused by mutations in both alleles of either ABCG5 or ABCG8 that nonetheless lead to indistinguishable phenotypes.[114,115]

The half-transporters ABCG5 and ABCG8 are encoded by two genes on chromosome 2. The genes are predominantly expressed in liver, intestine, and gallbladder.[116,117] Expression of ABCG5 and (to less extent) ABCG8 is regulated by the oxysterol-sensing nuclear receptor LXR-α, although the responsive element has not been identified.[118] In mice a high cholesterol diet as well as administration of the artificial LXR agonist T0901317 increases Abcg5/8 expression in the liver and increases biliary cholesterol secretion.[119] The intergenic promoter region also contains elements for LRH-1[120] as well as for GATA4 and HNF4-α, which seem to activate transcription of both genes.[121]

The role of the transporter couple ABCG5/8 was discovered by the fact that in patients with sitosterolemia, one of either gene is mutated. Sitosterolemia is a very rare inherited disorder characterized by up to 100-fold increased serum levels of plant sterols (phytosterols). In contrast to other inherited forms of hypercholesterolemia, sitosterolemia is characterized by increased sensitivity of serum cholesterol to dietary cholesterol (see Belamarich et al.[122] and references cited therein). In healthy individuals large changes in dietary cholesterol are associated with modest changes in serum cholesterol levels. In contrast, diets containing high cholesterol levels elicit severe hypercholesterolemia in sitosterolemic patients. Conversely, restriction of dietary cholesterol is able to normalize the serum cholesterol level in these patients. These observations indicate that intestinal ABCG5/8 functions to limit the amount of absorbed cholesterol, similar to its action in plant sterols.

It has now been firmly established that a large part of biliary cholesterol secretion depends on the action of the transporter ABCG5/8.[123] Biliary lipid secretion is also driven by bile salts. In the complete absence of bile salts there is no biliary phospholipid or cholesterol output and there is a curvilinear relationship between biliary bile salt and lipid secretion.[81] Hence, mixed micelles of bile salts and phospholipid serve as an acceptor for cholesterol that has been translocated by ABCG5/8. In line with this contention, Vrins and colleagues showed that cholesterol efflux from polarized epithelial cells transduced with ABCG5/8 depends on the presence of bile salts in the medium.[124]

The fact that an ABC transporter (ABCG5/8) is necessary for the large majority of cholesterol secretion strongly suggests that cholesterol cannot be extracted from the membrane nonspecifically. It may be assumed that the canalicular membrane does have substantial amounts of cholesterol in its outer leaflet even in the absence of the translocator ABCG5/8: cholesterol is essential to make the membrane sufficiently resistant towards bile salts, which are strong detergents. Membranes that lack cholesterol are highly sensitive to detergents, and the fact that patients with sitosterolemia as well as mouse models lacking Abcg5/8 do not have liver damage indicates that the outer leaflet of the canalicular membrane does contain cholesterol even in the absence of Abcg5/8. The question remains why a translocator such as Abcg5/8 is necessary for the efflux of cholesterol if sufficient cholesterol is already present in the outer leaflet and bile salts are present in the canalicular lumen to extract the cholesterol. In a seminal paper, Small[125] hypothesized that the principal function of ABCG5/8 is not in the actual translocation step (although it most likely functions as a translocator); instead, its primary purpose is to partially extrude the molecule from the lipid bilayer so that it can be accepted by bile salt micelles. In a membrane bilayer mostly composed of sphingomyelin, cholesterol is deeply buried in the outer leaflet and it requires substantial activation energy to lift it out of the leaflet. Hence, after translocation ABCG5/8 may lift cholesterol from the bilayer and the latter step may actually be the crucial rate-controlling step in secretion.

Other Hepatic ABC-Transporter Proteins

The *ABCA1* gene (also called ABC1) is mutated in patients with Tangier disease.[126] It appears that ABCA1 regulates plasma high-density lipoprotein (HDL) levels.[127] It promotes the efflux of cholesterol from macrophages and peripheral tissues to apolipoprotein A-I. Abca1 knockout mice secrete normal amounts of cholesterol in their bile, leading to the conclusion that Abca1 is not a cholesterol transporting protein.[128] It may be a phospholipid transporter that enables HDL to incorporate cholesterol.

Regulation of Bile Secretion

Hepatocytes are strictly polarized cells. They absorb substrates from the blood and secrete metabolites into the bile. Bile flow depends on the absorption of substrates and the secretion of metabolites, in particular bile salts. As mentioned earlier in this chapter, the supply of bile salts is variable. Absorption from the portal venous blood is nearly complete and in the fasting state occurs mainly in periportal hepatocytes. The main potential for regulation at the sinusoidal membrane is involvement of more hepatocytes, downstream in the liver acinus, when the bile salt concentration in portal venous blood suddenly increases, as occurs during feeding. It is important to note that Ntcp, the bile salt uptake transporter, is evenly distributed along the hepatic acinus.[28] Thus

perivenous hepatocytes, which are commonly exposed to low concentrations of bile salts, have a similar Ntcp expression as periportal hepatocytes, which are exposed to high bile salt concentrations. Bile salts are potentially cytotoxic and at high concentrations can induce apoptosis and necrosis.[129] Binding to intracellular binding proteins, storage in the ER, and activation of NFκB are possible defense mechanisms.[130] Most important, however, is a rapid canalicular secretion, which is balanced with sinusoidal absorption.

Many high-affinity ligands of the nuclear hormone receptor (NHR) family of transcription factors are also substrates for ABC transporters (see **Fig. 4-2**). This relationship is important for the physiologic regulation of ABC-transporter genes and other NHR-target genes in vivo. However, during liver disease this crosstalk may be disturbed because of the acute phase response–coupled down-regulation of NHRs and their target genes. Infection, inflammation, and trauma induce a wide array of metabolic changes in the liver that constitute the acute phase response, mediated by cytokines, particularly TNF-α, IL-1α, and IL-6. For example, in fulminant hepatic failure serum levels of TNF-α and TNF receptors are significantly increased. In livers of patients with fulminant hepatic failure, infiltrating mononuclear cells express high amounts of TNF-α and hepatocytes overexpress TNF receptor 1 (TNFR1).[131] The acute phase response is associated with a decrease in mRNAs coding for certain NHR proteins such as RXR, LXR, PPAR-α, and PPAR-γ.[132] Reduction of RXR levels, along with levels of other nuclear hormone receptors in the liver, could be a mechanism to coordinately down-regulate the expression of a large number of genes, including ABC transporters, during the acute phase response. Down-regulation of specific hepatic nuclear factors, such as HNF1 and HNF4, may play a key role in the regulation of certain negative acute phase proteins. For example, a decrease in HNF1 is thought to be responsible for the reduced transcription of albumin and Ntcp. The acute phase response also causes marked alterations in lipid metabolism in the liver. Many of the enzymes and transporters involved in these metabolic changes are known to be regulated by PPAR-α or LXR-α. It is possible that during the acute phase response, the reduced availability of RXR protein, and possibly of NHRs, represents a mechanism to coordinately regulate these metabolic changes. In addition, the importance of RXRs for liver gene expression has been demonstrated.[133] Biochemical parameters indicate that PPAR-α, CAR, PXR, LXR, and FXR coupled metabolic pathways in the liver were compromised in the absence of RXR-α. Thus RXR-α is integrated into a number of diverse physiologic pathways as a common regulatory component of cholesterol, fatty acid, bile salt, steroid, and xenobiotic metabolism and homeostasis.

BSEP (ABCB11) mediates the movement of bile salts from hepatocytes to bile. The unique organ specificity of this protein indicates the special position of the liver in bile salt metabolism. The liver plays a dominant role in the enterohepatic cycling of bile salts. Furthermore, in the liver bile salts are synthesized de novo from cholesterol via the so-called neutral and acid pathways. CYP7A1 (cholesterol 7α-hydroxylase) is the gatekeeper of the neutral pathway. This enzyme and an enzyme more downstream in the neutral pathway, CYP8B, are under the transcriptional control of the nuclear receptor FXR. In the regulation of these enzymes FXR acts indirectly through the action of at least two other transcription factors.[134] FXR is a ligand-activated transcription factor. Chenodeoxycholic acid, cholic acid, deoxycholic acid, and lithocholic acid bind and activate FXR. FXR forms complexes with the retinoid X receptor and this FXR/RXR heterodimer interacts with a highly conserved IR-1 motif (inverse repeat-1) in the promoter regions of BSEP and SHP-1, for example.[62,135] SHP-1 suppresses the transcription of CYP7A1 and CYP8B by binding to a transcription factor called liver receptor homologue 1.[15,136]

FXR acts as a bile salt sensor; it needs to be activated by its natural ligands—the bile salts. FXR controls several key steps in bile salt metabolism, not only bile salt synthesis but also transporter involvement in the enterohepatic cycle. Thus upon binding of bile salts, FXR suppresses the expression of NTCP via SHP-1. The presumed mechanism is by interfering with RXR/RAR binding to the NTCP promoter.[31] In contrast, FXR up-regulates the expression of BSEP in the liver and the bile salt binding protein in the ileum (iBABP). Studies in mice with a genetic disruption of FXR showed that the FXR response is particularly important in dealing with a bile salt load, as occurs when feeding mice a diet high in cholesterol or cholate. In FXR null mice the expression of Ntcp, CYP7A1, and CYP8B fails to be down-regulated and the expression of Bsep, iBABP, and SHP-1 is not enhanced as occurs in wild-type mice under these conditions.[137]

Cholestasis in rats is associated with a decreased expression of Ntcp.[138] This is most probably caused by enhanced expression of SHP-1 through activation of FXR by retained bile salts. Also in humans, NTCP expression in cholestatic liver disease is decreased.[44] Down-regulation of NTCP and CYP7A1 in cholestatic liver disease may be cytoprotective, reducing the entry and the synthesis of bile salts when intracellular bile salt levels are already elevated.

Recently a new hormone has been identified—fibroblast growth factor 19 (FGF19); it is synthesized in the terminal ileum upon activation of intestinal FXR by conjugated bile salts. This protein is secreted into the portal circulation, where it reaches maximal levels 3 to 4 hours after a meal. In the liver FGF19 binds to FGFR4, a receptor that is located on the surface of the hepatocyte. This binding initiates a signaling cascade in which the MAP kinases ERK1 and ERK2 are phosphorylated. Through a number of intermediate steps this down-regulates the expression of Cyp7a1 and CYP8B1, enzymes governing the classical and the so-called acidic bile salt biosynthetic pathway. In the mouse fgf15 (the mouse orthologue of human FGF19) is not produced in the liver; therefore serum fgf15 levels in mice with a ligated bile duct are very low and as a consequence Cyp7a1 in the liver is not down-regulated.[139] Consequently, in mice adaptation of liver metabolism during cholestasis is not optimal. Because mice are capable of detoxifying bile salts by hydroxylation, hepatotoxicity by bile salts during cholestasis remains limited. Because humans have more toxic bile salts, they show a very high hepatic expression of FGF19 during extrahepatic cholestasis, and as a consequence a very well repressed CYP7A1.[140] Humans with extrahepatic cholestasis also demonstrate a clear overexpression of OSTα/β, a transporter that together with MRP3 and MRP4 will help in the efflux of solutes from the liver when the route across the canaliculus is blocked. Thus humans show optimal adaptation during extrahepatic cholestasis by significant down-regulation of bile salt synthesis, thus reducing the intracellular concentration of toxic bile salts.

Canalicular Mrp2 is rapidly down-regulated in LPS-induced and bile duct ligation–induced cholestasis in rats while Bsep expression is maintained.[55,56,141] Also during cholestasis in humans MRP2 is down-regulated.[60] Mrp3 and Mrp4 in the basolateral membrane are up-regulated under these conditions.[93,95] Together these two proteins cover the entire spectrum of Mrp2 substrates; thus these proteins can fully compensate for the decreased canalicular Mrp2 activity. Mrp3 mediates the transport of non–bile salt glucuronides and glutathione conjugates and Mrp4 regulates the transport of bile salt sulfates. Mrp4 functions as a basolateral bile salt conjugate and glutathione co-transporter.[101] Up-regulation of Mrp3 and Mrp4 has a cytoprotective function. Metabolites are cleared from the hepatocyte via basolateral membrane pumps when exit via the canalicular membrane is not possible. The Mrp3 and Mrp4 genes are controlled and activated by PXR and CAR respectively.[102,142] CAR not only activates Mrp4 but also the sulfotransferase Sult2a, which mediates the sulfation of bile salts, the high-affinity substrates of Mrp4.[102]

Genetic Defects of Bile Secretion

The spectrum of diseases caused by defects of ABC-transporter proteins is diverse and includes the liver diseases progressive familial intrahepatic cholestasis (PFIC),[143] benign recurrent intrahepatic cholestasis (BRIC),[144] intrahepatic cholestasis of pregnancy (ICP),[145] cystic fibrosis–associated liver disease (CFALD),[146] adrenoleukodystrophy,[147] and Dubin-Johnson syndrome[148,149]; various eye disorders[150]; disorders of cholesterol and carbohydrate metabolism; and connective tissue diseases.[151-153]

Progressive familial intrahepatic cholestasis (PFIC) constitutes a group of autosomal recessive diseases characterized by cholestasis starting in infancy. For an initial differentiation of various PFIC subtypes, measurement of the serum γ-glutamyltransferase (γ-GT) activity is useful. Diseases associated with bile that has low bile salt concentration have a low serum γ-GT activity. These are PFIC types 1 and 2 and BRIC types 1 and 2. These diseases have a hepatocellular blockade of bile salt secretion and should be called hepatocellular cholestasis rather than intrahepatic cholestasis. γ-GT in human liver is mainly located in the membranes lining the biliary tree. Elevation of serum γ-GT activity results from a detergent, membranolytic effect of bile salts on these membranes. Thus either the blockade of bile flow downstream of the location of γ-GT or the presence of bile containing bile salts not antagonized by neutralizing phosphatidylcholine causes γ-GT to be released in the circulation under cholestatic conditions. Elevated serum γ-GT activity occurs in various forms of intrahepatic and extrahepatic cholestasis. In PFIC type 3, γ-GT activity is elevated.

Progressive Familial Intrahepatic Cholestasis Type 1

PFIC type 1 or Byler disease (**Table 4-2**) often begins with episodes of cholestasis progressing to permanent cholestasis with fibrosis, cirrhosis, and liver failure, necessitating liver transplantation in the first 2 decades of life.[154,155] Children with PFIC are small for their age and often have diarrhea. They may also have pancreatitis and can present with sensorineural deafness.[156] FIC1 is also expressed on the membranes of the organ

Table 4-2 Genetic Diseases of Hepatic Transport

DISEASE	CHROMOSOME	GENE/FUNCTION	DEFECT	PHENOTYPE	THERAPY
PFIC1 Progressive familial intrahepatic cholestasis type 1	18q21	FIC1/Aminophospholipid translocator	Hepatocellular cholestasis	First recurrent and later permanent and progressive cholestasis, no bile duct proliferation, normal GGT, deafness, diarrhea, pancreatitis, coarse granular bile on transmission EM	Partial external biliary diversion, liver transplantation
BRIC1 Benign recurrent intrahepatic cholestasis type 1	18q21	FIC1/Aminophospholipid translocator	Hepatocellular cholestasis	Episodic cholestasis with pruritus, weight loss and steatorhoea, normal GGT	Partial external biliary diversion
PFIC2 Progressive familial intrahepatic cholestasis type 2	2q24	ABCB11/Bile salt export pump (BSEP)	Hepatocellular cholestasis	Neonatal hepatitis, progressive cholestasis, lobular and portal fibrosis, normal GGT, amorphous bile on transmission EM, BSEP protein absent on IM	Partial external biliary diversion, liver transplantation
BRIC2 Benign recurrent intrahepatic cholestasis type 2	2q24	ABCB11/Bile salt export pump (BSEP)	Hepatocellular cholestasis	Episodic cholestasis with pruritus, weight loss and steatorhoea, normal GGT	Partial external biliary diversion
PFIC3 Progressive familial intrahepatic cholestasis type 3	7q21	ABCB4 (PGY3, MDR3)/ Phosphatidylcholine flippase	Intrahepatic cholestasis	Cholestasis, bile duct proliferation, periportal fibrosis, elevated GGT	Ursodeoxycholic acid, liver transplantation
ICP Intrahepatic cholestasis of pregnancy Intrahepatic gallstones	7q21	ABCB4 (PGY3, MDR3)/ Phosphatidylcholine flippase		Cholestasis in third trimester of pregnancy, elevated GGT	Ursodeoxycholic acid
Familial hypercholanemia	9q12-q13 9q22.3	TJP2/ZO-2/Tight junction protein BAAT/Bile salt CoA:amino acid N-acyltransferase	Leaky tight junctions, deficient bile salt conjugation	Elevated serum bile salts, pruritus, malabsorption	
Bile salt biosynthesis defects		3β-Δ5-C27-Hydroxysteroid oxidoreductase Δ4-3-Oxosteroid-5β reductase 3β-Hydroxy-C27-steroid dehydrogenase/ Isomerase oxysterol 7α-hydroxylase (CYP7B1)	Abnormal bile salts inhibit bile salt transport	Intrahepatic cholestasis, neonatal giant cell hepatitis	Cholic acid
Dubin-Johnson syndrome	10q24	ABCC2 (MRP2, cMOAT)/ Canalicular multispecific organic anion transporter	Deficient canalicular transport of bilirubin conjugates	Conjugated hyperbilirubinemia, increased urinary coproporphyrin isomer I, hepatic lysosomal pigment	Not needed

of Corti, and FIC1 deficiency leads to a progressive loss of cochlear hair cells and deafness.[157] In PFIC1, the larger bile ducts are anatomically normal and liver histologic analysis shows bland canalicular cholestasis with only slight duct proliferation, inflammation, fibrosis, or cirrhosis.[154,154] On electron microscopy there is a paucity of canalicular microvilli and a thickened pericanalicular network of microfilaments within the canaliculi coarse granular bile, referred to "Byler bile." Characteristically the serum γ-GT activity is not elevated even though the parameters of cholestasis, such as levels of alkaline phosphatase and serum primary bile salts (in particular, chenodeoxycholic acid), are strongly increased. Serum cholesterol levels are usually normal.

Patients belonging to the Byler kindred are descendants of Jacob Byler and Nancy Kaufmann, members of the Old Order Amish population who emigrated from Switzerland to the United States nearly 250 years ago. Many patients outside the United States are unrelated to the Old Order Amish. The PFIC syndrome has been described in families in The Netherlands, Sweden, and Greenland and in an Arab population.[154] In Amish and non-Amish families the genetic defect could be mapped to the FIC1 locus on chromosome 18q21-q22 encoding a P-type ATPase, ATP8B1. The function of this protein was discussed earlier in this chapter. A number of FIC1 mutations have been described, including the mutation causing Byler disease.[155] In humans FIC1 is highly expressed in pancreas, small intestine, urinary bladder, stomach, and prostate. This may explain the increased frequency of diarrhea and pancreatitis in these patients. Even after transplantation the patient exhibits a slow rate of catch-up growth, most likely attributable to the persistent malabsorption.[158] Dysfunction of FXR signaling has been reported in this disease.[159] This may be a secondary defect.

Children with PFIC type 1 may benefit from surgical partial external biliary diversion (PEBD).[160,161] In this procedure the gallbladder is connected to a stoma in the skin by a loop of small bowel. The mechanism of this therapy is not well understood. It may partially be explained by a decrease in the overall bile salt pool. In some patients an improvement of liver morphology and a normalization of biliary bile salt composition were seen, suggesting improved bile salt secretion.[162] Ursodeoxycholic acid, very helpful in the treatment of patients with PFIC type 3, is less effective in those with PFIC type 1. When PEBD fails, liver transplantation is the only effective solution. Because PFIC type 1 disease is not confined to the liver, extrahepatic manifestations may persist after transplantation, such as hearing loss, or may become worse, such as watery diarrhea. The diarrhea in this situation usually reacts to bile salt sequestrants.[163] Also, a few cases of pancreatitis have been reported in patients who have this disease.[164] Interestingly, liver steatosis (sometimes with progression to steatohepatitis) may develop in the liver graft.[158,165]

Benign Recurrent Intrahepatic Cholestasis Type 1

Recurrent familial intrahepatic cholestasis was a term introduced by Tygstrup and colleagues.[164] This disease is also known as benign recurrent intrahepatic cholestasis (BRIC) or Summerskill syndrome[166] (see **Table 4-2**). Despite recurrent attacks of cholestasis there is usually no progression to chronic liver disease. During the attacks the patients are severely jaundiced and have pruritus, steatorrhea, and weight loss. In analogy to PFIC1 the serum γ-glutamyltransferase activity is not elevated. Some patients also have renal stones, pancreatitis, and diabetes.[164] As in PFIC1 the gene involved in recurrent familial intrahepatic cholestasis has been mapped to the FIC1 locus.[144] This suggests that both diseases are genetically related. However, not all patients with benign recurrent intrahepatic cholestasis expressed chromosome 18 mutations.[167]

Ursodeoxycholic acid is of no benefit in BRIC.[168] Case reports indicate that rifampicin may reduce the number of cholestatic episodes.[169,170] In analogy to PFIC type 1, cholestasis may be improved and cholestatic episodes shortened by biliary drainage procedures.[171]

Progressive Familial Intrahepatic Cholestasis Type 2

Genetic studies revealed that the FIC1 locus is not involved in all patients with a PFIC type 1 phenotype and low serum γ-GT activity.[154] Moreover, in a large number of non-Amish patients the disease was mapped to a locus on chromosome 2q24 that later proved to be the ABCB11 (BSEP) gene (as described earlier in this chapter; see **Table 4-2**).[51,52,172] Antibodies directed against BSEP sequences enabled localization studies and it became clear that this protein not only is liver-specific but also is located in the canalicular domain of the hepatocyte's plasma membrane. Liver specimens of patients with PFIC type 2 stain negative for canalicular BSEP on immunohistochemistry using BSEP antibodies.[52] As in PFIC type 1, the serum γ-GT activity in these patients is not elevated and bile duct proliferation is absent. However, the disease differs from PFIC type 1 in several aspects: PFIC2 frequently presents as nonspecific giant cell hepatitis, which is indistinguishable from idiopathic neonatal giant cell hepatitis; patients are usually permanently jaundiced; and the disease rapidly progresses to persistent and progressive cholestasis requiring liver transplantation. Liver histologic studies show more inflammatory activity than in PFIC type 1, with giant cell transformation and lobular and portal fibrosis.[154] The bile of PFIC type 2 patients is amorphous or filamentous on transmission electron microscopy. This contrasts with the coarsely granular bile of PFIC type 1 patients. Extrahepatic manifestations are uncommon. In the majority of non-Amish patients, progressive familial intrahepatic cholestasis is type 2 rather than type 1. A particularly dreaded complication is cerebral or subdural hematoma at or shortly after birth as a result of vitamin K deficiency. Vitamin K therefore has to be supplemented without delay.

Bile salts are not completely absent in the bile of these patients. MRP2, the canalicular transporter of bilirubin, also transports glucuronidated or sulfated bile salts. This may also explain why these patients are jaundiced despite an intact bilirubin transporter: bilirubin transport may be inhibited by competition with bile salt conjugates.

PFIC type 2 patients usually need to undergo liver transplantation in the first 2 decades. Living related donor transplantation should be considered cautiously because parents may be carriers of the disease, which may manifest after transplantation. Partial bile diversion may provide symptomatic relief of pruritus in these patients, cause amelioration of liver functions, and induce catch-up growth.[161] The majority of PFIC type 2 patients do not respond to ursodeoxycholic acid therapy; in fact, administration of ursodeoxycholic acid to some of these patients led to very high serum bile salt levels (>1 mmol/L) without any increase of biliary bile salt secretion.[52]

Benign Recurrent Intrahepatic Cholestasis Type 2

Not all patients with benign recurrent intrahepatic cholestasis have mutations of ATP8B1. In a subset of patients with episodic cholestasis, mutations of BSEP were found. The disease was called BRIC type 2. It appears that these patients are particularly prone to the development of cholelithiasis and less to pancreatitis. This distinguishes them from patients with BRIC type 1. Serum γ-glutamyltransferase levels are low in both diseases. Patients with BRIC type 1 can be completely asymptomatic between attacks of cholestasis; however, if this is true for patients with BRIC type 2 is still under investigation.[173]

Familial Hypercholanemia

Familial hypercholanemia is characterized by elevated serum bile salt levels, severe pruritus, and fat malabsorption.[174] Thus far this disease has been identified among Amish individuals. It was originally believed to result from a sinusoidal uptake defect. Recently it has been reported to be caused by mutations of either one of two genes—a gene that encodes tight junction protein 2 (ZO-2) or a gene that encodes bile salt coenzyme A:amino acid N-acyltransferase. In these latter patients glycine and taurine bile salt conjugates cannot be formed.[175] The phenotype of these patients demonstrates that BSEP is not capable of transporting unconjugated bile salts to any significant extent.

Bile Salt Synthesis Defects

Defects of bile salt synthesis resemble PFIC type 2. Clayton and colleagues described a defect of 3β-Δ5-C27-hydroxysteroid oxidoreductase as a cause of giant cell hepatitis.[176] Deficiency of Δ4-3-oxosteroid-5β reductase and 3β-hydroxy-C27-steroid dehydrogenase/isomerase and mutations of the oxysterol 7α-hydroxylase gene may also be causes of neonatal hepatitis and cholestasis.[177-179] In these diseases toxic intermediates are formed that cause cholestasis by interaction with the hepatic bile salt transporter.[180] Bile salt synthesis defects are called PFIC type 4 by some authors.

Progressive Familial Intrahepatic Cholestasis Type 3

The third PFIC subtype, PFIC type 3, is quite different from the other PFIC subtypes. The serum γ-GT activity is markedly elevated in these patients and liver histologic analysis shows extensive bile duct proliferation and portal and periportal fibrosis.[145,181,182] Phenotypically PFIC type 3 resembles Mdr2(−/−) mice. In humans with PFIC type 3, mutations of the ABCB4 (MDR3) gene are the underlying cause.[145,181,183]

Phosphatidylcholine, the predominant phospholipid in bile, is washed from the canalicular membrane by bile salts. In contrast to PFIC type 2, in PFIC type 3 bile salt transport proceeds unimpaired, but this occurs without phospholipids because of the MDR3 deficiency. This has major pathophysiologic consequences. In normal bile the inherent toxicity of bile salts is quenched by phosphatidylcholine. In bile of patients with PFIC type 3 bile salt toxicity is unantagonized by phospholipids and this causes damage of bile duct epithelium with periportal inflammation and fibrosis and bile duct proliferation as a result. In humans this is even more extreme than in Mdr2(−/−) mice because human bile salts (e.g., chenodeoxycholic acid) are more toxic than those of the mouse, especially the very hydrophilic muricholate.

In patients with PFIC type 3 jaundice may be less apparent but pruritus is usually severe. Patients with a partial ABCB4 (MDR3) defect respond to ursodeoxycholic acid therapy.[184] The majority of patients, however, have to undergo liver transplantation. Mutations of the ABCB4 gene on chromosome 7q21 are the underlying cause of the disease. Although PFIC3 is discussed as a cholestatic disease, in a strictly physiologic sense there is no cholestasis because bile flow is not impaired.[78]

ABCB4 gene mutations have been associated with intrahepatic gallstones.[185,186] Liver disease in adults associated with ABCB4 mutations and ABCB4/MDR3 deficiency has been named low phospholipid associated cholelithiasis (LPAC). This disease is now recognized as a significant cause of rapidly progressive fibrosing cholestatic liver disease and portal hypertension that occurs in families.[187] Although the histopathology of Mdr2 knockout mice resembles to a certain extent that seen in human primary biliary cirrhosis and primary sclerosing cholangitis, no evidence has been obtained thus far that MDR3 is involved in these diseases.[61,188] An imbalance between bile salt and phospholipid secretion after liver transplantation was correlated with a transient imbalance between BSEP and MDR3 expression, and this may provide an explanation for the vulnerability of the bile ducts in the immediate period after transplantation.[189]

Intrahepatic Cholestasis of Pregnancy

Jacquemin and colleagues reported a high incidence of intrahepatic cholestasis of pregnancy (ICP) in families with PFIC type 3.[183] This suggests that in persons carrying one mutated ABCB4 gene, cholestasis may occur during pregnancy. Indeed, a study by Pauli-Magnus and others suggests that a substantial fraction of the ICP cases are attributable to mutations in ABCB4.[190] In contrast, ICP not related to MDR3 or ATP8B1 has been reported in a Finnish group of patients.[191] Mutations leading to single amino acid substitutions of the MDR3 protein may cause intracellular traffic mutants; that is, the protein is synthesized but does not reach its destination in the canalicular membrane.[192] One can hypothesize that in patients carrying these mutations, the hormones in the third trimester of pregnancy impair intracellular targeting, which causes the disease to clinically manifest.

ICP has also been described in families with other PFIC type 1.[193] BSEP (ABCB11) polymorphisms seem to be of less importance for ICP.[194] In contrast to ICP related to ABCB4, in ICP related to ATP8B1, serum γ-glutamyltransferase activity is not elevated. Ursodeoxycholic acid has been shown to benefit patients with ICP, resulting in improvement of serum liver tests and pruritus, prolongation of time to delivery, and decrease of intrauterine complications.[195,196]

Other Forms of Intrahepatic Cholestasis

More forms of intrahepatic cholestasis exist. Aagenaes syndrome is a combination of severe progressive lymphedema and episodic intrahepatic cholestasis.[197] The locus for this disease has been mapped to chromosome 15q.[198]

Dubin-Johnson Syndrome

Dubin-Johnson syndrome is caused by a mutation of ABCC2 encoding MRP2 (see **Table 4-2**).[149,199] Dubin-Johnson syndrome is characterized by conjugated hyperbilirubinemia without other serum enzyme abnormalities. Patients with Dubin-Johnson syndrome have a normal life span. A black or brownish lysosomal pigment in the hepatocytes is a characteristic histologic feature. Urinary coproporphyrin isomer I excretion is elevated in these patients.

TR− rats and EHBR rats are animal models for this disease. These animals have a decreased hepatobiliary secretion of organic anions because of a mutation of the Abcc2 gene.[86,200] Patients with Dubin-Johnson syndrome are homozygous carriers of ABCC2 gene mutations. Rapid degradation of mutated ABCC2 mRNA, or impaired MRP2 protein maturation and trafficking, may be the underlying cause of the disease.[201] The disease needs no treatment.

Key References

Ananthanarayanan M, et al. Human bile salt export pump promoter is transactivated by the farnesoid X receptor/bile acid receptor. J Biol Chem 2001;276(31):28857–28865. (Ref.62)

Assem M, et al. Interactions between hepatic Mrp4 and Sult2a as revealed by the constitutive androstane receptor and Mrp4 knockout mice. J Biol Chem 2004;279(21):22250–22257. (Ref.102)

Brewer HB Jr, et al. Regulation of plasma high-density lipoprotein levels by the ABCA1 transporter and the emerging role of high-density lipoprotein in the treatment of cardiovascular disease. Arterioscler Thromb Vasc Biol 2004; 24(10):1755–1760. (Ref.127)

Bustorff-Silva J, et al. Partial internal biliary diversion through a cholecystojejunocolonic anastomosis—a novel surgical approach for patients with progressive familial intrahepatic cholestasis: a preliminary report. J Pediatr Surg 2007;42(8):1337–1340. (Ref.160)

Cai SY, et al. ATP8B1 deficiency disrupts the bile canalicular membrane bilayer structure in hepatocytes, but FXR expression and activity are maintained. Gastroenterology 2009;136(3):1060–1069. (Ref.110)

Carlton VE, et al. Complex inheritance of familial hypercholanemia with associated mutations in TJP2 and BAAT. Nat Genet 2003;34(1):91–96. (Ref.175)

Chen F, et al. Progressive familial intrahepatic cholestasis, type 1, is associated with decreased farnesoid X receptor activity. Gastroenterology 2004;126(3):756–764. (Ref.159)

Claudel T, et al. The farnesoid X receptor: a novel drug target? Expert Opin Investig Drugs 2004;13(9):1135–1148. (Ref.63)

Cuperus FJ, et al. Acceleration of the gastrointestinal transit by polyethylene glycol effectively treats unconjugated hyperbilirubinemia in Gunn rats. Gut 2010;59(3):373–380. (Ref.25)

Dawson PA, et al. The heteromeric organic solute transporter alpha-beta, Ostalpha-Ostbeta, is an ileal basolateral bile acid transporter. J Biol Chem 2005;280(8):6960–6968. (Ref.22)

de Jong FA, et al. Irinotecan-induced diarrhea: functional significance of the polymorphic ABCC2 transporter protein. Clin Pharmacol Ther 2007;81(1):42–49. (Ref.88)

Dean M, Rzhetsky A, Allikmets R. The human ATP-binding cassette (ABC) transporter superfamily. Genome Res 2001;11(7):1156–1166. (Ref.49)

Denson LA, et al. The orphan nuclear receptor, shp, mediates bile acid-induced inhibition of the rat bile acid transporter, ntcp. Gastroenterology 2001;121(1):140–147. (Ref.31)

Donner MG, Keppler D. Up-regulation of basolateral multidrug resistance protein 3 (Mrp3) in cholestatic rat liver. Hepatology 2001;34(2):351–359. (Ref.94)

Egawa H, et al. Intractable diarrhea after liver transplantation for Byler's disease: successful treatment with bile adsorptive resin. Liver Transpl 2002;8(8):714–716. (Ref.163)

Eichelbaum M, Fromm MF, Schwab M. Clinical aspects of the MDR1 (ABCB1) gene polymorphism. Ther Drug Monit 2004;26(2):180–185. (Ref.72)

Eloranta JJ, Jung D, Kullak-Ublick, GA. The human Na+–taurocholate cotransporting polypeptide gene is activated by glucocorticoid receptor and peroxisome proliferator-activated receptor-gamma coactivator-1alpha, and suppressed by bile acids via a small heterodimer partner-dependent mechanism. Mol Endocrinol 2006;20(1):65–79. (Ref.33)

Folmer DE, Elferink RP, Paulusma CC. P4 ATPases—lipid flippases and their role in disease. Biochim Biophys Acta 2009;1791(7):628–635. (Ref.103)

Folmer DE, et al. Differential effects of progressive familial intrahepatic cholestasis type 1 and benign recurrent intrahepatic cholestasis type 1 mutations on canalicular localization of ATP8B1. Hepatology 2009;50(5):1597–1605. (Ref.113)

Freeman LA, et al. The orphan nuclear receptor LRH-1 activates the ABCG5/ABCG8 intergenic promoter. J Lipid Res 2004;45(7):1197–1206. (Ref.120)

Geier A, et al. Cytokine-dependent regulation of hepatic organic anion transporter gene transactivators in mouse liver. Am J Physiol Gastrointest Liver Physiol 2005;289(5):G831–G841. (Ref.36)

Geuken E, et al. Rapid increase of bile salt secretion is associated with bile duct injury after human liver transplantation. J Hepatol 2004;41(6):1017–1025. (Ref.189)

Ghose R, et al. Endotoxin leads to rapid subcellular re-localization of hepatic RXRalpha: a novel mechanism for reduced hepatic gene expression in inflammation. Nucl Recept 2004;2(1):4. (Ref.132)

Glaser SS, et al. Cholangiocyte proliferation and liver fibrosis. Expert Rev Mol Med 2009;11:e7. (Ref.27)

Goodwin B, et al. A regulatory cascade of the nuclear receptors FXR, SHP-1, and LRH-1 represses bile acid biosynthesis. Mol Cell 2000;6(3):517–526. (Ref.15)

Groen AK, et al. Hepatobiliary cholesterol transport is not impaired in Abca1-null mice lacking HDL. J Clin Invest 2001;108(6):843–850. (Ref.128)

Guo GL, et al. Complementary roles of farnesoid X receptor, pregnane X receptor, and constitutive androstane receptor in protection against bile acid toxicity. J Biol Chem 2003;278(46):45062–45071. (Ref.100)

Higuchi H, Gores GJ. Bile acid regulation of hepatic physiology: IV bile acids and death receptors. Am J Physiol Gastrointest Liver Physiol 2003;284(5):G734–G738. (Ref.129)

Huang L, et al. Farnesoid X receptor activates transcription of the phospholipid pump MDR3. J Biol Chem 2003;278(51):51085–51090. (Ref.85)

Inagaki T, et al. Fibroblast growth factor 15 functions as an enterohepatic signal to regulate bile acid homeostasis. Cell Metab 2005;2(4):217–225. (Ref.139)

Jacquemin E. Role of multidrug resistance 3 deficiency in pediatric and adult liver disease: one gene for three diseases. Semin Liver Dis 2001;21(4):551–562. (Ref.182)

Johnson BM, Zhang P, Schuetz JD, Brouwer KL. Characterization of transport protein expression in multidrug resistance-associated protein (Mrp) 2-deficient rats. Drug Metab Dispos 2006;34(4):556–562. (Ref.97)

Jung D, et al. Role of liver-enriched transcription factors and nuclear receptors in regulating the human, mouse, and rat NTCP gene. Am J Physiol Gastrointest Liver Physiol 2004;286(5):G752–G761. (Ref.32)

Jung D, Kullak-Ublick GA. Hepatocyte nuclear factor 1 alpha: a key mediator of the effect of bile acids on gene expression. Hepatology 2003;37(3):622–631. (Ref.40)

Kast HR, et al. Regulation of multidrug resistance-associated protein 2 (MRP2;ABCC2) by the nuclear receptors PXR, FXR, and CAR. J Biol Chem 2002;277(4):2908–2915.

Keitel V, et al. Expression and localization of hepatobiliary transport proteins in progressive familial intrahepatic cholestasis. Hepatology 2005;41(5):1160–1172. (Ref.41)

Keitel V, et al. A common Dubin-Johnson syndrome mutation impairs protein maturation and transport activity of MRP2 (ABCC2). Am J Physiol Gastrointest Liver Physiol 2003;284(1):G165–G174. (Ref.201)

Keppler D, Konig J. Hepatic secretion of conjugated drugs and endogenous substances. Semin Liver Dis 2000;20(3):265–272. (Ref.11)

Klomp LW, et al. Characterization of mutations in ATP8B1 associated with hereditary cholestasis. Hepatology 2004;40(1):27–38. (Ref.155)

Koepsell H. Polyspecific organic cation transporters: their functions and interactions with drugs. Trends Pharmacol Sci 2004;25(7):375–381. (Ref.47)

Kok T, et al. Peroxisome proliferator-activated receptor alpha (PPARalpha)-mediated regulation of multidrug resistance 2 (Mdr2) expression and function in mice. Biochem J 2003;369(Pt 3):539–547. (Ref.83)

Konig J, et al. Pharmacogenomics of human OATP transporters. Naunyn Schmiedebergs Arch Pharmacol 2006;372(6):432–443. (Ref.38)

Kosters A, et al. Relation between hepatic expression of ATP-binding cassette transporters G5 and G8 and biliary cholesterol secretion in mice. J Hepatol 2003;38(6):710–716. (Ref.123)

Kubo K, Sekine S, Saito M. Compensatory expression of MRP3 in the livers of MRP2-deficient EHBRs is promoted by DHA intake. Biosci Biotechnol Biochem 2009;73(11):2432–2438. (Ref.98)

Kullak-Ublick GA, et al. Hepatic transport of bile salts. Semin Liver Dis 2000; 20(3):273–292. (Ref.12)

Kurbegov AC, et al. Biliary diversion for progressive familial intrahepatic cholestasis: improved liver morphology and bile acid profile. Gastroenterology 2003;125(4):1227–1234. (Ref.162)

Lamireau T, et al. Epidemiology of liver disease in cystic fibrosis: a longitudinal study. J Hepatol 2004;41(6):920–925. (Ref.146)

Lankisch TO, et al. Gilbert's syndrome and irinotecan toxicity: combination with UDP-glucuronosyltransferase 1A7 variants increases risk. Cancer Epidemiol Biomarkers Prev 2008;17(3):695–701. (Ref.87)

Lee J, et al. Adaptive regulation of bile salt transporters in kidney and liver in obstructive cholestasis in the rat. Gastroenterology 2001;121(6):1473–1484. (Ref.92)

Link E, et al. SLCO1B1 variants and statin-induced myopathy—a genomewide study. New Engl J Med 2008;359(8):789–799. (Ref.45)

Lu K, et al. Two genes that map to the STSL locus cause sitosterolemia: genomic structure and spectrum of mutations involving sterolin-1 and sterolin-2, encoded by ABCG5 and ABCG8, respectively. Am J Hum Genet 2001;69(2): 278–290. (Ref.115)

Lykavieris P, et al. Progressive familial intrahepatic cholestasis type 1 and extrahepatic features: no catch-up of stature growth, exacerbation of diarrhea, and appearance of liver steatosis after liver transplantation. J Hepatol 2003; 39(3):447–452. (Ref.158)

Marzioni M, et al. Functional heterogeneity of cholangiocytes. Semin Liver Dis 2002;22(3):227–240. (Ref.17)

Mazzella G, et al. Ursodeoxycholic acid administration in patients with cholestasis of pregnancy: effects on primary bile acids in babies and mothers. Hepatology 2001;33(3):504–508. (Ref.195)

Mitic LL, Van Itallie CM, Anderson JM. Molecular physiology and pathophysiology of tight junctions I. Tight junction structure and function: lessons from mutant animals and proteins. Am J Physiol Gastrointest Liver Physiol 2000;279(2):G250–G254. (Ref.7)

Miyagawa-Hayashino A, et al. Allograft steatohepatitis in progressive familial intrahepatic cholestasis type 1 after living donor liver transplantation. Liver Transpl 2009;15(6):610–618. (Ref.165)

Nibbering CP, et al. Regulation of biliary cholesterol secretion is independent of hepatocyte canalicular membrane lipid composition: a study in the diosgenin-fed rat model. J Hepatol 2001;35(2):164–169. (Ref.106)

Nozawa T, et al. Role of organic anion transporter OATP1B1 (OATP-C) in hepatic uptake of irinotecan and its active metabolite, 7-ethyl-10-hydroxycamptothecin: in vitro evidence and effect of single nucleotide polymorphisms. Drug Metab Dispos 2005;33(3):434–439. (Ref.46)

Oswald M, et al. Expression of hepatic transporters OATP-C and MRP2 in primary sclerosing cholangitis. Liver 2001;21(4):247–253. (Ref.42)

Oude Elferink RP, Paulusma CC, Groen AK. Hepatocanalicular transport defects: pathophysiologic mechanisms of rare diseases. Gastroenterology 2006;130(3): 908–925. (Ref.107)

Painter JN, et al. Sequence variation in the ATP8B1 gene and intrahepatic cholestasis of pregnancy. Eur J Hum Genet 2005;13(4):435–439. (Ref.191)

Pauli-Magnus C, et al. BSEP and MDR3 haplotype structure in healthy Caucasians, primary biliary cirrhosis and primary sclerosing cholangitis. Hepatology 2004;39(3):779–791. (Ref.188)

Pauli-Magnus C, et al. Sequence analysis of bile salt export pump (ABCB11) and multidrug resistance p-glycoprotein 3 (ABCB4, MDR3) in patients with intrahepatic cholestasis of pregnancy. Pharmacogenetics 2004;14(2):91–102. (Refs.190, 194)

Paulusma CC, et al. Activity of the bile salt export pump (ABCB11) is critically dependent on canalicular membrane cholesterol content. J Biol Chem 2009; 284(15):9947–9954. (Ref.111)

Paulusma CC, et al. ATP8B1 requires an accessory protein for endoplasmic reticulum exit and plasma membrane lipid flippase activity. Hepatology 2008; 47(1):268–278. (Ref.109)

Paulusma CC, et al. Atp8b1 deficiency in mice reduces resistance of the canalicular membrane to hydrophobic bile salts and impairs bile salt transport. Hepatology 2006;44(1):195–204. (Ref.105)

Plosch T, et al. FAbcg5/Abcg8-independent pathways contribute to hepatobiliary cholesterol secretion in mice. Am J Physiol Gastrointest Liver Physiol 2006; 291(3):G414–G423. (Ref.119)

Repa JJ, et al. Regulation of ATP-binding cassette sterol transporters ABCG5 and ABCG8 by the liver X receptors alpha and beta. J Biol Chem 2002;277(21): 18793–18800. (Ref.118)

Rius M, et al. Cotransport of reduced glutathione with bile salts by MRP4 (ABCC4) localized to the basolateral hepatocyte membrane. Hepatology 2003; 38(2):374–384. (Ref.101)

Ros JE, et al. Induction of Mdr1b expression by tumor necrosis factor-alpha in rat liver cells is independent of p53 but requires NF-kappaB signaling. Hepatology 2001;33(6):1425–1431. (Ref.75)

Rosmorduc O, et al. ABCB4 gene mutation-associated cholelithiasis in adults. Gastroenterology 2003;125(2):452–459. (Ref.185)

Rosmorduc O, Hermelin B, Poupon R. MDR3 gene defect in adults with symptomatic intrahepatic and gallbladder cholesterol cholelithiasis. Gastroenterology 2001;120(6):1459–1467. (Ref.186)

Schaap FG, et al. High expression of the bile salt-homeostatic hormone fibroblast growth factor 19 in the liver of patients with extrahepatic cholestasis. Hepatology 2009;49(4):1228–1235. (Ref.140)

Schoemaker MH, et al. Resistance of rat hepatocytes against bile acid-induced apoptosis in cholestatic liver injury is due to nuclear factor-kappa B activation. J Hepatol 2003;39(2):153–161. (Ref.130)

Schonhoff CM, et al. Rab4 facilitates cyclic adenosine monophosphate-stimulated bile acid uptake and Na+-taurocholate cotransporting polypeptide translocation. Hepatology 2008;48(5):1665–1670. (Ref.35)

Schonhoff CM, et al. PKCε-dependent and -independent effects of taurolithocholate on PI3K/PKB pathway and taurocholate uptake in HuH-NTCP cell line. Am J Physiol Gastrointest Liver Physiol 2009;297(6): G1259–G1267. (Ref.37)

Schuetz EG, et al. Disrupted bile acid homeostasis reveals an unexpected interaction among nuclear hormone receptors, transporters, and cytochrome P450. J Biol Chem 2001;276(42):39411–39418. (Ref.142)

Shih DQ, et al. Hepatocyte nuclear factor-1 alpha is an essential regulator of bile acid and plasma cholesterol metabolism. Nat Genet 2001;27(4):375–382. (Ref.135)

Small DM. Role of ABC transporters in secretion of cholesterol from liver into bile. Proc Natl Acad Sci USA 2003;100(1):4–6. (Ref.125)

Smith NF, et al. Variants in the SLCO1B3 gene: interethnic distribution and association with paclitaxel pharmacokinetics. Clin Pharmacol Ther 2007; 81(1):76–82. (Ref.39)

Soroka CJ, Lee JM, Azzaroli F, Boyer JL. Cellular localization and up-regulation of multidrug resistance-associated protein 3 in hepatocytes and cholangiocytes during obstructive cholestasis in rat liver. Hepatology 2001;33(4):783–791. (Ref.95)

Stapelbroek JM, et al. ATP8B1 is essential for maintaining normal hearing. Proc Natl Acad Sci USA 2009;106(24):9709–9714. (Ref.157)

Stapelbroek JM, et al. Nasobiliary drainage induces long-lasting remission in benign recurrent intrahepatic cholestasis. Hepatology 2006;43(1):51–53. (Ref.171)

Sumi K, et al. Cooperative interaction between hepatocyte nuclear factor 4 alpha and GATA transcription factors regulates ATP-binding cassette sterol transporters ABCG5 and ABCG8. Mol Cell Biol 2007;27(12):4248–4260. (Ref.121)

Synold TW, Dussault I, Forman BM. The orphan nuclear receptor SXR coordinately regulates drug metabolism and efflux. Nat Med 2001;7(5): 584–590. (Ref.76)

Tauscher A, Kuver R. ABCG5 and ABCG8 are expressed in gallbladder epithelial cells. Biochem Biophys Res Commun 2003;307(4):1021–1028. (Ref.117)

Ujhazy P, et al. Familial intrahepatic cholestasis 1: studies of localization and function. Hepatology 2001;34(4 Pt 1):768–775. (Ref.108)

Uyama N, Geerts A, Reynaert H. Neural connections between the hypothalamus and the liver. Anat Rec A Discov Mol Cell Evol Biol 2004;280(1):808–820. (Ref.26)

van der Velden LM, et al. Folding defects in P-type ATP 8B1 associated with hereditary cholestasis are ameliorated by 4-phenylbutyrate. Hepatology 2010;51(1):286–296. (Ref.112)

van Mil SW, et al. Benign recurrent intrahepatic cholestasis type 2 is caused by mutations in ABCB11. Gastroenterology 2004;127(2):379–384. (Ref.173)

Vrins C, et al. The sterol transporting heterodimer ABCG5/ABCG8 requires bile salts to mediate cholesterol efflux. FEBS Lett 2007;581(24):4616–4620. (Ref.124)

Walters HC, et al. Expression, transport properties, and chromosomal location of organic anion transporter subtype 3. Am J Physiol Gastrointest Liver Physiol 2000;279(6):G1188–G1200. (Ref.21)

Wang R, et al. Compensatory role of P-glycoproteins in knockout mice lacking the bile salt export pump. Hepatology 2009;50(3):948–956. (Ref.54)

Wang R, et al. Targeted inactivation of sister of P-glycoprotein gene (spgp) in mice results in nonprogressive but persistent intrahepatic cholestasis. Proc Natl Acad Sci USA 2001;98(4):2011–2016. (Ref.53)

Ziol M, et al. ABCB4 heterozygous gene mutations associated with fibrosing cholestatic liver disease in adults. Gastroenterology 2008;135(1):131–141. (Ref.187)

Zollner G, et al. Adaptive changes in hepatobiliary transporter expression in primary biliary cirrhosis. J Hepatol 2003;38(6):717–727. (Refs.43, 61)

Zollner G, et al. Hepatobiliary transporter expression in percutaneous liver biopsies of patients with cholestatic liver diseases. Hepatology 2001;33(3): 633–646. (Refs.44, 60)

A complete list of references can be found at www.expertconsult.com.

Chapter 5

Hepatic Fibrosis and Cirrhosis

Don C. Rockey and Scott L. Friedman

ABBREVIATIONS

ADRP adipose differentiation related protein
ALT alanine aminotransferase
AST aspartate aminotransferase
AUROC area under the receiver operator characteristic
bFGF basic fibroblast growth factor
CCN2 connective tissue growth factor
CT computed tomography
CTGF connective tissue growth factor
CXCL4 platelet factor 4
ECM extracellular matrix
EGF epidermal growth factor
ET-1 endothelin-1
FGF fibroblast growth factor
GGT γ-glutamyltransferase
HA hyaluronic acid
HBV hepatitis B virus

HCV hepatitis C virus
HGF hepatocyte growth factor
HIV human immunodeficiency virus
HVPG hepatic venous pressure gradient
IL-10 interleukin-10
JI jejunoileal
LPS lipopolysaccharide
MRI magnetic resonance imaging
MMP matrix metalloproteinase
MEGX monoethylglycinexylidide
NASH non-alcoholic steatohepatitis
NGFR nerve growth factor receptor
NK natural killer
NO nitric oxide
PI 3-kinase phosphoinositol 3-kinase
PIIINP amino-terminal propeptide of type III collagen
PDGF platelet-derived growth factor

PPAR peroxisomal proliferator activated receptor
QTL quantitative trait loci
RAS renin-angiotensin system
RSK ribosomal S-6 kinase
STAT-1 signal transducers and activators of transcription
TIMP tissue inhibitor of metalloproteinases
TPN total parenteral nutrition
TGF transforming growth factor
TGF-β1 transforming growth factor-β1
TNF-α tumor necrosis factor-α
TRAIL TNF-related apoptosis-inducing ligand
VEGF vascular endothelial growth factor

Introduction

Hepatic fibrosis refers to the accumulation of extracellular matrix, or scar tissue, in response to acute or chronic liver injury. This response, or "fibrogenesis," represents a wound healing response to injury (**Fig. 5-1**), and ultimately leads to the clinical-pathologic syndrome known as cirrhosis. From a histologic standpoint, cirrhosis can be considered the end-stage consequence of fibrogenesis occurring in the hepatic parenchyma, resulting in nodule formation, which in turn may lead to altered hepatic function and blood flow, and the clinical sequelae typical of cirrhosis. Both fibrosis and cirrhosis are the consequences of a sustained wound healing response to chronic liver injury from a range of causes including viral, autoimmune, drug-induced, cholestatic, and metabolic diseases. The clinical manifestations of cirrhosis vary widely, from asymptomatic cirrhosis to liver failure, and are determined by both the nature and the severity of the underlying liver disease as well as the extent of hepatic fibrosis. Nearly 40% of patients with histologic cirrhosis are asymptomatic and may remain so for long periods of time. However, once complications (e.g., ascites, variceal hemorrhage, encephalopathy) develop, progressive deterioration leading to death or liver transplantation is typical. In such patients there is a 50% 5-year mortality, with approximately 70% of these deaths directly attributable to liver disease.[1] In asymptomatic individuals, cirrhosis may be first suggested during routine examination, although histologic analysis may be required to establish the diagnosis.

Cirrhosis affects hundreds of millions of patients worldwide. The overall burden of liver disease in the United States—the vast majority of which is due to chronic disease with fibrosis—continues to expand, exacting an increasing economic and social cost.[2] Indeed, in the United States cirrhosis is the most common non-neoplastic cause of death among hepatobiliary and digestive diseases, accounting for approximately 30,000 deaths per year. In addition, 10,000 deaths occur because of liver cancer, which typically develops in cirrhotic livers, consistent with a steadily rising mortality from hepatic cancer.[3] Notably, hepatocellular carcinoma is the most rapidly increasing neoplasm in the United States and Western Europe.[4]

Hepatic fibrosis is a highly relevant aspect of liver biology because of the significant progress in uncovering its mechanisms, combined with a growing realization that effective antifibrotic therapies may soon alter the natural history of chronic liver disease. Thus liver fibrosis can now be viewed as a clinical problem whose diagnosis and treatment will soon have rational, evidence-based approaches. This progress is very timely, since the continued "aging" of the hepatitis C virus (HCV)-infected cohort and the growing prevalence of obesity-related liver diseases are leading to precipitous increases in the current prevalence and predicted burden of advanced liver disease.[2,5] With these issues in mind, this chapter will review clinical

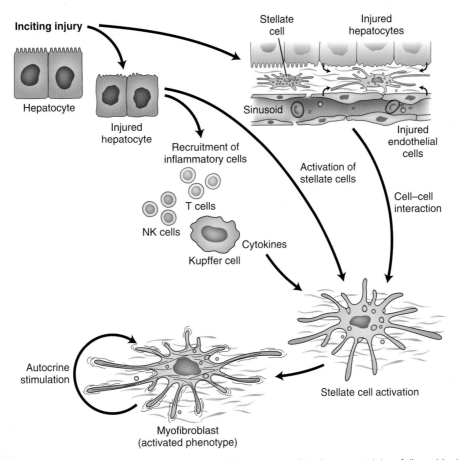

Fig. 5-1 The wound healing response to liver injury. Most forms of liver injury result in hepatocyte injury followed by inflammation, which in turn leads to activation of hepatic stellate cells. Inflammatory effectors are multiple and include T cells, NK cells, and NKT cells, as well as Kupffer cells. These cells produce growth factors, cytokines, and chemokines that play an important role in stellate cell activation. Additionally, injury leads to disruption of the normal cellular environment, including injury to endothelial cells, which may have paracrine effects on stellate cells. Overall, these events lead to activation of stellate cells *(right upper panel)* (or other fibrogenic effector cells). Once activated, stellate cells themselves produce a variety of compounds, including growth factors, cytokines, chemokines, and vasoactive peptides. These substances have pleiotrophic effects in the local environment, many of which have autocrine effects on stellate cells (or similar fibrogenic effector cells) themselves. Stellate cell activation has many effects (also see Fig. 5-4), the most prominent including synthesis of extracellular matrix as well as tissue contraction mediated by contractile myofibroblasts.

aspects of hepatic fibrosis including natural history, pathophysiologic mechanisms, current and future tools for diagnosing fibrosis, and emerging antifibrotic strategies.

Clinical Aspects of Hepatic Fibrosis
Natural History and Risk Factors

Fibrosis leading to cirrhosis can accompany virtually any chronic liver disease that is characterized by the presence of architectural disruption and/or inflammation. The vast majority of patients with liver disease worldwide have chronic viral hepatitis. Many other disorders may lead to fibrosis and cirrhosis, including steatohepatitis associated with either alcohol or obesity; autoimmune liver disease (including that affecting either hepatocytes or biliary epithelium); metabolic disorders including Wilson's disease, hemochromatosis, and a variety of storage diseases; parasitic infestation (e.g., schistosomiasis); neonatal liver disease; chronic inflammatory conditions (e.g.,

sarcoidosis); drug toxicity (e.g., methotrexate, hypervitaminosis A); and vascular derangements, either congenital or acquired.

Of the many causes of chronic liver disease, our understanding of the natural history of fibrosis is most extensive in patients with HCV infection, with some information about hepatitis B virus (HBV) and steatohepatitis, including alcoholic liver disease and non-alcoholic steatohepatitis (NASH). Information about fibrosis progression in other diseases is largely anecdotal, but the development of cirrhosis typically requires many years to decades. There are, however, some notable exceptions in which development of cirrhosis can be greatly accelerated, possibly occurring within months rather than years: (1) Neonatal liver disease—infants with biliary atresia may present at birth with severe fibrosis and marked parenchymal distortion; (2) HCV-infected patients after liver transplantation—a subset of patients who undergo liver transplantation for HCV cirrhosis may develop rapidly progressive cholestasis, fibrosis, and recurrent cirrhosis within months of transplantation[6]; (3) patients with human immunodeficiency virus (HIV)/HCV co-infection—these patients have relatively rapid fibrosis compared with those with HCV alone,[7] especially if the HIV is untreated (see below); (4) severe delta hepatitis[8]; and (5) some cases of drug-induced liver disease. These examples of more aggressive fibrogenesis likely reflect dysregulation of several pathways, including defective immunity, massive inflammation and necrosis, and/or altered matrix resorption. Together, they underscore the highly dynamic nature of scar accumulation and degradation. Moreover, these human diseases raise the possibility that when matrix accumulation is unopposed because degradation is ineffective, more rapid fibrosis may ensue.

Once cirrhosis and its complications develop, the prognosis is predicted by widely used systems including the Childs-Pugh score, PELD,[9] and MELD,[10] which are predictive independent of the cause of liver disease.

Hepatitis C Virus

Risk and natural history of fibrosis associated with HCV have been greatly clarified as a result of several large clinical studies incorporating standardized assessments of fibrosis combined with detailed historical and clinical information.[11] The disease can present a remarkably variable course, from decades of viremia with little fibrosis, to rapid onset of cirrhosis in 10 to 15 years. Factors other than those related to the virus itself appear to be most closely correlated with fibrosis progression in HCV. The data supporting this conclusion include the following: (1) There is no clear relationship between viral load or genotype and fibrosis severity even though these former factors affect response to antiviral therapy; (2) human gene polymorphisms appear to correlate with fibrosis risk,[12–17] and viral-related factors have yet to be clearly identified; and (3) the host immune phenotype may be critical because there is more rapid progression in immunosuppressed patients, whether attributable to HIV or immunosuppressive drugs.[7] In mice a Th2 phenotype strongly correlates with fibrogenic potential,[18] which has led to successful efforts to use quantitative trait loci (QTL) mapping to identify specific fibrosis risk genes in these animals[14,19] as well as studies emphasizing the role of lymphocytes and perhaps monocytes in modulating fibrogenesis.[20,21]

Other identified host risk factors for more rapid progression of HCV include the following: (a) older age at time of infection; (b) concurrent liver disease attributable to HBV or alcohol (>50 g/day); it is uncertain, however, whether lesser amounts of alcohol intake are additive towards fibrosis progression; recent studies suggest that less than 50 g/day of alcohol results in a negligible increased risk of hepatic fibrosis[22]; (c) male gender; (d) increased body mass index (BMI), associated with hepatic steatosis[23]; and (e) HIV infection or immunosuppression following liver transplantation (see Natural History and Risk Factors).

Given this information, several clinical variables are helpful in assessing fibrosis risk. Thus, for chronic HCV, if the time of infection is known and a biopsy is obtained at any time thereafter, the rate of progression per year based on either Ishak or Metavir scoring can be estimated.[24] Although initial analyses of this type suggested that fibrosis progression is truly linear, it is now increasingly clear that the progression rate accelerates as the disease advances[25]; for example, it takes less time to progress between Metavir stages 3 and 4 than from stage 1 to stage 2.

Assessment of fibrosis stage and rate of fibrosis progression can be valuable for at least three reasons: (1) Because advanced stages of fibrosis (F3 or F4) generally have a lower response rate to antiviral therapy, the stage of fibrosis plays a role in predicting the likelihood of response to interferon-α–based therapy.[26,27] (2) If little fibrosis progression has occurred over a long interval, then treatment with antiviral therapy may be deemed to be less urgent, and it may be safe to await more effective and/or better tolerated therapy. (3) The approximate time to the development of histologic cirrhosis can be estimated. This would not, however, indicate if or when clinical liver failure would occur because complications of liver disease may be delayed for up to a decade or more after the establishment of histologic cirrhosis. As genetic risk markers that predict a rapid fibrosis progression rate are developed, this information combined with the absolute stage of fibrosis may enable more accurate identification of patients at risk for disease and thus in need of antifibrotic therapy.

Hepatitis B Virus

Very few studies have assessed the progression rate of fibrosis in chronic HBV infection. In general, inflammatory activity, as influenced by viral factors including HBeAg status (which indicates active viral replication), correlates with fibrosis.[28,29] Fibrosis progression has been correlated with HBV genotype in at least one study.[30] In a subset of patients, a rapidly progressive "fibrosing cholestatic hepatitis" may occur,[31] but neither definitive risk factors for this condition nor unique etiologic, cellular, or molecular determinants have been identified. In addition, delta hepatitis superinfection or co-infection may greatly accelerate the risk of advanced fibrosis and cirrhosis.[8] What is striking, however, is that virologic suppression in response to potent antiviral regimens can lead to remarkable improvement not only in serum alanine aminotransferase (ALT) levels and histologic inflammation, but also in fibrosis as well.[8,32-34] Indeed, dramatic resolution of cirrhosis in a 10-year follow-up study has been reported in patients with delta hepatitis who were successfully treated with interferon-α.[8]

Alcoholic Liver Disease

Patients with fibrosis who continue to consume alcohol are virtually assured of disease progression. In addition, two clinical features commonly seen in steatohepatitis—elevated body mass index and elevated serum glucose level—also confer increased risk of fibrosis in alcoholic liver disease.[35] Pathologically, the presence of pericentral fibrosis (central hyaline sclerosis) carries a high risk of eventual panlobular cirrhosis, which is almost certain if alcohol intake continues.

Non-Alcoholic Steatohepatitis

There is a critical need for better data about natural history, risk factors for fibrosis, and rate of fibrosis progression in NASH, issues now being addressed in several multiinstitutional studies.[36] Patients with only steatosis and no inflammation appear to have a benign course when followed for up to 19 years[37]; however, it is unclear if this lesion is completely distinct from steatohepatitis or instead represents a precursor of NASH. It is instructive to remember that HCV fibrosis progression rates were underestimated shortly after the virus was first identified, because many patients had a relatively early fibrosis stage. With continued infection, however, a sizable fraction of HCV patients eventually have progressed to more advanced stages. In a parallel situation, the obesity epidemic in the United States and the developed world is only now fully appreciated, and a threshold level of obesity may have only begun to confer risk of liver disease that will become clinically significant in the next decade. In patients with sustained NASH, spontaneous histologic improvement is very uncommon, but better longitudinal data are needed to understand the natural history of this disease. In three combined studies of 26 patients with NASH followed with sequential biopsies for up to 9 years, 27% had progression of fibrosis and 19% advanced to cirrhosis; however, no patients exhibited reversal of fibrosis.[37] In obese patients with NASH undergoing Roux-en-Y gastric bypass surgery (RYGBP), the initial prevalence of hepatic pathology was as follows: steatosis, 89.7%; hepatocellular ballooning, 58.9%; and centrilobular/perisinusoidal fibrosis, 50%.[38] These data improved significantly after RYGBP (steatosis, 2.9%; ballooning, 0%; and centrilobular fibrosis, 25%). Fibrosis stage also declined, from 1.14 ± 1.05 to 0.72 ± 0.97 (p = 0.002).[38]

Risk of fibrosis and rate of progression are critical issues that will influence risk stratification and patient selection for clinical trials, because progression to cirrhosis is the most important clinical consequence of NASH. Recently developed systems to grade and stage liver disease in NASH[39] should allow for improved, prospective collection of standardized data that can further address these vital questions.

In general, increasing obesity (body mass index >28 kg/m^2) correlates with severity of fibrosis and risk of cirrhosis. Other risk factors include necroinflammatory activity with ALT values more than two times normal levels and/or AST/ALT >1, advanced age, elevated triglyceride levels, insulin resistance and/or diabetes mellitus, and systemic hypertension.[40] It is uncertain whether these features are comparable across the spectrum of disorders associated with NASH, including obesity with insulin resistance, jejunoileal (JI) bypass, total parenteral nutrition (TPN), and rapid weight loss, among others. Whether these factors represent surrogates for other risk factors (e.g., reduced antioxidant levels in older patients, increased renin-angiotensin activity in patients with hypertension) is unknown. A clinicobiologic score that combines age, BMI, and triglyceride and ALT levels and that reportedly has 100% negative predictive value for excluding significant fibrosis has been developed.[41]

Reversibility of Fibrosis and Cirrhosis

The evidence that fibrosis and even cirrhosis can be reversible is abundant. The feature common to essentially all situations in which fibrosis and/or cirrhosis improves is the elimination of the underlying cause of liver disease, ranging from eradication of HBV,[42] delta hepatitis,[8] or HCV[43]; to decompression of biliary obstruction in chronic pancreatitis[44]; to immunosuppressive treatment of autoimmune liver disease[45] or iron depletion in hemochromatosis[46]; or to reversal of the metabolic syndrome in NASH.[38] Moreover, there is ample evidence

of reversibility in animal models, which provide vital clues to underlying mechanisms.[47]

It remains unclear what distinguishes those patients whose cirrhosis is reversible from those in whom cirrhosis is fixed. The following factors may retard or even prevent reversibility: (1) A prolonged period of established cirrhosis, which could reflect a longer period of cross-linking of collagen, renders this collagen less sensitive to degradation by enzymes over time. Animal studies now clearly support this possibility.[48] (2) Another factor influencing reversibility is the total content of collagen and other scar molecules, which might lead to a large mass of scar tissue that is physically inaccessible to degradative enzymes. (3) A third factor that may prevent reversibility is reduced expression of enzymes that degrade matrix or sustained elevation of proteins that inhibit the function of these degradative enzymes, in particular elevated levels of tissue inhibitors of metalloproteinases (TIMPs), which block matrix proteases and also prevent apoptosis of activated stellate cells.[49,50] All three scenarios underscore the dynamic process of collagen deposition and collagen degradation.

Pathophysiology of Hepatic Fibrosis and Cirrhosis

Extracellular Matrix in the Normal and Fibrotic Liver

Extracellular matrix (ECM) refers to the array of macromolecules that comprise the scaffolding of normal and fibrotic liver. These macromolecules consist of three main types: collagens, glycoproteins, and proteoglycans (see Schuppan et al. [2001][51] for a review). The number of collagens identified in liver is rapidly growing and currently includes at least 20 subtypes. Glycoproteins include fibronectin, laminin, merosin, tenascin, nidogen, and hyaluronic acid, among others. Proteoglycans include heparan, dermatan sulfates, chondroitin sulfates, perlecan, dystroglycan, syndecan, biglycan, and decorin. There is tremendous heterogeneity of these matrix macromolecules with respect to their different isoforms, as well as variable combinations within different tissue regions and changes related to age.

In normal liver, the subendothelial space of Disse separates the epithelium (hepatocytes) from the sinusoidal endothelium. This space contains a basement membrane–like matrix that, unlike the typical basement membrane, is not electron-dense. The hepatic basement membrane is composed of non–fibril-forming collagens (including types IV, VI, and XIV), glycoproteins, and proteoglycans. This normal subendothelial ECM is critical for maintaining the differentiated functions of resident liver cells, including hepatocytes, stellate cells, and sinusoidal endothelium.

In contrast to basement membrane–type matrix, in normal liver the so-called interstitial ECM is largely confined to the capsule, around large vessels, and in the portal areas. It is composed of fibril-forming collagens (e.g., types I and III), together with cellular (EDA) fibronectin, undulin, and other glycoconjugates.

As the liver becomes fibrotic, the total content of collagens and noncollagenous components increases three-fold to

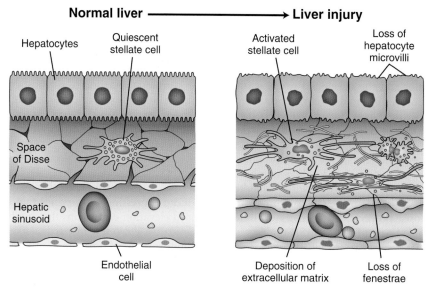

Fig. 5-2 Anatomy of hepatic sinusoid in normal and injured liver. On the left panel of the figure is shown the multiple key liver-specific cellular elements in the normal liver, including hepatocytes, endothelial cells, and stellate cells (although immune cells may be prominent in the liver, they are not shown). Stellate cells are located within the subendothelial space of Disse (i.e., between the sinusoidal endothelium and hepatocytes). The figure emphasizes the close physical relationships between the various cellular elements in the liver—all of which play a role in the normal functioning of hepatocytes as well as the maintenance of physiologic blood flow. After liver injury, changes in numerous cells occur; for example, stellate cells become activated, hepatocytes lose their microvilli, and endothelial cells lose their characteristic fenestrae. All of these features contribute to continued cell activation and injury as well as dysfunction at the whole organ level, including at the level of sinusoidal blood flow, which also becomes abnormal.

five-fold, accompanied by the shift in the type of ECM in the subendothelial space from the normal low-density basement membrane–like matrix to interstitial type matrix (see Schuppan et al. [2001][51] for a review). This "capillarization" leads to the loss of hepatocyte microvilli and the disappearance of endothelial fenestration (**Fig. 5-2**). The outcome of fibrogenesis is the conversion of normal low-density basement membrane–like matrix to high-density interstitial type matrix. A number of components are responsible for ECM remodeling (see Ramachandran and Iredale [2009][52] and Henderson and Iredale [2007][53] for reviews) (**Fig. 5-3**). These include a family of zinc-dependent enzyme matrix-metalloproteinases (MMPs)[54] and their inhibitors (TIMPs) as well as several converting enzymes such as MT1-MMP and stromelysin.

In human liver diseases, there is down-regulation of MMP1 (interstitial collagenase, collagenase I) and up-regulation of MMP2 (gelatinase A) and MMP9 (gelatinase B). Based on the differing substrate specificities of these enzymes, the result is increased degradation of basement membrane collagen and decreased degradation of interstitial collagens. These activated MMPs are regulated in part by their tissue inhibitors, TIMPs. TIMP1 and TIMP2 are up-regulated relative to MMP1 in progressive experimental liver fibrosis, which may explain decreased degradation of interstitial type matrix observed in experimental and human liver injury. In contrast, during the resolution of experimental liver injury, TIMP1 expression and TIMP2 expression are decreased, and collagenase expression is unchanged, resulting in a net increase in collagenase activity and increased resorption of scar matrix (see **Fig. 5-3**).

Stellate cells are a key source of MMP2 and stromelysin. They also express TIMP1 and TIMP2 mRNAs and produce TIMP1, MT1-MMP, and MMP9, which is a type IV collagenase locally secreted by Kupffer cells and that may also be produced by stellate cells in response to interleukin-1. The source of MMP1, which plays a crucial role in degrading the excess interstitial matrix in advanced liver disease, is still uncertain.[55] However, interstitial collagenase activity in liver may be attributable to either MT1-MMP or even MMP2, although further studies are required. There is elevated expression of MMP2 in cirrhosis. However, experimental animals that lack MMP2 have worsened fibrosis after toxic liver injury,[56] which suggests that MMP2 may normally limit liver injury—these findings complicate strategies aimed at simply inhibiting metalloproteinases to treat hepatic fibrosis.

ECM-Cell Interactions

Changes in the microenvironment of the space of Disse result in phenotypic changes in all resident liver cells. Hepatic stellate cells are activated by the surrounding increase in interstitial matrix.[57] Sinusoidal endothelial cells produce cellular fibronectin in very early liver injury, which also contributes to stellate cell activation. In addition, endothelial cells produce type IV collagen, proteoglycans, and factors (e.g., urokinase type plasminogen activator) that participate in the activation of latent cytokines such as TGF-β1. Activated Kupffer cells release cytokines and reactive oxygen intermediates that may stimulate stellate cells in a paracrine manner. Injury also leads to increased platelets, which are also an abundant source of cytokines, producing a rich array of important growth factors. Hepatocytes, the most abundant cells in the liver, generate lipid peroxides following injury that lead to stellate cell activation, a prerequisite for fibrogenesis (see below).

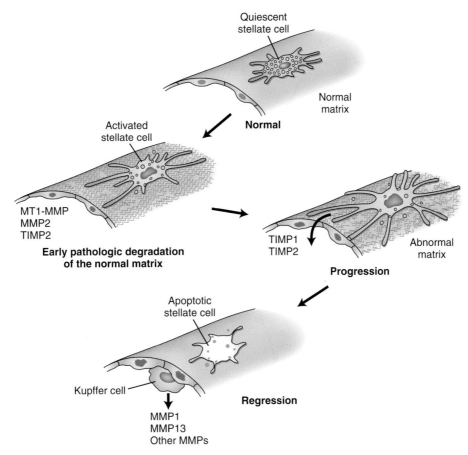

Fig. 5-3 **Mechanisms of pathologic matrix degradation, fibrosis progression, and fibrosis resolution in chronic liver disease.** Activation of stellate cells (*top left panel*) is a key event in hepatic fibrosis and is associated with pathologic matrix degradation attributable to increased production of membrane type 1 matrix metalloproteinase (MT1-MMP), matrix metalloproteinase-2 (MMP2), and tissue inhibitors of metalloproteinases (TIMPs), leading to replacement by interstitial collagen or scar matrix. As fibrosis progresses (*middle panel*), sustained expression of TIMPs prevents matrix degradation and apoptosis of activated stellate cells. Regression of fibrosis (*upper right panel*) is associated with increased apoptosis of activated stellate cells. Apoptosis requires decreased expression of tissue inhibitor of metalloproteinase-1 (TIMP1), yielding a net increase in protease activity. These events may occur coincident with production of matrix metalloproteinases, which could include MMP1 (in humans) and/or MMP13 (in rodents), although cellular sources of these enzymes (possibly including Kupffer cells) and clear evidence of their induction in vivo are still lacking. Validation of these events and further elucidation of mechanisms underlying fibrosis regression represent key challenges for future studies.

The dynamic interactions between fibrogenic cells in the liver and the ECM are an important determinant of fibrogenesis. The ECM is a reservoir for growth factors (e.g., platelet-derived growth factor [PDGF]).[51] Like all cytokines, PDGF signals by binding to membrane receptors. The PDGF receptor belongs to a receptor family known as receptor tyrosine kinases, which collectively are key transducers for many important cytokines, including hepatocyte growth factor (HGF), epidermal growth factor (EGF), vascular endothelial growth factor (VEGF), and fibroblast growth factor (FGF). Intracellular signaling cascades downstream of receptor tyrosine kinases and other receptors are pervasive (see Fernandez et al. [2009][58] for a review).

Integrins are another type of membrane receptor that transduce extracellular signals in liver. These are heterodimeric transmembrane proteins composed of an α subunit and a β subunit whose ligands are matrix molecules rather than cytokines.[59,60] Several integrins and their downstream effectors have been identified in stellate cells, including α1β1, α2β1, αvβ1, αvβ3, and α6β4.[61-63] Integrins may also form complexes with other receptor families in mediating cell motility and fibrogenesis (e.g., the tetraspanin family of receptors).[64]

Other adhesion proteins and cell matrix receptors have been characterized, including cadherins and selectins, which mediate interactions between inflammatory cells and the endothelial wall. ECM can also indirectly affect cell function through the release of soluble growth factors (cytokines), which is in turn controlled by local metalloproteinases. These include matrix-bound PDGF, HGF, connective tissue growth factor (CTGF), tumor necrosis factor-α (TNF-α), basic fibroblast growth factor (bFGF), and VEGF.[51]

Hepatic Stellate Cell Activation—The Common Pathway Leading to Hepatic Fibrosis

The identification of stellate cells as the key cellular source of extracellular matrix in liver has been a major scientific advancement. This distinct cell population, located in the

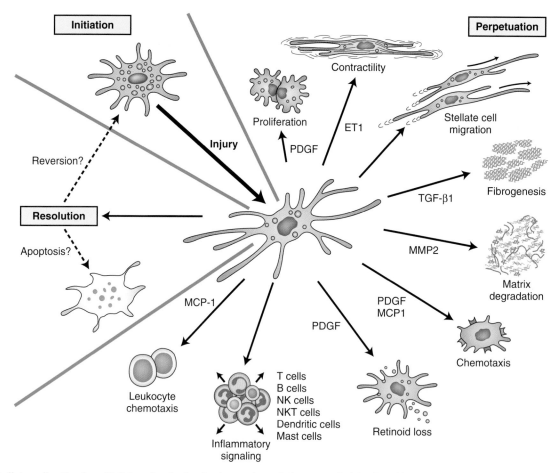

Fig. 5-4 **Stellate cell activation.** Stellate cell activation is a key pathogenic feature underlying liver fibrosis and cirrhosis. Multiple and varied stimuli contribute to the induction and maintenance of activation, including, but not limited to, cytokines, peptides, and the extracellular matrix itself. Key phenotypic features of activation include production of extracellular matrix, loss of retinoids, proliferation of up-regulation of smooth muscle proteins, secretion of peptides and cytokines (which have autocrine effects), and up-regulation of various cytokine and peptide receptors.

subendothelial space of Disse between hepatocytes and sinusoidal endothelial cells (see **Fig. 5-1**), represents one third of the non-parenchymal population, or approximately 15% of the total number of resident cells in normal liver.[65] In normal liver they are the principal storage site for retinoids (vitamin A metabolites), stockpiling 40% to 70% of the body's retinoids. Most of the retinoids are in the form of retinyl esters and are confined to cytoplasmic droplets. Preferential expression of extracellular matrix genes in stellate cells has been confirmed in mechanistically distinct experimental models of injury.

Recent findings implicate other mesenchymal cell types from a variety of sources that generate extracellular matrix, including classic portal fibroblasts[66] (especially in biliary fibrosis), bone marrow–derived cells,[67] and fibroblast-derived epithelial-mesenchymal transition (EMT) involving hedgehog signaling.[68,69] Moreover, experimental genetic "marking" of stellate cells by expression of fluorescent proteins downstream of either fibrogenic or contractile gene promoters illustrates the plasticity of fibrogenic populations in vivo.[70] In view of this capacity for "transdifferentiation" between different mesenchymal cell lineages and possibly even from epithelium,[69] the key issue is whether fibrogenic cells express target molecules such as receptors or cytokines in sufficient

concentrations in vivo to merit their targeting by diagnostic agents or antifibrotic compounds.

Following liver injury of any type, stellate cells undergo a process known as activation, which is characterized by the transition of quiescent vitamin A rich cells into proliferative, fibrogenic, and contractile myofibroblasts[57,71] (see **Figs. 5-1 to Fig. 5-4**). Stellate cell activation can be conceptually viewed as a two-stage process: initiation (also referred to as preinflammatory) and perpetuation[57] (see **Fig. 5-4**). Initiation refers to early changes in gene expression and phenotype that render the cells responsive to other cytokines and stimuli, and perpetuation results from the effects of these stimuli on maintaining the activated phenotype and generating fibrosis. Initiation is largely due to paracrine stimulation, whereas perpetuation involves autocrine as well as paracrine loops.

Initiation

Oxidant stress may be an early determinant of stellate cell activation.[72,73] Hepatocytes are a potent source of these fibrogenic lipid peroxides.[72] Moreover, steatosis in NASH and HCV correlates with increased stellate cell activation and fibrogenesis,[74] possibly because fat represents an enhanced source of lipid peroxides.

In hepatic injury, whether subclinical or overt, there is a perturbation of normal liver homeostasis, with extracellular release of either free radicals (i.e., "oxidant stress"), intracellular constituents, and/or cytokines and signaling molecules. Sources of these mediators may be circulating (i.e., endocrine), paracrine, or autocrine. In particular, oxidant stress-mediated necrosis leading to stellate cell activation may underlie a variety of liver diseases including hemochromatosis, alcoholic liver disease, viral hepatitis, and non-alcoholic steatohepatitis. Liver injury is typically associated with infiltration of inflammatory cells, but even in their absence, the liver contains sufficient resident macrophages (Kupffer cells) and natural killer cells (pit cells) to initiate local inflammation before the arrival of extrahepatic cells. In addition to oxidant stress, endothelial cells following early injury produce a splice variant of cellular fibronectin that is able to stimulate stellate activation. Sinusoidal endothelial cells may lose their fenestrations following injury and express proinflammatory molecules including intercellular adhesion molecule-1, VEGF, and adhesion molecules. Together with stellate cells, they activate angiogenic pathways in response to hypoxia associated with local injury or malignancy.[58]

Although necrosis is considered a classical inflammatory and fibrogenic stimulus, recent findings also suggest that apoptosis may provoke a fibrogenic response in stellate cells. Apoptotic fragments released from hepatocytes are fibrogenic towards cultured stellate cells,[75] and Fas-mediated hepatocyte apoptosis in vivo in experimental animals is also fibrogenic.[76] Apoptosis of hepatocytes is associated with enhanced stellate cell survival and up-regulation of NADPH oxidase, which further generates oxidant stress.[77,78]

Platelets in injured liver are a potent source of paracrine stimuli by generating multiple potentially important mediators including platelet-derived growth factor (PDGF), transforming growth factor-β1 (TGF-β1), epidermal growth factor (EGF), and the chemokine ligand CXCL4.[79] Additionally, activated stellate cells have been observed in primary and metastatic human tumors as well as in a murine model of metastatic melanoma to the liver.[80]

Gene Regulation in Hepatic Stellate Cells and Myofibroblasts

Advances in gene regulation have been increasingly applied to our understanding of hepatic stellate cell activation.[81] In addition to transcriptional regulation, epigenetic control by methylation,[82-84] mRNA stabilization,[85] and microRNA interactions[86-88] has been explored in models of stellate cell activation in culture and in vivo. These advances will generate new therapeutic strategies.[89]

Many transcription factors regulate gene expression through posttranslational modification of regulatory proteins, in particular phosphorylation. For example, stellate cell activation provokes phosphorylation of the RelA subunit of NF-κB at a specific serine residue (Ser536) that leads to its nuclear import, resulting in increased NF-κB transcriptional activity,[90] which increases survival of activated stellate cells. Angiotensin-converting enzyme inhibitors can reduce survival of activated stellate cells/myofibroblasts in experimental models and human diseases, leading to regression of fibrosis by inhibiting this phosphorylation.[90] Epigenetic regulation of

myofibroblast activity can also be controlled by a microRNA, miR132, that releases a translational block on the methyl-CpG binding protein, provoking repression of the PPAR-γ transcription factor.[88] Additionally, phosphorylation of the transcription factor C/EBPb by the ribosomal S-6 kinase (RSK) promotes stellate cell activation and can be inhibited by cell-permeable peptides that block RSK and stimulate apoptosis.[91]

Perpetuation

After initiation, activated stellate cells undergo a series of phenotypic changes that collectively lead to the accumulation of extracellular matrix. These changes include (1) proliferation; (2) contractility; (3) fibrogenesis; (4) chemotaxis; (5) matrix degradation; (6) retinoid loss; (7) chemokine, adipokine, and neuroendocrine signaling; and (8) inflammatory and immune signaling.

Proliferation

An increase in the number of stellate cells has been documented after both human and experimental liver injury, in large part attributable to local proliferation. Following liver injury, many mitogenic factors as well as their cognate tyrosine kinase receptors are unregulated, primarily through receptor tyrosine kinases.[64] PDGF is the best characterized and most potent mitogen towards stellate cells. Up-regulation of PDGF receptor following liver injury enhances the responsiveness to autocrine PDGF, whose expression is also increased. The downstream signaling pathways involve ERK/MAP kinase, phosphoinositol 3-kinase (PI 3-kinase), and STAT-1 (signal transducers and activators of transcription) (see Pinzani[92] for a review). PDGF-induced proliferation correlates with increased intracellular Ca^{2+} concentration and increased pH, raising the possibility that calcium channel blockers might modulate stellate cell mitogenesis or activation. Other stellate cell mitogens include endothelin-1 (ET-1), thrombin, FGF, and insulin growth factor (IGF), among others (see Magness et al.,[71] Parola and Pinzani,[73] Mann and Marra,[88] and Rockey[93] for reviews). There is also convergence with ephrin signaling[94] and involvement of the neuropilin receptor, which cooperates with the β-PDGF receptor.[95]

Contractility

Contraction by stellate cells may be a major determinant of early and late increases in portal resistance during liver fibrosis. Activated stellate cells impede hepatic blood flow both by constricting individual sinusoids and by contracting the cirrhotic liver, because the collagenous bands typical of end-stage cirrhosis contain large numbers of activated stellate cells (see Rockey[93] for a review). A key contractile stimulus towards stellate cells is ET-1.[93] Other contractile agonists include arginine vasopressin, adrenomedullin, and eicosanoids.[93]

Regulation of stellate cell contraction is complex. The endothelium-derived relaxing factor nitric oxide (NO) appears to be an important relaxing factor in the sinusoid (although other factors such as carbon monoxide also play a role). The net contractile activity of stellate cells in vivo, therefore, reflects the relative strength of each of these opposing activities. Current evidence suggests that intrahepatic portal hypertension likely results from diminished NO (and/or other vasodilators) activity as well as increased stimulation by ET-1 (or other constrictors).[93]

The expression of smooth muscle α-actin is increased during stellate cell activation. ET-1 and other vasoactive mediators increase their expression. Thus studies of contractile proteins in stellate cells may yield a therapeutic target for treatment of intrahepatic portal hypertension.

Fibrogenesis

Fibrogenesis is perhaps the key component of the stellate cell's contribution to hepatic fibrosis. TGF-β1 is the most potent fibrogenic factor, with some fibrogenic activity documented for chemokines,[96,97] connective tissue growth factor (CCN2),[98,99] interleukin-1β, tumor necrosis factor, lipid peroxides, acetaldehyde, and others (see Friedman,[57] Parola and Pinzani,[73] Henderson and Forbes,[100] and Dooley et al.[101] for reviews). Cross-talk with inflammatory signaling occurs through regulation of the TGF-β pseudoreceptor, BAMBI, by toll-like receptor 4.[102]

Because of its importance, TGF-β1 regulation has received considerable attention. TGF-β1 is up-regulated in experimental and human hepatic fibrosis. Although sources of this cytokine are multiple, autocrine expression is among the most important (see Mann and Marr[88] and Inagaki and Okazaki[103] for reviews). Several mechanisms underlie the increase in TGF-β1 expression by stellate cells during liver injury, including TGF-β transcriptional up-regulation, latent TGF-β1 activation, increased TGF-β receptor expression, and up-regulation of TGF-β signaling components. Signals downstream of TGF-β1 include a family of bifunctional molecules known as Smads, upon which many extracellular and intracellular signals converge to fine-tune and enhance TGF-β's effects during fibrogenesis.[103]

Chemotaxis

Stellate cells may accumulate both through proliferation and via directed migration into regions of injury, or chemotaxis. PDGF, the leukocyte chemoattractant MCP-1, and a growing family of chemokines have been identified as key stellate cell chemoattractants.[79,96,97,104]

Matrix Degradation

A greater understanding of matrix degradation in liver is emerging. Quantitative and qualitative changes in the activity of MMPs and their inhibitors play a vital role in extracellular matrix remodeling in liver fibrogenesis (see Extracellular Matrix in the Normal and Fibrotic Liver). As noted earlier in this chapter, the net effect of changes in matrix degradation is the conversion of the low-density subendothelial matrix to one rich in interstitial collagens.

Retinoid Loss and Nuclear Receptor Signaling

Activation of stellate cells is accompanied by the loss of the characteristic perinuclear retinoid (vitamin A) droplets. In culture, retinoid is released outside the cell during activation as retinol.[105] Adipose differentiation related protein (ADRP) coats lipid droplets and is increased as retinoids accumulate in stellate cells, whereas its knockdown by siRNA increases fibrogenesis in cultured stellate cells.[106] Despite the data from this study, it is unclear whether retinoid loss is required for stellate cells to be activated or whether these changes are linked to altered nuclear retinoid receptor signaling.

Chemokine, Adipokine, and Neuroendocrine Signaling

As noted previously, chemokines contribute significantly to the pathogenesis of hepatic fibrosis.[96,97] Both CCR1 and CCR5 are fibrogenic and are produced by different cellular sources.[96] Cell types generating CCR2 evolve with progressive liver injury—initially they are produced by bone marrow cells, but later they are derived from resident liver cells.[97] On the other hand, CXCL9 is antifibrotic following binding to its cognate receptor, CXCR3, and polymorphisms in CXCL9 may contribute to fibrosis progression risk in patients with chronic liver disease.[107]

Pathways stimulated by polypeptides derived from adipose, known as adipokines, are implicated in chronic liver disease.[108] Some adipokines are strictly derived from fat cells, whereas others are also produced by resident liver cells. Leptin and adiponectin are both derived from hepatic stellate cells, and both increased leptin levels and decreased adiponectin levels may amplify fibrogenesis following local paracrine signaling.[109]

Neuroendocrine activity is newly implicated in hepatic fibrogenesis as well,[110] in particular because of cannabinoids. Interruption of cannabinoid activity is an appealing therapeutic target, because CB1 receptor signaling is profibrogenic, and thus efforts to antagonize this molecule have met with significant success in animal models.[111] More importantly, recent studies using cannabinoid receptor antagonists that do not cross the blood–brain barrier are especially promising, because they avoid the possibility of untoward effects on mood and behavior associated with centrally active compounds.[112] Conversely, CB2 receptor signaling is antifibrogenic, and its stimulation by agonists is also rational for treatment of fibrosis[113]; however, they may amplify inflammation.[114] Neurotrophins have also been implicated in fibrogenesis,[115,116] in particular serotonin and opioids.[110]

Inflammatory and Immune Signaling

Stellate cells are central to inflammatory signaling in liver injury and fibrosis. Stellate cells interact with macrophages, traditional lymphocyte subsets (e.g., T and B cells), natural killer (NK) cells, NKT cells,[117,118] B cells,[119] dendritic cells,[120] and mast cells. Emerging roles for Toll-like receptors,[102,121-123] NF-κB signaling,[89] and the inflammasomes[124] have also been implicated. Interactions between stellate cells/myofibroblasts and immune cell subsets stimulate specific responses that alter the composition of inflammatory infiltrates and the rate of fibrogenesis.[125,126]

Disease-Specific Mechanisms Regulating Hepatic Fibrosis—HCV and NASH

In addition to generic mechanisms of fibrogenesis common to all experimental and human liver disease, there has been progress in elucidating disease-specific mechanisms, particularly in HCV and NASH. In HCV stellate cells might be capable of being infected by the virus because they express putative HCV receptors.[127,128] Moreover, adenoviral transduction of HCV nonstructural and core proteins induces stellate cell proliferation and release of inflammatory signals.[127,128] In HCV-infected liver, chemokines and their receptors are up-regulated, stimulating lymphocyte recruitment.[129] HCV proteins may also interact directly with sinusoidal endothelium.[130]

The rising prevalence of obesity in the United States and Western Europe is associated with an alarming increase in NASH,[131] leading to advanced fibrosis and cirrhosis. Increased signaling in stellate cells by leptin in conjunction with decreased activity of adiponectin contributes to an altered adipokine balance that favors fibrosis (see Chemokine, Adipokine, and Neuroendocrine Signaling; also see Marra and Bertolani[108] and Parekh and Anania[132] for reviews).

Resolution of Liver Fibrosis and the Fate of Activated Stellate Cells

During recovery from acute human and experimental liver injury the number of activated stellate cells decreases as tissue integrity is restored. Either reversion of stellate cell activation or selective clearance of activated stellate cells by apoptosis may explain the loss of activated cells in resolving liver injury. To date, evidence is strongest for stellate cell apoptosis and senescence in this setting.[52]

Apoptosis of hepatic stellate cells probably accounts for the decrease of activated stellate cells during resolution of hepatic fibrosis.[53,133] Following injury, apoptosis may be inhibited by soluble factors and matrix components that are present during injury, whereas an apoptotic pathway otherwise represents a "default" mode. Furthermore, cell death ligands including TRAIL and FAS are expressed in liver injury, and activated stellate cells are more susceptible to TRAIL-mediated apoptosis.[75,116,134] Another death receptor, nerve growth factor receptor (NGFR), is also expressed by activated hepatic stellate cells, and its stimulation with ligand drives apoptosis.[115,135] More recently, an elegant study has implicated senescence mediated by p53 as another pathway by which stellate cells may be cleared during fibrosis resolution.[136] The relationship between apoptosis and senescence has not been fully clarified.

Survival factors also regulate the net activity of stellate cell apoptosis. In particular, signaling by the NF-κB family potently regulates stellate cell survival (see Mann and Mann[81] and Watson et al.[137] for reviews). Studies using gliotoxin, a fungal toxin that induces apoptosis in hepatic stellate cells, emphasize the role of this pathway in stellate cell removal during resolution of liver fibrosis.[138,139]

Molecules regulating matrix degradation appear closely linked to survival and apoptosis. Active MMP2 correlates closely with apoptosis, and in fact may be stimulated by apoptosis.[139] Interactions between hepatic stellate cells and the surrounding matrix also influence their propensity towards apoptosis, and this might partly explain the anti-apoptotic activity of TIMP1. In particular, the stiffness of the extracellular matrix, rather than its chemical composition alone, has a significant impact on the behavior of stellate cells.[140] The fibrotic matrix may also provide important survival signals to activated stellate cells. For example, animals expressing a mutant collagen I resistant to degradation have more sustained fibrosis and less stellate cell apoptosis following liver injury,[141] and either transgenic animals expressing TIMP1 in liver[142] or animals treated with a TIMP1 neutralizing antibody[143] have delayed resolution of fibrosis.

It is unknown whether an activated stellate cell can revert to a quiescent state in vivo, although it has been observed in culture. When stellate cells are grown on a basement membrane substratum (Matrigel) they remain quiescent, and plating of highly activated cells on this substratum downregulates stellate cell activation.[144-146] In view of the findings that stiffness may regulate stellate cell activation,[140] the quiescent response to Matrigel may be a reflection of its more distensible physical state rather than its chemical composition.

Methods to Measure Liver Fibrosis

Measurement of fibrosis not only helps to stage the severity of disease but also allows serial determination of disease progression. The level of fibrosis may play an important role in clinical management and determine a patient's prognosis. For example, HCV-infected patients with advanced fibrosis/histologic cirrhosis are less likely to respond to interferon-based therapy than those with less advanced fibrosis. Furthermore, the fibrosis progression rate is an important predictor of the time to develop cirrhosis.[11]

Percutaneous liver biopsy has traditionally been considered to be the gold standard test to assess liver fibrosis. However, there are many issues surrounding liver biopsy (reviewed in Rockey et al.[147]), including that it is invasive and costly and, most importantly for the measurement of fibrosis, may be subject to sampling error. Thus a variety of noninvasive tests have emerged as potential alternatives to liver biopsy (**Fig. 5-5**). These include clinical signs, routine laboratory tests, quantitative assays of liver function, markers of extracellular matrix synthesis and/or degradation, and radiologic imaging studies. In addition to individual indicators of fibrosis, combinations of tests and a number of models for predicting liver fibrosis have been developed. Individual and combination tests are discussed in the following sections.

The ideal method to measure fibrosis would be simple, noninvasive, reproducible, inexpensive, accurate, and readily available. Unfortunately, at the time of publication of this book, none of the currently available approaches fulfills all of these criteria.

Bedside Diagnostic Tools

Clinical signs and symptoms of liver disease are frequently highlighted in assessing patients with liver disease, but these are of little value in detecting early, precirrhotic stages of liver fibrosis. In contrast, a number of clinical features can been used to assess whether cirrhosis with portal hypertension may be present. Signs of cirrhosis include spider angiomata, distention of abdominal wall veins, ascites, splenomegaly, muscle wasting, Dupuytren's contractures (especially with ethanol-associated cirrhosis), gynecomastia and testicular atrophy in males, and palmar erythema. However, it is important to emphasize that even in patients with histologic cirrhosis and even in those with portal hypertension, these physical signs may not be present.

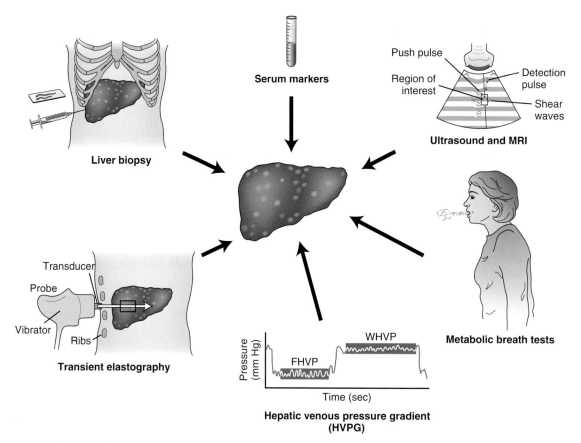

Fig. 5-5 **Diagnosis of hepatic fibrosis.** The diagnosis of liver fibrosis may be simple or complex, depending on its level. Advanced fibrosis and cirrhosis may be clinically evident in the patient with known chronic liver disease and symptoms and signs of portal hypertension. In other patients, however, fibrosis may be clinically silent and can only be detected using diagnostic tools. Routine laboratory tests may be used (e.g., the AST/platelet ratio) and panels of fibrosis markers may be used. Imaging techniques such as ultrasound, CT, or MRI may also provide information about fibrosis. Transient elastography uses pulsed-echo signals to measure the stiffness of the liver, which is theoretically proportional to the degree of fibrosis. More invasive tests include liver biopsy and determination of the hepatic venous pressure gradient (HVPG). Finally, the degree of liver fibrosis may be approximated by measuring the functional capacity of the liver (see text for details of all options).

Noninvasive Markers of Fibrosis

Blood-Based Markers—Overview

A key advantage of serum markers to detect fibrosis is their noninvasiveness. Additionally, it has been argued that serum markers overcome sampling problems associated with liver biopsy. Despite these important potential advantages, these approaches have several drawbacks. First, most of the studies examining serum markers have been performed in cohorts of patients that have been biased toward advanced fibrosis/cirrhosis. A further problem is that the currently proposed serum marker algorithms use dichotomous rather than continuous scales. The dichotomous nature of these variables would be less problematic if there were clear clinical associations (e.g., if prognosis or treatment response was highly linked to stages 0 to 1 versus stages 2 to 4). In the absence of clinical correlates between dichotomous variables and outcomes, it remains important to diagnose accurately the different stages of fibrosis (0 though 4). Unfortunately, current tests and algorithms are unable to do so with accuracy, and perhaps most importantly the tests do not differentiate between intermediate levels of fibrosis. Thus, although assessments of fibrosis with approaches that use serum markers have great appeal, further investigation is required to optimize these tests.

A wide variety of blood, serum, or plasma "markers" for fibrosis have been proposed and fall into several specific categories of markers or tests. For example, some detect abnormalities in serum chemistries or hematologic tests. Included are aspartate AST, ALT, γ-glutamyltransferase (GGT), bilirubin, albumin, α_2-macroglobulin, platelets, and others. Moreover, some of these individual tests have been incorporated into simple and/or complex mathematical models or algorithms (see below).

Another major category of tests includes those that are based specifically on the pathogenesis of fibrosis (see above). For example, proteins produced as a result of the fibrogenic process itself and that have been studied as markers of fibrosis include procollagen I, fibronectin, tenascin, laminin, hyaluronic acid, and others. Other markers have included cytokines (e.g., TGF-β1, CTGF, PDGF), matrix degrading enzymes (e.g., TIMP1) (**Table 5-1**).

Finally, groups of tests, including those that use markers of fibrosis in combination with each other or in combination with other types of tests, have been advanced in an attempt to detect and measure fibrosis.

Ideally, a blood-based test should have both high sensitivity and high specificity. Many of the available tests have a high specificity (>95%) for advanced fibrosis. However, few

Table 5-1 Cytokines, Growth Factors, Peptides, Proteases, and Other Components Important in Hepatic Fibrogenesis

CYTOKINES	GROWTH FACTORS	PEPTIDES
Transforming growth factor-β	Transforming growth factor-β	Endothelin-1
Transforming growth factor-α	Transforming growth factor-α	Norepinephrine
Interleukin-1	Insulin-like growth factor (I, II) †	Angiotensin II
Interleukin-4	Platelet-derived growth factor†	
Interleukin-6†	Fibroblast growth factor†	
Interleukin-10	Vascular endothelial growth factor	
Interleukin-13	Hepatocyte growth factor	
Monocyte chemotactic factor†	Connective tissue growth factor	
Proteases and Their Inhibitors	*Miscellaneous*	
Matrix metalloproteinase-1 (interstitial collagenase)	Thrombospondin (1,2) Leptin	
Matrix metalloproteinase-2 (gelatinase A)	Activin A	
Matrix metalloproteinase-3 (stromelysin-1)	Thrombin†	
Matrix metalloproteinase-7 (matrilysin)	Osteopontin	
Matrix metalloproteinase-8		
Matrix metalloproteinase-9 (gelatinase B)		
Matrix metalloproteinase-10 (stromelysin-2)		
Tissue inhibitor of metalloproteinase-1		

Compounds whose effect is largely via stimulation of proliferation.
†Agents may have direct effects on hepatic stellate cells, or indirect effects in the wounding environment.

(including algorithms) have great sensitivity to detect moderate levels of fibrosis. Moreover, a serum-based assay ideally should be linear over the full range of fibrosis, follow the natural history, and accurately reflect the effect of treatment.

Routine Laboratory Tests

A number of studies have used routine laboratory tests in an attempt to determine whether a patient may have advanced liver disease, in particular, to exclude or confirm portal hypertension and/or esophageal varices.[148,149] Although tests such as the prothrombin time, albumin level, and portal vein diameter (measured by ultrasound) have all been associated with varices, studies have been remarkably consistent in their identification of the platelet count as the best single predictor of esophageal varices. For example, in one study cirrhotic patients without splenomegaly on physical examination and with a platelet count of greater than 88,000/mm³ had a risk of large esophageal varices of 7.2%; however, the risk was 28% if the platelet count was less than 88,000/mm³.[148]

An AST/ALT ratio >1 has been proposed to indicate the presence of cirrhosis.[150] In one study of patients with HCV, a ratio >1 had 100% specificity and a positive predictive value for distinguishing cirrhotic from noncirrhotic patients, with a 53.2% sensitivity and 80.7% negative predictive value.[151] In addition, the ratio correlated positively with the stage of fibrosis but not with the grade of activity or other biochemical indices. Of cirrhotic patients, 17% had no clinical or biochemical evidence of chronic liver disease except for an elevated AST/ALT ratio. In another study, the AST/ALT ratio had 81.3% sensitivity and 55.3% specificity in identifying cirrhotic patients who died within 1 year of follow-up.[150,152]

Examples of combination type approaches include those that have used age, GGT and cholesterol levels, and platelet count[153] or simply the AST level and platelet count[154] (**Table 5-2**). The latter formula, termed the AST to platelet ratio index or APRI, uses the AST level/upper limit of normal (ULN) divided by the platelet count ($\times 10^9$/L) multiplied by 100. The sensitivity and specificity for fibrosis of the APRI value depended on the cut-offs used. Using an APRI value of 1.50, the positive and negative predictive values for significant fibrosis (Ishak score ≥3) were 91% and 65%, respectively; however, for cirrhosis with an APRI of 2.00, the positive and negative predictive values were 65% and 95%, respectively. Thus for a hypothetical patient with an AST of 90 IU/L (and an ULN of 45) and a platelet count of 100 ($\times 10^9$/L), the APRI would be 2.00. This means that the patient has essentially a 90% chance of having significant fibrosis, and somewhat less likelihood of having cirrhosis. However, cirrhosis could not be excluded with certainty. Although the APRI is attractive because of its simplicity, it can neither definitively diagnose nor exclude cirrhosis, and it does not readily differentiate patients with intermediate levels of fibrosis. Indeed, this has been an issue with many of the simple quantitative systems based on routine laboratory values. Essentially, the higher the sensitivity of the test, the lower the specificity, and vice versa.

More complicated algorithms based on commonly available laboratory tests include the FibroTest and others.[24] The FibroTest was developed with mathematical modeling in which an algorithm including five different markers to predict fibrosis was utilized (markers selected were α_2-macroglobulin, haptoglobin, GGT, apolipoprotein A$_1$, and total bilirubin).

Table 5-2 Combined Panels of Blood Markers Used to Detect Liver Fibrosis

PANEL	COMPONENTS
AST/ALT	AST/ALT
Forns*	Platelets, GGT, cholesterol
APRI	AST, platelets
PGA index	Platelets, GGT, apolipoprotein A
FibroTest	GGT, haptoglobin, bilirubin, apolipoprotein A, α_2-macroglobulin
FibroSpect	Hyaluronic acid, TIMP-1, α_2-macroglobulin
ELF†	ECM proteins
FPI	AST, cholesterol, HOMA-IR

*Also includes age in the panel.

†Components tested include collagen IV, collagen VI, amino-terminal propeptide of type III collagen (PIIINP), matrix metalloproteinase 2 (MMP2), matrix metalloproteinase-9 (MMP9), tissue inhibitor of matrix metalloproteinase-1 (TIMP1), tenascin, laminin, and hyaluronic acid (HA).

ALT, Alanine aminotransferase; APRI, AST to platelet ratio index; AST, aspartate aminotransferase; ECM, extracellular matrix; ELF, European liver fibrosis; FPI, fibrosis probability index; GGT, γ-glutamyltranspeptidase; HOMA-IR, insulin resistance by the homeostasis model assessment; TIMP-1, tissue inhibitor of metalloproteinase-1

This index predicted a specific biopsy category in 46% of patients[155] and has been validated in a number of hepatitis C patient cohorts, displaying an area under the receiver operator characteristic (AUROC) curve of 0.73 to 0.87.[156] Addition of ALT to the marker panel allows for prediction of Metavir necroinflammatory activity.[156] The panel has also been examined in other liver disease cohorts.[157,158] Limitations of this panel in fibrosis include false-positive results attributable to increases in bilirubin level or decreases in haptoglobin level (e.g., from hemolysis secondary to ribavirin therapy). Likewise, false-positive results may also occur in situations where there is hyperbilirubinemia, such as Gilbert's syndrome and cholestasis. Acute inflammation may also affect the results of the test because of reflex increases in α_2-macroglobulin level or increases in haptoglobin level. Although such panels have become popular in Europe, they remain less frequently utilized in the United States.

Others have attempted to use mixed algorithms. For example, by combining the APRI and FibroTest-FibroSure, an algorithm termed the sequential algorithm for fibrosis evaluation (SAFE) biopsy was developed.[159] This algorithm detects significant fibrosis (≥F2 by Metavir) and cirrhosis (F4) with slightly greater accuracy than either test alone.

Tests Using Extracellular Matrix/Fibrosis Markers

Analyses of serum markers of extracellular matrix/fibrosis have included many proteins important in fibrogenesis, ECM constituents (i.e., fibronectin, collagen I, collagen IV, collagen VI, amino-terminal propeptide of type III collagen [PIIINP], tenascin, hyaluronic acid), metalloproteinases (including many of those listed in **Table 5-1**), inhibitors of matrix metalloproteinases (e.g., TIMP1, TIMP2), and other proteins, peptides, and cytokines, as highlighted in **Table 5-1**. Although many tests have been studied individually, they generally are not associated with a high degree of sensitivity for detection of fibrosis[160,161] (see Afdhal and Nunes[162] for a review).

Tests Using Combinations of Extracellular Matrix and/or Routine Markers

A combination test including hyaluronic acid, TIMP1, and α_2-macroglobulin was examined in a cohort of 294 patients with HCV infection and subsequently validated in a second cohort of 402 patients[163] (FibroSpect, see **Table 5-2**). This had a combined AUROC of 0.831 for Metavir F2-F4 fibrosis. The positive and negative predictive values were 74.3 and 75.8%, respectively, with an accuracy of 75%. Another combination test was developed by the European Liver Fibrosis (ELF) study group.[164] This study group examined collagen IV, collagen VI, PIIINP, MMP2, MMP9, TIMP1, tenascin, laminin, and hyaluronic acid (HA). In a mixed cohort of patients, this panel detected the upper third of fibrosis groups (Scheuer stages 2, 3, 4) with a sensitivity of 90% and accurately detected the absence of fibrosis (Scheuer stages 0, 1) with a negative predictive value for this level of fibrosis of 92%. The AUROC plot was 0.804. The test also appeared to effectively predict clinical outcomes.[165]

Proteomics

Proteomic approaches have attempted to identify unique protein fingerprints in patients with liver disease. Various platforms are available, including those that measure protein expression, protein–protein interactions, or even enzymatic activity. The majority of approaches have used high-throughput technologies to identify novel protein expression patterns. For example, a study of 46 patients with chronic hepatitis B identified 30 proteomic features predictive of significant fibrosis (Ishak stage ≥3) and cirrhosis. The AUROC values for this analysis were 0.906 and 0.921 for advanced fibrosis and cirrhosis, respectively.[166] Another study in 193 patients with chronic hepatitis C identified 8 peaks that differentiated Metavir fibrosis stages with an AUROC of 0.88; this was compared with an AUROC of 0.81 for the FibroTest.[167] Another report in patients with HCV fibrosis identified several serum proteins to be differentially regulated.[168] Patients with advanced fibrosis had elevated levels of α_2-macroglobulin, haptoglobin, and albumin whereas levels of apolipoprotein A-I, apolipoprotein A-IV, complement C-4, and serum retinol binding protein were reduced. Another approach has included measurement of labeled N-glycans found in serum.[169] This approach appeared to be most sensitive and specific for cirrhosis. When combined with the commercially available FibroTest, it had 100% specificity and 75% sensitivity for diagnosing compensated cirrhosis.[169]

Radiographic Tests

A wide variety of radiographic tests have been used to image patients with fibrosis/cirrhosis. Included in this group are ultrasound, computed tomography (CT), and magnetic resonance imaging (MRI). In general, these tests are capable of detecting evidence of portal hypertension; thus they have the ability to detect advanced disease. As currently used in clinical practice, however, they are insensitive for detection of moderate degrees of fibrosis.

Transient elastography, which uses pulse-echo ultrasound acquisitions to measure liver stiffness and predict fibrosis stages, has gained interest as a method to quantitate fibrosis because it appears that liver "stiffness" may accompany the fibrogenic response.[170,171] In a prospective multicenter study of 327 chronic HCV patients, the AUROC values for Metavir stages F2-F4 and cirrhosis were 0.79 and 0.97, respectively.[172] In a separate study of 183 chronic HCV patients, transient elastography compared favorably with the FibroTest and APRI (AUROC for F2-F4 = 0.83, 0.85 and 0.78, for transient elastography, FibroTest, and APRI, respectively).[173] When transient elastography was combined with the FibroTest, the predictive value for fibrosis stages F2-F4 was improved, with an AUROC of 0.88.[173] Despite the attractiveness of transient elastography because of its noninvasive methodology, the depth of measurement from the skin surface is limited (to between 25 and 65 mm), raising the possibility that this technique may be difficult to use in obese patients or those with ascites. This examination suffers from many of the same issues as found for fibrosis markers, and it turns out to be very good at excluding advanced fibrosis or no fibrosis, but it is not highly accurate at delineating precise degrees of intermediate fibrosis.

Finally, it would theoretically be desirable to utilize advances in the molecular understanding of liver fibrosis to image the liver. For example, the number of activated stellate cells, which reflects fibrogenic activity, might be specifically identified by tagging them with cell-specific markers.[174] Alternatively, matrix or matrix turnover could be labeled using molecular tools. Although such approaches are appealing, they remain experimental at present.

Tests of Liver Function

A variety of bona fide liver tests have been used to assess liver fibrosis and cirrhosis. Such tests generally measure advanced disease and several depend on perfusion, such as indocyanine green, sorbitol, and galactose clearance tests; other tests, such as the ^{13}C-galactose breath test and ^{13}C-aminopyrine breath test, depend on the functional capacity of the liver.[175,177] Another test, the MEGX test, which measures monoethylglycinexylidide (MEGX) formation after administration of lidocaine, depends upon the activity of hepatic cytochrome P-450 3A4 isoenzyme (which catalyzes oxidative N-deethylation of lidocaine to MEGX).[178] The MEGX test has a sensitivity and specificity in the 80% range for distinguishing chronic hepatitis from cirrhosis in comparison with standard liver tests.[178] Unfortunately, although the MEGX test and other function tests may predict prognosis in cirrhotic patients, they are insensitive for quantifying fibrosis in patients with less advanced disease.[175-177]

Hepatic Venous Pressure Gradient (HVPG)

Although perhaps not a classic marker of liver fibrosis, the HVPG in fact may be an excellent surrogate for fibrosis and the best marker of clinical prognosis. Several studies have now emphasized that its level appears to correlate with the degree of fibrosis, and moreover has important prognostic value, particularly in patients after liver transplantation.[179-182] HVPG may also be an excellent predictor of clinical prognosis and decompensation; in patients with clinical cirrhosis at baseline those with a baseline HVPG of <10 mm Hg had approximately a 15% chance of having a clinical decompensation event; however, those with an HVPG >10 mm Hg had approximately a 70% risk of an event.[183] Unfortunately, this test is not routinely performed and considerable expertise is required to obtain accurate measurements.

Liver Biopsy

Percutaneous liver biopsy has traditionally been considered to be the "gold standard" test to measure fibrosis. Although there is great experience with liver biopsy, this procedure is time-consuming, inconvenient, uncomfortable, and invasive, and it makes both patients and physicians anxious. Furthermore, liver biopsy can be associated with substantial sampling error.[147] In a recent study in which 124 patients with chronic HCV infection underwent laparoscopic-guided biopsy of the right and left hepatic lobes, 33.1% had a difference of at least 1 histologic stage (modified Scheuer system) between the 2 lobes.[184] Furthermore, in 18 study subjects, a stage consistent with cirrhosis was found in 1 lobe, whereas stage 3 fibrosis was reported in the other. Finally, in 10% of subjects, stage 0-2 disease was identified in one lobe whereas stage 3-4 fibrosis was found in the other. In another study of patients with fatty liver disease, similar variability has been reported.[185]

There are several other limitations of liver biopsy. Quantitation of fibrosis in biopsies is subject to significant interobserver variation. In chronic hepatitis C, for example, standardized grading systems including Knodell, Metavir, Scheuer, or Ishak are concordant in only 70% to 80% of samples. Specimen quality is very important, with smaller samples leading to an underestimation of disease severity.[186] A recent study created digitized virtual image biopsy specimens of varying length from large liver sections, and revealed that 75% of 25-mm biopsy specimens were correctly classified using the Metavir staging system, compared with only 65% for biopsies 15 mm in length.[187] Interestingly, a recent study noted that the experience of the pathologist may have more influence on interobserver agreement than specimen length.[188]

Another major problem with using liver biopsy or serum markers to quantitate fibrosis is that all of the currently utilized grading systems use a simple linear numeric scoring approach, implying they represent linear changes in fibrosis content. Such an inference is likely to be inaccurate, because Metavir stage 4 fibrosis does not represent twice as much fibrosis as stage 2 fibrosis, but rather a much greater difference, perhaps 5- to 20-fold.

Treatment of Fibrosis

Treatment of liver fibrosis by itself has remained somewhat of an enigma. Although therapies directed at the underlying disease process (see following sections) have clearly emerged as effectively blocking, preventing, and even reversing fibrosis, a specific antifibrotic drug is still not available. That is to say, despite significant advances in the understanding of the basic mechanisms underlying fibrosis, a "silver bullet" antifibrotic remains elusive. The reasons underlying this are multifactorial and complex. First, although there are impressive data in animal models, it is likely that there are in fact differences between animal models and humans. Second, most if not all trials examining antifibrotic agents in humans have been of short duration (months) in comparison with the time that is required for the development of cirrhosis (years). Finally, as highlighted earlier in this chapter, the tools with which to measure fibrosis are problematic. Introduction of accurate and reliable measures of fibrosis will facilitate development of antifibrotic therapies.

Notwithstanding the lack of a specific antifibrotic compound available for clinical use, it is important to recognize that fibrosis itself appears to be a clinical end point. For example, several recent studies have now emphasized the importance of fibrosis—and its treatment—in clinical outcomes. In 1050 patients with compensated chronic hepatitis C who had failed combination peginterferon and ribavirin with generally advanced fibrosis, the 6-year cumulative incidence of first clinical decompensation event or hepatocellular cancer was 5.6% for stage 2, 16.1% for stage 3, 19.3% for stage 4, 37.8% for stage 5, and 49.3% for stage 6.[189] Patients with advanced fibrosis after liver transplantation for HCV were found to develop clinical complications at a higher rate than patients without advanced fibrosis.[179] In other studies in patients with HCV and advanced fibrosis or histologic cirrhosis who were sustained virologic responders, outcomes were improved.[190-193] Additionally, in HBV patients with advanced fibrosis or cirrhosis, continuous treatment with lamivudine significantly reduced the incidence of hepatic decompensation and the risk of hepatocellular carcinoma[34] (although actual histologic fibrosis was not measured, other studies have clearly demonstrated a reduction in fibrosis and even reversion of cirrhosis in HBV patients; see following text).

Therapies Directed at the Underlying Disease Process

The most effective antifibrotic therapies are currently those that treat or remove the underlying stimulus to fibrogenesis (**Table 5-3**). In many forms of liver disease, treatment of the underlying inciting lesion leads to improvement in fibrosis (**Table 5-4**), including its reversal (**Fig. 5-6**). Indeed, the data supporting this notion are now compelling. For example, eradication or inhibition of HBV[32,33,194,195] or HCV[43] leads to reversion of fibrosis, even in patients with histologic cirrhosis. Fibrosis reverts in patients with hemochromatosis during iron depletion,[196,197] in patients with autoimmune hepatitis after corticosteroid therapy,[196,197] and in patients with secondary biliary cirrhosis after decompression of bile duct obstruction.[44] In patients with NASH, weight loss and improvement in the metabolic syndrome lead to improvement in hepatic histologic results, including fibrosis,[38] whereas peroxisomal proliferator activated receptor (PPAR) γ-agonists may reduce both steatosis and fibrosis.[198-200]

Antifibrotic Therapies

Specific therapy for treatment of liver fibrosis is attractive because the scarring response leads to many if not all of the complications of chronic liver disease—in particular, impaired synthetic function, liver failure, and perhaps hepatocellular cancer. Fibrosis, particularly in its advanced

Table 5-3 Approaches to Treat Liver Fibrosis

APPROACH*	EXAMPLE
Remove injurious agent	Eradication of HBV or HCV
Antiinflammatory agents	Corticosteroids in AIH
Antioxidants	PPC in alcoholic hepatitis
Cytoprotective agents	Ursodeoxycholic acid
Inhibit stellate cell activation	Interferon-γ
Inhibit stellate cell activation phenotypes (fibrogenesis)	Colchicine

*Some approaches have not been demonstrated to be successful.
AIH, autoimmune hepatitis; PPC, polyenylphosphatidylcholine

Table 5-4 Diseases and Therapies in Which There Is Strong Evidence that Treatment Reduces Liver Fibrosis

DISEASE	THERAPY
Hepatitis B	Lamivudine
Hepatitis C	Interferon-α*
Bile duct obstruction	Surgical decompression
Autoimmune hepatitis	Corticosteroids
Hemochromatosis	Iron depletion
Alcoholic hepatitis	Corticosteroids

*Or PEG-interferon-α, with or without ribavirin.

stage, may also contribute to portal hypertension by preventing blood flow through the liver. Although attempts have been made previously to specifically treat the "fibrosis" component of liver disease, these approaches have generally been unsuccessful. Thus there remains a major unmet need for novel and effective antifibrotic therapy in patients in whom the underlying disease/lesion is not treatable. Advances in elucidating the pathogenesis of fibrosis have led to renewed efforts in this area. Additionally, data indicating that fibrosis is reversible have helped fuel this effort.

In addition, preclinical and human clinical studies have highlighted a number of therapies that may abrogate fibrogenesis without affecting the underlying disease by targeting specific steps in the fibrogenic response. Antiinflammatory therapies have been based on the knowledge that inflammation drives the fibrogenic cascade. Some treatments have attempted to inhibit cellular injury or have focused on stellate cell activation, whereas others have targeted collagen synthesis and matrix deposition. The following section highlights human studies in these areas.

Antiinflammatory Compounds

Many liver diseases such as HCV have an important inflammatory component. Inflammation in these disorders typically drives stellate cell activation and fibrogenesis, and these

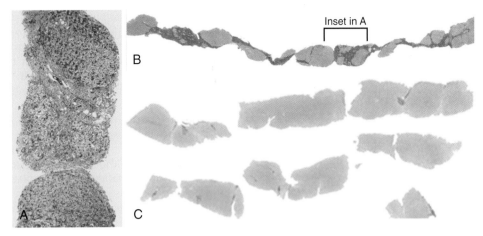

Fig. 5-6 Reversal of fibrosis. An example of reversal of advanced fibrosis (cirrhosis in this situation) is depicted. A liver biopsy before lamivudine treatment is shown *(upper panel and left panel)*. After treatment with lamivudine, liver biopsy was repeated, and shows almost complete dissolution of fibrosis. Data similar to these have been published in autoimmune liver disease, hepatitis C, alcoholic hepatitis, hepatitis B, and others. *(Reprinted with permission from Wanless IR, Nakashima E, Sherman M. Regression of human cirrhosis: morphologic futures and the genesis of incomplete septal cirrhosis. Arch Pathol Lab Med 2001;124:1599–1607.)*

diseases in particular have been studied in order to evaluate the efficacy of antiinflammatory drugs.

Corticosteroids

Classic examples of the benefits of steroids include the improvements seen in patients with autoimmune hepatitis and alcoholic hepatitis. It could be argued that these two diseases are driven largely by inflammation, and thus the antiinflammatory action of steroids serves to treat the underlying process. Notwithstanding, in patients with autoimmune hepatitis who respond to medical treatment (prednisone or equivalent), advanced fibrosis and cirrhosis are reversible.[45] Fibrosis may improve in patients with alcoholic liver disease who respond to corticosteroids.[201,202] Thus corticosteroids appear to have antifibrotic effects in patients with certain liver disorders.

Interleukin-10

Interleukin-10 (IL-10) has both antiinflammatory and immunosuppressive effects. IL-10 has been shown to reduce production of proinflammatory cytokines, such as TNF-α, IL-1, IFN-γ, and IL-2 from T cells. These cytokines belong to the TH1 family. Endogenous IL-10 reduces the intrahepatic inflammatory response, shifts the cytokine milieu toward a TH2 predominance, and reduces fibrosis in several in vivo models of liver injury.[203] A preliminary study was conducted of 30 patients with advanced HCV-mediated fibrosis who had failed standard IFN-α–based antiviral therapy and therefore received a 12-month treatment trial of subcutaneous IL-10 administered daily or three times per week. The results of this study revealed that although many patients had a reduction in hepatic inflammation and fibrosis score, serum HCV RNA levels increased during therapy.[204] For this reason, it has not been pursued as an antifibrotic compound because of putative detrimental virologic effects.

TNF Inhibitors

Because TNF-α amplifies inflammation in many diseases, and because TNF-α is up-regulated in liver diseases such as alcoholic hepatitis, an anti–TNF-α compound should theoretically reduce inflammation and the stimulus for fibrosis.[205–208] This concept has been tested in patients with alcoholic hepatitis, a condition believed to be primarily driven by inflammation; therefore these patients are considered ideal candidates for antiinflammatory treatment. Unfortunately, a recent study demonstrated that administration of the TNF-α neutralizing molecule etanercept to patients with moderate to severe alcoholic hepatitis was associated with a significantly higher death rate at 6 months than placebo.[209] This study has for all intents led to the abandonment of such treatments for patients with alcoholic hepatitis.

Miscellaneous Antiinflammatory Drugs

A number of other antiinflammatory approaches have gained attention as therapies for fibrosis. Penicillamine is a heavy metal chelating compound that has been proposed to have antiinflammatory and thus antifibrogenic effects.[210] However, this compound had no effect on fibrogenesis in patients with primary biliary cirrhosis.[211,212]

Methothrexate is thought to have antiinflammatory properties but, interestingly, has typically been considered to be profibrogenic in the liver for patients receiving methotrexate for treatment of rheumatologic diseases[213] (however, it is noteworthy that the risk of fibrosis progression may be less prominent than typically believed[213,214]). Methotrexate has been studied in patients with primary biliary cirrhosis. Although some investigators have reported highly favorable effects in this disease, including improvement of the disease and reversion of fibrosis,[215] the majority of the data on methotrexate have either been negative[216,217] or show that methotrexate's effects have been marginal, either alone[216] or in combination with ursodeoxycholic acid.[218]

Antioxidant Agents

Oxidative stress is thought to play an important role in injury, stellate cell activation, and stimulation of extracellular matrix production as described previously. Thus a wide variety of antioxidants have received attention as potential antifibrotics.

Vitamin E

Vitamin E is a lipid-soluble antioxidant that presumably protects cell membranes from oxidative injury, although the precise mechanism by which this occurs is unknown. Vitamin E has been studied in animal models[219] as well as in humans.[220-223] The vitamin E precursor D-α-tocopherol (1200 IU/day for 8 weeks) was shown to inhibit stellate cell activation in six patients with hepatitis C virus infection who failed to respond to interferon therapy. No affect on fibrosis was observed.[220] A randomized controlled trial examined the effect of vitamin E in patients with mild to moderate alcoholic hepatitis and found that vitamin E reduced serum hyaluronic acid levels, but did not lead to a change in type III collagen.[222] Finally, in a large randomized controlled trial including 247 adults with nonalcoholic steatohepatitis and without diabetes, vitamin E at a dose of 800 IU daily for 96 weeks led to a reduction in serum AST/ALT levels compared with placebo (P < 0.001), as well as reductions in hepatic steatosis (P = 0.005) and lobular inflammation (P = 0.02) but no improvement in fibrosis scores (P = 0.24).[224] Combined antioxidant therapy, including vitamin E, had no effect on outcome in patients with severe alcoholic hepatitis, although fibrosis was not specifically addressed.[223]

Silymarin

Silymarin is derived from the milk thistle *Silybum marianum*. This milk thistle extract has been shown to reduce lipid peroxidation and inhibit fibrogenesis in rodent animal models,[225,226] as well as in baboons.[227] It has been tested in several carefully performed human clinical trials, although fibrosis was not used as an end point. The compound has been found to be safe, but reportedly has mixed effects.[228,229] In one study examining silymarin use in alcoholics,[228] mortality was reduced; patients with early stages of cirrhosis also appeared to benefit. However, in another study in alcoholics, no survival benefit could be identified.[229] In both of these trials, silymarin appeared to be safe. Thus, although the agent is safe and is commonly used by patients with fibrosing liver disease, there is limited evidence of efficacy. Notwithstanding, because of its record of safety, studies of silymarin in patients with NASH or in those who have failed conventional antiviral treatment for HCV infection (*http://clinicaltrials.gov/*; Clinical Trials.gov Identifiers NCT00680407 and NCT00680342, respectively) have begun. Although fibrosis is not a primary outcome measure, histologic analyses are planned, and thus information about the effect of silymarin on liver fibrosis should be forthcoming.

Polyenylphosphatidylcholine

Polyenylphosphatidylcholine is a mixture of polyunsaturated phosphatidylcholine, extracted from soybeans. This compound has antioxidant properties, and oxidant stress is believed to be important in the inflammatory and fibrogenic response to injury, particularly in alcoholic liver disease. Because oxidative stress leads to lipid peroxidation, and lipid peroxidation is injurious at the level of the cell membrane, phosphatidylcholine has been proposed to be protective of injury to cell membranes, resulting in reduced cellular injury and fibrogenesis.[230]

A VA cooperative multicenter clinical trial examined the effect of polyenylphosphatidylcholine in 789 patients with alcoholic hepatitis who had extensive average alcohol intake (16 drinks/day).[231] Although subjects were randomized to either polyenylphosphatidylcholine or placebo for 2 years, the study failed to demonstrate an improvement in the treatment group. Notably, many subjects substantially reduced their ethanol consumption during the trial, which probably accounted for improvement in fibrosis in the control group, making it difficult to demonstrate an improvement in fibrosis in the polyenylphosphatidylcholine group. Results from a subsequent study examining the effect of polyenylphosphatidylcholine in patients with HCV are expected (*http://clinicaltrials.gov/*; Clinical Trials.gov Identifier NCT00211848).

Other Antioxidants

Malotilate is another potential cytoprotective agent, perhaps acting via inhibition of cytochrome P-450 2E1; in addition, this compound may have antiinflammatory properties. Although malotilate was found to diminish plasma cell and lymphocytic infiltrate and piecemeal necrosis in patients with primary biliary cirrhosis, it had no significant effect on fibrogenesis.[232]

Another agent used to antagonize oxidative stress is *S*-adenosylmethionine; this compound is important in the synthesis of the antioxidant glutathione. The enzyme responsible for its synthesis (methionine adenosyltransferase) is reduced in the injured liver[233]; thus it has been hypothesized that if *S*-adenosylmethionine was replaced, then injury and fibrogenesis might be slowed. *S*-Adenosylmethionine has been tested in a large randomized trial in patients with alcoholic cirrhosis.[234] There was an improvement in overall mortality/need for liver transplantation in the treatment arm, especially in patients with Child's A/B cirrhosis, although histologic assessment of fibrosis was not specifically measured.[234]

Propylthiouracil is an antithyroid drug that reacts with some of the oxidizing species derived from the respiratory burst and thus may be protective in alcoholic liver disease, a disease in which an increase in hepatic oxygen consumption may predispose the liver to ischemic injury. Thus propylthiouracil has been tested in a number of randomized clinical trials in patients with alcoholic liver disease. Unfortunately, a systematic review and meta-analysis found that propylthiouracil had no beneficial effect on fibrosis or on any other outcome measured.[235]

Cytoprotective Agents
Ursodeoxycholic Acid

Ursodeoxycholic acid binds to hepatocyte membranes, where it presumably stabilizes them and is thus cytoprotective. Such cytoprotective action theoretically reduces inflammation and may in turn have a beneficial effect on fibrogenesis.[236] Although the compound has been examined extensively, to date neither experimental data nor human studies indicate that ursodeoxycholic acid has a primary antifibrotic effect in the liver.[237-245]

Ursodeoxycholic acid has been studied in patients with a variety of liver diseases, including cystic fibrosis, primary biliary injury (primary biliary cirrhosis, primary sclerosing cholangitis, and progressive familial intrahepatic cholestasis), and miscellaneous liver diseases. Results with ursodeoxycholic acid in these conditions have been mixed. Both symptomatic and biochemical improvement have been observed in these diseases, in particular the biliary diseases; however, data on histologic improvement (and survival) have not been consistent. For example, in a randomized controlled trial in patients with primary biliary cirrhosis, ursodeoxycholic acid led to reduced fibrosis in those with mild disease, but had no effect on those with severe disease.[238] In another study survival was improved in patients treated with ursodeoxycholic acid, but fibrosis was not improved.[242] A combined analysis of the histologic effect of ursodeoxycholic acid on paired liver biopsies, including a total of 367 patients (200 ursodeoxycholic acid and 167 placebo), revealed that subpopulations of patients with initial early stages may benefit from therapy.[244] Results of meta-analyses examining ursodeoxycholic acid have been mixed, and have largely reported that ursodeoxycholic acid is not effective in primary biliary cirrhosis.[241] The aggregate data suggest that ursodeoxycholic acid may impede progression of fibrosis in primary biliary cirrhosis via effects on (bile duct) inflammation, particularly if administered early in the disease course. It should be emphasized that according to current data, ursodeoxycholic acid is extremely safe. Thus the available data justify its use in patients with primary biliary cirrhosis, including potentially as an antifibrotic.

Ursodeoxycholic acid has also been studied in children with progressive familial intrahepatic cholestasis,[239] in whom it appeared to improve fibrogenesis. Additionally, a small series indicated that 7 of 10 patients with cystic fibrosis treated with ursodeoxycholic acid had a reduction in liver fibrosis.[240] Although these effects are promising, it should be emphasized that the number of patients studied has been small. Finally, in a large randomized controlled trial of ursodeoxycholic acid in patients with non-alcoholic steatohepatitis that was conducted over 2 years, including 107 subjects who had paired biopsy data, there was no improvement in fibrosis.[245]

Miscellaneous Agents

Anabolic-androgenic steroids such as oxandrolone have been examined in randomized trials including patients with alcoholic liver disease, but have not been found to have significant effects on fibrosis (or other outcomes).[246]

Stellate Cell–Specific Compounds
Interferon-γ

A wealth of data support the antifibrotic potential of IFN-γ as an antifibrotic, in a variety of parenchymal organ diseases. The interferons consist of a family of three major isoforms. The three isoforms—α, β, and γ—are unique, not only in structure but also in their biologic actions. IFN-α and IFN-β bind to the same receptor whereas IFN-γ binds to a different receptor. IFN-α has more potent antiviral effects than does IFN-γ, whereas IFN-γ has been shown to specifically inhibit extracellular matrix synthesis in isolated cells, including stellate cells.[247,248] IFN-γ potently inhibits multiple aspects of stellate cell activation.[247,248] IFN-γ appears to have antifibrotic effects in patients with pulmonary fibrosis.[249] Such data have generated considerable enthusiasm about the use of IFN-γ in patients with hepatic fibrosis, although there is theoretical concern about its use because it is proinflammatory and, moreover, its overexpression in the liver leads to chronic hepatitis.[250] Nonetheless, it has now been tested in humans with fibrosing liver disease and appears to be safe.[251] Although this initial pilot study provided a firm foundation for use of this compound, and additionally underscored the potential of IFN-γ in humans with fibrosing liver disease, a larger study failed to demonstrate a therapeutic benefit, possibly because patients with advanced disease were studied and because the duration of therapy was too short.[252]

Peroxisome Proliferator Activated Receptor Agonists

Stellate cells possess each of the three major classes of PPAR.[253] Furthermore, the PPARs appear to be regulated during injury and stellate cell activation. PPAR-γ in particular is notable in that it is markedly down-regulated during activation.[254,255] Reversal of this reduction in PPAR-γ expression reverses the activated phenotype, in vitro or in vivo.[253] Furthermore, despite the fact that PPAR-γ is down-regulated, stimulation of this receptor with PPAR-γ ligands also reverses the activation process and phenotype.[255-258] In addition, PPAR-γ ligands, when administered to rats undergoing experimental liver injury, prevent fibrogenesis.[253,258,259]

Although the precise molecular mechanism(s) responsible for the effect of PPAR-γ ligands on stellate cells remain(s) controversial, preliminary data with a specific PPAR-γ agonist, GW570, demonstrated that it had significant effects on stellate cells[260] and led to a large clinical trial in patients with hepatitis C–induced fibrosis.[261] In this study patients with fibrosis of Ishak stages 2 to 4 (n = 265) were randomly assigned to groups given once-daily doses of 0.5 or 1.0 mg GW570 (also known as farglitazar) or placebo for 52 weeks. There were no significant differences between treatment groups in the ranked assessment of fibrosis score or Ishak stage on paired biopsy specimens. Furthermore, there was an increase in expression of smooth muscle α-actin and collagen during the treatment period. These data suggested that in patients with chronic hepatitis C and moderate fibrosis, 52 weeks of treatment with farglitazar did not affect stellate cell activation or fibrosis.

The Renin-Angiotensin System (RAS)

The angiotensin II system is an attractive antifibrotic target given the accessibility of clinically available compounds as well as the extensive experimental evidence pointing to a role for angiotensin II in the injured liver; furthermore, angiotensin II appears to directly stimulate stellate cell activation and fibrogenesis.[262,263] A number of studies have also demonstrated specific antifibrotic effects of angiotensin II inhibition in a variety of animal models.[264-266] Given its vasoactive actions, angiotensin II may also play a role in the pathogenesis of portal hypertension,[93] making its inhibition particularly attractive not only for use as an antifibrotic agent but also for treatment of portal hypertension.

To date, the angiotensin system has been evaluated in humans in small numbers of patients.[267-271] Human studies have examined the effects of angiotensin receptor blockers primarily in the setting of advanced liver disease—and most often in an attempt to reduce portal pressure (HVPG). The data to date in humans have been highly mixed, with some studies suggesting that blocking angiotensin II reduces HVPG and others showing limited effectiveness.

Given the particularly supportive preclinical data, the evidence suggests that there is likely to be some element of antifibrotic effect in humans when the angiotensin system is antagonized. Larger and longer studies appear to be warranted; many studies have recently been completed, are currently underway, or are planned (see *http://clinicaltrials.gov/*; Clinical Trials.gov Identifiers NCT00990639, NCT00298714, NCT00265642, NCT01051219).

Compounds That Inhibit Fibrogenesis

Colchicine

Colchicine is a plant alkaloid that inhibits polymerization of microtubules, a process that in turn is believed to be required for collagen secretion. On the basis of this concept, colchicine has been advanced as an antifibrotic agent. A sizeable body of literature indicates that colchicine has antifibrotic properties in experimental animal models.[272] This work has led to a number of human clinical trials.[273-276] A wide variety of liver diseases have been studied and include the following: (1) primary biliary cirrhosis, (2) alcoholic cirrhosis, (3) cryptogenic cirrhosis, and (4) miscellaneous other liver diseases. In a double blind, randomized, controlled trial examining colchicine in primary biliary cirrhosis, improvements were noted in a number of biochemical markers, but colchicine failed to reduce fibrosis.[273] In an often-cited, double-blind, randomized controlled trial of colchicine versus placebo in patients with various liver diseases, colchicine led to improved fibrosis as well as a dramatic improvement in survival.[274] However, this study has been extended to clinical practice with great caution because of a variety of methodologic concerns. First, many patients were lost to follow-up, and second, there was substantial unexplained excess mortality in the control group (unrelated to liver disease). A recent large VA cooperative multicenter study involving 549 patients compared colchicine (0.6 mg orally two times a day) with placebo in patients with alcoholic liver disease. Results showed that there was no apparent effect of active treatment on survival. Histologic data, which might have provided information on the antiinflammatory effects of colchicine, were not obtained.[275] A meta-analysis including 1138 subjects found that colchicine had no effect on hepatic fibrosis or mortality.[276] In summary, the data surrounding colchicine suggest that this compound is safe but is likely to be ineffective.

Future Antifibrotics

Given the major effort devoted to understanding the biology of hepatic fibrogenesis, it is not surprising that multiple pathways have been targeted as having therapeutic potential. Many compounds have been studied in experimental models and have been shown to have antifibrotic properties, including

Table 5-5 New Potential Antifibrotic Targets in Humans

AGENT	COMMENTS
Anti-TGF-β	Blocks stellate cell fibrogenesis
Anti-PDGF	Blocks stellate cell proliferation
Interferon-γ	Inhibits multiple features of stellate cell activation
PPAR ligands	? Stellate cell–specific effects

PDGF, platelet-derived growth factor; PPAR, peroxisome proliferator–activated receptor; TGF, transforming growth factor.

several with great potential for the treatment of human liver disease (**Table 5-5**).

Several important pathways merit discussion. One of the most important examples is the TGF-β pathway, because it plays a central role in the fibrogenic cascade. Several approaches to inhibit the action of TGF-β have been proposed and include use of molecules such as decorin (the protein core component of proteoglycan), which binds and inactivates TGF-β[277]; antibodies directed against TGF-β1; and soluble receptors, which typically encode for sequences that bind active TGF-β and prevent it from binding to its cognate receptors. The concept has been well established experimentally; indeed, the effect of inhibition of TGF-β in animal models of liver injury and fibrogenesis has been striking.[278,279] A limitation of approaches that target TGF-β is that TGF-β potently inhibits cellular proliferation, and inhibition of its effects in vivo could predispose to malignant transformation.

Another critical pathway involves PDGF. PDGF is the most potent stellate cell mitogen known[92,280] and additionally stimulates stellate cell migration.[281] A number of approaches have been used to inhibit the effect of PDGF. For example, kinase inhibitors that specifically inhibit PDGF signaling might be useful,[282] as could those with more general effects on tyrosine kinase receptors.

Additionally, stellate cells express endothelin receptors and their cognate ligands appear to be overproduced in the liver; furthermore, stimulation of stellate cells with their respective ligands leads to stellate cell activation.[93] A large body of evidence indicates that endothelin antagonism in the liver effectively inhibits fibrosis.[283] Thus, although inhibition of endothelin signaling may be clinically beneficial, studies in humans have not been undertaken.

Endotoxin or lipopolysaccharide (LPS), found on the outer wall of gram-negative bacteria, has received renewed attention lately. Studies performed many years ago suggested a role for LPS in the development of liver fibrosis.[284] More recently, studies in TLR4-deficient mice (TLR4 is the receptor for LPS) revealed that these mice are resistant to liver fibrosis, providing mechanistic insight into the TLR4-LPS pathway as a potential target for treatment of liver fibrosis.[102]

Angiogenesis appears to be important in liver fibrosis and may be important in the fibrogenic response. In one study, angiopoietin 1, an angiogenic cytokine important in angiogenesis, was found to be expressed by activated stellate cells. Moreover, when its signaling was blocked with an adenovirus expressing the extracellular domain of Tie2 (the cognate receptor for angiopoietin), angiogenesis and liver fibrosis induced by either CCl$_4$ or bile duct ligation were abrogated.[285] Additionally, sunitinib, a multitargeted receptor tyrosine kinase inhibitor, decreased hepatic vascular density, smooth muscle α-actin expression abundance, and fibrosis in cirrhotic rats,[286] suggesting that antiangiogenic factors could have direct effects on stellate cells.

As discussed previously, it appears that many different types of cells are involved in the pathogenesis of fibrosis. An area of great interest has focused on the possibility that bone marrow cells could play a role in either potentiating or inhibiting liver fibrosis. In one study, bone marrow cells administered to mice after established (total, 8 weeks) CCl$_4$-induced fibrosis led to reduced liver fibrosis and a significantly improved survival rate.[287] Follow-up study has begun to investigate the mechanisms underlying this effect, suggesting activation of MMP-9,[288] and possibly a direct effect on stellate cells. A limited number of data in humans suggest that such cell-based therapy may have profound effects in patients with cirrhosis.[289,290]

Miscellaneous Compounds

Among other agents, compounds such as pirfenidone,[291] halofuginone,[292] and farnesoid X receptor agonists appear to have direct effects on stellate cells and thus could evolve into effective antifibrotic compounds. Many others have been highlighted (see Rockey[293] for a review), and many are under investigation in humans (see *http://clinicaltrials.gov/*; Clinical Trials.gov Identifiers NCT00854087, NCT00119119, NCT00956098).

Summary and Future Directions for Antifibrotic Therapy

The wealth of new information about the pathogenesis of fibrogenesis has spawned a field dedicated to antifibrotics that is largely, but not entirely, focused on the activation of hepatic stellate cells. Stellate cell activation is characterized by a number of important features including enhanced matrix synthesis and a prominent contractile phenotype—processes that contribute to the dysfunction of the liver typically found in advanced disease. It should be emphasized that factors controlling activation are multifactorial, and thus multiple potential therapeutic interventions are possible. A further critical concept is that fibrosis, in particular the extracellular matrix component of fibrosis, is dynamic. Thus it is likely that fibrosis, including even advanced fibrosis, may be reversible under the appropriate conditions. Indeed, evidence from both animal and human studies supports this contention. Currently, effective therapy for hepatic fibrogenesis exists for several diseases in which the cause of the underlying disease is removed. In contrast, clearly effective therapy directed only at the fibrotic lesion is not currently available; the most effective therapies will most likely be directed at the stellate cell. However, given the multiple potential targets that have been identified, it is highly likely that specific, effective, safe, and inexpensive candidates will emerge.

Key References

Aithal GP, et al. Randomized, placebo-controlled trial of pioglitazone in nondiabetic subjects with nonalcoholic steatohepatitis. Gastroenterology 2008; 135:1176–1184. (Ref.200)

Asai K, et al. Activated hepatic stellate cells overexpress p75NTR after partial hepatectomy and undergo apoptosis on nerve growth factor stimulation. Liver Int 2006;26:595–603. (Ref.135)

Belfort R, et al. A placebo-controlled trial of pioglitazone in subjects with nonalcoholic steatohepatitis. New Engl J Med 2006;355:2297–2307. (Ref.199)

Blasco A, et al. Hepatic venous pressure gradient identifies patients at risk of severe hepatitis C recurrence after liver transplantation. Hepatology 2006;43: 492–499. (Ref.179)

Boetticher NC, et al. A randomized, double-blinded, placebo-controlled multicenter trial of etanercept in the treatment of alcoholic hepatitis. Gastroenterology 2008;135:1953–1960. (Ref.209)

Bourd-Boittin K, et al. CX3CL1/fractalkine shedding by human hepatic stellate cells: contribution to chronic inflammation in the liver. J Cell Mol Med 2009; 13:1526–1535. (Ref.104)

Buck M, Chojkier M. A ribosomal S-6 kinase-mediated signal to C/EBP-beta is critical for the development of liver fibrosis. PLoS One 2007;2:e1372. (Ref.91)

Cao S, et al. Neuropilin-1 promotes cirrhosis of the rodent and human liver by enhancing PDGF/TGF-beta signaling in hepatic stellate cells. J Clin Invest 2010;120:2379–2394. (Ref.95)

Chakraborty JB, Mann DA. NF-kappaB signalling: embracing complexity to achieve translation. J Hepatol 2010;52:285–291. (Ref.89)

Cheung O, Sanyal AJ. Recent advances in nonalcoholic fatty liver disease. Curr Opin Gastroenterol 2009;25:230–237. (Ref.131)

Choi SS, Diehl AM. Epithelial-to-mesenchymal transitions in the liver. Hepatology 2009;50:2007–2013. (Ref.88)

Connolly MK, et al. In liver fibrosis, dendritic cells govern hepatic inflammation in mice via TNF-alpha. J Clin Invest 2009;119:3213–3225. (Ref.120)

Debernardi-Venon W, et al. AT1 receptor antagonist Candesartan in selected cirrhotic patients: effect on portal pressure and liver fibrosis markers. J Hepatol 2007;46:1026–1033. (Ref.271)

Deveaux V, et al. Cannabinoid CB2 receptor potentiates obesity-associated inflammation, insulin resistance and hepatic steatosis. PLoS One 2009;4:e5844. (Ref.114)

Dooley S, et al. Hepatocyte-specific Smad7 expression attenuates TGF-beta-mediated fibrogenesis and protects against liver damage. Gastroenterology 2008;135:642–659. (Ref.101)

Dranoff JA, Wells RG. Portal fibroblasts: underappreciated mediators of biliary fibrosis. Hepatology 2010;51:1438–1444. (Ref.66)

Ebrahimkhani MR, Elsharkawy AM, Mann DA. Wound healing and local neuroendocrine regulation in the injured liver. Expert Rev Mol Med 2008; 10:e11. (Ref.110)

Farrell GC, Larter CZ. Nonalcoholic fatty liver disease: from steatosis to cirrhosis. Hepatology 2006;43:S99–S112. (Ref.36)

Fernandez M, et al. Angiogenesis in liver disease. J Hepatol 2009;50:604–620. (Ref.58)

Friedman SL. Mechanisms of hepatic fibrogenesis. Gastroenterology 2008;134: 1655–1669. (Ref.57)

Friedman SL. Evolving challenges in hepatic fibrosis. Nat Rev Gastroenterol Hepatol 2010;7:425–436. (Ref.71)

Friedman SL, Wei S, Blaner WS. Retinol release by activated rat hepatic lipocytes: regulation by Kupffer cell-conditioned medium and PDGF. Am J Physiol 1993; 264:G947–G952. (Ref.105)

Fritz D, Stefanovic B. RNA-binding protein RBMS3 is expressed in activated hepatic stellate cells and liver fibrosis and increases expression of transcription factor Prx1. J Mol Biol 2007;371:585–595. (Ref.85)

Gao B, Radaeva S, Jeong WI. Activation of natural killer cells inhibits liver fibrosis: a novel strategy to treat liver fibrosis. Expert Rev Gastroenterol Hepatol 2007;1:173–180. (Ref.20)

Gao B, Radaeva S, Park O. Liver natural killer and natural killer T cells: immunobiology and emerging roles in liver diseases. J Leukocyte Biol 2009;86: 513–528. (Ref.117)

Guo CJ, et al. miR-15b and miR-16 are implicated in activation of the rat hepatic stellate cell: an essential role for apoptosis. J Hepatol 2009;50:766–778. (Ref.86)

Guo J, et al. Functional linkage of cirrhosis-predictive single nucleotide polymorphisms of Toll-like receptor 4 to hepatic stellate cell responses. Hepatology 2009;49:960–968. (Ref.122)

Hagens WI, et al. Cellular targeting of the apoptosis-inducing compound gliotoxin to fibrotic rat livers. J Pharmacol Exp Ther 2008;324:902–910. (Ref.138)

Henderson NC, Forbes SJ. Hepatic fibrogenesis: from within and outwith. Toxicology 2008;254:130–135. (Ref.100)

Henderson NC, Iredale JP. Liver fibrosis: cellular mechanisms of progression and resolution. Clin Sci (Lond) 2007;112:265–280. (Ref.53)

Hirose A, et al. Angiotensin II type 1 receptor blocker inhibits fibrosis in rat nonalcoholic steatohepatitis. Hepatology 2007;45:1375–1381. (Ref.265)

Holt AP, et al. Liver myofibroblasts regulate infiltration and positioning of lymphocytes in human liver. Gastroenterology 2009;136:705–714. (Ref.126)

Huang H, et al. Identification of two gene variants associated with risk of advanced fibrosis in patients with chronic hepatitis C. Gastroenterology 2006; 130:1679–1687. (Ref.15)

Huang H, et al. A 7 gene signature identifies the risk of developing cirrhosis in patients with chronic hepatitis C. Hepatology 2007;46:297–306. (Ref.16)

Ikejima K, et al. Role of adipocytokines in hepatic fibrogenesis. J Gastroenterol Hepatol 2007;22(Suppl 1):S87–S92. (Ref.109)

Inagaki Y, Okazaki I. Emerging insights into transforming growth factor beta Smad signal in hepatic fibrogenesis. Gut 2007;56:284–292. (Ref.103)

Iredale JP. Models of liver fibrosis: exploring the dynamic nature of inflammation and repair in a solid organ. J Clin Invest 2007;117:539–548. (Ref.133)

Ishikawa T, et al. Administration of fibroblast growth factor 2 in combination with bone marrow transplantation synergistically improves carbon-tetrachloride-induced liver fibrosis in mice. Cell Tissue Res 2007;327:463–470. (Ref.288)

Jiang JX, et al. Apoptotic body engulfment by hepatic stellate cells promotes their survival by the JAK/STAT and Akt/NF-kappaB-dependent pathways. J Hepatol 2009;51:139–148. (Ref.78)

Jin H, et al. Telmisartan prevents hepatic fibrosis and enzyme-altered lesions in liver cirrhosis rat induced by a choline-deficient L-amino acid-defined diet. Biochem Biophys Res Commun 2007;364:801–807. (Ref.266)

Kalambokis G, et al. Clinical outcome of HCV-related graft cirrhosis and prognostic value of hepatic venous pressure gradient. Transpl Int 2009;22: 172–181. (Ref.180)

Kendall TJ, et al. p75 Neurotrophin receptor signaling regulates hepatic myofibroblast proliferation and apoptosis in recovery from rodent liver fibrosis. Hepatology 2009;49:901–910. (Ref.116)

Khan AA, et al. Safety and efficacy of autologous bone marrow stem cell transplantation through hepatic artery for the treatment of chronic liver failure: a preliminary study. Transplant Proc 2008;40:1140–1144. (Ref.289)

Krizhanovsky V, et al. Senescence of activated stellate cells limits liver fibrosis. Cell 2008;134:657–667. (Ref.136)

Kumar M, et al. Hepatic venous pressure gradient as a predictor of fibrosis in chronic liver disease because of hepatitis B virus. Liver Int 2008;28:690–698. (Ref.181)

Lee TF, et al. Downregulation of hepatic stellate cell activation by retinol and palmitate mediated by adipose differentiation-related protein (ADRP). J Cell Physiol 2010;223:648–657. (Ref.106)

Liu X, et al. Resolution of nonalcoholic steatohepatits after gastric bypass surgery. Obes Surg 2007;17:486–492. (Ref.38)

Mallet V, et al. Brief communication: the relationship of regression of cirrhosis to outcome in chronic hepatitis C. Ann Intern Med 2008;149:399–403. (Ref.191)

Mann DA, Mann J. Epigenetic regulation of hepatic stellate cell activation. J Gastroenterol Hepatol 2008;23(Suppl 1):S108–S111. (Ref.84)

Mann DA, Marra F. Fibrogenic signalling in hepatic stellate cells. J Hepatol 2010; 52:949–950. (Ref.88)

Mann J, et al. MeCP2 controls an epigenetic pathway that promotes myofibroblast transdifferentiation and fibrosis. Gastroenterology 2010;138: 705–714, 14 e1–4. (Ref.83)

Mann J, Mann DA. Transcriptional regulation of hepatic stellate cells. Adv Drug Deliv Rev 2009;61:497–512. (Ref.81)

Mann J, et al. Regulation of myofibroblast transdifferentiation by DNA methylation and MeCP2: implications for wound healing and fibrogenesis. Cell Death Differ 2007;14:275–285. (Ref.82)

Marra F, Bertolani C. Adipokines in liver diseases. Hepatology 2009;50:957–969. (Ref.108)

Mayo MJ, et al. Prediction of clinical outcomes in primary biliary cirrhosis by serum enhanced liver fibrosis assay. Hepatology 2008;48:1549–1557. (Ref.160)

McCall-Culbreath KD, Zutter MM. Collagen receptor integrins: rising to the challenge. Curr Drug Targets 2008;9:139–149. (Ref.50)

Mencin A, Kluwe J, Schwabe RF. Toll-like receptors as targets in chronic liver diseases. Gut 2009;58:704–720. (Ref.123)

Miele L, et al. The Kruppel-like factor 6 genotype is associated with fibrosis in nonalcoholic fatty liver disease. Gastroenterology 2008;135:282–291 e1. (Ref.17)

Morgan TR, et al. Colchicine treatment of alcoholic cirrhosis: a randomized, placebo-controlled clinical trial of patient survival. Gastroenterology 2005; 128:882–890. (Ref.275)

Morra R, et al. Diagnostic value of serum protein profiling by SELDI-TOF ProteinChip compared with a biochemical marker, FibroTest, for the diagnosis of advanced fibrosis in patients with chronic hepatitis C. Aliment Pharmacol Ther 2007;26:847–858. (Ref.167)

Muhanna N, et al. Activation of hepatic stellate cells after phagocytosis of lymphocytes: a novel pathway of fibrogenesis. Hepatology 2008;48:963–977. (Ref.125)

Muir AJ, Sylvestre PB, Rockey DC. Interferon gamma-1b for the treatment of fibrosis in chronic hepatitis C infection. J Viral Hepat 2006;13:322–328. (Ref.251)

Munoz-Luque J, et al. Regression of fibrosis after chronic stimulation of cannabinoid CB2 receptor in cirrhotic rats. J Pharmacol Exp Ther 2008;324: 475–483. (Ref.113)

Nabeshima Y, et al. Anti-fibrogenic function of angiotensin II type 2 receptor in CCl4-induced liver fibrosis. Biochem Biophys Res Commun 2006;346: 658–664. (Ref.264)

Notas G, Kisseleva T, Brenner D. NK and NKT cells in liver injury and fibrosis. Clin Immunol 2009;130:16–26. (Ref.118)

Novo E, Parola M. Redox mechanisms in hepatic chronic wound healing and fibrogenesis. Fibrogenesis Tissue Repair 2008;1:5. (Ref.72)

Oakley F, et al. Angiotensin II activates I kappaB kinase phosphorylation of RelA at Ser 536 to promote myofibroblast survival and liver fibrosis. Gastroenterology 2009;136:2334–2344 e1. (Ref.90)

Parekh S, Anania FA. Abnormal lipid and glucose metabolism in obesity: implications for nonalcoholic fatty liver disease. Gastroenterology 2007;132: 2191–2207. (Ref.132)

Parola M, Pinzani M. Hepatic wound repair. Fibrogenesis Tissue Repair 2009;2:4. (Ref.73)

Passino MA, et al. Regulation of hepatic stellate cell differentiation by the neurotrophin receptor p75NTR. Science 2007;315:1853–1856. (Ref.115)

Patsenker E, et al. Pharmacological inhibition of integrin alphavbeta3 aggravates experimental liver fibrosis and suppresses hepatic angiogenesis. Hepatology 2009;50:1501–1511. (Ref.61)

Pockros PJ, et al. Final results of a double-blind, placebo-controlled trial of the antifibrotic efficacy of interferon-gamma1b in chronic hepatitis C patients with advanced fibrosis or cirrhosis. Hepatology 2007;45:569–578. (Ref.252)

Rachfal AW, Brigstock DR. Connective tissue growth factor (CTGF/CCN2) in hepatic fibrosis. Hepatol Res 2003;26:1–9. (Ref.98)

Radbill BD, et al. Loss of matrix metalloproteinase-2 amplifies murine toxin-induced liver fibrosis by upregulating collagen I expression. Dig Dis Sci 2010;56:406–416. (Ref.56)

Ramachandran P, Iredale JP. Reversibility of liver fibrosis. Ann Hepatol 2009;8:283–291. (Ref.52)

Rockey DC. Antifibrotic therapy in chronic liver disease. Clin Gastroenterol Hepatol 2005;3:95–107. (Ref.293)

Rockey DC. Noninvasive assessment of liver fibrosis and portal hypertension with transient elastography. Gastroenterology 2008;134:8–14. (Ref.171)

Rockey DC, et al. Liver biopsy. Hepatology 2009;49:1017–1044. (Ref.147)

Sebastiani G, et al. SAFE biopsy: a validated method for large-scale staging of liver fibrosis in chronic hepatitis C. Hepatology 2009;49:1821–1827. (Ref.159)

Seki E, Brenner DA. Toll-like receptors and adaptor molecules in liver disease: update. Hepatology 2008;48:322–335. (Ref.121)

Seki E, et al. CCR1 and CCR5 promote hepatic fibrosis in mice. J Clin Invest 2009;119:1858–1870. (Ref.96)

Seki E, et al. CCR2 promotes hepatic fibrosis in mice. Hepatology 2009;50: 185–197. (Ref.97)

Seki E, et al. TLR4 enhances TGF-beta signaling and hepatic fibrosis. Nat Med 2007;13:1324–1332. (Ref.102)

Semela D, et al. Platelet-derived growth factor signaling through ephrin-b2 regulates hepatic vascular structure and function. Gastroenterology 2008;135: 671–679. (Ref.94)

Shafiei MS, Rockey DC. The role of integrin-linked kinase in liver wound healing. J Biol Chem 2006;281:24863–24872. (Ref.62)

Silva R, et al. Integrins: the keys to unlocking angiogenesis. Arterioscler Thromb Vasc Biol 2008;28:1703–1713. (Ref.60)

Tam J, et al. Peripheral CB1 cannabinoid receptor blockade improves cardiometabolic risk in mouse models of obesity. J Clin Invest 2010;120: 2953–2966. (Ref.112)

Taura K, et al. Hepatic stellate cells secrete angiopoietin 1 that induces angiogenesis in liver fibrosis. Gastroenterology 2008;135:1729–1738. (Ref.285)

Teixeira-Clerc F, et al. CB1 cannabinoid receptor antagonism: a new strategy for the treatment of liver fibrosis. Nat Med 2006;12:671–676. (Ref.111)

Tugues S, et al. Antiangiogenic treatment with sunitinib ameliorates inflammatory infiltrate, fibrosis, and portal pressure in cirrhotic rats. Hepatology 2007;46:1919–1926. (Ref.286)

Veldt BJ, et al. Sustained virologic response and clinical outcomes in patients with chronic hepatitis C and advanced fibrosis. Ann Intern Med 2007;147: 677–684. (Ref.190)

Venugopal SK, et al. Liver fibrosis causes down-regulation of miRNA-150 and miRNA-194 in hepatic stellate cells and their over-expression causes decreased stellate cell activation. Am J Physiol Gastrointest Liver Physiol 2009;298: G101–G106. (Ref.87)

Wasmuth HE, et al. Antifibrotic effects of CXCL9 and its receptor CXCR3 in livers of mice and humans. Gastroenterology 2009;137:309–319, 19 e1–3. (Ref.107)

Watanabe A, et al. Inflammasome-mediated regulation of hepatic stellate cells. Am J Physiol Gastrointest Liver Physiol 2009;296:G1248–G1257. (Ref.124)

Watson MR, et al. NF-kappaB is a critical regulator of the survival of rodent and human hepatic myofibroblasts. J Hepatol 2008;48:589–597. (Ref.137)

Wells RG. The role of matrix stiffness in regulating cell behavior. Hepatology 2008;47:1394–1400. (Ref.140)

Yang L, et al. Regulation of peroxisome proliferator-activated receptor-gamma in liver fibrosis. Am J Physiol Gastrointest Liver Physiol 2006;291:G902–G911. (Ref.253)

Zaldivar MM, et al. CXC chemokine ligand 4 (Cxcl4) is a platelet-derived mediator of experimental liver fibrosis. Hepatology 2010;51:1345–1353. (Ref.79)

Zeisberg M, et al. Fibroblasts derive from hepatocytes in liver fibrosis via epithelial to mesenchymal transition. J Biol Chem 2007;282:23337–23347. (Ref.69)

Zhan SS, et al. Phagocytosis of apoptotic bodies by hepatic stellate cells induces NADPH oxidase and is associated with liver fibrosis in vivo. Hepatology 2006; 43:435–443. (Ref.77)

A complete list of references can be found at www.expertconsult.com.

Chapter 6

Replication of Hepatitis B Virus

Nadia Warner and Stephen Locarnini

ABBREVIATIONS

BCP basal core promoter
ccc covalently closed circular
EnhI enhancer I
EnhII enhancer II
ER endoplasmic reticulum
HBcAg hepatitis B core protein or antigen
HBeAg hepatitis B e antigen
HBsAg hepatitis B surface antigen

HBSP hepatitis B splice protein
HBx hepatitis B x protein
HBV hepatitis B virus
LHB large hepatitis B surface protein
MHB medium hepatitis B surface protein
MHR major hydrophilic region
MUB multivescular body
NA nucleos(t)ide analogue
NLS nuclear localization signal

nt nucleotide
pg pregenomic
Pol polymerase
RNase H ribonuclease H
rt reverse transcriptase
SHB small hepatitis B surface protein
SVP subviral particles

Introduction

Hepatitis B virus (HBV) is the prototype member of the Hepadnaviridae family, which is subdivided into the genera *Orthohepadnavirus,* which infect mammals (e.g., human HBV, ground squirrel HBV, woodchuck HBV), and *Avihepadnavirus,* members of which infect birds (e.g., Shanghai duck HBV, Ross goose HBV, China duck HBV, heron HBV). A maximum sequence divergence of 25% is found among the avihepadnaviruses, compared with 35% for orthohepadnaviruses.[1]

HBV is an enveloped virus containing a circular, partially double-stranded DNA genome. There are three types of viral-associated particles found in serum; the virion, spherical subviral particles (SVPs), and filamentous SVPs (**Fig. 6-1**). Only the HBV virion is infectious because the spherical particles and filaments do not contain the HBV genome. The HBV virion is 42 to 47 nm in diameter, and consists of an outer envelope containing the three envelope proteins surrounding an inner nucleocapsid composed of the hepatitis B core protein or antigen (HBc), which forms a capsid around the viral genome and associated polymerase. The spherical SVPs are 17 to 25 nm in diameter and can occur in large numbers up to 10^{13}/ml. The filamentous or tubular SVPs are approximately 20 to 22 nm in diameter and are of variable length.

Despite its small size, the HBV genome is complex. The HBV genome is only 3.2 kb in length; to compensate for this limited coding potential, the HBV DNA is organized into a series of overlapping and co-terminal reading frames (**Fig. 6-2**) that encode proteins that are either multi-functional or have very different functions in the HBV lifecycle (**Fig. 6-3**) despite sharing similar amino acid residues. Furthermore, HBV has evolved unique strategies for genomic replication (**Fig. 6-4**) and is unique among animal DNA viruses because it replicates via reverse transcription. It is the intricacies of this replication strategy that this review will highlight, as well as new systems that have been developed to facilitate research into HBV replication and pathogenesis.

HBV Genotypes and Classification

Human HBV can be subdivided into eight genotypes, designated A-H, which differ by 8% to 17% at the nucleotide level. An additional two genotypes; I and J, have also been proposed but are yet to be widely accepted. These eight major genotypes can be further classed into subgenotypes that differ by at least 4%.[2] Prototypic HBV has a genome length of 3215 base pairs (bp) with genotypic variation due to characteristic insertions or deletions. Genotype A has a 6 nucleotide (nt) insertion in the polymerase terminal protein/core region, genotype D has a 33 nt deletion in PreS1, genotypes E and G have 3 nt deletions in the polymerase spacer/PreS1 region, and genotype G has a

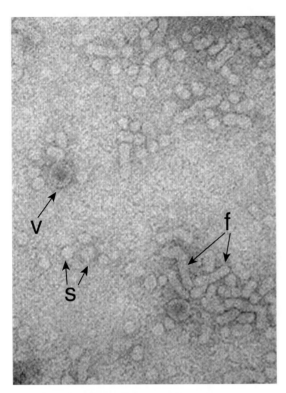

Fig. 6-1 Hepatitis B surface antigen (HBsAg). Electron micrograph of HBsAg secreted from hepatocytes showing virions (v), spherical (s), and filamentous (f) SVPs.

36 nt insertion in the core gene.[3] Different genotypes tend to have distinct geographic and ethnic distributions. Genotype A is common in parts of Africa, Europe, and North America; genotypes B and C are found predominantly throughout Asia. Genotype D has a vast distribution, but is mostly found in South Africa, India, parts of Europe, the Mediterranean basin, and Australia. Genotype E is mostly found in central Africa and South America, genotype F in South America, genotype G in Mexico, and genotype H in central America.[2] This geographic clustering is now starting to merge, reflecting the substantial population migrations that have occurred over the last 50 to 100 years. All HBV genotypes are present in Australia, with genotypes C and D being the most common. Recombinant genotypes have also been described, particularly between European genotypes A and D and Asian genotypes B and C.[4,5]

Differences in disease progression and selection of mutations exist among HBV genotypes. In general, genotype C HBV is associated with more severe liver disease than genotype B, and genotype D causes more severe liver disease than genotype A. The more severe genotypes C and D are also associated with a lower response to interferon therapy than genotypes A and B.[6] Differences in expression of viral products and cell stress also exist among genotypes, possibly contributing to disease severity.[7]

Historically, HBV has also been classified according to serologic subtypes, or serotypes, namely *adw, adr, ayw,* and *ayr.*[8] These are based on antibody reactivity to the amino acids at residues 122 and 160 in the S gene.[9-11] K122 confers *d* subtype whereas R122 confers *y* subtype. Similarly, K160 confers *w*

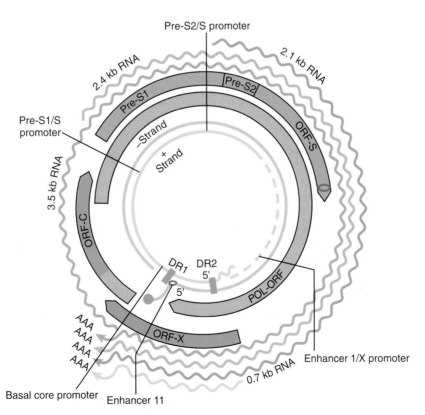

Fig. 6-2 Diagrammatic representation of the HBV genome. The inner circle represents the genomic DNA that is packaged within the virion, and the dashes represent the region of the positive-sense DNA, which is incompletely synthesized. The middle circle of boxes represents the four open reading frames corresponding to the precore, core, HBx, polymerase, and surface proteins. The outer circle of wavy lines represents the HBV RNAs. The promoter and enhancer regions are indicated.

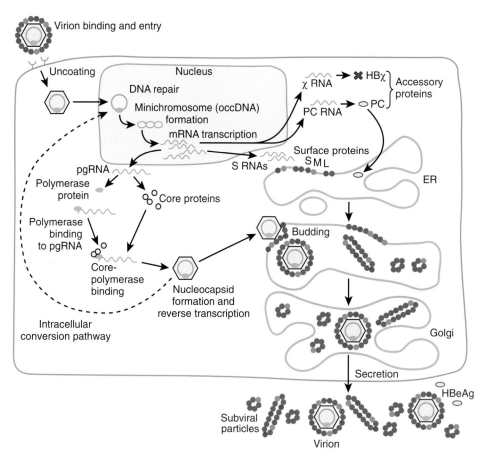

Fig. 6-3 **HBV lifecycle.** HBV binds to and enters the host hepatocyte via an unknown receptor complex, after which the envelope proteins are removed and the genome-containing nucleocapsid traffics to the nucleus where it releases the genome. Inside the nucleus, the partially double-stranded genome is repaired and converted to the minichromosome, or covalently closed circular DNA (cccDNA), which serves as the template for transcription of the viral mRNAs that encode the Pol, core, surface (L, M, and S), HBx, and precore (PC) proteins as depicted. Upon translation, the polymerase protein binds to the pgRNA. The core proteins then bind to the polymerase to form the nucleocapsid. Reverse transcription of the genome takes place inside the nucleocapsid to form the partially double-stranded genome. The interaction between the nucleocapsids and the surface proteins occurs at intracellular membranes, resulting in budding into multivescular bodies (MVBs) and eventual secretion as virions. The surface proteins can also bud at the ER/Golgi intermediate compartment in the absence of a nucleocapsid and be secreted as empty subviral particles. Nucleocapsids can also traffic back to the nucleus to release the HBV genome and replenish the pool of cccDNA (intracellular conversion pathway). The precore protein is also modified and secreted through the ER as HBeAg. The X protein is a nonstructural accessory protein.

subtype whereas R160 confers *r* subtype. The HBV serotypes can be further subdivided antigenically depending on further S mutations. Because the HBV serotype is based on variations at only two codons, it is limited in the overall classification of HBV strains and does not always reflect genotypic or geographic variation.[12] HBV genotypes are determined from the whole nucleotide sequence and are more suitable for studies on epidemiology, transmission, and geographic distribution. Hence, the HBV genotype has essentially replaced serotypes in the overall classification of HBV.

Cell Lines and Model Systems that Are Used to Investigate HBV Replication and Pathogenesis

Until recently, studies on the early steps of infection by HBV have been limited because there were no cell culture systems or small animal models available that were permissive to HBV binding and entry. Most studies on the replication of

HBV are performed by transfecting the HBV genome into hepatoma cell lines, including Huh7 and HepG2 cells and measuring products of HBV replication. Using transfected cells, most steps in the viral life cycle that occur post entry can be studied by measuring products of HBV replication using techniques such as Southern, Northern, and Western blotting. A number of new cell lines and cloning strategies have been developed to deliver HBV into cells and to investigate HBV replication, virus–host interactions, pathogenesis, and antiviral sensitivities. Recently, a cell line that is permissive to infection by HBV has been developed (HepaRG).[13] The wider availability of this cell line should facilitate research into the early events of HBV replication, including virus entry and the hunt for the elusive cellular receptor for HBV. Primary human and Tupaia[14] hepatocytes are also able to be infected with HBV.

A number of delivery systems have been developed to transport HBV DNA into cells. The most commonly used technique is transient transfection of circularized HBV genomes or plasmid DNA encoding a greater-than-genome-length HBV genome. HBV genomes can also be introduced into cells using

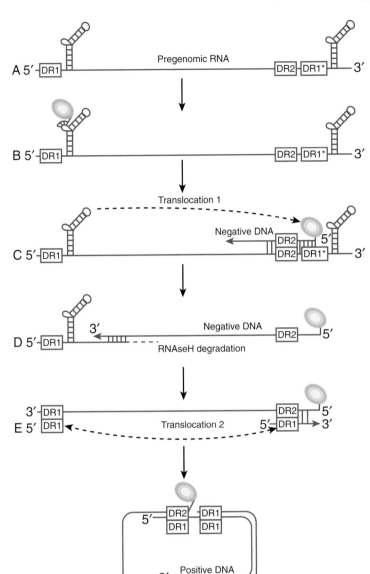

Fig. 6-4 **HBV replication strategy. A,** The blue line represents the greater-than-genome-length pgRNA. The identical ε-sequences at the 5' and 3' ends of the genome are shown as hairpin structures. The direct repeat elements are shown as boxes. The second copy of DR1 at the 3' end of the genome is indicated with an asterisk. **B,** The polymerase protein *(orange circle)* binds to the 5' ε and synthesizes a short oligonucleotide initiated using the terminal protein of the polymerase as a primer and the bulge region of ε as a template. Core protein dimers encapsidate this complex to form the nucleocapsid (not shown). **C,** The polymerase-oligonucleotide complex translocates to DR1 to initiate reverse transcription of the negative strand of the HBV genome. **D,** The RNA template is degraded by the RNAseH activity of the HBV polymerase, except for the 5' DR1 sequence. **E,** The 18 nt RNA sequence is then transferred to DR2 and used as a primer for positive-strand synthesis. **F,** Due to an 8 nt terminal redundancy, the genome can circularize.

the recombinant adenovirus[15] and the recombinant baculovirus systems.[16] There are several reference clones used by researchers around the world, and studies are performed by altering these clones (e.g., introduction of mutations observed clinically) and determining the phenotype conferred by the resulting strain. A number of groups have also developed strategies for the PCR amplification of full-genome-length (or near full genome length) HBV DNA directly from patient sera, and using these HBV strains for transfection into cells, usually after cloning the amplified product into vectors.[17] These patient-specific clones will enable HBV strains to be studied in the context of the entire authentic genetic framework and thus are extremely useful for determining phenotypically the antiviral resistance profile for a patient at a given time.[18–20]

HBV Particle Structure

Three types of HBV particles are found in the sera of patients infected with HBV: 42- to 47-nm virions, as well as 20 to 22 nm diameter spherical and filamentous SVPs (see **Fig. 6-1**). These three particle types contain an envelope consisting of host cell lipids and the L, M, and S surface proteins, which are present at different ratios for each particle type. The subviral particles contain no genetic material and are therefore noninfectious.

The least abundant HBV particle in the blood is the infectious 42- to 47-nm virion or Dane particle, consisting of the DNA-containing nucleocapsid, which is enveloped by the surface proteins.[21] The nucleocapsid is icosahedral with T = 4 symmetry, and consists of 120 core protein dimers. Inside the nucleocapsid is one copy of the partially double-stranded genome covalently linked to the HBV reverse transcriptase protein, as well as host cell proteins. HBV virion titres are variable and can reach up to 10^{10}/ml in patient sera.

The most abundant particles detected in patient sera are the smaller, spherical SVPs, which are composed mostly of S protein and can reach titres as high as 10^{12}/ml. The next most common are the filamentous SVPs, which are of variable length and are also composed mainly of S but contain a higher proportion of L protein than spherical particles.[22] The M protein can be detected in all types of secreted particles but is not necessary for their secretion. The SVPs can exceed the HBV virions by 100,000 fold in patient sera. The role of the SVPs is unknown, but they have been hypothesized to function as immune decoy molecules, adsorbing virus-neutralizing antibodies (see **Fig. 6-1**).

HBV Genome

HBV has a relatively small, partially double-stranded relaxed circular DNA (rcDNA) genome of approximately 3200 bp consisting of a minus-strand DNA with a terminal redundancy of 7 to 9 bases, and an incomplete plus-strand of variable length (see **Fig. 6-2**). Upon entry into the nucleus of the infected cell, the partially double-stranded HBV genome is repaired to form a completely double-stranded covalently closed circular DNA (cccDNA) genome, which serves as the transcriptional template. The HBV genome contains four overlapping reading frames (S, Pol, core, and X) that encode seven known proteins, of which spliced forms have also been identified[23,24] (see **Fig. 6-2**).

Products of the HBV Genome

The X gene is transcribed into a 0.9-kb mRNA initiated by the X promoter, which is then translated into the HBx regulatory protein. The P gene encodes the polymerase (Pol) protein, which does not have a unique mRNA, but is transcribed from the pregenomic RNA (pgRNA). The polymerase gene is the largest open reading frame and overlaps all six other genes. The core gene encodes both the core protein (HBc) and the N-terminally extended precore protein, which is trimmed and secreted from the cell as the hepatitis B e antigen (HBeAg). To express the core and precore proteins, the basal core promoter initiates transcription of two mRNAs, both of approximately 3.5 kb. The precore mRNA encodes only the precore protein, whereas the slightly shorter pgRNA encodes both the core and polymerase proteins and acts as the template for DNA replication (see later discussion). The polymerase protein is not translated from the precore mRNA despite having essentially the same sequence as the pgRNA. The surface gene encodes the surface proteins or hepatitis B surface antigen (HBsAg), and can be subdivided into three regions: PreS1, PreS2, and S. The S region encodes the small surface protein protein (S or SHBs), PreS2+S encodes the middle surface protein protein (M or MHBs), and PreS1+PreS2+S encodes the large surface protein protein (L or LHBs), all of which share a common C-terminus. L is translated from a 2.4-kb mRNA initiated by the PreS1 promoter, whereas M and S are translated from a common 2.1-kb transcript initiated by the PreS2/S promoter.

HBV Replication and Life Cycle
Attachment, Penetration, and Uncoating

HBV only productively infects hepatocytes, although there is some evidence that it can enter bile duct epithelium cells and some cells from the pancreas, kidneys, and the lymphoid system, presumably to ensure viral persistence.[25,26]

The first stage of infection involves attachment of the virion to a susceptible hepatocyte via an unknown receptor complex, followed by endocytosis[27] (see **Fig. 6-3**). The PreS1 region of the L protein on the surface of virions is required for binding to hepatocytes[28,29] and for the subsequent infection

process.[30-32] Monoclonal antibodies to the PreS1 region of L prevent virus attachment.[33] Interestingly, antisera to a conformational epitope within the S coding region can also prevent attachment; whereas monoclonal antibodies directed to the PreS2 coding region do not totally prevent virus attachment. Earlier studies have determined that the N-terminus region of the LHBs protein (codons 21 to 30) is critical for species specificity because all hepadnaviruses are highly species and cell-type specific.[34]

The search for the HBV receptor using the L protein has uncovered a large number of potential candidates, including the receptors for immunoglobulin A, interleukin 6, transferrin and asialoglycoprotein, glyceraldehyde-3-phosphate dehydrogenase, apolipoprotein H, and human liver Annexin V. Unfortunately, at the time of publication, none of these candidates have been unequivocally identified as the major receptor for the specific binding of HBV.[35] It is likely that a complex of cellular proteins, or a primary receptor and a number of co-factors are required for HBV attachment and penetration.

M is not necessary for infectivity, yet this region interacts with cellular proteins, which may enhance infection uptake and uncoating.[36] The PreS2 encoded region contains a binding site for polymerized human serum albumin (pHSA) and also the transferrin receptor that may facilitate attachment and penetration of HBV to target cells.[36]

After binding and entry, mature capsid containing the HBV genome are transported to the nucleus. This transport is mediated by a nuclear localization signal on the core proteins that comprise the HBV capsid. Nuclear transport is mediated by the importin pathway using nuclear transport receptors Imp-ß/Imp-α. The phosphorylation of the C-terminal sequences on the HBc protein is linked with capsid maturation and exposure of the nuclear localization signal. It has been demonstrated that it is only these mature capsids that are able to move through the nuclear pore into the collection of nuclear proteins referred to as the nuclear basket and the HBV rcDNA genome is released into the nucleus.[37] It is unclear at which of these steps the capsid dissociates to release the genome (see **Fig. 6-3**).

Conversion of Genomic rcDNA into cccDNA and Transcription of the Viral Minichromosome

In the nucleus, the partially double-stranded rcDNA HBV genome is converted into double-stranded cccDNA, which functions as a viral minichromosome (see **Fig. 6-3**), and is the major template of HBV used for the transcription of all the viral mRNAs involved in viral protein production and replication (see **Fig. 6-2**).[38,39]

The HBV viral genome is a circular partially double-stranded molecule containing a single-stranded "gap" region. The HBV viral polymerase may mediate the repair of the "gap," and in association with host cellular DNA repair enzymes, facilitate the conversion of viral genome into cccDNA. The conversion to cccDNA also requires the removal of the HBV polymerase protein and oligoribonucleotide, and ligation of DNA. Kock et al.[40] have demonstrated that the nucleos(t)ide analogues adefovir and lamivudine can inhibit the initial DNA repair process,[40] which suggests that an enzymatic activity of the HBV Pol protein is involved in this process. The HBV cccDNA is then chromatinized by cellular histone and nonhistone proteins and converted into a minichromosome[41] serving as the major transcriptional template.

Five promoters control the synthesis of the six viral transcripts of HBV (see **Fig. 6-2**). The HBV genome contains two enhancers, designated enhancer I (EnhI) and enhancer II (EnhII), which exhibit greater activity in hepatic cells than nonhepatic cells. Although the enhancers are located upstream of specific promoters, EnhI regulates all viral promoters and EnhII regulates the basal core promoter (BCP), as well as the transcription of the PreS2/S promoters. Doitsh and Shaul[42] have proposed that HBV may have both early and late transcriptional events in which EnhI may regulate the expression of the early transcripts of X and a long X-related transcript of 3.9 kb known as long-X RNA, whereas EnhII appears to regulate late gene transcription events.

All RNA molecules are transcribed by the host cell RNA polymerase II using the cccDNA template, and are capped and polyadenylated. The pgRNA and the precore mRNA are longer than genomic length, and their transcription is controlled by the basal core promoter (BCP). The bifunctional pregenomic mRNA is used as the genomic template for reverse transcription of the viral negative sense DNA and for translation of HBc and Pol proteins. Whereas the slightly longer precore mRNA encodes only the precore protein, which is subsequently processed and secreted as HBeAg. Three subgenomic RNAs are also transcribed that encode the X, L, and M+S proteins.

Viral Encapsidation and Reverse Transcription

HBV and the other members of the Hepadnaviridae family replicate their DNA genome by reverse transcription of a pgRNA template within the core particle. Mature nucleocapsids and virions contain the HBV 3.2-kb rcDNA genome with the Pol covalently attached to the 5′-end of the (−) DNA via the terminal protein region. The process of HBV DNA synthesis involves reverse transcription and a complicated process of three translocations of the polymerase and primer to complete double-stranded genome synthesis (see **Fig. 6-4**). The pgRNA contains critical stem loop structures (ε) at both the 5′ and 3′ ends. The HBV polymerase binds to the 5′ ε structure, which then signals the binding of core protein dimers that encapsidate the pgRNA-Pol complex, as well as cellular protein kinases and the putative chaperones heat shock proteins (HSP) HSP70 and HSP90, to form immature nucleocapsids. Although nucleocapsids contain host cell proteins, their precise role in replication has yet to be defined. Reverse transcription of the complementary negative strand is then initiated by the HBV polymerase via priming and synthesis of a short 3 nt oligomer (with the sequence GAA) complementary to the ε-region at the 5′ end of the genome (see **Fig. 6-4**). The Pol-oligomer complex is then translocated to the ε-region at the 3′ end of the genome where reverse transcription of the negative strand continues back toward the 5′ end of the pgRNA. During synthesis of the negative strand, the entire positive sense RNA template is degraded by the RNaseH activity of the HBV polymerase, except for the 5′ capped region, which contains the direct repeat element (DR1). This DR1 RNA then translocates and binds to the complementary DR2 sequence near the 5′ end of the newly

formed negative-strand DNA, acting as a primer for DNA synthesis, which continues for a short distance to the 5′ end of the genome. A further translocation then occurs whereby the 3′ end of the newly formed positive strand can jump to the 3′ end of the negative strand and continue synthesis, forming the double-stranded rcDNA. However, due to mechanisms not well understood, synthesis of the plus strand is terminated prematurely and reaches only approximately halfway around the genome; hence rcDNA molecules are only partially double stranded.[1] Mature rcDNA-containing nucleocapsids can then either traffic to the nucleus and release their DNA contents to replenish the pool of cccDNA, or can be enveloped and secreted as virions.

An alternative pathway of DNA synthesis also occurs in a small percentage of genomes where primer translocation does not occur, but rather, plus-strand formation is primed in situ. This results in a double-stranded linear DNA (dslDNA) molecule where the 18 nt primer exists in an RNA-DNA duplex at the 3' end of the negative strand. These dslDNA molecules can undergo nonhomologous recombination and become integrated into the host cell genome.[43]

Minus-strand DNA synthesis appears to be coupled to phosphorylation of the nucleocapsid, which is required for envelopment to occur. Incomplete dsDNA/RNA genomes that have completed minus-strand DNA synthesis and at least started plus-strand synthesis can readily be found in the blood as secreted virions.

Interestingly, significant amounts of unenveloped nucleocapsids are released from cell lines replicating HBV,[44,45] which may be an artifact of the cell culture models used, as this does not seem to be the case in vivo (see **Fig. 6-4**).

HBV Proteins
HBV Surface Proteins and Particle Formation

HBV encodes three membrane-associated proteins, all sharing the same stop codon, with translation initiating from different start codons (**Fig. 6-5**). The smallest of these proteins, S, is encoded by the S gene, which produces a 226 amino acid protein. The middle protein, M, contains a further N-terminal extension of 55 amino acids encoded by the upstream PreS2 gene. The largest of the envelope proteins, L, has yet another N-terminal extension of 108 to 119 amino acids, depending on the HBV genotype, encoded by the PreS1 gene. These proteins can self-assemble into SVPs or can interact with mature nucleocapsids to form virions (see **Figs. 6-3 and 6-5**).

The envelope proteins display a complex transmembrane topology. Translocation of S across the ER membrane is mediated by a hydrophobic signal sequence from amino acids 8 to 22 of the S domain (**Fig. 6-6, A**). The amino acid chain then translocates across the membrane a second time mediated by another hydrophobic signal sequence at amino acids 80 to 98 of S, forming a loop from amino acids 23 to 79, which is localized to the cytosol and required for virion formation presumably by interaction with the nucleocapsid[46]; this loop is eventually localized to the lumen of the virion.[47] The C-terminal region of S (amino acids 170 to 226) is highly hydrophobic and presumed to be membrane embedded, which would result in another loop from amino acids 99 to 169 localized to the ER lumen, resulting in eventual exposure on the surface of the virion. This latter loop forms the major hydrophilic region (MHR) that is found on the surface of

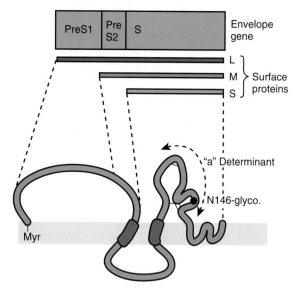

Fig. 6-5 The HBV surface proteins are encoded by the envelope or surface gene. They share a common termination codon, with translation initiating from different start codons, hence they share a common C-terminal region, which spans the entire S region. Depicted at the bottom of the diagram is the full-length L protein. The major antigenic region ("a" determinant) and glycosylation site at sN146 are indicated. A myristic acid (Myr) at the N-terminus is also depicted.

virions and subviral particles and contains a highly immunogenic region designated the "A" determinant, the major antibody neutralization domain of the virus. A number of cysteine bonds with the MHR are predicted to cause the formation of two loop structures; loop1 from amino acids 107 to 138 and loop2 from amino acids 139 to 147. Mutations within the "A" determinant can occur as a response to immune pressure resulting in decreased antibody binding, and subsequent vaccine or diagnostic escape. The most well-characterized vaccine escape mutation, sG145R, is also located within loop 2 of this region.

The M protein has the same topology as S,[48] but has an additional 55 amino acids at the ER-localized N-terminus (see **Fig. 6-6, B**). M can be incorporated into viral particles, despite not being necessary for their formation.[49] The M protein is considerably more immunogenic than S, and PreS2 containing HBs particles generated from animal cell lines have been used in some countries as a prophylactic vaccine.[50]

The L protein, which has yet another N-terminal extension of 108 to 119 amino acids, has two intracellular topologies. During protein translation, the first signal sequence is not been used and the PreS regions are located in the cytosol (see **Fig. 6-6, C**). Approximately half of the proteins then refold into the same topology as S and M, exposing the PreS regions to the ER lumen (see **Fig. 6-6, D**).[51-53] The N-terminus of L is myristoylated, which probably results in the membrane

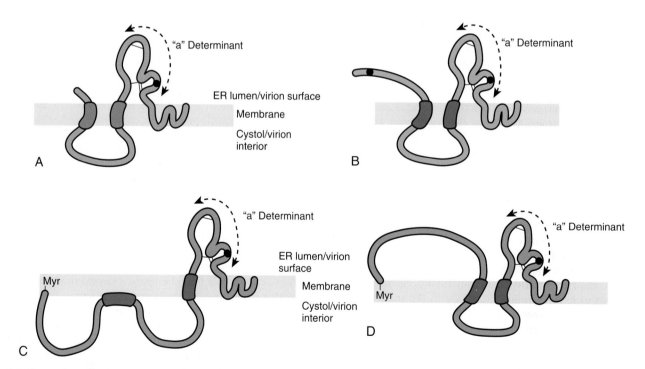

Fig. 6-6 Illustration of HBV surface proteins (A) S, (B) M, (C) L conformation 1, and (D) L conformation 2. Topology is illustrated with respect to the ER lumen (which corresponds to the surface of the secreted virion) and the cell cytosol (which corresponds to the internal part of the secreted virion). All numbers refer to amino acids and refer to their position in S, except where indicated by brackets. Black dots represent amino acids that have been referred to in the text. Transmembrane hydrophobic regions are depicted embedded in the membrane. Glycosylation sites (glyc.) at positions sN146 and mN4 are illustrated. The approximate location of the "a" determinant is also illustrated. The myristoylation site at the N-terminal of L is depicted, which is predicted to embed in the membrane.

association of this region[54] and is essential for the infection process.[55] The initial cytosolic localization of the PreS regions is probably necessary for interaction with nucleocapsids and subsequent virion formation,[56] whereas the secondary folding and exposure of the PreS regions to the ER lumen (which corresponds to the virion surface) is necessary for virus binding and entry during infection.[30,31,57]

The wild-type HBV envelope proteins exist in glycosylated (gp) and nonglycosylated (p) forms due to partial N-linked glycosylation at amino acid N146 in the S region (see **Fig. 6-6**). M has an additional N-linked glycosylation site at position amino acid N4 in the PreS2 region, which is completely glycosylated in all M molecules (see **Fig. 6-6, B**). This site was thought not to be glycosylated in the L protein; however, recent studies suggest this site may be used at low levels.[58] The M protein[59,60] and, to a smaller extent, the L protein[61] are also O-glycosylated at T37 in the PreS2 domain.[60] These glycosylation events result in species of varying molecular weight. The S protein exists in two forms, p24 and gp27. M is usually found as two glycosylated species; gp33 and twice glycosylated gp36, due to full glycosylation of amino acid N4 in PreS2 and partial glycosylation of amino acid N146 in the S region. The nonglycosylated form of M, p30, can usually only be observed when M is overexpressed. L is usually detected as nonglycosylated p39 and glycosylated gp42 species. However, it has recently been demonstrated that L has further posttranslational glycosylation events that occur at low levels at amino acids lN4 and lN112 (same residue as mN4).[58] The relevance of these glycosylation events in protein folding and regulation is yet to be fully elucidated (see **Fig. 6-6**).

Following their synthesis, the HBV surface proteins rapidly undergo dimer and multimer formation via extensive intermolecular and intramolecular disulphide bonding, eventually resulting in budding into a post-ER, pre-Golgi intermediate compartment as spherical or filamentous subviral particles, or they can interact with nucleocapsids in the cytosol to form virions (see **Fig. 6-3**). Recently, an alternative pathway for the generation of empty virions/defective particles, where the envelope proteins interact with a C-terminally truncated form of the precore protein, has also been described.[62] Each of these processes has different host cell protein requirements. The S and M proteins, when expressed alone, can be secreted as subviral particles,[63-65] whereas L is retained within the cell and can only be secreted in the presence of S. Not only is L dependent on S for secretion, but L can also inhibit the secretion of HBV particles when overexpressed.[66,67] HBV particles can consist of any combination of glycosylated and nonglycosylated L, M, and S proteins, depending on the abundance of the different glycoforms in the ER membrane.[68] When expressed in yeast, the S protein is also secreted as SVPs, which are the basis of the current HBV vaccine.[69]

HBV virion formation involves envelopment of nucleocapsids by L and S proteins at multivesicular bodies, which is mediated by host cell proteins. The L and S proteins can interact with genome-containing nucleocapsids formed in the cytoplasm, enveloping them to form virions before they are secreted.[70,71] Recruitment of HBV nucleocapsids to the L and S proteins at the site of budding is mediated by the host proteins γ2-adaptin and the ubiquitin ligase Nedd4. γ2-adaptin binds to a motif in L and then interacts with ubiquitin on either nucleocapsids or an accessory protein such as Nedd4.[72] Nedd4 binds to a motif in core and could interact with γ2-adaptin either directly or in conjunction with ubiquitin, hence recruiting nucleocapsids to L proteins at multivesicular bodies. These multivesicular bodies contain the cellular machinery required for viral budding and membrane fusion and are required for viral budding in HBV infected cells.[58,72]

Inhibition of these pathways inhibits the secretion of virions, whereas SVP secretion is unaffected, providing evidence that SVPs and virions are secreted by different pathways. For example, the HBV envelope proteins have been shown to co-localize with the cellular proteins VSP4B and AIP1, which are involved in multivesicular body formation and cargo protein sorting, disruption of which affects virion, but not SVP release.[73] Another study showed treatment of HBV-expressing cells with an inhibitor of glycosylation prevented virion, but not SVP release.[74] Therefore it is likely that the formation of virions is dependent on complex glycosylation events and involvement of host cell proteins at multivesicular bodies, whereas secretion of subviral particles has less stringent host cell requirements.

HBV Polymerase Protein

The HBV polymerase is a multifunctional protein that, besides having RNA- and DNA-dependent DNA polymerase activity, self-primes reverse transcription, acts as an RNase H, and coordinates intracellular assembly of viral nucleocapsids.[75,76] The Hepadnaviridae are the only animal DNA viruses that replicate using a reverse transcription step. The polymerase protein comprises four distinct structural/functional domains, namely (in order from the N-terminus): (1) the terminal protein (tp) used in priming HBV DNA synthesis; (2) a spacer domain; (3) the reverse transcriptase (rt) domain that has both RNA- and DNA-dependent DNA polymerase activities; and (4) an RNase H domain (see **Fig. 6-2**) that cleaves the RNA in RNA-DNA hybrids during reverse transcription (see **Fig. 6-4**). The HBV rt contains clusters of highly conserved amino acid motifs designated domains A to F, which are common to all RNA-dependent DNA polymerases and have specific functions essential for enzymatic activity. The HBV rt has not been crystallized; however, molecular models have been developed based on sequence homology with the human immunodeficiency virus rt.[77]

The specific antiviral agents used for the treatment of HBV are nucleos(t)ide analogues (NAs), which are targeted to the rt domains of the HBV Pol. Most of these NAs are also used in HIV therapy because the reverse transcriptase enzymes of these viruses are very similar. Like many other viral polymerase enzymes, the HBV Pol has no proofreading mechanism, which results in the rapid development of resistance mutations in the HBV reverse transcriptase domains. The reverse transcriptase region of the HBV polymerase gene overlaps with the HBV surface gene, hence NA resistance can also result in altered surface proteins, which can have dramatic effects on the life cycle.[78] Resistance to most NAs has now been detected, and new treatment strategies are needed.

Core Protein

The pgRNA serves as template for translation of both the polymerase protein and the 183 to 184 amino acids (21 kDa) core protein (HBc). The function of the core protein in the life cycle of HBV is to encapsidate the pgRNA-Pol complex, forming the nucleocapsid, which is in turn enveloped by the surface proteins to form the HBV virion. The HBc protein has been crystallized and the nucleocapsid has been studied using cryoelectron microscopy.[79]

Upon translation, the core protein initially forms homodimers mediated by disulphide bonding at cysteine residue 61, followed by multimerization of the dimers to encapsidate the pgRNA-Pol complex, forming the nucleocapsid. The HBc protein possesses two distinct domains[36]: the N-terminal domain (amino acid residues 1 to 144), which is involved in assembly of the nucleocapsid, and the arginine-rich C-terminal domain. The arginine-rich region is required for packaging of the pgRNA-Pol complex, and includes a potential nuclear localization sequence.

The core monomer is primarily α-helical. X-ray crystallography has shown that core protein dimers form a structure similar to an upside-down T. The horizontal bar of the T structure mediates polymerization of the dimers into nucleocapsids, which contain pores that allow diffusion of nucleotides during DNA synthesis. The vertical bar forms a spike that protrudes out from the capsid, which can be visualized using electron microscopy. The tip of the spike region contains the major B-cell epitope of the core protein. Mutations around the base of the spike region and at the capsid surface close to the pore structures have been shown to affect interactions with the surface proteins and subsequent envelopment.[80]

The core protein can also self-assemble into capsids when expressed in bacteria. Two icosahedral shells of different sizes are observed: particles with a T = 3 symmetry containing 90 homodimers of 30 to 32 nm, and particles with a T = 4 symmetry consisting of 120 homodimers of 34 to 36 nm.[81] Deletion of the arginine-rich domain at the C-terminus allows efficient expression of the protein in bacteria and favors the formation of T = 4 over T = 3 capsids. To date the preference of the T4 over the T3 in infected patients has not been determined.

Precore Protein (HBeAg)

The precore protein, or hepatitis B e antigen (HBeAg) is translated from its own mRNA (precore mRNA), which differs from the core-encoding mRNA (pgRNA) by an additional 33 nt at the 5′ end. Although the sequence of the precore protein is essentially the same as the core protein, with an additional 29 amino acids at the N-terminus, these two proteins are functionally very different. The precore protein, like HBx, is a nonstructural accessory protein whose function has yet to be clearly defined.

The first 19 amino acids of the precore protein comprise a secretion signal that induces the translocation of the precore protein into the lumen of the endoplasmic reticulum (ER) where the signal sequence is cleaved off by a host cell signal peptidase and the protein is secreted through the ER and Golgi apparatus. A further modification of the C-terminus results in the secretion of a heterogeneous population of 14 to 17 kDa proteins, serologically defined as HBeAg. The precore protein also expresses a nuclear transport signal for transport into the nucleus. The role of the HBeAg appears to be for establishment of persistent infection in vivo,[82] to serve an immunoregulatory role in natural infection via manipulation of the innate immune response (TLR2),[83] and to activate or tolerize T cells.[84]

X Protein

The 1.1-kb transcript encodes the 154 amino acid, 17-kDa X protein (HBx), the second accessory protein of HBV. There are conflicting reports on the necessity of HBx for in vitro HBV replication, but the equivalent protein is required for the establishment of hepadnaviral infection of woodchucks.[85] HBx is located in both the cytoplasm and the nucleus of the cell. The level of HBx expression can influence its cellular localization. It is predominantly nuclear when expressed in cells at very low levels but becomes largely cytoplasmic as its expression level increases. A number of conflicting in vitro studies have been reported about the role of the HBx protein that are probably related to variability in the expression levels of HBx, the cell line used, its ability to both be a substrate and an inhibitor of the proteasome complex, and its effect in the modulation of cytosolic calcium, which activates various signaling pathways involving Src kinases.[86-88]

HBx appears to be multifunctional. In the nucleus, HBx is a modest promiscuous transactivator that can regulate transcription through a direct interaction with different transcription factors and in some cases enhance their binding to specific transcriptional elements.[89] This regulation of viral and cellular genes affects viral replication and viral proliferation directly or indirectly, so it is not surprising that HBx can influence apoptosis and cell cycle regulatory pathways. However, the transactivational function of HBx is reduced in the presence of proteasome inhibitors. This interaction of HBx with the 26S proteasome complex may also affect immune evasion by suppressing viral antigen presentation.[90] HBx also affects cytosolic calcium possibly via alteration of the mitochondrial voltage-dependent anion channel,[88,91] thereby functioning in the cytoplasm to activate various signaling pathways. Overall, whether the HBx-induced activation of transcription or its effect on the cytoplasmic signaling pathways plays a significant role during natural infection with HBV remains an open question.

Splice Protein

In addition to the unspliced major HBV RNA transcripts described above, single- or double-spliced 2.2-kb RNAs have been detected in HBV-DNA–transfected hepatoma cells[92] and in infected human livers.[93] Sequencing of the singly spliced 2.2-kb HBV RNAs typically reveals a deletion from the last codon of the core gene to the middle of the S gene, which creates a new open reading frame, known as the hepatitis B splice protein (HBSP), which encodes truncated S and Pol proteins.[94] The in vivo expression of HBSP is associated with viral replication and, more importantly, liver fibrosis.[95] As well as pathogenesis, this alternative replication strategy may be a mechanism of viral persistence[96] and further studies are clearly required to determine its role in viral replication and its affect on the host.

Concluding Remarks

HBV is a DNA virus that infects the liver and can lead to fibrosis, cirrhosis, and hepatocellular carcinoma. It is estimated that around one third of the world's population has been infected with HBV, of whom 400 million are chronically infected. The HBV genome is compact and consists of overlapping reading frames. The early replication steps of receptor binding and entry have yet to be elucidated because there have been no suitable model systems available until recently. The establishment of a minichromosome or "cccDNA" within the infected cell nucleus ensures persistence of this virus, making viral elimination a difficult task. Replication involves reverse transcription of a greater-than-genome-length RNA (pgRNA) inside a nucleocapsid consisting of the HBV core protein. The virion is formed when the nucleocapsid buds into ER-Golgi derived membranes containing the HBV surface proteins. The surface proteins can also be secreted as noninfectious subviral particles, which are secreted in great excess over the virions. Nonstructural proteins encoded by HBV include X and HBeAg; several functions have been ascribed to these proteins, none of which have been conclusively accepted.

References

1. Seeger C, Zoulim F, Mason WS. Hepadnaviruses. In: Knipe DM, Howley PM, editors. Fields virology. Philadelphia: Lippincott Williams & Wilkins, 2007: 2977–3030.
2. Schaefer S. Hepatitis B virus taxonomy and hepatitis B virus genotypes. World J Gastroenterol 2007;13(1):14–21.
3. Stuyver L, et al. A new genotype of hepatitis B virus: complete genome and phylogenetic relatedness. J Gen Virol 2000;81(Pt 1):67–74.
4. Simmonds P, Midgley S. Recombination in the genesis and evolution of hepatitis B virus genotypes. J Virol 2005;79(24):15467–15476.
5. Yang J, et al. Identification of Hepatitis B virus putative intergenotype recombinants by using fragment typing. J Gen Virol 2006;87(Pt 8):2203–2215.
6. Kao JH, Liu CJ, Chen DS. Hepatitis B viral genotypes and lamivudine resistance. J Hepatol 2002;36(2):303–304.
7. Sugiyama M, et al. Influence of hepatitis B virus genotypes on the intra- and extracellular expression of viral DNA and antigens. Hepatology 2006;44(4):915–924.
8. Courouce-Pauty AM, Plancon A, Soulier JP. Distribution of HBsAg subtypes in the world. Vox Sang 1983;44(4):197–211.
9. Okamoto H, et al. Typing hepatitis B virus by homology in nucleotide sequence: comparison of surface antigen subtypes. J Gen Virol 1988;69 (Pt 10):2575–2583.
10. Norder H, Courouce AM, Magnius LO. Molecular basis of hepatitis B virus serotype variations within the four major subtypes. J Gen Virol 1992;73 (Pt 12):3141–3145.
11. Wallace LA, Carman WF. Surface gene variation of HBV: scientific and medical relevance. J Viral Hepat 1997;3(1):5–16.
12. Moriya T, et al. Distribution of hepatitis B virus genotypes among American blood donors determined with a PreS2 epitope enzyme-linked immunosorbent assay kit. J Clin Microbiol 2002;40(3):877–880.
13. Gripon P, et al. Infection of a human hepatoma cell line by hepatitis B virus. Proc Natl Acad Sci U S A 2002;99:15655–15660.
14. Walter EK, et al. Hepatitis B virus infection of Tupaia hepatocytes in vitro and in vivo. Hepatology 1996;24(1):1–5.
15. Ren S, Nassal M. Hepatitis B virus (HBV) virion and covalently closed circular DNA formation in primary Tupaia hepatocytes and human hepatoma cell lines upon HBV genome transduction with replication-defective adenovirus vectors. J Virol 2001;75(3):1104–1116.
16. Delaney WE IV, Isom HC. Hepatitis B virus replication in human HepG2 cells mediated by hepatitis B virus recombinant baculovirus. Hepatology 1998;28(4):1134–1146.
17. Durantel D, et al. A new strategy for studying in vitro the drug susceptibility of clinical isolates of human hepatitis B virus. Hepatology 2004;40(4):855–864.
18. Gunther S, et al. A novel method for efficient amplification of whole hepatitis B virus genomes permits rapid functional analysis and reveals deletion mutants in immunosuppressed patients. J Virol 1995;69:5437–5444.
19. Yang H, et al. In vitro antiviral susceptibility of full-length clinical hepatitis B virus isolates cloned with a novel expression vector. Antiviral Res 2004;61(1):27–36.
20. Delaney WE, et al. Combinations of adefovir with nucleoside analogs produce additive antiviral effects against hepatitis B virus in vitro. Antimicrob Agents Chemother 2004;48(10):3702–3710.
21. Ganem D, Schneider R. Hepadnaviridae: the viruses and their replication. In: Knipe DM, Howley PM, editors. Fields virology. Philadelphia: Lippincott-Raven, 2001: 2923–2970.
22. Heermann KH, et al. Large surface proteins of hepatitis B virus containing the pre-s sequence. J Virol 1984;52(2):396–402.
23. Gunther S, et al. Heterogeneity and common features of defective hepatitis B virus genomes derived from spliced pregenomic RNA. Virology 1997;238(2):363–371.
24. Soussan P, et al. In vivo expression of a new hepatitis B virus protein encoded by a spliced RNA. J Clin Invest 2000;105(1):55–60.
25. Lee JY, et al. Duck hepatitis B virus replication in primary bile duct epithelial cells. J Virol 2001;75(16):7651–7661.
26. Seeger C, Mason WS. Hepatitis B virus biology. Microbiol Mol Biol Rev 2000;64(1):51–68.
27. De Meyer S, et al. Organ and species specificity of hepatitis B virus (HBV) infection: a review of literature with a special reference to preferential attachment of HBV to human hepatocytes. J Viral Hepat 1997;4(3):145–153.
28. Pontisso P, et al. Identification of an attachment site for human liver plasma membranes on hepatitis B virus particles. Virology 1989;173(2):522–530.
29. Neurath AR, et al. Identification and chemical synthesis of a host cell receptor binding site on hepatitis B virus. Cell 1986;46(3):429–436.
30. Urban S, Gripon P. Inhibition of duck hepatitis B virus infection by a myristoylated pre-S peptide of the large viral surface protein. J Virol 2002;76(4):1986–1990.
31. Glebe D, et al. Mapping of the hepatitis B virus attachment site by use of infection-inhibiting preS1 lipopeptides and Tupaia hepatocytes. Gastroenterology 2005;129(1):234–245.
32. Gripon P, Cannie I, Urban S. Efficient inhibition of hepatitis B virus infection by acylated peptides derived from the large viral surface protein. J Virol 2005;79(3):1613–1622.
33. Glebe D, et al. Pre-s1 antigen-dependent infection of Tupaia hepatocyte cultures with human hepatitis B virus. J Virol 2003;77(17):9511-9521.
34. Chouteau P, et al. A short N-proximal region in the large envelope protein harbors a determinant that contributes to the species specificity of human hepatitis B virus. J Virol 2001;75(23):11565–11572.
35. De Falco S, et al. Cloning and expression of a novel hepatitis B virus-binding protein from HepG2 cells. J Biol Chem 2001;276:36613–36623.
36. Kann M, Gerlich W. Hepadnaviridae: structure and molecular virology. In: Zuckerman A, Thomas H, editors. Viral hepatitis. London: Churchill Livingstone, 1998: 77–105.
37. Rabe B, et al. Nuclear import of hepatitis B virus capsids and release of the viral genome. Proc Natl Acad Sci U S A 2003;100(17):9849–9854.
38. Bock CT, et al. Hepatitis B virus genome is organized into nucleosomes in the nucleus of the infected cell. Virus Genes 1994;8(3):215–229.
39. Newbold JE, et al. The covalently closed duplex form of the hepadnavirus genome exists in situ as a heterogeneous population of viral minichromosomes. J Virol 1995;69(6):3350–3357.
40. Kock J, et al. Inhibitory effect of adefovir and lamivudine on the initiation of hepatitis B virus infection in primary Tupaia hepatocytes. Hepatology 2003;38(6):1410–1418.
41. Newbold JE, et al. The covalently closed duplex form of the hepadnavirus genome exists in situ as a heterogeneous population of viral minichromosomes. J Virol 1995;69:3350–3357.
42. Doitsh G, Shaul Y. A long HBV transcript encoding pX is inefficiently exported from the nucleus. Virology 2003;309(2):339–349.
43. Yang W, Summers J. Illegitimate replication of linear hepadnavirus DNA through nonhomologous recombination. J Virol 1995;69(7):4029–4036.
44. Bruss V, Ganem D. The role of envelope proteins in hepatitis B virus assembly. Proc Natl Acad Sci U S A 1991;88(3):1059–1063.
45. Gerelsaikhan T, Tavis JE, Bruss V. Hepatitis B virus nucleocapsid envelopment does not occur without genomic DNA synthesis. J Virol 1996;70(7):4269–4274.
46. Loffler-Mary H, et al. Hepatitis B virus assembly is sensitive to changes in the cytosolic S loop of the envelope proteins. Virology 2000;270(2):358–367.
47. Eble BE, et al. Multiple topogenic sequences determine the transmembrane orientation of the hepatitis B surface antigen. Mol Cell Biol 1987;7(10):3591–3601.
48. Eble BE, Lingappa VR, Ganem D. The N-terminal (pre-S2) domain of a hepatitis B virus surface glycoprotein is translocated across membranes by downstream signal sequences. J Virol 1990;64(3):1414–1419.
49. Fernholz D, et al. Infectious hepatitis B virus variant defective in pre-S2 protein expression in a chronic carrier. Virology 1993;194(1):137–148.

50. Tron F, et al. Randomized dose range study of a recombinant hepatitis B vaccine produced in mammalian cells and containing the S and PreS2 sequences. J Infect Dis 1989;160(2):199–204.

51. Bruss V, et al. Post-translational alterations in transmembrane topology of the hepatitis B virus large envelope protein. EMBO J 1994;13(10):2273–2279.

52. Ostapchuk P, Hearing P, Ganem D. A dramatic shift in the transmembrane topology of a viral envelope glycoprotein accompanies hepatitis B viral morphogenesis. EMBO J 1994;13(5):1048–1057.

53. Prange R, Streeck RE. Novel transmembrane topology of the hepatitis B virus envelope proteins. EMBO J 1995;14(2):247–256.

54. Persing DH, Varmus HE, Ganem D. The preS1 protein of hepatitis B virus is acylated at its amino terminus with myristic acid. J Virol 1987;61(5):1672–1677.

55. Gripon P, et al. Myristylation of the hepatitis B virus large surface protein is essential for viral infectivity. Virology 1995;213(2):292–299.

56. Bruss V, Vieluf K. Functions of the internal pre-S domain of the large surface protein in hepatitis B virus particle morphogenesis. J Virol 1995;69(11):6652–6657.

57. Le Seyec J, et al. Infection process of the hepatitis B virus depends on the presence of a defined sequence in the pre-S1 domain. J Virol 1999;73(3):2052–2057.

58. Lambert C, Prange R. Posttranslational N-glycosylation of the hepatitis B virus large envelope protein. Virol J 2007;4(1):45.

59. Schmitt S, et al. Analysis of the pre-S2 N- and O-linked glycans of the M surface protein from human hepatitis B virus. J Biol Chem 1999;274(17):11945–11957.

60. Werr M, Prange R. Role for calnexin and N-linked glycosylation in the assembly and secretion of hepatitis B virus middle envelope protein particles. J Virol 1998;72(1):778–782.

61. Schmitt S, et al. Structure of pre-S2 N- and O-linked glycans in surface proteins from different genotypes of hepatitis B virus. J Gen Virol 2004;85(Pt 7):2045–2053.

62. Kimura T, et al. Hepatitis B virus DNA-negative dane particles lack core protein but contain a 22-kDa precore protein without C-terminal arginine-rich domain. J Biol Chem 2005;280(23):21713–21719.

63. Laub O, et al. Synthesis of hepatitis B surface antigen in mammalian cells: expression of the entire gene and the coding region. J Virol 1983;48(1):271–280.

64. Liu CC, Yansura D, Levinson AD. Direct expression of hepatitis B surface antigen in monkey cells from an SV40 vector. DNA 1982;1(3):213–221.

65. Persing DH, Varmus HE, Ganem D. A frameshift mutation in the pre-S region of the human hepatitis B virus genome allows production of surface antigen particles but eliminates binding to polymerized albumin. Proc Natl Acad Sci U S A 1985;82(10):3440–3444.

66. Ou JH, Rutter WJ. Regulation of secretion of the hepatitis B virus major surface antigen by the preS-1 protein. J Virol 1987;61(3):782–786.

67. Persing DH, Varmus HE, Ganem D. Inhibition of secretion of hepatitis B surface antigen by a related presurface polypeptide. Science 1986;234(4782):1388–1391.

68. Wounderlich G, Bruss V. Characterization of early hepatitis B virus surface protein oligomers. Arch Virol 1996;141(7):1191–1205.

69. Valenzuela P, et al. Synthesis and assembly of hepatitis B virus surface antigen particles in yeast. Nature 1982;298(5872):347–350.

70. Patzer EJ, et al. Intracellular assembly and packaging of hepatitis B surface antigen particles occur in the endoplasmic reticulum. J Virol 1986;58(3):884–892.

71. Huovila AP, Eder AM, Fuller SD. Hepatitis B surface antigen assembles in a post-ER, pre-Golgi compartment. J Cell Biol 1992;118(6):1305–1320.

72. Rost M, et al. Gamma-adaptin, a novel ubiquitin-interacting adaptor, and Nedd4 ubiquitin ligase control hepatitis B virus maturation. J Biol Chem 2006;281(39):29297–29308.

73. Watanabe T, et al. Involvement of host cellular multivesicular body functions in hepatitis B virus budding. Proc Natl Acad Sci U S A 2007;104(24):10205–10210.

74. Lu X, et al. Evidence that N-linked glycosylation is necessary for hepatitis B virus secretion. Virology 1995;213(2):660–665.

75. Will H, et al. Replication strategy of human hepatitis B virus. J Virol 1987;61(3):904–911.

76. Ganem D, Pollack JR, Tavis J. Hepatitis B virus reverse transcriptase and its many roles in hepadnaviral genomic replication. Infect Agents Dis 1994;3(2-3):85–93.

77. Bartholomeusz A, Tehan BG, Chalmers DK. Comparisons of the HBV and HIV polymerase, and antiviral resistance mutations. Antivir Ther 2004;9(2):149–160.

78. Warner N, Locarnini S. The antiviral drug selected hepatitis B virus rtA181T/sW172* mutant has a dominant negative secretion defect and alters the typical profile of viral rebound. Hepatology 2008;48(1):88–98.

79. Wynne SA, Crowther RA, Leslie AG. The crystal structure of the human hepatitis B virus capsid. Mol Cell 1999;3(6):771–780.

80. Ponsel D, Bruss V. Mapping of amino acid side chains on the surface of hepatitis B virus capsids required for envelopment and virion formation. J Virol 2003;77(1):416–422.

81. Zlotnick A, et al. Dimorphism of hepatitis B virus capsids is strongly influenced by the C-terminus of the capsid protein. Biochemistry 1996;35(23):7412–7421.

82. Hadziyannis SJ, Vassilopoulos D. Hepatitis B e antigen-negative chronic hepatitis B. Hepatology 2001;34(4 Pt 1):617–624.

83. Visvanathan K, et al. Regulation of Toll-like receptor-2 expression in chronic hepatitis B by the precore protein. Hepatology 2007;45(1):102–110.

84. Milich D, Liang TJ. Exploring the biological basis of hepatitis B e antigen in hepatitis B virus infection. Hepatology 2003;38:1075–1086.

85. Zoulim F, Saputelli J, Seeger C. Woodchuck hepatitis virus X protein is required for viral infection in vivo. J Virol 1994;68:2026–2030.

86. Starkman SE, et al. Geographic and species association of hepatitis B virus genotypes in non-human primates. Virology 2003;314(1):381–393.

87. Zhang Z, et al. Inhibition of cellular proteasome activities enhances hepadnavirus replication in an HBX-dependent manner. J Virol 2004;78(9):4566–4572.

88. Rahmani Z, et al. Hepatitis B virus X protein colocalizes to mitochondria with a human voltage-dependent anion channel, HVDAC3, and alters its transmembrane potential. J Virol 2000;74(6):2840–2846.

89. Bouchard MJ, Schneider RJ. The enigmatic X gene of hepatitis B virus. J Virol 2004;78(23):12725–12734.

90. Huang J, et al. Proteasome complex as a potential cellular target of hepatitis H virus X protein. J Virol 1996;70(8):5582–5591.

91. Bouchard MJ, Wang LH, Schneider RJ. Calcium signaling by HBx protein in hepatitis B virus DNA replication. Science 2001;294(5550):2376–2378.

92. Chen PJ, et al. Identification of a doubly spliced viral transcript joining the separated domains for putative protease and reverse transcriptase of hepatitis B virus. J Virol 1989;63(10):4165–4171.

93. Su TS, et al. Analysis of hepatitis B virus transcripts in infected human livers. Hepatology 1989;9:180–185.

94. Soussan P, et al. In vivo expression of a new hepatitis B virus protein encoded by a spliced RNA. J Clin Invest 2000;105:55–60.

95. Soussan P, et al. The expression of hepatitis B spliced protein (HBSP) encoded by a spliced hepatitis B virus RNA is associated with viral replication and liver fibrosis. J Hepatol 2003;38(3):343–348.

96. Rosmorduc O, et al. In vivo and in vitro expression of defective hepatitis B virus particles generated by spliced hepatitis B virus RNA. Hepatology 1995;22(1):10–19.

Chapter 7

Replication of Hepatitis C Virus

Darius Moradpour, François Penin, and Charles Rice

ABBREVIATIONS

ARF alternative reading frame
ARFP alternative reading frame protein
BVDV bovine viral diarrhea virus
cDNA complementary DNA
CRE *cis*-acting replication element
ER endoplasmic reticulum
GBV GB virus
HCC hepatocellular carcinoma
HCV hepatitis C virus
HCVDB Hepatitis C Virus Database

hVAP-A human vesicle-associated membrane protein–associated protein A
HVR hypervariable region
IRES internal ribosome entry site
ISDR interferon sensitivity-determining region
LDL low-density lipoprotein
LDLR low-density lipoprotein receptor
NCR noncoding region

NS nonstructural
PEG-IFN-α pegylated interferon-α
RdRp RNA-dependent RNA polymerase
SR-BI scavenger receptor class B type I
VLDL very-low-density lipoprotein
VSV vesicular stomatitis virus
YFV yellow fever virus

Introduction

Hepatitis C virus (HCV) infection is now the leading cause of chronic hepatitis, liver cirrhosis, and hepatocellular carcinoma (HCC) in many areas of the world. An estimated 120 to 180 million people are chronically infected with HCV.[1] A protective vaccine is not available and therapeutic options are still limited. Current standard therapy, pegylated interferon-α (PEG-IFN-α) combined with ribavirin, results in a sustained virologic response in approximately 50% of patients.[2] As a consequence, the number of patients presenting with long-term chronic hepatitis C sequelae, including HCC, is expected to increase further during the next 10 to 20 years.

HCV was identified in 1989 as the most common etiologic agent of posttransfusion and sporadic non-A, non-B hepatitis.[3] However, the virus was not visualized conclusively, the low titres in serum and liver tissue precluded biochemical characterization of native viral products, and, most important, it was not possible until recently to culture HCV efficiently in vitro, thus impeding elucidation of the viral life cycle and the development of preventive vaccines and specific antiviral agents. Despite these obstacles, great progress has been made over the past 20 years using heterologous expression systems,[4] functional cDNA clones that are infectious in vivo in chimpanzees,[5] the replicon system,[6] retroviral pseudoparticles displaying functional HCV glycoproteins,[7] and complete cell culture systems.[8-10] These and other selected milestones in HCV research, including the recent completion of large-scale phase II clinical studies of NS3-4A protease inhibitors[11,12] and the identification of polymorphisms in the *IL28B* gene that determine spontaneous and treatment-induced HCV clearance,[13-17] are listed in **Table 7-1**.

Classification and Genetic Variability

HCV and, more recently, GB virus B (GBV-B) have been classified in the *Hepacivirus* genus within the Flaviviridae family, which also includes the genera *Flavivirus* (e.g., yellow fever virus, dengue virus) and *Pestivirus* (e.g., bovine viral diarrhea virus), as well as the unassigned GBV-A and GBV-C.[9] HCV contains a 9.6-kb positive-strand RNA genome composed of a 5′ noncoding region (NCR), which includes an internal ribosome entry site (IRES), an open reading frame that encodes the structural and nonstructural proteins, and a 3′ NCR (**Fig. 7-1**). The structural proteins, which form the viral particle, include the core protein and the envelope glycoproteins E1 and E2. The nonstructural proteins include the p7 viroporin, the NS2-3 and NS3-4A proteases, the NS3 RNA helicase, the NS4B and NS5A proteins, and the NS5B RNA-dependent RNA polymerase (RdRp).

Table 7-1 **Milestones in HCV Research**	
1975	Description of non-A, non-B hepatitis
1989	Identification of HCV
1993	Delineation of HCV genome organization and polyprotein processing
1996	First three-dimensional structure of an HCV protein (NS3-4A protease)
1997	First infectious clone of HCV
1998	Interferon-α and ribavirin combination therapy
1999	Replicon system
2003	Functional HCV pseudoparticles
2003	Proof-of-concept clinical studies of an HCV protease inhibitor
2005	Production of recombinant infectious HCV in tissue culture
2009	First phase II studies of HCV protease inhibitors completed
2009	Polymorphisms of the *IL28B* gene determine HCV clearance

HCV infection is a highly dynamic process, with a viral half-life of only a few hours and production and clearance of approximately 10^{12} virions per day in a given individual.[18] This high replicative activity, together with the lack of a proofreading function of the viral RdRp, is the basis of the high genetic variability of HCV.

HCV isolates can be classified into genotypes and subtypes.[19] There are seven genotypes that differ in their nucleotide sequence by 30% to 35%. Patients infected with genotype 1 do not respond as well to IFN-α–based therapy as those infected with genotype 2 or 3. Within an HCV genotype, several subtypes (designated a, b, c, and so on) can be defined, which differ in nucleotide sequence by 20% to 25%. The term quasispecies refers to the genetic heterogeneity of the population of HCV genomes coexisting within an infected individual.

To date, more than 85,000 HCV sequences, including 770 full-length genomes, have been deposited in public databases. Three complementary databases are dedicated specifically to HCV: the European HCV Database (euHCVdb; http://euhcvdb.ibcp.fr),[20] the Los Alamos National Laboratory HCV Database (http://hcv.lanl.gov), and the Japanese Hepatitis Virus Database (http://s2as02.genes.nig.ac.jp).[21]

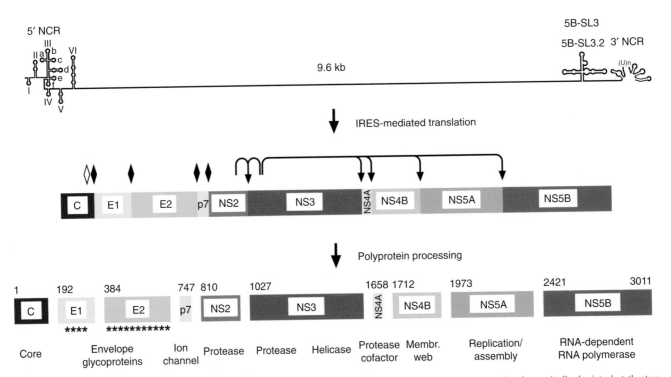

Fig. 7-1 Genetic organization and polyprotein processing of HCV. The 9.6-kb positive-strand RNA genome is schematically depicted at the top. Simplified RNA secondary structures in the 5′ and 3′ noncoding regions (NCRs) and the core gene, as well as the NS5B stem-loop 3 *cis*-acting replication element (5B-SL3), are shown. Internal ribosome entry site (IRES)-mediated translation yields a polyprotein precursor that is processed into the mature structural and nonstructural proteins. Amino acid numbers are shown above each protein (HCV H strain; genotype 1a; GenBank accession No. AF009606). *Solid diamonds* denote cleavages by the endoplasmic reticulum signal peptidase. The *open diamond* indicates further C-terminal processing of the core protein by signal peptide peptidase. *Arrows* indicate cleavages by the HCV NS2-3 and NS3-4A proteases. *Asterisks* in the E1 and E2 region indicate glycosylation of the envelope proteins. Note that polyprotein processing, illustrated here as a separate step for simplicity, occurs cotranslationally and posttranslationally.

<table>
<tr><td colspan="1">Table 7-2 In Vitro and in Vivo Models to Study HCV</td></tr>
</table>

In Vitro Models

- Transient cellular expression systems
- Stably transfected cell lines (constitutive or inducible expression)
- Replicons (subgenomic or full length; selectable or transient)
- Related viruses (e.g., GBV-B, BVDV)
- Retroviral pseudoparticles displaying functional HCV glycoproteins (HCVpp)
- Recombinant infectious HCV (cell culture–derived HCV, HCVcc)

In Vivo Models

- Chimpanzee *(Pan troglodytes)*
- Tree shrew *(Tupaia belangeri)*
- Transgenic mice
- Immunodeficient mice or hepatocellular reconstitution models
- Related viruses (e.g., GBV-B, BVDV)

BVDV, bovine viral diarrhea virus; GBV-B, GB virus B; HCV, hepatitis C virus

Model Systems

Different model systems have been used to study specific aspects of the viral life cycle[22,23] (**Table 7-2**).

In Vitro Models

In general, use of patient serum to inoculate primary hepatocytes or established cell lines in vitro yields only low-level replication, and often poorly reproducible results. In their present format, these systems may be useful (e.g., for neutralization assays) but they do not allow systematic investigation of the viral life cycle.[24]

The development of a replicon system for HCV was a particularly important breakthrough.[6] The prototype subgenomic replicon is a bicistronic RNA in which the portion of the HCV genome encoding the structural and part of the nonstructural proteins is replaced by the neomycin phosphotransferase gene (**Fig. 7-2**). Translation of the remaining nonstructural proteins 3-5B is initiated by a second, heterologous IRES. With this system it became possible for the first time to study

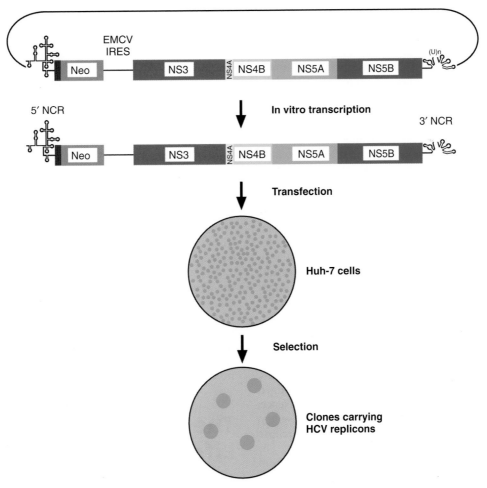

Fig. 7-2 Prototype subgenomic HCV replicon. RNA is transcribed in vitro from a plasmid containing the HCV 5′ noncoding region (NCR), which harbors an internal ribosome entry site (IRES), followed by a neomycin resistance cassette, a second heterologous IRES from encephalomyocarditis virus (EMCV), the HCV nonstructural region (NS3 to NS5B), and the HCV 3′ NCR. RNA is subsequently transfected into Huh-7 human hepatoma cells, followed by selection with G418 of clones harboring autonomously replicating subgenomic HCV RNA.

genuine HCV RNA replication in Huh-7 human HCC cells in vitro. Interestingly, selected amino acid substitutions (cell culture adaptive mutations or replication enhancing mutations) were found to increase the efficiency of replicon RNA amplification by several orders of magnitude.[25,26] In addition, the efficiency of replication was found to be dictated by the permissivity of a subset of Huh-7 cells within a given population.[27,28] Use of the replicon system has allowed the genetic dissection of HCV RNA elements and proteins, provided material for biochemical and ultrastructural characterization of the viral replication complex, and facilitated drug discovery and the investigation of antiviral resistance. Moreover, it has been exploited to study interactions between viral components and the host cell.

Since the original reports of functional genotype 1b replicons, replicons for genotypes 1a and 2a have also been constructed, as well as derivatives that express easily quantifiable marker enzymes. In addition, full-length replicons and HCV genomes that replicate efficiently in tissue culture have been developed, and the spectrum of permissive host cells has been expanded to other hepatic and nonhepatic cell lines. Finally, replicons have been established that harbor the green fluorescent protein in permissive sites within NS5A and allow tracking of functional HCV replication complexes in living cells.[29] Disappointingly, however, full-length HCV genomes with adaptive mutations were incapable of producing an infectious virus, and it became evident that the adaptive mutations required for efficient replication in tissue culture interfere with the productive packaging, assembly, or release of progeny particles.[30,31] On this background, the establishment of retroviral pseudoparticles displaying functional HCV glycoproteins (designated HCVpp for HCV pseudoparticles) as a robust model for the study of viral entry represented an important development.[7,32,33]

A major breakthrough became possible when an HCV genotype 2a clone isolated from a Japanese patient with a rare fulminant course of hepatitis C, designated JFH-1 (for *Japanese fulminant hepatitis 1*), was found to replicate in Huh-7 and other cell lines without requiring adaptive mutations.[34] Subsequently, cloned JFH-1 genomes transfected into Huh-7 cells were found to produce an infectious virus (designated HCVcc for cell culture-derived HCV), allowing for the first time studies of the complete life cycle of HCV in vitro.[8] Efficiency could be improved by using highly permissive Huh-7 sublines[35,36] and intragenotypic chimeras that consisted of the 5′ and 3′ NCRs and the NS3-5B region of JFH-1 and the C-NS2 region of a different genotype 2a isolate, designated J6.[35,37] Moreover, certain cell culture adaptive changes were found to further enhance virus yields.[38] Importantly, HCVcc particles were found to be infectious in vivo in chimpanzees[8,39] and immunodeficient mice with chimeric human livers,[39] and viral inocula derived from these animal models were infectious for naïve Huh-7 cells in vitro.[39] Hence, previously unexplored life cycle steps, including viral entry, genome packaging, virion assembly, maturation, and release can now be studied.

Low levels of infectious virus have also been obtained from the H77 genotype 1a isolate with five adaptive mutations.[40] In addition, JFH-1-based intergenotypic chimeras carrying the structural proteins from all major genotypes have been developed.[41] The challenge now remains to develop robust cell culture systems for primary HCV isolates.

In Vivo Models

The restricted host range of HCV has hampered the development of a suitable small animal model of viral replication and pathogenesis. Apart from a few reports showing transmission of the virus to tree shrews (*Tupaia belangeri*),[42] the chimpanzee (*Pan troglodytes*) is the only nonhuman species known to be susceptible to HCV infection. Indeed, the chimpanzee was essential in the early characterization of the agent responsible for non-A, non-B hepatitis and has allowed important aspects of HCV replication, pathogenesis, and prevention to be determined.[43] However, ethical and financial restrictions limit the use of primates to highly selected experimental questions.

Expression of HCV proteins in transgenic mice has provided some insights into the pathogenesis of virus-induced liver disease. However, expression of HCV proteins from chromosomally integrated cDNA does not appropriately reflect the viral life cycle and studies on viral entry and replication are hardly conceivable in this system.

GBV-B, the closest relative of HCV, can be transmitted to tamarins (*Saguinus* sp.) and common marmosets (*Callithrix jacchus*) and may represent a valuable surrogate model for HCV.[44] Remarkably, GBV-B can be cultured in tamarin hepatocytes in vitro. In addition, infectious cDNA clones and replicons have been established for GBV-B. However, GBV-B typically leads to self-limited infection and viral persistence is exceptional.

Progress in the development of a small animal model of HCV replication was achieved with the successful infection of immunodeficient mice reconstituted with human hepatocytes.[45,46] The properties of two different mouse strains, the *Alb-uPA*-transgenic and the immunodeficient SCID mouse, were combined to develop a model system that allows orthotopic engraftment of human hepatocytes (**Fig. 7-3**). Expression of the murine urokinase type of plasminogen activator under the transcriptional control of the albumin promotor (*Alb-uPA*) programs murine hepatocyte death, providing a suitable microenvironment for the engraftment and expansion of transplanted human hepatocytes. Inoculation with serum from patients with hepatitis C results in persistent HCV viremia in mice with high-level human hepatocyte engraftment, with viral titers similar to those found in infected humans.[45]

This model has been exploited successfully to investigate the in vivo phenotype of specific mutations introduced into the HCV genome, selected aspects of viral pathogenesis, neutralization of viral entry, and the evaluation of novel antiviral strategies.[31,38,39,47] The handling of these fragile mice, however, presents a nontrivial challenge and requires special expertise. More robust small animal models are therefore needed.[23]

The Virus and Its Life Cycle

The life cycle of HCV is illustrated in **Figure 7-4**. It includes (1) binding of the particle to a complex set of entry factors and internalization into the host cell, (2) cytoplasmic release of the viral RNA genome, (3) IRES-mediated translation and polyprotein processing by cellular and viral proteases, (4)

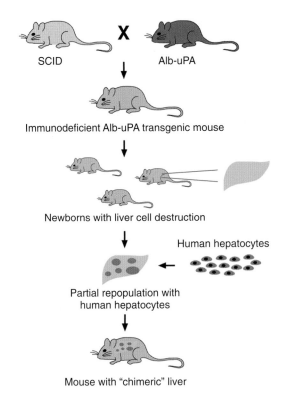

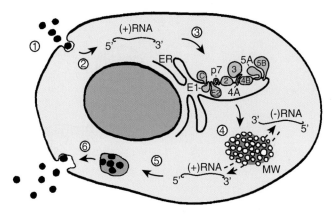

Fig. 7-4 **Life cycle of HCV.** *1,* Virus binding and internalization. *2,* Cytoplasmic release and uncoating. *3,* IRES-mediated translation and polyprotein processing. *4,* RNA replication. *5,* Packaging and assembly. *6,* Virion maturation and release. The topology of HCV structural and nonstructural proteins at the endoplasmic reticulum *(ER)* membrane is shown schematically. HCV RNA replication occurs in a specific membrane alteration, the membranous web *(MW)*. Note that IRES-mediated translation and polyprotein processing, as well as membranous web formation and RNA replication—illustrated here as separate steps for simplicity—may occur in a tightly coupled fashion.

Fig. 7-3 **A small animal model of HCV replication (see text for explanation).**

RNA replication, (5) packaging and assembly, and (6) virion maturation and release from the host cell.

Virion Structure

While exciting progress has been made toward determining virion structures of some of the related flaviviruses and alphaviruses (e.g., dengue virus),[48] HCV has not been definitively visualized and its structure remains obscure. Based on filtration and electron microscopic studies, HCV particles are 40 to 70 nm in diameter.[8] It is thought that the core protein and the envelope glycoproteins E1 and E2 represent the principal protein components of the virion. E1 and E2 are presumably anchored to a host cell–derived, double-layer lipid envelope that surrounds a nucleocapsid composed of multiple copies of the core protein and the genomic RNA. A growing body of evidence indicates that the infectious virus is associated with low-density (LDL) and very-low-density lipoproteins (VLDL), explaining the unusually heterogenous and low buoyant density of HCV (peak infectivity near 1.10 g/ml).[49] Indeed, apolipoproteins B, C1, and E have been reported to be present in HCV virions.[50]

Viral Entry

HCV is highly restricted in its tropism, with human hepatocytes representing the main target cell. Infection of B cells, dendritic cells, and other cell types has also been reported, but this remains controversial.

CD81, a tetraspanin protein found on the surface of many cell types including hepatocytes,[51] scavenger receptor class B type I (SR-BI),[52] and the tight junction proteins claudin-1

(CLDN1)[53] and occludin (OCLN)[54] have been identified as essential entry factors[55] (**Fig. 7-5**). These four factors are necessary and sufficient to confer HCV susceptibility to all cells tested so far. Interestingly, none of these molecules is exclusive to hepatocytes, although other cell types may not express the complete set at sufficient levels.[54] Complementation experiments using human and murine versions of these entry factors revealed that only CD81 and OCLN must be of human origin to support HCV entry,[54] thereby opening new avenues for the development of transgenic mice supporting HCV infection.[23]

In addition to the four specific entry factors, the low-density lipoprotein receptor (LDLR)[56,57] and glycosaminoglycans may serve as attachment factors that collect HCV particles for further targeting to SR-BI, CD81, and the tight junction components CLDN1 and OCLN (see **Fig. 7-5**). The mechanisms governing transit to and uptake via tight junctions in polarized hepatocytes are currently under intensive investigation. Interestingly, tight junction-associated molecules play key roles in the entry of other viruses (e.g., coxsackievirus B).[58] Of note, HCV has also been reported to undergo direct cell-to-cell transmission, which may represent a mechanism of escape from neutralizing antibodies and promote viral persistence.[59,60]

HCV enters the cell via clathrin-mediated endocytosis, with transit through an endosomal, low pH compartment and endosomal membrane fusion.[61] The structural basis for low pH-induced membrane fusion has been elucidated for related flaviviruses and alphaviruses.[62] The envelope proteins of these viruses have an internal fusion peptide that is exposed during low pH-mediated domain rearrangement and trimerization of the protein. The scaffolds of these so-called class II fusion proteins are remarkably similar, suggesting that entry of all viruses in the Flaviviridae family, including HCV, may include a class II fusion step. Recent evidence revealed a key role for

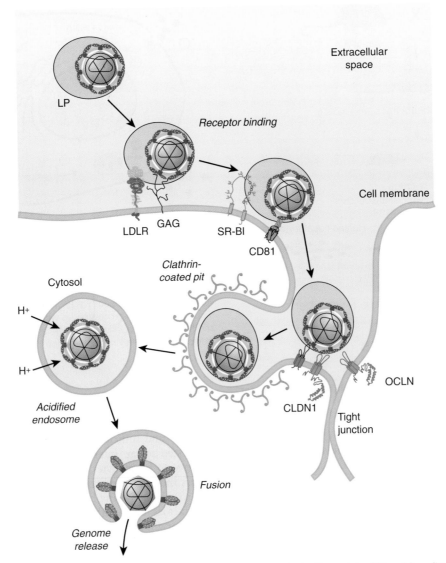

Fig. 7-5 HCV entry. Circulating infectious HCV particles are associated with very-low-density lipoproteins (LP) and form lipo-viro-particles (LVP). Virus binding to the cell surface and entry may involve glycosaminoglycans (GAG), the low-density-lipoprotein receptor (LDLR), the scavenger receptor class B type I (SR-BI), the tetraspanin protein CD81, claudin-1 (CLDN1), and occludin (OCLN). Acidification of the endosome induces HCV glycoprotein membrane fusion, leading to genome release. See http://ibcpdb.ibcp.fr/scripts/ibcp_resources.php?lang=fr&evene=Videos for a video animation.

E2 in the fusion process.[63,64] However, there is also evidence for the presence of fusion determinants in E1 and the E1-E2 heterodimer. Ongoing studies are aimed at elucidating the mechanisms involved in the activation of HCV for low pH-induced fusion, the fusion step itself, and the identity of the fusion peptide(s).

Genome Organization

HCV contains a 9.6-kb positive-strand RNA genome composed of a 5′ NCR, a long open reading frame encoding a polyprotein precursor of about 3000 amino acids, and a 3′ NCR (see **Fig. 7-1**). The mechanisms regulating the different fates of the genome (i.e., translation), replication, and packaging are only poorly understood.

It took 8 years from the discovery of HCV to the establishment of the first infectious cDNA clone[5] because in the absence of a robust tissue culture system, the only readout for infectivity was the direct inoculation of in vitro transcribed RNA into the liver of a chimpanzee. In addition, due to the variation present in the quasispecies and errors introduced by PCR amplification, construction of infectious cDNA clones required preparation of a consensus sequence from a number of clones. Functional cDNA clones now exist for genotypes 1a, 1b, 2a, 3a, and 4a.[65]

The 5′ NCR is highly conserved among different HCV isolates and contains an IRES that is essential for cap-independent translation of the viral RNA. The 5′ NCR is composed of four highly ordered domains numbered I to IV[66] (see **Fig. 7-1**). Domain I is not required for IRES activity, but domains I and II are both essential for HCV RNA replication.[67] Interestingly, an abundant liver-specific microRNA, miR-122, was found to bind the HCV 5′ NCR and to enhance viral RNA replication.[68] This finding provided the first example of a virus exploiting a cellular microRNA and uncovered a new angle for antiviral intervention.[69]

The 3′ NCR is composed of a short variable region, a poly(U/UC) tract with an average length of 80 nucleotides, and an almost invariant 98-nucleotide RNA element, designated the X-tail.[70,71] The conserved elements in the 3′ NCR, including a minimal poly(U) tract of about 25 bases, are essential for replication in cell culture and in vivo.[72]

Besides the 5′ and 3′ NCRs, essential *cis*-acting replication elements (CREs) have been identified in the sequences that encode the core[73,74] and the C-terminal region of NS5B.[75] An essential stem-loop, designated 5B-SL3.2, was identified within a larger cruciform RNA element, designated 5B-SL3, in the NS5B coding region (see **Fig. 7-1**). The upper loop of 5B-SL3.2 was found to interact with a stem-loop in the X-tail, suggesting that a pseudoknot is formed at the 3′ end of the HCV genome that is essential for RNA replication.[76] In addition, long-range RNA-RNA interactions between the 5′ NCR and the 5B-SL3.2 have been described, mediating circularization of the HCV genome.[77]

Of note, subgenomic HCV RNAs have been identified in several patients with chronic hepatitis C. These naturally occurring deletion mutants typically lack the envelope glycoprotein coding region, are capable of autonomous replication, and can be *trans*-packaged to generate infectious defective particles.[78]

IRES-Mediated Translation Initiation

Domains II, III, and IV of the 5′ NCR, together with the first 24 to 40 nucleotides of the core coding region, constitute the IRES. HCV translation initiation occurs through formation of a binary complex between the IRES and the 40S ribosomal subunit, followed by association of eukaryotic translation initiation factor 3 (eIF3) and ternary complex (eIF2•Met-tRNA$_i$•GTP) at the AUG initiation codon (48S-like complex). Finally, the rate limiting step is the GTP-dependent association of the 60S ribosomal subunit to form an 80S complex.[79]

Structural insights, coupled with biochemical studies, have revealed that the IRES substitutes for some activities of the translation initiation factors by binding and inducing conformational changes in the 40S ribosomal subunit.[80,81] Direct interactions of the IRES with initiation factor eIF3 are also crucial for efficient translation initiation.[66,82]

Polyprotein Processing

IRES-mediated translation of the HCV open reading frame yields a polyprotein precursor that is cotranslationally and posttranslationally processed by cellular and viral proteases into the mature structural and nonstructural proteins (see **Fig. 7-1**). The structural proteins and the p7 polypeptide are processed by the endoplasmic reticulum (ER) signal peptidase and signal peptide peptidase while the nonstructural proteins are processed by the viral NS2-3 and NS3-4A proteases.

The nonstructural proteins are cleaved in a preferential order.[83] The first cleavages occur cotranslationally at the NS2/NS3 and NS3/NS4A sites and liberate NS3 from the remainder of the polyprotein. Subsequent processing events can be mediated *in trans*, with rapid processing at the NS5A/NS5B site to produce a NS4A-5A intermediate. NS3-4A–mediated cleavage then occurs between NS4A and NS4B, to produce a relatively stable NS4B-5A precursor, and subsequently between NS4B and NS5A.

Structure and Function of the Viral Proteins

Core

The first structural protein encoded by the HCV open reading frame is the core protein, which forms the viral nucleocapsid. An internal signal sequence located between the core and E1 targets the nascent polypeptide to the ER membrane, followed by translocation of the E1 ectodomain into the ER lumen (**Fig. 7-6**). Cleavage of the signal sequence by signal peptidase yields an immature 191-amino acid core protein. Further C-terminal processing by signal peptide peptidase yields the mature 21-kDa core protein of 173 to 179 amino acids.[84]

The mature core is a dimeric α-helical membrane protein composed of two domains.[85] The N-terminal hydrophilic domain 1 (D1) contains a high proportion of basic amino acid residues and has been implicated both in RNA binding and homo-oligomerization. The C-terminal hydrophobic domain 2 (D2) mediates association with lipid droplets.[86]

When expressed in mammalian cells, the core is found on ER membranes, in seemingly ER-derived membranous webs (see later discussion), and on the surface of lipid droplets.[87] The association with lipid droplets[88-90] and interaction with NS5A[91] play central roles in viral assembly (see later discussion). In addition, it has been speculated that the interaction of the core with lipid droplets may affect lipid metabolism, contributing to the development of liver steatosis, which is often seen in hepatitis C, particularly in patients infected with genotype 3.

Little is known about the assembly of the core into nucleocapsids. Assembly of nucleocapsid-like structures has been reported with recombinant proteins and in cell-free translation systems.[92] In addition, the core has been reported to display RNA chaperone activity.[93] However, the signals and processes that mediate RNA packaging and nucleocapsid assembly during HCV replication are unknown.

Intriguingly, the core protein has been reported to interact with a variety of cellular proteins and to influence numerous host cell functions, including apoptosis, cell cycle control, gene expression, and many others. However, the relevance of these observations, derived mainly from heterologous overexpression experiments, for the natural course and pathogenesis of hepatitis C is presently unknown.

Envelope Glycoproteins

The envelope proteins E1 and E2 are glycosylated and form a noncovalent heterodimer, which is believed to represent the building block for the viral envelope. The ectodomains of E1 and E2 contain numerous highly conserved cysteine residues that may form four and nine disulfide bonds, respectively. In addition, E1 and E2 contain 4 and 11 glycosylation sites, respectively. Thus E1 and E2 maturation and folding is a complex and interdependent process that involves the ER chaperone machinery and disulfide bond formation, as well as glycosylation. E1 and E2 are anchored to the ER membrane by

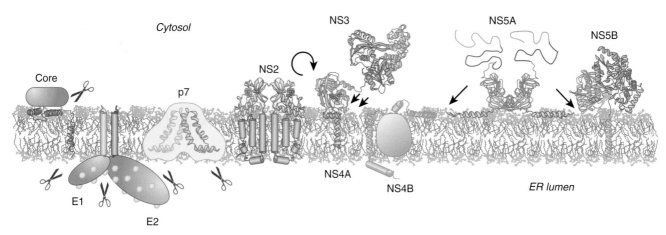

Fig. 7-6 Structures and membrane association of HCV proteins. *Scissors* indicate cleavages by the endoplasmic reticulum (ER) signal peptidase, except on the cytosolic side where it indicates the processing of the core protein by signal peptide peptidase (SPP). The *cyclic arrow* denotes cleavage by the NS2-3 protease. *Black arrows* indicate processing by the NS3-4A protease. Known protein structures are shown as *ribbon diagrams*. The structures and the membrane bilayer are shown at the same scale. Proteins or protein segments of unresolved structure are represented as *colored spheres* or *cylinders* with their approximate sizes. From left to right are shown: (i) Core protein *(red)* includes two amphipathic α-helices connected by a hydrophobic loop (D2 domain[86]) and the E1 signal peptide *(violet;* Penin F et al, unpublished data) cleaved by SPP. (ii) E1-E2 glycoprotein heterodimer associated by the C-terminal transmembrane domains. *Green spots* denote glycosylation of the envelope proteins. (iii) Tentative representation of two p7 monomers within the electron microscopy structure of the hexameric p7 ion channel.[101] A 180-degree rotation is applied between the two p7 monomers *(violet;* Penin F et al, unpublished data). (iv) NS2 catalytic domain (dimer subunits in *blue* and *magenta;* PDB entry 2HD0[105]) connected to their N-terminal membrane domains constituted of three putative transmembrane segments (PDB entry 2JY0[104]; Penin F et al, unpublished data). The active site residues His 143, Glu 163, and Cys 184 are represented as spheres. (v) NS3 serine protease domain *(cyan)* associated with the central protease activation and the N-terminal transmembrane domains of NS4A *(yellow).* The catalytic triad of the NS3 serine protease (His 57, Asp 81, and Ser 139) is represented as spheres *(magenta).* NS3 helicase domains I, II, and III are colored in *silver, red,* and *blue,* respectively. This representation of NS3 (derived from PDB entry 1CU1[109]) indicates that the helicase domain can no longer interact with the NS3 protease domain when the latter is associated with the membrane through its amphipathic α-helix 11-21 *(green)* and the transmembrane domain of NS4A (BMRB entry 15580[111]). (vi) NS4B with the N-terminal part, including two amphipathic α-helices of which the second has the potential to traverse the membrane bilayer (PDB entry 2KDR[121]), the central part harboring multiple predicted transmembrane segments, and the C-terminal cytosolic part, including a predicted highly conserved α-helix and an amphipathic α-helix interacting in-plane with the membrane (PDB entry 2JXF[122]). (vii) NS5A domain I dimer (PDB entry 1ZH1[139]; subunits colored in *magenta* and *ice blue*), as well as intrinsically unfolded domains II and III.[146-148] The N-terminal amphipathic α-helix in-plane membrane anchor (PDB entry 1R7E[138]; helices colored in *red* and *blue*) are shown in relative position to the phospholipid membrane (adapted from reference[139]). (viii) NS5B RNA-dependent RNA polymerase (RdRp) catalytic domain (PDB entry 1GX6[184]) associated with the membrane via its C-terminal transmembrane segment (Penin F et al, unpublished data). The fingers, palm, and thumb subdomains of the catalytic domain are colored in *blue, red,* and *green,* respectively. The catalytic site of the RdRp lies within the center of the cytosolic domain and the RNA template-binding cleft is located vertically on the right along the thumb subdomain β-loop *(orange)* and the C-terminal part of segment 545-562 *(silver),* connecting the cytosolic domain to the transmembrane segment *(magenta).* The membrane is represented as a simulated model of a 1-palmitoyl-2-oleoyl-3-*sn*-glycero-3-phospholcholine (POPC) bilayer (obtained from D.P. Tieleman, http://moose.bio.ucalgary.ca/). Polar heads and hydrophobic tails of phospholipids (stick structure) are colored in *light yellow* and *light gray,* respectively. The positions of the NS5A in-plane membrane helices at the membrane interface, as well as that of the transmembrane domain of NS5B, were deduced from molecular dynamics simulations in POPC bilayer (Penin F, Moradpour D et al, unpublished data). The positioning of the NS3-4A membrane segments and of the amphipathic α-helices in core and NS4B are tentative. The figure was generated from the structure coordinates deposited in the PDB using Visual Molecular Dynamics, VMD (http://www.ks.uiuc.edu/Research/vmd/) and rendered with POV-Ray (http://www.povray.org/).

C-terminal transmembrane domains, which are also involved in the heterodimerization and ER retention of the proteins.[94] A model of the structural organization of E2 was recently proposed, providing insights into antigenic determinants of the virus, the CD81 binding site, and the location of a putative fusion loop.[64] Determination of the three-dimensional structures of E1 and E2 will be key in elucidating the receptor binding and fusion processes mediated by these proteins.

The genes encoding the envelope glycoproteins E1 and E2 are particularly variable. A hypervariable region (HVR) of approximately 28 amino acids in the N-terminal domain of E2 has been termed HVR1 and differs by up to 80% among HCV isolates. Interestingly, despite high variability at the sequence level, the structural properties of this domain were found to be quite conserved.[95] Several observations indicate a role of HVR1 in virus entry.

p7

p7 is a hydrophobic 63-amino acid polypeptide comprising two transmembrane α-helices connected by a short cytoplasmic loop, while the N and C termini are oriented toward the ER lumen.[96] p7 is not required for RNA replication in vitro but is essential for the assembly and release of infectious HCV in vitro,[97,98] as well as productive infection in vivo.[99] However, its precise function is unknown.

p7 has been reported to form both hexamers and heptamers and to possess cation channel activity, indicating that it belongs to the viroporin family.[100,101] However, the relationship between ion channel activity and the role of p7 in viral assembly and release is unknown. Single-particle electron microscopy recently revealed the three-dimensional structure of the hexameric p7 channel at 16 Å resolution, revealing a flower-shaped protein architecture with six protruding petals oriented toward the ER lumen.[101] In the modeled structure, the first transmembrane α-helix lines the pore and the N and C termini occupy the "petal tips."

NS2-3 Protease

Cleavage of the polyprotein precursor at the NS2/NS3 junction is accomplished by a cysteine protease encoded by NS2 and whose function is strongly enhanced by the N-terminal one third of NS3.[102] This NS2-3 protease itself is dispensable for RNA replication, but cleavage at this junction is essential.[37,103] The catalytic activity resides in the C-terminal half of NS2 (amino acid residues 94-217, NS2^{pro}, with His 143, Glu 163, and Cys 184 representing the catalytic triad) while the N-terminal part represents a membrane domain with one to three transmembrane segments.[104] The crystal structure of NS2^{pro} revealed a dimer with two composite active sites[105] (see **Fig. 7-6**). Each active site is composed of residues from the two monomers (i.e., His 143 and Glu 163 are contributed by one monomer and Cys 184 by the other).

Solving the structure of the N-terminal membrane domain of NS2 should yield insights into additional functions of the protein. NS2 is known to play an essential role in HCV infectious virus assembly that is independent of its protease activity[97,104,106–108] but may involve a complex network of interactions with structural and other nonstructural viral proteins.[107]

NS3-4A Complex

NS3 is a multifunctional protein, with a serine protease located in the N-terminal one third (amino acids 1-180) and an RNA helicase/NTPase in the C-terminal two thirds (amino acids 181 to 631). Both enzyme activities have been well characterized, and high-resolution structures have been solved.[109]

The NS3-4A protease has emerged as a prime target for antiviral intervention.[11,12,110] It adopts a chymotrypsin-like fold with two β-barrel subdomains. The catalytic triad is formed by His 57, Asp 81, and Ser 139. The 54-amino acid NS4A polypeptide functions as a co-factor for the NS3 serine protease. Its central portion comprises a β-strand that is incorporated into the N-terminal β-barrel of NS3 while the hydrophobic N-terminal segment is required for membrane association[111] and the C-terminal acidic domain was shown to modulate RNA replication.[112] Determinants of substrate specificity include an acidic amino acid residue at the P6 position, a P1 cysteine (*trans*-cleavage sites) or threonine (*cis*-cleavage site between NS3 and NS4A), and an amino acid residue with a small side chain (i.e., alanine or serine) at the P1′ position (consensus cleavage sequence D/E-X-X-X-X-C/T | S/A-X-X-X).

Membrane association and structural organization of the NS3-4A complex are ensured in a sequential manner by two determinants: the N-terminal 21 amino acids of NS4A, which form a transmembrane α-helix, and an in-plane amphipathic α-helix at the N terminus of NS3, designated helix α$_0$.[111] Together, these determinants properly position the serine protease active site with respect to the membrane (**Fig. 7-7**).

Interestingly, it has been shown that the NS3-4A protease cleaves and thereby inactivates selected cellular proteins, including two crucial adaptor proteins in innate immune sensing—Cardif[113] (also known as MAVS, IPS-1 and VISA) and Trif[114]—as well as T-cell protein tyrosine phosphatase (TC-PTP).[115] Hence, the NS3-4A protease plays essential roles not only in the replication but also in the persistence and pathogenesis of HCV.

The NS3 helicase is a member of the superfamily 2 DExH/D-box helicases. It couples ATP hydrolysis to the unwinding of double-stranded RNA or of single-stranded RNA regions with extensive secondary structure. NS3 unwinds RNA in a ratchet-like fashion.[116] Similar to other HCV nonstructural proteins, the NS3 helicase has been proposed to form higher-order oligomers.[117] It is unknown why the serine protease and RNA helicase domains are physically linked, but evidence for cross-talk between these two essential enzymatic activities is emerging.[118,119]

NS4B

NS4B is a relatively poorly characterized, hydrophobic 27-kDa protein of 261 amino acids.[120] It is an integral membrane protein predicted to comprise an N-terminal part (amino acids 1 to approximately 69), a central region harboring four transmembrane passages (amino acids approximately 70 to approximately 190), and a C-terminal domain (amino acids approximately 191 to 261). The N-terminal portion comprises two amphipathic α-helices, the second of which has the potential to traverse the membrane bilayer, likely upon oligomerization.[121] The C-terminal part comprises a membrane-associated amphipathic α-helix[122] and two reported palmitoylation sites.[123]

NS4B induces the formation of the membranous web, the specific membrane alteration that serves as a scaffold for the HCV replication complex[124,125] (see later discussion). It interacts with other viral nonstructural proteins and has been reported to bind viral RNA.[126] In addition, NS4B was reported to harbor NTPase activity[127] and has recently been suggested to have a role in viral assembly.[128] Much work remains to be done to further dissection of these multiple functions, as well as refine the membrane topology and complete structure of NS4B.

NS5A

NS5A is a membrane-associated phosphoprotein that plays an important role in modulating viral RNA replication and particle formation. Comparative sequence analyses and limited proteolysis of recombinant NS5A have defined three domains separated by two low-complexity sequence (LCS) blocks.[129] Domains 1 (amino acids 36 to 213; genotype 1b Con1 strain) and 2 (amino acids 250 to 342) are primarily involved in RNA replication, whereas domain 3 (amino acids 356 to 447) is essential for viral assembly.[130,131]

HCV NS5A can be found in basally phosphorylated (56 kDa) and hyperphosphorylated (58 kDa) forms. Recent studies have shown that the α isoform of casein kinase I (CKIα)[132,133] and casein kinase II (CKII)[131] can phosphorylate NS5A on serine residues in the LCS between domains 1 and 2 and on Ser 457 (genotype 2 JFH-1 strain) in domain 3, respectively. However, it is unknown whether additional cellular kinases are involved in generating the different phosphoforms of NS5A.

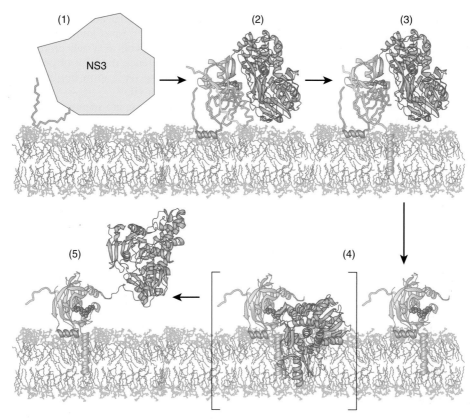

Fig. 7-7 Dynamic model for the membrane association and structural organization of HCV NS3-4A. Translation of NS3 occurs at the membrane (*Step 1*). An amphipathic α-helix at the N terminus of NS3 folds upon interaction with the membrane interface, followed by folding of the serine protease and helicase domains (*Step 2*). The hydrophobic N-terminal segment of NS4A is inserted into the membrane after processing at the NS3/NS4A site (*Step 3*). Complete folding and membrane association lock the serine protease in a strictly defined position onto the membrane (*Step 4*). At the same time, the helicase domain has to move away from the serine protease domain through a rotation of the linker segment connecting the two domains (*Step 5*). See http://ibcpdb.ibcp.fr/scripts/ibcp_resources.php?lang=fr&evene=Videos for a video animation. *(From Brass V, Berke JM, Montserret R, et al. Structural determinants for membrane association and dynamic organization of the hepatitis C virus NS3-4A complex. Proc Natl Acad Sci U S A 2008;105:14545–14550, with permission.)*

Cell culture–adaptive mutations often affect centrally located serine residues that are required for hyperphosphorylation, suggesting that the phosphorylation state of NS5A modulates the efficiency of HCV RNA replication.[134–136] According to one model, hyperphosphorylation of NS5A reduces its interaction with the human vesicle-associated membrane protein–associated protein A (hVAP-A).[134] This vesicle sorting protein has been implicated in directing nonstructural proteins to lipid rafts that may be involved in viral RNA replication.[137] More recently, CKII-mediated phosphorylation of Ser 457 was found to be essential for JFH-1 viral assembly and to regulate the production of an infectious virus.[131]

NS5A is a monotopic protein anchored to the membrane by an N-terminal amphipathic α-helix embedded in-plane into the cytosolic leaflet of the membrane interface.[138] The crystal structure of domain 1 immediately following this α-helix revealed a "clawlike" dimer with a groove that faces away from the membrane and could accommodate either single- or double-stranded RNA[139] (see **Fig. 7-6**). Indeed, the RNA binding properties of NS5A have been confirmed biochemically.[140] According to one hypothesis, multiple NS5A dimers may form a two-dimensional array on intracellular membranes, thereby creating a "basic railway" that would allow the

sliding of RNA.[141] This would allow NS5A to tether the viral RNA onto intracellular membranes and coordinate its different fates during HCV replication. It has been shown that only a small proportion of the HCV nonstructural proteins expressed in cells at a given time are actively engaged in RNA replication.[142,143] One can easily conceive, therefore, that these proteins may have additional structural functions as arrays or lattices on membranes. The formation of such higher-order structures may explain the extraordinary potency of small molecule inhibitors targeting the N-terminal region of NS5A.[144] Interestingly, a dimeric NS5A domain 1 structure with a different conformation of the two monomers was recently reported.[145] It is tempting to speculate that a switch between these alternative conformations may modulate the different roles of NS5A in viral RNA replication and particle assembly.

NS5A domains 2[146,147] and 3[148] have been found to be natively unfolded, suggesting that conformations with specific functions may be stabilized upon interaction with viral or host proteins. For example, domain 2 was found to interact with and serve as a substrate for cyclophilins A and B[147] (see later discussion).

HCV NS5A has attracted considerable interest because of its potential role in modulating the response to IFN-α therapy.

Studies performed in Japan first described a correlation between mutations within a discrete region of NS5A, termed interferon sensitivity determining region (ISDR), and a favorable response to IFN-α therapy.[149] However, this remains a controversial issue that has not translated thus far into clinically applicable predictors.[150] Numerous additional potential functions and interactions have been attributed to NS5A.[151,152] However, similar to the core protein, only very few of these postulated properties of NS5A have been validated in a meaningful context involving active HCV RNA replication or HCV infection in vivo.

NS5B

HCV replication proceeds via synthesis of a complementary negative-strand RNA using the genome as a template and the subsequent synthesis of genomic positive-strand RNA from this negative-strand RNA template. The key enzyme responsible for both of these steps is the NS5B RdRp. This viral enzyme has been extensively characterized,[153-155] and NS5B has emerged as a major target for antiviral intervention. NS5B contains motifs that are shared by all RdRps, including the hallmark GDD sequence within motif C, and the classical fingers, palm, and thumb subdomain organization of a right hand (see **Fig. 7-6**). A special feature of the HCV RdRp is that extensive interactions between the fingers and thumb subdomains result in a completely encircled active site. This feature is shared by other RdRps.[156] Similar to poliovirus RdRp,[157] oligomerization of HCV NS5B has been reported to be important for cooperative RNA synthesis activity.[158,159]

NS5B is a so-called tail-anchored protein. Membrane association is mediated by the C-terminal 21-amino acid residues, which are dispensable for polymerase activity in vitro but indispensable for RNA replication in cells.[160] (see **Fig. 7-6**). Molecular modeling of membrane-associated NS5B suggests that the RNA-binding groove is stacked onto the membrane interface, thereby preventing access to the RNA template. This inactive form of the RdRp may be activated by a conformational change of segment 545-562, which connects the catalytic domain and the C-terminal transmembrane segment of NS5B. Such a conformational change would liberate the RNA-binding groove and move the NS5B catalytic domain away from the membrane.

ARFP/F Proteins

An alternative reading frame (ARF) was identified in the genotype 1a core coding region that, as a result of a −2/+1 ribosomal frameshift, has the potential to encode a protein of up to 160 amino acids, designated ARFP (alternative reading frame protein) or F (frameshift) protein.[161] Amino acid sequencing indicated that the frameshift likely occurs at or near codon 11 of the core protein sequence. However, multiple and in part isolate-dependent frame shifting events, as well as internal translation initiation events, have also been reported. Detection of antibodies and T cells specific for the ARFP/F proteins in patients with hepatitis C suggests that these proteins are expressed during infection. However, the ARFP/F proteins are not required for RNA replication in vitro and in vivo.[73,74] More recently, alternative forms of the core protein, ranging in size from 8 to 14 kDa (minicores), have been described.[162] The functions, if any, of the ARFP/F proteins and minicores in the life cycle and pathogenesis of HCV remain to be elucidated.

The Viral Replication Complex

Formation of a membrane-associated replication complex, composed of viral proteins, replicating RNA, and altered cellular membranes, is a hallmark of all positive-strand RNA viruses investigated thus far.[163,164] Depending on the virus, replication may occur on altered membranes derived from the ER, Golgi apparatus, mitochondria, or even lysosomes. The role of membranes in viral RNA synthesis is not well understood. It may include (1) the physical support and organization of the RNA replication complex[157]; (2) the compartmentalization and local concentration of viral products; (3) tethering of the viral RNA during unwinding; (4) provision of lipid constituents important for replication; and (5) protection of the viral RNA from double-strand RNA-mediated host defenses or RNA interference.

A specific membrane alteration, designated the membranous web, was identified as the site of RNA replication in Huh-7 cells containing subgenomic HCV replicons[125] (**Fig. 7-8**). Formation of the membranous web was induced by NS4B alone and was very similar to the "spongelike inclusions" previously found by electron microscopy in the liver of HCV-infected chimpanzees.[124] It is currently believed that the membranous web is derived from ER membranes. Ongoing studies are aimed at characterizing the host factors and cellular processes involved in formation of the HCV replication complex. Life cell imaging and electron tomography have yielded insights into the dynamics and three-dimensional organization of the replication complexes of HCV and the related dengue virus, respectively.[165,166]

Recent studies demonstrate a complex interaction between HCV replication and the cellular lipid metabolism. Such observations suggest that pharmacologic manipulation of lipid metabolism may have therapeutic potential in hepatitis C.[167]

Additional host factors involved in HCV replication have been identified. Starting with the observation that cyclosporin A (CsA) inhibits viral RNA accumulation in vitro, cyclophilin B (CypB) was identified as target of CsA action.[168] More recently, cyclophilin A (CypA) was found to play an essential role in viral RNA replication and assembly through interactions with NS5A and NS2.[169-171] NS5A domain 2 was found to interact directly with the active sites of CypA and CypB, and nuclear magnetic resonance studies revealed that proline residues in domain 2 form a substrate for the peptidyl-prolyl *cis/trans* isomerase (PPIase) activity of both cyclophilins.[147] Based on these findings, nonimmunosuppressive CsA analogues are currently being developed as antivirals against hepatitis C.[172]

RNA interference has yielded important insight into host factors involved in HCV replication.[173] Intriguingly, siRNA screens performed by several independent groups led to the identification of phosphatidylinositol 4-kinase IIIα (PI4KIIIα) as an essential host factor involved in HCV RNA replication.[174-177] Knockdown of PI4KIIIα interferes with membranous web formation and inhibits HCV RNA replication. However, the precise mechanism by which PI4KIIIα is

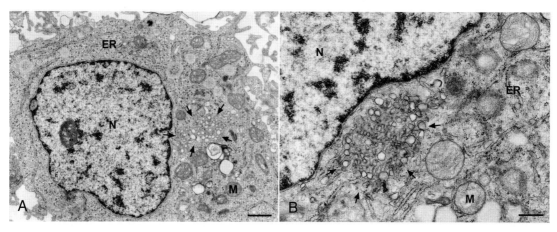

Fig. 7-8 **HCV replication complex.**[125] **A,** Low-power overview of a HuH-7 cell harboring a subgenomic HCV replicon. A distinct membrane alteration, named the membranous web *(arrows)*, is found in the juxtanuclear region. Note the circumscript nature of this specific membrane alteration and the otherwise unaltered cellular organelles. Bar, 1 μm. **B,** Higher magnification of a membranous web *(arrows)* composed of small vesicles embedded in a membrane matrix. Note the close association of the membranous web with the rough endoplasmic reticulum. Bar, 500 nm. The membranous web harbors all HCV nonstructural proteins and nascent viral RNA in HuH-7 cells harboring subgenomic replicons, and therefore represents the HCV RNA replication complex. ER, endoplasmic reticulum; M, mitochondria; N, nucleus.

involved in membranous web and HCV replication complex formation remains to be elucidated.

Packaging, Assembly, and Particle Release

The late steps of the viral life cycle have only recently become amenable to systematic study, with the introduction of the HCVcc system. Lipid droplets and the very-low-density lipoprotein (VLDL) pathway have been found to play central roles in HCV assembly and release.[88-90,178,179] By consequence, and as stated above, apolipoproteins B, C1, and E have been reported to be present in HCV virions.[50]

Interestingly, recent evidence indicates that most, if not all, HCV nonstructural proteins are involved in infectious particle assembly.[180] Current evidence indicates that NS5A might function as a "molecular switch" between translation, replication, and assembly,[130,131,134] possibly by tethering the viral RNA to membranes,[141] and/or by providing a physical link between replication complexes and viral assembly sites on lipid droplets. However, the mechanisms governing the assembly and release of newly formed viral particles are still poorly understood.

Implications for the Development of New Therapeutic Strategies

In principle, each step of the HCV life cycle (see **Fig. 7-4**) represents a target for antiviral intervention.[181] Specific inhibitors of the NS3-4A serine protease are the most advanced, with phase III clinical studies close to completion.[11,12,110] Nucleoside or nonnucleoside (allosteric) inhibitors of the NS5B RdRp have also shown great promise in early clinical trials. In addition, new targets have been uncovered by the recent studies highlighted above, including among others, the

HCV 5′ NCR, viral entry and fusion, the p7 viroporin, the NS2-3 protease, and NS5A. The latter is a particularly promising antiviral target.[144] Moreover, drugs affecting host factors, such as the cyclophilins,[172] involved in HCV replication are being explored as antiviral agents. Already at this early stage it is evident that the genetic variability of HCV, allowing the rapid development of antiviral resistance, represents a major challenge to the clinical development of specific inhibitors and that, similar to HIV, combination regimens will be necessary for therapeutic success.[182,183]

Conclusions and Perspectives

The development of increasingly powerful model systems has enabled dissection of the HCV life cycle and the identification of novel antiviral targets. Much work remains to be done with respect to the early and late steps, the virion assembly and structure, the mechanism and regulation of RNA replication, and the pathogenesis of HCV-induced liver disease. Ultimately, these efforts should result in innovative therapeutic and preventive strategies for one of the most common causes of chronic hepatitis, liver cirrhosis, and HCC worldwide.

Acknowledgments

Research in the authors' laboratories is supported by the Swiss National Science Foundation, the French Centre National de la Recherche Scientifique, the French National Agency for Research on AIDS and Viral Hepatitis (ANRS), the U.S. Public Health Service, the Greenberg Medical Research Institute, and the Starr Foundation.

Key References

Amako Y, et al. Pathogenesis of hepatitis C virus infection in Tupaia belangeri. J Virol 2009;84:303–311. (Ref.42)

Appel N, et al. Essential role of domain III of nonstructural protein 5A for hepatitis C virus infectious particle assembly. PLoS Pathog 2008;4:e1000035. (Ref.130)

Balfe P, McKeating J. The complexities of hepatitis C virus entry. J Hepatol 2009; 51:609–611. (Ref.55)

Beran RK, Lindenbach BD, Pyle AM. The NS4A protein of hepatitis C virus promotes RNA-coupled ATP hydrolysis by the NS3 helicase. J Virol 2009;83: 3268–3275. (Ref.118)

Berger KL, et al. Roles for endocytic trafficking and phosphatidylinositol 4-kinase III alpha in hepatitis C virus replication. Proc Natl Acad Sci U S A 2009;106:7577–7582. (Ref.174)

Borawski J, et al. Class III phosphatidylinositol-4 kinase alpha & beta are novel host factor regulators of hepatitis C virus replication. J Virol 2009;83: 10058–10074. (Ref.175)

Boulant S, et al. Structural determinants that target the hepatitis C virus core protein to lipid droplets. J Biol Chem 2006;281:22236–22247. (Ref.86)

Boulant S, Targett-Adams P, McLauchlan J. Disrupting the association of hepatitis C virus core protein with lipid droplets correlates with a loss in production of infectious virus. J Gen Virol 2007;88:2204–2213. (Ref.88)

Brass V, et al. Structural determinants for membrane association and dynamic organization of the hepatitis C virus NS3-4A complex. Proc Natl Acad Sci U S A 2008;105:14545–14550. (Ref.111)

Brenndörfer ED, et al. Nonstructural 3/4A protease of hepatitis C virus activates epithelial growth factor-induced signal transduction by cleavage of the T-cell protein tyrosine phosphatase. Hepatology 2009;49:1810–1820. (Ref.115)

Brillet R, et al. The nonstructural 5A protein of hepatitis C virus genotype 1b does not contain an interferon sensitivity-determining region. J Infect Dis 2007;195:432–441. (Ref.150)

Ciesek S, et al. Cyclosporine A inhibits hepatitis C virus nonstructural protein 2 through cyclophilin A. Hepatology 2009;50:1638–1645. (Ref.169)

Clarke D, et al. Evidence for the formation of a heptameric ion channel complex by the hepatitis C virus p7 protein in vitro. J Biol Chem 2006;281:37057–37068. (Ref.100)

Combet C, et al. euHCVdb: the European hepatitis C virus database. Nucleic Acids Res 2007;35:D363–D366. (Ref.20)

Coyne CB, Bergelson JM. Virus-induced Abl and Fyn kinase signals permit coxsackievirus entry through epithelial tight junctions. Cell 2006;124: 119–131. (Ref.58)

de Chassey B, et al. Hepatitis C virus infection protein network. Mol Syst Biol 2008;4:230. (Ref.152)

Delang L, et al. Statins potentiate the in vitro anti-hepatitis C virus activity of selective hepatitis C virus inhibitors and delay or prevent resistance development. Hepatology 2009;50:6–16. (Ref.167)

Dentzer TG, et al. Determinants of the hepatitis C virus nonstructural protein 2 protease domain required for production of infectious virus. J Virol 2009;83: 12702–12713. (Ref.106)

Dubuisson J, Helle F, Cocquerel L. Early steps of the hepatitis C virus life cycle. Cell Microbiol 2008;10:821–827. (Ref.61)

Einav S, et al. Discovery of a hepatitis C target and its pharmacological inhibitors by microfluidic affinity analysis. Nat Biotechnol 2008;26:1019–1027. (Ref.126)

Eng FJ, et al. Internal initiation stimulates production of p8 minicore, a member of a newly discovered family of hepatitis C virus core protein isoforms. J Virol 2009;83:3104–3114. (Ref.162)

Evans MJ, et al. Claudin-1 is a hepatitis C virus co-receptor required for a late step in entry. Nature 2007;446:801–805. (Ref.53)

Flisiak R, et al. The cyclophilin inhibitor Debio 025 combined with PEG IFNalpha2a significantly reduces viral load in treatment-naive hepatitis C patients. Hepatology 2009;49:1460–1468. (Ref.172)

Fraser CS, Doudna JA. Structural and mechanistic insights into hepatitis C viral translation initiation. Nat Rev Microbiol 2007;5:29–38. (Ref.66)

Fraser CS, Hershey JW, Doudna JA. The pathway of hepatitis C virus mRNA recruitment to the human ribosome. Nat Struct Mol Biol 2009;16: 397–404. (Ref.81)

Gastaminza P, et al. Cellular determinants of hepatitis C virus assembly, maturation, degradation, and secretion. J Virol 2008;82:2120–2129. (Ref.179)

Ge D, et al. Genetic variation in IL28B predicts hepatitis C treatment-induced viral clearance. Nature 2009;461:399–401.(Ref.13)

Ghany MG, et al. Diagnosis, management, and treatment of hepatitis C: an update. Hepatology 2009;49:1335–1374. (Ref.2)

Gottwein JM, et al. Novel infectious cDNA clones of hepatitis C virus genotype 3a (strain S52) and 4a (strain ED43): genetic analyses and in vivo pathogenesis studies. J Virol 2010;84:5277–5293. (Ref.65)

Gottwein JM, et al. Development and characterization of hepatitis C virus genotype 1-7 cell culture systems: role of CD81 and scavenger receptor

class B type I and effect of antiviral drugs. Hepatology 2009;49:364–377. (Ref.41)

Gouttenoire J, et al. Identification of a novel determinant for membrane association in hepatitis C virus nonstructural protein 4B. J Virol 2009;83: 6257–6268. (Ref.121)

Gouttenoire J, et al. An amphipathic alpha-helix at the C terminus of NS4B mediates membrane association. J Virol 2009;51:11378–11384. (Ref.122)

Gouttenoire J, Penin F, Moradpour D. Hepatitis C virus nonstructural protein 4B: a journey into unexplored territory. Rev Med Virol 2010;20:117–129. (Ref.120)

Gu M, Rice CM. Three conformational snapshots of the hepatitis C virus NS3 helicase reveal a ratchet translocation mechanism. Proc Natl Acad Sci U S A 2010;107:521–528. (Ref.116)

Haid S, Pietschmann T, Pecheur EI. Low pH-dependent hepatitis C virus membrane fusion depends on E2 integrity, target lipid composition, and density of virus particles. J Biol Chem 2009;284:17657–17667. (Ref.63)

Hanoulle X, et al. Hepatitis C virus NS5A protein is a substrate for the peptidyl-prolyl cis/trans isomerase activity of cyclophilins A and B. J Biol Chem 2009;284:13589–13601. (Ref.147)

Hanoulle X, et al. Domain 3 of non-structural protein 5A from hepatitis C virus is natively unfolded. Biochem Biophys Res Commun 2009;381:634–638. (Ref.148)

Hézode C, et al. Telaprevir and peginterferon with or without ribavirin for chronic HCV infection. N Engl J Med 2009;360:1839–1850. (Ref.11)

Huang H, et al. Hepatitis C virus production by human hepatocytes dependent on assembly and secretion of very low-density lipoproteins. Proc Natl Acad Sci U S A 2007;104:5848–5853. (Ref.178)

Icard V, et al. Secretion of hepatitis C virus envelope glycoproteins depends on assembly of apolipoprotein B positive lipoproteins. PLoS ONE 2009;4:e4233. (Ref.50)

Jennings TA, et al. NS3 helicase from the hepatitis C virus can function as a monomer or oligomer depending on enzyme and substrate concentrations. J Biol Chem 2009;284:4806–4814. (Ref.117)

Jirasko V, et al. Structural and functional characterization of nonstructural protein 2 for its role in hepatitis C virus assembly. J Biol Chem 2008;283: 28546–28562. (Ref.104)

Jones CT, et al. Hepatitis C virus p7 and NS2 proteins are essential for production of infectious virus. J Virol 2007;81:8374–8383. (Ref.97)

Jones DM, et al. The hepatitis C virus NS4B protein can trans-complement viral RNA replication and modulates production of infectious virus. J Virol 2009; 83:2163–2177. (Ref.128)

Kaul A, et al. Essential role of cyclophilin A for hepatitis C virus replication and virus production and possible link to polyprotein cleavage kinetics. PLoS Pathog 2009;5:e1000546. (Ref.170)

Kaul A, et al. Cell culture adaptation of hepatitis C virus and in vivo viability of an adapted variant. J Virol 2007;81:13168–13179. (Ref.38)

Kielian M, Rey FA. Virus membrane-fusion proteins: more than one way to make a hairpin. Nat Rev Microbiol 2006;4:67–76. (Ref.62)

Kneteman NM, Toso C. In vivo study of HCV in mice with chimeric human livers. Methods Mol Biol 2009;510:383–399. (Ref.47)

Krey T, et al. The disulfide bonds in glycoprotein E2 of hepatitis C virus reveal the tertiary organization of the molecule. PLoS Pathog 2010;6:e1000762. (Ref.64)

Kuiken C, et al. Hepatitis C databases, principles and utility to researchers. Hepatology 2006;43:1157–1165. (Ref.21)

Lanford RE, et al. Therapeutic silencing of microRNA-122 in primates with chronic hepatitis C virus infection. Science 2010;327:198–201. (Ref.69)

Lemm JA, et al. Identification of hepatitis C virus NS5A inhibitors. J Virol 2010;84:482–491. (Ref.144)

Li Q, et al. A genome-wide genetic screen for host factors required for hepatitis C virus propagation. Proc Natl Acad Sci U S A 2009;106:16410–16415. (Ref.176)

Liang Y, et al. Domain 2 of nonstructural protein 5A (NS5A) of hepatitis C virus is natively unfolded. Biochemistry 2007;46:11550–11558. (Ref.146)

Lindenbach BD, et al. Cell culture-grown hepatitis C virus is infectious in vivo and can be recultured in vitro. Proc Natl Acad Sci U S A 2006;103:3805–3809. (Ref.39)

Lindenbach BD, et al. The C-terminus of hepatitis C virus NS4A encodes an electrostatic switch that regulates NS5A hyperphosphorylation and viral replication. J Virol 2007;81:8905–8918. (Ref.112)

Lindenbach BD, Thiel HJ, Rice CM. Flaviviridae: the viruses and their replication. In: Knipe DM, Howley PM, editors. Fields virology, 5th ed. Philadelphia: Lippincott-Raven, 2007:1101–1152. (Ref.9)

Liu Z, et al. Critical role of cyclophilin A and its prolyl-peptidyl isomerase activity in the structure and function of the hepatitis C virus replication complex. J Virol 2009;83:6554–6565. (Ref.171)

Lorenz IC, et al. Structure of the catalytic domain of the hepatitis C virus NS2-3 protease. Nature 2006;442:831–835. (Ref.105)

Love RA, et al. Crystal structure of a novel dimeric form of NS5A domain I protein from hepatitis C virus. J Virol 2009;83:4395–4403. (Ref.145)

Luik P, et al. The 3-dimensional structure of a hepatitis C virus p7 ion channel by electron microscopy. Proc Natl Acad Sci U S A 2009;106:12712–12716. (Ref.101)

Masaki T, et al. Interaction of hepatitis C virus nonstructural protein 5A with core protein is critical for the production of infectious virus particles. J Virol 2008;82:7964–7976. (Ref.91)

McHutchison JG, et al. Telaprevir with peginterferon and ribavirin for chronic HCV genotype 1 infection. N Engl J Med 2009;360:1827–1838. (Ref.12)

McLauchlan J. Lipid droplets and hepatitis C virus infection. Biochim Biophys Acta 2009;1791:552–559. (Ref.87)

McMullan LK, et al. Evidence for a functional RNA element in the hepatitis C virus core gene. Proc Natl Acad Sci U S A 2007;104:2879–2884. (Ref.73)

Miller S, Krijnse-Locker J. Modification of intracellular membrane structures for virus replication. Nat Rev Microbiol 2008;6:363–374. (Ref.164)

Miyanari Y, et al. The lipid droplet is an important organelle for hepatitis C virus production. Nat Cell Biol 2007;9:1089–1097. (Ref.89)

Molina S, et al. The low-density lipoprotein receptor plays a role in the infection of primary human hepatocytes by hepatitis C virus. J Hepatol 2007;46:411–419. (Ref.57)

Moradpour D, Penin F, Rice CM. Replication of hepatitis C virus. Nat Rev Microbiol 2007;5:453–463. (Ref.10)

Murray CL, Jones CT, Rice CM. Architects of assembly: roles of Flaviviridae non-structural proteins in virion morphogenesis. Nat Rev Microbiol 2008;6:699–708. (Ref.180)

Pacini L, et al. Naturally occurring hepatitis C virus subgenomic deletion mutants replicate efficiently in Huh-7 cells and are trans-packaged in vitro to generate infectious defective particles. J Virol 2009;83:9079–9093. (Ref.78)

Phan T, et al. Hepatitis C virus NS2 protein contributes to virus particle assembly via opposing epistatic interactions with the E1-E2 glycoprotein and NS3-NS4A enzyme complexes. J Virol 2009;83:8379–8395. (Ref.107)

Pietschmann T, et al. Construction and characterization of infectious intragenotypic and intergenotypic hepatitis C virus chimeras. Proc Natl Acad Sci U S A 2006;103:7408–7413. (Ref.37)

Pietschmann T, et al. Production of infectious genotype 1b virus particles in cell culture and impairment by replication enhancing mutations. PLoS Pathog 2009;5:e1000475. (Ref.31)

Ploss A, et al. Human occludin is a hepatitis C virus entry factor required for infection of mouse cells. Nature 2009;457:882–886. (Ref.54)

Ploss A, Rice CM. Towards a small animal model for hepatitis C. EMBO Rep 2009;10:1220–1227. (Ref.23)

Quintavalle M, et al. Hepatitis C virus NS5A is a direct substrate of casein kinase I-alpha, a cellular kinase identified by inhibitor affinity chromatography using specific NS5A hyperphosphorylation inhibitors. J Biol Chem 2007;282:5536–5544. (Ref.133)

Randall G, et al. Cellular cofactors affecting hepatitis C virus infection and replication. Proc Natl Acad Sci U S A 2007;104:12884–12889. (Ref.173)

Rauch A, et al. Genetic variation in IL28B is associated with chronic hepatitis C and treatment failure: a genome-wide association study. Gastroenterology 2010 (in press). (Ref.17)

Romero-Lopez C, Berzal-Herranz A. A long-range RNA-RNA interaction between the 5′ and 3′ ends of the HCV genome. RNA 2009;15:1740–1752. (Ref.77)

Sarrazin C, Zeuzem S. Resistance to direct antiviral agents in patients with hepatitis C virus infection. Gastroenterology 2010;138:447–462. (Ref.183)

Schregel V, et al. Hepatitis C virus NS2 is a protease stimulated by cofactor domains in NS3. Proc Natl Acad Sci U S A 2009;106:5342–5347. (Ref.102)

Shavinskaya A, et al. The lipid droplet binding domain of hepatitis C virus core protein is a major determinant for efficient virus assembly. J Biol Chem 2007;282:37158–37169. (Ref.90)

Simister P, et al. Structural and functional analysis of hepatitis C virus strain JFH1 polymerase. J Virol 2009;83:11926–11939. (Ref.155)

Steinmann E, et al. Hepatitis C virus p7 protein is crucial for assembly and release of infectious virions. PLoS Pathog 2007;3:e103. (Ref.98)

Suppiah V, et al. IL28B is associated with response to chronic hepatitis C interferon-alpha and ribavirin therapy. Nat Genet 2009;41:1100–1104. (Ref.14)

Tai AW, et al. A functional genomic screen identifies cellular cofactors of hepatitis C virus replication. Cell Host Microbe 2009;5:298–307. (Ref.177)

Tanaka Y, et al. Genome-wide association of IL28B with response to pegylated interferon-alpha and ribavirin therapy for chronic hepatitis C. Nat Genet 2009;41:1105–1109. (Ref.15)

Tellinghuisen TL, Foss KL, Treadaway J. Regulation of hepatitis C virion production via phosphorylation of the NS5A protein. PLoS Pathog 2008;4:e1000032. (Ref.131)

Thomas DL, et al. Genetic variation in IL28B and spontaneous clearance of hepatitis C virus. Nature 2009;461:798–801. (Ref.16)

Thompson AA, et al. Biochemical characterization of recombinant hepatitis C virus nonstructural protein 4B: evidence for ATP/GTP hydrolysis and adenylate kinase activity. Biochemistry 2009;48:906–916. (Ref.127)

Timpe JM, et al. Hepatitis C virus cell-cell transmission in hepatoma cells in the presence of neutralizing antibodies. Hepatology 2008;47:17–24. (Ref.59)

Vassilaki N, et al. Role of the hepatitis C virus core+1 open reading frame and core cis-acting RNA elements in viral RNA translation and replication. J Virol 2008;82:11503–11515. (Ref.74)

Welsch S, et al. Composition and three-dimensional architecture of the dengue virus replication and assembly sites. Cell Host Microbe 2009;5:365–375. (Ref.166)

Witteveldt J, et al. CD81 is dispensable for hepatitis C virus cell-to-cell transmission in hepatoma cells. J Gen Virol 2009;90:48–58. (Ref.60)

Wölk B, et al. A dynamic view of hepatitis C virus replication complexes. J Virol 2008;82:10519–10531. (Ref.165)

Yi M, et al. Trans-complementation of an NS2 defect in a late step in hepatitis C virus (HCV) particle assembly and maturation. PLoS Pathog 2009;5:e1000403. (Ref.108)

Yi M, et al. Production of infectious genotype 1a hepatitis C virus (Hutchinson strain) in cultured human hepatoma cells. Proc Natl Acad Sci U S A 2006;103:2310–2315. (Ref.40)

You S, Rice CM. 3′ RNA elements in hepatitis C virus replication: kissing partners and long poly(U). J Virol 2008;82:184–195. (Ref.72)

Yu GY, et al. Palmitoylation and polymerization of hepatitis C virus NS4B protein. J Virol 2006;80:6013–6023. (Ref.123)

A complete list of references can be found at www.expertconsult.com.

Immune Pathogenesis of Viral Hepatitis B and C

Kyong-Mi Chang

ABBREVIATIONS

2'5'OAS 2'5' oligo adenylate synthetase
ADCC antibody-dependent cellular cytotoxicity
ALT alanine aminotransferase
anti-HBc antibody to hepatitis B virus core antigen
anti-HBs antibody to hepatitis B virus surface antigen
APC antigen-presenting cells
Bim Bcl-αinteracting mediator of cell death
CHB chronic hepatitis B
CTL cytolytic T lymphocyte
CTLA4 CTL-associated antigen 4
CXCL10 chemokine c-x-c motif ligand 10, IFN-inducible protein 10 or IP10
CXCL8 IL-8 or neutrophil chemotactic factor
DC dendritic cells
dsDNA double-stranded deoxyribonucleic acid
dsRNA double-stranded ribonucleic acid
HBcAg hepatitis B virus core antigen
HBeAg hepatitis B virus e antigen
HBsAg hepatitis B virus surface antigen
HBV hepatitis B virus
HCC hepatocellular carcinoma
HCV hepatitis C virus

HIV human immunodeficiency virus
HLA human leukocyte antigen
IFN interferon
Ig immunoglobin
IL interleukin
IPS-1 IFN-β promoter stimulator (also called MAVS, VISA, and CARDIF)
IRF1 IFN regulatory factor 1
IRF3 IFN regulatory factor 3
ISG IFN-stimulated gene
KIR killer cell immunoglobulin-like receptors
LAG-3 lymphocyte activation gene 3
LCMV lymphocytic choriomeningitis virus
LPS lipopolysaccharide
MDA5 melanoma differentiation associated gene 5
mDC myeloid dendritic cells
MHC major histocompatibility complex
MIG monokine induced by IFN-γ
NCR natural cytotoxicity receptor
NF-kB nuclear factor kappa-light-chain-enhancer of activated B cells
NK natural killer cells
NKT natural killer T cells
NLR NOD-like receptors
NOD nucleotide-binding oligomerization domain

PAMP pathogen-associated molecular patterns
PD-1 programmed death 1
pDC plasmacytoid dendritic cells
PGE2 prostaglandin E2
PKR protein kinase R
PRR pattern recognition receptors
RANTES regulated upon activation, normal T cells expressed and activated
RIG-I retinoic acid inducible gene-I
RLRs RIG-I–like receptors
RNA ribonucleic acid
SIV simian immunodeficiency virus
SNP single-nucleotide polymorphism
SOCS suppressors of cytokine signaling
ssRNA single-stranded ribonucleic acid
TGF-β transforming growth factor β
Th T helper
TIR Toll/interleukin-1 receptor
TLR Toll-like receptors
TNF-α tumor necrosis factor α
TRAIL TNF-related apoptosis-inducing ligand
TRIF TIR-domain-containing adapter-inducing interferon-β

Introduction

The balance between the virus and the host defense defines the course of viral infection and disease pathogenesis. Persistent viruses such as hepatitis B virus (HBV) and hepatitis C virus (HCV) are generally not directly cytopathic and have developed immune evasion mechanisms to survive without destroying the host. For the host, the goal is to prevent, eliminate, or at least control viral infection while limiting undue collateral damage. These interactions are influenced by various host, environmental, and viral factors. In this chapter, we will review the components of immune response during HBV and HCV infection, highlighting the immune mechanisms of viral clearance and persistence, as well as liver injury.

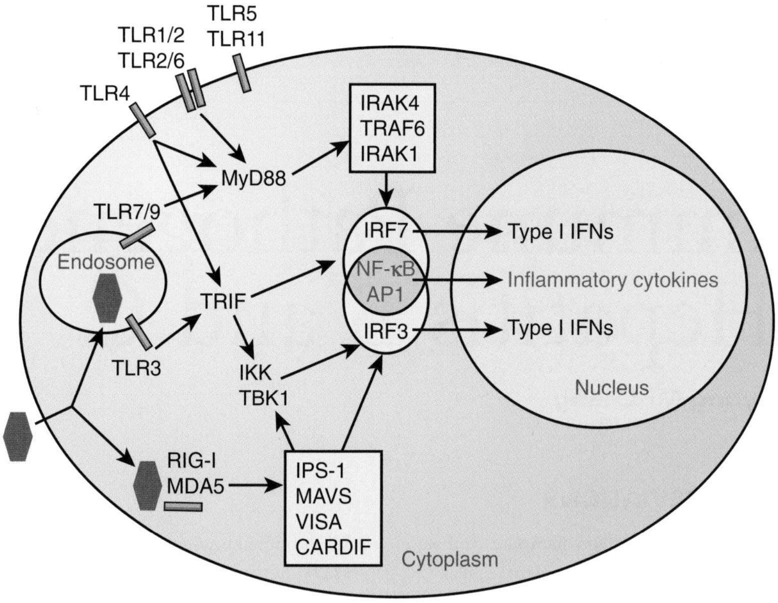

Fig. 8-1 **Activation of type I IFN and inflammatory cytokine transcription by TLR and RLR signaling.** Cell surface TLRs,[1,2,4,5,6,11] endosomal TLRs,[3,7,9] and cytoplasmic RLRs (RIG-I, MDA5) activate the IRF3/7 pathway, leading to type I IFN production, and the NF-κB/AP1 pathway for inflammatory cytokine production. HCV NS3/4A protease can cleave IPS-1 and TRIF, thereby inhibiting TLR3 and RIG-I pathways. (Adapted from Kawai T, Akira S. TLR signaling. Semin Immunol 2007;19:24–32; and Garcia-Sastre A, Biron CA. Type 1 interferons and the virus-host relationship: a lesson in detente. Science 2006;312:879–882.)

Innate and Adaptive Immune Response in Viral Infection

Innate Immune Response

As a foreign pathogen enters the host and its target cell, it immediately encounters and activates the host innate defense system by various pathogen sensing mechanisms.

Cell-Extrinsic and Cell-Intrinsic Induction of Innate Immune Response by PRRs

Innate immune and nonimmune cells express pattern recognition receptors (PRRs) that can bind pathogen-associated molecular patterns (PAMP) displayed by foreign pathogens.[1-4] Among the PRRs, endocytic receptors, such as LPS receptor, scavenger receptor, and C-type lectin receptors, can facilitate binding and internalization of microbial pathogens or their components. Secreted PRRs include opsonins such as collectins, ficolins, pentraxins that can bind microbial parts, sugars, and glycoproteins to enhance phagocytosis and complement activation. Signaling receptors include Toll-like receptors (TLRs) that are expressed on the cell surface (TLR1/2/4/5/6/11/12) or within the endosomal compartment (TLR3/7/9), as well as cytosolic receptors such as nucleotide-binding oligomerization domain (NOD)-like receptors (NLRs) and retinoic acid inducible gene-I (*RIG-I*) like receptors (RLRs).

Innate immune response can be cell-extrinsic, activated through extracellular mediators (e.g., secreted receptors), or PRRs expressed on the surface of noninfected cells (e.g., endocytic receptors or TLRs). For intracellular pathogens such as viruses, innate immune activation can occur in a cell-intrinsic manner within the infected cell. For example, intracellular PRRs such as RIG-I, melanoma differentiation associated gene 5 (MDA5), and endosomal TLRs (e.g.,TLR3/7/9) can be activated within the infected cells by ssRNA, dsRNA, and/or

dsDNA from the replicating virus. Sensing of viral nucleic acid by RLRs, such as RIG-I or MDA5, leads to the activation of proinflammatory (NF-κB) and antiviral (IFN regulatory factor 3 or IRF3) pathways through a common signaling adaptor molecule IPS-1 (also called MAVS, VISA, and CARDIF). IRF3 activation results in the production of type I IFN that can then bind type I IFN receptor with downstream antiviral effects. NLRs respond to various microbial products and stress, thereby mediating the formation of inflammasomes, which are multimolecular protein complexes that activate caspase 1 and induce the maturation of inflammatory cytokine IL-1β. **Figure 8-1** shows some of the TLR and RLR pathways that lead to production of type I IFNs and inflammatory cytokines.

Interferons

IFNs belong to the class II family of α-helical cytokines and can be divided into type I (IFN-α/ß), type II (IFN-γ) and type III (IFN-λ).[5-7] Most cells can make IFN-ß upon pathogen-sensing via the membrane-bound TLRs and cytoplasmic RLRs. Plasmacytoid dendritic cells (pDC) are the major producers of IFN-α (up to 1000-fold compared with other cells), although myeloid DC (mDC) can also up-regulate IFN-α production. Binding of IFN-α/ß to its cell surface receptor (IFNAR-1/IFNAR-2) activates the Jak/STAT IFN-signaling pathway that ultimately leads to the induction of numerous IFN-stimulated genes (ISGs) with pleiotropic biologic activities (e.g., antiviral, immune modulatory, antiproliferative, antiangiogenic, and antitumor effects).

Type I IFNs can affect all phases of viral life cycle including entry/uncoating, transcription, RNA stability, translation, maturation, assembly, and release.[5-7] Three of the major IFN-α/ß-induced antiviral pathways include the dsRNA-dependent protein kinase R-PKR), the 2′5′ oligo adenylate synthetase (2′5′OAS) system and the Mx proteins. In addition to direct antiviral activities, type I IFNs can exert an immune modulatory role by enhancing NK cell activity, up-regulate major histocompatibility complex MHC expression (especially class

I MHC relevant for CD8 T-cell response), influence T- and B-cell development (including B-cell isotype switching), and modulate DC function. These antiviral and immune modulatory activities provide the rationale for the use of exogenous IFN-α to treat HBV and HCV infection.

Type II IFN (IFN-λ) can be secreted by innate immune cells, including natural killer (NK) cells, and natural killer T (NKT) cells, although it is generally considered in the context of adaptive immunity as a T-cell cytokine. IFN-λ signals through the IFNGR-1/IFNGR-2 receptor complex. Type III IFN (IFN-λ) includes IFN-λ1 (IL-29), IFN-λ2 (IL-28A), and IFN-λ3 (IL-28B). IFN-λ signals through a distinct receptor composed of IFN-λR1 and IL-10R2, but ultimately activates the JAK/STAT pathway (similar to type I IFNs).[5,8] IFN-λ is expressed in various cell types including DCs, macrophages, and cancer cell lines, as well as the virus-infected liver. However, its target effect may be more restricted based on its receptor expression.[9] Our knowledge is still evolving for this relatively new cytokine, and genetic polymorphisms near the IL-28B locus may be relevant for natural history and treatment response in HCV-infected patients.[10-13]

Innate Immune Cell Subsets

The cellular components of the innate immune response include the monocytes/macrophages, DCs, NK and NKT cells.

Monocyte/Macrophages/Kupffer Cells

Monocytes are innate immune effector cells that circulate in the blood, spleen, and bone marrow.[14] Most human monocytes (90%) express CD14 (part of the LPS receptor complex), whereas a minority (10%) express CD16 (the FcγRIII). CD16+ monocytes display an inflammatory phenotype characterized by increased TNF-α in response to TLR stimulation and during infection.[15] Monocytes also express various chemokine receptors and adhesion molecules that mediate tissue entry during infection and inflammation. In the inflamed tissue, monocytes can differentiate into macrophages and inflammatory DCs. Macrophages are the primary tissue phagocytes in lymphoid and nonlymphoid tissue, clearing out apoptotic cells and producing cytokines and growth factor activities that are mediated by PRRs. Relevant for hepatitis, Kupffer cells are the resident macrophages in the liver with heterogeneous phenotype, size, and function based on their location within the liver.[16] Moving through the liver sinusoids, Kupffer cells phagocytose foreign particles and secrete inflammatory cytokines that promote leukocyte recruitment and retention.[17] Of note, the liver is continuously exposed to gut microbial products (e.g., LPS) from the portal circulation. Many cells in the liver also express receptors for LPS (e.g., TLR4, CD14), thereby removing LPS and preventing endotoxemia. With continuous LPS exposure, Kupffer cells and liver sinusoidal endothelial cells display LPS tolerance, thus avoiding immunopathology in physiologic conditions.[18,19] Kupffer cells may also present antigens to T cells. However, this could inhibit rather than stimulate T cells through PGE2, nitric oxide, and IL-10 in some cases.[19]

Dendritic Cells

DCs bridge the innate and adaptive immune response.[1,4,14,20,21] As professional antigen presenting cells (APC), DCs present foreign antigens to T cells and prime the adaptive immune response. They also secrete cytokines (e.g., IL-12, IL-10, IL-15, type I IFN) that shape both innate and adaptive immune responses. Circulating DCs include two major populations: myeloid DC (mDC) and plasmacytoid DC (pDC). MDCs express MHC class II and CD11c in addition to TLR 1-8 (greatest expression of TLR2/3). They enhance Th1 response and NK activity by producing IL-12 and transpresenting IL-15.[22-24] PDCs express BDCA2, BDCA4, and IL-3 receptor (CD123), in addition to TLR7 and TLR9 (+/− TLR1).[22-24] They produce large amounts of IFN-α with antiviral and immune modulatory effects. While monocytes can also develop DC-like characteristics in certain culture conditions (monocyte-derived DCs), DCs do not appear to be directly derived from monocytes in vivo based on murine adoptive transfer and genetic experiments.[14,21] Both pDC and mDC are found in the liver. While further studies are needed, hepatic pDC and mDC differ from their peripheral counterparts (e.g., greater IL-10 production and reduced APC function compared with splenic pDC and mDC).[19]

Natural Killer Cells

Natural Killer (NK) cells can directly lyse their target cells (e.g., virus-infected cells, tumor cells) by releasing cytotoxic granules that contain perforin and granzyme.[25] NK cells are highly abundant in the normal liver (up to 50% of liver infiltrating lymphocytes).[19,26] NK cells can be identified by their expression pattern of CD56 (the neural cell adhesion molecule also expressed in activated T cells and some neural tissues) and CD16. They also express inhibitory and activating receptors that interact with class I HLA molecules on target cells. NK inhibitory receptors include the C-type lectin receptor CD94/NKG2A, LIR1/ILT2 receptors, and killer cell immunoglobulin-like receptors (KIRs). NK activating receptors include CD16, NKG2D, the natural cytotoxicity receptors (NCRs) NKp44, NKp46, and NKp30 and truncated alleles of KIRs. The coordinated interactions of NK inhibitory and activating receptors with the target cell ligands determine the activation, viability, and cytotoxicity of NK cells. In addition, NK cells also express TLR (e.g., TLR3, 7, 8) that can modulate their function.[27] During viral infections, type I interferons (secreted by infected cells and pDC) and cytokines from activated DCs (e.g., IL-12, IL-15, IL-18) can activate NK cells.[28] Conversely, NK cells can modulate DC function via contact-dependent and cytokine-mediated mechanisms, leading to a cross-talk between NK cells and DC that can modulate the adaptive immune response.[24,29-31]

NKT Cells

Natural killer T cells are thymic-derived lymphocytes that express both NK (e.g., CD56) and T-cell markers (e.g., CD3+, CD4+, CD8+, CD4-CD8- double-negative).[32] Classical type I NKT cells express an invariant T-cell receptor (Vα24Jα18 in humans) and recognize glycolipid antigens (e.g., from bacterial cell walls) presented by the MHC class I-like molecule CD1d. Type II NKT cells are also CD1d-restricted but display a more diverse TCR repertoire without Vα24Jα18 expression. They recognize various hydrophobic antigens and may have immune regulatory function. Upon antigenic stimulation, NKT cells can secrete various cytokines (IFN-γ, IL-4, IL-10, IL-13, IL-17) that may contribute to autoimmunity, tumor immunity, and pathogen-specific immune response.[33-36] In humans, CD4+ NKT cells can secrete both Th1 and Th2 cytokines (e.g., IFN-γ, IL-4), whereas CD4- NKT cells produce primarily Th1 cytokines (e.g., IFN-γ). Relevant for the liver, NKT cells are enriched in the liver (approximately 10%)[26] and liver-derived CD4- NKT cells have greater antitumor activity than NKT cells from the spleen or thymus.[34] DC stimulation by TLRs (e.g., TLR4, TLR7/9) can further promote NKT cell activation.

Collectively, these innate immune components also modulate the adaptive T- and B-cell responses. In turn, T cells can modulate the level of innate immune activation.[37]

Adaptive Immune Response

Adaptive immune response is specific to antigenic sequence encoded by the infecting pathogen (epitopes). It is mediated by B and T cells with contributions from antigen presenting cells such as DC.

B-Cell Response

B cells produce antibodies and mediate the humoral adaptive immunity. Antibodies consist of an antigen-binding variable (V) region and a constant (C) region containing the Fc region that can bind cellular receptors and complements.[38,39] In a classical sense, neutralizing antibodies limit viral spread and promote resolution of infection by directly binding and eliminating the circulating virions or blocking their entry into target cells. In addition, antibodies can mediate opsonization, complement activation and antibody-dependent cellular cytotoxicity (ADCC). Protection afforded by neutralizing antibodies is the basis of successful vaccine strategy and passive immunization using hyperimmune globulins. Antibodies may also contribute to inflammatory response, enhance antigen presentation, and bind proinflammatory microbial products (e.g., LPS), thereby modulating T-cell and innate immune response. Regulatory B cells that produce immune regulatory cytokine IL-10 have been described.[40]

T-Cell Response

During viral infection, naive CD4 and CD8 T cells are initially activated (or primed) in the primary lymphoid organs upon encountering their target viral sequence presented on the surface of the professional antigen presenting cells (APC) as short peptides embedded within the major histocompatibility complex (MHC).[41] They can then migrate to the site of infection (e.g., the liver) to exert their antiviral activity. Alternatively, for hepatotropic pathogens such as HBV and HCV, priming of virus-specific T cells within the liver (e.g., by liver sinusoidal endothelial cells or hepatocytes) may lead to immune tolerance or activation.[42-44]

In general, a vigorous T-cell response is associated with viral clearance and disease resolution while a weak response is associated with viral persistence and disease progression. T cells can be classified by their cytokine profile as type 1 (IL-2, IFN-γ); type 2 (IL-4, 5, 10 and 13); type 3 (TGF-β); type 0 (IFN-γ and IL-4); Tr1 (IL-10); and Th17 (IL-17). Type I response with IFN-γ is typically associated with a more favorable outcome in viral infection.

CD4 T cells recognize exogenous peptide antigens presented by class II MHC molecules. Therefore, antigen recognition by CD4 T cells occurs only with class II-expressing cells (e.g., antigen presenting cells such as dendritic cells, B cells,

and macrophages) but not hepatocytes that generally do not express class II.[45-47] CD4 T cells play a key regulatory role by activating dendritic cells to prime CD8 T cells, producing cytokines and providing T cell help for B cells.[48,49]

CD8 T cells can recognize infected cells that display endogenously synthesized viral antigens presented on class I MHC molecules. This recognition can induce apoptosis of the infected cell through perforin/granzyme and/or fas/fasL pathway. However, these CD8 cytolytic T lymphocytes (CTLs) can also cure virus-infected cells in a noncytolytic manner by secreting potent antiviral cytokines.[50] Unlike CD4 T cells, CD8 T cells can recognize most cells including hepatocytes because class I MHC is expressed on most cells. Thus CD8 CTLs are the foot soldiers of the cell-mediated immune system.

The balance between immune effector and regulatory responses determines the extent of inflammation and viral clearance.[51] If the infection is cleared with sufficiently robust response, the antiviral effector cells undergo a contraction phase, resulting in a small number of polyfunctional memory T cells that persist. These memory T cells maintain efficient capacity to expand and perform effector function when rechallenged with the viral antigen, and they contribute to protective immunity after natural infection or vaccination. With prolonged antigenic stimulation (e.g., in chronic infection), the antiviral effector T cells become "exhausted" or "tolerized" with progressive loss of effector function. These immune exhaustion or tolerance mechanisms could limit severe immune-mediated damage in the face of ongoing viral infection. However, they also limit efficient virus control.

Mechanisms of T-Cell Dysfunction or Tolerance

There has been increasing appreciation for the complex mechanisms that regulate T-cell function and exhaustion in acute and chronic viral infection.

Immune Inhibitory Costimulatory Pathways

An intrinsic regulatory mechanism of T-cell function involves certain receptors that are directly expressed on T cells to suppress their activation, including programmed death 1 (PD-1) and CTL-associated antigen 4 (CTLA4).[52] Both PD-1 and CTLA-4 are inhibitory receptors within the CD28/B7 family of costimulatory molecules, and they are up-regulated on activated T cells and T cells that are exhausted by continued exposure to antigen-specific stimulation or high viral load. Binding of PD-1 on T cells to its ligands PD-L1 (B7-H1) and PD-L2 (B7-DC) can inhibit T-cells proliferation and cytokine secretion[53,54] and promote immune tolerance.[55,56] While PD-1 is up-regulated on exhausted virus-specific T cells during acute and chronic infection, blockade of PD-1/PD-ligand interaction can restore their effector function.[57-64]

Similarly, binding of CTLA4 to its ligands (B7-1, B7-2) can suppress T-cell function, whereas blockade of CTLA4 signaling can reverse T-cell dysfunction. Combined PD-1 and CTLA4 blockade can synergistically enhance intrahepatic HCV-specific T-cell function compared with individual PD-1 or CTLA4 blockade.[65] These findings raise the possibility that immune inhibitory blockade may have potential therapeutic application during chronic viral infection. Additional immune modulatory mechanisms for antiviral T-cell activation include the lymphocyte activation gene 3 (*LAG-3*)[66] and T-cell Ig and mucin proteins.[67,68]

Regulatory T Cells

An extrinsic mechanism involves the immune regulatory cells (e.g., CD25[+] Tregs and IL-10[+] Tr1 cells) that can suppress effector T-cell function. CD4[+]CD25[+] T cells (also termed CD25[+] Tregs) are naturally occurring, thymic-derived T cells that represent 5% to 10% of peripheral CD4 T cells and mediate immune tolerance via direct cell–cell contact. Their role in immune regulation is apparent by organ-specific auto-immune diseases that occur upon CD25[+] Treg depletion and reversed by their repletion.[69,70] CD25[+] Tregs also regulate immune response to pathogens, including chronic HCV, HBV, and HIV infection.[71] Another group of regulatory T cells include the IL-10 secreting Tr1 cells.[72] They are distinct from the CD25[+] Tregs, can include both CD4 and CD8 T cells, and mediate T-cell suppression via IL-10. IL-10 is a regulatory cytokine secreted by various cell subsets (e.g., monocytes, macrophages, dendritic cells) to limit the inflammatory responses.[73,74] IL-10 can inhibit IFN-α production by activated pDC,[75,76] induce a tolerogenic phenotype in DC that can be reversed by PD-1:PD-ligand blockade,[77] and mediate T-cell suppression during chronic viral infection that can be reversed by IL-10:IL-10R blockade.[78,79] Collectively, these immune regulatory pathways contribute to effector T-cell dysfunction in chronic viral infection and their counter-regulation could contribute to treatment response.

Immune Response and Hepatitis Viruses

Although there is no convenient, immunologically well-defined small animal model for HBV or HCV infection, significant progress has been made in our understanding of HBV and HCV immune pathogenesis, using alternate approaches including surrogate animal models (e.g., in vitro culture system; transgenic mice, chimpanzees, or woodchucks; infected patients).

Hepatitis B Virus

The clinical, virologic, and therapeutic aspects of HBV infection are discussed elsewhere. Briefly, HBV is a hepatotropic, partially double-stranded DNA virus that can cause acute and chronic liver disease worldwide. In many developed countries, HBV exposure typically occurs as adults via sexual transmission with a low chronicity rate (5%). In regions with high HBV prevalence (e.g., Asia, subsaharan Africa), HBV exposure tends to occur during the perinatal period (e.g., vertical transmission from mother to infant) with a high rate of persistence in the absence of timely vaccination.[80] The course of viral infection is defined by the interplay between the virus and host immune defense.

Innate Immune Response and HBV
HBV as a Stealth Virus Evading Innate Immune Recognition During Acute Infection

It is difficult to study innate immune responses in human viral hepatitis due to a lack of convenient small animal model to sample the relevant compartments (e.g., site of virus entry, draining lymph nodes, target cells) in a timely manner.[41] Nevertheless, a remarkable lack of early innate immune induction was demonstrated in acutely HBV-infected chimpanzees.[81] In these animals, HBV DNA and HBcAg became first detectable in the liver at 3 to 5 weeks after inoculation, but without associated liver injury or type I IFN response. The onset of acute hepatitis with elevated ALT activity occurred several weeks thereafter, coinciding with the detection of T-cell markers (CD3, IFN-γ) in the liver, followed subsequently by HBV clearance. These findings suggest that: (1) HBV is non-cytopathic; (2) T cells mediate liver injury; and (3) T cells also mediate viral clearance. Further analysis of global gene expression profile showed that no genes (including IFN-inducible genes) correlated with intrahepatic HBV DNA levels during acute hepatitis B, whereas 110 hepatic genes were associated with HBV clearance—the majority of which were associated with T cells. In acutely HBV-infected patients, type I IFN was barely detectable and no higher than those in uninfected controls.[82] These findings in chimpanzees and patients suggested that HBV is a "stealth virus" that spreads without detection by the innate sensing machinery during early infection (**Fig. 8-2, A-C**).

Despite the apparent stealth behavior, HBV infection is resolved in most acutely HBV-infected adults. Thus the ability for early innate immune avoidance cannot explain the long-term virologic outcome. However, it probably does allow for the initial establishment of HBV infection because HBV is readily suppressed by innate immune components including IFN-α,[83] TLR, NK, NKT, and antigen presenting cells.[36,50,84] On the other hand, HBV can activate the cellular components of innate immune response, such as Kupffer cells and NK/NKT cells.[85-87] For example, dynamic changes in NK and NKT cell activation and function were observed during acute HBV infection.[88] An early production of immune regulatory cytokine IL-10 was also observed in patients with acute hepatitis B in association with attenuated NK and T-cell response.[82] Thus HBV may be relatively but not absolutely invisible to the innate immune system, avoiding type I IFN but not other innate immune cells during acute infection.

HBV Can Activate Innate Cytokine Response Including Type I IFNs During Chronic Hepatitis B

Changes are observed in various innate immune parameters in patients with chronic hepatitis B (CHB). For example, NK cells from CHB patients displayed reduced cytotoxicity and antiviral cytokine production (IFN-γ and TNF-α) upon cytokine stimulation in one study.[89] Of interest, hepatitis flares during chronic hepatitis B coincided with increased serum IFN-α and IL-8 levels.[90] Hepatitis flares were also preceded by increased serum HBV DNA and IL-8 levels. **Figure 8-3** shows representative serum levels of HBV DNA, ALT activity, IL-8, and IFN-α longitudinally in CHB patients undergoing hepatitis flare, as well as a cross-sectional comparison of serum IL-8 and IFN-α levels in patients with or without elevated ALT activity. Collectively, these findings suggest that HBV can induce an innate immune response, including the type I IFN pathway, during chronic (although not acute) infection.

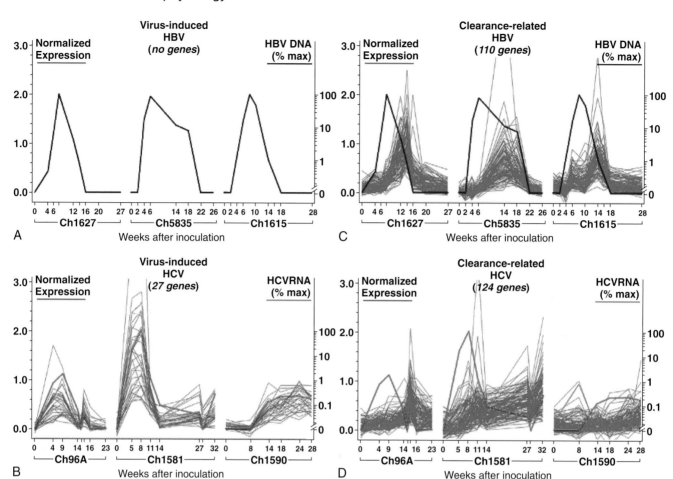

Fig. 8-2 Liver gene expression profile during HBV and HCV infection. A, Genes correlated with viremia in acutely HBV-infected chimpanzees. No genes correlated positively or negatively with intrahepatic HBV DNA during acute HBV infection. **B,** Intrahepatic gene expression correlated with viremia in three HCV-infected chimpanzees. **C,** Liver gene expression profile associated with viral clearance in three acutely HBV-infected chimpanzees; and **(D)** that associated with clearance in HCV-infected chimpanzees. Gene identities are described in reference 81 and in reference 116. *Blue and green lines* indicate the intrahepatic HBV DNA or serum HCV RNA as a percentage (% max) of the corresponding peak levels, respectively. Values on the x-axis represent weeks after inoculation with HBV. *(Adapted from Chisari FV, Isogawa M, Wieland SF. Pathogenesis of hepatitis B virus infection. Pathol Biol [Paris] 2010;58:258–266.)*

Adaptive Immune Response and HBV

The Onset of Adaptive Immune Response Is Delayed in Acute HBV Infection

Adaptive immune response to HBV is relatively delayed, detected several weeks after inoculation (rather than within days as seen in vaccinia or influenza virus infection).[50] While the precise mechanism for this apparent delay is not known, it is interesting that HBV and HCV are both hepatotropic viruses with similarly delayed onset of adaptive immune response. One potential explanation could be that the immune tolerance mechanisms activated in the liver might delay or tolerize the adaptive immune response.[43,44] However, the delay in adaptive immune response does not determine the virologic outcome because most HBV infection is resolved, whereas most HCV becomes chronic in acutely infected adults.

B-Cell Response to HBV

Antibody response to HBV envelope (anti-HBs) has virus-neutralizing capacity and is associated with HBV clearance.[91]

Anti-HBs also mediates long-term protective immunity after primary infection or upon vaccination by binding the circulating virions, removing them from circulation, and preventing their entry into hepatocytes. Accordingly, passive administration of hepatitis B immunoglobulin provides postexposure prophylaxis and prevents graft infection in HBV-infected liver transplant recipients. However, anti-HBs becomes detectable relatively late in the course of acute HBV infection as the circulating HBsAg level declines and acute clinical hepatitis resolves.[50] This suggests that antibody response to the HBV envelope is not critical for viral clearance in primary infection. Alternatively, anti-HBs may be induced early and contributes to HBV clearance but simply not detected by existing commercial assay while bound to saturating amount of circulating HBsAg—at least not until HBsAg drops sufficiently.

Unlike anti-HBs, antibody response to HBV nucleocapsid (anti-HBc) is not protective. However, anti-HBc is detectable in all phases of HBV infection (acute, chronic, and resolved), and it is a marker of HBV infection in vivo. The

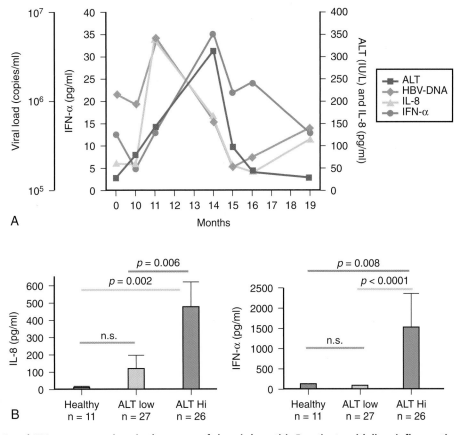

Fig. 8-3 **Increased IL-8 and IFN-α concentrations in the serum of chronic hepatitis B patients with liver inflammation. A,** Temporal relationship between serum IL-8 and IFN-α concentrations, HBV DNA, and serum ALT in a representative patient. **B,** Cross-sectional comparison of serum IL-8 and IFN-α concentrations in chronic HBV patients with low ALT (below 60 IU/L) and elevated ALT (>60 U/L) and healthy donors. *(Adapted from Dunn C, et al. Cytokines induced during chronic hepatitis B virus infection promote a pathway for NK cell-mediated liver damage. J Exp Med 2007;204:667–680.)*

immunogenicity of HBcAg may be mediated by its ability to enhance its antigen presentation by B cells and stimulate CD4 T-cell help.[92,93]

Role of T Cells in HBV Pathogenesis Defined in Mouse Model

The direct cytopathic potential of HBV-specific CD8 T cells was first demonstrated by the acute fulminant hepatitis that developed upon adoptive transfer of HBV-specific CD8 T cells into transgenic mice that express HBV envelope in the liver.[94] Subsequently, using transgenic mice that replicate HBV in the liver, adoptively transferred HBV-specific CD8 T cells were shown to suppress viral replication in a non-cytopathic manner by secreting antiviral cytokines (e.g., IFN-γ).[95,96] Thus, in different settings, HBV-specific CD8 T cells could mediate liver injury with severe consequences or inhibit viral replication with minimal damage by secreting antiviral cytokines.

As for CD4 T cells, the adoptive transfer of HBV-specific Th1-type CD4 T cells resulted in transient hepatitis and partial cytokine-mediated control of viral replication.[97] Further studies have revealed that HBV replication can be readily controlled in HBV replicating mice by cytokines induced in a non-HBV specific manner involving type I IFNs,

IFN-γ, NK/NKT cells, or immune responses to other liver pathogens.[91]

It is important to distinguish between the cytopathic and noncytopathic antiviral activity of virus-specific CD8 T cells in the setting of viral hepatitis. For example, HBV clearance by direct 1:1 CD8-mediated killing of infected hepatocytes is difficult to achieve. First, the number of HBV-infected cells (an estimated 10^{11} hepatocytes that can be infected) may greatly outnumber the achievable antiviral CD8 T cell number.[91] Second, if sufficient antiviral CD8 T cells can be induced, rapid killing of all infected hepatocytes could lead to fulminant liver failure. In this regard, the release of antiviral cytokines by HBV-specific CD8 T cells can terminate HBV gene expression and viral replication more efficiently from more hepatocytes with less overall injury. This duality of antiviral CD8 effector function is shown in **Figure 8-4**.[98]

Role of CD4 and CD8 T Cells in Chimpanzee Model of HBV Infection

A critical effector role for CD8 T cells in HBV clearance and liver disease pathogenesis was also shown by delayed viral clearance and onset of hepatitis in acutely HBV-infected chimpanzees that were depleted of CD8 T cells at 6 weeks

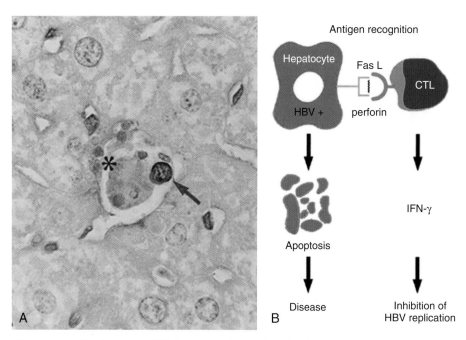

Fig. 8-4 **Direct lysis and noncytopathic clearance of HBV clearance by T-cell derived cytokines. A,** On antigen recognition, CD8⁺ CTL deliver an apoptotic signal to their target cells, killing them. The *arrow* points out the BrdU labeled CD8 T cell in the liver of a mouse after adoptive transfer. *Asterisk* indicates the apoptotic hepatocyte. *(Adapted from Chrisari FV. Rous-Whipple award lecture. Viruses, immunity, and cancer: lessons from hepatitis B, Am J Pathol 2000;98.)* **B,** In addition to direct cell kill, CD8 T cells can secrete IFN-γ and TNF-α, cytokines that abolish viral replication and HBV gene expression in vivo, potentially curing them. *(Adapted from Chisari FV, Isogawa M, Wieland SF. Pathogenesis of hepatitis B virus infection. Pathol Biol [Paris] 2010;58:258–266.)*

postinoculation.[99] Of note, CD4-depletion at 6 weeks postinoculation did not influence the course of liver disease or prevent viral clearance,[99] suggesting that CD4 T cells do not directly mediate viral clearance or liver injury. However, CD4 depletion before inoculation led to persistent infection with minimal pathology and without apparent detection of antiviral CD8 T-cell response.[100] In fact, the kinetics of antiviral CD4 T-cell priming (relative to viral spread also defined by the inoculum size) determined the virologic outcome. Thus CD4 T cells appear to regulate the overall antiviral immune response including the antiviral CD8 T-cell priming, whereas the CD8 T cells ultimately mediate liver injury, as well as viral clearance.[91-93,99]

CD4 and CD8 T-Cell Response to HBV Infected Patients

Hepatitis B–virus specific CD4 and CD8 T cells are detected in peripheral blood[101-103] and in the liver[104,105] of patients with acute, chronic, and resolved HBV infection. CD4 T-cell response to HBV is typically robust and multispecific in patients who clear HBV infection, whereas it is relatively weak and/or focused in patients with chronic infection.[50,91] HBV-specific CD4 T-cell response is also long-lasting after self-limited acute hepatitis B.[103] The association between virus-specific CD4 T-cell response and the outcome of HBV infection suggests a role for CD4 T cells in HBV clearance. Since CD4 T cells are activated in the context of class II MHC molecule as mentioned earlier, intrahepatic HBV-specific CD4 T cells are likely to be activated by nonhepatocytes that express class II (e.g., Kupffer cells, dendritic cells).

Similar to CD4 T cells, a vigorous and multispecific CD8 T-cell response to HBV is readily detected in blood from acutely HBV-infected patients that subsequently resolve their infection.[91,106-109] **Figure 8-5** shows a representative cytolytic CD8 T-cell response to multiple HBV epitopes relative to virologic status of HBV-infected patients. This response also persists indefinitely after the resolution of initial infection and may be maintained by minute amounts of HBV DNA that remain despite apparent serologic resolution.[108,110,111] HBV-specific CD8 T cells can target the viral envelope, core, and polymerase regions[106,109,112] with a particularly dominant response against an HLA A2-restricted epitope within HBcAg (HBc).[18-27] CD8 T-cell response targeting this epitope has been associated with flare of liver disease and immune escape mutation in HBV-infected patients.[113] Therapeutic vaccine targeting this single epitope was immunogenic in patients with chronic HBV infection. However it was not associated with viral clearance,[114] perhaps due to the limited scope of the immune response and immune tolerance mechanisms induced in chronic viral infection.[66,91]

Detailed analysis of intrahepatic HBV specific CD8 T-cell frequency, liver disease activity, and HBV DNA titers in chronic HBV patients suggested that antiviral activity of HBV-specific CD8 T cells can be independent of liver pathology.[101,115] Indeed, the balance between virus control and liver damage appeared to be defined by the functionality (rather than the sheer number) of HBV-specific CD8 T cells. Thus the failed attempt at viral clearance by the dysfunctional HBV-specific CD8 T cells mediate liver injury both directly and indirectly by promoting recruitment of other immune cells.

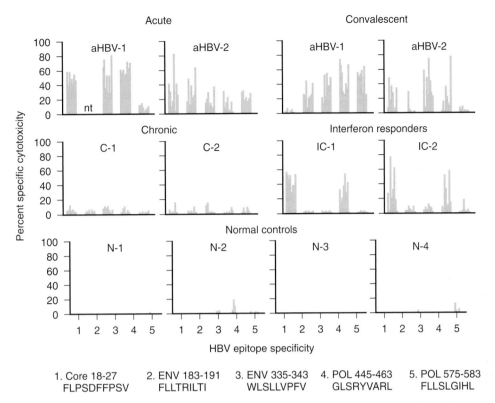

Fig. 8-5 **HBV-specific CTL response during acute and chronic infection.** The CTL response to 5 HLA A2-restricted epitopes derived from the viral core, envelope, and polymerase proteins is indicated by vertical bars. Each set of bars represents the cytolytic activity of eight replicate assays for each peptide in each patient. Acutely infected patients typically respond vigorously to multiple epitopes, as shown, and the response persists for many decades in patients who are convalescent from acute infection. In contrast, the CTL response is characteristically weak or undetectable in chronically infected patients. However, it is detectable in previously infected patients who clear the virus in response to interferon therapy, indicating CTLs are present in chronically infected patients but either too infrequently to be detected or functionally suppressed. *(Adapted from Chisari FV. Rous-Whipple award lecture. Viruses, immunity, and cancer: lessons from hepatitis B. Am J Pathol 2000;156:1117–1132.)*

Hepatitis C Virus

The clinical virologic, and therapeutic aspect of hepatitis C virus (HCV) infection is discussed in other chapters. Briefly, HCV is a hepatotropic, positive single-strand RNA virus that causes acute and chronic liver disease. HCV is highly persistent in an otherwise immune competent host (50% to 80%) and can cause progressive liver disease with cirrhosis and liver cancer. Similar to HBV, HCV is largely noncytopathic with immune-mediated disease pathogenesis and viral clearance.

Innate Immune Response and HCV
HCV Can Inhibit Type I IFN Induction and Its Downstream Antiviral Function

Hepatis C virus can interact with various components of the innate immune system. In a global gene expression profiling of three HCV-infected chimpanzees, various genes known to be stimulated with type I IFN were significantly up-regulated in the liver during acute HCV infection even before the onset of liver inflammation (see **Fig. 8-2, B** and **D**).[116] Similar induction of IFN-inducible genes was also described in other studies of HCV-infected chimpanzees in vivo.[117,118] Thus, HCV differs from HBV in that it is not transcriptionally silent and can induce a type I IFN response.

Paradoxical to the chimpanzee gene expression study, HCV NS3/4A protease can inhibit type I IFN induction via IRF3 by cleaving IPS-1 and TRIF (adaptor proteins involved in the RIG-I and TLR3 pathways) thereby preventing IRF3 activation and type I IFN induction.[119,120] This paradox may in part be explained by IFN production from HCV-uninfected hepatocytes and nonparenchymal cells in the setting of inflammation, despite limited IRF3 activation within HCV-infected hepatocytes.[121] The level of IFN induced in early infection may also be relevant for antigen processing and adaptive immune response because HCV-induced type I IFN can stimulate the generation of immunoproteasome.[122] On the other hand, greater ISG induction in the liver of chronically HCV-infected patients can predict resistance to IFN-α– based antiviral therapy.[123] Inhibitory effect of cell-culture produced HCV on TLR9-induced IFN-α production by pDC suggests that defective type I IFN response may extend to nonhepatocytes.[124]

Regardless of the source of type I IFN, HCV also evolved further mechanisms of IFN resistance. For example, HCV E2 and NS5A can bind and inhibit the dsRNA-dependent protein kinase PKR and IFN regulatory factor 1(IRF1) phosphorylation.[125,126] Sequence variations within HCV E2 and NS5A may influence responsiveness to IFN-based antiviral therapy in some but not all patients.[127]

Activation of Innate Cellular Immune Response in HCV Infection

Cellular components of innate immune response may contribute to HCV pathogenesis. For example, HCV E2 protein was initially suggested to suppress NK function in a study using recombinant HCV E2.[128] However, a subsequent study using the infectious virus showed no alteration in NK function by HCV exposure.[129] Potential relevance of NK cells in HCV clearance was suggested in a large genetic polymorphism study examining an inhibitory NK cell receptor and the HLA ligand.[130] In a subsequent study, NK cells were shown to be activated during acute hepatitis C irrespective of outcome, although with a tendency for functional difference associated with NK receptor expression.[131] In chronic HCV infection, NK cells are lower in frequency with variable phenotypic distributions and effector function.[89,132,133] Further studies of NKT and dendritic cell subsets suggest that functional differences in these cells may be relevant for outcome.[134-138]

Adaptive Immune Response and HCV

B-Cell Response to HCV

Antibody response to HCV can be detected within 7 to 8 weeks of inoculation,[139] targeting multiple HCV proteins but without associated viral clearance.[41] Nevertheless, HCV can induce neutralizing antibodies that target the viral envelope glycoproteins and prevent virus entry into hepatocytes. For example, in chimpanzees, HCV infection could be prevented when HCV-positive inoculum was neutralized with anti-HCV-containing plasma, although this protection was only isolate-specific.[140] However, HCV appears to continuously escape from the neutralizing antibody response through mutations, as demonstrated in one detailed study that monitored the antibody response and HCV sequence variation in a uniquely well-characterized chronically HCV-infected patient (HCV-H) over a 26-year period.[141] Moreover, neutralization-resistant antibody-escape variants were selected in vitro by broadly neutralizing monoclonal antibodies to HCV envelope glycoprotein.[142] In vivo, hypogammaglobulinemic patients lacking any antibodies (including those targeting HCV) display significantly less variability in the envelope HVR,[143] suggesting that antibodies can drive viral sequence heterogeneity. Taken together, antibody response with neutralizing capacity does occur during HCV infection. However, it is rendered ineffective during natural infection due to the rapid selection of antibody escape variants. Thus broadly neutralizing antibodies[144] are needed to prevent infection prophylactically in a high-risk population or as passive immunization (e.g., early infection, during liver transplantation for

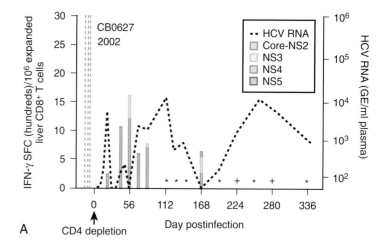

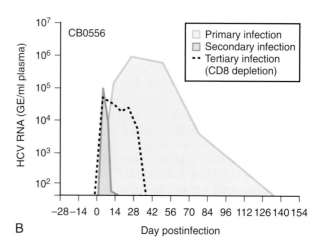

Fig. 8-6 **Course of HCV rechallenge in previously HCV-immune chimpanzees after antibody-mediated T-cell depletion.** **A,** Course of viremia *(dotted line)* and intrahepatic HCV-specific CD8 T-cell response *(stacked bar graph)* are shown after CD4 depletion and HCV reinoculation in chimpanzee CB0627. CD4 depletion resulted in persistent infection despite the detection of antiviral CD8 T-cell response. **B,** The kinetics of viremia in chimpanzee CB0556 is shown for three separate inoculations. Viremia persisted almost to day 140 in primary infection *(orange shade)*, whereas it was rapidly terminated before day 28 during the secondary infection. During the third infection associated with CD8 depletion *(dotted line)*, viremia persisted almost up to day 42 (two fold longer duration than secondary infection) until the return of CD8 T cells. *(Figures adapted from Grakoui A, et al. HCV persistence and immune evasion in the absence of memory T cell help. Science 2003;302:659–662; and Shoukry NH, et al. Memory CD8+ T cells are required for protection from persistent hepatitis C virus infection. J Exp Med 2003;197:1645–1655.)*

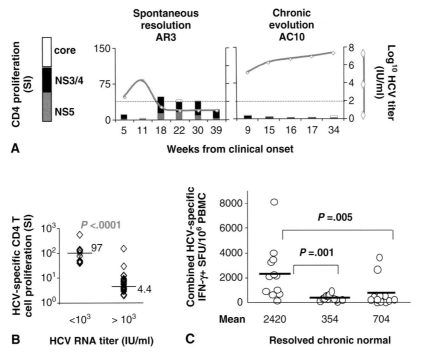

Fig. 8-7 **Inverse relationship between CD4 proliferative T-cell response and viremia. A,** Evolution of CD4 proliferative T-cell response to HCV core, NS3/4, and NS5 *(bar graphs)* relative to HCV RNA *(red line graph)* in two representative patients with acute hepatitis C with spontaneous resolution (AR3) and chronic evolution (AC10). **B,** HCV-specific CD4 proliferative T-cell response is greater with HCV RNA titer below 1000 IU/ml than above 1000 IU/ml in patients with acute hepatitis C. **C,** HCV-specific T-cell IFN-γ response is significantly greater in patients with resolved than chronic HCV infection in a cross-sectional analysis. *(A and B adapted from Kaplan DE, et al. Discordant role of CD4 T-cell response relative to neutralizing antibody and CD8 T-cell responses in acute hepatitis C. Gastroenterology 2007;132:654–666; C adapted from Sugimoto K, et al. Suppression of HCV-specific T cells without differential hierarchy demonstrated ex-vivo in persistent HCV infection. Hepatology 2003;38:1437–1448.[164])*

HCV-infected patients). Moreover, the interplay among HCV, lipoprotein components (to which it binds), and cellular receptors for virus entry should be considered.[145,146]

CD4 T-Cell Response to HCV

A critical role for CD4 T-cell help in protective immunity to HCV was shown in HCV-immune chimpanzees that developed chronic infection despite the induction of HCV-specific CD8 T-cell response when reinoculated after CD4-depletion[147] (**Fig. 8-6, A**). In HCV-infected patients, HCV-specific CD4 T cells are detectable in the liver and in peripheral blood.[148] In general, HCV-specific CD4 T-cell response in peripheral blood correlates with the clinical course. For example, control of HCV RNA titer in acute hepatitis C is associated with a vigorous and broad CD4 proliferative T-cell response (especially targeting the nonstructural proteins), whereas HCV persists with weak or transient antiviral CD4 T-cell response (usually targeting HCV core rather than the nonstructural proteins).[149-155] **Figure 8-7, A and B** shows the inverse association between HCV-specific CD4 T-cell proliferation and viremia.[152]

In general, HCV-specific CD4 proliferative T-cell response is detectable in less than a third of patients with chronic HCV infection compared with almost 90% in spontaneous HCV resolvers.[156] However, these T-cell responses are often directed toward viral isolates that have already been controlled,[157] whereas the T cells targeting the circulating virus are rendered dysfunctional by multiple immune regulatory mechanisms as discussed later in the chapter. Potential relevance of CD4 T cells in HCV infection is also suggested

by the associations between viral clearance and various class II HLA types.[158]

CD8 T-Cell Response to HCV

Hepatitis C virus–specific CD8 T cells are also detectable in the peripheral blood and liver during acute hepatitis C. HCV-specific CD8 T cells can target all viral proteins with numerous epitopes identified with various class I HLA restriction elements.[41] In HCV-infected chimpanzees, an early and multispecific intrahepatic CD8 cytolytic T-cell response has been associated with HCV clearance in one study.[159] Moreover, CD8 T-cell depletion before HCV inoculation resulted in prolonged viremia until the return of CD8 T cells in previously HCV-immune chimpanzees[160] (see **Fig. 8-6, B**). In another study, a vigorous and broadly specific IFN-γ⁺ CD8 and CD4 T-cell responses in the liver were associated with virus control.[161] These results suggest that CD8 T cells play a key effector role in controlling HCV viremia (similar to HBV), although CD4 help is needed to maintain their effectiveness.

In HCV-infected patients, HCV-specific CD8 T cells are highly activated during acute infection but unable to perform antigen-specific effector function such as IFN-γ production, proliferation or degranulation with a so-called/stunned/phenotype.[65,162,163] This dysfunction appears to occur irrespective of subsequent virologic outcome. In patients who subsequently clear viremia, CD8 T-cell dysfunction is resolved as HCV-specific CD8 T cells mature into protective CD127⁺ memory cells in the presence of functional CD4 T-cell response.[163] **Figure 8-7, C** shows the antiviral T-cell IFN-γ response in patients with resolved or chronic HCV infection.[164] In patients with chronic evolution, HCV-specific CD8 T-cell dysfunction persists via multiple immune inhibitory and regulatory mechanisms[61-65,165] and HCV-specific CD8 T cells are found in low frequency in peripheral blood but enriched in the liver.[64,166]

Vaccine Development in HCV

Based on the role of T cells in HCV clearance, it is believed that an effective vaccine approach for HCV should induce vigorous CD4 and CD8 T-cell responses. On the other hand, the development of effective prophylactic and therapeutic vaccine has been challenging despite much effort,[167,168] in part due to its high viral variability, weak immunogenicity, and potential immune evasion mechanisms. Among studies examining prophylactic vaccine in chimpanzees, adjuvanted recombinant envelope glycoprotein vaccine was able to protect up to 80% of vaccinated chimpanzees against chronic infection upon challenge with homologous or heterologous virus.[167,168] Protection could also be seen with T cell–based[169] and vaccinia virus–based[170] approaches. As for therapeutic vaccine, mechanisms of T–cell dysfunction and tolerance induced during chronic HCV infection may limit vaccine immunogenicity and efficacy in virus control.[171] Vaccine development is an important challenge that remains relevant, especially for highly endemic areas or high-risk populations to prevent further infection.

T Cells in Chronic HBV or HCV Infection and Therapy

Although HBV-specific CD8 T cells are weak in chronic HBV infection, an inverse relationship exists between HBV-specific CD8 T-cell response and HBV DNA. For example, HBV-specific CD8 T cells are more easily detected and functional in HBV carriers with lower viral titer than in highly viremic patients.[101,102] HBc-specific CD8 T-cell response (albeit low in frequency) showed a significant inverse association with HBV titer.[172] In the liver, HBV-specific CD8 T cells are found in similar number in patients displaying immune control and in patients with active disease.[115] However, in patients with active disease, HBV-specific CD8 T cells are effectively diluted in the liver by the massive inflammatory infiltrates. Thus ineffective HBV-specific CD8 T cells may contribute to cytopathology by recruiting nonspecific inflammatory cells (e.g., NK cells). Conversely, the level of viral antigen can influence CD8 T-cell function[173] and HBV-specific T-cell function can be enhanced in patients with therapeutic virus suppression.[108,174-176] It is likely that this is a dynamic process in patients with active chronic hepatitis B or flares.

In HCV, antiviral CD8 T cells follow a similar trend as HBV—weaker in persistence and stronger in clearance.[107] However, it differs from HBV in that therapeutic virus suppression does not always lead to enhanced antiviral T-cell function,[177,178] except in acute infection.[179] On the other hand, it is likely that T cells play a role in therapeutic response because treatment response is poor in patients with global T-cell dysfunction due to HIV infection or transplant immunosuppression.[180,181]

Viral persistence is also associated with the induction of various immune regulatory mechanisms. These inhibitory pathways may be reversed upon therapeutic virus suppression, thereby leading to enhanced antiviral effector T-cell response. With prolonged therapeutic virus suppression (with or without active immune modulatory therapy such as IFN-α or vaccination), the balance may ultimately tilt toward sustained virus control by dampening the immune regulatory pathways and enhancing the immune effector responses.

Immune Mechanisms of Viral Persistence

Innate Immune Evasion Mechanisms

As mentioned earlier, HBV can spread without triggering the innate type I IFN response during acute infection.[81,82] However, acute HBV infection is cleared in most adults despite this stealth capacity. For HCV, type I IFN pathway is inhibited at the level of induction via RIG-I and TRIF (within the infected cell although not globally)[81] and its downstream antiviral effect.[126,182,183] However, RIG-I and TRIF pathways are also inhibited by the hepatitis A virus, which does not generally persist.[184] Thus these innate immune evasion mechanisms do not completely explain the basis for HBV or HCV persistence. Nevertheless, they may contribute to the delayed onset of adaptive T-cell response that ultimately mediates viral clearance and liver injury.[99,147,160] Conceivably, with active viral spread and delayed adaptive immune induction, a number of immune regulatory pathways may be activated to limit liver damage while promoting viral persistence.

Mechanisms of T-Cell Regulation

Figure 8-8 shows some potential regulatory mechanisms of T-cell dysfunction or tolerance in HBV and HCV infection that are discussed below.

Inhibitory Costimulatory Pathways in Viral Infection

The balance between positive and negative immune costimulatory signals can influence virus-specific T-cell response. In particular, increased PD-1 expression is associated with

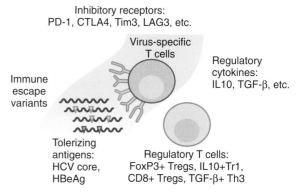

Fig. 8-8 **Potential regulatory mechanisms for virus-specific T cells in chronic HBV or HCV infection.**

virus-specific T-cell dysfunction during chronic viral infection. In chronic murine LCMV infection, in vivo blockade of PD-1 (but not CTLA4) promoted virus control and functionally restored exhausted virus-specific CD8 T cells lacking CD4 help ("helpless CD8 T cells").[57] In transgenic mice expressing HCV core in the liver, PD-1 blockade reversed the intrahepatic CD8 T-cell dysfunction and promoted the clearance of adenovirus infection.[185] In SIV-infected monkeys, PD-1 blockade enhanced T-cell immunity (also B-cell response) with improved survival and reduced viral load.[186] In humans, PD-1 expression on HIV-specific CD8 T cells was tightly associated with HIV-associated outcomes and effector dysfunction that was reversible by PD-1/PD-L blockade in vitro.[58,187,188] Collectively, these findings raise hope that modulation of inhibitory costimulatory pathways can have therapeutic benefit for chronic viral infection.

PD-1, CTLA4, and HBV

A role for PD-1 has been reported in HBV-infected patients. For example, during acute hepatitis B, HBV-specific CD8 T cells display increased PD-1 expression and impaired function,[189] followed by reduced PD-1 expression and increased CD127 (IL-7-receptor) expression as antigen-specific function improves with viral clearance. During chronic HBV infection, HBV-specific CD8 T cells are highly PD-1+ with impaired function that is restored by PD-1 blockade.[59] On the other hand, prolonged T-cell activation during chronic HBV infection can also lead to clonal deletion. For example, up-regulation of proapoptotic molecule Bim (Bcl-2-interacting mediator of cell death) in CD127-low HBV-specific CD8 T cells mediated their apoptosis.[190] In HBV transgenic mice, adoptively transferred HBV-specific CD8 T cells oscillate in their functionality in association with PD-1 expression, consistent with a regulatory role for PD-1 in T-cell function[191] and perhaps survival.

Interestingly, functional restoration with PD-1:PD-L1 blockade was observed for CD8 T-cell responses to HBV core and polymerase, but not envelope. On a related note, therapeutic vaccination with HBsAg during lamivudine therapy enhanced envelope-specific antibody and CD4 T-cell responses but without therapeutic efficacy,[192] suggesting that antibody and CD4 T-cell responses to HBV envelope are insufficient to clear viremia (perhaps due to lack of the effector CD8 T-cell responses and responses to core or polymerase). As for CTLA4, HBV persistence has been associated with CTLA4 single-nucleotide polymorphism (SNP).[193] However, its role has not been examined functionally in HBV.

PD-1, CTLA4, and HCV

In patients with chronic HCV infection, circulating HCV-specific CD8 T cells display increased PD-1 expression in direct association with their functional impairment, whereas PD-1 blockade can restore their function.[60-63] However, HCV-specific CD8 T cells from an HCV-infected liver show even greater PD-1 expression compared with those from peripheral blood.[61,63] Moreover, highly PD-1+ intrahepatic HCV-specific CD8 T cells are deeply impaired and refractory to PD-1 blockade alone.[64] Interestingly, combined PD-1/CTLA-4 blockade can synergistically enhance their effector function.[65] This differs from HIV in which CTLA4 blockade can augment CD4 T cells without a synergistic effect and does not augment CD8 T-cell function.[194] Thus the mechanisms of effector T-cell

dysfunction may differ between viruses (HIV vs. HCV), compartments (liver vs. blood) and T-cell subsets (CD4 vs. CD8). More recently, a role for Tim-3 has been reported in reversible HCV-specific T-cell dysfunction.[68]

Immune Regulatory T Cells and Cytokines

Relevance of CD25+ Tregs in viral infection has been reported for murine herpes simplex virus infection, as well as human HCV, HBV, and HIV infection.[71,195-197] A critical role for the IL-10/IL-10-receptor (IL-10R) pathway in viral pathogenesis was shown in chronic murine LCMV infection in which blockade of IL-10:IL-10R signaling resulted in viral clearance with increased IFN-γ^+ effector T-cell responses but no immune pathology.[78,79] Notably, IL-10R blockade also resulted in reduced PD-1-expression on antiviral CD8 T cells, thus linking IL-10/IL-10R and PD-1/PD-L pathways in LCMV infection.

Regulatory T Cells in HBV Infection

HBV persistence has been associated with increased circulating frequency of CD25+Tregs[198] that can suppress HBV-specific effector T cells.[199] In another study, CD25+ Tregs were increased in peripheral blood and the liver of HBV-infected patients while circulating CD25+ Treg frequency correlated with HBV titer.[200] In patients with HBV-associated hepatocellular carcinoma (HCC), circulating Treg frequency correlated with disease progression and mortality.[201] As for IL-10+ Tr1 response, a global cytokine deviation towards a Th0 rather than Th1 phenotype has been reported in chronic HBV infection[202] while T cells and monocytes from HBV-infected patients can secrete IL-10 in response to HBV core protein.[203,204]

Regulatory T Cells in HCV Infection

There is increasing evidence that immune regulatory T cells and cytokines contribute to HCV pathogenesis. First, patients with chronic HCV infection display increased circulating CD4+CD25+ Treg frequency.[164,197,205-207] Second, sorted CD25+ Treg are suppressive and their depletion can enhance HCV-specific effector T-cell function in vitro.[164,197,205-207] Third, CD25+ Tregs from HCV-infected patients display FoxP3 (the transcription factor generally accepted as a Treg marker) without any difference in phenotype, function, and gene expression profile compared with CD25+ Tregs from uninfected subjects,[208] consistent with the notion that HCV persists with increased FoxP3+ Tregs.

Because HCV-specific FoxP3+ and suppressive CD4 and CD8 Tregs can be expanded from HCV-infected patients,[208,209] it is conceivable that virus-specific FoxP3+ Tregs can be induced during viral infection with antigen-specific suppressive function. HCV-specific CD4 T cells expressing FoxP3 have been transiently detected ex vivo in the peripheral blood of acutely HCV-infected patients, although without a consistent association with immune effector function or virologic outcome.[210] FoxP3+ Tregs are detected in the HCV-infected liver,[211] suggesting that they can exert an immune regulatory effect at the site of viral replication. Intriguingly, Treg frequency is also increased in patients with liver cancer due to HBV or HCV, suggesting either a pathogenic role against tumor surveillance or an indicator of ongoing liver injury that contributes to carcinogenesis.[201,212]

As for Tr1 response, HCV gene products can induce IL-10 production in macrophages[213] and monocytes[214] promoting a cytokine milieu that favors Tr1 induction. HCV may promote DC dysfunction with increased IL-10 production by monocyte derived DC (mDC) and reduced IFN-α by plasmacytoid DC (pDC).[215] In fact, chronically HCV-infected patients display increased HCV-specific IL-10[+] Tr1 response[216,217] and serum IL-10 levels[218] that decrease with antiviral therapy. Relevant to immune regulation at the site of infection, HCV-specific IL-10[+] CD8 Tr1 cells in the liver of HCV-infected patients showed IL-10-dependent T-cell suppression.[219] HCV-specific CD4 T cells with TGF-β (and IL-10) secretion has been detected in chronic hepatitis C,[220] whereas HCV-specific CD8 T-cell cytotoxicity could be enhanced by TGF-β inhibition.[221] Tr1 response in HCV infection may have a dual role in promoting viral persistence during acute infection while limiting liver disease progression in established chronic infection. Consistent with this notion, exogenous IL-10 reduced liver fibrosis and increased HCV titer.[222,223]

In HCV, HCV-specific IL-10[+] Tr1 response has been associated with HCV persistence and decreased HCV-specific CD4 T-cell response. Interestingly, IL-10R blockade enhanced HCV-specific IFN-γ[+] T-cell response in vitro,[224] raising the possibility that blockade of IL-10 pathway may have therapeutic application.

Viral Immune Escape Mutation

As discussed earlier, neutralizing antibody response to the HCV envelope is readily evaded by ongoing selection of antibody escape variants.[41,141,225] Similarly, HCV also readily escapes virus-specific CD8 T cells by selection of immune escape variants in acute infection,[226] which is less common in established chronic infection with reduced immune selection pressure.[227,228] Evolution of escape mutations is also uncommon in established chronic HBV infection in the absence of immune selection pressure.[229] CD8 T-cells may be further tolerized in chronic HBV or HCV infection due to the emergence of epitope variants that not only escape CD8 T-cell recognition but also directly antagonize CD8 T-cell activation.[113,172,227]

Viral Antigens in Immune Regulation
HCV Core as an Immune Regulatory Protein

Hepatitis C virus core protein can be detected in the circulating blood of HCV-infected patients in direct association with HCV RNA titer and it is the most immunogenic protein targeted by T cells in chronically HCV-infected patients.[156,157] However, HCV core can also bind the complement receptor gC1qR on T cells and inhibit T-cell function in vitro by inhibiting IL-2 and IL-2Rα gene transcription and by inducing suppressors of the cytokine signaling (SOCS) pathway.[230-232] CD8 T cells may be more readily suppressed by the HCV due to greater gC1qR expression compared with CD4 T cells.[233] However, gC1qR is up-regulated by CD4 T cells during acute infection, thereby becoming more susceptible to core-mediated suppression.[234] While global T-cell dysfunction is not a feature of chronic HCV infection, HCV core may mediate a critical immune regulatory effect in early HCV infection by suppressing the antiviral T cells as they become activated.

HBVeAg as an Immunologic Tolerogen

In neonates, vertically transmitted HBV infection becomes invariably chronic. Potential mechanisms may include the immature immune system in the neonate and the tolerizing effect of HBV antigens[235,236] that may lead to T-cell exhaustion and/or clonal deletion. Nevertheless, timely passive and active immunization upon delivery can prevent chronic HBV infection, suggesting that a protective vaccine response can be induced even in newborns. In this setting, the soluble HBeAg is known to passively cross the placenta and mediate T-cell mediated tolerance to HBV. Clinical presentation of immune active chronic hepatitis B in HBeAg precore mutant patients may exemplify the loss of the immune tolerance mechanism.

Extrahepatic Site of Viral Replication

Hepatitis C virus replication has been reported in cells of nonhepatic origin. For example, immune cells such as T- and B-cell lines have been shown to harbor HCV replication in culture, although not in a very robust fashion.[237-240] Detection of HBV DNA in peripheral blood lymphocyte subsets has also been reported from HBV-infected and resolved subjects (including HBV RNA transcript in two subjects in the late convalescent phase of infection)[111,241] The clinical and pathogenetic relevance of these findings are not yet clearly defined.

Mechanisms of Liver Injury in HCV and HBV Infection

In acute hepatitis B and C, virus control is mediated by cytopathic and noncytopathic mechanisms that are largely mediated by CD8 T cells with further amplification nonspecific inflammatory recruitment. With chronic infection, the situation is more complex. For example, the virus has become better adapted and established within the liver (greater number of infected cells, immune escape mutation, inhibition of cellular antiviral pathways, potential extrahepatic reservoir). In some sense, the immune system recognizes this and appears to have developed mechanisms to prevent undue damage while maintaining some control of the virus. The balance between the virus and host immune response (driven by the host genetics and environment) will ultimately determine the course of liver disease.

Virus-Mediated Injury

Persistent viruses are generally noncytopathic since their continued survival requires a viable host (i.e., it does not burn down its own house). In fact, HBV and HCV replication in an experimental chimpanzee infection is unaccompanied by any biochemical or histologic evidence for liver injury until T cells are activated and recruited. Moreover, immunosuppression (e.g., by steroids) results in increased HBV and HCV replication without evidence of liver injury.[242,243]

For HBV, liver injury was observed in HBV envelope transgenic mice that accumulate the large envelope protein in high amounts within the endoplasmic reticulum,[244] but not in mice that replicate the virus in the liver without such high cellular protein retention.[245] A similar situation may occur in immunosuppressed patients with fibrosing cholestatic hepatitis B. In these patients, marked hepatocyte injury and ductular reactions occur without a significant inflammatory component in a setting of extremely high levels of HBV DNA and the so-called "ground glass hepatocytes" displaying massive viral antigen expression.[246] Similar cytopathic effect was also observed in some humanized chimeric mice harboring human hepatocytes with increased reactive oxygen species, TGF-β production and fibrosis that may differ among HBV strains or genotype in some[247,248] but not all studies.[249]

Similarly, HCV expression in the liver has been associated with hepatic injury, steatosis, and liver cancer development in some[250-252] but not all HCV transgenic or chimeric mice.[249,253,254] HCV may promote apoptosis of infected cells via TRAIL-mediated mechanisms in some studies,[255,256] whereas HCV may inhibit cytokine-mediated apoptosis in other studies.[257,258] Moreover, the course of liver disease is significantly accelerated in HIV/HCV co-infected patients[259,260] or HCV-infected liver transplant recipients,[261-263] suggesting a potential virus-mediated injury in the absence of immune-mediated virus control. Collectively, these findings point to the possibility that both HBV and HCV can be directly cytopathic in certain circumstances (particularly in the absence of immune control) but not in all cases.

Immune-Mediated Liver Injury

T Cell–Mediated Injury

A pathogenetic role for CD8 T cells was demonstrated by hepatocyte apoptosis and hepatitis upon adoptive transfer of HBV-specific CD8 T cells in HBV transgenic mice[50] and by reduced liver inflammation during acute experimental HBV infection in a CD8-depleted chimpanzee.[99] CD8-cytolytic activity involves both perforin and Fas death pathways. As shown in **Figure 8-9**, CD8-induced liver damage is further amplified by chemokines, neutrophils (and matrix metalloproteinases made by neutrophils) and platelets that mediate

recruitment of other immune cells (e.g., NK, NKT, T/B cells, macrophages, monocytes, DC) into the liver.[264] While CTLs (and the recruited inflammatory cells) contribute to liver cell injury, they also elaborate antiviral cytokines (e.g., IFN-γ) that can cure virus-infected hepatocytes, ultimately leading to viral clearance without fulminant liver failure.

A Role for Platelets in Virus-Specific CD8 T-Cell Recruitment into the Liver

Intrahepatic accumulation of virus-specific CD8 T cells and liver injury can be prevented by platelet depletion in various mouse models (HBV transgenic, LCMV, adenovirus).[264] Of interest, administration of antiplatelet agents (aspirin, clopidogrel) reduced the liver disease severity and inhibited viral clearance in mice with adenovirus-induced viral hepatitis.[265] It is not clear if this effect during acute liver injury is also relevant for progressive liver damage that occurs in chronic hepatitis B and C. Nevertheless, it highlights the relevance of immune recruitment signals in liver disease pathogenesis.

Chemokines in Recruitment of Immune Cells into the Liver

Chemokines are involved in leukocyte migration and inflammation. They can be divided into four subfamilies based on the position of the two N-terminal cysteine residues: CXC (divided into ELR-CXC or non-ELR-CXC based on preceding Glu-Leu-Arg residues), CC, C, and CX3C chemokines.

In HCV, viral gene products (e.g., core, NS5A) and antiviral cytokines (e.g., IFN-γ) can induce the production of chemokines such as RANTES (regulated upon activation, normal T cell expressed and activated), CXCL10 (IFN-inducible protein 10 or IP10) and MIG (monokine-induced by IFN-γ) by hepatocytes and sinusoidal endothelial cells.[266,267] Accordingly, T cells recruited to the HCV-infected liver display increased expression of chemokine receptor CXCR3 and CCR5, compared with those in the uninfected liver. Moreover, IP10 expression has been associated with the histologic marker of liver inflammation and fibrosis in HCV-infected patients.[268]

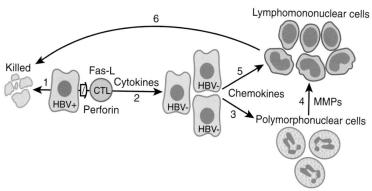

Fig. 8-9 **Mechanisms of cytotoxic T lymphocyte (CTL)–induced liver disease and viral clearance.** After antigen recognition, virus-specific CTLs kill a small number of hepatocytes via Fas L- and Perforin-mediated pathways and produce antiviral cytokines that inhibit HBV or HCV replication noncytopathically in many more cells. The same cytokines can activate parenchymal and nonparenchymal cells of the liver to produce chemokines that recruit antigen-nonspecific polymorphonuclear cells into the organ. Production of matrix metalloproteinases (MMPs) by these cells in addition to chemokine induction may contribute to the migration of antigen-nonspecific immune cells (e.g., natural killer cells, T cells, macrophages) into the liver and the amplification of the liver disease initiated by the CTL. (*Adapted from Guidotti LG, Chisari FV. Immunobiology and pathogenesis of viral hepatitis. Annu Rev Pathol 2006;1:23–61.*)

Similarly, HCV persistence and IFN-α treatment resistance have been associated with increased serum level of CXCL8 (IL-8 or neutrophil chemotactic factor), which can be produced by HCV-expressing hepatocytes via NS5A-dependent mechanism,[269] as well as other cells.

In HBV, a flare of chronic hepatitis B (with or without prior therapy) is preceded by a rise in serum IL-8 level[90,270] and temporally associated with increased CXCL9 and CXCL10 (both potent chemo-attractants of activated T cells). IL-8 can modify hepatocyte expression of the TRAIL receptor, thereby enhancing its susceptibility to TRAIL-mediated apoptosis upon exposure to activated NK cells.[90] Collectively, these findings support the role for chemokines and their receptors in liver injury and virus control in HCV and HBV infection.

NK Cells and Liver Injury

Interestingly, hepatitis flares correlated with increased NK activation and expression of TNF-related apoptosis inducing ligand (TRAIL).[90] A critical role for TRAIL in liver cell death and inflammation has been reported in murine models of hepatitis.[271] Importantly, NK cells stimulated with IFN-α displayed increased TRAIL expression and induced more apoptosis in liver-derived HepG2 cells. Conversely, HBV-infected patients with elevated sALT displayed greater hepatocyte expression of death-inducing TRAIL receptor. Both IL-8 and IFN-α could modulate the pattern of TRAIL receptor expression on liver-derived cells. Aside from NK cells, chronic hepatitis B is associated with mDC and/or pDC dysfunction that may be reversed by therapeutic virus suppression.[272,273]

In HCV, there is increasing support for the notion that HCV persists with activated NK cells[89,129,274] despite lower circulating frequency.[133] Expression of early NK activation marker CD69 is associated with increased serum ALT activity and HCV RNA in chronic HCV infection.[89] Moreover, activated NK cells from HCV-infected patients displayed a polarization toward cytolytic rather than noncytolytic antiviral activity.[274] IFN-α administration up-regulated TRAIL expression (both in vivo and in vitro) and the polarization towards cytolytic activity in vitro.[274] Finally, up-regulation of TRAIL expression on NK subset (CD56 bright) was associated with viral decline.[275] Collectively, these findings suggest that NK cells are likely to be involved in liver disease activity and virus control in HBV and HCV infection.

Summary

Hepatitis B and C virus can trigger a number of innate and/or adaptive immune responses that define the course of HBV infection. Despite limitations in available model system, there has been an enormous progress in our understanding of the host–virus interactions during infection with hepatitis B and C viruses. Both viruses have innate immune evasion mechanisms and the adaptive immune responses ultimately mediate viral clearance and protective immunity. CD4 T cells are needed to regulate the overall adaptive immune response whereas CD8 T cells are the critical effectors that mediate liver injury and viral clearance. During chronic infection, antiviral T cells are functionally exhausted, with impaired capacity for virus control, although they may contribute to hepatic recruitment of inflammatory cells that amplify liver injury.

Ultimately, these interactions that contribute to progressive fibrosis and hepatocarcinogenesis. While therapeutic options are evolving for HBV and HCV, better understanding of viral persistence and pathogenetic mechanisms will help develop new approaches to prevent and treat HBV and HCV infection and their considerable disease burden.

Key References

Adams DH, et al. Mechanisms of immune-mediated liver injury 1. Toxicol Sci 2010;115:307–321. (Ref.17)

Ahlenstiel G, et al. Natural killer cells are polarized toward cytotoxicity in chronic hepatitis C in an interferon-alfa-dependent manner. Gastroenterology 2010;138:325–335, e321–e322. (Ref.274)

Amadei B, et al. Activation of natural killer cells during acute infection with hepatitis C virus. Gastroenterology 2010;138:1536–1545. (Ref.131)

Asabe S, et al. The size of the viral inoculum contributes to the outcome of hepatitis B virus infection. J Virol 2009;83:9652–9662. (Ref.100)

Averill L, Lee WM, Karandikar NJ. Differential dysfunction in dendritic cell subsets during chronic HCV infection. Clin Immunol 2007;123:40–49. (Ref.215)

Badr G, et al. Early interferon therapy for hepatitis C virus infection rescues polyfunctional, long-lived CD8+ memory T cells. J Virol 2008;82: 10017–10031. (Ref.179)

Barber DL, et al. Restoring function in exhausted CD8 T cells during chronic viral infection. Nature 2006;439:682–687. (Ref.57)

Billerbeck E, et al. Determinants of in vitro expansion of different human virus-specific FoxP3+ regulatory CD8+ T cells in chronic hepatitis C virus infection. J Gen Virol 2009;90:1692–1701. (Ref.209)

Bissig KD, et al. Human liver chimeric mice provide a model for hepatitis B and C virus infection and treatment. J Clin Invest 2010;120:924–930. (Ref.249)

Blackburn SD, et al. Coregulation of CD8+ T-cell exhaustion by multiple inhibitory receptors during chronic viral infection. Nat Immunol 2009;10: 29–37. (Ref.66)

Boni C, et al. Characterization of hepatitis B virus (HBV)-specific T-cell dysfunction in chronic HBV infection. J Virol 2007;81:4215–4225. (Ref.59)

Bouaziz JD, Yanaba K, Tedder TF. Regulatory B cells as inhibitors of immune responses and inflammation. Immunol Rev 2008;224:201–214. (Ref.40)

Bryceson YT, Long EO. Line of attack: NK cell specificity and integration of signals. Curr Opin Immunol 2008;20:344–352. (Ref.25)

Casadevall A, Pirofski LA. A reappraisal of humoral immunity based on mechanisms of antibody-mediated protection against intracellular pathogens. Adv Immunol 2006;91:1–44. (Ref.39)

Chang KM. Regulatory T cells in hepatitis C virus infection. Hepatol Res 2007;37(Suppl 3):S327–S330. (Ref.197)

Chelbi-Alix MK, Wietzerbin J. Interferon, a growing cytokine family: 50 years of interferon research. Biochimie 2007;89:713–718. (Ref.5)

Chisari FV, Isogawa M, Wieland SF. Pathogenesis of hepatitis B virus infection. Pathol Biol (Paris) 2010;58:258–266. (Ref.91)

Crispe IN. The liver as a lymphoid organ. Annu Rev Immunol 2009;27:147–163. (Ref.19)

Cummings KL, Rosen HR, Hahn YS. Frequency of gC1qR+CD4+ T cells increases during acute hepatitis C virus infection and remains elevated in patients with chronic infection. Clin Immunol 2009;132:401–411. (Ref.234)

Day CL, et al. PD-1 expression on HIV-specific T cells is associated with T-cell exhaustion and disease progression. Nature 2006;443:350–354. (Ref.58)

Dunn C, et al. Cytokines induced during chronic hepatitis B virus infection promote a pathway for NK cell-mediated liver damage. J Exp Med 2007;204: 667–680. (Ref.90)

Dunn C, et al. Temporal analysis of early immune responses in patients with acute hepatitis B virus infection. Gastroenterology 2009;137:1289–1300. (Ref.82)

Durantel D, Zoulim F. Innate response to hepatitis B virus infection: observations challenging the concept of a stealth virus. Hepatology 2009;50: 1692–1695. (Ref.85)

Ebinuma H, et al. Identification and in vitro expansion of functional antigen-specific CD25+ FoxP3+ regulatory T cells in hepatitis C virus infection. J Virol 2008;82:5043–5053. (Ref.208)

Fisicaro P, et al. Early kinetics of innate and adaptive immune responses during hepatitis B virus infection. Gut 2009;58:974–982. (Ref.88)

Freeman GJ, et al. Reinvigorating exhausted HIV-specific T cells via PD-1-PD-1 ligand blockade. J Exp Med 2006;203:2223–2227. (Ref.56)

Fu J, et al. Increased regulatory T cells correlate with CD8 T-cell impairment and poor survival in hepatocellular carcinoma patients. Gastroenterology 2007;132: 2328–2339. (Ref.201)

Gal-Tanamy M, et al. In vitro selection of a neutralization-resistant hepatitis C virus escape mutant. Proc Natl Acad Sci U S A 2008;105:19450–19455. (Ref.142)

Ge D, et al. Genetic variation in IL28B predicts hepatitis C treatment-induced viral clearance. Nature 2009;461:399–401. (Ref.10)

Gehring AJ, et al. The level of viral antigen presented by hepatocytes influences CD8 T-cell function. J Virol 2007;81:2940–2949. (Ref.173)

Geissmann F, et al. Development of monocytes, macrophages, and dendritic cells. Science 2010;327:656–661. (Ref.14)

Godfrey DI, Stankovic S, Baxter AG. Raising the NKT cell family. Nat Immunol 2010;11:197–206. (Ref.32)

Golden-Mason L, et al. Phenotypic and functional changes of cytotoxic CD56pos natural T cells determine outcome of acute hepatitis C virus infection. J Virol 2007;81:9292–9298. (Ref.134)

Golden-Mason L, et al. Altered natural killer cell subset distributions in resolved and persistent hepatitis C virus infection following single source exposure. Gut 2008;57:1121–1128. (Ref.132)

Golden-Mason L, et al. Upregulation of PD-1 expression on circulating and intrahepatic hepatitis C virus-specific CD8+ T cells associated with reversible immune dysfunction. J Virol 2007;81:9249–9258. (Ref.63)

Golden-Mason L, et al. Negative immune regulator Tim-3 is overexpressed on T cells in hepatitis C virus infection and its blockade rescues dysfunctional CD4+ and CD8+ T cells. J Virol 2009;83:9122–9130. (Ref.68)

Grove J, et al. Identification of a residue in hepatitis C virus E2 glycoprotein that determines scavenger receptor BI and CD81 receptor dependency and sensitivity to neutralizing antibodies. J Virol 2008;82:12020–12029. (Ref.145)

Guidotti LG, Chisari FV. Immunobiology and pathogenesis of viral hepatitis. Annu Rev Pathol 2006;1:23–61. (Ref.50)

Guy CS, et al. Intrahepatic expression of genes affiliated with innate and adaptive immune responses immediately after invasion and during acute infection with woodchuck hepadnavirus. J Virol 2008;82:8579–8591. (Ref.87)

Harris RA, et al. Human leukocyte antigen class II associations with hepatitis C virus clearance and virus-specific CD4 T cell response among Caucasians and African Americans. Hepatology 2008;48:70–79. (Ref.158)

Heeg MH, et al. FOXP3 expression in hepatitis C virus-specific CD4+ T cells during acute hepatitis C. Gastroenterology 2009;137:1280–1288, e1281–e1286. (Ref.210)

Holz LE, et al. Intrahepatic murine CD8 T-cell activation associates with a distinct phenotype leading to Bim-dependent death. Gastroenterology 2008;135:989–997. (Ref.42)

Hosel M, et al. Not interferon, but interleukin-6 controls early gene expression in hepatitis B virus infection. Hepatology 2009;50:1773–1782. (Ref.86)

Houghton M. The long and winding road leading to the identification of the hepatitis C virus. J Hepatol 2009;51:939–948. (Ref.168)

Iannacone M, et al. Antiplatelet drug therapy moderates immune-mediated liver disease and inhibits viral clearance in mice infected with a replication-deficient adenovirus. Clin Vaccine Immunol 2007;14:1532–1535. (Ref.265)

Iwasaki A, Medzhitov R. Regulation of adaptive immunity by the innate immune system. Science 2010;327:291–295. (Ref.4)

Jeannin P, Jaillon S, Delneste Y. Pattern recognition receptors in the immune response against dying cells. Curr Opin Immunol 2008;20:530–537. (Ref.3)

Kaplan DE, et al. Peripheral virus-specific T-cell interleukin-10 responses develop early in acute hepatitis C infection and become dominant in chronic hepatitis. J Hepatol 2008;48:903–913. (Ref.224)

Kaplan DE, et al. Discordant role of CD4 T-cell response relative to neutralizing antibody and CD8 T-cell responses in acute hepatitis C. Gastroenterology 2007;132:654–666. (Ref.152)

Kaufmann DE, et al. Upregulation of CTLA-4 by HIV-specific CD4(+) T cells correlates with disease progression and defines a reversible immune dysfunction. Nat Immunol 2007;8:1246–1254. (Ref.194)

Kawai T, Akira S. TLR signaling. Semin Immunol 2007;19:24–32. (Ref.276)

Kim KD, et al. Adaptive immune cells temper initial innate responses. Nat Med 2007;13:1248–1252. (Ref.37)

Klade CS, et al. Therapeutic vaccination of chronic hepatitis C nonresponder patients with the peptide vaccine IC41. Gastroenterology 2008;134:1385–1395. (Ref.171)

Krieger SE, et al. Inhibition of hepatitis C virus infection by anti-claudin-1 antibodies is mediated by neutralization of E2-CD81-claudin-1 associations. Hepatology 2010;51(1):43–53. (Ref.146)

Kuntzen T, et al. Viral sequence evolution in acute hepatitis C virus infection. J Virol 2007;81:11658–11668. (Ref.228)

Lan L, et al. Hepatitis C virus infection sensitizes human hepatocytes to TRAIL-induced apoptosis in a caspase 9-dependent manner. J Immunol 2008;181:4926–4935. (Ref.255)

Lanier LL. Up on the tightrope: natural killer cell activation and inhibition. Nat Immunol 2008;9:495–502. (Ref.28)

Lau DT, et al. Interferon regulatory factor-3 activation, hepatic interferon-stimulated gene expression, and immune cell infiltration in hepatitis C virus patients. Hepatology 2008;47:799–809. (Ref.121)

Law M, et al. Broadly neutralizing antibodies protect against hepatitis C virus quasispecies challenge. Nat Med 2008;14:25–27. (Ref.144)

Liu K, Nussenzweig MC. Origin and development of dendritic cells. Immunol Rev 2010;234:45–54. (Ref.21)

Lopes AR, et al. Bim-mediated deletion of antigen-specific CD8 T cells in patients unable to control HBV infection. J Clin Invest 2008;118:1835–1845. (Ref.190)

Lucas M, et al. Dendritic cells prime natural killer cells by trans-presenting interleukin 15. Immunity 2007;26:503–517. (Ref.24)

Lukens JR, et al. Blockade of PD-1/B7-H1 interaction restores effector CD8+ T cell responses in a hepatitis C virus core murine model. J Immunol 2008;180:4875–4884. (Ref.185)

Manns MP, et al. The way forward in HCV treatment—finding the right path. Nat Rev Drug Discov 2007;6:991–1000. (Ref.167)

McCartney SA, Colonna M. Viral sensors: diversity in pathogen recognition. Immunol Rev 2009;227:87–94. (Ref.20)

Nakamoto N, et al. Synergistic reversal of intrahepatic HCV-specific CD8 T cell exhaustion by combined PD-1/CTLA-4 blockade. PLoS Pathog 2009;5: e1000313. (Ref.65)

Nakamoto N, et al. Functional restoration of HCV-specific CD8 T cells by PD-1 blockade is defined by PD-1 expression and compartmentalization. Gastroenterology 2008;134:1927–1937, e1921–e1922. (Ref.64)

Nemeth E, Baird AW, O'Farrelly C. Microanatomy of the liver immune system. Semin Immunopathol 2009;31:333–343. (Ref.16)

O'Brien TR. Interferon-alfa, interferon-lambda and hepatitis C. Nat Genet 2009;41:1048–1050. (Ref.8)

Oliviero B, et al. Natural killer cell functional dichotomy in chronic hepatitis B and chronic hepatitis C virus infections. Gastroenterology 2009;137:1151–1160, e1151–e1157. (Ref.89)

Palm NW, Medzhitov R. Pattern recognition receptors and control of adaptive immunity. Immunol Rev 2009;227:221–233. (Ref.1)

Penna A, et al. Dysfunction and functional restoration of HCV-specific CD8 responses in chronic hepatitis C virus infection. Hepatology 2007;45:588–601. (Ref.62)

Pham TN, et al. Hepatitis C virus replicates in the same immune cell subsets in chronic hepatitis C and occult infection. Gastroenterology 2008;134:812–822. (Ref.240)

Radziewicz H, et al. Unraveling the role of PD-1/PD-L interactions in persistent hepatotropic infections: potential for therapeutic application? Gastroenterology 2008;134:2168–2171. (Ref.165)

Radziewicz H, et al. Liver infiltrating lymphocytes in chronic human HCV infection display an exhausted phenotype with high PD-1 and low CD127 expression. J Virol 2006;81:2545–2553. (Ref.61)

Riley JL, June CH. The road to recovery: translating PD-1 biology into clinical benefit. Trends Immunol 2007;28(2):48–50. (Ref.55)

Schreibelt G, et al. Toll-like receptor expression and function in human dendritic cell subsets: implications for dendritic cell-based anti-cancer immunotherapy. Cancer Immunol Immunother 2010;59(10):1573–1582. (Ref.22)

Serbina NV, et al. Monocyte-mediated defense against microbial pathogens. Annu Rev Immunol 2008;26:421–452. (Ref.15)

Shiina M, Rehermann B. Cell culture-produced hepatitis C virus impairs plasmacytoid dendritic cell function. Hepatology 2008;47:385–395. (Ref.124)

Sommereyns C, et al. IFN-lambda (IFN-lambda) is expressed in a tissue-dependent fashion and primarily acts on epithelial cells in vivo. PLoS Pathog 2008;4(3):e1000017. (Ref.9)

Stegmann KA, et al. Interferon-alfa-induced tumor necrosis factor-related apoptosis-inducing ligand on natural killer cells is associated with control of hepatitis C virus infection. Gastroenterology 2010;138(5):1885–1897. (Ref.275)

Sugiyama M, et al. Direct cytopathic effects of particular hepatitis B virus genotypes in severe combined immunodeficiency transgenic with urokinase-type plasminogen activator mouse with human hepatocytes. Gastroenterology 2009;136(2):652–662, e3. (Ref.247)

Suppiah V, et al. IL28B is associated with response to chronic hepatitis C interferon-alpha and ribavirin therapy. Nat Genet 2009;41:1100–1104. (Ref.11)

Tan AT, et al. A longitudinal analysis of innate and adaptive immune profile during hepatic flares in chronic hepatitis B. J Hepatol 2010;52:330–339. (Ref.270)

Tanaka Y, et al. Genome-wide association of IL28B with response to pegylated interferon-alpha and ribavirin therapy for chronic hepatitis C. Nat Genet 2009;41:1105–1109. (Ref.12)

Thomas DL, et al. Genetic variation in IL28B and spontaneous clearance of hepatitis C virus. Nature 2009;461:798–801. (Ref.13)

Ueno H, et al. Dendritic cell subsets in health and disease. Immunol Rev 2007; 219:118–142. (Ref.23)

Urbani S, et al. CPD-1 expression in acute hepatitis C virus (HCV) infection is associated with HCV-specific CD8 exhaustion. J Virol 2006;80:11398–11403. (Ref.60)

Vandepapeliere P, et al. Therapeutic vaccination of chronic hepatitis B patients with virus suppression by antiviral therapy: a randomized, controlled study of co-administration of HBsAg/AS02 candidate vaccine and lamivudine. Vaccine 2007;25:8585–8597. (Ref.192)

Vasan S, Tsuji M. A double-edged sword: the role of NKT cells in malaria and HIV infection and immunity. Semin Immunol 2010;22:87–96. (Ref.33)

Velu V, et al. Enhancing SIV-specific immunity in vivo by PD-1 blockade. Nature 2009;458:206–210. (Ref.186)

Virgin HW, Wherry EJ, Ahmed R. Redefining chronic viral infection. Cell 2009;138:30–50. (Ref.51)

von Hahn T, et al. Hepatitis C virus continuously escapes from neutralizing antibody and T-cell responses during chronic infection in vivo. Gastroenterology 2007;132:667–678. (Ref.141)

Ward SM, et al. Quantification and localisation of FOXP3+ T lymphocytes and relation to hepatic inflammation during chronic HCV infection. J Hepatol 2007;47:316–324. (Ref.211)

Yoon JC, et al. Natural killer cell function is intact after direct exposure to infectious hepatitis C virions. Hepatology 2009;49:12–21. (Ref.129)

Youn JW, et al. Evidence for protection against chronic hepatitis C virus infection in chimpanzees by immunization with replicating recombinant vaccinia virus. J Virol 2008;82:10896–10905. (Ref.170)

Zhang SY, et al. Inborn errors of interferon (IFN)-mediated immunity in humans: insights into the respective roles of IFN-alpha/beta, IFN-gamma, and IFN-lambda in host defense. Immunol Rev 2008;226:29–40. (Ref.7)

Zhang Z, et al. Response to interferon-alpha treatment correlates with recovery of blood plasmacytoid dendritic cells in children with chronic hepatitis B. J Hepatol 2007;47:751–759. (Ref.273)

Zhu H, et al. Hepatitis C virus triggers apoptosis of a newly developed hepatoma cell line through antiviral defense system. Gastroenterology 2007;133: 1649–1659. (Ref.256)

Zipfel C. Pattern-recognition receptors in plant innate immunity. Curr Opin Immunol 2008;20:10–16. (Ref.2)

A complete list of references can be found at www.expertconsult.com.

Liver and Immune System

Percy Knolle

ABBREVIATIONS

APC antigen-presenting cell
IFN-γ interferon-γ
LSEC liver sinusoidal endothelial cell
MHC major histocompatibility complex

NKT natural killer T lymphocytes
PGE₂ prostaglandin E₂
TGF-β transforming growth factor-β
TLR toll-like receptor

TNF tumor necrosis factor
VAP-1 vascular adhesion protein 1

The liver has been recognized as a unique immune organ. First, immune responses within the liver are shaped by both organ-resident cells with extraordinary immune competence and by bone marrow–derived immune cells that are influenced in their function by the hepatic microenvironment. Liver-specific immune regulation is governed by strong innate immune responses but is also characterized by induction of antigen-specific immune tolerance toward antigens presented in the liver, which also has consequences for extrahepatic immune responses. Viral hepatitis and autoimmune hepatitis are important clinical entities where the liver serves as target for immune responses that cause tissue damage. This chapter sheds light on the molecular and cellular immune mechanisms active in the liver with respect to local regulation of immunity and immune tolerance.

Functions of the Immune System

The immune system is a remarkable defense mechanism to protect the organism against a constant challenge of facultative and obligatory pathogenic microorganisms. Genetically determined and acquired immune deficiencies that are associated with severe infections that are often not compatible with survival, clearly illustrate the central role of the immune response in protection of the organism. It is generally accepted that the interaction with microorganisms has shaped the immune system in evolutionary terms. While certain roles of the immune system, such as elimination of spontaneously arising tumor cells, have been debated, it has become clear that the immune defense against pathogens must avoid attacking host antigens to prevent autoimmunity and tissue damage. Such immune tolerance toward auto-antigens is an active process, which requires constant "education" of lymphocytes in several anatomically and functionally distinct compartments. To accomplish these complex features, the immune system consists of numerous highly specialized cell populations that closely cooperate to shape pathogen-specific immune responses.

One of the most eminent features of the immune system is its dynamic. Being of bone marrow origin, immune cells continuously circulate through the body to retrieve information (antigen) and/or to exert effector function. The immune system can be categorized into two parts: the innate immune response, which consists of cells such as natural killer (NK) cells, macrophages, granulocytes, dendritic cells and soluble molecules such as complement, which display fast and antigen-non-specific effector function. The adaptive immune response consists of cells bearing clonally restricted antigen-specific receptors, such as T lymphocytes and B lymphocytes. Activation of cells of the adaptive immune system requires a complex and cognate interaction with antigen-presenting cells (APCs).

APCs most importantly dendritic cells, patrol peripheral tissues and collect antigens. They migrate to secondary lymphoid tissue (lymph nodes) where in a unique microenvironment, major histocompatability complex I (MHC-I), MHC-II, or CD1-restricted presentation of antigen to naïve CD4 and CD8 T cells takes place. Depending on their activation status, dendritic cells will then either induce immune tolerance or stimulate T-cell immunity. In recent years it has become increasingly clear that different dendritic cell subpopulations exist,[1] which display different functional capacities in vitro—the relevance of which for the immune response in vivo is still unclear. Dendritic cells have been found that continuously sample antigens from mucosal surfaces. Contrary to the belief that epithelial cells in the mucosa constitute a tight barrier that prevents (commensal) bacteria from entering the body, dendritic cells breach this barrier by formation of transepithelial dendrites and continuously sample antigen and bacteria directly from the gut lumen or other mucosal surfaces.[2,3] Moreover, the dendritic cells collecting antigen may not be identical to the dendritic cells finally presenting the antigen to T cells. It has become clear that there is a "division of labor" among different dendritic cell subtypes. For instance, Langerhans cells reside in the skin, continuously collect antigen, and upon appropriate stimulation migrate into regional lymph nodes. However, it is not Langerhans cells that present skin-derived antigen to T cells but a lymph node resident CD8[+] dendritic cell population, indicating that Langerhans cells transfer antigen to this apparently more specialized dendritic cell population.[4] This presentation of exogenous antigens on MHC-I molecules is termed cross-presentation. Finally, antigens may directly gain access to the organism. Following oral ingestion of antigens, a rapid dissemination of antigen via the blood stream is observed that leads to systemic activation of the immune system toward gut-derived antigens.[5] Antigens may even directly gain access to lymph nodes using a conduit system that delivers antigens into certain anatomic compartments in the lymph node were interaction with specialized dendritic cells occurs.[6] All these observations strongly support the notion that in different anatomic compartments different dendritic cell subpopulations exist, which are shaped in their function by the unique microenvironment to fit the need to achieve local and systemic immune surveillance.

Immune tolerance in the organism is achieved by virtue of several different mechanisms. Clonal elimination of auto-reactive T cells occurs already early during T-cell ontogeny in the thymus. However, not all auto-reactive T cells are eliminated here and further control in the periphery is required. Many different mechanisms have been described to function in the maintenance of peripheral immune tolerance, such as clonal deletion, anergy, and regulation/deviation. Central to all these mechanisms are antigen-presenting cells. Under immature, steady-state conditions dendritic cells induce T-cell tolerance.[7] It is difficult to study the mechanisms involved in tolerance induction by dendritic cells because isolation and culture conditions already modify the functional phenotype of dendritic cells. Their capacity to induce T-cell tolerance in vivo under nonactivating conditions has been clearly demonstrated.[8] But what induces the switch from a tolerogenic to an immunogenic dendritic cell? Activation of the dendritic cell is the key to understanding their ability to trigger immunity. This activation can be achieved by a number of different molecular events, the most important probably being activation via CD40 ligation and via stimulation of pattern recognition receptors. CD40 ligation on dendritic cells or help from CD4 T cells is critical for induction of strong T-cell immunity by dendritic cells.[9,10] Conserved microbial patterns are recognized by pattern recognition receptors, such as toll-like receptors (TLR) or cytoplasmic pattern recognition receptors, and initiate strong activation of the dendritic cell.[11–13] Such activation is critical to license the dendritic cells to educate T cells for subsequent immune effector function.[14,15]

Upon priming of naïve T cells in lymphatic tissue by appropriately activated dendritic cells, activated antigen-specific T cells undergo clonal expansion and will eventually exit lymphoid tissue for recirculation via the blood stream. T cells that have undergone activation display a migratory pattern distinct from naïve T cells and will patrol peripheral tissues where they exert effector function after antigen-specific stimulation. Given the ubiquitous distribution of immune cells, one would assume that immune reactions occur in similar fashion regardless of anatomic localization. However, a wealth of experimental data rather supports the contrary: immune responses are strongly influenced by the local microenvironment.

Functional Hepatic Anatomy

The liver is optimally structured to function as metabolic organ (i.e., clearance of blood from macromolecules and release of metabolic products from hepatocytes into the blood stream). Blood from the gastrointestinal tract rich in nutrients and in microbial degradation products enters the liver via the portal vein, which drains after extensive ramifications into the so-called portal field composed of one portal venous vessel, one arterial vessel, and a bile duct surrounded by connective tissue. Portal-venous and arterial blood both drain into the hepatic sinusoids, which form a three-dimensional meshwork of vessels generating a mixed arterial-venous perfusion of the liver. This generates a microenvironment with a low oxygen pressure and metabolically active hepatocytes have adapted to this unique situation. It is assumed that the hepatic microenvironment is further characterized by the presence of gut-derived molecules such as microbial degradation products; for example endotoxins.[16,17]

Hepatic Cell Populations: Immune Phenotype and Function
Sinusoidal Cell Populations

Although hepatic sinusoidal cell populations (Kupffer cells, liver sinusoidal endothelial cells [LSEC], and stellate cells) contribute only to 6.3% of total liver volume, they represent approximately 40% of the total number of hepatic cells, 26% of the total membrane surface (mainly LSEC), 58% of total endocytotic vesicles (mainly LSEC), and 43% of the total lysosomal volume (mainly Kupffer cells and LSEC). (**Table 9-1**)[18]

Kupffer Cells

The hepatic macrophage population is named after the scientist Karl Wilhelm von Kupffer. Kupffer cells are located predominantly in the periportal area.[19] They originate from bone marrow as demonstrated by the detection of recipient-derived

Table 9-1 Hepatic Cell Populations

HEPATIC CELL POPULATION	PERCENT OF LIVER VOLUME*	PERCENT OF LIVER CELLS
Kupffer cells	2.1	15
LSEC	2.8	19
Stellate cells	1.4	5-8
Pit cells	n.d.	n.d.
Hepatocytes	78	60

Adapted from Blouin A, Bolender RP, Weibel ER. Distribution of organelles and membranes between hepatocytes and nonhepatocytes in the rat liver parenchyma. A stereological study. J Cell Biol 1977;72:441–455.

*Sinusoidal lumen 10.6%, space of Diss 4.9%.

LSEC, liver sinusoidal endothelial cells; n.d., not determined

macrophages in hepatic allografts.[20] The life span of Kupffer cells appears to be more than 3 months[21]; however, some Kupffer cells have an extremely long life span and are radiation resistant.[22] Under certain conditions proliferation of Kupffer cells is observed and can account for bone marrow independent amplification of Kupffer cells.[23] Depletion of Kupffer cells can be achieved through application of gadolinium chloride or liposome encapsulated chlodronate.[24] Kupffer cell depletion by itself does not lead to liver damage but affects certain hepatic immune functions (see later discussion).

Kupffer cells exert three complex functions: (1) phagocytosis of particulate matter and uptake of macromolecules, (2) presentation of antigen accompanied by immune regulation, and (3) release of soluble mediators. Kupffer cells form together with the liver sinusoidal endothelial cells—the reticulo-endothelial cell system of the liver. It is now recognized that Kupffer cells are not motile and exert their functions as a firmly adherent cell population.[25] They are efficient in phagocytosis of bacteria[25] and uptake of macromolecules via receptor-mediated endocytosis. Elimination of bacterial degradation products such as LPS is to a large extent achieved by Kupffer cells.[26] Kupffer cells further contribute to elimination of tumor cells,[27] apoptotic cellular material,[28] and bacterial degradation products.[29] As Kupffer cells are mainly situated in the periportal area, clearance of blood is achieved soon after entry into the hepatic microcirculation.[30] The localization of Kupffer cells correlates with their function.[31] Periportal Kupffer cells display high phagocytic capacity but low expression levels of MHC class II molecules and low release of mediators. In contrast, Kupffer cells located in the perivenous area show lower phagocytic capacity but express higher levels of MHC class II molecules.[32] Kupffer cells have been shown to be involved in induction of innate as well as pathogen-specific immunity and induction of immune tolerance.

It has been demonstrated that Kupffer cells function as antigen-presenting cells for CD4 T cells by MHC class II restricted antigen-presentation.[33–36] Kupffer cells are endowed with a large number of receptors (**Table 9-2**), which allow them to function as sentinel cells sensing infection. In response to activation, Kupffer cells release soluble mediators, such as IL-1 and IL-6, that trigger hepatocellular expression of acute phase proteins.[37] Further mediators released by Kupffer cells include reactive oxygen species, eicosanoids, cytokines, chemokines, proteinases, NO, and heme oxygenase (**Table 9-3**). The unique hepatic microenvironment, which is rich in bacterial degradation products and gut-derived antigens, appears to shape the immune function of Kupffer cells. Although Kupffer cells resemble macrophage populations in other anatomic sites, there is a clear difference of Kupffer cells with respect to release of soluble mediators after contact with pathogenic microorganisms.[38] As already mentioned, Kupffer cells contribute to clearance of blood-borne endotoxin. Different sets of receptors are involved in clearance and sensing of endotoxin by Kupffer cells. Scavenger receptors are functional in binding and endocytosis of endotoxin, whereas expression of the pattern recognition receptors CD14 and TLR4 in combination with the adaptor protein MD2 contribute to endotoxin-triggered Kupffer cell activation.[29] In contrast to macrophages obtained from the peritoneal cavity, CD14 is not required for Kupffer cell activation by endotoxin.[39] As portal venous blood contains bacterial degradation products,[17] it seems plausible that protective mechanisms have

Table 9-2 Phenotype of Kupffer cells

MOLECULE	FUNCTION	REFERENCE
CD54 (ICAM)	Cell adhesion	60
Fc-receptor	Uptake of pathogens coated with antibodies	34
CD14, TLR4, MD2	Receptors for endotoxin	61
CD11a/CD11b	Cell adhesion	34, 62
CD40	Co-stimulation	63
CD80	Co-stimulation	63, 64
CD86	Co-stimulation	63, 64
MHC-II	Antigen presentation	34
CD1	Antigen presentation	25

Table 9-3 Soluble Mediators Released by Kupffer Cells

MOLECULE	FUNCTION	REFERENCE
Prostanoids	Modulation of immune function	49
IL-1	Inflammation	50
IL-1RA	Blockade of IL-1 activity	51
IL-6	Inflammation	44, 52
IL-10	Antiinflammatory activity	43
IL-12	Induction of IFN-γ, immunity	53
IL-18	Induction of IFN-γ, immunity	54
TNF-α	Inflammation	55
TGF-β_1 and TGF-β_2	Fibrosis, antiinflammatory activity	56, 57
ROI	Effector function, inflammation	58
NO	Effector function, vasorelaxation	59

evolved to prevent inadvertent activation of innate immune reactions while conserving scavenger activity. Along this line, Kupffer cell activity toward endotoxin seems to be restricted. The high hepatic arginase activity, which results in low arginine concentrations locally in the liver, limits Kupffer cell reactivity towards endotoxin.[40] Furthermore, production of reactive oxygen species by Kupffer cells in contrast to macrophages derived from other locations is rather low.[41] In addition, Kupffer cells develop a refractory state after repetitive stimulation with endotoxin. After first contact with endotoxin, the release of soluble mediators such as TNF-α by Kupffer cells is dramatically decreased.[42] At the same time, scavenger activity as determined by increased phagocytosis activity is increased.[42] These results demonstrate that local populations of innate immune cells have adapted their function to physiologic needs. Further mechanisms operate to restrict Kupffer

Table 9-4 Different Populations of NKT Cells

	I	II	III	IV
Repertoire	Va14-Va18 Vb8.2	Va3.2-Ja9/Va8Vb8	Va diverse Vb diverse	Va diverse Vb diverse
Phenotype	CD4+ or DN	CD4+ or DN	CD8+, CD4+ or DN	CD4+ or CD8+
NK receptor	NK1.1	NK1.1+/−	DX5 +/− NK1.1	DX5 NK1.1+/−
Restriction	CD1d	CD1d	MHC I And others	MHC I MHC II
Reactivity	a-GalCer	Not determined	Self-agonist	Not determined

Adapted from Kronenberg M, Gapin L. The unconventional lifestyle of NKT cells. Nat Rev Immunol 2002;2:557–568.
DN, double negative

cell reactivity to endotoxins. Kupffer cells release IL-10 after contact with endotoxins.[43] IL-10 is known to have antiinflammatory effects and expression of IL-10 in Kupffer cells indeed controls reactivity to subsequent endotoxin challenge.[44] Expression of IL-10 thus functions as a negative auto-regulatory feedback loop. It is of interest to note that activation of Kupffer cells is not only achieved by direct contact with microbial products but may occur via the sympathetic nervous system, resulting in fast release of IL-10.[45] There is an increasing wealth of data that suggests contribution of the autonomic nervous system in control of immune responses in the liver. Adrenergic innervation appears to down-regulate inflammatory immune responses in the liver, whereas peptidergic innervation aggravates immune-mediated liver injury.[46]

While inadvertent reactivity of Kupffer cells to inflammatory stimuli appears to be controlled at multiple levels, effector function of Kupffer cells is critically linked to activation via TLR, because inability of Kupffer cells to react to TLR-4 ligands leads to failure to eliminate gram-negative bacteria from the liver.[47] Moreover, Kupffer cells that have phagocytosed bacteria activate invariant NKT cells in a CD1-restricted fashion that is required to achieve complete control of bacterial infection.[25] This establishes an important link of scavenging Kupffer cells with effector NKT cells in the liver in antibacterial immunity.

Kupffer cells may further engage in amplification of cell-mediated immune responses in the liver leading to organ pathology. Such a role has been described for ischemia-reperfusion injury, alcohol-induced liver injury, and neutrophil-induced liver injury. Central to the deleterious function of Kupffer cells is the release of TNF-α, which exerts deleterious affects in the liver via a TNF receptor expressed on parenchymal cells.[48] Clearly, the expression and release of pro-inflammatory mediators in the liver must be controlled in a precise manner to prevent unnecessary damage secondary to immune activation.

NKT Cells

The liver harbors a large number of lymphocytes, which share characteristics of T cells and NK cells. Characteristically, NKT cells express a T-cell receptor and a prototypical NK cell marker of the C type II lectin superfamily (i.e., NK1.1). Most NKT cells express an invariant T-cell receptor, Va14/Ja281 in

the mouse and Va24/JaQ in humans, together with a skewed repertoire of TCR-β chains, Vb8.2 in the mouse and Vb11 in humans.[65] However, NK1.1+ TCR+ cells are heterogeneous and can be classified according to their surface phenotype and their requirement for antigen-specific stimulation (**Table 9-4**).

The classical invariant NKT cells recognize their specific ligands in a CD1d-restricted fashion; the exact molecular structures of these ligands are still under investigation.[66] Most of NKT cells respond to CD1d-restricted presentation of a-GalCer with fast release of soluble mediators. Most NKT cells develop in the thymus; only certain subpopulations appear to originate from other sites.[67] Although the natural ligands for NKT cells are not known and their skewed expression of TCR genes imply a rather narrow ligand specificity of these cells, other ligands have been detected.[68] The distinct properties of glycosphingolipid antigen recognition by iNKT cells further suggests high ligand specificity.[69] In contrast to conventional T cells, NKT cells are more numerous in the liver than in other organs. Mechanistically, expression of CD54 and CD11a are required for homing of NKT cells to the liver.[70,71] Central to recruitment and survival of NKT cells in the liver is the chemokine receptor CXCR6.[72] For survival and expansion of NKT cells in the liver, one single cytokine is most important: IL-15. Interestingly, migration or retention of NKT cells to other organs is independent of CD11a.[71] The hepatic cell population most important for recruitment of NKT cells are NK cells.[73] In turn, Kupffer cells are operative in recruitment of NK cells[74] and dendritic cells[75] to the liver. The molecular mechanisms underlying recruitment of monocytes and hepatic differentiation of monocytes into organ-resident Kupffer cells are still not entirely resolved. After stimulation in vivo, NKT cells undergo a wave of proliferation in the liver, spleen, and bone marrow. Proliferation is accompanied by sustained and vast release of cytokines.

Functionally, NKT contribute to the unique immune regulatory microenvironment of the liver. Depending on the subtype, NKT cells may release large amounts of soluble mediators that influence development of Th1, Th2, or Th17 cells.[65,76] Expression of membrane-bound effector molecules such as FAS-ligand and CD40, as well as release of death-inducing mediators (granzyme B and perforin) from intracellular vesicles, are critical for the effector function of NKT cells in the liver.[76] They operate in functional maturation of dendritic cells and in direct execution of effector function that are important for clearance of bacterial and viral infection.[25,77] NKT cells have also been shown to contribute to antitumor immunity in the liver[78] and support liver regeneration.[79] However, under certain conditions, NKT cells also have deleterious effects as evidenced by their contribution to autoimmunity and development of hepatic fibrosis.[76,80] It is likely that the diverse subpopulations of NKT cells and the liver microenvironment influencing NKT cell function all contribute to modulating local immune responses and are thus responsible for observation of diverse functional phenotypes of NKT cells.

Liver Sinusoidal Endothelial Cells

Liver sinusoidal endothelial cells form a thin but continuous cell layer between leukocytes passing through the liver within the bloodstream and the hepatocytes.[81] In contrast to endothelial cells in other organs, they do not express tight junctions and are not separated from parenchymal tissue by a basement membrane. The space between hepatocytes and LSEC is called the space of Disse, which contains abundant extracellular matrix produced by LSEC and is populated by the stellate cells, which span around the LSEC and control sinusoidal blood flow by contraction—leading to reduction of the sinusoidal diameter.[82] LSEC possess enormous endocytotic capacity. Uptake of macromolecules from the blood is mainly achieved by receptor-mediated endocytosis and not pinocytosis or macropinocytosis in these cells. Via receptor-mediated binding, LSEC immobilize particulate material but are unable to internalize molecules larger than 200 nm in size.[83] The receptors active in endocytotic activity of LSEC and their main ligands are summarized in **Table 9-5**. The wide ligand range of these receptors ensures the effectiveness of LSEC scavenger function.[84] This scavenger function is not observed in endothelial cells from other vascular beds and emphasizes the notion that unique local cell populations define liver function.[84] Scavenged molecules are quickly degraded by LSEC or are transported across the cell to neighboring hepatocytes in a transcytotic fashion.[85,86] The molecular mechanisms determining lysosomal degradation or transcytosis in LSEC have not been identified yet. Scavenger function of LSEC may further be operative in the hepatotropism observed for certain viruses. Uptake of blood-borne viruses by LSEC has been demonstrated for duck hepatitis B virus[87] and for hepatitis C virus.[88] LSEC express receptors for these viruses. In analogy to what has been observed for human immunodeficiency viruses binding to dendritic cells through DC-SIGN,[89] binding of hepatotropic viruses to receptors on scavenger LSEC may target the virus to the liver and eventually lead to infection of hepatocytes in *trans*.

LSEC have pores, so-called fenestrae, approximately 100 to 150 nm in size,[81] which can be dynamically regulated by the actin cytoskeleton upon contact with substances such as alcohol or nicotine.[98] Blood cells passing through the narrow hepatic sinusoids exert a "sinusoidal massage," causing improved exchange of fluid between the sinusoidal lumen and the space of Disse.[81] Flexible macromolecules larger than 100 nm in diameter or rigid macromolecules larger than 12 nm are excluded from access to the space of Dissé via diffusion through fenestrate, resulting in a "sieve" function of LSEC.[81] Larger molecules, such as chylomicrons exceeding 100 nm in size, first have to be metabolized by

Table 9-5 Expression of Receptors Involved in Receptor-Mediated Endocytosis

RECEPTORS EXPRESSED ON LSEC	LIGANDS	REFERENCE
Hyaluronan/ Scavenger receptor	Hyaluronan, oxidized LDL, advanced glycation end products, aminoterminal propeptide of type I and III collagen	90-93
Mannose receptor	Lysosomal enzymes, tissue plasminogen activator, carboxyterminal propeptides, mannose-containing structures	94
Collagen-α chain receptor	Collagen-α chain	95
Fc-receptor (FcgR, FcRn)	Immunoglobulins	96, 97

membrane-associated lipase[99] before they can pass through fenestrae.[100] Interestingly, the infection rate of hepatocytes by blood-borne adenovirus has been demonstrated to depend critically on the diameter of LSEC fenestrae.[101] Alternatively, molecules may gain access to hepatocytes through receptor-mediated uptake by LSEC and subsequent transcytosis (see previous discussion).[102] LSEC constitutively express molecules necessary to establish interaction with passenger leukocytes. Expression levels of CD54 and CD106 are linked to bacterial colonization of the gut supporting the notion that bacterial degradation products derived from the gastrointestinal tract shape the hepatic microenvironment. LSEC further express two molecules that support adhesion of leukocytes (i.e., VAP-1, L-SIGN[103]). These molecules are expressed in the liver on LSEC and in lymphatic tissue. MHC class I and low levels of MHC class II molecules are constitutively expressed together with low levels of costimulatory molecules (CD80, CD86, and CD40).[64]

Liver Dendritic Cells

Dendritic cells are the prototypic antigen-presenting cells of the immune system. Depending on their maturation status—either immature, semimature, or mature—they are considered to shape the immune response either in direction of immune tolerance or immunity.[1,104,105] Dendritic cells are found in the liver under normal steady-state conditions. They are found primarily in the portal tract but are present in lower numbers in the periportal and perivenous area.[106] Being a strongly vascularized organ, immune surveillance of the liver by dendritic cells is different from immune surveillance in other sites such as the skin or the gut. Dendritic cells arrive via the blood stream in the liver and, as a consequence of the slow blood flow within hepatic sinusoids, have the opportunity to interact with sinusoidal lining cells. Within the liver, dendritic cells translocate from hepatic sinusoids to the lymph and finally accumulate in draining celiac lymph nodes.[107] The transition of dendritic cells from the blood stream into adherent cells within the hepatic sinusoid appears to be accompanied by changes in their ultrastructural characteristics, which are suggestive of a maturation step.[108] It is unclear whether changes in dendritic cell ultrastructure are paralleled by functional maturation. However, after transition from the hepatic sinusoid, dendritic cells loose their phagocytic capacity. The preferential accumulation of circulating dendritic cells in the liver implies that these dendritic cells will engage in antigen collection within the liver. Indeed, after translocation from the hepatic sinusoid into the space of Diss, dendritic cells are observed to engage in close physical contact with hepatocytes and stellate cells.[108]

Although the total number of dendritic cells in the liver is high compared with other parenchymal organs, the relative density of dendritic cells within the liver is much lower.[109] However, a fast turnover of dendritic cells may compensate for the lower cell number. As already mentioned, constant recruitment of dendritic cells from the marginating blood pool may result in different migration kinetics of dendritic cells in the tissue. The composition of dendritic cell subtypes in the liver appears to differ from those in other organs like the spleen.[110] The liver bears more plasmacytoid dendritic cells, characterized by CD8a B220+ expression than the spleen. However, it seems difficult to attribute functional capacity to dendritic cells purely on the basis of their phenotypic characteristics. It has become clear that subpopulations of dendritic cells are shaped by external factors and changes in the pattern of surface molecule expression may in fact reflect local influences rather than recruitment of lineage-dependent subpopulations of cells. A number of investigations were performed that yielded extensive information on the phenotype of hepatic dendritic cells.[110–112] A common result is that hepatic dendritic cells are rather immature when compared with dendritic cells from other organs.

In addition to the different distribution of dendritic cell subpopulation, hepatic dendritic cells show distinct immune-regulatory features.[111] Dendritic cells isolated from the liver show a reduced capacity to prime naïve allogeneic T cells compared with dendritic cells isolated from bone marrow. T cells primed by hepatic dendritic cells do not develop strong cytotoxic effector function.[113] Furthermore, adoptive transfer of these in vitro propagated hepatic dendritic cells leads to increased expression of IL-10 in lymphatic tissue.[113] Similar results were obtained by a number of other investigators.[110,112,114] Using a new technique to obtain dendritic cells from a human liver, it was possible to investigate the immune function of hepatic dendritic cells. Human hepatic dendritic cells were less effective in stimulating T cells compared with dendritic cells isolated from the skin. Moreover, hepatic dendritic cells expressed significant amounts of IL-10, a cytokine known to mediate potent antiinflammatory action.[115] T cells primed by hepatic dendritic cells release IL-10 and IL-4 but not IFN-γ, which is suggestive of their ability for induction of regulatory T cells. Because dendritic cells derived from other organs show different functional features, it is likely that dendritic cells entering the liver were modified by the microenvironment. Increasing the numbers of dendritic cells and NK cells by injection of flt3-ligand leads to modification of intrahepatic immune regulation. Liver transplants are typically well tolerated in rodent models of allotransplantation. However, if livers from flt3-ligand treated animals were transplanted,

increased transplant rejection was observed, which suggests that flt3 ligand-induced changes in hepatic cell populations tips the balance from a tolerogenic to an immunogenic milieu.[116]

Another important difference of hepatic dendritic cells is their low expression of TLR4. Stimulation of hepatic dendritic cells with low concentrations of endotoxins does not lead to strong activation and induction of a mature phenotype but rather results in reduced capacity to induce T-cell priming and proliferation as compared with dendritic cells isolated from the spleen.[117] Moreover, activation of NOD2—a cytoplasmic pattern recognition receptor—negatively regulates the stimulatory function of hepatic dendritic cells,[118] indicating that NOD2 plays a unique role in regulating innate and adaptive immunity in the liver. Given the continuous presence of bacterial degradation products in portal venous blood, it seems important to prevent inadvertent immune activation locally in the liver.

Dendritic cells in diseased liver are mainly found in the portal tract. Hepatic expression of the chemokine CCL21 stimulates increased recruitment of CCR7+ immune cells to the portal tract that resembles tertiary lymphoid tissue.[119] CCL21 recruits naïve T cells and dendritic cells, which both bear CCR7+, and thus promotes strong local interaction between these cell populations[120] similar to the role of CCR7 for recruitment of immune cells to lymphatic tissue.[121] So far, little is known on the ability of migratory hepatic dendritic cells to stimulate T cells in the draining lymph node. It is interesting to note that the composition of subpopulations of dendritic cells in the hepatic draining lymph node does not reflect the subpopulation composition in the liver.[122] In particular, dendritic cells in the draining hepatic lymph node had an activated mature phenotype and only a few cells had the surface phenotype characteristic of plasmacytoid dendritic cells.[122]

Stellate Cells

Stellate cells are located in the space of Diss between LSEC and hepatocytes. Stellate cells store 80% of retinoids in the whole body as retinyl palmitate within cytoplasmic vesicles. Following hepatic injury, stellate cells transdifferentiate into cells similar to myofibroblasts with a profibrogenic phenotype depositing large amounts of extracellular matrix.[123] They are further involved in regulating intrahepatic vascular resistance in response to a number of vasoactive substances.[124] Although stellate cells do not have direct contact with passenger leukocytes in the sinusoid, they release a number of mediators that are of importance for local immune control. Several chemokines, such as MCP-1, MIP-2, and IL-8, are produced by stellate cells upon activation by proinflammatory cytokines.[125] However, under resting conditions, few if any chemokines are expressed by these cells, suggesting that they contribute only in inflammatory situations to the recruitment of leukocytes from the blood into the hepatic parenchyma. In addition to their important scaffolding function, stellate cells have the capacity to take up antigens by fluid-phase endocytosis, receptor-mediated endocytosis, and phagocytosis.[126] They further express low levels of MHC class I and II molecules and costimulatory molecules (CD80 and CD40), which are further increased following incubation with proinflammatory mediators (**Table 9-6**). Whereas resting stellate

Table 9-6 Immune Phenotype of Stellate Cells

SURFACE MOLECULE	EXPRESSED IN RESTING/ACTIVATED STELLATE CELLS	REFERENCE
CD54 (ICAM-1)	– / +	129, 133
CD106 (VCAM-1)	– / +	129, 134
CD40	(+) / +	126
CD80	– / +	126
MHC class I	+ / ++	126
MHC class I	(+) / +	126
NCAM	+ / ++	135
CD1	+	127

cells fail to engage in cognate interaction with naïve T cells, cytokine-stimulated stellate cells support proliferation of CD4 T cells in a mixed lymphocyte reaction.[126] Stellate cells also function as antigen-presenting cells for T cells and for NKT cells.[127] This provides a very interesting and potentially important connection between immune responses and induction of fibrosis.[128]

Similar to Kupffer cells and LSEC, stellate cells express TLR4 and are thus responsive to stimulation by endotoxins, leading to release of chemokines.[129] However, upon activation stellate cells also release potent antiinflammatory mediators. Stellate cells treated in vitro with TNF or endotoxin or isolated from animals after bile duct ligation demonstrated a prominent increase in IL-10 release.[130] Moreover, stellate cell activation results in expression of transforming growth factor-β (TGF-β), one of the most potent antiinflammatory cytokines.[56] Latent TGF-β binding protein, expressed by trans-differentiating stellate cells, serves as a matrix to anchor latent TGF-β in hepatic tissue. Release of bioactive TGF-β then requires proteolytic cleavage of the binding protein.[131] TLR4-mediated stimulation of stellate cells leads to MyD88-dependent down-regulation of a TGF-β pseudoreceptor, thus rendering stellate cells more susceptible to TGF-β driven fibrosis.[132]

Hepatocytes

Hepatocytes constitute the vast majority of hepatic cells. They are situated behind a physical barrier constituted by LSEC and stellate cells. However, a large body of evidence suggests that hepatocytes have direct access to molecules contained in portal venous blood and to passenger leukocytes in the hepatic sinusoid. In a normal liver, hepatocytes express few MHC I molecules and are negative for MHC II. Other molecules relevant for interaction with T cells are either not expressed or expressed at very low levels (e.g., CD54, co-stimulatory molecules such as CD80 and CD86). The main function of hepatocytes is metabolism. Consequently, enormous amounts of molecules are generated within hepatocytes and subsequently released into serum or bile. Degradation of waste or toxic products occurs as well in hepatocytes and gives rise to modifications in the structure of protein antigens released by hepatocytes. Furthermore, hepatocytes metabolize nutrients,

which are extracted from portal venous blood. Given the huge metabolic function of hepatocytes, it seems plausible that mechanisms have evolved to protect these cells from an inadvertent immune attack. A detailed description of the metabolic function of hepatocytes is provided in the other chapters.

Characteristics of Blood Flow and Leukocyte–Liver Cell Interaction in the Liver

The liver holds a unique position with regard to blood circulation. It receives venous blood draining from almost the entire gastrointestinal tract via the portal vein and from the systemic circulation via the hepatic artery. More than 2000 liters of blood stream daily through the human liver. Even with an average circulation time of 1 hour, peripheral blood leukocytes pass through the liver more than 12 times per day. These simple facts clearly demonstrate that the liver is a "meeting point" for antigens and leukocytes circulating in the blood. Hepatic sinusoids are narrow channels with an average diameter ranging from 7 to 12 μm. Leukocytes, bearing a mean diameter of 10 to 12 μm, have to force their way through the sinusoidal meshwork in the liver.[136] Moreover, blood flow in the liver is slow due to low-pressure perfusion.

Interaction between passenger cells flowing through hepatic sinusoids and the sinusoidal cell populations is facilitated by these physical conditions.[137] Expression of selectins by endothelial cells is typically required to engage in interaction with leukocytes in the blood stream. Hepatic sinusoidal cell populations express little if any CD62E (E-selectin),[138] which is most instrumental in recruitment of leukocytes to endothelial cells. Despite the absence of CD62E, recruitment of leukocytes to sinusoidal cells can be observed even under inflammatory conditions.[139] Sinusoidal lining LSEC express other molecules that mediate interaction with passenger leukocytes, notably L-SIGN[140] and VAP-1.[103] Under noninflammatory conditions, naïve CD8 T cells can establish adhesion within the liver in an antigen-specific fashion,[141,142] which constitutes the first step in liver-specific immune regulation. Under inflammatory conditions, CD4 T helper cells use distinct molecular mechanisms for adhesion in the liver: Th1 cells use a_4b_1-integrin, whereas TH2 cells use VAP-1.[143] Thus T cells are not passively trapped in the liver by simple physical means but are actively recruited depending on expression of well-characterized molecular signals.

Immune Functions of the Liver

Immune Tolerance in the Liver

Among the many functions of the liver, clearance of the blood from macromolecules and its metabolization are important for the understanding of the liver as an immune-regulatory organ. Nutrients have to be extracted from portal venous blood and further used for hepatocellular metabolism, but at the same time the liver must eliminate toxic waste products and proinflammatory agents, such as endotoxins or other bacterial degradation products derived by translocation from the gut, or from blood without eliciting an immune response to all these antigens. Induction of immune tolerance in the liver has been reported already in 1967 by Cantor et al. and in 1969 by Calne et al.[144,145] and since then by many other groups. Three main points demonstrate the ability of the liver to induce antigen-specific immune tolerance: (1) Liver transplants are accepted by the recipients immune system despite MHC discrepancy and even in the absence of immune suppression.[144,145] (2) Simultaneous transplantation of the liver and another organ from the same donor leads to increased graft acceptance of the co-transplanted organ. Further organ-transplants from another donor led to graft rejection, demonstrating antigen-specific induction of immune tolerance by the transplanted liver.[146] (3) Drainage of an organ-transplant directly into the portal vein or direct application of donor cells into the portal vein led to increased acceptance of the graft.[147-150] Although for a long time, antigen-specific induction of immune tolerance in the liver was observed in the context of organ transplantation, it is clear from the physiologic function of the liver that immune tolerance needs to be established equally for circulating antigens. While the mechanisms involved in tolerance induction do not necessarily need to be different for antigens produced or taken up by hepatic cell populations, it is evident that immune tolerance toward circulating antigens requires the participation of cells conveying this specific information (i.e., antigen-presenting cells).

The Hepatic Microenvironment

Constitutive exposure to gut-derived bacterial degradation products in portal venous blood contributes to the unique hepatic microenvironment.[16,17] Endotoxins induce release not only of proinflammatory mediators from hepatic sinusoidal cell populations but at the same time lead to expression of a number of potent antiinflammatory, immune-suppressive mediators, such as IL-10,[43] TGF-β,[56] and certain prostanoids such as PGE$_2$.[151,152] This creates a local environment that suppresses rather than stimulates immune responses in the liver. IL-10, TGF-β, or PGE$_2$ are known to "educate" antigen-presenting cells such as dendritic cells and to induce a tolerogenic phenotype. Dendritic cells exposed to these mediators fail to induce immunity but rather support induction of tolerant T cells.[153] Moreover, the liver is rich in arginase, which metabolizes the essential amino acid arginine and thus deprives T cells of this critical growth factor. Depletion of arginine may contribute to the inability of the immune system to eliminate HBV infection.[154] However, it is difficult to separate the influence of specific hepatic antigen-presenting cell populations and the hepatic microenvironment on induction of immune tolerance from each other, as the microenvironment certainly has a role in shaping the functional phenotype of hepatic antigen-presenting cell populations.

Induction of T-Cell Tolerance by Antigen-Presenting Cells in the Liver

Different hepatic antigen-presenting cell populations contribute to antigen-specific induction of tolerance in T cells.[155] While the relevance of each of the antigen-presenting cell population has been described separately, more than one antigen-presenting cell population may be involved in tolerance induction in the liver. In fact, a number of determinants, such as origin of antigen and quantity of antigen, may strengthen or diminish the contribution of individual antigen-presenting cell populations for tolerance induction (see later discussion).

Hepatocytes

Hepatocytes can serve as antigen-presenting cells and induce stimulation of naïve CD8 T cells in a transgenic mouse setting, where hepatocytes express a transgenic MHC I molecule that is recognized together with an endogenous peptide. Although antigen-specific stimulation of T cells by hepatocytes even in the absence of co-stimulatory molecules CD80 and CD86 is rather effective during the first 3 days, T cells undergo apoptosis at later time points. Rather B7H1 expression, a member of the family of co-inhibitory molecules, is relevant for T-cell priming by hepatocytes.[156] Interestingly, previously activated T cells facilitate T-cell priming by hepatocytes,[157] which strengthens the notion that development of hepatic immune responses have to be viewed in the context of other ongoing immune reactions. Thus clonal elimination of T cells is involved in mediation of hepatic T-cell tolerance. As interaction with passenger T cells and antigen-presenting hepatocytes occurs even in the absence of local inflammation in the transgenic mouse model described above, hepatocytes may continuously contribute to shaping of the immune response.[158] The proapototic factor bim has been shown to be involved in hepatocyte-induced clonal elimination of T cells.[159,160] Taken together, hepatocytes play an important part in shaping the repertoire of T cells. However, as hepatocytes do not have the capacity to cross-present exogenous antigens on MHC I to CD8 T cells, tolerance induction by hepatocytes is limited to proteins expressed by hepatocytes and does not extend to antigens circulating with the bloodstream. Besides clonal elimination, hepatocytes also induce regulatory T cells, which are an important regulator of peripheral immune tolerance. It was found that hepatocyte-restricted expression of an antigen leads to induction and expansion of antigen-specific regulatory T cells that prevented induction of autoimmunity in the central nervous system (CNS).[161] This important finding also demonstrates that liver-specific immune regulation has a significant impact on extrahepatic immune responses.

Liver Dendritic Cells and Kupffer Cells

As already described previously, immature hepatic dendritic cells contribute to the induction of T-cell tolerance. Hepatic dendritic cells may either be involved directly in induction of T-cell tolerance by virtue of their tolerogenic phenotype, which may result from different subpopulations of dendritic cells being present, or from the influence of the local microenvironment.[110-112,114,115,117,162] On the other hand, dendritic cells may indirectly contribute to hepatic immune tolerance by release of soluble mediators or induction of regulatory T cells. Release of type I IFN from dendritic cells attenuates liver injury[163] and promotes at the same time induction of regulatory T cells.[164] It is of interest to note that liver dendritic cells do not functionally mature and induce T-cell immunity even after activation through pattern recognition receptors.[117,118] The molecular mechanisms determining this unique reaction pattern of liver dendritic cells has not been entirely resolved. Activated CD8 T cells are found to undergo apoptosis in the liver.[165] The trapping of CD8 T cells may occur antigen-specifically or through CD54/CD106-dependent mechanisms.[166-168] Using bone marrow chimeric animals, it was possible to demonstrate that antigen-specific recruitment of CD8 T cells was achieved by nonmyeloid organ-resident cells, whereas elimination of CD8 T cells occurred through a bone marrow dependent cell population.[166] In addition to liver dendritic cells, Kupffer cells also contribute to hepatic T-cell tolerance. Kupffer cells did not only express lower levels of MHC molecules and co-stimulatory molecules rendering them a poorly immune stimulator, but also suppressed dendritic cell–mediated T-cell activation through release of immune regulatory prostanoids.[169] Thus, bone marrow derived but liver-resident APC promote induction of immune tolerance rather than immunity.

Liver Sinusoidal Endothelial Cells

Similar to dendritic cells, LSEC bear the capacity to prime CD4$^+$ T cells (i.e., stimulation of cytokine release from naïve CD4$^+$ T cells that have not encountered their specific antigen before).[170] While dendritic cells require maturation and signals from the highly specialized lymphatic microenvironment to function as potent APC for naïve CD4$^+$ T cells,[171] LSEC do not require maturation or migration into lymphatic tissue to gain APC function.

This function of LSEC as sessile, organ-specific, and constitutively active antigen-presenting cell is not shared by endothelial cells from other organs. Microvascular endothelial cells from the skin or the gut are unable to act as antigen-presenting cells for naïve CD4$^+$ T cells unless stimulated with proinflammatory cytokines such as IFNg.[172-174] In contrast to antigen presentation by dendritic cells, however, CD4$^+$ T cells stimulated by antigen-presenting LSEC fail to differentiate into effector Th1 CD4$^+$ T cells but rather gain an immune-regulatory phenotype.[170] CD4$^+$ T cells primed by LSEC release large amounts of IL-4 and IL-10 following triggering via the T-cell receptor,[170] which efficiently down-regulate ongoing T-cell mediated immune responses (P. Knolle, unpublished results). Thus antigen presentation by LSEC to naïve CD4$^+$ T cells may rather down-regulate Th1 type of cell-mediated immune responses and at the same time stimulate Th2 type of immune responses, leading to increased production of antibodies. Indeed, ineffective cell-mediated immune responses despite the presence of efficient antibody responses are observed during persistent infection of the liver with noncytopathic viruses.[175]

Endothelial cells from other sites equally fail to lead to development of fully differentiated effector Th1 CD4$^+$ T cells.[174,176] It is important to note that these endothelial cells lack the capacity to actively engage in immune modulation as either endothelial cells or T cells have to be prestimulated to observe functional interaction, thus requiring other cell populations that drive the developing immune response. Together with the observation that intraportal injection of antigen leads to development of T cells, which release IL-4 and IL-10 upon restimulation,[177] it can be assumed that LSEC rather than endothelial cells in other organs are involved in tolerance induction to intraportally applied antigens.

Cytotoxic C8$^+$ T cells are of crucial importance for successful immune response against infection with intracellular pathogens and against development of cancer cells. Presentation of antigen on MHC class I molecules to CD8$^+$ T cells was believed to be restricted to those antigens synthesized de novo within the same cell. Although this allows for immune surveillance of parenchymal cells by CD8$^+$ T cells, it is difficult to envisage how professional antigen presenting cells, not

infected by the pathogenic microorganism or not transformed into a neoplastic cell, could induce in the first place a protective and efficient CD8$^+$ T-cell–mediated immune response. Thus presentation of exogenous antigens on MHC class I molecules (termed cross-presentation) obviously is required. Initially identified by Bevan et al.,[178] it was recently demonstrated that cross-presentation occurs in bone marrow–derived antigen-presenting cells, such as dendritic cells and macrophages, and in some instances in B cells.[179,180] Cross-presentation by dendritic cells was shown to be necessary to mount an efficient CD8$^+$ T-cell–mediated immune response against virus infection, although not infections by all viruses appear to require cross-presentation by myeloid APC for induction of immunity.[181]

It is therefore surprising to find that LSEC can efficiently cross-present exogenous antigens on MHC class I molecules to CD8$^+$ T cells.[182] Cross-presentation by LSEC is characterized by a number of features: efficient uptake of an antigen by receptor-mediated endocytosis, shuttling of an antigen from an endosome to cytosol for proteasomal degradation, TAP-dependent loading of processed peptides on de novo synthesized MHC class I molecules in the ER, and transport to the cell surface.[182] LSEC are more efficient in antigen uptake and cross-presentation than professional antigen-presenting cells.[183] LSEC not only cross-present antigen to armed effector CD8$^+$ T cells but have in fact the capacity to stimulate naïve CD8$^+$ T cells.[182] Following an encounter with cross-presenting LSEC, naïve CD8$^+$ T cells release cytokines and start proliferation in vitro. However, antigen-specific restimulation of these T cells revealed that they lost the ability to express effector cytokines, such as IL-2 and IFN-γ and that they lost their cytotoxic activity.[182] In vivo it has been demonstrated that LSEC cross-present antigen to naïve CD8$^+$ T cells outside the lymphatic system. So far, stimulation of naïve T cells was believed to occur exclusively in the highly specialized lymphatic microenvironment.

Following stimulation by cross-presenting LSEC, naïve CD8$^+$ T cells start to proliferate locally in the liver. However, the outcome of cross-presentation by LSEC in vivo is the induction of systemic immune tolerance. Similar to CD8$^+$ T cells stimulated by cross-presenting LSEC in vitro, CD8$^+$ T cells in vivo loose the capacity to express effector cytokines and to exert cytotoxic activity against their specific target antigens once stimulated by cross-presenting LSEC.[182] Deletion of antigen-specific CD8$^+$ T cells occurs to some extent but is not the main mechanism of immune tolerance induced by LSEC. Expression of the coinhibitory molecule B7H1 is essential and required for LSEC-induced T-cell tolerance.[184] Taken together, LSEC are the prototypic liver-resident APC with immune regulatory function.

Induction of Immunity in the Liver

The widespread distribution of pattern recognition receptors on the various immune cell populations of the liver attributes a strong capacity to induce innate immune reactions.[185,186] Thus antiinfective immunity appears to rely to a large extent on direct recognition of the pathogen and immediate elimination using rapidly acting immune effector mechanisms by innate immune cells. However, antigen-specific immunity needs to accompany initial innate immunity to achieve elimination of the pathogen.

For elimination of bacteria, phagocytic uptake through Kupffer cells is not sufficient; it requires recruitment of neutrophils.[187] It has been shown that platelets activated directly through TLR4 bind efficiently to neutrophils trapped in the hepatic sinusoid. This led to robust activation of neutrophils and formation of neutrophil extracellular traps, which ensnared bacteria within the sinusoidal vasculature.[188] CD1d-restricted NKT cells recognize bacterial antigens on antigen-presenting cells that have ingested infectious microorganisms and that release mediators promoting pathogen-specific immune responses.[189] Along this line, Kupffer cells also instruct NKT cells by CD1-restricted antigen presentation after phagocytosis of bacteria and thereby trigger pathogen-specific immunity.[25] Furthermore, hepatic dendritic cells interact with NKT cells to elicit sustained release of mediators promoting development of specific T-cell immunity.[190] Taken together, Kupffer cells and NKT cells play an important role in local generation of antiinfectious immunity in the liver.

Liver dendritic cells fail to functionally mature in response to activation of pattern-recognition receptors[117,118] and therefore appear to be incapable of eliciting adaptive immunity in conventional T cells. It is likely, however, that dendritic cells that were recently recruited to the liver as a consequence of increased chemokine expression by liver-resident cell populations bear immunogenic properties. Complex signaling involving chemokines and cytokines between sinusoidal cell populations and passenger leukocytes leading to hepatic recruitment of immune cells are operative in protective immune responses against viruses infecting the liver.[191,192] IL-12 released from pathogen-activated dendritic cells is sufficient to activate NKT cells in the vicinity for sustained release of soluble mediators.[193] CD1d-restricted NKT cells recognize lipid autoantigens[194] and function in a HBV-specific immunity.[77] Skewing of the microenvironment toward inflammation by local release of mediators from dendritic cells or Kupffer cells such as IL-12 may represent a pivotal point determining whether immune tolerance is locally maintained or whether immunity is induced.[193] On the other hand, interaction of dendritic cells with distinct CD1 reactive T cells leads to maturation of dendritic cells and may therefore contribute to early polarization of the immune response into immunity rather than immune tolerance.[194] LSEC, which are prototypic tolerogenic APC, also fail to functionally mature after isolated activation of pattern recognition receptors.[195] After viral infection, however, these cells gained full immune stimulatory function and induced strong CD8 T-cell immunity even in the absence of known co-stimulatory molecule expression.[195] These observations support the notion that local induction of T-cell immunity by liver-resident APC is possible in situations of true infections.

Concept of Organ-Resident Antigen-Presenting Cells (APC) in the Liver

The liver harbors a number of organ-resident cell populations that bear unique immune functions and thus critically influence immune responses. To establish organ-specific control of immune responses, local presentation of antigen by resident immune regulatory APC bears a number of advantages.

1. Dendritic cells take up antigen in the peripheral organs and following appropriate stimuli migrate to draining lymph nodes. During this journey they undergo functional maturation, rendering them potent APC once they arrive in the highly specialized and structured microenvironment of lymphatic organs. In contrast, liver-resident APC do not migrate and continuously interact with immune cells, thus achieving induction of immune responses within a short time frame.

2. Continuous culture of T cells or professional APC such as dendritic cells with immune suppressive mediators, such as IL-10 or TGF-β in vitro, gives rise to APC that induce T-cell tolerance rather than immunity.[196,197] Situated in the hepatic sinusoid, liver-resident APC are continuously exposed to the unique hepatic microenvironment, which is especially rich in immune suppressive mediators. Incorporation of signals from an organ-specific microenvironment is clearly more prominent in liver-resident than in conventional migratory APC, which stay only for short time periods in peripheral organs before migration into lymphatic tissue. The unique hepatic microenvironment may thus gain considerable influence on the way immune responses are modulated by liver-resident APC.

3. The various liver-resident cell populations cooperate in the modulation of local immune responses in a complex fashion. First, hepatocytes present antigens that are endogenously expressed in these cells, thus allowing development of immune tolerance against auto-antigens. Liver-resident APC capable of cross-presentation modulate immune responses against antigens that they have endocytosed (i.e., antigens secreted from hepatocytes or circulating within the blood stream). This allows them to locally establish immune tolerance toward a broad spectrum of antigens. Second, distinct expression of pattern recognition receptors on the various liver-resident APC allows the liver to sense infection in a complex fashion and to generate well-coordinated antiinfectious immunity. The unique responsiveness of liver-resident APC to functional maturation after activation through pattern-recognition receptors or infection allows detection of true infection of the liver, which is accompanied by induction of strong innate and adaptive immunity. At the same time, clearance of portal venous blood from bacterial degradation products and induction of the hepatic acute phase response, which constitute important physiologic functions of the liver, occurs without the induction of local immunity and thereby avoids the danger of causing autoimmunity or bystander damage.

Role of the Liver in Systemic Immune Surveillance

During viral hepatitis or autoimmune hepatitis, the liver becomes the target for immune responses generated in lymphatic tissue. However, the liver also actively contributes to modulation of immune responses. Such an active role of liver-shaping local and systemic immune responses involve both induction of immune tolerance[158,161,182] and induction of immunity.[198] Antigens and pathogens are not contained entirely by local immune cell populations in the skin or the gut. Following ingestion of antigens via the oral route, this antigen can be found within minutes in the systemic circulation and within a few hours, antigen-specific systemic activation of T cells is detected.[5] Within minutes after application of antigens to the skin, these antigens can be found in the liver, where they lead to induction of cytokine release from local hepatic cell populations.[198] The fact that antigens and pathogens overcome physical barriers and the hurdles of local immune surveillance operative at external body surfaces together with their rapid systemic dissemination necessitates a role of the liver in containment of immune responses toward these antigens.

The clearance function of the liver, which is mainly achieved by Kupffer cells and LSEC, is important to limit systemic dissemination of pathogens and antigens. The largest source of environmental antigens and commensal microorganisms is the gut and subsequently portal venous blood draining from the gastrointestinal tract into the liver. Within the liver, the immune system has to discriminate between nutrient or innocuous antigens and (potentially) pathogenic microorganisms. As hepatic antigen-presenting cells (i.e., Kupffer cells, dendritic cells, stellate cells, LSEC) take up antigens and present them to the immune system, it is unlikely that maintenance of a tolerant state toward blood-borne antigens is simply achieved by ignorance of the immune system toward these antigens. It rather seems that T cells with specificity for antigens presented locally in the liver are actively tolerized by hepatic antigen-presenting cells. Hepatic dendritic cells show considerable plasticity as they are activated upon encounter with microorganisms and subsequently induce pathogen-specific T-cell immunity.[199] Liver-resident APC may thus constitute a functional framework of local antigen-presenting cells, where local cell populations induce tolerance toward soluble blood-borne antigens in the absence of inflammatory signals. However, only hepatic dendritic cells upon sensing of "danger" or LSEC upon true viral infection will contribute to induction of specific T-cell immunity.

Antigen presentation by hepatic antigen-presenting cells has not only consequences for local control of immune responses in the liver, but even influences systemic immunity. Induction of antigen-specific T-cell tolerance by LSEC leads to outgrowth of tumor cells expressing the antigen initially presented by LSEC to T cells.[182] Adoptive transfer of hepatic dendritic cells equally modulates systemic immune responses rather favoring Th2 type of immune responses.[113,117] But it is not only the type and the functional status of the antigen-presenting cell itself that determines the outcome of immune responses. The decision to mount immunity or tolerance toward an antigen appears to depend on the anatomic localization where the antigen is first encountered by the immune system. The first encounter with the antigen in the liver leads to induction of specific T-cell tolerance, whereas first encounter in lymphatic tissue gives rise to strong immunity.[200] If the antigen is sequentially encountered first in lymphatic tissue and then in the liver, T cells are not tolerized but they mediate strong immunity, leading to hepatic tissue damage.[200] Similar observations were made if the antigen was selectively expressed in hepatocytes.[161] It is intriguing to speculate that such mechanisms may be operative in the immune-pathogenesis of persistent infection of the liver with viruses that show a strong hepato-tropism and therefore fail to be presented to the immune system first in lymphatic tissue. However, so far there are no definitive experimental data supporting the notion that local hepatic immune control is responsible for deviating immune responses toward

infectious microorganisms or hematogenously metastasizing tumor cells.

The liver appears not only to promote tolerance towards soluble antigens but under certain conditions even promotes local immunity at peripheral sites. Using a model of skin contact sensitivity it was demonstrated that the liver is involved to mediate recruitment of antigen-specific T cells to the site of initial antigen exposure (i.e., the skin). Minutes after application to the skin, antigen is found to stimulate NKT cells in the liver to release IL-4, which in turn stimulates peritoneal B-1 B cells to express IgM antibodies.[198] Circulating IgM antibodies form complexes with the antigen at the site of initial antigen application and trigger local complement activation and release of vasoactive mediators that finally lead to T-cell recruitment.[201] This example nicely illustrates the extraordinary position of the liver in scavenging antigens from the systemic circulation and its function as a sentinel organ to detect presence of foreign antigens. Central to this complex sentinel function is the concomitant presence of scavenger activity and sufficient numbers of lymphocytes that can engage in cognate interaction with local scavenger cells.

In conclusion, the liver not only serves as a target for the immune response during infection with microorganisms but is also involved constantly in modulation of local and systemic immune responses toward autoantigens and blood-borne antigens. Central to local and systemic modulation of immune responses is the scavenger activity of the various liver-resident APC populations in combination with their unique functional immune phenotype that is shaped by the hepatic microenvironment.

Key References

Ahmad N, et al. Regulation of cyclooxygenase-2 by nitric oxide in activated hepatic macrophages during acute endotoxemia. J Leukoc Biol 2002;71:1005–1011. (Ref.59)

Albert ML, Jegathesan M, Darnell RB. Dendritic cell maturation is required for the cross-tolerization of CD8+ T cells. Nat Immunol 2001;2:1010–1017. (Ref.9)

Allan RS, et al. Epidermal viral immunity induced by CD8alpha+ dendritic cells but not by Langerhans cells. Science 2003;301:1925–1928. (Ref.4)

Askenase PW, et al. Extravascular T-cell recruitment requires initiation begun by Valpha14+ NKT cells and B-1 B cells. Trends Immunol 2004;25:441–449. (Ref.201)

Baron JL, et al. Activation of a nonclassical NKT cell subset in a transgenic mouse model of hepatitis B virus infection. Immunity 2002;16:583–594. (Ref.77)

Bashirova AA, et al. A dendritic cell-specific intercellular adhesion molecule 3-grabbing nonintegrin (DC-SIGN)-related protein is highly expressed on human liver sinusoidal endothelial cells and promotes HIV-1 infection. J Exp Med 2001;193:671–678. (Ref.140)

Bertolino P, et al. Antigen-specific primary activation of CD8+ T cells within the liver. J Immunol 2001;166:5430–5438. (Ref.158)

Bertolino P, et al. Early intrahepatic antigen-specific retention of naive CD8+ T cells is predominantly ICAM-1/LFA-1 dependent in mice. Hepatology 2005;42:1063–1071. (Ref.141)

Bonder CS, et al. Rules of recruitment for Th1 and Th2 lymphocytes in inflamed liver: a role for alpha-4 integrin and vascular adhesion protein-1. Immunity 2005;23:153–163. (Ref.143)

Bowen DG, et al. The site of primary T cell activation is a determinant of the balance between intrahepatic tolerance and immunity. J Clin Invest 2004;114:701–712. (Ref.200)

Breiner K, Schaller H, Knolle P. Endothelial cell-mediated uptake of a hepatitis B virus: a new concept of liver-targeting of hepatotropic micro-organisms. Hepatology 2001;34:803–808. (Ref.87)

Breitkopf K, et al. Expression and matrix deposition of latent transforming growth factor beta binding proteins in normal and fibrotic rat liver and transdifferentiating hepatic stellate cells in culture. Hepatology 2001;33: 387–396. (Ref.131)

Brigl M, et al. Mechanism of CD1d-restricted natural killer T cell activation during microbial infection. Nat Immunol 2003;4:1230–1237. (Ref.193)

Bykov I, et al. Phagocytosis and LPS-stimulated production of cytokines and prostaglandin E2 is different in Kupffer cells isolated from the periportal or perivenous liver region. Scand J Gastroenterol 2003;38:1256–1261. (Ref.30)

Campos RA, et al. Cutaneous immunization rapidly activates liver invariant Valpha14 NKT cells stimulating B-1 B cells to initiate T cell recruitment for elicitation of contact sensitivity. J Exp Med 2003;198:1785–1796. (Ref.198)

Castellaneta A, et al. NOD2 ligation subverts IFN-alpha production by liver plasmacytoid dendritic cells and inhibits their T cell allostimulatory activity via B7-H1 up-regulation. J Immunol 2009;183:6922–6932. (Ref.118)

Clark SR, et al. Platelet TLR4 activates neutrophil extracellular traps to ensnare bacteria in septic blood. Nat Med 2007;13:463–469. (Ref.188)

Cormier EG, et al. L-SIGN (CD209L) and DC-SIGN (CD209) mediate transinfection of liver cells by hepatitis C virus. Proc Natl Acad Sci U S A 2004;101:14067–14072. (Ref.88)

Crispe IN. Hepatic T cells and liver tolerance. Nat Rev Immunol 2003;3: 51–62. (Ref.155)

Das A, et al. Functional skewing of the global CD8 T cell population in chronic hepatitis B virus infection. J Exp Med 2008;205:2111–2124. (Ref.154)

De Creus A, et al. Low TLR4 expression by liver dendritic cells correlates with reduced capacity to activate allogeneic T cells in response to endotoxin. J Immunol 2005;174:2037–2045. (Ref.117)

Diehl L, et al. Tolerogenic maturation of liver sinusoidal endothelial cells promotes B7-homolog 1-dependent CD8+ T cell tolerance. Hepatology 2008;47:296–305. (Ref.184)

Dikopoulos N, et al. Type I IFN negatively regulates CD8+ T cell responses through IL-10-producing CD4+ T regulatory 1 cells. J Immunol 2005;174: 99–109. (Ref.164)

Dikopoulos N, et al. Recently primed CD8+ T cells entering the liver induce hepatocytes to interact with naive CD8+ T cells in the mouse. Hepatology 2004;39:1256–1266. (Ref.157)

Emoto M, Kaufmann SH. Liver NKT cells: an account of heterogeneity. Trends Immunol 2003;24:364–369. (Ref.67)

Emoto M, et al. Participation of leukocyte function-associated antigen-1 and NK cells in the homing of thymic CD8+NKT cells to the liver. Eur J Immunol 2000;30:3049–3056. (Ref.73)

Fischer K, et al. Mycobacterial phosphatidylinositol mannoside is a natural antigen for CD1d-restricted T cells. Proc Natl Acad Sci U S A 2004;101: 10685–10690. (Ref.189)

Gao B, Jeong WI, Tian Z. Liver: an organ with predominant innate immunity. Hepatology 2008;47:729–736. (Ref.186)

Geijtenbeek TB, et al. DC-SIGN, a dendritic cell-specific HIV-1-binding protein that enhances trans-infection of T cells. Cell 2000;100:587–597. (Ref.89)

Geissmann F, et al. Intravascular immune surveillance by CXCR6+ NKT cells patrolling liver sinusoids. PLoS Biol 2005;3:e113. (Ref.72)

Goddard S, et al. Interleukin-10 secretion differentiates dendritic cells from human liver and skin. Am J Pathol 2004;164:511–519. (Ref.115)

Grant AJ, et al. Hepatic expression of secondary lymphoid chemokine (CCL21) promotes the development of portal-associated lymphoid tissue in chronic inflammatory liver disease. Am J Pathol 2002;160:1445–1455. (Ref.119)

Gregory SH, Wing EJ. Neutrophil-Kupffer cell interaction: a critical component of host defenses to systemic bacterial infections. J Leukoc Biol 2002;72: 239–248. (Ref.187)

Hemmi H, Akira S. TLR signalling and the function of dendritic cells. Chem Immunol Allergy 2005;86:120–135. (Ref.15)

Hoebe K, Janssen E, Beutler B. The interface between innate and adaptive immunity. Nat Immunol 2004;5:971–974. (Ref.14)

Holz LE, et al. Intrahepatic murine CD8 T-cell activation associates with a distinct phenotype leading to Bim-dependent death. Gastroenterology 2008; 135:989–997. (Ref.159)

Iwasaki A, Medzhitov R. Regulation of adaptive immunity by the innate immune system. Science 2010;327:291–295. (Ref.13)

Janssen EM, et al. CD4+ T cells are required for secondary expansion and memory in CD8+ T lymphocytes. Nature 2003;421:852–856. (Ref.10)

Johansson AG, Sundqvist T, Skogh T. IgG immune complex binding to and activation of liver cells. An in vitro study with IgG immune complexes, Kupffer cells, sinusoidal endothelial cells and hepatocytes. Int Arch Allergy Immunol 2000;121:329–336. (Ref.97)

Johansson C, Wick MJ. Liver dendritic cells present bacterial antigens and produce cytokines upon Salmonella encounter. J Immunol 2004;172: 2496–2503. (Ref.199)

John B, Crispe IN. Passive and active mechanisms trap activated CD8+ T cells in the liver. J Immunol 2004;172:5222–5229. (Ref.168)

Jomantaite I, et al. Hepatic dendritic cell subsets in the mouse. Eur J Immunol 2004;34:355–365. (Ref.112)

Jonuleit H, et al. Dendritic cells as a tool to induce anergic and regulatory T cells. Trends Immunol 2001;22:394–400. (Ref.197)

Kawai T, Akira S. Innate immune recognition of viral infection. Nat Immunol 2006;7:131–137. (Ref.11)

Kern M, et al. Virally infected mouse liver endothelial cells trigger CD8+ T-cell immunity. Gastroenterology 2010;138:336–346. (Ref.195)

Khanna A, et al. Effects of liver-derived dendritic cell progenitors on Th1- and Th2-like cytokine responses in vitro and in vivo. J Immunol 2000;164: 1346–1354. (Ref.113)

Klein I, et al. Kupffer cell heterogeneity: functional properties of bone marrow derived and sessile hepatic macrophages. Blood 2007;110:4077–4085. (Ref.22)

Knolle PA, Gerken G. Local control of the immune response in the liver. Immunol Rev 2000;174:21–34. (Ref.136)

Kronenberg M, Gapin L. The unconventional lifestyle of NKT cells. Nat Rev Immunol 2002;2:557–568. (Ref.65)

Laskin DL, Weinberger B, Laskin JD. Functional heterogeneity in liver and lung macrophages. J Leukoc Biol 2001;70:163–170. (Ref.38)

Lau AH, Thomson AW. Dendritic cells and immune regulation in the liver. Gut 2003;52:307–314. (Ref.111)

Lee WY, et al. An intravascular immune response to *Borrelia burgdorferi* involves Kupffer cells and iNKT cells. Nat Immunol 2010;11:295–302. (Ref.25)

Lievens J, et al. The size of sinusoidal fenestrae is a critical determinant of hepatocyte transduction after adenoviral gene transfer. Gene Ther 2004;11: 1523–1531. (Ref.101)

Lopes AR, et al. Bim-mediated deletion of antigen-specific CD8 T cells in patients unable to control HBV infection. J Clin Invest 2008;118:1835–1845. (Ref.160)

Lu L, et al. Liver-derived DEC205+B220+CD19-dendritic cells regulate T cell responses. J Immunol 2001;166:7042–7052. (Ref.114)

Luth S, et al. Ectopic expression of neural autoantigen in mouse liver suppresses experimental autoimmune neuroinflammation by inducing antigen-specific Tregs. J Clin Invest 2008;118:3403–3410. (Ref.161)

Lutz MB, Schuler G. Immature, semi-mature and fully mature dendritic cells: which signals induce tolerance or immunity? Trends Immunol 2002;23: 445–449. (Ref.105)

Maher JJ. Interactions between hepatic stellate cells and the immune system. Semin Liver Dis 2001;21:417–426. (Ref.125)

Matsuno K, et al. Kupffer cell-mediated recruitment of dendritic cells to the liver crucial for a host defense. Dev Immunol 2002;9:143–149. (Ref.75)

Mehal WZ, Azzaroli F, Crispe IN. Antigen presentation by liver cells controls intrahepatic T cell trapping, whereas bone marrow-derived cells preferentially promote intrahepatic T cell apoptosis. J Immunol 2001;167:667–673. (Ref.166)

Nakashima H, et al. Activation of mouse natural killer T cells accelerates liver regeneration after partial hepatectomy. Gastroenterology 2006;131:1573–1583. (Ref.79)

Neuhuber WL, Tiegs G. Innervation of immune cells: evidence for neuroimmunomodulation in the liver. Anat Rec 2004;280A:884–892. (Ref.46)

Niess JH, et al. CX3CR1-mediated dendritic cell access to the intestinal lumen and bacterial clearance. Science 2005;307:254–258. (Ref.3)

Notas G, Kisseleva T, Brenner D. NK and NKT cells in liver injury and fibrosis. Clin Immunol 2009;130:16–26. (Ref.80)

Oda M, Han JY, Yokomori H. Local regulators of hepatic sinusoidal microcirculation: recent advances. Clin Hemorheol Microcirc 2000;23:85–94. (Ref.82)

Paik YH, et al. Toll-like receptor 4 mediates inflammatory signaling by bacterial lipopolysaccharide in human hepatic stellate cells. Hepatology 2003;37: 1043–1055. (Ref.129)

Pillarisetty VG, et al. Liver dendritic cells are less immunogenic than spleen dendritic cells because of differences in subtype composition. J Immunol 2004;172:1009–1017. (Ref.110)

Politz O, et al. Stabilin-1 and -2 constitute a novel family of fasciclin-like hyaluronan receptor homologues. Biochem J 2002;362:155–164. (Ref.92)

Probst HC, et al. Resting dendritic cells induce peripheral CD8(+) T cell tolerance through PD-1 and CTLA-4. Nat Immunol 2005;6(3):280–286. (Ref.8)

Rescigno M, et al. Dendritic cells express tight junction proteins and penetrate gut epithelial monolayers to sample bacteria. Nat Immunol 2001;2:361–367. (Ref.2)

Reynaert H, et al. Hepatic stellate cells: role in microcirculation and pathophysiology of portal hypertension. Gut 2002;50:571–581. (Ref.124)

Salazar-Mather TP, Lewis CA, Biron CA. Type I interferons regulate inflammatory cell trafficking and macrophage inflammatory protein 1alpha delivery to the liver. J Clin Invest 2002;110:321–330. (Ref.192)

Salio M, Silk JD, Cerundolo V. Recent advances in processing and presentation of CD1 bound lipid antigens. Curr Opin Immunol 2010;22:81–88. (Ref.66)

Schumann J, et al. Parenchymal, but not leukocyte, TNF receptor 2 mediates T cell-dependent hepatitis in mice. J Immunol 2003;170:2129–2137. (Ref.48)

Schurich A, et al. Distinct kinetics and dynamics of cross-presentation in liver sinusoidal endothelial cells compared to dendritic cells. Hepatology 2009;50:909–919. (Ref.183)

Seki E, Brenner DA. Toll-like receptors and adaptor molecules in liver disease: update. Hepatology 2008;48:322–335. (Ref.185)

Seki E, et al. TLR4 enhances TGF-beta signaling and hepatic fibrosis. Nat Med 2007;13:1324–1332. (Ref.132)

Shortman K, Liu YJ. Mouse and human dendritic cell subtypes. Nat Rev Immunol 2002;2:151–161. (Ref.1)

Sidobre S, et al. The T cell antigen receptor expressed by Valpha14i NKT cells has a unique mode of glycosphingolipid antigen recognition. Proc Natl Acad Sci U S A 2004;101:12254–12259. (Ref.69)

Sixt M, et al. The conduit system transports soluble antigens from the afferent lymph to resident dendritic cells in the T cell area of the lymph node. Immunity 2005;22:19–29. (Ref.6)

Smedsrod B. Clearance function of scavenger endothelial cells. Comp Hepatol 2004;3(Suppl 1):S22. (Ref.84)

Steinman RM, et al. Dendritic cell function in vivo during the steady state: a role in peripheral tolerance. Ann N Y Acad Sci 2003;987:15–25. (Ref.7)

Steinman RM, Hawiger D, Nussenzweig MC. Tolerogenic dendritic cells. Annu Rev Immunol 2003;21:685–711. (Ref.104)

Steptoe RJ, et al. Comparative analysis of dendritic cell density and total number in commonly transplanted organs: morphometric estimation in normal mice. Transpl Immunol 2000;8:49–56. (Ref.109)

Swain MG. Hepatic NKT cells: friend or foe? Clin Sci (Lond) 2008;114:457–466. (Ref.76)

Swann JB, et al. CD1-restricted T cells and tumor immunity. Curr Top Microbiol Immunol 2007;314:293–323. (Ref.78)

Takeuchi O, Akira S. MDA5/RIG-I and virus recognition. Curr Opin Immunol 2008;20:17–22. (Ref.12)

Tanis W, et al. Human hepatic lymph nodes contain normal numbers of mature myeloid dendritic cells but few plasmacytoid dendritic cells. Clin Immunol 2004;110:81–88. (Ref.122)

Trobonjaca Z, et al. Activating immunity in the liver. II. IFN-beta attenuates NK cell-dependent liver injury triggered by liver NKT cell activation. J Immunol 2002;168:3763–3770. (Ref.163)

Trobonjaca Z, et al. Activating immunity in the liver. I. Liver dendritic cells (but not hepatocytes) are potent activators of IFN-gamma release by liver NKT cells. J Immunol 2001;167:1413–1422. (Ref.190)

van Oosten M, et al. Scavenger receptor-like receptors for the binding of lipopolysaccharide and lipoteichoic acid to liver endothelial and Kupffer cells. J Endotoxin Res 2001;7:381–384. (Ref.26)

Vazquez-Torres A, et al. Toll-like receptor 4 dependence of innate and adaptive immunity to Salmonella: importance of the Kupffer cell network. J Immunol 2004;172:6202–6208. (Ref.47)

Vinas O, et al. Human hepatic stellate cells show features of antigen-presenting cells and stimulate lymphocyte proliferation. Hepatology 2003;38:919–929. (Ref.126)

Vincent MS, et al. CD1-dependent dendritic cell instruction. Nat Immunol 2002;3:1163–1168. (Ref.194)

von Oppen N, et al. Systemic antigen cross-presented by liver sinusoidal endothelial cells induces liver-specific CD8 T-cell retention and tolerization. Hepatology 2009;49:1664–1672. (Ref.142)

Wahl C, et al. B7-H1 on hepatocytes facilitates priming of specific CD8 T cells but limits the specific recall of primed responses. Gastroenterology 2008;135:980–988. (Ref.156)

Winau F, et al. Ito cells are liver-resident antigen-presenting cells for activating T cell responses. Immunity 2007;26:117–129. (Ref.127)

Winau F, Quack C, Darmoise A, Kaufmann SH. Starring stellate cells in liver immunology. Curr Opin Immunol 2008;20:68–74. (Ref.128)

Wu D, et al. Bacterial glycolipids and analogs as antigens for CD1d-restricted NKT cells. Proc Natl Acad Sci U S A 2005;102:1351–1356. (Ref.68)

You Q, et al. Mechanism of T cell tolerance induction by murine hepatic Kupffer cells. Hepatology 2008;48:978–990. (Ref.169)

A complete list of references can be found at www.expertconsult.com.

Chapter 10

Epidemiology and Molecular Mechanisms of Hepatocarcinogenesis

Hashem B. El-Serag, André Lechel, and K. Lenhard Rudolph

ABBREVIATIONS

AFB₁ aflatoxin B1	**HCV** hepatitis C virus	**PTEN** phosphate and tensin homolog
ASR age-standardized rate	**HCC** hepatocellular carcinoma	**TERT** telomerase reverse transcriptase
BMI body mass index	**IL** interleukin	**TGF-β** transforming growth factor-β
C/EBP CCAAT-enhancer binding protein	**NAFLD** nonalcoholic fatty liver disease	**TNF-α** tumor necrosis factor-α
GST glutathione-*S*-transferase	**NASH** nonalcoholic steatohepatitis	**VEGFR1** vascular endothelial growth factor receptor 1
HBV hepatitis B virus	**OR** odds ratio	
HBeAg hepatitis B e antigen	**PGF3** placental growth factor 3	
HBsAg hepatitis B surface antigen	**PP2A** protein phosphatase 2A	

Introduction

The most unifying risk factors for the development of hepatocellular carcinoma (HCC) are chronic liver diseases and, in particular, the development of cirrhosis, which is characterized by loss of regenerative reserve, fibrosis, activation of liver progenitor cells, and increased inflammatory signaling. The increase in cancer risk at the cirrhosis stage involves intrinsic cellular alterations, including shortening of telomeres and the evolution of chromosomal instability. These alterations can, in turn, induce aberrations in gene expression, control of cell proliferation, and apoptosis. There is emerging evidence that extrinsic cell changes in the tissue microenvironment and possibly also alterations in the expression of systemically acting factors can contribute to the increasing risk for HCC in patients with cirrhosis. Relevant environmental changes at the cirrhosis stage include up-regulation of proinflammatory cytokines and growth factors and loss of proliferative competition of nontransformed hepatocytes. These environmental alterations increase the selection of abnormally proliferating hepatocytes and liver stem cells, which ultimately leads to the development of malignant clones at the cirrhosis stage. In addition, there are disease-specific mechanisms contributing to the increased risk for the development of HCC during chronic liver disease, including gene mutation induced by hepatitis viruses or chemical toxins, as well as the expression of oncogenic viral genes. This chapter summarizes the most important disease conditions that lead to the development of chronic HCC. Also discussed are some of the most important pathophysiologic and molecular mechanisms that contribute to the increased risk for HCC in the context of chronic liver diseases at the cirrhosis stage.

Epidemiology of Hepatocellular Carcinoma

Overview of Global Burden of Hepatocellular Carcinoma

Liver cancer is the fifth most common cancer in men (522,000 cases, 7.9% of the total) and the seventh in women (225,000 cases, 6.5% of the total). Most of the burden is in developing countries, where almost 85% of cases occur. Because of its high fatality (overall ratio of mortality to incidence, 0.93), liver cancer is the third most frequent cause of death from cancer worldwide.[1]

HCC is the most common (90% to 95%) type of primary liver cancer. There are considerable geographic variations in the incidence of HCC (**Fig. 10-1**). Differences in the prevalence of the major HCC etiologic factors, with more than 80% of cases of HCC arising in patients infected with hepatitis B virus (HBV) or hepatitis C virus (HCV),[2] explain most of its geographic variations. The highest age-standardized incidence rates (>20 cases per 100,000) were reported from countries in

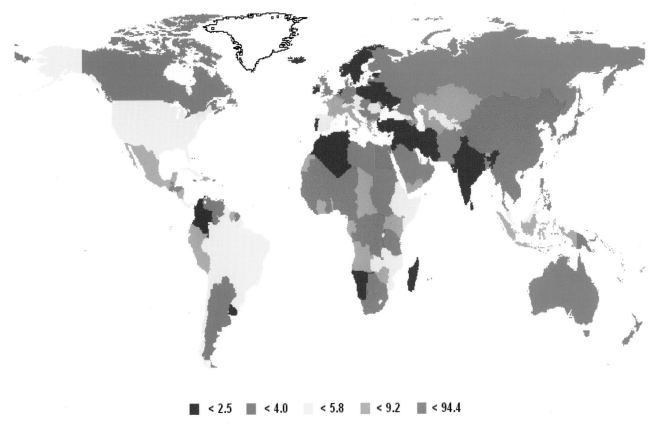

■ < 2.5   ■ < 4.0   □ < 5.8   ■ < 9.2   ■ < 94.4

Fig. 10-1 **Incidence of liver cancer.** Age-standardized incidence rates for primary liver cancer worldwide, estimated for 2008, are shown. The age-standardized rate is calculated using the 1960 world standard population in five age groups: 0 to 14, 15 to 44, 45 to 54, 55 to 64, and 65+. *(From Ferlay J, et al. GLOBOCAN 2008 Cancer Incidence and Mortality Worldwide, IARC Cancer Base No.10. Lyon, International Agency for Research on Cancer; 2010. Available from* http://globocan.iarc.fr.)

Southeast Asia (North and South Korea, China, Vietnam). Other high-incidence areas include sub-Saharan African countries such as Cameroon and Mozambique. These regions are endemic for HBV infection. In general, countries in southern Europe have medium to high HCC incidence rates. An exception to the predominance of HCC among primary liver cancer is the Khon Kaen region of Thailand, which had one of the world's highest rates of liver cancer (age-standardized rate [ASR] in 1993 to 1997 of 88.0 per 100,000 for males and 35.4 per 100,000 for females).[3] However, because of endemic infestation with liver flukes, the major type of liver cancer in this region is cholangiocarcinoma rather than HCC.[4]

There have been encouraging trends in the incidence of liver cancer in some areas with a high rate, such as China and Japan,[5] where HCC has been declining. Conversely, substantial increases in HCC incidence and mortality rates have been observed in areas previously considered to be low in incidence: North America, Europe, and Oceania. In these regions, HCV is the most frequent etiologic risk factor and accounts for 30% to 50% of cases of HCC. For example, the incidence of HCC has tripled in the United States during the past 2 decades[6] and has become the most rapidly increasing cause of cancer-related deaths.[7]

The median survival of patients with HCC is estimated to be less than 1 year.[8] Without effective treatment, the reported median survival is dismal, less than 5 months.[9,10] The main burden of HCC is due to premature mortality. Estimates from the Global Burden of Disease Study in 2004 revealed that HCC

caused nearly 7 million years of life lost—11.6% and 5.9% of the cancer-related years of life lost in men and women, respectively.

Demographic Features of Hepatocellular Carcinoma

Age

Hepatocellular carcinoma is rare before the age of 40 and reaches a peak at around the age of 70. In low-risk populations (e.g., United States, Canada, United Kingdom), the highest age-specific rates occur in persons 75 years and older (**Fig. 10-2**). However, in Qidong, China, where HCC rates are among the world's highest, age-specific incidence rates in males rise until the age of 45 and then plateau. In all regions, the peak age for females is 5 years older than the peak age for males. The variable age-specific patterns in different geographic regions are probably related to differences in the dominant hepatitis virus in the population, the age at viral infection, and the existence of other risk factors. For example, most HCV carriers become infected as adults, and most HBV carriers become infected at very young ages.

Sex

There is a striking male preponderance in HCC (**Fig. 10-3**), with the highest male-to-female ratios seen in areas with a

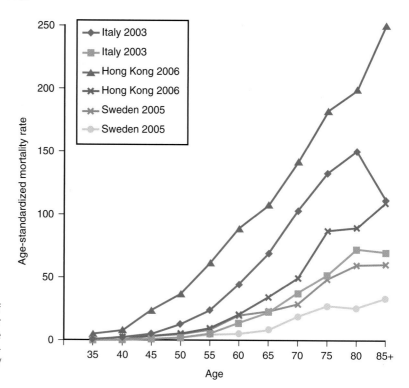

Fig. 10-2 Liver cancer mortality. The age distribution of primary liver cancer mortality (per 100,000) is shown for selected examples of high-, middle-, and low-incidence countries. *(From World Health Organization WHO mortality database. WHO Statistcal Information System 2008. Available at http://www.who.int/whosis.)*

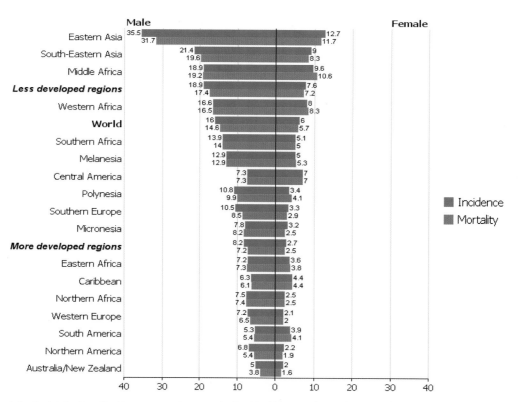

Fig. 10-3 Epidemiologic risk factors for liver cancer. Age-standardized incidence and mortality rates for primary liver cancer per 100,000 population at risk are shown. The age-standardized rate is calculated from the 1960 world standard population in five age groups: 0 to 14, 15 to 44, 45 to 54, 55 to 64, and 65+. *(From Ferlay J, et al. GLOBOCAN 2008 Cancer Incidence and Mortality Worldwider, IARC Cancer Base No.10. Lyon, International Agency for Research on Cancer; 2010. Available from http://globocan.iarc.fr.)*

high and medium incidence of HCC. HCC is more equally distributed among men and women in low-incidence countries in South and Central America. The prevalence of HBV, HCV, alcohol consumption, and cigarette smoking is higher in men than women. Some of the male preponderance seen in HCC can be explained by higher cancer rates in males in general. A possible role of sex hormones in the development of HCC has also been suggested.[11] High serum testosterone levels have been associated with risk for HCC in nested case-control studies of HBV carriers in Taiwan and Shanghai.[12]

Race/Ethnicity

Hepatocellular carcinoma incidence rates also vary substantially among different populations living in the same region. For example, ethnic Chinese populations in Singapore have considerably higher age-adjusted rates than do Indians in the same region.[3] Another example are the age-adjusted HCC incidence rates in individuals of Asian/Pacific Islander ethnicity, which are almost three times higher than those in whites (ASR of 11.7 and 3.9, respectively), with Hispanics and blacks being between these two extremes (ASR of 8.0 and 7.0, respectively).[13] Differences in prevalence of the main risk factors may explain some of these differences; for example, first-generation immigrants from Southeast Asia have high HBV infection rates, although differences in the risk for HCC may also vary among racial groups with the same risk factor (e.g., among HCV-infected individuals in the United States, blacks have higher risk for the development of HCC).

Risk Factors for Hepatocellular Carcinoma

The main risk factors for HCC are HBV, HCV, alcohol, aflatoxin, and possibly obesity and diabetes. Together, HBV and HCV account for 80% to 90% of all cases of HCC worldwide[2] (**Table 10-1**). Mendelian disorders (e.g., Wilson disease, α_1-antitrypsin deficiency, hemochromatosis) account for a very small proportion of cases of HCC. Cryptogenic or unknown cause of HCC accounts for 15% to 30% of cases. Most risk factors for HCC promote the development of cirrhosis, which is present in about 80% to 90% of patients with HCC.[14,15] The risk for development of HCC in patients with cirrhosis varies considerably with the underlying condition and severity of cirrhosis.[16] The highest 5-year cumulative risks are seen in

persons with HCV-induced cirrhosis (30% in Japan and 17% in the West), hemochromatosis (21%), HBV-induced cirrhosis (15% in Asia and 10% in the West), alcoholic cirrhosis (8%), and biliary cirrhosis (4%).[17] Patients with Child-Pugh stage B or C had a two-fold to three-fold increased risk for HCC in comparison with those with stage A.[18]

Hepatitis B Virus

Approximately 350 million people around the world are estimated to be chronically infected with HBV.[19] Worldwide, chronic HBV infection accounts for approximately 50% of HCC cases,[20] with considerable regional variation (70% in South Korea, 10% to 15% in Japan,[21] 3% in Sweden, 9% in the United States, and 55% in Greece[22]). HCC secondary to HBV results from chronic inflammation and repeated cellular regeneration, with HCC typically developing after 25 to 30 years of chronic infection.[23] The lifetime risk for HCC in a person with chronic HBV infection is between 10% and 25%.[24] The relative lifetime risk for HCC in HBV-infected individuals is 15- to 20-fold higher than noninfected controls.[25,26]

HBV is a notorious cause of HCC in the absence of cirrhosis; however, the great majority (70% to 90%) of HBV-related cases of HCC develop in livers already afflicted by cirrhosis.[27] HBV DNA is found in the host genome of both infected and malignant hepatic cells. HBV might thus exert its carcinogenic potential by increasing the likelihood of viral DNA insertion in or near proto-oncogenes or tumor suppressor genes. In addition, there is evidence that viral proteins can exert oncogenic actions. Along these lines it has been shown that the HBx gene product impairs p53.[28]

The increased risk for HCC associated with HBV infection applies particularly to areas where HBV infection is endemic. In these areas, HBV is usually transmitted from mother to newborn (vertical transmission), and up to 90% of infections follow a chronic course. This pattern is different in areas with low HCC incidence rates, where HBV is acquired in adulthood through sexual and parenteral routes (horizontal transmission), with more than 90% of acute infections resolving spontaneously. The annual incidence of HCC in chronic HBV carriers in Asia ranges between 0.4% and 0.6%, but it is considerably lower in white HBV carriers.[29]

Several additional factors increase the risk for HCC in HBV carriers, including male sex; older age; longer duration of infection; family history of HCC; exposure to aflatoxin,

Table 10-1 HBV- and HCV-Induced Hepatocarcinogenesis. Estimated Cases of Primary Liver Cancer in 2002 Attributable to HBV and HCV

	PRIMARY LIVER CANCER CASES	HBV		HCV		CASES ATTRIBUTABLE TO HBV OR HCV
		Attributable Fraction (%)	*Attributable Cases*	*Attributable Fraction (%)*	*Attributable Cases*	
Developed countries	110,800	23.3	25,800	19.9	22,000	48,000
Developing countries	515,300	58.8	303,000	33.4	172,000	475,000
Total	626,100	54.4	340,600	31.1	195,000	535,000

Adapted from Parkin DM. The global health burden of infection-associated cancers in the year 2002. Int J Cancer 2006;118:3030–3044.
HBV, hepatitis B virus; HCV, hepatitis C virus.

alcohol, or tobacco; or co-infection with HCV or delta hepatitis. Risk for HCC is also increased in patients with high levels of HBV hepatocellular replication, as indicated by high HBV DNA levels, the presence of hepatitis B e antigen (HBeAg),[30] or HBV genotype C.[31] HBV DNA can also be detected in hepatitis B surface antigen (HBsAg)-negative individuals, but it has an unclear association with risk for HCC. There is moderately strong evidence that effective antiviral therapy that controls HBV infection in viremic HBsAg-positive patients substantially reduces but does not eliminate the risk for HCC. One high-quality large randomized controlled trial involving Chinese patients with chronic HBV who had cirrhosis reported a significant reduction in the incidence of HCC in patients treated with lamivudine for several years versus placebo (3.9% vs. 7.4%; hazard ratio, 0.49; $P = .047$).[32]

Risk for HCC is substantially lower in persons who are immune to HBV. For example, in the seminal study by Beasley,[33] the incidence of HCC was significantly lower in immune persons than in carriers, 5 versus 495 per 100,000 per year.[33] With the use of sensitive amplification assays, many studies have shown that HBV DNA persists as "occult HBV infection" for decades in persons after serologic recovery (HBsAg negative) from acute infection.[34] Although some studies have linked the development of HCC in individuals with chronic HCV infection to occult HBV infection, others have not found such an association.

In 2006, more than 160 countries vaccinated infants against HBV in national immunization programs.[19] Frequently cited reports from Taiwan have described a reduction in HCC incidence rates in children 1 to 2 decades after the introduction of a universal vaccination program against HBV.[35]

Dietary Aflatoxin

Aflatoxins are naturally occurring potent hepatocarcinogenic mycotoxins produced by some *Aspergillus* species. They are molds that grow on grains, corn, cassava, peanuts, and fermented soybeans, particularly in the high-moisture conditions in parts of sub-Saharan Africa and eastern Asia. Animal experiments have demonstrated that AFB_1 is a powerful hepatocarcinogen, which led the International Agency for Research on Cancer to classify it as carcinogenic.[36] Once ingested, AFB_1 is metabolized to an active intermediate, AFB_1-*exo*-8,9-epoxide, which can bind to DNA and produce a characteristic mutation in the p53 tumor suppressor gene (p53 249[ser]).[37] This mutation has been observed in 30% to 60% of HCC tumors in areas endemic for aflatoxin.[38,39]

In most areas where AFB_1 exposure is a problem, chronic HBV infection is also highly prevalent. Individuals infected with HBV and exposed to aflatoxin have an even higher risk for liver cancer, thus suggesting a synergistic effect between HBV and aflatoxin.[40] Although HBV vaccination in these areas should be the major preventive tactic, persons already chronically infected will not benefit from vaccination. However, HBV carriers could benefit by eliminating exposure to AFB_1. Efforts have been launched to accomplish this goal in China[41] and Africa.[39]

Hepatitis C Virus

The global HCV prevalence is estimated to be 2% and is as high as 10% in Egypt.[42] It has been estimated that HCV began to infect large numbers of young adults in Japan in the 1920s, in southern Europe in the 1940s, and in North America in the 1960s and 1970s as a result of contaminated needles or injection drug use (or both).[43] The virus then migrated into national blood supplies and circulated until a screening test was developed in 1990, after which rates of new infection dropped dramatically.

The association between HCV infection and increased risk for HCC is well established and has been shown in case-control as well as cohort studies. Markers of HCV infection are found in a variable proportion of patients with HCC; for example, 45% to 65% of patients in Italy[44,45] and 80% to 90% of patients in Japan.[46] Risk for HCC was increased 17- to 20-fold in HCV-infected patients in comparison with HCV-negative controls.[47]

The rate of development of HCC in HCV-infected persons ranges from 1% to 3% after 30 years of chronic infection.[48] HCV increases risk for HCC by promoting fibrosis and eventually cirrhosis. Once cirrhosis is established, the annual incidence of HCC is 1% to 4%.[16] In HCV-infected patients, factors related to the host and environment/lifestyle appear to be more important than viral factors in determining progression to cirrhosis. Such factors include older age overall and older age at the time of acquisition of HCV infection, male sex, heavy alcohol intake (more than 50 g/day), diabetes, obesity, and co-infection with human immunodeficiency virus (HIV) or HBV.[49] In contrast, HCV viral load and HCV genotype have not been associated with risk for HCC. Evidence from one randomized controlled study and several nonrandomized studies of HCV-infected patients with and without cirrhosis indicated a 57% to 75% reduction in risk for HCC in those treated with interferon-based therapy who achieved a sustained viral response.[50,51] However, in patients with HCV-associated cirrhosis who do not achieve a sustained viral response with antiviral therapy, there is no further significant reduction in HCC with maintenance interferon therapy.[52]

Alcohol

Heavy alcohol intake, defined as the ingestion of more than 50 to 70 g/day for several years, is a well-established risk factor for HCC. It is unclear whether the risk for HCC is significantly altered in those with low or moderate alcohol intake. Most data indicate that alcohol does not have a carcinogenic effect in itself; rather, the increased risk is associated with the cirrhosis that prolonged alcohol intake can cause. There is evidence of a synergistic effect of heavy alcohol ingestion and HCV or HBV infection, with these factors presumably operating together to increase risk for HCC by more actively promoting cirrhosis.[47]

Fatty Liver Disease

Many studies conducted in Western countries fail to identify a major risk factor (HBV, HCV, alcohol) for chronic liver disease or HCC in a large proportion of patients (30% to 40%). Nonalcoholic fatty liver disease (NAFLD), including its more advanced form, nonalcoholic steatohepatitis (NASH), has been proposed as the etiologic factor for many cases of cryptogenic HCC. Insulin resistance has been suggested as the major pathogenic mechanism for this disorder, as well as its progression to NASH. Obesity and diabetes are the major clinical manifestations of insulin resistance syndrome.

There is epidemiologic evidence in support of a potential association between NAFLD/NASH and a modest increase in risk for HCC. The few available population-based cohort studies of patients with NAFLD/NASH provide modest support for this association[53,54]; however, given the few HCC cases, the data are too limited to identify subgroups at particularly increased risk for HCC. Cross-sectional and case-control studies are limited because the requisite histopathologic features for a confirmed diagnosis of NAFLD/NASH are less evident or even absent once cirrhosis is established. Indirect evidence of an NAFLD-HCC association is provided by multiple cross-sectional and case-control studies showing a significantly higher prevalence of obesity and diabetes in patients with cryptogenic cirrhosis than in controls with other causes of liver disease.[55-58] It is clear that the development of cirrhosis related to NASH signals a considerable increase in risk for HCC. Most studies that evaluated cryptogenic cirrhosis or documented NASH-related cirrhosis reported a high incidence of HCC that was generally lower than that of HCV-related cirrhosis. Although progression of NAFLD/NASH to cirrhosis and NAFLD/NASH-related HCC may very well occur infrequently, given their vast and increasing prevalence, obesity and diabetes could still contribute to a large number of cases of HCC.

Obesity

Most obese individuals (body mass index [BMI] >30 kg/m^2) and up to 70% of all people with type 2 diabetes have some degree of fatty liver.[59] Insulin resistance, which is strongly associated with obesity, especially abdominal obesity, contributes significantly to hepatic steatosis,[60,61] severe necroinflammatory activity,[62,63] and fibrosis.[62,64-69]

The increasing incidence of HCC has paralleled that of obesity in many countries. Obesity has been associated with a 1.5- to 3.0-fold increased risk for the development of HCC in population-based cohort studies in the United States, Scandinavia, Taiwan, and Japan.[70-72] In a large prospective U.S. cohort study including more than 900,000 individuals monitored for a 16-year period, liver cancer mortality rates were 4.5 higher in men with a BMI greater than 35 and 1.7 higher in women with a BMI greater than 35 relative to normal-weight individuals.[70]

Diabetes

Type 2 diabetes has been proposed as a moderately strong risk factor for chronic liver disease and HCC, possibly through the development of NAFLD and NASH. Several case-control studies have found a statistically significant association between diabetes and HCC. However, reverse causality is a concern in these studies because diabetes might be a result of cirrhosis. A few cohort studies, better suited to evaluate temporality, showed that individuals with type 2 diabetes had an increased risk for the development of HCC.[45,73] For example, a large U.S. cohort study of 173,643 patients with diabetes and 650,620 controls without diabetes reported that the incidence of HCC was approximately doubled in patients with diabetes and was even higher in those with a longer duration of diabetes.[73] Although other underlying risk factors such as HCV

infection may confound the association between diabetes and HCC, they do not seem to fully explain the observed associations between diabetes and HCC. The role of diabetes treatment is unclear.

Tobacco

The relationship between cigarette smoking and HCC has been examined in more than 50 studies in areas with both low and high rates of HCC. Given the concurrence of tobacco smoking and alcohol drinking, the confounding effect of alcohol cannot be completely excluded. In almost all countries, both a positive association and a lack of association have been reported. Taken together, the available evidence suggests that any effect of smoking on HCC is likely to be weak.

Diet

The role of diet in the etiology of HCC is largely unknown. Dietary antioxidants, including selenium, retinoic acid, and β-carotene, have been shown to inhibit hepatocarcinogenesis in animal experiments. However, epidemiologic data are limited and in some places conflicting. A weak protective effect of high intake of specific foods groups, including milk and yogurt, white meat, eggs, and fruits, and high intake of selected macronutrients, including β-carotene, was reported by a multicenter hospital-based case-control study in Italy.[74] In a cohort study of men in Taiwan, lower vegetable intake was significantly associated with increased risk for HCC. This effect was limited to chronic HBV carriers and cigarette smokers.[75] Another study of Japanese atomic bomb survivors reported an approximately 50% reduction in risk for HCC in those with high consumption of isoflavone-rich miso soup and tofu after adjusting for HBV and HCV infection.[76]

Coffee Drinking

Several epidemiologic studies have reported that coffee drinking reduces the risk for elevated liver enzymes, cirrhosis, and HCC. Animal studies suggest that coffee reduces liver carcinogenesis. Furthermore, coffee drinking has also been associated with reduced insulin levels, as well as reduced risk for type 2 diabetes, in itself a risk factor for HCC.[77] Meta-analyses of studies conducted in Japan and southern Europe have shown an approximately 25% reduction in risk with each additional cup of coffee consumed daily[78-80] (25% to 75% risk reduction with two to four cups of coffee per day as compared with none).[79,81-84] Three cohort studies reported on the association between coffee intake and future risk for HCC.[80,85,86] Two of these studies reported a significant reduction in risk for HCC with coffee intake of one or more cups, with one study showing a dose-response relationship (20% reduction with one to two cups and 75% reduction with five or more cups[85]). The third publication, which reported on two cohorts, showed reduced risk for HCC with coffee drinking that was of borderline significance.[80] Most of these studies had general population controls, which may not be an appropriate comparator given their low risk for HCC, as well as chronic liver disease. However, the inverse association between coffee consumption and HCC persisted in the studies that presented results stratified by liver disease[80,81,85,86] or used a second control group of patients with liver disease.[83]

Oral Contraceptives

There is experimental rationale for a possible role of oral contraceptives in liver neoplasia. Nuclear estrogen receptors exist in hepatocytes and are increased in those with HCC, thus suggesting hormonal responsiveness of hepatic neoplastic tissue. The estrogen and progesterone components of oral contraceptives have been shown to induce and promote liver tumors in animals.[87]

The epidemiologic evidence for an association between oral contraceptives and increased risk for HCC is unclear. The association between oral contraceptive use and risk for HCC was recently examined in a review of 12 case-control studies that included 739 patients and 5223 controls.[88] The pooled estimate of odds ratios (ORs), age and sex matched only, from these studies was 1.57 (95% confidence interval [CI], 0.96 to 2.54; $P = .07$). The pooled estimate from eight of the studies that reported adjusted ORs was 1.45 (95% CI, 0.93 to 2.27; $P = .11$). The evidence is inconclusive to establish a relationship between oral contraceptives and risk for HCC. Furthermore, there is no information on the newer, low-dose oral contraceptives.

Hemochromatosis

There are very few population-based risk estimates for HCC in individuals homozygous for known *HFE* mutations and no information on the risk in heterozygous carriers. A population-based study conducted in Sweden indicated a 1.7-fold increase in incidence of HCC in 1800 individuals with hereditary hemochromatosis (mostly homozygous for the C282Y mutation). Much higher HCC risk estimates were reported from selected samples of patients with hemochromatosis who were seen in referral centers. The proportion of patients with HCC who have *HFE* mutations is small for homozygous mutations (3% to 5%).[89,90] A higher than expected prevalence of *HFE* mutations in patients with HCC in the absence of cirrhosis has been suggested but remains unclear.[91] The proportion of patients with HCC who are heterozygous for *HFE* is larger, but it is not clear whether it is significantly greater than in controls. There is no evidence of an increased prevalence of H63D mutations in patients with HCC versus controls.[92]

Vinyl Chloride

An association has been established between vinyl chloride exposure in factory workers and angiosarcoma of the liver, but not with other histologic types of liver tumor. A meta-analysis reported a standardized mortality ratio for liver cancers other than angiosarcoma of 1.35 (95% CI, 1.04 to 1.77).[93] However, these nonangiosarcoma liver tumors included HCC, bile duct tumors, gallbladder cancer, and liver cancer of unknown histology. Given the small number of cancers, the potential for tumor misclassification, and the borderline statistical significance, a significant association between vinyl chloride exposure and HCC, as well as other nonangiosarcoma tumors, is highly unlikely.

Genetic Epidemiology of Hepatocellular Carcinoma

In most people with known environmental risk factors for HCC (e.g., HCV, HBV, alcohol), cirrhosis or HCC never develops, whereas a sizable minority of cases of HCC develop in individuals without any known risk factors. This led to a search for host genetic risk factors.

The majority of HCC studies have been case-control studies conducted in populations with a high rate of HCC (Asian, African) or a medium rate (European). Typically, they have examined only a few polymorphisms in a few selected genes because of (1) their role in the key liver function of detoxification, including phase I and phase II enzymes such as cytochrome P-450, *N*-acetyltransferase, and glutathione-S-transferase (GST); (2) their role in biologic pathways potentially relevant in chronic liver disease and carcinogenesis, including inflammatory response (e.g., interleukin-1β [IL-1β], interleukin receptor agonist [IRN]) and DNA repair (e.g., XRCC1); or (3) their role in mitigating or exacerbating the effects of exposure to specific etiologic risk factors for HCC such as alcohol or aflatoxin (e.g., ADH3, ALDH2, EPHX1). A meta-analysis evaluated the effect of the two most frequently evaluated polymorphisms on risk for HCC to date, the dual-deletion GST polymorphisms GSTM1 (14 studies) and GSTT1 (13 studies).[94] Pooled estimators suggested a possible small excess risk with either GSTM1 or GSTT1 null genotypes, although the findings approached significance only for GSTT1 ($OR_{GSTM1} = 1.16$; 95% CI, 0.89 to 1.53; $OR_{GSTT1} = 1.191$; 95% CI, 0.99 to 1.44). Results from other genetic association studies in HCC have largely been equivocal, with findings of a positive association, association only within a limited subset of the population, or no or negative associations.

Molecular Mechanisms of Hepatocarcinogenesis

Pathophysiology of Hepatocarcinogenesis at the Cirrhosis Stage

Hepatocellular carcinoma rarely develops in a healthy or noncirrhotic liver. In contrast, risk for HCC increases sharply at the cirrhosis stage to an annual incidence of 3% to 6%, depending on cause and ethnicity.[17] The following mechanisms could contribute to the increased cancer risk at the cirrhosis stage (**Fig. 10-4**).

Loss of Replicative Competition

Cirrhosis is characterized by a decrease in the regenerative capacity of the liver. As outlined later, telomere shortening and senescence impair the regenerative capacity of hepatocytes at the cirrhosis stage. In cancer studies there is emerging evidence that loss of replicative competence can increase risk for cancer in aging tissue or in continuously damaged tissues affected by chronic diseases.

Experimental animal studies have shown that leukemic cells do not lead to the development of leukemia in healthy, proliferation-competent bone marrow. In contrast, the same number of leukemic cells induced a rapid evolution of leukemia when implanted into proliferation-defective bone marrow, thus indicating that loss of replicative competition of nontransformed organ cells leads to stronger selection and the development of malignant clones.[95]

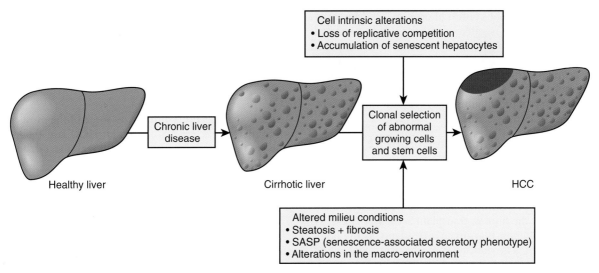

Fig. 10-4 **Pathophysiology of hepatocarcinogenesis at the cirrhosis stage.** Cirrhosis is characterized by regenerative exhaustion and an accumulation of senescent hepatocytes, steatosis, fibrosis, and inflammation. These conditions can increase the risk for cancer by selecting for activation and proliferation of aberrant liver cells, including stem cells. Regenerative exhaustion and the accumulation of senescent hepatocytes lead to loss of replicative competition, which can increase the selection of abnormally growing cells. In addition, the impairment in organ maintenance could lead to the activation of systemic-acting factors and stimulate the proliferation of aberrant cell clones. Moreover, senescence, steatosis, fibrosis, and inflammation induce changes in the tissue micromilieu by activating the secretion of proinflammatory cytokines and growth factors. These factors can also contribute to growth stimulation and selection of (premalignant) malignant cells and stem cells.

In accordance with these findings on leukemogenesis, it has been observed that a growth-restrained environment in the mouse liver enhances the clonal selection of cells and carcinogenesis. Specifically, it was shown that chemicals that inhibit hepatocyte proliferation also accelerate carcinogen-induced liver tumor formation in rats,[96] as well as the expansion and transformation of transplanted hepatocytes.[97] The enhancement of clonal cell selection in response to chemically induced damage involved activation of the p53 checkpoint.[96] There is evidence that this checkpoint is also active in response to accumulation of damage in human cirrhosis.

p53 plays a major role in restricting proliferation and cell survival in response to DNA damage and telomere dysfunction.[98] The cyclin-dependent kinase inhibitor p21 represents the major downstream target of p53, and cell cycle progression is halted in response to telomere dysfunction.[99] In primary human cells, activation of p21-dependent cell cycle arrest is required for induction of senescence.[100] In agreement with the data on telomere shortening in cirrhosis, up-regulation of p21 was observed in cirrhotic liver.[101,102] It is conceivable that the combination of telomere shortening, senescence, and growth restriction of hepatocytes at the cirrhosis stage leads to increased selection of abnormally growing cells and culminates in the expansion of malignant clones and carcinogenesis.

Altered Milieu Conditions

Different mechanism can change the microenvironment in a cirrhotic liver and possibly promote tumorigenesis.

Steatosis, Fibrosis, and Inflammation

These three processes represent key events in chronic liver disease that are associated with the formation of cirrhosis. Steatosis and fibrosis have been identified as independent risk factors for hepatocarcinogenesis in patients with chronic hepatitis.[103] Increased production of cytokines and growth factors, including placental growth factor 3 (PGF3), vascular endothelial growth factor receptor 1 (VEGFR1) and soluble VEGFR1, lymphotoxins, and IL-6, has been associated with fibrosis, steatosis, and increased risk for cancer at the cirrhosis stage.[104-106] Different cellular sources may contribute to the increased production of cytokines and growth factors in cirrhosis: (1) infiltration and activation of immune cells,[107] (2) stress responses in hepatocytes harboring abnormal lipid accumulations, and (3) stress responses in activated stellate cells and fibrotic scar tissue.[108,109] In addition to the increased production of cytokines and growth factors, there are profound changes in the extracellular matrix in persons with cirrhosis that can contribute to a protumorigenic environment, including alteration in integrin expression.[110]

Senescence-Associated Secretory Phenotype

Cirrhosis is characterized by telomere shortening and an accumulation of senescent hepatocytes. The accumulation of senescent hepatocytes could contribute to the increased production of cytokines and growth factors and accelerate the risk for cancer. It has been demonstrated that senescent human fibroblasts express abnormally high levels of proinflammatory cytokines and growth factors, including IL-6 and tumor necrosis factor-α (TNF-α).[111] A similar phenomenon also occurs in response to telomere dysfunction in telomerase knockout mice in vivo.[112] Studies on senescent human fibroblasts have shown that senescent cells stimulate the growth of epithelial tumors in xenotransplantation models.[113] It is conceivable that increased expression of proinflammatory cytokines and growth factors leads to a growth-stimulatory environment in tissues exhibiting an accumulation of senescent cells (e.g., cirrhosis). Interestingly, IL-6 and TNF-α production has been identified as key factors that accelerate hepatocarcinogenesis in the context of obesity.[103,105] Moreover, deletion of SOCS3—a negative regulator of IL-6–related cytokines—was shown to promote hepatitis-induced hepatocarcinogenesis in mice.[114] Together, these findings suggest that different cellular stress factors (e.g., telomere dysfunction, lipid accumulation, hepatitis) could cooperate to increase levels of expression of proinflammatory cytokines and thereby accelerate hepatocarcinogenesis.

Alterations in the Macroenvironment

Liver regeneration is a tightly regulated process that leads to exact restoration of organ mass in response to injury. In mouse models, it was observed long ago that liver regeneration after partial hepatectomy stops precisely when liver mass is restored. Also in the human transplant setting, it is a well-recognized phenomenon that organ size adapts to the body size of the recipient. The molecular mechanisms controlling regulation of liver mass have not been identified, however. Unlike the pancreas, liver size is not regulated by the size of the stem cell pool generated during development.[115] These findings indicate that liver size is controlled by an interplay of growth factors. A possible scenario for regulation of liver mass could be that hepatic metabolites activate some feedback mechanisms (growth factors) that induce growth or involution of the liver. In principle, it is possible that these mechanisms become activated in response to loss of liver cell mass during cirrhosis, thus creating a growth-stimulatory macroenvironment that could accelerate the progression of abnormal regenerative nodules and early cancer.

Aberrant Activation and Transformation of Liver Stem Cells

Twenty percent to 30% of human HCCs exhibit stem or progenitor cell features, including bilinear differentiation into hepatocytes and cholangiocytes[116] or stem cell–associated gene expression signatures.[117] These data fueled a debate whether liver stem and progenitor cells may represent the cell type of origin in at least a subset of human HCC.[118] In mouse models, it was shown that specific genetic lesions can result in abnormal activation and transformation of liver stem cells. Specifically, overactivation of cell proliferation resulted in chromosomal instability of hepatocytes and in activation and transformation of liver progenitor cells.[119,120]

In humans, there is evidence that liver stem cells become reactivated in response to fulminant liver injury and also at the cirrhosis stage.[116] Normally, liver regeneration does not require activation of liver stem cells but can be achieved by reentrance of hepatocytes into the cell cycle.[121] It is possible that activation of liver stem cells represents a backup system that is reactivated only in situations in which the regenerative capacity of hepatocytes does not suffice. At the cirrhosis stage, loss of regenerative competence of hepatocytes could represent the primary trigger leading to the activation of liver stem cells. The permanent reactivation of liver stem cells in a growth-restricted, cirrhotic liver may lead to increased risk for stem cell transformation. However, this hypothesis remains to be tested. The molecular mechanisms that increase the risk for liver stem cell transformation have yet to be delineated. In principle, these mechanisms could involve factors similar to those that induce the transformation of differentiated organ cells. The transformation of stem cells may also involve additional factors that control the self-renewal or genome stability of stem cells.

Molecular Mechanisms of Hepatocarcinogenesis at the Cirrhosis Stage

The following section summarizes some of the most common molecular characteristics of human HCC and their possible role in promoting cancer formation at the cirrhosis stage (**Fig. 10-5**).

Induction of Chromosomal Instability

Hepatocellular carcinoma is characterized by high rates of chromosomal instability.[122,123] Chronic liver diseases elevate the rate of hepatocyte death, which in turn increases the rate of cell division. It is possible that the chromosomal instability in chronic liver disease results from the accumulation of replication errors during elevated rates of cell division. However, this is unlikely to be the main cause of HCC because replication errors are rare in human HCC.[124] Instead, chromosomal imbalances and translocations represent the most prominent types of genetic instability in human HCC.[122] This type of instability can be induced by telomere dysfunction, which is known to accumulate during chronic liver disease.[125]

Telomeres form the ends of eukaryotic chromosomes and consist of small tandem DNA repeats that do not encode for a protein product.[126,127] The main function of telomeres is to cap the ends of chromosomes.[128-130] Telomere capping is required to distinguish the ends of chromosomes from DNA breaks within chromosomes.

Telomeres shorten during each round of cell division because of the "end replication problem" of DNA polymerase.[131] Telomere shortening limits the proliferative capacity of primary human cells (including hepatocytes) to a finite number of cell divisions.[131,132] In agreement with low rates of cell division, there is little telomere shortening in aging human liver.[125] In contrast, chronic liver diseases lead to an increased rate of liver cell proliferation, which is associated with an accelerated rate of telomere shortening.[125] Telomeres are significantly shorter in cirrhotic specimens than in samples from noncirrhotic liver.[125] Telomere shortening in cirrhosis correlates with the accumulation of senescent, cell cycle–arrested hepatocytes,[125] thus providing a plausible explanation for the decrease in liver regenerative capacity in patients with cirrhosis.[133]

It is conceivable that the accumulation of very short, dysfunctional telomeres in persons with cirrhosis also contributes to the induction of chromosomal instability. Telomere dysfunction (uncapping of chromosome ends) results in the activation of DNA repair responses that induce the formation of chromosomal fusion.[134,135] When cells with fused chromosomes enter the cell cycle, breakage of the chromosomal fusion can occur during anaphase, which results in chromosomal gains and losses in the daughter cells. In addition, the daughter cells acquire new telomere free ends at the break points that fuse and break again during the next round of cell division. This induction of repeated rounds of fusion-bridge-breakage cycles leads to an accumulation of chromosomal imbalances and translocations in telomere-dysfunctional cells.[134,135] An accumulation of chromosomal aberrations could contribute

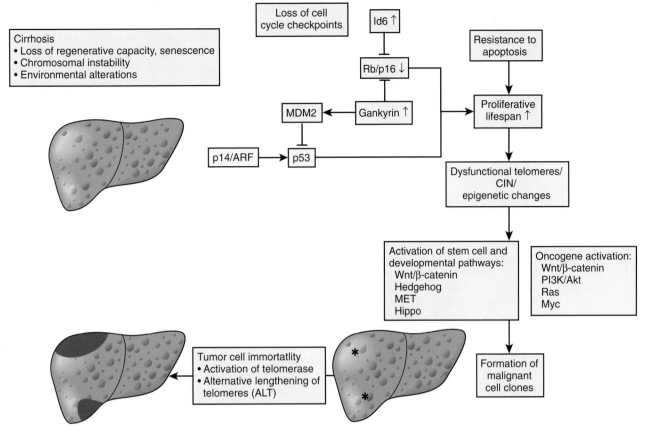

Fig. 10-5 Molecular mechanism of hepatocarcinogenesis at the cirrhosis stage. The most prominent molecular mechanisms that induce hepatocarcinogenesis include (1) induction of chromosomal instability by telomere dysfunction, (2) inactivation of cell cycle checkpoints, (3) inactivation of apoptosis checkpoints, (4) activation of developmental and stem cell pathways, and (5) activation of immortality pathways. It is conceivable that the growth-restricted environment at the cirrhosis stage will first select for repression of apoptosis and the cell cycle checkpoint. Prolonged survival of genetically instable cells with short telomeres can then aggravate the accumulation of chromosomal instability (CIN) and lead to aberrant activation of oncogenic pathways, including developmental and stem cell pathways. Formation of malignant cell clones are depicted as black stars. PI3K, phosphatidylinositol-3′-kinase.

to the transformation of hepatocytes and initiation of tumor development at the cirrhosis stage.

Studies on telomerase knockout mice have revealed that telomere shortening increases the rate of development of liver tumors.[136] A current hypothesis indicates that telomere shortening also contributes to the induction of HCC as a consequence of chronic liver diseases and cirrhosis in humans. In support of this model of telomere dysfunction–induced hepatocarcinogenesis, studies of human HCC have revealed significantly shorter telomeres in the vast majority of human HCC than in surrounding noncancerous liver tissue.[101,137] Moreover, a strong correlation between telomere shortening and aneuploidy was seen at the single-cell level in primary biopsy specimens from human HCC.[138]

Loss of Cell Cycle Checkpoints

Inactivation of cell cycle checkpoints represents a key event in human carcinogenesis, including hepatocarcinogenesis. Cell cycle checkpoints restrict the proliferation of cells in response to a variety of genomic insults, including DNA damage, telomere dysfunction, chromosomal aberrations, and oncogene activation and possibly also in response to epigenetic aberrations.[139] In addition, there is emerging evidence that cell cycle

checkpoints limit the self-renewal of tissue stem cells.[140-142] It is conceivable that loss-of-function mutations of cell cycle checkpoints would confer a growth advantage to cells at the cirrhosis stage, which is characterized by an accumulation of DNA damage, telomere dysfunction, activation of cell cycle checkpoints, and growth inhibition (see earlier). In line with this assumption, the inactivation of cell cycle checkpoints represents a hallmark feature of hepatocarcinogenesis. Among the most commonly affected checkpoints are the following (see **Fig. 10-5**).

p53 Checkpoint

p53 controls multiple checkpoints that can contribute to tumor suppression, including cell cycle arrest, senescence, apoptosis, and autophagy.[143-150] The relative contributions of these different p53-dependent checkpoints in the suppression of hepatocarcinogenesis remain to be determined. Studies on aging telomere-dysfunctional mice revealed that abolishment of p21-dependent cell cycle arrest improved the maintenance of stem cells and organs without increasing chromosomal instability or cancer risk.[99] These findings suggest that it might be a combined action of different p53-dependent checkpoint components that exert the antitumor effects of p53.

Mutation of p53 occurs at high frequency in aflatoxin-induced liver cancer but relatively rarely in other causes.[151,152] However, defects in the p53 pathway in HCC occur at multiple other levels, including microdeletion of the p53 inductor p14 (ARF) (15%),[153] as well as increased expression of negative regulators of p53 such as Mdm2[154] and gankyrin.[155,156] Gankyrin also inhibits Rb checkpoint function (see the next section).

At the cirrhosis stage, defects in p53 checkpoint function could confer a growth advantage to hepatocytes or liver stem cells harboring dysfunctional telomeres or other types of DNA damage. Studies on human fibroblasts have shown that p53 deletion can increase the life span of cells by eliminating induction of cellular senescence.[157] As a consequence, chromosomal instability increases, which can lead to the spontaneous immortalization of rare surviving clones that reactivate telomere maintenance mechanisms.[98] In vivo studies on mouse models have provided experimental evidence that p53 deletion cooperates with telomere dysfunction to induce chromosomal instability in tissue stem cells[158] and induction of epithelial cancers.[134] It is conceivable that the same mechanisms operate in telomere-dysfunctional liver cells at the cirrhosis stage. Recent studies have revealed experimental evidence that p53 also restricts the self-renewal of organ stem cells in response to other oncogenic lesions. It remains to be delineated whether p53-dependent restrictions in stem cell self-renewal contribute to hepatocarcinogenesis. This could be particularly interesting in tumors that exhibit mixed lineage differentiation, possibly originating from transformed liver stem or progenitor cells.[116,117]

Rb/p16

The p16/Rb checkpoint represents another major cell cycle checkpoint that inhibits the proliferation of cells in response to DNA damage, telomere dysfunction, or oncogene activation.[98] In human HCC, the p16/Rb pathway is disrupted in more than 80% of cases, and repression of p16 by promotor hypermethylation represents the most frequent alteration.[159] Moreover, overexpression of negative regulators of Rb/p16 checkpoint function occurs in HCC (e.g., gankyrin),[156] as well as in precancerous cirrhosis (e.g., Id1, an inhibitor of p16).[160] Similar to the results with p53 deletion, deletion of Rb/p16 can increase the proliferative life span of cells with dysfunctional telomeres, in addition to increasing the formation of malignant cell clones in response to oncogene activation.[161,162] It is conceivable that an impairment in the Rb checkpoint allows the expansion of hepatocytes with dysfunctional telomeres at the cirrhosis stage. In agreement with this hypothesis, p16 expression increases in liver cirrhosis but is inhibited in premalignant liver tumors (small cell changes) and HCC.[101]

Transforming Growth Factor-β

Transforming growth factor-β (TGF-β) has strong growth-inhibitory effects on liver cells, and activation of TGF-β is associated with the evolution of cirrhosis in response to telomere shortening.[163,164] It is conceivable that impairments in the TGF-β checkpoint would induce a strong positive selection of premalignant clones at the cirrhosis stage. In agreement with this assumption, loss of heterozygosity in the insulin-like growth factor 2 receptor (IGF2R) locus is a frequent and early event in human hepatocarcinogenesis that occurs in more than 60% of dysplastic nodules and HCC.[165]

IGF2R impairs cell proliferation by promoting degradation of the IGF2 mitogen and by activation of TGF-β signaling.[166] Impairments in TGF-β signaling could also inhibit the over-expression of cytokines, including IL-6.[167] Recent studies have demonstrated that an increase in IL-6 production contributes to the induction of cellular senescence in an autocrine manner.[168] Thus, in a cell autonomous manner, IL-6 may act as a tumor suppressor. Following this line of argumentation, elimination of TGF-β signaling could increase risk for cancer by inactivating induction of IL-6–dependent senescence.

Resistance to Apoptosis

Inhibition of apoptosis may contribute to the induction of HCC at the cirrhosis stage. Increased rates of apoptosis have been observed in chronic liver disease and at the cirrhosis stage.[164,169] Apoptosis is thought to act as a tumor suppressor by depleting damaged and mutant cells. However, this concept has recently been challenged by observations indicating that p53-dependent apoptosis is not required for tumor suppression but could also enhance tumorigenesis in irradiated mice.[170] It is possible that inhibition of apoptosis has different effects when occurring at the single-cell level or at the tissue level. At the single-cell level, elimination of apoptosis may enhance stress resistance and expansion of the mutant cell clone. In contrast, inhibition of apoptosis at the tissue level may lead to improved organ maintenance, thereby reducing environmental alterations that promote the selection of abnormally growing cell clones.

In human HCC, the most frequently affected apoptosis checkpoint is p53-dependent apoptosis. The p53 checkpoint is inactivated in the vast majority of human HCCs (see earlier). It is conceivable that loss of p53-dependent apoptosis contributes to the protumorigenic effects in p53 mutant cells. In agreement with this assumption, it was shown that hepatoma subtracted-cDNA library clone one (HSCO)—an inhibitor of p53-dependent apoptosis—is frequently overexpressed in human HCC.[171] Studies on telomerase knockout mice have shown that p53-independent apoptosis can contribute to the repression of HCC formation in response to telomere dysfunction.[172] Similarly, studies on human fibroblasts have shown that p53-independent apoptosis limits the survival of chromosomally unstable cells with dysfunctional telomeres at the crisis stage.[98] The nature of these p53-independent pathways remains to be defined. TGF-β/SMAD family member 4 (Smad4)–mediated B-cell leukemia/lymphoma 2 (BCL2) repression[173] and apoptosis-inducing genes that influence mitochondrial-induced apoptosis[174] could be relevant in this context. Apoptosis resistance could also involve insulin receptor signaling and activation of the Akt pathway.[175] It is conceivable that inhibition of p53-independent apoptosis could promote the progression of hepatic tumors with dysfunctional p53.

Activation of Oncogenic Pathways

A variety of oncogenic pathways have been implicated in hepatocarcinogenesis, thus indicating that activation of oncogenes is less uniform in HCC than in other cancers. A potential explanation is the high rate of chromosomal instability in HCC. It is possible that activation of oncogenes represents a late event in human HCC. The growth-inhibitory environment in cirrhosis and activation of intrinsic cell checkpoints limiting hepatocyte regeneration (senescence, apoptosis) induce a strong selection for the elimination of checkpoint genes. According to this hypothesis, the deletion of checkpoints may be an early event in hepatocarcinogenesis, followed by clonal expansion and chromosomal instability, which ultimately lead to oncogene activation and tumor growth. Among the most frequent oncogenic pathways in cirrhosis are the following.

Wnt/β-Catenin

The β-catenin pathway is temporarily up-regulated during early liver development.[176] Somatic mutations that lead to activation of the β-catenin pathway frequently occur in mouse and human HCC.[177] In addition, transcriptional repression of negative regulators of the Wnt pathway occurs in gastrointestinal cancers.[178-181] Studies in mouse models have revealed experimental evidence that hepatic deletion of adenomatosis polyposis coli (APC) with the consequent activation of β-catenin is sufficient to induce hepatocarcinogenesis.[182]

It is interesting to note that the Wnt/β-catenin pathway is one of the major pathways regulating the function of adult stem cells. Other developmental and stem cell–associated pathways that have been implicated in hepatocarcinogenesis are the Hedgehog pathway,[183] the MET pathway,[184] and the Hippo pathway.[185] The latter pathway has also been implicated in controlling liver size by regulating the proliferation of hepatocytes and liver stem cells.[186] Whether activation of stem cell pathways is associated with liver stem cell–derived hepatocarcinogenesis is currently unknown. It has been recognized that 20% to 30% of human HCCs exhibit bilinear differentiation into hepatocytes and cholangiocytes and the expression of stem cell markers.[116-118,187,188] Moreover, gene expression analysis has revealed that a subset of human HCC exhibits a stem cell gene expression signature.[188] It remains to be determined whether stem cells are indeed the cell type of origin of this type of HCC. Alternatively, hepatocytes may dedifferentiate to acquire stem cell–like properties during the transformation process.

PI3K/Akt

Activation of Akt signaling and impaired expression of PTEN (a negative regulator of Akt) have been reported in more than 40% of human HCCs.[189] Activation of the Akt pathway has prosurvival and growth-stimulatory effects involving the suppression of TGF-β–dependent apoptosis and blockage of the growth-inhibitory effect of C/EBPα through the protein phosphatase 2A (PP2A)-mediated dephosphorylation of C/EBPα on Ser193.[144,190] Both effects could promote tumor formation at the cirrhosis stage. Activation of the Akt pathway has been linked to activation of β-catenin signaling in intestinal stem cells.[191] It remains to be seen whether oncogenic activation of these pathways is also interconnected in hepatocarcinogenesis.

Ras

Activation of the *Ras* oncogene is a frequent event in human carcinogenesis in different organ compartments. In contrast to other types of cancer, human HCC rarely carries activating mutations in the *Ras* gene itself.[192] However, recent studies have provided compelling evidence that activation of the Ras signaling pathway occurs in the vast majority of human HCCs involving hypermethylation of the *Ras*-binding tumor suppressor genes *RASSF1A* and *NORE1A*.[193,194]

myc

Transgenic mouse models have provided experimental evidence that sustained activation of c-*myc* is sufficient to induce hepatocarcinogenesis.[195] In addition, it has been shown that *myc*-induced HCC remains *myc* dependent and that inactivation of the oncogene induces tumor regression. *myc* is also thought to be involved in human hepatocarcinogenesis, with activation of *myc* correlating with tumor size and prognosis.[196,197] One mechanism of *myc* activation in human HCC is amplification of the genomic *myc* locus.[122] These data indicate that chromosomal instability at the cirrhosis stage may select for chromosomal aberrations leading to the activation of *myc*. As outlined earlier, inactivation of checkpoint genes (e.g., *p53*) may enhance the induction of chromosomal instability by allowing clonal outgrow of unstable cells carrying dysfunctional telomeres and DNA damage. In agreement with this assumption, aneuploidy with an increased copy number of the *myc*-carrying chromosome represents a very frequent event in genetically unstable mouse HCC induced in the context of telomere dysfunction and p53 deletion.[172]

The similarities in mouse and human HCC indicate that the biology of control of liver cell proliferation is highly conserved across these species. Accordingly, an interspecies comparison could help identify novel oncogenes and tumor suppressor genes that are relevant for hepatocarcinogenesis. In principle, such approaches could include gene expression profiling, mapping of chromosomal aberrations, and functional genomic screens. Given the high rates of instability in HCC, interspecies comparisons could be particularly relevant to distinguish functional relevant lesions from bystander lesions. The initial reports on the identification of new antiapoptotic and oncogenic pathways in hepatocarcinogenesis support this concept.[198]

Tumor Cell Immortality

As described earlier, telomere shortening limits the proliferative capacity of human cells to a finite number of cell divisions by induction of cell cycle arrest (senescence) or apoptosis (crisis). To gain immortal growth capacity, tumor cells have to overcome this roadblock to cancer formation. Current data indicate that the vast majority of human HCCs reactivate the enzyme complex telomerase to stabilize telomeres and to gain immortal growth capacity. More than 90% of human HCCs show activation of telomerase, specifically, up-regulation of TERT (telomerase reverse transcriptase), which is the rate-limiting component of telomerase activity in most human cell types.[199] Telomerase activity is not detectable in normal human liver; however, significant telomerase activation occurs during the transition from premalignant lesions to HCC.[199] Experiments on primary human cells have shown that telomerase can immortalize human cells, including hepatocytes.[132] Moreover, activation of telomerase is an essential component for the generation of transformed human cells with unlimited proliferative potential.[200] In contrast, inhibition of telomerase was sufficient to shorten telomeres in human cancer cell lines and led to impaired proliferative capacity of tumor cells.[201] Pharmacologic inhibition of human telomerase was also sufficient to inhibit the growth of human HCC in xenotransplantation models.[202] Inhibition of tumor growth was associated with accumulating telomere dysfunction, chromosomal instability, and tumor cell death. Together, these data indicate that telomerase activation is an essential step in human hepatocarcinogenesis that is required for the gain of immortal growth capacity and tumor progression. According to these data, inhibition of telomerase could also represent a potential target for future therapies for HCC. Inhibitors of human telomerase are currently in clinical phase II trials for the treatment of other types of human cancer,[203] such as lymphoma. A possible limitation of telomerase-targeting therapies could be the reactivation of alternative lengthening of telomeres (telomerase-independent mechanisms).[204,205] Activation of alternative lengthening of telomeres leads to maintenance of telomere length by DNA recombination–based mechanisms. Studies on inhibition of telomerase in human cancer cell lines have shown that activation of alternative lengthening of telomeres could represent an escape mechanism leading to regain of immortal growth capacity in telomerase-inhibited tumor cells.[206]

Summary and Outlook

The pathophysiology of hepatocarcinogenesis is tightly linked to the prevalence of chronic liver disease and disease-specific risk factors. Moreover, the evolution of cirrhosis represents a unifying risk factor for the evolution of HCC in response to various chronic liver diseases. Several mechanisms appear to cooperate to induce hepatocarcinogenesis in this context. At the intrinsic cell level, chronic liver disease induces an increase in cell turnover that leads to telomere shortening, accumulation of DNA damage, dysfunctional telomeres, and an increase in chromosomal instability. Accumulation of damage in cells leads to the activation of cell cycle and apoptosis checkpoints that impair tissue regeneration and increase the selective pressure for abnormally growing cell and stem cell clones. In addition, hepatocyte senescence, regenerative dysfunction, infiltrating immune cells, fibrosis, and steatosis all contribute to increasing alterations in the microenvironment and macroenvironment, including increased production of locally and systemically acting cytokines and growth factors. These alterations in the environment lead to a further increase in the selection of aberrantly growing cell and stem cell clones. In this context, inactivation of the cell cycle and apoptosis checkpoints can represent an early lesion conferring a growth advantage to individual cell clones. However, clonal expansion of such unstable cells will ultimately lead to the activation of oncogenic pathways, cellular transformation, and eventually immortalization of malignant clones. Detailed analysis of the molecular chain of events that induce tumor initiation and progression at the cirrhosis stage will help in developing novel markers and therapeutic targets to improve surveillance, prevention, and treatment of HCC in patients with chronic liver disease and cirrhosis.

Key References

Abe H, et al. Etiology of non-B non-C hepatocellular carcinoma in the eastern district of Tokyo. J Gastroenterol 2008;43:967–974. (Ref.55)

Altekruse SF, McGlynn KA, Reichman ME. Hepatocellular carcinoma incidence, mortality, and survival trends in the United States from 1975 to 2005. J Clin Oncol 2009;27:1485–1491. (Ref.13)

Amann T, et al. Activated hepatic stellate cells promote tumorigenicity of hepatocellular carcinoma. Cancer Sci 2009;100:646–653. (Ref.108)

Asahina Y, et al. Effect of aging on risk for hepatocellular carcinoma in chronic hepatitis C virus infection. Hepatology 2010;52:518–527. (Ref.103)

Bantel H, et al. Detection of apoptotic caspase activation in sera from patients with chronic HCV infection is associated with fibrotic liver injury. Hepatology 2004;40:1078–1087. (Ref.169)

Bataller R, Brenner DA. Liver fibrosis. J Clin Invest 2005;115:209–218. (Ref.109)

Becker C, et al. TGF-beta suppresses tumor progression in colon cancer by inhibition of IL-6 trans-signaling. Immunity 2004;21:491–501. (Ref.167)

Begus-Nahrmann Y, et al. p53 deletion impairs clearance of chromosomal-instable stem cells in aging telomere-dysfunctional mice. Nat Genet 2009; 41:1138–1143. (Ref.158)

Bilousova G, et al. Impaired DNA replication within progenitor cell pools promotes leukemogenesis. PLoS Biol 2005;3:e401. (Ref.95)

Bosch FX, et al. Epidemiology of hepatocellular carcinoma. Clin Liver Dis 2005; 9:191–211, v. (Ref.2)

Bravi F, et al. Coffee drinking and hepatocellular carcinoma risk: a meta-analysis. Hepatology 2007;46:430–435. (Ref.78)

Budanov AV, Karin M. p53 target genes sestrin1 and sestrin2 connect genotoxic stress and mTOR signaling. Cell 2008;134:451–460. (Ref.149)

Calvisi DF, et al. Ubiquitous activation of Ras and Jak/Stat pathways in human HCC. Gastroenterology 2006;130:1117–1128. (Ref.193)

Chan DW, et al. Prickle-1 negatively regulates Wnt/beta-catenin pathway by promoting Dishevelled ubiquitination/degradation in liver cancer. Gastroenterology 2006;131:1218–1227. (Ref.181)

Chen CJ, Yang HI, Iloeje UH. Hepatitis B virus DNA levels and outcomes in chronic hepatitis B. Hepatology 2009;49:S72–S84. (Ref.30)

Chiba T, et al. Side population purified from hepatocellular carcinoma cells harbour cancer stem cell–like properties. Hepatology 2006;44:240–251. (Ref.187)

Choudhury AR, et al. Cdkn1a deletion improves stem cell function and lifespan of mice with dysfunctional telomeres without accelerating cancer formation. Nat Genet 2007;39:99–105. (Ref.99)

Cicalese A, et al. The tumor suppressor p53 regulates polarity of self-renewing divisions in mammary stem cells. Cell 2009;138:1083–1095. (Ref.140)

Colnot S, et al. Liver-targeted disruption of Apc in mice activates beta-catenin signaling and leads to hepatocellular carcinomas. Proc Natl Acad Sci U S A 2004;101:17216–17221. (Ref.182)

Crighton D, et al. DRAM, a p53-induced modulator of autophagy, is critical for apoptosis. Cell 2006;126:121–134. (Ref.148)

Davalos AR, et al. Senescent cells as a source of inflammatory factors for tumor progression. Cancer Metastasis Rev 2010;29:273–283. (Ref.111)

Di Bisceglie AM, et al. Prolonged therapy of advanced chronic hepatitis C with low-dose peginterferon. N Engl J Med 2008;359:2429–2441. (Ref.52)

Djojosubroto MW, et al. Telomerase antagonists GRN163 and GRN163L inhibit tumor growth and increase chemosensitivity of human hepatoma. Hepatology 2005;42:1127–1136. (Ref.202)

El-Serag HB. Hepatocellular carcinoma: recent trends in the United States. Gastroenterology 2004;127:S27–S34. (Ref.6)

El-Serag HB, Hampel H, Javadi F. The association between diabetes and hepatocellular carcinoma: a systematic review of epidemiologic evidence. Clin Gastroenterol Hepatol 2006;4:369–380. (Ref.77)

El-Serag HB, Rudolph KL. Hepatocellular carcinoma: epidemiology and molecular carcinogenesis. Gastroenterology 2007;132:2557–2576. (Ref.27)

El Serag HB, Tran T, Everhart JE. Diabetes increases the risk of chronic liver disease and hepatocellular carcinoma. Gastroenterology 2004;126:460–468. (Ref.73)

Farazi PA, DePinho RA. Hepatocellular carcinoma pathogenesis: from genes to environment. Nat Rev Cancer 2006;6:674–687. (Ref.139)

Fattovich G, et al. Hepatocellular carcinoma in cirrhosis: incidence and risk factors. Gastroenterology 2004;127(5 Suppl 1):S35–S50. (Ref.17)

Feng Z, et al. The coordinate regulation of the p53 and mTOR pathways in cells. Proc Natl Acad Sci U S A 2005;102:8204–8209. (Ref.147)

Galicia VA, et al. Expansion of hepatic tumor progenitor cells in Pten-null mice requires liver injury and is reversed by loss of AKT2. Gastroenterology 2010; 139:2170–2182. (Ref.119)

Gelatti U, et al. Coffee consumption reduces the risk of hepatocellular carcinoma independently of its aetiology: a case-control study. J Hepatol 2005;42: 528–534. (Ref.82)

Haybaeck J, et al. A lymphotoxin-driven pathway to hepatocellular carcinoma. Cancer Cell 2009;16:295–308. (Ref.104)

He XC, et al. PTEN-deficient intestinal stem cells initiate intestinal polyposis. Nat Genet 2007;39:189–198. (Ref.191)

Higashitsuji H, et al. The oncoprotein gankyrin binds to MDM2/HDM2, enhancing ubiquitylation and degradation of p53. Cancer Cell 2005;8:75–87. (Ref.156)

Huang XX, et al. Up-regulation of proproliferative genes and the ligand/receptor pair placental growth factor and vascular endothelial growth factor receptor 1 in hepatitis C cirrhosis. Liver Int 2007;27:960–968. (Ref.106)

Inoue M, et al. Influence of coffee drinking on subsequent risk of hepatocellular carcinoma: a prospective study in Japan. J Natl Cancer Inst 2005;97:293–300. (Ref.85)

Jablkowski M, et al. A comparative study of P53/MDM2 genes alterations and P53/MDM2 proteins immunoreactivity in liver cirrhosis and hepatocellular carcinoma. J Exp Clin Cancer Res 2005;24:117–125. (Ref.154)

Ju Z, et al. Telomere dysfunction induces environmental alterations limiting hematopoietic stem cell function and engraftment. Nat Med 2007;13:742–747. (Ref.112)

Kaposi-Novak P, et al. Met-regulated expression signature defines a subset of human hepatocellular carcinomas with poor prognosis and aggressive phenotype. J Clin Invest 2006;116:1582–1595. (Ref.184)

Karreth FA, Tuveson DA. Modelling oncogenic Ras/Raf signalling in the mouse. Curr Opin Genet Dev 2009;19:4–11. (Ref.192)

Kim SR, et al. Epidemiology of hepatocellular carcinoma in Japan and Korea. A review. Oncology 2008;75(Suppl 1):13–16. (Ref.21)

Kossatz U, et al. The cyclin E regulator cullin 3 prevents mouse hepatic progenitor cells from becoming tumor-initiating cells. J Clin Invest 2010;120:3820–3833. (Ref.120)

Kuilman T, et al. Oncogene-induced senescence relayed by an interleukin-dependent inflammatory network. Cell 2008;133:1019–1031. (Ref.168)

Kurozawa Y, et al. Coffee and risk of death from hepatocellular carcinoma in a large cohort study in Japan. Br J Cancer 2005;93:607–610. (Ref.86)

Lechel A, et al. Telomerase deletion limits progression of p53-mutant hepatocellular carcinoma with short telomeres in chronic liver disease. Gastroenterology 2007;132:1465–1475. (Ref.172)

Lee JS, et al. A novel prognostic subtype of human hepatocellular carcinoma derived from hepatic progenitor cells. Nat Med 2006;12:410–416. (Ref.188)

Liaw YF, et al. Lamivudine for patients with chronic hepatitis B and advanced liver disease. N Engl J Med 2004;351:1521–1531. (Ref.32)

Llovet JM, et al. A molecular signature to discriminate dysplastic nodules from early hepatocellular carcinoma in HCV cirrhosis. Gastroenterology 2006;131:1758–1767. (Ref.199)

Lu L, et al. Hippo signaling is a potent in vivo growth and tumor suppressor pathway in the mammalian liver. Proc Natl Acad Sci U S A 2010;107:1437–1442. (Ref.185)

Malhi H, Gores GJ. Cellular and molecular mechanisms of liver injury. Gastroenterology 2008;134:1641–1654. (Ref.164)

Marquardt JU, Thorgeirsson SS. Stem cells in hepatocarcinogenesis: evidence from genomic data. Semin Liver Dis 2010;30:26–34. (Ref.117)

Martin J, et al. Hint2, a mitochondrial apoptotic sensitizer down-regulated in hepatocellular carcinoma. Gastroenterology 2006;130:2179–2188. (Ref.174)

Matsuda Y, et al. Overexpressed Id-1 is associated with a high risk of hepatocellular carcinoma development in patients with cirrhosis without transcriptional repression of p16. Cancer 2005;104:1037–1044. (Ref.160)

Matsuzaki K, et al. Chronic inflammation associated with hepatitis C virus infection perturbs hepatic transforming growth factor beta signaling, promoting cirrhosis and hepatocellular carcinoma. Hepatology 2007;46:48–57. (Ref.107)

Michalak EM, et al. Apoptosis-promoted tumorigenesis: gamma-irradiation–induced thymic lymphomagenesis requires Puma-driven leukocyte death. Genes Dev 2010;24:1608–1613. (Ref.170)

Micsenyi A, et al. Beta-catenin is temporally regulated during normal liver development. Gastroenterology 2004;126:1134–1146. (Ref.176)

Moinzadeh P, et al. Chromosome alterations in human hepatocellular carcinomas correlate with aetiology and histological grade—results of an explorative CGH meta-analysis. Br J Cancer 2005;92:935–941. (Ref.123)

Montella M, et al. Coffee and tea consumption and risk of hepatocellular carcinoma in Italy. Int J Cancer 2007;120:1555–1559. (Ref.79)

Newell P, et al. Ras pathway activation in hepatocellular carcinoma and anti-tumoral effect of combined sorafenib and rapamycin in vivo. J Hepatol 2009;51:725–733. (Ref.195)

Nguyen VT, Law MG, Dore GJ. Hepatitis B–related hepatocellular carcinoma: epidemiological characteristics and disease burden. J Viral Hepat 2009;16:453–463. (Ref.8)

Ogata H, et al. Deletion of the SOCS3 gene in liver parenchymal cells promotes hepatitis-induced hepatocarcinogenesis. Gastroenterology 2006;131:179–193. (Ref.114)

Ohfuji S, et al. Coffee consumption and reduced risk of hepatocellular carcinoma among patients with chronic type C liver disease: a case-control study. Hepatol Res 2006;36:201–208. (Ref.84)

Ong JP, Pitts A, Younossi ZM. Increased overall mortality and liver-related mortality in non-alcoholic fatty liver disease. J Hepatol 2008;49:608–612. (Ref.53)

Park EJ, et al. Dietary and genetic obesity promote liver inflammation and tumorigenesis by enhancing IL-6 and TNF expression. Cell 2010;140:197–208. (Ref.105)

Parkin DM. The global health burden of infection-associated cancers in the year 2002. Int J Cancer 2006;118:3030–3044. (Ref.20)

Parrinello S, et al. Stromal-epithelial interactions in aging and cancer: senescent fibroblasts alter epithelial cell differentiation. J Cell Sci 2005;118:485–496. (Ref.113)

Plentz RR, et al. Hepatocellular telomere shortening correlates with chromosomal instability and the development of human hepatoma. Hepatology 2004;40:80–86. (Ref.137)

Plentz RR, et al. Telomere shortening and inactivation of cell cycle checkpoints characterize human hepatocarcinogenesis. Hepatology 2007;45:968–976. (Ref.101)

Plentz RR, et al. Telomere shortening correlates with increasing aneuploidy of chromosome 8 in human hepatocellular carcinoma. Hepatology 2005;42:522–526. (Ref.138)

Ratziu V, Trabut JB, Poynard T. Fat, diabetes, and liver injury in chronic hepatitis C. Curr Gastroenterol Rep 2004;6:22–29. (Ref.61)

Raza SA, Clifford GM, Franceschi S. Worldwide variation in the relative importance of hepatitis B and hepatitis C viruses in hepatocellular carcinoma: a systematic review. Br J Cancer 2007;96:1127–1134. (Ref.22)

Regimbeau JM, et al. Obesity and diabetes as a risk factor for hepatocellular carcinoma. Liver Transpl 2004;10:S69–S73. (Ref.58)

Ries L, et al. SEER cancer statistics review, 1975-2004. Bethesda, MD: National Cancer Institute, 2007. (Ref.7)

Roskams T. Liver stem cells and their implication in hepatocellular and cholangiocarcinoma. Oncogene 2006;25:3818–3822. (Ref.116)

Shachaf CM, et al. Related MYC inactivation uncovers pluripotent differentiation and tumour dormancy in hepatocellular cancer. Nature 2004;431:1112–1117. (Ref.195)

Shay JW, Wright WE. Telomerase therapeutics for cancer: challenges and new directions. Nat Rev Drug Discov 2006;5:577–584. (Ref.203)

Shepard CW, Finelli L, Alter MJ. Global epidemiology of hepatitis C virus infection. Lancet Infect Dis 2005;5:558–567. (Ref.42)

Shi J, et al. A meta-analysis of case-control studies on the combined effect of hepatitis B and C virus infections in causing hepatocellular carcinoma in China. Br J Cancer 2005;92:607–612. (Ref.26)

Shimazu T, et al. Coffee consumption and the risk of primary liver cancer: pooled analysis of two prospective studies in Japan. Int J Cancer 2005;116:150–154. (Ref.80)

Sicklick JK, et al. Dysregulation of the Hedgehog pathway in human hepatocarcinogenesis. Carcinogenesis 2006;27:748–757. (Ref.183)

Singal AG, et al. A sustained viral response is associated with reduced liver-related morbidity and mortality in patients with hepatitis C virus. Clin Gastroenterol Hepatol 2010;8:280–288. (Ref.50)

Singal AK, et al. Antiviral therapy reduces risk of hepatocellular carcinoma in patients with hepatitis C virus–related cirrhosis. Clin Gastroenterol Hepatol 2010;8:192–199. (Ref.51)

Stanger BZ, Tanaka AJ, Melton DA. Organ size is limited by the number of embryonic progenitor cells in the pancreas but not the liver. Nature 2007;445:886–891. (Ref.115)

Talamini R, et al. Food groups and risk of hepatocellular carcinoma: a multicenter case-control study in Italy. Int J Cancer 2006;119:2916–2921. (Ref.74)

Tanaka K, et al. Inverse association between coffee drinking and the risk of hepatocellular carcinoma: a case-control study in Japan. Cancer Sci 2007;98:214–218. (Ref.83)

Tasdemir E, et al. Regulation of autophagy by cytoplasmic p53. Nat Cell Biol 2008;10:676–687. (Ref.150)

Wang GL, et al. Liver tumors escape negative control of proliferation via PI3K/Akt-mediated block of C/EBP alpha growth inhibitory activity. Genes Dev 2004;18:912–925. (Ref.190)

Wilkens L, et al. Induction of aneuploidy by increasing chromosomal instability during dedifferentiation of hepatocellular carcinoma. Proc Natl Acad Sci U S A 2004;101:1309–1314. (Ref.122)

Willis G, et al. Hepatocellular carcinoma and the penetrance of HFE C282Y mutations: a cross sectional study. BMC Gastroenterol 2005;5:17. (Ref.90)

World Health Organization. Hepatitis B. 2008 (Fact Sheet No. 204). Geneva: WHO, 2010. (Ref.19)

Yang HI, et al. Associations between hepatitis B virus genotype and mutants and the risk of hepatocellular carcinoma. J Natl Cancer Inst 2008;100:1134–1143. (Ref.31)

Yang YA, et al. Smad3 reduces susceptibility to hepatocarcinoma by sensitizing hepatocytes to apoptosis through downregulation of Bcl-2. Cancer Cell 2006;9:445–457. (Ref.173)

Yeung YP, et al. Natural history of untreated nonsurgical hepatocellular carcinoma. Am J Gastroenterol 2005;100:1995–2004. (Ref.10)

Younossi ZM, Stepanova M. Hepatitis C virus infection, age, and Hispanic ethnicity increase mortality from liver cancer in the United States. Clin Gastroenterol Hepatol 2010;8:718–723. (Ref.54)

Yu MC, Yuan JM. Environmental factors and risk for hepatocellular carcinoma. Gastroenterology 2004;127:S72–S78. (Ref.87)

Yuan Y, et al. In vivo self-renewing divisions of haematopoietic stem cells are increased in the absence of the early G_1-phase inhibitor, p18INK4C. Nat Cell Biol 2004;6:436–442. (Ref.142)

Zender L, et al. Identification and validation of oncogenes in liver cancer using an integrative oncogenomic approach. Cell 2006;125:1253–1267. (Ref.198)

Zhou D, et al. Mst1 and Mst2 maintain hepatocyte quiescence and suppress hepatocellular carcinoma development through inactivation of the Yap1 oncogene. Cancer Cell 2009;16:425–438. (Ref.186)

A complete list of references can be found at www.expertconsult.com.

Stem Cells and Hepatocyte Transplantation

Sanjeev Gupta

ABBREVIATIONS

AFP α-fetoprotein
FAH fumaryl acetoacetate hydrolase
hESC human embryonic stem cells
LDLR low-density lipoprotein receptor

LEC Long-Evans cinnamon
MAPC multipotent adult progenitor cells
NAR Nagase analbuminemic rat
OLT orthotopic liver transplantation

T₃ triiodothyronine
VEGF vascular endothelial growth factor

Introduction

Identification of the hepatic stem cell will advance hepatology in many ways, including by facilitating insights into the development, regeneration, and repair of the liver. From an applied perspective, isolation of cells amenable to cryostorage, manipulation, and expansion in vitro, as well as survival in vivo following transplantation, will be highly appropriate. The common belief is that stem cells are capable of self-renewal. Through cells harboring extensive proliferation ability, often designated as transit-amplifying, lineage-restricted, or facultative progenitor cells, stem cells can produce progeny that may generate an entire animal (totipotency), all lineages (pluripotency), multiple lineages (multipotency), two lineages (bipotency), or even single lineages.

Most experts agree that stem/progenitor cells have a role to play in the liver.[1,2] However, the hepatic stem cell has neither been isolated nor been fully defined, although under specific circumstances activation of candidate liver stem cells has been shown. As discussed elsewhere, the liver is composed of multiple cell types that arise from separate germ layers; for example, epithelial cells, including hepatocytes, are endodermal in origin; liver sinusoidal endothelial cells, the next largest liver cell compartment, as well as Kupffer cells, are of mesodermal origin; and hepatic stellate cells exhibit features of the mesoderm and neuroectoderm. However, these concepts concerning germ-layer origins of cells may change in the future, while more is learned about mechanisms of lineage differentiation in pluripotential stem cells. Nonetheless, this embryologic diversity of cells produces unique, albeit incompletely defined, cell–cell interactions during both health and disease,[3] with further relevance for mobilization, recruitment, and expansion of endogenous stem–progenitor cells as well as for engraftment and proliferation of transplanted cells in the liver.

In contrast with the embryonic or the fetal liver, the normal adult liver is essentially a stable organ without significant cell turnover, and consequently it has generally been difficult to identify or to classify hepatic stem/progenitor cells in the conventional sense of cell lineages, as is understood for the hematopoietic system, for example. The fetal human liver develops quickly during the first two trimesters and contains rapidly cycling cells that exhibit properties of epithelial as well as mesenchymal cells, along with multilineage cell markers.[4,5] Under appropriate differentiation conditions, fetal liver cells can generate cells with properties of hepatocytes, cholangiocytes, endothelial cells, or even adipocytes,[5] which suggests that a common liver stem cell could potentially produce the entire organ. Although uncertainty in the location of the common liver stem cell has spawned numerous studies, this concept deserves further exploration. Among others, subsets of non-parenchymal liver epithelial cells, designated "oval cells," which were originally identified in the oncogenetically perturbed rat liver, have been assigned progenitor cell properties.[1-6] The molecular basis of lineage relationships between oval cells arising during carcinogenesis and those resembling oval cells in healthy fetal and adult livers is not well understood. Although the biology of healthy stem cells and cancer stem cells is of great interest, including for elucidating pathophysiologic mechanisms and developing therapies in liver cancer, these issues are beyond the scope of this chapter (see Sell and Leffert [2008][7] for a review). It should be pointed out that similar considerations apply to other organs (e.g., the pancreas, which is related to the liver by sharing its origin from the embryonic foregut endoderm).[8] Moreover, recent studies with isolated fetal pancreatic stem/progenitor cells established that these exhibited multilineage markers with epithelial and mesenchymal signatures that recapitulated the features of fetal liver stem/progenitor cells.[9] Although fetal liver, as well as pancreatic stem/progenitor cells, showed the capacity to proliferate considerably under culture conditions, compared with mature cells, this was not unlimited, and genetic manipulations were needed to enhance their

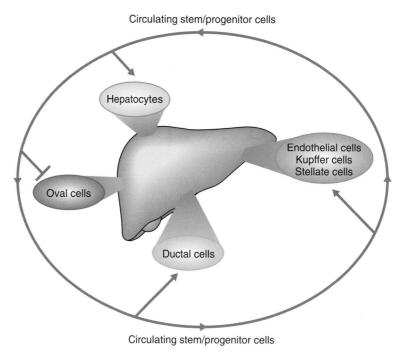

Fig. 11-1 Various sources of stem/progenitor cells in the adult liver. The adult liver is replicatively quiescent, but following injury to hepatocytes (e.g., liver resection) or bile ducts (e.g., biliary obstruction), these cell compartments can renew themselves, without recruiting stem/progenitor cells from elsewhere. However, in the presence of overwhelming parenchymal injury, resident facultative progenitor cells—"oval cells"—may appear, and these cells may replenish either hepatocytes or bile duct cells, as necessary. Evidence has also been provided for the capacity of hepatocytes to produce bile duct cells under certain circumstances. Circulating stem/progenitor cells do not contribute to the replenishment of parenchymal liver cells under physiologic circumstances, although hepatic stellate cells and Kupffer cells may be derived from stem/progenitor cells in the blood circulation. Whether liver sinusoidal endothelial cells could arise from circulating cells is uncertain. Bone marrow–derived cells do not generate hepatic oval cells and may generate only rare hepatocytes at best, although the role of cell fusion in this situation is controversial.

replication potential. On the other hand, under specific circumstances, adult hepatocytes demonstrate an indefinite stem cell–like replication potential in vivo.[10] The possibility that stem cells normally residing elsewhere in other organs may arrive through the circulation to generate liver cells captured considerable attention (**Fig. 11-1**), although experimental studies have led to uncertainties about the significance of this mechanism.

Because the supplies of donor human livers are limited, orthotopic liver transplantation (OLT) has been generally hampered, and improved utilization in recent years of donor livers for OLT has led to further decline in the number and quality of donor livers for cell isolation. Although hepatocytes have been transplanted in patients with many conditions, expansion of this early experience is currently restricted by the limited availability of donor human livers.[11] Therefore alternative sources of donor cells remain critical for advancing liver cell therapy. If stem cells are to meet this challenge, it will be helpful to obtain limitless supplies of undifferentiated stem/progenitor cells maintained and expanded without feeder cells or biologic products from other species; to have the ability to genetically manipulate stem/progenitor cells without deleterious perturbations or transformation; to efficiently and reproducibly differentiate stem/progenitor cells along lineages either before or after cell transplantation; and to identify stem/progenitor cells with the capacity to repopulate healthy or diseased organs without rejection. In parallel, optimal clinical protocols for cell transplantation, including strategies to

promote cell engraftment and proliferation, as well as to demonstrate the overall mass, function, and fate of transplanted cells in humans, will be most helpful.

Candidate Stem/Progenitor Cell Populations for Liver-Directed Cell Therapy

In principle, allogeneic stem/progenitor cells may be isolated from the liver as well as from extrahepatic sources, including embryonic, fetal, and adult organs. Although autologous stem cells can be readily harvested from the bone marrow or peripheral blood of individuals, isolation of hepatocytes requires surgery to obtain portions of the liver, which is an invasive procedure that deserves appropriate consideration.

In 1998 human embryonic stem cells (hESC) were first isolated from discarded embryos by dissociating the inner cell mass of blastocysts,[12] and these cells constituted a unique example of totipotent or pluripotent cells. Relatively few hESC lines were available for studies, as the policy of the United States was to restrict federally funded research to hESC lines created before August 9, 2001, although on March 9, 2009, some but not all barriers to research involving human stem cells were revised (to review the evolution of policies and qualified hESC cell lines for federally funded U.S. research, visit *http://stemcells.nih.gov/index.asp*). Most experts agree that large numbers of hESC lines are needed to study the biologic potential of hESC and to develop translational applications, such as for model development, drug discovery, and toxicity testing. With the recognition that hESC lines differed from one another for unknown reasons that alter requirements for growth, maintenance, and differentiation,[13] more cell lines have been created and examined without federal funds. Also, the states of California and New York assigned major public funds over 10-year spans to support stem cell research. These efforts are aimed at benefiting stem cell sciences, promoting the biotechnology industry, and advancing clinical applications, which will all be helped by large banks of hESC lines spanning the genetic diversity of human populations.

A major source of the excitement in stem cell research concerned generating indefinite supplies of autologous cells from individual donors, initially by somatic cell nuclear transfer, and later by the more efficient process of nuclear reprogramming of somatic cells by four transcriptional factors, as shown by the groups of Yamanaka and Thomson to generate "induced pluripotential stem (iPS) cells."[14,15] This fundamental discovery of nuclear reprogramming has been of enormous interest for defining basic mechanisms in the origin and maintenance of stem cells as well as the lineage differentiation and dedifferentiation of cells. Some have considered that the advent of iPS cells no longer requires hESC; more recently, however, careful studies of hESC and iPS cells have begun to demonstrate critical differences, including limitations in the overall replication potential of iPS cells compared with hESC.[10b] From a clinical perspective, the availability of autologous cells will obviously help avoid rejection after transplantation. Similarly, the availability of genetically-defined hESC or iPS cell lines will help define the basic biology of stem cells, including critical issues such as what imparts "stemness" to hESC and iPS cells; what regulates silencing and activation of specific genes and gene networks in hESC or iPS cells compared with other more differentiated cells; what underlies the capacity of hESC to replicate indefinitely without undergoing senescence or other deleterious changes, compared with iPS cells and other cells; and what mechanisms could induce differentiation in hESC or iPS cells, and other candidate stem/progenitor cells, along lineages of interest.

Progress has been made in understanding the potential of hESC and iPS cells, although much more needs to be accomplished. For instance, transplantation of undifferentiated hESC and of iPS cells results in formation of teratomas or teratocarcinomas, essentially by default, although this intrinsic teratogenic potential can be circumvented by the intermediary step of "embryoid body" formation before cell dissociation, particularly in hESC. Unique, albeit incompletely characterized, hepatic-like hESC subpopulations were selected initially through promoter regulation and expression of the endoderm-specifying Foxa2 (HNF-3β) transcription factor or chemicals (e.g., butyrate). Similarly, specific soluble signals were utilized to circumvent the requirement of embryoid body formation to obtain hepatic-like cells from stem cells. Early genome-wide transcription profiling of undifferentiated and differentiated stem cells identified changes in gene expression patterns under different states of hESC, including onset of fetal hepatic-enriched genes after formation of embryoid bodies. These types of studies initiated many other investigations into the activation of hepatic lineage-specific gene expression in stem cells, including the capacity

of hESC-derived and also iPS-derived cells to generate hepatocytes after transplantation in animals.[16-19]

The role of specific genetic pathways in the differentiation of hESC or iPS cells is being studied. Specific cell signaling pathways (e.g., the wnt pathway) were found to serve key roles in promoting and maintaining hESC in an undifferentiated state. The principles driving differentiation in stem cells along some lineages are now better understood, whereas regulation of stem cell differentiation along endodermal lineages (e.g., hepatic and pancreatic β-cell lineages) is less well defined.[9] Another restriction at present concerns expanding the number of differentiated cells derived from hESC or iPS cells because proliferation declines rapidly in differentiating cells. Moreover, scaling-up of hESC or iPS cells for clinical applications will be a major obstacle attributable to the cost of necessary hormones, sera, and additives. Also, it will be essential to eliminate or substitute animal products and feeder cells for transplanting stem cell–derived cells into humans. Because the selection of nontumorigenic subclones, especially in the case of iPS cells, will necessitate extensive efforts and prolonged culture, this may introduce further spontaneous genetic perturbations. Therefore considerable work lies ahead before hESC- or iPS-derived cells could become available for clinical testing.

Donor fetal tissues constitute an alternative source of stem cells or stem/progenitor cells with certain advantages. For instance, instead of being completely undifferentiated, fetal progenitor cells are already committed along given lineages, while retaining significant capacity for proliferation and ability to produce mature cells. Similarly, stem cells have been isolated from embryonic gonadal ridges. Because unique populations of stem/progenitor cells may be isolated from fetal liver subsequent to greater organ development, this provides access to donor cells that could mature rapidly. It should be noteworthy that fetal human liver develops rapidly during the first trimester, such that characteristic hepatic lobular architecture begins to be acquired within 7 to 8 weeks of gestation and bile is formed by 12 weeks.[4] However, during that period, the liver plate structure is not fully developed, and the liver simultaneously produces hematopoietic cells and parenchymal epithelial cells. Nonetheless, within 6 to 7 weeks of gestation, the parenchyma of the fetal human liver contains epithelial cells with evidence for maturation along hepatic and biliary lineages, although cells with a mixed hepatobiliary phenotype are also frequent. Most of these fetal parenchymal epithelial cells are in an active state of proliferation. Moreover, these cells express markers of multiple lineages, including markers expressed in hepatocytes (e.g., AFP, albumin, α$_1$-antitrypsin, α$_1$-microglobulin, glucose-6-phosphatase, glycogen), bile duct cells (e.g., CK-19, γ-glutamyltranspeptidase, dipeptidyl-peptidase IV), liver sinusoidal endothelial cells (e.g., von Willebrand factor), mesenchymal cells (e.g., desmin, vimentin, smooth muscle α-actin), and even in undifferentiated hESC (e.g., Oct-4, nanog).[5,20] Fetal stem/progenitor cells with such multilineage gene expression and extensive replication capacity should be of particular interest as alternative donor sources for cell therapy.

A critical element for cell therapy concerns prospective characterization of donor cells, which is greatly facilitated by the ability to cryopreserve cells. In general, mature hepatocytes are readily damaged during cell isolation procedures and it has been difficult to recover viable cells after cryopreservation of mature hepatocytes. By contrast, recent studies established that fetal human liver cells can be successfully thawed after cryopreservation with greater than 90% viability. After being thawed, fetal liver cells replicate extensively in culture conditions and can also be expanded enormously, such that cells isolated from a single midterm donor fetal human liver could potentially be sufficient for multiple recipients, although this proliferation capacity needs to be defined in vivo. Because fetal human liver cells have been amenable to genetic reconstitution with gene therapy vectors, including for permanent gene transfer through lentiviral vectors, this adds to their potential for cell/gene therapy applications.[21]

On the other hand, despite their capacity for significant proliferation, fetal liver cells behave differently from other stem cells (e.g., hESC) and undergo attrition of telomere length during cell culture, which gradually leads to decline in cell proliferation.[9,22] The loss of proliferation potential in fetal human liver or pancreatic cells was restored by genetic reconstitution of telomerase activity.

Transplantation studies of fetal liver cells isolated from rat or mouse verified that fetal cells mature rapidly, produce and secrete albumin, and proliferate extensively in the liver of syngeneic recipients, where cell rejection is not an issue.[23-25] Similarly, fetal human liver cells engraft and proliferate in the liver of immunodeficient animals.[19,21] Also, fetal human liver cells have been transplanted into patients with acute liver failure, although the precise therapeutic value of such therapy has been unclear because only few such patients have yet been studied.[26] Because candidate fetal liver stem/progenitor cell populations may be conveniently isolated by display of unique cell surface markers, and cells exhibit major histocompatibility antigens poorly, this should result in attenuated host immune responses,[27-34] although this concept requires further study.

During hepatic development, cell-cell signals, including those of embryonic endothelial cells, play significant roles in lineage differentiation.[3] The nature of these signals is best defined for the mouse liver, and knowledge of regulatory molecules and signals in humans is limited at present. Nonetheless, rapidly proliferating parenchymal cells in the fetal human liver demonstrate unique profiles of gene expression, as partly described earlier in this chapter, which is distinct from gene expression in mature liver cells. These findings introduce the possibility of stem/progenitor cells from the fetal liver being manipulated to express additional phenotypes. For instance, when Pdx-1, a homeobox regulator of pancreatic β-cell development and function, was expressed in fetal human liver cells, these cells expressed insulin and other pancreatic genes.[30] Therefore programs aimed at harvesting, storing, and using fetal liver cells for cell therapy will be appropriate. Use of fetal tissues will not interfere with the supply of donor livers for OLT. However, because of moral reservations, some scientists favor experimentation with adult stem cells, rather than with embryonic or fetal cells.

For the most part, stem/progenitor cells are neither readily visible nor necessarily recruited in most adult organs during the course of normal events, including in the liver.[1-4] Therefore undifferentiated stem cells are considered to be rare in adult life, although in some organs, typically the bone marrow and gastrointestinal tract, facultative progenitor cells participate in cell replenishment. On the other hand, stem/progenitor cells do appear to reside in the adult liver, as shown by many studies involving specific perturbations, such as oncogenic

manipulations, toxic injury, chronic hepatitis, or cell transplantation analysis. The so-called hepatic oval cells, which constitute a well-studied type of facultative stem/progenitor cell, were originally described by Farber in carcinogen-treated rats.[2] Subsequently, oval cells were identified to emanate from the canal of Hering, which is a specialized peribiliary structure in the liver.[31] Oval cells exhibit unique properties, including hybrid isoenzyme profiles, markers of both hepatic and biliary lineages, as well as the capacity to establish long-term cell cultures. Indeed, oval cell lines established from the rat liver have been studied in detail, including in cell transplantation assays, to establish their differentiation potential. These studies demonstrated that oval cells can produce mature hepatocytes as well as unrelated lineages (e.g., cardiomyocytes).[32] However, despite their capacity to replicate extensively in cell culture, oval cell lines have not shown the capacity to repopulate the liver, whereas primary oval cells isolated from the mouse liver or even the mouse pancreas can repopulate the liver, including in the fumaryl acetoacetate hydrolase (FAH) mutant mouse model of tyrosinemia type 1, the Long-Evans cinnamon (LEC) rat model of Wilson disease, and the Nagase analbuminemic rat (NAR). The evidence to date suggests that hepatic oval cells constitute an organ-specific stem cell niche, and that these cells do not arise from extrahepatic reservoirs of stem cells, such as from the bone marrow.[33] This raises the possibility that oval cells from the human liver might well be suitable for cell therapy applications. Of course, isolation of hepatic oval cells will require adult human livers, which are in short supply. However, the normal adult liver rarely contains oval cells (perhaps less than 0.001% of the total cell population) and diseased livers (e.g., livers explanted at OLT), which are normally discarded, might be a more suitable source of such cells. This has not been studied and should be investigated further.

It is well established that mature hepatocytes can restore the liver in many situations, including after partial hepatectomy or other types of limited hepatic injury.[1,2] The voluminous literature published over the past 70 years concerning the partial hepatectomy model has provided extensive insights into the capacity of hepatocytes to regenerate the liver.[34] More recently, in studies with adult mouse hepatocytes, using a transplantation system involving FAH mice burdened with progressive liver injury, it was found that transplanted hepatocytes possessed an indefinite replication potential, with the capacity to divide more than 90 times following transplantation across multiple generations of animals.[5] In contrast, primary adult hepatocytes undergo profound alterations and exhibit very limited proliferation capacity in vitro. This raises fundamental issues concerning how one defines the "stemness" of cells and the necessity of applying appropriate cell-specific models to elicit stem cell–like capacity. Despite the obvious liver-repopulating capacity of adult hepatocytes, there is little doubt that existing sources of donor livers are inadequate. The potential effectiveness of innovative solutions to this problem (e.g., using living-related donors, isolating cells from liver resections, using xenogeneic donors) is being studied.

Extrahepatic sources of cells (e.g., cells derived from bone marrow, umbilical cord blood, placenta, or amniotic fluid, which recently showed unimagined differentiation potential including the capacity to generate liver cells) have generated much interest. They offer the possibility of harvesting autologous cells (from bone marrow or peripheral blood) as needed or of preserving autologous cells for use in the future (from amniotic fluid, umbilical cord blood, or placenta).

The amniotic fluid has been shown to contain epithelial cells in animals, as well as humans. Surprisingly, a large proportion of amniotic epithelial cells demonstrate liver gene expression, including albumin and α_1-antitrypsin. These cells can be expanded in culture following growth factor stimulation and are amenable to gene transfer in vitro. Moreover, transplantation of amniotic epithelial cells in animals has been shown to result in the integration of transplanted cells in the liver parenchyma, long-term cell survival, and secretion of hepatic proteins. Significant numbers of amniotic epithelial cells can be harvested from individual donors, up to 2×10^8 cells. Also, it appears that these cells show poor expression of class I and class II histocompatibility antigens. Similarly, the human placenta is believed to represent a major additional source of stem cells, and the potential of multipotent cells resident in the placenta is currently being defined.[35]

The idea that circulating cells could contribute to organ repair during physiologic processes gained currency following early demonstrations of the differentiation potential of hematopoietic stem cells into hepatocytes.[36] Subsequently, specific subsets of bone marrow–derived mouse hematopoietic stem cells (particularly those with expression of c-kit and sca-1 antigens, low-level expression of Thy-1 antigen, and absence of lineage markers) and also bone marrow–derived mesenchymal cells, which were designated multipotent adult progenitor cells (MAPC), were capable of generating multiple cell lineages.[37,38] A large body of literature rapidly accumulated, verifying that such cells can produce mature hepatocytes both in vitro and in vivo. Analysis of the kinetics by which bone marrow–derived stem cells generated hepatocytes in the mouse liver indicated that 7 weeks elapsed after bone marrow transplantation before donor-derived hepatocytes first appeared.[39] Even a single bone marrow–derived mouse hematopoietic stem cell was sufficient for recapitulating multiple lineages additional to the liver.[40] Similarly, transplantation of MAPC into the inner cell mass of mouse blastocysts led to the appearance of mature cells in all three germ layers, verifying their multipotentiality.

Umbilical cord blood offers many advantages for use as a source of stem cells, including its well-established hematopoietic and mesenchymal potential, which has resulted in routine clinical applications. In addition, cells derived from umbilical cord blood have shown the capacity to produce hepatocytes in intact animals,[41] including after intrablastocyst or intrafetal injections. However, the overall frequency with which umbilical cord blood cells produced hepatocytes was low, similar to that of bone marrow–derived hematopoietic stem cells. On the other hand, umbilical cord blood may contain unique populations of epithelial-like cells, which can be expanded in vitro with soluble growth factors. Because umbilical cord blood cells are routinely harvested and banked for clinical use, these promising results need to be verified and strengthened.

Highly convincing demonstrations of the hepatic differentiation potential of bone marrow–derived cells were provided by studies in the FAH mutant mouse, where transplantation of healthy bone marrow–derived cells resulted in liver repopulation and correction of metabolic abnormalities.[37] Similar studies of therapeutic efficacy have not yet been performed with other types of extrahepatic stem cells. One difficulty

concerns the general lack of suitable animal models in which proliferation in human cells can be convincingly demonstrated. However, progress is being made in developing additional immunodeficient animals, where human cells can engraft, proliferate, and repopulate the liver to a better extent.[42,43]

The ability of extrahepatic stem cells to form hepatocytes is astounding and has far-reaching consequences. However, problems have also been encountered. First, it is now clear that conversion of bone marrow–derived cells into hepatocytes is a rare phenomenon.[39,44] For instance, bone marrow–derived hematopoietic cells generated hepatocytes infrequently in FAH mice with extensive liver injury—estimated at approximately 1 hepatocyte cell for 10^4 to 10^6 liver cells[39] and perhaps zero to fewer than 10 cells for the entire liver of healthy mice.[44] Similarly, although FAH mice showed significant liver repopulation and therapeutic correction, this was thought to result from only 50 to 500 "repopulation events" (i.e., the number of hepatocytes emanating from donor hematopoietic stem cells).[39] Second, during generation of mature hepatocytes, bone marrow–derived hematopoietic stem cells, as well as umbilical cord blood cells, have been shown to fuse with native cells, something peculiar to the myelomonocytic stem cell fraction. However, this observation is controversial because some studies have shown that such cell fusion may not be invariant. Nevertheless, one consequence of cell fusion is genetic instability (e.g., aneuploidy), which could lead to oncogenetic transformation in fused cells. On the other hand, it should be noteworthy that transplantation of mature hepatocytes does not result in cell fusion in the liver. Whether other types of stem cells (e.g., MAPC) generate hepatocytes via cell fusion is unknown. Third, hematopoietic stem cells may additionally—and possibly more efficiently—produce nonparenchymal liver cells, including Kupffer cells and hepatic stellate cells,[45,46] which could be mistaken for other cell types.

Another critical issue concerns the use of cells expanded in culture—either in their native state or after genetic manipulation (e.g., insertion of oncogenes or removal of cell cycle suppressor genes to induce proliferation). An example of the former is provided by MAPC, where cumbersome and incompletely understood cell culture requirements are necessary for expanding cells in culture. During this process, cells could potentially accumulate undesirable genetic lesions. Similarly, clinical use of cells immortalized with the simian virus 40 T antigen will probably raise issues of safety, although methods are available to genetically excise the oncogene after cell expansion is completed. The removal of cell cycle suppressor genes (e.g., p27^{kip}, p19^{ARF}) leads to accelerated cell proliferation, although this approach may not be safe because of concerns regarding malignant transformation of cells.[47]

This concise overview of the applied state-of-the-art of stem cell biology should indicate that liver-directed cell therapy in the near-term will most effectively utilize hepatocytes from adult human livers or stem/progenitor cells from fetal human livers, although cells from additional sources will probably become available at some time in the future.

Clinical Targets of Liver Cell Therapy

Several considerations should drive cell therapy applications in clinical disorders. A large number of genetic and acquired

Table 11-1 Useful Animal Models for Cell Therapy and Other Studies

ANIMAL STRAIN AND DISEASE MODEL DESIGNATION	DONOR CELLS	APPLICATIONS
Healthy wild-type, syngeneic or congeneic, or allogeneic mice, rats and larger animals, dogs, pigs, non-human primates, and fetal sheep	Genetically modified transgenic reporter containing cells, sex-mismatched cells	Analysis of transplanted cell biology, including cell engraftment, proliferation, tolerance, and function
Alb-uPA, Alb-HSV-TK transgenic, or AdMad-treated mice, rats, rabbits, pigs, or monkeys treated with chemicals or other agents to induce acute or chronic liver injury	Healthy hepatocytes or stem/progenitor cells	Studies of transplanted cell biology; cell therapy for acute liver failure, chronic liver failure, and complications of cirrhosis (e.g., hepatic encephalopathy)
Alb-uPA-Rag-2 mice, Alb-uPA-NOD-SCID mice, Tupaia	Woodchuck, human, tupaia hepatocytes	Hepadnavirus or HCV replication and pathogenesis, antiviral drug testing
DPPIV-deficient mutant F344 rats and mice	Healthy rat or mouse liver or stem/progenitor cells	Biology of transplanted hepatocytes and stem/progenitor cells
Eizai hyperbilirubinemic rats	Healthy hepatocytes	Restoration of biliary transport abnormality
FAH mutant mice	Healthy or genetically altered mouse hepatocytes, various stem/progenitor cells	Studies of stem cell biology and cell and gene therapy for hereditary tyrosinemia, type 1
Gunn rats	Healthy hepatocytes	Cell and gene therapy model for Crigler-Najjar syndrome, type 1
Hemophilia A knockout mice, hemophilia dogs	Healthy hepatocytes, endothelial cells, or stem/progenitor cells	Cell and gene therapies for hemophilia A
Histidinemia mice	Healthy hepatocytes	Restoration of amino acid metabolism
Long-Evans cinnamon rats, atp7b null mice, toxic milk mice	Healthy hepatocytes	Cell and gene therapies for Wilson disease
Mdr2 knockout mice	Healthy hepatocytes	Cell therapy model for progressive familial intrahepatic cholestasis
Nagase analbuminemic rats	Healthy hepatocytes	Cell and gene therapies for hypoalbuminemia
ODS$^{od/od}$ mutant rats	Healthy hepatocytes	Restoration of ascorbate synthesis
Purebred dalmatian dogs	Healthy hepatocytes	Cell transplantation for correcting purine metabolism and urate handling
Spf^{ash} mice	Healthy hepatocytes	Alleviation of ornithine transcarbamylase deficiency
Watanabe heritable hyperlipidemia rabbits, ApoE knockout mice	Normal hepatocytes	Cell and gene therapies for hypercholesterolemia

Modified from Gupta S, Rogler CE. Liver repopulation systems and study of pathophysiological mechanisms in animals. Am J Physiol Gastrointest Liver Physiol 1999;40:G1097–G1102.

Alb-uPA, urokinase-type plasminogen activator gene driven by the albumin promoter; DPPIV, dipeptidyl-peptidase IV; FAH, fumaryl acetoacetate hydrolase; HCV, hepatitis C virus; Mdr, multidrug resistance; ODS, osteogenic disorder Shionogi rats; Rag-2, recombination activation gene-2; Spf^{ash}, sparse fur mice

conditions are thought to be amenable to liver-directed cell therapy, based on a variety of studies in animal models (**Table 11-1**).

The therapeutic considerations extend to the replacement of deficient proteins in monogenetic disorders, including lack of circulating proteins such as coagulation factors, without organ injury or loss of function through genetic mutations (e.g., abnormal low-density lipoprotein receptor [LDLR] producing familial hypercholesterolemia with premature atherosclerosis and coronary artery disease, but not liver damage) or through abnormal intracellular proteins (e.g., the copper transporter ATP7B, which produces copper toxicosis and damage to the liver and brain, among other organs, in Wilson disease).

Acquired disorders represent the other end of the spectrum, including acute or chronic liver failure as well as other forms of liver damage. In general, animal models capable of mimicking acute liver failure in humans have been lacking for the study of cell therapy. A major problem in animals concerns extremely limited duration of survival after being exposed to hepatotoxins or rapid recovery in response to unrelated mechanisms, such as after subtotal liver resection. In acute liver failure the goal is that cell transplantation will offer critical metabolic support in the short term and promote regeneration of the native liver in the long term. The former should help in bridging patients to OLT, whereas the latter might help avoid OLT altogether, especially if cell transplantation could be coupled with bioartificial liver-assist devices to prolong survival. In chronic liver failure, the immediate expectation is that by providing additional synthetic or metabolic liver support cell therapy will ameliorate complications such as coagulopathy, hypoproteinemia, or encephalopathy, and thereby either improve quality of life or produce prolongation of survival. The potential for cell transplantation to help in regression of hepatic fibrosis and portal hypertension or portosystemic shunting in cirrhosis is less well defined.

At the conceptual level, these applications of cell therapy raise many issues concerning the route and site of cell transplantation, the number of cells needed for therapeutic effects, the rapidity by which transplanted cells will provide deficient function (particularly in acute liver failure), and the intrinsic mechanisms that would govern whether transplanted cells will overcome microenvironmental or systemic barriers to their engraftment, proliferation, and function. Many of these issues have been addressed in experimental studies. For instance, cells can be transplanted into the liver (most conveniently through catheters into the hepatic artery and less simply into the portal venous system) by approaches involving percutaneous transhepatic, intrasplenic, mesenteric veins, or portal vein branches. Alternatively, cells can be injected into extrahepatic sites, particularly the spleen or peritoneal cavity, although many other sites have been studied. Besides the technical ease of cell administration, one needs to consider the risk of potential complications and the fate of transplanted cells. The data indicate that injection of cells into arterial circulations, including hepatic, splenic, or pulmonary arteries, is ineffective because cells are entrapped in high-flow, high-pressure capillaries with embolic complications, including tissue infarction. Consequently, the transplanted cells are rapidly destroyed. On the other hand, injection of cells into the sinusoids of the spleen or liver offers better sanctuaries, and transplanted cells can then survive throughout the life of the recipients.[48] Use of the spleen as an extrahepatic reservoir of cells has interested many investigators because transplanted cells can be tracked more readily, although the capacity of splenic sinusoids for cells is relatively limited. The peritoneal cavity offers much larger space to accommodate cells; however, in view of their anchorage dependence and need for cell–cell interactions, survival of transplanted hepatocytes in this location requires the presence of extracellular matrix components or of non-parenchymal liver cells. Transplanted cells survive most effectively after injection into the portal venous system, which distributes cells in hepatic sinusoids throughout the liver. Injection of cells directly into the liver parenchyma leads to limited cell distribution, and transplanted cells may translocate into pulmonary capillaries upon accidental entry of the needle into the hepatic venous system. Injection of hepatocytes into the portal venous system results in transient, albeit significant, portal hypertension, because transplanted cells occlude portal vein radicles and sinusoids with perturbation of the hepatic microcirculation.[49] The larger size of hepatocytes (20 to 40 μm) compared with that of hepatic sinusoids (3 to 6 μm) leads to their retention in hepatic sinusoids, with occasional translocation of cells either into the pulmonary capillaries in the healthy liver or directly into the liver with an acutely injured organ. In the cirrhotic liver, portosystemic shunting may lead to extensive cell translocations into pulmonary capillaries. However, hepatic microcirculatory alterations regress within several hours after cell transplantation, and hepatocytes entering pulmonary capillaries caused only transient cardiovascular perturbations because these were rapidly destroyed—starting within minutes—in pulmonary capillaries. These considerations, and further issues discussed in the following paragraphs, are relevant for developing optimal strategies for clinical cell therapy.

To date, more than 80 patients with various clinical disorders have been treated with cell transplantation, including autologous hepatocytes from patients with cirrhosis or familial hypercholesterolemia, or allogeneic cells on one or more occasions. In the earliest studies, approximately 2×10^7 to 6×10^8 autologous hepatocytes were transplanted via the spleen, splenic artery, or portal vein in 10 patients with cirrhosis and ascites, and 9 of the patients exhibited no apparent benefits. However, 1 patient, in whom transplanted cells were detected in the spleen using an iminodiacetic acid radiotracer, improved and returned to work.[50] Several patients with advanced liver disease or cirrhosis have been treated in the United States with injection of hepatocytes into the splenic artery or the spleen.[51] Cell transplantation may have been beneficial in some of these patients; however, the data are difficult to interpret, partly because it is not possible to establish correlations between the number of transplanted cells that may have survived with disease outcomes.

In a small study from India of seven patients with acute liver failure and grade III to IV hepatic encephalopathy, 6×10^7 fetal human hepatocytes per kilogram body weight were transplanted intraperitoneally. Four of these patients died within 13 to 48 hours after cell transplantation, whereas three (43%) recovered. However, the fate of transplanted cells was not established and no further follow-up studies have been reported. More recently, these investigators treated another patient with acute liver failure caused by fatty liver of pregnancy and ascribed complete recovery to the intraperitoneal injection of 3×10^8 fetal human hepatocytes.[29]

In the United States, 20 patients (age range, 4 months to 69 years) with acute liver failure have been treated with approximately 3×10^7 to 4×10^{10} fresh or frozen adult human hepatocytes via the spleen or another route.[51] In some patients, intrapulmonary shunting of transplanted cells was observed, along with pulmonary infiltrates and transient hypoxia. After cell transplantation, 11 of these 20 patients died (55%); 7 subsequently received OLT (35%) and 2 (10%) recovered completely.[52] In some patients, the presence of transplanted cells was verified histologically by the in situ hybridization method to identify sex-mismatched donor cells. These early studies seemed promising, although disease in patients with acute liver failure is highly variable, which indicates that analysis of larger numbers of patients will be necessary, along with some measure of the transplanted cell mass, to fully define the benefits of cell therapy.

Patients with metabolic deficiency states constitute the most effective examples of cell therapy because transplanted cell functions can be verified in these conditions by specific assays. Several patients with genetic conditions have undergone hepatocyte transplantation (**Table 11-2**).[11] In six patients with familial hypercholesterolemia, $(1-3) \times 10^9$ autologous hepatocytes modified with a retrovirus vector to express LDLR were injected into the portal venous system, following the establishment of critical principles in a rabbit model of the disease.[53,54] These patients showed the presence of LDLR-expressing transplanted cells in the liver, as well as decreases in serum cholesterol levels in four of the patients. However, this therapeutic effect was limited, presumably a result of inferior gene transfer and poor survival of transplanted cells in the recipients.

Table 11-2 Genetic Disorders Amenable to Liver Cell Therapy

Disorders Already Treated in Humans

α_1-Antitrypsin deficiency with decompensated liver disease
Familial hypercholesterolemia
Citrullinemia
Crigler-Najjar syndrome, type 1
Ornithine transcarbamylase deficiency
Infantile Refsum's disease
Glycogen storage disease, type 1a
Coagulation factor VII deficiency
Progressive familial intrahepatic cholestasis

Additional Candidate Disorders

Additional hyperammonemia syndromes
Other glycogen storage disorders
Congenital hyperbilirubinemia syndromes
Hemophilia A
Apolipoprotein E deficiency
Maple syrup urine disease
Oxalosis
Protoporphyrias
Wilson disease

In a well-studied child with Crigler-Najjar syndrome type 1, intraportal transplantation of 7.5×10^9 adult human hepatocytes resulted in significant decreases in serum bilirubin levels and the appearance of detectable hepatic UGT1A1 activity along with conjugated bilirubin in bile, indicating the presence of functioning transplanted cells in the liver.[55] However, this patient eventually required an auxiliary liver transplant because the therapeutic benefit of cell transplantation was not sustained beyond several months.[52] Similarly, only transient improvements were observed in an infant with severe ornithine transcarbamylase deficiency following intraportal infusion of adult human hepatocytes, and OLT was eventually required.[56] In glycogen storage disease type 1a and severe fasting hypoglycemia, intraportal transplantation of 2×10^9 cells produced significant long-term improvement.[57] A 4-year-old girl with infantile Refsum's disease was treated with 2×10^9 fresh and cryopreserved adult hepatocytes over several sessions, resulting in decreased serum levels of total bile acids as well as of abnormal dihydroxycoprostanoic acid.[58] Survival of transplanted hepatocytes was verified by post-transplant liver biopsy and analysis of sex-mismatched chromosomal sequences. On the other hand, cell transplantation in two brothers with severe coagulation factor VII deficiency was less effective, and these patients were eventually treated with OLT.[59]

This clinical experience offers multiple insights. First, cells can be safely transplanted in patients ranging from those with acute liver failure to those with advanced cirrhosis, from infants to the elderly, and in patients with genetic as well as acquired disorders. Second, some methods have been developed to identify transplanted cells in recipients, such as sex-mismatched chromosomal markers, and more recently short tandem repeat sequences.[60,61] Novel technologies are being developed to permit identification of transplanted cells through noninvasive imaging modalities (e.g., by introducing genes capable of producing signals that can be imaged).[62]

Similarly, cells or cell surrogates have been labeled with radio-isotopes for short-term tracking in recipients.[63,64] These methods are useful for studying biodistribution of transplanted cells. The ability to verify the presence and abundance of transplanted cells will help develop correlations with therapeutic outcomes in patients, which is most necessary. Third, suitable immunosuppressive regimens have been identified,[57] although this area needs to be investigated further because mechanisms regulating rejection of allogeneic hepatocytes appear to be different from those involved in the rejection of solid organs.[65,66] Fourth, further insights are needed in transplanted cell engraftment and proliferation to improve the therapeutic results obtained so far, as discussed later in this chapter. Finally, careful and systematic studies in the future, perhaps in multiple centers using identical clinical protocols, including cell transplantation routes, dose of cells, as well as specific cell preparations, will probably be necessary to advance the potential of cell therapy.

The Biologic Basis of Transplanted Cell Engraftment, Proliferation, and Regulation of Liver Repopulation with Transplanted Cells

Investigations conducted over the past 2 decades generated novel insights into how transplanted cells engraft, function, and proliferate in the liver. These insights will be critical for using clinical applications, for studying the biology of stem/progenitor cells, and for developing chimeric animal models containing human cells for other applications (e.g., pharmaceutical development, toxicology testing of drugs).

To understand how cells engraft in the liver, working models have been developed that take into account the unique organization of the hepatic circulation, the potential for interactions between transplanted cells and various hepatic cell types in the recipient liver, and the need for reorganization of the liver plate structure during integration of transplanted cells in the hepatic parenchyma (**Fig. 11-2**).

The first of several critical steps in cell engraftment concerns deposition of transplanted cells in hepatic sinusoids. This culminates in a blood flow–dependent process of "cell embolization," where advancement of transplanted cells in sinusoids is determined by the difference in the sizes of cells and sinusoids.[49,67] Transplanted cells benefit by reaching distal sinusoids in the liver lobule because cells left behind in portal vein radicles are largely cleared by phagocytes. On the other hand, transplanted hepatocytes can recognize specific adhesion molecules and extracellular matrix receptors, such as fibronectin receptors, on liver sinusoidal endothelial cells. In the meantime, entrapment of transplanted cells in liver sinusoids rapidly results in the activation of microcirculatory perturbations and the onset of hepatic ischemia in affected regions.[67,68] For instance, video microscopy in live animals demonstrated that sinusoidal blood flow may cease immediately after cell transplantation, although blood flow begins to be restored after minutes to hours with some injury across the recipient liver.[68] This inevitable component of cell transplantation in the liver is accompanied by multiple perturbations, including activation of adjacent Kupffer cells and recruitment of neutrophils, hepatic stellate cells, endothelial cells, and native hepatocytes.[69-71] Ischemic damage to the hepatic

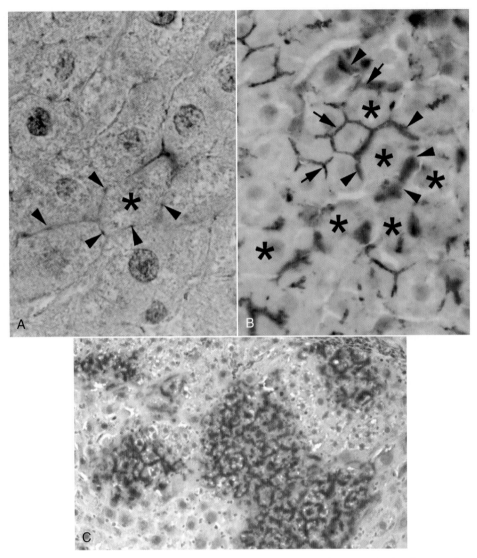

Fig. 11-2 **Illustration of transplanted cell engraftment and proliferation in the liver.** Shown are the key features of transplanted cell biology as demonstrated by studies using DPPIV-deficient F344 recipient rats. **A,** Integration of a transplanted cell *(asterisk)*, with the development of dotlike hybrid gap junctions *(arrowheads)* that join the transplanted cell with native cells in the liver parenchyma. **B,** Transplanted cells forming a network of hybrid bile canaliculi with contributions from DPPIV-positive domains (red color, *arrowheads*) and ATPase-positive domains from native hepatocytes (brown color, *arrows*). **C,** Expanding clusters of transplanted cells in a rat pretreated with retrorsine and partial hepatectomy. Note that some clusters of transplanted cells are far smaller than others. Also, proliferation in transplanted cells leads to progressive enlargement of confluent areas containing transplanted cells. Native hepatocytes exhibit megalocytosis and polyploid nuclei as evidence for liver injury induced by retrorsine and partial hepatectomy. Transplanted cells were identified in the liver with DPPIV histochemistry, seen with a red reaction product. Gap junctions were visualized by immunostaining for connexin using a diaminobenzidine substrate of peroxidase. Bile canaliculi in native cells were visualized by ATPase histochemical staining. **A** and **B,** Methylgreen counterstain; **C,** hematoxylin counterstain.

endothelium would help transplanted cells enter the space of Disse and then the liver parenchyma.[72] On the other hand, ischemia-reperfusion is a potent stimulus for neutrophil and Kupffer cell activation, which results in expression of multiple inflammatory chemokines and cytokines, including TNF-α and interleukin-6, for example.[73] Neutrophils and Kupffer cells can play important roles in engraftment of transplanted cells.[70] For instance, activation of Kupffer cells and generation of pro-oxidant stress in liver sinusoidal endothelial cells can help permeabilize the hepatic endothelial barrier, which would facilitate the entry of transplanted cells into the space of Disse.[72] On the other hand, activated neutrophils and Kupffer cells phagocytose and remove significant fractions of transplanted cells,[70] which impairs overall transplanted cell engraftment such that fewer than 20% of the transplanted cells eventually survive in the liver.[69]

The process of cell entry in the liver is facilitated by additional factors. For instance, activated hepatic stellate cells and hepatocytes release soluble factors—including vascular endothelial growth factor (VEGF), matrix-type metalloproteinases, and other molecules—that help permeabilize endothelial cells in the vicinity of transplanted cells.[69] Moreover, VEGF has hepatoprotective effects. VEGF is expressed rapidly after cell transplantation from both transplanted cells and native hepatocytes. This occurs before the demonstrated requirement of 16 to 20 hours for transplanted cells to penetrate through the endothelial barrier. During isolation of liver cells, plasma membrane structures, including tight junctions, gap junctions, and bile canaliculi, must be severed and subsequently restored. Therefore the next process in transplanted cell engraftment concerns restoration of cell polarity. Finally, integration of transplanted cells in the liver parenchyma must be completed. Analysis of these processes has shown that gap junctions and bile canaliculi are reconstituted over 3 to 7 days after cell transplantation, when transplanted cells and native hepatocytes begin to exhibit hybrid plasma membrane structures. This is a critical process, because transplanted cells then become indistinguishable from native hepatocytes and can begin to manifest normal functions, including bile excretion.[74,75]

Identification of this series of critical events following cell transplantation has provided ways to design specific manipulations aimed at enhancing transplanted cell engraftment. Initial deposition of transplanted cells in the liver lobule can be improved by the use of hepatic sinusoidal dilators (e.g., nitroglycerin, phentolamine, sodium nitroprusside).[67,76] This protects the liver from ischemia and microcirculatory disruption, helps accelerate the deposition of cells from the spleen into the liver, and promotes entry of transplanted cells into distal liver sinusoids. Similarly, Kupffer cell activation can be prevented by pharmacologic approaches.[70] Prior depletion of Kupffer cells significantly improved transplanted cell engraftment as well as the kinetics of liver repopulation. Similarly, depletion of neutrophils dampened the inflammatory response induced by cell transplantation.[73] As cytokine-chemokine responses may be inhibited by specific drugs, these mechanisms offer suitable strategies for clinical applications, which are currently being developed.

Another significant mechanism for improving cell engraftment concerns damage to the hepatic endothelium. In early studies, disruption of endothelial cells by cyclophosphamide accelerated entry of transplanted cells into the space of Disse and improved cell engraftment.[72] Subsequently, other drugs have been identified for this purpose (e.g., doxorubicin, which is suitable for clinical use; monocrotaline, a pyrrolizidine alkaloid, which is useful for animal studies). Additional mechanisms to facilitate transplanted cell engraftment include improved binding of transplanted cells to liver sinusoidal endothelial cells. Also, intrinsic differences in the properties of cells (e.g., the display of specific proteins on the cell surface, the greater capacity of cell subsets to proliferate) could be helpful in promoting cell engraftment or proliferation.[77-79] Moreover, genetic manipulation to introduce protective genes has been effective in some circumstances.[80,81] On the other hand, new ways to promote release of endogenous cytoprotective factors (e.g., drug-induced release of VEGF from hepatic stellate cells)[82] provide practical methods to approach this issue. A major advantage of superior transplanted cell engraftment concerns acceleration of the kinetics of liver repopulation, which will obviously be helpful for clinical applications.

It should be noted that transplanted hepatocytes are able to engraft and proliferate in the liver despite the presence of significant fibrosis or acute liver injury,[83,84] although

proliferation in transplanted cells is delayed in the acutely injured liver by several days because of the additional time required to complete cell engraftment.[84]

When cell engraftment is completed, transplanted cells can survive lifelong in syngeneic experimental animals, where cellular rejection is not an issue.[48,74] Throughout that period, transplanted cells exhibit normal hepatic functions and respond to mitogenic stimuli in a physiologic fashion. Moreover, in the normal liver, transplanted cells do not proliferate. These findings have practical implications for creating suitable masses of transplanted cells. For instance, transplantation of 1×10^7 cells in an adult rat or 1×10^{10} cells in an adult person is considered to be the equivalent of no more than 1% to 2% of total liver cells. Because only a fraction of this cell mass would engraft and survive long term, it is essential to find ways to augment the engraftment of the transplanted cell mass. This could potentially be accomplished by transplanting cells repeatedly; this process has been found to be safe and effective, with reconstitution of 5% to 7% of the liver mass following transplantation of cells on three separate occasions in rats.[85]

On the other hand, induction of proliferation in transplanted cells represents an alternative approach that will be particularly appropriate for using stem/progenitor cells in small numbers. A variety of animal studies indicated that instability in the liver parenchyma, such that native hepatocytes are burdened by survival or proliferation disadvantages compared with transplanted cells, promotes liver repopulation (see Shafritz and Oertel[86] for review). Several mouse models verified this principle, including alb-uPA mice, FAH mice, alb-HSV-TK mice, and AdMad mice, where toxic transgenes serve to deplete native hepatocytes, such that transplanted healthy cells can proliferate extensively and repopulate large areas of the liver. Similarly, when transgenic cells expressing the anti-apoptotic human *Bcl-2* gene are transplanted into mice susceptible to Fas ligand–mediated apoptosis, followed by administration of the mouse-specific J0-2 antibody, transplanted cells proliferated significantly.[87]

The principle of selective hepatic ablation also applies to chemical toxins, such as carbon tetrachloride, which induces proliferation in transplanted cells located in periportal areas of the liver lobule, away from perivenous areas susceptible to carbon tetrachloride injury.[88] Moreover, the chemical retrorsine, which is another DNA-binding pyrrolizidine alkaloid, similar to monocrotaline, was effective in inhibiting proliferation in hepatocytes, particularly when combined with additional manipulations, such as two-thirds partial hepatectomy and repeated administration of the thyroid hormone triiodothyronine (T_3) as well as carbon tetrachloride.[89,90] In these situations, proliferation in transplanted cells was markedly accelerated and the liver was extensively repopulated with transplanted cells. These manipulations were effective because genotoxic damage in retrorsine-treated hepatocytes produced susceptibility to additional oxidative injury produced by partial hepatectomy or by T_3 or carbon tetrachloride administration, leading to progressive repopulation with transplanted cells over several weeks. In contrast, when cells were not transplanted in retrorsine-treated animals, liver repopulation was completed by the activation of endogenous liver cell populations.[91] Studies with retrorsine or monocrotaline have provided further insights into the biology of transplanted cells. However, these chemicals are not suited to clinical applications in view of their potential for oncogenicity.

Recent studies of genotoxic damage with hepatic radiation showed efficacy in inducing transplanted cell proliferation.[92] In initial studies, radiation was found to induce extensive liver injury in animals subjected to partial hepatectomy, which again suggested the role of cumulative genotoxic damage in this process. However, additional studies demonstrated that the role of partial hepatectomy in this process was to activate oxidative DNA damage, thus adding ischemia-reperfusion injury to the radiation injury model.[93,94] Hepatic ischemia-reperfusion is a potent source of oxidative stress and has been used to treat liver cancer in humans. This combination of ischemia-reperfusion and radiation has been highly effective in promoting transplanted cell proliferation in the rat liver.[94] The process of liver repopulation is gradual, suggesting asynchronous loss of native hepatocytes in the rat over several weeks, during which time transplanted hepatocytes undergo an estimated nine population doublings (**Figs. 11-3 and 11-4**). Such a manipulation could be clinically applicable, and initial research in primates has been performed to study the safety and efficacy of radiation-based approaches.[92] Among the

problems is that radiation produces permanent changes in tissues with damage that may remain silent for years before serious issues arise.

Similarly, radiation-induced damage will obviously not be appropriate for transplanting cells on more than one discrete occasion (e.g., if cell transplantation became necessary again following loss of allogeneic cells). Therefore pharmacologic approaches will likely be most appropriate for clinical applications of cell therapy.

Further Considerations for Developing Cell Therapy Applications

Transplantation of human cells into immunodeficient mice offers ways to develop highly useful additional animal models, including for addressing the basic biology of stem cell populations, for characterizing and assessing the viability of human cell preparations, and also for developing chimeric mice for

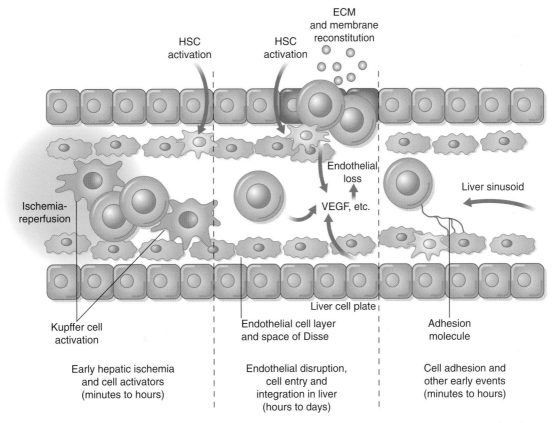

Fig. 11-3 **A working model outlining critical steps during transplanted cell engraftment in the liver.** Immediately after the arrival of transplanted cells in liver sinusoids (arrow; right) cells become entrapped in distal sinusoids (far left), which temporarily blocks sinusoidal blood flow, activates portal hypertension, and perturbs the hepatic microcirculation with the onset of ischemia-reperfusion. This promptly activates Kupffer cells and hepatic stellate cells, which release multiple cytokines and chemokines, including mediators of inflammation. Simultaneously, transplanted cells adhere to the hepatic endothelium through specific cell surface molecules and receptors (right). Activation of hepatic endothelial cells results from multiple mechanisms, including oxidative damage and permeabilization of cells through the release of VEGF, various matrix metalloproteinases, and other molecules. Hepatocytes begin to enter the space of Disse (center) 16 to 20 hours after cell transplantation and insinuate themselves between native hepatocytes in periportal areas. Cells entrapped in portal vein radicles or sinusoids are mostly cleared by 24 to 48 hours. Subsequently, transplanted cells begin to become integrated in the liver parenchyma, with remodeling of the liver plate structure, which is facilitated by the coordinated release of various matrix metalloproteinases as well as tissue inhibitors of matrix metalloproteinases (e.g., TIMP-1). Completion of plasma membrane reconstitution results in recovery of cell polarity and the formation of conjoint structures, such as gap junctions and bile canaliculi, which regain functional integrity 3 to 7 days after cell transplantation.

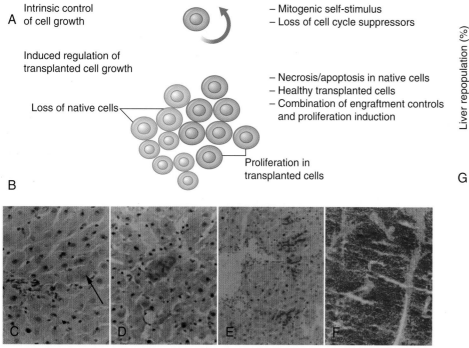

Fig. 11-4 Mechanisms regulating liver repopulation with cells. As discussed in the text, transplanted cell proliferation can be induced by regulating intrinsic cell cycling properties **A,** or by manipulating microenvironmental conditions **B,** which is more effective. Panels **C** to **F** show transplanted cells *(red color)* in the liver of syngeneic dipeptidyl-peptidase IV (DPPIV)-deficient F344 rats 3 months after cell transplantation. **C,** A control animal without any treatment before cell transplantation with occasional transplanted cells *(arrow).* **D,** A rat treated with liver ischemia-reperfusion before cell transplantation. **E,** A rat treated with 50 Gy liver irradiation, showing some transplanted cell proliferation. **F,** Treatment with ischemia-reperfusion plus radiation led to extensive liver repopulation. Tissues were subjected to DPPIV histochemistry with hematoxylin counterstaining. **G,** The chart shows liver repopulation kinetics with projected doublings of transplanted cells. The yellow area at the top shows liver repopulation after 50 Gy irradiation and ischemia-reperfusion, and the green area towards the bottom shows liver repopulation after 30 Gy irradiation and ischemia-reperfusion. The findings suggested nine doublings in the transplanted cell mass attributable to the asynchronous loss of native hepatocytes over 12 weeks. *(Modified from Malhi H et al. Cell transplantation after oxidative hepatic preconditioning with radiation and ischemia–reperfusion leads to extensive liver repopulation. Proc Natl Acad Sci USA 2002;99:13114–13119.)*

various studies. For instance, such mice will be most valuable[95-97] for use as models of hepatitis B or C viruses, including for testing drugs or biologic modifiers. Recent advances in repopulating the mouse liver with human cells will provide more information regarding species-specific needs for hepatotrophic factors or other mechanisms.[42,43]

It will be appropriate to contemplate whether cell therapy could be applied to large groups of patients, instead of small numbers of patients with less common or rare conditions. For instance, because viral hepatitis constitutes the single largest liver disease, affecting nearly 500 million people worldwide, a large number of whom will develop chronic liver disease, one should consider whether the benefits of cell therapy could be applied to this patient population. This would require cells that resist viral replication. Recently, genetic strategies have been developed to interrupt hepatitis B or C replication, which in principle could be applied to cells before transplantation (e.g., into patients at risk for disease recurrence after OLT).

Key References

Aldeguer X, et al. Interleukin-6 from intrahepatic cells of bone marrow origin is required for normal murine liver regeneration. Hepatology 2002;35:40–48. (Ref.45)

Alison MR. Characterization of the differentiation capacity of rat-derived hepatic stem cells. Semin Liver Dis 2003;23:325–336. (Ref.2)

Azuma H, et al. Robust expansion of human hepatocytes in Fah-/-/Rag2-/-/Il2rg-/- mice. Nat Biotechnol 2007;25:903–910. (Ref.42)

Baba S, et al. Commitment of bone marrow cells to hepatic stellate cells in mouse. J Hepatol 2004;40:255–260. (Ref.46)

Badve S, et al. An antigen reacting with das-1 monoclonal antibody is ontogenically regulated in diverse organs including liver and indicates sharing of developmental mechanisms among cell lineages. Pathobiology 2000;68:76–86. (Ref.21)

Basma H, et al. Differentiation and transplantation of human embryonic stem cell-derived hepatocytes. Gastroenterology 2009;136:990–999. (Ref.19)

Bilir BM, et al. Hepatocyte transplantation in acute liver failure. Liver Transpl 2000;6:32–40. (Ref.68)

Bissig KD, et al. Human liver chimeric mice provide a model for hepatitis B and C virus infection and treatment. J Clin Invest 2010;120:924–930. (Ref.43)

Bohnen NI, et al. Use of indium-111-labeled hepatocytes to determine the biodistribution of transplanted hepatocytes through portal vein infusion. Clin Nucl Med 2000;25:447–450. (Ref.63)

Bumgardner GL, et al. MHC-identical heart and hepatocyte allografts evoke opposite immune responses within the same host. Transplantation 2002;74:855–864. (Ref.65)

Cantz T, et al. Quantitative gene expression analysis reveals transition of fetal liver progenitor cells to mature hepatocytes after transplantation in uPA/RAG-2 mice. Am J Pathol 2003;162:37–45. (Ref.25)

Chen SJ, Tazelaar J, Wilson JM. Selective repopulation of normal mouse liver by hepatocytes transduced in vivo with recombinant adeno-associated virus. Hum Gene Ther 2001;12:45–50. (Ref.87)

Cheng K, Gupta S. Quantitative tools for assessing fate of transplanted human stem/progenitor cells in chimeric mice. Xenotransplantation 2009;16:145–151. (Ref.61)

Cheng K, et al. Switching of mesodermal and endodermal properties in hTERT-modified and expanded fetal human pancreatic progenitor cells. Stem Cell Res Ther 2010;1:6. (Ref.9)

Chinzei R, et al. Embryoid-body cells derived from a mouse embryonic stem cell line show differentiation into functional hepatocytes. Hepatology 2002;36:22–29. (Ref.16)

Dabeva MD, et al. Proliferation and differentiation of fetal liver epithelial progenitor cells after transplantation into adult rat liver. Am J Pathol 2000;156:2017–2031. (Ref.27)

Dandri M, et al. Repopulation of mouse liver with human hepatocytes and in vivo infection with hepatitis B virus. Hepatology 2001;33:981–988. (Ref.95)

Dandri M, et al. Chronic infection with hepatitis B viruses and antiviral drug evaluation in uPA mice after liver repopulation with tupaia hepatocytes. J Hepatol 2005;42:54–60. (Ref.97)

Darwish AA, et al. Permanent access to the portal system for cellular transplantation using an implantable port device. Liver Transpl 2004;10:1213–1215. (Ref.61)

Dhawan A, et al. Hepatocyte transplantation for inherited factor VII deficiency. Transplantation 2004;78:1812–1814. (Ref.59)

Duan Y, et al. Differentiation and enrichment of hepatocyte-like cells from human embryonic stem cells in vitro and in vivo. Stem Cells 2007;25:3058–3068. (Ref.17)

Enami Y, et al. Hepatic stellate cells promote hepatocyte engraftment in rat liver after prostaglandin-endoperoxide synthase inhibition. Gastroenterology 2009;136:2356–2364. (Ref.82)

Fausto N. Liver regeneration and repair: hepatocytes, progenitor cells, and stem cells. Hepatology 2004;39:1477–1487. (Ref.1)

Fisher RA, Strom SC. Human hepatocyte transplantation: worldwide results. Transplantation 2006;82:441–449. (Ref.11)

Fox IU, Roy Chowdhury J. Hepatocyte transplantation. J Hepatol 2004;40:878–886. (Ref.52)

Gagandeep S, et al. Transplanted hepatocytes engraft, survive and proliferate in the liver of rats with carbon tetrachloride-induced cirrhosis. J Pathol 2000;191:78–85. (Ref.84)

Gordon GJ, Coleman WB, Grisham JW. Temporal analysis of hepatocyte differentiation by small hepatocyte-like progenitor cells during liver regeneration in retrorsine-exposed rats. Am J Pathol 2000;157:771–786. (Ref.91)

Gorla GR, Malhi H, Gupta S. Polyploidy associated with oxidative DNA injury attenuates proliferative potential of cells. J Cell Sci 2001;114:2943–2951. (Ref.93)

Guo D, et al. Liver repopulation after cell transplantation in mice treated with retrorsine and carbon tetrachloride. Transplantation 2002;73:1818–1824. (Ref.90)

Gupta S, et al. Integration and proliferation of transplanted cells in hepatic parenchyma following D-galactosamine-induced acute injury in F344 rats. J Pathol 2000;190:203–210. (Ref.83)

Gupta S, et al. Cell transplantation causes loss of gap junctions and activates GGT expression permanently in host liver. Am J Physiol Gastrointest Liver Physiol 2000;279:G815–G826. (Ref.68)

Gupta S, et al. Entry and integration of transplanted hepatocytes in liver plates occur by disruption of hepatic sinusoidal endothelium. Hepatology 1999;29:509–519. (Ref.69)

Haridass D, et al. Repopulation efficiencies of adult hepatocytes, fetal liver progenitor cells, and embryonic stem cell-derived hepatic cells in albumin-promoter-enhancer urokinase-type plasminogen activator mice. Am J Pathol 2009;175:1483–1492. (Ref.18)

Held PK, et al. In vivo correction of murine hereditary tyrosinemia type i by varphiC31 integrase-mediated gene delivery. Mol Ther 2005;11:399–408. (Ref.80)

Horslen SP, et al. Isolated hepatocyte transplantation in an infant with a severe urea cycle disorder. Pediatrics 2003;111:1262–1267. (Ref.56)

Inada M, et al. Stage-specific regulation of adhesion molecule expression segregates epithelial stem/progenitor cells in fetal and adult human livers. Hepatol Int 2008;2:50–62. (Ref.4)

Inada M, et al. Phenotype reversion in fetal human liver epithelial cells identifies the role of an intermediate meso-endodermal stage before hepatic maturation. J Cell Sci 2008;121:1002–1013. (Ref.5)

Ise H, et al. Effective hepatocyte transplantation using rat hepatocytes with low asialoglycoprotein receptor expression. Am J Pathol 2004;165:501–510. (Ref.78)

Jang YY, et al. Hematopoietic stem cells convert into liver cells within days without fusion. Nature Cell Biol 2004;6:532–539. (Ref.55)

Jiang Y, et al. Pluripotency of mesenchymal stem cells derived from adult marrow. Nature 2002;418:41–49. (Ref.38)

Joseph B, et al. Kupffer cells participate in early clearance of syngeneic hepatocytes transplanted in the rat liver. Gastroenterology 2002;123:1677–1685. (Ref.70)

Katayama S, et al. Size-dependent in vivo growth potential of adult rat hepatocytes. Am J Pathol 2001;158:97–105. (Ref.77)

Keene CD, et al. Neural differentiation and incorporation of bone marrow-derived multipotent adult progenitor cells after single cell transplantation into blastocyst stage mouse embryos. Cell Transplant 2003;12:201–213. (Ref.48)

Khan AA, et al. Peritoneal transplantation of human fetal hepatocytes for the treatment of acute fatty liver of pregnancy: a case report. Trop Gastroenterol 2004;25:141–143. (Ref.26)

Kobayashi N, et al. Prevention of acute liver failure in rats with reversibly immortalized human hepatocytes. Science 2000;287:1258–1262. (Ref.58)

Krause DS, et al. Multi-organ, multi-lineage engraftment by a single bone marrow-derived stem cell. Cell 2001;105:369–377. (Ref.40)

Krohn N, et al. Hepatocyte transplantation-induced liver inflammation is driven by cytokines-chemokines associated with neutrophils and Kupffer cells. Gastroenterology 2009;136:1806–1817. (Ref.73)

Kubota H, Reid LM. Clonogenic hepatoblasts, common precursors for hepatocytic and biliary lineages, are lacking classical major histocompatibility complex class I antigen. Proc Natl Acad Sci USA 2000;97:12132–12137. (Ref.27)

Lagasse E, et al. Purified hematopoietic stem cells can differentiate into hepatocytes in vivo. Nature Med 2000;6:1229–1234. (Ref.37)

Lee JB, et al. Comparative characteristics of three human embryonic stem cell lines. Mol Cell 2005;19:31–38. (Ref.14)

Li H, et al. The Ink4/Arf locus is a barrier for iPS cell reprogramming. Nature 2009;460:1136–1139. (Ref.10b)

Malhi H, et al. Cyclophosphamide disrupts hepatic sinusoidal endothelium and improves transplanted cell engraftment in rat liver. Hepatology 2002;36:112–121. (Ref.72)

Malhi H, et al. Cell transplantation after oxidative hepatic preconditioning with radiation and ischemia–reperfusion leads to extensive liver repopulation. Proc Natl Acad Sci USA 2002;99:13114–13119. (Ref.94)

Malhi H, et al. Isolation of human progenitor liver epithelial cells with extensive replication capacity and differentiation into mature hepatocytes. J Cell Sci 2002;115:2679–2688. (Ref.20)

Mas VR, et al. Engraftment measurement in human liver tissue after liver cell transplantation by short tandem repeats analysis. Cell Transplant 2004;13:231–236. (Ref.60)

Menthena A, et al. Bone marrow progenitors are not the source of expanding oval cells in injured liver. Stem Cells 2004;22:1049–1061. (Ref.33)

Mercer DF, et al. Hepatitis C virus replication in mice with chimeric human livers. Nature Med 2001;7:927–933. (Ref.96)

Michalopoulos GK. Liver regeneration after partial hepatectomy: critical analysis of mechanistic dilemmas. Am J Pathol 2010;176:2–13. (Ref.34)

Mikula M, et al. Immortalized p19ARF null hepatocytes restore liver injury and generate hepatic progenitors after transplantation. Hepatology 2004;39:628–634. (Ref.47)

Muller-Borer BJ, et al. Adult-derived liver stem cells acquire a cardiomyocyte structural and functional phenotype ex vivo. Am J Pathol 2004;165:135–145. (Ref.32)

Muraca M, et al. Hepatocyte transplantation as a treatment for glycogen storage disease type 1a. Lancet 2002;359:317–318. (Ref.57)

Muraca M, et al. Intraportal hepatocyte transplantation in the pig: hemodynamic and histopathological study. Transplantation 2002;73:890–896. (Ref.49)

Nagata H, et al. Route of hepatocyte delivery affects hepatocyte engraftment in the spleen. Transplantation 2003;76:732–734. (Ref.63)

Newsome PN, et al. Human cord blood-derived cells can differentiate into hepatocytes in the mouse liver with no evidence of cellular fusion. Gastroenterology 2003;124:1891–1900. (Ref.41)

Nierhoff D, et al. Purification and characterization of mouse fetal liver epithelial cells with high in vivo repopulation capacity. Hepatology 2005;42:130–139. (Ref.29)

Ohashi K, et al. Functional life-long maintenance of engineered liver tissue in mice following transplantation under the kidney capsule. J Tissue Eng Regen Med 2010;4:141–148. (Ref.62)

Okita K, Ichisaka T, Yamanaka S. Generation of germline-competent induced pluripotent stem cells. Nature 2007;448:313–317. (Ref.15)

Penuelas I, et al. Positron emission tomography imaging of adenoviral-mediated transgene expression in liver cancer patients. Gastroenterology 2005;128:1787–1795. (Ref.62)

Petersen BE, et al. Bone marrow as a potential source of hepatic oval cells. Science 1999;284:1168–1170. (Ref.36)

Reddy B, et al. The effect of CD28/B7 blockade on alloreactive T and B cells after liver cell transplantation. Transplantation 2001;71:801–811. (Ref.66)

Sandhu JS, et al. Stem cell properties and repopulation of the rat liver by fetal liver epithelial progenitor cells. Am J Pathol 2001;159:1323–1334. (Ref.24)

Sato N, et al. Maintenance of pluripotency in human and mouse embryonic stem cells through activation of Wnt signaling by a pharmacological GSK-3-specific inhibitor. Nature Med 2004;10:55–63. (Ref.22)

Saxena R, Theise N. Canals of Hering: recent insights and current knowledge. Semin Liver Dis 2004;24:43–48. (Ref.31)

Schneider A, et al. Intraportal infusion of 99mtechnetium-macro-aggregated albumin particles and hepatocytes in rabbits: assessment of shunting and portal hemodynamic changes. Transplantation 2003;75:296–302. (Ref.64)

Sell S, Leffert HL. Liver cancer stem cells. J Clin Oncol 2008;26:2800–2805. (Ref.7)

Shafritz DA, Oertel M. Model systems and experimental conditions that lead to effective repopulation of the liver by transplanted cells. Int J Biochem Cell Biol 2011;43:198–213. [Epub ahead of print] (Ref.86)

Sigot V, et al. A simple and effective method to improve intrasplenic rat hepatocyte transplantation. Cell Transplant 2004;13:775–781. (Ref.76)

Si-Tayeb K, et al. Highly efficient generation of human hepatocyte-like cells from induced pluripotent stem cells. Hepatology 2010;51:297–305. (Ref.21)

Slehria S, et al. Hepatic sinusoidal vasodilators improve transplanted cell engraftment and ameliorate microcirculatory perturbations in the liver. Hepatology 2002;35:1320–1328. (Ref.67)

Sokal EM, et al. Hepatocyte transplantation in a 4-year-old girl with peroxisomal biogenesis disease: technique, safety, and metabolic follow-up. Transplantation 2003;76:735–738. (Ref.58)

Sokhi RP, Rajvanshi P, Gupta S. Transplanted reporter cells help in defining onset of hepatocyte proliferation during the life of F344 rats. Am J Physiol Gastrointest Liver Physiol 2000;279:G631–G640. (Ref.48)

Suzuki A, et al. Liver repopulation by c-Met-positive stem/progenitor cells isolated from the developing rat liver. Hepatogastroenterology 2004;51:423–426. (Ref.28)

Takashima S, et al. Human amniotic epithelial cells possess hepatocyte-like characteristics and functions. Cell Struct Funct 2004;29:73–84. (Ref.41)

Thomson JA, et al. Embryonic stem cell lines derived from human blastocysts. Science 1998;282:1145–1147. (Ref.12)

Wagers AJ, et al. Little evidence for developmental plasticity of adult hematopoietic stem cells. Science 2002;297:2256–2259. (Ref.44)

Walldorf J, et al. Expanding hepatocytes in vitro before cell transplantation: donor age-dependent proliferative capacity of cultured human hepatocytes. Scand J Gastroenterol 2004;39:584–593. (Ref.79)

Wang J, et al. Fas siRNA reduces apoptotic cell death of allogeneic-transplanted hepatocytes in mouse spleen. Transplant Proc 2003;35:1594–1595. (Ref.81)

Wang X, et al. The origin and liver repopulating capacity of murine oval cells. Proc Natl Acad Sci USA 2003;100(Suppl 1):11881–11888. (Ref.38)

Wang X, et al. Albumin-expressing hepatocyte-like cells develop in the livers of immune-deficient mice that received transplants of highly purified human hematopoietic stem cells. Blood 2003;101:4201–4208. (Ref.49)

Wang X, et al. Kinetics of liver repopulation after bone marrow transplantation. Am J Pathol 2002;161:565–574. (Ref.39)

Wege H, et al. Telomerase reconstitution immortalizes human fetal hepatocytes without disrupting their differentiation potential. Gastroenterology 2003;124:432–444. (Ref.23)

Wilhelm A, et al. Acute impairment of hepatic microcirculation and recruitment of nonparenchymal cells by intrasplenic hepatocyte transplantation. J Pediatr Surg 2004;39:1214–1219. (Ref.71)

Willenbring H, et al. Myelomonocytic cells are sufficient for therapeutic cell fusion in liver. Nature Med 2004;10:744–748. (Ref.54)

Yamanouchi K, et al. Hepatic irradiation augments engraftment of donor cells following hepatocyte transplantation. Hepatology 2009;49:258–267. (Ref.92)

Yen BL, et al. Isolation of multipotent cells from human term placenta. Stem Cells 2005;23:3–9. (Ref.35)

Yovchev MI, et al. Novel rat hepatic progenitor cell surface markers: the identity of oval cells. Hepatology 2007;45:139–149. (Ref.6)

Yu J, et al. Induced pluripotent stem cell lines derived from human somatic cells. Science 2007;318:1917–1920. (Ref.16)

Yuan RH, et al. p27Kip1 inactivation provides a proliferative advantage to transplanted hepatocytes in DPPIV/Rag2 double knockout mice after repeated host liver injury. Cell Transpl 2003;12:907–919. (Ref.59)

Zahler MH, et al. The application of a lentiviral vector for gene transfer in fetal human hepatocytes. J Gene Med 2000;2:186–193. (Ref.22)

Zalzman M, et al. Reversal of hyperglycemia in mice using human expandable insulin-producing cells differentiated from fetal liver progenitor cells. Proc Natl Acad Sci USA 2003;100:7253–7258. (Ref.30)

Zaret KS. Genetic programming of liver and pancreas progenitors: lessons for stem-cell differentiation. Nat Rev Genet 2008; 9:329–340. (Ref.8)

Zhao R, Duncan SA. Embryonic development of the liver. Hepatology 2005;41:956–967. (Ref.3)

A complete list of references can be found at www.expertconsult.com.

Section II

Approach to the Patient with Liver Disease

Liver Biopsy (Quality and Use of Gun)

Christian P. Strassburg and Michael P. Manns

ABBREVIATIONS

AFP α-fetoprotein	**HCC** hepatocellular carcinoma	**INR** international normalized ratio
CT computed tomography	**HIV** human immunodeficiency virus	**PSC** primary sclerosing cholangitis

Introduction

A liver biopsy specimen for histologic evaluation represents an important part of the clinical and laboratory workup for both the management of any chronic liver disease and the monitoring of liver transplant grafts.[1] Although biochemical, serologic, and molecular biologic tests and noninvasive procedures, such as elastography and laboratory scores,[2] have been constantly improved, histologic evaluation still remains the gold standard for answering the many questions regarding liver diseases. However, indications and techniques employed have changed considerably since the liver biopsy was first performed.[3] The first liver biopsy obtained by aspiration was performed by Paul Ehrlich in 1883 to assess hepatic glycogen content in a diabetic patient, and 12 years later by Lucatello to analyze a tropical abscess of the liver. Its first application for the diagnosis of cirrhotic liver disease in humans and rats was published in a series by Schüpfer in France in 1907, and the diagnostic potential was expanded by Bingel in Germany in 1923. Over the next 50 years the technique of obtaining liver biopsy samples was further developed in regard to the surgical approach used, the type of needle employed, and the integration of various diagnostic imaging modalities (e.g., ultrasound, computer tomography [CT], angiography, laparoscopy) into the procedure. Since the publication of *One-Second Needle Biopsy of the Liver* by Menghini in 1958,[4] the technique of hepatic needle biopsy has seen a broad introduction into clinical nonoperative medicine and is performed by experienced fellows and hepatologists on a daily basis in hepatologic centers.[3] Although the etiology of most chronic liver diseases can be diagnosed by currently available biochemical, serologic, immunologic, and molecular biologic tests, histologic evaluation remains firmly integrated into the management of chronic hepatic disease.[5] Histologic analysis is employed not only for the identification of undefined liver diseases but also, and most importantly, for the determination of inflammatory activity (grading) and degree of fibrosis/cirrhosis (staging). Grading and staging are relevant both for

the prognosis of the patient and for the indication for cost-intensive as well as potentially side effect prone therapies, such as the administration of interferon-α combination therapy in chronic hepatitis C virus infection.[6] The increasing number of liver transplant patients within the hepatologic spectrum requires that regular, safe, and high-quality biopsies, and also their appropriate assessment, be readily available.[7] In addition, the use of liver biopsy in the management of infectious diseases allows for a fast and sensitive discovery of mycobacteria or viruses in hepatic tissues (e.g., in HIV-infected patients, in patients with granulomatous diseases). The determination of copper and iron content in hepatic tissue can be achieved in biopsies from patients with hereditary storage diseases such as hemochromatosis and Wilson disease. In addition, biopsy can provide important clues to the etiology and further management of conditions such as α_1-antitrypsin deficiency, amyloidosis, unclear space-occupying lesions, or suspected drug toxicity.[8-11] In view of these considerations liver biopsies are of significant importance. In practical hepatology obtaining a liver biopsy involves not only consideration of the technique to be employed but also anticipation and appreciation of the potential side effects as well as the probability of obtaining information that will answer clinical questions and lead to a modification or initiation of a therapeutic approach.[12,13]

Definitions of a Percutaneous Liver Biopsy

From a technical point of view three important factors are considered when obtaining a liver biopsy. First, liver tissue can be obtained either by cutting or by aspiration (**Fig. 12-1**). Second, regarding the route of penetration, a liver biopsy can proceed transcutaneously via an intercostal or subcostal route. Third, ultrasound or computed tomography guidance as well as visual guidance during laparoscopy are further options.

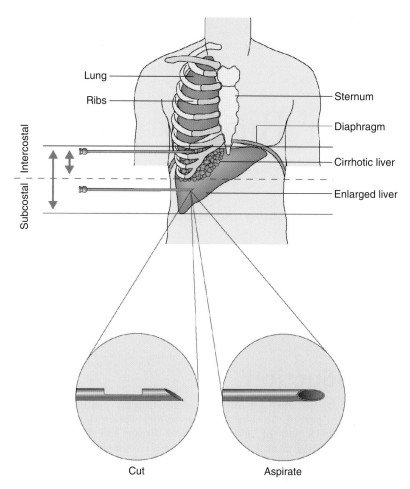

Lung
Ribs
Sternum
Diaphragm
Cirrhotic liver
Enlarged liver

Intercostal
Subcostal

Cut   Aspirate

Fig. 12-1 **Schematic of the approach to transcutaneous liver biopsies.** A transcutaneous biopsy of the liver is performed in complete expiration to limit accidental pulmonary injury. Because the liver is frequently cirrhotic and therefore small in size, an intercostal approach is necessary. However, in large livers a subcostal approach is preferred as a safer route of biopsy. The schematic illustrates the two principle types of needles used, cutting needles and aspiration needles; multiple models of these needles are commercially available and should be chosen on the basis of the patient's risk profile and the clinical indication for the biopsy (see text).

Transcutaneous Liver Biopsy

Transcutaneous liver biopsy is performed with the patient positioned prone with the right arm elevated behind the head. Percussion examines the extent of the liver. In our center every transcutaneous liver biopsy is preceded by an abdominal ultrasound, which confirms the absence of complicating factors (including dilated bile ducts, venous collaterals, Chilaiditi syndrome, very small cirrhotic livers, and abnormal vascular findings such as hemangiomas or echinococcal cysts) and the localization of the gallbladder. Ultrasound also corroborates the presence of an accessible mass of liver tissue in the envisioned path of penetration. However, conclusive evidence that ultrasound reduces morbidity and mortality has been debated in the literature.[14-17] Recent studies report reduced complications using ultrasound guidance[18] and an improvement of biopsy quality in hepatitis C patients,[19] and suggest that ultrasound guidance should be used routinely. Usually, an intercostal puncture site in the midaxillary line pointed at the xiphoid process is chosen. In very large livers, biopsy can be performed subcostally. Complications appear to favor a subcostal route (4.1%) to a transthoracic route (2.7%),[20] which is usually not possible in patients with small cirrhotic livers (see **Fig. 12-1**). After the thoracic wall and the liver capsule are anesthetized with a locally infiltrating anesthetic, a skin incision is made by scalpel (**Figs. 12-2 and 12-3**).

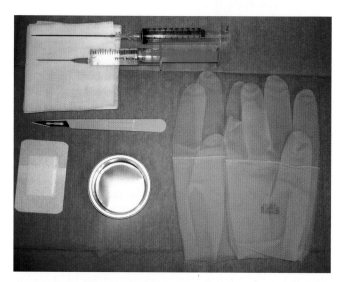

Fig. 12-2 **Typical setup of materials required for an aspiration transcutaneous liver biopsy.** The syringe is already connected to an aspiration needle (Menghini) biopsy set. The other syringe is used for the administration of local anesthetic.

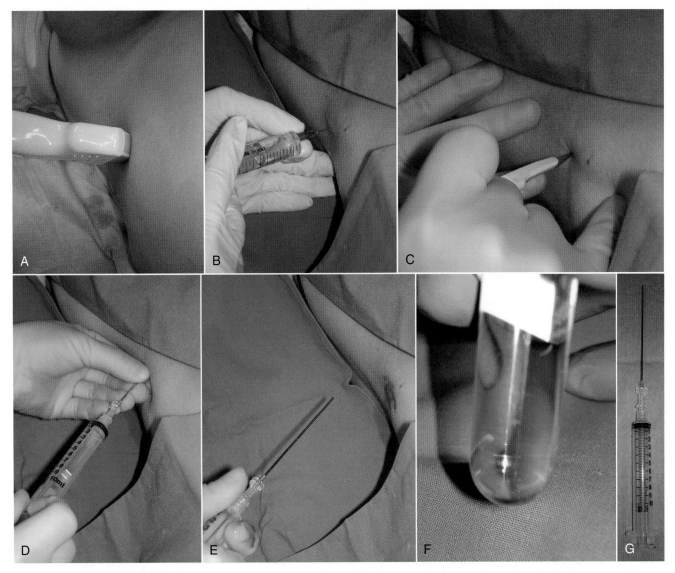

Fig. 12-3 Procedure of transcutaneous aspiration liver biopsy using a Menghini needle. Ultrasound is used to visualize the path of the biopsy needle (**A**); ultrasound is routinely performed in our center to minimize complications but is considered controversial because conclusive data suggesting a reduction of complications are not available. While the patient is holding her or his breath, the skin of the thoracic wall down to the liver capsule is locally anesthetized (**B**) before a small scalpel incision is made (**C**). Using sterile technique, the needle is positioned (**D**) in the incision canal and advanced to the liver capsule while the patient is holding her or his breath; suction is then applied with the connected syringe and the needle is rapidly advanced into the liver tissue. It is then withdrawn with the plunger still arrested in the suction position (**E**). The tissue cylinder is deposited in an appropriate specimen container (**F**). Menghini aspiration needle (**G**).

Depending upon the type of needle used, one of the two following procedures is then employed:

(1) Using a Menghini (aspiration) device, the needle (which is attached to a syringe optionally containing 10 ml of sterile normal saline) is advanced up to the pleural surface and flushed with 1 to 2 ml of saline. The patient is asked to hold his or her breath in complete expiration, suction is applied by retracting the plunger, and the needle is quickly advanced and withdrawn from the liver tissue. The specimen is visualized and deposited into the appropriate specimen container (see **Fig. 12-3**).

(2) When a Tru-Cut needle is used, a tissue specimen lodged in a niche in the obturator needle is excised by a second cylindrical needle sliding over it. To this end the needle is advanced into the liver and the sliding mechanism is triggered manually or automatically ("biopsy gun"); the needle is then withdrawn from the liver. The specimen is recovered from the obturator needle and placed in an appropriate specimen container.

Overall, the Tru-Cut needle remains in the liver for a longer time, increasing the possibility of patient movement and visceral injury. However, the Tru-Cut needle has been shown to produce superior tissue specimens. In a variation of the Tru-Cut needle technique a plugged biopsy can be performed. In this case the needle is withdrawn from the cutting sheath, which remains in the liver with the patient still holding his or her breath. It is replaced by a plastic cannula, which is used to embolize the puncture canal with gelatin. This procedure can be considered as an alternative to transvenous liver biopsy in selected patients.

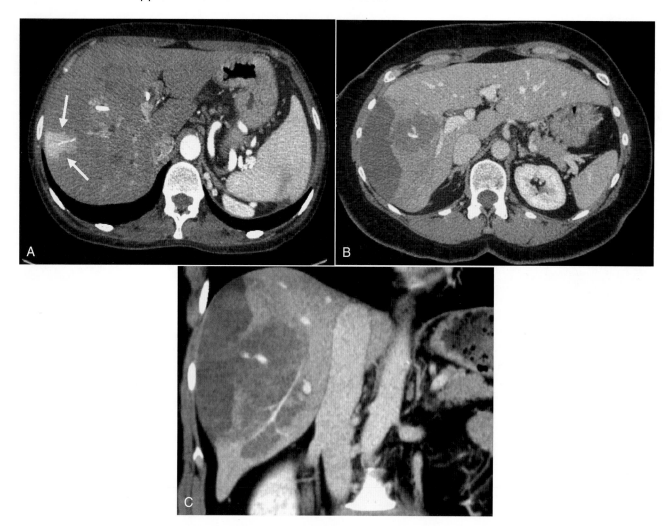

Fig. 12-4 **Hemorrhage as a complication of transcutaneous liver biopsy. A,** Computed tomography scan shows an arterial phase of a study performed incidentally after liver biopsy a few hours previously. The study demonstrates the extent of intrahepatic hemorrhage in a clinically inapparent patient with normal vital parameters and unchanged blood count following liver biopsy. **B** and **C,** These CT scans show a massive intrahepatic as well as subcapsular hemorrhage 24 hours after liver biopsy in a patient with normal coagulation studies; the patient was biopsied as a treatment decision for chronic hepatitis C. The scans show that hemorrhage can occur late after transcutaneous liver biopsy in individuals without coagulopathy.

Technique and Risk Assessment
Number of Passes

When a small or fragmented tissue cylinder is obtained the biopsy is repeated by a pass through the same incision.[13] The number of passes required to obtain a representative biopsy specimen has to be weighed against the increased risk of hemorrhage and other risks of biopsy. Irrespective of subcostal or transthoracic approach, one study found an increase of complications when more than three passes were performed.[20,21] However, the risk of hemorrhage in transcutaneous liver biopsy is also dependent on other factors, including patient age and the presence of malignant tumors[21] as well as renal impairment.[22,23] Hemorrhage can occur long after the needle biopsy has been performed.[24] Two passes during aspiration needle biopsy have been shown to increase diagnostic quality and minor complications in comparison with three passes.[25]

Experience

As noted in every invasive measure, complications are associated with the experience of the operator. The frequency of

complications was 3.2% in physicians with a history of fewer than 20 biopsies compared with 1.1% in physicians who had performed more than 100 procedures.[26] No differences were seen between gastroenterologists and general practitioners. It is important to realize that every needle biopsy leads to hemorrhage, which is usually minor and clinically irrelevant. This is best appreciated when laparoscopic biopsies are performed that allow for a direct visualization of the puncture site. If a CT scan is performed directly after a transcutaneous liver biopsy, hepatic hemorrhage can be demonstrated that is otherwise clinically inapparent and unnoticed by determinations of blood counts (**Fig. 12-4**).

Tru-Cut (Biopsy Gun) versus Aspiration Needle

In general, the accepted mortality rate from liver biopsy is between 0.1% and 0.01%. However, because most studies rely on retrospective data, these numbers have been found to vary considerably.[21,26,27] Estimating mortality rate is difficult for another reason. Patients subjected to liver biopsies usually suffer from advanced liver disease or malignancy with a high death rate, which is not influenced by the actual liver biopsy. The overall mortality in one study was shown to be 19% within 3 months after liver biopsy.[26] However, differences were also reported for the type of needle used. The overall complication rate in one series was 0.35% for Tru-Cut and 0.1% for Menghini needles.[26] This study identified a higher incidence of hemorrhage, pneumothorax, biliary leakage, and peritonitis with Tru-Cut needles; however, puncture of other internal organs and sepsis occurred more often with Menghini needles. In contrast, a study comparing Jamshidi suction needles with Tru-Cut Vim Silverman needles was unable to demonstrate such technique-related differences.[20,21] The relationship between the diameter of the needle and the degree of hemorrhage is still a subject of controversy. While in humans no differences were observed between the use of 1.6-mm versus 1.9-mm Menghini needles,[28] experiments on anesthetized pigs showed more bleeding in 2.1-mm versus 1.6-mm needles as well as 1.2-mm versus 1.6-mm needles.[23] Considerations weighing gauge as well as needle type (i.e., Menghini vs. Tru-Cut needles) should keep in mind that smaller needles and smaller specimens may increase the number of passes required[25] or necessitate repuncture to obtain representative tissue, increasing the bleeding risk.

Bacteremia

In normal and cirrhotic livers, biopsies have been documented to lead to bacteremia.[29-31] In patients with biliary enteric anastomoses the occurrence of septic complications following liver biopsy has been controversial.[32-35] Current data are not sufficient to recommend routine antibiotic prophylaxis. Antibiotics should, however, be administered to patients who have valvular heart disease, suspected cholangitis, or a documented history of septic complications following liver biopsy.

Transvenous (Transjugular) Liver Biopsy

Procedure

Because hemorrhage is the single most feared complication of transcutaneous liver biopsy and patients suffering from severe coagulation disorders attributable to hepatic and other diseases are common candidates for histologic assessment, transvenous liver biopsy was developed. It was described by Dotter in 1964.[36] During the past 20 years more than 60 studies have been published assessing transvenous liver biopsies, demonstrating an acceptable safety and quality profile for this method.[37] The transvenous liver biopsy is usually obtained through a right-sided puncture of the internal jugular vein, and rarely through a transfemoral route. Technically, it is a modified version of the aspiration needle (or Tru-Cut) biopsy procedure. However, transvenous liver biopsy requires a technically more complex operative setting, which includes fluoroscopy and contrast medium, the transvenous catheter and needle kit, and cardiac monitoring. The internal jugular vein is cannulated and a sheath inserted using the Seldinger technique. A catheter is then guided through the right atrium into the inferior vena cava. The transvenous biopsy needle is then advanced into one of the hepatic veins, which is visualized by the injection of contrast medium. However, previous surgery of the vena cava (e.g., following liver transplantation) can severely obstruct the cannulation of the hepatic veins. The

patient is asked to hold his or her breath and the needle is rapidly advanced 1 to 2 cm beyond the tip of the venous catheter; suction is then applied by a connected syringe during liver passage. Liver tissue can subsequently be recovered from the needle.

Technique and Risk Assessment
Complications and Alternatives

Transvenous liver biopsy is a second-line procedure limited to patients with significant coagulation disorders in whom liver histology is likely to alter therapeutic management. In patients with coagulation disorders, liver biopsy coupled with embolization of the puncture canal (plugged biopsy) is an alternative and has been shown to be a safe procedure.[38-40] Direct comparison of transvenous and embolization liver biopsy procedures showed that both methods were equally successful with low complication rates. Transcutaneous embolization biopsy yielded larger liver specimens, as expected with a cutting biopsy technique, but was also associated with a 3.5% rate of bleeding in one study.[41] However, cutting needles can also be employed in transvenous approaches and improve the quality of the liver specimen.[37,42] In our own experience comparing more than 100 percutaneous, mini-laparoscopic, and transvenous liver biopsies, the quality of the liver specimen was found to be higher with a mini-laparoscopic (Tru-Cut) and percutaneous (aspiration) technique than with a percutaneous (Tru-Cut) approach.[43] It would appear prudent to employ embolization liver biopsy in patients with coagulation abnormalities in the absence of tension ascites whenever a transjugular approach is impossible or has previously failed.[44] In impaired coagulation, mini-laparoscopic biopsy is also an option.

Technical Considerations

The main disadvantage of transvenous liver biopsy is the considerable effort incurred. While a standard transcutaneous liver biopsy can be performed in 15 minutes (including ultrasound visualization), a transvenous liver biopsy procedure takes 45 minutes to complete and requires a complex operative setup. There is a theoretical risk of arrhythmia and of contrast material–related reactions in addition to the proven risks associated with the use of x-rays. Compared with other liver biopsy procedures the transvenous approach is also more expensive, attributable to the costly catheter/needle kit and the longer physician presence required. This profile clearly limits its application to selected patients.

Laparoscopic Liver Biopsy

Laparoscopic liver biopsy is not an actual biopsy technique, but an alternative route of obtaining a liver biopsy specimen during visual assessment of the peritoneum and the abdominal organs.[45] Historically, minimally invasive abdominal procedures were developed by internists for diagnostic reasons. In the 1960s laparoscopy was routinely performed for the assessment of liver disease.[46,47] However, after the refinement of biochemical, serologic, and molecular biologic tests for the diagnosis of liver diseases, laparoscopy was employed less frequently and the considerable body of experience of macroscopic assessment of liver diseases has seen a significant decline. In recent years laparoscopic liver biopsy has again begun to attract increasing attention, primarily because of the development of the minimally invasive mini-laparoscopy for routine clinical practice[48] (**Fig. 12-5**). Mini-laparoscopy is distinguished from standard or midi-laparoscopy by the use of optical instruments with a diameter <2 mm and by the use of a sheathed Veress needle that allows for the application of a pneumoperitoneum and the abdominal introduction of the optical instrument through a single puncture (see **Fig. 12-5, B**). The abdomen is punctured at the so-called Kalk position 2 cm left and cranially of the umbilicus, and usually 3 to 4 L of N_2O are introduced to produce a sufficient pneumoperitoneum (see **Fig. 12-5, C**). An instrumentation sheath is subsequently positioned under direct sight, typically in the lateral upper right quadrant within reach of the liver (see **Fig. 12-5, D**). After a macroscopic assessment of the cranial and inferior liver surfaces including the edges, the gallbladder, and the hepatic ligament as well as the peritoneum, a liver biopsy can be performed either by the aspiration or by the Tru-Cut technique (see **Fig. 12-5, E**) with advancement of the respective biopsy device through the instrumentation sheath. This is preceded by macroscopically identifying a specific area of interest on the liver surface, thereby increasing the likelihood of a representative biopsy specimen relative to the original indication for the biopsy. The site of puncture can be monitored, and if prolonged hemorrhage occurs, monopolar electrical coagulation can be employed (**Fig. 12-6**) to induce hemostasis. In addition, the presence of ascites is not a limiting factor because ascitic fluid can be evacuated during laparoscopy before the liver biopsy procedure.

Technique and Risk Assessment

Mini-laparoscopy is less invasive than standard laparoscopy but has the disadvantage of using a zero-degree optical instrument of 1.9- to 2.0-mm diameter with decreased brightness, providing a diminished overview of the abdominal organs. For the representative diagnosis of liver cirrhosis a number of studies have suggested laparoscopy to be the gold standard.[45,48,49] In fact, when used in conjunction with a macroscopic diagnosis of nodular cirrhosis and increased tissue consistency, determined by direct palpation, laparoscopic procedures are relatively simple and have an increased sensitivity, as compared with "blind" biopsy or ultrasound visualization and biopsy. A recent study using Menghini aspiration needles has found cirrhosis sensitivity to be 96.4% for standard laparoscopy and 91.9% for mini-laparoscopy compared with 68% for histologic evaluation without laparoscopy.[48] Compared with transcutaneous liver biopsies the rate of complications appears not to be increased[50] for mini-laparoscopy. An important issue is the availability of this approach to patients with coagulation disorders. Mini-laparoscopy has been shown to be feasible in patients with prolonged international normalized ratios (INR >1.5) and thrombocytopenia (<50 platelets/mm³), and even in patients with von Willebrand disease or hemophilia without significant hemorrhage[51] (see **Fig. 12-6**). The risk assessment includes the inherent risks associated with the laparoscopy procedure—sedation, accidental vascular injection of N_2O, injury of the viscera, and hemorrhage of abdominal wall vessels. During 63,845 standard laparoscopies with 48,766 liver biopsies[46,47] the reported rate of hemorrhage was 0.09%, overall complications were 2.5%, and the mortality rate was 0.03%.

An important issue surrounding liver biopsies is the attempt to obtain a representative sample of the liver. Mini-laparoscopy combines direct visualization with histologic data obtained from a biopsy taken from a region of interest (**Fig. 12-7**). Many chronic liver diseases, including primary sclerosing cholangitis (PSC), viral hepatitis, and nodular regeneration, affect the liver in a zonal fashion. A "blind" biopsy is unlikely to accurately reflect the extent and variation of hepatic disease in these cases. Mini-laparoscopy offers the advantage of visual guidance of the biopsy needle to a region or multiple regions of interest, which considerably increases the accurate subsequent histologic assessment (**Fig. 12-8**). In addition, because laparoscopy includes the possibility of electrical hemostasis unclear hepatic masses can be directly biopsied, even in those cases in which vascular structures limit a transcutaneous approach. Finally, in diseases such as primary sclerosing cholangitis, cholangiocellular carcinoma, or hepatic metastases the peritoneum can be visualized, evidence of peritoneal carcinomatosis (see **Fig. 12-7**) documented, and specimens removed, which is important for the decision between operative and conservative treatment strategies such as resection, liver transplantation, and chemotherapy.

Ultrasound-Guided Fine Needle Aspiration

Ultrasound-guided fine needle aspiration is extensively used to obtain histologic or cytologic information regarding the diagnosis of focal hepatic lesions. It is not routinely employed to determine the grade of liver inflammation or the stage of hepatic fibrosis.[52] The indication for fine needle aspiration cytology of diffuse hepatic diseases is controversial. The hepatic lesion is visualized by ultrasound and a path for the needle aspiration is plotted to avoid intersecting vessels. Usually, an ultrasound array with an integrated needle guidance slot is employed. A needle with a diameter <1 mm is advanced into the lesion while the patient holds her or his breath; suction is then applied with a syringe connected to the needle and after three to five passes the needle is withdrawn from the liver. The aspirated material is spread on a glass microscopy coverslip, dried, and forwarded to the cytologist. Ultrasound-guided biopsy can also be performed with cutting needles. In general, a cirrhotic liver in a patient with a higher likelihood of bleeding would be a candidate for fine needle aspiration versus cutting needle biopsy. In addition, the biopsy of the liver can be performed under CT guidance.

Technique and Risk Assessment
Hemorrhage

Hemorrhage with fine needle aspiration using needles <1 mm is rare. The mortality rate has been estimated to range between 0.006% and 0.1%.[53] The lowest complication rate has been reported in an analysis of 2091 biopsies for the use of noncutting needles.[54]

Specificity

A number of studies have documented that the specificity of fine needle aspiration cytology is extremely accurate, with sensitivities and specificities approaching 100%.[55-57] Regarding biopsy size, it was suggested that fine needle aspiration versus

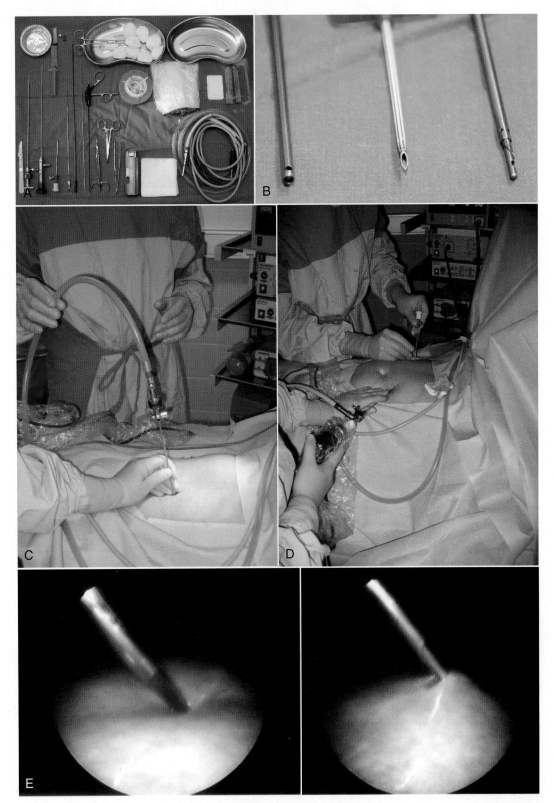

Fig. 12-5 A, Typical setup of materials required for a mini-laparoscopy and biopsy. Apart from the Veress needle and optical instruments, an instrumentation sheath is required, which is used to introduce the biopsy needle into the abdomen under direct vision and to obtain the liver biopsy sample. This figure shows an automatic biopsy gun for a Tru-Cut biopsy needle. **B,** Mini-laparoscopy in this figure uses equipment with a diameter of 2 mm. For comparison purposes, sizes of the fiberoptic instrument *(left)*, a 14-gauge venous cannula *(middle)*, and the Veress needle with the surrounding insertion sheath *(right)* are shown. **C,** Application of the pneumoperitoneum after puncture with a sheathed 2-mm Veress needle. The typical insertion point left and cranial of the umbilicus is visible. **D,** After generation of the pneumoperitoneum the 2-mm optical instrument is inserted. The image shows the situation before the insertion of the instrumentation. Images (**E**) show the liver surface and a visually guided cutting needle positioned on the superior liver surface of the right lobe. Direct visualization allows for the biopsy to proceed within an area of interest, thereby increasing the likelihood of obtaining a representative tissue sample.

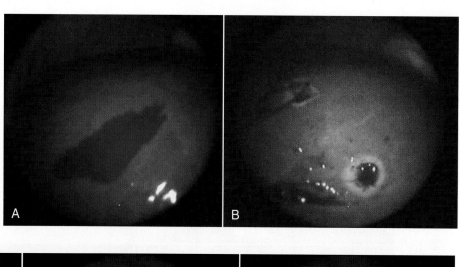

Fig. 12-6 Upon hemorrhage after mini-laparoscopic biopsy (**A**) hemostasis by monopolar electrocoagulation is possible (**B**), which expands the indication to patients with reduced coagulation studies.

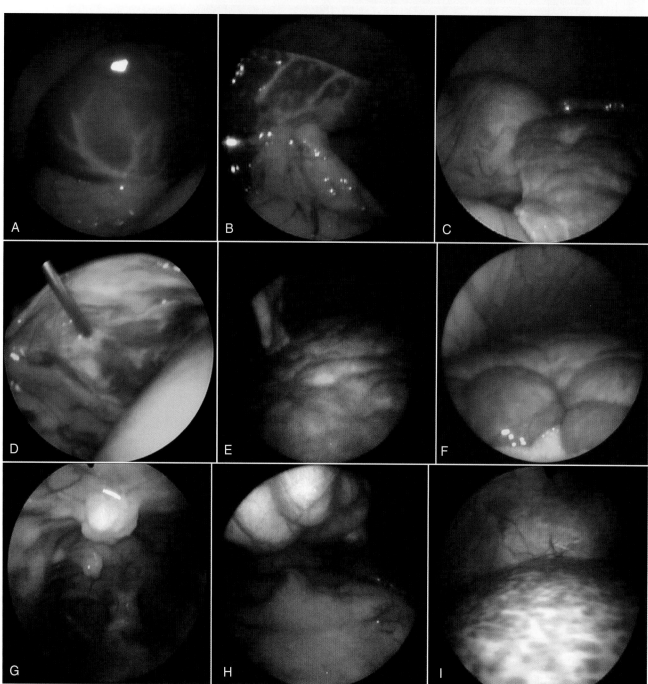

Fig. 12-7 **The advantage of the mini-laparoscopic biopsy is the visual evaluation of the liver before biopsy. A,** Aspect of minimal PSC with individual fibrotic duct structures; **B,** early PSC with more fibrotic duct structures; **C,** PSC that has advanced to cirrhosis; and **D,** PSC with cholangiocarcinoma revealed after histologic examination. Coarse nodular appearance of the liver in PBC (**E**) and autoimmune hepatitis (AIH) (**F**); the aspect of peritoneal carcinomatosis in cholangiocarcinoma (**G**); a patent umbilical vein in portal hypertension (**H**); and the appearance of Caroli's disease (**I**) are also shown.

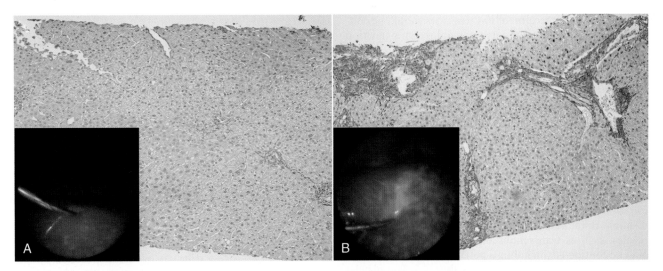

Fig. 12-8 Example of the variability of visually directed liver biopsies in a single patient with primary sclerosing cholangitis. Biopsy within an area with the appearance of mild fibrosis shows a histologic image with almost no changes of microscopic architecture (**A**). Biopsy of an area within the same liver that appears more affected leads to the histologic picture of advanced fibrosis (**B**). In this patient biopsies of the areas of interest led to an accurate assessment of histologic stage superior to a "blind" transcutaneous approach.

cutting needle aspiration both resulted in a diagnostic accuracy of 78%; however, when both techniques were combined the accuracy increased to 88%.[58] Based on these studies, fine needle aspiration cytology is a safe and sensitive diagnostic procedure.

Dissemination of Malignant Cells

One of the most controversial issues surrounding the biopsy of space-occupying lesions is the potential seeding of cancer cells following fine needle aspiration.[59] This is a valid problem because the diagnostic role of this technique is most often the assessment of suspect hepatic lesions. Seeding rates of biopsies obtained from all abdominal organs have been estimated to range between 0.0003% and 0.009%.[60,61] However, in a retrospective study by Takamori the seeding rate in hepatocellular carcinomas was 5.1%,[62] questioning the use of needle aspirations in hepatocellular carcinoma patients. When polymerase chain reaction for the detection of α_1-antitrypsin messenger RNA was employed, tumor cell dissemination after fine needle aspiration was suggested.[63] The evaluation of hepatic masses without fine needle biopsy in one study showed that standard imaging procedures resulted in a diagnostic accuracy of 99.6% and a sensitivity of 98.6% for hepatocellular carcinoma (HCC), similar to the accuracy and sensitivity values for liver metastases.[64] However, the issue of tumor cell seeding and its clinical relevance remains controversial[65-67] and varies with respect to the lesion to be biopsied.[68,69] Based on these considerations the biopsy of hepatocellular carcinomas or other suspected malignant lesions of the liver should be cautiously weighed against the risk of dissemination, the therapeutic consequences of the biopsy, and the probability of other imaging tests to provide sufficient information. In a recent study no negative impact of HCC biopsies for the indication for liver transplantation was reported.[7] Fine needle aspiration should be considered in patients with unclear hepatic lesions in whom the side effects of therapy outweigh the consequences of seeding. In HCC a lesion for cytology is typically <2 cm in diameter and lacks typical features of HCC observed from other imaging tests, including negative serum α-fetoprotein (AFP).

The Candidate Patient for Liver Biopsy

The technical aspects of a successful and therapeutically or diagnostically relevant liver biopsy can only be viewed in light of a general risk assessment of the patient and the observation of contraindications.

Informed Consent

Informed consent should always be obtained in writing on the day before the planned biopsy. Care should be taken to provide information in the patient's native language or through an interpreter.

Compliance

Most techniques (with the exception of laparoscopy) require a patient who is cooperative and is able to hold her or his breath for the required time. For a frightened patient, administration of midazolam (e.g., Versed) can be considered but should be weighed against the ability to cooperate.

Mechanical Biliary Obstruction

This is a relative contraindication. Biliary peritonitis, sepsis, and pain are possible consequences. If the benefit of the biopsy outweighs these complications a biopsy can be performed and a transvenous approach should be considered.

Cholangitis

Bacterial cholangitis is a relative contraindication and may actually provide useful bacteriologic information in some patients. In view of the risk of disseminating pathogens during the biopsy, antibiotic treatment in these cases should be considered, although data to support a general recommendation are lacking.

Hemostasis

A normal INR is desired for liver biopsies but frequently not present in patients requiring a liver biopsy. The fact that 90% of hemorrhages have been found in patients with an INR <1.3 reflects that although abnormal INR values predispose to bleeding, a normal INR does not represent an absolute reassurance that a hemorrhage will not occur[26] (see **Fig. 12-2**). Bleeding can also occur much later than anticipated.[24] Coagulation studies should be performed 24 hours before the biopsy and should result in an INR <1.4. If this is not the case other strategies, such as transvenous biopsy or mini-laparoscopy, should be considered, including a potential coagulation factor substitution to improve the coagulopathy.[39,51,70] The platelet counts are also a matter of controversy. In some patients, such as hemodialysis patients or patients with renal impairment as well as hematologic disorders or cholestasis, platelet function may be compromised despite normal numbers.[71] Evidence suggests that a liver biopsy can be safely performed when platelet levels are >60,000/mm^3.[21] The use of aspirin and other nonsteroidal antiinflammatory drugs 1 week before biopsy is a controversial issue but currently lacks data confirming an increased risk in these patients.

Ascites

There are no randomized controlled studies to suggest that ascites is a strict contraindication for a liver biopsy, although in many publications a potentially higher rate of postinterventional bleeding is assumed. Experience with CT-guided liver biopsies has not demonstrated an increase in complications in patients with ascites.[39,72,73]

References

1. Strassburg CP, Manns MP. Approaches to liver biopsy techniques—revisited. Semin Liver Dis 2006;26:318–327.
2. Carvalho-Filho RJ, et al. Optimized cutoffs improve performance of the aspartate aminotransferase to platelet ratio index for predicting significant liver fibrosis in human immunodeficiency virus/hepatitis C virus co-infection. Liver Int 2008;28:486–493.
3. Sheela H, et al. Liver biopsy: evolving role in the new millennium. J Clin Gastroenterol 2005;39:603–610.
4. Menghini G. One-second needle biopsy of the liver. Gastroenterology 1958;35:190–199.
5. Strassburg CP, Manns MP. Autoimmune tests in primary biliary cirrhosis. Baillieres Best Pract Res Clin Gastroenterol 2000;14:585–599.
6. Actis GC, et al. The practice of percutaneous liver biopsy in a gastrohepatology day hospital: a retrospective study on 835 biopsies. Dig Dis Sci 2007;52:2576–2579.
7. Durand F, Belghiti J, Paradis V. Liver transplantation for hepatocellular carcinoma: role of biopsy. Liver Transpl 2007;13:S17–S23.
8. Guido M, Rugge M. Liver biopsy sampling in chronic viral hepatitis. Semin Liver Dis 2004;24:89–97.
9. Li MK, Crawford JM. The pathology of cholestasis. Semin Liver Dis 2004; 24:21–42.
10. Brunt EM. Nonalcoholic steatohepatitis. Semin Liver Dis 2004;24:3–20.
11. Jevon GP, Dimmick JE. Histopathologic approach to metabolic liver disease: Part 1. Pediatr Dev Pathol 1998;1:179–199.
12. Storch IM, et al. Evaluation of fine needle aspiration vs. fine needle capillary sampling on specimen quality and diagnostic accuracy in endoscopic ultrasound-guided biopsy. Acta Cytol 2007;51:837–842.
13. Sporea I, et al. The quality of the fragment obtained by liver biopsy for staging chronic hepatitis. J Gastrointestin Liver Dis 2007;16:263–266.
14. Caturelli E, et al. Diagnosis of hepatocellular carcinoma complicating liver cirrhosis: utility of repeat ultrasound-guided biopsy after unsuccessful first sampling. Cardiovasc Intervent Radiol 2002;25:295–299.
15. Caturelli E, et al. Percutaneous biopsy in diffuse liver disease: increasing diagnostic yield and decreasing complication rate by routine ultrasound assessment of puncture site. Am J Gastroenterol 1996;91:1318–1321.
16. Stotland BR, Lichtenstein GR. Liver biopsy complications and routine ultrasound. Am J Gastroenterol 1996;91:1295–1296.
17. Vautier G, Scott B, Jenkins D. Liver biopsy: blind or guided? Br Med J 1994; 309:1455–1456.
18. Al Knawy B, Shiffman M. Percutaneous liver biopsy in clinical practice. Liver Int 2007;27:1166–1173.
19. Flemming JA, et al. Liver biopsies for chronic hepatitis C: should nonultrasound-guided biopsies be abandoned? Can J Gastroenterol 2009;23: 425–430.
20. Perrault J, et al. Liver biopsy: complications in 1000 inpatients and outpatients. Gastroenterology 1978;74:103–106.
21. McGill DB, et al. A 21-year experience with major hemorrhage after percutaneous liver biopsy. Gastroenterology 1990;99:1396–1400.
22. Ahmad A, et al. Transjugular liver biopsy in patients with end-stage renal disease. J Vasc Interv Radiol 2004;15:257–260.
23. Gazelle GS, Haaga JR, Rowland DY. Effect of needle gauge, level of anticoagulation, and target organ on bleeding associated with aspiration biopsy. Work in progress. Radiology 1992;183:509–513.
24. Yeo WT, et al. Delayed bleeding after liver biopsy: a dreaded complication. Singapore Med J 2008;49:76–80.
25. Maharaj B, Bhoora IG. Complications associated with percutaneous needle biopsy of the liver when one, two or three specimens are taken. Postgrad Med J 1992;68:964–967.
26. Gilmore IT, et al. Indications, methods, and outcomes of percutaneous liver biopsy in England and Wales: an audit by the British Society of Gastroenterology and the Royal College of Physicians of London. Gut 1995; 36:437–441.
27. Piccinino F, et al. Complications following percutaneous liver biopsy. A multicentre retrospective study on 68,276 biopsies. J Hepatol 1986;2: 165–173.
28. Forssell PL, et al. Intrahepatic hematoma after aspiration liver biopsy. A prospective randomized trial using two different needles. Dig Dis Sci 1981; 26:631–635.
29. Larson AM, et al. Infection complicating percutaneous liver biopsy in liver transplant recipients. Hepatology 1997;26:1406–1409.
30. Le Frock JL, et al. Transient bacteremia associated with percutaneous liver biopsy. J Infect Dis 1975;131(Suppl):S104–S107.
31. McCloskey RV, Gold M, Weser E. Bacteremia after liver biopsy. Arch Intern Med 1973;132:213–215.
32. Ben-Ari Z, et al. Liver biopsy in liver transplantation: no additional risk of infections in patients with choledochojejunostomy. J Hepatol 1996;24: 324–327.
33. Bubak ME, et al. Complications of liver biopsy in liver transplant patients: increased sepsis associated with choledochojejunostomy. Hepatology 1991; 14:1063–1065.
34. de Diego Lorenzo A, et al. Bacteremia following liver biopsy in transplant recipients with Roux-en-Y choledochojejunostomy. Rev Esp Enferm Dig 1997;89:289–295.
35. Galati JS, et al. The nature of complications following liver biopsy in transplant patients with Roux-en-Y choledochojejunostomy. Hepatology 1994;20:651–653.
36. Dotter CT. Catheter biopsy. Experimental technic for transvenous liver biopsy. Radiology 1964;82:312–314.
37. Kalambokis G, et al. Transjugular liver biopsy—indications, adequacy, quality of specimens, and complications—a systematic review. J Hepatol 2007;47:284–294.
38. Albeniz Arbizu E, et al. Fibrin-glue sealed liver biopsy in patients with a liver transplantation or in liver transplantation waiting list: preliminary results. Transplant Proc 2003;35:1911–1912.
39. Kamphuisen PW, et al. Plugged-percutaneous liver biopsy in patients with impaired coagulation and ascites. Pathophysiol Haemost Thromb 2002;32: 190–193.
40. Tobin MV, Gilmore IT. Liver biopsy with plugged needle track. Lancet 1984; 2:694.
41. Sawyerr AM, et al. A comparison of transjugular and plugged-percutaneous liver biopsy in patients with impaired coagulation. J Hepatol 1993;17:81–85.
42. Cholongitas E, et al. A systematic review of the quality of liver biopsy specimens. Am J Clin Pathol 2006;125:710–721.

43. Beckmann MG, et al. Clinical relevance of transjugular liver biopsy in comparison with percutaneous and laparoscopic liver biopsy. Gastroenterol Res Pract 2009;94 [Epub].

44. Jackson JE, Adam A, Allison DJ. Transjugular and plugged liver biopsies. Baillieres Clin Gastroenterol 1992;6:245–258.

45. Jalan R, et al. Laparoscopy and histology in the diagnosis of chronic liver disease. QJ Med 1995;88:559–564.

46. Bruhl W. Incidents and complications in laparoscopy and directed liver puncture. Result of a survey. Dtsch Med Wochenschr 1966;91:2297–2299.

47. Nord HJ. Complications of laparoscopy. Endoscopy 1992;24:693–700.

48. Weickert U, et al. The diagnosis of liver cirrhosis: a comparative evaluation of standard laparoscopy, mini-laparoscopy and histology. Z Gastroenterol 2005;43:17–21.

49. Nord HJ. Biopsy diagnosis of cirrhosis: blind percutaneous versus guided direct vision techniques—a review. Gastrointest Endosc 1982;28:102–104.

50. Helmreich-Becker I, Meyer zum Buschenfelde KH, Lohse AW. Safety and feasibility of a new minimally invasive diagnostic laparoscopy technique. Endoscopy 1998;30:756–762.

51. Denzer U, et al. Liver assessment and biopsy in patients with marked coagulopathy: value of mini-laparoscopy and control of bleeding. Am J Gastroenterol 2003;98:893–900.

52. Wee A. Fine needle aspiration biopsy of the liver: algorithmic approach and current issues in the diagnosis of hepatocellular carcinoma. Cytojournal 2005;2:7.

53. Pitman MB. Fine needle aspiration biopsy of the liver. Principal diagnostic challenges. Clin Lab Med 1998;18:483–506, vi.

54. Buscarini L, et al. Ultrasound-guided fine-needle biopsy of focal liver lesions: techniques, diagnostic accuracy and complications. A retrospective study on 2091 biopsies. J Hepatol 1990;11:344–348.

55. Fornari F, et al. Ultrasonically guided fine-needle aspiration biopsy: a highly diagnostic procedure for hepatic tumors. Am J Gastroenterol 1990;85:1009–1013.

56. Hertz G, et al. Fine-needle aspiration biopsy of the liver: a multicenter study of 602 radiologically guided FNA. Diagn Cytopathol 2000;23:326–328.

57. Jain D. Diagnosis of hepatocellular carcinoma: fine needle aspiration cytology or needle core biopsy. J Clin Gastroenterol 2002;35:S101–S108.

58. Franca AV, et al. Fine needle aspiration biopsy for improving the diagnostic accuracy of cut needle biopsy of focal liver lesions. Acta Cytol 2003;47:332–336.

59. Liu YW, et al. Needle tract implantation of hepatocellular carcinoma after fine needle biopsy. Dig Dis Sci 2007;52:228–231.

60. Cedrone A, et al. Neoplastic seeding complicating percutaneous ethanol injection for treatment of hepatocellular carcinoma. Radiology 1992;183:787–788.

61. Smith EH. Complications of percutaneous abdominal fine-needle biopsy. Review. Radiology 1991;178:253–258.

62. Takamori R, et al. Needle-tract implantation from hepatocellular cancer: is needle biopsy of the liver always necessary? Liver Transpl 2000;6:67–72.

63. Louha M, et al. Liver resection and needle liver biopsy cause hematogenous dissemination of liver cells. Hepatology 1999;29:879–882.

64. Torzilli G, et al. Accurate preoperative evaluation of liver mass lesions without fine-needle biopsy. Hepatology 1999;30:889–893.

65. Caturelli E, et al. Fine needle biopsy of focal liver lesions: the hepatologist's point of view. Liver Transpl 2004;10:S26–S29.

66. Ng KK, et al. Impact of preoperative fine-needle aspiration cytologic examination on clinical outcome in patients with hepatocellular carcinoma in a tertiary referral center. Arch Surg 2004;139:193–200.

67. Torzilli G, et al. Indication and contraindication for hepatic resection for liver tumors without fine-needle biopsy: validation and extension of an Eastern approach in a Western community hospital. Liver Transpl 2004;10:S30–S33.

68. Shah JN, et al. Melanoma seeding of an EUS-guided fine needle track. Gastrointest Endosc 2004;59:923–924.

69. de Sio I, et al. Subcutaneous needle-tract seeding after fine needle aspiration biopsy of pancreatic liver metastasis. Eur J Ultrasound 2002;15:65–68.

70. Shin JL, et al. A Canadian multicenter retrospective study evaluating transjugular liver biopsy in patients with congenital bleeding disorders and hepatitis C: is it safe and useful? Am J Hematol 2005;78:85–93.

71. Pihusch R, et al. Platelet function rather than plasmatic coagulation explains hypercoagulable state in cholestatic liver disease. J Hepatol 2002;37:548–555.

72. Little AF, et al. Image-guided percutaneous hepatic biopsy: effect of ascites on the complication rate. Radiology 1996;199:79–83.

73. Murphy FB, et al. CT- or sonography-guided biopsy of the liver in the presence of ascites: frequency of complications. AJR Am J Roentgenol 1988;151:485–486.

Chapter 13

Liver Biopsy Interpretation

Elizabeth M. Brunt

ABBREVIATIONS

AFLD alcoholic fatty liver disease	**FNH** focal nodular hyperplasia	**K7, K19** keratin 7, keratin 19
AIH autoimmune hepatitis	**GS** glutamine synthetase	**NAFLD** nonalcoholic fatty liver disease
AMA anti-mitochondrial antibody	**GVHD** graft-versus-host disease	**NASH** nonalcoholic steatohepatitis
ANA anti-nuclear antibody	**H&E** hematoxylin and eosin	**NRH** nodalar regenerative hyperplasis
BMI body mass index	**HAV** hepatitis A virus	**ORO** oil red O stain
CCa cholangiocarcinoma	**HCA** hepatocellular adenoma	**PASd** periodic acid–Schiff after diastase
CD68 cluster designation 68	**HCC** hepatocellular carcinoma	**PBC** primary biliary cirrhosis
CMV cytomegalovirus	**HCV** hepatitis C virus	**pCEA** polyclonal CEA
CRP C-reactive protein	**HHT** hereditary hemorrhagic telangiectasia	**pFIC** progressive familial intrahepatic
DILI drug-induced liver injury	**HPS** hepato-portal sclerosis	cholestasls
DM diabetes mellitus	**HSP** heat shock protein	**PSC** primary sclerosing cholangitis
DN dysplastic nodule	**HSV** herpes simplex virus	**SAA** serum amyloid A
EBV Epstein-Barr virus	**IAD** idiopathic adulthood ductopenia	**SLE** systemic lupus erythematosus
FFPE formalin fixed, paraffin embedded	**ICP** intrahepatic cholestasis of pregnancy	

"For the King of Babylon stood at the parting of the way… to use divination; he made his arrows bright, he consulted with images, he looked in the liver."

Ezekiel 21:21

Principles of Liver Biopsy Interpretation

Clinical-Pathologic Correlations

In current practices of hepatology, hepatobiliary surgery, and liver transplantation, hepatopathologic studies remain integral components in diagnosis and clinical decision making. Although many noninvasive tests have been developed (including combinations of serologic markers, imaging findings, and patient demographics), histopathologic studies are still the standard against which other test results are judged. An informed and informative pathologist can be an invaluable member of the medical, surgical, and transplant teams. Stereotypic histologic features are commonly zonal and can broadly categorize disease processes (e.g., the noninflammatory zone 3 necrosis of acetaminophen toxicity or shock), but rarely do the histologic features alone suffice for the determination of a final diagnosis. Rather, in most situations, a differential diagnosis exists for identified lesions; an example

is the "duct lesion" characterized by infiltration into the interlobular duct by lymphocytes. This lesion can occur in hepatitis C virus (HCV) infection (the Christoffersen-Poulsen lesion described in 1972), primary biliary cirrhosis (PBC), acute allograft rejection, drug-induced liver injury (DILI), and even in some cases of autoimmune hepatitis (AIH). Thus clinical information is necessary for, and often integrated into, a diagnosis. Without adequate clinical information, the pathologist reports only a descriptive list of lesions. In deriving a diagnosis for a well-differentiated hepatocellular neoplastic lesion, knowledge of the presence or absence of underlying liver disease and/or medication exposure is invaluable. It is a personal choice of the pathologist as to when in the course of liver biopsy interpretation the clinical indications for the biopsy and accompanying pertinent clinical information are known, but there is no argument that for the vast majority of liver biopsies, the final pathologic diagnosis rests on integration of the observed microscopic patterns with the clinical considerations. Thus, whether the biopsy tissue is procured by the treating clinician or by a radiologist, the interpreting pathologist needs ready access to this information.

Tissue Preparation and Stains

Immediate placement of a liver biopsy core into buffered formalin remains the fixation method of choice. Routine histochemical studies and an ever-increasing array of immunohistochemical, in situ hybridization, and nucleic acid retrieval–based studies have been optimized for use with formalin-fixed, paraffin-embedded (FFPE) tissues. Copper and iron quantitation studies are routinely performed from the tissue remaining in the paraffin block. The exceptions to the use of formalin include the need for fresh tissue (e.g., flow cytometry processing of a hematopoietic process, pediatric liver biopsies for enzymatic assays) and glutaraldehyde fixation for ultrastructural evaluation. On the other hand, the consideration of acute fatty liver of pregnancy can only be successfully addressed if the specimen has not previously been processed in paraffin. Formalin-fixed biopsies can be frozen and cut onto charged or albumin-coated glass slides, with the application of oil red O (ORO) stain used to identify microvesicular steatosis. Subsequently, the same core can be processed through paraffin embedding for routine evaluation as well as tissue preservation for possible future studies.

During submission for paraffin embedding and sectioning, embedding sponges and "ink" in liver biopsy preparation are not only unnecessary but also are detrimental to interpretation, and thus are both to be strongly discouraged. The former leads to distortion artifacts that create nonanatomic angled holes throughout the biopsy core[1]; the latter results in adherent pigment that may obscure cells and structures, or even be confused for bile.

Abundant information can be obtained from a careful, systematic review of the levels of hematoxylin- and eosin-stained (H&E) tissue; preferably three levels are available, one each from the beginning, middle, and end of the sectioned ribbons. Additional "special stains" utilized for evaluation can serve useful diagnostic purposes (**Table 13-1**). Hepatopathologists have their own preferences, but most employ stains for connective tissue and architectural assessment at the very least. Arguments in favor of periodic acid–Schiff after diastase (PASd) and iron stains include the many uses of PASd (e.g., ease of observation of periportal globules of α_1-antitrypsin [A1AT] PiZZ mutations; evaluation of bile duct basement membranes; visualization of enlarged, pigmented Kupffer cells) and iron (e.g., iron-free foci in cirrhosis with iron overloading can be a marker of dysplasia).[2]

Approach to Microscopy

Systematic review of liver biopsies assists in the identification of diagnostic patterns of injury. Pathologists often interchangeably use anatomic terminology based either on Rappaport's acinar concepts of vascular supplies or on Kiernan's hexagonal lobular architecture; in the former, the hepatocytes most proximal to portal tracts with portal venous and hepatic artery inflow are referred to as zone 1 and those most distal are zone 3. Zones 1 and 3 are pear shaped and starfish shaped, respectively. According to the lobular architecture described by Kiernan, the hepatocytes around the portal tract are referred to as periportal and those around the outflow vein as centrilobular or perivenular. Although both of these concepts are oversimplifications of the microarchitecture of the liver,[3] they can serve as aids in interpretation. It is well recognized that hepatocytes along the gradient from inflow to outflow have different functions as well as susceptibilities to pathologic insults. Thus recognition of zonal location of injury, pigment deposition, and/or fibrosis is often extremely useful in creating a differential diagnosis based on morphology. Prototypic zonal injuries are noted in **Table 13-2**.

The assessment of a medically indicated biopsy includes parenchymal architecture as assessed by presence and spacing of vascular structures (terminal hepatic venules and portal tracts) and cord architecture (atrophy, dropout, nodularity); presence, location, and types of cellular infiltrates (focal, panacinar, portal predominant; predominant cell types); hepatocellular injury patterns (zonality and types of alterations); and bile duct evaluation (presence, inflammation, features of cholestasis). Stereotypical patterns can provide diagnostic clues. The next step is to consider the broad injury patterns: hepatitic, cholestatic, vascular, and neoplastic diseases (**Table 13-3**).

For directed, lesional biopsies, the initial determination is the presence or absence of tissue consistent with a distinct, mass lesion; changes recognized as mass effect, such as sinusoidal dilatation with or without ductular reaction and portal chronic inflammation, suggest proximity to a lesion. If present these findings should not be misinterpreted as evidence of underlying liver disease. **Table 13-4** summarizes the morphologic features and associated diagnostic possibilities of hepatic injury and **Table 13-5** highlights unique histopathologic details for specific forms of acute and chronic liver diseases.

Morphologic Lesions of Hepatitis

Acute Hepatitis

Acute hepatitis is characterized by intraacinar-predominant findings of hepatocyte injury and inflammation and hepatocellular regeneration. The hepatocytes may be diffusely or zonally involved with swelling, cytoplasmic clearing, or lytic necrosis. Most types of acute hepatitis affect only zone 3, but hepatitides A and E are notable exceptions and may show zone 1 accentuation. Clusters of ceroid-pigmented Kupffer cells and/or mononuclear cells may be present diffusely; with resolution, PASd-pigmented Kupffer cells may be present in zone 3. Eosinophilic, rounded, apoptotic hepatocytes may be noted singly outside the cords. Hepatocellular necrosis is detected by foci of spotty necrosis, zone 3 or zone 1 confluent necrosis, submassive (bridging) necrosis, or massive hepatic necrosis. These types of necrosis may be clues to the underlying etiology. Necrosis of hepatocytes results in loss of plate architecture and reticulin collapse. Inflammatory cells may be present diffusely throughout the lobules; a notable exception is the restriction of lymphocytes to the sinusoidal spaces in Epstein-Barr virus (EBV) hepatitis. Inflammation is predominantly comprised of mononuclear cells. Polymorphonuclear leukocytes are uncommon in either lobules or portal tracts in acute hepatitis; microabscesses, however, can be indicative of cytomegalovirus (CMV) infection in the allograft liver and polymorphonuclear leukocytes surrounding individual hepatocytes (satellitosis) or accompanying ductular reaction in zone 1 are characteristic of alcoholic hepatitis (discussed later in this chapter). Subendothelial or transmural inflammation (phlebitis) of the outflow veins can be noted in cases of severe acute hepatitis. Chronic portal inflammation may be present in varying degrees. In acute hepatitis A or E, portal inflammation may be equal or predominant to the intraacinar findings, and may be dominated

Table 13-1 **Useful Histochemical and Immunohistochemical Stains for Liver Biopsy Interpretation**

HISTOCHEMICAL STAINS	USE	DISEASE PROCESSES
Reticulin	Collagen, type III	Hepatic plates
Trichrome	Collagen, type I	Native collagen and fibrosis; architecture evaluation; identification of small outflow veins
Sirius red	Several collagens	Architecture; abnormal connective tissue deposition
Periodic acid–Schiff after diastase (PASd; DPAS)	Globules of A1AT; bile duct basement membranes; activated Kupffer cells; periportal granules may be copper	Detection of periportal globules represents Z allele; does not distinguish zygosity
Periodic acid–Schiff (PAS)	Glycogen	Highlights portal tract architecture by absence of staining
Iron (modified Perls')	Iron granules (blue); identification of bile (yellow-brown) and lipofuschin (yellow granules)	Many diseases result in aberrant iron loading; iron stain documents cell types, acinar localization, and quantity
Rhodanine	Copper	Chronic cholestasis; Wilson disease, especially in advanced stages
Orcein, victoria blue	Copper binding protein	Chronic cholestasis; Wilson disease, especially in advanced stages
	HBV surface antigen	Chronic HBV
	Elastic fibers	Absence of elastic fibers in recent parenchymal collapse
Congo red, thioflavin T, crystal violet	Positive identification of amyloid*	Hepatic amyloidosis: intrasinusoidal, vascular walls
Verhoeff-van Gieson	Elastic fibers, smooth muscle vessel walls	Positive identification of obliterated outflow venules
Oil red O	Lipid	Confirmation of intrahepatocellular lipids in acute fatty liver of pregnancy

Immunohistochemical Stain/Antigen	*Pattern(s) of Reactivity*	*Disease Processes*
HB S Ag/hepatitis B surface antigen	Cytoplasmic; membranous; inclusion	Indicative of chronic hepatitis B; negative in acute HBV infection
HB C Ag/hepatitis B core antigen	Nuclear ± cytoplasmic in addition	Replicative HBV infection
Anti-A1AT/A1AT protein	Globules: rim positive, center negative or diffusely positive Cytoplasmic "blush"	A1AT mutation but not diagnostic of specific ZZ or MZ
CMV	Nuclear reactivity in infected cells	Confirmation of CMV
HSV1,2	Nuclear reactivity in infected cells	Confirmation of HSV
Adenovirus	Nuclear reactivity in infected cells	Confirmation of adenoviral infection
Anti-K8/18	Hepatocytes, ± biliary cells	Clearing of hepatocyte cytoplasm is indicative of "ballooning"; positive in Mallory-Denk bodies
Anti-K7	Biliary epithelium; hepatic progenitor cells; intermediate hepatocytes	Biliary differentiation; cholestatic metaplasia
Anti-K19	Biliary epithelium; hepatic progenitor cells; intermediate hepatocytes	Biliary differentiation; more specific for hepatic progenitor cells and "intermediate hepatocytes"
P62, ubiquitin, AE1/AE3	Positive identification of Mallory-Denk bodies	Alcoholic hepatitis; nonalcoholic steatohepatitis; chronic cholestatic liver diseases

Tumors

pCEA/polyclonal carcinoembryonic antigen	Canalicular reactivity in hepatocytes	HCC: canalicular Cholangiocarcinoma: cytoplasmic
Anti-CD10/CD10	Canalicular reactivity in hepatocytes	HCC: canalicular Renal cell cancer: cytoplasmic
Glypican-3	Membranous, inclusions, canalicular	Irregularly positive in HCC†

Table 13-1 Useful Histochemical and Immunohistochemical Stains for Liver Biopsy Interpretation—cont'd

Immunohistochemical Stain/Antigen	Pattern(s) of Reactivity	Disease Processes
Hepar/hepatocyte	Intracytoplasmic, granular reactivity in hepatocytes	May be positive in HCC
β-Catenin	Membranous or nuclear	Nuclear β-catenin is indicative of "activation"; membranous is present in normal liver; occasionally occurs in adenomas, HCC
Glutamine synthetase	Cytoplasmic in zone 3 hepatocytes	Loss of zonality of reactivity is abnormal; can occur in benign proliferations (FNH, adenoma) and malignant hepatocellular neoplasms
L-FABP	Cytoplasmic in normal hepatocytes	Absent in HNF-1α–mutated hepatocellular adenomas
K19/CK19	Biliary epithelium; marker of hepatic progenitor cells	Mixed HCC-Cca

*Use of amyloid stain and Masson's trichrome stain will enable positive identification of amyloid, because amyloid will result in a grayish discoloration of the trichrome.
†See text.

Table 13-2 Zonal Injury Patterns

ACINAR ZONE/ LOBULAR LOCATION	PATHOLOGIC FINDING (EXAMPLES OF POSSIBLE UNDERLYING CAUSES)
Zone 3/Perivenular	Canalicular cholestasis (large duct obstruction, drugs)
	Paucicellular necrosis (acetaminophen, carbon tetrachloride, mushroom toxicity, hypotensive shock)
	Ballooning (acute viral hepatitis B, C; steatohepatitis; ischemia in allograft)
	Cord atrophy (chronic venous outflow obstruction)
	Hepatocellular pigment (lipofuschin)
	Inclusions (fibrinogen)
	Perisinusoidal fibrosis (steatohepatitis, outflow obstruction)
	Sclerosing hyaline necrosis (alcoholic hepatitis)
Zone 1/Periportal	Ductular cholestasis (sepsis)
	Paucicellular necrosis (eclampsia, DIC, cocaine, phosphorus, ferrous sulfate)
	Feathery change (cholate stasis)
	Necroinflammatory (viral hepatitis A, E)
	Hepatocellular pigment (copper [chronic cholestasis], iron [multiple causes of iron accumulation])
	Inclusions (α$_1$-antitrypsin globules)
	Portal, periportal fibrosis (chronic hepatitis, most causes; methotrexate; chronic biliary diseases)

DIC, disseminated intravascular coagulation

by plasma cells. Spillover of inflammatory cells from portal tracts may be difficult to distinguish from interface activity. Evidence of hepatocellular regeneration is common in all but fulminant cases, and characterized by anisonucleosis of hepatocytes; bi- or trinucleated hepatocytes; and, rarely, mitotic figures in hepatocytes. Ductular structures may represent the only form of regeneration in fulminant liver failure.

Fibrosis is not present in acute hepatitis. In cases with marked collapse, the two-cell-thick regenerative cords of surviving hepatocytes surrounded by dense reticulin condensation may be confused with cirrhotic remodeling. The trichrome stain may or may not distinguish the deep, vibrant color of the native collagen of portal tracts from the paler and less well-defined dye retention of the collapsed parenchyma; reticulin stain highlights the collapse as well as regenerative cords. Elastic fiber stain, such as orcein, can be quite helpful because elastic fibers are absent in recent, "passive," collapse but are present in the true, "active," septa of fibrosis.[4]

Characteristic findings of particular entities that may result in lesions of acute hepatitis are presented in **Table 13-5**.

Massive or submassive hepatic necrosis, characterized by panacinar or bridging parenchymal necrosis, respectively, may be histologic features in clinical cases of hepatitis. CD68-positive, PASd-pigmented Kupffer cells are easily noted in the stroma. Ductular reaction, characterized by increased numbers of ductular elements and variable amounts of stroma and inflammation, may be noted in acute hepatitis when extensive necrosis is present. In massive hepatic necrosis, the only viable epithelial cells remaining are the K7, K19–positive bile ducts and the hepatic progenitor cells that characterize the ductular reaction.[5] Etiologic determination based on pathologic evaluation is typically not possible in massive hepatic necrosis. Zone 3 coagulative necrosis with very little inflammation characterizes both systemic shock and acetaminophen toxicity. Clusters of necrotic hepatocytes or massive necrosis may be seen with herpes simplex virus (HSV) or adenovirus hepatitis. Careful evaluation by light microscopy for the typical intranuclear inclusions of these viruses is suggested, particularly in cases of immunosuppression. The glassy nuclei, syncytial cell formation, and basophilic stippling of herpes simplex can be noted by routine stains.[6] Immunohistochemical stains are available to confirm both herpesvirus and the smudged nuclei of adenovirus.

Table 13-3 Morphologic Features of Normal and Abnormal Hepatic Parenchyma

Architecture	Vascular Structures of the Acinus

Vascular relationships normal
Portal tracts, outflow veins approximated
  Necrosis, collapse *(orcein, trichrome)*
  Fibrosis *(trichrome, reticulin)*
  Nodularity *(reticulin, trichrome)*
    With bridging fibrous septa
    With prominent sinusoids
    Without fibrous septa
	Terminal hepatic venules (central veins)
	  Present; normal size
	  Not visualizable without *trichrome, VVG*
	  Endophlebitis, endotheliitis
	  Dilated; several vascular channels
	  Perivenular fibrosis
	  Perisinusoidal fibrosis, ± "unaccompanied" artery present
	  Perivenular lipogranulomas with fibrosis

Portal Tracts	**Sinusoids and Lining Cells**

Normal connective tissue for size
Branches of hepatic artery, portal vein, bile duct identified
Rare mononuclear cells
Edematous; mild mixed inflammation present
Increased fibrosis *(trichrome, reticulin)*
  Periportal
  Bridging: portal-portal; portal-central
Increased ductular profiles at limiting plate: hepatocyte
  interface
  Ductal plate malformation
  Ductular reaction; types of inflammation
  Ductular cholestasis (cholangitis lenta)
	Not noticeable
	"Sinusoidal reaction" present
	Pigment in sinusoidal lining cells
	Fat droplets prominent in hepatic stellate cells
	Mononuclear cell inflammation confined to sinusoids
	Pigmented and/or enlarged Kupffer cells
	Erythrophagocytosis
	Dilated; zonal location
	  With cord atrophy, perisinusoidal fibrosis, red cell
	    extravasation
	  Loss of integrity of sinusoidal matrix *(reticulin, trichrome)*
	  Markedly enlarged and filled with blood: peliosis
	  Extramedullary hematopoiesis
	  Malignant infiltrates

Cellular Infiltrates	Deposition of amyloid Foam cell collections Loss of normal reticulin pattern: steatosis; HCC

Predominantly "chronic" inflammatory cells; ? interface activity
Plasma cells, eosinophils overrepresented
Pigmented portal macrophages
Polymorphonuclear infiltrates present
  Cholangitis
  Cholangiolitis
Granulomatous inflammation
Lipogranulomas
Neoplastic infiltrate
	Hepatocytes

	Normal cord and cellular structure
	  Cord atrophy: zonal location
	    Loss of normal cord architecture
	    Cellular infiltrates: mononuclear; microgranulomas;
	      microabscesses; epithelioid granulomas with or without
	      eosinophils
	    Hepatitic rosettes
	    Cholestatic rosettes
	    Ballooning
	    Apoptosis
	    Spotty necrosis, multifocal
	    Zonal necrosis: confluent necrosis; submassive (bridging)
	      necrosis; massive (panacinar) necrosis *(reticulin, orcein)*
	    Coagulative necrosis
	    Hepatocyte inclusions: types and zonal locations
	      Cytoplasmic: ground glass; steatosis, Mallory-Denk bodies,
	        pigments, viral organisms
	      Globules, granules
	      Canaliculi: dilated, bile plugs
	    Nuclear inclusions: glycogen, viral, pseudoinclusions, mitotic
	      figures
	    N/C ratio: regenerative small cells; large cell change; small cell
	      change

Bile Ducts	

Present (1:1 ratio with hepatic artery); absent
Lymphocytic, granulomatous, fibrous obliteration
Preserved architecture; loss of polarity, loss of nuclei, pyknotic
  alterations
Inflammation around and/or into biliary epithelium
  Chronic inflammatory cells
  Acute inflammatory cells
  Granulomatous
Inflammation in lumina of bile ducts (cholangitis)	

Portal Vein Branch	
Present; dilated; not identifiable Extruded from portal tract; direct contact with hepatocytes Larger portal tracts: subintimal fibrosis and muscle fibers replaced by scar Endotheliitis	
Hepatic Artery Branch	
Present; normal size for portal tract Eccentric thickening Concentric thickening; amyloid present Subendothelial "foam" cells noted	

Chronic Hepatitis

Chronic hepatitis is histologically characterized by the portal predominance of mononuclear or mixed chronic inflammation. In addition, PASd-pigmented portal macrophages are either more or equally prominent with intraacinar Kupffer cells; and lobular necroinflammatory activity ranges from that described for the previous lesions to nearly the absence of activity. In most diseases that result in chronic hepatitis, fibrosis occurs initially in and around the portal tracts. The most notable exception to these concepts is fatty liver disease, discussed in the following section. Interface activity, a defining lesion, is not specific to any disease entity, and is characterized by chronic inflammatory cells breaching the limiting plate of the portal tract and surrounding adjacent hepatocytes in zone 1; the older term for this was "piecemeal necrosis." Currently,

Table 13-4 Broad Morphologic Categorization of Diseases

DISEASE PROCESS	PATTERN OF LESIONS	COMMON DIFFERENTIAL DIAGNOSTIC POSSIBILITIES
Hepatitic	Acute: predominantly lobular	Viral A, B, D, E; AIH; drugs; toxins; EBV; HSV; CMV; adenovirus
	Chronic: predominantly portal or mixed lobular and portal	Viral B, C, D; AIH; drugs; toxins; metabolic diseases (A1AT, Wilson's disease, HH, ± alcoholic/nonalcoholic steatohepatitis*)
	Granulomatous	Opportunistic infection, drugs, chronic hepatitis, Hodgkin's disease, idiopathic granulomatous hepatitis, chronic granulomatous disease
Cholestatic	Acute: canalicular cholestasis; predominantly zone 3	Large duct obstruction, drugs, sepsis, ICP, PFIC
	Chronic: bile duct lesions, features of cholate stasis, predominantly zone 1	PBC, PSC, IAD, drugs, GVHD, sarcoidosis, other
	Granulomatous involvement of bile ducts	PBC, rarely in PSC, sarcoidosis
Vascular	Acute: zone 3 sinusoidal dilatation with red cell extravasation into cords	Large outflow vessel obstruction; right heart failure
	Chronic: various lesions of zone 3 cords, terminal hepatic venules, ± fibrosis in sinusoids; portal vein lesions; NRH	Large outflow vessel obstruction, right heart failure, chemotherapy injury, sinusoidal obstruction syndrome, hepatoportal sclerosis, noncirrhotic portal hypertension, NRH, HHT

*Lesions of alcoholic and nonalcoholic steatohepatitis are most commonly accentuated in zone 3.

actual necrosis is not required in the recognition of interface activity. The types and amounts of parenchymal necrosis and collapse depend on the specific disease. If the underlying disease is unchecked, fibrosis in chronic hepatitis may progress and may involve portal-portal bridging septa; portal-central approximation from loss of intervening parenchyma; and ultimately cirrhosis, defined not only by loss of hepatic parenchyma and replacement by septal scar tissue but also by vascular remodeling that results in (or from) intraparenchymal shunts. The extinct parenchyma, also known as fibrous septa, commonly contains not only collagens, but also ductular profiles, thin-walled vascular and lymphatic channels, and varying degrees of inflammatory infiltrates. Neither the inflammation nor the fibrosis is uniform throughout the organ in many cases; this lack of homogeneity can result in "sampling error" in liver biopsies, particularly if sufficiently large samples are not obtained.[7]

Figure 13-1 is an example of autoimmune hepatitis. AIH may manifest a variety of histopathologic findings, but rarely as an acute hepatitis. The most common lesions of AIH are marked overrepresentation of plasma cells in the otherwise mixed chronic portal infiltrates and at the portal–parenchymal interface. Plasma cells are also easily noted in foci of lobular necroses and/or infiltrates; swollen groups of hepatocytes form hepatitic rosettes; zone 3 confluent necrosis or bridging necrosis are commonly described. Eosinophils are a minor but common component of the portal inflammation. When cirrhosis occurs, there may be broad areas of extinction (septa). The untreated process is notable for more severe necroinflammatory activity and interface hepatitis than is seen with HCV. On the other hand, inactive cirrhosis with no other features may be due to AIH. Overlap of AIH and PBC may have either clinical and/or histologic features of both disease processes; treatment decisions will include consideration of the liver biopsy findings as well as biochemical and serologic tests.[8] It is important, however, to reiterate that no single finding distinguishes AIH and other forms of chronic hepatitis; thus

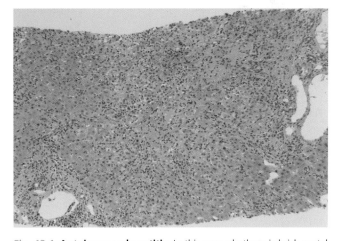

Fig. 13-1 **Autoimmune hepatitis.** In this example there is brisk portal and lobular inflammation; plasma cells are readily noted in both. There are hepatitic rosettes and a focus of acinar necrosis and collapse *(top right)*. (Hematoxylin and eosin, 20×)

careful clinical correlation (determination of total proteins and elevated globulins is as informative as measurement of autoantibodies) is needed.

Systems for semiquantitation of lesions of chronic hepatitis, initially developed for analysis of treatment effects, have evolved over the past 20 years into methods of evaluation in clinical practice.[9] Although each has subtle differences, they share a thorough evaluation of lesions with the separation of necroinflammatory lesions (portal and lobular) (grade) from evaluation of fibrosis amount and architectural alterations (stage). **Figure 13-2** is an example of the progression of fibrosis in chronic hepatitis due to HCV. Guidelines for application of scoring systems include knowledge of the clinical situation.[10,11]

Table 13-5 Histopathologic Features of Specific Acute and Chronic Hepatidides

ETIOLOGY	CLINICAL HEPATITIS		UNIQUE HISTOPATHOLOGIC FINDINGS
	ACUTE	CHRONIC	
Viral Hepatitis			
Hepatitis A, E	Yes	No	1. May be portal predominant; may have numerous plasma cells 2. May be cholestatic
Hepatitis C	Yes	Yes	1. May appear to have acute and chronic lesions simultaneously 2. Lymphoid aggregates and steatosis are common, but not exclusive to HCV 3. Sinusoidal infiltrates may predominate as in Dilantin toxicity 4. Duct injury and infiltration by lymphocytes and/or duct diverticuli may occur 5. Eosinophils are not uncommon in portal inflammation
Hepatitis B	Yes	Yes	1. Acute HBV: no specific characteristics; negative immunostains for surface and core antigens 2. Chronic HBV: may have ground glass inclusions of surface antigen; immunostains for surface positive; immunostains for core indicate replicative phase 3. Fibrosis in chronic HBV may have incomplete septal cirrhosis
Other Viral Infections			
CMV	Yes	No	1. In nonimmunosuppressed host, viral inclusions are not apparent; predominantly spotty necrosis or small collections of polymorphonuclear leukocytes 2. In immunosuppressed host, intranuclear and intracytoplasmic viral inclusions may be seen
HSV 1,2	Yes	No	1. Intranuclear viral inclusions noted around edges of nonzonal punched-out necrosis or in occasional cells in massive necrosis
EBV	Yes	No	1. Diffuse sinusoidal chronic inflammation; may have hemophagocytosis
Adenovirus	Yes	No	1. Intranuclear inclusions are noted; acute hepatitis to massive necrosis
Autoimmune hepatitis	Yes	Yes	1. Rarely may cause massive necrosis 2. Most commonly has features of chronic hepatitis with varying degrees of activity; plasma cells easily noted; hepatitic rosettes are common 3. Eosinophils may be present in portal inflammation 4. Duct lesion may occur; ductopenia is not a feature
Fatty Liver Diseases			
Alcoholic	Yes	Yes	1. ± Steatosis, zone 3 or panacinar 2. Ballooning 3. Mallory-Denk bodies: well-formed and marked satellitosis favors ALD 4. Zone 3 perisinusoidal (chickenwire) fibrosis: may be dense, complex; favors ALD ± ductular reaction 5. Sclerosing hyaline necrosis 6. Canalicular cholestasis
Nonalcoholic	?	Yes	1. Same as findings 1 through 5 for ALD
Metabolic Liver Diseases			
A1AT deficiency	No	Yes	1. Chronic hepatitis 2. Periportal PASd-positive globules, varying sizes
Hereditary hemochromatosis	No	Yes	1. Chronic hepatitis 2. Granular iron in hepatocytes; zone 1-3 gradient 3. ± Iron in reticuloendothelial cells 4. ± Iron in biliary epithelial cells
Wilson disease	No	Yes	1. Varying features: steatosis, chronic hepatitis 2. Periportal Mallory-Denk bodies 3. Atypical lipofuschin 4. Copper in hepatocytes; see text

Fatty Liver Diseases

The two most common diseases that are characterized by intrahepatocellular steatosis in some phase of their evolution are alcoholic fatty liver disease (AFLD) and nonalcoholic fatty liver disease (NAFLD). Although alcoholic liver disease (ALD) may exist as a clinical acute hepatitis but without steatosis (i.e., alcoholic hepatitis), to date no equivalent lesion (or clinical disease) has been described in nonalcoholic fatty liver. Likewise, the entity of alcoholic foamy degeneration has no equivalent in NAFLD. There may be substantial overlap of lesions in these two processes: mixed large and small droplet steatosis; zone 3 hepatocellular ballooning; presence of Mallory-Denk bodies[11]; zone 3 perisinusoidal fibrosis (**Fig. 13-3**). Both may progress to fibrosis in and around portal tracts; bridging septa between portal structures or outflow veins or portal-central

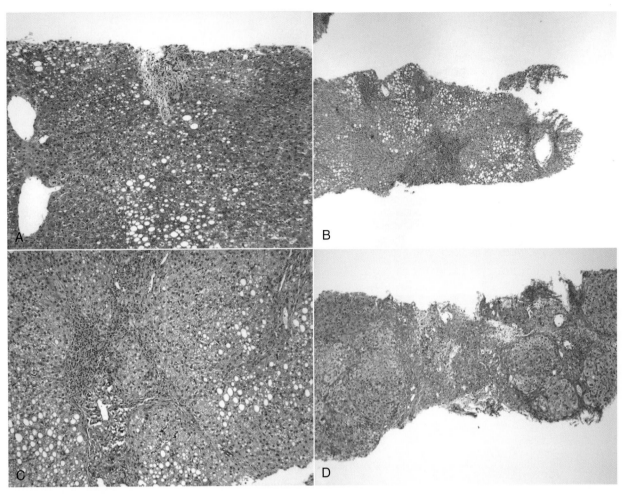

Fig. 13-2 **Chronic hepatitis C.** This figure contains images of trichrome-stained liver biopsies to illustrate the four Scheuer stages of fibrosis in a case of chronic hepatitis attributable to hepatitis C. **A,** Stage 1, portal expansion. **B,** Stage 2, portal expansion and periportal fibrosis. **C,** Stage 3, bridging fibrosis with nodularity. **D,** Stage 4, cirrhosis. (Masson's trichrome, 20×)

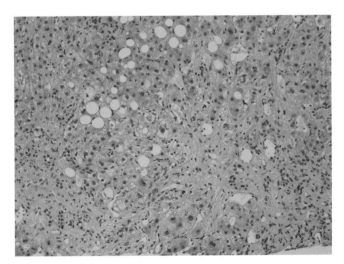

Fig. 13-3 **Alcoholic hepatitis.** An example of sclerosing hyaline necrosis, a lesion of alcoholic hepatitis, is shown. A group of hepatocytes *(center)* have steatosis, ballooning, and Mallory-Denk bodies; polymorphonuclear leukocytes are noted around some of the hepatocytes (satellitosis). The terminal hepatic venule is obliterated by the process. An expanded portal tract and ductular reaction are noted on the lower left portion of the image. (Hematoxylin and eosin, 20×)

bridging, (**Fig. 13-4**) and both may result in cirrhosis with or without features of the active disease. Thus distinguishing the two may be impossible without adequate clinical information. On the other hand, canalicular cholestasis, large and abundant Mallory-Denk bodies, pericholangitis, lesions of "alcoholic" hepatitis (nonsteatotic), the various occlusive lesions of the outflow veins (including sclerosing hyaline necrosis), and large regions of parenchymal extinction strongly favor alcohol abuse. Cryptogenic cirrhosis may be due to either of these entities. If, however, the prior disease process is known, cirrhosis cannot be considered cryptogenic.

Similar to the separation of necroinflammatory lesions (grade) from those of fibrosis and remodeling (stage) in chronic hepatitis, scoring systems for semiquantitative evaluation are commonly utilized for assessment and treatment trials of NAFLD.[12,13] A system has been proposed for alcoholic fatty liver disease as well.[14]

Hepatic steatosis and/or steatohepatitis may occur concurrently with other forms of chronic liver disease. Steatosis is noted in up to 70% of HCV biopsies; this is particularly common with genotype 3. Trichrome stain is essential to aid in diagnosis or exclusion of concurrent steatohepatitis.[15] Zone 3 perisinusoidal fibrosis, whether attributable to alcohol or obesity, is not a lesion associated with other forms of chronic

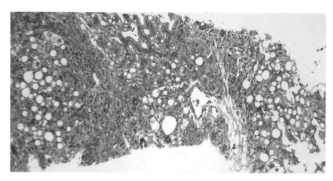

Fig. 13-4 Nonalcoholic steatohepatitis with perisinusoidal and bridging fibrosis. The trichrome-stained slide highlights the characteristic zone 3 perisinusoidal fibrosis as well as the central-portal septa. In this example, steatosis is still present; ballooning and poorly formed Mallory-Denk bodies can be seen in the upper left. The patient had a history of tamoxifen use. (Masson's trichrome, 20×)

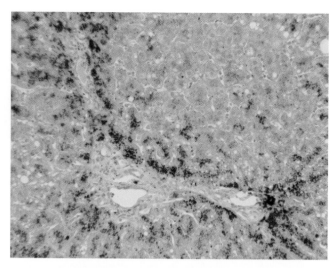

Fig. 13-6 C282Y homozygous hemochromatosis. The iron stain highlights the granules in hepatocytes with a notable gradient from the periportal to pericentral hepatocytes. (Modified Perls' stain, 40×)

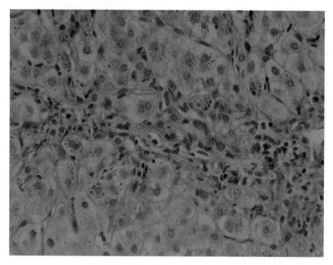

Fig. 13-5 α₁-Antitrypsin globules. High-power view of typical PASd-positive globules of α_1-antitrypsin. The globules are of varying shapes and sizes and are located in the periportal hepatocytes. (Periodic acid–Schiff after diastase, 40×)

hepatitis; thus its presence is necessary for diagnosing both causes of fatty liver.

Metabolic Liver Diseases

The three most commonly encountered adult metabolic liver diseases are α_1-antitrypsin (A1AT) deficiency, hereditary hemochromatosis (HH), and Wilson disease. Although each of these diseases is characterized by lesions associated with chronic hepatitis, each requires further clinical testing for a final diagnosis. The characteristic periportal/zone 1 PASd-positive globules of varying sizes of A1AT cannot distinguish the MZ from homozygous ZZ phenotype (**Fig. 13-5**).

HH liver biopsies may also have portal and lobular chronic inflammation and portal-based fibrosis, albeit initially "holly-leaf" shaped. However, HH cannot be diagnosed by histopathologic studies, because other causes of iron dysregulation may result in the characteristic pericanalicular deposition with a decreasing zonal gradient from 1 to 3 pattern of iron

loading in hepatocytes[16] (**Fig. 13-6**). Patients with untreated C282Y homozygous hemochromatosis have livers that contain sufficient iron to be visible without Prussian blue staining; however, the stain highlights the hepatocellular abundance as well as the presence of siderotic nodules (iron-loaded Kupffer cell aggregates) and bile duct iron. One unique form of hemochromatosis, type 4A (ferroportin disease), is characterized by iron granules solely deposited in the reticuloendothelial cells within the sinusoids. The current epidemic of obesity has highlighted the frequency with which hyperferritinemia occurs in settings outside of HH[17]; liver biopsy evaluation can be helpful in this differential.

Wilson disease is challenging to diagnose by biopsy. Steatosis, portal and lobular chronic inflammation, periportal Mallory-Denk bodies, glycogenated nuclei, atypical lipofuschin pigment deposition, and/or iron pigment may or may not be present. Copper stains are reliably positive in the diagnosis of cirrhotic Wilson disease, but typically not in noncirrhotic biopsies; thus hepatic copper measurement, the diagnostic test for Wilson disease, is best evaluated by quantitation from the paraffin block.

Cholestatic Lesions

Acute Cholestasis

Acute cholestasis (also referred to as bilirubinostasis) is characterized by zone 3 canalicular bile plugs. The hepatocytes may be deceptively unremarkable, or it may be swollen and have clarified cytoplasm (so-called feathery degeneration). In cases of severe obstruction, extravasated bile may lead to bile infarcts; this is not the classic ischemic coagulative necrosis, but rather foci of saponified hepatocytes with occasional remnants of polymorphonuclear leukocytes. They may be salmon colored, bile (yellow) colored, or transparent.

In addition, acute cholangitis has characteristic portal tract changes. Edema of the portal connective tissue imparts a rounded contour to the portal tract. Ductular reaction is noted and pericholangitis with polymorphonuclear leukocytes is characteristic. Neutrophilic clusters within the lumina of the interlobular bile ducts are evidence of ascending cholangitis. This is rarely encountered in routine practice because clinical diagnostic tests are reliable. Acute cholestasis is not associated with fibrosis (**Fig. 13-7**).

Cholestatic hepatitis, however, is a unique injury pattern that combines hepatocellular injury and canalicular cholestasis predominantly in zone 3, and is most often associated with drug-induced liver injury (DILI), as discussed later in this chapter.

Chronic Cholestasis

There are many histologic features common to all forms of chronic cholestatic liver disease. Chronic cholestatic injury,

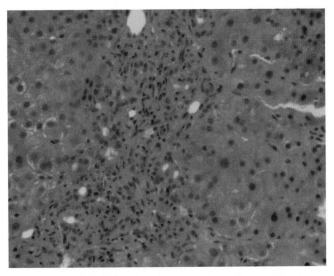

Fig. 13-7 **Sepsis.** Ductular cholestasis (*middle top* and *middle bottom*), known as cholangitis lenta, and hepatocellular cholestasis (*right*) are seen in this liver biopsy from a patient with sepsis. (Hematoxylin and eosin, 40×)

regardless of the cause, is characterized by several findings, most commonly in zone 1/periportal hepatocytes. There is pallor in the zone 1 hepatocytes and ductular cells; Mallory-Denk bodies may be present. Zone 1 hepatocytes may contain copper; the pigment is seen by H&E and PASd staining, but is best confirmed with copper stain. Ductular reaction is common in chronic cholestasis but may have subtle differences related to etiology; obstructive processes (e.g., primary sclerosing cholangitis [PSC]) may result in angulated anastomosing ductular profiles. In the sinusoids, collections of cells with pseudoxanthomatous transformation are a diagnostic aid, when present, in conditions of elevated levels of cholate salts. **Table 13-6** lists features that are unique to primary biliary cirrhosis (PBC), regardless of being AMA positive; sclerosing cholangitis (primary or secondary); idiopathic adulthood ductopenia (IAD)/small duct PSC; and chronic graft-versus-host disease (GVHD). Loss of the small interlobular ducts (ductopenia) is noted in advanced stages of chronic cholestatic liver diseases; the differential diagnosis for ductopenia, however, is not restricted to the classic forms of chronic cholestatic liver disease, and is noted in **Table 13-7**.

Parenchymal remodeling from chronic cholestasis occurs with portal-portal bridging fibrosis, but commonly with retention of the outflow vein in a central location. The periseptal pallor of cholestatic cirrhosis can result in the often-described "jigsaw" pattern. Hepatic cords within nodules may show the alterations typically described in nodular regenerative hyperplasia; interestingly, this feature may occur before complete cirrhotic remodeling. The presence of epithelioid granulomas in portal tracts and/or lobules may be suggestive—but not exclusive, necessary, or sufficient—for a diagnosis of PBC. Granulomas and features of chronic cholestasis are also indicative of involvement of the liver with sarcoidosis (**Figs. 13-8 and 13-9**).

Granulomatous Inflammation in Liver Biopsies

Various forms of granulomas may be seen in liver biopsies. A recent review summarizes the specific features and variety

Table 13-6 Histopathologic Features of Chronic Cholestatic Liver Diseases

ETIOLOGY	LESIONS OF CHOLATE STASIS	FLORID DUCT LESION	LOBULAR INFLAMMATION	PORTAL INFLAMMATION	DUCTS INVOLVED
PBC/AIC	✓	✓	Mononuclear cells; plasma cells; ± epithelioid granulomas	Mixed chronic inflammation; plasma cells; eosinophils; ± epithelioid granulomas	Small and medium ducts
PSC	✓	No	± Mild mononuclear	Mild mononuclear	Any portion of biliary tree: periductal fibrosis; obliterated ducts
IAD/small duct PSC	±	No	±	±	Smallest interlobular ducts; ± any ductular reaction; ductopenia
GVHD	±	No	±	Mild mononuclear	Small ducts; degenerative changes; obliteration

AIC, autoimmune cholangitis, characterized by AMA-negative ± ANA-positive serologies; clinical and histologic features are otherwise indistinguishable from AMA-positive PBC.

Table 13-7 Diseases that May Have Ductopenia

PBC, PSC/SSC, IAD
Autoimmune cholangitis
Chronic allograft rejection
Damage to hepatic artery: chemotherapy, surgical
GVHD
Sarcoidosis
Hodgkin disease
DILI
CMV infection

SSC, secondary sclerosing cholangitis

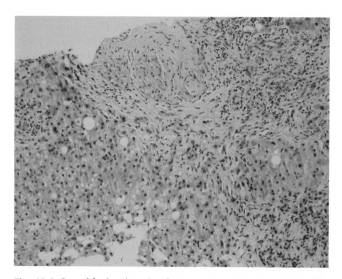

Fig. 13-8 Sarcoidosis. There is a large non-caseating, non-necrotizing epithelioid granuloma in the top center of the image; ductular reaction adjacent to it is brisk. Concentric fibrosis can be recognized around the granuloma. This biopsy is from a cholestatic patient with known sarcoidosis. (Hematoxylin and eosin, 20×)

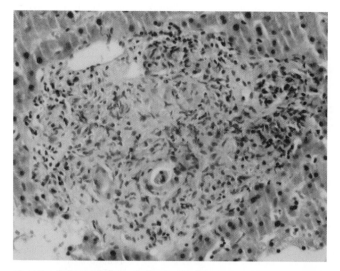

Fig. 13-9 Primary biliary cirrhosis. The bile duct profiles noted in this image are markedly abnormal; irregular spacing of the nuclei and eosinophilic cytoplasm are noted. The normal cuboidal shape has been simplified. A poorly formed granuloma is near the duct *(center)* among the mixed chronic inflammation that includes plasma cells and eosinophils. Ductular reaction is not seen in this image. (Hematoxylin and eosin, 40×)

of clinical associations of hepatic granulomas.[18] Of note, "incidental" epithelioid granulomas have been reported in hepatitis C and other forms of chronic liver disease including hepatitis B and AIH, and are not to be confused with granulomatous inflammation of PBC, infection, or drug-related granulomas. Some granulomas are manifestations of lobular activity (i.e., microgranulomas, composed of Kupffer cell aggregates; lipogranulomas, noted either in the lobules or in the portal tracts in association with active or inactive steatotic liver diseases). Larger lipogranulomas are often accompanied by fibrosis; when in a perivenular location, this may present confusion with the perisinusoidal fibrosis of nonalcoholic steatohepatitis (NASH). Fibrin-ring granulomas have been reported in a broad variety of disease processes, including EBV infection, Q-fever, hepatitis A virus (HAV), leishmaniasis, toxoplasmosis, allopurinol toxicity, vasculitis, systemic lupus erythematosus (SLE), and Hodgkin disease.[18] Hodgkin disease is also in the differential diagnosis of epithelioid granulomas with eosinophils. Most epithelioid granulomas, whether necrotizing or nonnecrotizing, represent an immune response to foreign material or antigen, and occur secondarily to certain types of particle deposition, infections, or drugs. Thus the initial description of granulomas in liver biopsies by the pathologist includes the following: epithelioid appearance, presence of caseation and/or necrotizing, and presence of polarizable material. The presence of eosinophils raises an important differential: both epithelioid granulomas in Hodgkin disease and drug-related epithelioid granulomas may be infiltrated with eosinophils. Immune deficiency syndromes may result in hepatic granulomas. Sarcoidosis may involve the liver in conjunction with other organs, or as a primary process.[19,20] The entire spectrum of cholestatic and duct lesions noted in PBC and PSC may occur in livers with primary or secondary sarcoidosis. The granulomas of sarcoid are coursed by reticulin fibers centrally and show concentric fibrosis peripherally; other features, including asteroid bodies, may be noted. These features are not noted in the epithelioid granulomas of PBC. Finally, idiopathic granulomatous hepatitis remains a clinical entity of unknown etiology. In this, disease entity, non-necrotizing, noncaseating, nonpolarizable epithelioid granulomas are found diffusely in the lobules; the process typically correlates with an inflammatory clinical presentation. For practical purposes, unless the patient is known to have PBC or sarcoidosis, it is reasonable for a pathologist to polarize the granulomas for identification of foreign material, and to routinely perform stains for fungal elements and mycobacteria when epithelioid granulomas are present.

Hepatic Parenchymal Manifestations of Vascular Lesions

Outflow Veins/Right-Sided Cardiac Dysfunction

The most recognizable vascular lesion in liver biopsies is that of large vein obstruction resulting from Budd-Chiari syndrome, or cardiac dysfunction with elevation of right-sided

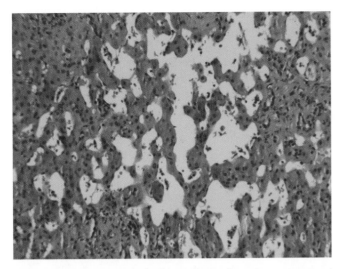

Fig. 13-10 **Large vessel outflow obstruction.** Hepatocyte cord atrophy and red cell extravasation are apparent. The sinusoids are markedly enlarged. Foci of ductular reaction can be seen (*middle, right,* and *left*). (Hematoxylin and eosin, 40×)

pressures. Acute venous outflow obstruction is characterized by irregularly spaced zone 3 sinusoidal dilatation, hepatic cord atrophy, and red cell extravasation into the hepatic cords. With time (chronicity), perisinusoidal fibrosis may occur along the atrophic cords; the red cell extravasation may or may not subside. Sinusoidal dilatation and ectatic sinusoids may be defined by fibrous replacement of the cords (**Fig. 13-10**). The smallest branches of outflow veins may become obliterated and difficult to observe without stains for the fibers in the walls. With intact portal tracts present, the remodeled liver adopts the appearance of reverse lobulation with a centrally located portal tract and the fibrous outflow veins at the periphery. When this occurs in the setting of chronic right-sided heart failure and results in bridging fibrosis, it may be referred to as cardiac sclerosis. Ductular reaction may emanate from portal areas and may be striking, and this may be confused with a primary cholestatic process.[21]

Inflow Vessels

Portal Vein

Acute obstruction of portal vein flow rarely results in parenchymal alterations. Chronic obstruction, on the other hand, may result in parenchymal atrophy, cord atrophy, nodular regenerative hyperplasia, Zahn infarction (a wedge-shaped region of atrophic parenchyma in which portal vein branches are obliterated), and hepato-portal sclerosis (HPS). The latter is defined as loss of portal vein branches within portal tract collagen; an obliterated vein may be present or a thin-walled open channel adjacent to the portal tract may be seen. Other lesions of HPS that may be present are non-zonal angiomatoid sinusoids/channels in the parenchyma and nodularity of the parenchyma. Fibrosis may occur, but is not common. Finally, cavernous transformation of the portal vein may result in ischemic biliopathy, a lesion identified by signs of damage to the bile ducts and best diagnosed by imaging.[22]

Hepatic Artery

Hepatic artery lesions rarely affect a normal liver because of the dual blood supply. However, thickening of the hepatic artery may occur with diabetes mellitus (DM).[23]

Arterio-Venous Malformations: Hereditary Hemorrhagic Telangiectasia (HHT)

HHT, or Osler-Weber-Rendu disease, may cause symptoms or imaging abnormalities that necessitate a liver biopsy. Detecting the subtleties of this entity on a core biopsy is challenging at best; wedge biopsies are preferable. The vascular alterations include clusters of ectatic sinusoids; randomly scattered fibrous bands that contain thick-walled, aberrantly shaped veins and arteries; and portal tracts with markedly distorted vascular structures. Nodular parenchymal changes are best appreciated by reticulin stain. There is no cirrhosis. Clinical history of recurrent epistaxis in the patient and family is helpful and worthy of inquiry.

Hepatic Sinusoids

Sinusoidal obstruction syndrome[24] is the modern moniker for venoocclusive disease. This is a process that first affects the sinusoidal lining cells and results in perivenular hepatocyte necrosis; sloughed sinusoidal lining can be appreciated with trichrome stain in some cases. Terminal hepatic venule subintimal fibrosis and obliteration may obscure the vein; special stains such as trichrome or Verhoeff-van Gieson (VVG) will aid in identification of the vein wall. This process occurs in the setting of allogeneic bone marrow transplant patients as well as in patients with neoadjuvant oxaliplatin-based therapy for hepatic metastases from colon cancer.[25] The lesions can range from focal sinusoidal dilatation, to sinusoidal destruction with focal hemorrhage and cord atrophy, to peliotic lesions. Perisinusoidal fibrosis and increased CD34 expression suggest capillarization. Severity is a clinicopathologic assessment and cannot be predicted from evaluation of frozen section of liver biopsies (**Fig. 13-11**).

Other lesions specific to the sinusoids include distortion by fat-filled stellate cells (vitamin A toxicity) or ruptured fat cysts; the presence of extramedullary hematopoietic cells (myeloid fibrosis); infiltration by benign (EBV hepatitis) or malignant (leukemia) hematopoietic cells; infiltration by other malignancies (e.g., small cell carcinoma, melanoma, breast carcinoma); and subendothelial fibrosis (diabetic hepatosclerosis) (**Fig. 13-12**) or amyloidosis (**Fig. 13-13**). Primary hepatic angiosarcoma may first be noted by a rare atypical, enlarged sinusoidal cell before mass lesion formation. All of these are relatively uncommon.

Mass Lesions

Most biopsies of mass lesions presented to pathologists for evaluation are the product of an image-guided procedure. The initial step in evaluation is determination of the presence or absence of an abnormal process that could account for the lesion. At times, discerning lesional versus nonlesional tissue is not straightforward, but adherence to the same structured

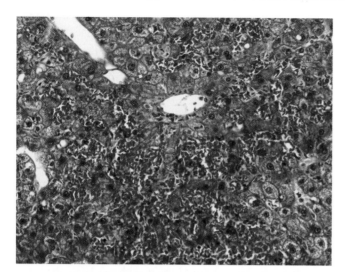

Fig. 13-11 **Oxaliplatin sinusoidal injury.** Note the clusters of sinusoids around the portal tract that are enlarged and filled with red blood cells. In several of these areas, the hepatic cords are atrophic and incomplete. (Masson's trichrome, 40×)

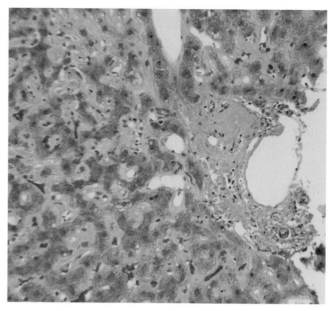

Fig. 13-13 **Amyloidosis.** The portal tract and the perisinusoidal spaces are filled with a dense, acellular material with a characteristic appearance on Masson's trichrome stain. (Masson's trichrome, 40×)

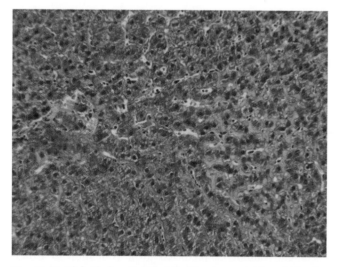

Fig. 13-12 **Diabetic hepatosclerosis.** The dense perisinusoidal collagen deposition is the characteristic lesion of this process. The hepatic cords do not appear atrophic and little to no inflammation is present. Steatosis, ballooning, and Mallory-Denk bodies are not seen in diabetic hepatosclerosis. (Masson's trichrome, 20×)

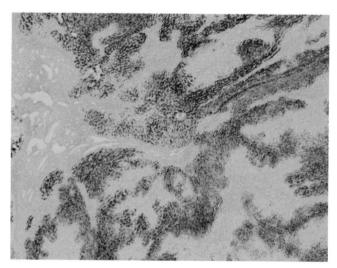

Fig. 13-14 **Focal nodular hyperplasia.** This is an illustration of the typical "map-like" glutamine synthetase reaction by immunohistochemistry with an FNH. (Glutamine synthetase immunohistochemistry, 20×)

evaluation as described previously for parenchymal injury can be helpful. The absence of portal tract structures and the presence of an unaccompanied arterial branch in hepatocellular lesions are strong guides to further assessment. Furthermore, knowledge of the status of the non-tumor liver (i.e., presence of cirrhosis) assists in further diagnostic evaluation; for example, hepatocellular adenoma is not a lesion found in a cirrhotic liver.

Benign Lesions/Tumors

Two French groups have developed a classification of benign hepatocellular lesions of the liver based on molecular and genotype-phenotype analyses of large numbers of cases.[26-28]

Focal nodular hyperplasia (FNH) is characterized by a central scar containing an abnormal vessel and close association of proliferating ductular structures. Copper is usually present. Immunohistochemical studies show that FNH has maplike deposition of glutamine synthetase (GS) (**Fig. 13-14**), in contrast to the perivenular restriction of this protein in normal liver.[29] Hepatocellular adenomas (HCA), once considered a single category of benign tumor, have been shown to have three identifiable subtypes. The first is related to mutation of hepatocyte nuclear factor 1α that results in loss of expression in the adenoma; these adenomas frequently have steatosis, and can be multiple (**Fig. 13-15**). The second is related to activation of β-catenin; immunohistochemical analysis permits

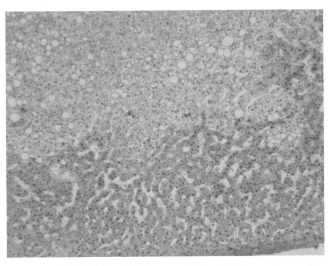

Fig. 13-15 HNF-1α mutated hepatic adenoma. The normal parenchymal expression of LFABP (liver fatty acid binding protein) can be seen in the lower portion of the slide; the steatotic adenoma lacks this reaction. This pattern is consistent with HNF-1α mutated adenoma. (LFABP immunohistochemistry, 20×)

documentation of the loss of normal membranous reactivity and the presence of diffuse cytoplasmic and nuclear reactivity. These tumors have a high rate of progression to hepatocellular carcinoma and are more common in men than the other forms of HCA. Histologically, they may show pseudoacini and more hepatocellular atypia than other forms of HCA. A third category is associated with elevated body mass index (BMI)[30] and may be associated with alcohol use and, in some cases, with elevated systemic inflammatory serum markers (serum amyloid A [SAA], C-reactive protein [CRP]). The moniker for this lesion has evolved from "telangiectatic FNH" to "telangiectatic adenoma" to the current nomenclature based on genetic studies: "gp130-mutated adenoma" or "inflammatory adenoma."[31,32] These lesions are challenging for the radiologist to distinguish from FNH, but recent guidelines may be helpful.[33] They are characterized by vascular ectasias, by thickened arterial branches, and by foci of portal-like fibrous septa (but no central scar) devoid of a bile duct but containing thickened vessels with a slight periseptal ductular reaction and, in some, mononuclear cell infiltrates. They may be steatotic and multiple. Immunohistochemical analysis shows production of serum amyloid A by the tumor cells. A fourth category is for HCA for which none of the other classifications applies. All adenomas may result in tumoral hemorrhage, and these lesions remain challenging to diagnose by liver biopsy. The genotyping and immunohistochemical studies developed to date have been performed on resection specimens of French patients, and their use in liver biopsy and in different patient populations has only been presented in abstract form from an urban hepatology practice[34] in which most of the findings described concurred with the French reports. However, the association of any form of adenoma with increased BMI was not noted because the majority of the patients in the series were overweight.

Other benign lesions and tumors of the liver are rarely encountered with the exception of the so-called bile duct adenoma in the setting of an unsuspected hepatic lesion found during surgery. This lesion is characterized by benign ductular structures embedded in a fibrous matrix. The differential diagnosis includes von Meyenburg complexes and, importantly, cholangiocarcinoma or metastatic pancreatic carcinoma. Angiomyolipomas may be confused for HCA if attention is not paid to the very large epithelioid eosinophilic cells that comprise the majority of the lesion; immunohistochemical analyses for melanoma markers are positive, whereas those for hepatocellular differentiation are not. Inflammatory pseudotumors are challenging to diagnose by liver biopsy because the lesion is predominantly a proliferation of spindle cells with scattered plasma cells and eosinophils; the concern that the tissue is from a pseudocapsule (adjacent to a tumor) remains, unless venular obliterative fibrosis and phlebitis are noted. A newer classification suggests that some may be a process related to steroid-sensitive IgG4 sclerosing pancreatitis/cholangitis.[35]

Malignant Tumors

The two most important primary malignant tumors of the liver are hepatocellular carcinoma (HCC) and cholangiocarcinoma (CCa). Currently, there is growing evidence that the division between these two epithelial neoplasms may not be as distinct as previously believed, and many examples of mixed HCC-CCa and variants of CCa with features of hepatic progenitor cells have been described.[36] Although HCC is more common in cirrhosis, it is increasingly recognized that both HCC and CCa, or their variants, may occur in either cirrhotic or noncirrhotic livers. HCC is characterized by neoplastic cells resembling hepatocytes in sheets intersected by branches of a small artery; it may be necessary to evaluate subtle features of the cord architecture (≥3 cells), the nuclear/cytoplasmic ratio, and CD34-reactive sinusoids to diagnose HCC. Bile production and identification of canaliculi by polyclonal carcinoembryonic antigen (pCEA) immunostaining are positive indications of the hepatocellular nature of the lesion. Distinction from high-grade dysplastic nodules (DN), especially in a liver biopsy, is a recognized challenge, and may not be possible.[37] When present, stromal invasion by tumor is considered diagnostic.[38,39] One group has proposed a combination of immunohistochemical analysis that includes Glypican-3, heat shock protein 70 (HSP-70), and glutamine synthetase (GS) to distinguish DN and HCC.[40] The panel was developed in resected specimens, and the application in a retrospective series of needle biopsies has recently been reported.[41]

Cholangiocarcinoma most often occurs in noncirrhotic livers, but is increasingly reported in cirrhosis attributable to viral hepatitis. Irregular gland formation by crowded, round cells with atypical nuclei and a high nuclear/cytoplasmic ratio characterize this tumor. Stromal desmoplasia is helpful, when present. Distinction from other forms of nonhepatic adenocarcinoma may be important, depending on the clinical setting. Algorithms for the use of immunohistochemistry are available.[21]

Primary angiosarcoma is a less common primary liver tumor, but one that can be deceivingly subtle to radiologists and pathologists alike because of its infiltrative nature. In a biopsy the only irregularity may be the occasional enlarged sinusoidal cell with a hyperchromatic nucleus. A high level of suspicion in the setting of an image description of an infiltrative mass may lead to the proper diagnosis.

Drug-Induced Liver Injury (DILI)

There are in-depth discussions[42] and overviews[43] of pathologic features of drug-induced liver injury. Because new drugs are introduced into the market regularly and patient populations typically have underlying co-morbidities, understanding and treating DILI is challenging and constantly evolving. Specifically, alcoholic liver injury and nonalcoholic fatty liver disease either may underlie liver test abnormalities or may be co-factors in a DILI response. Thus this is a field in which very close clinical and pathologic correlations are required, and a high level of suspicion that two conditions may co-exist is important. It is common to search PubMed for literature support that a particular drug causes liver abnormalities. DILI can manifest as hepatitic, cholestatic, steatosis/steatohepatitis, vascular, or neoplastic lesions. The injury pattern may be acute or chronic. DILI may cover the spectra of fulminant necrosis, chronic elevation of liver tests, duct injury or ductopenia, sinusoidal damage and peliosis, or fibrosis/cirrhosis. When inflammation is present, it may be granulomatous and eosinophilic; however, this is another variable of DILI. Some forms of DILI histologically mimic AIH. Hepatitis may be cholestatic, in which case DILI is highly suspected. In general, any time there is a concern of possible DILI, it is best to consult the literature so that a possible DILI will be neither overemphasized nor overlooked.

Liver Transplant Pathology

Liver transplant pathology continues to expand from the standard "acute rejection" and "chronic rejection" to include the more challenging areas of recurrent hepatitis C (versus acute rejection); perivenular necrosis and dropout with numerous plasma cells (acute rejection versus new-onset AIH); ischemic alterations of bile ducts (early "chronic rejection" and/or chronic arterial insufficiency); rapid development of fibrosis in recurrent HCV; cholestatic recurrent HCV; and steatosis in the liver allograft. Recurrent and de novo disease processes are part of the differential diagnosis of allograft dysfunction. Central necrosis with plasma cells and portal infiltrates dominated by plasma cells are findings that are becoming more widely recognized; the exact appellation of this "lesion" has not reached consensus, but treatment with immunosuppression is likely indicated.[44] There is also growing recognition of nonspecific "chronic hepatitis" and/or cirrhosis in allografts of long duration[45]; the importance of protocol biopsies regardless of time post-transplant or liver test values has been recently shown.[46] In biopsies of patients with normal liver tests, less than 33% of the biopsies were normal; in addition, 33% of all "late" protocol biopsies had evidence of idiopathic chronic hepatitis. Of those patients with chronic hepatitis, up to 33% responded to increased immunosuppression. As has always been the case in liver transplant pathology, consideration of opportunistic infections (CMV is most common), recurrence of the primary underlying disease, and vascular injury to the biliary tree and/or liver continue to be included in working differential diagnoses of liver transplant biopsies. The reader is referred to a recent, thorough review that begins with an algorithm for evaluation based on timing post-transplant.[47]

Pediatric Liver Biopsies

In addition to the entire spectra of diseases discussed for adults, liver biopsies in the pediatric age group include metabolic entities, some of which are inherited. In a large referral center study of 230 biopsies in a 36-month period, nearly 25%

Table 13-8 Liver Pathology Associated with Systemic Diseases

SYSTEMIC DISEASE	LIVER DISEASE	CLINICAL FEATURES	HISTOLOGIC DESCRIPTION
Type 1 DM	Diabetic hepatosclerosis	Elevated alkaline phosphatase; severe complications of DM in other organs	Nonzonal dense perisinusoidal fibrosis
	Glycogenic hepatopathy	Hepatomegaly; uncontrolled DM	Swollen, glycogen-filled hepatocytes without inflammation
Chronic granulomatous disease	May resemble PSC or inflammatory pseudotumor		Granulomas; abscesses; sclerosing duct lesions; obliterative fibrosis of veins
Graft versus host disease	Focused on bile ducts Unusual hepatitic form		Need to rule out infection
Pregnancy	Acute fatty liver of pregnancy	Third trimester; potential for liver failure	Microvesicular steatosis; need ORO to confirm; ± inflammation of acute hepatitis
	Toxemia Rupture		Zone 1 fibrin deposition
Celiac disease	None to various lesions	Elevated transaminases	Mononuclear cells in lobules, portal tracts; rarely associated with AIH or PBC
Hodgkin disease (HD)	Granulomatous inflammation	HD may not be clinically known	Epithelioid granulomas with eosinophils; differential diagnosis is DILI
	Ductopenia	HD may not be clinically known	Duct recovery has been reported in successfully treated HD

of biopsies were performed in children with either liver transplants or bone marrow transplants. Approximately 9% were for consideration of the differential diagnosis of infantile cholestasis; 7% were for hepatitis attributable to viral infection, autoimmune liver disease, or other causes (one third of the hepatitis cases); 4.5% were for metabolic liver diseases of childhood; and 9% were for neoplastic lesions; 4% of the biopsies had no diagnosis.[48] To obtain more information about lesions not discussed in this chapter, two recent authoritative reviews of diseases of infants and children are highly recommended.[48,49] The authors present critical clinicopathologic information and approaches to the metabolic diseases and tumors of infants and children.

Liver Biopsies in Systemic Disease

The liver can be affected by a variety of systemic disease processes. Two prime examples are (1) the close relationship between NAFLD and insulin resistance–related systemic disease and the higher proclivity for steatohepatitis and (2) the increased incidence of significant fibrosis in diabetic patients with NAFLD. The high occurrence rate of primary sclerosing cholangitis in patients with ulcerative colitis could be considered an example as well. Rheumatoid arthritis may result in hepatocellular unrest and lobular inflammation and lesions similar to those seen in methotrexate injury.[50] In contrast, systemic lupus erythematosis rarely is associated with nontherapy-related liver disease. In addition, clinical consideration of a mass lesion must include the possibility of metastasis from an otherwise unknown primary lesion. **Table 13-8** highlights clinical and histologic features of the liver affected by several systemic diseases.

References

1. Landas SK, Bromley CM. Sponge arteifact in biopsy specimens. Arch Pathol Lab Med 1990;114:1285–1287.
2. Deugnier YM, et al. Preneoplastic significance of hepatic iron-free foci in genetic hemochromatosis: a study of 185 patients. Hepatology 1993;18:1363–1369.
3. Roskams T, Desmet VJ, Verslype C. Development, structure and function of the liver. In: Burt AD, Portmann BC, Ferrell LD, editors. MacSween's pathology of the liver, 5th ed. Edinburgh: Churchill Livingstone Elsevier, 2007: 1–73.
4. Scheuer PJ, Lefkowitch JH. General considerations. In: Scheuer PJ, Lefkowitch JH, editors. Liver biopsy interpretation, 7th ed. Oxford: Elsevier Saunders, 2006: 1–19.
5. Katoonizadeh A, et al. Liver regeneration in acute severe liver impairment: a clinicopathological correlation study. Liver Int 2006;26(10):1225–1233.
6. Goodman ZD, Ishak KG, Sesterhenn IA. Herpes simplex hepatitis in apparently immunocompetent adults. Am J Clin Pathol 1986;85:694–699.
7. Colloredo G, et al. Impact of liver biopsy size on histological evaluation of chronic viral hepatitis: the smaller the sample, the milder the disease. J Hepatol 2003;39:239–244.
8. Dienes HP, et al. Autoimmune hepatitis and overlap syndromes. Clin Liv Dis 2002;6:349–362.
9. Brunt EM. Grading and staging the histopathological lesions of chronic hepatitis: the Knodell histology activity index and beyond. Hepatology 2000;31:231–236.
10. Scheuer PJ, Standish RA, Dhillon AP. Scoring of chronic hepatitis. Clin Liv Dis 2002;6:335–347.
11. Zatloukal K, et al. From Mallory to Mallory-Denk inclusion bodies: what, how and why? Exp Cell Res 2007;313:2033–2049.
12. Brunt EM, et al. Nonalcoholic steatohepatitis: a proposal for grading and staging the histological lesions. Am J Gastroenterol 1999;94:2467–2474.
13. Kleiner DE, et al. Design and validation of a histological scoring system for nonalcoholic fatty liver disease. Hepatology 2005;41(6):1313–1321.
14. Yip WW, Burt AD. Alcoholic liver disease. Semin Diag Pathol 2006;23:149–160.
15. Brunt EM, et al. Concurrence of histologic features of steatohepatitis with other forms of chronic liver disease. Mod Pathol 2003;16:49–56.
16. Brunt EM. Pathology of hepatic iron overload. Semin Liv Dis 2005;25:392–401.
17. Trombini P, Piperno A. Ferritin, metabolic syndrome and NAFLD: elective attractions and dangerous liaisons. J Hepatol 2007;46:549–552.
18. Kleiner DE. Granulomas in the liver. Semin Diag Pathol 2006;23:161–169.
19. Devaney K, et al. Hepatic sarcoidosis. Clinicopathologic features in 100 patients. Am J Surg Pathol 1993;17:1272–1280.
20. Ishak KG. Sarcoidosis of the liver and bile ducts. Mayo Clin Proc 1998;73:467–472.
21. Kakar S, et al. Best practices in diagnostic immunohistochemistry: hepatocellular carcinoma versus metastatic neoplasms. Arch Pathol Lab Med 2007;131:1648–1654.
22. Garcia-Pagan JC, et al. Extrahepatic portal vein thrombosis. Semin Liv Dis 2008;28:282–292.
23. Harrison SA, et al. Diabetic hepatosclerosis: diabetic microangiopathy of the liver. Arch Pathol Lab Med 2006;130:27–32.
24. DeLeve LD, Shulman HM, McDonald GB. Toxic injury to hepatic sinusoids: sinusoidal obstruction syndrome (veno-occlusive disease). Semin Liv Dis 2002;1:27–41.
25. Rubbia-Brandt L, Mentha G, Terris B. Sinusoidal obstruction syndrome is a major feature of hepatic lesions associated with oxaliplatin neoadjuvant chemotherapy for liver colorectal metastases. J Am Coll Surg 2006;202:199–200.
26. Bioulac-Sage P, et al. Hepatocellular adenoma subtype classification using molecular markers and immunohistochemistry. Hepatology 2007;46:740–748.
27. Zucman-Rossi J, et al. Genotype-phenotype correlation in hepatocellular adenoma: new classification and relationship with HCC. Hepatology 2006;43:515–524.
28. Dokmak S, et al. A single center surgical experience of 122 patients with single and multiple hepatocellular adenomas. Gastroenterol 2009;137:1698-1705.
29. Rebouissou S, Bioulac-Sage P, Zucman-Rossi J. Molecular pathogenesis of focal nodular hyperplasia and hepatocellular adenoma. J Hepatol 2008;48:163–170.
30. Paradis V, et al. Telangiectatic adenoma: an entity associated with incrased body mass index and inflammation. Hepatology 2007;46:140–146.
31. Paradis V, et al. Telangiectatic focal nodular hyperplasia: a variant of hepatocellular adenoma. Gastroenterol 2004;126:1323–1329.
32. Rebouissou S, et al. Frequent in-frame somatic deletions activate gp130 in inflammatory hepatocellular tumors. Nature 2009;457:200–204.
33. Laumonier H, et al. Hepatocellular adenomas: magnetic resonance imaging features as a function of molecular pathological classification. Hepatology 2008;48:808–818.
34. Kumari R, et al. Hepatocellular adenomas in a US center: Clinical-pathologic correlations utilizing a recently proposed classification. Lab Invest 2008;88:308A.
35. Zen Y, et al. Pathological classification of hepatic inflammatory pseudotumor with respect to IgG4-related disease. Mod Pathol 2007;20:884–894.
36. Komuta M, et al. Clinicopathological study on cholangiolocellular carcinoma suggesting hepatic progenitor cell origin. Hepatology 2008;47:1544–1546.
37. Kojiro M, Roskams T. Early hepatocellular carcinoma and dysplastic nodules. Semin Liv Dis 2005;25:133–142.
38. Park YN, et al. Ductular reaction is helpful in defining early stromal invasion, small hepatocellular carcinomas, and dysplastic nodules. Cancer 2007;109:915–923.
39. Kondo F. Histological features of early hepatocellular carcinomas and their developmental process: for daily practical clinical application. Hepatol Intern 2009;3:283–293.
40. Di Tommaso L, et al. Diagnostic value of HSP70, glypican-3 and glutamine synthetase in hepatocellular nodules in cirrhosis. Hepatology 2007;45:725–734.
41. Di Tommaso L, et al. The application of markers (HSP70 GPC3 and GS) in liver biopsies is useful for detection of hepatocellular carcinoma. J Hepatol 2009;50:746–754.
42. Lewis JH, Kleiner DE. Hepatic injury due to drugs, chemicals and toxins. In: Burt AD, Portmann BC, Ferrell LD, editors. MacSween's pathology of the liver, 5th ed. Edinburgh: Churchill Livingstone Elsevier, 2007: 649–760.
43. Goodman ZD. Drug hepatotoxicity. Clin Liv Dis 2002;6:381–397.
44. Demetris AJ, Sebagh M. Plasma cell hepatitis in liver allografts: variant of rejection or autoimmune hepatitis? Liver Transplant 2008;14:750–755.

45. Syn W-K, et al. Natural history of unexplained chronic hepatitis after liver transplantation. Liver Transplant 2007;13:984–989.

46. Mells G, et al. Late protocol liver biopsies in the liver allograft: a neglected investigation? Liver Transplant 2009;15):931–938.

47. Hubscher SG. Transplantation pathology. Semin Diag Pathol 2006;23: 170–181.

48. Finegold MJ. Common diagnostic problems in pediatric liver pathology. Clin Liv Dis 2002;6:421–454.

49. Ishak KG. Inherited metabolic diseases of the liver. Clin Liv Dis 2002;6: 455–479.

50. Farrell GC. Drug-induced hepatic fibrosis and cirrhosis. In: Farrell GG, editor. Drug induced liver disease. Edinburgh: Churchill Livingstone, 1994: 439–452.

Laboratory Testing for Liver Disease

Thierry Poynard and Françoise Imbert-Bismut

ABBREVIATIONS

AIDS acquired immunodeficiency syndrome
AIH autoimmune hepatitis
ALP alkaline phosphatase
ALT alanine aminotransferase
AMA antimitochondrial antibodies
ANA antinuclear antibodies
anti-LC1 liver specific cytosol antigen type 1
anti-LKM1 antibodies to liver/kidney microsome type 1
anti-SLA/LP antisoluble liver antigen/ liver pancreas
AST aspartate aminotransferase

AUROC area under the receiver characteristics curve
bDNA branched DNA
BSP bromsulphalein
ELISA enzyme-linked immunosorbent assay
GGT γ-glutamyl transferase
HBsAg hepatitis B surface antigen
HCV hepatitis C virus
HDL high-density lipoprotein
ICG indocyanine green
IL interleukin
INR international normalized ratio
LCAT lecithin-cholesterol acyltransferase

LDH lactate dehydrogenase
LFT liver function test
NAD nicotinamide adenine dinucleotide
pANCA perinuclear antineutrophil cytoplasmic antibodies
PBC primary biliary cirrhosis
PCR polymerase chain reaction
PDH pyruvate dehydrogenase
SGOT serum glutamic oxaloacetic transaminase
SGPT serum glutamic pyruvic transaminase
SMA smooth muscle antibodies
TNF tumor necrosis factor

Introduction

Because the liver performs multiple functions, no single laboratory test or even a battery of tests is sufficient to provide a complete estimate of the liver injury in every clinical situation. A broad array of biochemical tests is used to evaluate patients with suspected or established liver disease, but also for screening asymptomatic individuals.

Abnormal variations of serum liver chemistries may occur in 1% to 4% of the asymptomatic population.[1,2] As with the evaluation of all medical tests, liver tests must be interpreted in the context of the subject's risk factors for disease, symptoms, and historical and physical examination findings. There is an urgent need to replace invasive tests such as liver biopsy by noninvasive biomarkers.[3,4]

In approaching patients with liver disease, it is helpful to classify laboratory tests into several broad categories. These include (1) the common serum liver chemistry tests that reflect hepatocellular damage, cholestasis, or synthetic function; (2) tests or panels that reflect histologic features, such as fibrosis, steatosis, and steatohepatitis; (3) tests that contribute to accurate diagnosis in liver disease, including specific autoantibodies, genetic tests, and serologic tests for viral hepatitis; and (4) less common tests that measure the capacity of the liver to transport organic anions and clear endogenous or exogenous substances from the circulation, or that measure the capacity of the liver to metabolize drugs. Tests will not be analyzed separately for their prognostic values.

Common Serum Liver Chemistry Tests

Five laboratory assays are commonly called liver function tests (LFTs), although they are neither specific to the liver nor true measures of liver function: alanine aminotransferase (ALT or SGPT EC.2.6.1.2.), aspartate aminotransferase (AST or SGOT EC.2.6.1.1.), γ-glutamyl transferase (GGT EC. 2.3.2.2.), alkaline phosphatase (ALP EC.3.1.3.1.), and total bilirubin.

LFTs are used to screen people for the presence of liver disease, suggest the underlying cause, estimate the severity, assess prognosis, and monitor the efficacy of therapy. Abnormal LFTs may be the first indication of subclinical liver disease and may thereby guide further diagnostic evaluation.[2] After the existence of hepatic dysfunction is recognized, the specific pattern of liver test abnormalities may suggest the category of the underlying disease, such as hepatitis, biliary obstruction, or infiltrative liver disease (**Table 14-1**). Additional testing may permit an assessment of the severity of liver dysfunction, and certain tests, especially when performed repeatedly, may provide an estimate of prognosis. Prothrombin time and

Table 14-1 Common Serum Liver Chemistry Tests

LIVER CHEMISTRY TEST	CLINICAL IMPLICATION OF ABNORMALITY
Alanine aminotransferase	Hepatocellular damage
Aspartate aminotransferase	Hepatocellular damage
Bilirubin	Cholestasis, biliary obstruction, or impaired conjugation
γ-Glutamyltransferase	Cholestasis, biliary obstruction, infiltrative disease
Alkaline phosphatase	Cholestasis, biliary obstruction, infiltrative disease
Prothrombin time	Synthetic function
Albumin	Synthetic function
Bile acids	Cholestasis or biliary obstruction

serum albumin are the most common tests used as prognostic factors, together with serum bilirubin. For example, a rising bilirubin level is an adverse prognostic feature of primary biliary cirrhosis. Prolongation of the prothrombin time correlates with an adverse prognosis in acute hepatitis. Finally, sequential LFTs may be useful in assessing response to therapy, as in the case of declining serum aminotransferase levels after therapy for chronic viral hepatitis.

There are limitations to the use of LFTs in the diagnosis and management of liver disease. There are limitations in sensitivity; that is, the likelihood of an abnormal test result in patients known to have a disease. For example, patients with cirrhosis may have normal or minimally abnormal LFTs. Serum albumin, total bilirubin, and GGT decrease during a normal pregnancy.[5] There are also limitations in specificity; that is, the likelihood of a normal test result in a patient without the disease. At least one LFT is elevated in more than 20% of a general adult population.[2] Elevated serum aminotransferase levels may indicate liver disease or cardiac or muscle disease. LFT abnormalities rarely provide a specific diagnosis, but rather suggest a general category of liver disorder. Often, further specific diagnostic testing is required. In general, the multiple functions of the liver combined with the large number of LFTs available preclude simple diagnostic algorithms that are applicable to the evaluation of all patients with suspected liver disease. Therefore it is important for the physician evaluating a patient with suspected or known liver disease to have a firm understanding of the diverse tests available, their indications, and their limitations.

Aminotransferases [ALTE.C:2.6.1.2.] [ASTE.C:2.6.1.1.]

The aminotransferases, AST and ALT, are the most frequently used indicators of hepatic injury and represent markers of hepatocellular necrosis. These enzymes catalyze the transfer of the α-amino groups of aspartate and alanine to the α-keto group of ketoglutaric acid, resulting in the formation of oxaloacetic acid and pyruvic acid, respectively. The enzymes play a role in gluconeogenesis by facilitating the synthesis of glucose from noncarbohydrate sources. AST is present in both the mitochondria (80% of the total) and the cytosol (20%) of hepatocytes, but ALT is found only in the cytosol.[6] Whereas ALT is localized primarily to the liver, AST is present in a variety of tissues, including liver, heart, skeletal muscle, kidney, brain, pancreas, lungs, leukocytes and erythrocytes. Serum AST levels are typically elevated in cardiac and muscle diseases. Both AST and ALT are present in the serum as holoenzymes and apoenzymes, depending on whether or not they are associated with their co-factor pyridoxal 5'-phosphate. Thus potentially six different forms of AST and ALT can circulate in the serum: the apoenzymes and holoenzymes of ALT or AST, cytosolic AST, and mitochondrial AST.

The most sensitive and specific method for assaying the aminotransferases is enzymatic reduction of oxaloacetate and pyruvate to malate and lactate, respectively, coupled with oxidation of nicotinamide adenine dinucleotide, reduced form (NADH), to nicotinamide adenine dinucleotide (NAD). Because NADH absorbs light at 340 nm but NAD does not, the process can be followed spectrophotometrically. Aminotransferase's activity measurement has to be supplemented with pyridoxal phosphate to avoid falsely decreased activities in samples obtained from patients with low endogenous vitamin B_6 concentrations.[7-9]

The use of an international calibration guarantees harmonious results of enzyme activities between the different laboratories.[9] Thus the results of enzyme activity measurements are depending on the analytical conditions. They should no more be expressed in upper reference limit (URL), which still can differ from one laboratory to another, but in international units.[10,11] Moreover, the normal range should also be adjusted for sex and body index.[10,11]

Serum levels of AST and ALT are elevated to some extent in almost all liver diseases. On rare occasions, isolated elevations of AST in serum may be attributable to the formation of a macroenzyme with binding of AST to immunoglobulins (Ig).[12,13] The complex has a higher molecular mass and a delayed clearance that leads to an increase in the amount of the circulating enzyme. AST-IgA complexes in adult patients have been reported to be associated with liver malignancies or chronic liver disease. Macroenzymes are generally not considered pathologic, but the persistently increased enzyme values can lead to multiple or expensive diagnostic tests.[14]

In liver disease, the highest elevations occur in severe viral hepatitis, drug- or toxin-induced hepatic necrosis, and circulatory shock (ischemic hepatitis) (**Table 14-2**).[15,16] Although enzyme levels may reflect the extent of hepatocellular necrosis, they do not correlate with eventual outcome. In fact, declining AST and ALT levels may indicate either recovery or a poor prognosis because of a paucity of remaining hepatocytes in the latter case. Moderately elevated levels of serum aminotransferase are typical of acute or chronic hepatitis, including viral hepatitis and autoimmune, drug-induced and alcoholic hepatitis, whereas mild elevations are seen in fatty liver, nonalcoholic steatohepatitis, drug toxicity, and chronic hepatitis C.[17-21] In overweight people, mildly elevated levels of serum aminotransferase as a result of fatty liver may resolve with weight reduction of 10% or more.[22-27] It appears in some instances that mild elevations in the serum ALT (and the AST) level may result from myositis[28] or muscle injury after rigorous exercise.[29] In cirrhosis, cholestatic liver diseases, and hepatic

Table 14-2 Etiology of ALT or AST Elevations

MILD ALT OR AST ELEVATIONS, <200 IU/L	SEVERE ALT OR AST ELEVATIONS, >600 IU/L
Hepatic: ALT-Predominant	
Chronic hepatitis C	Acute viral hepatitis (A-E, herpes)
Chronic hepatitis B	Autoimmune hepatitis
Acute viral hepatitis (A-E, EBV, CMV)	Wilson disease
Steatosis/steatohepatitis	Acute bile duct obstruction
Hemochromatosis	Acute Budd-Chiari syndrome
Medications/toxins/illicit drugs/herbs	Hepatic artery ligation
Autoimmune hepatitis	
Sclerosing cholangitis	
Primary biliary cirrhosis	
Acute bile duct obstruction	
α_1-Antitrypsin deficiency	
Wilson disease	
Celiac disease	
Hepatic: AST-Predominant	
Alcohol-related liver injury	Medications/toxins/illicit drugs/herbs
Steatosis/steatohepatitis	Ischemic hepatitis
Cirrhosis	
Nonhepatic	
Hemolysis	
Myopathy	
Thyroid disease	
Strenuous exercise	
Sepsis	
Macro-AST	

ALT, alanine aminotransferase; AST, aspartate aminotransferase; CMV, cytomegalovirus; EBV, Epstein-Barr Virus

neoplasms, serum levels of AST and ALT may be elevated slightly. Acute biliary tract obstruction may result in elevations of AST and ALT of more than 300 U/L; these levels peak early and decline rapidly over 24 to 72 hours despite unresolved obstruction.[30]

Determinations of serum aminotransferase have proved useful as screening tests for subclinical liver disease in asymptomatic persons,[31,32] and an abnormal result may lead to a diagnosis of hemochromatosis,[33] Wilson disease, or α_1-antitrypsin deficiency and nonhepatic diseases such as anorexia nervosa[34,35] and celiac disease.[36,36a] In anorexia, starvation-induced hepatocyte autophagy has been suspected as the cause of liver necrosis.[35] Elevated serum aminotransferase levels have been found in as many as 54% of children[37] and 40% of adult patients with celiac disease,[38] but these prevalences were not observed in other studies.[39,40] Liver biopsy in these patients may show variable degrees of steatosis, inflammation, and fibrosis.[32] One recommendation is to assess anti-tissue transglutaminase antibodies in patients with abnormal liver tests, without frequent cause.[39]

The ratio of AST to ALT in serum has been associated with alcoholic liver disease but without high predictive values. An AST:ALT ratio of more than 2.0 is observed in alcoholic liver disease.[40] In this setting, the ALT is often normal or minimally elevated. High ALT levels (>500U/L) should suggest a diagnosis other than alcoholic liver disease, even when the AST:ALT ratio is greater than 2.0.[41] In viral hepatitis, the ratio of AST to ALT is usually less than 1.0. The ratio often rises, but not invariably[42,43] to more than 1.0 as cirrhosis develops.[44,45] The ratio of AST to ALT in patients with nonalcoholic fatty liver disease is typically less than 1.0 in the absence of fibrosis on liver biopsy; however, as in chronic viral hepatitis,[46] the ratio exceeds 1.0 in some patients with cirrhosis.[47] The lack of a substantial elevation in ALT levels in patients with alcoholic liver disease is thought to be related to pyridoxine deficiency. Pyridoxine deficiency decreases hepatic ALT more than hepatic AST, with corresponding changes in serum levels.[48] The ratio of mitochondrial AST to total AST may be useful in the diagnostic of specific liver diseases, but the isoenzyme activity is not assayed routinely in clinical practice.[49]

Under certain circumstances, the aminotransferase levels may be falsely diminished or inhibited. Markedly diminished serum levels of AST have been reported in patients on long-term hemodialysis and have been attributed either to dialysis of the enzyme or to pyridoxine deficiency, although neither possibility has been confirmed experimentally.[50]

Alkaline Phosphatase [ALPE.C:3.1.3.1.]

Alkaline phosphatase (ALP) is a family of isoenzymes that catalyze the hydrolysis of a number of phosphate esters at an alkaline pH optimum. This glycoprotein requires zinc for activity. ALP are coded by four genes,[51] including one that codes for ALP isoenzymes from liver, bone, first-trimester placenta, and kidney. Levels of ALP determined by different assay methods must be compared with caution because of the specific conditions of the different assays, the heterogeneity of the ALPs, and their overlapping but distinctly different specific activities with different substrates. Physiologic significance of ALP remains unclear. In the human body, ALP has been identified in liver, bone, intestine, placenta, kidney, and leukocytes. In the liver two distinct forms of ALP are found. Different methods of isoenzyme analysis can be used. The enzyme in the liver is associated with sinusoidal and canalicular membranes, also present in the cytosol, and secreted in bile in large amounts. Standardized analytical conditions for ALP activity measurement were described by the IFCC (International Federation of Clinical Chemistry) and reference intervals in the blood of adults and females at 37° C were determined.[52]

In healthy people, most circulating ALP originates from the liver or bone. In pregnant women, circulating placental ALP is often found. Average normal values of ALP vary with age: they are relatively high in childhood and puberty (correlating with the rate of growth of bone), lower in middle age (higher in men than in women), and higher again in old age (particularly in women). Serum levels of ALP correlate with a person's weight and the number of cigarettes smoked per day, and inversely with height.[53]

In patients with an elevated level of serum ALP, the source is the liver in a majority of cases; but in up to one third of such individuals no evidence of liver disease can be found. Even in hospitalized patients, nonspecific elevations of serum ALP are not uncommon and are often transient. Bone disease characterized by increased osteoblastic activity also may be the

Table 14-3 Causes of Elevated Serum Alkaline Phosphatase and γ-Glutamyltransferase

CAUSES OF ELEVATED SERUM ALKALINE PHOSPHATASE AND γ-GLUTAMYLTRANSFERASE	ELEVATED ALKALINE PHOSPHATASE ONLY
Hepatobiliary	
Bile duct obstruction	
Primary biliary cirrhosis	
Primary sclerosing cholangitis	
Medications	
Hepatocellular carcinoma	
Hepatic metastasis	
Hepatitis	
Cirrhosis	
Vanishing bile duct syndromes	
Benign recurrent cholestasis	
Infiltrating diseases of the liver	
Sarcoidosis	
Tuberculosis	
Fungal infection	
Other granulomatous diseases	
Amyloidosis	
Lymphoma	
Nonhepatic	
Chronic renal failure	Bone disease
Lymphoma and other malignancies	Pregnancy
Congestive heart failure	Childhood growth
Infection/inflammation	

source of an elevated serum ALP level, as may pregnancy. Only rarely is the intestine or kidney the source.

The highest elevations of serum ALP in patients with liver disease occur in cholestatic disorders (**Table 14-3**). Elevations occur as a result of both intrahepatic and extrahepatic obstruction to bile flow, and the degree of elevation does not help to distinguish the two. The mechanism by which cholestasis increases serum ALP levels is thought to involve the induction of ALP synthesis secondary to enhanced translation of the mRNA of ALP, not from a failure to clear or excrete circulating ALP.[54] That the passage of time is required for de novo synthesis of ALP after biliary obstruction is reflected in instances early in the course of acute suppurative cholangitis, in which serum ALP levels are normal but serum aminotransferase levels are markedly elevated. The serum ALP level may be normal in up to 3% of patients with primary sclerosing cholangitis.[55]

Elevated levels of serum ALP in patients with cancer may result from hepatic or bony metastases. In hepatic metastasis, elevation of the ALP in serum presumably results from localized biliary obstruction with induction of ALP and leakage into the serum. Elevated serum levels of ALP of hepatic origin also may result from other infiltrative liver diseases, such as abscesses, granulomatous liver disease, and amyloidosis. In hospitalized patients, the highest elevations of serum ALP (>1000 IU/L) occur in those with malignant biliary obstruction, sepsis, and acquired immunodeficiency syndrome (AIDS) combined with a systemic infection. Mildly elevated levels of serum ALP are nonspecific and may be seen in cirrhosis, hepatitis, or congestive heart failure.[55] Rarely, increased serum ALP occurs in a family on a genetic basis.[56]

Low levels of serum ALP may occur in hypothyroidism, pernicious anemia, zinc deficiency, and congenital hypophosphatasia, Wilson disease, or in severe hepatic insufficiency.

Finally, the place for ALP in first-line LFT is questionable as ALP is less sensitive than GGT and less specific than bilirubin for the diagnosis and prognosis of more frequent liver diseases.[2]

γ-Glutamyl Transferase (or transpeptidase) [E.C:2.3.2.2.]

γ-Glutamyl transferase (GGT) catalyzes the transfer of γ-glutamyl groups of peptides, such as glutathione, to other amino acids. GGT is widely distributed in membranes in a variety of tissues, including the kidney, seminal vesicles, pancreas, liver, spleen, heart, and brain, and is thought to function in amino acid transport via a γ-glutamyl cycle. GGT has also been shown to catalyze the metabolism of S-substituted glutathione conjugates of various xenobiotics, and is associated with oxidative stress.[57,58]

GGT has been localized to the entire hepatobiliary tree, from hepatocytes to the common bile duct, and to pancreatic acini and ductules. The greatest concentration of enzyme is in epithelial cells lining fine biliary ductules. GGT secreted into bile is primarily of two types. One corresponds to the particulate fraction of biliary ALP. The other is a complex of biliary ALP and lipoproteins. GGT occurs in the same membrane fragments that contain particulate ALP.[57,58]

Measurement of GGT activity is performed according to a standardized method against a IFCC reference method at 37°C.[59] As for aminotransferase's activity, GGT enzymatic measurement should be calibrated to minimize result variations between different laboratories.[9]

Serum levels of GGT depend on age and sex; normal values are greater in men than in women, and in adults increase with age.[57] Neonates may have values five to eight times higher than adults.[60]

GGT has been widely used as an index of liver dysfunction and marker of high alcohol intake.[57,61] The specific role of steatosis, or cholestasis in these levels have not been yet clarified. GGT levels are elevated in most acute and chronic liver diseases. GGT levels are also elevated in association with an array of pathologic states other than hepatobiliary disease; these include pancreatic disease, myocardial infarction, renal failure, chronic obstructive pulmonary disease, and diabetes.[57] GGT is inducible. Levels may be increased by a number of enzyme-inducing drugs, most notably alcohol and phenytoin, in the absence of other evidence of liver disease.[57] Associations between serum GGT and risk of coronary heart disease, type 2 diabetes, and stroke have been observed—all conditions also associated with liver steatosis.

In liver disease, GGT activity in serum correlates with serum ALP levels but is more sensitive. The accuracy of GGT has been challenged for its lack of specificity,[62-70] but the diagnostic interest of serum GGT is in its high sensitivity for hepatobiliary disease, particularly biliary tract disease, with an excellent negative predictive value (**Table 14-3**).[2,57] Rarely is the serum GGT level normal in intrahepatic cholestasis.[2,57,63,64] These exceptions tend to occur in infants or young children with some types of familial intrahepatic cholestasis such as progressive familial intrahepatic cholestasis type 1 and 2 but not in type 3 or in adenosine triphosphate-binding cassette

Table 14-4 Panels of Serum Biomarkers of Hepatic Fibrosis with at Least Two Validations

PANEL	YEAR FIRST PUBLICATION	COMPONENTS	LIVER DISEASE
Not Patented			
PGA	1991	Prothrombin, GGT, apoA1	ALD
AP	1997	Platelet, age	HCV
Bonacini	1997	Platelet, ALT, AST	HCV
Pohl	2001	Platelet, AST	HCV
Forns'	2002	Platelet, cholesterol, age	HCV
APRI	2003	Platelet, AST	HCV
MP3	2004	PIIINP, MMP1	HCV
FIB-4	2006	Platelet, AST, ALT, age	HCV/HIV
FibroIndex	2007	Platelet, AST, gamma globulins	HCV
Patented			
FibroTest/FibroSure	2001	A2M, haptoglobin, APOA1, bilirubin, GGT, age, gender	HCV, HBV, ALD, NAFLD, HIV
FibroSpect II	2004	A2M, HA, TIMP1	HCV
ELF	2004	HA, PIIINP, TIMP1	Mixed
FibroMeter	2005	Platelet, AST, A2M, HA prothrombin, age, gender	Mixed
HepaScore	2005	A2M, HA, GGT, age, gender	HCV

References are available in the recent published meta-analyses.

A1, apolipoprotein A1; ALT, alanine aminotransferase; AST, aspartate aminotransferase; ELF, Enhanced liver fibrosis; FM, FibroMeter; FS, FibroSure; FSII, FibroSpect II; FT, FibroTest; HA, hyaluronic acid; HOMA, homeostatic model assessment; MMP, matrix metalloproteinases; PI, prothrombin index; TIMP, tissue inhibitors of metalloproteinases

subfamily B, member 4 (ABCB4) mutations.[65-69] Benign recurrent intrahepatic cholestasis can progress to progressive familial intrahepatic cholestasis with low serum GGT.[68,69]

GGT is an "indirect" marker of liver fibrosis, at least due to associated biliary cell injury, and is included as a component of three panels of biomarkers used for the noninvasive assessment of liver fibrosis (**Table 14-4**).

Bilirubin

Bilirubin is an endogenous organic anion derived primarily from the degradation of hemoglobin released from aging red blood cells. Measurement of bilirubin levels in serum is important in the assessment of hepatic function. Serum levels of bilirubin may be determined by the photometric detection of the azo derivatives obtained by the reaction of plasma with the diazonium ion of sulfanilic acid (the so-called diazo or van den Bergh reaction).[71,72] The van den Bergh reaction separates bilirubin into two fractions: a water-soluble direct-reacting form representing conjugated bilirubin and a lipid-soluble indirect-reacting form representing unconjugated bilirubin.[73] Direct-reacting bilirubin is a mixture of bilirubin monoglucuronides and diglucuronide that results from the conjugation of bilirubin in the liver.

Bilirubin itself is insoluble in water and is bound to albumin; therefore it does not appear in urine. In contrast, bilirubin glucuronides are water soluble and appear in urine when plasma levels are increased. When serum bilirubin glucuronides are elevated, some of the conjugated bilirubin may be bound covalently to serum albumin-δ bilirubin. This last form of bilirubin is not filtered by the kidney and is the last pigment to clear from the serum following resolution of hepatobiliary disease. This mechanism accounts for the absence of bilirubinuria in some patients with conjugated hyperbilirubinemia, and for the slow resolution of jaundice in patients with otherwise normal liver function after recovery from acute liver disease.[74]

Measurement of bilirubin by the diazo method is not entirely accurate. At low serum levels, the measurement of direct bilirubin by the diazo method overestimates conjugated bilirubin because some unconjugated bilirubin reacts directly with the reagent. This may lead to misinterpretation of mild unconjugated hyperbilirubinemia, as in Gilbert syndrome and hemolysis. More accurate measurement of bilirubin and its conjugates by high-performance liquid chromatography reveals that conjugated bilirubin constitutes only about 4% to 5% of total bilirubin in normal sera. This corresponds to a serum level of less than 1 μmol/L. By such methods, the upper limit of normal for direct bilirubin is 3 μmol/L. Such methods to measure bilirubin are not routinely employed, but provide the most sensitive means of detecting hepatobiliary disease and distinguishing the true unconjugated hyperbilirubinemia of Gilbert syndrome and hemolysis from the mild conjugated hyperbilirubinemia of liver disease.[75]

Normal levels of total bilirubin in serum or plasma are between 3 and 15 μmol/L and are significantly higher in men

Table 14-5 Causes of Hyperbilirubinemia

ISOLATED UNCONJUGATED HYPERBILIRUBINEMIA	CONJUGATED HYPERBILIRUBINEMIA
Gilbert syndrome	Bile duct obstruction
Neonatal jaundice	Hepatitis
Hemolysis	Cirrhosis
Blood transfusion (hemolysis)	Medications/toxins
Resorption of a large hematoma	Primary biliary cirrhosis
Shunt hyperbilirubinemia	Primary sclerosing cholangitis
Crigler–Najjar syndrome	Total parenteral nutrition
Ineffective erythropoiesis	Sepsis, benign postoperative jaundice
Medications	Intrahepatic cholestasis of pregnancy
	Benign recurrent cholestasis
	Vanishing bile duct syndromes
	Dubin-Johnson syndrome
	Rotor syndrome

than in women. As previously indicated, hyperbilirubinemia is classified as either predominantly unconjugated or predominantly conjugated (**Table 14-5**). Levels between 17 and 70 μmol/L, representing unconjugated hyperbilirubinemia, may result from increased production of bilirubin, impaired transport of bilirubin into hepatocytes, or defective bilirubin conjugation in hepatocytes.

Even in cases of severe hemolysis, the total serum bilirubin level is rarely above 70 μmol/L (5mg/dl) in the presence of normal liver function. Serum bilirubin levels higher than 70 μmol/L or bilirubin levels between 17 and 70 μmol/L in association with other LFTs abnormalities usually signify the presence of liver disease. In these situations, at least 50% of the serum bilirubin is conjugated. Conjugated hyperbilirubinemia results from impaired intrahepatic excretion of bilirubin or extrahepatic obstruction. However, because of continued urinary excretion, maximum serum bilirubin levels plateau at around 500 μmol/L, even in complete bile duct obstruction. Extreme hyperbilirubinemia with levels above 500 μmol/L usually signifies severe parenchymal liver disease in association with hemolysis, as in sickle cell anemia or renal failure.

The serum bilirubin level has prognostic value in chronic liver disease,[76,77] particularly primary biliary cirrhosis and other cholestatic liver diseases,[78] and in hepatic failure, in which deep jaundice is associated with increased mortality.[79] Bilirubin is one of the validated prognostic score model for end-stage liver disease (MELD) together with prothrombin time and creatinine), widely used for liver transplantation decisions. Total bilirubin, in combination with other blood tests, is now proposed for one noninvasive biomarker of liver fibrosis (FibroTest) in patients with chronic liver diseases (see **Table 14-4**). In acute liver disease, such as acute viral hepatitis, however, even profound jaundice is typically followed by complete recovery.

Serum Bile Acids

Bile acids are synthesized from cholesterol in the liver, conjugated with glycine or taurine, and excreted by the liver.[80] Bile acid metabolism is mainly regulated by the farnesoid X receptor (FXR; also known as the bile acid receptor or BAR; gene symbol *NR1H4*) is a member of the nuclear receptor family of transcription factors.[81] As ligands for this nuclear receptor FXR, bile acids regulate their own synthesis, transport, and conjugation, thus protecting against bile acid toxicity. Recently the role of genetic variants in FXR itself, FXR target genes, and regulators of FXR in the pathophysiology of the liver have been demonstrated for cholestasis of pregnancy, cholesterol lithiasis, progressive familial intrahepatic cholestasis type 1, and benign recurrent intrahepatic cholestasis.[81] Whereas serum bilirubin levels are influenced by factors such as the rate of bilirubin production and hepatic perfusion that do not directly reflect the function of the liver, bile acids more specifically reflect hepatic excretory function.

Serum bile acids are more sensitive than bilirubin for detecting hepatobiliary disease. Fasting levels of serum bile acids are frequently elevated when the serum bilirubin level is normal.[82] The greater sensitivity of serum bile acids is due in part to the much larger pool of bile acids compared to bilirubin. Bile acids (but not bilirubin) undergo enterohepatic recycling and storage in the gallbladder. In patients with hyperbilirubinemia, fasting bile acid levels are usually elevated in serum, except in cases of hemolysis and congenital hyperbilirubinemia.

The highest concentrations of serum bile acids occur in viral hepatitis and extrahepatic obstruction.[80] Serum bile acids are markedly elevated in cholestatic liver diseases, including primary biliary cirrhosis, primary sclerosing cholangitis, and intrahepatic cholestasis of pregnancy. Concentrations of endogenous bile acids in serum decrease during treatment with ursodeoxycholic acid, which becomes the predominant bile acid, accounting for 50% of the serum bile acid concentration.[82]

Bile acid measurements are not as commonly used in clinical practice as GGT, despite its low specificity, is a simple first line biomarker of cholestasis.

Albumin

Albumin is quantitatively the most important plasma protein synthesized by the liver and is a useful indicator of hepatic function. In adults the average size of the albumin pool is approximately 500 g; 12 to 15 g are synthesized daily. Because the half-life of albumin in serum is as long as 20 days, the serum albumin level is not a reliable indicator of hepatic protein synthesis in acute liver disease.[83] Moreover, the serum albumin level at a single point in time may not reflect synthesis because the turnover of albumin can be affected by disturbances in distribution, catabolism, and synthesis. Albumin synthesis is affected not only by liver disease but also by nutritional status, hormonal balance, and osmotic pressure. In particular, albumin synthesis is exquisitely sensitive to the availability of amino acids, particularly tryptophan.[84] Hypergammaglobulinemia may also lead to a decrease in the serum albumin level by increasing the contribution of serum immunoglobulins to the total plasma oncotic pressure.[85]

Serum albumin levels are typically depressed in patients with cirrhosis and ascites. In patients with or without ascites, the serum albumin level correlates with prognosis.[86] In the presence of ascites decreased levels of serum albumin may be a reflection of increased volume of distribution and impaired synthesis, and the actual size of the exchangeable albumin pool may be normal or increased.[87] Albumin synthesis may also be depressed by heavy alcohol intake and poor dietary intake of protein. Other nonhepatic causes of hypoalbuminemia are nephrotic syndrome, protein-losing enteropathy, and burns.[88]

Prothrombin Time and Serum Coagulation Factor Levels

The liver synthesizes coagulation factors I (fibrinogen), II (prothrombin), V, VII, IX, and X.[89] Most of these are present in excess, and clotting abnormalities occur only when there is substantial impairment in the ability of the liver to synthesize these factors. The standard method of assessing impaired coagulation in liver disease is the one-stage prothrombin time of Quick,[90] which evaluates the extrinsic coagulation pathway by measuring the rate of conversion of prothrombin to thrombin in the presence of a tissue extract (thromboplastin) and Ca^{2+} ions. The prothrombin time is prolonged when factors I, II, V, VII, and X are deficient, either singly or in combination. Using the international normalized ratio (INR) rather than the prothrombin time itself in patients with liver disease is controversial. The use of plasma from patients with liver disease in the calibration model for thromboplastin could lead to a prothrombin time standardization specific for liver disease.[91,92]

In acute or chronic hepatocellular disease, the prothrombin time may serve as a useful prognostic indicator. In acute hepatocellular disease, a markedly prolonged and worsening prothrombin time suggests an increased likelihood of acute hepatic failure. The prognosis is particularly severe when the prothrombin time indicates decreases of clotting factors to 10% of control or less. Prolongation of the prothrombin time also suggests a poor long-term prognosis in chronic liver disease and an increased risk of mortality from portosystemic shunt surgery.[93,94]

Prolongation of the prothrombin time is not specific for liver disease. It may occur as a result of congenital deficiencies of coagulation factors,[95] acquired conditions such as consumptive coagulopathies, vitamin K deficiency, and the ingestion of drugs that antagonize the prothrombin complex (such as bishydroxycoumarin derivatives). Vitamin K deficiency primarily affects factors II, VII, IX, and X. Factor VII has the shortest half-life and decreases first, followed by factors X and IX. On the other hand, factor V is synthesized by the liver but not affected by vitamin K deficiency. Thus measurement of factor V levels can be used to distinguish hepatocellular injury from vitamin K deficiency, as occurs in obstructive jaundice or steatorrhea. In deficiency of vitamin K resulting from obstructive jaundice, steatorrhea, or therapeutic anticoagulation, coagulation factors are synthesized at the normal rate but lack procoagulant function because they have fewer of the γ-carboxyglutamic acid residues necessary for binding Ca^{2+} to phospholipids.[96] Vitamin K deficiency can be distinguished from impaired synthesis of coagulation factors by administering vitamin K parenterally.[97] If the prothrombin time returns to normal or improves by at least 30% within 24 hours of administration of a single 10-mg injection of vitamin K, hepatic function is intact with regard to the synthesis of clotting factors, and vitamin K deficiency can be presumed to be responsible for the prolongation of the prothrombin time. Acetylcysteine can artificially worsen prothrombin time in patients with uncomplicated paracetamol poisoning; a fall in this index might be misinterpreted as a sign of liver failure, leading to prolonged treatment time.[98]

Measurement of des-γ-carboxy prothrombin (also known as prothrombin produced in the absence or antagonism of vitamin K II) also is a marker of liver dysfunction,[99] and increased levels have been found in the plasma of patients with hepatocellular carcinoma.[100] The abnormal prothrombin is presumably produced by the tumor. As a marker for hepatocellular carcinoma, the plasma level of des-γ-carboxy prothrombin can be complementary with levels of α-fetoprotein. Unfortunately, with currently available assays, plasma levels of des-γ-carboxy prothrombin are elevated in fewer than 50% of patients with tumors smaller than 3 cm in diameter.[101-103] The test cannot be recommended for screening purposes.

Other Enzymes

5′-Nucleotidase catalyzes the hydrolysis of nucleotides by releasing inorganic phosphate from the 5′-position of the pentose ring. 5′-Nucleotidase is present in the intestines, brain, heart, blood vessels, endocrine pancreas, and liver.[104] In the liver, 5′-nucleotidase is associated primarily with canalicular and sinusoidal plasma membranes. Elevated serum levels of 5′-nucleotidase are thought to be hepatobiliary in origin despite the widespread distribution of the enzyme in other body tissues. Serum levels of 5′-nucleotidase correlate closely with serum ALP levels, and because serum 5′-nucleotidase is so specific for liver diseases, it is used to confirm the hepatic origin of elevated serum levels of ALP. Measurements of 5′-nucleotidase in serum can be useful in diagnosing liver disease in childhood and pregnancy. ALP is increased physiologically in these settings, but 5′-nucleotidase is not.[104]

Lactate dehydrogenase (LDH) is often included in liver biochemistry panels but has poor diagnostic specificity for liver disease. Markedly increased levels of LDH in serum may be seen in hepatocellular necrosis, shock liver, cancer, or hemolysis associated with liver disease.[105]

Glutamate dehydrogenase is a mitochondrial enzyme found particularly in centrilobular hepatocytes, whereas aminotransferases are distributed in a periportal location. It has been observed that serum glutamate dehydrogenase levels more closely reflect alcoholic hepatitis than do serum aspartate aminotransferase levels because the toxic effect of ethanol is directed primarily to the mitochondria in centrilobular hepatocytes.[106] However, elevated levels of glutamate dehydrogenase in serum fall rapidly after cessation of alcohol intake, and may not discriminate between fatty liver and alcoholic hepatitis.[107,108]

Carbohydrate Deficient Transferrin (CDT)

GGT, ALT, AST, and mean corpuscular volume of erythrocytes (MCV) are the traditional blood markers of chronic alcohol intake. CDT, a recently identified marker, exhibits a diagnostic usefulness for the detection of excessive alcohol consumption and the monitoring of sustained heavy drinking.[109,110] CDT corresponds to transferrin molecules that lack one or two complete N-glycan chains (asialo-, monosialo-, and disialotransferrin). Usually, the amount of CDT is reported as a relative amount of total transferrin (% CDT). The diagnostic sensitivity of CDT in detecting excessive alcohol consumption varies from 65% to 95%, while the diagnostic specificity is about 97%.[109,110] CDT and GGT have also been validated as markers of alcohol consumption in patients with HCV, HBV, and NAFLD, separately or in combination.[111] Liver fibrosis and steatosis can reduce %CDT and increase GGT activity results, features that are particularly important in heavy drinkers. Therefore, before interpreting %CDT and GGT activity results to validate the alcohol consumption declared by a patient, it is necessary to estimate the stage of fibrosis and the grade of steatosis.[112] A study of serum transferrin glycoform patterns on 1387 subjects has demonstrated that the adjustment of reference intervals for CDT in relation with ethnicity, age, gender, body mass index (BMI), and smoking is not required.[113]

Biomarkers of Liver Fibrosis

A new generation of liver tests has been studied for the diagnosis of liver fibrosis. There is a need of evaluation and management of the increasing numbers of patients with chronic liver disease, the four most frequent being patients infected with hepatitis C virus (HCV), hepatitis B virus (HBV), alcoholic liver disease (ALD), and nonalcoholic fatty liver disease (NAFLD).[114] Liver biopsy is still often recommended by guidelines but cannot be performed in millions of people.[114-120] Numerous studies strongly suggest that because of the limitations and risks of biopsy, as well as improvements in the diagnostic accuracy of biochemical markers, liver biopsy should no longer be considered mandatory.[4,114,121-123]

Because the reference standard even of 25 mm length has 25% of false positive or false negative, the methodology used for assessing the diagnosis performance of biomarkers must take into account this variability. Therefore quality of biopsy specimen, analysis of discordances, and long-term clinical endpoints must be used.[124,125]

Neither biomarkers nor biopsy are sufficient alone to make a definitive decision in a given patient and all the clinical and biologic data must be taken into account. Due to the evidence-based data, health authorities in some countries have already approved validated biomarkers as a first-line procedure for the staging of liver fibrosis.[121,122]

Isolated Biomarkers

In a review of 66 studies of tests predicting biopsy findings, Gebo and associates[126] concluded that panels of markers might have the greatest value in predicting the absence of, or no more than minimal, fibrosis upon taking a biopsy, and in predicting the presence of cirrhosis upon conducting a biopsy.

Serum ALT was the most commonly investigated marker, with sensitivity ranging from 61% to 71%. The diagnostic value was lower than that of a combination of markers.[127]

Among the extracellular matrix tests, hyaluronic acid correlated best with fibrosis stage overall, but has been demonstrated only for extensive fibrosis.[126] Elevated serum hyaluronic acid is not liver specific and may increase in cartilage disease such as osteoarthritis.[128] Markers of extracellular matrix degradation, such as tissue inhibitor of metalloproteinase-1-4, were less predictive than hyaluronic acid.[126]

Several cytokines and cytokine receptors were investigated, including tumor necrosis factors (TNF), TNF-R55, TNF-R75,

and TNF-α, as well as serum interleukin (IL)-10, and IL-2 receptors. They were associated with fibrosis, but were less predictive than panel tests. TNF-α was associated with hepatic inflammation, but not with fibrosis.[126,127]

Other tests were investigated, including glutathione, α-fetoprotein, prothrombin time, pseudocholinesterase, manganese superoxide dismutase, β-N-galactosidase, α₂-macroglobin, haptoglobin, β-globulin, albumin, glutamyl transpeptidase, bilirubin, apolipoprotein A1, lactate dehydrogenase, AST, ALP, white blood cell count, platelet count, creatinine, total bile acids, and immunoglobulin G. Isolated, these markers were less useful than the panel of markers.[114,122,126,127]

Panels of Fibrosis Biomarkers

Panels of markers have greater accuracy in comparison with isolated markers for the diagnosis of advanced fibrosis (bridging fibrosis) or fibrosis.[114,121,122,127,129-133]

Several overviews and meta-analysis have been performed, which summarized the advantages and the limits of the available combination of biomarkers of liver fibrosis. Among a total of 2237 references, a total of 14 validated serum biomarkers have been identified between 1991 and 2008.[133] Nine were not patented: PGA index, AP index, Bonacini index, Pohl score, Forns' index, APRI index, MP3 index, FIB4, and Fibro-Index. Five were patented: FibroTest, FibroSpect II, ELF, FibroMeter, and HepaScore. Among these panels, the number of components ranged from two to seven (see **Table 14-4**). A study using profiles of serum protein N-glycans found that a profile had a similar AUROC to FibroTest for the diagnosis of compensated cirrhosis.[134]

FibroTest was the most evaluated panel.[133] A total of 38 different populations including 7985 subjects with both FibroTest and biopsy (4600 HCV, 1580 HBV, 267 NAFLD, 524 ALD, and 1014 mixed). The mean diagnostic value for the diagnosis of advanced fibrosis assessed using standardized area under the ROC curves was 0.84 (95% confidence interval 0.83 to 0.86), without significant difference between the causes of liver disease, hepatitis C, B, alcoholic, or nonalcoholic fatty liver disease. High-risk profiles of false negative/false positive of FibroTest were present in 3% of patient populations, mainly Gilbert syndrome, hemolysis, and acute inflammation. In case of discordance between biopsy and FibroTest, half of the failures could be due to the taking of a biopsy and the prognostic value of a FibroTest was at least similar to that of a biopsy in HCV, HBV, and ALD.

For FibroSpect, a total of four published studies including 463 patients were identified; two studies for ELF included 1041 patients; three for FibroMeter included 1134 patients; and three for HepaScore included 757 patients.

To assess the performance of fibrosis biomarkers, the spectrum effect due to different prevalence of fibrosis among non-advanced and advanced fibrosis must be taken into account using the area under the receiver operating characteristic curve standardized for fibrosis stages prevalence (sAUROC).

For the other patented biomarkers, the mean AUROCs were similar to those observed for the FibroTest and FibroScan. Few studies have directly compared fibrosis serum biomarkers. FibroTest was significantly more effective than APRI. In six studies (1630 HCV patients), FT was directly compared with the ASAT/platelet ratio index (APRI), five being independent of the FibroTest inventor.[134] None of the meta-analyses of

Table 14-6 Prognostic Value of FibroTest in Patients with Chronic Hepatitis C and B and Alcoholic Liver Disease

LIVER DISEASE	NUMBER OF PATIENTS	MEAN DURATION OF FOLLOW-UP (yr)	NO DEATH AND NO LIVER COMPLICATION SAUROC (95% CI)	NO LIVER-RELATED DEATH	NO DEATH (OVERALL SURVIVAL)
Chronic hepatitis C	537	5	0.96 (0.75-0.79)	0.96 (0.75-0.79)	0.76 (0.81-0.85)
Chronic hepatitis B	1074	4	0.89 (0.84-0.93)	0.95 (0.91-0.97)	0.94 (0.89-0.96)
Alcoholic liver disease	262	10	Not performed	0.79 (0.68-0.86)	0.69 (0.61-0.76)

All AUROCS were significantly greater (P <.0001) than 0.50 (no prognostic value).

studies comparing directly patented biomarkers reached statistical significance.

Because of the absence of perfect gold standard, validation using strong clinical endpoints are needed to convince clinician and health authorities of the accuracy of biomarkers. Three studies have demonstrated similar prognostic values for the FibroTest in comparison with a liver biopsy for the prediction of death and liver-related death in patients with chronic hepatitis C and B, and alcoholic liver disease (**Table 14-6**).

Biomarkers of Steatosis

Clinicians often used ultrasonography in patients with elevated GGT, ALT, or AST for the diagnosis of steatosis.[135] Several biomarkers have been recently assessed to improve the accuracy of these standard tests. Serum retinol-binding protein 4 has been associated with steatosis in patients with hepatitis C.[136] SteatoTest is a patented test that combines 10 blood components (GGT, AST, ALT, apolipoprotein A1, α_2-macroglobulin, bilirubin, haptoglobin) with age, sex, and BMI.[137] The SteatoTest gives a quantitative estimate of steatosis of different origins: NAFLD (overweight, insulin resistance, hyperlipidemia, or diabetes mellitus), chronic viral hepatitis, and alcoholic liver disease (ALD). Several studies have observed the significant accuracy of the SteatoTest, with higher accuracy than classical markers of steatosis: GGT, ALT, and ultrasonography.[137-139] These biomarkers have permitted noninvasive assessment of steatosis in high-risk groups and the evaluation of treatment impact.[140-142]

Biomarkers of Nonalcoholic Steatohepatitis (NASH)

A liver biopsy is the usual reference for the diagnosis of NASH despite its limitations and the variability of the histologic diagnosis. Several biomarkers have been assessed with significant accuracy for the diagnosis of NASH: cytokeratin-18 serum levels, NashTest, and panels of other biomarkers.[143-147]

Biomarkers of Severe Alcoholic Hepatitis

Transvenous liver biopsy is the usual reference for the diagnosis of alcoholic hepatitis despite its limitations and the variability of the histologic diagnosis. Several biomarkers have been assessed with significant accuracy for the diagnosis of alcoholic hepatitis: serum laminin, type IV collagen, cytokeratin-18, and panels of biomarkers (AshTest).[148-150]

Plasma Lipids and Lipoproteins

The liver is important in the production and metabolism of plasma lipoproteins. The liver is the major source of plasma lipoproteins, with the exception of chylomicrons, which are synthesized by the intestine. Abnormalities in plasma concentrations of lipids and lipoproteins are common in liver disease.[151]

In acute hepatocellular injury, increased levels of plasma triglycerides, decreased levels of cholesterol esters, and abnormal electrophoretic patterns of lipoproteins are typically observed. Many of these abnormalities can be related to deficiencies of enzymes of hepatic origin, including lecithin-cholesterol acyltransferase (LCAT) and hepatic lipase.[152,153] Serum levels of apolipoprotein A1 decrease in acute viral hepatitis.[154]

In chronic liver disease, serum levels of apolipoprotein A1 decrease with fibrosis progression.[127] Apo A1 was also shown as a predictive factor for pure steatosis in alcoholic patients.[155] Low levels of cholesterol in serum may also reflect malnutrition. In genetic hepatic amyloidosis due to a mutation in apolipoprotein A1, the serum level is decreased and is associated with high γ-glutamyl transferase serum activity and a small increase in creatinine level.[156]

In patients with intrahepatic or extrahepatic cholestasis, levels of cholesterol and phospholipids are typically elevated, often strikingly in patients with chronic cholestasis. Factors contributing to these changes include increased hepatic synthesis of cholesterol, regurgitation of biliary cholesterol into the plasma, decreased plasma LCAT activity, and regurgitation of biliary lecithin into the plasma.[157,158] In addition, the serum of patients with obstructive jaundice contains an abnormal lipoprotein called lipoprotein X.[159] Lipoprotein X is thought to represent nonesterified cholesterol and phospholipid regurgitated from bile. In contrast to hepatocellular disease, LCAT deficiency is a late manifestation of cholestasis and reflects a long duration of disease and evidence of hepatocellular dysfunction.[159]

A marked increase in high-density lipoprotein (HDL) has been observed early in the course of primary biliary cirrhosis, presumably because of the release of an inhibitor of hepatic lipase. In advanced primary biliary cirrhosis, HDL levels are decreased and levels of low-density lipoproteins and lipoprotein X are increased.[160]

Cholesterol and triglycerides are associated in panels with other serum biochemical markers for the noninvasive assessment of liver steatosis (SteatoTest), alcoholic steatohepatitis (NashTest), and for the categorical diagnosis of nonalcoholic steatohepatitis.[137,147]

Tests that Contribute to Accurate Diagnosis in Liver Disease

Laboratory Tests for HCV

PCR Amplification

The polymerase chain reaction (PCR) can detect 10 to 50 IU/ml of HCV ribonucleic acid (RNA) using the previous methods. Testing for HCV RNA is a reliable way of demonstrating HCV infection and is the most specific test. Testing for HCV RNA is particularly useful when transaminases are normal, several causes of liver disease are possible (i.e., alcohol consumption), in immunosuppressed patients (i.e., after transplantation, in HIV co-infected patients), and in acute hepatitis C before the development of antibodies (4 to 10 weeks).[161]

Enzyme Immunoassay

Anti-HCV is detected by enzyme immunoassay. The third-generation test is usually very sensitive and very specific. In case of doubts about false-positive or false-negative results, the best test for confirmation of HCV infection is HCV RNA PCR. Immunosuppressed patients infected by HCV may test negative for anti-HCV. The antibody is usually present within 4 to 10 weeks after the onset of acute illness. Anti-HCV is still detectable during and after treatment, whatever the response, and must not be tested for again.[162]

Genotype and Serotype

There are six major genotypes of hepatitis C and more than 50 subtypes. Knowing the genotype or serotype (genotype-specific antibodies) is helpful for the interferon plus ribavirin combination treatment of choice. Genotypes do not change during the course of infection and must not be tested for again. HCV subtypes 1a versus 1b is becoming important with the use of the new HCV protease inhibitor–based triple therapies due to the differences in resistance profiles and efficacy. There is no relationship between the severity of the disease (fibrosis stage) and genotype.[162]

Quantification of HCV RNA in Serum

Methods measuring the level of virus in serum use quantitative PCR and a branched DNA (bDNA) test. They are currently less sensitive than qualitative assays.

An effort was made to define clinically relevant HCV RNA loads in standardized international units (IU) for use in routine clinical and research applications based on standardized quantitative assays validated with appropriate calibrated panels. The semiautomated quantitative RT-PCR SuperQuant assay (National Genetics Institute, Los Angeles) has a range from 50 to 1,470,000 IU/ml; the semiautomated Cobas Amplicor HCV Monitor assay version 2.0 (Cobas v2.0, Roche Molecular Systems, Pleasanton, Calif.) has a range from 600 to 2,630,000 IU/ml; the semiautomated HCV RNA quantitative assay LCx (Abbott Diagnostics, Chicago) has a range of 25 to 2,630,000 IU/ml; the semiautomated branched DNA signal amplification Versant HCV RNA 3.0 assay (bDNA) (Bayer Corp., Diagnostic Division, Tarrytown, N.Y.) has a range 615 to 7,700,000 IU/ml; the manual branched DNA signal amplification (Quantiplex) Versant HCV RNA 2.0 assay (bDNA) (Bayer Corp.) has a range 3200 to 19,000,000 IU/ml. In the more recent studies, the median viral load ranged from 800,000 IU/ml (5.9 $\log^{10}$ IU/ml) to almost 13,000,00 IU/ml (6.1 $\log^{10}$ IU/ml). Knowing the viral load is helpful in choosing the pegylated interferon plus ribavirin treatment. Patients with a high initial viral load have higher relapse rates and benefit more from a 48-week regimen than patients with a lower viral load. A 12-week stopping rule is also possible when the decrease in viral load is less than 2 logs compared with the baseline value.[162]

Unlike HIV infection, viral load does not correlate with the severity of hepatitis (fibrosis progression).

HCV Core Antigen Assays

HCV core antigen can be detected in serum and quantified (Total HCV-core Antigen Assay, Ortho-Clinical Diagnostics, Raritan, N.J.). This quantification can be used as an indirect marker of the HCV viral load but is less sensitive than molecular HCV RNA assays. However, it is stable and less expensive than quantitative HCV RNA testing.[163]

Laboratory Tests for HBV

Knowledge of the virus genome has permitted the development of several serologic markers for HBV infection.[164] Hepatitis B surface antigen (HBsAg), HbeAg, anti-Hbe, and anti-HBs are tested by enzyme-linked immunosorbent assay (ELISA). The presence of HBsAg in the serum for 6 months or more is indicative of chronic hepatitis B infection. The estimated annual incidence for clearance of HBsAg in chronically infected patients is low (0.1% to 0.8%) and usually due to a decrease in viremia rather than the emergence of HBsAg mutants. Preliminary studies in treated patients have suggested an interest of the quantification of HBsAg in the serum for predicting sustained response.[165]

To ensure comparison among different assays, it is recommended to express HBV viral load in international units. Serum HBV DNA levels are reported in many different units depending on the method used and the manufacturer of the assay (e.g., copies/ml, genome equivalents [Eq]/ml, mega-equivalents [MEq]/ml, or international units [IU]/ml). The World Health Organization has defined an international standard for HBV DNA amplification techniques that has been used to calibrate the IU/ml. Several HBV DNA quantification assays are available that have been normalized to the World Health Organization international standard. Serum HBV DNA levels now should be expressed universally in international units per milliliter in all available assays to ensure comparability between the assays, between different trials in which different assays have been used, and to allow the creation of guidelines that can be applied to whatever assay was used (in

Table 14-7 Interpretation of Hepatitis B Serologic Markers According to Symptoms, Transaminases, and Histologic Features

	HBSAG	HBSAB	HBEAG	HBEAB	ANTI-HBC-IGG	ANTI-HBC-IGM	HBV DNA	SYMPTOMS	ALT	HISTOLOGIC ACTIVITY AND FIBROSIS
Acute	+	−	+	+/−	+	+	+	+/−	++	+
Chronic carrier wild type	+	−	+	−	+	−/+	+	+/−	+/−	+
Chronic carrier precore mutant*	+	−	−	+	+	−/+	+	+/−	+/−	+
Asymptomatic carrier†	+	−	+	−	+	−	−	−	−	−
Immune–tolerance†	+	−	+	−	+	−	++	−	−	−
Recovery/immunity	−	+	−	+	+	−	−	−	−	−
Immunity from vaccination	−	+	−	−	−	−	−	−	−	−
Occult infection‡	−	+/−	−	−	+/−	−	+/−	+/−	+/−	+/−

*During flare-up, anti-HBc-IgM can be elevated.
†Carrier without symptoms, with normal transaminases and with normal biopsy are divided into "healthy carriers" with undetectable HBV DNA and subjects with detectable HBV DNA "immune tolerance." In these patients, a risk of cirrhosis or hepatocellular carcinoma cannot be excluded. Precore mutant can be detected.
‡HBV DNA can be detected in the liver in absence of serological markers.

general, an international unit is equivalent to approximately 5 to 6 copies, depending on the assay).

Commonly used commercial assays for HBV DNA levels are a branched DNA (bDNA) assay and a hybrid capture test. Commercially available PCR assays allow for the detection of less than 40 IU/ml. The interpretation of HBV serologic markers is described in **Table 14-7**.

In clinical practice, chronic HBV carriers may be divided into two easily identifiable serologic types: those that are positive for HBeAg (wild type) and those that are HBeAg negative and positive for anti-HBe.

Recently, genotype testing for HBV has been shown to be of value for treatment response and natural course. Despite the preliminary nature of HBV genotype testing, this may become important in the future because HBV genotype testing (major genotypes are A, B, C, D) will presumably become available.[164,165]

Laboratory Tests for HDV

All patients with positive HBsAg should be tested for co-infection with hepatitis D (delta virus). The best available test is anti-HDV antibody testing. The measurement of HDV RNA is limited to specialist laboratories.

Laboratory Tests for Other Liver Diseases

Hemochromatosis

In patients with serum GGT or ALT elevations without obvious origin, serum ferritin levels, serum iron, and total iron-binding capacity should be measured so that the iron saturation (serum iron/iron-binding capacity) can be calculated.[166] These tests, however, are not specific for hemochromatosis, and their specificity is particularly low in patients with other forms of liver disease. The serum tests that assay iron metabolism are age dependent and can be abnormal in the heterozygote state and in many other conditions. The genotype typically found in individuals of northern European descent can be diagnosed with a high degree of accuracy by detection of mutations in the HFE gene. The C282Y/C282Y homozygote is most likely to manifest the disease phenotype, whereas a minority of genotype C282Y/H63D (compound heterozygote) individuals may also develop the disease. A small population of patients have hemochromatosis due to genetic defects other than the HFE gene.[167-169]

Autoimmune Hepatitis (AIH)

Diagnosis requires the presence of characteristic features and the exclusion of other conditions that resemble AIH.[170] The conditions most likely to be confused with AIH are Wilson disease, drug-induced hepatitis, and chronic viral hepatitis, especially chronic hepatitis C. Autoantibodies are a diagnostic hallmark, and the conventional serologic markers of AIH are antinuclear antibodies (ANA), smooth muscle antibodies (SMA), and antibodies to liver/kidney microsome type 1 (anti-LKM1). Diagnostic criteria have been codified and updated by an international panel (**Table 14-8**).[171] Differences between a definite and a probable diagnosis of AIH relate mainly to the degree of serum γ-globulin or immunoglobulin G elevation, levels of ANA, SMA, or anti-LKM1, and exposure to alcohol, medications, or infections that could cause liver injury. There is no time requirement to establish chronicity, and cholestatic clinical, laboratory, and histologic changes

Table 14-8 Diagnostic Criteria for Autoimmune Hepatitis

	DEFINITE AUTOIMMUNE HEPATITIS	PROBABLE AUTOIMMUNE HEPATITIS
Positive Laboratory Testing		
Autoantibodies	SMA, ANA, or anti-LKM1, ≥1:80 in adults and ≥1:20 in children; no AMA	ANA, SMA, or anti-LKM1 ≥1:40 in adults or other autoantibodies*
Laboratory features	Predominant serum aminotransferase abnormality	
Globulin, γ-globulin, or immunoglobulin	Predominant serum aminotransferase abnormality	
G level ≥1.5 times normal		
Hypergammaglobulinemia of any degree		
Negative Laboratory Testing		
No active viral infection	No markers of current infection with hepatitis A, B, and C viruses	No markers of current infection with hepatitis A, B, and C viruses
No genetic liver disease	Normal α_1-antitrypsin phenotype	
Normal serum ceruloplasmin, iron, and ferritin levels	Partial α_1-antitrypsin deficiency	
Nonspecific serum copper, ceruloplasmin, iron, and/or ferritin abnormalities		
Other Criteria		
No toxic or alcohol injury	Daily alcohol ≤25 g/day and no recent use of hepatotoxic drugs	Daily alcohol ≤50 g/day and no recent use of hepatotoxic drugs
Histologic findings	Interface hepatitis; no biliary lesions, granulomas, or prominent changes suggestive of another disease	Interface hepatitis; no biliary lesions, granulomas, or prominent changes suggestive of another disease

Based on recommendations of the International Autoimmune Hepatitis Group.

*Includes perinuclear antineutrophil cytoplasmic antibodies and the not generally available antibodies to soluble liver antigen/liver pancreas, actin, liver cytosol type 1, and asialoglycoprotein receptor.

AMA, antimitochondrial antibodies; ANA, antinuclear antibodies; anti-LKM1 antibodies to liver/kidney microsome type 1; SMA, smooth muscle antibodies

preclude the diagnosis. The presence of liver-specific cytosol antigen type 1 (anti-LC1), soluble liver antigen/liver pancreas (anti-SLA/LP), actin (antiactin), and/or perinuclear antineutrophil cytoplasmic antibodies (pANCA), support a probable diagnosis if the other conventional markers are absent.[170-172]

Primary Biliary Cirrhosis (PBC)

The specific diagnostic features are serologic: elevated immunoglobulins, especially IgM, and disease-specific autoantibodies; antimitochondrial antibodies (AMA) and other autoantibodies reacting with nuclear pore complex, such as gp210; and histologic: bile duct damage and portal inflammation with granulomas. PBC is a chronic nonsuppurative destructive granulomatous cholangitis of uncertain etiology, affecting principally the medium-sized intrahepatic bile ducts. There is a female preponderance (>90%) and a strong association with other autoimmune conditions, particularly Sjögren syndrome and thyroid disease. PBC is unique among autoimmune diseases in that the condition has not been described in children. The diagnostic hallmark of PBC is the M2-AMA antibodies, the main target antigen of which is the E2 subunit of pyruvate dehydrogenase (PDH). Anti-PDH-E2 antibodies have a sensitivity of 95% and a specificity of close to 100% for PBC.[173,174]

Primary Sclerosing Cholangitis (PSC)

In contrast to AIH and PBC, there are no diagnostic immunologic features and biochemical, and serologic criteria define PSC only poorly. Bile ducts of all sizes may be affected by PSC, which also results in cholestasis and ultimately in cirrhosis. Unlike PBC and AIH, PSC affects predominantly men and is probably associated with inflammatory bowel disease in approximately 70% of cases (ranging from 40% to 98% in different series). The diagnosis rests on distinctive cholangiographic appearances showing large intrahepatic and extrahepatic bile duct involvement. The most prominent autoantibodies are ANCA, but are not specific of PSC.[175]

Miscellaneous Tests

Serum γ-Globulins

Autoimmune hepatitis is characterized by greatly increased serum γ-globulin levels, usually immunoglobulin (Ig) G.[170]

Increased levels of γ-globulins usually accompany alcoholic cirrhosis, specifically the so-called fast γ-fraction, which produces a characteristic bridging pattern on electrophoresis.[176] Alcoholic cirrhosis is associated with elevated levels of serum IgA. Primary biliary cirrhosis is associated typically with hyperglobulinemia, predominantly of the IgM class. Serum globulins are not usually elevated in drug-induced cholestasis or extrahepatic obstruction. The detection of hyperglobulinemia may be a clue to the presence of chronic liver disease but is less accurate than fibrosis biomarkers.[114]

Tests that Measure the Capacity of the Liver to Transport

Laboratory diagnosis of liver disease was introduced in 1913, when it was observed that a phthalein dye could be used to investigate hepatic function.[177] Subsequently, it was demonstrated that intravenously administered sulfobromophthalein (bromsulphalein; BSP), indocyanine green (ICG), or sorbitol were removed from the blood primarily by the liver, and that their rate of clearance was useful for evaluating liver function. The sensitivity of ICG for the detection of slight hepatic dysfunction is limited and less than for BSP. Clearance of sorbitol has also been used to measure hepatic blood flow, with the advantages of greater safety and less expense than ICG. These tests are usually not available in routine laboratories. ICG plasma disappearance rate can be measured reliably by the transcutaneous system in critically ill patients.[178-180]

Tests that Measure the Capacity of the Liver to Metabolize Drugs

Hepatic function may be assessed with substances that are metabolized selectively by the liver. The most widely performed tests assess hepatic drug metabolism, such as the determination of plasma clearance of antipyrine and the aminopyrine breath test.[181] Additional tests include the determination of caffeine clearance, galactose elimination, the maximum rate of synthesis of urea, and the formation of metabolites of lidocaine.[182-185] Their precise role in practice remains uncertain. Compared with common liver biochemical tests, "quantitative" tests are cumbersome, labor intensive, and expensive. They measure a specific function of a specific hepatic microsomal enzyme. In acute and chronic liver disease, the quantitative measurement of the function of an individual microsomal enzyme does not reflect a test for global liver function. Their prognostic performances in patients with cirrhosis have been suggested but must be compared with biochemical biomarkers and scoring systems in larger studies.[186-188]

Acknowledgment

Supported by grants from ARMHV.

Key References

Adams PC, Barton JC. Haemochromatosis. Lancet 2007;370:1855–1860. (Ref.171)

Afdhal NH. Biopsy or biomarkers: is there a gold standard for diagnosis of liver fibrosis? Clin Chem 2004;50:1299–1300. (Ref.3)

Ahlfors CE, et al. Unbound (free) bilirubin: improving the paradigm for evaluating neonatal jaundice. Clin Chem 2009;55:1288–1299. (Ref.75)

Alexander J, Kowdley KV. HFE-associated hereditary hemochromatosis. Genet Med 2009;11(5):307–313. (Ref.169)

Andersson KL, Chung RT. Monitoring during and after antiviral therapy for hepatitis B. Hepatology 2009;49:S166–S173. (Ref.167)

Bedossa P, Dargère D, Paradis V. Sampling variability of liver fibrosis in chronic hepatitis C. Hepatology 2003;38:1449–1457. (Ref.117)

Bellest L, et al. A modified international normalized ratio as an effective way of prothrombin time standardization in hepatology. Hepatology 2007;46:528–534. (Ref.92)

Bergstrom JP, Helander A. Influence of alcohol use, ethnicity, age, gender, BMI and smoking transferrin glycoform pattern: implication for use of carbohydrate-deficient transferring (CDT) as alcohol biomarker. Clin Chim Acta 2008;388:59–67. (Ref.113)

Bhvani M, et al. Screening for genetic haemochromatosis in blood samples with raised alanine aminotransferase. Gut 2000;46:707–710. (Ref.33)

Bravo AA, Sheth SG, Chopra S. Liver biopsy. N Engl J Med 2001;344:495–500. (Ref.116)

Callewaert N, et al. Noninvasive diagnosis of liver cirrhosis using DNA sequencer-based total serum protein glycomics. Nat Med 2004;10:1–6. (Ref.136)

Campos GM, et al. A clinical scoring system for predicting nonalcoholic steatohepatitis in morbidly obese patients. Hepatology 2008;47:1916–1923. (Ref.146)

Castera L. Non-invasive diagnosis of steatosis and fibrosis. Diabetes Metab 2008;34:674–679. (Ref.137)

Castera L, et al. Evolving practices of non-invasive markers of liver fibrosis in patients with chronic hepatitis C in France: time for new guidelines? J Hepatol 2007;46:528–529. (Ref.123)

Castera L, et al. Serum laminin and type IV collagen are accurate markers of histologically severe alcoholic hepatitis in patients with cirrhosis. J Hepatol 2000;32:412–418. (Ref.151)

Cholongitas E, et al. Review article: scoring systems for assessing prognosis in critically ill adult cirrhotics. Aliment Pharmacol Ther 2006;24:453–464. (Ref.189)

Chrostek L, et al. The diagnostic accuracy of carbohydrate-deficient transferrin, sialic acid and commonly used markers of alcohol abuse during abstinence. Clin Chim Acta 2006;364:167–171. (Ref.109)

Cibere J, et al. Association of biomarkers with pre-radiographically defined and radiographically defined knee osteoarthritis in a population-based study. Arthritis Rheum 2009;60:1372–1380. (Ref.129)

Colloredo G, et al. Impact of liver biopsy size on histological evaluation of chronic viral hepatitis: the smaller the sample, the milder the disease. J Hepatol 2003;39:239–244. (Ref.119)

Czaja AJ. Performance parameters of the diagnostic scoring systems for autoimmune hepatitis. Hepatology 2008;48:1540–1548. (Ref.174)

Davit-Spraul A, et al. Progressive familial intrahepatic cholestasis. Orphanet J Rare Dis 2009;4:1. (Ref.65)

Degré D, et al. Aminopyrine breath test compared to the MELD and Child-Pugh scores for predicting mortality among cirrhotic patients awaiting liver transplantation. Transpl Int 2004;17:31–38. (Ref.188)

Deugnier Y, Brissot P, Loréal O. Iron and the liver: update 2008. J Hepatol 2008;48(Suppl 1):S113–S123. (Ref.170)

Dienstag J. The role of liver biopsy in chronic hepatitis C. Hepatology 2002;36:S152–S160. (Ref.115)

Donnan PT, et al. Development of a decision support tool for primary care management of patients with abnormal liver function tests without clinically apparent liver disease: a record-linkage population cohort study and decision analysis (ALFIE). Health Technol Assess 2009;13:1–134. (Ref.2)

Eloranta JJ, Kullak-Ublick GA. The role of FXR in disorders of bile acid homeostasis. Physiology (Bethesda) 2008;23:286–295. (Ref.81)

Ercolani G, et al. The lidocaine (MEGX) test as an index of hepatic function: its clinical usefulness in liver surgery. Surgery 2000;127:464–471. (Ref.187)

Feldstein AE, et al. Cytokeratin-18 fragment levels as noninvasive biomarkers for nonalcoholic steatohepatitis: a multicenter validation study. Hepatology 2009;50:1072–1078. (Ref.145)

Fontaine H, et al. Guidelines for the diagnosis of uncomplicated cirrhosis. Gastroenterol Clin Biol 2007;31:504–509. (Ref.121)

Friedrich-Rust M, et al. Assessment of liver fibrosis and steatosis in PBC with FibroScan, MRI, MR-spectroscopy, and serum markers. J Clin Gastroenterol 2010;44:58–65. (Ref.141)

Gebo KA, et al. Role of liver biopsy in management of chronic hepatitis C: a systematic review. Hepatology 2002;36:S161–S172. (Ref.127)

Gonzalez-Quintela A, et al. Serum levels of keratin-18 fragments (tissue polypeptide-specific antigen [TPS]) are correlated with hepatocyte apoptosis in alcoholic hepatitis. Dig Dis Sci 2009;54:648–653. (Ref.152)

Halfon P, et al. A prospective assessment of the inter-laboratory variability of biochemical markers of fibrosis (FibroTest) and activity (ActiTest) in patients with chronic liver disease. Comp Hepatol 2002;2:3–7. (Ref.11)

Halfon P, Munteanu M, Poynard T. FibroTest-ActiTest as a non-invasive marker of liver fibrosis. Gastroenterol Clin Biol 2008;32:22–38. (Ref.134)

Hannuksela ML, et al. Biochemical markers of alcoholism. Clin Chem Lab Med 2007;45:953–961. (Ref.61)

Hickman IJ, et al. Modest weight loss and physical activity in overweight patients with chronic liver disease results in sustained improvements in alanine aminotransferase, fasting insulin, and quality of life. Gut 2004;53:413–419. (Ref.27)

Hietal H, et al. Comparison of the combined marker GGT-CDT and the conventional laboratory markers of alcohol abuse in heavy drinkers, moderate drinkers and abstainers. Alcohol Alcohol 2006;41:528–533. (Ref.111)

Hock B, et al. Validity of carbohydrate-deficient transferring (%CDT), γ-glutamyltransferase (γ-GT) and mean corpuscular erythrocyte volume (MVC) as biomarkers for chronic alcohol abuse: a study in patients with alcohol dependence and liver disorders of non-alcoholic and alcoholic origin. Addiction 2005;100:1477–1486. (Ref.110)

Hofmann AF. Bile acids: trying to understand their chemistry and biology with the hope of helping patients. Hepatology 2009;49:1403–1418. (Ref.80)

Imbert-Bismut F, et al. The diagnostic value of combining carbohydrate deficient transferrin, fibrosis and steatosis biomarkers for the prediction of excessive alcohol consumption. Eur J Gastroenterol Hepatol 2009;21:98–127. (Ref.112)

Imbert-Bismut F, et al. The diagnostic value of combining carbohydrate-deficient transferrin, fibrosis, and steatosis biomarkers for the prediction of excessive alcohol consumption. Eur J Gastroenterol Hepatol 2009;21:18–27. (Ref.140)

Imbert-Bismut F, et al. Biochemical markers of liver fibrosis in patients with hepatitis C virus infection: a prospective study. Lancet 2001;357:1069–1075. (Ref.128)

Imperiale TF, et al. Need for validation of clinical decision aids: use of the AST/ALT ratio in predicting cirrhosis in chronic hepatitis C. Am J Gastroenterol 2000;95:2328–2332. (Ref.44)

Ishii M, et al. Simultaneous measurements of serum α-fetoprotein and protein induced by vitamin K absence for detecting hepatocellular carcinoma. Am J Gastroenterol 2000;95:1036–1040. (Ref.101)

Jiao LR, et al. Effect of liver blood flow and function on hepatic indocyanine green clearance measured directly in a cirrhotic animal model. Br J Surg 2000;87:568–574. (Ref.182)

Kamath PS, Kim WR, Advanced Liver Disease Study Group. The model for end-stage liver disease (MELD). Hepatology 2007;45:797–805. (Ref.77)

Kaplan MM, Gershwin ME. Primary biliary cirrhosis. N Engl J Med 2005;353:1261–1273. (Ref.175)

Kew MC. Serum aminotransferase concentration as evidence of hepatocellular damage. Lancet 2000;355:591–592. (Ref.6)

Krawitt EL. Autoimmune hepatitis. N Engl J Med 2006;354(1):54–66. (Ref.172)

La Haute Autorité de Santé (HAS). The HAS recommendations for the management of the chronic hepatitis C using non-invasive biomarkers (website): http://www.has-sante.fr/portail/display.jsp?id 1/4c_476486. Accessed August 2008. (Ref.122)

Lo Iacono O, et al. Anti-tissue transglutaminase antibodies in patients with abnormal liver tests: is it always coeliac disease? Am J Gastroenterol 2005;100:2472–2477. (Ref.39)

Malik R, et al. The clinical utility of biomarkers and the nonalcoholic steatohepatitis CRN liver biopsy scoring system in patients with nonalcoholic fatty liver disease. J Gastroenterol Hepatol 2009;24:564–568. (Ref.147)

Manning DS, Afdhal NH. Diagnosis and quantitation of fibrosis. Gastroenterology 2008;134:1670–1681. (Ref.114)

McHutchison J, et al. Fibrosis as an end point for clinical trials in liver disease: a report of the international fibrosis group. Clin Gastroenterol Hepatol 2006;4:1214–1220. (Ref.130)

Mederacke I, et al. Performance and clinical utility of a novel fully automated quantitative HCV-core antigen assay. J Clin Virol 2009;46:210–215. (Ref.165)

Mugica F, et al. Prevalence of coeliac disease in unexplained chronic hypertransaminasemia. Rev Esp Enferm Dig 2001;93:707–714. (Ref.37)

Murayama H, Ikemoto M, Hamaoki M. Ornithine carbamyltransferase is a sensitive marker for alcohol-induced liver injury. Clin Chim Acta 2009;401:100–104. (Ref.108)

Myara A, et al. Harmonization of liver enzyme results: calibration for aminotransferases and gammaglutamyl transferase. J Hepatol 2004;41:501–502. (Ref.9)

Naveau S, et al. Predictive factors for pure steatosis in alcoholic patients. Alcohol Clin Exp Res 2009;33:1104–1110. (Ref.157)

Nyblom H, et al. High AST/ALT ratio may indicate advanced alcoholic liver disease rather than heavy drinking. Alcohol Alcohol 2004;39:336–339. (Ref.43)

Obici L, et al. Liver biopsy discloses a new apolipoprotein A-I hereditary amyloidosis in several unrelated Italian families. Gastroenterology 2004;126:1416–1422. (Ref.158)

Pawlotsky JM, et al. Standardization of hepatitis C virus RNA quantification. Hepatology 2000;32:654–659. (Ref.163)

Pawlotsky JM, et al. Virologic monitoring of hepatitis B virus therapy in clinical trials and practice: recommendations for a standardized approach. Gastroenterology 2008;134:405–415. (Ref.166)

Pawlotsky JM. Molecular diagnosis of viral hepatitis. Gastroenterology 2002;122:1554–1568. (Ref.164)

Petta S, et al. Retinol-binding protein 4: a new marker of virus-induced steatosis in patients infected with hepatitis C virus genotype 1. Hepatology 2008;48:28–37. (Ref.138)

Poynard T, et al. Liver biopsy: the best standard…when everything else fails. J Hepatol 2009;50:1267–1268. (Ref.4)

Poynard T, et al. Meta-analyses of FibroTest diagnostic value in chronic liver disease. BMC Gastroenterol 2007;7:40. (Ref.131)

Poynard T, et al. Assessment of liver fibrosis: noninvasive means. Saudi J Gastroenterol 2008;14:163–173. (Ref.135)

Poynard T, et al. Biomarkers of liver fibrosis. Adv Clin Chem 2008;46:131–152. (Ref.133)

Poynard T, et al. Prospective analysis of discordant results between biochemical markers and biopsy in patients with chronic hepatitis C. Clin Chem 2004;50:1344–1355. (Ref.125)

Poynard T, et al. Methodological aspects for the interpretation of liver fibrosis non-invasive biomarkers: a 2008 update. Gastroenterol Clin Biol 2008;32:8–21. (Ref.126)

Poynard T, Ratziu V, Bedossa P. Appropriateness of liver biopsy. Can J Gastroenterol 2000;14:543–548. (Ref.120)

Poynard T, et al. Diagnostic value of biochemical markers (NashTest) for the prediction of non alcoholic steato hepatitis in patients with non-alcoholic fatty liver disease. BMC Gastroenterol 2006;6:34. (Ref.149)

Poynard T, et al. The diagnostic value of biomarkers (SteatoTest) for the prediction of liver steatosis. Comp Hepatol 2005;4:10. (Ref.139)

Pratt DS, Kaplan MM. Evaluation of abnormal liver-enzyme results in asymptomatic patients. N Engl J Med 2000;342:1266–1271. (Ref.1)

Ratziu V, et al. Screening for liver disease using non-invasive biomarkers (FibroTest, SteatoTest and NashTest) in patients with hyperlipidemia. Aliment Pharmacol Ther 2007;25:207–218. (Ref.142)

Rautou PE, et al. Acute liver cell damage in patients with anorexia nervosa: a possible role of starvation-induced hepatocyte autophagy. Gastroenterology 2008;135:840–848. (Ref.35)

Regev A, et al. Sampling error and intraobserver variation in liver biopsy in patients with chronic HCV infection. Am J Gastroenterol 2002;97:2614–2618. (Ref.118)

Rivera-Nieves J, et al. Marked transaminase elevation in anorexia nervosa. Dig Dis Sci 2000;45:1959. (Ref.34)

Rosmorduc O, Poupon R. Low phospholipid associated cholelithiasis: association with mutation in the MDR3/ABCB4 gene. Orphanet J Rare Dis 2007;2:29. (Ref.66)

Rubio A, et al. Noninvasive procedures to evaluate liver involvement in HIV-1 vertically infected children. J Pediatr Gastroenterol Nutr 2010;51:685–686. (Ref.143)

Sakka SG. Assessing liver function. Curr Opin Crit Care 2007;13:207–214. (Ref.180)

Schmidt LE, et al. Effect of acetylcysteine on prothrombin index in paracetamol poisoning without hepatocellular injury. Lancet 2002;360:1151–1152. (Ref.98)

Schumann G, et al. IFCC primary reference procedures for the measurement of catalytic activity concentrations of enzymes at 37 °C. Part 5. Reference procedure for the measurement of catalytic concentration of alanine aminotransferase (L-Alanine:2-Oxoglutarate Aminotransferase [AST], EC 2.6.1.1). Clin Chem Lab Med 2002;40:718–724. (Ref.8)

Schumann G, et al. IFCC primary reference procedures for the measurement of catalytic activity concentrations of enzymes at 37 °C. Part 4. Reference procedure for the measurement of catalytic concentration of alanine aminotransferase (L-Alanine:2-Oxoglutarate Aminotransferase [ALT], EC 2.6.1.2). Clin Chem Lab Med 2002;40:718–724. (Ref.7)

Schumann G, et al. IFCC primary reference procedures for the measurement of catalytic activity concentrations of enzymes at 37 °C. Part 6. Reference procedure for the measurement of catalytic concentration of γ-Glutamyl transferase (γ-Glutamyl-Peptide: Amino Acid γ-Glutamyl transferase [GGT] EC 2.3.2.2). Clin Chem Lab Med 2002;40:718–724. (Ref.59)

Shaheen AA, Wan AF, Myers RP. FibroTest and FibroScan for the prediction of hepatitis C-related fibrosis: a systematic review of diagnostic test accuracy. Am J Gastroenterol 2007;102:2589–2600. (Ref.132)

Silveira MG, Lindor KD. Primary sclerosing cholangitis. Can J Gastroenterol 2008;22:689–698. (Ref.177)

Strømme JH, et al. Reference intervals for eight enzymes in blood of adult females and males measured in accordance with the International Federation of Clinical Chemistry reference system at 37 degrees C: part of the Nordic reference interval project. Scand J Clin Lab Invest 2004;64:371–384. (Ref.52)

Thabut D, et al. The diagnostic value of biomarkers (AshTest) for the prediction of alcoholic steato-hepatitis in patients with chronic alcoholic liver disease. J Hepatol 2006;44:1175–1185. (Ref.150)

Therapondos G, et al. Cerebral near infrared spectroscopy for the measurement of indocyanine green elimination in cirrhosis. Aliment Pharmacol Ther 2000;14:923–928. (Ref.181)

Tripodi A, et al. The international normalized ratio calibrated for cirrhosis (INR [liver]) normalizes prothrombin time results for model for end-stage liver disease calculation. Hepatology 2007;46:520–527. (Ref.91)

Van Ooteghem NA, et al. Benign recurrent intrahepatic cholestasis progressing to progressive familial intrahepatic cholestasis: low GGT cholestasis is a clinical continuum. J Hepatol 2002;36:439–443. (Ref.69)

Volta U, et al. Anti tissue transglutaminase antibodies as predictors of silent coeliac disease in patients with hypertransaminasaemia of unknown origin. Dig Liver Dis 2001;33:420–425. (Ref.38)

Whitehead MW, et al. A prospective study of the causes of notably raised aspartate aminotransferase of liver origin. Gut 1999;45:129–133. (Ref.16)

Whitfield JB. Gamma glutamyl transferase. Crit Rev Clin Lab Sci 2001;38: 263–355. (Ref.57)

Younossi ZM, et al. A novel diagnostic biomarker panel for obesity-related nonalcoholic steatohepatitis (NASH). Obes Surg 2008;18:1430–1437. (Ref.148)

Zelber-Sagi S, et al. Role of leisure-time physical activity in nonalcoholic fatty liver disease: a population-based study. Hepatology 2008;48:1791–1798. (Ref.144)

Ziol M, et al. ABCB4 heterozygous gene mutations associated with fibrosing cholestatic liver disease in adults. Gastroenterology 2008;135:131–141. (Ref.67)

A complete list of references can be found at www.expertconsult.com.

Imaging and Noninvasive Diagnosis of Liver Disease: Computerized Tomography, Ultrasound, Magnetic Resonance Imaging, and Emerging Techniques

Heather M. Patton, Benjamin F. Johnson, Emmanuil Smorodinsky, and Claude B. Sirlin

ABBREVIATIONS

ADC apparent diffusion coefficient
AUROC area under the receiver operator characteristic
AV arteriovenous
CC cholangiocarcinoma
CECT contrast-enhanced CT
CEUS contrast-enhanced ultrasound
CIN contrast-induced nephropathy
CKD chronic kidney disease
CT computed tomography
DLD diffuse liver disease
DWI diffusion-weighted imaging
FLL focal liver lesion
FNH focal nodular hyperplasia
GBCA gadolinium-based contrast agent

GFR glomerular filtration rate
HA hepatic adenoma
HBCA hepatobiliary contrast agent
HCC hepatocellular carcinoma
HG hemangioma
HU Hounsfield units
HVTT hepatic transit time
IOUS intraoperative ultrasound
IV intravenous
IVC intravenous contrast
MRCP magnetic resonance cholangiopancreatogram
MRE magnetic resonance elastography
MRI magnetic resonance imaging
MRS magnetic resonance spectroscopy

NECT nonenhanced computed tomography
NRH nodular regenerative hyperplasia
NSF nephrogenic systemic fibrosis
PET positron emission tomography
PSC primary sclerosing cholangitis
PV portal vein
RES reticuloendothelial system
SPIOs superparamagnetic iron oxides
SQUID superconducting quantum interference device
TE transient elastography
US ultrasound
VMC von Meyenburg complex

Introduction

In addition to the assessment tools reviewed elsewhere in this text, imaging plays a complementary role in the evaluation and management of patients with both diffuse liver disease (DLD) and focal liver lesions (FLLs). In some clinical settings, imaging may be able to provide a diagnosis without requirement for more invasive examinations (e.g., the diagnosis of hepatic hemangiomas). In other situations, imaging studies may help to guide the diagnostic workup (e.g., the identification of biliary dilatation in a patient with jaundice). Often, imaging is used to stage the severity or extent of disease

(e.g., staging of hepatocellular carcinoma) or to identify complications of disease (e.g., ascites or other evidence of portal hypertension in patients with cirrhosis). Finally, imaging may also play a role in measuring response to therapy (e.g., follow-up of patients who have undergone local ablative therapy for hepatocellular carcinoma).

Historically, imaging studies have served primarily to *detect* FLLs within the liver and some forms of DLD. More recently, the role of imaging has expanded beyond detection to include *characterization* of FLLs, in some cases providing a definitive, noninvasive diagnosis of FLLs. Additionally, emerging applications of imaging include the noninvasive assessment of histologic features of DLD, such as fat, iron, and fibrosis. The goal of this chapter is to familiarize the reader with the imaging modalities currently available to clinicians. This will include a discussion of the relative merits and shortcomings of current techniques in different clinical settings. A discussion of emerging imaging techniques will also be included.

Modalities

This section will focus on the most commonly employed imaging techniques: ultrasound (US), computed tomography (CT), and magnetic resonance imaging (MRI) (**Table 15-1**). We will briefly mention additional modalities that may have application in the assessment of patients with liver disease; however, a detailed discussion is beyond the scope of this chapter. For each of the imaging modalities, we will review the ability to assess tissue structure and function, and in some cases other tissue properties. General advantages and disadvantages of each modality will be discussed.

Ultrasound

Ultrasound (US) refers to sound with a frequency above the limits of human hearing. Sonographic imaging employs transmission of targeted high-frequency sound waves through tissues with computerized conversion of the reflected sound waves into anatomic images. The images produced are determined by the amount of reflection and scatter (affected by the interface between tissues of different densities) and attenuation (determined by US frequency and tissue density) of an US beam by tissue.[1] Doppler exploits the Doppler shift principle to determine the direction and estimate the velocity of blood flow within vessels and shunts. This can be used to generate waveforms or to display blood flow as an anatomic image with a color code (**Fig. 15-1**).

US remains an important imaging modality for the assessment of soft tissues, including the liver. US equipment is widely available, and portable. Portability is advantageous in bedside evaluation of patients or to assist in the operating room. US examinations are safe, with no known injury to sensitive tissues including the fetus if performed with appropriate parameters; therefore US can be used in the evaluation of pregnant patients. US can usually be completed quickly, requires no special preparation (aside from fasting for gallbladder assessment), may be performed without intravenous access, and involves only light application of pressure to the skin. US provides imaging in real time and thus can be used to guide diagnostic procedures such as biopsy or drainage of fluid collections.

Despite its many positive attributes, US has important limitations with which the clinician should be familiar. US is operator dependent and has limited reproducibility. The US beam does not readily cross tissue–gas or tissue–bone boundaries; therefore overlying ribs or gas-filled loops of bowel invariably generate blind spots within the liver. Additionally, overlying fat in obese patients may degrade images. Fat or fibrosis within the liver may scatter the US beam and fat may attenuate it, potentially obscuring lesions within the liver. These limitations reduce the ability of US to detect and characterize FLLs. This is particularly true in patients who are obese and in those with underlying fatty liver or cirrhosis. US also has a limited ability to characterize solid liver lesions as either benign or malignant and, except for simple cysts, rarely provides a definitive diagnosis for FLL (**Fig. 15-2**).

US is frequently used in the urgent evaluation of patients with acute right upper quadrant pain because this modality performs well in the detection of acute cholecystitis (estimated sensitivity, between 84% and 97%)[2] and acute extrahepatic biliary obstruction. US is also widely employed in the initial evaluation of patients with jaundice or persistent elevation of liver function studies.[3] However, it is important to be aware that US has limited sensitivity in detecting some of the common causes of DLD associated with abnormal liver function studies. The sensitivity of US in detecting hepatic steatosis is limited.[4,5] US is ineffective at differentiating fat from fibrosis.[5-7] US has no ability to detect hepatic iron deposition. Liver surface nodularity is the most common feature used to identify a cirrhotic liver by US.[8] In clinical studies, US-determined surface nodularity has a reported sensitivity

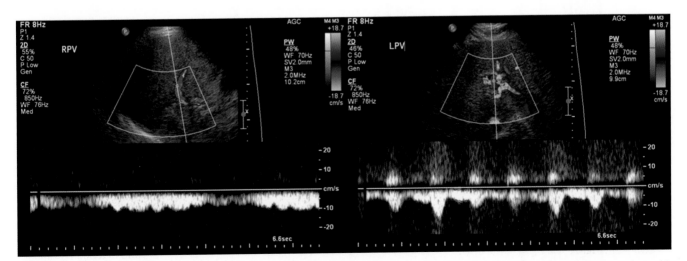

Fig. 15-1 Color Doppler ultrasound can be used to demonstrate both intra- and extrahepatic flow. This image, taken in a patient with cirrhosis caused by non-alcoholic fatty liver disease, demonstrates retrograde flow direction in the right portal vein *(RPV, left panel)* and left portal vein *(LPV, right panel)*.

Table 15-1 US, CT, MRI, or Elastography: Relative Merits of Various Imaging Modalities to Address Specific Clinical Questions

CLINICAL QUESTION	ULTRASOUND	CT	MRI AND MRS	US OR MR ELASTOGRAPHY
Acute right upper quadrant pain	Initial test of choice given ability to assess for gallstones and other biliary pathology without exposure to radiation or requirement for IV contrast. Limited sensitivity for common bile duct stones. No safety concerns in pregnant women for unenhanced ultrasound if appropriate parameters are used.	May be appropriate for follow-up of abnormality identified on US, but usually requires IVC for this purpose. Exposure to ionizing radiation.	No role for MRS. MRI may be appropriate for follow-up of abnormality identified on US, but may require IVC for this purpose. Excellent sensitivity for common bile duct stones. No exposure to ionizing radiation.	N/A
Abnormal liver function tests	May be useful as an initial screening examination for suspected fatty liver with caveat that failure to identify abnormalities with this modality does not exclude existence of diffuse or focal liver disease, particularly in setting of obesity or other factors that limit US diagnostic performance. Unable to detect iron overload.	Improved sensitivity for hepatic iron overload and more objective assessment of hepatic fat deposition compared with US, but involves exposure to ionizing radiation and not as accurate as advanced MRI or MRS techniques.	MRI and MRS techniques are more accurate than US or CT for assessment of fatty liver and iron overload, but quality of MR imaging studies may vary depending upon local expertise and patient cooperation. MRS is not widely available.	Although not usually used in initial evaluation of liver function test abnormalities, elastography may demonstrate elevated liver stiffness caused by acute hepatitis even in absence of fibrosis.
Biliary obstruction	US has good sensitivity for identification of biliary obstruction; however, may not always be able to identify cause of obstruction. Good choice for initial evaluation for biliary dilation.	CECT has higher sensitivity than US for identification of pancreatic abnormalities such as mass lesions or chronic pancreatitis that may result in biliary obstruction.	MRCP has excellent sensitivity for detection of both location and cause of biliary obstruction; however, requires patient cooperation to obtain quality images.	N/A
Hepatic steatosis	Most frequently used modality for assessment of steatosis, but has low sensitivity for mild steatosis, is operator-dependent, and lacks reproducibility. Fibrosis and steatosis can be difficult to differentiate at US. Objective analysis methods to quantify steatosis on US images are under development, but not yet validated.	Frequently used, but confounded by iron, glycogen, edema, and fibrosis. Shows correlation at population level, but has limited accuracy at individual level. Uses ionizing radiation whereas MRI is more accurate and does not use ionizing radiation. Use of CT solely to evaluate liver fat is difficult to justify.	MRS is most accurate method for steatosis quantification but requires expertise and is not widely available. MRS also only assesses a small proportion of total liver volume; sampling variability is common, which limits its efficacy in longitudinal monitoring. Conventional MRI uses out-of-phase and in-phase images. This provides qualitative information but can be confounded. Advanced techniques have recently been developed to address confounders and preliminary studies suggest these emerging techniques are highly accurate (will be clinically available soon).	In absence of inflammation or fibrosis, steatosis does not appear to affect liver stiffness measurements made by elastographic techniques.

	US	CT	MRI	Comments
Hepatic fibrosis	US lacks both sensitivity and specificity in detection of fibrosis. Changes of advanced cirrhosis may be detected, if present, but a normal exam does not exclude fibrosis. Increased echogenicity may be due to steatosis or infiltrative liver disease rather than fibrosis.	Conventional CT lacks both sensitivity and specificity in detection of fibrosis in precirrhotic stages of diffuse liver disease. Recent studies suggest that computer-based texture analysis of CT images may predict presence of fibrosis, but confirmatory studies are needed.	Conventional MRI lacks both sensitivity and specificity in detection of fibrosis in precirrhotic stages of diffuse liver disease. Recent studies suggest that contrast-enhanced MRI may detect parenchymal alterations associated with fibrosis but confirmatory studies are needed. Diffusion-weighted imaging is another promising technique that requires further refinement and validation.	Promising with many confirmatory studies performed in academic centers. Not yet fully validated in community setting. Major benefit seems to be in differentiating advanced from early fibrosis. Preliminary studies show modest ability to differentiate between early stages.
Cirrhosis	Has high specificity for cirrhosis but low sensitivity. US depiction of nodular liver surface, ascites, and splenomegaly have high PPV for cirrhosis. However, sensitivity is limited and normal US examination does not exclude presence of cirrhosis.	Improved sensitivity compared with US for identification of morphologic features of cirrhosis and portal hypertension; however, requires ionizing radiation. Absent features of cirrhosis does not exclude diagnosis.	Conventional MRI has higher sensitivity than US or CT for diagnosis of cirrhosis because of its greater soft tissue contrast, which permits delineation of regenerative nodules and fibrotic scars even in absence of surface nodularity. However, sensitivity for early cirrhosis remains limited and absent features of cirrhosis does not exclude diagnosis. Advanced MRI techniques with dual-contrast agents probably have high sensitivity for cirrhosis but confirmatory studies are needed.	Based on many independent published reports, both US and MR elastography have high sensitivity for cirrhosis. However, elevated stiffness may be observed in noncirrhotic but inflamed or cholestatic livers; therefore stiffness is not specific for cirrhosis.
HCC screening	Recommended by AASLD for routine surveillance but has low per-patient sensitivity for HCC. Probably most appropriate for screening lower-risk population, particularly if body habitus is amenable to US examination (e.g., slender individuals who are hepatitis B virus carriers).	Higher per-patient sensitivity for HCC than US. Low per-lesion sensitivity. Low staging accuracy for HCC.	Recent meta-analysis suggests that conventional MRI with single-contrast agents has higher per-patient sensitivity than CT. Per-lesion sensitivity and staging accuracy are low. Advanced MRI methods with double contrast may have higher per-lesion sensitivity and staging accuracy.	Use of elastography to detect liver lesions including HCC is in very early phases of development. However, with current resolution capability, it is not likely that these techniques will be useful for detection and characterization of small lesions in near future.
Characterization of benign FLL	CEUS provides excellent accuracy for noninvasive diagnosis of HGs and FNH, and differentiation of benign from malignant lesions; however, it requires expertise and is not widely available in North America. Can evaluate only a limited number of lesions per CEUS exam.	Because CEUS is not widely available in North America, CECT is most commonly used modality to workup nonspecific FLL identified at US. Multiphasic examination with IVC is required for appropriate assessment of FLL. Characterization is based almost entirely on lesion morphology and vascularity, which suffices for most but not all lesions.	MRI has superior soft tissue contrast compared with US or CT and assesses more tissue properties than CT; therefore it is often used as a problem-solving tool to characterize lesions that cannot be characterized adequately using US or CT. Another advantage over CT is lack of ionizing radiation, so patients can be followed over time if serial exams are needed.	Use of elastography to characterize benign FLL and to differentiate benign from malignant FLL is in very early phases of development. However, with current resolution capability, it is not likely that these techniques will be useful for characterization of small lesions in near future.
Detection of hepatic metastases	Standard US does not have adequate sensitivity for this purpose. CEUS is good for characterization of a limited number of lesions in a single liver, but not test of choice for detection of FLL because of its inability to scan entire liver parenchyma.	Multiphasic CECT has good sensitivity for detection of metastases >1 cm; however, requires exposure to ionizing radiation. May be advantageous modality if scans of other body regions are desired concurrently. Limited sensitivity for metastases <1 cm.	Conventional MRI with contrast has good sensitivity for detection of liver metastases >1 cm without exposure to ionizing radiation. MRI is not as practical for this purpose if multiple regions of body require concurrent screening. Advanced techniques including use of HBCAs show promise for detection of metastases <1 cm.	See comments for HCC screening.

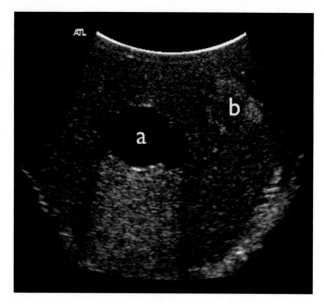

Fig. 15-2 Intraoperative ultrasound done on a 65-year-old man with known colorectal cancer metastases to the liver demonstrates two lesions. Lesion a can be diagnosed unequivocally as a benign simple cyst based on its US features: lack of internal echoes, sharply demarcated boundary, imperceptible walls, and posterior acoustic enhancement. Lesion b has a nonspecific US imaging appearance and is assumed to represent a metastasis based on clinical context.

of 87% to 91% to diagnose cirrhosis, using liver biopsy as the gold standard.[9,10] Assessment of liver surface nodularity by US to diagnose cirrhosis, however, requires meticulous technique and is performed in only select centers. Intraoperative US (IOUS) of the liver has application in hepatic segmental or lobar resection, resection of liver metastases, transplantation of live donor liver, evaluation of vessel patency, assessment of intrahepatic biliary disease, and performance of tumor ablation procedures.[11] IOUS may, in some cases, increase the sensitivity of lesion detection compared with preoperative cross-sectional imaging and provides real-time determination of the relation between FLLs and vessels to aid in resection (see **Fig. 15-2**). Disadvantages of IOUS include operator dependence, limited per-lesion sensitivity in patients with steatosis, and an inability to assess FLLs in advance of surgery.

Contrast-Enhanced Ultrasound

Contrast-enhanced ultrasound (CEUS) employs an intravascular microbubble contrast agent, a technique that was introduced in the early 1990s to assess myocardial perfusion.[12] The microbubbles consist of a gas, such as perfluorocarbon, sulfur hexafluoride, or air, encapsulated within a lipid or albumin shell. The microbubbles persist for about 5 minutes after intravenous (IV) injection and, unlike computed tomography (CT) or magnetic resonance (MR) contrast agents, can be injected repeatedly during a single examination. CEUS has the highest sensitivity to contrast compared with CT or MRI (uses the smallest volume of contrast) and has the unique advantage that the contrast is visualized in real time. Because the volume of contrast injected is small, it can be given via butterfly IV access. Although contrast bubbles are smaller than red blood

cells (2 to 3 μm in diameter), their intravascular behavior is similar and allows visualization of blood flow, particularly in highly vascular tumors.[13] Thus the addition of contrast extends to US many of the features of angiography while maintaining the other imaging properties of this modality.[1] CEUS is widely used throughout Europe, Asia, and Canada but its availability in the United States has been limited because of the reluctance of the Food and Drug Administration (FDA) to approve the use of contrast agents for clinical use.

CEUS shares many of the advantages of conventional grayscale US. In addition, it overcomes many of the disadvantages of imaging with US. CEUS offers markedly improved sensitivity and specificity in the visualization and characterization of several types of FLLs because of its capacity to assess vascularity and blood flow patterns.[13] Contrast begins to appear in the liver's arterial system 10 to 20 seconds after it is injected and this phase lasts up to 15 seconds. Subsequently, the portal venous phase lasts from 30 to 120 seconds after IV contrast injection. The late or delayed phase occurs approximately 3 to 4 minutes after injection and ends with the loss of contrast enhancement (contrast enhancement has usually dissipated by 5 minutes postinjection).

The primary advantage of CEUS is in the characterization of FLLs. CEUS can be helpful in characterizing hepatic hemangiomas, particularly in cases where gray-scale US features are noncharacteristic. CEUS also has excellent diagnostic accuracy for the detection of focal nodular hyperplasia (FNH) (87% to 95% in recent series).[14,15] CEUS has been reported to be superior to spiral CT in the detection (100% vs. 68%) and correct characterization (98% vs. 68%) of biopsy-proven malignant portal vein (PV) thrombosis.[16] One significant advantage offered by CEUS over CT or MRI is lack of nephrotoxicity and risk for nephrogenic systemic fibrosis (NSF). Finally, CEUS is the only way to obtain angiographic information at the bedside.

Although CEUS does offer several important advantages over conventional gray-scale US, it does have limitations. The lack of ionizing radiation would make an US-based technology attractive in populations requiring repetitive surveillance studies. It has been shown that CEUS may perform as well as contrast-enhanced CT, or better, for metastatic liver lesion detection, because metastases can be detected as a hypoechoic lesion in the portal venous phase.[17,18] On the other hand, hepatocellular carcinoma (HCC) is typically best seen in the arterial phase as a hypervascular (hyperechoic) lesion, but may not be seen as clearly as metastatic lesions in the portal venous phase. The short arterial phase makes it difficult to use CEUS for HCC surveillance. Although a single bolus injection can be used to assess only one or a few lesions with CEUS if they are in the same imaging plane, multiple injections of contrast agent may be possible if there are multiple lesions to be characterized. The number of injections administered during a single CEUS exam may vary with the particular contrast agent used (e.g., SonoVue [Bracco Diagnostics, Inc., Princeton, Nd] requires 2.3 to 4.6 ml per injection and thus only one or two injections may be given during an exam; Definity [Lantheus Medical Imaging, Inc. North Billerica, Mass.] requires only 0.2 ml per injection and six or seven injections may be given during a single exam). Thus this modality is most often used as a problem-solving technique, rather than as a surveillance tool. Currently, the primary disadvantage of CEUS is the lack of availability of this modality in clinical practice.

Computed Tomography

Computed tomography (CT) creates computer-generated images through detection of the transmission, attenuation, and scatter of photons produced by spinning in a helical fashion an x-ray source around the patient. Multidetector helical acquisition CT systems allow for rapid data acquisition as well as postacquisition reformatting.[1] Complete data acquisition from the upper abdomen may be obtained in as little as 5 to 10 seconds. Because of the speed with which data may be acquired, it is possible to obtain true multiphasic images with temporal separation of each contrast phase (nonenhanced, arterial, and venous). Furthermore, it is possible to obtain images of the entire liver, even in patients who may be dyspneic or uncooperative, with decreased motion artifact compared with magnetic resonance (MR). CT is a widely available and robust hepatic imaging technique, and consistently generates images with few visible artifacts. It is important to be aware, however, that lack of visible artifacts during CT does not always indicate diagnostic efficacy (i.e., the absence of image degradation from artifacts does not mean that an imaging study is of adequate quality to detect or characterize lesions).

Nonenhanced Computed Tomography

Nonenhanced computed tomography (NECT) is CT without intravenous contrast (IVC). NECT has few liver-specific applications but images of the liver are often obtained as part of other examinations (e.g., in evaluation of appendicitis, renal stones, vascular calcification, or CT colonography). NECT may have some value in evaluation of DLD such as fatty liver or iron overload, although magnetic resonance imaging (MRI) has improved sensitivity for both of these disease processes without ionizing radiation exposure. NECT may also rarely be used in assessing focal processes such as calcification or hemorrhage. The most common use of NECT for examining the liver is in acquisition of baseline, precontrast images during multiphase contrast-enhanced CT examinations (**Fig. 15-3**).

The advantages of NECT are that it is a precise modality that has high reproducibility for measuring attenuation. There is excellent agreement among different readers, scanners, and sites with NECT. Therefore attenuation values may be compared in serial images that were obtained at different scanners. Additionally, the lack of IVC in this imaging modality is advantageous in patients with chronic kidney disease (CKD), patients at risk for contrast-induced nephropathy (CIN) or contrast allergy, and patients with difficult IV access.

Despite the advantages noted, NECT has a limited role in evaluating either DLD or FLL. The most common forms of DLD assessed with cross-sectional imaging such as CT are cirrhosis, steatosis, and iron overload. CT is relatively insensitive to changes of early cirrhosis. As cirrhosis advances, NECT may demonstrate morphologic changes (decreased volume of the right lobe and medial segment of the left lobe with hypertrophy of the left lateral segment and caudate lobe), nodular surface contour, and evidence of portal hypertension (ascites and varices).[19] Fatty deposition lowers the attenuation value of hepatic parenchyma by CT and causes reversal of the attenuation relationship between the liver and spleen.[20] When accumulated in sufficient amount, iron attenuates the CT beam to an appreciable degree, resulting in increased

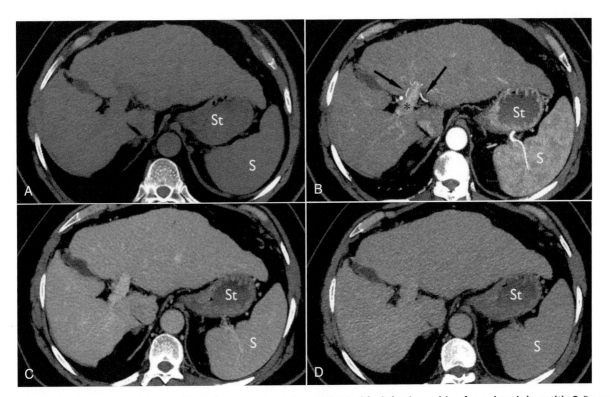

Fig. 15-3 Dynamic CT sequence with an iodinated contrast agent in a patient with cirrhosis resulting from chronic hepatitis C. Precontrast **(A)**, hepatic arterial phase **(B)**, portal venous phase **(C)**, and late venous phase **(D)** images are shown. Note that a properly timed hepatic arterial phase image shows enhancement of portal vein (*asterisk*) as well as hepatic artery branches (*arrows*). St, stomach; S, spleen

density of the liver.[1] The limitation of NECT in differentiating causes of DLD was demonstrated in a comparison of the distribution of attenuation values using density histograms. This study compared the hepatic attenuation of normal parenchyma and biopsy-proved steatosis, steatohepatitis, alcoholic cirrhosis, viral cirrhosis, and hemochromatosis and found no significant differences in the kurtosis and skewness of density histogram analysis between these causes of DLD.[21]

Contrast-Enhanced Computed Tomography

Contrast-enhanced CT (CECT) or multiphasic CT—CT performed following IV administration of water-soluble contrast medium—is widely used for the detection and characterization of FLL. CECT is often used as a problem-solving procedure and is routinely obtained as part of oncologic evaluations. Because of the very short time required to image the liver with CT, multiple acquisition phases may be obtained during contrast enhancement. These phases may include early and late arterial phases, portal venous phase, and late and delayed phases (see **Fig. 15-3**). The number of phases scanned depends upon the study indication. The basis for multiphasic CECT in identifying FLL lies in the fact that the majority of solid liver lesions have a predominantly arterial blood supply whereas the liver parenchyma itself receives 75% to 80% of its blood supply via the portal vein.

When used for HCC surveillance, CECT requires multiphasic imaging protocols. Hepatologists should be aware that not all HCC surveillance exams are done as multiphasic studies, either because the exam is incorrectly protocolled or because the exam was conducted for other purposes. Therefore in interpreting results of an abdominal CT in patients with risk factors for HCC, it is vital to be aware of whether the scan was done as a multiphasic study. Multiphasic CT is also important in characterization of metastatic liver lesions and, particularly, in differentiating these lesions from benign FLLs.

Similar to NECT, CECT may identify changes in liver morphology suggestive of cirrhosis as well as extrahepatic changes indicating portal hypertension. In contrast to NECT, CECT readily depicts portal vein thrombosis, which is relatively prevalent in patients with cirrhosis (10% to 25%) and is important to identify in the pretransplant population.[22] However, in the absence of portal hypertension, CT may not be a reliable modality in the diagnosis of early cirrhosis. Therefore a negative or normal CT scan should not be interpreted as an exclusion of cirrhosis. CECT may add slightly to the ability to see changes of cirrhosis, but the potential risk of IV contrast (IVC) is not justified by the small benefit provided by CECT if this is the sole purpose of the examination.

Use of CECT as an imaging modality in liver disease has several advantages. CT is a robust technology that routinely and rapidly produces artifact-free images, even in patients who may be limited in their ability to cooperate with examination. Spatial resolution with modern scanners is high, permitting three-dimensional reconstruction of the imaging data in planes of interest (**Fig. 15-4**). Radiology residents typically are well-trained in abdominal CT imaging because of the high volume of these studies performed in most medical centers. Additionally, most CT protocols produce acceptable quality scans with little or no manipulation. Because of the consistency of CT technology in producing acceptable quality

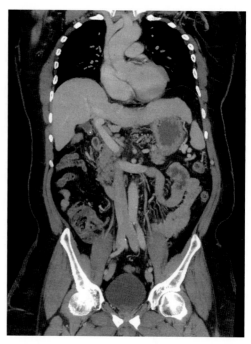

Fig. 15-4 High spatial resolution *and* rapid image acquisition are possible on modern CT scanners, making reformatting of images possible and practical. Shown here is a coronal re-formation of the portal venous phase images in the same patient whose axial images are shown in Figure 15-3. Such re-formations facilitate evaluation of multiple areas of the body with a single study, an advantage of CT over MRI. By comparison, MRI does not yet permit broad coverage of large body regions with both high spatial resolution *and* rapid image acquisition.

images as well as the widespread availability of radiologists with good training in this modality, the performance characteristics of CT cited in medical literature may be reasonably reproducible in clinical practice as long as an appropriate protocol is performed.

Limitations of CECT include the fact that this imaging modality only assesses two tissue properties: electron density or attenuation and vascularity. Electron density or attenuation approximates the physical density of the tissue being imaged and has a very low dynamic range (the physical density of soft tissue in the human body does not differ to a large extent). The low intrinsic soft tissue contrast results in images that consist of various shades of gray. IVC agents administered for CECT assess vascularity. This results in a limited ability to diagnose and characterize other tissue properties that may be relevant in the assessment of both benign and malignant diseases (e.g., in the assessment of fat or iron, in detecting solid lesions of similar density as the surrounding hepatic parenchyma). Any disease (focal or diffuse) that alters a tissue property in such a way that it does not manifest as a change in liver density or that alters vascularity may be undetectable by CT (e.g., inflammation fibrosis). For this reason, CECT does not generally play a role in the evaluation of DLL (IVC does not add clinically relevant information to NECT for DLL at this time), with the possible exception of cholestatic liver disease (peribiliary inflammation and biliary duct wall thickening can be appreciated with CECT). In addition, clinicians should understand that artifact-free images may not be synonymous with high-quality

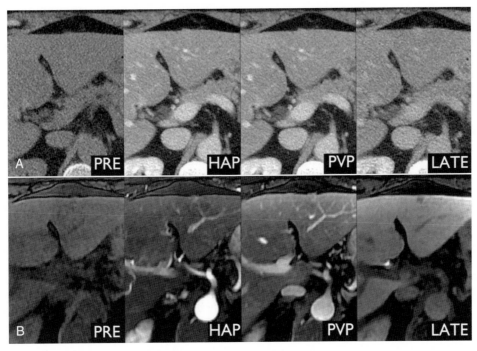

Fig. 15-5 CT (*top row,* **A**) is less sensitive to contrast agents than MRI (*bottom row,* **B**). A 4-mm colorectal cancer metastasis in the left lobe of the liver in a 67-year-old woman is barely visible with CT after administration of 150 ml of iodinated contrast material. By comparison, the metastasis is seen to better advantage with MR after administration of 10 ml of a gadolinium-based hepatobiliary contrast agent. MRI was performed 2 weeks after CT. The metastasis was resected and histologically; confirmed. PRE, precontrast image; HAP, hepatic arterial phase; PVP, portal venous phase; LATE, late venous phase; HCP, hepatocyte phase.

images: on occasion, CT images may appear clean but have inadequate soft tissue contrast to detect subtle but important pathologic conditions (i.e., the CT failure effect is not always obvious).

The risk of CT includes exposure to ionizing radiation. A typical CT scan of the abdomen or pelvis is equivalent to the exposure from 500 chest x-rays or 4.5 years of background radiation exposure.[23] In a study of CT exposure in 31,462 patients being treated at a tertiary care center, CT exposures were estimated to produce 0.7% of total expected baseline cancer incidence and 1% of total cancer mortality.[24] Therefore, particularly for cases in which multiple interval surveillance imaging studies are planned (e.g., HCC surveillance in patients with cirrhosis), the risk of cumulative exposure to ionizing radiation must be considered carefully in the risk/benefit ratio of the surveillance strategy. CT also carries the risk of exposure of the fetus to ionizing radiation in women who are pregnant. The mean and maximal radiation dose to a fetus during CT of the abdomen are 8.0 mGy and 49 mGy, respectively.[25] A recent review of imaging utilization during pregnancy, conducted at a single academic center from 1997 to 2006, found that the number of CT examinations increased by 25% per year over this time interval.[26] It is not recommended that exposure of the fetus to diagnostic levels of radiation should be cause for consideration for pregnancy termination, but efforts should be made to minimize radiation exposure in known pregnant or potentially pregnant women.[1]

CT has the lowest sensitivity to contrast compared with US and MRI; thus it requires administration of higher volumes of contrast at higher rates. This necessitates placement of larger bore IV access compared with other modalities. Despite

the use of large contrast agent doses, potentially important alterations in hepatic vascularity may be subtle and difficult to detect prospectively at CECT, potentially leading to false-negative interpretations in patients with small HCCs or metastases (**Fig. 15-5**).

IV-iodinated contrast media used in CECT may be associated with idiosyncratic anaphylactoid or nonidiopathic reactions, as well as combinations of these. Idiosyncratic anaphylactoid reactions occur unpredictably, usually without warning, are not presently preventable, and may be fatal. These reactions vary in severity and may mimic true allergic anaphylactic reactions (although no immunoglobulin E [IgE]-mediated antibody to contrast media has been identified). Fortunately, the incidence of severe adverse reactions to contrast media is rare (reported frequency, 0.004% to 0.22%[27,28]). Nonidiosyncratic reactions are dose dependent and may be responsive to substitution with low osmotic contrast media (nonionic). Vasomotor reactions may occur with idiosyncratic reactions or nonidiosyncratic reactions or may occur independently. These reactions may consist of hypotension with either bradycardia or tachycardia, sweating, anxiety, or significant reduction in cardiac output. Minor reactions (flushing, nausea, pruritus, urticaria, headache) may be seen in 5% to 10% of cases.[27] The incidence of contrast-induced nephropathy (CIN) from IVC for CECT is difficult to estimate because much of the literature is derived from patients undergoing coronary angiography. However, in a prospective trial in which the IV *N*-acetylcysteine was used in patients with a baseline creatinine level of 2.4 ± 1.3 mg/dl, 21% of patients in the placebo group developed an increase in serum creatinine level of at least 0.5 mg/dl 48 hours after the administration of

IVC.[27] Fortunately, CIN is usually reversible and a recent review of the literature suggests that its risk has largely been overestimated based on the quality of published literature on the topic.[27]

Magnetic Resonance Imaging and Spectroscopy

Magnetic resonance technology encompasses both magnetic resonance imaging (MRI) and magnetic resonance spectroscopy (MRS). MRI spatially encodes signals to generate anatomic images. MRS, in contrast, creates spectra or a frequency histogram, which shows the relative signal intensity at various resonance frequencies. Using prior knowledge of resonance frequencies, MRS can be used to deduct the relative content of lipids and metabolites in a tissue.

In MRI a powerful magnet aligns the protons in the body. A more powerful magnetic field is able to align the protons more strongly, providing higher potential for signal generation. Thus a 3-Tesla (T) magnet is able to generate greater signal than a 1.5-T magnet. Open magnets usually have weak field strengths that are rarely sufficient for liver imaging. Radiofrequency pulses (low energy in the form of radiowaves) and magnetic field gradients are turned on and off in various ways to generate images. The radiofrequency pulses interact with hydrogen protons in the body, which then release low energy in the form of radiowaves from the body. These emitted radiowaves are detected by antennas called coils that are placed on or near the patient's body and are the source of the images. The exact order of radiofrequency pulses and gradients defines the imaging sequence, or instructions for generating images. The image contrast produced in MR images is created through differences in several tissue properties (e.g., proton density, T_1, T_2, chemical shift, diffusion, susceptibility). These permit the development of imaging sequences with high soft tissue contrast that can improve tissue characterization in comparison with CT.

Contrast agents in MR work by altering the relaxation times of protons. The most common contrast agents in MRI are gadolinium based. These are compounds in which the gadolinium (Gd) atom is attached to a carrier molecule. Gd is a paramagnetic atom, that generally causes tissues to appear bright on T_1-weighted images and is useful for detecting vascular tissues such as tumors. Gd-based contrast agents (GBCA) are extracellular agents and are similar to contrast given for CT. MRI is more sensitive to contrast and therefore can identify subtle changes in vascular flow with lower doses of contrast (**Fig. 15-6**). Moreover, despite the use of lower contrast agent doses, MR imaging may be able depict alterations in vascularity that are difficult to detect at CECT. Reticuloendothelial system (RES)–specific contrast agents include superparamagnetic iron oxides (SPIOs), which are selectively absorbed by cells of the RES in the liver, spleen, and bone marrow. These particles result in disturbances in the local magnetic field, causing tissues that contain RES cells to lose signal strength. Superparamagnetic contrast agents, therefore, appear very dark on T_2-weighted images and may be particularly helpful in liver imaging because normal liver tissue will retain these particles whereas other tissues (scar, poorly differentiated HCC, metastases) will not. Unfortunately, the RES-specific contrast agent previously used most commonly for liver imaging in the United States (Feridex, Bayer HealthCare Pharmaceuticals) is no longer commercially available. Gadoxetic acid (Eovist, Bayer HealthCare Pharmaceuticals) is a hepatobiliary-specific contrast agent (HBCA). After bolus injection, gadoxetic acid is rapidly distributed in the intravascular and interstitial spaces (similar to GBCA). In the second phase (peaking at about 20 minutes after injection), approximately 50% of gadoxetic acid chelates are absorbed by hepatocytes and are then actively excreted by the biliary system. Because of this, late T_1-weighted sequence data provide both anatomic and functional information about the biliary system. Therefore on a multiphasic imaging study, gadoxetic acid (and similar HBCAs) may provide information

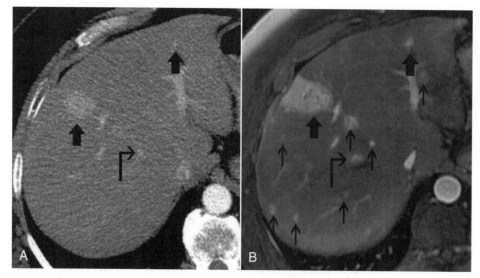

Fig. 15-6 **CT and MRI studies done within 10 days of each other on a patient with multiple leiomyosarcoma metastases to the liver.** A 150-ml aliquot of an iodinated contrast agent was used for the CT **(A)** and 15 ml of a gadolinium-based extracellular contrast agent was used for the MRI **(B)**. MRI is more sensitive to focal liver lesions than CT, with lesions evident in both scans *(block arrows)*, lesions evident by CT only retrospectively after identification by MRI *(curved arrows)*, and lesions evident by MRI but undetectable by CT *(straight arrows)*.

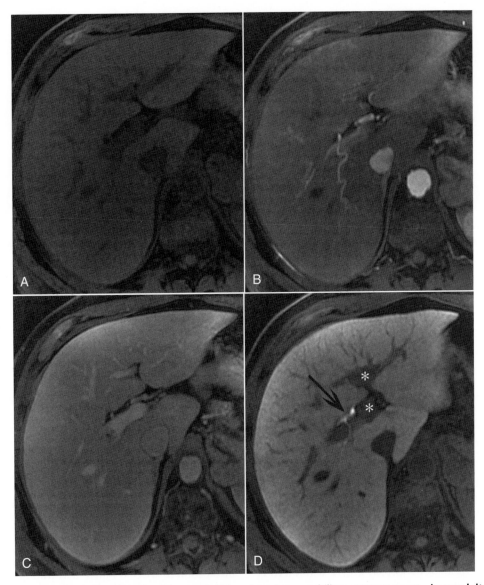

Fig. 15-7 **Dynamic MRI with 9.5 ml of gadoxetic acid—a gadolinium-based, hepatobiliary contrast agent—in an adult patient with well-compensated cirrhosis caused by chronic hepatitis C.** Precontrast **(A)**, 20 seconds postcontrast hepatic arterial phase **(B),** 1 minute postcontrast portal venous phase **(C),** and 20 minutes postcontrast hepatocellular phase **(D)** images are shown. Notice the intense enhancement of liver parenchyma and bile ducts *(arrow)* by 20 minutes; by comparison, the inferior vena cava, portal vein branches *(asterisks)*, and other intrahepatic vessels appear dark.

about vascularity and hepatocellular function and serve as a biliary contrast agent. The agent is not approved as a biliary contrast agent, however, and its use for this purpose is considered experimental at this time. Clinical experience with gadoxetic acid is currently limited, but emerging evidence suggests the agent may play an important role in select indications[29-31] (**Fig. 15-7**).

Diffusion-weighted imaging (DWI), a technique that historically has been used in imaging the brain, assesses the diffusion of protons within tissues measured as the apparent diffusion coefficient (ADC). Tissues with reduced water proton diffusion (lower ADC) appear brighter than those with "normal" water proton diffusion. Most solid liver lesions have reduced ADC and appear bright against a dark liver background on DWIs (**Fig. 15-8**). DWI techniques are used with increasing frequency in liver imaging, and emerging data

suggest that the additional information from DWI improves the sensitivity of MR protocols for FLL detection.[32] As opposed to the qualitative interpretation of DWI for lesion detection, the quantitative measurement of ADC for liver lesion or liver tissue characterization is more experimental (**Fig. 15-9**). ADC has been advocated as a way to predict tumor response to therapy or to monitor treatment response. ADC has also been advocated as a method to noninvasively evaluate liver fibrosis or inflammation. ADC in the liver has been reported to decrease as hepatic fibrosis increases (it is thought that collagen is not abundant in free water).[33-36] Both hepatic iron accumulation and hepatic steatosis may affect ADC values[36,37] and clinical experience with this quantitative evaluation of DWI technique remains limited. The authors do not recommend routine clinical implementation of quantitative DWI for lesion or tissue assessment at this time.

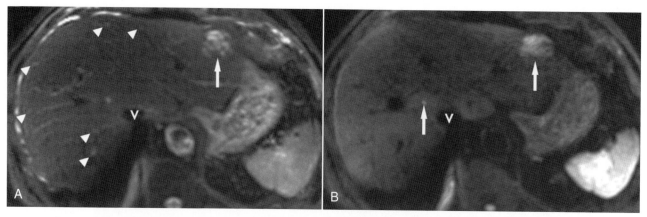

Fig. 15-8 Diffusion-weighted imaging of a patient with carcinoid metastases to the liver. Image **A** *(left)* has less diffusion weighting (b = 0 sec/mm^2) than image **B** *(right)* (b = 500 sec/mm^2). The image on the right shows two metastases *(arrows):* a 3-cm metastasis in the left lobe and a 5-mm metastasis at the junction of segments 8 and 4a near the inferior vena cava *(v)*. The image on the left prospectively shows only the 3-cm metastasis. The 5-mm metastasis is visible but not easily identified because of the presence of multiple distracting hyperintense vessels and bile ducts *(arrowheads)*. As illustrated in this example, diffusion weighting increases sensitivity to metastatic tumors by reducing the signal intensity of potentially distracting normal structures as well by other effects beyond the scope of this chapter.

Indications for use of MRI in evaluation of DLL and FLL are expanding. Until approximately 10 years ago, MRI was too slow to provide consistent high-quality images in the abdomen because of motion created by breathing, the beating heart, and peristalsis. Technologic improvements in MRI have resulted in image acquisition that can be completed during a reasonable breath-holding interval. The role for MRI in liver imaging has vastly expanded in recent years. MRI is frequently used as a problem-solving modality for FLL. With respect to evaluating the liver parenchyma, MRI is emerging as the modality of choice to measure liver fat noninvasively, is useful in the evaluation of hepatic iron overload, and is an experimental method in the quantification of hepatic fibrosis. MRI is often employed in the preoperative planning of patients undergoing hepatic resection. Finally, MRI allows for superior delineation of the biliary tree through magnetic resonance cholangiopancreatogram (MRCP), which can be performed with or without contrast agents (**Fig. 15-10**).

MRI has several advantages that make it a powerful tool in the assessment of FLL and DLD. As outlined previously, several data sets may be obtained during a single examination, thereby permitting assessment of multiple tissue properties and providing more comprehensive characterization of focal lesions and hepatic parenchyma. Images obtained with MR have high intrinsic soft tissue contrast, producing a wide dynamic range between white and black, which allows for detection of subtle soft tissue changes that may not be appreciable with CT. The MRI signal can be decomposed into its water and fat components (as opposed to CT, in which the content is inferred from the average tissue density, which is susceptible to confounding), allowing precise calculation of the fraction of signal derived from fat. Recent developments in MRI technique now permit accurate determination of fat content based on this property.[38-41] Tissue and lesion characterization is further enhanced by the use of various contrast agents noted earlier, all of which may be administered in lower volumes than IVC administered for CT. In some cases, characterization may be optimized by administration of more than one contrast agent. For these reasons, compared with high-quality CT, high-quality

MRI may provide superior detection and characterization of many focal and diffuse liver abnormalities (see **Figs. 15-5 and 15-6**).

The potential of MRI for comprehensive liver and lesion assessment through use of advanced sequences and contrast agents is a double-edged sword in that state-of-the-art MRI is not widely accessible. By comparison, adequate CT technology is available at most centers. MRI is generally more time-consuming to perform than CT. A diagnostic CECT examination can often be completed in 10 minutes whereas MRI exams may require 30 to 45 minutes. Most liver MR imaging sequences require breath-holding by the patient; thus complex studies with multiple sequences are cumbersome for patients and may be difficult to perform in those with dyspnea, agitation, or confusion. MRI can be particularly difficult for patients with anxiety or claustrophobia and may require premedication in selected individuals who may not otherwise be able to tolerate these exams. Because of the cooperation required for MRI, suboptimal examinations may also occur in patients with a language barrier or other limitation to following instructions. Young children may require conscious sedation or even general anesthesia to complete an MRI scan.

Depending on the scanner technology, MRI is not yet an ideal study for imaging large geographic regions of the body (e.g., to obtain images from the abdomen and pelvis during a single exam). Patient positioning with respect to the magnet is important; therefore repositioning to obtain images from two regions may considerably prolong examination time. Thus, if imaging of both the abdomen and the pelvis is required, CT may be a better technique (see **Fig. 15-4**). Because of the use of magnetic fields, MRI is contraindicated in patients with implantable electronic devices or metal in the eyes (appropriate screening of patients must be carried out before these exams and sometimes plain radiographs are required to exclude metallic fragments). Although MRI is largely believed to be safe during pregnancy, the U.S. FDA guidelines require labeling of MRI to indicate that safety with respect to the fetus "has not been established."[42] The major theoretical safety concerns with respect to the fetus are risk for teratogenic effect and acoustic damage. In general, human

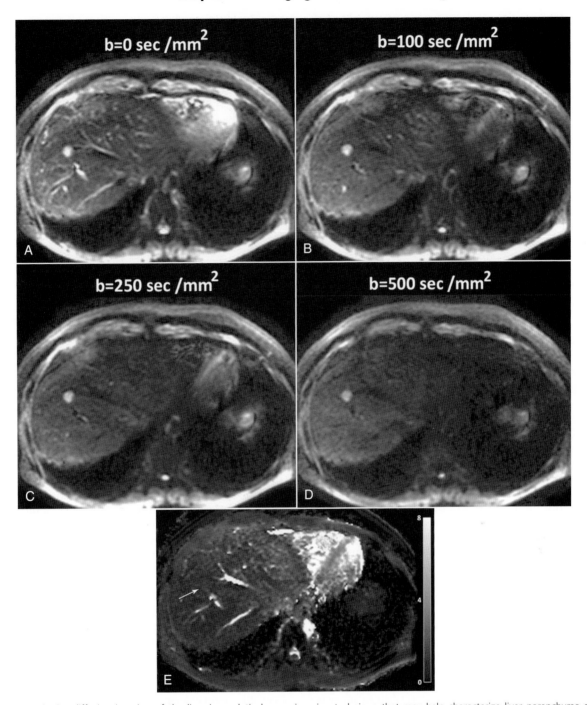

Fig. 15-9 Quantitative diffusion imaging of the liver is a relatively new imaging technique that may help characterize liver parenchyma and liver lesions. Shown here are diffusion-weighted images in a 44-year-old woman with FNH. Compared with background liver, the FNH has a high signal on the initial T_2-weighted image **(A)** acquired with minimal diffusion weighting (b = 0 sec/mm²). With progressively greater diffusion weighting—b = 100 **(B)**, b = 250 **(C)**, b = 500 **(D)**, b = 750 (not shown), and b = 1000 (not shown) sec/mm²—the lesion loses signal at a rate similar to that of background. Image **E** is an apparent diffusion coefficient (ADC) map that shows the ADC of every pixel on the image calculated from the source images *(top row)* assuming exponential signal decay. The FNH *(arrow)* is barely visible on the ADC map, indicating that it has similar ADC as background liver. The scale bar on the right ranges from 0 to 8 × 10³ mm²/sec. A malignant solid lesion would be expected to have lower ADC than background liver, and a benign cyst would be expected to have higher ADC. Preliminary results on the use of ADC to characterize focal liver lesions as benign or malignant, however, have been disappointing and further technical refinement likely will be necessary before quantitative diffusion imaging is used for this purpose in clinical practice.

studies do not support a teratogenic effect, but data are restricted to follow-up of the exam with 1.5-T scanners. Likewise, data have not demonstrated acoustic damage from MRI exposure in utero. GBCAs have been shown to be teratogenic in animal studies because they cross over to the placenta; they are categorized as Pregnancy Category C by the FDA. Although traditionally it has been recommended that lactating mothers discontinue breastfeeding for 24 hours after being exposed to iodinated contrast or GDCA, it appears that these agents likely pose no risk to the infant.[43]

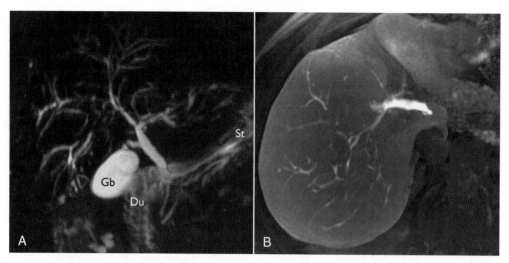

Fig. 15-10 A comparison of MRCP done conventionally using heavily T₂-weighted images without contrast agents (A) and using T₁-weighted images with a gadolinium-based hepatobiliary contrast agent (B) in a patient with primary sclerosing cholangitis. Peripheral biliary dilation and stricturing can be seen in both studies. Images are maximum intensity projections in the oblique coronal **(A)** and oblique axial **(B)** planes. Du, duodenum; Gb, gallbladder; St, stomach. Note that administration of hepatocellular agents for contrast-enhanced cholangiography is off-label use, because the agents are not approved by the FDA for this purpose.

Many factors are important determinants of the quality of images obtained with MRI, including the type of scanner, the experience of the radiologist protocolling and interpreting the study, the experience of the technician performing the study, protocol design and refinement capabilities, and patient variables (e.g., ability to hold breath, hold still, follow directions, and cooperate; presence of ascites). MRI is more prone to artifacts than CT, although the advantage of this limitation of MRI is that it is readily apparent when a poor-quality study has been performed (the MR failure effect is obvious; by comparison, the CT failure effect may be missed, as discussed earlier). MRI scans are operator dependent, although less so than US. MRI requires investment in maintaining protocols. Ascites may potentially result in image degradation with MRI, particularly if a 3-T scanner is used (ascites may require paracentesis before the examination; also, better-quality images may be obtained from a 1.5-T scanner).

In contrast to CT, MRI protocols usually require refinement. Therefore an applications specialist, radiologist (if local expertise exists), or physicist may be needed to create protocols that produce quality MRI examinations. Most radiologists are not trained in MR technical refinement and not all centers or hospitals have applications specialists or physicists available to perform MR refinement. As a result, the performance characteristics of MRI for characterization of DLL and FLL cited in the literature may not apply within individual institutions depending upon the local expertise available; in this respect, CT may be a better option than MRI in that it will typically produce good-quality images with little refinement of imaging protocols.

Initially recognized in 1997, a rare but potentially devastating complication of gadolinium termed nephrogenic systemic fibrosis (NSF) has been highlighted by the FDA to be of particular risk among patients with acute renal failure in the setting of chronic liver disease.[44-47] However, a recent review has demonstrated that patients with chronic liver disease (41 of 355 cases in the published literature between September 2000 and August 2008) are not at increased risk for NSF independent of the severity of their renal function, as estimated by glomerular filtration rate (GFR) approximated from creatinine values using the *Modification of Diet in Renal Disease*.[44] In this review, all but one patient with chronic liver disease who developed NSF had chronic kidney disease (CKD) stage IV or V with estimated GFR <30 ml/min/1.73 m² or required dialysis. The single patient with chronic liver disease and mild to moderate CKD (estimated GFR, 34.6 to 69.6 ml/min/1.73 m²) who developed NSF had undergone four MRI examinations with administration of double-dose gadolinium over a 10-week period. This would indicate that patients with chronic liver disease and estimated GFR (eGFR) >30 ml/min/1.73 m² have very low risk for NSF despite the well-known limitation of estimated GFR in reflecting renal function in this patient population. The American College of Radiology's Committee on Drugs and Contrast Media has released guidelines for the safe use of GBCA to help prevent NSF. The guidelines are updated periodically. The authors recommend that clinicians and radiologists follow the most current guidelines.

Magnetic Resonance Spectroscopy

Magnetic resonance spectroscopy (MRS) is a modality that allows for quantification of hepatocellular lipid content and other metabolites.[48,49] The advantage of this modality is that it is the most direct means of depicting the quantitative content of fat and other metabolites in the liver. Disadvantages of MRS include the fact that MRS is restricted in its spatial coverage. Only one cube of tissue (e.g., 2 × 2 × 2 cm area) is sampled during a study. This may result in inaccurate estimation of fat or other content in the entire liver and also makes it problematic to perform longitudinal studies because it is difficult to collect data from the identical region on serial exams. This technique is also time consuming and requires expertise both in conduct of the study and in interpretation of the data collected (usually a physicist with training in spectroscopy is required). In current clinical practice, therefore, MRS of the liver is not generally feasible.

Emerging Technologies

Transient Elastography

The principle underlying transient elastography is that the propagation velocity of a waveform through a homogeneous tissue is proportional to its stiffness. During transient elastography examination, a transducer is placed over the liver and transmits a low-frequency (50 Hz) mechanical wave that propagates through the liver; the velocity of the wave is then measured by pulse-echo ultrasound. If the liver is fibrotic, the mechanical waves propagate more rapidly than in a normal liver.[50] Stiffness is assessed at a depth of 25 to 65 mm below the skin surface and the volume measured is a cylinder 1 cm in diameter and 4 cm in length.[51] Typically 10 measurements are obtained during a single examination and the results of these measurements, if deemed valid by the machine, are used to determine a median value that is representative of the degree of hepatic fibrosis. In experienced hands, the examination takes 5 to 10 minutes, is painless for the examinee, and has no known adverse effects. Measurements may be invalid if the transducer is held incorrectly (over rib or lung tissue) or if the test is performed on patients who have ascites or who are overweight or obese. FibroScan was developed by the French company Echosens (Paris, France) and made commercially available in 2001. At the time of this book's publication, more than 600 of these machines had been distributed worldwide.

Magnetic Resonance Elastography

Magnetic resonance elastography (MRE) is an MR-based technique in which the stiffness of hepatic parenchyma may be assessed as an indicator of hepatic fibrosis.[52] MRE uses a modified phase-contrast technique to image the propagation characteristics of mechanical waves generated by an external mechanical or pneumatic driver within the liver. These studies can be performed using a conventional MRI scanner with addition of hardware necessary to generate propagating mechanical waves in the liver and software to analyze the data and generate images depicting tissue stiffness, called elastograms.[53] Potential advantages of MR elastography include the ability to obtain conventional MRI images during the examination, operator independence, no requirement for an acoustic window, ability to obtain quality measurements regardless of body habitus, and assessment of a large field (may include the entire liver).[53] The unit of measurement for elastography is kilopascals (kPa). TE estimates the Young elastic modulus. Higher elastic modulus connotes disease. MRE measures a different modulus—the shear elastic modulus. The shear elastic modulus is related to but not identical to the Young modulus measured by TE. Thus the results from these two modalities are not directly translatable, although recent in vitro data comparing results from these modalities using well-characterized phantom materials demonstrate good correlation ($r^2 = 0.93$).[54]

Future Directions in Elastography

The use of ultrasound and MR-based techniques to assess mechanical tissue properties such as stiffness is a rapidly evolving field. More advanced image acquisition and image analysis techniques are in development. For example, it is possible to model the acquired imaging data using sophisticated rheologic models to assess mechanical properties other than stiffness (e.g., shear viscosity, porosity). Studies are needed to assess the incremental diagnostic benefit of evaluating these additional properties.

Positron Emission Tomography (PET), PET/CT, and Scintigraphic Techniques

Visualization of metabolism with [18F]fluorodeoxyglucose positron emission tomography (FDG-PET) is a sensitive tool in the identification of primary and metastatic tumor sites throughout the body, although it is limited in its spatial resolution. Simultaneous PET/CT imaging has been developed to help overcome this limitation and allow more accurate anatomic location of malignant foci. Because metabolic activity in the liver may be heterogeneous, it may manifest patchy uptake on PET that may either mimic a malignant focus or obscure true malignant lesions. This heterogeneity is amplified in the cirrhotic liver; thus PET can be particularly difficult to interpret in this setting.

Focal Liver Lesions

Two goals in imaging focal liver lesions (FLLs) are detection and characterization. Detection refers to the identification of the presence of FLLs as well as the delineation of their location and number. Characterization of FLLs involves more than identifying liver lesions to provide a differential diagnosis and determining whether lesions are benign or malignant, and if malignant, whether they are primary or metastatic. Ideally, radiologic characterization of FLLs should produce the narrowest differential diagnosis possible and, in some cases, suggest a single diagnosis with high confidence. Experimental techniques in FLL imaging are being developed to help predict tumor biology, prognosis, and response to therapy; correlate lesions with gene expression; and describe specific histologic features. In this section, we will provide an overview of the role of various imaging modalities in FLL detection and characterization followed by a more detailed description of radiographic features of some of the more common or clinically important FLLs.

FLL Detection

US has reasonable sensitivity and accuracy in the detection of cystic lesions, but is limited in detection of solid liver lesions. As noted earlier, CEUS is significantly better at FLL detection but is limited in its ability to scan the entire liver. US is not able to demonstrate the location of FLLs with the same precision as CT or MRI. It is usually possible to identify the segmental location of FLLs with US, but FLL location with respect to relevant internal landmarks such as vessels, ducts, or other liver lesions or external landmarks such as adhesions, bowel, or abdominal wall varices can be difficult. For this reason, US is not an ideal modality for surgical planning. CT without contrast has markedly limited sensitivity to detect focal liver lesions. MRI without contrast has better sensitivity than CT or US for this purpose but is still limited. Therefore both CT and MRI require contrast administration for FLL detection. In comparison with US, both CT and MRI are better at depicting the location of FLLs, including relation to relevant internal and external landmarks.

FLL Characterization

Focal liver lesion characterization with US is limited with the exception of hepatic cysts and some typical hemangiomas.

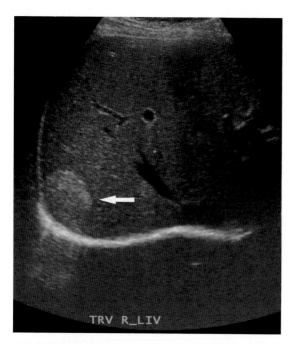

Fig. 15-11 **Transabdominal transverse ultrasound image of a hepatic hemangioma (arrow).** The hemangioma is hyperechoic (bright) compared with liver and associated with posterior acoustic enhancement (formerly called "through transmission") beyond the lesion.

Although US can be highly suggestive for the characterization of certain solid lesions such as metastatic lesions or HCC, this modality is not adequate for purposes of making a definitive diagnosis. Therefore, with the exception of cysts (see **Fig. 15-2**) and certain typical hemangiomas (**Fig. 15-11**), US is not considered to be accurate enough for FLL characterization and further imaging studies are required. In contrast, CEUS is superb in experienced hands for characterization of certain FLLs and can be very useful, for example, in the differential diagnosis of focal nodular hyperplasia versus hepatic adenoma[55] (**Fig. 15-12**). In centers with expertise in CEUS (rare in North America but more accessible in Europe) the use of CEUS is strongly advocated by the authors for FLL characterization. The key advantage of CEUS for this purpose is the real-time depiction of dynamic enhancement properties. For example, in FNH, CEUS allows visualization of contrast enhancement from the inside-out whereas enhancement in hepatic adenomas and HCC occurs from the outside-in; even tiny feeding and intralesional vessels may be depicted with high clarity. The sensitivity of US to the microbubble-based contrast agent is exquisite; even a single microbubble may be visualized. Thus lesions that may appear to be necrotic by CT or MRI may be demonstrated to be viable with CEUS if microbubbles are visualized within the ischemic cores.

CT and MRI have similar performance characteristics in lesion characterization with some exceptions. CT is able to identify calcification whereas MRI does not demonstrate this well (calcification is rarely present, so this is of limited usefulness for characterization of most liver lesions). MRI is able to demonstrate more tissue properties than CT, including the presence of fat, blood, and iron. As discussed earlier, the availability of both extracellular and hepatobiliary MR contrast agents may provide an additional advantage to MRI in that more biologic data can be obtained with which to characterize FLLs. Both modalities are able to demonstrate morphologic features of FLLs such as size, shape, and margination, with

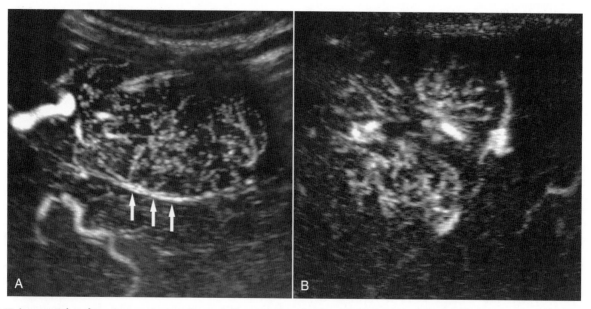

Fig. 15-12 **Images taken from two contrast-enhanced ultrasound studies demonstrating the difference between vascular characteristics of hepatic adenoma (A, left) and focal nodular hyperplasia (B, right).** In the hepatic adenoma, vascular flow is from the outside-in, as demonstrated to best advantage by real-time imaging, and intralesional vessels are arranged in an irregular pattern. By comparison, in the FNH, vascular flow is from the inside-out, and the vessels are arranged in a radiating spokewheel pattern.

the caveat that some lesions may be difficult to visualize with CT because of low-contrast resolution and other lesions may be difficult to visualize with MR if artifacts are present. Kinetic enhancement of FLLs with CT and MRI (enhancement of blood flow/perfusion) is similar to CEUS but with much lower temporal resolution: CEUS can generate 10 to 30 frames per second, in comparison with CT or MRI, which generate no more than one frame every 20 to 30 seconds (techniques are in development to capture images of the entire liver every 3 to 5 seconds, but these are not generally used in clinical practice). Thus images generated with CEUS versus CT or MRI are analogous to comparing video images with still-frame pictures.

Individual FLLs

In this section, we describe the imaging appearance of common or important liver lesions. The clinical, biologic, and histologic features of these FLLs are discussed in other chapters of this textbook. Characterization of FLLs depends on context, biologic stability, and imaging features. The influence of each is both lesion dependent and patient dependent. Parameters of biologic stability and clinical context are the same for imaging as for clinical hepatology. Here we focus on imaging features, but emphasize that the imaging features usually are interpreted within the context of the clinical scenario.

Cyst

On US, hepatic cysts appear as anechoic lesions with posterior acoustic enhancement and imperceptible walls (see **Fig. 15-2**). On CT and MRI, cysts demonstrate lack of enhancement with contrast agents, and are sharply demarcated with no nodularity of the wall (**Fig. 15-13**). Cysts are low density on NECT, have a low signal on T_1-weighted MRI, and appear very bright on T_2-weighted images (**Fig. 15-14**). Cysts may have septations and, rarely, blood or proteinaceous material on MRI. The presence of blood in cysts is not uncommon in polycystic liver disease, but its presence in isolated hepatic cysts may warrant further evaluation (need to distinguish from cystadenoma or cystadenocarcinoma[56,57]).

Cystic Biliary Hamartoma (von Meyenburg Complex)

On US, von Meyenburg complex (VMC) may demonstrate multiple hypoechoic to hyperechoic liver lesions that may not be clearly identified as cystic. On CT and MRI, VMC usually appear as multiple, tiny (2 to 10 mm), relatively uniformly sized cysts in a patchy or diffuse distribution. It is the multiplicity and uniformity of these lesions that distinguish them from simple cysts (**Fig. 15-15**). They may also display subtle ring enhancement on delayed images. MRI is superior in the detection and characterization of VMC.[58,59] Anecdotal experience at our institution has been that CT may demonstrate only a few lesions whereas MRI may reveal the presence of hundreds of lesions. The appearance of VMC may be confused with metastatic disease. Metastatic lesions typically have early ringlike arterial phase enhancement with dissipation of the contrast material on later phases. In contrast, VMC do not show early arterial enhancement but rather enhance slowly and progressively along their periphery; a subtle ring of enhancement may be visible on delayed images. T_2-weighted MR images are helpful in challenging cases; VMC are typically much brighter on T_2-weighted images than metastases.

Hemangioma

On US, hemangiomas typically appear as homogeneous hyperechoic nodules that are sharply demarcated with posterior acoustic enhancement and absent Doppler signal[60] (see **Fig. 15-11**). The appearance of HGs on US may be dynamic (the echotexture may change over the course of the sonogram). Most US findings are nonspecific and none of the US features are fully diagnostic in isolation. However, within the proper clinical context, US findings may be highly suggestive of this diagnosis. Using CEUS, HGs appear as a solitary, circular, nodular lesion without intralesional vessels on the arterial phase followed by a nodular fill-in pattern on the portal-venous phase. In one large series, CEUS was reported to have 82.2% accuracy in diagnosis of HG.[14]

On CT, HGs appear hypodense compared with the hepatic parenchyma with early nodular peripheral enhancement (puddling) followed by progressive, centripetal fill-in with isodensity to slight hyperdensity on delayed phase imaging.[61] On MRI with extracellular (Gd) contrast, typical HGs (in the 1- to 5-cm range) show peripheral nodular enhancement with progressive centripetal enhancement and fill-in on equilibrium phase[62,63] (**Fig. 15-16**). Because of its superior sensitivity to contrast agents, MRI may depict the characteristic enhancement pattern of HGs with greater clarity than CT, permitting a more definitive diagnosis. T_2-weighted MR imaging is also helpful; HGs appear very bright on such images (similar to benign cysts and VMC) (**Fig. 15-17**) in comparison with most malignant lesions, which are rarely very bright. With hepatocellular contrast agents, hemangiomas appear hypointense relative to the hepatic parenchyma in the delayed phase.[64]

Hepatic Adenoma (HA)

It is rare for a radiologist to be able to make a definitive diagnosis of HA. The classic radiologic features of HA (fat, blood, and sometimes calcium) are often not present and, even if present, do not exclude the possibility of HCC. Adenomas may appear isodense with peripheral enhancement on CECT. HAs may appear hyperintense on T_1-weighted MRI because of the presence of glycogen, fat (**Fig. 15-18**), or blood and have been reported to appear hypointense on T_2-weighted images related to the presence of fat, blood, or calcium.[65] Contrast agents can help in narrowing the differential diagnosis, often to either HCC or HA. Unfortunately, tissue is usually required to make a definitive diagnosis of HA because the imaging findings are rarely specific.

Focal Nodular Hyperplasia (FNH)

In contrast to HA, radiologists are able to make a definitive diagnosis of FNH if the lesion is large and classic in appearance. In these situations, further evaluation is probably not necessary, although periodic follow-up imaging may be performed to monitor growth. Lesions that are small are usually more difficult to characterize. If atypical in appearance,

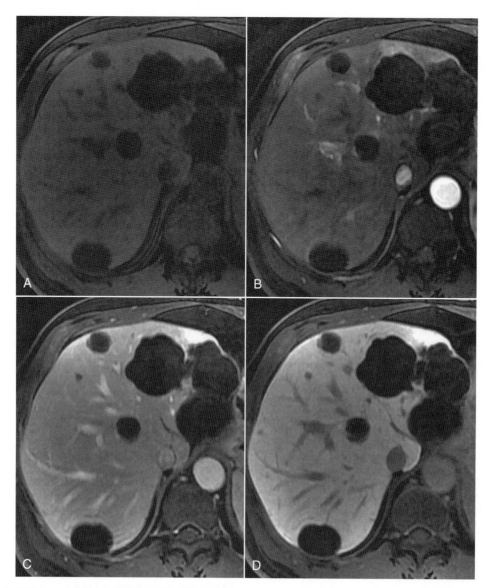

Fig. 15-13 Dynamic MRI done with a gadolinium-based hepatobiliary contrast agent in a patient with multiple hepatic cysts. The pre-contrast image **(A)** is T$_1$-weighted and demonstrates the characteristic low signal intensity of cysts on T$_1$ images. **B,** 25 seconds postcontrast, hepatic arterial phase; **C,** 80 seconds postcontrast, portal venous phase; and **D,** 20 minutes postcontrast, hepatocellular phase images are shown and demonstrate the lack of enhancement in all phases, characteristic of cysts.

findings may suggest a hepatocellular etiology and even benign nature, but further evaluation is usually necessary. Classic FNHs are hypervascular and homogeneous (with the exception of the central scar) and do not display a tumor capsule (**Fig. 15-19**). The central scar may have septations that carve the nodule into lobules. Because of its large extracellular spaces, the central scar of FNH typically appears bright on T$_2$-weighted MRI images and, if an extracellular agent is given, enhances late on dynamic or multiphasic contrast-enhanced imaging studies. Because the scar is not composed of hepatocytes, it appears dark on delayed images after administration of an HBCA (**Fig. 15-20**). For classic FNH, a multiphasic CECT or MRI with extracellular contrast agent (Gd-based) should suffice to make a definitive diagnosis. Atypical FNHs are missing one or more of the elements of classic FNH. They may also have additional elements present such as a

pseudocapsule (a rind of enhancement surrounding the nodule, probably composed of compressed hepatic parenchyma or vessels rather than a true capsule composed of fibrous tissue). Hemorrhage and fat are very rare and, when present, are not severe. In cases of atypical FNH, CEUS or MRI with liver-specific contrast agents (SPIO or gadoxetic acid) may be required for a definitive diagnosis.

Nodular Regenerative Hyperplasia (NRH)

Imaging studies may be able to detect some cases of NRH, but overall sensitivity and specificity is too poor to play a significant role in identification of this entity.[66] NRH does not typically display enhancing nodules, which is in contrast to large regenerative liver nodules.[67] Liver biopsy is currently required to make a definitive diagnosis of NRH.

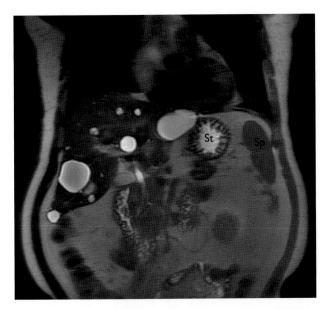

Fig. 15-14 A coronal, T₂-weighted, noncontrast study of the same patient from Figure 15-13 with multiple hepatic cysts demonstrates "lightbulb brightness" of cysts on T₂ images when compared with their dark appearance on T₁-weighted images as shown in Figure 15-13.

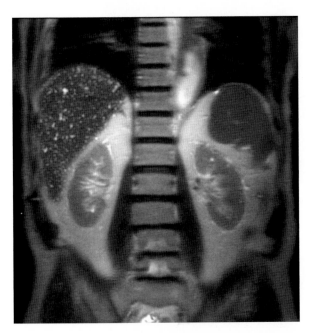

Fig. 15-15 **A coronal MR image of a patient with von Meyenburg complexes (VMCs).** Like simple cysts, VMCs appear bright on T₂-weighted images, as seen here. However, VMCs can be distinguished from simple cysts by their multiplicity and relative size uniformity.

Hepatocellular Carcinoma (HCC)

Multiphasic imaging is necessary to adequately detect and correctly characterize HCC. Most HCCs are hypervascular (**Fig. 15-21**). Small to moderately sized HCCs (e.g., ≤2 cm) tend to have homogeneous enhancement whereas large HCCs (e.g., ≥2 cm) *may* be homogeneous (**Fig. 15-22**); however, they are more likely to be mosaic in their enhancement. The two key characteristic features of HCC are (1) hyperenhancement on arterial phase imaging and (2) washout on delayed imaging phases (**Fig. 15-23**). When both features are present, the diagnosis can be established in the right clinical setting with nearly 100% positive predictive value (PPV). Because evaluation of features is more reliable with larger lesions than smaller lesions, emerging guidelines[68] allow for noninvasive diagnosis of HCC based on these two features alone for lesions larger than 2 cm but not for lesions smaller than 2 cm.

If both classic features are not present, then additional information is necessary to establish the diagnosis of HCC. One additional feature that can help in establishing a diagnosis in this case is growth, although there is no consensus as to what magnitude of growth over what time frame is adequate to implicate malignancy. In the absence of growth, hyperarterial enhancement, or washout, the diagnosis of HCC can be suggested, but not with complete certainty, according to published evidence by the presence of additional features. These features may include restricted diffusion, moderate high signal on T₂-weighted images, a disproportionately higher fat content compared with the rest of the liver, and the presence of a venous ring or "capsule"[69,70] (see **Fig. 15-23**).

In patients without cirrhosis or other known risk factors for HCC, a noninvasive diagnosis of HCC cannot be established with hyperenhancement, washout, and growth alone because these are nonspecific features of malignancy. In this setting, features that favor HCC over other malignancies include a well-formed capsule, the presence of internal arteries feeding the tumor (**Fig. 15-24**), mosaic architecture (see **Fig. 15-22**) (the random distribution of intralesional compartments with different imaging properties), and the presence of fat within the lesion (this virtually excludes metastatic disease).[70-72]

Nodules that do not meet all classic criteria for HCC (hyperenhancement, washout, and growth) may be malignant, but cannot be diagnosed as such noninvasively. In these cases, the differential diagnosis includes dysplastic nodule, regenerative nodule, and arteriovenous (AV) fistula, and close follow-up is usually recommended (**Fig. 15-25**). Although numerous studies have attempted to use imaging to differentiate among these benign or premalignant entities, no method is yet reliable.[72] Moreover, the clinical relevance of distinguishing these entities remains unclear. Clinically, these indeterminate nodules can usually be followed over time to allow for growth or other change in features that identify them as benign or malignant. A particular dilemma arises when there are definite HCCs and some indeterminate nodules, especially when there is desire for urgent management decisions without waiting for demonstration of growth. There is currently no evidence-based consensus on the appropriate strategy in these situations.

Another area that can be particularly problematic with respect to HCC imaging is identification of infiltrative HCC. Conventional CT and MRI techniques may both miss this particular variety of HCC. In the authors' experience, MRI with superparamagnetic iron oxides had high sensitivity for infiltrative HCC, but unfortunately these agents are no longer available. The presence of tumor thrombus surrounded by otherwise nonspecific parenchymal heterogeneity can be indicative of infiltrative HCC (**Fig. 15-26**). Tumor thrombus in the absence of a distinct nodule growing into the involved vessel should always raise suspicion for this entity.

CT and MRI have limited per-lesion sensitivity and per-patient specificity as well as poor staging accuracy for HCC.

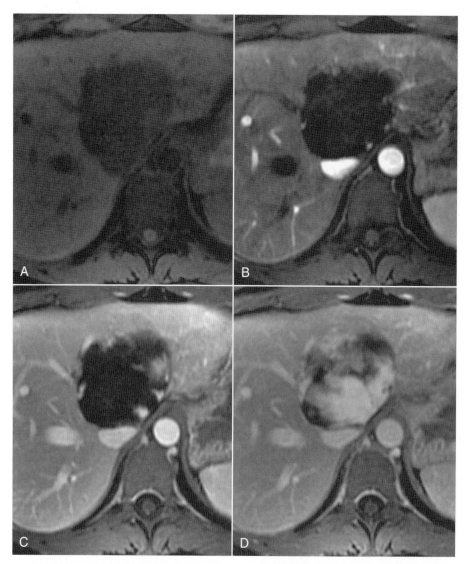

Fig. 15-16 A dynamic MRI study done with a gadolinium-based extracellular contrast agent demonstrates the presence of a large hemangioma in this woman. The lesion is dark in the precontrast T_1-weighted image **(A)**. Early nodular peripheral enhancement (puddling) can be seen in the hepatic arterial phase **(B)**, with subsequent progressive enhancement in the portal venous **(C)** and late venous **(D)** phases.

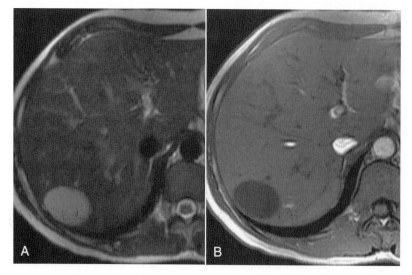

Fig. 15-17 **MR images of hepatic hemangioma in an adult woman.** Hemangiomas have high signal intensity on a T_2-weighted image **(A)** and low signal intensity on a T_1-weighted image **(B)**.

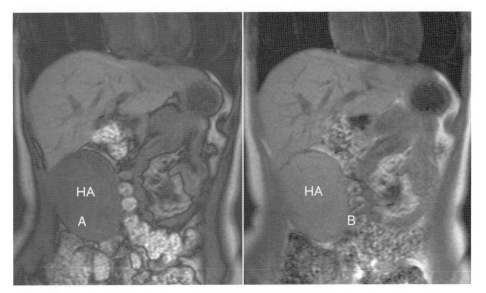

Fig. 15-18 **In-phase (B, *right*) and out-of-phase (A, *left*) coronal MR images in a woman with a large hepatic adenoma *(HA)* extending inferiorly from the liver.** The relatively high intralesional signal in the in-phase image suggests the presence of fat, a common finding in adenomas. The presence of fat is confirmed on the out-of-phase image, which signals loss of the HA relative to the liver. Note that the normal liver parenchyma does not change in signal intensity between the out-of-phase and in-phase images, suggesting little to no fat in the liver parenchyma. The presence of fat, blood, calcium, or glycogen in hepatic adenomas does not exclude HCC, and tissue sampling is often required to make a definitive diagnosis.

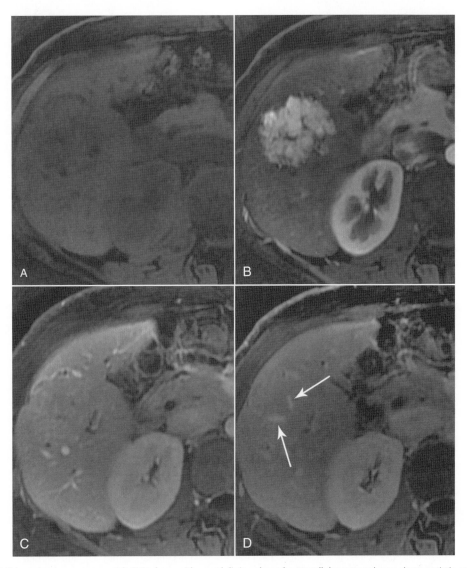

Fig. 15-19 Dynamic MR imaging in a woman with FNH done with a gadolinium-based extracellular agent shows characteristic arterial hypervascularity and dramatic contrast enhancement from the precontrast phase **(A)** to the hepatic arterial phase **(B)**. The central scar remains hypointense in the arterial phase. The lesion fades to isointensity with the background liver parenchyma in the portal venous phase **(C)**, and in the delayed-contrast phase **(D)** the central scar becomes hyperintense to the surrounding tissue *(arrows)*.

Overall, conventional CT and MRI have reported *staging* accuracies of about 40%.[73] In the pretransplant population, multiphasic CT has a reported per-lesion sensitivity of 49.4% to 61% for HCC when explant histopathologic analysis is used as the reference standard.[74-76] Lesions smaller than 2 cm pose a particular challenge to current imaging technology, and new techniques will need to be established to address this. These may include new sequences such as DWI, new contrast agents such as HBCA, or use of contrast agents in combination (double-contrast MRI). Preliminary data suggest that diffusion-weighted imaging may be superior to T_2-weighted images in the detection of small HCCs in patients with cirrhosis.[77] Diffusion-weighted imaging with MRI may also be able to distinguish bland thrombus from tumor thrombus[78]

(**Fig. 15-27**), but further work is needed to confirm these promising initial observations.

Further problems in HCC imaging include nonstandardized reporting techniques for these lesions, nonstandardized imaging techniques, and variability in the interpretation and recommendations made based on these techniques. National societies are working to develop standardized guidelines for the acquisition, interpretation, and reporting of scans obtained for purposes of HCC screening or in which lesions are identified with suspicion of HCC.

Cholangiocarcinoma (CC)

There are three types of cholangiocarcinoma (CC): mass-forming CC, periductal infiltrating CC, and intraductal

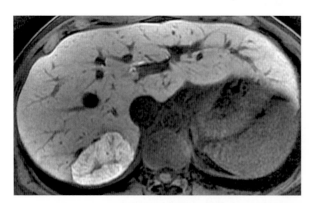

Fig. 15-20 **MR image, 20 minutes postcontrast hepatocyte phase, from a gadolinium-based hepatocellular contrast agent study in a woman with FNH.** The brightness of the lesion compared with the background normal liver demonstrates the ability of intralesional hepatocytes to take up the hepatocellular contrast agent, but an inability of the lesion to excrete it. The impaired excretion has been attributed to incomplete communication between intralesional bile ducts and the biliary system of the surrounding liver. The characteristic central scar is dark on hepatocyte phase images, because it is not composed of hepatocytes. Compare the dark appearance of the scar on this image with the bright appearance on the delayed image acquired after administration of an extracellular agent in Figure 15-19.

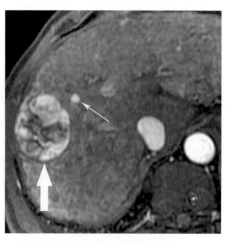

Fig. 15-22 An arterial phase gadolinium-based extracellular contrast MRI study demonstrates the mosaic architecture of moderate- to large-sized HCC. The mass *(block arrow)* is 5-cm in diameter and contains intralesional compartments with varying enhancement. Compare this mosaic enhancement with the more uniform enhancement of the 7-mm HCC satellite nodule in this figure *(arrow)* or the 1.8-cm HCC nodules in Figure 15-23.

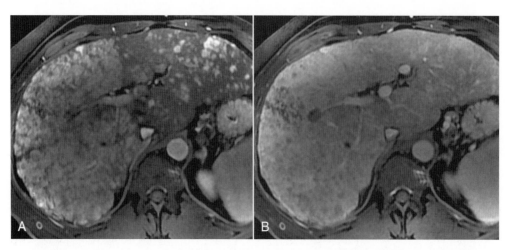

Fig. 15-21 Gadolinium-based extracellular contrast MRI study demonstrates the hypervascularity of HCC lesions. Notice innumerable hyperenhancing nodules in the hepatic arterial phase **(A)**. Although the nodules are present in both hepatic lobes, they are more densely concentrated in the right lobe, where they coalesce to form a conglomerate mass. The nodules fade to isointensity to background liver in the portal venous phase **(B)** and become more difficult to discern.

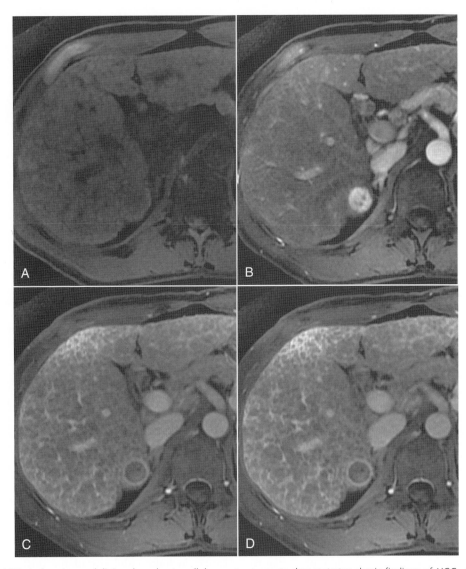

Fig. 15-23 Dynamic MRI study using gadolinium-based extracellular contrast agents demonstrates classic findings of HCC. A 1.8-cm HCC nodule enhances from precontrast phase **(A)** to arterial phase **(B)** and washes out to become hypointense to background liver in the portal venous **(C)** and late venous **(D)** phases. Notice a ring of enhancement surrounding the nodule in the portal venous and late phases; HCC nodules frequently manifest a venous phase ring or "capsule."

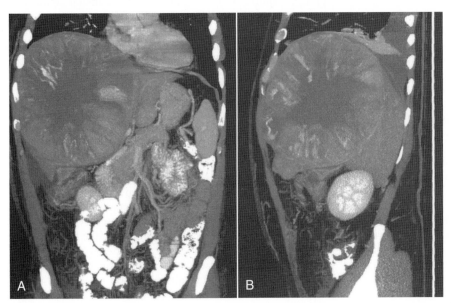

Fig. 15-24 Coronal and sagittal reformatted CT images demonstrate a large mosaic mass arising from the right lobe of the liver in a patient without underlying liver disease. Notice the presence of internal vessels within the tumor. The mosaic architecture and the presence of intralesional vessels are characteristic of large HCC and less commonly observed in metastases. Therefore an imaging diagnosis of HCC is favored over metastasis despite the absence of underlying liver disease.

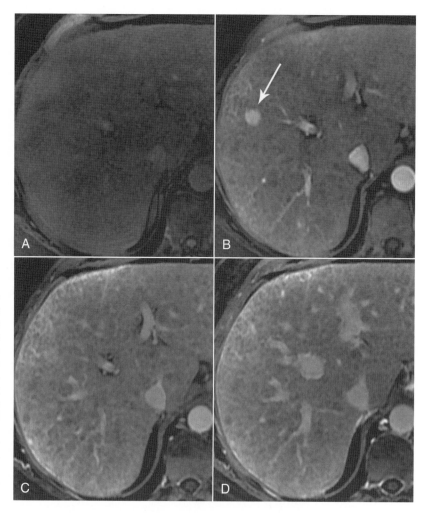

Fig. 15-25 This dynamic MRI study using a gadolinium-based extracellular contrast agent demonstrates enhancement of a 12-mm hepatic nodule (arrow) from the precontrast phase (A) to the hepatic arterial phase (B); however, in the portal venous phase (C) the lesion fades to isointensity with background liver, and remains isointense in the late venous phase image (D). Hypervascular nodules that fade to isointensity but do not wash out to hypointensity in the portal or late venous phase images usually cannot be definitively diagnosed as HCC based on a single imaging examination. Such nodules generally require close follow-up imaging or evaluation with a contrast agent that assesses a biologic property other than vascularity (e.g., a hepatocellular or, if available, reticuloendothelial agent). (See Figure 15-26.)

luminal CC (very rare). Mass-forming CC appears similar to a metastatic adenocarcinoma lesion with a ring or rind of enhancement. The enhancement washes out peripherally and fills in centrally because of the presence of a fibrotic core with large extracellular spaces in which the contrast agent pools (**Fig. 15-28**). Because these tend to be desmoplastic lesions, they may cause retraction of the overlying liver capsule.[79] Mass-forming CCs have a propensity to cause biliary ductal obstruction. Findings that favor diagnosis of a mass-forming CC over a metastatic lesion include presence of a solitary lesion, capsular enhancement, vascular invasion, and biliary obstruction, although these features are not always present and their presence does not exclude a diagnosis of metastatic disease. Therefore histologic confirmation with lesional biopsy is often required.

Periductal infiltrating CC may occur incidentally or can be associated with chronic inflammatory conditions of the bile ducts such as primary sclerosing cholangitis (PSC). This is a difficult lesion to differentiate from chronic inflammation. The findings consist of diffuse ductal thickening, hyperenhancement, and areas of stricturing with or without periductal enhancement, which may represent inflammation or neoplastic infiltration. It is often impossible on imaging to differentiate chronic inflammation from chronic inflammation with superimposed cancer. Findings that suggest

cancer include nodularity of the thickening, asymmetry of the thickening, and disproportionate progression focally.[80] If the diagnosis is not known, imaging can raise concern for cancer but cannot usually confirm the diagnosis; tissue sampling is required. If the diagnosis is known, then imaging may be used to stage the extent of the cancer to guide treatment options, but conventional imaging can be limited in this respect as well. In these cases, we recommend acquisition of delayed images up to 20 to 40 minutes after giving the contrast agent to fill up the extracellular spaces to the greatest extent possible. Experimental techniques may improve imaging performance characteristic in CC, including double-contrast and HBCA; however, there is no convincing evidence of this to date.

Metastases to the Liver

Metastases are classified into two groups based on arterial enhancement. Although all large metastases are supplied predominantly by the hepatic artery rather than the portal vein (PV) (regardless of original route into the liver), metastases differ in their propensity for arterial enhancement. Hypervascular metastases are those that enhance significantly in the arterial phase after administration of contrast agents (**Fig. 15-29**). These include breast cancer (even though

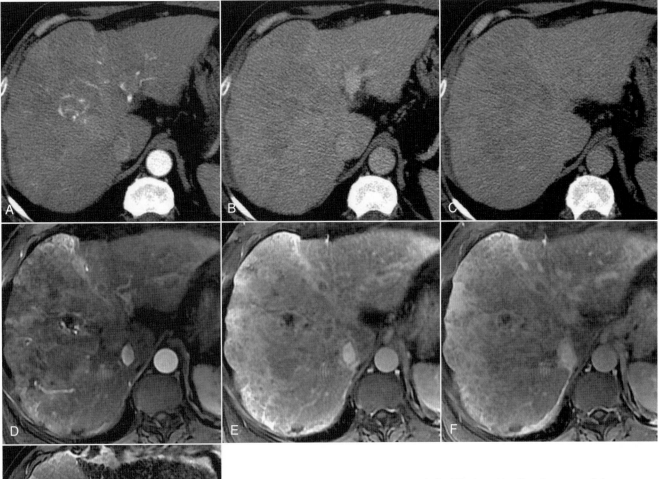

Fig. 15-26 Infiltrative HCC can be particularly difficult to identify using extracellular agents as illustrated by the images here. CT images with iodinated contrast (arterial phase **[A]**, portal venous phase **[B]**, late venous phase **[C]**) show a heterogeneous appearing liver but no discrete lesions. Dynamic MR images from a study done using a gadolinium-based extracellular contrast agent in the same patient 2 days later (arterial phase **[D]**, portal venous phase **[E]**, late venous phase **[F]**) show patchy arterial phase hyperenhancement in the right lobe and nonspecific heterogeneity in the venous phases. A huge infiltrative HCC occupies most of the right lobe of the liver but is difficult to visualize on the conventional CT or MR images because the vascularity of infiltrative cancer may not differ much from that of cirrhotic liver parenchyma. By comparison, an MR image from a study using superparamagnetic iron oxides (SPIO) **(G)** clearly delineates the cancer, which appears bright compared with the darker noncancerous tissue. This is because SPIO is taken up by Kupffer cells, leading to signal loss on the MR image from the paramagnetic effect of the SPIO, known as susceptibility. The cancerous region lacks Kupffer cells and cannot take up SPIO, and therefore does not have susceptibility-associated signal loss. As illustrated in this case, SPIO-enhanced imaging can help detect infiltrative cancers that may be difficult to identify using extracellular agents.

arterial phase enhancement is not always present, patients with breast cancer should initially be evaluated as if they have hypervascular metastases until imaging proves otherwise), renal cell carcinoma, melanoma, neuroendocrine tumors, sarcomas, choriocarcinoma, and thyroid carcinoma. Most other metastases are considered hypovascular because these do not enhance significantly in the arterial phase. These include gastrointestinal adenocarcinomas (colorectal, gastric, pancreas) and lung carcinoma (**Fig. 15-30**). The anticipated vascular enhancement pattern influences the protocols used for detection and staging of metastases. Hypervascular metastases are best visualized at arterial phase (bright) and late

venous phase (washout) and can be missed if only PV phase imaging is done (**Fig. 15-31**). Hypovascular metastases are best visualized at PV phase and this usually suffices for their detection and staging. Hepatologists should be aware that some metastases require multiphasic imaging whereas others can usually be visualized appropriately with monophasic imaging.

Classically, metastases show homogeneous enhancement if they are small and ring enhancement if they are large. Like HCCs, the enhancement washes out on venous phase images with the exception of some metastases with ischemic or fibrotic centers that will display peripheral washout (the

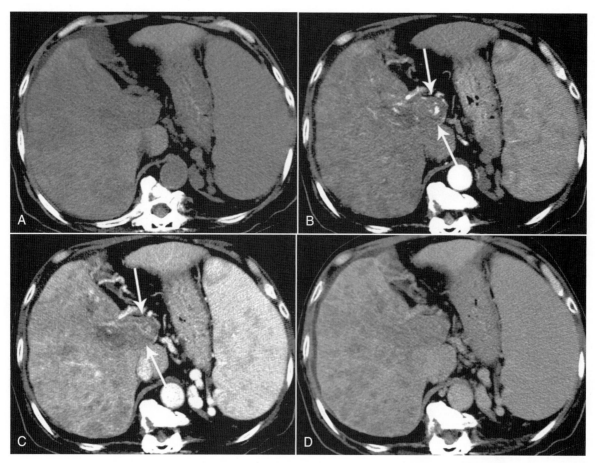

Fig. 15-27 As illustrated in this dynamic CT series of axial images taken in a patient with infiltrative HCC, the presence of a tumor thrombus *(arrows)* can help suggest the presence of infiltrative cancer. Tumor thrombus refers to the presence of tumor within the lumen of a vein. Imaging features that help differentiate tumor thrombus from bland thrombus include luminal expansion and presence of intraluminal material that hyperenhances in the arterial phase and washes out in the portal and late venous phases.

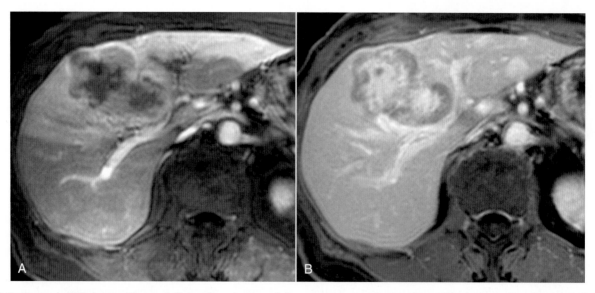

Fig. 15-28 Dynamic MRI done with a gadolinium-based extracellular contrast agent in a patient with the mass-forming type of cholangiocarcinoma (CC). This type of CC has a similar enhancement pattern as adenocarcinoma metastases. The contrast agent arrives in the outer part of the tumor first, resulting in a characteristic peripheral enhancement pattern in the hepatic arterial phase **(A)**. The contrast agent slowly clears from the outer part of the tumor and progressively accumulates in the central hypoxic or fibrotic core of the tumor. This results in the characteristic peripheral washout with central fill-in appearance in the delayed phase **(B)**.

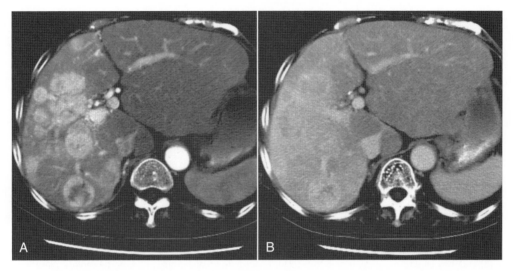

Fig. 15-29 Metastases of renal cell carcinoma, melanoma, neuroendocrine tumors, sarcomas, choriocarcinoma, thyroid cancer, and some breast cancers are hypervascular and enhance during the arterial phase **(A)** of contrast studies as shown in this contrast-enhanced CT study of a patient with neuroendocrine tumor metastases to the liver. These often fade to isointensity during the portal venous phase **(B)** and are not nearly as evident.

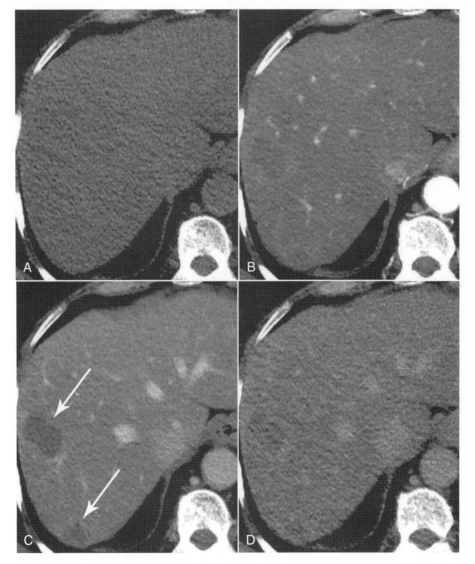

Fig. 15-30 Metastases of cancers other than those described in Figure 15-29 are considered hypovascular. These include gastrointestinal adenocarcinomas (colorectal, gastric, pancreatic) and lung. Precontrast **(A)**, arterial phase **(B)**, portal venous phase **(C)**, and delayed phase **(D)** images from a contrast-enhanced CT of a patient with colorectal adenocarcinoma metastases are shown. These lesions *(arrows)* are best seen in the portal venous phase, where the lesion appears hypointense to the background liver tissue.

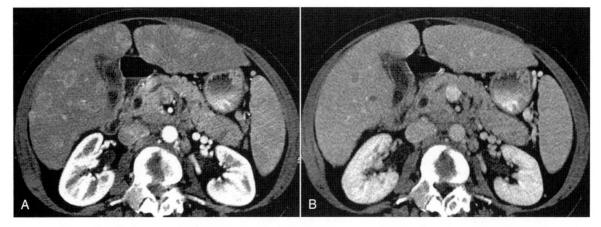

Fig. 15-31 Similar to the neuroendocrine metastases shown in Figure 15-29, breast cancer metastases to the liver are often hypervascular and enhance in the arterial phase of contrast studies, as shown by the arterial phase **(A)** of this contrast-enhanced CT study. The lesions fade to isointensity in the portal venous phase **(B)** and may be difficult or impossible to detect if images are obtained only in the portal venous phase.

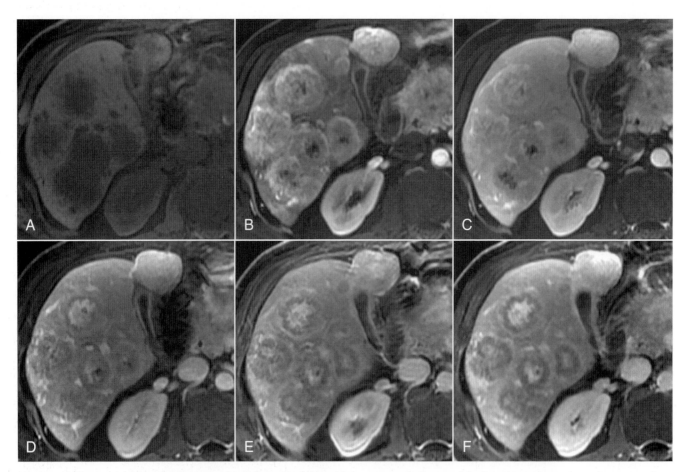

Fig. 15-32 This contrast-enhanced MR study of a patient with neuroendocrine metastatic disease of the liver demonstrates ring enhancement from precontrast **(A)** to arterial phase **(B)** and subsequent peripheral washout and central fill-in in the portal venous phase **(C)** and late venous phase images acquired at 3 **(D)**, 5 **(E)**, and 10 **(F)** minutes after administration of an extracellular gadolinium-based agent.

periphery washes out as the contrast works its way into the center of the tumor with progressive enhancement of the tumor center) (**Fig. 15-32**). Ringlike enhancement is visualized much better with MRI than CT, especially for hypovascular metastatic lesions. Metastases tend to be round or oval in shape. Ringlike enhancement may superficially mimic

abscesses, but abscesses tend to be irregular and heterogeneous in size and shape, whereas metastases tend to be smooth and more homogeneous in size and shape.

Distribution of metastases within the liver may reflect the underlying vascular flow pattern. Metastases transported to the liver via the portal system may preferentially occur in the right lobe or the left lobe depending on the streaming of blood flow in the main portal vein. In general, blood flow from the superior mesenteric vein preferentially enters the right portal vein and blood from the splenic vein preferentially enters the left portal vein, which may explain the predilection of colon cancer metastases to occur in the right lobe of the liver. In contrast, metastases that arrive in the liver from the hepatic artery are more likely to be diffusely distributed.

Pseudolesions

Pseudolesions are not true lesions but imaging findings that may be misinterpreted as lesions. Examples include focal fat deposition,[81] focal fat sparing,[82] and perfusion alterations attributable to arterio-portal shunts or vascular obstructions.[83] Key imaging features that help differentiate pseudolesions from true masses include absence of mass effect, straight rather than rounded borders, and shifting location on follow-up studies. In the authors' anecdotal experience, MRI can be particularly helpful as a problem-solving modality in patients with suspected pseudolesions identified at US or CT.

Diffuse Liver Disease

Although liver biopsy is the gold reference standard for clinical evaluation and diagnosis of diffuse liver disease (DLD), this diagnostic standard has practical limitations. Biopsy is invasive and thus is suboptimal for longitudinal surveillance, disease screening, or monitoring treatment response. Sampling variability is another potential limitation of liver biopsy. The liver tissue taken by biopsy, estimated to be approximately 1/50,000th of total liver volume,[84,85] may not represent the entire liver because hepatic steatosis, inflammation, and fibrosis may be distributed heterogeneously. Furthermore, there is demonstrated variability among pathologists with regard to histologic analysis.[86] Research has focused on developing imaging methods for evaluating DLD that address some of the drawbacks of biopsy and that provide complementary information to histologic analysis. Techniques in US, CT, and MR imaging have demonstrated varying ability to evaluate DLD. Although many of these techniques are either investigational or only of research utility, some are routinely employed for clinical purposes. In this section, we will discuss current and emerging imaging techniques for evaluation of hepatic steatosis, fibrosis, and iron overload.

Steatosis

There has been varying success in the radiographic detection and quantification of hepatic steatosis. Currently, US is the most widely used modality for evaluating steatosis, although new MR techniques in development have shown high accuracy across a wide range of liver fat in preliminary clinical studies. CT has also been used to quantify hepatic fat content; however, confounders and ionizing radiation exposure have made CT techniques less frequently used, particularly with safer, more accurate alternatives available. Current recommendations for evaluating hepatic steatosis are discussed by modality in the following sections. Many of these techniques are currently experimental, but are rapidly being adopted in clinical practice.

Ultrasound

Ultrasound is the most widely utilized modality in the evaluation of hepatic steatosis because of its ease of availability, low risk profile, and relative low cost. US techniques highlight the variation in tissue characteristics affecting wave propagation, allowing for differentiation of fatty tissue and normal hepatic tissue. Fat causes ultrasound beam scattering within the tissue, and the increased echoes returning to the US transducer lead to a brighter, more echogenic liver (**Fig. 15-33**). Hepatic echogenicity can be qualitatively compared

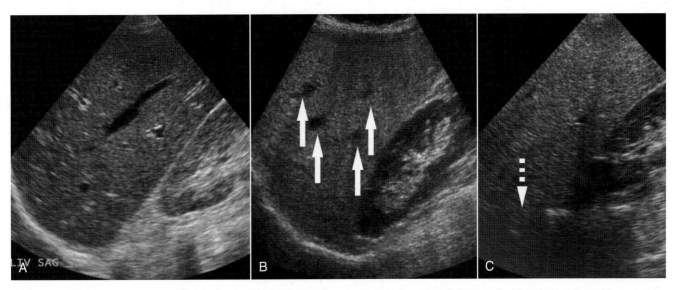

Fig. 15-33 Ultrasound can detect the presence of fat in the liver, as demonstrated in this series of three studies done in a patient with progressive steatosis over a period of 3 years. As the liver becomes more fatty (from image **A** to image **C**), the parenchyma becomes hyperechoic (brighter), vessels become blurred (*solid arrow*), and the diaphragm becomes dark and eventually disappears, a phenomenon known as posterior shadowing (*dashed arrow*).

with that of the kidney, because it is known to have an echogenicity similar to that of normal hepatic tissue.[87,88] Fat is also known to cause ultrasound beam attenuation. This attenuation results in nearly unnoticeable changes in echogenicity in cases of mild steatosis, but as the amount of liver fat increases, vessels and other intrahepatic structures become blurred and more difficult to visualize. With increasing levels of fat and further attenuation, far-field echogenicity loss and darkening of the liver–diaphragm interface lead to a depth-dependent phenomenon known as posterior shadowing[5,89] (see **Fig. 15-33**). US has reasonable sensitivity (73% to 90%[5,90,91]) for qualitatively detecting moderate to severe steatosis, but it is limited in its ability to detect liver fat less than 30%. Sensitivity declines further with obesity as subcutaneous fat causes beam attenuation before it reaches the liver. US techniques are also limited by confounding characteristics such as fibrosis and inflammation, which are often present along with steatosis and, like fat, increase hepatic echogenicity.[6,92,93] The qualitative nature of ultrasound evaluation of steatosis leads to decreased repeatability and reliability secondary to interoperator and interinterpreter variability. The development of computer-based ultrasound techniques to quantitatively estimate hepatic fat content based on beam backscatter and attenuation is in the experimental phase; such techniques are not currently available for clinical care.

Computed Tomography

Computed tomography techniques are more sensitive and specific than US in the detection of hepatic steatosis[94,95]; however, the additional expense of CT and its use of ionizing radiation make it less desirable than US for this purpose. Moreover, safer imaging modalities, such as MRI, estimate liver fat more accurately than CT; therefore CT is rarely used as a primary test for fatty liver. As with US, confounders such as iron, copper, glycogen, fibrosis, and edema affect the accuracy of CT estimates of liver fat content.[96] The radiodensity of hepatic tissue is inversely related to the degree of steatosis. This can be assessed qualitatively by comparing the liver with other organs such as the spleen or the kidneys, or quantitatively by measuring radiodensity using Hounsfield units (HU) (**Fig. 15-34**).

Magnetic Resonance Spectroscopy

Magnetic resonance spectroscopy (MRS) is currently the most accurate radiologic tool for estimating hepatic steatosis. MRS measures hydrogen proton precessional frequencies, which are determined by the electrochemical environments of the molecules in which they are located. The dominant frequency in the MR spectrum of hydrogen protons in water is 4.7 ppm, and in triglyceride is 1.2 ppm. Although the dominant frequency in triglyceride is 1.2 ppm, different hydrogen protons in triglyceride are subject to different electrochemical environments depending on their position in the molecule. These hydrogen protons produce a spectrum of fat frequency peaks on spectroscopy, whereas water protons produce a single large peak (**Fig. 15-35**). If no steatosis is present, the water peak is clear, with limited to no evidence of triglyceride peaks. In the presence of steatosis, the difference between the area under the water peak versus the area under the fat peaks can be used to estimate hepatic fat fraction. A unique strength of MRS is

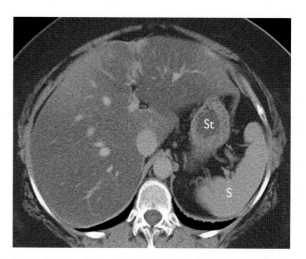

Fig. 15-34 **A nonenhanced, axial CT image in a patient with severe steatosis.** The liver tissue has lower attenuation (appears darker) than spleen (S), suggesting the presence of fat. In this case, the degree of hepatic fat deposition is so severe that the liver appears darker than unenhanced blood vessels. This resembles the appearance of a contrast-enhanced scan, but contrast agents were not administered. St, stomach.

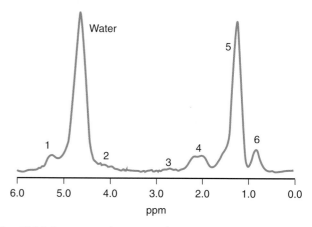

Fig. 15-35 **Representative magnetic resonance spectra collected by MRS demonstrating that hydrogen protons in water resonate at a single frequency, resulting in one large peak.** Triglyceride hydrogen protons, on the other hand, resonate at differing frequencies dependent on the electrochemical environment in which they reside within the molecule. This results in one dominant peak for the methylene moiety (peak 5) and five other peaks for other hydrogens within the molecule (peaks 1, 2, 3, 4, and 6).

its ability to accurately quantify fat fractions in livers with a wide range of steatosis, even in those with less than 10% fat. MRS-derived fat fraction has been used as a clinical measurement of steatosis in large adult and pediatric studies,[97-99] and is widely accepted as the noninvasive gold standard measure of liver fat.

Although MRS is able to estimate fat fractions across a spectrum of severity and has less operator dependence and variability compared with US, it does have a number of limitations. Many spectroscopy techniques do not address technical confounds, as discussed elsewhere,[100] and may lead to inaccurate estimates of hepatic steatosis severity. Additionally, like biopsy, MRS measurements are restricted by sampling variability. Current MRS techniques only analyze a single voxel, or about 0.5% of total liver volume. Two-dimensional MRS

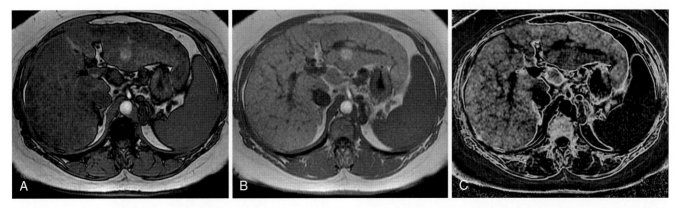

Fig. 15-36 Conventional out-of-phase/in-phase MRI imaging can detect the presence of fat in the liver based on the different precessional frequency of water and fat protons. On the out-of-phase image **(A)**, the liver appears darker than on the in-phase image **(B)**, because the fat proton signal subtracts from the water proton signal on the out-of-phase image and adds to it on the in-phase image. The change in signal intensity at each voxel can be evaluated algebraically to generate a fat signal fraction map **(C)** that shows the relative amount of fat in each voxel of the liver. On the map, higher signal in the liver corresponds to higher hepatic fat fraction. The patient in this example has cirrhosis attributable to chronic hepatitis C. Notice that the fat fraction map depicts low-signal reticulations throughout the liver parenchyma. These reticulations correspond to fibrotic scars. They appear dark because they are relatively devoid of fat. Intrahepatic vessels are also devoid of fat and appear dark as well.

imaging techniques that would allow whole liver analysis are being developed; however, at the time of publication of this book, they are not ready for clinical use. A final drawback of spectroscopy is that analysis of MR spectra is complicated and time consuming and few centers currently have adequate expertise to perform these studies.

Magnetic Resonance Imaging

Unlike MRS, which analyzes the frequency spectrum of protons in a single voxel to estimate hepatic fat content, MRI uses data from a complete anatomic image. MRI thus has a key advantage of being able to estimate steatosis throughout the entire liver. Since the mid-1980s researchers have been using MRI to evaluate fatty infiltration of the liver, using a technique first described by Dixon[101] and now commonly known as out-of-phase and in-phase imaging (other terms for this include "chemical-shift imaging," "dual-phase imaging," and "two-point imaging"). This technique exploits differences in the precessional frequency of water and fat protons to generate images in which fat and water signals are either entirely in-phase and additive (brighter image) or entirely out-of-phase and subtractive (darker image). In-phase and out-of-phase images can then be compared qualitatively to evaluate steatosis. Moreover, through simple algebraic manipulation, quantitative measurement of fat's contribution to the MRI signal can be used to estimate steatosis objectively[102-104] (**Fig. 15-36**). Out-of-phase and in-phase imaging has been refined over time to improve accuracy and decrease scan times, and studies have shown excellent correlation between MRI estimates of steatosis and fat measured by histologic analysis of biopsy and MRS-determined steatosis estimates.[41,102-105] Conventional out-of-phase and in-phase imaging is widely available on routine clinical scanners and is used frequently to evaluate steatosis qualitatively.

Because MRI estimates of fat fraction are determined by comparing water and fat MR signals, confounding variables that affect the measurement of either will lead to inaccurate estimates of liver fat. Recent research has shown that T_1 weighting, T_2^* relaxation, and signal interference from the multiple spectral components of fat molecules, particularly at low fat fractions or in the presence of iron, may lead to inaccurate estimates.[41,104,106] Techniques have been developed to address these confounders and have led to more accurate measurements of steatosis when compared with spectroscopic measurements.[39-41,107-110] Despite the mathematical complexity of these new techniques, they have the potential to be easily implemented with software that generates quantitative fat fraction maps on-line (**Fig. 15-37**). Currently, these techniques are available only at research centers. Once further large-scale validation studies are completed, they will likely be available on commercial scanners and ready for widespread clinical implementation.

Fibrosis

Conventional cross-sectional imaging techniques are limited in the diagnosis and staging of hepatic fibrosis. The cirrhotic liver may exhibit certain characteristic morphologic changes, including surface nodularity, segmental atrophy or enlargement, and extrahepatic manifestations of portal hypertension (**Fig. 15-38**). Because these are features of advanced disease, they are not present in all patients with cirrhosis and do not address lesser degrees of fibrosis. To address the need to noninvasively diagnose and grade hepatic fibrosis along its entire spectrum of severity, a number of new techniques are in development. The majority of these techniques focus on indirect markers of fibrosis, including liver stiffness (MRE and TE), water proton diffusivity (DWI), and tissue perfusion (perfusion MRI). Double-contrast MRI is a method that aims to evaluate fibrosis through direct visualization of textural abnormalities of the fibrotic liver (**Fig. 15-39**). In addition to a discussion of these emerging techniques, a brief overview of the uses and limitations of conventional imaging techniques will be included as well.

Ultrasound

Conventional ultrasound lacks both sensitivity and specificity in detection of hepatic fibrosis. Low specificity is derived from

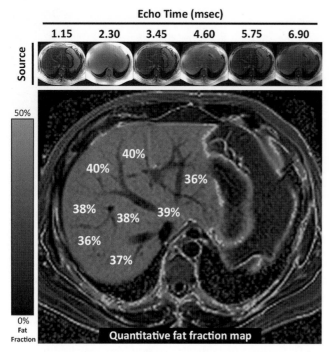

Fig. 15-37 Advanced MRI techniques are emerging that address confounders such as T_1 weighting, T_2^* decay, and the spectral complexity of triglycerides. One such technique is illustrated here, with source images at the stated echo times shown at the top, and a quantitative fat fraction map *(bottom)* generated through postprocessing of the source images. Fat fractions in various portions of the liver are shown as percentages.

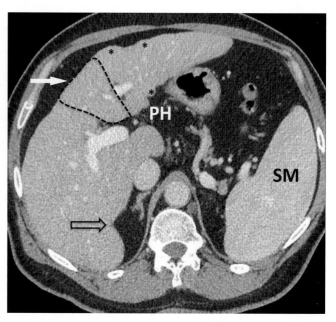

Fig. 15-38 Morphologic features of advanced cirrhosis can sometimes be appreciated with CT, as illustrated here. Morphologic features of cirrhosis include widened porta hepatis *(PH)*, flattened anterolateral margin *(solid arrow)*, surface nodularity *(asterisks)*, atrophy of segment 4 *(dashed contour)*, and posterior right hepatic notching *(hollow arrow)*. Notice also splenomegaly *(SM)* suggestive of portal hypertension.

the fact that the hyperechoic or "bright liver" seen on US from hepatic fibrosis is also seen in other diffuse liver pathologic conditions including steatosis and inflammation.[6,7] As in other conventional imaging techniques, morphologic abnormalities such as liver surface nodularity or lobar atrophy are only manifested in advanced stages of fibrosis,[36,111,112] making it an insensitive tool. Even in advanced disease, studies using surface nodularity by US to diagnose cirrhosis have reported limited sensitivities (87% to 91%).[9,10,113] Assessment of hepatic flow parameters with Doppler US has been studied extensively, but does not contribute substantially to sensitivity or specificity of conventional US examination.[114] Although it is most often used to evaluate focal liver lesions, CEUS has been studied for its ability to assess fibrosis by measuring the hepatic transit time (HVTT), which has been reported to correlate with fibrosis.[115] The use of CEUS to measure HVTT as a biomarker of liver fibrosis requires expertise, and this approach is currently utilized in only select centers.

Computed Tomography

Recent studies suggest that computer-based texture analysis of NECT images may predict the presence of fibrosis; however, confirmatory studies are needed.[116]

Ultrasound Elastography (Transient Elastography, FibroScan)

Several studies have compared the performance characteristics of transient elastography versus liver biopsy in various forms

of chronic liver disease, with most of these being performed in patients with chronic hepatitis C virus infection.[50] The first clinical study evaluating transient elastography was published in 2002; thus this is still a relatively new modality. A meta-analysis evaluating 50 studies in which transient elastography was compared with liver biopsy was recently published.[117] The mean AUROC (area under the receiver operator characteristic) values for the diagnosis of significant fibrosis (Metavir fibrosis stage 1 or less vs. stage 2 or greater), severe fibrosis (stage 2 or less vs. stage 3 or more), and cirrhosis (stage 3 or less vs. stage 4) were 0.84 (95% confidence interval [CI], 0.82 to 0.86), 0.89 (95% CI, 0.88 to 0.91), and 0.94 (95% CI, 0.93 to 0.95), respectively. Thus transient elastography performs best in distinguishing cirrhosis from lesser degrees of fibrosis, although it was unclear from the studies included in this meta-analysis in how many patients a clinical diagnosis of cirrhosis could have been made without need for transient elastography. Interestingly, data suggest that performance characteristics of transient elastography are better in alcohol-related disease and nonalcoholic steatohepatitis than in chronic viral hepatitis. It has been suggested that transient elastography is a robust tool for excluding cirrhosis as evidenced by high negative predictive values (NPV 99% at a cutoff of 11.9 kPa), which may be useful in triaging patients in need of liver biopsy.

The strengths of transient elastography are that it is rapid and painless, has no risk for complications, and has demonstrated excellent intraobserver and interobserver agreement in both adult and pediatric patients. Obesity (BMI >28 kg/m^2), narrow intercostal spaces, and ascites decrease the diagnostic performance of transient elastography and result in failure to obtain reliable measurements in 3% to 5% of patients.[118-121] The accuracy of this technique is further limited by factors other than fibrosis that alter liver

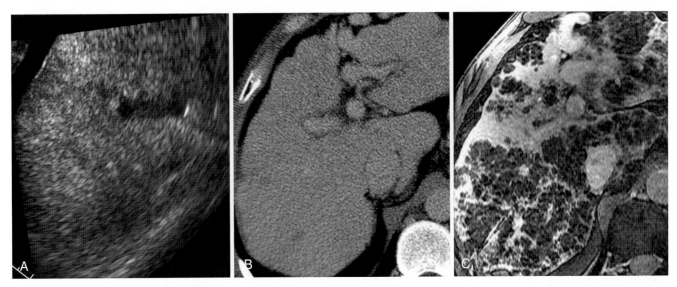

Fig. 15-39 Although all three main imaging modalities can detect hepatic abnormalities in cirrhotic patients, they do so to differing degrees. Here, a cirrhotic patient is imaged using US, CT, and MRI. US **(A)** shows only a coarse echotexture. CT **(B)** displays little more than abnormal liver morphology as described in Figure 15-38. Double-contrast (GBCA + SPIO) MRI **(C)** shows the abnormal liver morphology but can also illustrate abnormal internal architecture in cirrhosis.

stiffness, including necroinflammatory activity and congestive heart failure.

Conventional MRI

As previously discussed, morphologic abnormalities may become apparent with advanced fibrosis, and can be visualized by any conventional imaging technique, including MRI. In addition, MRI may be able to depict large fibrotic bridges and septa within the hepatic parenchyma. However, like US, MRI lacks the sensitivity to detect early stages of fibrosis. The liver parenchyma in precirrhotic and early cirrhosis usually has a normal appearance on conventional MRI or may exhibit only subtle abnormalities on unenhanced or single contrast agent–enhanced images. Because of this, advanced MRI techniques are required to more reliably evaluate hepatic fibrosis than those available in most clinical practice settings at this time.

Although single-contrast agents have limited efficacy in improving the visibility of fibrosis on MRI, multiple-contrast agents may act synergistically to enhance hepatic fibrosis. Two agents that depict fibrosis through different but complementary mechanisms are GBCA and SPIO (see **Fig. 15-39**). GBCAs freely diffuse into the extracellular space and as a result preferentially accumulate and cause signal enhancement of tissues with relatively large extracellular compartments, such as fibrotic liver tissue. In contrast, SPIO particles accumulate in Kupffer cells, which are present in normal liver tissue but are diminished or dysfunctional in fibrotic tissues. The iron oxide particles produce local magnetic field inhomogeneities that result in reduced signal in spared tissue with normal density of functional Kupffer cells; by comparison, tissues with reduced Kupffer cell density (e.g., fibrotic scars) do not accumulate the iron oxides, do not lose signal intensity, and appear relatively bright on MR images. Combined GBCA- and SPIO-enhanced MRI has been reported to detect advanced hepatic fibrosis and differentiate it from absent or mild fibrosis with up to 90% accuracy[120] (**Fig. 15-40**). Although most imaging

techniques rely on indirect markers of fibrosis, double contrast-enhanced MRI allows direct visualization of textural abnormalities without the need for specialized equipment. Furthermore, by imaging the entire liver, sampling variability is avoided and concurrent detection of other pathologic conditions is possible. Although the technique seems promising, further validation of this technique is required.

Magnetic Resonance Elastography (MRE)

Although both TE and MRE modalities are relatively early in their development, MRE appears at this time to have a number of advantages over transient elastography and to be superior in discriminating stages of fibrosis, particularly in milder disease (**Fig. 15-41**). Because MRE performance reportedly is not influenced by the presence of ascites or obesity, it has a higher technical success rate than transient elastography (94% vs. 84%).[53,122] Furthermore, MRE does not require an acoustic window or administration of contrast and it analyzes large volumes of liver, reducing the potential for sampling variability. Another advantage of MRE is that data acquisition is operator-independent. Finally, MRE can be included in a comprehensive MR examination that allows detection of morphologic abnormalities, hepatocellular carcinoma, and extrahepatic complications of liver disease. As with transient elastography, MRE measures an indirect marker of fibrosis and is therefore confounded by any process that affects liver stiffness. MRE cannot be performed on livers with iron overload because of signal-to-noise limitations. Although acquiring MR elastographic data requires several breath-holds, newer sequences should allow much faster acquisition times.

In a comparison of MRE and transient elastography performance in accuracy of staging fibrosis as compared with histologic analysis in a mixed population (N = 146) of chronic liver disease, MRE had greater AUROC values for all stages of fibrosis: F ≥ 1, F ≥ 2, F ≥ 3, F = 4 (0.962 vs. 0.803, 0.994 vs. 0.837, 0.985 vs. 0.906, and 0.998 vs. 0.930). With respect to diagnostic

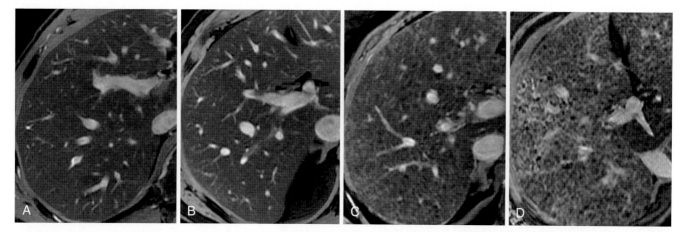

Fig. 15-40 Double-contrast MRI imaging (GBCAs + SPIO) of the liver is an experimental technique to noninvasively assess hepatic fibrosis. Shown are four patients with chronic HCV infection and histology-confirmed stage F1 **(A)**, F2 **(B)**, F3 **(C)**, and F4 **(D)** fibrosis. Notice progressively more conspicuous parenchymal reticulation and nodularity with more advanced stages of fibrosis. The sequential administration of SPIOs and GBCAs to generate double-contrast MR images is off-label, because these agents are not FDA approved for sequential administration.

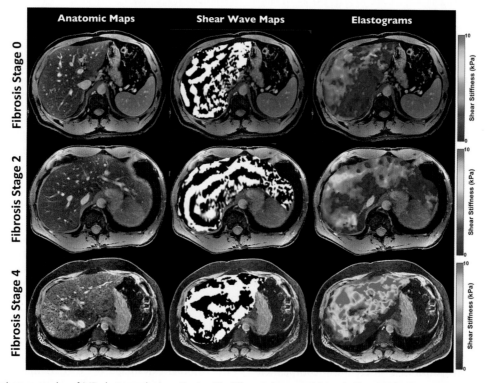

Fig. 15-41 Displayed are examples of MR elastography in patients with different degrees of hepatic fibrosis. The first column contains anatomic reference MR images. The second column contains shear wave maps, from which wave velocity can be measured and used to create the third column of images, elastograms, which estimate the shear stiffness of the liver tissue at each voxel. Fibrotic tissue is more stiff than normal tissue, and will have a higher stiffness measurement (more reds and oranges on the illustrated color code).

accuracy, the advantage of MRE appears most pronounced in the earlier stages of fibrosis where the difference in liver stiffness between stages is smaller. The AUROC value for MRE was 0.93 for F0 versus F1-F2 and 0.98 for F0-F1 versus F2, whereas the corresponding transient elastography values were 0.70 and 0.68, respectively. The ability to separate intermediate stages of fibrosis makes MRE a promising technique for noninvasive clinical assessment of hepatic fibrosis with potential for tracking disease progression and determining efficacy of therapeutic interventions.

Diffusion-Weighted Imaging

Diffusion-weighted imaging is a technique that has long been used for early detection of cerebral ischemia, but until recently, technical limitations such as physiologic motion of the abdomen limited its application in the liver. In DWI, the signal intensity varies inversely with the freedom of water proton diffusion. Imaging of liver fibrosis is based on the postulate that the molecular structure of collagen restricts diffusion of water protons. Several studies have demonstrated the ability of DWI to detect cirrhosis; however, studies

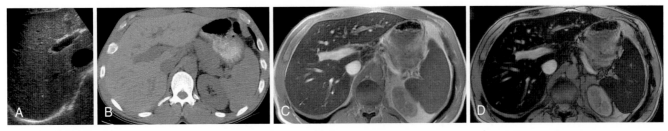

Fig. 15-42 Shown are different imaging studies of a patient with hepatic iron deposition. No abnormality can be detected with ultrasound **(A)**, because this modality is insensitive to the presence of iron. With CT **(B)** there is hyperattenuation in the liver, suggesting the presence of iron, but the degree of iron deposition is unknown. MR images taken at two sequential echo times **(C**, then **D)** illustrate a dramatic loss of signal diffusely throughout the liver in the later echo. This indicates the presence of paramagnetic components within the liver, consistent with iron deposition, but the degree of iron deposition is difficult to quantify based only on these two MR images.

evaluating the ability of DWI to stage fibrosis have shown mixed results.[34,36,37,115,123-127] Like other modalities, using diffusion as an indirect marker of fibrosis makes the technique susceptible to confounding factors such as necroinflammatory activity, steatosis, and significant iron deposits in liver tissue.

Iron Overload

There are a number of radiologic techniques being studied to noninvasively estimate hepatic iron concentration, most of which are based on the paramagnetic properties of iron and the influences those properties have on the MRI signal in the liver. US cannot detect iron deposition in the liver, and therefore there are currently no US-based techniques for this purpose. Although iron deposition can be seen as increased attenuation on CT, this is not readily seen with low levels of iron, and can be confounded by fat deposition, limiting the sensitivity of CT to detect hepatic iron deposits.[128] Furthermore, there are currently no CT-based techniques allowing for the quantification of hepatic iron levels. MR-based techniques focus on the finding that hepatic iron content leads to MRI signal loss, a property known as susceptibility, resulting from paramagnetic effects of iron. The superconducting quantum interference device (SQUID), which is built specifically to measure MR susceptibility, has demonstrated high sensitivity for measuring iron when compared with biopsy[129]; however, these devices are not widely available and require expert technicians to operate. MRI techniques have also been studied extensively as a means of measuring iron's paramagnetic effects, which lead to decreased T_2 and T_2^* relaxation times and decreased signal intensity, resulting in a dark-appearing image (**Fig. 15-42**). Gradient-recalled-echo sequences are highly sensitive to magnetic field inhomogeneity, and therefore tissue susceptibility, and have proven more effective than spin-echo sequences at qualitatively detecting hepatic iron levels[130] (**Fig. 15-43**). Using susceptibility imaging data, calibration curves can be empirically determined between signal loss measurements and iron concentration measurements, allowing for imaging-based hepatic iron quantification. Factors such as inflammation, fibrosis, and fat appear to confound iron measurement, but these confounders are not yet well understood. No single technique currently appears to be accurate across the entire iron spectrum severity, and further work is required before any can be implemented widely for clinical purposes.

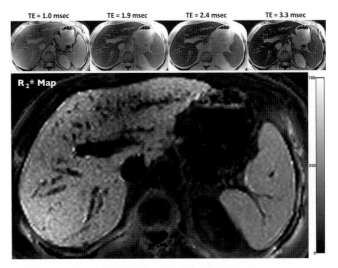

Fig. 15-43 Illustrated is a sequence of MR images designed to measure signal loss resulting from iron deposition. Signal loss can be appreciated as progressive darkening of liver as echo times increase (*left* to *right*). By quantifying this signal loss, postprocessing algorithms can generate R2* maps that, after calibration in patients with known liver iron concentration, can be used to make quantitative estimates of hepatic iron content at each voxel.

Clinical Scenarios: Algorithms for Workup of Focal Liver Lesions

General Principles

In general, there are few evidence-based guidelines to indicate the most effective imaging modality for various clinical scenarios, and even when such guidelines may exist there is likely to be controversy among experts. One factor that limits the creation of universally accepted guidelines is that few studies have assessed the reproducibility of diagnostic performance across institutions and radiologists spanning the spectrum from academic to community settings. Most studies have been done in academic centers by experts, often using specialized equipment with which they are proficient, and the results may not generalize to community practice. Thus the following scenarios are intended to provide general principles and not to be interpreted as rigid algorithms. Individual radiologists and institutions may have differing degrees of expertise and preferences. Thus it is recommended that practitioners (e.g., the hepatologist) consult the local radiologist(s) for guidance on selecting the appropriate workup for individual patients at their institutions.

Scenario 1: An Incidental Liver Lesion Is Found in an Asymptomatic Individual Without Underlying Liver Disease, Risk Factors for HCC, or Known Extrahepatic Malignancy

What Imaging Test(s) Should Be Ordered to Noninvasively Evaluate the Lesion?

Certain lesions may require no further workup. These include simple cysts identified on US, CT, or MRI; hemangiomas with definitive, classic features on US, CT, or MRI; and tiny lesions that are too small to characterize (TSTC) on CT. Lesions TSTC on CT are likely to be epithelial cysts or cystic hamartomas; confirmation could be achieved with MRI but this is rarely indicated because the chance of malignancy for TSTC lesions in this setting is vanishingly small. These TSTC lesions are described by some as "incidentalomas."

Lesions that are indeterminate at initial imaging do require additional workup. These include atypical hemangiomas on unenhanced US or monophasic CT; atypical cysts on monophasic CT; incidental hepatocellular nodules (FNHs, HAs); and some cases of focal fat or focal fat sparing. The appropriate workup depends on the suspected diagnosis based on initial imaging illustrating the size, location, and number of lesions. Atypical cysts on CT can be confirmed using US if the lesion is large enough (>1 cm), if there are only one or a few cystic lesions, and if the lesion is located in an area that is readily visualized by US (i.e., not in a blind spot). If small in size (<1 cm), multiple in number, or located in a blind spot, further evaluation with MRI is preferred.

Most other indeterminate lesions should be worked up with MRI because this technique is usually diagnostic and does not require ionizing radiation. When ordering an MRI for this purpose, hepatologists should indicate whether the suspected diagnosis is an atypical hemangioma or a hepatocellular lesion. Suspected hemangiomas are best evaluated with an extracellular Gd-based contrast agent whereas hepatocellular lesions may benefit from combined extracellular GBCA and HBCA. CEUS can be done as an alternate modality to evaluate atypical hemangiomas and hepatocellular lesions if there is local expertise. Although dynamic CECT may be helpful, it is rarely definitive and uses ionizing radiation; therefore it is not ideal if serial imaging studies are desired for longitudinal stability assessment. CT often requires MRI as a follow-up modality; therefore selecting MRI as the initial imaging study may be more cost effective, although this is an unstudied topic. In summary, unless local expertise with MRI is poor or access to MRI is limited, MRI is preferred to CT for the workup of most incidental lesions, particularly in children and young adults.

Scenario 2: A Patient Has an Extrahepatic Malignancy with a Propensity for Liver Metastasis (e.g., Colorectal Cancer, Breast Cancer, Gastric Cancer, Pancreatic Cancer)

What Imaging Test(s) Should Be Ordered to Noninvasively Determine if the Liver Contains Metastases?

If staging of the entire chest, abdomen, and pelvis is desired, then CT of these regions or PET-CT is recommended. CT is less sensitive in detecting sub-centimeter metastases, however. Therefore if it is critical to accurately identify these, the most accurate modality is probably MRI with a combined extracellular GBCA and HBCA, although there has been a paucity of comparative studies. Furthermore, combined GBCA and HBCA contrast agents may not be available at all imaging centers. In that case, a high-quality MRI with DWI and an extracellular GBCA is more accurate than CT in the authors' anecdotal experience (**Fig. 15-44**).

Scenario 3: A Patient Has Extrahepatic Malignancy Such as Colorectal Cancer with Known Liver Metastasis (e.g., Diagnosed by Scenario 2). The Patient Is Being Considered for Curative Hepatectomy

What Imaging Test(s) Should Be Ordered to Noninvasively Delineate the Number, Location, and Size of Metastases?

Workup of patients for curative hepatectomy requires detection of even tiny liver metastases. For this indication, the most accurate modality is probably MRI with a combined extracellular and hepatobiliary GBCA; however, few comparative studies have been conducted to prove this.

Scenario 4: A Patient Has Cirrhosis or Chronic HBV and Is Considered at Cisk for HCC. The Patient Needs HCC Screening

What Imaging Test(s) Should Be Ordered for Routine Screening for HCC in the At-Risk Population?

The screening guidelines for HCC established by the American Association for the Study of Liver Diseases (AASLD) can be summarized as follows[131]:
1. Surveillance for HCC should be performed using US. Measurement of α-fetoprotein (AFP) level alone should not be used for screening unless US is not available.
2. Screening for HCC should be performed at 6- to 12-month intervals. The surveillance interval does not need to be shortened for patients at higher risk for HCC.

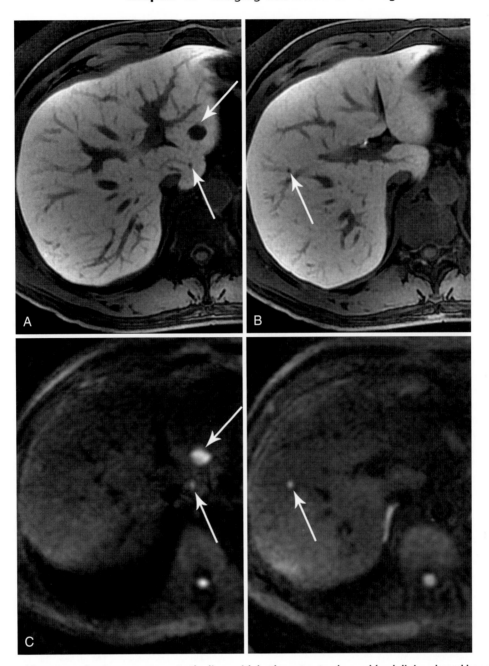

Fig. 15-44 **A patient with neuroendocrine metastases to the liver with both contrast-enhanced (gadolinium-based hepatobiliary contrast agent) and diffusion-weighted MR images.** Two slices with metastases *(arrows)* are shown for comparison between hepatocyte phase **(A, B)** and diffusion-weighted images **(C, D)**. Lesions can be seen with both techniques, because of focal hypointensities in the hepatocyte phase images (attributable to absence of functioning hepatocytes within the metastases) and focal hyperintensities on the diffusion-weighted images (attributable to restricted diffusion and prolonged T_2 relaxation).

The AASLD guidelines argue against the use of CT for HCC screening based upon the following concerns: a screening test is usually not the only diagnostic test of choice, the performance characteristics of CT in HCC surveillance are unknown, there is risk for significant radiation exposure, and there is risk for high false-positive rates. A fundamental flaw in HCC screening strategies that employ US is that this modality has limited per-patient sensitivity (<50% in patients with cirrhosis) and, in particular, the sensitivity for early stage disease (i.e., disease that is likely amenable to curative treatment) is quite low. Practitioners should be aware that patients enrolled in US screening strategies may not be diagnosed until they have progressed to a more advanced stage (and thus may no longer be candidates for curative therapies). Because of these limitations with US, there is a need to develop screening tests that are inexpensive, do not require repeated exposure to radiation, and have a higher sensitivity for early stage disease.

Scenario 5: A Patient Has Cirrhosis or Chronic HBV and a Screening Test Shows a Suspicious Nodule

What Imaging Test(s) Should Be Done to Evaluate the Nodule and Stage the Extent of HCC in the Liver?

The most recent recommendations by the AASLD state that a diagnosis of HCC can be made if a mass larger than 2 cm shows typical features of HCC (hypervascularity in the arterial phase and washout in the venous phase) at CECT or MRI or if a mass measuring 1 to 2 cm shows these features at both modalities. From a radiologic standpoint, the rationale for requiring congruent findings on CT and MRI for nodules that are 1 to 2 cm in size is difficult to justify. CECT and MRI with extracellular GBCA both assess lesion vascularity. As such, discrepant findings between CECT and MRI are more likely to reflect a technological failure of one or both of these modalities than to indicate benignity of the lesion itself. Thus a more rational approach would be to have strict, standardized criteria for a noninvasive diagnosis of HCC nodules using either CT or MRI, but not to require confirmation using both modalities. Such criteria are being developed by the United Network for Organ Sharing and the American College of Radiology. In difficult cases, use of a combined extracellular hepatobiliary contrast agent may be helpful in providing additional biologic information (evidence of hepatocellular uptake in addition to vascularity), but this premise has not been proven. The use of iron oxides to assess RES function and extracellular GBCA to assess vascularity may be the most accurate method in these cases; however, these tests can no longer be performed because iron oxides are not currently available.

Key References

Adam A, Dixon AK. Grainger & Allison's diagnostic radiology, 5th ed. London: Churchill Livingstone, 2007. (Ref.1)

Aguirre DA, et al. Liver fibrosis: noninvasive diagnosis with double contrast material-enhanced MR imaging. Radiology 2006;239(2):425–437. (Ref.120)

Ames JT, Federle MP, Chopra K. Distinguishing clinical and imaging features of nodular regenerative hyperplasia and large regenerative nodules of the liver. Clin Radiol 2009;64(12):1190–1195. (Ref.67)

Andersen ES, Christensen PB, Weis N. Transient elastography for liver fibrosis diagnosis. Eur J Intern Med 2009;20(4):339–342. (Ref.50)

Annet L, et al. Hepatic flow parameters measured with MR imaging and Doppler US: correlations with degree of cirrhosis and portal hypertension. Radiology 2003;229(2):409–414. (Ref.127)

Annet L, et al. Assessment of diffusion-weighted MR imaging in liver fibrosis. J Magn Reson Imaging 2007;25(1):122–128. (Ref.115)

Aube C, et al. Diagnosis and quantification of hepatic fibrosis with diffusion weighted MR imaging: preliminary results. J Radiol 2004;85(3):301–306. (Ref.36)

Bartolozzi C, Battaglia V, Bozzi E. HCC diagnosis with liver-specific MRI—close to histopathology. Dig Dis 2009;27(2):125–130. (Ref.69)

Borra RJ, et al. Nonalcoholic fatty liver disease: rapid evaluation of liver fat content with in-phase and out-of-phase MR imaging. Radiology 2009;250(1):130–136. (Ref.102)

Boulanger Y, et al. Diffusion-weighted MR imaging of the liver of hepatitis C patients. NMR Biomed 2003;16(3):132–136. (Ref.126)

Bruix J, Sherman M. Management of hepatocellular carcinoma. Hepatology 2005;42(5):1208–1236. (Ref.131)

Bugianesi E, et al. A randomized controlled trial of metformin versus vitamin E or prescriptive diet in nonalcoholic fatty liver disease. Am J Gastroenterol 2005;100(5):1082–1090. (Ref.97)

Bydder M, et al. Relaxation effects in the quantification of fat using gradient echo imaging. Magn Reson Imaging 2008;26(3):347–359. (Ref.39)

Carey DG, et al. Effect of rosiglitazone on insulin sensitivity and body composition in type 2 diabetic patients [corrected]. Obes Res 2002;10(10):1008–1015. (Ref.98)

Caseiro-Alves F, et al. Liver haemangioma: common and uncommon findings and how to improve the differential diagnosis. Eur Radiol 2007;17(6):1544–1554. (Ref.61)

Castera L, Forns X, Alberti A. Non-invasive evaluation of liver fibrosis using transient elastography. J Hepatol 2008;48(5):835–847. (Ref.51)

Catalano OA, et al. Differentiation of malignant thrombus from bland thrombus of the portal vein in patients with hepatocellular carcinoma: application of diffusion-weighted MR imaging. Radiology 2010;254(1):154–162. (Ref.78)

Chen MM, et al. Guidelines for computed tomography and magnetic resonance imaging use during pregnancy and lactation. Obstet Gynecol 2008;112(2 Pt 1):333–340. (Ref.42)

Chung YE, et al. Varying appearances of cholangiocarcinoma: radiologic-pathologic correlation. Radiographics 2009;29(3):683–700. (Ref.80)

Colli A, et al. Severe liver fibrosis or cirrhosis: accuracy of US for detection—analysis of 300 cases. Radiology 2003;227(1):89–94. (Ref.114)

Curvo-Semedo L, et al. The hypointense liver lesion on T2-weighted MR images and what it means. Radiographics 2010;30(1):e38. (Ref.65)

Fischer RF. Liver iron susceptometry. In: Andrä W, Nowak H, editors. Magnetism in medicine, a handbook, 2nd ed. Weinheim: Wiley-VCH, 2006. (Ref.129)

Fishbein M, et al. Hepatic MRI for fat quantitation: its relationship to fat morphology, diagnosis, and ultrasound. J Clin Gastroenterol 2005;39(7):619–625. (Ref.103)

Fraquelli M, et al. Reproducibility of transient elastography in the evaluation of liver fibrosis in patients with chronic liver disease. Gut 2007;56(7):968–973. (Ref.119)

Freeman RB, et al. Optimizing staging for hepatocellular carcinoma before liver transplantation: a retrospective analysis of the UNOS/OPTN database. Liver Transpl 2006;12(10):1504–1511. (Ref.73)

Friedrich-Rust M, et al. Assessment of liver fibrosis and steatosis in PBC with FibroScan, MRI, MR-spectroscopy, and serum markers. J Clin Gastroenterol 2010;44(1):58–65. (Ref.117)

Fritz GA, et al. Density histogram analysis of unenhanced hepatic computed tomography in patients with diffuse liver diseases. J Comput Assist Tomogr 2006;30(2):201–205. (Ref.21)

Furlow B. Contrast-enhanced ultrasound. Radiol Technol 2009;80(6):547S–561S. (Ref.13)

Genchellac H, et al. Hepatic pseudolesion around the falciform ligament: prevalence, aberrant venous supply, and fatty infiltration evaluated by multidetector computed tomography and magnetic resonance imaging. J Comput Assist Tomogr 2007;31(4):526–533. (Ref.82)

Gibson SE, Farver CF, Prayson RA. Multiorgan involvement in nephrogenic fibrosing dermopathy: an autopsy case and review of the literature. Arch Pathol Lab Med 2006;130(2):209–212. (Ref.45)

Girometti R, et al. Diffusion-weighted MRI in evaluating liver fibrosis: a feasibility study in cirrhotic patients. Radiol Med 2007;112(3):394–408. (Ref.37)

Girometti R, et al. Relevance of b-values in evaluating liver fibrosis: a study in healthy and cirrhotic subjects using two single-shot spin-echo echo-planar diffusion-weighted sequences. J Magn Reson Imaging 2008;28(2):411–419. (Ref.125)

Goyal N, et al. Non-invasive evaluation of liver cirrhosis using ultrasound. Clin Radiol 2009;64(11):1056–1066. (Ref.8)

Hagiwara M, et al. Advanced liver fibrosis: diagnosis with 3D whole-liver perfusion MR imaging—initial experience. Radiology 2008;246(3):926–934. (Ref.124)

Hamilton G, et al. Effect of PRESS and STEAM sequences on magnetic resonance spectroscopic liver fat quantification. J Magn Reson Imaging 2009;30(1):145–152. (Ref.100)

Hanna RF, et al. Cirrhosis-associated hepatocellular nodules: correlation of histopathologic and MR imaging features. Radiographics 2008;28(3):747–769. (Ref.72)

Health Protection Agency: Radiation CaEH. Diagnostic medical exposures. In: Agency HP, editor. Advice on exposure to ionizing radiation during pregnancy. Oxfordshire: Chilton, 2009. (Ref.25)

Hepburn MJ, et al. The accuracy of the report of hepatic steatosis on ultrasonography in patients infected with hepatitis C in a clinical setting: a retrospective observational study. BMC Gastroenterol 2005;5:14. (Ref.91)

Hines CD, et al. T1 independent, T2* corrected MRI with accurate spectral modeling for quantifcation of fat: validation in a fat-water-SPIO phantom. J Magn Reson Imaging 2009;30(5):1215-1222. (Ref.108)

Huppertz A, et al. Enhancement of focal liver lesions at gadoxetic acid-enhanced MR imaging: correlation with histopathologic findings and spiral CT—initial observations. Radiology 2005;234(2):468–478. (Ref.64)

Hussain HK, et al. Hepatic fat fraction: MR imaging for quantitative measurement and display—early experience. Radiology 2005;237(3): 1048–1055. (Ref.41)

Huwart L, et al. Magnetic resonance elastography for the noninvasive staging of liver fibrosis. Gastroenterology 2008;135(1):32–40. (Ref.122)

Jang HJ, Yu H, Kim TK. Contrast-enhanced ultrasound in the detection and characterization of liver tumors. Cancer Imaging 2009;9:96–103. (Ref.55)

Janica JR, et al. Contrast-enhanced ultrasonography in diagnosing liver metastases. Med Sci Monit 2007;13 Suppl 1:111–115. (Ref.18)

Kamura T, et al. Small hypervascular hepatocellular carcinoma versus hypervascular pseudolesions: differential diagnosis on MRI. Abdom Imaging 2002;27(3):315–324. (Ref.83)

Karahan OI, et al. Hepatic von Meyenburg complex simulating biliary cystadenocarcinoma. Clin Imaging 2007;31(1):50–53. (Ref.59)

Karcaaltincaba M, Akhan O. Imaging of hepatic steatosis and fatty sparing. Eur J Radiol 2007;61(1):33–43. (Ref.89)

Khan SA, et al. In vivo and in vitro nuclear magnetic resonance spectroscopy as a tool for investigating hepatobiliary disease: a review of H and P MRS applications. Liver Int 2005;25(2):273–281. (Ref.48)

Kim YK, et al. Detection and characterization of focal hepatic tumors: a comparison of T2-weighted MR images before and after the administration of gadoxectic acid. J Magn Reson Imaging 2009;30(2):437–443. (Ref.30)

Kinoshita H, et al. Clinical features and imaging diagnosis of biliary cystadenocarcinoma of the liver. Hepatogastroenterology 2001;48(37):250–252. (Ref.57)

Koinuma M, et al. Apparent diffusion coefficient measurements with diffusion-weighted magnetic resonance imaging for evaluation of hepatic fibrosis. J Magn Reson Imaging 2005;22(1):80–85. (Ref.35)

Koroglu M, et al. Biliary cystadenoma and cystadenocarcinoma: two rare cystic liver lesions. JBR-BTR 2006;89(5):261–263. (Ref.56)

Kruskal JB, Kane RA. Intraoperative US of the liver: techniques and clinical applications. Radiographics 2006;26(4):1067–1084. (Ref.11)

Laharie D, et al. Usefulness of noninvasive tests in nodular regenerative hyperplasia of the liver. Eur J Gastroenterol Hepatol 2010;22(4):487–493. (Ref.66)

Lazarus E, et al. Utilization of imaging in pregnant patients: 10-year review of 5270 examinations in 3285 patients—1997-2006. Radiology 2009;251(2): 517–524. (Ref.26)

Lee DH, et al. Diagnostic performance of multidetector row computed tomography, superparamagnetic iron oxide-enhanced magnetic resonance imaging, and dual-contrast magnetic resonance imaging in predicting the appropriateness of a transplant recipient based on Milan criteria: correlation with histopathological findings. Invest Radiol 2009;44(6):311–321. (Ref.74)

Lee JW, et al. Hepatic capsular and subcapsular pathologic conditions: demonstration with CT and MR imaging. Radiographics 2008;28(5): 1307–1323. (Ref.79)

Limanond P, et al. Macrovesicular hepatic steatosis in living related liver donors: correlation between CT and histologic findings. Radiology 2004;230(1): 276–280. (Ref.96)

Liu CY, et al. Fat quantification with IDEAL gradient echo imaging: correction of bias from T(1) and noise. Magn Reson Med 2007;58(2):354–364. (Ref.40)

Manduca A, et al. Magnetic resonance elastography: non-invasive mapping of tissue elasticity. Med Image Anal 2001;5(4):237–254. (Ref.52)

Marin D, et al. Hepatocellular carcinoma in patients with cirrhosis: qualitative comparison of gadobenate dimeglumine-enhanced MR imaging and multiphasic 64-section CT. Radiology 2009;251(1):85–95. (Ref.75)

Mathiesen UL, et al. Increased liver echogenicity at ultrasound examination reflects degree of steatosis but not of fibrosis in asymptomatic patients with mild/moderate abnormalities of liver transaminases. Dig Liver Dis 2002;34(7): 516–522. (Ref.93)

Mazhar SM, Shiehmorteza M, Sirlin CB. Noninvasive assessment of hepatic steatosis. Clin Gastroenterol Hepatol 2009;7(2):135–140. (Ref.44)

Mehta SR, et al. Non-invasive means of measuring hepatic fat content. World J Gastroenterol 2008;14(22):3476–3483. (Ref.84)

Nobili V, et al. Accuracy and reproducibility of transient elastography for the diagnosis of fibrosis in pediatric nonalcoholic steatohepatitis. Hepatology 2008;48(2):442–448. (Ref.118)

Olthof AW, et al. Non-invasive liver iron concentration measurement by MRI: comparison of two validated protocols. Eur J Radiol 2009;71(1):116–121. (Ref.130)

Oudry J, et al. Cross-validation of magnetic resonance elastography and ultrasound-based transient elastography: a preliminary phantom study. J Magn Reson Imaging 2009;30(5):1145–1150. (Ref.54)

Piscaglia F, et al. Real time contrast enhanced ultrasonography in detection of liver metastases from gastrointestinal cancer. BMC Cancer 2007;7:171. (Ref.17)

Pomfret EA, et al. Report of a national conference on liver allocation in patients with hepatocellular carcinoma in the United States. Liver Transpl 2010;16(3): 262–278. (Ref.68)

Qayyum A, et al. Accuracy of liver fat quantification at MR imaging: comparison of out-of-phase gradient-echo and fat-saturated fast spin-echo techniques—initial experience. Radiology 2005;237(2):507–511. (Ref.104)

Radiologists TRCo. Making the best use of a department of clinical radiology, guidelines for doctors, 5th ed. London: The Royal College of Radiologists, 2003. (Ref.23)

Raman SS, et al. Improved characterization of focal liver lesions with liver-specific gadoxetic acid disodium-enhanced magnetic resonance imaging: a multicenter phase 3 clinical trial. J Comput Assist Tomogr 2010;34(2): 163–172. (Ref.29)

Ratziu V, et al. Sampling variability of liver biopsy in nonalcoholic fatty liver disease. Gastroenterology 2005;128(7):1898–1906. (Ref.85)

Reeder SB, et al. Quantification of hepatic steatosis with MRI: the effects of accurate fat spectral modeling. J Magn Reson Imaging 2009;29(6):1332–1339. (Ref.109)

Roche SP, Kobos R. Jaundice in the adult patient. Am Fam Physician 2004;69(2): 299–304. (Ref.3)

Rossi S, et al. Contrast-enhanced ultrasonography and spiral computed tomography in the detection and characterization of portal vein thrombosis complicating hepatocellular carcinoma. Eur Radiol 2008;18(8):1749–1756. (Ref.16)

Saadeh S, et al. The utility of radiological imaging in nonalcoholic fatty liver disease. Gastroenterology 2002;123(3):745–750. (Ref.5)

Sandrin L, et al. Transient elastography: a new noninvasive method for assessment of hepatic fibrosis. Ultrasound Med Biol 2003;29(12):1705–1713. (Ref.121)

Schwimmer JB, et al. A phase 2 clinical trial of metformin as a treatment for non-diabetic paediatric non-alcoholic steatohepatitis. Aliment Pharmacol Ther 2005;21(7):871–879. (Ref.99)

Seale MK, et al. Hepatobiliary-specific MR contrast agents: role in imaging the liver and biliary tree. Radiographics 2009;29(6):1725–1748. (Ref.31)

Sodickson A, et al. Recurrent CT, cumulative radiation exposure, and associated radiation-induced cancer risks from CT of adults. Radiology 2009;251(1): 175–184. (Ref.24)

Solga SF, et al. Hepatic 31P magnetic resonance spectroscopy: a hepatologist's user guide. Liver Int 2005;25(3):490–500. (Ref.49)

Speliotes EK, et al. Liver fat is reproducibly measured using computed tomography in the Framingham Heart Study. J Gastroenterol Hepatol 2008;23(6):894–899. (Ref.94)

Strauss S, et al. Interobserver and intraobserver variability in the sonographic assessment of fatty liver. AJR Am J Roentgenol 2007;189(6):W320–323. (Ref.4)

Strobel D, et al. Tumor-specific vascularization pattern of liver metastasis, hepatocellular carcinoma, hemangioma and focal nodular hyperplasia in the differential diagnosis of 1,349 liver lesions in contrast-enhanced ultrasound (CEUS). Ultraschall Med 2009;30(4):376–382. (Ref.14)

Talwalkar JA, et al. Magnetic resonance imaging of hepatic fibrosis: emerging clinical applications. Hepatology 2008;47(1):332–342. (Ref.53)

Taouli B, et al. Chronic hepatitis: role of diffusion-weighted imaging and diffusion tensor imaging for the diagnosis of liver fibrosis and inflammation. J Magn Reson Imaging 2008;28(1):89–95. (Ref.123)

Taouli B, Ehman RL, Reeder SB. Advanced MRI methods for assessment of chronic liver disease. AJR Am J Roentgenol 2009;193(1):14–27. (Ref.106)

Taouli B, Koh DM. Diffusion-weighted MR imaging of the liver. Radiology 2010;254(1):47–66. (Ref.32)

Taouli B, et al. Diffusion-weighted MRI for quantification of liver fibrosis: preliminary experience. AJR Am J Roentgenol 2007;189(4):799–806. (Ref.34)

Ting WW, et al. Nephrogenic fibrosing dermopathy with systemic involvement. Arch Dermatol 2003;139(7):903–906. (Ref.46)

Trillaud H, et al. Characterization of focal liver lesions with SonoVue-enhanced sonography: international multicenter-study in comparison to CT and MRI. World J Gastroenterol 2009;15(30):3748–3756. (Ref.15)

Tsochatzis EA, et al. Systematic review: portal vein thrombosis in cirrhosis. Aliment Pharmacol Ther 2010; 31(3):366–374. (Ref.22)

Vuppalanchi R, et al. Effects of liver biopsy sample length and number of readings on sampling variability in nonalcoholic fatty liver disease. Clin Gastroenterol Hepatol 2009;7(4):481–486. (Ref.86)

Wang H, et al. Comparison of diffusion-weighted with T2-weighted imaging for detection of small hepatocellular carcinoma in cirrhosis: preliminary quantitative study at 3-T. Acad Radiol 2010; 17(2):239–243. (Ref.77)

Willatt JM, et al. MR imaging of hepatocellular carcinoma in the cirrhotic liver: challenges and controversies. Radiology 2008;247(2):311–330. (Ref.71)

Yokoo T, et al. Nonalcoholic fatty liver disease: diagnostic and fat-grading accuracy of low-flip-angle multiecho gradient-recalled-echo MR imaging at 1.5 T. Radiology 2009;251(1):67–76. (Ref.38)

Yu H, et al. Multiecho water-fat separation and simultaneous R2* estimation with multifrequency fat spectrum modeling. Magn Reson Med 2008;60(5):1122–1134. (Ref.110)

Zech CJ, Reiser MF, Herrmann KA. Imaging of hepatocellular carcinoma by computed tomography and magnetic resonance imaging: state of the art. Dig Dis 2009;27(2):114–124. (Ref.70)

Zhu NY, et al. Feasibility of diagnosing and staging liver fibrosis with diffusion weighted imaging. Chin Med Sci J 2008;23(3):183–186. (Ref.33)

A complete list of references can be found at www.expertconsult.com.

Transjugular Intrahepatic Portosystemic Shunt (TIPS)

Thomas D. Boyer

ABBREVIATIONS

ALT alanine aminotransferase	**HVPG** hepatic venous pressure gradient	**TIPS** transjugular intrahepatic
BCS Budd-Chiari syndrome	**INR** International Normalized Ratio	portosystemic shunt(s)
DSRS distal splenorenal shunt	**LVP** large-volume paracentesis	**VOD** veno-occlusive disease
FHVP free hepatic vein pressure	**MELD** Model for End-Stage Liver Disease	**WHVP** wedged hepatic vein pressure
GAVE gastric antral vascular ectasia	**PHG** portal hypertensive gastropathy	
HRS hepatorenal syndrome	**PTFE** polytetrafluoroethylene	

Introduction

Portal hypertension develops commonly in patients with cirrhosis and is manifested by the development of varices, ascites, or hepatic encephalopathy. Once it was realized that portal hypertension was the cause of many of the above problems, therapies were developed in an attempt to relieve the portal hypertension. The most effective way to lower portal pressure is by use of a surgical shunt that decompresses the portal circulation into the systemic circulation. Unfortunately, patients with cirrhosis are a poor surgical risk, especially if they are actively bleeding or have poor hepatic function. Thus alternatives to surgical shunts have been sought. In 1971 Rosch and colleagues[1] suggested that the creation of a portosystemic shunt within the liver itself may be a way to lower portal pressure. However, it was not until the development of stents to keep the intrahepatic tract open that transjugular intrahepatic portosystemic shunt(s) (TIPS) became a useful method for the treatment of portal hypertension.[2,3] Despite the ability to create an intrahepatic shunt, the role of TIPS in the management of most of the complications of cirrhosis was unclear as recently as 1995.[4] Variceal bleeding that was refractory to medical management was clearly an uncontroversial use of TIPS. However, the role of TIPS in the prevention of rebleeding and in the control of cirrhotic ascites was not well defined. Subsequently, a number of controlled trials have better defined the role of TIPS in the management of a variety of the complications of cirrhosis. Uncertainties, however, remain as to how TIPS should be used for the treatment of some complications of portal hypertension.

Procedure

TIPS are created in most cases by an interventional radiologist, or on occasion by a specially trained physician. The procedure is performed most commonly using conscious sedation, but if the procedure is going to be prolonged or the patient is unstable (actively bleeding varices) then general anesthesia may be required. Before the procedure, patency of the portal vein and the absence of a hepatoma should be ascertained by ultrasound. The success of achieving portal decompression is more than 90% in most series.[5-11] Recently the Society for Interventional Radiology has suggested that successful portal decompression should be achieved in more than 95% of cases, and if the success rate is lower than this number, then the program should review how they are performing the procedure.[12,13]

TIPS can be placed successfully in the sickest of patients, and yet many will die in the immediate postoperative period (30 days). The cause of death in most of these patients is due to disease progression and perhaps to diversion of portal vein flow (TIPS are a side-to-side shunt; **Fig. 16-1**) but is not usually due to complications of the procedure itself, such as intraperitoneal bleeding.[11,14-16] In one large series the incidence of fatal complications directly related to the procedure was 1.7% (range, 0.6% to 4.3%). Institutions performing fewer than 150 TIPS procedures had a higher rate of fatal complications than those with more experience.[11] The exact number of TIPS procedures that need to be performed by an individual before they are proficient has not been determined, but this is one of the more difficult procedures an interventional

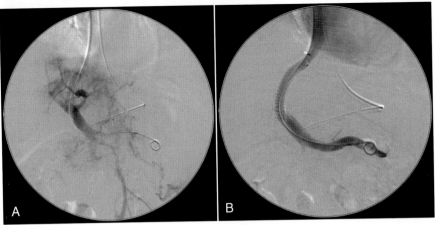

Fig. 16-1 A, Portogram of a patient before TIPS creation is shown with a liver parenchymal blush displaying portal perfusion. **B,** Following TIPS creation, all of the portovenous blood goes through the shunt and the liver is not perfused (i.e., a total shunt).

radiologist performs, and so extensive training and good support by physicians experienced in the management of patients with cirrhosis is required to achieve success.

The gold standard for successful reduction of the hepatic venous pressure gradient (HVPG) in the treatment of varices is to achieve a value of less than 12 mm Hg.[17-19] This goal has been used to define success with both pharmacologic therapy and use of TIPS. However, with pharmacologic therapy, even a 20% reduction of HVPG has a positive effect on the risk of bleeding. Similarly, in one series rebleeding following TIPS revision was 18% in those whose pressure failed to fall, 7% in those with a 25% to 50% decline in pressure, and 1% in those whose pressure fell by more than 50%.[19] In another series, a reduction of the pressure by at least 50% was associated with a rebleeding rate of 11%, whereas lesser falls in pressure were associated with rebleeding rates of 31%.[20] A gradient of less than 12 mm Hg is achievable in most patients, but this appears to increase the risk of hepatic encephalopathy.[20] If the shunts could be tailored to the patients (i.e., those with a high risk of encephalopathy might receive a smaller shunt), perhaps the outcome in these higher-risk patients could be improved.[20] Pending further studies, the goal of TIPS when used for bleeding varices is to lower the HVPG to less than 12 mm Hg. The HVPG that needs to be achieved when the indication is refractory ascites is unclear. This uncertainty is not surprising, as ascites forms in the cirrhotic patient not only because of the portal hypertension but also because of changes in renal and hepatic function. Thus simple decompression may not cure the ascites if hepatic and renal function fails to improve. One suggestion was that the gradient needs to be less than 8 mm Hg to achieve control of the ascites in many of these patients.[21] However, there is no widespread acceptance of this value and further study is required.

In the published studies, it has been difficult to correlate pressure changes with outcomes. One of the reasons consistent correlations have been difficult to obtain is because there is a lack of uniformity on how the pressure is measured preceding and following creation of TIPS. When determining portal pressure using the wedged hepatic vein pressure (WHVP), the pressure is measured in the wedged position and then the free hepatic vein pressure (FHVP) is determined. This allows for the measurement of the HVPG (WHVP-FHVP), which corrects for intraabdominal pressure.[17] After the

Table 16-1 **Contraindications to Placement of a TIPS**
Absolute
Primary prevention of variceal bleeding
Congestive heart failure
Multiple hepatic cysts
Uncontrolled systemic infection or sepsis
Unrelieved biliary obstruction
Severe pulmonary hypertension
Relative
Hepatoma, especially if central
Obstruction of all hepatic veins
Portal vein thrombosis
Severe coagulopathy (INR >5)
Bilirubin >5 mg/dl
Thrombocytopenia <20 000/cm³
Moderate pulmonary hypertension

creation of TIPS, the portal and hepatic veins are connected and most radiologists use the right atrial pressure to calculate the pressure gradient. The right atrium is in the chest, and thus the pressure gradient is influenced by the difference in pressure between abdomen and chest. A true HVPG is not determined when using the right atrial pressure. More accurate pressures would be obtained if the inferior vena cava pressure was used as the intraabdominal reference point, but this has not been accepted by the radiologic community.

Contraindications and Predictors of Survival

The contraindications to the creation of TIPS are shown in **Table 16-1.** Most of these contraindications must be considered relative rather than absolute. For example, patients with congestive heart failure or severe pulmonary hypertension (mean pulmonary artery pressure >45 mm Hg) are not candidates for TIPS because they are not candidates for liver transplantation, and may have worsening of their heart failure or pulmonary hypertension following a transjugular intrahepatic portosystemic shunt procedure (see Chapters 29 and 30). However, patients with mild pulmonary hypertension or a history of heart failure that is currently well controlled may well benefit from the procedure. Similarly, the presence of portal vein thrombosis or a large hepatic tumor is a relative contraindication, but in skilled hands TIPS can be safely created in these patients. When there are contraindications, it is important that experienced physicians are involved in the decision as to whether or not to create a TIPS in this difficult group of patients.

The level of hepatic and renal function is an important predictor of post-TIPS survival, and laboratory tests performed before the decision to create a TIPS should include serum electrolytes, BUN and creatinine, a complete blood count, serum bilirubin, albumin, AST, ALT, and prothrombin time. A Doppler ultrasound should be obtained to document hepatic and portal vein patency and the absence of liver masses. Although pulmonary hypertension and cardiac dysfunction are common in this group of patients, routine performance of a cardiac EKG is not required unless the patient has signs or symptoms suggestive of cardiac disease.

One-year survival rates for patients undergoing a TIPS procedure for bleeding varices vary from 48% to 90%. Survival rates following TIPS creation when the indication has been ascites are somewhat lower, at 48% to 76%.[22-27] A number of models have been created to predict the survival of patients before TIPS creation.[22-26] The modified Model for End-Stage Liver Disease (MELD) was the original model.[24] MELD uses serum bilirubin, International Normalized Ratio (INR) for prothrombin time, and serum creatine. The three variables are used in the following equation: $[3.8 \log_e (\text{bilirubin} [g/dl]) + 11.2 \log_e (\text{INR}) + 9.6 \log_e (\text{creatinine} [mg/dl])]$. Another model was developed based on the findings that four variables independently predicted survival following TIPS. These were: bilirubin greater than 3.0 mg/dl (1 point), ALT greater than 100 IU/l (1 point), pre-TIPS encephalopathy (1 point), and urgency of TIPS (2 points). Patients were divided into three groups (low risk: 0 points; medium risk: 1 to 3 points; high risk: 4 to 5 points) and survival was significantly worse in those who were considered high risk.[23] These two models and the Child-Pugh score were used to predict survival following TIPS in a subsequent study.[27] The concordance statistics for each of the models are shown in **Table 16-2**. All of the models are good at predicting 30-day mortality following a TIPS procedure, whereas MELD is better at predicting long-term survival. Short-term survival time has also been predicted using only bilirubin, the APACHE-II score, and the need for an emergency TIPS procedure.[28,29] Irrespective of which tests are used to determine mortality, the information should be used to decide whether or not the risk of death is too great to perform the procedure in any environment other than a transplant center. Also, patients with a poor 1-year survival prognosis should be referred to a transplant center following completion of the TIPS procedure.

Complications (Table 16-3)

Dysfunction is the most common complication of TIPS placement, and it is dysfunction that creates the need for frequent monitoring and reintervention to maintain shunt patency. TIPS dysfunction is said to occur when there is a loss of the portal system decompression that had been originally achieved by the shunt. Most physicians feel that when the HVPG rises to above 12 mm Hg or the complication for which the TIPS was originally created recurs, TIPS dysfunction is present and intervention is required.[30,31] TIPS dysfunction may be due to either thrombosis or endothelial hyperplasia. Thrombosis of the TIPS may occur within the first 24 hours after creation of the TIPS, and usually within the first few weeks. Thrombosis is observed in 10% to 15% of cases and is thought to

Table 16-2 Concordance Statistics for Prediction of Survival Following TIPS Using Three Models

MORTALITY	MELD (95% CI)	CHILD–PUGH (95% CI)	EMORY[25] (95% CI)
3 month	0.77 (0.61-0.94)	0.77 (0.63-0.91)	0.81 (0.68-0.94)
12 month	0.78*† (0.67-0.89)	0.67 (0.55-0.80)	0.65 (0.55-0.75)
36 month	0.79† (0.68-0.9)	0.70 (0.57-0.82)	0.64 (0.54-0.73)

Adapted from Schepke M, Roth F, Fimmers R, et al. Comparison of MELD, Child-Pugh, and Emory model for the prediction of survival in patients undergoing transjugular intrahepatic portosystemic shunting. Am J Gastroenterol 2003;98:1167–1174.

*MELD significantly better than Child-Pugh.
†MELD significantly better than Emory.

Table 16-3 Complications of TIPS

COMPLICATIONS	FREQUENCY (%)
TIPS Dysfunction	
Thrombosis	10-15
Occlusion/stenosis	18-78
Transcapsular puncture	33
Intraperitoneal bleed	1-2
Hepatic infarction	~1
Fistulas	Rare
Hemobilia	<5
Sepsis	2-10
Infection of TIPS	Rare
Hemolysis	10-15
Encephalopathy	
New/worse	10-44
Chronic	5-20
Stent migration or placement into portal vein or IVC	10-20*

Data from Boyer TD, Haskal ZJ. Transjugular intrahepatic portosystemic shunt (TIPS). Practice guidelines. Hepatology 2005;41:386–400.

*Data taken from experience at time of transplant; incidence probably overestimated.

be due to leakage of bile into the stent, hypercoagulable syndromes, or inadequate coverage of the TIPS tract with the stent.[32-34] The presence of the thrombosis is determined by Doppler ultrasound, and repeat catheterization is required to restore patency. There is little compelling evidence that the use of anticoagulation reduces the incidence of shunt thrombosis.[35,36]

Pseudointimal hyperplasia is common following a TIPS procedure and leads to stenosis or occlusion of the shunt. The reported incidence varies from 18% to 78%, and the latter is more reflective of the experience of most large centers.[6,8,9,37-41] The occluded stent is covered by a fibrinous exudate composed of connective tissue, mesenchymal cells, and a single layer of endothelial cells on the luminal surface.[33,34,42,43] Doppler ultrasound is commonly used to identify TIPS dysfunction due to pseudointimal hyperplasia. Unfortunately, the sensitivity of this test is not very good, varying between 10% and 26%. The specificity is better at 88% to 100%, and the positive and negative predictive values are poor to acceptable.[44,45] When the ultrasound findings are correlated with the presence or absence of TIPS insufficiency based on the pressure gradient, the sensitivity and specificity are even worse, being 86% and 48%, respectively.[46] The most predictive factor for TIPS dysfunction is the recurrence of the portal hypertension for which the TIPS was originally created, including the endoscopic reappearance of varices.[44] A normal ultrasound in the presence of recurrent ascites or varices, or rebleeding from the varices, does not rule out TIPS dysfunction and repeat catheterization of the shunt is required.

TIPS dysfunction has been the complication that has most limited the usefulness of TIPS in the treatment of complications of portal hypertension. In a recently completed controlled trial in which TIPS were compared to the distal splenorenal shunt for the prevention of rebleeding from varices, both TIPS and surgical shunt procedures were excellent methods, with similar rates of survival. However, only 11% of the surgical patients required reintervention to maintain patency, whereas 82% of the TIPS patients required a reintervention.[47] The development of covered stents may reduce the need for reintervention. In one series of 71 patients who received covered stents, the primary rates of patency at 6 and 12 months were 87% and 81%, respectively.[48] Primary patency rates with bare stents would be 30% to 50% at best. A randomized controlled trial has further clarified the role of covered stents in the prevention of TIPS insufficiency. Eighty patients were randomized to receive either bare or polytetrafluoroethylene (PTFE)-coated stent grafts and were followed at frequent intervals with Doppler ultrasound and venography. The probability of remaining free of TIPS dysfunction in the two groups is shown in **Figure 16-2**. Shunt dysfunction was seen in 12.8% of the covered shunts compared with 43.9% of the bare stents ($p < 0.001$). Recurrences of the complications of portal hypertension were also seen more commonly in those receiving bare rather than covered stents, but survival was the same.[30] The PTFE-coated stents are available in Europe and the United States. The use of the PTFE-covered stents does not mean that the shunts need not be monitored. Clearly, TIPS dysfunction will occur irrespective of the type of stent used, and if the patients are not monitored then failure will occur. At this time the sensitivity and specificity of Doppler

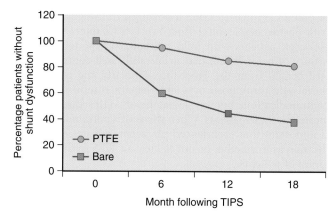

Fig. 16-2 Frequency of TIPS insufficiency using the polytetrafluoroethulene (PTFE)-coated stents versus the bare stents. *(Data from Bureau C, et al. Improved clinical outcome using polytetrafluoroethylene-coated stents for TIPS: results of a randomized study. Gastroenterology 2004;126: 469–475.)*

ultrasound for identifying TIPS dysfunction in patients with the covered TIPS stents are unknown.

Hepatic encephalopathy is another complication of TIPS procedures that has been of concern. De novo or worsening of preexisting encephalopathy is seen in 20% to 41% of cases.[22,30,49,50] Factors predictive of post-TIPS encephalopathy include female gender, hypoalbuminemia, increasing age, previous encephalopathy, and encephalopathy at the time of TIPS creation,[49,50] none of which is an absolute contraindication to TIPS placement. In addition, encephalopathy that occurred because of variceal bleeding is unlikely to recur if the TIPS successfully reduces the portal pressure, and therefore even severe encephalopathy following a variceal bleed should not be considered a contraindication to placing a TIPS. If encephalopathy develops following TIPS placement, most patients respond to standard treatment with lactulose or neomycin. If the patient develops refractory encephalopathy, then either the TIPS can be occluded or its diameter can be reduced to help with the encephalopathy.[51,52] Use of pharmacologic therapy to prevent development of encephalopathy post-TIPS does not appear to be warranted.[53]

During the initial stages of TIPS creation, it is common for the liver capsule to be punctured. Fortunately, serious intraperitoneal bleeding is uncommon at 1% to 2%. Creation of a biliary-venous or hepatic artery-portal vein fistula is rare, as is hepatic infarction due to injury of the hepatic artery.[54,55] Before the TIPS stent is covered with endothelial cells, red blood cells may be damaged during passage through the stent, leading to hemolysis.[56,57]

Indications for Tips

The indications for TIPS creation are shown in **Table 16-4**. The efficacy of TIPS is judged to be excellent if the complication of portal hypertension is controlled significantly better than with other therapies; good if the benefit is balanced by complications such as encephalopathy compared with other therapies; none if outcomes are no better or worse than with alternative therapies; and unknown if there are insufficient data to make a judgment.

Table 16-4 Indications for TIPS

INDICATION	EFFICACY
Primary prevention of variceal bleeding	None
Secondary prevention of variceal bleeding	Excellent (controlled trials)
Refractory cirrhotic ascites	Good (controlled trials)
Refractory acutely bleeding varices	Excellent
Portal hypertensive gastropathy	Good
Bleeding gastric varices	Excellent
Gastric antral vascular ectasia	None
Refractory hepatic hydrothorax	Good
Hepatorenal syndrome	
Type 1	Uncertain
Type 2	Good
Budd-Chiari syndrome	Good
Veno-occlusive disease	None
Hepatopulmonary syndrome	Uncertain

Primary Prevention of Variceal Bleeding

Treatments used to prevent bleeding in patients with varices that have never bled are termed primary prevention/prophylaxis, and β-blockers are currently considered the best therapy for this group of patients (see Chapter 26). Previously, when surgical shunts were developed for the treatment of portal hypertension it was thought that they would be an effective way to prevent bleeding in patients with varices that had never bled. Unfortunately, although less bleeding was seen in the patients who underwent surgical shunting, higher rates of mortality due to hepatic failure were observed compared with the control groups of patients. The increased incidence of hepatic failure was thought to be due to the diversion of portal venous blood away from the liver and into the shunt. As a TIPS is a side-to-side shunt (see **Fig. 16-1**) a similar diversion of portal blood will occur, thereby increasing the risk of hepatic failure. The use of TIPS to decompress the portal venous system before abdominal surgery such as a liver transplant is also without merit, as there is no evidence that this reduces operative time or the need for blood transfusion.[58,59] Thus the use of TIPS to prevent bleeding in patients who have never bled is not warranted.

TIPS in the Acutely Bleeding Patient Who Has Failed Medical Therapy

Acute variceal bleeding is one of the dreaded complications of portal hypertension and is associated with significant morbidity and mortality. Although progress has been made in salvaging this group of patients, 20% will die within 6 months of the variceal bleed.[60] One of the factors most predictive of death is continued bleeding despite medical therapy, or early

rebleeding in the hospital.[61] It has been in the patients who are medical failures that TIPS has been used as salvage therapy. In one report analyzing 15 studies in which TIPS was used to control acutely bleeding varices, bleeding was controlled in 94% of cases.[62] Unfortunately, mortality at 6 weeks was 36%. This high rate of mortality is not unexpected, as urgency is an independent predictor of postprocedure mortality from TIPS.[23] High mortality rates were also observed when surgical shunts were used to control acutely bleeding varices.[61] Preoperative tests of liver function can be used to predict postprocedure mortality (see previous discussion), and these determinations should be made before deciding whether or not a TIPS should be created in the actively bleeding patient. A high risk of death following a TIPS placement is not an absolute contraindication to the procedure in the patient bleeding to death from varices, but the risks should be conveyed to the patient and/or their family before undertaking the procedure. As a TIPS is effective in preventing rebleeding, if we could identify those patients at greatest risk for rebleeding, then perhaps TIPS creation would improve survival. A high HVPG (>20 mm Hg) is predictive of rebleeding and in a trial, patients with high HVPGs were randomized to urgently receive a TIPS or standard treatment. Patients undergoing TIPS placement had significantly better survival as compared with those receiving standard therapy, suggesting that a better understanding of portal hemodynamics may improve outcomes.[63] Most recently clinical characteristics were used to identify patients at high risk of rebleeding and in this population the use of TIPS improved survival compared to medically managed controls. [64]

Secondary Prevention of Esophageal Variceal Bleeding in Patients Who Have Failed Medical Therapy

The prevention of recurrent bleeding in the patient who has bled at least once from varices is termed secondary prevention or prophylaxis. It was this indication for which the TIPS was originally developed. The hope for TIPS compared with surgical shunt procedures was that both approaches would be effective in the prevention of rebleeding, but with lower rates of encephalopathy as the size of the TIPS could be varied to allow for portal decompression but with continued perfusion of the liver. Unfortunately, in most patients, to achieve a pressure of less than 12 mm Hg, 10-mm stents are required, and portal flow is diverted through the shunt. Results of a small controlled trials comparing outcomes according to the size of the stent suggested no advantage and perhaps decrease in efficacy when 8 mm versus 10 mm stents were used.[65] TIPS have been compared with surgical shunts in only one controlled trial and both TIPS and surgical shunts have been compared with endoscopic therapy in a large number of patients. It is useful to compare the two decompressive procedures to endoscopic therapy (**Table 16-5**).

Irrespective of whether a surgical shunt or a TIPS is used to decompress the portal venous system, the rebleeding rates with decompression were significantly better than those seen with endoscopic therapy, but at the cost of an increase in the incidence of encephalopathy and with no impact on survival (see **Table 16-5**).[61,66] The cost of TIPS was greater than

Table 16-5 Controlled Trials of Endoscopic Therapy vs. Surgical Shunt or TIPS and TIPS vs. Surgical Shunt

NUMBER OF PATIENTS	REBLEEDING RATE (%)		ENCEPHALOPATHY		MORTALITY	
	Endo	PCS	Endo	PCS	Endo	PCS
376	49.8	12.4*	8.6	17.2[†]	28.8	28.8
	Endo	TIPS	Endo	TIPS	Endo	TIPS
811	46.6	18.9*	18.7	34.0[†]	26.5	27.3
	DSRS	TIPS	DSRS	TIPS	DSRS	TIPS
140	5.5	9	37	24	38	36

Data from D'Amico G, Pagliaro L, Bosch J. The treatment of portal hypertension: a meta-analytic review. Hepatology 1995;22:332–353; Henderson JM, et al. DSRS vs TIPS for refractory variceal bleeding: a prospective randomized controlled trial; Hepatology 2004;40: presented as late breaking abstract AASLD; Papatheodoridis GV, et al. Transjugular intrahepatic portosystemic shunt compared with endoscopic treatment for prevention of variceal rebleeding: a meta-analysis. Hepatology 999;30:612–622.
*By meta-analysis rebleeding was significantly less with PCS or TIPS than with Endo.
[†]By meta-analysis the incidence of encephalopathy was greater with PCS or TIPS than with Endo.
DSRS, Distal splenorenal shunt; Endo, endoscopic therapy; PCS, Portocaval shunt.

endoscopic therapy because of the need for reintervention to maintain TIPS patency.[67] Similar results were observed when TIPS was compared with pharmacologic therapy. The risk of rebleeding was three times greater in those who received pharmacologic therapy, but the risk of encephalopathy was twofold less than in those who received a TIPS. Survival was the same in both groups, but the cost was significantly higher for TIPS.[68]

Most experts agree that TIPS should be used as salvage therapy for patients with variceal rebleeding who have failed medical therapy, and not as the initial approach to management. Therefore the most important issue with TIPS are how they compare with surgical therapies. There is one published trial in which TIPS were compared with H-graft shunts. Unfortunately, the patients were not randomized but done as pairs, which created a bias in the study. The investigators found rebleeding rates of 16% in the TIPS group and 3% in the shunted group, with no effect on survival.[69] A randomized controlled trial has been published in which TIPS were compared with distal splenorenal shunts (DSRS).[70] The results of the study are summarized in **Table 16-5**; rebleeding rates, the incidence of encephalopathy, and survival rates were the same in both groups. In both series[69,70] frequent reinterventions were required in the TIPS patients to ensure patency and thus prevent rebleeding. A cost-effectiveness analysis of the DSRS versus TIPS trial has been performed.[71] The average yearly costs were $16,363 for TIPS patients and $13,492 for the DSRS patients, values that are similar to what has been reported for endoscopic management of varices. TIPS were slightly more cost-effective than DSRS and use of covered stents had little impact on the cost-effectiveness of TIPS.[71] Both TIPS and surgical shunts are equally effective for the prevention of variceal rebleeding. The choice as to which approach to use should be based on the availability of physicians trained in the procedure and the cost.[72]

Secondary Prevention of Gastric Variceal Bleeding

Gastric varices are difficult to treat because standard therapies such as variceal band ligation and sclerotherapy are ineffective, and in many countries agents such as glue are not available. Using a TIPS has therefore been considered an excellent method for the management of gastric varices that have bled at least once. In a small published series, a TIPS was equally effective in controlling acute bleeding and preventing rebleeding when the indication was either esophageal or gastric variceal bleeding.[72-76] When TIPS was compared with glue, TIPS was more effective but the TIPS patients had an increased risk of hepatic encephalopathy.[77] Care must be exercised when using TIPS in the treatment of gastric varices. If after the creation of the TIPS there is persistent filling of the gastric varices, there is a risk of early rebleeding and the varices should be embolized, as shown in **Figure 16-3**.

Prevention of Rebleeding from Portal Hypertensive Gastropathy (PHG) and Gastric Antral Vascular Ectasia (GAVE)

PHG occurs commonly in patients with portal hypertension, is most prominent in the fundus and body of the stomach, and may be associated with acute and chronic blood loss. GAVE can be seen in patients with and without portal hypertension, is localized to the antrum, and can be associated with severe blood loss in the patient with portal hypertension.[78] TIPS have been used in patients with both PHG and GAVE, and have been associated with endoscopic improvement and a decrease in bleeding in those with PHG but not in those with GAVE.[79,80] Thus if patients have recurrent bleeding from PHG, they are candidates for creation of a TIPS, whereas with GAVE the only option is liver transplantation.

Cirrhotic Ascites

The development of ascites in the cirrhotic patient is due to both portal hypertension and disorders of renal function (see Chapters 25 and 28). Ascites can be controlled in most patients with a combination of diuretics and sodium restriction. However, about 10% will develop refractory ascites, defined as

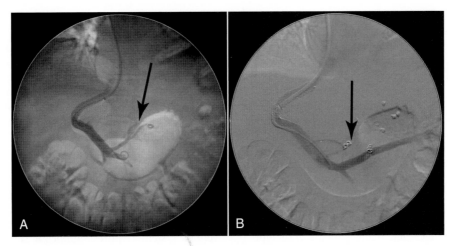

Fig. 16-3 A, Portogram following TIPS creation with continued filling of gastric varices *(arrow).* **B,** Following embolization of the collateral, no further flow into the gastric varices is seen *(arrow).*

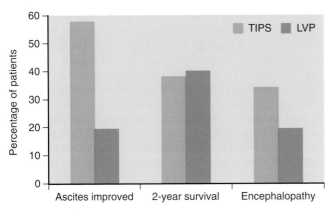

Fig. 16-4 Comparison of TIPS versus LVP in the treatment of refractory cirrhotic ascites. TIPS, transjugular portosystemic shunt; LVP, large-volume paracentesis. *(Data from Sanyal A, et al. The North American study for the treatment of refractory ascites. Gastroenterology 2003;124:634–631; Lebrec D, et al. Transjugular intrahepatic portosystemic shunts: comparison with paracentesis in patients with cirrhosis and refractory ascites: a randomized trial. J Hepatol 1996;25:135–144; Rossle M, et al. A comparison of paracentesis and transjugular intrahepatic portosystemic shunting in patients with ascites. N Engl J Med 2000;342:1701–1707; Gines P, et al. Transjugular intrahepatic portosystemic shunting versus paracentesis plus albumin for refractory ascites in cirrhosis. Gastroenterology 2002;123:1839–1847 and combined, and percent of patients who showed improvement in ascites, survival rates, and encephalopathy calculated.)*

a failure to respond to a high dose of diuretics (400 mg/day spironolactone plus 160 mg/day furosemide), or they develop complications of therapy, such as hyponatremia or renal insufficiency, that prevent a successful diuresis.[81] Once patients develop refractory ascites their prognosis is poor, with 50% dying within a year.[82] A number of approaches have been taken to manage these patients, including peritoneovenous shunts, repeated large-volume paracentesis (LVP), and TIPS. Peritoneovenous shunts have been abandoned because of a lack of efficacy and a high rate of complications. The efficacy of TIPS versus LVP in the control of refractory cirrhotic ascites has been compared in five controlled trials[21,83-86] (**Fig. 16-4**). Ascites was shown to improve in 38% to 84% of patients following a TIPS procedure, and in up to 43% following LVP.

Survival was unaffected irrespective of which treatment was selected, and encephalopathy tended to be slightly more common in those receiving a TIPS (see **Fig. 16-4**). None of the studies looked at cost as a variable. Meta-analyses of these trials have been performed and in one a survival advantage was seen for patients undergoing TIPS creation.[87] In conclusion, TIPS appear to be good at reducing the need for repeated LVP; however, there is no or a questionable improvement in survival and an increased risk of hepatic encephalopathy. Therefore the use of TIPS in patients with refractory cirrhotic ascites should be limited to those who can no longer tolerate LVP or who are developing renal insufficiency. TIPS should be considered a temporizing measure until the patient can undergo liver transplantation. Further studies using covered stents need to be performed to determine if this alters outcomes as to efficacy and survival.

Hepatic Hydrothorax Refractory to Medical Treatment

Ascitic fluid that enters the pleural space via pores in the diaphragm is termed hepatic hydrothorax. In the majority of patients, hepatic hydrothorax develops in the right lung and is responsive to diuretic therapy. Some patients, however, undergo repeated thoracenteses to control their symptoms despite the use of diuretics, and are said to have hepatic hydrothorax that is refractory to medical therapy.[88] Peritoneovenous shunts or thoracotomy, in an attempt to identify and repair the defect in the diaphragm, have had little success in this group of patients. TIPS have been used for the treatment of hepatic hydrothorax in a series of small studies.[89-91] All found that TIPS reduced or eliminated the need for thoracentesis as long as the shunts remained patent. Survival rates, however, were poor in this group of patients, and they should also be considered for liver transplantation irrespective of the ability of TIPS to control the hydrothorax.

Hepatorenal Syndrome

The development of renal insufficiency in the patient with cirrhosis is termed hepatorenal syndrome (HRS) (see Chapter

28) if there is no definable cause such as sepsis or exposure to nephrotoxic drugs. Patients with HRS have a very poor prognosis, and thus serum creatinine is one of the critical components of the MELD scoring system.[24] If the renal failure develops rapidly, over a period of 2 weeks or less, then the patient is said to have type 1 HRS and this group has a very poor prognosis. The more gradual development of HRS is termed type 2, and these patients have a better prognosis.[81,82] Creation of a TIPS is associated with improvements in glomerular filtration rates and renal plasma flow and falls in plasma renin activity and plasma aldosterone levels in patients with cirrhotic ascites, suggesting that TIPS may be an effective therapy for HRS.[92-94] However, despite the creation of a TIPS in patients with type 1 and 2 HRS, survival rates were still poor, being 20% and 45%, respectively, at 1 year.[92] Of greater concern is the fact that many patients with type 1 HRS have high MELD scores or are jaundiced, and thus have a high 30-day mortality following a TIPS procedure. To better define how TIPS should be used in the management of HRS, controlled trials comparing TIPS with other therapies are needed.

Budd-Chiari Syndrome

Budd-Chiari syndrome (BCS) develops because of obstruction to the venous outflow from the liver due to obstruction of the hepatic veins, the inferior vena cava, or both.[95,96] Previously it was believed that the best management of these patients was portal venous decompression using surgically placed side-to-side portacaval shunts. However, more recently it has become apparent that many patients can be managed with anticoagulation alone, whereas for those with more advanced disease, liver transplantation is the only option.[96] Thus the number of patients with BCS who require decompression is limited. Experience suggests that those with chronic BCS and refractory ascites are reasonable candidates for a TIPS. In contrast, in those who received a TIPS for acute hepatic failure caused by BCS, the rate of early mortality was 50%.[97,98] Given the rarity of BCS, it is unlikely that controlled trials will be performed in which TIPS is compared with alternative forms of therapy. Given this lack of data, TIPS should only be used in patients with an intermediate prognosis and refractory ascites, whereas those with less advanced disease can receive anticoagulation and those with more severe disease can receive a liver transplant. For patients with acute hepatic failure caused by BCS, liver transplantation is the best option, and TIPS should only be considered a bridge to transplantation.

Veno-Occlusive Disease

Veno-occlusive disease (VOD) or sinusoidal obstruction syndrome is seen most commonly following hematopoietic stem cell transplantation or after the ingestion of certain plants, such as bush tea. The syndrome varies in severity, with most patients having mild disorders of liver function and weight gain. For others, however, the disease is severe, with the development of ascites and hepatic failure. TIPS have been used in a few patients with severe disease, and in most cases ascites and liver tests improved but the patients still died of multiorgan system failure.[99,100] Thus TIPS are not considered an effective form of therapy for VOD.

Hepatopulmonary Syndrome

Patients with cirrhosis may develop hypoxemia because of the shunting of blood through arteriovenous fistulas in the lung (see Chapter 23). TIPS have been used in a few patients with hepatopulmonary syndrome, and oxygenation has improved.[101] Why creating a portosystemic shunt should reduce shunting in other organs is unclear, and the use of TIPS for hepatopulmonary syndrome is not warranted.

Conclusions

TIPS has become a useful therapy to control the complications of portal hypertension in patients with cirrhosis. The successful creation of a TIPS leading to decompression of the portal venous system requires significant skill on the part of the interventional radiologist. In addition, the decision to create a TIPS in a patient with cirrhosis should be made by a physician skilled in the management of patients with liver disease, in concert with the interventional radiologist. If the patient is at high risk of dying following a TIPS placement, a liver transplantation center should be contacted to determine his or her eligibility for a transplant before a TIPS procedure, except in an emergency. In controlled trials, TIPS have been shown to be as effective as surgical shunts in the prevention of rebleeding from esophageal varices. TIPS are also an excellent way to control acute bleeding in the patient who has failed medical therapy, to prevent rebleeding from gastric varices, and to control refractory bleeding from portal hypertensive gastropathy. TIPS are better than large-volume paracentesis in the control of refractory cirrhotic ascites, but this improvement has no impact on survival rates. TIPS are an effective form of management for some patients with Budd-Chiari syndrome and its effectiveness in hepatorenal syndrome is unclear. TIPS are not indicated in patients with varices that have never bled, for the control of bleeding from GAVE, and in patients with severe VOD or those with hepatopulmonary syndrome.

References

1. Rösch J, et al. Transjugular intrahepatic portocaval shunt. Am J Surg 1971;121:588–592.
2. Rösch J, Keller FS. Transjugular intrahepatic portosystemic shunt: present status, comparison with endoscopic therapy and shunt surgery, and future prospectives. World J Surg 2001;25:337–346.
3. Rössle M, et al. New non-operative treatment for variceal haemorrhage. Lancet 1989;2:153.
4. Shiffman ML, et al. Role of transjugular intrahepatic portosystemic shunt treatment of portal hypertension and its complication: conference sponsored by the National Digestive Diseases Advisory Board. Hepatology 1995;22:1591–1597.
5. Boyer TD. Transjugular intrahepatic portosystemic shunt: current status. Gastroenterology 2003;124:1700–1710.
6. Rössle M, et al. The transjugular intrahepatic portosystemic stent-shunt procedure for variceal bleeding. N Engl J Med 1994;330:165–171.
7. Luketic VA, Sanyal AJ. Esophageal varices. II. TIPS (transjugular intrahepatic portosystemic shunt) and surgical therapy. Gastroenterol Clin North Am 2000;29:387–421.
8. Cello JP, et al. Endoscopic sclerotherapy compared with percutaneous transjugular intrahepatic portosystemic shunt after initial sclerotherapy in patients with acute variceal hemorrhage. A randomized, controlled trial. Ann Intern Med 1997;126:858–865.
9. Sanyal AJ, et al. Transjugular intrahepatic portosystemic shunts compared with endoscopic sclerotherapy for the prevention of recurrent variceal hemorrhage. A randomized, controlled trial. Ann Intern Med 1997;126:849–857.

10. Cabrera J, et al. Transjugular intrahepatic portosystemic shunt versus sclerotherapy in the elective treatment of variceal hemorrhage. Gastroenterology 1996;110:832–839.

11. Barton RE, et al. TIPS: short- and long-term results: a survey of 1750 patients. Semin Intervent Radiol 1995;12:364–367.

12. Haskal ZJ, et al. Quality improvement guidelines for transjugular intrahepatic portosystemic shunts. J Vasc Interv Radiol 2001;12:131–136.

13. Haskal ZJ, et al. Quality improvement guidelines for transjugular intrahepatic portosystemic shunts. J Vasc Interv Radiol 2003;14:S265–S270.

14. Martin M, et al. Transjugular intrahepatic portosystemic shunt in the management of variceal bleeding: indications and clinical results. Surgery 1993;114:719–726.

15. Ring EJ, et al. Using transjugular intrahepatic portosystemic shunts to control variceal bleeding before liver transplantation. Ann Intern Med 1992;116:304–309.

16. Burroughs AK, Patch D. Transjugular intrahepatic portosystemic shunt. Semin Liver Dis 1999;19:457–473.

17. Groszmann R, Wongcharatrawee S. The hepatic venous pressure gradient: anything worth doing should be done right. Hepatology 2004;39:280–282.

18. Boyer TD. Changing clinical practice with measurements of portal pressure. Hepatology 2004;39:283–285.

19. Rossle M, et al. How much reduction in portal pressure is necessary to prevent variceal rebleeding? A longitudinal study in 225 patients with transjugular intrahepatic portosystemic shunts. Am J Gastroenterol 2001;96:3379–3383.

20. Casado M, et al. Clinical events after transjugular intrahepatic portosystemic shunt: correlation with hemodynamic findings. Gastroenterology 1998;114:1296–1303.

21. Sanyal A, et al. The North American study for the treatment of refractory ascites. Gastroenterology 2003;124:634–641.

22. Jalan R, et al. Analysis of prognostic variables in the prediction of mortality, shunt failure, variceal rebleeding and encephalopathy following the transjugular intrahepatic portosystemic stent-shunt for variceal haemorrhage. J Hepatol 1995;23:123–128.

23. Chalasani N, et al. Determinants of mortality in patients with advanced cirrhosis after transjugular intrahepatic portosystemic shunting. Gastroenterology 2000;118:138–144.

24. Malinchoc M, et al. A model to predict poor survival in patients undergoing transjugular intrahepatic portosystemic shunts. Hepatology 2000;31:864–871.

25. Patch D, et al. Factors related to early mortality after transjugular intrahepatic portosystemic shunt for failed endoscopic therapy in acute variceal bleeding. J Hepatol 1998;28:454–460.

26. Ferral H, et al. Evaluation of a model to predict poor survival in patients undergoing elective TIPS procedures. J Vasc Interv Radiol 2002;13:1103–1108.

27. Schepke M, et al. Comparison of MELD, Child-Pugh, and Emory model for the prediction of survival in patients undergoing transjugular intrahepatic portosystemic shunting. Am J Gastroenterol 2003;98:1167–1174.

28. Rajan DK, Haskal Z, Clark TW. Serum bilirubin as a predictor of early mortality after transjugular intrahepatic portosystemic shunt placement: a multivariate analysis. J Vasc Interv Radiol 2002;13:155–161.

29. Brensing KA, et al. Prospective evaluation of a clinical score for 60-day mortality after transjugular intrahepatic portosystemic stent-shunt. Eur J Gastroenterol Hepatol 2002;14:723–731.

30. Bureau C, et al. Improved clinical outcome using polytetrafluoroethylene-coated stents for TIPS: results of a randomized study. Gastroenterology 2004;126:469–475.

31. Haskal ZJ, et al. Sonography of transjugular intrahepatic portosystemic shunts: detection of elevated portosystemic gradients and loss of shunt function. J Vasc Interv Radiol 1997;84:549–556.

32. LaBerge JM, et al. Two-year outcome following transjugular intrahepatic portosystemic shunt for variceal bleeding: results in 90 patients. Gastroenterology 1995;108:1143–1151.

33. LaBerge JM, et al. Histopathologic study of stenotic and occluded transjugular intrahepatic portosystemic shunts. J Vasc Interv Radiol 1993;4:779–786.

34. Saxon RR, et al. Bile duct injury as a major cause of stenosis and occlusion in transjugular intrahepatic portosystemic shunts: comparative histopathologic analysis in humans and swine. J Vasc Interv Radiol 1996;7:487–497.

35. Sauer P, et al. Phenprocoumon for prevention of shunt occlusion after transjugular intrahepatic portosystemic stent shunt: a randomized trial. Hepatology 1996;24:1433–1436.

36. Siegerstetter V, et al. Platelet aggregation and platelet-derived growth factor inhibition for prevention of insufficiency of the transjugular intrahepatic

portosystemic shunt: a randomized study comparing trapidil plus ticlopidine with heparin treatment. Hepatology 1999;29:33–38.

37. Jalan R, et al. A randomized trial comparing transjugular intrahepatic portosystemic stent-shunt with variceal band ligation in the prevention of rebleeding from esophageal varices. Hepatology 1997;26:1115–1122.

38. Sauer P, et al. Transjugular intrahepatic portosystemic stent shunt versus sclerotherapy plus propranolol for variceal rebleeding. Gastroenterology 1997;113:1623–1631.

39. Cabrera J, et al. Transjugular intrahepatic portosystemic shunt versus sclerotherapy in the elective treatment of variceal hemorrhage. Gastroenterology 1996;110:832–839.

40. Merli M, et al. Transjugular intrahepatic portosystemic shunt versus endoscopic sclerotherapy for the prevention of variceal bleeding in cirrhosis: a randomized multicenter trial. Gruppo Italiano Studio TIPS (GIST). Hepatology 1998;27:48–53.

41. Garcia-Villarreal L, et al. Transjugular intrahepatic portosystemic shunt versus endoscopic sclerotherapy for the prevention of variceal rebleeding after recent variceal hemorrhage. Hepatology 1999;29:27–32.

42. Ducoin H, et al. Histopathologic analysis of transjugular intrahepatic portosystemic shunts. Hepatology 1997;25:1064–1069.

43. Sanyal AJ, et al. Development of pseudointima and stenosis after transjugular intrahepatic portosystemic shunts: characterization of cell phenotype and function. Hepatology 1998;28:22–32.

44. Sanyal AJ, et al. The natural history of portal hypertension after transjugular intrahepatic portosystemic shunts. Gastroenterology 1997;112:889–898.

45. Owens CA, et al. The inaccuracy of duplex ultrasonography in predicting patency of transjugular intrahepatic portosystemic shunts. Gastroenterology 1998;114:975–980.

46. Haskal ZJ, et al. Sonography of transjugular intrahepatic portosystemic shunts: detection of elevated portal systemic gradients and loss of shunt function. J Vasc Interv Radiol 1997;84:549–556.

47. Henderson JM, et al. Distal splenorenal shunt versus transjugular intrahepatic portal systemic shunt for variceal bleeding: a randomized trial. Gastroenterology 2006;130:1643–1651.

48. Hausegger KA, et al. Transjugular intrahepatic portosystemic shunt creation with the Viatorr expanded polytetrafluoroethylene-covered stent-graft. J Vasc Interv Radiol 2004;15:239–248.

49. Sanyal AJ, et al. Portosystemic encephalopathy after transjugular intrahepatic portosystemic shunt: results of a prospective controlled study. Hepatology 1994;20:46–55.

50. Somberg KA, et al. Hepatic encephalopathy after transjugular intrahepatic portosystemic shunts: incidence and risk factors. Am J Gastroenterol 1995;90:549–555.

51. Haskal ZJ, et al. Intentional reversible thrombosis of transjugular intrahepatic portosystemic shunts. Radiology 1995;195:485–488.

52. Kerlan RK Jr, et al. Successful reversal of hepatic encephalopathy with intentional occlusion of transjugular intrahepatic portosystemic shunts. J Vasc Interv Radiol 1995;6:917–921.

53. Riggio O, et al. Pharmacological prophylaxis of hepatic encephalopathy after transjugular intrahepatic portosystemic shunt: a randomized controlled study. J Hepatol 2005;42:674–679.

54. Pattynama PM, van Hoek B, Kool LJ. Inadvertent arteriovenous stenting during transjugular intrahepatic portosystemic shunt procedure and the importance of hepatic artery perfusion. Cardiovasc Intervent Radiol 1995;18:192–195.

55. Mallery S, et al. Biliary-shunt fistula following transjugular intrahepatic portosystemic shunt placement. Gastroenterology 1996;111:1353–1357.

56. Sanyal AJ, et al. The hematologic consequences of transjugular intrahepatic portosystemic shunts. Hepatology 1996;23:32–39.

57. Jalan R, et al. Prospective evaluation of haematological alterations following the transjugular intrahepatic portosystemic stent-shunt (TIPSS). Eur J Gastroenterol Hepatol 1996;8:381–385.

58. Moreno A, et al. Liver transplantation and transjugular intrahepatic portosystemic shunt. Transplant Proc 2003;35:1869–1870.

59. Tripathi D, et al. Transjugular intrahepatic portosystemic stent-shunt and its effects on orthotopic liver transplantation. Eur J Gastroenterol Hepatol 2002;14:827–832.

60. Chalasani N, et al. Improved patient survival after acute variceal bleeding: a multicenter, cohort study. Am J Gastroenterol 2003;98:653–659.

61. D'Amico G, Pagliaro L, Bosch J. The treatment of portal hypertension: a meta-analytic review. Hepatology 1995;22:332–353.

62. Vangeli M, Patch D, Burroughs AK. Salvage tips for uncontrolled variceal bleeding. J Hepatol 2003;37:703–704.

63. Monescillo A, et al. Influence of portal hypertension and its early decompression by TIPS placement on the outcome of variceal bleeding. Hepatology 2004;40:793–801.

64. Gracia-Pagan JC, et al. Early use of TIPS in patients with cirrhosis and variceal bleeding. N Engl J Med 2010;362:2370–2379.

65. Riggio O, et al. Clinical efficacy of transjugular intrahepatic portosystemic shunt created with covered stents with different diameters: Results of a randomized controlled trial. J Hepatol 2010;53:267–272.

66. Papatheodoridis GV, et al. Transjugular intrahepatic portosystemic shunt compared with endoscopic treatment for prevention of variceal rebleeding: a meta-analysis. Hepatology 1999;30:612–622.

67. Meddi P, et al. Cost analysis for the prevention of variceal rebleeding: a comparison between transjugular intrahepatic portosystemic shunt and endoscopic sclerotherapy in a selected group of Italian cirrhotic patients. Hepatology 1999;29:1074–1077.

68. Escorsell AM, et al. TIPS versus drug therapy in preventing variceal rebleeding in advanced cirrhosis: a randomized controlled trial. Hepatology 2002;35:385–392.

69. Rosemurgy AS, et al. Transjugular intrahepatic portosystemic shunt vs. small-diameter prosthetic H-graft portacaval shunt: extended follow-up of an expanded randomized prospective trial. J Gastrointest Surg 2000;4:589–597.

70. Henderson JM, et al. Distal splenorenal shunt versus transjugular intrahepatic portal systemic shunt for variceal bleeding: a randomized trial. Gastroenterology 2006;130:1643–1651.

71. Boyer TD, et al. Cost of preventing variceal rebleeding with transjugular intrahepatic portal systemic shunt and distal splenorenal shunt. J Hepatol 2008;48:407–414.

72. Boyer TD, Haskal ZJ. Transjugular intrahepatic portosystemic shunt (TIPS). Practice guidelines. Hepatology 2005;41:386–400.

73. Chau TN, et al. "Salvage" transjugular intrahepatic portosystemic shunts: gastric fundal compared with esophageal variceal bleeding. Gastroenterology 1998;114:981–987.[u2]

74. Rees CJ, et al. Do gastric and esophageal varices bleed at different portal pressures and is TIPS an effective treatment? Liver 2000;20:253–256.

75. Tripathi D, et al. The role of the transjugular intrahepatic portosystemic stent shunt (TIPSS) in the management of bleeding gastric varices: clinical and haemodynamic correlations. Gut 2002;51:270–274.

76. Barange K, et al. Transjugular intrahepatic portosystemic shunt in the treatment of refractory bleeding from ruptured gastric varices. Hepatology 1999;30:1139–1143.

77. Lo CH, et al. A prospective, randomized controlled trial of transjugular intrahepatic portosystemic shunt versus cyanoacrylate injection in the prevention of gastric variceal rebleeding. Endoscopy 2007;39:679–685.

78. Burak KW, Lee SS, Beck PL. Portal hypertensive gastropathy and gastric vascular ectasia (GAVE) syndrome. Gut 2001;49:866–872.

79. Kamath PS, et al. Gastric mucosal responses to intrahepatic portosystemic shunting in patients with cirrhosis. Gastroenterology 2000;118:905–911.

80. Urata J, et al. The effects of transjugular intrahepatic portosystemic shunt on portal hypertensive gastropathy. J Gastroenterol Hepatol 1998;13:977–979.

81. Runyon BA. Management of adult patients with ascites due to cirrhosis. Hepatology 2004;39:841–856.

82. Gines P, et al. Management of cirrhosis and ascites. N Engl J Med 2004;350:1646–1654.

83. Lebrec [u3]D, et al. Transjugular intrahepatic portosystemic shunts: comparison with paracentesis in patients with cirrhosis and refractory ascites: a randomized trial. J Hepatol 1996;25:135–144.

84. Rossle M, et al. A comparison of paracentesis and transjugular intrahepatic portosystemic shunting in patients with ascites. N Engl J Med 2000;342:1701–1707.

85. Gines P, et al. Transjugular intrahepatic portosystemic shunting versus paracentesis plus albumin for refractory ascites in cirrhosis. Gastroenterology 2002;123:1839–1847.

86. Salerno F, et al. Randomized controlled study of TIPS versus paracentesis plus albumin in cirrhosis with severe ascites. Hepatology 2004;40:629–635.

87. Salerno F, et al. Transjugular intrahepatic portosystemic shunt for refractory ascites: a meta-analysis of individual patient data. Gastroenterology 2007;133:825–834.

88. Strauss RM, Boyer TD. Hepatic hydrothorax. Semin Liver Dis 1997;17:227–232.

89. Strauss RM, et al. Transjugular intrahepatic portal systemic shunt (TIPS) for the management of symptomatic cirrhotic hydrothorax. Am J Gastroenterol 1994;89:1520–1522.

90. Gordon FD, et al. The successful treatment of symptomatic, refractory hepatic hydrothorax with transjugular intrahepatic portosystemic shunt. Hepatology 1997;25:1366–1369.

91. Siegerstetter V, et al. Treatment of refractory hepatic hydrothorax with transjugular intrahepatic portosystemic shunt: long-term results in 40 patients. Eur J Gastroenterol Hepatol 2001;13:529–534.

92. Brensing KA, et al. Long term outcome after transjugular intrahepatic portosystemic stent-shunt in non-transplant cirrhotics with hepatorenal syndrome: a phase II study. Gut 2000;47:288–295.

93. Wong F, et al. Transjugular intrahepatic portosystemic stent shunt: effects on hemodynamics and sodium homeostasis in cirrhosis and refractory ascites. Ann Intern Med 1995;122:816–822.

94. Guevara M, et al. Transjugular intrahepatic portosystemic shunt in hepatorenal syndrome: effects on renal function and vasoactive systems. Hepatology 1998;28:416–422.

95. Valla DC. The diagnosis and management of the Budd-Chiari syndrome: consensus and controversies. Hepatology 2003;38:793–803.

96. Murad SD, et al. Determinants of survival and the effect of portosystemic shunting in patients with Budd-Chiari syndrome. Hepatology 2004;39:500–508.

97. Garcia-Pagan JC, et al. TIPS for Budd-Chiari syndrome: long-term results and prognostic factors in 124 patients. Gastroenterology 2008;135:808–815.

98. Mancuso A, et al. TIPS for acute and chronic Budd-Chiari syndrome: a single center experience. J Hepatol 2003;38:751–754.

99. Fried MW, et al. Transjugular intrahepatic portosystemic shunt for the management of severe venoocclusive disease following bone marrow transplantation. Hepatology 1996;24:588–591.

100. Azoulay D, et al. Transjugular intrahepatic portosystemic shunts (TIPS) for severe venoocclusive disease of the liver following bone marrow transplantation. Bone Marrow Transplant 2000;25:987–992.

101. Paramesh AS, et al. Improvement in hepatopulmonary syndrome after transjugular intrahepatic portosystemic shunting: case report and review of literature. Pediatr Transplant 2003;7:157–162.

Section III

Clinical Consequence
of Liver Disease

Hepatic Encephalopathy

Jasmohan S. Bajaj

ABBREVIATIONS

BCAA branched-chain amino acids
BDT Block Design Test
CDR Cognitive Drug Research
DST Digit Symbol Test
EP evoked potentials
FDA Food and Drug Administration

HE hepatic encephalopathy
ICT inhibitory control test
LOLA L-ornithine-L-aspartate
LTT line tracing test
MHE minimal hepatic encephalopathy
NCT-A Number Connection Test-A

NCT-B Number Connection Test-B
OHE overt hepatic encephalopathy
PSE porto-systemic encephalopathy
RCT randomized controlled trial
SONIC spectrum of neurocognitive impairment in cirrhosis

Introduction

Hepatic encephalopathy (HE) is defined as "a condition which reflects a spectrum of neuropsychiatric abnormalities seen in patients with liver dysfunction after exclusion of other known brain disease."[1] In clinical practice, the prevalence of this disorder ranges from 30% to 50% in patients when diagnosed clinically.[2] Several other clinical conditions, such as alcoholic brain damage, extra-pyramidal consequences of liver disease, depression, and fatigue, are often diagnosed as HE given the nonspecificity of this clinical diagnostic pathway.[3] This is a formidable challenge in research and in clinical assessment of patients because there is immense subjectivity in the diagnostic strategies for hepatic encephalopathy clinically.[4]

Historical Background

The relationship between hepatic encephalopathy and ammonia has been noted since ancient Egypt.[5] The Egyptian god Amen was the source of the word "ammonia." A temple to Amen, known as "Ammona" to the Greek, had a cesspool consisting of camel urine, soot, and sea salt, which released heated vapors of ammonia believed to be the source of man and all life.

Hippocrates recognized HE and ammonia as well by describing that "yellow bile causes patients to thrash around." However, the original observation of interorgan ammonia metabolism in the context of HE was made by the landmark experiments of Marcel Nencki and Ivan Pavlov in 1893. Even the latest trend of associating infections with impaired brain function dates as far back as 2500 years ago and reiterated by William Osler in 1892.

Pathogenesis of Hepatic Encephalopathy

HE is considered a multifactorial disorder with several key players that determine the ultimate clinical manifestation.

There is an important role for ammonia in the pathogenesis of HE; however, the lack of consistent correlation between clinical manifestations and ammonia levels means that other factors are important in the development of HE (**Fig. 17-1**).[6] Toxins such as accumulation of manganese, inflammatory cytokines, or mercaptans may be implicated.[7-9] Autopsy and animal studies have implicated changes in neurotransmitter systems, such as neurosteroids, monoamines, and opioids in the hippocampus and frontal cortex in HE.[10-13] In addition to ammonia, the role of cerebral hyperemia has been evaluated in the pathogenesis of the increase in intracranial pressure in acute liver failure, although its effect in chronic liver disease is not as clear.[14] An important role of cerebral and systemic inflammation has been highlighted in recent studies. Sepsis is a frequently encountered precipitating factor for HE and there is evidence that there are worse outcomes and severity of HE in patients with marked inflammation, and in those patients with acute liver failure and those with cirrhosis.[15-17] The development of HE may also be critically dependent on the protein tyrosine nitration by benzodiazepines and reactive oxygen species production by inflammatory mediators. Ammonia-associated neurotoxicity can be modulated by oxidative stress, free radical production, and the activation of NMDA receptors.[18] The source of these free radicals may be caused by ammonia-induced mitochondrial dysfunction and can also result in deficiencies in the blood-brain barrier.[19,20]

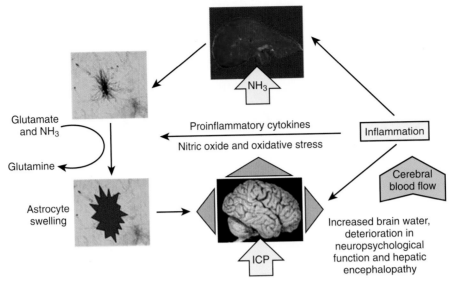

Fig. 17-1 **Pathogenesis of hepatic encephalopathy.**

Table 17-1 Classification of the Subtypes of Hepatic Encephalopathy

TYPE	DESCRIPTION	SUBCATEGORY	SUBDIVISION
A	Encephalopathy associated with acute liver failure	—	—
B	Encephalopathy with portosystemic bypass and no intrinsic hepatocellular disease	—	—
C	Encephalopathy associated with cirrhosis or portal hypertension/portosystemic shunts	Episodic HE	Precipitated Spontaneous Recurrent
		Persistent HE	Mild Severe Treatment dependent
		Minimal	—

Spectrum and Nomenclature of Hepatic Encephalopathy

The range of neurocognitive abnormalities in patients with cirrhosis forms a continuous spectrum that ranges from normal to those who have abnormalities only on specialized testing, known as minimal hepatic encephalopathy (MHE), and those with clinical signs of hepatic encephalopathy, called overt HE (OHE).[21-23] OHE is a syndrome that can be diagnosed by clinical examination and is the familiar "hepatic encephalopathy" that is known to clinicians.[24] These patients have mental status changes that are readily identifiable. However, there are studies indicating that there is a large percentage of patients that are normal by clinical examination but have significant abnormalities on specialized neuropsychometric or neurophysiologic tests. These patients have minimal hepatic encephalopathy (MHE). MHE used to be known as "subclinical HE," a term which has now fallen out of favor.[1]

The Working Group on Hepatic Encephalopathy published their recommendations in 2002 that delineated the major categories of HE for use in clinical and research scenarios.[1] The major categories are shown in **Table 17-1**. For this chapter, we will be discussing the type B and type C hepatic encephalopathy. The temporal and clinical course of persistent, episodic, and minimal HE is shown in **Figure 17-2**. Given the importance and relevance of MHE and OHE, each following section will be divided to reflect these two significant parts of the overall problem of hepatic encephalopathy.

Spectrum of Neurocognitive Impairment in Cirrhosis[4]

There is increasing evidence that the neurocognitive impairment in cirrhosis spans a continuum that ranges from normal cognition and mentation all the way to coma.[1,25] This poses several interesting questions regarding the current methods of diagnosis of HE in the patient population. There are several lines of evidence that spectrum of neurocognitive impairment in cirrhosis (SONIC) actually exists and all that is measurable by pure clinical scales such as the West-Haven criteria are the tip of a large iceberg of neurocognitive dysfunction.[26]

It is also useful to approach this syndrome as a continuum because it then avoids artificial and nonreproducible divisions of patients with cirrhosis into normal HE, MHE, and OHE. However, prospective evaluation of SONIC with respect to clinically relevant outcomes is required.

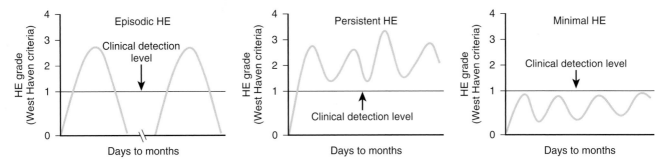

Fig. 17-2 **Temporal and clinical detection relationship of HE subtypes.** *(Adapted with permission from Bajaj JS. Review article: the modern management of hepatic encephalopathy. Aliment Pharmacol Ther 2010;31:537–547.)*

Importance of Hepatic Encephalopathy

The importance of HE lies in its overall prevalence, effect on daily life, and on survival.

Overt Hepatic Encephalopathy

The prevalence of OHE in the United States ranges from 30% to 45% of affected patients, with an annual incidence of 20%.[2] This incidence is associated with a high rate of hospitalization, which has continued to rise. Associated with this high rate of hospitalization is the rising charge per hospitalization. The estimated cost of HE-related disease in the United States between 1993 and 2003 was $932 million, which is a conservative estimate.[2] There is a substantial effect of overt HE on the patients' health-related quality of life (HRQOL), which affects patients mental and physical functioning.[27]

OHE is associated with poor survival rates in patients with cirrhosis.[28] Bustamante and colleagues showed that in those patients with the first episode of HE, the survival rate probability was 42% at 1 year and 23% at 3 years despite controlling for other factors associated with mortality in cirrhosis.[28] Stewart and colleagues found that advanced HE that required hospitalization remained a statistically significant predictor of mortality (hazard ratio, 2.6; 95% CI, 1.7 to 3.8; P <0.01), despite taking into account the MELD score.[29] Therefore, not only is HE an independent marker of mortality, its burden continues to rise in the United States.

Minimal Hepatic Encephalopathy

The estimated prevalence of MHE ranges from 30% to 84% of the patients tested worldwide.[22,30] These estimates vary because of the differing populations and tests used to classify patients as having MHE. MHE has a wide-ranging effect on patients' daily lives and their functioning as productive members of society.[31] Compared with healthy controls and patients without MHE, MHE patients exhibit severe impairments in the psychosocial aspects of social interaction, alertness, and emotional behavior, and on the physical domains of ambulation, mobility, body care, and movement.[32] MHE also adversely affects sleep, work, home management, recreation, pastimes, and eating behavior.[33] This leads to an overall reduction in all aspects of the HRQOL in MHE and engenders several complaints that are voiced in the hepatology clinic.

Earning capacity in patients with MHE is reduced compared with those cirrhotics who do not have MHE.[33] This is especially true for those who have blue collar jobs because the profile of impairment in MHE affects these professions.[33]

Driving skills are considered a balancing act among strategic, operational, and tactical strategies that employ most skills that are adversely affected in MHE.[34] Evaluation of driving skills is sensitive for patients because it could have medicolegal implications.[35] It can be performed using a driving simulator, on-road driving tests, and actual driving outcome results. Studies performed using on-road driving tests in Germany and Japan have shown that patients with MHE are unfit to drive in 52% to 100% of cases when a driving instructor, who was masked as to their underlying psychometric function, assessed their driving.[36,37] A study by Wein and colleagues showed that the instructor had to intervene to prevent an accident 10 times more frequently in MHE patients compared with cirrhotics without MHE.[36,37] Driving simulator assessment has consistently shown in several studies that MHE patients have a higher risk of collisions.[38-40] Their navigation skills on the simulator are also impaired compared with controls and cirrhotics without MHE (i.e., they got lost more frequently while driving).[38] A study of divided attention (i.e., when the patient has to perform two tasks at once, reminiscent of using a cell phone while driving) showed poor ability of MHE patients to "multitask" while driving.[38] Simulator studies also highlighted the difficulty with fatigue in patients with MHE in which there were significantly higher collisions during the second half of a 25-minute simulator task compared with the first half.[38,39]

Actual driving accidents and violations in cirrhosis were investigated using both anonymous and identified questionnaires.[41,42] Patients with MHE responding to anonymous questionnaires had a significantly higher rate of traffic accidents and violations over the last 1 and 5 years compared with those without MHE and those who were actively drinking alcohol.[41] A recent study citing data from the patient's own statements and department of transportation records showed that patients with cirrhosis who had an abnormal performance on the inhibitory control test (ICT) had a significantly higher risk of traffic accidents over the past 1 year compared with those who were normal. On prospective follow-up, patients diagnosed with MHE by the ICT and those with prior driving offenses were significantly more likely to be in traffic accidents.[42] Interestingly, there was no significant difference between the patient's admission of accidents and the official

Table 17-2 Use of Testing Modalities to Divide Patients with Cirrhosis into Normal, Minimal, and Overt Hepatic Encephalopathy

	NORMAL FUNCTION	MHE	EARLY OHE	LATE OHE
Psychometric testing	Normal	Abnormal	Abnormal	Not required
Neurophysiologic testing	Normal	Abnormal	Abnormal	Not required
Clinical examination	Normal	Normal	Abnormal	Abnormal

driving record.[42] Another aspect of the driving assessment is the lack of insight patients with MHE have regarding their driving skills; patients with MHE consider themselves to be significantly better drivers than adult observers who were familiar with their driving skills. In contrast, patients without MHE and controls had personal driving skill assessments similar to their adult observers.[40] [u1] Driving skills for those with MHE, therefore, are affected right from the simulator to the actual driving outcomes, and studies are needed to assess the effects of treatment on the skills of these individuals.

Diagnosis of Hepatic Encephalopathy

There are two levels of functional impairment in hepatic encephalopathy, both of which are important to diagnose[43]:

1. Impairment in mental status
2. Impairment in neuropsychological and neurophysiologic function

As the concept of SONIC, which treats HE as a continuum, demonstrates, there is some evidence that the process of HE is initially subclinical and purely in the neuropsychological domain. However, as liver disease progresses, it bursts onto the clinical realm and is diagnosable clinically.[4] The table shows the stages in which these tests (neuropsychometric and neurophysiologic) would be appropriate as opposed to simple clinical examination (**Table 17-2**).

Clinical Diagnosis of Hepatic Encephalopathy

Pure clinical diagnostic strategies for HE are flawed because of their inherent subjectivity.[44] The West-Haven Criteria, which are modifications of the original Parsons-Smith criteria, are the most recognized system for clinical classification of HE (**Table 17-3**).[4,44] They divide patients into grade 0, which is normal, through grade 4, which is a coma (**Fig. 17-3**).

Physical Examination in Patients with HE

There is considerable variation in the physical examination of patients with cirrhosis, and the depth of the examination can often reveal signs of extrapyramidal disorders or changes in ocular movements that are consistent with liver disease-associated cognitive impairment.[45] OHE tends to be a global process; therefore a previously unknown focal motor deficit is not considered typical. Hyperreflexia, positive Babinski sign,

Table 17-3 West-Haven Criteria for the Diagnosis of Hepatic Encephalopathy

STAGE	DISTINGUISHING FEATURES
0	No abnormality detected
I	Trivial lack of awareness Euphoria or anxiety Shortened attention span Impairment of addition or subtraction
II	Lethargy or apathy Disorientation for a time Obvious personality change Inappropriate behavior
III	Somnolence to semistupor Responsive to stimuli Confused Gross disorientation Bizarre behavior
IV	Coma, unable to test mental state

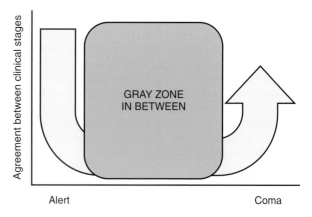

DIFFICULTIES WITH CLINICAL SYSTEMS

GRAY ZONE IN BETWEEN

Alert — Coma

Agreement between clinical stages

Fig. 17-3 Staging of hepatic encephalopathy and the means of diagnosis. *(Adapted with permission from Bajaj JS, Wade JB, Sanyal AJ. Spectrum of neurocognitive impairment in cirrhosis: implications for the assessment of hepatic encephalopathy. Hepatology 2009;50:2014–2021.)*

and asterixis are neurologic signs often found in overt HE.[46] Asterixis is defined as a flapping tremor associated with the disturbance in the oscillatory networks in the brain that is seen in the tongue, and in the upper and lower extremities.[24] Tremulousness due to alcohol abuse or withdrawal can be confused with asterixis, and the nonspecificity of asterixis, which can also be found in carbon dioxide intoxication and uremia, should always be kept in mind.[43]

Clinical Classification of HE into Normal and Overt HE

The West Haven Criteria are not consistent in their application and have poor reproducibility, apart from the extremes of consciousness.[47] For patients in coma, the Glasgow Coma Scale has been used to further analyze the patient's situation.[24] The clinical hepatic encephalopathy staging scale (CHESS)—a nine-question scale—and the hepatic encephalopathy scoring algorithm (HESA), a blended psychometric/question scale, are promising for mental status assessment but are currently in the process of validation.[47,48] However, a large intermediate area of uncertainty remains between the extremes of normal cognition and coma that is not resolved using pure clinical scales (**Fig. 17-4**).

Differentiation between Stage 0 and Stage 1 of the West-Haven Criteria

Stage 0, which consists of normal and MHE individuals (i.e., patients without any clinical signs of OHE), is difficult to differentiate from stage I of overt HE because of their nonspecificity. Therefore even the differentiation between clinically "normal" and early HE is difficult using pure clinical scales.

Diagnosis of MHE

The major modes of MHE diagnosis employ either neuropsychometric testing or neurophysiologic testing, or a combination of both (**Fig. 17-5**).

Neuropsychologic Examination and Psychometric Testing for the Diagnosis of MHE

MHE has a specific deficit profile on psychometric testing, which includes predominantly attention deficits.[26,49-51] The attentional hierarchy as described by Posner is impaired at all levels of vigilance, orienting, and executive functions. Attention deficits also result in learning impairment and difficulty in working memory.[37] There is also a defect in visuo-motor coordination and construction ability, and in the speed of mental processing.[52] Underlying most of these deficits is the impairment of response inhibition similar to patients with attention-deficit disorder, which has led to the use of the inhibitory control test.[53-55]

Neuropsychometric testing for HE concentrates on the evaluation of these specific spheres. There are several batteries for the diagnosis of HE that have been studied, all of which

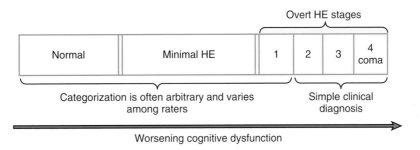

Fig. 17-4 **Problems with relying on clinical systems of classifying hepatic encephalopathy alone.** (Adapted with permission from Bajaj JS, Wade JB, Sanyal AJ. Spectrum of neurocognitive impairment in cirrhosis: implications for the assessment of hepatic encephalopathy. Hepatology 2009;50:2014–2021.)

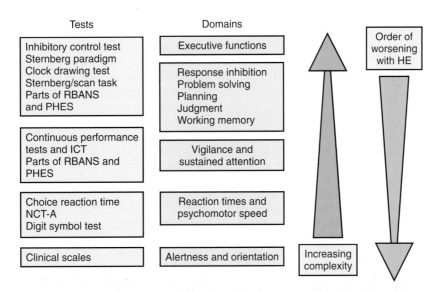

Fig. 17-5 **Tests for evaluation of hepatic encephalopathy and their worsening with progression of hepatic encephalopathy.** (Adapted with permission from Bajaj JS, Wade JB, Sanyal AJ. Spectrum of neurocognitive impairment in cirrhosis: implications for the assessment of hepatic encephalopathy. Hepatology 2009;50:2014–2021.)

are based on detecting deficits in attention and processing speed.[1]

The PSE syndrome test used by Weissenborn and colleagues has been validated for the diagnosis of MHE in Germany, Italy, and Spain.[26,52,56] It consists of six measures: Number Connection Test-A (NCT-A), Number Connection Test-B (NCT-B), Line Drawing Test errors and time, Serial Dotting Test, and Digit Symbol Test (DST). Test results within the ± 1 SD range are score 0; between 1 and 2 SD are -1 point; between 2 and 3 SD, -2 points; and beyond 3 SD is scored -3. Results better than the mean plus 1 SD are given 1 point; therefore $+6$ to -18 points is the range of scores. The cutoff between normal and pathologic results was found to be -4 points, which resulted in a sensitivity of 96% and 100% specificity. This battery has also been recommended by the Working Group on Hepatic Encephalopathy.[1] However, validation of this in the United States has not been performed to date.

The PSE syndrome test highlights different and complementary aspects of cognitive dysfunction that are found in MHE. The Digit Symbol Test is a test of associative learning; graphomotor speed, cognitive processing speed, visual perception, and working memory while the serial dotting and line tracing test evaluate motor speed and accuracy. The NCT-A test for deficits in visual scanning efficiency, sequencing, attention, and concentration. NCT-B analyzes attention, set shifting ability, psychomotor speed, visual scanning efficiency, sequencing, and concentration.[26]

The working group also recommended that if the PSE syndrome test was not available, a combination of two of the following four tests should be used: NCT-A, NCT-B, DST, or BDT. A convention for diagnosis of PSE is impairment in at least two of these tests that is two standard deviations below age- and education-matched healthy controls.[1]

A recent consensus statement of the thirteenth ISHEN meeting recommended the use of the Repeatable Battery for Assessment of Neuropsychological Status (RBANS), or the PSE syndrome test.[57] RBANS is a copyrighted set of tests consisting of five domains: immediate memory, delayed memory, attention, visuo-spatial skills, and language. This battery has been used for the evaluation of Alzheimer disease, schizophrenia, and traumatic brain injury, and in a selected population of patients with cirrhosis awaiting liver transplantation.[58] However, it has not been specifically validated in HE.[59]

Neurophysiologic Tests for the Diagnosis of MHE

Neurophysiologic tests are usually performed under the supervision of a neurologist and require specialized equipment, personnel, and time. Their relative advantages are the lack of learning effects and the relative specificity of the results.[1,4,56] However, the need for expensive equipment, low sensitivity, and the lack of accompanying behavioral information are drawbacks.[60] These tests can run the gamut from an electroencephalogram (EEG) to automated evoked potentials. The characteristic "triphasic waves" are noted on EEG only in advanced HE.[56] Techniques such as spectral EEG, mean dominant frequency, and peak power frequency of EEG have been studied but have demonstrated subjectivity.[61] In the earlier stages, the mean dominant frequency and spectral EEG analysis can predict the development of OHE. However, because EEG studies only cortical activity, there is limited concordance

among it and batteries such as the PSE syndrome test that rely on cortical and subcortical components.[62] The techniques that show the most promise are the evoked potentials (EP) that gauge the latency between application of a stimulus and the brain's ability to sense it. EPs studied in HE are visual, somatosensory, and auditory.[63] Visual evoked potentials that require active patient cooperation are insensitive to change in HE and therefore are only useful for early stages of HE. Abnormalities in somatosensory evoked potential are seen in 48% with abnormal interpeak latencies N20-N65, but there was no correlation with psychometric tests in later studies. Brain electrical responses in response to visual or auditory stimulus are also important means of gauging HE.[64] An auditory P300 is when a patient receives an infrequent stimulus embedded in other frequent stimuli ("oddball" paradigm). The brain shows a response typically 300 ms after the oddball stimulus; delay in brain response (i.e., after a 300-ms gap) signifies dysfunction. Auditory P300 does have good diagnostic potential and can be used when available for evaluation of neurophysiologic function in cirrhosis. Visual P300 responses, however, are not recommended due to their inconsistent results.[64]

Limitations of Currently Available Psychometric and Neurophysiologic Tests

The tests noted above, both psychometric and neurophysiologic, are available; however, they are copyrighted and need specialized personnel and equipment for administration and interpretation.[4] Therefore studies have been performed for tests that can be applied in the clinical setting by nonspecialized personnel. These tests are the critical flicker frequency (neurophysiologic test) and two computerized psychometric test systems: the Cognitive Drug Research (CDRS) and the inhibitory control tests.

Tests Applicable in the Clinical Setting that Do Not Require Psychological Expertise

Critical flicker frequency (CFF) is a test of retinal gliopathy (that occurs in patients with HE) that can be performed using a portable machine.[25] During this test, the patient is asked to indicate the maximum frequency at which they can still perceive the light as flickering while changing the frequency over time. A CFF threshold of 38 to 39 Hz has been shown to differentiate between manifest HE (i.e., early stages of OHE) and no HE; it was less sensitive in differentiating MHE from manifest HE. This test has been tested in Spain and India as well, with good results, but has not been validated for the U.S. population.[65] Encouragingly, it can be performed by clinic personnel without the need for a psychologist within a short period of time, and apart from the equipment, has minor costs.

The CDR consists of five psychometric subsets that test attention power, attention continuity, speed of memory, and quality of episodic and working memory. This battery has been developed by Cognitive Drug Research (CDR) Ltd. (Goring-on-Thames, United Kingdom).[66] These tests have 50 parallel forms and have population norms for the U.K. A recent study compared the CDR with the PSE syndrome test and showed improvement after liver transplantation and worsening after a nitrogen challenge. In this study, MHE patients were impaired in all subsets and there was worsening of the quality of working and episodic memory after a nitrogen challenge. CDR will be available from the U.K. at an assessment cost of £30 ($46).[66]

The inhibitory control test (ICT) is a computerized test that analyzes response inhibition, working memory, and sustained attention, which has been used in the description of traumatic brain injury, schizophrenia, and attention deficit disorder.[67] ICT consists of 1728 stimuli, 40 lures, and 212 targets that is presented within 13 minutes after a training run. A higher lure and lower target rate represents worse psychometric performance. ICT has been validated in the U.S. population with 88% sensitivity for the diagnosis of MHE.[55,68] ICT also predicted the development of OHE and changed appropriately with the clinical state of the patients (i.e., improved after therapy and worsened after shunting procedures) and it was also significantly associated with driving simulator performance and traffic accidents in the United States.[42,55,68] It may be appropriate for MHE testing at the clinic level in a U.S. population and is currently available for free download at www.hecme.tv.

An overview of available tests is shown in **Table 17-4**.

Treatment of Hepatic Encephalopathy

The management of HE has undergone relatively few changes for more than 30 years, until fairly recently when the influx of newer therapies rejuvenated the field with respect to therapeutic options. A review of current and past therapies is displayed below, and several new products are in the pipeline (**Tables 17-7 to 17-12**).

Goals for the Management of Hepatic Encephalopathy

Due to the multifaceted presentations of patients with HE, the goals of treatment differ between the management of an acute OHE episode and patients who have already recovered from an acute OHE episode (**Fig. 17-6**).

The goals in patients who have a current overt HE episode are:
1. Confirm the diagnosis of HE
2. Identify and treat possible precipitating factors
3. Reduce the duration of hospitalization
4. Consider evaluation for liver transplant

The goals in outpatients who have recovered from an overt HE episode are:
1. Prevent future recurrence of HE episodes
2. Improve quality of life and maximize productivity of the patient
3. Consider evaluation for liver transplant

Management of the Acute HE Episode

Based on the goals above, the overall therapeutic focus of an OHE episode should broadly progress on two fronts concurrently[43]:
1. Confirmation of the diagnosis of HE
2. Search for potential precipitating factors and therapy of those factors

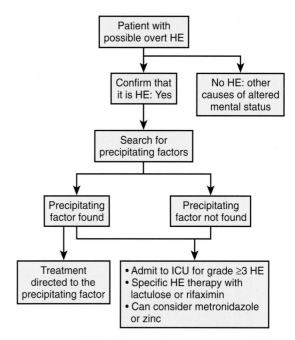

Fig. 17-6 **Proposed algorithm for the management of the acute episode of hepatic encephalopathy.** *(Adapted with permission from Bajaj JS. Review article: the modern management of hepatic encephalopathy. Aliment Pharmacol Ther 2010;31:537–547.)*

Complicating these situations are those in which the precipitating factor (e.g., sepsis can also mimic HE, including development of septic encephalopathy). Therefore the management of HE should be both aggressive and insightful.

It is also useful to devolve the management strategies of the episode into the following series of questions:
1. Is this HE or is there another reason for the altered mental status?
2. Are there any obvious precipitating factors?
3. Does the patient require hospital admission?
4. If hospitalized, should the patient be admitted to the floor or the intensive care unit?
5. Does the patient need intubation?
6. Should the lactulose be administered orally or by enema?
7. When should be therapies other than lactulose be considered?
8. How often should the ammonia levels be checked, if at all?

After it is confirmed that the patient has HE and while the search for a precipitating factor is going on, the patients should be assessed for consciousness, orientation, and ability to protect the airway (**Tables 17-5 and 17-6**). Patients that exhibit grade 3 or higher HE according to the West-Haven criteria should be transferred to the intensive care (ICU) or a step-down unit because by definition they are at risk from an airway standpoint. Patients with stage 2 (i.e., disorientation) should be admitted to the hospital in most cases to evaluate potential serious precipitating factors. There should be a low threshold for airway intubation in patients in the ICU, especially those with GI bleeding. A thorough evaluation for infections, including diagnostic paracentesis, culturing of urine and blood, chest x-ray, and skin examination for possible cellulitis, should be carried out. Patients with diarrhea could also benefit from stool analysis for *Clostridium difficile*. There is

Table 17-4 Logistic Issues with Currently Available Psychometric Tests

TEST	DOMAINS TESTED	U.S. NORMS	COPYRIGHT	SPECIALIZED EXPERTISE (PSYCHOLOGY/NEUROLOGY) NEEDED	TIME FOR ADMINISTRATION INTERPRETATION	SPECIFIC COMMENTS
Paper/Pencil Tests						
NCT-A (number connection test-A)	Psychomotor speed	+	No	No	30-120 sec	Poor specificity
NCT-B (number connection test-B)	Psychomotor speed, set shifting, divided attention	–	Yes	Yes	1-3 min	More specific than NCT-A but is not pathognomonic for any disorder
BDT (block design test)	Visuo-spatial reasoning, praxis, psychomotor speed	+	Yes	Yes	10-20 min	Can be used for dementia testing as well
DST (digit symbol test)	Psychomotor speed, attention	+	Yes	Yes	2 min	Tends to be very sensitive and is an early indicator
LTT (line tracing test)	Psychomotor speed, visuo-spatial	–	Yes	No	10 min	Outcomes are errors and time; tests a balance between speed and accuracy
SDT (serial dotting test)	Psychomotor speed	–	Yes	No	1-4 min	Only tests psychomotor speed
RBANS (Repeatable Battery for Assessment of Neuro-psychological Status)	Verbal/visual/working memory, visuo-spatial, language, and psychomotor speed	+	Yes	Yes	35 min	Has been primarily studied in dementia and brain injury, current trials with HE are underway
Computerized Tests						
ICT	Response inhibition, working memory, vigilance, attention	Limited norms	No	No	15 min	Need highly functional patients
CDRS	Attention, episodic and working memory	–	Yes	No	15-20 min	Familiarity with computers may be needed
Sternberg paradigm or scan test	Working memory, vigilance, attention	–	Yes	No	10-15 min	
Neurophysiologic Tests						
EEG MDF and spectral index	Generalized brain activity	Local norms	No	Yes	Different ranges	Can be performed in comatose patients
Visual evoked potentials	Interval between visual stimulus and activity	Local norms	No	Yes	Different ranges	Highly variable and poor overall results
Brainstem auditory evoked potentials	Response in the cortex after auditory click stimuli	Local norms	No	Yes	Different ranges	Inconsistent response with HE testing/prognostication
P300 cognitive evoked potentials	An infrequent stimulus embedded in irrelevant stimuli is studied	Local norms	No	Yes	Different ranges	Good diagnostic potential but requires patient cooperation
CFF	Visual discrimination and general arousal	–	No	No	10 min	Need highly functional patients

Adapted from Bajaj JS, Wade JB, Sanyal AJ. Spectrum of neurocognitive impairment in cirrhosis: implications for the assessment of hepatic encephalopathy. Hepatology 2009;50:2014-2021.

BDT, block design test; CDR, cognitive disease research; CFF, critical flicker fusion frequency; DST, digit symbol test; EEG, electroencephalogram; ICT, inhibitory control test; LDT, line drawing test; NCT-A, number connection tests A/B; MDF, mean dominant frequency; RBANS, Repeatable Battery for Assessment of Neuropsychological Status; SDT, serial dotting test. Expense for each test depends on local availability, and the need for copyrighted test materials and computers. Upfront costs may be minimal if these tests are used often.

Table 17-5 Differential Diagnosis of Altered Mental Status in Cirrhosis

Intracranial hematomas	Encephalitis
Thyroid dysfunction	Severe sepsisb
Acidosis	Uremia
Drug intoxication	Hypoxia
Hypoglycemia	Hypercapnia
Hyperglycemia	

Table 17-6 Precipitating Factors Associated with HE

Hyponatremia	Sedative drugs (including
Gastrointestinal bleeding	narcotics, sleep aids,
Infection	antihistaminics)
Surgery	Alkalosis
Dehydration	Azotemia
Fluid restriction	Hypokalemia
Diuretics	Excessive protein intake
Excessive paracentesis	Constipation
Vomiting	
Diarrhea	

Table 17-7 Treatment Summary

First Line

Lactulose or Lactitol

Episode of HE (Stage 2 or higher)—enemas: 300 ml in 1000 ml every 2 hours until clinical improvement
Episode of HE (able to tolerate oral)—oral: 45 ml each hour until bowel movement and clinical improvement
Outpatient therapy: 15-45 ml tid or bid until two to three bowel movements per day

Second Line

Rifaximin (Level I)

Outpatient therapy/episode of HE—oral: 400-550 mg PO bid
Neomycin (Level III)
Episode of HE—oral: 1 g every 6 hours for up to 6 days
Outpatient therapy—oral: 1-2 g/day
Metronidazole (Level III)
Outpatient therapy—oral: 250 mg bid

Third Line

Sodium benzoate (Level II-III)

Outpatient therapy—oral: titrate up to clinical improvement or a maximum dose of 5 g bid
Elemental zinc from zinc gluconate, zinc sulfate, and zinc acetate (Level II-III)
Outpatient therapy—oral: 11 mg in adult males and 8 mg in adult females every day

Bromocriptine (Level III)

Outpatient therapy—oral: 30 mg bid

Fourth Line

Outpatient therapy—surgical obliteration of large spontaneous portosystemic anatomoses, splenic artery embolization, or total colectomy

currently no role for prophylactic antibiotics in patients admitted with HE unless there is evidence of GI bleeding or sepsis. Metabolic abnormalities should be corrected as noticed and hydration should be gentle to prevent pulmonary fluid overload. A review of the patient's mental status should be performed at least three times especially in patients who are admitted to the floor.

The mainstay of the diagnosis in an acute episode of HE is essentially the exclusion of other known causes of cerebral dysfunction. As mentioned above, the diagnostic criteria are combinations of historical, clinical, and examination-based clues with assistance from laboratory and rarely, imaging modalities.

Specific Issues in Management of HE
Imaging for the Diagnosis of HE
BRAIN IMAGING

Patients with overt HE rarely require imaging of the head for diagnosis unless there are doubts about their clinical condition. Imaging is only advised for the diagnosis of HE if there are atypical features present (i.e., seizures, appearance of new focal changes) to exclude other diagnoses. It can also unearth consequences of falls in patients that can masquerade as HE.[60] Although a head CT can show loss of cerebral volume in HE, this is nonspecific and is often found in patients with cirrhosis without signs of HE as well.[24] In patients who are imaged though, the predominant finding on a MRI is hyperintensity of the basal ganglia on T1-weighted imaging.[69] This finding is probably related to manganese deposition and is often reversible after liver transplant.[70] Other modalities such as MR spectroscopy, PET scanning, and functional MRI are predominantly used for research purposes. MR spectroscopy shows an increase in glutamine and glutamate, and a compensatory decrease in brain myo-inositol.[71] There are characteristic changes in blood flow and cerebral activation seen on PET scan and functional MRI that mirror the ammonia

transport and assimilation in the brain.[72] However, due to the expense, time, and nonspecificity of these imaging findings, it is unlikely that they will be used for clinical practice for the diagnosis of HE.

IMAGING FOR INFECTIOUS WORK-UP

Chest imaging is a must for the evaluation of a possible chest infection. In patients with unremitting or intermittent HE, abdominal imaging may be required.

ABDOMINAL IMAGING

In patients with persistent HE, however, there is a role for a CT scan of the abdomen to evaluate the presence of collaterals that could sustain this condition despite adequate therapy. Large spontaneous portal-systemic shunts were detected in 71% of HE patients compared with only 14% of those without HE.[73] This is important because interventional radiologic embolization techniques can obliterate these shunts and improve the control of HE.[74]

Ammonia Levels for the Diagnosis of Hepatic Encephalopathy

There is considerable controversy regarding the need for obtaining ammonia levels in the routine clinical management of HE. Although it is well known that ammonia metabolism abnormalities play a key role in the pathogenesis of HE, it is inaccurate to assume a direct correlation between ammonia levels and consciousness levels for individual patients.[9,72] While this is true in groups of several hundred patients, the same cannot be said for an individual patient.[45] Clinical experience shows that there are patients who are severely obtunded with HE with normal ammonia levels and vice versa; however, the clinical decision to initiate therapy should always and only be based on the clinical and mental status rather than the ammonia level alone.

Complicating these assessments are the methods for drawing the ammonia sample, which should ideally be performed without a tourniquet, should be tested within 30 minutes, and should be kept on ice until testing.[75] Also the false elevation of ammonia after seizure activity adds another twist to the interpretation of ammonia levels. The specific situations where ammonia levels may help are in the rare patients with urea-cycle disorders or in the initial diagnosis of a patient with a coma who does not have a prior history of cirrhosis.[43]

Dietary Protein Restriction

The dictum for nutritional management in HE was to restrict dietary protein intake given the alterations in ammonia load in this population. Studies that first noted the role of protein loading and HE precipitation were in the 1950s and were not aimed at answering this question specifically, but at evaluating the efficacy of specific agents for HE therapy. Accordingly, in many trials a standard 40 g/day protein intake was adopted in addition to whatever therapies were being investigated for efficiency in the treatment of HE.[76]

Although protein restriction seems intuitively beneficial given the difficulty in converting nitrogenous substances into urea in these patients, the catabolic nature of cirrhosis needs to be underlined.[77] Dietary protein restriction below the maintenance level (e.g., 0.8 g/kg/day) may in fact lead to lean body mass catabolism and ultimately increase the nitrogen load to the systemic circulation.

An investigation into the role of dietary protein restriction in resolution of overt HE episodes did not reveal any significant difference in the protein-restricted versus normal protein diet group.[78] A subsequent study by this group, still only available in abstract form, again did not find any role of protein restriction in the prevention of overt HE recurrence, although the study was terminated prematurely due to sample size difficulties.

The current standard of care does not include protein restriction. If oral dietary protein intolerance is documented, then a vegetable protein diet with additional pectin or fiber may be recommended. In highly selected protein-intolerant patients, branched-chain amino acid–enriched supplements or formulations are still useful, but at a high expense.

Specific Treatment Strategies for the HE Episode

It is important to emphasize that these specific treatment strategies work in conjunction with reversing and investigating precipitating factors for the HE episode. The specific treatment strategies are broadly divided by their mechanisms of action and by and large, have not been adequately studied using well-designed randomized controlled trials.

The treatments for HE are divided according to their mechanisms of action into:

1. Reduction of nitrogenous load from the intestines
2. Promotion of nitrogen excretion
3. Neurotransmitter correction in the brain
4. Miscellaneous and newer medications

Reduction of Intestinal Nitrogenous Load

Given the prominent role played by ammonia in the pathogenesis of HE, the sources of nitrogen in the body are the leading targets of drugs aimed at control of HE. These are the most widespread group of therapies in HE and include nonabsorbable disaccharides and poorly absorbed antibiotics. These have been the mainstay of therapy in this field; however, the specific rationale for the use of some of these medications has not been proven.

Nonabsorbable Disaccharides

These medications are the first-line treatments for the HE episode and form the backbone of HE-directed therapy in most situations.[24] Lactulose and lactitol have been tested in several studies, most of which do not meet the current criteria for evidence-based research.[79]

The mechanisms of action of these agents are multifactorial and do not readily lend themselves to study. The primary mechanism appears to be an osmotic laxative effect; however, there are theoretical benefits proposed by the acidification of stool contents to increase ammonia fixation and possible inhibition of intestinal glutaminase to reduce small intestinal ammonia production.

The studies of lactulose and lactitol in HE have been poorly powered and therefore do not lend themselves to interpretation given the multitudes of patients who actually suffer from this complication[79] (**Table 17-8**). There has also been investigation of lactulose in the therapy of MHE (**Table 17-9**).

Ahls-Nielsen and colleagues questioned the overall validity of all poorly absorbed disaccharides as a standard of care for HE in a systematic review.[79] In the only placebo-controlled trials of lactulose in the treatment of HE, there was no statistical superiority of lactulose over the placebo. Although larger randomized controlled trials (RCTs) comparing lactulose with neomycin (usually with added sorbitol) have shown an

Table 17-8 RCTs of Lactulose vs. Placebo for Overt HE

STUDY	N	COMPARATOR	NUMBER IMPROVED/ TOTAL LACTULOSE VS. PLACEBO
Elkington	7	Sorbitol	Crossover no difference in efficacy
Simmons	26	Glucose	10/14 vs. 7/12
Rodgers	6	Sorbitol	Crossover no difference in efficacy
Germain	18	Saccharose	5/9 vs. 6/9

RCT, randomized controlled trial

equivalence, they are not powered to demonstrate this from a statistical standpoint. The call for placebo-controlled trials to clarify the efficacy of lactulose (or lactitol) in the treatment of HE awaits the resolution of the ethical constraints in performing such trials. Sharma and associates showed that in a randomized, un-blinded, placebo-controlled trial, lactulose was able to prevent a recurrent episode of HE.[80] A recent study also showed that outside of clinical trials, however, nonadherence with lactulose can lead to recurrent HE episodes.[81] Adding to this, it is often noted that correction of precipitating factors on their own may lead to improvement in HE.[82]

At this stage, there is insufficient evidence that lactulose is efficacious for the therapy of HE episodes; however, there is preponderance of anecdotal experience and comfort in the use of lactulose, which accounts for the lack of placebo-controlled trials in HE. Also an increased focus on patient and family member education to encourage adherence is needed.

Antibiotics

The role of antibiotics in HE has been investigated using both absorbable and poorly absorbable compounds. The poorly absorbable antibiotics have the advantage of fewer adverse events and possible development of resistance versus those that are absorbed. Unlike nonabsorbable disaccharides, there is a higher degree of scientific validity to their use as proven by RCTs.

NEOMYCIN

There is currently insufficient evidence that neomycin is better than a placebo; however, it is FDA-approved for the treatment of acute HE episodes. Although the mechanism is assumed to be its antibiotic action, there is also evidence of villous atrophy, resulting in inhibition of intestinal glutaminase after neomycin therapy. Studies by Conn and associates and Strauss and colleagues showed conflicting findings in relatively small sample sizes.[44,83] Treatment dose is typically 1 g qid for 6 days. Ototoxicity and nephrotoxicity can complicate neomycin therapy.[24]

RIFAXIMIN

Rifaximin is a nonabsorbable (<0.4%) antibiotic belonging to the rifamycin class. Its antibiotic action is due to the inhibition of chain formation in the RNA synthesis. It has a broad spectrum of action against several aerobic and anaerobic gram-positive and gram-negative bacteria and does not have any interactions with the cytochrome P450 enzyme substrates.

A number of studies have been performed comparing rifaximin with either other antibiotics or lactulose/lactitol in the treatment of the episode and the prevention of recurrence (**Table 17-10**). Enteric flora develop resistance to this antibiotic by a nonplasmid mediated mechanism, but the resistance is insufficient to prevent antibacterial action by the high levels of rifaximin in the gut.

The currently available dosing for rifaximin in the United States is based on a 200-mg tablet; it is used in a 400-mg PO TID dose based on a dose-ranging study. In several European countries, a cycling system of 2 weeks on and 2 weeks off rifaximin for 6 months has also been tested for long-term control of HE.[84] Apparently this works well, which may be useful for long-term treatment. However, most studies are for

Table 17-9 RCTs of Lactulose vs. Treatment for Minimal HE

STUDY	N	COMPARATOR	NUMBER IMPROVED/ TOTAL LACTULOSE VS. NO TX
Watanabe	36	No Tx	10/22 vs. 3/14*
Li	86	No Tx	26/48 vs. 11/38*
Dhiman	26	No Tx	8/14 vs. 0/12*
Prasad	61	No Tx	Number of psychometric tests improved in Lactulose group

*Lactulose significantly better than no treatment.
RCT, randomized controlled trial; Tx, treatment

Table 17-10 RCTs of Nonabsorbable Disaccharide vs. Antibiotics for Overt HE

STUDY	N	DISACCHARIDE/OTHER	ANTIBIOTIC/OTHER	NUMBER IMPROVED/TOTAL
Conn	33	Lact/placebo	Neomycin/sorbitol	15/18 vs. 13/15
Atterbury	47	Lact/placebo	Neomycin/sorbitol	19/23 vs. 20/24
Orlandi	190	Lactulose	Neomycin/MgSo₄	28/91 vs. 34/82
Russo	15	Lactulose	Ribostamycin	7/8 vs 5/7
Blanc	60	Lactitol	Vancomycin	20/29 vs. 21/31
Bucci	58	Lact/placebo	Rifaximin/sorbitol	Equivalent results
Fera	40	Lact/placebo	Rifaximin/placebo	16/20 vs. 20/20
Festi	21	Lactulose	Rifaximin	Equivalent results
Massa	40	Lact/placebo	Rifaximin/sorbitol	18/20 vs. 20/20
Song	64	Lactitol	Rifaximin	18/25 vs. 31/39
Longuerico	27	Lact/placebo	Rifaximin/placebo	2/13 vs. 8/14
Mas	103	Lact/placebo	Rifaximin/placebo	41/53 vs. 40/50

Lact, lactulose; MgSo₄, magnesium sulphate; RCT, randomized controlled trial

a comparatively shorter duration and study data indicate equivalence between rifaximin and neomycin or lactulose or lactitol. However, with small number of participants, these conclusions may not be statistically meaningful.[85–88] One study compared rifaximin with lactitol in more than 102 patients and confirmed the efficacy of rifaximin reported in earlier studies.[89] At this point it is important to state that although most treatments of HE have not been proved effective in placebo-controlled RCTs, this is not to say that they are without effect. The probability is that most have some efficacy, but deficiencies in study design have led to equivocal results in many trials. A phase III multicenter, randomized, double-blinded, placebo-controlled trial enrolled 299 patients using rifaximin 550 mg orally twice a day or placebo for 6 months was recently completed and showed that patients who received rifaximin for 6 months had highly statistically significant protection against clinical HE breakthrough episodes (58% risk reduction, $P < .0001$) compared with a placebo. Importantly, more than 90% of the study patients were on lactulose continually throughout the trial.[90]

Other Antibiotics Used to Treat HE

Metronidazole was first used in HE as a result of a study published by Morgan and associates.[91] Again the small sample size in this trial does not lend itself to widespread use, although in certain centers, metronidazole remains the drug to use after failure of lactulose. The recommended oral dose of metronidazole for chronic use is 250 mg bid. Metronidazole can result in CNS toxicity and irreversible peripheral neuropathy with chronic use, which has again detracted from its use.

Vancomycin was earlier used as third-line therapy for HE, but the reports of vancomycin-resistant enterococcus and the expense have again made it an unpopular choice for HE.[92]

Paromomycin is another nonabsorbable antibiotic currently approved for therapy of intestinal amebiasis. Rifaximin and paromomycin have been compared in three prospective open-label studies.[93,94] These studies enrolled approximately 20 to 32 subjects with duration between 5 and 15 days. Doses for rifaximin were 1200 mg/day while 1500 mg per day of paromomycin was used. Both groups demonstrated a trend toward lowered ammonia and Testa and colleagues showed a higher improvement in NCT-A with rifaximin, but there was no overall statistically significant difference.[95]

Promotion of Waste Nitrogen Excretion

Apart from prevention of nitrogenous by-products, another approach is to promote the excretion of waste nitrogen. This can be done by "fixing" ammonia or by enhancing the hepatic capacity for synthesis of urea and glutamine. More drugs working along these lines are being developed. Some of the existing data will be reviewed here.

L-ORNITHINE-L-ASPARTATE (LOLA)

LOLA promotes hepatic ureagenesis and glutamine synthetase activity, as well as promotion of glutamine synthesis and possibly protein anabolism in skeletal muscle.[96] It is available in an oral and parenteral form for HE in placebo-controlled randomized trials.[97-99] Several other trials have been performed with this agent versus a placebo in more than 300 patients.[100] The drug has not officially been released for treatment of HE in any country, which is unfortunate given the findings in the above studies. There may be a risk of

development of hyperammonemia following withdrawal of LOLA.

SODIUM BENZOATE

The prevalent therapy for urea-cycle disorders involves the fixation of ammonia using sodium benzoate to form hippurate and has been explored for the treatment of HE.[34] As is the case with several HE trials, the only published RCT compared sodium benzoate versus lactulose in overt HE, which judged them both to be equivalent in efficacy without the numbers to prove equivalency by today's standards.[101] While its low cost and availability in oral and parenteral form suggests that sodium benzoate should be studied further, it has an unpleasant taste and its sodium content is a concern in patients with cirrhosis. Currently, it is only commercially available and the usual dose is 5 g orally twice daily as a second-line drug. Newer options combining LOLA and phenylacetate include L-ornithine-phenyl-acetate, which has only undergone animal studies; human studies are pending at this time.[102]

Correction of Neurotransmitter Abnormalities in the Brain

As numerous abnormalities in brain chemistry were identified in HE, primarily in animal models, therapy was designed to try and connect these derangements. Some agents showed promise, but currently none is used frequently. Consequently, even though there is a large body of information on these potential approaches to the treatment of HE, only selective comments will be made.

FLUMAZENIL

The basis for the use of flumazenil was improvement of HE in animal models, which indicated that the accumulation of endogenous benzodiazepines might predispose to development of HE in those models.[103] This hypothesis was later supported by studies in several drug-free patients with cirrhosis.[104,105] Several studies have been performed with flumazenil, the majority of which have demonstrated improvement in overt HE rather than minimal HE.[106,107] However, this has not translated into widespread use because of several issues: lack of a long-acting oral preparation, only modest improvements in some patients (which is attributed to external benzodiazepine use), and the propensity to cause seizures (**Table 17-11**).

Branched-Chain Amino Acid (BCAA)-Enriched Formulations

Both the parenteral and enteral forms of BCAA therapy have been studied in great detail.[108-111] Although the enteral forms have some support by trials, results of these trials can be summarized by stating that the parenteral form of therapy has never been validated as a treatment for HE. In contrast, the enteral form of BCAA supplements has some reasonable evidence in its favor.[112,113] Whether the gains in preventing HE occurrences are worth the cost is debatable. As mentioned earlier, vegetable protein–based diets are now employed for patients with dietary intolerance to a typical American diet. The evidence in favor of this approach is not strong either. The extensive systematic review by Ahls-Nielsen and associates summarizes the experience with this approach in detail.[108]

Dopaminergic Agents

Because there are several patients with cirrhosis who have demonstrable extrapyramidal signs, this approach may be important to manage patients with HE.[114] A recent systematic review[115] showed a very limited role for dopaminergic agents in the management of HE. L-dopa and bromocriptine, the dopaminergic agents used in these trials, may have a role to play in the management of the apparently newly discovered cirrhotic patient with extrapyramidal symptoms and no overt signs of HE.[114,116] However, the data available do not preclude some benefit from this form of treatment.

Miscellaneous Agents

ZINC REPLETION

While prior studies showed positive results, there are no current recommendations for the supplementation of zinc in the therapy of HE.[117-119] The current role of zinc repletion is limited to supplementation in patients who are zinc deficient and who are resistant to therapy.[120]

DISACCHARIDASE INHIBITORS

Another intriguing application of the gut-milieu in the therapy of HE is the use of disaccharidase inhibitors, such as acarbose, which result in carbohydrate malabsorption and probably simulate the effect of lactulose. Two trials have been conducted that have demonstrated efficacy.[121,122] These were outpatient trials featuring patients with mild HE, but improvements were fairly well documented. Gentile and colleagues exclusively enrolled diabetic patients with HE and, not surprisingly, also demonstrated an improved glycemic control.[121] The strengths of these trials are the well documented endpoints and a placebo-controlled arm. However, acarbose can result in diarrhea and its use is contraindicated in cirrhosis according to its patient information sheet.

PROBIOTICS

Probiotic therapy has opened another vista of options in HE. Treatment studies using these agents again suffer from the same drawbacks as those of other agents (i.e., small participant numbers, inadequate duration). However, there are encouraging reports by Loguercio and associates, who demonstrated a reduction in ammonia levels and mental status using *Enterococcus faecium,* which was similar to that of lactulose.[123,124] There have been studies in MHE with probiotics and synbiotics. These have shown improvement in psychometric/neurophysiologic tests as well as improvement in the overall Child status.[125] Another small study of probiotic yogurt showed a statistically significant improvement in psychometric performance in patients randomized to yogurt compared with those who were not.[126] At this time, however, neither the mechanism nor the optimum probiotic organism has been identified. Adding to the problem is the lack of

Table 17-11 RCTs of Flumazenil vs. Placebo for Overt and Minimal HE

Study	n	Study design	Improvement in HE
Overt			
			Drug vs. placebo
Pomier-Layrargues	21	Crossover	5/11 vs. 0/11*
Cadranel	18	Crossover	6/10 vs. 0/8*
Gyr	49	Parallel	7/28 vs. 0/21*
Barbaro	527	Crossover	66/265 vs. 9/262*
Zhu	25	Parallel	3/13 vs. 0/12*
Lacetti	21	Parallel	5/11 vs. 0/10
Minimal			
Kapczinski	20	Crossover	No significant effect
Gooday	10	Crossover	Flumazenil superior
Amodio	13	Crossover	No effect
Dursun	40	Parallel	8/20 vs. 0/20*
			Flumazenil superior
			? All patients had minimal HE

*Signifies superior to placebo.
RCT, randomized controlled trial

Table 17-12 Newer Therapies for HE*

THERAPY	UNDERLYING MECHANISM	STAGE OF INVESTIGATION
AST-120	Adsorbent taken PO	Phase III for mild HE
L-carnitine	Stimulation of the urea cycle	Studies in MHE and OHE
L-ornithine phenylacetate	Stimulates fixation and excretion of ammonia	Animal studies only
Nitazoxanide	Gut-specific antibiotic	Small-scale study in MHE
Transdermal rivastigmine	Anticholinesterase	Small-scale study in MHE
Ammonul	Ammonia fixation	Phase II for OHE grades 3/4
Glycerol phenylbutyrate	Ammonia fixation	Phase II underway for OHE
Exercise training	Improvement of cognition	MHE trial underway
Probiotics: Lactobacillus GG (MHE) and Probiotics-Bio-plus (OHE)	Multiple mechanisms	OHE trial completed while MHE trial is underway

*As listed on www.clinicaltrials.gov and in latest abstracts.
MHE, minimal HE; OHE, overt HE; PO, by mouth

Table 17-13 Prevalent Reasons for HE Resistant to Treatment
End-stage liver disease only; still should be able to rouse Excessive purgation leading to dehydration/free water loss Failure to identify and treat sepsis Ileus, especially in association with azotemia (may need dialysis) Long-acting sedative drug intake Undiagnosed concomitant CNS problem (e.g., hypothyroidism) Too-effective portosystemic shunt procedure Profound zinc deficiency

Table 17-14 Issues of Liver Transplantation and HE
HE is not included in the MELD score. No priority is given to patients with severe recurrent or resistant HE. Older data on the failure of HE to predict survival in advanced liver disease patients may have occurred because of overstaging of HE to improve priority listing. New association of the independent predictive power of HE on survival may be more valid in the MELD era. However, HE status needs to be reported more exactly. How much HE is too much HE before transplant?

standardization of these agents because in the United States, they do not fall under the purview of the FDA.

A brief description of newer agents being investigated in HE is given in **Table 17-12.**

Hepatic Encephalopathy Resistant to Therapy

Resistant HE is fortunately relatively rare (**Table 17-13**). Arousing patients is usually not difficult, but it may be difficult to keep patients from again slipping into a state of altered mental status.

The usual precipitants of HE resistant to therapy are inadvertent dehydration and untreated/undiscovered sepsis. The former has already been mentioned and is a particular problem in patients with advanced liver disease and may be worsened by increased use of lactulose. Hyponatremia and hypernatremia can independently lead to resistant HE and may require slow correction. Untreated sepsis or undiagnosed sepsis (i.e., an intraabdominal abscess) can result in HE resistant to therapy and should be vigorously sought in all patients with severe HE who do not arouse after 3 to 4 days of treatment.

An additional vexing situation may be the combination of renal failure and ileus, together with severe spontaneous bacterial peritonitis or septicemia. In this situation, an aggressive approach to infection control and enemas for HE can be administered. Hemofiltration may be needed to control the situation until resumption of bowel function. Occasionally long-lasting metabolites of sedative drugs or sleep aids can lead to prolonged HE. Concomitant endocrinologic issues such as hypoadrenalism and hypothyroidism can appear as untreated HE and should definitely be considered. Sustained HE after a placement of a portosystemic shunt can be improved by measures that reduce the shunt size or flow as has been mentioned above. Finally, a severe loss or deficiency of zinc can result in resistant HE.[127]

Liver Support Systems

The ideal liver support system is lacking but there have been significant advances made in this field. The initial trials using these machines were promising but were mostly uncontrolled trials. Subsequently, most of the initial enthusiasm waned with the RCT results.[128-133] However, the molecular absorbent recirculating system (MARS) has emerged as a modality for patients with acute-on-chronic liver failure with HE. Heeman and colleagues reported an apparent benefit using this device in patients with acute or chronic liver failure; this study was terminated prematurely because the MARS-treated group were doing "too well."[134] Subsequently a large, multicenter trial of MARS in the United States has also demonstrated benefit of MARS in patients with grade III/IV HE when compared with standard medical therapy. This study showed a significantly faster improvement in mental status in the group randomized to MARS compared with the standard therapy group.[135]

Closure of Portosystemic Shunts

The vexing issue of persistent and/or recurrent HE in the absence of other precipitating factors could be due to the presence of large portosystemic shunts.[136,137] Specifically in this population, the problem of HE is out of proportion to the synthetic failure of the liver. In this situation it is prudent to image the abdomen to evaluate these shunts. It is possible to embolize or surgically alter these shunts to relieve the recurrent or persistent HE episodes, but it is always beneficial to consult the transplant surgeon and keep them as part of this team to prevent technical issues in a future transplant operation.[138,139] These manipulations, such as reduction of preexisting transhepatic stent diameters or closure of large collateral vessels, can dramatically improve the clinical course of HE.[140,141]

Liver Transplantation

Although it is not commonly the primary indication for liver transplantation, HE is generally improved by a successful graft. **Table 17-14** lists some of the current issues regarding HE and liver transplantation. Rather than reiterate these points in detail, the issue that will be discussed is the timing of referral for transplantation assessment in patients with drug and alcohol abuse problems. Successful completion of a rehabilitation program to qualify for liver transplantation requires well preserved cognitive skills, which may be limited because of HE. Recent evidence shows that patients with severe and multiple episodes of HE have worsened cognitive skills, therefore adding more impetus to listing these patients earlier.[142] Tragically, we see too many patients with drug problems referred when they already have difficult-to-control HE. At present, recurrent or persistent HE does not give patients priority for liver transplantation. However, more research needs to be performed to resolve these issues.

Ultimately, liver failure has to be addressed as a long-lasting approach to the correction of HE and the therapeutic and diagnostic criteria should always prepare the patient for possible transplant evaluation.

Key References

Ahboucha S, Butterworth RF. Role of endogenous benzodiazepine ligands and their GABA-A–associated receptors in hepatic encephalopathy. Metab Brain Dis 2005;20:425–437. (Ref.12)

Ali S, Stolpen AH, Schmidt WN. Portosystemic encephalopathy due to mesoiliac shunt in a patient without cirrhosis. J Clin Gastroenterol 2010 May-Jun; 44(5):381-383. (Ref.137)

Als-Nielsen B, Gluud LL, Gluud C. Dopaminergic agonists for hepatic encephalopathy. Cochrane Database Syst Rev 2004:CD003047. (Ref.115)

Als-Nielsen B, Gluud LL, Gluud C. Non-absorbable disaccharides for hepatic encephalopathy: systematic review of randomised trials. BMJ 2004;328: 1046–1052. (Ref.79)

Als-Nielsen B, et al. Branched-chain amino acids for hepatic encephalopathy. Cochrane Database Syst Rev 2003:CD001939. (Ref.108)

Amodio P, et al. Detection of minimal hepatic encephalopathy: normalization and optimization of the Psychometric Hepatic Encephalopathy Score. A neuropsychological and quantified EEG study. J Hepatol 2008;49:346–353. (Ref.56)

Amodio P, et al. Prevalence and prognostic value of quantified electroencephalogram (EEG) alterations in cirrhotic patients. J Hepatol 2001;35:37–45. (Ref.63)

Amodio P, et al. Characteristics of minimal hepatic encephalopathy. Metab Brain Dis 2004;19:253–267. (Ref.62)

Annas GJ. Doctors, drugs, and driving: tort liability for patient-caused accidents. N Engl J Med 2008;359:521–525. (Ref.35)

Arguedas MR, De Lawrence TG, McGuire BM. Influence of hepatic encephalopathy on health-related quality of life in patients with cirrhosis. Dig Dis Sci 2003;48:1622–1626. (Ref.27)

Bajaj JS. Management options for minimal hepatic encephalopathy. Expert Rev Gastroenterol Hepatol 2008;2:785–790. (Ref.21)

Bajaj JS. Minimal hepatic encephalopathy matters in daily life. World J Gastroenterol 2008;14:3609–3615. (Ref.31)

Bajaj JS. Review article: modern management of hepatic encephalopathy. Aliment Pharmacol Thera 2010;31:537–547. (Ref.43)

Bajaj JS. Review article: the modern management of hepatic encephalopathy. Aliment Pharmacol Ther 2010;31:537–547. (Ref.74)

Bajaj JS, et al. Inhibitory control test for the diagnosis of minimal hepatic encephalopathy. Gastroenterology 2008;135:1591–1600 e1. (Ref.68)

Bajaj JS, et al. Inhibitory control test for the diagnosis of minimal hepatic encephalopathy. Gastroenterology 2008;135:1591–1600 e1. (Ref.54)

Bajaj JS, et al. Minimal hepatic encephalopathy: a vehicle for accidents and traffic violations. Am J Gastroenterol 2007;102:1903–1909. (Ref.41)

Bajaj JS, et al. Navigation skill impairment: another dimension of the driving difficulties in minimal hepatic encephalopathy. Hepatology 2008;47:596–604. (Ref.38)

Bajaj JS, et al. Effect of fatigue on driving skills in patients with hepatic encephalopathy. Am J Gastroenterol 2009;104(4):898-905. (Ref.39)

Bajaj JS, et al. Probiotic yogurt for the treatment of minimal hepatic encephalopathy. Am J Gastroenterol 2008;103:1707–1715. (Ref.126)

Bajaj JS, et al. Patients with minimal hepatic encephalopathy have poor insight into their driving skills. Clin Gastroenterol Hepatol 2008;6:1135–1139; quiz 1065. (Ref.40)

Bajaj JS, et al. Minimal hepatic encephalopathy is associated with motor vehicle crashes: the reality beyond the driving test. Hepatology 2009;50:1175–1183. (Ref.42)

Bajaj JS, et al. Inhibitory control test is a simple method to diagnose minimal hepatic encephalopathy and predict development of overt hepatic encephalopathy. Am J Gastroenterol 2007;102:754–760. (Ref.55)

Bajaj JS, et al. Predictors of the recurrence of hepatic encephalopathy in lactulose-treated patients. Aliment Pharmacol Ther. 2010;31(9):1012-1017. (Ref.81)

Bajaj JS, et al. Persistence of cognitive impairment after resolution of overt hepatic encephalopathy. Gastroenterology 2010;138(7):2332-2340. (Ref.142)

Bass NM, et al. Rifaximin treatment in hepatic encephalopathy. N Engl J Med 2010;25;362(12):1071-1081. (Ref. 90)

Blei AT, Cordoba J. Hepatic encephalopathy. Am J Gastroenterol 2001;96: 1968–1976. (Ref.24)

Bustamante J, et al. Prognostic significance of hepatic encephalopathy in patients with cirrhosis. J Hepatol 1999;30:890–895. (Ref.28)

Cabre E, Gassull MA. Nutrition in liver disease. Curr Opin Clin Nutr Metab Care 2005;8:545–551. (Ref.77)

Cordoba J, et al. The development of low-grade cerebral edema in cirrhosis is supported by the evolution of (1)H-magnetic resonance abnormalities after liver transplantation. J Hepatol 2001;35:598–604. (Ref.71)

Cordoba J, et al. Normal protein diet for episodic hepatic encephalopathy: results of a randomized study. J Hepatol 2004;41:38–43. (Ref.78)

Das A, et al. Prevalence and natural history of subclinical hepatic encephalopathy in cirrhosis. J Gastroenterol Hepatol 2001;16:531–535. (Ref.30)

Davies NA, et al. L-ornithine and phenylacetate synergistically produce sustained reduction in ammonia and brain water in cirrhotic rats. Hepatology 2009;50: 155–164. (Ref.102)

de Waele JP, et al. Portacaval anastomosis induces region-selective alterations of the endogenous opioid system in the rat brain. Hepatology 1996;24:895–901. (Ref.11)

Ellis AJ, et al. Temporary extracorporeal liver support for severe acute alcoholic hepatitis using the BioLogic-DT. Int J Artif Organs 1999;22:27–34. (Ref.131)

Ferenci P, et al. Hepatic encephalopathy: definition, nomenclature, diagnosis, and quantification: final report of the working party at the 11th World Congresses of Gastroenterology, Vienna, 1998. Hepatology 2002;35:716–721. (Ref.1)

Garavan H, Ross TJ, Stein EA. Right hemispheric dominance of inhibitory control: an event-related functional MRI study. Proc Natl Acad Sci U S A 1999;96:8301–8306. (Ref.67)

Gentile S, et al. A randomized controlled trial of acarbose in hepatic encephalopathy. Clin Gastroenterol Hepatol 2005;3:184–191. (Ref.121)

Groeneweg M, et al. Subclinical hepatic encephalopathy impairs daily functioning. Hepatology 1998;28:45–49. (Ref.33)

Hassanein T, et al. Performance of the hepatic encephalopathy scoring algorithm in a clinical trial of patients with cirrhosis and severe hepatic encephalopathy. Am J Gastroenterol 2009;104:1392–1400. (Ref.47)

Hassanein TI, et al. Randomized controlled study of extracorporeal albumin dialysis for hepatic encephalopathy in advanced cirrhosis. Hepatology 2007;46: 1853–1862.(Ref.135)

Heemann U, et al. Albumin dialysis in cirrhosis with superimposed acute liver injury: a prospective, controlled study. Hepatology 2002;36:949–958. (Ref.134)

Huizenga JR, Gips CH, Tangerman A. The contribution of various organs to ammonia formation: a review of factors determining the arterial ammonia concentration. Ann Clin Biochem 1996;33(Pt 1):23–30. (Ref.75)

Jalan R, et al. Pathogenesis of intracranial hypertension in acute liver failure: inflammation, ammonia and cerebral blood flow. J Hepatol 2004;41:613–620. (Ref.16)

Jiang Q, et al. L-ornithine-l-aspartate in the management of hepatic encephalopathy: a meta-analysis. J Gastroenterol Hepatol 2009;24:9–14. (Ref.100)

Jover R, et al. Minimal hepatic encephalopathy and extrapyramidal signs in patients with cirrhosis. Am J Gastroenterol 2003;98:1599–1604. (Ref.114)

Kircheis G, et al. Therapeutic efficacy of L-ornithine-L-aspartate infusions in patients with cirrhosis and hepatic encephalopathy: results of a placebo-controlled, double-blind study. Hepatology 1997;25:1351–1360. (Ref.98)

Kircheis G, et al. Clinical efficacy of L-ornithine-L-aspartate in the management of hepatic encephalopathy. Metab Brain Dis 2002;17:453–462. (Ref.96)

Kircheis G, et al. Critical flicker frequency for quantification of low-grade hepatic encephalopathy. Hepatology 2002;35:357–366. (Ref.25)

Liu Q, et al. Synbiotic modulation of gut flora: effect on minimal hepatic encephalopathy in patients with cirrhosis. Hepatology 2004;39:1441–1449. (Ref.125)

Mardini H, Saxby BK, Record CO. Computerized psychometric testing in minimal encephalopathy and modulation by nitrogen challenge and liver transplant. Gastroenterology 2008; 135(5):1582-1590. (Ref.66)

Mas A, et al. Comparison of rifaximin and lactitol in the treatment of acute hepatic encephalopathy: results of a randomized, double-blind, double-dummy, controlled clinical trial. J Hepatol 2003;38:51–58. (Ref.89)

Master S, Gottstein J, Blei AT. Cerebral blood flow and the development of ammonia-induced brain edema in rats after portacaval anastomosis. Hepatology 1999;30:876–880. (Ref.14)

Miglio F, et al. Rifaximin, a non-absorbable rifamycin, for the treatment of hepatic encephalopathy. A double-blind, randomised trial. Curr Med Res Opin 1997;13:593–601. (Ref.84)

Mitzner SR, et al. Improvement of multiple organ functions in hepatorenal syndrome during albumin dialysis with the molecular adsorbent recirculating system. Ther Apher 2001;5:417–422. (Ref.128)

Mitzner SR, et al. Improvement of hepatorenal syndrome with extracorporeal albumin dialysis MARS: results of a prospective, randomized, controlled clinical trial. Liver Transpl 2000;6:277–286. (Ref.133)

Miwa Y, et al. Effect of ELAD liver support on plasma HGF and TGF-beta 1 in acute liver failure. Int J Artif Organs 1996;19:240–244. (Ref.132)

Montagnese S, Amodio P, Morgan MY. Methods for diagnosing hepatic encephalopathy in patients with cirrhosis: a multidimensional approach. Metab Brain Dis 2004;19:281–312. (Ref.64)

Montagnese S, Jackson C, Morgan MY. Spatio-temporal decomposition of the electroencephalogram in patients with cirrhosis. J Hepatol 2007;46:447–458. (Ref.61)

Mooney S, et al. Utility of the Repeatable Battery for the Assessment of Neuropsychological Status (RBANS) in patients with end-stage liver disease awaiting liver transplant. Arch Clin Neuropsychol 2007;22:175–186. (Ref.59)

Mullen K, et al. An algorithm for the management of hepatic encephalopathy. Semin Liver Dis 2007;27:32–48. (Ref.60)

Mullen KD. Hepatic encephalopathy after portosystemic shunts: any clues from tips? Am J Gastroenterol 1995;90:531–533. (Ref.136)

Mullen KD, Cole M, Foley JM. Neurological deficits in "awake" cirrhotic patients on hepatic encephalopathy treatment: missed metabolic or metal disorder? Gastroenterology 1996;111:256–257. (Ref.46)

Nishie A, et al. Treatment of hepatic encephalopathy by retrograde transcaval coil embolization of an ileal vein-to-right gonadal vein portosystemic shunt. Cardiovasc Intervent Radiol 1997;20:222–224. (Ref.138)

Olde Damink SW, et al. Interorgan ammonia metabolism in liver failure. Neurochem Int 2002;41:177–188. (Ref.6)

Ong JP, et al. Correlation between ammonia levels and the severity of hepatic encephalopathy. Am J Med 2003;114:188–193. (Ref.45)

Ong JP, Mullen KD. Hepatic encephalopathy. Eur J Gastroenterol Hepatol 2001;13:325–334. (Ref.139)

Ortiz M, et al. Development of a clinical hepatic encephalopathy staging scale. Aliment Pharmacol Ther 2007;26:859–867. (Ref.48)

Ortiz M, et al. Neuropsychological abnormalities in cirrhosis include learning impairment. J Hepatol 2006;44:104–110. (Ref.52)

Ortiz M, Jacas C, Cordoba J. Minimal hepatic encephalopathy: diagnosis, clinical significance and recommendations. J Hepatol 2005;42(Suppl 1):S45–S53. (Ref.22)

Poo JL, et al. Efficacy of oral L-ornithine-L-aspartate in cirrhotic patients with hyperammonemic hepatic encephalopathy. Results of a randomized, lactulose-controlled study. Ann Hepatol 2006;5:281–288. (Ref.99)

Poordad FF. Review article: the burden of hepatic encephalopathy. Aliment Pharmacol Ther 2007;25(Suppl 1):3–9. (Ref.2)

Prasad S, et al. Lactulose improves cognitive functions and health-related quality of life in patients with cirrhosis who have minimal hepatic encephalopathy. Hepatology 2007;45:549–559. (Ref.32)

Randolph C, et al. Neuropsychological assessment of hepatic encephalopathy: ISHEN practice guidelines. Liver Int 2009;29:629–635. (Ref.57)

Rao KV, Norenberg MD. Cerebral energy metabolism in hepatic encephalopathy and hyperammonemia. Metab Brain Dis 2001;16:67–78. (Ref.19)

Riggio O, et al. High prevalence of spontaneous portal-systemic shunts in persistent hepatic encephalopathy: a case-control study. Hepatology 2005;42:1158–1165. (Ref.73)

Rolando N, et al. The systemic inflammatory response syndrome in acute liver failure. Hepatology 2000;32:734–739. (Ref.15)

Schiff S, et al. Impairment of response inhibition precedes motor alteration in the early stage of liver cirrhosis: a behavioral and electrophysiological study. Metab Brain Dis 2005;20:381–392. (Ref.53)

Sharma BC, et al. Secondary prophylaxis of hepatic encephalopathy: an open-label randomized controlled trial of lactulose versus placebo. Gastroenterology 2009;137:885–891. (Ref.80)

Sharma P, et al. Critical flicker frequency: diagnostic tool for minimal hepatic encephalopathy. J Hepatol 2007;47:67–73. (Ref.65)

Shawcross DL, et al. Systemic inflammatory response exacerbates the neuropsychological effects of induced hyperammonemia in cirrhosis. J Hepatol 2004;40:247–254. (Ref.17)

Shawcross DL, et al. Ammonia and hepatic encephalopathy: the more things change, the more they remain the same. Metab Brain Dis 2005;20:169–179. (Ref.5)

Shawcross DL, et al. Role of ammonia and inflammation in minimal hepatic encephalopathy. Metab Brain Dis 2007;22:125–138. (Ref.9)

Sorrell JH, et al. Cognitive impairment in people diagnosed with end-stage liver disease evaluated for liver transplantation. Psychiatry Clin Neurosci 2006;60:174–181. (Ref.58)

Spahr L, et al. Magnetic resonance imaging and proton spectroscopic alterations correlate with parkinsonian signs in patients with cirrhosis. Gastroenterology 2000;119:774–781. (Ref.116)

Stauch S, et al. Oral L-ornithine-L-aspartate therapy of chronic hepatic encephalopathy: results of a placebo-controlled double-blind study. J Hepatol 1998;28:856–864. (Ref.97)

Stewart CA, et al. Hepatic encephalopathy as a predictor of survival in patients with end-stage liver disease. Liver Transpl 2007;13:1366–1371. (Ref.29)

Tan KH, et al. Peroxynitrite mediates nitric oxide-induced blood-brain barrier damage. Neurochem Res 2004;29:579–587. (Ref.20)

Uribe M, et al. Beneficial effect of carbohydrate maldigestion induced by a disaccharidase inhibitor (AO-128) in the treatment of chronic portal-systemic encephalopathy. A double-blind, randomized, controlled trial. Scand J Gastroenterol 1998;33:1099–1106. (Ref.122)

Wein C, et al. Minimal hepatic encephalopathy impairs fitness to drive. Hepatology 2004;39:739–745. (Ref.36)

Weissenborn K. Clinical features of hepatic encephalopathy. Philadelphia, Saunders, 2003. (Ref.3)

Weissenborn K, et al. Correlations between magnetic resonance spectroscopy alterations and cerebral ammonia and glucose metabolism in cirrhotic patients with and without hepatic encephalopathy. Gut 2007;56:1736–1742. (Ref.72)

Weissenborn K, et al. Neuropsychological characterization of hepatic encephalopathy. J Hepatol 2001;34:768–773. (Ref.26)

Weissenborn K, et al. Attention, memory, and cognitive function in hepatic encephalopathy. Metab Brain Dis 2005;20:359–367. (Ref.49)

Weissenborn K, et al. Attention deficits in minimal hepatic encephalopathy. Metab Brain Dis 2001;16:13–19. (Ref.50)

Weissenborn K, et al. Memory function in early hepatic encephalopathy. J Hepatol 2003;39:320–325. (Ref.51)

Williams R, et al. Evaluation of the efficacy and safety of rifaximin in the treatment of hepatic encephalopathy: a double-blind, randomized, dose-finding multi-centre study. Eur J Gastroenterol Hepatol 2000;12:203–208. (Ref.88)

Zeneroli ML, et al. Antibacterial activity of rifaximin reduces the levels of benzodiazepine-like compounds in patients with liver cirrhosis. Pharmacol Res 1997;35:557–560. (Ref.104)

Zidi SH, et al. Treatment of chronic portosystemic encephalopathy in cirrhotic patients by embolization of portosystemic shunts. Liver Int 2007;27:1389–1393. (Ref.141)

A complete list of references can be found at www.expertconsult.com.

Ascites

Guadalupe Garcia-Tsao

Introduction

Ascites is the pathologic accumulation of fluid in the peritoneal cavity, and its most common cause is cirrhosis. That fluid accumulates in the abdominal cavity has been known since ancient times, and it was Hippocrates who recognized that ascites (from the Greek *askos*, meaning a leather bag used to carry wine, water, or oil) was derived from a diseased liver and that it carried a grim prognosis.[1] The development of ascites is one of the complications of cirrhosis that marks the transition from compensated to decompensated cirrhosis. Other complications that mark this transition are variceal hemorrhage, hepatic encephalopathy, or jaundice; however, ascites is the most common.[2-4]

Epidemiology

Ascites is present in 20% to 60% of patients with cirrhosis at the time of diagnosis, depending on the referral pattern.[5] In prospective studies of patients with compensated cirrhosis of all causes, the cumulative probability of developing ascites ranges from 35% to 50% within 5 years (**Fig. 18-1**),[3,5] not unlike annual incidence rates between 5% and 6% in patients with viral cirrhosis.[6] In a large cohort of patients with HCV-related cirrhosis, ascites was the most frequent first decompensating event, occurring in 48% of the patients.[4]

Pathogenesis

In cirrhosis, leakage of ascites into the peritoneal space occurs as a result of sinusoidal hypertension that in turn results from

hepatic venous outflow block secondary to regenerative nodules and fibrosis. The other essential factor in the pathogenesis of cirrhotic ascites is plasma volume expansion, through sodium and water retention, that allows for the replenishment of the intravascular volume and maintains the formation of ascites (**Fig. 18-2**).

Sinusoidal Hypertension

Similar to gastroesophageal varices, in which a minimal portal pressure gradient of 10 to 12 mm Hg is needed for their development, ascites also seems to require a minimal portal pressure gradient of 12 mm Hg.[7,8] A portal pressure gradient of 10 mm Hg or more has been denominated "clinically significant portal hypertension" because it is the best predictor of the development of complications of cirrhosis such as ascites.[2,9]

Plasma Volume Expansion

Sinusoidal hypertension alone is not sufficient to maintain ascites formation. Without replenishment of the intravascular space, leakage of fluid into the peritoneal cavity would be a self-limited process. Replenishment of the intravascular space—that is, plasma volume expansion—is accomplished through sodium retention, which has been shown to precede the development of ascites.[10] Arterial (splanchnic and systemic) vasodilation is the most likely mechanism leading to sodium retention.[11] Arterial vasodilation results in reduction of the "effective" arterial blood volume, which in turn leads to stimulation of neurohumoral systems, specifically the renin-angiotensin-aldosterone system (RAAS), the sympathetic nervous system, and the nonosmotic release of antidiuretic hormone. Activation of RAAS and the sympathetic nervous system result in sodium retention and, in extreme cases, to renal vasoconstriction. Activation of antidiuretic hormone leads to free water retention and hyponatremia.[12] An increased production of the vasodilator nitric oxide (NO) is currently considered the main cause of vasodilation in cirrhosis. In experimental cirrhosis, NO blockade increases systemic blood pressure and sodium excretion, and decreases the volume of ascites while down-regulating the activation of the RAAS.[13,14] The administration of vasodilators, such as prazosin, angiotensin receptor blockers, and phosphodiesterase inhibitors to cirrhotic patients, leads to further activation of the RAAS[15-17] with associated sodium retention,[15,17] ascites,[15] and decreased creatinine clearance.[16]

The presence of normal or low levels of plasma renin activity in some patients with cirrhosis and ascites, suggests that in some cases sodium retention occurs unrelated to vasodilation. Another theory is that, early on in the process, there is primary renal sodium retention through an as yet unidentified hepatorenal reflex (overfill theory).[18]

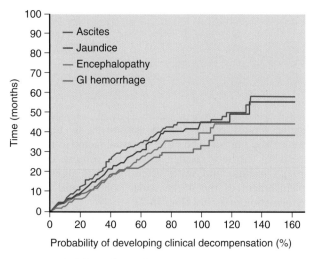

Fig. 18-1 Probability of developing decompensated cirrhosis in 257 patients with compensated cirrhosis of different causes. Of the complications of portal hypertension, ascites is the most frequent decompensating event. *(Modified from Gines P, Quintero E, Hrroyo V, Compensated cirrhosis: natural history and prognosis, Hepatology 1987;7:122–128.)*

Clinical Features

The most frequent symptoms associated with ascites are increased abdominal girth (described as tightness of the belt or garments around the waist) and recent weight gain.[19] Ascites induces abdominal distention but this sign in itself has a poor specificity[20] because it is present in other conditions such as obesity, gas, tumors, and pregnancy. Small to moderate amounts of ascites can be identified by bulging flanks, flank dullness, and shifting dullness. The last two are the most sensitive physical maneuvers in the diagnosis of ascites.[20,21] Ascites can be classified in three grades: (1) mild ascites only detectable by ultrasound examination; (2) moderate ascites manifested by moderate symmetric distention of abdomen; and (3) large or gross ascites with marked abdominal distention.[22]

Diagnosis

Abdominal ultrasonography is the most cost-effective and least invasive method to confirm or exclude the presence of ascites and is therefore considered the gold standard in the diagnosis of ascites. It can detect amounts as small as 100 ml[23] and even as small as 1 to 2 ml when the Morison pouch and the pelvic cul-de-sac are scanned.[24] Abdominal ultrasound is also useful in determining the best site to perform a diagnostic or therapeutic paracentesis, particularly in patients with a small amount of ascites or in those with loculated ascites. Additionally, findings on ultrasound (nodular surface, splenomegaly) can indicate the presence of cirrhosis, and Doppler ultrasound is the most useful initial test to investigate the presence of hepatic vein obstruction, an important and frequently overlooked cause of ascites.[24] Therefore, in patients with new onset of ascites, abdominal ultrasound should always be performed and should include Doppler examination of the hepatic veins.

Differential Diagnosis

Although cirrhosis is the cause of ascites in more than 75% of patients, other causes of ascites such as peritoneal malignancy (12%), cardiac failure (5%), and peritoneal tuberculosis (2%)[25] should be considered in the differential diagnosis of ascites.

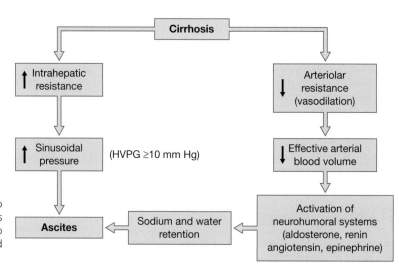

Fig. 18-2 Pathophysiology of cirrhotic ascites. Two main pathogenic mechanisms in the formation of ascites are sinusoidal hypertension and vasodilation leading to activation of neurohumoral systems and sodium and water retention.

A diagnostic paracentesis should be the first test performed in the diagnostic workup of a patient with ascites. It is a safe procedure with a very low incidence of serious complications, mostly transfusion-requiring hematomas that occur at a rate of 0.2% to 0.9%.[26,27] Renal dysfunction appears to be more predictive of bleeding complications than clotting abnormalities, and therefore coagulopathy is not a contraindication to perform a diagnostic paracentesis.[26,27] The preferred site for needle insertion is located in the left lower quadrant.[28] Care should always be taken to avoid abdominal wall collaterals and to avoid the area of the inferior hypogastric artery, which lies midway between anterior superior iliac spine and pubic tubercle.

Uncomplicated ascitic fluid is transparent, straw colored to slightly yellow. The presence of blood in a nontraumatic tap (in which blood does not clot) may indicate the presence of malignant ascites. Milky fluid is indicative of chylous ascites and although cirrhosis is the most common cause of nonsurgical chylous ascites, it represents only 0.5% to 1% of cases of cirrhotic ascites.[29]

Ascites total protein and serum ascites albumin gradient (SAAG) are two inexpensive tests that, taken *together*, are most useful in determining the cause of ascites and therefore in guiding the workup of patients with ascites. A high (>2.5 g/dl) ascites total protein occurs in peritoneal processes (malignancy, tuberculosis) because of leakage of high-protein mesenteric lymph from obliterated lymphatics and/or from an inflamed peritoneal surface. A high ascites total protein also occurs in cases of postsinusoidal or posthepatic sinusoidal hypertension when sinusoids are normal and protein-rich lymph "leaks" into the peritoneal cavity.[30] In hepatic cirrhosis, an abnormally low protein content of liver lymph has been demonstrated as a result of deposition of fibrous tissue in the sinusoids ("capillarization of the sinusoid") that renders the sinusoid less leaky to macromolecules.[31,32] On the other hand, the SAAG, which involves measuring the albumin concentration of serum and ascitic fluid specimens and subtracting the ascitic fluid value from the serum value, has been shown to correlate with hepatic sinusoidal pressure.[33,34] A SAAG cutoff value of 1.1 g/dl has been shown to be the best to distinguish patients in whom ascites is secondary to liver disease and those with malignant ascites.[35] Interestingly, this cutoff corresponds to a portal pressure gradient of 11 to 12 mm Hg,[33] the threshold pressure necessary for the development of ascites in cirrhotic patients (**Fig. 18-3**). Therefore the SAAG and the ascites total protein content can distinguish among the three main causes of ascites, cirrhosis, peritoneal pathology (malignancy or tuberculosis), and heart failure, and guide the further workup of the patient with ascites (**Fig. 18-4**). In cirrhosis, the SAAG is high and ascites total protein is low; in posthepatic or postsinusoidal causes of portal hypertension (e.g., heart failure, constrictive pericarditis), SAAG is high and ascites total protein is high; and in ascites secondary to peritoneal causes, SAAG is low and ascites total protein is high (**Fig. 18-5**).[36-38]

In patients with mixed ascites (e.g., cirrhosis with superimposed peritoneal malignancy), the SAAG is high and the ascites protein is low (i.e., the findings of ascites due to cirrhosis predominate).[38] Of note, massive hepatic metastasis can lead to the development of ascites but because the mechanism of ascites formation is sinusoidal hypertension, these cases of "malignant ascites" will have a high SAAG.[37]

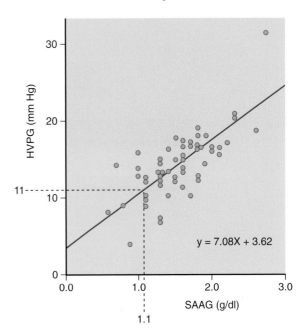

Fig. 18-3 **Correlation between serumascites albumin gradient (SAAG) and hepatic sinusoidal pressure.** A direct, very significant correlation between the SAAG and the hepatic venous pressure gradient (HVPG), a measure of sinusoidal pressure, is present. A cutoff SAAG of greater than 1.1 g/dl has been identified as one that distinguishes ascites secondary to sinusoidal hypertension from that secondary to peritoneal causes. This cutoff corresponds to an HVPG of 11 mm Hg, identified by other studies as the threshold pressure for the formation of ascites. *(Modified from Hoefs JC. Serum protein concentration and portal pressure determine the ascitic fluid protein concentration in patients with chronic liver disease. J Lab Clin Med 1983;102:260–273.)*

The definitive test to determine whether ascites is the result of sinusoidal hypertension is to actually perform measurements of hepatic sinusoidal pressure. The hepatic venous pressure gradient (HVPG), obtained by subtracting the free hepatic vein pressure (FHVP) from the wedged hepatic vein pressure (WHVP), is a measure of sinusoidal pressure. In cases of cirrhotic ascites, the HVPG will be 10 to 12 mm Hg or greater. In cases of cardiac ascites, both the WHVP and the FHVP will be elevated (reflecting elevated systemic pressures), and therefore the HVPG will be normal. In cases of peritoneal ascites (i.e., malignancy, tuberculosis), all hepatic venous pressure measurements (WHVP, FHVP, and HVPG) will be normal, unless the patient has coexisting cirrhosis or heart failure. When performed properly, HVPG measurements are reproducible and safe.[39] Additionally, hepatic vein catheterization for measurement of hepatic vein pressures allows for the performance, in the same procedure, of a transjugular liver biopsy that will further define the cause of ascites.

Associated Conditions

Hyponatremia develops in approximately 30% of cirrhotic patients with ascites and is defined as a serum sodium concentration of less than 130 mEq/L.[12] Hyponatremia in cirrhosis is dilutional and results mostly from the nonosmotic secretion of antidiuretic hormone that in turn is secondary to vasodilation. Although hyponatremia is usually asymptomatic, some

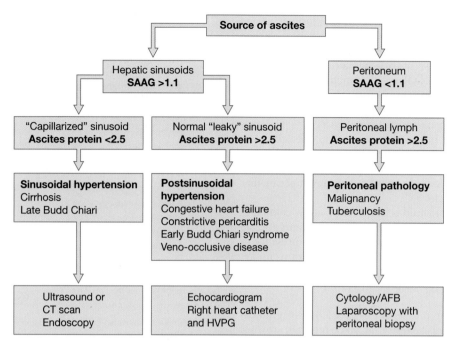

Fig. 18-4 **Differential diagnosis of ascites depending on the source of ascites.** The serum-ascites albumin gradient is high (>1.1 g/dl) when the source is hepatic sinusoids and is low when the source is other than the sinusoids. Ascites total protein is high (>2.5 g/dl) when ascites is coming either from normal sinusoids or from the peritoneum. Workup is directed accordingly.

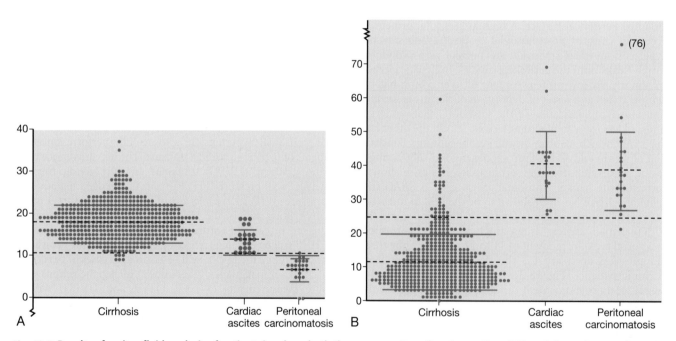

Fig. 18-5 **Results of ascites fluid analysis of patients in whom both the serum-ascites albumin gradient (5A) and the ascites total protein (5B) were determined.** As clearly shown, patients with cirrhosis have a high (>1.1 g/dl) SAAG and a low ascites protein (<2.5 g/dl); patients with cardiac ascites have high SAAG and high ascites protein; and patients with peritoneal carcinomatosis have a low SAAG and a high ascites protein. (Modified from Runyon BA, et al. The serum-ascites albumin gradient is superior to the exudate-transudate concept in the differential diagnosis of ascites. Ann Intern Med 1992;117:215–220.)

patients may complain of anorexia, nausea and vomiting, lethargy, and occasionally seizures. Hyponatremia appears to play a role in the pathogenesis of hepatic encephalopathy.[40]

Umbilical hernias develop in about 20% of cirrhotic patients with ascites (a rate significantly greater than 3% in patients without ascites) and may increase to up to 70% in patients with long-standing recurrent tense ascites.[41] The main risks of

these hernias are rupture[42] and incarceration, a complication that has been observed mostly in patients in whom ascites is resolved after paracentesis, peritoneovenous shunt, or transjugular intrahepatic portosystemic shunt.[43,44]

Hepatic hydrothorax develops in approximately 5% to 10% of patients with cirrhosis most probably as the result of the transdiaphragmatic movement of fluid from the peritoneum to the pleural space through diaphragmatic defects.[45,46] It usually develops in patients with ascites; however, hepatic hydrothorax may develop in patients without detectable ascites.[47] Although large amounts of ascites can accumulate in the peritoneal cavity before resulting in significant patient discomfort, the accumulation of smaller amounts of fluid (1 to 2 L) in the pleural space results in severe shortness of breath and hypoxemia. Pleural effusion is right sided in 85%, left sided in 13%, and bilateral in 2% of the cases.[48] The diagnosis of hepatic hydrothorax is established by radionuclide scanning of the chest after the intraperitoneal injection of Tc-99m–labeled sulfur colloid or macroaggregated serum albumin. In hepatic hydrothorax, presence of radiotracer in the pleural space is demonstrated generally within 2 hours of intraperitoneal injection.[49,50]

Disease Complication— Spontaneous Bacterial Peritonitis

Spontaneous bacterial peritonitis (SBP) is a potentially lethal complication of ascites. SBP is an infection of ascites that occurs in the absence of a contiguous source of infection (e.g., intestinal perforation, intraabdominal abscess) and in the absence of an intraabdominal inflammatory focus (e.g., abscess, acute pancreatitis, cholecystitis). Since its first description in the English literature in 1963-1964 as a "rarely recognized syndrome," great strides have been made in its recognition and therapy, leading to a decrease in its mortality from 80% or more in the initial series to a current mortality rate of 10% to 20%.[51]

Epidemiology

The most common type of infection in hospitalized cirrhotic patients, SBP occurs in 10%% to 20%[52,53] of the patients and accounting for about 25% of all bacterial infections.[53] The prevalence of SBP is much lower in the outpatient setting, ranging up to 3.5% in patients undergoing serial therapeutic paracenteses.[54-56] In prospective studies, the 1-year probability of developing a first episode of SBP in cirrhotic patients with ascites has ranged between 11%[57] and 29%,[58] incidence that is highly dependent on ascites total protein content (0% in patients with an ascites protein >1 g/dl vs. 20% in patients with an ascites protein <1 g/dl).[57] Spontaneous bacterial empyema is an entity akin to SBP in which hepatic hydrothorax becomes infected; it can occur in the absence of SBP or ascites and its diagnosis and management are the same as for SBP.[59]

Clinical Picture

The typical features of SBP consist of local symptoms and signs of a generalized peritonitis (i.e., diffuse abdominal pain, abdominal tenderness with rebound tenderness, decreased bowel sounds). Systemic symptoms consist of fever, encephalopathy, leukocytosis, and/or acute kidney injury. However, patients rarely have the complete picture, and the accuracy of the clinical picture in diagnosing or excluding SBP is low.[60]

Diagnosis

A diagnostic paracentesis is the mainstay in the diagnosis of SBP and should be performed not only in cirrhotic patients with ascites who have compatible clinical features (e.g., fever, abdominal pain, leukocytosis) but also in those admitted to the hospital for any other reason and in those with unexplained encephalopathy or renal dysfunction.[27,61]

Despite the use of more sensitive bacteriologic culture methods, such as inoculation of ascites into blood culture bottles, ascites culture is negative in up to 60% of patients with clinical manifestations suggestive of SBP and increased ascites PMN.[53,61] Therefore the diagnosis of SBP is established with an ascites PMN count greater than 250 per mm^3. This cutoff has been identified as the one with the greatest diagnostic accuracy.[52] In hemorrhagic ascites (i.e., ascites red blood cell count >10,000/mm^3), subtracting one PMN for every 250 red blood cells will correct for the excess blood in ascites.

To maximize the possibilities of isolating an infecting organism, both ascites and blood bacteriologic cultures should be performed whenever SBP is suspected.[61]

Treatment

Once an ascites PMN count greater than 250 per mm^3 is detected, empirical antibiotic therapy needs to be started before obtaining the results of ascites or blood cultures (**Fig. 18-6**). Antibiotic therapy is also justified in patients in whom ascites cultures are twice positive despite PMN counts less than 250 per mm^3.

The recommended initial antibiotics are intravenous (IV) cefotaxime or other third-generation cephalosporins and the combination of amoxicillin and clavulanic acid.[61] Doses of cefotaxime used range from 2 g IV every 4 hours to 2 g IV every 12 hours with equal efficacy.[62] Ceftriaxone is used at a dose of 1 to 2 g IV every 24 hours and ceftazidime at a dose of 1 g IV every 12 to 24 hours. Amoxicillin/clavulanic acid is used at a dose of 1 g/0.2 g IV every 8 hours.[63] Resolution of SBP with initial antibiotic therapy had been previously described as being approximately 85%, with the other 15% requiring antibiotic modification.[62-65] However, more recently, failure of initial antibiotic therapy has been described in about a third of patients[66,67] because of an increase in infections due to multidrug-resistant organisms.[68] These infections are more prevalent in hospital-acquired SBP[69] and are associated with a higher mortality.[67,68] Therefore broadest (carbapenems) or extended spectrum ß-lactam antibiotics (e.g., piperacillin/tazobactam) should be considered as initial empirical therapy in patients with hospital-acquired SBP, particularly in those who had been previously on antibiotics[68] (see **Fig. 18-6**).

After 5 days of antibiotic therapy, ascites PMN decreases below 250/mm^3 in the majority of patients with SBP.[70] In fact, 5-day antibiotic therapy has been shown to be as effective as 10-day therapy[64] and is therefore recommended as the minimum duration of therapy.[61]

Cirrhotic patients have an increased propensity to develop aminoglycoside-induced nephrotoxicity and therefore these antibiotics should be avoided.

Renal impairment, a main cause of death in SBP, occurs as a result of a further decrease in effective arterial blood volume that in turn probably results from a cytokine-mediated aggravation of vasodilation as occurs in sepsis, in addition to

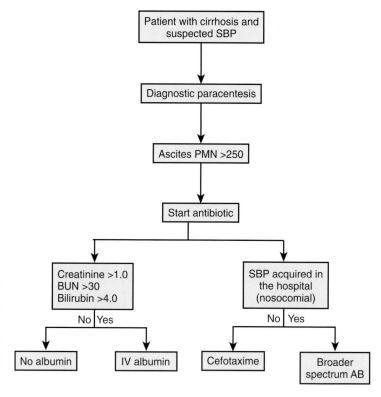

Fig. 18-6 **Treatment algorithm in a patient with suspected SBP.** Once a PMN count greater than 250/mm³ is detected, antibiotic treatment should be initiated. In patients with evidence of renal dysfunction or jaundice, concomitant IV albumin is recommended. In patients with hospital-acquired SBP, broadest (carbapenems) or extended spectrum ß-lactam antibiotics (e.g., piperacillin/tazobactam) should be considered, particularly in those who had been previously on antibiotics.

a possible impairment in cardiac function.[71] Intravenous albumin, as an adjunct to antibiotic therapy, has the objective of increasing effective blood volume and is associated with lower rates of renal dysfunction and in-hospital mortality.[65] The dose of albumin used is arbitrary, 1.5 g/kg of body weight during the first 6 hours, followed by 1 g/kg on day 3, to a maximum of 100 g/day. Patients that benefit from adjuvant albumin are those with evidence of renal impairment at baseline (BUN >30 mg/dl and/or creatinine >1.0 mg/dl) and/or with a serum bilirubin greater than 4 mg/dl.[65] It is this subgroup of patients in whom albumin can be recommended[72] (see **Fig. 18-6**). In the absence of these high-risk parameters, the risk of renal deterioration and death is almost negligible[73-75] and albumin is not indicated (see **Fig. 18-6**).

A control paracentesis performed 48 hours after starting therapy is recommended to assess the response to therapy and the need to modify antibiotic therapy (depending on the isolation of a causative organism) and/or to initiate investigations to rule out secondary peritonitis.[61] In the presence of obvious clinical improvement, this control paracentesis may not be necessary. Intravenous antibiotics can be safely switched to oral antibiotics after 2 days of therapy in patients who demonstrate an appropriate response to initial therapy.[76]

Prophylaxis

Because antibiotic prophylaxis is associated with a higher rate of infections by quinolone-resistant and trimethoprim-sulfamethoxazole–resistant organisms and by *Clostridium difficile*,[53,77,78] it should be restricted to patients with cirrhosis at the highest risk of developing SBP.

Patients who survive an episode of SBP have a very high probability of developing recurrent SBP (approximately 70% in 1 year). Recurrence, particularly from gram-negative

organisms, is significantly and markedly lower with the use of oral norfloxacin at a dose of 400 mg/day.[79,80] It is therefore essential that patients who survive an episode of SBP be started on antibiotic prophylaxis to prevent recurrence (**Fig. 18-7**). The use of weekly quinolones is not recommended because it has been shown to be less effective in preventing SBP recurrence and more likely to be associated with quinolone-resistant organisms.[80] Prophylaxis should be continuous until disappearance of ascites (i.e., patients with alcoholic hepatitis), death, or transplant.

Another group of patients in whom antibiotic prophylaxis should be used routinely is the group of patients admitted with GI hemorrhage, in which the rate of bacterial infection is as high as 45%. In these patients, short-term antibiotic prophylaxis has been shown to be effective not only in reducing the rate of bacterial infections, but also in reducing in-hospital mortality[81] and variceal rebleeding.[82] Although the recommended antibiotic is norfloxacin at a dose of 400 mg orally twice a day for up to 7 days,[61] a recent study shows that intravenous ceftriaxone (1 g/day) is more effective in preventing infection (including SBP) in patients with two or more of the following: malnutrition, ascites, encephalopathy, or serum bilirubin greater than 3 mg/dl.[83] However, in this study, six of seven gram-negative infections in the norfloxacin group were caused by quinolone resistant organisms.[83] Therefore the choice of antibiotic should be based on the local prevalence of quinolone resistance and perhaps on the severity of liver disease.

Although patients with ascites protein less than 1 g/dl who have never developed SBP are at higher risk of developing SBP than those with ascites protein greater than 1 g/dl, the overall risk is low at approximately 13% in a 12-month period.[77,84,85] However, a recent placebo-controlled study identified a subgroup of patients with a very high 1-year probability of developing SBP of approximately 60%. These were patients who, in

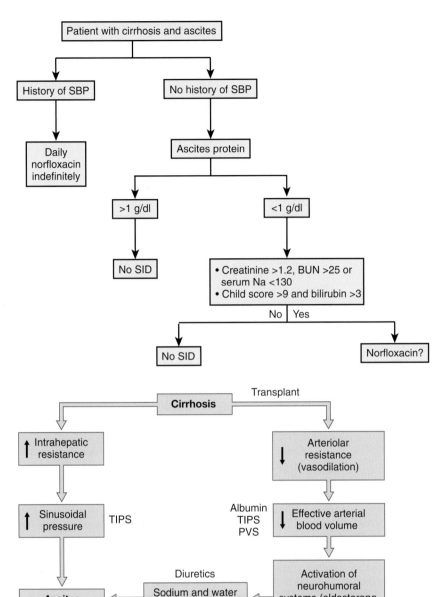

Fig. 18-7 **Prophylaxis of SBP.** Patients with a prior history of SBP should receive prophylactic norfloxacin as a means to achieve selective intestinal decontamination.[79] Prophylaxis may also be considered in patients without a history of SBP who have a low ascites protein (<1.5 g/dl) and who additionally have advanced liver failure (CTP score ≥9 and serum bilirubin ≥3 mg/dl) or evidence of circulatory dysfunction (serum creatinine of 1.2 mg/dl, blood urea nitrogen level of 25 mg/dl, or serum sodium level of 130 mEq/L).[86]

Fig. 18-8 **Different treatments of ascites placed in the context of its pathophysiology.**

addition to having a low (<1.5 g/L) ascites protein, had advanced liver failure (CTP score ≥9 and serum bilirubin ≥3 mg/dl) or evidence of circulatory dysfunction (serum creatinine of 1.2 mg/dl, blood urea nitrogen level of 25 mg/dl, or serum sodium level of 130 mEq/L).[86] Compared with a placebo, daily oral norfloxacin was associated with a significant reduction in SBP (to 7%), hepatorenal syndrome, and 3-month mortality.[86] It is in this selected subpopulation of patients with cirrhosis and ascites that prophylaxis with norfloxacin (400 mg PO qd) could be considered, although confirmatory studies are necessary before it can be firmly recommended (see **Fig. 18-7**).

Treatment of Ascites

The treatment of cirrhotic ascites is important, not only because it improves the quality of life of the cirrhotic patient

but because SBP, one of the most lethal complications of cirrhosis, does not occur in the absence of ascites. Therapies for ascites include sodium restriction, diuretics, large-volume paracentesis (LVP), the transjugular intrahepatic portosystemic shunt (TIPS), and the peritoneovenous shunt (PVS) (**Fig. 18-8**).[27,87] The development of ascites in a patient with cirrhosis denotes a poor prognosis and is an indication to initiate liver transplant evaluation. Therefore transplantation constitutes the ultimate treatment for ascites and its complications.

Ascites responds appropriately in 80% to 90% of the patients upon attainment of a negative sodium balance through the use of sodium restriction and/or diuretics. Even though this treatment takes longer and may have a higher complication rate than LVP, treatment based on sodium restriction and diuretics still constitutes the mainstay of therapy given its general applicability, low cost, and ease of administration. In fact, the categorization of cirrhotic patients with ascites is based on their response to diuretic therapy. In this scheme, uncomplicated ascites assumes an uninfected ascites with good response to diuretics and refractory ascites assumes either diuretic-resistant ascites (ascites that is not eliminated even with maximal diuretic therapy) or diuretic-intractable ascites (ascites that is not eliminated because maximal doses of diuretics cannot be reached given the development of renal and/or electrolyte abnormalities).[88]

Sodium Restriction

Sodium restriction is recommended in all cirrhotic patients with ascites. Although dietary sodium should be restricted to levels lower than urinary sodium excretion, sodium restriction to approximately 90 mEq/day (i.e., 2 grams of sodium per day or 5.2 g of dietary salt per day, considering that 1 mEq of sodium = 23 mg of sodium = 58.5 mg of dietary salt) is a realistic goal, particularly in the outpatient setting.[22] Further restriction of sodium is unrealistic and difficult to achieve. Patients with a baseline urinary sodium excretion greater than 50 mEq per 24 hours may respond to salt restriction alone, although this occurs in a minority of patients. There are virtually no complications associated with sodium restriction. However, clinicians should be cautious about the nutritional status of patients on sodium restriction because the nonpalatability of a salt-restricted diet may lead to an inadequate food intake. In these cases, liberalizing sodium restriction and adding diuretics is preferable to further compromising the already compromised nutrition of the cirrhotic patient with ascites.

Diuretics

Spironolactone is the diuretic of choice. Even though loop diuretics such as furosemide are more potent natriuretics, randomized trials have shown a significantly lower efficacy of furosemide used alone compared with spironolactone alone[89,90] or to the combination spironolactone/furosemide.[89] When furosemide is used alone, sodium that is not reabsorbed in the loop of Henle is taken up at the distal and collecting tubules as a result of the hyperaldosteronism present in most cirrhotic patients with ascites. Therefore furosemide should not be used as the sole agent in the treatment of cirrhotic ascites.

Diuretic therapy can be initiated with spironolactone alone or with spironolactone plus furosemide. Both schemes have their advocates and the choice may depend on the degree of ascites and the clinical setting.[91,92] The disadvantage of starting with spironolactone alone is the delay before its clinical effect and the associated hyperkalemia.[92] The disadvantage of starting with combination spironolactone/furosemide therapy is the need for more frequent monitoring and dose adjustments.[89,91] Spironolactone is initiated at a daily dose of 50 to 100 mg PO and increased in a stepwise fashion to a maximum of 400 mg/day. Because the effect of spironolactone takes several days, it can be administered in a single daily dose and dose adjustments should only be performed every 3 to 4 days. If spironolactone alone is initiated, furosemide should be added if and when weight loss is not optimal or hyperkalemia develops. Furosemide should be used with spironolactone and started at an initial single daily dose of 40 mg, increased in a stepwise fashion to a maximum of 160 mg/day. An insufficient diuretic response necessitating increases in the dose of diuretics is defined as a weight loss less than 1 kg in the first week

and less than 2 kg/week in subsequent weeks.[22] Before considering that ascites is refractory to diuretics, it is necessary to ascertain whether the patient has adhered to the prescribed sodium-restricted diet and has restrained from using nonsteroidal antiinflammatory drugs, known to blunt the response to diuretics. Nonadherence to dietary sodium restriction and/ or diuretics should be suspected if patients fail to lose weight despite an adequate 24-hour urine sodium excretion (>50 mEq/L or greater than daily sodium intake).

Complications

The more common complications of diuretic therapy are renal impairment due to intravascular volume depletion (25%), hyponatremia (28%), and hepatic encephalopathy (26%).[93-95] Diuretics should not be initiated in patients with a rising creatinine or in patients with concomitant complications of cirrhosis known to be associated with a decreased effective arterial blood volume, such as variceal hemorrhage and SBP. In patients who develop renal dysfunction (elevation in creatinine >50% to a creatinine >1.5 mg/dl), diuretics should be temporarily discontinued and restarted at a lower dose once creatinine returns to baseline. Patients who develop hyponatremia (serum sodium <130 mEq/L) while on diuretics should be managed with fluid restriction and a decrease in the dose of diuretics. To minimize the rate of complications, weight loss in patients without edema should be maintained at a maximum of 1 lb/day (0.5 kg/day), while patients with edema can safely lose up to 2 lb/day (1 kg/day).

Spironolactone is often associated with adverse events related to its antiandrogenic activity, mainly painful gynecomastia. Potassium canrenoate, one of the major metabolites of spironolactone, has a comparable diuretic effect and a lower antiandrogenic activity. However, this drug is not available in the United States. Amiloride, another potassium-sparing diuretic, does not produce gynecomastia and is recommended in patients with intolerable painful gynecomastia, but it has a significantly less natriuretic effect than spironolactone.[96] Amiloride is used at an initial dose of 20 mg/day and can be increased to 60 mg/day. In patients in whom natriuretic response on amiloride is suboptimal, it may be worthwhile to attempt retreatment with spironolactone.

Contraindications

Nonsteroidal antiinflammatory drugs or aspirin blunt the natriuretic effect of diuretics and should therefore not be used in cirrhotic patients with ascites.[97,98] Although selective cyclooxygenase-2 (COX-2) inhibitors have not been shown to impair natriuresis or to induce renal dysfunction in cirrhotic rats,[99] data in patients indicate that celecoxib may be related to a decrease in renal function[100] and therefore COX-2 inhibitor use should also be avoided.

Large Volume Paracentesis

Large volume paracentesis (LVP) associated with IV albumin has been shown to be as effective as standard therapy with diuretics but with a significantly faster resolution and with an equal or lower rate of complications.[93,94,101] Because this therapy is significantly more expensive and requires more resources than the administration of diuretics, it is reserved for patients who do not respond to diuretics. However, in patients with tense ascites and in order to ameliorate patient discomfort, it is reasonable to initiate therapy with an LVP followed by diuretics.

Currently, LVP is standard therapy for refractory ascites. Removal of all ascites in a single procedure (total paracentesis) accompanied by the concomitant infusion of 6 to 8 g of albumin per liter of ascites removed is as safe as repeated partial paracentesis[101] and is the recommended LVP modality.[22]

Because LVP is a local therapy that does not act on any of the mechanisms that lead to the formation of ascites, recurrence of ascites is the rule rather than the exception. The frequency of LVP is determined by the rate of ascites reaccumulation and ultimately on the need to relieve the patient's discomfort. The rate of ascites reaccumulation depends largely on the patient's compliance with salt restriction and diuretics, as well as the degree of sodium retention. The administration of diuretics after LVP is associated with a longer time to recurrence of ascites without any differences in complications.[102] Therefore sodium restriction and diuretics at the maximum tolerated dose should be used in conjunction with serial LVP. However, diuretics should be discontinued if associated with complications or if urinary sodium is less than 30 mEq/L.

Complications

One of the main complications of LVP is the development of postparacentesis circulatory dysfunction (PCD), defined as a significant increase in plasma renin activity (PRA) 6 days after LVP. Development of PCD is associated with a faster recurrence of ascites, development of renal dysfunction, and a higher mortality.[103,104] Two factors are independent predictors of the development of PCD: the amount of ascites extracted and the type of volume expander used in association with LVP,[103] with the lowest rates observed when less than 5 L are removed and/or when albumin is used as a plasma volume expander (rate approximately 16%) (see **Fig. 18-8**).[103,105-107] Albumin should be administered at a dose of 6 to 8 g of albumin IV per liter of ascites removed. For LVP less than 5 L, a synthetic plasma expander (Haemaccel, Dextran-70) or even a saline solution can be used instead of albumin, and it has been suggested that no plasma expansion may be necessary in this setting (**Fig. 18-9**).[22,103,107]

Procedure-related complications consist mainly of bleeding and ascites leakage.[108] Major bleeding occurs rarely but may be lethal[108,109] and although it is mostly related to puncture of mesenteric vessels, it has been recently suggested that a platelet count less than 50,000/mm[3] may be a predictor of severe complications and platelet transfusion before LVP may be recommended in these cases.[108] Leakage of ascitic fluid is rare and occurs with incomplete ascites removal. This complication can be solved by completing the LVP, preferably in a site remote from the leaking puncture site. Similarly, another complication of paracentesis that is rare but should be recognized is the development of sudden scrotal edema that results from subcutaneous tracking of peritoneal fluid into the scrotum and can be solved by elevation of the scrotum.[110]

Contraindications

The pathogenesis of PCD appears to be the worsening of the vasodilatory state of the cirrhotic patient with a consequent

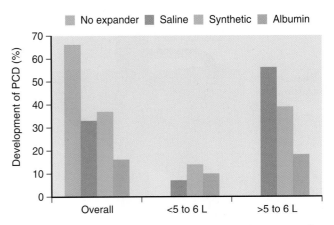

Fig. 18-9 **Summary of studies exploring plasma volume expansion and development of PCD.** Two factors are independent predictors of the development of PCD: the amount of ascites extracted and the type of volume expander used in association with LVP.[103] When no plasma volume expander is used, PCD occurs in the majority of patients[105]; when synthetic plasma volume expanders or saline are used, PCD occurs in about 30% of the patients[103,106,107]; and when albumin is used, the lowest rates of PCD (approximately 16%) occur after LVP.[103,107]

further decrease in effective arterial blood volume and marked activation of neurohumoral systems that lead to further sodium retention, renal vasoconstriction, renal dysfunction and death.[104] Therefore LVP should not be performed in the setting of conditions that have been associated with a worsening in the vasodilatory state of cirrhosis, such as SBP.

Transjugular Intrahepatic Portosystemic Shunt (TIPS)

Since the publication of the first uncontrolled study of TIPS for the treatment of refractory ascites in 1993,[111] advances have been made in our understanding of the effect of TIPS in patients with refractory ascites, including the publication of five prospective randomized trials comparing TIPS with LVP.[112-116] Meta-analyses of these trials show that TIPS are more effective in preventing recurrence of ascites.[117,118] This is not surprising because TIPS act on the pathophysiologic mechanisms responsible for ascites formation, whereas LVP does not (**Fig. 18-10**). TIPS placement is associated with a normalization of sinusoidal pressure and a significant improvement in urinary sodium excretion that correlates with suppression in plasma renin activity (indicative of an improvement in effective arterial blood volume).[119] However, compared with LVP, TIPS are associated with a higher risk for severe encephalopathy without differences in survival rates.[117,118] A recent meta-analysis of individual patient data of three trials[113,115,116] shows that TIPS are associated with a significantly lower mortality compared with LVP and identified a MELD score greater than 15 as being a strong predictor of post-TIPS death.[120] There are limitations in the trials performed so far, principally the use of uncovered TIPS stents in all of them. Uncovered stents obstruct frequently (18% to 78%)[121] and have been largely substituted by polytetrafluoroethylene-covered stents that are associated with a significantly lower obstruction rate and a decreased risk of encephalopathy.[122] Until results of ongoing trials using

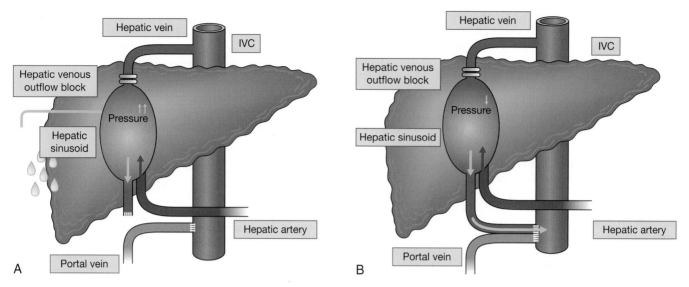

Fig. 18-10 Effects on ascites formation of an end-to-side portocaval shunt (A) and a side-to-side portocaval shunt (B). Although an end-to-side portocaval shunt **(A)** would decrease the development of ascites by decompressing splanchnic capillaries and decreasing blood flow into the sinusoids, it can also lead to greater ascites formation, particularly in patients with advanced cirrhosis in whom the outflow block is such that the portal vein becomes the outflow tract. On the other hand, the side-to-side portocaval shunt **(B)** (and the mesocaval shunt), by connecting the side of the portal vein (or the mesenteric vein) to the low-pressure inferior vena cava (IVC), effectively decompresses not only the collaterals but also the sinusoids. TIPS is physiologically a side-to-side portocaval shunt.

covered stents are available, TIPS should be considered second-line treatment for refractory ascites.[22] It is an option in patients who require frequent paracentesis and are good candidates for TIPS (bilirubin <3 mg/dl and/or MELD <15).

Complications

Long-term complications of TIPS are a new onset or worsening of prior hepatic encephalopathy and shunt dysfunction. Both occur in about a third of the patients in a mean follow-up of about 1 year.[119] The procedure-related complication rate is around 9%, with the most common being intraperitoneal hemorrhage.[121] Other important complications are heart failure and hemolysis that may develop in 10% to 15% of patients.

Contraindications

A poor liver function (a Child-Pugh score >11 and/or a MELD score >15 and/or a bilirubin >3 mg/dl) should be considered a contraindication for TIPS placement. TIPS should also be avoided in elderly patients (>70 years) and in those with heart dysfunction.[22] Patients with alcoholic cirrhosis who are drinking alcohol may improve with abstinence and therefore TIPS should be delayed in these patients.

Peritoneovenous Shunt

Peritoneovenous shunts (PVS) are an alternative to LVP. In randomized trials, PVS has been shown to be equally effective as LVP, with a similar rate of complications and a comparable survival rate.[123,124] However, due to its high obstruction rate, PVS requires frequent admissions for shunt revision or for the management of other more serious complications. The use of PVS has practically been abandoned because LVP is a simpler procedure that can be performed in the outpatient setting.

Additionally, placement of a PVS may hinder future placement of TIPS and may complicate liver transplant surgery given its ability to produce peritoneal adhesions. Therefore PVS is mostly indicated in patients who require LVP frequently and who are not candidates for TIPS or for transplant.

Treatment of Conditions Associated with Ascites
Treatment of Hyponatremia

Water restriction (1 to 1.5 L/day) prevents the progressive decrease in serum sodium but it does not correct hyponatremia. The administration of hypertonic saline solutions is not recommended because it will lead to further accumulation of ascites and edema. Because hyponatremia results primarily from a decrease in effective arterial blood volume, plasma volume expansion with albumin is a reasonable therapy, but its effect is transient.[125]

V2 receptor antagonists ("vaptans") have been the most investigated aquaretic agents. Although the short-term (7 to 14 days) use of lixivaptan[126,127] and satavaptan[128] was effective in increasing serum sodium in patients with cirrhosis, these drugs have been withdrawn because of severe side effects. Tolvaptan used for 30 days in patients with euvolemic or hypervolemic hyponatremia (of which 63 had cirrhosis), leads to rapid improvement in serum sodium and significant weight loss compared with a placebo, without significant side effects.[129] Longer-term trials targeting patients with cirrhosis are awaited.

Treatment of Hepatic Hydrothorax

Hepatic hydrothorax should be treated in the same manner as cirrhotic ascites (i.e., the mainstay of therapy is sodium restriction and diuretics). Before determining that hydrothorax is refractory, a trial of in-hospital diuretic therapy should be attempted. In patients with refractory hepatic hydrothorax, other therapeutic options, such as repeated thoracenteses, TIPS, or pleurodesis, should be considered. Regarding thoracentesis, and given that no more than 2 L be removed at a time because of the risk of reexpansion pulmonary edema, the procedure may need to be repeated very frequently. When thoracentesis is required every 2 to 3 weeks, alternative strategies such as TIPS should be considered. In a recent large series of 73 patients treated with TIPS, a good clinical response was observed in 75% with a median survival rate of 514 days.[130] A MELD score below 15 was once more identified as being a predictor of a better survival rate and should be used to select candidates for TIPS.[130] Placement of a chest tube should be avoided in patients with hepatic hydrothorax because it has been associated with multiple complications, mainly volume and electrolyte disturbances.

Prognosis and Natural History

The natural history of cirrhotic ascites progresses from diuretic-responsive (uncomplicated) ascites to the development of dilutional hyponatremia, refractory ascites, and finally, hepatorenal syndrome (HRS). While median survival time in patients with compensated cirrhosis is greater than 12 years,[2] once decompensation occurs, median survival time decrease to 1.6 to 1.8 years.[3,5] While the 1-year survival rate in patients who develop ascites is 85%, it decreases to 25% once it has progressed to hyponatremia, refractory ascites, or HRS.[131] In cirrhotic patients with moderate to tense ascites, four parameters have been found to be independent predictors of survival: impaired water excretion, mean arterial pressure, Child-Pugh class, and serum creatinine.[132] Except for the Child-Pugh score, which is a marker of liver function, all other parameters indicate a worsened hemodynamic status (a more vasodilated state) and are consistent with other studies that have shown that hyponatremia and renal dysfunction are predictors of a poor survival rate with cirrhosis.[133,134]

In patients with a low MELD score, persistent ascites and low serum sodium are the only parameters predictive of early mortality.[135,136]

HRS is a rare but severe complication that occurs in cirrhotic patients with ascites. From the time of first presentation with ascites, the 5-year probability of developing HRS is 11%,[131] with a higher probability in patients with hyponatremia or refractory ascites. Without liver transplantation and before recent studies using vasoconstrictors, recovery of renal function was unusual (<5% of patients) and prognosis was poor, with a median survival rate of 2 weeks.[137] With the use of vasoconstrictors, reversal of HRS occurs in about half the patients but the mortality is still high.[138]

Conclusions

Ascites is the most common decompensating event in cirrhosis and is associated with a poor prognosis. Mainstay of therapy is sodium restriction and diuretics. Patients in whom ascites is refractory to diuretic therapy should be treated with LVP accompanied by IV infusion of albumin. Until further studies are available evaluating the efficacy of covered stents,

TIPS should be reserved for patients who require frequent LVP. SBP is a complication of ascites with a high mortality. Prompt diagnosis and early therapy with antibiotics is essential. In patients with renal dysfunction or jaundice, IV albumin will prevent the development of renal dysfunction and death. Patients with ascites should initiate evaluation to determine liver transplant candidacy.

Key References

Albillos A, et al. A meta-analysis of transjugular intrahepatic portosystemic shunt versus paracentesis for refractory ascites. J Hepatol 2005;43:990–996. (Ref.118)

Albillos A, et al. Continuous prazosin administration in cirrhotic patients: effects on portal hemodynamics and on liver and renal function. Gastroenterology 1995;109:1257–1265. (Ref.15)

Andreu M, et al. Risk factors for spontaneous bacterial peritonitis in cirrhotic patients with ascites. Gastroenterology 1993;104:1133–1138. (Ref.58)

Angeli P, et al. Randomized clinical study of the efficacy of amiloride and potassium canrenoate in nonazotemic cirrhotic patients with ascites. Hepatology 1994;19:72–79. (Ref.96)

Angeli P, et al. Combined versus sequential diuretic treatment of ascites in nonazotemic patients with cirrhosis: results of an open randomized clinical trial. Gut 2010;59:10–11. (Ref.92)

Angeloni S, et al. Efficacy of current guidelines for the treatment of spontaneous bacterial peritonitis in the clinical practice. World J Gastroenterol 2008;14:2757–2762. (Ref.66)

Arnold C, et al. Acute hemoperitoneum after large-volume paracentesis. Gastroenterology 1997;113:978–982. (Ref.109)

Arroyo V, et al. Definition and diagnostic criteria of refractory ascites and hepatorenal syndrome in cirrhosis. Hepatology 1996;23:164–176. (Ref.88)

Bajaj JS, et al. Clostridium difficile is associated with poor outcomes in patients with cirrhosis: a national and tertiary center perspective. Am J Gastroenterol 2010;105(1):106–113. (Ref.78)

Bauer TM, et al. Daily norfloxacin is more effective than weekly rufloxacin in prevention of spontaneous bacterial peritonitis recurrence. Dig Dis Sci 2002;47:1356–1361. (Ref.80)

Belghiti J, Durand F. Abdominal wall hernias in the setting of cirrhosis. Semin Liver Dis 1997;17:219–226. (Ref.41)

Bernard B, et al. Antibiotic prophylaxis for the prevention of bacterial infections in cirrhotic patients with gastrointestinal bleeding: a meta-analysis. Hepatology 1999;29:1655–1661. (Ref.81)

Bhattacharya A, et al. Radioisotope scintigraphy in the diagnosis of hepatic hydrothorax. J Gastroenterol Hepatol 2001;16:317–321. (Ref.50)

Bosch-Marce M, et al. Selective inhibition of cyclooxygenase 2 spares renal function and prostaglandin synthesis in cirrhotic rats with ascites. Gastroenterology 1999;116:1167–1176. (Ref.99)

Boyer TD, Haskal ZJ. The role of transjugular intrahepatic portosystemic shunt in the management of portal hypertension. Hepatology 2005;41:386–400. (Ref.121)

Bureau C, et al. Improved clinical outcome using polytetrafluoroethylene-coated stents for TIPS: results of a randomized study. Gastroenterology 2004;126:469–475. (Ref.122)

Cardenas A, Kelleher T, Chopra S. Review article: hepatic hydrothorax. Aliment Pharmacol Ther 2004;20:271–279. (Ref.46)

Casado M, et al. Clinical events after transjugular intrahepatic portosystemic shunt: correlation with hemodynamic findings. Gastroenterology 1998;114:1296–1303. (Ref.8)

Castellote J, et al. Spontaneous bacterial peritonitis and bacterascites prevalence in asymptomatic cirrhotic outpatients undergoing large-volume paracentesis. J Gastroenterol Hepatol 2008;23:256–259. (Ref.56)

Cheong HS, et al. Clinical significance and outcome of nosocomial acquisition of spontaneous bacterial peritonitis in patients with liver cirrhosis. Clin Infect Dis 2009;48:1230–1236. (Ref.69)

Chinnock B, et al. Physician clinical impression does not rule out spontaneous bacterial peritonitis in patients undergoing emergency department paracentesis. Ann Emerg Med 2008;52:268–273. (Ref.60)

D'Amico G, Garcia-Tsao G, Pagliaro L. Natural history and prognostic indicators of survival in cirrhosis. A systematic review of 118 studies. J Hepatol 2006;44:217–231. (Ref.2)

D'Amico G, et al. Uncovered transjugular intrahepatic portosystemic shunt for refractory ascites: a meta-analysis. Gastroenterology 2005;129:1282–1293. (Ref.117)

De Gottardi A, et al. Risk of complications after abdominal paracentesis in cirrhotic patients: a prospective study. Clin Gastroenterol Hepatol 2009;7:906–909. (Ref.108)

Dhanasekaran R, et al. Transjugular intrahepatic portosystemic shunt for symptomatic refractory hepatic hydrothorax in patients with cirrhosis. Am J Gastroenterol 2010;105(3):635–641. (Ref.130)

Evans LT, et al. Spontaneous bacterial peritonitis in asymptomatic outpatients with cirrhotic ascites. Hepatology 2003;37:897–901. (Ref.54)

Fernandez J, et al. Bacterial infections in cirrhosis: epidemiological changes with invasive procedures and norfloxacin prophylaxis. Hepatology 2002;35:140–148. (Ref.53)

Fernandez J, et al. Primary prophylaxis of spontaneous bacterial peritonitis delays hepatorenal syndrome and improves survival in cirrhosis. Gastroenterology 2007;133:818–824. (Ref.86)

Fernandez J, et al. Norfloxacin vs ceftriaxone in the prophylaxis of infections in patients with advanced cirrhosis and hemorrhage. Gastroenterology 2006; 131:1049–1056. (Ref.83)

Fernandez-Esparrach G, et al. Diuretic requirements after therapeutic paracentesis in non-azotemic patients with cirrhosis. A randomized double-blind trial of spironolactone versus placebo. J Hepatol 1997;26: 614–620. (Ref.102)

Fernandez-Esparrach G, et al. A prognostic model for predicting survival in cirrhosis with ascites. J Hepatol 2001;34:46–52. (Ref.132)

Ferral H, et al. Refractory ascites: early experience in treatment with transjugular intrahepatic portosystemic shunt. Radiology 1993;189(3):795–801. (Ref.111)

Garcia-Tsao G. Bacterial infections in cirrhosis: treatment and prophylaxis. J Hepatol 2005;42(Suppl 1):S85–S92. (Ref.72)

Garcia-Tsao G. Spontaneous bacterial peritonitis. Gastroenterol Clin North Am 1992;21:257–275. (Ref.52)

Garcia-Tsao G. Spontaneous bacterial peritonitis: a historical perspective. J Hepatol 2004;41:522–527. (Ref.51)

Garcia-Tsao G. The transjugular intrahepatic portosystemic shunt for the management of refractory ascites. Nat Clin Pract Gastroenterol Hepatol 2006;3:380–389. (Ref.119)

Garcia-Tsao G, Lim JK. Management and treatment of patients with cirrhosis and portal hypertension: recommendations from the Department of Veterans Affairs hepatitis C resource center program and the national hepatitis C program. Am J Gastroenterol 2009;104:1802–1829. (Ref.87)

Gentilini P, et al. Long course and prognostic factors of virus-induced cirrhosis of the liver. Am J Gastroenterol 1997;92:66–72. (Ref.6)

Gerbes AL, et al. Therapy of hyponatremia in cirrhosis with a vasopressin receptor antagonist: a randomized double-blind multicenter trial. Gastroenterology 2003;124:933–939. (Ref.127)

Gines P, et al. Hyponatremia in cirrhosis: from pathogenesis to treatment. Hepatology 1998;28:851–863. (Ref.12)

Gines A, et al. Incidence, predictive factors, and prognosis of the hepatorenal syndrome in cirrhosis with ascites. Gastroenterology 1993;105:229–236. (Ref.137)

Gines A, et al. Randomized trial comparing albumin, Dextran-70 and polygeline in cirrhotic patients with ascites treated by paracentesis. Gastroenterology 1996;111:1002–1010. (Ref.103)

Gines A, et al. Treatment of patients with cirrhosis and refractory ascites by LeVeen shunt with titanium tip. Comparison with therapeutic paracentesis. Hepatology 1995;22:124–131. (Ref.124)

Gines P, et al. Transjugular intrahepatic portosystemic shunting versus repeated paracentesis plus intravenous albumin for refractory ascites in cirrhosis: a multicenter randomized comparative study. Gastroenterology 2002;123: 1839–1847. (Ref.114)

Gines P, et al. Effects of satavaptan, a selective vasopressin V(2) receptor antagonist, on ascites and serum sodium in cirrhosis with hyponatremia: a randomized trial. Hepatology 2008;48:204–213. (Ref.128)

Girgrah N, et al. Haemodynamic, renal sodium handling, and neurohormonal effects of acute administration of low dose losartan, an angiotensin II receptor antagonist, in preascitic cirrhosis. Gut 2000;46:114–120. (Ref.18)

Gluud LL, et al. Systematic review of randomized trials on vasoconstrictor drugs for hepatorenal syndrome. Hepatology 2010;51:576–584. (Ref.138)

Grange JD, et al. Norfloxacin primary prophylaxis of bacterial infections in cirrhotic patients with ascites: a double-blind randomized trial. J Hepatol 1998;29:430–436. (Ref.84)

Groszmann RJ, Wongcharatrawee S. The hepatic venous pressure gradient: anything worth doing should be done right. Hepatology 2004;39:280–283. (Ref.39)

Guevara M, Abecasis R, Terg R. Effect of celecoxib on renal function in cirrhotic patients with ascites. A pilot study. Scand J Gastroenterol 2004;39:385–386. (Ref.100)

Heuman DM, et al. Persistent ascites and low serum sodium identify patients with cirrhosis and low MELD scores who are at high risk for early death. Hepatology 2004;40:802–810. (Ref.135)

Hou MC, et al. Antibiotic prophylaxis after endoscopic therapy prevents rebleeding in acute variceal hemorrhage: a randomized trial. Hepatology 2004;39:746–753. (Ref.82)

Kim WR, et al. Hyponatremia and mortality among patients on the liver-transplant waiting list. N Engl J Med 2008;359:1018–1026. (Ref.136)

Lebrec D, et al. Transjugular intrahepatic portosystemic shunts: comparison with paracentesis in patients with cirrhosis and refractory ascites: a randomized trial. J Hepatol 1996;25:135–144. (Ref.112)

Lee FY, et al. Nw-nitro-L-arginine administration corrects peripheral vasodilation and systemic capillary hypotension, and ameliorates plasma volume expansion and sodium retention in portal hypertensive rats. Hepatology 1993;17:84–90. (Ref.14)

Llach J, et al. Incidence and predictive factors of first episode of spontaneous bacterial peritonitis in cirrhosis with ascites: relevance of ascitic fluid protein concentration. Hepatology 1992;16:724–727. (Ref.57)

Martin PY, et al. Nitric oxide synthase (NOS) inhibition for one week improves renal sodium and water excretion in cirrhotic rats with ascites. J Clin Invest 1998;101:235–242. (Ref.13)

McVay PA, Toy PT. Lack of increased bleeding after paracentesis and thoracentesis in patients with mild coagulation abnormalities. Transfusion 1991;31:164–171. (Ref.26)

Moore KP, et al. The management of ascites in cirrhosis: report on the consensus conference of the International Ascites Club. Hepatology 2003;38:258–266. (Ref.22)

Morali GA, et al. Is sinusoidal portal hypertension a necessary factor for the development of hepatic ascites? J Hepatol 1992;16:249–250. (Ref.7)

Navasa M, et al. Randomized, comparative study of oral ofloxacin versus intravenous cefotaxime in spontaneous bacterial peritonitis. Gastroenterology 1996;111:1011–1017. (Ref.73)

Novella M, et al. Continuous versus inpatient prophylaxis of the first episode of spontaneous bacterial peritonitis with norfloxacin. Hepatology 1997;25: 532–536. (Ref.77)

Planas R, et al. Natural history of decompensated hepatitis C virus-related cirrhosis. A study of 200 patients. J Hepatol 2004;40:823–830. (Ref.4)

Planas R, et al. Natural history of patients hospitalized for management of cirrhotic ascites. Clin Gastroenterol Hepatol 2006;4:1385–1394. (Ref.131)

Restuccia T, et al. Effects of dilutional hyponatremia on brain organic osmolytes and water content in patients with cirrhosis. Hepatology 2004;39:1613–1622. (Ref.40)

Reuben A. My cup runneth over. Hepatology 2004;40:503–507. (Ref.1)

Ricart E, et al. Amoxicillin-clavulanic acid versus cefotaxime in the therapy of bacterial infections in cirrhotic patients. J Hepatol 2000;32:596–602. (Ref.63)

Rimola A, et al. Diagnosis, treatment and prophylaxis of spontaneous bacterial peritonitis: a consensus document. J Hepatol 2000;32:142–153. (Ref.61)

Rimola A, et al. Two different dosages of cefotaxime in the treatment of spontaneous bacterial peritonitis in cirrhosis: results of a prospective, randomized, multicenter study. Hepatology 1995;21:674–679. (Ref.62)

Ripoll C, et al. Hepatic venous pressure gradient predicts clinical decompensation in patients with compensated cirrhosis. Gastroenterology 2007;133:481–488. (Ref.9)

Romney R, et al. Usefulness of routine analysis of ascitic fluid at the time of therapeutic paracentesis in asymptomatic outpatients. Results of a multicenter prospective study. Gastroenterol Clin Biol 2005;29:275–279. (Ref.55)

Rossle M, et al. Randomised trial of transjugular-intrahepatic-portosystemic shunt versus endoscopy plus propranolol for prevention of variceal rebleeding. Lancet 1997;349:1043–1049. (Ref.113)

Ruiz del Arbol L, et al. Paracentesis-induced circulatory dysfunction: mechanism and effect on hepatic hemodynamics in cirrhosis. Gastroenterology 1997;113:579–586. (Ref.104)

Ruiz-del-Arbol L, et al. Systemic, renal, and hepatic hemodynamic derangement in cirrhotic patients with spontaneous bacterial peritonitis. Hepatology 2003;38:1210–1218. (Ref.71)

Runyon BA. Ascites. In: Schiff L, Schiff ER, editors. Diseases of the liver. Philadelphia: Lippincott, 1993: 990–1015. (Ref.25)

Runyon BA. Management of adult patients with ascites due to cirrhosis: an update. Hepatology 2009;49:2087–2107. (Ref.27)

Runyon BA, et al. The serum-ascites albumin gradient is superior to the exudate-transudate concept in the differential diagnosis of ascites. Ann Intern Med 1992;117:215–220. (Ref.38)

Sakai H, et al. Choosing the location for non-image guided abdominal paracentesis. Liver Int 2005;25:984–986. (Ref.28)

Salerno F, et al. Transjugular intrahepatic portosystemic shunt for refractory ascites: a meta-analysis of individual patient data. Gastroenterology 2007;133: 825–834. (Ref.120)

Salerno F, et al. Randomized controlled study of TIPS versus paracentesis plus albumin in cirrhosis with severe ascites. Hepatology 2004;40:629–635. (Ref.116)

Santos J, et al. Spironolactone alone or in combination with furosemide in the treatment of moderate ascites in nonazotemic cirrhosis. A randomized comparative study of efficacy and safety. J Hepatol 2003;39:187–192. (Ref.91)

Sanyal AJ, et al. The North American study for the treatment of refractory ascites. Gastroenterology 2003;124:634–641. (Ref.115)

Schepke M, et al. Hemodynamic effects of the angiotensin II receptor antagonist irbesartan in patients with cirrhosis and portal hypertension. Gastroenterology 2001;121:389–395. (Ref.16)

Schrier RW, et al. Tolvaptan, a selective oral vasopressin V2-receptor antagonist, for hyponatremia. N Engl J Med 2006;355:2099–2112. (Ref.129)

Schuster DM, et al. The use of the diagnostic radionuclide ascites scan to facilitate treatment decisions for hepatic hydrothorax. Clin Nucl Med 1998;23:16–18. (Ref.49)

Sigal SH, et al. Restricted use of albumin for spontaneous bacterial peritonitis. Gut 2007;56:597–599. (Ref.74)

Sola R, et al. Total paracentesis with Dextran 40 vs diuretics in the treatment of ascites in cirrhosis: a randomized controlled study. J Hepatol 1994;20:282–288. (Ref.95)

Sola-Vera J, et al. Randomized trial comparing albumin and saline in the prevention of paracentesis-induced circulatory dysfunction in cirrhotic patients with ascites. Hepatology 2003;37:1147–1153. (Ref.107)

Song KH, et al. Clinical outcomes of spontaneous bacterial peritonitis due to extended-spectrum beta-lactamase-producing *Escherichia coli* and *Klebsiella* species: a retrospective matched case-control study. BMC Infect Dis 2009;9:41. (Ref.68)

Sort P, et al. Effect of intravenous albumin on renal impairment and mortality in patients with cirrhosis and spontaneous bacterial peritonitis. N Engl J Med 1999;341:403–409. (Ref.65)

Strauss RM, Boyer TD. Hepatic hydrothorax. Semin Liver Dis 1997;17:227–232. (Ref.48)

Terg R, et al. Oral ciprofloxacin after a short course of intravenous ciprofloxacin in the treatment of spontaneous bacterial peritonitis: results of a multicenter, randomized study. J Hepatol 2000;33:564–569. (Ref.76)

Terg R, et al. Ciprofloxacin in primary prophylaxis of spontaneous bacterial peritonitis: a randomized, placebo-controlled study. J Hepatol 2008;48:774–779. (Ref.85)

Terg R, et al. Serum creatinine and bilirubin predict renal failure and mortality in patients with spontaneous bacterial peritonitis: a retrospective study. Liver Int 2009;29:415–419. (Ref.75)

Thiesson HC, et al. Inhibition of cGMP-specific phosphodiesterase type 5 reduces sodium excretion and arterial blood pressure in patients with NaCl retention and ascites. Am J Physiol Renal Physiol 2005;288:F1044–F1052. (Ref.17)

Trotter JF, Suhocki PV. Incarceration of umbilical hernia following transjugular intrahepatic portosystemic shunt for the treatment of ascites. Liver Transpl Surg 1999;5:209–210. (Ref.44)

Umgelter A, et al. Failure of current antibiotic first-line regimens and mortality in hospitalized patients with spontaneous bacterial peritonitis. Infection 2009;37:2–8. (Ref.67)

Wong F, et al. A vasopressin receptor antagonist (VPA-985) improves serum sodium concentration in patients with hyponatremia: a multicenter, randomized, placebo-controlled trial. Hepatology 2003;37:182–191. (Ref.126)

Wong F, Liu P, Blendis L. Sodium homeostasis with chronic sodium loading in preascitic cirrhosis. Gut 2001;49:847–851. (Ref.10)

Xiol X, et al. Spontaneous bacterial empyema in cirrhotic patients: a prospective study. Hepatology 1996;23:719–723. (Ref.59)

A complete list of references can be found at www.expertconsult.com.

Chapter 19

Portal Hypertension and Bleeding Esophageal Varices

Patrick S. Kamath and Vijay H. Shah

ABBREVIATIONS

AIDS acquired immunodeficiency syndrome
ARPKD autosomal recessive polycystic kidney disease
BRTO balloon-occluded retrograde transvenous obliteration of varices
DSRS distal splenorenal shunt
EMT epithelial-mesenchymal transactivation
FHVP free hepatic vein pressure
GAVE gastric antral vascular ectasia

GVE gastric vascular ectasia
HHT hereditary hemorrhagic telangiectasia
HV hepatic vein
HVPG hepatic venous pressure gradient
ICG indocyanine green
IGV isolated gastric varices
IVC inferior vena cava
MELD Model for End-Stage Liver Disease
MRE magnetic resonance elastography
NO nitric oxide

NOS nitric oxide synthetase
NRH nodular regenerative hyperplasia
PBC primary biliary cirrhosis
PSC primary sclerosing cholangitis
PHG portal hypertensive gastropathy
TIPS transjugular intrahepatic portosystemic shunts
TLR4 Toll-like receptor 4
VEGF vascular endothelial growth factor
WHVP wedged hepatic vein pressure

The major cause of mortality in patients with decompensated cirrhosis, other than hepatocellular carcinoma, is complications of portal hypertension. Portal hypertension results in the formation of portosystemic collateral veins and leads to variceal bleeding, ascites, and hepatic encephalopathy. Approximately 20% of patients with an episode of variceal bleeding will die and thus portal hypertension is a serious sequela of chronic liver disease. In this chapter, the pathophysiology of portal hypertension and the diagnosis and management of portal hypertension–related bleeding are discussed.

Anatomy of the Portal Venous System

The liver is a derivative of the foregut that extends into the septum transversum. The portal vein is derived from the omphalomesenteric veins. As the yolk sac regresses, the principal tributaries of the portal vein arise from the intestine. The normal adult portal circulation is established soon after birth with the obliteration of the umbilical vein.[1]

The portal vein is formed behind the neck of the pancreas and anterior to the inferior vena cava by the confluence of the superior mesenteric vein and the splenic vein. The inferior mesenteric vein may drain into this confluence but usually drains into the splenic vein. The splenic vein is the vein of the foregut and drains the lower end of the esophagus, as well as the stomach, pancreas, and first portion of the duodenum. The superior mesenteric vein, the vein of the midgut, drains the entire small bowel from the second portion of the duodenum, the cecum and ascending colon, and the right two thirds of the transverse colon. The inferior mesenteric vein drains the remainder of the colon and the rectum. Additional tributaries of the portal vein are the left gastric or left coronary vein, gastro-epiploic veins, and pancreatic veins.

The portal vein arises at the level of the second lumbar vertebra and is about 8 cm in length before it divides in the hilum of the liver into the left and right branches. The portal vein is dorsal to the hepatic artery and common bile duct. The right and left branches of the portal vein serve the anatomic right and left lobes, respectively, and are accompanied in their course by the hepatic artery and its branches. The portal vein ramifies in the liver and ends in tiny capillary-like vessels termed sinusoids. In the hepatic sinusoids, portal venous blood mixes with hepatic arterial blood and the mixed blood drains into the hepatic veins. The right hepatic vein drains into the inferior vena cava adjacent to but separate from the left and middle hepatic veins, which typically enter the inferior vena cava via a common channel approximately 1 to 2 cm in length. In about a third of patients, the three major hepatic veins may drain separately into the inferior vena cava. The caudate lobe drains into the inferior vena cava separately from the right, middle, and left hepatic veins.[2]

Physiologic Principles of the Portal Circulation

The intrahepatic circulation has some unique features. One is the dual blood supply from portal vein and hepatic artery. Thirty percent of the flow and 30% to 60% of the oxygen consumed by the liver comes from the hepatic artery while the rest comes from the portal vein.[2] The dual hepatic blood supply makes the normal liver resistant to anoxia. Ligation of the portal vein, for example, will not cause hepatocellular necrosis. Similarly, accidental ligation of the hepatic artery or its major branches does not necessarily lead to hepatic failure, except in the transplant setting, where the organ is much more dependent on hepatic arterial blood flow.

There is also a unique interrelationship between hepatic artery and portal vein blood flow.[3] In both animals and humans, a decrease in portal venous flow or sinusoidal pressure causes a reflex increase in hepatic arterial flow. Conversely, an increase in sinusoidal flow or pressure causes a reflex decrease in hepatic arterial flow. This buffer response may be mediated by adenosine, and the response maintains a constant hepatic blood flow despite changes in portal venous flow that occur during digestion.

The liver also maintains a very low outflow resistance. Because of this, vasodilation causes a minimal rise in sinusoidal pressure because outflow resistance is low. Thus the sinusoidal pressure remains low despite changes in blood flow. In cirrhosis, however, increases in portal pressure increase vascular leak from the sinusoids, contributing to ascites. Another unique feature of the hepatic circulation relates to its microanatomy. The endothelial lining in the liver contains fenestrae that allow free passage of proteins between the sinusoidal lumen and the abluminal space of Disse.[4] Interestingly, these fenestrae are lost in response to liver injury and cirrhosis due to loss of the specialized phenotype of the sinusoidal endothelial cells. The presence of Kupffer cells and hepatic stellate cells in the hepatic microcirculation is also unique. In normal physiology, hepatic stellate cells store vitamin A and may contribute to low levels of sinusoidal constriction. Kupffer cells endocytose toxins and bacteria and are now well recognized as a mediator of innate immune responses by virtue of their expression of Toll-like receptor 4 (TLR4).

Portal Hypertension

Definition

The normal portal venous pressure is 5 to 10 mm Hg, and should be no greater than 5 mm Hg higher than the inferior vena cava (IVC) or hepatic vein (HV) pressure. A portal pressure-IVC or HV pressure difference determined by measuring the hepatic venous pressure gradient (HVPG) that is >6 mm Hg, indicates the presence of portal hypertension. Portal pressure is elevated usually secondary to increased resistance to portal blood flow, which may be at the prehepatic, intrahepatic, or suprahepatic level. Identification of portal hypertension requires further investigation to determine the cause. Cirrhosis, the major cause of portal hypertension, results in portal hypertension by increasing intrahepatic resistance.

Pathogenesis of Portal Hypertension

Physiologic Principles of Portal Hypertension

The pressure within a vessel is determined by the flow and resistance within that vessel. This relationship is expressed by Ohm's law: $\Delta P = Q \times R$, where P is pressure, and Q and R are flow and resistance, respectively. Therefore either increase in flow or resistance can lead to an increase in pressure. In the case of portal hypertension, the increase in pressure occurs through both an increase in flow (Q) and an increase in resistance (R). Resistance depends on a number of factors as defined by Poiseuille's law: $R = 8nL/\pi r,$[4] where n is the coefficient of viscosity, L the length of the vessel, and r the radius. Radius appears to be the most important factor, as small changes in radius are associated with large changes in resistance. These principles can be applied in relation to the development of portal hypertension and also for vascular regulation within each of the vascular beds in portal hypertension.

The vascular beds most salient for pathogenesis of portal hypertension include the intrahepatic circulation, the splanchnic circulation, and the portosystemic collateral circulation (**Fig. 19-1**). Changes in the intrahepatic circulation are thought to be the primary impetus in the development of portal hypertension. These changes are characterized by an increase in intrahepatic resistance, the mechanisms of which are described in further detail below. These changes not only initiate the development of portal hypertension but also result in secondary events that lead to a hyperdynamic circulatory state characterized by systemic and splanchnic vasodilation. Splanchnic vasodilation allows greater flow into the portal circulation, thereby further potentiating portal hypertension. At a critical level of portal pressure elevation, there is an expansion of the collateral circulation, which serves to decompress the portal circulation. As described further below, portal pressure reduction through collaterals comes at the expense of a number of complications of portal hypertension, including esophageal varices, and yet these collaterals fail to normalize portal pressure.

Increased Intrahepatic Resistance

Although it was previously thought that increased blood flow into the portal circulation may be the major driver of portal hypertension, current concepts indicate that an increase in vascular resistance is the major driver of most forms of portal hypertension.[4] In early studies of cirrhotic livers, distortion and reduction of the hepatic microcirculation were observed. These vascular changes, in concert with compression of portal and sometimes hepatic veins by regenerative nodules, were believed to be a major cause for the increase in vascular resistance observed in cirrhotic livers.[5] Portal hypertension may be found, however, without cirrhosis, and this observation has led investigators to question whether deposition of collagen alone is an important factor in increasing intrahepatic vascular resistance. Indeed, there also appears to be prominent changes in vascular structure and patency, which may precede actual fibrosis (**Fig. 19-2**). For example, thrombosis of the portal and hepatic veins is thought to lead to ischemia, loss of parenchyma, and worsening of the fibrosis, supporting the

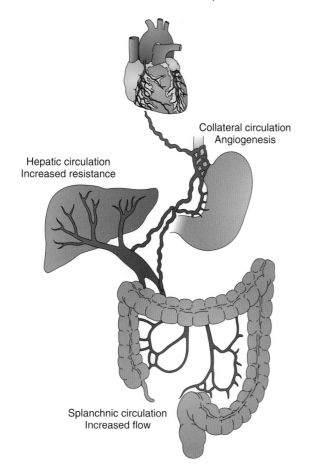

Fig. 19-1 Vascular beds implicated in pathogenesis of portal hypertension. Portal hypertension involves changes in multiple vascular beds including intrahepatic resistance, which is increased, and splanchnic circulation, which experiences increased flow. These changes lead to portal hypertension despite the collateral circulation that develops to try to decompress the increased portal pressure.

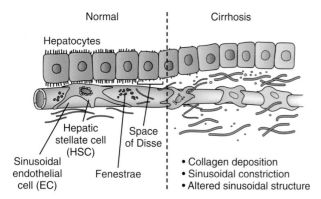

Fig. 19-2 Sinusoidal changes in the process of cirrhosis development. Hepatic microcirculation undergoes substantial changes in cirrhosis and portal hypertension. While endothelial cells lose their fenestrae and undergo endothelial dedifferentiation and dysfunction, hepatic stellate cells undergo activation with increased contractility, proliferation, and capacity to constrict the sinusoids.

idea that vascular change can precede and possibly promote cirrhosis.[6] Some of these observations led to the concept that increased intrahepatic resistance in cirrhosis may have an irreversible component relating to fibrosis and a reversible component that was more dynamic in nature. Experimentally, the concept of a reversible and dynamic component of increased intrahepatic resistance was further crystallized by studies by Bhathal and colleagues which demonstrated that a vasodilator, sodium nitroprusside, could reduce perfusion pressure in the isolated perfused rat liver preparation.[7,8] This observation was subsequently expanded in vivo and mechanistically and formed the basis for the concept that the nonfibrosis component of cirrhosis was an important aspect of portal hypertension and was amenable to therapeutic intervention. This is especially important because at the present time, the fibrotic component of portal hypertension is not amenable to pharmacologic modulation in humans.[9]

The cell biology of hepatic vascular cells and their paracrine regulation of vascular structure and function have emerged as important drivers of the pathogenesis of increased intrahepatic resistance in portal hypertension, as well as a site for therapeutic intervention. Paradigmatically, this is represented by the interplay of two cells, the sinusoidal endothelial cell and the hepatic stellate cell.[10] As previously mentioned, the sinusoidal endothelial cell is a unique endothelial cell in terms of its phenotype. It maintains fenestrae, which facilitate macromolecular transport across the space of Disse. While initially thought to be a cell that exclusively regulates such transport functions, more recent models indicate that this cell also maintains traditional vasoregulatory functions within the hepatic circulation, including paracrine regulation of adjacent hepatic stellate cells via production of a number of vasoregulatory molecules including the canonical vasodilator and vasoconstrictor, nitric oxide (NO), and endothelin, respectively.[11] Regulating mechanisms of NO are shown in **Figure 19-3**.

Hepatic stellate cells are interspersed within the hepatic sinusoids in the normal liver. However, in response to liver injury, these cells undergo a process termed activation, which is characterized by enhanced proliferation, migration, and collagen deposition capacity.[12,13] These changes enhance the ability of sinusoidal endothelial cells to regulate the sinusoidal structure and function through hepatic stellate cells, which thereby reach the critical mass and level of activation necessary to act as an effector cell for sinusoidal endothelial cell-derived molecules[14] (see Chapter 5). Although the hepatic stellate cell is the canonical cell type thought to mediate effector functions from endothelial cell–derived molecules, recent work suggests that the peribiliary fibroblast and other related mesenchymal cells can also activate to myofibroblasts and serve a similar function to the hepatic stellate cell.[15] One theory proposes that epithelial cells may also transactivate into myofibroblasts through a process termed epithelial-mesenchymal transactivation (EMT).[16] Thus the pool of contractile effector cells could be diverse in phenotype and may not be limited to hepatic stellate cells.

NO and endothelin are two prototypical vasoactive molecules that regulate interactions between SEC and HSC and are discussed in more detail below. Many other vasoactive signaling pathways also exist and are relevant for portal pressure regulation but will not be discussed here.

In the intrahepatic system it is believed that an underproduction of NO contributes to increased intrahepatic

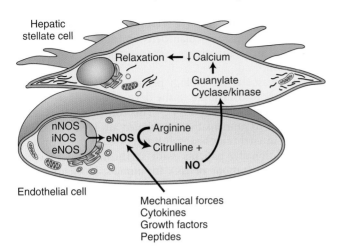

Fig. 19-3 Canonical pathways of nitric oxide generation and relaxation function. Nitric oxide is generated by various NOS isoforms, especially eNOS, in endothelial cells. Nitric oxide diffuses albuminally to contractile cells, such as stellate cells, to promote relaxation and other functions also.

vasoconstriction and increased intrahepatic resistance. This is in direct contradistinction to increases in NO generation in the splanchnic and systemic circulation that lead to the hyperdynamic circulation and increased portal inflow, which are discussed further below. The release of NO is reduced from the endothelial cells of cirrhotic animals, and the molecular mechanisms responsible for this hepatic endothelial dysfunction are an area of active investigation.[17] Some experimental therapeutic approaches have determined that if this relative NO deficiency could be corrected then there would be a fall in intrahepatic resistance and portal pressure, suggesting that targeted increases in NO levels in the hepatic circulation could be used to lower portal pressure. For example, if drugs, such as nitrates, can be developed that increase NO levels in the portal system without causing further vasodilation in the systemic circulation, then new therapeutic opportunities could be possible.[18] The most promising approaches at this time have included the statin class of medications, which appear to stimulate NO generation in the intrahepatic circulation without adverse NO generation in other vascular beds in both experimental models and in humans.[19,20] This class of drugs requires further investigation as a potential therapy that directly targets portal hypertension.

Endothelins are a group of compounds that are potent vasoconstrictors. They bind to two different types of receptors termed ET_A and ET_B. Binding of endothelins to ET_A receptors on vascular smooth muscle cells leads to vasoconstriction, whereas binding to ET_B receptors on endothelial cells leads to release of NO and vasorelaxation. A number of different studies in combination indicate that endothelins may increase portal pressure in liver disease by binding to hepatic stellate cells, leading to their contraction and a rise in resistance within the liver microcirculation.[21] In support of this idea are the findings that the acute administration of an $ET_{A/B}$ antagonist leads to a fall in portal pressure in cirrhotic rats.[21] Chronic administration of an $ET_{A/B}$ antagonist in

an animal model, however, failed to lower portal pressure.[22] Studies in humans using these receptor antagonists are awaited. Concerns about this pathway as a therapeutic target in human portal hypertension include the need for evidence of $ET_{A/B}$ antagonist safety profile in setting of liver dysfunction, better understanding of the effects of the various receptor subtypes, and the overall quantitatively small effect of modulation of this pathway that has been observed in animal and in vitro models.

Hepatic arterial flow also contributes to sinusoidal pressure because the arterial contribution to sinusoidal inflow is significant. Furthermore, with reduced portal blood flow into the cirrhotic liver there is a compensatory increase in hepatic arterial blood flow that aims to maintain total hepatic blood flow constant. Recent studies indicate that the hepatic artery participates in the generalized hyperdynamic arterial flow state that characterizes the systemic and splanchnic circulatory beds in portal hypertension, which is described in further detail below.[23,24] This could theoretically increase intrahepatic resistance and exacerbate portal hypertension. Overall, the role of the hepatic artery in increasing portal pressure requires further investigation.

Recently, there has been greater emphasis on the vascular structural changes that occur in parallel with cirrhosis and portal hypertension. This includes remodeling of the hepatic sinusoidal vasculature and angiogenesis, which is the proliferation of existing endothelial cells. Close links between the processes of angiogenesis and cirrhosis have been identified with both processes going hand in hand. These have suggested that angiogenesis could also be a new target for portal hypertension treatment, although more work is needed in this regard.[25-29] The sinusoidal remodeling changes in portal hypertension are also quite distinct. These include an increase in the mass of hepatic stellate cells that wrap around the endothelial cell tube. With regards to the endothelial cells themselves, they also undergo changes in phenotype characterized by dedifferentiation that includes loss of fenestrae, and development of basement membrane, termed capillarization. The pathologic significance of these changes is also anticipated to have therapeutic significance because reducing the contractile machinery and force of stellate cells should reduce intrahepatic resistance. Another prominent vascular structural change is the presence of "scar vessels" that transverse through dense cirrhotic scar. It has been postulated that these vessels may provide the metabolic and oxygen needs required for the scar to progress, akin to the role of angiogenesis required for tumors to continue to grow.[14] Thus the vascular changes of cirrhosis and portal hypertension may provide targets for therapies that not only target vasoregulation but also the related angiogenesis and sinusoidal structural changes that link intimately to the fibrotic process.[25-29]

The advances in molecular mechanisms of portal hypertension are leading to a number of potential therapeutic agents that can eventually be tested in humans. In addition to the advances targeting specific complications of portal hypertension that are discussed in other chapters, there are also a number of agents that can directly target the elevated portal pressure and increased intrahepatic resistance. Presently, some of these agents include liver specific NO donors, statin class of medicines that stimulate intrahepatic NO generation, blockers of the endothelin pathway, blockers of the angiotensin pathway, and blockers of growth factors including platelet-derived growth factor (PDGFR)/(TGF-β) pathways, especially receptor tyrosine kinase inhibitors, such as sorafenib and imatinib.[26,30,31] In total, most of these approaches are targeting hepatic stellate cell contractility, proliferation, migration, and activation, or alternatively are stimulating endothelial cell activation and its production of vasodilatory molecules such as NO.

Increased Splanchnic Blood Flow and the Hyperdynamic Circulatory State

Increased portal blood flow is an uncommon cause of portal hypertension in and of itself (aside from primary hypersplenism or arteriovenous shunts), but rather is usually a propagator of portal hypertension triggered by increased intrahepatic resistance. This is because there is little outflow resistance from the liver, and so the increase in flow must be quite large to raise sinusoidal pressure purely on an inflow basis. However, in the setting of increased intrahepatic resistance, increased flow into the portal circulation is an important propagator of portal hypertension and in fact represents the most widely used site of pharmacologic therapeutic intervention such as octreotide, vasopressin, somatostatin, and β-blockers.[32] Thus when the vascular resistance is increased, as is observed in cirrhosis, small increases in portal venous inflow may be associated with significant increases in portal vein pressure. Importantly, in cirrhosis, total flow entering the portal system does not equate to total flow entering the liver because the increase in pressure leads to portal-systemic collaterals that divert a significant component of the total flow entering the portal circulation, which are discussed in greater detail below.

With the development of portal hypertension, there is also the development of the *hyperdynamic circulation*, the pathogenesis of which is discussed in detail in Chapters 21 and 22. In brief, the following sequence of events appears to occur in the patient with portal hypertension, leading to circulatory disturbances.[33] Pressure in the portal circulation is increased either because of hepatic fibrosis or occlusion of the portal vein. Although portal blood flow into the liver declines, hepatic blood flow is partially maintained by an increase in hepatic arterial flow. In response to the rise in portal pressure, portal-systemic collaterals develop. Although this does not fully decrease portal hypertension, the shunting does cause vascular resistance to fall in the splanchnic bed, leading to the development of the hyperdynamic circulation. Splanchnic and portal venous inflow increase, causing portal pressure to continue to be elevated despite the opening of the collateral circulation. As resistance in the liver continues to increase, there is a further increase in portal pressure, a fall in liver perfusion by the portal vein, and an increasing percentage of blood that is shunted through the collateral circulation. The liver is therefore deprived of portal blood, which may, over time, accelerate the progression of liver disease even if the underlying cause of cirrhosis has been removed. Importantly, the hyperdynamic circulation contributes not only to the development of portal hypertension but also to the development of the hepatopulmonary syndrome (see Chapter 23), cirrhotic cardiomyopathy (see Chapter 22), and ascites and hepatorenal syndrome (see Chapters 18 and 21). Interestingly, the changes in the splanchnic circulation in portal hypertension may be viewed as a microchasm of the hyperdynamic systemic circulatory state observed in patients with cirrhosis, although there is controversy about this assertion because some vascular beds outside the splanchnic circulation may experience vasoconstriction rather than vasodilation.[34]

From a vascular cell biology perspective, NO overproduction appears to contribute to the development of the hyperdynamic circulation (**Fig. 19-4**).[33] This conclusion is based on the findings in humans that in exhaled air, levels of NO are increased in cirrhotics before but not after liver transplantation. Additionally, patients with cirrhosis have increased plasma concentrations of NO. In animals, blockade of NO synthesis ameliorates the hyperdynamic state. However, when portal hypertension was induced in knockout mice for both eNOS and iNOS, the hyperdynamic circulation still developed, indicating factors other than NO play an important role in the development of the hyperdynamic circulation (see Chapter 21). This remains unresolved because similar experiments conducted by a different group led to different results.[35] Nonetheless, it is increasingly clear that while NO is a major driver of the hyperdynamic circulatory state, there are numerous other redundant and compensatory pathways, many of which are under active investigation.

The primary driver of increased NO generation remains unclear. Two mechanisms have received the greatest experimental attention: VEGF and mechanical stress induced by hemodynamic forces. For example, VEGF production is increased in cirrhosis and is a well known stimulus of NO generation.[36] Similarly, biomechanical forces, such as shear stress and stretch, are known to stimulate NO generation from endothelial cells and are increased in the splanchnic circulation of cirrhosis.[36] However, a causal versus correlative relationship between these parameters continues to be actively debated.

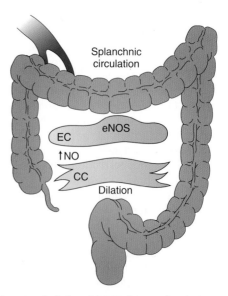

Fig. 19-4 Increased nitric oxide mediates splanchnic vasodilation. Splanchnic vasodilation occurs due to increased vasodilatory factors, including nitric oxide, which leads to increased flow into portal circulation.

Portosystemic Collateral Circulation in Portal Hypertension

Large portosystemic collaterals are seen in patients with portal hypertension and the higher the pressure the more extensive the collaterals. Indeed, these collaterals account for a significant component of morbidity and mortality attributable to patients with cirrhosis. For example, variceal formation and hemorrhage is directly attributable to gastroesophageal portosystemic collateral vessels that develop as a consequence of increased portal pressure. Although portosystemic collaterals that develop in response to the rise in portal pressure will tend to minimize the rate of rise in pressure, in the end the collateral circulation is insufficient to compensate for the factors that raise portal pressure.

Collateral vessels develop through several distinct but interrelated processes. These include vasodilation of existing collateral vessels, vascular remodeling of existing vessels, and angiogenesis; that is, the de novo formation of new vascular sprouts (**Fig. 19-5**).[29] Although vasodilation is a relatively rapid phenomenon, some of these other pathways require a longer timeframe of chronic portal hypertension that allows for the changes in vascular wall structure leading to remodeling of the vessel and sprouting of new endothelial sprouts. These interrelated processes are likely driven by both changes in growth factor levels in cirrhosis and mechanical factors related to increased pressure within the portal circulation that drives increased flow into the collateral bed.[37] Importantly, these mechanisms have potential therapeutic implications. For example, VEGF is a growth factor that has been demonstrated to mediate the angiogenic collateral vessel response in portal hypertension, with inhibition of VEGF attenuating collateral vessel formation in animal models.[38] Parallel strategies may be worthy of pursuit in humans with cirrhosis if safety of these drugs can be established.

Several factors eventually determine whether the collateral vessel will rupture as best exemplified by bleeding esophageal varices. These factors include the size of the varix, the thickness of the varix wall, and the pressure gradient between the variceal lumen and the esophageal lumen. The interplay of how these factors determine the risk of varix rupture is shown in **Figure 19-6**.

Clinical Features of Portal Hypertension

Portosystemic Collaterals

The portal venous system may decompress into the systemic venous system at several different sites. The most important site for this collateral circulation is within the mucosa of the proximal stomach and distal esophagus. When these collateral vessels dilate, gastric and esophageal varices develop. The normally obliterated umbilical vein, which lies in the *ligamentum teres,* is recanalized with increases in hepatic sinusoidal pressure and connects the left portal vein to systemic veins around the umbilicus. These veins then drain into the epigastric vessels and appear as *caput medusae*. Because the umbilical vein drains into the left portal vein, the presence of *caput medusae* rules out extrahepatic portal hypertension as the cause of portal hypertension. If the flow in the umbilical vein is high, an audible venous hum (Cruveilhier-Baumgarten murmur) may be heard over the course of the umbilical vein. When the inferior vena cava is occluded, as in Budd-Chiari syndrome, the veins in the flanks are more dilated and drain upward into the superior vena caval territory.[39] These veins may be best appreciated by examining the back.

Large venous shunts may also form between the splenic vein and the left renal vein (**Fig. 19-7**). These shunts are often large enough to decrease the risk of variceal bleeding, but may increase the risk of hepatic encephalopathy. Collaterals may also develop between the portal venous system and the abdominal wall in relation to surgical scars or surgically created ostomies (**Fig. 19-8**). Rectal varices (**Fig. 19-9**) develop from collaterals between the superior hemorrhoidal vein, which continues as the inferior mesenteric vein, and the inferior rectal vein, which drains into the systemic pudendal vein. The prevalence of hemorrhoids in patients with portal hypertension may not be increased, although occasionally hemorrhoidal bleeding can be severe.

Splenomegaly

There is poor correlation between portal venous pressure and the size of the spleen. Splenomegaly, which is common in portal hypertension, may be associated with hypersplenism;

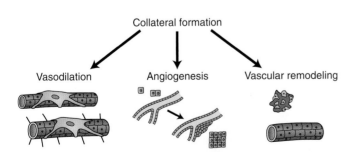

Collateral formation

Vasodilation   Angiogenesis   Vascular remodeling

Fig. 19-5 Mechanisms of portosystemic collateral formation. Collateral vessels develop from vasodilation of existing collaterals, angiogenesis from existing sprouts, and vascular remodeling of existing collateral vessels.

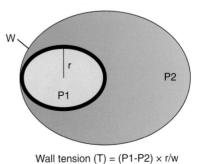

Wall tension (T) = (P1-P2) × r/w

Fig. 19-6 Mechanisms of variceal rupture. Variceal rupture is determined by wall tension that is regulated by the pressure gradient between the varix and esophageal lumen, as well as the width of the varix wall and varix radius.

that is, a reduction in one or more of the formed elements of platelets, white blood cells, and red cells. The degree of reduction in the formed elements is usually insufficient to cause clinical problems. Splenectomy is, hence, almost never recommended for hypersplenism resulting from portal hypertension. If the reduction in the formed elements is severe enough to be symptomatic, a cause other than hypersplenism, should be investigated.

Assessment of Portal Venous System

The most common method of assessing for esophageal varices is upper gastrointestinal endoscopy. However, there are several other methods, including radiological imaging and capsule endoscopy, to detect varices. An accurate comparison of the

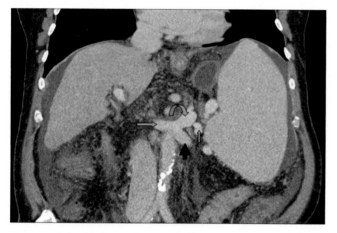

Fig. 19-7 Spontaneous splenorenal shunt. CT scan of the abdomen, coronal section, demonstrates a spontaneous splenorenal shunt *(arrow)* with communications between the splenic vein *(curved arrow)* and the renal vein *(arrowheads)*.

varying techniques to detect esophageal varices is difficult because the current gold standard for detecting varices, upper gastrointestinal endoscopy, may miss gastric varices, and considerable observer variation exists in assessing the size of esophageal varices.[40]

Esophageal varices develop in response to an increase in portal pressure. The correlation between the size of esophageal varices and portal hypertension is variable because there are several other beds where collaterals may form, and the degree of decompression into these beds is to variable degrees. In addition, valves are present in the perforating veins of the esophagus that may prevent the flow of blood from periesophageal veins into vessels within the esophageal mucosa. The valves may become incompetent in some patients with portal hypertension, which may lead to an increase in variceal size.

Upper Gastrointestinal Endoscopy

The most common method of identifying and determining the size of gastroesophageal varices is by upper endoscopy. Several different classifications are used to describe esophageal varices, namely size, form, and color. A simple method of grading esophageal varices is based on size: small or large. Small varices are less than 5 mm in diameter (**Fig. 19-10**), whereas large varices are greater than 5 mm in diameter. Large varices correspond to grade 2 and grade 3 varices in previous classifications.[41] The size of the varices should be described in the lower third of the esophagus with the esophagus completely insufflated with air and examined on withdrawal of the instrument. Additional descriptors of the varices include red signs. A cherry red spot on a varix is 3 mm in diameter or less, and a hematocystic spot or blood blister on the varix, is 4 mm in diameter or greater. The red wale sign describes a whiplike longitudinal mark on the varix (**Fig. 19-11**). The red wale sign is indicative of a weakness in the varix wall and is a marker of increased risk of bleeding, although not as predictive of bleeding as is the size of the varix.

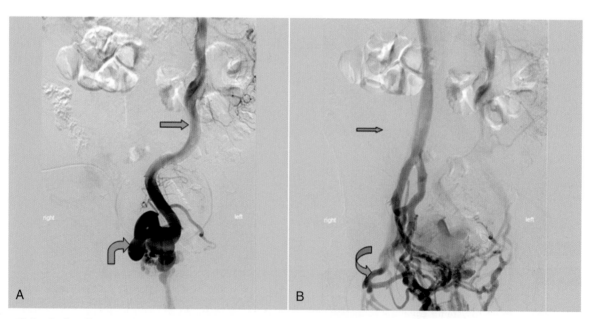

Fig. 19-8 Abdominal wall varices following an appendectomy. The patient had visible external bleeding from dilated veins in the abdominal wall. **A,** Abdominal wall varices *(curved arrow)* being fed by a large collateral vein *(arrow)*. **B,** Collaterals *(curved arrow)* connecting to superficial epigastric vein *(arrow)*.

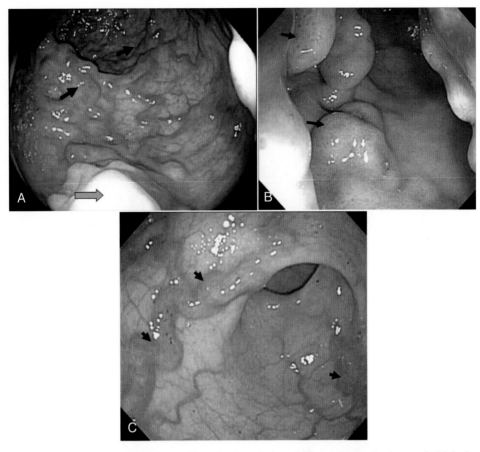

Fig. 19-9 **Endoscopic view of rectal varices, which are dilated veins of the middle and superior hemorrhoidal plexus. A,** Rectal varices *(short arrow),* hemorrhoids *(blue arrow).* **B** and **C,** Rectal varices. *(All endoscopic images in this chapter are courtesy Dr. L. M. Wong Kee Song and Dr. Nayantara Coehlo-Prabhu.)*

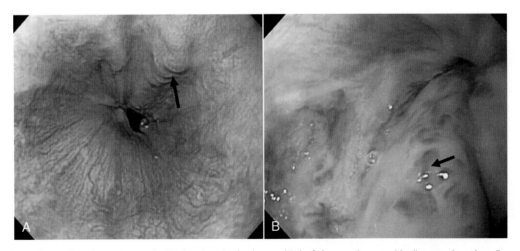

Fig. 19-10 **Small esophageal varices. A,** Longitudinal varices in the lower third of the esophagus with diameter less than 5 mm. **B,** Small varix with red wale sign *(arrow).*

Gastroesophageal varices are classified as follows: Type 1 gastroesophageal varices are in continuity with esophageal varices and extend for a variable distance into the lesser curvature of the stomach; type 2 gastroesophageal varices are again in continuity with esophageal varices but extend into the cardia of the stomach (**Fig. 19-12**). Isolated gastric varices can occur either in the fundus of the stomach (IGV type 1) or in the antrum of the stomach (IGV type 2). IGV type 2 varices are uncommon. Type 2 gastroesophageal varices are the most common site of bleeding from gastric varices, although the most severe bleeding is with IGV type 1 varices.[42]

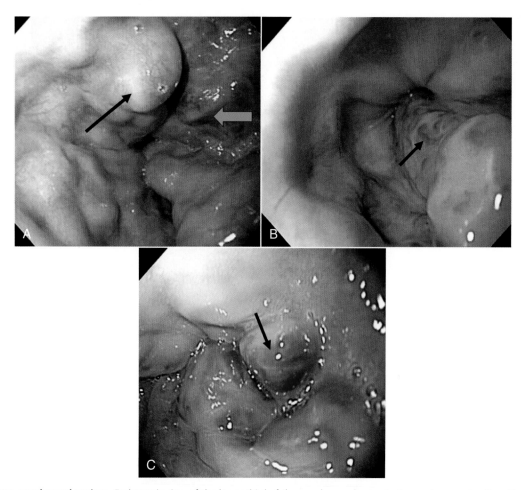

Fig. 19-11 **Large esophageal varices.** Endoscopic view of the lower third of the esophagus demonstrating varices greater than 5 mm in diameter. **A,** Large varix *(arrow)* with red wale sign. **B,** Red wale sign—longitudinal whip mark on varix *(arrow).* **C,** Large varix with hematocystic spot *(arrow).*

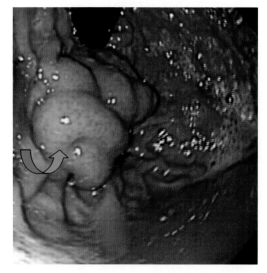

Fig. 19-12 **Gastric varices.** Tuft of varices noted in the fundus of the stomach on retroflexed views at endoscopy *(curved arrow).* These varices are in continuation with esophageal varices (type 2 gastroesophageal varices).

Capsule Endoscopy

Capsule endoscopy is a newer but yet investigational method to detect the presence of and the size of esophageal varices. Capsule endoscopy is less effective in determining the size of gastric varices. The potential advantage of capsule endoscopy over conventional endoscopy is that varices are graded without the esophagus being inflated, which reflects the normal physiologic state of the esophagus. Capsule endoscopy is not currently recommended to screen for varices, although it can be used in patients who are reluctant to undergo an endoscopic procedure.[43]

CT Scan

A computerized tomographic scan using multidetector arrays is another investigational modality to demonstrate esophageal varices (**Fig. 19-13**). The advantage of CT scans is that varices may be detected with accuracy close to that of endoscopy. In addition, the portal venous anatomy, liver masses, and extrahepatic pathology may be visible. Patients greatly prefer CT scans over upper endoscopy.[40] The risks of radiation with CT scans are minimal, but CT scans to screen for esophageal varices are probably best avoided in patients younger than 35 years in whom a minute risk of radiation exists. CT scan may be used to screen for varices in patients who do not wish to

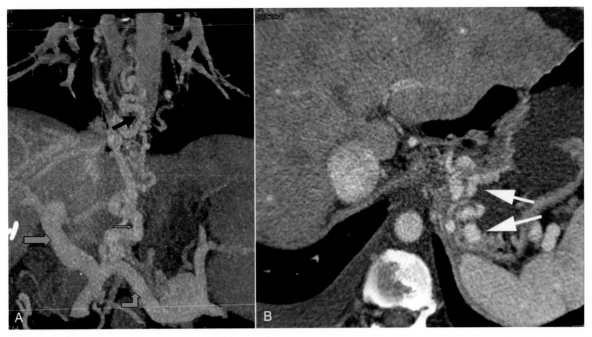

Fig. 19-13 **CT scan of the abdomen. A,** Coronal section demonstrates esophageal varices *(black arrow)*, left coronary vein *(thin blue arrow)*, portal vein *(thick arrow)*, and splenic vein *(bent arrow)*. **B,** Gastric varices *(white arrows)*.

undergo endoscopy, especially if they have had a history of dysphagia.

Magnetic Resonance Imaging

Magnetic resonance imaging is another investigational modality for detection of varices. Magnetic resonance imaging has the same advantages over endoscopy as the CT scan without the risk of radiation. There have been no studies that have compared upper endoscopy with magnetic resonance imaging in the detection of varices.

Magnetic resonance elastography (MRE) may determine the degree of hepatic fibrosis and possibly the degree of portal hypertension.[44] The advantage of MRE over ultrasound fibro-elastography is that the stiffness across the whole liver can be determined; with fibroelastography using ultrasound, stiffness is calculated across only a cylinder of liver approximately 1 cm in diameter and 2 to 4 cm in length. Spleen stiffness on MRE increases in patients with portal hypertension (**Fig. 19-14**).

Ultrasonography

Ultrasonography is the only imaging modality for use at the bedside to diagnose portal hypertension; the portal vein and collaterals can also be visualized and liver tumors detected. A diameter of the portal vein greater than 13 mm, the presence of collaterals, and the absence of respiratory variation in the diameter of the portal vein are all markers of portal hypertension.[45]

Endoscopic Ultrasound

Endoscopic ultrasonography uses radial or linear array echo-endoscopes or ultrasound mini probes passed through the biopsy channel of a conventional endoscope; it is still considered investigational in the evaluation of patients with portal hypertension. Endoscopic ultrasound allows measurement of

the cross-sectional area of varices (**Fig. 19-15**); the amount of blood flow in the varices and in the left gastric vein, azygos vein, portal vein, and splenic vein; and decrease in the size of varices following variceal ligation.[46,47] Endosonography combined with variceal pressure measurement can potentially allow for measurement of variceal wall tension because both the radius of the varix and the transmural variceal pressure are measurable. Measurement of variceal wall tension is important because it is the major determinant of variceal bleeding. Despite all of its potential uses, perhaps the most practical use of endoscopic ultrasound is in determining whether a submucosal mass in the fundus of the stomach in a patient with cirrhosis is a tumor or varices.

Ultrasound Fibroelastography

Ultrasound fibroelastography has been used primarily to determine liver stiffness as a surrogate for hepatic fibrosis. In a study of 61 consecutive patients with hepatitis C virus (HCV)–related chronic liver disease, there was a strong correlation between measurement of liver stiffness on fibroelastography and HVPG. The ROC AUC for prediction of HVPG of 10 and 12 mm Hg were 0.99 and 0.92; the cutoff values of 13.6 kPa and 17.6 kPa for liver stiffness had a sensitivity of 97% and 94%, respectively.[48] However, the correlation between HVPG and fibroelastography was imprecise when the HVPG was greater than 12 mm Hg. Therefore fibroelastography is not sufficient to replace HVPG monitoring in patients receiving pharmacologic treatment for portal hypertension.[49]

Measurement of Portal Venous Pressure
Hepatic Vein Catheterization

Catheterization of the hepatic vein is the usual technique used to measure HVPG. An end-hole catheter, or more commonly

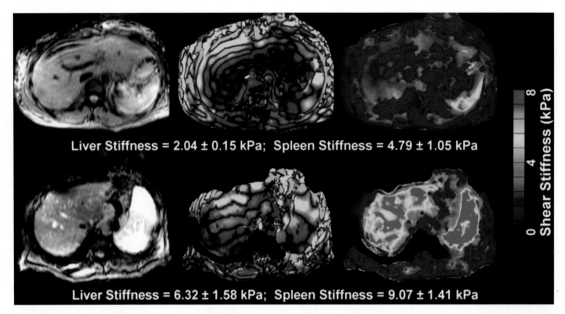

Liver Stiffness = 2.04 ± 0.15 kPa; Spleen Stiffness = 4.79 ± 1.05 kPa

Liver Stiffness = 6.32 ± 1.58 kPa; Spleen Stiffness = 9.07 ± 1.41 kPa

Fig. 19-14 **MRE demonstrating the appearance of a normal liver and spleen *(upper panel)*, and a cirrhotic liver with increased liver stiffness *(lower panel)*.** The *blue* color signifies the least stiffness and *red* significs the highest degree of stiffness within the liver and spleen *(right panels)*. Note the increased liver and spleen stiffness in cirrhosis. *(Image courtesy Dr. Jayant Talwalkar, Mayo Clinic, Rochester, Minn.).*

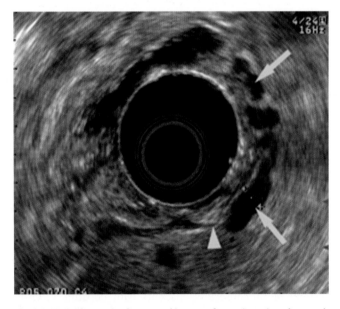

Fig. 19-15 **Endoscopic ultrasound image of gastric varices *(arrows)*.** The *arrowheads* point to the muscularis mucosa of the stomach.

a balloon catheter, is used to determine pressure via either the femoral or the transjugular route. In the presence of tense ascites, catheterization of the hepatic veins may be more difficult using the femoral approach; it may be necessary to use a deflector to enter the hepatic vein. Not only is catheterization of the hepatic vein using the transjugular route somewhat easier, it also allows right-sided cardiac pressure to be measured. Contrast is injected into the hepatic vein to confirm the balloon is in a wedged position. Total occlusion of the hepatic vein by the inflated balloon results in a sinusoidal pattern being demonstrated on contrast injection without a collateral

circulation to other hepatic veins. Once the balloon is deflated, the contrast washes out promptly. Additionally, there is a sharp increase in the pressure recorded on inflation of the balloon and a sharp drop when the balloon is deflated. When the balloon is correctly positioned and inflated, the pressure recorded is steady, with only respiratory variation. The HVPG should be measured at least three times to demonstrate reproducibility.[50] Procedure-related complications with HVPG measurement are uncommon.

Wedging of the catheter in the hepatic vein or inflation of the balloon to occlude the hepatic vein creates a stagnant column of blood, which represents hepatic sinusoidal pressure in patients with cirrhosis. In the normal situation, this pressure is rapidly dissipated via the other sinusoids. In sinusoidal causes of portal hypertension, as in alcoholic cirrhosis and HCV-related cirrhosis, the pressure is not dissipated and there is a continuous column of blood extending from the hepatic vein to the portal vein (**Fig. 19-16**). Thus wedged hepatic vein pressure (WHVP) represents portal pressure. Inferior vena caval pressure or the free hepatic vein pressure (FHVP) is measured at the junction of the hepatic vein and IVC, or with the balloon deflated in the hepatic vein. The FHVP is used as the reference standard and is recorded with the "zero" measured in the midaxillary line. The right atrial pressure should not be used as the reference standard.[51]

The major drawback of using an end-hole catheter in the wedged position for measurement of the WHVP is that the pressure over only a small area of the liver is measured. Because there is regional variation in the degree of fibrosis, pressures may be higher in some veins than in the others. On the other hand, if a balloon-occluding catheter is used in the main right hepatic vein, the pressures are averaged over a wide area of the liver. Thus the WHVP using a balloon catheter is more accurate. It is important to note in portal hypertension secondary to portal vein thrombosis that the hepatic sinusoidal pressure is normal, and therefore the HVPG is normal. In primary

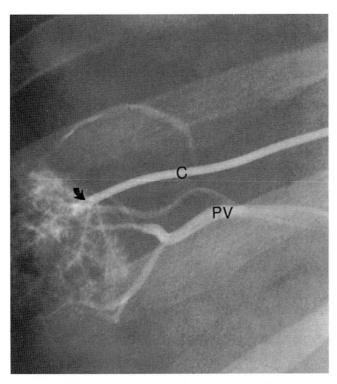

Fig. 19-16 The catheter (C) is in the wedged position. Contrast material has been injected, and beyond the tip of the catheter (arrow), the sinusoids are filled. There is no reflux of contrast material back along the catheter, confirming that it is properly wedged. There is reflux into the portal vein (PV).

biliary cirrhosis, a presinusoidal cause of portal hypertension, the HVPG is somewhat lower than the true hepatic sinusoidal pressure.[52]

At the current time, HVPG measurement is not routinely used to diagnose portal hypertension or to monitor therapy using pharmacologic agents. However, HVPG measurement may be used to determine whether the cause of portal hypertension is sinusoidal, presinusoidal, or postsinusoidal. HVPG measurement is particularly useful in combination with hepatic venography, transjugular liver biopsy, and right-sided heart pressure measurements to determine whether the cause of ascites is cardiac or hepatic in origin. HVPG has been used in patients with cirrhosis to assess the risk of hepatic resection as an end point in trials using pharmacologic agents, and as a prognostic marker.[53,54]

Direct Transhepatic Portal Venous Pressure Measurement

The portal venous pressure can be measured directly using either a transjugular approach to the portal vein via the hepatic veins, or by puncture of the portal vein through a percutaneous transhepatic route under ultrasound guidance. A catheter is then passed over a guidewire into the main portal vein. Because of the increasing experience with TIPS, most radiologists use a transjugular route for direct measurement of the portal vein pressure. Inferior vena caval pressure can also be measured at the same time, which allows for the determination of the portal vein to hepatic vein pressure gradient. Such measurements are useful in identifying patients with

presinusoidal portal hypertension and determining whether a surgical portosystemic shunt is feasible in patients with Budd-Chiari syndrome.[39] Portal venous pressure may be measured intraoperatively by cannulating the portal vein. Such measurements may not be accurate reflections of portal pressure because measurements are carried out under general anesthesia with the abdomen open.

Measurement of Variceal Pressure and Flow

Measurement of variceal pressure may be particularly important in patients with large varices and portal vein thrombosis in whom the HVPG does not accurately measure portal pressure. Variceal pressure can be measured during upper endoscopy by inserting into the varix a needle connected to a fluid-filled catheter connected to a pressure transducer. Measurement of pressure is followed by sclerotherapy of the varix because of the small risk of bleeding associated with variceal puncture. Because injection sclerotherapy is seldom used nowadays, measurement of esophageal variceal pressure by needle puncture is not recommended.

Esophageal variceal pressure can also be measured using miniature pneumatic pressure-sensitive gauges. These methods require not only considerable procedural skill but also stable intraesophageal pressure. The principle of the pneumatic pressure gauge is that varices are thin walled and quite elastic. Because they are elastic structures, the pressure required to compress and collapse the varix equals the venous pressure within the varix. Patients with previous variceal bleeding have higher variceal pressures than patients who have never bled.[55] A variceal pressure greater than 18 mm Hg in patients who have had a variceal bleed is associated with failure to control the bleed, as well as a predictor of early and subsequent rebleeding.

Measurement of Portal Venous and Hepatic Artery Blood Flow

Clearance studies measure only total hepatic blood flow; the relative contribution of the portal vein and hepatic artery to total blood flow cannot be determined. The most commonly used agent to measure total hepatic blood flow is indocyanine green (ICG) because it is cleared by the liver and is nontoxic. Following injection or infusion of ICG, the disappearance of the compound in both the peripheral vein and hepatic vein is measured. Using the Fick principle, hepatic blood flow is calculated.

Determining the relative contributions of the hepatic artery and portal vein to hepatic blood flow might be useful in selecting the patient who would benefit the most from a portosystemic shunt. It has been suggested that patients with normal portal venous blood flow might be poor candidates for portosystemic shunts because of rapid diversion of portal venous blood from the liver following creation of a shunt. However, the response of hepatic arterial blood flow to portal diversion may be more important. A poor outcome is likely following a portosystemic shunt if there is only a minimal increase in hepatic arterial blood flow in response to portal venous diversion. Additionally, decreased hepatic blood flow after liver transplantation may point to graft dysfunction.[56]

Measurement of portal venous blood flow alone and hepatic artery blood flow is possible during surgery using flow meters. Measuring portal venous flow without surgery is cumbersome and requires catheterization of the superior mesenteric artery, hepatic veins, and umbilical vein. Following injection into the umbilical vein of 99-mTc pertechnetate, rapid images are collected from the heart, kidney, lungs, spleen, and liver, and the portal venous fraction calculated. In patients with cirrhosis, the portal venous fraction of total hepatic blood flow varies from the normal 66% to essentially no flow.

Because measurements of total hepatic, hepatic artery, and portal vein blood flow are cumbersome and invasive, Doppler ultrasound has been used as an alternative modality. The velocity of flow of blood in the portal vein can be measured noninvasively using Doppler ultrasound. The velocity of flow multiplied by the cross-sectional area of the portal vein is then used to calculate the volume of blood flow in the portal vein. These results compare favorably with portal vein flow measured using flow meters. Technical problems associated with Doppler measurements, as well as body habitus, make it difficult to accurately estimate portal venous blood flow in some patients. Doppler is also used to measure hepatic arterial blood flow and resistance, and is a means of determining hepatic artery stenosis or thrombosis, especially following liver transplantation.

Classification of Diseases Causing Portal Hypertension

Diseases that cause portal hypertension have been classified traditionally into those causing presinusoidal, sinusoidal, and postsinusoidal portal hypertension. However, there is a considerable degree of variation among patients with the same disease as to the site of obstruction. In some patients with nonalcoholic cirrhosis, portal venous pressure exceeds WHVP, indicating a presinusoidal component, whereas in other patients, the portal venous pressure and the WHVP are identical, indicating sinusoidal hypertension. Consequentially, a simple way of classifying broadly diseases that cause portal hypertension is determining if the portal hypertension is caused principally by increased portal venous blood flow or by increased resistance to portal venous blood flow.

Portal Hypertension Secondary to Increased Portal Venous Blood Flow

Splanchnic arterio-venous fistula: The most common cause of increased portal venous blood flow is an arteriovenous fistula that may be intrahepatic or extrahepatic. A splenic artery–splenic vein fistula is an example of an extrahepatic splanchnic arteriovenous fistula (**Fig. 19-17**).[57] Fistulae may occur within the liver in hereditary hemorrhagic telangiectasia (HHT, Osler-Rendu-Weber syndrome), or may follow trauma such as a liver biopsy, or can result from a rupture of a hepatic artery aneurysm. Unlike patients with HHT with a hepatic artery–hepatic vein fistula who develop cardiac failure, patients with hepatic artery–portal vein fistula develop portal hypertension.[58] Because the portal venous system is exposed to arterial blood pressure in the presence of a hepatic artery–portal vein fistula, the rate of delivery of blood to the liver exceeds the outflow, resulting in a rise in portal pressure. With time, the high flow results in sinusoidal fibrosis and an increase in intrahepatic resistance, which propagates the portal hypertension, a phenomenon confirmed in animal studies using hepatic artery–portal vein anastomosis. It is important to recognize the contribution of intrahepatic resistance because ligation of the fistula may not always result in resolution of the portal hypertension. Moreover, creation of a portosystemic shunt without occlusion of the fistula in an effort to ameliorate portal hypertension will actually result in the creation of a systemic arteriovenous fistula, which could lead to high-output cardiac failure.

Splenomegaly

Portal hypertension with varices and ascites can develop in patients with hematologic disease, such as polycythemia vera and myelofibrosis, and agnogenic myeloid metaplasia. Rarely,

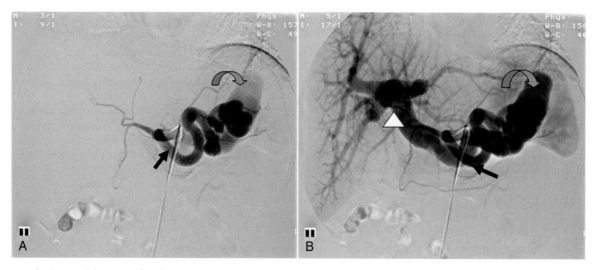

Fig. 19-17 Splenic arterial-venous fistula. A, Splenic arteriogram demonstrating splenic artery *(black arrow)* with simultaneous visualization of splenic vein *(curved arrow)*. The spleen is not outlined. **B,** Subsequent images demonstrate splenic artery *(black arrow)* with simultaneous visualization of splenic vein *(curved arrow)*, and portal vein *(arrowhead)*.

Gaucher disease, leukemia, and lymphoma may also cause portal hypertension. These patients have increased portal venous blood flow, elevated portal venous pressure, and either normal or elevated WHVP, suggesting an element of increased intrahepatic resistance. If the portal hypertension is a result purely of increased portal venous blood flow, splenectomy should be curative. On the other hand, if there is significant intrahepatic resistance, splenectomy would not reverse the portal hypertension as is often the case. It is increasingly recognized that in patients with hematologic disease, nodular regenerative hyperplasia within the liver contributes to portal hypertension and is the cause of increased intrahepatic resistance.

Portal Hypertension Secondary to Increased Resistance to Portal Blood Flow

Extrahepatic Portal Vein Thrombosis

Extrahepatic portal vein thrombosis (see Chapter 45) is a common cause of portal hypertension in children. The resistance to portal blood flow in this condition is presinusoidal. In children, umbilical vein sepsis may be a causal factor, but even in these children it is possible that an associated prothrombotic state predisposes to portal vein thrombosis. The most common causes of portal vein thrombosis in adults are polycythemia vera and other myeloproliferative disorders.[59,60] Intraabdominal infections, such as diverticulitis, Crohn disease, and pancreatitis are additional causes of portal vein thrombosis.[61] Cirrhosis, as well as splenectomy are associated with portal vein thrombosis.

Due to improved abdominal imaging, portal vein thrombosis is a much more common complication of cirrhosis than previously recognized. Thus the association between portal vein thrombosis and hepatocellular carcinoma is not as strong as previously thought. Patients with portal vein thrombosis present either with gastrointestinal bleeding or manifestations of hypersplenism. Bleeding is usually from gastroesophageal varices, but bleeding from duodenal varices can also occur. In addition, gallbladder varices (**Fig. 19-18**) and portal hypertensive cholangiopathy, which gives the appearance of pseudo-sclerosing cholangitis, can be present.

There are scanty data on primary prophylaxis against variceal bleeding, control of variceal bleeding, or prevention of rebleeding in patients with portal vein thrombosis. The management principles in these patients are similar to those in patients with cirrhosis in whom better data exist. However, the threshold for creating surgical portosystemic shunts in patients with extrahepatic portal vein thrombosis is much lower than in patients with cirrhosis. Placement of a TIPS might be technically feasible in some patients with chronic thrombosis limited to the portal vein.

Idiopathic Portal Hypertension

Idiopathic portal hypertension is diagnosed when portal hypertension and splenomegaly occur in the absence of portal vein obstruction or significant liver disease. The syndrome is sometimes termed Banti disease. Hepatopetal sclerosis and noncirrhotic portal fibrosis describe different stages of the same disease.

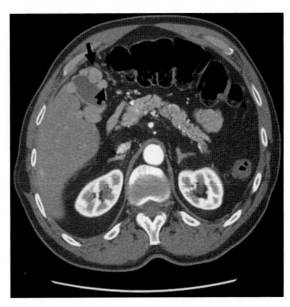

Fig. 19-18 **Gallbladder varices** *(arrowheads)* demonstrated on CT scan of the abdomen.

The pathogenesis of portal hypertension in this condition is not known but may result from an initial increase in portal blood flow secondary to splenomegaly. Endothelin has been localized to the portal tract in patients with idiopathic portal hypertension and entirely normal liver biopsies, suggesting that portal hypertension may be secondary to vasoconstriction in the early phases.[62] Collagen deposition in periportal areas and in the Space of Disse is noted later in the disease and subsequently the portal vein branches are reduced.

Splenic venous blood flow is higher than normal in all patients with idiopathic portal hypertension, but portal venous blood flow alone is elevated in only about 50% of patients. Patients with high portal flow have significantly lower portal pressures and presinusoidal resistance and less severe vascular changes in liver biopsy specimens. Therefore high portal flow is probably an early stage of the disease. With time, the intrahepatic resistance increases, initially probably related to local production of vasoactive substances. Subsequently, intrahepatic resistance increases due to fibrosis, which is the predominant cause of the high portal pressure later in the course of the disease. Before the pathogenesis of idiopathic portal hypertension can be firmly established, serial measurements of portal pressure and portal blood flow need to be made in a large number of patients.

Patients with idiopathic portal hypertension have splenomegaly, hypersplenism, or variceal hemorrhage. Ascites may develop late in these patients, typically in association with variceal bleeding and vigorous fluid resuscitation. Liver biochemical tests are normal except for mild elevation in the alkaline phosphatase, and hepatic failure, if it ever develops, is a late feature. The long-term prognosis is excellent. On liver biopsy, the appearances may be entirely normal. Moderate to marked portal fibrosis may be found, and sclerotic changes in the portal veins can be noted; ductopenia may also be seen. The surface of the liver can be nodular due to subcapsular fibrosis and may look cirrhotic. However, needle biopsies in these patients show that the deeper liver has a near normal architecture, unlike cirrhosis.

It is important on taking a liver biopsy to make certain that the biopsy specimen contains portal areas because an otherwise normal biopsy may represent a regenerative nodule in those with cirrhosis. Cross-sectional abdominal imaging is sufficient to exclude portal or splenic vein thrombosis. The WHVP in patients with idiopathic portal hypertension is normal or moderately elevated, but directly measured portal pressure is always greater than the WHVP.

Some investigators have linked idiopathic portal hypertension to environmental toxins, such as arsenic or vinyl chloride. However, the vast majority of patients with idiopathic portal hypertension have no evidence of these environmental toxin exposures.

Schistosomiasis

Schistosomiasis is probably the predominant cause of portal hypertension and bleeding esophageal varices worldwide. The major cause of death in patients with hepatosplenic schistosomiasis is portal hypertension–related bleeding. In infection with *Schistosoma mansoni* and *Schistosoma japonicum*, eggs are deposited in the presinusoidal portal venules. The resulting florid granulomatous inflammation leads to presinusoidal and periportal fibrosis termed pipe stem fibrosis.[63] Because the majority of the hepatocytes are preserved, liver function is well maintained. There is progressive obstruction to portal blood flow, which leads to portal hypertension and variceal bleeding. Splenomegaly and hypersplenism accompany the portal hypertension. In addition, coinfection with hepatitis B or hepatitis C infection can lead to rapid progression of fibrosis, hepatic failure, as well as hepatocellular carcinoma.[64] The WHVP is usually normal, confirming presinusoidal portal hypertension. It is thought that there is hepatitis B– or C–related liver disease in patients with hepatosplenic schistosomiasis who have elevated WHVP. Another possibility is that with more advanced disease there is extension of the fibrotic process into the sinusoids, which would explain the elevated WHVP. As a result of the decrease in portal venous flow, the hepatic artery is enlarged and hepatic arterial blood flow increases. Clamping the hepatic artery in such patients leads to a significant decline in WHVP without changing portal venous pressure. The increased hepatic arterial blood flow might be important in maintaining normal liver function in patients with hepatic schistosomiasis.

Alcoholic Liver Disease

The most common cause of portal hypertension in the western world is alcoholic cirrhosis. Portal hypertension is related to increased resistance to portal blood flow caused by fibrosis and distortion of the normal hepatic architecture with nodule formation. Zone 3 injury is most severe in alcoholic liver disease. In alcoholic hepatitis, there is sclerosis and obliteration of the terminal hepatic venules that results in a clinical picture similar to hepatic venous outflow tract obstruction. Thus portal hypertension with ascites and esophageal varices can develop even in the absence of cirrhosis. On the other hand, resolution of alcoholic hepatitis may result in delayed or only partial resolution of the portal hypertension because of the injury around the central vein. Alcoholic fatty liver may also cause portal hypertension secondary to compression of the sinusoids by the enlarged hepatocytes. Unlike in alcoholic hepatitis, complete recovery is the rule with abstention from alcohol in patients with alcoholic fatty liver disease.

In alcoholic cirrhosis, the WHVP and the portal vein pressure are equal irrespective of the stage of disease. This is because resistance to blood flow is along the entire sinusoid, along with reduction in collaterals between sinusoids. This creates a stagnant column that extends to the portal venules and therefore the pressure recorded in the occluded hepatic vein is equal to the pressure in the portal vein (**Fig. 19-16**).

Nonalcoholic Cirrhosis

Portal hypertension can develop in patients with cirrhosis secondary to causes other than alcohol, and include hepatitis B, hepatitis C, primary biliary cirrhosis (PBC), primary sclerosing cholangitis (PSC), Wilson disease, hemochromatosis, and autoimmune hepatitis. The risk of variceal bleeding is low in patients with autoimmune hepatitis. In patients with hemochromatosis, the severity of portal hypertension increases with iron deposition and phlebotomy may result in a decrease in portal pressure. In PBC, the risk of variceal bleeding increases with the stage of disease, but may occur even before cirrhosis has developed. The portal hypertension is predominantly presinusoidal in early stages of the disease, but a sinusoidal component develops in advanced stages of PBC. In patients with biliary obstruction secondary to a biliary stricture or PSC, the elevated portal pressure may regress with relief of biliary obstruction.

The portal vein pressure in patients with PBC and autoimmune hepatitis is higher than the WHVP.[52] This is because the resistance to flow is predominantly at the level of the portal venules because fibrosis is most severe in the portal areas. Even when the sinusoids are involved, there is sufficient collateral circulation between the sinusoids to dissipate the pressure with a catheter occluding the hepatic vein. Therefore the WHVP in patients with PBC underestimates portal pressure.[65]

Fibrocystic Liver Disease

The term fibrocystic liver disease encompasses congenital hepatic fibrosis, Caroli disease, and polycystic liver disease.[66] Congenital hepatic fibrosis causes portal hypertension in teenagers and young adults who have variceal bleeding, usually after the second decade of life. Congenital hepatic fibrosis is associated with autosomal recessive polycystic kidney disease (ARPKD) and Caroli disease of the liver. When Caroli disease occurs in the presence of congenital hepatic fibrosis, the term Caroli syndrome is used (**Fig. 19-19**). Clinical manifestations can be cholangitis, variceal bleeding, both cholangitis and variceal bleeding, or occasionally an asymptomatic presentation may occur. Patients with congenital hepatic fibrosis have normal or mildly elevated WHVP. Portal hypertension may rarely develop in patients with polycystic liver disease secondary to pressure on the portal vein by the cysts, or from portal vein thrombosis.

Nodular Regenerative Hyperplasia of the Liver

Nodular regenerative hyperplasia (NRH) is increasingly recognized as a cause of portal hypertension. Whereas the condition was previously described as being associated with rheumatoid arthritis, nowadays the most common association is with hematologic disease.[67] NRH is a histopathologic diagnosis in which there is hypertrophy of zone 1 hepatocytes and

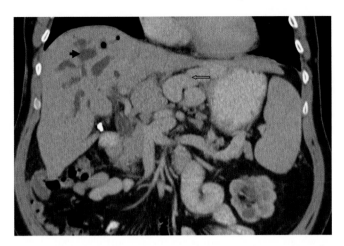

Fig. 19-19 Caroli disease with congenital hepatic fibrosis. Note the dilated bile ducts *(asterisk)* almost encircling the portal vein radicals *(arrowhead)*. Note also the presence of collaterals because of portal hypertension.

atrophy of zone 3 hepatocytes.[68] Significant fibrosis does not occur. The condition may be difficult to diagnose without a reticulin stain. NRH is well recognized in patients with Budd-Chiari syndrome and after liver transplantation, especially when azathioprine is used for immunosuppression. Ischemia may be a contributory factor. It is speculated that an imbalance between hyperperfused and hypoperfused areas of the liver results in regenerative nodules and areas of atrophy. This distortion of hepatic vascular architecture increases resistance to portal blood flow and results in portal hypertension. In addition, obliteration of the portal veins contributes to the portal hypertension. Liver biochemical tests are usually normal but mild elevation in the serum aminotransferases and alkaline phosphatase may occur. Patients with NRH may have variceal bleeding, ascites, or hypersplenism. Nodular regenerative hyperplasia is seen with common variable immunodeficiency and in patients with AIDS. The WHVP may be increased in these patients, signifying the presence of sinusoidal hypertension.

Partial Nodular Transformation of the Liver

Partial nodular transformation of the liver is rare but may lead to portal hypertension. In this condition, there are large nodules in the hilar region of the liver that may be visible on imaging studies. Partial nodular transformation of the liver is related to an imbalance in portal perfusion of the liver that is restricted to the larger hilar portal venous branches. Symptoms of partial nodular transformation of the liver include variceal bleeding and abdominal pain. Hepatocellular carcinoma has been known to develop in the regenerating nodules.

Hematologic Disease

Portal hypertension has been seen in patients with systemic mastocytosis, leukemias, and lymphomas. In patients with hematologic disease, the portal hypertension is related to portal vein thrombosis, NRH, or diffuse infiltration of the liver with malignant cells.[69] Treatment of the hematologic condition may result in regression of the portal hypertension.

Hepatocellular Carcinoma

Portal hypertension may be present in patients with hepatocellular carcinoma, even in the absence of cirrhosis. Portal pressure is elevated secondary to portal vein thrombosis, a hepatic artery–portal vein fistula, or compression of the portal vein by a large tumor.

Metastatic Carcinoma to the Liver

Ascites may develop in patients with widespread metastatic liver disease. In these patients who do not have peritoneal seeding by the tumor, the serum-ascitic fluid albumin gradient is high, indicating a portal hypertension cause for the ascites. Rarely, variceal bleeding may occur. Portal hypertension results from distortion of the hepatic vascular architecture by tumor, or is secondary to tumor thrombosis within the portal venules.

Hereditary Hemorrhagic Telangiectasia

Hereditary hemorrhagic telangiectasia (HHT), or Osler-Weber-Rendu syndrome, is diagnosed in patients who have epistaxis, a family history of HHT, visceral involvement by arteriovenous fistula (liver, lung, or brain), and mucocutaneous involvement noted as cherry red spots on the lip, tongue and palate, as well as the digits. The most common site of fistula formation is between the hepatic artery and hepatic vein, which results in high output cardiac failure.[58] A portal vein–hepatic vein fistula may result in hepatic encephalopathy, whereas a hepatic artery–portal vein fistula results in portal hypertension. In patients with HHT, NRH develops and may contribute to the portal hypertension. Though hepatic involvement occurs in the vast majority of patients with HHT, symptomatic involvement occurs in fewer than 10% of patients.

Sarcoidosis

Sarcoidosis is associated with portal hypertension, and when it occurs is an indication for steroid therapy. Patients with mild hepatic sarcoidosis have normal hepatic sinusoidal pressures, whereas those with severe involvement have elevated pressures. Portal hypertension may regress with steroid treatment. However, hepatic fibrosis and cirrhosis can develop in severe sarcoidosis and, in these patients steroid therapy may not decrease portal pressure.

Cystic Fibrosis

Secondary biliary cirrhosis may develop in patients with cystic fibrosis. Portal hypertension, which develops in about 2% of patients with cystic fibrosis, manifests with bleeding varices, hypersplenism, and ascites. Portal hypertension in patients with cystic fibrosis is an ominous sign. Whereas portosystemic shunts were used in patients with variceal bleeding, portal hypertension might be best treated long-term with liver transplantation.

Cardiac Disease

The pathophysiology of portal hypertension in patients with severe right heart failure is similar to those in patients with hepatic venous outflow tract obstruction. The liver biopsy shows centrilobular congestion identical to that seen early in liver biopsies from patients with Budd-Chiari syndrome. Portal hypertension may be seen in patients with constrictive pericarditis, severe tricuspid insufficiency, or in patients who have had the Fontan cardiac procedure as children. With many of the children with complex congenital heart disease reaching adulthood, variceal bleeding may be seen in patients with cardiac cirrhosis.

Portal Hypertension–Related Bleeding

Selection of Patients to Screen for Esophageal Varices

A low platelet count, splenomegaly, advanced liver disease, and an ultrasound demonstrating a portal vein diameter greater than 13 mm have all been used as surrogate markers for portal hypertension. Nonetheless, prognostic models based on a portal vein diameter greater than 13 mm, a platelet count less than 100,000, and prothrombin activity less than 70% have not been considered sensitive enough to be used to determine which patients would benefit from screening for esophageal varices.[70] The platelet count alone also is not predictive of the presence of varices, but the platelet count/spleen diameter might be. The platelet count is divided by the maximum spleen diameter (measured on ultrasound and expressed in millimeters).[71] A cutoff value for the platelet count/spleen diameter ratio of less than 909 corresponds to a positive and negative predictive value for the presence of varices of 96% and 100%, respectively. In validation studies, however, the positive and negative predictive values of this ratio of 909 were not sufficiently high to consider the platelet/spleen ratio as a valid method of screening for varices.

Risk Factors and Natural History of Portal Hypertension–Related Bleeding

In a patient with compensated cirrhosis, the presence of esophageal varices increases the 1-year risk of death from approximately 1% when no varices are noted to 3.4%. Variceal bleeding is a marker of decompensated cirrhosis and is associated with a greater than 50% risk of death within a year.[72] The HVPG, Model for End-Stage Liver Disease (MELD) score, and albumin are independent predictors for the development of clinical decompensation in patients with compensated cirrhosis. Patients with an HVPG less than 10 mm Hg have a greater than 90% probability of remaining compensated.[53] A 1-mm increase in HVPG, or a 1-point increase in MELD score, is associated with an 11% increase in the risk of clinical hepatic decompensation.

Esophageal varices are present in 30% to 40% of patients with compensated cirrhosis, and in 60% of patients with ascites. In patients who do not have varices, new varices develop at the rate of approximately 5% to 7% per year. An HVPG greater than 10 mm Hg is the strongest predictor of the development of varices.

Once small varices develop, the rate of progression from small varices to large varices is again approximately 5% to 10% per year, but can be as high as up to 30% per year with rapid worsening of liver disease as determined by the Child-Pugh class. Continued alcohol use increases the risk of developing large varices, while abstention from alcohol decreases the size of the varices and, in some cases, is associated with variceal disappearance. In patients with small varices, the risk of

variceal bleeding is approximately 7% in 2 years but, in patients with large varices, the risk of bleeding is 30% at 2 years. Esophageal variceal bleeding is only associated with an HVPG of 12 mm Hg.

When patients bleed from esophageal varices, in approximately one half of patients, the bleeding may stop spontaneously because hypovolemia results in reflex splanchnic vasoconstriction, which decreases portal pressure. With medical and endoscopic treatment, variceal bleeding is controlled in approximately 90% of patients. The presence of active bleeding at endoscopy, HVPG greater than 20 mm Hg, infection, advanced Child-Pugh class, and portal vein thrombosis complicating cirrhosis are associated with failure to control the initial bleed.[73] There is risk of rebleeding from esophageal varices within 6 weeks in up to one third of patients in whom variceal bleeding has been controlled, and almost one half of these patients will rebleed within 5 days of the initial bleed. Active bleeding at emergency endoscopy, bleeding from gastric varices, renal insufficiency, and an HVPG greater than 20 mm Hg are predictors of rebleeding. Patients with early rebleeding, especially if they have a MELD score greater than 18 and have required greater than 4 units of packed red cells for resuscitation, are at the highest risk of death.[74]

Approximately 25% of patients with portal hypertension have gastric varices. Type 1 gastroesophageal varices comprise 70% of all gastric varices.[42] When gastric varices occur in patients with cirrhosis, they are associated with more advanced liver disease. Bleeding is most common in patients with type 2 gastroesophageal varices and type 1 isolated gastric varices. Gastric varices bleed especially when their diameter is greater than 10 mm in patients with advanced cirrhosis as determined by the CTP score. It is important to note that gastric varices can develop and bleed, even when the HVPG is less than 12 mm Hg.

Portal Hypertensive Gastropathy and Gastric Vascular Ectasia

Two gastric lesions that are a source of bleeding in patients with portal hypertension are portal hypertensive gastropathy (PHG) and gastric vascular ectasia (GVE). Severe PHG is characterized by a background cobblestone appearance with superimposed red signs (**Fig. 19-20**). Both the cobblestone appearance of the mucosa and the presence of ectatic vessels can also be seen in the small intestine and colon. Mild PHG relates to a cobblestone appearance of the mucosa without superimposed red signs. GVE are recognized as dilated and ectatic blood vessels in the absence of a prominent background cobblestone appearance (**Fig. 19-21**). Gastric antral vascular ectasia (GAVE) defines aggregates of ectatic vessels in the antrum of the stomach. When the ectatic vessels are arranged in a linear pattern, they are termed "the watermelon stomach." A diffuse variety of GAVE also exists.

The pathogenesis of both PHG and GVE are poorly understood. Because bleeding from PHG subsides promptly with a decrease in portal pressure by creation of a TIPS, PHG is most likely related to elevation in portal pressure. On the other hand, bleeding from GVE does not respond to TIPS and, in fact, may increase following the procedure.[75] Therefore GVE is more likely related to increased vasodilation of the submucosal vessels in the stomach and intestine secondary to hepatic

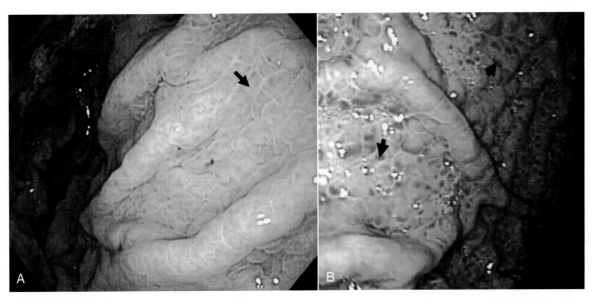

Fig. 19-20 **Endoscopic appearance of portal hypertensive gastropathy. A,** Cobblestone appearance *(arrowhead)* without red signs consistent with mild portal hypertensive gastropathy. **B,** Severe portal hypertensive gastropathy. Note the background mosaic pattern with prominent red signs *(arrows).*

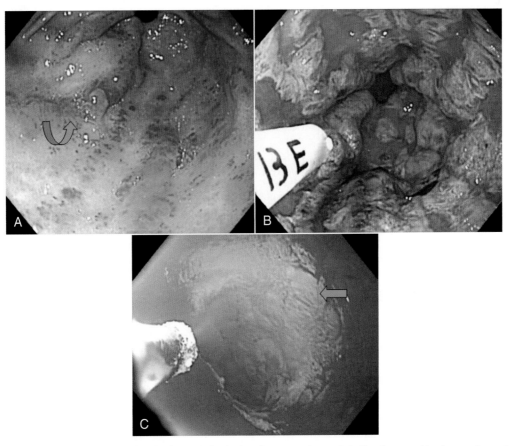

Fig. 19-21 **Endoscopic appearance of gastric vascular ectasia. A,** Prominent ectatic vessels in the absence of background mosaic pattern *(curved arrow).* **B,** Stomach in same patient after argon plasma coagulation. **C,** Antrum of stomach in a patient with diffuse gastric vascular ectasia following cryotherapy.

dysfunction rather than due to portal hypertension. The distribution of PHG is more proximal in the stomach, whereas GVE is normally in the antrum. The duration of cirrhosis seems to have an impact on the development of PHG, but the degree of liver dysfunction does not. PHG may be seen more commonly in patients who have undergone endoscopic treatment for esophageal varices, but this may only be a reflection of the longer duration of portal hypertension in such patients.[76]

Severe PHG accounts for approximately one fourth of all bleeding in patients with portal hypertension. The more common presentation is chronic and slow bleeding with iron deficiency anemia. However, approximately 10% of all acute bleeding episodes may be caused by severe PHG. The risk factors for bleeding from PHG and GVE are not known.

Bleeding from Other Sites in the Gastrointestinal Tract

Varices at sites other than the gastroesophageal junction are termed as ectopic varices.[77] Ectopic varices develop wherever the systemic circulation is in close contact with the portal circulation, especially at sites of previous surgery. Fewer than 5% of all portal hypertension–related bleeding episodes are secondary to ectopic varices. When ectopic varices occur associated with portal vein obstruction, the site of bleeding is usually in the duodenum. However, in the West, the usual cause of duodenal variceal bleeding is cirrhosis. Anorectal varices have been reported to occur in approximately 10% to 40% of patients with cirrhosis who undergo colonoscopy. Rectal varices are dilated superior and middle hemorrhoidal veins. On the other hand, hemorrhoids which are sometimes difficult to distinguish from anorectal varices are dilated vascular channels above the dentate line. Rectal varices can collapse with digital pressure; bleeding from rectal varices is infrequent.

Peristomal varices are a common site for ectopic variceal bleeding, typically in patients with inflammatory bowel disease and PSC who have undergone a proctocolectomy with an ileostomy. Stomal varices are recognized by a dark purple hue surrounding the stoma with friability of the stomal tissue.

The risk factors for ectopic variceal bleeding are uncertain.

Diagnosis of Portal Hypertension–Related Bleeding

Patients who bleed from gastric or esophageal varices may have hematemesis, hematochezia, or melena. Typically, there is painless, effortless, and recurrent hematemesis. Gastrointestinal bleeding from GVE or PHG typically tends to be slow, and patients have iron deficiency anemia. Severe PHG may also present as a more acute upper gastrointestinal bleed with hematemesis or melena. Patients with ectopic varices may have melena or hematochezia, depending on the severity of bleeding. In patients bleeding from stomal varices, the bleeding is obvious and patients describe spurting of blood from the edge of the stoma.

A portal hypertension source of bleeding should be considered in patients who have features of chronic liver disease, namely ascites, jaundice, spider nevi, hepatomegaly, parotid enlargement, and Dupuytren contracture. However, many patients may have no stigmata of chronic liver disease, and

patients may not even be aware that they have liver disease. On the other hand, patients with cirrhosis may have other causes of gastrointestinal bleeding, including ulcer disease and Mallory-Weiss tears, especially if they are actively consuming alcohol. Splenomegaly, in the presence of ascites, should point to the presence of portal hypertension. *Caput medusae* suggests a patent umbilical vein and therefore points toward an intrahepatic cause of portal hypertension. A bruit may be heard in the left upper quadrant in the presence of a splenic arteriovenous fistula, causing portal hypertension. A bruit also may be heard over the liver in patients with HHT. Laboratory abnormalities also point to portal hypertension as the potential cause for bleeding if there is thrombocytopenia, hypoalbuminemia, elevation in the bilirubin, or prolongation in the prothrombin time. Abdominal imaging can confirm splenomegaly, the abnormal configuration of the liver suggesting cirrhosis, obstruction of the extrahepatic portal venous system, and the presence of venous collaterals.

When a patient has gastrointestinal bleeding and portal hypertension is suspected to be the cause, the initial step is to establish the location, severity, and the nature of the hemorrhage. It is important to remember that an upper gastrointestinal source of bleeding should be considered, even in the presence of hematochezia because, with brisk bleeding, intestinal transit is so rapid that blood may not be altered in the intestines. The most accurate method of diagnosing bleeding gastroesophageal varices and excluding other lesions is upper endoscopy. Endoscopy is particularly important in diagnosing PHG as a cause of bleeding because this lesion is missed by radiological imaging.

Treatment Options for Portal Hypertension–Related Bleeding

Pharmacologic Treatment

Pharmacologic agents are available that are used in the control of acute variceal bleeding, and in the prevention of either the first variceal bleed or rebleeding. These agents are broadly classified into those that decrease splanchnic blood flow and those that may decrease intrahepatic vascular resistance. Vasopressin and its analogs, and somatostatin and its analogs are the agents typically used to decrease splanchnic blood flow as a means of controlling acute variceal bleeding. β-blockers also decrease portal blood flow but are currently used only in the prevention of variceal bleeding. There are several agents that may potentially decrease intrahepatic vascular resistance, such as α-adrenergic blocking agents, angiotensin receptor blockers, Simvastatin, and nitrates. Other agents that may decrease either plasma volume and therefore portal pressure, such as diuretics, or agents such as metoclopramide (which decrease intravariceal pressure by contracting the lower esophageal sphincter), are not currently recommended in the treatment of variceal bleeding.

Vasopressin and Its Analogs

Vasopressin, an endogenous peptide hormone, reduces portal venous inflow by causing splanchnic vasoconstriction and thereby reducing portal pressure. It is not currently used in the control of variceal bleeding because of serious systemic side effects. These include negative inotropic and chronotropic effects on the myocardium, leading to reduced cardiac output and bradycardia, as well as systemic vasoconstriction, which may result in bowel necrosis.

The vasopressin analog that is more commonly used is terlipressin or triglycl-lysine-vasopressin. Terlipressin is a long-acting synthetic vasopressin analog that has fewer cardiovascular side effects compared with vasopressin. Like vasopressin, terlipressin decreases cardiac output and causes splanchnic vasoconstriction, resulting in a decrease in portal blood flow. As a result of the increase in systemic vascular resistance, systemic arterial blood pressure may increase. The reduction in splanchnic blood flow decreases portal pressure by approximately 20%, even with a single dose of terlipressin. The portal pressure drops between 15 and 30 minutes following administration, and the reduction lasts for approximately 4 hours. The overall efficacy of terlipressin in controlling variceal bleeding is approximately 75% to 80%, especially when administered early. Meta-analysis suggests a decrease in mortality compared with a placebo (relative risk 0.66, 95% confidence interval, 0.49 to 0.88).[78] Because terlipressin is the only vasoactive treatment that has been shown to decrease mortality after variceal bleeding, and can improve renal function, it is the agent most frequently recommended for the control of acute bleeding. Terlipressin is administered in a dose of 2 mg every 4 hours for 2 to 5 days. After bleeding is controlled, it may be administered at a lower dose of 1 mg every 4 hours for up to 5 days. Side effects of terlipressin are similar to those with vasopressin and include myocardial and intestinal ischemia, but are less common. Terlipressin is not available in the United States.

Somatostatin and Its Analogs

Somatostatin is a 14-amino acid peptide, which works through somatostatin receptors. Because somatostatin has a half-life of less than 3 minutes, longer-acting analogs of somatostatin such as octreotide, lanreotide, and vapreotide have been synthesized. Somatostatin and its analogs decrease portal pressure by inhibiting the glucagon-mediated postprandial increase in portal blood flow. The usual dose of somatostatin is 250 μg as a bolus followed by an infusion of 250 μg/hr for 5 days. Octreotide is given in a bolus of 50 μg followed by an infusion of 25 to 50 μg/hr. The circulating half-life of octreotide is 80 to 120 minutes, but it does not have a prolonged affect in reducing portal pressure.

There is no clear evidence that somatostatin and its analogs are superior to placebo in the control of variceal bleeding. Some studies, however, demonstrate that somatostatin or octreotide may be equivalent to sclerotherapy or terlipressin in the control of acute variceal bleeding. A well-conducted study showed the early administration of vapreotide to be associated with better control of variceal bleeding, but without a reduction in the mortality rate.[79]

β-adrenergic Blocking Drugs

Nonselective β-blockers have been used extensively in the prevention of variceal bleeding. Only nonselective β-blockers should be administered because β_1-blockade alone decreases only cardiac output, whereas β_2-blockade inhibits splanchnic vasodilatation. The result of β_2-blockade is decreased portal blood flow, which reduces portal pressure. The nonselective β-blockers available are nadolol, propranolol, and timolol. Timolol needs to be administered four times a day and is not widely used in clinical practice. Nadolol is preferred to propranolol because it is less lipid soluble and is excreted mainly through the kidney. The decreased lipid solubility of nadolol probably results in fewer central side effects, such as depression and nightmares. β-blockers are most effective when they reduce the HVPG to below 12 mm Hg, or by 20% from the baseline. Ideally, monitoring of the HVPG in patients on nonselective β-blockers is required, but is not widely carried out in clinical practice.

When β-blockers are administered, a long-acting agent is preferable. The goal of treatment has traditionally been to reduce the resting heart rate to between 55 to 60 beats/min, or by 25% from the baseline. The heart rate decrease reflects only blockade of the β_1-receptor, whereas the β_2-blockade effect of decreasing portal blood flow may be more important in decreasing portal pressure. As long as there are no side effects, the dose of β-blockers may be increased every 3 to 5 days until a maximum tolerated dose is reached. The usual starting dose of propranolol is 60 mg once daily as a long-acting preparation, whereas nadolol is started at a dose of 40 mg once a day. In frail and older patients, especially older women with PBC, the starting dose of nadolol may be 20 mg once a day. The median maximum tolerated dose is approximately 80 mg for both long-acting propranolol and nadolol.

Approximately 15% of patients have contraindications to β-blocker use, including congestive heart failure, severe bronchial asthma, or severe chronic obstructive pulmonary disease, advanced heart blocks, as well as severe aortic stenosis and peripheral vascular disease. Side effects that limit use of β-blockers are mainly fatigue, lightheadedness, nightmares, and erectile dysfunction.[80]

Combined α- and ß-adrenergic Blockers

Carvedilol is a nonselective β-blocker which, in addition, has alpha vasodilatory effects by blockade of the α-receptor. Blockade of the α-receptor decreases intrahepatic vascular resistance, which results in a decrease in portal pressure. Carvedilol has, in addition, antioxidant, and antiproliferative effects. A recent randomized controlled trial demonstrated a possible benefit for carvedilol over endoscopic variceal ligation in the prevention of first variceal bleed.[81] In that study, among 152 patients with cirrhosis who were randomized to either carvedilol 12.5 mg once daily or endoscopic variceal ligation performed every 2 weeks, there was a lower rate of first variceal bleeding with carvedilol (10% versus 23%) without a significant decrease in overall or bleed related mortality. The study did not clearly demonstrate that the reduction in bleeding was related to a decrease in portal pressure because HVPG was not measured. It is possible that carvedilol looked promising because of the unusually high rate of bleeding in the variceal ligation group.[82]

Nitrates

Both short-acting nitrates such as nitroglycerin and long-acting nitrates such as isosorbide mononitrate have been used in the treatment of portal hypertension–related bleeding. Even though these agents were thought to decrease intrahepatic resistance, they act mainly by causing venodilation. The hypotension that the nitrates cause results in reflex splanchnic vasoconstriction, which decreases portal flow and reduces portal pressure. The experience with nitrates is far greater in Europe. In clinical practice within the United States, it is not common for patients to tolerate nitrates long-term because of side effects of headaches, dizziness, and hypotension. The only long-acting nitrate that has been adequately studied for the prevention of variceal bleeding is isosorbide mononitrate. Nitrates are not used either alone or in combination with a β-blocker for primary prophylaxis against variceal bleeding. Isosorbide mononitrate is, however, used to prevent variceal rebleeding in combination with a β-blocker, if β-blockers alone have not decreased the HVPG to target levels.

Drugs that Decrease Intrahepatic Vascular Resistance

An ideal drug to reduce portal pressure would be one that decreases intravascular resistance without compromising splanchnic blood flow or worsening systemic vasodilation. Potential agents that have been tried include the α_1-adrenergic blocker, prazosin; the combined α- and β-blocker carvedilol; angiotensin-2 receptor type 1 antagonist, losartan; endothelin receptor blockers; and liver selective NO donors. Long-term administration of prazosin has been associated with an increased risk of sodium retention and ascites. Neither losartan nor the angiotensin-2 receptor antagonist, irbesartan, have been clinically effective, and may worsen renal function.[83] Verapamil, the calcium receptor antagonist, has been associated with a decrease in the HVPG by approximately 14% with few systemic hemodynamic effects when used in patients with cirrhosis. The serotonin antagonist, ketanserin, has been used in only a small number of patients with reduction in the HVPG. Simvastatin may decrease intrahepatic resistance while maintaining hepatic blood flow and decreasing portal pressure, and should be the subject of future studies in the prevention of variceal bleeding.[19]

Endothelin-1 is a potential target to decrease portal pressure. However, administration of endothelin antagonists has been associated with a decrease in systemic blood pressure, which could worsen renal function. Thus, at the current time, there are no pharmacologic agents that can be used in clinical practice that decrease portal pressure predominantly by decreasing intrahepatic vascular resistance.

Endoscopic Therapy

The only modality that can be used for the spectrum of primary prevention of variceal bleeding, control of acute variceal bleeding, and prevention of variceal rebleeding is endoscopic therapy.

Sclerotherapy

The sclerotherapy technique involves intravariceal or paravariceal injection of a sclerosing agent, such as sodium tetradecyl sulfate, ethanolamine oleate, or sodium morrhuate. Because of the difficulty in determining whether an injection is intravariceal or paravariceal, most patients probably receive a combination of both paravariceal and intravariceal injections. Varices are injected in the lower third of the esophagus. Repeat injections are carried out at 1- to 4-week intervals until the varices are obliterated. Injection of varices at weekly intervals result in quicker obliteration of the varices, but a higher risk of sclerotherapy ulcers. Endoscopic sclerotherapy is seldom used nowadays except in the control of acute variceal bleeding when the presence of a large amount of blood in the esophagus prevents adequate visualization of the varix. Side effects of endoscopic sclerotherapy include ulceration with bleeding, strictures, and perforation. Both proton pump inhibitors and sucralfate may decrease the risk of variceal sclerotherapy ulcer-related bleeding. Postsclerotherapy dysphagia is due to a combination of stenosis as well as esophageal dysmotility. Postsclerotherapy strictures respond well to esophageal dilation.

Endoscopic Variceal Ligation

Endoscopic variceal ligation involves suctioning of the varix into a device at the tip of the endoscope, and application of rubber bands around the varix (**Fig. 19-22**). An overtube is no longer required with the advent of multiband ligators. The plastic device that holds the rubber bands is now transparent, which allows better visualization of the varix. Complications of endoscopic variceal ligation are less severe than following sclerotherapy, but include postbanding ulcers, hemorrhage, and esophageal strictures. Endoscopic variceal ligation is the preferred endoscopic therapy of esophageal varices.

Cyanoacrylate Glue Injection

Gastric varices may be obliterated by injection of polymers of cyanoacrylate. The cyanoacrylate most widely used worldwide is N-butyl-2-cyanoacrylate. This adhesive is not currently freely available within the United States. Within the United States, 2-octyl-cyanoacrylate, which is approved by the U.S. Food and Drug Administration for cutaneous wound closure, has been used "off label" for obturation of bleeding gastric varices.[84] It has a longer polymerization time than butyl cyanoacrylate due to a longer ester side chain and is, hence, used undiluted. The N-butyl-2-cyanoacrylate has to be diluted with Lipiodol to delay polymerization. Cyanoacrylates polymerize rapidly upon contact with weak bases such as blood. When injected intravascularly, cyanoacrylates solidify and form a cast of the vessel. Subtotal occlusion is immediate, whereas total occlusion occurs within hours. A prominent eosinophilic inflammation is seen in animal studies within the first day with tissue necrosis occurring by about the seventh day. The glue cast may either be extruded or remain in situ for months or years.

Glue therapy is used to control acute gastric variceal bleeding from isolated gastric varices or type 2 gastroesophageal varices. There are insufficient data to recommend the use of glue for prophylactic therapy to prevent gastric variceal bleeding. Glue injection is avoided in the presence of known large spontaneous splenorenal shunts because of the concern for risk of pulmonary embolization. With hepatopulmonary syndrome or intracardiac shunts, there is a risk of cerebral embolism.

Detachable Snares and Clips

There are a few reports of use of detachable snares for treatment of gastric varices. Detachable snares, available in varying diameters, have typically been used in the treatment of large polyps in the colon. Because detachable snares have "tails," they can interfere with visualization at endoscopy. Furthermore, traction of the varix during detachment of the snare can cause the varix to tear with an increase in bleeding.

There have been small studies have been carried out for the treatment of esophageal varices, as well as gastric varices with detachable snares. The data suggest that the snares are technically difficult to apply; thus there is a concern about widespread use. Snares are clearly not superior to endoscopic

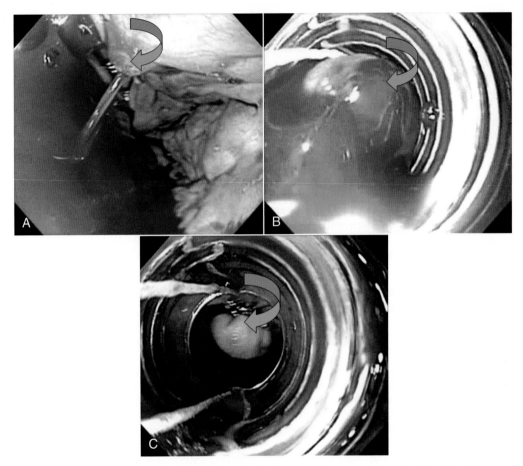

Fig. 19-22 Endoscopic images of actively bleeding esophageal varix (A, *arrow*), process of variceal ligation (B, *arrow*), and following ligation (C).

variceal ligation in the treatment of esophageal varices. There could be a potential role for detachable snares in the treatment of gastric varices, but the safety of this device should be demonstrated before detachable snares can be widely studied. Clips have also been used to treat large varices, especially at ectopic sites. Other than case reports or small series, the experience with this device is very limited and, again, widespread use in the treatment of variceal bleeding is not recommended.

Radiological Procedures
Transjugular Intrahepatic Portosystemic Shunts (TIPS) (see Chapter 16)

TIPS are currently used mainly for prevention of variceal rebleeding, but are also used in the control of refractory acute variceal bleeding.

A TIPS, which is created by interventional radiologists, is the most effective way of rapidly reducing resistance to portal blood flow, thereby decreasing portal pressure. A TIPS is effectively a side-to-side portocaval shunt that is used to treat not only bleeding-related complications of portal hypertension but also refractory ascites, hepatic hydrothorax, hepatorenal syndrome, and Budd-Chiari syndrome.

The goal of treatment with a TIPS is to reduce the portocaval pressure gradient (i.e., the difference in pressure between the portal vein and the inferior vena cava at the confluence of the hepatic veins) to below 12 mm Hg. Nowadays a coated stent

(Viatorr, Gore, Flagstaff, Ariz.) is used to bridge the tract between the portal vein and hepatic vein, usually from the right hepatic vein to the right portal vein. The uncoated portion of the stent anchors to the portal vein, whereas the polytetrafluoroethylene-coated portion lines the tract in the hepatic parenchyma. The major advantage of coated stents is that the frequency of shunt stenosis is reduced.[85] A TIPS can be successfully placed by an interventional radiologist in 95% to 98% of cases. Procedure-related mortality is usually 1% to 2% and is related to intraabdominal bleeding or pulmonary edema. The major long-term complications of the procedure include shunt occlusion and hepatic encephalopathy.[86]

TIPS is typically used in the prevention of variceal rebleeding when endoscopic and pharmacologic therapy have failed. TIPS can be used as salvage therapy to control acute variceal bleeding when two sessions of endoscopic treatment within a 24-hour period have failed to control the bleeding. Early TIPS, within 24 to 48 hours of control of bleeding, may be recommended in patients at high risk of rebleeding (Child Pugh Class C, or Child Pugh Class B with active bleeding at initial endoscopy). TIPS is also successful in better controlling and preventing gastric variceal bleeding. Meta-analysis of the 12 randomized control trials that have compared TIPS with endoscopic therapy have not demonstrated any survival benefit with TIPS. However, the rate of bleeding is lower in patients treated with TIPS but the frequency of encephalopathy is higher.

Ultrasound Doppler evaluation about every 6 months is used to monitor for shunt stenosis, but recurrence of complications of portal hypertension is a clear indication that the TIPS may have stenosed. This warrants venography of the shunt and measurement of the portocaval pressure gradient. Patients with a serum bilirubin greater than 3 mg/dl, especially if they have had previous hepatic encephalopathy, and an ALT greater than 100 U/L, and patients with a high Child-Turcotte-Pugh score are at a greater risk of mortality following TIPS. The Model for End-stage Liver Disease (MELD) was originally created from data obtained from patients undergoing TIPS. Those patients with a MELD score of 14 or less have an excellent survival rate post-TIPS, whereas those with a score greater than 24 have a mortality rate approaching 30% at three months.[87,88] In patients with a MELD between 15 and 24, TIPS placement requires careful discussion between the physician and patient, especially if liver transplantation is likely.

Balloon-Occluded Retrograde Transvenous Obliteration Of Varices (BRTO)

BRTO is a suitable treatment option for embolization of gastric varices and has also been used as a treatment option for refractory hepatic encephalopathy secondary to spontaneous splenorenal shunts. This procedure is only possible in patients with splenorenal shunts, which are visualized on CT angiography. A transfemoral route is used to access the left renal vein and then the gastrorenal shunt.[89] After the outflow vein of the shunt is occluded with a balloon, the varices can be injected with ethanolamine oleate or are coil embolized. Changes of portal hypertension, ascites, and splenomegaly can be aggravated following this procedure but, typically, there are no long-term problems. There is limited experience with this procedure and the long-term durability is uncertain.

Balloon Tamponade

Approximately 10% of patients with an acute variceal bleeding are refractory to pharmacologic and endoscopic treatment. Balloon tamponade is used as a temporizing measure in these patients until a TIPS can be carried out. Tamponade by a balloon is possible because the varices are superficial and thin-walled and the flow of blood is via submucosal vessels in the fundus of the stomach to the esophageal varices. Tamponade of either gastric or esophageal varices is appropriate and carried out by inflating a balloon either in the stomach or the esophagus, although inflation of the gastric balloon alone is preferred. The Sengstaken-Blakemore tube is a triple lumen tube, with one tube used for aspirating gastric contents; another leads to a gastric balloon with 200 to 400 ml in volume; and the third leads to an esophageal balloon. The Minnesota tube is a modification of the Sengstaken-Blakemore tube in that the gastric balloon is larger (500 ml) and there is an additional lumen for esophageal aspiration. The Linton-Nachlas tube has a 600-ml gastric balloon with lumens for aspirating both the stomach and esophagus. Balloon tamponade can control bleeding for up to 24 hours in approximately 90% of patients. In expert hands, the risk of pulmonary aspiration is low if endotracheal intubation precedes placement of the balloon. Inflation of the esophageal balloon should be avoided as much as possible, and instead attempts should be made to control bleeding by appropriate repositioning and traction on the gastric balloon.

Surgical Management of Portal Hypertension

The surgical procedures for managing portal hypertension fall into the following broad groups:
1. Decompressive shunts
   - Total
   - Selective
   - Partial
2. Nonshunt procedures
3. Mesenterico—portal venous bypass
4. Liver transplantation

Esophageal transaction, a nonshunt procedure, was previously used to control acute variceal bleeding but is seldom used nowadays. Devascularization procedures are carried out when a suitable vein is not available for shunting. Neither the nonshunt procedures nor liver transplantation will be discussed in this chapter.

Decompressive Shunts

The difference between total, partial, and selective shunts depends on which portions of the portal and superior mesenteric venous systems are decompressed (**Fig. 19-23**). In total portosystemic shunts, all parts of the portal venous system are decompressed and there is a significant loss to the liver of portal blood flow. In partial shunts, the varices are decompressed while maintaining some portal blood flow to the liver. Selective shunts decompress the spleen and gastroesophageal junction, but the portal and mesenteric venous systems are not decompressed. Portal hypertension is maintained while allowing antegrade hepatic blood flow.

Portocaval Shunts

The end-to-side and side-to-side portocaval shunts are total shunts. The side-to-side portocaval shunt is used to reduce portal pressure and to allow hepatic venous outflow in patients with Budd-Chiari syndrome. Any portocaval shunt greater than 12 mm in diameter results in total shunting of portal blood flow away from the liver. Such side-to-side portocaval shunts are an excellent way of treating variceal bleeding and controlling ascites because the hepatic sinusoids are decompressed. Following a side-to-side portocaval shunt, fewer than 10% of patients have recurrent variceal bleeding, but hepatic encephalopathy is seen in greater than 30% to 40% of patients. Moreover, when such patients undergo liver transplantation, there is an increased risk of operative morbidity and the requirement of transfusions. Therefore surgical portocaval shunts are best avoided in patients who are candidates for liver transplantation.

Selective Shunts

The Warren or distal splenorenal shunt (DSRS) is the most widely used surgical shunt. The surgical procedure aims at decompressing the spleen (Fig. 19-23, E) and varices at the gastroesophageal junction, whereas portal hypertension is maintained in other portions of the portal venous system. Following a distal splenorenal shunt, rebleeding rates are between 5% and 7% and hospital mortality is less than 10%. However, ascites persists because the hepatic sinusoids are not decompressed. Portoazygous disconnection, mobilization of the entire length of the pancreas, and ligation of the left adrenal vein is required before anastomosis between the

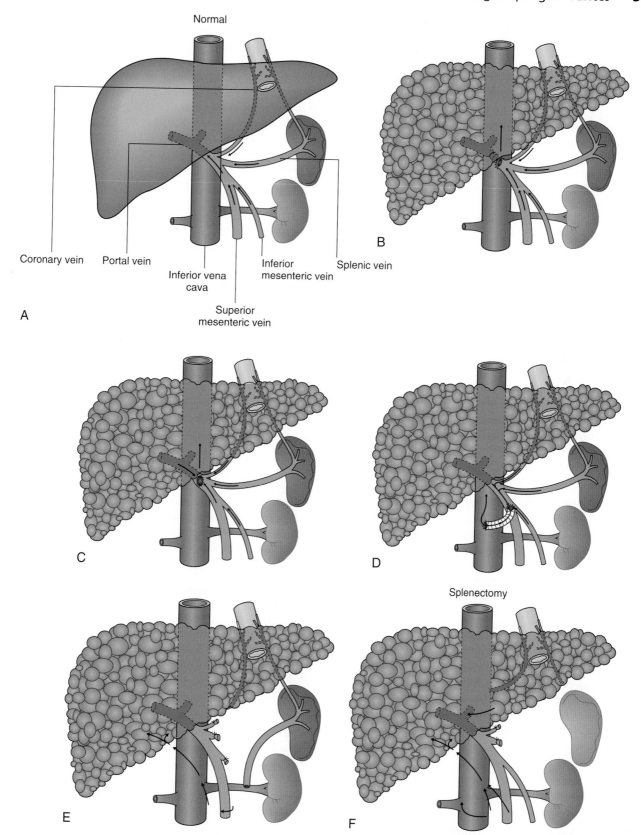

Fig. 19-23 **Total portal systemic shunts. A,** Normal. **B,** End-to-side portacaval shunt ligates the portal vein at the liver, so it does not decompress the liver sinusoids. **C,** Side-to-side portacaval shunt (>10 mm diameter) leaves the portal vein intact, so this shunt decompresses the liver as well as the varices. **D,** Mesocaval shunt requires an interposition graft—either PTFE (Gore-Tex) or autogenous jugular vein—to bridge the distance from the SMV to the IVC. Physiologically, this is the same as a side-to-side PCS. **Selective variceal decompression. E,** Distal splenorenal shunt decompresses the gastroesophageal junction and the spleen to control bleeding. The splanchnic and portal venous systems maintain hypertension and flow to the liver. **F,** Coronary caval shunt decompresses the gastroesophageal junction via the left gastric vein. Splenectomy is also performed. Portal hypertension and prograde portal flow is maintained.

splenic vein and the left renal vein is carried out to allow adequate decompression of the gastroesophageal junction.

Partial Portosystemic Shunts

When a synthetic 8-mm diameter interposition graft is used between the portal vein and the inferior vena cava, portal pressure can be reduced while allowing antegrade blood flow to the liver. Rebleeding and encephalopathy rates following creation of partial portosystemic shunts are similar to those with a distal splenorenal shunt, but ascites may occur because the hepatic sinusoidal pressure is not reduced.

Two large studies have compared surgical shunts to TIPS in the prevention of rebleeding in patients who have failed endoscopic and pharmacologic therapy. In the trial which compared TIPS with surgical 8-mm portocaval H interpositions grafts shunts, there was a benefit to surgical shunts compared to TIPS. Forty-six percent of these patients were of Child-Pugh Class C, and patients were not randomized.[90] In a well-conducted, randomized study carried out in patients with Child-Pugh Class A or B cirrhosis, the DSRS was compared with TIPS. The rebleeding rates were not significantly different (5.5% in the DSRS group and 10.5% in the TIPS group) and neither was there any difference in survival rate or the incidence of hepatic encephalopathy between the two groups.[91] The costs were higher in the long term in the TIPS group because of the need for surveillance and intervention in the presence of shunt stenosis. With the advent of coated stents, which have a lower rate of stenosis, the long-term costs of TIPS are likely to be reduced. Therefore there is no clear superiority of surgical shunts even in patients with Child-Pugh Class A cirrhosis. Surgical shunts might be best restricted to patients with noncirrhotic disease in whom the long-term prognosis is excellent.

Mensenterico—Portal Venous Bypass

The mesenterico-left portal venous bypass or Rex shunt is a recently described procedure carried out in patients with extrahepatic portal vein thrombosis in whom the intrahepatic portion of the portal vein is patent. The advantage of this shunt is that portal blood flow is restored to the liver, and there is no long-term risk of hepatic encephalopathy or learning disability in children. Typically, a jugular vein graft is used to bridge the obstruction in the portal vein via an anastomosis from the superior mesenteric vein to the intrahepatic portion of the left portal vein in the Rex recessus.[92] The Rex recessus is in the umbilical fissure where the left portal vein divides to supply segments III and IV of the liver. This surgery is probably the treatment of choice in children with extrahepatic portal vein thrombosis who have complications related to portal hypertension. The Rex shunt can also be carried out in patients in whom portal vein thrombosis has developed late after liver transplantation.

Approach to the Patient with Portal Hypertension–Related Bleeding

Esophageal Variceal Bleeding
Preprimary Prophylaxis of Variceal Bleeding

Preventing the development of varices in a patient who has been diagnosed with cirrhosis is termed preprimary prophylaxis. In experimental animal models, nonselective β-blockers can prevent or delay the development of collaterals. In a prospective study, 213 patients with cirrhosis and portal hypertension, but without varices, were randomized to treatment with a nonselective β-blocker, timolol, or a placebo for a median of 55 months.[93] In that study, the primary end point was development of esophageal varices or variceal hemorrhage. Unfortunately, the rate of development of varices in the two treatment groups was not different. Therefore β-blockers cannot be recommended for prevention of development of esophageal varices. A baseline HVPG lower than 10 mm Hg, a decrease in HVPG below 10 mm Hg, or a decrease of HVPG greater than 10% from baseline were independent predictors of remaining free of esophageal varices.

Primary Prophylaxis: Prevention of First Variceal Bleed
SMALL ESOPHAGEAL VARICES

Because patients with small varices with red signs or Child-Pugh Class C may have a bleeding risk similar to those with large varices, two studies addressed the role of nonselective β-blockers in these patients. In the French study, there was no benefit of propranolol in preventing variceal growth or bleeding.[94] On the other hand, an Italian study of 161 patients with cirrhosis with small varices showed a lower rate of increase in size of the varices in patients on nadolol as compared with a placebo.[95] Thus prophylactic therapy with nonselective β-blockers may be considered in Child-Pugh Class C patients with small esophageal varices.

LARGE ESOPHAGEAL VARICES

Patients with moderate and large varices should receive either pharmacologic or endoscopic treatment to prevent variceal bleeding. Either propranolol or nadolol may be used as pharmacologic therapy. In patients on pharmacologic treatment, a repeat endoscopy is not indicated unless patients are intolerant of treatment and require endoscopic variceal ligation; or if they have a variceal bleed in which case they require endoscopic treatment for control of the bleed. The acute hemodynamic response to β-blockers may predict the long-term outcome in patients undergoing primary prophylaxis of variceal bleeding.[96] In this study of 105 patients, who were administered propranolol intravenously, HVPG was measured before treatment and repeated 20 minutes later. A decrease of HVPG greater than 10%, during the acute study, was the best predictor of long-term response. Of those who had a greater than 10% response, only 4% had a bleed at 24 months. Of the nonresponders, 46% had a bleed at 24 months. Approximately 25% of patients with large varices may have contraindications to nonselective β-blockers, or do not tolerate the drugs. In such patients, endoscopic variceal ligation should be considered; long-acting nitrates are not recommended.

Endoscopic variceal ligation is the endoscopic treatment of choice for primary prophylaxis. Typically, 3 to 4 sessions are required before the varices can be obliterated. The interval between banding sessions varies between 2 to 4 weeks. Once varices are obliterated, repeat endoscopy is carried out every 6 to 12 months to look for variceal recurrence.

There have been 16 trials comparing endoscopic variceal ligation with β-blockers for primary prophylaxis; 10 of these studies have been published as full-length manuscripts. The meta-analysis favors endoscopic variceal ligation in prevention of bleeding without any difference in mortality. If

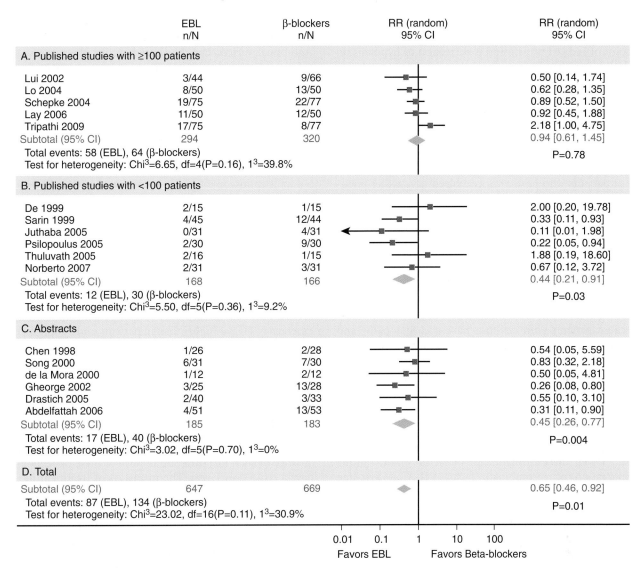

	EBL n/N	β-blockers n/N	RR (random) 95% CI	RR (random) 95% CI
A. Published studies with ≥100 patients				
Lui 2002	3/44	9/66		0.50 [0.14, 1.74]
Lo 2004	8/50	13/50		0.62 [0.28, 1.35]
Schepke 2004	19/75	22/77		0.89 [0.52, 1.50]
Lay 2006	11/50	12/50		0.92 [0.45, 1.88]
Tripathi 2009	17/75	8/77		2.18 [1.00, 4.75]
Subtotal (95% CI)	294	320		0.94 [0.61, 1.45]
Total events: 58 (EBL), 64 (β-blockers)				
Test for heterogeneity: Chi^2=6.65, df=4(P=0.16), I^2=39.8%				P=0.78
B. Published studies with <100 patients				
De 1999	2/15	1/15		2.00 [0.20, 19.78]
Sarin 1999	4/45	12/44		0.33 [0.11, 0.93]
Juthaba 2005	0/31	4/31		0.11 [0.01, 1.98]
Psilopoulus 2005	2/30	9/30		0.22 [0.05, 0.94]
Thuluvath 2005	2/16	1/15		1.88 [0.19, 18.60]
Norberto 2007	2/31	3/31		0.67 [0.12, 3.72]
Subtotal (95% CI)	168	166		0.44 [0.21, 0.91]
Total events: 12 (EBL), 30 (β-blockers)				
Test for heterogeneity: Chi^2=5.50, df=5(P=0.36), I^2=9.2%				P=0.03
C. Abstracts				
Chen 1998	1/26	2/28		0.54 [0.05, 5.59]
Song 2000	6/31	7/30		0.83 [0.32, 2.18]
de la Mora 2000	1/12	2/12		0.50 [0.05, 4.81]
Gheorge 2002	3/25	13/28		0.26 [0.08, 0.80]
Drastich 2005	2/40	3/33		0.55 [0.10, 3.10]
Abdelfattah 2006	4/51	13/53		0.31 [0.11, 0.90]
Subtotal (95% CI)	185	183		0.45 [0.26, 0.77]
Total events: 17 (EBL), 40 (β-blockers)				
Test for heterogeneity: Chi^2=3.02, df=5(P=0.70), I^2=0%				P=0.004
D. Total				
Subtotal (95% CI)	647	669		0.65 [0.46, 0.92]
Total events: 87 (EBL), 134 (β-blockers)				
Test for heterogeneity: Chi^2=23.02, df=16(P=0.11), I^2=30.9%				P=0.01

0.01   0.1   1   10   100
Favors EBL   Favors Beta-blockers

Fig. 19-24 **Meta-analyses of randomized controlled studies comparing endoscopic variceal ligation (EBL) with β-blockers (BB) in the prevention of variceal bleeding.** The meta-analyses favors EBL (lower risk of bleeding) when all studies are included; however, if only studies that included more than 100 patients are included, there is no statistically significant benefit of one treatment over the other. *(Modified from Bosch J, Garcia-Tsao G. Pharmacological versus endoscopic therapy in the prevention of variceal hemorrhage: and the winner is. Hepatology 2009;50:674–677.)*

only the four studies with 100 or more patients were considered, the superiority of endoscopic variceal ligation over β-blockers could not be demonstrated. Only if studies that included 62 or fewer patients were included did endoscopic ligation seem superior (**Fig. 19-24**).[82] Adverse events that warrant discontinuation of treatment are more frequent in patients undergoing β-blocker treatment (mainly fatigue and hypotension), but tend to be more severe in patients undergoing endoscopic variceal ligation (banding-related ulcers and occasional deaths). A recent study has suggested that nonbleed-related mortality may be lower in patients who receive β-blockers.[97]

Control of Acute Esophageal Variceal Bleeding
General Measures

The initial step in management of a patient suspected to have esophageal variceal bleeding is rapid assessment and correction of blood volume status. Because approximately 25% of blood volume may be lost without hypotension or tachycardia, determination of blood pressure and heart rate must be carried out, both in the supine and upright position in a patient who does not have supine hypotension. Replacement of blood volume is essential before endoscopy is carried out. Upper endoscopy carried out without correction of blood volume may miss esophageal varices because they collapse with significant hypotension. Overtransfusion should be avoided because it may increase portal pressure and the risk of variceal rebleeding. While blood is being typed and cross-matched, normal saline may be used to correct hypotension. Excessive use of saline can result in the rapid development of edema and ascites and, if glucose solutions are used, hyponatremia may develop. The routine measurement of central blood volume using central venous pressure or pulmonary capillary wedge pressure is not essential and, in fact, might be misleading. Because of the splanchnic vasodilation and increased pooling of blood in the splanchnic bed, correcting central venous pressure or pulmonary capillary wedge pressure often results in overcorrection of plasma volume. The endpoint of red cell transfusion is correction of hypotension and orthostatic changes, as well as improving urinary volume, with a hematocrit of 24% or so sufficing.

The current mortality at 6 weeks following esophageal variceal hemorrhage is approximately 15%. Though it is not entirely clear what accounts for the markedly decreased mortality from 50% about 2 decades ago, prophylactic antibiotics are certainly a major contributory factor. Bacterial infections are common in patients with cirrhosis and approximately 20% of patients who have a variceal bleed have either pneumonia, spontaneous bacterial peritonitis, or a urinary tract infection. Without antibiotics approximately 50% of patients with variceal bleeding are infected within a week. Therefore antibiotics should be administered to all patients with variceal bleeding irrespective of whether they have ascites or not.[98] The preferred antibiotic is norfloxacin 400 mg twice daily for 7 days. However, other options include ciprofloxacin, 400 mg every 12 hours; levofloxacin, 500 mg every 24 hours; or ceftriaxone, 1 g every 24 hours for a total of 7 days.

Because patients with cirrhosis have a coagulopathy and factor VII-A can normalize the coagulopathy even during bleeding, administration of recombinant factor VII-A has been studied in the control of variceal bleeding. Trials have evaluated the role of recombinant factor VII-A as adjuvant therapy to endoscopic and vasoactive treatment. Unfortunately, there was no benefit noted in control of the bleeding or rebleeding within the first 5 days. There was only a decrease in 42-day mortality in patients administered factor VII-A.[99] Given the exorbitant cost of factor VII-A, routine administration of recombinant factor VII-A as first-line treatment in the control of acute variceal bleeding is not recommended.

Specific Measures

A combination of pharmacologic therapy and endoscopic therapy is superior to either treatment alone in controlling variceal bleeding. The vasoactive agent should be started as early as possible, even as the patient is being brought by ambulance to the hospital. There are several vasoactive agents used, and the choice of treatment depends largely on availability. Terlipressin is the first choice in many centers in Europe and elsewhere because of evidence of improved survival rate associated with its use in controlling esophageal variceal bleeding. In the United States, octreotide is the agent used most commonly because terlipressin is not currently available. To prevent early rebleeding, pharmacologic treatment is continued for up to 5 days.

Endoscopic therapy should be initiated after the patient is hemodynamically stable, has had endotracheal intubation if there is active bleeding, and vasoactive agents have been infused for at least 30 minutes. At upper endoscopy, active bleeding from esophageal varices is confirmed: if active bleeding from a varix is noted (see **Fig. 19-22**); if there is a white fibrin plug or blood clot over a varix, especially if blood is noted in the stomach; or if there are varices noted with high-risk stigmata, such as a red wale sign. If varices are noted in the absence of any other lesion, then varices are the presumed source of the gastrointestinal bleeding.

Esophageal variceal ligation is carried out starting with the varix at or immediately below the bleeding site. No attempt should be made to band varices distal to the site of initial banding because this may cause dislodgement of the band. Additional varices may be ligated during the same session, proximal to the initial ligation, in a spiral fashion at approximately 2-cm intervals. In some patients, a large amount of blood in the lower esophagus can obscure visualization. In these patients, variceal ligation or sclerotherapy can be carried out blindly. Unfortunately, in these patients, there is a higher long-term risk of esophageal strictures.

Patients with acute variceal bleeding but without active bleeding at endoscopy have a lower risk of rebleeding within 5 days if endoscopic ligation is combined with terlipressin.[100] Failure to control bleeding is defined by the need for greater than 4 units of red cell transfusion to maintain the hematocrit above 25%, inability to increase the systolic blood pressure by 20 mm Hg or to greater than 70 mm Hg, or persistence of heart rate greater than 100 beats per minute. According to this definition, bleeding cannot be controlled in approximately 10% of patients despite two sessions of endoscopic treatment within a 24-hour period. In such patients, a TIPS should be carried out, but the mortality rate in patients undergoing an emergency TIPS is higher than in patients undergoing an elective TIPS. Until such time that a TIPS can be carried out, balloon tamponade is used to control the bleeding.

Secondary Prophylaxis: Prevention of Recurrent Esophageal Variceal Bleeding

All patients who have had esophageal variceal bleeding should receive treatment to prevent recurrent variceal bleeding. In the absence of such measures, up to 60% of these patients might have a rebleed in 1 year. The mainstays of treatment for secondary prophylaxis of esophageal variceal bleeding are pharmacologic treatment with nonselective β-blockers and/or endoscopic variceal ligation. Nonselective β-blockers have often been the first line of treatment. Meta-analysis have demonstrated a significant benefit in preventing rebleeding in patients on β-blockers with an approximately 20% lower risk of bleeding and 10% lower risk of bleed-related mortality.[101] The number of patients who need to be treated to prevent an episode of rebleeding is 5, and the number needed to prevent death is 14. There has been no significant difference in either prevention of rebleeding or reduction in mortality between patients on β-blockers and those treated with endoscopic variceal sclerotherapy. The addition of isosorbide mononitrate to propranolol or nadolol further reduces portal pressure. A combination of isosorbide mononitrate with nadolol has been shown to be superior to endoscopic sclerotherapy alone.[102] Meta-analysis comparing a combination of nonselective β-blockers and isosorbide mononitrate against endoscopic variceal ligation alone shows no significant difference in rebleeding or mortality. However, a combination of endoscopic variceal ligation and pharmacologic treatment is the best modality to prevent variceal rebleeding in patients with cirrhosis, according to a recent meta-analysis.[103] This meta-analysis of 23 trials, which included 1860 patients, showed a combination therapy with endoscopic variceal ligation and β-blockers reduced overall rebleeding more than endoscopic therapy alone (pooled relative risk 0.68 [95% 0.52 to 0.89]), or β-blocker therapy alone (pooled relative risk 0.71 [0.59 to 0.86]). Combination therapy, however, is not associated with reduction in mortality as compared with endoscopic therapy (pooled odds ratio 0.78 [0.58 to 1.07]), or drug therapy (pooled odds ratio 0.70 [0.46 to 1.06]).[104]

If patients have rebleeding on maximal treatment with β-blockers alone, then endoscopic variceal ligation should be added. Similarly, if patients have been only receiving endoscopic variceal ligation and have variceal rebleeding, then β-blockers should be added. If, however, variceal bleeding occurs despite of combined treatment with endoscopic variceal ligation and β-blockers, then a TIPS is considered. Patients with an HVPG greater than 20 mm Hg have an inferior response to both β-blockers and endoscopic variceal ligation. In these patients, TIPS may be considered early after control of the variceal bleed. When TIPS has been compared with either sclerotherapy or variceal ligation, the rebleeding rates with TIPS have been 9% to 23%; with endoscopic treatment, 21% to 66%. Thus TIPS is superior to endoscopic treatment in the prevention of variceal rebleeding. Similarly, a combination of propranolol and isosorbide mononitrate was inferior to TIPS in the prevention of rebleeding. However, TIPS was associated consistently with a higher risk of hepatic encephalopathy without any survival rate benefit. Consequently, TIPS cannot be recommended as the first choice of therapy in the prevention of variceal rebleeding. Surgical portosystemic shunts are seldom required for patients with cirrhosis, but are recommended in patients with noncirrhotic portal hypertension to prevent recurrent variceal bleeding.

Gastric Varices

There have been no randomized controlled studies that have addressed the role of primary prophylaxis to prevent gastric variceal hemorrhage. In the absence of data, current recommendations are to use β-blockers to prevent bleeding in patients with large gastric varices. The results of the studies comparing prophylactic cyanoacrylate obturation of gastric varices versus β-blockers are still awaited.

When a patient is diagnosed to have acutely bleeding gastric varices on endoscopy, obturation of the varices with cyanoacrylate glue is the treatment of choice. Initial management and resuscitation of these patients is no different than in patients with esophageal variceal hemorrhage. Gastric variceal hemorrhage is diagnosed when bleeding is noted from a gastric varix (**Fig. 19-25**); if blood is found at the gastroesophageal junction or fundus in the stomach; a white nipple sign is seen over gastric varices; or when gastric varices are noted in the absence of any other lesions that could explain upper gastrointestinal bleeding. Standard sclerosing agents are not effective in the control of gastric variceal bleeding and are associated with a high risk of rebleeding. In a randomized controlled trial,

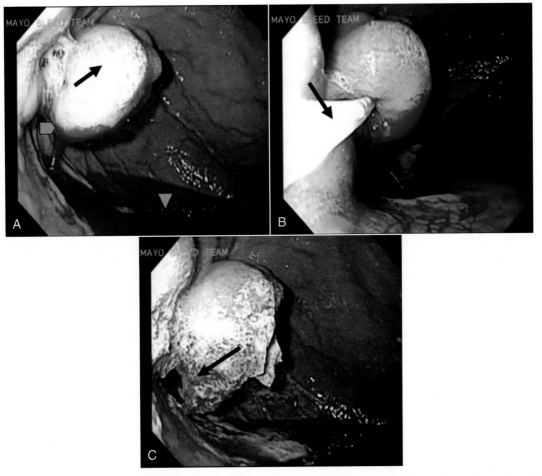

Fig. 19-25 Control of gastric variceal bleeding with cyanoacrylate glue injection. A, Actively bleeding (pentagon) gastric varix *(black arrow)* with large amount of blood *(arrowhead)* pooling in stomach. **B,** Injection *(arrow)* of bleeding gastric varix. **C,** Gastric varix after obliteration. Earlier appearance of cyanoacrylate casts *(arrow)*.

initial hemostasis up to 72 hours was achieved in 87% of patients treated with cyanoacrylate obturation but in only 45% of patients who were banded. There was significantly more rebleeding in the banded group (54% vs. 31% in the variceal obturation group).[105] Reports from within the United States demonstrate a similar level of hemostasis when 2-octyl cyanoacrylate is used.

If endoscopic variceal obturation is not available, or if rebleeding occurs despite of variceal obturation, then a TIPS is necessary. BRTO of gastric fundal varices may also be carried out in patients with spontaneous splenorenal shunts demonstrated on multidetector CT. TIPS can control gastric variceal bleeding in upwards of 95% of patients, with rebleeding in approximately 25% of patients. Because the control of bleeding and rebleeding rates between endoscopic variceal obturation and TIPS are similar, a head-to-head comparison of efficacy is necessary to demonstrate superiority of one procedure over the other. While patients are awaiting placement of an urgent TIPS, a Linton-Nachlas tube may be used to control active bleeding from gastric fundal varices.

The optimal reduction in pressure when a TIPS is used to treat gastric variceal bleeding is not clear because bleeding has been noted even when the portocaval pressure gradient is less than 12 mm Hg. Most operators will place a TIPS and expand the stent until the portocaval pressure gradient is less than 12 mm Hg. Any residual gastric varices will then be embolized.

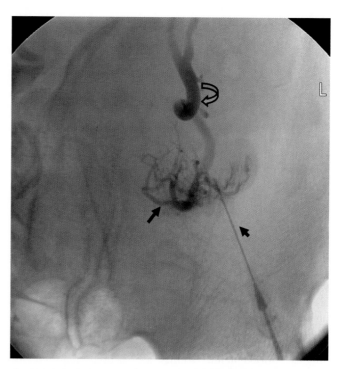

Fig. 19-26 **Percutaneous ultrasound-guided injection** *(short arrow)* of stomal varices *(long arrow)* being fed by abdominal wall collateral *(curved arrow)*.

Portal Hypertensive Gastropathy and Gastric Vascular Ectasia

Severe PHG is associated with iron deficiency anemia and chronic gastrointestinal blood loss, though acute variceal bleeding may also occur. Acute bleeding is treated with vasoactive agents similar to patients with esophageal variceal bleeding. To prevent rebleeding in patients with iron deficiency anemia, nonselective β-blockers are used, usually in combination with iron replacement. However, if patients continue to be transfusion-dependent despite iron and β-blocker therapy, then a TIPS can be carried out with excellent results. Thermo-ablative therapy should not be used.[75]

GVE do not respond to β-blockers or to TIPS. Rather, thermo-ablative therapy is required. Such therapy is possible in patients with a platelet count greater than 45,000 and an INR less than 1.4. There may be increased mucosal bleeding if the coagulation parameters are suboptimal. Cryotherapy using liquid nitrogen dioxide or liquid carbon dioxide has also been used to treat bleeding from GVE lesions, especially when such lesions are diffuse.[106] A combination of estrogen/progesterone oral contraceptive pills may be used when endoscopic therapy fails. Bleeding from GVE usually reverses with liver transplantation.

Ectopic Varices

Manifestations of ectopic variceal bleeding include hematemesis or melena, but hemobilia, hematuria, and intraperitoneal or retroperitoneal bleeding also occur. Patients with extrahepatic vein obstruction usually bleed from varices at the gastroesophageal junction, or in the duodenum. Patients with cirrhosis, on the other hand, tend to bleed from sites where

surgery has allowed the development of ectopic varices, usually peristomal varices.

Initial control of stomal variceal bleeding is local compression of the bleeding site with gauze soaked with a 1 : 10,000 epinephrine solution. To prevent rebleeding, patients with stomal varices may be treated with ultrasound-guided sclerotherapy of the ectopic varices (**Fig. 19-26**). In addition, transhepatic embolization of the varices may be carried out. TIPS are considered in patients in whom embolization fails to prevent rebleeding. It is important to note that selective shunts, such as the distal splenorenal shunt, are ineffective in preventing bleeding from stomal varices.

Bleeding from ectopic varices, other than stomal varices, is initially treated much the same way as varices at other sites. Endoscopic therapy includes band ligation, glue injection, and application of clips. In addition, surgical ligation may need to be considered for refractory bleeding varices, especially when associated with intraabdominal hemorrhage. TIPS may not be possible when ectopic variceal bleeding is secondary to extensive portal and mesenteric vein thrombosis. A surgical portosystemic shunt is considered in such situations.

Key References

Abraldes JG, et al. Simvastatin lowers portal pressure in patients with cirrhosis and portal hypertension: a randomized controlled trial. Gastroenterology 2009;136:1651–1658. (Ref.19)

Abraldes JG, et al. Mild increases in portal pressure upregulate vascular endothelial growth factor and endothelial nitric oxide synthase in the intestinal microcirculatory bed, leading to a hyperdynamic state. Am J Physiol Gastrointest Liver Physiol 2006;290:G980–G987. (Ref.36)

Abraldes JG, et al. Simvastatin treatment improves liver sinusoidal endothelial dysfunction in CCl4 cirrhotic rats. J Hepatol 2007;46:1040–1046. (Ref.20)

Bambha K, et al. Predictors of early re-bleeding and mortality after acute variceal haemorrhage in patients with cirrhosis. Gut 2008;57:814–820. (Ref.74)

Bataller R, Brenner DA. Liver fibrosis. J Clin Invest 2005;115:209–218. (Ref.12)

Bernard B, et al. Antibiotic prophylaxis for the prevention of bacterial infections in cirrhotic patients with gastrointestinal bleeding: a meta-analysis. Hepatology 1999;29:1655–1661. (Ref.98)

Bernard B, et al. Beta-adrenergic antagonists in the prevention of gastrointestinal rebleeding in patients with cirrhosis: a meta-analysis. Hepatology 1997;25:63–70. (Ref.101)

La Mura V, et al. Right atrial pressure is not adequate to calculate portal pressure gradient in cirrhosis: a clinical-hemodynamic correlation study. Hepatology 2010;51:2108–2116. (Ref.51)

Bosch J. Decreasing hepatic vascular tone by liver-specific NO donors: wishful thinking or a promising reality? J Hepatol 2003;39:1072–1075. (Ref.18)

Bosch J, Garcia-Tsao G. Pharmacological versus endoscopic therapy in the prevention of variceal hemorrhage: and the winner is. Hepatology 2009;50:674–677. (Ref.82)

Bosch J, et al. Recombinant factor VIIa for variceal bleeding in patients with advanced cirrhosis: a randomized, controlled trial. Hepatology 2008;47:1604–1614. (Ref.99)

Boyer TD, Haskal ZJ. The role of transjugular intrahepatic portosystemic shunt in the management of portal hypertension. Hepatology 2005;41:386–400. (Ref.86)

Brensing KA, et al. Endoscopic manometry of esophageal varices: evaluation of a balloon technique compared with direct portal pressure measurement. J Hepatol 1998;29:94–102. (Ref.22)

Brugge WR. EUS is an important new tool for accessing the portal vein. Gastrointest Endosc 2008;67:343–344. (Ref.47)

Bureau C, et al. Improved clinical outcome using polytetrafluoroethylene-coated stents for TIPS. Results of a randomized study. Gastroenterology 2004;126:469–473. (Ref.85)

Cales P, et al. Early administration of vapreotide for variceal bleeding in patients with cirrhosis. N Engl J Med 2001;344:23–28. (Ref.79)

Cales P, et al. Lack of effect of propranolol in the prevention of large oesophageal varices in patients with cirrhosis: a randomized trial. French-Speaking Club for the Study of Portal Hypertension. Eur J Gastroenterol Hepatol 1999;11:741–745. (Ref.94)

Cardenas A, Gines P. Portal hypertension. Curr Opin Gastroenterol 2009;25:195–201. (Ref.32)

Cho S, et al. Endoscopic cryotherapy for the management of gastric antral vascular ectasia. Gastrointest Endosc 2008;68:895–902. (Ref.106)

D'Amico G, de Franchis R. Upper digestive bleeding in cirrhosis. Post therapeutic outcome and prognostic indicators. Hepatology 2003;38:599–612. (Ref.73)

D'Amico G, Garcia-Tsao G, Pagliaro L. Natural history and prognostic indicators of survival in cirrhosis: a systematic review of 118 studies. J Hepatol 2006;44:217–231. (Ref.72)

de Franchis R. Evolving consensus in portal hypertension. Report of the Baveno IV consensus workshop on methodology of diagnosis and therapy in portal hypertension. J Hepatol 2005;43:167–176. (Ref.41)

de Franchis R, et al. Esophageal capsule endoscopy for screening and surveillance of esophageal varices in patients with portal hypertension. Hepatology 2008;47:1595–1603. (Ref.43)

DeLeve LD, Valla DC, Garcia-Tsao G. Vascular disorders of the liver. Hepatology 2009;49:1729–1764. (Ref.60)

Devarbhavi H, Abraham S, Kamath PS. Significance of nodular regenerative hyperplasia occurring de novo following liver transplantation. Liver Transpl 2007;13:1552–1556. (Ref.67)

de Ville de Goyet J, Clapuyt P, Otte JB. Extrahilar mesenterico-left portal shunt to relieve extrahepatic portal hypertension after partial liver transplant. Transplantation 1992;53:231–232. (Ref.92)

Escorsell A, et al. Predictive value of the variceal pressure response to continued pharmacological therapy in patients with cirrhosis and portal hypertension. Hepatology 2000;31:1061–1067. (Ref.55)

Escorsell A, et al. Increased intra-abdominal pressure increases pressure, volume, and wall tension in esophageal varices. Hepatology 2002;36:936–940. (Ref.46)

Feng HQ, Weymouth ND, Rockey DC. Endothelin antagonism in portal hypertensive mice: implications for endothelin receptor-specific signaling in liver disease. Am J Physiol Gastrointest Liver Physiol 2009;297:G27–G33. (Ref.21)

Fernandez M, et al. Reversal of portal hypertension and hyperdynamic splanchnic circulation by combined vascular endothelial growth factor and platelet-derived growth factor blockade in rats. Hepatology 2007;46:1208–1217. (Ref.37)

Fernandez M, et al. Anti-VEGF receptor-2 monoclonal antibody prevents portal-systemic collateral vessel formation in portal hypertensive mice. Gastroenterology 2004;126:886–894. (Ref.38)

Friedman SL. Mechanisms of hepatic fibrogenesis. Gastroenterology 2008;134:1655–1669. (Ref.13)

Garcia-Pagan JC, et al. Nadolol plus isosorbide mononitrate alone or associated with band ligation in the prevention of recurrent bleeding: a multicentre randomised controlled trial. Gut 2009;58:1144–1150. (Ref.104)

Garcia-Tsao G. Liver involvement in hereditary hemorrhagic telangiectasia (HHT). J Hepatol 2007;46:499–507. (Ref.58)

Garcia-Tsao G, Bosch J, Groszmann RJ. Portal hypertension and variceal bleeding: unresolved issues. Summary of an American Association for the Study of Liver Diseases and European Association for the Study of the Liver single-topic conference. Hepatology 2008;47:1764–1772. (Ref.54)

Giannini EG, et al. Platelet count/spleen diameter ratio for the noninvasive diagnosis of esophageal varices: results of a multicenter, prospective, validation study. Am J Gastroenterol 2006;101:2511–2519. (Ref.71)

Gonzalez R, et al. Meta-analysis: combination endoscopic and drug therapy to prevent variceal rebleeding in cirrhosis. Ann Intern Med 2008;149:109–122. (Ref.103)

Groszmann RJ. Hepatic venous pressure gradient: anything worth doing should be done right. Hepatology 2004;39:280–282. (Ref.50)

Groszmann RJ, et al. Beta-blockers to prevent gastroesophageal varices in patients with cirrhosis. N Engl J Med 2005;353:2254–2261. (Ref.93)

Henderson JM, et al. Distal splenorenal shunt versus transjugular intrahepatic portal systematic shunt for variceal bleeding: a randomized trial. Gastroenterology 2006;130:1643–1651. (Ref.91)

Huet PM, et al. Portal hypertension and primary biliary cirrhosis: effect of long-term ursodeoxycholic acid treatment. Gastroenterology 2008;135:1552–1560. (Ref.52)

Ioannou GN, Doust J, Rockey DC. Systematic review: terlipressin in acute oesophageal variceal haemorrhage. Aliment Pharmacol Ther 2003;17:53–64. (Ref.78)

Iwakiri Y. The molecules: mechanisms of arterial vasodilatation observed in the splanchnic and systemic circulation in portal hypertension. J Clin Gastroenterol 2007;41(Suppl 3):S288–S294. (Ref.33)

Iwakiri Y, Grisham M, Shah V. Vascular biology and pathobiology of the liver: report of a single-topic symposium. Hepatology 2008;47:1754–1763. (Ref.10)

Kamal SM, et al. Progression of fibrosis in hepatitis C with and without schistosomiasis: correlation with serum markers of fibrosis. Hepatology 2006;43:771–779. (Ref.64)

Kamath PS, et al. Hepatic localization of endothelin-1 in patients with idiopathic portal hypertension in cirrhosis of the liver. Liver Transpl 2000;6:596–602. (Ref.62)

Kamath PS, Kim WR. The model for end-stage liver disease (MELD). Hepatology 2007;45:797–805. (Ref.88)

Kamath PS, et al. Gastric mucosal responses to intrahepatic portosystemic shunting in patients with cirrhosis. Gastroenterology 2000;118:905–911. (Ref.75)

Kiyosue H, et al. Transcatheter obliteration of gastric varices: part 2. Strategy and techniques based on hemodynamic features. Radiographics 2003;23:921–937; discussion 937. (Ref.89)

Kumar S, Sarr MG, Kamath PS. Mesenteric venous thrombosis. N Engl J Med 2001;345:1683–1688. (Ref.61)

Langer DA, Shah VH. Nitric oxide and portal hypertension: interface of vasoreactivity and angiogenesis. J Hepatol 2006;44:209–216. (Ref.29)

Lazaridis KN, Abraham SC, Kamath PS. Hematological malignancy manifesting as ascites. Nat Clin Pract Gastroenterol Hepatol 2005;2:112–116; quiz 117. (Ref.69)

Lee JS, et al. Sinusoidal remodeling and angiogenesis: a new function for the liver-specific pericyte? Hepatology 2007;45:817–825. (Ref.14)

Levesque E, et al. Plasma disappearance rate of indocyanine green: a tool to evaluate early graft outcome after liver transplantation. Liver Transpl 2009;15:1358–1364. (Ref.56)

Lim JK, Groszmann RJ. Transient elastography for diagnosis of portal hypertension in liver cirrhosis: is there still a role for hepatic venous pressure gradient measurement? Hepatology 2007;45:1087–1090. (Ref.49)

Lo GH, et al. Improved survival in patients receiving medical therapy as compared with banding ligation for the prevention of esophageal variceal rebleeding. Hepatology 2008;48:580–587. (Ref.97)

Lo GH, et al. Low-dose terlipressin plus banding ligation versus low-dose terlipressin alone in the prevention of very early rebleeding of oesophageal varices. Gut 2009;58:1275–1280. (Ref.100)

Lo G, et al. A prospective, randomized trial of butyl cyanoacrylate injection versus band ligation in the management of bleeding gastric varices. Hepatology 2001;33:1060–1064. (Ref.105)

Lui HF, et al. Primary prophylaxis of variceal hemorrhage: a randomized controlled trial comparing band ligation, propranolol, and isosorbide mononitrate. Gastroenterology 2002;123:735–744. (Ref.80)

Mahadeva S, et al. Cost-effectiveness of N-butyl-2-cyanoacrylate (Histoacryl) glue injections versus transjugular intrahepatic portosystemic shunt in the management of acute gastric variceal bleeding. Am J Gastroenterology 2003; 98:2688–2693. (Ref.84)

Malinchoc M, et al. A model to predict poor survival in patients undergoing transjugular intrahepatic portosystemic shunts. Hepatology 2000;31:864–871. (Ref.87)

Mejias M, et al. Beneficial effects of sorafenib on splanchnic, intrahepatic, and portocollateral circulations in portal hypertensive and cirrhotic rats. Hepatology 2009;49:1245–1256. (Ref.31)

Menon KV, Shah VH, Kamath PS. The Budd-Chiari syndrome. N Engl J Med 2004;350:578–585. (Ref.39)

Merkel C, et al. A placebo-controlled clinical trial of nadolol in the prophylaxis of growth of small esophageal varices in cirrhosis. Gastroenterology 2004;127: 476–484. (Ref.95)

Norton ID, Andrews J, Kamath PS. Management of ectopic varices. Hepatology 1998;28:1154–1158. (Ref.77)

Novo E, et al. Proangiogenic cytokines as hypoxia-dependent factors stimulating migration of human hepatic stellate cells. Am J Pathol 2007;170:1942–1953. (Ref.28)

Omenetti A, et al. Hedgehog signaling regulates epithelial-mesenchymal transition during biliary fibrosis in rodents and humans. J Clin Invest 2008; 118:3331–3342. (Ref.16)

Pasha SF, et al. Splanchnic artery aneurysms. Mayo Clin Proc 2007;82:472–479. (Ref.57)

Patsenker E, et al. Pharmacological inhibition of integrin alphavbeta3 aggravates experimental liver fibrosis and suppresses hepatic angiogenesis. Hepatology 2009;50:1501–1511. (Ref.25)

Perri RE, et al. A prospective evaluation of computerized tomographic (CT) scanning as a screening modality for esophageal varices. Hepatology 2008;47: 1587–1594. (Ref.40)

Primignani M, et al. Natural history of portal hypertensive gastropathy in patients with liver cirrhosis. Gastroenterology 2000;119:181–187. (Ref.76)

Qamar AA, et al. Platelet count is not a predictor of the presence or development of gastroesophageal varices in cirrhosis. Hepatology 2008;47:153–159. (Ref.70)

Qian Q, et al. Clinical profile of autosomal-dominant polycystic liver disease. Hepatology 2003;37:164–171. (Ref.66)

Reshamwala PA, Kleiner DE, Heller T. Nodular regenerative hyperplasia: not all nodules are created equal. Hepatology 2006;44:7–14. (Ref.68)

Ripoll C, et al. Hepatic venous pressure gradient predicts clinical decompensation in patients with compensated cirrhosis. Gastroenterology 2007;133:481–488. (Ref.53)

Rockey DC, Shah V. Nitric oxide biology and the liver: report of an AASLD research workshop. Hepatology 2004;39:250–257. (Ref.17)

Rosemurgy AS, Goode SE, Swiebel BR. A prospective trial of TIPS versus small diameter prosthetic H graft portocaval shunt in the treatment of bleeding varices. Ann Surg 1996;224:378–386. (Ref.90)

Ross AJP, et al. Current concepts: schistosomiasis. N Engl J Med 2002;346: 1212–1220. (Ref.63)

Sarin SK, et al. Relevance, classification and natural history of gastric varices: a long-term follow-up study in 568 portal hypertension patients. Hepatology 1992;16:1343–1349. (Ref.42)

Schepis F, et al. Which patients with cirrhosis should undergo endoscopic screening for esophageal varices detection? Hepatology 2001;33:333–338. (Ref.45)

Schepke M, et al. Hemodynamic effects of the angiotensin II receptor antagonist irbesartan in patients with cirrhosis and portal hypertension. Gastroenterology 2001;121:389–395. (Ref.83)

Schuppan D, Afdhal NH. Liver cirrhosis. Lancet 2008;371:838–851. (Ref.9)

Semela D, et al. Platelet-derived growth factor signaling through ephrin-B2 regulates hepatic vascular structure and function. Gastroenterology 2008;135: 671–679. (Ref.26)

Shah V, et al. The hepatic circulation in health and disease: report of a single-topic symposium. Hepatology 1998;27:279–288. (Ref.4)

Shah V, et al. Liver sinusoidal endothelial cells are responsible for nitric oxide modulation of hepatic resistance. J Clin Invest 1997;100:2923–2930. (Ref.11)

Shah V, Kamath P, de Groen P. Physiology of the splanchnic circulation. In: Topol CJ, Lanzer F, editors. Theory and practice of vascular diseases. Berlin: Springer; 2002. (Ref.2)

Shah VH, Bruix J. Antiangiogenic therapy: not just for cancer anymore? Hepatology 2009;49(4):1066–1068. (Ref.30)

Talwalkar JA, et al. Magnetic resonance imaging of hepatic fibrosis: emerging clinical applications. Hepatology 2008;47:332–342. (Ref.44)

Theodorakis N, et al. The role of nitric oxide synthase isoforms in extrahepatic portal hypertension: studies in gene knock-out mice. Gastroenterology 2003; 124:1500–1508. (Ref.35)

Tripathi D, et al. Randomized controlled trial of carvedilol versus variceal band ligation for the prevention of the first variceal bleed. Hepatology 2009;50: 825–833. (Ref.81)

Tripathi D, Hayes PC. Review article: a drug therapy for the prevention of variceal haemorrhage. Aliment Pharmacol Ther 2001;15:291–310. (Ref.34)

Tugues S, et al. Antiangiogenic treatment with sunitinib ameliorates inflammatory infiltrate, fibrosis, and portal pressure in cirrhotic rats. Hepatology 2007;46:1919–1926. (Ref.27)

Valla DC. Thrombosis and anticoagulation in liver disease. Hepatology 2008;47: 1384–1393. (Ref.59)

Villanueva C, et al. Acute hemodynamic response to beta-blockers and prediction of long-term outcome in primary prophylaxis of variceal bleeding. Gastroenterology 2009;137:119–128. (Ref.96)

Villanueva C, et al. Nadolol plus isosorbide mononitrate compared with sclerotherapy for the prevention of variceal rebleeding. N Engl J Med 1996; 334:1624–1629. (Ref.102)

Vizzutti F, et al. Liver stiffness measurement predicts severe portal hypertension in patients with HCV-related cirrhosis. Hepatology 2007;45:1290–1297. (Ref.48)

Wanless IR, et al. Hepatic and portal vein thrombosis in cirrhosis: possible role in development of parenchymal extinction and portal hypertension. Hepatology 1995;21:1238–1247. (Ref.6)

Wells RG, Kruglov E, Dranoff JA. Autocrine release of TGF-beta by portal fibroblasts regulates cell growth. FEBS Lett 2004;559:107–110. (Ref.15)

Zipprich A, et al. The role of hepatic arterial flow on portal venous and hepatic venous wedged pressure in the isolated perfused CCl4-cirrhotic liver. Am J Physiol Gastrointest Liver Physiol 2008;295:G197–G202. (Ref.24)

Zipprich A, et al. Nitric oxide and vascular remodeling modulate hepatic arterial vascular resistance in the isolated perfused cirrhotic rat liver. J Hepatol 2008; 49:739–745. (Ref.23)

A complete list of references can be found at www.expertconsult.com.

Acute Liver Failure

R. Todd Stravitz and David J. Kramer

Introduction and Definition of the Syndrome

The syndrome of acute liver failure (ALF), characterized by jaundice, coagulopathy, and altered sensorium (hepatic encephalopathy), is among the most catastrophic afflictions of humans, and results in multiorgan system failure (MOSF) and death in the majority of patients (40% to 95%) unless orthotopic liver transplantation (OLT) is performed. Fortunately, ALF is uncommon, with approximately 2000 cases per year in the United States; unfortunately, the optimal management of ALF remains largely undefined because of its rarity, heterogeneity, and rapidity of evolution. Lucke and Mallory first described ALF in 1946 as three phases of liver disease: a prodromal/preicteric phase, an intermediate phase with the onset of jaundice, and a final phase of encephalopathy.[1] These and subsequent authors recognized that the interval between the onset of icterus and encephalopathy conveyed important etiologic and prognostic information. Accordingly, several groups have subcategorized patients with ALF by the time interval between the latter two phases. As most commonly defined, the term fulminant hepatic failure denotes the development of hepatic encephalopathy within 8 weeks of the onset of symptoms. A more gradually evolving "subfulminant" course of liver failure (also referred to as late-onset hepatic failure) was subsequently recognized by the King's College group, and defined as encephalopathy developing between 8 and 24 weeks of the onset of jaundice.[2] Subacute liver failure is characterized by a greater likelihood of developing signs of chronic liver disease, such as ascites and renal failure; a lower incidence of cerebral edema; but paradoxically, a higher mortality than the fulminant subtype (**Table 20-1**).

To better predict the clinical course, complications, and prognosis of patients with ALF, O'Grady and associates more recently proposed categorizing ALF into hyperacute (a jaundice to encephalopathy interval of less than 7 days), acute (interval of 8 to 28 days), and subacute (interval greater than 28 days) liver failure.[3] The somewhat arbitrary distinction was proposed after reviewing the cases of 538 patients seen in the Liver Failure Unit of King's College in London.[4] Patients with acetaminophen (APAP) hepatotoxicity universally progressed to hepatic encephalopathy within 7 days of the onset of jaundice, a hyperacute time course (**Table 20-2**), and regardless of cause, patients with hyperacute liver failure had a relatively favorable spontaneous survival rate (**Fig. 20-1**). In contrast, cryptogenic liver injury dominated as the cause of subacute liver failure, and was associated with a dismal survival rate (approximately 14%).[5] ALF due to viral hepatitis A and B usually followed a hyperacute time course, whereas idiosyncratic drug toxicity followed a more delayed course, with survival rates that were inversely proportional to the jaundice-to-encephalopathy interval.[3]

According to its strict definition, the diagnosis of ALF requires liver failure in a patient with a previously healthy organ. However, some patients have ALF superimposed on unrecognized chronic liver disease, such as acute Wilson disease and autoimmune hepatitis. Although not considered to represent true ALF by purists, patients with acute decompensation of previously subclinical liver disease should be considered under the umbrella of ALF for purposes of management.

Causes and Epidemiology

It is critical to identify the cause of ALF in order to administer appropriate antidotes and to better establish a prognosis, and thus the need for OLT. Many diverse insults to the liver may result in ALF, including viral infections, idiosyncratic drug reactions, toxins, metabolic abnormalities, and vascular catastrophes. In the multicenter U.S. ALF Study Group registry, APAP overdose accounts for nearly 45% of ALF cases reported since 1997, with indeterminate/cryptogenic and idiosyncratic drug reactions ranking second and third, causing 13% to 15% of cases each (**Fig. 20-2**). Globally, hepatitis B remains the most common cause of ALF. However, the relative contribution of different causes varies greatly by geography (**Table 20-3**). In developing nations, viral hepatitis (hepatitis A, B, and E) is the principal causes of ALF, whereas in the United Kingdom and United States, APAP toxicity is overwhelmingly the most common cause of ALF.[6] In the West, the cause of ALF remains unknown in a large proportion of cases,[7] up to 70% in a series specifically examining subacute liver failure, despite extensive serologic evaluation and polymerase chain reaction (PCR) testing of serum. Isoniazid hepatotoxicity is one of the most common drug-induced causes of ALF in regions where tuberculosis is endemic.[8]

Hepatotropic Viruses

All of the commonly recognized hepatotropic viruses (hepatitis A, B, C, B/D, and E) have been reported to cause ALF, although the relative risk of ALF in acute infection—the clinical course of ALF—and prognosis vary significantly (**Table 20-4**).

Hepatitis A

Acute infection with hepatitis A virus (HAV) remains an important cause of ALF because of its worldwide distribution, but is uncommon in the United States. The risk of ALF after acute hepatitis A infection ranges between 0.01% and 0.1%, and is higher in older patients and in patients living in, or traveling to, endemic areas.[9] ALF due to HAV is diagnosed by the presence of IgM antibodies, which are present in 95% of cases; repeat testing may be required in suspected cases of acute hepatitis A to detect the remaining 5%.[10] The prevalence

Table 20-1 Complications of ALF According to Traditional Classification

FEATURE	FULMINANT	SUBFULMINANT
Onset of encephalopathy after jaundice	<8 wk	8-24 wk
Patient age (yr)	25	45
Ascites (%)	7	62
Renal failure (%)	35	62
Cerebral edema (%)	67	9
Chronic liver disease	Rare	Infrequent

Adapted from Gimson AE, et al. Late onset hepatic failure: clinical, serological and histological features. Hepatology 1986;6(2):288–294.

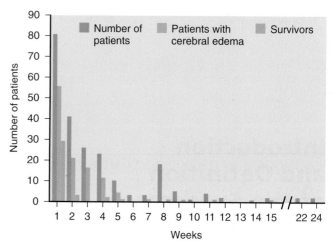

Fig. 20-1 Clinical outcome of 228 patients with non–acetaminophen-induced ALF according to the time between onset of jaundice and onset of hepatic encephalopathy in weeks. *(From O'Grady JG, Schalm SW, Williams R. Acute liver failure: redefining the syndromes. Lancet 1993; 342[8866]:273–275.)*

Table 20-2 Classification of ALF According to the Interval Between Onset of Jaundice and Development of Encephalopathy, and Relationship to Etiology

ETIOLOGY	Interval	HYPERACUTE LIVER FAILURE 0-7 days	ACUTE LIVER FAILURE 8-28 days	SUBACUTE LIVER FAILURE >28 days
	N	391	89	59
Acetaminophen (%)		100	0	0
Hepatitis A (%)		55	31	14
Hepatitis B (%)		63	29	8
Hepatitis non-A, non-B (%)		14	39	48
Drug (idiosyncratic; %)		35	53	12
Survival (%)		35	7	14

Adapted from O'Grady JG, Schalm SW, Williams R. Acute liver failure: redefining the syndromes. Lancet 1993;342(8866):273–275; and Williams R. Classification and clinical syndromes of acute liver failure. In: Lee WM, Williams R, editors. Acute liver failure. Cambridge, UK: Cambridge University Press, 1997:1–9.

of IgM antihepatitis A antibodies in ALF ranges between 2% and 6% in most series, although it has been reported as high as 20% to 31% in northwestern Europe.[11,12] The temporal pattern of ALF in acute hepatitis A is usually hyperacute, with only very rare subfulminant cases reported.[3,5] Accordingly, spontaneous survival among patients with ALF due to hepatitis A is relatively high (40% to 60%) as compared with ALF caused by hepatitis B or cryptogenic ALF.[13] Because the age of exposure to HAV has been delayed with improved sanitation and the mortality from HAV-associated ALF increases with age, the relative importance of HAV in ALF has increased in some areas of Europe. Acute hepatitis A is more likely to progress to ALF in patients over 40 years old, with a history of homosexuality or intravenous (IV) drug abuse, and with

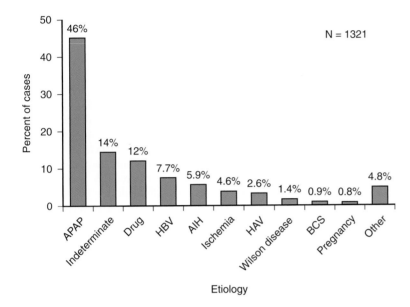

N = 1321

Fig. 20-2 Etiologies of ALF in the United States 1997-2008 reported to the Acute Liver Failure Study Group Registry. *(Data courtesy of W.M. Lee, P.I., ALF Study Group.)*

Table 20-3 Prevalence of ALF Etiologies According to Geography

COUNTRY	APAP (%)	HBV (%)	HAV (%)	DRUG (%)	INDETERMINATE (%)	OTHER (%)
UK	73	2	2	2	8	9
France	2	32	4	17	18	27
Denmark	19	31	2	17	15	13
Argentina	0	22	8	14	25	31
Japan	0	18	3	0	71	8
India	0	31	2	5	0	62

Adapted from Lee WM. Acute liver failure in the United States. Semin Liver Dis 2003;23:217–226.
APAP, acetaminophen; HAV, hepatitis A virus; HBV, hepatitis B virus

Table 20-4 ALF Due to Hepatotropic Viruses: Comparison of Clinical and Diagnostic Features

	HAV	HBV	HCV	HDV	HEV
Risk of ALF in acute infection	0.01%-0.1%	1.0%	Very rare	Co: 1%-10% Super: 5%-20%	Pregnant: 20%
Risk factors for ALF	HBV, HCV, age >40 yr, IVDA, EtOH	Females, HCV	HBV	Chronic HBV	Pregnancy
Clinical course	Hyperacute	Hyperacute/acute	Subacute	Acute	Acute
Spontaneous survival after ALF	40%-60%	15%-39%	–	31%-45%	–
Diagnostic tests	IgM-anti HAV	IgM-anti HBc, HBsAg, HBV DNA	Anti-HCV, HCV RNA	IgM-anti HDV; Co: IgM-anti HBc	IgM-anti HEV

Co, HBV/HDV co-infection; EtOH, ethanol; IVDA, intravenous drug abuse; OLT, orthotopic liver transplantation; Super, HDV superinfection of chronic HBV

underlying chronic viral hepatitis B or C, or alcoholic liver disease.[14,15] These observations support universal immunization against HAV in HBV- and HCV-infected patients, or in patients with alcoholic liver disease. Liver transplantation for HAV-induced ALF may uncommonly result in recurrence of hepatitis in the graft,[16] suggesting that HAV immunoglobulin should be administered in such patients.

Hepatitis B

The absolute risk of ALF after acute hepatitis B virus (HBV) infection is approximately 1%.[17] Women and older patients may be at greater risk for ALF from HBV.[18] Recent series from the United States have shown a marked reduction in HBV-induced ALF, comprising only 10% of cases, perhaps due to successful vaccination programs.[6] In areas of the world endemic for HBV, viral superinfection of chronic HBV carriers with HCV, HDV, or a cryptic viral agent may be the most common cause of ALF.[19] Preexisting HBsAg carriage greatly increases the risk of ALF after superinfection by other viruses, including the δ agent, especially in areas where HBV is endemic.[20] The overall spontaneous survival rate after HBV-induced ALF is poor, ranging between 15% and 36%.[6,18]

The diagnosis of HBV in ALF is frequently hampered by a vigorous immunologic response, which rapidly clears the virus.[21] Consequently, serum hepatitis B surface antigen (HBsAg), hepatitis B e antigen (HBeAg), and HBV DNA may be absent in ALF.[22] Because HBsAg may clear in as many as 30% to 50% of ALF patients within a few days of the onset of illness, the diagnosis of acute HBV often relies on detecting indirect serologic evidence of infection (IgM anti-HBc and/or anti-HBs).[23] The role of occult HBV infection in cryptogenic ALF remains uncertain. ALF occasionally follows withdrawal of immunosuppression or chemotherapy in patients with chronic HBV infection.[24] Presumably, immunosuppression in such patients increases HBV replication and hepatocyte infection, which may then provoke massive immune-mediated cytotoxicity after the restitution of immune competence.

Hepatitis D

Hepatitis D virus (HDV; the δ agent) is an adventitious RNA virus that requires concomitant HBV infection to complete its life cycle. HDV and HBV are acquired by similar parenteral means, and may infect a patient simultaneously with HBV (co-infection) or may superinfect a patient with preexisting HBV infection (superinfection); both forms of HDV infection frequently lead to ALF. Although both coinfection and superinfection with HDV increase the risk of ALF in hepatitis B by two-fold to five-fold, the risk appears to be highest in superinfected subjects (acute mortality 1% to 10% and 5% to 20%, respectively) in whom the replicative machinery of HBV is well established.[17,25,26] Paradoxically, the mortality from HDV/HBV co-infection may be less than for HBV alone,[22,26] suggesting mutual interference in replication between the viruses. The prevalence of HDV antibodies in patients with HBV-associated ALF is highest in endemic areas of the Mediterranean and Middle East. In the United States, it is most common in intravenous drug abusers (up to 34%), among whom epidemics of severe HDV hepatitis and ALF have been described.[17,26]

Hepatitis C

Whether hepatitis C virus (HCV) independently causes ALF remains controversial. Most series from centers in western nations report few or no cases of ALF attributable to HCV as the sole cause.[27] While HCV may be an uncommon cause of ALF in western nations, studies from Japan have detected HCV markers (antibody and/or RNA) in as many as 50% of non-A and non-B cases of ALF.[28,29] Chronic HCV infection probably plays an important role as a co-factor in ALF triggered by viral superinfection.[15,19,30]

Hepatitis E

Hepatitis E virus (HEV), a single-stranded RNA virus, has been identified as the agent responsible for enterically transmitted epidemic hepatitis. Infection with HEV occurs almost exclusively in developing nations and only rarely in the West, usually in émigrés or travelers from endemic areas.[31,32] Endemic areas of HEV infection include parts of northern Africa and southern Asia, where HEV is one of the two most common causes of ALF behind HBV.[8,31] Young adults and pregnant women appear to be particularly vulnerable to ALF after acute HEV infection, the latter usually presenting in their third trimester.[32] In such cases, the overall mortality approaches 20%.

Non–A-E Viruses

Other studies have attempted to identify nonhepatitis A-E viruses in patients with ALF of indeterminate cause. Putative agents have included togavirus, paramyxovirus, human papilloma virus 6, GB virus-C, transfusion-transmitted virus (TTV), and hepatitis G virus infection. Most studies refute a possible role of these viruses in non–A-E ALF because markers are equally as common in the general population, and none of these putative agents have rigorously fulfilled Koch's postulates.

Systemic Viral Infections

All members of the herpesvirus family have been anecdotally incriminated in ALF, usually in neonates and immunocompromised adults, including posttransplant patients. The clinical presentation of ALF due to varicella-zoster virus infection usually involves a vesicular rash, which may be delayed in comparison to abdominal symptoms. Similarly, herpes simplex viral (HSV) hepatitis can present as part of a disseminated infection including mucocutaneous vesicles, ALF, disseminated intravascular coagulation, and death.[33] Other reports emphasize the absence of systemic clues except for fever.[34] Rare reports of ALF due to other herpes viral infections (human herpesvirus-6, Epstein-Barr virus [EBV], and cytomegalovirus [CMV]), remain controversial. The diagnosis of ALF due to a herpesvirus is usually made by serologies, and detection of DNA in blood; liver biopsy specimens may be helpful in showing eosinophilic intranuclear inclusions. Prompt administration of IV acyclovir before confirmatory test results return has been advocated.[34] Other systemic viral infections, such as adenovirus, Coxsackie B, and hemorrhagic fever viruses (Ebola, Yellow fever, Lassa fever, Dengue) are rare causes of ALF in the appropriate geographic setting.

Table 20-5 Features of ALF Induced by Intrinsic vs. Idiosyncratic Drug Hepatotoxicity

FEATURE OF ALF	INTRINSIC HEPATOTOXIN	IDIOSYNCRATIC HEPATOTOXIN
Dose dependence	Yes	No
Incidence	High	Low
Latent period	Consistent, usually days	Variable, often weeks
Clinical course	Hyperacute	Subacute
Survival without transplantation	Relatively good	Poor

Adapted from Zimmerman HJ, editor. Hepatotoxicity: the adverse effects of drugs and other chemicals on the liver, 2nd ed. Philadelphia: Lippincott Williams & Wilkins, 1999:427–456.

Drug-Induced ALF

Drug hepatotoxicity accounts for 10% to 20% of ALF in developed nations, and a much higher proportion if acetaminophen is included. Almost 1000 drugs have been incriminated in liver injury, many of which can cause ALF.[35,36] Drugs that cause ALF may be intrinsic or idiosyncratic toxins. Intrinsic hepatoxins such as APAP cause ALF in a dose-dependent and predictable manner, while idiosyncratic hepatotoxins cause ALF rarely in a dose-independent manner[35] (**Table 20-5**).

Drug-induced ALF may be categorized by the primary pathologic lesion observed on liver biopsy[37] (**Table 20-6**). Most drugs cause hepatocellular necrosis, but others injure mitochondria and lead to microvesicular steatosis, whereas others damage endothelial cells of terminal hepatic venules, leading to veno-occlusive disease/sinusoidal obstruction syndrome. The clinical course of ALF caused by an idiosyncratic drug reaction often follows a subacute tempo, with high mortality without liver transplantation. In addition to ALF, drugs that cause microvesicular steatosis result in progressive lactic acidosis (e.g., fialuridine), and those that cause hepatic veno-occlusive disease result in acute right upper quadrant pain, tender hepatomegaly, and ascites. Age, gender, nutritional state, concomitant diseases, other drugs, ethanol consumption, and genetic polymorphisms of drug-metabolizing hepatic enzymes, most importantly the cytochrome P-450s, all contribute to the risk of idiosyncratic drug-induced ALF.[13,37] The risk of ALF after ingestion of some drugs increases in the presence of potentiating agents, often another drug (e.g., rifampin and trimethoprim, which enhance the hepatotoxic effects of isoniazid and sulfamethoxazole, respectively).[13,38]

Idiosyncratic drug reactions lead to ALF infrequently (approximately 1/10,000 prescriptions) or rarely (approximately 1/50,000 prescriptions). The most common drugs include nonsteroidal antiinflammatory drugs, antibiotics (especially sulfonamides, isoniazid, and rifampin), and anticonvulsants, particularly phenytoin.[39] ALF due to recreational drugs, such as cocaine and ecstasy (3,4-methyl-dioxymethamphetamine), appears to be increasing in Europe.[40] Dietary supplements have been incriminated in nearly 10% of drug-induced liver injury in the United States.[39]

Table 20-6 A Partial List of Drugs Causing ALF According to Primary Pathologic Findings

PATHOLOGIC LESION/DRUG	FREQUENCY OF ALF	POTENTIATING AGENTS
Hepatocellular Necrosis		
Acetaminophen	Dose dependent	EtOH isoniazid, barbiturates
Anesthetics: halothane	Infrequent	
Antiepileptics		
Phenytoin	Infrequent	
Carbamazepine	Rare	
Antibiotics		
Amoxicillin		Clavulanic acid
Isoniazid	Infrequent	Rifampin
Nitrofurantoin		
Ketoconazole	Rare	
Ofloxacin	Rare	
Sulfonamides	Infrequent	Trimethoprim
Antihypertensives		
α-Methyldopa		
Hydralazine		
Labetalol	Rare	
Nicotinic acid (slow release)	Rare	
Nonsteroidal Anti-Inflammatory Drugs		
Diclofenac	Infrequent	
Bromfenac	Infrequent	
Microvesicular Steatosis		
Amiodarone	Infrequent	
Fialuridine		
Tetracycline		
Valproate	Infrequent	
Veno-Occlusive Disease		
Azathioprine		
Busulfan		
Cyclophosphamide		
Dacarbazine		
6-Thioguanine		

Adapted from Sze G, Kaplowitz N. Drug hepatotoxicity as a cause of acute liver failure. In: Lee WM, Williams R, editors. Acute liver failure, 1st ed. Cambridge, UK: Cambridge University Press, 1997: 19–31; and Lee WM. Acute liver failure. N Engl J Med 1993;329:1862–1872.

Acetaminophen

The analgesic acetaminophen (APAP) is an intrinsic hepatotoxin with a narrow therapeutic window. When used in recommended doses (<4 g/day), APAP rarely causes hepatotoxicity. However, APAP overdose is the single most common cause of ALF in the United Kingdom, accounting for 60% to

70% of cases,[41] and in the United States, where the incidence has increased to nearly 45% in the last decade.[41,42] The intent of overdose also appears to have changed over the last 10 to 15 years, with a decrease in the proportion of ingestions with suicidal intent from more than 67% to 44%, and an increase in accidental overdoses from 33% to 48% in the United States.[42] A analysis of patient characteristics in those with intentional versus unintentional APAP ingestions has shown that the latter more often ingest multiple APAP-containing preparations usually bundled with narcotics over a longer period of time, while the former have more frequent histories of depression and ingest higher doses in single ingestions (**Table 20-7**).

The clinical presentation of ALF due to APAP includes a hyperacute progression from jaundice to hepatic encephalopathy and distinct patterns of laboratory abnormalities compared with ALF due to other causes (**Table 20-8**).[3] Hepatic transaminases rise within 12 to 24 hours of ingestion, often peaking at strikingly high levels with AST greater than ALT, significantly higher than for other causes of ALF.[6] Peak transaminases and prothrombin times are usually observed 3 days

after ingestion, and then rapidly resolve if the patient spontaneously recovers; peak bilirubin levels are lower than for other causes. The spontaneous survival rate is higher, and the need for liver transplantation is lower, than for ALF of other causes. Liver biopsy characteristically reveals centrilobular (zone 3) necrosis without inflammation.[43] Renal failure, usually due to acute tubular necrosis, develops in a higher proportion of patients (up to 70%) with ALF due to APAP overdose than other etiologies, usually within 24 to 72 hours of the ingestion.[44,45] The mechanisms of renal failure in APAP overdose are likely multiple, but direct nephrotoxicity by APAP metabolites seems primary.[45,46]

The mechanism of hepatic injury in APAP overdose and the rationale behind the use of its antidote, N-acetylcysteine (NAC), was elucidated in experimental animals by Mitchell and co-workers in 1973.[47] Under nontoxic conditions, 80% of an acetaminophen dose is glucuronidated and sulfated, and eliminated in urine (**Fig. 20-3**). A small fraction (<5%) is oxidized to the reactive intermediate N-acetyl-p-benzoquinone imine (NAPQI) by cytochrome P-450 enzymes, most importantly, cytochrome P-450 2E1. NAPQI may be rendered

Table 20-7 Characteristics of Intentional vs. Unintentional Acetaminophen Overdoses in 253 Patients with ALF

CHARACTERISTIC	INTENTIONAL N = 122	UNINTENTIONAL N = 131	P VALUE
Female (%)	74	73	NS
Total APAP dose (g)	25	20	NS
APAP dose/day (g)	25	7.5	0.001
ALT (mean IU/L)	5326	3129	0.001
Encephalopathy ≥grade 3 (%)	39	55	0.026
History of depression (%)	45	24	0.001
APAP-narcotic bundled (%)	18	63	0.001
Multiple APAP preparations (%)	5	38	0.001

Adapted from Larson AM, et al. Acetaminophen-induced acute liver failure: results of a United States multicenter, prospective study. Hepatology 2005;42(6): 1364–1372.

Table 20-8 Clinical and Laboratory Features of the 1321 Patients Enrolled in the Acute Liver Failure Study Group Registry, 1998-2008

VARIABLE	APAP (N = 605)	DRUG (N = 156)	INDETERMINATE (N = 180)	HAV/HBV (N = 34/102)	ALL OTHERS (N = 244)
Sex (% female)	75	68	57	44/43	73
Age (y)	36	46	38	49/42	42
Jaundice–encephalopathy (median days)	0	9	9	3/6.5	7
Encephalopathy stage III/IV (%)	51	37	49	53/53	41
Peak ALT (IU/L)	4016	626	846	2275/1702	668
Bilirubin (median mg/dl)	4.5	20.4	22.4	12.3/18.5	15.7
Transplanted (%)	9	44	44	29/44	31
Spontaneous survival (%)	64	27	25	56/26	37
Overall survival (%)	73	68	66	82/64	64

Data courtesy W.M. Lee, P.I., ALF Study Group.

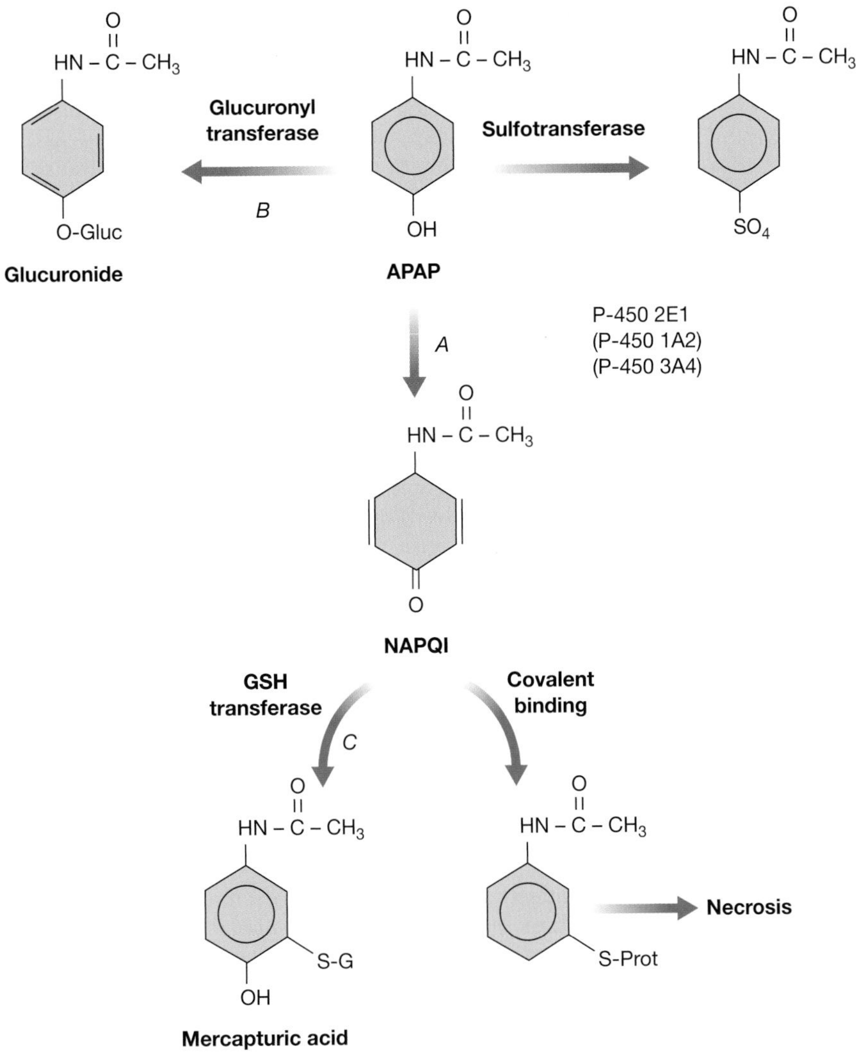

Fig. 20-3 **Pathways of acetaminophen (APAP) metabolism.** Pathway A, the pathway toward increased formation of the toxic APAP metabolite, NAPQI, is enhanced by larger doses of acetaminophen and inducers of cytochrome P-450 2E1 (ethanol, isoniazid, phenobarbital, phenytoin). Pathway A may also be enhanced by conditions that decrease glucuronidation (fasting, malnutrition). Pathway B is inhibited by fasting and glucuronyl transferase deficiency (Gilbert syndrome), leading to an increase in pathway A. Pathway C, a major pathway toward detoxification of NAPQI, is inhibited by conditions that deplete the hepatocyte of glutathione (GSH), such as fasting, malnutrition, and ethanol consumption. Inhibition of pathway C leads to increased covalent binding of NAPQI to hepatocyte proteins, and hence, necrosis. *(From Zimmerman HJ, editor. Hepatotoxicity: the adverse effects of drugs and other chemicals on the liver, 2nd ed. Philadelphia: Lippincott Williams & Wilkins, 1999.)*

harmless by binding to reduced glutathione (GSH), a reaction catalyzed by glutathione-S-transferase. However, under conditions where the supply of NAPQI exceeds available GSH, the former covalently binds hepatocellular proteins initiating hepatocyte necrosis.

In theory and common teaching, the hepatotoxicity of APAP may be enhanced by agents that either increase production of NAPQI or reduce the supply of GSH. High doses of APAP saturate the enzymes involved in conjugation, increasing the substrate for the oxidative pathway. Ethanol and certain drugs (e.g., isoniazid, barbiturates) induce the activity of cytochrome P-450s, thereby increasing NAPQI production; the increased toxicity of acetaminophen by ethanol appears to be predominantly from inducing cytochrome P-450 2E1.[48] In contrast, fasting and malnutrition such as that seen with chronic alcohol abuse decrease GSH synthesis, and theoretically deplete the hepatocyte's ability to detoxify NAPQI. In average-risk patients ingesting acetaminophen with suicidal intent, a minimal dose of 7 to 8 g of acetaminophen seems necessary to induce hepatocyte necrosis; 15-g ingestions often cause hepatotoxicity, while greater than 20 g consistently causes ALF.[42,49] Chronic alcohol consumption, however, has been associated with increased hepatotoxicity such that injury can occur at doses considered "therapeutic."[43,50,51] For example, in alcoholics with acute liver injury after ingestion of APAP for chronic pain, 40% ingested less than 4 g/day, the recommended dose, and 60% ingested less than 6 g/day, considered "nontoxic."[43] It should be noted, however, that the above risk factors for increased APAP hepatotoxicity are largely based upon retrospective data, and have been questioned.[52]

Biologic Toxins

ALF from ingestion of the mushrooms of the genus *Amanita* (*A. phalloides, verna,* and *virosa*) occurs occasionally in Europe (50 to 100 fatal cases per year) but rarely in the United States (usually in California and the Pacific Northwest) with fewer than 100 fatal cases between 1900 and 1994.[53] Three medium-sized mushrooms (50 g) contain sufficient toxin, α-amanitin and phalloidin, to cause ALF; the toxins are heat-stable and not degraded by cooking. Symptoms of gastroenteritis (abdominal pain, nausea, vomiting, and diarrhea) precede liver dysfunction, and renal failure and pancreatitis are common. A mitochondrial toxin isolated from the foodborne pathogen, *Bacillus cereus,* was also incriminated in a case of ALF in which an autopsy of the liver showed microvesicular steatosis.[54] ALF caused by herbal remedies has been reported with increasing frequency,[55] and all patients with ALF should be specifically queried about ingestion of alternative medicines.

Metabolic Causes of ALF

Acute Wilson disease (WD), a rare presentation of the autosomal recessive defect in canalicular copper transport, accounts for about 3% of ALF cases in the U.S. ALF Study Group registry and is a classical difficult diagnosis. Acute WD classically occurs in a young patient (first 2 decades of life) and is often accompanied by Coombs negative hemolytic anemia, the result of a massive copper release from necrotic hepatocytes and subsequent toxicity on erythrocyte membranes. Hypouricemia and low serum alkaline phosphatase accompany strikingly high serum bilirubin (largely indirect). A low serum ceruloplasmin concentration is insensitive for a diagnosis of acute WD; conversely, a high serum copper is sensitive but nonspecific.[56] The most diagnostic laboratory finding may be the alkaline phosphatase/total bilirubin ratio, which provided a 100% accuracy with a cutoff of less than 2 in one small series[57] and nearly as high for a cutoff of less than 4 in a larger series.[56] A suspicion of acute Wilson disease as the cause of ALF should immediately lead to liver transplant evaluation because spontaneous recovery rarely occurs.[56,58]

Reye syndrome, a disorder of hepatocyte mitochondrial metabolism, has become an extremely rare cause of ALF in the United States, with no more than 2 cases per year reported to the Centers for Disease Control between 1994 and 1997.[59] Reye syndrome usually presents in children with an influenza-like viral prodrome and a history of salicylate ingestion, and is followed by encephalopathy, cerebral edema, and frequently death. Liver biopsy shows characteristic microvesicular steatosis with little necrosis, reflecting mitochondrial injury, which impairs both urea cycle disposal of ammonium and β-oxidation of fatty acids.[60] Other metabolic causes of ALF in neonates or children include galactosemia, fructosemia, tyrosinemia, α_1-antitrypsin deficiency, and Niemann-Pick type II.[61,62]

ALF presenting in pregnant females may be caused by disease entities specific to pregnancy or nonspecific agents, such as viruses or drugs.[63] Acute fatty liver of pregnancy is a disorder of hepatocyte mitochondrial metabolism occurring in the late third trimester. The high mortality due to ALF for mother and fetus can usually be avoided by prompt delivery.[64] Studies have attributed acute fatty liver of pregnancy and the HELLP syndrome (*h*emolysis, *e*levated *l*iver chemistries, *l*ow *p*latelets) to concomitant defects in maternal and fetal mitochondrial long chain 3-hydroxyacyl-coenzyme A dehydrogenase.[65] The ability of delivery to reverse HELLP syndrome, which is associated with preeclampsia, may be less certain than for acute fatty liver of pregnancy, as a series of women transplanted for this indication has been described.[66]

Autoimmune Acute Liver Failure

Autoimmune hepatitis (AIH) may present as ALF in 5% of cases; conversely, approximately 5% of cases of ALF in the U.S. ALF Study Group Registry can be ascribed on clinical grounds to AIH. However, the latter statistic is based primarily upon clinical and serologic criteria rather than histology, an important criterion for the diagnosis of AIH. In a recent analysis of liver specimens from a large number of patients with ALF of indeterminate cause, the second largest group in the ALF Study Group registry behind APAP (19% of total cases), approximately half had histologic features of AIH.[67] The histologic hallmark of autoimmune ALF is central perivenulitis, often with a plasma cell–rich inflammatory infiltrate.[67,68] Whether the early administration of corticosteroids improves outcome in autoimmune ALF remains unproven.[69]

Ischemic Causes of ALF

Acute hepatic vein thrombosis, the Budd-Chiari syndrome, may present as ALF. The classical findings of chronic hepatic vein thrombosis, tender hepatomegaly and ascites, may be absent in patients with ALF. Pathologically, the liver shows extensive hemorrhagic infarction. Circulatory collapse, so-called "shock liver," may also evolve into ALF if hepatic ischemia is prolonged, often after sepsis or surgery, or in patients with severe heart failure. Severe intrahepatic sickling in patients with sickle cell anemia can also precipitate ischemic ALF, as can veno-occlusive disease (sinusoidal obstruction syndrome) after systemic chemotherapy, usually in preparation for bone marrow transplantation. In the early postliver transplant recipient, ALF may be a manifestation of hepatic artery or portal vein thrombosis. Finally, status epilepticus rarely may result in ALF due to ischemic liver injury.[70,71]

Diffuse Malignant Infiltration of the Liver

Rarely, massive hepatocellular necrosis may follow infiltration of the liver by several metastatic malignancies, most commonly, breast carcinoma and lymphomas. Other malignancies include melanoma, gastric carcinoma, small-cell lung carcinoma, pancreatic carcinoma, and leukemia.[72] Hepatic imaging by CT scan may not reveal nodular infiltration if there is diffuse intrasinusoidal spread. Pathologic examination of the liver most often reveals diffuse infiltration of the liver with tumor cells rather than nodular aggregates.

Primary nonfunction (PNF) after liver transplantation presents similarly to ALF, with coagulopathy, acidosis, and encephalopathy appearing within hours of allograft implantation, but it is generally not included in series of ALF. Thought to represent a form of preservation injury, PNF is the only non-ALF condition in the United States that allows listing for liver transplantation at the highest ("status 1") priority with ALF patients. The multiorgan systems failure of PNF may be abated by graft hepatectomy while a patient awaits retransplantation.[73]

Pathogenesis of the Syndrome of ALF

Early Presentation of the Acute Injury

Depending on the cause of ALF, the illness may either present without warning or be preceded by a prodromal illness. Patients often complain of nonspecific epigastric and upper abdominal distress accompanied by anorexia and nausea in the early stages of the illness, but marked liver pain should suggest acute Budd-Chiari syndrome.[74] On examination, the liver is usually normal or small in size, except for those with acute Budd-Chiari syndrome. Symptoms are accompanied by marked elevations of serum AST and ALT, with modest elevations of alkaline phosphatase.

Failure of Liver Function

Failure of Hepatobiliary Excretion

Notable impairment in hepatobiliary excretory function results in hyperbilirubinemia and jaundice. The canalicular excretion of bilirubin is the rate-limiting step in bilirubin excretion; consequently, ALF causes conjugated hyperbilirubinemia. The degree of hyperbilirubinemia is accentuated if hemolysis co-exists, which may result from the oxidant stress associated with the cause of ALF, or to ALF itself. For example, patients with ALF due to Wilson disease, which is often accompanied by hemolytic anemia,[75] experience marked hyperbilirubinemia.

Failure to Metabolize Toxic Substances

The liver metabolizes many potentially toxic endogenous substrates that accumulate with ALF, the most clinically important of which is ammonia. The increase in serum ammonia levels with ALF is primarily due to the failure of the liver to convert ammonia to urea via the urea cycle, and has been implicated in the pathogenesis of hepatic encephalopathy and intracranial hypertension.[76] Sources of ammonia in ALF include the intestine, and less importantly, the kidneys, while muscle can detoxify ammonia into glutamine (**Fig. 20-4**).

The metabolism of drugs is also drastically affected by ALF. Most drugs undergo some degree of hepatic modification, and because ALF impairs drug metabolism, their biologic half-life increases. Other sources of altered drug and drug metabolite disposal include alteration volume of distribution, and intravascular protein binding, and renal failure. These changes in pharmacokinetics enhance the probability of drug toxicity or worsened liver injury.[77] Therefore the use of all medications in the setting of ALF must be carefully considered in terms of necessity, dosage, and toxicity.

Failure of Intermediary Metabolism

The metabolic consequences of ALF include alterations in carbohydrate, lipid, and protein metabolism (**Table 20-9**). Spontaneous hypoglycemia frequently complicates ALF due to decreased glycogen stores, decreased ability to mobilize glycogen, and decreased gluconeogenesis within the liver. Serum concentrations of free fatty acids increase in ALF, resulting in a decrease in acetoacetate/3-ß-hydroxybutryate (arterial ketone body ratio), which may contribute to hepatic encephalopathy. ALF is also associated with negative nitrogen balance, which results from the enhanced catabolism of proteins, including muscle proteins.[78-81]

Failure of Biosynthetic Function of the Liver

The two most clinically relevant synthetic products of the liver include albumin and coagulation factors. Albumin has a

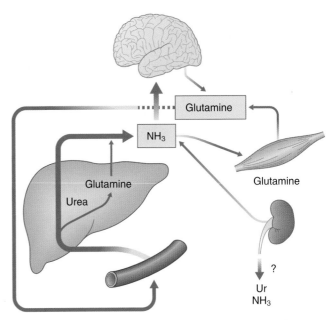

Fig. 20-4 Sources and metabolic fate of ammonia and glutamine in ALF. The primary source of ammonia is the gut, which under normal conditions is cleared by urea (major pathway) and glutamine (minor pathway) synthesis in the liver. Hepatocellular insufficiency in ALF results in the accumulation of ammonia in peripheral tissues, particularly brain and muscle, which detoxify ammonia by synthesizing glutamine from glutamate. In turn, glutamine released into blood is taken up by the intestines, liberating ammonia, or cleared by the kidneys. The capacity of renal excretion of glutamine in ALF is adversely affected by renal dysfunction, which often accompanies ALF. *(From Vaquero J, Chung C, Cahil M, Blei AT. Pathogenesis of hepatic encephalopathy in acute liver failure. Semin Liver Dis 2003;23:259–269.)*

Table 20-9 Metabolic Consequences of ALF

Carbohydrate metabolism:
- Hypoglycemia:
  - Decreased glycogen stores
  - Decreased gluconeogenesis
- Hyperglycemia (usually mild):
  - Insulin resistance

Lipid metabolism:
- Increased plasma free fatty acids:
  - Increased peripheral lipolysis
  - Decreased lipogenesis
- Altered arterial ketone body ratio:
  - Altered mitochondrial redox potential

Protein metabolism:
- Increased protein breakdown
- Increased plasma amino acid levels
- Relative decrease in branched chain amino acid levels

half-life of 15 to 20 days; consequently, serum concentrations decrease relatively late in the course of ALF. As part of the definition of ALF, elevated INR exists universally, but its significance in terms of predicting a bleeding diathesis remains unproven. Plasma activities of factors synthesized in the liver (factors II, V, VII, IX, and X), are reduced in all patients with ALF, as are liver-derived proteins involved in fibrinolysis.[82,83] The INR and activities of factors V and VII, which have the

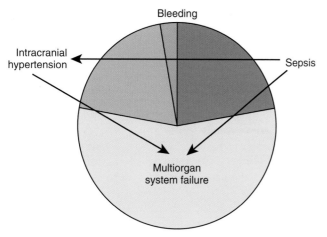

Fig. 20-5 **Proximate causes of death in patients with ALF.** Improvements in intensive care management and the widespread use of OLT to rescue patients with ALF have decreased the overall mortality from greater than 80% to 33% in the United States over approximately the last 25 years. Proximate causes of death have also changed over the same period, with the incidence of death from hemorrhage decreasing from approximately 25% to less than 5%, and intracranial hypertension/brainstem herniation decreasing to 20% from 25%. Currently, the most common cause of death in patients with ALF is multiorgan system failure, often triggered by sepsis, which may also exacerbate the bleeding diathesis and increase the risk of developing intracranial hypertension. *(Adapted from Stravitz RT, Kramer DJ. Management of acute liver failure. Nat Rev Gastroenterol Hepatol 2009;6[9]:542–553.)*

Table 20-10 Pathogenesis of Impaired Tissue Respiration in ALF

- Impaired pulmonary oxygenation of blood:
  - Decreased delivery (dysfunctional airway [e.g., mucous plugs])
  - Impaired ventilation
  - V̇/Q̇ mismatch
- Altered oxygen carriage and delivery capacity of blood:
  - Decreased hemoglobin concentration
  - Altered oxygen association-dissociation properties of hemoglobin:
    - Increased association:
      — Hypocarbia
      — Alkalosis
      — Decreased red cell DPG in stored blood
    - Increased dissociation:
      — Acidosis
      — Hypercarbia
      — Increased red cell DPG due to anemia and hypoxemia
- Altered ability to deliver oxygenated blood to tissues:
  - Decreased cardiac output (advanced ALF)
  - Changes in regional vascular resistance
  - Opening of peripheral arterio-venous shunts
- Impaired oxygen use by tissues:
  - Changes in transit time in peripheral microcirculation
  - Pathologic oxygen dependency

shortest half-lives, offer important prognostic information regarding the likelihood of spontaneous survival or death without OLT.[4,84]

Effects of ALF on Extrahepatic Systems

ALF affects the function of virtually all organ systems, not only from the direct consequences of hepatic necrosis and failure of liver function, but also from microcirculatory dysfunction, which causes inadequate oxygenation of peripheral tissues. As the function of one organ system declines, a domino effect occurs on other organ systems, often compounded by sepsis. MOSF represents the most common cause of death in recent studies of ALF (**Fig. 20-5**).

Microcirculatory Dysfunction (Table 20-10)

The pathogenesis of impaired peripheral tissue oxygenation in ALF includes defects in oxygenation of blood in the lungs, oxygen carriage in arterial blood, and oxygen extraction from the microcirculation. Decreased oxygenation of blood in the lungs may develop from atelectasis, volume overload, pneumonia, or the development of the adult respiratory distress syndrome (ARDS). Oxygen delivery to peripheral tissues within blood is adversely affected by decreased cardiac output and shifting of the oxygen dissociation curve of hemoglobin as a consequence of acid-base and ventilatory disturbances and altered 2,3-diphosphoglycerate levels. ALF also compromises peripheral tissue perfusion as a consequence of vasodilation of the microcirculation. Vasoactive factors such as nitric

oxide and tumor necrosis factor appear to be responsible for the microcirculatory dysfunction in ALF, which creates a functional diffusion barrier against oxygen delivery because of decreased contact time with tissue capillaries.[85-87]

Cardiovascular Consequences

The initial cardiovascular hallmark of ALF is a hyperdynamic state, characterized by an increased cardiac output and decreased systemic vascular resistance. The decrease in systemic vascular resistance results from peripheral arteriolar dilation, capillary recruitment in peripheral tissues, and arteriovenous shunting, predominantly the result of increased nitric oxide activity.[88] As a result, cardiac output often increases to values of 7 to 10 L/min, due to both tachycardia and increased stroke volume. In early ALF, central venous pressure usually remains low, reflecting decreased central blood volume, but hypervolemia usually follows due to infused intravenous fluids and the development of renal failure.[89] Similarly, mean arterial pressure is maintained by the increase in cardiac output in early ALF but drops once cardiac output succumbs to intravascular volume depletion, arrhythmias, or myocardial depression. The final stages of ALF are characterized by profound peripheral vasodilation, failing cardiac output, and eventually, hemodynamic collapse.

Pulmonary Consequences

Central hyperventilation with a respiratory alkalosis characterizes the initial pulmonary presentation of ALF. As intracranial pressure (ICP) rises, hyperventilation often progresses, and the development of sudden, severe hyperventilation may precede sudden respiratory arrest. Initially, oxygenation is relatively preserved in patients with ALF, but progressive hypoxemia supervenes due to ventilation/perfusion mismatch within the lungs, volume overload, left ventricular failure, intrapulmonary arteriovenous shunting, increased pulmonary capillary permeability, and pneumonia.[89] Pulmonary edema in the presence of a normal pulmonary capillary wedge pressure suggests the development of ARDS, which can also emerge as the pulmonary component of the systemic inflammatory response syndrome (SIRS).[90,91]

Renal and Electrolyte Disturbances (Table 20-11)

Acute renal failure occurs in 40% to 80% of patients with ALF, and is more common in patients with APAP-induced ALF.[92,93] The four major causes of acute renal failure in ALF include effective blood volume depletion, acute tubular necrosis, sepsis, and a syndrome of functional renal failure closely resembling the hepatorenal syndrome of cirrhosis.[45,92] Prerenal azotemia frequently results from marked systemic vasodilation, gastrointestinal bleeding, fluid loss due to inappropriately aggressive lactulose therapy, and inadequate volume replacement. Severe, prolonged hypovolemia, or the use of nonsteroidal anti-inflammatory drugs or aminoglycosides, can lead to acute tubular necrosis, a complication documented in 22% to 50% of patients with ALF.[44] Sepsis exacerbates peripheral vasodilation and may precipitate renal failure from circulatory collapse, or cause diffuse cortical necrosis by initiating disseminated intravascular coagulation (DIC). The functional renal failure associated with ALF appears to be initiated by pathophysiologic mechanisms similar to those present in cirrhotic individuals with hepatorenal syndrome.[45] The prognosis of patients with ALF and renal failure is very poor unless they receive a liver transplant, but spontaneous renal recovery can occur with recovery of liver function or liver transplantation.

Severe fluid and electrolyte abnormalities always accompany ALF. Free water retention occurs early, resulting in dilutional hyponatremia,[94] which can contribute to cerebral edema, mandating immediate correction. In general, the degree of hyponatremia is proportional to the severity of liver failure. Hypokalemia accompanies hyponatremia, due to gastrointestinal losses, diuretics, and alkalosis. Hypophosphatemia also occurs commonly, and results from a shift of phosphate from the extracellular to the intracellular compartment in response to glucose infusions and possibly due to use

in ATP synthesis by regenerating hepatocytes.[95] In the presence of oliguric renal failure, however, hyperkalemia and hyperphosphatemia usually develop. Finally, hypocalcemia can complicate the transfusion of large amounts of citrated blood products.

Hematologic Disturbances (Table 20-12)

Although disturbed hemostasis comprises a part of the definition of ALF, it would be inaccurate to conclude that elevated INR represents an assessment of the bleeding risk. Procoagulant and anticoagulant proteins decrease in parallel in ALF, and appear to generally maintain balanced hemostasis, similar to the case in cirrhosis.[96] Consequently, spontaneous, clinically significant bleeding is uncommon in patients with ALF (approximately 5%), and very rarely contributes to death.[97] When bleeding in patients with ALF occurs, the origin is most often from a mucosal (capillary-type) source, such as the gastric, pulmonary, or genitourinary systems, and rarely necessitates transfusion. Although portal hypertension accompanies ALF as a function of the architectural collapse of the liver,[98] bleeding from varices does not occur.

Disturbed hemostasis in patients with ALF results from decreased coagulation factor synthesis, increased factor consumption, and quantitative as well as qualitative platelet dysfunction.[82] The presence of disseminated intravascular coagulation (DIC) consumes coagulation factors and should be suspected in a patient with microangiopathic hemolytic anemia, increased fibrinogen degradation products and fibrin D-dimer levels, and decreased fibrinogen levels. The degree of hypofibrinogenemia reflects the severity of the DIC, and is most severe in ALF complicated by sepsis. Platelet defects, both qualitative and quantitative, are likely to compound the bleeding diathesis of ALF. Platelets from patients with ALF exhibit poor adhesion and aggregation, especially in the setting of renal failure.[99] Thrombocytopenia commonly accompanies ALF and probably results more from increased consumption rather than decreased production because thrombopoietin concentrations correlate poorly with platelet count.[100] Abnormal fibrinolysis accompanies ALF, but its contribution to a bleeding tendency remains unclear because decreases in liver-derived profibrinolytic proteins are offset by

---

Table 20-11 Mechanisms of Renal Failure in ALF

- Prerenal azotemia:
  - Increased GI losses (GI bleeding, nasogastric drainage, diarrhea from lactulose)
  - Inadequate volume replacement
- Acute tubular necrosis:
  - Volume depletion
  - Iatrogenic (aminoglycosides, NSAIDs)
  - Hepatotoxin-induced (APAP, amatoxin, TMP-SMZ)
- Sepsis-related:
  - Decreased renal perfusion
  - Cortical necrosis
  - Urinary tract infection
- Functional renal failure of ALF (hepatorenal syndrome)

Table 20-12 Abnormal Parameters of Coagulation in ALF

- Altered production of coagulation factors:
  - Decreased activity of factors II, V, VII, IX, and X
  - Increased activity of factor VIII (endothelial activation)
- Increased consumption of coagulation factors:
  - Disseminated intravascular coagulation (DIC)
  - Increased fibrinolysis (2 degrees decreased clearance of plasmin)
  - Bleeding
- Thrombocytopenia:
  - Sequestration
  - Consumption (bleeding, DIC)
  - Decreased production
- Qualitative platelet dysfunction:
  - de novo
  - Renal failure
  - Hypofibrinogenemia and acquired dysfibrinogenemia

increases in endothelial-derived profibrinolytic proteins; a similar balance has been observed for antifibrinolytic proteins.[83] Finally, endothelial cell injury and activation, which occurs as part of the SIRS in ALF, also contributes to abnormal hemostasis.[101] Indeed, alterations in both the systemic and hepatic microvasculature have been documented to decrease clot formation, and may also propagate liver injury by inducing a local hypercoagulable state within the liver, leading to ischemia.[102] In summary, abnormal hemostasis occurs in ALF, but mechanisms are complex and incompletely defined. Generally, a precarious state of balanced hemostasis remains, which may be upset by an appropriate trigger, such as infection.

Breakdown of Host Immune Defenses (Table 20-13)

Abnormalities in immune defense in patients with ALF greatly increase the susceptibility to infection, a major trigger of MOSF, intracranial hypertension, and death. More than 80% of patients with ALF have bacteriologic evidence of infection at some point during their illness.[103,104] Natural host barriers are breached by the process of caring for any critically ill patient. Abnormal antibacterial defenses further contribute to the susceptibility to infection, such as depressed complement concentrations, impaired opsonization of bacteria, and decreased neutrophil chemotaxis and superoxide production. Clinically, pneumonia, septicemia, and urinary tract infections are the most common types of infection encountered in patients with ALF.[103,104]

Gastrointestinal Consequences

Nausea and vomiting occur frequently early in the course of ALF, while an ileus may develop in later stages. The cause of ileus is often multifactorial, and includes electrolyte and acid-base disturbances, sepsis, and the use of narcotics to control agitation. Although pancreatic enzyme levels are elevated in a third of patients, clinically significant pancreatitis occurs infrequently.[105] Gastrointestinal bleeding from mucosal petechial lesions can also occur, especially in the setting of thrombocytopenia, DIC, and sepsis. The hepatic venous pressure gradient can become elevated, and both varices and ascites have been reported to develop late in ALF; however, variceal hemorrhage is distinctly rare.[98]

Neurologic Consequences

By definition, neurologic dysfunction follows liver injury in patients with ALF, but differs in several important respects to patients with cirrhosis. Seizures and agitation frequently complicate the hepatic encephalopathy of ALF, but occur rarely in patients with cirrhosis. Most importantly, patients with ALF develop cerebral edema and intracranial hypertension, significant degrees of which generally do not occur in patients with cirrhosis.[106,107]

Hepatic Encephalopathy (Tables 20-14 and 20-15)

The biochemical basis of hepatic encephalopathy in ALF remains incompletely understood, but certainly involves the accumulation of endogenous or gut-derived toxins within the central nervous system, which in turn alters energy balance and neurotransmission.[76] Circulating neurotoxins that have been incriminated in the genesis of hepatic encephalopathy include ammonia, endogenously derived benzodiazepine receptor agonists, and others. Ammonia has been most strongly implicated in the pathogenesis of hepatic encephalopathy in ALF (**Fig. 20-6**) because high serum and brain concentrations of ammonia, and brain concentrations of glutamine, the principal metabolic product of ammonia detoxification, are universal in patients with ALF.[76,108] Although circulating concentrations of ammonia weakly correlate with the degree of neurologic dysfunction, arterial rather than

---

Table 20-13 Factors Contributing to Infection in ALF

- Breakdown of natural barriers to infection:
  - Skin: intravenous lines
  - Airway:
    - Aspiration of pharyngeal and gastric contents
- Intubation
  - Urinary tract: indwelling catheters
  - Cranial: ICP monitors
  - GI tract: increased translocation from edematous and hemorrhagic mucosa
- Colonization:
  - Skin and pharynx: hospital flora
  - Stomach: use of antiacid therapy
  - Colon: use of antibiotics
- Impaired host defenses:
  - Decreased complement levels
  - Decreased neutrophil chemotaxis
  - Impaired ability of opsonize bacteria
  - Decreased neutrophil capacity to produce superoxide ions
  - Decreased reticulo-endothelial capacity to clear bacteria and bacterial products

---

Table 20-14 Clinical Stages of Hepatic Encephalopathy in ALF

GRADE	SYMPTOMS	SIGNS	EEG
1	Lack of awareness, short attention span, altered sleep pattern	Tremor, constructional apraxia, asterixis	Symmetric slowing
2	Agitation, lethargy seizures	Asterixis, hyperreflexia	Symmetric slowing, triphasic waves
3	Asleep, arousable by pain, confused when aroused	Hyperreflexia	triphasic waves
4	Unarousable	Babinski, ankle clonus, decerebrate posture	Delta (very slow) activity

Based on Conn HO. Quantifying the severity of hepatic encephalopathy. In: Conn HO, Bircher J, editors. Hepatic encephalopathy: syndromes and therapies. Medi-Ed Press, 1994.

Table 20-15 Proposed Mechanisms Underlying Hepatic Encephalopathy in ALF

- Circulating neurotoxins:
  - Ammonia
  - Gut-derived false neurotransmitters (e.g., octopamine)
  - γ-aminobenzoic acid (GABA)
  - Endogenous GABA receptor agonists
  - Miscellaneous: mercaptans, fatty acids, others
  - Amino acid imbalance (aromatic vs. branched-chain)
- Altered neurotransmission in brain:
  - Activation of GABA receptor complex (inhibitory)
  - Depletion of glutamate (excitatory)
- Altered cerebral energy homeostasis

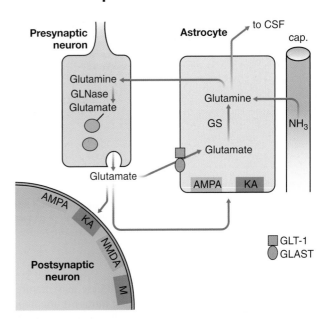

Fig. 20-6 Relationship of ammonia to hepatic encephalopathy in ALF. A cartoon demonstrating the relationship between arterial ammonia levels and glutamateric neurotransmission in cerebral neurons and astrocytes in the genesis of hepatic encephalopathy. *(From Butterworth RF. Hepatic encephalopathy: disorder of multiple neurotransmitter systems. In: Record C, Mardini H, editors. Advances in hepatic encephalopathy and metabolism in liver disease. Newcastle upon Tyne, UK: Ipswich, 1997.)*

venous concentrations may be more accurate.[78] Ammonia in the patient with ALF originates predominantly from the gut, from bacterial metabolism of urea and amino acids as well as use of glutamine as an energy source by the intestinal mucosa (see **Fig. 20-4**).

The accumulation of putative neurotoxins within the brain of patients with ALF causes encephalopathy by two interrelated mechanisms: altered brain metabolism and altered neurotransmission. Although early studies supported a role for altered brain energy homeostasis in the encephalopathy of ALF, more recent studies provide conflicting data; thus altered energy homeostasis may be a terminal rather than a primary mechanism. The two neurotransmitter systems that appear to be most adversely affected in ALF are the γ-aminobutyric acid (GABA) and the glutamatergic systems. The GABA receptor complex serves as the site of action of benzodiazepines and inhibits neurotransmission. Increased circulating endogenous ligands for GABA receptors have been detected in patients with ALF, and ammonia increases the affinity of such ligands for this receptor. Decreased turnover of GABA in the brain may also contribute to the increase in GABA-ergic tone in the brain. In contrast to the increased tone of the inhibitory GABA system, intracellular concentrations of glutamate, the major excitatory neurotransmitter of the mammalian brain, are decreased in ALF.[76,108] Diminished glutamate concentrations probably result from increased consumption rather than decreased production because glutamate is used to detoxify ammonia within astrocytes (see **Fig. 20-6**).

Intracranial Hypertension and Cerebral Edema

The adult cranium is a rigid compartment with low compliance. Increased blood volume (cerebral hyperemia), decreased elevation of cerebrospinal fluid, and cerebral swelling (edema) quickly result in intracranial hypertension. ALF results in compromised autoregulation, the normal response of cerebral blood flow to remain constant during variation in mean arterial pressure. Furthermore, regional variation in blood flow results in hyperperfusion of some areas and hypoperfusion of others, resulting in cerebral ischemia.[109] Initially, intracranial hypertension results from severe hyperemia, which gives way to osmotic swelling of cortical astrocytes and cerebral edema. Astrocytic swelling accounts for most of the increase in cerebral volume not only because they are quantitatively one of the major cell types in the brain, but they also regulate brain volume as the principal component of the blood–brain barrier.

Astrocyte swelling results from an increase in intracellular osmolarity (cytotoxic edema), which ensues with the accumulation of glutamine, in turn derived by the addition of ammonia to glutamate via glutamine synthetase.[110,111] Neurons normally adapt to increased intracellular osmolarity and cell volume by increasing export of inorganic ions and endogenous organic osmolytes such as myoinositol (**Fig. 20-7**).[112] The compensation of accumulating glutamine by exporting endogenous osmolytes from astrocytes also explains why patients with hyperacute liver failure frequently develop cerebral edema while those with subacute liver failure are relatively protected because patients with the former condition appear not to have time for compensation to occur.[113]

Management of Acute Liver Failure
General Management
Initial Evaluation and Triage (Table 20-16)

Every patient with acute hepatocellular necrosis can potentially progress to ALF. Once a patient's mental status begins to deteriorate, one may lose the opportunity to obtain vital information that could guide management, including the administration of life-saving antidotes. Therefore, upon initial contact with a medical team, a careful drug ingestion history should be obtained to include prescription medications, herbal remedies, over-the-counter medications, and recreational drugs. Confounding conditions, such as alcohol use, malnutrition, and drug–drug interactions, must be considered. Although by definition ALF occurs in a patient with

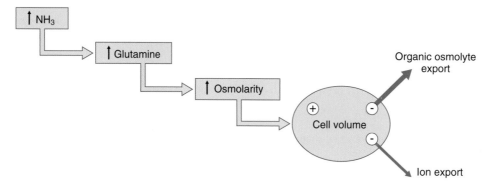

Fig. 20-7 Astrocyte swelling in the pathogenesis of cerebral edema in ALF: mechanisms of cell swelling and compensation. Intracerebral concentrations of ammonia are detoxified by the amidation of glutamate to glutamine, a reaction catalyzed by glutamine synthetase. Glutamine, an osmotically active solute, increases astrocyte cell volume, which may be attenuated by two mechanisms, exporting ions (minor pathway) or organic osmolytes (major pathway).

a previously normal liver, chronic liver disease may manifest initially as acute liver necrosis, including autoimmune hepatitis, Wilson disease, and in patients with underlying chronic liver disease who experience viral superinfections. Therefore past medical history should also include a search for signs, symptoms, and risk factors for chronic liver diseases. A travel history should be obtained because exposure to certain exotic causes of ALF may otherwise be overlooked. Finally, a detailed psychiatric history may provide clues about a possible surreptitious ingestion of hepatotoxins, particularly acetaminophen.

Initial laboratories should include tests to assess the degree of physiologic dysfunction, risk of mortality, and potential need for liver transplantation. Patients in whom the initial prothrombin time is more than 4 to 5 seconds prolonged should be admitted to the hospital for observation; the clinician should not be lulled into a false sense of security by a normal mental status in the presence of significant coagulopathy. Furthermore, patients with altered mental status, hemodynamic compromise, renal insufficiency, decreased oxygenation, acidosis, or hypoglycemia should be admitted to an intensive care facility, and the patient should be discussed with the nearest liver transplant center.

Whether to proceed with liver transplantation evaluation remains perhaps the most important decision in the initial evaluation of a patient with ALF.[46] Patients with grade 2 or higher encephalopathy should be evaluated unless contraindications exist. In subjects with lesser degrees of encephalopathy, profound coagulopathy (prothrombin time >50 seconds) or acidosis (pH <7.3) should also lead to early consideration for listing for transplant. Older subjects, those with idiosyncratic drug-induced ALF and patients with a subacute presentation, should be evaluated relatively early in the course of ALF in consideration of their poor prognosis for spontaneous recovery.

Therapies for Liver Injury (Table 20-17)
NAC for Acetaminophen Overdose

The use of an antidote may decrease hepatic injury and reverse ALF in specific circumstances. *N*-acetylcysteine (NAC) remains the treatment of choice for acetaminophen overdose, and in theory, may protect the liver from other toxins that cause hepatotoxicity by generating free radicals, such as carbon

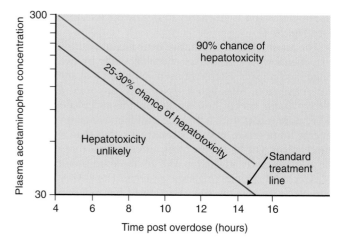

Fig. 20-8 Nomogram depicting the risk of hepatotoxicity from acetaminophen according to plasma acetaminophen concentration and time after ingestion. A standard treatment line for administering *N*-acetylcysteine (NAC) was derived empirically. Plots above the standard treatment line have significant risk of hepatotoxicity and should receive NAC immediately; plots below the line have a low risk of hepatotoxicity and do not require NAC. Such nomograms should be interpreted with caution, however (see text). *(From Makin A, Williams R. Acetaminophen-induced acute liver failure. In: Lee WM, Williams R, editors. Acute liver failure, 1st ed. Cambridge, UK: Cambridge University Press, 1997: 32–42.)*

tetrachloride or trichlorethylene.[114,115] The administration of NAC for APAP overdose replenishes GSH, thereby detoxifying NAPQI.[116] In addition, NAC improves oxygen delivery and consumption in ALF.[117] On presentation, the risk of APAP hepatotoxicity in an individual can be estimated by a nomogram plot of the initial plasma APAP concentration versus the time after ingestion (**Fig. 20-8**).[118] Patients with plots lying above an empirically derived treatment line have a high risk of hepatic necrosis and should definitely receive NAC. Below a zone of intermediate risk, a patient is unlikely to experience serious hepatotoxicity, and therefore does not require NAC. However, one must be aware of the potential pitfalls in the use of nomograms,[52] especially inaccurate assessment of the time since ingestion and the possibility of toxicity in individuals who accidentally ingest APAP over several days. It should also be obvious that the NAC nomogram is useful only in patients

Table 20-16 Initial Evaluation of ALF

History

Medications
Recreational drugs
Prodrome
Travel history
Alcohol
Past medical history, including psychiatric
Nutrition supplements
Mushrooms
Pregnancy

Physical Examination

Vital signs
Size of liver
Mental status
Rash/oropharyngeal lesions (HSV)
Stigmata of chronic liver disease

LABORATORY STUDIES	RATIONALE
Serology	1,4
Hepatis A (with IgM is screen positive) Hepatitis B surface antigen and antibody, core antibody (with IgM if positive) Hepatitis C antibody and quantitative RNA PCR Hepatitis D (if hepatitis B surface antigen is positive) Epstein-Barr virus (and EBV DNA PCR quantitative with high index of suspicion) Cytomegalovirus (and CMV DNA PCR if high index of suspicion) Herpes simplex virus Antinuclear antibody Antismooth muscle antibody HIV antibody	
White Blood Cell Count with Differential, Hemoglobin, Platelet Count	2,3,4
Chemistry	
Total and direct bilirubin, alkaline phosphatase, γ-glutamyl transpeptidase, AST, ALT	1,2,4
Albumin	1,4
Alkaline phosphatase	1
Electrolytes including sodium, potassium, chloride, total CO_2, phosphorus, calcium, magnesium	3
Blood urea nitrogen, creatinine	1,2,3,4
Plasma osmolality	3
Ceruloplasmin and serum copper	1
Lactate (arterial)	2,3
Ammonia (arterial)	2
β-hCG (females of childbearing potential)	1
α-fetoprotein	2
Arterial Blood Gas for pH	2,3
Coagulation	2,3
PT/INR, PTT Factor V and VII Thromboelastogram (TEG)	
Blood Type and Cross	
Urine Studies	
Urinalysis	2
Urine sodium and creatinine to calculate fractional excretion of sodium	2
24-hour urine collection for copper	1
Microbiology	
Blood and urine cultures	2
Imaging	
Chest x-ray	2
Doppler ultrasound of liver	1,3
Echocardiogram	

1, Identify etiology; 2, assess severity; 3, identify complications; 4, required for OLT

Table 20-17 General Management of ALF

- Administration of cause-specific therapy:
  - Acetaminophen: *N*-acetylcysteine (NAC)
  - Amanita: NAC, penicillin and silibinin
  - Carbon tetrachloride: NAC
  - Herpes simplex: acyclovir
  - Hepatitis B: lamivudine
  - Lassa fever, yellow fever: ribavirin
  - Malaria: quinine
  - Giant cell hepatitis: steroids
  - Autoimmune hepatitis: steroids
  - Wilson disease: high-dose penicillamine
  - Leptospirosis (Weil disease): penicillin or doxycycline
- Fluid and electrolyte disturbances requiring management:
  - Hyponatremia
  - Hypokalemia and hyperkalemia
  - Hypocalcemia and hypomagnesemia
  - Hypo-osmolarity
- Acid-base disturbances requiring management:
  - Respiratory acidosis and severe respiratory alkalosis
  - Metabolic acidosis with increased anion gap
- Nutrition:
  - Caloric goals: 35-40 kcal/kg/day
  - Protein: 40 g/day, titrate as necessary

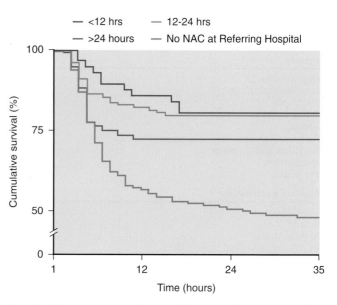

Fig. 20-9 **Survival of patients with acetaminophen overdose according to the time at which they received *N*-acetylcysteine (NAC).** Note that the survival of patients receiving NAC even greater than 24 hours after ingestion was significantly higher than for patients who were not treated with NAC before transfer to the liver failure unit at King's College Hospital (P <.0001). *(From Makin AJ, Wendon J, Williams R. A 7-year experience of severe acetaminophen-induced hepatotoxicity (1987-1993). Gastroenterology 1995;109:1907–1916.)*

who present with normal ALT; *any* patient with elevated ALT and a history of APAP ingestion should receive NAC regardless of plasma APAP levels. In the future, the determination of whether NAC should be administered may be made by detecting APAP-protein adducts, which have a longer half-life than APAP.[119]

The early administration of NAC (within 8 hours of overdose) minimizes hepatotoxicity regardless of the initial plasma concentration of APAP.[115,120] The time after which NAC administration is no longer effective, however, remains controversial, with some studies documenting benefit of administration up to 24 to 36 hours after ingestion.[121,122] Conversely, the worst survival rates after ALF because of acetaminophen overdose are observed in patients not given NAC at their referring hospital before transfer (**Fig. 20-9**).[121] Based upon these observations, it has been recommended that NAC "be used whenever there is any doubt concerning the timing, dose ingested, or plasma concentration because the use of the antidote is much less hazardous than the consequences of withholding it.[49]" In the United States, NAC is usually administered orally at a loading dose of 140 mg/kg followed by 70 mg/kg every 4 hours for a total of 17 doses. For patients who cannot tolerate oral administration, intravenous NAC administration has recently been approved in the same doses for a total of 48 hours.[123] NAC should be diluted 1:5 in 5% dextrose in a glass flask, and is equally effective.[123,124] In contrast to oral administration, intravenous NAC carries a small risk of allergic reaction, for which antihistamines are usually adequate therapy. The intravenous route is generally preferred in patients with greater than grade 1 hepatic encephalopathy, those intolerant of the putrid odor of the oral preparation, or in those with ileus.[125] The full course of NAC therapy should not be discontinued prematurely even after APAP levels have become undetectable; resolution of encephalopathy and correction of the INR to less than 1.5 have been advocated as criteria for discontinuation.[125]

NAC for Non-APAP ALF

Based upon experience in patients with ALF because of APAP overdose, three trials of NAC in non-APAP ALF have recently been completed, only one of which was randomized and placebo-controlled. The ALF Study Group trial concluded that IV NAC improved spontaneous (nontransplanted) survival compared with a placebo, but only in patients with grade 1 or 2 hepatic encephalopathy.[126] Suspected mushroom poisoning should be treated initially with ipecac and charcoal to decrease the *Amanita* toxin load, if the ingestion has occurred recently (within 30 minutes to a few hours).[53] NAC is also frequently advocated, although with scant supporting data.

Other Etiology-Specific Therapies

A combination of penicillin (300,000 to 1,000,000 units/kg/day, or 250 mg/kg/day IV) and silibinin (20 to 50 mg/kg/day IV) have been used as a specific antidote in those with evidence of liver injury due to *Amanita* poisoning.[127,128] These agents are hypothesized to interrupt the enterohepatic circulation of toxins and also to compete at the hepatocyte membrane for transmembrane transport.[53] Due to the rarity of this cause of ALF, the benefits of this regimen remain unproven. The use of corticosteroids for autoimmune ALF remains controversial but merits consideration in patients with early stage hepatic encephalopathy.[69] Nucleos(t)ide analogue inhibitors of hepatitis B virus replication were not found to improve outcome in a randomized, placebo-controlled trial of severe acute hepatitis B.[129] The use of acyclovir for herpes simplex hepatitis must be considered early in the course of acute liver injury, even before virologic confirmation.[34]

Management of Fluids, Electrolytes, and Acid-Base Abnormalities

Fluid and electrolyte abnormalities occur frequently in patients with ALF. Hyponatremia reflects free water excess and is often iatrogenic. Management requires isotonic intravenous fluid such as 0.9% saline (sodium 155 mmol/L) with or without dextrose. The target serum sodium concentration is 145 to 155 mmol/L, which has been associated with a reduced incidence of cerebral edema. Judicious use of hypertonic saline may facilitate correction of hyponatremia and has not been associated with pontine myelinolysis, in contrast to its use in patients with chronic liver failure and hyponatremia. Once renal failure sets in, severe hyponatremia is best treated in conjunction with renal replacement therapy.

Hypokalemic alkalosis occurs early in the course of ALF, whereas hyperkalemic acidosis dominates the late stages. The former condition requires intravenous infusion of potassium, whereas the latter mandates hemodialysis. Hypophosphatemia also occurs frequently in patients with ALF, and may be precipitated by dextrose infusions and respiratory alkalosis, which drives phosphate to the intracellular compartment. Hypophosphatemia may contribute to a worsening mental status and respiratory failure, and should therefore be corrected by intravenous repletion.[130] In the setting of renal failure and acidosis, the development of significant hyperphosphatemia requires dialysis. Hypocalcemia from repeated transfusions of citrated blood products may cause tetany or cardiac arrythmias.[131] Hypocalcemia and hypomagnesemia may present concurrently and interfere with the correction of hypokalemia; these abnormalities should be corrected by intravenous replacement.

Management of Nutrition

ALF is a catabolic state characterized by negative nitrogen balance, muscle wasting, and aminoaciduria.[132] While the clinical value of nutritional support in ALF has not been carefully studied, protein-calorie malnutrition adversely affects the immune system, thereby increasing susceptibility to infections, and impairs wound healing, suggesting that repletion may decrease the risk of infection and improve the outcome of liver transplantation, respectively. The enteral route is preferred for nutritional support in critically ill patients. Approximately 40 g/day of protein should be administered initially and the dose should be modified based on an assessment of the metabolic state.[133] However, increasing protein supplementation can contribute to hyperammonemia and hepatic encephalopathy, and arterial ammonia levels should be monitored during aggressive nutritional support and the protein load appropriately modified. Many studies have suggested that decreased levels of branched chain amino acids (BCAA) contribute to hepatic encephalopathy, forming the basis for the administration of enteral or parenteral nutritional products supplemented with BCAA. Although numerous studies have evaluated the utility of BCAA as a treatment of hepatic encephalopathy in cirrhosis, results remain inconclusive. Thus the routine use of BCAA-supplemented feeds or infusions in the management of ALF cannot be advocated. The initial caloric goal for the patient with ALF is approximately 35 to 40 kcal/day, preferably by the enteral route.[134] Patients with volume overload may meet caloric needs by the administration of lipid emulsions, which may be used safely in patients with ALF. Hypoglycemia is a common and potentially fatal complication of ALF, and blood glucose should be monitored at 2- to 3-hour intervals by finger stick, and 10% dextrose infused to maintain levels greater than 80 mg/dl.

Prevention and Management of Specific Complications of ALF

Bleeding

Patients with mild to moderate coagulopathy and absence of bleeding do not require specific intervention.[82] The administration of vitamin K will ensure that deficiency does not contribute to the bleeding diathesis. The use of fresh frozen plasma (FFP) in patients with severe, but asymptomatic, coagulopathy remains controversial and is usually discouraged because few data document efficacy in bleeding prevention, overzealous infusion of FFP may result in volume overload, a small but definite risk of transfusion-related acute lung injury exists, and the practice obscures important prognostic information regarding trends in the prothrombin time.[135] A more common clinical situation involves the patient with ALF who requires an invasive procedure, such as central venous catheter or ICP monitor. Guidelines for correction of the INR and platelet counts to minimize bleeding risk before procedures have not been developed, although goal values of 1.5 and 50,000/mm^3, respectively, have been advocated by consensus.[125] Strategies for correcting these laboratory abnormalities in patients with ALF who have fluid overload include exchange plasmapheresis and recombinant factor VIIa (rFVIIa).[136,137] DIC usually does not require specific intervention unless severe and accompanied by bleeding[97]; limited studies have shown that heparin may be used to treat DIC in patients with ALF, but the potential bleeding risks limit enthusiasm for this treatment. Gastrointestinal bleeding in a patient with ALF usually results from superficial gastric erosions and stress ulcers, which should be prophylaxed by the use of H$_2$ receptor antagonists or proton pump inhibitors.

Cardiovascular Derangements

ALF dramatically alters systemic hemodynamics, with the primary hemodynamic abnormality being systemic arterial vasodilation due to reduced precapillary sphincter tone, similar to sepsis. Volume status in a hypotensive patient with ALF can be difficult to assess. A normal saline challenge guided by changes in CVP should be administered before considering vasopressors. In hypotensive patients who do not respond to volume resuscitation, vasopressors should be titrated to achieve a mean arterial pressure (MAP) of greater than 75 mm Hg and cerebral perfusion pressure (CPP) of 60 to 80 mm Hg. Patients with liver disease manifest less vasoconstriction in response to α-adrenergic agents.[138] Although dopamine and norepinephrine increase hepatic blood flow in parallel with cardiac output,[139] the latter may be associated with fewer β-adrenergic–mediated side effects such as tachycardia for the same vasopressor response, and is often preferred. Dobutamine may be considered if left ventricular dysfunction is severe, but may increase arterial vasodilation and worsen hypotension. Vasopressin and its analogues potentiate the vasoconstricting effect of norepinephrine allowing for reduction in infusion rate of norepinephrine, but controversy about its potential to increase ICP in patients with ALF relegates it to a secondary role.[140] Persistently hypotensive patients with ALF despite vasopressors should be evaluated for adrenal insufficiency, which occurs frequently in patients with ALF and correlates with the severity of illness.[141]

In summary, the hypotensive patient with ALF should initially receive a normal saline bolus, later changing to 0.45% normal saline with 75 mEq/L sodium bicarbonate to maintain the infused sodium concentration at 152 mEq/L and to minimize the potential for hyperchloremic acidosis. Once cardiac filling pressures are optimized, norepinephrine is titrated to a MAP to keep CPP greater than 60 mm Hg. In patients without an ICP monitor, an ICP of 20 mm Hg can be assumed, mandating a target MAP of greater than 80 mm Hg. In the face of escalating norepinephrine requirements, or if side effects such as arrhythmias develop, vasopressin at a fixed dose of 0.04 units per minute can be added to permit downward titration of norepinephrine. Adrenal insufficiency is corrected with stress-dose hydrocortisone (200 to 300 mg/day in divided doses).

Pulmonary Complications and Ventilatory Support

A major decision in the management of a patient with ALF is the timing of endotracheal intubation. The indications for intubation include airway protection, provision of respiratory support, and management of intracranial hypertension. A less quantifiable indication includes extreme agitation, which risks exacerbating intracranial hypertension. The airway should be secured by endotracheal intubation after reaching grade 3 encephalopathy. A rapid sequence technique of intubation should be employed, with attention to avoiding exacerbating intracranial hypertension or cerebral underperfusion, including preoxygenation, prevention of hypercapnia, and avoidance of hypotension. Neuromuscular blockade with the nondepolarizing agent, *cis*-atracurium, may be preferable than the depolarizing agent, succinylcholine, which causes muscle contraction, which in turn increases ICP. Metabolism of *cis*-atracurium (by Hoffman elimination) is also independent of renal and hepatic function, and permits neurologic reassessment 40 to 60 minutes after the bolus. Initial ventilator settings should be selected to achieve a constant minute ventilation while minimizing lung trauma with low tidal volume ventilation (6 ml/kg, ideal body weight). The arterial carbon dioxide tension ($Paco_2$) is an important determinant of ICP in patients with ALF,[142] and an initial $Paco_2$ goal of 35 mm Hg after intubation allows for subsequent hyperventilation to address transient spikes in ICP without compromising cerebral blood flow.[143] $Paco_2$ can be later titrated to ICP by adjusting minute ventilation after placement of an ICP monitor. Acute lung injury and acute respiratory distress syndrome (ALI-ARDS) occur in approximately one third of patients with ALF and can contribute to death. The development of ALI-ARDS may result in increased dead space and a rising $Paco_2$, which leads to cerebral vasodilation and increased ICP. The temptation to lower $Paco_2$ by increasing tidal volume should be resisted because the consequences of worsening lung injury outweigh the potential of hypercapnia to increase ICP. The hypoxemia that results from ALI-ARDS should be managed with recruitment (a transient increase in mean

airway pressure to expand atelectatic lung) and positive end-expiratory pressure (PEEP) titrated to optimize compliance and minimize the decrease in venous return and cardiac output.

Prevention and Management of Infection

Sepsis remains one of the major causes of death in patients with ALF because of its frequency and subtle clinical presentation (**Fig. 20-10**). Bacteremia has been identified in up to 50% to 80% of patients with ALF, usually within the first few days after onset of ALF.[103,104] Compared with other patients undergoing orthotopic liver transplantation (OLT), patients with ALF are particularly vulnerable to bacterial infections.[144] The most common infections in patients with ALF are pneumonia followed by systemic bacteremia and urinary tract infections (**Fig. 20-11**). Of these, pneumonia accounts for half the cases of infection and is almost invariably accompanied by chest x-ray abnormalities. Gram-positive organisms account for the majority of bacterial infections, with *Staphylococcus aureus* the

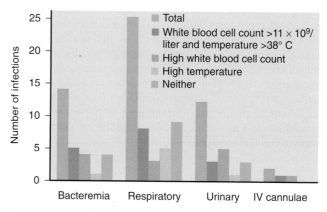

Fig. 20-10 **Clinical indicators of infection in patients with ALF.** *(From Rolando N, Philpott-Howard J, Williams R. Management of infection in acute liver failure. In: Lee WM, Williams R, editors. Acute liver failure. Cambridge, UK: Cambridge University Press, 1997:158–171.)*

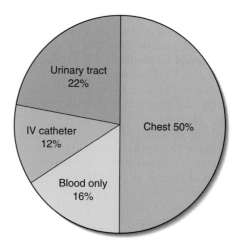

Fig. 20-11 **Sites of infection in patients with ALF.** *(From Rolando N, Philpott-Howard J, Williams R. Management of infection in acute liver failure. In: Lee WM, Williams R, editors. Acute liver failure. Cambridge, UK: Cambridge University Press, 1997:158–171.)*

most commonly isolated organism, and *Escherichia coli* the most commonly isolated gram-negative organism. Fungal infections, most commonly *Candida*, have been found in up to 32% of cases and contributed to death in 13%.[145]

Prevention of infection is thus an important objective of the medical management of ALF, and general guidelines to avoid nosocomial transmission of organisms should be strictly enforced (**Fig. 20-12**). Whether potentially infectious colonizing microbes should be monitored remains more controversial. Some authorities advocate obtaining daily blood and urine cultures especially early in the course of ALF to obtain antibiotic sensitivities in case of future infection.[103,104] Prophylactic antibiotics generally appear to decrease infections in patients with ALF. One study randomized patients with ALF and no evidence of infection on admission to the intensive care unit to a regimen of oral colistin, tobramycin, and amphotericin B, and a 4-day course of intravenous cefuroxime, or to a placebo.[146] This regimen significantly decreased the infection rate compared with patients who did not receive the antibiotics. Similarly, antibiotic prophylaxis was associated with an improved trend towards survival. Other regimens consisting of oral neomycin, colistin, and norfloxacin have also been effective.[147] Thus based on current literature, patients with ALF should receive

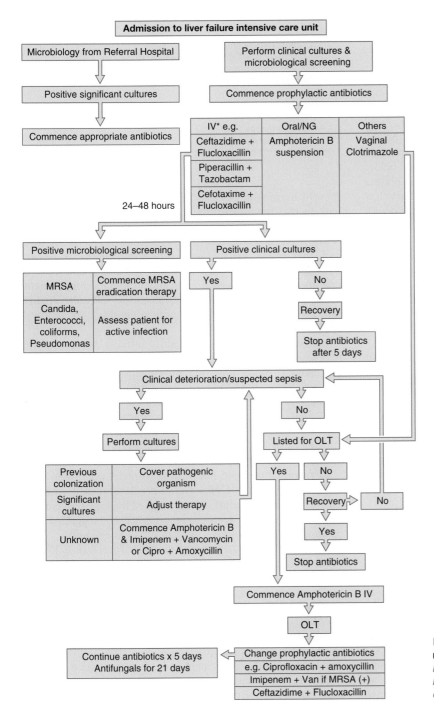

Fig. 20-12 **Algorithm for the prevention and treatment of infection in patients with ALF.** *(From Rolando N, Philpott-Howard J, Williams R. Management of infection in acute liver failure. In: Lee WM, Williams R, editors. Acute liver failure. Cambridge, UK: Cambridge University Press, 1997:158–171.)*

parenterally a third-generation cephalosporin in combination with amphotericin with or without additional antibiotics (e.g., norfloxacin) administered orally.

Once infection is suspected or documented, antibiotic coverage should be empirically administered according to results of surveillance cultures, or in their absence, adjustments made after definitive identification of the organism and its antibiotic sensitivities. Fungal infections should be suspected in patients with high fever unresponsive to antibiotics, profound leukocytosis, and acute renal failure. In such cases, amphotericin, fluconazole, or caspofungin should be administered. Granulocyte colony-stimulating factor has also been advocated to improve neutrophil function in patients with ALF.[148]

Management of Renal Insufficiency

The development of renal failure is a marker of poor prognosis and greatly complicates fluid and electrolyte, hemodynamic, and ventilatory management of the patient with ALF. The management of renal failure depends upon the underlying cause (see **Table 20-11**). Once oliguria develops, continuous arteriovenous or venovenous hemofiltration should be considered. Hemofiltration techniques minimize hypotension, rapid fluid shifts, and plasma osmolality changes, and thereby decrease the risk of cerebral edema as compared with standard hemodialysis.[149] Plasma osmolarity should be assessed before the institution of hemodialysis because a rapid drop in plasma urea levels may exacerbate cerebral edema in a patient with low osmolality before dialysis. Such patients may be managed with mannitol infusions to raise serum osmolarity before institution of dialysis. The functional renal failure associated with ALF usually requires hemodialysis and liver transplantation, but the use of vasopressors (e.g., norepinephrine) to improve effective renal blood flow may reverse this condition in cirrhotic patients, and should be considered.

Multiorgan System Failure

The microcirculatory disturbances associated with ALF lead to MOSF, which is characterized by noncardiogenic pulmonary edema, renal failure, gastrointestinal bleeding, ileus, and acidosis. Although sepsis usually precipitates this chain of events, a systemic inflammatory response syndrome (SIRS) commonly develops even in the absence of infection. In a retrospective analysis of 887 patients with ALF,[91] 40% of individuals without sepsis developed SIRS and MOSF. The development of SIRS and MOSF portend worsening intracranial hypertension and death.

Hepatic Encephalopathy, Cerebral Edema, and Intracranial Hypertension (Table 20-18)

Hepatic encephalopathy occurs in the presence or absence of cerebral edema, and often cannot be clinically distinguished even in some patients with marked elevations in intracranial pressure (ICP).[150] Complete neurologic recovery usually follows normalization of liver function whether spontaneous or following liver transplantation. However, severe cerebral ischemia, which results from cerebral edema, intracranial hypertension, or arterial hypotension with hypoperfusion, may result in permanent neurologic disability. The goals of treating intracranial hypertension are therefore to not only

Table 20-18 Management of Cerebral Edema in ALF

- Methods to modulate cerebral blood flow:
  - Elevate head of bed by 20-30 degrees
  - Correct volume overload
  - Maintain mean arterial pressure (MAP) ~50-60 mm Hg
  - Hyperventilate to keep Pco_2 25-30 mm Hg
- Correct factors that increase ICP:
  - Minimize head turning
  - Avoid bilateral internal jugular vein cannulation
  - Optimize PEEP
  - Intratracheal lidocaine before respiratory suctioning
  - Treat agitation with intubation and sedation (propofol); paralyze if necessary
  - Treat hypotension
  - Monitor for and treat seizures
  - Correct hypoxemia
- Direct measures:
  - Correct hypo-osmolarity
  - Mannitol (0.5-1 g/kg body weight IV bolus)
  - Induce hypernatremia to 150-155 mmol/L
  - Pentobarbital coma
- Liver transplantation
- Desperate measures:
  - Hypothermia
  - Indomethacin
  - Total hepatectomy

prevent herniation but also to optimize neurologic recovery. Risk factors for developing cerebral edema in patients with ALF include hyperacute compared with subacute liver failure,[76] serum ammonia concentrations greater than 150 to 200 μM, and high-grade hepatic encephalopathy (grade 3 or 4), although the relationship between ammonia and ICP is not linear.[41,110] The need for vasopressors, renal replacement therapy, and the presence of infection and/or SIRS, also predict the progression of hepatic encephalopathy and cerebral edema.[41,91,151]

Intracranial hypertension results initially from cerebral hyperemia and subsequently from cerebral edema. Monitoring cerebral blood flow, oxygen consumption, intracranial pressure offer the potential for optimizing perioperative medical management. However, noninvasive measures are inadequate as specialized techniques may not be widely available. CT imaging is insensitive to intracranial hypertension and demonstrates cerebral edema relatively late in the patient's course.

Intracranial pressure monitoring provides additional data to guide management. However, it remains unclear whether the risks of the procedure are outweighed by improved patient survival overall. Cerebral hypoperfusion suggested by prolonged (>2 hours) intracranial hypertension (ICP >25 mm Hg) or a low cerebral perfusion pressure (CPAP = mean arterial pressure minus ICP <40 mm Hg) portends a poor neurologic recovery and may contraindicate OLT. Certainly interventions in patients with ICP monitors are more frequent than in patients without ICP monitors. There is a 5% risk of clinically significant intracranial hemorrhage,[154,155] which varies in direct proportion to the invasiveness and reliability of the monitor. Furthermore, clinical endpoints are not standardized and management is not protocolized.

The medical management of intracranial hypertension requires optimization of cardiorespiratory parameters as detailed above, including intubation of the airway with progression to stage 3 or 4 encephalopathy. Hepatic encephalopathy with hyperammonemia can be treated with bowel cleansing by lactulose or saline enema,[125] and nonabsorbable antibiotics (rifaximin). Lactulose per os or via gastric or jejunal tube is problematic because it may result in gaseous distention of the bowel, which complicates transplant surgery. Simple measures should be undertaken to prevent unnecessary ICP increases. These include neutral position of the head with the patient elevated at 30 degrees and avoidance of bilateral jugular venous cannulation. Spontaneous hyperventilation with resulting hypocapnia may be protective by promoting cerebral vasoconstriction, controlling hyperemia, and decreasing intracranial pressure. Fever should be vigorously treated. Spontaneous hypothermia, which commonly accompanies ALF, reduces intracranial hypertension and restores cerebral autoregulation, and should not be corrected. Serum sodium should be maintained between 145 and 155 mmol/L.

The development of intracranial hypertension despite these prophylactic maneuvers should prompt urgent treatment. First-line therapy includes increasing blood osmolality with mannitol boluses (0.5 to 1 g/kg body weight), which draws water from swollen astrocytes back into the intravascular space. It should be appreciated, however, that the effectiveness of mannitol in treating cerebral edema in patients with ALF is based upon experience in only a few patients in nonrandomized studies.[152,153] Furthermore, mannitol is ineffective in returning ICP to an acceptably low level (<25 mm Hg) in subjects with severe intracranial hypertension (>40 to 60 mm Hg), and initial improvements in ICP usually wane, necessitating multiple doses, which can result in hyperosmolality (>320 mOsm/L). Mannitol will transiently expand circulating blood volume and increase central venous pressure (CVP), as well as ICP. In patients with renal failure, this may result in a paradoxical increase in ICP. Ultrafiltration with continuous renal replacement therapy (CRRT) can be increased to maintain intravascular volume and prevent increased CVP. Ultimately, mannitol administration may bridge a patient with ALF to OLT, but does not provide definitive therapy. Similar to other conditions characterized by cerebral edema, hypertonic saline (HTS) boluses have been advocated for established cerebral edema in patients with ALF,[154] although no studies yet have examined the efficacy of this practice. However, in ALF patients with normal ICP, the induction of prophylactic hypernatremia with HTS (serum sodium 145 to 155 mEq/L) effectively prevented the development of intracranial hypertension compared with "normonatremia" (135 to 145 mEq/L).[155] During transplant surgery, patients in whom ICP had been adequately controlled with mannitol and/or HTS are still susceptible to cerebral herniation during dissection of the native liver or reperfusion of the implanted graft; this risk persists through the early postoperative period. Consequently, monitoring of cerebral hemodynamics including ICP[156] should be continued until allograft function stabilizes. Therapeutic measures for intracranial hypertension should be weaned slowly to prevent rebound.

Patients with ALF who break through osmotic therapy for intracranial hypertension usually succumb to brainstem herniation if OLT does not immediately follow. Desperate measures considered under these conditions include the induction of deeper sedation with propofol[157] or barbiturates,[158,159] intravenous boluses of indomethacin[160] and therapeutic hypothermia. Of these, only hypothermia has been studied systematically, albeit in a small number of patients and not in a randomized fashion compared with normothermia.[161] Therapeutic hypothermia (core temperature 32° to 34° C) in patients with intracranial hypertension refractory to medical therapy effectively lowers ICP, restores autoregulation of cerebrovascular blood flow, and bridges patients with ALF to OLT. Furthermore, hypothermia continued during transplant surgery prevents spikes in ICP. Whether hypothermia bridges patients with ALF to spontaneous recovery without OLT has never been documented, and its safety in this critically ill population remains inadequately assessed.

Seizure activity in patients with ALF increase CBF and ICP, resulting in cerebral edema; if unremitting (status epilepticus), seizures exacerbate neuronal damage. In patients with ALF, seizures are often nonconvulsive and can be detected only by electroencephalography (EEG). Prophylaxis with phenytoin has been studied in two randomized, controlled cohorts with ALF and high-grade hepatic encephalopathy.[162,163] Unfortunately, the studies came to different conclusions regarding the efficacy of phenytoin in preventing seizures, cerebral edema, or improving outcome.

Methods to Protect the Liver from Injury and Promote Liver Regeneration

A successful outcome of ALF depends on both cessation of liver injury and regeneration of the injured liver, the "Holy Grail" of the management of ALF. While numerous possible modalities have been used to achieve these objectives, all have failed. These include infusions of insulin and glucagon, corticosteroids, human cross-circulation, extracorporeal liver perfusion, exchange transfusions, hemodialysis, prostaglandin infusion, and charcoal hemoperfusion. High-volume plasmapheresis improved cerebral hemodynamics and was associated with a favorable spontaneous survival rate in patients with ALF,[164] and is undergoing multicenter evaluation in Europe.

Orthotopic Liver Transplantation

Liver transplantation remains the "definitive treatment" of patients with severe ALF, and clearly improves both short- and long-term survival in patients with grade III or grade IV encephalopathy, especially in patients with non–APAP-induced ALF.[165] Because ALF due to APAP overdose usually resolves spontaneously with the early administration of NAC and with meticulous ICU care, only approximately 10% of affected individuals undergo OLT for this indication in the United States compared with 30% to 50% with ALF from other causes.[166] In addition, patients with ALF due to APAP often have psychosocial barriers to OLT, such as substance abuse and a history of suicidal behavior.[42] Overall, approximately 5% of OLTs performed in the United States are for ALF, and 25% to 30% of all patients with ALF undergo OLT.[167] The success of liver transplant mandates that patients with ALF be transported to a transplant center whenever feasible. The challenge remains to identify patients with a high risk of mortality with medical management and a high probability of survival with transplant (see Assessment of Prognosis section). It is equally important to decide when not to proceed with liver transplantation. Patients with a poor prognosis for neurologic recovery, such as a sustained increase in ICP greater than

40 mm Hg or a decrease in CPP less than 40 mm Hg, may not benefit from liver transplantation even if technically successful. The presence of septicemia or advanced multiorgan failure are also contraindications to liver transplantation.

Patients with ALF listed for OLT in the United States receive priority above all with cirrhosis according to the rules of the United Network for Organ Sharing (UNOS), so-called "status 1A" priority.* Status 1A criteria include a life expectancy without transplant of less than 7 days, onset of encephalopathy within 8 weeks of the first symptom of liver injury, care within an ICU, and absence of preexisting liver disease. Objective criteria include being at least 18 years old, and at least one of the following: ventilator-dependence, receiving RRT, or INR greater than 2.0. Listing a patient status 1A also broadens the geographic area from which a liver may originate, such that waiting times are typically short (mean of approximately 2 to 4 days).[168] Nevertheless, patients listed status 1A have extremely high death rates on the liver transplant waiting list compared with patients with cirrhosis.

The challenges in transplanting patients with ALF differ markedly from those in patients with cirrhosis. In the relative absence of portal hypertension, bleeding rarely poses a major problem despite abnormal coagulation parameters, and the preoperative degree of "coagulopathy" does not predict post-OLT outcome.[168] Patients with ALF who die after OLT usually succumb to MOSF, but a significant fraction herniate intraoperatively or within the first 24 hours after transplantation. Not surprisingly, the primary cause of graft loss after OLT for ALF is patient death, but primary nonfunction seems much more common in this population than patients transplanted for cirrhosis.[168] Long-term patient survival after OLT for ALF is generally lower than for patients transplanted for cirrhosis, but remains favorable (70% to 75% at 3 years). In contrast to patients with cirrhosis, most of the deaths occur within the first month posttransplant, reflecting the severity of the acute liver injury.

Many liver transplant centers have reported average survival after transplantation for ALF of about 65%, which compares favorably with medical management.[165,169-171] In one of the largest studies,[172] a number of static and dynamic variables were evaluated as predictors of outcome after liver transplant in 100 patients with ALF. In patients with ALF unrelated to acetaminophen (n = 79), the cause was an important predictor of survival. Of the dynamic variables, an elevated serum creatinine predicted poor outcome, as did grade 3 or 4 encephalopathy (80% survival for those with grade 1 or 2 vs. 56% for 3 or 4). Survival after liver transplantation is also adversely influenced by the use of suboptimal organs (fatty liver, ABO-incompatible liver).[170] The outcome of liver transplantation in children is similar to that in adults.[61] Although experience worldwide with adult-to-adult living donor liver transplantation is limited, the procedure has been used occasionally in patients with ALF, and outcomes are similar to using deceased-donor grafts.[173] The major hindrance to its widespread use in ALF, however, will likely remain the amount of time required to evaluate a potential donor, which often requires several days. Auxiliary liver transplantation, in which a donor liver (whole or partial) is heterotopically implanted below the native liver to provide support while regeneration of the native liver occurs, has also been explored in patients with ALF.[174] Withdrawal of immunosuppression after regeneration of the native liver causes rejection and atrophy of the donated liver, and obviates the need for long-term immunosuppression.

Assessment of Prognosis: When to Initiate OLT Evaluation

Patients with ALF have one of three outcomes: spontaneous recovery, liver transplantation, or death. As of October 2008, the U.S. Acute Liver Failure Study Group registry of more than 1300 patients recorded that roughly 45% spontaneously recovered, 25% underwent liver transplantation (of whom 11% died), and 30% died without transplantation. The overall survival, with or without liver transplantation and for all major causes, has steadily improved with time, and is currently 69% in the U.S. ALF Study Group Registry. The ability to predict which patient with ALF will recover spontaneously with medical management, and who will succumb without liver transplantation, remains the question of paramount importance. Although liver transplantation offers hope of survival from ALF, the decision to transplant introduces the need for lifelong immunosuppression, an operative mortality of up to 30%, and the use of a scarce resource.[175] Thus universal liver transplantation for ALF cannot be endorsed. Although mortality from all causes of ALF parallels the depth of hepatic encephalopathy (>80% mortality rates for grade 3 or 4 encephalopathy), spontaneous recovery occasionally follows even the deepest hepatic coma[176]; thus more accurate predictors of outcome are needed.

Several groups have proposed guidelines with which to select a patient for liver transplantation (**Table 20-19**). The most widely accepted were proposed by O'Grady and colleagues in 1989, and have become known as the King's College criteria.[4] Based upon a retrospective review of 588 patients with ALF who were medically managed between 1973 and 1985, these authors identified poor prognostic variables in patients with ALF due to acetaminophen overdose and other causes by multivariate analysis, and then applied the variables to a test group of 175 patients who were seen between 1986 and 1987. For patients with acetaminophen overdose, acidosis (arterial pH <7.30) on admission or the combination of a peak prothrombin time of greater than 100 seconds, serum creatinine greater than 3.4 mg/dl, and grade 3 or 4 hepatic encephalopathy was highly associated with mortality without liver transplantation. Fulfillment of one of these criteria predicted 77% of the total deaths in the test group. In the group with ALF from nonacetaminophen causes, three static variables obtained on admission (etiology, age, and duration of jaundice to onset of encephalopathy >7 days) and two dynamic variables obtained during the evolution of liver failure (peak bilirubin and prothrombin time) predicted a poor prognosis. The presence of a prothrombin time of greater than 100 seconds or, in patients with a prothrombin time less than 100 seconds, any three of the following: (age <10 or >40 years, non-A, non-B viral or idiosyncratic drug etiology, evolution from jaundice to encephalopathy of >7 days, prothrombin time >50 seconds, bilirubin >17.4 gm/dl) predicted more than 96% of the fatalities in the test group. Although the predictive

---

*Policy 3.6 available at UNOS.ORG.

Table 20-19 Schemes for Predicting Mortality and Need for Liver Transplantation in ALF

TEST	CAUSE OF ALF	CRITERIA FOR LIVER TRANSPLANTATION	REFERENCE
King's College Criteria	APAP	Arterial pH <7.30 or all of the following: 1. PT >100 sec (INR >6.5) 2. Creatinine >3.4 mg/dl 3. Grade 3/4 encephalopathy	O'Grady, 1989 (4)
	Non-APAP	PT >100 sec (INR >6.5) or any three of the following: 1. NANB/drug/halothane etiology 2. Jaundice to encephalopathy >7 days 3. Age <10 or >40 yr 4. PT >50 sec 5. Bilirubin >17.4 mg/dl	
Factor V (Clichy criteria)	Viral	Age <30 yr: factor V <20% or Any age: factor V <30% and grade 3/4 encephalopathy	Bernuau, 1986; 1991 (18, 181)
Liver biopsy	Mixed	Hepatocyte necrosis >70%	Donaldson, 1993 (185)
Arterial phosphate	APAP	>1.2 mmol/L	Schmidt, 2002 (95)
Serum lactate	APAP	>3.5 mmol/L	Bernal, 2002 (183)
APACHE II score	APAP	Score >15	Mitchell, 1998 (180)

APAP, acetaminophen; HBV, hepatitis B virus; NANB, non-A, non-B viral hepatitis; mixed, mixed causes

accuracy of the King's College criteria has been substantiated by other groups,[177,178] the *failure* to fulfill the King's College criteria did not predict survival without liver transplant in another study,[179] and in the ALF Study Group Registry, the King's College criteria predicted patient mortality with a sensitivity of only 12%.[6]

Other indices have been developed to improve the predictive accuracy of the King's College criteria (see **Table 20-19**). An APACHE (Acute Physiology and Chronic Health Evaluation) II score greater than 15 was highly predictive of death or the need for liver transplantation in patients with APAP overdose, even though prothrombin time and bilirubin, the two most important indicators of hepatic necrosis, are not part of the score.[180] Coagulation parameters also have an important role in assessing prognosis. The degree of prothrombin time elevation, and in particular, a continued rise 4 days after APAP ingestion, is associated with a 93% mortality without transplant.[135] Levels of factor V, a liver-derived coagulation factor with short half-life (12 to 24 hours), may be a more accurate indicator of the need for liver transplantation than the prothrombin time, which tends to become more markedly elevated in certain etiologies of ALF (APAP).[18,175] Based upon experience with HBV-induced ALF, the "Clichy criteria" based upon factor V levels were later refined in a prospective study of patients with viral ALF. In patients with stage 3 or 4 hepatic encephalopathy, a factor V level of less than 20% in patients less than 30 years old, or a level of less than 30% in patients greater than 30 years old, predicted very high mortality (90%) and thus the need for liver transplantation.[181] Although factor V levels fared nearly as well as other prognostic indicators in two subsequently studied groups of patients with non-APAP ALF, no level of factor V discriminated patients with APAP-induced ALF who lived or died.[178,182] In contrast to factor V,

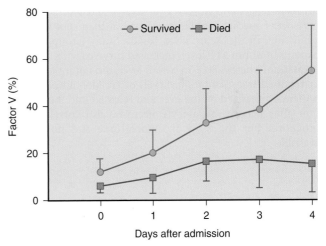

Fig. 20-13 Sequential factor V levels in 22 patients with acetaminophen-induced ALF according to prognosis. Factor V levels recovered to within a normal range (60% to 150%) within 4 days of admission in survivors, while patients who died had no significant recovery of factor V levels. *(From Pereira L, et al. Coagulation factor V and VIII/V ratio as predictors of outcome in paracetamol induced fulminant hepatic failure: relation to other prognostic indicators. Gut 1992;33:98–102.)*

factor VIII levels are routinely elevated in ALF and reflect the degree of endothelial cell activation during evolution of the SIRS. A factor VIII/V ratio of less than 30 provided high predictive value for spontaneous survival.[84] The same study found low factor V concentrations useful in predicting mortality from APAP-induced ALF when levels do not recover over the first 3 days of hospitalization (**Fig. 20-13**).

Other readily available laboratory parameters also appear to have prognostic value. In a multivariate, retrospectively analyzed group of more than 100 patients with APAP-induced ALF, arterial lactate concentration was identified as a predictor of death (8.5 mmol/L in those who died vs. 1.4 mmol/L in those who survived).[183] In a subsequent prospectively studied patient sample, a threshold of arterial lactate before volume expansion of 3.5 mmol/L had a sensitivity of 67% and specificity of 95% in predicting early death from acetaminophen-induced ALF. Serum phosphate also may improve standard prognostic criteria.[95] In patients with APAP-induced ALF, serum phosphate concentrations 48 to 72 hours after the overdose were significantly higher in patients who died than in survivors (mean 2.65 vs. 0.68 mmol/L, respectively), and a threshold value of 1.2 mmol/L provided 89% sensitivity and 100% specificity.

The role of liver biopsy in determining prognosis in ALF remains controversial. An early study advocated the use of hepatocyte necrosis to estimate prognosis, but found coagulation parameters reflected the likelihood of regeneration nearly as well, and that biopsy offered no prognostic information in many patients.[184] Despite bias introduced by sampling variation, a subsequent study showed that the prognosis was dismal in patients with greater than 70% hepatocyte necrosis[185]; others have not found that the extent of necrosis predicts outcome, however.[186,187]

Other proposed prognostic criteria include serum α-fetoprotein (AFP) levels, a marker of liver regeneration that tends to be higher in patients who recover spontaneously.[188] An increasing trend in AFP over days 1 and 3 of admission may better predict spontaneous survival than spot levels on admission; in the Acute Liver Failure Study Group, 71% of patients in whom AFP levels increased survived without transplantation, whereas 80% in whom levels did not increase died or required transplantation. Levels of Gc globulin, a plasma protein synthesized by the liver and released into the circulation after massive hepatocyte necrosis, also correlate with prognosis, but the assay is cumbersome and not widely available.

Key References

Acharya SK, et al. Fulminant hepatitis in a tropical population: clinical course, cause, and early predictors of outcome. Hepatology 1996;23(6):1448–1455. (Ref.8)

Anand AC, Nightingale P, Neuberger JM. Early indicators of prognosis in fulminant hepatic failure: an assessment of the King's criteria. J Hepatol 1997;26(1):62–68. (Ref.177)

Andreu V, et al. Ecstasy: a common cause of severe acute hepatotoxicity. J Hepatol 1998;29(3):394–397. (Ref.40)

Baudouin SV, et al. Acute lung injury in fulminant hepatic failure following paracetamol poisoning. Thorax 1995;50(4):399–402. (Ref.90)

Belay ED, et al. Reye's syndrome in the United States from 1981 through 1997. N Engl J Med 1999;340(18):1377–1382. (Ref.59)

Bernal W, et al. Intensive care management of acute liver failure. Semin Liver Dis 2008;28(2):188–200. (Ref.154)

Bernal W, et al. Blood lactate as an early predictor of outcome in paracetamol-induced acute liver failure: a cohort study. Lancet 2002;359(9306):558–563. (Ref.183)

Bernal W, et al. Arterial ammonia and clinical risk factors for encephalopathy and intracranial hypertension in acute liver failure. Hepatology 2007;46(6):1844–1852. (Ref.41)

Bhatia V, Batra Y, Acharya SK. Prophylactic phenytoin does not improve cerebral edema or survival in acute liver failure: a controlled clinical trial. J Hepatol 2004;41(1):89–96. (Ref.163)

Bismuth H, et al. Orthotopic liver transplantation in fulminant and subfulminant hepatitis. The Paul Brousse experience. Ann Surg 1995;222(2):109–119. (Ref.170)

Bismuth H, et al. Liver transplantation in Europe for patients with acute liver failure. Semin Liver Dis 1996;16(4):415–425. (Ref.171)

Blei AT. The pathophysiology of brain edema in acute liver failure. Neurochem Int 2005;47(1-2):71–77. (Ref.76)

Broussard CN, et al. Mushroom poisoning: from diarrhea to liver transplantation. Am J Gastroenterol 2001;96(11):3195–3198. (Ref.53)

Butterworth RF. Hepatic encephalopathy and brain edema in acute hepatic failure: does glutamate play a role? Hepatology 1997;25(4):1032–1034. (Ref.111)

Campsen J, et al. Outcomes of living donor liver transplantation for acute liver failure: the adult-to-adult living donor liver transplantation cohort study. Liver Transpl 2008;14:1273–1280. (Ref.173)

Castro MA, et al. Reversible peripartum liver failure: a new perspective on the diagnosis, treatment, and cause of acute fatty liver of pregnancy, based on 28 consecutive cases. Am J Obstet Gynecol 1999;181(2):389–395. (Ref.64)

Chalasani N, et al. Causes, clinical features, and outcomes from a prospective study of drug-induced liver injury in the United States. Gastroenterology 2008;135(6):1924–1934. (Ref.39)

Clemmesen JO, et al. The effect of increasing blood pressure with dopamine on systemic, splanchnic, and lower extremity hemodynamics in patients with acute liver failure. Scand J Gastroenterol 1999;34(9):921–927. (Ref.139)

Clemmesen JO, Kondrup J, Ott P. Splanchnic and leg exchange of amino acids and ammonia in acute liver failure. Gastroenterology 2000;118(6):1131–1139. (Ref.78)

Clemmesen JO, et al. Cerebral herniation in patients with acute liver failure is correlated with arterial ammonia concentration. Hepatology 1999;29(3):648–653. (Ref.110)

Cordoba J, Gottstein J, Blei AT. Glutamine, myo-inositol, and organic brain osmolytes after portocaval anastomosis in the rat: implications for ammonia-induced brain edema. Hepatology 1996;24(4):919–923. (Ref.112)

Davern TJ, et al. Measurement of serum acetaminophen-protein adducts in patients with acute liver failure. Gastroenterology 2006;130(3):687–694. (Ref.119)

Devlin J, et al. Pretransplantation clinical status and outcome of emergency transplantation for acute liver failure. Hepatology 1995;21(4):1018–1024. (Ref.172)

Ellis AJ, et al. Late-onset hepatic failure: clinical features, serology and outcome following transplantation. J Hepatol 1995;23(4):363–372. (Ref.5)

Ellis AJ, Wendon JA, Williams R. Subclinical seizure activity and prophylactic phenytoin infusion in acute liver failure: a controlled clinical trial. Hepatology 2000;32(3):536–541. (Ref.162)

Farmer DG, et al. Liver transplantation for fulminant hepatic failure: experience with more than 200 patients over a 17-year period. Ann Surg 2003;237(5):666–675. (Ref.168)

Gane E, et al. Clinical recurrence of hepatitis A following liver transplantation for acute liver failure. J Med Virol 1995;45(1):35–39. (Ref.16)

Hamid SS, et al. Fulminant hepatic failure in pregnant women: acute fatty liver or acute viral hepatitis? J Hepatol 1996;25(1):20–27. (Ref.63)

Hanau C, Munoz SJ, Rubin R. Histopathological heterogeneity in fulminant hepatic failure. Hepatology 1995;21(2):345–351. (Ref.187)

Harry R, Auzinger G, Wendon J. The clinical importance of adrenal insufficiency in acute hepatic dysfunction. Hepatology 2002;36(2):395–402. (Ref.141)

Hofer H, et al. Centrilobular necrosis in autoimmune hepatitis: a histological feature associated with acute clinical presentation. J Clin Pathol 2006;59(3):246–249. (Ref.68)

Ibdah JA, et al. A fetal fatty-acid oxidation disorder as a cause of liver disease in pregnant women. N Engl J Med 1999;340(22):1723–1731. (Ref.65)

Ichai P, et al. Herpes simplex virus-associated acute liver failure: a difficult diagnosis with a poor prognosis. Liver Transpl 2005;11(12):1550–1555. (Ref.34)

Ichai P, et al. Usefulness of corticosteroids for the treatment of severe and fulminant forms of autoimmune hepatitis. Liver Transpl 2007;13(7):996–1003. (Ref.69)

Ichai P, et al. Fulminant hepatitis after grand mal seizures: mechanisms and role of liver transplantation. Hepatology 2003;38(2):443–451. (Ref.71)

Iwai H, et al. Removal of endotoxin and cytokines by plasma exchange in patients with acute hepatic failure. Crit Care Med 1998;26(5):873–876. (Ref.85)

Izumi S, et al. Coagulation factor V levels as a prognostic indicator in fulminant hepatic failure. Hepatology 1996;23(6):1507–1511. (Ref.182)

Korman JD, et al. Screening for Wilson disease in acute liver failure: a comparison of currently available diagnostic tests. Hepatology 2008;48(4):1167–1174. (Ref.56)

Kumar M, et al. A randomized controlled trial of lamivudine to treat acute hepatitis B. Hepatology 2007;45(1):97–101. (Ref.129)

Lake JR, Sussman NL. Determining prognosis in patients with fulminant hepatic failure: when you absolutely, positively have to know the answer. Hepatology 1995;21(3):879–882. (Ref.175)

Larsen FS, et al. Functional loss of cerebral blood flow autoregulation in patients with fulminant hepatic failure. J Hepatol 1995;23(2):212–217. (Ref.109)

Larsen FS, Wendon J. Prevention and management of brain edema in patients with acute liver failure. Liver Transpl 2008;14 Suppl 2:S90–S96. (Ref.108)

Larson AM, et al. Acetaminophen-induced acute liver failure: results of a United States multicenter, prospective study. Hepatology 2005;42(6):1364–1372. (Ref.42)

Lee WM, et al. Intravenous N-acetylcysteine improves transplant-free survival in early stage non-acetaminophen acute liver failure. Gastroenterology 2009;137(3):856–864. (Ref.126)

Lee WM. Acute liver failure in the United States. Semin Liver Dis 2003;23(3):217–226. (Ref.6)

Lee WM. Etiologies of acute liver failure. Semin Liver Dis 2008;28(2):142–152. (Ref.166)

Leithead JA, et al. The systemic inflammatory response syndrome is predictive of renal dysfunction in patients with non-paracetamol-induced acute liver failure. Gut 2009;58(3):443–449. (Ref.93)

Liou IW, Larson AM. Role of liver transplantation in acute liver failure. Semin Liver Dis 2008;28(2):201–209. (Ref.165)

Losser MR, Payen D. Mechanisms of liver damage. Semin Liver Dis 1996;16(4):357–367. (Ref.77)

Mahler H, et al. Fulminant liver failure in association with the emetic toxin of Bacillus cereus. N Engl J Med 1997;336(16):1142–1148. (Ref.54)

Makin A, Williams R. Acetaminophen-induced acute liver failure. In: Lee WM, Williams R, editors. Acute liver failure, 1st ed. Cambridge, UK: Cambridge University Press, 1997: 32–42. (Ref.49)

Makin AJ, Wendon J, Williams R. A 7-year experience of severe acetaminophen-induced hepatotoxicity (1987-1993). Gastroenterology 1995;109(6):1907–1916. (Ref.121)

Makin AJ, Williams R. Acetaminophen-induced hepatotoxicity: predisposing factors and treatments. Adv Intern Med 1997;42:453–483. (Ref.122)

Manyike PT, et al. Contribution of CYP2E1 and CYP3A to acetaminophen reactive metabolite formation. Clin Pharmacol Ther 2000;67(3):275–282. (Ref.48)

McConnell JR, et al. Proton spectroscopy of brain glutamine in acute liver failure. Hepatology 1995;22(1):69–74. (Ref.113)

Mitchell I, et al. Earlier identification of patients at risk from acetaminophen-induced acute liver failure. Crit Care Med 1998;26(2):279–284. (Ref.180)

Moore K. Renal failure in acute liver failure. Eur J Gastroenterol Hepatol 1999;11(9):967–975. (Ref.92)

Munoz SJ, Stravitz RT, Gabriel DA. Coagulopathy of acute liver failure. Clin Liver Dis 2009;13(1):95–107. (Ref.97)

Murphy N, et al. The effect of hypertonic sodium chloride on intracranial pressure in patients with acute liver failure. Hepatology 2004;39(2):464–470. (Ref.155)

O'Grady J. Clinical disorders of renal function in acute liver failure. In: Gines P, Arroyo V, Rodes J, Schrier R, editors. Ascites and renal dysfunction in liver disease, 2nd ed. Malden, Mass: Blackwell, 2005: 383–393. (Ref.45)

Oldhafer KJ, et al. Rescue hepatectomy for initial graft non-function after liver transplantation. Transplantation 1999;67(7):1024–1028. (Ref.73)

Ostapowicz G, et al. Results of a prospective study of acute liver failure at 17 tertiary care centers in the United States. Ann Intern Med 2002;137(12):947–954. (Ref.167)

Oswiecimski P, et al. Profound hypocalcemia in fulminant hepatic failure. Am J Gastroenterol 2000;95(3):824–825. (Ref.131)

Pereira SP, Langley PG, Williams R. The management of abnormalities of hemostasis in acute liver failure. Semin Liver Dis 1996;16(4):403–414. (Ref.82)

Perry HE, Shannon MW. Efficacy of oral versus intravenous N-acetylcysteine in acetaminophen overdose: results of an open-label, clinical trial. J Pediatr 1998;132(1):149–152. (Ref.124)

Rolando N, et al. Granulocyte colony-stimulating factor improves function of neutrophils from patients with acute liver failure. Eur J Gastroenterol Hepatol 2000;12(10):1135–1140. (Ref.148)

Rolando N, Philpott-Howard J, Williams R. Bacterial and fungal infection in acute liver failure. Semin Liver Dis 1996;16(4):389–402. (Ref.103)

Rolando N, et al. The systemic inflammatory response syndrome in acute liver failure. Hepatology 2000;32(4 Pt 1):734–739. (Ref.91)

Rumack BH. Acetaminophen misconceptions. Hepatology 2004;40(1):10–15. (Ref.52)

Schiodt FV, et al. Etiology and outcome for 295 patients with acute liver failure in the United States. Liver Transpl Surg 1999;5(1):29–34. (Ref.58)

Schiodt FV, et al. Thrombopoietin in acute liver failure. Hepatology 2003;37(3):558–561. (Ref.100)

Schiodt FV, et al. Alpha-fetoprotein and prognosis in acute liver failure. Liver Transpl 2006;12(12):1776–1781. (Ref.188)

Schiodt FV, et al. Acetaminophen toxicity in an urban county hospital. N Engl J Med 1997;337(16):1112–1117. (Ref.50)

Schmidt LE, Dalhoff K. Serum phosphate is an early predictor of outcome in severe acetaminophen-induced hepatotoxicity. Hepatology 2002;36(3):659–665. (Ref.95)

Shakil AO, et al. Acute liver failure: clinical features, outcome analysis, and applicability of prognostic criteria. Liver Transpl 2000;6(2):163–169. (Ref.179)

Shami VM, et al. Recombinant activated factor VII for coagulopathy in fulminant hepatic failure compared with conventional therapy. Liver Transpl 2003;9(1):138–143. (Ref.137)

Shawcross DL, et al. Worsening of cerebral hyperemia by the administration of terlipressin in acute liver failure with severe encephalopathy. Hepatology 2004;39(2):471–475. (Ref.140)

Squires RH Jr. Acute liver failure in children. Semin Liver Dis 2008;28(2):153–166. (Ref.61)

Squires RH Jr, et al. Acute liver failure in children: the first 348 patients in the pediatric acute liver failure study group. J Pediatr 2006;148(5):652–658. (Ref.62)

Stedman C. Herbal hepatotoxicity. Semin Liver Dis 2002;22(2):195–206. (Ref.55)

Strauss G, et al. Hyperventilation restores cerebral blood flow autoregulation in patients with acute liver failure. J Hepatol 1998;28(2):199–203. (Ref.142)

Stravitz RT, et al. Intensive care of patients with acute liver failure: recommendations of the U.S. acute liver failure study group. Crit Care Med 2007;35(11):2498–2508. (Ref.125)

Stravitz RT, Kramer DJ. Management of acute liver failure. Nat Rev Gastroenterol Hepatol 2009;6(9):542–553. (Ref.46)

Stravitz RT, Larsen F. Therapeutic hypothermia for acute liver failure. Crit Care Med 2009;37:S258–S264. (Ref.161)

Stravitz RT, et al. Autoimmune acute liver failure: proposed clinical and histological criteria. Hepatology 2010 Nov. 18 (Epub ahead of print). (Ref.67)

Sze G, Kaplowitz N. Drug hepatotoxicity as a cause of acute liver failure. In: Lee WM, Williams R, editors. Acute liver failure, 1st ed. Cambridge, UK: Cambridge University Press, 1997: 19–31. (Ref.37)

Tofteng F, Larsen FS. The effect of indomethacin on intracranial pressure, cerebral perfusion and extracellular lactate and glutamate concentrations in patients with fulminant hepatic failure. J Cereb Blood Flow Metab 2004;24(7):798–804. (Ref.160)

Tripodi A, et al. Evidence of normal thrombin generation in cirrhosis despite abnormal conventional coagulation tests. Hepatology 2005;41(3):553–558. (Ref.96)

van Hoek B, et al. Auxiliary versus orthotopic liver transplantation for acute liver failure. EURALT study group. European Auxiliary Liver Transplant Registry. J Hepatol 1999;30(4):699–705. (Ref.174)

Vaquero J, et al. Pathogenesis of hepatic encephalopathy in acute liver failure. Semin Liver Dis 2003;23(3):259–269. (Ref.107)

Vaquero J, et al. Infection and the progression of hepatic encephalopathy in acute liver failure. Gastroenterology 2003;125(3):755–764. (Ref.151)

Vento S, et al. Fulminant hepatitis associated with hepatitis A virus superinfection in patients with chronic hepatitis C. N Engl J Med 1998;338(5):286–290. (Ref.15)

Wade JJ, et al. Bacterial and fungal infections after liver transplantation: an analysis of 284 patients. Hepatology 1995;21(5):1328–1336. (Ref.144)

Wijdicks EF, Nyberg SL. Propofol to control intracranial pressure in fulminant hepatic failure. Transplant Proc 2002;34(4):1220–1222. (Ref.157)

Williams AM, et al. Hyaluronic acid and endothelial damage due to paracetamol-induced hepatotoxicity. Liver Int 2003;23(2):110–115. (Ref.101)

Yamaguchi M, et al. Decreased protein C activation in patients with fulminant hepatic failure. Scand J Gastroenterol 2006;41(3):331–337. (Ref.102)

Zarrinpar A, et al. Liver transplantation for HELLP syndrome. Am Surg 2007;73(10):1013–1016. (Ref.66)

Zimmerman HJ, Maddrey WC. Acetaminophen (paracetamol) hepatotoxicity with regular intake of alcohol: analysis of instances of therapeutic misadventure. Hepatology 1995;22(3):767–773. (Ref.43)

Zimmerman HJ. Drug-induced liver disease. Clin Liver Dis 2000;4(1):73–96. (Ref.36)

Zimmerman HJ. In: Zimmerman HJ, editor. Hepatotoxicity. The adverse effects of drugs and other chemicals on the liver, 2nd ed. Philadelphia: Lippincott Williams & Wilkins, 1999. (Ref.35)

A complete list of references can be found at www.expertconsult.com.

Renal Failure in Cirrhosis, Hepatorenal Syndrome, and Hyponatremia

Arun J. Sanyal and Thomas D. Boyer

ABBREVIATIONS

AKI acute kidney injury
Akt serine/threonine protein kinase
Ang angiotensin
ATP adenosine triphosphate
cAMP cyclic adenosine monophosphate
CB cannabinoid
cGMP cyclic guanosine monophosphate
CNTs concentrative nucleoside transporters
CO carbon monoxide
eNOS endothelial nitric oxide synthetase
GFR glomerular filtration rate

HRS hepatorenal syndrome
H₂S hydrogen sulfide
HVPG hepatic venous pressure gradient
iNOS inducible nitric oxide synthetase
MDRD Modification of Diet in Renal Disease
MELD Model for End-Stage Liver Disease
NHE Na⁺/H⁺ exchanger
nNOS neuronal nitric oxide synthetase
NO nitric oxide
NSAIDs nonsteroidal antiinflammatory drugs

PGI₂ prostacyclin (prostaglandin I₂)
PTH parathyroid hormone
SBP spontaneous bacterial peritonitis
SLK simultaneous liver/kidney (transplantation)
TGF tubuloglomerular feedback (tubuloglomerular reflex)
TIPS transjugular intrahepatic portosystemic shunt
TNF tumor necrosis factor
VEGF vascular endothelial growth factor

Introduction

Hepatorenal syndrome (HRS) is a clinical condition characterized by the development of renal dysfunction in the absence of histologically obvious renal disease in patients with advanced liver disease (**Table 21-1**). The hallmarks of HRS include severe renal vasoconstriction, which decreases renal perfusion and the glomerular filtration rate (GFR) and thus causes renal dysfunction.[1] HRS develops in about 50% of subjects with cirrhosis and ascites and is often the harbinger of death.[2] Clinically, two forms of HRS with varying rates of progression of renal dysfunction are seen. Type 1 HRS progresses relatively rapidly and is usually associated with death without specific intervention, whereas type 2 HRS follows a more subacute to chronic course. HRS typically occurs in subjects with cirrhosis and ascites. The progression from cirrhosis with ascites to refractory ascites and HRS represents a pathophysiologic continuum that is driven by the presence of sinusoidal portal hypertension and severe systemic arterial vasodilation. Given the clinical significance of HRS, a clear understanding of its pathogenesis, clinical and diagnostic features, and treatment is a cornerstone of the management of cirrhosis.

Pathophysiology of Hepatorenal Syndrome

The pathophysiology of HRS is closely linked to the hemodynamic consequences of cirrhosis with sinusoidal portal hypertension and the ability of the heart and kidneys to compensate for these changes (**Fig. 21-1**). It is therefore germane to review these changes and their impact on renal function.

Sinusoidal Portal Hypertension and Its Role in Development of Hepatorenal Syndrome

It has been appreciated for many years that HRS typically develops in patients with cirrhosis and ascites. Ascites caused by peritoneal infections and tumors is not associated with HRS. In addition, HRS is rarely if ever seen in subjects with cirrhosis who do not have ascites. The development of ascites in patients with cirrhosis requires the presence of clinically significant portal hypertension.[1] Normal portal venous pressure, as measured by the hepatic venous pressure gradient

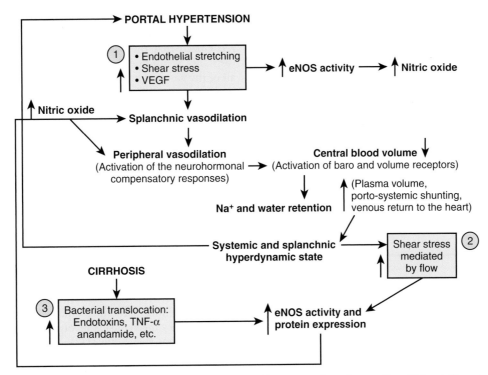

Fig. 21-1 **Overview of the pathophysiology of portal hypertension and hepatorenal syndrome.** Sinusoidal portal hypertension leads to shear stress and endothelial activation in the splanchnic vascular bed, thereby resulting in splanchnic arteriolar dilation. Simultaneously, increased gut permeability because of congestion of the intestines from increased portal venous backpressure causes increased bacterial translocation, which results in a systemic inflammatory state and further worsening of arteriolar dilation. These actions decrease the effective circulating volume and result in the activation of renal Na and water-retentive mechanisms. When renal autoregulation fails to maintain the glomerular filtration rate, renal function declines. eNOS, endothelial nitric oxide synthase; TNF-α, tumor necrosis factor-α; VEGF, vascular endothelial growth factor. *(With permission from Iwakiri Y, Groszmann RJ. The hyperdynamic circulation of chronic liver diseases: from the patient to the molecule. Hepatology 2006;43(2 Suppl 1):S121–S131.)*

Table 21-1 Definition of Hepatorenal Syndrome

Cirrhosis with ascites
Serum creatinine >1.5 mg/dl (133 µmol/L)
No improvement in serum creatinine (<1.5 mg/dl) after at least 2 days of diuretic withdrawal and volume expansion with albumin (1 g/kg)
Absence of shock
No current or recent treatment with nephrotoxic drugs
No proteinuria (<500 mg/day), microhematuria (>50 red blood cells per high-power field), and normal renal ultrasound findings

From Salerno F, et al. Diagnosis, prevention and treatment of hepatorenal syndrome in cirrhosis. Gut 2007;56:1310–1318.

(HVPG), is 5 mm Hg or less. Ascites and varices do not develop until the HVPG rises to levels greater than 10 to 12 mm Hg.[3]

The development of sinusoidal portal hypertension in those with cirrhosis is a function of architectural disruption of the normal hepatic microvasculature and functional changes in sinusoidal blood flow on one hand and increased inflow into the portal vein because of dilation of arterioles in the splanchnic vascular bed on the other.[4] Structural disruption of the hepatic microvasculature begins with the development of advanced fibrosis (bridging fibrosis) in subjects with chronic liver disease and is part and parcel of the vascular remodeling that occurs concomitantly with the progression to cirrhosis.

For the past decade it has been well recognized that the hepatic microcirculation is not simply a passive conduit for blood flow but is actively regulated locally. Regulation of the hepatic microcirculation has been reviewed in depth elsewhere[5,6] and is beyond the scope of this chapter. Briefly, about 30% of the vascular resistance to flow through the liver is determined by a balance between vasoconstrictive and vasodilatory factors that regulate sinusoidal blood flow. Hepatic stellate cells, which wrap themselves around the hepatic sinusoids, play a key role in this process via their contractile properties, which allow them to constrict or dilate the sinusoids.[7] Normally, nitric oxide (NO), a potent vasodilatory molecule, is a key regulator of sinusoidal vascular resistance (**Table 21-2**).[7] Release of NO into the sinusoidal vasculature has recently been shown to be linked to the enterohepatic circulation of bile acids, which activate NO synthesis by endothelial nitric oxide synthetase (eNOS) via specific G protein–coupled (TGR5) receptors.[8] eNOS activity is also affected by circulating high-density lipoproteins.[9,10] In subjects with cirrhosis, several mechanisms leading to impaired eNOS activation have been identified, including impairment of serine/threonine protein kinase (Akt)-dependent phosphorylation of eNOS, which is partially reversible by statins; increased caveolin expression, particularly in cholestatic states; and deficiency of tetrahydrobiopterin.[7,11,12] The availability of NO may be further impaired by its utilization for nitrosylation reactions driven by oxidative stress and increased phosphodiesterase activity. Other factors that have been implicated in intrahepatic vasoconstriction include increased endothelin activity,

Table 21-2 Mechanisms of Sinusoidal Portal Hypertension

Increased Intrahepatic Resistance

Fixed architectural disruption
Dynamic modulation of intrahepatic resistance to flow
   Decreased NO production by sinusoidal endothelial cells
   Increased thromboxanes

Increased Splanchnic Arteriolar Vasodilation

Increased NO
Increased CO
Increased prostacyclins
Increased endogenous cannabinoids
Cytokines that promote vasodilation, such as tumor necrosis
   factor-α
VEGF
Adrenomedullin

CO, carbon monoxide; NO, nitric oxide; VEGF, vascular endothelial growth factor

enhanced angiotensinogen activation or sensitivity, and increased thromboxane A_2 and leukotriene production.[13] These factors may be counteracted by increased vasodilatory NO and carbon monoxide (CO) production.[14] The role of adrenergic tone, endotoxemia, and inflammatory cytokines is currently under investigation. It is hoped that improved understanding of the dynamic regulation of sinusoidal blood flow in patients with cirrhosis will provide novel "druggable" targets for the correction of sinusoidal portal hypertension and prevention, as well as treatment of its consequences, including HRS.

Sinusoidal portal hypertension contributes to the pathophysiologic cascade that leads to the development of ascites and eventually HRS in several ways. It is linked to the systemic arterial vasodilatory state, which in turn has several downstream effects that contribute to Na and water retention initially and renal dysfunction in later stages. Sinusoidal hypertension also directly leads to increased renal sympathetic nervous system activity, which causes renal vasoconstriction and thus diminishes renal perfusion.[15] Furthermore, portal vein distention as a result of sinusoidal portal hypertension also contributes to increased renal sympathetic nerve activation.[16]

It has been shown that thoracic duct constriction, which increases sinusoidal pressure, increases renal efferent sympathetic nerve activity.[17,18] These effects are mediated by hepatic baroreceptors, which increase hepatic afferent nerve activity, rather than by volume receptors.[18,19] The renal hemodynamic effects are further affected by the specific nerve bundles activated.[20] There are also osmoreceptors and volume receptors within the liver that can modulate renal hemodynamics via hepatic humoral responses.[21] Section of the hepatic afferents to the vagus nerve does not affect these responses.

The Systemic Hemodynamic Response to Sinusoidal Portal Hypertension

The hallmark of the cirrhotic state is systemic arterial vasodilation. It has long been recognized that subjects with cirrhosis and advanced liver failure have a hyperdynamic circulation

characterized by a marked decrease in systemic vascular resistance and an increase in cardiac output.[13,22,23] It is further recognized that the observed decrease in systemic vascular resistance is not due to an equal decrease in the resistance of all of the vascular beds and that there are differential changes in different vascular beds. For example, femoral and brachial artery flow is not significantly altered in subjects with cirrhosis, whereas there is profound dilation in the splanchnic arterial circulation. This has been verified experimentally by both direct measurements and measurement of the resistive index of the superior mesenteric artery via sonographic methods.[24] Thus splanchnic arterial dilation with relative sequestration of the circulating blood volume within the splanchnic bed is a major hemodynamic consequence of cirrhosis.

Drivers of Systemic Arterial Vasodilation

Several neurohumoral mechanisms have been found to be activated in subjects with cirrhosis and contribute to the state of systemic arterial vasodilation. The humoral mechanisms act via systemic, paracrine, and autocrine pathways (**Fig. 21-2**). The key mechanisms involved are discussed in the following sections (see **Table 21-2**).

The Nitric Oxide Pathway

Nitric oxide is an endothelium-derived factor with potent vasodilatory properties. It activates soluble guanylate cyclase, thereby increasing cyclic guanosine monophosphate (cGMP), which causes smooth muscle relaxation.[25] Three isoforms of nitric oxide synthetase (NOS) are involved in the production of NO. Endothelial NOS (eNOS) is constitutively expressed and is the principal source of excess NO in the splanchnic vascular bed.[26] Inducible NOS (iNOS) is expressed in a variety of cell types, including macrophages and vascular smooth muscle cells. It can be induced by a number of cytokines, such as tumor necrosis factor-α (TNF-α) or bacterial lipopolysaccharide (endotoxin).[5,13] Surprisingly, despite increased endotoxemia, iNOS activity is not increased in the splanchnic arteries of cirrhotic animals.[27] Increased iNOS expression has, however, been reported in the aortic rings in animal models of cirrhosis.[28] The third form of NOS is neuronal NOS (nNOS). It has also been shown to be up-regulated in neurons and vascular smooth muscle in the superior mesenteric artery in models of cirrhosis.[29] Of these isoforms, increased eNOS activity is considered to be the dominant form that contributes to the splanchnic arterial vasodilation and hyperdynamic circulation seen in cirrhotics.

There are several mechanisms by which eNOS activity is increased in patients with cirrhosis. Expression of eNOS itself is regulated by several posttranslational modifications, including phosphorylation and S-nitrosylation.[30,31] eNOS synthesis is Ca^{2+}/calmodulin dependent and requires tetrahydrobiopterin as a co-factor. The increased endotoxemia in cirrhotics generates tetrahydrobiopterin, which is associated with enhanced eNOS activity.[32] Moreover, increased portal pressure causes shear stress, which induces Akt/protein kinase B and thus activates eNOS.[33] This may be particularly important in the early stages of arterial vasodilation in the splanchnic circulation. Vascular endothelial growth factor (VEGF) is yet another cytokine that activates Akt and thus eNOS.[34] VEGF signaling is currently under evaluation as a potential therapeutic target in

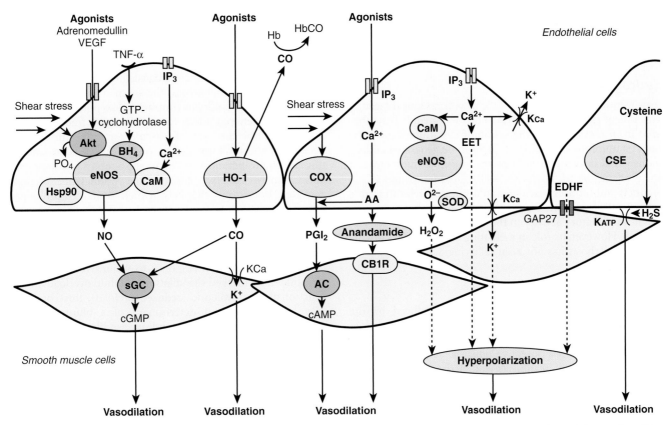

Fig. 21-2 Factors modulating endothelial dysfunction and arteriolar dilation in subjects with cirrhosis. A variety of metabolites and cytokines act in an endocrine, paracrine, and autocrine manner to promote arteriolar dilation in the splanchnic and other systemic arterial beds. In the arterial splanchnic circulation *(right panel)*, agonists such as adrenomedullin, vascular endothelial growth factor (VEGF), and tumor necrosis factor-α (TNF-α) or physical stimuli such as shear stress stimulate Akt, which directly phosphorylates and activates endothelial nitric oxide (NO) synthase (eNOS). eNOS is calcium (Ca^{2+})/calmodulin (CaM) dependent and requires co-factors such as tetrahydrobiopterin (BH_4) for its activity. Heat shock protein 90 (Hsp90) is one of the positive regulators of eNOS. In the intrahepatic circulation *(central panel)*, decreased NO and increased thromboxane A_2 (TXA_2) production in sinusoidal endothelial cells causes vasoconstriction by removing the normal vasodilatory effects of NO. This is compounded by the direct constrictive effects of endothelin-1 (ET-1) in cirrhosis. AA, anachidonic acid; AC, adenyl cyclase; cAMP, cyclic adenosine monophosphate; cGMP, cyclic guanosine monophosphate; CO, carbon monoxide; COX, cyclooxygenase; CSE, cystathionine-y-lyase; EDHF, endothelium-derived hyperpolarizing factor; EET, epoxyeicosatrienoic acid; GTP, guanosine triphosphate; HO-1, heme oxygenase-1; IP_3, inositol triphosphate; PGI_2, prostaglandin I_2 (prostacyclin); sGC, soluble guanylate cyclase; SOD, superoxide dismutase. *(With permission from Iwakiri Y, Groszmann RJ. Vascular endothelial dysfunction in cirrhosis. J Hepatol 2007;46:927–934.)*

patients with cirrhosis and portal hypertension. Activation of Akt can also result from the actions of adrenomedullin, levels of which are increased in patients with cirrhosis.[13] Finally, it has recently been shown that the subcellular localization of eNOS profoundly affects its function. It is normally located mainly in the perinuclear region and within the Golgi apparatus[35]; activation of eNOS is associated with transport of it to a more cytoplasmic location in proximity to the plasma membrane.[36] Palmitoylation of eNOS is important for this process and underscores the impact of the metabolic changes in cirrhosis as a determinant of the hemodynamic responses to this condition.[37]

Carbon Monoxide

Carbon monoxide is the end product of the heme oxygenase pathway and also causes vasodilation. Heme oxygenase catalyzes the conversion of heme to biliverdin and releases CO in the process.[13] It exists in a constitutive and inducible form. Inducible heme oxygenase-1, also known as heat shock protein-32, is up-regulated in the systemic and splanchnic

circulation in subjects with cirrhosis.[38] CO also increases cGMP and synergizes with NO to produce splanchnic arterial vasodilation.

Endocannabinoids

Endocannabinoids are endogenous ligands for the cannabinoid (CB) receptors. CB1 receptors have been identified in the splanchnic circulation and in the liver vasculature.[39] Binding of appropriate ligands to these receptors produces severe vascular smooth muscle relaxation and vasodilation.[40] The endogenous ligands for these receptors are derived from membrane phospholipids, and anandamide is considered to be the prototypic ligand for CB1 receptors, where it functions as an inverse agonist. Anandamide production is enhanced in circulating macrophages and platelets in subjects with cirrhosis.[41] Infusion of *met*-anandamide, a long-acting analogue of anandamide, produces marked splanchnic arterial vasodilation and induces a hyperdynamic circulation characterized by decreased systemic vascular resistance and increased cardiac output.[40] In animal models of cirrhosis, infusion of a CB1 receptor antagonist increases systemic vascular resistance and arterial blood pressure and corrects several features of the hyperdynamic circulation that is present.[41]

Hydrogen Sulfide

Hydrogen sulfide (H_2S) is one of the newest gaseous molecules with potent signaling properties to be identified. It is synthesized from L-cysteine via the action of cystathionine-β-lyase and cystathionine-β-synthase.[42] H_2S can be generated endogenously and is also produced by the intestinal microbiota. It opens adenosine triphosphate (ATP)-gated potassium (K_{ATP}) channels and induces vascular smooth muscle relaxation in a non–cGMP-dependent manner.[43] It has been shown to have potent vasodilatory activity in the splanchnic and hepatic circulation. However, its role in mediating the circulatory disturbances in cirrhosis has not been fully elucidated.

Prostacyclins

These cyclooxygenase-derived lipids are produced by the metabolism of polyunsaturated fatty acids. Prostacyclin (prostaglandin I_2 [PGI_2]) increases cyclic adenosine monophosphate (cAMP) and is a potent vasodilator.[44] Circulating levels of PGI_2 are increased in subjects with cirrhosis.

Endothelium-Derived Hyperpolarizing Factor

There are other endothelium-derived factors that also cause hyperpolarization of vascular smooth muscle cell membranes and prevent contraction that have yet to be characterized. Current candidates for this factor include other arachidonic acid–derived factors, potassium itself, gap junction–associated proteins, and hydrogen peroxide.[13]

Tumor Necrosis Factor-α

This key cytokine is produced by cells of the innate immune system, especially macrophages, in response to a variety of activators such as endotoxin and free fatty acids. It activates iNOS, and by increasing the synthesis of tetrahydrobiopterin, it increases the synthesis of eNOS. TNF-α promotes vasodilation, and inhibition of TNF-α blunts the hyperdynamic circulation in models of cirrhosis.[45,46]

Endothelial Dysfunction and Systemic Arterial Vasodilation in Cirrhosis

It is now recognized that the vascular endothelium and its derived factors play a key role in the regulation of vascular tone in various circulatory beds. There is substantial evidence that endothelial dysfunction plays an important role in genesis of the systemic vasodilated state in patients with cirrhosis.[5] This is reflected by increased levels of circulating asymmetric dimethyl arginine.

The Cardiovascular Response to Systemic Arterial Vasodilation
Altered Arterial Compliance and Afterload

The arterial vasodilation in subjects with cirrhosis produces immediate functional changes in the vasculature and in the

long term induces vascular remodeling that also alters arterial compliance and the functional characteristics of the systemic arterial vasculature. In animal models of cirrhosis, it was observed that the conductive vessels undergo an intense process of vascular remodeling consisting of a decrease in the thickness and the total area of the vascular wall and a reduction in the vessels' ability to contract.[47] Two potential explanations have been put forth to explain these findings: (1) a decrease in the amount of vascular smooth muscle cells because of the inhibitory effect of NO on vascular smooth muscle cell proliferation and increased apoptosis of these cells and (2) increased expression of large-conductance calcium-activated potassium channels, which leads to prolonged hyperpolarization of vascular smooth muscle.[48] These changes are partially reversible and closely associated with the arterial vasodilation that is present. Arterial compliance is an important determinant of afterload because the heart autoregulates cardiac performance in response to venous return. Because cirrhotics have marked vasodilation and fluid overload but are functionally hypovolemic (reduced preload), this condition may be an important determinant of a blunted cardiac response to severe and long-standing vasodilation, which may trigger HRS.

Volume Expansion

An important consequence of arterial vasodilation is an increase in total blood volume. Blood volume tends to increase as early as in pre-ascitic cirrhosis.[49,50] It is related to renal Na and water retention. This excess blood volume is not distributed uniformly throughout the body and is largely accounted for by the increased vascular space in the splanchnic circulatory bed as a result of splanchnic arterial vasodilation.[51,52] In fact, the distribution of blood volume is decreased in the heart, lung, and central arterial tree, whereas it is increased in the abdomen, liver, and spleen. This leads to a state of effective hypovolemia, and despite the hypervolemia, there is activation of central volume receptors and baroreceptors that trigger Na-retentive pathways in subjects with progressive cirrhosis and ascites.

The Cardiac Response and the Role of Cirrhotic Cardiomyopathy

In the early phases of cirrhosis, the decrease in systemic vascular resistance is compensated by the increase in heart rate and cardiac output (hyperdynamic circulation).[53,54] Such compensation allows maintenance of renal perfusion and the GFR. However, as the disease state progresses with increasing peripheral arterial vasodilation, the cardiac response to the vasodilation is blunted and there is a modest drop in cardiac output (**Table 21-3**). This hyporesponsiveness of the myocardium is also referred to as cirrhotic cardiomyopathy and is discussed in depth elsewhere.[54] Cirrhotic cardiomyopathy is characterized by "chronic cardiac dysfunction in patients with cirrhosis characterized by blunted contractile responsiveness to stress and/or altered diastolic relaxation with electrophysiologic abnormalities, in the absence of known cardiac disease."[54]

Initially, a hyperdynamic circulation may appear or is enhanced in the supine position because of translocation of volume to the central circulation and concomitant arterial

Table 21-3 Key Features of Cardiac Dysfunction in Patients with Cirrhosis
Physiologic
Blunted cardiac response to stress
Diastolic dysfunction
Systolic dysfunction
Electrophysiologic
Prolonged QT interval
Impaired excitation-contraction coupling
Echocardiographic
E/A ≤1
Prolonged deceleration time (>200 ms)
Prolonged isovolumetric relaxation (>80 ms)
Decrease in resting ejection fraction with severity
Prolongation of the ratio of preejection to left ventricular ejection time (>0.44 s, rate corrected)

E/A, early-to-late diastolic filling ratio

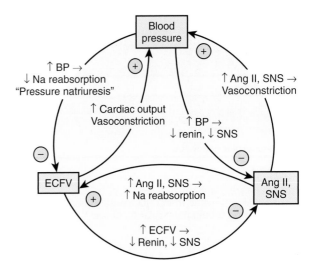

Fig. 21-3 Feedback relationship between blood pressure (BP), angiotensin II (Ang II), the sympathetic nervous system (SNS), and extracellular fluid volume (ECFV). *(With permission from McDonough et al. Am J Physiol Renal Physiol 2007;292:F1105-F1123.)*

hyporesponsiveness to physiologic vasoconstrictors.[55] Subsequently, autonomic dysfunction contributes to the myocardial hyporeactivity to precipitants of the hyperdynamic circulatory state.[56,57] These impair normal baroreceptor reflexes in response to arterial vasodilation and thus lead to blunting of the cardiac response. The autonomic dysfunction along with the altered cytokine milieu and abnormal electrolytes contributes to electrophysiologic abnormalities, electrical-mechanical dyssynchrony, and inotropic and chronotropic incompetence, all of which contribute to the blunted cardiac response to vasodilation in patients with advanced cirrhosis, liver failure, and ascites. A key consequence of this worsening of the effective hypovolemia is intense activation of renal Na- and water-retentive pathways, such as renal sympathetic nerve activity, plasma renin, angiotensin, aldosterone, and antidiuretic hormone.

The Renal Response to the Hemodynamic Changes in Advanced Cirrhosis

The key consequence of the systemic hemodynamic changes for the kidney is an alteration in renal perfusion and the GFR. This is accompanied by an inability to excrete Na and water.[2] These changes represent one extreme of a pathophysiologic cascade of events that start as early as the pre-ascitic stage of cirrhosis and progress through the clinical stages of ascites, refractory ascites, type 2 HRS, and finally type 1 HRS.

Changes in Renal Perfusion

The kidney is composed of the cortical region, which is enriched with glomeruli and renal tubules, and the medulla, which is enriched with loops of Henle and collecting ducts. Blood flow in the kidneys is closely regulated by intrarenal mechanisms to maintain effective renal perfusion (mean arterial pressure [MAP] – inferior vena cava pressure). Thus, over a substantial range of renal perfusion pressure, renal blood

flow remains relatively unchanged. This autoregulation is maintained by a number of intrarenal pathways, of which prostaglandins play an important role. In addition to overall renal perfusion, a balance between cortical and medullary flow is also maintained to protect renal function.

The GFR is a function of glomerular perfusion pressure, the glomerular surface available for filtration, and the permeability characteristics of the glomerulus. Glomerular perfusion pressure is determined by the balance in arterial tone of the afferent arteriole, which brings blood into the glomerulus, and the efferent arteriole, which drains the glomeruli. These arterioles act as a buffer between systemic renal perfusion pressure (i.e., MAP) and actual glomerular perfusion. This buffer allows renal filtration of plasma to proceed relatively unimpeded despite fluctuations in systemic blood pressure. This is critically important for both Na homeostasis and survival. Because changes in GFR are a major abnormality that drives the development of HRS, it is germane to review some key aspects of its regulation.

Mechanisms of Autoregulation of Renal Blood Flow and Hepatorenal Syndrome

Renal blood flow is regulated at two levels: (1) systemic factors, which include MAP, sympathetic nervous system output to the kidneys, and humoral factors such as renin-angiotensin and catecholamines, and (2) intrarenal factors, which can be further broadly categorized as myogenic responses and tubuloglomerular feedback (TGF) (**Fig. 21-3 and Table 21-4**).[58] In subjects with cirrhosis and profound systemic arterial vasodilation, MAP is reduced and there is activation of renal sympathetic nerve outflow and circulating renin-angiotensin and catecholamines. The renal sympathetic nerves and circulating angiotensin tend to induce renal arteriolar constriction at the efferent arteriolar level and thus preserve glomerular filtration. However, when HRS sets in, afferent arteriolar constriction occurs and the GFR drops.[59,60] The afferent arterioles are

Table 21-4 Factors Involved in Autoregulation of the Glomerular Filtration Rate

Myogenic Tone

Basal tone
Response to stretch (myogenic reactivity)
Postconstrictive dilation

Tubuloglomerular Feedback

Macula densa:
  Adenosine
  Adenosine triphosphate
  Nitric oxide (NO) of neuronal NO synthetase origin
Factors affecting tubuloglomerular feedback:
  Angiotensin
  Interleukin-6
  Prostaglandins
  Na intake
  Na$^+$ and Cl$^-$ content of tubular fluid

particularly sensitive to the intrarenal pathways, which are considered in the following sections.

MYOGENIC MECHANISMS

It is known that small arteries, specifically those with a relaxed internal diameter smaller than 300 µm, respond to changes in perfusion pressure independent of neurohumoral influences.[61] This is called the myogenic reflex and is mediated by mechanoreceptors that sense stretch and changes in blood vessel wall tension.[62] These receptors are analogous to those found elsewhere in the body, including the gastrointestinal tract and the acid-sensitive anion channels. In the kidney, the myogenic reflex has been shown to provide a fast autoregulatory response to rapid changes in perfusion pressure and is not dependent on tubular function. Mechanotransduction of changes in wall tension leads to depolarization of the cell membrane of vascular smooth muscle cells and activation of L-type calcium channels.[63]

The cellular events that regulate smooth muscle arterial tone and contractility are well known and beyond the scope of this chapter, and the reader is referred to several excellent reviews of the subject.[64,65] Briefly, calcium influx as a result of the opening of L-type calcium channels on the plasma membrane causes Ca^{2+}/calmodulin–mediated phosphorylation of myosin light chain kinase, thus increasing actin-myosin cross-linkage and contraction. These contractile responses are countered by independently regulated relaxant pathways, including the constitutively activated myosin light chain phosphatase, which is regulated by phosphorylation by rho kinase.[58,66,67] The key point is that renal arteriolar contraction and relaxation are both active processes and are independently regulated. Unfortunately, despite the highly characterized information on the cellular mechanisms regulating renal arteriolar tone and contractility, there is a paucity of knowledge regarding changes in these pathways in patients with cirrhosis and HRS.

In persons with a consistent and long-term change in renal perfusion, additional myogenic adaptive mechanisms come into play.[58] In the first phase, myogenic tone is reset. This is associated with changes in membrane potential and

intracellular calcium fluxes via L-type voltage-gated calcium channels. In the second phase, sensitization of the intracellular pathways to a given calcium level occurs and results in enhanced constriction when perfusion pressure is consistently increased. It is unclear whether a consistent decrease in MAP, as seen in cirrhosis, would result in desensitization to intracellular calcium. Finally, remodeling of blood vessels takes place. In the hypertensive state, which has been studied extensively, two forms of remodeling are seen: an increase in wall thickness with either a reduction in the lumen (eutrophic remodeling) or preservation of the lumen (hypertrophic remodeling).[58,61,68,69] Once again, virtually nothing is known about the cellular changes in the renal afferent and efferent arterioles in subjects with cirrhosis, and this remains an area begging to be studied.

TUBULOGLOMERULAR REFLEX

Tubuloglomerular reflex provides another mechanism for the kidney to adapt to more long-term changes in renal perfusion pressure. The anatomic basis for this mechanism involves the thick ascending limb of the loop of Henle and the distal tubule, which loop back and make contact with the upstream glomerulus, specifically the afferent arteriole (**Fig. 21-4**). This juxtaglomerular apparatus is composed of the macula densa, which mediates cross-talk between the luminal contents in the distal tubule and the afferent arteriole. Increased Na content in the distal tubule enhances afferent arteriolar constriction and reduces the GFR, whereas decreased Na content relaxes the afferent arteriole and enhances the GFR.[70] It has also been suggested that the macula densa senses the osmolality of the distal tubule luminal contents.

Purinergic Regulation of Tubuloglomerular Feedback Reflex

The macula densa mediates afferent arteriolar constriction by the release of adenosine, which acts via adenosine-1 receptors.[71] Adenosine-1 receptors mediate vasoconstriction by G protein–coupled receptors. There is synergy between the vasoconstrictive effects of adenosine and angiotensin II (Ang II),[72] which is likely to be related to activation of phospholipase C and mobilization of intracellular calcium.[72] Recently, ATP was also shown to be an important mediator of the vasoconstrictive effects of the macula densa. ATP receptors (P2 purinergic receptors) of both the P2X and P2Y class have been found in renal afferent arterioles.[73] Adenosine and ATP have been shown to be present in the interstitial fluid of the kidney. There is, however, some controversy as to whether the adenosine is produced intracellularly and then transported by concentrative nucleoside transporters (CNTs) or whether it is produced by cleavage of phosphates from ATP in the interstitium by ecto-ATPases. It is highly likely that dysregulated TGF plays a role in the profound renal vasoconstriction and decreased GFR in patients with HRS. Once again, there is unfortunately a marked paucity of direct experimental evidence of this.

Nitric Oxide and Regulation of Tubuloglomerular Feedback

There are high levels of nNOS in the macula densa.[74,75] NO mediates vasorelaxation in response to decreased tubular Na content. Subjects given NOS inhibitors as well as nNOS knockout mice are unable to mount this response. It is not

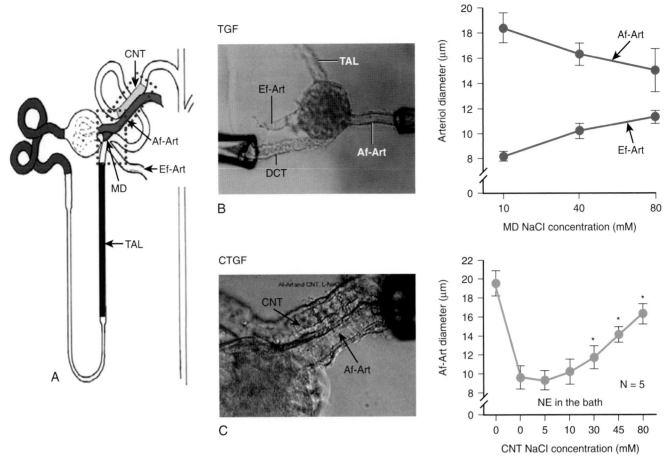

Fig. 21-4 **Cross-talk between tubule and arteriole. A,** Schematic representation of the relationship of the nephron to the vasculature. **B,** Microperfusion of a microdissected rabbit afferent arteriole (Af-Art) and macula densa (MD) shown on the left and the effects of varying tubular concentrations of Na on Af-Art or the efferent arteriole (Ef-Art). **C,** Microperfusion of microdissected rabbit Af-Art with attached connecting duct (CNT), as shown on the left, reveals the effects of connecting duct Na concentration on Af-Art. CTGF, connecting tubule glomerular feedback; DCT, distal convoluted tubule; NE, norepinepherine; TAL, thick ascending limb; TGF, tubuloglomerular feedback. *(With permission from Ren Y, Garvin JL, Liu R, Carretero OA. Cross-talk between arterioles and tubules in the kidney. Pediatr Nephrol 2009;24:31–35.)*

known whether there is a paucity of macula densa NOS activity in patients with cirrhosis and whether this plays a role in the genesis of afferent arteriolar vasoconstriction in those with HRS.

Other Mediators of Tubuloglomerular Feedback

The angiotensin system is a key mediator of TGF and modulates the sensitivity of TGF to various stimuli. It also modulates the myogenic response to changes in perfusion pressure. Renal production of various prostaglandin derivatives, especially 20-hydroxyeicosatetraenoic acid, also plays an important role in the regulation of renal blood flow.[76,77] Recently, it has been shown that there is cross-talk between the intestine and the kidney, where osmolality and the nutritional and Na content of the intestinal lumen affect changes in renal blood flow.[78] This has been particularly characterized with respect to calcium and phosphate content and with changes in parathyroid hormone (PTH) levels, which also alter renal blood flow.[79] This may be relevant in patients with HRS once renal insufficiency develops.

The Connecting Tubule and the Tubuloglomerular Reflex

The portion of the nephron that connects the distal tubule to the collecting duct is often referred to as the connecting tubule.[80] This segment is also in apposition to the afferent arteriole and affects afferent arteriolar tone. Interestingly, in contrast to classic TGF, increased Na content in this segment results in arteriolar dilation and increased GFR.[81,82] The role of this phenomenon and pathway remains completely unexplored in HRS.

Renal Tubular Dysfunction and Hepatorenal Syndrome

A key pathophysiologic hallmark of HRS is renal Na reabsorption. There is avid Na reabsorption in the proximal tubules, which results in the delivery of a low volume of isotonic filtrate into the loop of Henle.[83] The bulk of the Na reabsorption, as in the normal state, occurs in the proximal tubule. Three sets of transporters play an important role in this process. The first is the Na^+/H^+ exchanger (NHE); of the various isoforms,

NHE3 is expressed in the greatest abundance in the proximal tubule and is an important mediator of Na and bicarbonate reabsorption. The Na^+-phosphate cotransporter-2 helps reabsorb Na, phosphate, glucose, and amino acids. Aquaporin receptors are involved in the water transport that accompanies Na and solute transport.[84] Several isoforms have been described, and renal aquaporin 2 (AQP2) is decreased in patients with cirrhosis. AQP1 levels in urine are decreased in those with type 1 HRS.[84]

These transporters are regulated by both circulating cytokines and hormones, as well as by paracrine factors.[85] Conditions associated with decreased Na reabsorption involve retrieval of these transporters from the cell surface into the cytoplasm, which is regulated by several transport proteins and cellular trafficking pathways. These pathways are also sensitive to intracellular calcium, and PTH is an important regulator of this process. The renin-angiotensin system is the most important intrarenal mechanism for the regulation of proximal tubular function.

The Intrarenal Renin-Angiotensin System

The role of the renin-angiotensin system in Na and volume homeostasis has been recognized for many decades. Ang II is the most studied and one of the most biologically active angiotensins. Ang II directly causes smooth muscle contraction, enhances myocardial contractility, stimulates release of catecholamines from the adrenal medulla, and stimulates thirst. The systemic increase in levels of Ang II thus has several effects that have a direct impact on the pathophysiology of HRS.

The kidney has specific mechanisms for the intrarenal production of Ang II, where it acts in a paracrine manner and modulates renal function (**Table 21-5**).[86] All of the components of the renin-angiotensin system are present in the kidney. Intrarenal concentrations of Ang II are often higher than those in circulation and are regulated independently from systemic Ang II. Historically, the site of action of Ang II has been considered to be the efferent arteriole. However, it is now known to constrict both afferent and efferent arterioles.[87] Ang II is also a modulator of the sensitivity of the response arm of TGF and the myogenic responses to changes in renal perfusion. In addition, Ang II is a powerful stimulator of renal Na reabsorption. This is mediated by aldosterone production, which enhances distal tubular Na^+/H^+ exchange. In fact, the major effect of Ang II on Na homeostasis is due to increased tubular reabsorption rather than a change in GFR. Ang II also directly enhances proximal tubular Na reabsorption. Although the role of circulating Ang II in the pathogenesis of HRS has been recognized for many decades,[50,88] the role of the intrarenal renin-angiotensin system remains relatively unexplored. Recently, it has been proposed that the I/I allele of Ang II rather than the I/D or D/D alleles increases susceptibility to HRS.[89]

Failure to Regulate the Glomerular Filtration Rate and the Development of Hepatorenal Syndrome

The pathophysiologic hallmark of HRS is a decrease in GFR with consequent enhancement of Na and water reabsorption. The drop in GFR is clearly associated with altered renal autoregulation of blood flow, with the flow-to-MAP relationship being shifted to the right.[90] Thus, with smaller changes in MAP, there are changes in renal perfusion and GFR. Moreover, the drop in MAP further contributes to the drop in GFR. Unfortunately, even though much is now known about the mechanisms of renal blood flow autoregulation, the specific changes in these pathways in cirrhotics and how they contribute to the observed decrease in GFR remain to be defined.

Hepatorenal Syndrome and the Systemic Inflammatory State

It is recognized that HRS is associated with high mortality. This mortality, however, is not a simple function of azotemia because dialysis does not consistently prolong life in such cases. On the other hand, HRS is often associated with development of multiorgan failure as a preterminal event. At this stage, sepsis is also frequently present. These observations have led to emergence of the concept that HRS may represent one aspect of a systemic disturbance that leads to HRS as its renal manifestation and multiorgan failure in its full-blown form.[91,92] Recently, it has been shown that a systemic inflammatory response state is often present in subjects with HRS.[92] The systemic inflammatory state affects organ function by altering the microcirculation and is associated with widespread endothelial dysfunction. These effects worsen the hemodynamics that drives HRS. In addition, the proinflammatory cytokine milieu associated with the systemic inflammatory response affects renal endothelial, vascular, mesangial, and tubular function, thus further contributing another layer of complexity to the pathophysiology of HRS.[93,94] The inflammatory state resolves after liver transplantation.[95]

The Intestinal Microbiome and Gut-Derived Infections and Hepatorenal Syndrome

Spontaneous bacterial peritonitis (SBP) is a well-known precipitant of HRS. SBP is usually caused by gut-derived bacteria. The human intestine contains more than 100 trillion microorganisms representing thousands of species.[96] It is now known that more than 70% of the species in the intestine cannot be cultured by traditional methods.[97] There is also both an axial and radial gradient in terms of the quality and quantity of microbes in the intestine; whereas the upper part of the small intestine is relatively sparsely populated by bacteria, the colon contains 10^{13} to 10^{14} microorganisms.[96] Cumulatively, the number of genes within the microbial pool exceeds

---

Table 21-5 Sites of Action of Angiotensin II within the Kidney Causing Effects on the Glomerular Filtration Rate

Direct vasoconstrictor of afferent and efferent arterioles

Reabsorption of Na from the proximal tubule, which affects the Na content in the lumen of the tubule

Modulation of the magnitude of response by the macula densa—especially affects the afferent arteriole

At low perfusion pressure, angiotensin II maintains the glomerular filtration rate by efferent arteriolar constriction (direct effect) and afferent arteriolar dilation via tubuloglomerular feedback

those of the human genome by 100-fold.[96] Although four phyla (Firmicutes, Bacteriodetes, Actinobacteria, and Proteobacteria) represent the great majority of the intestinal microbiome, the microbial makeup of a given individual is relatively unique at a species and strain level.[98] Numerous studies have confirmed the presence of small intestinal bacterial overgrowth in subjects with cirrhosis.[99-106] These studies have used both quantitative bacterial culture techniques and breath hydrogen content. The latter technique is, however, mired with many limitations and does not represent an optimal way to evaluate alterations in the intestinal microbiome in the current era.[107] The presence of small intestinal bacterial overgrowth is associated with changes in intestinal motility and gut permeability.[108-111] It is hypothesized that increased ingress of intestinal bacteria or bacteria-derived products elicits a systemic inflammatory reaction that may be important for development of the systemic inflammatory response state observed in patients with SBP and HRS.

Summary of the Pathogenesis of Hepatorenal Syndrome

Hepatorenal syndrome is a key complication of cirrhosis and results from progressive vasodilation and cirrhotic cardiomyopathy, which produce a critical degree of effective hypovolemia, altered cytokine milieu, and activation of the renal sympathetic nervous system, as well as key Na homeostatic systems that result in profound renal afferent arteriolar vasoconstriction. This diminishes the GFR and contributes to marked Na reabsorption by the kidneys, thereby resulting in impaired overall clearance of toxins by the kidney and the development of renal failure. HRS is often precipitated by infections, especially SBP, and the role of the intestinal microbiome and development of the systemic inflammatory response state following SBP in the genesis of HRS is an important area of current investigation. Relatively little is known of the molecular mechanisms of intrarenal failure to autoregulate renal blood flow and preserve the GFR in patients with HRS.

Clinical Features of Hepatorenal Syndrome

Acute Kidney Injury in Liver Disease

Before discussion of HRS it is important to review all of the causes of acute kidney injury (AKI) in patients with liver disease (**Table 21-6**). AKI is now the preferred term for acute renal failure. There are also causes of renal failure in patients with cirrhosis that will not be discussed, including membranoproliferative glomerulonephritis in patients with hepatitis B and C, diabetic nephropathy in patients with metabolic syndrome, and fatty liver and IgA nephropathy in alcoholics. These chronic forms of kidney disease can be associated with acute rises in serum creatinine. It can be difficult to determine in a patient with cirrhosis and chronic renal disease whether it is the underlying liver disease or HRS that has led to a sudden rise in serum creatinine. In general, we assume that it is the underlying renal disease. AKI is defined as an abrupt

Table 21-6 Causes of Acute Kidney Injury in Patients with Cirrhosis

CAUSE	FREQUENCY
Prerenal	68% (of total population with AKI)
Volume responsive	66% (of those who are prerenal)
Infection	
Hypovolemia	
Vasodilators	
Other	
Not volume responsive	34%
HRS type 1	25%
HRS type 2	9%
Intrarenal (ATN, GMN)	32%
Obstructive	<1%
Nephrotoxic drugs	
NSAIDs, aminoglycosides, contrast agents	

Data from Garcia-Tsao G, Parikh CR, Viola A. Acute kidney injury in cirrhosis. Hepatology 2008;48:2064–2077.

ATN, acute tubular necrosis; GMN, glomerulonephritis; HRS, hepatorenal syndrome; NSAIDs, nonsteroidal antiinflammatory drugs

(within 48 hours) increase in serum creatine of at least 0.3 mg/dl or a 1.5-fold increase from baseline associated with oliguria. The severity of the increase is used to separate patients into three stages.[112] The frequency of the different causes of AKI in patients hospitalized with cirrhosis is shown in **Table 21-6**. The most common cause of AKI is prerenal, and it is usually volume responsive. Only about a third of patients will have HRS. Other causes of AKI in this patient population are the use of nephrotoxic drugs such as nonsteroidal antiinflammatory drugs (NSAIDs) or aminoglycoside antibiotics and contrast agents for computed tomography. Shown in **Table 21-7** are the urinary findings for the most common causes of AKI in hospitalized patients with cirrhosis. The two most common causes of AKI in these patients are acute tubular necrosis and HRS. Examination of the urinary sediment is the quickest way to distinguish these two causes of AKI and to institute appropriate therapy.

Serum Creatinine as a Measure of Renal Function in Cirrhosis

The diagnosis of AKI is based on a rise in the serum creatinine level and the development of oliguria. There is reason to be concerned about the accuracy of serum creatinine in measuring the GFR. Patients with cirrhosis have been shown to have normal serum creatinine levels and low GFRs.[113] Given the marked muscle wasting seen in cirrhotics, it is not surprising that serum creatinine is an inaccurate measure of GFR. More recently, the GFR has been estimated by using a formula called the Modification of Diet in Renal Disease (MDRD), in which age, sex, race, blood urea nitrogen, and albumin, in addition to serum creatinine, are used to estimate the GFR. Recently, the GFR was measured and that result compared with the value estimated by using a modified GFR formula that included age, race, and sex in 660 patients listed for liver

Table 21-7 Urinary Findings in Patients with Renal Dysfunction and Cirrhosis

CAUSE	OSMOLALITY (mOsm/kg)	URINE NA (mmol/L)	SEDIMENT	PROTEIN (mg/dl)
Prerenal				
Hypovolemia	>500	<20	Normal	<500
HRS	>500	<20*	Nil†	<500
Intrinsic				
ATN	<350	>40	Granular	500-1500
AIN	<350	>40	Casts	500-1500
AG	Variable	Variable	WBCs	
			RBC and casts	>2000

*May be higher if the patient received diuretics.
†May have a few hyaline casts.

AG, acute glomerulonephritis; AIN, acute interstitial nephritis; ATN, acute tubular necrosis; HRS, hepatorenal syndrome; RBC, red blood cell; WBCs, white blood cells

transplantation.[114] There was a significant but relatively poor relationship (R^2 = 0.63) between measured and estimated GFR. At GFRs higher than 50 ml/min/1.73 m², estimated GFR values were scattered equally above and below the measured value. When the measured GFR was lower than 50 ml/min/1.73 m², the estimated GFR was almost always higher than the measured value. Thus, in patients with more advanced liver disease, serum creatinine or the MDRD is most likely to underestimate the severity of the renal insufficiency. In addition, small rises in serum creatinine may reflect more severe reductions in GFR than are estimated based on serum creatinine alone.

Approach to Cirrhosis with Acute Kidney Injury

Shown in **Figure 21-5** is an algorithm for the approach to patients with cirrhosis and AKI. If the patient has no ascites, the cause of the renal failure is not HRS but one of the other causes shown in **Table 21-6**. If the patient has ascites, HRS is possible and urinalysis with a careful examination of the urine sediment should be performed. In addition, the use of diuretics is stopped and the patient queried about exposure to nephrotoxic drugs, especially NSAIDs.[115] If the urine sediment is clear, a fluid challenge of saline plus albumin (1 g/kg) is given. If there is a decrease in serum creatine of greater that 10% and an improvement in urine output, HRS is excluded.[116] If there is no response, the patient is thought to have HRS.

Definition, Prognosis, and Prevention of Hepatorenal Syndrome

Criteria for the diagnosis of HRS are shown in **Table 21-1**. These criteria were agreed to by a group of experts and are widely used both in clinical practice and for the design of studies.[1,117] The diagnosis rests on the level of serum creatinine and response to a volume challenge. It is critical in this group of patients that infection be excluded because patients with

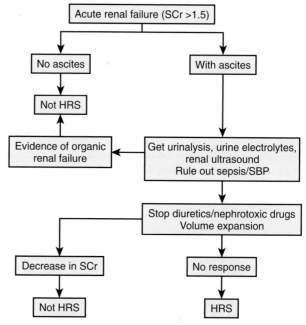

Fig. 21-5 Approach to a patient with cirrhosis and acute kidney injury. HRS, hepatorenal syndrome; SBT, spontaneous bacterial peritonitis; SCr, serum creatinine.

cirrhosis are commonly infected and yet lack many of the signs and symptoms of bacteremia. For example, in a recent series of 104 cirrhotic patients with ascites, 44.6% were infected. Pneumonia and urinary tract infections were most common, followed by SBP. Spontaneous bacteremia was observed in 6% of the patients.[118] The presence of an infection more than doubled the risk for the development of renal failure. Finally, if the renal failure did not improve with treatment, a diagnosis of HRS was made, and this was associated with progressive renal failure and a high likelihood of death.[118]

HRS is separated into two groups, types 1 and 2. Type 1 is defined as a doubling in serum creatinine to greater than 2.5 mg/dl in less than 2 weeks, and in type 2 this rise occurs over a period of more than 2 weeks and usually peaks between

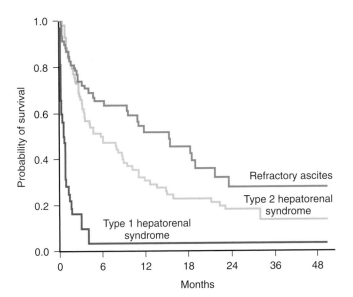

Fig. 21-6 **Survival of patients with refractory ascites and types 1 and 2 hepatorenal syndrome.** *(Adapted from Gines P, et al. Management of cirrhosis and ascites. N Engl J Med 2004;350:1646–1654, with permission.)*

1.5 and 3.0 mg/dl.[119] In addition, in those with type 2 HRS the rise frequently plateaus, whereas in those with type 1 the rise continues and progressive renal failure develops. Given the lack of accuracy of serum creatinine in reflecting GFR in patients with cirrhosis and ascites (see earlier), those with HRS clearly have advanced renal failure when the diagnosis is made. Patients in whom HRS type 1 develops generally have a precipitating cause such as SBP or have a form of acute on chronic liver disease, such as alcoholic hepatitis. The prognosis for those with type 1 HRS is poor, with a median survival of less than a month, and almost all patients are dead within 6 months of diagnosis (**Fig. 21-6**).[120] In contrast, survival of patients with type 2 is better, with a median survival of longer than 6 months. However, their survival is still significantly worse than that in patients with refractory ascites but a normal serum creatinine level (see **Fig. 21-6**). The prognostic significance of serum creatinine in predicting survival in cirrhotics is demonstrated by its inclusion as one of the three independent variables in the Model for End-Stage Liver Disease (MELD) scoring system.[121]

The risk for HRS is dependent on the presence of ascites (essentially zero in its absence), on the severity of the liver disease, and finally, on complications of cirrhosis that increase risk for the development of HRS. In one report, 263 patients with cirrhosis and ascites were observed for a mean of 41 months. Renal failure developed in 49%. Most of the renal failure was due to volume depletion or associated with infection but was reversible. HRS developed in 7.6% of the patients. The 1-year probability of survival was 91% in those in whom renal failure did not develop but fell to 46.9% in those in whom it did.[2]

The most common complication of cirrhosis associated with the development of HRS is SBP. In one series, HRS developed in 33% of patients with SBP who were treated appropriately with antibiotics. This risk could be reduced to 10% if the patients received intravenous albumin in addition to antibiotics. The patients who benefited most from the use of albumin were cirrhotics with the most advanced liver disease or those who had evidence of renal dysfunction at baseline. Intravenous albumin administration lowered plasma renin activity, thus suggesting that its benefit was on the abnormal hemodynamics seen in patients with cirrhosis and HRS.[122] In support of this belief that infection increases the risk for development of HRS by making the hyperdynamic circulation worse is a study in which patients with low-protein ascites and advanced liver disease were given a placebo or norfloxacin. The risk for development of HRS was significantly reduced in those who received norfloxacin versus placebo.[120,123]

The other clinical situation in which the prophylactic use of antibiotics reduces the risk for SBP and perhaps HRS is acute variceal bleeding. Renal failure occurs in 11% of patients admitted to the hospital with variceal bleeding. The severity of the bleeding and liver disease was predictive of the development of renal failure.[124] Many of the patients were also infected, and this may have contributed to the risk for development of renal failure. Use of prophylactic antibiotics in this patient population reduces the risk for all types of bacterial infection, including SBP, and improves their prognosis.[125,126] Because infections, especially SBP, are known to increase the risk for development of HRS, the use of prophylactic antibiotics in cirrhotics with gastrointestinal bleeding should reduce the risk for HRS.

The last risk factor for the development of HRS is the development of acute on chronic liver disease, specifically alcoholic hepatitis. In one series, HRS (mostly HRS type 1) developed in 24 of 52 patients with severe alcoholic hepatitis. Ninety-two percent of those in whom HRS developed died. When an effective therapy for alcoholic hepatitis was given to the patients, in this case pentoxifylline, the risk for development of HRS was reduced and outcome improved.[127]

Prevention of the development of HRS is likely to improve outcomes. The use of albumin in association with antibiotics in patients with SBP appears to be warranted based on current data, but only in patients who are jaundiced or have renal insufficiency. The prophylactic use of antibiotics in cirrhotics with gastrointestinal bleeding also appears to be warranted because the use of antibiotics is associated with a reduced incidence of infections, improved survival, and less rebleeding. Risk for HRS is also likely to be reduced. Prophylactic use of antibiotics in patients with low-protein ascites and advanced liver disease is not warranted because the use of antibiotics in this patient population increases the risk for *Clostridium difficile* infection and bacterial resistance. New therapies to treat diseases such as alcoholic hepatitis are needed because improvements in liver function are likely to be associated with improvements in renal function. Finally, new treatments to slow progression of the hyperdynamic circulation are needed because the hyperdynamic circulation is the driving force behind the development of refractory cirrhotic ascites and HRS.[119]

Management of Patients with Hepatorenal Syndrome

General management of patients with AKI is no different from that in any other patient with advanced liver disease. First and foremost, the presence of a bacterial infection must be sought by cultures of blood, urine, and ascitic fluid. If infection is considered likely, antibiotics should be started pending the results of culture. Gram-negative enteric organisms are most common, and appropriate antibiotics should be selected. A history of the use of nephrotoxins such as NSAIDs should be sought. Diuretics should be withdrawn and the patient should undergo volume expansion with albumin, 1 g/kg intravenously. Urinalysis should be performed and the urine sediment examined by a nephrologist to exclude other causes of AKI. Once all of these measures have been completed and there is no improvement in renal function, the patient is considered to have HRS (see **Table 21-1**).

Renal Replacement Therapy and Liver Transplantation

Acute progressive renal failure leading to symptoms of uremia is seen most commonly with HRS type 1. In patients with HRS type 2, serum creatinine infrequently exceeds 3 mg/dl, but when it does, the increase is usually due to overdiuresis of a patient with refractory cirrhotic ascites. Therefore an acute rise in serum creatinine in a patient with HRS type 2 will usually respond to volume replacement therapy. In contrast, in patients with HRS type 1 and especially in those with alcoholic hepatitis, the rise in serum creatinine is rapid and progressive and leads to the question of hemodialysis. The general consensus is that dialysis in these patients does not improve their survival and should not be performed unless they are candidates for a liver transplant.[120]

Patients with HRS who undergo liver transplantation clearly benefit from the liver transplant and have improved survival relative to those who do not undergo liver transplantation.[128-130] In one series of patients treated with terlipressin in whom HRS was reversed before transplantation, the frequency of renal insufficiency was similar at 6 months in those who did and did not have HRS before transplantation.[128] In a second series of 32 patients with HRS type 1 who underwent liver transplantation, 30 recovered renal function over a median time of 24 days (range, 1 to 234 days). The two other patients died of renal insufficiency. Dialysis was required after transplantation in eight patients.[129] In a third series, renal function improved in patients with HRS (type not specified) who underwent liver transplantation. Renal function 1 year following transplantation was similar in those who did and did not have HRS before transplantation.[131]

With the advent of MELD for allocating organs for liver transplantation, the number of patients undergoing simultaneous liver/kidney (SLK) transplantation has increased 300%. At issue are which patients should receive an SLK transplant and which should receive a liver-only transplant despite the presence of renal dysfunction. It is clear that there is no uniformity of opinion on this issue inasmuch as rates of SLK transplantation vary widely.[132] In one series, 22 patients with HRS who were maintained on dialysis for more than 30 days and who underwent SLK transplantation were compared with 148 HRS patients, 80 of whom were maintained on dialysis for less than 30 days and received a liver-only transplant. Renal function recovered in essentially all of those who received a liver-only transplant. Outcomes were similar in the two groups regarding survival and recovery of renal function.[133] Hence, it would appear that most patients with HRS will recover their renal function following a liver-only

transplant. SLK transplantation for patients with AKI should be reserved for those who have been undergoing renal replacement therapy for a minimum of a month and probably 2 months preceding liver transplantation. In addition, those who have intrinsic renal disease, such as seen with diabetes, and have significant renal insufficiency are best served by SLK transplantation.[132]

Transjugular Intrahepatic Portosystemic Shunt

Creation of a transjugular intrahepatic portosystemic shunt (TIPS) leads to improvements in GFR and decreases in plasma renin activity and aldosterone levels.[134] A small number of patients with type 1 and 2 HRS have received a TIPS, and renal function improved. However, the prognosis remains poor, especially in those with HRS type 1.[135,136] Recently, a small number of patients with HRS type 1 received midodrine, octreotide, and albumin, and if they responded to vasoconstrictor therapy, they received a TIPS. Five patients who responded to vasoconstrictor therapy demonstrated further improvement in renal function following the creation of a TIPS.[137] Given the small number of patients studied and the lack of a control group, it is difficult to conclude that patients who respond to vasoconstrictor therapy should proceed to TIPS creation in the hope of preserving their renal function. Patients who respond to vasoconstrictor therapy in general have a sustained improvement in renal function, and the added benefit of a TIPS is unclear (see later). In addition, in patients with HRS type 1, the risk associated with creation of a TIPS is significant because they frequently have advanced liver disease and after the TIPS procedure are at risk for multiorgan failure. Urgent liver transplantation in a suitable candidate is more likely to be of benefit in this patient population than is creation of a TIPS.

Vasoconstrictor Therapy

It was recognized many years ago that the so-called effective plasma volume was reduced in patients with HRS, and this led to attempts to expand the patient's plasma volume in the hope of improving renal function. In addition, active renal vasoconstriction was recognized as being present in these patients, and vasodilators were infused. Both approaches lead to improvement in renal function; however, the improvement was not maintained when the therapy was discontinued. More recently, clarification of the role of hyperdynamic circulation and vasodilation in the splanchnic bed in the pathogenesis of HRS has led to the use of vasoconstrictors in the treatment of HRS (see earlier). Small case series have been followed by randomized controlled trials, and it is clear that vasoconstrictor therapy improves renal function in these patients and that the improvement in many is long lasting.

The drug used most widely is terlipressin, and the efficacy of this agent in the reversal of HRS type 1 has been subjected to controlled trials as shown in **Table 21-8**.[138-141] The largest study was a randomized, double-blind, placebo-controlled trial that was performed largely in the United States. One hundred twelve patients with HRS type 1 were randomized to terlipressin, 1 mg every 6 hours, plus albumin versus placebo plus albumin. The patient characteristics in the two arms were similar. Thirty-four percent of the terlipressin-treated

Table 21-8 Controlled Trials of Terlipressin plus Albumin in the Treatment of Hepatorenal Syndrome

AUTHOR	TREATMENT GROUP	N	COMPLETE RESPONSE (%)	HRS TYPE 1 (%)
Solanki et al.[138]	Terlipressin	12	42	100
	Control	12	0	
Neri et al.[139]	Terlipressin	26	81	100
	Control	26	19	
Sanyal et al.[140]	Terlipressin	56	34	100
	Control	56	13	
Martin-Llahi et al.[141]	Terlipressin	23	39	56
	Control	23	4	

patients and 13% of controls ($P = .008$) achieved reversal of HRS, defined as a serum creatinine level of 1.5 mg/dl or less. Mean serum creatinine levels rose in the placebo-treated patients and fell in those who received terlipressin. Overall survival was the same in both groups, but survival was significantly better in those who achieved HRS reversal than in those who did not. Although serious adverse events were similar in the treated and control groups, ischemic events were seen only in those receiving terlipressin.[140] All of the trials showed a beneficial effect of terlipressin on renal function in comparison with controls (see **Table 21-8**). Most remarkable was the fact that about 90% of patients maintained HRS reversal for several weeks after discontinuation of treatment. Although none of the controlled trials demonstrated a survival advantage for terlipressin, a meta-analysis suggested that treatment with terlipressin plus albumin versus albumin alone reduces mortality (relative risk, 0.81; 95% confidence interval, 0.68 to 0.97).[142] Factors predictive of a response to terlipressin included baseline serum bilirubin, increase in MAP following terlipressin administration, and baseline serum creatinine.[143,144] Baseline serum creatinine, the presence of alcoholic hepatitis, and Child-Pugh score were predictive of survival.[144]

Other drugs used to treat HRS include midodrine, octreotide, and noradrenaline. Terlipressin was compared with noradrenaline in a small open-label controlled trial, and the outcomes were similar.[145] Midodrine plus octreotide appeared to improve renal function in some patients with HRS but has not been subjected to controlled trials.[146,147] All of these trials suggest that vasoconstrictive drugs improve renal function by causing splanchnic vasoconstriction, which increases effective arterial blood volume and hence improves renal blood flow and kidney function. In Europe, terlipressin plus albumin is used most commonly, whereas in the United States, where terlipressin is not approved, octreotide and midodrine in addition to albumin is most used for the treatment of HRS.

All of these studies provide some guidance on how to use vasoconstrictors in patients with HRS. First, the diagnosis of HRS must be based on the criteria shown in **Table 21-1**. There are multiple causes of AKI in this patient population, and use of vasoconstrictors in those with low plasma volume or intrinsic renal disease is likely to lead to a deterioration in renal function. In patients with HRS, the more severe the renal failure, the less likely they are to respond to vasoconstrictors.

For example, in one report the likelihood of responding to terlipressin was 50% in those with a creatinine level lower than 3.0 mg/dl, 33% in those with a creatinine level of 3 to 5 mg/dl, and 9% in those with a creatinine level higher than 5 mg/dl.[144] There are no data supporting the use of vasoconstrictors in patients undergoing renal replacement therapy. Although it is unclear whether one can predict a response to terlipressin based on a rise in blood pressure following the infusion, it is clear that if the patients are to respond to terlipressin, a rise in MAP is required.[143,144] Finally, the response to vasoconstrictor therapy appears to be rapid, with a fall in serum creatinine seen within 48 to 72 hours of initiation of therapy. If serum creatinine does not begin to fall after 3 days, either the dose of the vasoconstrictor should be increased or the treatment is ineffective. Finally, the role of vasoconstrictors in the treatment of HRS type 2 is unclear because there are too few studies from which to draw any firm conclusions. Because patients with HRS type 2 are clinically stable and the use of vasoconstrictors is associated with side effects, their use in this group of patients should probably be limited to controlled trials.

Hyponatremia

Disorders of water metabolism are common in patients with cirrhosis, especially in those with HRS. The development of hyponatremia reflects the inability of the kidney to excrete free water. The primary reason for this inability to excrete solute-free water in cirrhotics is an increase in levels of arginine vasopressin (AVP). The nonosmotic secretion of AVP in these patients is due to the same mechanism that leads to renal failure: arterial splanchnic vasodilation and arterial underfilling leading to activation of baroreceptors that regulate the release of AVP.[148,149] Hyponatremia is common in cirrhotics, and the severity of hyponatremia is a marker of more advanced disease. The prevalence of hyponatremia (serum Na^+ <135 mmol/L) was high in inpatients (57%) and outpatients (40%). Twenty-one percent of cirrhotics had a serum sodium level of 130 mmol/L or lower. The presence of hyponatremia was associated with refractory ascites, hepatic encephalopathy, and HRS. The use of diuretics was frequently stopped in those with more severe hyponatremia, thus adding to the difficulty of controlling their ascites.[150] Once hyponatremia develops, a patient's risk for dying increases, and this is independent of the MELD score.[151,152] Finally, hyponatremic patients undergoing liver transplantation appear to be at increased risk for neurologic injuries, renal failure, and infections in the immediate post-transplant period.[153]

The most common approach to the treatment of hyponatremia is fluid restriction. Both patients and physicians find this form of treatment difficult because it is hard for patients to do, the rate of rise in serum sodium is slow, and hospitalization is prolonged. In addition, if diuretics are continued, the serum sodium level may fail to increase.[154] Infusion of hypertonic saline will correct the hyponatremia more quickly but will put the patient at risk for the development of hypernatremia and osmotic demyelination. A number of other agents, including demeclocycline, urea, and κ-opioids, have been used in the past, but complications and ineffectiveness have led to their abandonment.[155] The development of a new class of drugs that block the effects of AVP on the renal tubule has led to hope that a new and effective therapy is now available for cirrhotics with hyponatremia.

The effect of AVP on water homeostasis is mediated via its effect on water transport by principal cells in the collecting duct. AVP binds to the V2 receptor on the basolateral membrane of principal cells and leads to activation of the G_s-coupled adenylyl cyclase system and an increase in levels of cAMP. Stimulation of protein kinase A by cAMP leads to phosphorylation of preformed AQP2, which is then translocated to the apical membrane and makes the cells more water permeable.[156] An increase in AVP, as is seen in cirrhosis, causes more AQP2 to move to the apical membrane and makes the cells more permeable to water, thus decreasing solute-free water clearance and leading to the development of hyponatremia. Drugs such as tolvaptan and satavaptan bind to the V2 receptor and block the effect of AVP, which results in an increase in solute-free water clearance and correction of the hyponatremia. In addition, this group of drugs also induces a mild natriuresis, increases urine output, and causes more rapid weight loss than in patients not receiving the drug.[157,158]

The Food and Drug Administration (FDA) has approved tolvaptan for use in the treatment of hyponatremia in cirrhotics based on two randomized controlled trials comparing placebo with tolvaptan in patients with hyponatremia (**Fig. 21-7**).[158] The majority of the patients in the study suffered from congestive heart failure, and only 63 cirrhotic patients received tolvaptan. Patients with a Child-Pugh score higher than 10 or sodium level lower than 120 mmol/L were excluded. Patients were treated for up to 30 days, and during the first 4 days the dose of tolvaptan could be increased, depending on the response to treatment. Serum sodium rose quickly in those receiving tolvaptan and was 135 mmol/L or higher by day 20. Discontinuation of treatment was associated with a fall in serum sodium. No mention is made of the use of diuretics in this group of patients. No difference in survival was seen with tolvaptan versus placebo, but the patients were treated for a maximum of 30 days.[158]

The other oral V2 receptor antagonist that has been investigated more extensively in patients with cirrhosis is satavaptan.[157] In a recent report, 151 cirrhotic patients with recurrent ascites, with or without hyponatremia, were randomized to receive different doses of satavaptan or placebo. The use of satavaptan was associated with a decrease in the need for paracentesis. In addition, urine volume increased with

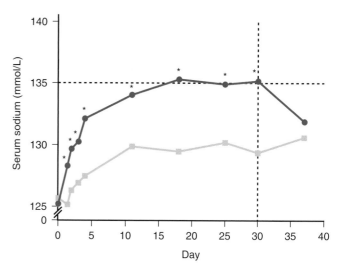

Fig. 21-7 **Response to tolvaptan versus placebo in patients with severe hyponatremia.** Patients received tolvaptan *(blue circles)* or placebo *(yellow squares)* for 30 days. *Asterisk,* significant difference between tolvaptan-treated patients and controls. *(From Schrier RW, et al. Tolvaptan, a selective oral vasopressin V2-receptor antagonist, for hyponatremia. N Engl J Med 2006;355:2099–2112, with permission.)*

satavaptan. Somewhat surprising was observation that serum sodium remained the same in all of the groups, including placebo. Survival and side effects were similar in the two groups.[159] Another study of satavaptan given in combination with diuretics to patients with cirrhosis found an increase in mortality in those receiving satavaptan.[160] The reason for the increase in mortality is unclear, but the company making satavaptan (Sanofi-Aventis) has withdrawn the drug.

The adverse event most feared with the use of these drugs is too rapid a rise in serum sodium (>12 mmol/L/24 hr) leading to hypernatremia, osmotic demyelination, and central nervous system injury. The FDA has included a black box warning that therapy with tolvaptan should be instituted in an inpatient setting with close monitoring of serum sodium. Patients with cirrhosis tolerate hyponatremia with minimal neurologic sequelae, and therefore the use of tolvaptan should be limited to those with a serum Na^+ concentration of less than 120 mmol/L. How to use tolvaptan and other V2 receptor antagonists in combination with diuretics is unclear. Based on the experience with satavaptan it appears that better control of the patient's ascites may be possible, but until the increase in mortality seen with satavaptan is explained, use of this class of drugs in combination with diuretics in an outpatient setting should be limited to controlled trials.[161]

Key References

Abraldes JG, et al. Mild increases in portal pressure upregulate vascular endothelial growth factor and endothelial nitric oxide synthase in the intestinal microcirculatory bed, leading to a hyperdynamic state. Am J Physiol Gastrointest Liver Physiol 2006;290:G980–G987. (Ref.34)

Akriviadis E, et al. Pentoxifylline improves short-term survival in severe acute alcoholic hepatitis: a double-blind, placebo-controlled trial. Gastroenterology 2000;119:1637–1648. (Ref.127)

Aller MA, et al. Inflammation: a way to understanding the evolution of portal hypertension. Theor Biol Med Model 2007;4:44. (Ref.91)

Almeida J, et al. Gut flora and bacterial translocation in chronic liver disease. World J Gastroenterol 2006;12:1493–1502. (Ref.103)

Ancel D, et al. [Intestinal permeability and cirrhosis.] Gastroenterol Clin Biol 2006;30:460–468. (Ref.109)

Angeli P, et al, for the CAPPS Investigators. Hyponatremia in cirrhosis: results of a patient population survey. Hepatology 2006;44:1535–1542. (Ref.150)

Arroyo V, Fernandez J, Gines P. Pathogenesis and treatment of hepatorenal syndrome. Semin Liver Dis 2008;28:81–95. (Ref.23)

Batkai S, et al. Endocannabinoids acting at vascular CB1 receptors mediate the vasodilated state in advanced liver cirrhosis. Nat Med 2001;7:827–832. (Ref.41)

Bauer TM, et al. Diagnosis of small intestinal bacterial overgrowth in patients with cirrhosis of the liver: poor performance of the glucose breath hydrogen test. J Hepatol 2000;33:382–386. (Ref.107)

Bauer TM, et al. Small intestinal bacterial overgrowth in patients with cirrhosis: prevalence and relation with spontaneous bacterial peritonitis. Am J Gastroenterol 2001;96:2962–2967. (Ref.105)

Beierwaltes WH. Cyclooxygenase-2 products compensate for inhibition of nitric oxide regulation of renal perfusion. Am J Physiol 2002;283:F68–F72. (Ref.76)

Bell PD, Komlosi P, Zhang ZR. ATP as a mediator of macula densa cell signalling. Purinergic Signal 2009;5:461–471. (Ref.73)

Biggins SW, et al. Serum sodium predicts mortality in patients listed for liver transplantation. Hepatology 2005;41:32–39. (Ref.152)

Boyer TD, et al. Liver transplant affects survival outcomes in patients with type 1 hepatorenal syndrome treated with terlipressin vs. placebo. Am J Transplant 2009;9:s450. (Ref.130)

Brensing KA, et al. Long-term outcome after transjugular intrahepatic portosystemic stent-shunt in non-transplant cirrhotics with hepatorenal syndrome: a phase II study. Gut 2000;47:288–295. (Ref.136)

Cardenas A, et al. Renal failure after upper gastrointestinal bleeding in cirrhosis: incidence, clinical course, predictive factors, and short-term prognosis. Hepatology 2001;34:671–676. (Ref.124)

Castrop H. Mediators of tubuloglomerular feedback regulation of glomerular filtration: ATP and adenosine. Acta Physiol (Oxf) 2007;189:3–14. (Ref.71)

Chen YC, et al. Increased vascular heme oxygenase-1 expression contributes to arterial vasodilation in experimental cirrhosis in rats. Hepatology 2004;39:1075–1087. (Ref.38)

Cheng Y, et al. Hydrogen sulfide–induced relaxation of resistance mesenteric artery beds of rats. Am J Physiol Heart Circ Physiol 2004;287:H2316–H2323. (Ref.42)

Cupples WA, Braam B. Assessment of renal autoregulation. Am J Physiol 2007;292:F1105–F1123. (Ref.58)

Cupples WA. Interactions contributing to kidney blood flow autoregulation. Curr Opin Nephrol Hypertens 2007;16:39–45. (Ref.61)

Dagher L, Moore K. The hepatorenal syndrome. Gut 2001;49:729–737. (Ref.90)

de Lisle RC, Sewell R, Meldi L. Enteric circular muscle dysfunction in the cystic fibrosis mouse small intestine. Neurogastroenterol Motil 2010;22:341–e87. [Epub] (Ref.108)

Eason JD, et al. Proceedings of consensus conference on simultaneous liver kidney transplantation (SLK). Am J Transplant 2008;8:2243–2251. (Ref.132)

Eckburg PB, et al. Diversity of the human intestinal microbial flora. Science 2005;308:1635–1638. (Ref.98)

Esrailian E, et al. Octreotide/midodrine therapy significantly improves renal function and 30-day survival in patients with type 1 hepatorenal syndrome. Dig Dis Sci 2007;52:742–748. (Ref.147)

Esteva-Font C, et al. Aquaporin-1 and aquaporin-2 urinary excretion in cirrhosis: relationship with ascites and hepatorenal syndrome. Hepatology 2006;44:1555–1563. (Ref.84)

Fasolato S, et al. Renal failure and bacterial infections in patients with cirrhosis: epidemiology and clinical features. Hepatology 2007;45:223–229. (Ref.118)

Fernandez J, et al. Primary prophylaxis of spontaneous bacterial peritonitis delays hepatorenal syndrome and improves survival in cirrhosis. Gastroenterology 2007;133:818–824. (Ref.123)

Fernandez-Varo G, et al. Nitric oxide synthase 3–dependent vascular remodeling and circulatory dysfunction in cirrhosis. Am J Pathol 2003;162:1985–1993. (Ref.47)

Fulton D, et al. Localization of endothelial nitric-oxide synthase phosphorylated on serine 1179 and nitric oxide in Golgi and plasma membrane defines the existence of two pools of active enzyme. J Biol Chem 2002;277:4277–4284. (Ref.35)

Gallis B, et al. Identification of flow-dependent endothelial nitric-oxide synthase phosphorylation sites by mass spectrometry and regulation of phosphorylation and nitric oxide production by the phosphatidylinositol 3-kinase inhibitor LY294002. J Biol Chem 1999;274:30101–30108. (Ref.33)

Garcia N Jr, et al. Systemic and portal hemodynamic effects of anandamide. Am J Physiol Gastrointest Liver Physiol 2001;280:G14–G20. (Ref.40)

Garcia-Tsao G, Nathanson MH. Portal hypertension: from the patient to the molecule and back: a symposium honoring Roberto J. Groszmann, MD. J Clin Gastroenterol 2007;41(Suppl 3):S243–S244. (Ref.4)

Garcia-Tsao G, Parikh CR, Viola A. Acute kidney injury in cirrhosis. Hepatology 2008;48:2064–2077. (Ref.116)

Gill SR, et al. Metagenomic analysis of the human distal gut microbiome. Science 2006;312:1355–1359. (Ref.96)

Gines P, Cardenas A. The management of ascites and hyponatremia in cirrhosis. Semin Liver Dis 2008;28:43–58. (Ref.155)

Gines P, et al. Management of cirrhosis and ascites. N Engl J Med 2004;350:1646–1654. (Ref.120)

Gines P, Schrier RW. Renal failure in cirrhosis. N Engl J Med 2009;361:1279–1290. (Ref.119)

Gines P, et al. Effects of satavaptan, a selective vasopressin V2 receptor antagonist, on ascites and serum sodium in cirrhosis with hyponatremia: a randomized trial. Hepatology 2008;48:204–213. (Ref.157)

Gluud LI, et al. Systematic review of randomized trials on vasoconstrictor drugs for hepatorenal syndrome. Hepatology 2010;51:576–584. (Ref.142)

Goh BJ, et al. Nitric oxide synthase and heme oxygenase expressions in human liver cirrhosis. World J Gastroenterol 2006;12:588–594. (Ref.14)

Gunnarsdottir SA, et al. Small intestinal motility disturbances and bacterial overgrowth in patients with liver cirrhosis and portal hypertension. Am J Gastroenterol 2003;98:1362–1370. (Ref.110)

Hansen PB, et al. Vasoconstrictor and vasodilator effects of adenosine in the mouse kidney due to preferential activation of A1 or A2 adenosine receptors. J Pharmacol Exp Ther 2005;315:1150–1157. (Ref.67)

Hayashi H, Sakamoto M, Benno Y. Phylogenetic analysis of the human gut microbiota using 16S rDNA clone libraries and strictly anaerobic culture-based methods. Microbiol Immunol 2002;46:535–548. (Ref.97)

Heuman DM, et al. Persistent ascites and low serum sodium identify patients with cirrhosis and low MELD scores who are at risk for early death. Hepatology 2004;40:802–810. (Ref.151)

Iwakiri Y, Groszmann RJ. The hyperdynamic circulation of chronic liver diseases: from the patient to the molecule. Hepatology 2006;43(2 Suppl 1):S121–S131. (Ref.13)

Iwakiri Y, Groszmann RJ. Vascular endothelial dysfunction in cirrhosis. J Hepatol 2007;46:927–934. (Ref.5)

Iwakiri Y, et al. Phosphorylation of eNOS initiates excessive NO production in early phases of portal hypertension. Am J Physiol Heart Circ Physiol 2002;282:H2084–H2090. (Ref.31)

Jun DW, et al. Association between small intestinal bacterial overgrowth and peripheral bacterial DNA in cirrhotic patients. Dig Dis Sci 2010;55:1465–1471. (Ref.99)

Kamath PS, Kim WR. The Model for End-Stage Liver Disease (MELD). Hepatology 2007;45:797–805. (Ref.121)

Keitel V, et al. The G-protein coupled bile salt receptor TGR5 is expressed in liver sinusoidal endothelial cells. Hepatology 2007;45:695–704. (Ref.8)

Khavandi K, et al. Myogenic tone and small artery remodelling: insight into diabetic nephropathy. Nephrol Dial Transplant 2009;24:361–369. (Ref.68)

Kobori H, et al. The intrarenal renin-angiotensin system: from physiology to the pathobiology of hypertension and kidney disease. Pharmacol Rev 2007;59:251–287. (Ref.86)

Kumar S, Berl T. Vasopressin antagonists in the treatment of water-retaining disorders. Semin Nephrol 2008;28:279–288. (Ref.156)

Lakshmi CP, et al. Frequency and factors associated with small intestinal bacterial overgrowth in patients with cirrhosis of the liver and extra hepatic portal venous obstruction. Dig Dis Sci 2010;55:1142–1148. (Ref.100)

Lee RF, Glenn TK, Lee SS. Cardiac dysfunction in cirrhosis. Best Pract Res 2007;21:125–140. (Ref.53)

Lim Y-S, et al. Serum sodium, renal function, and survival of patients with end-state liver disease. J Hepatol 2010;52:523–528. (Ref.114)

Liu J, et al. Functional CB1 cannabinoid receptors in human vascular endothelial cells. Biochem J 2000;346 Pt 3:835–840. (Ref.39)

Londono MC, et al. Hyponatremia impairs early posttransplantation outcome in patients with cirrhosis undergoing liver transplantation. Gastroenterology 2006;130:1135–1143. (Ref.153)

Martin-Llahi M, et al. Terlipressin and albumin vs. albumin in patients with cirrhosis and hepatorenal syndrome: a randomized study. Gastroenterology 2008;134:1352–1359. (Ref.141)

Mehta RL, et al. Acute Kidney Injury Network: report of an initiative to improve outcomes in acute kidney injury. Crit Care 2007;11:R31. (Ref.112)

Ming Z, et al. Contribution of hepatic adenosine A1 receptors to renal dysfunction associated with acute liver injury in rats. Hepatology 2006;44:813–822. (Ref.21)

Minshall RD, et al. Caveolin regulation of endothelial function. Am J Physiol Lung Cell Mol Physiol 2003;285:L1179–L1183. (Ref.11)

Mohammadi MS, et al. Possible mechanisms involved in the discrepancy of hepatic and aortic endothelial nitric oxide synthases during the development of cirrhosis in rats. Liver Int 2009;29:692–700. (Ref.10)

Moller S, Henriksen JH. Cirrhotic cardiomyopathy: a pathophysiological review of circulatory dysfunction in liver disease. Heart 2002;87:9–15. (Ref.56)

Nazar A, et al. Predictors of response to therapy with terlipressin and albumin in patients with cirrhosis and type 1 hepatorenal syndrome. Hepatology 2010;51: 219–226. (Ref.143)

Pande C, Kumar A, Sarin SK. Small-intestinal bacterial overgrowth in cirrhosis is related to the severity of liver disease. Aliment Pharmacol Ther 2009;29: 1273–1281. (Ref.101)

Ren Y, et al. Crosstalk between the connecting tubule and the afferent arteriole regulates renal microcirculation. Kidney Int 2007;71:1116–1121. (Ref.81)

Ren Y, et al. Cross-talk between arterioles and tubules in the kidney. Pediatric Nephrol 2009;24:31–35. (Ref.82)

Restuccia T, et al. Effects of treatment of hepatorenal syndrome before transplantation on posttransplantation outcome. A case-controlled study. J Hepatol 2004;40:140–146. (Ref.128)

Ripoll C, et al. Hepatic venous pressure gradient predicts clinical decompensation in patients with compensated cirrhosis. Gastroenterology 2007;133:481–488. (Ref.3)

Ruiz R, et al. Long-term analysis of combined liver and kidney transplantation at a single center. Arch Surg 2006;141:735–742. (Ref.133)

Salerno F, et al. Diagnosis, prevention and treatment of hepatorenal syndrome in cirrhosis. Gut 2007;56:1310–1318. (Ref.1)

Sanchez E, et al. Role of intestinal bacterial overgrowth and intestinal motility in bacterial translocation in experimental cirrhosis. Rev Esp Enferm Dig 2005;97: 805–814. (Ref.104)

Sanyal AJ, et al. A randomized, prospective, double-blind, placebo-controlled trial of terlipressin for type 1 hepatorenal syndrome. Gastroenterology 2008; 134:1360–1368. (Ref.140)

Satou R, et al. IL-6 augments angiotensinogen in primary cultured renal proximal tubular cells. Mol Cell Endocrinol 2009;311:24–31. (Ref.85)

Schneider AR, et al. Application of the glucose hydrogen breath test for the detection of bacterial overgrowth in patients with cystic fibrosis—a reliable method? Dig Dis Sci 2009;54:1730–1735. (Ref.102)

Schrier RW, et al. Tolvaptan, a selective oral vasopressin V2-receptor antagonist, for hyponatremia. N Engl J Med 2006;355:2099–2112. (Ref.158)

Sessa WC. Regulation of endothelial derived nitric oxide in health and disease. Mem Inst Oswaldo Cruz 2005;100(Suppl 1):15–18. (Ref.30)

Shah V. Molecular mechanisms of increased intrahepatic resistance in portal hypertension. J Clin Gastroenterol 2007;41(Suppl 3):S259–S261. (Ref.7)

Sharma P, et al. An open label, pilot, randomized controlled trial of noradrenaline versus terlipressin in the treatment of type 1 hepatorenal syndrome and predictors of response. Am J Gastroenterol 2008;103: 1689–1697. (Ref.145)

Soares-Weiser K, et al. Antibiotic prophylaxis of bacterial infections in cirrhotic inpatients: a meta-analysis of randomized controlled trials. Scand J Gastroenterol 2003;38:193–200. (Ref.126)

Solanki P, et al. Beneficial effects of terlipressin in hepatorenal syndrome: a prospective, randomized placebo-controlled clinical trial. J Gastroenterol Hepatol 2003;18:152–156. (Ref.138)

Tazi KA, et al. Norfloxacin reduces aortic NO synthases and proinflammatory cytokine up-regulation in cirrhotic rats: role of Akt signaling. Gastroenterology 2005;129:303–314. (Ref.28)

Thabut D, et al. Model for End-Stage Liver Disease score and systemic inflammatory response are major prognostic factors in patients with cirrhosis and acute functional renal failure. Hepatology 2007;46:1872–1882. (Ref.92)

Thabut D, et al. High-density lipoprotein administration attenuates liver proinflammatory response, restores liver endothelial nitric oxide synthase activity, and lowers portal pressure in cirrhotic rats. Hepatology 2007;46: 1893–1906. (Ref.9)

Thomas L, Kumar R. Control of renal solute excretion by enteric signals and mediators. J Am Soc Nephrol 2008;19:207–212. (Ref.78)

Wang JY, Liu HY, Liu P. [Expression of type I inositol 1,4,5-triphosphate receptor on rat glomerular and afferent arterioles in a model of liver cirrhosis.] Zhonghua Gan Zang Bing Za Zhi 2004;12:609–611. (Ref.60)

Wiest R, et al. Bacterial translocation up-regulates GTP-cyclohydrolase I in mesenteric vasculature of cirrhotic rats. Hepatology 2003;38:1508–1515. (Ref.32)

Wong F, et al, Blendis. A vasopressin receptor antagonist (VPA-985) improves serum sodium concentration in patients with hyponatremia: a multicenter, randomized placebo-controlled trial. Hepatology 2003;37:182–191. (Ref.154)

Wong F, et al. Double-blind placebo-controlled study of satavaptan in the management of recurrent ascites. Hepatology 2009;50:448A. (Ref.160)

Wong F, et al. Effects of a selective vasopressin V2 receptor antagonist, satavaptan, on ascites recurrence after paracentesis in patients with cirrhosis. J Hepatol 2010;53:283–290. (Ref.159)

Wong F, Pantea L, Sniderman K. Midodrine, octreotide, albumin, and TIPS in selected patients with cirrhosis and type 1 hepatorenal syndrome. Hepatology 2004;40:55–64. (Ref.137)

Wu XX, et al. [Correlative study between angiotensin-converting enzyme gene polymorphism and hepatorenal syndrome.] Zhongguo Wei Zhong Bing Ji Jiu Yi Xue 2005;17:121–123. (Ref.89)

Xu X, et al. Neuronal nitric oxide synthase and systemic vasodilation in rats with cirrhosis. Am J Physiol 2000;279:F1110–F1115. (Ref.29)

Xu X, et al. Outcome of patients with hepatorenal syndrome type 1 after liver transplantation: Hangzhou experience. Transplantation 2009;87:1514–1519. (Ref.129)

Yokomori H, et al. Elevated expression of caveolin-1 at protein and mRNA level in human cirrhotic liver: relation with nitric oxide. J Gastroenterol 2003;38: 854–860. (Ref.12)

Zhang Q, et al. Functional relevance of Golgi- and plasma membrane–localized endothelial NO synthase in reconstituted endothelial cells. Arterioscler Thromb Vasc Biol 2006;26:1015–1021. (Ref.36)

Zhao W, et al. The vasorelaxant effect of H(2)S as a novel endogenous gaseous K(ATP) channel opener. EMBO J 2001;20:6008–6016. (Ref.43)

A complete list of references can be found at www.expertconsult.com.

Cardiovascular Complications of Cirrhosis

Samuel S. Lee and Soon Koo Baik

ABBREVIATIONS

ANP atrial natriuretic peptide
BDL bile duct–ligated
BNP brain or B-type natriuretic peptide
CNS central nervous system
CO carbon monoxide
dP/dT first time derivative of peak ventricular pressure rise
E/A ratio early diastolic filling wave velocity/late diastolic filling wave velocity ratio

G-protein guanosine triphosphate binding protein
HO heme oxygenase
LV left ventricle
NF-κB nuclear factor kappa B
NO nitric oxide
NOS nitric oxide synthase
NTS nucleus of the solitary tract
ROK Rho kinase
SR sarcoplasmic reticulum

SVR systemic vascular resistance
TIPS transjugular intrahepatic portosystemic shunt
TNF-α tumor necrosis factor-alpha
VEGF vascular endothelial growth factor.

You raise
and gather
the threads and the grams
of life, the final
distillate,
the intimate essences.
Submerged
viscus,
measurer
of the blood

Pablo Neruda, *Ode to the Liver*

Introduction

Until relatively recently in history, the liver was considered to play the dominant role in blood circulation. Indeed, the belief that the liver controlled a separate venous circulation was not dispelled until 1628, when William Harvey demonstrated that the blood circulation is a continuous circuit controlled by the heart. In the latter half of the twentieth century, with the development of techniques for accurately measuring cardiovascular phenomena, Kowalski and Abelmann confirmed that cirrhosis is associated with cardiovascular disturbances.[1]

Specifically, the cardiac output was increased and the systemic vascular resistance and blood pressure decreased in their patients with alcoholic cirrhosis. They ascribed this hyperdynamic circulation to the presence of a circulating vasodilator produced by the diseased liver. This work was followed by many others that confirmed the presence of hyperdynamic circulation in cirrhosis (reviewed in Laleman et al.,[2] Liu et al.,[3] Henriksen and Moller,[4] and Cardenas and Gines[5]). Almost as an afterthought, Kowalski and Abelmann also reported that the electrocardiographic QT interval was prolonged in some patients. This repolarization phenomenon went essentially unnoticed and was "rediscovered" more than 4 decades later. This seminal paper, dating back more than 5 decades, launched the modern era of "cardio-hepatology"—the study of cardiovascular disturbances in liver disease. This area of inquiry, from its early days as an obscure scientific curiosity, has evolved into a clinically important entity. Currently it is recognized that these cardiovascular derangements contribute to the pathogenesis of several complications of liver disease including variceal bleeding, ascites, and hepatorenal syndrome; hepatopulmonary syndrome; and increased susceptibility to peri- and postoperative complications. In the remainder of this chapter, all aspects of cardiovascular function and dysfunction in liver disease will be reviewed, including the peripheral vasculature and the heart as well as their regulatory mechanisms.

Table 22-1 Clinical Consequences of Hyperdynamic Circulation and Cirrhotic Cardiomyopathy

TISSUE OR VASCULAR BED	CLINICAL SYNDROME	PUTATIVE MECHANISM	CLINICAL SIGNIFICANCE
HDC, lung	Hepatopulmonary syndrome	Pulmonary vasodilatation causes hypoxemia	Dyspnea, limited exercise tolerance
HDC, gut	Gastroesophageal varices	Mesenteric vasodilatation increases portal venous flow	Increased risk of variceal bleeding
HDC, kidney	Sodium and water retention	Peripheral vasodilatation produces decreased effective volume?	Peripheral edema and ascites
HDC, brain	Encephalopathy?	Decreased cerebral blood flow; regional redistribution of flow in CNS; autonomic insufficiency	Unknown
HDC, skeletal muscle	Muscle wasting?	Hypoperfusion in late stages? Abnormal blood flow autoregulation	Muscle wasting and weakness
Heart, endocardium	Infective endocarditis	Defective immune cell phagocytosis, opsonization, bacterial killing	Triples risk of endocarditis compared to controls; still rare
Heart, pericardium	Small pericardial effusions	Manifestation of generalized systemic fluid overload	None
Cardiomyocyte repolarization	Prolonged QT interval	Abnormal potassium-channel function causing delayed repolarization	Probably none; torsade de pointes arrhythmia very rare
CCM, after TIPS (short-term)	Precipitate overt heart failure	Abrupt increase in preload severely aggravates diastolic dysfunction	Uncommon and usually transient
CCM, after TIPS (long-term)	Associated with increased mortality within first year	Diastolic dysfunction response to TIPS increases stress on heart?	Presence of diastolic dysfunction at day 28 predicts risk of 1-yr mortality
CCM, after liver transplantation	Precipitate acute heart failure	Afterload normalization stresses ventricular function	Usually transient but more common than suspected in first week
CCM, kidney	Precipitate hepatorenal syndrome in SBP?	Blunted cardiac response to sepsis reduces renal perfusion?	Strong circumstantial evidence
CCM, kidney	Sodium and water retention?	Inadequate LV function decreases effective circulating volume and renal perfusion?	Circumstantial evidence

CCM, cirrhotic cardiomyopathy; CNS, central nervous system; HDC, hyperdynamic circulation; LV, left ventricle; SBP, spontaneous bacterial peritonitis; TIPS, transjugular intrahepatic portosystemic shunt

Hyperdynamic Circulation

Introduction

Since the initial description of hyperdynamic circulation in cirrhosis, much progress has been made in understanding the pathophysiology and pathogenesis of this phenomenon. The hyperdynamic circulation is characterized by increased cardiac output and heart rate, and decreased systemic vascular resistance (SVR) with low arterial blood pressure.[1-5] These hemodynamic alterations arise as a complication of portal hypertension, although the exact mechanisms that lead to hyperdynamic circulation remain unclear.

However, it is clear that many aspects of the cardiovascular system are abnormal in portal hypertension or cirrhosis. The heart itself functions abnormally in several respects, which will be detailed in the following section. Abnormalities in several regional vascular beds including the hepatic, mesenteric/splanchnic, renal, pulmonary, skeletal muscle, and cerebral circulations have been documented (**Table 22-1**).

Clinical Features of Hyperdynamic Circulation

Hyperdynamic circulation is readily evident when well established. The patient with tachycardia, hypotension, and bounding pulses is easily recognized. Although hyperdynamic circulation alone is not distressing to the patient, the clinical relevance of this phenomenon is its propensity to aggravate or precipitate some of the complications of portal hypertension. The degree of hyperdynamic circulation is correlated with advancing liver failure—patients with end-stage liver failure generally show the greatest extent of peripheral vasodilatation and increased cardiac output.[2-6] Thus virtually all patients with decompensated cirrhosis demonstrate evident hyperdynamic circulation. However, the presence of portal hypertension, rather than liver failure, is a "sine qua non" for development of hyperdynamic circulation. Patients with prehepatic portal hypertension attributable to portal vein obstruction, hepatic schistosomiasis, and noncirrhotic portal fibrosis have normal or near-normal hepatocellular function and hyperdynamic circulation.[2-5] Animal models of portal vein stenosis or ligation also confirm this finding.[7,8]

Hyperdynamic splanchnic circulation causes problems. The gut and liver receive approximately 33% of the entire cardiac output, and abnormalities in this vascular bed directly or indirectly contribute to two of the most troublesome complications of cirrhosis: ascites and variceal bleeding. In concert with the increased total cardiac output, mesenteric blood flow also increases.[7,8] Moreover, studies of cirrhosis or portal hypertension both in humans and in animal models confirm that mesenteric hyperemia is not only due to a passive increase in blood flow as part of the increased cardiac output but also due to mesenteric vasodilatation (i.e., the percentage of overall cardiac output perfusing the mesenteric organs also increases).[3-5,7,8] Because portal venous pressure is the product of resistance times flow rate, this mesenteric hyperemia contributes to portal hypertension (the "forward flow" mechanism). Moreover, the portal hypertension induces creation of portosystemic collaterals (gastroesophageal varices), which may not only bleed but also affect the local and systemic circulations.

Recently, bacterial infection has been recognized as a risk factor for precipitating variceal bleeding.[9] The underlying mechanism of this curious observation remains unknown; however, it has been suggested that humoral substances released during the course of sepsis, including endotoxins and cytokines such as tumor necrosis factor-alpha (TNF-α), intensify the hyperdynamic circulation, and thus increase blood flow through varices.

Complications and management of hyperdynamic circulation in different organs or vascular beds such as the lung, kidney, and portal circulation are discussed in detail elsewhere (see Chapters 18, 19, 21, 23). Peripheral vasodilatation has also been proposed to be the main pathogenic determinant leading to renal sodium and water retention, the "primary peripheral vasodilatation" hypothesis.[10] Vasodilatation in the pulmonary vasculature produces the hepatopulmonary syndrome.

Pathogenesis

The exact pathogenic mechanisms of hyperdynamic circulation should be definitively determined. Several factors to date have been postulated to play a role, including humoral substances, central neural activation, tissue hypoxia, and hypervolemia. A proposed schema is outlined as follows (**Fig. 22-1**).

Because portal venous hypertension is a prerequisite for developing hyperdynamic circulation, consideration should begin there. Portal hypertension by itself, or an associated problem such as mesenteric congestion or portosystemic collateralization, starts a chain of events that eventually lead to hyperdynamic circulation. The congested gut favors translocation of bacteria or endotoxin to the portal circulation, and these substances access the systemic circulation by intrahepatic or extrahepatic portosystemic collateral shunts. Moreover, these factors stimulate other vasoactive substances such as cytokines, nitric oxide (NO), carbon monoxide (CO), and endocannabinoids. Portal or mesenteric venous hypertension also leads to neuronal activation in the brainstem and hypothalamic central cardiovascular-regulatory areas such as the ventrolateral medulla and nucleus of the solitary tract (NTS). These subcortical regions then activate the circulation by neurohormonal mechanisms such as the sympathetic nervous system and arginine vasopressin.

Intrahepatic or portal hypertension also leads to expansion of total blood and plasma volume, by a direct signal from the liver/gut either to the kidney or to the vessels to produce peripheral vasodilatation. The vasodilatation decreases the effective circulating volume, thus inducing renal sodium and water retention, which expands extracellular fluid volume. The expanded volume remains ineffective because of pooling in the mesenteric venous reservoir. The decreased effective circulating volume, in concert with humoral factors such as NO and cytokines, induces tissue hypoxia. Hypoxia along with other humoral substances stimulates oxidative stress (i.e., reactive oxygen, nitroxy intermediates). Moreover, the tissue hypoxia and decreased effective volume are sensed by the central neural centers, which stimulate further activating signals to the heart and vasculature. The signal from the gut to the central neural centers is carried by vagal afferent nerves.

Therefore, in this schema, the hyperdynamic circulation starts as a reactive compensatory attempt by the central nervous system (CNS) to relieve mesenteric congestion and/or tissue hypoxia. With progression of liver failure, hyperdynamic alterations become more profound, associated with hyporesponsiveness to vasoconstrictors, increased shunt formation, and autonomic neuropathy. The spleen also contributes to cardiovascular regulation in portal hypertension, via splenic venous baroreceptors as well as a splenorenal interaction. Thus several positive-feedback loops involving humoral factors and neurohormonal substances accentuate the cardiovascular changes. The evidence on which this schema is based is briefly discussed in the next sections.

Nitric Oxide

Nitric oxide (NO) is a powerful endogenous vasodilator released from many different sources including vascular endothelial cells. It is synthesized from L-arginine by three distinct isoforms of NO synthase: neuronal or brain NOS (nNOS, bNOS, NOS1), inducible NOS (iNOS, NOS2), and endothelial NOS (eNOS, NOS3). In 1991 Vallance and Moncada proposed that in cirrhosis, gut-derived endotoxemia up-regulates iNOS, and the overproduction of NO causes hyperdynamic circulation.[11] This hypothesis was subsequently tested by numerous studies. At present, there is abundant evidence that NO contributes to the development or maintenance of hyperdynamic circulation.[12-15] For example, many studies have demonstrated an increased synthesis of NO in humans and in animal models of cirrhosis, and that inhibition of NOS suppresses the hyperdynamic circulation.[16-18] Increased levels of NO also blunt the activity of vasoconstrictor influences such as endothelin and vasopressin in cirrhosis. The exact origin of the increased NO is still unknown. Most evidence indicates that iNOS is not pathogenically involved in hyperdynamic circulation.[19-22]

An alternative hypothesis of eNOS up-regulation is supported by much evidence. Rats with prehepatic portal hypertension show enhanced eNOS activity and protein expression.[20-22] A major mechanism of eNOS up-regulation is

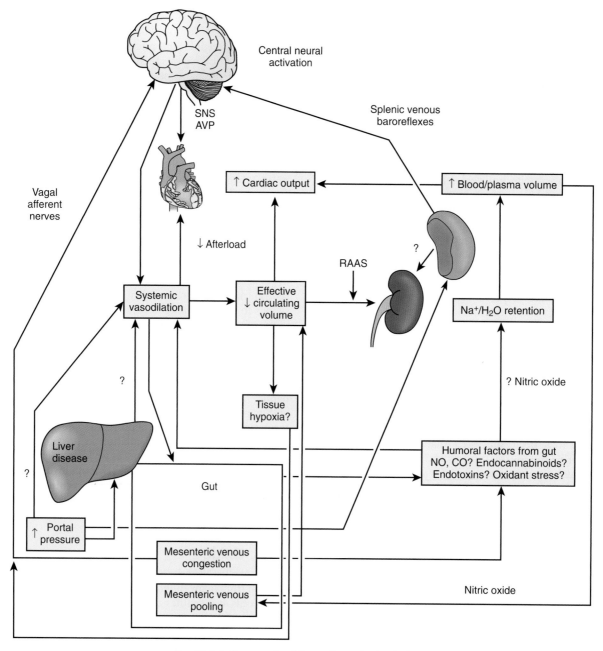

Fig. 22-1 **Pathogenesis of hyperdynamic circulation.**

increased shear stress in vascular endothelial cells. However, this raises a chicken-and-egg paradox because the shear stress is due to peripheral vasodilation and increased blood flow. Proponents of the eNOS hypothesis point to other up-regulatory mechanisms including heat shock protein-90, endocannabinoids, and bacterial translocation with subsequent increased TNF-α production and elevated tetrahydrobiopterin levels.[23-25] Studies in gene-knockout mice lacking the eNOS gene have produced conflicting results. Theodorakis and colleagues reported that such mice do not develop most features of hyperdynamic circulation after portal vein stenosis[26] or CCl4-induced liver fibrosis.[27] However, Iwakiri and co-workers showed that portal-stenosed knockout mice lacking eNOS as well as other mice lacking both iNOS and eNOS still develop hyperdynamic circulation (**Fig. 22-2**).[28]

Several studies indicate a role for RhoA, a small GTPase, and its downstream effector Rho kinase (ROK), which phosphorylates the intracellular signaling protein moesin. Activation of the RhoA/ROK pathway sensitizes the contractile proteins to the effects of calcium, leading to a stronger contraction of vascular smooth muscle. In animal models of portal hypertension and cirrhosis,[29] as well as in human hepatic arteries from cirrhotic patients,[30] RhoA/ROK signaling is defective, leading to a reduced pressor effectiveness of the angiotensin-1 receptor and other constrictor influences. This German group has shown in several studies that abnormal RhoA/ROK signaling thus plays an important role in the reduced constrictor responsiveness to substances such as angiotensin, endothelin, and catecholamines in cirrhosis. Such a reduced pressor response thus contributes to the net

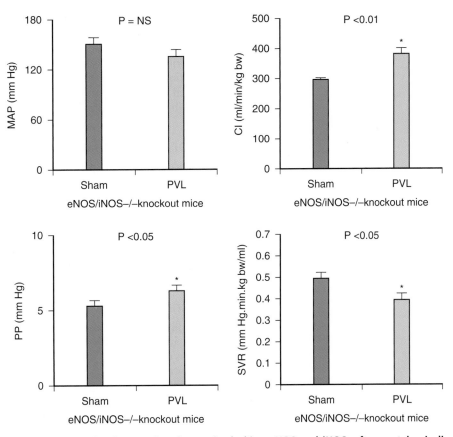

Fig. 22-2 **Hyperdynamic circulation persists in gene-knockout mice lacking eNOS and iNOS, after portal vein ligation.** *(Reproduced from Iwakiri Y, Cadelina G, Sessa WC, et al. Mice with targeted deletion of eNOS develop hyperdynamic circulation associated with portal hypertension. Am J Physiol Gastrointest Liver Physiol 2002;283:G1074–G1081 [orig Fig. 5, p. G1078].)*

vasodilatation, which is a key component of hyperdynamic circulation. A recent study also showed that norfloxacin antibiotic treatment of bile duct–ligated (BDL) cirrhotic rats decreased mesenteric lymphatic bacterial counts and measures of eNOS activity, including the activity of the NO second messenger protein kinase G, but failed to change hyperdynamic circulation and any indices of RhoA/ROK activity.[31] This study thus suggests that the RhoA/ROK system is more important than NO in regulation of hyperdynamic circulation in cirrhosis.

Another isoform of NO synthase, nNOS, may compensate for eNOS in situations where eNOS is inhibited or downregulated. In the aortas of eNOS-knockout mice, increased levels of nNOS partially compensate for the absence of eNOS.[32] A pathogenic role for up-regulated nNOS in cirrhosis is also supported by other studies.[3,5,33] Xu and co-workers treated rats with CCl$_4$-induced cirrhosis with the selective nNOS inhibitor 7-nitroindazole for 1 week.[33] This treatment reverses the hyperdynamic circulation in these rats, without affecting renal function (**Fig. 22-3**). All these results indicate that in portal hypertension and cirrhosis, the source of the increased NO levels is likely eNOS, but nNOS may also contribute, especially in situations where eNOS is inhibited.

Endocannabinoids

The psychotropic properties of exogenous cannabinoids derived from the plant *Cannabis sativa* were discovered centuries ago, but only relatively recently has it been recognized that endogenous cannabinoids or endocannabinoids are found in mammals, including humans. Endocannabinoids exert a vasodilatory effect by means of a ligand-specific G-protein–coupled receptor, the CB1 receptor. In cirrhosis, endocannabinoid levels are increased and vascular CB1 receptors activated.[34-36] Additionally, the CB1 receptor antagonist SR141716A increases the arterial pressure, and reduces the elevated mesenteric blood flow and portal pressure in a cirrhotic rat model.[34,35] An increase in monocyte-derived endocannabinoids was demonstrated in human and rat cirrhosis compared with controls.[34,35] Endocannabinoids such as anandamide may also activate vanilloid receptor 1 (VR1).[37,38] A VR1 antagonist, capsazepine, decreased cardiac output and mesenteric arteriolar diameter and flow, and increased systemic vascular resistance in cirrhotic rats.[38] Therefore the presence of increased levels of endogenous cannabinoids and the activation of vascular cannabinoid CB1 and VR1 receptors in mesenteric vasculature may well contribute to splanchnic vasodilation in portal hypertension. However, not all studies support this notion; one recent study found elevated endocannabinoid levels in patients with cirrhosis, but no correlation between these levels and any hemodynamic measurement.[39] This result only weakly weighs against the endocannabinoid hypothesis, because the multiple cardiovascular-regulatory systems would tend to compensate for changes induced by any one system, and thus would render a simple correlational analysis unreliable.

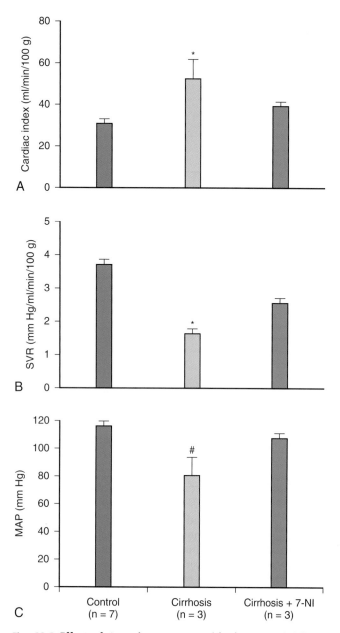

Fig. 22-3 Effect of 1-week treatment with the nNOS inhibitor 7-nitroindazole (7-NI) in rats with CCl₄-induced cirrhosis. Cirrhotic rats treated with 7-NI normalized cardiac index, systemic vascular resistance, and mean arterial pressure. *(Reproduced from Xu L, Carter EP, Ohasa M, et al. Neuronal nitric oxide synthase and systemic vasodilation in rats with cirrhosis. Am J Physiol 2000;279: F1110–F1115 [orig Fig. 2, p. F1112].)*

Heme Oxygenase and Carbon Monoxide

The enzyme heme oxygenase (HO), which exists in inducible (HO-1) and constitutive (HO-2) isoforms, catalyzes the oxidation of heme to the following biologically active molecules: iron, biliverdin, and carbon monoxide (CO). Like NO, CO is a short-lived gas that vasorelaxes by stimulating guanylate cyclase to generate cGMP. Some circumstantial evidence implicates a role for the HO/CO pathway in modulation of vascular tone in portal hypertension. HO-1 up-regulation is observed in cirrhosis with portal hypertension.[39-42] The HO/CO pathway is activated in patients with cirrhosis, and the degree of its activation is greater in those with more severe

disease.[42] In portal-hypertensive rats, NOS inhibition does not completely abolish relaxation of isolated arterial smooth muscle cells and hyporeactivity to vasoconstrictors, suggesting a contribution by a NO-independent local mechanism. HO inhibition partially restores the depressed reactivity to KCl-induced vasoconstriction of isolated perfused mesentery in portal-hypertensive rats.[39]

Other Humoral Factors

Evidence of a possible pathogenic role for several other vasoactive humoral substances has been published. This list includes adrenomedullin, glucagon, adenosine, prostaglandins, substance P, calcitonin gene–related peptide, and bile acids.[2-5,43-46] Patients or animal models of cirrhosis or portal hypertension have elevated levels of all these substances. However, whether this represents cause or effect in terms of hyperdynamic circulation remains unsettled.

Central Neural Mechanisms

Normally, the cardiovascular system is regulated by specific nuclei in the brainstem and hypothalamus, including the nucleus of the solitary tract (NTS), the ventrolateral medulla, the supraoptic nucleus, and the paraventricular nucleus. These areas serve as processing and integration centers for the afferent and efferent nerve traffic that directly controls cardiac and peripheral vascular tone. *c-fos* is an immediate-early gene, which has important roles in cellular signal transduction and transcriptional regulation.[47] Immunohistochemical detection of the *c-fos* protein product, Fos, has been well established as a marker to identify neurons and neuronal pathways that have been activated by physiologic and pathophysiologic stimuli.[47] Recent studies show that central neural activation through a *c-fos*–mediated pathway is a crucial initiating factor in the genesis of the hyperdynamic circulation in cirrhotic and portal-hypertensive animal models.[48-51] Fos immunoreactivity in several central nuclei precedes the development of hyperdynamic circulation in a portal-hypertensive rat model (**Figs. 22-4 and 22-5**).[48] Even more compelling, inhibition of Fos-mediated neuronal activation in the NTS by local microinjections of *c-fos* antisense oligonucleotides completely eliminates the hyperdynamic circulation in portal-hypertensive rats.[48] Therefore it appears that the activation of central cardiovascular-regulatory nuclei, through a *c-fos*–dependent pathway, is necessary for development of hyperdynamic circulation in portal-hypertensive rats.

Several questions remain unanswered, including the following: Which central neurons are activated? The obvious ones, sympathetic catecholaminergic neurons, proved to be only modestly activated (**Fig. 22-6**).[50,53] Perhaps more importantly, what is the cause of this central neural activation? Administration of capsaicin to neonatal animals, which denervates sensory afferent nerves, significantly reduces the baseline central Fos expression in adult portal-hypertensive and cirrhotic rats,[51] and also blocks the development of both ascites and hyperdynamic circulation.[52] In other words, interruption of the peripheral-to-central afferent signaling, from the gut to the cardiovascular-regulatory nuclei, blocks the central neuronal activation and also normalizes the deranged hemodynamics. The peripheral signal is carried to central nuclei by vagal afferent nerves because local capsaicin treatment of the

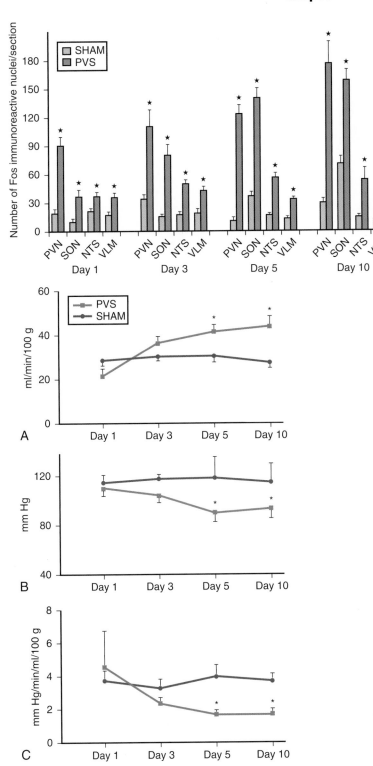

Fig. 22-4 **Central neural activation and hemodynamics following portal vein stenosis *(PVS)* or sham operation in rats.** *Top panel*, Numbers of Fos-positive neurons in paraventricular nucleus *(PVN)*, supraoptic nucleus *(SON)*, solitary tract nucleus *(NTS)*, and ventrolateral medulla *(VLM)* at postoperative days 1, 3, 5, 10. Fos-positive neurons are significantly increased in all areas at all time points in the PVS group. **A,** Cardiac output; **B,** mean arterial pressure; **C,** systemic vascular resistance. *Asterisks*, Significantly different from corresponding sham-control value. Note that central neuronal activation precedes development of hyperdynamic circulation. *(Reproduced from Song D, Liu H, Sharkey KA, et al. Hyperdynamic circulation in portal-hypertensive rats is dependent on central c-fos gene expression. Hepatology 2002;35: 159–166 [orig Figs. 2 (top panel) and 4 (ABC), p. 162].)*

vagal nerves blocked central Fos activation and also partially abrogated the hyperdynamic circulation.[54] In that study, acute portal hypertension caused by inflation of a balloon occlusion around the portal vein resulted in intense vagal afferent nerve electrical activity after a delay of about 4 minutes, suggesting that some factor associated with mesenteric/portal ischemia rather than venous distention is the initiating signal carried to the central areas (**Fig. 22-7**).[54] However, the exact nature of the peripheral signal remains unclear. All these studies demonstrate that central cardiovascular dysregulation plays a crucial initiating role in the genesis of hyperdynamic circulation in portal hypertension and cirrhosis.

Role of the Spleen

This organ is generally ignored by cardiovascular physiologists; however, several studies by the Kaufman laboratory over the past 15 years have elegantly demonstrated that the spleen

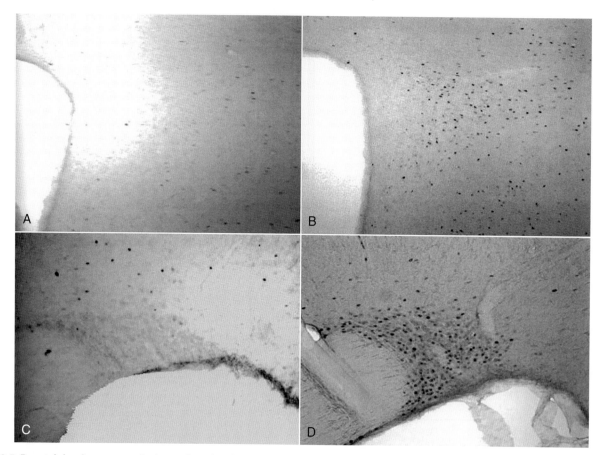

Fig. 22-5 **Fos staining in paraventricular nucleus (PVN) and supraoptic nucleus (SON) of rats at day 1 after portal vein stenosis or sham operation. A,** PVN of sham-control shows virtually no Fos-staining neurons *(small oval dark spots).* **B,** PVN of portal-hypertensive rat shows increased Fos staining. **C,** SON of sham-control shows scant Fos staining. **D,** SON of portal-hypertensive rat shows intense Fos staining.

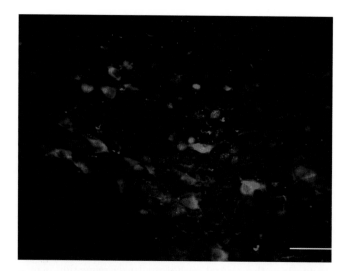

Fig. 22-6 Dual-labeled immunofluorescence staining for tyrosine hydroxylase–containing neurons *(green)* and Fos-positive neurons *(orange)* in NTS of portal-hypertensive rat. Cytoplasmic TH stain indicates a catecholaminergic neuron. Nuclear Fos stain indicates activated neuron. Note that most activated neurons are not TH positive. Day 18 after portal vein stenosis surgery. Calibration bar = 25 μm.

contributes to cardiovascular regulation in the normal state and also in portal hypertension.[55-57] Before the work of Kaufman and colleagues, it was known that the spleen serves as a venous blood reservoir in some animals and volume depletion results in forceful contraction of the organ to help defend the circulating volume. This phenomenon is prominent in cats and dogs[58] but is thought to play little, if any, role in humans.

Kaufman's studies have firmly established that the spleen functions as more than a blood reservoir. Using rats in which, like humans, the spleen does not contract in response to volume depletion, they have shown several pathways by which it helps regulate the cardiovascular system (**Fig. 22-8**).[55-57] First, intrasplenic fluid extravasation from capillaries into the lymphatics is controlled by precapillary and postcapillary sphincters under the control of local mediators such as atrial natriuretic peptide (ANP), NO, and adrenomedullin. Second, and more importantly in portal hypertension, splenic venous hypertension or congestion activates splenic afferents to the hypothalamic cardiovascular-regulatory areas such as the paraventricular and supraoptic nuclei, as well as renal sympathetic efferents (see **Figs. 22-1 and 22-8**). The renal efferent stimulation induces sodium and water retention. The exact mechanism by which splenic venous hypertension leads to renal efferent activation remains unclear but presumably is similar to the peripheral afferent/CNS/efferent arc described

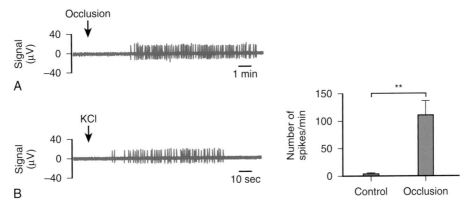

Fig. 22-7 **Effect of acute portal vein occlusion on vagal afferent nerve electrical activity in normal rats. A,** Vagal afferent electrical activity markedly increases starting about 4 min after portal vein occlusion. **B,** After deflation of occluder, KCl depolarization confirms that vagal afferents remain intact and can quickly respond to appropriate stimuli. *(Reproduced from Liu H, Schuelert N, McDougall JJ, et al. Central newal activation of hyperdynamic circulation in portal hypertensive rats depends on vagal afferent nerves. Gut 2008;57:966–973.)*

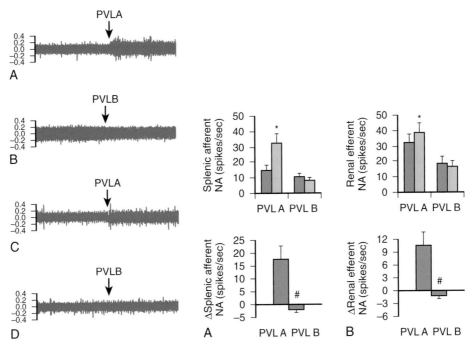

Fig. 22-8 **Splenic afferent and renal efferent nerve electrical activity with portal vein ligation in rats.** *Left panel* shows four representative tracings from splenic afferents (**A** and **B**) and renal efferents (**C** and **D**) with acute portal vein ligation above *(PVLA)* and below *(PVLB)* the porto-splenic junction. *Right panel* shows (**A**) splenic afferent activity as absolute values *(top)* and change from baseline *(bottom)* and (**B**) renal efferents in absolute *(top)* and change from baseline *(bottom)*. *Asterisk,* Significantly different from baseline. #, Significantly different from PVLA group. Note that splenic venous hypertension *(PVLA)* but not mesenteric venous hypertension *(PVLB)* increases splenic afferent and renal efferent nerve activity. *(Reproduced from Hamza SM, Kaufman S. Effect of mesenteric vascular congestion on reflex control of renal blood flow. Am J Physiol 2007;293:R1917–R1922 [Figs. 4, 5; pp. R1920–R1921].)*

previously for the mesenteric/portal system. Finally, the spleen itself may release a vasoactive or neuroactive humoral substance, although this remains conjectural.

Increased Blood and Plasma Volume

It is indisputable that plasma volume and total blood volume are expanded as a result of renal sodium and water retention in cirrhosis. Many other issues about hypervolemia remain highly controversial, in particular the mechanism underlying the renal dysfunction. The debate about the "overload" theory versus the "underfill" or "peripheral vasodilatation" theory has

continued for more than 3 decades. Depending on the theory, the central blood volume, defined as the volume in the heart, aorta, and lungs, should be either expanded or low. Studies have reported both high and low central volume, and this point also remains very controversial.[59,60] Further discussion of this topic is beyond the scope of this chapter (see Chapter 18), but some aspects of hypervolemia merit discussion here.

In patients with cirrhosis, there is evidence of volume-dependent effects on systemic and splanchnic circulation. During acute volume expansion by head-out water immersion, hypervolemia and consequent natriuresis are more pronounced in well-compensated cirrhotic patients than in controls.[61] In contrast, depletion of circulating volume after furosemide administration reduces the portal pressure and hyperdynamic circulation.[62] These observations indicate that significant volume expansion or depletion may regulate the hyperdynamic circulation in well-compensated cirrhosis. In other words, hypervolemia might be involved in the development of hyperdynamic circulation in early cirrhosis. In this regard, a two-phase pathogenesis of hyperdynamic circulation has been proposed.[63] First, the initial event in early preascitic cirrhosis may be extracellular volume expansion attributable to subclinical sodium retention and subsequent passive relaxation of the vasculature in order to accommodate the increased volume. Sodium retention either could be due to a direct hepatorenal interaction acting through sinusoidal portal hypertension and/or hepatic dysfunction (overload theory) or could be a secondary result of peripheral vasodilation, and thus decreased effective volume (peripheral vasodilatation theory). In the second phase, worsening vasodilatation secondary to hyporesponsiveness to vasoconstrictors; activation of neurohormonal systems such as the renin-angiotensin-aldosterone, sympathetic, and endothelin systems; and increased portosystemic shunting may explain the greater degree of hyperdynamic circulation in advanced stages of cirrhosis.[63]

If blood volume is increased, why are SVR and arterial pressure so low? Three possible reasons are (1) tremendous arterial dilatation, (2) pooling of blood volume in the circulation, and (3) inadequate pump function (discussed in the next section). There is ample evidence for the first reason, as detailed previously. Accumulating evidence also supports the second factor. The obvious site for volume pooling is the capacity reservoir of the body—the veins—especially in the splanchnic region. A Danish study using whole-body scintigraphy with indicator dilution methods confirmed that the expanded volume is indeed sequestered in the mesenteric veins of patients with cirrhosis.[64]

In the BDL rat model of cirrhosis, we recently demonstrated that both the hepatic and the mesenteric veins/venules inadequately constrict to mobilize the blood reservoir with normal constrictive stimuli such as vasoconstrictor catecholamines and hemorrhage (i.e., a "sump" effect).[65,66] Moreover, the compliance or the pressure/volume relationship of the mesenteric veins was abnormal in the cirrhotic rat. These venous abnormalities were found to be caused by excess NO produced from the nNOS isoform, because treatment with a specific nNOS inhibitor restores the ability of the cirrhotic mesenteric venules to constrict and thereby mobilize the blood volume reserve to defend arterial perfusion pressure (**Fig. 22-9**).[66] These results partly explain the previously puzzling paradox of "decreased effective circulating volume" in the face of a significantly increased total blood volume.

Tissue Hypoxia and Oxidative Stress

Another adverse effect of the three factors discussed in the preceding section, or perhaps other mechanisms, is latent or overt tissue hypoxia. A significant number of patients have hepatopulmonary syndrome with hypoxemia. Furthermore, even those without overt hypoxemia may suffer from a latent type of tissue hypoxia. Moreau and colleagues noted that patients with cirrhosis show a supply-dependent oxygen consumption.[67,68] In patients with a relatively normal mean Pao_2

level of 92 mm Hg, whole-body oxygen delivery was changed by vasoactive drugs.[68] When O_2 delivery was decreased, oxygen extraction increased to preserve oxygen uptake. However, when O_2 delivery was increased, oxygen consumption increased linearly without an apparent plateau.[68] A normal nonhypoxic individual will not consume any superfluous oxygen, whereas those in a hypoxic state, such as patients with septic shock, avidly consume extra delivered oxygen. Interestingly, patients with cirrhosis show the same delivery-dependent oxygen uptake as those with hypoxic shock syndromes. This suggests the existence of a latent or subclinical hypoxic state in these patients. The intriguing speculation that hyperdynamic circulation is a compensatory reaction to this latent tissue hypoxia[69] was tested by Moller and colleagues in 1996.[70] The administration of 100% oxygen for 20 minutes to cirrhotic patients significantly decreased cardiac output by 11% and increased SVR by 15%. These results suggest that tissue hypoxia does not entirely explain hyperdynamic circulation but may contribute in part.[70]

A related issue is oxidative stress in cirrhosis. In addition to hypoxia, many other factors such as bile acids, endotoxin, NO, sympathetic activation, angiotensin, inflammation, ischemia-reperfusion, and cellular necrosis can generate reactive oxygen and nitroxy intermediates such as O_2^- and $ONOO^-$.[71] There is little doubt about the presence of oxidative stress in liver disease, because many markers such as isoprostanes are elevated in serum and most tissues in cirrhosis.[71] The key question is whether oxidative stress contributes to the genesis of the circulatory dysfunction. Moore and co-workers have shown that treatment of portal-hypertensive rats with the antioxidants N-acetylcysteine and lipoic acid abrogates the hyperdynamic circulation.[72,73] In addition, it has been reported that hyporeactivity to vasoconstrictors in patients with alcoholic cirrhosis of the liver can be reversed by antioxidants.[74] Although these data are suggestive, a definitive pathogenic role for oxygen and nitroxy intermediates is not yet confirmed.

Complications of Hyperdynamic Circulation

Autonomic Dysfunction

The autonomic nervous system plays a critical role in modulating cardiac performance and vasomotor activity. Patients with cirrhosis show an impairment of autonomic cardiovascular reflexes.[75-77] The prevalence and severity of autonomic dysfunction increase with advancing hepatic dysfunction in cirrhosis.[78] Up to 80% of patients with advanced cirrhosis show some evidence of autonomic dysfunction.[77-79] The presence of vagal neuropathy has been reported to be a predictor of reduced survival in patients with compensated cirrhosis.[75-77] An equal prevalence of autonomic neuropathy in alcoholic and nonalcoholic cirrhosis is observed, which strongly suggests that this is not simply a type of alcoholic neurotoxicity.[79] Recent studies confirm the presence of autonomic neuropathy in patients with primary biliary cirrhosis[80] and chronic hepatitis C.[81] In all types of cirrhosis, the parasympathetic system seems to be more commonly affected than the sympathetic system. Vagal dysfunction is reported in 30% to 60% of patients, whereas only 10% to 20% show sympathetic dysfunction.[75-78]

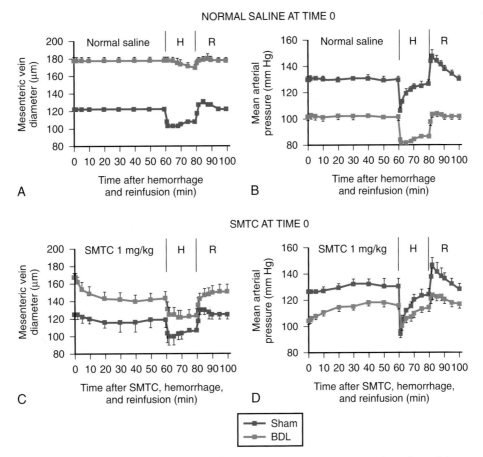

NORMAL SALINE AT TIME 0

SMTC AT TIME 0

Sham
BDL

Fig. 22-9 **Demonstration of in vivo "sump" effect in cirrhotic rat mesenteric venules and restoration of arterial pressure homeostasis by the nNOS inhibitor S-methyl-L-thiocitrulline (SMTC).** In sham-operated control rats *(purple squares)* subjected to graded hemorrhage, mesenteric veins constrict to expel their blood reserve and defend arterial pressure, which after the initial fall is quickly restored. The BDL cirrhotic rat *(blue squares)* veins only slightly constrict and thus arterial pressure remains low during the period of hemorrhage. Pretreatment of the BDL rat with the nNOS inhibitor SMTC restores the ability to constrict mesenteric veins to defend arterial pressure. *(Reproduced from Li Y, Liu H, Gaskari SA, et al. Altered mesenteric venous capacitance and volume pooling in cirrhotic rats are mediated by nitric oxide. Am J Physiol 2008;295:G252–G259 [Fig. 6, p. G255].)*

Autonomic reflex function can be evaluated by standardized cardiovascular tests that quantify the changes in heart rate and blood pressure during a Valsalva maneuver, deep breathing, posture change, sustained hand grip, and pharmacologic stimulation.[75-82] Baroreceptor function can also be quantified by using intravenous phenylephrine to rapidly increase the patient's blood pressure. The abrupt hypertension stimulates baroreceptors to transmit afferent signals to the brainstem cardiovascular centers, which then increase parasympathetic traffic via vagal efferents to reduce heart rate and contractility. This baroreflex function is known to be depressed in cirrhotic patients awaiting liver transplantation.[75,76]

It has been shown that autonomic dysfunction is associated with hyperdynamic circulation.[78,82] Because some patients without autonomic dysfunction have hyperdynamic circulation, such dysfunction is not a prerequisite for the appearance of circulatory abnormalities. However, autonomic dysfunction may amplify the hyperdynamic circulatory abnormalities.[63,82] Furthermore, the severity of hyperdynamic circulation is correlated with the degree of autonomic dysfunction.[3,63,82] Thus autonomic dysfunction can contribute to circulatory abnormalities in several ways. Parasympathetic dysfunction reduces inhibitory vagal tone, thus allowing unfettered cardioacceleration. Moreover, defective sympathetic function may

contribute to the blunted cardiovascular response to vasoconstrictors. Clinical consequences of baroreflex dysfunction include postural hypotension and diminished ability to maintain circulatory homeostasis with cardiovascular insult. This may partially explain the relative fragility of patients with advanced cirrhosis to infection, hemorrhage, and volume depletion.

Cerebral Circulation

Cerebral blood flow, measured by various methods, appears to be decreased in patients with cirrhosis.[83-85] Moreover, virtually all studies have also documented regional redistribution of blood flow, generally from cortical to subcortical regions. Although the exact subcortical regions of such redistribution still need to be definitively determined, most studies have found that the basal ganglia, thalamus, and cerebellum enjoy more blood flow relative to cortical areas such as the frontal and temporal lobes.[83-85] In part, disparities in the literature may reflect heterogeneity in patient populations. Alcohol is a well-known neurotoxin and patients with alcoholic cirrhosis generally have more frontal cortical atrophy and thus decreased blood flow in that region, compared with nonalcoholic patients.

As a result of a high degree of vascular autoregulation the cerebral circulation is normally protected from changes in systemic hemodynamics. For example, cerebral perfusion is unaffected by arterial hypertension or hypotension within a broad range. Such autoregulation appears to be generally intact in patients with cirrhosis, but some studies have found defective autoregulation in those with severe liver failure or with hepatic encephalopathy.[84,85] Even more controversial is whether the cerebral blood flow changes are related to functional neurologic problems such as encephalopathy, abnormal cerebral ammonia metabolism, or altered permeability of the blood–brain barrier. Evidence supporting and rejecting these notions has been reported, and no clear consensus is available at present. For example, Newton and colleagues have suggested that autonomic neuropathy with impaired cerebral vascular autoregulation may cause fatigue and other symptoms in patients with primary biliary cirrhosis.[77,80]

Management

Many attempts to alter hyperdynamic circulation have been reported, although the aim of most such studies is to investigate pathogenesis, rather than treatment. Current pharmacotherapy focused on hyperdynamic circulation includes drugs such as vasopressin, terlipressin, somatostatin, octreotide, and β-blockers such as propranolol and nadolol, all of which exert systemic and splanchnic effects.[5,86,87] Because these drugs are administered for specific effects in the splanchnic circulation such as control of variceal bleeding (Chapter 19), or to treat hepatorenal syndrome (Chapter 21), discussion here will be limited to other treatments relevant to hyperdynamic circulation.

Because NO is a key mediator of circulatory dysfunction, this approach has been studied. Acute administration of the nonspecific NOS inhibitor N^G-monomethyl-L-arginine

(L-NMMA) corrected the altered systemic hemodynamics and improved renal function in one study,[18] whereas in another study arterial pressure increased but renal function remained unchanged.[88] All studies with NOS inhibitors have been acute; therefore chronic effects remain unknown. A theoretical concern of chronic NOS inhibitors is worsening of portal hypertension by aggravating the deficiency of NO in the hepatic microcirculation. However, a study by the Edinburgh group showed no effect of an acute L-NMMA dose on portal pressure in cirrhotic patients.[89] The ideal therapeutic mode of manipulating NO would be a selective NOS blockade of a specific vascular bed or selective delivery of NO to hepatic microcirculation. NO-selective delivery by NOS gene transfer to the liver has been demonstrated in animal models, with promising results.[90]

The oral antibiotic norfloxacin has been used in cirrhotic patients in two studies to reduce bacterial endotoxin levels. In a Spanish study,[91] 42% of 71 patients showed high levels of lipopolysaccharide binding protein (LBP), putatively a marker of endotoxin activation (although 60% of those with high LBP levels had normal endotoxin levels). Norfloxacin treatment for 4 weeks improved SVR and cardiac output only in the high-LBP subgroup (**Fig. 22-10**).[91] An Australian study treated 14 patients with alcoholic cirrhosis, also for 4 weeks.[92] These patients showed a decreased forearm blood flow and increased SVR and arterial pressure, associated with a significant decrease in endotoxin levels. In neither study did renal function change. These studies suggest an important role of gut bacteria in the genesis of hyperdynamic circulation,[5,93] and also highlight the need to confirm these results by larger randomized studies.

Recent studies have disclosed that angiogenesis plays a key pathogenic role in portal hypertension.[93,94] In this regard, vascular endothelial growth factor (VEGF) and platelet-derived growth factor stimulate increased splanchnic

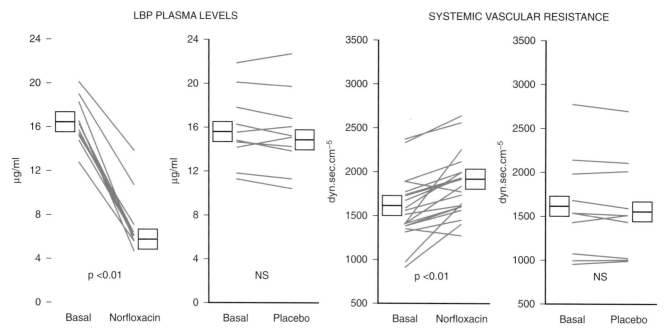

Fig. 22-10 **Effect of norfloxacin treatment or placebo on LBP levels and systemic vascular resistance in patients with ascites.** *LBP,* Lipopolysaccharide binding protein. (*Reproduced from Albillos A, de la Hera A, Gonzálet M, et al. Increased lipopolysaccharide binding protein in cirrhotic patients with marked immune and hemodynamic derangement. Hepatology 2003;37:208–213 [orig Fig. 3, p. 213].)*

neovascularization, and have been shown to be a crucial mechanism in hyperdynamic circulation and portosystemic collateral formation.[93-97] Sorafenib, a tyrosine kinase inhibitor of vascular endothelial growth factor receptor 2 (VEGFR-2), has beneficial effects in rat models of portal hypertension by decreasing splanchnic neovascularization, leading to attenuation of the hyperdynamic circulation.[96,97] However, as a result of their high cost and adverse effects, the tyrosine kinase inhibitors, which have shown promise in patients with advanced hepatocellular carcinoma, have not yet been meaningfully studied in patients with portal hypertension.

The Heart in Cirrhosis

Introduction

Despite all the attention focused on the peripheral circulation, the heart itself was relatively ignored until 1969. This was probably because the increased basal cardiac output as part of the hyperdynamic circulation seemed to be undisputable evidence of normal contractile function. However, in that year, two pioneering studies found similar results. Regan and colleagues carefully studied cardiac contractile function under angiotensin stress in patients with alcoholic liver disease.[98] With angiotensin infusion in the alcoholic patients, left ventricular end-diastolic pressure increased dramatically, almost tripling from the basal value (**Fig. 22-11**). This markedly increased pressure indicated a large increment in ventricular diastolic filling. A normal response to increased diastolic filling would be a significant augmentation of stroke volume. However, on average, stroke volume only rose slightly and

even decreased in some patients, thus indicating a significantly attenuated ventricular contractile response. A few months later, Gould and colleagues subjected patients with alcoholic cirrhosis to exercise stress and noted a similar result: ventricular end-diastolic pressure increased but stroke work index remained unchanged.[99] Five years later, Limas and colleagues again showed that patients with alcoholic cirrhosis had blunted contractile responsiveness to stimuli, and the short-acting cardiac glycoside ouabain was ineffective in increasing contractility.[100] Over the next 1 or 2 decades, many further studies confirmed attenuated cardiac responsiveness to physiologic and pharmacologic challenges in cirrhotic patients, a phenomenon ascribed by every study to the presence of mild or latent alcoholic cardiomyopathy.[2,3,69,101-105]

The idea that these blunted contractile responses are due to cirrhosis rather than alcohol remained unimaginable until the late-1980s. In 1986 Caramelo and colleagues infused physiologic saline into rats with CCl_4-induced cirrhosis and found an astounding 50% decrease in cardiac output.[106] This landmark study was completely ignored by the scientific community at the time, probably because there was no plausible explanation for this unexpected result. In 1989 Lee[69] proposed that the blunted cardiac responsiveness is not due to alcohol, but to cirrhosis itself, an idea subsequently confirmed by numerous studies over the next decade.[101-105] The term cirrhotic cardiomyopathy was coined to describe this phenomenon. The dominant feature of this syndrome is normal or increased baseline ventricular contractility with an attenuated cardiac response to stress. These stresses can include pharmacologic stress, exercise, volume expansion and contraction, and procedures such as placement of transjugular intrahepatic portosystemic stent-shunts (TIPS) and liver transplantation.[77-81]

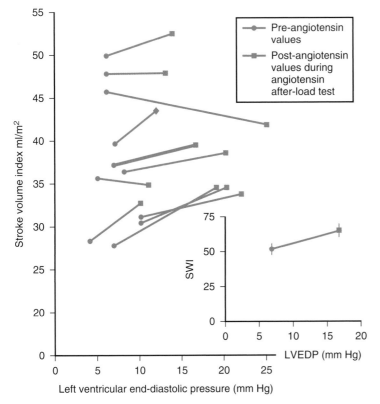

Fig. 22-11 **Effect of angiotensin infusion in patients with alcoholic cirrhosis.** The small inset displays mean values for stroke work index (SWI) and left ventricular end-diastolic pressure (LVEDP). The thicker line represents mean values of stroke volume index and LVEDP. Modest increase in SVI and SWI despite tripling of LVEDP indicates ventricular dysfunction. *(From Regan TJ, Levinson GE, Oldewurtel HA, et al. Ventricular function in noncardiacs with alcoholic fatty liver: role of ethanol in the production of cardiomyopathy. J Clin Invest 1969;48:397–407 [orig Fig. 2, p. 400].)*

The next sections describe the clinical features and pathogenesis of this syndrome and other features of the heart in cirrhosis.

Diagnosis of Cirrhotic Cardiomyopathy

Because no widely accepted, specific diagnostic criteria yet exist, the exact prevalence of the syndrome remains unknown at present. An expert working group is formulating consensus recommendations about specific diagnostic criteria, with a report expected soon. In the absence of these consensus specific criteria, cirrhotic cardiomyopathy can currently be defined by the following general criteria: (1) normal or increased left ventricular systolic contractility at rest, but attenuated systolic or diastolic responses to stress stimuli; (2) electrophysiologic abnormalities such as prolonged electrocardiographic QT interval; (3) structural or histologic changes in cardiac chambers; and (4) serum markers suggestive of cardiac stress. Not all features need be present to suspect the presence of the syndrome.

Systolic and Diastolic Function

Ventricular contraction during systole can be quantified in several ways. These include measurement of stroke volume, end-diastolic and end-systolic volumes, and ejection fraction, which is calculated by the following formula: EF (%) = (stroke volume/end-diastolic volume) × 100. Maximal or submaximal exercise provides the "purest" stress test of cardiac function. Pharmacologic manipulations such as angiotensin to "normalize" the afterload have the inevitable drawback of possible direct drug effects on the heart. Gould and colleagues[99] were the first to use exercise stress in patients with alcoholic cirrhosis. These authors found that with exercise, indices of left ventricular systolic function such as the stroke index, mean systolic ejection rate, stroke-work, and stroke-power showed a markedly blunted response. Many years later, with more sophisticated methods available to study ventricular function, Kelbaek and colleagues[107] examined patients with alcoholic cirrhosis by echocardiography and radionuclide angiocardiography. Although the baseline ejection fraction in cirrhotic patients was similar to that in controls, with submaximal exercise this variable increased 14% in controls but only 6% in cirrhotic patients. In addition, echocardiography demonstrated reduced ventricular wall compliance in the patients with cirrhosis, along with enlarged left atrial dimensions.

In 1995 Grose and colleagues[108] examined maximal exercise responses in patients with both alcoholic and nonalcoholic cirrhosis. Compared with healthy controls that increased their left ventricular ejection fractions and tripled their cardiac output from resting values, cirrhotic patients showed no change in ejection fraction and only doubled cardiac output. Alcoholic and nonalcoholic patients showed virtually identical exercise responses. More recently, Wong and colleagues showed that patients with all types of cirrhosis exhibit impaired systolic function with exercise.[109] Again in this study, increments in maximal ejection fractions and cardiac outputs during exercise were limited in cirrhotic patients, with ascitic patients showing greater dysfunction than those lacking ascites (**Fig. 22-12**).[109]

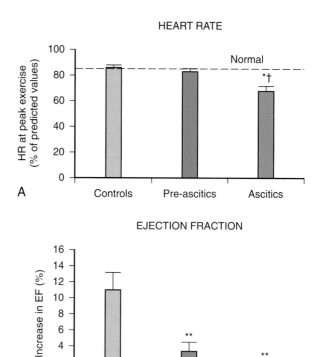

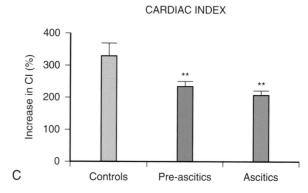

Fig. 22-12 **Cardiac function with maximal exercise in controls and cirrhotic patients with and without ascites. A,** Heart rate (HR) expressed as percent of predicted value. **B,** Increase in ejection fraction. **C,** Increase in cardiac index. Significantly different from controls: *p < 0.05, **p < 0.01. *Dagger,* Significant difference between preascitic and ascitic groups, p < 0.05. (*Reproduced from Wong F, Girgrah N, Graba J, et al. The cardiac response to exercise in cirrhosis. Gut 2001;49:268–275 [orig Fig. 1, p. 271].*)

Despite the aforementioned potential drawbacks of studying vasoactive drug responses, such studies have provided much useful information. The pioneering study of Regan and co-workers used angiotensin to increase afterload stress.[98] Limas and colleagues also normalized the peripheral vascular resistance by infusing angiotensin.[100] This maneuver did not change cardiac output despite a doubling of pulmonary capillary wedge pressure (a measurement of left ventricular end-diastolic pressure), indicating ventricular dysfunction. Since this study, many others have also shown similar systolic dysfunction under pharmacologic stress, equally in alcoholic and nonalcoholic cirrhosis.[69,101-105]

Because the major function of diastole is to quickly refill the ventricle with blood, the factors that determine diastolic function are pressure, volumes, and mechanical forces in the ventricle. Normal diastolic refilling has both passive and active components. Hypertrophy causes the ventricle to become stiff and noncompliant, thus hindering passive elastic recoil and active relaxation in early diastole. Incomplete or slow refilling places added importance on the "atrial kick" of late diastole, which contributes relatively little in the normal ventricle. Echocardiographically, these components can be measured as the E wave, representing the velocity of blood movement in early diastolic filling, and the A wave, the velocity of atrial contraction in late diastole. The E/A ratio is a commonly used parameter of diastolic function. The deceleration time of the mitral E wave also is a measure of the ventricular compliance during the early rapid phase.

In noncirrhotic types of heart failure, such as ischemic or hypertensive cardiomyopathy, diastolic dysfunction usually precedes the more clinically overt systolic dysfunction. A similar chronology appears to be present in cirrhotic cardiomyopathy. In virtually every study to examine diastolic function in cirrhosis, evidence of a stiff, hypertrophic left ventricle has been found, even at rest.[101-105] The E/A ratio is invariably reduced, although some studies reported that this is due to increased A-wave velocity only, whereas others found a combination of both reduced E-wave and increased A-wave velocities[101-105,110,111] (**Fig. 22-13**). E-wave deceleration time is generally prolonged. In many of these studies, indices of systolic function are unimpaired, even increased, and a strong stress is required to show some blunted systolic response. These results suggest that some element of diastolic dysfunction is present in most if not all patients with cirrhosis, whereas systolic dysfunction only manifests under significant stress, and then only in some individuals.

Insertion of transjugular intrahepatic portosystemic stent-shunts (TIPS) represents a significant cardiac stressor because it shunts an important portal venous volume to the right side of the heart. Not unexpectedly, ventricular contractility, particularly diastolic function, can deteriorate following TIPS insertion.[112-114] The cardiac response seems to depend at least partly on the effective volume status of the patient at the time of the procedure.[115] Overt left ventricular failure has been reported after TIPS insertion. Indeed, in a large randomized trial of TIPS versus large-volume paracentesis to treat ascites, overt congestive heart failure (CHF) was precipitated in 12% of the TIPS patients compared with none of the paracentesis group.[116] By a similar mechanism, creation of a surgical portosystemic shunt in patients with cirrhosis also stresses ventricular function, allowing indices of contractile dysfunction to manifest.[117]

Recent studies have shown that the cardiac response to TIPS may be a major, if not the most important, determinant of medium-term survival. Cazzaniga and colleagues demonstrated that the E/A ratio measured at day 28 after TIPS insertion and the baseline MELD score both predicted 1-year survival on univariate analysis; however, on multivariate analysis, only the day-28 E/A ratio remained a significant predictor of survival (**Fig. 22-14**).[118] Rabie and colleagues reported that 40 of 101 patients undergoing TIPS had a baseline E/A <1. This group with diastolic dysfunction not only showed lower survival but also demonstrated impaired diuresis following the TIPS insertion.[119]

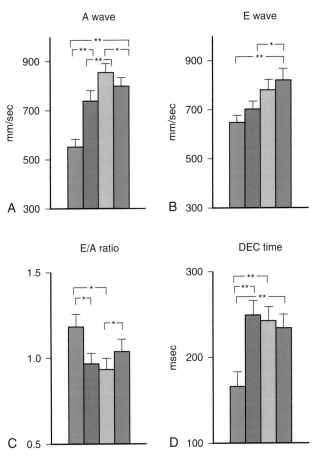

Fig. 22-13 Left ventricular function measured by echocardiography in patients with cirrhosis and controls. A, A wave: velocity of blood filling in late diastole. **B,** E wave: velocity of blood filling in early diastole. **C,** E/A ratio: ratio of early to late filling velocities. **D,** DEC: deceleration time of E-wave velocity. *Green bars,* controls; *blue,* all cirrhotic patients; *orange,* ascitic patients before paracentesis; *turquoise,* ascitic patients after paracentesis. Significantly different, *p < 0.05, **p < 0.01. (*Reproduced from Pozzi M, Carugo S, Boari G, et al. Evidence of functional and structural cardiac abnormalities in cirrhotic patients with and without ascites. Hepatology 1997;26:1131–1137 [original Fig. 3, p. 1135].*)

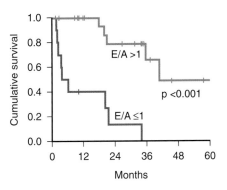

Fig. 22-14 Cumulative survival in patients with TIPS insertion according to their E/A ratio measured at day 28 post-TIPS. (*Reproduced from Cazzaniga M, Salern F, Pagnozzi G, et al. Diastolic dysfunction is associated with poor survival in patients with cirrhosis with transjugular intrahepatic portosystemic shunt. Gut 2007;56:869-875 [orig Fig. 1, p. 872].*)

Cardiac Chamber Dimensions and Histology

Cardiac chamber sizes can be increased volumetrically and by wall thickness. The previous concept that volume overload induces dilatation whereas pressure overload induces hypertrophy is now considered an oversimplification. An example is the cardiac chamber dimensions in cirrhosis, with its hyperdynamic circulation being a low-pressure, volume-overloaded state. There is universal agreement that the left atrium is enlarged, consistent with volume overload and hyperdynamic circulation. Most studies in both cirrhotic patients and animal models have documented slight but significant left ventricular hypertrophy. Echocardiography in cirrhotic patients shows increased wall thickness in the left ventricle and interventricular septum, as well as increased relative wall thickness, defined as LV wall plus septal thickness relative to the LV internal dimensions.[84-87] Right heart chamber sizes remain controversial. The right ventricle has been reported as decreased, normal, or increased in size.[101-105] Animal data are similar. In rats with biliary cirrhosis attributable to chronic bile duct ligation, the left ventricle shows eccentric hypertrophy, whereas the right ventricle is normal.[120]

Antemortem cardiac tissue is very difficult to obtain in the cirrhotic patient. Although there are several large histologic series in patients with cirrhosis, all are autopsy studies and almost all only included patients with alcoholic cirrhosis.[69,101-105] These studies showed myocardial hypertrophy, subendocardial and myocyte edema, patchy fibrosis, exudation, nuclear vacuolation, and unusual pigmentation. Whether these changes truly reflect cirrhotic cardiomyopathy or alcoholic cardiotoxicity remains uncertain. The only study to date to examine antemortem endomyocardial and liver biopsies from the same patients is limited by a relatively small sample size and possible referral/selection bias.[121] Notwithstanding these drawbacks, however, the cardiac samples demonstrated patchy fibrosis and hypertrophy, generally similar to the autopsy studies. Further research is needed before firm conclusions can be drawn.

Electrophysiologic Abnormalities

The three manifestations of electrophysiologic abnormalities in cirrhosis are (1) QT prolongation, (2) chronotropic incompetence, and (3) asynchrony of electromechanical coupling. After the almost incidental finding of prolonged electrocardiographic QT interval by Kowalski and Abelmann,[1] case reports and series of cardiac arrhythmias in cirrhosis have sporadically appeared.[69,101-105] Cases of atrial fibrillation and flutter, ectopic atrial and ventricular beats, and ventricular arrhythmias have been reported. As with much of the older literature in cirrhosis, interpretation of these results is enormously complicated because most patients had alcoholic cirrhosis; therefore potentially arrhythmogenic effects of alcohol cannot be excluded. In other words, it remains unclear if these arrhythmias are due to alcohol or to cirrhosis itself.

QT prolongation was investigated further by Kempler and colleagues in 1993.[122] These authors suggested that QT prolongation is a manifestation of autonomic dysfunction in patients with primary biliary cirrhosis. Subsequently, several more studies conclusively showed that the rate-corrected QT interval (QTc; normal up to 440 msec) is prolonged in

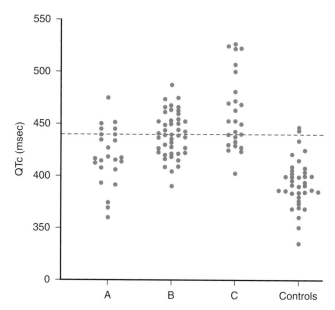

Fig. **22-15** **Electrocardiographic QTc prolongation in patients with cirrhosis (Child-Pugh classes A, B, C) and controls.** *Dotted line* represents the accepted value for the normal limit (440 msec). *(Reproduced from Bernardi M, Calandra S, Colantoni A, et al. Q-T interval prolongation in cirrhosis: prevalence, relationship with severity, and etiology of the disease and possible pathogenetic factors. Hepatology 1998;27:28–34 [orig Fig. 1, p. 31].)*

approximately 30% to 60% of patients with cirrhosis of all etiologies.[123-125] The wide range of the percentage of patients with QTc prolongation is partly due to different methods of correcting the QT for heart rate. The commonly used Bazett method should be avoided in patients with cirrhosis. A careful analysis of several methods of QTc correction in patients with cirrhosis by Zambruni and colleagues showed that the Bazett method incompletely corrected the QT interval for heart rate and thus led to the largest values of QTc.[126] Their study suggests that the Fridericia correction and a cirrhosis-specific correction method are the most reliable and valid correction techniques.[126]

Most studies show that the prevalence of QT prolongation increases with advancing degrees of liver failure (**Fig. 22-15**),[123-126] and is reversible after liver transplantation.[123-125] In other cardiac conditions, delayed repolarization evidenced by QTc prolongation is thought to be a risk factor for a type of ventricular tachycardia called torsade de pointes. However, whether patients with cirrhosis and QT prolongation are truly at risk of this tachycardia remains unclear. Although cases of torsade de pointes have been reported in cirrhotic patients, in every case other potential causes of torsade such as electrolyte disturbance, shock, and the presence of torsadogenic drugs were present. Moreover, sudden cardiac death is not considered to be increased in patients with cirrhosis.

Chronotropic incompetence refers to an inability of the cirrhotic heart to respond to stimuli with the appropriate degree of tachycardia. The clearest demonstration of this is the blunted tachycardic response to exercise (**Fig. 22-11**)[107,109] or vasoactive drug infusion in patients and in animal models of cirrhosis. The most obvious clinical consequence of this phenomenon would be limited exercise capacity.

Finally, Henriksen and colleagues showed that in cirrhotic patients, the time interval between the electrocardiographic and actual mechanical onset of systole is significantly more variable than in controls.[127] In other words, the normally tightly regulated time between the QRS complex and actual onset of ventricular systole becomes abnormally shortened or prolonged. Most patients with prolonged QTc in their study also had prolonged electromechanical time intervals.[127] The clinical significance of this curious phenomenon remains unknown at present.

Serum Markers

Several serum markers, such as cardiac troponin I and the family of natriuretic peptides, appear to reflect myocardial strain or distress. These differ from traditional markers of necrosis/injury, such as CK-MB, in that cardiac muscle stretching or strain without necrosis is sufficient to increase levels. Atrial natriuretic peptide (ANP) is released mainly by the atria in response to stretch, and brain or B-type natriuretic peptide (BNP) is released by the ventricles. They are released as pre-prohormones and cleaved in the circulation. A cardiology consensus committee agreed that BNP and proBNP are excellent markers of a ventricle distressed by pressure/volume overload.[128] Many disease states resulting in volume expansion increase levels of these natriuretic peptides, including renal and heart failure, and cirrhosis. For troponin I, conditions leading to ventricular hypertrophy or dilatation increase levels. Therefore some studies suggest that these markers in cirrhosis merely reflect hyperdynamic circulation and volume overload rather than true cardiac distress.

The available evidence, however, does not support that view. A French study documented increased serum troponin I levels in about one third of cirrhotic patients.[129] Elevated levels correlated with decreased ventricular stroke volume index, rather than any hemodynamic measure of hyperdynamic circulation, portal hypertension, or stage of cirrhosis. In cirrhotic patients, BNP levels correlate with left ventricular size and diastolic dysfunction,[130] and both BNP and proBNP levels are associated with QT interval and degree of liver failure, rather than measures of hyperdynamic circulation such as cardiac output and peripheral vascular resistance.[131,132] These results indicate the potential usefulness of these serum markers to diagnose myocardial distress in cirrhosis, but specific criteria such as exact diagnostic cutoff values remain to be determined.

Complications of Cirrhotic Cardiomyopathy

A possible relationship among ventricular dysfunction, peripheral vasodilatation, and sodium retention in cirrhosis has been postulated. Regardless of whether one believes in the "primary peripheral vasodilatation" or the "overload" theory of salt and fluid retention, renal blood perfusion is dependent on the cardiovascular system. Irregardless of the status of the vessels or fluid inside them, it is intuitive that the pump function be adequate for proper renal perfusion. However, definitively demonstrating that depressed pump function contributes to the pathogenesis of renal sodium retention in cirrhosis is difficult. A study subjected patients with preascitic cirrhosis to a high-sodium diet for 7 days.[133] As expected, these patients started retaining sodium and fluid during this challenge. Whereas healthy controls showed the normal cardiac response, increasing the slope of the peak systolic pressure to end-systolic volume relationship, about half the preascitic cirrhotic patients showed an abnormal inverse relationship (i.e., a reduction of systolic pressure with increasing end-systolic volume). In other words, cardiac contractility was already abnormal at baseline and worsened under sodium loading challenge, in conjunction with renal sodium retention.[133] Another piece of evidence is the aforementioned TIPS-diastolic dysfunction study of Rabie and colleagues,[119] wherein those with diastolic dysfunction (E/A <1) showed an impaired diuresis after the TIPS insertion, compared to cirrhotic patients without diastolic dysfunction (E/A >1). These studies therefore offer compelling circumstantial evidence suggesting that inadequate ventricular contractility contributes to the renal salt and water retention in cirrhosis.

An intriguing study examined cardiovascular and renal function in 23 patients admitted with spontaneous bacterial peritonitis.[134] All patients successfully resolved their infection with appropriate antibiotics. However, during the admission, 8 patients subsequently developed hepatorenal syndrome (HRS) whereas 15 showed unimpaired renal function. In those who developed HRS, compared with those with normal renal function, cardiac output at admission was lower and declined even further with infection resolution, along with a drop in arterial pressure. In contrast, cardiac output did not change in those who had unimpaired kidneys. SVR, a measure of peripheral vascular tone, remained unchanged, indicating that the reduced cardiac output directly translated to decreased renal perfusion. These observations clearly imply, as detailed in a commentary,[135] that inadequate ventricular contractility may contribute to the pathogenesis of hepatorenal syndrome associated with spontaneous bacterial peritonitis.

A longitudinal study from the same Spanish group showed that those with lower cardiac output tended to have worse outcomes in terms of eventually developing HRS.[136] Recently Krag and colleagues demonstrated that the subgroup of patients with cirrhosis and ascites with a low cardiac index (and therefore reduced systolic function [<1.5 L/min/m²]) had significantly worse 1-year survival and renal function parameters, including lower renal blood flow and decreased glomerular filtration rate (**Fig. 22-16**).[137] These studies therefore demonstrate that the extent of cardiac systolic and diastolic dysfunction is associated with worse outcomes as well as a greater degree of renal dysfunction. Whether this relationship is merely associational or causal remains unknown at present.

Pathogenesis of Cirrhotic Cardiomyopathy

Because of the difficulty in obtaining antemortem cardiac tissue or performing invasive research protocols in humans, most pathogenic studies have been done in animal models, particularly the bile duct–ligated (BDL) rat, which develops biliary cirrhosis 3 to 4 weeks after surgery. BDL rats show almost all the characteristics of human cirrhosis including portal hypertension, ascites, jaundice, encephalopathy, and cardiovascular disturbances, including hyperdynamic circulation, hepatopulmonary syndrome, and cirrhotic cardiomyopathy (**Fig. 22-17**).[138-140]

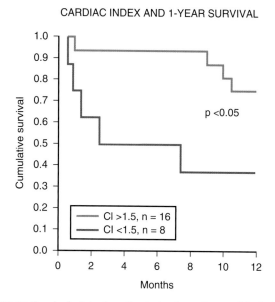

CARDIAC INDEX AND 1-YEAR SURVIVAL

Fig. 22-16 **Survival plot of cardiac index in patients with cirrhosis and ascites.** Patients with low cardiac index (<1.5 L/min/m^2) showed poorer survival compared with those with higher cardiac index. *(Reproduced from Krag A, Bendtsen F, Henriksen JH, et al. Low cardiac output predicts development of hepatorenal syndrome and survival in patients with cirrhosis and ascites. Gut 2010;59:105–110 [Fig. 2, p. 108].)*

Cardiomyocyte Membrane Mechanisms

Myocardial contractility is primarily regulated by the stimulatory β-adrenergic receptor system (**Fig. 22-18**). When the β-adrenoceptor is occupied by a catecholamine ligand, it undergoes conformational change to couple with guanosine triphosphate (GTP) binding protein (G-protein), activating adenylate cyclase to produce the second messenger cAMP. cAMP then stimulates protein kinase A–catalyzed phosphorylation of intracellular calcium-regulatory proteins that eventually leads to calcium fluxes and cell contraction by actin-myosin cross-linking. The major G-protein type associated with the β-adrenergic receptor, Gs (G-stimulatory), is a heterotrimer with α, β, and γ subunits. The β-adrenoceptor-ligand complex couples with oligomeric Gs and eventually dissociates, leaving the Gsα-GTP subunit that then stimulates adenylate cyclase to generate cAMP. A physiologic counterbalance is the muscarinic μ$_2$ receptor coupled to Gi, which inhibits adenylate cyclase. No direct human heart data are available; however, Gerbes and colleagues examined lymphocyte β$_2$-adrenoceptors in patients with cirrhosis.[141] Generally, lymphocyte β$_2$-adrenoceptors reflect the status of cardiac β-receptors (which are predominantly β$_1$ subtype). Gerbes and co-workers reported that lymphocyte β-adrenoceptor density is significantly reduced only in a subgroup of patients with decompensated cirrhosis.

In myocardial membranes from BDL and other rat models of cirrhosis, several defects in β-adrenergic receptor signaling leading to reduced cAMP-generating ability are present.[138-140,142-144] Compared with controls, β-adrenoceptor density[138,142] and Gs-protein content and function[142] are significantly reduced. The presence of jaundice impairs the activity of the adenylate cyclase enzyme.[140] Finally, abnormal membrane biophysical properties affect β-adrenoceptor signaling.[139,143]

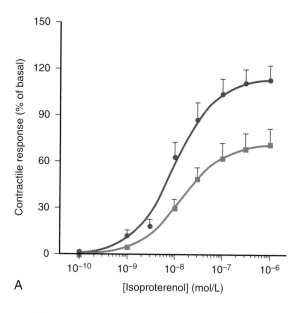

A

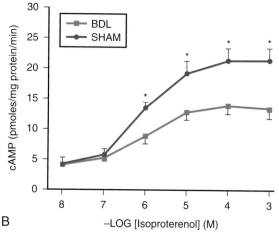

B

Fig. 22-17 **Isoproterenol-stimulated dose-response effects. A,** isolated left ventricular papillary muscles. *Purple line,* controls, *blue line,* bile duct–ligated (BDL) rats. Maximal contractility (Rmax) in BDL muscles is significantly decreased. **B,** cAMP generation in cardiomyocyte plasma membranes from BDL rats and controls. *Asterisk,* Significantly different from corresponding BDL value. These data indicate the presence of ventricular hyporesponsiveness to β-adrenergic stimulation. *(Panel A reproduced from Ma Z, Miyamoto A, Lee SS. Role of altered beta-adrenoceptor signal transduction in the pathogenesis of cirrhotic cardiomyopathy in rats. Gastroenterology 1996;110:1191–1198 [original Fig. 1, p. 1194]. Panel B reproduced from Ma Z, Meddings JB, Lee SS. Membrane physical propertics determine cardiac beta-adrenergic receptor function in cirrhotic rats. Am J Physiol 1994;267:G87–G93 [orig Fig. 4, p. G90].)*

Cellular plasma membranes are composed of a lipid bilayer. Rather than a static arrangement of phospholipids, cholesterol, and other lipids aligned in a neat bilayer, both the lipids and various protein receptors embedded in the membrane are in constant motion. Such motions—including lateral diffusion, rotation, and wobbling—can be quantified by measuring the movement of signals generated by fluorescent lipid probes inserted in the membrane. The biophysical term for this movement ability is membrane fluidity; decreased fluidity implies restricted motional ability. When occupied by the appropriate ligand, receptor proteins undergo conformational change; hence normal membrane fluidity is required for such

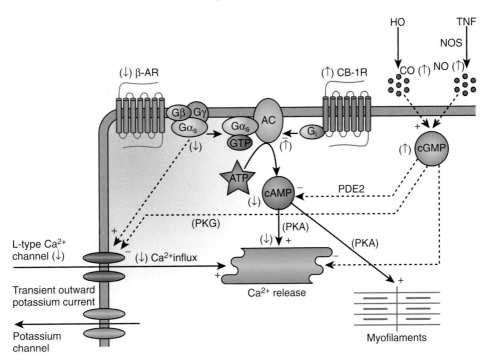

Fig. 22-18 **Regulation of contractility in cirrhotic cardiomyocytes.** *Plus signs* indicate stimulatory effect. *Minus signs* indicate inhibitory effect. *Arrows in parentheses* indicate increased or decreased activity in cirrhosis. AC, adenylyl cyclase; β-AR, β-adrenergic receptor; cAMP, cyclic AMP; CB-1R, cannabinoid receptor 1; cGMP, cyclic GMP; CO, carbon monoxide; Gαs, Gβ, and Gγ, heterotrimeric components of a stimulatory G-protein; Gi, inhibitory G-protein; HO, heme oxygenase; NO, nitric oxide; NOS, nitric oxide synthase; PDE2, phosphodiesterase 2; PKA, cyclic AMP-dependent protein kinase; PKG, cyclic GMP-dependent protein kinase; SR, sarcoplasmic reticulum; TNF, tumor necrosis factor. *(Reproduced from Gaskari SA, Honar H, Lee SS. Therapy insight: cirrhotic cardiomyopathy. Nature Clin Pract Gastroenterol Hepatol 2006;3:329–337.)*

receptors to function properly. Membrane fluidity is predominantly determined by the lipid composition of the bilayer, especially the cholesterol/phospholipid ratio, with higher ratios indicating decreasing fluidity. Cardiomyocyte plasma membranes from BDL rats show increased cholesterol content, and thus decreased fluidity (**Fig. 22-19**).[139] When an in vitro membrane-fluidizing fatty acid analogue (A_2C) is incubated with isolated BDL cardiomyocyte membrane preparations, fluidity is restored to values seen in normal membranes, and concomitantly the cAMP-generating ability is restored.[139] To identify the mechanism whereby decreased fluidity impairs β-adrenergic signaling function, Ma and colleagues used A_2C and other drugs in cirrhotic membranes to directly stimulate the β-adrenergic signaling pathway at different levels (receptor, G-protein, and adenylate cyclase).[143] The results suggest that in the cirrhotic cardiomyocyte, decreased fluidity suppresses cAMP generation by hindering the coupling between the β-adrenoceptor-ligand complex and G-protein, which is undoubtedly a conformation-dependent process.

The inhibitory muscarinic cholinergic system has also been examined. In the cirrhotic rat heart, muscarinic μ2 receptor density and binding affinity are unchanged, but overall muscarinic function is blunted.[145] Membrane Gi-protein content is dramatically reduced, explaining the attenuated muscarinic function. This attenuation is very likely a compensatory effort to balance the blunted stimulatory β-adrenergic system.

Cellular Calcium Kinetics

Intracellular free calcium is the crucial element in contractility. The sources of Ca^{2+} include entry through plasma

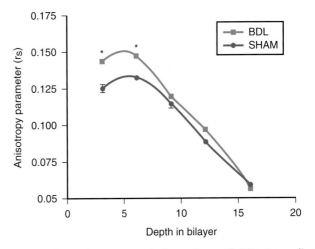

Fig. 22-19 **Dynamic component of membrane fluidity in cardiac sarcolemmal plasma membranes from BDL cirrhotic rat ventricles and sham-operated controls.** Fluidity expressed as anisotropy parameter (r_s) is significantly decreased (higher r_s) in BDL membranes at the superficial depths of the bilayer. *(Reproduced from Ma Z, Meddings JB, Lee SS. Membrane physical properties determine cardiac beta-adrenergic receptor function in cirrhotic rats. Am J Physiol 1994;267:G87–G93. [orig Fig. 2, p. G89].)*

membrane calcium channels and release from intracellular stores in the sarcoplasmic reticulum (SR). SR stores of Ca^{2+} are rapidly released by signals such as depolarization of adjacent transverse tubules (invaginations of the sarcolemmal plasma membrane), free Ca^{2+} that has entered the cell through Ca^{2+}

channels, or drugs such as caffeine or ryanodine (the SR calcium release channel is sometimes termed the ryanodine receptor). Ward and colleagues demonstrated a significant reduction of the elicited inward current of the plasma membrane L-type calcium channel in BDL cardiomyocytes, at baseline and also after isoproterenol stimulation.[145] Western blotting showed that L-type calcium channel protein expression is decreased in BDL ventricles compared with controls.[146]

On the other hand, intracellular SR calcium handling is intact. Several methods to examine SR function and the structure of its component proteins showed no differences between BDL and control hearts. For example, Ca^{2+} reuptake and binding and ryanodine receptor binding characteristics are all unimpaired in the cirrhotic heart.[146] mRNA and protein expression of the proteins controlling SR calcium reuptake and release, the SR Ca^{2+}-ATPase pump (SERCA2) and ryanodine receptor, respectively, are similarly intact.[146] These results indicate that defects in calcium kinetics are not inside the cell, but are concentrated in the plasma membrane.

cGMP-Mediated Mechanisms

Nitric oxide helps regulate contractility by inhibiting certain β-adrenergic functions or calcium kinetics. The exact sites of NO action are still not established but evidence indicates that it may directly inhibit adenylate cyclase, or its intracellular messenger cGMP might inhibit L-type Ca^{2+} channels or the ryanodine receptor.

Systemic or local cardiac overproduction of NO, from any of the three isoforms of NOS, may also play a role in the cardiodepression of cirrhosis.[147-149] Two studies have examined this issue. Van Obbergh and colleagues treated isolated working hearts from BDL rats with the NOS inhibitor N^G-monomethyl-L-arginine and noted increased left ventricular systolic pressure and dP/dT, whereas control hearts were unaffected.[148] Liu and colleagues documented increased iNOS mRNA and protein expression in BDL ventricles, but no change in eNOS mRNA and protein.[149] Immunohistochemical staining localized the iNOS mainly to cardiomyocytes. In control hearts, the NO donor S-nitrosoacetylpenicillamine reduced isolated LV papillary muscle contractility. Administration of the NOS inhibitor L-NAME normalized the attenuated papillary muscle contractility in cirrhotic rats, but did not affect control muscles.[149] These studies therefore strongly suggest that NO generated by local cardiac iNOS up-regulation plays a role in the pathogenesis of contractile dysfunction in cirrhosis. It is interesting that in cirrhosis, eNOS seems to be involved in the peripheral arteries and resistance vessels, nNOS predominates in the veins, and iNOS plays a role in the heart. This highlights the tremendous variability in pathophysiologic mechanisms of NO in different organs and tissues.

Compared with NO, the impact of CO on cardiac physiology and pathophysiology has received much less attention. Liu and colleagues demonstrated increased HO-1 mRNA and protein expression in BDL hearts compared with controls.[150] BDL left ventricular cGMP levels were also elevated, but these levels normalized by treatment with the HO inhibitor zinc protoporphyrin IX (ZnPP). Incubation of cirrhotic papillary muscles with ZnPP also restored the blunted contractile response to isoproterenol, but had no effect in control muscles.[150] These data suggest a pathogenic role for the HO/CO/cGMP system; however, further studies are needed before accepting this notion. A critical unanswered question is the possible interaction of the NO and CO systems in the cirrhotic heart. The relative magnitude of the cGMP generated by each gas also needs clarification, because NO generally is a significantly stronger generator of cGMP than CO.

An Inflammatory Phenotype: NF-κB, TNF-α, and Endocannabinoids

Some of the previously described pathways also link into a complex interrelated system that produces a systemic and local cardiac inflammatory phenotype. According to this schema, increased gut translocation and other factors, including the immunosuppressed condition of cirrhosis, allow bacteria and toxins to access the systemic circulation. The inflammatory cascade is then driven by key mediators such as nuclear factor kappa B (NF-κB). This nuclear transcription factor regulates the transcription of hundreds of genes including most of the key mediators of inflammation such as the cytokines, TNF-α, and interleukins. Our lab has shown a key role of NF-κB in cirrhotic cardiomyopathy. The regulation of this transcription factor is complex; there are multiple regulatory κB subunits. Levels of NF-κB in the cirrhotic rat heart are increased and administration of two different NF-κB antagonists improved the depressed contraction and relaxation velocities of isolated cardiomyocytes excised from cirrhotic rats.[151] TNF-α is a known cardiodepressant and it also interacts with endocannabinoids, which are themselves cardiodepressant.

In cirrhotic rats TNF-α mediates its negative inotropic effects via multiple signaling pathways including interaction with endocannabinoids.[152] Several groups have shown that the cannabinoid CB1 system is activated in rat models of cirrhosis, leading to a suppressive effect on cardiac contractility.[153,156] Treatment with CB1 antagonists such as AM251 improves contractility (**Fig. 22-20**).[155] Preliminary evidence suggests that the source of cannabinoids is local cardiac macrophages and monocytes, with anandamide as the main cannabinoid released by these cells. The excess levels of anandamide may contribute to several adverse effects including a blunted cardiovascular response to hemorrhage.[153-156]

Mechanism of Delayed Repolarization

The underlying mechanism of the QT prolongation is suggested by animal studies. Ward and colleagues examined BDL rat ventricular myocytes and observed significant reduction of two types of K^+ currents: the Ca^{2+}-independent transient outward K^+ current (I_t) and the sustained delayed rectifier current (I_{sus}).[157] Such a reduction in K^+ currents should prolong the action potential and thus the QT interval. However, extrapolating these rat data to humans should be done cautiously because of species variability in subtypes of myocardial K^+ channels.

Coronary Artery Disease in Cirrhosis

A pervasive view dating back to the early twentieth century, and perhaps even earlier, is that patients with cirrhosis are somehow protected from coronary atherosclerosis. Autopsy

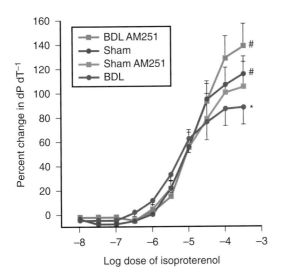

Fig. 22-20 Effect of cannabinoid-1 receptor antagonist AM251 on papillary muscle contractility of cirrhotic rats. CB1 blockade with AM251 treatment increased contractility in BDL cirrhotic rat hearts but did not affect the sham-operated controls. *(Reproduced from Gaskari SA, Liu H, Moezi L, et al. Role of endocannaboids in the pathogenesis of cirrhotic cardiomyopathy in bile duct-ligated rats. Br J Pharmacol 2005;146: 315–323.)*

studies from the first half of the twentieth century generally support this idea. Several theoretical considerations underpin this notion. Serum cholesterol levels are low in patients with noncholestatic cirrhosis. Moderate chronic alcohol intake may somehow decrease atherogenesis. Finally, a major risk factor for coronary artery disease (CAD)—arterial hypertension—is distinctly uncommon once advanced cirrhosis supervenes. On the other hand, moderate or excessive alcohol consumption is a well-known risk factor for precipitating or aggravating hypertension, and type 2 diabetes, another coronary risk factor, is prevalent in patients with cirrhosis. Moreover, the prevalence of nonalcoholic fatty liver disease (NAFLD) is increasing globally, and such patients are at high risk of coronary atherosclerosis because of the metabolic risk factor profile.[158]

The literature suggests that in the early to middle stages of cirrhosis/liver dysfunction, very-low-density lipoprotein levels are normal whereas cardioprotective high-density lipoprotein (HDL) levels are high; as liver failure progresses, low-density lipoprotein (LDL) levels increase and HDL levels decline. Large epidemiologic surveys indicate a U-shaped mortality curve for alcohol consumption: more coronary events in teetotallers compared with moderate (10 to 30 g of ethanol daily) drinkers, whereas heavy drinkers show excess mortality from accidents, liver disease, and certain cancers.[159]

Only a few studies have used the gold standard test, coronary angiography, in patients with advanced cirrhosis being evaluated for transplantation.[160-162] Three studies showed a 3% to 6% prevalence of significant coronary atherosclerosis, whereas two reported a 20% to 27% prevalence of moderate or severe lesions in patients with advanced cirrhosis. In one of the largest series of 167 patients, some degree of coronary atherosclerosis was noted in 60% of the patients, and 20% showed severe stenosis.[162] In that study CAD was similarly prevalent regardless of the etiology of cirrhosis (viral hepatitis, alcoholic, or NAFLD).[162] Limitations of these studies include lack of noncirrhotic control groups, referral and selection bias, and variability in the definitions of significant atherosclerosis.

The belief that alcoholics have less CAD is also prevalent. Coronary angiography studies performed on 100 consecutively admitted male American veterans with a clinical diagnosis of "alcoholism," based on the presence or history of either pancreatitis or cirrhosis, and presenting with chest pain were compared with those of 200 age-matched nonalcoholic controls with chest pain, in a retrospective analysis.[163] CAD was found in a significantly lower number of the alcoholics (42% vs. 58%). However, this study has a number of limitations related to the uncertainty of the diagnosis of "alcoholism," the high prevalence of CAD and alcoholism in a male veteran population, and also the retrospective nature of the study.

Studies have also used less accurate methods of diagnosing CAD. A recent study did not perform routine angiography but instead labeled patients according to a clinical definition of CAD, which included angina pectoris symptoms or previous diagnosis either by a cardiologist or by noninvasive and invasive tests.[164] Compared with an age-, gender-, and smoking-matched control group, cirrhotic patients had increased CAD prevalence (20% vs. 12% in controls). A multivariate analysis determined that cirrhosis alone was not an independent risk factor for CAD; rather, diabetes emerged as the major risk factor, and CAD was more prevalent in cirrhotic patients because this group had more diabetes. Subgroup analysis also showed that in the patients with cirrhosis, older age and alcoholic etiology of cirrhosis were associated with CAD.[164]

The weight of evidence is now sufficient to firmly dispel the myth that cirrhosis protects against CAD. With the increasing global prevalence of NAFLD as a cause of cirrhosis, it is clear that coronary artery disease is a major problem in all patients with cirrhosis. If patients with NAFLD cirrhosis are excluded, then do the other cirrhotic patients show CAD? Most studies suggest that such patients have at least an equal if not greater risk of CAD compared with the noncirrhotic population matched for age and risk factor profile. Although not incontrovertible, it appears that heavy drinking also does not protect against CAD. Finally, not unexpectedly, cardiac surgery in cirrhotic patients with CAD carries higher risks of death and surgical complications.[165]

Endocarditis and Pericarditis

Patients with cirrhosis are immunosuppressed. Defective opsonization, phagocytosis, and bacterial death in immune cells have been demonstrated. A population-based Scandinavian study revealed a 10-fold increased risk of bacterial infections in patients with cirrhosis compared with healthy controls.[166] It is unsurprising then to find a modestly increased risk of bacterial endocarditis in cirrhosis. Snyder and co-workers reviewed the records of more than 41,000 autopsies in Yale-affiliated hospitals, and found a three-fold increase in endocarditis (0.1% in noncirrhotic patients vs. 0.34%).[167]

Small pericardial effusions are very common in patients with ascites. These effusions are rarely clinically symptomatic, and presumably reflect the generalized edematous state of the patient with advanced cirrhosis.

Cardiovascular Function and Liver Transplantation

Liver transplantation is arguably the longest and most strenuous (to both patient and surgeon) routine surgical procedure. Accordingly, it places great stress on the cardiovascular system. Approximately 7% to 15% of early and late mortality after liver transplantation is due to cardiac causes.[168-170] The peripheral vasodilatation of advanced cirrhosis usually improves quickly, increasing the ventricular afterload. Even during the first postoperative day, some parameters of cardiovascular function are improving, although patients with viral cirrhosis improve faster than those with alcoholic cirrhosis.[171] By the third postoperative day, systemic vascular resistance increased by 28% and cardiac output decreased 26% in one study.[172] Given the prevalence of diastolic dysfunction in end-stage cirrhosis, it is not surprising that pulmonary congestion and edema are common in the immediate postoperative period, affecting 47% to 56% of patients.[168,169] Fortunately these episodes are often subclinical and transient. Clinically overt severe heart failure is much less common, afflicting approximately 1% to 4% of patients in the early postoperative period. In part, this relatively small percentage may be due to careful selection: patients with significant coronary disease or overt heart failure are excluded from transplantation.

Emerging interest in the transplant literature focuses on prediction of cardiovascular events after liver transplantation. Commonly used tests to monitor cardiac function such as the dobutamine stress test and radionuclide methods do not accurately predict the occurrence of postoperative ventricular dysfunction or other cardiac events.[173] In a study using intraoperative hemodynamic monitoring, factors including hyponatremia, lower central venous and pulmonary capillary wedge pressures, and longer postoperative intubation times were associated with development of ventricular dysfunction immediately after reperfusion.[174] In another study of the pre- and perioperative factors that predict cardiovascular events, preexisting heart disease, severity of underlying liver disease as estimated by the integrated MELD score, and intraoperative cardiovascular complications predicted later cardiovascular complications.[175]

Later complications potentially include ischemic heart disease attributable to the antirejection drugs that induce hypertension and hyperlipidemia. Several studies of the incidence of ischemic heart disease after transplantation show conflicting results[169,170]; therefore this issue remains undecided.

Whether hyperdynamic systemic circulation and splanchnic circulation completely reverse after transplantation also remains unclear. Several studies have examined cardiac output, SVR, and arterial pressure, as well as splanchnic measurements such as portal pressure and azygos venous blood flow (index of portosystemic collaterals). Some have found no or only minimal changes posttransplantation whereas others determined complete or near-complete resolution. The contention that reversal is a gradual process, and therefore the discrepancy is due to the timing of the follow-up hemodynamic study, does not entirely explain the controversy. For example, Henderson and colleagues followed patients up to 2 years after transplantation who remained hyperdynamic[176] whereas Park[177] and Torregrosa[178] reported essentially complete normalization by 6 months. Gadano and co-workers performed regression analysis of factors affecting hyperdynamic circulation posttransplantation, finding that infection, anemia, rejection, time after transplant, and persistence of portosystemic shunts are significant.[179]

Management of Cirrhotic Cardiomyopathy

Specific management recommendations are currently unclear because of the lack of definitive diagnostic criteria for cirrhotic cardiomyopathy. Moreover, there are very few human studies on treatment of any manifestations of this syndrome.[180-185] Fortunately, in the absence of co-existing alcoholic cardiomyopathy, severe overt heart failure is uncommon. This is likely due to the peripheral vasodilatation of cirrhosis, which "unloads" the left ventricle, as well as compensatory reduction in myocardial inhibitory systems such as the muscarinic system. Nevertheless, some management points should be noted. First, because a hallmark of this syndrome is attenuated ventricular response to stimuli, situations that significantly stress the heart should elicit extra vigilance by treating physicians. Such conditions include major surgery, hemorrhage, infection, rapid volume expansion, paracentesis, TIPS insertion, and vasoactive drug administration. Second, if uncertain about the presence of cardiac dysfunction, imaging studies such as magnetic resonance imaging (MRI), radionuclide scans, or echocardiography in the resting unstressed patient may not reveal any defects; a stress test such as exercise or drug challenge is needed. Third, if overt severe congestive failure appears, then the same general treatment principles of noncirrhotic CHF still apply, with two important caveats. The first is that digitalis compounds are likely ineffective. The evidence for this is a study from 1974 that showed no effect of ouabain in patients with alcoholic cirrhosis.[100] However, this conclusion is still tentative because some patients in that study may have had alcoholic cardiomyopathy. The second caveat is that afterload reduction, a mainstay of CHF treatment in noncirrhotic patients, should be done cautiously in cirrhotic patients. Many already have significant hypotension, and aggressively administering large doses of vasodilators may precipitate vascular collapse and renal shutdown. The treatment of severe CHF should include standard measures such as bed rest, salt restriction, diuretic administration, preload reduction, oxygen supplementation, and *cautious* use of vasodilators to reduce afterload.

Animal studies of cirrhosis imply that inotropic-stimulating drugs based on β-adrenergic stimulation may not be effective, because of the multiple defects in the signaling of this system. The scant available human data support this idea. Patients with cirrhosis show attenuated chronotropic or vascular responses to dobutamine and isoproterenol.[69,101] Phosphodiesterase antagonists such as amrinone inhibit cAMP degradation and thus might be useful because many of the β-adrenergic signaling defects are upstream of adenylate cyclase. Unfortunately, the only available study with this type of drug did not show efficacy. Cirrhotic patients undergoing partial hepatectomy for hepatocellular carcinoma were given amrinone, attempting to decrease perioperative ischemia-reperfusion injury.[182] This drug did not affect cardiac output or arterial pressure in these patients.

In noncirrhotic heart failure, current consensus suggests blocking the potentially cardiotoxic effects of the sympathetic cardiac overdrive by drugs such as β-blockers. This somewhat paradoxical idea has been examined in two studies in patients with cirrhosis. The Copenhagen group administered propranolol to patients with cirrhosis, some of whom had QT prolongation.[183] This drug significantly reduced the prolonged QTc from a mean value of 460 msec to 440 msec. However, the response was different with chronic β-blockade. Zambruni and colleagues administered nadolol for 1 to 3 months to 30 cirrhotic patients, of whom 10 had baseline-prolonged QTc.[184] Interestingly, QTc was shortened only when measured by the unreliable Bazett formula; with the other rate-correction methods, it remained unchanged. By all correction methods, nadolol tended to prolong QT in those with normal QTc and shorten QT in those with a baseline-prolonged QTc. Both studies have limitations including the use of the Bazett correction in the Danish study and the small sample sizes in both. At present, the efficacy of β-blockade in the electrophysiologic complications of cirrhotic cardiomyopathy remains unclear.

The cardiac fibrogenic influence of the angiotensin-aldosterone system has been recently recognized. In this regard, Pozzi and colleagues reported that 6 months of chronic treatment with the aldosterone receptor antagonist potassium canrenoate in cirrhotic patients significantly reduced left ventricular wall thickness and end-diastolic volumes, and showed a nonsignificant tendency to improve the E/A ratio.[185] It is possible that a longer period of drug administration may have eventually improved the diastolic dysfunction. This promising avenue should be further investigated.

Liver transplantation of course is the ultimate curative therapy for cirrhosis and virtually all its complications. In this regard, unlike the controversial reversal of hyperdynamic circulation, transplantation eventually appears to completely reverse the major aspects of cirrhotic cardiomyopathy within 6 to 9 months[178] (discussed under Natural History). However, transplantation is not universally available, and some patients are not suitable transplant candidates. Thus there is a pressing need for further research on treatment of cirrhotic cardiomyopathy.

Natural History

Even though each of the myriad cardiovascular abnormalities in cirrhosis is unique in many ways, they also share a few common features. One such commonality relates to the natural history. Specifically, the magnitude of the cardiovascular disorder is correlated to the degree of liver failure. In other words, patients with mild cirrhosis tend to have the mildest perturbation, whereas those with severe end-stage liver disease show the greatest derangement of the cardiovascular changes.[2-6,69,101-105] This relationship appears to hold in every organ or tissue examined to date, including the brain, kidneys, lungs, gut, and heart, as well as the overall hyperdynamic circulation. For example, cerebral blood flow is generally normal or only slightly decreased in the well-compensated patient, but decreases as liver function deteriorates. The extent of cirrhotic cardiomyopathy also tends to increase with decreasing liver function: ventricular contractile response to exercise or other stress progressively diminishes as cirrhosis worsens, and QT prolongation is accentuated as liver function deteriorates.

Similar to other biologic systems, however, the relationship between these parameters is not infinitely linear—a plateau effect is observed for cardiovascular changes. For example, the extent of peripheral vasodilatation reaches a plateau when the mean arterial pressure drops to the 55 to 60 mm Hg range. No matter how severe the liver failure, mean arterial pressures below this range are rare in the cirrhotic patient (in the absence of acute problems such as bleeding or sepsis). Presumably the plateau effect represents the point at which the cardiovascular disturbance triggers new or previously inadequate compensatory mechanisms, thus allowing continued existence of the organism.

The relationship between circulatory change and liver failure continues to hold when liver function is improved. An example is the decrease in indices of hyperdynamic circulation in patients with alcoholic cirrhosis who stop drinking and gradually improve their liver function. However, the alternative explanation could be that this is due to relief from the many direct toxic effects of alcohol itself, rather than to any improvement in liver function. The strongest evidence in favor of the notion comes from studies of liver transplantation, the ultimate way to improve liver function. Many studies have examined various types of cardiovascular abnormalities before and after transplantation, and although there are a few contrary reports, the weight of evidence indicates that most circulatory disturbances revert to normal or improve dramatically after transplantation. Hepatopulmonary syndrome, cerebral hypoperfusion, hepatorenal syndrome, splanchnic hyperemia, and cirrhotic cardiomyopathy[178] all normalize or disappear at some point after successful liver transplantation. Thus transplantation appears to be the ultimate treatment for cardiovascular complications of cirrhosis.

Conclusion

Hyperdynamic circulation is characterized as increased cardiac output and decreased peripheral vascular resistance with low arterial pressure. Despite the increased baseline cardiac output, the ventricular systolic and diastolic response to stimuli is blunted, a condition termed cirrhotic cardiomyopathy. Other features include abnormal left heart chamber dimensions, electrophysiologic abnormalities, and serum markers suggestive of ventricular strain. Both conditions exert widespread effects in different organs and vascular beds. Moreover, a complex interplay of multifactorial pathogenic mechanisms probably underlies these phenomena, including some factors common to both hyperdynamic circulation and cirrhotic cardiomyopathy such as NO and neurohumoral activation. Extensive research has improved our understanding of pathogenic mechanisms, thus allowing the possibility of novel treatment modalities. Future studies should focus on pharmacologic and genetic approaches to modulate cardiovascular-regulatory systems, and thereby ameliorate complications related to hyperdynamic circulation and cirrhotic cardiomyopathy.

Key References

Albillos A, et al. Increased lipopolysaccharide binding protein in cirrhotic patients with marked immune and hemodynamic derangement. Hepatology 2003;37:208–213. (Ref.91)

Al-Hamoudi WK, et al. Hemodynamics in the immediate post-transplantation period in alcoholic and viral cirrhosis. World J Gastroenterol 2010;16:608–612. (Ref.171)

Baik SK, Fouad TR, Lee SS. Cirrhotic cardiomyopathy: causes and consequences. Orphanet J Rare Dis 2007;2:15. (Ref.104)

Baik SK, et al. Acute hemodynamic effects of octreotide and terlipressin in patients with cirrhosis: a randomized comparison. Am J Gastroenterol 2005;100:631–635. (Ref.87)

Bal JS, Thuluvath PJ. Prolongation of QTc interval: relationship with etiology and severity of liver disease, mortality and liver transplantation. Liver Int 2003;23:243–248. (Ref.125)

Batkai S, et al. Endocannabinoids acting at vascular CB1 receptors mediate the vasodilated state in advanced liver cirrhosis. Nat Med 2001;7:827–832. (Ref.34)

Batkai S, Pacher P. Endocannabinoids and cardiac contractile function: pathophysiological implications. Pharmacol Res 2009;60:99–106. (Ref.154)

Batkai S, et al. Endocannabinoids acting at CB1 receptors mediate the cardiac contractile dysfunction in vivo in cirrhotic rats. Am J Physiol Heart Circ Physiol 2007;293:H1689–H1695. (Ref.156)

Biecker E, et al. Nitric oxide synthase 1 is partly compensating for nitric oxide synthase 3 deficiency in nitric oxide synthase 3 knock-out mice and is elevated in murine and human cirrhosis. Liver Int 2004;24:345–353. (Ref.32)

Blei AT, et al. Hemodynamic evaluation before liver transplantation: insights into the portal hypertensive syndrome. J Clin Gastroenterol 2007;41(Suppl 3):S323–S329. (Ref.162)

Butterworth RF. Pathogenesis of hepatic encephalopathy: new insights from neuroimaging and molecular studies. J Hepatol 2003;39:278–285. (Ref.85)

Cardenas A, Gines P. Portal hypertension. Curr Opin Gastroenterol 2009;25:195–201. (Ref.5)

Cazzaniga M, et al. Diastolic dysfunction is associated with poor survival in patients with cirrhosis with transjugular intrahepatic portosystemic shunt. Gut 2007;56:869–875. (Ref.118)

Ceolotto G, et al. An abnormal gene expression of the β-adrenergic system contributes to the pathogenesis of cardiomyopathy in cirrhotic rats. Hepatology 2008;48:1913–1923. (Ref.144)

Domenicali M, et al. Increased anandamide induced relaxation in mesenteric arteries of cirrhotic rats: role of cannabinoid and vanilloid receptors. Gut 2005;54:522–527. (Ref.36)

Fernandez M, Lambrecht RW, Bonkovsky HL. Increased heme oxygenase activity in splanchnic organs from portal hypertensive rats: role in modulating mesenteric vascular reactivity. J Hepatol 2001;34:812–817. (Ref.39)

Fernandez M, et al. Reversal of portal hypertension and hyperdynamic splanchnic circulation by combined vascular endothelial growth factor and platelet-derived growth factor blockade in rats. Hepatology 2007;46:1208–1217. (Ref.95)

Fernandez M, et al. Angiogenesis in liver disease. J Hepatol 2009;50:604–620. (Ref.94)

Fernandez-Rodriguez CM, et al. Circulating endogenous cannabinoid anandamide and portal, systemic and renal hemodynamics in cirrhosis. Liver Int 2004;24:477–485. (Ref.38)

Feslitsch A, et al. Vasoconstrictor hyporeactivity can be reversed by antioxidants in patients with advanced alcoholic cirrhosis of the liver and ascites. Crit Care Med 2005;33:2028–2033. (Ref.74)

Fouad TR, et al. Prediction of cardiac complications after liver transplantation. Transplantation 2009;87:763–770. (Ref.174)

Frith J, Newton JL. Autonomic dysfunction in chronic liver disease. Liver Int 2009;29:483–489. (Ref.77)

Garcia-Estan J, Ortiz MC, Lee SS. Nitric oxide and renal and cardiac dysfunction in cirrhosis. Clin Sci 2002;102:213–222. (Ref.147)

Garcia-Tsao G, Wiest R. Gut microflora in the pathogenesis of the complications of cirrhosis. Best Pract Res Clin Gastroenterol 2004;18:353–372. (Ref.25)

Gaskari SA, Honar H, Lee SS. Therapy insight: cirrhotic cardiomyopathy. Nature Clin Pract Gastroenterol Hepatol 2006;3:329–337. (Ref.181)

Gaskari SA, et al. Anandamide mediates hyperdynamic circulation in cirrhotic rats via CB1 and VR1 receptors. Brit J Pharmacol 2006;149:898–908. (Ref.37)

Gaskari SA, et al. Role of endocannabinoids in the pathogenesis of cirrhotic cardiomyopathy in bile duct-ligated rats. Br J Pharmacol 2005;146:315–323. (Ref.155)

Geerts AM, et al. Increased angiogenesis and permeability in the mesenteric microvasculature of rats with cirrhosis and portal hypertension: an in vivo study. Liver Int 2006;26:889–898. (Ref.93)

Genovesi S, et al. QT interval prolongation and decreased heart rate variability in cirrhotic patients: relevance of hepatic venous pressure gradient and serum calcium. Clin Sci (London) 2009;116:851–859. (Ref.124)

Gines P, et al. Transjugular intrahepatic portosystemic shunting versus paracentesis plus albumin for refractory ascites in cirrhosis. Gastroenterology 2002;123:1839–1847. (Ref.116)

Gonzalez-Abraldes J, Garcia-Pagan JC, Bosch J. Nitric oxide and portal hypertension. Metab Brain Dis 2002;17:311–324. (Ref.12)

Hamza SM, Kaufman S. Effect of mesenteric vascular congestion on reflex control of renal blood flow. Am J Physiol Regul Integr Comp Physiol 2007;293:R1917–R1922. (Ref.56)

Hamza SM, Kaufman S. Role of spleen in integrated control of splanchnic vascular tone: physiology and pathophysiology. Can J Physiol Pharmacol 2009;87:1–7. (Ref.57)

Hennenberg M, et al. Defective RhoA/Rho-kinase signaling contributes to vascular hypocontractility and vasodilation in cirrhotic rats. Gastroenterology 2006;130:838–854. (Ref.30)

Hennenberg M, et al. Vascular dysfunction in human and rat cirrhosis: role of receptor-desensitizing and calcium-sensitizing proteins. Hepatology 2007;45:495–506. (Ref.29)

Hennenberg M, et al. Lack of effect of norfloxacin on hyperdynamic circulation in bile duct-ligated rats despite reduction of endothelial nitric oxide synthase function: result of unchanged vascular Rho-kinase? Liver Int 2009;29:933–941. (Ref.31)

Henriksen JH. Volume adaptation in chronic liver disease: on the static and dynamic location of water, salt, protein and red cells in cirrhosis. Scand J Clin Lab Invest 2004;64:523–533. (Ref.59)

Henriksen JH, et al. Acute non-selective β-adrenergic blockade reduces prolonged frequency-adjusted Q-T interval (QTc) in patients with cirrhosis. J Hepatol 2004;40:239–246. (Ref.183)

Henriksen JH, et al. Dyssynchronous electrical and mechanical systole in patients with cirrhosis. J Hepatol 2002;36:513–520. (Ref.127)

Henriksen JH, et al. Increased circulating pro-brain natriuretic peptide (proBNP) and brain natriuretic peptide (BNP) in patients with cirrhosis: relation to cardiovascular dysfunction and severity of disease. Gut 2003;52:1511–1517. (Ref.132)

Henriksen JH, Moller S. Cardiac and systemic haemodynamic complications of liver cirrhosis. Scand Cardiovasc J 2009;43:218–225. (Ref.4)

Inserte J, et al. Left ventricular hypertrophy in rats with biliary cirrhosis. Hepatology 2003;38:589–598. (Ref.120)

Iwakiri Y, et al. Mice with targeted deletion of eNOS develop hyperdynamic circulation associated with portal hypertension. Am J Physiol 2002;283:G1074–G1081. (Ref.28)

Jimenez W, Arroyo V. Origins of cardiac dysfunction in cirrhosis. Gut 2003;52:1392–1394. (Ref.131)

Johnston SD, et al. Cardiovascular morbidity and mortality after orthotopic liver transplantation. Transplantation 2002;73:901–906. (Ref.170)

Jones DE, et al. Impaired cardiovascular function in primary biliary cirrhosis. Am J Physiol Gastrointest Liver Physiol 2010 Feb 4 (Epub ahead of print). (Ref.80)

Kalaitzakis E, et al. Coronary artery disease in patients with liver cirrhosis. Dig Dis Sci 2010;55:467–475. (Ref.164)

Kiszka-Kanowitz M, et al. Blood volume distribution in patients with cirrhosis: aspects of the dual-head gamma-camera technique. J Hepatol 2001;35:605–612. (Ref.64)

Kokolis S, et al. Effects of alcoholism on coronary artery disease and left ventricular dysfunction in male veterans. J Invasive Cardiol 2006;18:304–307. (Ref.163)

Krag A, et al. Low cardiac output predicts development of hepatorenal syndrome and survival in patients with cirrhosis and ascites. Gut 2010;59:105–110. (Ref.137)

La Villa G, et al. Hemodynamic, renal, and endocrine effects of acute inhibition of nitric oxide synthase in compensated cirrhosis. Hepatology 2001;34:19–27. (Ref.18)

Laleman W, et al. Portal hypertension: from pathophysiology to clinical practice. Liver Int 2005;25:1079–1090. (Ref.2)

Lee SS. Cardiac dysfunction in spontaneous bacterial peritonitis: a manifestation of cirrhotic cardiomyopathy? Hepatology 2003;38:1089–1091. (Ref.135)

Li Y, et al. Hepatic venous dysregulation contributes to blood volume pooling in cirrhotic rats. Gut 2006;55:1030–1035. (Ref.65)

Li Y, et al. Altered mesenteric venous capacitance and volume pooling in cirrhotic rats are mediated by nitric oxide. Am J Physiol Gastrointest Liver Physiol 2008;295:G252–G259. (Ref.66)

Li Y, et al. Effect of neonatal capsaicin treatment on haemodynamics and renal function in cirrhotic rats. Gut 2003;52:293–299. (Ref.51)

Liu H, Gaskari SA, Lee SS. Cardiac and vascular changes in cirrhosis: pathogenic mechanisms. World J Gastroenterol 2006;12:837–842. (Ref.3)

Liu H, Lee SS. Nuclear factor-kappaB inhibition improves myocardial contractility in rats with cirrhotic cardiomyopathy. Liver Int 2008;28:640–648. (Ref.151)

Liu H, et al. Central neural activation of hyperdynamic circulation in portal hypertensive rats depends on vagal afferent nerves. Gut 2008;57:966–973. (Ref.53)

Makino N, et al. Altered expression of heme oxygenase-1 in the livers of patients with portal hypertensive diseases. Hepatology 2001;33:32–42. (Ref.41)

Mandell MS, et al. Cardiac evaluation of liver transplant candidates. World J Gastroenterol 2008;14:3445–3451. (Ref.172)

McAvoy NC, et al. Prevalence of coronary artery calcification in patients undergoing assessment for orthotopic liver transplantation. Liver Transpl 2008;14:1725–1731. (Ref.161)

Mejias M, et al. Beneficial effects of sorafenib on splanchnic, intrahepatic, and portocollateral circulations in portal hypertensive and cirrhotic rats. Hepatology 2009;49:1245–1256. (Ref.97)

Merli M, et al. Modifications of cardiac function in cirrhotic patients treated with transjugular intrahepatic portosystemic shunt (TIPS). Am J Gastroenterol 2002;97:142–148. (Ref.114)

Mirbagheri SA, et al. Liver: an alarm for the heart? Liver Int 2007;27:891–894. (Ref.158)

Moezi L, Gaskari SA, Lee SS. Endocannabinoids and liver disease. V. Endocannabinoids as mediators of vascular and cardiac abnormalities in cirrhosis. Am J Physiol Gastrointest Liver Physiol 2008;295:G649–G653. (Ref.153)

Moller S, Henriksen JH. Cardiovascular complications of cirrhosis. Gut 2008;57:268–278. (Ref.103)

Moncrief K, Hamza S, Kaufman S. Splenic reflex modulation of central cardiovascular regulatory pathways. Am J Physiol Regul Integr Comp Physiol 2007;293:R234–R242. (Ref.55)

Moreau R. Heme oxygenase: protective enzyme or portal hypertensive molecule? J Hepatol 2001;34:936–939. (Ref.40)

Ocel JJ, et al. Heart and liver disease in 32 patients undergoing biopsy of both organs, with implications for heart or liver transplantation. Mayo Clin Proc 2004;79:492–501. (Ref.121)

Osztovits J, et al. Chronic hepatitis C virus infection associated with autonomic dysfunction. Liver Int 2009;29:1483–1489. (Ref.81)

Pozzi M, et al. Cardiac, neuroadrenergic and portal hemodynamic effects of prolonged aldosterone blockade in postviral Child A cirrhosis. Am J Gastroenterol 2005;100:1110–1116. (Ref.185)

Rabie RN, et al. The use of E/A ratio as a predictor of outcome in cirrhotic patients treated with transjugular intrahepatic portosystemic shunt. Am J Gastroenterol 2009;104:2458–2466. (Ref.119)

Rasaratnam B, et al. The effect of selective intestinal decontamination on the hyperdynamic circulatory state in cirrhosis. A randomized trial. Ann Intern Med 2003;139:186–193. (Ref.92)

Reiberger T, et al. Sorafenib attenuates the portal hypertensive syndrome in partial portal vein ligated rats. J Hepatol 2009;51:865–873. (Ref.96)

Reynaert H, Geerts A. Pharmacological rationale for the use of somatostatin and analogues in portal hypertension. Aliment Pharmacol Ther 2003;18:375–386. (Ref.86)

Ripoll C, et al. Cardiac dysfunction during liver transplantation: incidence and preoperative predictors. Transplantation 2008;85:1766–1772. (Ref.173)

Ros J, et al. Endogenous cannabinoids: a new system involved in the homeostasis of arterial pressure in experimental cirrhosis in the rat. Gastroenterology 2002;122:85–93. (Ref.35)

Ruiz-del-Arbol L, et al. Circulatory function and hepatorenal syndrome in cirrhosis. Hepatology 2005;42:439–447. (Ref.136)

Ruiz-del-Arbol L, et al. Systemic, renal, and hepatic hemodynamic derangement in cirrhotic patients with spontaneous bacterial peritonitis. Hepatology 2003; 38:1210–1218. (Ref.134)

Salerno F, et al. Humoral and cardiac effects of TIPS in cirrhotic patients with different "effective" blood volume. Hepatology 2003;38:1370–1377. (Ref.115)

Salqahtani SA, Fouad TR, Lee SS. Cirrhotic cardiomyopathy. Semin Liver Dis 2008;28:59–69. (Ref.102)

Shah V, et al. Regulation of hepatic eNOS by caveolin and calmodulin after bile duct ligation in rats. Am J Physiol 2001;280:G1209–G1216. (Ref.23)

Shaheen AA, et al. Morbidity and mortality following coronary artery bypass graft surgery in patients with cirrhosis: a population-based study. Liver Int 2009;29:1141–1151. (Ref.165)

Silver MA, et al. BNP Consensus Panel 2004: A clinical approach for the diagnostic, prognostic, screening, treatment monitoring, and therapeutic roles of natriuretic peptides in cardiovascular diseases. Congest Heart Fail 2004;10 (5 Suppl 3):1–30. (Ref.128)

Song D, et al. Hyperdynamic circulation in portal-hypertensive rats is dependent on central c-fos gene expression. Hepatology 2002;35:159–166. (Ref.48)

Song D, et al. Disordered central cardiovascular regulation in portal hypertensive and cirrhotic rats. Am J Physiol 2001;280:G420–G430. (Ref.50)

Spahr L, et al. Clinical significance of basal ganglia alterations at brain MRI and 1H MRS in cirrhosis and role in the pathogenesis of hepatic encephalopathy. Metab Brain Dis 2002;17:399–413. (Ref.83)

Tarquini R, et al. Increased plasma carbon monoxide in patients with viral cirrhosis and hyperdynamic circulation. Am J Gastroenterol 2009;104: 891–897. (Ref.42)

Theodorakis NG, et al. The role of nitric oxide synthase isoforms in extrahepatic portal hypertension: studies in gene-knockout mice. Gastroenterology 2003; 124:1500–1508. (Ref.26)

Theodorakis NG, et al. Role of endothelial nitric oxide synthase in the development of portal hypertension in the carbon tetrachloride induced liver fibrosis model. Am J Physiol Gastrointest Liver Physiol 2009 June 12 (ePub ahead of print). (Ref.27)

Therapondos G, et al. Cardiac morbidity and mortality related to orthotopic liver transplantation. Liver Transpl 2004;10:1441–1453. (Ref.169)

Thiesson HC, et al. Nitric oxide synthase inhibition does not improve renal function in cirrhotic patients with ascites. Am J Gastroenterol 2003;98: 180–186. (Ref.88)

Torregrosa M, et al. Cardiac alterations in cirrhosis: reversibility after liver transplantation. J Hepatol 2005;42:68–74. (Ref.178)

Wiest R, Groszmann RJ. The paradox of nitric oxide in cirrhosis and portal hypertension: too much, not enough. Hepatology 2002;35:478–491. (Ref.13)

Wong F. Cirrhotic cardiomyopathy. Hepatol Int 2009;3:294–304. (Ref.105)

Wong F, Blendis L. The hyperdynamic circulation in cirrhosis: an overview. Pharmacol Ther 2001;89:221–231. (Ref.63)

Yang YY, et al. Mechanisms of TNFα-induced cardiac dysfunction in cholestatic bile duct-ligated mice: interaction between TNF? and endocannabinoids. J Hepatol 2010;53:298–306. (Ref.152)

Zambruni A, et al. QT interval correction in patients with cirrhosis. J Cardiovasc Electrophysiol 2007;18:77–82. (Ref.126)

Zambruni A, et al. Effect of chronic beta-blockade on QT interval in patients with liver cirrhosis. J Hepatol 2008;48:415–421. (Ref.184)

A complete list of references can be found at www.expertconsult.com.

Chapter 23

Pulmonary Complications in Patients with Liver Disease

Moises I. Nevah R. and Michael B. Fallon

ABBREVIATIONS

CBDL common bile duct ligation
CO carbon monoxide
CT computerized tomography
CXR chest radiography
DLCO diffusing capacity for carbon monoxide
ET-1 endothelin-1

HO-1 heme oxygenase-1
HPS hepatopulmonary syndrome
iNOS inducible nitric oxide synthase
L-NAME N^G-nitro-L-arginine methyl ester
mPAP mean pulmonary artery pressure
PAH pulmonary artery hypertension
PFT pulmonary function test(s)

PPHTN portopulmonary hypertension
PVR pulmonary vascular resistance
TIPS transjugular intrahepatic portosystemic shunt
TNF-α tumor necrosis factor alpha

Introduction

Pulmonary symptoms and gas exchange abnormalities occur commonly in patients with chronic liver disease, and a variety of causes have been identified. These include intrinsic cardiopulmonary disorders as well as unique problems associated with the presence of liver disease and/or portal hypertension. Over the last 2 decades, two distinct pulmonary vascular disorders have emerged as important clinical complications in patients with liver disease: hepatopulmonary syndrome (HPS) and portopulmonary hypertension (PPHTN). This chapter will highlight the epidemiology, clinical features, and management of these unique pulmonary vascular complications of liver disease (**Fig. 23-1**).

The Spectrum of Pulmonary Abnormalities in Liver Disease

Between 50% and 70% of cirrhotic patients undergoing evaluation for liver transplantation complain of dyspnea if questioned.[1] In addition, gas exchange abnormalities and abnormal pulmonary function test results occur in as many as 50% of patients. The common causes of pulmonary abnormalities in liver disease are outlined in **Table 23-1**. Chronic obstructive pulmonary disease and congestive heart failure are pulmonary complications that can be present in patients both with and without liver disease. In patients with cirrhosis and portal hypertension, the presence of ascites and/or hepatic hydrothorax may result in pulmonary restriction. In addition, the

deconditioning and muscle wasting associated with advanced liver disease may also cause dyspnea. In a small subset of patients, specific liver diseases are associated with unique pulmonary parenchymal abnormalities, including pulmonary granulomas or fibrosing alveolitis in primary biliary cirrhosis and panacinar emphysema in α_1-antitrypsin deficiency. Finally, two unique pulmonary vascular complications—microvascular dilatation in HPS or vasoconstriction and remodeling in resistance vessels in PPHTN—may develop in 20% to 30% and 6% to 8%, respectively, of patients with liver disease being evaluated for liver transplantation.[2-5]

Hepatopulmonary Syndrome
Definition

Hepatopulmonary syndrome results from intrapulmonary microvascular alterations, dilatation, and/or angiogenesis that develop in a subgroup of patients with liver disease and/or portal hypertension. It is commonly defined by the presence of hepatic dysfunction or portal hypertension, a widened age-corrected alveolar-arterial oxygen gradient on room air with or without hypoxemia, and intrapulmonary vasodilatation.[6,7] Although the association between pulmonary dysfunction and liver disease has been recognized for more than 100 years,[8] the term hepatopulmonary syndrome was not used until 1977[9] when the concept emerged that intrapulmonary vasodilatation caused the gas exchange abnormalities in these patients. Currently, studies demonstrate that as many as 40% to 60% of cirrhotic patients have detectable intrapulmonary vasodilatation[10-12] and that up to 30% will develop impaired

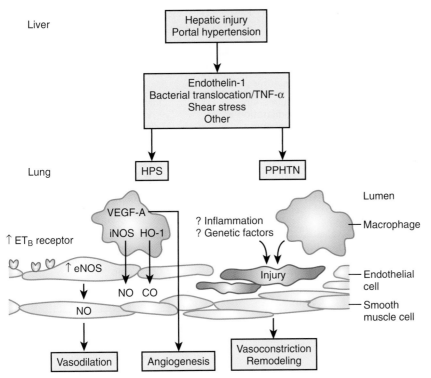

Fig. 23-1 Potential mechanisms of pulmonary vascular alterations in HPS and POPH. Hepatic injury and/or portal hypertension influence the production and release of vasoactive mediators and cytokines and modulate vascular shear stress. In experimental HPS pulmonary vasodilatation results when endothelin-1, produced in the liver, is released into the circulation and stimulates pulmonary vascular eNOS-derived nitric oxide (NO) production through an increased number of endothelin B (ET_B) receptors. Macrophages also accumulate in the vascular lumen and produce NO from inducible nitric oxide synthase (iNOS) and carbon monoxide (CO) from heme oxygenase-1 (HO-1), contributing to vasodilatation. In addition, intravascular macrophages also produce vascular endothelial growth factor A (VEGF-A), which may contribute to angiogenesis in HPS. In POPH similar events, possibly modified by genetic factors and the inflammatory response, may cause endothelial injury, resulting in smooth muscle proliferation and vascular remodeling.

Table 23-1 Pulmonary Abnormalities in Chronic Liver Disease

Intrinsic Cardiopulmonary Disease

Chronic obstructive pulmonary disease
Interstitial lung disease
Congestive heart failure
Pneumonia
Asthma

Related to Liver Disease

Associated with specific liver diseases
   Panacinar emphysema (α_1-antitrypsin deficiency)
   Fibrosing alveolitis, pulmonary granulomas (primary biliary cirrhosis)
Associated with complications from cirrhosis and/or portal hypertension
   Ascites
   Hepatic hydrothorax
   Muscular wasting/debilitation
Specific pulmonary vascular abnormalities
   Hepatopulmonary syndrome
   Portopulmonary hypertension

oxygenation leading to significant functional limitations.[3-5] Early definitions emphasized the need to exclude intrinsic cardiopulmonary disease or hepatic hydrothorax in order to make the diagnosis of HPS.[13] However, it is now clear that HPS may occur in the setting of other cardiopulmonary abnormalities[6,14] and contribute significantly to gas exchange abnormalities in these patients.

A recent task force has graded the severity of HPS based on the degree of hypoxemia as mild ($Pao_2 \geq 80$ mm Hg), moderate ($Pao_2 \geq 60$ to <80 mm Hg), severe ($Pao_2 \geq 50$ to <60 mm Hg), and very severe (Pao_2 <50 mm Hg).[6]

Epidemiology

Hepatopulmonary syndrome is most commonly diagnosed in subjects with cirrhosis and portal hypertension. However, no specific etiology of cirrhosis has been found to increase the risk of developing HPS. Also, conflicting reports regarding whether the presence or severity of HPS correlates with the degree of hepatic synthetic dysfunction and portal hypertension have been published.[3,11,12,15,16] However, a recent prospective multicenter cohort study did not find an association between severity of liver disease and HPS. This study also determined that smokers were less likely to develop HPS.[4] The spectrum of hepatic abnormalities associated with the development of HPS has also recently broadened to include portal hypertension without cirrhosis (prehepatic portal hypertension, nodular regenerative hyperplasia, congenital hepatic fibrosis, and hepatic venous outflow obstruction)[17-19] and hepatic dysfunction in the absence of established portal hypertension (acute and chronic hepatitis).[20-22] Two cases of intrapulmonary shunting and HPS have been reported in patients with metastatic carcinoid and normal liver function but with no evidence of portal hypertension,[23] suggesting that tumor-derived vasoactive substances may have triggered intrapulmonary vasodilatation. Finally, a syndrome similar to HPS has been found in children with congenital cardiovascular abnormalities that result in reduced hepatic venous drainage to the lungs.[24-26] This observation supports the belief that factors normally produced or metabolized in the liver modulate vascular tone and/or angiogenesis.

Pathology and Pathogenesis

One key underlying structural alteration in HPS is dilatation of the precapillary and postcapillary pulmonary vasculature, which leads to impaired oxygenation of venous blood while it passes through the lung.[2] More recent studies in experimental HPS induced by common bile duct ligation (CBDL) in rats demonstrate that angiogenesis also contributes to the pathogenesis of the syndrome.[7,27]

The recognition that angiogenesis also contributes to splanchnic vascular alterations in cirrhosis suggests that similar mechanisms may be involved in both vascular beds. However, splanchnic alterations occur in most patients with cirrhosis whereas HPS is seen in a minority of patients. In addition, HPS may develop in the absence of cirrhosis, and possibly in the absence of portal hypertension. These findings suggest that patients who develop HPS may have a unique susceptibility. In humans, increased systemic and pulmonary production of nitric oxide (NO) occurs in HPS, but inhibition of nitric oxide production does not reliably improve HPS despite improving systemic hemodynamics.[28-31] Therefore the precise role of NO in changes in vascular tone and structure in HPS and the possibility of other mediators contributing to this process have not yet been studied.[32,33]

The development of experimental HPS after CBDL is unique among rodent models of cirrhosis and/or portal hypertension in that other common models, such as thioacetamide-induced cirrhosis and partial portal vein ligation, do not trigger similar molecular or physiologic changes in the lung.[34-36]

Increased pulmonary vascular activation of endothelial nitric oxide synthase (eNOS) increases NO production early after CBDL.[35] The eNOS increase is due in part from a combination of enhanced hepatic production and release of endothelin-1 (ET-1) and a shear-mediated increase in pulmonary endothelial endothelin B (ET_B) receptor expression,[37-39] which signals through eNOS. Later, intravascular macrophages accumulate and produce inducible nitric oxide synthase (iNOS),[35,36] heme oxygenase-1 (HO-1),[35,40] and vascular endothelial growth factor A (VEGF-A).[7] These events contribute to vasodilatation and angiogenesis through the production of iNOS-derived NO, HO-1–derived carbon monoxide (CO), and VEGF-A.[7,35,41,42] Both increased tumor necrosis factor alpha (TNF-α) production and ET-1 itself appear to contribute to endothelial alterations and macrophage accumulation and activation.[37,42,43] Accordingly, in CBDL animals TNF-α inhibition with intestinal decontamination and pentoxifylline administration and the use of selective ET_B receptor antagonists ameliorate HPS and angiogenesis.[37,42,44] **Figure 23-1** summarizes the current understanding of the pathophysiologic mechanisms of hypoxia in experimental HPS. However, whether similar mechanisms are operative in human disease is unknown.

Clinical Features

The majority of patients with HPS either are asymptomatic or develop the insidious onset of dyspnea (**Table 23-2**).[1] Classically, an increase in dyspnea with standing (platypnea) and hypoxemia exacerbated in the upright position (orthodeoxia) have been described in HPS, attributed to the predominance of vasodilatation in the lung bases and the increased blood flow through these regions when the patient is upright.[45] However, these findings are uncommon and are of limited diagnostic utility.[46,47] Several other clinical signs, including spider angiomas, digital clubbing, and cyanosis, are commonly described in subjects with HPS but also have not been

Table 23-2 Characteristics of HPS and PPHTN

HEPATOPULMONARY SYNDROME	PORTOPULMONARY HYPERTENSION
Key Features	
Intrapulmonary vasodilatation and/or angiogenesis	Intrapulmonary vasoconstriction and arterial remodeling
Develops with hepatic synthetic dysfunction and/or portal hypertension	Develops in setting of portal hypertension
Present in 8-30% of patients with cirrhosis	Present in 3-16% of patients with advanced liver disease
Liver transplantation generally curative	Liver transplant only beneficial in limited and selected cases; often contraindicated
Symptoms	
May be asymptomatic	Often asymptomatic
Dyspnea	Dyspnea (most common)
Platypnea	Chest pain
	Syncope
Signs	
Spider angiomas	Jugular distention
Digital clubbing	Accentuated P2
Cyanosis	Tricuspid regurgitation murmur
	Anasarca
Arterial Blood Gases	
Widened AaPO2 common Hypoxemia	Widened AaPO2 uncommon
Pulmonary Function Tests	
Decreased DLCO	Normal
Chest Radiography	
Normal or basilar interstitial changes	Normal or prominent PA/right heart chambers

$AaPO_2$, alvcolar-arterial oxygen gradient; DLCO, carbon monoxide diffusion in the lungs; P2, pulmonic second sound

prospectively evaluated as diagnostic indicators. In addition, because respiratory symptoms are common and may co-exist with poor physical condition, smoking, ascites, and/or intrinsic lung disease in cirrhosis, the diagnosis of HPS may be delayed and identified only after severe arterial hypoxemia has ensued. Finally, sleep-time oxygen desaturation also appears to occur commonly in patients with HPS and may worsen hypoxemia at night.[48]

Chest radiography (CXR) and pulmonary function tests (PFT) are often performed to evaluate dyspnea. In HPS the CXR is most commonly normal, but may reveal lower lobe interstitial changes that may be confused with pulmonary fibrosis.[3] PFT typically demonstrate well-preserved spirometry and lung volumes in HPS. However, the diffusing capacity for carbon monoxide (DLCO) is often significantly reduced and may suggest the diagnosis. Unfortunately, the DLCO is also commonly decreased in cirrhosis in the absence of HPS, and the diagnostic utility of a reduced value is not established.[49,50]

Diagnosis

A high index of suspicion is needed to identify HPS in patients with chronic liver disease and/or portal hypertension. An

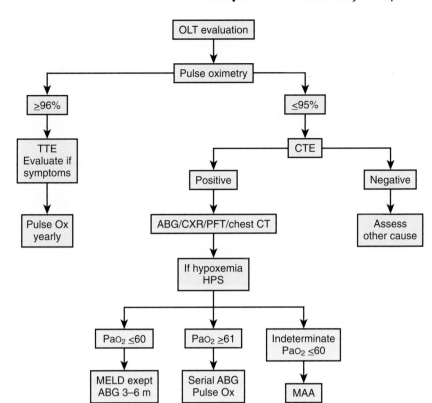

Fig. 23-2 Diagnostic approach to HPS. See text for details. ABG, arterial blood gases; CT, computed tomography; CTE, contrast transthoracic echocardiogram; CXR, chest x-ray; MAA, technetium-labeled macroaggregated albumin scan; MELD, Model for End-Stage Liver Disease; OLT, orthotopic liver transplantation; Pao$_2$, partial pressure of oxygen in arterial blood; PFT, pulmonary function test; TTE, transthoracic echocardiogram.

overview of the evaluation for HPS is outlined in **Figure 23-2**. The threshold for pursuing the diagnosis may be influenced by a number of factors, including the presence of specific signs and symptoms and/or risk factors for intrinsic cardiopulmonary disease as well as the consideration of liver transplantation. Specifically, evaluation is appropriate in all patients complaining of dyspnea and/or displaying clubbing or cyanosis. In patients with specific risk factors (smoking and other cardiovascular risk factors, occupational exposure, liver diseases associated with intrinsic lung disease) assessment of the presence and severity of intrinsic cardiopulmonary disease is crucial. In patients being considered for liver transplantation, regardless of the presence of symptoms, screening is important and cost effective.[51] In this latter group it is particularly important to diagnose and differentiate HPS and PPHTN, given that the presence of these disorders may influence treatment and transplant candidacy and priority.

The diagnosis of HPS relies on documentation of the presence of arterial gas exchange abnormalities resulting from intrapulmonary vasodilatation in the appropriate clinical setting. Gas exchange abnormalities are generally detected by arterial blood gas (ABG) measurements and have been defined as a widened alveolar-arterial oxygen gradient (Aapo$_2$ >5-20 mm Hg) with or without hypoxemia (Pao$_2$ <70 mm Hg) in HPS.[6] The inclusion of mild gas exchange abnormalities in the definition of HPS detects "early" disease and may be important based on recent findings that mortality is increased in HPS relative to non-HPS cirrhotic patients, even when gas exchange abnormalities are mild.[4,12] The Aapo$_2$ value normally widens with age and therefore should be corrected for age (normal = 10 + 0.43[age − 20]) to avoid overestimation of the prevalence of HPS. Obtaining arterial blood gases in the sitting position may enhance the detection of arterial deoxygenation in HPS because of the predominance of

vasodilatation in the lower lung fields. Pulse oximetry is an alternative noninvasive screening modality that indirectly measures oxygen saturation and can screen for arterial hypoxemia. Recent studies demonstrate that using a pulse oximetry threshold Spo$_2$ value of ≤96% is highly sensitive (100%) and specific (88%) in detecting all patients with HPS and a Pao$_2$ of <70 mm Hg.[52,53]

Intrapulmonary vasodilatation can be detected using contrast echocardiography, lung perfusion scanning, pulmonary angiography, and high-resolution chest CT scanning. Two-dimensional transthoracic contrast echocardiography is the most sensitive and most commonly employed screening technique. Typically, agitated saline is used as a contrast agent because the microbubbles are visible on echocardiography (**Fig. 23-3**). A positive test for intrapulmonary vasodilatation occurs when intravenously administered microbubbles are visualized late (more than three cardiac cycles) in the left cardiac chambers.[10,54,55] Immediate visualization of injected contrast in the left heart indicates intracardiac shunting. Transesophageal contrast echocardiography may increase the sensitivity of detecting intrapulmonary vasodilatation compared with transthoracic echocardiography, but is invasive and more expensive.[10,54,55] Echocardiography can also assess cardiac function and estimate pulmonary arterial systolic pressure, and is useful to screen for cardiac dysfunction and PPHTN. As many as 40% to 60% of patients with cirrhosis and normal arterial blood gases may have a positive contrast echocardiogram, suggesting that mild intrapulmonary vasodilatation insufficient to alter gas exchange is common in patients with cirrhosis.[10-12] Also, a positive result on contrast echocardiography in a hypoxemic patient with concomitant pulmonary dysfunction (pleural effusion, chronic obstructive pulmonary disease) does not establish HPS as a cause of gas exchange

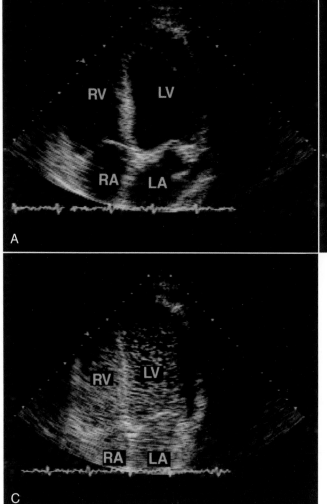

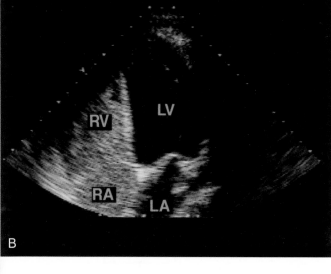

Fig. 23-3 **Contrast echocardiogram for detecting intrapulmonary vasodilatation. A,** Parasternal four-chamber view of the heart (RA, right atrium; RV, right ventricle; LA, left atrium; LV, left ventricle) before the administration of agitated saline contrast. **B,** Four-chamber view immediately after the administration of contrast, demonstrating the presence of echogenic microbubbles in the right atrium and ventricle immediately after injection of agitated saline into the antecubital vein. **C,** Three cardiac cycles after visualization on the right side of the heart, echogenic microbubbles are seen in the left atrium and ventricle because of intrapulmonary vasodilatation in a patient with hepatopulmonary syndrome. Intracardiac shunting results in the immediate passage of microbubbles from the right to left chambers without a three-cycle delay and can be excluded using this technique.

abnormalities, because either intrapulmonary vasodilatation or the underlying pulmonary process could be responsible. In these patients additional testing with radionuclide lung perfusion scanning may be useful.

Radionuclide lung perfusion scanning using technetium-labeled macroaggregated albumin particles (^{99m}TcMAA scan) is another method for detecting intrapulmonary vasodilatation (**Fig. 23-4**). In this test, macroaggregated albumin particles 20 µm in size are injected intravenously. Normally, all particles are trapped in the lung microvasculature. In HPS, some particles escape through abnormal capillaries and lodge in downstream capillary beds. Quantitative imaging of the lung and brain using a standardized methodology allows the calculation of a shunt fraction.[10,27,56] The ^{99m}TcMAA scan offers one significant advantage over contrast echocardiography: a positive scan (shunt fraction >6%) is specific for the presence of HPS even in the setting of co-existing intrinsic lung disease.[10,56] In addition, it can be used to quantify intrapulmonary shunting and is useful for following the progression and/or resolution of the disease prospectively. However, as a screening test, ^{99m}TcMAA scanning is less sensitive than contrast echocardiography in detecting intrapulmonary vasodilatation, and cannot evaluate cardiac function or intracardiac shunting, or estimate pulmonary artery pressures.

Pulmonary angiography is an invasive and insensitive diagnostic modality for detecting intrapulmonary vasodilatation in HPS and is not useful as a screening test. Two types of angiographic findings have been reported: type 1, a diffuse "spongiform" appearance of pulmonary vessels during the arterial phase; and type 2, small discrete arteriovenous communications. The great majority of patients with HPS have either normal angiograms or type 1 findings even when hypoxemia is severe. Therefore angiography has a very limited diagnostic and therapeutic role in HPS.[57,58]

Recent studies and case reports have demonstrated that high-resolution chest computed tomography (CT) may be a less invasive radiologic method to detect dilated pulmonary vessels and intrapulmonary shunting in HPS.[23,59,60] The degree of dilatation observed on CT was found to correlate with the severity of gas exchange abnormalities in several studies, suggesting that CT may be useful in assessing the presence and severity of HPS.

Therapy

No clearly effective medical therapy for HPS is available. Somatostatin, almitrine, indomethacin, inhaled (nebulized) L-NAME, aspirin, and plasma exchange have all been tried

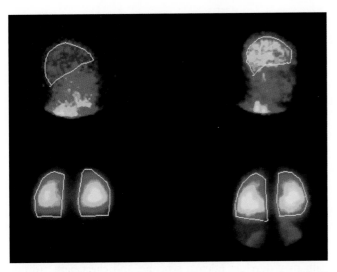

Fig. 23-4 Technetium-labeled macroaggregated albumin (MAA) scanning to detect and quantify intrapulmonary shunting in HPS. *Left,* Normal MAA scan with regions of interest drawn around the lungs and cerebrum. In the absence of intrapulmonary vasodilatation, little of the intravenously administered labeled albumin passes through the lungs and signal intensity is low in the cerebrum. Shunting is quantified by comparing the relative signal intensity in the lung versus that in the brain. *Right,* An abnormal MAA scan in HPS demonstrates significant cerebral uptake attributable to the passage of labeled albumin through the dilated pulmonary microvasculature. *(Reproduced from Abrams GA et al. Use of macroaggregated albumin lung perfusion scan to diagnose hepatopulmonary syndrome: a new approach. Gastroenterology 1998;114:308.)*

without clear benefit.[3,27] A single open labeled clinical trial and case reports using garlic have shown some benefit in HPS.[61,62] In one trial, garlic powder was administered for a minimum of 6 months; 6 of the 15 (40%) patients demonstrated a significant improvement in Pao_2 (>10 mm Hg) and 1 patient showed resolution of hypoxemia (Pao_2, 46 to 80 mm Hg) over a 1.5-year period. Recently, pentoxifylline (PTX), a phosphodiesterase inhibitor with known mild tumor necrosis factor alpha (TNF-α) and NO inhibitory properties, has been linked to improved oxygenation in experimental HPS.[43,63,64] However, in human subjects HPS results with PTX are conflicting. In one study, tolerability of the drug was poor and no oxygenation benefit was observed.[63] In the other study, tolerability to PTX was not a limiting factor and there was an overall improvement in Pao_2 of more than 10 mm Hg.[64] These reports highlight the need to target likely pathogenetic mechanisms in randomized multicenter trials in order to recruit sufficient numbers of patients to achieve adequate statistical power.

Eight case reports have evaluated the effects of transjugular intrahepatic portosystemic shunt (TIPS) on HPS in cirrhosis; five found a degree of improvement in oxygenation. However, the short duration of follow-up in the first two reports[65] and the presence of co-existent hepatic hydrothorax in the third study[66] limit evaluation of the utility of TIPS in these cases. In the fourth report, 6 months after TIPS placement arterial oxygenation clearly improved by 20 mm Hg.[67] However, based on radionuclide lung perfusion scanning, significant intrapulmonary shunting persisted and the cardiac output increased after TIPS. These findings suggest that improved oxygenation may not have been due to reversal of intrapulmonary vasodilatation. Fifth and sixth reports in a 11-year-old girl with biliary

atresia and in a 46-year-old woman with alcoholic liver disease revealed significantly improved oxygenation and decreased intrapulmonary shunting sustained over 8 months and 3 years, respectively, after TIPS placement.[68] The seventh and most recent case report is of a 46-year-old female with HPS presenting with severe dyspnea, hypoxemia, and orthodeoxia. After TIPS placement the patient experienced complete resolution of her symptoms and a 12 mm Hg improvement in the Pao_2. Six months later, recurrence of symptoms coincided with a 50% reduction in TIPS caliber, which later improved after dilatation of the shunt. One year after placement of the TIPS, the patient underwent successful liver transplantation. An eighth report showed failure of TIPS to improve oxygenation in one patient, and identification of two patients where HPS developed in the setting of a functioning TIPS.[69] Together, these findings document the considerable uncertainty regarding the utility of TIPS in HPS. Currently, TIPS should be considered an experimental treatment and its use confined to the setting of clinical trials so that its efficacy may be judged.

Prognosis and Natural History

The natural history of HPS is incompletely characterized, although quality of life and survival are adversely affected by its presence.[4] Over time, most patients appear to develop progressive intrapulmonary vasodilatation and worsening gas exchange, and spontaneous improvement is rare. Mortality is significant in patients with HPS and is significantly increased relative to unaffected cirrhotic patients.[4,16,70] In addition, many patients with moderate to severe HPS have comparatively well-preserved hepatic synthetic function, making it likely that the presence of HPS will contribute to poor outcomes.[4,15,70]

Currently, liver transplantation is the only effective treatment for patients with HPS.[27,71] An early prospective study in 24 patients with HPS found that mortality after liver transplantation was markedly increased in severe HPS, in part because of the development of unique postoperative complications recognized in HPS patients. A perioperative Pao_2 value of ≤50 mm Hg, either alone or in combination with a macroaggregated albumin shunt fraction ≥20%, was the strongest predictor of postoperative mortality. Hence, the presence of HPS may adversely affect survival after orthotopic liver transplantation (OLT) in patients with cirrhosis. Since this initial study several other cohorts and studies have evaluated the outcomes of cirrhotic patients with HPS undergoing transplantation and have found 1- to 3-year mortality after OLT to range from 5% to 42%.[16,70,72-76] These studies highlight the need to more precisely define the influence of HPS on OLT outcomes.

Portopulmonary Hypertension
Definition

The unusual association between pulmonary arterial hypertension and portal hypertension was initially described in 1951.[77] Over the last several decades, portal hypertension has become recognized as a common secondary cause of pulmonary arterial hypertension. PPHTN is defined by the World Health Organization and the European Respiratory Society

Task Force as a mean pulmonary artery pressure (mPAP) >25 mm Hg at rest, or >30 mm Hg during exercise; a mean pulmonary capillary wedge pressure <15 mm Hg; and elevated pulmonary vascular resistance (PVR) (>240 dyne-sec/cm^{-5}) occurring in the setting of portal hypertension.[2,6,78,79] The presence of portal hypertension may manifest as thrombocytopenia, splenomegaly, and portosystemic shunts, and may be confirmed by hemodynamic measurements. Cirrhosis itself is not necessary for the development of PPHTN, because some prehepatic portal hypertension may also be associated with the development of PPHTN.[78,80]

The severity of PPHTN is classified by the elevation in mPAP as mild (mPAP between 25 and 35 mm Hg), moderate (mPAP between 35 and 45 mm Hg), and severe (mPAP >45 mm Hg). Patients with moderate and severe PPHTN (mPAP >35 mm Hg) appear to have higher operative mortality and are targeted for medical therapy.[6,79,81]

Epidemiology

Portopulmonary hypertension occurs most commonly in patients with cirrhosis and portal hypertension, but is also observed in patients with portal hypertension in the absence of cirrhosis. These observations support that portal hypertension is the predisposing condition.[2] Retrospective studies in patients referred for liver transplantation have found a prevalence of 6% to 16%.[79,81-84] Although there are no definitive clinical predictors of PPHTN in patients with portal hypertension, a recent multicenter study has found an increased risk of developing PPHTN in female patients with autoimmune hepatitis and a decreased risk in patients with hepatitis C as the cause of liver disease.[85] The prevalence and severity of PPHTN do not appear to correlate with the degree of hepatic synthetic dysfunction or the severity of portal hypertension.[85]

Pathology and Pathogenesis

The pulmonary abnormalities of PPHTN occur in the resistance arterial vessels and mimic those in primary pulmonary hypertension (see **Fig. 23-1**). These abnormalities include smooth muscle hypertrophy and hyperplasia, concentric intimal fibrosis, plexogenic arteriopathy, and necrotizing vasculitis.[86] The underlying mechanisms in PPHTN remain incompletely understood and no animal models have been developed. To date, all patients with PPHTN have been found to have portal hypertension, suggesting that some consequence of elevated portal pressures is critical for the development of pulmonary hypertension. Accordingly, the hyperdynamic circulatory state, which causes increased vascular shear stress and portosystemic shunting that lead to altered production or metabolism of vasoactive substances, has been hypothesized to contribute to the vascular changes present in PPHTN.[2]

A number of specific endothelial and circulating factors (prostacyclin, thromboxane, endothelin-1) as well as genetic polymorphisms in genes regulating vascular proliferative responses (TGF-β receptor superfamily) might contribute to PPHTN, but have not been directly evaluated in PPHTN. Elevated free plasma serotonin levels and genetic polymorphism in serotonin handling predispose to pulmonary artery hypertension (PAH), but a recent publication has demonstrated that the presence of these factors is not associated with the risk of developing PPHTN.[87] Similarly, mutations in the gene that codes for the bone morphogenetic protein receptor type II cause some forms of PAH, but have not been reported in PPHTN.[88]

Finally, a recent multicenter study evaluating genetic risk factors for PPHTN identified that genetic variations in estrogen signaling and rising levels of both estradiol and cell growth regulators increase the risk of developing PPHTN, suggesting that PPHTN may develop in patients with select genetic susceptibilities.[89]

Clinical Features

Symptoms are nonspecific in PPHTN and many patients are asymptomatic.[83] The most common symptom, as in HPS, is dyspnea on exertion. As the disease advances, progressive fatigue, dyspnea at rest, peripheral edema, syncope, and chest pain may develop. Edema, syncope, and chest pain are not characteristic of HPS (see **Table 23-2**). On physical examination elevated jugular pressure, a loud pulmonary component of the second heart sound, a systolic murmur resulting from tricuspid regurgitation, and lower extremity edema are common features of pulmonary hypertension but their frequency in PPHTN is not defined. Electrocardiographic abnormalities seen in patients with pulmonary hypertension may also be present in PPHTN, and consist of right atrial enlargement, right ventricular hypertrophy, right axis deviation, and/or right bundle branch block. Radiographic findings are generally subtle, but in advanced cases a prominent main pulmonary artery or cardiomegaly attributable to prominent right cardiac chambers may be appreciated. Gas exchange abnormalities are generally mild and less severe than in HPS. An increased AaPo$_2$ with mild hypoxemia and hypocarbia may be seen, particularly in more severe disease.[2,90]

Other causes of dyspnea in patients with cirrhosis and portal hypertension, including intrinsic lung disease, deconditioning, muscle wasting, ascites, hepatic hydrothorax, and HPS, should be considered when the diagnosis of PPHTN is entertained. In addition, other causes of elevated pulmonary pressures and/or right heart failure, including left ventricular dysfunction, volume overload, and chronic obstructive lung disease, may present with clinical features similar to those of PPHTN.

A recent small retrospective analysis documented nocturnal oxygen desaturation that was unrelated to lung function or sleep apnea in patients with moderate to severe PPHTN, suggesting the need for overnight screening and oxygen supplementation in those patients with moderate to severe PPHTN.[91]

Diagnosis

Because patients with PPHTN may be asymptomatic and the diagnostic utility of various clinical features (systemic hypertension, accentuated P2, electrocardiographic and chest radiographic abnormalities) is low,[92] the diagnosis requires a high index of suspicion. In general, in patients not being evaluated for liver transplantation, the presence of "compatible" symptoms and signs, in the absence of other cardiopulmonary disease, signals the need for screening for PPHTN. In all patients being evaluated for liver transplantation, regardless of signs or symptoms, screening is warranted because the presence of PPHTN may influence transplant candidacy.[93,94]

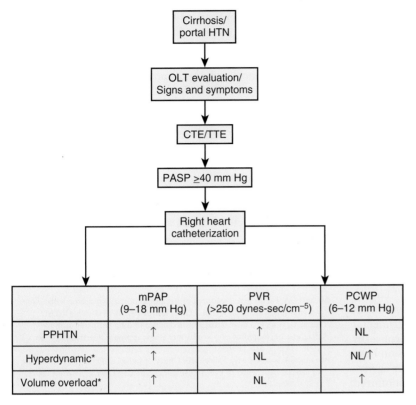

	mPAP (9–18 mm Hg)	PVR (>250 dynes-sec/cm⁻⁵)	PCWP (6–12 mm Hg)
PPHTN	↑	↑	NL
Hyperdynamic*	↑	NL	NL/↑
Volume overload*	↑	NL	↑

Fig. 23-5 **Diagnostic approach to PPHTN.** See text for details. The difference between the hyperdynamic state and volume overload is an elevated cardiac index in the hyperdynamic state. CTE, Contrast transthoracic echocardiography; HTN, hypertension; mPAP, mean pulmonary arterial pressure; OLT, orthotopic liver transplantation; PASP, pulmonary artery systolic pressure; PCWP, pulmonary capillary wedge pressure; PVR, pulmonary vascular resistance; TTE, transthoracic echocardiography.

Transthoracic Doppler echocardiography is the best noninvasive screening study to detect PPHTN (**Fig. 23-5**). If combined with intravenous contrast injection, screening for HPS and PPHTN can be accomplished simultaneously. The presence of pulmonary hypertension is suggested by an increased estimated pulmonary artery (PA) systolic pressure (derived by measuring the velocity of the tricuspid regurgitant jet), pulmonic valve insufficiency, right atrial enlargement, and/or right ventricular hypertrophy or dilatation. Several studies have evaluated the utility of estimated PA systolic pressure measurements in the diagnosis of PPHTN.[79,81,83,84,92,95] However, the precise methods for estimating PA systolic pressures are not standardized among studies and affect the operating characteristics of echocardiographic screening. From a practical perspective, finding an estimated PA systolic pressure of >40 to 45 mm Hg, particularly if right atrial and/or right ventricular abnormalities are also present, should trigger further evaluation. The most common causes for a false-positive echocardiogram are elevated pulmonary venous pressures caused by the hyperdynamic circulatory state of cirrhosis and volume overload.[83]

Patients with suggestive echocardiographic findings should undergo right heart catheterization to confirm elevated mean PA pressure and to exclude pulmonary venous hypertension. Direct measurement of PA pressures, pulmonary capillary wedge pressure, and cardiac output and calculation of systemic and pulmonary vascular resistance should be done. Responsiveness to a number of vasodilator agents, most frequently nitric oxide and/or epoprostenol, may be measured in those with confirmed PPHTN in an effort to predict a favorable response to long-term vasodilator therapy. However, the utility of vasodilator testing in the management of PPHTN is not established.

Treatment

Medical treatment for PPHTN is based largely on experience in primary pulmonary hypertension. Treatment with vasodilators is the mainstay of therapy and can reverse the vasoconstriction associated with PPHTN, but does not appear to influence fibrotic and proliferative remodeling changes. In PAH the administration of calcium channel blockers improves cardiac hemodynamics,[96] but they are not recommended in patients with PPHTN because of the possibility of increasing portal pressures. The use of β-adrenergic blockers in patients with PPHTN is controversial, based on the potential risk for cardiac depression, worsening pulmonary hemodynamics, and decreased exercise capacity.[97] Therefore variceal prophylaxis may require endoscopic intervention.

Diuretics are often required to control fluid retention in cirrhosis and portal hypertension, and this requirement may be significantly increased in the setting of right heart failure attributable to PPHTN. However, diuretics should be used with particular caution in PPHTN, because intravascular volume depletion may critically reduce the cardiac output by decreasing right ventricular preload. Oral anticoagulation therapy is not recommended in PPHTN because of the increased risk of bleeding in the presence of thrombocytopenia, coagulopathy, and varices.

Prostacyclin PGI_2 (epoprostenol) is a potent vasodilator and platelet aggregation inhibitor that results in clinical improvement and increased survival in patients with primary pulmonary hypertension, and is useful as a bridge to lung transplantation. Although randomized controlled trials have not been performed in PPHTN, several studies and case reports using continuous epoprostenol infusion indicate it improves pulmonary hemodynamics and symptoms.[98,99]

Reports of the use of newer prostacyclin analogs, including treprostinil (subcutaneous injection) and iloprost (inhalation), suggest that these agents may be easier to administer and may also be useful to improve pulmonary hemodynamics in PPHTN.[100-103]

A number of newer orally administered agents used in PAH may also be useful in patients with PPHTN. These include endothelin (ET) receptor antagonists (bosentan and ambrisentan), phosphodiesterase inhibitors (sildenafil and tadalafil), L-arginine, and tyrosine kinase inhibitors (imantinib). Bosentan is a dual ET antagonist (both ET_A and ET_B receptors) that improves pulmonary hemodynamics in portopulmonary hypertension.[100,102] However, this agent may increase liver enzymes by inhibiting hepatocyte bile acid transport,[104] and may lower systemic blood pressure. The safety of this agent in advanced cirrhosis is not fully established. Sitaxsentan, a selective ET_A receptor blocker, has been associated with severe cases of acute hepatitis and should be avoided in PPHTN.[105] Ambrisentan is a selective ET_A receptor blocker that also appears to be effective and well tolerated in preliminary studies.[106] Finally, recent case series support that sildenafil also improves mean PA pressure in patients with PPHTN without detrimental effects on systemic hemodynamics,[100,107-109] although concerns regarding potential exacerbation of portal hypertension have been raised.[110] The safety and efficacy of these newer agents, alone or in combination, have not been studied in randomized controlled studies for PPHTN.

The efficacy of liver transplantation as a treatment for PPHTN also remains controversial. Based on retrospective and clinical experience, severe PPHTN (mean pulmonary artery pressure >45 mm Hg) is a contraindication to transplantation because of a perioperative mortality of 40% and lack of reversibility of pulmonary hypertension.[93] Patients with mild PPHTN (mean pulmonary artery pressure <35 mm Hg) appear to have no increase in perioperative cardiopulmonary mortality after liver transplantation, although long-term outcomes have not been reported. Recent case series have reported favorable short-term outcomes after OLT in patients with moderate or severe PPHTN, with these patients demonstrating improved PAP values to <35 mm Hg when OLT was used in conjunction with medical therapies.[81,111,112] However, the percentage of patients with PPHTN who improve enough to undergo OLT and how often PPHTN reverses in this situation are not known.

Recent guidelines and some United Network for Organ Sharing (UNOS) regions provide MELD exception points for patients whose mean pulmonary arterial pressure decreases below 35 mm Hg for 3 months, if the PVR improves and right ventricular function is normal, on medical therapy.[94] Although case reports have demonstrated successful outcome after combination lung-liver or heart-lung-liver transplantation, limited organ availability and the technical challenges limit the feasibility of such approaches for PPHTN.

Prognosis and Natural History

PPHTN may be complicated by the development of progressive right ventricular dysfunction and cor pulmonale as well as by complications of cirrhosis. Survival in PAH correlates with the severity of right-sided cardiac dysfunction, as assessed by the degree of elevation in the right-sided cardiac pressures and the degree of decline in cardiac output. In PPHTN, survival appears to be worse than in PAH and correlates with the presence and severity of cirrhosis. These observations may be due to exacerbation of portal hypertension by elevated right-sided cardiac pressure. Perioperative mortality is increased significantly in those patients with moderate to severe PPHTN, precluding liver transplantation in this setting.[81,113,114] Compared with primary pulmonary hypertension, survival data in patients with PPHTN appear to be controversial. However, the reported mortality at 1 and 5 years ranges between 15% and 50% and between 50% and 70%, respectively, with a median survival of 2 years.[115,116] To date, no studies have demonstrated that medical therapy for PPHTN improves survival, although combined medical therapy and liver transplantation has the potential to improve outcomes in selected patients and should be studied in clinical trials.

Key References

Abrams GA, Fallon MB. Treatment of hepatopulmonary syndrome with *Allium sativum* L (garlic): a pilot trial. J Clin Gastrol 1998;27:232–235. (Ref.61)

Abrams G, et al. Use of macroaggregated albumin lung perfusion scan to diagnose hepatopulmonary syndrome: a new approach. Gastroenterology 1998;114:305–310. (Ref.56)

Abrams GA, Sanders MK, Fallon MB. Utility of pulse oximetry in the detection of arterial hypoxemia in liver transplant candidates. Liver Transplant 2002; 8:391–396. (Ref.52)

Akyüz F, et al. Is there any medical therapeutic option in hepatopulmonary syndrome? A case report. Eur J Intern Med 2005;16:126–128. (Ref.62)

Aller R, et al. Diagnosis of hepatopulmonary syndrome with contrast transesophageal echocardiography: advantages over contrast transthoracic echocardiography. Dig Dis Sci 1999;44:1243–1248. (Ref.54)

Arguedas M, et al. Prospective evaluation of outcomes and predictors of mortality in patients with hepatopulmonary syndrome undergoing liver transplantation. Hepatology 2003;37:192–197. (Ref.72)

Arguedas MR, et al. Carboxyhemoglobin levels in cirrhotic patients with and without hepatopulmonary syndrome. Gastroenterology 2005;128:328–333. (Ref.41)

Arguedas M, et al. Utility of pulse oximetry screening for hepatopulmonary syndrome. Clin Gastroenterol Hepatol 2007;5:749–754. (Ref.53)

Ashfaq M, et al. The impact of treatment of portopulmonary hypertension on survival following liver transplantation. Am J Transplant 2007;7:1258–1264. (Ref.111)

Austin MJ, et al. Safety and efficacy of combined use of sildenafil, bosentan, and iloprost before and after liver transplantation in severe portopulmonary hypertension. Liver Transplant 2008;14:287–291. (Ref.100)

Barst RJ, et al. Clinical efficacy of sitaxsentan, an endothelin-a receptor antagonist, in patients with pulmonary arterial hypertension: open-label pilot study. Chest 2002;121:1860–1868. (Ref.105)

Benjaminov FS, et al. Portopulmonary hypertension in decompensated cirrhosis with refractory ascites. Gut 2003;52:1355–1362. (Ref.82)

Binay K, et al. Hepatopulmonary syndrome in inferior vena cava obstruction responding to cavoplasty. Gastroenterology 2000;118:192–196. (Ref.18)

Brussino L, et al. Effect on dyspnoea and hypoxaemia of inhaled NG-nitro-L-arginine methyl ester in hepatopulmonary syndrome. The Lancet 2003;362: 43–44. (Ref.32)

Budhiraja R, Hassoun PM. Portopulmonary hypertension: a tale of two circulations. Chest 2003;123:562–576. (Ref.2)

Carter EP, et al. Regulation of heme oxygenase-1 by nitric oxide during hepatopulmonary syndrome. Am J Physiol Lung Cell Mol Physiol 2002;283: L346–L353. (Ref.40)

Cartin-Ceba R, Swanson K, Krowka MJ. Safety and efficacy of ambrisentan for the therapy of portopulmonary hypertension. Hepatology 2009;50:348A. (Ref.106)

Colle I, et al. Portopulmonary hypertension in candidates for liver transplantation: diagnosis at evaluation comparing Doppler echocardiography with cardiac catheterization and incidence on the waiting list. Hepatology 2003;37:401–409. (Ref.83)

Deberaldini M, et al. Hepatopulmonary syndrome: morbidity and survival after liver transplantation. Transplant Proc 2008;40:3512–3516. (Ref.73)

Degano B, et al. Nitric oxide production by the alveolar compartment of the lungs in cirrhotic patients. Eur Respir J 2009;34:138–144. (Ref.29)

Duncan BW, Desai S. Pulmonary arteriovenous malformations after cavopulmonary anastomosis. Ann Thorac Surg 2003;76:1759–1766. (Ref.26)

Fallon M, Abrams G. Pulmonary dysfunction in chronic liver disease. Hepatology 2000;32:859–865. (Ref.3)

Fallon MB, et al. Impact of hepatopulmonary syndrome on quality of life and survival in liver transplant candidates. Gastroenterology 2008;135:1168–1175. (Ref.4)

Fattinger K, et al. The endothelin antagonist bosentan inhibits the canalicular bile salt export pump: a potential mechanism for hepatic adverse reactions. Clin Pharmacol Ther 2001;69:223–231. (Ref.104)

Ferreira PP, et al. Prevalence of hepatopulmonary syndrome in patients with decompensated chronic liver disease and its impact on short-term survival. Arquiv Gastroenterol 2008;45:34–37. (Ref.5)

Fix O, et al. Long-term follow-up of portopulmonary hypertension: effect of treatment with epoprostenol. Liver Transplant 2007;13:875–885. (Ref.98)

Fuhrmann V, et al. Hepatopulmonary syndrome in patients with hypoxic hepatitis. Gastroenterology 2006;131:69–75. (Ref.20)

Gomez F, et al. Gas exchange mechanism of orthodeoxia in hepatopulmonary syndrome. Hepatology 2004;40:660–666. (Ref.46)

Gough MS, White RJ. Sildenafil therapy is associated with improved hemodynamics in liver transplantation candidates with pulmonary arterial hypertension. Liver Transplant 2009;15:30–36. (Ref.107)

Gupta S, et al. Improved survival after liver transplantation in patients with hepatopulmonary syndrome. Am J Transplant 2009;10:354–363. (Ref.74)

Gupta LB, et al. Pentoxifylline therapy for hepatopulmonary syndrome: a pilot study. Arch Intern Med 2008;168:1820–1823. (Ref.64)

Gupta D, et al. Prevalence of hepatopulmonary syndrome in cirrhosis and extrahepatic portal venous obstruction. Am J Gastroenterol 2001;96: 3395–3399. (Ref.19)

Halank M, et al. Nocturnal oxygen desaturation is a frequent complication in portopulmonary hypertension. Z Gastroenterol 2008;46:1260–1265. (Ref.91)

Hemnes AR, Robbins IM. Sildenafil monotherapy in portopulmonary hypertension can facilitate liver transplantation. Liver Transplant 2009;15: 15–19. (Ref.108)

Hino T, et al. Portopulmonary hypertension associated with congenital absence of the portal vein treated with bosentan. Int Med 2009;48:597–600. (Ref.80)

Hoeper MM, et al. Bosentan therapy for portopulmonary hypertension. Eur Respir J 2005;25:502–508. (Ref.101)

Hoeper MM, Krowka MJ, Strassburg CP. Portopulmonary hypertension and hepatopulmonary syndrome. The Lancet 2004;363:1461–1468. (Ref.90)

Hoeper MM, et al. Experience with inhaled iloprost and bosentan in portopulmonary hypertension. Eur Respir J 2007;30:1096–1102. (Ref.102)

Kawut S, et al. Clinical risk factors for portopulmonary hypertension. Hepatology 2008;48:196–203. (Ref.85)

Kawut S, et al. Hemodynamics and survival of patients with portopulmonary hypertension. Liver Transplant 2005;11:1107–1111. (Ref.115)

Koksal D, et al. Evaluation of intrapulmonary vascular dilatations with high-resolution computed thorax tomography in patients with hepatopulmonary syndrome. J Clin Gastroenterol 2006;40:77–83. (Ref.59)

Krowka MJ. Portopulmonary hypertension: diagnostic advances and caveats. Liver Transplant 2003;9:1336–1337. (Ref.79)

Krowka MJ, et al. Model for end-stage liver disease (MELD). Exception for portopulmonary hypertension. Liver Transplant 2006;12:S114–S116. (Ref.94)

Krowka MJ, et al. Hepatopulmonary syndrome and portopulmonary hypertension: a report of the multicenter liver transplant database. Liver Transplant 2004;10:174–182. (Ref.71)

Krowka M, et al. Pulmonary hemodynamics and perioperative cardiopulmonary-related mortality in patients with portopulmonary hypertension undergoing liver transplantation. Liver Transplant 2000;6:443–450. (Ref.93)

Krowka M, et al. Hepatopulmonary syndrome: a prospective study of relationships between severity of liver disease, Pao2 response to 100% oxygen, and brain uptake after 99mTc MAA lung scanning. Chest 2000;118:615–624. (Ref.15)

Laving A, et al. Successful liver transplantation in a child with severe portopulmonary hypertension treated with epoprostenol. J Pediatr Gastroenterol Nutr 2005;41:466–468. (Ref.99)

Le Pavec J, et al. Portopulmonary hypertension: survival and prognostic factors. Am J Respir Crit Care Med 2008;178:637–643. (Ref.114)

Lee D, Lepler L. Severe intrapulmonary shunting associated with metastatic carcinoid. Chest 1999;115:1203–1207. (Ref.23)

Lima B, et al. Frequency, clinical characteristics, and respiratory parameters of hepatopulmonary syndrome. Mayo Clin Proc 2004;79:42–48. (Ref.49)

Ling Y, et al. The role of endothelin-1 and the endothelin B receptor in the pathogenesis of experimental hepatopulmonary syndrome. Hepatology 2004; 39:1593–1602. (Ref.37)

Luo B, Abrams GA, Fallon MB. Endothelin-1 in the rat bile duct ligation model of hepatopulmonary syndrome: correlation with pulmonary dysfunction. J Hepatol 1998;29:571–578. (Ref.34)

Luo B, et al. Increased pulmonary vascular endothelin B receptor expression and responsiveness to endothelin-1 in cirrhotic and portal hypertensive rats: a potential mechanism in experimental hepatopulmonary syndrome. J Hepatol 2003;38:556–563. (Ref.38)

Makisalo H, et al. Sildenafil for portopulmonary hypertension in a patient undergoing liver transplantation. Liver Transplant 2004;10:945–950. (Ref.109)

Martinez G, et al. Hepatopulmonary syndrome associated with cardiorespiratory disease. J Hepatol 1999;30:882–889. (Ref.14)

Martinez G, et al. Hepatopulmonary syndrome in candidates for liver transplantation. J Hepatol 2001a;34:756–758. (Ref.11)

Martinez G, et al. Hepatopulmonary syndrome in candidates for liver transplantation. J Hepatol 2001b;34:651–657. (Ref.47)

Møller S, et al. Pulmonary dysfunction and hepatopulmonary syndrome in cirrhosis and portal hypertension. Liver Int 2009;29:1528–1537. (Ref.50)

Murray K, Carithers RA. ASLD practice guidelines: evaluation of the patient for liver transplantation. Hepatology 2005;41:1407–1432. (Ref.95)

Nunes H, et al. Role of nitric oxide in hepatopulmonary syndrome in cirrhotic rats. Am J Respir Crit Care Med 2001;164:879–885. (Ref.36)

Palma DT, et al. Oxygen desaturation during sleep in hepatopulmonary syndrome. Hepatology 2008;47:1257–1263. (Ref.48)

Paramesh A, et al. Improvement of hepatopulmonary syndrome after transjugular intrahepatic portasystemic shunting: case report and review of literature. Pediatr Transplant 2003;7:157–162. (Ref.68)

Pietra GG, et al. Pathologic assessment of vasculopathies in pulmonary hypertension. J Am Coll Cardiol 2004;43:S25–S32. (Ref.86)

Pilatis N, et al. Clinical predictors of pulmonary hypertension in patients undergoing liver transplant evaluation. Liver Transplant 2000;6:85–91. (Ref.92)

Provencher S, et al. Deleterious effects of [beta]-blockers on exercise capacity and hemodynamics in patients with portopulmonary hypertension. Gastroenterology 2006;130:120–126. (Ref.97)

Rabiller A, et al. Prevention of gram-negative translocation reduces the severity of hepatopulmonary syndrome. Am J Respir Crit Care Med 2002;166:514–517. (Ref.42)

Regev A, et al. Transient hepatopulmonary syndrome in a patient with acute hepatitis A. J Viral Hep 2001;8:83–86. (Ref.21)

Roberts DN, Arguedas MR, Fallon MB. Cost-effectiveness of screening for hepatopulmonary syndrome in liver transplant candidates. Liver Transplant 2007;13:206–214. (Ref.51)

Roberts KE, et al. Serotonin transporter polymorphisms in patients with portopulmonary hypertension. Chest 2009;135:1470–1475. (Ref.87)

Roberts KE, et al. Genetic risk factors for portopulmonary hypertension in patients with advanced liver disease. Am J Respir Crit Care Med 2009;179: 835–842. (Ref.89)

Rodriguez-Roisin R, Krowka MJ. Hepatopulmonary syndrome—a liver-induced lung vascular disorder. New Engl J Med 2008;358:2378–2387. (Ref.27)

Rodriguez-Roisin R, et al. ERS Task Force PHD Scientific Committee. Pulmonary-hepatic vascular disorders (PHD). Eur Respir J 2004;24:861–880. (Ref.6)

Rolla G, Brussino L, Colagrande P. Exhaled nitric oxide and impaired oxygenation in cirrhotic patients before and after liver transplantation. Ann Intern Med 1998;129:375–378. (Ref.30)

Ryu JK, Oh JH. Hepatopulmonary syndrome: angiography and therapeutic embolization. Clin Imaging 2003;27:97–100. (Ref.57)

Saad NEA, et al. Pulmonary arterial coil embolization for the management of persistent type i hepatopulmonary syndrome after liver transplantation. J Vasc Interven Radiol 2007;18:1576–1580. (Ref.58)

Sakai T, et al. Initial experience using continuous intravenous treprostinil to manage pulmonary arterial hypertension in patients with end-stage liver disease. Transplant Int 2009;22:554–561. (Ref.103)

Schenk P, et al. Hepatopulmonary syndrome: prevalence and predictive value of various cut offs for arterial oxygenation and their clinical consequences. Gut 2002;51:853–859. (Ref.12)

Schenk P, et al. Methylene blue improves the hepatopulmonary syndrome. Ann Int Med 2000;133:701–706. (Ref.33)

Schenk P, et al. Prognostic significance of the hepatopulmonary syndrome in patients with cirrhosis. Gastroenterology 2003;125:1042–1052. (Ref.16)

Schiffer E, et al. Hepatopulmonary syndrome increases the postoperative mortality rate following liver transplantation: a prospective study in 90 patients. Am J Transplant 2006;6:1430–1437. (Ref.75)

Simonneau G, et al. Clinical classification of pulmonary hypertension. J Am Coll Cardiol 2004;43:S5–S12. (Ref.78)

Sood G, et al. Utility of a dyspnea-fatigue index for screening liver transplant candidates for hepatopulmonary syndrome. Hepatology 1998;28:2319 [abstract]. (Ref.1)

Suga K, et al. Findings of hepatopulmonary syndrome on breath-hold perfusion SPECT-CT fusion images. Ann Nucl Med 2009;23:413–419. (Ref.60)

Sussman NV, et al. Successful liver transplantation following medical management of portopulmonary hypertension: a single-center series. Am J Transplant 2006;6:2177–2182. (Ref.112)

Swanson K, McGoon M, Krowka MJ. Survival in portopulmonary hypertension. Am J Respir Crit Care Med 2003;167:A683. (Ref.116)

Swanson K, Wiesner R, Krowka M. Natural history of hepatopulmonary syndrome: impact of liver transplantation. Hepatology 2005;41:1122–1129. (Ref.70)

Swanson KRH, et al. Survival in portopulmonary hypertension: Mayo Clinic experience categorized by treatment subgroups. Am J Transplant 2008;8:2445–2453. (Refs.81,113)

Sztrymf B, et al. Prevention of hepatopulmonary syndrome by pentoxifylline in cirrhotic rats. Eur Respir J 2004;23:752–758. (Ref.44)

Taille C, et al. Liver transplantation for hepatopulmonary syndrome: a ten-year experience in Paris, France. Transplantation 2003;79:1482–1489. (Ref.76)

Tanikella R, et al. Pilot study of pentoxifylline in hepatopulmonary syndrome. Liver Transplant 2008;14:1199–1203. (Ref.63)

Teuber G, et al. Pulmonary dysfunction in non-cirrhotic patients with chronic viral hepatitis. Eur J Intern Med 2002;13:311–318. (Ref.22)

The International PPHC, et al. Heterozygous germline mutations in BMPR2, encoding a TGF-[beta] receptor, cause familial primary pulmonary hypertension. Nat Genet 2000;26:81–84. (Ref.88)

Torregrosa M, et al. Role of Doppler echocardiography in the assessment of portopulmonary hypertension in liver transplantation candidates. Transplantation 2001;71:572–574. (Ref.84)

Wang Y-W, et al. Sildenafil decreased pulmonary arterial pressure but may have exacerbated portal hypertension in a patient with cirrhosis and portopulmonary hypertension. J Gastroenterol 2006;41:593–597. (Ref.110)

Zhang J, et al. Analysis of pulmonary heme oxygenase-1 and nitric oxide synthase alterations in experimental hepatopulmonary syndrome. Gastroenterology 2003;125:1441–1451. (Ref.35)

Zhang J, et al. Pentoxifylline attenuation of experimental hepatopulmonary syndrome. J Appl Physiol 2007;102:949–955. (Ref.43)

Zhang J, et al. Pulmonary angiogenesis in a rat model of hepatopulmonary syndrome. Gastroenterology 2009;136:1070–1080. (Ref.7)

Zhang M, et al. Endothelin-1 stimulation of endothelial nitric oxide synthase in the pathogenesis of hepatopulmonary syndrome. Am J Physiol 1999;277:G944–G952. (Ref.39)

Zierer A, et al. Impact of calcium-channel blockers on right heart function in a controlled model of chronic pulmonary hypertension. Eur J Anaesthesiol 2009;26:253–259. (Ref.96)

A complete list of references can be found at www.expertconsult.com.

Hematopoietic Abnormalities and Hemostasis

Sammy Saab

ABBREVIATIONS

ADP adenosine 5′-diphosphate
ATG antithymocyte globulin
ATIII antithrombin III
CFU-GM colony-forming unit, granulocyte macrophage
DIC disseminated intravascular coagulation
ELT euglobulin clot lysis time
EPO erythropoietin
FDP fibrin degradation product
FFP fresh frozen plasma
FHF fulminant hepatic failure

G-CSF granulocyte colony-stimulating factor
GM-CSF granulocyte-macrophage colony-stimulating factor
GVHD graft-versus-host disease
HCV hepatitis C virus
HLA human leukocyte antigen
INR international normalized ratio
ITP immune thrombocytopenic purpura
MELD Model for End-Stage Liver Disease
pRBC packed red blood cell
PSC primary sclerosing cholangitis

PT prothrombin time
rhFVIIa recombinant human factor VIIa
TAFI thrombin-activatable fibrinolysis inhibitor
TF tissue factor
TFPI tissue factor pathway inhibitor
tPA tissue plasminogen activator
TPO thrombopoietin
vWF von Willebrand factor
Xa activated factor X

Introduction

There is an integral relationship between the liver and the hemostasis and hematopoietic systems. The liver is the source of most of the clotting factors that are needed for hemostasis, and the liver produces thrombopoietin (TPO), which is required for platelet production and maturation. Not only is the liver the source of the features responsible for hemostasis, but coagulation abnormalities also is associated with the severity of liver disease and patient survival.

From the anemia encountered in the treatment of viral hepatitis to gastrointestinal bleeding, the hematopoietic system and hemostasis are relevant areas when treating patients with liver disease. Although abnormalities in these fields are often managed by internists and hematologists, hepatologists typically take a lead role when these conditions are the result of liver disease. The intricacies of bone marrow function and the coagulation cascade can be found in hematology textbooks; this chapter focuses on issues of practical importance to the hepatologist and provides only a brief description of the coagulation pathways.

Epidemiology

Abnormalities in hematopoiesis and hemostasis in patients with liver disease have been described since the early part of the 20th century.[1-3] All hematopoietic cell lines can be affected in patients with liver disease. For instance, one of the most clinically important aberrations is anemia. Anemia in the setting of liver disease is multifactorial and can be related to decreased erythrocyte production and survival, renal insufficiency, splenic sequestration, medications, and blood loss.[4] Defining incidence and prevalence data is difficult, and the existing studies describe a wide prevalence of anemia between 4.3% and 28.2%.[5] This range is so broad because studies in children and adults that include such data vary with respect to their definitions of anemia.[6,7] Thrombocytopenia is also commonly seen in patients with liver disease.[8,9] Like anemia, the causes of thrombocytopenia are multifactorial. Thrombocytopenia can reflect the severity of liver disease by decreased production of TPO and the development of splenomegaly, which promotes platelet sequestration.[10] However, medications also contribute to thrombocytopenia.[10,11]

Pathogenesis
Hematopoiesis

Hematopoiesis refers to the production of peripheral blood cells by bone marrow. Growth factors stimulate hematopoietic stem cells to give rise to progenitor cells (**Fig. 24-1**). These progenitor cells further differentiate into mature circulating cells. The blood islands of the yolk sac are the first

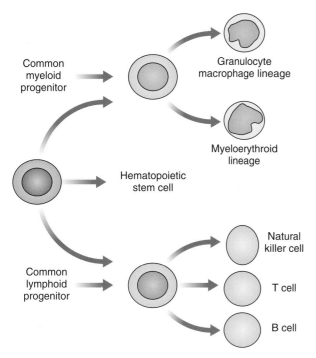

Fig. 24-1 **Hematopoiesis.** Normal hematopoiesis involves differentiation of pluripotential hematopoietic stem cells expressing the CD34 surface protein (CD34⁺) into two main committed progenitors: common myeloid and common lymphoid progenitors. Common myeloid progenitors can differentiate into all cells of the myeloerythroid lineage (granulocytes, macrophages, megakaryocytes, erythroid cells), and common lymphoid progenitors can differentiate into T cells, B cells, and natural killer cells. (*Reproduced from McCormack MP, Rabbitts TH. Activation of the T-cell oncogene LMO2 after gene therapy for X-linked severe combined immunodeficiency. N Engl J Med 2004;350:913, with permission.*)

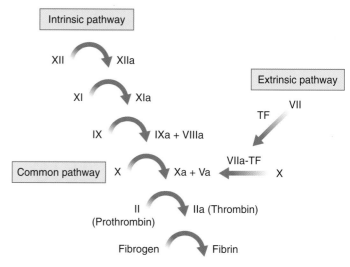

Fig. 24-2 **Simplified coagulation cascade.** After endothelial cell injury, platelets adhere to the subendothelial matrix, and the coagulation cascade is initiated. Tissue factor (TF) binds factor VII to form the activated TF-VIIa complex. Thrombin eventually cleaves fibrinogen to fibrin, which leads to stabilization of the platelet plug. (*Reproduced from Roberts HR, Monroe DM, Escobar MA. Current concepts of hemostasis: implications for therapy. Anesthesiology 2004;100:723, with permission.*)

developmental site of hematopoiesis.[12] However, by the end of the first trimester, the liver becomes the primary site of hematopoiesis in the embryo.[13,14] As the embryonic and fetal bone marrow develops, the hematopoietic responsibility gradually shifts from the liver to the bone marrow.

After birth, the bone marrow is the primary site of hematopoiesis. Hematopoietic growth factors are produced in different parts of the body. In adults, erythropoietin (EPO) production becomes predominantly a function of the kidneys, whereas TPO is produced in the liver.[14,15] EPO production is stimulated by tissue hypoxia and regulates the differentiation of erythroid precursor cells. Finally, hematopoietic-specific proteins called granulocyte colony-stimulating factor (G-CSF) and granulocyte-macrophage colony-stimulating factor (GM-CSF) drive granulopoiesis.[16,17] These growth factors stimulate granulocyte and macrophage colony-forming units (CFU-GM) and, ultimately, granulocyte differentiation.[17]

Platelet Plug Formation and the Coagulation Cascade

Other than von Willebrand factor (vWF), most proteins involved in the coagulation cascade and ultimately hemostasis are produced in the liver.[18] Therefore it should not be surprising that patients with compromised liver function often manifest a clinically significant coagulopathy. A delicate balance of

platelet aggregation, fibrin clot formation, and fibrinolysis is part of the normal hemostatic mechanism.[19] Endothelial cell damage is the initial key stimulus for platelet adherence to the subendothelial matrix, platelet aggregation, and ultimately, formation of the platelet plug.[20] vWF, a protein product of the endothelium, facilitates the adherence of platelets to subendothelial components. This adherence is responsible for the commencement of hemostasis. Before platelet activation, glycoprotein Ib on the platelet's surface facilitates binding to vWF. In this manner, platelets bind to exposed subendothelial collagen until a sheet of platelets is in place. Platelets then become activated by substances such as adenosine 5′-diphosphate (ADP) and serotonin. These activated platelets then bind fibrinogen via an integrin assembly of glycoproteins IIb and IIIa (GPIIb/IIIa).[21] Thromboxane A₂, released from activated platelets, stimulates platelet aggregation until, ultimately, the platelet plug is formed.[3]

Concurrent activation of the coagulation cascade results in fibrin formation, cross-linking, and stabilization of the platelet plug. The same endothelial cell injury that causes platelet adhesion allows tissue factor (TF) to be exposed and bind factor VII to form an activated complex (TF-VIIa).[22] **Figure 24-2** summarizes the consequent pathway toward activation of factors IX and X that leads to thrombin formation (IIa). Thrombin further activates platelets; activates factors VIII, V, and XI; and cleaves fibrinogen to fibrin to stabilize the platelet plug.[2] Although a small amount of thrombin is produced initially, activation of clotting factor accelerates thrombin formation, thereby leading to further hemostatic plug stabilization.[23]

Endogenous inhibition mechanisms are also activated after initiation of the hemostasis process to focus clot formation at the site of injury and prevent diffuse, catastrophic thrombosis. Tissue factor pathway inhibitor (TFPI) contributes to this process by binding activated factor X (Xa) and the TF-VIIa complex and inhibiting their aforementioned roles in the coagulation cascade.[24] Protein C, protein S, and antithrombin III (ATIII) are also produced in the liver and make important intrinsic contributions to anticoagulation. Thrombin likewise contributes to anticoagulation by binding a protein on endothelial cells called thrombomodulin. This thrombin-thrombomodulin complex activates protein C. Activated protein C and the co-factor protein S mutually inhibit activated factors Va and VIIIa, thus inhibiting key stimulators of thrombin production.[25] ATIII is a circulating protein synthesized by the liver that inhibits thrombin formation and inactivates factors IXa, Xa, and XIa.[26] Heparin and glycosaminoglycans on the endothelium stimulate the anticoagulation activity of ATIII.[27]

A system of fibrinolysis acts in concert with coagulation and the aforementioned prothrombotic system. This interplay is also regulated by feedback mechanisms to prevent excessive activity of any one system. During fibrinolysis, plasminogen binds fibrin. Plasminogen is subsequently cleaved and activated by tissue plasminogen activator (tPA) to form plasmin. Plasmin, the powerful enzyme that drives this process, then lyses fibrin to form fibrin degradation products (FDPs).[28] Plasminogen activator inhibitor and α_2-antiplasmin serve as regulatory agents limiting the activity of this system.[29,30]

Clinical Features and Disease Complications
Anemia in Patients with Liver Disease

Anemia is one of the most common hematopoietic abnormalities in patients with liver disease. However, the causes of anemia are multifactorial but can be stratified according to mean corpuscular volume (MCV): microcytic, normocytic, or macrocytic.

Microcytic Anemia

Microcytic anemia secondary to iron deficiency is common in patient with cirrhosis. Iron deficiency from gastrointestinal blood loss is usually due to complications of portal hypertension. Although bleeding from esophageal and gastric varices is striking, subtle blood loss may go unnoticed. Less rapid bleeding as a result of portal hypertensive gastropathy can be occult and contribute to iron deficiency.[31,32] Patients with cirrhosis may also have intestinal blood loss from non–portal hypertensive causes. Daily minute amounts of blood loss from gingival bleeding after tooth brushing and from epistaxis may also have eventual cumulative effects on body iron stores. This gradual blood loss may be due to thrombocytopenia or to the coagulopathy.[33,34]

Transferrin and ferritin are important components of iron metabolism that are synthesized in the liver, thus making the liver a critical organ in iron transport and storage.[35,36] Transferrin is a protein that binds iron after absorption in the proximal part of the small bowel to enable transport to tissues, and ferritin is a key protein for iron storage in hepatocytes, bone marrow, spleen, and other tissues. However, interpretation of ferritin values in patients with cirrhosis can be unclear. Ferritin is an acute phase reactant, and its specificity with respect

to functioning as a marker of iron overload is low.[37] Ferritin levels can be elevated in patients with a variety of inflammatory disorders, infections, malignancies, and liver-specific injuries ranging from viral hepatitis to true iron overload states. Patients with cirrhosis and elevated serum ferritin levels often undergo evaluation for hereditary hemochromatosis. Our increasing understanding of the genetic features of hereditary hemochromatosis and the development of testing strategies can assist the clinician in make this differentiation.[38,39] Transferrin is made in the liver, and in advanced disease its levels are generally low.

Sideroblastic anemia is another common cause of microcytic anemia in patients with alcoholic liver disease.[40] Alcohol inhibits steps in the heme biosynthetic pathway, with consequent deposition of iron in mitochondria, but these findings often resolve after the toxic effects of alcohol are no longer present.[41]

Macrocytic Anemia

The most common causes of macrocytic anemia in patients with liver disease are megaloblastic anemia related to cobalamin (vitamin B_{12}) and folic acid (folate) deficiency and normoblastic anemia related to erythrocyte membrane pathology.[42] Both deficiencies contribute to impaired DNA synthesis and macrocytic erythrocytes (macrocytes) with excessive nuclear/cytoplasmic ratios and frequently hypersegmented neutrophils.[43] However, even in the presence of these deficiencies the classic peripheral smear findings may not always be present.[44]

Cobalamin is synthesized exclusively by bacteria and is found primarily in meat, eggs, and dairy products. Although the stomach and small bowel are classically involved in the binding and absorption, respectively, of cobalamin, the liver has an important storage role. Transcobalamin I and III (R-binders) are present in gastric secretions and bind cobalamin. Cobalamin eventually undergoes absorption in the terminal ileum, transport to the liver, secretion into bile, and reabsorption in the terminal ileum.[45] Nutritional cobalamin deficiency is less common in industrialized countries than in the developing world, but patients with alcoholism are particularly susceptible to this deficiency, which makes this issue clinically relevant in hepatology.[46-48] Hepatic dysfunction negatively affects the enterohepatic pathway of cobalamin metabolism. Excess cobalamin can be released from the liver after hepatic injury of various causes. Cirrhosis, viral hepatitis, and hepatocellular carcinoma (HCC) can all be associated with decreased cobalamin stores and increased circulating levels.[49] Thus serum cobalamin levels may overestimate true body stores and may not be the best method for screening at-risk patients. Measurement of methylmalonic acid levels in serum is more reliable in this setting.[50]

Folate is a water-soluble vitamin that is predominantly found in green, leafy vegetables. It is also found in meats and a variety of other foods. Folate plays a critical role in single-carbon metabolism, methionine metabolism, and other important biosynthetic pathways.[51-53] As with cobalamin, folate is stored in the liver, and its metabolism depends on the enterohepatic circulation. Patients with cirrhosis and even diminished hepatic function because of noncirrhotic liver disease can exhibit disturbances in this circulation. The poor nutritional state of the alcoholic contributes to folate deficiency and other global nutritional deficiencies.[54,55] In the

Table 24-1 **Causes of Macrocytosis Seen in Patients with Liver Disease**
Cobalamin deficiency
Folate deficiency
Alcohol use
Cirrhosis
Aplastic anemia
Hemolytic anemias
Drugs (e.g., antiviral agents)

setting of alcoholic liver disease, folate metabolism is affected by the impaired liver function and the toxic effects of alcohol itself.[56] The enterohepatic circulation of folate depends on its excretion into bile by hepatocytes, and alcohol plays a direct role in inhibiting the normal workings of this process and also affects folate metabolism in general.[57-62]

Nonmegaloblastic, or normoblastic, anemia and macrocytosis without anemia are also common in patients with liver disease.[63] The exact cause is unclear, but in patients with alcoholic cirrhosis, a direct effect of alcohol on red cells is also a potential contributing factor.[64,65] This effect may be related to a modification of the lipid composition in erythrocyte membranes.[66,67] In addition, anemia of chronic disease (also known as the anemia of acute and chronic inflammation) and renal disease are often present in patients with liver disease. The confluence of these factors may drop MCV from a baseline high value to a normal or low value. **Table 24-1** lists common causes of macrocytosis in patients with liver disease.

Despite the strong association between anemia and liver disease, erythrocytosis can also occur in these patients. Erythrocytosis is most frequently associated with HCC, but it can rarely be seen in other forms of liver disease.[68-70] A constellation of factors such as hypoxia, anemia, and thrombocytopenia may stimulate dysregulated EPO synthesis in the diseased liver.[71]

Normocytic Anemia

An important cause of normocytic anemia is hemolysis. Structural abnormalities on erythrocyte membranes in patients with liver disease can also contribute to hemolysis and hemolytic anemia.[72,73] Because of the crucial role of the liver in lipid metabolism, erythrocytes in patients with liver disease may have abnormalities in lipid membrane composition that may contribute to hemolysis.[74,75] Spur cell anemia is an important form of hemolytic anemia that is associated with both alcoholic and nonalcoholic liver disease.[75] Acanthocytes are large erythrocytes with a spiculed appearance because of an abnormal free cholesterol/phospholipid ratio in the outer leaflet of the erythrocyte lipid bilayer. These cells have decreased membrane fluidity, irregular osmotic fragility, and a predisposition to splenic sequestration and destruction. Acanthocytes are not exclusive to spur cell anemia in liver disease but have also been associated with other disorders such as abetalipoproteinemia; however, the pathophysiology differs depending on the underlying disorder.[76,77] Several reports document improvement of acanthocytosis and spur cell anemia with liver transplantation, thus suggesting a relationship between liver function and the erythrocyte abnormality.[78,79] Furthermore, erythrocytes transfused into a patient

with liver disease and spur cell anemia can become acanthocytes, and acanthocytes may revert to a normal morphology when incubated with normal serum.[80,81]

Wilson disease is associated with hemolytic anemia and should be considered in patients with liver disease and hemolysis.[82,83] In fulminant disease, patients can experience intravascular hemolysis. In this acute setting, plasma exchange can be an effective bridging treatment to subsequent chelation therapy or liver transplantation.[84,85] Finally, Zieve syndrome is a rare entity that includes alcoholic hepatitis, hyperlipidemia, hemolytic anemia, jaundice, and abdominal pain.[86] Although there is no specific treatment, alcohol cessation can result in resolution of the hemolytic anemia that is a hallmark feature of the syndrome.

Special Circumstances
Anemia Associated with Viral Hepatitis and Its Treatment

Hematologic complications may arise from the different forms of viral hepatitis, as well as their treatments. Aplastic anemia is a condition in which hematopoiesis is compromised and there is a paucity of normal bone marrow components. Although congenital forms of this hypocellular bone marrow state exist, the majority of cases are acquired. It is thought to have an immune-mediated pathophysiology and has also been associated with viral hepatitis. The precise mechanism of this association is the subject of ongoing study.[87] T-cell–mediated destruction of important hematopoietic cells has been described.[88,89] In hepatitis-associated aplastic anemia, a gender-specific factor may be involved inasmuch as most cases have been described in young males, and patients typically have pancytopenia within 3 months after the onset of hepatitis.[90,91] There has been concern that the EPO used to treat ribavirin-associated hemolytic anemia may in rare cases be associated with aplastic anemia. This condition is potentially fatal, but combinations of immunosuppressive regimens have been successful. Approximately half the patients with severe cases treated with antithymocyte globulin (ATG) and cyclosporine exhibit sustained recovery.[92] Despite the effectiveness of immunosuppressive therapy, corticosteroids have not been effective and are not recommended.[78] If human leukocyte antigen (HLA)-matched donors exist, survival rates are even higher with bone marrow transplantation, and the results are generally better in younger patients.[93]

Viral hepatitis has also been associated with abnormalities in individual hematopoietic cell lines. Descriptions exist of different forms of viral hepatitis causing pure red cell aplasia, but this is a rare clinical association.[94,95] Viral hepatitis in general has also been associated with both neutropenia and thrombocytopenia.[96,97] Hepatitis C virus (HCV) has been suggested to cause hemolytic anemia, neutropenia, and thrombocytopenia in the absence of other clear causes.[98,99]

Although the mechanism of the direct virologic effect of hepatitis viruses on hematopoietic cell lines requires further study, adverse hematologic effects have been reported with antiviral therapy. Pegylated interferon alfa and ribavirin therapy for HCV is associated with significant decreases in hemoglobin concentrations.[100,101] Both drugs have specific mechanisms by which they cause these side effects. Interferon alfa has a direct myelosuppressive effect, whereas ribavirin is associated with a dose-dependent hemolytic anemia.[102,103] This hemolysis can be severe, and clinically evident hemoglobin-uria may occur.[104] A recent report also implicates ribavirin itself in causing a pure red cell aplasia.[105] Recently, a variant has been described that predicts hemolytic anemia in patients treated with pegylated interferon and ribavirin.[106]

Hematologic Issues in Liver Transplantation

Patients awaiting liver transplantation have complex medical problems, as well as anemia.[4] Hemolysis, gastrointestinal bleeding, drug side effects, renal insufficiency, and hematopoi-etic abnormalities may all play a role. Although figures vary depending on the definition of anemia, posttransplant anemia has been described in up to 28.2% of these patients.[5,107] Post-transplant immunosuppressive regimens are clear contribu-tors to these abnormalities.[108,109]

As mentioned previously, aplastic anemia refers to mark-edly reduced numbers or the absence of precursors of all cell lines in the bone marrow. Though classically associated with parvovirus B19 infection, aplastic anemia has also been reported after liver transplantation, and a higher incidence is seen in patients who undergo liver transplantation for fulmi-nant viral hepatitis.[110,111] Despite being rare, with a reported incidence of approximately 1%, graft-versus-host disease (GVHD) should likewise be considered in patients in whom pancytopenia develops following both cadaveric and living donor transplantation.[112,113] Increased fibrinolysis may also be seen in the perioperative period, and antifibrinolytic therapy with aprotinin and tranexamic acid has been used with success in reducing blood product requirements.[114-116] However, more evidence and well-designed studies are needed before wide-spread use can be advocated.

Similar to the treatment of other complications of cirrhosis, orthotopic liver transplantation is considered to be the ulti-mate therapy for some disorders of hematopoiesis and hemo-stasis in patients with cirrhosis. Liver transplantation is discussed extensively elsewhere in this book, but from hemo-philia to fibrinolysis, evidence exists that derangements in the coagulation cascade and their complications improve after transplantation of a healthy liver.[117,118] Recent evidence cites improvement in hypersplenism with living donor transplanta-tion as well.[119]

Alcohol and Anemia

Alcohol is an important cause of hematopoietic abnormalities in patients with liver disease. It has a broad suppressive effect on bone marrow and can result in anemia, leukopenia, and thrombocytopenia.[120,121] Severe pancytopenia is not common in alcoholics, but production of all three cell lines can be impaired, and this impairment is reversible with cessation of alcohol.[122] The aforementioned nutritional deficiencies that are common in alcoholics can also contribute to anemia in these patients. Furthermore, if alcoholic cirrhosis, portal hypertension, and splenic sequestration of platelets develop, thrombocytopenia may likewise be present. Alcohol is also a toxin that has a selective influence on the suppression of megakaryocytes.[123-125] In addition, it has been suggested that platelet function is impaired by alcohol in vitro.[126]

Leukocyte Abnormalities

Patients with liver disease commonly exhibit leukopenia and atypical leukocyte function. Leukopenia may result from a combination of decreased leukocyte production, splenic sequestration, and impaired survival. Neutrophil survival appears to be shortened via apoptosis.[127,128] In the setting of both decreased leukocyte counts and suboptimal leukocyte function, patients with cirrhosis are susceptible to bacterial infections. Ineffective neutrophil recruitment to sites of infec-tion may be an important component of this reduced leuko-cyte function.[129,130] Evidence also exists that the compromised phagocytic function of neutrophil granulocytes may contrib-ute to this susceptibility to bacterial infections.[131,132] Further-more, any bone marrow suppressive effects of toxins, drugs, and viral infections at play in patients with liver disease will negatively affect this cell line as well.

Thrombocytopenia

Thrombocytopenia is one of the most common laboratory abnormalities found in patients with cirrhosis, and it is associ-ated with complications of portal hypertension, such as esophageal varices and splenomegaly.[133] TPO is produced pre-dominantly in the liver and is the primary regulator of platelet production.[134] Acquired TPO deficiency may be a contributing factor to the thrombocytopenia seen in cirrhotic patients. Evi-dence suggests that patients with cirrhosis have lower TPO levels than do those with noncirrhotic liver disease.[135] More-over, TPO production appears to be related to the amount of functional liver cell mass, and some describe decreased TPO levels in proportion to the severity of the liver disease.[136,137] However, the correlation between liver disease severity and TPO levels is controversial.[138] After orthotopic liver transplan-tation, patients experience an increase in TPO production and a subsequent increase in bone marrow production of plate-lets.[139] Autoantibodies to GPIIb/IIIa are also implicated in the immune thrombocytopenic purpura (ITP) occurring in patients with cirrhosis.[140] ITP is seen in association with viral hepatitis and specifically with HCV infection.[141,142] Further evidence of an immune-mediated component of the throm-bocytopenia in patients with liver disease is the increased levels of platelet-associated immunoglobulins in these patients.[123]

Hypersplenism refers to cytopenia, such as thrombocytope-nia or leukopenia, as a result of platelet and leukocyte destruc-tion or sequestration in the spleen (or both).[143] Hypersplenism has also been reported to be an independent risk factor for complications of portal hypertension, such as variceal bleed-ing.[144] The prevalence of hypersplenism in patients with cir-rhosis ranges from 2% to 61%, depending on the definitions of leukopenia and thrombocytopenia.[145] Decompression of portal hypertension, such as by creation of a transjugular intrahepatic portosystemic shunt (TIPS) or by liver transplan-tation, can improve the consequences of hypersplenism, though not predictably. **Table 24-2** lists common causes of hypersplenism in patients with liver disease.

Coagulopathy

The abnormal coagulation in patients with liver disease often facilitates bleeding because of the accompanying thrombo-cytopenia and other potential contributing factors, such as disseminated intravascular coagulation (DIC) and fibrinoly-sis. However, spontaneous hemorrhage is uncommon, and most of the bleeding is from the gastrointestinal tract or

Table 24-2 Causes of Hypersplenism Related to Liver Disease
Cirrhosis
Congestive hepatopathy
Budd-Chiari syndrome
Acute viral hepatitis
Amyloidosis
Portal vein thrombosis
Hepatic schistosomiasis

related to complications of invasive procedures. Coagulation disorders are possible but uncommon in patients with uncomplicated acute hepatitis. Furthermore, the results of coagulation tests are usually normal until levels of clotting factors fall to 30% to 40% of normal values.[18] In sepsis, not only may coagulopathy be related to the impaired synthesis of clotting factors, but consumption of clotting factors may also be present.[146]

Vitamin K is a fat-soluble vitamin and a co-factor required for γ-carboxylation of clotting factors II, VII, IX, and X. Bile salts are an important component of fat-soluble vitamin metabolism, and biliary obstruction and small bowel bacterial overgrowth can contribute to vitamin K deficiency.[147] Factor VII has the shortest half-life of all of the clotting factors, and recombinant factor VII, as discussed later, may be a useful adjunct to conventional therapies when managing the coagulopathy of liver disease.

Indices of coagulation have been demonstrated to measure the severity of liver disease and assess the need for liver transplantation. The prothrombin time (PT) and international normalized ratio (INR) are the most commonly used tests used to assess the production of coagulation factors by the liver and to diagnose vitamin K deficiency. The PT/INR is also included in both the Model for End-Stage Liver Disease (MELD) and Child-Pugh classifications to assess the severity of liver disease.[148] In addition, PT/INR values are used in the King's College criteria for predicting prognosis in patients with fulminant hepatic failure (FHF).[149] Administration of vitamin K may gradually improve the PT and INR in the setting of vitamin K deficiency, but this treatment is not likely to be helpful during acute bleeding in a patient with liver disease and a coagulopathy.[150]

Thrombotic Disorders

Because patients with liver disease commonly have many of the derangement in the coagulation cascade that lead to coagulopathy, some patients may be at risk for the development of thrombotic disorders.[151] Endogenous anticoagulation proteins C, S, and ATIII are also produced in the liver, and synthetic dysfunction impairs normal production.[152] Although levels of these anticoagulant proteins in patients with liver disease may be as low as those seen in persons with inherited deficiencies, thrombosis is uncommon in patients with advanced liver disease. Low levels of these proteins may contribute to intrahepatic venous thrombosis and inflammation, which will accelerate fibrosis in patients with liver disease.[153] Patients with cholestatic liver disease, such as primary sclerosing cholangitis (PSC), also demonstrate a potential for

hypercoagulability. A difference in platelet function in comparison to noncholestatic liver disease may contribute to this association.[154] Patients with HCC have a hypercoagulable potential similar to that of patients with other solid organ malignancies. Furthermore, HCC is associated with a higher incidence of portal and hepatic vein thrombosis.[155] Finally, other gene mutations, such as mutation 20210 of the prothrombin gene, cause thrombophilia and are reported to be an independent risk factor for portal vein thrombosis.[156,157] Multiple prothrombotic factors may cumulatively increase the risk for venous thrombosis when present in a patient with liver disease.

Gastrointestinal Bleeding

Despite the potential risk for bleeding as a result of abnormalities in the platelet count and coagulopathy, the risk for hemorrhage is not universal and tends to be localized to the gastrointestinal tract through the development of varices, arteriovenous malformations, and gastropathy. In particular, variceal bleeding is one of the most serious complications of cirrhosis. Variceal bleeding can be life-threatening if not treated on an urgent basis.[158] Although varices are covered extensively elsewhere in this book, abnormalities in hematopoiesis and hemostasis are intimately involved in the clinical scenarios giving rise to esophageal, gastric, small bowel, and rectal varices.[159] An acutely bleeding patient is often coagulopathic and thrombocytopenic, and resuscitation with blood products is frequently a necessary prerequisite for endoscopic management.

Disseminated Intravascular Coagulation and Primary Fibrinolysis

Disseminated intravascular coagulation refers to intravascular fibrin deposition in small and medium-sized vessels secondary to systemic activation of the coagulation cascade.[160] No specific set of coagulation findings is pathognomonic for DIC, but patients typically have a prolonged PT and partial thromboplastin time (PTT), elevated FDPs, and a low fibrinogen level.[161] Hyperbilirubinemia in this setting may be related to hemolysis, an underlying liver disease, or a combination of both. Patients with cirrhosis frequently have the same laboratory abnormalities as those with DIC, thus leading to a debate as to whether DIC is part of the natural history of cirrhotic coagulopathy.[162] However, patients with cirrhosis are certainly at risk for development of the known causes of DIC, such as sepsis and shock, and as with DIC in other patients, treatment of the underlying cause is the prevailing recommendation. Although infusion of fresh frozen plasma (FFP) is helpful in transiently improving the PT and PTT in this setting, fibrinogen levels usually stay low. Cryoprecipitate transfusion is useful in increasing the serum fibrinogen level when it is less than 100 mg/dl.[163,164] However, cryoprecipitate can be misused, and it should not be transfused to treat a coagulopathy secondary to liver disease in the absence of hypofibrinogenemia.[165]

tPA and α$_2$-antiplasmin play an important role in the endogenous fibrinolytic system. Accelerated fibrinolysis has long been described in patients with cirrhosis. Fibrinolysis is suggested by a shortened whole blood euglobulin clot lysis time (ELT) and a low fibrinogen level. When severe, fibrinolysis can also cause increased levels of D-dimers and FDPs. One study reported hyperfibrinolysis in 31% of patients with cirrhosis and correlated the degree of abnormality with the severity of liver disease.[166] Decreased hepatic clearance of tPA in patients with cirrhosis, combined with decreased levels of regulatory agents such as α_2-antiplasmin and thrombin-activatable fibrinolysis inhibitor (TAFI), contribute to the fibrinolysis, although not everyone agrees on their importance.[167-174] ε-Aminocaproic acid has been used for fibrinolysis associated with bleeding in cirrhotic patients, but unlike its application in cardiac surgery, there is insufficient evidence for its widespread use.

Treatment Options
Transfusion of Blood Products

Packed red blood cell (pRBC), FFP, cryoprecipitate, and platelet transfusions are important aspects of treatment when combating hematopoietic and hemostatic abnormalities. When performing procedures as diverse as percutaneous liver biopsy and gastrointestinal endoscopy, clinicians often have concern about bleeding in patients with liver disease. Because patients who require paracentesis often have cirrhosis, as well as abnormal results on coagulation tests, exclusion of these patients because of the coagulopathy would mean that a number of important diagnostic procedures would not be performed. The information obtained from these procedures may be critical to patient management, and the use of alternative approaches, such as transjugular liver biopsy or resuscitation with blood products to temporarily improve the coagulopathy, may be necessary.[168]

A recent study supports increasing the number of FFP units used in the initial management of coagulopathy in patients with chronic liver disease.[169] However, in the absence of bleeding, pending invasive procedures, or other indications, clinicians must remember that adverse effects are possible with any transfusion and that these resources should be used judiciously.[170] The effect of FFP on coagulation studies is rapid but transient and usually lasts 12 to 24 hours.[15] Numerous reports have detailed the use of recombinant human factor VIIa (rhFVIIa) to treat bleeding or correct coagulopathy before performing invasive procedures, but controlled trials are lacking.[171-174]

Because of an increased risk for complications, clinical judgment should be exercised when considering invasive procedures such as surgery and percutaneous liver biopsy in patients with coagulopathy, thrombocytopenia, or both. Administration of subcutaneous vitamin K is helpful in improving the PT and INR in patients with vitamin K deficiency, and this improvement may be all that is necessary before an elective outpatient liver biopsy. However, in a bleeding patient and in the absence of vitamin K deficiency, FFP transfusion should be the treatment of choice to correct this coagulopathy. Resuscitation with platelet transfusions and FFP should be considered to increase the platelet count to greater than 50,000 and to lower the INR to less than 1.5 before performing invasive procedures.[175] Transjugular liver biopsy by an interventional radiologist can be considered as an alternative when the INR cannot be easily corrected and liver biopsy is indicated.[176-179]

Other Therapies

A number of specific hematopoietic growth factors are available, with each growth factor targeting a specific hematopoietic cell line. The need for hematopoietic growth factors varies according to the cause of the defect. For instance, patients with hepatitis C are treated with interferon and ribavirin.[180] Some of the potential complications with antiviral therapy are decreased production of white blood cells and platelets and increased destruction of red blood cells. Hematopoietic growth factors may have a role in management of the hematologic abnormalities associated with treatment of HCV infection with interferon alfa and ribavirin.[181] Reductions in ribavirin doses may hinder efforts to obtain a sustained virologic response, but the use of epoetin-α appears to be effective in combating the anemia associated with ribavirin therapy.[182] However, the improvement in sustained viral responses with EPO appears to be best when administered during the first 8 weeks of therapy.[183] A recent prospective double-blind randomized controlled trial has demonstrated improved quality of life in patients receiving epoetin-α in comparison to placebo controls.[184]

Although epoetin-α is helpful in correcting the hemolytic anemia associated with ribavirin therapy, further study is needed to evaluate its use for posttransplant anemia. Indeed, a major adherence-related limiting step in liver transplant recipients receiving antiviral therapy for HCV infection is ribavirin-induced anemia.[185] Before transplantation, cirrhotic patients demonstrate an inappropriate EPO response to anemia that may improve after transplantation.[186]

Recombinant human TPO may also be a useful option when treating thrombocytopenia in patients with bleeding or impending invasive procedures. Although the use of TPO growth factors showed initial promise, safety concerns have limited wide use in clinical practice.[187] DDAVP (1-deamino-8-D-arginine vasopressin), also known as desmopressin, is likewise used to facilitate hemostasis in cirrhotic patients with coagulopathy. Although the mechanism is still not well defined, administration of desmopressin can increase levels of vWF and factor VIII and shorten the bleeding time.[188] Nonetheless, there are conflicting case series on the clinical impact of DDAVP on bleeding in patients with cirrhosis, and more rigorous studies are needed.[189]

Key References

Ades L, et al. Long-term outcome after bone marrow transplantation for severe aplastic anemia. Blood 2004;103:2490–2497. (Ref.93)

Afdhal N, et al. Thrombocytopenia associated with chronic liver disease. J Hepatol 2008;48:1000–1007. (Ref.10)

Afdhal NH, et al. Proactive Study Group. Epoetin alfa maintains ribavirin dose in HCV-infected patients: a prospective, double-blind, randomized controlled study. Gastroenterology 2004;126:1302–1311. (Ref.184)

Alcindor T, Bridges KR. Sideroblastic anaemias. Br J Haematol 2002;116:733–743. (Ref.40)

Amitrano L, et al. Coagulation disorders in liver disease. Semin Liver Dis 2002;22:83–96. (Ref.18)

Amitrano L, et al. Risk factors and clinical presentation of portal vein thrombosis in patients with liver cirrhosis. J Hepatol 2004;40:736–741. (Ref.157)

Anantharaju A, et al. Use of activated recombinant human factor VII (rhFVIIa) for colonic polypectomies in patients with cirrhosis and coagulopathy. Dig Dis Sci 2003;48:1414–1424. (Ref.172)

Antony AC. Vegetarianism and vitamin B-12 (cobalamin) deficiency. Am J Clin Nutr 2003;78:3–6. (Ref.48)

Aref SE, et al. Assessment of neutrophil apoptosis ex vivo in hepatosplenic patients with neutropenia pre and post splenectomy. Hematology 2003;8: 265–272. (Ref.128)

Basu S, Dunn A, Ward A. G-CSF: function and modes of action. Int J Mol Med 2002;10:3–10. (Ref.17)

Bergheim I, et al. Nutritional deficiencies in German middle-class male alcohol consumers: relation to dietary intake and severity of liver disease. Eur J Clin Nutr 2003;57:431–438. (Ref.46)

Bosch J, Abraldes JG. Management of gastrointestinal bleeding in patients with cirrhosis of the liver. Semin Hematol 2004;41(Suppl 1):8–12. (Ref.169)

Caprini JA, et al. Laboratory markers in the diagnosis of venous thromboembolism. Circulation 2004;109:I4–I8. (Ref.25)

Chagraoui J, et al. Fetal liver stroma consists of cells in epithelial-to-mesenchymal transition. Blood 2003;101:2973–2982. (Ref.14)

Chak E, Saab S. Pegylated interferon and ribavirin dosing strategies to enhance sustained virologic response. Curr Hepat Rep 2010;9:147–154. (Ref.181)

Cheng TI, et al. Dermatomyositis and erythrocytosis associated with hepatocellular carcinoma. J Gastroenterol Hepatol 2002;17:1239–1240. (Ref.70)

Comar KM, Sanyal AJ. Portal hypertensive bleeding. Gastroenterol Clin North Am 2003;32:1079–1105. (Ref.160)

Dalmau A, et al. The prophylactic use of tranexamic acid and aprotinin in orthotopic liver transplantation: a comparative study. Liver Transpl 2004;10: 279–284. (Ref.115)

Danesi R, Del Tacca M. Hematologic toxicity of immunosuppressive treatment. Transplant Proc 2004;36:703–704. (Ref.109)

Dieterich DT, et al. Once-weekly epoetin alfa improves anemia and facilitates maintenance of ribavirin dosing in hepatitis C virus–infected patients receiving ribavirin plus interferon alfa. Am J Gastroenterol 2003;98: 2491–2499. (Ref.180)

Ermens AA, Vlasveld LT, Lindemans J. Significance of elevated cobalamin (vitamin B_{12}) levels in blood. Clin Biochem 2003;36:585–590. (Ref.49)

Federal Drug Administration: FDA warns against eltrombopag use in patients with chronic liver disease. WWW.FDA.Gov. Posted 05/12/2010. Accessed 11/15/10. (Ref.187)

Fellay J, et al. ITPA gene variants protect against anaemia in patients treated for chronic hepatitis C. Nature 2010;464:405–408. (Ref.106)

Fiuza C, et al. Granulocyte colony-stimulating factor improves deficient in vitro neutrophil transendothelial migration in patients with advanced liver disease. Clin Diagn Lab Immunol 2002;9:433–439. (Ref.130)

French CJ, Bellomo R, Angus P. Cryoprecipitate for the correction of coagulopathy associated with liver disease. Anaesth Intensive Care 2003;31: 357–361. (Ref.165)

Gaeta GB, et al. Premature discontinuation of interferon plus ribavirin for adverse effects: a multicentre survey in "real world" patients with chronic hepatitis C. Aliment Pharmacol Ther 2002;16:1633–1639. (Ref.100)

Garfia C, Garcia-Ruiz I, Solis-Herruzo JA. Deficient phospholipase C activity in blood polymorphonuclear neutrophils from patients with liver cirrhosis. J Hepatol 2004;40:749–756. (Ref.132)

Giannini E, et al. Serum thrombopoietin levels are linked to liver function in untreated patients with hepatitis C virus–related chronic hepatitis. J Hepatol 2002;37:572–577. (Ref.137)

Giannini E, et al. Relationship between thrombopoietin serum levels and liver function in patients with chronic liver disease related to hepatitis C virus infection. Am J Gastroenterol 2003;98:2516–2520. (Ref.135)

Giannini EG. Review article: thrombocytopenia in chronic liver disease and pharmacologic treatment options. Aliment Pharmacol Ther 2006;23: 1055–1065. (Ref.9)

Grattagliano I, et al. Low membrane protein sulfhydrils but not G6PD deficiency predict ribavirin-induced hemolysis in hepatitis C. Hepatology 2004;39: 1248–1255. (Ref.103)

Halsted CH, Villanueva JA, Devlin AM. Folate deficiency, methionine metabolism, and alcoholic liver disease. Alcohol 2002;27:169–172. (Ref.51)

Halsted CH, et al. Metabolic interactions of alcohol and folate. J Nutr 2002; 132(Suppl):2367S–2372S. (Ref.61)

Halsted CH, et al. Folate deficiency disturbs hepatic methionine metabolism and promotes liver injury in the ethanol-fed micropig. Proc Natl Acad Sci U S A 2002;99:10072–10077. (Ref.56)

Hanslik T, Prinseau J. The use of vitamin K in patients on anticoagulant therapy: a practical guide. Am J Cardiovasc Drugs 2004;4:43–55. (Ref.151)

Iglesias-Berengue J, et al. Hematologic abnormalities in liver-transplanted children during medium- to long-term follow-up. Transplant Proc 2003;35: 1904–1906. (Ref.107)

Itterbeek P, et al. Aplastic anemia after transplantation for non-A, non-B, non-C fulminant hepatic failure: case report and review of the literature. Transpl Int 2002;15:117–123. (Ref.111)

Kahl BS, Schwartz BS, Mosher DF. Profound imbalance of pro-fibrinolytic and anti-fibrinolytic factors (tissue plasminogen activator and plasminogen activator inhibitor type 1) and severe bleeding diathesis in a patient with cirrhosis: correction by liver transplantation. Blood Coagul Fibrinol 2003;14:741–744. (Ref.118)

Kajihara M, et al. A role of autoantibody-mediated platelet destruction in thrombocytopenia in patients with cirrhosis. Hepatology 2003;37:1267–1276. (Ref.140)

Kaneko J, et al. Spleen volume and platelet number changes after living donor liver transplantation in adults. Hepatogastroenterology 2004;51:262–263. (Ref.119)

Kaushansky K. Thrombopoietin: a tool for understanding thrombopoiesis. J Thromb Haemost 2003;1:1587–1592. (Ref.134)

Kim AI, Saab S. Treatment of hepatitis C. Am J Med 2005;118:808–815. (Ref.180)

Kovacs TO, Jensen DM. Recent advances in the endoscopic diagnosis and therapy of upper gastrointestinal, small intestinal, and colonic bleeding. Med Clin North Am 2002;86:1319–1356. (Ref.159)

Laffi G, Tarquini R, Marra F. Thrombocytopenia in chronic liver disease: lessons from transplanted patients. J Hepatol 2007;47:625–629. (Ref.11)

Latvala J, Parkkila S, Niemela O. Excess alcohol consumption is common in patients with cytopenia: studies in blood and bone marrow cells. Alcohol Clin Exp Res 2004;28:619–624. (Ref.121)

Levi M, de Jonge E, van der Poll T. New treatment strategies for disseminated intravascular coagulation based on current understanding of the pathophysiology. Ann Med 2004;36:41–49. (Ref.161)

Levi M, et al. Safety of recombinant activated factor VII in randomized clinical trials. N Engl J Med 2010;363:1791–1800. (Ref.173)

Levi MM, Vink R, de Jonge E. Management of bleeding disorders by prohemostatic therapy. Int J Hematol 2002;76(Suppl 2):139–144. (Ref.188)

Liangpunsakul S, Ulmer BJ, Chalasani N. Predictors and implications of severe hypersplenism in patients with cirrhosis. Am J Med Sci 2003;326:111–116. (Ref.144)

Lijnen HR. Elements of the fibrinolytic system. Ann N Y Acad Sci 2001;936: 226–236. (Ref.29)

Lisman T, Leebeek FWG, de Groot PG. Haemostatic abnormalities in patients with liver disease. J Hepatol 2002;37:280–287. (Ref.20)

Lu J, et al. Analysis of T-cell repertoire in hepatitis-associated aplastic anemia. Blood 2004;103:4588–4593. (Ref.89)

Luo JC, et al. Clinical characteristics and prognosis of hepatocellular carcinoma patients with paraneoplastic syndromes. Hepatogastroenterology 2002;49:1315–1319. (Ref.68)

Maheshwari A, Mishra R, Thuluvath PJ. Post–liver-transplant anemia: etiology and management. Liver Transpl 2004;10:165–173. (Ref.5)

Malik P, et al. Spur cell anemia in alcoholic cirrhosis: cure by orthotopic liver transplantation and recurrence after liver graft failure. Int Surg 2002;87:201–204. (Ref.79)

Massoud OI, Yousef WI, Mullen KD. Hemoglobinuria with ribavirin treatment. J Clin Gastroenterol 2003;36:367–368. (Ref.104)

Mitra B, et al. The safety of recombinant factor VIIa in cardiac surgery. Anaesth Intensive Care 2010;38:671–677. (Ref.174)

Nosari A, et al. Bone marrow hypoplasia complicating tacrolimus (FK506) therapy. Int J Hematol 2004;79:130–132. (Ref.108)

O'Shaughnessy DF, et al, for the British Committee for Standards in Haematology, Blood Transfusion Task Force. Guidelines for the use of fresh-frozen plasma, cryoprecipitate and cryosupernatant. Br J Haematol 2004; 126:11–28. (Ref.171)

Pantanowitz L, Kruskall MS, Uhl L. Cryoprecipitate. Patterns of use. Am J Clin Pathol 2003;119:874–881. (Ref.166)

Papatheodoridis GV, et al. Thrombotic risk factors and extent of liver fibrosis in chronic viral hepatitis. Gut 2003;52:404–409. (Ref.154)

Patt CH, Fairbanks KD, Thuluwath PJ. Renal insufficiency may partly explain chronic anemia in patients awaiting liver transplantation. Dig Dis Sci 2004;49:629–632. (Ref.4)

Pietrangelo A. Hereditary hemochromatosis—a new look at an old disease. N Engl J Med 2004;350:2383–2397. (Ref.38)

Pihusch R, et al. Platelet function rather than plasmatic coagulation explains hypercoagulable state in cholestatic liver disease. J Hepatol 2002;37:548–555. (Ref.155)

Plessier A, et al. Coagulation disorders in patients with cirrhosis and severe sepsis. Liver Int 2003;23:440–448. (Ref.146)

Pockros PJ, et al. Immune thrombocytopenic purpura in patients with chronic hepatitis C virus infection. Am J Gastroenterol 2002;97:2040–2045. (Ref.141)

Porte RJ. Antifibrinolytics in liver transplantation: they are effective, but what about the risk-benefit ratio? Liver Transpl 2004;10:285–288. (Ref.116)

Poujol-Robert A, et al. Genetic and acquired thrombotic factors in chronic hepatitis C. Am J Gastroenterol 2004;99:527–531. (Ref.153)

Qamar AA, et al. Incidence, prevalence, and clinical significance of abnormal hematologic indices in compensated cirrhosis. Clin Gastroenterol Hepatol 2009;7:689–695. (Ref.8)

Ramos-Casals M, et al. Severe autoimmune cytopenias in treatment-naive hepatitis C virus infection: clinical description of 35 cases. Medicine (Baltimore) 2003;82:87–96. (Ref.99)

Rand ML, et al. Ethanol enhances the inhibitory effect of an oral GPIIb/IIIa antagonist on human platelet function. J Lab Clin Med 2002;140:391–397. (Ref.126)

Roberts EA, Schilsky ML; American Association for Study of Liver Diseases (AASLD). Diagnosis and treatment of Wilson disease: an update. Hepatology 2008;47:2089–2111. (Ref.83)

Roberts HR, Monroe DM, Escobar MA. Current concepts of hemostasis. Anesthesiology 2004;100:722–730. (Ref.19)

Roberts LN, Patel RK, Arya R. Haemostasis and thrombosis in liver disease. Br J Haematol 2010;148:507–521. (Ref.147)

Roemisch J, et al. Antithrombin: a new look at the actions of a serine protease inhibitor. Blood Coagul Fibrinol 2002;13:657–670. (Ref.27)

Rosenfeld S, et al. Antithymocyte globulin and cyclosporine for severe aplastic anemia: association between hematologic response and long-term outcome. JAMA 2003;289:1130–1135. (Ref.92)

Saab S, et al. Same day outpatient transjugular liver biopsies in haemophilia. Haemophilia 2004;10:727–731. (Ref.179)

Saab S, et al. Anemia in liver transplant recipients undergoing antiviral treatment for recurrent hepatitis C. Liver Transpl 2007;13:1032–1038. (Ref.185)

Sakuraya M, et al. Steroid-refractory chronic idiopathic thrombocytopenic purpura associated with hepatitis C virus infection. Eur J Haematol 2002;68:49–53. (Ref.142)

Samonakis DN, et al. Hypercoagulable states in patients with hepatocellular carcinoma. Dig Dis Sci 2004;49:854–858. (Ref.158)

Sandoval C, et al. Clinical and laboratory features of 178 children with recurrent epistaxis. J Pediatr Hematol Oncol 2002;24:47–49. (Ref.34)

Slofstra SH, Spek CA, ten Cate H. Disseminated intravascular coagulation. Hematol J 2003;4:295–302. (Ref.162)

Smith DM, et al. Liver transplant–associated graft-versus-host disease. Transplantation 2003;75:118–126. (Ref.112)

Sobhonslidsuk A, Reddy KR. Portal vein thrombosis: a concise review. Am J Gastroenterol 2002;97:535–541. (Ref.156)

Soejima Y, et al. Graft-versus-host disease following living donor liver transplantation. Liver Transpl 2004;10:460–464. (Ref.113)

Soza A, et al. Neutropenia during combination therapy of interferon alfa and ribavirin for chronic hepatitis C. Hepatology 2002;36:1273–1279. (Ref.102)

Stieltjes N, et al. Interest of transjugular liver biopsy in adult patients with haemophilia or other congenital bleeding disorders infected with hepatitis C virus. Br J Haematol 2004;125:769–776. (Ref.178)

Sulkowski MS, et al. Hepatitis C virus treatment–related anemia is associated with higher sustained virologic response rate. Gastroenterology 2010;139:1602–1611. (Ref.183)

Sulkowski MS, et al. Changes in haemoglobin during interferon alpha-2b plus ribavirin combination therapy for chronic hepatitis C virus infection. J Viral Hepatol 2004;11:243–250. (Ref.101)

Tacke F, et al. Analysis of factors contributing to higher erythropoietin levels in patients with chronic liver disease. Scand J Gastroenterol 2004;39:259–266. (Ref.71)

Tanaka N, Ishida F, Tanaka E. Ribavirin-induced pure red-cell aplasia during treatment of chronic hepatitis C. N Engl J Med 2004;350:1264–1265. (Ref.105)

Thomopoulos KC, et al. Non-invasive predictors of the presence of large oesophageal varices in patients with cirrhosis. Dig Liver Dis 2003;35:473–478. (Ref.133)

Thuluvath PJ, Yoo HY. Portal hypertensive gastropathy. Am J Gastroenterol 2002;97:2973–2978. (Ref.31)

Trevisani F, et al. Impaired tuftsin activity in cirrhosis: relationship with splenic function and clinical outcome. Gut 2002;50:707–712. (Ref.31)

Trotter JF, Cohn A, Grant R. Erythrocytosis in a patient with hepatocellular carcinoma. J Clin Gastroenterol 2002;35:365–366. (Ref.69)

Wells PS. Safety and efficacy of methods for reducing perioperative allogeneic transfusion: a critical review of the literature. Am J Ther 2002;9:377–388. (Ref.114)

Witters P, et al. Review article: blood platelet number and function in chronic liver disease and cirrhosis. Aliment Pharmacol Ther 2008;27:1017–1029. (Ref.138)

Wong AY, et al. Desmopressin does not decrease blood loss and transfusion requirements in patients undergoing hepatectomy. Can J Anaesth 2003;50:14–20. (Ref.189)

Young NS. Acquired aplastic anemia. Ann Intern Med 2002;136:534–546. (Ref.87)

Youssef WI, et al. Role of fresh frozen plasma infusion in correction of coagulopathy of chronic liver disease: a dual phase study. Am J Gastroenterol 2003;98:1391–1394. (Ref.170)

A complete list of references can be found at www.expertconsult.com.

Section IV

Toxin-Mediated Liver Injury

Drug-Induced Liver Injury

Herbert L. Bonkovsky, Dean P. Jones, Mark W. Russo, and Steven I. Shedlofsky

ABBREVIATIONS

ADR adverse drug reaction
AERS Adverse Events Reporting System
ALF acute (or subacute) liver failure
ALT alanine aminotransferase
ANT adenine nucleotide translocase
AP alkaline phosphatase
ARE antioxidant response element
AST aspartate aminotransferase
CAM complementary and alternative medications
CYP cytochrome P450
DILI drug-induced liver injury
ER endoplasmic reticulum
ERCP endoscopic retrograde cholangiopancreatography
FDA Food and Drug Administration
5-FU 5-fluorouracil
GSH glutathione

HAART highly active antiretroviral therapy
HIPAA Health Insurance Portability and Accountability Act
LT Liver test
MMPT mitochondrial membrane permeability transition
6-MP 6-mercaptopurine
MTX methotrexate
NAPQI N-acetyl-p-benzoquinoneimine
NIDDK National Institute of Diabetes and Digestive and Kidney Diseases
NNRTI nonnucleoside reverse transcriptase inhibitor
NRTI nucleoside analogue reverse transcriptase inhibitor

PAPS 3′-phosphoadenosine-5′-phosphosulfate
PI protease inhibitor
PPAR peroxisome proliferator–activated receptor-γ
PXR pregnane X receptor
RNS reactive nitrogen species
ROS reactive oxygen species
RUCAM Roussel-Uclaf Causality Assessment Method
SLE systemic lupus erythematosus
SOS sinusoidal obstruction syndrome
TNF-α tumor necrosis factor alpha
UDPGA uridine diphosphoglucuronic acid
ULN upper limit of normal
VDAC voltage-dependent anion channel
WHO World Health Organization

Introduction

In humans and other higher organisms the liver is the principal site for the metabolism of foreign substances. It is responsible for absorbing, detoxifying, and excreting an astonishing array of chemical substances, encountered both from outside the organism (i.e., xenobiotics) and from within the organism, including many substances synthesized by the liver itself. In the toxicology literature, there is a distinction between "toxins," which are naturally occurring poisons, and "toxicants," which can be derived from any source. In general, the liver and kidneys are chiefly responsible for maintenance of the internal milieu of chemicals within narrow concentration gradients. These organs also function to remove potentially toxic compounds from organisms. In general, toxic compounds of lower molecular weight and higher water solubility are excreted chiefly by the kidneys through glomerular filtration and/or tubular secretion. In contrast, larger, more lipophilic substances must be absorbed and undergo initial metabolism by the liver before their excretion either in the bile and feces or in the urine.

The multistep process for the metabolism of drugs and chemicals is summarized in **Figure 25-1**. Most such chemicals are ingested orally and absorbed, chiefly in the proximal small intestine. Some of them undergo initial metabolism within the gastrointestinal tract. Parent compounds and/or metabolites then enter the splanchnic blood, from which they are eventually delivered by the portal circulation to the liver. Depending upon the xenobiotic in question, cells within the liver absorb a variable proportion of the compound. This initial removal of compounds from the portal blood, which is the chief blood supply to the liver, is called the "first-pass effect" of the liver.

The uptake into liver cells occurs primarily, but not solely, into hepatocytes. During the past several years a number of transporters of cations and anions have been described and have been identified as important in the uptake of endogenous chemicals and xenobiotics (drugs, foreign chemicals) by liver cells. Once inside hepatocytes, these chemicals undergo further intracellular binding and transport. The intracellular mechanisms responsible for such transport are less well understood. It is likely that highly lipophilic compounds dissolve readily into the membranes of cells and diffuse widely and quickly within and across such membranes. In contrast, more hydrophilic compounds require protein binding and other means for transport.

As shown in **Figure 25-1**, many (but certainly not all) drugs and chemicals require an initial oxidation reaction, termed

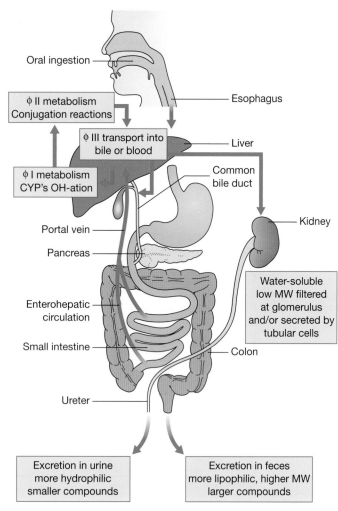

Fig. 25-1 Disposition of xenobiotics in humans.

Labels in figure:
- Oral ingestion
- φ II metabolism Conjugation reactions
- φ III transport into bile or blood
- φ I metabolism CYP's OH-ation
- Esophagus
- Liver
- Common bile duct
- Kidney
- Portal vein
- Pancreas
- Enterohepatic circulation
- Small intestine
- Colon
- Ureter
- Water-soluble low MW filtered at glomerulus and/or secreted by tubular cells
- Excretion in urine more hydrophilic smaller compounds
- Excretion in feces more lipophilic, higher MW larger compounds

eventual excretion of water-soluble hydrophilic products in the urine; alternatively, drugs can be transported across the apical membrane domain of hepatocytes into bile canaliculi (secretion into the bile), with eventual excretion in the feces. Subsequent metabolism of drug conjugates can be complex, with some undergoing metabolism in the intestines and further metabolism in the liver in a process dependent upon enterohepatic circulation. Others are metabolized in other organs; for instance, glutathione conjugates are metabolized by hydrolysis and acetylation to mercapturic acids, which are the primary excreted product.

Drug-induced liver injury (DILI) is the major toxic effect of drugs. It is the principal reason for abandonment of the development of possible new drugs, for the failure of new drugs to achieve approval by the U.S. Food and Drug Administration (FDA), and for the withdrawal of new drugs from the market after initial approval. Adverse drug reactions (ADRs), which are detected in preclinical studies in cells or experimental animals, usually lead to abandonment of the drug as a candidate for further development, unless there is a unique and highly important desirable effect of such compounds. Those new drugs that survive this initial level of scrutiny then proceed through phases 1 to 3 of clinical development and testing. In these phases, only a limited number of highly selected subjects, typically between 2000 and 10,000, receive the medication. As a result, clinically significant but relatively rare ADRs usually are not detected until after drugs have been approved and are in use by a larger number of persons. These ADRs are often associated with other underlying problems or conditions, which may increase the risk of development of ADRs. Thus continued monitoring of new drugs during phase 4 (postapproval surveillance) is now recognized by the FDA and by the pharmaceutical industry to be of paramount importance.

As described previously, DILI is a rare event, occurring in only a small percentage of persons who take drugs. The reasons for this are not fully understood. However, based on a combination of experimental results in cell models and whole-animal models and careful clinical observations, and by analogy to numerous other disorders, drug-induced liver injuries are caused and modulated by an interplay of at least the following three factors: (1) the drug, (2) the host (i.e., the person ingesting the drug), and (3) the environment of the host. This interaction is depicted in **Figure 25-2**.

It is difficult to establish a diagnosis of DILI. This is because there are numerous other potential causes of liver injury, and because there is no single pathognomonic test to establish that a given drug in a given subject is the cause of liver injury. Furthermore, the clinical and laboratory manifestations of DILI vary markedly, from asymptomatic laboratory abnormalities, which may resolve even though the drug is continued (so-called "adaptation"), to severe, life-threatening acute (or subacute) liver failure (ALF). Because of these factors, a diagnosis of DILI is frequently delayed or may be missed entirely. Similar considerations also apply to "herbal remedies" and complementary and alternative medications (CAM), which are not regulated with the same rigorous standards as prescription medications. The scope of this chapter is to provide a review and update of drug-induced liver injury attributable to over-the-counter and prescription drugs. The hepatic effects and toxicities of herbal remedies and CAM are considered elsewhere (see Chapter 26).

phase I metabolism. The most common example is hydroxylation catalyzed by 1 of the 57 varieties of cytochrome P450 (CYP). Many of these CYPs are found in hepatocytes, and they carry out hydroxylation reactions in concert with NADPH (as a source of electrons) and cytochrome P450 reductase; for some chemicals, cooperation with another heme-containing protein called cytochrome b_5 is also required. These enzymes and reactions occur principally in the smooth endoplasmic reticulum.

Following the initial hydroxylation reaction, one of several additional reactions leads to the addition of more water-soluble moieties to the initial hydroxylated product. The enzymes responsible for this so-called phase II metabolism are chiefly glucuronosyl transferases, sulfotransferases, and enzymes that add glutathione or products of the reduced thiol form of glutathione (e.g., GSH transferases). The key substrates for these conjugation reactions are uridine diphosphoglucuronic acid (UDPGA), 3′-phosphoadenosine-5′-phosphosulfate (PAPS), and reduced glutathione (GSH, the tripeptide L-γ-glutamyl-L-cysteinyl-glycine).

The third phase of hepatic drug metabolism—the transport of the parent drug and/or its metabolites out of hepatocytes—can occur in one of the following ways: drugs and/or metabolites can be transported across the plasma membrane, with

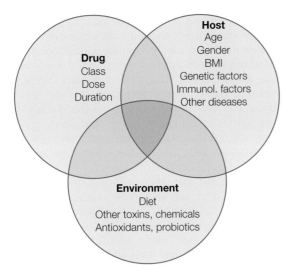

Fig. 25-2 **Factors believed to be involved in pathogenesis of DILI.**

Epidemiology: Scope of the Problem

Although the occurrence of drug toxicities, and in particular hepatotoxicities, should be an expected consequence of the widespread use of complex and potent medications, the U.S. public generally expects the FDA to keep toxic drugs off the market. Regulatory agencies in Europe, Australia, and other developed countries serve a similar function to protect their populations. However, there are many drugs with known, well-described hepatotoxicities, including acetaminophen, isoniazid, valproate, phenytoin, and propylthiouracil, that remain available because their medical benefits are deemed to outweigh the risks. Nevertheless, between 1990 and 2002, acute liver failure from these five drugs accounted for 15% of all liver transplantations in the United States, with 51% of the cases attributable to ADRs after drugs were taken with therapeutic intent, not to suicide attempts from acetaminophen overdose.[1] ADRs were estimated to be the fourth to sixth most common cause of U.S. in-hospital mortality in the 1990s.[2]

For drugs that have been introduced into the market since the FDA began stringent regulatory control in 1962, the required animal toxicity studies and/or human trials eliminated most new chemical entities that were likely to cause predictable and dose-related organ toxicity.[3] However, some drugs that appeared "safe" were withdrawn in the postmarketing period because of serious ADRs that became apparent only after many more patients were exposed to the drug (**Table 25-1**). These withdrawals represented huge economic setbacks for the pharmaceutical companies that had developed the drugs, and they sometimes frustrated patients and their providers who were satisfied with, and depended on the availability of, the withdrawn drugs. Hepatotoxicity was the reason for withdrawal in almost half the cases. Noteworthy is that drug withdrawals attributable to hepatotoxicity were the most common reasons before 1990, and have occurred less frequently since 1990, suggesting improved preclinical assessment of risk.

If a new medication causes a serious ADR with risk of mortality in as few as 1 in 10,000 exposed persons, society

Table 25-1 Drugs Approved by the U.S. FDA but Withdrawn in the Postmarketing Setting

DRUG	TOXICITY	YEAR WITHDRAWN
Iproniazid (Marsalid)	Hepatotoxicity	1956
Thalidomide (Thalomid)	Limb deformities	1961*
Ibufenac§ (in Europe)	Hepatotoxicity	1975
Ticrynafen (Selacryn)	Hepatotoxicity	1979
Benoxaprofen (Oraflex)	Hepatotoxicity	1982
Perihexilene§ (in France)	Hepatotoxicity	1985
Dilevalol§ (in Ireland, Portugal)	Hepatotoxicity	1990
Encainide (Enkaid)	Excessive mortality	1991
Temafloxacin (Omniflox)	Hemolytic anemia	1992
Flosequinan (Manoplex)	Excessive mortality	1993
Bromfenac (Duract)	Hepatotoxicity	1998
Mibefradil (Posicor)	Multiple drug interactions	1998
Terfenadine (Seldane)	Cardiac arrhythmias	1998
Troglitazone (Rezulin)	Hepatotoxicity	2000
Cisapride (Propulsid)	Cardiac arrhythmias	2000†
Alosetron (Lotronex)	Ischemic colitis	2001‡
Cerivastatin (Baycol)	Rhabdomyolysis	2001
Rofecoxib (Vioxx)	Cardiac mortality	2004

*Made available again on a severely restricted basis in 1998.
†Made available again on a severely restricted basis in 2000.
‡Made available again on a severely restricted basis in 2002.
§Drugs not approved in United States and withdrawn in other countries.

deems this unacceptable, especially if there are alternative drugs available. Phase 1 to 3 trials generally include fewer than 10,000 carefully selected subjects. Although this is a large number, it is not large enough to reliably identify serious idiosyncratic ADRs that occur less frequently than 1 to 2 times in 10,000 subjects. Therefore postmarketing surveillance has become critically important in identifying ADRs. In January 2002 the FDA organized an Office of Drug Safety, which oversees a large database of ADRs entered into its Adverse Events Reporting System (AERS) at its MedWatch website (www.fda.gov/medwatch/safety/3500.pdf) or by fax or post. Similar pharmacovigilance efforts have been mounted in Europe. The World Health Organization (WHO) maintains the Uppsala Monitoring Centre (www.who-umc.org) that receives and analyzes ADRs from around the world, including reports from the U.S. FDA.[4]

With these efforts, it would seem possible to accurately report epidemiologic trends in ADRs and identify offending medications quickly. However, most of the reporting systems rely on voluntary submission of information. Also, even though submission of personal health data to MedWatch is exempt from Health Insurance Portability and Accountability Act (HIPAA) privacy restrictions,[5] very few healthcare providers take the time to submit reports. It is estimated that only about 1% to 10% of ADRs are reported.[5] Furthermore, the databases consist of large numbers of reports (184,702 were submitted to the FDA's AERS in 2002) varying in both quality and detail and submitted by pharmaceutical companies (as required by law) or by physicians.[4] Because of the potential economic impact on pharmaceutical companies, and because of complex legal liabilities, the raw data from all of these ADRs are not easily available in the public domain. The FDA allows public access to extracts of AERS data through the National Technical Information Service report. The WHO's Uppsala Monitoring Centre has contracted with VigiBase Services (www.umc-products.com), which can provide customized data but at a substantial cost. This service is chiefly designed for regulatory agency professionals and pharmaceutical companies who study drug safety and utilize data mining techniques.

Currently, the incidence and impact of ADRs from specific agents remain largely unknown. Many healthcare providers now use one or more of the available web-based drug information services such as the *Physicians' Desk Reference* (www.pdr.net) or *Epocrates* (www.epocrates.com) to review drug toxicity data. However, such sources do not provide specific information regarding the incidence and types of hepatotoxicity caused. We therefore rely upon regulatory agencies such as the FDA to monitor ADRs and either issue "black box" warnings or recommend voluntary withdrawal of the drug. Because of medicolegal liabilities, most pharmaceutical companies voluntarily withdraw their products when evidence of hepatotoxicity or other toxicities begins to mount. However, it is likely that if physicians and other healthcare providers were more conscientious in suspecting and reporting ADRs, the collective data would lead to better patient care and fewer ADRs. With current electronic web-based reporting systems, such reports are now relatively easy and quick to submit. Furthermore, there is an expectation that high-throughput technologies will allow individualized therapeutics to become a central component of developing capabilities in personalized medicine.

Causality Assessment

A continuing challenge in the study of adverse effects of drugs and chemicals on the liver (and other organs) is that of causality assessment, the process whereby the likelihood of the diagnosis DILI is determined. This process of deduction involves analysis of the relevant data and should include an assessment of the temporal relationship, clinical features, laboratory data, histologic data (if available), and current knowledge about the drug in question. From a statistical standpoint the most scientifically sound approach is to use Bayes' theorem. Using this technique, an attempt is made to estimate the overall probability of a particular adverse event occurring in a particular individual in a particular situation (posterior probability), given the probability of this event occurring in a group of individuals similarly exposed (prior probability). Individual and situational details considered include the subject's clinical history, temporal relationships, histologic pattern of injury, and

resolution with discontinuation of the agent, as well as whether rechallenge with the agent resulted in recurrence of the adverse event. These details are used to develop a likelihood ratio; the product of this ratio and the prior probability is a measure of the posterior probability. The major problems that limit the application of Bayes' theorem in practice are that it is time-consuming and data needed to compute the likelihood ratio (e.g., background incidence) are often unavailable.

Although several scoring systems and tools for assessing whether drugs are the cause of liver injury have been developed,[6-9] they are not widely used in practice because they take time to complete and because key information is often lacking. Probably, the best known and most widely used of these is RUCAM—the *Roussel-Uclaf Causality Assessment Method*.[6,7] However, numerous ambiguities and problems with application of RUCAM have been found, and its reproducibility, even among experts in DILI, has been poor.[10] Thus there is need for a more robust evidence-based instrument. Until this is developed, the Delphic approach, using a structured process, appears to produce higher agreement rates and likelihood scores.[11]

A major problem is that data needed to assess causality, especially to exclude other possible causes of DILI, often are missing. Elements that should be included in reports of DILI have been proposed recently[12] (**Table 25-2**). Often missing are records of the presence of underlying diseases; history of alcohol, herbal, or other drug use; tests to exclude viral hepatitis (especially hepatitides A, B, and C; cytomegalovirus [CMV]; Epstein-Barr virus [EBV]; herpes simplex virus [HSV]); tests to exclude autoimmune hepatitis (antinuclear antibody [ANA], anti–smooth muscle antibody [ASMA]); and abdominal imaging studies to exclude biliary tract disease. Based on the degree of certainty of a causal interaction between drug intake and hepatic injury, different terms are used to describe the strength of the relationship. "Definite" is usually supported by a "signature" clinical pattern, a strong temporal correlation, including a positive rechallenge, and exclusion of all other potential causes. Weaker relationships are termed "very likely," "probable," "possible," and "unlikely" in descending order of strength; these terms are used when the relevant evidence is judged to be less compelling.[11]

One problematic issue is whether the subject in question has DILI or autoimmune hepatitis, because the former may trigger the latter and because subjects with autoimmunoallergic diatheses are probably more prone to develop DILI of the immunoallergic type. In all cases of suspected cholestatic DILI, it is important to exclude biliary tract disease and/or biliary obstruction.

Mechanisms of Hepatic Injury Due to Drugs and Chemicals
Apoptosis and Necrosis

Necrosis and apoptosis are terms used to describe patterns of morphologic changes associated with cell death. Both morphologies include a spectrum of biochemical processes, can occur concomitantly, and often vary in appearance, depending on the unique properties of the toxic agent, the time course

Table 25-2 Minimal Elements for Reporting Drug-Induced Liver Injury

Patient gender and age

Drug and its dose

Primary disease (for which drug was prescribed)

Concomitant diseases (with special attention to heart failure or episodes of hypotension, sepsis, or receipt of parenteral nutrition)

Pertinent medical history (including previous exposure to drug, previous reaction to drug or other drugs, history of liver disease, and risk factors for liver disease)

History of alcohol use

Dates of start and discontinuation of therapy (or time from onset of event)

Symptoms

    Date of onset

    List of pertinent symptoms (fatigue, weakness, nausea, anorexia, abdominal pain, dark urine, jaundice, pruritus, rash, and fever)

Pertinent physical findings at the time of presentation (with special mention of whether or not there is fever, rash, jaundice, hepatic tenderness, or signs of chronic liver disease)

Medication history (other medications taken in 3 months before onset of liver injury with dose, generic name, and duration)

Laboratory tests

    Date and time of first abnormal laboratory test result

    Laboratory test results from before drug exposure (specifically liver tests)

    Initial laboratory results at presentation (bilirubin, ALT, AP,* INR, or PT, and eosinophil count or percentage)

    Laboratory results needed to exclude other causes (IgM anti-HAV, IgM anti-HBc, HBsAg, anti-HCV, HCV RNA, and ANA)

    Course of serum bilirubin, ALT, AP, and INR levels (preferably in a table with entries dated from time of starting and stopping drug and until resolution)

Imaging studies (abdominal ultrasound, CT, or MR)

Liver histologic results (if obtained and date of procedure in relation to episode of drug-induced liver injury)

Whether rechallenge with same medication as performed and, if so, results of challenge

From Agrawal VK, et al. Important elements for the diagnosis of drug-induced liver injury. Clin Gastroent Hepatol 2010;8:463–470.

ANA, antinuclear antibody; AP, alkaline phosphatase; CT, computed tomography; HAV, hepatitis A virus; HBc, hepatitis B core antibody; HBsAg, hepatitis B surface antigen; HCV, hepatitis C virus; Ig, immunoglobulin; INR, International normalized ratio; MR, magnetic resonance; PT, prothrombin time

and dose dependence of exposure, and the interactions with other host and environmental factors (see **Fig. 25-2**). The most common recognized morphologic form of cell death in the liver is necrosis, which is characterized by cellular and organellar swelling and membranal lysis with release of cytoplasmic contents. After the occurrence of such changes, the outlines of cells are often indistinct and cells have an amorphous or coarsely granular appearance.

Detailed morphologic studies of pathologic as well as normal tissues revealed a second, distinct morphology of cell death, originally termed "shrinkage necrosis"[13] and now termed apoptosis.[14] These distinct morphologies are now recognized to represent two general cellular phenomena that can occur concomitantly. In apoptosis, typical changes include cell shrinkage, organellar compaction, nuclear condensation, fragmentation of cells into smaller "apoptotic bodies," and the appearance of phagocytosis signals on the cell surface.[15] Apoptotic cells are rapidly removed by phagocytosis. Necrosis generally represents a loss of osmotic regulation and cell lysis, whereas apoptosis represents activation of an enzyme-mediated autolytic cell disposal system. Both are often linked to bioenergetic changes, mitochondrial failure, and oxidative stress. Thus consideration of the distinctions between necrosis and apoptosis is important not only for pathologic evaluation of hepatotoxicity but also for investigation of underlying mechanisms of cell injury.

Although apoptosis is defined morphologically, it is generally used to refer specifically to a series of cellular changes that result from the activation of a family of highly conserved enzymes termed caspases. These enzymes are proteases that cleave specific target amino acid sequences, resulting in characteristic morphologic changes and leading to cell elimination by phagocytosis.[16] Activation occurs through plasma membrane–associated death receptor activation of caspase-8,[17] through mitochondria-mediated activation of caspase-9,[18] and through endoplasmic reticulum–mediated activation of caspase-12.[19] These activation mechanisms normally function in homeostatic control of the liver and represent a mechanism to eliminate damaged cells and allow replacement by mitosis. Chemicals that alter the expression and function of the death receptor components, disrupt mitochondrial function, or disturb the secretory pathway can therefore be expected to activate apoptosis (**Fig. 25-3**). In addition, disruption of the cell cycle and inhibition of proteosomes also activate apoptosis. Thus many agents previously believed to kill cells by disruption of homeostatic processes are now believed to do so by activation of apoptosis. Of critical importance is that an increase in apoptosis is often a more sensitive indicator of tissue injury than necrosis. However, because the liver is always undergoing renewal and this process involves apoptosis, definition of the lower limit of toxicity in terms of an increase in apoptosis can be difficult without detailed examination of a large number of cells.

An extension of this concept to higher doses and increased activation of apoptosis reveals that a true distinction between necrosis and apoptosis as causative mechanisms in liver toxicity may not be possible. If apoptosis occurs at a rate that exceeds the capacity of phagocytic cells (itself variable) to remove the apoptotic cells, large fields of contiguous cells will swell and lyse, producing characteristics of necrosis. On the other hand, if the toxic insult causes rapid loss of ionic homeostasis, cells may rapidly swell and lyse (i.e., undergo necrosis), even though the apoptotic cascade has been activated.

Many toxicants show a dose-dependent switch between apoptosis and necrosis attributable to differential effects on mitochondrial function and energy metabolism. Disruption of only a fraction of mitochondria can result in sufficient cytochrome *c* release to activate the caspase-9/caspase-3 pathway without disrupting cellular energetics. Under these conditions, cells maintain osmotic regulation and undergo apoptosis. However, with greater disruption of mitochondria, cellular energetics are impaired, osmotic regulation is lost, and cells undergo swelling and lysis. Because of this, the mechanisms involved in activation of caspases and/or loss of osmotic regulation are key to understanding chemical-induced liver disease.

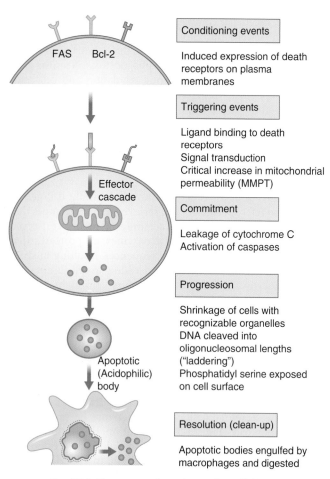

Conditioning events

Induced expression of death receptors on plasma membranes

Triggering events

Ligand binding to death receptors
Signal transduction
Critical increase in mitochondrial permeability (MMPT)

Commitment

Leakage of cytochrome C
Activation of caspases

Progression

Shrinkage of cells with recognizable organelles
DNA cleaved into oligonucleosomal lengths ("laddering")
Phosphatidyl serine exposed on cell surface

Resolution (clean-up)

Apoptotic bodies engulfed by macrophages and digested

Fig. 25-3 **The apoptotic pathway for cell death.**

During the past decade, rapidly developing knowledge about the mechanisms of apoptosis has dramatically changed the perception of how chemicals induce hepatic injury. In the past, injury was considered to be due to failure of critical cell machinery, especially that controlling Ca^{2+} homeostasis. Now, however, attention has shifted to mechanisms of apoptosis, which is executed by the caspase proteolytic cascade that is activated by specific signaling involving death receptors or disruption of mitochondria, endoplasmic reticulum (ER), or nuclei, for example. Central features of chemical-induced liver injury remain the same; however, death is now viewed as occurring through targeted cleavage of specific proteins rather than generalized failure. Bioactivation of organic compounds to reactive electrophiles occurs prominently in the liver because of the presence of high concentrations of enzyme systems designed to aid in the elimination of foreign compounds (see **Fig. 25-1**). Electrophilic agents covalently modify macromolecules, disrupting normal functions, including protein–protein interactions and protein degradation by proteosomes. Oxidants alter the expression of death receptor machinery, enhancing death receptor–mediated apoptosis, and target the MMPT pore, triggering mitochondria-mediated apoptosis. Protection against reactive electrophiles and oxidants occurs through systems that depend upon GSH, and maintenance of GSH is a key mechanism for protection against chemical-induced liver injury. As mass spectrometry and proteomic techniques become widely used in toxicologic research, the possibility of applying systems biology approaches to define toxicity improves. By incorporating a broad spectrum of potential targets into the toxicologic models, this approach is likely to yield a more nearly complete and accurate understanding of the mechanisms of hepatotoxicity.

Mitochondria are a common target of toxicity in liver and play a central role in both apoptosis and necrosis. A recent model integrates major features of energy metabolism, oxidative stress, and apoptosis through central regulatory functions of complex III and aconitase. In oxidative phosphorylation, essentially all electrons flow from coenzyme Q to cytochrome *c* through complex III to drive the production of adenosine triphosphate (ATP). The electron flow through this complex is partitioned between reduction of cytochrome *c* and 1-electron reduction of O_2 to produce the reactive oxygen species superoxide ion. The superoxide ion provides an oxidant source for the regulation of aconitase, a key enzyme in the citric acid cycle; for oxidation of cardiolipin, a key step in the release of cytochrome *c* and activation of the caspase-9/caspase-3 cascade; and for opening of the mitochondrial membrane permeability transition (MMPT) pore, a generalized trigger for both cytochrome *c* release and loss of ATP production. This complex can therefore serve as a sensor for energetic and redox homeostasis, integrating ATP supply requirements, the efficacy of GSH and other antioxidant systems, calcium homeostasis, and nutritional supply of oxidizable substrates. Consequently, physiologic variations such as food supply and hepatic O_2 supply (e.g., hypoxia) can function as important modulators of the biochemical mechanisms and morphology associated with specific toxicant exposures.

Bioactivation of Xenobiotic Agents

Some compounds are not toxic to the liver in the parent form but are bioactivated to reactive species. One of the more common mechanisms of bioactivation involves conversion to compounds with electron-seeking properties (i.e., to electrophiles). In most cases, these electrophiles are the result of phase I metabolism by CYP-dependent reactions. Epoxides are an important class of toxic electrophiles. Bromobenzene and aflatoxin B1 are metabolized by hepatic mixed-function oxidases to the epoxide intermediates bromobenzene-3,4-oxide[20,21] and aflatoxin B1-8,9-oxide,[22] respectively. Other electrophilic species include alkyl and aryl halides, carbonium and diazonium ion intermediates, aldehydes, esters, α,β-unsaturated carbon compounds, and compounds containing double-bonded nitrogen (e.g., isothiocyanates, isocyanates, quinazolines).[23] Phase II metabolism also may result ultimately in toxic electrophiles, exemplified by toxic GSH S-conjugates, glucuronides, and sulfates[24,25]; these metabolites may be toxic to the liver as well as to extrahepatic organs.

Reactive electrophiles generated during bioactivation react with specific macromolecules or sites to cause toxicity.[26] For instance, earlier research showed that calcium transport systems in the plasma membrane[27] and endoplasmic reticulum[28,29] contain reactive cysteine thiol groups that are critical for function. More recent studies show that molecular chaperones, proteolytic systems, and transcription factors are susceptible to redox modifications.[30-32] DNA may be a target of electrophiles, in which case the lesion may cause acute hepatocellular death or lead to carcinogenicity. The epoxide of aflatoxin B1 formed during hepatic biotransformation binds guanine residues in DNA at the N-7 position, which may ultimately result in hepatocarcinogenesis.[22,33] Covalent modification of proteins may result in the formation of a neoantigen against which an immune response is mounted, giving rise to immunoallergic DILI. Metabolites of halothane, phenytoin, and numerous other drugs may cause liver injury by this type of idiosyncratic mechanism.[34,35]

Role of Glutathione in Chemical Detoxification of Reactive Electrophiles

Glutathione (GSH) is a major low-molecular-weight thiol compound that constitutes more than 90% of the acid-soluble thiol pool in hepatocytes and accounts for about 30% of the total thiol groups in liver.[36] GSH serves many important functions, including detoxifying peroxides and electrophiles (see Oxidative Stress and Free Radical Reactions in Hepatotoxicity), maintaining protein thiols in a reduced state, serving as a nontoxic storage form of cysteine, and participating in the synthesis of leukotrienes and prostaglandins as well as the reduction of ribonucleotides to deoxyribonucleotides.[36] The liver is very active in synthesis of GSH, not only for detoxification functions but also to provide a reservoir of cysteine through an interorgan transport mechanism.[37] Sulfur amino acid homeostasis also depends on the presence of the cystathionine pathway in the liver, which provides the major site for conversion of methionine to cysteine.[38] Cirrhotic changes in the liver therefore not only affect the sensitivity of the liver to toxicity, but also affect the sensitivity of other organ systems to toxicity attributable to impaired cysteine supply and glutathione regulation.

Of great relevance to chemical toxicity is that GSH is a key compound involved in the detoxification of electrophiles. The thiol group of GSH is a nucleophilic center that undergoes S-conjugation with electrophiles; in most cases this leads to detoxification. Many electrophiles form GSH S-conjugates nonenzymatically to some extent, which is a function of charge localization of both electrophile and nucleophile.[39] Hepatocytes and other cells do not rely on nonenzymatic conjugation of electrophiles; instead, they contain enzymes termed GSH S-transferases that catalyze S-conjugation of GSH to electrophiles. Four major classes of cytosolic GSH S-transferase (i.e., α, μ, π, δ) and one microsomal enzyme have been characterized in mammalian tissues.[40] The cytosolic GSH S-transferases have been studied in the greatest detail and have been shown to be a multigene family of enzymes. Each cytosolic GSH S-transferase is a dimer, a discrete gene codes for each subunit, only subunits of the same class form dimers, and dimers may contain identical subunits (homodimers) or different subunits (heterodimers). The cytosolic enzymes are expressed to various extents in different tissues and are important in detoxification of several groups of xenobiotics, including polycyclic aromatic hydrocarbons, aflatoxins, aromatic amines, and alkylating agents.[41] The liver is most active in GSH-dependent detoxification of electrophiles, and human liver is particularly rich in GSH S-transferases of the α class; in other species, such as rat, the μ class of GSH S-transferases also is abundant in liver.

The generation of large quantities of electrophiles in liver ultimately depletes cellular GSH pools, resulting in enhanced covalent binding to critical macromolecules and cell death. Because GSH and the GSH S-transferases play such an integral role in detoxification of electrophilic species in liver, physiologic or pathophysiologic conditions that either decrease or elevate levels or activities in liver would be expected to affect chemical detoxification in the anticipated direction. Experimentally, this has been demonstrated for a variety of electrophiles. For example, depletion of hepatocellular GSH exacerbates hepatotoxicity associated with electrophiles, including metabolites of acetaminophen[42] and bromobenzene.[21] Fasting for 1 or 2 days decreases hepatic GSH content by 30% to 50%[43] and enhances liver injury caused by many electrophilic agents. Diurnal variation in hepatic GSH stores of about 25% to 30%[44] may influence hepatotoxicity as a result of the availability of GSH for detoxification. Diurnal variation in plasma GSH levels also occurs, but a larger variation is observed in plasma cysteine levels,[45] and acetaminophen at therapeutic levels alters plasma cysteine level without affecting plasma GSH level.[46] Cysteine prodrugs (N-acetylcysteine or oxothiazolidine-4-carboxylate) and GSH esters[47] can increase hepatic GSH levels and protect against the hepatotoxicity caused by acetaminophen overdose.[48]

Similar to the CYPs, the GSH S-transferases have relatively broad and overlapping substrate specificities and their activities may be increased following exposure to certain drugs, environmental chemicals, and dietary components. This occurs chiefly through a well-characterized transcription enhancer system, consisting of an antioxidant response element (ARE)-binding sequence in the DNA and the Nrf-2/Maf transcription factor system.[49,50] Nrf-2 is normally present as an inactive complex with Keap-1, bound to cytoskeletal components in the cytoplasm. Keap-1 has several cysteine thiols that are sensitive to oxidation and alkylation. Modification of these thiols results in the release of Nrf-2, which translocates to the nucleus, interacts with small Maf proteins and binds to the ARE, and activates transcription of a broad range of phase 2 detoxification systems (**Fig. 25-4**). Dietary inducers contained in cruciferous vegetables induce GSH S-transferases and other protective phase 2 enzymes without having a significant effect on the CYPs.[51-54] These results suggest that increased intake of foods containing these agents may provide a simple and effective means to prevent toxicity as well as cancer caused by toxicants.

A prototypic example of bioactivation and covalent binding in hepatotoxicity is provided by the analgesic acetaminophen (N-acetyl-p-aminophenol; paracetamol). In overdose, acetaminophen results in severe hepatocellular necrosis in zone 3 of the hepatic acini (centrilobular necrosis) (**Fig. 25-5**).[55] Bioactivation occurs via hepatic CYP to the electrophilic intermediate N-acetyl-p-benzoquinoneimine (NAPQI)[56] (see **Fig. 25-4**). In humans, CYPs 2E1 and 1A2 account for the largest fraction of this conversion.[57] At low rates of production, NAPQI is detoxified by S-conjugation with GSH; however, at higher rates of NAPQI production, hepatocellular GSH pools are depleted and extensive covalent binding to cellular macromolecules occurs.[58,59] Ultrastructural and functional studies

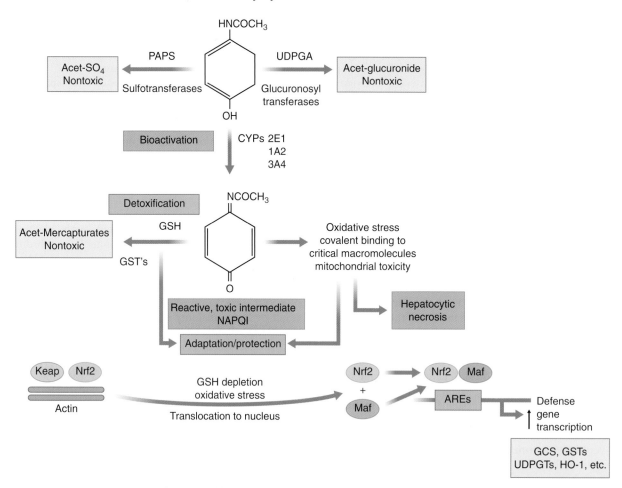

Fig. 25-4 **Hepatic metabolism and effects of acetaminophen and the Nfr2, Maf, ARE system for cytoprotection.**

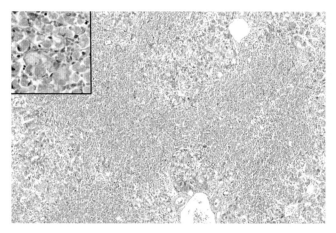

Fig. 25-5 **Submassive (zone 3) coagulative necrosis attributable to an overdose of acetaminophen.** Viable hepatocytes surround the portal areas, and the terminal hepatic venules are surrounded by necrotic tissue. Inset shows the necrotic hepatocytes at high magnification.

have shown that mitochondria are an early target in the hepatocellular necrosis caused by acetaminophen[60-63]; however, acetaminophen metabolites also form adducts to hepatic proteins in the cytosol, microsomes, nuclei, and plasma membranes.[35] Arylation of specific proteins has been reported[64-66]; however, large numbers of adducted proteins have also been detected, and other mechanisms of toxicity have also been suggested.[67-73]

Oxidative Stress and Free Radical Reactions in Hepatotoxicity

Oxidative stress is an imbalance between oxidants and antioxidants in favor of the oxidants, leading to a disruption of redox signaling and control and/or molecular damage.[74] Although it was earlier viewed as a global balance, increasing knowledge of redox signaling mechanisms indicates that toxicants can disrupt redox signaling and control without necessarily altering major systems that control overall redox balance, indicating a specificity in mechanisms.[75] Key mechanisms involve reactive oxygen species (ROS), reactive nitrogen species (RNS), and a range of free radicals generated by bioactivation of xenobiotics. All of the classes of cellular macromolecules can be the target of oxidant-induced liver injury. As discussed previously for covalent modification, proteins are most often considered the critical targets in acute necrosis, but oxidants also are genotoxic. Nonradical oxidants, such as hydrogen peroxide and lipid hydroperoxides, are quantitatively most important under most conditions[75]; however, free radicals can also be important in medicating hepatotoxicity.

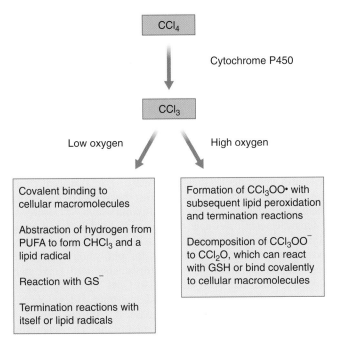

Fig. 25-6 **Hepatic metabolism and oxygen-dependent effects of carbon tetrachloride (CCl$_4$). •CCl$_3$, trichloromethyl radical.** GS$^-$, glutathione thiolate anion; GSH, glutathione; PUFA, polyunsaturated fatty acid.

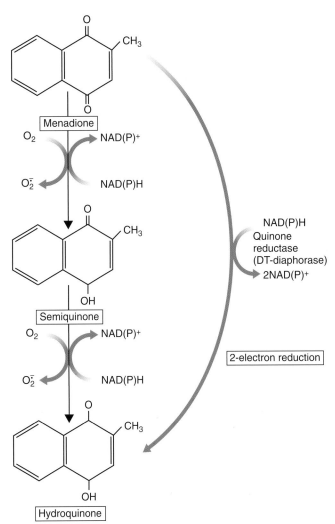

Fig. 25-7 **Redox cycling of menadione, an example of a hepatotoxic drug that produces superoxide (O$_2^-$).** NAD$^+$, nicotinamide adenine dinucleotide; NADH, nicotinamide adenine dinucleotide (reduced form); NAD(P)$^+$, nicotinamide adenine dinucleotide phosphate; NADPH, nicotinamide adenine dinucleotide phosphate (reduced form).

Free radicals can be generated in the liver in several ways. CYP enzymes generate radicals from xenobiotics by three different mechanisms: 1-electron oxidation to form a cation radical (R $\rightarrow$ •R$^+$ + e$^-$); 1-electron reduction to yield an anion radical (R + e$^-$ $\rightarrow$ •R$^-$); or homolytic bond scission to yield a neutral radical (R–R $\rightarrow$ •R + •R).[76] Hepatotoxicants of occupational/environmental (e.g., CCl$_4$) as well as of clinical importance (e.g., halothane) are bioactivated in liver to free radical species. CCl$_4$ toxicity provides a useful model and is representative of a large number of halogenated hydrocarbons that can be similarly activated.

CCl$_4$ is a prototypical hepatotoxin that causes centrilobular necrosis and associated fatty liver. Caspase-3 is activated and released into the plasma with a time course suggesting initial activation of apoptosis followed by secondary necrosis.[77] A primary event in the pathogenesis is the reductive dehalogenation of CCl$_4$ to the trichloromethyl free radical (•CCl$_3$) by hepatic mixed function oxidases (**Fig. 25-6**). The free radical •CCl$_3$ can initiate lipid peroxidation, and in the presence of oxygen it forms the more reactive trichloromethylperoxy free radical (CCl$_3$OO•), which also decomposes to phosgene (CC$_2$O). The lipid peroxidation in liver associated with CCl$_4$ has been viewed as a critical event because it occurs early and is associated with reductions of enzyme activities[78] and inactivation of the Ca^{2+} sequestering capacity of endoplasmic reticulum.[79,80] Elevation of cellular Ca^{2+} concentration establishes conditions for activation of the mitochondrial permeability transition, with associated cytochrome c release and caspase activation (see **Fig. 25-3**).

In addition to free radicals of the parent compound, other reactive oxygen and reactive nitrogen species are often involved in hepatotoxicity. Reactive oxygen species such as the hydroxyl radical (•OH) are generated during redox cycling of several xenobiotics, following activation of the respiratory burst in host phagocytic cells, and during exposure to ionizing radiation. Reactive nitrogen species can also be involved in these toxic processes because of the formation of the free radical nitric oxide (NO•), an important signaling agent that reacts with superoxide anion (•O$_2^-$) to generate peroxynitrite.[81-83]

Redox cycling refers to a pathway whereby a compound undergoes a series of cyclic 1-electron reductions and oxidations with concomitant generation of toxic oxygen species. A variety of flavoproteins catalyze 1-electron reductions. In the presence of oxygen, the reduced product can spontaneously oxidize back to the parent compounds, and this oxidation is coupled to the reduction of molecular oxygen to the superoxide radical ion •O$_2^-$ (**Fig. 25-7**). Many redox cycling agents cause toxicity to hepatocytes in vitro, but also usually cause toxicity to other organ systems when administered in vivo. Examples are the lung injury associated with paraquat[84] and the cardiotoxicity caused by adriamycin.[62] This probably reflects a relative resistance of liver parenchyma, attributable to the large capacity of the liver to detoxify reactive oxygen species.

Menadione (2-methyl-l,4-naphthoquinone; vitamin K_3) is a therapeutic quinone compound that can cause liver injury attributable to redox cycling. Menadione undergoes 1-electron reduction to the semiquinone free radical, which is catalyzed by many flavoenzymes, including NADPH:cytochrome P450 reductase.[76] In hepatocytes and other cells, it can also undergo a 2-electron reduction to the hydroquinone in a reaction catalyzed by NADPH:quinone reductase, a cytosolic enzyme also known as DT-diaphorase (see **Fig. 25-7**). This 2-electron reduction provides a detoxification reaction because the hydroquinone can be conjugated by sulfotransferases or uridine diphosphoglucuronic acid glucuronosyltransferases (UDPGT). DT-diaphorase knockout mice are more sensitive to the hepatotoxicity of menadione.[85]

The oxidative stress caused by redox cycling of menadione leads to irreversible cell injury via a complex interplay between oxidation of soluble thiols (e.g., GSH) and that of protein thiols, causing a sustained rise in Ca^{2+} concentration that is critical to the activation of mitochondria-mediated apoptosis. Oxidation of critical protein thiols decreases microsomal Ca^{2+} sequestering capacity[28,29] and plasma membrane extrusion of Ca^{2+} from cells.[27] Oxidation of soluble thiols precedes this and is a contributing factor in inhibition of the microsomal Ca^{2+} pump because GSH keeps the protein thiols in a reduced and functional form. In the presence of elevated Ca^{2+} concentration mitochondria load Ca^{2+}, and this loading sets conditions appropriate for activation of the mitochondrial membrane permeability transition (MMPT).[86]

The GSH system is complemented by thioredoxin-dependent antioxidant proteins termed peroxiredoxins.[87] Thioredoxin 1 is present in the nucleus and cytoplasm and serves to support peroxide elimination by peroxiredoxins 1 and 2. Thioredoxin 2 is present in the mitochondria and supports peroxide metabolism by peroxiredoxins 3 and 5. These systems are very active, and some estimates indicate that a majority of peroxide may be eliminated by peroxiredoxins rather than by GSH peroxidases.[88] Thioredoxins also bind to apoptosis-regulating kinase-1 (Ask-1), inhibiting activity. When thioredoxin becomes oxidized, Ask-1 is released and signals apoptosis.[89] In this way, toxicants that cause oxidation of either mitochondrial or cytoplasmic thioredoxin can activate cell death without causing macromolecular damage.

The MMPT occurs in response to the opening of a high-conductance channel in the mitochondrial inner membrane.[86] Ordinarily, the inner membrane is highly impermeable to solutes. However, in the presence of matrix Ca^{2+}, certain agents trigger the opening of the high-conductance MMPT pore. The prevailing interpretation is that the pore is a protein complex containing adenine nucleotide translocase (ANT, inner membrane), voltage-dependent anion channel (VDAC, outer membrane), cyclophilin D (associated with ANT), and peripheral benzodiazepine receptor (associated with VDAC). Sensitivity to oxidants and thiol reagents, especially arsenicals, indicates that the pore contains thiols, probably vicinal thiols, which control opening. Thus, in the presence of elevated Ca^{2+} levels, oxidants trigger opening of the MMPT pore, with resulting swelling and release of cytochrome c[90] and other pro-apoptotic components.[69,91,92] Cytochrome c binds to APAF-1, an assembly protein that allows the recruitment and activation successively of procaspase-9 and procaspase-3 (see **Fig. 25-3**).[18]

Lipid peroxidation can occur as a consequence of activation of any of the aforementioned free radical processes. Lipid peroxidation decreases membrane fluidity and is associated with inactivation of membrane-bound receptors and enzymes, increased permeability of membranes, and generation of toxic degradation products of lipid peroxidation.[78,93] GSH plays a central role in protection against lipid peroxidation through enzyme-catalyzed reactions and through nonenzymatic reduction of other antioxidants (vitamins C and E). GSH is required for degradation of lipid hydroperoxides and other hydroperoxides in reactions catalyzed by the selenium-dependent GSH peroxidase. For this reduction, the fatty acid hydroperoxides must be released first from the bulk lipid by the action of phospholipase A_2.[94,95] However, a separate selenium-dependent phospholipid hydroperoxide GSH peroxidase that directly detoxifies phospholipid hydroperoxides without a requirement for phospholipase A_2 has been characterized.[96,97] A selenium-independent GSH peroxidase, which has been ascribed to GSH S-transferases of the α class,[98] also detoxifies lipid hydroperoxides; like the selenium-dependent GSH peroxidase, it requires release of the fatty acid peroxide from the membrane. The selenium-independent form also is active in detoxification of cumene hydroperoxide and nucleic acid hydroperoxides.[99] GSH also detoxifies toxic degradation products of lipid hydroperoxides, most notably the 4-hydroxyalkenals (e.g., 4-hydroxynonenal) via S-conjugation. 4-Hydroxynonenal is an extremely toxic product of lipid peroxidation, with submicromolar concentrations causing genotoxic lesions to cultured rat hepatocytes.[100] Its conjugation with GSH is catalyzed by a specific form of glutathione S-transferase,[101,102] suggesting that this reaction may be fundamentally important in the prevention of free radical–mediated liver injury.

Clinicopathologic Patterns of Drug-Induced Liver Injury

Drugs and foreign chemicals produce manifold and varied damage and changes to the liver. Although not absolute, drugs typically produce patterns of injury that are characteristic for each individual drug. It is been found useful to categorize these patterns as hepatocellular (or hepatitic), cholestatic, mixed, or steatotic. Some key features of these four patterns are summarized in **Table 25-3**.

Hepatocellular (Hepatitic) Pattern of Injury

The majority of drugs that cause DILI produce principally a pattern of hepatocellular type injury.[1,50,103-109] Most of these instances are asymptomatic and mild. When they are unusually severe, patients typically develop symptoms similar to those manifested in acute viral hepatitis—fatigue, loss of appetite (especially for smoking), and nausea. Patients with very severe cases may suffer from vomiting, which can be intractable, and hypersomnia; usually a complaint of abdominal pain, primarily in the epigastrium and right upper quadrant, is given.

Table 25-3 Clinicopathologic Patterns of Drug-Induced Liver Injury

	PATTERNS OF INJURY			STEATOSIS	
FEATURES	**Hepatocellular (Hepatitic)**	**Cholestatic**	**Mixed**	**Microvesicular**	**Mixed Micro-/Macrovesicular**
Typical clinical presentation	Nausea, anorexia (vomiting) Loss of taste for food, smoking Upper abdominal pain	Jaundice; pruritus; nausea, anorexia, when very severe	Jaundice; pruritus; nausea, anorexia, when very severe	Nausea, anorexia Vomiting Confusion Somnolence (hepatic encephalopathy)	Asymptomatic Upper abdominal discomfort, heaviness Nausea, anorexia
Typical laboratory findings	Serum ALT, AST > 5 × ULN Serum AP < 2 × ULN Serum TBR, DBR variable May resemble acute ischemic or viral hepatitis	Serum ALT, AST < 5 × ULN Serum AP > 2 × ULN Serum TBR, DBR > 2 × ULN (often >5 × ULN) Resembles biliary obstruction or cholestatic phase of acute hepatitis A	Serum ALT, AST > 3 × ULN Serum AP > 2 × ULN Serum TBR, DBR > 2 × ULN Features of both hepatocellular and cholestatic patterns	Serum ALT, AST 5-25 × ULN Serum AP 1-3 × ULN Serum TBR, DBR variable, often normal Resembles acute viral hepatitis	Serum ALT, AST 1-5 × ULN Serum AP 1-3 × ULN Serum TBR, DBR variable, usually normal Resembles alcoholic hepatitis
Value of *R*	>5	<2	2-5	>5	2-5
Typical hepatobiliary-pancreatic imaging findings	Normal liver or diffuse, homogeneous hepatomegaly, perhaps with changes compatible with diffuse fatty change or phospholipidosis No biliary dilation Pancreatic swelling may be present	Normal liver or diffuse, homogeneous hepatomegaly No biliary dilation No pancreatic abnormalities No changes to suggest chronic liver disease or cholecystitis	Normal liver or diffuse, homogeneous hepatomegaly No biliary dilation No pancreatic abnormalities No changes to suggest chronic liver disease or cholecystitis	Normal liver No biliary dilation Normal pancreas Normal spleen No PHT No changes to suggest chronic liver disease or cholecystitis	Diffuse, generalized hepatomegaly Increased echogenicity (US) Decreased attenuation (CT) No biliary dilatation Normal or "fatty" pancreas No changes to suggest chronic liver disease or cholecystitis
Major considerations for differential diagnosis	Acute viral hepatitis Ischemic hepatitis Acute congestive hepatitis Budd-Chiari syndrome Hepatic decompensation due to Wilson disease Autoimmune hepatitis	Biliary obstruction due to gallstones, tumors, strictures, pancreatic diseases Primary biliary cirrhosis Primary sclerosing cholangitis "Overlap" syndromes of autoimmune cholangitis/ hepatitis	Biliary obstruction due to gallstones, tumors, strictures, pancreatic diseases Primary biliary cirrhosis Primary sclerosing cholangitis "Overlap" syndromes of autoimmune cholangitis/ hepatitis	Reye's syndrome Acute fatty liver of pregnancy Inborn or other acquired defects in mitochondrial function—fatty acid oxidation and/or ATP production	Alcoholic liver disease Liver disease associated with metabolic syndrome: NAFL, NASH Inborn or other acquired defects in normal hepatic lipid metabolism

Continued

Table 25-3 Clinicopathologic Patterns of Drug-Induced Liver Injury—cont'd

	PATTERNS OF INJURY			STEATOSIS	
FEATURES	Hepatocellular (Hepatitic)	Cholestatic	Mixed	Microvesicular	Mixed Micro-/Macrovesicular
Typical findings on liver biopsy	Acute zone 3 necrosis Findings indistinguishable from acute viral hepatitis Increased eosinophils and/or acute granulomas may be present Fat (usually mainly in zone 3) may be present; steatohepatitis may be present	Cholestasis without acute cholangitis or pericholangitis Zone 3 hepatocytic swelling No bile lakes or other features typical of extrahepatic obstruction	Cholestasis without acute cholangitis or pericholangitis Zone 3 hepatocytic swelling No bile lakes or other features typical of extrahepatic obstruction Acute zone 3 necrosis Findings indistinguishable from acute viral hepatitis Increased eosinophils and/or acute granulomas may be present Fat (usually mainly in zone 3) may be present; steatohepatitis may be present	Hepatocytic "swelling" with foamy appearance of cytoplasm and centrally located nuclei Apoptotic bodies—hepatocyte dropout with minimal inflammation No or minimal fibrosis	Variable amounts of neutral fat accumulation in hepatocytes, usually mainly in zones 3 and 2 Hepatocyte nuclei pushed to periphery of cells by macrovesicular steatosis Apoptotic bodies, hepatocyte dropout Variable inflammation Variable fibrosis, usually pericellular Lipogranulomas common in zone 3
Typical course after inciting agent stopped	Rapid improvement in symptoms, signs, and lab tests, with >50% decreases within 8-30 days	Protracted course with symptoms, signs, and labs worsening or remaining for 30-60 days Gradual improvement thereafter, but may require >180 days to resolve	Variable course Usually more protracted than hepatocellular, but less than cholestatic	Rapid improvement in symptoms, signs, and labs with >50% decreases within 8-30 days	Variable, depending upon drug accumulation, half-life Often, underlying alcohol or metabolic syndrome effects persist
Usual therapy	Stop offending drug N-Acetylcysteine for acetaminophen; prednisolone 20-30 mg/d, azathioprine 1-2 mg/kg/d for severe immunoallergic disease	Stop offending drug Ursodeoxycholic acid 20-30 mg/kg/d Cholestyramine, phenobarbital (rifampicin) for severe pruritus	Stop offending drug Prednisolone 20-30 mg/d, azathioprine 1-2 mg/kg/d for severe immunoallergic disease Ursodeoxycholic acid 20-30 mg/kg/d Cholestyramine, phenobarbital (rifampicin) for severe pruritus	Stop offending drug Supportive care, nutrition Urgent liver transplant for severe disease with grade 3-4 encephalopathy	Stop offending drug Supportive care, nutrition Consider prednisone 20-40 mg/d, pentoxifylline 400 mg tid for severe disease (DF > 32 or renal insufficiency)
Course and long-term prognosis	Follow "Hy's rule": ≈10% develop jaundice ≈10% of those who develop jaundice die If FHF develops, case-fatality rate for non-acetaminophen cases is ≈75% For acetaminophen cases is ≈25% A minority (perhaps ≈15-30%) with smoldering presentations may develop bridging fibrosis or cirrhosis Triggering of ongoing AI hepatitis by drugs is very rare (<0.5%)	Protracted cholestatic syndrome lasting weeks to months Severity often increases even after offending drug has been stopped Great majority of patients recover, apparently nearly completely (although few follow-up biopsies are done) Small minority (perhaps ≈1%) develop vanishing bile duct syndrome or course that resembles sclerosing cholangitis or biliary cirrhosis	A mixture of prognoses listed for cholestatic	Full recovery No progression to chronic liver disease	Variable, depending upon underlying conditions and duration and nature of prior injury

AI, autoimmune; ALT, alanine aminotransferase; AP, alkaline phosphatase; AST, aspartate aminotransferase; DBR, direct-reacting bilirubin; FHF, fulminant hepatic failure; R, ratio of serum ALT/ULN for ALT to serum AP/ULN for AP; TBR, total bilirubin; ULN, upper limit of normal

The laboratory features of this type of injury typically include a normal complete blood count, although a mild increase in white blood cell count may occur, and a minority of patients with immunoallergic-type reactions will show peripheral eosinophilia. Because the underlying pathogenesis involves primarily apoptosis and/or necrosis of hepatocytes, serum alanine aminotransferase (ALT) and aspartate aminotransferase (AST) levels are markedly elevated. In the case of acute poisoning with intrinsic hepatotoxins, such as acetaminophen, carbon tetrachloride, or other halogenated hydrocarbons, the elevations in levels of serum aminotransferases may be extreme (more than 100 times the upper limit of normal [ULN]). For the larger number of drugs that produce idiosyncratic, unpredictable, non–dose-dependent DILI, the degree of elevation of serum ALT and AST levels generally is less marked (10 to 25 times the ULN). The serum alkaline phosphatase (AP) level is generally normal or mildly elevated (less than twice the ULN). Serum total and direct bilirubin levels are variable. They may remain normal, although with the more severe forms of injury they are invariably increased. The degree of increase in serum bilirubin level may be extreme, and it is one of the negative prognostic factors for hepatocellular type injury. R is defined as the ratio of serum ALT/ULN of ALT divided by serum AP/ULN of AP, with ALT and AP concentrations in units per liter. In hepatocellular DILI, R is >5, by definition.

Hepatobiliary-pancreatic imaging in such injury shows a normal liver or diffuse homogeneous hepatomegaly. For some drugs, changes compatible with diffuse fatty change (**Table 25-4**), Mallory-Denk bodies (**Table 25-5**), or phospholipidosis (**Table 25-6**) may be present. Of particular importance, especially when patients are jaundiced, is the lack of evidence of dilatation of the biliary tree or cholecystitis. Of course, preexisting gallstones may be present, making it somewhat more difficult to arrive at a correct diagnosis. Some drugs, such as acetaminophen, can also cause acute pancreatic, myocardial, or renal injury. If pancreatitis occurs, the pancreas on imaging studies generally shows diffuse enlargement or edema. Typically, changes suggestive of chronic underlying liver disease are absent, although there is nothing about preexisting liver disease that prevents patients from developing DILI. Therefore such changes may be present.

The major considerations for the differential diagnosis of acute hepatocellular injury attributable to drugs include acute ischemic liver injury; acute viral hepatitis, which may be due to any of the agents that are capable of causing this syndrome (see Chapters 29 to 34); acute congestive hepatitis, including Budd-Chiari syndrome; autoimmune hepatitis; or hepatic decompensation caused by Wilson disease.

When liver biopsy is performed on patients with acute hepatocellular injury caused by drugs, typical findings are variable and highly dependent upon the offending agent. The most common hepatotoxic drug (namely, acetaminophen) causes acute necrosis first and foremost in zone 3 of the hepatic acinus. When very severe, necrosis extends into and through zone 2 as well (see **Fig. 25-5**).

Other common histologic findings include variable inflammation of the portal tracts, often with a considerable number of polymorphonuclear or eosinophilic forms. Acute granulomas may also occur. Indeed, drug-induced liver injury is one of the common causes of granulomas in the liver.[110-112] Some drugs and chemicals are well-known to produce fatty change in the liver. Usually this is primarily in zone 3, although it is certainly not restricted to this zone. All of the features of steatohepatitis may sometimes be present.

In most instances of hepatocellular injury, particularly when it has been sudden and acute in onset, there is a rapid improvement in symptoms, signs, and laboratory features when the offending agent is discontinued. This does not always occur, however, and in rare individuals drugs appear to be capable of triggering the development of self-perpetuating autoimmune hepatitis.[109,113]

Table 25-5 Some Drugs and Chemicals that May Produce Mallory-Denk Bodies

Amiodarone	Glucocorticoids
Diethylstilbestrol	Griseofulvin
4,4′-Diethylaminoethoxyhexestrol	Nifedipine
Ethanol	Tamoxifen

Table 25-4 Some Drugs and Chemicals that Produce Hepatic Steatosis

MICROVESICULAR	MACROVESICULAR OR MIXED MICRO-/ MACROVESICULAR
Aflatoxin β_1	Fialuridine [FIAU]
Amiodarone	Halothane
L-Asparaginase	Methotrexate
Aspirin	Minocycline
Chloroform	Mitomycin
Cocaine	Tamoxifen
Coumadin	Tetraethylene, trichloroethylene
Deferoxamine	Tetracyclines
Didanosine	Valproic acid
Ethanol	

Table 25-6 Some Drugs that Produce Phospholipidosis

All amphiphilic drugs	Gentamicin
Amantadine	Imipramine
Amikacin	Iprindole
Amiodarone	Ketoconazole
Amitriptyline	Mepacrine
Chloramphenicol	Promethazine
Chlorcyclizine	Propranolol
Chloripramine	Sulfamethoxazole-trimethoprim
Chloroquine	Thioridazine
Chlorpheniramine	Trimipramine
Chlorpromazine	Tripelennamine
Desipramine	

The short-term and long-term prognosis of hepatocellular type injury follows "Hy's rule." This was popularized by Hyman Zimmerman, a clinical hepatologist with special interest in drug-induced liver injury.[103] Hy's rule states that about 10% of patients with drug-induced liver injury of the hepatocellular type develop jaundice and that among those who develop jaundice, approximately 10% will die of drug-induced liver injury. Several recent reports have confirmed the accuracy of Hy's rule.[104-108] The case fatality rate for persons who develop fulminant hepatic failure attributable to drugs is very high (around 75%) for drugs other than acetaminophen. In contrast, the case fatality rate for acetaminophen-induced fulminant hepatic failure is much lower, with only about 25% of patients dying and/or requiring liver transplant.

For the most part there is no specific therapy for drug-induced liver injury beyond identifying the offending agent and discontinuing its use. It is clear that acute acetaminophen overdose should be treated immediately with *N*-acetylcysteine. For adults with acetaminophen ingestion less than 24 hours before presentation, an *N*-acetylcysteine loading dose of 140 mg/kg/body weight should be given, followed by 70 mg/kg every 4 hours for 17 doses, starting 4 hours after the loading dose. It has been suggested that *N*-acetylcysteine may be of benefit in other forms of fulminant hepatic failure, and indeed there seems little to be lost by administering it in other forms of acute hepatitic failure.

Particularly when hepatocellular type injury is severe, and/or when it is accompanied by evidence of immunoallergic features, a corticosteroid, such as prednisolone (20 to 30 mg/day), and azathioprine (1 to 2 mg/kg body weight per day) often are administered as well.

Cholestatic Pattern of Injury

The typical presentation of cholestatic hepatitis attributable to drugs is jaundice and pruritus. Nausea, anorexia, or vomiting typically occurs only when the reaction is very severe. The typical laboratory features are those of any cholestatic syndrome, with elevations primarily in serum AP level, which is more than twice the ULN, and serum total and direct bilirubin levels, which also are at least twice the ULN. In the pure cholestatic case, levels of serum aminotransferases are normal or only mildly elevated, and certainly less than three times the ULN. *R* is <2.

The typical hepatobiliary-pancreatic imaging findings in cholestatic DILI are primarily important because they show no evidence of biliary dilatation and no pancreatic abnormalities. The liver is usually normal or nearly normal, and there is nothing to suggest chronic liver disease or cholecystitis (see **Table 25-3**).

The major differential diagnosis for cholestatic DILI includes biliary obstruction (resulting from gallstones, tumors, strictures, or pancreatic diseases) and autoimmune disorders that affect chiefly the bile ducts, such as primary biliary cirrhosis or primary sclerosing cholangitis. There are also "overlap" syndromes of autoimmune cholangitis and autoimmune hepatitis. These are considered in greater detail in Section VI (Immune Diseases of the Liver).

Typical findings on liver biopsy in cholestatic DILI are the presence of bile in hepatocytes, bile plugs in canaliculi, and hepatocyte swelling in zone 3 (**Fig. 25-8**). Bile lakes or other

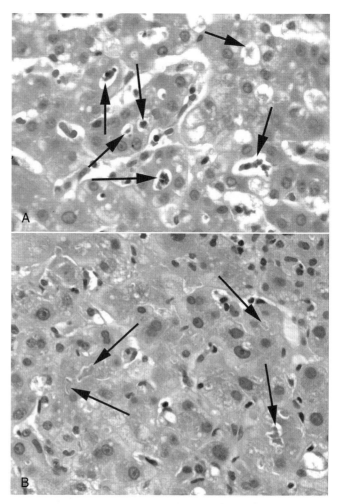

Fig. 25-8 A, Cholestatic injury. This biopsy, from a patient who became jaundiced while taking the NSAID nabumetone, shows relatively "bland" cholestasis with numerous canalicular bile plugs *(arrows)* but relatively little hepatocellular injury. The peak serum bilirubin level in the patient was 110 mg/dl. **B,** Cholestatic injury. This biopsy, from a patient who became jaundiced after a course of amoxicillin, shows a combined hepatocellular and cholestatic injury with canalicular bile plugs *(arrows)* as well as hepatocyte injury, apoptosis, and dropout with Kupffer cell hypertrophy and lymphocytic inflammation, producing disarray of the liver cell plates.

features of extrahepatic obstruction are absent, and as a rule there are no findings of acute cholangitis or pericholangitis, such as one would expect to see in bacterial ascending cholangitis.

The typical course of cholestatic hepatitis is quite different from that of hepatocellular DILI in being more protracted. In fact, it is not uncommon for signs and laboratory worsening to continue after the offending drug has been discontinued, sometimes for as long as 30 to 180 days. There is gradual improvement thereafter, unless the offending agent or another like it is readministered. There are rare instances in which the disease does not resolve but instead evolves to produce the adult vanishing bile duct syndrome, sometimes with progression to secondary biliary cirrhosis.[112]

The usual therapy for cholestatic DILI is to stop the offending drug and administer ursodeoxycholic acid. It is our recommendation that ursodeoxycholic acid be given at a dosage of 20 to 30 mg/kg/day in two divided doses. If pruritus is severe the usual treatment is cholestyramine; however, this must be given at times other than when ursodeoxycholic acid or other drugs are administered, because it will bind the drugs and prevent their absorption. We generally recommend that the cholestyramine be administered in the morning, when there is maximal turnover of the biliary pool. Other helpful measures to control pruritus include plasmapheresis and administration of phenobarbital, rifampicin, or naltrexone, although all of these drugs, especially rifampicin, may also cause hepatotoxicity on their own.

"Mixed" Pattern of Injury

This pattern, as the name implies, involves features of both hepatocellular and cholestatic injury (see **Table 25-3**). The typical clinical presentation is nausea, anorexia, and vomiting when severe. Jaundice and pruritus may also be present.

The typical laboratory findings are for serum aminotransferase levels to be greater than three times the ULN and for serum AP and total and direct bilirubin levels to be more than twice the ULN. The biopsy features are also a mixture of the features described previously for the other two types of injury. R is between 2 and 5.

The considerations for differential diagnosis must include ischemic hepatitis, acute congestive hepatitis, acute viral hepatitis, autoimmune hepatitis, or overlap syndromes of autoimmune cholangitis and hepatitis; hepatic decompensation caused by Wilson disease, primary biliary cirrhosis, primary sclerosing cholangitis, and biliary obstruction attributable to gallstones, tumors, strictures, or primary pancreatic diseases should also be included in the differential diagnosis.

The typical treatments are the same as those already described for hepatocellular and cholestatic injuries. The typical course is somewhat longer than for hepatocellular injury, but somewhat shorter than for typical cases of pure cholestatic DILI.

Steatotic (Fatty Liver) Pattern of Injury

As shown in **Table 25-3**, there are two major types of disease that produce primarily fatty change in the liver: microvesicular steatosis results in changes in pure small-droplet fat particles whereas macrovesicular steatosis is associated with alterations in fewer large-droplet fat molecules. Typically, however, macrovesicular steatosis is present with at least a mild degree of microvesicular steatosis.

Microvesicular steatosis is due principally to mitochondrial toxicity, leading both to a deficiency in mitochondrial β-oxidation of free fatty acids and to critical compromise of mitochondrial ATP production. Patients with these defects commonly present with nausea, anorexia, vomiting, confusion, or coma, the latter attributable to hepatic encephalopathy with prominent and severe hyperammonemia. They often have significant lactic acidosis because of the critical defect in mitochondrial respiration and oxidative phosphorylation. The typical laboratory features are moderate to marked increases in levels of serum aminotransferases; serum AP level

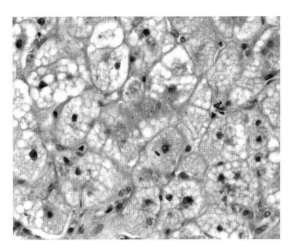

Fig. 25-9 **Microvesicular steatosis in a child taking valproic acid.** Most of the hepatocytes have small vacuoles of fat, and liver cell dropout with Kupffer cell hypertrophy and a mild lymphocytic infiltrate are visible.

is normal or only slightly increased, and serum bilirubin levels are variable, depending on the severity of the injury. R is >5.

Typical hepatobiliary-pancreatic imaging studies in patients with microvesicular steatosis show a normal liver, pancreas, and spleen as well as the absence of biliary dilatation or any imaging findings to suggest portal hypertension or chronic liver disease. The major differential diagnosis is Reye's syndrome or inborn or other acquired defects in mitochondrial function, particularly fatty acid metabolism or ATP production.

The findings on liver biopsy are remarkably mild (**Fig. 25-9**). To clearly visualize the lipid, it may be necessary to perform oil red O staining on frozen sections. The reason is that there is diffuse lipid accumulation in very small droplets, often smaller than the limit of resolution by light microscopy. There is no displacement of hepatocytic nuclei, such that the lipid may not be apparent in formalin-fixed tissue stained in the routine way. There is minimal inflammation, although apoptotic bodies and evidence of hepatocytic dropout may be present, and there is usually no fibrosis.

The usual course is one of rapid improvement if the inciting agent is discontinued. However, some patients have such severe defects that they may be unable to recover unless they receive urgent liver transplantation. Certainly, all such patients who might be transplant candidates and who develop higher grades of hepatic encephalopathy should rapidly be transferred to a transplant center. If patients can be nursed successfully through the acute phase of disease, complete recovery with no progression to chronic liver disease will ensue. Examples of drugs that produce microvesicular steatosis are summarized in **Table 25-4**.

Macrovesicular or Mixed Microvesicular and Macrovesicular Steatosis

The accumulation of fat is probably the most common liver abnormality. Potential causes of fatty liver are manifold and discussed in greater detail in Chapter 53. Drugs and chemicals

Table 25-7 Some Drugs and Chemicals that May Produce Peliosis Hepatis

Anabolic steroids	Glucocorticoids
Arsenic	Medroxyprogesterone
Azathioprine	Tamoxifen
Contraceptive steroids	Thioguanine
Danazol	Thorotrast
Diethylstilbestrol	Vinyl chloride
Estrone	Vitamin A excess

are among the important causes of fatty liver. Indeed, if one considers ethanol as a drug, they are probably the most common causes. Most people with fatty liver attributable to alcohol or other conditions that produce macrovesicular steatosis are asymptomatic. When the fatty deposition is severe, hepatomegaly ensues, and patients may have upper abdominal discomfort and a sense of heaviness. It is rare for more severe symptoms, such as nausea, anorexia, vomiting, or jaundice, to occur. Laboratory studies may be entirely normal or may show mild increases in levels of serum aminotransferases. Although serum AP levels may be slightly increased, γ-glutamyltranspeptidase levels are usually more elevated. Typical findings on hepatobiliary-pancreatic imaging are diffuse, generalized hepatomegaly. Ultrasound shows evidence of increased echogenicity, whereas CT scanning shows a decrease in hepatic attenuation. There is generally no biliary dilatation and the pancreas appears normal or may show increased echogenicity indicative of a fatty deposition in the pancreas.

In addition to heavy alcohol use, macrovesicular steatosis is commonly caused by liver disease associated with metabolic syndrome (nonalcoholic fatty liver and nonalcoholic steatohepatitis; see Chapter 53). The typical findings on liver biopsy in patients with drug-induced macrovesicular steatosis are indistinguishable from those caused by alcohol or by nonalcoholic fatty liver. It is common for patients to have these changes because of an element of alcohol and nonalcoholic fatty liver plus one or more drugs. Mallory-Denk bodies may develop as a result of alcoholic or nonalcoholic steatohepatitis, and have been associated with several drugs (see Table 25-5). The usual therapy is to stop the offending drug. However, if the fatty change is mild and asymptomatic and if the drug is essential for other reasons, such as methotrexate for the management of rheumatoid arthritis or psoriasis, the decision may be made to continue the drug with careful monitoring. In addition to the histopathologic features already described, drugs can cause the accumulation of phospholipids in hepatocytes and other cells (see Table 25-6), vascular lesions in the liver (including peliosis hepatis) (Table 25-7), sinusoidal obstruction or venoocclusive disease, and arterial vascular compromise, which is manifest as a syndrome that resembles sclerosing cholangitis.

Predictable versus Unpredictable DILI

Another useful way to categorize DILI is as predictable or "intrinsic" injury versus unpredictable or "idiosyncratic." By far the most important example of the former is acetaminophen, which, by mechanisms already described, will produce liver injury in virtually everyone who takes a sufficient dose. Examples of other drugs or toxins that act similarly are listed in **Table 25-8**.

Most drugs, however, cause DILI unpredictably and in only a small percentage of subjects. Such reactions are called idiosyncratic reactions and are further subdivided according to the accompanying presence or absence of immunoallergic manifestations. Such manifestations include symptoms such as fever, peripheral eosinophilia, skin rash, arthralgia, and arthritis. As shown in **Table 25-8**, many drugs are recognized as capable of causing idiosyncratic DILI either with or without an immunoallergic phenotype, stressing the importance of genetic host factors in modulating the response to injury (see **Fig. 25-2**).

The mechanisms that probably lead to immunoallergic injury are summarized in **Figure 25-10**. According to this figure, drugs may produce antigens by binding to host proteins (perhaps altering them), which are recognized as foreign and against which the host's immune system mounts a T- or B-lymphocyte response. Because such neoantigens are displayed on hepatocytes, where most drug metabolism occurs, the net effect may resemble autoimmune hepatitis. Indeed, ingestion of drugs appears to trigger autoimmune hepatitis in rare individuals.[109,113] The importance of host immune responses in pathogenesis of DILI is emphasized by the fact that nearly all genetic associations with risks of DILI thus far identified, mostly from genomewide or candidate-gene association studies, have been to HLA alleles (**Table 25-9**). In several cases (amoxicillin/clavulanic acid, carbamazepine, flucloxacillin) the causative drugs result in immunoallergic disease, whereas in others (isoniazid [INH], ximelagatran) they do not. This suggests that immune reactions are important in most cases of clinically important DILI, even in the absence of classical immunoallergic features.

DILI Due to Specific Agents
Anesthetics

Of the agents currently in use to induce and maintain anesthesia, only the halogenated volatile agents have clinically significant hepatotoxicity. Beginning with halothane in the 1950s, the halogenated anesthetics replaced the routine use of ether and chloroform. Halothane, besides being nonflammable, had much better pharmacokinetics than ether, and had fewer respiratory and cardiac side effects than chloroform. However, postoperative liver injury was soon recognized, especially in patients reexposed to halothane,[103,128,129] and it was also an occupational hazard for those administering the anesthetic.[130] The development of other halogenated agents, such as enflurane, isoflurane, desflurane, and sevoflurane, was associated with less hepatotoxicity, most likely because these agents underwent less hepatic metabolism. However, all have been reported to cause liver injury,[131-134] and although sevoflurane may be the safest,[135] reports still appear of hepatotoxicity.[136] The incidence of hepatotoxic reactions after halothane administration has been estimated between 1:3,000 and 1:30,000.[137] The incidence after enflurane use has been estimated to be

Table 25-8 Classification of DILI: Comparison of Intrinsic (Predictable) vs. Idiosyncratic (Unpredictable) DILI

	TYPE OF DRUG-INDUCED LIVER INJURY		
		IDIOSYNCRATIC	
VARIABLE	**INTRINSIC**	**WITH IMMUNOALLERGIC FEATURES**	**WITHOUT IMMUNOALLERGIC FEATURES**
Predictability/ dose dependence	High/yes All subjects given high doses will develop hepatotoxicity Regularly produced in experimental animals	Low/slight or nil Most subjects will not develop hepatotoxicity, regardless of dose Not reproducible in experimental animals	Low/slight or nil Most subjects will not develop hepatotoxicity, regardless of dose Not reproducible in experimental animals
Associated features	Toxic damage to other tissues also occurs Drug-induced renal, pancreatic injury common	Fever, skin rash, peripheral adenopathy, eosinophilia Development of autoantibodies (ANA, ASMA), hyperglobulinemia	No extrahepatic manifestations of immunoallergic responses
Underlying risk factors	Induction (without inhibition) of enzymes that increase formation of toxic intermediates Conditions that decrease metabolism, detoxification, and removal of toxic intermediates	Allergic diathesis Other host genetic factors presumed to play a role such as presence of certain HLA types, factors that influence Th1 vs. Th2 phenotypes Women more susceptible than men (like most autoimmune diseases)	Other host genetic factors presumed to play a role, such as genetic variations that influence expression of phase I-II enzymes of drug metabolism Presence of underlying liver disease, especially chronic viral hepatitis in subjects receiving HAART and fatty liver in subjects receiving methotrexate or dugs implicated in producing steatohepatitis
Typical pattern of injury	Hepatocellular, acute	Hepatocellular, acute Less often, cholestatic or mixed	Hepatocellular, acute Less often, cholestatic or mixed
Response to rechallenge	Reproduced promptly and dependably	Very rapid recurrence (1-3 doses)	Variable—may be delayed for several weeks, usually more rapid than initial episode
Examples of inciting agents	Acetaminophen *Amanita* toxins Bromobenzene Carbon tetrachloride Chloroform Halothane White phosphorus	Amoxicillin/clavulanic acid α-Methyldopa Diclofenac Doxycycline Fenofibrate Halothane Hydralazines Minocycline Nitrofurantoin Penicillins Phenlbutazone Phenytoin Quinidine Statins (very rarely)	Amoxicillin/clavulanic acid Chlorpromazine (other phenothiazines) Enflurane Fluroxene Glitazones (rosi-, pio-, troglitazone) Isoniazid Nifedipine Penicillins Phenelzine Phenylbutazone Propylthiouracil Statins (rarely) Sulfonylureas Quinidine
Typical duration of exposure, before onset	Very brief (<1 week) (e.g., acetaminophen overdose in attempted suicide)	Brief (1-5 weeks) (e.g., development of allergic reaction to phenytoin)	Valproic acid Highly variable, depending upon poorly defined host susceptibility factors (1-100 weeks) (e.g., variable onset of glitazone-induced DILI)

approximately 1:800,000.[138] The newer agents have an even lower incidence.

Studies of pathogenesis support an immune mechanism for liver injury,[109,139] with identification of halothane metabolite–modified neoantigens in injured livers[140] and IgG antibodies to neoantigens in sera of patients.[141] CYP2E1 appears to be the cytochrome P450 responsible for the oxidative generation of the reactive metabolite.[142] When halothane, isoflurane, and sevoflurane were administered to dogs,[143] all caused elevations in aminotransferase levels postoperatively, but halothane caused toxicity much earlier and to a greater degree than the other agents.

The clinical features of halogenated anesthestic liver injury were reviewed both years ago[103,128,130] and more recently.[144,145] Most individuals had undergone anesthesia on multiple occasions and there can be cross-sensitization between agents. Nonspecific symptoms, including fever and malaise, occur days to weeks postoperatively and are followed by marked elevations of aminotransferase levels and then jaundice. Onset is variable, with jaundice occasionally taking more than 1

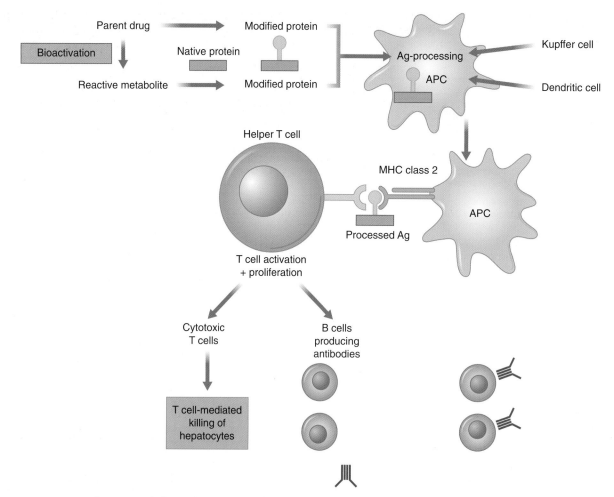

Fig. 25-10 Likely mechanisms for pathogenesis of drug-induced immunoallergic hepatitis.

month to develop. The usual histologic pattern of liver injury is centrilobular necrosis[146]; however, cholestatic features can also occur.[147] The most frequently affected patients are obese women between 40 and 60 years old. A small percentage of patients proceed to fatal fulminant liver failure, with some rescued by transplantation. However, complete resolution without residual liver dysfunction occurs in the majority of cases. Patients who have survived such reactions should not be reexposed to any halogenated anesthetics.

Anesthetic agents not reported to cause DILI include the barbiturates (thiopental [Pentothal], methohexital [Brevital]), ketamine (Ketalar), propofol (Diprivan), the opioids (alfentanil [Alfenta], fentanyl [Sublimaze], remifentanil [Ultiva], sufentanil [Sufenta]), etomidate (Amidate), dexmedetomidine (Precedex), and all the topical "-caines."

Anticonvulsants

Many anticonvulsants have potential hepatotoxic effects (**Table 25-10**), including agents that have been in use for decades (e.g., phenytoin, valproic acid, carbamazepine) as well as newer drugs such as felbamate and lamotrigine. Because of the clinical importance of seizure control, all of these agents remain in use despite their potential toxicities. Felbamate is considered an "adjunct" second-line agent, to be used only if

other agents are ineffective. Vigabatrin (i.e., vinyl-GABA) has restricted use in the U.S. market because it has caused visual field defects.[148,149] However, the drug may be useful for treating methamphetamine and cocaine addiction.[150] Many other anticonvulsant agents will probably become available in the future,[149] and careful postmarketing monitoring will be required to elucidate their toxicities.

Phenytoin has been known for decades to cause hepatotoxicity in association with hypersensitivity reactions.[151-153] The majority of patients taking phenytoin develop mild elevations of AP and gamma glutamyl transpeptidase (GGTP) levels within the first few months of therapy that normalize with continued use of the drug. These changes are part of hepatic adaptation and generally do not require cessation of therapy. It is the hypersensitivity reaction that is most worrisome.[154] The formation of the reactive arene oxide metabolite by CYP2C9, followed by formation of the o-quinone by CYPs 2C9, 2C19, and 3A4, leads to haptens and immune activation. The incidence of this idiosyncratic non–dose-related hepatotoxicity is estimated to be <1 : 10,000, and 56% of phenytoin hypersensitivity is associated with some hepatotoxicity.[154] Liver failure necessitating transplantation still occurs.[1]

The clinical symptoms usually manifest within 1 to 8 weeks of drug exposure and include fever, malaise, lymphadenopathy, splenomegaly, and rash. Serum aminotransferase levels

Table 25-9 Reported Genetic Associations with Risk of DILI

DRUG; REFERENCE	ALLELE	NO. OF CASES/ NO. OF CONTROLS	ALLELE FREQUENCY, CASES/ CONTROLS (%)	OR (95% CI)	COMMENT
HLA Genes					
Abacavir; 114, 115 Haplotype	DRB*5701 DRB*5701, DR7, DQ3	18/167 18/167	78/2 72/0	117 (29-481) 822 (43-15,675)	
Amoxicillin/ clavulanic acid; 116	DRB1*1501	35/60	57/12	N/A	
117	DRB1*1501	22/134	70/20	9.2 (N/A)	
118	DRB1*15	52/228	50/30	2.45 (1.37-4.8)	
119	DRB1*0602	27/635	74/41	4.14 (1.73-9.95)	Most significant association observed for haplotype A*201-B*0702-DRB1*1501-DQB1*0602 (OR's 13-20)
120	DQB1*0602	201/532	NR	2.8 (2.1-3.8)	
Flucloxacillin; 121	DRB1*5701	72/346	83/6.3	80.6 (22.8-285)	
INH; 122	DQB*0201 DRA*0103	56/290 56/290	52/23 6/39	2.1 (1.0-4.18) 0.2 (0.04-0.69)	Study among Asian Indians Protective allele
Lapatinib; 123	DQA1*0201	99/275	10/1.1	9.0 (2-53)	For ALT > 5 × ULN
Lumiracoxib; 124	DRB1*1501 (GWAS rs3129900)	139/581	41/10	6.3 (4.1-9.7)	Part of haplotype DRB1*1501-DQA1*0102-DQB1*0602-DRB5*0101 associated with amoxicillin/clavulanic acid DILI and multiple sclerosis
Ticlopidine; 124	A*3303 (Japanese)	22/85	68/14	13 (4.4-38.6)	
Ximelagatran; 125	DRB1*07 DQA1*02	74/130 74/130	26/8.5 26/8.5	4.41 (2.22-8.87) 4.41 (2.21-8.80)	
Non-HLA Genes					
INH; 126	CYP2E1 [c1/c1] (wild type) CYP2E1 [c1/c1] + NAT2 slow acetylator	21/318	20/9	2.52 (NR) 7.43 (NR)	
INH; 127	NAT2 slow acetylator	18/114	36.8/9.7	5.41 (1.76-16.59)	No association between CYP2E1 genotype and anti-Tb drug DILI

ALT, serum alanine aminotransferase; CI, confidence interval; HLA, human leukocyte antigen; NAT, N-acetyltransferase; NR, not reported; OR, odds ratio; ULN, upper limit of normal

are elevated 2- to 100-fold (ALT > AST) and AP levels 2- to 8-fold.[152,154,155] Leukocytosis and atypical lymphocytes suggesting mononucleosis and eosinophilia are common, with a lupus-like syndrome and pseudolymphoma reported occasionally. Other organ system toxicities can include interstitial nephritis, myositis and rhabdomyolysis, pneumonitis, and marrow suppression. The clinical presentation can also simulate viral hepatitis. When liver biopsies are performed, the histologic analysis shows a panlobular mixed mononuclear and polymorphonuclear infiltrate with prominent eosinophilia. In 10% of cases cholestasis is the predominant finding. The findings are not specific, however.

Therapy is discontinuation of the drug, which in most cases leads to resolution of toxicity. However, once liver failure develops, the case/fatality ratio can be as high as 40%. Because of cross-reactivity with carbamazepine and oxcarbazepine,[153,156] these latter agents should not be used to replace phenytoin for seizure control in patients who have

experienced symptomatic phenytoin toxicity. A phosphate ester prodrug of phenytoin, fosphenytoin, developed for parenteral administration[157] should also be avoided.

Carbamazepine, like phenytoin, can also cause asymptomatic mild elevations in serum GGTP (64%) and AP (14%) levels that do not require discontinuation of therapy.[154] However, increases in aminotransferase levels, seen in 22% of patients, may indicate susceptibility to develop the more serious idiosyncratic hypersensitivity reaction. A Swedish analysis[158] estimated the risk to be about 1 in 6000, which is more common than with phenytoin. The hypersensitivity reaction is also due to formation of a reactive metabolite, probably an unstable epoxide formed by CYP3A4.[159] Drug toxicity usually occurs within 8 to 16 weeks of therapy and presents with fever, rash, and peripheral eosinophilia. Marrow suppression, nephritis, and pneumonitis can also occur. Carbamazepine is more likely than phenytoin to cause a pure cholestatic pattern of hepatotoxicity, which occurs in 30% of

Table 25-10 Anticonvulsants and DILI

DRUG	COMMENTS
Reported to Cause DILI	
Phenytoin (Dilantin) Fosphenytoin (Cerebyx)	Immunoallergic; hepatitic > cholestatic
Valproic acid, divalproex sodium (Depakote)	Mitochondrial
Clonazepam (Klonopin)	Very rare idiosyncratic (one case report[174])
Carbamazepine (Tegretol, Carbatrol)	Idiosyncratic
Oxcarbazepine (Trileptal)	
Felbamate (Felbatol)	Hepatitic > cholestatic
Lamotrigine (Lamictal)	Cholestatic > hepatitic
Topiramate (Topamax)	
Levetiracetam (Keppra)	1 case fulminant failure
Zonisamide (Zonegran)	1 case vanishing bile ducts
Not Reported to Cause Hepatotoxicity	
Ethosuximide (Zarontin), phenobarbital,* primidone (Mysoline), tiagabine (Gabitril)	

*Phenobarbital activates the orphan nuclear receptor CAR and exerts well-known proliferative effects on hepatocytes.

reactions. A mixed pattern of liver injury with elevations in AP, bilirubin, and aminotransferase levels occurs in 50% of cases. A predominantly hepatocellular injury may have a worse prognosis.[154] Consistent with the cholestatic clinical picture, histopathologic study commonly demonstrates a granulomatous reaction with eosinophilia.[160] Resolution of injury takes several weeks after drug withdrawal. Because the injury is immune mediated, rechallenge is not recommended, and both phenytoin and oxcarbamazepine should also be avoided.[156,161] The keto analogue of carbamazepine, **oxcarbazepine,** was first introduced in 1990 in Denmark and has recently become available in most countries, including the United States. It is considered to be a safe and useful anticonvulsant[162] with fewer P450-related drug interactions than carbamazepine.[149] However, it has also been reported to cause acute liver failure as a result of hypersensitivity,[163] with a similar clinical presentation to that of carbamazepine and phenytoin.[161]

Valproic acid (VPA) may be the most widely prescribed anticonvulsant worldwide,[164] and in general is considered very safe, with the incidence of hepatotoxicity in adults and children older than 2 years being approximately 1 in 35,000.[165] However, in children younger than 2 years, especially those taking other anticonvulsants, the incidence may be as frequent as 1 in 600. It is also clear that patients with genetic mitochondrial enzyme defects are at greater risk,[166,166a] most likely because of valproate's depletion of coenzyme A levels and its metabolism via mitochondrial oxidation. Persons with the Alpers-Huttenlocher syndrome are at especially high risk, and this is related to mutations in the mitochondrial polymerase gamma gene.[166a] Hepatotoxicity usually occurs within the first 3 to 6 months of therapy,[154] although delays as long as 2788 days have been reported.[166a]

Valproate's hepatotoxicity is most likely dose related,[166] although epidemiologic studies have suggested that other host factors and polypharmacy may be more important.[165] Up to 40% of patients have transient, asymptomatic elevations in ALT concentration that improve with dose reduction.[154] High doses of drug, in addition to young age and polypharmacy, are significantly associated with higher excretion of thiol conjugates of the toxic valproate metabolite (E)-2,4-diene-VPA.[167] Therefore ALT monitoring is recommended for the first 6 months of therapy and after dose increases. Patients taking olanzepine in addition to valproate had higher ALT level elevations than with either drug alone.[168] Although no specific degree of ALT level elevation has been identified as an indicator of impending hepatic failure, a greater than three-fold elevation should prompt drug cessation. If fever, nausea, vomiting, and abdominal pain accompany laboratory evidence of developing hepatic failure and poor seizure control, then liver failure will probably become irreversible.

The characteristic histopathology of valproate hepatotoxicity is that of microvesicular steatosis, similar to Reye's syndrome, seen mainly in zones 2 and 3.[154] These changes may occur without toxicity. In one recent report 61% of patients receiving long-term valproate had sonographic evidence of fatty liver,[169] with the majority having normal concentrations of serum aminotransferases. Valproate therapy has also been reported to decrease serum albumin concentrations by up to 30% without apparent toxicity in a small study of children with severe neurologic disabilities.[170]

Because of the potential for valproate to damage mitochondrial function, L-carnitine was suggested as a protective agent[171] and may improve survival with severe valproate hepatotoxicity,[172] especially if administered intravenously. Oral supplementation of 100 mg/kg/day is recommended for infants and young children taking valproate, and for patients with symptomatic hyperammonemia or multiple risk factors for hepatotoxicity.[173] Prophylactic use of L-carnitine decreases the risk of valproate hepatotoxicity and is recommended.

Newer Anticonvulsants

Felbamate was approved for use in 1993; it was the first new anticonvulsant approved in the United States since the introduction of valproate in 1978. However, during its first year of use an incidence of hepatic failure of 1 in 6000 (and an aplastic anemia incidence of 1 in 3000) prompted restriction of its use to severe epilepsy not responding to other agents.[149] However, felbamate is still considered an important drug, with more than 8000 patients treated annually in the United States. By 1996, 36 cases of hepatotoxicity had been collected by the FDA, with 5 deaths.[175] However, since then no further cases of hepatotoxicity have been reported and it is considered very safe.[176] The mechanism of toxicity appears to involve the formation of an aldehyde monocarbamate[177] that is activated to atropaldehyde.[154,178,179] Because felbamate is usually given with other anticonvulsants and is a CYP3A4 substrate, studies of drug interactions have been carried out. A recent in vivo study[179] suggests that felbamate may heteroactivate CYP3A4 to promote the formation of carbamazepine-10,11-epoxide when these agents are used together. The paucity of reported cases makes it difficult to describe the clinical characteristics and histopathology of felbamate hepatotoxicity. However, presentation occurs between 3 weeks and 6 months of initiation of therapy, with a possible female preponderance.[154]

Clonazepam is listed in www.epocrates.com and www.pdr.net as having hepatotoxicity as a serious adverse event. However, only one case report could be found in the literature.[180]

Lamotrigine is a chlorinated phenyltriazine anticonvulsant that has been in use for more than a decade. The first case of fulminant hepatic failure attributable to its use was reported in 1995.[181] Another severe case of an 8-year-old boy who recovered was reported in 1998.[182] Despite more than 2 million prescriptions written,[149] only 9 cases of hepatotoxicity have been reported so far in the literature[183] and most of these were polytherapy patients. The most common adverse event of lamotrigine is a skin rash,[184,185] which occurs in 3% to 10% of patients[154] and can be severe. Whether the metabolism of lamotrigine to a reactive arene oxide[186] is responsible for both the cutaneous toxicity and the rare hepatotoxicity is not yet clear.

Topirimate, also marketed to prevent migraines, is related to carbonic anhydrase inhibitors and can cause metabolic acidosis. It has been considered very safe with few side effects (the majority involving the CNS), especially if started at low doses and increased slowly (<50 mg/week).[187] Only one case of acute liver failure necessitating a transplant has been reported, in a woman also taking carbamazepine.[188] Five additional cases of reversible hepatotoxicity in three children and two adults, all of whom were also taking valproate, have since been reported.[189-191]

Levetiracetam is minimally metabolized (only 34%)[192] with few long-term side effects[193]; however, it did appear to cause fulminant liver failure in an Australian patient, who required a transplant.[194] Unfortunately, inadvertent reexposure to the drug injured the new liver.

Zonisamide is hepatically metabolized, but has few drug interactions.[195] A case of vanishing bile duct syndrome has been reported.[196]

Psychotropic Drugs
Attention-Deficit/Hyperactivity Disorder

Methylphenidate is a commonly used and possibly overused stimulant agent that can cause liver test (LT) abnormalities, but has only been reported to cause hepatotoxicity with IV abuse in high doses.[197] It has also been reported to precipitate an autoimmune hepatitis.[198] However, these hepatic adverse events appear to be very rare.

Atomoxetine is a non–stimulant-selective norepinephrine reuptake inhibitor often used instead of methylphenidate because it is not a controlled substance. It is metabolized by CYP2D6 and has been reported to rarely cause serious hepatotoxicity in postmarketing surveillance.[199] CYP2D6 rapid metabolizers may have fewer ADRs.

Antipsychotics—First Generation

The phenothiazine neuroleptics, including **chlorpromazine, prochlorperazine, perphenazine,** and **thioridazine,** are well-known to cause both hepatocellular and cholestatic injury, most likely by immunoallergic mechanisms.[200] **Fluphenazine, thioproperazine,** and **trifluoperazine** appear to cause cholestasis only. In a pharmacovigilance study using a British database,[201] chlorpromazine was found to be the agent most often associated with drug-induced liver injury, with an adjusted odds ratio of 416. If serial LFTs are drawn, 42% of patents receiving chlorpromazine show abnormalities. The butyrophenone **haloperidol** can also rarely cause cholestasis, which is sometimes prolonged.

Antipsychotics—Second Generation

The second-generation antipsychotics have largely replaced the first-generation agents because of greater efficacy and fewer side effects, including less hepatotoxicity. However, **clozapine** commonly causes abnormal LT results, in up to 40% of patients,[202] but only two cases of fatal fulminant liver failure have been reported.[203] When clozapine was compared with **ziprasidone** in an 18-week study of 147 patients, no hepatotoxicity was found for either drug.[204] **Olanzapine,** which has become popular because it is well tolerated, causes transiently abnormal LT results in 10% of patients, and three cases of reversible hepatitis with jaundice have been reported.[205] However, in the last case report,[205] the patient had also been taking **risperidone,** for which there are numerous case reports of acute hepatitis from the 1990s.[200] Interestingly, the Epocrates database does not mention hepatotoxicity as an adverse event for risperidone. **Quetiapine** is listed as causing abnormal LT results, and there is one case report of cholestatic injury.[206] No reports of liver injury have yet been submitted for **aripiprazole, paliperidone, pimozide,** and **iloperidone.** Therefore although these agents all have numerous serious side effects, hepatotoxicity appears to be rare and monitoring of LT results has not been recommended for any of them.

Antidepressants

The *tricyclic antidepressants,* especially **amitriptyline** and **imipramine,** cause transient elevations in aminotransferase levels in up to 10% to 20% of patients, but only rarely cause fulminant hepatitis and prolonged cholestasis.[200] In fact, hepatitis is listed as a possible ADR in the Epocrates database for many tricyclic antidepressants, including **amoxapine, clomipramine, desipramine, doxepin, nortriptyline,** and **trimipramine.** The tricyclics are metabolized by CYP2D6 and toxicity is more common in 2D6-poor metabolizers. **Amineptine,** no longer marketed, could also be metabolized by CYP3A4 to reactive metabolites that were more likely to cause an immunoallergic reaction. It was shown that amitriptyline and its *N*-dealkylated metabolite, nortriptyline, can be bioactivated by CYPs 2D6 and 3A4 to an arene oxide intermediate.[207]

The *monoamine oxidase inhibitors* **phenelzine** and **tranylcypromine** are also listed as causing "hepatitis"; however, no case reports of significant liver injury were found. Phenelzine, in particular, is a potent inhibitor of hepatic P450s, especially CYPs 3A4 and 2C19.[208] **Iproniazid,** withdrawn from the U.S. market in 1956 due to hepatotoxicity, was associated with an antimitochondrial antibody against a different antigen than what is seen in primary biliary cirrhosis.[200]

Selective serotonin reuptake inhibitors (SSRIs) rarely cause liver injury and they are not mentioned in the Epocrates database. However, **paroxetine** has been reported to cause acute hepatitis in a small number of cases[209] and **fluoxetine, citalopram, escitalopram, fluvoxamine,** and **sertraline** have all had a few case reports of liver damage, with only 2 out of 30 being fatal.[209]

Two newer *serotonin and norepineprine reuptake inhibitors (SNRIs)*—**duloxetine** and **venlafaxine**—have been reported[209-211] to cause DILI. Although duloxetine was estimated to have a likelihood of producing severe hepatic injury in only 0.7/100,000,[212] in an analysis of 17,615 subjects, the incidence of serum ALT levels >5 × ULN was 500/100,000.[213] Postmarketing surveillance identified 406 cases of presumed DILI from duloxetine, of which 58 were judged to be clinically significant, with 2 fatalities: 1 in a woman also taking mirtazapine and the second in a man with chronic alcohol abuse.[212] This led to a warning in the package insert that duloxetine "should ordinarily not be prescribed to patients with substantial alcohol use or evidence of chronic liver disease." Seven additional cases of clinically important DILI attributable to duloxetine have been described from the U.S. Drug-Induced Liver Injury Network (DILIN) Registry. Five of the cases were hepatocellular; two were cholestatic, and three occurred in subjects with preexisting chronic liver disease. In two patients, acute renal failure also occurred. Venlafaxine was associated with fatal fulminant failure in two cases, although the first was an overdose[210] and the other case was in association with trazodone[211]—an "atypical" antidepressant with far more reported hepatotoxicity.[209]

The other *atypical antidepressants*, besides **trazodone,** include **bupropion** (also FDA approved for nicotine addiction), **mirtazapine,** and **nefazodone.** All of these drugs have hepatotoxicity listed in the Epocrates database. Nefazodone, a phenylpiperazine, appears to be more hepatotoxic than the rest[209] with an estimated incidence of liver failure 1:250,000 patient years of use and 5 of 10 reported cases requiring transplant or causing death. Trazodone, a chemical congener of nefazodone, also causes primarily a hepatocellular injury, but mixed-type and immunoallergic injuries can occur. Mirtazapine has not had any new reports of hepatotoxicity since the two cases in 2002, and it is therefore probably not very hepatotoxic.

Anxiolytic and Soporific Agents

The *anxiolytic benzodiazepines* have been in use since the 1950s and significant hepatotoxicity is rare. There is no liver toxicity listed in the Epocrates database for **alprazolam, midazolam, triazolam, lorazepam,** or **temazepam.** Diazepam, **chlordiazepoxide, flurazepam,** and **oxazepam** have all rarely been reported to cause various types of liver injury.[200] Although hepatotoxicity is listed as the first serious ADR in Epocrates for **clorazepate,** this appears to be based on only one 1979 case report. Similarly, **clonazepam** has hepatotoxicity listed as the second most serious ADR; however, this appears to be based on only one 1988 case report. In general, all benzodiazepines appear not to cause DILI. This is also the case for the *nonbenzodiazepine anxiolytics* **buspirone** and **hydroxyzine.**

Of the four agents used in the treatment of *insomnia*— **zaleplon, zolpidem, eszopiclone,** and **ramelteon**—there is only one case of hepatotoxicity reported in 1999 for zolpidem.[214]

Agents Used in the Treatment of Parkinson's Disease, Migraines, and Alzheimer's Disease

In 1998 **tolcapone,** a catechol-O-methyltransferase (COMT) inhibitor, was the first of its drug class to be approved for adjunctive therapy with levodopa in Parkinson's disease (**Table 25-11**).[215] Although no DILI was reported before its approval, subsequent clinical trials noted ALT level elevations more than three times normal in about 1% of patients receiving 100 mg/day tolcapone, and 3% of those patients taking 200 mg/day.[216] Three fatal cases of acute liver failure occurred in 1998 out of 60,000 patients administered the drug, which led to the drug's withdrawal in Europe and Canada, and restrictions on its use in the United States.[215,216] More than 90% of cases of serious toxicity occurred within 6 months of starting therapy. Tolcapone, but not the subsequently approved COMT inhibitor entacapone, was shown to uncouple oxidative phosphorylation in rat liver mitochondria.[217] Oxidative metabolism by CYPs 1A2 and 2E1 may activate a tolcapone amine or acetylamine metabolite to a reactive species.[218] In 2000 an expert panel suggested that tolcapone was safe to use with frequent ALT concentration monitoring during the first 6 months of therapy, and that the drug should be discontinued if the ALT level was two-fold to three-fold elevated;[219] this approach was reaffirmed more recently.[220]

Pergolide is a dopamine agonist approved for adjunctive treatment of Parkinson's disease, and is also useful in the

Table 25-11 Anti-Parkinson's, Antimigraine, Anti-Alzheimer's, Other Neurologic Drugs and DILI

DRUGS	COMMENTS
Reported to Cause DILI	
Tolcapone (Tasmar)	↑ALT, acute liver failure (4 cases)
Methazolamide	Only one 1981 case report
Pergolide (Permax)	"Hepatitis" in database, but no citations
Tacrine (Cognex)	↑ALT common and must discontinue or acute liver failure
Glatiramer (Copaxone)	"Hepatotoxicity" in database, but no citations
Riluzole (Rilutek)	↑ALT, 3 cases of acute hepatitis
Modafinil (Provigil)	↑ALT in database, but no citations
Gabapentin (Neurontin)	1 case of cholestasis
Pregabalin (Lyrica)	1 case of hepatitis
Varenicline (Chantix)	1 case of acute hepatitis
Not Reported to Cause Liver Injury	
Amantidine (Symmetrel), benztropine (Cogentin), biperiden (Akineton), bromocriptine (Parlodel), carbidoba/levodopa (Sinemet), donepezil (Aricept), entacapone (Comtan), galantamine (Reminyl), memantine (Nameda), pramipexole (Mirapex), rivastigmine (Exelon), ropinirole (Requip), selegiline (Eldepryl), trihexyphenidyl (Artane), all the "-triptans"	

treatment of restless leg syndrome[221] and prolactinomas.[222] Both the Epocrates database (www.epocrates.com) and the medication's package insert (www.pdr.net) mention abnormal ALT levels and hepatitis as possible ADRs. However, no literature reports of liver toxicity were found.

Methazolamide, a carbonic anhydrase inhibitor used in the treatment of glaucoma, can also be used for therapy of essential tremor. The Epocrates database lists hepatic necrosis and dysfunction as ADRs. However, only one possible case of hepatitis in association with red blood cell aplasia was reported in 1981.[223]

Tacrine is an acetylcholinesterase inhibitor that has a mild beneficial effect on Alzheimer's disease, but can cause severe hepatocellular injury.[224,225] Analysis of multicenter clinical trials in the United States, France, and Canada[226,227] demonstrated that 25% of patients who take tacrine develop asymptomatic ALT elevations more than three times normal, usually within the first 6 to 12 weeks of therapy. Hepatic abnormalities are usually reversible, and only one fatal case of hepatotoxicity has been reported—a 75-year-old woman who had taken tacrine for 14 months.[225] Tacrine is metabolized by CYP1A2 and its mechanism of toxicity has been suggested to involve a hypoxia-reoxygenation injury mediated via the sympathetic nervous system[228] and an alteration in membrane fluidity that is not related to lipid peroxidation.[229]

Glatiramer is an injectable preparation of synthetic polypeptides related to myelin basic protein. It may have some efficacy in slowing the progression of relapsing-remitting multiple sclerosis,[230] although a recent Cochrane Review has not supported this claim.[231] The Epocrates database mentions hepatotoxicity in its long list of adverse events. However, no citation could be found, and liver injury was not mentioned in the Cochrane Review.

Riluzole is a centrally acting glutamate antagonist. It has been used in Europe since 1995 and was the first drug to be approved by the FDA for amyotrophic lateral sclerosis (ALS). It appears to prolong survival in ALS patients by approximately 1 month.[232] It is regarded as relatively safe, although three cases of acute hepatitis have been reported[233,234] and biopsies showed inflammation and microvesicular steatosis. No deaths attributable to hepatic failure have been reported. Recent reviews[232,235] list ALT level elevation as one of the most frequent adverse events, and serum ALT levels more than three times normal are observed in 10% to 15% of patients.[236] This last report recommends strict ALT level monitoring of patients, and avoiding the drug if ALT levels are already elevated.

Modafinil is approved for narcolepsy and sleep apnea, and this drug is listed in the Epocrates database as causing elevated levels of aminotransferases. However, no citation could be found, and a study of 151 patients did not report any instances of liver test abnormalities.[237]

Varenicline is an agent now very widely used for smoking cessation. Only one case of reversible acute liver injury was reported after 4 weeks of therapy in a patient with alcohol and hepatitis C–induced liver disease.[238]

Gabapentin[239] and **pregabalin**[240] have each been rarely reported to cause acute reversible liver injury.

Antidiabetic Agents

As a group, the **sulfonylureas** have a very low incidence of hepatotoxicity. The Epocrates database lists rare cholestatic events as occurring after glipizide, glyburide, and chlorpropamide use, which is most likely due to a hypersensitivity reaction.[241] Although tolbutamide, glimepiride, and tolazamide are not listed in the database, reports of acute cholestatic hepatitis, chronic vanishing bile duct syndrome, and granulomas have been submitted for all of these agents.[155,242]

Repaglinide is a benzoic acid derivative that is listed in the Epocrates database as causing rare hepatic dysfunction. However, a review of five large long-term trials did not mention liver toxicity[243] (and in addition found no liver toxicity with glyburide). Despite these data, there was one report of acute hepatotoxicity.[244] Because repaglinide is metabolized by CYP2C8, caution is advised when also using inhibitors of this CYP, such as trimethoprim.[245]

Metformin is the only remaining biguanide medication available for use. The other two agents in this class, buformin and phenformin, were withdrawn in the 1950s because of a high incidence of lactic acidosis.[246] Metformin's risk of lactic acidosis is lower, and the drug is considered safe as long as dose adjustments are made for renal impairment, liver impairment, surgery, and the use of radiologic contrast.[247] Although the Epocrates database does not mention hepatotoxicity due to metformin, several cases of acute cholestatic hepatitis have been reported.[248,249] The mechanism of toxicity is not known. Metformin is believed to have added risks when used in patients with liver disease,[241,246] because it increases insulin sensitivity at the receptor level,[250,251] nevertheless, it is often used in patients with nonalcoholic steatohepatitis.

Thiazolidinediones are peroxisome proliferator–activated receptor-γ (PPAR) agonists that have complex metabolic effects on adipose cells, myocytes, and hepatocytes to improve overall insulin sensitivity.[252] **Troglitazone** was the first of this class to reach the market, in 1997, but was withdrawn in 2000 after a large number of cases of serious hepatotoxicity, a number of which were fatal or required liver transplantation.[252] Analysis of postmarketing and other data by FDA reviewers estimated a high risk of liver failure (1:600 to 1:1500) at 26 months of troglitazone use.[252] The other two agents, **pioglitazone** and **rosiglitazone,** have a lesser tendency to cause hepatotoxicity, although cases have been reported.[252-256] In an analysis of 13 clinical trials,[257] the frequency with which troglitazone caused increases in serum ALT levels more than three times the ULN was 1.91%, compared with only 0.26% for pioglitazone and 0.17% for rosiglitazone. Furthermore, 0.68% of the subjects taking troglitazone developed serum ALT levels more than 10 times ULN, whereas no one developed such increases while taking the other agents.

The mechanism of liver injury for troglitazone is unknown. The drug does undergo metabolism, probably by CYP3A4 and to a lesser extent CYP2C8, to a reactive sulfonium ion that covalently binds to microsomal protein and GSH. A reactive metabolite may also adversely affect basolateral organic anion transporters.[257] However, the parent drug is also hepatotoxic. The clinical presentation of hepatotoxicity in the reported cases was generally delayed, with a mean presentation after 4 months of use.[252] Therefore current recommendations relating to glitazone use include avoiding starting the drug if the baseline serum ALT level is more than 2.5 times the ULN and monitoring the ALT level every 2 months for the first year. In addition, the drug should be stopped and immediate medical care obtained if unexplained nausea, vomiting, abdominal pain, fatigue, anorexia, or dark urine develops, or if the ALT level becomes more than three times the ULN. These recommendations notwithstanding, the value of regular monitoring of serum ALT level has not been established, and for troglitazone 19 of 94 patients progressed from normal tests to irreversible liver injury within 1 month.[252]

Antimicrobial Agents

Antimicrobials—Antifungals/Antiparasitics/Antimalarials/Antituberculars

Antimicrobial agents are among the most common drugs associated with DILI. In the U.S. DILIN Registry, antimicrobial agents (antibacterial, antiviral, antituberculosis drugs) were the most common class of drugs, accounting for 45.5% of cases.[106] Similarly, in the Spanish prospective study antimicrobial agents were the most common class of drugs, accounting for 32% of cases, with amoxicillin-clavulanate as the single most common drug.[105] Although serious DILI from antimicrobial agents is rare (estimated incidence of 0.03%), patients who develop jaundice requiring hospitalization from DILI caused by antimicrobial agents have a high mortality.[258] Severe DILI led to black box warning or removal from the market of telithromycin and trovafloxacin in the United States.[259]

Amphotericin B

Significant hepatotoxicity is very unlikely based on this drug's widespread use for so many years and the paucity of reports (a total of three documented cases[260]) describing DILI. In animal studies features of hepatotoxicity on liver biopsy include macrophage vacuolation, hepatocellular necrosis, foamy macrophage accumulation, and fatty infiltration.[261] One study of 64 severely immunocompromised patients conducted over a 10-year period reported that none of the patients developed evidence of serious hepatotoxicity on liver biopsy.[261] A study of bone marrow transplant recipients reported that one third of recipients developed marked increases in bilirubin levels after treatment with liposomal amphotericin, compared to 8% of recipients treated with flucanazole.[262] Nevertheless, nephrotoxicity from amphotericin is its most important toxic side effect (**Table 25-12**).

Ketoconazole and Other Azoles

Ketoconazole is an imidazole oral antifungal drug and a potent competitive inhibitor of hepatic CYP3A.[263,264] This latter property has probably led to more adverse drug reactions than to direct hepatotoxicity. However, shortly after its introduction in 1981, ketoconazole was noted to cause an acute hepatitic or mixed form of acute liver injury, often with jaundice, which was more common in women and elderly patients.[265-267] Pure cholestatic injury occurred in 10% of cases. Evidence of allergy was rare. Injury was noted on average after 8 weeks of therapy. Fatalities were uncommon, and usually associated with continuation of the drug. A more recent prospective cohort study[268] showed that 18% of patients

Table 25-12 Antifungal, Antiparasitic, Antitubercular Drugs and DILI

DRUGS	COMMENTS
Reported to Cause DILI	
Antifungals	
Ketoconazole (Nizoral)	Hepatitic > cholestatic
Fluconazole (Diflucan)	Hepatitic, ?Cholestatic
Itraconazole (Sporanox)	Cholestatic, hepatitic
Voriconazole (Vfend)	Too new, incidence unknown
Terbinafine (Lamisil)	Cholestatic > hepatitic
Griseofulvin	Very low incidence
Caspofungin (Cancidas IV)	Too new, incidence unknown
Flucytosine (Ancobon)	Hepatitic
Antiparasitics	
Thiabendazole (Mintezol)	Cholestatic > hepatitic
Mebendazole (Vermox)	↑ALT
Albendazole (Albenza)	↑ALT
Antimalarials	
Pyrimethamine/sulfadoxine (Fansidar)	Very rare
Amodiaquine (not available in U.S.)	Very rare
Antituberculars	
Isoniazid	Idiosyncratic hepatitic
Rifampicin	Idiosyncratic hepatitic
Pyrazinamide	Idiosyncratic hepatitic
Ethambutol (Myambutol)	Doubtful
Dapsone	↑ALT
Rifapentine (Priftin)	Idiosyncratic hepatitic
Ethionamide (Trecator-SC)	Idiosyncratic hepatitic
Not Reported to Cause Hepatotoxicity	
Antifungals	
Amphotericin (only mild ↑ALT), clotrimazole (Mycelex), miconazole (Monistat), nystatin (Mycostatin)	
Antimalarials	
Chloroquine (Aralen), hydroxychloroquine (Plaquenil), primaquine, mefloquine (Lariam ±↑LFTs), atovaquone/proguanil (Malarone ±↑LFTs), pyrimethamine (Deraprim)	
Antiparasitics	
Pentamidine (Pentam), atovaquone (Mepron), praziquantel (Biltricide), pyrantel (Antiminth), ivermectin (Stromectol ±↑LFTs), nitazoxanide (Alinia)	
Antituberculars	
Streptomycin, rifabutin (Mycobutin), cycloserine (Seromycin ±↑LFTs)	

have transient asymptomatic elevations of serum ALT levels that normalize with continued therapy (adaptation), but 3% develop clinical hepatitis. Another recent cohort study[269] tracked acute liver injury in more than 69,000 patients taking various oral antifungal drugs and found the following incidences: ketoconazole, 1 in 750 person-months; itraconazole, 1 in 10,000; terbinafine, 1 in 40,000. Although ketoconazole's idiosyncratic injury is not considered immune-mediated, a recent report of a woman developing severe hepatitis just 48 hours after an unintentional rechallenge suggests that an immune reaction can occur.[270] Another case report suggests that cirrhosis may develop despite withdrawal of the drug and resolution of acute liver injury.[271]

The mechanism of ketoconazole liver injury appears to involve formation of an *N*-deacetyl metabolite that is converted to a toxic dialdehyde by the flavin-containing monooxygenases.[272,273] Treatment is drug cessation, and ursodeoxycholate may help prevent progressive cholestatic injury.[274]

Itraconazole, a less potent CYP3A inhibitor than ketoconazole,[264] also causes less hepatotoxicity.[269] In a pharmaceutical database study of >54,000 itraconazole and fluconazole users,[275] "serious adverse liver events" were reported in only 1 in 30,000 prescriptions for either drug. If itraconazole was given as "pulse" therapy (1 week/month × 3), then no serious hepatotoxicity was found.[276] However, three cases of cholestatic liver injury were reported in patients taking itraconazole long term. These patients presented with jaundice, and ductopenia was noted in two of the three biopsies.[277] Focal nodular hyperplasia has been linked to itraconazole in one patient who had been taking the drug for 4 months.[278] **Fluconazole** is considered very safe, with only 5% of 562 children developing transient elevations of serum ALT levels.[279] In some reports of DILI, fluconazole was found to have been administered with nitrofurantoin[280] or amphotericin B.[281] **Voriconazole** is probably still too new for its incidence of hepatotoxicity to be known, and no literature citations have been found. However, recent safety reviews suggest that both liver tests and visual changes should be monitored in patients using voriconazole.[282,283]

Terbinafine

This allylamine antifungal has replaced pulse itraconazole for the treatment of onychomycosis, and is widely advertised. The incidence of hepatobiliary dysfunction in postmarketing surveillance has been reported to be as low as 1 in 40,000.[269,284] However, recent case reports,[285-287] and many others too numerous to cite, suggest a higher incidence with a predominance of cholestatic reactions, including one liver transplant patient who was initially thought to have acute rejection 5 years after his transplant.[288] Toxicity can be seen as early as after 1 week of use.[287] The mechanism of injury might be the formation of an *N*-dealkylated allylic aldehyde that is conjugated with GSH and transported across the canalicular membrane.[286,289]

Griseofulvin

This older antifungal agent has been the mainstay of therapy for tinea capitis, but may now be supplanted by the newer antifungals that require only 2 to 3 weeks of therapy instead of 6 weeks.[290] Although gastrointestinal side effects of the drug are common, only one case report from 1976 described griseofulvin hepatotoxicity.[291] A more recent prospective study[268] showed no liver test abnormalities in 74 patients treated for 3 months.

Caspofungin

This echinocandin antifungal is the first of its kind to be approved and is only available for intravenous use. It can be used by itself or with liposomal amphotericin B, or with voriconazole for refractory invasive aspergillosis and candidiasis in immunosuppressed patients[282,292-294]; however, it is not an effective agent in the treatment of cryptococcus infection. The drug inhibits fungal cell wall β-(1,3)-glucan synthesis. It appears to be metabolized by hepatic P450s and may inhibit CYP3A4.[295] Caution is therefore required when it is used with cyclosporin A[296] and other calcineurin inhibitors. However, nelfinavir did not alter its pharmacokinetics.[297] Because of a paradoxic loss of efficacy against *Candida* spp. at high concentrations,[295] it may best be used for complicated infections in combination with other drugs. Because phase 1 and 2 trials commonly reported elevated levels of liver enzymes,[292] its long-term safety and incidence of hepatotoxicity are still to be determined.

Flucytosine

This oral antifungal, available since the 1970s, is known to cause elevations of serum ALT levels in 5% to 15% of patients.[260] Its mechanism of hepatic injury is unknown, but appears to be dose related.[298] Its main use currently is for the treatment of severe fungal infections. It has been used successfully in combination with fluconazole[299] for cryptococcosis in a liver transplant patient. Because its use is so limited, it is doubtful that its mechanism of hepatotoxicity will ever be known.

Antimalarials

The toxicities of most antimalarials, such as chloroquine and hydroxychloroquine, are chiefly neurologic and hematologic. However, pyrimethamine/sulfadoxine[300,301] and amodiaquine[300,302] have been associated with DILI and ALF when the drugs have been continued after the onset of jaundice. The incidence of serious hepatotoxicity is estimated to be 1 in 11,000 to 15,000.[300] Amodiaquine is not available in the United States, but is widely used in countries with endemic malaria where drug-resistant strains are a problem.[303,304]

Benzimidazole Antiparasitics

Thiabendazole, mebendazole, and albendazole all seem to occasionally cause elevations of serum ALT levels[305]; however, only thiabendazole, available since 1964, has been reported to cause a cholestatic hepatitis that has led to ductopenia and cirrhosis.[306-309] The incidence appears to be low, but has not been determined, and no recent case reports have appeared.

Isoniazid, Rifampicin, and Pyrazinamide

Isoniazid (INH), available since the 1960s, is well-known to be a hepatotoxic drug that causes an idiosyncratic hepatitic reaction leading to overt clinical hepatitis in 0.3% to 1.0% of patients when used as monotherapy.[310,311] It is the second most common drug responsible for ALF requiring liver transplantation in the United States.[1] Hepatotoxicity increases when used in combination with other agents, such as rifampicin[311] and pyrazinamide.[312] Despite the risks, INH continues to be used because it is still the most effective agent for *Mycobacterium tuberculosis* therapy.[310] For patients with latent tuberculosis (TB) infection, the use of INH monotherapy for 6 or 9 months is considered the therapy of choice,[313] but compliance is often low[314] (<65%). A 2-month course of INH, rifampicin, and pyrazinamide, given twice weekly, was shown to improve compliance, but was three times more likely to cause serious hepatotoxicity than INH alone.[315-318] Therefore this drug combination is unlikely to supplant INH. Of patients taking INH alone, 10% develop elevations of serum ALT levels, most of which normalize with continued therapy, but 0.6% progress to overt clinical hepatitis that requires drug cessation.[311] With INH and rifampicin, serum ALT level increases occur in 35% of patients and 2.73% develop overt, clinical hepatitis.

Overt hepatotoxicity usually presents within 6 weeks of INH monotherapy, and with INH and rifampicin usually in the first 2 weeks,[319] but can be as early as a few days.[311] When INH is used with rifampicin and pyrazinamide, hepatotoxicity beginning after 4 weeks is more ominous than early toxicity.[319] Histologic changes resemble those of acute hepatitis A or B, and include diffuse lobular inflammation with ballooning or confluent necrosis, and occasionally macrovesicular fat.[320]

The mechanism of INH hepatotoxicity involves the formation of acetylisoniazid that is hydrolyzed to monoacetylhydrazine. It is hypothesized that CYP2E1 then activates the monoacetylhydrazine to a toxic metabolite. The exact mechanism of toxicity remains unclear, and is complicated by the fact that INH is often used with other agents. INH itself appears to inhibit a number of human CYPs, including 1A2, 2A6, 2C19, and 3A4,[321,322] whereas rifampicin is a potent inducer of CYPs 2B6,[323] 2C8,[324] 2C9,[325] 3A4, and 3A5,[326] as well as some phase II enzymes, all via activation of the pregnane X receptor (PXR). Pyrazinamide does not appear to inhibit CYPs[321]; the mechanism employed by pyrazinamide to enhance toxicity with INH or rifampicin also remains unknown. A study in which patients were receiving multiple antituberculosis drugs in addition to isoniazid also reported that the NAT2 polymorphism associated with slow acetylator status was associated with DILI from isoniazid.[327] In both of these studies the NAT2*6/*6 and NAT2*6/*7 genotypes were associated with slow acetylation and DILI from isoniazid. Shimizu and colleagues also reported that the NAT2 genotype associated with slow acetylation was associated with DILI from isoniazid. A total of 80% of slow acetylators and 9.1% of rapid acetylators developed AST or ALT level elevations more than twice the upper limit of normal ($p < 0.05$).[328] Similar findings were reported by others.[329] Polymorphisms in GSTT1 and GSTM1 have been associated with DILI from isoniazid.[330] In a study of 37 subjects there was a higher prevalence of the null mutation for GSTM1 in patients who developed DILI from INH compared with controls (52% vs. 24%; $p < 0.05$).

Besides slow acetylator status, age is the next most important predictor of hepatotoxicity. Although DILI attributable to INH is rare in patients younger than age 20 and increases to 2.3% in those older than age 50,[310] pediatric Japanese patients younger than 5 years had an unexpectedly high rate of severe hepatotoxicity[331] (>8%), to which the use of pyrazinamide may have contributed. A study from India also implicated the use of pyrazinamide.[312] Other variables—including female sex; underlying liver disease

related to alcohol, hepatitis B, and hepatitis C; and malnutrition—have all been variably implicated in increasing the incidence of severe hepatotoxicity.[310,312] A case of hyperacute liver failure in a young patient also receiving carbamazepine was recently reported.[332]

In an effort to avoid overt hepatitis, complex algorithms have been developed[313] that include baseline laboratory testing for all but the most healthy young (<35 years) non–HIV-infected adults, and monitoring at monthly intervals if the patient is taking INH alone. If the patient is also taking rifampicin and/or pyrazinamide, more intense monitoring is recommended[319] (e.g., twice weekly for 2 weeks, then every 2 weeks up to 2 months, and then monthly). INH should be stopped if ALT levels become more than three times the ULN with symptoms, or more than five times the ULN without symptoms. Patients must be advised to observe for side effects and report them immediately. If overt clinical hepatitis develops, all therapy must be stopped. Because antitubercular therapy must usually be resumed, some experts[333] recommend a stepwise reintroduction of drugs, starting with INH at a low dose, then pyrazinamide, and finally rifampicin, with careful monitoring. Only 7% of patients rechallenged in this way developed subsequent hepatotoxicity.

Ethambutol

This agent is added to INH, rifampicin, and pyrazinamide to treat active TB when INH resistance is suspected. Although fatal hepatotoxicity is listed as a rare adverse event in the drug databases, no specific citations could be found to suggest this agent has significant hepatotoxicity. Because it is almost always given as part of a multidrug regimen with known hepatotoxic agents, liver injury ascribed to ethambutol would be difficult to identify and characterize.

Dapsone

Dapsone is a second-line agent for TB and is used for other disorders such as dermatitis herpetiformis, leprosy, malaria, and *Pneumocystis carinii* pneumonia in HIV-infected patients. It is metabolized by CYPs 2E1 and 2C isoforms[334] to a hydroxylamine that can cause hemolysis, methemoglobinemia, and agranulocytosis.[335] A cutaneous syndrome is also described[336] that is often associated with mild hepatotoxicity. When dapsone is given with pyrimethamine, the rate of serious hepatotoxicity has been estimated to be low, only 1 in 75,000.[300]

Rifapentine

It is hoped that this long-acting cyclopental derivative of rifampicin, which can be given once weekly, will improve adherence to antitubercular treatment regimens. It has been shown to be safe and effective in HIV-negative pulmonary TB patients,[337,338] and no dosage adjustments are required in patients with cirrhosis.[339] However, in one study of its use with INH, adverse events were twice as high with rifapentine as compared with rifampicin.[340] Because rifapentine is also an inducer of CYPs, it has significant drug interactions. Hepatotoxicity is listed in the drug databases, with an incidence of serum ALT level elevations during combination TB therapy being slightly less than that found with rifampicin.

Ethionamide

This agent is rarely used, but hepatotoxicity was recognized and reported in the 1960s.[341] Because it is related to INH, its toxicity is probably attributable to an idiosyncratic hepatitis.

The American Thoracic Society statement on hepatotoxicity of antituberculosis therapy recommends monitoring of ALT levels during treatment of latent TB in individuals who chronically consume alcohol; take concomitant hepatotoxic drugs; have viral hepatitis or other preexisting liver disease, abnormal baseline ALT levels, or a history of prior INH hepatitis; are pregnant or within 3 months postpartum; or are co-infected with HIV. It is also recommended that monitoring be considered in individuals older than 35 years.[342] The committee recommends that treatment should be interrupted in individuals with ALT level elevations more than three times the upper limit of normal in the presence of hepatitis symptoms and/or jaundice, or five times the upper limit of normal in the absence of symptoms.

Antimicrobials—Antivirals

Anti-HIV Agents

With the development of effective antiviral agents for HIV and the dramatic decrease in mortality from AIDS in the 1990s, primarily attributable to the development of highly active antiretroviral therapy (HAART), liver disease in HIV patients has emerged as an important cause of morbidity and mortality. The main culprits in promoting liver disease in this population are believed to be sequelae of co-infection with HIV and hepatitis viruses B and/or C.[343-346] Different algorithms have been proposed for monitoring patients on HAART, depending on whether there is preexisting liver disease or co-infection with hepatitis B or C.[347] The mechanism by which co-infection increases DILI and mortality is still a subject of controversy. Some studies suggest that hepatitis C hampers the effectiveness of HAART.[348,349] Others suggest that hepatitis C has no impact on survival.[350] Liver damage by hepatitis B was probably controlled with lamivudine, which was a component of most HAART regimens, and now other effective agents are available for lamivudine-resistant strains. Therefore the increasing incidence of liver failure in HIV patients could be drug related (**Table 25-13**).[351,352]

Serious or severe drug-related ADRs occurred in 16% of patients in one large study,[353] but very few of these were liver related, despite 20% of patients being noted to have asymptomatic increases in serum ALT levels. Characterizing DILI is difficult in this complex patient population; typically, these patients not only take multiple therapeutic drugs and herbal remedies but also have a high incidence of alcoholism (in those patients with a history of IV drug abuse) and hepatitis C co-infection (32% to 68%)[343,349,350] concomitant with frequent opportunistic infections. Several recent comprehensive reviews of the hepatic injury from these agents have been published.[354-357]

Regular monitoring of liver function tests is considered mandatory for patients beginning HAART,[347,352] with monthly testing for the first 3 months and then every 3 months thereafter. Avoidance of alcohol should always be recommended. Asymptomatic increases in serum ALT levels that are less than five times the ULN are considered relatively

Table 25-13 Antiviral Drugs and DILI

DRUG	COMMENTS
Anti-HIV, NRTIs	
Lamivudine (Epivir)	Mitochondrial (low incidence)
Zidovudine (Retrovir)	Mitochondrial (low incidence)
Didanosine (Videx)	Mitochondrial (higher incidence)
Stavudine (Zerit)	Mitochondrial (higher incidence)
Emtricitabine (Emtriva)	Mitochondrial (low incidence)
Abacavir (Ziagen)	Mitochondrial (low incidence)
Zalcitabine (Hivid)	Mitochondrial (higher incidence)
Anti-HIV, PIs	
Amprenavir (Agenerase)	↑ALT
Lopinavir (Kaletra, with ritonavir)	↑ALT
Saquinavir (Fortovase, Invirase)	↑ALT
Indinavir (Crixivan)	↑ALT and inhibits UDPGT
Atazanavir (Reyataz)	↑ALT
Nelfinavir (Viracept)	↑ALT
Ritonavir (Norvir)	↑ALT and most potent CYP3A4 inhibitor
Fosamprenavir (Lexiva)	↑ALT
Anti-HIV, NNRTIs	
Efavirenz (Sustiva)	↑ALT
Nevirapine (Viramune)	↑ALT
Delavirdine (Rescriptor)	↑ALT, ?immune features
Anti-HIV, Anti-HBV NRTIs	
Tenofovir (Viread)	Very rare
Adefovir (Hepsera)	Very rare
Anti-CMV	
Cidofovir (Vistide)	Very rare
Not Reported to Cause DILI	
Anti-CMV: ganciclovir (Cytovene ±↑LFTs), foscarnet (Foscavir), valganciclovir (Valcyte)	
Anti-herpes: acyclovir (Zovirax), famciclovir (Famvir), valacyclovir (Valtrex)	
Anti-influenza: amantidine (Symmetrel), rimantadine (Flumadine), zanamivir (Relenza), oseltamivir (Tamiflu)	

ALT, alanine aminotransferase; CMV, cytomegalovirus; HIV, human immunodeficiency virus; NNRTI, nonnucleoside reserve transcriptase inhibitor; NTRI, nucleoside analogue reserve transcriptase inhibitor

"safe," but must be checked monthly until resolved, and other causes of hepatitis should be investigated. If serum ALT levels are more than five times the ULN without symptoms, monitoring should be every 2 weeks. However, if clinical symptoms exist, or if serum ALT levels are >10 times the ULN, especially with lactic acidosis, HAART and other potentially hepatotoxic drugs must be discontinued.

Nucleoside Analogue Reverse Transcriptase Inhibitors

The most ominous toxic effect of nucleoside analogue reverse transcriptase inhibitors (NRTIs) is the development of mitochondrial toxicity that leads to lactic acidosis and liver failure, similar to Reye's syndrome.[356] It is thought that depletion of mitochondrial DNA (mtDNA) by NRTIs causes the mitochondrial dysfunction. This supposition was strengthened by findings that stavudine, didanosine, and zalcitabine, which are known to deplete mtDNA in cultured hepatocytes,[358] are associated with lower mtDNA levels in liver biopsy samples and higher serum lactate levels in HIV/HCV co-infected patients, compared with patients taking zidovudine, lamivudine, and abacavir, which do not deplete mtDNA levels.[359] DILI from NRTIs usually occur within the first 9 months although liver test elevations may occur later. Hepatitis C infection by itself might cause mitochondrial dysfunction;[360] however, it is not yet clear whether co-infection increases the risk of mitochondrial toxicity. Stavudine is associated with more cases of lactic acidosis than other NRTIs,[361] but all have been associated with cases of microvesicular steatosis and liver failure.[354] Some experts[343,356,361,362] advise the use of coenzyme Q (30 to 60 mg three times daily), carnitine (1 to 3 g/day), riboflavin (50 mg/day), and/or thiamine (100 mg/day) in the event of lipoatrophy or severe lactic acidosis, but most of these interventions have not been studied in the setting of liver failure. Abacavir has been associated with a hypersensitivity reaction characterized by fever and generalized rash. There has been an association with HLA-B*5701. This class of drugs should not be used with ribavirin.

Protease Inhibitors

The introduction of protease inhibitors (PIs) in the 1990s marked the beginning of HAART and control of HIV. All of the PIs (see **Table 25-13**) are used in combination with other antivirals, and increased serum ALT or AST levels more than five times the ULN occurred in 1% to 9.5% of patients during the original registration trials.[355] Ritonavir used in higher doses caused liver injury more frequently than the other agents, and is now given in lower doses in combination with other PIs to boost drug levels. A characteristic of all PIs is that they are metabolized by and are inhibitors of hepatic CYPs, primarily 3A4, and ritonavir is the most potent.[363] Furthermore, all PIs, except possibly indinavir, appear to be mechanism-based inhibitors of P450, which means they irreversibly inactivate the enzyme. Nelfinavir may also affect CYP2C19.[364] Indinavir also causes a reversible inhibition of UDPGT that leads to benign unconjugated hyperbilirubinemia in 12% of patients. Because ritonavir inhibits CYP3A so well, it is given with lopinavir in one of the more commonly used PI combinations, to prevent lopinavir's metabolism. Liver toxicity with this combination is not greater than that found with nelfinavir-based HAART.[365]

The mechanism whereby PIs cause liver injury is not yet known.[355] Whether asymptomatic ALT level elevations promote more rapid progression of fibrosis in patients co-infected with hepatitis B or C is another source of debate. Because PIs are always given in combination with other agents to patients, sorting this out will be complex. However, inhibition of CYPs by PIs causes the most important clinically relevant ADRs. One example is the effect of lopinavir/ritonavir therapy on HIV in liver transplant patients who are receiving tacrolimus; these patients need profound dose reductions in tacrolimus.[366]

Nonnucleoside Reverse Transcriptase Inhibitors

Of the three available nonnucleoside reverse transcriptase inhibitors (NNRTIs), nevirapine and efavirenz have been utilized to a much greater extent than delavirdine, possibly because delavirdine is an inhibitor of several CYPs.[367] A number of large cohort studies have shown that, when administered with NRTIs and/or PIs, nevirapine is two to three times as likely as efavirenz to cause increases in serum ALT levels more than five times the ULN.[353,368-373] The incidence across multiple studies with nevirapine was 10%,[370] with clinical symptoms in 4.9%. The hepatotoxicity with both nevirapine and efavirenz was often delayed, being recognized 3 to 9 months (median 5.5 months) after therapy began,[373] and was more common in patients co-infected with hepatitis B and hepatitis C. Another study has suggested that HAART regimens that contain nevirapine are associated with more rapid progression of hepatic fibrosis in hepatitis C patients,[374] and that co-infected patients receiving PIs do better than those being administered NNRTIs. Nevirapine has also been reported to cause severe hepatotoxicity and cutaneous reactions, both when used alone and when used with other antivirals for postexposure prophylaxis in non-HIV patients.[375] These authors recommended avoiding nevirapine in prophylaxis regimens. The mechanism of hepatotoxicity for the NNRTIs may involve an idiosyncratic response with immune features, and this may explain why the hepatotoxicity is worse in non-HIV subjects and is delayed in HIV patients. Nevirapine has been associated with a hypersensitivity reaction, and individuals with HLA-DRB*0101 may be at increased risk for this reaction.

Nucleotide Reverse Transcriptase Inhibitors

Tenofovir is effective against HIV and does not appear to deplete mitochondrial DNA.[376] Both tenofovir and adefovir are effective against hepatitis B.[377,378] Although the Epocrates database lists hepatotoxicity as a serious reaction for both drugs, no citations could be found and adverse liver effects are not mentioned in the package inserts for either drug.

Fusion Inhibitors and Integrase Inhibitor

The fusion inhibitors (enfuviritide, selzentry, vicriviroc, ibalizumab) have been associated with a 5% rate of elevation of liver tests. The development of aplaviroc was abandoned because of grade 2 or higher elevations in ALT levels in 6% of subjects and grade 2 or higher elevations in total bilirubin levels in 10% of subjects. Drug-induced liver injury from raltegravir appears to be less common compared with ART, but this may be because it is not as frequently prescribed and a newer agent.

Cidofovir

This anti-CMV agent, approved to treat CMV retinitis in HIV patients, causes nephrotoxicity and neutropenia as its major side effects (www.pdr.net). Hepatotoxicity is mentioned in the Epocrates database, but no citations could be found. Almost all of the anti-CMV agents appear to be devoid of hepatotoxicity.

Antimicrobials—Antibacterials

Penicillins and Cephalosporins

In general, the β-lactam antibiotics and structurally related cephalosporins have a very low incidence of hepatotoxicity, most of which is idiosyncratic with immune features that can manifest as either primarily hepatic, primarily cholestatic, mixed, and/or granulomatous (**Table 25-14**).[260,305] The ability of the same agent to present in several ways suggests that host factors must dictate the type of allergic injury. β-Lactamase-resistant agents and penicillins with β-lactamase inhibitors, such as sulbactam and clavulanate, more often cause a cholestatic response,[379-382] occasionally with a prolonged clinical course.[383] The incidence of DILI with amoxicillin alone is 1 in 30,000, but with clavulanate it is 1 in 6000.[382] If older patients are given repeated courses, the incidence may be as high as 1 in 1000. Piperacillin with another β-lactamase inhibitor, tazobactam, was noted to cause only mild increases in serum ALT levels in clinical trials,[384] and no reports of cholestatic injury have yet been made. Flucloxacillin, one of the earlier β-lactamase-resistant agents, had a very high incidence of chronic cholestasis[385,386] and is no longer used in the United States. Only oxacillin and dicloxacillin are available in the United States, with no serious hepatotoxicity listed for either of these agents in the Epocrates database. Yet, recent reports[385,387] have indicated that IV oxacillin use in children should be monitored for hepatotoxicity.

Amoxicillin-Clavulanic Acid

Amoxicillin-clavulanic acid is the most common antibiotic reported to cause DILI in the U.S. DILIN Registry and the Spanish Registry.[105,106] Typical presenting symptoms are jaundice and pruritus with cholestatic DILI. Immunoallergic features, including rash and eosinophilia, may be present. Resolution of liver test abnormalities may take months and chronic liver injury with ductopenia can occur.

Because the HLA complex is inherited and involved in antigen presentation several studies have been performed on the association between HLA polymorphisms and susceptibility to DILI (see **Table 25-9**).[116,119,388-393] One of the best examples of an association of HLA and DILI is a study of 35 patients with amoxicillin-clavulanate hepatotoxicity.[116] This study is unique because it includes a large number of patients with DILI from a single drug that was biopsy proven and all of the patients developed jaundice. HLA-A and HLA-B were typed using lymphocytotoxicity assays and HLA-DRB and HLA-DBQ were typed by polymerase chain reaction (PCR)-line probe assay. Cases were more likely to have HLA class II antigen DRB1*1501-DRB5*0101-DQB1*0602 haplotype, $p < 0.0002$,

Table 25-14 Antibacterial Drugs and DILI

Reported to Cause Hepatotoxicity		Sulfisoxazole (Gantrisin)	Cholestatic > hepatitic
Penicillins		Sulfadiazine	Cholestatic > hepatitic
Ampicillin	Hepatitic > cholestatic Cholestatic + sulbactam (Unasyn) > hepatitic	**Tetracyclines**	
		Tetracycline	Mitochondrial in high doses
Amoxicillin + clavulanic acid (Augmentin)	Hepatitic > cholestatic Cholestatic, granulomatous	Doxycycline	Hepatitic
		Demeclocycline (Declomycin)	None reported
Oxacillin	Cholestatic, granulomatous	Minocycline (Minocin, Vectrin)	Autoimmune hepatitis, hepatitic
Ticarcillin (Ticar) + clavulanic acid (Timentin)	Unknown Cholestatic	**Other Antimicrobials**	
Piperacillin ± tazobactam (Zosyn)	↑Hepatitic or mixed	Nitrofurantoin	Acute hepatitic and chronic fibrosis
Cephalosporins		Nalidixic acid	Possible cholestasis (one case)
Cefaclor (Ceclor)	Possibly cholestatic	Quinupristin/dalfopristin (Synercid)	Possible cholestasis
Cefdinir (Omnicef)	Possibly hepatitic	Fosfomycin (Monurol)	↑ALT
Ceftriaxone	Biliary sludge	**Not Reported to Cause Significant Hepatotoxicity**	
Macrolides		**Penicillins**	
Erythromycin	Cholestatic	Pen Vee K, ampicillin, nafcillin, mezlocillin (Mezlin)	
Clarithromycin (Biaxin)	Cholestatic	**Cephalosporins**	
Azithromycin (Zithromax)	Cholestatic	Almost all first-, second-, and third-generation agents	
Telithromycin (Ketek)	Cholestatic	**Other Antimicrobials**	
Quinolones		Chloramphenicol, aztreonam (Azactam, ±↑ALT), ertapenem (Invanz, ±↑ALT), meropenem (Merrem), clindamycin, metronidazole, tinidazole (Tindamax), furazolidone (Furoxone, not available in U.S.), vancomycin, daptomycin (Cubicin, ±↑ALT), imipenem/cilastin (Primaxin, ±↑ALT), linezolid (Zyvox), iodoquinol (Yodoxin), rifaximin (Xifaxan)	
Trovafloxacin (Trovan)	Immune-mediated FHF		
Probably all others	Hepatitic or mixed		
Sulfonamides			
Trimethoprim/ sulfamethoxazole	Immune hepatitic (especially HIV)		

compared with controls, and they were more likely to have cholestatic injury. Of interest is that the DRB5*0101 haplotype has also been associated with primary sclerosing cholangitis, a cholestatic disorder, and the injury from amoxicillin-clavulanate is cholestatic.[394] Others have speculated that neo-antigens presented on bile duct epithelium are part of the mechanism of liver injury from amoxicillin-clavulanate.[394] Studies have demonstrated an association between HLA alleles and DILI from flucloxacillin. In a genome-wide association study the HLA allele HLA-B*5701 was associated with an 80-fold increased risk of DILI from flucloxacillin.[121] A separate proposed mechanism of action is as a pregnane X receptor agonist. Subjects who developed DILI from flucloxacillin were more likely to have the PXR polymorphism (rs3814055;C-25385-T) compared with controls and were 3.37 times more likely to have developed DILI.[395]

For the cephalosporins, most of the reports of hepatotoxicity are from the 1980s.[260] Ceftriaxone, which is excreted into bile, has been associated with the formation of biliary sludge and stones.[396] Up to 3% of patients treated with ceftriaxone may develop elevations in the levels of aminotransferases.[397] In general, the cephalosporins have only a minor risk of hepatotoxicity. Although cefaclor and cefdinir are listed in the Epocrates database as causing cholestatic jaundice and hepatitis, no literature citations were found.

Macrolides

Hepatotoxicity from **erythromycin** has been known for decades and can occur with either erythromycin base or any of the salts.[260] Erythromycin toxicity is predominantly cholestatic, owing to an idiosyncratic immunoallergic reaction. Often the clinical presentation will occur well after treatment has ended. Fever, jaundice, right upper quadrant pain, and nausea can present like acute cholecystitis. Eosinophilia is often present. Fortunately the incidence is low (1 in 30,000).[398] Although recovery can take many weeks, rarely is it fatal. Similar cholestatic presentations, including occasional fatalities, have been reported recently for clarithromycin,[399-410] azithromycin,[402,403] and roxithromycin.[404] However, the incidence of hepatotoxicity appears to be lower with the newer macrolides.[405] Telithromycin, a new ketolide antibiotic that is a structural analogue of erythromycin, was FDA approved in April 2004 to treat resistant *Streptococcus pneumoniae* respiratory tract infections and sinusitis.[406,407] No reports of hepatotoxicity have appeared, although increased serum ALT levels and hepatic dysfunction are listed as adverse reactions in the Epocrates database, and two instances have been entered into the U.S. DILIN Registry.

Erythromycin and troleandomycin, a related macrolide no longer available, are well-known to be potent inhibitors of CYP3A species and the P-glycoprotein transporter. Clarithromycin is also such an inhibitor.[408,409] In fact, erythromycin and clarithromycin cause adverse drug interactions much more frequently than they cause cholestatic liver injury, especially with immunosuppressive agents such as cyclosporin A[410,411] and tacrolimus,[412] which require CYP3A metabolism. Azithromycin, roxithromycin, and dirithromycin are much weaker inhibitors of CYP3A.[413] A potential link between CYP3A inhibition and cholestatic liver injury was identified when erythromycin and troleandomycin were found to block canalicular bile acid efflux in human hepatocytes much more effectively than the newer macrolides.[414]

Quinolones

The fluoroquinolones are considered to be relatively safe antibiotics,[415] with only trovafloxacin identified as having an incidence of hepatotoxicity (1 in 7000)[260] appreciable enough to limit its use to serious infections in hospitalized patients. With trovafloxacin, the patients who developed ALF appeared to have a hypersensitivity reaction and were taking medication for more than 14 days. However, case reports of hepatic failure have been published for most of the fluoroquinolones,[416-419] and the Epocrates database lists increased serum ALT levels as occurring with all fluoroquinolones.

Sulfonamides

All the sulfonamides have been associated with reports of hepatotoxicity, usually considered idiosyncratic with immunoallergic features.[260] A cholestatic clinical presentation is most common, usually with rash, fever, and eosinophilia. One case of intrahepatic cholestasis with phospholipidosis has been reported.[420] **Trimethoprim/sulfamethoxazole (TMP/SMX)** is one of the oldest and most widely prescribed antibiotic combinations. The incidence of hepatotoxicity in the general population must be very low, because only occasional reports of hepatitis, ALF, and cholestatic disease appeared in the literature in the 1970s and 1980s.[260] However, several recent case reports of liver failure[421-423] serve to remind us of this potential. In the U.S. ALF study, sulfonamides were the second largest class causing ALF.[424]

In HIV patients, the use of TMP/SMX has been noted to lead to a much higher incidence of allergic reactions ($\approx$20%) than in non-HIV patients.[260,425-427] Because TMP/SMX is considered the best therapy for the treatment and prevention of *Pneumocystis jiroveci* pneumonia, desensitization protocols were developed[428] and efforts made to determine the cause of hypersensitivity. A slow acetylator status may contribute[429] by allowing more drug to be activated by CYPs to sulfamethoxazole hydroxylamine.[260] Co-treatment with CYP3A inducers leads to more measurable hydroxylamine, and inhibitors decrease this metabolite.[430] No consensus has yet been reached to explain HIV-induced sensitivity. Interestingly, TMP/SMX is widely used in developing countries as chronic prophylaxis against opportunistic infections, with some success,[431-433] and no mention is made of severe allergic or hepatotoxic reactions with the use of the drug in these populations.

Tetracyclines

The original descriptions of hepatotoxicity attributable to tetracyclines were in patients receiving high doses intravenously.[260,305] The clinical presentation was similar to that seen in Reye's syndrome, with ALF, renal failure, and acidosis. Serum ALT levels were generally not very high (<1000 units/ml), and histologic findings were of microvesicular steatosis with minimal necrosis. The mechanism of the steatosis and toxicity appeared to be inhibition of mitochrondrial fatty acid oxidation[434] and was probably dose related. Intravenous tetracycline is rarely used today, and the incidence of hepatotoxicity from oral low-dose tetracyclines is extremely low.[435] However, reversible hepatic failure[436] and prolonged cholestasis with paucity of bile ducts[437] have been reported. **Minocycline,** which has been widely used as chronic therapy for acne in adolescents, was reported to cause both acute hepatitis[438] and chronic autoimmune hepatitis, with positive ANA and anti–smooth muscle antibodies.[97-99,439-441] No reports of liver injury have been submitted for demeclocycline, used mainly for treatment of syndrome of inappropriate antidiuretic hormone (SIADH), but the Epocrates database lists hepatotoxicity as a serious reaction.

Other Antibiotics

Nitrofurantoin, still used as a chronic urinary tract infection antimicrobial, was reported in 1980 to cause acute and chronic liver disease.[442] It is considered relatively safe to use as prophylaxis in children,[443] but authors continue to report the occurrence in elderly women of DILI resembling autoimmune hepatitis; DILI may or may not improve with drug withdrawal.[444,445] It is still a common cause of increased serum ALT level that prompts referral to hepatologists,[446] and caution with its use is warranted. **Nalidixic acid** is also used as a chronic urinary tract infection antimicrobial and is listed as possibly causing cholestatic hepatitis, based on one case report from 1974.[447] Whether it is safer than nitrofurantoin to use as a chronic medication is unclear.

Quinupristin/dalfopristin is a relatively new streptogramin antibiotic for vancomycin-resistant enterococci (VRE) and resistant staphylococcal infections[448] that caused hyperbilirubinemia when given to liver transplant recipients.[449] Although that study suggested that the cholestatic changes were not drug related, another study[450] suggested that elevated AP values might be drug related. The drug's main side effect appears to be a myalgia/arthralgia syndrome.

Fosfomycin, an epoxide low-molecular-weight antibiotic introduced in the early 1990s also for VRE and methicillin-resistant *Staphylococcus aureus* (MRSA),[451] was noted to frequently cause increases in serum ALT levels and *Clostridium difficile* colitis.[452] One case of acute hepatotoxicity with repeated use in a cystic fibrosis patient has been reported.[453]

Cardiovascular Agents

Antiplatelet/Anticoagulant/Thrombolytic Agents

A fixed dose of dipyridamole 200 mg and aspirin 25 mg (Aggrenox) taken twice daily has been shown to be effective in the secondary prevention of strokes,[454,455] although there is still controversy regarding its benefit over aspirin alone. Hepatic dysfunction is listed as an adverse reaction in the Epocrates database, but no literature citations could be found. On the other hand, ticlopidine, a thienopyridine inhibitor of platelet ADP-induced aggregation with thrombolytic effects,[456] is more effective than aspirin in preventing stroke.[457] Ticlopidine was first reported in 1993[458] to cause hepatitis, and subsequent reports from many countries[459-463] have confirmed that the drug causes a primarily cholestatic injury. Presentation was between 2 and 13 weeks and was not correlated with the degree of platelet inhibition.[463] The hepatotoxicity can be associated with red cell aplasia,[460] and an

immune mechanism is therefore likely. Because of these side effects, another antiplatelet drug, clopidogrel, has become more popular[464] and was used successfully in one patient with ticlopidine hepatotoxicity.[465] This was despite the fact that clopidogrel is also a thienopyridine and has been reported to cause fatal liver injury.[466] However, clopidogrel requires hepatic activation,[467] and variable resistance to its efficacy has been found because of lack of activation by CYP3A4.[468] Besides monitoring for antiplatelet effects, it is important to review medications that might inhibit CYP3A4 in patients using clopidogrel therapy. So far, only one case report of a mixed hepatocellular and cholestatic injury has appeared, in 2000.[469] Therefore clopidogrel probably has low hepatotoxicity (**Table 25-15**).

Hepatotoxicity attributable to warfarin is exceedingly rare, with only two case reports in the past decade,[470,471] and in both cases the patients had been taking phenprocoumon before the warfarin was administered. Cross-reactivity and rechallenge confirmed the sensitivity. Phenprocoumon, not available in the United States, led to at least eight cases of severe hepatitis in Germany between 1992 and 2002, with one death and two patients requiring liver transplantation.[472]

Although no significant hepatotoxicity is reported with heparin, a number of the low-molecular-weight heparins are listed in the Epocrates database as causing increased serum ALT levels. For tinzaparin, cholestatic hepatitis is listed. However, only one citation[473] could be found that reported increased ALT levels for tinzaparin, and a more recent report[474] suggested that attribution of such increases is often erroneous (e.g., more careful investigation of a reaction attributable to dalteparin determined that it was instead attributable to ranitidine). Enoxaparin has been reported to cause elevated levels of transaminases,[475] including one recent case. Of presumed hepatotoxicity.[476] No literature citation for liver toxicity could be found for the direct thrombin inhibitor lepirudin, and a recent review including postmarketing surveillance did not mention hepatotoxicity.[477]

Angiotensin-Converting Enzyme Inhibitors

All of these drugs have an excellent safety profile, although hepatotoxicity and increased serum ALT levels are listed in the Epocrates database. Many of the angiotensin-converting enzyme (ACE) inhibitors have been shown to have a low incidence of causing cholestatic hepatitis,[155,241] including captopril,[478,479] lisinopril,[480] fosinopril,[481] and ramipril.[482] Patients who developed cholestasis were generally middle-aged and had been taking the drug for between 4 and 8 weeks. Most cases displayed a long recovery time. The sole fatality was a patient who had been continued on lisinopril for 3 weeks after developing jaundice and whose death was attributed to a perforated ulcer while his cholestasis was improving.[480] Currently there are no known risk factors for developing cholestasis.

Angiotensin II Receptor Blockers

These agents, best characterized by losartan, can cause an idiosyncratic hepatitic reaction,[483,484] and candesartan,[485] irbesartan,[486] and valsartan[487] have been reported to cause cholestatic hepatitis. Onset of clinical illness was always just a few weeks after starting therapy and resolution was relatively rapid

Table 25-15 Cardiovascular Drugs and DILI

Reported to Cause Liver Injury

Antiplatelets/Anticoagulants/Thrombolytics

Dipyridamole/ASA (Aggrenox)	±Hepatic dysfunction
Ticlopidine (Ticlid)	Definite cholestatic
Warfarin (Coumadin)	±Hepatitis/cholestatic jaundice
Dalteparin (Fragmin)	±↑ALT
Tinzaparin (Innohep)	±Cholestatic hepatitis
Enoxaparin (Lovenox)	±↑ALT
Lepirudin (Refludan)	±↑ALT

ACE Inhibitors

All the "-prils"	Reports of cholestatic jaundice

Angiotensin Receptor Blockers

All the "-sartans"	Hepatotoxicity, ↑ALT

Antiarrhythmics

Amiodarone (Cordarone, Pacerone)	↑ALT, phospholipidosis
Quinidine (Quinidex)	Immune mixed with granulomas
Procainamide	Immune cholestasis with granulomas
Propafenone (Rythmol)	Rare cholestasis

β-Blockers

Labetatolol (Trandate, Normodyne)	↑ALT, hepatitic, nonimmune

Ca2+ Channel Blockers

Nifedipine	Rare hepatitic, immune
Diltiazem (Cardizem)	Rare hepatitic, rare granulomas
Verapamil	Rare hepatitic or cholestatic

Cholesterol Lowering

All statins	↑ALT, rare hepatitic, cholestatic
Fenofibrate	Rare autoimmune picture
Niacin (slow release > crystalline)	Rare acute hepatitic/cholestatic

Other Antihypertensives

Hydralazine	Very rare immune hepatitic, granulomas
Bosentan (Tracleer)	↑ALT, too new to characterize

Not Reported to Cause Significant Liver Injury

Antiplatelets/Anticoagulants/Thrombolytics

Alteplase (Activase), clopidogrel (Plavix), anagrelide (Agrylin), dipyridamole (Persantine), eptifibatide (Integrilin), cilostazol (Pletal), tirofiban (Aggrastat), abciximab (ReoPro), fondaparinux (Arixta), bivalirudin (Angiomax), argatroban, antithrombin III (ATnativ), anistreplase (Eminase), streptokinase (Kabikinase), urokinase (Abbokinase), reteplase (Retevase), tenecteplase (TNKase)

Antiarrhythmics

Adenosine, bretylium, sotalol (Betapace), ibutilide (Corvert), moricizine (Ethmozine), mexiletine (Mexitil), disopyramide (Norpace), flecanide (Tambocor), dofetilide (Tikosyn)

β-Blockers

Almost all except labetolol appear without significant toxicity

Ca2+ Channel Blockers

All but verapamil and diltiazem appear safe

Cholesterol Lowering

Gemfibrazole (Lopid), ezetimibe (Zetia)

Diuretics

All loop and thiazide diuretics appear without significant hepatotoxicity

Other Antihypertensives

Minoxidil (Loniten), eplerenone (Inspra), treprostinil (Remodulin), epoprostenol (Flolan), fenoldopam (Corlopam), doxazosin (Cardura), clonidine (Catapres), terazosin (Hytrin), guanabenz (Wytensin), prazosin (Minipress), nesiritide (Natrecor)

ALT, alanine aminotransferase.

after discontinuation of the drug. The incidence of this reaction appears to be low.

Antiarrhythmic Drugs

Amiodarone is a highly effective and widely used iodinated benzofuran antiarrhythmic that has long been known to cause liver injury.[241] Its pulmonary toxicity is more serious, but elevations in serum aminotransferase or AP levels are common.[488,489] Amiodarone was the drug most commonly associated with liver injury in one tertiary hepatology referral center.[446]

The spectrum of amiodarone liver injury is broad. An acute hepatitis can occur within 24 hours of starting parenteral therapy,[490] but the incidence of this is difficult to assess because the drug is usually used during cardiac arrests and the majority of patients do not survive. Asymptomatic elevations of liver enzyme levels occur in about 25% of patients using oral therapy, usually detected 10 months after exposure, with the mean ALT level (104 units/ml) greater than the mean AST level (89 units/ml) and generally normal AP and bilirubin levels. Although adaptation may occur, with normalization of values on continued use, the drug is often stopped because of toxicities to other organs and death from heart disease.[488] Between 1% and 3% of patients develop symptomatic hepatitis, with hepatomegaly that resolves relatively quickly on drug withdrawal. The drug and its metabolite remain in liver and plasma for long periods and can cause persistent abnormalities for many months after cessation of therapy.[488]

The most ominous form of liver injury with amiodarone is the development of cirrhosis that has been termed pseudoalcoholic based on the findings of Mallory bodies, polymorphonuclear leukocytes, and steatosis,[491] and this can occur even with low doses of the drug.[494] Regular monitoring of serum ALT level is recommended, especially if doses greater than 400 mg/day are used. Decreasing the dose or discontinuing the drug if ALT levels are more than three times the ULN and performing a liver biopsy if elevations persist are also recommended. A recent prospective study of serum amiodarone levels in 125 patients suggested that only 6% will have serum ALT levels more than three times the ULN if amiodarone levels are <2.5 mg/L, and there should be no ALT level elevations if amiodarone levels are <1.5 mg/L.[493]

Amiodarone is metabolized by CYP3A4 and CYP2C8[494] to N-desethylamiodarone.[494] The drug and metabolite accumulate in the liver because they are amphiphilic, becoming trapped in lysosomes and subsequently inhibiting phospholipases.[241] Even in patients without liver injury, intralysosomal inclusions are found with a characteristic lamellar structure on electron microscopy that is the hallmark of phospholipidosis.[495] Because of amiodarone's iodine content, hepatic accumulation can be demonstrated on noncontrast CT scans.[496] The drug can also accumulate in mitochondria and cause lipid peroxidation and steatohepatitis in animal models.[497] However, the mechanism that amiodarone (or a metabolite) employs to cause hepatic injury is still unclear. The drug is also an inhibitor of the organic anion transporter oatp2 in rats.[498]

Quinidine remains an important antiarrhythmic despite many case reports from the 1970s describing idiosyncratic hypersensitivity hepatotoxic reactions that occurred within a month of therapy,[241] often with granulomas on histologic analysis.[499] No recent case reports have appeared, and the incidence of hepatotoxicity is not really known. Another important effect of quinidine recently recognized is its ability to heteroactivate CYP3A4 activity for other substrates.[500,501] Therefore complex drug interactions should be expected when using quinidine.

Although only mild abnormalities of liver tests are listed in the Epocrates database for procainamide, the drug has been reported to cause intrahepatic cholestasis in a number of cases,[241] often with granulomas. The drug is much more likely to cause a systemic lupus-like reaction than hepatotoxicity. Propafenone is not listed to have any hepatotoxicity, but seven cases of cholestatic jaundice have been reported in the literature since 1980.[502]

β-Blockers

All of these widely used agents have a very low incidence of hepatotoxicity, with the possible exception of labetalol.[503,504] Labetalol causes mild asymptomatic ALT level increases in 8% of patients, usually within the first few weeks of therapy. Although ALT levels usually normalize with continued therapy (a poorly understood phenomenon that has sometimes been dubbed "adaptation"), they may worsen in 2% of patients, requiring drug withdrawal. Three fatalities have been reported,[503] and the RR-stereoisomer of labetalol, dilevalol, was withdrawn in postmarketing surveillance outside the United States in 1990 because of hepatotoxicity (see **Table 25-1**). The mechanism of injury appears to be idiosyncratic without immune features. Only one case report (of an acute hepatitis) was found for DILI ascribed to metoprolol.[505] More recently, a case of severe cholestasis was reported for carvedilol,[506] which recurred 1 year later when the patient began taking metoprolol. Considering the wide use of these agents, it appears that hepatotoxicity is very rare.

Ca²⁺ Channel Blockers

These agents appear to have a very low incidence of hepatotoxicity, with only verapamil and diltiazem listed in the Epocrates database. Still, nifedipine has been reported to cause acute hepatitis with immune features,[507] with the last report published in 1992.[508] The cases of acute hepatic injury described after diltiazem[509] were both in patients who had been taking nifedipine before their exposure to diltiazem. Diltiazem has been reported to cause granulomatous hepatitis.[510] Verapamil has been reported to cause a few cases of both hepatitic and cholestatic injury.[511]

Diuretics

Although rare hepatotoxicity is listed in the Epocrates database for **hydrochlorothiazide, ethacrynic acid,** and **spironolactone,** no citations could be found. Considering the widespread use of these agents in relatively sick patients, including those with liver disease, it is clear that they have very little hepatotoxicity. The uricosuric diuretic **tienilic acid** was withdrawn from the market in 1979 because of a large number of cases of acute and chronic hepatitis, most likely the result of an immune-mediated process.[512]

Other Antihypertensive Agents, Including Prescription Drugs for Pulmonary Hypertension

Hydralazine is not listed in the Epocrates database to cause any form of hepatotoxicity. However, its congener, **dihydralazine** (no longer available in the United States), is a classic drug that causes immune-mediated drug-induced toxicity[109] attributable to mechanism-based inactivation of CYPs 1A2 and 3A4,[513] which then creates a neoantigen and the development of antimicrosomal antibodies. Most case reports of hepatotoxicity from dihydralazine[514] and hydralazine[515] are from the 1980s and show classic centrilobular necrosis. Granulomatous hepatitis attributable to hydralazine has also been reported.[516] Apparently, hydralazine must not inactivate CYPs to the extent of dihydralazine, and the incidence of hepatotoxicity is low.

From a historical perspective, **α-methyldopa** (Aldomet) was one of the first drugs in widespread use that was noted to have hepatotoxicity, but with a low enough incidence that it was not withdrawn from the market. It was introduced in 1960, remains available in the United States, and continues to cause serious DILI, even though there now are many more effective and less risky antihypertensives. All forms of liver injury, including acute hepatitis, chronic hepatitis, cholestatic hepatitis, fulminant liver failure, and cirrhosis, have been associated with its use.[241]

Bosentan is an orally available benzenesulfonamide designed to potently inhibit both endothelin receptor A and endothelin receptor B.[517] It has been FDA approved to treat pulmonary hypertension[518,519] but has significant hepatotoxicity that occurs in 2% to 18% of patients, is dose related, and is reversible with drug withdrawal.[520] It is interesting that blocking endothelin receptors with the drug was initially shown to protect the livers of experimental animals from warm ischemia,[521] and it was beneficial in portal-hypertensive rats.[522] When the drug was studied in humans, it became apparent that it was extensively metabolized by CYPs 2C9 and 3A4, and its induction of these same enzymes caused a drop in initial steady-state concentrations for as long as 3 to 5 days.[519] It was also found to have important interactions with 3A4 and 2C9 substrates such as cyclosporin and warfarin.[519] Although the mechanism of hepatotoxicity is still not certain, bosentan's ability to inhibit the canalicular bile salt export pump may cause intracellular accumulation of cytotoxic bile salts.[520] Despite its potential for hepatotoxicity, it has been used successfully for the treatment of portopulmonary hypertension.[523-525] **Sildenafil** has become more popular for treatment of portopulmonary hypertension. It can rarely cause cholestatic liver injury.[526] **Epoprostenol** infusions, used for pulmonary hypertension, do not appear to cause hepatotoxicity, but inhaled **iloprost** is listed in the Epocrates database as causing LFT abnormalities.

Cholesterol-Lowering Agents

Hydroxymethylglutaryl-Coenzyme A Reductase Inhibitors (Statins)

The introduction of the statins has made a major impact on the therapy of hypercholesterolemia and heart disease, making these agents among the most widely prescribed medications.

However, because these are long-term medications, there was early concern about ocular, muscle, and liver toxicities that had been seen with previous inhibitors of cholesterol synthesis.[241,527] Ocular toxicity did not occur, but asymptomatic increases in serum ALT levels more than twice the ULN were found in 1% to 3% of subjects in early studies, which was 10 to 30 times more frequent than rhabdomyolysis.[527] The increases occurred within 3 months and there was a dose dependence. There were also a number of severe cases of acute hepatitis and cholestatic injury reported.[155] Therefore recommendations were to avoid the use of statins in patients with almost any liver disease. Unfortunately, following these recommendations would deny many patients with high cholesterol levels the benefit of these drugs, because these patients often have increased levels of serum aminotransferases as part of their metabolic syndrome.

Postmarketing surveillance studies of the statins have shown that asymptomatic ALT level increases occur in 0.2% to 1.14% of patients[528,529] and that the majority of patients have adaptation and normalization of ALT levels with continued therapy. Studies in specific groups, including children with familial hypercholesterolemia,[530] obese patients,[531] elderly patients,[532] and patients with increases before therapy,[533] showed that all tolerated statin therapy with a low incidence of side effects. It is still recommended that liver tests and creatine kinase (CK) levels be monitored at baseline, 3 months, and then every 6 months,[534] although it has not been demonstrated that this will identify those patients at risk of, nor reduce the occurrence of, severe liver or muscle toxicity.[155] Serum ALT levels more than three times the ULN should be monitored every 2 to 4 weeks, and the drug discontinued if adaptation fails to occur or clinical symptoms develop. The dose should be adjusted as low as possible to control cholesterol. When using a statin that is metabolized by CYP3A4 (simvastatin, lovastatin, and atorvastatin), caution is necessary if prescribing other medications that inhibit this CYP (e.g., ketoconazole, erythromycin). Fluvastatin is metabolized by CYP2C9, and pravastatin and rosuvastatin are not metabolized by the P450 system. There are also warnings concerning the combination of statins with gemfibrozil, niacin, amiodarone, and verapamil.[534] Cerivastatin was withdrawn from the market in 1991 because of a high frequency of rhabdomyolysis, not because of liver injury.

Serious DILI from statins seems to be rare based upon their widespread chronic use and results from large databases or cohorts.[104,107,108,535] In a retrospective study of DILI leading to death or transplantation from the Swedish Adverse Drugs Reaction Advisory Committee (SADRAC) database, there were 151 cases with a fatal outcome and 17 patients who underwent liver transplantation from 1966 to 2002.[535] There was one case each of DILI attributed to atorvastatin and simvastatin. Among 4690 suspected DILI cases reported from 1968 to 2003 to the WHO Collaborating Center for Drug Monitoring, a statin was not one of the top 20 drugs associated with fatality from DILI.[104] A population-based study was conducted over a 3-year period in a region of France with a population of 81,301; 34 cases of DILI were reported.[107] A statin (atorvastatin) was the single implicated drug in two cases or one of mutiple implicated drugs (both atorvastatin and ticlodipine). The Spanish drug-induced liver injury study is a prospective study of DILI from centers in Spain.[105] The investigators for the Spanish Registry reported 461 cases collected over a 10-year period. Statins were incriminated in 11 cases with a mean serum total bilirubin level of 6.1 mg/dl, mean ALT level of 15.8 times the ULN, and mean alkaline phosphatase level of 2.8 times the ULN.

In a systemic review of serious DILI from statins, 40 cases of statin hepatotoxicity were identified.[536] In 11 cases, autoantibodies were detected with or without DILI. Given the vast number of prescriptions written for this class of drug, more than 142 million in the United States in 2008 alone, the relatively small number of published case reports is a testament to the hepatic safety of statins.[537] The majority of these reports have occurred with lovastatin, simvastatin, and atorvastatin, probably reflecting their time on the market and numbers of prescriptions written. Despite differences in pharmacokinetics, lipophilicity, and degree of hepatic metabolism,[538] all statins appear capable of causing rare but significant hepatotoxicity. Presenting symptoms have generally been consistent with an acute hepatitis, including jaundice, anorexia, nausea, abdominal pain, fatigue, and pruritus. Mortality secondary to statin-induced DILI is exceedingly uncommon and identified in only two of the case reports.[539,540]

Among the reported cases identified in the systematic review the duration of statin therapy before the development of symptomatic hepatotoxicity from statins is highly variable, ranging from 5 days to 4 years.[536] In more than half the cases, DILI occurred within 4 months of instituting statin therapy. The time from cessation of statin use until resolution of hepatotoxicity ranges from several weeks to 6 months. The most common pattern of liver injury is hepatocellular, with peak ALT levels varying from 39 to 8275 units/L, although a mixed injury pattern with prolonged symptomatic cholestasis may occur. In cases of mixed injury, the peak serum total bilirubin level has been reported as high as 25 mg/dl, but most cases report total bilirubin levels of 5 to 10 mg/dl.

On liver biopsy the most frequent histologic features of DILI from statins are portal inflammation with mononuclear cells with or without cholestasis. The portal inflammation typically includes lymphocytes, and although eosinophils were noted in a few cases, they are not commonly prominent. Changes on liver biopsy may not be due to statins, however, because these patients may have preexisting underlying fatty liver disease and/or liver fibrosis. Statin-induced liver injury may occasionally present with an autoimmune phenotype.[542] This pattern of liver injury on biopsy was reported with atorvastatin, rosuvastatin, and simvastatin. These cases could represent sporadic autoimmune hepatitis (AIH) presenting in someone who happened to be prescribed a statin, although the evidence for statins serving as a trigger is strong. High titers of autoantibodies, suchs as ANA, anti–smooth muscle antibody, antihistone antibodies, and acetylcholine-binding antibodies, may be seen in patients with DILI from statins.

The pathogenesis of this type of DILI remains to be elucidated, but proposed mechanisms include the drug serving as a hapten for cellular targets in genetically predisposed hosts with specific HLA haplotypes (DR3,4) who are reexposed to the same statin or another statin.[541] The exact mechanism of liver injury is not known, but studies in guinea pigs administered 125 mg/kg/day of simvastatin suggest toxicity is a result of inhibition of hydroxymethylglutaryl-coenzyme A (HMG-CoA) reductase and mevalonate synthesis.[540] The mevalonate pathway is important for production of cell membrane proteins, anchoring of proteins, and biosynthesis of steroids.

As a drug class, statins are remarkably safe, including in patients with chronic liver disease or a history of elevated liver tests. A randomized, double-blind, placebo-controlled study of 326 subjects with underlying liver disease treated with 80 mg of pravastatin or placebo demonstrated no significant difference in serum ALT level elevations between the 2 groups.[543] The rate either of the serum ALT level elevation exceeding two times the ULN or of doubling of the baseline ALT level (if the baseline ALT level was already elevated) was 5% in the pravastatin group and 7% in the placebo group. No statistical differences in ALT level doubling were demonstrated in the pravastatin group or placebo group regardless of whether the baseline ALT level was elevated. Most of the subjects in the study had chronic liver disease from nonalcoholic fatty liver disease (NAFLD) (64.1%) or chronic hepatitis C (24.8%). The U.S. DILIN Registry prospective study reported the results of the first 300 enrolled cases in 2008.[106] Lipid-lowering agents were reported to be the causative agent in 3.4% of cases. One patient with cirrhosis treated with ezetimibe and simvastatin died and one patient with rheumatoid arthritis treated with leflunomide and lovastatin underwent a liver transplant.

The following are recommendations from The National Lipid Association Safety Task Force regarding the safety of statins with a focus on patients with chronic liver disease[544]: (1) chronic liver disease is not a contraindication to statin therapy; (2) compensated cirrhosis is not a contraindication to statin therapy; (3) statins can be prescribed safely to patients with nonalcoholic fatty liver disease (NAFLD). Based upon expert opinion, the authors also concluded that statins should not be used in patients with decompensated cirrhosis or acute liver failure. Furthermore, patients should not reinitiate statin therapy if they experienced prior liver test elevations presumably attributable to statin use.

Fenofibrate has been used for decades and is effective for the management of hypertriglyceridemia. It has been reported to rarely cause an autoimmune hepatitis with ductopenia and fibrosis.[155] Mild ALT level increases occur rarely, and routine monitoring of liver tests is not considered necessary.[545] Although the fibrates are potent peroxisomal proliferator agents in rodents, this effect is not seen in humans based on analysis of liver histologic findings.[241] The fibrates can also increase the lithogenicity of bile, but this effect does not appear to be clinically significant.[545]

Niacin has also been shown to cause an acute hepatitis[241] that occurs more frequently with the sustained-release form, usually after a relatively short time (2 days to 7 weeks),[546] and often immediately after changing from the crystalline formulation that was well tolerated.[547,548] A cholestatic picture has also been described.[549] Overall, the incidence of hepatotoxicity must be low. There is some indication that toxicity may be dose related,[241] but the mechanism of liver injury has never been clarified.

Nonsteroidal Antiinflammatory Drugs and Acetaminophen

Nonsteroidal antiinflammatory drugs (NSAIDs) as a class are important causative agents of hepatotoxicity. Although the incidence of hepatotoxicity varies for different agents, the overall incidence of overt dysfunction is low (less than 0.1%).[550] However, because of the large number of people who use NSAIDs on a regular basis (approximately 20 million in the United States alone), the actual number of cases that occur is ultimately substantial.[550] In the U.S. DILIN Registry, NSAIDs and muscle relaxants accounted for 5% of serious DILI cases.[106] It is estimated, from Medicaid billing data, that acute hepatitis, probably related to NSAID use, results in about 2.2 hospitalizations per 100,000 people.[551] In a retrospective Canadian study of 228 adult patients who contributed 645 person-years, the age- and gender-matched risk ratio for hospitalization for acute liver injury related to NSAID use was 1.7, or about 5 episodes per 100,000 patient-years.[552] A systematic review of population-based studies reported the risk of serious liver injury in NSAID users was 3.1 to 23.4 per 100,000 patient-years.[553] Risk factors for the development of hepatotoxicity from NSAIDs include advanced age, renal insufficiency, multiple drug use, and high doses.[554] Different NSAIDs have different propensities to cause hepatotoxicity. Benoxaprofen proved to be an agent that caused liver injury with a high incidence and fatalities, prompting its withdrawal from medical use. Other agents have minimal potential for hepatotoxicity. NSAIDs that are capable of causing hepatotoxicity are listed in **Table 25-16**. In a systematic review of 67 articles and 65 studies from the FDA archives, diclofenac and

rofecoxib had the highest rates of elevations of aminotransferase levels—more than three times the upper limit of normal.[555] The most common mechanism of injury appears to be idiosyncratic, probably as a result of metabolic abnormalities, and the most common type of injury appears to be hepatocellular. Polymorphisms in glutathione S-transferase have been reported to be associated with DILI from antibacterials and NSAIDs.[556] Cross-reactivity between different classes of NSAIDs may occur.[557]

The primary risk factor for **aspirin**-induced hepatotoxicity appears to be the dose of the drug, and hence frequency correlates with the serum salicylate levels.[550] Most patients with hepatotoxicity, as evidenced by elevated aminotransferase levels, are taking 2 to 6 g of aspirin daily and have serum levels of salicylates exceeding 25 mg/dl, although toxicity has been seen at levels as low as 10 mg/dl.[558] Predisposing conditions have also been suggested as being risk factors. These include the connective tissue disorders rheumatoid arthritis, systemic lupus erythematosus (SLE), and juvenile rheumatoid arthritis. However, the increased incidence in this subgroup is probably explained largely by the higher doses used in treating these conditions, rather than an intrinsic susceptibility, although the cytokine milieu in systemic inflammatory diseases may predispose to hepatotoxicity.[559] The same explanations are likely for the increased incidence seen in cases of rheumatic fever.

Table 25-16 Nonsteroidal Antiinflammatory Drugs and DILI

CLASS/AGENT	TYPE OF INJURY	PROPOSED MECHANISM	CLASS/AGENT	TYPE OF INJURY	PROPOSED MECHANISM
Salicylates			Fenoprofen	Hepatocellular/cholestatic	Idiosyncratic
Aspirin	Hepatocellular	Toxic	Flurbiprofen	Hepatocellular	Idiosyncratic-metabolic
Diflunisal	Cholestatic	Idiosyncratic-metabolic	Ibufenac	Hepatocellular	Idiosyncratic-metabolic
Benorilate	Hepatocellular	Toxic	Ibuprofen	Hepatocellular	Idiosyncratic-metabolic
Salicylates	Hepatocellular	Toxic	Ketoprofen	Hepatocellular	Idiosyncratic-immune
Acetic Acid Derivatives			Naprosyn	Hepatocellular/cholestatic	Idiosyncratic-immune
Amfenac	Hepatocellular	Idiosyncratic-metabolic	Oxaprozin	Hepatocellular	Idiosyncratic-immune
Clometacin	Hepatocellular	Idiosyncratic-metabolic	Pirprofen	Hepatocellular	Idiosyncratic-metabolic
Diclofenac	Hepatocellular	Idiosyncratic-metabolic	**Fenamates**		
Etodolac	Hepatocellular	Idiosyncratic	Cinchophen	Hepatocellular	Idiosyncratic-metabolic
Fenclofenac	Hepatocellular	Idiosyncratic-metabolic	Glafenine	Hepatocellular	Idiosyncratic-metabolic
Fenclofenamic acid	Hepatocellular	Idiosyncratic-metabolic	Meclofenamic acid	Hepatocellular	Idiosyncratic-metabolic
Fenclozic acid	Cholestatic	Idiosyncratic-metabolic	Mefenamic acid	Hepatocellular	Idiosyncratic-metabolic
Fentiazac	Hepatocellular	Idiosyncratic-metabolic	Niflumic acid	Hepatocellular	Idiosyncratic-immune
Indomethacin	Hepatocellular	Idiosyncratic	Tolfenamic acid	Hepatocellular	Idiosyncratic-metabolic
Isoxepac	Hepatocellular	Idiosyncratic-metabolic	**Oxicams**		
Nabumetone	Cholestatic	Idiosyncratic	Droxicam	Hepatocellular/cholestatic	Idiosyncratic
Sulindac	Cholestatic	Idiosyncratic-immune	Isoxicam	Cholestatic	Idiosyncratic-metabolic
Tolmetin	Hepatocellular	Idiosyncratic	Piroxicam	Hepatocellular/cholestatic	Idiosyncratic
Propionic Acid Derivatives			Sudoxicam	Hepatocellular	Idiosyncratic-metabolic
Benoxaprofen	Cholestatic	Idiosyncratic-metabolic			
Carpofen	Hepatocellular	Idiosyncratic-metabolic			
Fenbufen	Hepatocellular	Idiosyncratic-metabolic			

In patients who develop Reye's syndrome, aspirin intake appears to be one of the most common—if not the most common—triggers for the development of its characteristic features, namely, a microvesicular hepatic steatosis and acute encephalopathy. This occurs in the setting of a febrile illness in children, most commonly induced by a viral infection. The underlying predisposing condition is as yet unclear, but may involve congenital mitochondrial enzyme defects or deficiencies, the effect of which is exacerbated by the use of aspirin.[550,560] In experimental animals, salicylic acid inhibits mitochondrial β-oxidation of long-chain fatty acids,[561] and up to one third of children who develop Reye's syndrome have inborn errors of metabolism in this pathway.[562] The incidence of Reye's syndrome is decreasing, mirroring the decline in use of aspirin for childhood viral illnesses.[550] In this dose-dependent type of hepatotoxicity the mechanism is probably related to an intrinsic ability to injure the hepatocyte. Based on the ultrastructural histology, the site of injury appears to be the mitochondria. Other mechanisms that have been postulated include lipid peroxidation, hydroxyl radical scavenging, and injury to the hepatocyte membrane.[550]

Apart from the features of the disease condition necessitating the use of aspirin, findings are minimal. Tender hepatomegaly may occur. Liver injury is most often recognized by determining elevated serum AST and ALT levels, and, less commonly, ammonia and bilirubin levels. Up to 50% of individuals with serum levels of salicylate greater than 15 mg/dl have elevated AST and ALT levels.[558] Acute liver failure, characterized by coagulation abnormalities and hepatic encephalopathy, is rare.[563] The classic histologic description of liver injury from aspirin is a nonspecific focal hepatitis. Ballooning degeneration that is more prominent in zone 3 is a typical finding. Hepatocyte necrosis is also seen, and inflammatory cell infiltration is minimal. Steatosis is unusual in the hepatotoxicity associated with high doses of aspirin. However, in Reye's syndrome microvesicular steatosis is the hallmark. Aspirin hepatotoxicity is rapidly reversible when the drug is discontinued. Fatalities are very rare but have been reported.[564] There is no conclusive evidence that aspirin can cause chronic hepatitis.

Aspirin overdose is managed by discontinuation of the drug, with supportive care in the rare individual who has severe hepatotoxicity. If aspirin is absolutely essential in the individual's management, an attempt may be made to restart the drug at a lower dose after the liver tests have returned to normal. Close monitoring of the liver tests in this rechallenge is necessary.

Diflunisal (Dolobid) is a difluorophenyl derivative of salicylic acid that has been reported to cause a cholestatic and mixed hepatocellular type injury.[565,566]

Indomethacin (Indocin), an indole-containing acetic acid derivative, is probably the most frequently used NSAID of this class. There are relatively few reports of indomethacin-related hepatic injury compared with other organ toxicities caused by this drug.[550,567] In one series, although indomethacin accounted for relatively fewer instances of hepatotoxicity (compared with other NSAIDs), the incidence of fatalities was higher.[567] Case fatalities have been reported.[567-569] Children may be more susceptible to severe injury, and therefore the drug is not recommended for use in the pediatric age group.[550]

Based on the few case reports available, the mechanism of toxicity appears to be metabolic idiosyncrasy. Features are usually nonspecific, with laboratory values suggesting hepatocellular injury, and much less often concomitant cholestasis. Massive hepatocellular necrosis, primarily centrally located,[568] is typical. Microvesicular steatosis and cholestasis may occur. Discontinuation of the drug and supportive measures should be instituted. A good outcome is expected with early detection and withdrawal. However, case fatalities have been reported.

Sulindac (Clinoril) is also an indole derivative of acetic acid and therefore has some structural similarities to indomethacin. There are many reported cases of hepatotoxicity related to this drug, which is a potent analgesic and has relatively fewer gastrointestinal side effects than other NSAIDs. However, it is still considered one of the most likely NSAIDs to produce hepatic injury.[550] In an analysis of 91 cases reported to the FDA, the ratio of females to males was $3:5$.[570] Based on the reported cases, the mechanism for most appeared to be a generalized immunoallergic hypersensitivity reaction, which included liver involvement. Metabolic idiosyncrasy may account for a minor subset.[570] Patients present with features of a hypersensitivity reaction, including fever, skin rash, pruritus, and tender hepatomegaly. Stevens-Johnson syndrome may occur. The onset is usually within 4 weeks of starting the drug.[571-573] Jaundice occurs in about two thirds of cases.[570] Laboratory tests often reveal significant hepatocellular damage. Eosinophilia tends to be more common when the pattern of injury is cholestatic than when it is primarily hepatocellular.[570] Pancreatitis may occur in some cases.[574] Cholestasis is prominent in most cases, with only about 25% showing hepatocellular injury.[570] Five percent (4 cases of 91) of patients with sulindac-associated jaundice died.[570] Although the cause of death in most cases was attributable to systemic hypersensitivity, death from liver failure secondary to massive hepatocellular necrosis can occur.[570] Rechallenge with the drug may result in the reappearance of the hypersensitivity reaction after only a few doses.[572]

Diclofenac (Arthrotec, Voltaren) is a phenylacetic acid derivative that has been in use for some time. Although the most common manifestation of hepatotoxicity is asymptomatic elevations in liver tests, there are numerous reports in the literature of significant hepatotoxicity and even fatalities attributable to the use of this drug.[575,576] It is estimated that up to 5 of 100,000 individuals have significant hepatotoxicity. The onset is from 3 weeks to 12 months after starting the drug.[575,576] Elderly women with osteoarthritis seem to be more susceptible.[575] Among 17,829 patients treated with diclofenac for arthritis over a mean of 18 months, 0.5% developed AST or ALT levels more than 10 times the upper limit of normal, 0.023% of patients required liver-related hospitalization, and none of the patients died or required liver transplant. Aminotransferase level elevations occurred primarily during the first 4 to 6 months of therapy.[555] Data from the reports suggest that in most cases the cause is immunologic idiosyncrasy. However, metabolic idiosyncrasy has seemed to be the more logical explanation in other cases. Polymorphisms in the genes encoding UDPGT2B7, CYP2C8, and ABCC2 have been reported to be associated with diclofenac DILI. The strongest association was seen with the UDPGT2B7*2 allele, which was 8.5 times more common in individuals who developed DILI from diclofenac compared with controls.[577]

Symptoms are nonspecific in most cases, with nausea, vomiting, abdominal discomfort, and jaundice being hallmarks of more severe hepatitis. Rash and fever occur in a minority of cases. The liver test abnormalities favor hepatocellular damage. In rare cases the ANA titers may be elevated and care should be taken to rule out autoimmune chronic hepatitis.[576,578] Zone 3 or spotty acute hepatocellular necrosis is the most common histologic finding. Other features may include granulomas, cholestasis, hepatic eosinophilia, and chronic hepatitis. Overdose is managed by withdrawal of the agent and supportive care. With early withdrawal the prognosis is good, even with severe hepatitis. Rarely, the use of diclofenac has been thought to trigger development of autoimmune hepatitis.[578] Similar occurrences and features have been described also for **meloxicam** (Mobic), and likely occur with all drugs of this class.[579]

Although there have been cases of serious DILI from **ibuprofen,** both hepatocellular and cholestatic patterns of injury, its rarity as an implicated cause of DILI and almost ubiquitous use suggest ibuprofen rarely if ever causes serious DILI.[580-582]

Acetaminophen is a widely used analgesic, and compared with other drugs that are associated with liver injury, acetaminophen is available over-the-counter. Of the 76% of Americans who reported using nonprescription products in the Third National Health and Nutrition Examination Survey (NHANES III), 36% reported using acetaminophen.[582] Annual costs associated with acetaminophen toxicity are estimated at $51.5 million.[583] Acetaminophen is the most common cause of drug-induced acute liver failure in the United States.[584] Acetaminophen is the nonnarcotic analgesic of choice in patients with significant co-morbidities, such as impaired renal function, gastrointestinal disease, and bleeding disorders.

Animal studies demonstrate acetaminophen-induced liver injury is mediated through reactive oxygen species and hepatocyte apoptosis. During phase I metabolism acetaminophen undergoes oxidation, reduction, or hydrolysis by cytochrome P450 enzymes. During phase II metabolism acetaminophen metabolites are conjugated with glucuronic acid, sulfates, or glutathione. Acetaminophen is metabolized by the cytochrome CYPs and CYP2E1 is the major source of the toxic metabolite N-acetyl-p-benzoquinone (NAPQI) that depletes hepatic glutathione stores and leads to oxidative injury (see **Fig. 25-4**). NAPQI covalently binds to hepatocyte proteins and leads to cell death. Reactive oxygen species are associated with mitochondrial damage and the activation of caspases.[585] This sequence of events leads to premature apoptosis of hepatocytes. Further support of the role of the oxidative stress response as an important mechanism in acetaminophen hepatotoxicity is demonstrated in a study of metallothionein knockout mice (MT null mice).[586] MT null mice were more susceptible to acetaminophen liver injury as demonstrated by markedly elevated liver enzyme levels and hepatic necrosis compared with control mice. More lipid peroxidation was present in MT null mice based upon immunohistochemical localization of 4-hydroxynonenal and malondialdehyde protein adducts. Other transcription factors that protect against oxidative injury have been reported to be associated with acetaminophen toxicity in mice. Other enzymes and pathways associated with acetaminophen DILI include activation of the glycogen synthase kinase-3β and c-Jun-N-terminal kinase (JNK) pathways.[587] Increased mitochondrial-derived reactive oxygen species as a result of GSH depletion in mitochondria was implicated in liver injury from acetaminophen. The innate immune system and natural killer (NK) cell activation and increase in interferon-γ level have been shown to play a role in progression and severity of acetaminophen

hepatotoxicity.[588] Risk factors for acetaminophen hepatotoxicity include age, alcohol use, tobacco use, and nutritional status.[584]

Novel methods for early detection of drug-induced liver injury are needed to try to avoid serious DILI or the development of jaundice or high levels of aminotransferases. In a study of healthy volunteers administered a single 4-g dose of acetaminophen, changes in the blood transcriptome were seen 48 hours after the dose even though there were no significant increases in serum liver chemistries.[589] Genes in oxidative phosphorylation and mitochondrial function are downregulated in subjects administered acetaminophen compared with subjects administered placebo ($p < 1.66 \times 10^{-9}$). Corresponding changes were seen in the serum metabolome with an increase in lactate concentration from 24 to 72 hours after dosing.

Antineoplastic and Immunosuppressive Agents

These agents produce a large number of hepatic abnormalities (**Table 25-17**). Causality assessment of hepatotoxicity in the setting of cancer chemotherapy is often difficult for the following reasons:

1. Abnormal liver tests may result from metastasis or infiltration of the liver parenchyma or biliary tree by tumor. A Budd-Chiari–like picture may resemble sinusoidal obstruction syndrome and may occur as a result of the procoagulant state caused by many tumors.
2. Immunosuppression may result in sepsis and shock, with its attendant cytokine-induced effects on the liver, such as cholestasis. Occasionally the liver itself may be opportunistically infected, or transfusion may result in viral hepatitis.
3. Multiple drugs are often used in overlapping schedules, making it difficult to assign causality of DILI to a single drug.
4. Other modalities of treatment (i.e., nonchemotherapy) may also lead to hepatotoxicity. Examples include the direct effects of radiation and graft-versus-host disease in patients undergoing bone marrow or stem cell transplants.
5. Drugs that have minimal hepatotoxic potential when used alone may produce severe liver disease when used in combination with other chemotherapeutic agents or with radiation therapy.
6. Liver biopsy, which might help in differential diagnosis, is often contraindicated because of thrombocytopenia and coagulation abnormalities caused by treatment.
7. Toxicity in other organ systems may result in abnormal liver tests (e.g., adriamycin-induced cardiac failure may result in hepatic congestion and its resultant liver test abnormalities).

Antimetabolites

Methotrexate (MTX), a derivative of aminopterin, is a folate analogue that inhibits dihydrofolate reductase, which causes the arrest of rapidly dividing cells in the S-phase of the cell

Table 25-17 Antineoplastic and Immunosuppressive Agents and DILI

MANIFESTATION OF HEPATOTOXICITY	AGENT

Sinusoidal obstruction syndrome	Mitomycin
	6-Thioguanine
	Azathioprine
	Cytarabine
	Dacarbazine
	Indicine-*N*-oxide
	Daunorubicin
	Combination chemotherapy
	Radiation therapy plus
	  Cyclophosphamide
	  Busulfan
	  Carmustine
	  Mitomycin C
	  Other regimens

Hepatocellular necrosis	Common
	  Mithramycin
	  L-Asparaginase
	  Streptozocin
	  Methotrexate (high dose)
	Rare
	  Nitrosoureas
	  6-Thioguanines
	  Cytarabine
	  Adriamycin
	  5-Fluorouracil
	  Cyclophosphamide
	  Etoposide
	  Vinca alkaloids

Hepatic steatosis	L-Asparaginase Actinomycin D Mitomycin C Bleomycin Methotrexate
Cholestasis	6-Mercaptopurine Azathioprine Busulfan Amsacrine
Fibrosis	Methotrexate Azathioprine
Sclerosing cholangitis	Floxuridine
Peliosis hepatis	Androgens Hydroxyprogesterone Azathioprine Hydroxyurea Tamoxifen
Nodular regenerative hyperplasia	Azathioprine 6-Thioguanine Androgens Estrogens
Hepatic neoplasms	Estrogens Androgens Methotrexate

cycle. This property has been used in the treatment of leukemias and other neoplasms, and also as a disease-modifying agent in several chronic inflammatory conditions, including psoriasis, rheumatoid arthritis, and chronic idiopathic inflammatory bowel disease. Hepatotoxicity has been recognized as a potential major adverse reaction that can occur with long-term use. Case reports describing cirrhosis as a result of MTX

use first appeared in the 1960s.[590] The pathogenesis of MTX hepatotoxicity is poorly understood. It has been hypothesized that the drug can activate hepatic stellate (Ito) cells, which leads to increased collagen deposition. Others have speculated that the drug itself, and its metabolites (polyglutamates), may accumulate, leading to prolonged folate inhibition with resultant impairment of nucleotide and methionine synthesis that in turn leads to hepatocyte injury.[590] Patients with preexisting liver disease seem to be more susceptible to toxicity.[591] Factors associated with increased risk of MTX toxicity include heavy alcohol use, preexisting liver disease (especially fatty liver), daily dosing, duration of therapy more than 2 years, cumulative dose >1500 mg, and obesity with diabetes mellitus.[590] Acute symptoms are rare. With advanced toxicity and cirrhosis, clinical features will reflect these changes and are therefore nonspecific. Minor elevations in liver tests may occur in many who take methotrexate (20% to 50%), but this does not necessarily imply significant toxicity.[592] Conversely, liver tests may be normal in the setting of severe fibrosis. With advanced disease, the laboratory findings reflect those associated with cirrhosis and its complications.

In 1982 the Psoriasis Task Force (Roenigk and colleagues) devised a classification scheme for the liver biopsy findings in methotrexate hepatotoxicity (**Table 25-18**). This is probably the most popular classification scheme, despite its subjective nature. Ultrastructural changes precede microscopic changes and include the deposition of fibrous tissue in the space of Disse and an increase in the size and number of hepatic stellate (Ito) cells in the perisinusoidal space.[590] Microscopic changes include macrovesicular steatosis; nuclear variability; infiltration with chronic inflammatory cells; focal liver cell necrosis; fibrosis in the perivenular, pericellular, and portal regions; and eventually cirrhosis. Many of these findings may also be a result of other underlying conditions, many of which have been identified as being risk factors for hepatotoxicity. A systematic review of medical databases unearthed 426 references relevant to MTX use in rheumatoid or psoriatic arthritis, of which 47 were included.[593] Among persons with rheumatoid arthritis, the 3-year incidence rate of increased liver tests was 13/100 patient-years with cumulative incidence of 31%. After 4 years, liver biopsies show mild fibrosis in 15% (vs. 9% at baseline), severe fibrosis in 1.3% (vs. 0.3%), and cirrhosis in 0.5% (vs. 0.3%). The manner in which therapy should be adjusted if liver tests or biopsies are abnormal is unresolved.

There is no antidote for MTX toxicity. Patients with cirrhosis have sometimes required transplantation. Prevention of significant toxicity requires close monitoring of patients who are taking the drug long term. In cases where a preexisting liver disease is strongly suspected, a baseline, pre-MTX liver biopsy should be performed. In those with appreciable preexisting liver disease, liver tests should be monitored every 4 to 8 weeks for the first year and every 3 to 6 months thereafter for as long as the patient is taking MTX. Subjects should avoid alcohol and should take folic acid supplements. Patients with diabetes mellitus should maintain strict control of glucose levels and obese patients strongly advised to lose weight. Patients with no history of liver disease but who develop abnormal liver tests early after starting MTX (within a few months) should have a liver biopsy before continuing with further treatment. Otherwise, when the patient has received a predetermined cumulative dose (the American College of

Table 25-18 Roenigk Histopathologic Classification of Methotrexate Hepatotoxicity

	FATTY INFILTRATION	NUCLEAR VARIABILITY	PORTAL INFLAMMATION AND NECROSIS	FIBROSIS
Grade I	Mild or none	Mild or none	Mild or none	None
Grade II	Moderate to severe	Moderate to severe	Moderate to severe	None
Grade IIIa	May or may not be present	May or may not be present	May or may not be present	Mild
Grade IIIb	May or may not be present	May or may not be present	May or may not be present	Moderate to severe
Grade IV	May or may not be present	May or may not be present	May or may not be present	Cirrhosis

Rheumatology recommends after 1.5 g initially, and thereafter every 1 to 1.5 g), liver biopsies should be performed. If the Roenigk classification is used (see **Table 25-18**), the finding of grade IIIb or grade IV fibrosis is grounds to discontinue the drug.

Leflunomide is a pyrimidine synthesis inhibitor that was approved for treatment of rheumatoid arthritis in 1998 and has also been prescribed for a small number of psoriasis patients. At the time of this drug's approval, it was known that mild transient aminotransferase level elevations commonly occurred. However, in 2001, when the European EMEA reported 129 liver-related ADRs with 15 cases of ALF, subsequent careful transaminase monitoring was mandated.[594] In a recent large U.S. study,[595] elevated levels of transaminases more than twice the ULN were found in 1% to 2% of patients prescribed leflunomide or MTX monotherapy, and in 5% of patients prescribed both agents. However, no cases of ALF were mentioned and several other series have found little evidence of significant DILI.[594,596] Therefore DILI attributable to leflunomide appears to be very low.

Similar to MTX, **6-mercaptopurine (6-MP)** and **azathioprine** are probably used more frequently as immunosuppressive agents in the treatment of chronic inflammatory disorders and in the posttransplant setting than as antineoplastic agents. 6-MP has been in use for the last 60 years. It is a thiopurine analogue of the natural purine bases. Its potential to cause hepatotoxicity is well recognized. Cholestatic liver injury appears to be the most common manifestation of this toxicity and may occur in 6% to 40% of recipients.[597-599] The effect appears to be dose dependent. Doses exceeding 2.5 mg/kg have the highest likelihood of toxicity.[598,600,601] The latent period between commencement of the drug and the onset of toxicity is anywhere from 1 to 18 months. Adults appear to be more susceptible to injury than children.[602] 6-MP is metabolized extensively in the liver, and this probably relates to its hepatotoxic potential. The mechanism of toxicity appears to be intrinsic. Evidence in support of this conclusion includes the paucity of evidence that would suggest a hypersensitivity mechanism (i.e., the long lag time before the onset of symptoms, the lack of hypersensitivity features such as rash and eosinophilia). Other supporting facts include the relatively high incidence and dose dependence. Jaundice and pruritus are the main presenting features. The laboratory studies reflect a mixed hepatocellular and cholestatic injury with moderate elevations in serum AST, ALT, AP, and bilirubin levels.[600,601] Hepatic histopathology shows a mixed picture, with features of both cholestasis and hepatocellular necrosis. Management consists of discontinuing the agent. Cases of fatal hepatic necrosis, in the setting of continued use despite evidence of toxicity, have been described. Rechallenge has led to recurrent hepatotoxicity in some cases.[601]

Azathioprine is a prodrug of 6-MP and appears to be less hepatotoxic than its metabolite. This notwithstanding, it is capable of causing DILI with a spectrum of toxicity that is wider than that of 6-MP. In addition to the cholestatic injury seen with 6-MP,[603,604] other patterns have been recognized. Predominant cholestasis, with evidence of a hypersensitivity reaction, has been reported,[605] as has a primarily hepatocellular type of injury, especially in post–renal transplant patients.[606] More recently, several other lesions with a common pathogenesis, in that they involve an insult to the vascular endothelium, have been appreciated. These conditions include striking sinusoidal dilation, peliosis hepatis,[607] nodular regenerative hyperplasia,[608,609] hepatoportal sclerosis,[608] and sinusoidal obstruction syndrome (SOS).[610-612] These observations were all made in the post–renal transplant setting, and in one report about such patients the incidence of SOS was estimated to be 2.5%.[612] The onset of SOS occurs from 2 months to as long as 9 months after transplantation. There is a male preponderance. In one series co-infection with a hepatotrophic virus was suggested as a probable contributing factor in the pathogenesis of SOS.[612] Clinically, signs of portal hypertension with minimal elevations of the liver tests in a nonspecific pattern are noted. Portal hypertension may progress, which may have an effect on future morbidity and mortality.[612] The hepatotoxicity appears to be primarily an idiosyncratic reaction, although azathioprine is converted to 6-MP in vivo and direct toxicity may also play a role. As alluded to previously, patients may display features of a hypersensitivity reaction in some instances of toxicity attributable to azathioprine. Histologic features are usually classic for SOS or the other pathologies described.

6-Thioguanine is also a purine analogue, used primarily in the treatment of acute and chronic leukemia. As with azathioprine, this agent also appears to result in endothelial dysfunction leading to manifestations of SOS, nodular regenerative hyperplasia, and hepatoportal sclerosis.[598,613,614] In one study the incidence of portal hypertension in patients with chronic myeloid leukemia who were treated with busulfan alone or busulfan with 6-thioguanine was determined. In the latter group, 18 of 675 patients, compared with none in the busulfan-only group, developed portal hypertension. Histologically, idiopathic portal hypertension with minimal morphologic abnormalities or nodular regenerative hyperplasia was the major finding; three patients developed cirrhosis and its attendant complications.[613] Other studies have described SOS in patients treated with 6-thioguanine and cytosine arabinoside.[615,616]

5-Fluorouracil (5-FU) is used in the treatment of malignancies of the digestive system, breast, and ovary. It is a pyrimidine-based analogue that is metabolized by the liver with little hepatotoxicity when used orally. Floxuridine, a derivative of 5-FU, is administered by continuous intravenous infusion or by direct infusion into the hepatic artery for the treatment of hepatic metastasis from colon cancer.[617,618] This leads to higher remission rates and improved survival, but at the cost of increased hepatic injury. Damage appears to be more common with direct hepatic artery infusions,[598] which cause a chemical hepatitis in more than half of the patients treated.[619] Liver tenderness and elevations in serum AST, ALT, AP, and bilirubin levels characterize the reaction. In a smaller subset of patients sclerosing cholangitis may develop.[619-622] This is usually heralded by the onset of jaundice and marked elevations in serum AP level. In one study of intraarterial infusion all 35 patients developed a predominantly cholestatic pattern of liver tests. Seven patients receiving intraarterial therapy were studied with cholangiography, which in all cases demonstrated sclerosis of the intrahepatic or extrahepatic bile ducts. In addition, liver biopsies showed cholestasis and pericholangitis, with minimal hepatocytic damage. It was suggested that biliary sclerosis is probably more common than the often-described chemical hepatitis.[619] Chemical hepatitis usually resolves after therapy is complete or discontinued. Fatal cirrhosis has been reported to result from the more serious sclerosing cholangitis.[623] Cases with sclerosing cholangitis are managed with endoscopic retrograde cholangiopancreatography (ERCP) and stenting versus surgical therapy if complications develop or are impending. The biliary tree is highly dependent on the hepatic arterial supply for oxygenation and delivery of nutrients, and it is thought that damage or dysfunction of the arteries caused by the chemotherapeutic agent leads to the biliary sclerosis.

Cytosine arabinoside is also a pyrimidine analogue. Hepatotoxicity appears to be dose related and ranges from mild increases in serum AST, ALT, and AP levels to more significant elevations with frank jaundice.[624-627] These changes are usually reversible.

L-Asparaginase is an enzyme that catalyzes the hydrolysis of L-asparagine to aspartic acid and ammonia. Because leukemic cells cannot produce L-asparagine, whereas normal cells can, L-asparaginase is used to treat acute lymphocytic leukemia and T-cell lymphoblastic lymphoma. Abnormal liver tests have been reported in up to 75% of recipients.[628] Hypersensitivity-type reactions, especially after repeated doses, are common and have been reported in 43% of recipients, although anaphylactic-like reactions occur in only about 10% of recipients.[629,630] Steatosis, a finding more typical of a metabolic aberration, is common, occurring in 50% to 90% of recipients.[631] This is probably a result of impaired mitochondrial protein synthesis. Given the frequency of its occurrence, DILI attributable to L-asparaginase is likely to be a direct toxic effect of the drug itself (rather than metabolic idiosyncrasy). The clinical features of reactions to L-asparaginase usually develop within 1 hour after administration and include pruritus, dyspnea, urticaria, swelling at the injection site, angioedema, rash, abdominal pain, laryngospasm, nasal stuffiness, bronchospasm, and hypotension.[629] The liver test abnormalities include modestly elevated serum AST, ALT, bilirubin, and AP levels. The serum albumin levels and also levels of several other proteins that are synthesized by the liver are decreased. These proteins include factors I, II, VII, IX, and X; ceruloplasmin; haptoglobin; transferrin; and lipoproteins.[628] Coagulopathy may be a prominent feature. Elevated ammonia levels may, abnormal liver tests are common, and it is often difficult to differentiate hepatotoxicity from other toxic effects of the drug. Fatal outcomes can occur. A less immunogenic form of the drug (pegaspargase) has been developed and is reportedly less likely to result in hypersensitivity reactions.[629]

Mithramycin (plicamycin) is an antibiotic that can intercalate with DNA and thus inhibit RNA synthesis. In addition to its use as an anticancer agent, it is sometimes used in the treatment of hypercalcemia and Paget disease. Abnormal liver tests occur in almost all patients treated.[632,633] Levels of serum aminotransferases may be quite elevated, and correlate with dose. Depression of coagulation factor production and thrombocytopenia may result in a bleeding diathesis. Hepatocellular necrosis (zone 3) and steatosis have been observed in liver biopsies.[633] The lower doses used to treat hypercalcemia and Paget disease are reportedly associated with less frequent hepatotoxicity.[607] All of these features imply that mithramycin is an intrinsic hepatotoxin.

Adriamycin (doxorubicin) is also an antibiotic. It has rarely been implicated as the cause of hepatic injury. In six cases of acute lymphoblastic leukemia it was thought to have caused acute or chronic hepatitis.[634] It has also been postulated that adriamycin potentiates the hepatotoxicity of 6-MP. It may increase the incidence of radiation-induced injury when used before radiation therapy.[635] Adriamycin has a high propensity to produce cardiomyopathy that can result in congestive heart failure. The resultant liver congestion can sometimes be misleading, but reverses with appropriate treatment of the heart failure.

Dactinomycin (actinomycin D) has been used for many years without much evidence of hepatotoxicity. A few cases of severe hepatic injury have been described when the agent is used alone or with vincristine.[636-638] Cases of SOS have also been described, especially in the setting of concomitant irradiation for treatment of Wilms' tumor.[639-642]

Vinca alkaloids are derived from the periwinkle plant. Their antitumor effects are dependent on their ability to disrupt cellular microtubule function. Vincristine appears to increase liver toxicity when used with radiation therapy.[598] Rarely it may result in a mild increase in serum aminotransferase levels outside the setting of radiation.[643] Otherwise, these agents do not appear to be significant hepatotoxins.

The alkaloid **etoposide (VP-16)** is a derivative of podophyllotoxin. The drug disrupts the formation of the mitotic spindle. Acute hepatocellular necrosis has been reported.[644] In combination with ifosfamide severe hepatotoxicity has been described.[645]

Alkylating Agents

Cyclophosphamide is commonly used in treatment regimens for leukemia, lymphoma, and solid tumors. It is also used in the treatment of a few chronic inflammatory conditions, such as Wegener's granulomatosis and systemic lupus erythematosus (SLE). It is metabolized to its active form by CYPs. The alkylating species usually are formed only in cells with high turnover rates. However, hepatotoxicity may result from a metabolic idiosyncrasy in some individuals who form toxic amounts of these species in the hepatocytes. Hepatotoxicity appears to be a rare complication of therapy. There are case reports of hepatocellular necrosis that were possibly related to the use of cyclophosphamide.[646] In patients with collagen vascular diseases cyclophosphamide rarely has caused hepatic injury, including mild hepatitis to massive hepatocellular necrosis.[647] A convincing case of toxicity with resolution after withdrawal and recurrence on rechallenge was seen in a patient with SLE, who exhibited jaundice and marked elevation in serum ALT levels.[648] There are increasing reports of SOS in patients undergoing bone marrow transplantation who receive a conditioning regimen containing cyclophosphamide and busulfan.[649-652] There is a report of SOS in the nontransplant setting related to the use of cyclophosphamide.[653] **Busulfan** appears to be a contributing factor in the causation of SOS, as described previously. **Ifosfamide** has been reported to cause cholestasis when this agent is used in combination with etoposide (VP-16).[645] **Chlorambucil** rarely causes hepatotoxicity, but there is a recent report of an acute cholestatic hepatitis with its use. Older, sparse reports focus more on hepatocellular injury.[654]

Nitrosoureas (Carmustine [BCNU], Lomustine, Semustine, Streptozocin)

These compounds can all cause what appears to be reversible hepatic dysfunction, with jaundice and an elevated AST level in up to 25% of cases. Higher doses have been noted to increase the AST levels in up to 40% of patients.[655,656] With high doses of BCNU, fatal hepatic necrosis can occur. Pericholangitis and intrahepatic cholestasis accompany mild hepatic necrosis in most cases. Recent animal studies provide evidence that lipid peroxidation and alterations in the antioxidant system may significantly contribute to BCNU-induced hepatotoxicity, and some antioxidant agents may be of benefit in reducing the incidence of cholestasis.[657] **Dacarbazine** is used primarily to treat malignant melanoma and some lymphomas. Recent case reports implicate this drug in the causation of acute hepatocellular necrosis secondary to SOS.[658-660] This seems to occur within a few days of the second dose, and eosinophilia may be a feature, raising the possibility of an immunologically mediated process. Massive elevations in AST and ALT levels occur, and histologic results are consistent with those of SOS. There tends to be minimal inflammatory infiltration.[658] Management is supportive. It has been recommended that if eosinophilia develops after the first dose of dacarbazine, subsequent doses should be avoided.[658]

Immunosuppressives for Solid Organ Transplantation

Cyclosporin A, a calcineurin inhibitor extracted from *Tolypocladium inflatum,* revolutionized solid organ transplantation in the 1980s by effectively controlling organ rejection. It has a narrow therapeutic window that requires monitoring of trough serum levels, and because it is metabolized by CYP3A4, care must be taken with regard to drug interactions. Problems with erratic bioavailability led to the need for microemulsion preparations and careful twice-daily dosing. With regard to DILI, cyclosporin has been reported to cause a mild, dose-dependent cholestatic injury[594,661,662] with a highly variable frequency, and most of these cases were reported before there

were reliable assays available for monitoring cyclosporin levels. In many patients hepatotoxicity is subclinical, with liver tests revealing mild, often transient increases in AP levels, occasionally accompanied by slight elevations in serum bilirubin and aminotransferase levels. In the setting of liver transplantation, there are often multiple other potential causes of liver dysfunction (e.g., infection, organ rejection, hepatic artery thrombosis), confounding conditions that must be ruled out with imaging studies and liver biopsy. Nephrotoxicity, hypertension, dyslipidemia, and neurotoxicity are much more common problems.

Tacrolimus, formerly known as FK-506, is another calcineurin inhibitor and has become more popular than cyclosporin A because of better bioavailability and fewer cases of ADRs such as hypertension and dyslipidemia. However, it is also metabolized by CYP3A4 and requires therapeutic monitoring, and compared to cyclosporin, it causes just as much nephrotoxicity and may cause more diabetes and neurotoxicity. DILI is extremely rare, but has been reported.[594,663]

Sirolimus (rapamycin) and the related drug **everolimus** (also used in higher doses for advanced renal cell cancer) are macrocyclic lactone compounds that cause immunosuppression by binding to m-TOR (mammalian target of rapamycin). They cause less nephrotoxicity than the calcineurin inhibitors and can be used when transplant patients develop kidney injury. However, they are not used initially after transplantation because they inhibit wound healing and sirolimus may promote hepatic artery thrombosis in liver transplant patients.[594] A few cases of cholestatic DILI have been reported[663,664] but these appear to be rare events.

Mycophenolate mofetil is an antimetabolite that inhibits inosine monophosphate and has largely replaced azathioprine in solid organ transplantation because of fewer side effects. Although elevated levels of aminotransferases were reported in 14% of Turkish renal transplant patients,[665] no other significant reports of DILI from mycophenolate have been found. It appears to be unlike the thiopurines (see Antimetabolites) that can cause cholestatic, mixed cholestatic-hepatocellular, and sinusoidal obstruction syndrome.

Tyrosine Kinase Inhibitors

Imatinib (Gleevec) was the first of this class of drugs, which includes busutinib, dasatinib, INNO-406, lapatinib, and nitotinib, to be used for the treatment of leukemia. There have been major advances in long-term management of Philadelphia chromosome-positive acute lymphoblastic or chronic myelogenous leukemia, gastrointestinal stromal tumors, and others. Unfortunately, imatinib may cause DILI. About 5% of subjects develop moderate to marked increases in serum ALT levels, which rarely progresses to acute massive hepatic necrosis and fulminant liver failure.[666] Cholestatic hepatitis has also been reported.[667]

Biologic Response Modulators

Alpha-interferons (IFN-α) are used in the treatment of chronic viral hepatitis (C and B), some solid tumors (e.g., Kaposi sarcomas in patients with HIV disease), melanoma, and certain leukemias. Hepatotoxicity is extremely rare with the low percutaneous doses used to treat hepatitis. However, a few cases that probably represent induction of autoimmune hepatitis by IFN-α–induced enhancement of the immune system have been described.[668] In addition, a small subset of patients being treated for chronic hepatitis C often have mild elevations in AST and ALT levels, despite a good virologic response. These return to normal levels when the interferon is discontinued, suggesting that IFN-α plays a role in their elevation. The incidence of liver enzyme abnormalities seems somewhat more common with the pegylated than with the standard interferons.[669] Elevations of serum aminotransferase levels are more frequent with administration of the higher doses of IFN-α used in therapy of malignancies.[670,671] Rare cases of jaundice and hepatic failure have been reported with interferon alfa-2b.[671] Beta-Interferons are used increasingly in the treatment of multiple sclerosis and may cause DILI of varying severity, ranging from asymptomatic elevation of liver tests to fatal DILI.[672] A population-based review of 844 Canadian patients with multiple sclerosis who were prescribed beta-interferon showed 40% developed new elevations of serum ALT levels.[673] **Tumor necrosis factor-α (TNF-α)** is a biologic agent that is produced in response to several types of injury, such as alcoholic liver disease and chronic inflammatory bowel disease. It has been implicated in the pathogenesis of cholestasis,[674] and therefore it is not surprising that it has been found to cause profound cholestasis when it is used as treatment in advanced colorectal cancer.[675] **Anti–TNF-α drugs,** including infliximab and etanercept, have been found to reactivate latent infections, such as chronic hepatitis B or tuberculosis, and to lead to enhanced rates of replication of the hepatitis C virus. Infliximab use has been associated with severe hepatotoxicity, leading to death or the need for liver transplant. Clinical features have been variable, ranging from severe, prolonged cholestatic hepatitis (that sometimes progresses to hepatic failure and need for liver transplant[676,677]) to autoimmune hepatitis (that improved with cessation of infliximab and initiation of therapy with prednisone plus azathioprine).[677] The mechanism of injury is uncertain, but an immunoallergic reaction may be involved.

Interleukin-2 (IL-2) immunotherapy is associated with the development of profound reversible cholestasis and hyperbilirubinemia in a large proportion of patients (up to 85%) who receive it.[678-684] There is evidence to suggest that this reversible cholestasis is a direct result of IL-2–dependent reduced excretion of bile.[678] Clinical features include jaundice, right upper quadrant pain and tenderness, nausea, pruritus, and hepatomegaly. Surprisingly, the administration of total parenteral nutrition has been noted to reduce the incidence of this phenomenon.[679] Several other biologic response modifiers, including **lenalidomide** (Revlimid)[680] and **leflunomide** (Arava),[681,682] have been reported to cause severe DILI.

Summary and Conclusions

Drug-induced liver injury is underdiagnosed and underappreciated as a cause or contributor to liver injury. Drugs and toxins should be considered in virtually all types of liver injury occurring in subjects of all ages, although the risks are higher in older subjects (and probably increase progressively with age [it is not clear whether this is due to increased intrinsic risk or to the fact that older people take more drugs and therefore have more opportunities to experience ADRs]).

A goal that now appears attainable within the next generation is to define the environmental and host factors that underlie the development of idiosyncratic DILI. However, this will require the establishment of a national registry of subjects with bona fide, well-characterized DILI and the discovery of the genetic polymorphisms and other factors that distinguish these subjects from those with similar demographics and drug exposure who do not develop DILI. Such an effort has begun in the United States, thanks to funding provided by the NIDDK of the National Institutes of Health (NIH). There is a National DILI Network comprising eight clinical centers and regional consortia. More information is available at http://dilin.dcri.duke.edu/. Healthcare providers are encouraged to contact one of these centers for advice or to refer subjects to the National DILIN Registry of patients. It is only through careful phenotype-genotype correlation in DILI subjects versus suitable controls that we will realize the promise implicit in the sequencing of the human genome and the analytical advances that have made metabolomics and metabonomics emerging fields of science.

Acknowledgments

This work was supported by the following grants and contracts from the U.S. Public Health Service (USPHS) of the NIH: DK38825 and DK065201. The opinions expressed herein are those of the authors. They do not necessarily reflect the official views of the USPHS or the Universities of Connecticut, Iowa, or Kentucky, nor of Emory University. We thank Melanie McDermid for much help in preparing the manuscript.

Key References

Aithal GP, Day CP. Nonsteroidal anti-inflammatory drug-induced hepatotoxicity. Clin Liver Dis 2007;11:563–575. (Ref.580)

Alla V, et al. Autoimmune hepatitis triggered by statins. J Clin Gastroenterol 2006;40:757–761. (Ref.542)

Andrade RJ, et al. HLA class II genotype influences the type of liver injury in drug-induced idiosyncratic liver disease. Hepatology 2004;39:1603–1612. (Ref.119)

Andrade RJ, et al. Drug-induced liver injury: an analysis of 461 incidences submitted to the Spanish registry over a 10-year period. Gastroenterology 2005;129:512–521. (Ref.105)

Andrews E, et al. A role for the pregnane X receptor in flucloxacillin-induced liver injury. Hepatology 2010;51:1656–1664. (Ref.395)

Andrews E, Daly AK. Flucloxacillin-induced liver injury. Toxicology 2008;254:158–163. (Ref.386)

Anselmino M, et al. Clopidogrel treatment in a patient with ticlopidine-induced hepatitis following percutaneous coronary stenting. Minerva Cardioangiol 2010;58:277–280. (Ref.465)

Baker EL, et al. Probable enoxaparin-induced hepatotoxicity. Am J Health Syst Pharm 2009;66:638–641. (Ref.477)

Bjornsson E, et al. Fulminant drug-induced hepatic failure leading to death or liver transplantation in Sweden. Scand J Gastroenterol 2005;40:1095–1101. (Ref.535)

Bjornsson E, Olsson R. Suspected drug induced liver fatalities reported to the WHO database. Dig Liver Dis 2006;38:33–38. (Ref.104)

Blanco RA. Diurnal variation in glutathione and cysteine redox status in human plasma. Am J Clin Nutr 2007;86:1016–1023. (Ref.45)

Bohan TP, et al. Effect of L-carnitine treatment for valproate-induced hepatotoxicity. Neurology 2001;56:1405–1409. (Ref.172)

Brinker AD, et al. Telithromycin-associated hepatotoxicity: clinical spectrum and causality assessment of 42 cases. Hepatology 2002;49:250–257. (Ref.259)

Brown SJ, Desmond PV. Hepatotoxicity of antimicrobial agents. Semin Liver Dis 2002;22:157–167. (Ref.305)

Campos-Franco J, Gonzalez-Quintela A, Alende-Sixto MR. Isoniazid-induced hyperacute liver failure in a young patient receiving carbamazepine. Eur J Intern Med 2004;15:396–397. (Ref.332)

Chalasani N, et al. Causes, clinical features, and outcomes from a prospective study of drug-induced liver injury in the United States. Gastroenterology 2008;135:1924–1934. (Ref.106)

Chang A, et al. Clozapine-induced fatal fulminant hepatic failure: a case report. Can J Gastroenterol 2009;23:376–378. (Ref.203)

Chitturi S, George J. Hepatotoxicity of commonly used drugs: nonsteroidal anti-inflammatory drugs, antihypertensives, antidiabetic agents, anticonvulsants, lipid-lowering agents, psychotropic drugs. Semin Liver Dis 2002;22:169–183. (Ref.254)

Cho HJ, et al. Genetic polymorphisms of NAT2 and CYPE2E1 associated with antituberculosis drug-induced hepatotoxicity in Korean patients with pulmonary tuberculosis. Tuberculosis (Edinb) 2007;87:551–556. (Ref.127)

Daly AK, et al. Genetic susceptibility to diclofenac-induced hepatoxicity: contribution of UGT2B7, CYP2C8, and ABCC2 genotypes. Gastroenterology 2007;132:272–281. (Ref.577)

Daly AK, et al. HLA-B*5701 genotype is a major determinant of drug-induced liver injury due to flucloxacillin. Nat Genet 2009;41:816–821. (Ref.121)

Davern TJ. Hepatotoxicity of immunomodulating agents and the transplant situation. In: Kaplowitz N, DeLeve LD, editors. Drug induced liver disease, 2nd ed. New York: Informa Healthcare, 2007:663–681. (Ref.594)

de Abajo FJ, et al. Acute and clinically relevant drug-induced liver injury: a population based case-control study. Br J Clin Pharmacol 2004;58:71–80. (Ref.201)

DeSanty KP, Amabile CM. Antidepressant-induced liver injury. Ann Pharmacother 2007;41:1201–1211. (Ref.209)

Detry O, et al. Fulminant hepatic failure induced by venlafaxine and trazodone therapy: a case report. Transplant Proc 2009;41:3435–3436. (Ref.211)

Dieckhaus CM, et al. Mechanisms of idiosyncratic drug reactions: the case of felbamate. Chem Biol Interact 2002;142:99–117. (Ref.179)

Einarsdottir S, Björnsson E. Pregabalin as a probable cause of acute liver injury. Eur J Gastroenterol Hepatol 2008;20:1049. (Ref.240)

Fisher MA, et al. The hepatotoxicity of antifungal medications in bone marrow transplant recipients. Clin Infect Dis 2005;41:301–307. (Ref.262)

Franck AJ, Sliter LR. Acute hepatic injury associated with varenicline in a patient with underlying liver disease. Ann Pharmacother 2009;43:1539–1543. (Ref.238)

Gahimer J, et al. A retrospective pooled analysis of duloxetine safety in 23,983 subjects. Curr Med Res Opin 2007;23:175–184. (Ref.213)

Galan MV, et al. Hepatitis in a United States tertiary referral center. J Clin Gastroenterol 2005;39:64–67. (Ref.446)

Galindo PA, et al. Anticonvulsant drug hypersensitivity. J Invest Allergol Clin Immunol 2002;12:299–304. (Ref.184)

Garnock-Jones KP, Keating GM. Atomoxetine: a review of its use in attention-deficit hyperactivity disorder in children and adolescents. Paediatr Drugs 2009;11:203–226. (Ref.199)

Goodman ZD. Drug hepatotoxicity. Clin Liver Dis 2002;6:381–397. (Ref.112)

Hirata K, et al. Ticlopidine-induced hepatotoxicity is associated with specific human leukocyte antigen genomic subtypes in Japanese patients: a preliminary case-control study. Pharmacogen J 2008;8:29–33. (Ref.124)

Huang YS, et al. Cytochrome P450 2E1 genotype and the susceptibility to antituberculosis drug-induced hepatitis. Hepatology 2003;37:924–930. (Ref.126)

Hussain S, Parekh S. Lenalidomide-induced severe hepatotoxicity. Blood 2007; 15(110):3814. (Ref.680)

Kastalli S, et al. Fatal liver injury associated with clopidogrel. Fundam Clin Pharmacol 2009 Nov 5 (Epub ahead of print). (Ref.466)

Kenna JG. Mechanism, pathology, and clinical presentation of hepatotoxicity of anesthetic agents. New York: Marcel Dekker, 2003. (Ref.145)

Kindmark A, et al. Genome-wide pharmacogenetic investigation of a hepatic adverse event without clinical signs of immunopathology suggests an underlying immune pathogenesis. Pharmacogen J 2008;8:186–195. (Ref.125)

Kong JH, et al. Early imatinib-mesylate-induced hepatotoxicity in chronic myelogenous leukaemia. Acta Haematol 2007;118:205–208. (Ref.667)

Kontorinis N, Dieterich DT. Hepatotoxicity of antiretroviral therapy. AIDS Rev 2003;5:36–43. (Ref.352)

Kontorinis N, Dieterich DT. Toxicity of non-nucleoside analogue reverse transcriptase inhibitors. Semin Liver Dis 2003b;23:173–182. (Ref.357)

Laine L, et al. How common is diclofenac-associated liver injury? Analysis of 17289 arthritis patients in a long-term prospective clinical trial. Am J Gastroenterol 2009;104:356–362. (Ref.555)

Larrey D. Hepatotoxicity of psychotropic drugs and drugs of abuse. In: Kaplowitz N, DeLeve LD, editors. Drug induced liver disease, 2nd ed. NewYork: Informa Healthcare, 2007: 507–526. (Ref.200)

Laurent S, et al. Subfulminant hepatitis requiring liver transplantation following ibuprofen overdose. Liver 2000;20:93–94. (Ref.581)

Leeder JS, Pirmohamed M. Anticonvulsant agents. In: Kaplowitz N, DeLeve LD, editors. Drug induced liver disease. New York: Marcel Dekker, 2003: 425–446. (Ref.154)

Legrass A, Bergemer-Fouquet AM, Jonville-Bera AP. Fatal hepatitis with leflunomide and itraconazole. Am J Med 2002;113:352–353. (Ref.681)

Lewis JH, et al. Efficacy and safety of high-dose pravastatin in hypercholesterolemic patients with well-compensated chronic liver disease: results of a prospective, randomized, double-blind, placebo-controlled, multicenter trial. Hepatology 2007;46:1453–1463. (Ref.543)

Lewis JJ, Iezzoni JC, Berg CL. Methylphenidate-induced autoimmune hepatitis. Dig Dis Sci 2007;52:594–597. (Ref.198)

Lin NU, et al. Fatal hepatic necrosis following imatinib mesylate therapy. Blood 2003;102:3455–3456. (Ref.666)

Longin E, et al. Topiramate enhances the risk of valproate-associated side effects in three children. Epilepsia 2002;43:451–454. (Ref.191)

Lucena I, et al. Susceptibility to amoxicillin-clavulanate-induced liver injury is influenced by multiple HLA class I and class II alleles. New Engl J Med 2010;in press. (Ref.120)

Lucena MI, et al. Glutathione S-transferase m1 and t1 null genotypes increase susceptibility to idiosyncratic drug-induced liver injury. Hepatology 2008;48: 588–596. (Ref.556)

Luef GJ, et al. Valproate therapy and nonalcoholic fatty liver disease. Ann Neurol 2004;55:729–732. (Ref.169)

Lui SY, et al. Possible olanzapine-induced hepatotoxicity in a young Chinese patient. Hong Kong Med J 2009;15:394–396. (Ref.205)

Mallal S, et al. Association between presence of HLA-B*5701, HLADR7, and HLADQ3 and hypersensitivity to HIV-1 reverse-transcriptase inhibitor abacavir. Lancet 2002;359:722–723. (Ref.115)

Mallal S, et al. HLA-B*5701 screening for hypersensitivity to abacavir. New Engl J Med 2008;358:568–579. (Ref.114)

McNeill L, et al. Pyrazinamide and rifampin vs isoniazid for the treatment of latent tuberculosis: improved completion rates but more hepatotoxicity. Chest 2003;123:102–106. (Ref.316)

Menghini VV, Arora AS. Infliximab-associated reversible cholestatic liver disease. Mayo Clin Proc 2001;76:84–86. (Ref.676)

Montessori V, Harris M, Montaner JS. Hepatotoxicity of nucleoside reverse transcriptase inhibitors. Semin Liver Dis 2003;23:167–172. (Ref.356)

Ogedegbe AO, Sulkowski MS. Antiretroviral-associated liver injury. Clin Liver Dis 2003;7:475–499. (Ref.351)

Olanow CW, Watkins PB. Tolcapone: an efficacy and safety review (2007). Clin Neuropharmacol 2007;30:287–294. (Ref.220)

Pelli N, et al. Autoimmune hepatitis revealed by atorvastatin. Eur J Gastroenterol Hepatol 2003;15:921–924. (Ref.113)

Perger L, et al. Fatal liver failure with atorvastatin. J Hepatol 2003;39:1096–1097. (Ref.541)

Pizarro AE, et al. Acute hepatitis due to ticlopidine. A report of 12 cases and review of the literature. Rev Neurol 2001;33:1014–1020. (Ref.463)

Polasek TM, et al. An evaluation of potential mechanism-based inactivation of human drug metabolizing cytochromes P450 by monoamine oxidase inhibitors, including isoniazid. Br J Clin Pharmacol 2006;61:570–584. (Ref.208)

Polson JE. Hepatotoxicity due to antibiotics. Clin Liver Dis 2007;11:549–561. (Ref.424)

Ramakrishna J, Johnson AR, Banner BF. Long term minocycline use for acne in healthy adolescents can cause severe autoimmune hepatitis. J Clin Gastroenterol 2009;43:787–790. (Ref.441)

Rochon J, et al. Reliability of the Roussel Uclaf Causality Assessment Method for assessing causality in drug-induced liver injury. Hepatology 2008;48: 1175–1183. (Ref.10)

Rockey DC, et al. Causality assessment in drug-induced liver injury using a structured expert opinion process: comparison to the Roussel-Uclaf Causality Assessment Method. Hepatology 2010;51:2117–2126. (Ref.11)

Roy B, et al. Increased risk of antituberculosis drug-induced hepatotoxicity in individuals with glutathione S-transferase M1 'null' mutation. J Gastroenterol Hepatol 2001;16:1033–1037. (Ref.329)

Russo MW, et al. Liver transplantation for acute liver failure from drug induced liver injury in the United States. Liver Transpl 2004;10:1018–1023. (Ref.1)

Russo MW, Scobey M, Bonkovsky HL. Drug-induced liver injury associated with statins. Semin Liver Dis 2009;29:412–422. (Ref.536)

Sacchetti E, et al. Ziprasidone vs clozapine in schizophrenia patients refractory to multiple antipsychotic treatments: the MOZART study. Schizophr Res 2009; 113:112–121. (Ref.204)

Saukkonen JJ, et al. An official ATS statement: hepatotoxicity of antituberculosis therapy. Am J Respir Crit Care Med 2006;174:935–952. (Ref.342)

Shaw MW, Sheard JD. Fatal venlafaxine overdose with acinar zone 3 liver cell necrosis. Am J Forensic Med Pathol 2005;26:367–368. (Ref.210)

Spraggs C. HLA-DQA1*0201 is a major determinant of lapatinib-induced hepatotoxicity risk in women with advanced breast cancer. Presented at AASLD-FDA Workshop 24 March 2010; available at www.aasld.org/

conferences/Documents/PresentationLibrary/2010Hepatoxicity_SessionII_Spraggs.pdf. (Ref.123)

Suissa S, et al. Newer disease-modifying antirheumatic drugs and the risk of serious hepatic adverse events in patients with rheumatoid arthritis. Am J Med 2004;117:87–92. (Ref.682)

Sulkowski MS. Hepatotoxicity associated with antiretroviral therapy containing HIV-1 protease inhibitors. Semin Liver Dis 2003;23:183–194. (Ref.355)

Tahaoglu K, et al. The management of anti-tuberculosis drug-induced hepatotoxicity. Int J Tuberc Lung Dis 2001;5:65–69. (Ref.333)

Tan TC, et al. Levetiracetam as a possible cause of fulminant liver failure. Neurology 2008;71:685–686. (Ref.194)

Tietz A, et al. Fulminant liver failure associated with clarithromycin. Ann Pharmacother 2003;37:57–60. (Ref.399)

Tobon GJ, et al. Serious liver disease induced by infliximab. Clin Rheumatol 2007;26:578–581. (Ref.677)

Treeprasertsuk S, et al. The predictors of complications in patients with drug induced liver injury caused by antimicrobial agents. Aliment Pharmacol Ther 2010;31:1200–1207. (Ref.258)

Tremlett H, Oger J. Hepatic injury, liver monitoring and the beta-interferons for multiple sclerosis. J Neurol 2004;251:1297–1303. (Ref.672)

Tremlett HL, Yoshida EM, Oger J. Liver injury associated with the beta-interferons for MS: a comparison between the three products. Neurology 2004;62:628–631. (Ref.673)

van Hest R, et al. Hepatotoxicity of rifampin-pyrazinamide and isoniazid preventive therapy and tuberculosis treatment. Clin Infect Dis 2004;39:488–496. (Ref.318)

Visser K, van der Heijde DM. Clin Exp Rheumatol 2009;27:1017–1025. (Ref.593)

Vittorio CC, Muglia JJ. Anticonvulsant hypersensitivity syndrome. Arch Intern Med 1995;155:2285–2290. (Ref.153)

Volbeda F, et al. Liver cirrhosis due to chronic use of nitrofurantoin. Ned Tijdschr Geneeskd 2004;148:235–238. (Ref.444)

Wernicke J, et al. Hepatic effects of duloxetine-II: spontaneous reports and epidemiology of hepatic events. Curr Drug Saf 2008;3:143–153. (Ref.212)

White JR, et al. Long-term use of felbamate: clinical outcomes and effect of age and concomitant antiepileptic drug use on its clearance. Epilepsia 2009;50:2390–2396. (Ref.176)

Wilfong AA, Willmore LJ. Zonisamide—a review of experience and use in partial seizures. Neuropsychiatr Dis Treat 2006;2:269–280. (Ref.195)

Wright TM, Vandenberg AM. Risperidone- and quetiapine-induced cholestasis. Ann Pharmacother 2007 41:1518–1523. (Ref.206)

Yki-Jarvinen H. Thiazolidinediones. New Engl J Med 2004;351:1106–1118. (Ref.252)

Zapata Garrido AJ, Romo AC, Padilla FB. Terbinafine hepatotoxicity. A case report and review of literature. Ann Hepatol 2003;2:47–51. (Ref.287)

A complete list of references can be found at www.expertconsult.com.

Chapter 26

IV

Hepatotoxicity of Herbal Preparations

Doris B. Strader, Victor J. Navarro, and Leonard B. Seeff

ABBREVIATIONS

AIH autoimmune hepatitis
ALT alanine aminotransferase
ATR atractyloside
CAM complementary and alternative medicine

INR international normalized ratio
NCCAM The National Institute of Health's National Center for Complementary and Alternative Medicine

NDGA nordihydroguaiaretic acid
OLT orthotopic liver transplantation
VOD (SOS) venoocclusive disease; sinusoidal obstruction syndrome

Introduction

The use of "complementary and alternative" medicine (CAM) to treat a variety of ailments is increasing in the United States and elsewhere.[1-3] The National Institute of Health's National Center for Complementary and Alternative Medicine (NCCAM) divides CAM into five categories: (1) *alternative* therapy, which includes homeopathic and naturopathic methods; (2) *mind-body interventions*, including prayer, meditation, art, and dance; (3) *biologically based* therapy, to which herbals and dietary supplements belong; (4) *manipulative and body-based* methods, including chiropractic, osteopathic, and massage therapy; and (5) *energy* therapies, including gi-gong, Reiki, and electromagnetic field methods. Biologically based therapies, particularly herbal preparations, are the most common variety of CAM in the United States. Herbal preparations are part of a broader category of products commonly referred to as dietary supplements. In 1994, Congress defined a dietary supplement in the Dietary Supplement Health and Education Act (DSHEA) of 1994 as a product intended to supplement the diet that is taken by mouth and contains any of the following ingredients: vitamins, minerals, herbs or other botanicals, and extracts or concentrates thereof.[4]

It is estimated that since 1997, at least 42% of Americans have used some form of CAM within the previous year, with herbals being most common.[1] Furthermore, surveys of hepatology clinics across the United States reveal that 20% to 40% of patients with liver disease use herbal remedies.[5,6] Based on a U.S. survey, 21% of adult prescription drug users report the concurrent use of dietary supplements.[7] Demographically, dietary supplement users in this survey were more likely to be Hispanic, non-Hispanic Asian, uninsured, younger, female, highly educated, living in the West, having a high self-perceived health status, being a former smoker, using a fitness center, and having no usual course of primary care. Menopause,

chronic gastrointestinal disorders (including liver disease), and severe headache or migraine were the most common chronic health conditions among dietary supplement users. Importantly, 69% of respondents who took dietary supplements did not disclose such use to their conventional medical provider. Given these data and the high frequency of undisclosed use of dietary supplements, the true prevalence of their use in the general population, including nonprescription drug users, is likely to be higher.

In the United States, dietary supplements are not subjected to the same regulatory policies that govern manufactured pharmaceuticals. Specifically, manufacturers of these products are not required to perform preclinical toxicology assessments or human safety, tolerability, and clinical trials, which are mandatory for a pharmaceutical drug placed on the market. Rather, before marketing, a manufacturer need only attest to a dietary supplement's safety, purity, and contents as expressed on the label. Manufacturers may not make claims to diagnose, treat, cure, or prevent disease without a disclaimer that the product was not evaluated by the U.S. Food and Drug Administration (FDA). Manufacturers must report adverse events as they become known; however, the burden of proof of safety (or toxicity) of a marketed dietary supplement falls on the FDA. The U.S. regulatory environment is different from that in the European Union, in which the published literature can be used to make claims of safety and efficacy. Criteria have also been promulgated in the European Union that allow dietary supplements to be approved for specific indications.[8]

The purpose of this chapter is to discuss single ingredients, such as black cohosh, and complex mixtures of herbs and other botanicals marketed under a single label that have been associated with liver injury. Unlike conventional medications, which generally consist of a standardized formulation of a specific agent in a known concentration, herbal preparations often consist of mixtures of ingredients, frequently in impure form and varying concentration.[9] Herbal medications are available in a variety of forms, including roots, seeds, leaves, teas, powders, oils, capsules, and tablets. The form that a patient receives is dependent on geography, season, and culture, as well as the expertise and preference of the practitioner. For example, in rural areas of some developing countries, patients are more likely to receive leaves, seeds, and teas "in season," whereas in the West, capsules and tablets are the preferred form and are available throughout the year. In developed and developing countries alike, the purity of a particular herbal is uncertain because standards for harvesting, extracting, and storing herbal agents do not exist. In a report in which 12 samples of red peony root (*Paeonia lactiflora*) were purchased in London and analyzed, the concentration of the active ingredient, paeoniflorin, ranged from 0.01% to 4.5%.[10] There are also reports of contamination with ingredients such as conventional medications, other substances, or pathogenic microorganisms. In one trial, corticosteroids, nonsteroidal antiinflammatory drugs, and benzodiazepines were found in "ethnic" remedies of Asian origin.[11] Other studies have identified heavy metals, such as arsenic, mercury, and lead, in ayurvedic remedies.[12-14] Finally, there are reports of product substitution or adulteration, microbial contamination, and lack of compound stability.[9,15] It is probable that these factors may increase the likelihood of toxicity, result in diagnostic delay, and lead to difficulty in identifying the causal agent.

Diagnosis of Hepatotoxicity from Herbal Preparations

Attribution of overt liver dysfunction to the use of any medication, be it a conventional drug or a herbal product, can be problematic. Even in well-accepted instances of so-called idiosyncratic hepatotoxicity, the frequency of such an occurrence is rare. Confidence in such an association increases when there are a large number of reported cases and when the manifestations of the hepatotoxic response generally breed true. That is to say, that the resulting liver disease is consistently necroinflammatory in character, simulating hepatitis; is consistently cholestatic, simulating biliary obstruction; or is consistently a mixed pattern, although emerging data indicate that this may not always be the case. The difficulty is compounded by the fact that many instances of presumed herbal-related hepatotoxicity are based on only a single case or on a very small number of cases and are not always adequately evaluated, such that the validity of the association may be suspect. Nonetheless, there are clearly herbals that have caused liver disease, sometimes very serious in nature, and others in which the observed liver dysfunction seems very likely to have been associated with the use of a particular agent. It is therefore imperative to maintain continuing careful surveillance and to undertake sophisticated diagnostic evaluation and appropriate reporting of probable instances of herbal-related hepatotoxicity to fully establish the frequencies and patterns of liver disease provoked by these products. Contrary to the views of many proponents, herbals are no safer than conventional medications, and assessment of causality is more complex

because of the frequent uncertainty of the purity of the product or its contents.

A diagnosis of herbal hepatotoxicity is predicated on the provider's suspicion that such a product, or products, may be responsible for the injury. Therefore it is incumbent on the provider to query a patient with unexplained liver enzyme abnormalities about herbal use. A complete diagnostic evaluation should be undertaken that is sufficient to exclude other causes of liver injury, including viral hepatitis and autoimmune hepatitis, inherited and metabolic diseases, and space-occupying lesions or biliary tract disease. A formal causality assessment process can be applied to cases of suspected herbal-induced hepatotoxicity[16-19]; however, given the complex mixtures found in many available dietary supplement and herbal products, it can be nearly impossible to identify the specific ingredient that is responsible for injury.

Herb–Drug Interactions

Most consumers of herbal remedies regard them as safe and, moreover, rarely consider the possibility that herbals may interact with their prescribed medications. However, herb–drug interactions have been reported in a number of publications and can be significant.[11,20-27] Most reports focus on herbals used in Western countries and describe an increased international normalized ratio (INR) or altered platelet function leading to bruising or bleeding, a reduction in the concentration of immunosuppressant drugs resulting in decreased immune suppression and possible graft loss, and an increase in toxic metabolites producing abnormalities in liver biochemistry.[25-30] **Table 26-1** provides a list of the most common herb–drug interactions.

Types of Liver Injury

A wide variety of liver injuries have been associated with herbal use, including abnormal liver associated test results, acute and chronic hepatitis, cirrhosis, and liver failure.[29-33] Histologic studies of herbal hepatoxicity are relatively sparse, but evidence of zonal/bridging necrosis, fibrosis, steatosis, and venoocclusive disease (VOD), now known as sinusoidal obstructive syndrome (SOS), have been reported.[34,35] Some herbals are associated with a specific type of histologic injury, but in most cases the histologic appearance of herbal hepatotoxicity is indistinguishable from that of toxic liver injury of other causes. The form of histologic hepatic injury reported for several herbal remedies is shown in **Table 26-2**.

Herbal and Botanical Preparations Associated with Hepatotoxicity
Atractylis gummifera and *Callilepsis laureola*

A. gummifera is a thistle indigenous to the Mediterranean region, where 26 species have been identified. The plants secrete a whitish-yellow gluelike substance often used by children as chewing gum. Intoxication often occurs by accident,

Table 26-1 Hepatotoxic Herb–Drug Interactions

DRUG	HERB	INTERACTION	CLINICAL SIGN
Anticoagulants	Danshen	Increased INR	Bleeding risk
	Devil's claw	Unknown	Purpura
	Dong quai	Increased INR	Bleeding risk
	Feverfew	Platelet dysfunction	Bleeding risk
	Garlic	Increased INR	Bleeding risk
	Gingko	Platelet dysfunction	Bleeding risk
	Ginseng	Decreased INR	Clotting risk
	Papaya	Increased INR	Bleeding risk
	St. John's wort	Decreased INR	Clotting risk
	Tamarind	Inc. aspirin conc.	Bleeding risk
Cyclosporine	St. John's wort	CYP3A4 induction	Rejection risk
CYP34A drugs	Pyrrolizidines	CYP3A4 induction	Hepatotoxicity
	Germander	CYP3A4 induction	Hepatotoxicity
Prednisolone	Licorice	Reduced clearance	Hypokalemia
	Sho-saiko-to	Reduced clearance	Low prednisolone conc.
Spironolactone	Licorice	Mineralocorticoid	Low spironolactone conc.

Adapted from Stedman C. Herbal hepatotoxicity. Semin Liver Dis 2002;22:195–206.
conc., concentration; CYP, cytochrome P; INR, international normalized ratio

Table 26-2 Herbs and Associated Liver Injury

HERBAL REMEDY	HISTOLOGIC LIVER INJURY
Atractylis gummifera	Diffuse hepatic necrosis
Black cohosh	Elevated LFT values, liver failure
Camphor	Elevated LFT values, Reye syndrome
Cascara	Bridging fibrosis, bile duct proliferation
Chaparral	Cholestasis, zone 3 necrosis
Chaso (and Onshido)	Elevated LFT values, liver failure
Greater celandine	Cholestasis
Germander	Zone 3 necrosis, cirrhosis
Impila	Hepatic necrosis
Ju bu huan	Periportal fibrosis, steatosis
Kava	Elevated LFT values, liver failure
Ma huang	Elevated LFT values, hepatic necrosis
Mistletoe (skullcap, valerian)	Elevated LFT values, acute hepatitis
Pennyroyal	Acute hepatitis, liver failure
Pyrrolizidine (comfrey, mate, bush tea)	Venooclusive disease
Sho-saiko-to (dai-saiko-to, TJ-9)	Bridging fibrosis, steatosis

LFT, liver function test

because of confusion with wild artichoke, after ingestion of the roots, where the toxins are concentrated.[33,36] Traditionally, *A. gummifera* has been used as a purgative, emetic, diuretic, abortifacient, and antipyretic. Almost 100 cases of poisoning have been attributed to this plant, frequently involving children.

The onset of hepatitis is usually acute and begins a few hours after ingestion.[37,38] Headache, vomiting, and abdominal pain are characteristic, with neurovegetative symptoms, hepatorenal failure, and profound hypoglycemia rapidly ensuing. Fulminant hepatic failure and death have been reported.[38-40] Toxicity is thought to be due to atractylosides (ATRs) and gummiferin, which have been shown to inhibit mitochondrial function.[41-43] ATRs competitively inhibit the transport of adenosine diphosphate (ADP) and adenosine triphosphate (ATP), thereby blocking oxidative phosphorylation. ATR is also thought to lead to apoptosis by inducing activation of the mitochondrial membrane permeability transition pore, which leads to the release of cytochrome *c* and caspase-activating proteases.[41-43] No specific therapy is available, although efforts to develop immunotherapy are in progress.

Impila, *C. laureola*, is a plant indigenous to the Natal region of South Africa. For years it has been used as a remedy for stomach ailments, tapeworm infestation, impotence, and cough; as a fertility enhancer; and to ward off "evil spirits." Several cases of fulminant hepatic failure and renal tubular necrosis have been reported. The clinical features begin abruptly and include abdominal pain, vomiting, diarrhea, convulsions, acute liver and renal failure, and profound hypoglycemia. A mortality rate of greater than 60% is reported within 24 hours and 91% by 5 days.[39] Interestingly, the toxic components of impila have been identified as ATR and carboxyatractyloside, which decomposes to ATR. Antioxidant therapies, including *S*-adenosyl-L-methionine and betaine, have been suggested for the management of toxicity caused by either herb but are of unproven benefit at present.

Black Cohosh

Black cohosh, *Cimicifuga racemosa*, is a leafy, cylindrical black rhizome with white flowers that is native to Canada and the United States and cultivated in Europe. The medicinal portions are in the fresh and dried roots. Black cohosh has many common names, including black snake root, rattleroot, rattleweed, squaw root, bugbane, bugwort, cimicifuga, and richweed. It is used primarily for the relief of menopausal symptoms, but also to treat rheumatism and bronchitis and as a weight loss aid.

There are a number of reported instances of hepatotoxicity from this product,[44-47] even some manifested as autoimmune hepatitis,[48] although some reports have been viewed with skepticism.[49,50] Indeed, in a recent careful assessment of the 69 cases of suspected black cohosh hepatotoxicity—36 assembled by the European Medicines Agency,[51] 22 by the U.S. Pharmacopeia, and 11 case reports—68 of the 69 were regarded by the authors as questionable instances of drug-induced liver injury.[52] This conclusion was reached after applying a more sophisticated assessment of causality involving use of the structured method developed by the Council for International Organizations of Medical Sciences (CIOMS). Among the many reasons for uncertainty regarding the 68 cases were poor descriptions of the signs and symptoms, thereby confounding other forms of underlying liver disease, co-mixtures with other drugs or herbals that might have been responsible, missing data, and uncertainty about the dose and contents of the product used. The authors concluded that in only one instance did the evaluation include appropriate assessment tools.

This case was a 54-year-old woman in whom fulminant hepatic failure developed 8 months after beginning treatment with levothyroxine for hypothyroidism and with black cohosh for menopausal symptoms.[46] Her primary complaints were fatigue for 8 weeks, forgetfulness, and unintentional weight loss. She had no history of blood transfusions, tattoos, illicit drug use, or alcohol abuse, although she did admit drinking two glasses of wine nightly for years. The only physical finding was right upper quadrant tenderness. Her laboratory values on admission included the following: aspartate transaminase (AST), 1014 U/L; alanine transaminase (ALT), 1003 U/L; alkaline phosphatase, 266 U/L; γ-glutamyltransferase, 504 mg/dl; total bilirubin, 2.4 mg/dL; and INR, 1.4. The results of other blood tests were unremarkable. Viral serology, autoimmune antibodies, α_1-antitrypsin level, and hemochromatosis gene testing were all negative. No abnormalities were noted on imaging, and a liver biopsy revealed predominantly lymphocytic panlobular inflammation, bridging necrosis, and moderate piecemeal necrosis. The patient was treated with prednisone for possible autoimmune hepatitis, but 2 weeks later, encephalopathy and worsening biochemical test results ensued (AST, 2000 U/L; ALT, 1400 U/L; total bilirubin, 20.6 mg/dL; INR, 2.6). She underwent orthotopic liver transplantation (OLT) 39 days after initial evaluation but expired in the operating suite because of uncontrolled hemorrhage. On postmortem examination the liver was found to be shrunken with large areas of firm, micronodular tissue, bridging fibrosis and necrosis, and severe canalicular and ductular cholestasis. The authors assessed the case as representing direct hepatotoxicity from black cohosh, thus raising the possibility that her moderate alcohol consumption placed her at increased risk for injury from black cohosh.

A similar conclusion regarding the validity of many reported cases of black cohosh hepatotoxicity was reached in another systematic review.[53] These authors examined data from 13 clinical trials, 3 postmarketing surveillance studies, 4 case series, and 8 single case reports. They found no supporting evidence of hepatotoxicity in the clinical and postmarketing surveillance studies and also expressed concern about causal attribution in the case reports of drug-induced liver injury. They concluded, as do the present authors, that although black cohosh has been associated with serious safety concerns, future reported cases must include more complete data recording and improved assessment of causality to determine the true potential for liver injury from this product.

Camphor Oil

Camphor oil is extracted from the camphor tree, *Cinnamomum camphora*, which is indigenous to Vietnam and an area extending from southern China to southern Japan. It is used externally as a bronchial secretolytic and hyperemic for cough and bronchitis, rheumatism, and arrhythmia. One case of hepatotoxicity involving a 2-month-old girl treated with a camphor-containing cold remedy applied to the skin has been reported.[54] In this case, the infant, with recent swelling in her right inguinal area, was taken to the local hospital. She was noted to be malnourished because of the use of an improperly diluted infant formula and was admitted for nutritional support. During routine laboratory evaluation to monitor for refeeding syndrome, abnormal aminotransferase values were noted. On physical examination, a soft liver edge was palpated 1.5 cm below the costal margin. Viral hepatitis was ruled out as a cause. On questioning, the mother admitted to applying generous amounts of Vicks VapoRub to the baby's chest and neck three times a day for 5 days. Liver test results returned to normal after application of the rub was discontinued. A second report by Jimenez and associates involved a case of oral ingestion of camphor that resulted in toxicity resembling Reye syndrome.[55] In this report a 6-month-old child was evaluated for a 2-day history of cough and fever, pneumonia was diagnosed, and the child was treated with ampicillin by his private physician. The following day the infant was lethargic, with worsening pulmonary manifestations and radiographic evidence of bilateral diffuse interstitial infiltrates. Six hours later the infant was not arousable, the liver was palpated 3 cm below the costal margin, and a diagnosis of Reye syndrome was suspected. On transfer to a tertiary care center the infant was comatose and had an elevated white blood cell count with bandemia, aminotransferase levels of 750 to 1000 U/L, an elevated serum bilirubin level, and a prolonged prothrombin time. Liver biopsy did not show the characteristic pleomorphic, greatly swollen mitochondria with absent dense bodies and stranding of mitochondrial matrix typically seen in fatal Reye syndrome; however, given the clinical and neurologic syndrome, a presumptive diagnosis of Reye syndrome was made. On questioning the family it was learned that the infant was treated regularly with a home remedy containing camphor and alcohol. Although the infant's liver function improved over the next few days, his neurologic status did not and electroencephalographic studies revealed an absence of electrical activity. The infant died on the fifth hospital day as a result of cardiac arrest.

Camphor is a cyclic terpene compound that is a constituent of several medications, including salves, ointments, and oral cold remedies. When rubbed on the skin, camphor is a rubefacient that causes local irritation of the skin, thereby blocking pain by "counterirritation" (affects the same segmental central nervous system level as that inducing the original pain).[56,57] Camphor can be absorbed through the skin, mucous membranes, and placenta and lead to significant hepatoneurotoxicity, occasionally culminating in hepatic encephalopathy.[58,59] Ingestion of small doses of camphor, characterized by an abrupt onset of nausea and vomiting followed by agitation and seizures, can be fatal in young children. The mechanism by which camphor leads to hepatotoxicity is unclear. Ordinarily, camphor is metabolized in the liver and excreted in urine as an inactive glucuronide compound. Although the exact hepatotoxic metabolite is unknown, it is thought that infants are particularly susceptible to camphor hepatotoxicity because of their immature hepatic detoxification mechanisms.[60,61] As a result, it has been recommended that camphor-containing cold remedies (Vicks VapoRub, Ben-Gay, Afrin saline mist) not be used in children younger than 2 years.

Cascara

Cascara sagrada is derived from the dried bark of the bush or tree *Rhamnus purshiana*. The plant is indigenous to the western part of North America and is also cultivated in Canada and eastern Africa. Cascara is used for the relief of constipation and hemorrhoids and as a rectoanal postoperative treatment. The active constituent is an anthracene derivative (O- and C-glycosides). Right upper quadrant pain, jaundice, ascites, and portal hypertension were reported in a 48-year-old man 3 days after ingesting *C. sagrada* for laxative purposes.[62] Liver biopsy revealed moderate portal inflammation with eosinophils and plasma cells and mild portal-portal bridging fibrosis without cirrhosis. Bile duct proliferation and bile stasis were also noted. The patient recovered fully 3 months after discontinuation of cascara. No other cause of hepatotoxicity was identified, and a presumed diagnosis of cascara hepatotoxicity was made.

The pathogenesis of cascara hepatotoxicity is unknown, but it is assumed that anthracene glycosides are involved. Temporal association of the ingestion of cascara with symptoms and liver biopsy evidence of moderate inflammation with lymphocytes, plasma cells, and eosinophils suggest an immune-mediated process. Two anthraquinones, the first, Doxidan (a combination of danthron-1,8-hydroxyanthraquinone and dioctyl calcium sulfosuccinate), and the second, a senna alkaloid, have also been associated with the development of chronic hepatitis.[63,64] Interestingly, in the first report the authors attributed the hepatotoxicity to the dioctyl sulfosuccinate component rather than the anthraquinone. Cascara is approved by the FDA for use as a laxative and is widely used in the United States without hepatic sequelae. Nevertheless, it appears that cascara has, in extremely rare instances, caused cholestatic hepatitis.

Chaparral

Chaparral leaf, *Larrea tridentate*, is commonly known as creosote bush or greasewood. It is a desert plant indigenous to the southwestern region of the United States and Mexico. Native Americans grind the leaf and use it as a tea for a variety of ailments, including the common cold, bone and muscle pain, chicken pox, cancer, tuberculosis, venereal diseases, and snake bites.[9] Currently, chaparral is packaged as capsules, tablets, or balms and used as a "liver tonic" and for the treatment of skin lesions. Sheikh and colleagues reviewed all 18 cases of chaparral-induced injury reported to the FDA since 1990.[65] Thirteen patients displayed hepatic injury ranging from mild hepatitis to cirrhosis and even fulminant hepatic failure. Although the hepatic manifestations were heterogeneous, the predominant pattern of liver injury was cholestatic, with elevations in serum aminotransferase, bilirubin, and alkaline phosphatase levels. Only a few patients progressed to cirrhosis, and two required OLT for hepatic failure. The latter two patients had used chaparral for more than a year, whereas in the remainder it had been used for 1 to 6 months. A subsequent report of a 22-year old woman describes the development of deep jaundice and markedly increased aminotransferase levels 8 weeks after taking chaparral.[66] The biochemical values improved after stopping the drug but recurred when she started using the product again. An initial liver biopsy showed features of acute necroinflammatory disease, and a follow-up biopsy 9 months later revealed minimal inflammation but bridging fibrosis.

The pathophysiology of chaparral toxicity is unknown. It contains a mixture of flavonoids, amino acids, lignans and volatile oils.[67] The active ingredient is nordihydroguaiaretic acid (NDGA), which may inhibit cyclooxygenase or cytochrome P-450 activity or act via an immune-mediated mechanism.[68,69] In addition, chaparral metabolites exhibit estrogen activity, which may contribute to the hepatotoxicity.[70,71]

Comfrey and Pyrrolizidine Alkaloids

Comfrey, *Symphytum officinale*, is a plant indigenous to Europe and temperate Asia. The medicinal portions are the leaves and fresh roots, which are used externally for bruises, sprains, rheumatism, and pleuritis. The active ingredients, pyrrolizidine alkaloids (PAs), are the most important plant toxins associated with liver disease. There are several hundred varieties of PAs. *Heliotropium*, *Senecio*, *Crotalaria*, and t'u-sanchi' (Compositae) species are most often responsible for liver injury, but PAs have also been identified in other plant families such as Boraginaceae and Leguminoseae. Indeed, there has been a recent report of liver injury from ingestion of the Gynura root, which contains PAs (*Gynura segetum*).[72]

Hepatotoxicity related to PAs was first described 70 years ago as Senecio (mate tea) disease in South Africa.[73-76] Reports of hepatomegaly developing in Jamaican children and evidence of decompensated cirrhosis with ascites after the ingestion of "bush tea" soon followed.[77,78] Later, epidemics were reported from India and Afghanistan.[79,80] PAs are dose-dependent hepatotoxins that typically cause VOD, currently referred to as SOS. VOD (SOS) may be manifested as an acute illness with ascites, hepatomegaly, and jaundice; as a subacute illness identified by persisting hepatomegaly; or as chronic liver injury characterized by histologic features resembling cardiac cirrhosis. Pathophysiologically, nonthrombotic obliteration of terminal centrilobular veins develops, reminiscent of Budd-Chiari syndrome, and leads to disruption of hepatic blood flow.[78] High doses of PAs are often responsible for acute liver injury, and the long-term use of relatively low-dose PAs has been associated with insidious hepatotoxicity.

Children exposed to PAs are at risk for particularly severe liver injury,[81,82] as exemplified by a report from South Africa.[83] This report involved 20 children admitted to two hospitals with SOS after the administration of a traditional remedy that contained PAs. The major clinical findings were massive ascites and hepatomegaly. Mortality was high, and among those who survived, there was a significant rate of progression to cirrhosis and portal hypertension. Also concerning is a report of intrauterine SOS caused by the maternal ingestion of an herbal used for cooking that contained PAs.[84] The preterm neonate, delivered via cesarean section, was noted to have ascites and hepatomegaly. Postmortem evaluation of the liver revealed SOS and the presence of PAs in hepatic tissue.

The mechanism of PA-induced hepatotoxicity has been unclear. Numerous reports have suggested a toxic mechanism that is reproducible in animals and related to biotransformation of alkaloids by cytochrome P-450, with pyrrole derivatives being formed that serve as alkylating agents.[85,86] Toxicity can be augmented by the concomitant use of phenobarbital via the induction of cytochrome P-450. More recently, evidence has emerged to indicate that the process begins with damage to sinusoidal endothelial cells that leads to partial obstruction of the sinusoidal lumen, thereby allowing red cells to enter the space of Disse and ultimately obstructing blood flow.[87] This finding was the basis for changing the name of the pathologic condition from VOD to SOS. Discontinuing use of the herbal can result in the resolution of symptoms in some patients, but those with acute or chronic liver failure may require liver transplantation.

Dai-Saiko-To (Sho-Saiko-To, TJ-9, Xiao-Chai-Hu-Tang)

Dai-saiko-to is a Japanese kampo formula consisting of seven herbs that has been used since 100 AD for the treatment of fatigue, fever, dyspepsia, gallstones, and recently, chronic liver disease.[88] Like germander (discussed next), these compounds contain diterpenoids, which have been associated with hepatotoxicity. Dai-saiko-to differs from Sho-saiko-to only in the proportion of herbal constituents, which include bupleurum, pinellia, jujube, ginseng, ginger rhizome, glycyrrhiza, and scutellaria.[88] Itoh and co-authors reported four cases of acute drug-induced liver injury following a latent period of 1.5 to 3 months, which improved with cessation of the drug and recurred with rechallenge.[89] In 1997 a case of autoimmune hepatitis was reported that was possibly induced by Dai-saiko-to.[32] The patient was a 55-year-old woman with fatigue, fever, and abnormal liver test values (ALT, 866 IU/L; total bilirubin, 13 mg/dl; alkaline phosphatase, 317 IU/L). Autoimmune markers and hepatitis serologic tests were negative; liver histology revealed chronic hepatitis. Within 4 weeks the symptoms and biochemical abnormalities had resolved spontaneously, and the ALT values remained normal for 5 years. Subsequently, an increase in the ALT level to 300 IU/L was noted and liver histology revealed chronic hepatitis with severe steatosis and a lipogranuloma. The patient was treated with Dai-saiko-to, and 2 weeks later, fatigue, fever, an elevated ALT level of 390 IU/L and an antinuclear antibody (ANA) titer of 1:2560 developed. An International Autoimmune Hepatitis Group diagnostic score of 18 supported the diagnosis of autoimmune disease, and a strongly positive lymphocyte stimulation test for Dai-saiko-to (340%) suggested that this herb was responsible.[90] Abnormalities in the ALT values returned to normal after treatment with prednisolone.

The mechanism by which the hepatic abnormalities occur is unclear. It has been suggested that either scutellaria or glycyrrhizin, both implicated in other cases of hepatic injury, may be the culprits.[91]

Germander

The genus *Teucrium* consists of more than 300 plant species. Germander, *Teucrium chamaedrys*, is a subshrub with a short-lived main root from which long-reaching thin branched roots grow. It is indigenous to the Mediterranean region as far as the Urals. The active ingredients are diterpenes, iridoid monoterpenes, caffeic acid derivatives, and flavonoids. Germander is thought to have cholagogic and antiseptic properties and is ingested as a capsule or tea to treat dyspepsia, fever, gout, and obesity. Following large-scale marketing as a weight loss aid in France in 1992, 30 cases of acute, chronic, and fulminant hepatitis were reported.[29,92] Affected patients were predominantly women attempting to lose weight, most of whom ingested 600 to 1600 mg daily. The clinical syndrome, characterized by markedly elevated levels of aminotransferases and bilirubin and impaired hepatic synthetic function, began approximately 2 months after ingestion. The range of histologic findings included mild chronic hepatitis, fibrosis, cirrhosis, and in some cases, acute midzonal hepatocellular necrosis. The patients without cirrhosis recovered completely after discontinuation of the herb.

Teucrium species used for indications other than weight loss have been implicated as the cause of hepatic injury. One presumptive case of *Teucrium* hepatotoxicity was reported in Greece in 2002.[93] The patient, a 62-year-old man with hypercholesterolemia and diabetes, consumed *Teucrium capitatum* in his daily cup of tea. Four months later, jaundice and symptoms of acute hepatitis developed. All other causes of liver disease were excluded, and liver biopsy revealed bridging necrosis with active inflammation. *Teucrium* was discontinued and the clinical and laboratory abnormalities returned to normal within 9 weeks. In 2008, another case of presumed *Teucrium* hepatoxicity secondary to *Teucrium viscidum* was described.[94] In this instance, a 51-year-old woman was admitted to the hospital with a 3-day history of nausea, jaundice, vomiting, and tea-colored urine. Three days before these symptoms developed she had consumed 60 g of a medicinal herb, crushed and suspended in rice wine daily to treat low back pain. She had used this same medicinal in a similar fashion 3 months earlier without sequelae. The results of her physical examination were normal with the exception of jaundice. Biochemical tests revealed a total bilirubin level of 11.4 mg/dl, ALT of 2620 U/L, AST of 1876 U/L, and alkaline phosphatase of 186 U/L. Viral hepatitis serology and autoimmune markers were negative. The herbal remedy was discontinued, her symptoms resolved, and blood test results returned to normal within 9 weeks. Unused herb was obtained and identified as *T. viscidum*, a species closely related to germander.

Analysis of *T. chamaedrys* revealed the presence of a number of furan-containing neoclerodane diterpenoids, which are well-known powerful carcinogens.[95-97] In rat hepatocytes, these constituents are oxidized by cytochrome P-450 3A4 to reactive metabolites that bind to proteins, deplete cellular glutathione and protein thiols, and cause plasma membrane blebbing and cell disruption.[96] Two cell culture studies suggest that germander induces apoptosis after the formation of reactive metabolites.[98,99] These reports suggest a reactive metabolite as the mechanism of injury for germander; however, an autoimmune mechanism was proposed after antimicrosomal epoxide hydrolase autoantibodies were found in the sera of some patients.[100]

Greater Celandine

Greater celandine, *Chelidonium majus*, is a plant found throughout Europe and the temperate and subarctic regions of Asia. The plant belongs to the poppy family Papaveraceae. The root is harvested between August and October. Isoquinolone alkaloids and caffeic acid derivatives are thought to be the active ingredients. Celandine is believed to have mild analgesic, central sedative, cholagogic, and antimicrobial effects and is used to treat biliary colic, cholelithiasis, jaundice, gastroenteritis, and diffuse liver and gallbladder complaints.

A recent review of the literature, based on a MEDLINE and EMBASE search, identified 16 reported cases, to which was added 1 additional newly identified case.[101] Causality was assessed by using the Naranjo probability scale. Fourteen of the 17 cases involved women. In most instances, symptoms of fatigue, pruritus, and jaundice developed 2 or more months after starting the drug. A cholestatic pattern was noted in eight patients; moderate- to low-titer ANAs were noted in eight of the nine patients tested for these antibodies, and portal inflammation with bridging fibrosis and eosinophilic infiltrates was seen on liver biopsy in most of them. Liver chemistry returned to normal 2 to 6 months after cessation of the herb. Two patients had a flare-up of liver disease after inadvertent reexposure to the herb. The new reported case involved a patient in whom a mixed pattern of liver injury developed as indicated by extremely high levels of both aminotransferases and alkaline phosphatase, as well as serum bilirubin.

The mechanism of action of celandine hepatotoxicity is unknown but it is considered to be idiosyncratic in nature as a result of the variable latency period and the lack of dose dependence.[31,34] Some have suggested an immune response because of the presence of serum autoantibodies and eosinophilic infiltrates on liver biopsy, but these findings can be nonspecific. More than 20 alkaloids with biologic activity have been identified in celandine; however, the toxic component has yet to be identified.

Green Tea (Camellia sinensis)

Tea is the most commonly consumed beverage in the world, second only to water, and the fourth most commonly used dietary supplement in the United States.[102] Tea has been available for thousands of years, and the most popular forms are the green, black, and oolong varieties. Green tea is prepared by stabilizing the leaves with dry heat or steam to inactivate enzymes, rolled, dried rapidly, and roasted. Unlike black or oolong tea, green tea is not fermented. Unfermented teas contain polyphenols, primarily catechins in the form of (−)-epigallocatechin gallate (EGCG) and (−)-epicatechin

gallate (ECG). Studies of green tea suggest that it contains antioxidants, which can be associated with a reduced risk for cardiovascular disease and cancer and may help in the management of diabetes and body weight.

When used as a dilute infusion for drinking, no hepatic adverse events occur, but there have been a number of reports of liver injury from concentrated supplements of green tea.[103-108] Another publication reported that over a period of 2 years, five cases of drug-induced liver injury attributed to a weight loss supplement called Cuur were reported to the Swedish Adverse Drug Reactions Advisory Committee.[109] This is a weight loss supplement in which 82% of the product consists of ethanolic dry extract of green tea. Similarly, the Spanish Liver Toxicity Registry reported that among 521 submitted cases of drug-induced liver injury, 13 (2%) were a consequence of herbal remedies or dietary supplements, the most common product being *C. sinensis*.[110] Concern regarding reports of liver injury from this popular product and the fact that French and Spanish authorities in 2003 suspended market authorization of Exolise, a weight loss product that contains a hydroalcoholic extract of green tea, prompted two recent extensive reviews of the literature.[102,111] Sarma and colleagues, on behalf of the U.S. Pharmacopeia, performed a wide search of U.S. and international databases and identified 34 reports of liver injury associated with green tea extracts.[102] Products implicated were Exolise (13 cases); Tealine (4 cases); Hydroxycut (2 cases); The Right Approach: TRA Complex (1 case); Camiline Arkocaps tea leaf powder (1 case); and Green Lite Polyphenol (1 case). Assessment of causality found probable causality in 7 cases and possible causality in the remaining 27 cases. Pharmacologic and animal toxicologic studies determined that adverse effects were more common when the products were taken on an empty stomach. The review by Mazzanti and co-workers also focused on 34 published cases of hepatitis following the consumption of green tea.[111] The cases occurred between 1999 and October 2008 and involved 6 men and 28 women. In 15 cases, the herbal preparation contained only green tea; in the others, multiple herbals were present. All were taken to promote weight loss. Laboratory analysis revealed that serum aminotransferase values were up to 140-fold the upper limit of normal, alkaline phosphatase values were 8.3-fold higher than normal, and total bilirubin levels increased by 25-fold. Viral hepatitis, autoimmune disease, and alcohol abuse was excluded. Fifteen patients were consuming other medications in addition to the herbal preparation; 7 were not. Histologic evaluation revealed inflammatory hepatitis, cholestasis, necrosis, and occasional steatosis. In 29 cases, laboratory abnormalities resolved completely within 4 to 13 weeks after discontinuation of the green tea supplement. A positive rechallenge was demonstrated in seven patients, four of whom were taking no other medications.

The authors also reported two unpublished cases of elderly women consuming the green tea herbal Epinerve, prescribed by their ophthalmologist to treat glaucoma.[111] Both women were admitted to the hospital with jaundice, bilirubin levels higher than 18 mg/dl, and elevated aminotransferase values within 1 to 3 months of beginning the herbal. Imaging studies excluded biliary or pancreatic disease, and no other cause of liver disease was identified. One woman had been taking simvastatin daily for several years. Discontinuation of the herbal preparation resulted in complete resolution of the symptoms and laboratory abnormalities within 3 months in one woman.

In the other woman, liver biopsy suggested granulomatous cholangitis, and treatment with ursodeoxycholic acid and glutathione, in addition to drug discontinuation, led to resolution of the laboratory abnormalities before discharge. In 80% of the published cases of liver injury attributed to green tea extract, no concomitant medication was believed to contribute to the hepatic injury, thus suggesting that green tea was indeed the causative agent. In the two unpublished cases, the association between green tea and hepatotoxicity was scored as "possible."

Polyphenols, such as those found in green tea, may behave as prooxidants, as well as antioxidants. Although the bioavailability of green tea catechins is low, serum concentrations of EGCG may reach toxic levels under certain conditions, including fasting and repeated administration. High concentrations of green tea extract and subsequent increases in the toxic compound EGCG are believed to induce cytotoxicity primarily by the formation of reactive oxygen species and depletion of glutathione.[111,112] Inhibitors of NAD(P)H:quinone oxidoreductase 1 (a detoxifier of O-quinone metabolites) and catechol-O-methylase (a hepatocyte methylator) have been shown to increase the susceptibility of hepatocytes to EGCG cytotoxicity.[113] Of interest, one group of investigators has suggested a sex susceptibility to EGCG hepatotoxicity by demonstrating that hepatic injury is more likely to develop in female Swiss Webster mice after the consumption of green tea extracts.[114]

These data, in addition to the widespread use of green tea products and the fact that a green tea extract was withdrawn from the market in April 2003 because of 13 cases of liver damage associated with its use (www.afssaps.sante.fr), suggest that further monitoring and surveillance of these products may be necessary to ensure their safety.

Hydroxycut is an herbal slimming aid that has been reported in several publications to cause severe liver injury.[115-120] The first account consisted of two cases, part of a series of reported instances of herbal-associated hepatotoxicity, in which it was suggested that the ingredient probably responsible for the liver injury was ma huang. Because ma huang is a recognized hepatotoxin that was restricted for use by the FDA in 2004, the manufacturer continued marketing Hydroxycut but with ma huang removed. Nevertheless, as noted earlier, cases of liver injury continued to be reported. Most recently, 17 new instances of Hydroxycut hepatotoxicity have been reported, 8 identified at several academic centers and 9 that had been submitted to the FDA via the MedWatch reporting system.[121] After a latency period of 1 to 8 weeks, nausea and vomiting, fatigue, deep jaundice, and markedly elevated aminotransferase levels developed; four patients had a positive ANA test. All were hospitalized, three underwent liver transplantation, and one patient died of liver failure. Causality assessment scored eight cases as definite, five as highly likely, two as probable, and two as possible. These cases, all manifested as hepatocellular injury, were similar in pattern to those previously reported.

The precise basis for the liver injury is uncertain. Hydroxycut products contain numerous ingredients, but the specific item responsible for the liver disease is unknown. The authors of the 17 reported cases focused attention on *Garcinia cambogia*, *Cissus quadrangularis*, and caffeine or green tree extract and suggested that green tea was the most likely culprit, but they did not rule out the possibility of a toxic contaminant as

the cause.[121] Because of the numerous instances of severe hepatotoxicity attributed to Hydroxycut, the FDA issued a warning to the public on May 1, 2009, to stop using the product, which prompted the manufacturer to recall all of their products.

Herbalife

Launched in a small number of countries in 1980 as a nutritional supplement, Herbalife has since grown to become one of the most popular supplements worldwide. Moreover, its product line has expanded markedly so that it targets not only nutrition but also weight loss, energy and fitness, dermatologic personal care, and immunity boosting. Each product is formulated differently, with some being used as a nutritional drink, some as herbal extracts and powders, and some as tablets. In 2007 two reports were published that between them identified a total of 24 apparently implicated or potential instances of Herbalife hepatotoxicity, although 2 of the cases were eliminated for lack of significant documentation.[122,123] Investigators of both reports evaluated the cases by using either the CIOMS or World Health Organization criteria for determining hepatotoxicity, most being defined as either certain or probable cases. The pattern of injury was hepatocellular in 20 cases and mixed in the remaining 2, which were also reflected in the liver biopsy findings. Five patients had a positive rechallenge response. Although all but one patient recovered after discontinuing the product, fulminant hepatitis developed in several individuals, two of whom underwent liver transplantation and one subsequently died of complications of surgery. No single product could be identified as the cause of the injury because most of the affected persons had been taking multiple supplements.

At least two other reports of hepatotoxicity have since appeared.[15,124] In one of these reports, two patients are described whose disease was manifested as cholestatic and lobular/portal hepatitis with cirrhosis in one of them and biliary fibrosis with ductopenia in the other.[15] Unable to identify the specific causative ingredient, the authors sought contaminants that might have been responsible. Careful study revealed the presence of *Bacillus subtilis* in some of the products taken by both patients that was considered possibly responsible for the injury because they determined that the bacteria created dose-dependent leakage of lactate dehydrogenase from HepG2 cells. The other publication reported three cases of apparent Herbalife hepatotoxicity, with the authors noting an additional case in a letter to the editor.[125]

The mechanism of liver injury is not known, in part because the actual constituent responsible for the injury among the many ingredients making up these products remains uncertain. Some apparently contain ma huang, some contain nitrosofenfluramine, and some include *C. sinensis* (green tea). Others have suggested immune-mediated liver toxicity or, as noted earlier, a contaminant.

Ju (Jin) Bu Huan

Ju (jin) bu huan, *Lycopodium serratum*, is a plant found worldwide. It is believed to have sedative, analgesic, and antispasmodic effects and has been used for more than a millennium as a sleeping aid. Several cases of acute and chronic hepatitis associated with ju bu huan have been published in the literature.[126,127] The largest report describes seven patients in whom hepatitis developed a mean of 20 weeks after ingestion.[126] Abdominal pain, constitutional symptoms, jaundice, hepatomegaly, and pruritus were characteristic, as were elevations in aminotransferase and alkaline phosphatase levels. Liver histology generally revealed periportal necrosis and cholestasis. Eosinophilic inflammation was noted in one patient, and in another, moderate periportal fibrosis, lymphocytic inflammation, focal hepatocellular necrosis, and microvesicular steatosis were present. The symptoms and abnormal laboratory test results resolved within 8 weeks after discontinuation of the herb.

A recent report describes a 46-year-old woman who was admitted to the hospital because of nausea, anorexia, and abdominal pain.[128] She had been taking 50 drops of *Lycopodium similiaplex* solution (containing *L. serratum* and eight other herbals) daily for insomnia. She had no significant past medical history, was not taking any other medications, and reported no risk factors associated with liver disease. Her physical examination was within normal limits. Laboratory analysis revealed an ALT level of 2364 U/L, AST of 737 U/L, total serum bilirubin of 3.2 mg/dl, alkaline phosphatase of 255 U/L, and a normal INR. Viral serology and autoimmune markers were negative. Liver biopsy revealed a portal mixed inflammatory infiltrate with eosinophils and pigmented macrophages. Two months after discontinuation of the preparation, the laboratory abnormalities returned to normal.

The mechanism of ju bu huan hepatotoxicity is not fully understood. An L-alkaloid, L-tetrahydropalmatine, structurally similar to pyrrolizidine and berberine alkaloids, may be the toxic agent. Long-term berberine use is associated with hyperbilirubinemia in animals, which may be caused by displacement of bilirubin from albumin or disruption of bilirubin conjugation.[34,126] Although the exact mechanism of action of ju bu huan is unknown, the presence of fever, rash, and eosinophilia in some patients suggests an immune-mediated mechanism.

Kava

Kava is a rhizome of the pepper plant *Piper methysticum*. The plant is a 2- to 3-m-tall bush indigenous to the South Sea islands. An extract of the dried rhizome contains kava lactones, which have central muscle relaxant, anticonvulsive, and antispasmodic effects. The herb also has hypnotic/sedative, analgesic, and psychotropic effects, which explains its worldwide use in industrialized countries as therapy for anxiety and tension. For more than 2000 years, however, the leaves and roots of the pepper plant have been used in the South Pacific to prepare beverages for ceremonial purposes (kava kava), as well as for informal social drinking. The traditional beverages are aqueous extracts of kava, whereas the herbal remedies, marketed as capsules and tablets, are ethanolic or acetonic kava extracts.[129] Used as a ceremonial beverage, kava was seen as a safe product.

With the achievement of great popularity of kava as an antidepressant in Western countries, Germany and Switzerland in particular, reports of liver injury began to appear. In 2003, a critical assessment was made of 36 cases of potential kava hepatotoxicity (27 reported to the German Department of Pharmacovigilance, 2 seen by the authors, and 7 published cases).[130] Assessment involved the use of a clinical diagnostic scale. The pattern of injury was both hepatocellular and cholestatic; the majority of affected persons were women; the cumulative dose and latency were variable; fulminant hepatitis developed in nine patients, eight of whom underwent liver transplantation; three patients died; and the rest recovering after withdrawal of kava. The majority of cases were assessed as probably related. In the same year, the U.S. Centers for Disease Control and Prevention summarized 11 reported cases and added 2 more patients in whom liver failure had developed following the use of kava and thus required liver transplantation.[131] This prompted the U.S. FDA to issue a customer advisory about the potential dangers of the product. In addition, the use of kava was banned in Germany, the United Kingdom, and France. These decisions led to a worldwide debate on the legitimacy of these judgments, some questioning whether the reports of hepatotoxicity were appropriate.

A critical analysis of the 26 cases of kava hepatotoxicity previously assessed by the German regulatory agency (20 from Germany and 6 from Switzerland) was undertaken and reported in 2008.[132] The affected individuals had all received ethanolic or acetonic kava extracts. The authors, who reassessed the cases by using the CIOMS system, thus challenged the previous conclusions. They claimed that only 8 of 26 patients were evaluable for causality, the others being excluded for lack of temporal association, the presence of concomitant significant liver disease, or both. They indicated that only one of the eight patients "adhered to the regulatory recommendations for kava use regarding a daily dose of up to 120 mg kavapyrones for not longer than 3 months." The others had used kava beyond the recommended dosage or duration or were also taking other medications with known hepatotoxicity. They thus concluded that if taken in recommended doses, kava is rarely associated with hepatotoxicity. Shortly thereafter, the lead author of this critical analysis extended the evaluation to the patients who had not been enrolled by the German authorities to include additional worldwide reports of kava, some following the use of aqueous extracts of kava.[133-136] Again, analysis was performed with use of the CIOMS strategy. Assessment focused on five reported patients with the addition of nine from Germany and Switzerland whom they considered to have had verified kava hepatotoxicity. Three of the five new patients had received an aqueous extract, whereas the other two had received a kava–herb mixture. They graded all 5 patients as having possible instances of hepatotoxicity and thus concluded that among all reported cases, they were willing to grant kava-associated liver injury to a total of 14 patients. Clearly, as is the case for many reported instances of herbal hepatotoxicity, a careful and sophisticated approach to assessment of causality, often not performed, is mandatory to obtain convincing data on hepatotoxicity.

The exact mechanism of kava hepatotoxicity is unknown. Lactone hydrolases are involved in the degradation of kavapyrones, and kavapyrones inhibit most of the isoenzymes of human cytochrome P-450 in vitro.[137] It is unclear whether this inhibition results in a direct pathogenic effect of kava. Rather, it is possible that inhibition of cytochrome P-450 is relevant to kava-drug interactions by leading to increases in the plasma concentrations of potentially hepatotoxic metabolites of co-administered drugs.[138,139] Some have suggested that a relatively common genetic polymorphism of drug metabolism, CYP2D6 deficiency, may predispose to kava hepatotoxicity.[140,141] However, further study is required before this mechanism can be considered definitive.

Ma Huang

Ma huang, *Ephedra sinica,* is a 30-cm-tall, lightly branched shrub found mainly in Mongolia and the bordering area of China. The dried young branchlets, which are harvested in the autumn, are considered the medicinal parts. Ma huang is generally used as a tea for cough and bronchitis, as a weight loss aid, and as an energy enhancer. Instances of ma huang hepatotoxicity have been reported. In the first case, a 33-year-old woman experienced nausea, vomiting, jaundice, and abdominal pain 3 weeks after taking a herbal preparation containing ma huang.[142] She reportedly continued use of the preparation despite symptoms, until jaundice developed. Serum aminotransferase and bilirubin levels were elevated without signs of chronic liver disease, and the presumptive diagnosis was acute viral hepatitis. She was admitted to the hospital 1 week later with increasing jaundice, worsening aminotransferase levels, and evidence of autoimmune disease with an ANA titer of 1:160 and an anti–smooth muscle antibody titer of 1:80. Viral hepatitis serology was negative. Liver biopsy demonstrated diffuse hepatic necrosis with occasional eosinophils and plasma cells in the portal tracts. On further questioning, the patient admitted taking another dose of the herbal preparation after her first hospital visit. Her symptoms resolved and the liver panel returned to normal 4 months after discontinuation of ma huang.

In a second case, a 58-year-old woman with obesity had a history of 4 months of jaundice, fatigue, nausea, and abdominal pain of unclear etiology.[141] Initial evaluation revealed elevated aminotransferases levels, elevated bilirubin, negative viral hepatitis serologic findings, negative ANA, an anti–smooth muscle antibody titer of 1:320, and normal findings on abdominal computed tomography (CT). Her medication history revealed that she had used ma huang as a weight loss aid for 4.5 months. Liver biopsy revealed severe infiltration with polymorphonuclear leukocytes, moderate fibrosis, and lobular necrosis. She was treated with steroids for presumed autoimmune hepatitis, but encephalopathy subsequently developed and she was referred for liver transplant evaluation. While awaiting liver transplantation, her status improved and she was discharged in stable condition.

Several other cases of hepatotoxicity from ma huang have been reported, including 10 cases seen in transplant centers in the United States in 2004.[143-145] Seven of the patients recovered within 8 weeks despite marked increases in bilirubin and severe coagulopathy. Three patients progressed to grade 4 encephalopathy, two underwent liver transplantation, and the third patient died. Liver explants revealed panacinar and centrilobular necrosis.

The active ingredient in ma huang is ephedrine, a sympathomimetic used in Western medicine to treat asthma and also used as a central nervous system stimulant. Well-known side effects include nervousness, palpitations, headache, and insomnia. The exact mechanism by which ephedrine induces hepatotoxicity is unknown, but the presence of autoimmune markers in both cases suggests an immune-mediated process, either as a primary effect or through unmasking of an underlying autoimmune diathesis. In the first case presented earlier, the concomitant use of other plant extracts in the preparation raises the possibility of herb–herb interaction or other contamination. In both cases the women were obese, and it is possible that nonalcoholic fatty liver disease may have contributed to the liver injury.

Margosa Oil (Neem)

Antelaea azadirachta (neem) and *Azadirachta indica* (margosa oil) are indigenous to the woods of India and Sri Lanka. The bark, leaves, and seeds of the deciduous tree are the medicinal portions. *A. indica* and *A. azadirachta* are commonly used in India, Sri Lanka, Burma, Indonesia, Thailand, and Malaysia for inflammatory and febrile illnesses, as well as for dyspeptic symptoms and worm infestations. There have been several case reports of toxic encephalopathy developing in infants and young children given small amounts of oral margosa oil.[146] Although the oil is generally used externally, some traditional practices include giving small amounts orally to infants and children. Several children were seen by physicians because of vomiting, drowsiness, tachypnea, and recurrent seizures. Laboratory studies revealed leukocytosis, abnormal liver test values (albumin, bilirubin, INR), severe metabolic acidosis, and hepatic lesions consistent with Reye syndrome. Supportive care and control of seizure activity led to resolution of the symptoms in most children, but neurologic deficits developed in a few and some died as a result of hepatic failure.

Animal studies of the ingestion of margosa oil indicate that the sequence of injury begins with the rapid development of mitoses and binucleated cells, followed by mitochondrial injury, swelling, and pleomorphism within the nuclei of hepatocytes.[147,148] Proliferation and hypertrophy of the endoplasmic reticulum and subsequent microvesicular steatosis have also been noted. It has been suggested that margosa oil is a mitochondrial uncoupler that increases mitochondrial respiration and decreases intramitochondrial ATP.[146] These effects may be due to alterations in fatty acid metabolism that result in a change in the proportion of acid-soluble and acid-insoluble coenzyme A esters. Even though some suggest that supplementary therapy with L-carnitine and coenzyme A may be useful in the management of margosa oil–induced Reye syndrome, avoidance of oral use of this herbal product is clearly prudent.[146]

Mistletoe

Mistletoe, *Viscum album,* is a semiparasitic round bush that grows on deciduous trees found primarily in Europe. The medicinal portions include the leaves, stem, and pea-sized berries. Mistletoe has been used widely to treat many illnesses, including degenerative inflammation of the joints, hypertension, asthma, vertigo, diarrhea, epilepsy, and nervousness. One case of presumed mistletoe-associated hepatitis was reported in a 49-year-old woman with nausea, general malaise, and right upper quadrant pain.[149] Aminotransferase levels were elevated, hepatitis B surface antigen was not detected, cholecystographic findings were normal, and liver biopsy revealed mild inflammation. Two years later she had a similar illness, and questioning revealed that both episodes were preceded by the ingestion of an herbal remedy containing kelp, motherwort, skullcap, and mistletoe.[149] A challenge test established that the herb was responsible for the symptoms. At the time, mistletoe was the only herb known to contain a potential toxin, lectin, and it was therefore singled out as the causative agent. Later evaluation of the herbal compound suggested that mistletoe was probably not an ingredient, thus casting doubt on the association between mistletoe and hepatitis. This attests to the uncertainty of attributing liver injury to a herbal when only a single case report exists and assessment of causality is incomplete.

Noni Juice (Morinda citrifolia)

Noni juice comes from a tropical fruit called noni and has been used for centuries as a remedy for a large array of illnesses.[150] The product has recently achieved popularity in the West.[151] The first case of hepatotoxicity attributed to the product, reported in 2005, involved a 45-year-old man with nausea, fatigue, and anorexia who was found to have biochemical dysfunction suggestive of hepatitis.[152] He underwent an extensive workup that failed to identify a cause. Liver biopsy revealed hepatocellular injury with numerous eosinophils. He then gave a history of drinking noni juice every day for several weeks. He was told to discontinue this practice, and the symptoms abated and his biochemical dysfunction normalized.

There have been four further reports of hepatotoxicity attributed to noni juice, thus accounting for at least six cases of drug-induced liver injury.[153-156] Three of the patients were men, latency ranged from 1 to 4 weeks, and markedly elevated aminotransferase levels developed in most. Four were jaundiced, two deeply so, and five recovered after discontinuing the drink, but fulminant hepatitis requiring liver transplantation developed in one.[156] The suggested hepatotoxic components are anthraquinones. That noni juice is hepatotoxic has, however, been disputed based on a human clinical safety study and the relatively small quantities of *M. citrifolia* used.[157] Clearly, identifying additional cases, should they occur, will provide further support for the potential hepatotoxicity of this product.

Pennyroyal

Pennyroyal, *Mentha pulegium*, is a downy perennial that grows in western, southern, and central Europe; Asia; Iran; and Ethiopia. It is naturalized in North America. The medicinal portion, the essential oil, is extracted from the fresh plant or dried aerial parts. For centuries it was used as an abortifacient and as a pesticide against fleas, and because it is a source of intoxication, it continues to be used widely.[158] Current medical applications include its use in individuals with digestive disorders, liver and gallbladder disease, amenorrhea, gout, colds, and skin disease. Most cases of hepatotoxicity have been reported in women who use pennyroyal to induce menstruation or abortion.[158] In one instance, a 24-year-old woman ingested pennyroyal extract and black cohosh root for 2 weeks in an attempt to induce abortion. When this failed, she ingested additional, unknown amounts of these herbals over a short period. Soon after ingestion, abdominal cramping, chills, vomiting, and syncope developed, with difficulty being roused. Paramedics discovered the patient to be in cardiopulmonary arrest an estimated 7.5 hours after acute ingestion. She was intubated, successfully resuscitated, and admitted to the intensive care unit. CT of the abdomen revealed a possible ruptured ectopic pregnancy. Aminotransferase levels, bilirubin, and the prothrombin time were elevated, and over the next 36 hours

signs of multiorgan failure and disseminated intravascular coagulation developed. The patient was comatose and unresponsive to all stimuli, anoxic encephalopathy was confirmed by CT, life support was discontinued, and she died within 48 hours of acute ingestion. Multiorgan failure developed in two infants after the ingestion of mint tea containing pennyroyal, one with confluent hepatic necrosis noted at autopsy.[159]

Unlike most herbal preparations, the mechanism of pennyroyal hepatotoxicity is well known. The main constituent is R-(+)-pulegone, which is oxidized by cytochrome P-450 to menthofuran.[160] Pulegone depletes hepatic glutathione by the formation of electrophilic metabolites, whereas menthofuran is directly toxic to hepatocytes. As a result of the loss of glutathione, replacement of sulfhydryl groups by administering N-acetylcysteine has been advocated as a therapy. Because menthofuran toxicity is not greatly affected by glutathione loss, the benefits of this therapy may be evident only in the early phases of pennyroyal poisoning. Nonetheless, N-acetylcysteine is recommended in cases in which more than 10 ml of pennyroyal has been ingested.

Skullcap (Scutellaria) and Valerian (Centella asiatica)

Skullcap, *Scutellaria*, is a perennial herb 60 cm in height and thickly covered with simple and glandular hairs that is indigenous to North America and cultivated in Europe. The herb is pulverized and used as a sedative, an antispasmodic, and an antiinflammatory agent, and it is thought to inhibit lipid peroxidation. Valerian, *Valeriana officinalis*, is a short, cylindrical rhizome with bushy round roots that is indigenous to Europe and the temperate regions of Asia. It is widely cultivated in England, France, Japan, and the United States and is used to treat conditions such as nervousness, insomnia, lack of concentration, headache, and nervous stomach cramps. Frequently, both valerian and skullcap are contained in the same preparation used to relieve stress. Several cases of acute hepatitis have been reported with the use of herbal preparations containing skullcap and valerian. Four cases of jaundice, abdominal pain, and dark urine have been reported in women taking two different herbal preparations, Kalms and Neurelax, for relief of stress.[91] In one woman, ascites and encephalopathy developed and necessitated intensive medical support. Available liver biopsy tissue revealed a range of abnormalities from moderate acute hepatitis to bridging fibrosis, advanced fibrosis, and cirrhosis. In all four women the aminotransferase levels returned to normal and symptoms resolved with discontinuation of the herbal compound. Several other cases of jaundice have been reported to the Welsh Drug Information Centre after the ingestion of preparations containing skullcap, valerian, or both.[91]

In 2008, the first case of potential valerian hepatotoxicity in 20 years was described.[161] In this report, a young Nicaraguan woman was evaluated by her physician because of epigastric pain, nausea, and fatigue for 2 weeks. She had no other symptoms, no contact with sick people, and no recent travel. Her medications included valerian root in 300-mg tablets, which she had taken twice daily over the previous 3 months. Physical examination showed only hepatomegaly and epigastric tenderness. Biochemical tests revealed serum aminotransferases in the 600- to 800-U/L range, mildly elevated alkaline phosphatase, and normal bilirubin. Amylase, lipase, albumin, the prothrombin time, viral hepatitis serology, and autoimmune antibodies were within normal limits. Valerian was discontinued and improvement in liver test values was noted as early as 3 days. Within 4 weeks, she was asymptomatic with normal liver test results and normal findings on physical examination.

C. asiatica is an ayurvedic medicine used as a slimming aid and to treat leprosy and skin lesions. Three cases of acute hepatitis in middle-aged women using the medication as a slimming aid have been described.[162] All three women used the medicine for 3 to 8 weeks, and all had clinical and biochemical evidence of an acute hepatocellular process and elevation of autoimmune markers. Histologic examination revealed granulomatous hepatitis in two specimens and cirrhosis in the third. The woman with cirrhosis recalled having abnormal liver associated test results during consumption of *C. asiatica* 1 year previously. All three were treated with ursodeoxycholic acid, prednisone, or both, and all recovered completely. The authors note that it is unclear whether treatment in these cases was indicated. *C. asiatica* contains pentacyclic triterpenic saponosides, which may induce germander-like reactive metabolites and lead to immune-mediated injury.

In all of these cases, with the exception of *C. asiatica* in which previous use had caused similar symptoms, the association with hepatitis is presumed; direct experimental evidence is lacking.

Weight Loss Aids—Chaso/Onshido/LipoKinetix: *N*-Nitrosofenfluramine–Containing Products

Chaso and Onshido are two widely available Chinese herbal weight loss aids. The manufacturers report that Chaso contains green tea, cassia torae semen, leaves of lotus, *Fructus lycii*, *Fructus crataegi*, and chrysanthemum flowers. Onshido contains extract of *Gynostemma pentaphyllum makino*, green tea, aloe, *F. crataegi*, and raphani semen. In 2002, 12 Japanese patients (6 using Chaso and 6 using Onshido) exhibited symptoms of severe fatigue and anorexia 5 to 40 days after ingesting the herbs.[163] Most mistook their symptoms for those associated with weight loss and did not seek immediate medical attention. On evaluation, aminotransferase and bilirubin levels were increased, and the INR was significantly elevated. Hepatic encephalopathy developed in two patients, and one underwent liver transplantation 8 days after admission. Another patient died 45 days after admission secondary to intestinal bleeding and infection; the remaining 10 patients improved after discontinuation of the herbals, with the liver biochemical test results all returning to normal.[163] On analysis of the ingredients contained in the preparations, *N*-nitrosofenfluramine was detected. Fenfluramine was once prescribed for weight loss but was withdrawn from clinical use because of severe cardiac complications. Although fenfluramine was not identified in either Chaso or Onshido, data suggest that *N*-D-nitroso compounds have been linked with hepatic carcinogenesis.[164] The mechanism of injury is thought to be direct hepatotoxicity. In vitro studies of rat hepatocytes have demonstrated increased mitochondrial permeability and uncoupled oxidative phosphorylation resulting in intracellular depletion of ATP and cell death.[165]

Since publication of this report, 21 cases of Chaso-induced hepatitis and 135 cases of Onshido-induced hepatitis were reported to the Ministry of Health, Labor, and Welfare in Japan, most occurring between April and August 2002.[166] Other *N*-nitrosofenfluramine–containing compounds have been implicated in the causality of hepatotoxicity, including Sennomotokounou and LipoKinetix.[167] LipoKinetix is a dietary supplement that contains sodium usniate, norephedrine, yohimbine, and caffeine, in addition to *N*-nitrosofenfluramine. Favreau and colleagues reported seven patients in whom acute hepatitis developed after the use of LipoKinetix. Within 1 month of use, most patients reported jaundice, fatigue, and abdominal pain.[168] Serum aminotransferase levels peaked at 14,000 U/L, along with a moderate rise in bilirubin of 38 to 250 µmol/L. Complete recovery was noted within 3 months after drug discontinuation in all patients. Unfortunately, liver biopsy data were not available from any of the cases. The herbals have subsequently been removed from the market in the United States. Although making a definitive case for causality is difficult, LipoKinetix also contains sodium usniate or usnic acid, a compound previously implicated in severe liver injury. In one instance, acute liver failure necessitating liver transplantation developed in a 28-year-old woman 1 month after beginning usnic acid.[169] Extensive parenchymal collapse was noted during examination of the explant. In another case, panacinar hepatitis and bridging necrosis were noted.[170] Usnic acid is also found in Kombucha tea, which is made by brewing the Manchurian mushroom Kombucha in sweet black tea. In the 1990s, a few cases of acute hepatitis associated with drinking this tea were reported.[171] As with *N*-nitrosofenfluramine, in vitro testing of usnic acid has demonstrated uncoupling of oxidative phosphorylation with the subsequent generation of oxidative stress.[172]

Conclusion

The use of herbal preparations to treat various medical conditions is increasing. In most consumers of herbals there is an implicit assumption of safety, and therefore physician consultation is not sought. Over the past decade, as the popularity of herbal remedies has increased, so have reports of toxicity. The scope of hepatotoxicity ranges from asymptomatic elevations in liver biochemistry panels to chronic hepatitis, cirrhosis, and fulminant hepatic failure. Unfortunately, herbal preparations are neither regulated nor standardized, thereby making precise identification and quantification of ingredients or possible contaminants extremely challenging. This shortcoming significantly hampers the ability to definitively assign causality to a particular herb when evidence of hepatic injury is observed. In most instances of reported toxicity, no attempt at phytochemical analysis is made; rather, a presumptive association is based on temporal relationships and, occasionally, unintentional rechallenge. Despite these drawbacks, the volume of consistent reporting of herb-related hepatotoxicity mandates serious consideration. It is essential that increased public awareness regarding the potential toxicity of herbals be maintained, as well as improved agricultural monitoring, appropriate regulatory systems, and improved scientific evaluation of the potential benefits and hazards of herbal preparations.

Key References

Adachi M, et al. Hepatic injury in 12 patients taking the herbal weight loss AIDS Chaso or Onshido. Ann Intern Med 2003;139:488–492. (Ref.163)

Bjornsson E, Olsson R. Serious adverse liver reactions associated with herbal weight-loss supplements. J Hepatol 2007;47:295–297. (Ref.109)

Bonkovsky HL. Hepatotoxicity associated with supplements containing Chinese green teas (*Camellia sinensis*). Ann Intern Med 2006;144:68–69. (Ref.106)

Borrelli F, Ernst E. Black cohosh (*Cimicifuga racemosa*). A systematic review of adverse events. Am J Obstet Gynecol 2008;199:455–466. (Ref.53)

Borum ML. Fulminant exacerbation of autoimmune hepatitis after the use of ma huang. Am J Gastroenterol 2001;96:1654–1655. (Ref.142)

Bressler R. Herb-drug interactions: interactions between kava and prescription medications. Geriatrics 2005;60:24–25. (Ref.139)

Centers for Disease Control and Prevention (CDC). Hepatic toxicity possibly associated with kava-containing products—United States, Germany and Switzerland, 1999-2002. MMWR Morb Mortal Wkly Rep 2002;51(47):1065–1067. (Ref.131)

Chitturi S, Farrell GC. Herbal hepatotoxicity: an expanding but poorly defined problem. J Gastroenterol Hepatol 2000;15:1093–1099. (Ref.35)

Chow EC, et al. Liver failure associated with the use of black cohosh for menopausal symptoms. Med J Aust 2008;188:420–422. (Ref.47)

Cohen DL, Del Toto Y. A case of valerian-associated hepatotoxicity. J Clin Gastroenterol 2008;42:961–962. (Ref.161)

Cohen SM, et al. Autoimmune hepatitis associated with the use herbal preparations containing black cohosh. Menopause 2004;11:575–577. (Ref.48)

Conti E, et al. *Lycopodium similiaplex*–induced acute hepatitis: a case report. Eur J Gastroenterol Hepatol 2008;20:468–471. (Ref.128)

Dai N, et al. Gynura root induces hepatic veno-occlusive disease: a case report and review of the literature. World J Gastroenterol 2007;13:1628–1631. (Ref.72)

Daniele C, et al. *Atractylis gummifera* L. poisoning—an ethnopharmacologic review. Ethnopharmacology 2005;97:175–162. (Ref.37)

Dara L, Hewett J, Lim K. Hydroxycut hepatotoxicity: a case series and review of liver toxicity from herbal weight loss supplements. World J Gastroenterol 2008;14:6999–7004. (Ref.118)

De Berardinis V, et al. Human microsomal epoxide hydrolase is the target of germander-induced autoantibodies on the surface of human hepatocytes. Mol Pharmacol 2000;58:542–551. (Ref.100)

DeLeve LD, et al. Embolization by sinusoidal lining cells obstructs the microcirculation in rat sinusoidal obstruction syndrome. Am J Physiol Gastrointest Liver Physiol 2003;125:882–890. (Ref.87)

DeLeve LD, Shulman HM, McDonald GB. Toxic injury to hepatic sinusoids: sinusoidal obstruction syndrome (veno-occlusive disease). Semin Liver Dis 2002;22:27–42. (Ref.36)

De Smet PA. Herbal medicine in Europe—relaxing regulatory standards. N Engl J Med 2005;352:1176–1178. (Ref.3)

Directive 2004/24/EC of the European Parliament and of the council amending, as regards traditional herbal medicinal products, Directive 2001/83 EC on the community code relating to the medicinal products for human use. Official Journal of the European Union; Available at http://www.mhra.gov.uk/home/groups/es-herbal/documents/websiteresources/con009359.pdf. (Ref.8)

Dourakis SP, et al. Acute hepatitis associated with herb (*Teucrium capitatum* L.) administration. Eur J Gastroenterol Hepatol 2002;14:693–696. (Ref.93)

Duque JM, et al. Hepatotoxicity associated with the consumption of herbal slimming products. Med Clin (Barc) 2007;128:238–239. (Ref.124)

Durazo FA, et al. Fulminant liver failure due to usnic acid for weight loss. Am J Gastroenterol 2004;99:950–952. (Ref.169)

Elinav E, et al. Association between Herbalife nutritional supplements and acute hepatotoxicity. J Hepatol 2007;47:514–520. (Ref.123)

Estes JD, et al. High prevalence of potentially hepatotoxic herbal supplement use in patients with fulminant hepatic failure. Arch Surg 2003;138:852–858. (Ref.145)

European Medicines Evaluation Agency. Assessments of case reports connected to herbal medicinal products containing *Cimicifigae racemosae* rhizome (black cohosh root). Available at http://www.emaeuropa.eu/pdfs/human/hmpe/26925806.pdf. Accessed Nov 15, 2008. (Ref.51)

Favreau JT, et al. severe hepatotoxicity associated with the dietary supplement LipoKinetix. Ann Intern Med 2002;136:590–595. (Ref.168)

Fong T-L, et al. Hepatotoxicity due to Hydroxycut 2010; a case series. Am J Gastroenterol 2010;105:1561–1566. (Ref.121)

Fu PP, et al. Toxicity of kava-kava. J Environ Sci Health C Environ Carcinog Ecotoxicol Rev 2008;26:89–112. (Ref.137)

Fugh-Berman A. Herb-drug interactions. Lancet 2000;355:134–138. (Ref.23)

Galati G, et al. Cellular and in-vivo hepatotoxicity caused by green tea phenolic acids and catechins. Free Radic Biol Med 2006;40:570–580. (Ref.112)

Garcia-Cortez M, et al. Liver injury induced by "natural remedies": an analysis of cases submitted to the Spanish Liver Toxicity Registry. Span J Gastroenterol 2008;100:688–695. (Ref.110)

Gardiner P, et al. Factors associated with dietary supplement use among prescription medication users. Arch Intern Med 2006;166:1968–1974. (Ref.7)

Gloro R, et al. Fulminant hepatitis during self-medication with hydroalcoholic extract of green tea. Eur J Gastroenterol Hepatol 2005;17:1135–1137. (Ref.105)

Goodin MG, Bray BJ, Rosen RJ. Sex- and strain-dependent effects of epigallocatechin gallate (EGCG) and epicatechin gallate (ECG) in the mouse. Food Chem Toxicol 2006;44:1496–1504. (Ref.114)

Gow PJ, et al. Fatal fulminant hepatic failure induced by a natural therapy containing kava. Med J Aust 2003;178:442–443. (Ref.134)

Han D, et al. Usnic acid–induced necrosis of cultured mouse hepatocytes: inhibition of mitochondrial function and oxidative stress. Biochem Pharmacol 2004;67:439–451. (Ref.172)

Humbertson CL, Akhtar J, Krenzelok EP. Acute hepatitis induced by kava kava. J Toxicol Clin Toxicol 2003;41:109–113. (Ref.135)

Jiminez-Saenz M, Martinez-Sanchez MDC. Acute hepatitis associated wit the use of green tea infusions. J Hepatol 2006;44:616–617. (Ref.107)

Jones FJ, Andrews AH. Acute injury associated with the herbal supplement Hydroxycut in a soldier deployed in Iraq. Am J Gastroenterol 2007;102:2357–2358. (Ref.117)

Jorge OA, Jorge AD. Hepatotoxicity associated with the ingestion of *Centella asiatica*. Rev Esp Enferm 2005;97:115–124. (Ref.162)

Karliova H, et al. Interaction of *Hypericum perforatum* (St John's wort) with cyclosporin A metabolism in a patient after liver transplantation. J Hepatol 2000;33:853–855. (Ref.21)

Kauma H, et al. Toxic acute hepatitis and hepatic fibrosis after consumption of chaparral tablets. Scand J Gastroenterol 2004;39:1168–1171. (Ref.66)

Kawaguchi T, et al. Severe hepatotoxicity associated with *N*-nitrosofenfluramine–containing weight-loss supplement: report of three cases. J Gastroenterol Hepatol 2004;19:349–350. (Ref.167)

Laczek J, Duncan M. Three cases of acute hepatitis in patients taking Hydroxycut bodybuilding supplement. Am J Gastroenterol 2008;103(S1):143. (Ref.119)

Levitsky J, et al. Fulminant liver failure associated with the use of black cohosh. Dig Dis Sci 2005;50:538–539. (Ref.45)

Lopaz-Capero Andrada JM, et al. Hepatotoxicity caused by a Noni (*Morinda citrifolia*) preparation. Rev Esp Enferm Dig 2007;99:179–181. (Ref.155)

Lynch CR, Hutson WR. Fulminant hepatic failure associated with the use of black cohosh. Liver Transpl 2006;12:989–992. (Ref.46)

Manso G, et al. Spanish reports of hepatotoxicity associated with Herbalife products. J Hepatol 2008;49:289–290. (Ref.125)

Mazzanti G, et al. Hepatotoxicity from green tea: a review of the literature and two unpublished cases. Eur J Clin Pharmacol 2009;65:331–341. (Ref.111)

Millonig G, Stadlmann S, Vogel W. Herbal hepatotoxicity: acute hepatitis caused by a Noni preparation (*Morinda citrifolia*). Eur J Gastroenterol Hepatol 2005;17:445–447. (Ref.152)

Ministry of Health, Labor, and Welfare. Hepatic injury in cases taking self-imported healthfoods or non-approved drugs [press release]. Ministry of Health, Labor, and Welfare, 12 July 2002. Accessed at www.mhlw.go.jp/houdou/2002/07/bo712-1.html. (Ref.166)

Molinari M, et al. Acute liver failure induced by green tea extracts: case report and review of the literature. Liver Transpl 2006;12:1892–1895. (Ref.108)

Moro PA, et al. Hepatitis from greater celandine (*Chelidonium majus* L.): review of literature and report of a new case. J Ethnopharmacol 2009;124:328–332. (Ref.101)

Nadir A, et al. Acute hepatitis associated with the use of a Chinese herbal product, ma-huang. Am J Gostroenterol 1996;91:1436–1438. (Ref.115)

Nadir A, Reddy D, Van Thiel DH. *Cascara sagrada*–induced intrahepatic cholestasis causing portal hypertension: case report and review of herbal hepatotoxicity. Am J Gastroenterol 2000;95:3634–3637. (Ref.62)

Nakagawa Y, et al. ATP-generating glycolytic substrates prevent *N*-nitrosofenfluramine–induced cytotoxicity in isolated rat hepatocytes. Chem Biol Interact 2006;164:93–101. (Ref.165)

Neff GW, et al. Severe hepatotoxicity associated with the use of weight loss diet supplements containing ma huang or usnic acid. J Hepatol 2004;41:1062–1064. (Ref.143)

Pedros C, et al. Liver toxicity of *Camellia sinensis* dried ethanolic extract. Med Clin 2003;121:598–599. (Ref.104)

Poon WT, et al. Hepatitis induced by *Teucrium viscidum*. Clin Toxicol 2008;46:819–822. (Ref.94)

Popat A, et al. The toxicity of *Callilepis laureola*, a South African traditional herbal medicine. Clin Biochem 2001;34:229–236. (Ref.39)

Popat A, et al. Mechanism of impila (*Callilepis laureola*)-induced cytotoxicity in Hep G2 cells. Clin Biochem 2002;35:57–64. (Ref.40)

Rasenack R, et al. Veno-occlusive disease in a fetus caused by pyrrolizidine alkaloids of food origin. Fetal Diagn Ther 2003;18:223–225. (Ref.84)

Russmann S, et al. Hepatic injury due to traditional aqueous extracts of kava root in New Caledonia. Eur J Gastroenterol Hepatol 2003;15:1033–1036. (Ref.133)

Russmann S, Lauterburg BH, Helbling A. Kava hepatotoxicity. Ann Intern Med 2001;135:68–69. (Ref.140)

Sanchez W, et al. Severe hepatotoxicity associated with the use of the dietary supplement containing usnic acid. Mayo Clin Proc 2006;81:541–544. (Ref.170)

Saper RB, et al. Heavy metal content of ayurvedic herbal medicine products. JAMA 2004;292:2868–2873. (Ref.12)

Sarma DN, et al. Safety of green teas extracts: a systematic review of the US Pharmacopeia. Drug Saf 2008;31:469–484. (Ref.102)

Schmidt M, et al. Toxicity of green tea extracts and their constituents in primary culture. Food Chem Toxicol 2005;43:307–314. (Ref.113)

Schoepfer AM, et al. Herbal does not mean innocuous: ten cases of severe hepatotoxicity associated with dietary supplements from Herbalife products. J Hepatol 2007;47:521–526. (Ref.122)

Seeff LB, et al. Herbal product use by persons enrolled in the Hepatitis C Antiviral Long-Term Treatment against Cirrhosis (HALT-C) Trial. Hepatology 2008;47:605–612. (Ref.6)

Shim M, Saab S. Severe hepatotoxicity due to Hydroxycut: a case report. Dig Dis Sci 2009;54:406–408. (Ref.120)

Shimizu I. Sho-saiko-to: Japanese herbal medicine for protection against hepatic fibrosis and carcinoma. J Gastroenterol Hepatol 2000;15(Suppl):D84–D90. (Ref.88)

Singh YN. Potential for interaction of kava and St John's wort and prescription medications. J Ethnopharmacol 2005;100:108–113. (Ref.138)

Skoulidid F, Alexander G, Davies SE. Ma huang associated liver failure requiring liver transplantation. Eur J Gastroenterol Hepatol 2005;17:581–584. (Ref.144)

Stadlbauer V, et al. Hepatotoxicity of noni juice: report of two cases. World J Gastroenterol 2005;11:4758–4760. (Ref.153)

Stadlbauer V, et al. Herbal does not mean innocuous: the sixth case of hepatotoxicity associated with Morinda citrifolia (noni). Am J Gastroenterol 2008;103:2406–2407. (Ref.156)

Stedman C. Herbal hepatotoxicity. Semin Liver Dis 2002;22:195–206. (Ref.9)

Steenkamp V, Stewart MJ, Zuckermam M. Clinical and analytic aspects of pyrrolizidine poisoning cause by South African traditional medicines. Ther Drug Monit 2000;22:303–306. (Ref.83)

Stevens T, Qadri A, Zein NN. Two patients with acute liver injury associated with the use of the herbal weight-loss supplement Hydroxycut. Ann Intern Med 2005;142:477–478. (Ref.116)

Stewart MJ, Steenkamp V. The biochemistry and toxicity of atractyloside: a review. Ther Drug Monit 2000;22:641–649. (Ref.42)

Stickel F, et al. Hepatitis induced by kava (Piper methysticum rhizome). J Hepatol 2003;39:62–67. (Ref.130)

Stickel F, et al. Severe hepatotoxicity following ingestion of Herbalife nutritional supplements contaminated with Bacillus subtilis. J Hepatol 2009;50:111–117. (Ref.15)

Stickel F, Egerer G, Seitz HK. Hepatotoxicity of botanicals. Public Health Nutr 2000;3:113–124. (Ref.38)

Strader DB, et al. Use of complementary and alternative medicine in patients with liver disease. Am J Gastroenterol 2002;97:2391–2397. (Ref.5)

Teschke R, et al. Suspected black cohosh hepatotoxicity—challenges and pitfalls of causality assessment. Maturitas 2009;63:302–314. (Ref.52)

Teschke R, Gaus W, Loew D. Kava extracts: safety and risks including rare hepatotoxicity. Phytomedicine 2003;10:440–446. (Ref.141)

Teschke R, Genthner A, Wolff A. Kava hepatotoxicity: comparison of aqueous, ethanolic, acetonic kava extracts and kava-herb mixtures. J Ethnopharmacol 2009;123:378–384. (Ref.129)

Teschke R, Schwarzenboeck A, Hennermann K-H. Kava hepatotoxicity: a clinical survey and critical analysis of 26 suspected cases. Eur J Gastroenterol Hepatol 2008;20:1182–1193. (Ref.132)

Thomsen M. Hepatotoxicity of Cimicifuga racemosa? Recent Australian case not sufficiently substantiated. J Altern Med 2003;9:337–340. (Ref.50)

Uc A, Bishop WP, Sanders KD. Camphor hepatotoxicity. South Med J 2000;93:596–598. (Ref.54)

Vial T, et al. Acute hepatitis due to Exolise, a Camellia sinensis–derived drug. Gastroenterol Clin Biol 2003;27:1166–1167. (Ref.103)

Vitetta L, Thomsen M, Sali A. Black cohosh and other herbal remedies associated with acute hepatitis. Med J Aust 2003;178:411–412. (Ref.49)

Wang MY, et al. Morinda citrifolia (Noni): a literature review and recent advances in Noni research. Acta Pharmacol Sin 2002;23:1127–1141. (Ref.150)

Wang X, Kanel GC, DeLeve LD. Support of sinusoidal endothelial cell glutathione prevents hepatic veno-occlusive disease in the rat. Hepatology 2000;31:428–434. (Ref.86)

Weise B, et al. Toxic hepatitis after intake of kava-kava. Verdauungskrankheiten 2003;4:166–169. (Ref.136)

West BJ, Jensen JJ, Westendorf J. Noni juice is not hepatotoxic. World J Gastroenterol 2006;12:3616–3619. (Ref.157)

Whiting PW, Clouston A, Kerlin P. Black cohosh and other herbal remedies associated with acute hepatitis. Med J Aust 2002;177:440–443. (Ref.44)

Wilson KM, et al. Use of complementary medicine and dietary supplements among U.S. adolescents. J Adolesc Health 2006;38:385–394. (Ref.2)

Yuce B, et al. Hepatitis induced by Noni juice from Morinda citrifolia: a rare cause of hepatotoxicity or the tip of the iceberg? Digestion 2006;73:167–170. (Ref.154)

A complete list of references can be found at www.expertconsult.com.

Chapter **27**

Occupational and Environmental Hepatotoxicity

Matt Cave, Keith Cameron Falkner, and Craig McClain

ABBREVIATIONS

2,4-D 2,4-dichlorophenoxyacetic acid
2,4,5-T 2,4,5-trichlorophenoxyacetic acid
AhR aryl hydrocarbon receptor
AP-1 activator protein-1
ATSDR Agency for Toxic Substances and Disease Registry
BPA bisphenol A
CAR constitutive androstane receptor
CAS Chemical Abstracts Service
CCl$_4$ carbon tetrachloride
CERM cumulative exposure rank month
CFC chlorofluorocarbon
DCA dichloroacetate
DDT dichlorodiphenyltrichloroethane
DEHP di(2-ethylhexyl)phthalate
DILI drug-induced liver injury
DMAC dimethylacetamide
DMF dimethylformamide
EPA Environmental Protection Agency
FDA U.S. Food and Drug Administration
FIFRA Federal Insecticide, Fungicide, and Rodenticide Act

FHH focal hepatocytic hyperplasia
FMH focal mixed hyperplasia
HPV high production volume
IARC International Agency for Research on Cancer
IRIS Integrated Risk Information System
LPS lipopolysaccharide
MDA methylenedianiline
MeHg methylmercury
NCTR National Center for Toxicological Research
NF-κB nuclear factor κB light-chain enhancer of activated B cells
NHANES National Health and Nutrition Examination Survey
NIEHS National Institute of Environmental Health Sciences
NIOSH National Institute for Occupational Safety and Health
NOES National Occupational Exposure Survey

nrf-2 nuclear factor (erythroid-derived 2)-like 2
NTP National Toxicology Program
OSHA Occupational Safety and Health Administration
PCBs polychlorinated biphenyls
PCE perchloroethylene (tetrachloroethylene)
PPAR-α peroxisome proliferator–activated receptor-α
PVC polyvinyl chloride
SAMe S-adenosylmethionine
SECs sinusoidal endothelial cells
SOT Society of Toxicology
TASH toxicant-associated steatohepatitis
TCA trichloroacetate
TCDD 2,3,7,8-tetrachlorodibenzodioxin
TCE trichloroethylene
TNT trinitrotoluene
TSCA Toxic Substances Control Act
VC vinyl chloride

Introduction

As of December 2009, more than 50 million unique chemicals were registered with the Chemical Abstracts Service (CAS). Notably, only 9 months had passed since registration of the 40 millionth chemical. With the rapid commercialization of many new chemicals, it is virtually impossible to fully understand the potential impact of these compounds on the human liver. The National Institute for Occupational Safety and Health (NIOSH) issues the *Pocket Guide to Chemical Hazards*, which contains information on 677 chemicals commonly found in the work environment. Hepatotoxicity has been documented for approximately a third of these chemicals.[1] In the United States, the Toxic Substances Control Act (TSCA) and the Federal Insecticide, Fungicide, and Rodenticide Act (FIFRA) regulate toxic chemicals and pesticides, respectively. The TSCA is enforced by the Environmental Protection Agency (EPA), which must assess and approve all toxic

chemicals before they may be marketed. Despite these regulations, as late as 1997, basic toxicity data were unavailable for nearly 75% of high production volume (HPV) chemicals. The EPA has addressed this gap through initiatives such as the HPV Challenge Program, which challenges companies to post health and environmental data on all chemicals used in excess of 1 million pounds per year. In addition to the *Pocket Guide to Chemical Hazards*, the EPA's Integrated Risk Information System (IRIS), the National Toxicology Program (NTP), and the International Agency for Research on Cancer (IARC) have searchable databases containing hepatotoxicity data for selected industrial chemicals. **Table 27-1** contains internet addresses for these and other relevant agencies involved in chemical toxicity.

The rapid pace of chemical discovery outstrips current toxicity screening assays. Therefore it remains impossible to completely understand the potential hepatotoxicity of many chemicals. However, in the future, high-throughput in silico analysis, such as that currently being developed through the EPA's Virtual Liver Project (v-Liver), may enable rapid liver toxicity screening. This chapter reviews the principles of toxicity from industrial and environmental chemicals and describes specific examples of well-documented industrial hepatotoxicants (**Table 27-2**). A comprehensive list of the 228 hepatotoxic industrial chemicals from the NIOSH *Pocket Guide to Chemical Hazards* may be found in the review article by Tolman and Sirrine.[1]

Clinical Features, Patterns of Liver Injury, and Treatment

Occupational and environmental liver diseases may be accompanied by a wide spectrum of liver injury ranging from asymptomatic elevation of liver enzymes to acute liver failure, cirrhosis, and cancer (**Table 27-3**; also see Table 27-2). In some cases, such as with vinyl chloride (VC), the Occupational Safety and Health Administration (OSHA) mandates that a medical surveillance program to monitor serial liver enzymes

be implemented in highly exposed workers. Unusual pathognomonic lesions such as zonal necrosis or vascular lesions such as hemangiosarcoma or sinusoidal damage may raise suspicion for chemical-induced liver disease. However, in most cases the pathologic findings are nonspecific, thus making a high degree of clinical suspicion and a thorough occupational history critically important. From an occupational and public health standpoint, the burden of chemical-induced chronic liver disease may be underappreciated because it may be associated with normal liver enzyme levels.[2,3] In fact, steatohepatitis with normal serum transaminase levels appears to be one of the most common forms of chemical hepatitis (**Table 27-4**). Therefore occupational and environmental liver diseases are likely to largely be underrecognized by clinicians because of a lack of suspicion compounded by a lack of effective serologic biomarker tests. Until proved otherwise, occupational and environmental liver disease must be considered in the differential diagnosis of all forms of liver disease, and a thorough occupational history must be taken with special consideration given to high-risk occupations (**Table 27-5**) and household exposures. Furthermore, synergies between industrial chemicals and other liver diseases such as viral hepatitis and alcoholic liver disease have been described.

In most cases, treatment involves removal from the workplace and supportive care. However, following some acute ingestions, gastric decontamination is indicated. Liver transplantation has been performed in rare situations (e.g., VC-related hepatic hemangiosarcoma, industrial chemical–related fulminant failure). In general, there are no validated specific treatments of occupational and environmental liver disease. However, chelation therapy has been performed in some instances of metal toxicity with variable results. Cholestyramine and the nonabsorbable dietary lipid olestra have been demonstrated to reduce the burden of persistent organic pollutants that undergo enterohepatic circulation (including organochlorine pesticides, polychlorinated biphenyls [PCBs], and dioxin) by increasing their elimination through the gastrointestinal tract.[4,5] Although weight loss mobilizes lipophilic-persistent pollutants stored in adipose tissue for potential elimination, this may also lead to increased damage to nonadipose tissues such as skeletal muscle and potentially the liver. Because oxidative stress appears to be a conserved mechanism for many forms of occupational liver disease, antioxidants, such as *N*-acetylcysteine, warrant further study for the prevention and treatment of chemical liver disease.

Similarities and Differences Between Occupational and Environmental Liver Diseases and Drug-Induced Liver Injury

Occupational liver diseases are, in most cases, quite different from drug-induced liver injury (DILI). First, the typical routes of exposure are different. Apart from anesthetic gases such as

Table 27-2 Selected Hepatotoxic Industrial Chemicals, Their Uses, and Toxicities

CHEMICAL	USES	HEPATIC RESPONSES
Arsenic	Pesticides, wood preservatives, semiconductors, drugs, environmental pollutant	Acute hepatitis, steatosis, hepatocellular necrosis, cirrhosis, hemangiosarcoma, hepatocellular carcinoma (possible), portal hypertension
Carbon tetrachloride	Chemical intermediate; formerly used as a solvent, as a refrigerant, and in fire extinguishers	Acute liver failure, steatosis, hepatocellular necrosis, cirrhosis, hepatocellular carcinoma (possible)
Chlordecone	Insecticide	Hepatomegaly, steatosis, portal inflammation
Di(2-ethylhexyl)phthalate (DEHP)	Plasticizer	Total parenteral nutrition–related cholestatic liver disease
Dimethylacetamide (DMAC)	Solvent, synthetic fibers	Abnormal liver enzymes
Dimethylformamide (DMF)	Solvent	Abnormal liver enzymes, acute hepatitis, steatosis, hepatocellular necrosis
Dioxin	Herbicide contaminant	Porphyria cutanea tarda
Lead	Environmental pollutant	Lead-induced hepatic hyperplasia
Methylenedianiline (MDA)	Solvent	Acute cholestatic hepatitis/cholangitis
Methylmercury	Environmental pollutant	Steatosis, mitochondrial abnormalities
Nitrobenzene	Chemical intermediate	Steatosis, centrilobular necrosis, bile stasis
2-Nitropropane	Solvent, chemical intermediate, explosives	Acute liver failure, steatosis, hepatocellular necrosis
Paraquat	Herbicide	Acute cholestatic hepatitis/cholangitis
Polychlorinated biphenyls (PCBs)	Environmental pollutant; formerly used in transformers, capacitors, and hydraulic fluids	Toxic hepatopathy, cirrhosis, hepatocellular carcinoma
Tetrachloroethane	Solvent	Subacute liver failure, steatosis, hepatocellular necrosis
Tetrachloroethylene (perchloroethylene [PCE])	Solvent, dry-cleaning fluid	Steatosis, hepatocellular necrosis, hepatocellular carcinoma (probable)
Trichloroethane	Solvent	Steatosis, hepatocellular necrosis, cirrhosis
Trichloroetheylene (TCE)	Solvent, degreaser	Acute liver failure, steatohepatitis, autoimmune hepatitis, cirrhosis hepatocellular carcinoma (probable)
Toluene, benzene, xylene	Solvents, chemical intermediates	Steatohepatitis
Trinitrotoluene (TNT)	Explosives	Subacute liver failure, cirrhosis, hepatocellular carcinoma
Vinyl chloride	Plastics, solvent production, chemical intermediate	Steatohepatitis, cirrhosis, hemangiosarcoma, hepatocellular carcinoma
Yellow phosphorus	Matches, fireworks, rodenticides	Acute hepatitis, periportal steatosis, hepatocellular necrosis

Adapted from Schiano D, Hunt K. Occupational and environmental hepatotoxicity. In: Zakim D, Boyer TD, editors. Hepatology: a textbook of liver disease, 5th ed. Philadelphia: WB Saunders, 2006.

halothane, most medications associated with DILI are administered orally. In contrast, most occupational exposures occur via inhalation and may also be associated with skin, eye, and mucous membrane irritation. Many volatile industrial chemicals are hydrophobic organic chemicals and may be absorbed transdermally, even across some "protective" gloves. Inhalational exposure of many industrial chemicals is regulated by OSHA. In contrast, environmental liver disease, similar to DILI, typically involves the ingestion of chemical pollutants,

such as methylmercury (MeHg) and PCBs, which bioconcentrate in the food chain.

Mechanistically, as in DILI, the hepatotoxicity of many industrial chemicals depends on their bioactivation by cytochrome P-450. However, in contrast to DILI, where the majority of reactions are idiosyncratic, most cases of occupational liver disease are believed to be mediated by dose-dependent cytotoxic agents. Furthermore, industrial chemicals are more likely than prescription medications to be carcinogenic.

Table 27-3 Chemical-induced Liver Disease Patterns in Humans or Animal Models

CATEGORY	SELECTED EXAMPLES
Steatohepatitis	Petrochemical mixtures, vinyl chloride, others (see Table 27-4)
Necrosis	Carbon tetrachloride and other halogenated aliphatic hydrocarbons, haloaromatic compounds, nitroaromatic compounds, arsenic, yellow phosphorus
Cholestasis	Beryllium, copper, di(2-ethylhexyl) phthalate, methylenedianiline, paraquat, toxic rapeseed oil
Cirrhosis	Arsenic, carbon tetrachloride, polychlorinated biphenyls, trichloroethane, trichloroethylene, trinitrotoluene, vinyl chloride
Peliosis hepatitis	Thorotrast, urethane, vinyl chloride
Granulomas	Beryllium, copper
Pigment deposition	Anthracite, Thorotrast, titanium
Cholangiocarcinoma	Thorotrast, polychlorinated biphenyls (rodents)
Hepatocellular carcinoma	Arsenic, carbon tetrachloride, polychlorinated biphenyls, tetrachloroethylene (rodents), Thorotrast, trichloroethylene, trinitrotoluene, vinyl chloride
Hemangiosarcoma	Vinyl chloride, butoxyethanol (rodents), chloronitrobenzene (rodents), polyhexamethylene biguanine (rodents), urethane, tetrafluoroethylene (rodents)

Adapted from Schiano D, Hunt K. Occupational and environmental hepatotoxicity. In: Zakim D, Boyer TD, editors. Hepatology: a textbook of liver disease, 5th ed. Philadelphia: WB Saunders, 2006.

Table 27-4 Selected Chemicals Associated with Steatohepatitis in Humans or Animal Models with Either Normal or Elevated Serum Transaminase Levels

STEATOHEPATITIS WITH NORMAL TRANSAMINASE LEVELS	STEATOHEPATITIS WITH ELEVATED (OR UNKNOWN) TRANSAMINASE LEVELS
Lead	Arsenic
Nitrobenzene	Carbon tetrachloride
Nitromethane	Dimethylformamide (DMF)
Tetrachloroethylene (perchloroethylene [PCE])	Methylmercury
1,1,1-Trichloroethane	Pesticides: chlordecone, atrazine, paraquat
Toluene	Petrochemical mixtures: benzene, toluene, xylene, etc.
Vinyl chloride	Polychlorinated biphenyls (PCBs)
	Thallium
	Yellow phosphorus

Table 27-5 Selected Occupations that May Entail Exposure to Hepatotoxicants

Airplane hangar employees	Lacquer makers and lacquerers
Artificial pearl makers	Leather workers
Burnishers	Linoleum makers
Cement makers	Paint remover makers and users
Chemical industry workers	Paraffin workers
Chemists	Perfume makers
Chlorinated rubber makers	Pesticide makers
Cobblers	Petrochemical refiners and workers
Color makers	Pharmaceutical workers
Core makers	Photographic material workers
Degreasers	Plastics workers
Dry cleaners	Polish (metal) makers and users
Dye makers	Printers
Dyers	Refrigerator workers
Electrical equipment manufacturers	Resin makers
Electroplaters	Rubber workers
Enamel makers	Semiconductor makers
Extractors, oil and fats	Shoe factory workers
Fire extinguisher makers	Soap makers
Galvanizers	Straw hat makers
Garage workers	Synthetic fabric makers
Gardeners and farmers (pesticides)	Thermometer makers
Gas (illuminating) workers	Tobacco denicotizers
Glass makers	Varnish workers
Glue workers	Waterproofers
Ink makers	Wax makers
Insulators (wire)	

Adapted from Zimmerman HJ. Occupational hepatotoxicity. In: Zimmerman HJ, editor. Hepatotoxicity: the adverse effects of drugs and other chemicals on the liver, 2nd ed. Philadelphia: Lippincott Williams & Wilkins, 1999.

Multiple factors, including the setting, timing, magnitude, route, and co-exposures, are potential determinants of exposure severity. However, it has become increasingly clear that individuals have differing susceptibilities to occupational and environmental liver disease. An individual's susceptibility is determined, in part, by polymorphisms in genes of xenobiotic metabolism, age of the employee, concomitant use of alcohol or prescription medications, nutritional factors, and obesity inasmuch as many organic chemicals are lipid soluble.[6,7] Recently, it was demonstrated that hypertriglyceridemia is a risk factor for greater absorption of inhalational organic chemicals because it changes the blood-air partition coefficient to increase the solubility of these molecules in the bloodstream.[8]

Halogenated Aliphatic Compounds

Haloalkenes, including VC, and other compounds, such as carbon tetrachloride (CCl_4), represent for historical purposes the paradigm for occupational liver disease. These and other relevant haloalkenes such as trichloroethylene (TCE) and tetrachloroethylene are discussed subsequently. Many of these agents remain important from either industrial/environmental health or mechanistic research perspectives. Although a wide spectrum of liver diseases have been associated with these compounds, steatohepatitis and liver cancer remain hallmarks of their hepatotoxicity. Importantly, in cases of chronic liver disease induced by these chemicals, routine liver enzymes may be normal. Thus their potential hepatotoxicity in the industrial setting is probably underestimated.

Haloalkenes

Vinyl Chloride

Vinyl Chloride (VC) (monochloroethylene) is a colorless gas with a sweet, mild odor. Occupational VC exposure has been associated with both malignant and benign liver disease. However, the recognition of VC-related hemangiosarcoma is perhaps the most important sentinel event in occupational hepatology. This initial report occurred in 1974, when Creech and Johnson described the occurrence of the unusual liver tumor hemangiosarcoma in three workers at a single B.F. Goodrich chemical plant in Louisville, Kentucky.[9] However, VC remains a relevant hepatotoxicant, and emerging data suggest that this problem could represent more than a historical curiosity. VC production was recently estimated at 27 million metric tons annually, valued at U.S. $19 billion. VC is most often polymerized into the ubiquitous plastic polyvinyl chloride (PVC). To date, more than 80,000 American chemical workers have been exposed to VC. In addition to its use in PVC, VC is currently used to synthesize chlorinated solvents. Before it was banned by the Consumer Product Safety Commission, VC was used as an aerosol propellant in household consumer products such as hairspray from approximately 1962 through 1974.[10] Furthermore, VC has been identified as a solvent degradation product, and it is present in landfill leachate, where it potentially places surrounding populations at risk. Exposure typically occurs through the dermal and inhalational routes.

VC is listed as class 1 (definite) human carcinogen by the IARC. Of the malignant liver diseases associated with VC exposure, hemangiosarcoma (**Fig. 27-1**), a vascular tumor believed to originate from sinusoidal endothelial cells (SECs), has classically been described.

However, hepatocellular carcinoma has become a more recent concern.[6] Importantly, ethanol appears to be a strongly synergistic risk factor for both cirrhosis and hepatocellular carcinoma in highly exposed VC workers.[6] Although hemangiosarcoma may occur spontaneously with some frequency in other mammalian species, it is exceptionally rare in humans.[11] To date, hepatic hemangiosarcoma has developed in 25 B.F. Goodrich workers from the Louisville plant, and this is probably the largest single-site cluster worldwide.[12] All Louisville cases to date came from a group of approximately 100 highly exposed chemical workers and helpers who entered and manually cleaned PVC batch reactor vessels (polys or autoclaves). These workers were exposed to exceptionally high concentrations of VC and lower concentrations of approximately 30 other chemicals. These VC exposures may have been in excess of 1000 ppm and occurred during the manual scraping and chipping of resins from the reactor walls from the onset of plant operations in 1942 until implementation of the modern time-weighted VC exposure limit of 1 ppm in 1975.

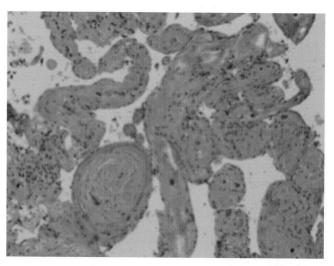

Fig. 27-1 Photomicrograph (100×, hematoxylin-eosin stain) of a well-differentiated vinyl chloride–related hepatic hemangiosarcoma.

Importantly, hepatic hemangiosarcoma occurred only in workers with high cumulative VC exposure. Although cancer did not develop in the majority of the most highly exposed workers, their risk remains high because of a long latency period. In the Louisville experience, hemangiosarcoma was diagnosed at a mean of 30.7 ± 12.2 years after the first VC exposure.[12] Large epidemiologic studies of more than 10,000 North American and 12,000 European VC workers have confirmed excess mortality from hemangiosarcoma in VC workers.[13,14] In accord with the Louisville data, the duration of exposure, cumulative exposure, and employment as an autoclave cleaner were risk factors for hemangiosarcoma mortality. At cumulative exposures below 1500 ppm/yr, mortality from hemangiosarcoma approached that of the entire cohort, again demonstrating the dose dependence of this cancer.[14] Recently, a case series documented the occurrence of hepatic hemangiosarcoma in a barber and cosmetologist with hairspray propellant–related VC exposures in excess of 1000 ppm.[10] Hemangiosarcoma occurred in these hairdressers following a prolonged latency period in excess of 30 years, which is consistent with the chemical worker cases.

Hepatic hemangiosarcoma in VC workers remains a diagnostic dilemma. Liver enzymes are insensitive for the diagnosis of hemangiosarcoma, and even modern cross-sectional imaging techniques such as magnetic resonance imaging do not reliably distinguish cavernous hemangioma (benign) from hemangiosarcoma (malignant) unless metastasis has occurred (**Fig. 27-2**). Fatal hemorrhage has occurred following biopsy of VC-induced hemangiosarcoma, similar to cases of sporadic hepatic cavernous hemangioma. Once the diagnosis is made, there are no standardized effective therapies for this tumor, which has uniformly been fatal in the Louisville experience. Excluding one subject who had prolonged survival following resection, the mean survival was 1.24 years after diagnosis.[12] Prolonged survival after complete surgical resection in some early cases has also been reported by other authors.[15] Importantly, because of a high early recurrence rate, liver transplantation is contraindicated in patients with hepatic hemangiosarcoma.[16] Chemotherapy with doxorubicin-based regimens has had limited success in treating advanced disease.[17]

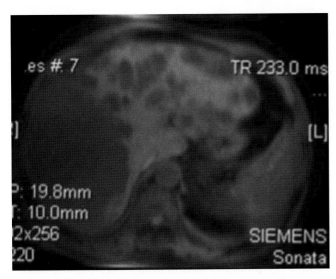

Fig. 27-2 T1-weighted magnetic resonance image of a vinyl chloride worker demonstrating a hypointense liver mass (hemangiosarcoma) that could not be distinguished from cavernous hemangioma.

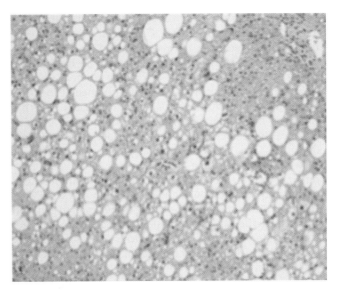

Fig. 27-3 Photomicrograph of a liver biopsy specimen (100×, hematoxylin-eosin stain) from a vinyl chloride worker with toxicant-associated steatohepatitis demonstrating extensive steatosis with a mild inflammatory infiltrate.

The mode of action of VC-related hemangiosarcoma has been attributed to the genotoxicity of several VC metabolites. VC is metabolized in a strikingly similar fashion to ethanol. At concentrations of up to approximately 220 ppm, VC is metabolized by CYP2E1 to the highly reactive genotoxic epoxide chloroethylene oxide. CYP2E1 polymorphisms were associated with fibrosis in VC workers from Taiwan and possibly with hemangiosarcoma at the Louisville plant.[7] Chloroethylene oxide is converted either spontaneously or enzymatically to chloroacetaldehyde. Other liver insults such as viral hepatitis, aflatoxin, and ethanol may potentiate malignant—and possibly benign—VC-related liver diseases.[6,18]

The initial report of VC-related hemangiosarcoma sparked the rapid development of medical surveillance by the chemical plant in association with the University of Louisville and several governmental agencies. Importantly, in 1975 OSHA implemented a time-weighted VC exposure limit of 1 ppm and mandated medical surveillance of VC workers. Although this has virtually eliminated the development of hemangiosarcoma in employees hired after 1975, some cases of VC-related hemangiosarcoma still occur today in the population of VC workers hired before 1975. It is potentially important to note that in the Louisville experience, routine liver enzymes were usually normal at the time of diagnosis of hemangiosarcoma, and the development of serologic biomarkers is ongoing.[12]

Multiple benign liver lesions have been associated with occupational VC exposure. VC or its metabolites appear to be toxic to SECs, and SECs are believed to be the progenitor cell for hemangiosarcoma. Sinusoidal dilation, ranging from mild to peliosis hepatitis, is a relatively common finding in VC workers. Multiple changes in hepatocytes have also been observed, such as foci of enlarged hepatocytes with increased amounts of cytoplasm and large, hyperchromatic nuclei. These changes were described as focal hepatocytic hyperplasia (FHH).[19] When these hepatocyte changes were observed in association with sinusoidal changes, the term focal mixed hyperplasia (FMH) was used historically.[19] However, it is becoming increasing clear that steatohepatitis may be the most characteristic benign liver lesion in VC workers. As early

as 1975 it was recognized that "fatty changes" similar to those observed in alcoholic liver disease were present in about half of biopsy specimens from chemical workers with high cumulative exposure.[20] In fact, in his final paper addressing FHH and FMH, Hans Popper noted that FHH and FMH were often obscured by "fatty infiltration and/or chronic disease (hepatitis/granuloma)."[19] Our group became interested in this topic following the publication of a report documenting nonalcoholic steatohepatitis in lean Brazilian petrochemical workers exposed to a multitude of chemicals, including VC.[21] Subsequently, 25 liver biopsies from the Louisville plant were reviewed and revealed an 80% prevalence of biopsy-proven steatohepatitis in highly exposed VC workers (**Fig. 27-3**).[2] Subsequently, we coined the term toxicant-associated steatohepatitis (TASH) to describe this condition, which occurred in the absence of obesity or alcohol use. Fibrosis was present in 55% of TASH cases. Remarkably, serum transaminase levels were normal in most cases. TASH was associated with insulin resistance, reduced serum adiponectin levels, marked elevation of proinflammatory cytokines, and reduced serum antioxidants. Although these cases are of historical interest, several ultrasound studies published within the last decade have noted a high incidence of hepatomegaly, steatosis, and fibrosis in modern-day VC workers.[22,23] Unfortunately, these studies were uncontrolled and histologic confirmation was not provided. Clearly, more work needs to be done to determine whether TASH remains a problem for modern-day VC workers with lower occupational exposure.

Trichloroethylene

Trichloroethylene is a colorless liquid that has been used for multiple industrial and medical applications. It was developed and used as an alternative anesthetic agent to chloroform. Although it was initially believed to be safer than chloroform, its use was subsequently abandoned because of toxicity concerns. However, TCE is an excellent solvent, and it was used as a degreasing agent for dry cleaning and is still being used today to clean metals. A total of 197,000 metric tons were used in the United States and Europe combined in 1997, and an estimated 685,000 workers have potentially been exposed.[24] TCE was extensively used by the U.S. military to clean weapons and aircraft. Importantly, TCE is an environmental contaminant at many Superfund sites and military bases. TCE has become an increasingly recognized contaminant of groundwater near these sites, thus potentially exposing surrounding populations, and this has sparked recent legislation in the U.S. Senate. TCE exposure may occur through inhalation, ingestion, or the dermal route. The hepatic metabolism of TCE is exceptionally complex, but similar to VC, it involves CYP2E1-dependent oxidation with subsequent conjugation to glutathione.[25] Along the way many important reactive metabolites such as dichloroacetate (DCA) and trichloroacetate (TCA) are formed and are thought to be mediators of hepatotoxicity.[25]

TCE is listed as a class 2A (probable) human carcinogen by the IARC. TCE induces hepatocellular carcinoma in mice but not rats.[26] Some, but not all, epidemiologic studies show an association between TCE exposure and liver cancer in human populations.[26] However, no association could be demonstrated in a recent metaanalysis.[27] The mode of hepatocarcinogenesis of TCE and its metabolites in mice is complex but involves genotoxicity, activation of peroxisome proliferator–activated receptor-α (PPAR-α), and modulation of cell growth and death.[26]

In contrast to hepatocellular carcinoma, benign liver disease is relatively well established for TCE in human populations. Both acute liver failure and chronic hepatitis have been reported following occupational exposure and recreational abuse (sniffing).[28] Although steatosis has been reported in humans, the majority of recent cases have been associated with a rash, thus suggesting similarity to a drug hypersensitivity reaction.[3] Cirrhosis following chronic exposure has also been reported.[29] Animal studies frequently demonstrate hepatic steatosis with necrosis following TCE exposure, although recent reports demonstrate autoimmune hepatitis.[3] Even though the mechanisms remain to be elicited, these reports suggest that TCE may cause both cytotoxic and immune-mediated forms of liver disease.

Tetrachloroethylene

Tetrachloroethylene (perchloroethylene [PCE]) is a colorless liquid that is widely used today as a dry-cleaning fluid and for metal degreasing. A total 263,000 metric tons were used in the United States and Europe in 1997, and more than 1.5 million workers were potentially exposed.[24] It is a common contaminant at Superfund waste sites and a surface water and groundwater pollutant. PCE is volatile, and approximately 85% of the PCE that is used annually is lost to the atmosphere, thus making it an airborne pollutant as well. Therefore PCE is an extremely common potential occupational and environmental hepatotoxicant. Exposures occur through inhalation, ingestion, and the dermal route. As with TCE, the metabolism of PCE is exceptionally complex, with multiple competing pathways leading to the formation of DCA and TCA.[30]

Although PCE is regarded as relatively nontoxic, hepatic injury has been documented in humans, as well as in animal models. Biopsy-proven liver disease has been documented in the setting of high occupational exposure.[3] Interestingly, chronic occupational PCE exposure appears to be associated with liver disease with normal liver enzyme levels.[3,30] Findings on hepatic ultrasound were abnormal in 62% of PCE-exposed laundry workers with normal liver enzymes versus only 39% of nonexposed laundry workers.[31] Although pathologic confirmation was lacking, the ultrasound appearance was consistent with fatty liver.[31] PCE is listed as a 2A (probable) human carcinogen by the IARC. Like TCE, PCE is a well-documented hepatocarcinogen in mice. However, liver tumors have not been documented in humans. Chronic inhalation studies conducted by the NTP demonstrated both benign (hepatocellular necrosis) and malignant liver disease.[32]

Haloalkanes

Carbon Tetrachloride

Carbon tetrachloride is a colorless liquid with an etherlike odor. Although human cases of acute CCl_4 poisoning seldom occur today, it remains the classic experimental model of occupational hepatotoxicity. CCl_4 was in widespread use as a solvent, vermicide, refrigerant, and ingredient in fire extinguishers. However, its use for these applications was limited after several hundred cases of its toxicity were reported in the early to mid-twentieth century.[33] It has continued to be used as a feedstock for the synthesis for chlorofluorocarbon (CFC) gases. However, following adoption of the Clean Air Act and the Montreal Protocol banning CFCs, U.S. CCl_4 production has been reduced to 130 million pounds per year.[34] CCl_4 is a stable molecule and a persistent environmental pollutant, which importantly does not appear to bioconcentrate in animals. Nonetheless, CCl_4 is a ubiquitous ambient air pollutant and may also contaminate groundwater supplies. The estimated daily intake by the U.S. general population from air and water ranges from 12 to 511 µg/day and from 0.2 to 60 µg/day, respectively.[34]

The primary route of acute CCl_4 poisoning is via inhalation, although accidental ingestion has occurred. An interesting and early observation was the fact that chronic alcoholics had increased susceptibility to CCl_4 poisoning, although alcoholism was certainly not required.[33] Multiorgan failure progressed in a fairly predictable clinical sequence and resulted in death in 25% of cases.[33] Following a 1- to 2-day prodromal phase consisting of dizziness, headache, confusion, nausea, vomiting, and diarrhea, symptoms subsided for 1 to 2 days before the onset of acute liver failure. The liver injury followed a hepatocellular pattern typified by extremely high transaminase levels. Aspartate transaminase (AST) was typically greater than alanine transaminase (ALT) and in one case reached 27,000 U/L. Jaundice developed in half of the cases. Hepatic coma and ascites developed in severe cases. Oliguric renal failure ensued and was the usual cause of death because most cases occurred before the advent of hemodialysis. When death occurred, it was typically within 10 days of exposure. Liver histopathology consisted of zone 3 steatosis and necrosis, and necrosis was also observed in the renal tubular epithelium in most fatal cases. Similar to acetaminophen overdose, recovery was typically rapid in those who survived. Treatment was supportive, although some reports attributed benefit to intravenous N-acetylcysteine or hyperbaric oxygen.[33] Cirrhosis has been reported in cases of chronic exposure. CCl_4 is an IARC group 2B (possible) human carcinogen, and three cases of liver cancer have been documented in workers following recovery from acute CCl_4 poisoning.[34]

After ethanol, CCl$_4$ is the most widely studied hepatotoxicant, and it continues to be investigated today. In multiple models, CCl$_4$ induces liver injury (steatosis, necrosis, fibrosis, and hepatocellular carcinoma) similar to that observed in humans. As with other chlorinated aliphatic compounds, bioactivation of CCl$_4$ by CYP2E1 to reactive metabolites is critical for its toxicity.[35] In the case of CCl$_4$, the critical intermediates appear to be the trichloromethyl radical and the even more highly reactive trichloromethyl peroxy free radical. The trichloromethyl radical may form DNA adducts, whereas the trichloromethyl peroxy free radical attacks membrane-bound polyunsaturated fatty acids. This lipid peroxidation unleashes a chain of events leading to glutathione depletion, generation of reactive aldehydes, increased membrane permeability, disrupted calcium homeostasis, increased proinflammatory and profibrotic cytokines, disrupted lipid homeostasis, hypomethylation, and altered cell cycling.[35] These events lead to the cytotoxicity and carcinogenesis observed in animal models. Protection has been demonstrated by agents that block steps in this pathway, such as cytochrome inhibitors, antioxidants, calcium chelators, and Kupffer cell depleters, and by administration of the methyl donor S-adenosylmethionine (SAMe).[35]

1,1,2,2-Tetrachloroethane

Tetrachloroethane is a clear liquid and is among the most potent solvents ever developed. Unfortunately, it is also a powerful hepatotoxicant, and for this reason, tetrachloroethane is essentially no longer used in the United States. Before TCE, tetrachloroethane was used by the military to clean aircraft. However, human cases of severe hepatic toxicity were reported during World War I and again in World War II.[33] Liver injury consisted of hepatic steatosis and necrosis, similar to CCl$_4$, but followed a subacute rather than an acute course.[33] Indeed, the syndrome of subacute hepatic necrosis was a major problem in both world wars and was caused by trinitrotoluene (TNT) and PCB-chloronaphthalene mixtures, as well as by tetrachloroethane.[33]

1,1,1-Trichloroethane

Trichloroethane (methyl chloroform) is a clear liquid that was considered to be the least toxic haloalkane solvent. Therefore it was widely used as an industrial solvent until it was banned by the Montreal Protocol on Substances That Deplete the Ozone Layer. Although it was considered to have little hepatotoxic potential, benign liver disease associated with this chemical has been described in both humans and animal models. Similar to other chlorinated aliphatic compounds, it produces hepatic steatosis and necrosis in animal models.[36] Both fatty liver and cirrhosis have been reported in chronically exposed workers.[29,36]

Nonhalogenated Aromatic Hydrocarbons

Toluene, benzene, xylene, and styrene are colorless liquids that continue to be mass-produced in the United States (several billion pounds per year each) and have multiple industrial applications, including use as solvents and in the production of synthetic rubber and plastic. In comparison with the halogenated aliphatic solvents, these agents are associated with limited acute human hepatic toxicity. However, it appears that chronic occupational exposure, particularly to mixtures of these agents, may result in steatohepatitis. Petrochemical workers are frequently exposed to these and other hydrocarbons. A recent study of petrochemical workers from Brazil demonstrated a 29.4% prevalence of abnormal liver enzyme levels in workers exposed to benzene, toluene, and xylene, even after significant alcohol use and diabetes were excluded.[37] Fifty-two percent of affected workers were found to have fatty liver on ultrasound. Multiple other recent studies have documented a relatively high prevalence of abnormal liver enzymes and even biopsy-proven steatohepatitis in petrochemical workers.[38,39] However, because the workers were exposed to a multitude of chemicals in most cases, it is impossible to know the identity of the agent or agents responsible. Furthermore, obesity and alcohol consumption were not controlled for in some of these studies. Likewise, biopsy-proven steatohepatitis occurring in the absence of obesity or ethanol abuse was reported in eight toluene-exposed printing workers with mild transaminase elevations.[40] Abnormal transaminase levels were found in 44% of shoe repairmen who, like petrochemical workers, were exposed to a mixture of chemicals, including toluene.[41] Painters are another group potentially at risk for solvent-induced liver injury. Although data in the literature are mixed, biopsy-proven steatohepatitis was documented in several cases of suspected acute solvent poisoning occurring in chronically exposed workers.[33,42] A recent National Health and Nutrition Examination Survey (NHANES) analysis found a positive correlation between the levels of six volatile organic compounds, including benzene, toluene, and xylene, which were detected by passive exposure monitors, and alkaline phosphatase and γ-glutamyltransferase (GGT).[43] In particular, more data are needed on the development of steatohepatitis in petrochemical workers and the potential effects of chronic low-level exposure to these chemicals on liver disease in the general population.

Halogenated Aromatic Hydrocarbons
Polychlorinated Biphenyls

Polychlorinated biphenyls are polyhalogenated aromatic hydrocarbons consisting of up to 10 chlorine atoms attached to a biphenyl group. PCB congeners are odorless, tasteless, and clear to pale yellow viscous liquids. The more highly chlorinated forms of PCBs are more hydrophobic, less volatile, and more viscous. Although there are 209 theoretic PCB congeners, only about 130 were manufactured between 1929 and 1977. PCBs were manufactured as mixtures and sold as a function of their chlorine content. For example, Monsanto marketed Aroclors 1221, 1231, and 1242 up to 1268, which contain 21%, 31%, and 42% up to 68% chlorine by weight, respectively. Aroclors were used in multiple industrial applications and were components in dielectric insulating fluids for transformers and capacitors, hydraulic fluids, plastics, and paints. An estimated 1.3 million tons of PCBs was manufactured, for use almost exclusively (97%) in the northern hemisphere. Although PCBs were banned in the United States in the late

1970s, their high thermodynamic stability makes them resistant to biodegradation, and they are thus persistent organic pollutants. Animal studies demonstrate that PCBs concentrate in both the liver and adipose tissue.[44] Like organochlorine pesticides, PCBs are members of the "dirty dozen" chemicals that were officially banned by the Stockholm Convention on Persistent Environmental Pollutants in 2001.

Because they are banned, acute PCB poisoning should no longer occur in humans. However, acute PCB poisoning was previously associated with fatigue, anorexia, nausea, and jaundice.[45,46] Severe zone 2 and 3 necrosis was observed on liver biopsy specimens, and cirrhosis was documented in some subjects who survived the acute event.[45,46] Jaundice was also observed in approximately 10% of cases following the "yusho" incident in Japan, where rice oil had been contaminated by PCBs and polychlorinated dibenzofurans (PCDFs).[47] The chronic effects of PCB exposure on liver disease in humans are poorly understood. However, the mortality rate secondary to cirrhosis was 2.7-fold higher than expected in victims of the "yucheng" incident, where cooking oil had been contaminated by PCBs and PCDFs in Taiwan.[48] Following the yusho epidemic, increased mortality risk from liver cancer was observed only in male subjects (Standardized mortality ratio [SMR] = 5.59).[47] Mild liver enzyme elevation and hepatomegaly were reported in workers at an electrical capacitor plant who were chronically exposed to PCBs.[49] We recently reported that 20 PCBs were associated with up to 14.7-fold dose-dependent increased odds ratios for liver enzyme elevation in American adults in NHANES 2003-2004. Although limited epidemiologic data suggest a potential role for PCBs in chronic liver disease, histologic confirmation has generally been lacking.

The NTP has performed 2-year toxicity studies on PCB 126 and PCB 153 in female Harlan Sprague-Dawley rats.[44] These studies demonstrated that the liver was the principal target organ for these compounds. Both benign (toxic hepatopathy) and malignant (hepatocellular carcinoma and cholangiocarcinoma) liver lesions were observed at high frequencies in a dose-dependent fashion, particularly in animals treated with PCB 126 alone or in combination with PCB 153. Even though acute PCB poisoning should no longer occur, more research is need on the possible effects of chronic low-level environmental PCB exposure on chronic liver diseases and possibly liver cancer.

Miscellaneous Chemicals in Plastics

Other chemicals in plastics such as bisphenol A (BPA) and di(2-ethylhexyl)phthalate (DEHP) are emerging mediators of liver disease. In contrast to VC monomer, these agents leach from plastics and result in widespread low-level exposure in the general population.

Di(2-ethylhexyl)phthalate

Plastic made from VC (PVC), such as that found in home plumbing, is hard and brittle. Plasticizers such as DEHP, a colorless and viscous liquid, are often used in plastic production to make PVC softer and more pliable. PVC is one of the most widely used plastics in health care, and many of these products contain DEHP. DEHP can be found in bags used for intravenous fluids, medications, and total parenteral nutrition (TPN), as well as in intravenous tubing, including hemodialysis and extracorporeal membrane oxygenation (ECMO) circuits; enteral feeding tubes; and examination gloves.[50] In the home setting, DHEP is frequently found in PVC toys, shower curtains, car seats, and floor coverings, in addition to the cabins of automobiles.[50] Occupational exposure also occurs at some PVC manufacturing facilities.

Importantly, DEHP may leach from medical devices and be infused intravenously, and it may "outgas" in the home setting and be inhaled. DEHP may contaminate food and water, and ingestion is the most likely route of exposure for most humans.[51] DEHP has been intensively studied in the neonatal intensive care unit, where babies may unintentionally receive several milligrams of DEHP daily.[50] DEHP has been reported to leach from plastic bags and tubing into parental etoposide, cyclosporine, and particularly TPN fluids. Because DEHP is lipid soluble, lipid-containing TPN increases the amount of DEHP delivered. Other factors affecting DEHP leaching include temperature, storage time, flow rate, volume, pH, and agitation. DEHP metabolism varies by route of exposure but initially involves the formation of mono(2-ethylhexyl)phthalate and 2-ethylhexanol by esterases. The subsequent metabolism of these biologically active metabolites is complex and has been reviewed.[51]

DEHP exposure primarily affects the development of the liver and reproductive system, but other organ systems may also be affected.[50,52] In newborn infants receiving TPN, cholestatic liver disease developed in 50% of infants in whom DEHP-plasticized PVC lines were used versus 13% of infants in whom PVC-free lines were used.[52] In rodents, DEHP induces multiple histopathologic changes, including hepatomegaly secondary to both hepatocyte hypertrophy and hyperplasia, midzonal to periportal steatosis, bile duct changes, and hepatocellular carcinoma.[51] The modes of action of DEHP include activation of nuclear receptors (including PPAR-α, the constitutive androstane receptor [CAR], and the aryl hydrocarbon receptor [AhR]), Kupffer cell activation, oxidative stress, endocrine disruption, epigenetic changes, and induction of cell proliferation with suppression of apoptosis.[51] These issues led to a U.S. Food and Drug Administration (FDA) Public Health Notification in 2002 addressing the use of DEHP in medical devices, particularly in high-risk populations, including young males.

Bisphenol A

In contrast to DEHP, less is known about the potential hepatotoxicity of BPA. A white powder, BPA is widely used primarily in the synthesis of polycarbonate plastic, which is used in reusable containers such as baby bottles, and in the synthesis of epoxy resins, which are used to line metal beverage cans. It has also been widely used as an antioxidant in some plasticizers and as a polymerization inhibitor in PVC. BPA is one of the highest volume chemicals produced, with global production exceeding 6 billion pounds per year.[53] BPA may leach from beverage containers and be ingested orally, but other routes of exposure exist. BPA is an endocrine disrupter with estrogenic activity,[53] and BPA in baby bottles has garnered recent media attention because of concern regarding endocrine disruption. BPA exposure has been associated with diabetes, cardiovascular disease, and abnormal liver enzyme levels in population-based studies.[54] However, documenting these associations remains problematic because BPA, as well as other endocrine disrupters, may follow nonmonotonic dose-response curves.[53] Despite concerns raised by the public and the NTP, the FDA has advised that consumers not discontinue BPA-containing products while it performs its own risk assessment. Because most studies focus on the effects of BPA on growth and development, more data on the potential role of BPA on human liver disease are needed.

Pesticides

The major categories of pesticides include insecticides, herbicides, and fungicides. The first recorded account of pesticide use occurred nearly 3000 ago in Homer's *Odyssey*, where it is stated that Odysseus burned sulfur "...to purge the hall and the house and the court." However, it was not until the twentieth century that pesticides were in widespread use, primarily for agricultural and antimalarial purposes. Over the past 20 years, total pesticide use in the United States has reached a plateau.[55] In 2000, 1234 million pounds of pesticides were used in the United States, with an estimated cost exceeding $11 billion.[55] Pesticide use is not limited to commercial operations, and 74% of U.S. households use pesticides.[55] Pesticide exposure occurs through the oral, dermal, and inhalational routes. Although virtually all Americans are subject to chronic low-level pesticide exposure, higher occupational exposure does occur in the pesticide production and agricultural (sprayers and harvesters) sectors. Pesticides are tightly regulated because they are associated with 3 million acute poisonings and 250,000 deaths per year, and some agents are possibly associated with cancer. In the United States, pesticides are primarily regulated by the EPA, which requires that all pesticides be registered after a large number of toxicity studies have been performed at an estimated cost of $50 to $100 million per product. Acute pesticide poisoning is associated with liver enzyme elevation in many instances; however, significant liver injury does not typically occur except in cases of paraquat and perhaps organochlorine pesticide poisoning. Emerging epidemiologic data suggest a possible role for organochlorine pesticides in chronic liver disease. The remainder of this section focuses on the potential hepatotoxicity of insecticides and herbicides.

Insecticides

Insecticides are used primarily for insect control in developing countries. Indeed, U.S. insecticide use accounted for only 9% of total worldwide use, which is in contrast to herbicides, for which the United States accounted for 46% of worldwide use.[55] Although there have been multiple recent reports of liver enzyme elevations occurring in agricultural workers exposed to combinations of insecticides, histologic confirmation was generally lacking.[56,57] Major insecticide categories discussed here include organochlorine and organophosphorus insecticides.

Organochlorine Insecticides

Organochlorine insecticides include dichlorodiphenyltrichloroethane (DDT); cyclodienes such as chlordane, dieldrin, aldrin, endrin, and heptachlor; caged structures such as mirex and chlordecone; and others. Sodium channel activation is believed to be the insecticidal mechanism of action. DDT is a colorless, crystalline solid with a weak chemical odor. The insecticidal activity of DDT was discovered by the Swiss scientist Paul Mueller in 1939, who was later awarded the Nobel Prize for this discovery. Subsequently, DDT was marketed in 1944, followed by the other organochlorine insecticides in the late 1940s and 1950s. Primarily because of adverse effects on wildlife and carcinogenicity in animal models, most of these chemicals have been banned for more 30 years. However, these lipid-soluble and highly thermodynamically stable molecules are persistent environmental pollutants that have bioaccumulated in living organisms. Indeed, there is now not a single living organism on the planet that does not contain DDT.[58] These chemicals, members of the so-called dirty dozen, were officially banned for most uses by an international treaty, the Stockholm Convention on Persistent Environmental Pollutants, under the direction of the United Nations in 2001; therefore acute organochlorine pesticide–related toxicity should no longer occur except in Africa, where DDT application is still permitted. Although neurotoxicity was the most prominent feature of acute poisoning, hepatic necrosis did occur in some cases.[59] The most complete data on the hepatic effects of organochlorine pesticide exposure in human subjects stem from the miniepidemic of chlordecone intoxication in 32 plant workers in Virginia. Although liver enzymes were repeatedly normal in these workers, many had hepatomegaly, which eventually led to liver biopsy in 12 cases. These biopsies revealed mild steatosis, mild portal inflammation and fibrosis, glycogenated nuclei, and lipofuscin accumulation.[60] A notable aspect of this outbreak was the successful use of cholestyramine to promote elimination of chlordecone, which appears to undergo enterohepatic circulation.[4] Although DDT is carcinogenic in rodents, organochlorine pesticides have only inconsistently been linked to liver cancer (hepatocellular, biliary, and hemangiosarcoma) in pesticide applicators and farmers.[58,61] Recently, we used the NHANES 2003-2004 database to investigate the effects of chronic low-level organochlorine pesticide exposure on liver enzyme elevation in American adults. We found that multiple pesticides, including dieldrin, *trans*-nonachlor (component of chlordane), and heptachlor epoxide (metabolite of heptachlor), were associated with dose-dependent increased odds ratios for ALT elevation.[62] These data suggest but do not prove that organochlorine pesticides may play a previously unsuspected role in liver disease several decades after they were banned. Although the mechanisms of hepatotoxicity are not clearly defined in animal models, organochlorine pesticides induce cytochrome P-450, and emerging data suggest that they may be endocrine disrupters.[58]

Organophosphorus Insecticides

Organophosphorus insecticides inhibit acetylcholinesterases and are rapidly degraded by hydrolysis on exposure to sunlight, thus making them an attractive alternative to organochlorine pesticides. Malathion and chlorpyrifos are currently the most heavily used insecticides in the U.S. agricultural sector, whereas diazinon is the single most heavily used insecticide in home gardens.[55] These compounds appear to be relatively nonhepatotoxic in humans, but liver injury, including steatosis, has been reported in animal models exposed to both chlorpyrifos and diazinon.[63,64] Recently, the caspase-cleaved fragment of cytokeratin-18 was reported to be elevated in the serum of humans following occupational exposure to chlorpyrifos, with improvement over time following removal from the exposure.[65] Unfortunately, histopathologic confirmation was lacking. Animal models of chorpyrifos hepatotoxicity implicate zinc deficiency as a possible mechanism of action.[63]

Herbicides

In contrast to pesticides, herbicides are used extensively in the U.S. agricultural sector. The hepatotoxicity of the major categories of herbicides, including chlorophenoxy compounds, bipyridil compounds, chloracetanilides, triazines, and phosphonomethyl amino acids, is subsequently discussed.

Chlorophenoxy Herbicides

Chlorophenoxy herbicides are structurally characterized by an aliphatic carboxylic acid moiety attached to a chlorine- or methyl-substituted ring, and they mimic auxins, the plant growth-regulating hormones. 2,4-Dichlorophenoxyacetic acid (2,4-D) is a white to yellow powder developed during World War II. It was the first successful selective herbicide and is still one of the most widely used herbicides worldwide. Although the use of 2,4,5-trichlorophenoxyacetic acid (2,4,5-T) was halted by the U.S. EPA in 1985, it remains important for historical reasons. Acute chlorophenoxy herbicide poisoning usually occurs following ingestion, and it represented the second most common form of death from herbicide poisoning in Wales between 1945 and 1989.[66] Although liver enzyme elevation was present, it represented a relatively minor component of the poisoning.[66] However, biopsy-proven acute hepatitis was attributed to 2,4-D in a golfer who habitually licked his golf ball on sprayed putting greens.[67] The potential risks associated with chronic human exposure are even less well defined but do not seem significant. For example, the risk for liver-related death was not increased in plant workers involved in 2,4-D manufacturing.[68] However, liver enzyme elevation was noted in rodents chronically exposed to 2,4-D.[69] Other potential modes of action include uncoupling of oxidative phosphorylation, interference of pathways involving acetylcoenzyme A, and plasma membrane effects.[66]

An estimated 12 million gallons of Agent Orange, a mixture of 2,4-D and 2,4,5-T, was sprayed during Operation Ranch Hand in the Vietnam Conflict. Liver disease has inconsistently been reported in U.S. veterans exposed to Agent Orange.[70] Most of the potential toxicities of Agent Orange have been assigned to 2,3,7,8-tetrachlorodibenzodioxin (TCDD, or dioxin), which is a potent AhR agonist. TCDD contaminated 2,4,5-T in Agent Orange. Although TCDD is a classic hepatocarcinogen in rodents, no definitive link has been shown between TCDD and liver cancer in humans. During 1976 in Seveso, Italy, several kilograms of dioxin was inadvertently released into the atmosphere. Recently, it was demonstrated that exposed residents had no increase in mortality secondary to either cirrhosis or hepatobiliary cancer.[71] However, GGT and transient aminotransferase elevations of uncertain significance have been inconsistently observed in multiple cohorts with high TCDD exposure.[72] Biopsy-proven

liver disease, in general, was lacking. Porphyria cutanea tarda has inconsistently been linked to TCDD exposure.

Bipyridil Herbicides

This class includes paraquat (1,1′-dimethyl-4,4′-bipyridinium dichloride) and diquat (6,7-diydrodipyridol pyrazidinium dibromide). Among herbicides, paraquat, a viologen, is perhaps the most acutely toxic to animals, including humans. Although it is heavily used worldwide, because of toxicity it is licensed in the United States only for use by licensed applicators. Paraquat is hydrophilic and forms large particles when aerosolized.[73] Therefore paraquat poisoning from the dermal and inhalational routes is rare. However, since its introduction, there have been thousands of cases of paraquat poisoning, mostly from ingestion, and many of these cases resulted in death.[73] Although many of these ingestions represented suicide attempts, in some cases paraquat was mistaken for beverages such as coffee or soft drinks.[73] Paraquat was subsequently reformulated and is now blue-green in color and contains stanching and emetic agents. In humans, acute paraquat toxicity is associated primarily with severe lung disease, but liver, renal, and cardiovascular disease has also been reported.[33] Death may occur within several days following ingestion. Although hepatic necrosis is the earliest observed hepatic lesion, cholestasis subsequently ensues with prominent bile duct injuries.[33] Hepatic steatosis has also been observed. Paraquat generates superoxide radicals leading to lipid peroxidation and depletion of reduced nicotinamide adenine dinucleotide phosphate (NADPH), and redox cycling is its proposed mechanism of both plant and animal toxicity.[73]

Chloracetanilide Herbicides

Acetochlor, alachlor, and metolachlor are among the most widely used herbicides in the U.S. agricultural industry and work by disrupting enzymes of the *gibberellin* pathway. Although liver enzyme elevation was not a prominent component of acute human chloracetanilide poisonings, the potential hepatotoxicity of these compounds has been demonstrated in rodent models, as well as in human cell lines.[74] Because of environmental persistence, alachlor has been banned in the European Union since 2006.

Triazine Herbicides

Triazine herbicides, including atrazine (2-chloro-4-ethylamine-6-isopropylamino-S-triazine) and simazine, were banned in the European Union, but widespread use continues in the United States. In fact, atrazine was the second most commonly used pesticide in the U.S. agricultural industry.[55] However, widespread atrazine contamination of community water supplies, particularly in the United States during the summer months, has been a recent public health concern. Atrazine inhibits the electron transport chain in chloroplasts. Chronic atrazine treatment induces mitochondrial toxicity, visceral adiposity, and fatty liver in Sprague-Dawley rats, possibly because of similarity between chloroplasts and mammalian mitochondria.[75] Although confirmatory human data are lacking, this study suggests a potential role for triazine herbicides in patients with obesity, metabolic syndrome, and nonalcoholic fatty liver disease. More research on triazine herbicides is clearly needed.

Phosphonomethyl Amino Acids

Glyphosate (Roundup, Monsanto) disrupts amino acid synthesis in plants and is currently used as an alternative to paraquat. Human poisoning has been encountered with increasing frequency following intentional ingestion as a suicide attempt. Although poisoning victims are usually initially seen with multisystem disease, mild serum transaminase elevations do occur and are predictive of mortality.

Nitrogen-Containing Organic Compounds
Nitro Compounds

Nitro compounds are organic molecules that contain one or more nitro ($-NO_2$) functional groups. They are often highly explosive. Nitro compounds may be classified as either nitroaromatic or nitroaliphatic. Even though hepatotoxicity occurs with both types, nitroaromatic compounds are generally believed to be more toxic.

Nitroaromatic Compounds
Trinitrotoluene

Trinitrotoluene, a yellow solid, is a widely used explosive that is often combined with other explosive compounds in synergistic blends. The proposed route of exposure is dermal, although other routes may exist. Improved handling techniques have led to a decline in TNT-related toxicity. A wide spectrum of TNT-related hepatotoxicity ranging from acute liver failure to cirrhosis has been reported in munitions workers and military personnel.[33] Hepatotoxicity has been confirmed in animal models.[76] TNT-associated liver toxicity may occur in the context of other, more common TNT-related hematologic diseases, including methemoglobinemia and aplastic anemia. Rash and cataracts may also occur. During detonation, not all of the TNT in a bomb explodes, and thus TNT may be an environmental contaminant at some sites. Biomonitoring of TNT-exposed workers at ammunition waste sites has become a recent concern. Although the IARC was unable to classify the carcinogenicity of TNT because of limited human and animal data, hepatocellular carcinoma has been reported. In chronically exposed Chinese munitions workers, liver cancer mortality was 3.97 times that of controls.[77] The incidence of liver cancer was related to cumulative TNT exposure, and alcohol use was synergistic.

TNT hepatotoxicity was a significant problem in both world wars. During World War I, 474 cases of TNT-related liver disease (with a 25% fatality rate) were observed in munitions workers.[33] TNT hepatotoxicity typically occurred after several months of regular exposure.[33] Subacute hepatotoxicity followed this latent period, and liver injury developed in some individuals, even after removal from the exposure. Next, after a period of vague constitutional symptoms, jaundice with minimal liver enzyme elevation developed. Some

individuals then progressed rapidly to hepatic necrosis and death, whereas others survived and exhibited macronodular cirrhosis. Importantly, hepatic disease, though oftentimes severe, occurred in only a minority of exposed workers ranging from 0.01% to 5% of those exposed.[33] Susceptibility to TNT toxicity has been the subject of several recent studies. Alcohol consumption and the N-acetyltransferase rapid acetylator polymorphism appear to be risk factors.[77,78] Several modes of action have been proposed, including oxidative stress; altered amino acid, zinc, and copper metabolism; and hypersensitivity reactions.

Nitrobenzene

Nitrobenzene is a water-insoluble, pale yellow oil with an almond-like odor. Nitrobenzene is used as an intermediate primarily for the synthesis of aniline but also in specialty chemicals, including acetaminophen. In 2002, nitrobenzene production capacity in the United States was 2.96 billion pounds. Occupational exposure may occur through the inhalational and dermal routes, and nitrobenzene has been found in surface water and groundwater. Nitrobenzene induces liver cancer in rats and is an IARC group 2B (possible) human carcinogen.[79] Similar to TNT, nitrobenzene is associated with hematologic affects such as methemoglobinemia, and liver injury has been described in human case reports supported by animal studies.[80] Liver injury ranges from bile stasis with isolated hyperbilirubinemia to steatosis and severe centrilobular necrosis.[80] Importantly, as in other forms of occupational liver disease, routine liver enzymes are not a good biomarker for nitrobenzene-related liver disease.[80] The proposed mode of action of nitrobenzene involves free radicals, inflammation, and epigenetic changes.

Nitroalkanes
Nitromethane

Nitromethane is a colorless, slightly viscous, highly polar liquid. Most of the 16 million pounds of nitromethane produced yearly in the United States is used for the synthesis of derivatives used as pharmaceuticals, fumigants, and industrial antimicrobials.[81] It is also used as a fuel or fuel additive for high-performance race cars and as a solvent. Occupational exposure occurs through the inhalational and dermal routes. In the early 1980s alone more than 175,000 workers were exposed.[81] Nitromethane is also a by-product of cigarette smoke and internal combustion engines and is an environmental pollutant. In animal models, nitromethane exposure leads to hepatic steatosis with mild zone 3 necrosis.[33] However, the effects of nitromethane, if any, on human populations are not well characterized. Based on animal data, nitromethane is an IARC class 2B (possible) human carcinogen, and hepatocellular carcinoma has been reported in chronically exposed female mice.

Nitroethane

Nitroethane, a colorless oily liquid with a fruity odor, is another HPV nitroalkane. It is used as a solvent, as an intermediate for the production of multiple products, including pharmaceuticals, and as a fuel additive. As with nitromethane, minor degrees of steatosis and zone 3 necrosis have been reported in animal models,[33] but human hepatotoxicity has not definitively been documented.

2-Nitropropane

In contrast to other nitroalkanes, human hepatotoxicity secondary to nitropropane has been relatively well documented. Worldwide nitropropane production has been estimated to be 5 to 6 million pounds. Like other nitroalkanes, it is used primarily as a solvent, chemical intermediate, and fuel/explosive. The National Occupational Exposure Survey (NOES) estimated that 10,000 U.S. workers were exposed between 1980 and 1983. Nitropropane is also a food and cooking oil contaminant, thus exposing the general population. Animal studies document hepatic steatosis, degenerative change, and necrosis.[33] Nine deaths have been attributed to acute liver failure following occupational exposure to nitropropane.[82] All cases involved the application of paint coatings in poorly ventilated areas. Massive hepatocellular necrosis was described following a prodromal phase consisting of headache, nausea, and vomiting. Although the mode of action is not entirely understood, it appears that hepatic nitropropane metabolism generates acetone, nitrite, and NO radicals, with decreased catalase activity resulting in lipid peroxidation.[83] Nitropropane is an IARC class 2B (possible) human carcinogen based on rodent studies documenting hepatocellular carcinoma.

N-Substituted Amide Solvents

Dimethylformamide

Dimethylformamide (DMF) is a colorless liquid that is miscible with both water and many organic liquids. It has been called the "universal solvent" and has been used as such in many commercial applications. Production of DMF was estimated at 125,000 tons.[84] In addition to its synthesis, occupational exposure to DMF may occur in the production or use of many resins, inks, and adhesives, as well as in the leather and aircraft repair industries. Data from NOES indicate that as many as 125,000 U.S. workers were exposed between 1980 and 1983.[84] Acute, high-level exposure to DMF causes hepatotoxicity as its major effect.[84] Occupational exposure typically occurs through the dermal or inhalational route. A high prevalence of abnormal liver enzyme levels has been reported in workers exposed to DMF.[85-87] More recently, an outbreak of acute hepatitis occurred in five industrial waste disposal workers exposed to DMF and resulted in one death.[88] Other associated symptoms included dizziness, anorexia, nausea, and abdominal pain. An unusual disulfiram-like alcohol intolerance has been noted on multiple occasions in exposed workers.[84] Liver biopsy specimens from exposed workers revealed focal hepatocellular necrosis and microvesicular steatosis with prominence of smooth endoplasmic reticulum, complex lysosomes, and pleomorphic mitochondria with crystalline inclusions.[85] Fibrosis was not seen on biopsy of workers with long-term exposure.[85] Hepatitis B, elevated body mass index, and alcohol use appear to have synergistic effects on DMF hepatotoxicity.[86,87] Hepatic necrosis has been documented in multiple animal models with high-level acute exposure.[33]

Dimethylacetamide

Dimethylacetamide (DMAC) is a colorless, polar solvent similar to DMF. Multiple case reports have documented DMAC-associated hepatotoxicity, mainly in synthetic fiber workers. Acute DMAC poisoning is primarily manifested as neuropsychiatric illness, including psychosis, delirium, and seizures, and as systemic disease, including acute hepatitis. The primary route of exposure appears to be dermal absorption of DMAC vapor. Subclinical ALT elevations appear to occur not infrequently in new synthetic fiber workers (within the first 7 months of employment) in a dose-dependent fashion.[89,90] The elevation in ALT improved by 50% within 30 days in 90% of persons after DMAC exposure was halted.[89] Interestingly, transaminitis appears to occur much less frequently, if at all, in workers exposed longer than 7 months, thus suggesting adaptation to chronic exposure.[89-91] However, animal models have documented liver injury following both acute and chronic DMF exposure.[92]

Anilines

Methylenedianiline

Methylenedianiline (MDA, or 4′,4′-diaminophenylmethane, DAPM) is an aromatic amine and a classically described mediator of occupational and environmental liver disease. U.S. production was estimated at 600 million pounds in 1987.[81] Currently, more than 90% of the MDA produced in the United States is used in the closed-system production of a variety of isocyanates, which are used primarily in the synthesis of polymers, elastomers, and resins.[81] The primary route of industrial exposure is dermal, and prompt (within 30 minutes) washing of contaminated skin appears to reduce systemic exposure. Trace amounts of MDA may leach from synthetic fibers, polyurethane, epoxy-containing products, and medical devices. Such exposure is thought to pose no human risk.[81] In the early 1980s, as many as 15,000 workers were potentially exposed.[81] In 1987, the Methylenedianiline Mediated Rulemaking Advisory Committee convened by OSHA estimated that in the worst-case scenario, approximately 5000 workers were exposed.[81] Acute hepatitis with jaundice has been documented in MDA workers.[33] However, MDA is best known for the outbreak of Epping jaundice. In 1965, jaundice developed in at least 84 people in Epping, Essex, U.K.[93] This outbreak was traced to the ingestion of bread made from flour that had been contaminated by MDA. Contamination occurred during transport when a plastic container carrying MDA spilled onto the floor of a van also carrying flour. Liver disease developed in roughly 25% of exposed subjects and was more common in those who consumed more heavily contaminated loaves. A prodromal phase consisting of abdominal pain resembling biliary colic was usually followed by flulike symptoms with an occasional rash that was followed by jaundice. In addition to hyperbilirubinemia, modest aminotransferase elevations typically developed later in the course of the disease. Alkaline phosphatase elevation occurred in only 20% of cases, whereas 50% of cases were associated with eosinophilia.[59] The histologic features on liver biopsy varied according to the stage of the disease, but the most important findings were intense portal inflammation, often with significant numbers of eosinophils, centrilobular cholestasis, and necrosis of biliary epithelial cells. The unusual combination of acute cholestatic hepatitis/cholangitis with severe bile duct injury has also been reported with paraquat and toxic rapeseed oil exposure and rarely with prescription medications. Destruction of biliary epithelial cells has likewise been noted in many animal models. Proposed modes of action include biotransformation of MDA into toxic metabolites with biliary excretion, glutathione depletion, mitochondrial dysfunction, and disrupted biliary epithelial cell tight junctions.[94,95] In animal studies, gender and *N*-acetyltransferase 2 polymorphisms modulated toxicity.[96] Based on animal studies demonstrating the development of tumors, including hepatocellular carcinoma, MDA is an IARC group 2B (possible) human carcinogen. Furthermore, genotoxicity has been noted in experimental studies. However, hepatocellular carcinoma has not been documented in exposed humans. Long-term mortality was no different from controls in the Epping jaundice cohort.[97] As several other authors have noted, Epping jaundice was remarkable for the fact that although MDA is an intrinsic (predictable) toxin, its clinical manifestation resembled the hypersensitivity reactions observed in many forms of idiosyncratic DILI.[33,59]

Toxic Oil Syndrome (Aniline)

Toxic oil syndrome, also called toxic epidemic syndrome, was a widespread systemic disease that occurred in Spain in 1981. The epidemic was believed to be caused by the ingestion of rapeseed cooking oil that had been denatured with 2% aniline (phenylamine) and illicitly sold as olive oil. Aniline is a colorless, liquid, volatile, aromatic amine with a putrid odor that is currently used in urethane production. A cooking oil specimen bank was created and subsequent analysis revealed an association between toxicity and the presence of fatty acid (typically oleic acid) esters of 3-(*N*-phenylamino)-1,2-propanediol (PAP).[98] The epidemic was massive. Approximately 100,000 individuals were exposed, and clinical disease occurred in 20,000 people, 10,000 of whom were hospitalized.[98] Clinical disease developed more frequently in females. More than 300 victims died and many more were left with chronic disease. Vasculitis was a prominent feature of the acute phase of the disease, and scleroderma developed in 20% of survivors. Liver disease occurred in about 25% of exposed individuals and jaundice in 8% of them.[33] Nearly all cases of liver injury featured elevations of alkaline phosphatase and GGT.[33] Liver biopsy demonstrated cholestatic or mixed cholestatic/hepatocellular disease with prominent portal inflammation and eosinophilic infiltrates.[33] The liver disease resembled MDA toxicity. Despite relatively intense research on the potential role of the identified ester, disease pathogenesis remains unclear.

Metals
Mercury

Methylmercury is the principal form of organic mercury historically associated with organ toxicity. Though not widely appreciated as hepatotoxic, MeHg may be an underrecognized mediator of environmental liver disease. However, since the outbreak of Minamata disease (MeHg intoxication) in a Japanese fishing village in the 1950s, MeHg has been recognized as one of the most hazardous environmental pollutants. Coal-fired power plants have been identified as the primary source of current mercury emissions, and atmospheric mercury may be converted into MeHg in water body sediment and subsequently enter the aquatic food chain and bioaccumulate in fish.[99] The primary route of human MeHg exposure is consumption of contaminated fish and shellfish, and PCB

co-exposure may occur.[99] MeHg has well-characterized toxic effects on the human nervous system, developing fetus, and kidney.[99] We recently showed that whole blood total mercury, but not urinary total (inorganic plus elemental) mercury, was associated with dose-dependent increased odds for ALT elevation in the NHANES adult population 2003-2004. These results suggest that the organic form of mercury was associated with liver disease.[62] Furthermore, mercury was commonly found, and whole blood mercury was detectable in 92.5% of subjects.

MeHg concentrates considerably within the liver because of enterohepatic recirculation, and several animal studies have examined the potential role of MeHg in liver disease. Both acute and chronic toxicity studies conducted in rats and cats have demonstrated that mercury exposure results in depletion of body fat with the development of centrilobular hepatic steatosis and increased lipid peroxidation products, proliferation of the endoplasmic reticulum, and floccular degeneration of the mitochondria with extrusion of diseased organelles into the sinusoidal space.[100,101] Many of these changes were irreversible following discontinuation of MeHg exposure. The primary mechanism of MeHg hepatotoxicity may be related to its high affinity for sulfhydryl residues and consequent poisoning of cysteine-containing proteins and glutathione depletion. Previous human epidemiologic studies have inconsistently linked mercury contamination in Japanese fishing villages to increased liver-related mortality in villagers.[102]

Lead

Although lead paint was banned in 1977, significant lead exposure continues to occur in the general population. In the NHANES adult population 2003-2004, the detection rate was nearly universal at 99.6%.[62] Lead exposure in the NHANES population was associated with a dose-dependent increased odds for liver disease. The classic liver disease caused by lead has been called "lead-induced hepatic hyperplasia" and was recently reviewed.[103] However, lead may have other effects that may be particularly relevant to alcoholic liver disease. Lead has been found to contaminate moonshine, and importantly, lead worsens endotoxin-mediated liver disease by priming Kupffer cells.[104]

Lead exposure most commonly occurs through the respiratory or gastrointestinal system. Regardless of the route of exposure, the liver is the largest lead repository in the body.[103] Although acute lead poisoning is characterized by nephrotoxicity, neurotoxicity, and anemia, chronic lead exposure may result in hepatotoxicity. Even though a cholestatic pattern of liver enzyme elevation was reported in one series of lead-exposed industrial workers with a mean blood lead level of 78 μg/dl, this finding was not reproduced in a longitudinal study of battery workers with mean blood levels ranging from 60 μg/dl in 1989 to 30 μg/dl in 1999.[105,106] In a Spanish study, liver biopsy findings, including steatosis with centrilobular hepatitis, correlated with lead levels in exposed patients.[107] However, liver enzymes were an unreliable indicator of disease.

Multiple molecular events have been described in association with lead-induced liver disease. In both animal and human studies, lead exposure decreased hepatic phase I metabolism while inconsistently increasing phase II metabolic enzyme activity in animal studies.[103] Oxidative stress, proinflammatory cytokine production/sensitivity, and liver/serum cholesterol levels were all increased by lead.[103,104]

Arsenic

Arsenic is a well-characterized hepatotoxin. High chronic arsenic exposure is linked with several nonmalignant abnormalities such as hepatomegaly, fibrosis, and noncirrhotic portal hypertension. Although hepatic malignancies such as hepatic hemangiosarcoma and hepatocellular carcinoma are observed in humans, the majority (75% to 80%) of arsenic-induced hepatotoxicity leading to mortality results from the complications of cirrhosis and ascites.[108,109] The effects of high arsenic consumption on noncirrhotic portal hypertension may be underestimated because it may be diagnosed as idiopathic portal hypertension (Banti syndrome). Indian patients in whom Banti syndrome has been diagnosed have been shown to have a higher body burden of arsenicals than unaffected individuals.[110]

Arsenic exposure is most common through the ingestion of well water. High levels of arsenic can be found naturally in some water sources such as in West Bengal, an area with an unexpectedly high level of nonalcoholic fatty liver disease in nonobese individuals, or as a consequence of mining activity, where arsenic frequently contaminates mine tailings and then leaches into the water supply.[111] Acute hepatotoxicity has been observed in patients undergoing arsenite therapy for acute promyelocytic leukemia. Hepatotoxicity from the treatment has been reported in up to 38% of patients.[112]

Three mechanisms of toxicity have been proposed to explain the hepatotoxicity of arsenic, including direct interaction with critical protein thiols, induction of oxidative stress, and methyl group depletion leading to hypomethylation of DNA. The direct interaction of arsenic with protein thiols includes a wide range of proteins, such as enzymes involved in redox regulation, DNA methylation, and repair; tubulin-related genes; and transcription factors, including the redox-sensitive transcription factors nuclear factor (erythroid-derived 2)-like 2 (nrf-2), activator protein-1 (AP-1) family, nuclear factor κB light-chain enhancer of activated B cells (NF-κB), and zinc finger–containing transcription factors, including the steroid receptors.[113] Arsenite interacts with glutathione, which is found to be depleted in acute exposure studies.[114]

The hepatotoxic action of arsenicals is often attributed to the ability of either arsenite or a metabolic product, such as dimethylarsine, to induce oxidative stress. Arsenite binds lipoic acid in mitochondria, which leads to inhibition of pyruvate dehydrogenase with resultant mitochondrial uncoupling and an increase in hydrogen peroxide production.[115] The minor arsenic metabolite dimethylarsine can react with oxygen to form the dimethlyarsenic radical and superoxide and be further metabolized to a peroxy radical. By either mechanism, free radicals or reactive oxygen species are generated. Increases in free radical production, lipid peroxidation products, and oxidized DNA damage have been reported in multiple studies. Arsenite and other prooxidizing stimuli have been shown to cause SEC proliferation with increased capillarization.[116] The proangiogenic stimulation also induces cells to up-regulate cell adhesion molecules and the formation of a basement membrane limiting appropriate hepatic fenestration. This effect may limit sinusoidal vessel resistance and is a precursor for hepatic fibrosis.

The primary method of arsenite detoxication/elimination is by methylation to form dimethyl arsenous acid. The methylation reactions use SAMe as a methyl donor. Arsenic exposure is thus linked to SAMe depletion. Such depletion may lead to global hypomethylation of DNA, even though specific genes may be hypermethylated. These epigenetic changes may be linked to cancer.

Conclusion

More than 50 million chemicals are currently registered with CAS, and it is impossible to fully understand the potential hepatotoxicity of all of them. Although extensive research has been conducted by industry and multiple governmental agencies, clinical and translational research in this area lags far behind most other areas in hepatology. Nonetheless, both malignant and nonmalignant liver diseases have been associated with industrial chemical exposure. Importantly, routine liver enzymes may be normal in individuals with occupational and environmental liver disease, and there are no FDA-approved medications indicated for the prevention or treatment of these conditions. More research—particularly clinical and translational research—is needed in this area.

Key References

Agency for Toxic Substances and Disease Registry. Toxicological profile for carbon tetrachloride. Atlanta: U.S. Department of Health and Human Services, 2005. (Ref.34)

Alexander DD, et al. A meta-analysis of occupational trichloroethylene exposure and liver cancer. Int Arch Occup Environ Health 2007;81:127–143. (Ref.27)

Al-Neamy FR, et al. Occupational lead exposure and amino acid profiles and liver function tests in industrial workers. Int J Environ Health Res 2001;11: 181–188. (Ref.105)

Anthony J, Banister E, Oloffs PC. Effect of sublethal levels of diazinon: histopathology of liver. Bull Environ Contam Toxicol 1986;37:501–507. (Ref.64)

Antov G, et al. [Biochemical and histological changes after acute oral poisoning with the acetanilide herbicide acetochlor.] J Toxicol Clin Exp 1991;11:349–356. (Ref.74)

Barberino JL, et al. [Liver changes in workers at an oil refinery and in a reference population in the state of Bahia, Brazil.] Rev Panam Salud Publica 2005;17: 30–37. (Ref.39)

Bashir S, et al. Arsenic-induced cell death in liver and brain of Straub, A.C., experimental rats. Basic Clin Pharmacol Toxicol 2006;98:38–43. (Ref.114)

Bond GG, et al. Cause specific mortality among employees engaged in the manufacture, formulation, or packaging of 2,4-dichlorophenoxyacetic acid and related salts. Br J Ind Med 1988;45:98–105. (Ref.68)

Borges LP, et al. Acute liver damage induced by 2-nitropropane in rats: effect of diphenyl diselenide on antioxidant defenses. Chem Biol Interact 2006;160: 99–107. (Ref.83)

Bradberry SM, et al. Mechanisms of toxicity, clinical features, and management of acute chlorophenoxy herbicide poisoning: a review. J Toxicol Clin Toxicol 2000;38:111–122. (Ref.66)

Brautbar N, Williams J 2nd. Industrial solvents and liver toxicity: risk assessment, risk factors and mechanisms. Int J Hyg Environ Health 2002;205: 479–491. (Ref.3)

Brodkin CA, et al. Hepatic ultrasonic changes in workers exposed to perchloroethylene. Occup Environ Med 1995;52:679–685. (Ref.31)

Bull RJ. Mode of action of liver tumor induction by trichloroethylene and its metabolites, trichloroacetate and dichloroacetate. Environ Health Perspect 2000;108(Suppl 2):241–259. (Ref.26)

Cave M, et al. Toxicant-associated steatohepatitis in vinyl chloride workers. Hepatology 2010;51:474–481. (Ref.2)

Cave M, et al. Elevated serum hyaluronic acid may identify vinyl chloride workers at high risk for the subsequent development of hepatic angiosarcoma [abstract 427]. Hepatology 2007;46(4). (Ref.12)

Charnley G. Assessing and managing methylmercury risks associated with power plant mercury emissions in the United States. Med Gen Med 2006;8:64. (Ref.99)

Cheong HK, et al. Grand rounds: an outbreak of toxic hepatitis among industrial waste disposal workers. Environ Health Perspect 2007;115:107–112. (Ref.88)

Cocco P, et al. Long-term health effects of the occupational exposure to DDT. A preliminary report. Ann N Y Acad Sci 1997;837:246–256. (Ref.61)

Cohen SM, et al. Hemangiosarcoma in rodents: mode-of-action evaluation and human relevance. Toxicol Sci 2009;111:4–18. (Ref.11)

Consonni D, et al. Mortality in a population exposed to dioxin after the Seveso, Italy, accident in 1976: 25 years of follow-up. Am J Epidemiol 2008;167:847–858. (Ref.71)

Cotrim HP, et al. Nonalcoholic steatohepatitis: a toxic liver disease in industrial workers. Liver 1999;19:299–304. (Ref.38)

Cotrim HP, et al. Clinical and histopathological features of NASH in workers exposed to chemicals with or without associated metabolic conditions. Liver Int 2004;24:131–135. (Ref.21)

Das K, et al. Nonobese population in a developing country has a high prevalence of nonalcoholic fatty liver and significant liver disease. Hepatology 2010;51:1593–1602. (Ref.111)

Dimethylformamide. IARC Monogr Eval Carcinog Risks Hum 1999;71(Pt 2):545–574. (Ref.84)

Dinis-Oliveira RJ, et al. Paraquat poisonings: mechanisms of lung toxicity, clinical features, and treatment. Crit Rev Toxicol 2008;38:13–71. (Ref.73)

Farrell G. Drug-induced liver disease. New York: Churchill Livingstone, 1994:511–549. (Ref.59)

Futatsuka M, et al. Long-term follow-up study of health status in population living in methylmercury-polluted area. Environ Sci 2005;12:239–282. (Ref.102)

Gelpi E, et al. The Spanish toxic oil syndrome 20 years after its onset: a multidisciplinary review of scientific knowledge. Environ Health Perspect 2002;110:457–464. (Ref.98)

Goel A, Chauhan DP, Dhawan DK. Protective effects of zinc in chlorpyrifos induced hepatotoxicity: a biochemical and trace elemental study. Biol Trace Elem Res 2000;74:171–183. (Ref.63)

Guzelian P, Mills S, Fallon HJ. Liver structure and function in print workers exposed to toluene. J Occup Med 1988;30:791–796. (Ref.40)

Hall AG. Nurses: taking precautionary action on a pediatric environmental exposure: DEHP. Pediatr Nurs 2006;32:91–93. (Ref.50)

Harrison R, et al. Fulminant hepatic failure after occupational exposure to 2-nitropropane. Ann Intern Med 1987;107:466–468. (Ref.82)

Hernandez AF, et al. Influence of exposure to pesticides on serum components and enzyme activities of cytotoxicity among intensive agriculture farmers. Environ Res 2006;102:70–76. (Ref.57)

Hodgson MJ, Heyl AE, Van Thiel DH. Liver disease associated with exposure to 1,1,1-trichloroethane. Arch Intern Med 1989;149:1793–1798. (Ref.36)

Holder JW. Nitrobenzene potential human cancer risk based on animal studies. Toxicol Ind Health 1999;15:458–463. (Ref.76)

Honchel R, et al. Lead enhances lipopolysaccharide and tumor necrosis factor liver injury. J Lab Clin Med 1991;117:202–208. (Ref.104)

Hsiao CY, et al. A longitudinal study of the effects of long-term exposure to lead among lead battery factory workers in Taiwan (1989-1999). Sci Total Environ 2001;279:151–158. (Ref.106)

Hsiao TJ, et al. Liver fibrosis in asymptomatic polyvinyl chloride workers. J Occup Environ Med 2004;46:962–966. (Ref.22)

Hsieh HI, et al. Effect of the CYP2E1 genotype on vinyl chloride monomer–induced liver fibrosis among polyvinyl chloride workers. Toxicology 2007;239:34–44. (Ref.7)

Hsieh HI, et al. Synergistic effect of hepatitis virus infection and occupational exposures to vinyl chloride monomer and ethylene dichloride on serum aminotransferase activity. Occup Environ Med 2003;60:774–778. (Ref.18)

Husted TL, et al. Liver transplantation for primary or metastatic sarcoma to the liver. Am J Transplant 2006;6:392–397. (Ref.16)

Infante PF, et al. Vinyl chloride propellant in hair spray and angiosarcoma of the liver among hairdressers and barbers: case reports. Int J Occup Environ Health 2009;15:36–42. (Ref.10)

Jung SJ, et al. Dimethylacetamide-induced hepatic injuries among spandex fibre workers. Clin Toxicol (Phila) 2007;45:435–439. (Ref.89)

Kanz MF, et al. Glutathione depletion exacerbates methylenedianiline toxicity to biliary epithelial cells and hepatocytes in rats. Toxicol Sci 2003;74:447–456. (Ref.94)

Kennedy GL Jr, Sherman H. Acute and subchronic toxicity of dimethylformamide and dimethylacetamide following various routes of administration. Drug Chem Toxicol 1986;9:147–170. (Ref.92)

Khan DA, et al. Adverse effects of pesticides residues on biochemical markers in Pakistani tobacco farmers. Int J Clin Exp Med 2008;1:274–282. (Ref.56)

Kiely T, Donaldson D, Grube A. Pesticide industry sales and usage. 2000 and 2001 market estimates. Washington, DC: U.S. Environmental Agency, 2004. (Ref.55)

Kim HR, et al. Clinical features and treatment outcomes of advanced stage primary hepatic angiosarcoma. Ann Oncol 2009;20:780–787. (Ref.17)

Kitchin KT, Wallace K. The role of protein binding of trivalent arsenicals in arsenic carcinogenesis and toxicity. J Inorg Biochem 2008;102:532–539. (Ref.113)

Lang IA, et al. Association of urinary bisphenol A concentration with medical disorders and laboratory abnormalities in adults. JAMA 2008;300:1303–1310. (Ref.54)

Lash LH, et al. Metabolism of trichloroethylene. Environ Health Perspect 2000;108(Suppl 2):177–200. (Ref.25)

Lash LH, Parker JC. Hepatic and renal toxicities associated with perchloroethylene. Pharmacol Rev 2001;53:177–208. (Ref.30)

Lee CY, et al. Incidence of dimethylacetamide induced hepatic injury among new employees in a cohort of elastane fibre workers. Occup Environ Med 2006;63:688–693. (Ref.90)

Leonard C, et al. "Golf ball liver": Agent Orange hepatitis. Gut 1997;40:687–688 (Ref.60)

Levine BS, et al. Subchronic toxicity of trinitrotoluene in Fischer 344 rats. Toxicology 1984;32:253–265. (Ref.76)

Li J, Jiang QG, Zhong WD. Persistent ethanol drinking increases liver injury induced by trinitrotoluene exposure: an in-plant case-control study. Hum Exp Toxicol 1991;10:405–409. (Ref.78)

Lim S, et al. Chronic exposure to the herbicide, atrazine, causes mitochondrial dysfunction and insulin resistance. PLoS One 2009;4:e5186. (Ref.75)

Lin YS, et al. Association of the blood/air partition coefficient of 1,3-butadiene with blood lipids and albumin. Environ Health Perspect 2002;110:165–168. (Ref.8)

Liu J, et al. Examination of the relationships between environmental exposures to volatile organic compounds and biochemical liver tests: application of canonical correlation analysis. Environ Res 2009;109:193–199. (Ref.43)

Lu T, et al. Application of cDNA microarray to the study of arsenic-induced liver diseases in the population of Guizhou, China. Toxicol Sci 2001;59:185–192. (Ref.109)

Luo JC, et al. Abnormal liver function associated with occupational exposure to dimethylformamide and hepatitis B virus. J Occup Environ Med 2001;43:474–482. (Ref.86)

Manibusan MK, Odin M, Eastmond DA. Postulated carbon tetrachloride mode of action: a review. J Environ Sci Health C Environ Carcinog Ecotoxicol Rev 2007;25:185–209. (Ref.35)

Maroni M, et al. Periportal fibrosis and other liver ultrasonography findings in vinyl chloride workers. Occup Environ Med 2003;60:60–65. (Ref.23)

Mastrangelo G, et al. Increased risk of hepatocellular carcinoma and liver cirrhosis in vinyl chloride workers: synergistic effect of occupational exposure with alcohol intake. Environ Health Perspect 2004;112:1188–1192. (Ref.6)

Mathews V, et al. Hepatotoxicity profile of single agent arsenic trioxide in the treatment of newly diagnosed acute promyelocytic leukemia, its impact on clinical outcome and the effect of genetic polymorphisms on the incidence of hepatotoxicity. Leukemia 2006;20:881–883. (Ref.112)

Matthaei H, et al. Long-term survival after surgery for primary hepatic sarcoma in adults. Arch Surg 2009;144:339–344; discussion 344. (Ref.15)

Michalek JE, Ketchum NS, Longnecker MP. Serum dioxin and hepatic abnormalities in veterans of Operation Ranch Hand. Ann Epidemiol 2001;11:304–311. (Ref.70)

Moser GA, McLachlan MS. A non-absorbable dietary fat substitute enhances elimination of persistent lipophilic contaminants in humans. Chemosphere 1999;39:1513–1521. (Ref.5)

Mudipalli A. Lead hepatotoxicity & potential health effects. Indian J Med Res 2007;126:518–527. (Ref.103)

Mundt KA, et al. Historical cohort study of 10 109 men in the North American vinyl chloride industry, 1942-72: update of cancer mortality to 31 December 1995. Occup Environ Med 2000;57:774–781. (Ref.113)

Neuman M, Lehotay D. Soluble cytokeratin (CK 18-M30) as a bio-marker of environmental herbicide cytotoxicity and subsequent repair [abstract]. Hepatology 2008;48:505A. (Ref.65)

Nichols L. The Epping jaundice outbreak: mortality after 38 years of follow-up. Int Arch Occup Environ Health 2004;77:592–594. (Ref.95)

NTP toxicology and carcinogenesis studies of tetrachloroethylene (perchloroethylene) (CAS No. 127-18-4) in F344/N rats and B6C3F1 mice (inhalation studies). Natl Toxicol Program Tech Rep Ser 1986;311:1–197. (Ref.32)

NTP. NTP toxicology and carcinogenesis studies of a binary mixture of 3,3',4,4',5-pentachlorobiphenyl (PCB 126) (CAS No. 57465-28-8) and 2,2',4,4',5,5'-hexachlorobiphenyl (PCB 153) (CAS No. 35065-27-1) in female Harlan Sprague-Dawley rats (gavage studies). Natl Toxicol Program Tech Rep Ser 2006;530:1–258. (Ref.44)

Patel M, et al. Pesticide and heavy metal exposures are associated with ALT elevation in American adults: NHANES 2003-2004 [abstract].Gastroenterology 2009;136(5 Suppl 1):289. (Ref.62)

Patrick L. Toxic metals and antioxidants: Part II. The role of antioxidants in arsenic and cadmium toxicity. Altern Med Rev 2003;8:106–128. (Ref.115)

Paulino CA, et al. Acute, subchronic and chronic 2,4-dichlorophenoxyacetic acid (2,4-D) intoxication in rats. Vet Hum Toxicol 1996;38:348–352. (Ref.69)

Perez CA, et al. [Liver damage in workers exposed to hydrocarbons.] Gastroenterol Hepatol 2006;29:334–337. (Ref.37)

Redlich CA, et al. Clinical and pathological characteristics of hepatotoxicity associated with occupational exposure to dimethylformamide. Gastroenterology 1990;99:748–757. (Ref.85)

Report on Carcinogens. Research Triangle Park: U.S. Department of Health and Human Services, Public Health Service, National Toxicology Program, 2005. (Ref.81)

Ruder AM. Potential health effects of occupational chlorinated solvent exposure. Ann N Y Acad Sci, 2006;1076:207–227. (Ref.24)

Rusyn I, Peters JM, Cunningham ML. Modes of action and species-specific effects of di-(2-ethylhexyl)phthalate in the liver. Crit Rev Toxicol 2006;36: 459–479. (Ref.51)

Sanchez J, de la Fuente J, Castrillo J. Hepatotoxicidad por plomo inorganico: resultados en 85 casos de saturnismo agudo. Gastroenterol Hepatol 1985; 8:24–29. (Ref.107)

Santa Cruz V, Dugas TR, Kanz MF. Mitochondrial dysfunction occurs before transport or tight junction deficits in biliary epithelial cells exposed to bile from methylenedianiline-treated rats. Toxicol Sci 2005;84:129–138. (Ref.95)

Spies GJ, et al. Monitoring acrylic fiber workers for liver toxicity and exposure to dimethylacetamide. 2. Serum clinical chemistry results of dimethylacetamide-exposed workers. J Occup Environ Med 1995;37:1102–1107. (Ref.91)

Straub AC, et al. Arsenic stimulates sinusoidal endothelial cell capillarization and vessel remodeling in mouse liver. Hepatology 2007;45:205–212. (Ref.116)

Sweeney MH, Mocarelli P. Human health effects after exposure to 2,3,7,8-TCDD. Food Addit Contam 2000;17:303–316. (Ref.72)

Takaki A, et al. A 27-year-old man who died of acute liver failure probably due to trichloroethylene abuse. J Gastroenterol 2008;43:239–242. (Ref.28)

Tolman KG, Sirrine R. Occupational hepatoxicity. Clin Liver Dis 1998;2: 563–589. (Ref.1)

Tomei F, et al. Liver damage among shoe repairers. Am J Ind Med 1999;36: 541–547. (Ref.41)

Turusov V, Rakitsky V, Tomatis L. Dichlorodiphenyltrichloroethane (DDT): ubiquity, persistence, and risks. Environ Health Perspect 2002;110:125–128. (Ref.58)

Vandenberg LN, et al. Bisphenol-A and the great divide: a review of controversies in the field of endocrine disruption. Endocr Rev 2009;30:75–95. (Ref.53)

von Rettberg H, et al. Use of di(2-ethylhexyl)phthalate–containing infusion systems increases the risk for cholestasis. Pediatrics 2009;124:710–716. (Ref.52)

Ward E, et al. Update of the follow-up of mortality and cancer incidence among European workers employed in the vinyl chloride industry. Epidemiology 2001;12:710–718. (Ref.14)

Wrbitzky R. Liver function in workers exposed to N,N-dimethylformamide during the production of synthetic textiles. Int Arch Occup Environ Health 1999;72:19–25. (Ref.87)

Yan C, et al. [The retrospective survey of malignant tumor in weapon workers exposed to 2,4,6-trinitrotoluene.] Zhonghua Lao Dong Wei Sheng Zhi Ye Bing Za Zhi 2002;20:184–188. (Ref.77)

Yoshimura T. Yusho in Japan. Ind Health 2003;41:139–148. (Ref.47)

Yu ML, et al. Increased mortality from chronic liver disease and cirrhosis 13 years after the Taiwan "yucheng" ("oil disease") incident. Am J Ind Med 1997;31:172–175. (Ref.48)

Zhang X, et al. 4,4'-Methylenedianiline–induced hepatotoxicity is modified by N-acetyltransferase 2 (NAT2) acetylator polymorphism in the rat. J Pharmacol Exp Ther 2006;316:289–294. (Ref.96)

Zimmerman H. Hepatotoxicity: the adverse effects of drugs and other chemicals on the liver. 2nd ed. Philadelphia: Lippincott Williams & Wilkins, 1999.(Ref.33)

A complete list of references can be found at www.expertconsult.com.

Alcoholic Liver Disease

Stephen F. Stewart and Chris P. Day

ABBREVIATIONS

ADH alcohol dehydrogenase
AMPK adenosine monophosphate–activated protein kinase
ALD alcoholic liver disease
ALDHs aldehyde dehydrogenases
ALT alanine transaminase
AP-1 activator protein-1
poB apolipoprotein B
AST aspartate transaminase
ATP adenosine triphosphate
Bax Bcl-2-associated x protein
Bid BH3 interacting domain death agonist
COX-2 cyclooxygenase-2
CT computed tomography
CTLA-4 cytotoxic T-lymphocyte antigen-4
CYP2E1 cytochrome P450 2E1
ER endoplasmic reticulum
DF discriminant function
DISC death-inducing signaling complex
ECM extracellular matrix
FFA free fatty acids
G-3P glycerol-3-phosphate
GSH mitochondrial glutathione

HCC hepatocellular cancer
HERs hydroxyethyl radicals
HRS hepatorenal syndrome
HSC hepatic stellate cells
IgA immunoglobulin A
IL-6 interleukin-6
iNOS inducible NO synthase
LBP LPS binding protein
LPS lipopolysaccharide
LSP liver-specific membrane lipoprotein
MAA MDA-acetaldehyde
MARS molecular adsorbents recycling system
MAT methionine adenosyltransferase
MDA malondialdehyde
MEOS microsomal ethanol-oxidizing system
MMPs matrix metalloproteinases
mRNA messenger RNA
MS methionine synthase
MTP microsomal triglyceride transfer protein
NO nitric oxide
NK natural killer

NKT natural killer T
PAP phosphatidate phosphohydrolase
PT prothrombin time
PPAR-α peroxisome proliferator-activated receptor-α
PUFA polyunsaturated fatty acid
PTX pentoxifylline
RA retinoic acid
ROS reactive oxygen species
SAH S-adenosylhomocysteine
SAMe S-adenosylmethionine
SOD2 superoxide dismutase
SREBP-1c sterol response element binding protein-1c
TAG triacylglycerol
TGF-β transforming growth factor-β
TLR4 Toll-like receptor 4
TNF-α tumor necrosis factor-α
TNFR1 TNF-α receptor 1
TRAIL tumor necrosis factor–related apoptosis-inducing ligand
UPR unfolded protein response
VLDL very-low-density lipoproteins

Introduction

Alcohol is consumed by a large percentage of the world's population and is an effective anxiolytic and social lubricant. A small proportion of consumers become dependent, and a moderate proportion of these, and many who are not dependent, develop clinically significant liver disease. These problems are not new. Alcohol was recognized to be a cause of liver damage by the ancient Greeks, and is currently a common cause of liver disease in the Western world. The magnitude and range of the health and socioeconomic problems attributable to alcohol abuse are enormous. Cirrhosis, predominantly alcoholic, is now the fourth commonest cause of death between the ages 25 and 64 in the United States and alcohol may also make a significant contribution to cardiovascular-related mortality. The overall socioeconomic cost of alcohol abuse in the United States in terms of healthcare, crime, and loss of work capacity has been estimated at more than $180

million per year. It is therefore a significant drain on limited healthcare resources. In common with all alcohol-related disease, abstinence is the cornerstone of management in patients with alcoholic liver disease (ALD). The development of specific therapies has, however, been hampered by a continued lack of a clear understanding of the mechanisms through which ethanol causes liver injury. Intense research efforts have now highlighted several important metabolic and immunologic consequences of excessive alcohol consumption that may contribute to disease pathogenesis, and it is hoped that further defining these disease mechanisms may lead to the development of novel treatment strategies. It has also become increasingly clear that individuals are not "all equal" in their susceptibility to ALD. Although cumulative alcohol dose undoubtedly plays a role in determining disease risk, only a small proportion of heavy drinkers go on to develop the more advanced forms of ALD—hepatitis, fibrosis, and cirrhosis. Elucidating the genetic and environmental factors associated with disease progression would be a major step toward disease prevention. This chapter will focus on the pathogenetic mechanisms of alcoholic liver disease and the current treatments available.

Epidemiology

Several independent studies have demonstrated a close correlation between deaths from cirrhosis and per capita alcohol consumption. Perhaps the best example of this is the effect of wine rationing in France during World War II, which was associated with an 80% reduction in cirrhosis deaths, followed by a return to prewar levels when restrictions were removed.[1] A similar effect was observed during Prohibition in the United States. **Figure 28-1** shows the decline in cases after the act was passed in 1916 and a gradual increase following the repeal of the act in 1932.

The worldwide increase in mortality from cirrhosis observed during the 1950s and 1960s was associated with a similar rise in alcohol consumption, attributed largely to the falling price of alcohol relative to income.[2] Conversely, the reduction in per capita alcohol intake that has occurred in several countries since the late 1970s (including the United States) and has been reflected in the reduction of deaths due to cirrhosis. More recently, this decline has leveled off and, once again, there has been a rise in ALD mortality rates in some countries.[3] This may be associated with a rise in alcohol consumption, but may also be due in part to the increased prevalence of obesity, now recognized to be an important risk factor for the development of ALD.[4]

In 2005 liver cirrhosis was the twelfth leading cause of death in the United States, and 45.9% of the cases of cirrhosis were alcohol related. These figures translate to around 28,200 deaths from cirrhosis, of which 12,900 are alcohol related.[5] These deaths occur in an estimated total population of 2 million individuals with ALD of varying severities that represent approximately 1 in 7 of the estimated 14 million heavy drinkers in the United States. The potential environmental and genetic explanations for this clear interindividual variation in susceptibility to ALD will be discussed later. First it is important to review the putative mechanisms through which this injury occurs. Most of the studies producing the data presented next were driven by the question of how alcohol leads to liver injury. With few exceptions they fail to address the fact that most individuals appear to be remarkably resistant to the deleterious effects of ethanol on the liver.

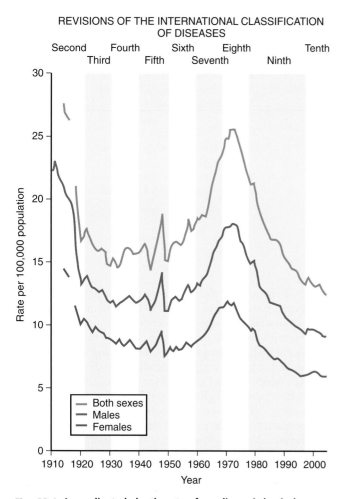

REVISIONS OF THE INTERNATIONAL CLASSIFICATION OF DISEASES

Fig. 28-1 **Age-adjusted death rates from liver cirrhosis by sex.** States with death registration 1910-1932 and all United States 1933-2005. *(Reproduced with permission from National Institute on Alcohol Abuse and Alcoholism, www.niaaa.gov.)*

Pathogenesis

Although there is good epidemiologic evidence that heavy ethanol intake can result in liver disease in some individuals, there is still much debate about the main pathogenetic mechanisms through which this occurs. Several mechanisms have been proposed, and data from human and animal studies support the fact that more than one is likely to be important. The first and most direct is the effect of ethanol metabolism on liver biochemistry and the resulting steatosis and oxidative stress. The second is the indirect release of cytokines as a result of the increase in gut-derived endotoxin transported to the liver via the portal vein. The third is the liver-directed adaptive immune responses generated as a result of the development of new antigens formed by the reactive intermediates produced by the first two mechanisms. Many of these mechanisms have been elucidated using a variety of animal models. The intragastric ethanol-fed rat model designed by Tsukomoto and French has proven to be the most useful; however, there have also been mouse, guinea pig, hamster, and primate models, each producing their own challenges. As with all animal work, there is often difficulty in interpreting the data with regard to humans. Attempts to minimize this problem lead to studies in the baboon, and, using this model, Lieber and colleagues described lesions resembling alcoholic hepatitis and cirrhosis.[6] Working with animals so closely related to humans has obvious benefits, however, difficulty replicating the experiments and cost and ethical implications have somewhat limited the usefulness of this approach.[7] Later sections of this chapter attempt to describe the putative mechanisms of ethanol-induced liver injury in detail and offer some theories as to how they may interact. First, however, there is a brief description of the absorption, distribution, metabolism, and elimination of alcohol. Alcohol metabolism will be discussed in terms of the fate of a unit of alcohol following ingestion.

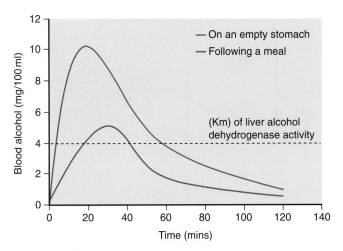

Fig. 28-2 **The typical time course of blood alcohol concentration following the ingestion of 1 unit either following a meal (continuous line) or on an empty stomach (dotted line).**

One unit is equivalent to 10 g or 12.5 ml of absolute alcohol that is present in approximately half a pint (284 ml) of beer, and 1 standard measure of wine (114 ml) or liquor (24 ml).

Absorption, Distribution, and Excretion

The typical time course of blood alcohol concentration following the ingestion of one unit is shown in **Figure 28-2**. The peak level occurs approximately 20 minutes after ingestion and reaches between 10 and 15 mg/l00 ml. The rate of rise and height of peak is a function of alcohol absorption and tissue distribution. In addition, it has been suggested that the peak value may be influenced by first-pass metabolism of alcohol by alcohol dehydrogenase activity within the gastric mucosa, however, the biologic importance of this effect is controversial. Alcohol is absorbed from the gastrointestinal tract by simple diffusion.[8] Because of slow absorption of ethanol in the stomach, 50% to 80% of absorption occurs in the duodenum and upper jejunum. The rate of absorption is delayed following a meal and increases in proportion to the alcohol concentration of the drink consumed. Because absorption is more rapid from the intestine than the stomach, any pathologic condition, drug, or surgical intervention that delays or increases gastric emptying will also affect alcohol absorption accordingly.

Following absorption, the tissue distribution of alcohol is determined principally by blood flow and water content. Thus in organs with a rich vasculature, such as the brain, lungs, and liver, alcohol levels rapidly equilibrate with the blood. Alcohol is poorly soluble in lipids, which will take up only 4% of the amount of ethanol that can be dissolved in a corresponding volume of water. As a result, tissues with a high fat/water ratio attain much lower levels than organs such as the kidneys, where the high water content results in urinary alcohol levels 1.3 times higher than those in blood. The low lipid solubility of alcohol also explains why, following the ingestion of the same amount of alcohol per unit weight, an obese person attains a higher level of blood alcohol than a thin person.

Furthermore, the higher fat content of female body composition compared with a male has been invoked as part of the explanation for their higher alcohol levels following the ingestion of similar amounts of alcohol per unit of weight.[9] More than 90% of circulating alcohol is oxidatively metabolized, primarily in the liver, and excreted as carbon dioxide and water. The remainder is eliminated unchanged in the urine (<1%) and breath (1% to 5%).

In view of the negligible renal and pulmonary excretion, the rate of alcohol elimination is largely determined by the body's capacity for alcohol oxidation. The rate of alcohol metabolism does not vary widely in the population and above a concentration of 10 mg/100 ml occurs at a constant rate of approximately 100 mg/kg body weight per hour; so-called zero-order kinetics. A 70-kg man, therefore, eliminates one unit of alcohol in about 90 minutes. An important implication of this type of kinetics is the absence of a rapid feedback mechanism to increase the rate of alcohol oxidation in response to its concentration. Heavy, repeated alcohol consumption can, however, increase the rate of elimination by up to 100%.

Alcohol Metabolism

Site of Alcohol Oxidation

Alcohol metabolism is performed almost entirely by the liver, which contains several different high-affinity (low K_m) enzyme systems capable of oxidizing alcohol (**Fig. 28-3**). Other organs, including kidney, intestine, and bone marrow, also possess alcohol oxidizing capacity, but because of the low affinity of the alcohol dehydrogenase (ADH) activities present in these tissues, they make an insignificant contribution to overall alcohol oxidation at the concentrations attained following normal "social" drinking. The possible exception is the ADH activity present in the gastric mucosa, where the very high gastric levels of alcohol following ingestion may render the affinity of the enzyme(s) present less critical and the resulting alcohol oxidation significant. This effect has been claimed to contribute to a significant first-pass metabolism of alcohol determining both its bioavailability and its toxic effects.[10] This gastric "barrier" may be lower in females and further contribute to their increased susceptibility to alcohol.[11] The increased first pass metabolism due to gastric ADH seems to be primarily a function of men under 40, with older men having similar or lower activity than their female counterparts.[12] In addition certain drugs, such as H_2-receptor antagonists, may also influence the activity of gastric ADH[13] as they have been shown to influence the bioavailability of ethanol by reducing first-pass metabolism.[14] A study showing that gastritis results in a reduction in gastric ADH activity without affecting ethanol bioavailability casts doubt on the clinical role of this gastric first-pass effect.[15]

Oxidation of Alcohol to Acetaldehyde

Alcohol oxidation in the liver takes place via three steps. First alcohol is oxidized, principally within the cytosol, to acetaldehyde. Then acetaldehyde is further oxidized to acetate, primarily within the mitochondria, and finally, acetate is released into the blood and oxidized to carbon dioxide and water in peripheral tissues. At least three enzyme systems with the capacity to oxidize alcohol to acetaldehyde are present within the liver,

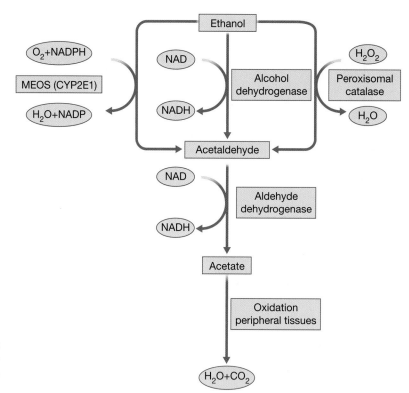

Fig. 28-3 **The three pathways of alcohol oxidation: alcohol dehydrogenase (ADH), microsomal ethanol-oxidizing system (MEOS), and catalase.** *NADPH,* nicotinamide-adenine dinucleotide phosphate.

although in normal individuals only the alcohol dehydrogenase enzymes are important.

The Alcohol Dehydrogenase (ADH) Pathway

Alcohol dehydrogenase catalyzes the oxidation of a variety of alcohols to aldehydes and ketones. This includes catalyzing the oxidation of ethanol to acetaldehyde and transferring hydrogen to the cofactor nicotinamide adenine dinucleotide (NAD), which is converted to its reduced form, NADH. The resulting increase in the ratio of NADH/NAD, which is further increased by acetaldehyde oxidation, is partly responsible for the metabolic imbalances that occur following alcohol ingestion and has been considered to play a major role in the initial pathogenesis of alcohol-induced fatty liver.

Human ADH exhibits multiple isoenzymes that have been divided into five major classes on the basis of their electrophoretic mobility, kinetic properties and inhibition by pyrazole.[16] They are encoded by at least seven different gene loci, *ADH1* to *ADH7*, encoding the α-, β-, γ-, π-, χ-, σ-, and μ-subunits, respectively. The class I isoenzymes are formed by random association of the α-, β-, and γ- subunits to form the active homodimeric or heterodimeric isoenzymes, whereas the others are all homodimers. The *ADH2* and *ADH3* genes are polymorphic, encoding three different β and two different γ subunits with different kinetic properties resulting in isoenzymes with different rates of alcohol oxidation in vitro.[17] Expression of the ADH genes is tissue specific. The liver contains the highest levels of class I activity, while class III activity is present equally in all tissues. In humans, the class II isoenzyme, π-ADH has been found only in the liver while the class IV enzyme, σ-ADH, is present only in the stomach.[18] The class I isoenzymes have by far the lowest K_m and highest V_{max} for alcohol and accordingly are thought to be responsible for the major part of hepatic alcohol oxidation. The overall K_m of liver

ADH activity is in the order of 1 mmol (4 mg/100 ml), which explains why alcohol follows zero-order kinetics at anything above very low blood levels. Experiments performed both in vivo and in vitro suggest that the principal regulatory mechanism for the ADH pathway is the capacity of the mitochondria to reoxidize NADH back to NAD.[19]

The Microsomal Ethanol-Oxidizing System (MEOS) Pathway

In addition to ADH, alcohol is metabolized by the MEOS; an accessory pathway that principally involves a specific alcohol-inducible form of cytochrome P450 designated CYP2E1.[20] The enzyme is located on the endoplasmic reticulum, is present in greater amounts in perivenular than periportal hepatocytes and requires oxygen and NADPH. The CYP2E1 protein has been purified and the human gene cloned, sequenced, and localized to chromosome 10.[21] The overall contribution of MEOS to alcohol oxidation in vivo is not yet fully clear. Its K_m for alcohol is in the order of 50 to 80 mg/100 ml, so it appears to play an important role at high blood alcohol levels or following chronic alcohol abuse, in view of its inducibility. Alcohol induction of CYP2E1, and microsomal enzyme systems in general, has also been implicated in the tolerance to various drugs commonly observed in alcoholics, and may explain their increased susceptibility to hepatotoxicity by other drugs and xenobiotics that are converted to toxic metabolites by microsomal enzyme systems. An important example of this phenomenon is the increased susceptibility of heavy drinkers to the toxic effects of acetaminophen, where severe liver damage has been reported in alcoholics taking large, but previously considered safe, doses.[22,23] More recent data suggests that this effect may, at least in part, be due to an acetaminophen-induced reduction in antioxidants that subsequently renders the hepatocyte sensitive to apoptosis induced by tumor necrosis factor-α (TNF-α), a cytokine found at higher concentrations in the livers of heavy drinkers than abstainers.[24] Nevertheless, it is likely that increased metabolism plays a significant role in the increased sensitivity of drinkers to acetaminophen. Enhanced microsomal enzyme activity may also lead to an increased rate of testosterone breakdown, contributing to low blood levels of hormone already decreased due to inhibition of testosterone production by the direct toxic effects of alcohol on the testes.[25] The methods by which ethanol induces CYP2E1 are not entirely clear but are likely to be multifactorial including increased transcription, increased mRNA stabilization, increased translation and reduced degradation.

The Catalase Pathway

The third pathway for alcohol oxidation is catalyzed by the enzyme, catalase. This enzyme is located in the peroxisomes of most tissues and requires the presence of hydrogen peroxide. The reaction is limited by the availability of hydrogen peroxide, which in normal circumstances is low and suggests that the catalase pathway accounts for less than 2% of overall in vivo alcohol oxidation.[26]

Oxidation of Acetaldehyde to Acetate

More than 90% of the acetaldehyde formed from alcohol oxidation is further oxidized in the liver to acetate by aldehyde dehydrogenases (ALDHs). ALDH, like ADH, uses NAD as a co-factor and further increases the NADH/NAD ratio. Human ALDHs are encoded at four independent loci on four different chromosomes.[27] *ALDH2* on chromosome 12 encodes the major mitochondrial enzyme, which has a low K_m for acetaldehyde and is responsible for the majority of acetaldehyde oxidation. The *ALDH2* gene exists in at least two allelic forms, *ALDH2*1* and *ALDH2*2*.[28] Isoenzymes present in individuals homozygous for the *ALDH2*2* allele have little or no catalytic activity, while those present in heterozygotes have measurable although reduced activity compared with the isoenzymes present in *ALDH2*1* homozygotes.[29] The inactive form of ALDH2 is present in about 50% of Asians but has not been found in Caucasian populations. Increased levels of acetaldehyde are thought to be the mechanism through which homozygotes for the *ALDH2*2* allele develop the "flushing" reaction after alcohol. Interestingly, heterozygotes for the allele appear to develop advanced liver disease with lower levels of ethanol consumption.[30] This, too, is putatively secondary to increased concentrations of acetaldehyde and adds to the extensive evidence that acetaldehyde is centrally involved in the pathogenesis of ALD. The cytosolic form of ALDH, ALDH1 has a higher K_m for acetaldehyde than ALDH2 and may play a role following the ingestion of large doses of alcohol. ALDH inhibitors such as disulfuram (Antabuse) have been used in the treatment of alcoholism to sensitize alcoholics to the unpleasant effects of alcohol intake secondary to high levels of acetaldehyde.

Alterations in Alcohol Metabolism Following Chronic Consumption

Many studies have shown that chronic alcohol consumption increases the rate of alcohol elimination except in the presence of severe liver damage. This increase is due both to alcohol induction of the MEOS and to adaptive changes in the ADH pathway. The basis for the increased activity of the ADH pathway is probably increased mitochondrial reoxidation of NADH to NAD, which, as discussed previously, is the important rate-limiting step. It has been suggested that the increased mitochondrial NADH-reoxidation rate is secondary to alcohol-induced stimulation of Na+, K+-ATPase activity, leading to enhanced ATP and oxygen consumption.[31] This so-called hypermetabolic state of the liver has also been implicated in the pathogenesis of alcohol-related liver injury. Alcohol elimination is decreased in jaundiced patients with alcoholic cirrhosis and animals with non–alcohol-related liver disease[32]; this probably reflects decreased ADH activity.[33] An important consequence of the increased rate of alcohol oxidation in alcoholics is that, following alcohol ingestion, levels of acetaldehyde in both blood and tissues are higher than those seen after similar ingestion in nonalcoholic controls.[34,35] This increase is potentiated by a reduction in the capacity of the mitochondria to oxidize acetaldehyde, at least in alcohol-fed rats, and a reduction in total hepatic ALDH activity, observed in chronic alcoholic patients with and without liver disease.[36] As discussed, this may have important implications for disease pathogenesis. Having discussed the pathways of ethanol metabolism, the next sections will review the evidence for how this impacts on disease pathogenesis.

Alcohol Metabolism and the Pathogenesis of ALD

Many studies have focused on the downstream effects of ethanol metabolism in an effort to explain the biochemical and histologic features of ALD. These studies have yielded several mechanisms through which this metabolism may result in the generation of fatty liver (steatosis), oxidative stress/lipid peroxidation, and acetaldehyde, all of which are thought to be important in disease pathogenesis.

The Pathogenesis of Fatty Liver

The accumulation of triacylglycerol (TAG), synthesized via the sequential esterification of glycerol-3-phosphate within the liver is an early and reversible effect of alcohol consumption in humans and animal models of ALD. It is the consequence of increased substrate supply (glycerol and free fatty acids [FFA]), increased esterification, and decreased export of TAG from the liver.[37] The molecular mechanisms that contribute to these three main effects have recently been elucidated (**Fig. 28-4**).

The Role of Dietary Fat

It is intuitive to suspect that dietary fat will have a role in the development of hepatic steatosis, and indeed rat models of ALD have shown that the rate of development of fatty liver is proportional to the fat content of the diet.[38] Further studies in these rats in conjunction with human epidemiologic data have also highlighted the role that different types of dietary fat may play in influencing the severity of the more advanced forms of ALD, such as necroinflammation and fibrosis. These will be discussed in the section on oxidative stress. Although the quantity of dietary fat can increase the supply of fat to the liver, alcohol intake also increases the lipolysis of adipose

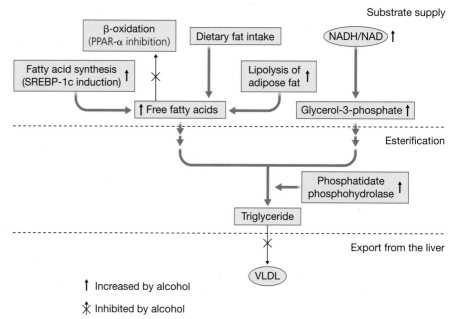

Fig. 28-4 The multiple mechanisms by which ethanol metabolism can result in fatty liver. Ethanol metabolism contributes to fatty liver by increasing substrate supply, increasing fat esterification to triglyceride, and reducing the export of very-low-density lipoprotein (VLDL) from the liver. *PPAR*, peroxisome proliferator-activated receptor; *SREBP-1c*, sterol regulatory element-binding protein 1c.

tissue, further increasing the concentration of circulating FFA. These are then taken up by the liver and provide the substrate for TAG synthesis. The high concentrations of FFA further promote the synthesis of TAG by increasing the activity of the enzyme phosphatidate phosphohydrolase (PAP), which is the rate limiting step for TAG synthesis catalyzing the dephosphorylation of phosphatidic acid to diacylglycerol.[37,39]

Altered Redox State

Of the three well-characterized metabolic pathways discussed previously, two appear to be of clinical and pathogenetic importance; the alcohol dehydrogenase pathway and the MEOS. The first of these involves the oxidation of ethanol to acetaldehyde by cytosolic alcohol dehydrogenases, and subsequent oxidation to acetate by predominantly mitochondrial aldehyde dehydrogenase. Both of these steps are coupled to the reduction of NAD to NADH.

The increased NADH/NAD ratio has profound effects on the metabolism of carbohydrates and lipids. Gluconeogenesis is impaired and substrate flow through the citric acid cycle is diminished, with acetyl CoA diverted toward ketogenesis and fatty acid synthesis. In addition to increased fatty acid synthesis, the altered redox state also directly inhibits fatty acid oxidation. Through these two mechanisms, the altered redox state can contribute toward increased substrate supply. The altered NADH/NAD ratio also increases the production of the other key component of TAG, glycerol-3-phosphate (G-3P), thereby again promoting TAG synthesis.

The Role of PPAR-α Inhibition

Recent evidence suggests that ethanol also has an effect on fatty acid oxidation through the transcriptional factor peroxisome proliferator-activated receptor-α (PPAR-α). This ligand-activated receptor/transcription factor is a critical component in the regulation of mitochondrial, microsomal, and peroxisomal fatty acid oxidation systems in the liver.[40] As FFA are ligands for this receptor, ethanol consumption, which increases

hepatic fatty acid levels via the mechanisms outlined, would be expected to result in an induction of enzymes in the oxidation systems and a subsequent increase in fatty acid oxidation. In fact, ethanol feeding results in a decrease in transcription and activity of many of these enzymes due to an inhibition of the transcriptional and DNA binding activity of PPAR-α.[41] This effect was replicated with acetaldehyde, and inhibited by inhibiting ethanol metabolism, implicating acetaldehyde as the factor leading to the PPAR-α inhibition.[41] Treatment with the PPAR-α agonists WY14,643 and clofibrate reversed the effects of ethanol-feeding and the resulting abnormalities in hepatic lipid metabolism in rodent models[42,43] while alcohol-fed PPAR-α null mice develop more steatosis, hepatocyte injury, and fibrosis than their wild-type litter mates.[44] It appears, therefore, that PPAR-α inhibition plays a critical role in the accumulation of fatty acids in the liver after ethanol feeding, which will then promote TAG synthesis and potentially necroinflammation and fibrosis. It also seems likely that acetaldehyde is a key component of this inhibition. The precise mechanism of acetaldehyde-induced PPAR-α inhibition is still unclear.

Mechanisms of Altered Triglyceride Export

In addition to increased substrate supply and esterification resulting in increased levels of TAG in the liver, a decrease in the export of TAG from the liver also appears to contribute to the generation of ethanol-induced steatosis. Usually fat is exported into the circulation in the form of very-low-density lipoproteins (VLDL). With chronic ethanol ingestion, this export mechanism becomes defective for reasons that are not entirely clear but appear to involve the Golgi complex. Acetaldehyde produced during ethanol metabolism can bind α-tubulin[45] and disrupt microtubule dynamics.[46] Possibly as a result of this, fat accumulates in the Golgi complex and mainly, or at least initially, in the perivenular hepatocytes. This situation is compounded by ethanol-induced down-regulation of microsomal triglyceride transfer protein (MTP).[47] MTP is the principal enzyme responsible for packaging TAG and apolipoprotein B (apoB) into VLDL particles. In the absence of effective lipidation apoB is degraded in the proteosome.

Role of TNF-α in the Pathogenesis of Steatosis

The putative role of TNF-α in the pathogenesis of necroinflammation in ALD is described in the section on endotoxin later. This cytokine has also been linked to the development of hepatic steatosis. Interest in this area stemmed from a study showing that TNF-α receptor 1 (TNFR1)-deficient mice developed considerably less steatosis than their wild-type litter mates when fed ethanol.[48] Recently, the mechanisms for this TNF-α induced steatosis have been better elucidated. They include the down-regulation of MTP (discussed previously), the increased expression of sterol response element binding protein-1c (SREBP-1c),[49] a transcription factor critical in controlling de novo hepatic lipogenesis, and inhibition of adiponectin, an antisteatotic adipocytokine.[50] Because one of adiponectin's antisteatotic effects is via PPAR-α, the inhibition of adiponectin by TNF-α provides a potential mechanism for ethanol's inhibition of PPAR-α activity discussed previously.

Inhibition of the Methionine Cycle and Endoplasmic Reticular Stress

Studies, predominantly in micropigs, have demonstrated that the inhibition of transmethylation reactions by ethanol is the major mechanism leading to the well-established abnormal methionine metabolism associated with ethanol consumption.[51] The principal enzyme inhibited by ethanol is methionine synthase (MS),[52] and a significant effect of this appears to be the development of hyperhomocysteinemia.

Hyperhomocysteinemia has been implicated in the pathogenesis of atherosclerosis and Alzheimer disease through a phenomenon known as endoplasmic reticulum (ER) stress. The ER is the main site of protein synthesis from messenger RNA (mRNA), and is also involved in protein transport and some posttranslational modifications.[53] When abnormally folded or unfolded proteins build up in the ER, this acts as a marker to the cell that the quantity of "client" protein exceeds the ability of the ER to process it and results in a set of responses termed the unfolded protein response (UPR) or ER stress.[54] This response, which can be triggered by homocysteine, has three main arms. The first results in the increased transcription of ER proteins and chaperone proteins that aid processing. The second is to reduce the biosynthesis of other proteins to reduce the unfolded client load. The third is to up-regulate proapoptotic protein synthesis so that, in extreme circumstances, the cell will apoptose. In addition, ER stress triggered by homocysteine increases the gene expression of SREBP-1c.[55] Previous studies have shown that ethanol induces SREBP-1c in rat hepatoma cell lines and mouse liver with a concomitant increase in the expression of lipogenic genes,[56] and that this induction may be related to inhibition of AMP-activated protein kinase (AMPK).[57] Whether this inhibition of AMPK by ethanol is related to ER stress is unknown, however, studies with the intragastric ethanol-fed mouse have shown that ethanol induces hyperhomocysteinemia, triggers ER stress, and promotes the features of ALD including steatosis. Furthermore, feeding mice betaine, a methyl donor converting homocysteine to methionine, significantly inhibits the development of steatosis, implying that it is the inhibition of methylation and resulting hyperhomocysteinemia that is responsible.[58] It has recently been shown that the effect of ethanol on the development of hyperhomocysteinemia is independent of TNF-α, and that these two mechanisms induce steatosis independently and in parallel.[59]

The Role of Steatosis in the Pathogenesis of Advanced ALD

These described mechanisms all appear to promote the rapid and reproducible accumulation of hepatic TAG. This has been shown in humans and several animal models of alcoholic liver injury. The next question is whether this fat accumulation is harmful or benign. A growing body of evidence suggests that, rather than being an epiphenomenon of excessive alcohol intake, steatosis may play a direct role in progression to more advanced disease.[60] In several prospective studies of heavy drinkers the severity and pattern of steatosis on index biopsy predicts the subsequent risk of fibrosis and cirrhosis.[61,62] These and other studies have led to steatosis being considered as the "first hit," increasing the sensitivity of the liver to a variety of "second hits" that result in injury and inflammation. These "second hits" could be gut-derived endotoxin, oxidative stress or, indeed, immune mechanisms. In support, studies in animal models have shown that steatosis increases endotoxin-mediated necroinflammation[63] and the degree of lipid peroxidation in ethanol- and other drug-induced steatosis.[64] Furthermore, genetically obese mice with steatosis have altered proportions of intrahepatic lymphocyte subpopulations. The normal liver contains significant numbers of T cells, B cells, natural killer (NK) cells, and natural killer T (NKT) cells, many of which differ phenotypically and functionally from circulating lymphocytes. Leptin-deficient ob/ob mice have steatotic livers and interestingly a selective reduction in the number of NKT cells. Although these mice are not a model of alcohol-induced steatosis, this finding does raise questions about whether steatosis itself may alter the intrahepatic immune milieu.[65]

Oxidative Stress and Lipid Peroxidation

Oxidative stress describes a situation where the generation of prooxidant species within or outside the cell overwhelms the endogenous antioxidant systems. One of the most important consequences of cellular oxidative stress is the peroxidation of the polyunsaturated fatty acid (PUFA) constituents of membrane and lipoprotein lipids, which can lead directly to cell death[66] and to the release of reactive aldehydes with potent proinflammatory, profibrotic, and proimmune properties.[67] An accumulating body of evidence now supports a role for oxidative stress and lipid peroxidation in the pathogenesis of ethanol-induced liver injury that can be summarized as follows: (1) products of lipid peroxidation can be detected in the peripheral blood of heavy drinkers[68] and in the livers of patients with ALD,[69] and the magnitude of lipid peroxidation correlates with the degree of liver injury[70]; (2) in patients and animal models of ALD, lipid peroxidation is most prominent in the perivenular region where the liver injury is typically most severe; (3) a variety of sources of oxidative stress have been identified in patients with ALD and in animal models of

Table 28-1 Evidence for the Role of Oxidative Stress in the Pathogenesis of ALD

Presence of lipid peroxidation products	Found in serum and liver of patients with ALD and correlates with histologic severity
Site of lipid peroxidation products	Found in perivenular region where ALD starts and is most severe
Multiple potential sources of reactive oxygen species in heavy drinkers	Hepatocyte microsomes and mitochondria, Kupffer cells
Depletion of antioxidant defenses	Depletion of glutathione, selenium, and coenzyme Q is found in heavy drinkers
Manipulating oxidative stress in animal models influences disease severity	Prooxidant diets worsen disease while overexpression or underexpression of antioxidant enzymes affects the degree of liver injury

disease; (4) ethanol consumption results in the depletion of endogenous antioxidant capabilities and patients with ALD have evidence of antioxidant deficiencies; (5) in animal models of ALD, dietary and genetic manipulations that increase oxidative stress increase the severity of liver injury and reducing oxidative stress ameliorates injury (**Table 28-1**).

Sources of Oxidative Stress in ALD

The principal prooxidant species considered to be important in the pathogenesis of ALD are the reactive oxygen species (ROS), the superoxide anion, hydrogen peroxide and hydroxyl, and hydroxyethyl radicals. Considerable controversy remains over the most important source of these ROS in ALD, but the most likely appear to be microsomal CYP2E1 (the only source of hydroxyethyl radicals[71,72]), the mitochondrial electron transport chain,[73] inducible nitric oxide synthase, and Kupffer cells.

CYP2E1

In the presence of iron, isolated microsomes can generate sufficient oxidizing species to initiate lipid peroxidation. Most of the ROS in this system come from the ethanol-inducible microsomal ethanol oxidizing system (MEOS). The major component of this system is CYP2E1, which can also oxidize alcohol to acetaldehyde and subsequently to acetate, while concomitantly oxidizing NADPH to NADP. It appears that most ROS in the ethanol-fed rat model appear to be generated by CYP2E1. Spin-trapping studies, experiments that allow the identification of highly reactive radicals produced during reactions for very short periods of time to be identified, have revealed that the hydroxyethyl radical is the main radical formed when CYP2E1 metabolizes ethanol. The best in vivo evidence for the important role of CYP2E1 metabolites comes from experiments in the ethanol-fed rat discussed previously, where enzyme inhibition with diallyl sulfide resulted in decreased lipid peroxidation and amelioration of liver injury.[74,75]

MITOCHONDRIA

The mitochondrial respiratory electron transport chain generates superoxide radicals during the reoxidation of NADH arising during ethanol metabolism. The superoxide anions are subsequently converted to hydrogen peroxide by mitochondrial SOD2. Although the hydrogen peroxide is further metabolized to carbon dioxide and water by mitochondrial glutathione peroxidase, the increased rate of production after ethanol consumption results in a significant production of ROS.[76] As discussed in detail later, TNF-α may play an important role in the mitochondrial production of ROS through inhibition of electron flow in the respiratory chain. Perhaps the best evidence that mitochondria are involved in the pathogenesis of ALD are the ultrastructural changes that occur in these organelles in human and experimental ALD.[77] These changes are almost certainly related to mitochondrial oxidative stress and its downstream effects.

INDUCIBLE NITRIC OXIDE SYNTHASE

Nitric oxide (NO) has recently emerged as a critical regulator of certain aspects of mitochondrial function.[78] In particular, NO can bind to cytochrome-c oxidase and increase the rate of superoxide production.[79] After ethanol consumption, liver mitochondria are much more susceptible to NO-dependent inhibition of respiration. Furthermore, mice deficient in the inducible enzyme that synthesizes NO, inducible nitric oxide synthase (iNOS), develop much milder liver disease after ethanol consumption.[80] The fact that these iNOS$^{-/-}$ mice have dramatically reduced levels of liver lipid peroxidation end products and reactive nitrogen species provides compelling evidence for the role of this enzyme in oxidative stress-related injury. As with the mitochondrial production of ROS, TNF-α is likely to play a critical role in the generation of oxidative stress via iNOS due to its NF-κB dependent up-regulation of iNOS gene transcription.

KUPFFER CELLS

In addition to playing a central role in the generation of proinflammatory cytokines in response to endotoxin (see later discussion), activated Kupffer cells also act as a rich source of free radicals during ethanol-induced liver injury. Inhibition of Kupffer cells with gadolinium chloride during alcohol exposure has a profound inhibitory effect on the magnitude of lipid peroxidation,[81] and mice deficient in Kupffer cell NADPH-oxidase have no increase in free radical production and develop no liver pathology after 4 weeks exposure to ethanol.[82]

Depletion of Antioxidant Defenses in ALD

Ethanol consumption undoubtedly results in a depletion of endogenous antioxidant capabilities. Consumption of glutathione (GSH) during oxidative stress and inhibition of two enzymes involved in the synthesis of its precursor, S-adenosylmethionine (SAMe), methionine synthase, and methionine adenosyltransferase (MAT), contribute to the decreased levels of hepatic SAMe and GSH observed in patients with ALD[83] (**Fig. 28-5**). Depletion of mitochondrial GSH precedes and promotes the progression of alcoholic liver injury in animal models[84] with one mechanism of action being an increased sensitivity of hepatocytes to TNF-α induced cytotoxicity.[85] A recent study has suggested that, rather than reduced GSH levels, a high S-adenosylhomocysteine (SAH)/

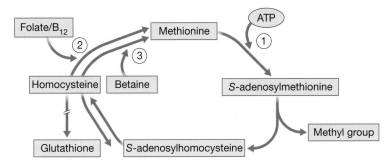

Fig. 28-5 **The methionine cycle.** (*1*) Methionine adenosyl-transferase catalyzes the synthesis of *S*-adenosyl-L-methionine (SAMe) from methionine and adenosine triphosphate. After donation of a methyl group, SAMe becomes *S*-adenosyl-homocysteine, which, through homocysteine, acts as a precursor for glutathione. (*2*) Methionine synthase regenerates methionine from homocysteine in a reaction that requires normal levels of folate and vitamin B$_{12}$, and (*3*) betaine-homocysteine methyltransferase regenerates methionine from homocysteine in a reaction that requires betaine. Ethanol inhibits reactions (1) and (2).

SAMe ratio may be responsible for the ethanol-induced enhanced sensitivity of hepatocytes to TNF-α killing, possibly by increasing the activity of caspase-8, a key initiator of the apoptotic cascade.[86] Heavy drinkers, including those with ALD, are deficient in the antioxidant trace element selenium,[87] which is required for the activity of the antioxidant enzyme GSH peroxidase, the antioxidant vitamins A, C, and E[88,89] and coenzyme Q.[90] This latter compound is present in plasma and mitochondrial matrix membranes and has emerged as one of the most important, natural free radical scavengers. It is partly derived from the diet, but is also synthesized in the liver. Whether these deficiencies are a cause or an effect of ALD remains unclear, although the fact that antioxidant supplementation appears to be of no benefit in patients with ALD is perhaps more in favor of the latter explanation.[91]

Manipulating Oxidative Stress in Animal Models Influences Disease Severity

Diets that promote oxidative stress increase the severity of ALD in animal models. Perhaps the best example of this comes from studies in which animals were fed a diet supplemented with different types of dietary fat in addition to alcohol. The degree of liver injury depends on whether the animals had their diet supplemented with beef fat, lard, or corn oil, with beef fat resulting in the least injury and corn oil the most.[92] A hypothesis that liver injury correlated with the amount of linoleic acid in the diet was supported by a study in which beef fat was supplemented with linoleic acid. These rats, like the corn oil–fed rats, developed severe liver disease when fed ethanol.[93] Severe liver injury was also seen when fish oil was used as the source of dietary fat, implying that polyunsaturated fats, which are much more vulnerable to attack from ROS, have a role in promoting liver injury.[94] The mechanisms through which polyunsaturated fats promote ethanol-induced liver injury are not entirely clear, but appear to involve up-regulation of CYP2E1 and an increase in lipid peroxidation.[94] In addition, polyunsaturated fats are the precursors of eicosanoids, powerful mediators of inflammation. Interestingly, cyclooxygenase-2 (COX-2), the key enzyme involved in the generation of eicosanoids, is inducible by both endotoxin and TNF-α.[95] Dietary iron supplementation also leads to an increase in the concentration of the aldehyde end products of lipid peroxidation within the liver. The addition of this prooxidant to the diet in the intragastric ethanol infusion model exacerbates hepatocyte damage and promotes liver fibrogenesis.[96] Studies employing genetic manipulation to increase the degree of oxidative stress provide further support for its role as an important disease mechanism in

ALD. Cytosolic superoxide dismutase (SOD-1) knockout mice develop more significant liver injury compared with wild-type litter mates following ethanol feeding,[97] whereas MAT knockout mice have reduced hepatic glutathione levels and develop spontaneous steatohepatitis even without alcohol.[98]

Further evidence supporting the role of oxidative stress in ALD comes from studies aimed at reducing its levels during ethanol feeding. Reduction of oxidative stress by supplementation with the GSH precursor and methyl donor SAMe reduced cell and mitochondrial injury in the baboon model of ALD[99] and led to the pilot study in humans discussed later. Inhibiting the prooxidant effect of iron with the oral chelator 1,2-dimethyl-3-hydroxypyrid-4-one reduced hepatic-free iron, lipid peroxidation, and fat accumulation in chronically ethanol-fed rats[100] and inhibiting the induction of CYP2E1 with diallyl sulfide (DAS) and phenylethyl isothiocyanate (PIC) resulted in the production of fewer free radicals and end products of lipid peroxidation and ameliorated liver injury in the same model.[74,75] Amelioration of liver injury could also be achieved using an adenovirus to deliver the mitochondrial, manganese-dependent superoxide dismutase-2 (SOD2) to rats fed ethanol,[101] and, as discussed previously, NADPH-oxidase deficient mice have also been used to show the importance of this source of oxidants in the development of early alcohol-induced hepatitis.[82]

Acetaldehyde

It is widely considered that acetaldehyde, the first metabolite of ethanol, has a central role in the pathogenesis of ALD, but precisely what role is still unclear. It has been known for some time that acetaldehyde can bind covalently to albumin,[102] tubulin,[103] hemoglobin,[104] plasma proteins,[105] collagen,[106] and microsomal enzymes[107] and results in both stable and unstable adduct formation. These reactions are likely to involve the formation of Schiff bases between the aldehyde and valine, and lysine and tyrosine residues on the carrier protein.[104] This binding may affect protein function, and this disruption has been implicated in the pathogenesis of ALD.[108] Defects in assembly of microtubules,[109] protein excretion,[110] and enzymatic activity[108] have all been attributed to acetaldehyde; however, no firm evidence exists for these mechanisms as disease pathways. With regard to disruption of enzymatic activity, an interesting study identified a 37 kDa protein-acetaldehyde adduct in the liver of alcohol-fed rats to be the enzyme Δ^4-3-Ketosteroid 5β-reductase.[111] This was felt to be important because children having inborn errors in this enzyme develop intrahepatic cholestasis and in some cases liver failure. Although this may be just one of many proteins that adduct to acetaldehyde, it raises questions about whether the binding of acetaldehyde may indeed alter enzyme activity. Along with potentially disrupting protein function, the formation of protein-acetaldehyde adducts results in the production of immunodominant antigenic determinants. The consequence of this is discussed in detail in the Adaptive Immune System section.

More recently, a further and more complex role for acetaldehyde has been suggested. Hepatocytes are resistant to TNF-α–induced cytotoxicity unless they have been previously exposed to ethanol.[112] As discussed previously, selective depletion of mitochondrial glutathione can induce this sensitization, and is postulated to be the mechanism through which it happens in vivo. When HepG2 cells are exposed to acetaldehyde, there is a selective reduction in mitochondrial glutathione and increased sensitization to TNF-α.[85] This has been shown to occur even when further metabolism of acetaldehyde is inhibited, and recent evidence suggests it is due to an inhibition of glutathione transport into the mitochondria secondary to an increased proportion of cholesterol in the mitochondrial membrane and a resulting increase in viscosity.[113] It is postulated that acetaldehyde induces this increase in cholesterol through the unfolded protein and ER stress response via SREBP-1c up-regulating the transcription of cholesterol-synthesizing enzymes. This effect on GSH transport will exacerbate the GSH depletion resulting from decreased SAMe synthesis and consumption during oxidative stress. In this way, the induction of SREBP-1c by TNF-α and by acetaldehyde and homocysteine-induced ER stress can induce a viscous cycle resulting not only in steatosis, but also in sensitization to the cytotoxic effects of TNF-α. This is particularly significant in view of the role of endotoxin in ALD, which acts predominantly as a stimulus to the release of TNF-α from hepatic Kupffer cells.

Acetate

Acetate is the end product of ethanol metabolism in the liver and can be incorporated into acetyl CoA in a reaction catalyzed by the enzyme acetyl CoA synthetase. While acetyl CoA is an important donor of carbon atoms to the citric acid cycle for oxidation, it may also have an important role in the control of inflammation. Recent data suggests that acetyl CoA may have a key role in the acetylation of histones, the protein spools in chromatin around which the DNA is wound. The acetylation of histones unwinds the chromatin and allows polymerases to transcribe DNA. Macrophages exposed to ethanol developed an enhanced IL-6, IL-8, and TNF-α response to lipopolysaccharide with time-dependent increases in histone acetylation that could be prevented by inhibition of ethanol metabolism and knockout of the acetyl CoA synthetase enzyme.[114]

This novel finding may explain the perpetuation of the inflammatory response in acute alcoholic hepatitis.

The Innate Immune System and the Pathogenesis of ALD

A considerable body of evidence supports a role for the innate immune system in the pathogenesis of ALD. Enhancement of

cytokine production and perpetuation of the inflammatory response appear to be key to the progression of alcoholic hepatitis. As discussed previously, ethanol metabolism and the production of acetate may have an important role in this. Increased translocation and an augmented response to endotoxin are also central.

Endotoxin

Endotoxin, which refers collectively to the lipopolysaccharide (LPS) components of the cell wall of all gram-negative bacteria, appears to play a central role in the development of ALD. Ethanol ingestion increases intestinal permeability and increases the translocation of endotoxin from the gut lumen.[115] This appears to occur through more than one mechanism. Acetaldehyde can cause redistribution of tight and adherens junctions, and affect epithelial cell–cell adhesion. Alcohol also increases the expression of inducible nitric oxide synthase, which can result in the nitration and oxidation of tubulin and result in barrier disruption.[116] Interestingly, treatment with lactobacillus can ameliorate alcohol-induced liver injury in a rat mode by improving gut integrity.[117]

When endotoxin translocates to the portal circulation, it is recognized by intrahepatic macrophages (Kupffer cells). Endotoxinemia has been found in drinkers with varying degrees of liver disease;[118] in the ethanol-fed rat, the level of plasma endotoxin correlated with the degree of liver injury.[119] When Kupffer cells encounter the LPS component of endotoxin in conjunction with lipopolysaccharide binding protein (LBP),[120] they respond by releasing cytokines and ROS. Although this can be blocked in vitro by the addition of anti-CD14 monoclonal antibodies,[121] implying the importance of this constitutively expressed and inducible receptor, CD14 does not have a transmembrane component, and therefore must rely on alternative receptors for signal transduction. Experiments on mice hyporesponsive to LPS have helped to identify the Toll-like receptor 4 (TLR4) as an important concomitant signal,[122] and current data suggest that LPS signaling occurs through activation clusters of these two receptors along with other membrane proteins. The importance of TLRs has been further highlighted recently by the discovery that they control activation of adaptive immune responses as well as innate responses. This occurs through an IL-6 dependent pathway, resulting in suppression of CD4+CD25+T regulatory cells that normally specifically inhibit adaptive immune responses.[123] This has profound implications for the role of endotoxin in ALD.

The role of endotoxin and Kupffer cells in the pathogenesis of ALD has been suggested largely by studies in the rodent model of continuous intragastric feeding developed by Tsukamoto and French.[124] As discussed previously, these animals develop lesions similar to human alcoholic hepatitis when fed a diet high in ethanol and fat. The eradication of gram-negative fecal flora with antibiotics reduces endotoxin levels to those of controls not fed alcohol, and prevents liver injury.[125] Recent data reveal that this injury is also attenuated in CD14 and TLR4 knockout mice, highlighting the importance of these receptors.[126,127] Alcohol can also affect Kupffer cell function directly. Rodents fed alcohol initially become more tolerant of endotoxin; however, with time, this response converts to one of sensitization.[128] An early suppressive effect of alcohol on Kupffer cell function and a later induction of CD14 may partly explain the time course of this response. Acetate-mediated histone acetylation may also contribute. Interestingly, when Kupffer cells are inactivated in the ethanol-fed rat model using gadolinium chloride, disease is ameliorated and the steatosis is diminished. This highlights that these cells also have a role in the TAG accumulation, most likely through TNF-α production, as discussed previously.

Sinusoidal endothelial cells are also actively involved in the response to endotoxin. These cells constitutively express all the surface molecules necessary for antigen presentation, and may induce tolerance or immunity depending on the local microenvironment. This environment may be dictated by Kupffer cell release of immunomodulatory cytokines in response to varying doses of portal endotoxin, with a high-dose endotoxin resulting in potentially harmful immunity, and low-dose endotoxin resulting in tolerance through the secretion of IL-10.[129]

The Role of TNF-α

Kupffer cells are the primary intrahepatic source of TNF-α, a cytokine believed to be central to the pathogenesis of ALD. Peripheral blood mononuclear cells produce more basal and lipopolysaccharide induced TNF-α than controls,[130] and plasma levels are higher in patients with more severe disease.[131] Furthermore, mice lacking TNFR1 fail to develop liver injury in the Tsukamoto-French model.[48] More recently it has been suggested that these mice develop an ameliorated form of ALD rather than none at all,[59] nevertheless, the findings suggest an important role for the cytokine (**Fig. 28-6**). How TNF-α contributes to hepatocyte cytotoxicity in ALD, and whether this is via necrosis or apoptosis is an area of dispute; however, recent studies showing a correlation between the degree of apoptosis and clinical indices of severity in patients with alcoholic hepatitis suggest that apoptosis plays an important role.[132,133] The interaction of TNF-α with its receptor TNFR1 (via the death-inducing signaling complex [DISC]) activates procaspase-8 into caspase-8, which cuts Bid (BH3 interacting domain death agonist).[134] Truncated Bid can enter the outer mitochondrial membrane to make this membrane leaky, and it also induces a conformational change in Bax (Bcl-2–associated x protein), which translocates to mitochondria

and associates with its analogue Bak, to form channels in the outer mitochondria membrane.[135] Increased permeability of the outer mitochondrial membrane releases cytochrome C from the intermembrane space of mitochondria, thus partially blocking the flow of electrons into the respiratory chain and increasing mitochondrial ROS formation.[136] The resulting ROS then acts on the same or other mitochondria to open an inner membrane pore, the mitochondrial permeability transition pore. This causes an influx of water into the mitochondrial matrix, leading to mitochondrial swelling and eventually rupture of the unfolded outer membrane. This leads to the leakage of apoptosis-inducing factors (predominantly cytochrome C) into the cytosol, where they can activate caspase-9, which initiates the apoptotic cascade.

Given the role of ROS in this cascade, it is easy to see how the oxidative stress-related mechanisms of alcohol-induced cell injury can synergize with TNF-α to induce apoptosis and/or necrosis. TNF-α–induced apoptosis is increased by alcohol, an effect that is exaggerated in HepG2 cells with high CYP2E1 activity presumably related to increased oxidative stress.[112] As discussed, the depletion of glutathione by alcohol will also increase the sensitivity of hepatocytes to the mitochondrial effects of TNF-α.[24,85] It has recently been shown that the mechanism of TNF-α–induced cell death, necrosis, or apoptosis depends on the degree and site of glutathione depletion.[137] Mitochondrial depletion leads to necrosis due to profound loss of mitochondrial function,[85] whereas less severe, predominantly cytosolic, depletion of glutathione leads to apoptosis due to inhibition of the NF-κB–induced transactivation of survival genes that normally follows TNF-α binding to its receptor. As also discussed previously, in addition to TNF-α and oxidative stress, the apoptotic cascade may also be initiated in response to ER stress.

Natural Killer Cells

A further, less well understood, arm of the innate immune system that appears to be involved in the pathogenesis of ALD is the natural killer (NK) and natural killer T (NKT) cell population. These cells are abundant in the liver[138] and both populations have been reported to increase in the peripheral blood of heavy drinkers.[139] Recent evidence points to an

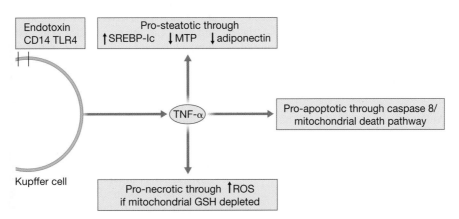

Fig. 28-6 **Tumor necrosis factor-α (TNF-α), a central cytokine in alcoholic liver injury.** TNF-α induces steatosis through the up-regulation of sterol response element-binding protein-1c (SREBP1-c), the down-regulation of microsomal triglyceride transfer protein (MTP), and the inhibition of adiponectin. Depending on the degree of oxidative stress and the availability of mitochondrial glutathione (GSH), TNF-α can also induce either necrosis or apoptosis through the death-inducing signaling complex, with subsequent activation of caspase-8 and the mitochondrial death pathway.

increase in the number of NKT cells in the livers of mice after alcohol consumption and augmenting their activation using a marine sphingolipid during ethanol feeding results in fatal hepatotoxicity.[140] The relevance of this to clinical liver disease is as yet unclear and is made more complicated by the fact that acute ethanol consumption inhibits innate immunity by suppressing TLR3 signalling,[141] and inhibits NK cell killing of activated stellate cells, which would have marked profibrogenic effects.[142]

The Adaptive Immune System and the Pathogenesis of ALD

Several clinical features suggest that adaptive immune mechanisms may have a role in the pathogenesis of ALD. Abstinent patients that return to drinking have a rapid and aggressive recurrence of their disease that may imply an immunologic anamnestic response. There is a partial response to immunosuppressive steroids in selected groups with severe disease.[143] Patients receiving interferon therapy for hepatitis C, which can trigger autoimmune thyroid disease, can rapidly develop alcoholic hepatitis with no increase in their daily alcohol intake.[144] Lymphocyte infiltration is a well-recognized histologic feature of advanced disease[145] and hypergammaglobulinemia is common. These features have led researchers to look at the importance of antigen-specific immune responses and how they might lead to liver injury.

Humoral Immune Responses in ALD

Although nonspecific liver cell membrane antibodies have been implicated in ALD pathogenesis for some time,[146,147] recent studies have focused on determining the antigen specificity of this humoral response.

Antibodies to Acetaldehyde Adducts

Acetaldehyde can adduct to host proteins and this can result in the formation of immunogenic epitopes.[148] Acetaldehyde-modified proteins have been found in the liver cytosol, membranes, and mitochondria of rats chronically fed ethanol, and their decline over several weeks after ethanol withdrawal has been investigated.[149] They accumulate particularly in hepatocytes in the perivenular region, which is also the main area of distribution of the ethanol metabolizing enzyme CYP2E1, the main site of lipid peroxidation and the first area to be injured in ALD.[150] Interestingly, extracellular and not intracellular acetaldehyde-adduct staining correlates with fibrosis progression in humans regardless of whether the patients abstained from alcohol or not.[151]

Antiacetaldehyde (Anti-AcA) adduct antibodies have been found in the sera of heavy drinkers by several groups.[151-153] Their relationship to the presence and severity of liver disease is controversial.

Antibodies to the Other Products of Ethanol Metabolism

Other targets for the humoral immune response in ALD include the hydroxyethyl radical (HER; a reactive intermediate formed by the action of CYP2E1 during ethanol metabolism[154]) and aldehydes generated as a result of prolonged oxidative stress, such a malondialdehyde (MDA) and 4-hydroxynonenal (4-HNE).[155] Anti-HER antibodies have been found in significantly higher titer in patients with alcohol-induced cirrhosis than in non–alcohol-induced cirrhosis or normal controls.[156] The third, and final, antigen that has been studied in detail is a combination of acetaldehyde and malondialdehyde called malondialdehyde-acetaldehyde (MAA) adducts. Antibodies to these hybrid conjugates have now been detected in sera from patients with alcohol-induced liver cirrhosis and alcoholic hepatitis but not in heavy drinkers with no liver disease or healthy controls.[157]

Autoantibodies

When ethanol is metabolized by CYP2E1, the hydroxyethyl radical is produced,[156] which can form immunogenic adducts with the cytochrome. It has now been demonstrated that a significant proportion of patients with ALD have antibodies reactive with the hydroxyethyl radical complexed with CYP2E1.[158] Furthermore, both patients with ALD and rats fed ethanol have been shown to develop anti-CYP2E1 specific autoantibodies.[159] Interestingly, in humans with ALD, the presence of these autoantibodies is predicted by the presence of antibodies to hydroxyethyl radicals, suggesting a potential mechanism for tolerance breakdown.[160]

Whether the humoral immune response is a cause or a consequence of liver disease remains an important question. Antibody dependent cell cytotoxicity (ADCC) has been observed when sera from patients with ALD positive for anti-HER antibodies were co-cultured with ethanol-treated rat hepatocytes and peripheral blood mononuclear cells from healthy controls.[161] Further studies are required to provide evidence for the role of this mechanism of disease in vivo.

Cellular Immune Responses in ALD

Both mice and human livers have significant numbers of T cells and some B cells, which recirculate from the peripheral pool; however, in contrast to peripheral blood, there are more CD8[+] cells than CD4[+] cells.[138] In addition there are high frequencies of what appear to be resident liver lymphocytes that are found in very low frequencies in peripheral blood. These are natural killer (NK) cells, recognized by CD56 in humans and NK1.1 in mice, and NKT cells that express these proteins along with the T-cell receptor. In normal liver, these cell types are distributed throughout the parenchyma. In liver disease, this situation changes, and in alcoholic cirrhosis expanded portal tracts contain large numbers of classical CD4[+] and CD8[+] lymphocytes.[145] No work has been done to determine the antigen specificity of these intrahepatic lymphocyte populations; however, peripheral blood mononuclear cell responses to malondialdehyde (MDA) have been detected in a significant proportion of patients.[162]

A further population of T cells appears to have a role in disease progression. IL-17–secreting T cells are found at increased concentration in the liver and peripheral blood of patients with ALD. In chronic liver disease, the numbers correlate with the model of end-stage liver disease score, and in acute alcoholic hepatitis they correlate with the discriminant function. These cells can induce chemokine secretion and aid neutrophil recruitment, and may therefore represent a link between adaptive and innate immune responses.[163]

Further work is required to determine whether antigen-specific cellular immune responses are an important part of disease progression in ALD.

Mechanisms of Alcohol-Induced Fibrosis

Fibrosis and ultimately cirrhosis is the final common pathway of most chronic liver disease, and the mechanisms underlying it are discussed elsewhere in this book. It is, however, important to briefly review these and to discuss the factors that are particularly relevant to the pathogenesis of the fibrosis seen in ALD.

Hepatic stellate cells (HSC) are found in the space of Disse, between hepatocytes and sinusoidal endothelial cells, and are responsible for producing the majority of the extracellular matrix (ECM).[164] In a normal liver, the space of Disse contains little collagen; however, when these stellate cells become "activated" during liver injury by cytokines and ROS, the composition of the ECM changes as more collagen, glycoproteins, proteoglycans, and glycosaminoglycans are produced (**Fig. 28-7**). In particular, there is a shift in the type of proteoglycans produced and an increase in collagen types I, III, and IV.[165] In addition, these changes are associated with an up-regulation in numerous integrins, selectins, and soluble growth factors, which modulate cell–cell and cell–ECM interactions. Sinusoidal endothelial cells[166] and lymphocytes[167] may also play important roles in fibrogenesis. More recently, there has been increasing evidence that fibrosis can be reversible, and the discovery of matrix metalloproteinases (MMPs) that degrade collagen has implications for most liver diseases. These MMPs are activated by proteolytic cleavage and are inactivated by tissue inhibitors of metalloproteinases (TIMPs).

In ALD, fibrosis starts in the perivenular area and may progress to bridging fibrosis and, ultimately, cirrhosis. This early fibrosis occurs at the site of maximal alcohol-induced hepatocyte injury. The principal cell types involved in the activation of HSC in ALD are Kupffer cells and hepatocytes. Kupffer cells are stimulated to release cytokines by endotoxin in ALD, and in turn these cells can lead to the activation and proliferation of stellate cells through the production of transforming growth factor-ß (TGF-ß), TNF-α, and ROS. Hepatocytes are rich sources of ROS, lipid peroxidation products, and acetaldehyde during alcohol-induced injury, all of which have been shown to enhance collagen production by HSC.[67,77] CYP2E1 may be particularly important in this regard given its inducibility by alcohol and a high-fat diet and its perivenular distribution. HSC grown in the presence of hepatocyte cell lines that overexpress CYP2E1 increase their production of collagen, an effect that is prevented by antioxidants or a CYP2E1 inhibitor.[168] Hepatocyte apoptosis is a notable feature of alcoholic hepatitis,[132] and apoptosing hepatocytes express Fas, which can promote stellate cell initiation through the tumor necrosis factor–related apoptosis-inducing ligand (TRAIL).[169] Furthermore, apoptosing hepatocytes may also be ingested by Kupffer cells and HSC, which subsequently release TGF-β capable of activating HSC.[169,170] Alcohol can also be profibrotic by attenuating the antifibrotic effects of interferon-γ (IFN-γ). It does this by reducing expression of IFN-γ by NK cells and impairing downstream signaling in HSCs (**Table 28-2**).[142]

Mechanisms of Hepatocellular Cancer

Epidemiologic studies reveal that alcohol plays a major contributory role in the development of hepatocellular cancer (HCC); however, the primary mechanisms through which this occurs are not clearly defined. Cirrhosis itself is a precancerous condition, and alcohol-related HCC without preexisting cirrhosis is rare. Nevertheless, three features indicate that alcohol may be a co-carcinogen. The first is that heavy alcohol consumption is associated with several extrahepatic cancers (discussed later). The second is that when the incidence of incidental HCCs in liver explants from patients with alcoholic

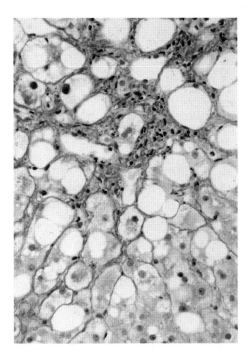

Fig. 28-7 **Alcohol-induced hepatic fibrosis.**

Table 28-2 The Primary Mechanisms Thought to Be Involved in Ethanol-Induced Hepatic Fibrosis and Hepatocellular Carcinoma

Fibrosis
Kupffer cell production of profibrotic cytokines
Kupffer cell production of profibrotic reactive oxygen species
Hepatocyte production of profibrotic reactive oxygen species
Hepatocyte production of acetaldehyde
Kupffer cell and hepatic stellate cell production of transforming growth factor-β after ingestion of apoptotic hepatocytes

Hepatocellular Carcinoma
Lipid peroxidation and DNA mutagenesis
Activation of carcinogenic xenobiotics
Antiapoptotic effect of tumor necrosis factor-α
DNA hypomethylation
Immunosuppression

cirrhosis is compared with that from other causes, it lies between that of immune-mediated liver disease and viral hepatitis.[171] It appears therefore that the incidence of HCC is above that of the "baseline" expected because of pure cirrhotic risk. The third is that there are several plausible mechanisms through which alcohol could promote carcinogenesis.

Lipid Peroxidation and DNA Mutagenesis

Malondialdehyde (MDA), an end product of lipid peroxidation, can bind to DNA and form adducts as it does with other endogenous compounds.[172] These adducts were found to be highly mutagenic in *E. coli*[173] and are repaired by nucleotide excision repair. They are also found at significant levels in healthy humans and can induce cell cycle arrest.[174] This latter property results in an increase in the number of hepatic progenitor cells (oval cells)[175] that are more resistant to oxidative stress than fully differentiated hepatocytes. It has been suggested that this may promote HCC because the oval cells survive through oxidative damage but remain susceptible to mutagenesis.[175]

Activation of Xenobiotics

Another mechanism proposed for the increased rate of HCC seen in alcoholic cirrhosis is the increased production of carcinogenic metabolites from other environmental carcinogens (xenobiotics) that are metabolized through the MEOS and other metabolic pathways upregulated in heavy drinkers. This mechanism has been suggested to explain the increased cancer risk seen with tobacco smoking,[176] aflatoxin,[177] and other chemicals.[178] In addition, CYP2E1 is responsible for the metabolism of retinoic acid (RA) in the liver.[179] Up-regulation of CYP2E1 by ethanol therefore synergizes with its inhibition of RA synthesis and results in reduced RA levels, increased expression of the AP-1 transcriptional complex, and increased hepatocyte proliferation.[180] Supplementation with RA reverses this effect.[179]

TNF-α Induced Survival Factors

As discussed previously, TNF-α has both proapoptotic and antiapoptotic properties and the balance of these appears to depend on the local microenvironment and the disease. Although apoptosis may reduce the risk of HCC, increased cell survival through TNF-α–induced NF-κB activation could have the opposite effect, particularly in combination with the mutagenic effects of lipid peroxidation products.

Reduced DNA Methylation

DNA methylation is an important negative regulator of gene expression and hypomethylation of oncogenes has been shown in human and rat HCC.[181] Chronic ethanol consumption results in reduced concentrations of SAMe, the main methyl donor (as discussed previously) and dietary depletion of SAMe increases the risk of HCC in rats.[182]

Immunosuppression

Malnutrition, vitamin deficiencies, and acute ethanol per se can all result in reduced immunosurveillance. Of particular relevance is the effect on natural killer cells, thought to be central to tumor surveillance. The primary functional effect appears to be one of suppression.[139,183] In addition, there are other, more widespread effects on the innate and adaptive immune responses that could all have knock-on effects on tumor surveillance (discussed in Associated Conditions and Extrahepatic Manifestations section). A reduction in immunosurveillance, and a subsequent increase in viral replication may also be the mechanism through which alcohol leads to an increased rate of HCC in hepatitis C cirrhosis.[184]

Susceptibility to Alcoholic Liver Disease

Although the majority of heavy drinkers will develop some degree of steatosis (fatty liver), only around a third go on to develop alcoholic hepatitis and only between 1 in 4 and 1 in 12 ever progress to cirrhosis (**Fig. 28-8**).[185] This leads to the obvious question: what factors determine whether or not a heavy drinker develops advanced ALD?

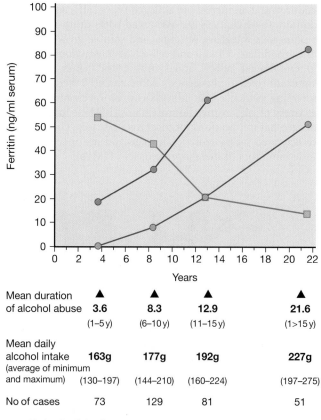

Mean duration of alcohol abuse	▲ 3.6 (1–5 y)	▲ 8.3 (6–10 y)	▲ 12.9 (11–15 y)	▲ 21.6 (1>15 y)
Mean daily alcohol intake (average of minimum and maximum)	163g (130–197)	177g (144–210)	192g (160–224)	227g (197–275)
No of cases	73	129	81	51

—●— Cirrhosis of the liver
—●— Cirrhosis and potentially precirrhotic lesions (severe steatofibrosis with inflammatory reactions, chronic alcoholic hepatitis)
—■— Moderate to severe fatty infiltration

Fig. 28-8 **Frequency of cirrhotic and precirrhotic liver lesions according to dose and duration of alcohol consumption in 334 drinkers.** *(Reproduced from Lelbach WK. Cirrhosis in the alcoholic and its relation to the volume of alcohol abuse. Ann N Y Acad Sci 1975;252:85–105 with permission of New York Academy of Science.[202])*

Dose of Ethanol

The observation that only a minority of heavy drinkers develop ALD was first reported 30 years ago by Lelbach and colleagues. They showed that although the risk of disease increased in proportion to the duration of intake, only 20% of consumers of more than 200 g of ethanol (around 20 standard "drinks") per day develop cirrhosis after 13 years and fewer than 50% after 20 years.[186] Further work from around this time showed that women appeared to develop ALD at lower doses of alcohol consumption than men.[187] More detailed studies examining the precise dose-response relationship between alcohol intake and risk of ALD, the gender effect and the risk threshold have been reported in the last 10 years.

A large cohort study from Italy involving 6917 subjects between the ages of 12 and 65 reported that the risk of developing ALD begins at 30 g/day of ethanol.[185] However, only 5.5% of the individuals drinking this amount showed signs of liver disease. The risk increased according to daily dose, reaching 10% at 60 g per day. The study also reported that the risk is higher among those older than 50 years of age if alcohol is drunk outside mealtimes or consumed in a variety of different beverages rather than one "tipple of choice." Interestingly, this study showed no sex effect. Further evidence for a dose-response relationship and a risk threshold came from an even larger study from Copenhagen involving 13,285 subjects between the ages of 30 and 79.[188] A self-administered questionnaire assessed intake, and incidence of disease was taken from death certificates and hospital medical records. This study revealed a dose-dependent increase in risk with women having a significant risk above 7 to 13 units per week, and men 14 to 27 units per week. This group updated their data analysis recently by looking at the type of alcohol consumed.[189] Their results suggest that the highest risk is seen in drinkers that do not include wine in their drinking repertoire. Furthermore the relative risk of cirrhosis fell as the proportion of wine increased. This association between wine intake and ALD risk may be confounded by other factors associated with wine drinking such as a lower prevalence of obesity compared with beer and spirit drinkers. One study following the eating habits of beer drinkers compared with wine drinkers has shown that the former tend to buy more unhealthy items at the supermarket.[190]

Although all these studies have their flaws, with data collection being the most obvious, they do allow a number of conclusions to be drawn. No dose of alcohol confers a guarantee of developing cirrhosis regardless of the period it is consumed for, and relatively low doses can cause problems.

Diet

The data discussed previously from ethanol-fed rats linking a diet high in polyunsaturated fats with an increased risk of alcoholic liver injury are supplemented by an epidemiologic study linking cirrhosis mortality with pork (high in linoleic acid) consumption and dietary intake of unsaturated fats.[191] A further case-control study from France has reported that the risk of cirrhosis is increased by diets high in fat and alcohol and low in carbohydrate.[192] A more obvious role for diet in ALD risk has been suggested by two studies showing that obesity and associated hyperglycemia increase the incidence of all stages of ALD in heavy drinkers.[4,193]

Although these studies have provided evidence that dose, pattern, and type of alcohol consumption and dietary (and presumably exercise-related) factors play a role in determining ALD risk, they have also demonstrated that other, "endogenous" factors are likely to be equally if not more important.

Sex and Risk of ALD

The most obvious endogenous or "genetic" factor determining ALD risk is female sex. It has long been appreciated that women develop ALD at a lower intake of alcohol than men. The traditional explanation has been that women develop higher blood alcohol concentrations per unit of alcohol consumed due to their lower volume of distribution for alcohol. This in turn is attributed to their lower body mass index and to fat constituting a higher percentage of their body mass than in men. Thurman and colleagues have demonstrated in the rat model that estrogen increases gut permeability to endotoxin and accordingly up-regulates endotoxin receptors on Kupffer cells, leading to an increased production of tumor necrosis factor in response to endotoxin.[194] These exciting data suggest several new directions for research into human sex-specific susceptibility to ALD.

Non–Sex-Linked Genetic Factors and Risk of ALD

Evidence for non–sex-linked genetic susceptibility to ALD comes principally from a twin study showing that the concordance rate for alcoholic cirrhosis was three times higher in monozygotic than in dizygotic twin pairs.[195] This difference in concordance rates was not entirely explained by the difference in concordance rates for alcoholism per se. Further indirect evidence of a genetic component to disease risk comes from the observation that the death rate from ALD is subject to wide interethnic variation that is not entirely explained by variations in the prevalence of alcohol abuse.[196,197] Hispanics appear to be at particularly high risk, for example. Difficulties in performing family linkage studies in ALD have resulted in almost all of the relevant information thus far coming from classical case-control, candidate gene, allele association studies. Accordingly these studies are subject to all the common pitfalls of this type of study design and must be interpreted with caution.[198] Many early reports of positive associations are likely to be subject to type I errors (chance findings), while negative reports may be subject to type II errors (false negatives) attributed to small underpowered studies. Given that the most likely mechanisms of hepatocyte injury in excessive drinkers are related to fat accumulation, oxidative stress, endotoxin-mediated release of proinflammatory cytokines, and immunologic damage, the majority of studies reported thus far have focused on genes encoding proteins involved in these various pathways.

Genes Influencing the Severity of Steatosis

Recognition of the role played by steatosis in the pathogenesis of more advanced liver disease[60] suggests that factors determining its severity may play a key role in determining the risk of cirrhosis. Clearly genetic and environmental factors determining the degree of obesity would fall into this category, as would functional polymorphisms of genes encoding enzymes involved in hepatic lipid metabolism. Most recently a striking association has been demonstrated between a polymorphism in the *PNPLA3* gene, encoding adiponutrin, and ALD in Mexican subjects[199] and Europeans.[200] This rs738409 polymorphism was identified as a susceptibility gene for nonalcoholic fatty liver disease in two independent genomewide association studies (GWAS).[201,202] The precise biologic function of adiponutrin is unknown but the polymorphism appears to disrupt triglyceride hydrolysis to cause fatty liver.

Genes Influencing Oxidative Stress and Risk of ALD

The principal class of genes that influences the oxidant load in heavy drinkers are those genes encoding enzymes involved in alcohol metabolism. Polymorphisms have been identified in two of the seven genes encoding alcohol dehydrogenases (*ADH2* and *ADH3*), in the promoter region of the *CYP2E1* gene and in the coding region of the gene encoding the mitochondrial form of aldehyde dehydrogenase (ALDH2). The genes encoding ADH2 and ALDH2 undoubtedly play a role in determining the risk of alcoholism and, to a lesser extent, ALD in Asian populations.[203-205] Previously reported associations with *ADH3* probably reflect linkage disequilibrium with *ADH2*.[206] In Caucasians, results from studies reported to date support a role for the *ADH2* polymorphism in determining the risk of alcoholism but not ALD.[207] Several studies have looked for an association between the c2 promoter *(Rsa I)* polymorphism of the *CYP2E1* gene and ALD with no consistent results emerging in any population, although one study did report that the cumulative lifetime alcohol intake of patients with ALD heterozygous for the c2 (more transcriptionally active) allele was almost half that of patients with ALD homozygous for the c1, wild-type allele.[208] The HFE gene is another obvious candidate gene for ALD because liver iron promotes oxidative stress and iron deposition is common in ALD. Unfortunately, a case-control study of more than 400 patients and controls found no evidence of an association between ALD and either of the HFE mutations associated with hemochromatosis.[209] This lack of association was explained by the observation that hepatic iron content did not differ between patients with and without the mutations.

The lack of any striking associations between polymorphisms in genes encoding proteins involved in the generation of reactive oxygen species and ALD has recently turned attention towards polymorphisms in genes encoding proteins involved in the body's antioxidant defenses. Manganese-dependent SOD2 is the most important mitochondrial antioxidant enzyme and a polymorphism altering its mitochondrial targeting sequence has been associated with ALD in a small French study,[210] although not confirmed in a larger study from the United Kingdom.[211] This and other polymorphisms affecting the function of antioxidant defense systems are clearly worthy of further study.

Endotoxin Receptor and Cytokine Genes and Risk of ALD

Evidence supporting a role for endotoxin-mediated cytokine release in the pathogenesis of ALD, together with the identification of promoter polymorphisms in genes encoding endotoxin receptors, cytokines, and cytokine receptors, has recently suggested an alternative set of "candidates" to explain genetic susceptibility to ALD. CD14, an LPS receptor on monocytes, macrophages, and neutrophils, has no intracellular domain but enhances signaling through another LPS receptor, Toll-like receptor 4 (TLR4). A C/T polymorphism is present at position -159 in the CD14 promoter, with the TT genotype associated with increased levels of soluble and membrane CD14.[212] A study from Finland has recently reported an association between possession of the TT CD14 genotype and advanced ALD[127]; however, this has not been observed in a larger study in northeast England.[213] This latter study also showed no association between ALD and possession of the $Asp_{299}Gly$ polymorphism in the *TLR4* gene, previously reported to be linked to hyporesponsiveness to LPS.[214]

With respect to polymorphisms in the cytokine genes, the first such association was reported between alcoholic hepatitis and a polymorphism at position -238 in the TNF-α promoter region.[215] The functional significance of this polymorphism is, however, unclear and the association may well be either spurious or due to linkage disequilibrium with another true "disease-associated polymorphism" on chromosome 6. An association with ALD has also been reported for a promoter polymorphism in interleukin-10 (IL-10). IL-10 is the classical antiinflammatory cytokine that inhibits: (1) the activation of CD4$^+$ T-helper cells, (2) the function of cytotoxic CD8$^+$ T-cells and macrophages, (3) class II HLA/B7 expression on antigen-presenting cells, and (4) hepatic stellate cell collagen synthesis. A variant C→A substitution at position -627 in the IL-10 promoter has been associated with decreased reporter gene transcription, decreased IL-10 secretion by peripheral blood monocytes, and an increased response to α-interferon in patients with chronic hepatitis C—all consistent with the polymorphism being associated with *lower* IL-10 production. A strong association between possession of the A allele and ALD has been reported from a study of more than 500 heavy drinkers with and without advanced liver disease.[216] This is consistent with low IL-10 favoring inflammatory and immune-mediated mechanisms of disease as well as hepatic stellate cell collagen production.

Immune Response Genes and Risk of ALD

In view of the immunoregulatory functions of IL-10, the association between ALD and a low-activity promoter polymorphism in IL-10 may be considered as further evidence that immune mechanisms are involved in the pathogenesis of ALD. Further evidence supporting a role for immune mechanisms in determining individual susceptibility to ALD has come from a recent study showing that, compared with drinkers with no evidence of ALD, patients with ALD are more likely to have high titres of autoantibodies against CYP2E1[160] and to have T-cell responses against oxidative stress-derived adducts.[162] Cytotoxic T lymphocyte antigen-4 (CTLA-4) is a T-cell surface molecule that normally acts to "damp down" the immune response to antigens either directly, by competing with CD28 on the surface of CD4$^+$ Th cells for the antigen-presenting cell costimulatory molecule B7, or indirectly by activating T regulatory cells that act to inhibit CD4$^+$ Th cell function.[217] CTLA-4 knockout mice develop lethal autoreactive lymphoproliferative disease, and an A→G polymorphism in exon 1 leading to a Thr→Ala substitution has recently been associated with autoimmune liver diseases, insulin-dependent diabetes, and autoimmune thyroid disease. These associations strongly suggest that this polymorphism is associated with impaired CTLA-4 function, although recent data suggest that other tightly linked CTLA-4 polymorphisms may be responsible for the functional effect.[218] Although the exon 1 polymorphism has been associated with the titre of anti-CYP2E1 antibodies in one study[160] and with ALD in another,[219] this has yet to be confirmed as an ALD susceptibility allele in large studies examining the full CTLA-4 gene haplotype.

In future, the choice of candidate genes for detailed study as ALD risk factors is likely to be guided by: (1) genome and proteome expression studies in tissue from patients with various stages of ALD, (2) whole-genome single nucleotide polymorphism (SNP) scans of cases and controls; and (3) mouse mutagenesis studies. Most importantly, however, as with other so-called complex diseases, establishing reliable genetic associations is critically dependent on the collection of large numbers of well-phenotyped cases and controls, which almost certainly requires national and multinational collaborations. Only then are we likely to come up with associations that are robust enough to guide targeted treatment and prevention strategies.

Clinical Features
Diagnosis

Chronic alcohol abuse produces a wide range of morphologic changes in the liver, the most frequent being fatty liver (steatosis), alcoholic hepatitis, and cirrhosis.[220,221] For ease of presentation, the three principal lesions will be discussed separately in terms of their pathology, clinical features, and prognosis, but it is important to appreciate that alcohol-related liver damage is a spectrum, with the various lesions occurring more commonly in combination than in isolation. Significantly, the clinical manifestations of each of these histologic lesions are extremely variable, ranging from completely asymptomatic forms to a first presentation with severe hepatic failure. Patients with none or minimal symptoms are, however, more likely to have the earlier, more reversible, forms of liver disease and therefore the early recognition of these patients is critical to allow intervention at a stage when it is likely to be of most benefit.

Patients most commonly have symptoms unrelated to the liver, typically nonspecific digestive symptoms, or vague psychiatric complaints. The patient may seek advice concerning the social effects of alcohol abuse on family life or work performance. Often, physical examination will be normal, other than occasional plethora, suffused conjunctivae, tremulousness, and aggressive behavior. Up to 30% of patients with alcoholic liver disease have no symptoms related to excessive alcohol intake and may "present" following the chance finding of hepatomegaly or abnormal blood tests at routine medical examination. The key to the early recognition of patients with alcohol-related disease is a high index of suspicion. Once the diagnosis is suspected, it is usually easy to confirm by direct questioning for alcohol history and alcohol-related symptoms, careful clinical examination, and supportive laboratory investigations.

History

Features in the history important for both the confirmation of alcohol abuse and to aid in its subsequent management include the amount and duration of alcohol intake, the pattern of intake, precipitating factors of drinking bouts, and evidence of physical dependence such as early morning tremor, blackouts, and morning drinking. Confirmation of the history should be sought from a family member or close associate. Specific liver-related symptoms, such as jaundice and hematemesis, should be inquired about but are uncommon, even in patients with established disease. In addition, because not all alcohol-dependent patients with liver disease necessarily have disease caused by alcohol,[222] inquiries should be made concerning other risk factors for liver disease, including family history, foreign travel, blood transfusions, or intravenous drug use.

Clinical Examination

Important features to note on examination are the signs of chronic liver disease including hepatomegaly and signs indicative of alcohol-related pathology in other organs such as hypertension, atrial fibrillation, and a cushingoid appearance. It is important to understand that many of the classical signs of chronic liver disease, including spider nevi, Dupuytren contractures, palmar erythema, and parotid swelling, can occur in alcoholics in the absence of cirrhosis. Clinical signs and history cannot be relied upon to distinguish the various histologic subtypes of alcoholic liver disease because patients with cirrhosis can be asymptomatic while patients with hepatocellular failure may have only severe fatty change.[223]

Laboratory Investigations

Biochemical and hematologic tests can confirm the presence of alcohol abuse and indicate the presence of liver damage, but are not useful in determining the severity of the histologic lesion. Blood alcohol estimations are an often underused method of confirming a suspicion of excess drinking, with levels greater than l00 mg/l00 ml at a morning clinic, or levels greater than 150 mg/100 ml without obvious intoxication, strongly suggestive of alcohol abuse. Elevation of γ-glutamyl transferase (γGT) has been reported in up to 90% of patients abusing alcohol.[224] The rise is mainly due to hepatic microsomal induction and is independent of the presence of liver disease, although hepatocellular necrosis and cholestasis may contribute. It is not specific for alcohol abuse and is raised in other forms of liver injury and in patients taking other enzyme-inducing drugs.[225] Its main clinical use is probably in monitoring a period of supposed abstinence because it falls within a week of cessation of drinking. Other biochemical markers of alcohol abuse rather than liver disease include elevated serum uric acid[226] hypertriglyceridemia and desialylated transferrin.[227] The classical hematologic marker of alcohol abuse is a raised mean corpuscular volume (MCV), which has been reported to occur in 80% to 100% of alcoholics with and without liver disease,[228] and may be more common in alcoholic women. It is due to a direct toxic effect of alcohol on the marrow, although nutritional folate and B_{12} deficiencies may contribute in some patients. With regard to biochemical markers of alcohol-related liver damage, a rise in serum aspartate transaminase activity (AST) of up to five times normal is common in patients abusing alcohol and reflects the presence, but not the severity, of liver damage.[229] However, unlike nonalcoholic liver disease, alanine transaminase (ALT) activity is raised less often than AST, and the AST/ALT ratio has been suggested as a means of distinguishing liver disease of alcoholic and nonalcoholic cause.[230] Recently, however, it has been appreciated that an AST greater than the ALT can also be a marker of severe nonalcoholic liver disease.[231] Biochemical markers of the stage of liver disease have so far proved elusive. Possible exceptions include plasma IgA, which is twice normal in fewer than 30% of alcoholics with early disease and greater than three times normal in 60% of patients with cirrhosis[232] and the procollagen peptides. Levels of procollagen III in particular have been shown to distinguish advanced from early alcoholic liver disease.[233]

Liver Biopsy

Liver biopsy is a mandatory investigation in all patients chronically abusing alcohol who have hepatomegaly and/or abnormal liver blood tests. First, it is used to establish the diagnosis of alcohol-related liver disease. This is important because it has been shown that up to 20% of liver disease in alcoholics with abnormal liver function is due to an alternative cause.[222] Second, it is the only way of accurately staging the disease, which cannot be achieved by any combination of clinical or laboratory data.[234] Without knowledge of the histologic severity, no prognostic information can be given to the patient and no rational treatment plan can be devised.

Alcohol-Induced Fatty Liver

Pathology

Fatty liver is the earliest lesion seen in ALD. The classical appearance is of a single large fat droplet displacing the nucleus occurring predominantly in perivenular hepatocytes (macrovesicular steatosis). Very rarely, the steatosis is panacinar and may be associated with severe cholestasis, cholangiolitis, and clinical presentation with hepatic failure.[223] Inflammation is rare in simple fatty liver although occasional lipogranulomata may be seen as a response to the extrusion of cellular lipid. Mild fibrosis may occur in response to lipogranulomata and is usually considered reversible; however, the presence of marked perivenular fibrosis in an otherwise uncomplicated fatty liver may be a marker of high risk of progression to cirrhosis.[235] Microvesicular steatosis, in the form of finely dispersed lipid droplets, may also occur in some patients (alcoholic foamy degeneration) and is associated with bilirubinostasis and focal liver necrosis.[236] This lesion resolves with abstention. Alcoholic fatty liver is histologically indistinguishable from nonalcoholic fatty liver (NAFLD) associated with the metabolic syndrome (hyperlipidemia, hypertension, type II diabetes, and obesity).

Clinical Features

Patients with fatty liver are usually asymptomatic or present with nonspecific digestive symptoms. Rarely fatty liver may be associated with hyperlipidemia, hemolytic anemia, and jaundice (Zieve syndrome, see later discussion) or hepatic failure.

Smooth, nontender hepatomegaly is usually the only clinical finding, although signs of portal hypertension may be observed if perivenular fibrosis (central hyaline sclerosis) is present. All, or none, of the laboratory investigations discussed may be abnormal, most commonly, the γGT, AST, and MCV are mildly raised.

Prognosis

It is widely considered that fatty liver is an entirely benign lesion reversible with abstention from alcohol. Fat starts to accumulate in the liver after as little as one weekend of heavy drinking in nonalcoholic human volunteers.[237] Fortunately the reverse seems to hold true, and in the majority of patients with fatty liver who stop drinking, the laboratory abnormalities quickly return to normal[238] and the histologic abnormality rapidly regresses.[239] Accordingly, no treatment options have been evaluated in patients with fatty liver other than abstention and a well-balanced diet. However, there are reports that alcoholic fatty liver per se is not always benign, with occasional mortality due to hepatic failure, fat emboli, and hypoglycemia. Furthermore, fatty liver may be a precursor of alcoholic cirrhosis. In a study by Sorenson and colleagues,[61] it was found that the extent of fatty liver on initial liver biopsy was a better predictor of subsequent progression to cirrhosis 10 years later than alcohol history. Furthermore, a more recent study revealed that even "pure" fatty liver can progress to fibrosis and cirrhosis in a proportion of patients.[62] In this study, the presence of mixed macrovesicular and microvesicular fat and giant mitochondria were associated with disease progression. This suggests, as discussed previously, that fatty liver may be causative in the development of cirrhosis rather than simply an epiphenomenon of alcohol abuse.

Alcoholic Hepatitis

Pathology

Alcoholic hepatitis consists of a constellation of histologic abnormalities (**Fig. 28-9**). The features obligatory for diagnosis are[220] (**Fig. 28-10**).

1. Liver cell damage typified by ballooning degeneration that progresses to necrosis with or without Mallory bodies. Ballooning degeneration is characterized by hepatocyte swelling, a pale granular cytoplasm, and a small hyperchromatic nucleus. Mallory bodies are intracytoplasmic inclusions staining purplish-red with hematoxylin and eosin, and consisting of aggregates of intermediate filament proteins reflecting impaired function of the microtubular system.
2. Inflammatory cell infiltrate, predominantly neutrophils, that are typically arranged around necrotic hepatocytes that contain Mallory-Denk bodies ("satellitosis").
3. Pericellular fibrosis that produces a "chicken wire" appearance. In addition, there is often fibrous thickening around the hepatic vein radicals and eventual obliteration of the veins, a process referred to as central hyaline sclerosis.
4. Perivenular distribution, unless cirrhosis is present, in which lesions occur at the periphery of nodules. As the severity increases the damage extends to involve the whole lobule.

   Other features, which are often present but are not obligatory for diagnosis include: fatty change, bridging necrosis, bile

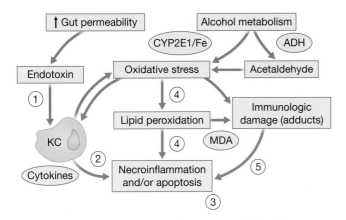

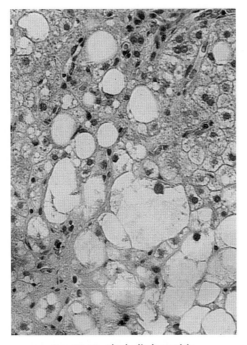

Fig. 28-9 Putative mechanisms of hepatocyte injury in alcoholic hepatitis with potential targets for therapy.
(*1*) Antiendotoxin therapy: antibiotics, probiotics, enteral nutrition; (*2*) anticytokine therapy: corticosteroids, pentoxifylline, infliximab; (*3*) antiapoptotic therapy: caspase inhibitors; (*4*) antioxidants; (*5*) immune-based therapy: corticosteroids. CYP2E1/Fe, cytochrome P450 2E1; ADH, alcohol dehydrogenase; MDA, malondialdehyde; KC, Kupffer cells.

Fig. 28-10 Alcoholic hepatitis.

duct proliferation, apoptotic bodies, cholestasis, and giant mitochondria. Histologic features considered to indicate a high risk of progression to cirrhosis are: the extent and degree of fibrosis (central hyaline sclerosis is the worst sign), a panlobular distribution, and widespread Mallory-Denk body formation. It is important to highlight that this pattern of lesions can also occur in other conditions including diabetes mellitus, obesity, jejunal-ileal bypass, total parenteral nutrition, and following treatment with various drugs, when it is referred to as nonalcoholic steatohepatitis (NASH).

Clinical Features

There is no good correlation between the severity of the histologic lesion and the clinical presentation, which can range from asymptomatic to life-threatening hepatic decompensation.[240] However, patients with the milder histology are more likely to present with nonspecific symptoms, incidental hepatomegaly or raised transaminases, while patients with severe histology usually have symptoms specifically related to hepatocellular failure, such as jaundice, ascites and encephalopathy, or variceal bleeding. The episode of decompensation leading to clinical presentation may be precipitated by vomiting, diarrhea, anorexia, increased alcohol intake, or intercurrent infection. The majority of patients have tender, smooth, hepatomegaly with an arterial bruit in severe cases. Signs of chronic liver disease may be present, even without co-existing cirrhosis, and the more advanced cases may also have signs of portal hypertension and encephalopathy. Nonliver signs commonly present include pyrexia, signs of associated vitamin deficiency and malnutrition, a hyperdynamic circulation, and cyanosis due to intrapulmonary arteriovenous shunting. Abnormalities of liver-related blood tests are always present and include decreased albumin and increased γGT, AST, bilirubin, alkaline phosphatase, and prothrombin time (PT). In addition, blood urea and serum sodium and potassium are all low, unless hepato-renal syndrome supervenes, and hypoglycemia may be present. Macrocytic anemia, neutrophil leukocytosis, and thrombocytopenia are present in all but the mildest cases. A peculiar clinical feature of patients with severe alcoholic hepatitis is that they often rapidly deteriorate in the days immediately following hospital admission.[241] This has been observed in up to 40% of patients and varies from deteriorating blood tests to increasing encephalopathy or variceal bleeding. The pathophysiologic basis of this is not clear but suggestions have included the nutritional implications of withdrawing an alcoholic from the principal source of calorific intake and a reduction in hepatic blood flow consequent upon a reduction in levels of acetaldehyde, which, via conversion to adenosine, has vasodilatory actions.

Prognosis

The short-term outcome in patients with alcoholic hepatitis is associated with the severity of the initial histologic lesion but liver biopsy is invasive and often precluded on the grounds of coagulopathy. Although transjugular liver biopsy is an alternative, it is not always locally available. In view of this difficulty, many clinical and laboratory variables have been suggested as indicators of histologic severity and therefore of potential use in predicting short-term mortality in alcoholic hepatitis. Based on these variables, there have been several prognostic indices developed to aid the clinician. First is the modified Child's criteria, which combines the presence of encephalopathy and ascites, with serum albumin, bilirubin, and PT.[242] Second is a more complex system combining 12 different variables to derive a combined clinical and laboratory index (CCLI).[243] Third is the discriminant function (DF) of Maddrey and colleagues, which is based on PT and bilirubin only.[244] This has been confirmed as a useful predictor of mortality prospectively and to determine patients most suitable for therapy. In view of its simplicity, it is probably the most clinically useful index at present. A fourth scoring system, the Glasgow alcoholic hepatitis score (GAHS) incorporates renal function (an important predictor of survival) white cell count and age as well. Although this scoring system needs validation in large numbers prospectively, initial work suggests that it is more sensitive and specific than the Maddrey score at determining prognosis.[245] Finally, the Lille score has been developed to determine survival on treatment (with corticosteroids). This score takes into account the poor prognosis in those patients that do not get a drop in bilirubin after 7 days of steroid therapy. It is particularly useful in determining those patients that are steroid "nonresponders" and in whom alternative therapies should be considered.[246]

If the patient survives to hospital discharge, then the long-term prognosis is determined by the initial histology, the progression to cirrhosis, and the subsequent drinking behavior. Thus the 5-year survival rate is 70% in those with mild histologic features and 50% in those with severe histologic feature.[247] In the Veterans Administration study, patients with mild hepatitis who developed cirrhosis had a 71%, 2-year survival rate compared with 81% for those who did not develop cirrhosis.[248] In addition, the 7-year survival rate has been reported to fall from 80% to 50% in patients who continue to drink compared with abstainers,[247] which is presumably due, at least in part, to the influence of intake on the risk of progression to cirrhosis. In men with mild histology, drinking behavior is the major factor determining progression to cirrhosis, whereas in women and men with severe histology, progression can occur independently of drinking behavior.[249]

Cirrhosis
Pathology

With progressive injury, the features of cirrhosis—namely fibrous septa linking hepatic and portal veins, and regenerative nodules—eventually appear. The cirrhosis is usually micronodular, possibly reflecting the inhibition of regenerative activity by alcohol, and frequently reverts to a macronodular cirrhosis with abstention.[250] The coexistence of steatosis and hepatitis is common and usually indicates continued consumption. In contrast, alcohol withdrawal at the cirrhotic stage can make the histologic determination of etiology almost impossible.

Clinical Features

As with other forms of cirrhosis, the clinical presentation of alcoholic cirrhosis can range from asymptomatic hepatomegaly to hepatic failure and the complications of portal hypertension, such as ascites or variceal bleeding. Severe hepatic decompensation usually implies the presence of continued drinking and superimposed alcoholic hepatitis, but may signal the development of hepatocellular carcinoma (HCC) or portal

vein thrombosis. The clinical findings will depend on the presence of portal hypertension or encephalopathy and do not differ significantly from those observed in other forms of cirrhosis. Patients with compensated cirrhosis, particularly if abstinent from alcohol, can have completely normal laboratory investigations, whereas patients with continued intake will have a similar range of abnormal laboratory investigations compared with those seen in patients with alcoholic hepatitis. In addition, a raised α-fetoprotein suggests the presence of HCC and indicates the need for further investigations.

Prognosis

The survival of patients with alcoholic cirrhosis is determined by the clinical and histologic severity of the disease at presentation and the patient's subsequent drinking behavior. It has also been shown in some studies that sex[251] and ethnicity[252] may influence survival. Several studies have shown that patients who have decompensated disease do significantly worse than those with a compensated disease.[253,254] The influence of drinking behavior on this trend is best illustrated by the seminal study of Klatskin and Powell.[255] They showed that in patients with compensated disease, continued drinking reduced the 5-year survival rate from 89% to 68%. Abstaining patients with ascites or jaundice had lower survival rates than compensated patients, but higher survival rates than patients with ascites or jaundice who continued to drink. The lowest survival rate was seen in patients with variceal bleeding; alcohol habits had no effect on their mortality. The presence of coexisting alcoholic hepatitis on initial biopsy also adversely effects prognosis.[256] HCC develops in 5% to 15% of patients with alcoholic cirrhosis.[257] It is most common in abstaining men and the majority of patients die within a few months of diagnosis.[254,258]

Associated Conditions and Extrahepatic Manifestations
Introduction

The range of health problems associated with excess alcohol consumption extends beyond the liver, with virtually every system in the body affected (**Fig. 28-11 and Table 28-3**). As with alcoholic liver disease, the pathogenetic pathways are not always clear, but are more complex than the direct effect of

Table 28-3 Important Extrahepatic Gastrointestinal Conditions Associated with Excess Alcohol Consumption

SALIVARY GLANDS AND OROPHARYNX	ESOPHAGUS	SMALL BOWEL	COLON	PANCREAS
Parotid enlargement	Gastroesophageal reflux disease	High-transit diarrhea	High-transit diarrhea	Acute and chronic pancreatitis
Glossitis/stomatitis Oropharyngeal malignancy	Mallory-Weiss tears Esophageal malignancy	Malabsorption		Exocrine and endocrine pancreatic insufficiency

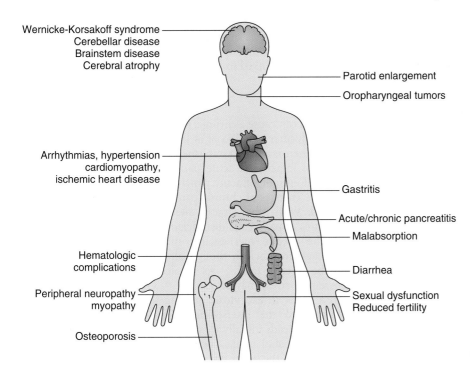

Wernicke-Korsakoff syndrome
Cerebellar disease
Brainstem disease
Cerebral atrophy

Parotid enlargement
Oropharyngeal tumors

Arrhythmias, hypertension
cardiomyopathy,
ischemic heart disease

Gastritis

Acute/chronic pancreatitis

Malabsorption

Hematologic
complications

Diarrhea

Peripheral neuropathy
myopathy

Sexual dysfunction
Reduced fertility

Osteoporosis

Fig. 28-11 Extrahepatic complications of excess alcohol consumption.

ethanol per se. This chapter will give an overview of these problems.

Gastrointestinal Effects

As the first site of exposure after ethanol ingestion, the gastrointestinal system is a prime candidate for toxicity. In addition to the liver, alcohol can affect most parts of the gastrointestinal system (see later discussion).

Salivary Glands and Oropharynx

Parotid enlargement is frequently observed in heavy drinkers with and without chronic liver disease. A histologic study at necropsy demonstrated an increase in adipose tissue at the expense of acinar tissue in the salivary glands of patients with alcoholic cirrhosis compared with the control group.[259] It may be this that contributes to the reduction in both basal and stimulated parotid gland salivary flow reported in these patients.[260] Whether the reduced secretion and altered gland structure in patients with alcoholic cirrhosis is primarily associated with the liver disease or the effects of prolonged alcohol consumption per se is not clear. However, reports of *increased* resting salivary flow in heavy drinkers without liver disease would suggest that the development of liver disease is the important factor leading to reduced secretion.

The prevalence of glossitis and stomatitis is higher in alcoholics than control groups,[261] presumably reflecting the alcoholics' poor nutritional status, including deficiencies in B vitamins and iron. In addition, heavy drinkers have a very significant increase in the incidence of oropharyngeal tumors. Tobacco and alcohol are the principal causal factors associated with the development of head and neck malignancies and appear to act in synergy. One study has reported a history of alcohol and tobacco use in more than 75% of patients with

tumors of the oropharynx.[262] As these tumors are more common in Asians carrying the null *ALDH2* gene, it has been suggested that acetaldehyde, which has been shown to accumulate in the saliva of these individuals, plays a role in the pathogenesis.[263] A history of alcoholism or alcohol-related disease is also associated with a worse prognosis in patients with head and neck malignancy.

Esophagus

Acute alcohol ingestion alters esophageal motor function by reducing lower esophageal sphincter pressure and inhibiting the primary peristaltic movement of the distal esophageal body.[264] This reduces esophageal clearance and increases gastroesophageal reflux. Chronic ethanol consumption also results in reduced esophageal clearance, but lower sphincter pressures are increased unless the patient has concomitant autonomic neuropathy. Although ethanol is associated with heartburn, there is no good evidence that drinkers are more prone to esophagitis. Nausea and vomiting are frequent in chronic alcoholics and may induce Mallory-Weiss tears.[265]

Esophageal cancer is the sixth most common cancer in the world, and alcohol has been identified as a major risk factor since 1962. This association is dose related, and there is no dose below which there is no increased risk. Smoking is an important co-factor. Alcohol-associated nutritional deficiencies and the enhanced bioactivation of dietary mycotoxins and nitrosamines and tobacco-related carcinogens may be important co-factors.[266]

Stomach

The effects of ethanol on gastric motility have been inconclusive, but tend towards an inhibitory effect on gastric emptying. Gastric acid secretion is greatly increased by beer and less so by wine. Most spirits do not lead to an increase in gastric acid secretion, leading to the suggestion that it is other products of fermentation that have this effect.[267] Acute alcohol consumption causes an acute erosive hemorrhagic form of gastritis, with loss of surface epithelial cells and neutrophil infiltration. This peaks at 60 minutes and lasts at least 24 hours. Both nonsteroidal antiinflammatory drugs (NSAIDs) and portal hypertensive gastropathy are risk factors. Chronic heavy drinkers are more likely to develop a superficial or atrophic type of gastritis. Whether alcohol abuse per se induces this classical chronic gastritis with a mononuclear cell infiltrate and glandular atrophy is unclear. This may be due to the increased incidence of *Helicobacter pylori* infection in the gastrointestinal tract of heavy drinkers.[268]

Although there is some debate over whether chronic ethanol consumption increases the risk of duodenal ulcers,[269] there is no evidence that the incidence of gastric ulceration is higher than in the general population.

Small Intestine

Alcohol is one of the main causes of malnutrition in the Western world. It can be severe and is associated with neurologic problems, skin abnormalities, and glossitis, and may also contribute to increased susceptibility to infection and malignancy. Malnutrition in a dependent drinker can be both primary, due to inadequate nutrient intake, and secondary due to malabsorption or maldigestion resulting from gastrointestinal complications. Although pancreatic and hepatic dysfunction can play a role, particularly in fat malabsorption, a major cause of malabsorption is probably altered small bowel function. Several factors contribute to alcohol-related intestinal dysfunction, including the effects of alcohol on gut motility, cellular structure and function, and blood flow. Significant increases in motility have been reported, the most obvious clinical manifestation of which is reduced transit time and diarrhea.[270] Cellular changes observed in the jejunoileal epithelium of alcoholics include abnormal mitochondria, dilated endoplasmic reticulum, altered membrane fluidity, and focal cytoplasmic degradation.[271] These changes are manifest macroscopically by a decrease in villous height,[272] biochemically by a decrease in the activity of mucosal disaccharidases,[273] and functionally by an increased permeability to water and solutes.[274] Intraluminal ethanol also causes regional changes in blood flow within the jejunal mucosa.[275] Together, these various effects of alcohol intake impair the absorption of a variety of nutrients and minerals including glucose, amino acids, trace elements, and vitamins such as thiamine, B_{12}, B_6, and folic acid. This intestinal malabsorption can lead to overall weight loss and multiple deficiencies of micronutrients. The role of oxidative stress in the pathogenesis of many alcohol-related diseases highlights the importance of micronutrient deficiencies in antioxidant vitamins and trace elements, such as zinc, manganese, and selenium.[276]

Colon

Alcohol has been shown to have direct effects on colonic motility with alcohol increasing propulsive activity and contributing to alcohol-induced diarrhea. This effect can be observed following alcohol withdrawal when colorectal transit time increases significantly from approximately 25 to 33 hours.[277] There is a weak association between the dose of alcohol and the incidence of colorectal cancer. This seems to be primarily linked to beer consumption.[278]

Pancreas

Alcohol can cause a chronic, recurrent, calcifying pancreatitis, typically after a period of at least 6 years of heavy consumption. There is also an established association between excessive alcohol intake and acute pancreatitis. In practice, the first clinical episode of acute pancreatitis will occur after the histologic changes of chronic pancreatitis have been well established. With time, attacks often become less severe as the features of pancreatic insufficiency set in.

The precise mechanisms of alcohol-related pancreatic damage are unclear, though alcohol per se does not seem to be directly toxic.[279] As in alcohol-induced liver disease, oxidative stress may play a role.[280] Oxidative injury can lead to a block in exocytosis, leading to the shunting of secretions into the interstitium. The resulting inflammatory response leads initially to acute pancreatitis and, if the insult (excess alcohol intake) persists, eventually to chronic pancreatitis as the acini dedifferentiate into tubular structures, losing their secretory capacity and fibrosing. The fibrosis is particularly prominent in areas of fat necrosis,[281] presumably reflecting the direct fibrogenic effect of lipid peroxidation products.

If alcohol abuse continues after the first episode of pancreatitis, the majority of patients will suffer from recurrent attacks of pain occurring at intervals of weeks or months. Eventually, with progressive loss of acinar tissue, patients develop clinical features of chronic pancreatitis. These include diabetes mellitus, reflecting impaired endocrine function, and malabsorption associated with steatorrhea because of impaired exocrine function. It remains controversial whether or not alcohol abuse is a risk factor for pancreatic cancer.

Cardiovascular System

Acute and chronic alcohol ingestion lead to a variety of beneficial as well as deleterious effects on the heart and cardiovascular system. There now seems little doubt that moderate alcohol intake is associated with a decreased risk of ischemic heart disease,[282] whereas excessive alcohol intake can lead to hypertension; disordered cardiac rhythm, including sudden cardiac death; cardiomyopathy; and cerebrovascular accidents. This dual effect of alcohol on the cardiovascular system is thought to be responsible for the well-known U- or J-shaped curve describing the relationship between alcohol intake and total, as well as cardiovascular-related mortality.[283] This curve shows that mortality among light (1 to 9 drinks per week) and moderate (10 to 34 drinks per week) drinkers is lower than in abstainers and heavy drinkers. The left-hand part of the curve is due to an inverse relationship between death from coronary artery disease and alcohol intake, while the right-hand portion is attributable to a greater risk of nonischemic cardiovascular and noncardiovascular deaths (accidents, suicide, cancer, liver disease) in heavy drinkers. Importantly, contrary to popular belief, almost 50% of the excess deaths occurring in heavy drinkers are attributable to circulatory diseases rather than to liver disease.[284] Concerns have been that the cardiovascular risk curve may be J shaped because the abstainers are previous heavy drinkers that have now stopped drinking. A more recent study using a comparator of "lifelong abstainers" has helped to clarify that low-dose alcohol really does have a protective effect.[285]

Hypertension

A number of epidemiologic studies, controlling for variables such as diet and smoking, have established a dose-response relationship between blood pressure and alcohol consumption.[286-288] It has been estimated that 30% of all cases of hypertension may be attributable to alcohol, with females apparently less susceptible.[289] The threshold for alcohol-associated hypertension appears to be around three standard drinks per day, with some studies showing a dose-response relationship with higher levels of intake.[290] Findings from short-term studies have suggested that cessation of alcohol consumption in hypertensive patients results in a decrease in blood pressure.[289] Whether alcohol-induced hypertension remains reversible in the long term is unknown. The mechanisms underlying the association between alcohol and hypertension are unclear.

Coronary Artery Disease

As discussed, in recent years a number of epidemiologic studies have demonstrated a negative correlation between moderate consumption of alcohol and fatal coronary artery disease.[291] Case-control studies have also shown a lower incidence of myocardial infarction in moderate drinkers compared with abstainers.[292] In these studies, "moderate" drinking was no more than two drinks per day in men and one drink per day in women. Supportive evidence for a protective effect of alcohol on ischemic heart disease is provided by its biologic plausibility.[293] Moderate alcohol consumption increases the plasma levels of the protective high-density lipoprotein cholesterol by as much as 33%.[294] The mechanism is likely to be a result of altered hepatic synthesis and secretion of lipoproteins. Alcohol intake is also associated with impaired platelet aggregation[295,296] and lower levels of fibrinogen, thereby reducing the risk of thrombo-occlusive events.

Cerebrovascular Disease

All types of strokes have been associated with alcohol consumption. This is perhaps not surprising in view of the association between alcohol and most of the established stroke risk factors, including hypertension, cardiomyopathy, arrhythmias, diabetes, and cigarette smoking.[297] In view of its negative association with coronary heart disease, it might be expected that moderate consumption would be associated with a reduced risk of ischemic strokes. The consumption of one drink per day has been associated with a reduced risk of ischemic stroke in one study,[298] but this has not been confirmed in other similar studies, with some reporting a positive association between heavy alcohol intake and cerebral infarction in young men following alcohol "binges."[299] This may be attributed either to dehydration or to the occurrence of alcohol-related supraventricular arrhythmias with resulting embolic events. The expected positive association with hemorrhagic strokes has been reported,[300] but it remains unclear whether this association is independent of alcohol's effect on other risk factors, particularly hypertension.

Cardiomyopathy

It has been recognized since the early 1960s that long-term, heavy alcohol consumption is the main cause of a nonischemic, dilated cardiomyopathy. Postmortem and endomyocardial biopsy studies performed in chronic alcoholics both with and without cardiac symptoms have shown dilation of the atria and ventricles, increased myocardial mass, interstitial fibrosis, and small vessel coronary artery disease.[301] Although subclinical alcoholic cardiomyopathy, characterized by left ventricular hypertrophy and mild systolic and diastolic dysfunction, appears to be relatively common in heavy drinkers, clinical presentation is relatively uncommon and appears to require at least 5 years of more than 90 g of ethanol per day. Interestingly the duration of drinking seems to be more important than the dose over this threshold, with the mean duration in symptomatic patients being 25 years of heavy drinking compared with 16 years in asymptomatic patients.[302] The onset is usually insidious with nonspecific fatigue and chest pain associated with palpitations, most commonly due to atrial fibrillation. As the disease progresses, features of biventricular failure develop. With continued drinking, death from cardiac failure or arrhythmias usually occurs within 4 years of presentation, although in the early stages of disease dramatic recovery can occur with abstention.[303]

Arrhythmias and Sudden Cardiac Death

Heavy drinking increases the risk of cardiac arrhythmias whether or not heart disease is present. This evidence has come from clinical observations, retrospective case-control studies, controlled studies of consecutive admissions for supraventricular tachyarrhythmias and prospective epidemiologic studies.[304] The association is best established for atrial fibrillation, although in one study individuals drinking more than six drinks per day had a higher risk of all supraventricular tachyarrhythmias than those drinking less than one drink per day when matched for age, sex, and smoking.[305] The tendency of these arrhythmias to present following weekend or holiday "binges" has led to the term "holiday heart syndrome." Alcohol has also been shown to promote the onset of ventricular tachyarrhythmias[306] and this presumably explains the increased incidence of sudden cardiac death observed in heavy compared with occasional or light drinkers.[307]

The mechanism of alcohol-related arrhythmogenesis is almost certainly multifactorial. Factors that may play a role include subclinical cardiomyopathy producing conduction delays, potassium and magnesium depletion, the hyperadrenergic state accompanying alcohol withdrawal, autonomic neuropathy, and a direct effect of ethanol on cardiac conduction.[306] The mechanism of ventricular tachyarrhythmias is most likely early afterdepolarizations provoked by catecholamine release and potassium depletion during withdrawal in the presence of a prolonged action potential due to the autonomic neuropathy. In support, patients with a prolonged action potential, manifest on the surface electrocardiogram as QT interval prolongation, have been shown to be at risk of sudden cardiac death.[308]

Effects on the Nervous System

Acute and chronic alcohol intake is associated with a wide range of effects on the nervous system. The depressant effect of alcohol means that acute heavy consumption can lead to blackouts and even coma. After a sudden reduction in alcohol consumption, tremulousness and agitation are common, whereas the full-blown syndrome of delirium tremens, including hallucinations and seizures, is less frequently seen but is more serious. Alcohol and its metabolite acetaldehyde are almost certainly directly neurotoxic, but associated nutritional deficiencies undoubtedly contribute to the pathogenesis of some, if not all, alcohol-related neurologic diseases.[309]

The Wernicke-Korsakoff Syndrome

The Wernicke-Korsakoff syndrome is a nutritional disorder caused by thiamine deficiency predominantly observed in alcoholics. Wernicke encephalopathy represents its acute phase, whereas Korsakoff psychosis represents the chronic continuation of the disease. The major pathologic changes of this syndrome are predominantly in the paraventricular parts of the thalamus and hypothalamus, the mammillary bodies, the periaqueductal gray matter, and the floor of the fourth ventricle. An abrupt onset and the triad of oculomotor disturbances, cerebellar ataxia, and mental confusion characterize classical Wernicke encephalopathy. The most common ocular abnormality is nystagmus (vertical or horizontal), but bilateral sixth nerve palsy, palsies of conjugate gaze, and complete ophthalmoplegia are also seen. Ptosis and pupillary abnormalities may also occur. Mental inattention is characterized by disorientation, inattention, and unresponsiveness that progresses to coma if untreated. Treatment is with parenteral thiamine. The disease can be aggravated by giving intravenous dextrose before thiamine supplementation is administered. Patients usually recover within 48 to 72 hours or progress to Korsakoff psychosis. Korsakoff psychosis is characterized by various degrees of both retrograde and anterograde amnesia, with relative preservation of other intellectual functions. The Korsakoff state is potentially reversible by early intervention with thiamine and prompt treatment of Wernicke encephalopathy. Unfortunately recovery is incomplete in more than 50% of cases and individuals may be left with devastating chronic memory deficits.

Cerebellar Disease

Alcoholic cerebellar degeneration is characterized clinically by an ataxic gait and truncal ataxia, while typically the upper limbs are unaffected.[310] Pathologically there is degeneration of the cerebellar cortex, predominantly of the anterior and superior vermis and anterior lobes. In most cases the syndrome evolves over a period of several weeks or months, after which it remains unchanged for years. Acute cerebellar degeneration may respond to large doses of thiamine and abstinence, but patients usually present long after the onset of their symptoms. At this stage the likelihood of improvement is small, and probably occurs as a result of an improvement

in the peripheral neuropathy that is present in around half the patients.

Brainstem Disease

Central pontine myelinolysis (CPM) is a rare demyelinating disease characterized by neuronal dysfunction centered on the pons. It is encountered predominantly in malnourished alcoholics with disordered electrolytes. Cerebral edema associated with either severe hyponatremia or the rapid correction of hyponatremia during electrolyte replacement may play a role in the pathogenesis. Clinical features include the subacute onset of a progressive quadriparesis, pseudobulbar palsy affecting speech and swallowing, and paralysis of horizontal eye movements. More extensive brainstem dysfunction may result in pupillary abnormalities, decerebrate posturing, altered level of consciousness, and respiratory paralysis. Not surprisingly, the prognosis of this condition is poor with the diagnosis often only made at postmortem. CPM may be associated with Marchiafava-Bignami syndrome, which is a rare demyelinating disease of the corpus callosum also predominantly occurring in alcoholics. This has acute bilateral hemispheric dysfunction and a poor prognosis.

Alcoholic Dementia

Although some studies suggest that a high level of alcohol consumption may be a contributing factor in some cases of dementia, this is an area of great controversy. One study of moderate drinkers in Bordeaux, France, revealed that consumption of between 250 and 500 ml of wine per day resulted in a significant reduction in the risk of dementia and Alzheimer disease in later life.[311] Computed tomography (CT) studies have shown a substantially higher incidence of cerebral cortical atrophy in alcohol-dependent patients, and brain weights at autopsy are less than half that of age-matched control subjects. However, no correlation has been demonstrated between either the CT or histologic changes and the neuropsychological impairment frequently seen in chronically dependent patients. For example, ventricular and sulcal enlargements are often seen on CT with no clinical evidence of cerebral dysfunction. Furthermore, there is little firm evidence of any histologic abnormality in the brains (of study cadavers) other than that related to the complications of alcohol dependence, such as Wernicke encephalopathy, posttraumatic changes, and chronic hepatocerebral degeneration. Thus cerebral atrophy is common in alcohol dependence, and dementia may occur as a result of the direct toxic effect of ethanol on the brain, but there is no defined clinicopathologic entity that constitutes "alcoholic dementia." The mental disturbances are more likely to be related to other established complications of alcohol abuse.

Neuropathies

Peripheral neuropathy is another common nutritional complication in alcoholics. The precise mechanism is unclear but histology reveals a noninflammatory degeneration of myelin sheaths and axon cylinders, which is more intense in distal segments. In advanced cases, degeneration may also be observed in the anterior and posterior roots of the spinal cord. Patients with electrophysiologic evidence of peripheral neuropathy can be asymptomatic, or more typically present with pain and paresthesia initially affecting the lower limbs. In severe cases, weakness and atrophy may be seen. With continued drinking, the symptoms progress relentlessly, such that in advanced cases significant distal motor deficits with atrophy may be seen. Treatment consists of abstinence and nutritional supplementation, particularly with B vitamins. Recovery is slow and often incomplete.

An association between alcoholism and autonomic neuropathy was first reported in 1980.[312] The subsequent observation that it was more common in alcoholics with liver disease than those without suggested that the liver disease rather than alcohol might be the primary cause.[313] This hypothesis was supported by a report that the incidence of autonomic neuropathy (45%) was similar in liver disease regardless of etiology.[314] More recently, evidence for a reversible metabolic effect of liver disease on autonomic function has been provided by a study demonstrating an improvement in autonomic function 3 months after successful liver transplantation.[315] Importantly, autonomic neuropathy is associated with an adverse prognosis in patients with liver disease, attributed either to an impaired response to stresses or to the associated QT interval prolongation and subsequent risk of ventricular arrhythmias.[308] As many as 50% of patients with liver disease experience typical symptoms of autonomic neuropathy, including postural dizziness, abnormal sweating, and impotence.[314]

Alcoholic Myopathy

Alcoholic myopathy can occur in an acute form with variable severity. In the mild form, it may represent a mild rise in muscle enzymes, while at its most severe there may be rhabdomyolysis. In the severe form the patient presents, often after a heavy bout of drinking, with muscle pain and weakness. Muscle enzymes are markedly raised and electromyography is abnormal. Occasionally the rhabdomyolysis can be severe enough to cause myoglobinuria and acute renal impairment. The condition improves in most cases over days.

Alcoholic myopathy also has a more common, chronic form, which has progressive, painless weakness, and wasting of the proximal muscle groups. The condition is associated with chronic alcohol consumption, and histology reveals a loss of type IIb muscle fibers.

Although ethanol may partly induce myopathy through well-characterized neuropathy, there appears to be an additional impact of ethanol and its metabolism on muscle. These mechanisms remain unclear, but are likely to involve the generation of oxidative stress, mirroring other end-organ damage.

Fetal Alcohol Syndrome

A conservative estimate for the incidence of fetal alcohol syndrome (FAS) has been put at 0.33 per 1000 live births with many more children suffering from various alcohol-related effects not amounting to the full syndrome.[316] A similar per capita frequency is likely to occur in other industrialized countries, but little data are available on the magnitude of this problem in the developing or third world. FAS is caused by excessive alcohol consumption during pregnancy, which results in a variety of abnormalities in the fetus thought to be caused by the direct effect of alcohol and its metabolite acetaldehyde, rather than by associated nutritional deficiencies or other drugs. The severity of the syndrome depends on both the timing and severity of maternal alcohol consumption during gestation. The diagnostic criteria include features of growth retardation and developmental delay, central nervous system involvement, and characteristic facial dysmorphology in the presence of maternal alcohol consumption of more than two drinks per day. The central nervous system involvement typically presents as behavioral dysfunction and mental retardation. The characteristic facial features include short palpebral fissures, an elongated midface, an indistinct philtrum, a thin vermilion, and a foreshortened maxilla.

Alcohol and Cancer

Results from several large epidemiologic studies have firmly established that alcohol is associated with a higher cancer incidence and mortality[317] (**Table 28-4**). Alcohol consumption is most strongly associated with cancers of the esophagus (as discussed previously), oropharynx, and larynx, with the increased risk particularly prominent in smokers. The controversy over the association between alcohol and breast cancer has been resolved by two large meta-analyses. The first was a meta-analysis of six prospective cohort studies.[318] This has clearly demonstrated that for intakes less than 60 g per day, breast cancer risk increases linearly with intake. A daily intake of 30 to 60 g was associated with a relative risk of 1.41[318] when compared with nondrinkers, and this risk was independent of other known risk factors. The second, more recent study had very similar findings.[319]

The mechanisms underlying alcohol-related cancers are unclear but several factors have been suggested to play a role. Alcohol may be important in the initiation of cancer, either by increasing the expression of certain oncogenes or by impairing the cell's ability to repair DNA, thereby increasing the likelihood that oncogenic mutations will occur. Alcohol may act as a co-carcinogen by enhancing the effect of direct carcinogens, such as those found in tobacco and the diet. This effect of alcohol may be in part via induction of the cytochrome P450 family of enzymes that are found in the liver, lung, and intestine, and which are capable of metabolizing various tobacco and dietary constituents into cancer promoting free radicals. Because reduced levels of iron, zinc, and vitamins A, B, and E have been experimentally associated with some cancers, the nutritional deficiencies associated with chronic alcohol intake may also play a role in alcohol-related cancers, possibly by increasing the magnitude of free radical–related oxidative stress. Finally, alcoholism is associated with immunosuppression, which makes chronic alcoholics more

Table 28-4 Cancers Confirmed to Be Associated with Excess Alcohol Consumption	
Mouth	Esophagus
Pharynx	Breast
Larynx	Liver

susceptible to infection and theoretically reduces immune surveillance of early tumors.

Hematologic Complications

Heavy alcohol consumption, with or without liver disease, can have profound effects on the hematologic system. Although the earliest and most obvious effects are on erythrocytes, derangements in production, function, and consumption of leukocytes, platelets, and coagulation can also have important consequences.

Erythrocytes

It has long been recognized that many alcoholics have increased mean corpuscular volume. This simple macrocytosis can occur in the absence of vitamin deficiency and is thought to be a direct effect of alcohol, or the products of its metabolism, on the development of the red cell. In line with this, the corpuscular volume returns to normal several weeks after abstinence.

In true folate deficiency, there may also be a macrocytic, megaloblastic anemia. This is quite common in alcoholics, who may also suffer from B_{12} deficiency, which can cause a similar picture. Alcohol can also promote a sideroblastic anemia in which heme synthesis is impaired. In this condition, serum ferritin is raised and the red cells are hypochromic in the peripheral blood, and have ring sideroblasts in the marrow.

Heavy drinkers also suffer from the anemias associated with some degree of alcohol-induced liver injury. Zieve syndrome is a condition described in 1958,[320] typically found in middle-aged male heavy drinkers with alcoholic fatty liver and severe hyperlipidemia. It is rare, and improves with abstinence. This is in contrast to the more concerning spur cell anemia, which tends to be associated with advanced alcoholic cirrhosis, though it can occur occasionally in other types of cirrhosis. Spur cells, or acanthocytes, are caused by the equilibration of the outer lipid layer of the cell membrane with the cholesterol-rich abnormal lipoproteins in the plasma. The problem is compounded by the reduced fluidity of the red cell membrane seen in cirrhosis because of a reduction in the proportion of polyunsaturated versus saturated fatty acids. The acute development of spur cell anemia is a poor prognostic indicator in alcoholic cirrhosis, and has been considered an indication for transplantation, which may be curative. Finally, red cell consumption can occur as a result of congestive hypersplenism resulting from liver disease and portal hypertension.

Leucocytes

Chronic alcohol-dependent patients are more prone to a variety of infections[321] and malignancies.[322] This sensitivity has often been attributed to defects in innate and acquired immunity caused by alcoholic liver disease and ethanol consumption. Although the effects of ethanol on neutrophil[323,324] and macrophage function[130,325,326] have been well investigated, revealing in particular a disruption in phagocytosis[327] and antigen processing and presentation,[328] studies into the effects on lymphocyte functioning have been less conclusive. A uniform finding, however, in both chronic alcoholics and chronically ethanol-fed animals is a reduction in circulating T-cell numbers, and, in mice, a reduction in spleen and lymph node size.[329,330] Whether this reduction in numbers is primarily due to a failure of proliferation or an increase in apoptotic rates is, however, unclear. It appears therefore that chronic, or even acute, ethanol consumption may alter the host's ability to mount an appropriate magnitude immune response.[331]

Platelets

Although an acute single dose of ethanol may not affect platelet number or function, chronic heavy drinking does. The changes that occur can do so in the absence of folate deficiency or hypersplenism, although these problems can compound the condition. The thrombocytopenia seen as a consequence of alcohol ingestion appears to be a direct myelosuppressive effect of ethanol on bone marrow megakaryocytes, and is usually mild, and rarely of clinical consequence.[332] In addition, ethanol can also affect platelet function, even in the absence of thrombocytopenia. Chronic heavy drinkers have been found to have prolonged bleeding times and platelets that are significantly less responsive to standard platelet aggregation tests and have decreased thromboxane A2 release. When these patients have been followed up during an in hospital period of abstinence, these abnormalities returned to normal during 2 to 3 weeks of alcohol withdrawal.

Coagulation

One of the difficult problems in patients with alcoholic liver disease is the derangement in coagulation that can compound acute episodes of gastrointestinal bleeding. These disturbances are common and complex. Liver synthesis of clotting factors can be impaired by hepatocellular dysfunction or inadequate absorption of vitamin K, which is required for the synthesis of factors II, VII, IX, and X. These abnormalities have an abnormal prothrombin time. Treatment requires replacement of the factors plus vitamin K. In many cases of cirrhosis, there will also be a reduced fibrinogen level.

Effects on the Endocrine System

The pathogenesis of decreased libido and impotence in heavy drinkers is not fully understood. There is evidence from human and rat studies that chronic alcohol consumption reduces testosterone synthesis. Although dependent drinkers may develop the resulting hypoandrogenization, there is not the expected rise in gonadotrophins that normally accompanies this end-organ failure.[333] This in turn suggests a problem with the hypothalamic and pituitary feedback mechanisms. These problems are compounded by the hyperestrogenization seen in liver disease and manifested by spider nevi and gynecomastia. Heavy alcohol consumption may also induce changes in peripheral testosterone and estrogen metabolism, as well as changes in estrogen receptors.

Even in patients without liver disease, alcohol can affect fertility. In men, abnormal spermatogenesis is more frequent, with decreased numbers and motility of sperm. In women, amenorrhea, anovulation, and accelerated onset of menopause have all been associated with alcohol intake.

Alcohol-induced pseudo-Cushing syndrome has the same characteristics as classical Cushing, namely moon face, central obesity, muscle wasting, abdominal striae, fatigue, easy bruising, and hypertension.[334] This syndrome can be indistinguishable from true Cushing syndrome, except for the fact that it resolves with abstinence and may recur when heavy drinking is resumed. Whether pseudo-Cushing is a true identity or simply a syndrome combining several of the clinical features of alcohol abuse is presently in debate.

In addition to the endocrinologic associations of heavy drinking described previously, there are also more subtle effects resulting in a reduction in growth hormone and a rise in prolactin. The first of these has no direct impact apart from enhancing hypoglycemia (see later discussion). The second can exacerbate the effects of hypogonadism and hyperestrogenism.

Hypoglycemia and Ketoacidosis

Inhibition of hepatic gluconeogenesis, depleted hepatic glycogen stores, and deranged glucocorticoid secretion may all contribute to the presentation of the alcoholic with severe hypoglycemia. These often-malnourished patients are prone to episodes of ketoacidosis that, when compounded with starvation and vomiting, can be life threatening.

Hyperuricemia

Hyperuricemia is caused by a decrease in the excretion of uric acid, secondary to hyperlactacidemia. Lactate competitively inhibits uric acid clearance by the proximal renal tubule, and consequently reduces its excretion. This situation is exacerbated by the alcohol-induced increase in urate synthesis secondary to accelerated degradation of adenine nucleotides.

Osteoporosis

Even in the absence of liver disease, alcohol can cause osteopenia,[335] possibly through a direct toxic effect on osteoblasts and bone remodeling. This loss of bone can result in increased incidence of fractures in alcoholics. Although the pathogenesis of this problem may involve the influence of endocrine factors, such as pseudo-Cushing or hypogonadism, nutritional deficiencies associated with alcoholism, and low levels of osteocalcin, which rapidly rises on abstinence, point to a more direct effect of alcohol itself on bone formation.[336]

Treatment

The age-adjusted death rate from all-cause cirrhosis, the greatest percentage of which is alcohol related, fell by 48.3% in the United States between 1970 and 2005. This greatly exceeded the age-adjusted all-cause mortality that fell by 34.7%. The total annual per capita ethanol consumption rose steadily from 2 gallons to 2.8 gallons between 1955 and 1980 and then dropped back to around 2.31 gallons in the following 27 years. In crude terms, it appears, therefore, that the improvement in alcoholic cirrhosis mortality exceeds the reduction in ethanol consumption. This may be due to the fact that there are fewer individuals drinking heavily and more drinking within healthy levels. It may also reflect improvements in the management of patients with alcoholic liver disease. Clearly, any improvement in the treatment of the complications of cirrhosis will have a beneficial effect on the management of patients with end-stage ALD. However, this section focuses on treatment

strategies that have been specifically directed at mechanisms involved in the pathogenesis of alcohol-related liver injury and considers their current and future role in the management of patients with the various stages of ALD.

Achieving Abstinence

Because cessation or a marked reduction in alcohol intake has been shown to improve the histology and/or survival of patients with all stages of ALD,[247,249,255] measures aimed at establishing and maintaining abstinence are critical in the management of patients with ALD. This is best achieved by close liaison between liver physicians and addiction psychiatrists, with support from specialist alcohol nurses and trained counselors.[337] Available treatments for alcohol-dependent patients can be divided into psychological and pharmacologic (**Table 28-5**). So-called "brief interventions" are the simplest form of psychological therapy and can be implemented by nonpsychiatric staff. This involves educating and informing the patients about the nature of their problem and providing them with advice on how to go about changing their behavior. Despite the apparent simplicity of this form of management, brief interventions have been shown to significantly increase the chances of heavy drinkers significantly reduced drinking at 6 and 12 months in an outpatient setting.[338,339] With only minimal training, medical and nursing staff can also deliver a variety of manual-guided psychosocial treatments including cognitive-behavioral therapy and motivational enhancement therapy, both of which have been shown to reduce drinking in dependent patients in a randomized controlled trial.[340]

As an alternative, or an addition, to psychological therapies, some patients may derive benefit from pharmacologic therapy. Both acamprosate and naltrexone have been shown to reduce drinking days and increase abstinence rates in more than one randomized controlled trial and a recent meta-analysis.[341-343] Acamprosate is derived from taurine and its beneficial effect is thought to be via binding to the γ-amino butyric acid (GABA) receptor with a reduction in the neuronal excitation that is normally observed during alcohol craving. Importantly for patients with ALD, acamprosate, unlike naltrexone, is well tolerated in all but patients with Childs-Pugh C cirrhosis,[344] and its benefit seems to persist for at least 1 year after treatment withdrawal. The only pharmacotherapy in a trial study in patients with advanced liver disease is baclofen.[345] This drug was well tolerated and effective at promoting abstinence in

Table 28-5 Nonpharmacologic and Pharmacologic Therapies to Obtain and Maintain Abstinence
Nonpharmacologic
• Brief intervention • Cognitive therapy • Motivational enhancement therapy • Psychotherapy
Pharmacologic
• Acamprosate • Naltrexone • Disulfiram • Baclofen

alcohol-dependent patients. Disulfiram, an inhibitor of acetaldehyde dehydrogenase, has been used for many years in the management of alcohol-dependent patients. As discussed previously, it induces an acetaldehyde-mediated adverse reaction to alcohol intake characterized by nausea and flushing. Trials of effectiveness, however, have given conflicting results.[346,347] The drug also requires compliance and its potential for hepatotoxicity has limited its use in patients with established ALD.[348]

Importantly, there have been no formal trials of either psychological or pharmacologic therapies in drinkers with ALD. However, previous evidence that the severity of alcohol dependence in ALD patients is less than that observed in an unselected group of alcohol-dependent patients,[349] suggests that these treatments may be even more beneficial in the ALD population. Consistent with the low level of dependency, up to 50% of ALD patients will either abstain completely or achieve a significant reduction in intake after being given simple advice by physicians during their initial presentation, with a significant improvement in survival compared with continued heavy drinkers.[350]

Alcoholic Hepatitis

Alcoholic hepatitis (AH) covers a spectrum of disease from subclinical to a severe, life-threatening disorder. Independent predictors of survival in these patients are serum bilirubin, PT, and the presence of hepatic encephalopathy. As discussed, the two laboratory indices have been combined to derive a discriminant function (bilirubin [mg/dl] + 4.6 [PT prolongation]), and a value of 32 or greater has been shown to predict a high short-term mortality in several prospective studies.[244,351-353] Accordingly almost all treatment trials in patients with AH have been short term (usually 1 month) and restricted to patients with a discriminant function greater than 32 and/or encephalopathy. Patients with less severe disease appear to have a good short-term prognosis even when jaundiced.[248] Accordingly, in these patients and the severe patients surviving their initial presentation, treatment is focused on achieving abstinence, which has been convincingly shown to improve long-term outcome.[247,249,255] Reports that some patients with AH can progress to cirrhosis even with abstention,[249] and that patients with co-existing AH and cirrhosis have a worse long-term survival rate than patients with cirrhosis only,[256] suggest the need for longer term treatment trials in patients with AH.

Progress in developing specific treatments for acute alcoholic hepatitis has been hampered by a poor understanding of disease pathogenesis. Reflecting this paucity of information, many treatment modalities have been tried in patients with AH; however, none have been consistently shown to have a beneficial effect and, accordingly, none have achieved consensus status among practicing hepatologists.

Corticosteroids

Of all the treatments available for patients with severe AH, corticosteroids are the most intensively studied, and probably the most effective. Steroids are aimed at suppressing or "switching off" the hepatic inflammatory response seen in liver biopsies from patients with severe AH. The mechanism of this effect is, at least in part, through the inhibition of NF-κB transcriptional activity.[354] The transcription of many inflammatory cytokines, chemokines, and adhesion molecules is dependent on the NF-κB signaling cascade.[355] Two important side effects of steroids used in medium dose include poor wound healing and susceptibility to infection, both of which can lead to life-threatening complications in this group of patients. Concern over these adverse effects coupled with a continued uncertainty over efficacy has contributed to the reluctance of many clinicians to prescribe steroids for patients with AH.

Patients with alcoholic hepatitis form a heterogeneous population, both in severity, and probably in disease pathogenesis. Without a liver biopsy it is difficult to differentiate a patient with severe acute inflammatory AH from one with alcohol- or non–alcohol-induced cirrhosis that has decompensated while drinking. Many initial trials of steroids were poorly designed and included patients with a variety of disease severities and almost certainly patients without AH. Most of these trials showed no treatment benefit. However, two randomized controlled trials focused only on patients that had the worst prognosis, defined by a DF of greater than or equal to 32 and/or encephalopathy, and both showed a survival benefit in the steroid-treated patients.[244,352] Interestingly, one of these studies required biopsy confirmation of alcoholic hepatitis, whereas the other did not. Nevertheless, the results were remarkably similar, suggesting that a clinical diagnosis (without biopsy) may be adequate to determine the group that gets benefit from treatment, provided the DF is greater than 32. Several meta-analyses have attempted to resolve the steroid controversy, and although most have shown a survival benefit,[356-358] this has not been a universal finding.[359] Rather than performing a further conventional meta-analysis, the authors of the last three large randomized controlled trials have pooled their individual patient data, only including patients with encephalopathy and/or a discriminant function greater than 32.[143] This study showed that steroids improved survival time versus the placebo (85% vs. 65%), with placebo treatment, increasing age, and creatinine independent predictors of mortality on multivariate analysis. A weakness of this study is that two of the three original trials included gastrointestinal bleeding as a contraindication, whereas one did not and only one trial required a liver biopsy for diagnosis. Nonetheless, the large numbers (102 on placebo, 113 on steroids) make this the most robust meta-analysis to date. The same group has now published evidence to support the withdrawal of steroids if the bilirubin has not fallen by the seventh day of steroid treatment. This simple clinical observation significantly reduces the length of treatment in nonresponders.[360]

Traditionally, sepsis has been a contraindication to the use of steroids in patients with acute alcoholic hepatitis. This is partly because of initial studies showing that it was "nonseptic" patients that benefited and partly due to concerns about increasing the risk of sepsis in treated patients. A recent study has shown that while sepsis is common in patients with alcoholic hepatitis, those with infection before steroid treatment had similar 2-month survival rates compared with those who did not have an infection. These data suggest that a treated infection should not be a contraindication to the use of steroids.[361]

Despite 13 randomized controlled trials and 6 meta-analyses, the debate over the use of steroids continues. It appears that they are probably beneficial in patients with severe disease; however, mortality on treatment remains high, particularly when renal impairment is present, and treatment is relatively contraindicated in the large number of patients with concomitant infection and gastrointestinal bleeding. There are also significant numbers of patients that can be classed as "nonresponders." It is because of these limitations that alternative therapeutic strategies have been sought.

Pentoxifylline

As discussed in the section on pathogenesis, there is good evidence from animal models that tumor necrosis factor-α (TNF-α) plays an important role in acute alcohol-mediated liver injury. Pentoxifylline (PTX) is a nonselective phosphodiesterase inhibitor that is approved for use in claudication at a dose of 400 mg three times a day because of its effect on red blood cell deformability. In the late 1980s, PTX was observed to have an anticytokine effect, later attributed to a reduction in TNF-α gene transcription[362] and, accordingly, to reduced levels of important downstream TNF-α effectors including other proinflammatory cytokines, chemokines, and adhesion molecules. The first randomized controlled trial of PTX in 101 patients with AH was reported in 2000.[363] The effective claudication dose was given for 28 days to patients with a DF greater than 32 and lead to a 40% reduction in mortality compared with a placebo. The secondary end point of hepatorenal syndrome (HRS) was reduced in the treated population by 65%. Importantly, almost all of the improvement in the survival rate was due to a fall in mortality from HRS, suggesting that PTX may have a specific beneficial effect in AH patients developing this ominous complication.[364] Clearly, further trials are needed to determine whether PTX should become standard treatment for patients with AH. In particular, comparisons should be made with steroids and a placebo (in patients in whom steroids are contraindicated), and trials of PTX in combination with steroids should be performed. Pentoxifylline has been shown to be ineffective as a salvage treatment in steroid nonresponders.[365]

Nutritional Supplementation

Trials investigating the role of nutritional supplementation have been prompted by the degree of protein calorie malnutrition seen in patients having acute AH and the correlation between the severity of malnutrition and mortality.[366] Initial trials with parenteral amino acid therapy yielded conflicting results[367,368]; however, more consistent and promising results have been reported from two randomized controlled trials of enteral tube feeding. The first compared enteral tube feeding of an energy-dense formula supplying 2115 kcal/day with an isocaloric standard oral diet.[369] The enteral feed contained whole protein plus branched-chain amino acids, medium- and long-chain triglycerides, and maltodextrin. Thirty-five severely malnourished cirrhotics were randomized and the in-hospital mortality was 12% in the tube-fed group compared with 47% in the oral group. This prompted a further study 10 years later comparing enteral feeding to steroids in 71 patients with acute severe AH. In this trial, while there was no difference in mortality between the groups during the 28-day treatment period, deaths occurred earlier in the steroid-treated patients and the mortality rate was lower in the enterally fed group in the year following treatment. The overall mortality rate at 1 year was 61% and 38%, in steroid- and enteral-treated groups, respectively. Although this difference did not reach significance ($P = .26$), it must be appreciated that this treatment was being compared with what is currently considered to be the best available treatment.

In summary, nutritional supplementation may have a role in improving medium- to long-term survival in patients with severe AH. Which patients benefit the most and the mechanisms by which they derive benefit are, as yet, unclear. There is no doubt, however, that this form of treatment deserves further investigation.

Antioxidants

Interest in the potential value of antioxidant therapy in the treatment of AH has arisen as a result of the growing body of evidence, discussed previously, implicating oxidative stress as a key mechanism in alcohol-mediated hepatotoxicity. These considerations have recently led to three trials investigating the effect of antioxidant supplementation in patients with severe AH. In the first study, 56 patients were randomized to receive vitamin E, selenium, and zinc supplementation or placebo.[370] Although treated patients had an in-hospital mortality of 6.5% compared with 40% in the placebo group, the entry criteria and patient details were not clear. The second trial compared steroids with an antioxidant cocktail (vitamins A, C, E, selenium, allopurinol, desferrioxamine, and N-acetylcysteine) and was stopped after an interim assessment found steroid treatment to be associated with a significantly higher survival rate.[371] This trial did not examine whether antioxidants conferred any benefit in patients in whom steroids were contraindicated, or in combination with steroids. The most recent study investigated the role of antioxidants in patients with severe AH stratified by gender and steroid treatment. The active group received a loading dose of N-acetylcysteine of 150 mg/kg followed by 100 mg/kg/day for 1 week, and vitamins A-E, biotin, selenium, zinc, manganese, copper, magnesium, folic acid, and coenzyme Q daily for 6 months. The decision to treat with steroids was made by the supervising clinician according to conventional criteria.[91] Although white blood cell count and bilirubin at trial entry were both associated with increased mortality, antioxidant therapy showed no benefit either alone or in combination with steroids. In summary, on the basis of the data available thus far, high-dose antioxidant therapy confers no survival benefit in patients with severe AH.

Hepatic Mitogens

The observation that survival time in patients with severe AH correlates with the intensity of hepatocyte staining for proliferating cell nuclear antigen[372] implies that the liver's capacity for regeneration is an important determinant of outcome and suggests that therapy directed at enhancing proliferation might be beneficial. An infusion of insulin and glucagon has been shown to improve liver regeneration in a rat partial hepatectomy model,[373] and to improve survival time in a mouse model of fulminant hepatitis.[374] These observations were the stimulus to several trials investigating the role of insulin and glucagon therapy in the treatment of patients with severe AH. Although the first trial showed a significant reduction in mortality in the treated group,[375] two subsequent larger studies showed no benefit, with one reporting a high incidence of hypoglycemia.[376,377] At present, therefore, this form of therapy cannot be recommended. Anabolic steroids have also been shown to promote hepatocyte regeneration; however, three large randomized controlled trials with either testosterone or oxandrolone in males with AH have reported no treatment benefit.[378]

Propylthiouracil

Centrilobular hypoxia is a feature of animal models of ALD and has been postulated to play a role in the liver injury, which is characteristically most severe in the centrilobular acinar zone 3.[379] The hypoxia has been attributed to the hypermetabolic state induced by ethanol, which is similar to the hypermetabolic state associated with hyperthyroidism, and can be attenuated in the rodent model of ALD by the antithyroid drug PTU.[379] Two trials have evaluated the role of this drug in improving short-term mortality in patients with AH. Although the first trial reported a more rapid improvement in clinical and laboratory indices, neither trial showed any survival benefit.[380,381]

Experimental Therapies

In addition to the treatments described previously, several novel therapies for acute AH are currently undergoing investigation. The one that initially showed the most promise was the anti–TNF-α antibody, infliximab. This chimeric human/mouse monoclonal antibody binds to TNF-α and blocks its biologic effects. Its potential use in AH has been suggested by its reported benefit in several other inflammatory conditions, the putative role of TNF-α in the pathogenesis of ALD, and a report that anti-TNF-α antibodies ameliorate the liver injury in a mouse model of ALD.[382] Three initial reports demonstrated an improvement in biochemistry and a satisfactory safety profile when used alone[383,384] or in combination with steroids.[385] A further pilot study using a "sister" molecule, etanercept, also showed a satisfactory safety profile, though only 7 of 13 patients had a DF greater than 32.[386] The safety aspect is important because experience with infliximab in other diseases has raised concerns over the risk of infection.[387] This could potentially limit the number of patients with AH suitable for treatment and was the rationale for excluding patients with severe disease (DF >55) from one of the initial trials.[385] The beneficial role of TNF-α in promoting liver regeneration is another potential problem for anti–TNF-α treatments in patients with AH for the reasons discussed previously.[388] To date, one clinical trial has examined the role of infliximab in combination with steroids in patients with acute severe alcoholic hepatitis. Infliximab was used at twice the dose given for Crohn disease and at 0, 2, and 4 weeks. The study was stopped after 36 patients were randomized because of the high mortality in the treated group. Most of the deaths were infection related, and the Maddrey scores were not found to be different in the treated group after a mean of 2 months.[389] There has also been one randomized controlled trial of etanercept versus a placebo.[390] Patients with a MELD score of greater than 15 were included and the drug was compared with a placebo. Survival at 6 months was significantly lower in the etanercept group and serious infectious adverse events were higher. These studies are likely to have put a halt to further trials of anti–TNF-α antibodies.

A further experimental therapy that may benefit patients with AH is the molecular adsorbents recycling system (MARS). The primary aim of this treatment is to support impaired liver function while the liver recovers or the patient undergoes liver transplantation. It may therefore have a role in patients with AH either alone or in combination with other pharmacologic therapies. The principal of the MARS procedure is to dialyze blood against an albumin solution aimed at removing albumin-bound toxins, including bilirubin and bile salts. Clinical improvement and a drop in portal pressure have been reported with MARS in a small series of patients with severe alcoholic hepatitis.[391,392] Recently, MARS has been studied as a follow-up therapy to steroids in those patients who do not have a drop in bilirubin at day 7; the so-called nonresponders. Although there were improvements in bilirubin and creatinine on treatment, 1- and 2-month survival rates were similar to the placebo.[393]

Treatment of HRS in AH

As alluded to previously, in patients with severe AH, the development of renal failure is associated with a survival of less than 10%, even with intensive management and renal support.[364] Perhaps the most significant advance in the management of patients with advanced liver disease over the past decade has been the introduction of albumin infusions combined with splanchnic vasoconstrictor agents for patients with HRS. This combination appears to significantly improve the survival of patients with cirrhosis who have this life-threatening complication.[394-396] Although no randomized trials have specifically examined this form of therapy in patients with AH, the previously reported high mortality in AH patients with HRS suggests that it will have a significant and beneficial impact on patient survival.

Alcoholic Cirrhosis

Although the high mortality of severe AH, coupled with the young age of many of the patients, makes it an important area for therapeutic trials, the vast majority of patients with ALD in clinical practice have advanced fibrosis or cirrhosis. These patients may be asymptomatic or have symptoms related to portal hypertension, advanced liver failure, or the development of hepatocellular carcinoma. As discussed previously, the most important therapy is achieving and maintaining abstinence because this has been shown to improve survival in both well-compensated and decompensated patients.[255] Unfortunately, as with AH, no adjunctive pharmacotherapies have been consistently shown to improve survival time in more than one randomized controlled trial, although some have shown promise and will be reviewed later. Potential reasons for the lack of progress thus far include: (1) a lack of a clear understanding of disease pathogenesis; (2) problems with compliance in long-term treatment trials; and (3) the confounding effect of drinking behavior during the duration of the trial. As a result, at present the management of patients with advanced fibrotic ALD is directed primarily at preventing and treating the complications of portal hypertension, liver failure, and hepatocellular carcinoma and deciding if and when to consider patients for orthotopic liver transplantation.

Pharmacologic Therapy
Propylthiouracil

In contrast to its lack of effect in patients with acute AH, PTU may improve the long-term survival of patients with alcoholic cirrhosis. There has, however, been only one trial reported thus far.[397] In this study, the investigators went to great lengths to assess drinking behavior and compliance by checking daily urine samples for alcohol and a drug biomarker. Treatment for 2 years improved mortality in the patient group as a whole, particularly in patients who continued to drink moderately during the trial. No improvement was seen in abstinent patients who had an excellent prognosis on the drug or placebo or in continued heavy drinkers who had a universally bad prognosis. Although the patient numbers were high (310), a large percentage of patients were either noncompliant or dropped out of the study. For this reason and the lack of any confirmatory studies, PTU has not been widely adopted by the liver community. In view of the promising results, however, it does seem surprising that no centers have attempted to repeat the study, which remains an excellent model of how to perform a randomized controlled trial in this potentially difficult group of patients.

Colchicine

This antiinflammatory drug has been evaluated in the treatment of patients with alcohol and non–alcohol-related cirrhosis because of its antifibrotic effect in vitro.[398,399] To date, clinical results have been conflicting. The most convincing evidence supporting the use of colchicine comes from a study including 100 patients followed for up to 14 years. The survival rate was 75% and 34% in treated and placebo groups, respectively. Some patients appeared to have a resolution of their cirrhosis to either minimal fibrosis or normal histology.[400] Three further trials, however, with median follow-ups of 1,[401] 6,[402] and 40[403] months, have all shown no benefit. A recent meta-analysis has also reviewed 14 randomized controlled trials and found no benefit of colchicine treatment on mortality or liver histology.[404] This has been confirmed by a further large randomized study.[405]

Antioxidants

In addition to trials in patients with AH, the accumulating evidence that oxidant stress is involved in the pathogenesis of ALD has prompted trials of antioxidants in patients with chronic disease. Two trials have evaluated the drug silymarin, which is the active component of the herb milk thistle and has potent antioxidant properties in vitro[406] and in vivo.[407,408] The first trial in 170 patients with cirrhosis (92 had ALD) followed up for between 2 and 6 years reported a beneficial effect on survival time.[409] In contrast, a later, larger study of 200 patients with cirrhotic ALD, followed up for 5 years, showed no benefit.[410] SAMe, which acts as both an antioxidant by replenishing GSH and a methyl donor maintaining cell membrane fluidity, has also been evaluated in patients with alcoholic cirrhosis. Using death or liver transplantation as a combined end point, Mato and colleagues reported a significant beneficial effect of SAMe treatment in patients with Child's A and B cirrhosis.[411] Clearly further trials with this agent are awaited with interest.

Phosphatidylcholine

Phosphatidylcholine (PPC) is an essential component of all cell membranes and is vulnerable to attack by lipid peroxidation. Through mechanisms that are, as yet, unclear, dietary supplementation with phosphatidylcholine has been shown to attenuate ethanol-induced fibrosis in baboons.[412] Potential mechanisms of action include stimulation of collagenase[413] and acting as a "sink" for free radicals.[414] A long-term trial in patients with alcoholic cirrhosis has just been completed in the United States. Although there was a trend to improvement in transaminases and bilirubin in the PPC group in certain patient subgroups (heavy drinkers and those with hepatitis C), overall there was no improvement in liver histology as determined by liver biopsies 24 months apart. The potential benefits of the drug may not have been evaluated appropriately because of the dramatic reduction in drinking seen in the treated and placebo groups of patients that were followed up to completion.[415]

Liver Transplantation for Advanced ALD

Since the initial report of its success in 1988,[416] liver transplantation has become an increasingly common treatment for ALD cirrhosis in both Europe[417] and North America.[418] However, transplantation for ALD remains controversial, principally due to concerns over the risk of posttransplant recidivism and its effect on outcome and public opinion at a time of increasing donor shortage. This issue, coupled with a perception that these patients are more likely to have contraindications to transplantation due either to extrahepatic complications of excessive alcohol abuse or to an associated lack of self-care, has contributed to a continued reluctance of many centers to offer transplantation to patients with ALD. An accumulating number of reports of transplantation in patients with ALD have now provided a firm evidence base from which these issues can now be addressed.

Outcome of Liver Transplantation for ALD

Several studies have convincingly demonstrated that the survival of patients transplanted for cirrhotic ALD is comparable with or better than patients with cirrhosis of alternative etiologies, with 5- and 10-year survival rates lying somewhere between those of patients transplanted for cholestatic and viral hepatitis–related liver disease.[419] Recent figures for ALD transplantation in Europe reveal a 1-, 3-, 5-, and 10-year patient survival rate of 84%, 78%, 73%, and 54%, respectively.[420] There is no evidence that patients with ALD have a higher frequency of immediate postoperative complications or resource use compared with patients transplanted for other indications despite being transplanted at a more advanced stage of disease.[421] Patients transplanted for ALD are, however, more likely to die from cardiovascular disease and de novo malignancy than patients transplanted for other causes.[420] The improvement in quality of life following transplantation also compares favorably with other indications in the short term,[422,423] although not after 3 years following the transplant.[421] The reason for this decline is unclear, but does not seem to be related to a return to problem drinking.

As with other indications, the decision to offer transplantation to a patient with ALD is based on his or her expected survival with and without transplantation. Without transplantation, survival depends on the severity of the liver disease and subsequent drinking behavior. Patients with Child C cirrhosis have a 1-year survival rate of 50% to 85% compared with 75%

to 95% in patients with Child B.[424] This suggests that in the absence of other predictors of high mortality, such as a history of spontaneous bacterial peritonitis, recurrent variceal hemorrhage or the development of hepatocellular carcinoma, transplantation should be restricted to patients with Child C cirrhosis. In support of this policy, Poynard and colleagues demonstrated that ALD patients with a Child-Pugh score of 11 or higher had a significantly improved 2-year survival rate when transplanted compared with matched controls who were not.[425] The potential effect of abstinence on prognosis of these transplant patients has led most units to adopt a policy of offering transplantation to patients whose Child-Pugh score remains high after a period of abstinence.

Posttransplant Recidivism

Perhaps the greatest concern when considering transplantation for patients with ALD is the risk of recidivism and its effect on outcome and public opinion. With respect to the frequency of recidivism, this depends critically on its definition. Studies that have considered any alcohol use posttransplantation as a "relapse" have reported recidivism rates as high as 49%,[426-428] whereas those that have restricted the definition to heavy or problem drinking have reported lower rates of 10% to 15%.[422,429-433] With respect to the influence of recidivism on outcome, so far there are few data on which to base firm conclusions. From the information available, the incidence of graft dysfunction related to recidivism ranges up to 17% and mortality ranges up to 5%.[428,429,431,432] In a study from 2001, the recidivism rates were 30% with many showing evidence of recurrent disease on their protocol biopsies. Neither recidivism nor histology affected 84-month survival rates.[434] Despite this apparently reassuring report, there is now evidence that if the follow-up is prolonged to 10 years, mortality in recidivists is significantly higher than in abstainers.[435] It is therefore imperative that patients are monitored carefully for relapse following transplantation, with relapsers offered appropriate counseling. It is important that this is done for all ALD patients because at present few factors have been identified that reliably predict the risk of posttransplant recidivism before transplantation. Efforts to minimize the risk of posttransplant recidivism are important not only for the individual patient, but also to avoid the likely adverse effect this has on the organ-donating public.

Public Opinion

With organ shortage as a significant problem and while the decision to be an organ donor remains voluntary in most of the Western world, it is imperative that the public is convinced that donated livers are being given to the most deserving patients. A U.K. study clearly demonstrated that the general public, primary care physicians, and gastroenterologists all place patients with ALD well down their list of patients most deserving a liver transplant.[436] The perception that patients with ALD have played a significant role in their disease and the widely held belief that "once a drinker, always a drinker" seem likely to be the most important factors contributing to this negative view of ALD patients. It is therefore vital that the public are made aware that patients are only offered transplantation if they fail to recover after a period of abstinence and that the incidence of significant posttransplant recidivism is low.

Comorbidity

Excessive alcohol consumption can, and often does, affect many organ systems apart from the liver and this can potentially give rise to contraindications to surgery. An increased risk of pancreatitis, cardiomyopathy, osteoporosis, cerebrovascular disease, dementia, and malnutrition might all be expected to limit the number of patients fit for surgery. In practice, however, although most transplant units routinely screen ALD patients for cardiac and cerebral complications of excessive alcohol intake, this results in the exclusion of very few patients.[433] Similarly, despite the increased risk of psychiatric comorbidity in heavy drinkers, this rarely, if ever, leads to the exclusion of patients at the stage of transplant assessment.[433] This seems likely to be attributable either to patients with significant physical or psychiatric comorbidities not being referred for formal transplant assessment and/or to the tendency of many alcohol-related morbidities to improve during the period of abstinence required by most units before assessment.

Preoperative Abstinence

In light of the previous considerations, it is perhaps not surprising that most centers require patients to have been abstinent for a period of time before assessment. This is primarily to give the liver a chance to recover spontaneously; however, it also allows time for other alcohol-related morbidities to recover, thereby improving the patient's fitness for surgery and, importantly, satisfies public opinion. During this period, the patient can also be put in contact with alcohol treatment services for support both before and following transplantation. Although there is broad consensus on the need for a period of pretransplant abstinence, there is far less agreement on the requirement for a minimum duration. Many units have previously insisted on a 6-month period of abstinence, possibly attributable to early reports that this was a positive predictor of posttransplant abstinence.[422] Although a recent study confirms a 6-month period of abstinence to be associated with reduced rates of recidivism at 1 and 2 years posttransplant,[437] other studies have shown this period of abstinence to have little if any predictive power for subsequent drinking habits.[432] It is likely that other factors along with abstinence are important and one study has found the period of drinking, the amount of drinks per day, social situation, and psychiatric comorbidity to also be important. They suggest a score that includes these factors and abstinence to predict recidivism.[438] This is obviously a very important question as the price of insisting on a fixed abstinence period may be death for some patients. A recent study demonstrating that the chance of recovery in patients with decompensated ALD can be predicted in as early as 3 months,[439] has led some observers to suggest that, if required at all, the minimum period of abstinence could safely be reduced to 3 months from 6 months.[440] Currently, it appears that most centers do not adhere strictly to a fixed period of abstinence, instead preferring to assess each case on an individual basis and listing the patient when it is considered that recovery is unlikely.[419]

Transplantation for AH

Clearly, many of these issues are pertinent when it comes to considering the possibility of giving a transplant to patients with severe acute AH. A reasonable period of abstinence is not possible to assess the liver's potential for spontaneous recovery; significant comorbidities are common and formal psychiatric assessment and pretransplant counseling is often precluded by the severity of the illness. Accordingly, although these patients undoubtedly have a poor prognosis without transplantation, most clinical centers do not consider these patients to be transplant candidates. Nonetheless, there have been isolated reports of survival following transplantation of these patients.[364,441] Histologic AH in the explanted liver of patients receiving a transplant for apparently chronic stable ALD is not associated with a worse prognosis or an increased risk of recidivism.[442] A recent report from France has evaluated the role of liver transplantation in patients treated with steroids for alcoholic hepatitis who do not have a drop in bilirubin at day 7. These nonresponders were considered for transplantation if they fulfilled strict criteria. They had to be at their first presentation with liver disease, be socially integrated, have supportive family members, have no comorbidities, and have the support of all medical and paramedical staff. Six-month survival was 83% in the transplanted cohort, which was significantly higher than the 44% in the nontransplanted control cohort.[443] Although these data are promising in very selected patients, it challenges the principle of a period of abstinence before transplantation. Liver transplant units need to assess whether they, and the public, feel that this is an appropriate use of the donor organ pool.

Conclusions

The short-term social and psychological benefits of alcohol have meant that its use and abuse have been widespread in many societies. End-stage liver disease is the result of prolonged heavy alcohol intake among a small proportion of users. Nevertheless, alcoholic liver disease still accounts for around half the total number of deaths from cirrhosis in the United States, and a great many more patients with fibrosis and alcoholic hepatitis. It therefore makes up a significant proportion of the workload of most liver units. The interaction between the physical and psychological dependence of the drug and the complexity of disease susceptibility makes this patient population a fascinating group. The multiple potential mechanisms of pathogenesis make it an intriguing disease to study, made all the more interesting considering the gray areas around the relative importance of each mechanism. Animal work is slowly improving this knowledge. This is filtering down into human trials of novel treatments, but improvements are slow considering the high mortality of acute alcoholic hepatitis, and liver transplantation remains the mainstay of treatment for advanced cirrhosis. Further research to understand the basics of hepatocyte injury are required to fuel further clinical trials hopefully leading to significant improvements in patient survival.

Key References

Addolorato G, et al. Effectiveness and safety of baclofen for maintenance of alcohol abstinence in alcohol-dependent patients with liver cirrhosis: randomised, double-blind controlled study. Lancet 2007;370(9603): 1915–1922. (Ref.345)

Becker U, et al. Lower risk for alcohol-induced cirrhosis in wine drinkers. Hepatology 2002;35(4):868–875 (see comment). (Ref.189)

Boetticher NC, et al. A randomized, double-blinded, placebo-controlled multicenter trial of etanercept in the treatment of alcoholic hepatitis. Gastroenterology 2008;135(6):1953–1960. (Ref.390)

Boitard J, et al. Tolerance and efficacy of the MARS system in patients with severe alcoholic hepatitis non-responder to steroids. Hepatology 2007; 46(Suppl 1):327A. (Ref.393)

Burra P, et al. Longitudinal prospective study on quality of life and psychological distress before and one year after liver transplantation. Acta Gastroenterol Belg 2005;68(1):19–25. (Ref.423)

Burra P, et al. Liver transplantation for alcoholic liver disease in Europe: a study from the ELTR (European Liver Transplant Registry). Am J Transplant 2010; 10(1):138–148. (Ref.420)

Canbay A, et al. Apoptotic body engulfment by a human stellate cell line is profibrogenic. Lab Invest 2003;83(5):655–663. (Ref.169)

Castel H, et al. Early transplantation improves survival of non-responders to steroids in severe alcoholic hepatitis: challenge to the 6 month rule of abstinence. Hepatology 2009;50(4 Suppl):307A. (Ref.443)

Cortez-Pinto H, et al. Lack of effect of colchicine in alcoholic cirrhosis: final results of a double blind randomized trial. Eur J Gastroenterol Hepatol 2002;14(4):377–381. (Ref.403)

Cuadrado A, et al. Alcohol recidivism impairs long-term patient survival after orthotopic liver transplantation for alcoholic liver disease. Liver Transpl 2005;11(4):420–426. (Ref.435)

De Gottardi A, et al. A simple score for predicting alcohol relapse after liver transplantation: results from 387 patients over 15 years. Arch Intern Med 2007;167(11):1183–1188. (Ref.438)

Elabbadi N, et al. Relationship between the inhibition of phosphatidic acid phosphohydrolase-1 by oleate and oleoyl-CoA ester and its apparent translocation. Biochimie 2005;87(5):437–443. (Ref.39)

Enomoto N, et al. Estriol enhances lipopolysaccharide-induced increases in nitric oxide production by Kupffer cells via mechanisms dependent on endotoxin. Alcohol Clin Exp Res 2002;26(8 Suppl):66S–69S. (Ref.194)

Fischer M, et al. Peroxisome proliferator-activated receptor alpha (PPARalpha) agonist treatment reverses PPARalpha dysfunction and abnormalities in hepatic lipid metabolism in ethanol-fed mice. J Biol Chem 2003;278(30): 27997–28004. (Ref.42)

Forrest EH, et al. The Glasgow Alcoholic Hepatitis Score identifies patients likely to benefit from corticosteroids. Gut 2004;53(Suppl 3):A13. (Ref.245)

Forsyth CB, et al. Lactobacillus GG treatment ameliorates alcohol-induced intestinal oxidative stress, gut leakiness, and liver injury in a rat model of alcoholic steatohepatitis. Alcohol 2009;43(2):163–172. (Ref.117)

Galli A, et al. The transcriptional and DNA binding activity of peroxisome proliferator-activated receptor alpha is inhibited by ethanol metabolism. A novel mechanism for the development of ethanol-induced fatty liver. J Biol Chem 2001;276(1):68–75. (Ref.41)

Hamajima N, et al. Alcohol, tobacco and breast cancer: collaborative reanalysis of individual data from 53 epidemiological studies, including 58,515 women with breast cancer and 95,067 women without the disease. Br J Cancer 2002; 87(11):1234–1245. (Ref.319)

Hirano K, et al. Expression of a mutant ER-retained polytope membrane protein in cultured rat hepatocytes results in Mallory body formation. Histochem Cell Biol 2002;117(1):41–53. (Ref.84)

Jalan R, et al. Extracorporeal liver support with molecular adsorbents recirculating system in patients with severe acute alcoholic hepatitis. J Hepatol 2003;38(1):24–31 (see comment). (Ref.391)

Jarvelainen HA, et al. Promoter polymorphism of the CD14 endotoxin receptor gene as a risk factor for alcoholic liver disease. Hepatology 2001;33(5): 1148–1153 (see comment). (Ref.127)

Jeong WI, Park O, Gao B. Abrogation of the antifibrotic effects of natural killer cells/interferon-gamma contributes to alcohol acceleration of liver fibrosis. Gastroenterology 2008;134(1):248–258. (Ref.142)

Ji C, Deng Q, Kaplowitz N. Role of TNF-alpha in ethanol-induced hyperhomocysteinemia and murine alcoholic liver injury. Hepatology 2004; 40(2):442–451. (Ref.59)

Ji C, Kaplowitz N. Hyperhomocysteinemia, endoplasmic reticulum stress, and alcoholic liver injury. World J Gastroenterol 2004;10(12):1699–1708. (Ref.58)

Johansen D, et al. Food buying habits of people who buy wine or beer: cross sectional study. BMJ 2006;332(7540):519–522. (Ref.190)

Kendrick SF, et al. Acetate, the key modulator of inflammatory responses in acute alcoholic hepatitis. Hepatology 2010;51(16):1988–1997. (Ref.114)

Kessova IG, et al. Alcohol-induced liver injury in mice lacking Cu, Zn-superoxide dismutase. Hepatology 2003;38(5):1136–1145. (Ref.97)

Kirkland RA, et al. A Bax-induced pro-oxidant state is critical for cytochrome C release during programmed neuronal death. J Neurosci 2002;22(15):6480–6490. (Ref.136)

Kollerits B, et al. A common variant in the adiponutrin gene influences liver enzyme values. J Med Genet 2010;47(2):116–119. (Ref.202)

Lemmers A, et al. The interleukin-17 pathway is involved in human alcoholic liver disease. Hepatology 2009;49(2):646–657. (Ref.163)

Lieber CS, et al. Veterans Affairs cooperative study of polyenylphosphatidylcholine in alcoholic liver disease. Alcohol Clin Exp Res 2003;27(11):1765–1772. (Ref.415)

Lieber CS. S-adenosyl-L-methionine and alcoholic liver disease in animal models: implications for early intervention in human beings. Alcohol 2002; 27(3):173–177. (Ref.99)

Lluis JM, et al. Acetaldehyde impairs mitochondrial glutathione transport in HepG2 cells through endoplasmic reticulum stress. Gastroenterology 2003; 124(3):708–724. (Ref.113)

Louvet A, et al. Early switch to pentoxifylline in patients with severe alcoholic hepatitis is inefficient in non-responders to corticosteroids. J Hepatol 2008; 48(3):465–470. (Ref.365)

Louvet A, et al. The Lille model: a new tool for therapeutic strategy in patients with severe alcoholic hepatitis treated with steroids. Hepatology 2007;45(6): 1348–1354. (Ref.246)

Louvet A, et al. Infection in patients with severe alcoholic hepatitis treated with steroids: early response to therapy is the key factor. Gastroenterology 2009; 137(2):541–548. (Ref.361)

Lu SC, et al. Methionine adenosyltransferase 1A knockout mice are predisposed to liver injury and exhibit increased expression of genes involved in proliferation. Proc Natl Acad Sci U S A 2001;98(10):5560–5565. (Ref.98)

Lucey MR. Is liver transplantation an appropriate treatment for acute alcoholic hepatitis? J Hepatol 2002;36(6):829–831. (Ref.440)

Mandayam S, Jamal MM, Morgan TR. Epidemiology of alcoholic liver disease. Semin Liver Dis 2004;24(3):217–232. (Ref.3)

Marnett LJ. Oxy radicals, lipid peroxidation and DNA damage. Toxicology 2002;181-182:219–222. (Ref.172)

Mathurin P, et al. Early change in bilirubin levels is an important prognostic factor in severe alcoholic hepatitis treated with prednisolone. Hepatology 2003;38(6):1363–1369. (Ref.360)

Mathurin P, et al. Corticosteroids improve short-term survival in patients with severe alcoholic hepatitis (AH): individual data analysis of the last three randomized placebo controlled double blind trials of corticosteroids in severe AH. J Hepatol 2002;36(4):480–487. (Ref.143)

Matsumaru K, Ji C, Kaplowitz N. Mechanisms for sensitization to TNF-induced apoptosis by acute glutathione depletion in murine hepatocytes. Hepatology 2003;37(6):1425–1434. (Ref.137)

McClain CJ, et al. Monocyte activation in alcoholic liver disease. Alcohol 2002;27(1):53–61. (Ref.326)

McKim SE, et al. Inducible nitric oxide synthase is required in alcohol-induced liver injury: studies with knockout mice. Gastroenterology 2003;125(6): 1834–1844. (Ref.80)

Menon KV, et al. A pilot study of the safety and tolerability of etanercept in patients with alcoholic hepatitis. Am J Gastroenterol 2004;99(2):255–260. (Ref.386)

Miguet M, et al. Predictive factors of alcohol relapse after orthotopic liver transplantation for alcoholic liver disease. Gastroenterol Clin Biol 2004;28(10 Pt 1):845–851. (Ref.437)

Minagawa M, et al. Activated natural killer T cells induce liver injury by Fas and tumor necrosis factor-alpha during alcohol consumption. Gastroenterology 2004;126(5):1387–1399. (Ref.140)

Morgan TR, et al. Colchicine treatment of alcoholic cirrhosis: a randomized, placebo-controlled clinical trial of patient survival. Gastroenterology 2005; 128(4):882–890. (Ref.405)

Mottaran E, et al. Lipid peroxidation contributes to immune reactions associated with alcoholic liver disease. Free Radic Biol Med 2002;32(1):38–45. (Ref.155)

Moyer A, et al. Brief interventions for alcohol problems: a meta-analytic review of controlled investigations in treatment-seeking and non-treatment-seeking populations. Addiction 2002;97(3):279–292. (Ref.339)

Mukamal KJ, et al. Alcohol consumption and cardiovascular mortality among U.S. adults, 1987 to 2002. J Am Coll Cardiol 2009;55(13):1328–1335. (Ref.285)

Mukamal KJ, et al. Roles of drinking pattern and type of alcohol consumed in coronary heart disease in men. N Engl J Med 2003;348(2):109–118. (Ref.282)

Nagai H, et al. Reduced glutathione depletion causes necrosis and sensitization to tumor necrosis factor-alpha-induced apoptosis in cultured mouse hepatocytes. Hepatology 2002;36(1):55–64. (Ref.24)

Nair S, et al. Is obesity an independent risk factor for hepatocellular carcinoma in cirrhosis? Hepatology 2002;36(1):150–155 (erratum appears in Hepatology 2002;36(3):774). (Ref.171)

Nakajima T, et al. Peroxisome proliferator-activated receptor alpha protects against alcohol-induced liver damage. Hepatology 2004;40(4):972–980 (see comment). (Ref.44)

Nanji AA, et al. Alcoholic liver injury in the rat is associated with reduced expression of peroxisome proliferator-alpha (PPARalpha)-regulated genes and is ameliorated by PPARalpha activation. J Pharmacol Exp Ther 2004;310(1):417–424. (Ref.43)

Natori S, et al. Hepatocyte apoptosis is a pathologic feature of human alcoholic hepatitis. J Hepatol 2001;34(2):248–253. (Ref.132)

Naveau S, et al. A double-blind randomized controlled trial of infliximab associated with prednisolone in acute alcoholic hepatitis. Hepatology 2004; 39(5):1390–1397 (see comment). (Ref.389)

Nelson S, Kolls JK. Alcohol, host defence and society. Nat Rev Immunol 2002;2(3):205–209. (Ref.321)

Neuberger J, et al. Transplantation for alcoholic liver disease. J Hepatol 2002;36(1):130–137. (Ref.419)

Niemela O, et al. Effect of Kupffer cell inactivation on ethanol-induced protein adducts in the liver. Free Radic Biol Med 2002;33(3):350–355. (Ref.81)

Nieto N, Friedman SL, Cederbaum AI. Cytochrome P450 2E1-derived reactive oxygen species mediate paracrine stimulation of collagen I protein synthesis by hepatic stellate cells. J Biol Chem 2002;277(12):9853–9864. (Ref.168)

Ortega R, et al. Terlipressin therapy with and without albumin for patients with hepatorenal syndrome: results of a prospective, nonrandomized study. Hepatology 2002;36(4(1)):941–948. (Ref.394)

Parlesak A, et al. Gastric alcohol dehydrogenase activity in man: influence of gender, age, alcohol consumption and smoking in a Caucasian population. Alcohol Alcohol 2002;37(4):388–393. (Ref.12)

Parola M, Robino G. Oxidative stress-related molecules and liver fibrosis. J Hepatol 2001;35(2):297–306. (Ref.67)

Pasare C, Medzhitov R. Toll pathway-dependent blockade of CD4+CD25+ T cell-mediated suppression by dendritic cells. Science 2003;299(5609): 1033–1036 (comment). (Ref.123)

Pedersen A, Johansen C, Gronbaek M. Relations between amount and type of alcohol and colon and rectal cancer in a Danish population based cohort study. Gut 2003;52(6):861–867. (Ref.278)

Pessayre D, Fromenty B. NASH: a mitochondrial disease. J Hepatol 2005;42(6): 928–940. (Ref.134)

Pessione F, et al. Five-year survival predictive factors in patients with excessive alcohol intake and cirrhosis. Effect of alcoholic hepatitis, smoking and abstinence. Liver Int 2003;23(1):45–53. (Ref.258)

Pruett SB, et al. Suppression of innate immunity by acute ethanol administration: a global perspective and a new mechanism beginning with inhibition of signaling through TLR3. J Immunol 2004;173(4):2715–2724. (Ref.141)

Rambaldi A, Iaquinto G, Gluud C. Anabolic-androgenic steroids for alcoholic liver disease: a Cochrane review. Am J Gastroenterol 2002;97(7):1674–1681. (Ref.378)

Raynard B, et al. Risk factors of fibrosis in alcohol-induced liver disease. Hepatology 2002;35(3):635–638. (Ref.193)

Romeo S, et al. Genetic variation in PNPLA3 confers susceptibility to nonalcoholic fatty liver disease. Nat Genet 2008;40(12):1461–1465. (Ref.201)

Roskams T, et al. Oxidative stress and oval cell accumulation in mice and humans with alcoholic and nonalcoholic fatty liver disease. Am J Pathol 2003;163(4):1301–1311. (Ref.175)

Safadi R, et al. Immune stimulation of hepatic fibrogenesis by CD8 cells and attenuation by transgenic interleukin-10 from hepatocytes. Gastroenterology 2004;127(3):870–882. (Ref.167)

Sen S, et al. Albumin dialysis reduces portal pressure acutely in patients with severe alcoholic hepatitis. J Hepatol 2005;43(1):142–148. (Ref.392)

Seth D, et al. Patatin-like phospholipase domain containing 3: a case in point linking genetic susceptibility for alcoholic and nonalcoholic liver disease. Hepatology 2010;51(4):1463–1465. (Ref.200)

Sharma P, et al. Infliximab monotherapy for severe alcoholic hepatitis and predictors of survival: an open label trial. J Hepatol 2009;50(3):584–591. (Ref.384)

Song Z, et al. S-adenosylhomocysteine sensitizes to TNF-alpha hepatotoxicity in mice and liver cells: a possible etiological factor in alcoholic liver disease. Hepatology 2004;40(4):989–997. (Ref.86)

Spahr L, et al. Combination of steroids with infliximab or placebo in severe alcoholic hepatitis: a randomized controlled pilot study. J Hepatol 2002; 37(4):448–455. (Ref.385)

Stewart SF, et al. Valine-alanine manganese superoxide dismutase polymorphism is not associated with alcohol-induced oxidative stress or liver fibrosis. Hepatology 2002;36(6):1355–1360. (Ref.211)

Stewart SF, et al. A trial of antioxidant therapy alone or with corticosteroids in acute alcoholic hepatitis. J Hepatol 2002;36(Suppl 1):16. (Ref.91)

Stewart SF, et al. Oxidative stress as a trigger for cellular immune responses in patients with alcoholic liver disease. Hepatology 2004;39(1):197–203. (Ref.162)

Sugimoto T, et al. Decreased microsomal triglyceride transfer protein activity contributes to initiation of alcoholic liver steatosis in rats. J Hepatol 2002; 36(2):157–162. (Ref.47)

Szabo G, Bala S. Alcoholic liver disease and the gut-liver axis. World J Gastroenterol 2010;16(11):1321–1329. (Ref.116)

Tian C, et al. Variant in PNPLA3 is associated with alcoholic liver disease. Nat Genet 2009;42(1):21–23. (Ref.199)

Tome S, et al. Influence of superimposed alcoholic hepatitis on the outcome of liver transplantation for end-stage alcoholic liver disease. J Hepatol 2002; 36(6):793–798 (see comment). (Ref.442)

Ueda H, et al. Association of the T-cell regulatory gene CTLA4 with susceptibility to autoimmune disease. Nature 2003;423(6939):506–511. (Ref.218)

Ueki K, et al. Central role of suppressors of cytokine signaling proteins in hepatic steatosis, insulin resistance, and the metabolic syndrome in the mouse. Proc Natl Acad Sci U S A 2004;101(28):10422–10427. (Ref.49)

Uesugi T, et al. Toll-like receptor 4 is involved in the mechanism of early alcohol-induced liver injury in mice. Hepatology 2001;34(1):101–108. (Ref.126)

Valenti L, et al. Cytotoxic T-lymphocyte antigen-4 A49G polymorphism is associated with susceptibility to and severity of alcoholic liver disease in Italian patients. Alcohol Alcohol 2004;39(4):276–280. (Ref.219)

Veldt BJ, et al. Indication of liver transplantation in severe alcoholic liver cirrhosis: quantitative evaluation and optimal timing. J Hepatol 2002; 36(1):93–98. (Ref.439)

Vidali M, et al. Genetic and epigenetic factors in autoimmune reactions toward cytochrome P4502E1 in alcoholic liver disease. Hepatology 2003;37(2): 410–419. (Ref.160)

Villanueva JA, Halsted CH. Hepatic transmethylation reactions in micropigs with alcoholic liver disease. Hepatology 2004;39(5):1303–1310. (Ref.51)

Wheeler MD, et al. Overexpression of manganese superoxide dismutase prevents alcohol-induced liver injury in the rat. J Biol Chem 2001;276(39): 36664–36672. (Ref.101)

Xu A, et al. The fat-derived hormone adiponectin alleviates alcoholic and nonalcoholic fatty liver diseases in mice. J Clin Invest 2003;112(1):91–100. (Ref.50)

Yoon YH, Hsiao-ye Y. Liver cirrhosis mortality in the United States, 1970-2005. NIAAA surveillance report #83 2008. (Ref.5)

You M, et al. Ethanol induces fatty acid synthesis pathways by activation of sterol regulatory element-binding protein (SREBP). J Biol Chem 2002;277(32):29342–29347. (Ref.56)

You M, et al. The role of AMP-activated protein kinase in the action of ethanol in the liver. Gastroenterology 2004;127(6):1798–1808. (Ref.57)

A complete list of references can be found at www.expertconsult.com.

Section V

Liver Diseases Due to Infectious Agents

Hepatitis A

Daniel Shouval

History

The hepatitis A virus (HAV) has been infecting humans for more than 2000 years. Descriptions of a clinical illness resembling hepatitis have been found in Greek, Roman, and Talmudic scripts dating back to the fifth century BC and in ancient Chinese texts.[1] Nine outbreaks of so-called "epidemic jaundice," later referred to as "catarrhal jaundice," "epidemic hepatitis," and "campaign jaundice," among other terms, were reported in the eighteenth century.[1] The initial evidence for the viral cause of hepatitis was established during the second world war by successive transmission experiments to human volunteers, first in Germany[2] and then in Palestine.[3] The terms epidemic hepatitis and homologous serum jaundice were introduced in 1947,[4] enabling the subsequent distinction between hepatitis A (MS-1) and B (MS-2), respectively, in the 1960s and 1970s.[5] In 1973, HAV was first identified by immune electron microscopy in fecal suspensions collected from infected human volunteers.[6] This breakthrough enabled the development of serologic immunoglobulin G (IgG) and immunoglobulin M (IgM) immunoassays for diagnosis of hepatitis A. Following propagation of HAV in cell culture in 1979,[7] a cDNA copy of the reverse-transcribed HAV-RNA was cloned in 1987 and used for HAV infection of mammalian cells.[8] The ability to propagate HAV in a culture has finally lead to development of efficacious and safe hepatitis A vaccines.[9,10]

Genomic Organization of HAV

The "Wild-Type" HAV

HAV is classified as a *Hepatovirus* of the Picornaviridae family. HAV is a 27- to 32-nm, nonenveloped, icosahedral positive single-stranded linear RNA virus with an approximately 7.5-kb genome. The genome contains three regions, namely a 5′ untranslated region with 734 to 742 nucleotides; a single open reading frame encoding a polyprotein; and a 3′ noncoding region of 40 to 80 nucleotides.[11-13] Upon hepatocyte cell entry, host cell ribosomes bind to the viral uncoated RNA. HAV-RNA is then translated into a major protein of 2225 amino acids. This large polyprotein is divided into three regions: the P1 region encoding for the structural proteins VP1, VP2, and VP3, and the P2 and P3 regions, which encode for nonstructural proteins involved in viral replication. The HAV polyprotein appears to possess a very short VP$_4$ polypeptide segment at its amino terminus. However, this putative moiety was never detected in a purified virus.

HAV-RNA can be detected in body fluids and feces using nucleic acid amplification and sequencing techniques. Such methods, mainly used by research laboratories, have been used for studies on the genetic organization and molecular epidemiology of HAV infection (**Fig. 29-1**). There are six known HAV genotypes. Sequence variations within the VP1/P2A junction are used to define genotypes and subgenotypes. Genotypes have a nucleotide sequence variability of approximately 15% to 25% as compared with up to 7.5% in subgenotypes. Three genotypes, namely I, II, and III, were identified in infected humans, while genotype IV, V, and VI have been found in infected nonhuman primates. All HAV genotypes share a common serotype, irrespective of their origin and whether they derive from wild-type or attenuated strains. The identification of the various HAV genotypes has enhanced the ability to investigate the molecular epidemiology of hepatitis A outbreaks with special emphasis on transmission routes.[11,13] An attempt to correlate specific genomic variations in 5′NTR, 2B, and 2C of HAV with HAV virulence, severity of viral hepatitis A, and development of fulminant hepatitis[14] has not been confirmed so far.[15]

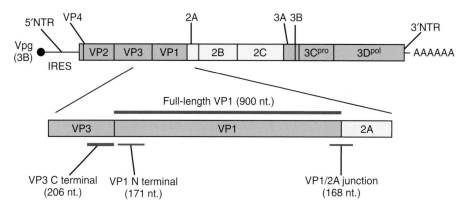

Fig. 29-1 Hepatitis virus genome regions used for studies on genetic analysis and molecular epidemiology of HAV infection. The thick red lines below the genome scheme indicate the different genomic regions used to characterize the different HAV isolates. *(Reproduced by permission from Cristina J, Costa-Mattioli M. Genetic variability and molecular evolution of hepatitis A virus. Virus Res 2007;127:151–157.)*

Table 29-1 Attenuated Hepatitis A Virus Strains Used for Production of Formaldehyde-Inactivated Hepatitis A Virus Vaccines

ATTENUATED HAV STRAIN	TRADE NAME	ADJUVANT	HAV ANTIGEN DOSE/INJECTION		MANUFACTURERS	REFERENCE
			Pediatric	*Adult*		
HM-175	Havrix	Alum hydroxide	720 EU	1440 EU	GSK	10
CR-326	Vaqta	Alum hydroxide	25 U	50 U	MSD	9
GBM	Avaxim	Alum hydroxide	80 U	160 U	Aventis Pasteur	16
TZ84	Healive	Alum hydroxide	250 U	500 U	Sinovac Biotech	18
RG-SB	Epaxal	Virosome	24 U	24 U	Crucell/Berna Biotech	17

Attenuated HAV Strains

Successful propagation of HAV in a culture[7] led to development of several attenuated hepatitis A virus strains that were subsequently used for generation of inactivated HAV vaccines. Vaccine prototypes were tested initially in nonhuman primates and then in human clinical trials.[9,10,16-18]

All HAV vaccines contain HAV antigens derived from cell cultures of attenuated hepatitis A virus strains (**Table 29-1**). Comparison of the nucleotide sequence of cDNA cloned from a wild-type virus (propagated in a marmoset's liver in vivo). with an attenuated HM-175 strain (propagated in tissue culture) revealed a 95% identity with only a small number of nucleotide changes. These were distributed throughout the genome and some are apparently associated with growth adaptation in culture and attenuation.[19]

Epidemiology

Approximately 1.5 million cases of acute hepatitis A are reported annually worldwide with an assumed underreporting rate of up to 80%.[20-25] Thus the reported rates do not reflect the true global burden of disease (GBD). A recent estimate of the GBD by the World Health Organization suggests that tens of millions of individuals are infected each year worldwide (www.who.int/vaccines-documents).

Traditionally, the global spread of HAV infection can be assessed through monitoring of overall and age-specific prevalence or incidence of HAV infection rates. Historically, overall prevalence has been classified into high, intermediate, and low levels of endemicity based on detection of anti-HAV (IgG) antibodies in selected populations. High endemicity of HAV infection is found in countries with poor sanitary and socioeconomic conditions, where infection typically occurs before the age of 5 years. Intermediate endemicity of HAV is typically found in countries in transition from a low socioeconomic status to improved housing and hygienic conditions, mainly in segments of the middle class population. In such countries, the pediatric population may escape HAV infection in early childhood and as a result, older children and young adults become susceptible to HAV infection, which may occur during outbreaks or through person-to-person contact. In countries with low HAV endemicity, the risk for acquiring HAV infection is low or very low.

An epidemiologic shift from high to intermediate endemicity of HAV is now being observed worldwide. As a result, more adults in such areas of transition escape exposure to HAV in early childhood, but become susceptible to infection during outbreaks. This change in susceptibility to HAV infection is paradoxically associated with an increase in disease incidence rates in the presence of improved socioeconomic and sanitary conditions. Data on the global incidence of acute HAV infection are incomplete. A new classification is emerging regarding endemicity of HAV worldwide based on the reported incidence of confirmed acute HAV cases. Thus nowadays endemicity to HAV may be classified as very low, with an estimated incidence of less than 5 cases/10^5; low, 5 to 15 cases/10^5; intermediate, 15 to 150 cases/10^5, and high, greater than 150 cases/10^5. HAV infection is mainly spread through the fecal–oral route, as well as through contaminated water and food. Shellfish are able to ingest and concentrate HAV and as a result become a reservoir for spread of the virus.[26,27] Transmission occurs mainly through common source outbreaks (i.e., food and water borne) and person-to-person contact. HAV is very rarely transmitted through blood products or medical procedures. Epidemiologic risk groups include: populations of low socioeconomic status living under crowded conditions, household contacts with infected individuals, children visiting day care centers and kindergartens, international travelers from countries with low endemicity to areas with intermediate or high endemicity, men who have sex with men (MSM), intravenous drug users, patients with chronic liver disease, food handlers, caretakers of nonhuman primates, and patients with blood clotting disorders. The major risk groups reported by the U.S. Centers for Disease Control and Prevention (CDC) for the year 2007 are shown in **Figure 29-2**.[25]

Pathogenesis

Infection usually occurs through a fecal–oral transmission route following ingestion of food or fluid(s) contaminated by HAV. HAV is shed in the feces for 3 to 6 weeks during the incubation period, extending to the early phase of hepatocellular injury in symptomatic as well as in asymptomatic infected patients. Fecal shedding is maximal at the onset of hepatocellular injury, during a time when the infected individual is most infectious (**Fig. 29-3**). The virus is extremely stable in the environment and survives heating of 60° C for 60 minutes but becomes inactivated at 81° C after 10 minutes.[28,29] Thus the virus may survive in feces, in soil, in food, and in contaminated fresh water, as well as seawater, for a prolonged period. HAV is also resistant to detergents and low pH during transition through the stomach. Upon ingestion, HAV penetrates the gut mucosa where it apparently starts to replicate in intestinal epithelial crypt cells[30] and then reaches the liver via the portal blood. HAV has a special tropism for liver cells. Some cell-culture adopted HAV strains are cytopathic but "wild-type" HAV is noncythopatic in infected human hepatocytes. The mechanism of virus–host cell interaction is not fully understood. A putative HAV surrogate receptor embedded in a cell membrane mucinlike glycoprotein has been identified

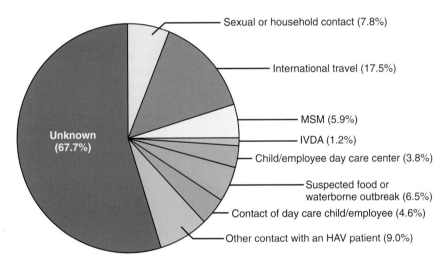

Fig. 29-2 The epidemiologic risk groups for acute hepatitis A virus infection obtained from reported cases in the USA in 2007. Percentage of cases for which a specific risk factor was reported was calculated on the basis of the total number of cases for which any information for that exposure was reported. Percentages dot not total 100% because multiple risk factors have been reported for a single case. MSM, men who have had sex with men; IVDA, intravenous drug abuse. (*Adopted from Daniels D, Grytdal S, Wasley A. Surveillance for acute viral hepatitis—United States, 2007. MMWR Surveill Summ 2009;58:1–27.*)

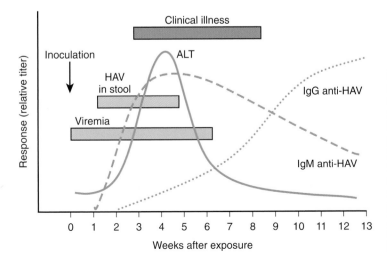

Fig. 29-3 Timeline of clinical and laboratory manifestations of acute hepatitis A. Symptoms and signs of the acute infection usually occur within 2 to 4 weeks of exposure. The sequence of events includes HAV viremia (*green-blue*), shedding of infectious HAV in feces (*orange bar*), followed by increases in serum alanine aminotransferase (ALT) (*green line*), and the appearance of IgM (*blue dashed line*) and total, mainly IgG anti-HAV antibody responses (*blue dotted line*). IgM antibodies decline within 3 months but can be detected in some patients as late as 6 to 12 months postinfection by sensitive assays. Data were obtained during the course of experimental infection in chimpanzees inoculated by IV with human strain HLD2. (*Adopted by permission from Margolis HS, et al. Appearance of immune complexes during experimental hepatitis A infection in chimpanzees. J Med Virol 1988;26:315–326.*)

in African green monkey kidney cells.[31] A human homolog receptor, HAVcr-1, has been described as well.[32,33] However, this protein is not expressed selectively by hepatocytes and therefore does not provide proof for the selective hepatotropism of HAV. Another study suggests that HAV enters the liver cell as a virus-IgA complex through the hepatocellular asialoglycoprotein receptor.[34] Following entry into the hepatocyte cytoplasm, the virus replicates in the liver and then is shed mainly into the feces through the biliary canaliculi and at a lesser degree into the blood stream.

Infection with HAV leads to a cellular immune response, which is involved in the immunopathogenesis of HAV infection and the induction of hepatocyte injury.[35] Liver cell injury occurs through activation of HAV specific cytolytic T cells. Inflammatory cell infiltrates isolated from liver biopsies of patients with hepatitis A contain CD8[+] T cells that can specifically lyse hepatitis A virus–infected target cells in an HLA class I restricted manner.[36] Limited evidence for involvement of the innate immune system in HAV infection suggests that secretion of interferon-γ by activated T cells facilitates expression of HLA class 1 determinants on the surface of infected liver cells.[37] Cytolytic T-cell epitopes residing on the structural protein of HAV may be involved in cytolysis of HAV infected hepatocytes.[37-39] Little is known on the role of T-helper cells in mounting an immune response to HAV. One putative CD4 T-cell helper lymphocyte epitope was identified on the VP3 102 to 121 sequence.[40] There is also some evidence that nonspecific immune mechanisms, including natural killer cells (NK) and lymphokine activated killer cells (LAK), are involved in the induction of hepatocellular injury even before the initiation of cytotoxic T-lymphocyte injury.[41] Finally impaired function of CD4[+]/CD25[+] regulatory T cells has been linked to the frequent resolution of acute hepatitis A with spontaneous recovery.[42]

Diagnosis

Acute HAV infection cannot be distinguished from other causes of hepatitis based on clinical symptoms alone. HAV infection generates a humoral immune response, directed mainly against structural HAV proteins. Diagnosis of acute hepatitis A is confirmed through detection of IgM anti-HAV antibodies. Postinfection and postvaccination immunity is established through detection of total (mainly IgG) anti-HAV antibodies.[43] In the absence of detectable anti-HAV IgM, presence of total anti-HAV antibodies at a titer above 10 to 20 mIU/ml, (depending on immunoassay) signifies immunity against HAV and exclusion of acute HAV infection.

Anti-HAV IgM antibodies are detectable in symptomatic and asymptomatic patients alike. In symptomatic patients, IgM anti-HAV antibodies appear within 5 to 10 days before symptoms or at the early phase of ALT elevation and persist for a period of about 4 months (range 30 to 420 days) (**Fig. 29-3**).[44,45] In patients with relapsing hepatitis A (3% to 20% of patients), IgM anti-HAV, viremia, and shedding of HAV in the feces may reappear intermittently for a period up to 6 months and rarely even longer.[46,47] False-positive IgM anti-HAV may infrequently be present more than 1 year postinfection.[44,48]

Total anti-HAV, IgG antibodies, are usually detectable at the onset of symptoms and their titer rises slowly in parallel to the decrease in titer of anti-HAV, IgM antibodies (see **Fig. 29-1**). IgG anti-HAV antibodies established through natural

infection, provide protection against rechallenge with hepatitis A virus and signify immunity against hepatitis A for life.

In most patients HAV-RNA can be detected during the acute phase by the polymerase chain reaction (PCR) for a limited period of approximately 3 weeks in blood and at higher concentration in stools (for approximately 3 to 6 weeks). In a similar manner, HAV-RNA is detectable in patients with relapsing hepatitis A.[11,46,47,49-51]

Clinical Course of Acute Hepatitis A

Acute hepatitis A virus infection causes an acute necroinflammatory process in the liver, which normally resolves spontaneously without chronic sequelae.[52-54] The incubation period of acute HAV usually lasts between 14 to 28 days and up to 50 days. The likelihood of symptoms during acute HAV infection is age related. In approximately 70% of children beyond the age of 6 years, the disease is mild and asymptomatic and the remaining patients are usually unicteric.[55] In children above the age of 6 years and especially in adults, more than 70% develop jaundice and symptoms that last between 2 and 8 weeks. Prodromal symptoms of acute hepatitis include malaise, fatigue, anorexia, vomiting, abdominal discomfort, diarrhea and, at a later stage and less commonly, fever, headaches, arthralgia, and myalgia[53] (**Table 29-2**). The prodromal symptoms usually regress upon development of jaundice.

Five clinical patterns of hepatitis A are recognized: (1) asymptomatic HAV infection, often present in children under the age of 5 to 6 years; (2) symptomatic HAV infection with the appearance of dark urine and sometimes clay-colored stools, often accompanied or followed by jaundice; (3) cholestatic hepatitis characterized by a protracted course associated with pruritus, prolonged elevation of alkaline phosphates, γ-glutamyl transpeptidase, bilirubinemia, and weight loss[56]; (4) relapsing hepatitis A infection manifested by reappearance

Table 29-2 Most Frequently Reported Symptoms by Patients with Hepatitis A

SYMPTOMS	REPORTED RANGES (%)
Jaundice	40-80
Dark urine	68-94
Fatigue, lassitude	52-91
Loss of appetite, anorexia	42-90
Abdominal pain/discomfort	37-65
Clay-colored (acholic) stools	52-58
Nausea and vomiting	26-87
Fever or chilliness	32-73
Headache	26-73
Arthralgia	11-40
Myalgia	15-52
Diarrhea	16-25
Sore throat	0-20

From Koff RS. Clinical manifestations and diagnosis of hepatitis A virus infection. Vaccine 1992;10(Suppl 1):S15–S17.

of some or all the clinical, biochemical virologic and serologic markers of acute hepatitis A after initial resolution;[46,47] and (5) fulminant hepatitis, which is rare and frequently resolves spontaneously but may be fatal or require liver transplantation.[57,58]

According to one report, the most common signs on physical examination include hepatomegaly and jaundice present in 78% and 71% of symptomatic adult patients respectively. Splenomegaly and lymphadenopathy, are less common.[59]

Extrahepatic and atypical manifestations of acute hepatitis A are relatively rare[60] and include skin involvement (rash), leukocytoclastic vasculitis, pancreatitis, carditis, glomerulonephritis, pneumonitis, hemolysis (especially in patients with glucose-6 phosphate dehydrogenase deficiency), thrombocytopenia, aplastic anemia, cryoglobulinemia, arthritis, neurologic findings including mononeuritis, encephalitis, Guillain-Barré syndrome, and transverse myelitis. A posthepatitic syndrome may occur in a minority of patients who develop prolonged fatigue, right upper quadrant discomfort, fat intolerance and indigestion, weight loss, emotional instability, and prolonged indirect bilirubinemia. Acute HAV infection resolves spontaneously in more than 99% of infected individuals (overall case fatality ratio approximately 0.3% to 0.6%). Relapsing hepatitis A may develop in 3% to 20% of cases.[46,47] The cholestatic and relapsing forms of hepatitis A resolve spontaneously with few exceptions.[61] Fulminant hepatitis is very rare with a wide range of estimated rates up to 1:10,000 or more in immunocompetent, healthy individuals. Mortality in fulminant hepatitis A is declining mainly because of availability of better intensive care and liver transplantation,[57] and is linked to age greater than 50 years (case fatality rate is approximately 1.8%). However, in recent years a rising number of cases with fulminant hepatitis A has been reported in children in South America[58,62,63] and Korea.[23,64] Major risk factors associated with fulminant hepatitis A include age, underlying chronic liver disease,[65,66] intake of paracetamol, co-infection with other viruses such as hepatitis C (HCV),[67] and co-infection with other viral agents.

The outcome of viral hepatitis A in pregnancy is usually unaltered and favorable although the clinical course may be more severe in older women. Cases of vertical transmission from infected mothers to their newborns or perinatal transmission are very rare,[68-71] but premature labor and increased gestational complications have been reported in the second and third trimesters of pregnancy.[72-74]

Differential Diagnosis

The most common differential diagnosis of acute hepatitis A includes, among others, acute viral infections such as hepatitis B, C, and E; Epstein-Barr and cytomegalic viruses; measles; varicella; Q fever; reaction to hepatotoxic drugs, as well as to herbal medicines; bacterial infections and sepsis; and alcoholic and autoimmune hepatitis.

Treatment and Prevention

There are no specific medications for treatment of hepatitis A. Symptomatic treatment and appropriate hydration are essential parts of management. Care must be taken to avoid potentially hepatotoxic drugs with special emphasis on paracetamol. Hand washing and disinfection are necessary means for

patients as well as their close contacts and their healthcare workers.

Immunization Against Hepatitis A

Hepatitis A is a vaccine-preventable disease.[66] Protection is achieved either by passive or active immunization.

Passive Immunization

Between the late 1940s and the 1990s, preexposure and postexposure prophylaxis against hepatitis A was based on administration of hepatitis A immunoglobulin (IG).[75,76] IG is prepared from pooled human plasma by ethanol fractionation.[77] IG is given for preexposure prophylaxis through intramuscular injection at a dose of 0.02 to 0.06 ml/kg body weight and provides protection against HAV within a few hours of injection, lasting for 12 to 20 weeks, respectively. Postexposure prophylaxis is effective in 80% to 90% of cases if given within 14 days of exposure.[78,76] The mechanism of protection against hepatitis A conferred by IG is not fully understood but most probably involves neutralization of the circulating virus and possibly prevention of uptake of the virus through the gut mucosa and by hepatocytes.

Administration of IG is considered very safe, but is contraindicated in patients with IgA deficiency, who may develop an anaphylactic reaction to IG. Interference with live attenuated vaccines, such as MMR and varicella, requires special caution. Co-administration of IG with a hepatitis A vaccine may blunt the anti-HAV antibody response after the first vaccine dose, but this effect is abolished by a booster injection.[79] Although administration of IG for preexposure and postexposure prophylaxis is highly efficacious, the use of IG worldwide is now declining for a number of reasons: (1) Nonspecific IG preparations increasingly fail to contain adequate amounts of anti-HAV (IgG).[80] (2) Cost of specific HAV IG preparation is high.[81] (3) Duration of IG-mediated protection against HAV infection lasts only several months as compared with hepatitis A vaccines.[76] (4) Hepatitis A vaccines have been shown to induce very rapid protection against HAV following the first of two recommended doses.[82]

Active Immunization
PREEXPOSURE PROPHYLAXIS

Formaldehyde-inactivated HAV vaccines derived from attenuated HAV strains were developed in the United States, Belgium, Switzerland, and China (see **Table 29-1**). A live attenuated HAV vaccine is available in China. Efficacy of three inactivated HAV vaccines, HAVRIX, VAQTA, and EPAXAL, was evaluated in controlled clinical trials conducted in Thailand,[10] the United States,[9] and Nicaragua,[83] respectively. Formaldehyde-inactivated hepatitis A vaccines are highly immunogenic and safe.[66] Protection against hepatitis A following the first dose develops rapidly, reaching anti-HAV (IgG) levels of greater than 20 mIU/ml in up to 70% of children within 2 weeks and in 94% to 100% of healthy children and adults within 4 weeks of primary immunization. The booster dose is given at a flexible interval of 6 to 12 or 18 months. Based on clinical data and mathematical modeling, protection against HAV afforded by two doses of inactivated HAV vaccines is estimated to last for decades and possibly for life, and a booster vaccination is unnecessary.[84] Nonresponse to HAV immunization is

Table 29-3 Recommended Doses of Hepatitis A Vaccines*

VACCINE	AGE (yr)	DOSE	VOLUME	SCHEDULE
Havrix	1-18	720 EL.U	0.5 ml	0, 6-12 mo
Havrix	>18	1440 EL.U	1.0 ml	0, 6-12 mo
Vaqta	1-18	25 U	0.5 ml	0, 6-18 mo
Vaqta	>18	50 U	1.0 ml	0, 6-18 mo
Twinrix	>18	720 EL.U, 20 μg HBsAg	1.0 ml	0, 1, 6 mo
Ambirix	1-5	720 El.U 20 μg HBsAg	1.0 ml	0, 16 mo

Modified from Sjogren MH. Hepatitis A. In: Zakim D, Boyer TD, editors: Hepatology: a textbook of liver disease, 5th ed. Philadelphia; Saunders, 2006: 627–634.
Vaccines injected IM in the deltoid area.
EL.U, Elisa units

extremely rare.[85] However, there are a number of factors that may lead to a blunted humoral immune response to inactivated HAV vaccines. Acquired anti-HAV antibodies through passive immunization with IG or following maternal placental transfer from HAV immune mothers to their neonates may suppress the quantitative anti-HAV(IgG) antibody response to active immunization.[86-88] Yet, the somewhat lower level of total anti-HAV (IgG) antibodies measured following primary immunization in such vaccinees has no significant biologic consequences and a booster dose will lead to a similar anamnestic response as in naïve recipients of the active vaccines. Other factors that may attenuate the anti-HAV antibody response to active immunization include age, overweight, smoking, HIV infection, and immune suppression (i.e., transplanted patients, and chronic liver disease).[66]

Infection with live, wild-type HAV involves virus replication in liver cells and is associated with an active cellular and humoral immune response against the virus, which induce hepato-cellular injury. In contrast, viral replication does not occur after immunization with a killed HAV vaccine and protection against HAV is primarily antibody based.[89] Experience with IG and active immunization initially suggested that vaccine-induced protective immunity against hepatitis A is mainly humoral with little involvement of the cellular immune system.[76,82] However, evidence has by now been obtained that immunization against HAV with a killed vaccine also leads to a measurable cellular protective immune response that lasts for at least 6 years and may be boosted to revive the immune memory.[85,90-92]

The monovalent hepatitis A vaccines HAVRIX and VAQTA are licensed worldwide for pediatric and adult use (**Table 29-3**). Combined, bivalent HAV and HBV vaccines are available worldwide for adult use (Twinrix) and for children 1 to 15 years old in Canada and several European countries (Ambirix). Other HAV vaccines formulated with alum hydroxide (Avaxim)[16] or virosomes (Epaxal)[17] are available in many countries on the globe.

Almost 200 million doses of HAV vaccines have been distributed between 1995 and early 2006 worldwide. Based on the cumulative experience gained during these years, the overall safety profile of all formaldehyde-inactivated hepatitis A vaccines administered to children and adults has been excellent, irrespective of manufacturer.[16,17,66]

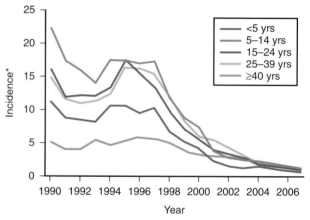

* Per 100,000 population.

Fig. 29-4 U.S. CDC report on decline of hepatitis A incidence between 1990 and 2007. *(Reproduced by permission from Wasley A, Grytdal S, Gallagher K. Surveillance for acute viral hepatitis—United States, 2006. MMWR Surveill Summ 2008;57:1–24.)*

POSTEXPOSURE PROPHYLAXIS

Cumulative experience obtained since 1992 suggests that postexposure immunization against hepatitis A is in general as effective as IG in prevention of HAV infection.[9,93-95] Effectiveness of postexposure prophylaxis with an inactivated HAV vaccine has recently been reported from Kazakhstan.[78] In this controlled trial, 1090 household and daycare contacts (2 to 40 years old) with acute hepatitis A were randomized to receive the hepatitis A vaccine or IG. Transmission of HAV confirmed by anti-HAV IgM testing occurred in 4.4% and 3.3% of the study groups, respectively (RR, 1.35; 95% CI, 0.70 to 2.67). Thus the CDC now recommends this strategy for postexposure prophylaxis in 2 to 40 year olds.[96]

Immunization Strategies

Early strategies for preexposure prophylaxis that are still valid include immunization of defined risk groups, including international travelers to areas with intermediate endemicity, MSM, intravenous drug users, patients with chronic liver

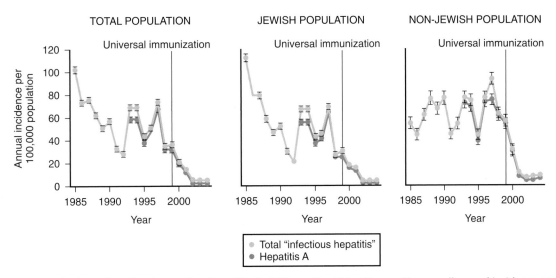

Fig. 29-5 **The impact of universal vaccination against hepatitis A of 18-month-old toddlers on the overall annual incidence rates in Israel.** Data obtained by passive surveillance. Between 1985 and 2004, cases were classified as "infectious hepatitis" (A, B, C, and nonspecified). Afterward, between 1993 and 2004, data include only confirmed hepatitis A cases. *(Reproduced by permission from Dagan R, et al. Incidence of hepatitis A in Israel following universal immunization of toddlers. JAMA 2005;294:202–210.)*

disease, food handlers, day care center staff, caretakers of non-human primates, and patients with blood clotting disorders. Although this policy provided individual protection to vaccinees at risk, it had little public health impact on reduction of disease incidence and herd immunity. The extraordinary immunogenicity, effectiveness, and safety of hepatitis A vaccines, proven repeatedly worldwide,[66,97] has led to a shift in immunization strategies and recommendations from the CDC Advisory Committee on Immunization Practices (ACIP). In 1999, ACIP recommended that routine vaccination against HAV should be implemented in 11 U.S. states with an average annual HAV rate greater than 20 cases per 100,000. Following the impressive reduction in the incidence of HAV in these states, ACIP expanded the recommendation to all children in 50 U.S. states. The results of this effort lead to a massive drop in incidence of hepatitis A in the United States in all age groups up to age 39 years as shown in **Figure 29-4**.[98] Similar experience was gained in Israel following introduction of universal vaccination in toddlers. Israel was a country in transition with an intermediate endemicity of HAV and an overall annual incidence of 33 to 70 cases/100,000 in all age groups. During 1992 to 1998 most HAV infections occurred between the age of 1 and 9 years (annual incidence, 105.7 to 181.2 cases/100,000). In 1999, two doses of an HAV vaccine were given to toddlers at age 18 and 24 months. Within 2 to 3 years from initiation of the program, the incidence of HAV infection dropped by 95% in all pediatric and adult age groups reaching an overall annual rate of approximately 2.5 cases/100,000[99] (**Fig. 29-5**). Although universal vaccination against HAV of toddlers and young children using a two-vaccine dose schedule was shown to be highly effective in the United States and in Israel, a new public health strategy is now being evaluated in Argentina where universal vaccination against hepatitis A was introduced using a single dose in toddlers and children.[100] So far, the incidence of HAV infection using this protocol has dropped by approximately 80%. Duration of protection following single-dose immunization is still not established.

In summary, hepatitis A vaccines have been shown to be highly immunogenic and safe in children and in adults and are used successfully for control of hepatitis A.

Key References

ACIP. Update: prevention of hepatitis A after exposure to hepatitis A virus and in international travelers. Updated recommendations of the Advisory Committee on Immunization Practices (ACIP). MMWR Morb Mortal Wkly Rep 2007;56:1080–1084. (Ref.96)

Akriviadis EA, Redeker AG. Fulminant hepatitis A in intravenous drug users with chronic liver disease. Ann Intern Med 1989;110:838–839. (Ref.65)

Andre FE. Universal mass vaccination against hepatitis A. Curr Top Microbiol Immunol 2006;304:95–114. (Ref.97)

Anonychuk AM, et al. Cost-effectiveness analyses of hepatitis A vaccine: a systematic review to explore the effect of methodological quality on the economic attractiveness of vaccination strategies. Pharmacoeconomics 2008;26:17–32. (Ref.8)

Armstrong GL, Bell BP. Hepatitis A virus infections in the United States: model-based estimates and implications for childhood immunization. Pediatrics 2002;109:839–845. (Ref.21)

Asher LV, et al. Pathogenesis of hepatitis A in orally inoculated owl monkeys (Aotus trivirgatus). J Med Virol 1995;47:260–268. (Ref.30)

Baba M, et al. The role of natural killer cells and lymphokine activated killer cells in the pathogenesis of hepatic injury in hepatitis A. J Clin Lab Immunol 1992;38:1–14. (Ref.4)

Bower WA, et al. Duration of viremia in hepatitis A virus infection. J Infect Dis 2000;182:12–17. (Ref.45)

Cederna JB, Klinzman D, Stapleton JT. Hepatitis A virus-specific humoral and cellular immune responses following immunization with a formalin-inactivated hepatitis A vaccine/ Vaccine 1999;18:892–898. (Ref.90)

Centeno MA, Bes DF, Sasbon JS. Mortality risk factors of a pediatric population with fulminant hepatic failure undergoing orthotopic liver transplantation in a pediatric intensive care unit. Pediatr Crit Care Med 2002;3:227–233. (Ref.62)

Ciocca M, et al. Hepatitis A as an etiologic agent of acute liver failure in Latin America. Pediatr Infect Dis J 2007;26:711–715. (Ref.63)

Cohen JI, et al. Complete nucleotide sequence of an attenuated hepatitis A virus: comparison with wild-type virus. Proc Natl Acad Sci U S A 1987;84: 2497–2501. (Ref.19)

Cohen JI, et al. Hepatitis A virus cDNA and its RNA transcripts are infectious in cell culture. J Virol 1987;61:3035–3039. (Ref.8)

Cohn EJ, et al. Chemical, clinical, and immunological studies on the products of human plasma fractionation. I. The characterization of the protein fractions of human plasma. J Clin Invest 1944;23:417–432. (Ref.77)

Cristina J, Costa-Mattioli M. Genetic variability and molecular evolution of hepatitis A virus. Virus Res 2007;127:151–157. (Ref.13)

Dagan R, et al. Immunization against hepatitis A in the first year of life: priming despite the presence of maternal antibody. Pediatr Infect Dis J 2000;19: 1045–1052. (Ref.86)

Dagan R, et al. Incidence of hepatitis A in Israel following universal immunization of toddlers. JAMA 2005;294:202–210. (Ref.99)

Daniels D, Grytdal S, Wasley A. Surveillance for acute viral hepatitis—United States, 2007. MMWR Surveill Summ 2009;58:1–27. (Ref.25)

Dotzauer A, et al. Hepatitis A virus-specific immunoglobulin A mediates infection of hepatocytes with hepatitis A virus via the asialoglycoprotein receptor. J Virol 2000;74:10950–10957. (Ref.34)

Elinav E, et al. Acute hepatitis A infection in pregnancy is associated with high rates of gestational complications and preterm labor. Gastroenterology 2006;130:1129–1134. (Ref.74)

Feigelstock D, et al. The human homolog of HAVcr-1 codes for a hepatitis A virus cellular receptor. J Virol 1998;72:6621–6628. (Ref.32)

Feinstone SM, Kapikian AZ, Purceli RH. Hepatitis A: detection by immune electron microscopy of a viruslike antigen associated with acute illness. Science 1973;182:1026–1028. (Ref.6)

Ferreira CT, et al. Hepatitis A acute liver failure: follow-up of paediatric patients in southern Brazil. J Viral Hepat 2008;15(Suppl 2):66–68. (Ref.58)

Fiore AE, Wasley A, Bell BP. Prevention of hepatitis A through active or passive immunization: recommendations of the Advisory Committee on Immunization Practices (ACIP). MMWR Recomm Rep 2006;55:123. (Ref.66)

FitzSimons D, et al. Hepatitis A and E: update on prevention and epidemiology. Vaccine 2010;28:583–588. (Ref.24)

Fujiwara K, et al. Phylogenetic analysis of hepatitis A virus in sera from patients with hepatitis A of various severities. Liver Int 2009;29:838–845. (Ref.14)

Garner-Spitzer E, et al. Correlation between humoral and cellular immune responses and the expression of the hepatitis A receptor HAVcr-1 on T cells after hepatitis A re-vaccination in high and low-responder vaccinees. Vaccine 2009;27:197–204. (Ref.85)

Glikson M, et al. Relapsing hepatitis A. Review of 14 cases and literature survey. Medicine (Baltimore) 1992;71:14–23. (Ref.47)

Gordon SC, et al. Prolonged intrahepatic cholestasis secondary to acute hepatitis A. Ann Intern Med 1984;101:635–637. (Ref.56)

Gust ID. Epidemiological patterns of hepatitis A in different parts of the world. Vaccine 1992;10(Suppl 1):S56–S58. (Ref.20)

Hadler SC, et al. Hepatitis A in day-care centers. A community-wide assessment. N Engl J Med 1980;302:1222–1227. (Ref.55)

Halliday ML, et al. An epidemic of hepatitis A attributable to the ingestion of raw clams in Shanghai, China. J Infect Dis 1991;164:852–859. (Ref.27)

Hashimoti E, et al. Immunohistochemical characterization of hepatic lymphocytes in acute hepatitis A, B, and C. J Clin Gastroenterol 1996;23: 199–202. (Ref.36)

Hayney MS, Buck JM, Muller D. Production of interferon-gamma and interleukin-10 after inactivated hepatitis A immunization. Pharmacotherapy 2003;23:431–435. (Ref.91)

Hendrickx G, et al. Has the time come to control hepatitis A globally? Matching prevention to the changing epidemiology. J Viral Hepat 2008;15(Suppl 2): 1–15. (Ref.23)

Hieber JP, et al. Hepatitis and pregnancy. J Pediatr 1977;91:545–549. (Ref.73)

Howell D, Barbara JA, Brennan M. Hepatitis A virus, blood donors, and immunoglobulin preparations. Lancet 1991;337:1165. letter. (Ref.80)

Innis BL, et al. Protection against hepatitis A by an inactivated vaccine. JAMA 1994;271:1328–1334. (Ref.10)

Jacobsen KH, Koopman JS. Declining hepatitis A seroprevalence: a global review and analysis. Epidemiol Infect 2004;132:1005–1022. (Ref.22)

Jeong SH, Lee HS. Hepatitis A: clinical manifestations and management. Intervirology; 2010;53:15–19. (Ref.64)

Jiang WP, et al. Immunogenicity and safety of three consecutive lots of a new preservative-free inactivated hepatitis A vaccine (Healive): a double-blind, randomized and controlled trial. Vaccine 2008;26:2297–2301. (Ref.18)

Kao HW, Ashcavai M, Redeker AG. The persistence of hepatitis A IgM antibody after acute clinical hepatitis A. Hepatology 1984;4:933–936. (Ref.48)

Kaplan G, et al. Identification of a surface glycoprotein on African green monkey kidney cells as a receptor for hepatitis A virus. EMBO J 1996;15:4282–4296. (Ref.3)

Koff RS. Clinical manifestations and diagnosis of hepatitis A virus infection. Vaccine 1992;10(Suppl 1):S15–S17. (Ref.53)

Krugman S, Giles JP. Viral hepatitis. New light on an old disease. JAMA 1970; 212:1019–1029. (Ref.52)

Krugman S, Giles JP, Hammond J. Infectious hepatitis. Evidence for two distinctive clinical, epidemiological, and immunological types of infection. JAMA 1967;200:365–373. (Ref.5)

Kurane I, et al. Human lymphocyte responses to hepatitis A virus-infected cells: interferon production and lysis of infected cells. J Immunol 1985;135: 2140–2144. (Ref.37)

Lednar WM, et al. Frequency of illness associated with epidemic hepatitis A virus infections in adults. Am J Epidemiol 1985;122:226–233. (Ref.54)

Lees D. Viruses and bivalve shellfish. Int J Food Microbiol 2000;59:81–116. (Ref.26)

Leikin E, et al. Intrauterine transmission of hepatitis A virus. Obstet Gynecol 1996;88(4 Pt 2):690–691. (Ref.69)

Lemon SM. Immunologic approaches to assessing the response to inactivated hepatitis A vaccine. J Hepatol 1993;18(Suppl 2):S15–S19. (Ref.89)

Lemon SM. Type A viral hepatitis: epidemiology, diagnosis, and prevention. Clin Chem 1997;43(8 Pt 2):1494–1499. (Ref.43)

Liaw YF, Yang CY, Chu CM, Huang MJ. Appearance and persistence of hepatitis A IgM antibody in acute clinical hepatitis A observed in an outbreak. Infection 1986;14:156–158. (Ref.44)

Lieberman JM, et al. Kinetics of maternal hepatitis A antibody decay in infants: implications for vaccine use. Pediatr Infect Dis J 2002;21:347–348. (Ref.87)

Liu JP, Nikolova D, Fei Y. Immunoglobulins for preventing hepatitis A. Cochrane Database Syst Rev 2009:CD004181. (Ref.76)

Lysy Y, et al. Fatal relapsing viral hepatitis A infection during pregnancy. Isr J Med Sci 1988;24:681–683. (Ref.6)

MacCallum F. Homologous serum jaundice. Lancet 1947;2:691–692. (Ref.4)

Margolis HS, et al. Appearance of immune complexes during experimental hepatitis A infection in chimpanzees. J Med Virol 1988;26:315–326. (Ref.101)

Martin A, Lemon SM. Hepatitis A virus: from discovery to vaccines. Hepatology 2006;43(2 Suppl 1):S164–S172. (Ref.12)

Mayorga Perez O, et al. Efficacy of virosome hepatitis A vaccine in young children in Nicaragua: randomized placebo-controlled trial. J Infect Dis 2003;188:671–677. (Ref.83)

McCaustland KA, et al. Survival of hepatitis A virus in feces after drying and storage for 1 month. J Clin Microbiol 1982;16:957–958. (Ref.28)

Nainan OV, et al. Diagnosis of hepatitis A virus infection: a molecular approach. Clin Microbiol Rev 2006;19:63–79. (Ref.11)

Normann A, et al. Time course of hepatitis A viremia and viral load in the blood of human hepatitis A patients. J Med Virol 2004;72:10–16. (Ref.51)

Oren R, Shouval D, Tur-Kaspa R. Detection of hepatitis A virus RNA in serum from patients with acute hepatitis. J Med Virol 1989;28:261–263. (Ref.49)

Perrella A, et al. Impaired function of CD4+/CD25+ T regulatory lymphocytes characterizes the self-limited hepatitis A virus infection. J Gastroenterol Hepatol 2008;23(7 Pt 2):e105–e110. (Ref.42)

Prikazsky V, et al. Interruption of an outbreak of hepatitis A in two villages by vaccination. J Med Virol 1994;44:457–459. (Ref.93)

Provost PJ, Hilleman MR. Propagation of human hepatitis A virus in cell culture in vitro. Proc Soc Exp Biol Med 1979;160:213–221. (Ref.7)

Ranger-Rogez S, Alain S, Denis F. Hepatitis viruses: mother to child transmission. Pathol Biol (Paris) 2002;50:568–575. (Ref.68)

Rezende G, et al. Viral and clinical factors associated with the fulminant course of hepatitis A infection. Hepatology 2003;38:613–618. (Ref.15)

Sagliocca L, et al. Efficacy of hepatitis A vaccine in prevention of secondary hepatitis A infection: a randomised trial. Lancet 1999;353:1136–1139. (Ref.94)

Sanchez G, Pinto RM, Bosch A. A novel CD4+ T-helper lymphocyte epitope in the VP3 protein of hepatitis A virus. J Med Virol 2004;72:525–532. (Ref.40)

Schiff ER. Atypical clinical manifestations of hepatitis A. Vaccine 1992;10(Suppl 1):S18–S20. (Ref.60)

Schmidtke P, et al. Cell mediated and antibody immune response to inactivated hepatitis A vaccine. Vaccine 2005;23:5127–5132. (Ref.92)

Shouval D, et al. Single and booster dose responses to an inactivated hepatitis A virus vaccine: comparison with immune serum globulin prophylaxis. Vaccine 1993;11(Suppl 1):S9–S14. (Ref.82)

Siegl G, Weitz M, Kronauer G. Stability of hepatitis A virus. Intervirology 1984; 22:218–226. (Ref.29)

Sjogren MH, et al. Hepatitis A virus in stool during clinical relapse. Ann Intern Med 1987;106:221–226. (Ref.46)

Sjogren MH, Hepatitis A. In: Zakim D, Boyer TD, editors: Hepatology: a text book of liver disease, 5th ed. Philadelphia: Philadelphia; Saunders, 2006: 627–634. (Ref.102)

Stokes J Jr, et al. Methods of protection against homologous serum hepatitis: studies on the protective value of gamma globulin in homologous serum hepatitis Sh virus. JAMA 1948;138:336–341. (Ref.75)

Tami C, et al. Immunoglobulin A (IgA) is a natural ligand of hepatitis A virus cellular receptor 1 (HAVCR1), and the association of IgA with HAVCR1 enhances virus-receptor interactions. J Virol 2007;81:3437–3446. (Ref.33)

Taylor RM, et al. Fulminant hepatitis A virus infection in the United States: incidence, prognosis, and outcomes. Hepatology 2006;44:1589–1597. (Ref.57)

Tong MJ, el-Farra NS, Grew MI. Clinical manifestations of hepatitis A: recent experience in a community teaching hospital. J Infect Dis 1995;171(Suppl 1):S15–S18. (Ref.59)

Tong MJ, et al. Studies on the maternal-infant transmission of the viruses which cause acute hepatitis. Gastroenterology 1981;80(5 Pt 1):999–1004. (Ref.70)

Usonis V, et al. Antibody titres after primary and booster vaccination of infants and young children with a virosomal hepatitis A vaccine (Epaxal). Vaccine 2003;21:4588–4592. (Ref.88)

Vacchino MN. Incidence of Hepatitis A in Argentina after vaccination. J Viral Hepat 2008;15(Suppl 2):47–50. (Ref.100)

Vallbracht A, et al. Cell-mediated cytotoxicity in hepatitis A virus infection. Hepatology 1986;6:1308–1314. (Ref.39)

Vallbracht A, et al. Liver-derived cytotoxic T cells in hepatitis A virus infection. J Infect Dis 1989;160:209–217. (Ref.35)

Van Damme P, et al. Hepatitis A booster vaccination: is there a need? Lancet 2003;362:1065–1071. (Ref.84)

Van Der Wielen M, et al. Immunogenicity and safety of a pediatric dose of a virosome-adjuvanted hepatitis A vaccine: a controlled trial in children aged 1-16 years. Pediatr Infect Dis J 2007;26:705–710. (Ref.17)

Vento S, et al. Fulminant hepatitis associated with hepatitis A virus superinfection in patients with chronic hepatitis C. N Engl J Med 1998;338:286–290. (Ref.67)

Victor JC, et al. Hepatitis A vaccine versus immune globulin for postexposure prophylaxis. N Engl J Med 2007;357:1685–1694. (Ref.78)

Vidor E, et al. Aventis Pasteur vaccines containing inactivated hepatitis A virus: a compilation of immunogenicity data. Eur J Clin Microbiol Infect Dis 2004;23:300–309. (Ref.16)

Walter EB, et al. Concurrent administration of inactivated hepatitis A vaccine with immune globulin in healthy adults. Vaccine 1999;17:1468–1473. (Ref.79)

Wasley A, Grytdal S, Gallagher K. Surveillance for acute viral hepatitis—United States, 2006. MMWR Surveill Summ 2008;57:1–24. (Ref.98)

Watson JC, et al. Vertical transmission of hepatitis A resulting in an outbreak in a neonatal intensive care unit. J Infect Dis 1993;167:567–571. (Ref.71)

Werzberger A, et al. A controlled trial of a formalin-inactivated hepatitis A vaccine in healthy children. N Engl J Med 1992;327:453–457. (Ref.9)

Willner IR, et al. Serious hepatitis A: an analysis of patients hospitalized during an urban epidemic in the United States. Ann Intern Med 1998;128:111–114. (Ref.72)

Wunschmann S, et al. Cytolytic T-lymphocyte epitopes are present on hepatitis A virus structural proteins. Turin, Italy: Minerva Medica, 1997. (Ref.38)

Yotsuyanagi H, et al. Duration of viremia in human hepatitis A viral infection as determined by polymerase chain reaction. J Med Virol 1993;40:35–38. (Ref.50)

Zamir C, et al. Control of a community-wide outbreak of hepatitis A by mass vaccination with inactivated hepatitis A vaccine. Eur J Clin Microbiol Infect Dis 2001;20:185–187. (Ref.95)

Zuckerman A. The history of viral hepatitis from antiquity to the present. In: Deinhardt F, Deinhard J: Viral hepatitis: laboratory and clinical science, 1st ed. New York: Marcel Dekker, 1983:3–32. (Ref.1)

A complete list of references can be found at www.expertconsult.com.

Hepatitis B

Henry Lik-Yuen Chan and Vincent Wai-Sun Wong

ABBREVIATIONS

AFP α-fetoprotein	**BMI** body mass index	**HCC** hepatocellular carcinoma
ALT alanine aminotransferase	**GGT** γ-glutamyl transpeptidase	**HCV** hepatitis C virus
ALP alkaline phosphatase	**HBIG** hepatitis B immunoglobulin	**HDV** hepatitis D virus
anti-HBc hepatitis B core antibody	**HBcAg** hepatitis B core antigen	**HIV** human immunodeficiency virus
anti-HBe hepatitis B e antibody	**HBeAg** hepatitis B e antigen	**PCR** polymerase chain reaction
anti-HBs hepatitis B surface antibody	**HBsAg** hepatitis B surface antigen	
AST aspartate aminotransferase	**HBV** hepatitis B virus	

Introduction

Approximately 350 million people in the world are chronically infected by hepatitis B virus (HBV), which is a major cause of liver cirrhosis and hepatocellular carcinoma (HCC). The diagnosis of HBV infection was revolutionized by the discovery of Australia antigen, now called hepatitis B surface antigen (HBsAg), by Blumberg in 1965.[1] During the ensuing decade, serologic assays for HBsAg, as well as other HBV antigens and antibodies, were identified and serologic assays for their detection were established. HBV vaccination was first introduced in 1980s for prevention of new HBV infection. Advances in molecular biology techniques in the 1980s led to the development of hybridization assays for direct determination of virus replication and polymerase chain reaction (PCR) assays that permitted the detection of as little as 10 molecules of HBV DNA per milliliter of serum. Interferon treatment for chronic hepatitis B was available in the mid-1980s, but its use was not popular because of its limited effectiveness, inconvenient route of administration, and multiple adverse effects. No new medical treatment was available for more than 10 years, until the late 1990s, when lamivudine was registered as the first oral antiviral agent against HBV. It was followed by an explosion in the development of anti-HBV therapy, with numerous antiviral agents flooding the market in the last decade. Interferon was also upgraded with pegylation to allow weekly injection of the medication. All these medical advances have changed chronic hepatitis B from a dreadful, incurable disease into a preventable and treatable condition.

Epidemiology
Burden of Disease

Seventy-five percent of the chronic HBV-infected patients reside in Asia and the western Pacific. HBV-related end-stage liver disease or HCC accounts for more than 1 million deaths per year. In Asia excluding Japan, chronic HBV infection is the cause for 60% to 80% of the cases of HCC, and HBV-related liver disease is the major reason for liver transplantation. In an U.S. national survey performed from 1988 to 1994, it was estimated that approximately 800 million people were suffering from ongoing infection with HBV.[2] However, this was probably a serious underestimate as the high-risk populations, such as Asians, Pacific Islanders, and the Alaskan Natives as well as the institutionalized, homeless, or incarcerated individuals, were underrepresented in the survey.

Universal HBV vaccination to newborns was started in the mid-1980s in Taiwan followed by several Southeast Asian countries. In 1991, the World Health Organization recommended integration of HBV vaccination into the neonatal programs in countries with a hepatitis B carrier prevalence of 8% or higher. In the United States, universal vaccination of all newborns was implemented in 1992. HBV vaccination is currently part of the National Infant Immunization Program in more than 160 countries and the global infant vaccine coverage reached 65% in 2007. Universal vaccination has dramatically reduced the prevalence of HBV infection in the vaccinated population. The prevalence of adult chronic HBV infection is expected to fall in countries or regions such as Korea, Hong Kong, Thailand, Malaysia, Singapore, and Taiwan that adopted infant HBV immunization in the mid to late 1980s. Reduction in childhood HCC has been demonstrated in Taiwan after the launching of the vaccination program, but its benefit in adult HCC may take more time to become evident.[3] Nonetheless, there is still a wide variation in the infant coverage rate in different parts of Asia, and some Asian countries such as the Philippines, India, and Cambodia have not yet implemented universal HBV vaccination for newborns.

In the United States, the age-adjusted mortality rate for HBV-infected individuals increased throughout the 1980s and 1990s but started to fall after 2000.[2] Similarly, the waiting list for liver transplantation due to end-stage liver disease peaked in 2000 and fell by 37% by 2006. Hospitalization due to HBV-related diagnoses also rose in the early 1990s and seemed to reach a plateau in 2004 to 2006. All these observations are probably related to the introduction of antiviral therapy, which may have decreased the number of patients developing complications of end-stage liver disease due to HBV in the mid to late 1990s.

Prevalence of HBV Infection

The prevalence of HBV infection varies in different geographic areas (**Table 30-1**). The HBV carrier rate is about 0.1% to 2% in low-prevalence areas, such as the United States, western Europe, Australia, and New Zealand. It increases to approximately 3% to 5% in intermediate-prevalence areas such as the Mediterranean countries, Japan, India, and Singapore and 10% to 20% in high-prevalence areas such as Southeast Asia and sub-Saharan Africa. The lifetime risk of being exposed to HBV infection is approximately 20% in low-risk areas, 20% to 60% in intermediate-risk areas, and 60% to 80% in high-risk areas. Within the United States, the prevalence of HBV infection is higher among African Americans, Hispanics, and Asians than in the white population. The majority of the non-white HBV-infected population are immigrants born outside America coming from Asia, Central America, the Caribbean, Africa, and Eastern Europe.[2] Several communities have been reported to have higher carrier rates than their neighboring regions, namely Alaskan Eskimos, Asian-Pacific Islanders, and Australian Aborigines.

In most high-prevalence areas such as China, perinatal transmission is the major mode of spread, accounting for 40% to 50% of chronic HBV infection. Horizontal spread during the first 2 years of life is the major mode of transmission in other endemic areas, including Africa and the Middle East. The preponderance of perinatal transmission among Asians is probably related to the high prevalence of hepatitis B e antigen (HBeAg) among Asian carriers of reproductive age. The risk of HBV transmission by an HBeAg-positive carrier mother to the offspring is about 60% to 90%, while that of an HBeAg-negative mother is only 15% to 20%. Approximately 90% of infected infants will develop a chronic infection after acquiring HBV at birth. In intermediate-prevalence areas, transmission occurs at all age groups but early childhood infection accounts for most cases of chronic infection. In low-prevalence areas, most infections are acquired in early adult life through unprotected sexual intercourse or intravenous

drug abuse. The risk of developing a chronic infection decreases with age, from 25% to 50% in children infected between the age of 1 and 5 years to less than 5% in those infected during adult life.

Mode of HBV Transmission

The exclusion of paid donors and the application of hepatitis B serologic screening have almost eliminated the risk of HBV transmission by blood transfusion. The major modes of HBV transmission are through perinatal, percutaneous, and sexual routes.

Perinatal Transmission

In high-endemic areas, the rate of perinatal infection can be as high as 90% without vaccination to the newborn, particularly when the pregnant woman is HBeAg or serum HBV DNA positive. Maternal–infant transmission takes place at the time of delivery by maternal–fetal transfusion or exposure to maternal blood during passage through the birth canal. HBV transmission can also take place at infancy through intimate mother–baby contact, and cases of possible father–to–baby transmission have been reported. Intrauterine transmission is uncommon because the detection of HBsAg in infants is frequently delayed. Cesarean section cannot reduce the risk of perinatal HBV transmission. Although HBsAg can be detected in breast milk, there is no evidence that HBV infection can be transmitted by breastfeeding.

Percutaneous Transmission

Hepatitis B virus is efficiently transmitted by percutaneous and mucous membrane exposure to infectious blood and body fluids. HBV is approximately 100 times more infectious than the human immunodeficiency virus (HIV) and 10 times more infectious than hepatitis C virus. HBV DNA has been demonstrated in most body fluid by PCR, but only semen and saliva have been consistently shown to harbor infectious virions.

Needle sharing by intravenous drug users is an important route of transmission of HBV. Reuse of contaminated needles for tattoos, acupuncture, and ear piercing also provide opportunities for percutaneous transmission. In the healthcare environment, needlestick injury, exposure to contaminated medical instruments, hemodialysis, and exposure to infected

Table 30-1 Prevalence of HBV Infection in Different Geographic Areas

Prevalence	Geographic distribution	Route of transmission	Age of infection
High (10%-20%)	Southeast Asia China Sub-Saharan Africa Alaska	Perinatal Percutaneous	Perinatal and early childhood
Intermediate (3%-5%)	Mediterranean Central Asia Middle East Japan Latin and South America	Percutaneous Sexual	Early childhood
Low (0.1%-2%)	North America Western Europe Australia New Zealand	Sexual Percutaneous	Adult

healthcare workers, particularly during invasive and surgical procedures, can also be sources of HBV infection. In the recent European practice guideline, healthcare workers who have high HBV viremia involved in exposure-prone procedures are recommended to receive antiviral agents to reduce the risk of transmitting the virus.[4] In endemic areas, horizontal transmission among children may result from close bodily contact, leading to transfer of the virus across minor skin breaks and mucous membranes. Direct inoculation of HBV through saliva by human bite has been documented to cause acute HBV infection. Bloodfeeding insects such as mosquitoes can serve as vectors for HBV transmission in animal models but firm evidence for this mode of transmission in humans is lacking. Because HBV remains stable for a long time outside the human body, transmission via contaminated environmental surfaces and daily articles, such as toothbrushes, razors, eating utensils, or even toys, may also be possible.

Sexual Transmission

Sexual transmission accounts for approximately 30% of acute HBV infection in the United States. A high prevalence of chronic HBV infection has been reported in homosexuals and in heterosexuals with multiple sex partners. The risk of sexual transmission of HBV infection is proportional to the number of lifetime sex partners, low education level, paid sex, and history of sexually transmitted diseases. Since the late 1980s, the rate of sexual transmission of HBV has dropped to less than 10%, probably as a result of modification of high-risk sexual behavior secondary to the HIV epidemic.

Clinical Manifestations
Acute HBV
Symptoms and Signs

The incubation period of acute HBV infection lasts 1 to 4 months. During the prodromal period, a serum sickness-like syndrome manifested as fever, skin rash, arthralgia, and arthritis may develop. This is followed by insidious onset of constitutional symptoms including malaise, anorexia, nausea, and occasionally vomiting, low-grade fever, myalgia, and easy fatigability. Patients may have disordered gustatory acuity and smell sensation. Some patients may experience intermittent mild to moderate right upper quadrant or epigastric pain. Approximately 70% of patients have subclinical or anicteric hepatitis and only 30% have icteric hepatitis. Jaundice, if present, usually begins within 10 days after the onset of constitutional symptoms. Serum sickness-like syndrome and constitutional symptoms generally subside after the peak of aminotransferases and the development of jaundice. Patients may have hepatic encephalopathy and multiorgan failure if fulminant hepatic failure occurs. Clinical symptoms and jaundice usually disappear after 1 to 3 months, but some patients may have persistent fatigue after normalization of the aminotransferase levels. Physical examination can be unrevealing. The most common findings include low-grade temperature, clinical icterus, and soft, mildly tender hepatomegaly. Splenomegaly may be found in approximately 5% to 15% of patients. Mild lymph node enlargement may be present. Rarely palmar erythema or spider nevi can be detected.

Laboratory Findings

Elevation of alanine and aspartate aminotransferases (ALT and AST) up to 1000 IU/L to 2000 IU/L is typically seen, with ALT being higher than AST. The increase in bilirubin usually lags behind the increase in ALT. The peak ALT level has no correlation with prognosis. Because of the short half-life of clotting factors (6 hours for factor VII), prothrombin time is the best indicator of prognosis. Mild leucopenia with relative lymphocytosis is common. In patients who recover, ALT usually returns to normal after 1 to 4 months followed by normalization in serum bilirubin.

Sequelae

The risk of chronicity is inversely proportional to the age at infection. Chronic infection will develop in fewer than 5% of immunocompetent adults but in up to 95% of those infected during infancy. Fewer than 1% of patients with acute hepatitis B develop fulminant hepatic failure. Acute HBV infection is estimated to account for 35% to 70% of all virally related cases of fulminant hepatitis. It accounts for 5% of all cases of acute liver failure and approximately 400 deaths annually in the United States. The spontaneous survival rate from fulminant hepatitis B is approximately 20% without liver transplantation. Liver transplantation has resulted in a 50% to 60% survival rate. Reinfection of the liver graft after liver transplantation is uncommon due to the prophylaxis with hepatitis B immunoglobulin and antiviral agents.

Chronic Hepatitis B
Symptoms and Signs

In areas of low or intermediate prevalence, approximately 30% to 50% of cases of chronic HBV infection are preceded by a classical clinical acute hepatitis. A history of acute or symptomatic hepatitis is often lacking in the vast majority of chronic hepatitis B patients in high-prevalence areas where perinatal infection is the predominant mode of transmission. Most patients with chronic HBV infection are asymptomatic. Occasionally, nonspecific symptoms, such as fatigue or mild right upper quadrant or epigastric pain, may be present. Physical examination may be unrevealing or there may be stigmata of chronic liver disease and a mild hepatomegaly. Among patients with liver cirrhosis, splenomegaly may be detected. Hepatic decompensation may present as variceal bleeding, ascites, jaundice, peripheral edema, and hepatic encephalopathy. Patients with chronic HBV infection may experience spontaneous acute exacerbations that may mimic acute hepatitis with fatigue, anorexia, nausea, and jaundice and, in rare instances, progress to hepatic decompensation.

Laboratory Findings

Laboratory tests including ALT levels and blood counts can be entirely normal in chronic hepatitis B patients, as well as in patients with compensated cirrhosis. In other patients, mild to moderate liver enzyme elevation may be the only biochemical abnormality. ALT levels are generally higher than AST levels. During spontaneous acute exacerbation of chronic

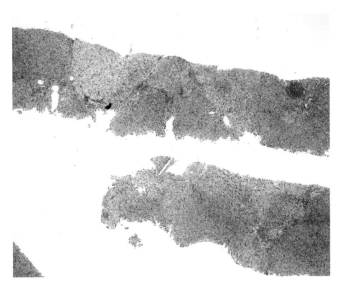

Fig. 30-1 Low (×40) magnification of the Masson Trichrome stained sections shows portal inflammation and significant portal–portal fibrosis but no regenerative nodules. *(Photo courtesy Dr. Paul Choi, Department of Anatomical and Cellular Pathology, Prince of Wales Hospital, Hong Kong.)*

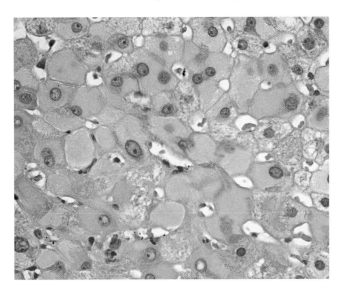

Fig. 30-2 High magnification shows that most of the hepatocytes have the homogenous "ground glass" appearance. (H&E ×40, ×60). *(Photo courtesy Dr. Paul Choi, Department of Anatomical and Cellular Pathology, Prince of Wales Hospital, Hong Kong.)*

hepatitis B, very high ALT levels, up to 1000 IU/ml, may be seen. Some patients, particularly those with underlying liver cirrhosis, may develop hepatic decompensation during exacerbation with elevated serum bilirubin and deranged clotting profiles. The increase in α-fetoprotein (AFP) levels may parallel the rise in ALT levels, and it often creates false alarms at HCC surveillance. Low platelet and leukocyte counts may indicate hypersplenism and liver cirrhosis should be suspected. Hypoalbuminemia, hyperbilirubinemia, and prolongation in prothrombin time are features of hepatic decompensation in advanced liver cirrhosis.

Histologic Findings

The predominant histologic findings include inflammatory cell infiltration in the portal tracts and periportal necrosis. The inflammatory infiltrate consists mainly of mononuclear cells. Periportal necrosis may be mild or severe, leading to disruption of the limiting plate (referred to as interface hepatitis). As the liver damage progresses, fibrous tissue is deposited initially within the portal tracts, later extending into the centrilobular areas and adjacent portal tracts forming bridging fibrosis and eventually cirrhosis (**Fig. 30-1**). In some patients, "ground glass" hepatocytes that stain positive for HBsAg can be found (**Fig. 30-2**). Abundance of "ground glass" hepatocytes often indicates a state of active viral replication. Hepatitis B core antigen (HBcAg) is usually seen inside the nucleus of the hepatocytes. Persistence of nuclear HBcAg staining after successful nucleos(t)ide analog treatment indicates persistence of the closed covalently circular (ccc) DNA template.

Extrahepatic Manifestations

Extrahepatic manifestations occur in about 10% to 20% of patients with chronic HBV infection. The exact pathogenesis of these manifestations has not been fully elucidated. They are believed to be mediated by circulating immune complexes. It is important to recognize these manifestations because they may occur without clinically apparent liver disease.

Polyarteritis Nodosa

Approximately 10% to 50% of patients with polyarteritis nodosa are found to be HBsAg positive. Circulating immune complexes containing HBsAg are believed to trigger the vascular injury. Vasculitis may affect large-, medium-, and small-sized vessels in multiple organs, including cardiovascular (pericarditis, hypertension, cardiac failure), renal (hematuria, proteinuria, renal failure), gastrointestinal (abdominal pain, mesenteric vasculitis), musculoskeletal (arthralgia, arthritis), neurologic (polyneuropathy or mononeuritis, intracranial hemorrhage, central nervous system involvement), and dermatologic (tender subcutaneous nodules, livedo reticularis, angioedema, urticaria, ulceration) systems. The clinical course is highly variable. There is no apparent relationship between the severity of vasculitis and the severity of liver disease. Despite combination treatment with corticosteroid, immunosuppressive drugs, and plasma exchange, the mortality is high: 20% to 45% in 5 years. Preliminary data suggest a possible role for interferon monotherapy or in combination with plasma exchange, but further studies are required to confirm the efficacy of these therapies.[5]

Glomerulonephritis

Hepatitis B virus–related glomerulonephritis is more often found in children. Membranous glomerulonephritis is the most common type, especially among children, but membranoproliferative glomerulonephritis and immunoglobulin A (IgA) nephropathy have also been reported. Nephrotic syndrome is the commonest presentation. The diagnosis of HBV-related glomerulonephritis is usually established by serologic evidence of chronic hepatitis B, the presence of immune complex glomerulonephritis on renal biopsy, and the demonstration of immune complexes of hepatitis B surface, core, and/or e antigens in the glomerular basement membrane and mesangium by immunohistochemistry. Liver disease tends to be mild in patients who have HBV-related glomerulonephritis. Approximately 30% to 60% of children with HBV-related membranous glomerulonephritis undergo spontaneous remission. Remission accompanying HBeAg seroconversion has also been reported. Corticosteroids are usually ineffective and may potentiate HBV replication. Interferon has been reported to induce remission of HBV-related renal disease in small clinical trials, but the response is less satisfactory in Asians and in adults. A significant proportion (30%) of these patients may progress to renal failure and as many as 10% will require maintenance dialysis.[6]

Papular Acrodermatitis (Gianotti Disease)

Papular acrodermatitis is a rare skin disorder associated with acute hepatitis B in children, particularly among those under the age of 4 years. Circulating HBsAg and anti-HBs immune complexes is thought to play a role in the pathogenesis. It manifests as symmetric, erythematous, maculopapular, non-itchy eruptions over the face, buttocks, limbs, and occasionally the trunk, lasting for 15 to 20 days. Mucous membranes are spared. Lymphadenopathy, particularly in the axillary and inguinal regions, is common. Evidence of acute hepatitis may coincide with the onset of the skin eruption or more commonly begin as the dermatitis starts to wane.

Diagnosis and Investigations

Clinical tests for patients with chronic hepatitis B serve three purposes: (1) to confirm the diagnosis; (2) to assess the disease activity; and (3) to assess the degree of liver damage. This is the basis for the decision of treatment and hepatocellular carcinoma surveillance. In patients on antiviral treatment, further investigations are required to monitor treatment response and detect drug resistance.

Serologic Markers of HBV Infection

The meaning and interpretation of various serologic markers of HBV infection are summarized in **Table 30-2**.

HBsAg and Antibodies

In acute hepatitis B, HBsAg appears in the serum 2 to 10 weeks after exposure to the virus and before symptom onset and elevation of serum ALT (**Fig. 30-3**). In most adult patients, HBsAg disappears in 4 to 6 months. Hepatitis B surface antibody (anti-HBs) may appear several weeks after HBsAg seroclearance. After recovery with seroconversion of HBsAg to anti-HBs, HBV DNA may still be detectable in the liver, and HBV-specific T-cell response can still be demonstrated decades later.[7] It indicates persistent immune control over the residual

Table 30-2 Interpretations of Serologic Markers of HBV Infection

SEROLOGIC MARKERS		INTERPRETATION
HBsAg	Hepatitis B surface antigen	Current HBV infection (acute or chronic)
Anti-HBs	Hepatitis B surface antibody	Past HBV infection or vaccination
HBeAg	Hepatitis B e antigen	Positive in (1) immune tolerant phase or (2) HBeAg-positive chronic hepatitis B with active disease
Anti-HBe	Hepatitis B e antibody	Positive in (1) inactive HBsAg carrier state or (2) HBeAg-negative chronic hepatitis B with active disease
IgM anti-HBc	IgM antibody against hepatitis B core antigen	Positive in (1) acute hepatitis B or (2) acute exacerbation of chronic hepatitis B
IgG anti-HBc	IgG antibody against hepatitis B core antigen	Past or present HBV infection

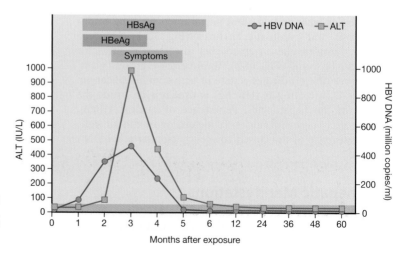

Fig. 30-3 Relationship of serologic, biochemical, and clinical profiles in a typical case of acute hepatitis B. There is a brief period of viremia preceding the onset of symptoms and ALT elevation.

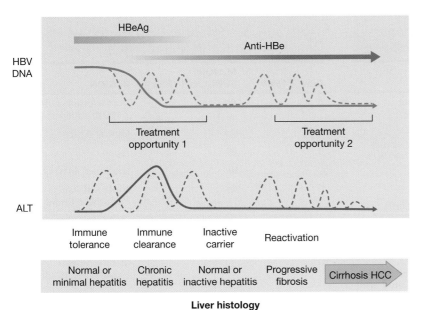

Fig. 30-4 **Natural history of perinatally acquired chronic HBV infection.** Treatment opportunities exist during the immune clearance phase and the reactivation phase when there is elevation of ALT and AST indicative of host immune response to HBV. *(Adapted from Perriool R, Nair S. Hepatitis B and D. In: Feldman M, Friedman L, editors. Sleisenger and Fordtran's gastrointestinal and liver disease, 8th ed. Philadelphia: Elsevier, 2005.)*

HBV infection that is present indefinitely after clinical recovery of the acute infection. On rare occasions, patients with positive anti-HBs can be infected by HBV again because of incomplete protection of the anti-HBs to another HBV serotype. Thus the development anti-HBs after acute HBV infection can only be regarded as a marker of past exposure to HBV. Anti-HBs are a marker of immunity only in the setting of HBV vaccination.

Persistence of HBsAg for more than 6 months indicates development of chronic hepatitis B. HBsAg and anti-HBs may co-exist in the same individual in 10% to 25% of cases. This phenomenon occurs more often in patients with chronic hepatitis B than those with acute hepatitis B.[8] The antibody titer is usually low. The underlying mechanism of this phenomenon is not completely understood but may be due to infection by HBV of more than one serotype. In most instances, the antibodies in these individuals are directed against one of the subtypic determinants (not the common "a" determinant) and are unable to neutralize the circulating virions. These patients are managed as having an HBV infection and the presence of anti-HBs does not alter the disease activity and clinical outcome.

HBV DNA has been demonstrated in the serum and liver tissue of HBsAg-negative patients suffering from chronic hepatitis, liver cirrhosis, and HCC (i.e., occult HBV infection). In these cases, determination of HBV DNA would be mandatory, particularly among patients suffering from liver disease with undetermined cause in areas where HBV infection is prevalent. This is equally important in patients with fulminant hepatitis B, who may have cleared HBsAg by the time they present.

HBeAg and Antibodies

Hepatitis B e antibody is a soluble viral protein. It is found early in the course of acute hepatitis B and disappears soon after ALT peaks. Persistence of HBeAg beyond 3 months after the onset of illness is unusual and may suggest progression to chronic infection.

In patients with chronic hepatitis B, the presence of positive HBeAg usually indicates a high level of viral replication and thus infectivity. HBeAg is positive in the immune tolerant phase and in the early immune clearance phase. HBeAg seroconversion is the disappearance of HBeAg and appearance of hepatitis B e antibody (anti-HBe). Most patients enter the inactive HBsAg carrier state after HBeAg seroconversion (**Fig. 30-4**). This state is associated with low HBV DNA, normal ALT, and little hepatic necroinflammation. However, some patients continue to have active liver disease and detectable serum HBV DNA. This can be due to either a wild-type virus or the presence of precore stop codon mutation and/or basal core promoter mutations that impair HBeAg secretion.[9]

Hepatitis B Core Antibodies

In acute hepatitis B, the period between the disappearance of HBsAg and the appearance of anti-HBs is called the window period. During this period, HBeAg is negative and HBV DNA is usually undetectable. The only positive marker is the IgM antibody against hepatitis B core antigen (IgM anti-HBc), which is thus the most important serologic marker of acute hepatitis B (**Table 30-3**). IgM anti-HBc usually lasts 4 to 6 months during acute hepatitis B, and rarely persists up to 2 years. Although IgM anti-HBc is a marker of acute hepatitis B, it may be also positive during acute exacerbation of chronic hepatitis B.

On the other hand, IgG anti-HBc is a marker of HBV exposure and is positive in both chronic hepatitis B patients and those recovered from acute hepatitis B. In the latter case, it usually co-exists with anti-HBs antibodies. Isolated presence of IgG anti-HBc in the absence of HBsAg and anti-HBs has been reported in 0.4% to 1.7% among blood donors in low-prevalence areas and in 10% to 20% of the population in endemic countries. Transmission of HBV infection from blood and organ (nonliver) donors with isolated anti-HBc is very rare. Transmission of HBV infection due to extrahepatic organ transplantation, such as the kidney, heart, and cornea, may be related to residual blood in the vascular pedicles due

Table 30-3 Interpretation of HBV Serologic Markers in Patients with Acute Hepatitis

HBSAG	IGM ANTI-HBC	INTERPRETATION
+	+	Acute hepatitis B or acute exacerbation of chronic hepatitis B
+	−	Chronic hepatitis B (may or may not explain the abnormal liver function tests)
−	+	Acute hepatitis B
−	−	Abnormal liver function tests not due to HBV

Table 30-4 Geographic Distribution of HBV Genotypes and the Major Subgenotypes

GENOTYPES	MAJOR SUBGENOTYPES	REGION
A	Ae	Northwestern Europe, North America
	Aa	Central Africa
B	Bj	Japan
	Ba	Southeast Asia, China
C	Cs	Southeast Asia, southern China
	Ce	East Asia (Japan, Korea), northern China
D		Mediterranean countries, Middle East, India
E		West Africa
F		Central and South America, Polynesia, American natives
G		United States, France
H		Central and South America

to inadequate flushing or the presence of infectious virions in the organ. On the contrary, the rate of HBV transmission through liver transplantation from donors with isolated anti-HBc ranged from 33% to 78% without antiviral prophylaxis. It suggests that the virus may persist in the liver despite serologic resolution of the infection. Routine screening of isolated anti-HBc for liver donors and antiviral and/or hepatitis B immunoglobulin prophylaxis to recipients can prevent the HBV transmission, but the optimal prophylactic regimen and its cost-effectiveness remain uncertain.[4,10]

Molecular Tests of HBV Infection

Serum HBV DNA

Serum HBV DNA is a measurement of viral load. Its major clinical uses are (1) determination of viral activity and prognosis; (2) monitoring the effectiveness of antiviral treatment; and (3) early detection of drug resistance.

The older-generation HBV DNA tests are mainly based on hybridization and signal amplification technology. Examples include hybrid-capture amplification assay (Digene Hybrid Capture II, Qiagen, Hilden, Germany), branched DNA assay (Bayer Versant 1.0, Bayer Diagnostics, Berkeley, Calif.) and DNA cross-linking assay (NAXCOR XLnt, NAXCOR, Palo Alto, Calif.). The lower limits of detection of these assays fall between 100,000 and 1,000,000 copies/ml. The low sensitivity makes them unsuitable for clinical use in the era of antiviral therapy.

Nowadays, newer HBV DNA assays have detection limits of 10 to 100 copies/ml. Examples are PCR-based assays (Roche Cobas Amplicor, Roche Molecular Diagnostics, Pleasanton, Calif.), 5′ nuclease technology based assay (Roche Cobas TaqMan, Roche Molecular Diagnostics), and newer-generation branched DNA assay (Bayer Versant 3.0).

Different commercial tests may report the results in different units (e.g., copies per milliliter, picograms per milliliter) and are not directly comparable. Therefore 22 laboratories around the world participated in a collaborative study to establish a World Health Organization international standard for HBV DNA nucleic acid amplification techniques in 2001.[11] Using three standard samples, most laboratories have good accuracy and agreement using different HBV DNA assays. At present, it is encouraged to report HBV DNA levels in international units per milliliter. In general 1 IU/ml is roughly equivalent to 5 copies/ml.

HBV Genotyping

Hepatitis B virus can be divided into eight genotypes (A-H) based on a difference in genomic sequence of 8% or more. Different HBV genotypes are found in different geographic regions (**Table 30-4**). Some HBV genotypes can be further subdivided into different subgenotypes. HBV genotype may influence the natural history of chronic HBV infection. For example, genotype C HBV is associated with delayed HBeAg seroconversion, more active disease, higher risk of liver cirrhosis, and HCC as compared with genotype B HBV.[12,13] However, the exact role of HBV genotyping in treatment decision or HCC surveillance remains uncertain.

The most appealing use of HBV genotyping is patient selection for peginterferon treatment. Patients infected by genotype A HBV tend to respond best to peginterferon.[14] Otherwise, HBV genotyping has no role in nucleos(t)ide analog treatment because patients with different HBV genotypes have similar responses. A number of assays can be used to determine HBV genotypes, including direct sequencing, restriction fragment length polymorphism, line probe assay, and enzyme-linked immunosorbent assay.

Drug Resistance Testing

In patients on oral nucleos(t)ide analogs, the first sign of drug resistance is virologic breakthrough (i.e., a rise in HBV DNA level by 10-fold or more). To confirm and characterize the viral mutations conferring resistance, two types of commercial assays are available—direct sequencing (TruGene HBV, Siemens Healthcare Diagnostic Solutions, Deerfield, Ill.; Affigene HBV DE/3TC Assay, Sangtec Molecular Diagnostics AB, Cepheid, Sunnyrate, Calif.) and reverse hybridization (INNO-LiPA DR Version 2.0, Innogenetics, Gent, Belgium).

Direct sequencing of the polymerase gene has the advantage of identifying both known and previously unreported mutations. However, the test may be falsely negative if the mutants constitute less than 20% of the whole viral population. Besides, the detection of previously unreported mutations may not necessarily represent drug resistance. In vitro phenotypic analysis is required to confirm decreased susceptibility to treatment.

In contrast, hybridization assays are more sensitive and can detect mutants that constitute only 5% of the whole viral population. Nevertheless, one major limitation of hybridization assays is that only known mutations can be detected. When new drug-resistant mutations are reported, the test needs regular updating.

Mass spectroscopy represents an inexpensive and sensitive method that may detect mutant population that represents 5% of the overall population.[15] Ultradeep pyrosequencing is another more sensitive technique. These new technologies may overcome the limitations of existing assays and warrant further validation.

Assessment of Liver Fibrosis

Liver fibrosis is the natural response to liver injury. Accumulation of fibrous tissue eventually results in distortion of liver architecture and the development of cirrhosis. Chronic hepatitis B patients with advanced liver fibrosis or cirrhosis are at increased risk of HCC and other liver-related complications. Accurate assessment of liver fibrosis is therefore an important part of patient evaluation in chronic hepatitis B.

Liver Biopsy

Liver biopsy is the gold standard for the assessment of liver fibrosis. A number of histologic scoring systems are commonly used to describe the necroinflammatory activity (grading) and fibrosis (staging) in chronic hepatitis B. Each system is an ordinal scale ranging from no fibrosis to cirrhosis (e.g., Knodell's system [0, 1, 3, 4], Metavir system [0 to 4], Ishak's system [0 to 6]). These scoring systems can facilitate statistical comparisons among patients in clinical studies but they cannot supersede the overall interpretation of an experienced pathologist.

The major limitation of liver biopsy is its invasive nature. Significant bleeding may occur in approximately 3 in 1000 cases and mortality may occur in 3 in 10,000 cases. Recently, the accuracy of liver biopsy as the gold standard has been put under scrutiny. As a usual biopsy specimen represents only 1 of 50,000 of the liver volume, histologic assessment is subject to sampling bias. By computer modeling, the accuracy of histologic staging was approximately 65% when the length of a biopsy specimen is 15 mm and 75% when the biopsy specimen is 25 mm.[16]

Imaging Studies

Ultrasound scan, computerized tomography, and magnetic resonance imaging are common imaging studies of the hepatobiliary system. Definitive diagnosis of cirrhosis by imaging is only made when the liver is shrunken or there are features of portal hypertension (e.g., ascites, varices). Imaging tests are insensitive to detect liver fibrosis and early cirrhosis. The main role of imaging tests is surveillance and diagnosis of HCC.

Clinical Models and Serum Tests

Because of the limitations of liver biopsy, various noninvasive tests for liver fibrosis have been developed. In general, these models are composed of (1) clinical factors or routine laboratory parameters associated with fibrosis, (2) biomarkers of fibrogenesis or fibrinolysis, and (3) a combination of the above. **Table 30-5** shows a number of models that predict significant fibrosis in chronic hepatitis B. FibroTest (Biopredictive, Paris) in Europe, or FibroSure (LabCorp, Burlington, N.C.) in the United States, is composed of five serum biomarkers and commercially available for the prediction of fibrosis and cirrhosis. In a meta-analysis, the area under the receiver operating characteristics curve of FibroTest for chronic hepatitis B was 0.80.[17] Most of these clinical models have not been independently validated in different patient cohorts by different investigators. More validation studies are required before they can be recommended for routine clinical use.

Transient Elastography

Transient elastography by Fibroscan (Echosens, Paris) measures liver stiffness by detecting the velocity of an elastic shear wave that propagates through the liver parenchyma by pulse-echo ultrasound acquisitions. The technique has been

Table 30-5 Combined Panels of Clinical and Serum Markers of Significant Fibrosis in Chronic HBV

AUTHOR	FORMULAS
Hui et al.	$\exp(1.23 + 0.167 \times BMI + 1.191 \times ALP[/ULN] + 0.081 \times bilirubin[\mu M] - 0.139 \times albumin[g/l] - 0.017 \times platelet[10^9/l]/(1 + \exp(1.23 + 0.167 \times BMI + 1.191 \times ALP[/ULN] + 0.081 \times bilirubin[\mu M] - 0.139 \times albumin[g/l] - 0.017 \times platelet[10^9/l]))$
Liu et al.	Age-plateletUAST; GGT∩Age-platelet
Mallet et al.	$Age \times AST[/ULN]/platelet[10^9/l] \times \sqrt{ALT[U/l]}$ (FIB-4 index)
Mohamadnejad et al.	$10 + (0.771 \times HBV\ DNA[\log_{10}\ copies/ml]) + (3.828 \times \log_{10}\ ALP[/ULN]) - (1.066 \times albumin[g/dl]) - (0.011 \times platelets[/1000\ \mu l])$ (HBeAg-negative patients)
Myers et al.	Bilirubin, GGT, α_2-macroglubulin, apolipoprotein A1, haptoglobin (formula protected by patent [FibroTest])
Zeng et al.	$-13.995 + 3.220 \log (\alpha_2\text{-macroglobulin}) + 3.096 \log (age) + 2.254 \log (GGT) + 2.437 \log (hyaluronic\ acid)$

Data from Hui AY, et al. Identification of chronic hepatitis B patients without significant liver fibrosis by a simple noninvasive predictive model. Am J Gastroenterol 2005;100(3):616–623; Mallet V, et al. The accuracy of the FIB-4 index for the diagnosis of mild fibrosis in chronic hepatitis B. Aliment Pharmacol Ther 2009;29(4):409–15; Mohamadnejad M, et al. Noninvasive markers of liver fibrosis and inflammation in chronic hepatitis B-virus related liver disease. Am J Gastroenterol 2006;101(11):2537–2545; Myers RP, et al. Prediction of liver histological lesions with biochemical markers in patients with chronic hepatitis B. J Hepatol 2003;39(2):222–230; Zeng MD, et al. Prediction of significant fibrosis in HBeAg-positive patients with chronic hepatitis B by a noninvasive model. Hepatology 2005;42(6):1437–1445.

ALP, alkaline phosphatase; ALT, alanine aminotransferase; AST, aspartate aminotransferase; BMI, body mass index; GGT, γ-glutamyl transpeptidase; ULN, upper limit normal

validated in different liver diseases including chronic hepatitis C, alcoholic liver disease, and cholestatic liver diseases.[18] Validation studies in chronic hepatitis B are relatively scanty. In general, transient elastography is more accurate to detect liver cirrhosis (Metavir F4) than early fibrosis (Metavir F2). One point of caution is that liver stiffness is increased by hepatic necroinflammation as reflected by elevated serum ALT levels. Therefore liver stiffness measurement should be interpreted in the context of ALT level.[19] In patients with very high ALT levels, liver stiffness can increase to cirrhotic range despite the lack of underlying cirrhosis. Clinicians should be cautious when selecting the appropriate patients for this noninvasive test.

Natural History of Chronic HBV Infection

The natural course of chronic hepatitis B infection is generally described in four phases: immune tolerant, immune clearance, low or nonreplicative (also known as inactive carrier stage), and reactivation phases (see **Fig. 30-4**). Patients may progress from one phase to the next or reverse backwards. Active viral replication is the hallmark of the immune tolerant, immune clearance, and reactivation phases. The different phases represent the interaction between the host immune system and the virus. The natural history is modified by gender, alcohol consumption, and co-infection by other viruses. In general, the outcome of HBV infection depends on the duration and severity of liver injury. The earlier HBV replication is arrested, the less is the cumulative liver injury.

Phases of Chronic HBV Infection

Replicative Phase—Immune Tolerant Phase

In patients who acquire HBV infection during the perinatal period or early childhood, the initial phase is characterized by high HBV replication and no or little immune response. Serum HBV DNA is high and HBeAg is positive, whereas the patients are asymptomatic and ALT level is normal. No or minimal necroinflammation and fibrosis is observed on liver biopsy. Spontaneous HBeAg seroconversion (loss of HBeAg and emergence of anti-HBe) is uncommon at this stage. HBeAg is positive in 90% of children below the age of 5 years and in 80% of teenagers.[20] Therefore many women with chronic hepatitis B remain HBeAg positive and have a high viral load at their reproductive age. This explains the high rate of perinatal transmission in Asian and African countries before the introduction of universal vaccination.

The exact mechanism of immune tolerance is unclear. Studies in transgenic mice suggest that exposure to HBeAg results in a state of immune tolerance. Helper T cells become unresponsive to both HBeAg and hepatitis B core antigen because of cross-reactivity.[21] Thus cytotoxic T-cell response to hepatitis B core antigen is rendered ineffective. Moreover, after stimulation by recombinant hepatitis B core antigen, peripheral blood mononuclear cells fail to proliferate and produce interleukin-2 receptors.[22]

Replicative Phase—Immune Clearance Phase

The second phase of perinatally acquired chronic HBV infection typically occurs from the second to fourth decades. The immune clearance phase is characterized by an elevated ALT level, a decrease in HBV DNA, and an increased rate of spontaneous HBeAg seroconversion. At this phase, the annual rate of HBeAg seroconversion is 10% to 20%.[23] Immune-mediated lysis of infected hepatocytes accounts for ALT elevation.

The duration of the immune clearance phase is highly variable. Successful immune clearance early in life leads to resolution of hepatitis activity and transition to the nonreplicative phase. Some patients may not have notable hepatitis exacerbations before HBeAg seroconversion. This is likely due to mild hepatitis activity escaping medical attention. In other patients, exacerbations of hepatitis B may not result in HBeAg seroconversion because of unsuccessful immune clearance. Chronic or intermittent necroinflammation leads to ongoing liver injury, which may progress to cirrhosis and liver failure. Patients who have progressed to cirrhosis are at substantial risk of liver-related complications even if the virus may be finally under control afterward.

The mechanism causing the transition to the immune clearance phase is not completely understood. An increase in serum HBV DNA and the translocation of hepatitis B core antigen from the nucleus to the cytoplasm have been suggested to be the triggering events.[24]

Low or Nonreplicative Phase (Inactive Carrier State)

In patients with successful immune clearance, HBeAg seroconversion occurs and HBV DNA is suppressed to low or undetectable levels. Serum ALT level is normalized. Histologic necroinflammation is reduced and fibrosis may regress. Intrahepatic hepatitis B core antigen is reduced or absent.

After successful HBeAg seroconversion, some patients go on to develop HBsAg seroclearance. The annual rate of HBsAg seroclearance is estimated to be 0.5% to 1% in patients below the age of 30 years, but increases to 1.5% to 2% after the age of 40.[25] Patients achieving HBsAg seroclearance have an excellent prognosis. The risk of developing hepatocellular carcinoma is minimal in patients who achieve HBsAg seroclearance before the age of 50 years, before the development of liver cirrhosis, and without concurrent hepatitis C virus (HCV) or delta virus infection.[26,27]

Reactivation Phase

In 20% to 30% of patients with HBeAg seroconversion, HBV may become active again. This may or may not be accompanied by HBeAg reversion (HBeAg becomes positive again). At this phase, HBV DNA is high and ALT is elevated. In 30% to 50% of cases, fluctuation of ALT with periods of normal levels is observed. HBeAg-negative chronic hepatitis B is usually due to HBV mutants with defective HBeAg production (e.g., precore stop codon mutation, basal core promoter mutations). Patients who have fluctuating HBeAg status tend to have a high risk of developing liver cirrhosis and its related complications.

Difference Between Perinatal and Adulthood Infection

The four phases of chronic HBV infection apply to patients who acquire the infection perinatally or during early childhood. In adults with acute hepatitis B, more than 95% develop spontaneous HBsAg seroclearance within 6 months. Among the minority of adult patients who progress to chronic hepatitis B, the immune tolerant phase is typically absent. Successful immune clearance occurs more readily.

Sequelae of Chronic HBV Infection

Various outcomes may occur in patients with chronic hepatitis B. Some patients remain inactive carriers with no significant liver injury and have normal life expectancy. Other patients may develop cirrhosis, hepatic decompensation, and HCC possibly followed by death.

Liver Cirrhosis and HCC

Long-term follow-up studies show that the majority of chronic hepatitis B patients with normal ALT, negative HBeAg, and positive anti-HBe at the baseline remain asymptomatic and have low incidence of cirrhosis and HCC.[28] On the other hand, patients with active hepatitis are at high risk of disease progression (**Fig. 30-5**). The survival rate is notably reduced once cirrhosis occurs. In one study, the 5-year survival rate was 86% in patients with chronic active hepatitis and 55% in patients with cirrhosis.[29] The presence of jaundice and ascites is further associated with increased mortality. Overall, up to 40% of men and 15% of women with perinatally acquired chronic hepatitis B eventually die from cirrhosis or HCC.[30] HBV carriers have more than a 200-fold increase in the risk of HCC.

The duration of the replicative phases is a strong determinant of the final outcome. Patients with delayed HBeAg seroconversion and viral control have prolonged and cumulative liver injury. In addition, acute exacerbations of chronic hepatitis B are more common in patients with positive HBeAg.[31] Repeated episodes of hepatic necroinflammation and regeneration predispose the liver to progressive liver fibrosis and hepatocarcinogenesis. Positive HBeAg and high HBV DNA are independent factors associated with HCC and adverse outcomes.[32,33] In a study of 3653 chronic hepatitis B patients

with a mean follow-up of 11.4 years, the incidence of HCC was 108 per 100,000 person-years for an HBV DNA level of less than 300 copies/ml and 1152 per 100,000 person-years for an HBV DNA level of 1 million copies/ml or more.[33] Other risk factors of hepatocellular carcinoma are listed in **Table 30-6**.

Severe Acute Exacerbation and Liver Failure

Severe acute exacerbation of chronic hepatitis B is a special presentation of chronic hepatitis B. Vigorous immune pressure leads to excessive necroinflammation. During biochemical exacerbation of chronic hepatitis B, 23% to 38% may develop jaundice and hepatic decompensation.[31] This may progress to fulminant or subfulminant hepatic failure (i.e., acute or chronic liver failure).

Severe acute exacerbation is characterized by jaundice and very high ALT level. Sometimes, the presentation is preceded by a period of constitutional symptoms. If a patient does not have a known history of chronic hepatitis B, severe acute exacerbation can be indistinguishable from acute hepatitis B. Although IgM anti-HBc is the hallmark of acute hepatitis B, this marker is also positive in some cases of severe acute exacerbation.[34] However, an IgM anti-HBc titer of 1:1000 or less makes the diagnosis of acute hepatitis B less likely. The presence of cirrhosis at presentation as well as basal core promoter or precore stop codon mutations also support the diagnosis of severe acute exacerbation instead of acute hepatitis B. In indeterminate cases, the final diagnosis is made when HBsAg remains positive at 6 months. The prognosis of severe acute exacerbation is poor if a patient has underlying cirrhosis or develops features of hepatic decompensation, such as hyperbilirubinemia, prolonged prothrombin time, and ascites.

Special Groups with Altered Natural History

Alcoholism

The prevalence of alcoholism varies widely among different countries. In a study in France, excessive alcohol consumption was associated with higher mortality among chronic hepatitis

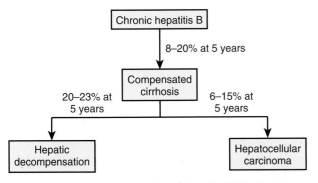

Fig. 30-5 **Long-term sequelae of chronic HBV infection.**

Table 30-6 Risk Factors of HCC in Patients with Chronic HBV	
Host factors	Male sex Older age Family history of HCC
Disease factor	Liver cirrhosis
Viral factors	High HBV DNA Positive HBeAg Genotype C (in particular subgenotype Ce) HBV Basal core promoter mutations Co-infection with hepatitis C virus or delta virus
Chemical exposure	Alcoholism Aflatoxin

B patients.[35] Excessive alcohol consumption was observed in 15% of chronic hepatitis B patients who died. The mean age of death for chronic hepatitis B patients with excessive alcohol consumption was 52 years, compared with 64 years for those with low or moderate alcohol consumption.

The mechanism of alcohol in increasing liver injury is not completely understood. Histologically, excessive alcohol consumption is associated with increased portal inflammation and piecemeal necrosis.[36] This results in increased risk of cirrhosis.[37] In transgenic mice, alcohol increases HBV gene expression and replication and enhances HCC development.[38]

The safety limit of alcohol consumption is uncertain. According to current evidence, drinking less than the World Health Organization's recommendations of 21 units per week in men and 14 units per week in women appears to be safe even in patients with viral hepatitis.[35]

Co-Infection with Other Viruses

Owing to shared modes of transmission, co-infection of HBV and other parenterally transmitted viruses is commonly observed. In a survey in Taiwan, co-infection with HCV was observed in 10% to 15% of chronic hepatitis B patients.[39] Co-infection with HBV and HCV is associated with increased morbidity and mortality. Compared with monoinfection with either virus alone, the standardized mortality ratio of co-infected patients is two to three times higher.[40]

Although co-infection increases disease activity and fibrosis progression, it is generally observed that the replicative levels of the two viruses have an inverse relationship. In chronic hepatitis B patients, superimposed acute hepatitis C results in a drop in HBV DNA.[41] Similarly, acute hepatitis B in patients with chronic HCV infection also results in a drop in HCV RNA.[42] After successful eradication of chronic HCV infection by peginterferon and ribavirin, reactivation of HBV with hepatitis flares has been reported.[43] During chronic HBV and HCV co-infection, HCV is usually the dominant virus, with HBV relatively suppressed. Recent cell line studies suggest that HBV replication does little to interfere with HCV replication and vice versa.[44] Thus the observation of reciprocal replication is likely because of interference with host immune response and/or competition for residing hepatocytes.

The hepatitis delta virus (HDV) is a subviral agent whose life cycle is dependent on HBV. It is estimated that 20 million people worldwide suffer from chronic HDV infection.[45] Superinfection of HDV in patients with chronic hepatitis B increases the risk of fulminant liver failure substantially. Chronic co-infection is also associated with more rapid disease progression.

In HIV-infected patients who are first exposed to HBV in adulthood, the clinical presentation is often more subtle and may be silent. ALT is usually lower and jaundice is infrequently seen. This reflects reduced immune response in these patients. Nevertheless, HIV-positive individuals are less likely to clear the virus and more prone to develop a chronic infection. In a study in Australia, 23% of the HIV-infected patients developed chronic HBV infection after acute hepatitis B, compared with 4% of non–HIV-infected patients.[46] The chance of seroconversion to anti-HBs was proportional to the CD4 count.

HIV-infected patients with chronic hepatitis B commonly have high viral load and positive HBeAg. This translates into more rapid disease progression and adverse outcomes. In a multicenter study involving 5293 homosexual men, liver-related mortality was 14.2 per 1000 person-years in HBV-HIV co-infected cases, compared with 1.7 per 1000 in those infected with HIV alone and 0.8 per 1000 in those infected with HBV alone.[47]

Immunosuppressive or Anticancer Therapy

Hepatitis B virus reactivation is common in patients receiving immunosuppressive or anticancer therapy. In patients with HCC, hepatitis after systemic chemotherapy occurs in up to 60% of cases, most of which is attributed to HBV reactivation.[48] In patients receiving hematopoietic stem cell transplantation, HBV reactivation also occurs in up to 50% of HBV-infected patients.[49] HBV reactivation may result in liver decompensation and death. In addition, cessation of anticancer therapy is often necessary during HBV reactivation and it may interfere with successful cancer treatment.

HBV reactivation during immunosuppressive or anticancer therapy is characterized by a rise in HBV DNA, followed by ALT flares. ALT flares commonly occur after the withdrawal of immunosuppressive or anticancer therapy because of the combined effect of rising viral load and immune restitution. When icteric hepatitis occurs, the mortality rate is between 5% and 40%.[48]

Young patients, male sex, high pretreatment ALT, and HBV DNA are risk factors of HBV reactivation.[50] Although HBeAg is associated with high HBV DNA in general, HBeAg-negative patients with precore and/or basal core promoter mutants are also at risk of reactivation.[51] The risk of reactivation is also associated with the intensity of immunosuppression. Systemic corticosteroids and anthracyclines are most commonly associated with HBV reactivation.[48] Recent studies also reported a high risk of HBV reactivation with the use of rituximab.

Antiviral Therapy for Chronic HBV
Indications for Treatment

The aim of antiviral treatment for chronic hepatitis B is to reduce the risk of HCC and liver-related complications. Therefore treatment should be initiated in patients who are at risk of developing complications and who have already developed significant liver injury (**Table 30-7**). In a meta-analysis of 17 studies including 5031 patients, interferon and lamivudine were found to reduce the risk of HCC by 34% and 78%, respectively, as compared with a placebo or no treatment.[52] Treatment guidelines have been issued by the American Association for the Study of Liver Diseases, the European Association for the Study of the Liver, and the Asian-Pacific Association for the Study of the Liver.[4,10,53] In general, a combination of clinical, biochemical, virologic, and histologic factors should be considered together before the decision on treatment. Because treatment is often prolonged and drug compliance is important, proper patient counseling is essential.

The evidence of the benefit of antiviral therapy is strongest in patients with liver cirrhosis. In the largest randomized controlled trial using clinical outcomes as study endpoints, 651 chronic hepatitis B patients with histology-confirmed severe

Table 30-7 Indications of Treatment for Chronic HBV

Significant liver injury
Moderate to severe hepatic necroinflammation
Advanced liver fibrosis or cirrhosis
Liver decompensation

Active disease
Persistently abnormal serum ALT
High HBV DNA

Patients on immunosuppressive or cytotoxic therapy

Prophylactic treatment for liver transplantation

ALT, alanine aminotransferase; DNA, deoxyribonucleic acid; HBV, hepatitis B virus

fibrosis or early cirrhosis were randomized to receive lamivudine or a placebo.[54] At a median follow-up of 32 months, the composite endpoint of time to disease progression, defined by hepatic decompensation, HCC, spontaneous bacterial peritonitis, bleeding varices, or liver-related death occurred in 7.8% of the patients receiving lamivudine and in 17.7% of those receiving the placebo ($P = .02$). Therefore, in all regional guidelines, patients with compensated early cirrhosis should be considered for antiviral treatment if the HBV DNA is higher than 2000 IU/ml (10,000 copies/ml) regardless of the ALT levels.

Patients with decompensated liver cirrhosis have a high mortality rate and should be considered for liver transplantation. However, weak evidence suggests that antiviral therapy in this setting may improve the survival time. Some patients may even have significant improvement in liver function, allowing them to be removed from the transplant list.[55] Antiviral therapy is recommended by all regional guidelines when HBV DNA is detectable among decompensated cirrhotic patients.

Other than liver cirrhosis, the guidelines also recommend treatment in chronic hepatitis B patients with HBV DNA greater than 2000 to 20,000 IU/ml (10,000 to 100,000 copies/ml) and serum ALT persistently elevated, especially if it is at least twice the upper limit of normal. In large prospective studies, high HBV DNA has been confirmed to be a strong factor associated with subsequent development of HCC.[33,56] However, it should be noted that the association between HBV DNA and HCC only applies in patients who have started immune clearance but not in those in the immune tolerant phase. Similarly, elevated ALT is associated with adverse liver outcomes. At present, the best ALT threshold for treatment is unclear. Chronic hepatitis B patients with high normal or mildly elevated ALT are also at risk of liver-related complications.[57] As some patients who have normal ALT levels may still harbor advanced fibrosis or cirrhosis, liver biopsy should be considered in borderline cases, especially in patients aged 40 years or above. Because liver biopsy is invasive and may not be acceptable to all patients, there is a growing interest in the use of noninvasive measures of liver fibrosis to complement or avoid a liver biopsy.[4]

On the other hand, treatment is not recommended in patients in the immune tolerant phase or in the inactive HBsAg carrier state. This is based on the observation that disease progression and liver-related complications are rare in these individuals. In addition, patients in the immune tolerant phase have a very high viral load due to little host immune control, which increases the risk of drug resistance and the difficulty of sustained virologic response.

More than 95% of adults with acute hepatitis B recover spontaneously. Antiviral therapy does not alter the clinical outcome or increase the chance of HBsAg seroclearance, and is generally not indicated.[58] However, antiviral therapy has been suggested as useful because of its minimal side effects if the acute hepatitis is severe and protracted.[53]

Currently Available Antiviral Agents

Seven antiviral agents for chronic hepatitis B have been registered in the United States and Europe. They can be divided in two broad categories: interferon-based therapy (conventional interferon alpha and peginterferon alpha) and oral nucleos(t)ide analogs (lamivudine, adefovir dipivoxil, entecavir, telbivudine, and tenofovir disoproxil fumarate) (**Table 30-8**).

Interferon Alpha

Interferon works by dual action: a direct antiviral effect and an immunomodulatory effect. It enhances human leukocyte antigen class I antigen expression on the surface of infected hepatocytes and augments CD8$^+$ cytotoxic T-cell activity. Interferon can be given for a finite period (4 to 6 months) and does not have the problem of drug resistance. On the other hand, side effects are common during interferon treatment (**Table 30-9**).

In HBeAg-positive patients, approximately 33% can achieve HBeAg seroconversion after a course of interferon treatment, compared with 12% of controls.[59] Similarly, the rate of HBsAg seroclearance (7.8% vs. 1.8%) and undetectable HBV DNA by hybridization assay (37% vs. 17%) is higher in treated patients. Once HBeAg seroconversion is achieved, the durability is up to 80%. A number of observational studies suggested that responders to interferon treatment have a lower incidence of cirrhosis, HCC, and mortality.

In HBeAg-negative patients, 60% to 90% of treated patients can achieve undetectable HBV DNA by hybridization assay and normalization of ALT at the end of treatment, but the relapse rate is high.[60] Overall, approximately 20% of patients have sustained response after the cessation of treatment.

Because interferon is an immunomodulatory agent, ALT flares may occur during treatment. In general, ALT flares are benign and transient, and are associated with a higher rate of HBeAg seroconversion.[61] However, ALT flares can result in clinical deterioration in patients with advanced cirrhosis or preexisting liver decompensation.

Peginterferon Alpha

Peginterferon alpha is constructed by the addition of polyethylene glycol to interferon through a process called pegylation. This process prolongs the half-life of the drug. As a result, peginterferon can be given less frequently (see **Table 30-8**), and the efficacy is higher than that of conventional interferon. There are two types of peginterferon on the market: peginterferon alfa-2a (40 kD) and peginterferon alfa-2b (12 kD). Existing data suggest that the performance of both drugs is largely similar. At present, peginterferon alfa-2a is registered

Table 30-8 Comparison of Antiviral Therapies for Chronic HBV

GENERIC NAME	ROUTE	DOSAGE	DURATION	SIDE EFFECTS	SAFETY IN PREGNANCY	DRUG RESISTANCE
Interferon Alpha	Subcutaneous	10 mU 3 times per week	4 to 6 months	Frequent	Category C	Nil
Peginterferon Alfa-2a	Subcutaneous	180 μg weekly	12 months	Frequent	Category C	Nil
Peginterferon Alfa-2b	Subcutaneous	1.5 μg/kg/wk	12 months	Frequent	Category C	Nil
Lamivudine	Oral	100 mg daily	Prolonged	Negligible	Category C	~20% at year 1 ~70% at year 5
Adefovir Dipivoxil	Oral	10 mg daily	Prolonged	Potential nephrotoxicity	Category C	None at year 1 29% at year 5
Entecavir	Oral	0.5 mg daily (1 mg daily for lamivudine resistance)	Prolonged	Negligible	Category C	0.2% at year 1 1.2% at year 5
Telbivudine	Oral	600 mg daily	Prolonged	Potential myopathy	Category B	5% at year 1 25% at year 2
Tenofovir Disoproxil Fumarate	Oral	300 mg daily	Prolonged	Potential nephrotoxicity	Category B	<1% at year 2

Table 30-9 Side Effects of Interferon Alpha and Peginterferon Alpha

Flulike symptoms	Fever Myalgia
Hematologic	Anemia Leukopenia Thrombocytopenia
Thyroid	Hyperthyroidism Hypothyroidism
Metabolic	Hyperglycemia Hypertriglyceridemia
Psychiatric	Depression Anxiety Alopecia
Gastrointestinal	Diarrhea Abdominal pain Nausea and vomiting
Allergy	Injection site reactions

for chronic hepatitis B in most parts of the world. Peginterferon alfa-2b is only registered for chronic hepatitis B in a few countries outside the United States.

After peginterferon treatment for 6 to 12 months in HBeAg-positive patients, HBeAg seroconversion can be achieved in approximately 30% to 35% of cases.[14,62,63] A similar proportion of patients have ALT normalization and HBV DNA suppressed to 10,000 copies/ml or less 6 months after treatment cessation. Similar to conventional interferon, more than 80% of patients who have achieved HBeAg seroconversion with peginterferon treatment have sustained virologic response up to 3 years.[64,65] Approximately 43% to 58% of patients who can achieve sustained HBeAg seroconversion will have HBV DNA undetectable by PCR at 3 years after treatment stopped. In a European series, 9% of patients achieved HBsAg clearance 3 years posttreatment.[65] The response to peginterferon is genotype-specific, with the best response observed in patients infected with genotype A HBV.[14,62] The intrahepatic level of covalently closed circular (ccc) DNA is also significantly reduced among responders to peginterferon.[66] This likely explains the durability of treatment.

In HBeAg-negative patients, peginterferon treatment for 12 months results in ALT normalization in 60%, HBV DNA suppression to below 20,000 copies/ml in 43%, and HBV DNA suppression to below 400 copies/ml in 20% of patients.[67] Three years after stopping treatment, ALT remains normal in 31%, HBV DNA remains below 10,000 copies/ml in 25% to 28%, and HBV DNA is below 400 copies/ml in 13% to 18% of patients.[68] Enhanced HBsAg seroclearance appears to be a unique feature of peginterferon treatment and may occur even after cessation of treatment. HBsAg seroclearance occurs in 8.7% of patients 3 years after the completion of peginterferon treatment.[68]

The combination of peginterferon and lamivudine enhances on-treatment viral suppression but does not increase the rate of sustained off-treatment response.[14,62,63,67] Therefore peginterferon is currently only recommended as monotherapy for chronic hepatitis B. Moreover, combination of peginterferon and telbivudine leads to severe peripheral neuropathy in more than 10% of treated patients and should be avoided.[69]

Lamivudine

Lamivudine was the first nucleoside analog registered for the treatment of chronic hepatitis B. After treatment for 1 year, ALT is normalized in 41% to 72% and HBeAg seroconversion occurs in 16% to 17%.[70,71] HBV DNA decreases by 4 to 4.5 log copies/ml. Extension of treatment to 2 and 3 years further increases the rate of HBeAg seroconversion to 27% and 40%, respectively.[72,73] However, long-term use of lamivudine is associated with high risk of drug resistance. The incidence of lamivudine resistance at 1, 2, 3, 4, and 5 years is 23%, 46%, 55%, 71%, and 65%, respectively.[74] Lamivudine resistance is most commonly caused by amino acid mutation from methionine to valine or isoleucine at the HBV polymerase (rtM204V/I). Development of drug resistance is associated with hepatitis flares, loss of histologic benefits, and occasionally liver decompensation, and death.[73,74] Because lamivudine has cross-resistance with other nucleoside analogs, such as telbivudine, emtricitabine, and entecavir, it is no longer recommended as the first-line treatment in the United States and Europe.[4,53]

Adefovir Dipivoxil

Adefovir dipivoxil is the acyclic analog of dAMP. It has efficacy in both treatment-naïve patients and patients with lamivudine resistance. In HBeAg-positive treatment-naïve patients, adefovir dipivoxil treatment for 1 year reduces HBV DNA by 3.5 to 4.8 log copies/ml.[75] HBeAg seroconversion occurs in 12% to 14%, and ALT is normalized in 48% to 55% of patients. In HBeAg-negative patients, 1-year treatment reduces HBV DNA by 3.9 log copies/ml, and ALT is normalized in 72% of patients.[76] Extension of the original HBeAg-negative study confirmed that viral suppression could be maintained with continuous treatment but was lost if adefovir dipivoxil was discontinued.[77]

Common mutations conferring adefovir dipivoxil resistance include rtN236T and rtA181T/V. Cumulative incidence of genotypic resistance to adefovir dipivoxil in treatment-naïve HBeAg-negative patients at 1, 2, 3, 4, and 5 years is 0, 3%, 11%, 18%, and 29%, respectively.[78]

De novo combination treatment with lamivudine and adefovir dipivoxil does not increase viral suppression but reduces the risk of lamivudine resistance and thus virologic breakthrough.[79] At 2 years, rtM204V/I occurs in 43% of patients on lamivudine monotherapy and 15% of those on combination of lamivudine and adefovir dipivoxil. Nevertheless, the resistance rate of combination treatment still compares less favorably with entecavir or tenofovir. Owing to the high cost and significant risk of drug resistance, de novo combination treatment of lamivudine and adefovir cannot be recommended.

One specific side effect of adefovir dipivoxil is nephrotoxicity. At 5 years, 3% of treated patients have an increase in serum creatinine of 0.5 mg/dl or more.[78] Most cases of nephrotoxicity are mild and resolve spontaneously with continued adefovir dipivoxil or cessation of treatment.

Entecavir

Entecavir is a deoxyguanine nucleoside analog that is more potent than lamivudine and adefovir in viral suppression.[80,81] In HBeAg-positive patients treated with entecavir for 1 year, HBV DNA decreases by 6.9 log, and 67% have undetectable HBV DNA by PCR.[80] HBeAg seroconversion occurs in 21% and ALT is normalized in 68%. In HBeAg-negative patients, entecavir treatment for 1 year results in HBV DNA reduction by 5.0 log and undetectable HBV DNA in 90%.[82]

Entecavir is an antiviral drug with a high genetic barrier of resistance. Drug resistance requires at least three mutations including rtM204V and rtL180M, plus another mutation at rtT184, rtS202, or rtM250. Because concurrent development of three mutations is a rare event, the incidence of entecavir resistance in treatment-naïve patients is low. The cumulative incidence of genotypic entecavir resistance at year 1, 2, 3, 4, and 5 is 0.2%, 0.5%, 1.2%, 1.2%, and 1.2%, respectively.[83]

Telbivudine

Telbivudine is the L-nucleoside analog of L-deoxythymidine. After 1 year of treatment, HBV DNA is undetectable by PCR in 60% of HBeAg-positive patients and 88% of HBeAg-negative patients.[84] ALT is normalized in more than 70%. In HBeAg-positive patients, HBeAg seroconversion occurs in 23% at year 1 and 30% at year 2.[84,85]

Telbivudine has also shown to have more potent viral suppression than lamivudine and adefovir by head-to-head comparisons.[84,86] Unfortunately, telbivudine is a drug with a low genetic barrier of resistance. A single mutation at rtM204I confers resistance to telbivudine. Telbivudine resistance occurs in 5% and 25% at 1 and 2 years, respectively, in HBeAg-positive patients.[84,85] Corresponding rates in HBeAg-negative patients are 2% and 11%, respectively.

Symptomatic myopathy with muscle pain and weakness has been rarely reported with telbivudine, but it usually resolves with cessation of the drug. It is uncertain if the risk would be increased if telbivudine is administered together with other drugs known to cause myopathy (e.g., statins).

Tenofovir Disoproxil Fumarate

Tenofovir is an acyclic nucleotide inhibitor of HBV polymerase and has close chemical similarity with adefovir dipivoxil. It is superior to adefovir dipivoxil in viral suppression.[87] In HBeAg-positive patients, 1 year of tenofovir treatment reduces HBV DNA to below 400 copies/ml in 76% and HBeAg seroconversion in 21%. ALT normalization occurs in 68%. In HBeAg-negative patients treated with tenofovir for 1 year, 93% have HBV DNA below 400 copies/ml and 76% have normal ALT. The rate of maintained response is high in patients continuing tenofovir treatment for 2 years.

Up to 2 years, no tenofovir-resistant mutants have been identified in treatment-naïve patients. However, the response to tenofovir is slower in patients with preexisting adefovir dipivoxil resistance (rtN236T and rtA181V).[88] These patients respond favorably to the addition of emtricitabine (Truvada). On the other hand, tenofovir remains effective against lamivudine-resistant mutants.

Clevudine

Clevudine is a pyrimidine analog with potent HBV suppression. Although initial studies only involved 24 weeks of treatment and showed promising results in both HBeAg-positive and HBeAg-negative patients, long-term use of clevudine is associated with a high risk of myopathy due to depletion of mitochondrial DNA.[89] Clevudine has been registered in Korea but the global phase III trial of this drug was terminated in 2009.

Choice of Treatment

The selection of antiviral therapy should be a joint decision between the clinician and the patient. The pros and cons of various treatments, patient characteristics, and preference should be considered (see **Table 30-8**).

The advantage of interferon-based therapy is the finite course of treatment and lack of drug resistance. This is particularly important in young patients, especially women with childbearing potential. On the other hand, peginterferon treatment is limited by its side effects, the need of subcutaneous administration, and its relatively high cost. Some patients may not tolerate the side effects of interferon. The drug may cause ALT flare, which may lead to further deterioration in patients with hepatic decompensation.

In contrast, oral nucleos(t)ide analogs are given orally and easily administered. Side effects are rare and mild. Nucleos(t)ide analogs have a potent antiviral effect by inhibiting replication of HBV. They are the drug of choice in older patients and patients with hepatic decompensation. On the other hand, the relative lack of immunomodulation renders their effect less sustained than interferon after stopping treatment. Many patients require long-term treatment and the emergence of drug resistance would negate the beneficial effect. This has major implications in young patients who may need to continue the drug for decades.

Predictors of Treatment Response for Peginterferon

It would be desirable if peginterferon is prescribed only to patients who have a high chance to respond, whereas nonresponders can be identified so that peginterferon can be avoided or stopped early during the course of therapy. As liver-related complications take decades to develop, most treatment trials use short-term surrogate markers of response as the outcome measures.

Surrogate Outcome for Peginterferon

The most commonly used surrogate outcome for peginterferon treatment is HBeAg seroconversion. HBeAg seroconversion after interferon therapy reduces the risk of hepatic decompensation and improves survival. Ten to thirty percent of patients may still have active liver disease after HBeAg seroconversion and 10% to 20% of inactive carriers may have reactivation of HBV replication and exacerbations of hepatitis after years of quiescence. Most hepatitis reactivation post-HBeAg seroconversion occurred within 6 months after stopping interferon treatment. Therefore HBeAg seroconversion is usually assessed 6 to 12 months after stopping treatment. HBsAg clearance is the best definition of virologic response, but it is usually a delayed phenomenon.

Baseline Predictors of Response to Peginterferon

Asian patients are less likely to respond to peginterferon treatment as compared with Caucasians. This is partly related to the long duration of infection and partly to the HBV genotype. Asians usually acquire the infection at infancy and have a long immune tolerant phase, which may render immune modulation less effective with interferon-based therapy. It is therefore not recommended to use peginterferon therapy in young Asian patients in the immune tolerant phase. Genotype A HBV, which is prevalent in western Europe and America, is associated with a higher rate of response to interferon treatment. In the Asia-Pacific region, genotype B and C HBV are prevalent. There is some suggestion that genotype B HBV responds better to conventional interferon, but it is controversial whether any difference exists on their response to peginterferon. The best timing for peginterferon therapy is at the immune clearance phase when the patient has elevated ALT,

lower HBV DNA, and higher necroinflammatory activity on histology.

On-Treatment Predictors of Response to Peginterferon
Serum HBV DNA

In general, HBV DNA tends to fall faster during treatment among sustained responders. One way of using serum HBV DNA as an on-treatment predictor of response is to identify the nonresponders so that peginterferon treatment can be stopped earlier. However, there is no consensus on the best timing and cutoff of HBV DNA to predict response to peginterferon treatment. There are reports using serum HBV DNA at week 8 to week 24 to predict sustained virologic response to peginterferon with a negative predictive value of approximately 90%. This may assist in the decision of treatment cessation, particularly among patients who do not tolerate the peginterferon treatment well. Another potential limitation of using HBV DNA to predict treatment response is its failure to differentiate sustained responders from relapsers. In a French study using peginterferon alfa-2a to treat HBeAg-negative chronic hepatitis B, the on-treatment viral kinetics of patients who had initial viral suppression on treatment, but subsequently relapsed after stopping treatment, was almost identical to that of the sustained virologic responders.[90]

Quantitative HBsAg

There is increasing evidence that changes of serum HBsAg titer during antiviral treatment correlates with changes in ccc DNA level. Monitoring of serum HBsAg titer becomes a reasonable on-treatment predictor of response to peginterferon therapy. Recent emerging data suggests that HBsAg titer at week 12 to 24 of peginterferon treatment can predict sustained virologic response. However, there is some controversy whether the absolute HBsAg level or reduction in HBsAg titer during treatment serves as a better predictor of response. More studies are required to validate the use of HBsAg titer as an on-treatment response predictor and to define how treatment can be individualized.

Quantitative HBeAg

Measurement of on-treatment HBeAg level may predict the chance of HBeAg seroconversion to peginterferon alfa-2a therapy. Among 271 HBeAg-positive patients received peginterferon alfa-2a monotherapy in the global study, high levels of HBeAg (>100 PEIU/ml) had a greater negative predictive value (96%) of sustained virologic response than that of serum HBV DNA levels (86%).[91] Unfortunately, the methodology of HBeAg quantification is not standardized and it is not useful in HBeAg-negative patients.

Predictors of Treatment Response for Nucleos(t)ide Analogs

A major concern with long-term nucleos(t)ide analog treatment is the selection of drug-resistant mutations. According to American and European recommendations, nucleos(t)ide analogs with a high genetic barrier of resistance (entecavir and tenofovir) should be used as the first-line agents.[4,53] However, the high cost of these drugs is a major concern in Asian countries where the relatively inexpensive antiviral drugs with a lower genetic barrier of resistance (lamivudine, adefovir, and telbivudine) are also accepted as first-line agents.[10] In this scenario, prediction of response becomes important as one may need to modify the treatment regimen among patients who have a higher risk of developing drug resistance. Even using drugs with a high genetic barrier of resistance, it may be useful to predict the potential nonresponders for closer surveillance of resistance and possible intensification of treatment.

Surrogate Outcome for Nucleos(t)ide Analogs

Hepatitis B e antigen seroconversion is much less durable for nucleos(t)ide analogs than peginterferon therapy, particularly among Asian patients for whom the infection has persisted since early childhood. Up to 50% of patients may experience hepatitis relapse after HBeAg seroconversion within 3 years posttreatment.[92] Therefore HBeAg seroconversion is not an ideal surrogate marker of response for nucleos(t)ide analogs, particularly if the posttreatment follow-up is not long enough. As HBsAg clearance is rarely observed with nucleot(s)ide analogs, evaluation of predictors for HBsAg clearance may be difficult and less clinically useful.

Although nucleos(t)ide analogs can achieve potent viral suppression, viral relapse will occur in most HBeAg-positive patients who fail to lose HBeAg, as well as most HBeAg-negative patients after stopping treatment. The durability of drug-induced viral suppression after 1 year of lamivudine or adefovir treatment in HBeAg-negative patients is less than 10%. Therefore the use of HBV DNA as a surrogate marker for response is valid only if viral suppression is maintained during nucleot(s)ide analog treatment. As viral resistance may develop with ongoing viral replication activity, undetectable HBV DNA by PCR is needed to prevent the development of drug resistance. In other words, although there is no evidence to suggest that undetectable HBV DNA is needed for a better prognosis, it is required to prevent the development of drug resistance and should therefore be the surrogate marker of response in nucleot(s)ide analog treatment.

Baseline Predictors of Response to Nucleos(t)ide Analogs

A stronger host immune clearance, as reflected by a lower serum HBV DNA and higher ALT level, can generally facilitate the viral suppression by nucleos(t)ide analogs. The rate of HBeAg loss was particularly high in lamivudine-treated patients when the ALT level was greater than 5 times the upper limit of laboratory normal. In a posthoc analysis of the GLOBE study, baseline ALT greater than 2 times the upper limit of normal and HBV DNA lower than 9 log copies/ml can predict good maintained response to telbivudine treatment among HBeAg-positive patients at year 2.[93] Similarly, baseline HBV DNA lower than 7 log copies/ml can predict a good maintained response to telbivudine in HBeAg-negative patients. Most data on the prediction of response by baseline HBV DNA and ALT comes from studies including lamivudine, telbivudine, and adefovir. Other clinical factors including HBV genotypes have no relationship with the chance of response to nucleos(t)ide analogs.

On-Treatment Predictors of Response to Nucleos(t)ide Analogs
HBV DNA

In general, a faster and complete suppression of HBV DNA by an antiviral drug is associated with a lower risk of drug resistance. The key evidence comes from the randomized controlled study comparing telbivudine versus lamivudine in both HBeAg-positive and HBeAg-negative chronic hepatitis B (GLOBE study), in which complete viral suppression at 24 weeks of therapy could predict reduced risk of subsequent drug resistance in either treatment arms.[84,93] Among HBeAg-positive patients, 45% of patients on telbivudine and 32% of patients on lamivudine had HBV DNA undetectable at week 24. Among HBeAg-negative patients, 80% of patients on telbivudine and 71% patients on lamivudine achieved undetectable HBV DNA at week 24. Patients on lamivudine who could achieve undetectable HBV DNA at week 24 only had a 2% to 3% risk of resistance at year 1 and a 5% to 9% risk of resistance at year 2. Patients on telbivudine who could achieve undetectable HBV DNA at week 24 had a 0% to 1% risk of resistance at year 1 and a 2% to 4% risk of resistance at year 2. Adefovir has a slower HBV DNA suppression as compared with lamivudine and telbivudine, and week 48 is a more appropriate time point to evaluate its effectiveness. In a long-term follow-up study of HBeAg-negative patients on continuous adefovir therapy, patients who could achieve HBV DNA suppression to below 1000 copies/ml at week 48 had only 6% risk of adefovir-resistance over 192 weeks, whereas 49% of patients with HBV DNA greater than 1000 copies/ml at week 48 had adefovir resistance at week 192.[78] The data on the use of early HBV DNA suppression to predict drug resistance or long-term response to entecavir and tenofovir is lacking.

As HBV DNA suppression at week 24 to 48 can predict the subsequent risk of drug resistance, a roadmap model with on-treatment monitoring of HBV DNA has been proposed.[94] In this model, the HBV DNA at week 24 is used to classify the virologic responses as complete (undetectable HBV DNA), partial (HBV DNA <2000 IU/ml or 4 $\log_{10}$ copies/ml), or inadequate (HBV DNA levels $\geq$ 2000 IU/ml or 4 $\log_{10}$ copies/ml). Patients with a complete virologic response are recommended to continue therapy with the same drug with regular monitoring of HBV DNA because these patients have a lower risk of developing drug resistance in the subsequent years. Patients with partial or inadequate response may need to change to, or add on, another antiviral agent(s), and the strategies will depend on the genetic barrier of resistance of the current nucleos(t)ide analog. However, clinical trials on how to modify the antiviral drug regimen among partial or inadequate responders are lacking, and the current recommendations are largely based on expert opinions. The aim of the roadmap model is to identify patients who have a higher risk of drug resistance for preemptive intensification of treatment, while patients who have lower risk of drug resistance can remain on the original treatment with greater confidence. It is particularly relevant when drugs with lower genetic barrier of resistance are used.

Quantitative HBsAg

The evidence concerning the predictive value of quantitative HBsAg levels in patients receiving nucleos(t)ide analogs is evolving. The ability of nucleos(t)ide analogs to reduce serum HBsAg titer and cccDNA is not as prominent as peginterferon. As the data on the use of quantitative HBsAg to predict response for nucleos(t)ide analogs is still very preliminary, it cannot be recommended for clinical use at this stage.

Management of Drug Resistance

Selection of Drug-Resistance Mutants

Replication of HBV by reverse transcriptase through a RNA intermediate is an error prone process with no proofreading mechanism. If viral replication cannot be suppressed completely by nucleos(t)ide analogs, persistent HBV replication may lead to mutations at the HBV polymerase. Under the natural selection process, viral strains that are resistant to the nucleos(t)ide analog can survive and replicate better than the wild-type virus and hence will be selected as the predominant species. Furthermore, compensatory mutations at other parts of the polymerase gene may emerge subsequently. These compensatory mutations will not directly confer resistance to the drug but they will improve the replication efficacy of the drug resistant mutant. For examples, rtM204V/I is the primary mutation that confers resistance to lamivudine, whereas mutations rtL80I/V, rtV173L, and rtL180M are compensatory mutations that occur commonly with the rtM204V/I mutation. However, compensatory mutations to one drug can cause cross-resistance to another. The best example is rtL180M mutant, which is partially resistant to entecavir. Therefore sequential antiviral treatment with inadequate viral suppression should be avoided because it may nurture the emergence of a multidrug resistant HBV (**Fig. 30-6**).

Detection of HBV Drug Resistance

The first clinical evidence of drug resistance is the emergence of genotypic resistance, which is defined by the detection of mutations in the HBV genome that confer resistance to the drug (**Fig. 30-7**). At this phase, the HBV DNA is still very low and drug resistance is difficult to detect. Drug resistance can only be detected by molecular assays, such as sequencing or hybridization, and these assays are usually employed in clinical

trials for surveillance of resistance. On continued antiviral treatment, virologic breakthrough will follow, defined as an increase of serum HBV DNA by at least 1 log copies/ml (10-fold) from the nadir value. It is recommended to confirm the virologic breakthrough by repeating the HBV DNA testing 1 month later. The HBV DNA levels at virologic breakthrough tend to be lower than the pretreatment level initially, but they may rise with time as the replication fitness of the drug-resistant mutant is enhanced by the emergence of compensatory mutations. The increase in HBV DNA level at virologic breakthrough may be very slow with rtA181T mutation, which causes a stop codon change in the overlapping surface gene at amino acid 172 (sW172*) resulting in truncation of the last 55 amino acid of the C-terminal hydrophobic region of the surface protein.[95] This truncated surface protein has a negative effect on virion secretion and obviates a classical virologic rebound. One important differential diagnosis of drug resistance is poor drug compliance, which should be excluded before genotypic resistance is tested or salvage therapy is commenced. If no salvage therapy is given and the original antiviral drug is continued, biochemical breakthrough, defined as raised ALT, may occur a few months after the virologic breakthrough. Some patients may experience severe hepatitis flare

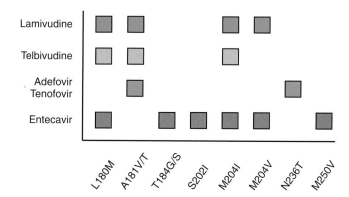

Fig. 30-6 Common HBV drug resistance mutation sites. Rt204 mutation will confer cross-resistance to all L-nucleoside analogs. rtA181V/T is a common mutation pathway between L-nucleoside analogs and acyclic phosphonates. L180M is a compensatory mutation to L-nucleoside analogs, but it will confer cross-resistance to entecavir.

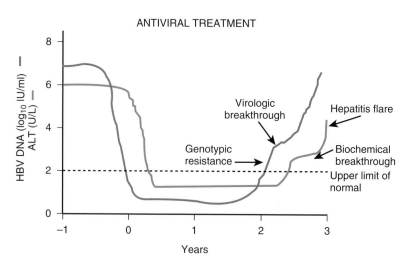

Fig. 30-7 Serial changes of serum HBV DNA and ALT levels in association with emergence of HBV drug resistance. *(Adapted from Lok AS, McMahon BJ. Chronic hepatitis B. Hepatology 2007;45:507–539.)*

or even hepatic decompensation at biochemical breakthrough. Once drug resistance has developed, the resistant HBV mutants will be retained in the viral population inside the liver. Stopping treatment may lead to disappearance of the resistant virus from the blood, but reintroduction of the original antiviral drug will rapidly reselect the drug resistant HBV mutant as the predominant species.

Treatment of HBV Drug Resistance
L-nucleoside Analog Resistance

The most commonly used nucleoside analogs are lamivudine and telbivudine. All L-nucleoside analogs share the same loci of drug resistance mutation at amino acid 204 of the reverse transcriptase. Although lamivudine resistant mutation comprises both rtM204I and rtM204V, whereas only the former mutant is resistant to telbivudine, the treatment strategy for lamivudine resistance should be applicable to telbivudine resistance. Most data on the treatment of L-nucleoside analog resistance are from lamivudine resistance. The drugs of choice for the treatment of rtM204V/I mutants are acyclic phosphonates (i.e., adefovir dipivoxil, tenofovir). Adefovir has proven effectiveness in suppressing viral replication of lamivudine-resistant HBV both in vitro and in vivo. Tenofovir has a more potent viral suppression than adefovir for lamivudine-resistant HBV, and it has become the drug of choice for the treatment of L-nucleotide analog resistance.

Direct switching or add-on adefovir in patients with lamivudine resistance can reduce the HBV DNA by approximately 4 log copies/ml in 1 year. Among patients with decompensated liver cirrhosis, treatment of lamivudine resistance with adefovir can improve the liver function and some patients can be taken off the transplant waiting list. The risk of transient hepatitis flare on direct switching to adefovir from lamivudine is very low, and it is safe to switch the drugs even among cirrhotic patients.

The major drawback of direct switching from lamivudine to adefovir is the high rate of adefovir resistance. In several Asian series, the rate of adefovir resistance after switching from lamivudine is up to 18% in 1 year and 25% in 2 years. In contrary, add-on adefovir to lamivudine can greatly reduce the rate of adefovir resistance. In an Italian series, the rate of adefovir resistance 4 years after adding on to lamivudine was only 4%.[96] All patients who have resistance to add-on adefovir therapy harbored the rtA181V/T mutant, which is cross-resistant to both lamivudine and adefovir. Nonetheless, adding on, rather the switching to, adefovir is the standard strategy for the treatment of lamivudine resistance. There are little data comparing direct switching versus add-on tenofovir in the treatment of lamivudine resistance, though add-on tenofovir is the recommended strategy by most treatment guidelines.

Another crucial factor for the treatment of lamivudine resistance is the timing of the addition of adefovir. The best timing for starting add-on adefovir is when the HBV DNA concentration is less than 6 log copies/ml and the ALT level is normal; nearly all patients can achieve a complete viral suppression within 3 months if salvage adefovir therapy is started promptly.[97] On the contrary, if add-on adefovir is started when HBV DNA is higher than 6 logs and ALT is elevated, less than 50% of patients can achieve undetectable HBV DNA in 2 years. Regular HBV DNA monitoring every 3 to 6 months is therefore very important for patients on lamivudine (or

telbivudine) so that salvage treatment can be administered as soon as genotypic resistance develops.

Entecavir also has antiviral activity against lamivudine-resistant HBV, but entecavir 1 mg daily is required to achieve better viral suppression than the usual dose of 0.5 mg daily. Nonetheless, entecavir resistance still develops in 51% and virologic breakthrough occurs in 43% of lamivudine-resistant patients in 5 years.[83] This is related to the partial cross-drug resistance shared by lamivudine and entecavir. Lamivudine resistance is caused by rtM204I/V mutation, which is usually accompanied by the compensatory mutation rtL180M. For entecavir resistance to develop, one additional mutation at amino acid 184, 202, or 250 will suffice when rtL180M and rtM204I/V are present. In other words, lamivudine has reduced the genetic barrier of resistance to entecavir. Therefore entecavir monotherapy is not a satisfactory option for the treatment of lamivudine-resistant HBV.

Acyclic Phosphonate Resistance

Both L-nucleoside analog and entecavir can be used to treat rtN236T adefovir resistance. Entecavir is the drug of choice because the rtA181V/T mutant also has resistance to lamivudine. Although tenofovir shares partial resistance to adefovir, it has been shown to have some antiviral effect to adefovir resistance. Combination of emtricitabine (Truvada) has better viral suppression than tenofovir monotherapy in treating patients with adefovir resistance. There are no data on the management of tenofovir resistance.

Entecavir Resistance

Adefovir and tenofovir have been shown to have antiviral activity against entecavir resistant HBV in vitro. The clinical efficacy of treatment for entecavir resistance is only documented in small case series.

Treatment of Special Patient Groups
Severe Acute Exacerbation of Chronic HBV

Severe acute exacerbation of chronic hepatitis B can occur spontaneously or on withdrawal of immunosuppressive therapy. At present, there is no evidence that antiviral therapy can reduce the short-term mortality, particularly among patients who develop acute-on-chronic liver failure. Short-term mortality depends on the severity of immune response and hepatic necrosis. Hepatic encephalopathy is the sign of hepatic failure and liver transplantation should be considered. During severe acute exacerbation, the HBV DNA level is often reduced because of heightened immune response. Nevertheless, antiviral therapy is still recommended for viral prophylaxis in case liver transplantation is required and for the prevention of future severe exacerbations. Interferon is contraindicated because of the risk of hepatic decompensation. Among the oral nucleos(t)ide analogs, lamivudine has the most extensive data in this situation. The risk of drug resistance appears to be lower in patients with severe acute exacerbation, probably because of a more potent viral clearance. When lamivudine is used, the cumulative incidence of drug resistance is 23% in 5 years for HBeAg-positive cases and 25% in 4 years for HBeAg-negative cases.[98,99]

Prophylactic Treatment for Immunosuppressive or Anticancer Therapy

As the risk of HBV reactivation among patients on immunosuppressive and anticancer therapy is significant, prophylaxis with oral nucleoside analogs is generally recommended.[53] In a meta-analysis of 21 studies, lamivudine prophylaxis reduced clinical and virologic reactivation by more than 90%.[100] All cause mortality was also reduced (odds ratio, 0.36). The number needed to treat to prevent one death was 11. Because interferon may have a bone marrow suppressive effect, oral nucleos(t)ide analogs should be used in this setting. The duration of prophylactic treatment depends on the original need for antiviral therapy. If a patient does not require antiviral therapy and the baseline HBV DNA is below 2000 IU/ml, an antiviral drug should be given for 6 months after completion of immunosuppressive or anticancer therapy. If a patient has indications for antiviral therapy or high HBV DNA greater than 2000 IU/ml, an antiviral drug should only be stopped if treatment endpoints are reached as in immunocompetent patients.

Liver Transplantation

Without prophylactic treatment, reinfection of the liver graft by HBV is universal and is associated with accelerated fibrosis, liver decompensation, and graft loss. Before the era of prophylactic treatment, the 5-year survival rate for transplantation of hepatitis B was only 50%, which was considerably lower than the survival for transplantation of other liver diseases.[101]

At present, combination treatment with hepatitis B immunoglobulins (HBIG) and oral nucleos(t)ide analogs is the standard of care to prevent HBV reinfection. Though these treatments are highly effective, the optimal dosage and duration of HBIG, and the optimal combination therapy regimen, have not been defined. Experience in Australia suggests that low-dose HBIG can be used when concomitant lamivudine is provided.[102] In some Asian centers, lamivudine monotherapy has been tried with various success.[103] Nevertheless, lamivudine resistance is associated with reinfection and adverse outcomes. HBV DNA should be monitored closely.

High HBV DNA and the presence of drug-resistant mutants are associated with increased risk of infection and the requirement of higher doses of HBIG.[104] Thus the use of antiviral drugs with a high genetic barrier to resistance in patients with decompensated liver cirrhosis, especially potential transplantation candidates, cannot be overemphasized.

HBV and HIV Co-Infection

There are insufficient data to determine the threshold to start treatment for chronic hepatitis B in HIV co-infected patients. Because HIV co-infection speeds up disease progression and results in more severe liver injury, it is prudent to consider treatment when HBV DNA is above 2000 IU/ml and liver biopsy shows more than mild disease. Few studies examined the performance of noninvasive tests of liver fibrosis in co-infected patients and their role is undefined.

Some oral nucleos(t)ide analogs have activities against both HBV and HIV. In the management of HBV and HIV co-infection, it is important to determine if HBV, HIV, or both require treatment. When highly active antiretroviral therapy (HAART) is required, a regime including tenofovir and emtricitabine provides strong antiviral effect on both HBV and HIV. Compared with lamivudine treatment, tenofovir and emtricitabine are more likely to suppress HBV DNA to less than 1000 copies/ml.[105] When tenofovir cannot be used, entecavir, adefovir dipivoxil, telbivudine, and peginterferon are possible options. Entecavir treatment is associated with a 4 to 5 log drop in HBV DNA in co-infected patients.[106] Recent data also showed that entecavir had modest activity against HIV.[107] It remains to be seen if entecavir is associated with increased HBV and/or HIV drug resistance in co-infected patients.

When HAART is not required, antiviral drugs with no activity on HIV should be used to treat chronic hepatitis B so that the risk of HIV drug-resistant mutants is reduced. The possible choices include adefovir dipivoxil, telbivudine, and peginterferon. Although telbivudine is more potent than adefovir dipivoxil, it has a high risk of drug resistance. Peginterferon does not cause drug resistance in HBV and HIV, but its efficacy in co-infected patients is unclear.

In the first 4 to 8 weeks of HAART, there is a rapid rise in CD4+ T cells. This may induce an immune response to HBV, causing hepatic damage. The condition is termed immune reconstitution inflammatory syndrome. Therefore adequate HBV control has been suggested before HAART, though high-quality evidence is lacking.[108]

HBV and HCV Co-Infection

In patients co-infected with HBV and HCV, HCV is usually the more active virus. Standard treatment with peginterferon and ribavirin appears effective in this condition. In a multicenter cohort study in Taiwan, 161 patients with HBV and HCV co-infection received peginterferon and ribavirin.[43] The overall rate of sustained virologic response was 72% for genotype 1 infection and 83% for genotype 2 and 3 infections. The response rate was similar to that in patients with HCV monoinfection. Although HBV DNA would become detectable in 36% in those with negative HBV DNA before peginterferon/ribavirin treatment, this was not associated with significant hepatitis. HBsAg seroclearance also occurred in 11%.

HBV and HDV Co-Infection

The optimal treatment for HBV and HDV co-infection is undefined. Small cohort studies showed that a minority of patients had undetectable HDV RNA after a course of peginterferon or conventional interferon treatment.[109,110] There were conflicting data regarding histologic improvement and survival. Ribavirin and lamivudine do not have effect on HDV.

Pregnancy

There are limited safety data on the use of antiviral therapy during pregnancy. At present, tenofovir and telbivudine are "Category B" drugs, indicating that they are safe in animal models and there are limited data in humans (see **Table 30-8**). Lamivudine, adefovir dipivoxil, and entecavir are "Category C" drugs, indicating that their safety has not been adequately demonstrated in animal models and humans. On the other hand, interferon has antiproliferative actions and is contraindicated during pregnancy. Based on the safety data in HIV patients, it is reasonable to use oral nucleos(t)ide analogs, especially those in "Category B," if the benefits of treatment outweigh the theoretical risk.

Despite prophylactic treatment with HBIG and HBV vaccine, 5% of infants born to HBV-infected mothers still acquire the infection. Thus various groups have evaluated the use of lamivudine before delivery. Overall, the risk of vertical transmission appears to be reduced with lamivudine treatment among carrier mothers with very high HBV DNA levels (>9 log copies/ml) in small cohort studies and a randomized controlled trial.[111,112] Unfortunately, the results of the randomized trial were jeopardized by the high dropout rate, precluding an accurate assessment of the rate of vertical transmission.[112] Thus further data are required before antiviral therapy for the prevention of vertical transmission can be recommended.

Children

Most children with chronic HBV infection are in the immune tolerant phase and can be safely observed. Long-term follow-up studies confirmed that the risk of liver-related complications is low even when the children are left untreated.[113] In some children who develop active disease with high ALT or histologic evidence of liver damage, both interferon and oral nucleos(t)ide analogs have been shown to be safe and effective. In children, 1 year of lamivudine treatment was associated with HBeAg seroconversion in 22%, undetectable HBV DNA in 61%, and ALT normalization in 55%.[114] In adolescents, a composite endpoint of normal ALT and HBV DNA below 1000 copies/ml was achieved in 23% of those receiving adefovir dipivoxil for 48 weeks, compared with 0% of those receiving a placebo.[115] Similarly, HBeAg seroclearance and negative HBV DNA were achieved in 26% of children treated with interferon alpha-2b for 24 weeks, compared with 11% of controls.[116] HBsAg seroclearance also occurred in 10% of interferon-treated patients and 1% of controls.

HCC Surveillance

Rationale

The majority of HCC develops in a background of liver cirrhosis in chronic hepatitis B patients. However, approximately 15% of HBV-related HCC can develop without the presence of underlying liver cirrhosis. There is no precancerous state that can be detected to predict or prevent HCC. Most HCC is asymptomatic in the early stage and the prognosis is grave once the tumor is big enough to cause symptoms. Thus the main objective of surveillance protocol is early detection of small HCCs that are amendable to curative treatment, either by surgical resection, loco-regional therapy, or liver transplantation. Although most studies on HCC surveillance are case control studies and the results of the few randomized trials are subjected to various limitations, it is generally agreed that HCC surveillance can increase the chance of detecting small HCCs and improve patient survival.[117]

Surveillance Tools

The most common tests used for HCC surveillance are ultrasonography and AFP measurement. The sensitivity and specificity of AFP for HCC is at the range of 41% to 65% and 80% to 95%, respectively, when an AFP cutoff of 20 ng/mL is used. Up to 50% of patients with HCC have an AFP lower than

20 ng/ml, and the HCC is associated with significant false-positive results related to hepatitic activities. AFP greater than 400 ng/ml is more diagnostic of HCC, but the HCC is usually advanced at this high AFP level.

Ultrasound is the most popular imaging method for HCC surveillance because it is widely available, inexpensive, and noninvasive. The sensitivity and specificity of ultrasound to detect HCC is approximately 44% to 76%, and 95% to 98%, respectively.[118] Cirrhotic liver with nodular echogenicity may increase the difficulty of the ultrasonic examination. Computerized tomography is not recommended for routine HCC surveillance because of its high cost and significant radiation exposure.

Surveillance Strategy

All patients who are at risk of developing HCC with potential curative treatment available are recommended for regular HCC surveillance. Ultrasound examination every 6 months, with or without AFP, seems to be the most optimal and cost-effective measure for HCC surveillance.

In general, older age, male sex, positive family history of HCC, presence of liver cirrhosis, persistently high viral load, and active hepatitis are risk factors for HCC. All chronic hepatitis B patients with liver cirrhosis that does not preclude curative treatment of HCC should undergo HCC surveillance. Among patients with advanced liver cirrhosis, HCC surveillance should still be carried out as long as liver transplantation remains a treatment option. On the other hand, HCC surveillance should not be conducted among patients with advanced liver cirrhosis who are not liver transplant candidates. For noncirrhotic patients, males older than 40 and females older than 50 (for African Americans, older than 20), those with positive family history of HCC, and those with persistently high serum HBV DNA levels are also suitable cases for HCC surveillance.[53] Whether HBV genotypes and basal core promoter mutations should be considered in the HCC surveillance program remains to be studied.

Prevention of HBV Infection

To prevent the transmission of HBV, three strategies can be employed: (1) suppressing HBV in the host, (2) blocking the transmission routes, and (3) immunization of susceptible subjects. General measures to block the transmission routes include safe sex, avoidance of needle sharing, and universal precaution in the handling of blood products and body fluid. Active immunization can be achieved by vaccination against HBsAg, which provides long-term immunity. Passive immunization by HBIG provides short-term protection for 2 to 4 months.

Hepatitis B Vaccines

In 1982, two subunit vaccines containing 22-nm HBsAg particles were licensed. The vaccines were prepared from plasma of patients with chronic HBV infection. Despite a good safety record, the potential risk of using human blood products results in the development of newer vaccines using DNA recombinant technology. At present, two recombinant vaccines are registered in the United States for the prevention of HBV infection: Recombivax HB (Merck) and Engerix-B (GlaxoSmithKline, Brentford, UK). Another registered preparation, Twinrix (GlaxoSmithKline), is a combination vaccine for hepatitis A virus (HAV) and HBV. Each 1-ml dose contains 720 EL.U. of inactivated HAV and 20 µg of HBsAg.

The recombinant vaccines are produced by introducing the HBsAg gene (S gene) into yeast called *Saccharomyces cerevisiae*. These vaccines induce HBsAg-specific T-helper cells and T cell–dependent B cells to produce neutralizing antibodies against the epitope a (aa124 to 148) of HBsAg as early as 2 weeks after the first immunization.[119] Aluminum hydroxide is added as an adjuvant. Nowadays, owing to the concern about mercury content, thimerosal preservative-free vaccines are available.

Because recipients are only exposed to recombinant HBsAg, the response is reflected by the development of anti-HBs. The presence of anti-HBc indicates prior infection. Anti-HBs titers greater than 100 mIU/ml confer 100% protection against hepatitis B. After receiving all three doses of HBV vaccines, 94% to 98% of recipients develop protective antibodies. The anti-HBs titer decreases rapidly in the first year after vaccination and then more gradually. Although anti-HBs frequently turns negative with time, immunologic memory is maintained for at least 12 years.[120] On the other hand, immunologic memory appears to decrease beyond 15 years.[121] However, because there is no increase in cases of acute or chronic hepatitis B even among subjects vaccinated more than 20 years ago, routine booster doses are not recommended in immunocompetent adults and children.[122] In patients undergoing hemodialysis, anti-HBs should be checked annually and a booster dose given when the titer is below 10 mIU/ml.

Factors associated with decreased response to HBV vaccination include smoking, obesity, chronic liver disease, chronic kidney disease, older age, and immunosuppression. Patients with chronic kidney disease should receive vaccination before the disease progresses to a more advanced stage to improve the response. Other methods that may increase the response include intradermal injection, higher dosage, and more frequent dosing. A meta-analysis of 13 randomized controlled trials with 734 patients showed that the addition of a granulocyte macrophage colony-stimulating factor as an adjuvant significantly increases the response to HBV vaccination.[123] Other new methods under investigations include hepatitis B DNA vaccination with plasmid DNA encoding HBsAg and the administration of HBsAg pulsed blood dendritic cells.

The vaccines have an excellent safety record. Mild fever occurs in 1% to 6% of recipients, pain at the injection site occurs in 3% to 30%, and anaphylaxis occurs in 1.1 per million. Although rare adverse events such as multiple sclerosis, rheumatoid arthritis, type 1 diabetes, leukemia, aseptic meningitis, and Guillain-Barré syndrome have been reported, the incidence is not higher than the general population and the causal relationship has not been established.

Target Group

High-risk individuals who may benefit from HBV vaccination are listed in **Table 30-10**. However, targeted vaccination for people other than healthcare workers is difficult to implement. Universal vaccination for newborns is easier and cost-effective,

Table 30-10 High-Risk Groups Requiring Consideration for HBV Vaccine

Healthcare workers
Public safety workers with likelihood of exposure to blood
Staff and clients of institutions for developmentally disabled
Hemodialysis patients
Patients who are likely to require multiple transfusion with blood or blood products
Household contacts and sex partners of HBV carriers or patients with acute hepatitis B
Travelers to endemic areas who may have intimate contact with local population
Injecting drug users
Unsafe sexual practice
Inmates of correctional facilities
Patients with chronic liver disease
Potential organ recipients

and has been adopted by the United States and many countries.

Vaccination Regimen

The vaccines are given intramuscularly in the deltoid area of adults and the anterolateral thigh in infants or neonates. The dosage and schedule of HBV vaccine are listed in **Table 30-11**. The first two doses are important in the recruitment of responders and the third acts as a booster. In immunocompromised patients and those on hemodialysis, an extra booster dose is recommended. If a vaccination series is interrupted, the second dose should be administered as soon as possible. If the third dose is interrupted, it can be resumed when convenient. The second and third doses should be separated by at least 2 months.

Vaccine Escape Mutants

Mutations in the HBV genome encoding for HBsAg can result in mutant HBV strains that escape neutralization by anti-HBs. The mutation involves the "*a* determinant" and the most common is a glycine to arginine change at amino acid position 145 (sG145R). This results in decreased binding to monoclonal anti-*a* epitope antibodies. Such mutants are more commonly seen in HBV endemic areas, and have been implicated in failed prophylaxis against perinatal transmission. In Taiwan, the prevalence of escape mutants among children with positive HBsAg rose from 8% to 20% after the universal vaccination program, but there was no further rise in the subsequent decade.[124] At present, there is no evidence that the mutant virus causes rising HBV infection in the community. Studies in chimpanzees also suggest that the present vaccines are protective against the "*a* determinant" variants.[125]

Hepatitis B Immunoglobulins

HBIG contains high titers of anti-HBs antibody. The licensed HBIG in the United States has anti-HBs titer of 1:100000. HBIG is safe with rare anaphylactic reactions, particularly when given intravenously. Myalgia, skin rash and arthralgia have been reported, but are believed to be due to

Table 30-11 Recommended Dosing for the Currently Available HBV Vaccines*

GROUP	RECOMBIVAX HB (10 µg/ml)	ENGERIX-B (20 µg/ml)
Infants[†] and children <11 yr	2.5 µg	10 µg
Adolescents (11-19 yr)	5 µg	20 µg
Adults (≥20 yr)	10 µg	20 µg
Hemodialysis patients	40 µg (1 ml)[‡]	40 µg (2 ml)[§]
Immunocompromised patients	40 µg (1 ml)[‡]	40 µg (2 ml)[§]

*The standard schedule is 0, 1, and 6 months.
[†]Infants born to HBsAg-negative mothers.
[‡]Special formulation.
[§]Two 1 ml doses administered at one site in four-dose schedule (0, 1, 2, 6 months).

Table 30-12 Hepatitis B Prophylaxis for Infants Born to an HBsAg-Positive Mother

	VACCINE (EITHER ONE)		HBIG	TIME
	Recombivax HB (5 µg)	Engerix B (10 µg)	(0.5 ml)	
First dose	✓	✓	✓	Within 12 hr of birth
Second dose	✓	✓	—	1 mo
Third dose	✓	✓	—	6 mo

Table 30-13 Postexposure Prophylaxis if the Source Is HBsAg Positive

VACCINATION STATUS OF EXPOSED PERSON	IMMUNE PROPHYLAXIS
Unvaccinated	HBIG (0.06 ml/kg) and initiate HBV vaccination series
Previously vaccinated	
Known responder (Anti-HBs >10 mIU/ml)	No treatment
Known nonresponder	HBIG × 2 doses or HBIG × 1 dose and initiate revaccination
Unknown response	Check anti-HBs If >10 mIU/ml, no treatment If <10 mIU/ml, HBIG × 1 dose and give vaccine booster

antigen-antibody complexes that occur in HBsAg positive patients who are mistakenly given HBIG.

Perinatal Prophylaxis

Infants of mothers with HBeAg-positive chronic hepatitis B are at high risk of contracting the virus. To provide adequate protection, both passive immunization by HBIG and active immunization by HBV vaccine should be given within 24 hours after birth. The purpose of HBIG is to clear the circulating virus before the infant can produce protective antibodies. HBIG and HBV vaccine should be given at different locations to prevent interference. When both are given, the efficacy of protection is more than 90%.[126] If HBIG is skipped, the efficacy is around 83%.[127] Therefore, checking HBsAg and/or

HBeAg in mothers and providing HBIG selectively to infants will be more effective. On the other hand, providing universal HBV vaccination alone to infants without maternal HBsAg testing is a reasonable and cheaper strategy in developing countries. The perinatal prophylaxis regime is listed in **Table 30-12**.

Postexposure Prophylaxis

Postexposure prophylaxis should be considered after any percutaneous, ocular, or mucous membrane exposure. The most common scenario is a healthcare worker with needlestick injury. **Table 30-13** outlines the postexposure prophylaxis if the source is HBsAg positive.

Key References

Amin J, et al. Causes of death after diagnosis of hepatitis B or hepatitis C infection: a large community-based linkage study. Lancet 2006;368:938–945. (Ref.40)

Bedossa P, Dargere D, Paradis V. Sampling variability of liver fibrosis in chronic hepatitis C. Hepatology 2003;38:1449–1457. (Ref.16)

Buster EH, et al. Sustained HBeAg and HBsAg loss after long-term follow-up of HBeAg-positive patients treated with peginterferon alpha-2b. Gastroenterology 2008;135:459–467. (Ref.65)

Chan HL, et al. Treatment of hepatitis B e antigen positive chronic hepatitis with telbivudine or adefovir: a randomized trial. Ann Intern Med 2007;147: 745–754. (Ref.86)

Chan HL, et al. Genotype C hepatitis B virus infection is associated with an increased risk of hepatocellular carcinoma. Gut 2004;53:1494–1498. (Ref.12)

Chan HL, et al. Long-term follow-up of peginterferon and lamivudine combination treatment in HBeAg-positive chronic hepatitis B. Hepatology 2005;41:1357–1364. (Ref.64)

Chan HL, et al. A randomized, controlled trial of combination therapy for chronic hepatitis B: comparing pegylated interferon-alpha2b and lamivudine with lamivudine alone. Ann Intern Med 2005;142:240–250. (Ref.63)

Chan HL, et al. Hepatitis B e antigen-negative chronic hepatitis B in Hong Kong. Hepatology 2000;31:763–768. (Ref.9)

Chan HL, et al. High viral load and hepatitis B virus subgenotype ce are associated with increased risk of hepatocellular carcinoma. J Clin Oncol 2008; 26:177–182. (Ref.56)

Chan HL, et al. Alanine aminotransferase-based algorithms of liver stiffness measurement by transient elastography (Fibroscan) for liver fibrosis in chronic hepatitis B. J Viral Hepat 2009;16:36–44. (Ref.19)

Chan HL, et al. Long-term lamivudine treatment is associated with a good maintained response in severe acute exacerbation of chronic HBeAg-negative hepatitis B. Antivir Ther 2006;11:465–471. (Ref.98)

Chang TT, et al. A comparison of entecavir and lamivudine for HBeAg-positive chronic hepatitis B. N Engl J Med 2006;354:1001–1010. (Ref.80)

Chen CJ, et al. Risk of hepatocellular carcinoma across a biological gradient of serum hepatitis B virus DNA level. JAMA 2006;295:65–73. (Ref.33)

Chen YC, et al. Prognosis following spontaneous HBsAg seroclearance in chronic hepatitis B patients with or without concurrent infection. Gastroenterology 2002;123:1084–1089. (Ref.26)

Chu CM, Liaw YF. HBsAg seroclearance in asymptomatic carriers of high endemic areas: appreciably high rates during a long-term follow-up. Hepatology 2007;45:1187–1192. (Ref.25)

Colli A, et al. Accuracy of ultrasonography, spiral CT, magnetic resonance, and alpha-fetoprotein in diagnosing hepatocellular carcinoma: a systematic review. Am J Gastroenterol 2006;101:513–523. (Ref.118)

Corrao G, et al. Exploring the combined action of lifetime alcohol intake and chronic hepatotropic virus infections on the risk of symptomatic liver cirrhosis. Collaborative groups for the study of liver diseases in Italy. Eur J Epidemiol 1998;14:447–456. (Ref.37)

Cruciani M, et al. Granulocyte macrophage colony-stimulating factor as an adjuvant for hepatitis B vaccination: a meta-analysis. Vaccine 2007;25:709–718. (Ref.123)

Dickson RC, et al. Protective antibody levels and dose requirements for IV 5% Nabi hepatitis B immune globulin combined with lamivudine in liver transplantation for hepatitis B-induced end stage liver disease. Liver Transpl 2006;12:124–133. (Ref.104)

Dienstag JL, et al. Lamivudine as initial treatment for chronic hepatitis B in the United States. N Engl J Med 1999;341:1256–1263. (Ref.71)

Ding C, et al. Quantitative subtyping of hepatitis B virus reveals complex dynamics of YMDD motif mutants development during long-term lamivudine therapy. Antivir Ther 2006;11:1041–1049. (Ref.15)

Drake A, Mijch A, Sasadeusz J. Immune reconstitution hepatitis in HIV and hepatitis B coinfection, despite lamivudine therapy as part of HAART. Clin Infect Dis 2004;39:129–132. (Ref.108)

European Association for the Study of the Liver. EASL clinical practice guidelines: management of chronic hepatitis B. J Hepatol 2009;50:227–242. (Ref.4)

Eyre NS, et al. Hepatitis B virus and hepatitis C virus interaction in Huh-7 cells. J Hepatol 2009;51:446–457. (Ref.44)

Farci P, et al. Long-term benefit of interferon alpha therapy of chronic hepatitis D: regression of advanced hepatic fibrosis. Gastroenterology 2004;126:1740–1749. (Ref.109)

Fontana RJ, et al. Determinants of early mortality in patients with decompensated chronic hepatitis B treated with antiviral therapy. Gastroenterology 2002;123:719–727. (Ref.55)

Fried MW, et al. HBeAg and hepatitis B virus DNA as outcome predictors during therapy with peginterferon alfa-2a for HBeAg-positive chronic hepatitis B. Hepatology 2008;47:428–434. (Ref.91)

Friedrich-Rust M, et al. Performance of transient elastography for the staging of liver fibrosis: a meta-analysis. Gastroenterology 2008;134:960–974. (Ref.18)

Gane EJ, et al. Lamivudine plus low-dose hepatitis B immunoglobulin to prevent recurrent hepatitis B following liver transplantation. Gastroenterology 2007; 132:931–937. (Ref.102)

Hadziyannis SJ, et al. Adefovir dipivoxil for the treatment of hepatitis B e antigen-negative chronic hepatitis B. N Engl J Med 2003;348:800–807. (Ref.76)

Hadziyannis SJ, et al. Long-term therapy with adefovir dipivoxil for HBeAg-negative chronic hepatitis B for up to 5 years. Gastroenterology 2006;131:1743–1751. (Ref.78)

Hadziyannis SJ, et al. Long-term therapy with adefovir dipivoxil for HBeAg-negative chronic hepatitis B. N Engl J Med 2005;352:2673–2681. (Ref.77)

Hsu HY, et al. Survey of hepatitis B surface variant infection in children 15 years after a nationwide vaccination programme in Taiwan. Gut 2004;53:1499–1503. (Ref.124)

Iorio R, et al. Long-term outcome in children with chronic hepatitis B: a 24-year observation period. Clin Infect Dis 2007;45:943–949. (Ref.113)

Janssen HL, et al. Pegylated interferon alfa-2b alone or in combination with lamivudine for HBeAg-positive chronic hepatitis B: a randomised trial. Lancet 2005;365:123–129. (Ref.14)

Jonas MM, et al. Safety, efficacy, and pharmacokinetics of adefovir dipivoxil in children and adolescents (age 2 to <18 years) with chronic hepatitis B. Hepatology 2008;47:1863–1871. (Ref.115)

Jonas MM, et al. Clinical trial of lamivudine in children with chronic hepatitis B. N Engl J Med 2002;346:1706–1713. (Ref.114)

Katz LH, et al. Lamivudine prevents reactivation of hepatitis B and reduces mortality in immunosuppressed patients: systematic review and meta-analysis. J Viral Hepat 2008;15:89–102. (Ref.100)

Keeffe EB, et al. A treatment algorithm for the management of chronic hepatitis B virus infection in the United States: 2008 update. Clin Gastroenterol Hepatol 2008;6:1315–1341; quiz 1286. (Ref.94)

Kim WR. Epidemiology of hepatitis B in the United States. Hepatology 2009; 49(5 Suppl):S28–S34. (Ref.2)

Kim WR, et al. Outcome of liver transplantation for hepatitis B in the United States. Liver Transpl 2004;10:968–974. (Ref.101)

Kumar M, et al. A randomized controlled trial of lamivudine to treat acute hepatitis B. Hepatology 2007;45:97–101. (Ref.58)

Lai CL, et al. Telbivudine versus lamivudine in patients with chronic hepatitis B. N Engl J Med 2007;357:2576–2588. (Ref.84)

Lai CL, et al. Entecavir versus lamivudine for patients with HBeAg-negative chronic hepatitis B. N Engl J Med 2006;354:1011–1020. (Ref.82)

Lampertico P, et al. Low resistance to adefovir combined with lamivudine: a 3-year study of 145 lamivudine-resistant hepatitis B patients. Gastroenterology 2007;133:1445–1451. (Ref.96)

Lampertico P, et al. Adefovir rapidly suppresses hepatitis B in HBeAg-negative patients developing genotypic resistance to lamivudine. Hepatology 2005; 42:1414–1419. (Ref.97)

Larkin J, et al. Chronic ethanol consumption stimulates hepatitis B virus gene expression and replication in transgenic mice. Hepatology 2001;34(4 Pt 1):792–797. (Ref.38)

Lau GK, et al. Peginterferon alfa-2a, lamivudine, and the combination for HBeAg-positive chronic hepatitis B. N Engl J Med 2005;352:2682–2695. (Ref.62)

Leung N, et al. Early hepatitis B virus DNA reduction in hepatitis B e antigen-positive patients with chronic hepatitis B: a randomized international study of entecavir versus adefovir. Hepatology 2009;49:72–79. (Ref.81)

Leung NW, et al. Extended lamivudine treatment in patients with chronic hepatitis B enhances hepatitis B e antigen seroconversion rates: results after 3 years of therapy. Hepatology 2001;33:1527–1532. (Ref.73)

Liaw YF, et al. Impact of acute hepatitis C virus superinfection in patients with chronic hepatitis B virus infection. Gastroenterology 2004;126:1024–1029. (Ref.41)

Liaw YF, et al. 2-Year GLOBE trial results: telbivudine is superior to lamivudine in patients with chronic hepatitis B. Gastroenterology 2009;136:486–495. (Ref.85)

Liaw YF, et al. Asian-Pacific consensus statement on the management of chronic hepatitis B: a 2008 update. Hepatol Int 2008;2:263–283. (Ref.10)

Liaw YF, et al. Effects of extended lamivudine therapy in Asian patients with chronic hepatitis B. Asia hepatitis lamivudine study group. Gastroenterology 2000;119:172–180. (Ref.72)

Liaw YF, et al. Lamivudine for patients with chronic hepatitis B and advanced liver disease. N Engl J Med 2004;351:1521–1531. (Ref.54)

Limquiaco JL, et al. Lamivudine monoprophylaxis and adefovir salvage for liver transplantation in chronic hepatitis B: a seven-year follow-up study. J Med Virol 2009;81:224–229. (Ref.103)

Liu CJ, et al. Peginterferon alfa-2a plus ribavirin for the treatment of dual chronic infection with hepatitis B and C viruses. Gastroenterology 2009; 136:496–504, e3. (Ref.43)

Livingston SE, et al. Clearance of hepatitis B e antigen in patients with chronic hepatitis B and genotypes A, B, C, D, and F. Gastroenterology 2007;133:1452–1457. (Ref.13)

Lok AS, et al. Long-term safety of lamivudine treatment in patients with chronic hepatitis B. Gastroenterology 2003;125:1714–1722. (Ref.74)

Lok AS, McMahon BJ. Chronic hepatitis B. Hepatology 2007;45:507–539. (Ref.53)

Lu CY, et al. Humoral and cellular immune responses to a hepatitis B vaccine booster 15-18 years after neonatal immunization. J Infect Dis 2008;197:1419–1426. (Ref.121)

Lui YY, Chan HL. A review of telbivudine for the management of chronic hepatitis B virus infection. Expert Opin Drug Metab Toxicol 2008;4:1351–1361. (Ref.69)

Manesis EK, Hadziyannis SJ. Interferon alpha treatment and retreatment of hepatitis B e antigen-negative chronic hepatitis B. Gastroenterology 2001; 121:101–109. (Ref.60)

Marcellin P, et al. Sustained response of hepatitis B e antigen-negative patients 3 years after treatment with peginterferon alpha-2a. Gastroenterology 2009; 136:2169–2179 e1–e4. (Ref.68)

Marcellin P, et al. Adefovir dipivoxil for the treatment of hepatitis B e antigen-positive chronic hepatitis B. N Engl J Med 2003;348:808–816. (Ref.75)

Marcellin P, et al. Tenofovir disoproxil fumarate versus adefovir dipivoxil for chronic hepatitis B. N Engl J Med 2008;359:2442–2455. (Ref.87)

Marcellin P, et al. Peginterferon alfa-2a alone, lamivudine alone, and the two in combination in patients with HBeAg-negative chronic hepatitis B. N Engl J Med 2004;351:1206–1217. (Ref.67)

Marcellin P, et al. Mortality related to chronic hepatitis B and chronic hepatitis C in France: evidence for the role of HIV coinfection and alcohol consumption. J Hepatol 2008;48:200–207. (Ref.35)

Matthews GV, et al. A randomized trial of combination hepatitis B therapy in HIV/HBV coinfected antiretroviral naive individuals in Thailand. Hepatology 2008;48:1062–1069. (Ref.105)

McMahon MA, et al. The HBV drug entecavir: effects on HIV-1 replication and resistance. N Engl J Med 2007;356:2614–2621. (Ref.107)

Moucari R, et al. Early serum HBsAg drop: a strong predictor of sustained virological response to pegylated interferon alfa-2a in HBeAg-negative patients. Hepatology 2009;49:1151–1157. (Ref.90)

Nair S, Perrillo RP. Serum alanine aminotransferase flares during interferon treatment of chronic hepatitis B: is sustained clearance of HBV DNA dependent on levels of pretreatment viremia? Hepatology 2001;34:1021–1026. (Ref.61)

Ni YH, et al. Two decades of universal hepatitis B vaccination in Taiwan: impact and implication for future strategies. Gastroenterology 2007;132:1287–1293. (Ref.122)

Niro GA, et al. Pegylated interferon alpha-2b as monotherapy or in combination with ribavirin in chronic hepatitis delta. Hepatology 2006;44:713–720. (Ref.110)

Ogata N, et al. Licensed recombinant hepatitis B vaccines protect chimpanzees against infection with the prototype surface gene mutant of hepatitis B virus. Hepatology 1999;30:779–786. (Ref.125)

Pessoa MG, et al. Efficacy and safety of entecavir for chronic HBV in HIV/HBV coinfected patients receiving lamivudine as part of antiretroviral therapy. AIDS 2008;22:1779–1787. (Ref.106)

Poynard T, et al. Meta-analyses of FibroTest diagnostic value in chronic liver disease. BMC Gastroenterol 2007;7:40. (Ref.17)

Radjef N, et al. Molecular phylogenetic analyses indicate a wide and ancient radiation of African hepatitis delta virus, suggesting a deltavirus genus of at least seven major clades. J Virol 2004;78:2537–2544. (Ref.45)

Sagnelli E, et al. HBV superinfection in HCV chronic carriers: a disease that is frequently severe but associated with the eradication of HCV. Hepatology 2009;49:1090–1097. (Ref.42)

Saldanha J, et al. An international collaborative study to establish a World Health Organization international standard for hepatitis B virus DNA nucleic acid amplification techniques. Vox Sang 2001;80:63–71. (Ref.11)

Seok JI, et al. Long-term therapy with clevudine for chronic hepatitis B can be associated with myopathy characterized by depletion of mitochondrial DNA. Hepatology 2009;49:2080–2086. (Ref.89)

Sung JJ, et al. Lamivudine compared with lamivudine and adefovir dipivoxil for the treatment of HBeAg-positive chronic hepatitis B. J Hepatol 2008;48:728–735. (Ref.79)

Sung JJ, et al. Meta-analysis: treatment of hepatitis B infection reduces risk of hepatocellular carcinoma. Aliment Pharmacol Ther 2008;28:1067–1077. (Ref.52)

Sung JJ, et al. Intrahepatic hepatitis B virus covalently closed circular DNA can be a predictor of sustained response to therapy. Gastroenterology 2005;128:1890–1897. (Ref.66)

Tan J, et al. Tenofovir monotherapy is effective in hepatitis B patients with antiviral treatment failure to adefovir in the absence of adefovir-resistant mutations. J Hepatol 2008;48:391–398. (Ref.88)

Tenney DJ, et al. Long-term monitoring shows hepatitis B virus resistance to entecavir in nucleoside-naive patients is rare through 5 years of therapy. Hepatology 2009;49:1503–1514. (Ref.83)

Thio CL, et al. HIV-1, hepatitis B virus, and risk of liver-related mortality in the multicenter cohort study (MACS). Lancet 2002;360:1921–1926. (Ref.47)

van Nunen AB, et al. Durability of HBeAg seroconversion following antiviral therapy for chronic hepatitis B: relation to type of therapy and pretreatment serum hepatitis B virus DNA and alanine aminotransferase. Gut 2003;52:420–424. (Ref.92)

van Zonneveld M, et al. Lamivudine treatment during pregnancy to prevent perinatal transmission of hepatitis B virus infection. J Viral Hepat 2003;10:294–297. (Ref.111)

Warner N, Locarnini S. The antiviral drug selected hepatitis B virus rtA181T/sW172* mutant has a dominant negative secretion defect and alters the typical profile of viral rebound. Hepatology 2008;48:88–98. (Ref.95)

Wong VW, Chan HL. Severe acute exacerbation of chronic hepatitis B: a unique presentation of a common disease. J Gastroenterol Hepatol 2009;24:1179–1186. (Ref.34)

Wong VW, et al. Long-term follow-up of lamivudine treatment in patients with severe acute exacerbation of hepatitis B e antigen (HBeAg)-positive chronic hepatitis B. Antivir Ther 2008;13:571–579. (Ref.99)

Xu WM, et al. Lamivudine in late pregnancy to prevent perinatal transmission of hepatitis B virus infection: a multicentre, randomized, double-blind, placebo-controlled study. J Viral Hepat 2009;16:94–103. (Ref.112)

Yang HI, et al. Hepatitis B e antigen and the risk of hepatocellular carcinoma. N Engl J Med 2002;347:168–174. (Ref.32)

Yeo W, et al. Hepatitis B reactivation in patients with hepatocellular carcinoma undergoing systemic chemotherapy. Ann Oncol 2004;15:1661–1666. (Ref.48)

Yeo W, et al. Sequence variations of precore/core and precore promoter regions of hepatitis B virus in patients with or without viral reactivation during cytotoxic chemotherapy. J Viral Hepat 2000;7:448–458. (Ref.51)

Yuen MF, et al. HBsAg seroclearance in chronic hepatitis B in Asian patients: replicative level and risk of hepatocellular carcinoma. Gastroenterology 2008;135:1192–1199. (Ref.27)

Yuen MF, et al. Prognostic determinants for chronic hepatitis B in Asians: therapeutic implications. Gut 2005;54:1610–1614. (Ref.57)

Zeuzem S, et al. Baseline characteristics and early on-treatment response predict the outcomes of 2 years of telbivudine treatment of chronic hepatitis B. J Hepatol 2009;51:11–20. (Ref.93)

Zhang BH, Yang BH, Tang ZY. Randomized controlled trial of screening for hepatocellular carcinoma. J Cancer Res Clin Oncol 2004;130:417–422. (Ref.117)

A complete list of references can be found at www.expertconsult.com.

Chapter 31

Hepatitis C

Hans L. Tillmann and John G. McHutchison

ABBREVIATIONS

ALT alanine aminotransferase
AST aspartate aminotransferase
bDNA branched-chain DNA
CDC Centers for Disease Control and Prevention
cEVR complete early virologic response (HCV RNA negative at week 12 of therapy)
CI confidence interval
CIA chemiluminescent immunoassay
CMIA chemiluminescent microparticle immunoassay
EIA enzyme immunoassay
EMEA European Medicines Evaluation Agency
eRVR extended rapid virologic response (HCV RNA negative at weeks 4 and 12)
ETR end-of-treatment response
EVR early virologic response
FDA Food and Drug Administration
GWAS genomewide association study
HAART highly active antiretroviral therapy

HAV hepatitis A virus
HBV hepatitis B virus
HCC hepatocellular carcinoma
HCV hepatitis C virus
HIV human immunodeficiency virus
IDU injection drug use
IFN interferon
IL28b interleukin-28b (one of the λ or type III interferons), a genomic region that has been identified to be associated with response to interferon and ribavirin therapy
INR international normalized ratio
ISDR interferon sensitivity determining region
LIA line immunoassay
LP lichen planus
MC essential mixed cryoglobulinemia
MELD Model for End-Stage Liver Disease
MEIA microparticle immunoassay
MPGN membranoproliferative glomerulonephritis
MSM men who have sex with men
NAT nucleic acid testing

NHANES National Health and Nutrition Examination Survey
NHL non-Hodgkin lymphoma
PCR polymerase chain reaction
PCT porphyria cutanea tarda
PEG-IFN pegylated interferon
pEVR partial early virologic response (≥2-log reduction in HCV RNA, but HCV RNA still detectable at week 12 of therapy)
RF rheumatoid factor
RIBA recombinant immunoblot assay
RVR rapid virologic response
SNP single nucleotide polymorphism
SOC standard of care
STAT-C specifically targeted antiviral therapy for HCV
SVR sustained virologic response
TMA transcription-mediated amplification
TSH thyroid-stimulating hormone

Introduction

When hepatitis C virus (HCV) was identified in the late 1980s and the data first published in April 1989, it became clear that most patients with non-A, non-B hepatitis were infected with HCV. A great deal of information about this viral infection and its consequences has been learned within the 2 decades since the virus was first reported.

Based on clinic cohorts from hepatology centers, it is estimated that liver cirrhosis develops in 20% to 30% of patients infected with HCV within 20 years, a figure that was later found to be somewhat lower in prospective cohorts. Still, HCV is one of the leading causes of death from liver cirrhosis and hepatocellular carcinoma (HCC) and is now the most common indication for liver transplantation in the western world. HCV is estimated to kill more people per infected individual than chronic hepatitis B does.[1]

Importantly, overall treatment response rates have improved from less than 10% to greater than 50%, and prediction of treatment response can be based on individual characteristics and on "on-treatment" response. Since the last edition, further progress has been achieved, with direct antivirals now being at the brink of entering the clinic and a genetic marker (IL28B) predictive of response to treatment having been identified. This genetic marker is referred to as IL28B because of its location within the area of the *IL28B* gene. At present, we are on the verge of an era in which new treatment regimens using multidrug modalities and prediction of response will allow progressively higher response rates and a personalized approach to the treatment of patients with HCV infection.[2]

This chapter focuses on our current knowledge with regard to the clinical aspects of HCV, whereas virology and immunopathogenesis are discussed in detail in Chapters 7 and 8. The clinical importance of HCV relates to the complications of long-standing infection that lead to the development of cirrhosis and its consequences, along with HCC, but physicians are increasingly recognizing clinical consequences that occur outside the liver. These so-called extrahepatic manifestations range from mild to disabling fatigue, from asymptomatic cryoglobulinemia to vasculitis and membrano-proliferative glomerulonephritis (MPGN).

Notably, with several new treatments on the horizon, there is hope that eventually all or at least most patients can be cured of hepatitis C.

Epidemiology
Prevalence

The uncertainty in the exact estimates of the worldwide prevalence of HCV infection is best reflected by the different numbers published by the World Health Organization (WHO). The most recent estimates published in 2004 indicated that 2.2%, or 120 to 130 million people, are infected with HCV worldwide.[3] Still, the WHO's current fact sheet concerning hepatitis C quotes 170 million based on estimates published in 1999.[4] There is no doubt, however, that the prevalence of HCV infection varies globally, with the highest prevalence being reported in Egypt, especially in the Nile delta, and with more than 50% of the people born before 1962 being HCV positive and the overall prevalence reported at well above 10%.[5] The lowest prevalence was reported from northern Europe, with 0.003% in Sweden and 0.02% in Finland according to the 1999 WHO document.[6] Despite differences between countries, the overall prevalence is mostly between 1% and 5%, with an estimated 1% in Europe, 1.7% in the Americas, 2.2% in Southeast Asia, 3.9% in the western Pacific, 4.6% in the eastern Mediterranean, and 5.3% in Africa. The WHO data listed the following countries with an estimated HCV prevalence of higher than 5%: Surinam, 5.1%; Thailand, 5.6%; Vietnam, 6.1%; Democratic Republic of Congo, 6.4%; Gabon, 6.5%; Zimbabwe, 7.7%; Libyan Arab Jamahiriya, 7.9%; Guinea, 10.7%; Mongolia, 10.7%; Burundi, 11.1%; Bolivia, 11.2%; Cameroon, 12.5%; Rwanda, 17.0%; and Egypt, 18.1% (**Fig. 31-1**).

In the United States, studies conducted by the Centers for Disease Control and Prevention (CDC) suggest that more than 2.7 million individuals in the United States and potentially upward of 5 million are infected with HCV. The most recent 1999 to 2002 National Health and Nutrition Examination Survey (NHANES) data estimated that 1.6% (confidence interval [CI], 1.3% to 1.9%) of people have been exposed to HCV (anti-HCV positive), which is not significantly different from the earlier 1.8% estimate from the period 1994 to 1998.[7] However, because incarcerated and homeless people were excluded from all these NHANES studies, the true prevalence is probably about 5 million given the higher prevalence of HCV in these groups.[8] Especially worrisome is the high prevalence of alcohol use in people with HCV infection, because of the fact that they are most likely unaware of their infection. It has been shown that awareness of HCV infection can be associated with reduced alcohol consumption, even in those with a history of injection drug use (IDU).[9,10]

HCV infection is most prevalent in people born between 1940 and 1965. Accordingly, the NHANES 1999-2002 and 1994-1998 data indicate a shift in the age of infected people. Both studies highlight the important role of drug abuse as a risk factor for HCV infection (**Table 31-1**). A history of IDU has been associated with the highest risk for HCV positivity, with an odds ratio of almost 150 in the NHANES 1999-2002 population who were 20 to 59 years of age. Importantly, persons of low socioeconomic status had the next highest odd ratio, though substantially lower. The epidemiologic relevance of HCV is also highlighted by the estimated 10,000 deaths and 2000 liver transplantations annually in the United States that are attributed to HCV-related liver disease.

People with abnormal alanine transaminase (ALT) levels, any illicit drug use (except marijuana), transfusion before 1992, or more than 20 lifetime sexual partners reflect 98.7% of all estimated HCV-positive people in the United States. However, they also account for more than 40% of the general

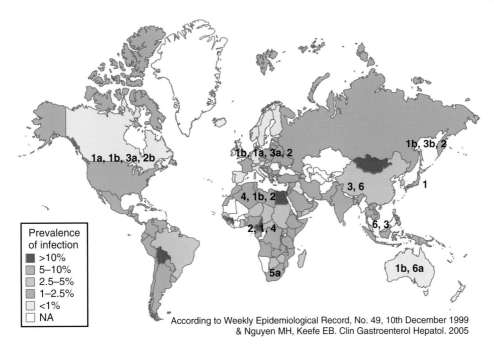

Prevalence of infection
- ■ >10%
- ▨ 5–10%
- ▨ 2.5–5%
- ▨ 1–2.5%
- ▨ <1%
- □ NA

According to Weekly Epidemiological Record, No. 49, 10th December 1999
& Nguyen MH, Keefe EB. Clin Gastroenterol Hepatol. 2005

Fig. 31-1 Prevalence of infection with hepatitis C virus according to the World Health Organization 1999 Weekly Epidemiological Record, No 49 December 10, 1999.

Table 31-1 Odds Ratio for Being HCV Positive with Various Risk Factors According to NHANES Studies

ALTER ET AL.[7]		ARMSTRONG ET AL.[8]	
Poverty Index			
Below poverty level	2.37 (1.50-3.75)	Below poverty level	9.1 (4.5-18.2)
At or above poverty level	1	1.0 to 1.9 times poverty level	3.5 (1.9-6.4)
		>2 times poverty level	1
Drug Use			
		IDU, ever	148.9 (44.9-494)
Cocaine use, ever	4.70 (2.49-8.87)	Drug use (not intravenous, not marijuana)	3.7 (1.7-7.9)
Marijuana use, 1-99 times	2.99 (1.69-5.27)		
Never	1	Never	1
No. of Lifetime Sexual Partners			
≥50	5.16 (1.80-14.73)	>20	5.2 (1.5-18.2)
2-49	2.54 (1.14-5.66)	2-19	1.4 (0.3-6.0)
0-1	1	0-1	1

IDU, injection drug user; NHANES, National Health and Nutrition Examination Survey

population.[8] As in most countries, HCV infection remains undiagnosed in most affected people at present. Still, the U.S. Preventive Services Task Force did not recommend screening for HCV in 2004. This was based on the assumption that HCV-infected patients who feel healthy would not change their behavior after becoming aware of their infection and the lack of data confirming improved outcome with screening. Hepatologists in general oppose this recommendation because there is increasing evidence that HCV-infected patients change their behavior when aware of their infection status,[9,10] and there are also emerging data that treatment intervention with a successful outcome improves long-term survival. With the significant increase in success of antiviral therapy, the reason for screening for HCV increases, and the discussion regarding screening will undoubtedly again swing toward screening and treatment. In line with this, the Institute of Medicine in its most recent statement concerning hepatitis (released January 2010) advocates screening for risk factors for viral hepatitis, followed by testing for viral hepatitis in individuals with identified bona fide risk factors.

In some countries there is a predominance of HCV infection in females.[11] In others such as the United States, there is a clear male preponderance, with an approximate 1:2 ratio. Another interesting finding is that being born in the United States is associated with a higher risk for HCV positivity than being born outside the United States.[8] Most patients with chronic HCV infection have a stable viral load of between 100,000 and 10,000,000 IU/ml.

Incidence

Estimates of the incidence of hepatitis C are difficult to make because the majority of patients with acute HCV infection do not experience symptoms severe enough to seek medical attention. Since 1989, the number of estimated new infections in the United States has declined by more than 80% to fewer than 30,000 estimated new infections per year (**Fig. 31-2**).[12] A similar

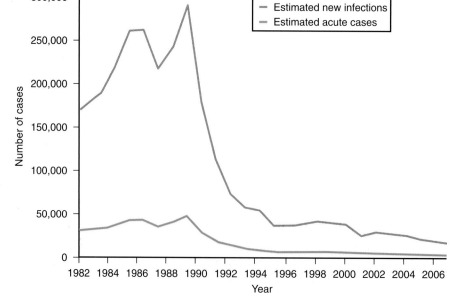

Fig. 31-2 Estimated incidence of hepatitis C virus infection in the United States according to data published by the Centers for Disease Control and Prevention. *(Modified from http://www.cdc.gov/hepatitis/Statistics.htm#section3, accessed September 16, 2009).* The green line *(lower line)* indicates the estimated cases with infection and hepatitis, whereas the blue line *(upper line)* indicates all estimated cases of new infection (with and without concomitant hepatitis).

pattern can be expected in the developed world because of general screening of blood for the virus with anti-HCV testing and, more recently, nucleic acid testing (NAT), as well as education and needle exchange programs in IDU populations.

The decline in the incidence of HCV infection will eventually be reflected in a decrease in complications from such infection in the future. However, the incidence of complications is expected to rise in most countries in the interim because of the delay between infection, disease progression, and development of complications. For example, in Japan a decline in the incidence of HCC is expected soon[13] or may have already started.[14]

HCV Genotypes

Currently, six different HCV genotypes and more than 50 subtypes have been identified. The six major genotypes are numbered 1 to 6, which differ in their nucleotide sequence by 31% to 33%.[15] Each genotype is composed of different subtypes with sequence diversity of 20% to 29%. Some genotypes, such as genotypes 3 and 6, harbor such different subtypes that it was suggested that they be named clade 3 with genotypes 3 and 10 and clade 6 with genotypes 6, 7, 8, 9, and 11. However, at present these clades are still referred to as genotypes 3 and 6, respectively.

HCV genotypes have thus far not been convincingly associated with different outcomes regarding the natural history of hepatitis C, although there is emerging evidence that genotypes differ in their relationship to insulin resistance and hepatic steatosis. Given the relative high divergence of the different genotypes, this is not surprising.

The greatest importance of the HCV genotypes relates to treatment—both in regard to response to current standard of care (SOC) and in regard to response to some of the newer agents (see Treatment).

An accurate nomenclature concerning mutations will be important in the future with direct antivirals entering the clinic. Similar to antiviral treatment of hepatitis B virus (HBV) and human immunodeficiency virus (HIV), individual genotypes and subtypes might differ in the length of individual viral proteins; therefore a numbering system according to the HCV isolate, such as H77 (GenBank accession number AF009606), has been proposed.[16]

Genotype Distribution

The six major genotypes differ in their geographic location.[17] For example, there is a predominance of genotype 1b in western Europe and 1a in North America. Among western

European IDU patients, genotype 3 predominates. Genotype 4 is closely related to Egypt and northern Africa. Genotype 5 is common in southern Africa, and genotype 6 is common in Southeast Asia and in Southeast Asian immigrants in Australia (see **Fig. 31-1**).[15,18]

Transmission

Transmission of infection can be divided into percutaneous/parenteral (blood transfusion, blood or virus transmission via needlestick inoculation) and nonpercutaneous transmission routes (sexual contacts, perinatal exposure, airborne, enteral [oral] or vector-based transmission). Hepatitis C is predominantly or almost exclusively acquired through percutaneous exposure to blood. HCV infections have been proven only in settings in which trauma allowing HCV access to the circulation is at least likely (see Nonpercutaneous Transmission). There is no evidence of HCV transmission via vectors or oral or airborne transmission. HCV is considered more infectious than HIV in cases of needlestick injury or needle sharing and less infectious than HBV in the setting of household and sexual contacts. HCV is also less infectious than HIV in the context of sexual contacts and significantly less infectious than HBV.

There is a very high frequency of markers of past or present HBV infection in partners and household members of hepatitis B surface antigen (HBsAg)-positive individuals (see Chapter 30), but only rarely does HCV transmission occur between stable monogamous partners.

Percutaneous Transmission

Needlestick Injury and Heathcare Workers

Although hepatitis B was the most common occupationally acquired disease before the availability of the HBV vaccine, the prevalence of HCV in healthcare providers is similar to that in the general population.[19,20] Still, there is molecular proof of transmission via needlestick injury, which, however, is again relatively uncommon. In a review of 22 studies on needlestick injury, only 52 of a total of 7112 (0.73%) exposed individuals demonstrated seroconversion to anti-HCV (**Table 31-2**).[21-25] In the absence of injury, there have been individual cases in which the combination of broken skin and failure to use gloves was associated with HCV transmission.[26]

HCV Transmission in the Setting of Drug Abuse

In the NHANES epidemiologic data, occasional marijuana consumption was not associated with HCV, whereas cocaine

Table 31-2 Risk for Seroconversion after Exposure to an Infected Source

	HCW EXPOSURE	NEEDLE SHARING	INTIMATE CONTACTS	HOUSEHOLD CONTACTS
HBeAg negative	1.9% (CI, 0.0-4.1)[21]	Very high	High	High
HBeAg positive	19% (CI, 13.8-23.8)[22]	Very high	Very high	Very high
Hepatitis C	0.73% (CI, 0.53-0.93%)[23]	Very high	Very low	Very low
HIV	0.31%[24]	High	High	Very low

CI, confidence interval; HBeAg, hepatitis B e antigen; HCW, health care worker; HIV, human immunodeficiency virus

use was. This could be due to transmission of HCV via damaged nasal mucosa or to undeclared IDU inasmuch as cocaine use in the absence of co-occurring IDU is rare in patients with acute HCV.[7]

Preventing needle sharing reduced but did not eliminate HCV transmission in IDU patients. Drug use paraphernalia are also important transmission factors.[27] Thus, besides not sharing needles, IDU patients need to be educated to also use their own paraphernalia (cookers, cotton, spoon, and rinse water).

Transmission of Infection to Patients in the Healthcare Setting

Unlike HBV, HCV transmission outbreaks have rarely been reported in patients who were operated on or cared for by HCV-positive surgeons or physicians, and in any such reports few patients actually became infected.[28-30] If more patients are documented to be infected in this setting, it is likely that some blatant disregard for infection control procedures has occurred, as in the case of an anesthetist who infected more than 200 patients between 1988 and 1997 to save anesthetic medicine for personal use.

Infections in the healthcare setting are mostly associated with inappropriate multivial use and poor adherence to universal precautions, especially hand hygiene in dialysis units.[31-33] With adherence to universal precautions, nosocomial transmission should be preventable.[34] Most HCV transmissions in the healthcare setting have not been attributed to any HCV-infected healthcare provider but, instead, to inappropriate infection control procedures. For example, the most recent outbreak of acute HCV infection in an endoscopy clinic in Nevada was attributed to unsafe injection practices rather than an HCV-infected healthcare provider or contaminated endoscopes.[35]

Nonetheless, HCV transmission in the healthcare setting is still possible, with 15% to 67% of patients in some studies with acute hepatitis C reporting medical procedures or a recent hospital admission as the probable cause of infection.[36,37]

Infection via Organ Transplantation, Immunoglobulin Preparations, and Blood Transfusions

Pereira and colleagues[37a,37b] demonstrated in a retrospective study as early as 1991 and 1992 that transmission of HCV via transplantation of organs from HCV RNA–positive donors is almost universal. Hemophiliac patients treated before 1986 with pooled clotting factor concentrates also experienced a nearly 100% risk for infection with HCV. Likewise, women exposed to contaminated batches of anti–D immunoglobulin exhibited evidence of HCV infection in more than 95% of instances. Interestingly, some exposed women never showed signs of infection.[38]

Nonpercutaneous Transmission

Vertical or perinatal transmissions have been well documented. The perinatal transmission rate is estimated to be around 3% to 10%. Surprisingly, up to 50% of HCV-infected newborns were shown to clear HCV RNA by 1 year

of age and another 25% between year 1 and year 2 to 3 of age.[39]

A study involving twin pregnancies revealed HCV infection in the second twin in three of four twin pregnancies, thus fitting with the concept that labor of longer duration and thereby a higher risk for mucosal and skin damage might be a factor contributing to HCV transmission.[40] Breastfeeding has not been associated with transmission of HCV as long as the breast and nipple are intact and without injury (http://www.cdc.gov/BREASTFEEDING/disease/hepatitis.htm).

Sexual Transmission

There is little evidence to support transmission of HCV during sexual intercourse in the absence of risk factors for significant mucosal trauma. In two prospective studies involving 216 and 895 monogamous couples, no HCV seroconversion was observed.[41,42] Still, there are two case reports from monogamous couples in whom acute hepatitis C developed after more than 20 years of a long-term relationship.[43] In some cases this could potentially be attributed in part to older age and thereby lower lubrication, which again could predispose to mucosa trauma.

The role of mucosa trauma is supported by the NHANES studies in that these surveys found a higher prevalence of HCV in those with multiple partners.[8] The higher number of lifetime partners (>50) increases the likelihood of additional sexually transmitted infections, which would also enable viral entry via injured mucosa. This concept of the vulnerable mucosa as a prerequisite for HCV transmission would likewise be supported by the recent epidemic of HCV infection in high-risk groups of men who have sex with men (MSM). In these settings, sexual transmission of HCV seems to be associated with HIV infection, IDU, bleeding during unprotected traumatic anal sex (i.e., "fisting"), and the use of "party drugs" (i.e., γ-hydroxybutyrate) and is further facilitated by sexually transmitted disease–associated mucosal lesions,[44,45] especially when drugs are applied via the mucosa. **Table 31-3** presents recommendations for preventing sexual transmission of HCV.[46]

Household Spread of HCV Infection

There have been cases of supposed household spread of HCV infection. However, iatrogenic exposure seems more likely than intrafamilial or sexual transmission.[47,48] Transmission might occur in the setting of shared razors or toothbrushes, so any instrument that might become contaminated with blood should not be shared with any HCV-positive individuals.

Unknown or Sporadic Infection

In some cases, no clear risk can be identified. However, it would be impossible to exclude all potential exposures because almost everyone has received some form of iatrogenic exposure such as a vaccination, previous injection of an antibiotic or other drug, or medical treatment. This could theoretically have been a risk factor, especially before the implementation of general precautions. Furthermore, patients may be unaware that an exposure has occurred, or finally, they might simply not wish to communicate a known exposure for a variety of reasons.

Table 31-3 Recommendations for Prevention of Sexual Transmission of HCV Infection	
RELATIONSHIP	**RECOMMENDATION**
HCV-positive individuals in relationships	No change in sexual practices in long-term monogamous couples. If couples wish to reduce the low risk for sexual transmission, barrier methods should be used. Partners may be considered for anti-HCV testing
HCV-infected individuals with multiple or short-term sexual partners	Barrier methods or abstinence recommended. Routine testing of partners not recommended
Other STDs present, sex during menses, after surgery on the genital tract, sexual practices that might traumatize the genital mucosa	Barrier precautions
Couples regardless of stability of their relationship	Avoid sharing razors, toothbrushes, and nail-grooming equipment

From Terrault NA. Sexual activity as a risk factor for hepatitis C. Hepatology 2002;36:S99–S105.
HCV, hepatitis C virus; STDs, sexually transmitted diseases

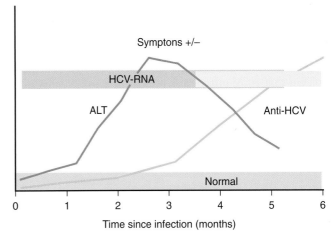

Fig. 31-3 Schematic graph of the course of acute hepatitis C. Hepatitic C virus (HCV) RNA becomes detectable within days and remains for some variable time or persists. Transaminase levels rise only after a few weeks and usually decline during the first 6 months back toward normal values. Symptoms may be present as well. ALT, alanine transaminase.

Natural History
Acute Hepatitis C

After percutaneous exposure to HCV, viremia develops in most people within days (**Fig. 31-3**). Some patients may have typical prodromal flulike symptoms, but most patients remain asymptomatic. Some clear the infection without anti-HCV or a strong T-cell response ever developing.[49] Usually, the T-cell response is stronger in patients with spontaneous clearance of HCV infection.[50]

New HCV infections are best identified by surveillance of persons at risk for acute HCV infection because only some patients become symptomatic or icteric (or both) during the acute infectious period.[51,52] From such studies it recently became evident that the serum viral load fluctuates more during the acute phase of HCV infection than it does during the chronic phase.[53] In the setting of symptomatic acute hepatitis, the anti-HCV IgM titer and anti-HCV IgG antibody avidity may be useful for discriminating acute HCV infection from exacerbation of chronic hepatitis C.[54] These assays are, however, not routinely available. Although these characteristics could be used for diagnosing acute hepatitis C in the rare instances of absence of an earlier negative anti-HCV result, serial viral load determinations have also been suggested to predict acute viral clearance without treatment intervention.[53]

Fulminant hepatitis is rare with HCV infection.[53] In more recent years, very few HCV infections have been seen in patients with fulminant hepatitis, both in the United States (0 of 354 cases[55]) and in Japan (only 3 of 127 cases of fulminant hepatitis in Japan were due to HCV in 2002 and 0 of 94 cases in 2003; Kojiro Michitaka, personal communication). Although fatal cases have been reported,[56] many patients recover before the need for liver transplantation,[57] including the patient whose viral sequence was used to derive the highly replicative JHF-1 HCV-2a clone.[58,59]

Chronic Hepatitis C
Chronicity

Once HCV RNA has persisted for more than 6 months, HCV infection is defined as chronic. Spontaneous clearance occurs within the first 6 months in only about 20% to 50% of patients. This outcome also probably depends partially on the clinical findings: patients with jaundice are more likely to clear acute HCV infection (**Fig. 31-4**).[38] The strength of the HCV-targeting immune response likewise plays a crucial role in controlling HCV infection.[60]

Clearance is most likely also influenced by genetic factors.[61,62] Some genetic markers have been identified in several studies but were subsequently not confirmed in others. Because of these conflicting study results, no genetic testing for predicting outcome has been established at present. A promising single nucleotide polymorphism (SNP), however, was recently identified. This SNP was identified in a genome-wide association study (GWAS) to predict treatment response (see Treatment)[63-65] and was subsequently found to also be associated with spontaneous clearance in cohorts with acute HCV infection.[66,67] This polymorphism (rs12979860) is 3 kilobases (kb) upstream of the *IL28B* gene. Its function is currently unknown.

Outcome of Liver Disease

Although liver disease from HCV seems to be mild in most prospective cohorts, epidemiologic data from mortality information indicate substantial mortality from HCV. Similar to the estimates on prevalence and spontaneous clearance, accurate estimates of the natural history of hepatitis C are difficult because acute HCV infection is mostly mild and subclinical and chronic HCV infection does not produce specific symptoms until the disease reaches more advanced stages of liver disease. When HCV was identified in 1989, it became evident that HCV infection is present in most patients with so-called non-A, non-B hepatitis in the western world.[68,69] Based on these initial studies from tertiary referral centers, it was estimated that liver cirrhosis will develop in about 15% to 30% of HCV-infected patients within 10 to 20 years. Some initial estimates have calculated the time to cirrhosis and HCC

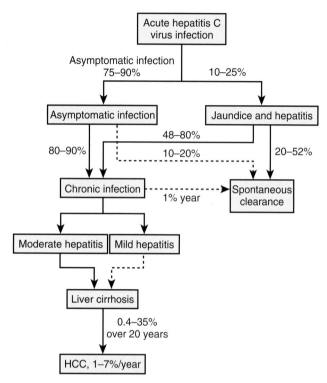

Fig. 31-4 Estimated percentages of the different outcomes of acute infection. HCC, hepatocellular carcinoma.

to be about 20 to 30 years after infection.[70] Prospective studies in immunosuppressed individuals such as HIV-infected patients[71] or in patients with hypogammaglobulinemia[72] have found even higher rates of development of cirrhosis after the acquisition of HCV infection.

However, prospective studies involving immunocompetent adults show mostly mild disease during the first 20 years. In the prospective cohort with HCV infection and the highest rate of cirrhosis after 25 years, it is interesting to note that (1) overall survival did not differ in relation to HCV infection, (2) cirrhosis developed in 35% of HCV RNA–positive patients with elevated liver enzyme levels (**Table 31-4**),[38,68,73-78] and (3) importantly, in none of the patients with normal liver enzyme levels did cirrhosis develop.

This relatively mild picture of liver disease is in contrast to the high number of liver transplants required for HCV-infected patients, as well as estimates of death as a result of HCV infection. Given the current HCV prevalence estimates and death rates, an estimated 360,000 of the 130 to 170 million HCV-infected people (0.21% to 0.28%) die annually of HCV-associated liver disease.[1,3] Although this appears moderate, it translates to 10% to 13% of HCV-infected patients dying of HCV-associated liver disease (based on an estimated 50-year infection duration). This is well within the range of an estimated lifetime risk for cirrhosis of 15% to 20% in immunocompetent patients,[79] especially if one considers that inaccurate coding of liver-related death leads to an underrepresentation of the true burden of HCV.[80] However, not only liver-related but also overall mortality has been reported to be increased in HCV-positive patients.[81,82] Actually, to put HCV into perspective with HBV, more patients die of HCV per infected person than of HBV in that an estimated 560,000 of the 350 million HBV-infected people (0.16%) die annually of HBV (**Fig. 31-5**).[1]

How can we explain the high liver mortality rate on one hand and mild disease in several prospective studies on the other? HCV probably requires co-factors that are prevalent in the normal population. Several risk factors have been identified (**Table 31-5**), age being especially crucial.[83] Age at the time of biopsy is strongly related to the presence of fibrotic changes

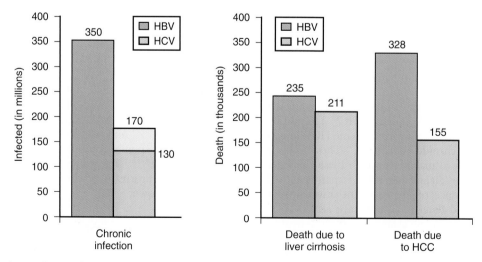

Fig. 31-5 Estimated prevalence of hepatitis B virus (HBV, 350 million) and hepatitis C virus (HCV, 130 to 170 million) infection and estimated death from liver cirrhosis and hepatocellular carcinoma (HCC). Note that the scale for prevalence is in millions for chronic infection but in thousands for death and HCC.

Table 31-4 Summary of Prospective and Retrospective/Prospective Long-Term Natural History Studies

PATIENT GROUP	N	FOLLOW-UP (yr)	CHRONICITY RATE	CIRRHOSIS RATE	MORTALITY	RISK FACTOR FOR CIRRHOSIS
American adult transfusion recipients[68]	222 90/220	25 20	ND 77%	ND 22% overall 35% in those with elevated ALT	67.1% vs. 65.2% and 4.1% vs. 1.3% for liver related	Alcohol or elevated ALT
Irish women infected by anti-D prophylaxis[73]	704 376 viremic	20	55%	ND 2% (in the viremic)	0 0	ND
German women infected by anti-D prophylaxis[74]	1018	20	55%*	0.4%	0.2% with alcohol or fulminant hepatitis B	ND
German women infected by anti-D prophylaxis[38]	1980	25	55%	2%		ND
Australian patients monitored after acute hepatitis[75]	150 98 living	25	54%	8%	12% vs. 8% Liver-related mortality, 1% vs. 0%	Only when ALT elevated Higher alcohol consumption in HCV group 8 times more likely to die of overdoses or suicide than liver disease
American soldiers[76]	17	45 to 50	ND	1/17 (5.9%)	41% vs. 26% Of those who died, liver-related mortality was 16.7% vs. 6.3%	More likely to die of diseases unrelated to HCV
American IDU patients[77]	207	20.7 mean	ND	1.5%		ALT, GGT, age
Austrian plasma donors with elevated ALT[77b]	485 (439 males)	31 mean	ND	34%	16%	Alcohol abuse and diabetes

*About 15% lost antibody response.
ALT, alanine transaminase; GGT, γ-glutamyltransferase; HCV, hepatitis C virus; IDU, injection drug use; ND, not determined

in the liver.[84] In line with this assumption, death attributable to HCV occurs relatively late in life. A French study found a mean age at death of 70 years for HCV patients versus 64 years for patients with HBV infection and 75 years in the normal population.[85] Furthermore, this study highlights the deleterious effect of alcohol consumption, with a mean age of 58 years at death for patients with HCV infection and alcoholic liver disease versus 70 years for those with HCV disease alone. It might well be that HCV increases the sensitivity to additional damage induced by alcohol, diabetes, and other factors (see **Table 31-5**).

The aspect of the development of liver complications relatively late in life is important when considering initiation of treatment. If everyone could be cured of HCV infection with few or no side effects, one would probably universally recommend treatment. Given the drawback of current SOC and the promising development of new treatment strategies, waiting for optimized treatment might be worthwhile in certain patients. This approach does not hold true for patients with more advanced disease, however.

HCV in Children

Parenteral transmission of HCV has become a rarity since the early nineties. Thus at present hepatitis C is mostly acquired vertically in the perinatal period. Maternal HCV RNA levels and HIV co-infection have been attributed to be risk factors for transmission of HCV in this setting.

HCV infection initially appeared as a rather mild disease, with a 45% to 50% viral clearance rate observed in a prospective study of children analyzed almost 20 years after their presumed tainted transfusion while undergoing heart surgery.[86] Progressive liver damage was seen only in patients with additional risk factors: congestive heart failure in two and HBV co-infection in one. However, with more studies available, the picture has become more complex (**Table 31-6**).[86-94] Clearance was seen in 20% to 52%, and progression of fibrosis to stage 2 or higher occurs in a substantial number of patients. Stage 2 fibrosis at an age younger than 25 years is certainly a poor long-term prognosticator. Several children have also required liver transplantation in the setting of HCV infection.[95-97] Unfortunately, their

Table 31-5 Risk Factors for Progressing Liver Disease in the Setting of HCV Infection

Definite Risk Factors

Age (accelerated course with aging likely)
Duration of infection
Obesity
Diabetes
Heavy alcohol consumption (>50 g/day)
Steatosis
Fibrosis stage at earlier biopsy
HIV infection with CD4$^+$ cell count <200 (nadir might be crucial)
Male gender
Concomitant liver disease (HBV co-infection, NASH, ASH)

Probable Risk Factors

Smoking
Absence of coffee consumption[83]
Moderate alcohol intake

Unclear Risk Factors

Heterozygosis for hemochromatosis
Viral load (proven relevant in the setting of liver transplantation)
Mode of acquisition of HCV
HCV genotype

Modifiable risk factors are listed in boldface.
ASH, alcoholic steatohepatitis; HBV, hepatitis B virus; HCV, hepatitis C virus; HIV, human immunodeficiency virus; NASH, nonalcoholic steatohepatitis

prognosis after liver transplantation seems to be relatively poor, with 71.6% and 55.0% patient and graft survival rates, respectively, at 5 years.[97] Thus there is increasing evidence that HCV infection needs to be investigated thoroughly in children, will require monitoring, and may require treatment intervention.[98]

HCV-HAV Superinfection

Acute hepatitis A virus (HAV) infection in adults may require hospitalization and may lead to fulminant hepatitis with high mortality rates, especially in patients older than 50 years.[99] In 1998 it was reported that 7 of 17 HCV-positive patients with HAV superinfection progressed to fulminant hepatitis and that 6 of the 7 died.[100] However, such adverse outcomes were not confirmed in subsequent studies. That is, although 8 of 4591 patients (0.17%) with acute HAV infection but without co-existing liver disease died of acute hepatitis A, none of 199 HCV-infected patients died of acute hepatitis A infection in Switzerland between 1988 and 1998.[101] During an outbreak involving 144 Norwegian drug abusers, of whom 101 of 125 tested positive for anti-HCV, 1 patient died. This patient was anti-HCV positive and had underlying cirrhosis because of heavy alcohol abuse.[102] Other series have also confirmed a rather more benign course.[103-106] Still, vaccination to prevent HAV superinfection is recommended in light of the higher than expected mortality in some series, especially in patients with more severe liver disease.[107,108] In individual cases of acute

Table 31-6 Liver Disease in Children: Prospective Cohorts of Transfused Children and from Liver Clinics

COHORT	COUNTRY	CHRONICITY	NO. VIREMIC CHILDREN EVALUATED HISTOLOGICALLY	FIBROSIS STAGE		MEAN DURATION OF FOLLOW-UP
				F0/F0-1/F2	F3/F4	
Heart surgery	China[87]	8/10 (80%)	NA	NA	NA	NA
Heart surgery	Taiwan[88]	14/29 (48%)	14	2/6*/5[†]	1[‡]/0	6.9 yr
Heart surgery	Germany[86]	30/67 (55%)	17	14/0/2[§]	0/1[¶]	21.2 ± 4.6 yr
Heart surgery	Japan[89]	12/20 (60%)	38	4/8	0/0	≈10 yr
Malignancy	Japan[88]	30/35 (80%)		18/8	0/0	≈10 yr
Failure to thrive	Italy[90]	16/31 (52%)	16	14/1	1/0	35 yr
Liver clinic	Italy[91]	NA	112	25/81	5/1	8.04 ± 5.3 yr
Liver clinic	Egypt[92]	74/105 (58%)	26[¶]	20/3/1	1/1**	NA
Liver clinic	Spain[93]	NA	17	7/9	0/1[††]	11.2 ± 5.6 yr
Liver clinic	Australia[94]	25/31 (81%)	41	0/4	0/0	age 10.6 ± 0.8 yr

*Chronic persistent hepatitis.
[†]Chronic active hepatitis, mild.
[‡]Chronic active hepatitis, severe.
[§]Two patients had congestive heart failure.
[¶]Patient with anti-HBs, anti-HBc, and anti-HEV antibodies.
[¶]Some patients were co-infected with HBV or had secondary iron overload (or both).
**This 12-year-old cirrhotic patient was not thalassemic, and HBV markers were negative.
[††]This leukemic patient was infected with HCV and was also receiving chemotherapy concurrently.
NA, not applicable

HAV infection, clearance of chronic HCV infection has also rarely been observed.[106]

HCV-HBV Co-Infection

Only a few studies have been conducted on the prevalence of HBV coinfection in HCV-infected patients and vice versa, and the data available are another interesting example of the limitation of prevalence estimates determined from liver clinic–derived data. Given that more people are infected with HBV than with HCV, one would expect a higher frequency of co-infection in patients with HCV than in those with HBV. However, studies on the prevalence of HCV in patients with chronic HBV infection indicate an estimated greater than 10% prevalence of HCV in HBsAg-positive patients (**Table 31-7**).[109-115] This translates into an estimated greater than 35 million HBV-HCV co-infected people. Given the estimated 130 to 170 million HCV-infected people, one would expect a 20% to 26% prevalence of HBV in HCV-infected patients, which is clearly lower than reported.[111] A recent paper from Canada involving all persons identified as either HBV infected, HCV infected, or co-infected with HBV and HCV reported a 3.1% HBV infection rate in HCV-infected individual and a 5.2% HCV infection rate in HBV-infected individuals.[114]

Even though the prevalence data are not well established, the finding of more severe liver disease in the setting of co-infection is well established. The frequency of liver cirrhosis appears to be two to four times higher in the setting of HBV co-infection than in the setting of HCV monoinfection. The risk for HCC is especially increased.[116] Acute HBV superinfection might also be associated with higher mortality and morbidity than in the absence of underlying HCV infection.[117]

Treatment in this situation depends on the "dominance" of HCV or HBV. In either situation, monitoring of HBV viral load during HCV treatment is advised because a reduction in HCV viral load can be associated with an increase in HBV viral load.[118,119] Although interferon (IFN) monotherapy has had disappointing results in curing HCV infection, in HBV-HCV co-infected patients, this has changed with pegylated interferon (PEG-IFN) plus ribavirin. Two prospective studies, one from Taiwan and one from Germany, achieved a sustained 70% HCV clearance rate in patients with HCV-HBV co-infection.[118,119] In contrast, Italian and Turkish retrospective observational studies found a poor response.[120,121]

Some patients not only clear HCV viremia but also HBsAg. Therefore it seem worthwhile to evaluate these patients for appropriate treatment judiciously.

HCV-HBV Co-Infection in the Setting of Liver Transplantation

Some early studies indicated a more benign course of HBV infection after transplantation in patients with HCV co-infection,[122] but the prognosis of HCV infection also seems to be better in the setting of HBV co-infection than with HCV monoinfection alone.[123]

HCV-HIV Co-Infection

About 30% of HIV-infected patients are co-infected with HCV; specifically, it is estimated that there are 300,000 HIV-HCV–co-infected people in the United States. This translates to about 10% of HCV-positive patients being co-infected with HIV. Therefore all HCV-positive patients should be screened for HIV infection.

Early after the discovery of HCV it became evident that patients with HCV infection have an impaired prognosis when HIV co-infection is present. Co-infected patients die relatively early as a result of cirrhosis-associated complications when compared with patients infected with HCV alone.[71,124] However, in the mid-1990s it was also demonstrated that cirrhosis and mortality associated with cirrhosis develop only once immune competence is suppressed as indicated by a CD4$^+$ cell count below 100/μl.[125,126] Within the Data Collection on Adverse Events of Anti-HIV Drugs dataset, which reflects 23,441 patients between 1998 and 2004, liver-related death was the most frequent cause of death not attributed to acquired immunodeficiency syndrome, and it was associated with both HCV and lower CD4$^+$ cells.[127] However, some data indicate that liver-related mortality is decreasing in people initiating HIV-directed therapy earlier, when CD4$^+$ cell counts are still high.[128] Thus highly active antiretroviral therapy (HAART) has to some degree made HCV-directed intervention somewhat less urgent. Whether higher HCV viral load in HIV-infected than in non–HIV-infected individuals plays a role is unclear. Because of the probable relevance of the CD4$^+$ cell count nadir, earlier HIV treatment intervention is recommended in the setting of HIV-HCV co-infection.

There is insufficient evidence that HCV itself accelerates the progression of HIV disease. However, there is evidence that drug-induced liver injury is more frequent and more pronounced in HIV patients co-infected with HCV. This is one of the reasons why elimination of HCV in the setting of HIV is desirable, though more difficult to achieve.

Eradication of HCV is beneficial in this population. To initiate therapy, one should address the likelihood of achieving a sustained virologic response (SVR). SVR is more likely in patients with genotype 2 or 3, higher CD4$^+$ cell count, higher cholesterol values, and HCV RNA viral load lower than

Table 31-7 Frequency of HCV in Patients with Chronic HBV Infection and Frequency of HBV in Patients with Chronic HCV Infection

HCV in Patients with Chronic HBV

103/712 (14.5%) in China[109]
15/82 (18.3%) in Japan[110]
139/518 (26.8%) in Germany[111]
59/754 (7.8%) in Italy[112]
378/3588 (10.5%) in Asian Pacific region[113]
169/883 (19.1%) in Western countries[113]
1810/32,895 (5.5%) in British Columbia, Canada[114]

HBV in Patients with Chronic HCV

1% of anti-HCV viremic[111]
11.9% in anti-HCV nonviremic patients[111]
1810/58,157 (3.1%) in British Columbia, Canada[114]

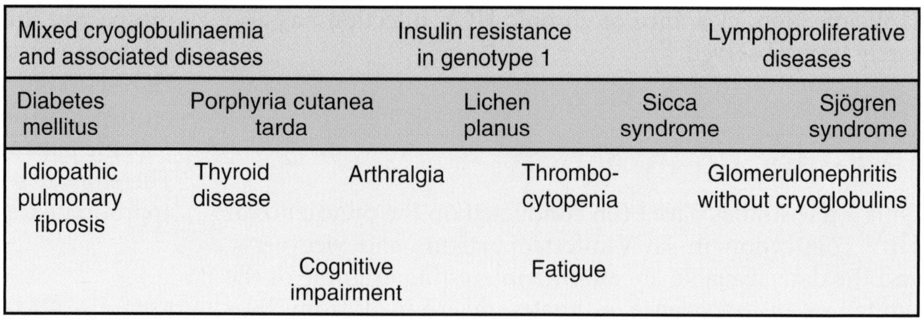

Mixed cryoglobulinaemia and associated diseases		Insulin resistance in genotype 1		Lymphoproliferative diseases
Diabetes mellitus	Porphyria cutanea tarda	Lichen planus	Sicca syndrome	Sjögren syndrome
Idiopathic pulmonary fibrosis	Thyroid disease	Arthralgia	Thrombo-cytopenia	Glomerulonephritis without cryoglobulins
		Cognitive impairment	Fatigue	

Fig. 31-6 **Different diseases have been associated with hepatitis C virus infection with varying strength of association.** The *yellow* field indicates those with a very strong link and pathogenetic evidence, the *green* field indicates diseases with a strong epidemiologic link, and the *blue* field represents diseases with a weaker link.

100,000 IU/ml. SVR rates range between 24% and 62% in those with genotype 2 or 3 and between 9% and 38% in those infected with genotype 1 or 4.[129] Thus, in patients with mild liver disease who are unlikely to respond, awaiting newer treatment options may be an alternative and is considered by some. Prediction of response in this population may be further improved with IL28B testing (see Genetics in the section Predicting Response). Some of the new direct antivirals are also under evaluation for HIV co-infected population, but drug-drug interaction will be a greater challenge in this population.

Clinical Manifestations
Signs and Symptoms

Hepatitis is diagnosed in only a minority of patients without screening because the infection is not associated with any specific complaints in either the acute or chronic phase. Acute infection rarely causes jaundice, is mostly subclinical, and is infrequently diagnosed unless patients are in a screening or surveillance setting, such as IDU patients or after known exposure such as needlestick injury. In the chronic phase, symptoms are usually absent (in about 30% to 70%) or at best nonspecific.

The overwhelming symptom is fatigue. Other frequent nonspecific manifestations include arthralgia, paresthesia, myalgia, pruritus, sicca syndrome, depression, nausea, anorexia, abdominal discomfort, and difficulty concentrating. The severity of these symptoms is not clearly related to the severity of the HCV-induced liver disease.

HCV-infected patients frequently display fluctuating or slightly elevated ALT levels. In about a third, serum ALT values will be persistently normal despite persistent detectable viremia. It has been documented that these patients can still have significant fibrosis. Whether cirrhosis ever develops in such patients remains uncertain given the absence of cirrhosis in HCV viremic patients with normal transaminase levels in the 25-year follow-up study of Seeff and associates.[130] However, some patients with normal transaminase values actually do have fluctuating transaminase levels that are detected only with closer, more regular follow-up testing.

Once advanced fibrosis develops, patients are at risk for the development of HCC. Thus these patients should undergo surveillance for HCC. When cirrhosis has developed, patients are also at risk for the development of portal hypertension and its complications (ascites, gastrointestinal bleeding, and encephalopathy). Jaundice is usually seen only in the setting of significant hepatic decompensation. Referral for liver transplantation should be considered in any patient with decompensated cirrhosis: ascites, varices of grade II or greater, hepatic encephalopathy, or deteriorated liver function (Child stage B or Model for End-Stage Liver Disease [MELD] score higher than 10; see Chapter 47).

Extrahepatic Manifestations

Early after the discovery of HCV, its association with multiple extrahepatic manifestations was recognized, including essential mixed cryoglobulinemia (MC), MPGN, leukocytoclastic vasculitis, porphyria cutanea tarda (PCT), focal lymphocytic sialadenitis, Mooren corneal ulcers, lichen planus (LP), arthralgia, non-Hodgkin lymphoma (NHL), and diabetes mellitus. The strength of these associations with HCV is variable (**Fig. 31-6**).

Extrahepatic Manifestations with Strong Association Based on Pathogenetic Evidence or Improvement with Viral Clearance
Mixed Cryoglobulinemia

Cryoglobulins are antibodies that precipitate in the cold and their detection requires blood to be transported and centrifuged at 37° C (98.6° F) to prevent their precipitation before serum/plasma separation. The pathologic consequence of cryoglobulinemia is precipitation into tissues at low temperatures. This induces inflammation and tissue damage.

There are three type of cryoglobulinemia, one monoclonal type (I) and two different mixed types (II and III). Type I is caused by a monoclonal antibody, most frequently IgM and sometimes IgG, IgA, or light chains. Type I is usually associated with hematologic diseases.[131] Types II and III are caused by a mixture of antibodies and differ by the presence of a monoclonal rheumatoid factor (RF) in type II and polyclonal RF in type III cryoglobulinemia. Type II cryoglobulinemia was also called "essential mixed cryoglobulinemia" until its strong association with HCV was discovered; 90% of type II cryoglobulinemic patients are HCV positive.[131]

Mixed cryoglobulinemia (or MC syndrome) is clinically characterized by a triad of symptoms—purpura, weakness, arthralgias—and association with different pathologic conditions (MPGN, peripheral neuropathy, skin ulcers, diffuse vasculitis, xerostomia and xerophthalmia, and less frequently, lymphatic malignancies). Although clinically overt MC occurs infrequently in patients with chronic HCV infection, a meta-analysis of 19 studies published between 1994 and

2001 found that about 44% of a total of 2323 patients with chronic hepatitis C have detectable cryoprecipitate when tested with sensitive and adequate methods. Furthermore, although cirrhosis was present in 40% of patients with MC, cirrhosis was present in only 17% of patients without MC (P < .001).[132]

Survival of HCV-infected patients with clinically evident cryoglobulinemia is impaired, especially if there is renal involvement.[133] Therefore, an attempt to eradicate HCV is worthwhile, but one should be aware of the potential of IFN to trigger an exacerbation of any underlying autoimmune condition. In some patients, the symptoms of MC might improve during IFN therapy but deteriorate after the end of therapy despite successful eradication of HCV. This indicates that the immune-modulating action of IFN itself may contribute to the amelioration of MC in some individuals.[134]

Membranoproliferative Glomerulonephritis

Even though there was an age-dependent association between HCV seropositivity and albuminuria within the NHANES III data set of 15,029 patients, there was no evidence of a general increased frequency of impaired renal function as determined by estimation of the glomerular filtration rate in HCV-positive individuals.[135] Thus overall renal disease is relatively rare in HCV-infected patients.

Nonetheless, there is strong evidence for a relationship between HCV and MPGN in epidemiology studies[136] and with the association of renal improvement with control of HCV. The presence of MPGN is highly related to the presence of cryoglobulinemia. PEG-IFN plus ribavirin has been associated with SVR in 8 of 18 (44%) receiving 1.0 μg/kg PEG-IFN-α-2b plus 1000 mg ribavirin in one study.[137] Treatment may be less effective in patients with MPGN than in patients without MPGN.[138,139] This may be due to the fact that MPGN tends to be present in older patients or those with more advanced liver disease. If antiviral therapy fails, immunosuppressive approaches, including plasma exchange, rituximab, or both, have been used when the severity of the underlying renal disease mandates such approaches.[140]

Vasculitis

Patients with MC-associated vasculitis may also benefit from antiviral therapy, with seven of nine (78%) in a French study achieving SVR and five eliminating all detectable cryoglobulinemia.[141] In 72 consecutive patients from the same center, PEG-IFN was also found to be more effective than standard IFN.[142]

Lymphoproliferative Diseases

There is the perception of an increased frequency of lymphomas in HCV-infected patients. Two large U.S. Veterans Administration studies consisting of 32,000 and 146,000 HCV-positive individuals found an adjusted odds ratio of 1.22 (CI, 1.01 to 1.39) and 1.28 (CI, 1.12 to 1.45), respectively. Although the overall frequency is only mildly increased, there is a significant increase, especially for B-cell NHL, in patients with type II cryoglobulinemia.[133] Also in noncryoglobulinemic patients, B-cell–originated lymphomas are increased. Cure of the lymphoma by antiviral therapy

has been achieved in patients with follicular splenic lymphoma,[143] which is the first line of treatment of such diseases.[144]

Extrahepatic Manifestations that Show a Strong Epidemiologic Link to HCV
Porphyria Cutanea Tarda

Porphyria cutanea tarda is clearly associated with HCV as indicated by the significantly higher prevalence of HCV in patients with PCT than in the general population. Except for one study from New Zealand (1/25; 4%) and one from Germany (9/111; 8.1%), all studies reported an HCV prevalence of greater than 10% in patients with PCT. In all studies the prevalence of HCV was significantly higher than in the respective general population.[145] The improvement in symptoms associated with phlebotomy indicates a role of iron overload, as in other forms of PCT. HCV is most likely involved in iron accumulation via oxidative stress followed by suppressed hepcidin expression leading to increased iron absorption.[146] A combined phlebotomy and antiviral therapy approach is recommended for these patients.

Lichen Planus

An association between LP, mainly the oral type, and HCV has been reported, with higher frequency noted in Japan and southern Europe. The incidence of LP has been reported to be increased in HCV-infected groups. A large Veterans Administration study found a 0.3% prevalence of LP in 34,204 HCV-positive veterans versus only a 0.13% prevalence in 136,816 controls (adjusted odds ratio of 2.3 for HCV-positive vs. HCV-negative veterans).[136] This result is well in line with a 2.5 odds ratio found in a recent meta-analysis.[147] HCV sequences have been detected in LP lesions, and a recent study suggested a link to HCV-associated IFN induction.[148] This might explain why worsening of oral lesions occurs in some patients during IFN therapy.[149] However, LP is not an absolute contraindication to IFN therapy, but in patients with worsening disease during therapy, treatment should clearly be stopped.

Diabetes Mellitus

There are numerous reports on the role of HCV in diabetes. White and co-workers performed a meta-analysis of 34 studies and found an odds ratio of 1.6 for an increased prevalence of diabetes in HCV patients.[150] Similar results were found in relation to new-onset diabetes in liver transplant recipients.[151]

A recent study reported the changes in homeostatic model assessment (HOMA) levels, a measure of insulin resistance, in patients with hepatitis C treated within the hepatitis C albuferon studies. Interestingly, there was an improvement in insulin resistance for genotype 1 patients achieving SVR, and no improvement was observed in either nonresponder or genotype 2/3 patients with SVR.[152]

Sjögren Syndrome and Sicca Syndrome

Anti-HCV–associated Sjögren syndrome somehow differs from primary Sjögren syndrome in that patients with HCV-associated Sjögren syndrome are older and mostly have cryoglobulins.[153,154] The term pseudo-Sjögren syndrome has therefore been suggested to indicate the difference from primary Sjögren syndrome.[155] The prevalence of Sjögren syndrome has been reported to be between 18% and 50% in HCV-infected cohorts.[156,157] An association is further supported by experimental animal data in which expression of HCV envelope protein was associated with Sjögren-like disease in mice.[158] Sicca syndrome alone can be observed more frequently than complete Sjögren syndrome.[156]

Extrahepatic Manifestations that Are Epidemiologically Linked with HCV but Not Clearly Understood
Thyroid Disease

Thyroid dysfunction and thyroid-directed autoantibodies and autoimmune thyroid disease are increased in patients with hepatitis C.[159] There is also a substantial incidence of thyroid disease during IFN therapy.[160] Women are at higher risk, as are older patients; however, life-threatening thyrotoxic crises can even occur in young men. Severe events are fortunately rare, and if the liver disease requires treatment, this supersedes concerns related to the thyroid. Screening for autoantibodies and serum thyroid-stimulating hormone (TSH) is recommended before and at 3-month intervals during and after IFN-α treatment,[161] and patients need to be informed of the risk for thyroid dysfunction. The hypothyroidism induced by IFN can easily be treated by hormone substitution, and the hypothyroidism is usually reversible[162] but less commonly permanent.

Arthralgia

Arthralgia is common with any acute or chronic viral infection. In HCV-infected patients this may be due to autoimmune phenomena, be a consequence of endogenous IFN production in response to the presence of HCV, or be due to IFN treatment itself. In the Irish anti-D cohort, 38% of women reported arthralgia.[73] The clinical picture may mimic rheumatoid arthritis because RF is present in 50% to 80% of HCV-infected patients.[163] Real rheumatoid arthritis associated with anti–cyclic citrullinated peptide antibodies (anti-CCP), however, is rare in patients with hepatitis C.[164]

Management of HCV-associated arthritis is poorly standardized. When the arthritis is associated with cryoglobulinemia, it usually responds to antiviral treatment. Symptomatic approaches include glucocorticoid therapy, hydroxychloroquine, and methotrexate, but systematic evidence-based data are lacking. HCV in the setting of rheumatoid arthritis can sometimes be treated with Interferon using a preemptive anti-TNF therapy to shield the arthritis. Anti-TNF might be additionally helpful to achieve SVR.

Fatigue Syndrome

Fatigue might be one of the most underestimated and least understood conditions in relation to HCV infection inasmuch as in some studies (e.g., the anti-D cohorts from Ireland and Germany), there is a high frequency of fatigue but no correlation with viral replication.[165] It is unclear at present whether HCV has a causal role or is merely an associated factor. At present, no treatment has proved effective,

although there have been some reports of the usefulness of ondansetron.[166] The efficacy of ondansetron is fitting with the observation of altered monoaminergic neurotransmission in HCV-infected patients with fatigue.[167] However, to date there has been only one randomized study and one case report.

Autoimmune Hepatitis and HCV Infection

When HCV was discovered initially, many patients with autoimmune hepatitis tested anti-HCV positive. It was later shown that this was mostly related to false-positive anti-HCV test results in the presence of hypergammaglobulinemia—a hallmark of autoimmune hepatitis (see Chapter 40).

Rare cases of both HCV infection and autoimmune hepatitis have been reported, as well as exacerbations of hepatitis in the setting of IFN therapy. However, most such patients had a specific anti-LKM (liver-kidney microsomal) antibody.

Serologic markers of autoimmunity such as antinuclear and smooth muscle antibodies are frequent but rarely indicate true autoimmune disease. Monitoring of patients with autoantibodies during immune-modulating therapy is advised, however, to detect deteriorating liver disease early.

Immunopathogenesis

Hepatitis C virus is frequently considered to be a noncytopathic virus, and the immune response rather than the virus itself is believed to be central to the pathogenesis of liver disease. This, however, does not easily fit with the observation of more aggressive liver disease in patients with immunodeficiencies such as HIV co-infection or hypogammaglobulinemia.

Diagnosis and Testing
Diagnosis

Given the absence of signature symptoms, the diagnosis of HCV relies on virologic assays. There are two different principal types of HCV testing: serologic assays and NATs. Serologic assays detect antibodies against HCV protein (anti-HCV) or HCV antigen (i.e., HCV core antigen). Nucleic acid detection is based on different methods of signal or target amplification.

Diagnosis of chronic HCV infection requires proof of HCV replication; such confirmation can be achieved by detecting either viral nucleic acid or HCV core antigen. Determination of past infection or past exposure might be feasible only with anti-HCV testing, which is still the primary screening tool. In locations where HCV core antigen assays have become available, such as in Europe and different regions of Asia, HCV core antigen might be an appropriate alternative but is not currently broadly available.

Serologic Assays
Anti-HCV Screening Assays

Anti-HCV tests have become highly reliable, but it should be noted that anti-HCV is not related to protective immunity but instead is a marker of past or remote infection, analogous to the presence of anti-HBc following HBV

Table 31-8 Signal-to-Cutoff Ratio Predictive of a True-Positive Result 95% or More of the Time

SCREENING TEST KIT NAME	MANUFACTURER	ASSAY FORMAT	SIGNAL-TO-CUTOFF RATIO PREDICTIVE OF A TRUE-POSITIVE ≥95% OF THE TIME
Ortho HCV Version 3.0 ELISA Test System	Ortho	EIA	≥3.8
Abbott HCV EIA 2.0	Abbott	EIA	≥3.8
VITROS Anti-HCV	Ortho	CIA	≥8.0
AxSYM Anti-HCV	Abbott	MEIA	≥10.0
Architect Anti-HCV	Abbott	CMIA	≥5.0
Advia Centaur HCV	Bayer	CIA	≥11.0

CIA, chemiluminescent immunoassay; CMIA, chemiluminescent microparticle immunoassay; EIA, enzyme immunoassay; ELISA, enzyme-linked immunosorbent assay; HCV, hepatitis C virus; MEIA, microparticle immunoassay

infection. The first-generation HCV screening tests were associated with a relatively high degree of inaccuracy.[168] Second-generation assays included recombinant antigens from the core (C22) and the NS3 region (C33c), in addition to the NS4 region (C100),[169] whereas today's highly accurate third-generation assays frequently include an NS5 protein in addition to the other antigens/protein. The presence of anti-HCV indicates exposure to the virus but does not differentiate among acute, persistent, resolved, or remote infection. A positive screening test result must therefore be confirmed by either proof of infection (detection of HCV antigens or HCV RNA) or the use of a confirmatory antibody test. Antibodies against HCV persist when the infection has resolved spontaneously or induced following treatment. However, titers may decrease over time and might eventually disappear.[170]

High signal-to-cutoff ratios have been recognized as being predictive of positive confirmatory assay results (**Table 31-8**). Accordingly, the CDC recently stated, "*Signal-to-cut-off ratios are calculated by dividing the optical density (OD) value of the sample being tested by the OD value of the assay cut-off for that run. Analysis of enzyme immunoassay and chemiluminescence assay data indicates that s/co ratios can be used to predict supplemental test-positive results. A specific s/co ratio can be identified for each test that would predict a true antibody-positive result (as defined by the results of supplemental testing) ≥95% of the time, regardless of the anti-HCV prevalence or characteristics of the population being tested.*"[171] This should, however, not be applied to settings with a low prevalence of HCV infection.

Confirmatory Assays to Complement Anti-HCV Screening

Confirmation of anti-HCV in the setting of elevated liver enzyme levels may not be required. However, confirmation is still thought to be advisable to prove infection via detection of nucleic acid or HCV core antigen. In general, there are five different principal methods for confirming infectious diseases (**Table 31-9**). In HCV infection, specialized serologic assays are used, such as recombinant immunoblot assay (RIBA) and Inno-Lia (a line immunoassay). These assays use recombinant or synthetic peptides different from those used for the screening assay. RIBA and Inno-Lia are the most widely used.

Table 31-9 Confirmatory Antibody Assays for Diagnosing Infectious Diseases

Use of different screening assays, for example, based on different methods and/or antigens
Specific neutralization
Testing of the sample for additional markers of infection
Use of specialized serologic assays, for example, Western blot, line assays
Use of molecular techniques to detect nucleic acids

HCV Core Antigen Assay

An HCV core antigen assay was evaluated (trak-C, Ortho Clinical Diagnostics, Raritan, N.J.,) in early 2000. It has been shown to be a useful additional diagnostic tool, and HCV core antigen showed good correlation with different HCV RNA assays, but this assay was never marketed. Recently, a novel, fully automated chemiluminescent microparticle immunoassay (CMIA) for quantitative detection of HCV core antigen with an improved sensitivity of 0.06 pg/mL (3 fmol/L) (Architect HCV Ag, Abbott, Germany) has become available in Europe and Asia. This assay detected acute HCV infection at the same time as NAT testing did, thus indicating similar sensitivity and detectability and 99.8% specificity.[172] A comparison with polymerase chain reaction (PCR)-based quantification assays showed a correlation coefficient (r) of 0.7 for quantification.[172,173] However, its place in the diagnostic armamentarium is not established and will require further solid scientific evaluation.

HCV RNA Assays/Nucleic Acid Tests/Viral Load Quantification

Whereas serologic assays are typically used for screening and initial diagnosis, HCV RNA assays are needed to confirm an infection and monitor response to treatment. HCV-RNA is considered more sensitive and is the current gold standard for confirming the diagnosis and monitoring viral load during and after therapy.

In the past, individual laboratories developed their own HCV RNA assays; this practice is considered obsolete at present. Several commercial assays are available, all of which are based on either one of three amplification methods: PCR or real-time PCR, branched-chain DNA (bDNA), and target-mediated amplification (TMA) (**Table 31-10**).[174-181] TMA is a qualitative assay only. The up-to-date quantitative assays show good correlation with each other and usually have a lower limit of detection of 10 IU/ml, with the exception of the bDNA assay, which has lower sensitivity with a lower limit of detection of 615 IU/ml.[182] This limits its utility during antiviral therapy. Treatment monitoring needs a lower limit of detection below 50 IU/ml; thus today's quantification is based on real-time PCR assays.

Because HCV is an RNA virus, the stability of HCV is an issue, and adequate sample preparation is essential for accurate assessment of viral load. Inadequate sample preparation can lead to a significant reduction in HCV RNA levels.[183] Separation of serum/plasma from the cellular component of blood within 2 hours plus freezing within 6 hours is advised. When optimal handling cannot be guaranteed, tubes with RNA stabilizers can be used. Accurate sample preparation is more important than the specific assay used because response to treatment is determined by viral load undetectability or log reduction (see treatment response definitions in **Figures 31-7 and 31-8**).

Table 31-10 Sensitivity of Different Viral Load Assays for Serum and Plasma

TEST	PRINCIPLE*	SENSITIVITY; LIMIT OF DETECTION (IU/ml)	LIMIT OF QUANTIFICATION (IU/ml)	LINEAR RANGE (IU/ml)
Versant 3.0[174]	bDNA	615	615	615 (2.8 log) to 7,690,000 (6.9 log)
Versant TMA[175]	TMA	5.3		
COBAS AmpliPrep/COBAS TaqMan HCV Test[176]		43	43 (1.63 log)	43 (1.6 log) to 69,000,000 (7.8 log)
COBAS TaqMan HCV Test, v2.0 for use with the High Pure System[177†]		10 to 20[178]	25 (1.4 log)	25 (1.4 log) to 390,000,000 (8.6 log)
UltraQual 1000 (2X) HCV RT-PCR (NGI)[179]		6.9		
HCV SuperQuant PCR by NGI[180]			100 (2 log)	100 to 5,000,000
Abbott RealTime HCV 0.5 ml[181‡]		12	12 (1.08 log)	12 (1.08 log) to 100 million (8.0 log)
Abbott RealTime HCV 0.2 ml[180‡]		30		

*Most tests are real-time PCR unless indicated otherwise.

†Available as a registered in vitro diagnostic (IVD) in Europe, the United States, and Canada.

‡The CE mark is the official marking required by the European community. CE marking is not available in the United States.

bDNA, branched-chain DNA; HCV, hepatitis C virus; NGI, National Genomics Institute/LabCorp; RT-PCR, reverse transcriptase polymerase chain reaction; TMA, transcription-mediated amplification;

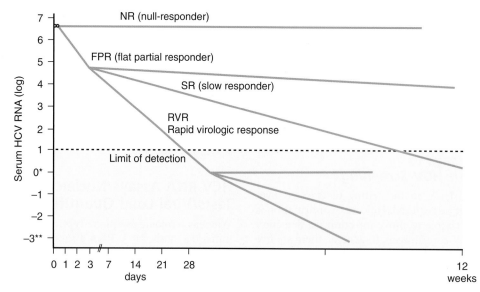

Fig. 31-7 Different scenarios for response of hepatitis C virus (HCV) to interferon are indicated as nullresponse (NR; <2 log reduction till week 12), flat partial response (FPR) with an initial decline but then no further reduction, slow response (SR), and rapid virologic response (RVR). The limit of detection is indicated at 10 IU/ml. Asterisk, Reflects 1 IU/ml, which is currently not detectable. Double asterisk, Reflects 1 IU/1 L of plasma.

Genotyping and Serotyping of HCV

Hepatitis C genotyping is helpful in defining the epidemiology of hepatitis C, but on an individual patient basis, genotyping is crucial in regard to treatment recommendations and duration. Genotyping is based on sequence analysis by sequencing or reverse hybridization. Although viral load can vary within a 0.5- to 1-log range, HCV genotype does not change during the course of infection. In case of suspected superinfection, another genotype might rarely be detected. For reliable genotyping, 5′URT (5′untranslated region) alone is insufficient, including parts of the core sequence enhance genotyping reliability. Sequencing of NS5b is the gold standard.

Serotyping is the only other option to test for the type of HCV in cases of remote infection. This, however, is relevant for epidemiologic studies only and is not used clinically.

Selection for Antiviral Therapy and Pretreatment Assessments

All patients with confirmed, chronic HCV infection should be evaluated for antiviral therapy. However, initiation of treatment is advised only after adequate assessment given the limitations of efficacy and the potential of current antiviral therapies for toxicity. Careful assessment should weigh the potential risks and benefits. Furthermore, pretreatment assessment helps in the decision-making process with regard to beginning therapy immediately, delaying therapy until a later time (because of no immediate need), or deferring treatment indefinitely (because of contraindications). Pretreatment evaluations include the following: (1) clinical assessment, (2) laboratory tests, and (3) liver biopsy.

Clinical Assessment

It is important to assess medical comorbid conditions that might be a contraindication or may worsen with treatment. Ribavirin-induced anemia occurs in almost everyone, though to varying degrees. With the addition of the first generation protease inhibitors, anemia will get even worse. This may lead to worsening of cardiac ischemia during antiviral therapy. IFN-enhanced immunity might lead to exacerbation of diseases such as autoimmune hepatitis, autoimmune rheumatoid arthritis, or sarcoidosis. Thyroid disease and diabetes may also worsen during therapy. However, none of these diseases are absolute contraindications but may increase the risks associated with treatment. Given the usually slowly progressive nature of HCV infection, life expectancy should also be considered. In patients with life-limiting underlying diseases, the risk related to treatment probably outweighs the potential benefits of viral clearance. In such cases, patients may prefer their life not being burdened with a side effect–loaded additional therapy.

All patients should be evaluated for underlying psychiatric disorders, particularly depression. Uncontrolled depression or a history of significant aggressive behavior is especially difficult in light of IFN-based therapies. However, patients with well-controlled psychiatric disorders may receive antiviral therapy. Involvement of mental health professionals throughout the course of therapy should be encouraged in such cases.

Substance abuse should be addressed. Heavy alcohol use is known to limit the effectiveness of therapy. With active IDU, the benefit of therapy has to be evaluated carefully because such patients are more likely to die of diseases unrelated to the liver.[184] Referral to an addiction specialist is encouraged.

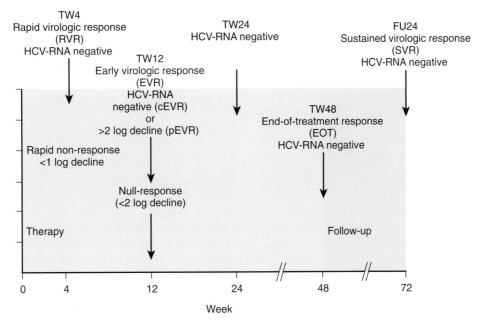

Fig. 31-8 **Cornerstone of current standard of care for hepatitis C virus (HCV) infection, which helps in predicting eventual treatment outcome.** FU24, follow-up 24; TW4, treatment week 4.

Establishing abstinence from drugs and alcohol before initiating treatment is also recommended.

A baseline ophthalmic examination should be performed in patients with risk factors for retinal disease (e.g., hypertension, diabetes) to identify any ophthalmologic condition that might be worsened by IFN and to provide a reference point should any ophthalmic symptoms occur later during therapy.

Laboratory Tests and Imaging Studies, Including Elastography

Laboratory tests are helpful in managing patients with hepatitis C. Serial determination of liver function (international normalized ratio [INR], bilirubin, albumin), liver inflammation (ALT and aspartate transaminase [AST]), and total blood cell count at 6-month intervals helps in monitoring disease progression. Decreasing platelet counts or albumin levels, or both, as well as increasing prothrombin time, are clear signs of progressive disease.

In some areas of the world, different methods to assess the elasticity of the liver are used to assess the stage or degree of liver fibrosis. Most fibrosis is associated with a decrease in elasticity and an increase in liver stiffness, the latter being measured with noninvasive ultrasound-based systems. Liver stiffness, however, also increases with bile duct obstruction[185]; with increased blood flow to the liver, as in the setting of acute liver inflammation[186,187]; and after a meal.[188] Still, taking these limitations into consideration, liver elastography is rapidly becoming a validated and accepted valuable tool to assess and monitor progression of liver disease.

Noninvasive laboratory-based blood tests such as the FibroTest, FibroSure, and enhanced liver fibrosis (ELF) panel are being evaluated and also show promising reliability in predicting patients with minimal or advanced degrees of fibrosis.[189,190] When serologic noninvasive fibrosis tests and imaging fibrosis assessments (e.g., ultrasound, magnetic resonance elastography) are available and show concordant results, biopsy will probably not be required to assess the stage of liver disease in the future.[191,192]

Liver Biopsy

Liver biopsy is still the gold standard for determining the severity of liver injury (grade of inflammation and stage of fibrosis), and liver biopsy may also be helpful in excluding other causes of liver disease in HCV-infected patients. However, liver biopsy has limitations because of sampling error.[193] Liver biopsy is indicated only if the results of such biopsy may alter the management of a patient. Thus, when a short course of a treatment with moderate or mild side effects clears the infection, in most patients liver biopsy is not generally required. Accordingly, in patients with genotype 2 or 3 infection and no contraindications to therapy, biopsy seems of little value because the likelihood of SVR is high. An exception might be a patient who plans to become pregnant or father a child, in which case biopsy might help in determining whether therapy can wisely be deferred. Biopsy is also helpful if one suspects an additional underlying liver disease that cannot be otherwise excluded.

In patients with genotype 1 and other genotypes with lower response rates, biopsy helps identify those with immediate need of treatment, even with moderate or little chance of clearance. There is no absolute threshold. Fibrosis stage 2 of 4 has been used as a threshold by several countries in the past (i.e., Australia, Belgium) to reimburse treatment. Although this strategy has been abandoned, stage 2 probably reflects a reasonable threshold by most authorities.

There are a variety of histologic scoring systems that differ in the numerical range of scores for defining degrees of inflammation and stage of liver fibrosis (see Chapter 13). The most commonly used currently is the METAVIR system, which grades inflammation from 0 to 4 and stages fibrosis from 0 to 4.[194] In addition, biopsy specimens can be scored for the amount of hepatic steatosis because steatosis is linked to risk for fibrosis, as well as reduced response to therapy.

With increasing response rates, the role of liver biopsy might becomes less relevant.

Therapy for Hepatitis C

Treatment of hepatitis C, previously "non-A, non-B hepatitis," started before the discovery of HCV. A regimen of IFN given subcutaneously three times a week (3 to 5 million units) for 24 weeks resulted in a 6% to 10% SVR rate. Extending therapy from 24 to 48 weeks did not lead to substantial increases in response rates. When ribavirin was added to IFN, a substantial increase in response rate to approximately 40% was achieved, which was further incrementally improved with the pegylation of IFN. PEG-IFNs were developed to improve the pharmacokinetic profile and efficacy and provide a more convenient once-weekly dosing schedule for IFN therapy. PEG-IFN-α-2b and PEG-IFN-α-2a in combination with ribavirin (1000/1200 mg daily for genotype 1 for 48 weeks and 800 mg daily for genotype 2/3 for 24 weeks) were noted to improve overall SVR rates to 54% to 56%, thus leading to regulatory approval as SOC for patients with HCV in 2001/2002. Since 2001, further progress has been made in individualizing therapy, but no overall improvement has really occurred. until the licensing of the protease inhibitors "telaprevir" and "boceprevir," which increased the overall response rates for treatment naive patients to 70% (**Fig. 31-9**).

Viral Kinetics and Definition of Treatment Response

Viral kinetics represents the change in viral load over time. Analyzing such change in viral load during IFN-based therapy led to an estimation that 10^{12} HCV are produced daily.[195] The first phase of the decline in viral load during therapy likely reflects blocking of viral production and secretion. The magnitude of decline correlates with a given drug's efficacy in blocking efficient virus production. Because there is never 100% efficacy, a second, slower phase of viral decline becomes evident and reflects the rate of death of infected cells or clearance of infection from a cell. The second phase of decline is likely to reflect the time needed for eventual viral eradication. It is important to note that HCV kinetics can be assessed only in serum or plasma at present, which sets a limitation (see **Fig. 31-7**). There could also be potential extrahepatic reservoirs that limit the predictability of viral load assessment in plasma. Given the high efficacy of some of the newer agents, it might

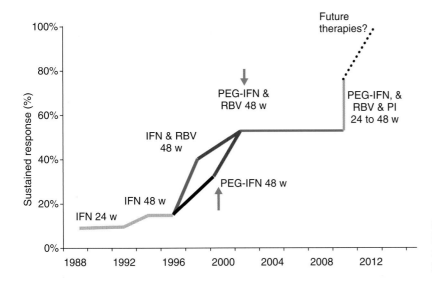

Fig. 31-9 Improvement of therapy for infection with hepatitis C virus (HCV) until 2001 and expected improvement with the licensing of protease inhibitors. PEG-IFN, pegylated interferon. P1, protease inhibitor.

Table 31-11a Response Criteria for HCV at the End of and after Therapy

End-of-treatment (EOT) response	HCV RNA undetectable at end of treatment
Sustained virologic response (SVR)	HCV RNA undetectable 24 weeks after end of treatment
Relapse	HCV RNA recurrence after having become undetectable

Table 31-11b Response Criteria for HCV during Therapy and Potential Consequences

	DURING THERAPY	POTENTIAL CONSEQUENCES
Rapid virologic response (RVR)	HCV RNA undetectable by week 4	Consider shorter treatment duration
Early virologic response (EVR)	HCV RNA showing a ≥2-log drop by week 12	If not achieved, consider stopping therapy because SVR unlikely
Complete early virologic response (cEVR)	HCV RNA undetectable by week 12	
Partial early virologic response (pEVR)	HCV RNA showing a 2-log drop by week 12, but virus is detectable	Consider stopping therapy because SVR unlikely
Breakthrough	HCV RNA showing a ≥1-log increase during treatment	If occurring, consider stopping therapy because SVR unlikely
Nullresponse	HCV RNA showing a ≤2-log decline by week 12 or never undetectable during a treatment course	Consider stopping therapy because SVR unlikely
Flat nonresponse	HCV-RNA showing a <1-log decline by week 12	Predicts lower chance of viral clearance even with newer agents

be that the second-phase decline might not be evaluable in treatments with such newer agents. For the current management of patients with PEG-IFN and ribavirin therapy or triple therapy including protease inhibitors, the slope of viral decay has not become part of routine clinical practice, whereas achievement of certain threshold levels has become an integrated part of HCV treatment management.

For understanding response to HCV therapy, it is important to know the definitions of response. A definition of biochemical response has become obsolete. Different virologic responses are classified according to different time points during treatment and by decline in viral load or by undetectability of HCV (**Tables 31-11a and 31-11b**; also see **Fig. 31-8**). Undetectability should currently reflect a viral load of less than 10-15 IU/ml. Thus, highly sensitive assays need to be used.

Given the efficacy of protease inhibitors, many patients are HCV RNA negative by week 4. Thus additional response criteria might be needed in the future, such as HCV RNA not being detectable at week 2 or perhaps even week 1. These time points could possibly be classified as fast and immediate rapid virologic response (RVR), respectively. It might additionally be reasonable to classify patients not responding to treatment with at least a 1-log drop by week 4 as rapid nonresponders.

Predicting Response

Genetics

There is a significant difference in response to PEG-IFN-α-2a and PEG-IFN-α-2b plus ribavirin with regard to ethnicity,

with only approximately 20% to 28% of African Americans achieving SVR as compared with 40% to 52% of white patients with genotype 1 infection[196-198] and 57% versus 82% for genotype 2/3.[199] This racial difference was strongly suggestive of a genetic influence on HCV outcome. Recently, a team of scientists and clinicians performed a GWAS and compared patients

Table 31-12 Host and Viral Predictors of Sustained Virologic Response

Before Treatment

Host Factors

IL28B polymorphism C/C
Female sex
Non–African American
Age <40 years
Normal body mass index
No insulin resistance

Viral Factors

Genotype 2 or 3
Low HCV RNA levels (<600,000 IU/ml)

Biochemical Parameters

High cholesterol
Low γ-glutamyltransferase
High ALT

Histologic Criteria

Absence of bridging fibrosis or cirrhosis
Absence of steatosis

During Treatment

Rapid virologic response (week 4)
Early virologic response (week 12)
Adherence to therapy*
Absence of alcohol abuse*

*Factors that can be influenced by patients themselves during treatment.

achieving SVR with patients not achieving SVR. A key role was identified for a genetic variation in the IL28B gene region on chromosome 19 for predicting response to PEG-IFN and ribavirin therapy in patients chronically infected with genotype 1 HCV infection.[63] This finding has since been confirmed in other independent cohorts.[64,65] In addition, the most strongly associated SNP for treatment response, rs12979860, has also been shown to be significantly associated with spontaneous clearance of HCV after acute infection.[66]

Clinical and Virologic Predictors

During the 1990s, several factors were associated with achieving SVR: HCV genotype (genotype 2 or 3), low baseline viral load, elevated ALT, low γ-glutamyltransferase (GGT), and early stages of fibrosis. Patients infected with genotypes 2 and 3 responded significantly better to treatment than did those with genotype 1. Parameters known to be associated with achieving SVR are presented in **Table 31-12**. They do not accurately predict response in an individual but rather indicate the likelihood of response in a group of individuals with similar criteria, and some of these factors have been identified in multivariate models.

Laboratory Tests

Before Therapy
Total Blood Cell Count

Interferon therapy leads a reduction in neutrophils and platelets,[200] whereas ribavirin leads to a reduction in hemoglobin

because of hemolysis, which is even more pronounced with the addition of protease inhibitors. Thus, when initiating treatment, adequate platelet counts (>75,000/μl), neutrophils (absolute neutrophil count >1500/μl), and hemoglobin (>13 g/dl for men and >12 g/dl for women) are desirable for patients to tolerate therapy. Patients with neutrophil and platelet counts below these recommended levels can begin therapy but may require dose reductions of IFN. The development of neutropenia is especially common in African Americans,[201] who usually have a lower chance of response. Patients with neutrophil or platelet counts (or both) below these thresholds generally have more serious liver disease, should be referred for transplant evaluation, and might best be treated after being evaluated and listed for transplantation.

Clinical Chemistry

Renal function should be normal or only moderately impaired (creatinine <1.5 mg/dl or creatinine clearance >50 ml/min). In patients with impaired renal function, the tolerability of treatment may be impaired and the dose of ribavirin must be adjusted. Patients should have evidence of normal hepatic synthetic function (serum bilirubin, albumin, and prothrombin time). Patients with impaired hepatic function may be treated cautiously, potentially with lower doses and in the setting of a potential liver transplantation backup. For estimating treatment response, cholesterol, GGT, and ALT levels may also be determined.

Pregnancy Test

A pregnancy test is crucial because HCV treatment is absolutely contraindicated in pregnant women due to the teratogenicity of ribavirin.

Virologic Assays

Hepatitis C genotyping is required for planning treatment, and determination of viral load is required for both planning and monitoring treatment. Viral load and genotype may aid in counseling patients regarding their likelihood of response. Those with low pretreatment viral loads (<400,000 to 800,000 IU/ml) are more likely to respond to treatment than are those with higher baseline viral loads. For consistency, the same quantitative assay should be used to evaluate changes in viral load during and after therapy.

During Therapy

Total blood cell count, ALT, blood glucose, bilirubin, and creatinine should be monitored at weeks 2, 4, 6, 8, 12, 24, 36, and 48. Viral load needs to be determined at weeks 4, 12, and 24; at the end of therapy; and at 12 or 24 weeks, or both, after the end of therapy. Pregnancy testing is required monthly, and TSH monitoring is recommended every 3 months (**Fig. 31-10**). When using telaprevir, the viral load for weeks 4 and 12 must be assessed with highly sensitive assays to determine eligibility for a shortened 24- versus 48-week course of therapy. When using boceprevir, week 8 must be assessed in addition, because the protease inhibitor is added after week 4, and undetectability from weeks 8 to 24 is required for a shortened 28-versus 48-week therapy.

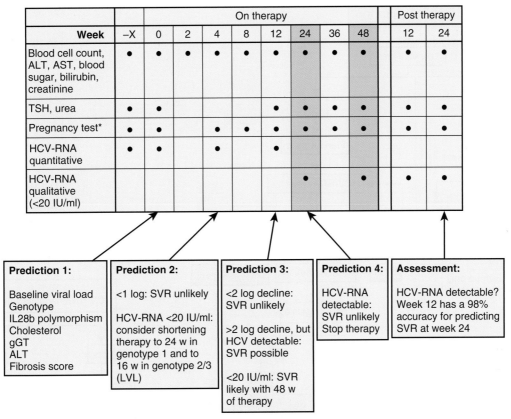

		On therapy								Post therapy	
Week	−X	0	2	4	8	12	24	36	48	12	24
Blood cell count, ALT, AST, blood sugar, bilirubin, creatinine	●	●	●	●	●	●	●	●	●	●	●
TSH, urea	●	●				●	●	●	●	●	●
Pregnancy test*	●			●	●	●	●	●	●	●	●
HCV-RNA quantitative	●	●		●		●					
HCV-RNA qualitative (<20 IU/ml)							●		●	●	●

Prediction 1:

Baseline viral load
Genotype
IL28b polymorphism
Cholesterol
gGT
ALT
Fibrosis score

Prediction 2:

<1 log: SVR unlikely

HCV-RNA <20 IU/ml: consider shortening therapy to 24 w in genotype 1 and to 16 w in genotype 2/3 (LVL)

Prediction 3:

<2 log decline: SVR unlikely

>2 log decline, but HCV detectable: SVR possible

<20 IU/ml: SVR likely with 48 w of therapy

Prediction 4:

HCV-RNA detectable: SVR unlikely Stop therapy

Assessment:

HCV-RNA detectable? Week 12 has a 98% accuracy for predicting SVR at week 24

−X: Pretreatment evaluation shall include: HBsAg, HIV, ferritin, transferrin saturation, INR, electrolytes, serum albumin or serum protein-electrophoresis, ophthalmologic exam, HCV genotype, cholesterol, gGT, urea, bilirubin, urine analysis, autoantibodies (ANA, LKM, SLA)
*: Monthly pregnancy test

Fig. 31-10 **Schematic overview of the tests recommended during pegylated interferon and ribavirin therapy.** ALT, alanine transaminase; ANA, antinuclear antibody; AST, aspartate transaminase; GGT, γ-glutamyltransferase; HCV, hepatitis C virus; INR, international normalized ratio; LKM, liver-kidney microsomes; LVL, low viral load (<600,000 IU/ml); SLA, soluble liver antigen; SVR, sustained virologic response; TSH, thyroid-stimulating hormone; −X, evaluation before initiation of treatment.

Pegylated Interferon And Ribavirin Therapy
Treatment-Naïve Patients

Pegylated interferon (PEG-IFN) and ribavirin will remain the backbone of HCV for years to come. There are two PEG-IFNs (PEG-IFN-α-2a and PEG-IFN-α-2b).[202,203] IFNs are a group of naturally occurring cytokines that exhibit a range of immunomodulatory, antiproliferative, and antiviral effects. Pegylation refers to the covalent attachment of an inert, water-soluble polymer of polyethylene glycol (PEG) to the IFN molecule in either a linear-chain (PEG-IFN-α-2b [PEG-Intron], Schering Corp., a subsidiary of Merck & Co., Inc., white house station, N.J.) or a branched-chain configuration (PEG-IFN-α-2a [Pegasys], Hoffmann-La Roche, Basel, Switzerland). PEG-IFNs exhibit improved pharmacokinetic profiles and a prolonged elimination half-life in comparison with standard IFN-α, thus allowing increased efficacy and a convenient once-weekly subcutaneous dosing schedule (PEG-IFN-α-2b: 1.5 µg/kg/wk, PEG-IFN-α-2a: 180 µg/wk). Licensing trials for either of the PEG-IFNs showed substantially increased response rates in comparison with standard IFN

and ribavirin. Overall SVR rates increased from 47% to 54% and from 44% to 56%; the increase was 9% for patients infected with genotype 1 in both studies, 42% versus 33% and 46% versus 37%, respectively. Because the clinical registration trials differed slightly, there are slightly different labels for each of the PEG-IFNs related to ribavirin dosing (**Table 31-13**) by the two major registration authorities, the Food and Drug Administration (FDA) in the United States

Table 31-13 Recommended Doses of Pegylated Interferon and Weight-Based Ribavirin According to Label

PEGINTERFERON ALFA-2A (180 µg/wk s.c.)		PEGINTERFERON ALFA-2B (1.5 µg/kg/wk)	
Body Weight (kg)	**Ribavirin (orally)**	**Body Weight (kg)**	**Ribavirin (orally)**
<75	1000 mg	<65	800 mg
≥75	1200 mg	≥65-80	1000 mg
		≥80-105	1200 mg
		≥105	1400 mg

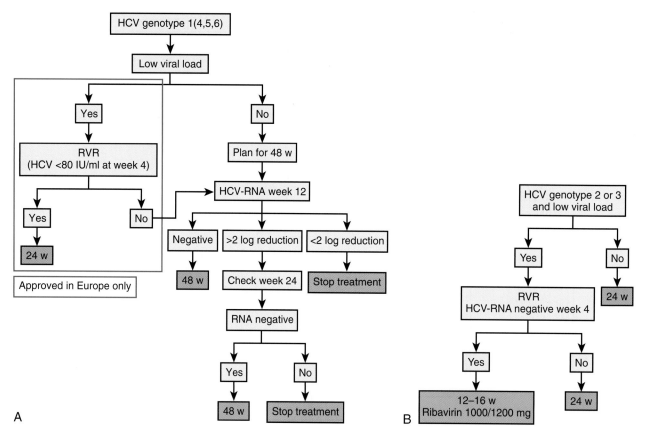

Fig. 31-11 **A,** Flow chart of treatment of genotype 1 (and 4 to 6) hepatitis C virus (HCV). In patients with a low viral load (<600,000 IU/ml), a shortened treatment duration can be considered when a rapid virologic response (RVR) (HCV RNA negative at week 4) is achieved. **B,** Flow chart of treatment of genotype 2 and genotype 3. A shortened treatment duration can be considered when RVR (HCV RNA negative at week 4) is achieved in genotype 2 and genotype 3 patients with a low viral load (<600,000 IU/ml).

and the European Medicines Evaluation Agency (EMEA) in the European Union.

The slightly different response rates in different trials raised speculation whether one IFN was better than the other in terms of efficacy. Two small prospective studies from Italy reported higher SVR rates with PEG-IFN-α-2a than with PEG-IFN-α-2b[204,205] despite higher relapse rates with PEG-IFN-α-2a. In contrast, a large and very well-controlled postapproval commitment study for PEG-IFN-α-2b did not show a difference in SVR, but it did in relapse rates. This "IDEAL" study (Individualized Dosing Efficacy vs. Flat Dosing to Assess Optimal Pegylated Interferon Therapy) compared PEG-IFN-α-2b, 1.5 μg/kg/wk, with PEG-IFN-α-2b, 1.0 μg/kg/wk, each combined with ribavirin, but also compared both PEG-IFN-α-2b arms with an arm consisting of PEG-IFN-α-2a, 180 μg/wk, and demonstrated very comparable results in terms of SVR for all three arms: 40%, 38%, and 41% SVR rates, respectively.[206] Within the IDEAL trial there was no significant difference in SVR between the 1.0-μg/kg arm (38%) and the 1.5-μg/kg arm of PEG IFN-α-2b (40%).

The difference between the Italian and American studies could in part be due to smaller sample sizes in the Italian studies, potential misbalance of the IL28B genotype, and differences in the distribution of genotype 1a and 1b. The later seems relevant in light of a French study reporting a significant difference in SVR rates depending on the HCV genotype 1 subtype, independent of either form of PEG-IFN.[207] Likewise,

the briefing documents form Merck for boceprevir and from Vertex for telaprevir to the FDA showed differences in response in favor for 1b over 1a. An advantage for PEG-IFN-α-2b is a lower relapse rate. Thus patients can be more accurately identified during therapy with regard to their prospect for eventual cure of hepatitis C or, on the other hand, with regard to stopping treatment in event of achievement of SVR being unlikely. Therefore fewer patients treated with PEG-IFN-α-2b need to be treated unnecessarily long without an eventual successful outcome. With newer treatment regimens in development that will be combined with long-acting IFNs, it will be important to evaluate whether these differences translate into differences in SVR with these newer compounds.[208]

There is general consensus that patients infected with genotype 1 should be treated for 48 weeks (**Fig. 31-11, A**) whereas patients infected with genotype 2 or 3 need only 24 weeks of treatment in most circumstances. In selected patients infected with genotype 2/3 and with low baseline viral load and minimal fibrosis who achieve RVR, shortening the treatment duration can be considered.[209] In Europe, a shortened course of 24 weeks has been licensed for genotype 1 patients with low viral load and undetectable viral load (RVR) at week 4 of treatment. The recently updated American Association for the Study of Liver Diseases (AASLD) practice guideline suggests that one can "consider" shortening the course for patients with RVR at week 4 but does not recommend shortening treatment.[203]

For PEG-IFN-α-2a the recommended dose is 180 μg. According to the IDEAL study results, one could consider using a reduced dose of PEG-IFN-α-2b, 1.0 μg/kg body weight, instead of the current label, which indicates a dose of 1.5 μg/kg body weight of PEG-IFN-α-2b. Similarly, a smaller study evaluating PEG-IFN-α-2a monotherapy did not find a difference in SVR with 180 μg PEG-IFN-α-2a versus 135 μg PEG-IFN-α-2a. Each arm showed a 28% SVR rate.[210] Each of the PEG-IFNs is administered subcutaneously weekly and combined with oral ribavirin. According to the prescribing information, there is a slight variation in ribavirin dosing, depending on the respective PEG-IFN used (see **Table 31-13**). Both licensed PEG-IFNs plus ribavirin have been evaluated in combination with protease inhibitors, and any PEG-IFNs can be used with either protease inhibitor according to the label.

To minimize side effects, as well as cost, an "early stopping rule" may be applied to patients infected with genotype 1 who fail to achieve an early virologic response (EVR). This means that quantitative HCV RNA measurement should be performed before treatment and at weeks 4 and 12 of treatment. If there is less than a 2-log decline in viral load at week 12,[202,203] treatment should be stopped because further treatment is unlikely to lead to SVR. In one study it was suggested that a combination of a decline in viral load and threshold values can predict both SVR and non-SVR in some patients as early as 2 or 4 weeks.[211]

With few exceptions, patients experience side effects during therapy, which can vary from mild flulike symptoms to severe adverse events requiring interruption of treatment (**Table 31-14**). The majority of side effects are mild. Constitutional symptoms can frequently be treated with low-dose paracetamol/acetaminophen. As long as a low dose is used, this regimen is superior to other nonsteroidal antiinflammatory drugs (NSAIDs).[212]

Arthralgia, muscle pain, flulike symptoms, fever, and other side effects are common. Leukopenia, granulocytopenia, and thrombocytopenia are important and need to be monitored. For ribavirin, anemia is the most prominent adverse event and leads to a significant decline in hemoglobin (median of about 3.5 g/dl) within the first 4 to 8 weeks of treatment (Pegasys prescribing information). In patients with coronary artery disease, careful evaluation of the risk/benefit ratio of this treatment is essential. In individual patients, IFN-related adverse events may occur and require specific management and, in some cases, termination of therapy. Among the most important side effects are depression, autoimmune thyroid disease, alopecia, and worsening of diabetes (see **Table 31-14**). Patients and physicians must be aware of these adverse events and need to react appropriately.

Management of side effects is important to prevent premature discontinuation of treatment or dose reductions. Patients able to take more than 80% of both drugs for more than 80% of the planned duration of therapy had an optimized response rate of 63% in a secondary analysis as compared with 48% in the overall intent-to-treat analysis of the PEG-IFN-α-2b licensing trial.[213]

Treatment of patients with persistently normal ALT levels is safe, and viral responses are comparable with those with abnormal ALT levels.[214] Thus elevated ALT values are not a prerequisite for therapy.[202] In patients with normal ALT levels, biopsy should be performed and treatment initiated if the fibrosis score and activity indicate significant liver disease and injury.

Because ribavirin is eliminated through the kidneys, dose adaptations are required for those with impaired renal function.

Management of Side Effects

The most difficult and most important part of treatment is management of side effects. Compliance or the amount of drug received correlates with the success of therapy; therefore management of side effects and preemptive education of patients concerning side effects are of utmost importance. The most common and most important side effects are listed in **Table 31-14**.

General Side Effects

Endogenous IFN production is the natural response of the host to viral infection. Thus experiencing flulike symptoms is relatively common, particularly in the first few weeks of therapy. Headache, fever, and myalgia are mostly related to flulike symptoms and are best treated with acetaminophen/paracetamol. There are no systematic data on these versus other NSAIDs in the treatment of hepatitis C, but in IFN-β treatment of patients with multiple sclerosis, acetaminophen/paracetamol has been found to be superior to other NSAIDs.[212] Acetaminophen/paracetamol can be recommended safely as long as doses remain below 2 to 3 g daily.

Mental and Mood Status

Although systemic flulike side effects usually improve after the first weeks of treatment, the central effects of IFN on mental status frequently increase gradually during the first 12 weeks of treatment and remain thereafter. There is also a high prevalence of preexisting mental health illness in HCV-infected patients.[215,216] Patients with preexisting depression or a history of depression may require preemptive treatment with antidepressive agents because their condition will probably worsen during IFN therapy; all other patients should be monitored carefully and prescribed antidepressants if such symptoms occur or worsen. The same holds true for irritability, which might require treatment intervention with, for example, a selective serotonin reuptake inhibitor (SSRI).[217] Increased irritability, another common side effect, should be clearly discussed with patients and their caregivers. Depressive symptoms are reported in almost a third of HCV-infected patients but in only 3% to 6% of HBV-infected patients treated with PEG-IFN.[218]

Insomnia, one of the most frequent complaints during IFN-based therapy, can and should be treated with standard approaches such as the short-term use of sedative-hypnotics.

Other central symptoms range from cognitive deficits to psychosis and suicidal ideation, the latter of which fortunately occurs rarely. Psychoses, mania, and suicidal ideation need more immediate consultation or hospitalization (or both) with psychiatric care.

Hematologic Side Effects
Anemia

Ribavirin leads to different degrees of hemolysis in practically all patients and results in various declines in the hemoglobin

Table 31-14 Common Side Effects of Interferon-α and Ribavirin Therapy and Potential Therapies to Alleviate the Side Effects

SIDE EFFECTS	TREATMENT OPTIONS TO ALLEVIATE THE SIDE EFFECTS	COMMENTS
Constitutional		
Flulike symptoms	Paracetamol/acetaminophen, other NSAIDS	Beware of liver toxicity, <2 g/day best
Fatigue	SSRI	
Headache	Paracetamol/acetaminophen, other NSAIDS	Beware of liver toxicity, <2 g/day best
Fever	Paracetamol/acetaminophen, other NSAIDS	Beware of liver toxicity, <2 g/day best
Myalgias	Paracetamol/acetaminophen, other NSAIDS	Beware of liver toxicity, <2 g/day best
Gastrointestinal		
Nausea	Antiemetics (metoclopramide, ondansetron)	
Anorexia	NA	
Diarrhea	Loperamide	
Dyspepsia	PPI	
Mental		
Insomnia	Sleep medication	
Irritability	Mood stabilizer	Depending on severity, consult with psychiatrist
Depression	Antidepressants such as SSRI	Consult with psychiatrist
Dermatologic		
Alopecia	Topical steroids	
Effluvium	NA	Mostly reversible after end of therapy
Rash	Topical steroids such as triamcinolone cream	
Dry skin	Lotions, lipid cream	
Skin itching	Antihistamines	
Stomatitis	Mouth wash	
Dry mouth	Saliva substitute	
Dry eyes	Artificial teardrops	
Reaction at injection site	Clobetasol	
Lichen ruber cutis	PUVA or retinoid	
Lichen ruber mucosae	Local steroids or systemic cyclosporine	
Psoriasis	Local steroids, PUVA therapy; consider stopping therapy	
Ophthalmologic		
Vision impairment	Stop therapy	Risk in patients with diabetes and/or hypertension, require evaluation before therapy
Endocrine		
Hypothyroidism	Levothyroxine substitution	Improves after end of IFN therapy. No need to interrupt therapy
Hyperthyroidism	β-Blocker, antithyroid drugs (methimazole and propylthiouracil)	Consider stopping therapy
Worsening of diabetes	Adapt insulin requirement	Usually improves after end of therapy
Pneumologic		
Cough	Antitussive	
Interstitial pneumonitis	Steroids	Stop therapy. Can be life-threatening, and might not reverse despite stopping IFN

Table 31-14 Common Side Effects of Interferon-α and Ribavirin Therapy and Potential Therapies to Alleviate the Side Effects—cont'd

SIDE EFFECTS	TREATMENT OPTIONS TO ALLEVIATE THE SIDE EFFECTS	COMMENTS
Laboratory		
Anemia	Erythropoietin	Probably does not improve SVR but improves quality of life during therapy
Neutropenia	GM-CSF sargramostim (Leukine), G-CSF filgrastim (Neupogen) or pegfilgrastim (Neulasta)	Dose reduction according to label. Probably indicated only in life-threatening situations
Thrombocytopenia	Eltrombopag, romiplostim	Dose reduction according to label. Bleeding complication likely only if drops below 30,000/μl Safety of eltrombopag and romiplostim has not been evaluated, nor has its efficacy in this situation

G-CSF, granulocyte colony-stimulating factor; GM-CSF, granulocyte-macrophage colony-stimulating factor; IFN, interferon; NA, not available; NSAIDs, nonsteroidal antiinflammatory drugs; PPI, proton pump inhibitor; PUVA, psoralen and ultraviolet A light; SSRI, selective serotonin reuptake inhibitor; SVR, sustained virologic response

level, which is of potential concern in patients with preexisting cardiorespiratory disease. Usually, the peak of anemia is reached by week 4 to 8 and stabilizes thereafter at the decreased hemoglobin level.[219] The decline is mostly in the range of 2 to 3 g/dl. IFN also inhibits the ability of bone marrow to compensate for ribavirin-induced hemolysis. Anemia is somewhat more pronounced with the protease inhibitors telaprevir and boceprevir. Although erythropoietin may not significantly improve SVR rates, the associated increase in hemoglobin improves quality of life during therapy.[220] Given the recent warnings regarding these agents, debate exists on when, at what dose, the target hemoglobin level, and for how long erythropoietin-stimulating agents should be given, if at all, in the setting of HCV antiviral therapy.

Neutropenia

The risk for serious infection remains low even with severe neutropenia (<500/mm³).[201] Still, IFN dose reduction is recommended in patients with decreasing neutrophil counts.[50] Recombinant granulocyte colony-stimulating factor (G-CSF) is often used to stimulate granulopoiesis but is associated with significant expense, bone pain, and uncertain benefit.

Lymphopenia

Lymphopenia below 500/mm³ occurs in few patients, but infections on treatment with PEG-IFN plus ribavirin were recently found to be associated with minimal lymphocyte count on treatment. Lymphopenia is more pronounced by adding protease inhibitors; however, whether that translates into higher risk of infection remains unclear at present.[201a]

Thrombocytopenia

Likewise, thrombopenia is relatively frequent during treatment, but life-threatening thrombocytopenia is fortunately rare. Nonetheless, dose reduction according to the product labeling is recommended as required. Whether thrombopoietic drugs may prove helpful in allowing completion of treatment is currently under investigation after an initial promising study.[221]

Thyroid Dysfunction

There is good evidence to suggest an association of HCV infection with autoimmune thyroid disease and hypothyroidism. PEG-IFN–induced thyroid dysfunction with or without thyroid antibodies may be observed in up to 3% to 5% of patients.[29] Patients should be screened for thyroid disease at baseline, every 3 months during treatment, and at least once following completion of antiviral therapy. IFN can also augment other nonspecific preexisting subclinical autoimmune responses.[222]

Gastrointestinal

Nausea has been observed in many patients with hepatitis C during therapy (about 30% in each of the different arm of the IDEAL trial).[206] No systematic evaluation has been performed to determine the efficacy of antiemetics; however, taking the higher of the daily divided ribavirin doses in the evenings and with food may be helpful. If this is not sufficient, proton pump inhibitors (PPIs) can be added. In patients with persistent symptoms, metoclopramide and rarely ondansetron may be used. Diarrhea usually responds to loperamide.

Most patients experience some form of anorexia and weight loss during therapy, which abates within weeks after the end of therapy. Occasionally, dose adjustments are required for profound weight loss, but ingestion of drinks with high caloric energy should be advised when appropriate.

Cutaneous Side Effects

Rashes can be seen in about a third of patients during IFN therapy. Most frequently they consist of injection site reactions, pruritus, dry skin, and loss of hair, mostly as diffuse effluvium and in some instances as alopecia areata.

Effects of Sustained Virologic Clearance on Clinical Outcomes

Clearance of HCV is only a surrogate for improved clinical outcomes. It has now been shown that some patients with cirrhosis still progress to HCC despite viral clearance.[223,224] However, the frequency of development of HCC is significantly lower.[225,226] In a Greek epidemiologic study that included 1727 patients, 993 of whom were treated and 734 remained untreated, there was a significantly lower rate of liver decompensation and development of HCC in patients who achieved SVR, and additionally, there was an observed trend toward fewer clinical events, even in the absence of SVR.[227] The majority of patients with SVR also achieve improvement in their histologic fibrosis score,[227-229] which can even lead to reversal of advanced liver fibrosis.[228] In addition, SVR is associated with a reduced risk for the development of end-stage liver disease[230,231] and with improved quality of life.[232]

Retreatment Options for Nonresponders or Relapsers after Previous Treatment

With the increasing use of PEG-IFN and response rates between 40% and 85% to 90%, depending on HCV genotype, there is an increasing number of patients who do not respond or who relapse while awaiting newer, more effective treatment options. Patients who relapsed with previous standard IFN-based or shorter-duration treatments should in general be retreated with 48 weeks of PEG-IFN and ribavirin if they previously tolerated treatment.

Retreatment with either PEG-IFN or consensus interferon can be undertaken, but SVR rates are low (**Table 31-15**),[233-236] usually less than 10% unless the previous course of therapy had to be shortened or stopped because of side effects, which would now be manageable, or unless treatment duration or

dose was inadequate for other reasons. Induction therapy has little effect, but extending the duration of treatment from 48 to 72 weeks holds some promise. However, these longer, more intensive regimens are often poorly tolerated and result in more frequent withdrawal of treatment.

Histologic benefits have been noted in patients with virologic responses during treatment, but long-term therapy without viral suppression does not reduce disease progression. Three independent studies failed to show histologic or significant clinical benefits with long-term, low-dose maintenance IFN. Lifestyle measures such as weight loss and reduction of alcohol intake should be encouraged in all patients to reduce the risk for disease progression. In addition, coffee consumption has been associated with decreased progression of disease.[77]

Given the poor prospects of current retreatment with PEG-IFN and ribavirin alone, adding one of the recently licensed protease inhibitors or awaiting further improved options is advisable. Based on evidence of inhibition of progression of liver fibrosis by angiotensin receptor blockers,[237,238] some early reports in HCV-infected patients have emerged.[239,240] A phase III clinical trial was initiated in 2006 in France to evaluate the effect of irbesartan on hepatic fibrosis in patients with chronic hepatitis C (NCT00265642).

Optimizing the Interferon and Ribavirin Regimen

Optimization of the current standard treatment regimen is based on the principles of managing side effects and individualizing treatment to allow the shortest duration needed to cure hepatitis C or identify patients who are unlikely to eventually respond and eradicate the virus long-term. After the licensing of protease inhibitors, this remains important in settings where protease inhibitors are unavailable or prohibitively expensive. Patients who do not exhibit a 2-log reduction at week 12 have a very low likelihood of achieving SVR[206,210]; in addition,

Table 31-15 Response in Nonresponders to a Previous Course of Peginterferon

STUDY (PATIENTS)	POPULATION	DURATION	THERAPY	SVR
Control arm, Boceprevir NR Study[233]	Nonresponder (null response) to PEG-IFN/ribavirin	48 wk	1.5 μg/kg PEG-IFN-α-2b + 800-1400 mg ribavirin	2%
EPIC3[234]	Nonresponder to PEG-IFN/ribavirin	48 wk	1.5 μg/kg PEG-IFN-α-2b + 800-1400 mg ribavirin	6% 4% (genotype 1) 36% (genotype 2/3)
REPEAT[235]	Nonresponder to PEG-IFN-α-2b/ribavirin	48 wk	180 μg PEG-IFN-α-2a + 1000/1200 mg ribavirin	9%
REPEAT[234]	Nonresponder to PEG-IFN-α-2b/ribavirin	48 wk (induction)	360/180 μg PEG-IFN-α-2a + 1000/1200 mg ribavirin	7%
REPEAT[234]	Nonresponder to PEG-IFN-α-2b/ribavirin	72 wk	180 μg PEG-IFN-α-2a + 1000/1200 mg ribavirin	14%
REPEAT[234]	Nonresponder to PEG-IFN-α-2b/ribavirin	72 wk (induction)	360/180 μg PEG-IFN-α-2a + 1000/1200 mg ribavirin	16%
DIRECT[236]	Nonresponder to PEG-IFN/ribavirin	48 wk	Consensus IFN, 3 × 9 μg/wk	6.9%
DIRECT[235]	Nonresponder to PEG-IFN/ribavirin	48 wk	Consensus IFN, 3 × 15 μg/wk	10.7%

PEG-IFN, pegylated interferon; SVR, sustained virologic response

patients with either a 1-log decline by week 4 or a 2-log decline at week 4 and a viral load of less than 5.5 log or a viral load that does not decline by 2 logs at week 12 have a very low likelihood of achieving SVR.[206,210] Early discontinuation of therapy at week 4 or 12 should then be considered. Likewise, in patients with a rapid response at week 4, genotype 2 or 3, and a low viral load, the infection is frequently cured with a 12- to 16-week course of treatment when the dose of ribavirin is based on weight instead of using a fixed 800-mg dose.[209] Moreover, a shorter duration of 24 versus 48 weeks is justifiable in some instances for patients infected with genotype 1 who have a low baseline viral load.[241-243] It should be noted that a shortened treatment duration of PEG-IFN plus ribavirin has led to slightly lower SVR rates and higher relapse rates than seen with treatment of standard duration. Thus an individual decision should be made regarding these different strategies, the tolerability of the treatment, and all other factors.

Protease Inhibitors Plus Peg-IFN/RBV

Telaprevir and Boceprevir
Treatment-Naïve Patients

We are in an era in which new treatment options are being licensed to be used with PEG-IFN and ribavirin. Two protease inhibitors, telaprevir and boceprevir, have been successfully evaluated in phase II and phase III clinical trials. When protease inhibitors became available for HIV therapy, the deadly disease became a somewhat controllable infection. It is expected that similar improvement in HCV therapy will be achieved with the introduction of HCV-specific protease inhibitors. The different phase II studies have shown SVR rates between 60% and 74%, which is greater than a 20% increase in SVR rates over SOC in the respective studies (**Fig. 31-12**).[244-246]

In the PROVE 2 study (Protease Inhibition for Viral Eradication), in which one arm was treated without ribavirin, we have learned that ribavirin cannot be omitted from telaprevir and PEG-IFN treatment strategies without impairing the response. Importantly, the risk for resistance is significantly higher in the absence of ribavirin. Breakthrough during the first 12 weeks developed in 24% of patients treated with PEG-IFN plus telaprevir as compared with 0.5% and 1.2%, respectively, in either of the PEG-IFN/ribavirin plus telaprevir arms ($P < .0012$).

Interestingly, both drugs, telaprevir and boceprevir, increase the rate and severity of adverse events during therapy and, in addition, have another distinguished side effect: dysgeusia (distorted sense of taste) with boceprevir and rash, which can be severe, with telaprevir. The dysgeusia and rashes resolved after discontinuation of treatment, and a rash management plan was implemented in the phase III trials of telaprevir.[244,245]

Sixty percent of patients from the European PROVE 2 trial cleared their HCV infection and achieved SVR with only 12

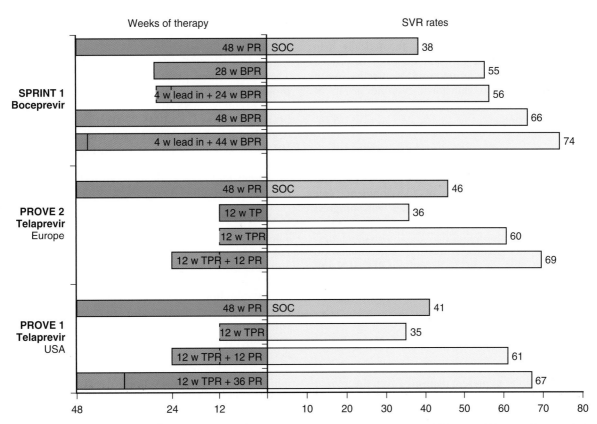

Fig. 31-12 **Treatment scheme (left side) and sustained virologic response (SVR) rates (right side) for the different phase II clinical trials of boceprevir and telaprevir (protease inhibitors).** BPR, boceprevir, pegylated interferon (PEG-IFN), and ribavirin; PR, PEG-IFN and ribavirin; SOC, standard of care; TP, telaprevir and PEG-IFN without ribavirin; TPR, telaprevir, PEG-IFN, and ribavirin.

weeks of triple therapy. Because of the potency of these protease inhibitors, many patients have undetectable HCV RNA by week 4; thus, evaluation of virologic response at week 1 or 2 might be more predictive of treatment response and tailored treatment duration in the future.

Data from the phase III studies confirmed the expected improvement in SVR, and both protease inhibitors were licensed in May 2011 in the United States. Approval by EMEA is pending as of mid June 2011. The duration of treatment will be 24, 28, or 48 weeks, depending on the early treatment response and PI.

In the telaprevir phase II study, nonresponder and relapse patients received either SOC for 48 weeks, PEG-IFN and ribavirin for 24 weeks plus telaprevir for 12 or 48 weeks, or SOC plus telaprevir for 24 weeks. The SOC arm achieved SVR in 9% of patients as compared with 39% and 38% in the two arms of previous nonresponders receiving telaprevir plus PEG-IFN and ribavirin. Patients with relapse after a previous regimen of PEG-IFN plus ribavirin responded significantly better (69% and 76%) in the telaprevir-containing arms than in the SOC arm (20%). The difference between relapse patients (60% and 76%) and previous nonresponder patients (39% and 38%) was significant ($P < .05$).

In the boceprevir phase II study, only 14% of nonresponders achieved SVR, but this study recruited well-defined true nonresponders, in whom the SVR rate in those receiving SOC was just 2%. This clearly indicated that patients who had been compliant and were true nonresponders during an earlier course of PEG-IFN therapy may have a relatively small benefit in terms of SVR rates with these new direct antiviral–based regimens. Because protease inhibitors can select for resistance mutations within days in the absence of a solid IFN response, such patients might best be advised to await additional treatment options. This may theoretically help prevent the development of protease inhibitor–associated mutations, which may in the future limit the effective use of this class of drugs in this difficult-to-respond group of patients. See "The Pivotal Trials for Protease Inhibitors" online www.expertconsult.com.

Other Protease Inhibitors

Multiple other protease inhibitors are in phase II trials and many more in earlier phases of development (see www.hcvdrugs.com); which of these drugs will progress through the different phases of clinical development is unknown. One protease inhibitor, RG7227 (formerly ITMN-191), is discussed later because it was used in combination with a polymerase inhibitor (RG7128) without PEG-IFN and ribavirin.

Alternative Approaches and Novel Therapies

Numerous other therapies are in development, but it is beyond the scope of this chapter to present them all. Given the myriad targets and compounds in development, this section should be considered an overview to give some feel for the activity in current anti-HCV drug development. It is unknown which of these therapies will eventually proceed into the clinic and, if so, at what time point.

Viral Enzyme–Targeting Approaches
Protease Inhibitors
NS3 PROTEASE INHIBITORS

Examples of protease inhibitors have been discussed earlier. The principle of protease inhibitors is inhibition of viral maturation. Maturation requires the viral protease to cleave proteins from the polyprotein and can be inhibited by blocking the function of the protease. There will probably be a genotype dependence inasmuch as a small study consisting of patients infected with genotype 2/3 found a beneficial effect on genotype 2 but not on genotype 3 when NS3 protease inhibitors were given with the SOC regimen. This study, however, included only 49 patients and was not controlled for IL28B.[247]

NS4A PROTEASE INHIBITORS

NS3 is the major protease inhibitor, but it requires the NS4a protein as a co-factor for optimal function.[248] This requirement of NS4a enables drugs to target NS4a specifically and thus to inhibit HCV synergistically with protease and polymerase inhibitors.[249] A theoretic advantage could be the use of protease inhibitors without overlapping resistance profiles.

NS3 Helicase Inhibitors

Part of the NS3 protein is a helicase in addition to the protease. The helicase is likewise required for the viral life cycle and could possibly be a potential drug target.[250]

NS4b RNA-Binding Inhibitors

The nonstructural protein NS4b binds to the 3′ terminus of the HCV RNA negative strand, which was recently identified and can be inhibited by clemizoles.[251]

NS5a Pleiotropic Protein and Its Inhibition

The nonstructural protein NS5a is considered a pleiotropic protein; it was found to be involved in RNA replication and virus assembly.[252] NS5a could be targeted by inhibition of protein function (i.e., BMS-790052)[253] or by increasing its degradation.[254] BMS-790052 used with a protease inhibitor (BMS-650032) was shown to successfully clear HCV in 4 of 11 patients treated with an all oral agent approach and in 10 of 10 non-responder patients when BMS-790052 and BMS-650032 were combined with PEG-IFN and ribavirin.[254a]

NS5b Polymerase Inhibitors

The HCV NS5b protein corresponds to HCV polymerase. Polymerase inhibitors are some of the most widely used antivirals (i.e., ganciclovir for cytomegalovirus, acyclovir for herpes simplex virus, entecavir or tenofovir for HBV). Polymerase inhibitors target the viral polymerase, but high specificity for the viral polymerase is required to prevent interaction with human polymerases. No HCV polymerase inhibitor is currently licensed, but multiple polymerase inhibitors are in development. Some are nucleotide-like and some are non-nucleotides. One example is RG7128, a nucleoside polymerase inhibitor that is currently being developed in combination with a protease inhibitor (RG7227, formerly known as ITMN-191). Except for the lowest-dose groups, more than 50% of patients treated with 1000 mg RG7128 plus 100 mg RG7227 three times daily to 900 mg RG7227 twice daily achieved viral decline to below 43 IU/ml and about 25% of patients to below the level of detection (15 IU/ml) within 14 days. This study proved that potentially a non–IFN-ribavirin–based therapy might be feasible. However, the study was limited to 14 days, and patients eventually received PEG-IFN plus ribavirin for 48 week thereafter.[255]

New Generations of Type I Interferons, Interferon Inducers, Other Cytokines, and Growth Factors
Consensus Interferon

Consensus INF was designed from the consensus sequence of different IFN sequences. Consensus IFN is approved in many countries. Because a pegylated formulation is not yet available, daily injections of consensus IFN may be necessary to achieve an optimal response. No head-to-head study comparing consensus IFN and PEG-IFN has been published, and potentially a long-acting consensus IFN will become available in the future.

Albuferon

Protein coupling to albumin is an alternative to pegylation for prolonging half-life. IFN-α-2b linked to albumin (albuferon [Zalbin]) has completed two phase III studies: one in patients infected with genotype 1 and the other in those infected with genotype 2 or 3. In both studies, albuferon plus ribavirin was equivalent to PEG-IFN-α-2a plus ribavirin. SVR was achieved in 48.2% (213/442) of patients receiving 900 μg albinterferon-α-2b biweekly versus 51.0% (225/441) of patients receiving PEG-IFN-α-2a weekly for genotype 1 (P = .0008 for noninferiority) and 79.8% (249/312) and 84.8% (263/310; P = .009 for noninferiority) for genotypes 2 and 3, respectively.[256,257] Despite achieving non-inferiority in the clinical trials, Human Genome Sciences and Novartis stopped further development of albinterferon-α-2b.

Interferon Beta

Interferon-β is the current standard treatment for patients with multiple sclerosis but is not licensed for the treatment of HCV in most countries. IFN-β is, however, used for the treatment of hepatitis C in Japan.[258] Three forms of IFN-β are available, one natural human IFN-β (nIFN-β) and two recombinant IFN-βs. nIFN-β is produced from human fibroblasts and is currently used in Japan for the treatment of chronic hepatitis C. Recombinant human IFN-β-1a (rhIFN-β-1a) is procured from mammalian cells and is identical to the IFN-β that occurs naturally in humans. rhIFN-β-1b contains an altered amino acid sequence with a serine substitution for cysteine at position 17 and is produced in *Escherichia coli*. IFN-β might hold additional promise when combined with cyclosporine according to a small study from Japan.[259] A potential concern is the high frequency of liver enzyme elevation in patients with multiple sclerosis receiving IFN-β,[212] including fulminant hepatic failure.[260]

Several other IFNs or IFN deliveries are under investigation. Duros interferon omega (IFN-ω) is an implant device in which IFN-ω is applied via the device to achieve a constant level of drug. IFN-ω shares about 70% homology with IFN-α and IFN-β and also binds to same receptors.[261] Locteron is another controlled-release IFN administered via biweekly or monthly injections and is currently in clinical trials.

Several cytokines have been evaluated with limited or no success, among them IFN-γ, interleukin-10 (IL-10), and IL-12. Thymosin alpha is still under evaluation in combination with PEG-IFN or administered alone.

Interferon Lambda

Although the type I IFNs were discovered more than 5 decades ago, the type III IFNs (also known as IFN-λ or IL-28/29) were discovered only in the last decade. IFN-λ represent a new class of cytokines with biologic activities similar to those of type I IFNs.[262] However, in contrast to the type I IFNs receptors, the receptor for IFN-λ is not universally expressed.[263] Given its more restricted expression, IFN-λ has the potential to have fewer side effects, to be less active in clearing HCV infection, or both.[264]

A 4-week phase I study involving PEG-IFN-λ-1a (PEG-IFN-λ/PEG-rIL-29) found no hematologic toxicity in 18 patients, but 2 of the 18 patients experienced an increase in transaminases and bilirubin. Thirty-three percent, 50%, and 100% of patients in the 1.5-μg/kg biweekly, 3.0-μg/kg biweekly, and 1.5-μg/kg weekly dosing arms achieved a 2-log decline in HCV load.[265] The drug is currently in phase II clinical development.

Ribavirin Analogues

Anemia is a major problem with PEG-IFN and ribavirin combination therapies. Reduction of the ribavirin dose impairs treatment outcomes, particularly in patients infected with genotype 1. Given ribavirin's universal side effect of hemolysis, attempts have been made to develop less toxic ribavirin analogues. Levovirin, an *l*-enantiomer of ribavirin, was not further developed because of low bioavailability. Viramidine (also known as taribavirin) is a prodrug of ribavirin and should therefore have a beneficial liver-to-body drug ratio. Even though this translated into a lower frequency of hemolysis and anemia, it did not translate into equivalent SVR rates. The ViSER1 and ViSER2 (Viramidine's Safety and Efficacy versus Ribavirin) studies reported 54.6% and 54.3% lower hemoglobin events with viramidine versus 83.7% and 80.2% with ribavirin, but also impaired SVR rates of 38% and 40% versus 52% and 55%, respectively.[266,267]

Host-Targeting Drugs
Cyclophilin Inhibitors

In an attempt to ameliorate liver inflammation, Japanese investigators first reported a synergy between cyclosporine and IFN, which they subsequently demonstrated in a prospective study.[268] In a similar approach, investigators from the United States did not see a substantial effect of adding cyclosporine to IFN in patients who failed a previous course of IFN.[269]

However, in vitro studies confirmed the concept that cyclophilins are involved in HCV replication, and their interaction with HCV might be a target for inhibiting viral replication. Several cyclophilin inhibitors without the immunosuppressive action of cyclosporine are currently under development (i.e., Debio-025, NIM811). It has been shown that these substances can select for resistance mutations, thus further supporting their antiviral potential.[270,271] They also hold promise for being combined with other HCV therapies.[271,272]

Debio-025 is a synthetic cyclophilin inhibitor. A phase Ib study in HIV/HCV–co-infected patients demonstrated a 3.6-log reduction in HCV RNA when Debio, 1200 mg, was given as monotherapy for 15 days and a 1-log decline in HIV viral load.[273] A phase IIa study involving the use of Debio-025 in HCV-monoinfected patients found a 1.72-log and a 3.59-log reduction in HCV RNA for genotypes 1 or 4 and 2 or 3, respectively. The effect was more pronounced when combined with PEG-IFN (3.92 and 4.73 log after 15 days, respectively, and 4.75 and 5.89 log after 4 weeks, respectively).[274]

NIM811 is also another cyclophilin inhibitor currently in phase II testing (NCT00983060).

HCV Receptor Blockade

HCV has a high replication rate, and infection of uninfected cells appears to be a crucial part of the life cycle. Thus targeting the receptors required for viral uptake into cells is theoretically an attractive strategy. This aim might be achievable after the identification of four co-receptors required for entry of HCV: CD-81, SR-BI, claudin-1, and occludin.[275,276] Several of these receptors are currently targeted for antiviral approaches.

Statins

HCV leads to lipid disturbances, thus suggesting that HCV requires lipid machinery for efficient viral replication.[277] Indeed, some in vitro data have suggested that disturbance in the lipid machinery results in reduced HCV replication by depletion of geranylgeranyl lipids when HCV replicon cells are cultivated with lovastatin, one of several cholesterol-lowering statins.[278] In a similar study comparing the effect of five different statins on viral replication in vitro, fluvastatin was found to be the most effective, atorvastatin and simvastatin somewhat less, lovastatin only a little active, and pravastatin inactive.[279] In another study, mevastatin and simvastatin exhibited the strongest anti-HCV activity in vitro, lovastatin and fluvastatin had moderate inhibitory effects, and pravastatin was devoid of antiviral activity, similar to the earlier study.[280] Interestingly, both studies found a synergistic effect with either IFN or direct antivirals and noted the emergence of delayed resistance in the presence of a statin with antiviral activity.[280] This synergistic effect with IFN might explain why a retrospective study involving HCV-infected veterans did not see any effect with regard to statins and viral load[281] whereas an analysis of the IDEAL trial and statin use indicated an increased SVR rate in patients taking statins.[282] Importantly, several statins are contraindicated for when telaprevir or boceprevir are used.

Therapeutic Vaccines

In studies attempting to induce sterilizing immunity in chimps, it has not been possible to prevent infection, but the severity of disease can be ameliorated and infection duration shortened.[283] Therefore it seems likely that therapeutic vaccines could eventually become a feasible treatment option. An HCV-E1–based vaccine with 14 vaccinations of 20 μg administered over a period of 62 weeks suggested some trend in improvement of fibrosis, but a subsequent larger study failed to document any further efficacy.[284] Several other trials

are underway. GI-5005 is a vaccine based on a yeast vector that expresses hepatitis C NS3 and core proteins. A phase IIb study with 140 patients randomized to either SOC or SOC plus GI-5005 found a 59% versus a 74% increase in end-of-treatment response (ETR), respectively, but it is not yet known whether this will translate into increased SVR rates. However, a reduction in viral load corresponding to the strength of the TG4040 (a therapeutic vaccine)-induced immune response after therapeutic vaccination has recently been reported.[285]

Various Drugs with Therapeutic Potential against HCV
Silymarin

Silymarin is a mixture of flavolignans, with silibinin being the main component and extracted from milk thistle (*Silybum marianum* Gaertneri). Although some data affirmed its efficacy in patients with alcohol-induced liver cirrhosis,[286] silymarin never became SOC because of insufficient data to support any real benefit for oral sylimarin.[287] However, when more recently evaluated as an intravenous formulation, Austrian investigators surprisingly observed anti-HCV activity with up to a 3-log decline after the infusion of 20 mg/kg of silymarin over a period of 4 hours on 7 consecutive days.[288] The same group reported a successful decline in HCV viral load when silymarin was given to patients who were still HCV RNA positive at week 24 of PEG-IFN/ribavirin therapy.[289] One promising case report has also been provided from another center.[290] Analyzing the different components of silibinin in more detail, it also appears that silibinin A and B interact with HCV polymerase.[291]

Nitazoxanide

Nitazoxanide is a first-line choice for treating *Cryptosporidium parvum* or *Giardia lamblia* infection in immunocompetent adults and children. It can also be considered as treatment of infections with other protozoa or helminths.[292]

By chance, the antiviral activity of nitazoxanide was detected in HIV-infected patients co-infected with HCV or HBV when it was used in patients with HIV infection. After its antiviral potency was confirmed in vitro,[293] phase II studies of patients with chronic hepatitis C genotype 4 received nitazoxanide combined with PEG-IFN-α-2a and ribavirin. Increased SVR rates of 79% to 80% versus 50% for PEG-IFN plus ribavirin were observed. Patients receiving nitazoxanide combined with PEG-IFN-α-2a without ribavirin also had a better response (61%) than did patients receiving SOC.[294] Randomized, controlled studies of treatment-naïve and nonresponder patients with chronic hepatitis C genotype 1 and patients with chronic hepatitis B are underway, and newer second-generation thiazolides are currently under development.

Treatment-Induced Resistance of HCV to Antivirals

Resistance is a major concern in the treatment of any virus infection. When IFN was the only treatment option, this was less of a concern since no resistance to IFN emerged during treatment. Rather, preexisting mutations in the HCV genome (*NS5A*) have been associated with some degree of responsiveness to IFN therapy.[295] Sequencing of this so-called interferon sensitivity determining region (ISDR) of 40 amino acids within the *NS5A* gene has never become ingrained in clinical practice,[296] mostly likely because differences in the ISDR region could not explain differences in IFN response in patients from Western countries, where the prevalence of viruses with more than three mutations was rare.[297] Resistance to IFN might also be on a cellular level based on the following three observations: (1) there is substantial difference in responsiveness to IFN that is not explained by viral but rather by host factors (see Predictors of Response), (2) there is in vitro evidence that resistance to IFN can be induced at the cellular level while the virus remains sensitive to IFN,[298] and (3) no mutation in the HCV genome could be linked to viral breakthrough during IFN therapy. This is similar to HBV, where no resistance mutation of the virus in relation to IFN therapy has been identified.

However, with the use of direct antivirals for HBV it became evident that resistance emerges during treatment (see Chapter 30). The same is now observed with HCV as we move into the era of specifically targeted antiviral therapy for HCV (STAT-C).[299] With these direct antiviral agents (DAA) resistance has become an issue, and it can be detected within days of exposure to an HCV-specific protease inhibitor. Resistance actually emerges more rapidly in HCV than in either HIV or HBV,[300] probably because (1) HCV has no overlapping reading frames within its genome, (2) HCV replication does not depend on a DNA intermediate, and (3) HCV has a very high replication rate of 10^{12}.[301] The emergence of resistance seems to be rapid specifically within the protease region as compared with the polymerase region when patients are treated with protease or polymerase inhibitors, respectively.[302] Resistance has become detectable within 2 weeks of therapy with either of the two most advanced protease inhibitors, telaprevir[303] and boceprevir, but not with the polymerase inhibitors R1626 (prodrug of R1479) or NM283 within 2 weeks.[301] Mutations conferring resistance to protease inhibitors have been reported to be detectable as a preexisting dominant strain in a small minority of patients.[304,305] In addition, one study analyzing 2700 clones from 30 patients found that 70% of these treatment-naïve patients had 1% to 3% of clones harboring protease inhibitor resistance.[302]

With combination therapy, the problem of resistance is likely to be overcome when different drugs with nonoverlapping resistance profiles are combined, which has become the standard therapy for HIV infection.[306]

When analyzing resistance patterns to different direct antivirals, it is clear that there is a great variety of potential combinations without overlapping resistance mutations. **Figure 31-13** shows the position of the respective mutation in relation to the HCV polyprotein, and **Figures 31-14 and 31-15**

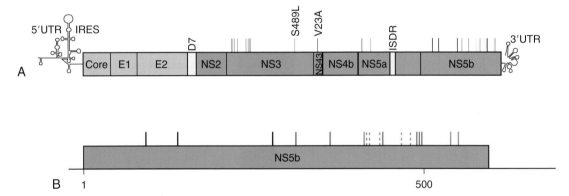

Fig. 31-13 **A** and **B,** The vertical lines over the hepatitis C virus polyprotein depict the position of the identified mutation in relation to its position on the respective proteins. There is no known cross-resistance between NS3b-targeting and NS5a- or NS5b-targeting therapies. Likewise, the different colors over the NS5b protein indicate targets with different resistance profiles, thus making combination of drugs targeting the different areas interesting for the prevention of resistance. IRES, internal ribosome entry site; ISDR, interferon sensitivity determining region; 5′UTR, 5′ untranslated region; 3′UTR, 3′ untranslated region.

	V36M/A	Q41R	F43C/S	T54S/A	V55A	Q80R/K	S138T	R155K/ Q/T	A156S/ V/T	D168V/ A/t/H	V170A
Telaprevir	■			■				■	■		■
Boceprevir	■			■				■	■		
Narlaprevir	■				■			■	■		
R7227 (ITMN 191)		■					■	■	■	■	
BILN 2061										■	
MK-7009										■	
TMC435350						■				■	
BI-201335										■	

Red indicates the linear NS3 protease inhibitors; *green* indicates the macrocyclic NS3 protease inhibitors.

Fig. 31-14 **Resistance-associated amino acid variants (RAV) in the NS3 region associated with NS3 proteases.**

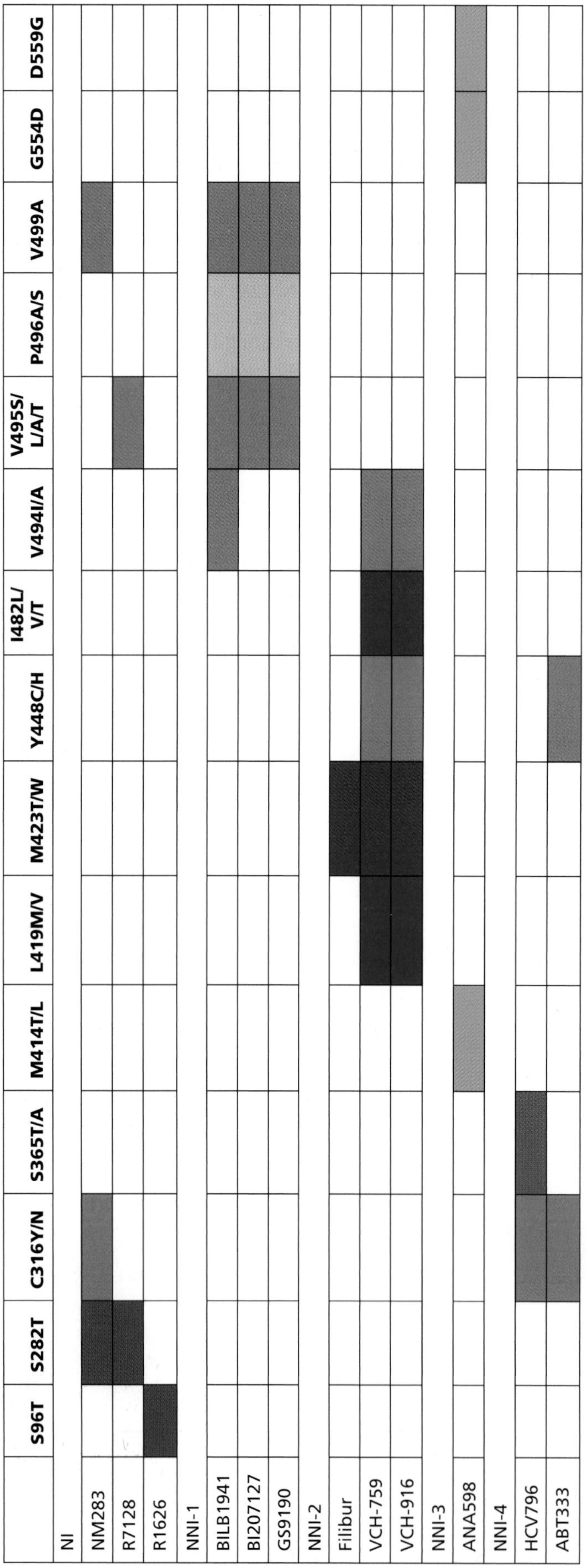

Fig. 31-15 **Resistance-associated amino acid variants (RAV) in the NS5b region associated with nucleoside analogues.** *Red* indicated variants with cross resistance across different classes; *brown* indicates resistance-associated amino acid variants (RAV) associated with nucleoside inhibitors; *orange* indicates RAV associated with non-nucleoside inhibitors 1 (NNI-1); *blue* indicates RAV associated with NNI-2; *light green* indicates RAV associated with NNI-3; *dark green* indicates RAV associated with NNI-4. NI, nucleoside analogue polymerase inhibitor; NNI, nonnucleoside polymerase inhibitor.

HEPATITIS C THERAPY STATE OF DEVELOPMENT 2010

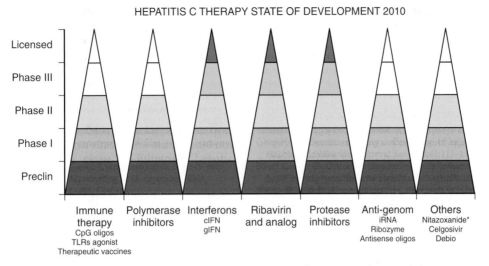

Fig. 31-16 The future of hepatitis C virus therapy will probably be built on several different types of principal alternative options. IFN, interferon; iRNA, inhibitory RNA; TLR, toll-like receptors; *, Nitazoxanide is in clinical trials for HCV, but licensed for certain infectious diarrhea.

show the resistance mutation according to different drug classes. There will be a class effect with regard to HCV resistance. However, given the existence of different targets within the HCV genome, it is hoped that we can overcome antiviral resistance for HCV more effectively than for HIV for several reasons: HCV does not integrate into the genome, and persistence of HCV requires ongoing replication. Alone, the polymerase offers five different target structures. Although each class targeting one of these sites will probably have some cross-resistance, there is little or no cross-resistance between different classes as of today.

The Future of Therapy for Hepatitis C

There are many different treatment options for HCV at different stages of development. It is currently unpredictable which new treatments will become available at what time point and in which combinations. We envision a variety of options eventually for the treatment of hepatitis C (**Fig. 31-16**), but at present only three of the principal options are licensed, IFN, ribavirin, and protease inhibitors. Once several of these different treatment alternatives are available, one might theoretically envision that IFN or ribavirin can be omitted from the regimen.

Patients with a favorable IL28B polymorphism predicting response to interferon may still receive IFN, but only to enable a shorter overall treatment course. In contrast, there might not be added benefit for those with a predictable less favorable response to IFN, and these patients might then be theoretically treated with alternative regimens, similar to the situation with HBV, where the role of IFN has diminished with the availability of more effective and safer alternatives. Nonetheless, for those with a very high likelihood of response to IFN, it will remain a valuable treatment option. However, some recent data suggest that direct antiviral might be so strong that IFN will not have any added benefit.

Proof of concept cure from HCV with an all oral regimen has been presented at EASL 2011 for a combination of a protease inhibitor plus NS5a inhibitor.[254a]

Special Patient Populations

Hepatitis C virus infection disproportionally affects certain populations in the United States. Fortunately, children are currently rarely positive, whereas vulnerable populations with a higher prevalence of HCV include individuals who inject drugs, the incarcerated, the homeless, and the poor. Furthermore, there is a high prevalence of HCV in veterans and people with HIV infection. Many of these patient groups have been excluded from registration trials of therapy with PEG-IFN and ribavirin.

African Americans

The highest prevalence of HCV in any ethnic group in the United States is found in those of African-American descent. They do respond less favorably to PEG–IFN/RBV therapy, independent of HCV genotype.[196,199,206] This can be partially explained by a significantly lower frequency of the beneficial IL28B polymorphism than in other ethnicities. There is some indication, though, that HCV might be associated with a slightly milder course of disease in African Americans.[307,308] Yet complications in the form of HCC also appear more frequently in African Americans.[309] Clearly, treating these patients more effectively is an important future priority. With the addition of protease inhibitors, African Americans show still lower response than Caucasians, but they were found to achieve SVR in up to 60% compared with about 20% with PEG-IFN/RBV alone.

Patients with Cirrhosis

Patients with cirrhosis have the greatest need for effective therapy. Unfortunately, the likelihood of response decreases with progression of fibrosis. Still, in a prospective PEG-IFN study specifically targeting cirrhotic patients, up to 30% achieved SVR even without ribavirin, but with a significant difference depending on HCV genotype.[310] Patients with high and low genotype 1 viral loads had SVR rates of 10% and 16%, respectively. Furthermore, there was a difference with genotype 1a (9%) versus 1b (20%). In contrast, 20 of 50 (40%) non–genotype 1 patients in that study achieved SVR with 180 μg PEG-IFN-α-2a.[309]

Because of the risk for decompensation in the setting of advanced liver disease, such treatment is best planed with transplant availability in mind in the event of decompensation. The presence of cirrhosis or advanced fibrosis is associated with risk for the development of HCC. The annual incidence of HCC in patients with cirrhosis is about 2% to 6%.[22] Low-dose maintenance therapy has not proved effective in reducing the complications of cirrhosis. It is hoped that more people with cirrhosis can be cured of HCV infection when newer, more effective agents become available. Elimination of the virus would also, one hopes, improve survival and will be documented in future long-term follow-up studies. A caveat is that current protease inhibitors are less effective in cirrhotic patients. Furthermore, although drug exposure with boceprevir increases in patients with hepatic impairment, it decreases with telaprevir.

Patients with Renal Disease

Patients with renal disease, especially those requiring hemodialysis, should be screened for HCV and be considered for treatment.[178] When considering treatment, one needs to judge the stage of liver disease and overall life expectancy. HCV infection has been shown to have an overall negative impact on survival, especially after renal transplantation. Because IFN carries the risk of promoting rejection after kidney transplantation, effort should be made to clear HCV infection before transplantation. The ribavirin dose must also be adjusted to as low as 200 mg every other day in patients with end-stage renal disease. There is no uniform consensus to use ribavirin in this population because of poor tolerability, severe anemia, and the associated risks. Side effects with IFN are more common, but SVR rates in patients who can tolerate therapy appear to be equivalent or even higher than those in non-renally impaired patients.

Pregnant Women, Women of Childbearing Age, and Men Who Plan to Become Fathers

Current therapy is contraindicated in pregnant women because of unpredictable toxicity in the unborn.[203] Therapy is also contraindicated in both women and men who are unable or unwilling to comply with adequate contraception because of the teratotoxicity of ribavirin.

Key References

Amin J, et al. Causes of death after diagnosis of hepatitis B or hepatitis C infection: a large community-based linkage study. Lancet 2006;368:938–945. (Ref.184)

Antaki N, et al. The neglected hepatitis C virus genotypes 4, 5 and 6: an international consensus report. Liver Int 2010;30:342–355. (Ref.18)

Armstrong GL, et al. The prevalence of hepatitis C virus infection in the United States, 1999 through 2002. Ann Intern Med 2006;144:705–714. (Ref.8)

Ascione A, et al. Peginterferon alpha-2a plus ribavirin is more effective than peginterferon alpha-2b plus ribavirin for treating chronic hepatitis C virus infection. Gastroenterology 2010;138:116–122. (Ref.205)

Aus dem Siepen M, et al. Interferon-alpha and ribavirin resistance of Huh7 cells transfected with HCV subgenomic replicon. Virus Res 2007;125:109–113. (Ref.298)

Barshes NR, et al. The natural history of hepatitis C virus in pediatric liver transplant recipients. Liver Transpl 2006;12:1119–1123. (Ref.97)

Castera L, Forns X, Alberti A. Non-invasive evaluation of liver fibrosis using transient elastography. J Hepatol 2008;48:835–847. (Ref.192)

Chen T, et al. New onset diabetes mellitus after liver transplantation and hepatitis C virus infection: meta-analysis of clinical studies. Transpl Int 2009; 22:408–415. (Ref.151)

Coppola N, et al. Improvement in the aetiological diagnosis of acute hepatitis C: a diagnostic protocol based on the anti-HCV-IgM titre and IgG avidity index. J Clin Virol 2009;46:222–229. (Ref.54)

Cox AL, et al. Rare birds in North America: acute hepatitis C cohorts. Gastroenterology 2009;136:26–31. (Ref.51)

Delang L, et al. Statins potentiate the in vitro anti–hepatitis C virus activity of selective hepatitis C virus inhibitors and delay or prevent resistance development. Hepatology 2009;50:6–16. (Ref.280)

de Lédinghen V, Vergniol J. Transient elastography (FibroScan). Gastroenterol Clin Biol 2008;32(6 Suppl 1):58–67. (Ref.187)

Deterding K, et al. The German Hep-Net acute hepatitis C cohort: impact of viral and host factors on the initial presentation of acute hepatitis C virus infection. Z Gastroenterol 2009;47:531–540. (Ref.36)

Dienstag JL, McHutchison JG. American Gastroenterological Association technical review on the management of hepatitis C. Gastroenterology 2006; 130:231–264. (Ref.202)

Duberg AS, et al. Cause of death in individuals with chronic HBV and/or HCV infection, a nationwide community-based register study. J Viral Hepat 2008; 15:538–550. (Ref.81)

Einav S, et al. Discovery of a hepatitis C target and its pharmacological inhibitors by microfluidic affinity analysis. Nat Biotechnol 2008;26:1019–1027. (Ref.251)

El-Serag HB, et al. Extrahepatic manifestations of hepatitis C among United States male veterans. Hepatology 2002;36:1439–1445. (Ref.136)

Fang L, Yu A, Buxton JA. Identification of chronic hepatitis B and hepatitis C co-infection in British Columbia from 1991 to 2007. Can J Public Health 2009;100:349–352. (Ref.114)

Fattovich G, et al. Hepatocellular carcinoma in cirrhosis: incidence and risk factors. Gastroenterology. 2004;127(5 Suppl 1):S35–S50. (Ref.116)

Ferenci P, et al. Silibinin is a potent antiviral agent in patients with chronic hepatitis C not responding to pegylated interferon/ribavirin therapy. Gastroenterology 2008;135:1561–1567. (Ref.288)

Ferri C, et al. Mixed cryoglobulinemia: demographic, clinical, and serological features, and survival in 231 patients. Semin Arthritis Rheum 2004;33: 355–374. (Ref.133)

Flisiak R, et al. The cyclophilin inhibitor Debio 025 combined with PEG IFNalpha2a significantly reduces viral load in treatment-naïve hepatitis C patients. Hepatology 2009;49:1460–1468. (Ref.274)

Francis GS, et al. Hepatic reactions during treatment of multiple sclerosis with interferon-b-1a. Incidence and clinical significance. Drug Saf 2003;26:815–827. (Ref.212)

Friedrich-Rust M, et al. Assessment of liver fibrosis and steatosis in PBC with FibroScan, MRI, MR-spectroscopy, and serum markers. J Clin Gastroenterol. 2010;44:58–65. (Ref.190)

Gaeta GB, et al. Multiple viral infections. J Hepatol 2006;44(1 Suppl):S108–S113. (Ref.112)

Galossi A, et al. Extrahepatic manifestations of chronic HCV infection. J Gastrointest Liver Dis 2007;16:65–73. (Ref.155)

Gane EJ, et al. Combination therapy with a nucleoside polymerase (RG7128) and protease (RG7227/ITMN-191) inhibitor in HCV: safety, pharmacokinetics, and virologic results from INFORM-1. Hepatology 2009;50(Suppl):394A.(Ref.255)

Ge D, et al. Genetic variation in IL28B predicts hepatitis C treatment–induced viral clearance. Nature 2009;461:399–401. (Ref.63)

Ghany MG, et al. Diagnosis, management, and treatment of hepatitis C: an update. Hepatology 2009;49:1335–1374. (Ref.203)

Girou E, et al. Determinant roles of environmental contamination and noncompliance with standard precautions in the risk of hepatitis C virus transmission in a hemodialysis unit. Clin Infect Dis 2008;47:627–633. (Ref.31)

Gisbert JP, et al. Prevalence of hepatitis C virus infection in porphyria cutanea tarda: systematic review and meta-analysis. J Hepatol 2003;39:620–627. (Ref.145)

Haushofer AC, et al. Hepatitis B virus activity in patients with anti–hepatitis C virus antibody positivity and hepatitis B antigen positivity. J Clin Virol 2002; 25(Suppl 3):S99–S102. (Ref.111)

Hermine O, et al. Regression of splenic lymphoma with villous lymphocytes after treatment of hepatitis C virus infection. N Engl J Med 2002;347:89–94. (Ref.143)

Hézode C, et al. Telaprevir and peginterferon with or without ribavirin for chronic HCV infection. N Engl J Med 2009;360:1839–1850. (Ref.245)

Hofmann WP, Zeuzem S, Sarrazin C. Hepatitis C virus–related resistance mechanisms to interferon α-based antiviral therapy. J Clin Virol 2008;32: 86–91. (Ref.295)

Holtzman D, et al. The influence of needle exchange programs on injection risk behaviors and infection with hepatitis C virus among young injection drug users in select cities in the United States, 1994-2004. Prev Med 2009;49:68–73. (Ref.27)

Hou W, et al. Zinc mesoporphyrin induces rapid proteasomal degradation of hepatitis C nonstructural 5A protein in human hepatoma cells. Gastroenterology 2010;138:1909–1919. (Ref.254)

Kaplan DE, et al. Discordant role of CD4 T-cell response relative to neutralizing antibody and CD8 T-cell responses in acute hepatitis C. Gastroenterology 2007;132:654–666. (Ref.60)

Kayali Z, et al. Hepatitis C, cryoglobulinemia, and cirrhosis: a meta-analysis. Hepatology 2002;36(4 Pt 1):978–985. (Ref.132)

Kubitschke A, et al. Verletzungen mit hepatitis-C-virus-kontaminierten nadeln. Wie hoch ist das risiko einer serokonversion bei medizinischem personal wirklich? Internist (Berl) 2007;48:1165–1172. (Ref.23)

Kuiken C, Simmonds P. Nomenclature and numbering of the hepatitis C virus. Methods Mol Biol 2009;510:33–53. (Ref.16)

Kuntzen T, et al. Naturally occurring dominant resistance mutations to hepatitis C virus protease and polymerase inhibitors in treatment-naïve patients. Hepatology 2008;48:1769–1778. (Ref.304)

Kwo P, et al. HCV Sprint-1: boceprevir plus peginterferon alfa-2B/ribavirin for treatment of genotype 1 chronic hepatitis C in previously untreated patients. Hepatology 2008;48(4 Pt 2):1027A. (Ref.246)

Labus B, et al. Acute hepatitis C virus infections attributed to unsafe injection practices at an endoscopic clinic—Nevada 2007. JAMA 2008;299:2738–2740. (Ref.35)

Landau DA, et al. Relapse of hepatitis C virus–associated mixed cryoglobulinemia vasculitis in patients with sustained viral response. Arthritis Rheum 2008;58:604–611. (Ref.134)

Legrand-Abravanel F, et al. Influence of the HCV subtype on the virological response to pegylated interferon and ribavirin therapy. J Med Virol 2009;81: 2029–2035. (Ref.207)

Liaw YF, et al. Impact of acute hepatitis C virus superinfection in patients with chronic hepatitis B virus infection. Gastroenterology 2004;126:1024–1029. (Ref.117)

Liu CJ, et al. Peginterferon alfa-2a plus ribavirin for the treatment of dual chronic infection with hepatitis B and C viruses. Gastroenterology 2009;136: 496–504. (Ref.119)

Manesis EK, et al. Natural course of treated and untreated chronic HCV infection: results of the nationwide Hepnet.Greece cohort study. Aliment Pharmacol Ther 2009;29:1121–1130. (Ref.227)

Marcellin P, et al. Mortality related to chronic hepatitis B and chronic hepatitis C in France: evidence for the role of HIV coinfection and alcohol consumption. J Hepatol 2008;48:200–207. (Ref.85)

Martínez-Bauer E, et al. Hospital admission is a relevant source of hepatitis C virus acquisition in Spain. J Hepatol 2008;48:20–27. (Ref.37)

Mathy JE, et al. Combinations of cyclophilin inhibitor NIM811 with hepatitis C virus NS3-4A protease or NS5B polymerase inhibitors enhance antiviral activity and suppress the emergence of resistance. Antimicrob Agents Chemother 2008;52:3267–3275. (Ref.271)

Mazzaro C, et al. Treatment with peg-interferon alfa-2b and ribavirin of hepatitis C virus–associated mixed cryoglobulinemia: a pilot study. J Hepatol 2005;42: 632–638. (Ref.137)

McGovern BH, et al. Improving the diagnosis of acute hepatitis C virus infection with expanded viral load criteria. Clin Infect Dis 2009;49:1051–1060. (Ref.53)

McHutchison JG, et al. Eltrombopag for thrombocytopenia in patients with cirrhosis associated with hepatitis C. N Engl J Med 2007;357:2227–2236. (Ref.221)

McHutchison JG, et al. Telaprevir with peginterferon and ribavirin for chronic HCV genotype 1 infection. N Engl J Med 2009;360:1827–1838. (Ref.244)

McHutchison JG, et al. Peginterferon alfa-2b or alfa-2a with ribavirin for treatment of hepatitis C infection. N Engl J Med 2009;361:580–593. (Ref.206)

Mederacke I, et al. Performance and clinical utility of a novel fully automated quantitative HCV-core antigen assay. J Clin Virol 2009;46:210–215. (Ref.173)

Meyer MF, et al. Clearance of low levels of HCV viremia in the absence of a strong adaptive immune response. Virol J 2007;4:58. (Ref.49)

Morota K, et al. A new sensitive and automated chemiluminescent microparticle immunoassay for quantitative determination of hepatitis C virus core antigen. J Virol Methods 2009;157:8–14. (Ref.172)

Nakayama H, et al. Molecular investigation of interspousal transmission of hepatitis C virus in two Japanese patients who acquired acute hepatitis C after 40 or 42 years of marriage. J Med Virol 2005;75:258–266. (Ref.43)

Ndong-Atome GR, et al. Absence of intrafamilial transmission of hepatitis C virus and low risk for sexual transmission in rural central Africa indicate a cohort effect. J Clin Virol 2009;45:349–353. (Ref.47)

Nelson D, et al. Efficacy and safety results of albinterferon alfa-2b in combination with ribavirin in interferon-alfa treatment naïve patients with genotype 2 or 3 chronic hepatitis C. J Hepatol 2009;50(Suppl 1):S378. (Ref.257)

Perz JF, et al. The contributions of hepatitis B virus and hepatitis C virus infections to cirrhosis and primary liver cancer worldwide. J Hepatol 2006;45: 529–538. (Ref.1)

Piche T, et al. Effect of ondansetron, a 5-HT₃ receptor antagonist, on fatigue in chronic hepatitis C: a randomised, double blind, placebo controlled study. Gut 2005;54:1169–1173. (Ref.166)

Pockros PJ, et al. Epoetin alfa improves quality of life in anemic HCV-infected patients receiving combination therapy. Hepatology 2004;40:1450–1458. (Ref.220)

Posthouwer D, et al. Antiviral therapy for chronic hepatitis C in patients with inherited bleeding disorders: an international, multicenter cohort study. J Thromb Haemost 2007;5:1624–1629. (Ref.230)

Potthoff A, et al. The HEP-NET B/C co-infection trial: a prospective multicenter study to investigate the efficacy of pegylated interferon-alpha2b and ribavirin in patients with HBV/HCV co-infection. J Hepatol 2008;49:688–694. (Ref.118)

Pradat P, et al. Progression to cirrhosis in hepatitis C patients: an age-dependent process. Liver Int 2007;27:335–339. (Ref.84)

Rehermann B, Nascimbeni M. Immunology of hepatitis B virus and hepatitis C virus infection. Nat Rev Immunol 2005;5:215–229. (Ref.50)

Rifai K, et al. Longer survival of liver transplant recipients with hepatitis virus coinfections. Clin Transplant 2007;21:258–264. (Ref.123)

Rossignol JF, et al. Improved virologic response in chronic hepatitis C genotype 4 treated with nitazoxanide, peginterferon, and ribavirin. Gastroenterology 2009;136:856–862. (Ref.294)

Rumi M, et al. Randomized study of peginterferon-alpha2a plus ribavirin versus peginterferon-alpha2b plus ribavirin in chronic hepatitis C. Gastroenterology 2010;138:108–115. (Ref.204)

Sarrazin C, et al. Dynamic hepatitis C virus genotypic and phenotypic changes in patients treated with the protease inhibitor telaprevir. Gastroenterology 2007;132:1767–1777. (Ref.303)

Schiødt FV, et al. Viral hepatitis–related acute liver failure. Am J Gastroenterol 2003;98:448–453. (Ref.55)

Seeff LB, et al. Long-term mortality and morbidity of transfusion-associated non-A, non-B, and type C hepatitis: a National Heart, Lung, and Blood Institute collaborative study. Hepatology 2001;33:455–463. (Ref.78)

Shebl FM, et al. Prospective cohort study of mother-to-infant infection and clearance of hepatitis C in rural Egyptian villages. J Med Virol 2009;81:1024–1031. (Ref.39)

Shengyuan L, et al. Hepatitis C virus and lichen planus: a reciprocal association determined by a meta-analysis. Arch Dermatol 2009;145:1040–1047. (Ref.137)

Simmonds P, et al. Consensus proposals for a unified system of nomenclature of hepatitis C virus genotypes. Hepatology 2005;42:962–973. (Ref.15)

Singal AK, Anand BS. Management of hepatitis C virus infection in HIV/HCV co-infected patients: clinical review. World J Gastroenterol 2009;15:3713–3724. (Ref.129)

Soriano V, Perelson AS, Zoulim F. Why are there different dynamics in the selection of drug resistance in HIV and hepatitis B and C viruses? J Antimicrob Chemother 2008;62:1–4. (Ref.300)

Suppiah V, et al. IL28B is associated with response to chronic hepatitis C interferon-alpha and ribavirin therapy. Nat Genet 2009;41:1100–1104. (Ref.64)

Tahan V, et al. Sexual transmission of HCV between spouses. Am J Gastroenterol 2005;100:821–824. (Ref.42)

Tanaka Y, et al. Genome-wide association of IL28B with response to pegylated interferon-alpha and ribavirin therapy for chronic hepatitis C. Nat Genet 2009;41:1105–1109. (Ref.65)

Taura N, et al. Long-term trends of the incidence of hepatocellular carcinoma in the Nagasaki prefecture, Japan. Oncol Rep 2009;21:223–227. (Ref.14)

Thomas DL, et al. Genetic variation in IL28B and spontaneous clearance of hepatitis C virus. Nature 2009;461:798–801. (Ref.66)

Thompson AJ, McHutchison JG. Antiviral resistance and specifically targeted therapy for HCV (STAT-C). J Viral Hepat 2009;16:377–387. (Ref.299)

Tillmann HL, et al, for the German anti-D study group. A polymorphism near IL28B is associated with spontaneous clearance of acute hepatitis C virus and jaundice. Gastroenterology 2010;139:1586–1592. (Ref.67)

Toda T, et al. Molecular analysis of transmission of hepatitis C virus in a nurse who acquired acute hepatitis C after caring for a viremic patient with epistaxis. J Med Virol 2009;81:1363–1370. (Ref.26)

Tomer Y. Hepatitis C and interferon induced thyroiditis. J Autoimmun. 2010;34: J322–J326. (Ref.159)

Tsui JI, et al. Risk behaviors after hepatitis C virus seroconversion in young injection drug users in San Francisco. Drug Alcohol Depend 2009;105: 160–163. (Ref.10)

Tsui JI, et al. Relationship between hepatitis C and chronic kidney disease: results from the Third National Health and Nutrition Examination Survey. J Am Soc Nephrol 2006;17:1168–1174. (Ref.135)

Urbanus AT, et al. Hepatitis C virus infections among HIV-infected men who have sex with men: an expanding epidemic. AIDS 2009;23:F1–F7. (Ref.44)

Vandelli C, et al. Lack of evidence of sexual transmission of hepatitis C among monogamous couples: results of a 10-year prospective follow-up study. Am J Gastroenterol 2004;99:855–859. (Ref.41)

Weissenborn K, et al. Monoaminergic neurotransmission is altered in hepatitis C virus infected patients with chronic fatigue and cognitive impairment. Gut 2006;55:1624–1630. (Ref.167)

White DL, Ratziu V, El-Serag HB. Hepatitis C infection and risk of diabetes: a systematic review and meta-analysis. J Hepatol 2008;49:831–844. (Ref.150)

Wiegand J, et al. Autologous blood donor screening indicated a lower prevalence of viral hepatitis in East vs West Germany: epidemiological benefit from established health resources. J Viral Hepat 2009;16:743–748. (Ref.11)

Wiese M, et al. Outcome in a hepatitis C (genotype 1b) single source outbreak in Germany—a 25-year multicenter study. J Hepatol 2005;43:590–598. (Ref.38)

Zeuzem S, et al. Efficacy and safety of albinterferon alfa-2b in combination with ribavirin in treatment naïve, chronic hepatitis C genotype 1 patients. J Hepatol 2009;50(Suppl 1):S377. (Ref.256)

A complete list of references can be found at www.expertconsult.com.

Hepatitis D

Mario Rizzetto and Alessia Ciancio

ABBREVIATIONS

ALT alanine aminotransferase	**HCC** hepatocellular carcinoma	**L-HDAg** large HD antigen
anti-HD antibody to the HD antigen	**HDV** hepatitis delta virus	**LKM** liver-kidney microsomal
HBIg hyperimmune serum against HBsAg	**IFN** interferon	**PCR** polymerase chain reaction
HBsAg hepatitis B surface antigen	**IgM** immunoglobulin M	**Pol II** RNA polymerase II
HBV hepatitis B virus	**IgM anti-HDV** IgM antibody to HDV	**S-HDAg** small HD antigen

---

Introduction

The hepatitis delta virus (HDV, or hepatitis D virus) is a defective RNA pathogen that is dependent on the obligatory helper functions provided by the hepatitis B virus (HBV) for replication.[1,2] HDV is the only member of the genus *Deltavirus*. It is currently divided into eight genotypes that differ as much as 40% in nucleotide sequence.[3] Other hepadnaviruses can support HDV; for example, infection was also established in the Eastern woodchuck carrying the woodchuck HBV.[4]

Virology

Each virion is approximately 36 nm in diameter and is contained within a hepatitis B surface antigen (HBsAg) envelope. The genome is composed of a molecule of single-stranded circular RNA of approximately 1.7 kilobases (kb); each genome assumes a rodlike structure as a result of extensive base-pairing and two related structural phosphoproteins sharing a common antigenic reactivity (the hepatitis delta antigen [HDAg]). Because the genome contains only about 1700 nucleotides, it is the smallest among animal viruses, resembling viroid RNAs of plants.

The hepatitis D virus needs only the hepatitis B surface antigen (HBsAg) coat from HBV for binding to hepatocytes and for virion assembly.[5] Hepatocyte nuclear extracts can replicate the entire genomic and antigenomic HDV without any extraneous factor; cDNA constructs of HDV and the RNA injected into the tail vein of mice elicited typical HDV replication in several tissues of the rodent.[5]

Transcriptional run-off experiments using low-dose amanitin,[5] a toxin that selectively blocks the transcription of RNA polymerase II (Pol II), have confirmed that HDV-RNA undergoes replication by the host Pol II[6]; presumably Pol II is deceived by the rodlike structure of HDV-RNA and becomes redirected to read and copy the viral RNA as if it were an endogenous DNA.

Both the genomic and the antigenomic strands of HDV-RNA contain a segment of less than 100 bases that acts like a ribozyme[7]—it retains the genetic information but is also able to self-cleave and self-ligate the circular HDV genome without any enzymatic assistance.

HDV replicates by a rolling-circle mechanism similar to that involved in the replication of viroids of plants. Redirected host Pol II elongates a multimeric linear transcript of either the genome or the antigenome over the viral RNA circular template of the other; thereafter the viral ribozymes first cleaves the redundant linear multimeric strand to genome-size monomer and then ligates the monomeric strand into the infectious circular form.

The life cycle of HDV is regulated by the HD antigen, the only protein expressed by HDV. The HD antigen is edited by a cellular double-stranded adenine deaminase into a small HDAg (S-HDAg, 195 amino acid residues) and a large HDAg (L-HDAg, 214 amino acid residues), with S-HDAg promoting replication and L-HDAg supporting virion assembly.[8]

The HD proteins undergo several posttranslational modifications. Phosphorylation,[9,10] acetylation,[11] methylation,[12] and prenylation[13] provide molecular switches to the many functions of the HD proteins necessary to orchestrate the synthesis and assembly of HDV[14]; prenylation (farnesylation) of the L-HDAg is essential to target the HDAg to the HBsAg in order to trigger viral assembly.[15]

Transmission

Hepatitis delta virus is transmitted by the same route as helper HBV—by the parenteral route, either overt or covert. The highest rates of hepatitis D infection were reported in parenteral drug addicts; in contrast, vertical transmission from mother to newborn is rare.[16]

Transmission can occur by sexual contact, in particular mercenary heterosexual contact, as attested by the higher prevalence of HDV in prostitutes and sexual partners of HDV-infected persons; however, the spread of HDV has not been evident among homosexual men.[16]

Household transmission was frequent in the 1970s and 1980s in endemic areas in southern Europe, and co-habitation of HBsAg carriers with HDV-infected family contacts was a major risk factor for the acquisition of the virus.[17] Molecular studies have confirmed sexual and household dissemination of HDV.[18]

The efficiency of HDV transmission is primarily determined by the HBsAg carrier status of the exposed individual. In normal (i.e., HBsAg-negative) persons, HDV cannot be transmitted unless HBV infection was previously established; in this setting HDV is acquired simultaneously with HBV (i.e., by HBV/HDV co-infection) (**Fig. 32-1, A**) and transmission efficiency depends on the infectious titer of the co-infecting HBV.[16] In HBsAg-positive individuals the preexisting HBV state acts as a selective magnet to activate HDV, and this infection is therefore rapidly established and amplified—there is HDV superinfection on prior HBV infection (see **Fig. 32-1, B**). A titer of HDV as low as that contained in 10^{-11} serum dilutions was sufficient to establish infection in chimpanzees carrying the HBsAg.[19] Because the chronic HBsAg state provides the HDV with continued biologic support, superinfected HBsAg carriers often also become chronic carriers of HDV; therefore HBsAg carriers are the selective victims of HDV and the main epidemiologic reservoir and source of the virus.

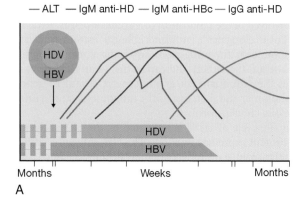

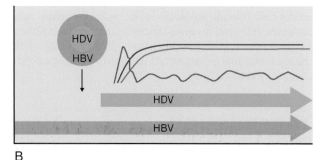

Fig. 32-1 A, Course of co-infection with hepatitis B virus (HBV) and hepatitis D virus (HDV). **B,** Course of hepatitis D viral superinfection. ALT, alanine aminotransferase; IgM, immunoglobulin M

Epidemiology

Hepatitis D was endemic in the 1980s in many areas of the world; however, its distribution and ratio relative to the local prevalence of HBV varied widely. Overall frequency rates were higher in tropical and subtropical areas with a high prevalence of HBV, compared to North America and northern Europe, where the prevalence of HBV was low. In northern Europe and North America HDV infection was mostly confined to intravenous drug addicts.[16,20] In countries with intermediate HBV prevalence, such as southern Europe and Taiwan, there was a composite pattern of infection, resulting from an endemic pattern in the general population and an epidemic pattern within drug addicts.

Because helper HBV infection has been restricted in the last 20 years, the circulation of HDV declined significantly in the developed world in the 1990s, in particular in Europe.[21] In Italy the rate of anti-HD in HBsAg carriers diminished from 24.6% in 1983 to 8.3% in 1997,[22] and consistent declines were reported from Spain,[23] Taiwan,[24] and Turkey.[25] However, no further decline of HDV infection was observed in Europe after the end of the twentieth century.

In 1179 HBsAg carriers with liver disease surveyed in Italy in 2006, the prevalence of anti-HD was 8.1%,[26] similar to the prevalence found in 1997; a distinct proportion of new HDV entries in Italy are immigrants from Romania and Albania. Likewise, in London[27] the prevalence of HDV remained stable (around 8.5%) between 2000 and 2006; most HDV patients were from southern or eastern Europe, Africa, and the Middle East, and their mean age was 36 years. In Hannover, Germany,[28] the prevalence declined from 18.6% in 1992 to 6.8% in 1997; no further decrease has been recorded since 1999, with 8% to 14% of the HBsAg carriers being positive for anti-HD, the majority immigrants from Turkey and the former Soviet Union. In France[29] there is a residual HDV population represented mostly by African immigrants, within which the rate of infection is increasing.

The residual pool of HDV in Europe is thus composed of the aging domestic pool that survived the brunt of the hepatitis D epidemic in the 1970s and 1980s and by a population of young immigrants from areas where HDV remains endemic.[30]

HDV still represents a major health problem in the developing world where HBV remains unchecked. In recent years, a significant presence of hepatitis D has been observed in several areas of the developing world, such as Pakistan,[30,31] India, Mongolia, Iran, Vietnam, Tajikistan, Tunisia, Gabon,[32] Mauretania (F. Lunel, personal communication), and Turkmenistan (Dr. B. Nepesova, personal communication).

Diagnosis

On exposure to HDV, immunocompetent patients raise and increase the concentration of IgG antibody to HDAg (anti-HD)[33]; the antibody response may be weakened in immunocompromised patients, in particular in those with HIV infection. Detection of anti-HD is the first step in the diagnosis of HDV infection; it should be determined in all HBsAg carriers with liver disease.

Detection of intrahepatic HDAg by immunohistochemistry was initially the standard for diagnosing active HDV infection. Sensitivity is limited; in a liver biopsy sample it is detectable only in about 50% of patients with ongoing HDV infection; it is often undetectable in patients with advanced fibrosis.

The determination of HDV-RNA in serum by polymerase chain reaction (PCR) is the most specific and sensitive test to diagnose active HDV infection.[33] PCR can detect as few as 10 copies of the virus per milliliter; with these assays HDV-RNA is detectable in virtually all patients with an ongoing HDV infection. Quantitative assays were developed[34,35]; however, the levels of HD viremia do not appear to correlate with the degree of severity of hepatitis D.

Quantitative real-time PCR assays are of use in the evaluation of patients undergoing treatment, with the degree of the decline of HDV-RNA (and of HBsAg) during early therapy predicting the response to interferon (IFN) treatment.[35,36] The HDV genotype may be determined in serum by restriction fragment length polymorphism analysis of PCR amplification products or by sequencing; genotyping has no clinical significance but is of use in epidemiologic studies.

When access to HDV-RNA assay is limited, the commercially available IgM antibody to HDV (IgM anti-HDV) provides a useful surrogate tool for monitoring HDV disease. This antibody is raised to high titers together with anti-HD during acute HDV infections; it then declines in a few weeks in patients whose infection resolves whereas the IgG antibody may persist for a while; it persists at high titer together with the IgG antibody in patients in whom hepatitis D progresses to chronicity. The decrease of IgM anti-HD titer correlates with the response to antiviral therapy.[21,36]

The IgG antibody to HDAg may persist in serum as a serologic scar to past HDV infection in both HBsAg-positive and HBsAg-negative individuals.

Clinical Features

Acute hepatitis D acquired by HBV/HDV co-infection runs a clinical course similar to that of ordinary acute hepatitis B (see **Fig. 32-1, *A***); diagnosis is made by the finding of HDV markers superimposed on markers of acute HBV infection. Acute co-infections may run a biphasic course with two peaks of alanine aminotransferase (ALT) several weeks apart. Recovery is the rule, with no more than 2% of the patients progressing to chronic HDV infection.[20] Primary HDV superinfection on HBsAg carriers (see **Fig. 32-1, *B***) usually runs a severe clinical course; outbreaks of severe acute hepatitis D acquired by superinfection have been described worldwide.[20]

Superinfection may appear as acute hepatitis B if the superinfected HBsAg carrier is unaware of his/her HBV infection. In carriers with prior chronic hepatitis B, primary HDV superinfection may be mistaken for a recrudescence of the underlying HBV infection. Superinfection usually results in chronic hepatitis D.

Studies in the 1980s indicated that HDV usually induced a severe liver disease leading rapidly to cirrhosis. In Italy 41% of 75 patients without cirrhosis in the initial biopsy developed cirrhosis within 2 to 6 years of follow-up and 13% died of liver disease.[37] In a retrospective European study,[38] HDV infection increased the risk of decompensation and of mortality by a factor of 2.2 and 2.0, respectively, compared with HBsAg-positive HDV-negative cirrhosis. In a German study,[39] 26 of

50 HDV patients (52%) progressed to advanced cirrhosis within 14 years of follow-up and in Taiwan[40] the cumulative adverse outcomes' rate (cirrhosis, hepatocellular carcinoma [HCC], and mortality) of HDV genotype I patients was 52% in an 11-year follow-up study.

The changes in the epidemiology of HDV infection have been accompanied by important changes in the clinical features of hepatitis D. The histologic and clinical features of 122 chronic hepatitis D patients recruited from 1987 to 1996 in Italy were compared with 162 such patients collected in the previous decade.[41] The proportion of severe chronic hepatitis was higher in the early (65%) than the late cohort (17%), and overt cirrhosis was higher in the late (44%) than the early cohort; disease had been asymptomatic and nonprogressive in 10% of the cases but had rapidly advanced to a cirrhosis that stabilized over the long-term in the others.

In a survey from a single center in Spain[42] the features of 326 HDV patients recruited from 1983 to 1995 were compared with those of 72 patients recruited from 1996 to 2008. Those in the early cohort were younger, mainly intravenous drug addicts; many had concomitant HIV and HCV infection. Acute self-limited hepatitis was virtually limited to the early cohort. Among the patients with chronic liver disease, 18% became decompensated, 3% developed HCC, and 8% cleared the HBsAg. Liver-related death was observed in 13% and occurred mainly in the early cohort. These studies indicate that the outbreak of HDV in the 1980s was accompanied by clinical severity and significant mortality. With the decline in the circulation of HDV, fresh forms of hepatitis D have no longer occurred; most patients recruited in the last 2 decades appear to represent cohorts with residual burnt-out disease who survived the medical brunt of the HDV epidemic of the 1980s. The pattern of florid disease described in southern Europe in the 1980s is currently recapitulated in immigrants presenting with chronic hepatitis D and is still the predominant pattern in the many areas of the developing world where HDV remains unchecked.

A single center report of 299 patients followed for 28 years in Milano[43] has shown a relatively low propensity to evolve to cirrhosis (4% per year) and to progress to HCC (2.8% per year). The discrepancy with the other studies might be due to different referral criteria or changes in the virulence of HDV; among drug addicts in an infectious unit in Milano in the early 1980s,[44] 10 of 33 carriers of HBsAg superinfected with HDV developed histologic evidence of cirrhosis 18 to 59 months after the primary HDV infection.

The risk of HCC remains controversial. In a European multicenter study,[38] HDV infection increased the risk of HCC threefold (5-year risk in compensated HDV cirrhosis of 13% vs. 4% in HBV cirrhosis). In other studies HDV did not appear to increase the risk of HCC over HBV. In Greece[45] 40% of the HDV patients who escaped death from liver failure developed HCC within 12 years of follow-up; in Milano[43] the annual rate of HCC in HDV patients was 2.8%; and in London[27] a retrospective analysis of 962 HBsAg-positive patients showed similar rates of HCC in the 82 HDV-infected and in the 880 HDV-noninfected patients. HCC has developed in 17 (9%) of 127 cirrhotic HDV patients enrolled from 1991 to 2005 in Italy (G.A. Niro, personal communication).

The course of disease may be influenced by the genotype of the HDV.[30] Genotype I, the most frequent worldwide, has variable pathogenicity. In Taiwan chronic HDV disease patients infected with genotype I HDV had a lower remission rate and more adverse outcomes than those with HDV genotype II. Genotypes II and IV are found predominantly in East Asia and were associated with mild disease. Genotype III was associated with fulminant hepatitis in South America.[46]

HDV disease may be in part an immune-mediated disease. The level of HDV viremia does not directly correlate with the stage of liver disease, and studies on the cellular immune responses against HDV have suggested that the quantity and quality of T-cell responses may be associated with control of the infection.[47] In HDV genotype I hepatitis D patients, the response frequencies both of cytotoxic CD4+ T cells and of HBV-specific T cells were higher than those determined in individuals with HBV or HCV infections.[48,49] More intriguing, the participation of HDV in the regulation of cellular gene expression could trigger HDV-related liver damage. The L-HD Ag is sensitive to tumor necrosis factor-α induced NF-κB signaling[50] and isoprenylation of L-HD Ag appears to regulate transforming growth factor-β induced signal transduction; through these mechanisms, the virus might induce liver fibrosis.[51]

In the 1980 and 1990s the majority of the patients with chronic hepatitis D in the Mediterranean area were HBsAg carriers superinfected in adolescence or early adulthood, and presented with active cirrhosis at age 40 to 50. The prototype patient with florid HDV disease had persistently elevated ALT levels, histologic evidence of a chronic active hepatitis, anti-HD of IgG and IgM types, HDV-RNA in serum, and HDAg detectable in the liver; HBV-DNA in serum was lacking or barely detectable, HBsAg and IgM anticore were absent, and anti-HBe was present. The discrepancy between a florid HBsAg-positive disease and lack of replicative markers of HBV was the best diagnostic harbinger to the suspicion of an underlying presence of hepatitis D.

The histologic features of chronic HDV disease were not specific and not distinctive from those of ordinary hepatitis B. A proportion of these patients generated autoantibodies, the most frequent of which was a liver-kidney microsomal (LKM3) antibody that displayed a pattern of tissue immunofluorescence similar to that shown by the LKM1 antibody of autoimmune type 2 hepatitis. The reactivity is directed against uridine diphosphate glucuronytransferase type 1.[20]

Co-infection of HDV with HCV was often observed in drug addicts. It may result in different patterns of reciprocal inhibition.[27] In studies conducted in Spain, France, and Germany HDV acted as the dominant virus suppressing HCV; however, in a study in Taiwan HCV was dominant, suppressing HDV, and in Germany less than one fifth of the HBsAg anti-HD–positive individuals with anti-HCV were positive also for HCV-RNA.[52] HDV co-infection diminished survival in HIV-infected patients in Taiwan[53] and increased the risk of liver cirrhosis in HBV/HIV/HCV co-infected patients versus HDV-negative HBV/HIV/HCV patients.[54]

Prevention and Treatment

Vaccination against HBV provides protection against HDV.

No effective HDV vaccine has been developed to protect the HBsAg carrier; natural anti-HD co-exists with disease and

vaccine-induced anti-HDV was not protective in the woodchuck model.[55]

The problem confronting HDV therapy is that there is no specific enzymatic function of the virus to target for therapy, such as the polymerases and proteases of HBV and HCV. The hepatitis D virus depends on HBsAg and not on HBV replication; therefore its synthesis is not influenced by the level of HBV-DNA in serum; the secretion of HDV in vitro and the levels of HDV-RNA in vivo are directly correlated to the amount of serum HBsAg, not to the titer of HBV-DNA.[56]

The HBV/HDV interactions and the fact that in most HDV patients HBV is spontaneously repressed explain why synthetic antivirals against HBV were not efficacious; no virologic or clinical improvement of HDV disease was obtained with famciclovir, lamivudine, adefovir, and ribavirin either in monotherapy or in combination with IFN.[30,57-60]

Interferon-alfa (IFN) was first used empirically 25 years ago and still remains the only licensed therapy. In clinical trials the rate of response to IFN (normalization of ALT level and clearance of serum HDV-RNA) has varied, occurring at different times from the beginning of treatment.[61] The response was proportional to the dose of IFN. In one study[62] patients given 9 million units of IFN three times per week responded better than patients given lower dosages. Overall, standard treatment given for 1 year to patients with active chronic hepatitis D resulted in disease remission in about 20% to 25% of patients; however, the rates of HDV-RNA clearance were distinctly lower. Prolonging therapy with conventional IFN up to 2 years did not increase the rate of sustained response over 1 year of treatment.[63] Of note, the number of patients included in all series treated with conventional IFN is small and it is therefore difficult to distinguish a true therapeutic advantage from a benign spontaneous course. In particular, no controlled study has been carried out to determine whether IFN induces a significant long-term effect. Although an anecdotal study demonstrated resolution of HBV/HDV infections and even of fibrosis in HDV patients treated with IFN,[64] disease resolution may occur in the natural history of HDV infections and in a follow-up over many years the rate of spontaneous clearance of HBsAg was higher in HDV-positive than in HDV-negative carriers of HBsAg.[65]

Peginterferon (Peg-IFN) may be a more rewarding treatment option.[66] Of 14 patients treated with Peg-IFN alfa-2b 1.5 μg/kg weekly for 12 months, 6 (43%) achieved a sustained clearance of serum HDV-RNA.[67] However, in two other series of patients treated with the same Peg-IFN,[59,68] a sustained viral response was obtained only in 17% and 21%. In the largest therapeutic trial conducted so far, the Hep-Net International Delta Hepatitis Intervention Trial (HIDIT-1),[60] 90 patients from Germany, Turkey, and Greece were randomized to receive either 180 μg/kg Peg-IFN alfa-2a each week plus 10 mg of adefovir (31 patients), 180 μg/kg Peg-IFN alfa-2b plus placebo (29 patients), or adefovir alone (30 patients). By week 48 of therapy the reduction of HDV-RNA was significantly higher and similar in the two groups using Peg-IFN, HDV-RNA becoming negative in 28% of the patients given Peg-IFN and in only 8% of the patients administered adefovir alone. Long-term Peg-IFN may be more efficacious.[69] Of 13 patients with advanced disease treated for a mean of 131 weeks (range, 6 to 240 weeks) with an average dose of 184 mg of Peg-IFN alfa-2a, 5 lost HDV-RNA and 3 lost HBsAg.[69]

Parameters predictive of response are still unidentified. Because response can be delayed, IFN should be given for at least 1 year before a patient is regarded as a nonresponder; loss of HBsAg is the only reliable marker of resolution of hepatitis D.

A potential target to therapy is the process of HD virion assembly, which requires the integrity of critical regions of HBsAg[70]; their disruption may therefore prevent HDV virion synthesis. The deletion of residues 24 to 28 on the small HBsAg led to an envelope HBV mutant deficient for production of HD virions[71]; likewise, the substitution of phenylalanine for tryptophan at positions 196, 199, or 201 of the small HBsAg[72] and conformational changes in the cysteines on the antigenic loop of HBsAg (which bears the conserved a determinant and is involved in HDV infectivity) created a block to the entry of HDV into cells.[73] Lamivudine-induced changes in SW196L/S of the small HBsAg, carried out by M204I overlap mutation in the reverse transcriptase of HBV, were found to inhibit the secretion of HDV particles in cell cultures, suggesting that lamivudine therapy may indirectly abrogate an underlying HDV infection.[74] Also critical to the interaction of L-HDAg with the HBV envelope protein is farnesylation (prenylation) of the last four amino acids on the L-HDAg (the so-called CXXX box). By preventing the association of the HDV ribonucleoprotein with HBsAg and, therefore, virion assembly, disruption of L-HDAg prenylation might form the basis of a new therapeutic strategy against HDV; experiments in vitro and in vivo have shown that prenylation inhibitors were effective in preventing HD virion assembly and in clearing HD viremia in a mouse model of HDV infection.[75]

Liver Transplantation

The spontaneous risk of graft reinfection is distinctly lower for HDV than for HBV. In chronic hepatitis D, HBV replication is usually strongly diminished; because HBV reinfection of the graft is precluded by its low infectious titer, the satellite HDV cannot be transmitted.

Current prophylaxis regimens with hyperimmune serum against HBsAg (HBIG) and antivirals (lamivudine) protect virtually every HDV transplant patient from reinfection, with very good survival rates.[76]

References

1. Rizzetto M, et al. Immunofluorescence detection of a new antigen–antibody system (delta/anti-delta) associated to hepatitis B virus in liver and in serum of HBsAg carriers. Gut 1977;18:997–1003.
2. Murphy FA. Virus taxonomy. In: Fields BN, Knipe DM, Howley PM, editors. Fields virology, 3rd ed. New York: Raven Press, 1996.
3. Dény P. Hepatitis delta virus genetic variability: from genotypes I, II, III to eight major clades? Curr Top Microbiol Immunol 2006;307:151–171.
4. Ponzetto A, et al. Transmission of the hepatitis B virus-associated delta agent to the eastern woodchuck. Proc Natl Acad Sci 1984;81:2208–2212.
5. Taylor JM. Chapter 3. Replication of the hepatitis delta virus RNA genome. Adv Virus Res 2009;74:103–121.
6. Lai MM. RNA replication without RNA-dependent RNA polymerase: surprises from hepatitis delta virus. J Virol 2005;79:7951–7958.
7. Been MD. HDV ribozymes. Curr Top Microbiol Immunol 2006;307: 47–65.
8. Casey JL. RNA editing in hepatitis delta virus. Curr Top Microbiol Immunol 2006;307:67–89.
9. Mu JJ, et al. Characterization of the phosphorylated forms and the phosphorylated residues of hepatitis delta virus delta antigens. J Virol 1999; 73:10540–10545.
10. Chen YS, et al. ERK1/2-mediated phosphorylation of small hepatitis delta antigen at serine 177 enhances hepatitis delta virus antigenomic RNA replication. J Virol 2008;82:9345–9358.
11. Huang WH, Mai RT, Lee YH. Transcription factor YY1 and its associated acetyltransferases CBP and p300 interact with hepatitis delta antigens and modulate hepatitis delta virus RNA replication. J Virol 2008;82: 7313–7324.
12. Li YJ, Stallcup MR, Lai MM. Hepatitis delta virus antigen is methylated at arginine residues, and methylation regulates subcellular localization and RNA replication. J Virol 2004;78:13325–13334.
13. Glenn JS, White JM. Identification of a prenylation site in delta virus large antigen. Science 1992;256:1331–1333.
14. Huang WH, et al. Post-translational modification of delta antigen of hepatitis D virus. Curr Top Microbiol Immunol 2006;307:91–112.
15. O'Malley B, Lazinski DW. Roles of carboxyl-terminal and farnesylated residues in the functions of the large hepatitis delta antigen. J Virol 2005; 79:1142–1153.
16. Rizzetto M, Ponzetto A, Forzani I. Hepatitis delta virus as a global health problem. Vaccine 1990;8(Suppl):S10–S14.
17. Sagnelli E, et al. The epidemiology of hepatitis delta infection in Italy. J Hepatol 1992;15:211–215.
18. Niro GA, et al. Intrafamilial transmission of hepatitis delta virus: molecular evidence. J Hepatol 1999;30:564–569.
19. Ponzetto A, et al. Serial passage of hepatitis delta virus in chronic hepatitis B virus carrier chimpanzees. Hepatology 1988;8:1655–1661.
20. Smedile A, Rizzetto M, Gerin JL. Advances in hepatitis D virus biology and disease. In: Boyer JL, Ockner RK, editors. Progress in liver disease, Vol. XII. Philadelphia: Saunders, 1994: 157–175.
21. Hadziyannis SJ. Decreasing prevalence of hepatitis D virus infection. J Gastroenterol Hepatol 1997;12:745–746.
22. Gaeta GB, et al. Chronic hepatitis D: a vanishing disease? An Italian multicenter study. Hepatology 2000;32: 824–827.
23. Navascués CA, et al. Epidemiology of hepatitis D virus infection: changes in the last 14 years. Am J Gastroenterol 1995;90:1981–1984.
24. Huo TI, et al. Changing seroepidemiology of hepatitis B, C, and D virus infections in high-risk populations. J Med Virol 2004;72:41–45.
25. Değertekin H, Yalçin K, Yakut M. The prevalence of hepatitis delta virus infection in acute and chronic liver diseases in Turkey: an analysis of clinical studies. Turk J Gastroenterol 2006;17:25–34.
26. Gaeta GB, et al. Hepatitis delta in Europe: vanishing or refreshing? Hepatology 2007;46:1312–1313.
27. Cross TJS, et al. The increasing prevalence of hepatitis delta virus (HDV) infection in South London. J Med Virol 2008;80:277–282.
28. Wedemeyer H, Heidrich B, Manns MP. Hepatitis D virus infection—not a vanishing disease in Europe! Hepatology 2007;45:1331–1332.
29. Le Gal F, et al. Hepatitis D virus infection–not a vanishing disease in Europe! Hepatology 2007;45:1332–1333.
30. Rizzetto M. Hepatitis D: thirty years after. J Hepatol 2009;50:1043–1050.
31. Mumtaz K, et al. Epidemiology and clinical pattern of hepatitis delta virus infection in Pakistan. Gastroenterol Hepatol 2005;20:1503–1507.
32. Makuwa M, et al. Prevalence and molecular diversity of hepatitis B virus and hepatitis delta virus in urban and rural populations in northern Gabon in central Africa. J Clin Microbiol 2009;47:2265–2268.
33. Farci P. Delta hepatitis: an update. J Hepatol 2003;39(S):212–219.
34. Le Gal F, et al. Quantification of hepatitis delta virus RNA in serum by consensus real-time PCR indicates different patterns of virological response to interferon therapy in chronically infected patients. J Clin Microbiol 2005; 43:2363–2369.
35. Manesis EK, et al. Quantitative analysis of hepatitis D virus RNA and hepatitis B surface antigen serum levels in chronic delta hepatitis improves treatment monitoring. Antivir Ther 2007;12:381–388.
36. Hughes S, et al. Hepatitis delta virus RNA level and IgM antibody titer predict response to Peg-Interferon therapy. Hepatology 2009;50:735A.
37. Rizzetto M, et al. Chronic HBsAg hepatitis with intrahepatic expression of the delta antigen. An active and progressive disease unresponsive to immunosuppressive treatment. Ann Intern Med 1983;98:437–441.
38. Fattovich G, et al. Influence of hepatitis delta virus infection on morbidity and mortality in compensated cirrhosis type B. The European concerted action on viral hepatitis. Gut 2000;46:420–426.
39. Serrano B, et al. Long-term outcome of hepatitis delta: a 14-year single center experience. Hepatology 2009;50:737A.
40. Su CW, et al. Genotypes and viremia of hepatitis B and D viruses are associated with outcomes of chronic hepatitis D patients. Gastroenterology 2006;130:1625–1635.
41. Rosina F, et al. Changing pattern of chronic hepatitis D in Southern Europe. Gastroenterology 1999;117:161–166.

42. Buti M, et al. Clinical outcome of acute and chronic hepatitis delta over time: a long-term follow up study. J Viral Hepat 2011;18:434–442.

43. Romeo R, et al. A 28-year study of the course of hepatitis delta infection: a risk factor for cirrhosis and hepatocellular carcinoma. Gastroenterology 2009;136:1629–1638.

44. Caredda F, et al. Course and prognosis of acute HDV hepatitis. Prog Clin Biol Res 1987;234:267–276.

45. Hadzyiannis SJ. Hepatitis delta: an overview. In: Rizzetto M, Purcell RH, Gerin JL, Verme G, editors. Viral hepatitis and liver disease. Torino: Minerva Medica 1997: 283–289.

46. Gomes-Gouvêa MS, et al. Hepatitis D and B virus genotypes in chronically infected patients from the Eastern Amazon Basin. Acta Trop 2008;106:149–155.

47. Aslan N, et al. Analysis and function of delta-hepatitis virus-specific cellular immune responses. J Hepatol 2003;38(Suppl):15–16.

48. Aslan N, et al. Cytotoxic CD4+ T cells in viral hepatitis. J Viral Hepat 2006;13:505–514.

49. Grabowski J, et al. HDV and HBV specific T cell response patterns in patients with delta hepatitis. Hepatology 2009;50:733A (Abstr 910).

50. Park C-Y, et al. Hepatitis delta virus large antigen sensitizes to TNF-α-induced NF-κB signaling. Mol Cells 2009;28:49–55.

51. Choi SH, Jeong SH, Hwang SB. Large hepatitis delta antigen modulates transforming growth factor-beta signaling cascades: implication of hepatitis delta virus-induced liver fibrosis. Gastroenterology 2007;132:343–357.

52. Heidrich B, et al. Virological and clinical characteristics of delta hepatitis in Central Europe. J Viral Hepat 2009;16:883–894.

53. Sheng WH, et al. Impact of hepatitis D virus infection on the long-term outcomes of patients with hepatitis B virus and HIV coinfection in the era of highly active antiretroviral therapy: a matched cohort study. Clin Infect Dis 2007;44:988–995.

54. Castellares C, et al. Liver cirrhosis in HIV-infected patients: prevalence, aetiology and clinical outcome. J Viral Hepat 2008;15:165–172.

55. Fiedler M, et al. Immunization of woodchucks (Marmota monax) with hepatitis delta virus DNA vaccine. Vaccine 2001;19:4618–4626.

56. Shih HH, et al. Hepatitis B surface antigen levels and sequences of natural hepatitis B virus variants influence the assembly and secretion of hepatitis D virus. J Virol 2008;82:2250–2264.

57. Niro GA, et al. Lamivudine therapy in chronic delta hepatitis: a multicentre randomized-controlled pilot study. Aliment Pharmacol Ther 2005;22:227–232.

58. Yurdaydin C, et al. Treatment of chronic delta hepatitis with lamivudine vs lamivudine + interferon vs interferon. J Viral Hepat 2008;15:314–321.

59. Niro GA, et al. Pegylated interferon alpha-2b as monotherapy or in combination with ribavirin in chronic hepatitis delta. Hepatology 2006;44:713–720.

60. Wedemever H, et al. Peginterferon plus adefovir versus either drug alone for hepatitis delta. N Engl J Med 2011;364:322–331.

61. Niro GA, Rosina F, Rizzetto M. Treatment of hepatitis D. J Viral Hepat 2005;12:2–9.

62. Farci P, et al. Treatment of chronic hepatitis D with interferon alfa-2a. New Engl J Med 1994;330:88–94.

63. Yurdaydin C, et al. A pilot study of 2 years of interferon treatment in patients with chronic delta hepatitis. J Viral Hepat 2007;14:812–816.

64. Farci P, et al. Long-term benefit of interferon alpha therapy of chronic hepatitis D: regression of advanced hepatic fibrosis. Gastroenterology 2004;126:1740–1749.

65. Niro GA, et al. Clearance of hepatitis B surface antigen in chronic carriers of hepatitis delta antibodies. Liver 2001;21:254–259.

66. Yurdaydin C, et al. Efficacy of pegylated interferon-based treatment in patients with cirrhosis due to chronic delta hepatitis: comparison with non-cirrhotic patients. Hepatology 2009;50:736A (Abstr 916).

67. Castelnau C, et al. Efficacy of peginterferon alpha-2b in chronic hepatitis delta: relevance of quantitative RT-PCR for follow-up. Hepatology 2006;44:728–735.

68. Erhardt A, et al. Treatment of chronic hepatitis delta with pegylated interferon-alpha2b. Liver Int 2006;26:805–810.

69. Heller T, et al. Long-term, high-dose peginterferon alfa 2a is an effective treatment for chronic hepatitis D. Hepatology 2009;50:734A (Abstr 911).

70. Shih H, et al. Hepatitis B surface antigen levels and sequences of natural hepatitis B virus variants influence the assembly and secretion of hepatitis D virus. J Virol 2008;82:2250–2264.

71. Jenna S, Sureau C. Effect of mutations in the small envelope protein of hepatitis B virus on assembly and secretion of hepatitis delta virus. Virology 1998;251:176–186.

72. Komla-Soukha I, Sureau C. A tryptophan-rich motif in the carboxyl terminus of the small envelope protein of hepatitis B virus is central to the assembly of hepatitis delta virus particles. J Virol 2006;80:4648–4655.

73. Abou-Jaoudé G, Sureau C. Entry of hepatitis delta virus requires the conserved cysteine residues of the hepatitis B virus envelope protein antigenic loop and is blocked by inhibitors of thiol-disulfide exchange. J Virol 2007;81:13057–13066.

74. Vietheer PT, et al. Failure of the lamivudine-resistant rtM204I hepatitis B virus mutants to efficiently support hepatitis delta virus secretion. J Virol 2005;79:6570–6573.

75. Glenn JS. Prenylation of HDAg and antiviral drug development. Curr Top Microbiol Immunol 2006;307:133–149.

76. Samuel D, et al. Report of the monothematic EASL conference on liver transplantation for viral hepatitis (Paris, France, Jan 12-14, 2006). J Hepatol 2006;45:127–143.

Hepatitis E

S.K. Sarin and Manoj Kumar

Introduction

Hepatitis E is caused by infection with hepatitis E virus (HEV), the most recently discovered of the five well-recognized hepatotropic viruses, named hepatitis A to hepatitis E. HEV is an enterically transmitted (other routes of transmission may exist) RNA virus that causes an acute, self-limiting hepatitis in immunocompetent subjects, but may also cause chronic infection in immunosuppressed subjects. Infection with HEV may be asymptomatic or may cause varying degrees of hepatitis, ranging from mild cases to fulminant disease. Fulminant hepatitis E has been reported with increased frequency in pregnant women. The inability to reproducibly culture hepatitis E virus makes it impossible to develop traditional live or inactivated vaccines. However, significant progress has been made in developing and testing recombinant subunit vaccines based on the viral capsid protein.

History

The earliest well-documented report of this disease was a large epidemic of water-borne hepatitis in New Delhi, India, during 1955 to 1956. Although it was initially believed to be related to hepatitis A, subsequent testing of stored sera from this epidemic and another outbreak during 1978 to 1979 in Kashmir, India, failed to demonstrate specific serologic markers for hepatitis A and hepatitis B. A new agent for viral hepatitis was implicated and provisionally named as enterically transmitted non-A, non-B hepatitis (ET-NANBH) virus.[1] In 1983 Balayan and colleagues provided the first proof of the existence of a newly identified form of acute viral hepatitis by transmitting hepatitis to a volunteer from a patient involved in an ET-NANBH outbreak in central Asia.[2] The volunteer, who had preexisting antibody to hepatitis A virus (HAV), developed a severe hepatitis, shed 27- to 30-nm viruslike particles in his feces (detected by immune electron microscopy [IEM]), and developed antibodies to the viruslike particles during convalescence. The researchers also inoculated cynomolgus monkeys with the new virus; again, the monkeys developed hepatitis, shed viruslike particles, and developed an immune response to the particles. In 1990 Reyes and colleagues cloned and sequenced a part of the genome of the virus.[3] This new form of non-A, non-B hepatitis was referred to as epidemic non-A, non-B hepatitis or enterically transmitted non-A, non-B hepatitis (ET-NANBH), and later the name of the disease was changed to hepatitis E.

Virology
Classification

Hepatitis E virus was originally classified in the Caliciviridae family because of its structural similarity to other *Caliciviruses;* however, it is now the sole member of the Hepeviridae family.[4]

Structure
Physiochemical Characteristics

Hepatitis E virus is a spherical, nonenveloped particle that is approximately 27 to 34 nm in diameter and has an icosahedral symmetry. The buoyant density of HEV is 1.35 to 1.40 g/cm^3 in CsCl with a sedimentation coefficient of 183 S.[5] The virus is relatively stable to environmental and chemical agents. In a recent study comparing the thermal stability of virulent HEV and HAV, HEV was found to be less stable than HAV, although some HEV would most likely survive the internal temperatures of rare-cooked meat.[6]

Morphology

Hepatitis E virus has an indefinite surface structure that is intermediate between that of the Norwalk agent (a member of the Caliciviridae family) and that of HAV (a member of the Picornaviridae family). HEV contains an RNA genome enclosed within a capsid. The viral capsid protein is encoded by open reading frame 2 (ORF2) near the 3′ end. The ORF2 capsid protein contains a total of 660 amino acid (aa) residues. The viral capsid protein induces neutralizing antibodies by its immunization or during the course of infection. A typical signal sequence at the N-terminus and three potential N-glycosylation sites (Asn-X-Ser/Thr) are well-conserved in the capsid protein derived from all mammalian genotypes. The receptor-binding site has been mapped to the second half of the polypeptide chain.[7] As an alternative to in vitro propagation of HEV, the baculovirus expression system opens the prospect of studying HEV capsid assembly, as HEV-like particles (HEV-LPs) with protruding spikes on the surface can be formed in insect cells infected with a recombinant baculovirus expressing the capsid protein of a genotype 1 strain.[8] Cryo-electron microscopic (cryoEM) analysis has revealed that HEV-LP is a $T = 1$ icosahedral particle composed of 60 copies of truncated products of ORF2.[8] HEV-LP did not appear to contain RNA because of its lack of significant density.[8] The HEV-LP, which displays $T = 1$ symmetry with a diameter of 270 Å, is smaller than the native HEV particle, which displays $T = 3$ symmetry with an estimated diameter of 350 to 400 Å.[9] The surface of the HEV-LP is dominated by 30 dimeric protrusions, and each capsid subunit appears to have 2 domains.[9] Recently the crystal structure of HEV-LP determined to 3.5-Å resolution has been reported. Each HEV capsid protein contains the following three linear domains: S (aa 118-313), P1 (aa 314-453), and P2 (aa 454 to end), the final two of which are linked by a long, flexible hinge linker. The S domain forms a continuous capsid shell that is reinforced by three-fold protrusions formed by P1 and by two-fold spikes formed by P2. It adopts the jelly-roll β-barrel fold that is most closely related to plant $T = 3$ viruses. P1 and P2 contain compact, six-stranded β-barrels that resemble the β-barrel domain of phage sialidase

and the receptor-binding domain of *Calicivirus*, respectively, both of which are capable of polysaccharide binding. The highly exposed P2 domain likely plays an important role in antigenicity determination and virus neutralization. Structural modeling shows that the assembly of the native $T = 3$ capsid requires flat capsid protein dimers with less curvature than those found in the $T = 1$ viruslike particle (VLP), suggesting that additional N-terminal sequences may be involved in particle size regulation.[10] However, the HEV-LP retained the antigenicity and capsid formation of the native HEV particles and is therefore a promising candidate for use in vaccine development.

Genome Organization

Genome and Proteins

The HEV genome consists of a single-stranded, positive-sense RNA approximately 7.3 kilobases (kb) in length. It contains a short 5′ untranslated region (UTR), three open reading frames (ORFs: ORF1, ORF2, and ORF3), and a short 3′ UTR that is terminated by a poly(A) tract.[11] The genome is organized as 5′-ORF1-ORF3-ORF2-3′, with ORF3 and ORF2 largely overlapping (**Fig. 33-1**). Although a single serotype has been proposed, extensive genomic diversity has been observed among HEV isolates.

The 5′ and 3′ untranslated regions are highly conserved and are likely to play roles in RNA replication and encapsidation. The 5′ end of the genome has a 7-methylguanosine cap. ORF1, the largest ORF, begins at the 5′ end of the viral genome after a 27-bp noncoding sequence and extends 5079 bp to the 3′ end (in the Burmese prototype strain); it encodes approximately 1693 amino acids encompassing nonstructural, enzymatically active proteins probably involved in viral replication and protein processing. Based on the identification of characteristic amino acid motifs, the following genetic elements have been identified, in order, from the 5′ to the 3′ end of the open reading frame (ORF): (1) a methyltransferase, presumably involved in capping the 5′ end of the viral genome; (2) the "Y" domain, a sequence of unknown function that is found in certain other viruses, including rubella virus; (3) a papain-like cysteine protease, a type of protease found predominantly in alphaviruses and rubella virus; (4) a proline-rich "hinge" that may provide flexibility and that contains a region of hypervariable sequence; (5) an "X" domain of unknown function

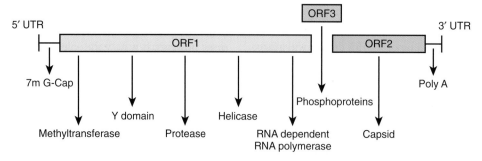

Fig. 33-1 **Genome organization and proteins of HEV.** The positive-strand RNA genome of HEV is capped at the 5′ end and polyadenylated at the 3′ end. It contains short stretches of untranslated regions *(UTR)* at both ends. There are three open reading frames (ORFs). *ORF1* encodes the nonstructural polyprotein *(nsp)* that contains various functional units—methyltransferase, papain-like cysteine protease, RNA helicase, and RNA-dependent RNA polymerase. *ORF2* encodes the viral capsid protein. *ORF3* encodes a small regulatory phosphoprotein.

that has been found adjacent to papain-like protease domains in the polyproteins of other positive-strand RNA viruses; (6) a domain containing helicase-like motifs similar to those found in viruses containing type I (superfamily 3) helicases; and (7) an RNA-dependent polymerase, with motifs most closely related to those found in viruses containing an RNA polymerase of superfamily 3.[12] In vitro expression of the HEV ORF1 produced a polyprotein that was processed into two products following extended incubation.[13] When expressed in insect cells, ORF1 was processed and this was partially blocked by a cell-permeable cysteine protease inhibitor.[14] The presence of methyltransferase motifs in ORF1 suggested HEV had a capped RNA genome. A 5′-methylguanosine residue in the HEV genome is essential for infectivity and replication. The GDD motif in RNA-dependent RNA polymerases (RdRp) is also important for HEV replication. Two predicted stem-loop (SL) structures at the 3′ NCR and the poly(A) tract were necessary for RdRp binding during HEV genome replication.[15] Except for the methyltransferase,[16] none of the other putative components of ORF1 have been expressed, purified, and biochemically characterized.

ORF2, approximately 2000 nucleotides in length, begins approximately 40 nucleotides after the termination of ORF1 and consists of a 5′ signal sequence; a 300-nucleotide region rich in codons for arginine, probably representing an RNA-binding site; and three potential glycosylation sites. ORF2 encodes a 660-aa protein, most likely representing one or more structural or capsid protein(s) of HEV. Polyprotein open reading frame 2 (pORF2) is an 80-kilodalton (kDa) glycoprotein with a potential endoplasmic reticulum directing signal at its N-terminus (a region containing high concentrations of arginine and lysine). The ORF2 protein enters the endoplasmic reticulum (ER), but a fraction retrotranslocates to the cytoplasm to trigger a stress pathway.[17] When pORF2 is expressed in mammalian cells, a large proportion of the nascent protein is modified by N-glycosylation. Mutations in the pORF2 glycosylation sites prevented the formation of infectious virus particles and had low infectivity in macaques.[18] When pORF2 is expressed in insect cells, it is cleaved at a site between amino acids 111 and 112 and at various other sites within the C-terminus of the protein. Some of these truncated forms of pORF2 have the ability to self-assemble into HEV-LPs or subviral particles. The structure of a self-assembled HEV-LP was determined by cryoelectron microscopy and showed the capsid to be dominated by dimers. This dimerization property may not be amino acid sequence–dependent but instead is a complex formation of a specific tertiary structure that imparts to pORF2 its property to self-associate. The ORF2 protein also contains RNA-binding activity and specifically binds to the 5′ end of the HEV genome. A 76-nucleotide region at the 5′ end of the HEV genome was responsible for binding the ORF2 protein. This interaction may be responsible for bringing the genomic RNA into the capsid during assembly, thus playing a role in viral encapsidation.[19]

ORF3, less than 400 nucleotides in length, overlaps ORF1 by 1 nucleotide at its 5′ end and overlaps ORF2 by more than 300 nucleotides at its 3′ end. It codes for a 123-aa, 13.5-kDa nonglycosylated protein (pORF3), which is a very basic protein ($pI = 12.5$), and is the most variable protein among the HEV strains. Recently it was proposed to be translated from a bicistronic subgenomic RNA and to be nine amino acids shorter at its N-terminus.[20] Although ORF3 was dispensable for

replication in vitro,[21] it is required for infection in monkeys inoculated with HEV genomic RNA.[22] Expression of pORF3 in mammalian cells showed it to interact with various cellular proteins. It co-localizes with the cytoskeleton and binds a MAP kinase phosphatase.[23] It also interacts with hemopexin, an acute-phase plasma glycoprotein.[24] The P1 region contains the phosphorylated serine residue that is conserved in all HEV strains except the Mexican isolate, and the P2 region contains a motif that binds several proteins containing src-homology 3 (SH3) domains.[25] ORF3 protein of hepatitis E virus also interacts with the Bbeta chain of fibrinogen, resulting in decreased fibrinogen secretion.[26] The ORF3 protein is likely used to regulate the host cell environment through its interaction with various intracellular pathways (Fig. 33-2).[4] It activates the extracellularly regulated kinase (ERK) by binding and inhibiting its cognate phosphatase.[23] Prolonged activation of ERK would generate a survival and proliferative signal (see Fig. 33-2). Higher levels of hexokinase and oligomeric voltage-dependent anion channel (VDAC) were found in ORF3-expressing cells, which displayed attenuated mitochondrial death signaling.[27] Recently ORF3 protein has been shown to interact with microtubules and interfere with their dynamics, which might be needed for establishment of an HEV infection.[28] The ORF3 protein might act as an adaptor to link intracellular transduction pathways and this might promote HEV replication and assembly. pORF3 localized to early and recycling endosomes, and delayed postinternalization trafficking of epidermal growth factor receptor (EGFR). This ineraction is likely to prolong endomembrane signaling and promote cell survival[4] (see Fig. 33-2). Another effect of this interaction is reduced nuclear translocation of pSTAT3 and attenuation of the acute-phase response. Thus pORF3 might reduce the host inflammatory response, further creating an environment favorable for viral replication (see Fig. 33-2). The α1-microglobulin and bikunin precursor protein (AMBP) and its constituents—α1-microglobulin and bikunin—were also identified as pORF3-binding partners.[29] There was increased secretion of α1-microglobulin from ORF3-expressing cells.[30] Because α1-microglobulin is immunosuppressive, this is proposed to protect virus-infected cells (see Fig. 33-2). Recently it has been shown that hepatitis E virus ORF3 protein stabilizes hypoxia-inducible factor (HIF)-1α and enhances HIF-1-mediated transcriptional activity through p300/CBP, which leads to increased activity of the glycolytic pathway, thus promoting survival of the host cell.[31]

Two broad roles are thus predicted for pORF3 in HEV pathogenesis (see Fig. 33-2).[4] The first is promotion of cell survival through ERK activation, prolonged endomembrane signaling, and attenuation of the intrinsic death pathway (see Fig. 33-2). The second is to down-regulate innate host responses through reduced expression of acute-phase proteins and increased secretion of α1-microglobulin (see Fig. 33-2).[4] A recent study has shown that ORF3 protein is responsible for virion egress from infected cells and is present on the surface of released HEV particles, which may be associated with lipids.[32]

Replication Cycle

Little is known about the cellular receptors for HEV or its entry process. A recent study showed that truncated peptide p239 spanning aa 368-606 of pORF2 formed 23-nm particles

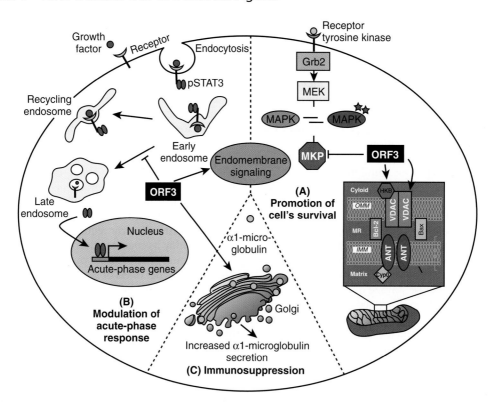

Fig. 33-2 **Role of the ORF3 protein in HEV pathogenesis.** Three broad functions for the ORF3 protein have been proposed. **A,** Promotion of cell survival. The ORF3 protein activates MAP kinase by binding and inactivating its cognate phosphatase (MKP). Additionally, it up-regulates and promotes homooligomerization of the outer mitochondrial membrane porin (VDAC) and increases hexokinase levels, thus reducing mitochondrial depolarization and inhibiting intrinsic cell death. **B,** Modulation of the acute-phase response. The ORF3 protein localizes to early and recycling endosomes, and inhibits the movement of activated growth factor receptors to late endosomes. This prolongs endomembrane growth factor signaling and contributes to cell survival. Through this mechanism, pORF3 also reduces the nuclear transport of pSTAT3, a critical transcription factor for the expression of acute-phase response genes. **C,** Immunosuppression. The ORF3 protein promotes the secretion of α_1-microglobulin, an immunosuppressive protein that could act in the immediate vicinity of the infected cell. *(From Chandra V, Taneja S, Kalia M, Jameel S. Molecular biology and pathogenesis of hepatitis E virus. J Biosci 2008;33:451–464.)*

that bind and penetrate HepG2, Huh-7, PLC/PRF5, and A549 cells[33] and prevent further infection of these cells. The cell surface molecules that bind HEV or its capsid protein are not known. A model for HEV replication and gene expression was proposed based on similarities and sequence homology to better characterized positive-strand RNA viruses.[4] This is shown in **Figure 33-3**. Following entry into a permissive cell (step a), the viral genomic RNA is uncoated (step b) and translated in the cytosol of infected cells to produce the ORF1-encoded nonstructural polyprotein (nsP) (step c). Cleavage of the ORF1 nsP is achieved by cellular proteases, possibly with help from the viral PCP. The viral replicase (RdRP) replicates the genomic positive strand into the negative-strand replicative intermediates (step d1). Endoplasmic reticulum has been identified as the site of replicase localization and possible site of replication.[34] The RdRp copies the input genome to yield full-length minus-strand RNAs, followed by subgenomic plus-strand RNAs and full-length plus-strand RNAs (new viral genomes) (step d2). This process is similar to that of alphaviruses, and a region homologous to alphavirus junction sequences is proposed to serve as the subgenomic promoter. The subgenomic RNA can then be translated into the structural protein(s) (step e). The capsid proteins package the viral genome to assemble progeny virions (step f) that exit the cell through an undefined pathway. Direct experimental confirmation of this replication scheme is still needed but several

findings support this model.[4] In experimentally infected rhesus monkeys and pigs, HEV-positive and HIV-negative strand RNAs are observed in the liver. Because in vitro transcripts of full-length cDNA clones are infectious for nonhuman primates and pigs, the subgenomic RNAs are not required to initiate an infection, and must be synthesized as part of the replication process. Replicons have shown mixed results with respect to detection of negative-stranded replicative intermediates.[4,35]

Genomic Variability of HEV

Although several classification schemes have been proposed, the most accepted scheme classifies HEV isolates into four major genotypes: 1 to 4.[36] HEV was discovered by immune electron microscopy in 1983.[2] Eight years after its discovery, the full genomic sequence of HEV was first determined for a strain from Myanmar (formerly Burma),[37] which had greater than 88.2% nucleotide identity across the entire genome to isolates obtained from other developing countries both in Asia (including China, India, Nepal, and Pakistan) and in Africa (including Chad and Morocco). In 1992 a Mexican strain, implicated in an outbreak that occurred in Mexico in 1986, was reported.[38] The Mexican strain is distinct from the Burmese variants, and constituted a second genotype. In 1997 an HEV isolate of sporadic acute hepatitis E from a U.S.

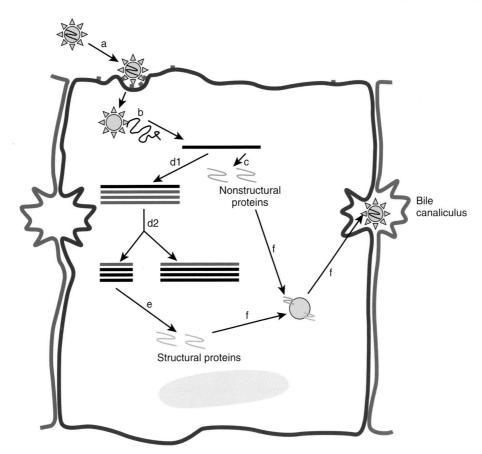

Fig. 33-3 Replication cycle of HEV. (*a*) The virus enters the hepatocyte via a cellular receptor, the identity of which remains uncertain. (*b*) This is followed by uncoating of the viral particle and release of the positive-sense RNA genome into the cell. (*c*) The genomic RNA is translated in the cytoplasm into nonstructural proteins encoded by ORFI, which can then be processed into individual functional units including methyltransferase, protease, helicase, and replicase activities. (*d*) The replicase thus synthesized replicates the positive-strand genomic RNA into negative-strand RNA intermediates (*d1*) and genomic and subgenomic positive-strand RNAs are synthesized from the negative-strand RNA intermediates (*d2*). (*e*) The positive-strand subgenomic RNA is translated into structural proteins. (*f*) The capsid protein packages the genomic RNA to assemble new virions. Newly assembled HEV particles are secreted by the cell across the apical membrane of the hepatocyte into the biliary canaliculus, from which they are passed into the bile and small intestine.

patient who had no history of travel abroad was reported,[39] and it constituted a third genotype, which was subsequently found to be widely distributed throughout the world.[40] In 1999 HEV isolates distinct from the original Chinese isolates of genotype 1 were recovered from Chinese patients with acute hepatitis, and they constituted a fourth group.[41] HEV isolates classifiable into the fourth group have also been identified from sporadic cases of HEV infection not only in China but also in Taiwan and Japan.[40] HEV genotypes are further classified into the following subtypes: genotype 1 into 5 subtypes (1a to 1e); genotype 2 into 2 subtypes (2a and 2b); genotype 3 into 10 subtypes (3a to 3j); and genotype 4 into 7 subtypes (4a to 4g).[40]

Distribution of HEV Genotypes

Genotype 1 is distributed in various countries including Bangladesh, Cambodia, China, India, Kyrgyzstan, Myanmar, Nepal, Pakistan, Uzbekistan, and Vietnam in Asia and Algeria, the Central African Republic (CAR), Chad, Djibouti, Morocco, Sudan, Tunisia, Namibia, Egypt, and South Africa in Africa. HEVs that are commonly found in Asia and Africa have been classified as the Asian and African subgenotypes of genotype

1, respectively.[40] Genotype 2 has been represented by the prototype sequence from an epidemic in Mexico[38] and new variants were recently identified from endemic cases in African countries including CAR, Chad, Democratic Republic of the Congo (DRC), Egypt, Namibia, and Nigeria.[40] HEVs of genotypes 1 and 2 have caused epidemics and outbreaks of hepatitis E in tropical and some subtropical regions, usually attributable to transmission by fecal contamination of water supplies.[40] In contrast, HEVs of genotypes 3 and 4 were found in sporadic acute hepatitis E cases in the United States, European countries, China, and Japan, and these cases were most likely zoonotic in origin.[40] Genotype 3 accounts for the largest number of isolates among all HEV sequences archived in the GenBank/EMBL/DDBJ databases, and many of them were identified in the United States or Japan.[40] However, genotype 3 HEV is widely distributed and has been isolated from sporadic cases of acute hepatitis E and/or domestic pigs in many countries including Argentina, Australia, Austria, Cambodia, Canada, France, Germany, Greece, Hungary, Italy, Japan, Korea, Kyrgyzstan, Mexico, the Netherlands, New Zealand, Russia, Spain, Taiwan, Thailand, the United Kingdom, and the United States. In contrast, genotype 4 is restricted to Asian countries and contains strains from humans and/or domestic

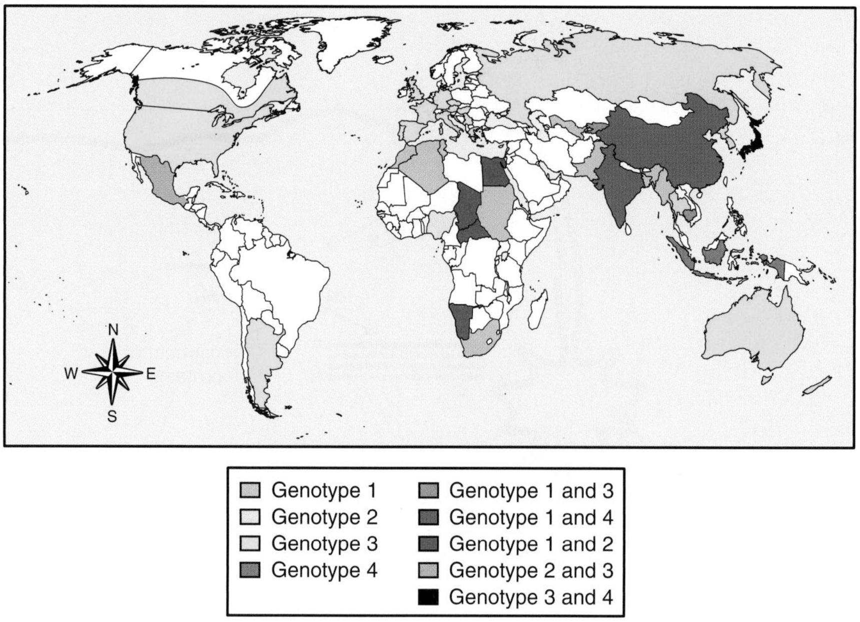

Fig. 33-4 **Geographic distribution of HEV isolates according to genotypes.** HEV genotypes 1 and 2 are epidemic strains causing human infection. HEV genotypes 3 and 4 are zoonotic strains isolated from humans and a variety of animals, particularly pigs. In some countries, different genotypes co-circulate in distinct ecologic niches: for example, genotypes 1 and 4 in China, India, and Vietnam; genotypes 1 and 2 in several African countries; genotypes 3 and 4 in Japan; genotypes 1 and 3 in Cambodia; and genotypes 2 and 3 in Mexico.

☐ Genotype 1   ☐ Genotype 1 and 3
☐ Genotype 2   ■ Genotype 1 and 4
☐ Genotype 3   ■ Genotype 1 and 2
■ Genotype 4   ☐ Genotype 2 and 3
                ■ Genotype 3 and 4

pigs in China, India, Indonesia, Japan, Taiwan, and Vietnam. Among 38 countries where HEV strains have been isolated from infected patients, HEVs of a single genotype were isolated from infected patients in 28 countries (genotype 1 in 12 countries, genotype 2 in 3 countries, genotype 3 in 12 countries, and genotype 4 in 1 country) and HEVs of 2 distinct genotypes were isolated from infected patients in 8 countries (genotypes 1 and 2 in 4 countries, genotypes 1 and 3 in 2 countries, and genotypes 1 and 4 in 2 countries). Japan is unique in that three distinct genotypes (1, 3, and 4) of HEV strains have been identified in infected patients, although genotype 1 HEV is most likely imported.[40]

Thus genotype 1 consists of epidemic strains in developing countries in Asia and Africa; genotype 2 has been described in Mexico and Africa; genotype 3 HEV is widely distributed and has been isolated from sporadic cases of acute hepatitis E and/or domestic pigs in many countries in the world, except for countries in Africa; and genotype 4 contains strains from humans and/or domestic pigs exclusively in Asian countries.[40]

In some countries, different genotypes co-circulate in distinct ecologic niches: for example, genotypes 1 and 4 in China, India, and Vietnam; genotypes 1 and 2 in several African countries; genotypes 3 and 4 in Japan; genotypes 1 and 3 in Cambodia; and genotypes 2 and 3 in Mexico.

Figure 33-4 shows the worldwide distribution of HEV genotypes.

Quasi-Species Nature and Evolution of HEV

A high degree of conservation of the amino acid sequence of the capsid protein among distinct genotypes is observed, which correlates with the small degree of antigenic diversity; thus there is only a single serotype of HEV. However, despite this limited amino acid heterogeneity, a significant degree of nucleic acid variability has been observed among different isolates from different regions of the world.[40] The molecular basis of this genetic variability may be the high error rate of the viral RNA-dependent RNA polymerase (RdRp) and

the absence of proofreading mechanisms. Based on the assumption that JKK-Sap00 (isolation date: 10 November 2000), JYW-Sap02 (30 August 2002), and JTS-Sap02 (14 September 2002) are descendants of JSM-Sap95 (28 March 1995), all of which were isolated in Hokkaido and differed from each other by 0.056% to 1.050%, the mutation rate of HEV has been estimated to be $(1.40\text{-}1.72) \times 10^{-3}$ base substitutions per site per year.[42]

Quasi-species have mainly been described in persistent viral infections such as those attributable to human immunodeficiency virus type 1 and hepatitis C virus during which virus populations develop a high degree of sequence variation within each infected individual. They are less common in viruses causing acute self-limited infections, such as dengue virus and hepatitis A virus.[40] HEV epidemics are mainly caused by a common source of contamination, usually drinking water resources. Although the spread of HEV among humans is assumed to be clonal according to a "one outbreak, one strain" scheme, the quasi-species nature of epidemic HEV was demonstrated in a retrospective analysis of both inter- and intrapatient diversity using 23 serum samples collected during a water-borne outbreak that occurred from 1986 to 1987 in Algeria.[43] However, the extent of the sequence variation of HEV in vivo and its relationship to disease severity remain unknown. The reason why HEV strains of genotypes 1 and 2 have less genomic variability than HEV strains of genotypes 3 and 4 remains to be elucidated. HEV strains of genotypes 1 and 2 often cause outbreaks or epidemics of hepatitis as a result of efficient transmission via the fecal–oral route, usually by contaminated water or food supply.[44] In contrast, HEV variants of genotypes 3 and 4 are predominantly maintained among animal species such as domestic pigs and only occasionally infect humans; this is most likely due to inefficient cross-species transmission of these variants. Maintenance of HEV strains of genotypes 3 and 4 among animal species would contribute to the long-term circulation of HEV in particular geographic regions and the independent evolution of the virus in specific animal species. Therefore differences in the degree of viral divergence among genotypes of HEV may reflect different transmission patterns.[40]

To investigate the genetic changes in HEV strains in the community, Shrestha and colleagues compared the 412-nt sequence within ORF2 of HEV among HEV isolates recovered from 48 patients in 1997, 16 patients in 1999, 14 patients in 2000, and 38 patients in 2002 in Kathmandu valley of Nepal.[45] All 116 HEV-viremic samples were typed as genotype 1, and further as subgenotype 1a ($n = 85$, 73%), 1c ($n = 29$, 25%), and mixed infection of 1a and 1c ($n = 2$, 2%); subgenotype 1c was detected only in 1997. Genetic variability was observed among HEV strains and even among HEV strains of the same subtype (1a) obtained each year for 1997, 1999, 2000, and 2002. When phylogenetic analysis of the 87 subtype 1a isolates was performed, they further segregated into 5 clusters, with 2 predominant clusters of 1a-2 and 1a-3: the annual frequency of cluster 1a-2 isolates decreased from 63% in 1997, to 50% in 1999, to 7% in 2000, to no cases in 2002; cluster 1a-3 isolates were observed in all 4 years and their annual frequency increased from 5% in 1997 to 95% in 2002. Of the remaining three clusters, cluster 1a-1 was detectable only in 1997 and clusters 1a-4 and 1a-5 emerged in 2000 and 2002, respectively. These results indicate that the genetic changes and invasion of HEV strains may contribute to the genetic variability of HEV in the community. The fact that no significant amino acid substitutions were recognized in the HEV strains isolated during a 5-year period suggests that genomic mutations of HEV may occur naturally in infected individuals without immunologic pressure from the host, and that selective forces that do not allow amino acid substitutions may be involved in the observed pattern of divergence. Taking into account that partial sequencing of a selected genomic region was employed, a definitive depiction of the biologic significance of these and other possible changes in the entire genome needs to be obtained from more in-depth studies.[40]

Serotypes and Antigenicity

Despite the presence of genetically different isolates of HEV, there appears to be only one serotype. Antigenic variations have important implications for the serologic detection of HEV infection. Antibody responses to individual viral antigens are highly variable, both because of strain-specific differences in some epitopes and because of differences in response to single antigens among individual patients. For example, pORF3 varies greatly among strains, and many experimentally infected animals and some patients fail to develop antibodies to ORF3 protein. This variable reactivity contributes to the poor sensitivity and concordance of HEV diagnostic tests based on such antigens.[40] Conversely, all isolates of HEV share some important cross-reactive antigens. Immunization of prehuman primates with recombinant pORF2 proteins conferred immunity to both homologous and heterologous challenge, suggesting that major protection epitopes are common among HEV genotypes.

Animal Models and in Vitro Culture

Studies of HEV transmission have mostly been conducted in nonhuman primates such as cynomolgus, rhesus, and owl monkeys as well as chimpanzees.[46,47] These have provided important information regarding the biology and pathogenesis of HEV, and are indispensable tools for vaccine and drug testing. Experimental transmission studies have also been conducted in pigs, an established reservoir for HEV.[48] Recently, Mongolian gerbils and Balb/c nude mice have been found to be useful animal models for studying the pathogenesis of HEV.[49,50]

There has been only limited success in generating suitable tissue culture replication systems for HEV. Early studies reported propagation of HEV in 2BS,[38] A549,[51] and FRhK[52] cells. Infection of primary cynomolgus hepatocytes and PLC/PRF/5 cells has been shown, but replication was inefficient.[53] Recently, HEV genotype 3 from a high-titer stool suspension was successfully passaged for multiple generations in PLC/PRF/5 cells[54] and these cells were used to assess the infectivity of HEV shed in patients' stools.[55] The replication of HEV has been observed in cell lines transfected with transcripts of infectious cDNA clones and with a replicon derived from the clones.[56] Monkeys inoculated with culture media or lysates of HEV replicon-transfected cells developed infection, but viral titers were low. Some species barrier for HEV replication might exist because replicons did not function in nonprimate cell lines. However, sufficient amounts of viral particles cannot be obtained for studies of the structure, life cycle, and pathogenesis of HEV.[40]

Epidemiology
Incidence and Prevalence and Worldwide Disease Patterns

Worldwide, two geographic patterns can be differentiated: (1) endemic regions or areas of high HEV prevalence, in which major outbreaks and a substantial number of sporadic cases occur; and (2) non–endemic regions, in which HEV accounts for a few cases of acute viral hepatitis, mainly among travelers to endemic regions (**Fig. 33-5**).

HEV in Endemic Regions

In such regions epidemics of hepatitis E occur frequently. These epidemics are usually separated by a few years. Such outbreaks have been observed in the Indian subcontinent, China, Southeast and Central Asia, the Middle East, and the northern and western parts of Africa. In North America (Mexico), two small outbreaks were reported during 1986 to 1987, but no further outbreaks have since been reported. The outbreaks are often large, and affect several hundred to several thousand persons.[1] Most reported outbreaks have been related to consumption of fecally contaminated drinking water. Their time course varies from unimodal outbreaks, which last a few weeks, to prolonged, multipeaked epidemics, with a duration of more than 1 year. The latter represent continuing water contamination. The outbreaks frequently follow heavy rainfall and floods, which create conditions that favor mixing of human excreta with sources of drinking water. Some outbreaks have occurred in hot and dry summer months, possibly a result of diminished water flow in rivers leading to an increased concentration of fecal contaminants. In Southeast Asia, recurrent epidemics have been shown to be associated with disposal of human excreta into rivers and subsequent use of water from the same river for drinking, cooking, and

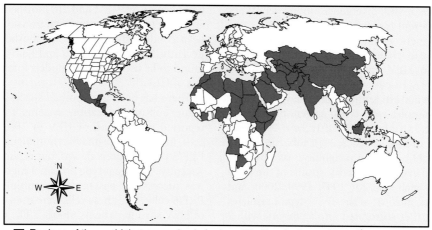

■ Regions of the world that are endemic for hepatitis E and where >25% of acute viral hepatitis is due to HEV.

Fig. 33-5 **Geographic distribution of hepatitis E.**

personal hygiene.[57] These practices provide conditions that allow continuous fecal contamination of water. Outbreaks of hepatitis E have occurred in underdeveloped urban areas with leaky water pipes passing through soil that is contaminated with sewage. Intermittent water supply in these areas leads to a negative pressure in pipes during periods of no flow, allowing inward suction of contaminants.[58] Although the dissemination of HEV infection through contamination of food may be possible, few outbreaks related to food-borne transmission have been reported from disease-endemic areas. This may be due to a relatively long incubation period, which makes it difficult to establish a relationship between consumption of a particular food and occurrence of disease.[59]

Overall attack rates during hepatitis E outbreaks have ranged from 1% to 15%. The rates are highest among young adults (3% to 30%); the reason for this is not clear. Lower attack rates among children are related probably to a higher proportion of asymptomatic infections than to rarity of infection. Males outnumber females in most outbreaks; this may be due either to their greater risk of exposure to HEV infection or to a greater propensity for clinical disease once infected.[59] Hepatitis E outbreaks have characteristically been associated with a high attack rate and mortality among pregnant women. The rate of development of acute liver failure among those with symptomatic hepatitis E was also higher among pregnant women. Once acute liver failure appears, the death rate may be no different among pregnant women with hepatitis E than in those with other causes of severe liver injury (see Pregnant Women later). Because HEV infection during pregnancy is associated with a high attack rate and risk of severe disease, pregnant women are overrepresented among case series of women with liver failure in the endemic areas, and also among fatal cases during hepatitis E outbreaks.[59]

In disease-endemic areas, HEV infection accounts for a large proportion of acute sporadic hepatitis in all age groups. In India HEV infection is the most common cause of acute sporadic hepatitis and accounts for up to 70% of such cases among adults.[59] In these regions, patients with sporadic hepatitis E closely resemble those of epidemic hepatitis E in age distribution, severity and duration of illness, propensity for

worse prognosis among pregnant women, and absence of chronic sequelae. The route of acquisition of infection in most patients with sporadic hepatitis E is unclear. However, given the high potential for fecal contamination of water and food in these areas, these sources are most likely. HEV genomic sequences could be isolated from nearly 40% of sewage specimens obtained through all seasons from a large drain in a large Indian city.[60] This indicates ubiquitous circulation of HEV in the population, even in the absence of a disease outbreak.

Unlike several other enterically transmitted infections, person-to-person transmission of HEV from either epidemic or sporadic cases is distinctly uncommon.[61] The exact reason for this is unknown. During outbreaks, secondary attack rates among household contacts of patients with hepatitis E have been as low as 0.7% to 2.2%. This is much lower than the 50% to 75% infection rate among susceptible household contacts of hepatitis A cases. Even with multiple cases in one family, the time interval between cases is short, indicating a shared primary water-borne infection rather than person-to-person transmission.[59]

Maternal–fetal transmission of HEV infection has been reported (see Modes of Transmission, later). In regions endemic for hepatitis E, the presence of HEV viremia among healthy blood donors and transmission of this infection to transfusion recipients have been documented. However, the contribution of such transmission to the overall disease burden remains unclear.

Reservoirs of HEV in Endemic Regions

In disease-endemic areas, the reservoir of HEV responsible for maintaining the disease in a population has not been clearly determined. Protracted viremia and prolonged fecal shedding of HEV have been suggested. However, viral shedding in feces lasts for a short period, making this possibility unlikely. Another potential reservoir of the virus may be a continuously circulating pool of individuals with subclinical HEV infection. In an experimental cynomolgus macaque model, HEV-infected animals that lacked biochemical evidence of liver injury were found to excrete large amounts of viable and infectious HEV.[62] Similar fecal shedding of the virus by persons with subclinical HEV infection could lead to continuous maintenance of a source of infection in a disease-endemic area, somewhat similar to the situation that existed with poliovirus in areas where it was endemic. This pool of infection could, in turn, lead to periodic contamination of drinking water supplies.

The issue regarding the existence of an animal reservoir in disease-endemic regions remains unresolved. The zoonotic hypothesis for transmission of HEV is based primarily on the following factors: (1) the high prevalence of anti-HEV antibodies in several animal species; (2) the isolation of HEV genomic sequences from pigs; and (3) the genomic sequence homology between human and animal HEV isolates. However, most of the supporting genomic data have been from non–endemic regions. In contrast, data from endemic regions are conflicting. Isolates from animals and sporadic human cases have belonged to the same genotype (genotype 4) in China and Vietnam. In India, however, animal isolates have all been members of genotype 4 and human isolates genotype 1. Genotype 1 HEV, which is responsible for the large majority of cases in all endemic countries, has never been isolated from pigs. Also, in experimental studies, genotype 1 virus is unable to infect pigs. Thus zoonotic transmission may not be a major mode of distribution in these areas, in particular for the widely prevalent genotype 1 HEV.[59]

Thus it appears that in the regions where hepatitis E is endemic, the infection is acquired from either an environmental or a human reservoir through poor general sanitation, contaminated drinking water supplies, and lack of attention to personal hygiene. Further data are necessary before zoonotic transmission of HEV can be implicated in these regions.

HEV in Non-Endemic Regions

In non-endemic regions, where outbreaks have not been reported, the disease accounts for only a minority of reported cases of acute viral hepatitis. Until a few years ago, most such cases were found to be related to travel to disease-endemic areas. However, in recent years isolated cases or small series of cases related to autochthonous transmission of hepatitis E in these regions have been recorded in the United States, Europe (including the United Kingdom, France, the Netherlands, Austria, Spain, and Greece), and developed countries of Asia-Pacific (Japan, Taiwan, Hong Kong, Australia). In a series of 40 cases with hepatitis E identified in the United Kingdom, the disease showed seasonal variations with peaks in spring and summer and no cases during November and December.[63] In the United Kingdom, the disease appeared to be more common among residents of coastal and estuarine areas.[64] The mode of transmission in most of these cases could not be identified, although zoonotic distribution has been proposed (see HEV Infection as a Zoonosis, later). **Table 33-1** shows epidemiologic differences in hepatitis E in disease-endemic and non-endemic regions.

Seroprevalence Data

The presence of anti-HEV immunoglobulin G (IgG) antibody has generally been considered evidence of prior exposure to HEV. The duration of persistence of circulating IgG anti-HEV antibodies remains unclear. In one study, nearly half of those

Table 33-1 Epidemiologic Differences in Hepatitis E in Disease-Endemic versus Non-Endemic Regions

FEATURE	ENDEMIC REGIONS	NON-ENDEMIC REGIONS
Geographic locations	Underdeveloped countries, mostly in Asia and Africa	Developed countries in Europe, North America, parts of Asia, Australia
Epidemiologic patterns	Large epidemics, small outbreaks, and sporadic cases	Only sporadic cases
Water-borne transmission	Most common route	Unknown
Animal reservoir	No	Yes
Animal-to-human transmission	Not reported	Yes; a likely mode of transmission
Virus genotype	Mostly genotypes 1 and 2, in China	Mostly genotype 3
Age group	Young men mostly affected	Usually elderly

who had been affected during a hepatitis E outbreak 14 years previously had no detectable anti-HEV.[65] In another study of serial sera from patients with acute hepatitis E, total anti-IgG titers showed a rapid decline, although titers remained above the detection threshold 14 months later.[66] Anti-HEV antibodies have been found in healthy subjects living in all geographic areas, although the prevalence varies widely. In general, prevalence rates are higher in developing countries where hepatitis E is common than in countries where clinical cases attributable to hepatitis E are uncommon. In endemic countries, despite the common occurrence of clinical cases and outbreaks of hepatitis E, the age-specific seroprevalence rates of anti-HEV are much lower than those for hepatitis A virus (HAV) and other enterically transmitted infections, such as *Helicobacter pylori*.[67] These unexpectedly low seroprevalence rates are particularly perplexing when compared with the situation in Egypt, with anti-HEV detection rates among adults of greater than 70% despite the absence of disease outbreaks.[68] In developed countries, anti-HEV antibody prevalence rates ranging from 1% to above 20% have been reported.[69,70] These appear to be higher than those expected from the low rate of clinically evident hepatitis E disease in these areas. Some of these variations may be related to differences in the assays used. In a direct comparison using a panel of coded sera, various anti-HEV antibody assays showed sensitivity rates varying from 17% to 100%, and concordance rates among reactive sera of 0% to 89% (median 32%).[71] Thus the relative contributions of subclinical HEV infection, serologic cross-reactivity with other agents, and false-positive serologic tests to seroprevalence rates in non-endemic areas remain unclear. In developed countries, veterinarians and swine farm workers who come in close contact with pigs have higher anti-HEV seroprevalence rates than the general population.

Modes of Transmission

Hepatitis E virus infection has four documented routes of transmission: (1) water-borne; (2) food-borne, from the consumption of raw or undercooked meat of infected wild animals such as boar and deer and domestic animals such as pigs; (3) blood-borne, or parenteral transmission; and (4) vertical transmission from mother to child.

HEV may be transmitted by the fecal–oral route. The most common vehicle of transmission during epidemics has been the ingestion of fecally contaminated water. Outbreaks in endemic areas occur most frequently during the rainy season, after floods and monsoons, or following recession of flood waters.[72,73] These climatic conditions in conjunction with inadequate sanitation and poor personal hygiene lead to epidemics of HEV infection when the sewage waters gain access to open-water reservoirs. In several regions of HEV endemicity, a pattern of recurrent epidemics has been observed, which is probably related to the permanent existence of conditions in which drinking water is fecally contaminated. In Southeast Asia the disposal of human excreta into rivers and the subsequent use of river water for drinking, cooking, and personal hygiene have been shown to be significantly associated with a high prevalence of HEV infection; the use of river water over years for various activities can lead to recurrent epidemics.[57]

Both in epidemic and in sporadic cases of HEV there is a low rate of clinical illness among household contacts of infected patients. Even when multiple cases occur among members of a family, such occurrence is related to exposure to a common source of contaminated water rather than to person-to-person transmission (see HEV in Endemic Regions, earlier). The mode of transmission responsible for sporadic HEV infections is unclear. Contaminated water is probably responsible for most of the cases in this setting. However, food-borne hepatitis E infection after ingestion of uncooked liver of pig or wild boar and meat of wild deer has been reported (see later).

More recent findings have led to speculation of an additional route of transmission for hepatitis E virus. Higher HEV seroprevalence levels in specific groups such as paid blood donors positive for other blood-borne viruses and in repeatedly transfused hemodialysis patients have led to suggestions that HEV could be acquired parenterally. There is also a risk of posttransfusion hepatitis E, and this should be considered in non-endemic areas (see Transfusions and Other Healthcare Settings, later).

Presumed nosocomial distribution of HEV has been reported in South Africa, where acute hepatitis developed in three healthcare workers 6 weeks after they treated a patient with fulminant hepatic failure (FHF) attributable to HEV infection.[74]

In an experimental study, pregnant rhesus monkeys failed to transmit the virus to their offspring.[75] However, vertical transmission of HEV infection from mother to infant has been shown to occur. In one study, six of eight babies born to mothers who had either acute uncomplicated hepatitis or FHF attributable to HEV infection in the third trimester of pregnancy were found to have evidence of HEV infection. Of these, five had HEV RNA in samples of their blood taken at birth, suggesting that infection was transmitted transplacentally.[76] More recent studies have shown that mother-to-infant transmission occurred in 50% to 100% of HEV RNA-positive mothers during pregnancy.[77,78]

Specific Groups and Settings

Persons Having Contact with Swine and Untreated Waste Water

Recently, a high prevalence of antibodies to HEV was found among persons who work with swine. Human populations with occupational exposure to certain animals have an increased risk of HEV infection. However, whether infection with swine HEV leads to clinical illness is unclear (see Symptoms, later).

Recently HEV RNA has been identified in a substantial proportion of untreated sewage samples in both non-endemic and endemic areas. However, sewage does not appear to be a source of HEV occupational infection in trained sewage workers who wear personal protective equipment and work in a region with good sanitation. However, this may not be true in other areas. One group found that 43.5% (20/46) of urban sewage samples collected in Barcelona, Spain, from 1994 to 2002 tested positive for HEV RNA.[79] In a study from India, anti-HEV IgG positivity was significantly higher among staff members of a sewage treatment plant (56.5%) when compared with controls (18.9%). A seven-fold higher risk of hepatitis E infection was recorded in sewage workers working in close proximity to sewage, whereas a 3.9-fold higher risk was noted in staff members not having frequent contact with sewage.[80]

HIV-Infected Persons

An association between anti-HEV seropositivity and human immunodeficiency virus (HIV) infection has been suspected. Up to one third of HIV-infected homosexual men are positive for IgG anti-HEV.[81] However, contrary observations have also been reported, showing that HEV infection does not seem to be prevalent in the HIV population.[82]

Transfusions and Other Healthcare Settings

Even in developed countries a small but significant proportion of blood donors with or without elevated alanine aminotransferase (ALT) levels are viremic and potentially able to cause transfusion-associated hepatitis E.[83] A few cases of transfusion transmission of hepatitis E virus (HEV) have been reported so far.[84] Thus precautions are needed to prevent transfusion-transmitted HEV infection. The safety of plasma-derived products with respect to HEV may be an important issue and each product should be evaluated for safety against HEV contamination. The sensitivity of HEV to heat has been shown to vary greatly depending on the heating conditions. On the other hand, the HEV particles are completely removed using 20-nm filters. However, each inactivation/removal step should be carefully evaluated with respect to the HEV inactivation/removal capacity, which may be influenced by processing conditions such as the stabilizers used for blood products.[85]

Anti-HEV IgG antibody prevalence has been found to be significantly higher in patients with hemophilia as compared with blood donors. HEV antibody was not detected in patients <20 years of age and in patients who had received only virus-inactivated coagulation factors. Thus parenteral transmission of HEV may occur in patients with hemophilia via non–virus-inactivated coagulation factors.[86] A higher prevalence of IgG anti-HEV in various other groups has been found, including patients with sickle cell anemia and beta-thalassemia major as well as persons working in emergency departments or in operating rooms, as determined in a German study.[87]

The prevalence rates of IgG anti-HEV are variably reported in hemodialysis patients and asymptomatic blood donors.[88] A significantly higher risk of HEV infection has been shown among patients subjected to chronic hemodialysis in endemic regions.[89]

HEV Infection as a Zoonosis

In addition to human beings, virologic evidence of mammalian HEV has been found in domestic pigs, wild boar, deer, mongoose, horse, and bivalves.[90] In most of these animals, the HEV identified was either genotype 3 or genotype 4. Antibodies to HEV (but not HEV RNA) have been detected in a wide range of domestic and feral mammals including cats, dogs, cattle, sheep, goats, macaques, donkeys, wild deer, rats, and mice.[90]

Evidence for differences in genotype virulence is not abundant. Based on experimental cross-infection data,[91] the genotype 3 strains are considered by some to be attenuated for human beings. There is little published evidence to date, however, of comparative assessments of the relative morbidity and mortality of travel-associated (genotype 1 or 2) and autochthonously acquired (genotype 3 or 4) hepatitis E. In reciprocal cross-infection trials using nonhuman primates and pigs, genotype 1 strains produced more severe pathology than genotype 3 strains.[91] There is also evidence from India that subtype differences might be responsible for the apparent inability of the genotype 4 HEV strains to infect human beings.[92] Investigators showed 26 amino acid substitutions of Indian HEV genotype 4 strains, compared with genotype 4 strains found in pigs and humans in China, Japan, and Taiwan.

The first evidence of a zoonotic source of autochthonous hepatitis E resulted from the observation in the United States that the partial nucleotide sequences of two pig and two human HEV strains were very closely related genotype 3 strains.[93,94] In many developed countries, compared with travel-related cases, the human autochthonously acquired cases showed the closest genetic homology to pig strains from the same region.[90] Additionally, high seroprevalences of HEV were reported in the pig herds of many countries, both developed and developing. Occupational exposure to pigs was also identified as a risk factor for hepatitis E in human beings. This evidence was not based on clinical cases, as there are only a few documented, but on reports of veterinarians and other pig industry workers who had a high HEV IgG seroprevalence.[90] The available data show that at any one time, more than 20% of pigs in pig production units are excreting HEV in feces,[95] and large quantities of HEV most probably enter watercourses as a consequence of runoff from outdoor pig farms. HEV has been detected in slurry lagoons on pig farms, from urban sewage works, and from pig slaughterhouses.[90] The risks of spreading untreated slurry on farmland remain unknown. However, HEV recovered from sewage and slurry has been shown to infect rhesus monkeys.[96]

The strongest evidence of zoonotic transmission of hepatitis E is from Japan, where consumption of uncooked or poorly cooked wild boar and deer meat resulted in hepatitis E infection in which identical viruses were recovered from the meat and from the patients.[97,98] Contamination of retail pig liver with HEV has been reported in many countries.[90] HEV has been found to be infective after heating to 56° C for 1 h, but was inactivated at an internal liver temperature of 71° C for 5 minutes,[99] which means that light cooking might not eliminate the risk of infection from contaminated meat. A provisional report using data from 1990 to 2000 shows that there is a relation between pork consumption and mortality from chronic liver disease in 18 developed countries.[100] Multivariate regression analysis showed that alcohol consumption, pork consumption, and hepatitis B virus (HBV) seroprevalence were all independent risk factors for death from chronic liver disease, but beef consumption was not. The reason for these observations is uncertain. It could be a result of factors in pig meat (e.g., pork fat) that cause cirrhosis. Another possible explanation is that an infectious agent found in pig meat causes increased mortality in patients with preexisting chronic liver disease.[100] A candidate for the latter hypothesis is HEV, because viable HEV has been found in pig meat in the human food chain,[101] and HEV superinfection in patients with chronic liver disease carries a high mortality (see Acute HEV Superinfection in Patients with Cirrhosis, later).

Despite the serologic, clinical, and molecular genetic evidence suggesting that autochthonous hepatitis E might be a porcine zoonosis, a direct connection between the disease and either consumption of pig meat or exposure to pigs is sparse.[102] Ingestion of infected animal tissue is one zoonotic transmission route, but the evidence indicates that several routes could be contributing to the burden of human HEV infections.[102]

Pathogenesis
Incubation Period

The incubation period from exposure to the onset of clinical disease is approximately 28 to 40 days, based on analysis of water-borne epidemics in which the time of exposure was identified.[103] In experimental HEV transmission studies in humans, liver enzyme values peak 42 to 46 days after ingestion of the virus.[2] In experimental infection of pregnant rhesus monkeys, the incubation period varied from 1 to 2 weeks to 4 to 5 weeks.[104,105]

Viral Replication

Knowledge of HEV replication is poor, because of the lack of practicable cell culture systems for the virus. Several strategies for experimental propagation and production of HEV to study the molecular biology have been reported, but their reproducibility and feasibility need confirmation (see Animal Models and in Vitro Culture, earlier).

Because HEV does not replicate well in cell culture, the mechanisms of HEV pathogenesis and replication are not fully understood. Our understanding of the replication and expression of HEV is based largely on recognized conservative motives of nonstructural domains and analogies with other positive-stranded RNA viruses. Studies in rats and swine suggest that extrahepatic tissues such as peripheral blood monocytes, spleen, lymph nodes, and the small intestine are involved in the replication of HEV.[48]

However, the main target cells are hepatocytes. A small amount of HEV is found in plasma during infection, consistent with the release of progeny virus through the basolateral domain of hepatocytes, leading to distribution through the liver. However, most of the virus appears to be excreted through the biliary system to complete the replication cycle, consistent with the release of the virus through the apical domain of hepatocytes. Bile appears to be the principal source of HEV in the feces.

Disease Progression

The incubation period in human volunteers after oral exposure is 4 to 5 weeks.[106] HEV can first be detected in stools approximately 1 week before the onset of illness and persists for an initial few weeks; however, in some patients positive reverse transcriptase polymerase chain reaction (RT-PCR) results persist for as long as 52 days.[107] HEV RNA has regularly been found in serum by RT-PCR in virtually all patients in the first 2 weeks after the onset of illness. Periods of HEV RNA positivity in serum range from 4 to 16 weeks.[107]

Although exposure to HEV is thought to occur usually via the oral route, the virus can be transmitted parenterally. Infection of nonhuman primates via the oral route has been successful in some (but not all) studies. In one study in which quantitative data were available, the infectivity titer of HEV as measured by intravenous inoculation was at least 10,000-fold higher than that obtained by oral administration.[108] Infection transmitted by the intravenous route is more reproducible than the oral route. After the intravenous inoculation of HEV in cynomolgus macaques, the average incubation period for acute hepatitis is about 3 weeks. After exposure (regardless of route), the first evidence of infection with HEV is found in the liver. Shortly thereafter, virus is detected in the blood, bile, and feces. The expression of hepatitis E antigen (HEAg) in hepatocytes, indicative of viral replication, first appears about day 7 after infection. HEAg can be detected simultaneously in hepatocytes, bile, and feces during the second or third week after inoculation, and before and concurrently with the onset of alanine aminotransferase (ALT) elevation and histopathologic changes in the liver.[109] The antigen can be detected in 70% to 90% of hepatocytes at peak expression and begins to decline after peak ALT activity has been reached. The peak shedding of virus into the blood and bile occurs before onset of clinical disease. The onset of clinical disease usually coincides with first detection of the humoral immune response, diminished replication of the virus, and the start of resolution of the infection. Both IgG and IgM class anti-HEV can usually be detected by the time liver enzymes become elevated and hepatic pathology becomes detectable.

Although a site of replication in the intestinal tract has not been identified, it is believed to exist. Nevertheless, bile is probably responsible for the distribution of virus in the intestinal tract. HEV replication in the liver is the initial event and a rise in serum ALT level and the presence of mild histologic injury at this time would be consistent with a direct cytopathic effect of the virus or an early immune-mediated effect. Later, hepatic HEAg becomes undetectable, indicating that viral replication has stopped, and during this time the histologic changes are more pronounced, suggesting that the injury at this time is primarily immune mediated. In support of this idea is the finding of infiltrating lymphocytes in the liver that have a cytotoxic immunophenotype.[110] The delayed appearance of anti-HEV (if true and not the result of insensitivity of antibody testing) suggests that antibody is not essential for initiating hepatocyte injury but may be important in perpetuating it. It is also possible that development of an antibody response occurs independently of hepatocyte injury. In summary, the mechanism of cell death is not known; however, early in the course of infection the mechanism may be predominantly direct cytopathic and later predominantly immune mediated.

In experimental infections of nonhuman primates, the clinical presentation of hepatitis E is dose dependent. Thus the severity of infection is directly related to the infectivity titer of the challenge virus, and consistent demonstration of hepatitis in experimentally infected nonhuman primates has required challenge doses at least 1000 times greater than the minimum dose needed for infection in humans.[111] It is not known whether such a clinical-to-infectious dose relationship exists for naturally infected humans; however, cycles of inapparent infection resulting from exposure to low doses of virus could explain how HEV can be maintained in a population with little or no clinical disease.

The disease is self-limiting and no chronic sequelae have been reported in general. However, recent reports present biochemical, histologic, and genetic evidence of chronic HEV infection in transplant patients (see Chronicity, later). It would be interesting to test other immunosuppressed persons, such as those with HIV infection, for their ability to resolve acute hepatitis E. Hepatitis E has a mortality rate of 0.2% to 1% in the general population. Increased morbidity and mortality is observed in chronic liver disease patients superinfected with HEV (see Acute HEV Superinfection in Patients with Cirrhosis, later). A unique clinical feature is HEV's increased incidence and severity in pregnant women, with mortality rates of 15% to 20% (see Pregnant Women, later). A role of endotoxin-mediated hepatocyte injury was proposed[112]; however, the precise cellular/molecular mechanisms are not clear. A shift in the Th1/Th2 balance towards Th2 has been observed in pregnant women infected with HEV compared with nonpregnant women[113]; however, the manner in which this influences the severity of HEV infection is not clear. Pregnant women with jaundice and acute viral hepatitis attributable to HEV showed higher mortality rates and worse obstetric and fetal outcomes than those with other types of viral hepatitis.[114] There were increased levels of estrogen, progesterone, and the β-subunit of human chorionic gonadotropin in HEV-positive pregnant patients with fulminant hepatitis compared with HEV-negative patients and controls.[115] Selective suppression of nuclear factor kappa B (NF-κB) p65 in pregnant compared with nonpregnant fulminant hepatitis patients has also been proposed to cause liver degeneration, severe immunodeficiency, and multiorgan failure.[116]

Immune Response

Specific IgM and IgG immune responses to HEV occur early in the infection, usually by the onset of clinical illness. In this respect, hepatitis E resembles hepatitis A, and a serologic diagnosis can usually be made at the time of presentation of the patient. In patients with hepatitis E, IgM anti-HEV begins to develop just before the peak of ALT activity and reaches a maximal titer around the time of maximal ALT activity. IgM anti-HEV disappears approximately 4 to 5 months into the convalescent phase of the disease. Of samples of sera collected from patients during various outbreaks of hepatitis E at 1 and 40 days, at 3 and 4 months, and at 6 and 12 months after the onset of jaundice, 100%, 50%, and 40%, respectively, were positive for IgM anti-HEV.[117] IgG antibodies develop shortly after the IgM antibodies, and the titers increase throughout the acute phase into the convalescent phase, remaining high from 1 to 5 years after resolution of the illness. IgG anti-HEV appears to diminish in titer at a more rapid rate than does antibody to hepatitis A, raising questions about the duration of immunity following acute hepatitis E. Anti-HEV has been detected as long as 13 to 14 years after infection; however, the possibility of repeated exposure cannot be dismissed.[118]

Antibody responses to individual viral antigens are highly variable, due to both strain-specific differences in some epitopes and differences in response to single antigens between individual patients. For example, after reaching high levels during the acute phase, HEV pORF2-specific IgG declines rapidly over 6 to 12 months and might not persist at protective levels for life.

Conversely, the responses to pORF3 are highly variable, with a proportion of patients mounting no detectable response to the antigen while others maintain reactivity to pORF3 for many years. Anti-HEV of the IgA class (as a correlate of mucosal immunity) has also been detected in the serum of about 50% of naturally infected individuals. These antibodies rapidly decline to undetectable levels and the significance of such antibodies is unknown. Because passive immunization with IgG appears to be sufficient for protection, it is likely that IgA is not essential.[119]

All isolates of HEV are serologically related, and convalescent antibody produced in response to infection with one strain of HEV probably protects against subsequent exposure to all other strains. Little is known about the cell-mediated immune response to HEV in humans. Recent evidence suggests that cellular immune responses do occur in patients with acute HEV infection. Lymphocytes of patients with acute hepatitis E show sensitization to HEV peptides. The specific T-cell response decreases along with convalescence and may play a role in the pathogenesis of acute hepatitis E and recovery.[120] A recent study assessed the frequency and activation status of natural killer (NK) and natural killer T (NKT) cells and the cytotoxic activity of NK cells in the peripheral blood mononuclear cells (PBMCs) obtained from patients with hepatitis E ($n = 41$) and healthy controls ($n = 61$). In 14 patients, the studies were repeated during the convalescence period. Patients had fewer median (range) NK cells (8.9% [2.4-47.0] vs. 11.2% [2.6-35.4]) and NKT cells (8.7% [2.8-34.1] vs. 13.6% [2.3-36.9]) than controls (P < 0.05 each). Activation markers were present on a large proportion of NK cells (43.5% [11.2-58.6] vs. 15.5% [3.0-55.8]) and NKT cells (41.5% [17.4-71.1] vs. 12.8% [3.3-63.2]; P < 0.05 each) from patients. NK cell cytotoxicity was similar in patients and controls. During convalescence, all the parameters normalized. Thus reversible alterations in NK and NKT cell number and activation status during acute hepatitis E suggest a role of these cells in the pathogenesis of this disease.[121]

Pathology

Studies of ET-NANBH epidemics occurring in developing countries have provided most of the information about the pathology of acute HEV infection.[122] The morphologic findings are of two main types: (1) typical acute hepatitis and (2) a cholestatic variant. In the latter, prominent features include bile stasis in canaliculi, glandlike transformation of hepatocytes, and extensive proliferation of small bile ductules. There is also prominent cholestasis in the centroacinar zone. Degenerative changes in hepatocytes and focal areas of necrosis are less common than in the noncholestatic type. Kupffer cells that contain lipofuscin granules are prominent. Portal tracts are expanded; polymorphonuclear leukocytes are conspicuous in the portal tract infiltrates, but lymphocytes predominate. Phlebitis of portal and central veins may be seen. Intralobular infiltrates consist mainly of polymorphonuclear leukocytes and macrophages. With the noncholestatic type of HEV infection, focal hepatocyte necrosis, ballooned hepatocytes, acidophilic degeneration of hepatocytes, and acidophilic body formation are common. An important morphologic feature is focal intralobular areas of hepatocyte necrosis with prominent accumulations of macrophages and activated Kupffer cells in the presence of lymphocytes. The histologic severity of the hepatitis is variable, but in one well-documented epidemic, 78% of biopsy specimens were graded as at least moderately severe. In fatal cases, severe acute hepatitis with submassive or massive hepatocyte necrosis is observed. No chronic histologic manifestations have been described in immunocompetent subjects.

In acute but nonfulminant cases of HEV infection, electron microscopy reveals considerable hepatocyte polymorphism. Some hepatocytes show ballooning degeneration and vesiculation of the perinuclear envelope and rough endoplasmic reticulum, whereas other hepatocytes show shrinking and condensation of cytoplasm and cell organelles to form a weblike pattern. The bile canaliculi are dilated, and intracanalicular and intracytoplasmic bile stasis is seen. In fulminant cases of HEV infection, hepatocytes display extensive organelle damage.

Recently some insight has been obtained on the pathology of autochthonous hepatitis E. Most patients with autochthonous hepatitis E do not require a liver biopsy because they have a self-limiting illness. A few patients will have more severe hepatitis with worsening liver blood tests and therefore a liver biopsy is sometimes helpful. There are few data on the hepatic histopathology of acute autochthonous hepatitis E, and such reports are limited to patients with severe disease. Liver histologic analysis of acute autochthonous hepatitis E in the noncirrhotic liver is similar to that seen in acute viral hepatitis, with lobular disarray with reticulin framework distortion. Portal tracts are expanded by a severe mixed polymorphic and lymphocytic inflammatory infiltrate. Moderate to severe interface hepatitis and cholangiolitis are also present.[123,124] In one study of three patients with autochthonous hepatitis E, polymorphs were shown to be concentrated at the periphery and interface of the liver, with lymphocytes—including aggregates—concentrated centrally.[125] These findings might be helpful in distinguishing autochthonous hepatitis E from other causes of hepatitis—for example, autoimmune hepatitis—but are based on a small number of cases and require confirmation. In patients with hepatitis E who have underlying cirrhosis, the liver histology is nonspecific and could easily be mistaken for alcoholic hepatitis in the context of established ethanolic cirrhosis.[126] These changes were much more marked than those seen in patients with HEV infections from endemic areas. In the small number of immunosuppressed transplant patients who have developed chronic infection with HEV, liver histologic examination displays progressive fibrosis and portal hepatitis with lymphocytic infiltration and piecemeal necrosis, with progression to cirrhosis.[127,128]

Clinical Features
Symptoms

Acute icteric hepatitis is the most common recognizable form of illness associated with HEV infection. Two phases of illness have been described: (1) a prodromal and preicteric phase and (2) an icteric phase. The prodromal phase, lasting about 1 to 4 days, is characterized by a variable combination of flulike symptoms, including fever, chills, abdominal pain, anorexia, nausea, aversion to smoking, vomiting, diarrhea, arthralgias, asthenia, and urticarial rash. These symptoms are followed within a few days by the appearance of jaundice. The onset of the icteric phase is usually heralded by the appearance of darkening of urine, and may be accompanied by pruritus or lightening of stool color. With the onset of jaundice, the fever and other prodromal symptoms tend to diminish and may entirely disappear. The exception is gastrointestinal symptoms, which may persist. The physical examination reveals jaundice and a mildly enlarged, soft, and slightly tender liver. Splenomegaly is seen in about 25% of patients.

In acute hepatitis, classical biochemical abnormalities are seen. Laboratory test abnormalities include a variable increase in serum bilirubin (predominantly conjugated) levels, markedly elevated levels of aminotransferases, and increased γ-glutamyltransferase levels, as well as a mild rise in serum alkaline phosphatase activity. An elevated ALT level often precedes the onset of symptoms by as much as 10 days and reaches a peak by the end of the first week, coinciding with the onset of the icteric phase. As the illness subsides, the ALT levels decrease significantly, followed by a decrease in serum bilirubin levels, which are usually normal by 6 weeks[128] (**Fig. 33-6**).

HEV RNA can be detected in the stool for up to 10 days after the onset of the icteric phase, although viral shedding for up to 52 days after the onset of icterus has been described.[107] HEV RNA can be detected in the serum during the preicteric phase and before the detection of virus in stool but becomes undetectable after the peak in serum aminotransferase activity. The detection of HEV RNA in the serum during the preicteric phase suggests that sporadic transmission of the virus may occur via the parenteral route.

The IgM antibody to HEV becomes detectable just before the peak ALT activity; peak antibody titers occur at approximately the same time as peak ALT levels and decline rapidly thereafter. In the majority of patients, IgM anti-HEV is undetectable 5 to 6 months after the onset of illness. IgG anti-HEV is detectable shortly after IgM anti-HEV becomes detectable, increases in titer throughout the acute and convalescent phases of infection, and remains detectable in most patients 1 year

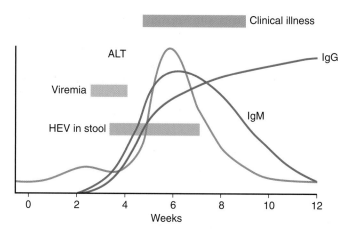

Fig. 33-6 Timeline of hepatitis E manifestations.

after acute infection. The duration of the IgG anti-HEV response is unknown, but high titers have been measured up to 14 years after acute infection.[118] The duration of protective immunity is not known; however, in the short term, there appears to be protection from reinfection. In nonfatal cases, acute hepatitis is followed by complete recovery without chronic sequelae. No evidence of chronic hepatitis or cirrhosis has been detected in immunocompetent patients who were followed clinically or underwent liver biopsy after being diagnosed with acute hepatitis E.[129]

Anicteric Hepatitis and Asymptomatic Infection

Some infected persons may develop nonspecific symptoms that resemble those of an acute viral febrile illness without jaundice (anicteric hepatitis). Liver involvement in these patients is only recognized after laboratory studies are performed. In its most benign form, HEV infection is entirely inapparent and asymptomatic and passes unnoticed. The exact frequency of anicteric hepatitis and asymptomatic infection is unknown, although it probably far exceeds that of icteric hepatitis. In areas of endemicity, anti-HEV is present in a large proportion of the population; most of these seropositive individuals do not recall being jaundiced and may have sustained an asymptomatic or anicteric infection. In most of the outbreaks of hepatitis E, the highest rate of clinically evident disease is among persons 15 to 40 years of age—a pattern that contrasts with HAV infection, in which children have the highest attack rates. The lower rate of disease among children may be the result of a higher frequency of asymptomatic or anicteric HEV infection in this age group.

Chronicity

Until very recently, chronic infection with HEV was considered nonexistent. The first indication of chronic infection with HEV was a recent report describing a Japanese patient with T-cell lymphoma receiving chemotherapy who was found to have persistent HEV viremia.[130] Chronic hepatitis E infection has been documented in patients receiving immunosuppressive therapy following organ transplantation.[126,127] In a French study of hepatitis E infection in solid organ transplant recipients, of the 14 patients who developed hepatitis E infection posttransplantation, 8 patients later developed chronic liver disease with a persistently raised transaminase concentration, persistent viremia, and progressive inflammation and fibrosis on liver biopsy.[127] The patients who developed chronic infection with HEV had more profound immunosuppression (lower levels of serum leukocytes, total lymphocytes, and CD4 lymphocytes) compared with the patients who did not progress to chronic infection. Several case reports have been presented on the occurrence of chronic hepatitis and cirrhosis caused by HEV infection in organ transplant recipients.[126,131] Recent case reports have appeared about persistent infection of hepatitis E virus in patients with lymphomas.[132] Chronic infection with hepatitis E virus may also occur in patients with HIV infection and may be associated with active hepatitis.[133] Chronic hepatitis E may also develop in post–liver transplant settings and needs to be considered in the differential diagnosis of posttransplant hepatitis.[134] Serologic testing may be unreliable in these contexts; PCR-based detection of hepatitis E viral RNA is essential to establish the diagnosis.[133]

Several issues deserve consideration before we add chronic hepatitis to the spectrum of diseases associated with HEV infection. First, the persistent HEV infection was observed in immunosuppressed patients. Such patients are known to have persistence of viral agents that are associated with a self-limited course in otherwise healthy persons, such as Epstein-Barr virus and cytomegalovirus. Thus the occurrence of chronic HEV infection in immunosuppressed patients may reflect a similar phenomenon, and may not occur in nonimmunosuppressed individuals. Also, finding persistent HEV viremia in such patients does not necessarily imply that HEV infection led to ALT level elevation or chronic liver disease. Future studies on persistent HEV infection in immunosuppressed patients should not only include patients with ALT level elevation and chronic liver injury but also incorporate patients with immunosuppression but normal ALT levels and no chronic liver injury, with the latter group serving as a comparison group to clarify the role of HEV infection in causing liver injury.[135]

Complications
Prolonged Cholestatic Hepatitis

In a few patients, the course of hepatitis E is prolonged, with marked cholestasis, persistent jaundice, and pruritus. In these cases, laboratory tests show an increase in alkaline phosphatase level and a persistent increase in bilirubin level, even after the concentrations of transaminases have returned to normal. The prognosis is good because the jaundice resolves spontaneously after 2 to 6 months. Recurrent (bimodal) hepatitis E has not been reported, except in experimentally infected nonhuman primates. In contrast, recurrent hepatitis A is relatively common.

Fulminant Hepatic Failure

The case-fatality rate in reports based on hospital data has ranged from 0.5% to 4%. However, the hospital-based data may overestimate mortality. Studies based on data obtained from population surveys during outbreaks have reported lower mortality rates, ranging from 0.07% to 0.6%.[136] In a small proportion of patients, the disease is more severe and associated with subfulminant or fulminant hepatic failure, which can be rapidly fatal. In regions of endemicity, HEV infection is an important cause of FHF.

Acute HEV Superinfection in Patients with Cirrhosis

Acute HEV superinfection in patients with cirrhosis produces decompensation and is associated with a high death rate. An Indian study[137] documented high rates of HEV superinfection in patients with cirrhosis, and these infections were a common cause of hepatic decompensation of otherwise stable cirrhotic patients in endemic areas. The mortality in these patients was higher at 4 weeks and 12 months when compared with cirrhotic patients without HEV superinfection. In another study,[138] HEV superinfection was a common cause of acute exacerbations in patients with an otherwise stable and asymptomatic chronic hepatitis B carrier state. In a study conducted in India,[139] acute on chronic liver failure occurred in 121 (3.75%) of 3220 patients (mean age, 36.3 ± 18.0 years; M/F ratio 85:36) with liver cirrhosis admitted from January 2000 to June 2006. Liver failure was due to HEV in 80 (61.1%), HAV in 33 (27.2%), and both HEV and HAV in 8 (6.1%) patients. Three-month mortality was 54 patients (44.6%).[140] In areas of high endemicity, the large majority of adult chronic liver disease patients are vulnerable to infection with HEV, but are protected against hepatitis A. This group would be an ideal candidate for an HEV vaccine. In developed countries also, locally acquired hepatitis E infection in a cirrhotic patient can result in liver failure and death.[125]

Pregnant Women

Pregnant women, particularly those in the second and third trimesters, are more frequently affected during hepatitis E outbreaks and have a worse outcome. In fact, the major cause of mortality in epidemics is the high rate of FHF in pregnant women. In a recent study from India,[114] pregnant women with HEV infection had higher maternal mortality rates and worse obstetric and fetal outcomes than did pregnant women with jaundice and acute hepatitis caused by other hepatitis viruses (Table 33-2). This confirmed earlier observations of increased incidence and severity of HEV infection in pregnancy, in which death rates approach 15% to 20%. In an earlier study,[140] pregnant women with fulminant hepatitis caused by HEV had shorter duration of illness, lower serum bilirubin levels, shorter preencephalopathy period, and high occurrence of disseminated intravascular coagulation (DIC). Considering the explosive nature of HEV in pregnancy with DIC, it was postulated to represent a severe manifestation of a Schwartzman-like phenomenon. Several studies have documented high rates of vertically transmitted intrauterine and newborn HEV infections causing high fetal mortality attributable to fulminant hepatitis. The disease in this age group presented with hypoglycemia, hypothermia, and death. In another study,[141] data pointed to a relationship between severity of HEV infection in the mother and the fetus. It was postulated that severe fetal infections and fetal death may produce toxins that overload maternal circulation, causing severe maternal

Table 33-2 Maternal Mortality and Medical Complications in Acute HEV–Infected Pregnant Women

VARIABLE	HEV-INFECTED WOMEN (n = 132), n/n (%)	NON–HEV–INFECTED WOMEN (n = 88), n/n (%)	RELATIVE RISK (95% CI)	P VALUE
Maternal mortality rate				
Overall	54/132 (41)	6/88 (7)	6.0 (2.7–13.3)	<0.001
Patients with fulminant hepatic failure	54/73 (74)	6/18 (33)	2.2 (1.1–4.3)	0.001
Second trimester	18/27 (66)	0/7 (0)	–	0.002
Third trimester	36/46 (78)	6/11 (54)	1.4 (0.8–2.5)	0.11
Patients without fulminant hepatic failure	0/59 (0)	0/70 (0)	–	1.00
Medical complications				
Coagulation defect*	104/132 (79)	32/88 (36)	2.2 (1.6–2.9)	<0.001
Nasal or gastrointestinal hemorrhage	25/132 (19)	4/88 (4)	4.2 (1.5–11.6)	0.002
Leukocyte count ≥11 × 10⁹ cells/L	86/132 (65)	31/88 (35)	1.8 (1.4–2.5)	<0.001
Serum creatinine concentration ≥34 μmol/L (≥2 mg/dL)	39/132 (30)	4/88 (4)	6.5 (2.4–17.5)	<0.001
Ascites	33/132 (25)	5/88 (6)	4.4 (1.8–10.8)	<0.001
Clinical signs of increased intracranial tension	27/132 (20)	1/88 (1)	18.0 (2.5–130.1)	<0.001

From Patra S, et al. Maternal and fetal outcomes in pregnant women with acute hepatitis E virus infection. Ann Intern Med 2007;147:28–33.
*International normalized ratio >2.0.
HEV, hepatitis E virus

disease. Mothers who delivered infected babies within the first few days of infection recovered from fulminant disease, and those in whom pregnancy continued with fetal death often had a fatal outcome.

Co-Infection of HEV with Other Hepatotropic Viruses

Co-infection with multiple hepatotropic viruses occurs in various combinations in 7% to 24% of all cases of sporadic acute viral hepatitis (AVH). The most common combination is HAV and HEV co-infection.[142,143] Simultaneous infection with multiple hepatotropic viruses in the disease states of both AVH and FHF does not adversely affect the outcome. Total serum bilirubin level is significantly lower with multiple infections than with single infection for both AVH and FHF. Multiple hepatotropic viral infection thus seems to produce less cholestatic illness and equal, if not better, outcomes as compared with single virus infection. Whether this represents a phenomenon of mutual viral suppression or viral restitution occurring in multiple virus infections requires further studies.[143] Another study reported that dual infection with hepatotropic viruses was associated with greater elevation of both aspartate aminotransferase and alanine aminotransferase levels.[144]

Other Complications

Other reported complications include Guillain-Barré syndrome, transverse myelitis, Bell's palsy, hemolysis (both immune and nonimmune), thrombocytopenia, and acute pancreatitis, which can be severe.

Autochthonous HEV in Developed Countries

The clinical features of autochthonous hepatitis E infection range from asymptomatic infection to mild hepatitis to subacute liver failure.[102] In a United Kingdom hospital-based study of patients with unexplained hepatitis, 40 patients with autochthonous hepatitis E were identified, of whom 75% were icteric.[63] The incubation period of autochthonous hepatitis E infection ranges from 2 to 9 weeks. The presentation of HEV in individuals infected in developed countries seems to be similar to that shown by infected individuals from endemic regions; however, the mortality rate is higher, ranging from 8% to 11%. Peak viremia occurs during the incubation period and the early acute phase of disease. Immediately before the onset of clinical symptoms HEV RNA can be detected in the blood and stool. The concentration of serum liver enzymes rises, with a predominant transaminitis, peaking at about 6 weeks' postexposure before falling to normal levels by week 10. The abnormality in serum liver enzyme concentrations at presentation is variable; with the exception of the few patients who develop liver failure, the increase in levels of serum transaminases and bilirubin usually peaks at presentation. A few days to weeks after the onset of clinical symptoms, HEV RNA is cleared from the blood; however, the virus continues to be shed in stool for another 2 weeks.[102] The period of viremia can be very brief in some patients. It is probable that most infections are asymptomatic or anicteric, or both. This would account for the discrepancy between the perceived rarity of clinically apparent infections and the relatively high anti-HEV IgG seroprevalence in some developed countries.

Compared with hepatitis E infections in the developing world, in developed countries most autochthonous hepatitis

E infections are reported in middle-aged and elderly men.[102] Similar to endemic regions, secondary and intrafamilial distribution has rarely been reported. Most autochthonous HEV infections are self-limiting; however, comprehensive follow-up studies showed that approximately 15% of patients developed complications.[145] Moreover, 8% to 11% of HEV-infected patients develop fulminant hepatitis and liver failure. The outcome can be poor in those individuals with underlying chronic liver disease, with mortality approaching 70%.[146,147] Autochthonous hepatitis E in developed regions is frequently misdiagnosed as drug-induced liver injury, a common problem that occurs with increased frequency in elderly people. A retrospective analysis showed that 21% of 28 patients who met the standard criteria for drug-induced liver injury did not have the condition, but instead suffered from autochthonous hepatitis E.[148]

Clinical Significance of HEV Genotype

It is generally believed that the severity of hepatitis E infection depends on host factors of the infected patient, such as pregnancy, chronic liver disease, and advancing age. However, similar to other known hepatitis viruses, viral factors may play a role in the pathogenesis of HEV-associated fulminant hepatitis. Recent studies in Japan suggest that the severity of hepatitis E is affected by the genotype of HEV, based on the finding that patients infected with genotype 4 HEV tend to have more severe disease, including FHF, than those infected with genotype 3 HEV.[149] It has been suggested that genotype 4 had a higher HEV load in the circulation than genotype 3, based on a case with co-infection with both genotypes.[150] If this is common for HEV virions circulating in humans, it may explain why patients with genotype 4 appear to have a higher incidence of fulminant hepatitis than those with genotype 3. However, more data will be needed with studies conducted in other countries to draw a plausible conclusion regarding the relationship between the severity of hepatitis E and the genotype of the virus.

Diagnosis and Detection of HEV

Diagnosis of HEV infection in individual patients remains problematic. Although HEV particles have been visualized by electron microscopy in the stools of infected humans and there has been recent progress with cell culture, the routine laboratory diagnosis of hepatitis E depends on serologic and nucleic acid amplification techniques. Tests for the diagnosis of HEV infection are based either on the detection of the virus or viral components or on serologic tests determining a virus-specific immune response in the host.

Approaches to HEV Detection

Virus or Viral Component Detection

Virus isolation is not appropriate for HEV because it is largely refractory to routine isolation in cell culture. The first assay for detection of HEV infection used IEM to detect viral particles in feces.[151] This provides a specific diagnostic marker but has very poor sensitivity and is technically demanding.

Conventional and real-time RT-PCR assays have been used to detect HEV RNA in clinical specimens (mainly blood) and seem to be more sensitive than serologic studies for hepatitis E diagnosis.[152] Assuming that contamination can be excluded, a positive result proves HEV infection and allows for further study, including sequencing and genotyping of the infecting virus. However, the window of detectable HEV viremia is narrow, continuing for a mean of 28 days (range, 17 to 48 days) after the onset of symptoms.[55] Because patients might not present until some time after the onset of illness, a negative result does not exclude infection. Two highly sensitive and specific real-time PCR assays (TaqMan chemistry and primer-probe energy transfer [PriProEt] techniques) have been developed to detect a wide range of HEV variants and simultaneous detection of all known four genotypes.[153] HEV antigen may have a role for diagnosis during the window period before seroconversion to anti-HEV occurs.[154]

Serologic Assays

Most primary serologic testing uses an enzyme immunoassay (EIA) format, although rapid immunochromatographic assays have been developed,[155] which make it feasible to perform testing at a location close to the patient or field. A small number of commercial EIA assays are in general use and several "in-house" EIA assays have been developed. These assays use recombinant antigens derived from different strains of HEV. This diversity of strains should not affect the accuracy of the assays because different genotypes appear to constitute a single serotype upon serologic testing.

Enzyme-linked immunosorbent assay (ELISA) kits based on ORF2 of HEV have been reported to have broad activity and reproducible results and are better than kits using a combination of ORF2 and ORF3. The presence of anti-HEV IgM is the marker of recent HEV infection, but the sandwich and indirect ELISA methods for detecting anti-HEV IgM have two disadvantages. One is the reduced sensitivity caused by competition among virus-specific IgM, IgA, and IgG for antigen-binding sites. Another disadvantage is that IgM-rheumatoid factor in sera from patients with rheumatoid arthritis presumably induced false-positive results. A class-capture enzyme immunoassay that eliminates the competing IgG and IgA antibodies at the beginning of the assay, enhancing the reaction between anti-HEV IgM and HEV antigen, has been introduced.[156] Although the IgG class of antibody against HEV (anti-HEV IgG) is generally only used as the postinfectious index, detection of newly elicited anti-HEV IgG also can be the proof needed to diagnose acute HEV infection. Specific IgG is usually produced early in infection and concentrations rise rapidly afterwards. Estimates of the duration of the IgG response and immunity to subsequent infection vary, with durations from 6 months to 14 years having been reported. Anti-HEV IgG is generally used in epidemiologic investigation and as the postinfectious index because of its long duration. However, anti-HEV IgG does not exist throughout an individual's lifetime; thus the positive rate of anti-HEV IgG in a population cannot completely reflect the postinfection rate.

The anti-HEV IgG avidity index has also been suggested for differentiation between acute infection and previous exposure to HEV, especially in countries of low endemicity. Defined as the strength with which the IgG attaches to antigen, IgG avidity matures with the length of time following primary infection. Thus, IgG produced with the first few months following primary infection exhibits low avidity, whereas IgG produced several months or years later exhibits high avidity. The IgG avidity index was high (>60%) in patients with previous infection or polyclonal activation but was low (<40%) in patients with acute infection. The IgG avidity index can therefore be used to exclude primary infection. This method should improve the diagnosis of acute hepatitis E.[157]

Anti-HEV IgA can be a useful supplementary marker for recent HEV infection. In one study[158] it was found that the duration of anti-HEV IgA was longer than that of anti-HEV IgM. The positive rate of anti-HEV IgA in acute HEV infection patients was 100%, 100%, 97%, 93%, 63%, and 30% in the second week and in months 1, 2, 3, 4, and 5 after disease onset, respectively. The positive rate of anti-HEV IgM was 100%, 100%, 77%, 57%, 20%, and 3% in the second week and in months 1, 2, 3, 4, and 5, respectively.[158] In another study, the specificity of anti-HEV IgA assay was 99.6%. Among 245 acute hepatitis E patients, 84 samples from 84 patients were positive for HEV RNA. The positive rate of anti-HEV IgA, anti-HEV IgM, and anti-HEV IgG in 84 samples positive for HEV RNA was 96.3%, 97.6%, and 88.1%, respectively, and no sample was negative for anti-HEV IgA and anti-HEV IgM simultaneously. Among 245 acute hepatitis E patients, 9 samples collected from 9 patients in the acute period were negative for anti-HEV IgM but positive for anti-HEV IgA and 2 samples were positive for HEV RNA. Anti-HEV IgM and anti-HEV IgA may individually be falsely positive but the specificity of combined detection was 100%.[159] However, 84 serum samples positive for HEV RNA in this study all were of genotype 4 HEV. The significance of anti-HEV IgA in other genotype HEV infection remains to be clarified. Herremans and colleagues[160] reported IgA responses were more prominent in the patients with genotype 1 HEV infection compared with those with genotype 3 infection, but the differences between genotype 1– and genotype 3–infected patients could be explained by the use of the homologous genotype 1 antigens in the assay.

Although only one serotype of HEV has been reported, the immunoreactivities of polypeptides from various HEV genotype isolates are different.[161] Therefore it is necessary to synthesize various polypeptides from various HEV genotype isolates to clarify the significance of anti-HEV antibodies. Thus detection of anti-HEV IgA can be a useful supplement for diagnosis of acute HEV infection, especially in patients negative for anti-HEV IgM.[159]

Laboratory Diagnosis

The diagnosis of acute hepatitis E infection thus relies on demonstration of the presence of specific IgM, rising levels of IgG, or detection of HEV RNA. A pragmatic case definition of acute hepatitis E is a patient who has one or more of these features and a substantially raised serum transaminase concentration, similar to that shown for acute hepatitis.[102] This definition will miss some cases but is easy to apply and is rarely falsely positive. Other strategies under evaluation include IgA serology, anti-HEV IgG avidity index, and confirming positive EIA serology with an immunoblot assay,[162] although this produces some equivocal results.

Differential Diagnosis

Acute hepatitis E cannot be clinically distinguished from other forms of acute viral hepatitis. As a result of their identical clinical presentations and modes of transmission, hepatitis E may be suspected in the same circumstances as hepatitis A. Although hepatitis A is more common than hepatitis E in developed countries, in endemic areas HEV is often the most common cause of acute hepatitis. In a patient with symptoms and biochemical evidence of acute hepatitis, serologic tests for excluding acute hepatitis A (IgM anti-HAV), hepatitis B (hepatitis B surface antigen [HbsAg], IgM, and hepatitis B core antibody [anti-HBc]), hepatitis C (anti-HCV), cytomegalovirus, and Epstein-Barr virus are performed. In non-endemic areas, suspicion of acute HEV should be heightened by a history of travel to areas endemic for HEV. In endemic areas, an outbreak may be associated with a common contaminated water source, and such information should be obtained. In endemic areas, infection with HEV may be seen in association with other hepatotropic viruses (A, B, and C), and in the absence of specific anti-HEV testing, the diagnosis of acute HEV co-infection or superinfection may be missed.

Natural History

In nonfatal cases, acute hepatitis is followed by complete recovery without chronic sequelae. Under certain circumstances chronicity can occur (see earlier section, "Chronicity"). There appears to be protection from reinfection for a time; however, the duration of this protection is unknown. Long-term serologic studies will be needed to determine the duration of protective immunity and the nature of the anamnestic response.

Therapy and General Management

Like other forms of acute viral hepatitis, the mainstay of therapy is to monitor for the development of complications and provide good nutrition. The HEV infection is usually self-limited, and no specific therapeutic interventions are available. Rarely, if fulminant hepatitis develops intensive management and options of liver transplantation should be considered.

Currently there is no antiviral treatment that is effective against HEV. RNA interference (RNAi) is a natural mechanism for suppressing or silencing expression of aberrant or foreign genes. It is a powerful antiviral strategy that has been widely employed to protect hosts from viral infection. The nonstructural polyprotein region of HEV possesses an RNA-dependent RNA polymerase (RdRp) that is responsible for the replication of the viral RNA genome. RdRp is therefore regarded as an attractive candidate for RNA interference (RNAi). HEV-specific siRNA (siRNA-RdRp-1) is capable of inhibiting the HEV expression and replication both in vitro in A549 cells and in vivo in piglets. In piglets treated with a shRNA-RdRp-1 expression plasmid before HEV inoculation, levels of HEV antigens were significantly reduced in the liver, spleen, and kidneys, and the activities of alanine aminotransferase (ALT), aspartate aminotransferase (AST), and total bilirubin were clearly decreased. These results suggest that RNAi is a potentially effective antiviral strategy against HEV replication and infection.[163]

Prevention

General Measures

Improved sanitation is important in controlling diseases that have fecal–oral transmission as a prominent part of their epidemiology. Industrialized countries with a generally high level of public sanitation do not experience epidemics of waterborne hepatitis E. Effective prevention relies primarily on maintaining a clean drinking water supply and paying strict attention to sewage disposal, because immunoprophylaxis is not currently available. Many epidemics in developing countries have occurred as a result of leakage of sewage pipes into municipal water supply pipes laid in the same or adjacent trenches. A barrier between these two supplies is essential for long-term prevention. During an epidemic, steps to improve water quality can lead to rapid abatement of the occurrence of new cases. During an epidemic in India, failure to chlorinate water was followed by a rapid rise in the number of cases, and reinstitution led to rapid abatement of the epidemic.[73] Because the virus is transmitted by the fecal–oral route, it must withstand exposure to bile salts during excretion and low pH during ingestion, but it is generally considered to be more labile than hepatitis A. Boiling water appears to inactivate HEV effectively. Chlorination may be ineffective in the presence of large amounts of organic matter (e.g., in water contaminated with feces).

Travelers to endemic areas must take precautions against the consumption of contaminated water. They should be advised to avoid drinking water or beverages from sources of unknown purity. Only boiled or bottled water should be used. Although infection via food is much less common for hepatitis E than for hepatitis A, it is important to maintain caution about contaminated food and avoid eating uncooked shellfish, or eating uncooked and unpeeled fruits and vegetables. Women should avoid unnecessary travel to endemic areas during pregnancy. Isolation of affected persons is not indicated because person-to-person transmission is uncommon. However, infected persons should not be involved in food preparation or handling until their symptoms have fully resolved.[12]

Passive Immunoprophylaxis

Although four genotypes of HEV have been identified, only one serotype has been described. In experimental studies in primates, passive transfer of anti-HEV has been shown to reduce virus shedding in feces and abrogate disease when given to nonhuman primates challenged with a high dose of homologous HEV.[164] Thus immunoglobulin (Ig) preparations similar to those used for protection against hepatitis A would be efficacious against hepatitis E. However, no reduction in disease rates could be shown in pre- or postexposure prophylaxis studies among recipients of Ig preparations manufactured in hepatitis E endemic areas.[165] Failure of Ig preparations to protect against HEV in humans may reflect the low titers of IgG anti-HEV in Ig preparations derived from persons living in endemic areas. Ig prepared in non-endemic countries would be expected to have even lower levels of anti-HEV and hence would be of little benefit as preexposure prophylaxis for travelers to endemic areas. Therefore pooled normal human Ig is unlikely to be useful as an immunoprophylactic agent against HEV and the protective role of anti-HEV antibodies in humans requires further study. The occurrence of large hepatitis E epidemics among adults in disease-endemic areas suggests either that anti-HEV antibody may not be fully protective or that antibody levels decline with time and gradually reach an unprotective level.

As an alternative, an Ig preparation consisting of HEV-neutralizing monoclonal antibodies (MAbs) might protect against hepatitis E.[166] Clinical trials of MAbs have not been conducted and further work is necessary before a definitive role of immune serum globulin can be discerned.

Active Immunoprophylaxis

Although four HEV genotypes and significant geographic genome variability have been described, all HEV subtypes share major cross-reactive epitopes, prompting the development of a recombinant HEV (rHEV) vaccine based on the capsid protein.[71] The HEV genome contains three ORFs. ORF1 encodes nonstructural protein(s); therefore ORF1 protein(s) would not be a target for humoral immunity. ORF3 overlaps with ORF1 and ORF2 and encodes a small protein of unknown function but significant antigenicity. However, unlike antibody to ORF2, antibodies to ORF3 do not neutralize virus in in vitro assays. ORF2 encodes the capsid protein and, because the ORF2 protein is the major protein in the virion, it has been the focus of vaccine development.

The various options for a vaccine include attenuated or killed virus vaccine, recombinant protein–based vaccine, and nucleic acid–based vaccines. The development of an attenuated or killed virus vaccine is not currently feasible, because an efficient cell culture system for HEV does not exist. Therefore either a recombinant protein–based or a nucleic acid–based vaccine is needed. Most work has focused on recombinant vaccines.

Recombinant Protein Vaccines

Several recombinant ORF2 antigens of different lengths have been expressed using a variety of expression systems and have been shown to induce anti-ORF2 antibody responses. Although many truncated versions of the ORF2 protein have been expressed, purified, and tested for immunogenicity and efficacy, the size and nature of the native protein in HEV virions remain elusive.

Proteins Expressed in *Escherichia coli*

Only two of the proteins expressed in *E. coli* have shown promise as vaccine candidates, the rest being useful as diagnostic reagents.

The first of these, TrpE-C2, contained a 221- to 660-aa carboxy-terminal fragment of the ORF2 protein of a Burmese strain (genotype 1) of HEV fused to tryptophan synthetase.[167] In preclinical challenge experiments, two cynomolgus macaques vaccinated with the recombinant TrpE-C2 protein were challenged with wild-type homologous (genotype 1) or heterologous (genotype 2) HEV. The animal receiving homologous challenge showed no evidence of HEV infection.

However, the animal challenged with a heterologous Mexican strain of HEV became infected as demonstrated by viremia, viral excretion, and increase in anti-HEV antibody levels; however, the animal did not develop biochemical or histologic evidence of hepatitis.

Another candidate, pE2, was expressed as a glutathione-*S*-transferase (GST) fusion protein containing amino acids 394-660 of the ORF2 protein from a Chinese isolate.[168] Following its purification and cleavage from the GST partner, the pE2 polypeptide was found to self-associate into a dimer. The dimeric form of the protein was efficiently recognized by convalescent human sera from patients with hepatitis E, and antibodies to it successfully recognized HEV in an immune capture assay.[168] Cynomolgus macaques vaccinated with pE2, but not control animals, showed efficient seroconversion and no infection following challenge with the homologous virus.[169]

Another candidate, called HEV239, contains ORF2 amino acids 376-606.[170] This consists of 23-nm particles that dissociate under mild denaturing conditions into homodimers that react strongly with acute and convalescent sera of hepatitis E patients and HEV-specific monoclonal antibodies. In primate studies, this vaccine was found to provide protection against HEV genotypes 1 and 4, and sera from vaccinated animals neutralized infectivity of HEV in vitro.[170]

Proteins Expressed in Insect Cells

The recombinant ORF2 proteins produced using baculovirus vectors in insect cells have been pursued vigorously as candidate vaccines. In this system, the 72-kDa ORF2 protein of a Pakistani HEV strain (SAR55) is rapidly processed into smaller proteins of 63, 56, and 53 kDa. Of these, the 56-kDa form accumulates in the cytoplasm of insect cells, whereas the 53-kDa form is secreted as viruslike particles (VLPs).[171] The recombinant 56-kDa ORF2 protein was found to be an efficient immunogen in monkeys when given with an alum adjuvant.[111] Furthermore, the vaccinated animals were protected from intravenous challenges with high doses of both homologous and heterologous strains of HEV.[111]

A 62-kDa recombinant ORF2 protein from a Burmese HEV strain produced in insect cells has also been tested in monkeys.[172] Two 20-μg doses of an alum-adjuvanted preparation were shown to protect cynomolgus macaques against challenge by a heterologous HEV strain. Similarly, insect cells expressing the ORF2 protein of the Burmese strain of HEV secreted VLPs consisting of a 50-kDa protein.[173] Whether this protein and the 53-kDa secreted protein produced from insect cells expressing the SAR55 ORF2 protein are identical is not known. These VLPs have been found to induce both systemic and mucosal anti-HEV responses when administered orally to mice.[174] Cynomolgus macaques orally vaccinated with these VLPs, without any added adjuvant, have recently been shown to raise systemic and mucosal anti-HEV antibody responses.[175] Furthermore, these animals were fully protected against infection and hepatitis following an intravenous challenge with HEV.[175] These results raise the possibility of developing an oral recombinant hepatitis E vaccine.

All the baculovirus-mediated ORF2 protein expression and purification studies have been carried out in either Sf21 or Tn5 insect cell lines. Recently intact *Spodoptera litura* larvae have also been used for this purpose.[176] A recombinant baculovirus was engineered to express a truncated ORF2 antigen from an Indian strain of HEV. This contained amino acids 112-660 with an inframe deletion of a hydrophobic region between residues 585 and 610. High levels of the recombinant ORF2 antigen were expressed and found to accumulate in the larval fat bodies within 5 days of virus injection into fourth-instar *S. litura* larvae. The recombinant protein could be purified to homogeneity in an estimated yield of 0.2 mg per larva.[176]

Proteins Expressed in Other Systems

A C-terminal peptide of ORF2 encompassing amino acids 551-607 has been expressed on chimeric VLPs formed by the hepatitis B surface antigen (HBsAg) in the methylotropic yeast *Pichia pastoris*.[177] The VLPs showed reactivity to human sera containing antibodies against HBV as well as those with anti-HEV antibodies, and are being explored as a recombinant HBV/HEV bivalent vaccine candidate. ORF2 antigens 69-660 and 112-660 have also been expressed independently in *P. pastoris*, and the purified proteins have been shown to induce high-titer antibodies in rhesus monkeys.[178]

The 23-kDa ORF2 antigen (pE2; residues 394-604) has also been expressed in transgenic tomato plants.[179] The expression levels of the protein in this system were, however, quite low.[179]

DNA Vaccines

Direct injection of plasmid DNA has been shown to cause intracellular synthesis of immunizing viral antigens, as well as induction of humoral and cellular immune responses. Vaccination with HEV ORF2 expression constructs has been shown to elicit anti-HEV antibodies[180] and immunologic memory in mice.[181] These antibody responses can be augmented by co-delivery of genes for the immunomodulatory cytokines interleukin 2 and granulocyte-macrophage colony stimulating factor.[180] Cynomolgus macaques vaccinated with an ORF2 expression construct were protected from virus challenge only when the DNA was administered with a gene gun and not when it was given as an intradermal injection.[181] Although DNA vaccines have obvious advantages of stability and ease of preparation, much work remains on the mode of delivery and characterization of immune responses.[182]

Neutralizing Antibody Assays

An enzyme-linked immunosorbent assay (ELISA) for putative neutralizing antibodies to HEV has been developed that detects antibodies to all four genotypes of the virus.[183] Although this test has been used with sera from experimentally inoculated macaques, it remains to be evaluated in a human field situation. An ELISA based on truncated forms of the ORF2 protein has also been developed to differentiate between vaccination and infection.[182] At this time, vaccination of cynomolgus or rhesus macaques and their subsequent challenge with homologous and heterologous HEV strains appear to be the best model for assaying the potential efficacy of a candidate vaccine. The in vitro assays for neutralizing antibodies against HEV and the full-length infectious clones of HEV may, in the future, provide tools for quicker and easier assessment of the protective efficacy of the induced antibodies.[182]

Clinical Trials

Two candidate HEV vaccines produced with truncated structural proteins have reached clinical trials. One of the vaccines (aa 112-607) is expressed in insect cells.[184] A genotype 1 HEV recombinant protein (rHEV) vaccine, which provided protection in nonhuman primates, was found to be immunogenic in humans. These results prompted a phase II clinical trial of the vaccine's efficacy in volunteers from the Nepalese Army, a population at high risk for hepatitis E. A total of 1794 subjects (898 in the vaccine group and 896 in the placebo group) received 3 vaccine doses; the total vaccinated cohort was followed for a median of 804 days. After 3 vaccine doses, hepatitis E developed in 69 subjects, of whom 66 were in the placebo group. The vaccine efficacy was 95.5% (95% confidence interval [CI], 85.6 to 98.6). In an intention-to-treat analysis that included all 87 subjects in whom hepatitis E developed after the first vaccine dose, 9 subjects were in the vaccine group, with a vaccine efficacy of 88.5% (95% CI, 77.1 to 94.2). Thus this vaccine was found to be safe and immunogenic for humans and could also protect against hepatitis E.[185] Yet, some questions about the "true" efficacy remain unanswered. Studies from rhesus monkeys revealed that rHEV may protect from clinical disease, but not from HEV infection.[186] Similar to the study conducted by Shrestha and colleagues, only symptomatic subjects were screened for HEV infection; the potential number of asymptomatic cases, who could potentially carry and spread the virus, is unknown.[187] The duration of protection by the rHEV vaccine is also unclear; whereas 100% of screened rHEV-vaccinated subjects had high antibody titer 1 month after the third vaccination (81% after the second vaccination), only about 56% had HEV antibodies at the end of the study, about 1.5 years after the third dose.[188]

The other vaccine is expressed in bacteria (HEV239 vaccine) and it is more extensively truncated (aa 376-606) than the insect cell–expressed vaccine.[189] The vaccine consists of 23-nm viruslike particles that are strongly reactive with acute and convalescent sera from hepatitis E patients and are recognized by a panel of HEV-specific murine monoclonal antibodies, including at least two neutralizing antibodies.[190] It evoked a vigorous T-cell–dependent antibody response in mice, and this was partly attributed to its particulate nature and at least two T-cell epitopes locating to aa 533-552.[191] The vaccine was found to confer protection on nonhuman primates against infection by genotypes 1 and 4 HEV, and sera from vaccinated animals were found to neutralize infectivity of the virus for the animals.[192] A randomized controlled phase II clinical trial of the vaccine was conducted in southern China and it was found that the vaccine is safe and immunogenic for humans. A course consisting of three 20-μg doses of the vaccine induced 100% seroconversion. The mean antibody level of 15.9 units/ml induced by the vaccine was lower than that of 43.4 units/ml determined for the pooled serum from hepatitis E patients, but markedly higher than that of 0.76 unit/ml in the pooled sera from seropositive subjects. The results reflect the response by subjects who had not been previously infected by HEV and had not been significantly confounded by new HEV infection occurring during the course of the study. The significant reduction in frequency of new infection occurring after receipt of the second vaccine dose suggests that vaccination could prevent HEV infection.[193]

Recently, a randomized, double-blind, placebo controlled, phase 3 trial that assessed the efficacy and safety of the recombinant HEV vaccine (HEV 239), in the general population (men and women 16-65 years) has been reported from China.[194] Three doses of vaccine or placebo were given intramuscularly at 0, 1, and 6 months. Participants were randomly assigned to vaccine (n = 56 302) or placebo (n = 56 302) and were followed up for 19 months. Vaccine efficacy for participants who received at least one dose was 95.5% (95% CI 66.3 – 99.4). Vaccine efficacy after two doses was 100%. Of the 13 patients with acute hepatitis E whose viruses were isolated for sequencing, 12 had genotype 4 and one had genotype 1. Thus, in this study, vaccine was effective in general population of healthy men and women (aged 16–65 years). The vaccine cross protected against genotype 4 in human beings, and the cross protection may also extend to other genotypes as well, because they belong to the same serotype as the vaccine strain. However, many issues still remain unanswered. The authors did not study the HEV infection rate, the focus was instead on clinical disease rate. The duration of protection afforded by this vaccine also remains unknown. Safety in pregnant women, people younger than 15 years or older than 65 years and chronic liver disease remains to be seen.

Even if HEV vaccine becomes available, there are several issues to be considered. First issue is which group of subjects could benefit from such a vaccine. The majority of HEV-related diseases are benign. However, HEV infection in patients with chronic liver disease can cause severe hepatic decompensation. Also, pregnant women and children older than 2 years of age have worse outcomes. Therefore, vaccination of these patients would be desirable. Also, international travelers to endemic regions would likely benefit from the vaccine. Vaccination could also have a role in HEV outbreaks. Vaccination has been found to be beneficial under less than perfect circumstances (i.e., when participants do not receive all three doses). Vaccine efficacy after two doses is 100.0%. Therefore, during a hepatitis E outbreak, or for travelers to an endemic area, protection can be quickly obtained by two vaccine doses given within 1 month. The second issue is the length of the vaccine-mediated protection. Whether long-term immunity to hepatitis E is achieved through vaccination when it wanes off following natural infection, is unknown. Also, the titre of the protective antibodies remains unanswered. The third issue is whether the vaccine offers protection only against symptomatic disease or also against HEV infection. If the vaccine does not protect against HEV infection, then the vaccine is not expected to make any major impact on the epidemiology of HEV infection in the endemic regions. However, in clinical situations, protection from symptomatic disease and the resulting liver damage (that may lead to fulminant hepatic failure or acute on chronic liver failure), may be a desirable goal. In such situations, the vaccine may still be useful despite its failure to prevent the infection. It is also not known whether the vaccine can be used for post-exposure prophylaxis. This assumes importance, if the vaccine is to be offered for controlling an outbreak of HEV infection. In outbreaks, the exposure to the infection may have has already occurred, before the identification of the outbreak. An issue which relates more to public health and policy issue is the availability and distribution of the vaccine especially in resource poor countries which may need the vaccine the most. Experience in resource-poor countries has shown that hepatitis B vaccine is not readily available to the population at risk even decades after its introduction. The cost of vaccine, infrastructure and manpower for delivery and maintenance of a cold chain will remain critical issues.[195]

Improved sanitation is important in controlling diseases that have fecal–oral transmission as a prominent part of their epidemiology. Industrialized countries with a generally high level of public sanitation do not experience epidemics of waterborne hepatitis E. Effective prevention relies primarily on maintaining a clean drinking-water supply and paying strict attention to sewage disposal. Vaccines should never be considered a substitute for, or reason to delay, basic improvements in overall sanitation. However, the rates of improvement of sanitary conditions in many areas of Asia and Africa have been dismal, and HEV vaccine might be helpful in the interim.[195]

Summary, Conclusions, and Perspective for the Future

Hepatitis E is an emerging disease. It is estimated that about 2 billion people live in areas endemic for this disease. The virus has four genotypes with one serotype: genotypes 1 and 2 exclusively infect humans, whereas genotypes 3 and 4 also infect other animals, particularly pigs. In endemic areas, both large outbreaks of acute hepatitis as well as sporadic cases occur frequently. These cases are usually due to genotype 1 or 2 HEV and are predominantly caused by fecal–oral transmission, usually through contamination of drinking water; contaminated food, maternal–fetal (vertical spread), and parenteral routes are less common modes of infection. The acute hepatitis caused by this virus has the highest attack rates in young adults and the disease is particularly severe among pregnant women. HEV superinfection can occur among persons with preexisting chronic liver disease. In non-endemic regions, locally acquired disease was believed to be extremely uncommon. However, in recent years, an increasing number of cases, mostly attributable to genotype 3 or 4 HEV, have been recognized. These are more often elderly men who have other co-existing illnesses, and appear to be related to zoonotic transmission from pigs, wild boars, and deer, either foodborne or otherwise. Also, chronic infection with genotype 3 HEV has been reported among immunosuppressed persons in these regions.

Molecular epidemiologic studies suggested that the genetic changes and invasion of particular HEV strains may contribute to the genetic variability of HEV in the community. However, further clinical, epidemiologic, and virologic studies are needed to elucidate the extent of genomic heterogeneity of HEV strains circulating in the world, the various and possibly region-dependent modes of HEV transmission, and the association of HEV genotype with disease severity and its underlying mechanism.

The inability to reproducibly culture hepatitis E virus makes it impossible to develop traditional live or inactivated vaccines. However, significant progress has been made in developing and testing recombinant subunit vaccines based on the viral capsid protein, and a vaccine is likely to be available soon. It would be a boon for select groups of individuals such as pregnant women, patients with preexisting liver disease, and foreign travelers. HEV infection remains a major health problem worldwide. It has only recently received adequate attention, and we anticipate that the next decade will provide major developments in our understanding of both its pathogenesis and its prevention/treatment with specific antiviral drugs and vaccines.

Key References

Aggarwal R. Hepatitis E: does it cause chronic hepatitis? Hepatology 2008;48: 1328–1330. (Ref.135)

Aggarwal R, Jameel S. Hepatitis E vaccine. Hepatol Int 2008;2:308–315. (Ref.182)

Aggarwal R, Naik S. Epidemiology of hepatitis E: current status. J Gastroenterol Hepatol 2009;24:1484–1493. (Ref.59)

Arankalle VA, et al. Challenge studies in Rhesus monkeys immunized with candidate hepatitis E vaccines: DNA, DNA-prime-protein-boost and DNA-protein encapsulated in liposomes. Vaccine 2009;27:1032–1039. (Ref.186)

Bigaillon C, et al. Use of hepatitis E IgG avidity for diagnosis of hepatitis E infection. J Virol Methods 2010;164:127–130. (Ref.157)

Bouwknegt M, et al. Bayesian estimation of hepatitis E virus seroprevalence for populations with different exposure levels to swine in the Netherlands. Epidemiol Infect 2008;136:567–576. (Ref.96)

Chandra V, et al. Molecular biology and pathogenesis of hepatitis E virus. J Biosci 2008;33:451–464. (Ref.4)

Chen HY, et al. Comparison of a new immunochromatographic test to enzyme-linked immunosorbent assay for rapid detection of immunoglobulin M antibodies to hepatitis E virus in human sera. Clin Diagn Lab Immunol 2005;12:593–598. (Ref.155)

Chobe LP, Lole KS, Arankalle VA. Full genome sequence and analysis of Indian swine hepatitis E virus isolate of genotype 4. Vet Microbiol 2006;114:240–251. (Ref.92)

Dalton HR, et al. Hepatitis E: an emerging infection in developed countries. Lancet Infect Dis 2008;8:698–709. (Ref.102)

Dalton HR, et al. Persistent carriage of hepatitis E virus in patients with HIV infection. New Engl J Med 2009;361:1025–1027. (Ref.133)

Dalton HR, Bendall RP, Pritchard C. Pig meat consumption and mortality from chronic liver disease. Gut 2008;57(Suppl 1):A76. (Ref.100)

Dalton HR, et al. The role of hepatitis E virus testing in drug-induced liver injury. Aliment Pharmacol Ther 2007;26:1429–1435. (Ref.148)

Dalton HR, et al. Locally acquired hepatitis E in chronic liver disease. Lancet 2007;369:1260. (Ref.146)

Dalton HR, et al. Autochthonous hepatitis E in Southwest England: natural history, complications and seasonal variation, and hepatitis E virus IgG seroprevalence in blood donors, the elderly and patients with chronic liver disease. Eur J Gastroenterol Hepatol 2008;20:784–790. (Refs.63,145)

Emerson SU, Arankalle VA, Purcell RH. Thermal stability of hepatitis E virus. J Infect Dis 2005;192:930–933. (Ref.6)

Emerson SU, et al. ORF3 protein of hepatitis E virus is not required for replication, virion assembly, or infection of hepatoma cells in vitro. J Virol 2006;80:10457–10464. (Ref.21)

Feagins AR, et al. Detection and characterization of infectious hepatitis E virus from commercial pig livers sold in local grocery stores in the USA. J Gen Virol 2007;88:912–917. (Ref.101)

Feagins AR, et al. Inactivation of infectious hepatitis E virus present in commercial pig livers sold in local grocery stores in the United States. Int J Food Microbiol 2008;123:32–37. (Ref.99)

Galiana C, et al. Occupational exposure to hepatitis E virus (HEV) in swine workers. Am J Trop Med Hyg 2008;78:1012–1015. (Ref.95)

Graff J, et al. The open reading frame 3 gene of hepatitis E virus contains a cis-reactive element and encodes a protein required for infection of macaques. J Virol 2005;79:6680–6689. (Ref.22)

Graff J, et al. A bicistronic subgenomic mRNA encodes both the ORF2 and ORF3 proteins of hepatitis E virus. J Virol 2006;80:5919–5926. (Ref.20)

Graff J, et al. Mutations within potential glycosylation sites in the capsid protein of hepatitis E virus prevent the formation of infectious virus particles. J Virol 2008;82:1185–1194. (Ref.18)

Guu TS, et al. Structure of the hepatitis E virus-like particle suggests mechanisms for virus assembly and receptor binding. Proc Natl Acad Sci USA 2009;106:12992–12997. (Ref.10)

Gyarmati P, et al. Universal detection of hepatitis E virus by two real-time PCR assays: TaqMan and primer-probe energy transfer. J Virol Methods 2007;146: 226–235. (Ref.153)

Haagsma EB, et al. Chronic hepatitis E virus infection in liver transplant recipients. Liver Transpl 2008;14:547–553. (Ref.126)

Hagedorn CH. Phylogenetic analysis of global hepatitis E virus sequences: genetic diversity, subtypes and zoonosis. Rev Med Virol 2006;16:5–36. (Ref.36)

He S, et al. Putative receptor-binding sites of hepatitis E virus. J Gen Virol 2008; 89:245–249. (Ref.7)

He S, et al. Putative receptor-binding sites of hepatitis E virus. J Gen Virol 2008; 89:245–249. (Ref.33)

Herremans M, et al. Use of serological assays for diagnosis of hepatitis E virus genotype 1 and 3 infections in a setting of low endemicity. Clin Vaccine Immunol 2007;14:562–568. (Ref.162)

Herremans M, et al. Detection of hepatitis E virus-specific immunoglobulin A in patients infected with hepatitis E virus genotype 1 or 3. Clin Vaccine Immunol 2007;14:276–280. (Ref.160)

Huang F, et al. Effective inhibition of hepatitis E virus replication in A549 cells and piglets by RNA interference (RNAi) targeting RNA-dependent RNA polymerase. Antiviral Res 2009;83:274–281. (Ref.163)

Huang F, et al. Experimental infection of Balb/c nude mice with hepatitis E virus. BMC Infect Dis 2009;9:93. (Ref.50)

Ijaz S, et al. Non-travel-associated hepatitis E in England and Wales: demographic, clinical, and molecular epidemiological characteristics. J Infect Dis 2005;192:1166–1172. (Ref.64)

Ippagunta SK, et al. Presence of hepatitis E virus in sewage in Northern India: frequency and seasonal pattern. J Med Virol 2007;79:1827–1831. (Ref.60)

Jilani N, et al. Hepatitis E virus infection and fulminant hepatic failure during pregnancy. J Gastroenterol Hepatol 2007;22:676–682. (Ref.115)

Jothikumar N, et al. A broadly reactive one-step real-time RT-PCR assay for rapid and sensitive detection of hepatitis E virus. J Virol Methods 2006;131: 65–71. (Ref.152)

Kamar N, et al. Hepatitis E virus and chronic hepatitis in organ-transplant recipients. New Engl J Med 2008;358:811–817. (Ref.127)

Kannan H, et al. The hepatitis E virus open reading frame 3 product interacts with microtubules and interferes with their dynamics. J Virol 2009;83(13): 6375–6382. (Ref.28)

Khuroo MS, Khuroo M. Association of severity of HEV infection in the mother and vertically transmitted infection in fetus (letter to Editor, rapid response). Ann Intern Med 2007;147:33. (Ref.141)

Krawczynski K. Hepatitis E vaccine—ready for prime time? New Engl J Med 2007;356:949–951. (Ref.187)

Kumar AS, et al. Hepatitis E virus (HEV) infection in patients with cirrhosis is associated with rapid decompensation and death. J Hepatol 2007;46:387–394. (Ref.137)

Kumar AS, et al. Does co-infection with multiple viruses adversely influence the course and outcome of sporadic acute viral hepatitis in children? J Gastroenterol Hepatol 2006;21:1533–1537. (Ref.143)

Kumar M, Sharma BC, Sarin SK. Hepatitis E virus as an etiology of acute exacerbation of previously unrecognized asymptomatic patients with hepatitis B virus-related chronic liver disease. J Gastroenterol Hepatol 2008;23:883–887. (Ref.138)

Lee CC, et al. Prevalence of antibody to hepatitis E virus among haemodialysis patients in Taiwan: possible infection by blood transfusion. Nephron Clin Pract 2005;99:c122–c127. (Ref.89)

Li SW, et al. A bacterially expressed particulate hepatitis E vaccine: antigenicity, immunogenicity and protectivity on primates. Vaccine 2005;23:2893–2901. (Refs.170,189)

Li TC, et al. Essential elements of the capsid protein for self-assembly into empty virus-like particles of hepatitis E virus. J Virol 2005;79:12999–13006. (Ref.8)

Li W, et al. Experimental infection of Mongolian gerbils by a genotype 4 strain of swine hepatitis E virus. J Med Virol 2009;81:1591–1596. (Ref.49)

Lockwood GL, et al. Hepatitis E autochthonous infection in chronic liver disease. Eur J Gastroenterol Hepatol 2008;20:800–803. (Ref.125)

Madejón A, et al. Lack of hepatitis E virus infection in HIV patients with advanced immunodeficiency or idiopathic liver enzyme elevations. J Viral Hepat 2009;16:895–896. (Ref.82)

Malcolm P, et al. The histology of acute autochthonous hepatitis E virus infection. Histopathology 2007;51:190–194. (Ref.124)

Mansuy JM, et al. High prevalence of anti-hepatitis E virus antibodies in blood donors from South West France. J Med Virol 2008;80:289–293. (Ref.83)

Matsubayashi K, et al. A case of transfusion-transmitted hepatitis E caused by blood from a donor infected with hepatitis E virus via zoonotic food-borne route. Transfusion 2008;48:1368–1375. (Ref.84)

Meng XJ. Hepatitis E virus: animal reservoirs and zoonotic risk. Vet Microbiol 2010;140:256–265. (Ref.90)

Mitsui T, et al. Distinct changing profiles of hepatitis A and E virus infection among patients with acute hepatitis, patients on maintenance hemodialysis and healthy individuals in Japan. J Med Virol 2006;78:1015–1024. (Ref.88)

Mizuo H, et al. Possible risk factors for the transmission of hepatitis E virus and for the severe form of hepatitis E acquired locally in Hokkaido, Japan. J MedVirol 2005;l76:341–349. (Ref.149)

Moin SM, et al. The hepatitis E virus ORF3 protein stabilizes HIF-1alpha and enhances HIF-1-mediated transcriptional activity through p300/CBP. Cell Microbiol 2009;11:1409–1421. (Ref.31)

Moin SM, Panteva M, Jameel S. The hepatitis E virus Orf3 protein protects cells from mitochondrial depolarization and death. J Biol Chem 2007;282: 21124–21133. (Ref.27)

Myint KS, et al. Hepatitis E antibody kinetics in Nepalese patients. Trans R Soc Trop Med Hyg 2006;100:938–941. (Ref.66)

Okamoto H. Genetic variability and evolution of hepatitis E virus. Virus Res 2007;127:216–228. (Ref.40)

Ollier L, et al. Chronic hepatitis after hepatitis E virus infection in a patient with non-Hodgkin lymphoma taking rituximab. Ann Intern Med 2009;150: 430–431. (Ref.132)

Pal R, et al. Immunological alterations in pregnant women with acute hepatitis E. J Gastroenterol Hepatol 2005;20:1094–1101. (Ref.113)

Patra S, et al. Maternal and fetal outcomes in pregnant women with acute hepatitis E virus infection. Ann Intern Med 2007;147:28–33. (Ref.114)

Peron JM, et al. Fulminant liver failure from acute autochthonous hepatitis E in France: description of seven patients with acute hepatitis E and encephalopathy. J Viral Hepat 2007;14:298–303. (Ref.147)

Peron JM, et al. Liver histology in patients with sporadic acute hepatitis E: a study of 11 patients from southwest France. Virchows Arch 2007;450:405–410. (Ref.123)

Pischke S, et al. Hepatitis E virus infection as a cause of graft hepatitis in liver transplant recipients. Liver Transpl 2010;16:74–82. (Ref.134)

Prusty BK, et al. Selective suppression of NF-κBp65 in hepatitis virus-infected pregnant women manifesting severe liver damage and high mortality. Mol Med 2007;13:518–526. (Ref.116)

Radha Krishna Y, et al. Clinical features and predictors of outcome in acute hepatitis A and hepatitis E virus hepatitis on cirrhosis. Liver Int 2009;29: 392–398. (Ref.139)

Ratra R, Kar-Roy A, Lal SK. The ORF3 protein of hepatitis E virus interacts with hemopexin by means of its 26 amino acid N-terminal hydrophobic domain II. Biochemistry 2008;47:1957–1969. (Ref.24)

Ratra R, Kar-Roy A, Lal SK. ORF3 protein of hepatitis E virus interacts with the Bbeta chain of fibrinogen resulting in decreased fibrinogen secretion from HuH-7 cells. J Gen Virol 2009;90(Pt 6):1359–1370. (Ref.26)

Rehman S, et al. Subcellular localization of hepatitis E virus (HEV) replicase. Virology 2008;370:77–92. (Ref.34)

Sailaja B, et al. Outbreak of waterborne hepatitis E in Hyderabad, India, 2005. Epidemiol Infect 2009;137:234–240. (Ref.58)

Sarin SK, Kumar M. Hepatitis E. In: Boyer T, Manns M, Wright TL, editors. Zakim & Boyer's hepatology: a textbook of liver disease, 5th ed., Philadelphia: Saunders, 2007: 693–724. (Ref.12)

Schildgen O, Müller A, Simon A. Chronic hepatitis E and organ transplants. New Engl J Med 2008;358:2521–2522. (Ref.131)

Sehgal D, et al. Expression and processing of the hepatitis E virus ORF1 nonstructural polyprotein. Virol J 2006;3:38 (Ref.14)

Shrestha MP, et al. Safety and efficacy of a recombinant hepatitis E vaccine. New Engl J Med 2007;356:895–903. (Ref.185)

Srivastava R, et al. Alterations in natural killer cells and natural killer T cells during acute viral hepatitis E. J Viral Hepat 2008;15:910–916. (Ref.121)

Stoszek SK, et al. Hepatitis E antibody seroconversion without disease in highly endemic rural Egyptian communities. Trans R Soc Trop Med Hyg 2006;100: 89–94. (Ref.68)

Surjit M, Jameel S, Lal SK. The ORF2 protein of hepatitis E virus binds the 5′ region of viral RNA. J Virol 2004;78:320–328. (Ref.19)

Surjit M, Jameel S, Lal SK. Cytoplasmic localization of the ORF2 protein of hepatitis E virus is dependent on its ability to undergo retrotranslocation from the endoplasmic reticulum. J Virol 2007;81:3339–3345. (Ref.17)

Surjit M, et al. Enhanced alpha1 microglobulin secretion from hepatitis E virus ORF3-expressing human hepatoma cells is mediated by the tumor susceptibility gene 101. J Biol Chem 2006;281:8135–8142. (Ref.30)

Tacke F, Trautwein C. Efficient recombinant hepatitis E virus vaccine: mission accomplished? Hepatology 2007;46:941–943. (Ref.188)

Takahashi M, et al. Prolonged fecal shedding of hepatitis E virus (HEV) during sporadic acute hepatitis E: evaluation of infectivity of HEV in fecal specimens in a cell culture system. J Clin Microbiol 2007;45:3671–3679. (Ref.55)

Tamura A, et al. Persistent infection of hepatitis E virus transmitted by blood transfusion in a patient with T-cell lymphoma. Hepatol Res 2007;37:113–120. (Ref.130)

Tanaka T, et al. Development and evaluation of an efficient cell-culture system for hepatitis E virus. J Gen Virol 2007;88:903–911. (Ref.54)

Tian DY, Chen Y, Xia NS. Significance of serum IgA in patients with acute hepatitis E virus infection. World J Gastroenterol 2006;12:3919–3923. (Ref.158)

Toyoda H, et al. Prevalence of hepatitis E virus IgG antibody in Japanese patients with hemophilia. Intervirology 2008;51:21–25. (Ref.86)

Tyagi S, Surjit M, Lal SK. The 41-amino-acid C-terminal region of the hepatitis E virus ORF3 protein interacts with bikunin, a kunitz-type serine protease inhibitor. J Virol 2005;79:12081–12087. (Ref.29)

Wu T, et al. Difference of T cell and B cell activation in two homologous proteins with similar antigenicity but great distinct immunogenicity. Mol Immunol 2007;44:3261–3266. (Ref.191)

Wu T, et al. Specific cellular immune response in hepatitis E patients. Intervirology 2008;51(5):322–327. (Ref.120)

Yamada K, et al. ORF3 protein of hepatitis E virus is essential for virion release from infected cells. J Gen Virol 2009;90(Pt 8):1880–1891. (Ref.32)

Yunoki M, et al. Extent of hepatitis E virus elimination is affected by stabilizers present in plasma products and pore size of nanofilters. Vox Sang 2008;95:94–100. (Ref.85)

Zaki Mel S, et al. Hepatitis E virus coinfection with hepatotropic viruses in Egyptian children. J Microbiol Immunol Infect 2008;41:254–258. (Ref.144)

Zhang J, et al. Analysis of hepatitis E virus neutralization sites using monoclonal antibodies directed against a virus capsid protein. Vaccine 2005;23:2881–2892. (Ref.190)

Zhang J, et al. Randomized-controlled phase II clinical trial of a bacterially expressed recombinant hepatitis E vaccine. Vaccine 2009;27:1869–1874. (Ref.193)

Zhang S, et al. Clinical significance of anti-HEV IgA in diagnosis of acute genotype 4 hepatitis E virus infection negative for anti-HEV IgM. Dig Dis Sci 2009;54:2512–2518. (Ref.159)

Zhang S, et al. Clinical significance of anti-HEV IgA in diagnosis of acute genotype 4 hepatitis E virus infection negative for anti-HEV IgM. Dig Dis Sci 2009;54:2512–2518. (Ref.119)

Zhao C, et al. Relationships among viral diagnostic markers and markers of liver function in acute hepatitis E. J Gastroenterol 2009;44:139–145. (Ref.154)

A complete list of references can be found at www.expertconsult.com.

Liver Disease Associated with Viral Infections

Ulrich Spengler, Hans-Peter Fischer, and Wolfgang H. Caselmann

ABBREVIATIONS

AIDS acquired immunodeficiency syndrome
ALT alanine aminotransferase
AST aspartate aminotransferase
CCHF Crimean-Congo hemorrhagic fever
CMV cytomegalovirus
DEN1 to DEN4 dengue virus serotypes 1 through 4
DHF dengue hemorrhagic fever

DSS dengue shock syndrome
EBV Epstein-Barr virus
ELISA enzyme-linked immunosorbent assay
HAART highly active antiretroviral therapy
HHV human herpesvirus
HIV human immunodeficiency virus
HSV herpes simplex virus

IgG immunoglobulin G
IgM immunoglobulin M
PTLD posttransplant lymphoproliferative disease
RT-PCR reverse transcription polymerase chain reaction
SARS severe acute respiratory syndrome
TTV torquetenovirus
VZV varicella-zoster virus

The liver is a major blood-filtering organ and consequently is predisposed to blood-borne infections causing infectious hepatitis. Viral infections tend to affect the liver in particular, and because of their high affinity for the liver, a subgroup of viruses is termed hepatitis viruses. This group is covered in separate chapters of this book. Here, we summarize other viral infections that do not primarily target the liver but can cause viral hepatitis as part of a systemic infection or lead to hepatic complications under certain conditions, such as immunodeficiency. Of course, this chapter cannot replace a clinical textbook on viral infections but instead focuses on the hepatic aspects of viral infections.

Infections caused by viruses other than the hepatitis viruses can roughly be classified into three major categories: liver disease in patients with fever returning from tropical and subtropical areas, which is frequently caused by exotic agents; severe liver damage in patients with immunodeficiency as a result of de novo infection or exacerbations of common agents such as herpesviruses or adenoviruses; and liver involvement in patients with respiratory and systemic infections, frequently mediated via immunologic mechanisms.

Viral Hemorrhagic Fevers

Approximately 8% of travelers to the developing world require medical care during or after travel, and fever is the underlying problem in 28% of them.[1,2] Physicians evaluating returned travelers with fever frequently suspect rare or exotic diagnoses. Travel-associated liver disease caused by exotic infections such as Ebola virus, Rift Valley fever, or Lassa fever has been reported sporadically in the literature but currently does not represent a frequent health problem. Of the identified causes, dengue is among the top three etiologic agents, and it accounts for approximately 6% of febrile illnesses in travelers.[2] Of note, although malaria is the leading cause of systemic febrile illness worldwide, travelers from every tropical or subtropical region except sub-Saharan Africa and Central America have confirmed or suspected dengue more frequently than malaria. Chikungunya is an emerging novel viral infection that has recently been reported in Asia and Africa to cause fever with prominent myalgia, arthralgia, and rash in increasing numbers of patients.[3]

Viral hemorrhagic fevers share some epidemiologic and clinical features and cause rather similar liver pathology. Most viruses are transmitted via arthropod vectors. The various viruses cause damage to small vessels in multiple organs, which frequently leads to overt hemorrhage. The spectrum of diseases and their geographic distribution are listed in **Table 34-1**. Much attention has been paid to abnormal liver function and altered hepatic pathology. Nevertheless, clinically significant liver disease and death from liver failure are rare complications except in patients with yellow fever.

Dengue Fever

The dengue virus complex consists of four antigenically related but distinct flaviviruses termed dengue virus serotypes 1 through 4 (DEN1 to DEN4).[4] Dengue viruses are transmitted by *Aedes aegypti* mosquitos in epidemic and endemic

Table 34-1 Viral Hemorrhagic Fevers Affecting the Liver

DISEASE	VIRUS GROUP	GEOGRAPHIC REGION
Dengue	Flaviviridae	Africa, Asia, tropical America
Yellow fever	Flaviviridae	Africa, South America
Lassa fever	Arenaviridae	West Africa
Argentine hemorrhagic fever (Junin virus)	Arenaviridae	Argentina
Ebola fever	Filoviridae	Central and western Africa
Marburg fever	Filoviridae	Central and southern Africa
Rift Valley fever	Bunyaviridae	East and central Africa
Congo-Crimea hemorrhagic fever	Bunyaviridae	Former Soviet Union, central-western Asia, Africa
Hemorrhagic fever with renal syndrome	Bunyaviridae	Northern Eurasia
Chikungunya	Togaviridae	West Africa, Asia, Oceania, southern Europe

outbreaks and cause acute infections. Three to 6 days after a mosquito bite the virus spreads via the bloodstream, and among the various organs it can be isolated frequently from liver samples,[5] where dengue viral antigens have been detected in Kupffer cells, sinusoidal endothelial cells, and hepatocytes.[6,7] Dengue virus infection usually causes a flulike illness with a rash—dengue fever. Hepatomegaly and elevated serum aminotransferases, which are usually mild, are common in dengue virus infections.[8,9] Clinically more severe diseases, such as dengue hemorrhagic fever (DHF) and dengue shock syndrome (DSS), can follow secondary infection with dengue virus of a different serotype, thus suggesting that immune responses generated during previous exposure to dengue viruses may enhance the damage triggered by secondary dengue infection. In DHF there are widespread petechial hemorrhages together with multiple organ damage; in DSS, which mostly affects children younger than 15 years, there is extensive capillary leakage and severe fluid depletion leading to hypovolemic shock. If untreated, mortality approaches 50%. In fatal cases of DHF the liver is enlarged, is pale as a result of steatosis, and shows multifocal hemorrhages. Microscopically, focal hepatocellular necrotic areas are seen, as well as coalescent perivenular and midzonal necrosis with Councilman bodies, but relatively little inflammatory cell infiltration.[10,11] It is supposed that liver injury is mediated by dengue virus infection of hepatocytes and Kupffer cells, as in vitro infection of a human hepatoma cell line with dengue virus has been shown to induce apoptotic cell death.[12]

Currently, a vaccine against dengue virus is not available, and treatment is supportive, with DSS requiring intensive care.

Yellow Fever

Yellow fever is the prototype member of the Flaviviridae family, a group of plus-strand, single-stranded RNA viruses. The yellow fever virus has a single conserved serotype and seven major genotypes reflecting distinct regions in western Africa, central-east Africa, and South America.[13,14] Yellow fever virus is transmitted by a variety of different *Aedes* vectors and causes endemic and epidemic outbreaks in Africa and South America. Approximately 200,000 cases of yellow fever are currently still reported per year, with 90% occurring in Africa. Yellow fever in travelers to Africa and South America has become rare since the introduction of routine vaccination.

The spectrum of infection with yellow fever virus ranges from subclinical infection to a life-threatening disease with fever, jaundice, renal failure, and hemorrhage. Usually, yellow fever initially appears as an acute, flulike illness of sudden onset with fever, myalgia, and headache that cannot easily be distinguished from other acute infections.[15] Between 48 and 72 hours after onset, serum aminotransferases start to rise, thus heralding the development of jaundice. The degree of liver abnormalities at this stage predicts the severity of liver disease later during the course of the illness.[16] Next, a period of remission lasting up to 48 hours may follow the initial infection. Patients with abortive infection recover at this stage, but approximately 15% of patients will enter the third stage of intoxication, which is characterized by the return of fever, prostration, and organ dysfunction leading to nausea, vomiting, epigastric pain, jaundice, oliguria, and a hemorrhagic diathesis. Yellow fever differs from all other viral causes of hepatitis by the fact that serum aspartate aminotransferase (AST) levels exceed those of alanine aminotransferase (ALT). Aminotransferase levels are proportional to the severity of disease.[16] Direct bilirubin levels range between 5 and 10 mg/dl, with levels being higher in those with fatal infection than in recovering patients. The diagnosis of yellow fever is confirmed by the serologic demonstration of specific IgM by enzyme-linked immunosorbent assay (ELISA), by polymerase chain reaction (PCR), or by isolation of the virus from blood. Liver biopsy is not recommended because of a high risk for hemorrhage.

The outcome of infection with yellow fever virus is determined during the second week after onset, when many patients recover rapidly, but between 20% and 50% of the patients who have progressed to the stage of intoxication will ultimately die of circulatory shock. Convalescence may be associated with fatigue for several weeks, and in some cases jaundice and elevated aminotransferase levels may persist for months.

Liver pathology varies according to the stage of the disease. In fatal cases, approximately 80% of hepatocytes undergo coagulative necrosis. The midzone of the liver lobule is affected, with sparing of cells neighboring the central vein and portal tracts.[17] Very high viral loads have been detected in liver samples from patients who died, and viral antigen is located at the midzone of the hepatic lobule, thus indicating that this is the site of direct viral injury.[18] Liver injury is characterized by eosinophilic degeneration and the presence of Councilman bodies. Rarely, intranuclear inclusion bodies (Torres bodies) are present. Fatty changes may be prominent. In specimens from surviving patients, the liver shows ballooned hepatocytes and regenerative hyperplasia with multiple multinucleated hepatocytes and some portal inflammation consisting mainly of CD4[+] T cells and smaller numbers of natural killer and CD8[+] T cells.[19,20] Biopsy specimens from survivors during the recovery phase may show a nonspecific acinar hepatitis.[21] However, the hepatic reticular architecture is not disrupted, and in nonfatal cases healing is complete without any residual postnecrotic fibrosis.

Antiviral activity against yellow fever has been demonstrated for several nucleosides and plant alkaloids.[22] Ribavirin inhibits yellow fever virus in vitro, but only at extremely high concentrations that cannot be achieved in vivo. Thus treatment is supportive. A highly active attenuated live vaccine is available that induces seroconversion rates of greater than 95% and provides a high level of protection. This vaccine should not be given to pregnant women and immunosuppressed individuals because of concern about the risk associated with live attenuated virus vaccines. Infrequently, two serious vaccine-related complications may also occur in immunocompetent persons: a form of encephalitis termed yellow fever–associated neurotropic disease and a syndrome resembling natural infection that is designated yellow fever vaccine–associated viscerotropic disease.

Lassa Fever

Lassa virus is an enveloped, single-stranded, bisegmented RNA virus that belongs to the Arenaviridae family. Its natural reservoir is the multimammate rat, *Mastomys natalensis*, which excretes the virus through urine, saliva, and other secretions.[23] Humans presumably become infected directly via contact with infected rodent excreta through the fecal–oral route or inhalation of contaminated air.[24] The risk of human–human transmission is low.[25,26] Serologic evidence demonstrates that the infection is widespread in western Africa, but clinically overt disease occurs in fewer than 10% and overall mortality is 1%. Increasing international travel has sporadically resulted in importation of Lassa fever to Western countries, which challenges the diagnostic skills of physicians.[27]

At onset, the infection is insidious, with fever, myalgia, headache, and malaise.[28] More specific features include ulcerations in the oral cavity, bleeding from the gums, sore throat, cough, pleurisy, and watery diarrhea. There is lymphadenopathy and swelling of the liver and kidney, which become painful on palpation.[29] Serum aminotransferase levels rise, but jaundice is not present. In Lassa fever the liver has a mottled appearance, and liver histology shows necrosis without inflammation. Single hepatocytes or groups of cells stain acidophilic and are found to harbor abundant arenaviruses under electron microscopy. There is no steatosis or cholestasis, whereas lipofuscin deposits are conspicuous.

ELISAs for Lassa virus antigen and immunoglobulins M and G (IgM and IgG)antibodies are sensitive and specific and in Africa have largely replaced indirect fluorescent antibody testing.[30] In Western countries, the diagnosis can be established reliably by reverse transcription PCR (RT-PCR).[31]

Supportive therapy is often necessary. In addition, the antiviral drug ribavirin is effective against Lassa virus infection, but only if administered early in the course of illness.[32] A study from Sierra Leone in patients at high risk for mortality confirmed the efficacy of ribavirin in the treatment of Lassa fever: only 1 of 20 patients died if intravenous ribavirin administered over a period of 10 days had been started within the first 6 days after the onset of fever, whereas mortality was 26% in

the 43 patients whose treatment had begun later.[33] However, because of its toxicity and teratogenicity, the need for intravenous application, and its expense, empiric therapy with ribavirin is not advised.[33]

Junin virus is another arenavirus that in Argentina can cause a viral hemorrhagic fever similar to Lassa fever.[34] Ribavirin, as well as ribavirin-interferon combination therapy, has been attempted with some success in this disease.[35]

Ebola and Marburg Hemorrhagic Fever

Marburg and Ebola viruses are nonsegmented, negative-sense, single-stranded RNA viruses that belong to the Filoviridae virus family.[36] They are among the most virulent pathogens and cause severe hemorrhagic fever and fulminant septic shock. No approved therapy is currently available to treat the devastating infections with Ebola and Marburg viruses.

All isolates of Marburg virus represent members of a single family, whereas Ebola isolates can be divided into different species (Zaire, Sudan, Ivory Coast, Reston, and probably Uganda 2007) that differ in their virulence.[37,38] The natural reservoirs of these viruses still remain a mystery, although it is suspected that both viruses are maintained in small animals, with bats heading the list of suspects.[39-43] Retrospective analyses of African epidemics suggest that person–person transmission can occur through contact with virus-contaminated fluids (e.g., blood, vomitus, feces, urine).

Marburg virus fever was first detected in 1967, when people had come in contact with African green monkeys imported from Uganda. Mortality in this first outbreak was 25%. Meanwhile, natural outbreaks of Marburg virus and Ebola fever have been reported repeatedly from several western and central African regions (**Fig. 34-1**). Ebola and Marburg virus

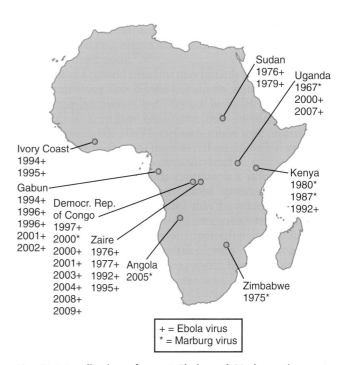

Fig. 34-1 **Localization of recent Ebola and Marburg virus outbreaks in Africa.**

infections are still relevant. In 1989, monkeys imported into the United States from the Philippines died of Ebola virus infection. Outbreaks still occur in western Africa, and the risk of undiagnosed patients arriving in industrialized countries remains real. Information on current outbreaks is available on the World Health Organization website (www.who.int/topics/haemorrhagic_fevers_viral/en).

The disease caused by the various Marburg and Ebola virus isolates results in similar syndromes that differ only in severity and case fatality rates. The incubation period is 5 to 10 days but may exceed 20 days. Symptomatic persons have high levels of virus in their blood and must be considered contagious, so appropriate safety precautions should be taken.[44] Marburg and Ebola infections typically begin with an abrupt onset of fever, chills, and general malaise. Other features include weakness, severe headache, pain in the muscles of the trunk and lower part of the back, nausea, vomiting, diarrhea, and abdominal pain.[37,45,46] A nonproductive cough, pharyngitis, and a maculopapular rash on the upper half of the body are also frequent findings. Symptoms persist with worsening of prostration, stupor, and hypotension; disseminated intravascular coagulation eventually leads to conjunctival hemorrhages, easy bruising, and bleeding from venipuncture sites. Marked laboratory abnormalities include a striking leukopenia with immature granulocytes and abnormal lymphocytes, as well as thrombocytopenia. Filoviruses cause multifocal hepatic necrosis. Thus AST and ALT levels rise rapidly in the first days. Hypoproteinemia and proteinuria may also be present. The hepatic pathology is similar to that seen with Lassa virus infection: spotty to widespread necrosis of hepatocytes and minimal hepatic inflammation, but no cholestasis.[47-49] Abundant filovirus particles are found in blood, phagocytes, endothelial cells, and hepatocytes. In lymph nodes, the reticular network is damaged.

Survivors of Marburg and Ebola hemorrhagic fever require prolonged convalescence and suffer from marked weakness, fatigue, and failure to regain weight. Marked sloughing of the skin and hair loss are commonly observed.[50]

Rift Valley Fever

Rift Valley fever is an acute vector-borne zoonotic disease caused by the Rift Valley fever virus, which belongs to the Bunyaviridae family and genus Phlebovirus. The virus was initially described in sheep and was first isolated from humans in Kenya.[51] The disease is widespread in sub-Saharan Africa and also occurs in Egypt, Mauretania, Senegal, Saudi Arabia, and Yemen. Rift Valley virus is transmitted by several mosquito species or by direct contamination from infected animals. Patients with Rift Valley fever have symptoms and signs of an influenza-like illness. Fewer than 8% of patients progress to severe disease, including hepatitis, encephalitis, retinitis, and a generalized hemorrhagic syndrome.[52]

Crimean-Congo Hemorrhagic Fever

Crimean-Congo hemorrhagic fever (CCHF) is a tick-borne viral infection that occurs in parts of Africa, Asia, eastern Europe, and the Middle East.[53] The virus belongs to the genus Nairovirus in the Bunyaviridae family. Isolates from different regions show considerable genetic diversity. Farmers and healthcare workers are particular at risk for this infection, but

fortunately, CCHF develops in only one of five people infected. The disease has four stages: incubation, prehemorrhagic, hemorrhagic, and convalescence. Incubation takes 3 to 7 days, and then fever, headache, myalgia, and dizziness develop suddenly. Facial hyperemia, conjunctivitis, and occasionally diarrhea are also noted. This stage lasts 4 to 5 days. The hemorrhagic period is short (2 to 3 days). The most common bleeding sites are in the nose, the gastrointestinal tract, the genitourinary tract, and the respiratory tract. In survivors, the convalescence phase begins about 10 to 20 days after the onset of disease. RT-PCR is the method of choice for rapid laboratory confirmation of CCHF viral infection.[54] Leukopenia and thrombocytopenia are consistent laboratory features, and raised levels of AST, ALT, and lactate dehydrogenase and prolonged coagulation tests are other common findings. Aminotransferase levels seem to correlate with the severity of disease.[55,56] Microscopic examination of liver tissue reveals variable degrees of hepatocellular necrosis with hemorrhage and Councilman bodies, fatty changes, Kupffer cell hyperplasia, and mild mononuclear portal inflammatory infiltrates.[57]

Treatment options are limited, but ribavirin has demonstrated antiviral activity against CCHF virus in vitro and in an animal model.[58,59] However, thus far, clinical effectiveness of ribavirin has been demonstrated only in observational studies.[55,60-62] In a recent outbreak, patients with severe disease were treated successfully with ribavirin for 10 days (30 mg/kg body weight as an initial loading dose, then 15 mg/kg every 6 hours for 4 days, and then 7.5 mg/kg every 8 hours for 6 days).[53]

Hantaviruses

Hantaviruses are prime examples of emerging viruses and are members of the genus Hantavirus within the Bunyaviridae family. They are negative-sense single-stranded RNA viruses that are carried primarily in rodents, which shed the virus in their urine, saliva, and feces. The virus is inhaled by humans as aerosols from dried rodent excreta or, in unusual circumstances, is transmitted via rodent bites.[63] Hantaviruses exist in multiple serotypes worldwide, which differ in their virulence. Some are considered nonpathogenic, whereas certain isolates can produce two distinct severe syndromes in humans: Hantavirus cardiopulmonary syndrome, mostly caused by isolates in the Americas, and hemorrhagic fever with renal syndrome, caused by isolates (Seoul virus, Dobrava virus, Puumala virus, Hantaan virus) in Europe and Asia.[64] In some instances, patients with Hantavirus hemorrhagic fever have suffered from severe acute hepatitis, whereas renal damage was rather mild.[65,66] Furthermore, a significantly increased prevalence of Hantavirus antibodies has been reported in patients with acute hepatitis of unknown cause from southwestern China[67] and in patients with chronic hepatitis from Japan.[68] However, the latter study failed to detect any Hantavirus antibodies in patients with acute hepatitis, thus implying a rather indirect pathogenetic role of Hantaviruses. Of note, Hantavirus infection has been observed to trigger acute exacerbations of autoimmune liver disease, and this mechanism has been proposed to contribute to community-acquired hepatitis.[69] Nevertheless, the precise role of Hantavirus infections in human liver disease still awaits clarification. Analogous to other bunyaviruses, Hantavirus is sensitive to ribavirin, which, although not approved by the Food and Drug Administration, can be used as emergency treatment.[70]

Chikungunya Fever

Chikungunya is an arthropod-borne togavirus initially endemic to western Africa that in recent years has spread to the Indian Ocean islands and Southeast Asia.[71] Although traditionally considered a disease of tropical and subtropical regions, in 2007 a local outbreak of chikungunya was even recorded in northern Italy.[72] Because of international travel, chikungunya infections have also been exported from Southeast Asia and Indian Ocean islands to other Western countries. The infection begins abruptly with high fever, symmetric polyarthralgia, and macular or maculopapular rash.[73] Pruritus and bullous skin lesions have also been described. Previously, chikungunya fever has been considered a self-limited disease. However, severe complications, including acute viral hepatitis and death, have been reported in recent outbreaks, particularly in elderly patients (>65 years) and people with chronic medical problems. Clinically, chikungunya fever must be differentiated from dengue fever, which shares many symptoms and features. Serology is the primary diagnostic tool in clinical practice, and chikungunya IgM antibodies become detectable by ELISA 5 days after the onset of symptoms. Viral culture and molecular techniques are valuable tools in a research setting. Although interferon alfa and ribavirin exhibit in vitro activity against chikungunya virus,[74] an effective specific antiviral therapy does not exist. Thus treatment is primarily supportive. Chikungunya infection cannot currently be prevented by vaccination.

Viral Liver Disease Associated with Immunodeficiency

The establishment of organ transplantation as a routine therapeutic procedure, the growing use of anticancer chemotherapy, and the recent pandemics of human immunodeficiency virus (HIV) infection have resulted in increasing awareness of unusual manifestations of viral infections as complications of immunosuppression. Such infections occur either as acute disease during primary infection or as severe exacerbation of a latent viral persistence. Cytomegalovirus is the most common opportunistic pathogen that causes hepatitis in both patients with drug-induced immunosuppression and HIV-infected patients with advanced immunodeficiency, but the other members of the herpes family, as well as common community-acquired agents such as adenovirus, are also important causes in this setting.

Liver Disease Attributable to HIV

In approximately half of patients, a faint rash and an infectious mononucleosis–like syndrome develop 3 weeks to 6 months after a primary HIV infection. Several case reports have described a hepatitis-like syndrome in such patients that could not be explained by other concomitant infections.[75,76] Patients complained of vomiting, upper abdominal pain, and hepatomegaly. There was a rise in aminotransferases, but jaundice or elevated serum alkaline phosphatase was not present. The liver disease resolved spontaneously, and no histologic reports are available for this condition.

At autopsy, hepatomegaly was found in approximately two thirds of patients with acquired immunodeficiency syndrome (AIDS).[77] In liver biopsy specimens, macrovesicular steatosis has been a common finding, which in rare instances could become excessive.[78] HIV has repeatedly been detected in the liver, particularly in Kupffer cells and endothelial cells, both by in situ hybridization and by p24 immunohistochemical staining,[79-81] thus suggesting that the liver might be an important site of HIV replication. A moderate chronic lymphocytic portal inflammation can be encountered in liver specimens and is thought to reflect HIV-associated reactive hepatitis. These nonspecific changes associated with HIV infection can then become superseded by further liver pathology caused by opportunistic infections and tumors (**Fig. 34-2**), illicit drug

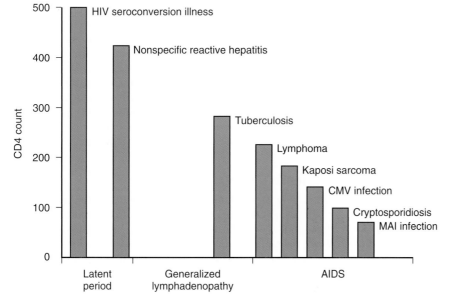

Fig. 34-2 **Overview of opportunistic diseases associated with human immunodeficiency virus (HIV) infection and their relationship to progressing immunodeficiency.** AIDS, acquired immunodeficiency syndrome; CMV, cytomegalovirus; MAI, *Mycobacterium avium-intracellulare* complex.

Table 34-2 Human Herpesviruses

SYSTEMATIC NAME	COMMON NAME	HERPESVIRUS SUBFAMILY	ESTIMATED PREVALENCE	ROUTE OF TRANSMISSION
Human herpesvirus 1	Herpes simplex virus 1 (HSV1)	α-Herpesvirinae	75% to >95%	Oral secretions Close contact
Human herpesvirus 2	HSV2	α-Herpesvirinae	4% to 95%	Genital secretions Close contact
Human herpesvirus 3	Varicella-zoster virus (VZV)	α-Herpesvirinae	>90%	Aerosol Close contact
Human herpesvirus 4	Epstein-Barr virus (EBV)	γ-Herpesvirinae	70% to 95%	Oral secretions
Human herpesvirus 5	Human cytomegalovirus (CMV)	β-Herpesvirinae	40% to 95%	Oral secretions Genital secretions
Human herpesvirus 6	Human herpesvirus 6 (HHV6)	β-Herpesvirinae	>85%	Oral secretions
Human herpesvirus 7	Human herpesvirus 7 (HHV7)	β-Herpesvirinae	>85%	Oral secretions
Human herpesvirus 8	Kaposi sarcoma–associated herpesvirus	γ-Herpesvirinae	10% to 25%	Oral secretions Genital secretions

abuse, and currently, also the side effects of HIV antiretroviral therapy.[82]

The Herpesvirus Group

The herpesviruses form a large family of DNA viruses, and eight members cause disease in humans (**Table 34-2**). Herpes simplex virus (HSV), varicella-zoster virus (VZV), Epstein-Barr virus (EBV), cytomegalovirus (CMV), and human herpesvirus type 6 (HHV6) can directly affect the liver and are infections that in humans are usually acquired during childhood or adolescence. Herpesviruses persist lifelong and can reactivate and induce aggressive liver disease in immunosuppressed patients. Unlike the other herpesviruses, the prevalence of Kaposi sarcoma–associated virus, or HHV8, is more limited. HHV8 is found in saliva, which may serve as a source for transmission both sexually and probably also vertically from mother to child. Apart from Kaposi sarcoma, HHV8 can cause Castleman disease and body cavity lymphoma in severely immunosuppressed patients.

Herpes Simplex Virus

Primary herpes simplex infection produces characteristic oral (HSV1) or genital (HSV2) vesicular lesions on an erythematous base. The symptoms can be severe, with fever and malaise, but many primary infections are asymptomatic. Once primary infection has been established, the virus adopts a latent state and persists in the nerve cell bodies of the dorsal ganglia, from where it can reactivate under immunosuppression.

Fulminant hepatitis is a complication of both HSV1 and HSV2 infection.[83] Organ transplantation and treatment of hematologic malignancies are the most frequent underlying predispositions.[84-86] Other individuals at risk include neonates, patients taking steroids, HIV-infected patients, and patients with cancer or myelodysplastic syndromes.[83,85-90] Fatal HSV-related hepatitis has also rarely been reported in immunocompetent adults.[91] HSV-related hepatitis has high mortality (>80%) and resembles septic endotoxic shock; jaundice is not always present.[85,87] Clinical features include fever, anorexia with

nausea and vomiting, abdominal pain, leukopenia, and coagulopathy. Typical oral or genital vesicular lesions occur in only about a third of patients.[83] Some patients also have disseminated extrahepatic involvement of the lung, lymph nodes, spleen, and adrenal glands. The diagnosis of HSV-related hepatitis must be established rapidly via detection of HSV by either viral isolation,[92] immunofluorescence staining, or preferentially, PCR[92,93]; serologic assays have rather limited application.

In fatal cases the liver is enlarged and congested at autopsy and has a mottled appearance with multiple white and yellow foci. Microscopy reveals irregular parenchymal necrosis with little inflammation. At the margins of necrotic areas multinucleated hepatocytes may be found, and hepatocytes may contain purple nuclear inclusion bodies with a surrounding halo.[88]

After organ transplantation, none of the patients survived once the liver was diffusely involved, whereas three of seven patients with more focal disease had survived with acyclovir therapy.[85] Prompt systemic treatment with acyclovir has also been shown to reduce HSV-associated morbidity and the risk for serious complications in HIV-infected patients.[94] In addition, anti-HSV prophylaxis with acyclovir at organ transplantation has markedly reduced HSV reactivation after surgery.[95,96] Acyclovir resistance occurs in about 5% of immunocompromised patients and is negligible (<0.5%) in immunocompetent subjects.[97] Valacyclovir, a prodrug of acyclovir, and famciclovir, a prodrug of penciclovir, have similar antiviral mechanisms as acyclovir, and thus HSV isolates resistant to acyclovir are also resistant to these drugs.[98] Cidofovir and foscarnet are alternative choices to treat acyclovir-resistant HSV, but side effects are greater with these drugs than with acyclovir.[99]

Varicella-Zoster Virus

Varicella-zoster virus causes chickenpox, as well as shingles when latent infection is reactivated. In a first viremic phase after infection, VZV replicates in the epithelia of the gut, respiratory tract, liver, and endocrine glands. A secondary viremia leads to infection of the skin, which results in the usual rash. Liver disease is rare and limited to patients with severe immunodeficiency. Anticancer chemotherapy and corticosteroid treatment are risk factors for this complication.[100] In severe VZV infection, hepatic lesions are similar to herpes simplex hepatitis, with massive liver necrosis and inclusion bodies but little inflammation. Electron microscopy and immunohistochemistry reveal abundant VZV. The diagnosis is best made by PCR,[93] and treatment and prophylaxis are similar to that for HSV, with acyclovir also being effective against VZV. In addition, VZV has been reported to trigger severe autoimmune hepatitis.[101]

Epstein-Barr Virus

Epstein-Barr virus is the agent that accounts for 90% of acute infectious mononucleosis syndromes. It persists lifelong in a latent state, which results from a dynamic interplay between viral evasion strategies and the host's immune responses. However, unlike other herpesviruses, reactivation-associated disease is not a prominent feature in chronic EBV disease. Still, EBV is a potent cause in a variety of malignancies, such B- and T-cell lymphomas, Hodgkin lymphoma, and nasopharyngeal carcinoma. In transplant patients, EBV has been associated with an aggressive lymphoproliferative disease.

EBV is shed in oral secretions, and most primary EBV infections originate in the oropharynx. Based on genetic differences in the EBV nuclear antigen-3 genes, two types of EBV have been identified[102] that show divergent prevalence throughout the world: in Western countries, EBV1 is 10 times more prevalent than EBV2, whereas in Africa, the two EBV genomes are distributed equally.[103]

Because few pregnant women are susceptible, intrauterine EBV infection is rare but in isolated cases may lead to diverse congenital anomalies, including biliary atresia.[104] In infants and young children, primary infection is common and frequently asymptomatic, whereas in adults, it results in the infectious mononucleosis syndrome, which begins with malaise, headache, and low-grade fever before more specific symptoms such as pharyngitis/tonsillitis, swelling of the cervical lymph nodes, and moderate to high-grade fever develop.[105] Patients have peripheral blood lymphocytosis with characteristic large abnormal lymphocytes in their blood smears. Nausea, vomiting, and anorexia are common findings and probably reflect the mild hepatitis that accompanies infectious mononucleosis fever in approximately 90% of patients. Liver histology shows diffuse lymphocytic infiltrates in the sinusoids, and focal apoptotic hepatocytes can occasionally be seen (**Fig. 34-3, A**).[106,107] These infiltrates may be atypical and must then be carefully differentiated from leukemia/lymphoma. Nonnecrotic hepatic granulomas are occasionally detected in

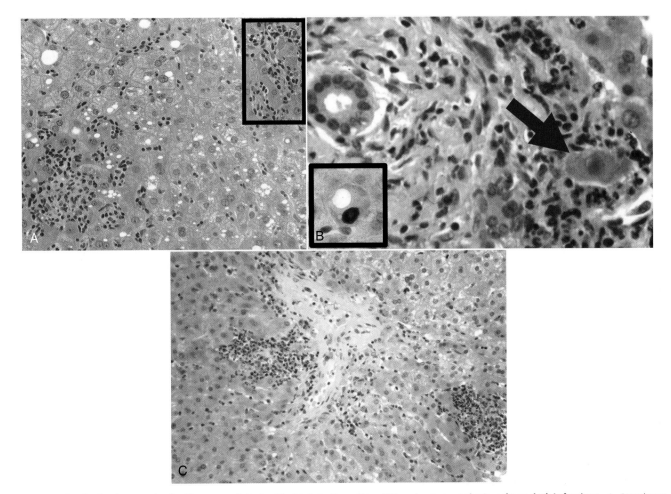

Fig. 34-3 **Histologic changes in the liver associated with Epstein-Barr virus (A) and cytomegalovirus (B and C) infections. A,** Prominent sinusoidal infiltration of lymphocytes into the sinusoidal space. **B,** Cytomegalovirus inclusion bodies *(arrow)* and immunohistochemical nuclear staining for cytomegalovirus antigen. **C,** Microabscesses in early cytomegalovirus infection.

patients with infectious mononucleosis. Splenomegaly is found in about half of patients, but hepatomegaly and jaundice are uncommon findings. The vast majority of patients recover over a period of 2 to 4 weeks, but fatigue may persist for several months after infection.

Patients with X-linked lymphoproliferative disease, which is caused by a mutation in the *SH2D1A* gene on the X chromosome, are particularly vulnerable to EBV[108] and may suffer fatal infections with extensive liver necrosis.[109] In patients with severe immunodeficiency, lymphomatoid granulomatosis is a further unusual complication of EBV infection that leads to granuloma formation in multiple organs, including the liver, and may require interferon alfa antiviral therapy.[110] An EBV-associated lymphoproliferative disorder with hepatic infiltration of immunoblasts[111] and a hemophagocytic syndrome[112] have also been reported in patients with HIV infection.

EBV is also the major causative agent of the so-called post-transplant lymphoproliferative disease (PTLD), which after organ transplantation may result in lymphocytic infiltration of the liver and other organs ranging from benign polyclonal B-cell proliferation to malignant B-cell lymphoma.[113] PTLD occurs more commonly in children than in adults and is related to the type and degree of immunosuppression. It is a particularly common complication in EBV-negative individuals who receive a graft from an EBV-positive donor, with primary EBV infection developing as a result of immunosuppression.[114] Clinical suspicion of EBV infection is confirmed by detection of heterophilic or EBV-specific antibodies in patients with infectious mononucleosis and quantitative PCR assays in those with lymphoproliferative disorders.[115,116]

Treatment of EBV infection is primarily supportive. Corticosteroid therapy can ameliorate the symptoms but is not generally recommended because EBV infection is usually a self-limited disease and there are theoretic concerns of suppression of immune responses with a viral infection, which can potentially cause malignant disease. Nevertheless, corticosteroids should be considered in individuals with life-threatening complications such as imminent liver failure. Acyclovir inhibits EBV DNA polymerase, and antiviral therapy with this drug has shortened viral shedding but failed to demonstrate a convincing clinical benefit even in patients with severe acute EBV infection.[117] Acyclovir does not affect latent EBV infection. Thus anticancer chemotherapy,[118,119] B-cell monoclonal antibodies,[120-122] and if possible, a reduction in immunosuppression[123] are needed to treat EBV-related lymphoproliferative disorders, but antiviral therapy in general is not effective.

Cytomegalovirus

In immunocompetent hosts, CMV infection is asymptomatic or causes only transient, minimally symptomatic acute disease. Newborns and immunocompromised patients, such as those with HIV infection, cancer, and solid organ or bone marrow transplantation, are commonly infected with CMV and may be susceptible to the development of serious disease.

In about 10% of immunocompetent subjects, primary CMV infection produces an infectious mononucleosis–like syndrome that is associated with elevated serum aminotransferase levels and a mild hepatitis. Liver histology may show focal hepatocyte and bile duct damage with lymphocytic infiltration into the sinusoids.[124] In other patients, epithelioid granulomas

without necrosis were present, but CMV inclusion bodies or CMV immunostaining were rarely detectable.[124,125]

Congenital CMV infection is observed in fewer than 2% of newborns and commonly occurs when mothers have primary CMV infection or reactivation of CMV during pregnancy. Approximately 10% of such neonates have symptoms at birth, including hepatosplenomegaly and jaundice.[126] Fetal CMV infection has also been associated with obstructive biliary disease and neonatal hepatitis with giant cell transformation, cholestasis, and viral inclusion bodies.[127] In CMV infection of the liver, endothelial cells, Kupffer cells, and hepatocytes become swollen and may contain basophilic granules in their cytoplasm. A typical intranuclear amphophilic inclusion body surrounded by a clear halo resembling an owl's eye may also be present (see **Fig. 34-3, *B***). Both nuclear and cytoplasmic inclusions are full of virions.[128]

CMV-related liver disease is the most common cause of acute viral hepatitis in patients after organ transplantation. Infection may result from reactivation of endogenous virus because of immunosuppression, transmission from the transplanted organ of a CMV-positive donor, or transfusion of blood and blood products. In liver transplantation, most CMV disease occurs after 1 and 4 months, and CMV infection is also discussed as a potential risk factor for the subsequent development of acute and chronic rejection. On the other hand, rejection therapy with corticosteroid boluses may trigger reactivation of endogenous CMV. Liver biopsy specimens from patients with posttransplant CMV hepatitis usually show scanty CMV inclusion bodies, which may be associated with small foci of necrosis and inflammation (microabscesses) (see **Fig. 34-3, *C***).

Although reactivation of CMV is also a common severe complication in HIV-positive patients with advanced immunodeficiency (usually CD4$^+$ counts <50/μl), hepatic involvement seems to be rather minor.[129] Occasionally, CMV causes severe bile duct necrosis, and it is also a major cause of HIV cholangiopathy, a sclerosing cholangitis that is encountered rarely in patients with terminal HIV-related immunodeficiency.[130-132]

De novo appearance of CMV antibodies of the IgM class or a four-fold rise in IgG antibodies is considered indicative of active CMV infection in immunocompetent individuals. However, serology is unreliable in immunocompromised patients and is being replaced by quantitative molecular DNA amplification assays.[133-136] Currently, most transplant centers perform CMV surveillance by weekly quantitative determination of CMV DNA and also administer hyperimmune antibodies or antiviral drugs for CMV prophylaxis to transplant recipients at high risk for acquiring CMV disease.[137,138] However, CMV infection and disease may still develop. In patients with immunodeficiency, CMV hepatitis should be treated promptly. At present, intravenous ganciclovir or oral valganciclovir for 3 weeks is the treatment of choice. Treatment can be continued in reduced doses as chemoprophylaxis if prolonged immunosuppression is anticipated.[139] Fortunately, ganciclovir resistance seems to be a rather rare event,[140] so the toxic alternatives cidofovir and foscarnet can largely be avoided.

Human Herpesvirus 6 and Human Herpesvirus 7

There are two variants of HHV6, HHV6A and HHV6B, which infect not only T cells but also other cells types expressing the

CD46 receptor.[141] Though genetically clearly distinct from HHV6, HHV7 is another β-herpesvirus that shares many features with HHV6. Primary infection with either virus commonly occurs at a young age and can lead to a febrile illness known as exanthema subitum or roseola infantum.[142] Pityriasis rosea reflects primary infection with HHV7. Although the spectrum of diseases caused by HHV6 and HHV7 later on is not fully known, these viruses have been linked to a variety of different syndromes such as encephalitis, multiple sclerosis, pneumonitis, an infectious mononucleosis–like condition, and postinfectious drug hypersensitivity, as well as lymphoproliferative disorders and systemic disease in immunocompromised patients.[143]

HHV6 can also cause hepatitis, which has occasionally resulted in liver failure in neonates and young infants.[144-145] Moreover, HHV6 DNA and antigens have been detected in a significant proportion of children and adults who underwent transplantation for acute liver failure of unknown cause.[146-149] Of note, in two patients with HHV6 infection and imminent liver failure, HHV6 infection was controlled successfully with valganciclovir and with liver transplantation plus ganciclovir, respectively.[150] Hepatitis caused by HHV6 and HHV7 also complicates organ transplantation.[151-153] HHV6-induced acute liver failure and co-infection with hepatitis B and C viruses have been identified as risk factors for reactivation of HHV6 in patients after liver transplantation.[154,155] Of note, HHV6 reactivation seems to significantly increase mortality in living related liver transplant recipients.[155] HHV6 and HHV7 can reactivate each other[156,157] and can also reactivate CMV infection and lead to symptomatic disease in liver transplant patients.[158] In addition, HHV6 has been associated with autoimmunity and postinfantile giant cell hepatitis,[159,160] as well as giant cell transformation of bile duct cells.[161]

Seroconversion with at least a four-fold rise in IgG antibody titer between paired samples is considered diagnostic of HHV6 infection, but serology does not distinguish between HHV6A and HHV6B variants and may also be cross-reactive with HHV7. HHV6 IgM antibodies develop within a week after infection but are an unreliable marker because approximately 5% of healthy subjects may have a positive IgM test at any given time.[162] HHV6 can be detected in tissue samples by virus-specific monoclonal antibodies, but the preferred method for diagnosing HHV6 and HHV7 infection is by quantitative DNA amplification assays.[163-165]

In most immunocompetent patients, HHV6 and HHV7 cause a benign self-limited infection that does not require specific antiviral treatment. Nevertheless, foscarnet is active against HHV6A, HHV6B, and HHV7 in vitro, whereas unlike HHV6B, both HHV6A and HHV7 may be relatively resistant to ganciclovir.[166-169] Cidofovir may be a therapeutic alternative, but some resistant HHV6 isolates have been identified.[170] Although in vitro studies and anecdotal reports in the transplant setting seem to suggest some beneficial effects in human infections,[150,169] antiviral therapy against HHV6 or HHV7 has not yet been evaluated in controlled trials.

Human Herpesvirus 8

HHV8 is a γ-herpesvirus that has the potential for malignant transformation. Although primary HHV8 infection can cause rash and fever in children and immunocompromised individuals, the onset of HHV8-related diseases usually occurs several years after the acquisition of HHV8. Kaposi sarcoma, body cavity lymphoma, and multicentric Castleman disease are the typical manifestation of HHV8 infection, but bone marrow aplasia and multiple myeloma have also been described in association with this infection.[171] T lymphocytes play an important role in the control of HHV8 infection, which explains why the incidence of HHV8-related diseases is increased in patients with a transplant or AIDS. This concept is also supported by the observation that regression of Kaposi sarcoma is achieved when immunosuppression is reduced in patients with a transplant[172,173] and when highly active antiretroviral therapy (HAART) has improved immune function in subjects with AIDS.[174] Other risk factors for Kaposi sarcoma, the predominant manifestation of HHV8-associated disease, are multiple homosexual contacts in HIV-infected men[175] and, in the transplant setting, male sex, old age, and lung transplantation.[176]

In autopsy studies, Kaposi sarcoma has involved the liver in approximately 20% of subjects with AIDS, but its prevalence is declining with HAART. Hepatic Kaposi sarcoma is usually part of widespread cutaneous and visceral disease but may rarely be the primary manifestation.[177] Fulminant hepatic Kaposi sarcoma has also been observed in the first few weeks after liver transplantation (**Fig. 34-4, _A_ to _E_**). Macroscopically, dark red tumors 0.5 to 2 cm in diameter may be seen on the skin, the liver capsule, and the parenchyma. At the microscopic level, the typical lesion is a mesh of spindle cell–like tumour cells and dilated thin-walled vessels.[178] Diffuse plasma cells, infrequent mitosis, and clusters of intracytoplasmic eosinophilic inclusions resembling small erythrocytes are further characteristic features. Hepatosplenomegaly, fever, and weight loss are typical features of multicentric Castleman disease, a noncancerous proliferation of B lymphocytes (see **Fig. 34-4, _F_**). Lymphocytes in patients with multicentric Castleman disease and Kaposi sarcoma seem to cooperate with each other, and thus the two HHV8-related lesions can occasionally be found within the same lymph node.[179,180]

Ascites and pleural effusions may initially raise suspicion of some underlying liver disease in patients with HHV8-related body cavity lymphoma, but they can be differentiated by the presence of abundant lymphoma cells in aspirated fluid (see **Fig. 34-4, _G_**). HHV8 can also cause solid organ lymphoma, which in the liver leads to diffuse sinusoidal accumulation of HHV8-infected B lymphocytes.[181]

Reconstitution of immune function is a primary goal in the treatment of HHV8-associated diseases and, apart from HAART in HIV infection, may be achieved with the use of antiproliferative m-TOR (mammalian target of rapamycin) inhibitors for immune suppression in transplantation[182,183] or immune stimulation with imiquimod and interferon alfa.[184,185] Chemotherapy with liposomal anthracyclines or paclitaxel for Kaposi sarcoma[186,187] and rituximab for Castleman disease and lymphoma are further potent treatment options.[188] Ganciclovir, cidofovir, foscarnet, adefovir, and lobucavir, but not acyclovir, show some in vitro activity in blocking replication of HHV8-infected cell lines, and in a double-blind, placebo-controlled crossover trial, valganciclovir reduced oropharyngeal shedding of HHV8 by 80%.[189]

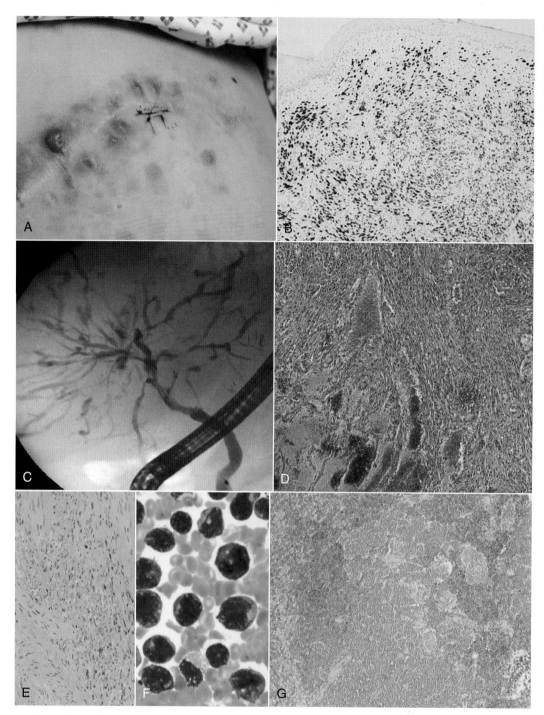

Fig. 34-4 **Human herpesvirus 8 (HHV8)-associated manifestations. A,** Cutaneous Kaposi sarcoma developing in a surgical scar 4 weeks after liver transplantation. **B,** Detection of HHV8 latency-associated nuclear antigen-1 in a skin section from the patient in **A. C,** Endoscopic retrograde cholangiopancreatography demonstrates compressed and partially blocked biliary ducts as a result of multifocal hepatic tumor infiltration (same patient as in **A**). **D,** Liver histology illustrating typical Kaposi sarcoma with abundant spindle cells and dilated vascular spaces (same patient as in **A**). **E,** High-power field of hepatic Kaposi sarcoma. **F,** Multicentric Castleman disease in a perihepatic lymph node. Histology shows many atypical follicle-like structures and abnormal vessels. **G,** Plasma cell–like lymphoma cells in an HIV-infected patient with HHV8-associated body cavity lymphoma.

Adenoviruses

Adenoviruses have a worldwide distribution and cause febrile diseases in infants and young children. More than 50 serotypes can be distinguished and are further subdivided into six subgroups, A through F. Typical syndromes include conjunctivitis, upper respiratory tract infections such as pharyngitis and

coryza, pneumonia, and otitis media. In young children, an acute diarrheal illness is caused by subgroup F type 40 and 41 adenoviruses. Adenoviruses can persist in human tissue over prolonged periods[190,191] and can cause a variety of clinical syndromes in immunocompromised individuals, including serious hepatitis.[192] Adenoviral hepatitis occurs in congenital and acquired immunodeficiency syndromes and may be fatal

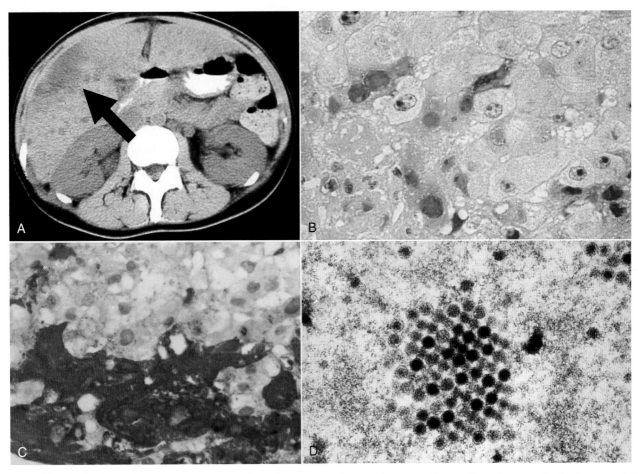

Fig. 34-5 Fulminant adenoviral hepatitis in an HIV-infected woman. A, Computed tomographic scan illustrating extensive focal necroses in the liver *(arrow)*. **B,** Necrosis and enlarged hepatocytes with adenoviral inclusions (same patient as in **A**). **C,** Immunohistochemistry demonstrates the presence of abundant adenoviral antigens (same patient as in **A**). **D,** Intracellular adenoviral virions seen on electron microscopy (same patient as in **A**).

in these individuals.[193-196] Adenoviral hepatitis is a particular problem in pediatric liver transplantation and was identified in 14 (3%) of 484 pediatric liver transplant recipients[197]; 6 of the 14 patients died, 4 required retransplantation, and only 4 patients recovered with a decrease in immunosuppressive therapy. Transmission of latent adenovirus with the donated organ seems to be a potential risk factor for this complication.[198] The signs and symptoms of adenoviral hepatitis resemble those of HSV infection and consist of massively elevated aminotransferase levels and severe coagulopathy. There are extensive areas of liver cell necrosis with little inflammation and intranuclear inclusion bodies (**Fig. 34-5, *A* to *D***). To date, a proven therapy for adenoviral hepatitis does not exist, but ribavirin may be helpful in selected cases.[199]

Liver Disease Associated with Systemic Viral Infections

The liver can be affected as part of a generalized infection with viruses that primarily target tissues other than liver, such as adenovirus and influenza. Liver involvement can range from

asymptomatic deranged biochemistry to fulminant hepatic failure. Loss of immune control is considered responsible for hepatitis associated with opportunistic viral infections, and rather similar mechanisms may operate in severe acute respiratory syndrome (SARS)-associated hepatitis, which is characterized by focal lobular lymphocytic infiltrates. Finally, "collateral damage" has been proposed in influenza infection and reflects expansion of virus-specific CD8[+] T cells generated outside the liver that may trigger T-cell–dependent hepatitis even when viral antigens are apparently absent in the liver.[200] Kupffer cells play a pivotal role in this process because they can take up and present viral antigens, coordinate lymphocyte recruitment, or possibly become activated by lymphocytes to induce hepatocellular apoptosis.[201] Because T-cell expansion occurs with many viral infections,[202] this bystander mechanism may contribute to hepatitis in many extrahepatic infections, with important implications for liver pathobiology.

Influenza

Influenza viruses represent three genera in the Orthomyxoviridae family. Generally, influenza A viruses are associated with more severe disease in humans than are influenza B and C viruses. Influenza A is further subdivided with respect to genetic variation in its hemagglutinin (H) and neuraminidase

(N) genes. Influenza viruses commonly cause a self-limited acute respiratory infection manifested as fever, rhinorrhea, sore throat, and occasionally, gastrointestinal symptoms. Therefore aminotransferase levels are not monitored routinely. In the 2004 H1N5 influenza outbreak, however, about 60% of patients with pneumonia had deranged liver function test values and gastrointestinal symptoms such as vomiting, abdominal pain, or diarrhea on initial evaluation.[203] Of note, among other extrahepatic abnormalities, autopsy revealed hepatic centrolobular necrosis, although neither viral antigen detection nor RT-PCR could provide evidence of viral liver disease.[204] Thus liver damage in patients dying of influenza has been considered immune mediated, in particular because high cytokine levels were detected.[205] Of note, in 4 of 15 volunteers infected intranasally with influenza A/Kawasaki/86 (H1N1), markedly elevated aminotransferase levels also transiently developed.[200] This experimental observation is remarkable because the rise in liver enzymes occurred after pyrexia had settled, thus suggesting that the liver damage was mediated by the host's immune response rather than viral infection of the liver. It has been proposed that immune-mediated liver damage may also be the cause of elevated aminotransferases in other viral respiratory infections such as respiratory syncytial virus,[206] although cardiovascular effects and hepatic ischemia must be considered in these severely ill patients as well.[207]

Coronavirus (Severe Acute Respiratory Syndrome)

A novel coronavirus (SARS-coronavirus [SARS-CoV]), causes SARs, and it resulted in an outbreak of severe infection of the lung and gastrointestinal tract in the Far East and Canada.[208,209] There was also involvement of other organs; approximately 25% of patients had elevated liver enzymes at the onset of infection, and elevated levels developed later in an additional 45% of patients with normal liver enzymes at initial evaluation, so overall, up to 70% of patients had elevated liver enzyme levels during their illness.[210-215] Jaundice was observed in less than 10% of patients. In most patients, aminotransferase levels started to rise toward the end of the first week and peaked at the end of the second week. With resolution of SARS, aminotransferases normalized spontaneously in the majority of patients. Severe liver damage (ALT more than five times the upper limit of normal) was observed more frequently in male patients and those with significant other co-morbid conditions or elevated serum creatinine levels.[215] The role of concomitant hepatitis B in disease severity is controversial.[214,215] However, there was a close relationship between the severity of hepatic dysfunction and degree of pulmonary damage and the outcome of SARS.[214] Thus high ALT levels appeared to be an independent predictor of more severe disease and a worse outcome.

Histopathologic studies revealed marked apoptosis of hepatocytes and conspicuous (presumably compensatory) mitotic activity.[216] Hepatocytes also showed some ballooning, and mild to moderate lymphocytic infiltrates were described in the portal tracts and liver lobules. Although SARS-CoV RT-PCR was consistently positive in liver specimens, immunohistochemistry and electron microscopy failed to detect viral antigens and viral particles in several biopsy and postmortem studies.[216-218] Thus only small amounts of SARS-CoV seem to be present in the liver, and analogous to influenza infection, the host's immune response may contribute to the liver damage.[219] In the recent SARS outbreak, both ribavirin and Kaletra (baby-dose ritonavir/lopinavir) were used as experimental therapy with limited success.

Measles (Rubeola)

Measles is caused by Morbillivirus of the Paramyxoviridae family. It is an acute febrile illness with a typical rash that is currently preventable by vaccination. Measles is associated with diverse complications such as pneumonitis or subacute sclerosing panencephalitis and causes significant mortality in third-world countries and in patients with immunodeficiency.[220] Liver dysfunction has increasingly been recognized as a complication of measles in children and adults[221-223] and may become a prominent feature in patients with atypical measles and partial immunity to the measles virus.[224,225] Hepatic abnormalities have been noted to occur more frequently in adult patients with primary infection (up to 66%) than in children.[226] Two patterns of hepatic dysfunction are encountered: asymptomatic elevations of aminotransferases, which resolve within a few days, and rarely, prolonged cholestasis and jaundice, which may appear when measles begins to recede.[227] In liver tissue, steatosis, portal inflammation, and focal necrosis have been reported.[228] Viral inclusions and giant cells are rarely seen but have been observed in a child with congenital immunodeficiency.[229] In addition, measles has been incriminated in triggering autoimmune hepatitis.[230] Paramyxovirus particles have also been reported in several patients with syncytial giant cell hepatitis.[231-234] However, the very nature of these particles has thus far remained elusive.

Rubella

Childhood rubella is apparently not associated with significant liver disease. Nonetheless, this virus has been proposed as a cause of neonatal giant cell hepatitis, which may also be accompanied by necrosis, cholestasis, and lymphocytic infiltrates on histologic examination.[235]

Enteroviruses

Group B coxsackievirus infection can cause liver disease as part of a serious multisystem infection in young children and also rarely in adults.[236-238] Liver histology shows hemorrhagic necrosis in neonates, whereas in adults, swollen hepatocytes, bile stasis, and a mixed infiltrate of mononuclear and polymorphic leukocytes in the portal tracts and sinusoids have been observed.

Parvovirus

Human parvovirus B19 is a nonenveloped, single-stranded DNA virus that belongs to the Erythrovirus genus of the Parvoviridae family. Humans are the only known host, in whom it can produce a wide range of different syndromes. Most immunocompetent people with B19 infection will be asymptomatic or suffer only nonspecific malaise, muscle pain, and fever, which in the second week may be followed by rash, arthralgia, pancytopenia, and edema in about a quarter of infected patients.[239-240] Erythema infectiosum occurs in school-aged children and occasionally also in adults. Arthropathy and aplastic anemia are further complications in adults. Fetal infection during gestation is a cause of hydrops fetalis, which is associated with marked damage to the liver[241]; hepatocytes have ballooned, swollen nuclei that harbor eosinophilic nuclear inclusion bodies. In addition, erythroid-myeloid precursors are greatly expanded in the sinusoids. Parvovirus B19 has also been identified as a cause of acute hepatitis[242] and has been incriminated as the underlying cause in acute liver failure with anemia.[243] However, a subsequent study could not confirm parvovirus B19 as a cause of fulminant hepatic failure.[244]

Torquetenovirus and Other Anelloviruses

Torquetenovirus (TTV) was initially identified as a novel virus in three of five patients in whom posttransfusion hepatitis developed but were found to be negative for all known hepatitis viruses.[245] TTV is classified in the genus Anellovirus, which is not attached to any family. Torquetenominivirus and related viruses with smaller genomes, provisionally designated as small anelloviruses, are further members of this genus. TTV can be subdivided into five phylogenetic groups, 1 to 5, and co-infection with several genotypes is common. Some TTV variants have their own designation, such as SEN virus, named after the patient from whom it had been isolated.

Soon after its discovery, it became clear that TTV viremia occurs frequently in the healthy general population worldwide. Thus the clinical significance of TTV infections remains uncertain. Inoculation of chimpanzees with TTV led to viremia but did not cause hepatitis.[246] Moreover, several studies on TTV transmission failed to establish any consistent relationship between TTV viremia and elevated serum aminotransferase levels.[247-249] Nevertheless, it cannot be excluded that TTV is responsible for acute hepatitis in some subsets of patients,[247,250] and if so, TTV seems to cause a rather mild form of hepatitis.[251]

Likewise, most studies also could not confirm any consistent associations between persistence of TTV and the presence of biochemical and histologic hepatic abnormalities in a variety of different clinical settings.[248,252-254] TTV infection does not seem to trigger autoimmune hepatitis,[255] and a case-control study failed to establish TTV as an independent risk for factor hepatocellular carcinoma.[256]

Taken together, it seems most likely that the initial reports of an increased TTV prevalence in patients with chronic liver disease[257,258] reflect shared risk factors for infection and liver damage rather than TTV as the cause of the liver disease.

Key References

Alexopoulou A, et al. A fatal case of postinfantile giant cell hepatitis in a patient with chronic lymphocytic leukaemia. Eur J Gastroenterol Hepatol 2003;15:551–555. (Ref.234)

Al-Hoamoudi WK. Severe autoimmune hepatitis triggered by varicella zoster infection. World J Gastroenterol 2009;15:1004–1006. (Ref.101)

Alsop Z. Ebola outbreak in Uganda "atypical," say experts. Lancet 2007;370:2085. (Ref.38)

Babel N, et al. Development of Kaposi's sarcoma under sirolimus-based immunosuppression and successful treatment with imiquimod. Transpl Infect Dis 2008;10:59–62. (Ref.184)

Bae HG, et al. Analysis of two imported cases of yellow fever infection from Ivory Coast and The Gambia to Germany and Belgium. J Clin Virol 2005; 33:274–280. (Ref.18)

Barnett ED. Yellow fever: epidemiology and prevention. Clin Infect Dis 2007;44: 850–856. (Ref.15)

Barozzi P, et al. Indirect antitumor effects of mammalian target of rapamycin inhibitors against Kaposi sarcoma in transplant patients. Transplantation 2009; 88:597–598. (Ref.183)

Bonnafous P, et al. Characterization of a cidofovir-resistant HHV-6 mutant obtained by in vitro selection. Antiviral Res 2008;77:237–240. (Ref.170)

Briolant S, et al. In vitro inhibition of chikungunya and Semliki Forest viruses replication by antiviral compounds: synergistic effect of interferon-alpha and ribavirin combination. Antiviral Res 2004;61:111–117. (Ref.74)

Booth CM, et al. Clinical features and short term outcome of 144 patients with SARS in the greater Toronto area. JAMA 2003;289:2801–2809. (Ref.211)

Bower M, et al. Brief communication: rituximab in HIV-associated multicentric Castleman disease. Ann Intern Med 2007;147:836–839. (Ref.188)

Cacheux W, et al. HHV-6–related acute liver failure in two immunocompetent adults: favourable outcome after liver transplantation and/or ganciclovir therapy. J Intern Med 2005;258:573–578. (Ref.150)

Caliendo AM, et al. Comparison of molecular tests for detection and quantification of cell-associated cytomegalovirus DND. J Clin Microbiol 2003; 41:3509–3513. (Ref.135)

Campistol JM, Schena FP. Kaposi's sarcoma in renal transplant recipients—the impact of proliferation signal inhibitors. Nephrol Dial Transplant 2007; 22(Suppl 1):17–22. (Ref.182)

Capello D, et al. Analysis of immunoglobulin heavy and light chain variable genes in post-transplant lymphoproliferative disorders. Hematol Oncol 2006; 24:212–219. (Ref.114)

Casper C, et al. Valganciclovir for suppression of human herpesvirus-8 replication: a randomized, double-blind, placebo-controlled, crossover trial. J Infect Dis 2008;198:23–30. (Ref.189)

Centers for Disease Control and Prevention (CDC). Imported Lassa fever—New Jersey, 2004. MMWR Morb Mortal Wkly Rep 2004;53:894–897. (Ref.27)

Centers for Disease Control and Prevention (CDC). Rift Valley fever outbreaks—Kenya November 2006-January 2007. MMWR Morb Mortal Wkly Rep 2007; 56:73–76. (Ref.52)

Centers for Disease Control and Prevention (CDC). Update: chikungunya fever diagnosed among international travelers—United States, 2006. MMWR Morb Mortal Wkly Rep 2007;56:276–277. (Ref.3)

Chan HL-Y, et al. Clinical significance of hepatic derangement in severe acute respiratory syndrome. World J Gastroenterol 2005;11:2148–2153. (Ref.215)

Chang YL, et al. Human herpesvirus 6–related fulminant myocarditis in an immunocompetent adult with fatal outcome. Hum Pathol 2009;40:740–745. (Ref.149)

Charrel RN, de Lamballerie X, Raoult D. Chikungunya outbreaks—the globalization of vector-borne diseases. N Engl J Med 2007;356:769–771. (Ref.71)

Chau TN, et al. SARS-associated viral hepatitis caused by a novel coronavirus: report of three cases. Hepatology 2004;39:302–310. (Ref.216)

Chevret L, et al. Human herpesvirus-6 infection: a prospective study evaluating HHV-6 DNA levels in liver from children with acute liver failure. J Med Virol 2008;80:1051–1057. (Ref.146)

Choi KW, et al. Outcomes and prognostic factors in 267 patients with severe acute respiratory syndrome in Hong Kong. Ann Intern Med 2003;139:715–723. (Ref.213)

Choquet S, et al. Efficacy and safety of rituximab in B-cell post-transplantation lymphoproliferative disorders: results of a prospective multicentre phase 2 study. Blood 2006;107:3053–3057. (Ref.122)

Colebunders R, et al. Marburg hemorrhagic fever in Durba and Watsa, Democratic Republic of the Congo: clinical documentation, features of illness, and treatment. J Infect Dis 2007;196(Suppl 2):S148–S153. (Ref.40)

Deback C, et al. Detection of human herpesviruses HHV-6, HHV-7 and HHV-8 in whole blood by real-time PCR using the new CMV, HHV-6, 7, 8 R-gene kit. J Virol Methods 2008;149:285–291. (Ref.163)

Di Trolio R, et al. Role of pegylated liposomal doxorubicin (PLD) in systemic Kaposi's sarcoma: a systematic review. Int J Immunopathol Pharmacol 2006; 19:253–263. (Ref.186)

Drosten C, et al. Identification of a novel coronavirus in patients with severe acute respiratory syndrome. N Engl J Med 2003;348:1967–1976. (Ref.209)

Drosten C, et al. Molecular diagnostics of viral haemorrhagic fevers. Antiviral Res 2003;57:61–87. (Ref.54)

Eisenhut M. Ischemic hepatitis and collateral damage to the liver in severe viral respiratory tract infections. Am J Pathol 2006;169:1100. (Ref.207)

Eisenhut M, Thorburn K, Ahmed T. Transaminase levels in ventilated children with respiratory syncytial virus bronchiolitis. Intensive Care Med 2004;30:931–934. (Ref.206)

Engelmann I, et al. Rapid quantitative PCR assay for the simultaneous detection of herpes simplex virus, varicella zoster virus, cytomegalovirus, Epstein-Barr virus, and human herpesvirus 6 DNA in blood and other clinical specimens. J Med Virol 2008;80:467–477. (Ref.164)

Engles EA, et al. Risk factor for human herpesvirus 8 infection among adults in the United States and evidence for sexual transmission. J Infect Dis 2007;196:199–207. (Ref.175)

Enria DA, Briggiler AM, Sánchez Z. Treatment of Argentine hemorrhagic fever. Antiviral Res 2008;78:132–139. (Ref.35)

Ergönül Ö. Crimean-Congo haemorrhagic fever. Lancet Infect Dis 2006;6:203–214. (Ref.53)

Ergönül Ö, et al. Analysis of the mortality among the patients with Crimean Congo hemorrhagic fever virus infection: severity criteria revisited. Clin Microbiol 2006;12:551–554. (Ref.56)

Ergönül Ö, et al. The characteristics of Crimean-Congo hemorrhagic fever in a recent outbreak in Turkey and the impact of oral ribavirin therapy. Clin Infect Dis 2004;39:285–289. (Ref.55)

Finström N, et al. Analysis of varicella-zoster virus and herpes simplex virus in various clinical samples by the use of different PCR assays. J Virol Methods 2009;150:193–196. (Ref.93)

Flamand L, et al. Multicentre comparison of PCR assays for detection of human herpesvirus 6 DNA in serum. J Clin Microbiol 2008;46:2700–2706. (Ref.165)

Fohrer C, et al. Long-term survival in post-transplant lymphoproliferative disorders with a dose-adjusted ACVBP regimen. Br J Haematol 2006;134:602–612. (Ref.119)

Frederick DM, Bland D, Gollin Y. Fatal disseminated herpes simplex virus infection in a previously healthy pregnant woman. J Reprod Med 2002;47:591-596. (Ref.90)

Freeman DO, et al. Spectrum of disease and relation to place of exposure among ill returned travelers. N Engl J Med 2006;354:119–130. (Ref.1)

Garnett CT, et al. Latent species C adenoviruses in human tonsil tissues. J Virol 2009;83:2417–2428. (Ref.191)

Gross TG, et al. Low dose chemotherapy of Epstein-Barr virus–positive post-transplantation lymphoproliferative disease in children after solid organ transplantation. J Clin Oncol 2005;23:6481–6488. (Ref.118)

Haas WH, et al. Imported Lassa fever in Germany: surveillance and management of contact persons. Clin Infect Dis 2003;36:1254–1258. (Ref.26)

Härmä M, et al. Pre-transplant human herpesvirus 6 infection of patients with acute liver failure is a risk factor for post transplant human herpesvirus 6 infection of the liver. Transplantation 2006;81:367–372. (Ref.154)

Härmä M, Höckerstedt K, Lautenschlager I. Human herpesvirus-6 and acute liver failure. Transplantation 2003;76:536–539. (Ref.147)

Hayakawa H, et al. A clinical study of adult human parvovirus B 19 infection. Intern Med 2007;41:295–299. (Ref.239)

Hsiao CH, et al. Immunohistochemical study of severe acute respiratory syndrome–associated coronavirus in tissue sections of patients. J Formos Med Assoc 2005;104:150–156. (Ref.218)

Isegawa Y, et al. Human herpesvirus 6 ganciclovir-resistant strain with amino acid substitutions associated with the death of an allogeneic stem cell transplant recipient. J Clin Virol 2009;44:15–19. (Ref.167)

Jessie K, et al. Localization of dengue virus in naturally infected human tissues, by immunohistochemistry and in situ hybridization. J Infect Dis 2004;189:1411–1418. (Ref.7)

Kojaoghlanian T, Flomenberg P, Horwitz MS. The impact of adenovirus infection on the immunocompromised host. Rev Med Virol 2003;13:155–171. (Ref.192)

Koreishi A, et al. Synchronous follicular lymphoma, Kaposi sarcoma, and Castleman's disease in a HIV-negative patient with EBV and HHV-8 coinfection. Int J Surg Pathol 2009, Aug 5 [Epub ahead of print].(Ref.180)

Ksiazek TG, et al. A novel coronavirus in patients with severe acute respiratory syndrome. N Engl J Med 2003;348:1953–1966. (Ref.208)

Kuntzen T, et al. Postinfantile giant cell hepatitis with autoimmune features following a human herpesvirus 6–induced adverse drug reaction. Eur J Gastroenterol Hepatol 2005;17:1131–1134. (Ref.160)

Kylat RI, Kelly EN, Ford-Jones EL. Clinical findings and adverse outcome in neonates with symptomatic congenital cytomegalovirus (SCCMV) infection. Eur J Pediatr 2006;165:773–778. (Ref.126)

Lee N, et al. A major outbreak of severe acute respiratory syndrome in Hong Kong. N Engl J Med 2003;348:1986–1994. (Ref.210)

Lee WM, et al. Brief report: no evidence for parvovirus B19 or hepatitis E as a cause of acute liver failure. Dig Dis Sci 2006;51:1712–1715. (Ref.244)

Leroy EM, et al. Fruit bats as reservoir of Ebola virus. Nature 2005;438:575–576. (Ref.39)

Levin MJ, Bacon TH, Leary JJ. Resistance of herpes simplex virus infections to nucleoside analogues in HIV-infected patients. Clin Infect Dis 2004;39(Suppl 5):S248–S257. (Ref.98)

Lledó L, et al. Hantavirus infections in Spain: analysis of sera from the general population and from patients with pneumonia, renal disease and hepatitis. J Clin Virol 2003;27:296–307. (Ref.66)

Lo AW, Tang NLS, To KF. How the SARS coronavirus causes disease: host or organism? J Pathol 2006;208:142–151. (Ref.219)

Mahanty S, Bray M. Pathogenesis of filoviral haemorrhagic fevers. Lancet Infect Dis 2004;4:487–498. (Ref.37)

Mardani M, et al. The efficacy of oral ribavirin in the treatment of Crimean-Congo hemorrhagic fever in Iran. Clin Infect Dis 2003;36:1613–1618. (Ref.61)

Martin BK, et al. Change over time in incidence of ganciclovir resistance in patients with cytomegalovirus retinitis. Clin Infect Dis 2008;44:1001–1008. (Ref.140)

Nakazibwe C. Marburg virus outbreak leads scientists to suspected disease reservoir. Bull World Health Organ 2007;85:654–656. (Ref.41)

Naresh KN, Rice AJ, Bower M. Lymph nodes involved by multicentric Castleman disease among HIV-positive individuals are often involved by Kaposi sarcoma. Am J Surg Pathol 2008;32:1006–1012. (Ref.179)

Nobili V, et al. Acute liver failure as presenting feature in tyrosinemia type 1 in a child with primary HHV-6 infection. J Gastroenterol Hepatol 2006;21:339. (Ref.148)

Oertel SH, et al. Effect of anti-CD20 antibody rituximab in patients with post-transplant lymphoproliferative disorder (PTLD). Am J Transplant 2005;5:2901–2906. (Ref.121)

Ogbu O, Ajuluchukwu E, Uneke CJ. Lassa fever in West African subregion: an overview. J Vector Borne Dis 2007;44:1–11. (Ref.28)

Ohashi M, et al. Human herpesvirus 6 infection in adult living related liver transplant recipients. Liver Transpl 2008;14:100–109. (Ref.155)

Peiris JS, et al. Re-emergence of fatal human influenza A subtype H5N1 disease. Lancet 2004;363:617–619. (Ref.205)

Peters CJ. Marburg and Ebola—arming ourselves against the deadly filoviruses. N Engl J Med 2005;352:2571–2573. (Ref.36)

Piaggio F, et al. Torque Teno virus—cause of viral liver disease following liver transplantation: a case report. Transplant Proc 2009;41:1378–1379. (Ref.250)

Pinna AD, et al. Five cases of fulminant hepatitis due to herpes simplex virus in adults. Dig Dis Sci 2002;47:750–754. (Ref.83)

Piselli P, et al. Risk of Kaposi sarcoma after solid-organ transplantation: multicenter study in 4,767 recipients in Italy, 1970-2006. Transplant Proc 2009;41:1227–1230. (Ref.176)

Polakos NK, et al. Kupffer cell–dependent hepatitis occurs during influenza infection. Am J Pathol 2006;168:1169–1178. (Ref.200)

Potenza I, et al. HHV-6A in syncytial giant-cell hepatitis. N Engl J Med 2008;359:583–602. (Ref.159)

Pourrut X, et al. Spatial and temporal patterns of Zaire Ebola virus antibody prevalence in the possible reservoir bat species. J Infect Dis 2007;196(Suppl 2):S176–S183. (Ref.42)

Poutanen SM, et al. Identification of severe acute respiratory syndrome in Canada. N Engl J Med 2003;348:1995–2005. (Ref.212)

Quaresma JA, et al. Reconsiderations of histopathology and ultrastructural aspects of the human liver in yellow fever. Acta Trop 2005;94:116–127. (Ref.17)

Quaresma JA, et al. Immunohistochemical examination of the role of Fas ligand and lymphocytes in the pathogenesis of human liver yellow fever. Virus Res 2006;116:91–97. (Ref.20)

Quaresma JA, et al. Revisiting the liver in human yellow fever: virus-induced apoptosis in hepatocytes associated with TGF-beta, TNF-alpha and NK cell activity. Virology 2006;345:22–30. (Ref.19)

Rezza G, et al. Infection with chikungunya virus in Italy: an outbreak in a temperate region. Lancet 2007;370:1840–1846. (Ref.72)

Shi X, et al. Severe acute respiratory syndrome–associated coronavirus is detected in intestinal D tissues of fatal cases. Am J Gastroenterol 2005;100:169–176. (Ref.217)

Sidwell RW, Smee DF. Viruses of the Bunya- and Togaviridae families: potential as bioterrorism agents and means of control. Antiviral Res 2003;57:101–111. (Ref.70)

Spengler U. Hepatic toxicity of antiviral agents. In: Kaplowith N, De Leve LD, editors. Drug induced liver disease. New York: Informa Health Care USA, 2007;567–591. (Ref.82)

Stebbing J, et al. Paclitaxel for anthracycline-resistant AIDS-related Kaposi's sarcoma: clinical and angiogenic correlations. Ann Oncol 2003;14:1660–1666. (Ref.187)

Tasdelen NF, et al. The role of ribavirin in the therapy of Crimean-Congo hemorrhagic fever: early use is promising. Eur J Clin Microbiol Infect Dis 2009;28:929–933. (Ref.62)

Taubitz W, et al. Chikungunya fever in travelers: clinical presentation and course. Clin Infect Dis 2007;45:e1–e4. (Ref.73)

Towner JS, et al. Marburg virus infection detected in a common African bat. PLoS One 2007;2:e764. (Ref.43)

Van der Ende M, et al. Complete clinical and virological remission of refractory HIV-related Kaposi's sarcoma with pegylated interferon alpha. AIDS 2007;21:1661–1662. (Ref.185)

Vasconcelos PF, et al. Genetic divergence and dispersal of yellow fever virus, Brazil. Emerg Infect Dis 2004;10:1578–1584. (Ref.14)

Waza K, Inoue K, Matsumura S. Symptoms associated with parvovirus B19 infection in adults: a pilot study. Intern Med 2007;46:1975–1978. (Ref.240)

Weinberger B, et al. Quantitation of Epstein-Barr virus mRNA using reverse transcription and real-time PCR. J Med Virol 2004;74:612–618. (Ref.116)

Wilder-Smith A, Schwartz E. Dengue in travelers. N Engl J Med 2005;353:924–932. (Ref.4)

Wilson ME, et al. Fever in returned travelers: results from the GeoSentinel Surveillance Network. Clin Infect Dis 2007;44:1560–1568. (Ref.2)

Wong WM, et al. Temporal pattern of hepatic dysfunction and disease severity in patients with SARS. JAMA 2003;290:2663–2665. (Ref.214)

A complete list of references can be found at www.expertconsult.com.

Chapter 35

Parasitic Liver Disease

Gamal Esmat and Naglaa Zayed

ABBREVIATIONS

ALA amebic liver abscess	**ERCP** endoscopic retrograde cholangiopancreatography	**PAIR** puncture, aspiration, injection, reaspiration
CAA circulating anodic antigen	**GASP** gut-associated schistosome proteoglycan	**PCR** polymerase chain reaction
CCA circulating cathodic antigen		**PPF** periportal fibrosis
CIE counterimmunoelectrophoresis	**HCV** hepatitis C virus	**PZQ** praziquantel
EDHS Egypt Demographic and Health Survey	**HIV** human immunodeficiency virus	**T$_H$1** T helper 1 cell
	IFA indirect immunofluorescence assay	**T$_H$2** T helper 2 cell
ELISA enzyme-linked immunosorbent assay	**IHA** indirect hemagglutination	**WHO** World Health Organization

Introduction

Parasitic diseases continue to be a major cause of morbidity and mortality, with more than 3 billion people infected worldwide, especially in the developing world, where improved measures to prevent infection require considerable investments in the public health infrastructure.[1]

Liver parasites span a wide range of complexity, and different species mature and reproduce within hepatocytes, reticuloendothelial cells, the portal venous system, and the bile ducts. Successful well-adapted parasites can accommodate the immune responses of normal hosts and cause minimal acute injury as they generate enormous numbers of progeny with the potential to infect other hosts, whereas hosts with abnormal or compromised responses are at risk for severe disease manifestations.[2] Long-lived parasites such as helminths are more remarkable for their ability to down-regulate host immunity to protect them from elimination and minimize severe pathology in the host.[3] Helminths that infect the liver and hepatobiliary system include nematodes (roundworms), cestodes (tapeworms), and trematodes (flatworms or flukes).[4] The infection is often chronic and can cause insidious or frank disease that leads to considerable morbidity; however, the risk for mortality is low.[5] The majority of morbidity and mortality from these infestations is caused by the host immune response to the larvae or adult worm.[4] They establish numerous strategies and diverse molecular mechanisms for evading host immunity that can promote persistence and facilitate their establishment, growth, and reproduction, in addition to chronicity factors that favor completion of the life cycle inside an immunologically hostile environment and transmission of parasites. The generation of protective immunity to helminth parasites is critically dependent on the development of a CD4$^+$ T helper type 2 (T$_H$2) cytokine response (**Fig. 35-1**).[6] Helminth products appear to be inherently adjuvantized in that they can promote strong T$_H$2 responses to themselves and to bystander antigens in the absence of any additional adjuvant. Dendritic cells, the primary interface between infection and induction of adaptive immune responses, play a central role in the modulation of helper T cells with the initiation of T$_H$2 responses through the production of cytokines and expression of certain surface molecules.[7] Furthermore, host–parasite interactions specifically involve interactions between helminth excretory/secretory products and host Toll-like receptors and lectins, as well as the putative functions of helminth proteases in activating and recruiting innate immune cells. The development of adaptive antiparasitic T$_H$2 cytokine responses may prevent strong immune responses against parasitic worms, thereby allowing their long-term survival and restricting pathology.[8] Interestingly, both parasitic infections and cancer have complex natural histories and long latent periods during which numerous exogenous and endogenous factors interact to conceal causality. Although only urinary bladder carcinoma and cholangiocarcinoma have been definitely known to develop as a result of *Schistosoma haematobium* and the hepatobiliary parasites (*Clonorchis sinensis*, *Opisthorchis viverrini*, and *Opisthorchis felineus*), respectively, other parasites have been implicated in facilitating malignant transformation through chronic inflammation, modulation of the host immune system, disruption of proliferation-antiproliferation pathways, induction of genomic instability, and stimulation of malignant stem cell progeny.[9] Liver parasites can either affect the liver parenchyma itself, such as schistosomiasis, hydatid liver disease, or amebiasis, or have a hepatobiliary effect and affect both the liver and the biliary system, such as fascioliasis, clonorchiasis, and opisthorchiasis.

Stool studies, radiologic imaging, and serologic testing are the mainstays in diagnosis. However, having a high index of

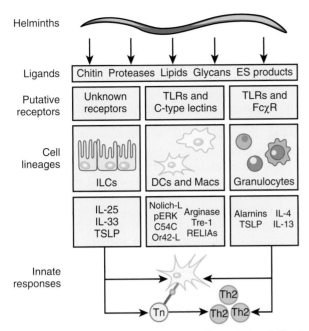

Helminths

Ligands | Chitin | Proteases | Lipids | Glycans | ES products

Putative receptors | Unknown receptors | TLRs and C-type lectins | TLRs and FcχR

Cell lineages | ILCs | DCs and Macs | Granulocytes

| IL-25 IL-33 TSLP | Nolich-L pERK C54C Or42-L | Arginase Tre-1 RELIAs | Alarnins TSLP | IL-4 IL-13 |

Innate responses

Tn → Th2 Th2 Th2

Fig. 35-1 Orchestration of CD4⁺ T_H2 cell differentiation following innate immune cell recognition and response to helminth-derived products. DCs, dendritic cells; ES, excretory/secretory; IL-25, interleukin-25; Macs, macrophages; pERK, protein extracellular signal-regulated kinase; TLR, Toll-like receptors; TSLP, thymic stromal lymphopoietir

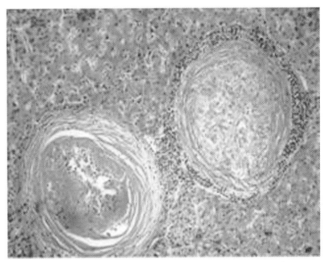

Fig. 35-2 **Schistosomiasis: cicatricial granulomas with lamellar walls and a perifocal lymphohistiocytic inflammatory rim (hematoxylin-eosin stain).**

suspicion is a critical step in the diagnosis and management of patients with hepatic helminthiasis. Researchers and clinicians alike are moving forward with chemoprophylactic and vaccine preventive strategies in an effort to decrease the morbidity and mortality caused by helminthic infestation worldwide.[4]

Schistosomiasis

Schistosomiasis is a multifactorial disease caused by the trematode *Schistosoma* that involves environmental, behavioral, parasitic, vector, and host factors. It continues to be a significant cause of morbidity and mortality worldwide[10] and the second leading parasitic disease after malaria. Four of the five *Schistosoma* species infecting humans may cause liver disease: *S. mansoni, S. japonicum, S. intercalatum,* and *S. mekongi.*[11] Approximately 300 million people are affected by schistosomiasis in 74 countries worldwide, with a high concentration in Asia, Africa, and South America[12]; annual deaths are reported to total 280,000.[13] The Nile River has been an epicenter for schistosomiasis since ancient Egypt. In 1980, an estimated 10% of the 200 million persons infected with *Schistosoma* were Egyptians.[14] Two species of *Schistosoma*—*S. haematobium,* which primarily causes disease in the urinary tract, and *S. mansoni,* which principally causes morbidity in the gut and liver—are endemic in Egypt. Infection takes place when the free-swimming larval forms of the parasite, known as cercariae, are shed into fresh water by the snail intermediate host and enter the body by penetration of the skin. Larvae migrate to the portal venous system; sexual reproduction occurs in the portal vein, where adult worms reside and eggs

are laid. Eggs pass from blood vessels into tissues, including intestinal or bladder mucosa, from which they are shed in feces or urine.[15] Hepatic schistosomiasis results from the host's granulomatous cell–mediated immune response to the soluble egg antigen of *S. mansoni,* which eventually progresses to irreversible fibrosis and, consequently, severe portal hypertension.[16] Eggs remain viable in the liver for about 3 weeks. The eggs cause a primarily T_H1 immune response with later recruitment of eosinophils and granuloma formation.[17] Granuloma formation (**Fig. 35-2**) is a helper T cell–mediated delayed hypersensitivity reaction driven by T_H2 cytokines such as interleukin-4 (IL-4) and IL-13, whereas IL-10, interferon-γ, and a subset of regulatory T cells can limit the schistosome-induced pathology. In addition, a variety of cell types have also been implicated, including hepatic stellate cells, activated macrophages, and regulatory T cells.[10] The balance between T_H1- and T_H2-type cytokines influences the extent of the pathology and the development of fibrosis.[18] Eggs are detectable inside the granulomas with the subsequent formation of marked portal and perilobular fibrosis, which is most pronounced with *S. mansoni* and *S. japonicum.* The final result of hepatic schistosomiasis with a heavy *S. mansoni* burden is severe portal fibrosis and greatly enlarged fibrotic portal tracts, which resemble clay pipestems thrust through the liver (termed Symmers pipestem fibrosis).[19] Interestingly, normal liver architecture is preserved, lobular architecture is retained, nodular regenerative hyperplasia is not observed, and thus the fibrosis could be reversible, at least in part.

Co-infection with viral hepatitis, either hepatitis B virus (HBV) or hepatitis C virus (HCV), is very common since the regions with a high prevalence of schistosomiasis usually have a high endemicity of chronic viral hepatitis as well. Egypt is endemic for both *S. mansoni* and *S. haematobium,* with community prevalence often ranging between 15% and 45%,[20] in addition to having the highest worldwide prevalence of HCV, with an estimated 8 to 10 million in a population of 68 million exposed to the virus and 5 to 7 million with active infection. An important cause of the high exposure to HCV was the establishment of a large reservoir of infection as a result of extensive schistosomiasis control programs that used intravenously administered tartar emetic 20 to 50 years ago.[21] In 2008, the Egypt Demographic and Health Survey (EDHS) conducted on behalf of the Ministry of Health revealed that an overall 15% of EDHS respondents had HCV antibodies in their blood, thus indicating that they had been exposed to the virus at some point, whereas 10% were found to have an active infection with higher levels of infection in older cohorts because of their exposure to the schistosomiasis treatment programs during the 1960s to 1980s.[22] The association between both schistosomiasis and HCV is known to cause earlier liver deterioration and more severe illness. The liver is the principal site for both HCV replication and egg deposition, which down-regulates the local immune responses in the liver[23] and results in suppression of the intrahepatic bystander immune response to HCV. This may also occur during inactive schistosomal infection, as the ova remain in the hepatic portal tracts and their soluble antigens could influence the host's cell-mediated immunity for a considerable time.[24] Co-infection can also produce a unique clinical, virologic, and histologic pattern manifested by viral persistence with high HCV RNA titers, higher necroinflammatory and fibrosis scores in liver biopsy specimens in addition to poor response to interferon therapy, and accelerated progression of hepatic fibrosis.[25]

Clinical Manifestations

The disease has an incubation period of 4 to 6 weeks. A maculopapular eruption may arise at the site of skin penetration by the cercarial form of the parasite in the early stage. A potentially fatal, acute form of schistosomiasis that is common in areas with high transmission rates, termed Katayama fever, may occur. It is manifested by fever, chills, headaches, arthralgia, epigastric pain, diarrhea with blood-flecked mucus, loss of weight, lymphadenopathy, and urticarial skin reactions. The liver and the spleen are moderately enlarged, especially in the case of *S. japonicum* and *S. mansoni* infection.[11] In chronic schistosomiasis, advanced hepatic disease is characterized by signs and symptoms related to the portal fibrosis and the presinusoidal portal hypertension: esophageal and gastric variceal bleeding and splenomegaly with preserved hepatocellular synthetic function until the last stage of the disease. Growth retardation and late development are specifically associated with schistosomiasis in heavily infected children. When present, laboratory evidence may include peripheral eosinophilia, anemia, hypoalbuminemia, and hypergammaglobulinemia, in addition to pancytopenia because of splenic sequestration. A syndrome caused by chronic persistent infection with one of the *Salmonella* species has been described in association with schistosomal infection. It is characterized by a long history of an indolent febrile illness and bacteremia, as well as hepatosplenomegaly, edema, and lower limb petechial rash.[26]

Diagnosis

Identification of *Schistosoma* ova in excreta or in mucosal biopsy specimens is the most appropriate method for diagnosis of schistosomal infection, to determine whether there is an indication for chemotherapy, for evaluation of antischistosomal drugs, and for monitoring in epidemiologic surveys.[27] No single stool examination procedure is totally reliable;

sensitivity varies between 50% and 80%, depending on the patient's intensity of infection, the number of eggs in the sample examined, and the care taken by the examiner. Multiple (three to four) specimens should be examined, and sedimentation, filtration, and centrifugation procedures are better than floatation because schistosome eggs are relatively heavy. The Kato-Katz technique, a semiquantitative stool examination technique, is the standard method recommended by the World Health Organization (WHO) for the field diagnosis of intestinal schistosomiasis and is generally recommended for the diagnosis and evaluation of *S. mansoni* infection by schistosome experts. However, there is increasing concern that this technique has low diagnostic sensitivity.[28] Rectal biopsy is considered the most sensitive technique and is valuable when stool examination is negative in patients with light and partially treated infections. In contrast, serologic tests have many disadvantages in that they become positive too late after infection, become negative too late after cure, can cross-react with other infections (e.g., fascioliasis), and are unrelated to the intensity of infection. However, they are useful when parasitologic tests are negative, in nonendemic situations, and in epidemiologic surveys, especially in eradicated controlled areas where prevalence is expected to be low.[29] Indirect hemagglutination (IHA) and enzyme-linked immunosorbent assay (ELISA) are the most commonly used methods, but other techniques, including complement fixation, flocculation, indirect fluorescent antibody testing, and radioimmunoassay, have highly variable sensitivity and specificity because of the wide range of types and purity of schistosome antigens used, in addition to lack of standardization.[30] Schistosomal antigen detection tests can alternatively be used because they measure parasite-derived substances and therefore would be more comparable with the worm burden and more indicative of active infection. The best studied antigens are the secretory-excretory antigens of the adult worm, also known as gut-associated antigens; the circulating anodic antigen (CAA), also known as gut-associated schistosome proteoglycan (GASP); and the circulating cathodic antigen (CCA), also known as M antigen. An ELISA test for another circulating antigen derived from *S. mansoni*—soluble egg antigen—had a sensitivity of 91% in serum and 97% in urine.[31] A dipstick assay that detects CCA in the urine of *S. mansoni*–infected patients with 92% sensitivity has been of great value in monitoring large-scale interventions such as chemotherapy and vaccination programs. In addition, polymerase chain reaction (PCR), which can detect *S. mansoni* DNA in human serum and feces, yielded high sensitivity because it can detect fecal egg counts as low as 2 to 4 eggs/g, with no cross-reaction with other helminthic infections.[32]

Ultrasound (US) is a well-established tool for the diagnosis and grading of hepatic periportal fibrosis (PPF), a major pathologic consequence of *S. mansoni* infection and a hallmark in its diagnosis.[33] The typical "bull's-eye" appearance on US is characteristic and represents an anechoic portal vein surrounded by an echogenic mantle of fibrous tissue.[34] A US grading system for hepatic PPF in patients with pure schistosomiasis that involves the thickness of portal tracts has been proposed: grade I, 3 to 5 mm; grade II, 5 to 7 mm; and grade III, greater than 7 mm (**Fig. 35-3**).[33] This score provides a simple, inexpensive, accurate, noninvasive means of screening individuals with hepatosplenic schistosomiasis for esophageal varices. This score strongly correlates with previous

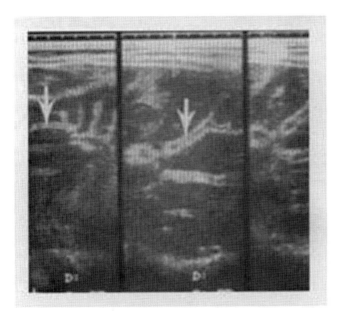

Fig. 35-3 **Moderate periportal fibrosis of the liver demonstrated by ultrasonography.** The *arrows* point to the typical lesions.

gastrointestinal hemorrhage[35] and thus accurately reflects the hemodynamic changes and provides a good estimate of the clinical status of patients. However, the finding of PPF by sonographic examination has been questioned when magnetic resonance imaging (MRI) was used to confirm the diagnosis of hepatic PPF.[36] A significant number of patients in whom PPF was diagnosed by US were shown by MRI to have fat infiltration of the periportal tracts. Thus a more accurate clinical diagnosis of hepatosplenic *S. mansoni* could be based on the information obtained by clinical, US, and MRI examination (whenever possible).[37]

Treatment

Schistosomal infections can be cured with inexpensive drugs, but people living in endemic countries usually become reinfected. The first effective therapy for schistosomiasis, in which multiple intravenous injections of tartar emetic were used, was introduced in 1918 and remained the standard therapy for *S. mansoni* and *S. japonicum* infection for more than 60 years.[29] Three effective schistosomicidal drugs are now in use[38]: metrifonate (for *S. haematobium*), oxamniquine (for *S. mansoni*), and praziquantel (PZQ) (for all human species).

Praziquantel

Praziquantel is an isoquinoline compound that is used to treat human schistosomiasis on a large scale. It is a safe, nontoxic drug that is given orally in a single dose of 40 mg/kg of body weight and is highly effective against all human schistosomes, with cure rates of 80% to 90%. PZQ produces instantaneous contraction of the muscles of the parasite, followed by spastic paralysis of the worm, which is swept to the liver for phagocytosis; thus the host's immune response appears to be strongly implicated in the mode of action of PZQ.[39] Minor side effects may occur in the form of epigastric discomfort, abdominal colic, nausea, vomiting, headache, dizziness, pruritus, and

transient skin eruptions. An impending danger with serious implications for the health protection of millions of people infested with schistosomiasis is the development of drug resistance, which has occurred in Brazil and Kenya. Cure rates have decreased in the last decade and were found to be very low in Senegal because of drug resistance.[40] This concern is reflected by the recent proposal of a new class of compounds that could represent a novel source of drugs against schistosomiasis.[41] Another problem with PZQ is that it does not kill schistosomula that are 3 to 12 days old.

New Drugs

Mirazid is an herbal drug derived from myrrh (purified *Commiphora molmol* Engier) that was developed in Egypt. The drug was found to be safe with no serious side. However, its efficacy has been debated; some studies showed high efficacy in the treatment of schistosomiasis and fascioliasis,[42] with a cure rate of 91.7%, whereas other authors have found it to have a much lower cure rate than PZQ in their studies.[43] Therefore Botros and colleagues did not recommend mirazid as an agent to control schistosomiasis.[44]

Artemether (an antimalarial drug) can kill these organisms and can prevent new infection with a dose given every 2 weeks, but it should not be used in malaria-endemic areas to prevent the selection of artemether-resistant *Plasmodium falciparum*.[45] Artemether has been tried in *S. japonicum*–endemic areas in southern China to prevent new infections[46]; it was found to be active against other human schistosomes and appears to be synergistic to PZQ in killing adult worms.

Ultimately, prevention and control programs of schistosomiasis should be multifaceted; that is, they should include chemotherapy, reduction of water contact and contamination, snail control, and vaccination.[29] More than 10 important antigens with strong potential as vaccines candidates were developed; however, most of them have been difficult to move forward.[47] A recombinant antigen vaccine against *S. mansoni* remains elusive, in part because the parasite deploys complex defensive and offensive strategies to combat immune attack. A successful vaccine will probably require a cocktail of antigens rather than a single recombinant protein.[48]

Echinococcosis (*Echinococcus granulosus/Echinococcus multilocularis*)
Introduction

The most important zoonotic *Echinococcus* species, from a public health standpoint, are *E. granulosus* and related species that cause cystic echinococcosis and *E. multilocularis*, the cause of alveolar echinococcosis. The WHO has included both echinococcosis and cysticercosis as part of a neglected zoonosis subgroup for its 2008-2015 strategic plans for the control of neglected tropical diseases.[49] Geographically distinct strains of *E. granulosus* exist with different host affinities. Molecular studies using mitochondrial DNA sequences have identified 10 distinct genetic types (G1 to G10) within *E. granulosus*. The sheep strain (G1) is the most cosmopolitan form and is the one most commonly associated with human infection.[50]

Immune Response

A combined T_H1 and T_H2 cytokine profile appears to be crucial for prolonged parasitic growth and survival. T_H1 cytokines promote the initial cell recruitment around the parasite vesicles by inducing a chronic cell infiltrate and the formation of organized periparasitic granuloma, fibrosis, and necrosis. T_H2 cytokines could be responsible for the ineffective immune response.[51]

Humans are infected by ingesting eggs shed in the feces of definitive canine hosts. The eggs hatch into slow-growing larval cysts and penetrate through the mucosa, thereby leading to blood-borne distribution of the organism.[52] The liver is the most commonly affected organ (60%), followed by the lungs (30%), kidneys, brain, spleen, bone, mesocolon, and potentially any other viscera.[53] The right lobe (80%) of the liver is affected more than the left lobe, and in a third of cases the cysts are multiple.[54] Pathologically, a hydatid cyst is a fluid-filled structure delimited by three layers in *E. multilocularis* infection; the cysts are less well limited because there is no sharp separation between the parasitic tissue and the liver parenchyma.[55] The poor vascularization of the parasitic mass and superimposed bacterial infection often lead to necrosis in the central part of the cyst.

Clinical Manifestations

Clinical signs associated with echinococcosis usually develop as a result of mass effect, allergic reactions, or tissue necrosis/fibrosis. Symptoms can take 5 to 10 years to occur following the initial infestation.[56] The initial phase of primary infection is always asymptomatic and may be maintained for many years even if the infection was acquired in childhood. The clinical manifestations are variable and determined by the site, size, and condition of the cysts.[52] Hepatic echinococcosis is usually manifested as hepatomegaly (with or without a palpable mass in the right upper quadrant), right epigastric pain, nausea, and vomiting. In the event of a ruptured cyst, allergic reactions ranging from mild to fatal anaphylaxis may occur. Common complications include rupture into the biliary tree with secondary cholangitis, biliary obstruction or extrinsic compression, subphrenic abscess formation, and intraperitoneal rupture with anaphylaxis.[57]

Diagnosis

The diagnosis is usually made at a stage when a fully developed and still proliferating cyst has already induced an immune response in the host.[58] In addition to the history and clinical examination, the diagnosis is based on a combination of imaging techniques. Thus clinical findings such as a space-occupying lesion and residence in an endemic region are suggestive of cystic hydatid disease.[59] Serologic tests (hemagglutination, immunoelectrophoresis, and enzyme immunoassay) are positive and confirm the presumptive radiologic diagnosis.[53] However, a detectable immune response does not develop in some patients with cystic echinococcosis.[60] Hepatic cysts are more likely than pulmonary cysts to elicit an immune response; it appears, however, that regardless of location, the sensitivity of serologic tests is inversely related to the degree of sequestration of the echinococcal antigens inside cysts.[61] In seronegative individuals, a presumptive diagnosis can be confirmed by the demonstration of protoscolices or hydatid membranes in the liquid obtained by percutaneous aspiration of the cyst.[62]

Imaging techniques such as abdominal US, computed tomography (CT), and MRI are used to determine the location, number and size, morphology, and vitality of the cysts; the status of the biliary tree and involvement of adjacent or distal organs; and the diagnosis of deep-seated lesions in all organs.[63,64] Chest roentgenography permits the detection of echinococcal cysts in the lungs, and CT is very helpful, especially for the diagnosis of nontypical lesions.[59] A standardized classification system for hepatic cysts detected by US has been developed by the WHO.[65] The most common sonographic appearance of hepatic hydatid cysts reported in 362 Egyptians patients with 558 cysts was a noncomposite anechoic pattern in 91% of the cysts, with the remaining cysts having either a rosette or honeycomb appearance.[66]

Treatment

Surgery was considered the only option for the treatment of echinococcal cysts; however, chemotherapy with benzimidazole compounds and treatment by cyst puncture, aspiration, injection of chemicals, and reaspiration (PAIR) has been introduced and, increasingly, has supplemented or even replaced surgery as the preferred treatment.[64] Surgical excision of intact hydatid cysts, when possible, may be the best treatment to remove cysts and lead to complete cure with avoidance of the adverse consequences of spilling the contents. Both albendazole (10 to 15 mg/kg/day) and mebendazole (40 to 50 mg/kg/day) have demonstrated efficacy; however, the results of albendazole have been superior, probably because of its pharmacokinetic profile, which favors intestinal absorption and penetration into the cyst. Small (<7 mm in diameter), isolated cysts surrounded by minimal adventitial reaction respond best, whereas complicated cysts with multiple compartments or daughter cysts or those with thick or calcified surrounding adventitial reactions are relatively refractory to treatment.[62]

Another option for the treatment of hepatic hydatid cysts is the PAIR technique.[67] PAIR is indicated for patients who cannot undergo surgery and for those who refuse surgery and have single or multiple cysts in the liver, abdominal cavity, spleen, or kidney. The PAIR technique is contraindicated for inaccessible or superficially located liver cysts and for calcified lesions. PAIR was found to be a safe, effective, and inexpensive therapeutic modality. Follow-up by US after 1 year revealed cyst collapse in 88%, and repeated US showed a continued decrease in the size of all remaining and organized lesions (pseudosolid pattern) in 26% of patients after 5 years of follow-up.[66]

Amebiasis
Introduction

Amebiasis, a disease caused by the intestinal protozoan parasite *Entamoeba histolytica*, is the third leading parasitic cause of death in humans after malaria and schistosomiasis. Globally, it is responsible for 40,000 to 100,000 deaths per year.[68,69] It is distributed throughout the world and occurs in almost all countries in which the barriers between human feces and food or water are insufficient. Africa, Central and South America, and India have the highest morbidity and mortality.[68] The genus *Entamoeba* contains many species, some of which (*E. histolytica, E. dispar, E. moshkovskii, E. polecki, E. coli, E. hartmanni*) can reside in the human interstitial lumen. *E. histolytica* is the only *Entamoeba* species definitely associated with disease; the others are considered nonpathogenic.[70] *E. dispar,* one of the noninvasive, nonpathogenic, nonantigenic species, is responsible for more than 90% of amebic infections, whereas *E. histolytica* (invasive and pathogenic) can cause invasive disease and remains an important cause of morbidity and mortality in developing countries.[71] Both are genetically distinct but microscopically indistinguishable[72]; however, advances in molecular technology have allowed clear characterization of the aforementioned *Entamoeba* species. Interestingly, only a few strains are responsible for approximately one case of disease per four asymptomatic infected individuals, which may be based on the genetic background of *E. histolytica* strains.[73]

Ingestion of cysts from fecally contaminated food or water initiates infection, and the trophozoite may remain confined to the intestinal lumen as a simple boarder and feed on bacteria and cellular debris. A great number of patients infected with *E. dispar* and some strains of *E. histolytica* are asymptomatic, whereas only a relatively small proportion of infected individuals suffer from amebic colitis. Intestinal invasion may occur, depending on the parasite's genetic[74] and immunoenzymatic[75] profile, in addition to its ability to produce proteolytic enzymes and to resist complement-mediated lysis. Trophozoites invading the portal circulation disseminate systemically and reach the liver, where they cause hepatic amebiasis and its distinctive lesion, the amebic liver abscess (ALA). Amebic lysis of neutrophils at the edge of the lesion releases mediators that lead to hepatocyte death and can extend the damage to distant hepatic cells.[76] Eventually, the small lesions coalesce into a larger hepatic lesion, which is unsuitably named the amebic abscess. ALA is surrounded by a well-circumscribed region with completely unaffected adjacent liver parenchyma. The cavity contains a thick, nearly sterile material that varies in color from creamy white to dirty brown and pink, similar to "anchovy sauce." Amebae are rarely present in this material.

Clinical Manifestations

Asymptomatic Patients

In most *E. histolytica* infections, symptoms are absent or very mild and represent "noninvasive" disease. Asymptomatic patients never become symptomatic; they may excrete cysts for a short period until they clear the infection. These patients should be treated to eliminate the organism and prevent further transmission.[69]

Symptomatic Patients

In only a small proportion of people infected with *E. histolytica* will clinical disease eventually develop, the most frequent manifestations being amebic colitis and ALA.[69]

Amebic Colitis

Patients often have a history of several weeks of abdominal pain and diarrhea (usually characterized by blood, mucus, and fecal leukocytosis). Fever occurs in fewer than 40% of patients.[69]

Amebic Liver Abscess

Amebic liver abscess is the most common extraintestinal manifestation of amebiasis. Some days or months after the onset of diarrhea, or even without a history of intestinal amebiasis, the clinical manifestations of hepatic abscess can appear. Patients are usually seen initially within 5 months of contracting the disease; however, prolonged latency may also occur.[77] The hepatic lesion is generally solitary and located in the right lobe, close to the capsule. Clinical symptoms include fever (in 87% to 100% of patients), malaise, right upper quadrant pain with no concomitant colitis (in 60% to 70% of patients), hepatic tenderness, and hepatomegaly.[76] If the abscess compresses the diaphragm, cough and dyspnea may be present, along with dullness and rales in the right lung base.[78] Ruptured abscess will cause abdominal pain with guarding and rigidity. Jaundice is very uncommon and is associated with a worse prognosis.

Several laboratory findings are usually abnormal but nonspecific, including moderate leukocytosis without eosinophilia; mild anemia, either normochromic or hypochromic; increased levels of alkaline phosphatase; and an increased erythrocyte sedimentation rate.[79]

Diagnosis

The diagnosis of amebiasis is established either by detecting *E. histolytica* parasites in feces or by detecting an antibody response to the parasite in serum.[80] *E. histolytica* cysts and trophozoites are found in fixed fecal smears stained with a permanent stain (iron hematoxylin or trichrome). Multiple samples are required because the organism is shed intermittently. The sensitivity of microscopy is poor, and it cannot distinguish between the *Entamoeba* species; thus further testing is required for a correct diagnosis.[72] Colonoscopy and flexible sigmoidoscopy are useful in patients with acute colitis when *E. histolytica* infection is suspected on clinical grounds but not detected in stool samples. Examination of scrapings and biopsy specimens for trophozoites has higher sensitivity than does examination of fecal specimens.[80] Culture techniques can detect *E. histolytica*; however, they are time-consuming, laborious, and often unrewarding, with a sensitivity of only about 50%. Antigen detection methods using monoclonal antibodies directed against various proteins of *E. histolytica* were reported to be an essential adjunctive method for examination of stool that has improved sensitivity and specificity.[81] Molecular methods using the PCR technique can amplify *E. histolytica* genes from extracted fecal DNA and from pus aspirated from ALA, and such tests are highly sensitive and specific[82] and can reliably differentiate between nonpathogenic and pathogenic *Entamoeba* species. However, these tests are expensive and require a high level of expertise.[80]

Serologic tests are specific but have varying sensitivity. They are reported to be about 100% specific for ALA[70] and 84% for invasive intestinal disease.[68] Serologic tests are helpful in places where infection with *E. histolytica* is not common; however, they are unable to distinguish past from current infection in endemic areas. Detection of antibodies can be helpful in the case of ALA when patients do not have detectable parasites in stool. Many different assays have been developed, such as IHA, latex agglutination, immunoelectrophoresis, counterimmunoelectrophoresis (CIE), the amebic gel diffusion test, immunodiffusion, complement fixation, indirect immunofluorescence assay (IFA), and ELISA. The latter is the most popular assay in diagnostic laboratories for studying the epidemiology of asymptomatic amebiasis and making the diagnosis of symptomatic amebiasis after fecal examination.[70] The sensitivity of ELISA approaches 95% with no cross-reaction with other, non–*E. histolytica* parasites.

The diagnosis of ALA relies on the identification of a space-occupying lesion in the liver and positive amebic serology. Definitive confirmation is based on demonstration of trophozoites in aspirated pus, which can be further supported by recovering trophozoites and cysts in the feces of these patients. Cyst aspiration is not usually required for diagnosis in a patient with the clinical findings of ALA and in whom serologic evaluation is positive. Liver tests are not very helpful, presumably because too little liver tissue is affected.[71] Moderate elevation of alkaline phosphatase, as well as hypoalbuminemia and mildly increased transaminase levels, would suggest the possibility of a large abscess. US and CT are the imaging tests of choice; both methods are very sensitive, but neither provides absolute specificity for ALA. US is the most widely used initial imaging procedure because of its low cost, accessibility, and ability to rapidly detect hepatic lesions at the different stages of the disease. On US, hepatic lesions tend to be round or oval and hypoechoic, with well-defined margins. Abdominal CT is another valuable imaging procedure that has greater resolution and sensitivity in detecting hepatic lesions, especially smaller ones, and thus is useful in early diagnosis.[71] In a series of 52 patients with ALA diagnosed by US and serologic tests, US revealed that most abscesses were solitary (81%), in the right lobe (71%), rounded or oval (78%), and cystic (57%) and had a mean abscess diameter of 9.2 cm with a well-defined wall (53%). All patients survived and were cured completely with medications. Drainage of large abscesses was performed in only four patients.[83]

Treatment

Asymptomatic carriers of *E. histolytica* should be treated with a luminal agent to minimize the spread of disease and the risk for development of invasive disease. Amebic colitis is first treated with a nitroimidazole derivative (metronidazole followed by a luminal agent to eradicate colonization).[69]

Most uncomplicated ALAs can be treated successfully with tissue amebicides to eradicate the invasive trophozoite forms in the liver, followed by luminal amebicides for eradication of the asymptomatic colonization state. Metronidazole is given at a dose of 500-750 mg three times a day orally for 10 days and has cure rates of 90%. Alternatively, tinidazole, a closely related, well-tolerated nitroimidazole, may be administered once daily and appears to be at least as effective as metronidazole, with a clinical cure rate of greater than 90%. Luminal agents with proven efficacy include diloxanide furoate, iodoquinol, and paromomycin. A second course of a luminal amebicide may be required in a few weeks if the first course fails to eradicate the intestinal carriage.[71] Metronidazole is the standard of care for uncomplicated ALAs (complicated liver abscesses are those localized in the left lobe, multiple, or pyogenic). Therapeutic aspiration in addition to metronidazole to hasten clinical or radiologic resolution of uncomplicated ALA cannot be supported or refuted.[84] Aspiration of ALA may be performed in patients with no clinical improvement in 48 to 72 hours, a left lobe abscess because of concern for rupture into the pericardium, a thin rim of liver tissue around the abscess (<10 mm), seronegative abscesses,[85] a large abscess at risk for rupture, and an uncertain diagnosis.[86] The clinical response to antiamebic drugs is usually evident within 48 to 72 hours and should be fairly rapid, especially in endemic areas. Follow-up US or CT is unnecessary after the cessation of symptoms and signs because resolution on imaging may take several months to years to become apparent and does not correlate with clinical resolution. Therefore clinical criteria rather than US should be used to monitor the result of therapy, and a follow-up stool examination is recommended after completion of therapy.[85] Alternatively, surgery for cyst drainage is limited to patients with complications of invasive disease and very severe or therapy-resistant cases.[87]

Hepatobiliary Parasites

Parasitic infection of the biliary tree is caused by liver flukes, namely, *C. sinensis, O. viverrini,* and *O. felineus,* in addition to human infection with *Fasciola hepatica,* a cattle fluke, which may occur inadvertently.

Fascioliasis

Fascioliasis, a frequent cause of liver disease in endemic areas, is caused by the trematode *F. hepatica,* and *Fasciola gigantica* affects sheep and cows in particular. It was considered a secondary zoonotic disease until the mid-1990s. Human fascioliasis is emerging or reemerging in many countries, including increases in prevalence and intensity and geographic expansion.[88] It is estimated that 2.4 to 17 million people are infected throughout the world[89] and that 91.1 million are at risk for infection.[90]

Humans are infected accidentally by ingesting contaminated watercress or water containing encysted larvae. In the stomach, the excysted larvae are liberated, escape into the peritoneal cavity, and then penetrate the capsule of Glisson, after which they enter the liver parenchyma. In the liver, the flukes slowly migrate randomly through the hepatic parenchyma until they reach the larger bile ducts and penetrate into the lumen of the bile ducts.[91] The migratory larval and resting adult stages correspond to two clinical stages of the life cycle, called the hepatic and biliary stages. The hepatic stage lasts 2 to several months.[89]

The biliary phase may last for a decade or more. The pathogenesis of fascioliasis is due to larval migration through the hepatic parenchyma and chronic inflammatory changes such as marked local inflammatory reaction, hepatocyte necrosis, hemorrhage, and abscess formation, followed by fibrosis within the biliary tract.[92] The adult fasciola and its ova, in addition to causing chronic intermittent obstruction, form a nidus for recurrent cholelithiasis, which can lead to secondary biliary cirrhosis and sclerosing cholangitis.[93] Previous studies have shown a strong association between fascioliasis and liver fibrosis, depending on the duration and burden of infection. The pathogenesis of injury may be due to cathepsin L1 and its collagenolytic function associated with tissue invasion mediated by the parasite's proteolytic activity. These injuries lead to collagen type I expression and ultimately hepatic fibrosis.[94]

Clinical Manifestations

Infection with *F. hepatica* has two distinct clinical phases corresponding to the migratory stages of its life cycle (acute—hepatic) and to the presence of worms in their final habitat in the bile ducts (chronic—biliary). In 50% of cases, the initial manifestation is subclinical. The acute hepatic phase begins within 12 weeks of exposure and is characterized by low-grade fever, tender hepatomegaly, anorexia, nausea, and pruritus. Mild to moderate peripheral eosinophilia is common but can become marked during larval migration through the liver. Elevated levels of alkaline phosphatase and γ-glutamyltranspeptidase are typical, with high aminotransferase levels seen only with significant hepatocellular necrosis. During the chronic biliary phase, patients may be asymptomatic or complain of such nonspecific symptoms as dyspepsia, dull right upper quadrant discomfort, or diarrhea. Patients may have classic biliary colic, ascending cholangitis, acute pancreatitis, or cholecystitis in obstructed biles ducts. In the chronic phase of infestation, peripheral eosinophilia may be mild or absent.[94]

Diagnosis

The diagnosis should be considered in any patient who lives or has traveled to endemic areas and has a history of ingesting freshwater plants or drinking untreated water in conjunction with fever, right upper quadrant pain, intrahepatic cystic lesions, and absolute peripheral blood eosinophilia.[91] Detection of eggs in feces, bile, or duodenal aspirate is the definitive test. However, multiple stool specimens and concentration techniques are often necessary in light infestations because egg production and shedding may be low.[93] In a patient with the typical clinical findings and travel history, a negative stool examination does not rule out fascioliasis. Immunodiagnostic tests using every available technique from skin to antibody and antigen detection assays targeting somatic and excretory/secretory antigens of adult worms are helpful.[95] Serologic diagnosis using ELISA-based tests greatly aids in diagnosis because of their extremely high sensitivity (>95%) and specificity (97% to 100%).[93,96] Serologic tests are considered less useful during acute infection because of cross-reactions with other helminthic antigens, which may confuse interpretation of the results. However, because symptoms develop 1 to 2 months before eggs or antibodies are detectable in stool or serum, respectively, serologic tests may be an alternative method of confirming early fascioliasis, in addition to extrabiliary infestation. A Fas2 ELISA was found to be more specific than Western blot and Arc II.[95] Furthermore, serologic titers should decline after successful therapy and can therefore be used to monitor response to treatment.

Imaging techniques are also helpful in establishing the diagnosis, particularly in the chronic biliary phase. Hepatic US may demonstrate adult flukes in the bile ducts or gallbladder, as well as hyperechoic lesions. The most common findings on CT or MRI include multiple hepatic metastatic-like lesions

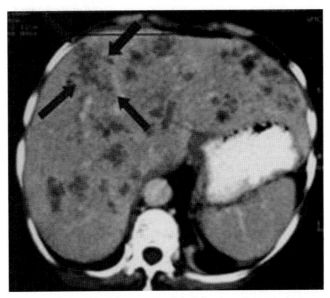

Fig. 35-4 **Late stage of acute *Fasciola* infection.** Computed tomography after venous contrast enhancement shows a variety of changes, including nodular, perivascular, some serpiginous *(arrows)*, tracklike, and subcapsular peripheral lesions.

that change in position, attenuation, and shape in time; tracklike hypodense lesions with a subcapsular location; low-density, serpiginous, tortuous tunnel-like branching lesions ranging from 2 to 10 mm; or subcapsular hematomas (**Fig. 35-4**).[97] Endoscopic retrograde cholangiopancreatography (ERCP) is useful to confirm the location of the trematode in the extrahepatic biliary tract.[98] Another clue to suspecting acute fascioliasis is the presence of hypergammaglobulinemia.[97] Finally, a diagnostic criterion is significant clinical improvement and decreasing levels of eosinophils in the 3 to 5 days after a trial of triclabendazole.

Treatment

Treatment of fascioliasis remains highly problematic, in contrast to other nematode infections, because it requires high or multiple doses of drugs with significant side effects.[99] Triclabendazole remains the drug of choice for treating *F. hepatica* in humans and livestock, as well for both phases, and it has a cure rate exceeding 90% for acute stages after a single dose of 10 mg/kg and similar results in chronic infections.[100-102] The most common adverse event is biliary colic caused by the passage of dead or dying parasites through the bile ducts. In biliary obstruction, ERCP and anthelmintic therapy are recommended in patients with light infestation, whereas in those with a heavy fluke burden that is resistant to oral therapy, intraductal endoscopic treatment with a fasciolicidal agent has been successful.[89,103]

Clonorchiasis and Opisthorchiasis

Clonorchiasis is an infection caused by *C. sinensis*, whereas opisthorchiasis is caused by *O. viverrini* and *O. felineus*. The geographic distribution of these liver flukes is largely in Asia and eastern Europe.[104] People living along rivers are prone to infection with these flukes because they have a habit of eating uncooked freshwater fish. Cercariae that emerge from freshwater snails encyst in the muscle of certain freshwater fish species. Humans acquire the infestation when they ingest raw, undercooked, or pickled fish that carry the metacercariae. Larvae excyst from the ingested metacercariae and migrate into the biliary system through the ampulla of Vater. Once the larvae reach the intrahepatic bile ducts, they mature into adult liver flukes over a period of approximately 1 month and begin producing eggs.[105] The pathogenesis of liver fluke–mediated tissue damage may be directly via mechanical or chemical irritation or immune-mediated injury (or both).[106]

The organisms reside in the bile ducts and give rise to chronic inflammation, dilation, and mechanical obstruction of the bile duct. Repeated infestation or chronicity can lead to recurrent pyogenic cholangitis, as well as secondary biliary cirrhosis or sclerosing cholangitis, and may lead to cholangiocarcinoma.[106,107]

Clinical Manifestations

The signs and symptoms depend on the number of flukes and the presence of complications. The majority of patients are asymptomatic during the acute infestation, but up to 10% of patients have fever, malaise, dull right upper quadrant pain, jaundice, lymphadenopathy, and tender hepatomegaly, in addition to nonspecific abdominal complaints such as abdominal discomfort and indigestion.[92,93,108] With obstruction from parasite eggs or recurrent pigment stones, patients may have classic biliary colic, ascending cholangitis, or acute pancreatitis, in addition to the symptoms of cholecystitis. Laboratory evaluation may be suggestive of pancreatobiliary obstruction with or without cholangitis; peripheral eosinophilia is typically absent in chronic liver fluke infestation.[92] Cholangiocarcinoma should be considered in all patients from endemic regions with weight loss, anorexia, and jaundice.

Diagnosis

Detection of eggs in feces, bile, or duodenal aspirate is the definitive test for diagnosis. However, multiple stool specimens and concentration techniques are often necessary in light infestations because egg production may be low.[93,105] The Kato-Katz method is accepted as the best for fecal examination, although the eggs may sometimes not be detected because of biliary obstruction or intermittent egg excretion, similar to fascioliasis. In light infections with fewer than 10 adult worms in the biliary tract, PCR to detect the DNA of the adult parasite in stool may be helpful.[109]

Serologic tests may be helpful but cannot distinguish between recent and past infection. Serologic tests are available for *C. sinensis* (immunoblot antigen assay and ELISA) and *O. viverrini* (ELISA) but are not routinely used except as an adjunct to stool studies or cholangiography.[96,105] The sensitivity and specificity of the ELISA-based tests range from 81.3% to 96% and 92.6% to 96.2%, respectively.[110,111] US reveals intrahepatic duct dilation in 76% of patients, with increasing periductal echogenicity and gallbladder sludge seen only in patients with heavy infection.[112] Flukes are difficult to visualize because they are packed within the small bile ducts, whereas in heavy infection, flukes or aggregate of flukes can be seen as a nonshadowing echogenic focus or cast within the bile ducts. Flukes in the gallbladder are easy to visualize as floating or dependent, discrete echogenic foci.[96] Flukes can be visualized in the larger bile ducts or extrahepatic ducts with CT and MRI as well.[113]

Treatment

Praziquantel is the drug of choice for the treatment of *O. viverrini*, *O. felineus*, and *C. sinensis*. For *O. viverrini*, a single dose (40 to 50 mg/kg) of PZQ is indicated, with a cure rate between 91% and 97%. For clonorchiasis, the recommended dose of PZQ is 25 mg/kg three times at 5-hour intervals in 1 day (total dose, 75 mg/kg), with a cure rate of 83% to 85%.[104,114] Chronic complications include recurrent stones, biliary strictures, and cholangiocarcinoma, which can be managed endoscopically or surgically as an adjunct to medical therapy.

Capillaria hepatica

C. hepatica infection is a rare cause of human liver disease.[107] The pathogenesis of disease is related to the host immune response, with the larvae or eggs producing an eosinophilic granulomatous reaction in the portal tracts.[115] Infection with *C. hepatica* may be mild or asymptomatic or lead to weight loss, general malaise, fever, edema, and eosinophilia, as well as hepatomegaly with an increase in transaminases and alkaline phosphatase. A definitive diagnosis is made by finding of *C. hepatica* in percutaneous liver biopsy samples. Mebendazole, 200 mg twice daily for 20 days, and albendazole, 400 mg twice daily for 10 days, are two options that may prove efficacious.

Ascaris lumbricoides

A. lumbricoides is widely distributed in tropical and subtropical regions and in other humid areas. Humans are permanent hosts, and infection occurs by the ingestion of eggs. After lung and tracheal migration, the worms reside in the small intestine, and occasionally, worms migrate through the ampulla of Vater into the biliary tree and gallbladder and cause bile duct obstruction, cholangitis, and pancreatitis. A sonographic findings is nonshadowing, echogenic tubular structures within the bile ducts, sometimes with a longitudinal central echo-free line representing the gastrointestinal tract of the worm. ERCP shows a long tubular filling defect in the bile duct or gallbladder, and magnetic resonance cholangiography may show intraductal worms as a linear low-intensity filling defect in the bile ducts.[116] Mebendazole, albendazole, and pyrantel pamoate are the most widely used agents for treating ascariasis.[117]

Human Immunodeficiency Virus and Parasitic Infections

Parasites are endemic in many regions of the world, including sub-Saharan Africa, where the largest burden of human immunodeficiency virus/acquired immunodeficiency syndrome (HIV/AIDS) exists.[118] The same factors, including poverty and malnutrition, could promote the transmission of both infections, and several studies have investigated the interaction between these agents.[119] Parasitic infections, particularly helminths, cause chronic activation of the immune system, in addition to skewing the immune response toward T_H2 immune responses, which has been shown to increase host susceptibility and thereby promote HIV infection and progression of disease.[120,121] Thus chronic activation of the immune system was suggested as one factor that has adversely influenced epidemics of HIV/AIDS in Africa.[122] On the other hand, with the emergence of AIDS, the epidemiology and the outcome of diseases caused by opportunistic parasites were significantly modified.[123] Overall, either because of HIV co-infection or independently, parasitic infections have continued to be a major cause of morbidity and mortality in humans.[124]

Amebiasis has been greatly associated with HIV, and patients with advanced HIV disease represent one of the highest risk groups for invasive amebiasis.[125] Studies from Japan, Taiwan, and the Republic of Korea, areas where *E. histolytica* endemicity is generally low, suggest that amebiasis is an emerging parasitic infection that occurs exclusively in men who have sex with men, especially those infected with HIV.[126] Host factors, such as dysregulation of T-cell activity, was suggested to play an important role in HIV-infected patients who are susceptible to invasive amebiasis.[127] Moreover, ALA is an emerging parasite infection in HIV-infected patients, even in areas where the disease is not endemic. ALA should be considered in HIV-infected patients with space-occupying lesions in the liver, and HIV screening is strongly recommended in areas where ALA is not endemic, especially in those with no history of travel to a disease-endemic area.[126] Both fever and abdominal pain are less frequent in HIV-infected ALA patients with significantly lower white blood cell counts than HIV-negative patients. CD4[+] T-cell counts vary greatly from 14/μl to 798/μl, thus suggesting that ALA is not caused by an opportunistic infection.[128]

Schistosomiasis is a highly prevalent parasitic infection that causes significant morbidity and mortality in sub-Saharan Africa, where HIV is also endemic.[129] Schistosomal infection is often asymptomatic for many years, and therefore recommended screening for schistosomiasis should be offered to HIV-infected patients along with subsequent PZQ treatment.[130] The exact number of persons co-infected with HIV and schistosomiasis is not known, but in some areas the prevalence can reach high proportions.[131] There are very few studies of the interaction of the two pathogens, but it is speculated that either infection enhances progression of the other, with reports from uncontrolled studies showing no or even negative effects of schistosomiasis treatment.[132,133] Circulating IL-10 involved in the systemic inflammation induced by *S. mansoni* was reduced after treatment with PZQ in co-infected persons, and the production of other proinflammatory cytokines was also be affected by schistosomiasis co-infection.[133,134] Moreover, studies from Kenya showed significantly lower egg excretion with impaired periovular granuloma formation in HIV-positive schistosomal cases than in HIV-negative patients. The reduction in egg excretion, which may be due to the immune dependence of egg excretion, was correlated with decreasing CD4[+] cell counts and resulted in more severe pathology. HIV-positive schistosomiasis patients have higher levels of alanine transaminase than do HIV-negative patients.[135] On the other hand, HIV replication and progression of AIDS may be enhanced in schistosomal patients because of nonspecific activation of the immune system and the preferential T_H2

environment, which inhibits cytotoxic T-cell responses.[136] Nevertheless, HIV-positive patients were found to respond normally to PZQ therapy irrespective of their CD4[+] cell counts.[137]

Thus it is apparent that HIV infection has been modifying both the epidemiology and the outcome of parasitic infections, and therefore raising patient immune status, as well as screening HIV-positive patients for these treatable parasites, is important.[119]

Finally, parasites are the most common infectious agents of humans in developing countries and produce a global burden of disease that exceeds that of better-known conditions. New insight into the fundamental biology and dynamics of parasite transmission, in addition to the mechanisms of their induced T_H2 immune response, has increased significantly, but more is still needed. Ultimately, advances in molecular and medical biology should one day translate into a new and robust pipeline of drugs, diagnostics, and vaccines for targeting parasitic worms that infect humans.[5]

Key References

Agaoglu N, Turkyilmaz S, Arslan MK. Surgical treatment of hydatid cysts of the liver. Br J Surg 2003;90:1536–1541. (Ref.63)

Ali IK, Clark CG, Petri WA Jr. Molecular epidemiology of amebiasis. Infect Genet Evol 2008;8:698–707. (Ref.73)

Ali IK, et al. *Entamoeba moshkovskii* infections in children, Bangladesh. Emerg Infect Dis 2003;9:580–584. (Ref.72)

Oto A, et al. Infection with *Fasciola hepatica*. Clin Microbiol Infect 2005;11:859–861. (Ref.99)

Assefa S, et al. Intestinal parasitic infections in relation to HIV/AIDS status, diarrhea and CD4 T-cell count. BMC Infect Dis 2009;9:155. (Ref.119)

Barakat R, Elmorshedy H, Fenwick A. Efficacy of myrrh in the treatment of human schistosomiasis mansoni. Am J Trop Med Hyg 2005;73:365–367. (Ref.43)

Berhe N, et al. Variations in helminth faecal egg counts in Kato-Katz thick smears and their implications in assessing infection status with *Schistosoma mansoni*. Acta Trop 2004;92:205–212. (Ref.28)

Borkow G, Bentwich Z. Chronic immune activation associated with chronic helminthic and human immunodeficiency virus infections: role of hypo-responsiveness and anergy. Clin Microbiol Rev 2004;17:1012–1030. (Ref.120)

Botros S, et al. Efficacy of mirazid in comparison with praziquantel in Egyptian *Schistosoma mansoni*–infected school children and households. Am J Trop Med Hyg 2005;72:119–123. (Ref.44)

Brown M, et al. Treatment of *Schistosoma mansoni* infection increases helminth-specific type 2 cytokine responses and HIV-1 loads in coinfected Ugandan adults. J Infect Dis 2005;191:1648–1657. (Ref.133)

Bukhari AJ. Ruptured amoebic liver abscess. J Coll Physicians Surg Pak 2003;13:159–160. (Ref.79)

Burke ML, et al. Immunopathogenesis of human schistosomiasis. Parasite Immunol 2009;31:163–176. (Ref.10)

Carmena D, Benito A, Eraso E. Antigens for the immunodiagnosis of *Echinococcus granulosus* infection: an update. Acta Trop 2006;98:74–86. (Ref.60)

Carvalho L, et al. Review series on helminths, immune modulation and the hygiene hypothesis: mechanisms underlying helminth modulation of dendritic cell function. Immunology 2009;126:28–34. (Ref.7)

Chavez-Tapia NC, et al. Image-guided percutaneous procedure plus metronidazole versus metronidazole alone for uncomplicated amoebic liver abscess. Cochrane Database Syst Rev 2009;1:CD004886. (Ref.84)

Choi MS, et al. Correlation between sonographic findings and infection intensity in clonorchiasis. Am J Trop Med Hyg 2005;73:1139–1144. (Ref.112)

Cioli D, et al. Will new antischistosomal drugs finally emerge? Trends Parasitol 2008;24:379–382. (Ref.41)

Diaz Granados CA, Duffus WA, Albrecht H. Parasitic diseases of the liver. In: Zakim D, Boyer TD, editors. Hepatology: a textbook of liver disease. Philadelphia: WB Saunders, 2002: 1073–1107. (Ref.107)

Doenhoff MJ, Cioli D, Utzinger J. Praziquantel: mechanisms of action, resistance and new derivatives for schistosomiasis. Curr Opin Infect Dis 2008;21: 659–667. (Ref.39)

Duenngai K, et al. Improvement of PCR for detection of *Opisthorchis viverrini* DNA in human stool samples. J Clin Microbiol 2008;46:366–368. (Ref.109)

Dunn MA. Parasitic diseases. In: Schiff ER, Sorrell MF, Maddrey WC, editors. Schiff's diseases of the liver. Philadelphia: Lippincott Williams & Wilkins, 2003: 1509–1527. (Ref.96)

EDHS. El-Zanaty F, Way A. 2008 Egypt Demographic and Health Survey. Cairo, Egypt: Ministry of Health, El-Zanaty and Associates, and Macro International, 2009. (Ref.22)

El-Tantawy WH, Salem HF, Mohammed Safwat NA. Effect of fascioliasis on the pharmacokinetic parameters of triclabendazole in human subjects. Pharm World Sci 2007;29:190–198. (Ref.102)

Erikstrup C, et al. Schistosomiasis and infection with human immunodeficiency virus 1 in rural Zimbabwe: systemic inflammation during co-infection and after treatment for schistosomiasis. Am J Trop Med Hyg 2008;79:331–337. (Ref.129)

Esmat G, El Raziky M. Antischistosomal therapy: current status and recent developments. ARG 2009;10:1–3. (Ref.38)

Espinoza JR, et al. Evaluation of FAS2-ELISA for the serological detection of *Fasciola hepatica* infection in humans. Am J Trop Med Hyg 2007;76:977–982. (Ref.95)

Evering T, Weiss LM. The immunology of parasite infections in immunocompromised hosts. Parasite Immunol 2006;28:549–565. (Ref.1)

Fairweather I. Triclabendazole progress report, 2005-2009: an advancement of learning? J Helminthol 2009;83:139–150. (Ref.100)

Farid A, et al. *Schistosoma* infection inhibits cellular immune responses to core HCV peptides. Parasite Immunol 2005;27:89–96. (Ref.24)

Fincham JE, Markus MB, Adams VJ. Could control of soil-transmitted helminthic infection influence the HIV/AIDS pandemic? Acta Trop 2003;86: 315–333. (Ref.122)

Fotedar R, et al. Laboratory diagnostic techniques for *Entamoeba* species. Clin Microbiol 2007;20:511–532. (Ref.70)

Furrows SJ, Moody AH, Chiodini PL. Comparison of PCR and antigen detection methods for diagnosis of *Entamoeba histolytica* infection. J Clin Pathol 2004; 57:1264–1266. (Ref.81)

Georgescu SO, et al. Minimally invasive treatment of hepatic hydatid cysts. Rom J Gastroenterol 2005;14:249–252. (Ref.53)

Gryseels B, et al. Are poor responses to praziquantel for the treatment of *Schistosoma mansoni* infections in Senegal due to resistance? An overview of the evidence. Trop Med Int Health 2001;6:864–873. (Ref.40)

Gulsen MT, et al. Fascioliasis: a report of five cases presenting with common bile duct obstruction. Neth J Med 2006;64:17–19. (Ref.98)

Habtamu B, Kloos H. Intestinal parasitism. In: Berhane Y, Hailemariam D, Kloos H, editors. Epidemiology and ecology of health and diseases in Ethiopia. Addis Ababa, Ethiopia: Shama Books, 2006: 519–538. (Ref.124)

Harms G, Feldmeier H. Review: HIV infection and tropical parasitic diseases: deleterious interactions in both directions. Trop Med Int Health 2002;7: 479–488. (Ref.132)

Hotez PJ, et al. Helminth infections: the great neglected tropical diseases. J Clin Invest 2008;118:1311–1321. (Ref.5)

Hsieh SM, et al. Aberrant induction of regulatory activity of CD4+CD25+ T cells by dendritic cells in HIV-infected persons with amebic liver abscess. J Acquir Immune Defic Syndr 2007;44:6–13. (Ref.127)

Hsu M-S, et al. Association between amebic liver abscess and human virus infection in Taiwanese subjects. BMC Infect Dis 2008;8:48–52. (Ref.128)

Kaewpitoon N, Kaewpitoon SJ, Pengsaa P. Opisthorchiasis in Thailand: review and current status. World J Gastroenterol 2008;14:2297–2302. (Ref.114)

Kallestrup P, et al. HIV in Africa—still a major matter of unsafe sex. Int J STD AIDS 2004;15:709–710; author reply 710–711. (Ref.131)

Kamal SM, et al. Progression of fibrosis in hepatitis C with and without schistosomiasis: correlation with serum markers of fibrosis. Hepatology 2006;43:771–779. (Ref.25)

Keiser J, et al. Triclabendazole for the treatment of fascioliasis and paragonimiasis. Expert Opin Investig Drugs 2005;14:1513–1526. (Ref.101)

Keiser J, Utzinger J. Emerging foodborne trematodiasis. Emerg Infect Dis 2005; 11:1507–1514. (Ref.90)

Kelly P, et al. Susceptibility to intestinal infection and diarrhoea in Zambian adults in relation to HIV status and CD4 count. BMC Gastroenterol 2009;9:7. (Ref.123)

Kern P. *Echinococcus granulosus* infection: clinical presentation, medical treatment and outcome. Langenbecks Arch Surg 2003;388:413–420. (Ref.57)

Kershenobish D, Corona DL. Amibiasis hepática. In: Sociedad Mexicana de Parasitología, editor. Amibiasis en el siglo XXII. DISA Press, Mexico; 2008: 44–56. (Ref.86)

Lebbad M, Svard SG. PCR differentiation of *Entamoeba histolytica* and *Entamoeba dispar* from patients with amoeba infection initially diagnosed by microscopy. Scand J Infect Dis 2005;37:680–685. (Ref.82)

Lundy SK, Lerman SP, Boros DL. Soluble egg antigen stimulated T helper lymphocyte apoptosis and evidence for cell death mediated by FasL+ T and B cells during murine *Schistosoma mansoni* infection. Infect Immun 2001;69: 271–280. (Ref.23)

MacLean JD, Graeme-Cook FM. Case records of the Massachusetts General Hospital. Weekly clinicopathological exercises. Case 12-2002. A 50-year-old man with eosinophilia and fluctuating hepatic lesions. N Engl J Med 2002;346: 1232–1239. (Ref.91)

Mairiang E, Mairiang P. Clinical manifestation of opisthorchiasis and treatment. Acta Trop 2003;88:221–227. (Ref.108)

Maizels RM, Yazdanbakhsh M. Immune regulation by helminth parasites: cellular and molecular mechanisms. Nat Rev Immunol 2003;3:733–744. (Ref.3)

Marcos LA, et al. Natural history, clinico-radiologic correlates and response to triclabendazole in acute massive fascioliasis. Am J Trop Med Hyg 2008;78:222–227. (Ref.97)

Marinho CC, et al. Clinical versus ultrasound examination in the evaluation of hepatosplenic schistosomiasis mansoni in endemic areas. Mem Inst Oswaldo Cruz 2006;101(Suppl 1):317–321. (Ref.37)

Mas-Coma S. Epidemiology of fascioliasis in human endemic areas. J Helminthol 2005;79:207–216. (Ref.88)

Mayer DA, Fried B. The role of helminth infections in carcinogenesis. Adv Parasitol 2007;65:239–296. (Ref.9)

McElroy MD, et al. Coinfection with *Schistosoma mansoni* is associated with decreased HIV-specific cytolysis and increased IL-10 production. J Immunol 2005;174:5119–5123. (Ref.134)

McManus DP, Loukas A. Current status of vaccines for schistosomiasis. Clin Microbiol Rev 2008;21:225–242. (Ref.47)

McManus DP, Thompson RC. Molecular epidemiology of cystic echinococcosis. Parasitology 2003;127(Suppl):S37–S51. (Ref.50)

Medici V, et al. Innate and adaptive immune responses to bacterial and parasitic infections. Clinicopathological consequences. In: Gershwin ME, Vierling JM, Manns MP, editors. Liver immunology: principles and practice. Totowa, NJ: Humana Press, 2008: 153–162. (Ref.2)

Moro P, Schantz PM. Echinococcosis: a review. Int J Infect Dis 2009;13:125–133. (Ref.62)

Mortelé KJ, Segatto E, Ros PR. The infected liver: radiologic-pathologic correlation. Radiographics 2004;24:937–955. (Ref.34)

Nagano I, et al. Molecular expression of a cysteine proteinase of *Clonorchis sinensis* and its application to an enzyme-linked immunosorbent assay for immunodiagnosis of clonorchiasis. Clin Diagn Lab Immunol 2004;11: 411–416. (Ref.110)

Park WB, et al. Amebic liver abscess in HIV-infected patients, Republic of Korea. Emerg Infect Dis 2007;13:516–517. (Ref.126)

Pawlowtski Z, et al. Echinococcosis in humans: clinical aspects, diagnosis and treatment. In: Eckert J, Gemmell MA, Meslin FX, et al, editors. WHO/OIE manual on echinococcosis in humans and animals. Paris: Office International des Épizooties, 2001: 20–71. (Ref.64)

Perrigoue JG, Marshall FA, Artis D. On the hunt for helminths: innate immune cells in the recognition and response to helminth parasites. Cell Microbiol 2008;10:1757–1764. (Ref.6)

Pockros PJ, Capozza TA. Helminthic infections of the liver. Curr Infect Dis Rep 2005;7:61–70. (Ref.4)

Pontes LA, Dias-Neto E, Robello A. Detection by polymerase chain reaction of *Schistosoma mansoni* DNA in human serum and feces. Am J Trop Med Hyg 2002;66:157–162. (Ref.32)

Rim HJ. Clonorchiasis: an update. J Helminthol 2005;79:269–281. (Ref.104)

Roig GV. Hepatic fascioliasis in Americas: a new challenge for therapeutic endoscopy. Gastrointest Endosc 2002;56:315–317. (Ref.89)

Ross AGP, Bartley PB, Sleigh AC. Schistosomiasis. Review. N Engl J Med 2002;346:1212–1220. (Ref.15)

Ryan ET, Wilson ME, Kain KC. Illness after international travel. N Engl J Med 2002;347:505–516. (Ref.92)

Salles JM, Moraes LA, Salles MC. Hepatic amebiasis. Braz J Infect Dis 2003;7:96–110. (Ref.76)

Salles JM, et al. Invasive amebiasis: an update on diagnosis and management. Expert Rev Anti Infect Ther 2007;5:893–901. (Ref.71)

Secor WE, et al. Increased density of human immunodeficiency virus type 1 co-receptors CCR5 and CXCR4 on the surfaces of CD4+ T cells and monocytes of patients with *Schistosoma mansoni* infection. Infect Immun 2003;71:6668–6671. (Ref.121)

Sheir Z, et al. A safe, effective, herbal antischistosomal therapy derived from myrrh. Am J Trop Med Hyg 2001;65:700–704. (Ref.42)

Siles-Lucas S, Gottstein B. Molecular tools for the diagnosis of cystic and alveolar echinococcosis. Trop Med Int Health 2001;6:463–475. (Ref.58)

Silva LCS, et al. Disagreement between ultrasound and magnetic resonance imaging in the identification of schistosomal periportal fibrosis. Mem Inst Oswaldo Cruz 2006;101(Suppl I):279–282. (Ref.36)

Smego RA, et al. Percutaneous aspiration-injection-reaspiration-drainage plus albendazole or mebendazole for hepatic cystic echinococcosis: a meta-analysis. Clin Infect Dis 2003;37:1073–1083. (Ref.67)

Smith C, et al. Seroprevalence of schistosomiasis in African patients infected with HIV. HIV Med 2008;9:436–439. (Ref.130)

Sripa B. Pathobiology of opisthorchiasis, an update. Acta Trop 2003;88:209–220. (Ref.106)

Stack CM, et al. The major secreted cathepsin L1 protease of the liver fluke, *Fasciola hepatica*: a leu-12 to pro-12 replacement in the nonconserved C-terminal region of the prosegment prevents complete enzyme autoactivation and allows definition of the molecular events in prosegment removal. J Biol Chem 2007;282:16532–16543. (Ref.94)

Stadecker MJ, et al. The immunobiology of Th1 polarization in high pathology schistosomiasis. Immunol Rev 2004;201:168–179. (Ref.18)

Stanley SL. Amoebiasis. Lancet 2003;361:1025–1034. (Ref.69)

Torgerson PR, Budke CM. Echinococcosis: an international public health challenge. Res Vet Sci 2003;74:191–202. (Ref.56)

van der Kleij D, et al. A novel host parasite lipid cross-talk. Schistosomal lyso-phosphatidylserine activates toll-like receptor 2 and affects immune polarization. J Biol Chem 2002;277:48122–48129. (Ref.16)

van der Werf MJ, et al. Quantification of clinical morbidity associated with schistosome infection in sub-Saharan Africa. Acta Trop 2003;86:125–139. (Ref.13)

van Hal SJ, et al. Amoebiasis: current status in Australia. Med J Aust 2007;186:412–416. (Ref.80)

van Riet E, Hartgers FC, Yazdanbakhsh M. Chronic helminth infections induce immunomodulation: consequences and mechanisms. Immunobiology 2007;212:475–490. (Ref.8)

Vuitton DA. The ambiguous role of immunity in echinococcosis: protection of the host or of the parasite? Acta Trop 2003;85:119–132. (Ref.51)

Wilson RA, Coulson PS. Immune effector mechanisms against schistosomiasis: looking for a chink in the parasite's armour. Trends Parasitol 2009;25:423–431. (Ref.48)

World Health Organization (WHO). Prevention of schistosomiasis and soil transmitted helminthiasis: report of WHO Expert Committee. WHO Technical Report Series 912. Geneva: WHO, 2002. (Ref.118)

World Health Organization. International classification of ultrasound images in cystic echinococcosis for application in clinical and field epidemiological settings. Acta Trop 2003;85:253–261. (Ref.65)

World Health Organization. The control of neglected zoonotic diseases: a route to poverty alleviation. In: Global plan to combat neglected tropical diseases. Geneva: WHO, 2007: 2008–2015. (Ref.49)

Wynn TA, et al. Immunopathogenesis of schistosomiasis. Immunol Rev 2004; 201:156–167. (Ref.17)

Yagci G, et al. Results of surgical, laparoscopic, and percutaneous treatment for hydatid disease of the liver: 10 years experience with 355 patients. World J Surg 2005;29:1670–1679. (Ref.54)

Yang YR, et al. Community surveys and risk factor analysis of human alveolar and cystic echinococcosis in Ningxia Hui Autonomous Region, China. Bull World Health Organ 2006;84:9714–9721. Erratum in Bull World Health Organ 2006;84:840. (Ref.59)

Zhang W, McManus DP. Recent advances in the immunology and diagnosis of echinococcosis. FEMS Immunol Med Microbiol 2006;47:24–41. (Ref.61)

Zhao QP, et al. Evaluation of *Clonorchis sinensis* recombinant 7-kilodalton antigen for serodiagnosis of clonorchiasis. Clin Diagn Lab Immunol 2004;11:814–817. (Ref.111)

A complete list of references can be found at www.expertconsult.com.

Bacterial and Miscellaneous Infections of the Liver

Helmut Albrecht

Entities covered in this chapter include pyogenic liver abscess, pyelophlebitis, parainfectious hepatitis, bacterial hepatitis, fungal hepatitis, and infectious peliosis hepatis. Parasitic infections including amebic liver abscess (see Chapter 35) are reviewed separately.

Pyogenic Liver Abscess

Four centuries BC liver abscesses were already known to Hippocrates, who reported an association between prognosis and the type of fluid contained within the lesion:

"When abscess of the liver is treated by cautery or incision, if the pus which is discharged be pure and white the patients recover (for in this case it is situated in the coats of the liver) but if it resembles the lees of oil as it flows they die."[1]

Despite an apparent recent increase in incidence, pyogenic liver abscesses remain a relatively uncommon clinical entity responsible for 7 to 20 per 100,000 hospital admissions.[2-14] The prevalence in autopsy series ranges from 0.29% to 1.47%.[3,13] In contrast to amebic liver abscess, no significant gender differences have been reported in patients with pyogenic liver abscess.

Almost 50% of patients will have more than one abscess. Solitary abscesses involve the right lobe in 75%, the left in 20%, and the caudate in approximately 5%. Multiple abscesses follow a similar pattern of distribution. While this is likely due to the relative mass of each lobe, it remains unclear if other factors such as hepatic blood flow contribute to this distribution.

Over the last 20 to 30 years significant changes in epidemiology, pathogenesis, microbiology, diagnostics, therapies, and outcome have been documented.[2-14] There is a perceived increase in incidence in recent decades, which at least partially is likely due to improved quality and availability of imaging methods. Additionally, prolonged survival of patients with increased susceptibility such as iron overload states, sickle cell disease, diabetes mellitus, advanced cardiovascular disease, or metastatic cancer may also contribute to the growing patient load. The increasing number of immunocompromised patients has added another new dimension to this problem. Hepatic abscesses have been reported in patients with a multitude of immunodeficiency states, including primary immunodeficiencies, especially patients with neutrophil deficiencies such as Job's syndrome or chronic granulomatous disease; acquired immunodeficiencies, such as HIV infection; and iatrogenic immunodeficiencies, such as patients undergoing chemotherapy. Patients undergoing orthotopic liver transplantation are also at risk for the formation of hepatic abscesses post transplant. In these patients liver abscesses commonly develop secondary to hepatic arterial thrombosis.[15]

While the incidence seems to be on the increase, mortality has decreased dramatically from close to 100% to now 5% to 31% despite greater numbers of patients with underlying diseases in recent case series.[4-14]

In recent studies underlying malignancies (especially cholangiocarcinoma), severe hepatic dysfunction, and multiple versus singular abscesses were associated with an increased mortality.[6,9,14,16-18] In a large study from John Hopkins compared with earlier cases, however, the reduction of mortality was most apparent for patients with multiple abscesses (88% vs. 44%; *P* <.05) and patients with a biliary etiology (90% vs. 38%; *P* <.05).[10] Mortality of patients with cryptogenic liver abscesses was as low as 5%.

Pathogenesis

Bacterial pathogens can reach the liver by five different routes: portal vein, hepatic artery, biliary tract, penetrating trauma, and direct extension from a contiguous, usually intraabdominal, rarely pleural focus. Infection via any of these routes can potentially lead to formation of liver abscesses but the associated scope of pathogens may be quite different. Furthermore, since the classic report of Ochsner in 1938,[2] the etiology of hepatic abscesses has changed significantly. In the preantibiotic era, liver abscesses were typically encountered in patients with appendicitis and associated pyelophlebitis (i.e., infective suppurative thrombosis of the portal vein). Incidence was highest in the third to fourth decade of life. Mortality, especially in patients who did not undergo prompt surgical drainage, approached 100%.[2] Pylephlebitis has become rare but is still observed. Diverticulitis has surpassed appendicitis as the most common cause of septic portal vein thrombosis. Other rare causes include pancreatitis, inflammatory bowel disease, postoperative infections, omphalitis (especially in infancy), suppurative thrombophlebitis, and others. Most abscesses that have their source in the portal system are right sided and single.

The peak incidence of hepatic abscess has shifted into the older age group with most recent case series reporting an average patient's age at over 60 years. Cryptogenic and biliary tract–associated liver abscesses are dominating more recent case series.[9-14]

While cholelithiasis is by far the most common cause of biliary tract–derived pyogenic abscess disease, patients with Caroli disease and sclerosing cholangitis are also at increased risk. In developing countries biliary ascariasis is not infrequently a cause of liver abscesses. Patients with biliary disease as the cause of liver abscesses often have multiple abscesses. Several changes in medical practice, including the use of invasive therapeutic approaches for benign and malignant hepatobiliary and pancreatic disorders, the insertion of stents and other foreign bodies into biliary and pancreatic ducts, and surgical resection and reconstruction of the hepatobiliary system, predispose to liver abscess formation.

Liver abscesses for which no source of infection is identified are termed cryptogenic. Cryptogenic abscesses now account for up to 60% in recent series.[4,9,12-14] The reason for this observation is not entirely clear. Improved diagnostic modalities resulting in earlier intervention and the early use of empiric antibiotic therapy may allow eradication of infectious foci before they become clinically apparent. On the other hand, improved management of biliary tract disease, including ERCP and stent placement, may have reduced the incidence of biliary-derived abscesses resulting in proportionally more cryptogenic cases. Host factors predisposing patients to pyogenic abscess development may also increase the likelihood of cryptogenic abscesses. In patients with iron overload states, sickle cell disease, diabetes mellitus, cirrhosis, advanced cardiovascular disease, metastatic cancer, or immunodeficiency states, trivial bacterial insults may manifest as hepatic abscesses. Because these patients are becoming more frequently seen, cryptogenic abscesses may become more common.

Any bacteremic episode including line-associated septicemia or endocarditis may seed the liver via the hepatic artery. The discovery of multiple microabscesses is not an infrequent finding at autopsy, especially in patients succumbing to overwhelming sepsis. These patients, however, have traditionally been excluded from most case series of patients with pyogenic liver abscesses unless they also had evidence of macroscopic abscesses.

Spread from a contiguous focus has been associated with subphrenic, paracolic or perinephric abscesses, empyema, cholecystitis, and necrotizing pancreatitis. Pyogenic abscess formation associated with penetrating trauma often involves skin flora but may be associated with intestinal flora if the gastrointestinal tract was lacerated at the same time. The initial insult may be as trivial as the incidental ingestion of toothpicks or fish bones.[19-22] Children and patients with psychiatric disorders, such as pica or suicidal ideation, are at highest risk because they are more likely to swallow sharp items.[21,23,24] In rare cases, liver abscesses have even been observed following blunt trauma to the abdomen, presumably as a result of secondary superinfection of liver hematomas.[25,26]

Modern therapeutic interventions such as transarterial chemoembolization, percutaneous ethanol injection, or radiofrequency ablation have added new risk factors for liver abscesses. Patients with biliary tract disease or bilioenteric anastomosis are at particular risk.[17,27-30]

Hepatic abscesses are also observed as a late complication of endoscopic sphincterotomy for biliary duct stones. Case series have shown rates of up to 2% of patients undergoing sphincterotomy.[31] Most cases were associated with recurrent stones. Biliary-intestinal anastomosis has also been described as a risk factor for the subsequent development of pyogenic liver abscesses.[32] Patients who underwent anastomosis with subsegmental bile ducts or had vascular reconstruction were at highest risk. In all affected patients, surgery was performed to resect a malignant lesion, and mortality, while significant, was often due to an underlying illness.

Microbiology

The organisms recovered from patients with pyogenic liver abscesses vary greatly (**Table 36-1**). This is not surprising given the diverse pathogenesis discussed above. Results of single studies should not be generalized because they are highly dependent on the culture methods used and the patient population studied. Despite these difficulties, recent studies have improved our understanding of the microbiology of pyogenic liver abscesses. Early studies reported a high rate of "sterile" abscesses, often exceeding 50%. Despite the increased use of empiric and more effective antibiotic therapy, recent studies commonly report positive abscess cultures in 80% to 100% of patients with pyogenic liver abscesses.[5,7,14,33,34] Gram stains are mandatory and may provide the only clue to a mixed infection in a patient heavily pretreated with antibiotics; 35% to 70% of patients will also have positive blood cultures. Because blood cultures are often the only cultures obtained before antibiotic administration, they provide the only positive culture data in 5% to 10% of patients.

Using strict anaerobic techniques, recent studies have found that 45% to 75% of hepatic abscesses are caused by anaerobic or mixed aerobic/anaerobic infections, with *Bacteroides* and *Fusobacterium* species as the most frequent anaerobes cultured from liver abscesses.[33-38] Even reports indicating anaerobic infections in greater than 50% of patients may represent underestimates secondary to the fastidious nature of some

Table 36-1 Microbial Pathogens Isolated from Pyogenic Liver Abscesses

Gram-negative aerobic bacteria	***Escherichia coli*** ***Klebsiella pneumoniae*** *Pseudomonas aeruginosa* *Proteus* sp. *Enterobacter* sp. *Citrobacter freundii* *Morganella* sp. *Serratia* sp. *Haemophilus* sp. *Legionella pneumophila* *Yersinia* sp.
Gram-positive aerobic bacteria	***Viridans streptococci*** ***Staphylococcus aureus*** ***Enterococcus sp.*** Beta-hemolytic streptococci *Streptococcus pneumoniae* *Listeria monocytogenes*
Anaerobes	***Anaerobic streptococci*** ***Bacteroides sp.*** *Fusobacterium* sp. *Peptostreptococcus* sp. *Prevotella* sp. *Actinomyces* (Fig. 36-4) *Eubacterium* *Propionibacterium acnes* *Clostridium* sp. *Lactobacillus* sp. *Peptococcus* sp. *Eubacterium* sp. *Sphaerophorus* sp. *Capnocytophaga* sp. (facultatively anaerobic)
Microaerophilic organisms	*Streptococcus milleri* group
Miscellaneous	***Mycobacterium sp.*** *Chlamydia* sp. *Candida* sp. *Cryptococcus* sp. *Verticillium* sp.

Bold entries are commonly isolated pathogens (>5% of cases).

anaerobes. Anaerobes are especially common in polymicrobial abscesses. It is generally believed that many abscesses are polymicrobial, but culture-based estimates range from 10% to 75%.

Escherichia coli and *Klebsiella pneumoniae* are the most common specific pathogens isolated. Whereas *E. coli* dominated virtually all early series, *K. pneumoniae* has emerged as a major cause of pyogenic liver abscesses, and is currently dominating all reviews of case series, especially in patients with monomicrobial abscesses. In one of the first series to point out the emergence of this new threat, the authors compared 160 patients in whom *K. pneumoniae* was believed to be the sole etiologic factor with those with polymicrobial abscesses.[39] In the group of patients with *Klebsiella* pneumonia liver abscesses, there was a striking increase in diabetes or glucose intolerance (75% vs. 4.5%), a lower rate of coexisting intraabdominal infection (0.6% vs. 95.5%), a lower death rate (11.3% vs. 41%), and a lower relapse rate (4.4% vs. 41%). Alkaline phosphatase and bilirubin levels were higher in patients with polymicrobial abscesses, but on other grounds

(i.e., signs, symptoms) the groups were indistinguishable, except for the fact that a number of patients with *Klebsiella* pneumonia abscesses had other foci of infection, including pneumonia, skin lesions, meningitis, or endophthalmitis. The predilection for diabetic patients and the impression that liver abscesses caused by *K. pneumoniae* represent a unique clinical entity characterized by a relatively benign course has been confirmed in subsequent studies.[40,41] The illness was initially described in series from Southeast Asia, but the disease has now reached the United States.[41-43]

Capsular serotypes K1 and K2, a mucoid phenotype, as well as expression of magA and rmpA have been documented in high prevalence in *K. pneumoniae* strains associated with liver abscesses.[41-49] Many isolates display a so-called hypermucoviscosity phenotype, which is associated with phagocytic resistance.

While most isolates appear sensitive to the most commonly used antibiotics, including third generation cephalosporins, isolates with extended-spectrum β-lactamases (ESBLs) have been described.[50] Preimmunization with certain class I mutant strains protected mice against a challenge from wild-type strains, implying the possibility that a vaccine may be feasible for prophylaxis against *K. pneumoniae* infections associated with liver abscesses.[51]

Of the gram-positive pathogens, staphylococci are more commonly found in monomicrobial abscesses, whereas streptococci and especially enterococci are most often associated with polymicrobial abscesses.

In one large series, isolation of *S. aureus* and β-hemolytic streptococci were associated with trauma; Streptococcus group D, *K. pneumoniae*, and *Clostridium* sp. with biliary disease; and *Bacteroides* and *Clostridium* spp. were associated with colonic disease.[33]

Disturbingly, highly resistant and difficult to treat nosocomial pathogens, such as multidrug-resistant *Pseudomonas* isolates,[5] vancomycin-resistant enterococci, and even vancomycin-intermediate *Staphylococcus aureus* have been isolated from hepatic abscesses.[52] Other disturbing trends include the increased frequency of fungal or mixed bacterial and fungal abscesses, probably reflecting recent shifts in the causes of nosocomial infections.[5,53] In one large series, mortality was significantly increased (50%) in patients with mixed bacterial and fungal abscesses (P < .02).[5]

Clinical Features

Timely diagnosis of pyogenic liver abscesses is challenging and requires a high degree of suspicion because presenting symptoms are varied and frequently nonspecific. The spectrum of presenting symptoms and signs ranges from long-standing fever of unknown origin to an acute abdomen requiring emergency surgical evaluation. Only 10% of patients will have the "characteristic" symptom triad of fever, jaundice, and right upper quadrant (RUQ) tenderness. The most common presentation is a mildly symptomatic patient with fever and other nonspecific constitutional symptoms including malaise, anorexia, and weight loss (**Table 36-2**). Localizing symptoms such as nausea/vomiting, diarrhea, and abdominal pain may be present but are not specific to this diagnosis. Some patients have only respiratory symptoms including pleuritic pain and cough. Pain may be felt in the left upper quadrant by patients with abscesses of the left lobe or may be diffuse in patients

Table 36-2 **Symptoms Associated with Pyogenic Liver Abscess**	
Fever/chills	45%-100%
Anorexia/weight loss	28%-100%
Malaise/weakness	11%-97%
Abdominal pain	27%-91%
Nausea/vomiting	9%-53%
Diarrhea	8%-48%
Cough	4%-28%
Chest pain	2%-%24%

Data from references 2-15.

Table 36-3 **Physical Signs Associated with Pyogenic Liver Abscess**	
Hepatomegaly	7%-91%
RUQ tenderness	14%-71%
Jaundice	4%-54%
Chest findings	11%-52%
Splenomegaly	1%-21%
Sepsis	3%-18%
Ascites	2%-6%

Data from references 2-15.

Table 36-4 **Laboratory Findings Associated with Pyogenic Liver Abscess**	
Elevation of alkaline phosphatase	66%-100%
Leukocytosis	65%-99%
Anemia	45%-91%
Prolonged prothrombin time	44%-87%
Albumin <3.0 g/dl	20%-87%
Bilirubin elevation	21%-74%
Hypergammaglobulinemia	33%-66%
Transaminase elevation	15%-60%

with secondary peritonitis. Patients with peripheral subphrenic abscesses may have referred right shoulder pain.

None of the aforementioned symptoms are specific. Patients with necrotic hepatocellular carcinomas may have classic symptoms and signs of pyogenic liver abscess, namely fever, chills, abdominal pain, leukocytosis, and hepatomegaly.[16,17] The pathogenesis is presumed to involve spontaneous tumor necrosis and/or biliary obstruction caused by tumor thrombi with or without bacterial superinfection. Major clues to the possibility of underlying hepatocellular carcinoma in a series of 10 patients were the presence of hepatitis B surface antigen in 7 of 10 patients and pronounced liver dysfunction, including Child B or C liver dysfunction, in 9 of 10 patients.[17] Because significant underlying liver disease is uncommon in patients with uncomplicated pyogenic (or amebic) liver abscess, impairment of liver function should result in a workup to rule out malignancy.

Diagnostic Approach

Patients with hepatic abscesses commonly have nonspecific symptoms, are often elderly, or have underlying illnesses that may mask their symptoms. Empiric antibiotic therapy may prevent timely recovery of the etiologic pathogen. The diagnosis of liver abscess in one study was made in fewer than 20% of emergency room patients before admission despite a fairly high number of patients with a past medical history of orthotopic liver transplantation or biliary tract disease drawing attention to the right upper quadrant.[54] Diagnosis is therefore often delayed. Symptoms are present an average of 2 weeks before the diagnosis is made, although one third of patients may be symptomatic for more than a month. The availability of modern imaging, however, has enabled physicians to streamline the diagnostic workup of patients significantly. In a study comparing the period from 1981 to 1989 with 1990 to 1998, there was a clear reduction in time to diagnosis (13 vs. 3 days), which was explained by the earlier and more frequent use of modern imaging modalities.[7]

Hepatomegaly is the most common finding on physical examination (**Table 36-3**). Other clues may include a palpable liver mass and RUQ tenderness. Abnormal physical findings on chest examination are common and may include an upwardly displaced and fixed lower pulmonary border on the right, evidence of consolidation or pleural effusions, friction rubs, or rales. Jaundice is noted in 10% to 50% of patients and

is associated with a biliary etiology or advanced disease. Splenomegaly has become uncommon in recent series.

Leukocytosis is detected in most patients and can be high. Anemia is also common. Although liver tests, bilirubin, albumin level, and prothrombin time are often abnormal, these aberrations are seldom marked. Normal results do not exclude the diagnosis. Alkaline phosphatase levels are commonly elevated and tend to be farther out of range than other liver tests. In summary, laboratory studies may suggest liver abnormalities but are neither sensitive nor specific for the diagnosis of pyogenic liver abscess (**Table 36-4**).

Chest x-ray findings may be abnormal in up to 80% of patients with pyogenic liver abscess. Findings include pneumonitis, consolidation, pleural effusions, and elevation and/or immobility of the right diaphragm. Air fluid levels may be visible on plain films of the abdomen. Radionuclide scanning with ^{99m}Tc sulfur colloid was commonly used in early studies. Sensitivity for lesions greater than 2 cm was 50% to 90%, but specificity was low.[4,5,11,32]

Ultrasonography and computed tomography (<7) have replaced radionuclide scanning because they are the diagnostic procedures of choice for liver imaging.[4,5] Both modalities offer excellent sensitivity and may be used for guidance of percutaneous drainage procedures.

Features identified on ultrasound can be highly variable and nonspecific, ranging from hypoechoic to hyperechoic lesions with a varying degree of internal echoes and debris. However, in most cases, hepatic abscesses are usually less echogenic than the surrounding liver tissue on ultrasound.[55] Sensitivity of ultrasonography ranges from 65% to 95%, with higher detection rates in patients with larger lesions. Limitations are a lack of sensitivity for microabscesses and singular lesions high in the dome of the liver.

In CT images, hepatic abscesses are generally less dense than surrounding liver tissue (**Figs. 36-1 and 36-2**). Administration of contrast medium often enhances these attenuation differences. Contrast-enhanced CT scanning offers improved sensitivity over ultrasonography (range, 75% to 100%) and is superior for guiding complex drainage procedures.

Available technologies for imaging of the liver are rapidly evolving. The introduction of new contrasting agents, spiral CT scanning, and rapid magnetic resonance imaging are among the promising technologies that continue to improve the diagnostic evaluation of patients with suspected hepatic abscesses.[56,57] Characteristic imaging features on MRI are based on the abscess cavity and wall, perilesional signal, and the dynamic enhancement pattern noted with gadolinium. The abscess cavity is usually hypointense on T1-weighted and hyperintense on T2-weighted images. The most distinctive feature of liver abscesses on MRI is the enhancement of the abscess wall on dynamic postgadolinium images.[5,56] A limiting factor for MRI is the fact that it may not be used to guide therapeutic drainage procedures. As further experience with these newer techniques is gained, further improvements in diagnostic capabilities are anticipated.

Whether and to what extent patients should be evaluated in an attempt to identify an underlying lesion is another controversial area.[58] In a study in California, 53% of patients without an obvious source of infection underwent invasive examination of the colon. Colonoscopy failed to detect lesions in any of these patients. Likewise, in patients without jaundice, elevated bilirubin, or dilated biliary ducts, ERCP revealed cholecystolithiasis in only 3 of 10 patients examined. No other abnormality was detected in any of the 10 patients examined.[4] Some authors have suggested that a complete evaluation of the colon and the biliary tract is indicated in patients with cryptogenic liver abscesses because these patients frequently have underlying biliary tract disease not identified by laboratory evaluation or diagnostic imaging, but evidence suggests that appropriate and, if necessary, invasive evaluations should be restricted to patients with localizing clinical or laboratory findings.

Therapy

Untreated hepatic abscesses carry a mortality rate approaching 100%. Before modern imaging techniques became available, the treatment of choice consisted of open surgical drainage plus antibiotics. Initial management has notably shifted from a primarily surgical approach[2] to antibiotic management with or without the use of percutaneous modalities.[5]

In a large series from the University of California hospitals, the rate of patients treated with a primary surgical approach dropped from 92% for the time from 1972 and 1973 to 0% for the period from 1990 to 1994. During the latter period all patients had percutaneous aspiration with or without drainage. In this series the success rate of this approach was excellent, with complete resolution in 90% and a mortality rate of 5%.[4] A retrospective meta-analysis concluded that percutaneous drainage is safe and associated with a success rate of 90%, comparable with open drainage.[59] Several modern case series have documented a lower mortality in patients undergoing open surgical as opposed to percutaneous abscess drainage, but the numbers were generally small and the lack of randomization may have resulted in allocation bias.[5,60]

Surgical intervention is therefore usually reserved for patients failing percutaneous drainage or for patients with multiloculated abscesses (**Fig. 36-3**), who tend to pose problems for both drainage and aspiration.

Laparoscopic drainage of complicated abscesses has been used successfully[61-63] and offers a viable alternative for some patients who are poor surgical candidates. Initially continuous drainage became the mainstay of therapy, and drainage catheters were left in place until drainage had subsided, which usually required 5 to 10 days. Relative contraindications to percutaneous drainage include large amounts of ascites and severe coagulopathy. Potential complications include hemorrhage, sepsis, catheter dislodgement, leakage, and perforation of other organs. In recent series, most centers have switched

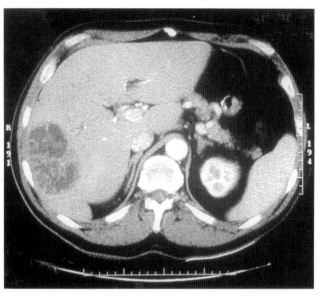

Fig. 36-1 **CT image of an early pyogenic abscess.**

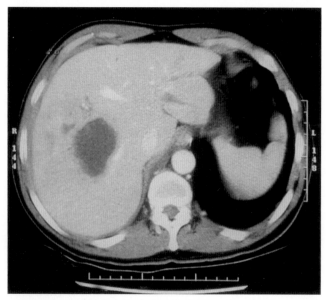

Fig. 36-2 **CT image of a mature abscess resulting from Klebsiella pneumoniae infection.**

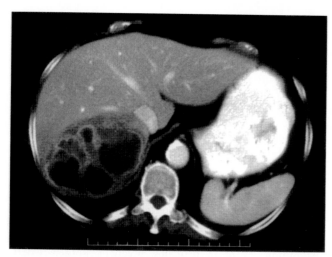

Fig. 36-3 **CT image of a multiloculated abscess resulting from** *Staphylococcus aureus* **infection.**

to repeated percutaneous aspiration without drainage. In combination with antibiotic therapy, success rates ranging from 58% to 96% have been reported, similar to what has been communicated for percutaneous drainage.[4-6,9,14]

Before a randomized trial comparing drainage with aspiration, a number of case series had confirmed high success rates using aspiration alone. Giorgio reported success in 113 of 115 consecutive patients with 147 abscesses.[27] Only two patients with large viscous abscesses required open drainage. Repeat aspiration was required in a majority of patients, but no complications or deaths were reported. In large abscesses, aspiration alone is less likely to succeed, but overall success rates in experienced hands may approach 100%.[9] In a recent randomized study, needle aspiration was considered at least as effective as catheter drainage.[64]

The use of antibiotics without drainage has remained controversial but has become the treatment of choice in up to 20% of cases. While this approach may not be sufficient in many cases, it has proven highly effective in selected patients, with reported success rates ranging from 75% to 85%.[4,8,9] A major problem of empiric antibiotic therapy without aspiration is the lack of microbiologic data, which allows for a more targeted selection of antimicrobial agents. Although conservative medical therapy may be a reasonable option for certain patients, most patients will benefit from a combined approach. Because there are no prospective trials comparing antibiotics alone to the more conventional combined approach, this approach should be reserved for patients with small abscesses not amenable to drainage or those in whom drainage is associated with an unacceptable risk.

Initial antibiotic therapy should provide coverage against aerobic gram-negative bacilli, microaerophilic streptococci, and anaerobes including *Bacteroides fragilis* such as ertapenem, beta-lactam/beta-lactamase inhibitor combinations (ampicillin-sulbactam, ticarcillin-clavulanic acid, piperacillin-tazobactam) or combination of metronidazole with either quinolones (ciprofloxacir, levofloxacin) or ceftriaxone.[65] Metronidazole offers the advantage of good coverage of anaerobes and *Entamoeba histolytica* while these possibilities are still evaluated. Empiric coverage for enterococci is not generally recommended unless clinical or epidemiologic factors suggest otherwise.[65] Blood cultures and, if at all possible, a diagnostic aspiration should be performed before or shortly after initiating therapy. The suspected source and origin of infection should be considered when choosing initial antibiotic therapy because these will help predict the most likely pathogens. Empiric antibiotic coverage should respect local resistance patterns and should be adjusted once culture results become available.

Optimal duration of therapy depends on the size of the abscesses, extent of prior drainage, virulence of the organism, response to therapy, and immune status of the affected patient. In general, parenteral antibiotics should be given at least until defervescence is achieved followed by a prolonged course of oral therapy. Follow-up ultrasound or CT scans are often helpful in determining required length of treatment. Complete resolution of the abscess cavity is not required for cure, and may not be achievable in up to 50% of patients.[10,64] If the remaining cavity is stable on serial imaging studies and the patient is asymptomatic, antibiotic therapy can be discontinued with close follow-up observation.

Pylephlebitis

Pylephlebitis or septic thrombophlebitis of the portal vein used to be common in the pre-antibiotic era and was frequently associated with appendicitis. In early series pylephlebitis was the most common cause of hepatic abscesses. In recent years it has become a very uncommon entity with approximately 75 cases reported since 2000. Nowadays, a precipitating focus of infection, most commonly diverticulitis, can be identified in approximately two thirds of affected patients.[66-68] Bacteremia (often polymicrobial) was present in most recent cases. The most common blood isolate was *B. fragilis*. Overall mortality was 32%, but most of the patients who died had severe refractory sepsis before initiation of antibiotic therapy. Heparin was used in one fourth of the patients, all of whom survived, but no clear benefit of this compound could be detected because of the small number of evaluable patients.

Parainfectious Hepatitis

Jaundice and liver function abnormalities are well-described complications of severe bacterial infections ("bilirubin of bacterial badness"). This is especially common in neonates and infants, but has also been documented in adults with severe bacterial infections. The exact incidence of this phenomenon remains unknown, but Franson reported bilirubin elevations in 54% of 82 consecutive bacteremic patients.[69]

Another study of 84 bacteremic patients found bilirubin levels elevated in only 6%, but elevated aspartate aminotransferase was present in 53% of patients.[70]

Elevated serum bilirubin levels are frequently out of proportion to the serum alkaline phosphatase and aminotransferase levels, and hyperbilirubinemia is usually more severe among patients with underlying hepatobiliary disease.

While neither sensitive nor specific for bacterial infection, parainfectious hepatitis with persistent or increasing hyperbilirubinemia was in retrospective studies associated with high mortality (up to 100%) and was therefore deemed prognostically important.[71] In prospective studies comparing patients suffering from severe extrahepatic infection with or without jaundice, however, the presence of jaundice did not seem to correlate with decreased survival.[72,73]

Sepsis-associated cholestasis should always be considered in the differential diagnosis of jaundice in hospitalized and critically ill patients. Parainfectious hepatitis appears to be caused by the systemic effects of the release of inflammatory mediators, such as tumor necrosis factor-α and interleukin-1 (IL-1), IL-2, IL-6, and IL-8, in response to inciting antigens including bacterial lipopolysaccharide (LPS).[74]

Implicated primary infection sites are diverse and include entities such as endocarditis, pneumonia, appendicitis, diverticulitis, pyelonephritis, distant abscesses, septic abortion, and myriad other infections.[75] Jaundice associated with lobar pneumonia ("pneumonia biliosa") was reported as early as 1836.[76]

Jaundice secondary to generalized sepsis syndrome must be differentiated from primary infections of the liver. Clinical manifestations and laboratory findings are sufficiently characteristic to distinguish the underlying disease from jaundice due to other causes.

In sepsis-associated jaundice, hepatomegaly may be present, but pruritus and abdominal pain are rare. Bilirubin levels are commonly elevated to a level of less than 10 mg/dl but may be much higher in neonates, reflecting their immature biliary excretory mechanisms. Most of the bilirubin is conjugated. Alkaline phosphatase and aminotransferase levels may also be elevated, but elevations exceeding 400% of the upper limit of normal are rare unless prolonged hypotension occurred. Histologically, there is intrahepatic cholestasis but little or no necrosis of hepatocytes is seen. Kupffer cell hyperplasia, mild to moderate nonspecific inflammatory cell infiltrates predominantly in portal areas, and mild fatty changes have been described. Electron microscopy shows dilation of bile canaliculi, flattening and diminution of microvilli, prominent bile-containing Golgi complexes, and peculiarly enlarged mitochondria.[77]

Organic anion transport may be impaired, whereas synthetic, cytosolic, and microsomal functions remained preserved.[73]

Bacterial and Fungal Hepatitis

A variety of bacteria and fungi are capable of directly infecting the liver[78] (see **Table 36-1**). The signs and symptoms of bacterial and fungal hepatitides may be indistinguishable from those of viral hepatitis, and thus individuals with elevated liver-associated enzymes or jaundice with fever should be evaluated with blood cultures and appropriate serologies.

Gram-Positive Bacteria

Staphylococcal and Streptococcal Toxic Shock Syndromes

Staphylococci and streptococcal infections may directly infect the liver or, more commonly, induce parainfectious hepatitis via inflammation and/or toxin release, as noted earlier. A scarlatiniform rash, hypotension, fever or hypothermia, vomiting, and rapid progression to multiorgan failure are hallmarks of the staphylococcal and streptococcal toxic shock syndromes. Etiologic agents possess superantigens capable of eliciting an unusually broad and potentially fatal immune response. Hepatic involvement is almost universally present and may be extensive with high transaminase levels and deep jaundice. In one study deposition of teichoic acid on hepatocyte membranes was demonstrated using indirect immunofluorescent staining.[79] The authors speculated that teichoic acid, a common component of the bacterial cell wall, might exert an endotoxin-like effect on hepatocytes.

Listeriosis

Listeria monocytogenes is a zoonotic gram-positive bacterium, which may cause meningoencephalitis, endocarditis, gastrointestinal disease, and pneumonitis in humans. Infection is uncommon except in neonates, pregnant women, elderly individuals, transplant recipients, and others with impaired cell-mediated immunity. The propensity of *L. monocytogenes* to affect the liver is well documented in animals and human neonates. Interestingly, one of the initial names proposed for the organism was *Listerella hepatolytica* in recognition of the characteristic focal hepatic necrosis it causes in some animals.[80] Hepatic involvement in adults is rare but may be severe with transaminase levels in excess of 5000 IU/ml reported in the literature.[66] Most patients with clinically significant liver involvement have underlying liver disease. Histology shows microabscesses and granulomas.[81-83]

Clostridial Infections

Jaundice is detected in 20% of patients with *Clostridium perfringens* infection but is mostly due to intravascular hemolysis secondary to toxin release. Liver involvement with abscess formation and gas in the portal vein or biliary tract has been described, but bacterial hepatitis is rare.[84]

Actinomycosis

Actinomycosis caused by *Actinomyces israelii* and rarely by other anaerobic or microaerophilic actinomycetales may involve the liver.[85-88] Up to 20% of reported cases of actinomycosis involve the abdomen, and hepatic infection is present in approximately 10% to 20% of cases of abdominal actinomycosis.

Most patients with hepatic disease will develop frank pyogenic abscesses[88] but some have chronic indolent infection mimicking malignant liver disease. The typical patient is male and between 30 and 50 years of age. Common presenting symptoms include fever, abdominal pain, and anorexia with weight loss. Findings on physical examination include fever, RUQ pain, and hepatomegaly. Leukocytosis with a left shift, anemia, an elevated erythrocyte sedimentation rate, and an elevated level of alkaline phosphatase are almost universally present. Many patients undergo exploratory laparotomy to rule out malignancy, but most recent cases have been diagnosed with percutaneous biopsy. Histologically characteristic sulfur granules and the characteristic gram-positive filamentous rods may be seen (**Fig. 36-4**). Anaerobic cultures usually result in growth of the organism. Treatment consists of prolonged administration of penicillin or tetracycline and is associated with complete recovery in the majority of cases.

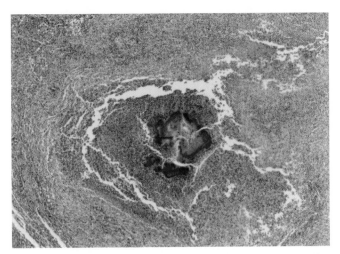

Fig. 36-4 **Hepatic necrosis and sulfur granules in actinomycosis.**

Table 36-5 Differential Diagnosis of Typhoid Versus Viral Hepatitis

	TYPHOID HEPATITIS (n = 27)	VIRAL HEPATITIS (n = 27)	P
Jaundice	33%	89%	<.0001
Fever >104° F	44%	4%	<.0001
Relative bradycardia	42%	4%	<.002
Rigors	44%	33%	n.s.
Hepatomegaly	44%	66%	n.s.
Splenomegaly	7%	11%	n.s.
Peak ALT	296 U/L	3234 U/L	<.0001
Peak AST	535 U/L	2844 U/L	<.0003
AP	500 U/dl	228 U/dl	<.004
Admission ALT/LDH ratio (expressed as multiples of upper limit of normal value)	100% <4	100% >5	<.0001
Left shift	83%	37%	<.004
Hospitalization (in days)	14.8	6.5	<.0001

Data from El-Newihi HM, Alamy ME, Reynolds TB. Salmonella heptitisi analysis of 27 cases and comparison with acute viral hepatitis. Hepatology 1996;24:516–519.

ALT, alanine aminotransferase; AP, alkaline phosphatase; AST, aspartate aminotransferase; LDH, lactate dehydrogenase; n.s., not specified.

Gram-Negative Bacteria

Melioidosis

Burkholderia pseudomallei is a water- and soil-borne gram-negative bacterium that is predominantly found in Southeast Asia, Madagascar, and regions of Central America. It is the causative agent of melioidosis.[89-92] The clinical spectrum of melioidosis may range from asymptomatic infection to fulminant overwhelming multiorgan disease involving the liver.[92] Chronic indolent courses have also been described and *B. pseudomallei*, like tuberculosis, has the potential for reactivation from a latent focus. Latency periods have been documented to be up to 29 years. Hepatic involvement may manifest as microabscesses, inflammatory infiltrates with or without focal necrosis, and occasionally granulomatous hepatitis. Diagnosis is usually made through culture, but immunohistochemistry and serologic testing may aid in localized or chronic disease.

Salmonellosis

Hepatocellular injury resembling viral hepatitis has been described in patients with acute salmonellosis, especially with *Salmonella typhi*.[93,94] "Typhoid hepatitis" was first described by William Osler as early as 1899.[95] Patients usually have a chief complaint of fever. A history of recent travel or the finding of relative bradycardia may provide diagnostic clues. The clinical symptoms may be indistinguishable from acute viral hepatitis. Differentiating features are listed in **Table 36-5**.[93] Hepatomegaly and tender splenomegaly are common, as are abnormal liver tests. Bilirubin levels are elevated in one fifth of affected patients, but frank jaundice is present in fewer than 10% of patients with typhoid fever. Transaminase levels are usually not as high as in viral hepatitis, but in rare cases may exceed 1000 U/L, with aspartate aminotransferase (AST) levels exceeding alanine aminotransferase (ALT) levels in 66% of affected patients. Periportal thickening may be detectable on ultrasound.

Liver histology shows hepatocyte swelling, nonspecific inflammatory changes, and occasionally steatosis. The term Mallory or typhoid nodule refers to a rare but characteristic focal area of hepatocyte necrosis, with aggregation of hyperplastic Kupffer cells with eosinophilic cytoplasm. Salmonella are relatively resistant to phagocytosis and reticuloendothelial cell killing, and *S. typhi* antigens and intact *Salmonella* organisms have been demonstrated in liver tissue.[96] Prolonged exposure to endotoxins is the likely pathogenesis for the observed hepatic injury. Unrecognized typhoid hepatitis carries a mortality rate of 20%. Mortality is low, however, with appropriate antibiotic therapy, including quinolones, ampicillin, or third-generation cephalosporins.[93,94]

Shigellosis

Cholestatic hepatitis is not uncommon in severe shigellosis. Histologic findings include portal and periportal polymorphonuclear inflammatory infiltrates, cholestasis, and hepatocyte necrosis.[97-99]

Yersiniosis

Diabetes and conditions associated with iron-overload predispose to *Yersinia enterocolitica* extraintestinal infections. Abscess formation is not uncommon in these patients. Yersiniosis is also an underappreciated cause of granulomatous hepatitis.[100,101]

Brucellosis

Several species of brucella, small gram-negative coccobacilli, cause brucellosis. Brucellosis is a universal zoonosis, most prevalent in the Mediterranean basin, the Indian subcontinent, and in parts of Mexico and Central and South America.

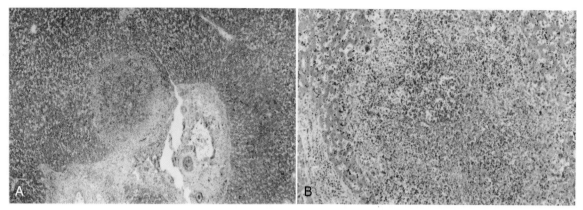

Fig. 36-5 **A and B, Granulomatous hepatitis from *Brucella abortus* infection.**

Typically, patients with brucellosis have prolonged, recurrent, and classically undulating fevers. Headache, malaise, arthralgia, backache, and night sweats are common. Hepatic abnormalities are common but often subclinical. The presence of jaundice correlates with the severity of the illness. Hepatosplenomegaly is detected in more than half of affected patients.[102,103] Imaging may show typical lesions characterized by central calcification surrounded by a necrotic rim.[104] Infection with *Brucella abortus* is associated with formation of noncaseating or necrotizing hepatic granulomas (**Fig. 36-5, *A and B***). Focal mononuclear infiltrates may be detected in portal tracts or lobules.[102,103] Positive blood or tissue cultures are diagnostic. Serum agglutination tests are helpful in chronic disease. Prolonged treatment with rifampin and doxycycline results in a cure in most cases.

Legionellosis

About half of the patients with documented *Legionella pneumophila* infection will have elevated transaminase and alkaline phosphatase levels; few will have frank jaundice.[105-107] Liver histology shows microvesicular steatosis and focal necrosis; organisms can occasionally be detected.[106] In one fatal case, peculiar margination of mitochondria in hepatocytes was demonstrated.[106]

Q Fever

Q fever is a zoonotic infection caused by the gram-negative intracellular rickettsial organism, *Coxiella burnetii*. The animal reservoirs include cattle, sheep, and goats and the most common mode of infection is inhalation of aerosolized bacteria, ingestion of contaminated milk, and tick bites. *C. burnetii* is found worldwide but is most prevalent in developing nations with significant livestock populations. Q fever is characterized by myalgia, headache, relapsing fevers, pneumonitis, and occasionally culture-negative endocarditis. Ten percent of patients progress to chronic disease, and liver abnormalities are found in 11% to 65% of such cases.[107-110] Hepatitis was reported to be the most common manifestation of Q fever in France[109] and in another study of 72 patients, 85% had abnormal liver tests and 65% had hepatomegaly.[110] Although histology may show a nonspecific reactive hepatitis and steatosis, the typical finding in Q fever is fibrin ring granulomas (or so-called doughnut granuloma). This granuloma has a clear central space felt to represent a lipid vacuole. In many cases, a fibrin ring is present that either surrounds the lipid vacuole or the periphery of the entire granuloma. Although fibrin ring granulomas are considered characteristic for Q fever, they are not seen in all such patients and are not specific for this disease. Isolated case reports have described similar granulomas in liver biopsies from patients with Hodgkin disease, hepatitis A virus infection, temporal arteritis, Epstein-Barr virus infection, cytomegalovirus infection, systemic lupus erythematosus, leishmaniasis, and allopurinol-induced hepatitis. It is, however, imperative to rule out Q fever serologically, whenever fibrin ring granulomas are found on histology. Confirmation of diagnosis usually requires serologic testing. The treatment of choice is doxycycline 100 mg twice daily or fluoroquinolones for 14 days unless endocarditis is present, which requires prolonged therapy.

Other Rickettsial Infections

Several rickettsial species cause spotted fevers, the most notable of which is Rocky Mountain spotted fever (RMSF). RMSF is caused by *Rickettsia rickettsii*. The classic triad of fever, headache, and characteristic rash occurring 1 to 2 weeks after a tick bite or a potential exposure in an endemic area should raise suspicions for RMSF. Jaundice is common and is in up to 60% of cases accompanied by various degrees of increases of transaminases and alkaline phosphatase.[111,112] The diagnosis is clinical and treatment empiric. Laboratory tests are usually not helpful because antibodies are often detected only in convalescence, and immunohistologic methods for detection of rickettsiae are unavailable in most clinics.

The basic hepatic lesion in RMSF is portal triaditis in which large mononuclear cells and neutrophils predominate. Sinusoidal erythrophagocytosis and portal vasculitis can be demonstrated in severe cases, but hepatocellular necrosis is uncommon. In two series of fatal cases, rickettsiae were identified in the portal tracts of 8 of 9 adults, and 7 of 16 pediatric patients.[113,114]

Rickettsia prowazekii causes epidemic typhus, which is transmitted by lice, and causes devastating epidemics associated with conditions of poor personal hygiene such as war, poverty, and natural disasters. Patients have fever, headache, and myalgia, usually accompanied by a rash. *Rickettsia typhi* causes murine typhus and is most prevalent in tropical and subtropical regions where the vectors (fleas) and reservoirs (rats) are most common. Scrub typhus (caused by *Orientia tsutsugamushi*) is transmitted by chigger bites and is found in a triangular region of the world bordered by Japan, Australia, and India.

Epidemic, murine, and scrub typhus may have severe multisystem illness, commonly with neurologic signs, pneumonia, fever, and rash. Jaundice and elevated liver-associated enzymes are present in up to 24% of patients with murine typhus and may suggest viral hepatitis.[115] In severe cases multiple organ failure, including hepatic failure and hemorrhage, may ensue. Doxycycline is the treatment of choice for all rickettsial diseases.

Ehrlichiosis

Human ehrlichioses are tick-borne, zoonotic infections caused by members of the genera *Ehrlichia, Anaplasma,* and *Neorickettsia* within the family Anaplasmataceae, which can affect multiple organs including the gastrointestinal tract and liver.[116,117] *Ehrlichia* are rickettsia-like, obligate intracellular, gram-negative bacteria. Human monocytic ehrlichiosis (HME) is caused by *Ehrlichia chaffeensis,* whereas human granulocytic anaplasmosis (HGA; previously human granulocytic ehrlichiosis) is caused by *Anaplasma phagocytophilum.*

Signs and symptoms include abdominal pain, nausea, vomiting, diarrhea, jaundice (40%), hepatosplenomegaly, leukopenia, thrombocytopenia, and rarely a faint macular rash. Patients usually have rapidly increasing transaminase elevations. Even with successful therapy transaminase levels normalize slowly. Bilirubin elevations may exceed 10 mg/dl. Immunocompromised and asplenic patients are at risk for more severe and protracted disease.

Both diseases can be diagnosed by detection of intracytoplasmic morulae, in either monocytes or neutrophils, which are occasionally visualized on Wright-stained peripheral smears. The diagnosis can be confirmed by demonstrating seroconversion, positive polymerase chain reaction (PCR), or growth in tissue culture, however, treatment should not be deferred pending diagnosis. If not treated in a timely fashion, ehrlichiosis can progress to multiorgan failure, which is associated with significant mortality. Doxycycline provides rapid and effective treatment.

Gonorrhea

The liver is commonly involved in gonococcal bacteremia with more than 50% of patients manifesting abnormal liver tests.[118] Frank jaundice is rare (<10%) but increased levels of transaminases (approximately 33%) and alkaline phosphatase (50% to 100%) are relatively common. Liver biopsy often shows a dense inflammatory infiltrate most pronounced in portal areas and focal necrosis of hepatocytes. Perihepatitis (Fitz-Hugh-Curtis syndrome) is the most common hepatic complication of disseminated gonococcal infection.[119,120] This syndrome has a striking sex predilection for women. Abrupt onset of sharp RUQ pain is the typical presenting symptom. Most patients are febrile. The liver tends to be tender and a friction rub may be present. Most patients have an occasionally remote history of pelvic inflammatory disease. Laparoscopic detection of violin string–like adhesions between the liver capsule and peritoneal wall are highly suggestive of the diagnosis. CT scans have been found to be more sensitive than ultrasound examinations.[120] While gonococcal infection tends to respond

dramatically to antimicrobial therapy, abnormal liver tests may initially exacerbate during therapy. Within a month, however, all laboratory markers tend to normalize. A similar perihepatitis can accompany chlamydial infections.[121,122]

Other Bacterial Pathogens

Mycobacterial Infections

Most mycobacterial infections including *Mycobacterium tuberculosis, Mycobacterium avium,* and Bacille Calmette-Guérin (BCG) cause a granulomatous hepatitis, which is described in more detail in Chapter 37.

Liver involvement in tuberculosis is well documented and may have protean presentations.[123-126] In miliary tuberculosis, liver involvement was present in up to 50% of patients dying from pulmonary tuberculosis. Ascites may be present in patients with peritoneal involvement. Jaundice is rare and usually caused by adenopathy in the porta hepatis obstructing the common bile duct or postinflammatory strictures. Localized lesions such as tuberculomas or tuberculous abscesses are much less common and frequently misdiagnosed initially.[123-127]

Symptoms are often nonspecific (**Table 36-6**). RUQ pain is not uncommon; generalized pain usually indicates concurrent peritoneal involvement. In these patients a "doughy" feel is described on abdominal examination. Elevation of alkaline phosphatase and transaminases are common. Hyperbilirubinemia is present in fewer than 25% of patients. Hypoalbuminemia and hyponatremia are noted in 88% and 65% of patients, respectively.

The presence of hepatic calcification and evidence of concurrent pulmonary disease are helpful in distinguishing hepatic tuberculosis from other liver diseases. Radiological evidence of pulmonary disease, however, may be absent in as many as a third of affected patients.[124,125] Because signs and symptoms of hepatic tuberculosis are nonspecific, diagnosis requires histologic or bacteriologic confirmation. Percutaneous, laparoscopic, or open biopsies have all been used successfully. In rare cases bile fluid obtained via ERCP is diagnostic. Hepatitis is also a common complication of antituberculous medications.[128]

The most common nontuberculous mycobacteria to affect the liver belong to the *Mycobacterium avium-intracellulare* complex (MAI). MAI dissemination with liver involvement is commonly seen in HIV-positive individuals and less commonly in organ transplant recipients, patients receiving

Table 36-6 **Clinical Features in Hepatic Tuberculosis**	
Hepatomegaly	91%
Fever	75%
Weight loss	64%
Abdominal pain	52%
Splenomegaly	39%
Digestive symptoms	33%
Night sweats	25%
Jaundice	12%

chronic steroids, or children with congenital defects in the interferon-gamma and IL-12 receptor. Hepatic MAI infection is characterized by a disproportionate elevation of serum alkaline phosphatase (up to 40 times the upper limits of normal) that may be seen in up to 5% of patients. The other liver-associated enzymes may be remarkably normal or minimally elevated.[129]

Leptospirosis

Leptospirosis is presumed to be the most widespread zoonosis in the world and has a wide range of domestic and wild animal reservoirs. Leptospires are tightly coiled spirochetes. Humans usually acquire the spirochete from water contaminated with urine from an infectious animal. The incidence is higher in warmer and humid climates, presumably due to prolonged survival of the organisms in the environment.[130]

A majority of infections are subclinical or mild enough not to result in medical attention. Anicteric leptospirosis accounts for 90% of all recognized cases. Affected patients characteristically suffer a biphasic illness. The first phase (leptospiremic or acute stage) is characterized by the abrupt onset of an influenza-like illness with fever, myalgia, headache, and malaise. Conjunctival suffusion, if present, may provide an early diagnostic clue. Following a brief period of improvement, the second phase (leptospiuric or immune stage)—characterized by myalgia, potentially severe headache, abdominal pain, nausea, vomiting, and occasionally aseptic meningitis—commences. During this phase elevations of transaminase and bilirubin levels are rare, but hepatomegaly is not uncommon. A maculopapular rash and iridocyclitis may be present. Mortality is extremely rare in anicteric leptospirosis.

Five percent to 10% of infected patients develop the more severe icteric form, which is often referred to as Morbus Weil or Weil syndrome. The first phase, which may last for weeks, is characterized by jaundice. During the second phase, which commonly follows without interceding improvement, high fevers ensue. Hepatic and renal injury predominate this phase. Jaundice may be marked with bilirubin levels in excess of 80 mg/dl as reported in the literature. Most bilirubin is conjugated. Aminotransferase levels are usually only mildly or moderately elevated. Acute tubular necrosis is common and may result in acute renal failure. Hemorrhagic complications are common and probably immune complex mediated.

Hepatic histology is generally nonspecific. Intrahepatic cholestasis, hypertrophy and hyperplasia of Kupffer cells are frequently found. Erythrophagocytosis has been documented in severe or fatal cases.[130] Electron microscopy shows mitochondrial alterations and disruption of the hepatocyte membrane. Frank hepatocyte necrosis, however, is uncommon. Diagnosis can be made by positive blood (first phase) or urine (second phase) cultures. More commonly, serologic or molecular tests are used to confirm the diagnosis of leptospirosis.

A recent review concluded that there is insufficient evidence to recommend antibiotic treatment of leptospirosis but that there is a suggestion that penicillin may cause more good than harm.[131] There is also a significant collection of anecdotal data suggesting that doxycycline is effective if administered early, as is prophylaxis before or following exposure in high-risk environments or laboratory accidents. Long-term sequelae in survivors are extremely rare.

Borreliosis

This arthropod-transmitted infection is caused by several spirochetal organism of the genus *Borrelia*. Diseases include relapsing fever and Lyme disease.

Incubation time of relapsing fever is 3 to 15 days. Onset of symptoms is usually abrupt with high fevers, headache, and myalgia. Epistaxis, profound prostration, bronchial symptoms, a rash, and/or conjunctival injection may be present. In severe attacks jaundice and tender hepatosplenomegaly may develop. Defervescence may be dramatic, with fatal collapses reported in the literature.

Borrelia multiply in organs of the reticuloendothelial system. They invade liver cells causing focal necrosis. Before a crisis, Borrelia coil tightly and are ingested by cells of the reticuloendothelial system where they may survive and cause relapsing infection. Several relapses may occur in weekly intervals. Spirochetes may be visualized in thick blood films, cutaneous biopsies, or lymph node aspirates but diagnosis is often established using agglutination or complement fixation-based serologic tests. Treatment with doxycycline is curative.

Hepatic involvement has also been described in Lyme disease, which is caused by infection with the tick-transmitted spirochete *Borrelia burgdorferi*.[132-134] Liver test abnormalities are common in patients with erythema migrans, but are usually mild, asymptomatic, and improved or resolved by 3 weeks after the onset of antibiotic therapy in most patients. In a prospective study of patients with early Lyme disease, 40% of patients had at least one liver test abnormality compared with 19% of controls. γ-Glutamyl transpeptidase (28%) and ALT (27%) levels were the most frequently elevated liver tests. Patients with early disseminated Lyme disease were more likely to have elevated liver studies (66%) compared with patients with localized disease (34%). Gastrointestinal symptoms, including anorexia, nausea, or vomiting, were reported by 30% of patients, but were not associated with elevated liver tests.[132] In later stages of the illness, presumably following invasion of the reticuloendothelial system, hepatitis type of illnesses have been described.[134] These are rare and usually overshadowed by other manifestations of the disease but may become diagnostic pitfalls.

Syphilis

Jaundice complicating early syphilis was first described by Paracelsus in 1510.[135]

Liver disease has been reported accompanying congenital, primary, secondary, and tertiary syphilis during treatment of syphilis (Jarisch-Herxheimer reaction),[136] as well as Lues maligna, even though some early reports must be viewed with caution because testing for concurrent hepatitis C virus infection was not available.

Congenital syphilis is associated with formation of small epithelioid granulomas and variable but occasionally significant portal and interstitial fibrosis.[137,138] Coiled treponemes are usually easily detected in vascular structures, fibrous tissue, and liver parenchyma using a silver stain, such as Warthin-Starry. Extensive granulomatous disease can cause hepatomegaly ("hepar lobatum"), portal hypertension, and ascites. Hepatic calcifications may be extensive.

Patients with secondary syphilis often have a maculopapular rash involving palms and soles, and nonspecific symptoms including malaise, weight loss, fever, and anorexia. Jaundice,

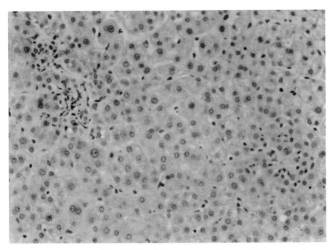

Fig. 36-6 **Portal triaditis in secondary syphilis.**

RUQ tenderness, or hepatomegaly have been described[139,140] and, while uncommon, may be severe.[141] Laboratory testing usually shows an isolated or disproportionate elevation of alkaline phosphatase levels.

Lymphocytic infiltration in and around portal tracts is common (**Fig. 36-6**); in some patients there is evidence of focal intralobular necrosis. Kupffer cell hyperplasia may be seen. Spirochetes have been demonstrated on silver staining in up to 50% of affected patients.

Syphilitic hepatitis appears to be especially common in patients with concurrent HIV infection,[143,144] and in a recent study was found in 38% of such patients.[143] Tertiary syphilis with the exception of CNS disease is now rare. Patients may be asymptomatic or have nonspecific symptoms, including malaise, anorexia, weight loss, abdominal pain, or fever. Tender nodular hepatomegaly has been reported resulting in a workup for suspected malignancy.[144] The characteristic lesion is the gumma, a centrally necrotic granuloma of rubbery consistency. Histologically extensive scarring surrounding granulation tissue, consisting of a lymphoplasmacytic infiltrate, can be seen. In most cases syphilis is diagnosed serologically. Penicillin is effective for all stages. Desensitization, tetracyclines, and cephalosporins may be used in penicillin-allergic patients.

Bartonellosis (Peliosis Hepatis)

Peliosis hepatis is characterized by cystic, blood-filled spaces in the liver. While it may be seen in patients with chronic infections, it has also been described in patients with advanced cancer and as a consequence of therapy with certain medication including anabolic steroids. In children, patients with HIV infection, and rarely other immunocompromised patients, most cases of peliosis hepatis are now due to infection by *Bartonella henselae*.[145-148] *B. henselae* infection is epidemiologically linked to cat and flea exposure. In immunocompetent patients bartonellosis manifests as cat-scratch disease, trench fever, bacteremia, or endocarditis. In immunocompromised patients, complications include bacillary angiomatosis, peliosis, bacteremia, and endocarditis. *B. henselae* has been cultured from peliotic liver lesions.

Affected patients have prolonged fever and hepatomegaly, which in 75% of cases is accompanied by splenomegaly. Other symptoms or findings may include the presence of bony lesions, lymphadenopathy, and abdominal or RUQ pain. Concurrent cutaneous lesions of bacillary angiomatosis are seen in 40% of the cases.

Anemia is common, and thrombocytopenia or pancytopenia has been reported. Transaminase levels are rarely elevated, but alkaline phosphatase levels are increased by an average of five-fold in many patients.

On CT scans peliotic lesions appear as scattered hypodense lesions. Pathologically the lesions are formed by dilated capillaries and larger, occasionally macroscopically visualized cystic, blood-filled spaces scattered throughout the hepatic parenchyma. The lining of these cystic spaces is often thin. Peliosis hepatis associated with *Bartonella* infection, but not in unrelated cases, is additionally characterized by a myxoid stroma and clumps of a granular purple material, which on Warthin-Starry staining and electron microscopy can be identified as bacilli. As culture remains difficult, serologic tests have become the mainstay of diagnosis. PCR-based tests are being evaluated.

Peliosis hepatis due to *Bartonella* responds to treatment with macrolides and doxycycline. Other drugs with in vitro activity against *Bartonella* species, but with no established clinical efficacy, include rifampin, third-generation cephalosporins, trimethoprim-sulfamethoxazole, and quinolones. Results of in vitro susceptibility tests do not necessarily correlate with clinical efficacy as treatment failures with penicillins and first-generation cephalosporins are common despite several in vitro reports documenting in vitro susceptibility.[149] Patients with hepatic bartonellosis should be treated for at least 4 months. Relapsing patients should receive lifelong treatment. Jarisch-Herxheimer–like reactions have been reported following the first dose of antibiotics in patients with *Bartonella* peliosis hepatis.[149]

Fungal Hepatitis

Many fungal infections affect the liver. Some, such as *Histoplasma capsulatum*, are taken up by the reticuloendothelial system. In fungemic patients, organisms reach the liver via the hepatic artery. Disruption of the gastrointestinal lining may result in invasion of the portal venous system by *Candida* species that are part of the normal human intestinal flora. Most fungal infections of the liver occur in immunocompromised patients. HIV-infected patients suffer from opportunistic mycoses, including histoplasmosis, blastomycosis, cryptococcosis, histoplasmosis, penicilliosis, coccidioidomycosis, and paracoccidioidomycosis. Patients with prolonged neutropenia following transplantation or chemotherapy are at risk for candidiasis including hepatosplenic candidiasis, aspergillosis, mucormycosis, trichosporonosis, and other rare fungal infections. This section reviews fungal pathogens affecting the liver of immunocompetent patients.

Candidiasis

Candida species are currently the fourth most common cause of nosocomial bloodstream infections. Patients with indwelling lines, abdominal surgery, or neutropenia are at highest risk. Seeding of the liver is common but in immunocompetent patients is usually not clinically apparent, even though microabscesses are found in virtually all organs including the liver at autopsy. In contrast, patients with impaired neutrophil function or severe neutropenia develop microabscesses in the liver that may progress to frank hepatic candidiasis.[150,151] Because *Candida* species are part of the normal intestinal flora, disruption of the intestinal wall may also result in hepatic candidiasis.

Cryptococcosis

Infection with the yeast *Cryptococcus neoformans* usually presents as a self-limited pneumonia, fever of unknown origin, or most commonly as meningitis. Hepatic cryptococcosis is rare with the exception of patients suffering from AIDS. In non–HIV-infected patients, liver infiltration may result in focal granulomatous hepatitis; liver abscess, which may clinically mimic viral hepatitis; and very rarely in widespread infiltrates resulting in hepatic failure.[152] Other rare presentations include hepatic abscess[153] and obstructive jaundice secondary to sclerosing cholangitis with recovery of yeast from the common bile duct.[154]

Microscopic examination of affected tissues or body fluids may suggest the correct diagnosis. Staining with India ink or nigrosin-based stains emphasize the capsule of the organism. Confirmation requires a positive culture or the detection of antigen using latex agglutination. Treatment varies based on immune status and should include attempts to restore host immunity. Most commonly a combination of amphotericin (aqueous or liposomal) and flucytosine is used, frequently followed by oral azole therapy.

Coccidioidomycosis and Paracoccidioidomycoses

Coccidioides immitis is endemic in the southwest United States and the San Joaquin Valley. Males, especially African Americans and immigrants, as well as immunocompromised patients, appear more susceptible to infection. In the disseminated form, hepatic involvement is common, occurring in 40% to 60% of cases. In many patients liver disease is asymptomatic but some manifest a hepatitis-like picture, which is characterized by a disproportionate elevation of alkaline phosphatase. Hepatic granulomas may be found on biopsy.[155]

Paracoccidioides brasiliensis is found in South and Central America. Infection is common in endemic areas but clinical disease is rare and most commonly affects adult men. Evidence of hepatic involvement in immunocompetent patients is largely based on an autopsy series in which up to 50% of patients who die of paracoccidioidomycosis are found to have liver involvement.[156,157] Hepatomegaly is reported in 40% of patients with clinical disease, but jaundice is found in fewer than 6% of affected patients. Aminotransferase levels are commonly elevated, whereas bilirubin and alkaline phosphatase levels are only elevated in patients with severe disease. Biopsy specimens show lesions ranging from small granulomas to diffuse infiltration of yeast forms and fibrosis. Bile ducts are commonly involved. Diagnosis of both dimorphic fungal infections relies on detection of organisms through a biopsy, serologic tests detecting antibodies or fungal antigens, or PCR-based methods. Treatment is amphotericin or azole based.

Histoplasmosis

Histoplasma capsulatum is a dimorphic fungus that can be found in soil contaminated with bird or bat excreta. Histoplasmosis is endemic in the east and central United States, Central and South America, Africa, India, and the Far East.

Infection occurs via inhalation but subsides without clinical disease in most patients. Occasionally the infection may disseminate from the lungs to involve organs of the reticulo-endothelial system including the liver. In nonimmunocompromised hosts infection is commonly self-limiting. In many patients from endemic areas, unaware of a primary infection, hepatic calcifications—some of which may contain *H. capsulatum organisms*—may be detected in routine examinations. Progressive dissemination is not uncommon in immunocompromised patients but may rarely occur in normal hosts.[158]

Affected patients have hepatosplenomegaly, high fever, and abnormal liver function tests. Ferritin levels are usually grossly elevated. Several reports have also documented histoplasmosis as a common cause of infection-associated hemophagocytic syndrome[159] and in rare cases histoplasmosis may present as an isolated liver lesion.[160] The most common histologic finding is a portal lymphohistiocytic inflammation; discrete hepatic granulomas were seen in fewer than 20% of involved livers in one study.[161] Diagnosis is based on demonstration of the organism in histologic specimens, growth in fungal culture media or detection of fungal antigen in urine. Serologic tests are only helpful in non-endemic settings. Treatment of patients with severe disease consists of amphotericin B in doses of 0.8 to 1 mg/kg daily followed by prolonged treatment with itraconazole.

Key References

Ahsan N, et al. Peliosis hepatis due to *Bartonella henselae* in transplantation: a hemato-hepato-renal syndrome. Transplantation 1998;65:1000–1003. (Ref.148)

Alvarez SZ. Hepatobiliary tuberculosis. J Gastroenterol Hepatol 1998;13:833–839. (Ref.126)

Baddley JW, et al. Crohn's disease presenting as septic thrombophlebitis of the portal vein (pylephlebitis): case report and review of the literature. Am J Gastroenterol 1999;94:847–849. (Ref.67)

Barakate MS, et al. Pyogenic liver abscess: a review of 10 years' experience in management. Aust N Z J Surg 1999;69:205–209. (Ref.8)

Barrio J, et al. Pyogenic liver abscesses of bacterial origin. A study of 45 cases. Rev Esp Enferm Dig 2000;92:232–239. (Ref.11)

Brook I, Frazier EH. Microbiology of liver and spleen abscesses. J Med Microbiol 1998;47(12):1075–1080. (Ref.33)

Chemaly RF, et al. Microbiology of liver abscesses and the predictive value of abscess Gram stain and associated blood cultures. Diagn Microbiol Infect Dis 2003;46:245–248. (Ref.34)

Cheng HC, et al. Long-term outcome of pyogenic liver abscess: factors related with abscess recurrence. J Clin Gastroenterol 2008;42:1110–1115. (Ref.14)

Chong VH. Changing spectrum of microbiology of liver abscess: now *Klebsiella*, next *Burkholderia pseudomallei*. J Emerg Med 2010; doi:10.1016/j.jemermed. 2009.10.027. (Ref.89)

Chong VH. Hepatobiliary tuberculosis: a review of presentations and outcomes. South Med J 2008;101:356–361. (Ref.123)

Chou FF, et al. Single and multiple pyogenic liver abscesses: clinical course, etiology, and results of treatment. World J Surg 1997;21:384–389. (Ref.9)

Chu KM, et al. Pyogenic liver abscess. An audit of experience over the past decade. Arch Surg 1996;131:148–152. (Ref.6)

Clarençon F, et al. Recurrent liver abscess secondary to ingested fish bone migration: report of a case. Surg Today 2008;38:572–575. (Ref.19)

Corredoira Sanchez JC, et al. Pyogenic liver abscess: changes in etiology, diagnosis and treatment over 18 years. Rev Clin Esp 1999;199:705–710. (Ref.7)

Crum-Cianflone N, Weekes J, Bavaro M. Syphilitic hepatitis among HIV-infected patients. Int J STD AIDS 2009;20:278–284. (Ref.142)

Cunha BA. Clinical features of legionnaires' disease. Semin Respir Infect 1998;13:116–127. (Ref.105)

Dadamessi I, et al. Hepatic disorders related to Lyme disease. Study of two cases and a review of the literature. Gastroenterol Clin Biol 2001;25:193–196. (Ref.134)

Dance DA. Melioidosis as an emerging global problem. Acta Trop 2000;74:115–119. (Ref.90)

de Baere T, et al. Adverse events during radiofrequency treatment of 582 hepatic tumors. AJR Am J Roentgenol 2003;181:695–700. (Ref.28)

Drnovsek V, et al. Gastrointestinal case of the day. Pyogenic liver abscess caused by perforation by a swallowed wooden toothpick. Radiographics 1999;19(3):820–822. (Ref.22)

El-Newihi HM, Alamy ME, Reynolds TB. Salmonella hepatitis: analysis of 27 cases and comparison with acute viral hepatitis. Hepatology 1996;24:516–519. (Ref.93)

Fang CT, et al. *Klebsiella pneumoniae* genotype K1: an emerging pathogen that causes septic ocular or central nervous system complications from pyogenic liver abscess. Clin Infect Dis 2007;45:284–293. (Ref.44)

Fang FC, Sandler N, Libby SJ. Liver abscess caused by magA+ *Klebsiella pneumoniae* in North America. J Clin Microbiol 2005;43:991–992. (Ref.42)

Foo NP, et al. Characteristics of pyogenic liver abscess patients with and without diabetes mellitus. Am J Gastroenterol 2010;105:328–335. (Ref.37)

Gaskin DA, Bodonaik NC, Williams NP. Hepatic abscesses at the University Hospital of the West Indies. A 24-year autopsy review. West Indian Med J 2003;52:37–40. (Ref.13)

Giorgio A, et al. Complications after interventional sonography of focal liver lesions: a 22-year single-center experience. Am Inst Ultrasound Med 2003;22:193–205. (Ref.27)

Guidugli F, et al. Antibiotics for treating leptospirosis. Cochrane Database Syst Rev 2010;1:CD001306. (Ref.131)

Hageman JC, et al. Vancomycin-intermediate *Staphylococcus aureus* in a home health-care patient. Emerg Infect Dis 2001;7:1023–1025. (Ref.52)

Halimi C, et al. Hepatic brucelloma: 2 cases and a review of the literature. Gastroenterol Clin Biol 1999;23:513–517. (Ref.104)

Hansen PS, Schonheyder HC. Pyogenic hepatic abscess. A 10-year population-based retrospective study. APMIS 1998;106:396–402. (Ref.12)

Hernandez JL, Ramos C. Pyogenic hepatic abscess: clues for diagnosis in the emergency room. Clin Microbiol Infect 2001;7:567–570. (Ref.54)

Hickey N, et al. Acute hepatobiliary tuberculosis: a report of two cases and a review of the literature. Eur Radiol 1999;9:886–889. (Ref.124)

Horowitz HW, Dworkin B, Forseter G. Liver functions in early Lyme disease. Hepatology 1996;23:1412–1417. (Ref.132)

Hsieh CH. Comparison of hepatic abscess after operative and nonoperative management of isolated blunt liver trauma. Int Surg 2002;87:178–184. (Ref.26)

Hsieh CH, Hsu YP. Early-onset liver abscess after blunt liver trauma: report of a case. Surg Today 2002;33:392–394. (Ref.25)

Hsieh HF, et al. Aggressive hepatic resection for patients with pyogenic liver abscess and APACHE II score > or = 15. Am J Surg 2008;196:346–350. (Ref.60)

Huang CJ, et al. Pyogenic hepatic abscess. Changing trends over 42 years. Ann Surg 1996;223:600–609. (Ref.5)

Huang CY, et al. Gas-forming pyogenic liver abscess. QJM 2009;102:885–888. (Ref.38)

Huang SF, et al. Liver abscess formation after transarterial chemoembolization for malignant hepatic tumor. Hepatogastroenterology 2003;50:1115–1118. (Ref.29)

Jan YY, Yeh TS, Chen MF. Cholangiocarcinoma presenting as pyogenic liver abscess: is its outcome influenced by concomitant hepatolithiasis? Am J Gastroenterol 1998;93:253–255. (Ref.16)

Janbon F. The liver and brucellosis. Gastroenterol Clin Biol 1999;23:431–432. (Ref.103)

Johannsen EC, Sifri CD, Madoff LC. Pyogenic liver abscesses. Infect Dis Clin North Am 2000;14:547–563. (Ref.10)

Joshi V, et al. Actinomycotic liver abscess: a rare complication of colonic diverticular disease. Ann Hepatol 2010;9:96–98. (Ref.88)

Kawamoto S, et al. Nonneoplastic liver disease: evaluation with CT and MR imaging. Radiographics 1998;18:827–848. (Ref.56)

Kim JK, et al. Risk factor analysis of invasive liver abscess caused by the K1 serotype *Klebsiella pneumoniae*. Eur J Clin Microbiol Infect Dis 2009;28:109–111. (Ref.48)

Kok KY, Yapp SK. Isolated hepatic tuberculosis: report of five cases and review of the literature. J Hepatobiliary Pancreat Surg 1999;6:195–198. (Ref.125)

Ku YH, Chuang YC, Yu WL. Clinical spectrum and molecular characteristics of *Klebsiella pneumoniae* causing community-acquired extrahepatic abscess. J Microbiol Immunol Infect 2008;41:311–317. (Ref.47)

Kubo S, et al. Risk factors for and clinical findings of liver abscess after biliary-intestinal anastomosis. Hepatogastroenterology 1999;46:116–120. (Ref.32)

Kumar N, Jain S, Singh ZN. Disseminated histoplasmosis with reactive hemophagocytosis: aspiration cytology findings in two cases. Diagn Cytopathol 2000;23:422–424. (Ref.159)

Kumar R, et al. Antituberculosis therapy-induced acute liver failure: magnitude, profile, prognosis, and predictors of outcome. Hepatology 2010;51:1665–1674. (Ref.128)

Lamps LW, et al. The pathologic spectrum of gastrointestinal and hepatic histoplasmosis. Am J Clin Pathol 2000;113:64–72. (Ref.161)

Lederman ER, Crum NF. Pyogenic liver abscess with a focus on *Klebsiella pneumoniae* as a primary pathogen: an emerging disease with unique clinical characteristics. Am J Gastroenterol 2005;100:322–331. (Ref.41)

Lee SS, et al. Predictors of septic metastatic infection and mortality among patients with *Klebsiella pneumoniae* liver abscess. Clin Infect Dis 2008;47:642–650. (Ref.49)

Levett PN. Leptospirosis. Clin Microbiol Rev 2001;14:296–326. (Ref.130)

Lipsett PA, et al. Fungal hepatic abscesses: characterization and management. J Gastrointest Surg 1997;1:78–84. (Ref.53)

Liu PY, Yang Y, Shi ZY. Cryptococcal liver abscess: a case report of successful treatment with amphotericin-B and literature review. Jpn J Infect Dis 2009;62:59–60. (Ref.153)

Lo JO, Harrison RA, Hunter AJ. Syphilitic hepatitis resulting in fulminant hepatic failure requiring liver transplantation. J Infect 2007;54:115–117. (Ref.141)

Maincent G, et al. Tertiary hepatic syphilis. A treatable cause of multinodular liver. Dig Dis Sci 1997;42:447–450. (Ref.144)

Marks J, et al. Laparoscopic liver surgery. A report on 28 patients. Surg Endosc 1998;12:331–334. (Ref.61)

Martin RC II, Edwards MJ, McMasters KM. Histoplasmosis as an isolated liver lesion: review and surgical therapy. Am Surg 2001;67:430–431. (Ref.160)

Martin-Vivaldi Martinez R, et al. Pseudotumorous hepatic tuberculosis: laparoscopic appearance. Gastroenterol Hepatol 1996;19:456–458. (Ref.127)

Mosely RH. Sepsis and cholestasis. Clin Liver Dis 2004;8:83–94. (Ref.74)

Mullick CJ, et al. Syphilitic hepatitis in HIV-infected patients: a report of 7 cases and review of the literature. Clin Infect Dis 2004;39:100–105. (Ref.143)

Nicolas X, et al. Lyme borreliosis hepatitis. Presse Med 2002;31:319. (Ref.133)

Nutt AK, Raufman J. Gastrointestinal and hepatic manifestations of human ehrlichiosis: 8 cases and a review of the literature. Dig Dis 1999;17:37–43. (Ref.117)

Perkins M, Lovell J, Gruenewald S. Life-threatening pica: liver abscess from perforating foreign body. Australas Radiol 1999;43:349–352. (Ref.24)

Peter NG, Clark LR, Jaeger JR. Fitz-Hugh-Curtis syndrome: a diagnosis to consider in women with right upper quadrant pain. Clevel Clin J Med 2004;71:233–239. (Ref.120)

Pope JV, et al. *Klebsiella pneumoniae* liver abscess: an emerging problem in North America. J Emerg Med 2008; doi:10.1016/j.jemermed.2008.04.041. (Ref.43)

Pramoolsinsap C, Viranuvatti V. *Salmonella* hepatitis. J Gastroenterol Hepatol 1998;13:745–750. (Ref.94)

Rabkin JM, et al. Hepatic allograft abscess with hepatic arterial thrombosis. Am J Surg 1998;175:354–359. (Ref.15)

Ralls PW. Inflammatory disease of the liver. Clin Liver Dis 2002;6:1–18. (Ref.55)

Raoult D. Rickettsial diseases. Medicine (Baltimore) 1996;24:71–75. (Ref.110)

Runge VM, Wells JW, Williams NM. Hepatic abscesses. Magnetic resonance imaging findings using gadolinium-BOPTA. Invest Radiol 1996;31:781–788. (Ref.57)

Saxena R, et al. Pylephlebitis: a case report and review of outcome in the antibiotic era. Am J Gastroenterol 1996;91:1251–1253. (Ref.68)

Seeto RK, Rockey DC. Pyogenic liver abscess. Changes in etiology, management, and outcome. Medicine (Baltimore) 1996;75:99–113. (Ref.4)

Sharma M, Briski LE, Khatib R. Hepatic actinomycosis: an overview of salient features and outcome of therapy. Scand J Infect Dis 2002;34:386–391. (Ref.87)

Shibata T, et al. Cholangitis and liver abscess after percutaneous ablation therapy for liver tumors: incidence and risk factors. J Vasc Interv Radiol 2003;14:1535–1542. (Ref.30)

Siu WT, et al. Laparoscopic management of ruptured pyogenic liver abscess. Surg Laparosc Endosc 1997;7:426–428. (Ref.62)

Solomkin JS, et al. Guidelines for the selection of anti-infective agents for complicated intra-abdominal infections. Clin Infect Dis 2003;37:997–1005. (Ref.65)

Spach DH, Koehler JE. *Bartonella*-associated infections. Infect Dis Clin North Am 1998;12:137–155. (Ref.149)

Su SC, et al. Community-acquired liver abscess caused by serotype K1 Klebsiella pneumoniae with CTX-M-15-type extended-spectrum beta-lactamase. Antimicrob Agents Chemother 2008;52:804–805. (Ref.50)

Tanaka M, et al. Long-term consequence of endoscopic sphincterotomy for bile duct stones. Gastrointest Endosc 1998;48:465–469. (Ref.31)

Taniguchi Y, et al. Subclinical syphilitic hepatitis, which was markedly worsened by a Jarisch-Herxheimer reaction. Am J Gastroenterol 1999;94:1694–1696. (Ref.136)

Trauner M, Fickert P, Strauber RE. Inflammation-induced cholestasis. J Gastroenterol Hepatol 1999;14:946–959. (Ref.75)

Tsai JL, et al. Liver abscess secondary to fish bone penetration of the gastric wall: a case report. Chung Hua I Hsueh Tsa Chih 1999;62:51–54. (Ref.20)

Tsui BC, Mossey J. Occult liver abscess following clinically unsuspected ingestion of foreign bodies. Can J Gastroenterol 1997;11:445–448. (Ref.21)

Tu YC, et al. Genetic requirements for *Klebsiella pneumoniae*–induced liver abscess in an oral infection model. J Infect Immun 2009;77:2657–2671. (Ref.51)

Walker DH, Paddock CD, Dumler JS. Emerging and re-emerging tick-transmitted rickettsial and ehrlichial infections. Med Clin North Am 2008;92:1345–1361. (Ref.118)

Wang JH, et al. Primary liver abscess due to *Klebsiella pneumoniae* in Taiwan. Clin Infect Dis 1998;26:1434–1438. (Ref.39)

Weng W, et al. Laparoscopic drainage of pyogenic liver abscesses. Surg Today 2004;34:323–325. (Ref.63)

Woo SY, et al. Clinical outcome of Fitz-Hugh-Curtis syndrome mimicking acute biliary disease. World J Gastroenterol 2008;14:6975–6980. (Ref.121)

Yang CC, et al. Comparison of pyogenic liver abscess caused by non-*Klebsiella pneumoniae* and *Klebsiella pneumoniae*. J Microbiol Immunol Infect 2004;37:176–184. (Ref.40)

Yeh KM, et al. MagA is not a specific virulence gene for *Klebsiella pneumoniae* strains causing liver abscess but is part of the capsular polysaccharide gene cluster of *K. pneumoniae* serotype K1. J Med Microbiol 2006;55:803–804. (Ref.45)

Yeh KM, et al. Capsular serotype K1 or K2, rather than magA and rmpA, is a major virulence determinant for *Klebsiella pneumoniae* liver abscess in Singapore and Taiwan. J Clin Microbiol 2007;4:466–471. (Ref.46)

Yeh TS, et al. Hepatocellular carcinoma presenting as pyogenic liver abscess: characteristics, diagnosis, and management. Clin Infect Dis 1998;26:1224–1226. (Ref.17)

Yeom JO, et al. A case of hepatocellular carcinoma combined with liver abscess. Korean J Gastroenterol 2009;53:378–382. (Ref.18)

Yu SC, et al. Treatment of pyogenic liver abscess: prospective randomized comparison of catheter drainage and needle aspiration. Hepatology 2004;39:932–938. (Ref.64)

Zakout R, et al. Colonoscopy for "cryptogenic" pyogenic liver abscess? Colorectal Dis 2010;12:71–72. (Ref.58)

Zangerl B, et al. Coccidioidomycosis as the cause of granulomatous hepatitis. Med Klin 1998;93:170–173. (Ref.155)

Zysk G, Splettstosser WD, Neubauer H. A review on melioidosis with special respect on molecular and immunological diagnostic techniques. Clin Lab 2000;46:119–130. (Ref.91)

A complete list of references can be found at www.expertconsult.com.

Granulomatous Diseases of the Liver

Helmut Albrecht

Introduction

Hepatic granulomas are associated with a wide variety of underlying conditions and are found in 1% to 15% of patients undergoing liver biopsies.[1-13] They may also be an incidental finding on otherwise normal liver biopsy specimens. An isolated granuloma therefore does not reliably indicate the presence of granulomatous liver disease. While most liver granulomas do not cause structural liver injury, their detection may be the first indication of a systemic disease.

Histopathology

A granuloma is a circumscribed and organized lesion, which is distinct from nearby uninvolved tissue and characterized by a central accumulation of mononuclear cells, primarily activated macrophages, with a surrounding rim consisting of lymphocytes and fibroblasts. As activated macrophages loosely resemble epithelial cells, they are commonly and somewhat erroneously referred to as epithelioid cells. Epithelioid cells have elongated and often large nuclei and abundant pale cytoplasm, which is rich in endoplasmic reticulum and has fewer phagolysosomes than regular macrophages. These characteristics are consistent with the cytokine-secreting function of epithelioid cells as opposed to the primarily phagocytic function of most macrophages. Based on these differences, it is possible to distinguish an epithelioid cell granuloma from an aggregate of macrophages using the periodic acid–Schiff (PAS) stain. Epithelioid cell granulomas are PAS negative, in contrast to an aggregate of macrophages, which may contain PAS-positive debris. Macrophages within an aggregate are also always separate from one another, whereas adjacent macrophages in a true granuloma may fuse, forming multinucleated giant cells.

Early in the development of a granuloma, lesions may be ill-defined and appear as punched-out clusters of histiocytes or lymphocytes. Persistent secretion of a variety of cytokines allows more defined granulomas to form.

There are several classification schemes that address types of granulomas but regardless of the classification used, the morphology of the granulomas and their location may be helpful for narrowing the differential diagnosis. Several histologic variants of hepatic granulomas have been recognized, the first two of which are most common in the United States.

- Epithelioid granulomas (noncaseating) such as seen with sarcoidosis may also be associated with a large number of other diseases and may be an incidental finding of no clinical significance in patients undergoing liver biopsies for other reasons. Nonnecrotizing granulomas are generally small (100 to 300 μm), but may coalesce to form large, at times macroscopically visible lesions. As granulomas can incite an inflammatory response, many such lesions are surrounded by dense, scarlike fibrous tissue with variable numbers of lymphocytes, plasma cells, and eosinophils.
- Epithelioid granulomas (caseating), characterized by central necrosis, are most commonly seen in tuberculosis, but can be found in other disease states, most commonly infectious causes. Necrotizing granulomas may range from small

lesions to large cavitating abscesses. The epithelioid layer may be thin and only one to two cells thick. The necrotic material is generally eosinophilic, may be granular, and may contain calcifications.

- Fibrin-ring granulomas (also known as doughnut granulomas) have a distinctive appearance in which epithelioid cells surround a vacuole that has an encircling eosinophilic fibrin ring, which can be visualized with the Masson trichrome stain. Conditions associated with the usually well formed fibrin-ring granulomas include Q fever and less commonly Hodgkin lymphoma, cytomegalovirus (CMV), leishmaniasis, hepatitis A, toxoplasmosis, giant cell arteritis, rickettsial disease, and use of allopurinol.
- Lipogranulomas contain a central lipid vacuole, which may be stained with Oil Red O stains. These granulomas are quite distinctive but are often inconsequential. Lipogranulomas are composed of lipid-laden histiocytes, lipid vacuoles, and a variable number of chronic inflammatory cells. They are usually located around the central vein, though they may be present in the portal areas. The surrounding hepatic parenchyma may be normal or steatotic.[14,15] In nonsteatotic livers, these granulomas appear to develop in response to exogenous mineral oils that are used in food processing. Some authors have reported that the incidence of lipogranulomas has increased with time and have speculated that this increase is consistent with the widespread use of mineral oils in the food industry.[15]

Granulomas can be located throughout the hepatic lobule. However, a tendency to be located in specific sites is recognized in some disorders. Examples include the portal or periportal location of granulomas in sarcoidosis, and the portal location in primary biliary cirrhosis.

Special stains for fungal and mycobacterial pathogens, silver stains, and examination under polarized light may help elucidate the pathophysiology of a granuloma. Foreign material, such as talc, may be birefringent under polarized light.[16] In the absence of acid-fast organisms, fungi, parasites, or foreign material, it is not possible to reliably identify the cause of a granuloma on morphologic grounds. Some morphologic features, however, may help narrow down the differential diagnosis. Granulomas associated with infection commonly have a mixed infiltrate of macrophages, lymphocytes, neutrophils, and eosinophils, whereas immunologically mediated entities usually display a dense lymphocytic infiltrate. Eosinophilic predominance increases the odds that the granulomas are associated with parasitic disease, malignancy, or drug reaction. Foreign tissue, such as a schistosomal egg remnant, may provide additional clues to the diagnosis.

Immunology

Granuloma formation can be classified as a component of a type IV delayed hypersensitivity reaction, which is triggered by exposure to chronic presentation of an antigen not eliminated by the humoral immune system. The antigen may be a substance resistant to degradation, such as talc or mineral oil, or an infectious agent, which due to its intracellular location or protective virulence factors cannot be eliminated by "first-responder" inflammatory cells such as neutrophils and eosinophils.

The two key cellular immunologically active components in a granuloma are macrophages and CD4$^+$ T-lymphocytes. Without effective intercellular cytokine-mediated communication between the cell types, granulomas may fail to form, may not be sustained, or may not be able to eliminate the target antigen. Unactivated macrophages are capable of phagocytosis but in order for macrophages to form granulomas, they must be immunologically activated. This activation can be induced by lymphocytes secreting either type 1 (T_H1) or type 2 (T_H2) cytokines.

Secretion of T_H1 type cytokines including interferon-gamma (IFN-γ) as well as interleukin-2 (IL-2) and IL-12 is an important response against intracellular pathogens and in sarcoidosis. Activation by T_H1 type cytokines (mainly IFN-γ) primes macrophages via a JAK1/2-STAT1 pathway to display more MHC class II molecules, up-regulate respiratory burst, and secrete proinflammatory cytokines, including tumor necrosis factor alpha (TNF-α), IL-1, and IL-6.[17]

TNF-α up-regulates the expression of intercellular adhesion molecules (ICAM), allowing inflammatory cells to adhere to endothelial cells and localize to the antigenic stimulus. TNF-α also stimulates T-cell proliferation and, in a positive feedback loop, increases secretion of IFN-γ. Granulomas that develop under the influence of a T_H1 response tend to form slower, are larger, poorly formed, and more destructive than those that develop in response to T_H2 cytokines.

T_H2 responses are characterized by secretion of IL-4, IL-5, IL-6, IL-10, and IL-13 and tend to be triggered primarily by extracellular antigens. Schistosomal ova, for instance, induce a T_H2 response against soluble egg antigens. In this pathway, macrophages are stimulated to up-regulate the mannosyl receptor, MHC class II antigens, and growth factors, resulting in fusion of activated macrophages. T_H2 type cytokines are also potent attractors of eosinophils.

T_H1 and T_H2 cytokine response patterns are not mutually exclusive. In schistosomiasis, for instance, an initial type 1 response usually evolves into a type 2 response.[18-20] Which response predominates depends on the antigen and the timing of the cytokines secreted in relation to the chronologic evolution of the granuloma. Both cytokine pathways are capable of activating macrophages but IFN-γ appears to be an absolute requirement for the aggregation of activated macrophages into granulomas. IFN-γ–deficient knock-out mice and human patients who are deficient for the IFN-γ receptor fail to form granulomas. TNF-α and lymphotoxin-α are also required for the formation and more importantly maintenance of granulomas, as well as the fusion of macrophages into giant cells. TNF-α receptor blockers, commonly used for certain autoimmune conditions, cause regression of granulomas but increase susceptibility for certain infections including mycobacterial diseases.

Incidence

The incidence of granulomas detected in liver biopsies varies from 0.8% to 15%.[1-13] The incidence in autopsy studies tends to be higher than in cohorts undergoing liver biopsy, reflecting the amount of tissue sampled as well as the ability to select grossly abnormal areas for sampling in autopsy material.[2] The likelihood of finding granulomas increases with the number of biopsies obtained.[21,22]

Table 37-1 Selected Reported Causes and Associated Conditions in Patients with Hepatic Granulomas

Unclassified	Viral
Idiopathic **Incidental**	Cytomegalovirus Epstein-Barr virus Hepatitis A virus Hepatitis B virus Hepatitis C virus HIV
Autoimmune	
Blau syndrome Churg-Strauss syndrome Crohn's disease Eosinophilic gastroenteritis Graves' disease Lupus erythematosus **Primary biliary cirrhosis** Rheumatoid arthritis **Sarcoidosis**	**Drug Induced**
	Allopurinol Amoxicillin-clavulanic acid Aprindine Aspirin with codeine **Carbamazepine** Chlorpromazine Chlorpropamide Clofibrate Dicloxacillin Didanosine Diltiazem **Diphenylhydantoin** Glyburide Halothane Hydralazine Interferon Mebendazole Mesalamine Methyldopa Norfloxacin Oral contraceptives Paracetamol **Phenylbutazone** **Phenytoin** Procainamide Pyrazinamide **Quinidine** **Quinine** Rosiglitazone Sulfadoxine/pyrimethamine Sulfasalazine Ticlopidine
Infections	
Mycobacterial	
M. tuberculosis (including Bacillus Calmette-Guérin [BCG]) **M. avium/intracellulare** *M. kansasii* *M .chelonae* *M. leprae* *M. mucogenicum* *M. scrofulaceum*	
Parasitic	
Ascaris *Enterobius* *Fasciola* *Giardia* *Leishmania* *Linguatula* ***Schistosomiasis*** *Strongyloides* *Toxocara* *Toxoplasma*	
Fungal	**Neoplasms**
Blastomyces *Candida* *Coccidioides* *Cryptococcus* *Histoplasma* *Trichosporon*	Hairy cell leukemia Hodgkin disease Non-Hodgkin lymphoma Renal cell carcinoma
	Miscellaneous Other Diseases
Bacterial	
Bartonella *Borrelia burgdorferi* ***Brucella*** *melitensis* **Coxiella burnetii (Q fever)** *Listeria monocytogenes* *Rickettsial* sp. *Treponema pallidum* *Tropheryma whippelii* *Yersinia enterocolitica*	Cardiopulmonary bypass surgery **Chronic granulomatous disease** **Common variable immunodeficiency** Exposure to aluminum, copper, gold Ileal bypass surgery

Highlighted entities are discussed in detail because they are either common or important causes of hepatic granulomas or entities for which granulomas are considered pathognomonic.

Causes of Hepatic Granulomas

Table 37-1 provides a list of established causes and diseases associated with hepatic granulomas. Several of the associations reported stem from case reports and small case series.

The emboldened diseases are entities in which granulomas are either frequent or typical. The relative frequency of various etiologies will vary depending on practice location and referral population (**Table 37-2**).

Several broad etiologic categories and a myriad of specific causes of granulomas need to be considered. Diagnostic and therapeutic considerations for specific causes of hepatic

Table 37-2 Cause of Hepatic Granulomas in Recent Series with Greater Than 50 Cases (1990-2009)

COHORT	COUNTRY	YEAR	TOTAL BIOPSIES	NUMBER OF CASES	PERCENTAGE	PRIMARY BILIARY CIRRHOSIS	SARCOID	TUBER-CULOSIS	HEPATITIS C	DRUGS	SCHISTOSO-MIASIS	OTHER ENTITIES	IDIOPATHIC/ UNKNOWN
Satti	Saudi Arabia	1990	404	59	14.6%	0%	0%	34%	0%	3%	54%	9%	0%
Sartin	United States	1991	NA	88	NA	4.5%	22%	3%	0%	6%	0%	14.5%	50%
McCluggage	Northern Ireland	1994	4124	163	4%	55%	18%	1%	0%	1%	0%	14%	11%
Mert	Turkey	2001	NA	74	1.6%	0%	36%	20%	1%	1%	0%	22%	20%
Gaya	Scotland	2003	1662	63	3.7%	36%	11%	4%	9%	9%	0%	20%	11%
Dourakis	Greece	2007	1768	66	3.7%	68%	7.5%	1.5%	4.5%	3%	1.5%	8%	6%
Drebber	Germany	2008	12161	442	3.6%	48.6%	8.3%	0.7%	0%	2.5%	0%	3.9%	36%

granulomas will be discussed according to the following classification:

- Unclassified (incidental/idiopathic)
- Autoimmune disorders
- Infections
- Drugs
- Malignancies

Unclassified (Incidental/Idiopathic)

Incidental

Hepatic granulomas may be an incidental finding on otherwise normal liver biopsies. Incidental granulomas can also be seen in virtually any chronic liver disease. Incidental granulomas have been documented in patients who undergo liver biopsy for the grading and staging of chronic hepatitis B and hepatitis C infection, and the reported incidence varies from 0.73% to 13%.[23-29] In one large study of 435 patients,[29] nonnecrotizing granulomas of unknown significance were observed in 4.5% of biopsies from 155 patients with HCV infection. This was significantly higher than in the control groups of hepatitis B infection (0.66% of 151 patients) and alcoholic liver disease (0 of 129 patients). The cause of granulomas in this setting remains unclear, and patients do not appear to have symptoms attributable to this finding.

Incidental granulomas are also a common finding in explanted livers of patients with primary sclerosing cholangitis.[30] In this study, 7% of explanted livers had evidence of well-formed, nonnecrotizing granulomas that were quite dissimilar from the typical primary biliary cirrhosis (PBC)-like granulomatous lesions that are intimately associated with interlobular bile duct damage.[31] An isolated granuloma therefore does not necessarily indicate the presence of significant pathology.

Idiopathic

After all common causes of fever or abnormal liver tests have been excluded in patients with granulomatous inflammation of the liver, a significant percentage of patients remain without a specific etiologic diagnosis, summarized by the descriptive term idiopathic granulomatous hepatitis. Depending on locality, intensity of diagnostic workup, and whether cases were collected prospectively or identified through chart review, the reported range for idiopathic granulomatous hepatitis varies from 0% to 50%[1-13] (see **Table 37-2**). Although the cause, by definition, remains unclear, most of the series that report high rates of idiopathic disease tend to be older, are retrospective, have limited follow-up, and do not specifically address the question of an autoimmune cause or hepatitis C.[3,12,32-37]

Many of the patients with idiopathic disease have high fever and abnormal liver enzyme tests that are often associated with chills, rigors, and significant weight loss. The duration of symptoms varies from months to years. A liver biopsy is usually performed as part of the workup for a fever of unknown origin (FUO) and for abnormal liver tests. Most patients receive but do not respond to empiric antituberculous therapy, which is presented as evidence against tuberculosis as a cause of this disease. In some patients there is spontaneous resolution of symptoms, whereas others require treatment with steroids, to which most patients tend to show a dramatic response. Although some are cured with short-term steroids, others must be maintained on medication for long periods to avoid relapse upon withdrawal. The duration of steroid treatment depends on the response to withdrawal and can vary from months to years. In those patients who have undergone sequential liver biopsies, the granulomas disappear with therapy and reappear when the patient again becomes symptomatic.[33,34] A recommended steroid dose for patients who do not recover spontaneously is equivalent to prednisone 0.5 to 1 mg/kg/day.[37] Several authors have recommended a prophylactic course of antituberculous medication (isoniazid 5 mg/kg for 9 months), particularly in anergic patients or patients with a positive tuberculin skin test or in vitro IFN-γ–based assays before receiving steroid therapy.[33,37] Indomethacin[36] or methotrexate[38] have been used successfully in steroid-resistant patients.

A likely related entity, the so-called GLUS syndrome (granulomatous lesions of unknown significance), describes patients who have fever, abdominal pain, and weight loss, who are found to have multiorgan granulomatous inflammation that appears to be primarily subdiaphragmatic, mainly involving the liver, spleen, and lymph nodes.[39] The granulomas differ from sarcoidal granulomas in that they are rich in B rather than T lymphocytes. Because none of the other studies discussed under idiopathic granulomatous hepatitis have examined the phenotype of the inflammatory cells within the granulomas, it is possible that all these entities form a spectrum of likely autoimmune-related granulomatous hepatitides of unknown cause.

Autoimmune Disorders

Among diseases thought to have an autoimmune cause, sarcoidosis and primary biliary cirrhosis are the most common diagnoses associated with hepatic granulomas in recent series. Other autoimmune diseases that have been associated with hepatic granulomas include Crohn's disease,[40] Blau syndrome,[41] eosinophilic gastroenteritis,[42] Churg-Strauss syndrome,[43] giant cell arteritis including polymyalgia rheumatica,[44,45] Graves' disease,[46] lupus erythematosus,[47] rheumatoid arthritis,[48] and Sjögren syndrome.[49]

Primary Biliary Cirrhosis

Primary biliary cirrhosis predominantly affects middle-aged Caucasian women who may be diagnosed during the investigation of nonspecific symptoms such as fatigue, or in whom PBC is suspected because of cholestatic symptoms and signs such as pruritus and jaundice. The laboratory investigations show a two-fold to five-fold increase in alkaline phosphatase and the presence of diagnostic antimitochondrial antibodies. The principal feature of PBC is a progressive, inflammatory destruction of medium-sized intrahepatic bile ducts involving a dense lymphocytic infiltrate in the portal tracts (florid duct lesions). The inflammation may organize into noncaseating granulomas composed of lymphocytes, histiocytes, plasma cells, and occasionally eosinophils.[30] The histiocytes may form multinucleated giant cells and lesions resembling sarcoid granulomas. As in other hepatic granulomatous diseases that primarily involve the portal tract, portal hypertension may be seen before the development of cirrhosis.[50,51] Although granulomatous inflammation may cause complications even in early

disease, it does appear to be associated with less ductal damage and a better prognosis.[52] PBC is discussed more extensively in Chapter 41.

Sarcoidosis

Sarcoidosis is a systemic granulomatous disease characterized by a T_H1 response presumed to be directed against an unknown antigen causing an autoimmune reaction. Clustering of patients suggests a temporal and spatial relationship as would be expected if the cause was a transmissible agent or a shared environmental factor. The fact that the clustering has been shown to be greater between relatives of patients than among their spouses suggests a genetic predisposition, as the latter would be considered most susceptible if contact or a shared environment were the only factors involved in the clustering of cases.[53-56]

This disease predominantly affects patients in the 20- to 40-year age groups. Patients of African American and Scandinavian descent have the highest prevalence rates. The clinical course is quite variable and ranges from asymptomatic to a fatal disease. A worse outcome is associated with African American race, older age at diagnosis, and involvement of greater than two organ systems.[57,58]

Although the disease most commonly affects lungs and the lymphatic system, the liver is involved in 24% to 75% of patients with sarcoidosis, mostly depending on whether estimates are based on biopsy or autopsy data.[59-62] Hepatic involvement, however, is usually silent and signs and symptoms suggestive of hepatic involvement such as abdominal pain, hepatomegaly, jaundice, and portal hypertension is uncommon even in patients with extensive granulomatous involvement and is seen in approximately 4% to 7% of patients[58,59,63-70] If clinical evidence of hepatic disease is present, however, granulomatous inflammation is found in 100% of biopsies.[71] In a review of 1436 patients with sarcoidosis, increased risk of hepatic disease was associated with splenomegaly and male sex.[59]

The granulomas are characteristically noncaseating, tight, and well formed. Despite a predilection for the periportal area, they can be found anywhere in the liver. Lobular hepatitis, when present, usually consists of spotty inflammation. Portal triaditis with lymphocyte predominance may be present.[71] Injury to the biliary tree with lesions that are histologically indistinguishable from PBC-or PSC-associated duct lesions are seen in up to 10% of biopsies.[72] Presinusoidal portal hypertension secondary to scarring and obliteration of small portal and hepatic veins by portal granulomas, and arteriovenous shunts within the granulomas have been described.[63,66,69,71,73,74] Budd-Chiari syndrome due to obliteration of hepatic veins by granulomas are uncommon.[75]

The diagnosis is one of exclusion. Clinical history and physical examination must exclude other occupational or environmental factors that can cause granulomas. Other tests including chest x-ray, pulmonary function testing, electrocardiogram, liver tests, ophthalmic examination, serum angiotensin-converting enzyme levels, and tuberculin skin testing can screen for involvement of the lung, heart, liver, and eye, and rule out tuberculosis, the main differential diagnosis. Elevations of serum angiotensin-converting enzyme levels are not specific for sarcoidosis and levels are normal in approximately 25% of patients.[76] As stated before, frank hepatitis is uncommon and liver tests are most commonly characterized by a disproportionate elevation in alkaline phosphatase, which is seen in up to a third of patients, as compared with usually minor increases of amino transaminase levels.

Ursodeoxycholic acid has been used to alleviate cholestatic symptoms.[77,78] Whether corticosteroids can prevent hepatic disease progression or the development of complications is unknown. Corticosteroids are therefore not recommended for asymptomatic hepatic disease alone, but they may be considered in patients with severe cholestasis or portal hypertension.[59] Although patients with hepatic involvement may improve symptomatically and biochemically when placed on steroids, structural damage, particularly ductopenia, can become irreversible requiring a liver transplant.[67,68,75] Recurrence of the disease following liver transplantation has been documented, but is considered unusual.[79-81]

Infections

The spectrum of infections that have been associated with hepatic granulomas is extensive (see **Table 37-1**). The most common infectious causes of liver granulomas vary considerably by geographic location. Whereas tuberculosis, acquired immunodeficiency syndrome-related infections (*Mycobacterium avium*, CMV, *Cryptococcus neoformans*), and dimorphic fungal infections, such as histoplasmosis and coccidioidomycosis, are prevalent in the United States, additional infections including schistosomiasis, brucellosis, leprosy, and Q fever are common in other parts of the world.

Mycobacterial Infections

Mycobacterium tuberculosis

Hepatic granulomas are present in more than 90% of patients with miliary tuberculosis, approximately 70% of patients with extrapulmonary tuberculosis, and up to 25% of patients with what clinically appears to be isolated pulmonary tuberculosis.[59,82-85] Typical symptoms such as fever, night sweats, fatigue, anorexia, and weight loss are nonspecific and may be present in granulomatous disease from other causes.

While caseating granulomas are considered pathognomonic of tuberculosis, only approximately 50% of cases show evidence of such necrosis.[82] Patients with HIV infection may have an even lower rate of caseation.[86] In one study of 36 patients with miliary tuberculosis, granulomas were present in 91% of the liver biopsies, but only in 53% of the bone marrow biopsies performed on the same patients. Moreover, hepatic granulomas were present in 78% of cases without granulomas in bone marrow biopsies, indicating a higher diagnostic yield from liver biopsies in miliary tuberculosis cases.[82]

While an acid-fast stain should be performed in all cases of febrile granulomatous inflammation, it is a highly insensitive test. In one study, acid-fast bacilli were only identified in 9% of hepatic granulomas in patients with miliary tuberculosis.[83] Similarly, culture of material taken during a biopsy yields organisms in fewer than 10% of cases. PCR for *M. tuberculosis* can now be performed on formalin-fixed paraffin embedded tissue samples. Although it has a specificity of 96%, the sensitivity is only 53%, resulting in a 90% positive and 76% negative predictive value.[87] Standard antituberculous therapy is indicated but may be poorly tolerated in patients with tuberculous liver disease.[88] The role of adjunctive corticosteroids remains unclear.[89]

Bacille Calmette-Guerin (BCG) is an attenuated bovine *Mycobacterium tuberculosis* strain that is used for the intravesical immunotherapy of transitional cell bladder carcinoma. Hepatic dysfunction and granulomatous hepatitis is a rare complication of intravesical BCG therapy.[90-93] In a large series of 2602 patients, tuberculous hepatitis developed in 18 (0.7%) patients,[90] although the frequency of asymptomatic hepatic granulomas is probably higher.[91] As culture and acid-fast stains are negative in more than 90% of cases, the distinction between hypersensitivity reaction and systemic infection remains difficult to make. Patients with symptoms or signs of hepatic dysfunction should be covered for both diagnoses, which includes a 6-month course of rifampin and isoniazid, accompanied by steroids if indicated, and possibly cessation of immunotherapy.[90]

Nontuberculous Mycobacteria

In immunocompetent persons, hepatic infection with nontuberculous mycobacteria is exceptionally rare. Infection is characterized by well-formed noncaseating granulomas in the liver and spleen. In these patients, it is unusual to demonstrate acid-fast organisms in the tissue sections and confirmation is by culture.[94,95]

In immunocompromised patients and children, the hallmark of nontuberculous infection is the presence of collections of foamy macrophages filled with acid-fast organisms. High-risk groups include patients with HIV or genetic receptor defects, patients treated with anti-TNF inhibitors, and posttransplant patients. Granulomas tend to be ill defined without evidence of necrosis. This can change dramatically when AIDS patients with subclinical mycobacterial infection are treated with antiretroviral drugs. A rapid increase of CD4 cells can result in a dramatic immune reconstitution inflammatory syndrome (IRIS) characterized by fever and large necrotizing abscesses. Mycobacterial cultures are often negative even though residual bacteria may be detectable by staining or PCR testing.

While most nontuberculous mycobacterial infections are caused by the *Mycobacterium avium*/intracellulare complex, infection with other mycobacteria such as *Mycobacterium kansasii, Mycobacterium genavense, Mycobacterium chelonae, Mycobacterium mucogenicum, Mycobacterium scrofulaceum* and even *Mycobacterium leprae* have been described.[95-99]

M. leprae typically affects nerves, skin, and the lymphatic systems, but while usually asymptomatic and without consistent liver test abnormalities, liver involvement is not uncommon.[100-102] Host immunity to *M. leprae* determines the diversity of clinical manifestations seen in affected patients. On one end of the spectrum is tuberculoid leprosy with robust production of T_H1 type cytokines, significant and at times detrimental inflammation, and a low organism load. On the other end of the spectrum is lepromatous disease, characterized by elevated levels of T_H2 type cytokines, a suboptimal proinflammatory response and very high numbers of organisms. The T_h response pattern in leprosy is not only a host function, but M. leprae actively modulates the host's cytokine response system to suppress the natural T_H1 response by providing both positive and negative regulatory signals via multiple signaling pathways.[103] Not surprisingly, the spectrum of immune response to *M. leprae* is reflected in the hepatic granulomas observed. In tuberculoid leprosy, well-organized epithelioid granulomas with rare acid-fast organisms are seen, but in lepromatous leprosy typically ill-defined granulomas mainly composed of foamy histiocytes laden with acid-fast bacilli are found.

Bacterial Infections

Many bacterial infections have been associated with granuloma formation. Examples include *Borrelia burgdorferi* (Lyme disease),[104] *Listeria monocytogenes*,[105-107] different rickettsial species,[108-110] *Treponema pallidum* (syphilis),[111] *Tropheryma whippelii* (Whipple disease),[112] and *Yersinia enterocolitica*.[113-115] Except for listeriosis, which causes necrotizing granulomas associated with a neutrophilic inflammatory infiltrate, the other associations are documented too rarely to consider granulomatous hepatitis a typical reaction in these relatively common infections. On the other hand, hepatic granulomas are certainly a very common finding in patients with bartonellosis, brucellosis, and Q fever.

Bartonellosis

Bartonella henselae classically causes cat-scratch disease. The organism is introduced into the skin through a kitten's scratch or bite and produces a papule at the site of inoculation within 3 to 5 days. Within 3 weeks, lymphadenopathy develops in the regional lymph nodes draining the primary inoculation site. Organisms can be identified using the Warthin-Starry silver stain. In rare cases, however, *B. henselae* causes isolated visceral disease. In immunocompromised patients, a disease entity called bacillary angiomatosis can affect all organs including the liver.[116] The lesions have angioproliferative features, resembling Kaposi sarcoma, but frank granulomas are rare.

Some apparently healthy children have hepatic involvement in the absence of peripheral lymphadenopathy.[117-121] On performing a biopsy, necrotizing granulomas and organisms are identified. Most of these patients will also have some histologic evidence of peliosis hepatis, characterized by the presence of blood-filled spaces within the hepatic parenchyma. While peliosis is not specific for bartonellosis, the presence of peliosis and necrotizing granulomas warrants special staining (Warthin-Starry) to rule out infection with *B. henselae*. It is not clear why only few children develop this syndrome. Some authors have postulated that the cause is an underlying T lymphocyte abnormality, but this has not been consistently demonstrated.[122] Blood tests show mild but nonspecific abnormalities in liver tests. A CT scan may show filling defects suspicious for a malignant neoplasm. Symptoms and findings often resolve spontaneously, but visceral disease is often treated with macrolides, rifampin, or fluoroquinolones.

Brucellosis

Brucellosis is a zoonotic infection found in a variety of farm animals, including goats, pigs, cattle, and dogs. Human infection is caused by *Brucella abortus* (cattle), *Brucella suis* (pigs), *Brucella canis* (dogs), and *Brucella melitensis* (goats) and

occurs through contact with animals or animal products, such as cheese made from unpasteurized milk. Patients have recurrent and undulating fever; drenching sweats; frontal and occipital headaches; body, chest, and abdominal pains; and anorexia. Physical examination reveals splenomegaly and variable hepatomegaly. Resolution is slow and may take weeks or months.

Although hepatic involvement is not typical, symptoms of liver disease were noted in 40 of 82 patients in one series.[123] Most patients had hepatomegaly (65%) and mild elevations of transaminases and alkaline phosphatase. The main finding in a liver biopsy was a nonspecific reactive hepatitis. Small nonnecrotizing granulomas were noted in 28 patients. The development of granulomas appears to be an early event based on the observation that of the 28 patients with granulomas only 3 had had symptoms for longer than 100 days. As these granulomas are smaller than those usually associated with sarcoidosis or tuberculosis, their appearance may suggest this diagnosis in a patient being investigated for an FUO.[123,124] The diagnosis is confirmed by serologic testing and, if suspected, through a prolonged culture of blood and bone marrow specimens. Treatment requires combination therapy with doxycycline and rifampin for at least 6 weeks.

Q Fever

Q fever is a zoonotic infection caused by the gram-negative intracellular rickettsial organism, *Coxiella burnetii*. The animal reservoirs include cattle, sheep, and goats and the most common mode of infection is inhalation of aerosolized bacteria, ingestion of contaminated milk, and tick bites. *C. burnetii* is found worldwide but is most prevalent in developing nations with significant livestock populations. Most infected patients are asymptomatic. Of the patients who develop disease after an incubation period of 2 to 6 weeks, 90% will have a self-limited illness characterized by hectic fever, malaise, headache, and in many cases pneumonia. The remaining 10% develop chronic Q fever, which often includes endocarditis.

Liver abnormalities are found in 11% to 65% of cases.[125-134] Hepatitis was reported to be the most common manifestation of Q fever in France[133] and in another study of 72 patients, 85% had abnormal liver tests and 65% had hepatomegaly.[128] Although nonspecific granulomas may be seen against a background of nonspecific reactive hepatitis and steatosis, the typical granuloma in Q fever is a fibrin-ring granuloma (or so-called doughnut granuloma). This granuloma has a clear central space believed to represent a lipid vacuole. In many cases a fibrin ring is present that either surrounds the lipid vacuole or the periphery of the entire granuloma.[129-132] Although fibrin-ring granulomas are considered characteristic for Q fever, they are not seen in all such patients[132] and are not specific for this disease. Isolated case reports have described similar granulomas in liver biopsies from patients with Hodgkin disease, hepatitis A virus infection, temporal arteritis, Epstein-Barr virus infection, cytomegalovirus infection, systemic lupus erythematosus, leishmaniasis, and allopurinol-induced hepatitis. It is, however, imperative to rule out Q fever serologically whenever fibrin-ring granulomas are found on histology. In some patients who underwent a repeat liver biopsy following successful therapy, resolution of liver pathology was noted. Confirmation of the diagnosis usually requires serologic testing. The treatment of choice is doxycycline 100 mg twice daily or fluoroquinolones for 14 days unless endocarditis is present, which requires prolonged therapy.

Parasitic Infections

Several parasitic infections have been associated with hepatic granulomas. Many of these include single case reports, raising the possibility of incidental granulomas. In several instances, however, evidence of the parasite is found in the center of the granulomas.[135,136]

Parasites that have been associated with granulomas include *Ascaris*,[137] *Capillaria*,[135] *Enterobius*,[138-140] *Fasciola*,[141,142] *Giardia*,[143] *Leishmania*,[144] *Linguatula*,[145,146] *Strongyloides*,[147,148] *Toxocara*,[135,149] and *Toxoplasma*.[136] Characteristically, most of these pathogens are associated with eosinophilic granulomas. This is true for all helminthic organisms but not for unicellular protozoa, such as *Giardia* and *Toxoplasma*.

Schistosomiasis

Schistosomiasis, also known as bilharziasis, is a parasitic disease caused by several species of flukes belonging to the genus *Schistosoma*. (See also Chapter 35.) Although it has a low mortality rate, schistosomiasis causes significant, and at times devastating, chronic illness, affecting 200 million people in the developing world. Through travel and migration 400,000 people with schistosomiasis are believed to live in the United States. *Schistosoma mansoni*, *Schistosoma intercalatum*, *Schistosoma japonicum*, and *Schistosoma mekongi* are the species known to cause hepatic disease. *S. mansoni* is found in parts of South America, the Caribbean, Africa, and the Middle East; whereas *S. japonicum* resides in the Far East. *S. mekongi* and *S. intercalatum* are found in geographic pockets in Southeast Asia and central West Africa, respectively.[150-156]

The life cycle of all human schistosomes includes the release of parasite eggs from infected individuals into the environment, hatching on contact with fresh water to release free-swimming miracidia. Miracidia infect freshwater snails and eventually transform into cercariae, which are small motile larvae that are released into the water and capable of infecting humans by direct penetration of intact skin. Following migration and further transformation, the parasites reach the liver sinusoids where they develop into mature worms. Mature worms pair and eventually relocate to the mesenteric or rectal veins where they begin to produce 200 to 4000 eggs per day, depending on the species. Worm pairs can live in the body for an average of 4 to 5 years, but may persist up to 20 years. Mature eggs are capable of crossing into the digestive tract, but a significant proportion of the eggs released by the worm pairs become trapped in mesenteric veins, or will be washed back into the liver, where they will become lodged.

Adult worms are not immunogenic, but *Schistosoma* ova are highly antigenic. Trapped eggs mature normally and secrete antigens that elicit a vigorous immune response. While the eggs themselves do not cause damage, the resulting immune response with its cellular infiltration causes the pathology classically associated with schistosomiasis. The ova elicit a T_H2 cytokine response, resulting in the development of eosinophil-rich granulomas in the portal tracts. In early stages, the schistosomal egg is visible in the center of the granuloma.[156-166]

Complications within the liver include portal fibrosis due to the release of fibrogenic cytokines such as IL-4. Granulomas

and fibrosis cause obliteration or compression (or both) of the portal veins, resulting in presinusoidal portal hypertension, which at times is severe. In a small proportion of patients, an extensive, quite distinctive pattern of fibrosis develops that tracks along the portal venous system and is known as pipe-stem fibrosis.[158,167-170]

Hepatic fibrosis does not develop in all patients. Early infection, prolonged illness, and a genetic predisposition appear to modulate the extent of the disease. Immune response appears tightly regulated, with minimal deviations resulting in destructive response patterns.[160,171-173]

Schistosomiasis should be suspected in persons who have a history of freshwater exposure in endemic areas. Persons living in endemic regions are usually asymptomatic. In contrast, visitors to endemic areas develop fever, chills, cough, diarrhea, malaise, and arthralgias 4 to 10 weeks after infection. The physical examination of acute schistosomiasis is characterized by hepatosplenomegaly, and the blood workup shows peripheral blood eosinophilia. Liver tests demonstrate a mild elevation of aminotransferases. Current diagnostic tests for schistosomiasis include serologic tests and microscopic examination of stool, urine, or tissue for eggs. Simple microscopy can detect heavy infections, but intermittent shedding often requires concentration procedures and repeated examinations. Serologic tests for antibodies to schistosomes are available at the Centers for Disease Control and Prevention (CDC) in Atlanta, and some commercial laboratories. The CDC uses a combination of tests with purified adult worm antigens with a specificity of 99% for all species and a sensitivity of 99% for *S. mansoni* infection, but less than 50% for *S. japonicum*. Serologic tests cannot distinguish active from past infections but are useful for screening previously unexposed travelers and expatriates.[174]

The preferred treatment is with praziquantel in a single dose in expatriates, or given once yearly in endemic areas. With the global attention given to schistosomiasis in recent years and the availability of effective therapy, prolonged infection is less common than before. Even in high-prevalence areas, the incidence of late disease including liver disease is decreasing, resulting in lower rates of schistosomiasis in recent case series of hepatic granulomas from developing countries.[175]

Fungal Infections

Several fungal infections have been associated with hepatic granulomas including blastomycosis,[2,176] candidiasis,[177,178] coccidioidomycosis,[179,180] cryptococcosis,[181,182] histoplasmosis,[183-185] and infection with *Trichosporon*.[186,187]

Silver- or PAS-based stains can usually detect organisms within the hepatic parenchyma of infected patients, most of which are severely immunocompromised. The geographic restriction of blastomycosis (Mississippi and Ohio river basins, around the Great Lakes, Canada, and Africa), coccidioidomycosis (southwestern United States, northern Mexico, and parts of Central and South America), and histoplasmosis (central United States, specifically the Ohio and Mississippi river valleys, Central and South America, the Caribbean, Africa, and Asia) can be helpful in identifying patients at risk.

According to a pathology-based study, only 19% of cases of hepatic histoplasmosis are associated with granulomas.[185] Granuloma formation is associated with clearance of infection.[183] Granulomas may be large and contain abundant lymphocytes and macrophages, with only a few epithelioid cells and histoplasma organisms found in the center of the lesion.[183,185]

Viral Infections

Hepatic granulomas have been described in patients with CMV,[12,188-192] Epstein-Barr virus infection,[192,193] hepatitis A virus infection,[194-196] hepatitis B virus infection, and HIV, even in the absence of opportunistic infections.[197] CMV and hepatitis A have been associated with fibrin-ring granulomas.

Hepatitis C

Asymptomatic hepatic granulomas have been documented in patients who undergo liver biopsy for the grading and staging of their hepatitis C infection (HCV), and the reported incidence varies from 0.73% to 13%.[23-29,198-200] In one large study of 435 patients, nonnecrotizing granulomas were observed in 4.5% of biopsies from 155 patients with HCV infection and no alternative causes. This was significantly higher than in the control groups of hepatitis B infection (0.66% of 151 patients) and alcoholic liver disease (none of 129 patients).[29] The cause of these granulomas is unclear, and patients do not appear to have symptoms attributable to this finding. Some authors have argued that their presence correlates with the response, but this has not been confirmed in larger studies.[25-27,199]

Several reports have demonstrated development of liver granulomas during interferon therapy, possibly indicating an immune reconstitution effect.[26,201-203] Others have argued that interferon may unmask subclinical sarcoidosis in patients with hepatitis C,[204] an association that had been described previously.[205]

Drugs

Numerous drugs have been associated with hepatic granulomas. Unequivocal determination of causality (resolution upon cessation, recurrence upon rechallenge) is often difficult as it requires multiple liver biopsies and reexposure to potentially dangerous medications. There is consensus that drug-induced granulomatous disease is likely underrecognized; the incidence of drug-induced hepatic granulomas is estimated to be around 10%.[206]

Certain drugs are either well established or common causes of hepatic granulomas or granulomas represent the typical response to these drugs. Examples include allopurinol,[207-211] carbamazepine,[212-215] diphenylhydantoin,[216] phenylbutazone,[217] phenytoin,[218,219] quinidine,[220-223] and quinine.[224-226]

Other drugs that have been implicated in the development of granulomas in the liver include acetaminophen,[227] amoxicillin-clavulanate,[228,229] aprindine,[230] aspirin with codeine,[231] chlorpromazine,[232] chlorpropamide,[233] clofibrate,[234] dicloxacillin,[235] didanosine,[236] diltiazem,[237,238] glyburide,[239] halothane,[240] hydralazine,[241] mebendazole,[242] mesalamine,[243] methyldopa,[244-246] norfloxacin,[247] oral contraceptives,[248] procainamide,[249] pyrazinamide,[250] rosiglitazone,[251] sulfadoxine/pyrimethamine,[252] sulfasalazine,[253] and ticlopidine.[254]

Therapeutically administered and environmental gold, copper, and aluminum have been demonstrated in granulomas using spectroscopic methods.[255-257]

As mentioned above, hepatitis C has been associated with hepatic granulomas and some authors have argued that their presence correlates with response. This is compatible with several reports demonstrating development of liver granulomas during interferon therapy, possibly indicating an immune reconstitution effect.[26,201-203]

Drug-induced granulomas are usually seen on a background of lobular hepatitis and/or portal triaditis. Cholangitis is a more variable finding, and eosinophils may or may not be a prominent component of the inflammatory infiltrate. Physical examination may reveal jaundice and hepatomegaly, and liver tests show abnormalities in transaminases and alkaline phosphatase or isolated elevations of alkaline phosphatase. Hyperbilirubinemia is an inconstant finding and peripheral blood eosinophilia is not seen in all patients, but if present is suggestive of drug-induced hepatitis when parasitic infections have been ruled out.

Malignancies

Noncaseating and rarely caseating hepatic granulomas have been identified in patients with malignancies, most commonly Hodgkin and non-Hodgkin lymphoma.[258-263] They are usually discovered as a part of the staging procedure and not because of liver dysfunction. The presence of granulomas is not synonymous with involvement by lymphoma, although their presence warrants a careful examination of the lymphoid cells intermixed in the granuloma and within the adjacent parenchyma.

Whether the observed granulomas indicate a host response to the lymphoma or are incidental is debatable.[261] It appears that their incidence is too high to be incidental. In one study more than half of the liver biopsies examined as a part of the staging protocol for Hodgkin disease showed granulomas in the absence of hepatic involvement by the disease.[258] In another report, a hypodense lesion was noted on a CT scan of the liver in a patient with Hodgkin disease. The liver biopsy showed the lesion to be composed of a necrotizing granulomatous reaction. An abnormal lymphoid infiltrate was also noted in the adjacent portal tracts within the biopsy. No microorganisms were identified and the lesion resolved with treatment of the lymphoma.[259] Examples of both B- and T-cell lymphomas have been described in which involvement of the liver by the non-Hodgkin lymphoma has been associated with a granulomatous reaction, either separate from or intimately admixed with the abnormal lymphoid infiltrate.[260,263] Other cancers that have been associated with hepatic granulomas include hairy cell leukemia[264] and renal cell carcinoma.[265]

Miscellaneous Other Diseases

Hepatic granulomas have been reported following invasive surgery including cardiopulmonary bypass procedures[266] and ileal bypass operations.[267-269] Exposure to gold, copper, and aluminum can result in granuloma formation, as can the exposure to mineral oils—the latter resulting in characteristic lipogranulomas.

Patients with chronic granulomatous disease have a defect in the NADPH-oxidase complex, which prevents macrophages from producing hydrogen peroxidase. The liver is commonly involved. In a study of 368 patients, the liver was the second most commonly involved organ (27%) following the skin.[270]

Affected patients have variable granulomas from small, poorly formed histocytic aggregates to large, multiloculated, irregularly shaped granulomatous abscesses. The granulomas tend to be surrounded by a thick and dense fibro-inflammatory scar tissue.[271] Another characteristic finding is the presence of heavily pigmented macrophages, which are found even in macroscopically uninvolved liver sections.

Common variable immunodeficiency and other hypogammaglobulinemic disorders are other immunodeficiencies commonly associated with hepatic granulomas. The granulomas resemble sarcoid granulomas but are typically steroid resistant, progressive, and associated with increased mortality.[272-276]

Clinical Manifestations and Diagnostic Approach

Clinical manifestations of liver granulomas depend on the underlying cause and the severity of associated illness. Fever is the most common associated symptom (see later discussion), especially in patients with tuberculosis, sarcoidosis, and infectious causes. Hepatomegaly and minor elevations of transaminases and/or alkaline phosphatase are common.

A thorough history and physical examination, combined with judicious laboratory testing (**Table 37-3**) can provide specific clues to the cause of liver granulomas. Hypercalcemia secondary to ACE-secreting granulomas can be indicative of sarcoid, whereas eosinophilia may provide a clue that drugs or parasites are involved. Pruritus may indicate the presence of primary biliary cirrhosis. Multiple infections may indicate presence of an immunodeficiency and concurrent autoimmune disorders increase the likelihood of autoimmune hepatitis. While portal hypertension is rare in granulomatous hepatitis, its presence may favor sarcoid, primary biliary cirrhosis, or schistosomiasis. Histopathologic features (see Histopathology) including type and location of granulomas may also aid in the differential diagnosis.

A detailed exposure and travel history is imperative because it may help narrow the differential diagnosis. In the United States, sarcoidosis, tuberculosis, drug reactions, and primary biliary cirrhosis account for the majority of cases but if a patient has spent time in Asia or sub-Saharan Africa the differential diagnosis must include other infectious diseases.

Table 37-3 Suggested Laboratory Evaluation in Patients with Liver Granulomas

Chest x-ray
Test for latent TB (skin testing or IFN-γ testing)
Blood cultures (including fungal and mycobacterial pathogens in immunocompromised patients)
Serum antimitochondrial antibodies
Liver biopsy:
  Fungal and AFB staining
  Polarizing light microscopy
  Special stains (silver, immunohistochemistry) or molecular testing (PCR) depending on differential diagnosis
Serology (e.g., HIV, *Brucella*, Q fever, *Bartonella*, syphilis)
Discretionary: serum angiotensin-converting enzyme concentration

---

Imaging is not useful in delineating causes of hepatic granulomas; the presence of calcification usually correlates with the age of the lesion, not its cause.[277]

Fever of Unknown Origin

Many patients with FUO undergo percutaneous liver biopsies during workup, even though the diagnostic utility of a blind liver needle biopsy remains arguable in this setting. In both immunocompetent and immunocompromised patients the diagnostic yield for fungi and mycobacterial infections, however, is greater in liver biopsy than in bone marrow biopsy.[82,278] Overall, in immunocompetent patients, the diagnostic yield on liver biopsy for informative granulomas such as mycobacterial or fungal infection is quite low and varies from 0% to 18%.[279-281] In immunocompetent patients, liver biopsies should therefore be limited to patients with hepatomegaly and abnormal liver tests. In contrast, hepatic granulomas are found in 16% to 75% of HIV-infected patients being investigated for the cause of an FUO and elevated liver tests or hepatomegaly.[181,278,282-287] In one study[286] liver biopsy was diagnostic in 43.1%, and helpful in 22.4%. The presence of hepatomegaly or splenomegaly was the most useful factor in predicting the usefulness of liver biopsy, with a positive predictive value of 86.1% and negative predictive value of 68.2%. As this study was done in Spain with a high incidence of tuberculosis and leishmaniasis, results may not be applicable to other parts of the world.

Complications

Granulomas other than those associated with primary biliary cirrhosis, sarcoidosis, and schistosomiasis are rarely destructive and generally not associated with consistent derangements of liver tests. Damage to bile ducts is seen in primary biliary cirrhosis and less frequently in sarcoidosis. Destruction of hepatic and portal veins with subsequent obliteration and scarring is implicated as a mechanism of portal hypertension that can develop in patients with granulomatous hepatitis. Granuloma-induced hypercalcemia is rare. Hepatic vein compression can result in a Budd-Chiari–like picture.[75] Biliary ductopenia with subsequent intrahepatic cholestasis and biliary strictures, histologically resembling sclerosing cholangitis, are rare but seen in patients with immune mediated diseases[72] End-stage liver disease resulting from hepatic granulomatous disease resulting from hepatic granulomatous disease is rare and therefore an uncommon indication for liver transplantation. In a recent small series of patients with sarcoidosis, graft survival rates were 100% at 1 year and 86% at 5 years, comparable with other indications.[288]

Key References

Akritidis N, et al. The liver in brucellosis. Clin Gastroenterol Hepatol 2007;5: 1109–1112. (Ref.126)

Alam I, et al. Diffuse intrahepatic biliary strictures in sarcoidosis resembling sclerosing cholangitis. Case report and review of the literature. Dig Dis Sci 1997;42:1295–1301. (Ref.73)

Ardeniz O, Cunningham-Rundles C. Granulomatous disease in common variable immunodeficiency. Clin Immunol 2009;133:198–207. (Ref.277)

ATS, ERS, WASOG. Statement on sarcoidosis. The joint statement of the American Thoracic Society (ATS), the European Respiratory Society (ERS) and the World Association of Sarcoidosis and other granulomatous disorders (WASOG). Am J Respir Crit Care Med 1999;160:736–755. (Ref.59)

Baratta L, et al. Ursodeoxycholic acid treatment in abdominal sarcoidosis. Dig Dis Sci 2000;45:1559–1562. (Ref.79)

Barcena R, et al. Posttransplant liver granulomatosis associated with hepatitis C? Transplantation 1998;65:1494–1495. (Ref.24)

Becheur H, et al. Effect of ursodeoxycholic acid on chronic intrahepatic cholestasis due to sarcoidosis. Dig Dis Sci 1997;42:789–791. (Ref.78)

Bhardwaj SS, Saxena R, Kwo PY. Granulomatous liver disease. Curr Gastroenterol Rep 2009;11:42–49. (Ref.208)

Bica I, Hamer DH, Stadecker MJ. Hepatic schistosomiasis. Infect Dis Clin North Am 2000;3:583–604. (Ref.159)

Björnsson E, Olsson R, Remotti H. Norfloxacin-induced eosinophilic necrotizing granulomatous hepatitis. Am J Gastroenterol 2000;95:3662–3664. (Ref.248)

Bjøro K, et al. The spectrum of hepatobiliary disease in primary hypogammaglobulinaemia. J Intern Med 1999;245:517–524. (Ref.274)

Bonnet F, et al. Sarcoidosis-associated hepatitis C virus infection. Dig Dis Sci 2002;47:794–796. (Ref.207)

Boros DL. T helper cell populations, cytokine dynamics, and pathology of the schistosome egg granuloma. Microbes Infect 1999;1:511–516. (Ref.161)

Braun M, et al. Mesalamine-induced granulomatous hepatitis. Am J Gastroenterol 1999;94:1973–1974. (Ref.244)

Brooklyn TN, et al. Churg-Strauss syndrome and granulomatous cholangiopathy. Eur J Gastroenterol Hepatol 2000;12:809–811. (Ref.44)

Burke ML, et al. Immunopathogenesis of human schistosomiasis. Parasite Immunol 2009;31:163–176. (Ref.163)

Chevillard C, et al. INF-gamma polymorphisms (INF-gamma +2109 and INF-gamma +3810) are associated with severe hepatic fibrosis in human hepatic schistosomiasis (Schistosoma mansoni). J Immunol 2003;171:5596–5601. (Ref.174)

Chong VH. Hepatobiliary tuberculosis: a review of presentations and outcomes. South Med J 2008;101:356–361. (Ref.89)

Colle I, et al. Granulomatous hepatitis due to mebendazole. J Clin Gastroenterol 1999;28:44–45. (Ref.243)

de la Serna-Higuera C, et al. Cytomegalovirus granulomatous hepatitis in an immunocompetent patient. Gastroenterol Hepatol 1999;22:230–231. (Ref.190)

Delfosse V, et al. Budd-Chiari syndrome complicating hepatic sarcoidosis: definitive treatment by liver transplantation: a case report. Transplant Proc 2009;41:3432–3434. (Ref.76)

Dessein AJ, et al. Severe hepatic fibrosis in Schistosoma mansoni infection is controlled by a major locus that is closely linked to the interferon-gamma receptor gene. Am J Hum Genet 1999;65:709–721. (Ref.173)

Dhawan M, et al. Rosiglitazone-induced granulomatous hepatitis. J Clin Gastroenterol 2002;34:582–584. (Ref.252)

Diaz ML, et al. Polymerase chain reaction for the detection of Mycobacterium tuberculosis DNA in tissue and assessment of its utility in the diagnosis of hepatic granulomas. J Lab Clin Med 1996;127:359–363. (Ref.88)

Dourakis SP, et al. Hepatic granulomas: a 6-year experience in a single center in Greece. Eur J Gastroenterol Hepatol 2007;19:101–104. (Ref.13)

Drebber U, et al. Hepatic granulomas: histological and molecular pathological approach to differential diagnosis: a study of 442 cases. Liver Int 2008;28:828–834. (Ref.12)

Elliot DE. Schistosomiasis. Pathophysiology, diagnosis and treatment. Gastroenterol Clin North Am 1996;25:599–625 (review). (Ref.158)

Elzouki AN, Lindgren S. Granulomatous hepatitis induced by aspirin-codeine analgesics. J Intern Med 1996;239:279–281. (Ref.233)

Engels D, et al. The global epidemiological situation of schistosomiasis and new approaches to control and research. Acta Trop 2002;82:139–146. (Ref.153)

Fenwick A, Rollinson D, Southgate V. Implementation of human schistosomiasis control: challenges and prospects. Adv Parasitol 2006;61:567–616. (Ref.152)

Fidler HM, et al. Recurrent hepatic sarcoidosis following liver transplantation. Transplant Proc 1997;29:2509–2510. (Ref.81)

Fiel MI, et al. Development of hepatic granulomas in patients receiving pegylated interferon therapy for recurrent hepatitis C virus post liver transplantation. Transpl Infect Dis 2008;10:184–189. (Ref.205)

Fogaça HS, et al. Liver pseudotumor: a rare manifestation of hepatic granulomata caused by Ascaris lumbricoides ova. Am J Gastroenterol 2000;95:2099–2101. (Ref.139)

García-Ordoñez MA, et al. Diagnostic usefulness of percutaneous liver biopsy in HIV-infected patients with fever of unknown origin. J Infect 1999;38:94–98. (Ref.287)

Gaya DR, et al. Hepatic granulomas: a 10 year single centre experience. J Clin Pathol 2003;56:850–853. (Ref.11)

Goldblatt MR, Ribes LA. Mycobacterium mucogenicum isolated from a patient with granulomatous hepatitis. Arch Pathol Lab Med 2002;126:73–75. (Ref.102)

Goldin RD, et al. Granulomas and hepatitis C. Histopathology 1996;28:265–267. (Ref.30)

Gross JW, Kan VL. Trichosporon asahii infection in an advanced AIDS patient and literature review. AIDS 2008;22:793–795. (Ref.189)

Gryseels B, et al. Human schistosomiasis. Lancet 2006;368:1106–1118. (Ref.155)

Harada K, Minato H, Hiramatsu K, et al. Epithelioid cell granulomas in chronic hepatitis C: immunohistochemical character and histological marker of favourable response to interferon-alpha therapy. Histopathology 1998;33:216–221. (Ref.28)

Heninger E, et al. Characterization of the Histoplasma capsulatum–induced granuloma. J Immunol 2006;177:3303–3313. (Ref.185)

Hoffman RM, et al. Sarcoidosis associated with interferon-alpha therapy for chronic hepatitis C. J Hepatol 1998;28:1058–1063. (Ref.206)

Hoffmann KF, Wynn TA, Dunne DW. Cytokine-mediated host responses during schistosome infections: walking the fine line between immunological control and immunopathology. Adv Parasitol 2002;52:265–307. (Ref.168)

Hou M, et al. Multiple quinine-dependent antibodies in a patient with episodic thrombocytopenia, neutropenia, lymphocytopenia, and granulomatous hepatitis. Blood 1997;90:4806–4811. (Ref.226)

Hunt J, et al. Sarcoidosis with selective involvement of a second liver allograft: report of a case and review of the literature. Mod Pathol 1999;12:325–328. (Ref.82)

Ishak KG. Sarcoidosis of the liver and bile ducts. Mayo Clin Proc 1998;73:467–472. (Ref.71)

Kahi CJ, et al. Hepatobiliary disease in sarcoidosis. Sarcoidosis Vasc Diffuse Lung Dis 2006;23:117–123. (Ref.60)

Kahr A, et al. Visceral manifestation of cat scratch disease in children. A consequence of altered immunological state? Infection 2000;28:778–784. (Ref.124)

Kaplan KJ, Goodman ZD, Ishak KG. Eosinophilic granuloma of the liver: a characteristic lesion with relationship to visceral larva migrans. Am J Surg Pathol 2001;25:1316–1321. (Ref.137)

Kaplan MM. Primary biliary cirrhosis. N Engl J Med 1996;335:1570–1580. (Ref.32)

Kibria R, et al. "Ohio River Valley fever" presenting as isolated granulomatous hepatitis: a case report. South Med J 2009;102:656–658. (Ref.186)

Kikichi L, et al. Images of interest. Hepatobiliary and pancreatic: hepatic granulomas and hepatitis C. J Gastroenterol Hepatol 2005;20:792. (Ref.278)

Knobel B, et al. Pyrazinamide-induced granulomatous hepatitis. J Clin Gastroenterol 1997;24:264–266. (Ref.251)

Lamp LW, Gray GF, Scott MA. The histologic spectrum of hepatic cat scratch disease. A series of six cases with confirmed Bartonella henselae infection. Am J Surg Pathol 1996;20:1253–1259. (Ref.123)

Lamps LW, et al. The pathologic spectrum of gastrointestinal and hepatic histoplasmosis. Am J Clin Pathol 2000;113:64–72. (Ref.187)

Levine S, et al. Histopathological features of chronic granulomatous disease (CGD) in childhood. Histopathology 2005;47:508–516. (Ref.272)

Lindgren A, et al. Paracetamol-induced cholestatic and granulomatous liver injuries. J Intern Med 1997;241:435–439. (Ref.229)

Lipson EJ, et al. Patient and graft outcomes following liver transplantation for sarcoidosis. Clin Transplant 2005;19:487–491. (Ref.288)

Liston TE, Koehler IE. Granulomatous hepatitis and necrotizing splenitis due to Bartonella henselae in a patient with cancer: case report and review of hepatosplenic manifestations of Bartonella infection. Clin Infect Dis 1996;22:951–957. (Ref.120)

Luther VP, Bookstaver PB, Ohl CA. Corticosteroids in the treatment of hepatic tuberculosis: case report and review of the literature. Scand J Infect Dis 2010;42:315–317. (Ref.90)

Ma J, et al. Regulation of macrophage activation. Cell Mol Life Sci 2003;60:2334–2346. (Ref.17)

Malphettes M, et al. Granulomatous disease in common variable immunodeficiency. Rev Med Interne 2008;29:28–32. (Ref.276)

Mandel J, Weinberger SE. Clinical insights and basic science correlates in sarcoidosis. Am J Med Sci 2001;1:99–107. (Ref.57)

Mayo MJ. Natural history of primary biliary cirrhosis. Clin Liver Dis 2008;12:277–288. (Ref.52)

Mayo MJ. Portal hypertension in primary biliary cirrhosis: a potentially reversible harbinger of demise. Gastroenterology 2008;135:1450–1451. (Ref.51)

McKerrow JH. Cytokine induction and exploitation in schistosome infections. Parasitology 1997;115:S107–S112. (Ref.160)

Mert A, et al. The etiology of hepatic granulomas. J Clin Gastroenterol 2001;32:275–276. (Ref.6)

Mert A, et al. Hepatic granulomas in chronic hepatitis C. J Clin Gastroenterol 2001;33:342–343. (Ref.201)

Miller EB, et al. Granulomatous hepatitis and Sjögren's syndrome: an association. Semin Arthritis Rheum 2006;36:153–158. (Ref.50)

Moreno-Merlo F, et al. The role of granulomatous phlebitis and thrombosis in the pathogenesis of cirrhosis and portal hypertension in sarcoidosis. Hepatology 1997;26:554–560. (Ref.74)

Morimoto Y, Routes JM. Granulomatous disease in common variable immunodeficiency. Curr Allergy Asthma Rep 2005;5:370–375. (Ref.275)

Musso C, et al. Visceral larva migrans granulomas in liver and central nervous system of children who died of bacterial or viral meningitis. Clin Neuropathol 2006;25:288–290. (Ref.151)

Mwatha JK, et al. High levels of TNF, soluble TNF receptors, soluble ICAM-1 and IFN-gamma, but low levels of IL-5, are associated with hepatosplenic disease in human schistosomiasis mansoni. J Immunol 1998;160:1992–1999. (Ref.175)

Nakanuma Y, et al. Hepatic sarcoidosis with vanishing bile duct syndrome, cirrhosis, and portal phlebosclerosis. Report of an autopsy case. J Clin Gastroenterol 2001;32:181–184. (Ref.75)

Newman LS, Rose CS, Maier LA. Sarcoidosis. N Engl J Med 1997;336:1224–1234. (Ref.58)

Ozaras R, et al. The prevalence of hepatic granulomas in chronic hepatitis C. J Clin Gastroenterol 2004;38:449–452. (Ref.27)

Pearce EJ, MacDonald AS. The immunobiology of schistosomiasis. Nat Rev Immunol 2002;2:499–511. (Ref.164)

Raoult D. Rickettsial diseases. Medicine (Baltimore) 1996;24:71–75. (Ref.135)

Ruiz A, Mederos L, Capó V. Isolation of *Mycobacterium avium-intracellulare* from a hepatic biopsy. Rev Cubana Med Trop 2002;54:161–163. (Ref.96)

Rupali P, et al. Granulomatous hepatitis following open heart surgery with cardiopulmonary bypass. Natl Med J India 2008;21:222–224. (Ref.267)

Saab S, Venkataramani A, Yao F. Possible granulomatous hepatitis after dicloxacillin therapy. J Clin Gastroenterol 1996;22:163–164. (Ref.236)

Saini SK, Rose CD. Liver involvement in familial granulomatous arthritis (Blau syndrome). J Rheumatol 1996;23:396–399. (Ref.42)

Sanai FM, et al. Hepatic granuloma: decreasing trend in a high-incidence area. Liver Int 2008;28:1402–1407. (Ref.177)

Saw D, et al. Granulomatous hepatitis associated with glyburide. Dig Dis Sci 1996;41:322–325. (Ref.240)

Sinsimer D, et al. *Mycobacterium leprae* actively modulates the cytokine response in naive human monocytes. Infect Immun 2010;78:293–300. (Ref.105)

Snyder N, Martinez JG, Xiao SY. Chronic hepatitis C is commonly associated with hepatic granulomas. World J Gastroenterol 2008;14:6366–6369. (Ref.200)

Stadecker MJ. The development of granulomas in schistosomiasis: genetic backgrounds, regulatory pathways, and specific egg antigen responses that influence the magnitude of disease. Microbes Infect 1999;1:505–510. (Ref.162)

Tahan V, et al. Prevalence of hepatic granulomas in chronic hepatitis B. Dig Dis Sci 2004;49:1575–1577. (Ref.29)

Tsang VC, Wilkins PP. Immunodiagnosis of schistosomiasis. Immunol Invest 1997;26:175–186. (Ref.176)

Vakiani E, et al. Hepatitis C–associated granulomas after liver transplantation: morphologic spectrum and clinical implications. Am J Clin Pathol 2007;127:128–134. (Ref.202)

Veerabagu MP, Finkelstein SD, Rabinovitz M. Granulomatous hepatitis in a patient with chronic hepatitis C treated with interferon-alpha. Dig Dis Sci 1997;42:1445–1448. (Ref.204)

Vercelli-Retta J, Lagios MD, Chandrasoma P. *Fasciola hepatica* and parasitic eosinophilic granuloma of the liver. Am J Surg Pathol 2002;26:1238–1240. (Ref.143)

Wainwright H. Hepatic granulomas. Eur J Gastroenterol Hepatol 2007;19:93–95. (Ref.87)

Wilson MS, et al. Immunopathology of schistosomiasis. Immunol Cell Biol 2007;85:148–154. (Ref.165)

Winkelstein JA, et al. Chronic granulomatous disease. Report on a national registry of 368 patients. Medicine (Baltimore) 2000;79:155–169. (Ref.271)

Wynn TA, Cheever AW. Cytokine regulation of granuloma formation in schistosomiasis. Curr Opin Immunol 1995;7:505–511. (Ref.20)

Yamamoto S, et al. Epithelioid granuloma formation in type C chronic hepatitis: report of two cases. Hepatogastroenterology 1995;42:291–293. (Ref.25)

Yazici P, et al. Visceral leishmaniasis as a rare cause of granulomatosis hepatitis: a case report. Turkiye Parazitol Derg 2008;32:12–15. (Ref.146)

Zanchi AC, et al. Necrotizing granulomatous hepatitis as an unusual manifestation of Lyme disease. Dig Dis Sci 2007;52:2629–2632. (Ref.106)

Zangerl B, et al. Coccidioidomycosis as the cause of granulomatous hepatitis. Med Klin 1998;93:170–173. (Ref.181)

A complete list of references can be found at www.expertconsult.com.

HIV Co-Infection Drug Toxicity

Barbara H. McGovern, Mark S. Sulkowski, and Richard K. Sterling

ABBREVIATIONS

ACTG AIDS Clinical Trials Group
AHR abacavir hypersensitivity reaction
AIDS acquired immunodeficiency syndrome
ALT alanine aminotransferase
ALP alkaline phosphatase
APC antigen-presenting cell
ART antiretroviral therapy
AST aspartate aminotransferase
AZT zidovudine
BMI body mass index
CT computed tomography
DILI drug-induced liver injury
FDA Food and Drug Administration
HAART highly active antiretroviral therapy

HBsAg hepatitis B surface antigen
HBV hepatitis B virus
HCV hepatitis C virus
HIV human immunodeficiency virus
HLA human leukocyte antigen
HR hazard ratio
MHC major histocompatibility complex
mtDNA mitochondrial DNA
NA nucleoside analogue
NAFLD nonalcoholic fatty liver disease
NASH nonalcoholic steatohepatitis
NNRTI nonnucleoside reverse transcriptase inhibitor
NRTI nucleoside reverse transcriptase inhibitor
PEP postexposure prophylaxis

PI protease inhibitor
PREDICT-1 Prospective Randomized Evaluation of DNA Screening in a Clinical Trial
PT prothrombin time
RADAR Research on Adverse Drug Events and Reports
ROS reactive oxygen species
RR relative risk
SNP single-nucleotide polymorphism
UGT uridine diphosphate-glucuronosyltransferase
ULN upper limit of normal

Introduction

Background

Human immunodeficiency virus (HIV) infection is a global health concern with an estimated 1 million persons infected in the United States and 42 million worldwide (www.UNAIDS.org). Since the introduction of potent antiretroviral therapy (ART) in 1996, there has been a dramatic reduction in HIV-associated morbidity and mortality in those living with HIV infection.[1,2] Classes of antiretroviral agents include nucleoside reverse transcriptase inhibitors (NRTIs), nonnucleoside reverse transcriptase inhibitors (NNRTIs), protease inhibitors (PIs), integrase inhibitors, chemokine receptor 5 (CCR5) receptor antagonists, and fusion inhibitors, which act at various stages of the HIV life cycle (**Table 38-1**).

Many of these potent drugs have been associated with elevations of aminotransferases and have warnings in their product labeling regarding potential drug-induced liver injury (DILI). Hepatotoxicity from DILI can lead to liver-related morbidity and mortality, and discontinuation of needed HIV treatment. The likelihood of ART-associated liver injury is increased in those who have concomitant infection with hepatitis B or C viruses.[3-7] Because co-infection with viral hepatitis is common in this patient population, drug toxicity remains a clinical challenge. Clinicians caring for patients with HIV need to understand the clinical importance, limitations of existing literature, risk factors, mechanisms, and management of DILI in this population.[7]

Definitions and Patterns of Drug-Induced Liver Injury

DILI can lead to three patterns of liver injury defined as hepatocellular, cholestatic, or mixed. In hepatocellular injury, elevations in alanine aminotransferase (ALT) and aspartate aminotransferase (AST) predominate, with ALT characteristically greater than AST. In cholestatic injury, elevations in alkaline phosphatase (ALP) predominate. In some cases, both hepatocellular and cholestatic enzymes are equally elevated, which is referred to as mixed injury. In severe cases, there is also impairment of liver function with increases in total and conjugated bilirubin and prothrombin time (PT). These cytolytic reactions usually resolve within weeks after drug discontinuation but may lead to life-threatening hepatic injury. The severity of hepatic injury is reflected by increases in prothrombin time and total bilirubin, which reflects severe limitation in liver function.[8] Cholestatic reactions are

Table 38-1 Drugs Used to Treat HIV and Their Risk for Hepatotoxicity

CLASS	DRUG	HEPATIC SAFETY PROFILE
NRTI	Didanosine (ddI)	Caution
	Stavudine (d4T)	Caution
	Zidovudine (AZT)	Intermediate
	Abacavir (ABV)	Safe*
	Lamivudine (LAM)	Safe
	Emtricitabine (FTC)	Safe
	Tenofovir (TDF)	Safe
NNRTI	Nevirapine NVP)	Caution
	Efavirenz (EFV)	Safe
	Etravirine	Pending
PI	Ritonavir (full dose, RTV)	Caution†
	Tipranavir (TPV)	Caution
	Fosamprenavir (AMP)	Safe
	Darunavir (DRV)	Safe
	Atazanavir (ATV)	Safe
	Indinavir (IDV)	Safe
	Lopinavir (LPV)	Safe
	Saquinavir (SQV)	Safe
	Nelfinavir (NFV)	
Entry inhibitor	Enfuvirtide (T-20)	Safe
Integrase inhibitor	Raltegravir (RAL)	Safe*
CCR5 antagonist	Maraviroc (MVC)	Safe*

*Hypersensitivity reactions can occur.
†At full doses, not when used to boost PIs.
CCR5, chemokine receptor 5; NNRTI, nonnucleoside reverse transcriptase inhibitors; NRTI, nucleoside reverse transcriptase inhibitors; PI, protease inhibitor

usually not life-threatening but tend to resolve slowly over months.[9]

Interpretation of increases in liver enzymes must take into account patterns that are commonly seen in association with ART administration, but are of no clinical significance. For example, some PIs (see later discussion) act as inhibitors of uridine diphosphate-glucuronosyltransferase (UGT)1A1, an enzyme of the glucuronidation pathway that transforms small lipophilic molecules such as steroids, bilirubin, hormones, and drugs into water-soluble metabolites. Genetic variations in the UGT1A1 enzyme have been linked to hyperbilirubinemia.[10-12] Similarly, two PIs, indinavir and atazanavir, inhibit UGT1A1 and may be associated with clinically apparent increases in bilirubin. Furthermore, polymorphisms in genes encoding for UGT1A1 are strongly associated with the development of unconjugated hyperbilirubinemia during therapy with atazanavir or indinavir,[13-15] especially in those with underlying Gilbert syndrome.[16,17] These elevations of bilirubin can be cosmetically concerning for the patient, but do not infer significant liver disease. In contrast, patients with marked impairment of hepatic synthetic function, with increases in direct conjugated bilirubin along with elevations of aminotransferases, are at risk for liver-related mortality.

Prevalence of Elevated Liver Enzymes

Many studies also suggest that elevated liver enzymes are common and occur in 40% to 60% of patients on ART regimens.[18-22] In a recent large study of almost 6000 HIV patients, the prevalence of abnormal ALT and AST in those without alternative etiologies (e.g., viral hepatitis) was 55% and 76%, respectively.[23] This high proportion is far greater than expected in the general population of 8%[24] and may be due to drugs used in HIV or other factors, such as alcohol use. Among individual antiretroviral drugs, exposure to full-dose ritonavir, ritonavir-boosted tipranavir, stavudine and/or nevirapine have been identified in some studies as independent risk factors for the development hepatotoxicity.[25-28] In two of the largest cohort studies to report this association, the risk attributed to full-dose ritonavir was independent of co-infection with chronic hepatitis B or C.[25,26] Wit and co-workers found that the use of full dose ritonavir was independently associated with 5.8-fold increased risk of developing grade 4 liver enzyme elevations, and full-dose ritonavir was associated with 23 of 35 (66%) of the grade 4 hepatotoxicity cases observed.[25] Importantly, low-dose ritonavir (defined as 200 mg twice daily) used to boost other PIs, such as lopinavir, fosamprenavir, and darunavir, has not been independently associated with an increased risk of liver injury.

Clinical Importance of Drug-Induced Liver Injury
Morbidity and Mortality Related to Drug-Induced Liver Injury

Two major consequences of DILI are of great clinical relevance in HIV-infected patients: DILI can lead to discontinuation of needed ART and to liver-related morbidity and mortality. Discontinuation of antiretroviral agents due to recurrent hepatotoxicity can also lead to profound immunosuppression and risk of AIDS-related opportunistic infections. Drug-associated hepatotoxicity also adds to the economic burden of already strained medical budgets because additional visits and hospital admissions may be required for appropriate patient care and management.[29]

The spectrum of manifestations of DILI in HIV-infected patients can range from asymptomatic elevations of aminotransferases to hepatic failure and death. In a study of 755 HIV patients starting ART, clinical outcomes were separated into "relevant hepatotoxicity" (transaminases of >5 times the upper limit of normal [ULN] or 2.5 times baseline) and severe hepatotoxicity (10 times ULN or 5 times baseline). Twenty-six patients developed severe hepatotoxicity leading to the clinically important outcome of drug discontinuation.[30] Furthermore, seven of these patients subsequently developed liver failure 3 to 25 days after the peak ALT occurred. In a large AIDS Clinical Trial Group cohort of nearly 3000 patients initiating ART, the most common grade 4 adverse events were liver related.[31] These data, and multiple other studies, suggest that hepatotoxicity can lead to serious morbidity and mortality among HIV-infected patients.

Symptoms of Drug-Induced Liver Injury

The two most common clinical presentations of drug-induced liver disease include acute icteric hepatitis or cholestatic liver disease, each with their own individual pattern of laboratory abnormalities, as discussed previously. Symptoms of drug-induced liver injury are similar to those seen with acute viral hepatitis and include nausea, vomiting, right upper quadrant pain, fatigue, and anorexia. Symptoms of cholestatic injury include pruritus. One specific syndrome is related to mitochondrial toxicity (see later discussion). Clinically, this is manifested by nausea, vomiting, and abdominal pain, which can progress to severe acidosis. In addition to elevated lactate levels, there are often increases in pancreatic enzymes and liver enzymes with an AST greater than ALT.[32] The most common NRTIs associated with mitochondrial toxicity are didanosine (ddI) and stavudine (d4T), which are now uncommonly used in resource-rich countries.

Hy's Law

Continued administration of a drug after onset of symptomatic hepatitis (i.e., isoniazid) increases the risk of severe liver injury and death.[33] Drug-induced hepatocellular injury associated with jaundice carries a mortality rate of 10% or more.[34] Known as Hy's law, elevations of aminotransferases (three times ULN), which are accompanied by a serum bilirubin level of two times the ULN, have been advocated by the U.S. Food and Drug Administration (FDA) for use in the assessment of drug-induced hepatotoxicity.[35]

Limitations of Data on ART-Associated Hepatotoxicity from Clinical Trials

Definitions of Drug-Induced Liver Toxicity

Because of varying definitions of antiretroviral DILI, the AIDS clinical trials group (ACTG) developed a grading system of 1 to 4 based on baseline serum aminotransferase levels (**Table 38-2**) to define the severity of hepatotoxicity (http://www.actg.org). In this system, the degree of hepatotoxicity

depends on the increase in liver enzymes over the baseline values where the upper limit of normal for ALT and AST is 40 IU/ml. The ACTG adverse event grading scheme has separate criteria for mild, moderate, and severe toxicity based on whether baseline transaminases are normal or not.[26,36-38] In another study, ACTG criteria were used but the authors did not factor in an increase in aminotransferases among those patients who already had baseline abnormalities of transaminases.[39] Some investigators also account for fold changes over an abnormal baseline while other researchers have used an arbitrary increase of 200 IU/ml to define significant hepatotoxicity. Some researchers have interpreted an increase of transaminases as little as two-fold over baseline as significant.[40,41] Whether these mild increases in transaminases are of clinical relevance is unknown. Because of the varying criteria, frequency of monitoring, and length of follow-up, it is often difficult to compare study outcomes. Furthermore, few of these studies have histologic data to correlate with laboratory abnormalities.[42]

Incomplete Data on Clinical Events in Association with Hepatotoxicity

Some studies have not specified whether patients with severe elevations of transaminases had symptomatic or asymptomatic hepatitis, each of which has different degrees of clinical concern. Also some studies have not fully characterized whether drug-associated hepatotoxicity reactions are cytotoxic or cholestatic and do not include information about bilirubin, alkaline phosphatase, or measures of synthetic function (prothrombin time).

Of the 23 HIV seropositive patients who developed severe drug-associated hepatotoxicity in an initial cohort of 1080 subjects, 11 patients (48%) had at least one clinical manifestation. This was characterized by mainly jaundice (6 patients) and abdominal pain (5 patients).[43] However, jaundice was not differentiated in this study between that seen with expected medication-induced increases in indirect hyperbilirubinemia versus hepatocellular or cholestatic injury, all of which have very different clinical implications for prognosis and management.

Lack of Histopathology

Most studies infer drug-induced liver injury but pathology is available for few of the subjects with severe hepatotoxicity.[30,39,41] In a study of 751 patients, severe hepatotoxicity developed in a subset of 26 subjects.[30] Sixteen underwent a liver biopsy, which demonstrated significant inflammatory changes and piecemeal necrosis. Nine subjects also had some evidence of eosinophilic infiltrate. Without systemic biopsy sampling, the pathologic mechanism remains speculative in the vast majority of subjects.

Lack of Information of Other Causes of Acute Hepatitis

Many studies have not examined the potential role of other causes of acute hepatitis. A careful review of patient charts in one large cohort found that 9 of 44 cases of elevated transaminases (20.4%) were related to causes other than drug toxicity, including acute viral hepatitis, secondary syphilis, and

Table 38-2 Grading Hepatotoxicity

GRADE OF HEPATOTOXICITY				
0	1	2	3	4
Patients with Normal Baseline AST/ALT				
<1.25 × ULN	1.25-2.5 × ULN	2.6-5.0 × ULN	5.1-10 × ULN	>10 × ULN
Patients with Elevated Baseline AST/ALT				
<1.25 × BL	1.25-2.5 × BL	2.6-3.5 × BL	3.6-5 × BL	>5 × BL

Grades of hepatotoxicity will be consistent with the NIH-NIAI Guidelines (AIDS Clinical Trial Group. Grading Severity of Adult Adverse Experiences. Rockville, MD: Division of AIDS, NIAI, 1996).

ALT, alanine aminotransferase; AST, aspartate aminotransferase; BL, baseline; ULN, upper limit of normal

rhabdomyolysis.[25] After this thorough investigation, the overall incidence of drug-associated toxicity subsequently declined from 7.9% to 6.3%. Few studies have examined the role of other ancillary medications, such as sulfonamides or fluconazole, in the development of hepatotoxicity.[43,44]

Drug Registration Trials

In randomized, controlled trials, the incidence of significant, grade 3 (>5 times the ULN) and grade 4 (>10 times the ULN) elevations in serum ALT or AST levels associated with the use of combination ART has varied between approximately 1% and approximately 14%.[29] The incidence of hepatotoxicity in such studies typically reflects not only the toxicity associated with the ART of interest but also that of concurrently administered ARTs. In addition, the population studied may have profound effects on the incidence of severe hepatotoxicity (e.g., treatment-experienced vs. treatment-naive). Given the substantial heterogeneity in patient populations and drug regimens, comparison of hepatotoxicity incidence rates for individual ARTs across clinical trials is difficult.

Observational Studies

Limitations of current observational studies include lack of standardized follow-up leading to bias in ascertainment and poor measures of medication adherence or alcohol use, which could have differential effects on toxicity profiles.[18]

Risk Factors for Drug-Induced Liver Injury

Role of Co-Infection with Hepatitis Viruses B or C (or Both)

Although concomitant viral hepatitis has not been described as a risk factor for DILI in immunocompetent patients,[34] several studies in HIV-infected patients demonstrate that chronic infection with hepatitis B and C viruses are major risk factors for ART-associated hepatotoxicity.[30,45] In fact, in most studies, co-infection with hepatitis C and/or B virus has been identified as the most significant risk factor for the development of significant liver enzyme elevations following ART. For example, after adjustment for higher baseline liver enzymes, den Brinker and co-workers found that HCV-infected patients had a 2.46-fold greater risk of developing severe hepatotoxicity compared with HCV-uninfected patients.[46] In a United States cohort, Sulkowski and colleagues reported that HCV co-infection was independently associated with a greater than two-fold increased risk of severe hepatotoxicity after adjusting for the type of medication received and baseline liver enzyme levels.[47] While baseline abnormalities of ALT/AST have been demonstrated to be important predictors of drug-associated hepatotoxicity in most of these studies,[25,46,48] in one study fibrosis stage was the strongest predictor of liver injury; the greatest risk of hepatotoxicity was observed in persons with underlying cirrhosis.[49] In a study from Italy, HCV genotype 3 infection was more frequently associated with hepatotoxicity than genotype 1.[50]

In chronic hepatitis B, the pathogenesis of such elevations may be related to immunologic response to HBV rather than drug-induced liver injury. For example, Manegold and colleagues recently reported the reactivation of chronic HBV in two HIV-infected patients receiving PIs.[51] Conversely, Velasco and co-workers reported the resolution of chronic hepatitis B in an HIV-infected patient treated with ritonavir.[52] Similarly, den Brinker and colleagues reported that 38% of patients with chronic HBV lost HBeAg following the administration of ART.[46] In addition, the discontinuation of ART regimens that contain drugs active against HBV (e.g., lamivudine and/or tenofovir) has been associated with significant liver enzyme flares in HIV-infected patients co-infected with chronic hepatitis B.[25,53] Thus available data suggest that mechanisms of liver injury in the setting of hepatitis B may be quite different from that observed in HCV-infected patients.

These observations hold great significance because chronic HCV and HBV are highly prevalent among HIV-infected patients. Due to shared routes of transmission, co-infection with hepatitis B and C viruses is common among HIV-infected patients. One series found that in a cohort of 232 HIV-infected patients, 9% had chronic HBV infection and 86% of these patients were viremic (hepatitis B surface antigen [HBsAg] positive). In addition, approximately 30% of patients infected with HIV in the United States and Europe are also hepatitis C seropositive.[54-56] However, the prevalence is much higher (70% to 90%) among those who acquired HIV through injection drug use than through sex (5% to 15%).[57] The vast majority of these HCV seropositive patients are viremic.

However, it is important to emphasize that the majority of patients with underlying chronic viral hepatitis tolerate ART without significant liver injury.[26] Consequently, ART should not be withheld from a patient due to the presence of underlying chronic viral hepatitis.

Additional Factors Predicting Susceptibility to Liver Injury

The liver is under constant stress with potentially toxic metabolites normally being produced during the biotransformation process. The vulnerability of an individual to liver injury is dependent on the delicate balance between toxification and detoxification processes involved in drug metabolism. Many factors can up-regulate specific isoenzymes of the cytochrome P-450 (CYP) system, which then increase production of certain toxic metabolites. If the detoxification process of the individual is overwhelmed by increased harmful products or cannot handle oxidative stress due to glutathione deficiency, the individual's risk of liver injury increases.[34]

Because most examples of drug-induced liver disease occur in a very small proportion of patients using any given agent, it is likely that the individual risk is determined by various combinations of host, environmental, and genetic variations.[34] Risk factors are listed below with illustrative examples.

- **Gender:** Women are more likely to develop drug-related toxicity than men.[58,59] Some data suggest that gender may play a role in nevirapine toxicity.[25,60]
- **HIV infection:** The presence of HIV is associated with lower plasma and hepatic glutathione levels, which increase the risk of oxidative stress and drug toxicity.[61,62]
- **Genetic polymorphisms:** Multiple mutations of the CYP system have been recognized, therefore explaining

individual susceptibility to administration of the same drug.[63] As an example, deficiencies in CYP2D6 activity are found in 5% to 10% of Caucasians and have been correlated with marked interpatient variability in drug plasma levels of antiretroviral medications.[64-66]

- **Metabolic:** Obesity enhances acetaminophen toxicity, probably through induction of CYP2E1.[67]
- **Drug interactions:** When administered alone, isoniazid is converted to a toxic metabolite, which subsequently undergoes detoxification. However, when INH is co-administered with rifampin, CYP isoenzymes are induced and the metabolism of isoniazid is accelerated. This leads to an imbalance between the rate of production of toxic metabolites and their detoxification, which increases the risk of DILD.[68] Administration of certain antiretroviral medications, which induce or inhibit isoenzymes of the CYP system, can also significantly impact the plasma concentrations of other administered drugs.[66]
- **Alcohol use:** Chronic alcohol use increases oxidative damage to mitochondrial DNA and decreases glutathione stores.[69]
- **Drug levels:** The development of elevated aminotransferase levels appears to be related to the dose of amiodarone and to the plasma level of the drug.[67] It is not clear as to whether elevated plasma levels of antiretroviral medications cause elevated transaminases, although some provocative data have been published[70] (see Therapeutic Management of Drug-Induced Liver Injury).
- **Acetylator status:** Patients with a slow acetylator phenotype have a higher risk of hypersensitivity to sulfonamides, which are frequently used in prophylaxis of opportunistic infections.[71]
- **Duration of treatment:** The risk for mitochondrial toxicity increases with long-term administration of nucleoside analogues.[72]
- **Nutritional status:** Nutritional deficiencies can lead to depleted glutathione stores and the inability to detoxify certain reactive metabolites.[59]
- **Age:** Aging results in a decline in the ability to eliminate drugs as a result of decreased hepatic blood flow.[73] Older adults are more susceptible to liver injury from isoniazid than children.[33]

Mechanisms of Drug-Induced Liver Injury

The mechanisms of DILI can be idiosyncratic or predictable.[8] Predictable DILI is dose dependent and host independent, with the classic example being acetaminophen toxicity. Early onset toxicity (within a few days) is strong evidence for direct drug toxicity, particularly if there has been no previous exposure. Most predictable hepatotoxins are recognized during animal testing or early clinical phases of drug development.

Idiosyncratic DILI is usually host dependent and not dose related and can result from biotransformation of drugs to intermediary metabolites that are either directly toxic or provoke an immunologic response.[8] Unfortunately, the vast majority of drug reactions are unpredictable. The latency period of unpredictable reactions is either "intermediate" (1 to 8 weeks) or "long" (2 to 12 months). Intermediate latency is characteristic of hypersensitivity reactions; long latency is characteristic of host-dependent metabolism reactions. Unpredictable reactions are often not identified until well into the postmarketing experience of the drug.

Antiretroviral DILI can be divided into four broad categories: direct drug toxicity, hypersensitivity, mitochondrial toxicity, and immune reconstitution (**Table 38-3**). Unfortunately, these are not mutually exclusive and can co-exist within the same person. Additionally, patients can have underlying hepatic pathology, such as steatosis or advanced fibrosis, which might affect drug metabolism and risk of DILI.

Direct Drug Toxicity

Most drugs are metabolized in the liver, which converts them through oxidized intermediary metabolites via the CYP system, which then are conjugated for elimination. Host differences in drug metabolism may lead to an excess of potentially harmful reactive drug metabolites via aberrant metabolic pathways. This process is affected by genetic polymorphisms, which can cause accumulation of a toxic metabolite. Examples of this include certain NNRTIs, such as nevirapine.[74-76] Other medications can promote liver injury via cytokine-mediated hepatocyte apoptosis[77] or increased oxidative stress.

Table 38-3 Mechanisms of Drug-Induced Liver Injury with Antiretroviral Agents

MECHANISM	EXAMPLE	CHARACTERISTIC	TIME OF ONSET
Idiosyncratic reaction or intrinsic toxicity	NVP	Dose dependent for intrinsic	Can vary by agent
Hypersensitivity reaction	NVP* > ABV*	Often associated with rash	Usually within 8 weeks
Mitochondrial toxicity	ddI > d4T > AZT > ABV = TDF = LAM = FTC	Lactic acidosis	Tends to occur after prolonged exposure
Immune reconstitution	Any	More common in those with low CD4⁺ count and chronic HBV	Usually within the first few months
Steatosis	NRTIs PIs	Metabolic syndrome, lipodystrophy, HCV (especially GT3)	Usually with prolonged exposure

*Increased with certain polymorphisms.
ABV, abacavir; AMP, amprenavir; AZT, zidovudine; FTC, emtricitabine; GT, genotype; LAM, lamivudine; NRTI, nucleoside reverse transcriptase inhibitor; NVP, nevirapine; PI, protease inhibitor; TDF, tenofovir

Hypersensitivity Reaction

Hypersensitivity reactions are idiosyncratic allergic reactions to the drug or its hepatic-derived metabolite. They can occur almost immediately after initiation of the drug or weeks later.

Two separate theories have been proposed to explain the basis of hypersensitivity reactions.[71] The "hapten hypothesis" suggests that formation of a reactive metabolite is not sufficient to induce an immunologic reaction, but rather must be bound to a macromolecule, such as the specific cytochrome enzyme that generated it. The covalent binding of these two components is perceived as foreign by both arms of the immune system, leading to production of autoantibodies and activation of the cellular immune response. T cells recognize this neoantigen, which is expressed on the surface of the hepatocyte in the context of major histocompatibility complex class I molecules. "Hepatic sensitization" occurs along with flares of transaminases. However, the hapten hypothesis would suggest that immune-mediated reactions should occur more frequently than they do. The "danger hypothesis" suggests that the immune system only responds to a foreign antigen if it is associated with a "danger signal." The nature of the danger signal is unknown, but cellular stress or chronic infections, such as hepatitis C or HIV, have been proposed as potential triggers.[78]

The incidence of hypersensitivity reactions is more common in those with HIV compared with the general population.[61] Symptoms include fever, skin rash, fatigue, nausea, vomiting, diarrhea, abdominal pain, and eosinophilia. Hypersensitivity reactions must promptly be identified because they can result in severe life-threatening illness. Hypersensitivity reactions have been reported for trimethoprim-sulfamethoxazole, abacavir, nevirapine, atazanavir, enfuvirtide, fosamprenavir, and maraviroc[79] and may be related to genetic predisposition of drug metabolism.

The term pharmacogenetics refers to the effects of polymorphisms within human genes on drug therapy outcomes.[80] By definition, single-nucleotide polymorphisms (SNPs) are defined as sequence variations that occur in human DNA, with single nucleotide changes occurring at an allele frequency greater than 1%.[81] Nucleotide changes occurring with a frequency lower than this are referred to as mutations. Numerous associations have been reported between host genetic polymorphisms and responses to ART drugs, and include drug pharmacokinetics and pharmacodynamics that affect the rates of hepatotoxicity.

Abacavir Hypersensitivity

Interest in HLA background as a potential risk factor for certain drug reactions has only become well defined over the past few years. Associations have been drawn between severe hypersensitivity reactions to particular drugs and specific class I MHC backgrounds. The association between HLA type HLA-B*5071 and abacavir hypersensitivity reaction is by far the best example of casual genotype-phenotype correlation in HIV medicine. A strong body of evidence suggests that abacavir hypersensitivity is exquisitely HLA-B*5701 restricted and mediated via CD8+ T lymphocytes.[82,83] It is currently theorized that a "danger signal" initiates the hypersensitivity reaction through the innate immune system. Abacavir is metabolized and undergoes classic MHC class-I processing. This is followed by presentation of the peptide-HLA complex on an antigen-presenting cell (APC) to the receptor of an abacavir-specific CD8+ T cell. This process activates the CD8+ T cell to release inflammatory cytokines, resulting in the clinical syndrome of abacavir hypersensitivity reaction (AHR).

Clinically AHR is characterized by fever, constitutional symptoms, such as malaise and headache, and gastrointestinal disturbance, such as nausea, vomiting, and diarrhea.[84,85] In one retrospective study, respiratory symptoms including dyspnea, occurred in approximately one third of patients.[84] The median time to onset of symptoms in confirmed cases is approximately 7 days; rash is often a late symptom. Signs may include tachycardia and hypotension; severe morbidity and even death have been reported in patients with symptoms of hypersensitivity who were reexposed to abacavir.

Screening for HLA-B*5701 represents a major advance in the care of HIV-infected patients and remains the mainstay in preventing the abacavir hypersensitivity reaction, which occurs in approximately 4% of patients.[86] The Prospective Randomized Evaluation of DNA Screening in a Clinical Trial (PREDICT-1) was a double-blinded study enrolling 1956 predominantly Caucasian patients initiating an abacavir-containing regimen.[85] This was the first study of its kind to examine the clinical effectiveness of a genetic screening test to prevent a specific drug toxicity. Immunologically confirmed abacavir hypersensitivity, which occurred in 2.7% of the control arm, was eliminated in the screened arm. A retrospective, case-control study in a racially diverse population showed 100% sensitivity of HLA-B*5701 for confirmed AHR, suggesting a 100% negative predictive value of HLA-B*5701 testing for abacavir hypersensitivity in both Caucasian and African American patients.[87] This study supported broad applicability of genetic screening for AHR in HIV-infected patients. Subsequently, HIV treatment guideline committees have endorsed the use of abacavir only in patients who have tested negative for HLA-B*5701.[88]

Skin patch testing helps to define those patients with a history of possible AHR with true immunogenetically mediated disease versus a false positive clinical diagnosis.[89] Experience to date suggests that only those genetically susceptible patients who are "immunologically primed" by prior ingestion of abacavir exposure will develop a positive patch test. Thus skin patch testing can only be reliably performed to characterize patients with a history of "possible AHR," and patch testing is not helpful for predicting risk of AHR in unexposed patients. Skin patch testing has also helped to reinforce the strong association between HLA-B*5701 and AHR. For example, of 95 patients with clinically suspected abacavir hypersensitivity and positive patch tests described in three studies, 100% have carried HLA-B*5701.[90] However, a negative abacavir patch test result can neither rule out AHR nor be used to justify rechallenge with abacavir in a patient with a compatible history.[85]

The presence of the HLA class II allele *HLA-DRB* 0101* is associated with increased risk for nevirapine-associated hypersensitivity reaction and hepatotoxicity, and the risk is attenuated by a low CD4+ cell count. NNRTI hepatotoxicity is also associated with an *MDR1* gene polymorphism, because the 3435 CT genotype appears to confer a reduced risk.[74,75]

Mitochondrial Toxicity

Mitochondria are important in energy production and fat and glucose metabolism, and serve as the main source of reactive oxygen species (ROS). NRTIs used to treat HIV can cause mitochondrial toxicity by inhibiting mitochondrial DNA polymerase-gamma, which is responsible for replication of mitochondrial DNA (mtDNA). Significant decreases in mitochondrial function can result in decreased oxidative phosphorylation leading to increased lactate production.[91,92] Impaired oxidation may also lead to a decrease in fatty acid oxidation. Free fatty acids subsequently accumulate and are metabolized to triglycerides. These excess triglycerides reside in the liver, causing hepatic steatosis.[93] Fortunately, in 2010, first-line NRTIs for treatment-naïve patients include tenofovir and either emtricitabine or lamivudine, which are not associated with mitochondrial toxicity (http://www.aidsinfo.nih.gov/Guidelines/).

This risk of mitochondrial toxicity is increased in HCV co-infected patients[94,95] due to the additional oxidative stress from the chronic HCV core protein.[96-98] In both the APRICOT and RIBAVIC HCV treatment trials, mitochondrial toxicity was identified in approximately 3% of patients.[99,100] In a prospective analysis of 113 co-infected patients, Laguno and associates identified evidence of this disorder in 12% of patients treated with combination therapy for HCV plus ART, although most patients were asymptomatic.[101]

One of the major risk factors for mitochondrial toxicity in HIV-infected patients on combination interferon/ribavirin therapy is the co-administration of didanosine.[102,103] Ribavirin monophosphate inhibits IMPDH, the primary phosphate donor to didanosine.[104] This inhibition increases the intracellular concentrations of didanosine triphosphate and the occurrence of resultant toxicities such as lactic acidosis. Therefore didanosine should not be co-administered with ribavirin therapy.

Immune Reconstitution

Patients infected with HIV who commence ART when they have advanced immunodeficiency are susceptible to immune reconstitution disorders.[105-107] Immune restoration is associated with recovery of pathogen-specific responses, but may also cause significant morbidity and negatively affect quality of life.[108] Inflammatory reactions following immune restoration can occur in up to 40% of individuals who begin ART at low baseline CD4$^+$ counts.[105,109,110]

The pathogenesis of immune restoration syndromes is not well understood, but may be related to an unmasking of a previously latent infection precipitated by ART-induced immunologic recovery of CD4$^+$ and CD8$^+$ T-cell function.[111] The immunologic changes associated with ART have been linked to a change in the T_H1/T_H2 balance to a predominantly T_H1 cytokine environment,[110] which may produce increased inflammation.

Immune restoration syndromes associated with several pathogens have been described[108-110,112-115] and patients who are co-infected with HBV or HCV are at particular risk for this syndrome.[116] In a study of 352 subjects starting ART, 81 (23%) developed increased liver enzymes. This observation was more commonly seen in those with HBV and/or HCV co-infection versus those with HIV alone (51% vs. 14%). Another risk factor for IRS in this study included a higher absolute increase in CD4$^+$ cell count.[116]

Because the pathogenesis of HBV-associated liver injury includes cell-mediated immunity, it is not unexpected that immune restoration from ART can result in liver cell injury. In those with advanced immunodeficiency, HBV DNA levels are usually higher whereas hepatic inflammation is lower than in patients with relatively preserved immunity.[117] However, after ART is initiated, improved cellular immunity can result in "flares" in hepatic enzymes[118] and even seroconversion[119] in the absence of specific HBV therapy.[120] Besides immune reconstitution, the clinician must also be aware that increases in aminotransferases in those co-infected with HIV/HBV can be due to multiple other causes including: (1) idiosyncratic drug reactions, (2) hypersensitivity reactions, (3) seroconversion or reactivation of HBV, or (4) co-infection with other viruses, such as HDV or HCV.

Although there were several early reports of elevated aminotransferases in HIV/HCV co-infected patients initiating ART,[115,121] evidence of immune reconstitution secondary to HCV infection is less well established than in HIV/HBV co-infected patients. There have been conflicting reports on whether increases in CD4$^+$ cells after initiation are associated with liver enzyme elevations and the role of cellular immunity in hepatocyte cytolysis is less clear than in HBV infection.[26,30,122,123] In the only study with paired biopsies, liver histology worsened in 31 HIV/HCV co-infected patients who developed hepatotoxicity after initiating ART.[42]

Hepatic Steatosis

Patients with HIV are at particular risk of steatosis, which may also play an important role in facilitating liver injury.[17] Several studies have shown increased risk of DILI in those patients with underlying steatosis.[30,32,124] Additionally, steatosis associated with HCV genotype 3 has also been associated with increased risk of DILI.[37,50,125] These studies suggest that the presence of steatosis may predispose HIV-infected patients for DILI.[17]

Nonalcoholic fatty liver disease (NAFLD) is also prevalent in patients with HIV infection. In addition to traditional risk factors, such as obesity, the lipodystrophy syndrome is highly prevalent among HIV-infected patients.[126] This syndrome includes multiple components such as hyperlipidemia, visceral adiposity, and glucose intolerance, all of which are well-known risk factors for hepatic steatosis in the general population. In addition, many antiretroviral medications associated with mitochondrial toxicity (e.g., didanosine, stavudine) are strongly associated with the development of hepatic steatosis.[127]

Several studies have examined the prevalence of steatosis in those with HIV. One study using CT imaging found liver-spleen attenuation, consistent with hepatic steatosis, in 37% of HIV-infected persons.[128] Factors associated with the presence of hepatic steatosis have included a higher serum ALT/AST ratio, male gender, increased waist circumference, and long-term NRTI use compared with HIV-uninfected controls Another study showed HIV-infected subjects with NAFLD have a lower BMI and a lower percentage of fat mass when compared with HIV-uninfected subjects with NAFLD.[129] Severe steatosis (>30%) assessed by ultrasound (US) was found in 13% of patients and related to BMI, alcohol consumption, lipohypertrophy, and higher HIV RNA levels.[130] Similarly, steatosis by US was seen in 13% of a cohort from Nigeria.[131] Conversely, in another study using US in 216 HIV subjects without HCV, 31% had steatosis, which was associated with increased waist circumference, higher triglyceride, and lower HDL levels but not HIV levels.[132] Finally, a recent study of 30 HIV subjects with elevated liver enzymes without alcohol or viral hepatitis found a high prevalence of histologic abnormalities (22/30) with steatosis present in 18 (9 severe) 16 of whom had histology consistent with nonalcoholic steatohepatitis NASH.[133] In this small study, presence of NASH was associated with insulin resistance (IR). Hepatic steatosis has been shown to progress rapidly to cirrhosis in HIV-infected persons despite effective control of HIV replication, even in the absence of HCV co-infection.[134] Taken together, these studies show that similar to the general population, hepatic steatosis is an important liver disease in those living with HIV.

Several studies have shown that a significant proportion of HIV-infected patients with HCV co-infection have steatosis.[135-140] The prevalence of hepatic steatosis in different studies has varied widely, which may be related to race. For example, the prevalence of hepatic steatosis was 69% in one study of mainly Caucasian and Hispanic patients; in contrast, in another study hepatic steatosis was only present in 17%, but the vast majority of patients were African American.[138,141] Notably, in one study, cytologic ballooning, a pathognomonic feature of steatohepatitis, was associated with increased hepatic inflammation and fibrosis.[140]

Nucleoside Reverse Transcriptase Inhibitors and Drug-Induced Liver Injury

Nucleoside reverse transcriptase inhibitors have been the cornerstone of HIV therapy since the approval of zidovudine (AZT) in 1987. Within a few months of its approval, reports began to emerge of a possible association with elevated liver enzymes. In a population-based study, all HIV patients seen from July 1989 through July 1994 (n = 1836) were screened for evidence of steatosis and liver disease by assessment of hospital discharge diagnoses, pathology reports, out- and in-patient laboratory data, and clinic records. A total of 322 (18%) patients had evidence of liver test abnormalities. In these patients, viral hepatitis and alcohol-induced liver disease were the most common diagnoses. The incidence of the mitochondrial toxicity syndrome was 1.3 per 1000 person-years of follow-up in antiretroviral users in our cohort (95% confidence interval: 0.2, 4.5 per 1000 person-years).[142] In 1993 the FDA and the drug manufacturer issued a warning related to hepatic steatosis and AZT use. Similar reports of hepatic steatosis, elevated liver enzymes, and lactic acidosis were subsequently reported with most nucleoside analogues (NA), notably didanosine, stavudine, and fialuridine, a now discontinued agent that had been developed to treat chronic hepatitis B.[143-145] The proposed mechanism on the basis of several in vitro studies is inhibition of mitochondrial DNA polymerase gamma, which in turn is thought to interfere with energy production and fatty acid catabolism within cells. The ability of NRTIs to inhibit mitochondrial DNA synthesis in vitro is in the following order: (greatest) zalcitabine, didanosine, stavudine, zidovudine, lamivudine = emtricitabine = abacavir = tenofovir (least).[146]

A major risk factor for NA-related liver toxicity occurring in the context of hyperlactatemia is the use of stavudine-containing ART regimens. This risk appears to be further accentuated in regimens that include didanosine in addition to stavudine. While some retrospective studies have implicated female gender and obesity as additional predisposing factors, neither has been substantiated in prospective analyses. The combination of ribavirin, a guanosine nucleoside analogue, and didanosine has also been linked to severe liver injury. Ribavirin potentiates the intracellular activity of didanosine through inhibition of inosine monophosphate dehydrogenase. Multiple reports have indicated that the interaction between ribavirin and didanosine may lead to clinically significant inhibition of mtDNA polymerase gamma, resulting in severe pancreatitis, lactic acidosis, and, in some patients, death. The combination of ribavirin and didanosine is strictly contraindicated[147] (http://aidsinfo.nih.gov/contentfiles/AdultandAdolescentGL.pdf).

Another potential hepatic manifestation of chronic NRTI "toxicity" is the development of steatosis. Sulkowski and co-workers observed steatosis in 40% of 112 HIV/HCV co-infected patients who underwent liver biopsy; the presence of steatosis was associated with Caucasian race, weight greater than 86 kg, hyperglycemia, and stavudine use.[135] In addition, patients with steatosis also were more likely to have greater hepatic fibrosis and necroinflammatory activity. Similarly, McGovern and colleagues found steatosis in 69% of 183 HIV/HCV co-infected persons who underwent liver biopsy.[138] Factors associated with steatosis in this study included use of dideoxynucleoside analogues didanosine and stavudine. Lipodystrophy related to ART has also been linked to the finding of hepatic steatosis in HIV/HCV co-infected patients.[148] Although data regarding the prevalence of steatosis are more limited in patients without chronic HCV, several case series have reported cryptogenic cirrhosis or nodular regenerative hyperplasia in the setting of chronic dideoxynucleoside analogue therapy. Taken together, these preliminary data suggest that ART may contribute to the development of chronic hepatic steatosis; however, the long-term significance of this observation is unknown.

HIV-Associated Noncirrhotic Portal Hypertension or Nodular Regenerative Hyperplasia

As early as 2001, rare, unexplained, serious cases of liver disease have been reported in HIV-infected patients without hepatitis co-infection.[149-152] Reported rates have ranged from 1% (32 of 3200 patients) of HIV-infected patients from three clinics to 8% (8 of 97 patients) of HIV-infected patients presenting to a French liver disease center. Findings have included abnormal liver function tests, portal hypertension, and nodular regenerative hyperplasia. While no single etiology or characteristic histological finding has been identified, researchers have suggested the chronic exposure to nucleoside analogues with significant mitochondrial toxicity (e.g., didanosine, stavudine) may play a role in the etiopathogenesis of liver disease. For example, in one study, didanosine use appeared to play an important role; all but 3 of 32 HIV-infected patients with cryptogenic liver disease in one series had been exposed to didanosine. Most of these patients (27/29) were withdrawn from didanosine treatment; nearly half (13/27) showed clinical improvement 1 year later. Mean ALT levels fell significantly (75 to 49 IU/mL; P = .001).[149] Although no single cause has been identified, several studies have found an association with cumulative didanosine exposure; this has led the FDA in 2010 to issue a warning linking didanosine with this serious hepatopathy.[149,152] Further research is needed to better define this condition and to elucidate the role, if any, of antiretroviral drugs other than didanosine.

Nonnucleoside Reverse Transcriptase Inhibitors and Drug-Induced Liver Injury

Nonnucleoside reverse transcriptase inhibitors include nevirapine, efavirenz, delavirdine, and etravirine. Although registration trials of all four drugs demonstrated acceptable toxicity profiles, postmarketing reports of severe DILI related to nevirapine focused attention on this particular agent from the early introduction of this medication into clinical practice.[153] Delavirdine is infrequently used because of dosing frequency and numerous drug interactions. There are much less data on etravirine due to its relatively recent availability and restricted use in patients with drug-resistant HIV infection.[154]

Nevirapine and Immunologic Idiosyncrasy

The incidence of drug hypersensitivity reactions is about 1:1000 in the general population, but is more common in patients with HIV.[61] Hypersensitivity reactions have been reported with nevirapine, abacavir (as discussed previously) and less frequently with amprenavir, both in HIV-infected patients and in subjects receiving HIV prophylaxis after potential exposure.

Nevirapine-induced drug reactions follow the classic description for immune-mediated hypersensitivity reactions including intermediate latency (within 8 weeks of initiation) and association with constitutional symptoms (fever, rash, and eosinophilia).[155] In drug-induced hypersensitivity, T cells participate in the pathogenesis of these reactions by reacting to a drug metabolite or "neoantigens."[71,156]

There are several observations that suggest that relatively preserved CD4+ counts may be a risk factor for DILI.[157] For example, in one trial that compared nevirapine-containing ART to efavirenz-containing ART, grade 4 elevations in aminotransferases were observed in 36 (9.4%) of nevirapine patients and in none of the subjects receiving efavirenz; most of these reactions predominated in female patients.[27] Thirty-three of 36 cases of hepatotoxicity occurred within the first 4 weeks of therapy and one third of these patients had a concomitant rash. In the original randomization scheme, patients with higher CD4+ counts were stratified to the nevirapine arm versus the efavirenz arm. It has been postulated that this randomization scheme may have contributed to the higher rates of drug-associated liver injury that were seen in this trial.

Severe hepatotoxicity has also been reported in HIV-seronegative patients who took nevirapine for postexposure prophylaxis (PEP) against HIV infection leading to warnings against the use of nevirapine for PEP.[28] In another study, adverse event reports were identified from pharmaceutical manufacturers, the FDA, peer-reviewed journals, and the Research on Adverse Drug Events and Reports (RADAR project).[158] Among 151 persons who received nevirapine for 5 days or more, the risk of grade 3 or 4 hepatotoxicity was 13.3%. The median time to onset of elevated aminotransferases has been longer with efavirenz compared with nevirapine

(20 vs. 14 weeks), suggesting that most drug-induced liver injury with efavirenz does not involve immune-mediated mechanisms.[47]

Nucleoside Reverse Transcriptase Inhibitors and Drug-Induced Liver Injury in Large Cohorts

Because of concern regarding potential hepatotoxicity, several researchers investigated the incidence of DILI relative to NNRTI use in several large cohorts. One U.S.-based cohort study found that the rate of occurrence of grade 3 or 4 elevations of aminotransferases was more common in patients receiving nevirapine (15.6%) than those prescribed efavirenz (8.0%).[47] The risk of hepatotoxicity was increased in association with viral hepatitis, abnormal baseline aminotransferases, and the concomitant use of protease inhibitors. In contrast, a retrospective cohort study of predominantly homosexual white men found grade 3 or 4 elevations in aminotransferases in only 1.1% of patients with a similar rate among all three NNRTI treatment groups.[159] This low incidence of hepatotoxicity across the nevirapine, efavirenz, and delavirdine arms may have also been related to low rates of chronic viral hepatitis in this cohort.

A subsequent analysis was performed in 1731 patients who had taken nevirapine in various clinical trials and 1900 control patients to assess risk factors for nevirapine-related toxicity.[60] Women with higher CD4+ counts were at a 12 times higher risk of developing potentially fatal hepatitis compared with controls (11% vs. 0.9%). Similarly, men with higher CD4+ counts were also at higher risk than controls (6.3% versus 1.2%). The risk of asymptomatic hepatotoxicity was greatest during the first 6 weeks of therapy in this combined analysis. The pharmaceutical company that markets nevirapine, Boehringer-Ingelheim, subsequently released a warning on the risk of severe liver toxicity—on some occasions with fatal outcome—and currently only recommends the use of NVP in women with a CD4+ T-cell count less than 250 cells per microliter and in men with less than 400 cells per microliter.

Interestingly, more recent data suggest that nevirapine use is associated with overall low rates of hepatotoxicity when prescribed to patients with HIV RNA suppression, regardless of the CD4+ cell count. In a collaboration of seven observational clinical cohorts, risk factors for treatment-limiting toxicities in both antiretroviral naïve and experienced patients starting nevirapine-containing ART were explored.[160] In adjusted Cox analyses, treatment-experienced patients with high CD4+ cell counts and HIV viremia had a significantly increased risk for hypersensitivity reactions compared with naïve patients with a low CD4+ cell count (hazard ratio, 1.45; 95% CI, 1.03 to 2.03). In contrast, treatment-experienced patients with a high CD4+ cell count and viral suppression had no increased risk for developing a hypersensitivity reaction. In another cohort study of 3752 patients receiving nevirapine-based therapy, 6.2% discontinued therapy because of rash and/or hepatotoxicity.[161] However, the risk of hepatotoxicity was 50% lower among treatment-experienced patients who had viral suppression at the time of switching therapy compared with those with detectable viremia. These combined data suggest that using nevirapine in a "switch strategy" may be well tolerated provided there is no detectable viremia. However, in similar patients with a detectable viral load, it is prudent to continue to adhere to current CD4$^+$ cell count thresholds, as described previously.

Protease Inhibitors and Drug-Induced Liver Injury

Since their introduction in the mid-1990s, protease inhibitors (PIs) have become one of the integral parts of ART regimens. However, shortly after their widespread use, the following warning was incorporated into product labeling approved by the U.S. Food and Drug Administration for HIV-1 PIs: (1) hepatitis, including cases resulting in hepatic failure and death, has been reported in patients taking PIs; and (2) there may be an increased risk for alanine aminotransferase and/or aspartate aminotransferase (ALT/AST) elevations in patients with preexisting liver disease or underlying hepatitis B virus (HBV) or hepatitis C virus (HCV) infection. An increased frequency of AST/ALT monitoring should be considered for these patients. Thus research has focused on relative safety and the spectrum of liver abnormality linked to the PIs.

Unconjugated Hyperbilirubinemia Associated with Specific PIs: Indinavir and Atazanavir

In clinical trials, indinavir and atazanavir were associated with increases in unconjugated bilirubin in 6% to 40% of patients.[12,162] However, this phenomenon was not associated with signs or symptoms of hepatocellular injury, such as increases in serum liver enzyme levels; in addition, levels of bilirubin returned to normal after the discontinuation of the drug in all subjects. Research by Zucker and colleagues[13] demonstrated that indinavir directly inhibits the activity of the hepatic enzyme UDP glucuronosyltransferase (UGT), leading to the development of a reversible, asymptomatic, indirect hyperbilirubinemia that clinically resembles Gilbert syndrome. Not surprisingly, the effect of indinavir on serum levels of unconjugated bilirubin is most pronounced in persons with a polymorphism in the gene *UGT1*, which is associated with Gilbert syndrome. In indinavir-treated HIV-infected patients lacking the Gilbert polymorphism, serum bilirubin levels were increased by a mean of 0.34 mg/dl, whereas in those patients who were either homozygous or heterozygous for the polymorphism, serum bilirubin levels were increased by a mean of 1.45 mg/dl. More recently, studies of atazanavir have demonstrated potent inhibition of the activity of UGT similar to that observed with indinavir.[162] In clinical trials, significant increases in the total bilirubin level (>2.5 times ULN) were observed in 22% to 47% of patients treated with atazanavir; however, clinical jaundice or scleral icterus was observed in only 7% to 8% of subjects, and discontinuation of therapy because of unconjugated hyperbilirubinemia was rare (<1%). Nonetheless, the manufacturer of atazanavir, Bristol-Meyers Squibb, recommends that alternative therapies be considered if jaundice or scleral icterus presents cosmetic concerns for patients (see product label for Reyataz [atazanavir]). Taken together (although increases in unconjugated or indirect bilirubin are commonly seen in HIV-infected patients who receive atazanavir and indinavir)

this phenomenon does not reflect hepatocellular injury and should not be considered in the spectrum of hepatotoxicity related to PIs.

Early during the era of PI-based HAART, a prospective cohort study of ART therapy among 298 patients prescribed a new ART regimen found the incidence of severe hepatotoxicity (grade 3 to 4) was 10.4% (95% CI, 7.2% to 14.4%).[26] However, the incidence of severe hepatotoxicity was higher in patients who received full-dose ritonavir than in those who received dual NRTIs, indinavir, nelfinavir, or saquinavir (without concurrent ritonavir). Ritonavir (full-dose) use was associated with 48% of all cases of severe hepatotoxicity and with the highest incidence of toxicity (incidence, 30%; 95% CI, 17.9% to 44.6%). In this study, the risk of severe hepatotoxicity with the use of NRTIs was similar to that with use of indinavir, nelfinavir, or saquinavir (without the concurrent use of ritonavir). Hepatotoxicity of any grade was higher (54%) in patients infected with HCV, compared with 39% of uninfected patients. However, no severe hepatotoxicity developed in 139 (88%) of 158 patients with evidence of chronic HBV or HCV infection. In a multivariate analysis, only full-dose ritonavir use and a CD4$^+$ cell count increase of greater than 50 mm^3 cells were associated with severe hepatotoxicity. Among individuals who did not receive ritonavir-containing regimens, HCV and/or HBV co-infection was associated with an increased risk of severe hepatotoxicity (relative risk [RR], 3.7; 95% CI, 1.0% to 11.8%). However, most co-infected patients (88%) did not experience significant hepatotoxicity.[26]

Studies in Europe have had similar findings. In the Swiss HIV Cohort Study cohort,[25] grade 4 liver enzyme elevations occurred in 35 (6.3%) of 560 patients, of whom 6 (17.1%) were symptomatic and 12 (34%) discontinued ART. In multivariate analysis, independent risk factors for grade 4 liver injury were higher baseline ALT levels (hazard ratio [HR], 1.05 for each 10 U increase), chronic HBV infection (HR, 9.2), chronic HCV infection (HR, 5.0), the use of first-line potent ART combination regimens in patients without prior NRTI treatment (HR, 2.8), recent start of nevirapine (HR, 9.6) or ritonavir (HR, 4.9) therapy, and female sex (HR, 2.8). Furthermore, among patients chronically co-infected with HBV, discontinuing the use of lamivudine (3TC) was associated with the development of grade 4 liver enzyme elevations (HR, 6.8).

Of significance, in the study by Wit and colleagues, the use of low-dose ritonavir-based ART (i.e., <200 mg/day) was not associated with any cases of grade 4 hepatotoxicity. Furthermore, in a randomized controlled trial that compared lopinavir therapy boosted with low-dose ritonavir and nelfinavir, only 4.5% of lopinavir/ritonavir recipients developed an AST or ALT level greater than five times the ULN, which was similar to the incidence observed in nelfinavir recipients (5.2%).[163] Similarly, Sulkowski and associates[19] reported that in a prospective cohort analysis of 1161 PI-naïve, HIV-infected patients receiving RTV-boosted (lopinavir, indinavir, and saquinavir) and unboosted PI-based ART (indinavir, nelfinavir), the incidence of severe liver enzyme elevations among PI-naïve patients was: nelfinavir, 11%; lopinavir/RTV (200 mg/day), 9%; indinavir, 13%; indinavir/RTV (200 to 400 mg/day), 12.8%; and saquinavir/RTV (800 mg/day), 17.2%. Importantly, the analysis suggested that low-dose RTV used to boost PI concentration did not appear to alter the risk of liver injury beyond that of the parent PI.[19] Taken together, these studies indicate that the use of ART with full-dose ritonavir (i.e., >400 mg of ritonavir daily) was associated with an increased risk of liver injury compared with other PI-based ART regimens. However, the use of low-dose ritonavir to boost other PIs has not been associated with a greater risk of liver injury compared with other nonboosted PIs. This is important because current HIV treatment guidelines recommend the use of ritonavir-boosted PIs (PI/r) due to the favorable pharmacokinetic profile and documented effectiveness.

Newer PIs may also carry the same risks. Tipranavir (TPV) is approved by the FDA for use in combination with low-dose ritonavir for treatment experienced patients with HIV strains resistant to first-generation PIs. In the phase II and III TPV/ritonavir trials ($N = 1299$), 11.1% of TPV/r patients receiving 500/200 mg bid developed grade 3 or 4 ALT/AST elevations through 96 weeks of TPV/r-based ART treatment in the studies.[164] In a multivariate Cox regression model, the risk of developing grade 3 or grade 4 hepatotoxicity was related to the use of tipranavir, HBV/HCV co-infection, baseline abnormalities of aminotransferases, and a pretreatment CD4 count greater than 200 cells/mm^3.[165] Thus, among currently available PIs, full-dose ritonavir and tipranavir boosted with ritonavir has been associated with a markedly higher incidence of significant drug-induced liver injury, whereas other PI regimens have had similar rates of DILI in most settings.

Hepatotoxicity of Later-Generation Antiretroviral Agents

In addition to the nucleoside analogs, nonnucleoside reverse transcriptase inhibitors, and protease inhibitors, integrase inhibitors and CCR5 antagonists have been developed for HIV treatment.

CCR5 Antagonists

CCR5 antagonists block HIV cell entry through competitive binding to the CCR5 receptor present on the surface of CD4$^+$ T cells. Concern about hepatotoxicity with CCR5 antagonists was heightened when the development of aplaviroc (another drug in this class) was halted because of severe hepatotoxicity, raising the possibility of a class effect side effect.[166]

Subsequently, maraviroc was developed; this agent is moderately metabolized in the liver, primarily via the CYP3A4 isozyme.[167] Although clinical trial data among treatment-experienced patients demonstrate overall safety, there was low representation of patients with chronic viral hepatitis.[168] Furthermore, severe hepatotoxicity occurred in one of 1300 patients who were enrolled in the phase 2b/3 clinical program.[164] However, this patient was also taking other known hepatotoxic agents (i.e., isoniazid, trimethoprim-sulfamethoxazole). Thus, while data is still emerging regarding the hepatic safety of CCR5 antagonists, the available data do not indicate any unique toxicity with maraviroc.

Integrase Inhibitors

Raltegravir is an integrase inhibitor with potent in vitro activity against both wild-type and multidrug-resistant HIV. Raltegravir was associated with high rates of virologic suppression and immunologic improvements in both treatment-naïve and treatment-experienced patient populations.[169,170] In comparative clinical trials, the overall adverse event profile of raltegravir has been similar to a placebo. It is metabolized by hepatic glucuronidation and has no effect on cytochrome 3A4. Dosing adjustments are not necessary in patients with renal or mild to moderate hepatic dysfunction.[171]

Fusion Inhibitors

Enfuvirtide, the only approved fusion inhibitor, has demonstrated a consistent safety record in terms of liver toxicity.[172]

Other Drugs and Drug-Induced Liver Injury in HIV-Infected Patients

HIV patients often require treatment for co-morbid conditions (e.g., fungal infections, *Pneumocystis pneumoniae*, herpes, cytomegalovirus, tuberculosis, hyperlipidemia) with medications that may also cause hepatotoxicity, independent of ART[173] (**Table 38-4**). Antituberculosis drugs (isoniazid, rifampicin, and pyrazinamide) can cause direct hepatotoxicity and immune-mediated hepatic necrosis.[174,175] Several studies have examined the risk of hepatotoxicity of antituberculosis therapy in patients who are co-infected with HCV or HBV. In one study, the risk of DILI in HIV-infected patients with concomitant HCV was increased 14.4-fold compared with TB patients with either viral infection.[176] However, another study from India suggested that antituberculosis therapy was safe in co-infected patients.[177]

Table 38-4 Non-HIV Drugs Associated with Drug-Induced Liver Injury

DRUG	EXAMPLE	HEPATOTOXICITY
Antifungal agents	Ketoconazole	Increased AST and ALT Inhibits cytochrome P-450 and may increase PI levels
Macrolide antibiotic	Erythromycin	Increased ALP Inhibits cytochrome P-450 and may increase PI levels
Antituberculosis agents	Isoniazid Rifampicin Pyrazinamide	Increased AST and ALT
Antipneumocystis agents	Trimethoprim-sulfamethoxazole	Increased AST, ALT, and ALP possible
Antiherpes and cytomegalovirus	Acyclovir	Rare elevations in AST and ALT, bilirubin
Lipid-lowering agents	Statins	Increased AST and ALT
Anabolic steroids	Nandrolone	Increased ALP, bilirubin

ALP, alkaline phosphatase; ALT, alanine aminotransferase; AST, aspartate aminotransferase; PI, protease inhibitor

Therapeutic Management of Drug-Induced Liver Injury

When Should a Medication Be Discontinued?

Clinical decision-making regarding drug discontinuation has important clinical consequences. By stopping medications at the very first sign of mild injury, one can prevent serious consequences; however, this approach can unnecessarily sacrifice needed HIV antiretroviral therapy with subsequent deleterious immunologic consequences. On the other hand, continued therapy in the face of DILI can lead to untoward outcomes, such as liver failure.

For patient safety, several important principles need to be emphasized. In general, symptomatic hepatitis is much more concerning than asymptomatic elevations of aminotransferases and should prompt discontinuation of ART in most patients because the longer a patient continues to ingest a drug after onset of symptomatic hepatitis, the higher the likelihood of an untoward outcome.[17] Drug-induced hepatitis associated with overt jaundice and increased levels of direct bilirubin carries a high mortality rate (Hy's law); medications should be immediately discontinued in this clinical scenario.[178] If the patient has symptoms consistent with drug hypersensitivity such as a fever or rash (e.g., abacavir or nevirapine hypersensitivity), the medication should be stopped immediately; readministration can be fatal. In addition, the diagnosis of clinically significant mitochondrial toxicity due to NRTIs (e.g., hepatomegaly, steatosis, lactic acidosis) should prompt the immediate discontinuation of ART.

Most authorities agree that medications should be discontinued promptly if ALT or AST levels are greater than 10 times the upper limit of normal, even if the patient is asymptomatic.[179] For patients with advanced liver disease, more conservative management should be exercised to prevent hepatic decompensation.[30] Special caution should be exercised with newly marketed medications because the true hepatotoxic potential of the drug may not have been recognized in premarketing clinical studies.

Alternative causes for elevations of aminotransferases, including viral hepatitis (e.g., acute hepatitis A, hepatitis B flare, and hepatitis D superinfection), cholecystitis, alcohol, cocaine, and opportunistic infections, should also be considered. Interpretation of elevated aminotransferases in patients with HIV/HBV co-infection can be challenging. HBV reactivation and seroconversion following the introduction of ART have been reported.[46,51,52] In addition, the discontinuation of ART regimens that contain drugs active against HBV (e.g., lamivudine) has been associated with significant liver enzyme flares in HIV-infected patients co-infected with chronic hepatitis B.[25,53] Thus available data suggest that there are multiple potential causes for increased liver function test results in HIV/HBV–co-infected patients in addition to DILI. Furthermore, while HBV co-infected patients can be safely treated with ART, which includes dually active drugs, such patients should be closely monitored for changes in their HBV replication status.[180-182]

An algorithm for managing liver injury related to antiretroviral therapy is shown in **Figure 38-1**. Clinical management

of antiretroviral-associated hepatotoxicity must be individualized. In addition, serious hepatotoxicity has been associated with the use of most of the currently available antiretroviral medications; the optimal use of these medications in persons with underlying liver disease has also not been well established. Patients with grade 3 or 4 hepatotoxicity and no symptoms of acute hepatitis that do not discontinue antiretroviral therapy should be monitored closely.[183]

Of note, although a specific drug may be suspected, in most cases of ART-associated DILI, all medication in the regimen should be discontinued simultaneously to prevent the emergence of HIV drug resistance and because absolute certainty regarding the relationship of a specific drug and DILI is often elusive.

Spontaneous Improvement in Aminotransferases with Drug Continuation

In clinical trials of new drugs, mild elevations of aminotransferases are commonly seen after treatment initiation and often improve despite administration of the same drug, a process referred to as adaptation.[184] The same observation has been noted for many antiretroviral medications, particularly the protease inhibitor class. For example, in several studies, marked declines in ALT/AST have occurred after severe elevations despite continuation of the same drug.[25,48] Based upon these data, some authors have suggested that PI-containing ART does not need immediate adjustment but simply careful monitoring.[46] It should be emphasized that most of these patients had *asymptomatic* elevations of transaminases. This could imply that either there is an adjustment or adaptation in hepatic metabolism after induction of various enzyme systems, or that the drug did not cause the original flare of transaminases, as in occult alcohol use.

At this point in time, it is not clear which patients with significant asymptomatic aminotransferase elevations can safely continue medications. If a decision is made to continue the same ART regimen, patients need to be closely monitored. Furthermore, the patient should be educated about clinical symptoms of hepatitis and medications should be discontinued immediately if symptoms arise.

It should be emphasized that this strategy applies to specific agents, such as PI-containing ART only. The occurrence of hepatotoxicity in association with signs of hypersensitivity syndrome (e.g., fever, rash) in patients taking known culprit drugs, such as nevirapine or abacavir, should lead to immediate withdrawal of the drug. Ongoing exposure in this situation can lead to a fatal outcome. Similarly, if the patient has symptoms consistent with mitochondrial toxicity (e.g., nausea, vomiting, fatigue, abdominal bloating), medications should be immediately discontinued pending results of testing for lactic acid. Drugs with a high risk of mitochondrial toxicity include stavudine and didanosine, which are less commonly used in the United States, but commonly given in developing countries.[185]

Cumulative Effects of Liver Injury

Another aspect of antiretroviral therapy that requires much more research is the issue of cumulative liver injury. In one study where the same antiretroviral medications were reintroduced in 17 patients with severe hepatotoxicity after a 4-month

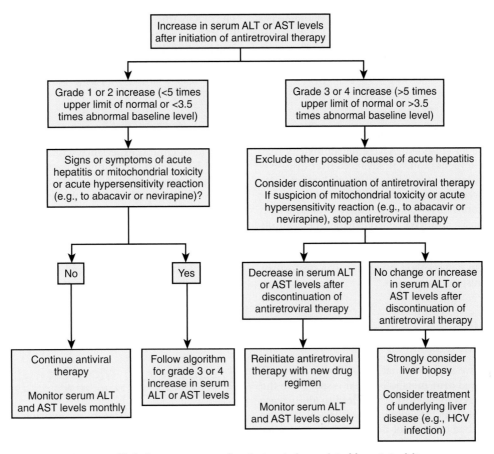

Fig. 38-1 **Clinical management of antiretroviral-associated hepatotoxicity.**

"wash-out" period, 59% successfully tolerated their medications. However, it is important to note that 41% had another episode of hepatotoxicity, limiting the success of this approach.[30] Whether there are long-term implications of recurrent liver injury in HIV-infected patients is unknown.

A related issue concerns patients who already have inflammatory changes from chronic viral hepatitis who then develop DILI. In one study, patients with chronic viral hepatitis determined by a biopsy underwent treatment with a PI-containing regimen. A subset of patients who subsequently developed severe hepatotoxicity had repeat biopsies that demonstrated a dramatic worsening of liver pathology compared with the specimen taken before ART.[42] Whether recurrent DILI can exacerbate underlying chronic viral hepatitis is unknown.

Unfortunately, the liver biopsy often does not contribute substantially to patient management or assigning causality. On occasion, histology can be helpful if eosinophils or granulomas are found, which suggest drug hypersensitivity. If mitochondrial toxicity is suspected, then histology and electron microscopy can help determine if microvesicular steatosis and evidence of mitochondrial injury is present.[186]

Use of Interferon in Patients with History of Drug-Induced Liver Injury

As discussed earlier, patients with chronic viral hepatitis have an increased risk of developing hepatotoxicity related to ART. If this occurs, strategies include continuation of medications with careful monitoring or drug discontinuation with retrial of alternative regimens.

However, an alternative approach may be to obtain a liver biopsy and treat the underlying chronic viral hepatitis before any further attempts to administer ART. The benefit of using interferon to treat underlying hepatitis C in order to reintroduce ART was demonstrated in two small case series.[30,187] In one case series, 12 patients attained notable improvement in aminotransferases and continued to receive ART treatment during a mean follow-up regimen of 27 months, with subsequent suppression of HIV RNA and significant immunologic reconstitution. However, only one patient maintained HCV suppression after completion of treatment with interferon/ribavirin therapy. The authors concluded that the beneficial effects of IFN-based therapy may be modulated through the suppression of proinflammatory cytokines (e.g., tumor necrosis factor), even in virologic nonresponders.[187] Whether this strategy will prove to be a useful adjunct in treatment of patients with a history of drug-induced liver injury will need further study.

Prevention of Drug-Induced Hepatic Injury

The most effective therapy for drug-induced liver disease is primary prevention. Unfortunately, most drug-induced hepatotoxicity is difficult to predict. Therefore the clinician must be aware of the patient's predisposing risk factors for DILI, which may help guide monitoring and management.

Patients with Suspected Advanced Liver Disease

The treatment of patients with cirrhosis must be carefully undertaken because an episode of severe hepatotoxicity may lead to hepatic decompensation.[30] If advanced liver disease is suspected, a liver biopsy or a noninvasive evaluation (e.g., serum fibrosis markers) may be considered in select cases before drug initiation. The rationale would be to make a firm diagnosis of cirrhosis and give antiretroviral medications dosed appropriately for advanced liver disease.[188] If mitochondrial toxicity is suspected, then histology and electron microscopy can help determine if microvesicular steatosis or paracrystalline inclusions are present.[186]

Potential Role of Therapeutic Drug Monitoring

Some researchers have suggested that elevated transaminases are the result of altered drug metabolism that is specific to the individual host. Altered metabolism could lead to an increase in serum drug levels, which theoretically could lead to liver injury. A well-described example of this type of drug toxicity model is the relationship between abnormal aminotransferases and elevated plasma levels of amiodarone.[34]

Altered metabolism of antiretroviral medications has also been described in the setting of virally mediated liver disease.[188] In one case control study, 70 patients taking nevirapine were separated into two groups based on whether they had developed any grade of hepatotoxicity. The median nevirapine plasma concentrations were significantly higher in subjects who developed aminotransferase elevations than in controls. In subjects with chronic hepatic C, nevirapine plasma levels above 6 μg/ml were associated with a 92% risk of liver toxicity, suggesting a potential role for therapeutic drug monitoring in this patient subgroup.[70] However, other studies of nevirapine did not support this finding of altered pharmacokinetics in the setting of viral hepatitis.[189]

In contrast, another drug within the same NNRTI category, efavirenz, has been associated with elevated serum concentrations among patients with advanced liver disease in several studies. In one pharmacokinetic study, 268 HIV/HCV co-infected patients underwent plasma drug concentration monitoring while taking ART regimens including either lopinavir/ritonavir, atazanavir/ritonavir, efavirenz, or nevirapine.[190] The study results demonstrated that hepatic clearance of efavirenz was particularly impaired in patients with cirrhosis. No similar effect was seen for the protease inhibitor class in this or other studies.[191] Another study of 134 HIV-infected patients also demonstrated that efavirenz levels were excessively high in those with concomitant viral hepatitis and advanced fibrosis.[192] In summary, therapeutic drug monitoring to prevent liver injury is not supported in most patient populations, with the potential exception of efavirenz in patients with cirrhosis.

Ritonavir is a powerful inhibitor of CYP3A, which metabolizes many antiretroviral agents. In the presence of chronic viral hepatitis, ritonavir-based therapy further reduces CYP3A activity by half,[193] which may partly explain the high incidence of hepatotoxicity seen in the past when ritonavir was used in high doses.[26] In contrast, use of low-dose ritonavir for pharmacokinetic boosting of other protease inhibitors appears safe.[19]

Patient Education

Long-term clinical experience with medications such as isoniazid has shifted the emphasis away from laboratory monitoring to renewed focus on patient education. The best strategy is to educate the patient about the symptoms of drug-induced liver injury, including fatigue, nausea, vomiting, right upper quadrant pain, and jaundice. Patient education is particularly important when considering hypersensitivity reactions, which occur early and rapidly and can be devastating if the offending drug is continued. Patients need to be instructed to contact their medical provider immediately should these symptoms occur. In resource-poor countries, regular laboratory monitoring is usually not feasible and patient education takes on even greater importance.

Frequency of Monitoring: A Patient-Tailored Approach

The frequency of laboratory monitoring is uncertain. Some authors have suggested that testing of aminotransferases should be done quarterly along with routine tests for HIV RNA and CD4+ T-lymphocyte counts. Others have recommended once-monthly monitoring of liver function tests for the first 3 months and less frequent monitoring if stable.[194] Others have pointed out that cases of acute liver failure with subsequent death have occurred suddenly without warning despite regular follow-up.[41] These authors suggested that laboratory monitoring has poor predictability.

A strategy that incorporates more frequent monitoring in patients with risk factors for drug-induced liver injury has been employed in the treatment of tuberculosis.[195] A similar model for HIV patients undergoing antiretroviral therapy should be considered where more frequent monitoring is focused on those at higher risk of DILI.[25] For example, more vigilant monitoring should be considered in patients with abnormal aminotransferases before treatment, because this factor has been identified as a major risk factor for DILI. Patients with a history of DILI need careful monitoring because of the risk of recurrent hepatotoxicity, even if all medications in the regimen are changed. Frequent monitoring should also be employed in those with a history of alcohol use.

In patients with preexisting liver disease and cirrhosis, bimonthly monitoring after initiation of ART followed by monthly evaluations has been proposed by some experts.[196] Laboratory surveillance in this patient subset should also include measurements of prothrombin and albumin in order to follow synthetic function.

Frequency and timing of monitoring may also be guided by drug selection. For example, a patient who is prescribed nevirapine should be educated about hypersensitivity reactions and be monitored within 1 to 6 weeks because most reactions occur early after medication initiation.

Decreasing the Risk for Drug-Induced Liver Injury

As noted above, one of the most consistent risk factors for onset of hepatotoxicity is underlying chronic viral hepatitis. One retrospective study of 132 co-infected patients identified 49 episodes of drug-related toxicity during a mean of 35 months of follow-up after interferon-based therapy for hepatitis C infection. The yearly incidence of hepatic events was significantly greater in patients who did not achieve a sustained virologic response compared with those who did, suggesting that viral eradication of hepatitis C decreased the risk of drug-induced liver injury.[197]

Counseling patients about other potential hepatotoxins, such as alcohol, cocaine, and other over-the-counter drugs (e.g., acetaminophen, herbal remedies) is also important. Chronic use of alcohol is especially pertinent; alcohol can predispose to hepatocyte injury by increasing oxidative damage to mitochondrial DNA, further depleting stores of glutathione, an important scavenger of free oxygen radicals.[198]

Is There a Role for Antiretroviral Therapy in Preventing Disease in HIV-Infected Persons?

Despite their potential liver toxicity, ARTs usually are safe for the vast majority of co-infected patients. In one series, 84% of 568 HIV-infected patients with HBV or HCV co-infection did not develop severe hepatotoxicity.[47] Another evaluation found no evidence that ART caused severe histologic liver disease in HIV/HCV co-infected patients. In fact, in this series, suppression of HIV replication to undetectable levels was associated with less liver necrosis and inflammation.[100]

Furthermore, in many studies, advanced immunosuppression (e.g., CD4$^+$ cell count <200 cells per microliter) has been independently associated with an increased risk of advanced histologic and/or clinical liver disease in persons with HIV/HCV co-infection.[199] This inverse relationship between CD4$^+$ cell count and liver disease supports the hypothesis that reversal or prevention of immunosuppression by means of ART will decrease the rate of HCV-related fibrosis progression and the risk of cirrhosis and its clinical consequences (end-stage liver disease, hepatocellular carcinoma, and death) in HIV-infected patients. For example, Benhamou and colleagues[200] reported that HIV/HCV–co-infected patients who received PI-based ART had a significantly decreased rate of fibrosis progression compared with those who did not receive treatment or who received less-effective ART regimens. Similarly, Macías and associates[201] reported that HCV-infected patients exposed to PI-based HAART had less fibrosis than those who did not receive treatment or who received other ARTs.

More recently, the liver histology findings for HIV/HCV co-infected patients receiving ART as their only therapy were comparable with those for HCV monoinfected patients.[202] The mean fibrosis stage for co-infected patients who did not receive therapy or who received NRTIs only or who received ART after NRTIs was significantly more advanced than that for HCV monoinfected patients. The rate of fibrosis progression in those receiving only ART was similar to that in HCV monoinfected patients but was significantly faster than that in other HIV/HCV co-infected patients. In another study, ART that led to an undetectable HIV RNA (<400 copies/ml) in HIV/HCV co-infected patients was found to be associated with rates of fibrosis progression similar to those in HCV monoinfected patients. In addition, co-infected patients with an undetectable HIV RNA level had rates of fibrosis progression that were slower than those in patients with any detectable HIV RNA level.[203] Finally, decreased liver disease–related mortality among HIV-infected persons who had received ART has been reported.[204,205] Therefore the benefit of ART clearly outweighed its toxicity.

The mechanism of improved outcomes of ART is not clear. It may mediate its beneficial effects through the restoration of Kupffer cells, which may play a central role in controlling microbial translocation.[206] Microbial translocation may be a mechanism through which HIV accelerates fibrosis progression in patients with co-existing HCV.[207]

Conclusion

Although life-saving, antiretroviral medications can lead to significant drug-induced liver injury. Fortunately, advances in drug development have led to later-generation antiviral medications that have better overall hepatic safety profiles within existing drug classes (e.g., nucleotide reverse transcriptase inhibitor, tenofovir). Agents within new classes of drugs, such as integrase inhibitors, have exhibited excellent hepatic safety records to date. There are also data suggesting that control of HIV itself may lead to a decrease in risk of drug injury with known hepatotoxic agents, such as nevirapine. This observation may lead to new insights into mechanisms of hepatic injury. Finally, although drug-induced hepatotoxicity can lead to significant morbidity and mortality among certain individuals, the benefits of potent antiretroviral medications far outweigh their risk.

Key References

Anderson PL, et al. Pharmacogenetic characteristics of indinavir, zidovudine, and lamivudine therapy in HIV-infected adults: a pilot study. J Acquir Immune Defic Syndr 2006;42:441–449. (Ref.11)

Aranzabal L, et al. Influence of liver fibrosis on highly active antiretroviral therapy-associated hepatotoxicity in patients with HIV and hepatitis C virus coinfection. Clin Infect Dis 2005;40:588–593. (Ref.49)

Armstrong GL, et al. The prevalence of hepatitis C virus infection in the United States, 1999-2002. Ann Intern Med 2006;144:705–714. (Ref.24)

Balagopal A, et al. Human immunodeficiency virus–related microbial translocation and progression of hepatitis C. Gastroenterology 2008;135:226–233. (Ref.207)

Balagopal A, et al. Kupffer cells are depleted with HIV immunodeficiency and partially recovered with antiretroviral immune reconstitution. AIDS 2009;23:2397–2404. (Ref.206)

Bani-Sadr F, et al. Hepatic steatosis in HIV-HCV coinfected patients: analysis of risk factors. AIDS 2006;20:525–531. (Ref.136)

Bani-Sadr F, et al. Risk factors for symptomatic mitochondrial toxicity in HIV/hepatitis C virus–coinfected patients during interferon plus ribavirin-based therapy. J Acquir Immune Defic Syndr 2005;40:47–52. (Ref.100)

Barreiro P, et al. Influence of liver fibrosis stage on plasma levels of antiretroviral drugs in HIV-infected patients with chronic hepatitis C. J Infect Dis 2007;195:973–979. (Ref.190)

Björnsson E. Drug-induced liver injury: Hy's rule revisited. Clin Pharmacol Ther 2006;79:521–528. (Ref.35)

Braitstein P, et al. Special considerations in the initiation and management of antiretroviral therapy in individuals coinfected with HIV and hepatitis C. AIDS 2004;18:2221–2234. (Ref.5)

Bräu N, et al. Slower fibrosis progression in HIV/HCV-coinfected patients with successful HIV suppression using antiretroviral therapy. J Hepatol 2006;44: 47–55. (Ref.203)

Cammett AM, et al. Pharmacokinetic assessment of nevirapine and metabolites in human immunodeficiency virus type 1–infected patients with hepatic fibrosis. Antimicrob Agents Chemother 2009;53:4147–4152. (Ref.189)

Crum-Cianflone N, et al. Nonalcoholic fatty liver disease among HIV-infected persons. J Acquir Immune Defic Syndr 2009;50:464–473. (Ref.132)

Davis CM, Shearer WT. Diagnosis and management of HIV drug hypersensitivity. J Allergy Clin Immunol 2008;121:826–832. (Ref.79)

de Mendoza C, et al. Mitochondrial DNA depletion in HIV-infected patients is more pronounced with chronic hepatitis C and enhanced following treatment with pegylated interferon plus ribavirin. Antivir Ther 2005;10: 557–561. (Ref.95)

de Mendoza C, Soriano V. The role of hepatitis C virus (HCV) in mitochondrial DNA damage in HIV/HCV-coinfected individuals. Antivir Ther 2005;10(Suppl 2):M109–M115. (Ref.94)

Drugs for HIV infection. Med Lett Drugs Ther 2008;50:2–3. (Ref.171)

Forna F, et al. Clinical toxicity of highly active antiretroviral therapy in a home-based AIDS care program in rural Uganda. J Acquir Immune Defic Syndr 2007;44:456–462. (Ref.185)

French AL, et al. Longitudinal effect of antiretroviral therapy on markers of hepatic toxicity: impact of hepatitis C coinfection. Clin Infect Dis 2004;39:402–410. (Ref.123)

French MA. HIV/AIDS: immune reconstitution inflammatory syndrome: a reappraisal. Clin Infect Dis 2009;48:101–107. (Ref.105)

Fulco PP, McNicholl IR. Etravirine and rilpivirine: nonnucleoside reverse transcriptase inhibitors with activity against human immunodeficiency virus type 1 strains resistant to previous nonnucleoside agents. Pharmacotherapy 2009;29:281–294. (Ref.154)

Gaslightwala I, Bini EJ. Impact of human immunodeficiency virus infection on the prevalence and severity of steatosis in patients with chronic hepatitis C virus infection. J Hepatol 2006;44:1026–1032. (Ref.139)

Guaraldi G, et al. Nonalcoholic fatty liver disease in HIV-infected patients referred to a metabolic clinic: prevalence, characteristics, and predictors. Clin Infect Dis 2008;47:250–257. (Ref.128)

Gulick RM, et al. Maraviroc for previously treated patients with R5 HIV-1 infection. N Engl J Med 2008;359:1429–1441. (Ref.168)

Haas DW, et al. Pharmacogenetics of nevirapine-associated hepatotoxicity: an adult AIDS clinical trials group collaboration. Clin Infect Dis 2006;43: 783–786. (Ref.74)

Hammer SM, et al. Antiretroviral treatment of adult HIV infection: 2008 recommendations of the International AIDS Society-USA panel. JAMA 2008;300:555–570. (Ref.88)

Ingiliz P, et al. Liver damage underlying unexplained transaminase elevation in human immunodeficiency virus-1 mono-infected patients on antiretroviral therapy. Hepatology 2009;49:436–442. (Ref.133)

Jain MK. Drug-induced liver injury associated with HIV medications. Clin Liver Dis 2007;11:615–639. (Ref.124)

Kesselring AM, et al. Risk factors for treatment-limiting toxicities in patients starting nevirapine-containing antiretroviral therapy. AIDS 2009;23: 1689–1699. (Ref.160)

Knox TA, et al. Ritonavir greatly impairs CYP3A activity in HIV infection with chronic viral hepatitis. J Acquir Immune Defic Syndr 2008;49:358–368. (Ref.193)

Kottilil S, Polis MA, Kovacs JA. HIV infection, hepatitis C infection, and HAART: hard clinical choices. JAMA 2004;292:243–250. (Ref.22)

Kovari H, et al. Association of noncirrhotic portal hypertension in HIV-infected persons and antiretroviral therapy with didanosine: a nested case-control study. Clin Infect Dis 2009;49:626–635. (Ref.151)

Labarga P, et al. Hepatotoxicity of antiretroviral drugs is reduced after successful treatment of chronic hepatitis C in HIV-infected patients. J Infect Dis 2007;196:670–676. (Ref.197)

Laguno M, et al. Incidence and risk factors for mitochondrial toxicity in treated HIV/HCV-coinfected patients. Antivir Ther 2005;10:423–429. (Ref.101)

Lankisch TO, et al. Gilbert's disease and atazanavir: from phenotype to UDP-glucuronosyltransferase haplotype. Hepatology 2006;44:1324–1332. (Ref.16)

Lennox JL, et al. Safety and efficacy of raltegravir-based versus efavirenz-based combination therapy in treatment-naive patients with HIV-1 infection: a multicentre, double-blind randomised controlled trial. Lancet 2009;374: 796–806. (Ref.169)

Lesi OA, Soyebi KS, Eboh CN. Fatty liver and hyperlipidemia in a cohort of HIV-positive Africans on highly active antiretroviral therapy. J Natl Med Assoc 2009;101:151–155. (Ref.131)

Lieberman-Blum SS, Fung HB, Bandres JC. Maraviroc: a CCR5-receptor antagonist for the treatment of HIV-1 infection. Clin Ther 2008;30:1228–1250. (Ref.168)

Loulergue P, et al. Hepatic steatosis as an emerging cause of cirrhosis in HIV-infected patients. J Acquir Immune Defic Syndr 2007;45:365. (Ref.134)

Macias J, et al. Antiretroviral therapy based on protease inhibitors as a protective factor against liver fibrosis progression in patients with chronic hepatitis C. Antivir Ther 2006;11:839–846. (Ref.201)

Maida I, et al. Liver enzyme elevation in hepatitis C virus (HCV)-HIV–coinfected patients prior to and after initiating HAART: role of HCV genotypes. AIDS Res Hum Retroviruses 2006;22:139–143. (Ref.125)

Mallal S, et al. HLA-B*5701 screening for hypersensitivity to abacavir. N Engl J Med 2008;358:568–579. (Ref.85)

Mallet V, et al. Nodular regenerative hyperplasia is a new cause of chronic liver disease in HIV-infected patients. AIDS 2007;21:187–192. (Ref.149)

Marks KM, et al. Histologic findings and clinical characteristics associated with hepatic steatosis in patients coinfected with HIV and hepatitis C virus. J Infect Dis 2005;192:1943–1949. (Ref.137)

Martin AM, et al. Immune responses to abacavir in antigen-presenting cells from hypersensitive patients. AIDS 2007;21:1233–1244. (Ref.83)

Martin AM, et al. Predisposition to abacavir hypersensitivity conferred by HLA-B*5701 and a haplotypic Hsp70-Hom variant. Proc Natl Acad Sci U S A 2004;101:4180–4185. (Ref.82)

Mayer H. Case study of a patient with serious hepatotoxicity in maraviroc IIB/III trial. Presented at Targeting HIV Entry—First International Workshop. Bethesda, MD, Dec 3, 2005. (Ref.164)

McCabe SM, et al. Antiretroviral therapy: pharmacokinetic considerations in patients with renal or hepatic impairment. Clin Pharmacokinet 2008;47: 153–172. (Ref.188)

McGovern B. Hepatic safety and HAART. J Int Assoc Physicians AIDS Care (Chic). 2004;3(Suppl 2):S24–S40. (Ref.78)

McGovern BH, et al. Managing symptomatic drug-induced liver injury in HIV-hepatitis C virus–coinfected patients: a role for interferon. Clin Infect Dis 2007;45:1386–1392. (Ref.187)

McGovern BH, et al. Hepatic steatosis is associated with fibrosis, nucleoside analogue use, and hepatitis C virus genotype 3 infection in HIV-seropositive patients. Clin Infect Dis 2006;43:365–372. (Ref.138)

McKoy JM, et al. Hepatotoxicity associated with long- versus short-course HIV-prophylactic nevirapine use: a systematic review and meta-analysis from the research on adverse drug events and reports (RADAR) project. Drug Saf 2009;32:147–158. (Ref.158)

Mehta SH, et al. The effect of antiretroviral therapy on liver disease among adults with HIV and hepatitis C coinfection. Hepatology 2005;41:123–131. (Ref.204)

Meraviglia P, et al. Lopinavir/ritonavir treatment in HIV antiretroviral-experienced patients: evaluation of risk factors for liver enzyme elevation. HIV Med 2004;5:334–343. (Ref.20)

Meynard JL, et al. Influence of liver fibrosis stage on plasma levels of efavirenz in HIV-infected patients with chronic hepatitis B or C. J Antimicrob Chemother 2009;63:579–584. (Ref.192)

Micheli V, et al. Lopinavir/ritonavir pharmacokinetics in HIV/HCV-coinfected patients with or without cirrhosis. Ther Drug Monit 2008;30:306–313. (Ref.191)

Mikl J, et al. Hepatic profile analyses of tipranavir in phase II and III clinical trials. BMC Infect Dis 2009;9:203. (Ref.165)

Mohammed SS, et al. HIV-positive patients with nonalcoholic fatty liver disease have a lower body mass index and are more physically active than HIV-negative patients. J Acquir Immune Defic Syndr 2007;45:432–438. (Ref.129)

Molina JM, et al. Once-daily atazanavir/ritonavir versus twice-daily lopinavir/ ritonavir, each in combination with tenofovir and emtricitabine, for management of antiretroviral-naive HIV-1–infected patients: 48 week efficacy and safety results of the CASTLE study. Lancet 2008;372:646–655. (Ref.162)

Nathwani RA, Kaplowitz N. Drug hepatotoxicity. Clin Liver Dis 2006;10:207–217. (Ref.76)

Nichols WG, et al. Hepatotoxicity observed in clinical trials of aplaviroc (GW873140). Antimicrob Agents Chemother 2008;52:858–865. (Ref.166)

Norris W, Paredes AH, Lewis JH. Drug-induced liver injury in 2007. Curr Opin Gastroenterol 2008;24:287–297. (Ref.178)

Núñez MJ, et al. Impact of antiretroviral treatment–related toxicities on hospital admissions in HIV-infected patients. AIDS Res Hum Retroviruses 2006;22:825–829. (Ref.29)

Ofotokun I, et al. Liver enzymes elevation and immune reconstitution among treatment-naïve HIV-infected patients instituting antiretroviral therapy. Am J Med Sci 2007;334:334–341. (Ref.116)

Padmapriyadarsini C, et al. Hepatitis B or hepatitis C co-infection in individuals infected with human immunodeficiency virus and effect of anti-tuberculosis drugs on liver function. J Postgrad Med 2006;52:92–96. (Ref.177)

Peters MG. Diagnosis and management of hepatitis B virus and HIV coinfection. Top HIV Med 2007;15:163–166. (Ref.6)

Phillips EJ, et al. Clinical and immunogenetic correlates of abacavir hypersensitivity. AIDS 2005;19:979–981. (Ref.89)

Poveda E, Briz V, Soriano V. Enfuvirtide, the first fusion inhibitor to treat HIV infection. AIDS Rev 2005;7:139–147. (Ref.172)

Puoti M, et al. HIV-related liver disease: ART drugs, coinfection, and other risk factors. J Int Assoc Physicians AIDS Care (Chic) 2009;8:30–42. (Ref.7)

Ritchie MD, et al. Drug transporter and metabolizing enzyme gene variants and nonnucleoside reverse-transcriptase inhibitor hepatotoxicity. Clin Infect Dis 2006;43:779–782. (Ref.75)

Rockstroh JK, et al. Influence of hepatitis C virus infection on HIV-1 disease progression and response to highly active antiviral therapy. J Infect Dis 2005;192:992–1002. (Ref.23)

Rodriguez-Novoa S, et al. Influence of 516G greater than T polymorphisms at the gene encoding the CYP450-2B6 isoenzyme on efavirenz plasma concentrations in HIV-infected subjects. Clin Infect Dis 2005;40:1358–1361. (Ref.15)

Rodríguez-Nóvoa S, et al. Genetic factors influencing atazanavir plasma concentrations and the risk of severe hyperbilirubinemia. AIDS 2007;21:41–46. (Ref.10)

Rodríguez-Torres M, et al. Hepatic steatosis in HIV/HCV co-infected patients: correlates, efficacy and outcomes of anti-HCV therapy: a paired liver biopsy study. J Hepatol 2008;48:756–764. (Ref.140)

Rotger M, et al. Gilbert syndrome and the development of antiretroviral therapy-associated hyperbilirubinemia. J Infect Dis 2005;192:1381–1386. (Ref.12)

Ryan P, et al. Predictors of severe hepatic steatosis using abdominal ultrasound in HIV-infected patients. HIV Med 2009;10:53–59. (Ref.130)

Saag M, et al. High sensitivity of human leukocyte antigen-B*5701 as a marker for immunologically confirmed abacavir hypersensitivity in white and black patients. Clin Infect Dis 2008;46:1111–1118. (Ref.87)

Sabin CA. Pitfalls of assessing hepatotoxicity in trials and observational cohorts. Clin Infect Dis 2004;38(Suppl 2):S56–S64. (Ref.18)

Saifee S, et al. Noncirrhotic portal hypertension in patients with human immunodeficiency virus-1 infection. Clin Gastroenterol Hepatol 2008;6:1167–1169. (Ref.152)

Sanne I, et al. Severe hepatotoxicity associated with nevirapine use in HIV-infected subjects. J Infect Dis 2005;191:825–829. (Ref.27)

Saukkonen JJ, et al. An official ATS statement: hepatotoxicity of antituberculosis therapy. Am J Respir Crit Care Med 2006;174:935–952. (Ref.174)

Servin-Abad L, et al. Liver enzymes elevation after HAART in HIV-HCV co-infection. J Viral Hepat 2005;12:429–434. (Ref.121)

Shear NH, et al. A review of drug patch testing and implications for HIV clinicians. AIDS 2008;22:999–1007. (Ref.90)

Soriano V, et al. Antiretroviral drugs and liver injury. AIDS 2008;22:1–13. (Ref.17)

Soriano V, et al. Care of HIV patients with chronic hepatitis B: updated recommendations from the HIV-Hepatitis B Virus International Panel. AIDS 2008;22:1399–1410. (Ref.3)

Steigbige RTL, et al. Raltegravir with optimized background therapy for resistant HIV-1 infection. N Engl J Med 2008;359:339–354. (Ref.170)

Sterling RK, et al. The prevalence and risk factors for abnormal liver enzymes in HIV-positive patients without hepatitis B or C coinfections. Dig Dis Sci 2008;53:1375–1382. (Ref.21)

Sterling RK, et al. Steatohepatitis: risk factors and impact on disease severity in HIV-HCV coinfection. Hepatology 2008;47:1118–1127. (Ref.141)

Sulkowski MS. Management of hepatic complications in HIV-infected persons. J Infect Dis 2008;197(Suppl 3):S279–S293. (Ref.179)

Sulkowski MS, et al. Hepatotoxicity associated with protease inhibitor-based antiretroviral regimens with or without concurrent ritonavir. AIDS 2004;18:2277–2284. (Ref.19)

Sulkowski MS, et al. Hepatic steatosis and antiretroviral drug use among adults coinfected with HIV and hepatitis C virus. AIDS 2005;19:585–592. (Ref.135)

Torriani FJ, et al. Peginterferon Alfa-2a plus ribavirin for chronic hepatitis C virus infection in HIV-infected patients. N Engl J Med 2004;351:438–450. (Ref.99)

Torti C, et al. Influence of genotype 3 hepatitis C coinfection on liver enzyme elevation in HIV-1-positive patients after commencement of a new highly active antiretroviral regimen: results from the EPOKA-MASTER cohort. J Acquir Immune Defic Syndr 2006;41:180–185. (Ref.50)

Tostmann A, et al. Antituberculosis drug-induced hepatotoxicity: concise up-to-date review. J Gastroenterol Hepatol 2008;23:192–202. (Ref.175)

Tozzi V. Pharmacogenetics of antiretrovirals. Antiviral Res 2010;85:190–200. (Ref.80)

Verma S, et al. Do type and duration of antiretroviral therapy attenuate liver fibrosis in HIV-hepatitis C virus–coinfected patients? Clin Infect Dis 2006;42:262–270. (Ref.202)

Wit FW, et al. Discontinuation of nevirapine because of hypersensitivity reactions in patients with prior treatment experience, compared with treatment-naive patients: the ATHENA cohort study. Clin Infect Dis 2008;46:933–940. (Ref.161)

Zhang D, et al. In vitro inhibition of UDP glucuronosyltransferases by atazanavir and other HIV protease inhibitors and the relationship of this property to in vivo bilirubin glucuronidation. Drug Metab Dispos 2005;33:1729–1739. (Ref.14)

A complete list of references can be found at www.expertconsult.com.

Chapter 39

Hepatitis B and C in Non–Liver Transplant Patients

Hari S. Conjeevaram and Anna S.F. Lok

ABBREVIATIONS

ALT alanine aminotransferase
anti-HBc hepatitis B core antibody
anti-HBs hepatitis B surface antibody
AST aspartate aminotransferase
ASTP American Society of Transplant Surgeons
BMT bone marrow transplantation

FCH fibrosing cholestatic hepatitis
HBeAg hepatitis B e antigen
HBsAg hepatitis B surface antigen
HBV hepatitis B virus
HCC hepatocellular carcinoma
HCV hepatitis C virus
IFN interferon

NAT nucleic acid testing
PEG-IFN pegylated interferon
SOS sinusoidal obstruction syndrome
SVR sustained virologic response
VOD veno-occlusive disease

Introduction

Chronic hepatitis B and C infections can have an impact on the outcomes of non–liver transplant patients, including bone marrow and solid organ transplants such as the kidneys, heart, and lungs. Immunosuppressive therapy associated with transplantation may lead to reactivation of hepatitis B (HBV) and C (HCV) virus replication and acceleration of progression of the underlying liver disease. In addition, patients with hepatitis B and C may be at greater risk of developing sinusoidal obstruction syndrome (SOS), formerly called veno-occlusive disease (VOD), after bone marrow transplantation (BMT).

Reactivation of hepatitis virus replication may be prevented by the administration of antiviral therapy before or after transplantation. Oral antiviral therapy has been shown to be safe and effective in preventing reactivation of hepatitis B. Reactivation of hepatitis C in transplant patients is less common than reactivation of hepatitis B, but antiviral therapy for hepatitis C is difficult to implement in transplant patients because interferon is associated with many side effects, including bone marrow suppression and increased risk of graft rejection. In addition, ribavirin is excreted by the kidneys and contraindicated in patients with renal failure.

Transmission of HBV and HCV through bone marrow or non-liver solid organ transplantation has been reported, but serologic screening of organ donors has made this a rare event.

This review will discuss the effect of immunosuppression associated with transplantation on the outcomes of hepatitis B and C, the impact of underlying hepatitis B and C on the outcomes of bone marrow and non-liver solid organ transplants, the role of antiviral therapy in improving these outcomes, and the risks of transmission of HBV and HCV through bone marrow and non-liver solid organ transplantation.

Hepatitis B

The outcome of hepatitis B in transplant patients depends on several factors including the status of hepatitis B before initiation of immunosuppression and the type of immunosuppression used after transplantation. Among patients who are hepatitis B surface antigen (HBsAg) positive, those who are hepatitis B e antigen (HBeAg) positive or have high levels of serum HBV DNA are more likely to experience reactivation of hepatitis B than patients who are HBeAg negative or have low or undetectable serum HBV DNA before immunosuppression. Reactivation of HBV replication with reappearance of HBsAg can also occur in patients with serologic evidence of past infection (presence of hepatitis B core antibody [anti-HBc] with or without hepatitis B surface antibody [anti-HBs]), and is referred to as reverse seroconversion or seroreversion (**Fig. 39-1**).

Reactivation of hepatitis B after bone marrow or solid organ transplantation can manifest in several forms: (1) acute hepatitis that usually recovers but occasionally can lead to liver failure and death; (2) worsening of underlying chronic hepatitis with accelerated progression to cirrhosis; and (3) rise in serum HBV DNA without overt evidence of liver injury.[1] Prophylactic antiviral therapy has been shown to prevent reactivation of hepatitis B but controversy remains regarding which transplant patients require antiviral prophylaxis and when antiviral therapy can be stopped.

All patients being evaluated for bone marrow or non-liver solid organ transplantation should be screened for HBV infection by testing for HBsAg, anti-HBs, and anti-HBc.[2] In patients who are HBsAg positive, antiviral prophylaxis is recommended before or at the onset of immunosuppression, regardless of HBeAg or HBV DNA status. Initiation of antiviral therapy

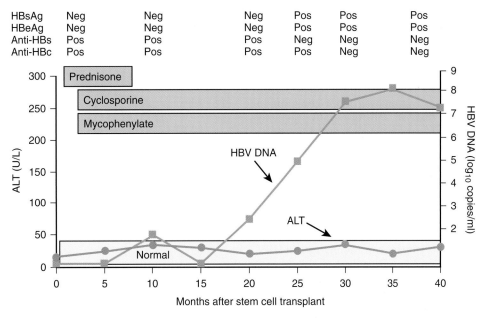

Fig. 39-1 Reverse seroconversion after bone marrow transplantation. The patient was HBsAg negative but anti-HBs positive and anti-HBc positive before transplantation *and* became HBsAg positive with high HBV DNA levels after transplantation. *(From Hoofnagle JH. Reactivation of hepatitis B. Hepatology 2009;49:S156–S165.)*

when clinical hepatitis is evident may not be effective because it will take several weeks before adequate HBV DNA suppression occurs and even longer for hepatitis to resolve. In patients with serologic markers of prior exposure to hepatitis B (anti-HBc ± anti-HBs), reactivation of HBV replication is less common and it is unclear whether antiviral therapy should be administered prophylactically in all patients or only when an increase in serum HBV DNA is observed. Because reactivation of HBV replication can occur many years after transplantation, the latter approach will require long-term monitoring of serum HBV DNA.

Screening of organ donors for HBsAg and anti-HBc has decreased the risk of HBV transmission from bone marrow and non-liver solid organ transplantation to negligible levels, especially when individuals test negative for both markers. Whether the addition of nucleic acid testing (NAT) will reduce this risk further is unclear. In a recent analysis of the efficacy of serologic marker screening in detecting HBV infection in organ, tissue, and cell donors, the prevalence of HBV DNA in organ donors who were seronegative for HBV markers (HBsAg, anti-HBc, and anti-HBs negative) or had isolated anti-HBs (immunity after vaccination) was found to be 0.07% (95% confidence interval [CI], 0.01% to 0.40%)[3]; however, the risk of transmission of HBV infection may be higher if one considers the donation of multiple organs or tissues from the same donor.

Bone Marrow Transplantation

Incidence and Risk Factors Associated with Reactivation of Hepatitis B

The prevalence of HBsAg among patients undergoing BMT is comparable to that in the general population in the region of study. Immunosuppression associated with BMT can result

not only in reactivation of HBV replication in patients who are chronically infected with HBV but also in those with immunity to HBV. Among patients with a history of resolved hepatitis B before undergoing BMT, it has been shown that anti-HBs titers decline and serum HBV DNA may become detectable following transplantation.[4] In some patients, serum HBV DNA persist at low levels with no obvious evidence of liver injury, but other patients may have high levels of HBV DNA and reappearance of HBsAg, as well as elevated aminotransferases and even liver failure. Among HBsAg carriers, high serum HBV DNA before BMT is associated with an increased risk of reactivation of HBV replication. Although reactivation of HBV replication usually occurs during the first few months after BMT, it can be delayed for up to several years.

The chemotherapy used before BMT may also influence HBV infection. In one of the earliest reports of reactivation of hepatitis B, Lok and colleagues reported on 100 Chinese patients undergoing chemotherapy for lymphoma.[5] They found that development of biochemical hepatitis attributed to HBV occurred in 13 of 27 (48%) HBsAg-positive patients; 2 of 51 (3.9%) HBsAg-negative, anti-HBc-positive patients; and none of 22 (0%) HBsAg-negative, anti-HBc-negative patients. In a recent systematic review of 14 studies on reactivation of hepatitis B during cancer chemotherapy, Loomba and colleagues found that the incidence of HBV reactivation was 24% to 88% and the average rate was 37% (156 of 424) when the results of all studies were combined.[6] Liver failure attributed to hepatitis B reactivation was seen in 13% (21 of 162) and deaths related to HBV in 7% (27 of 394) of patients. These studies indicate that morbidity and mortality associated with reactivation of hepatitis B is substantial in HBsAg-positive patients undergoing cytotoxic therapy. Furthermore, reactivation of hepatitis B may be associated with more frequent disruption of chemotherapy regimens and an increased rate of cancer-related deaths.

In a study by Lau and colleagues,[7] 137 consecutive patients undergoing autologous hematopoietic cell transplantation were followed prospectively (23 HBsAg-positive, 37 anti-HBs-negative, and 77 seronegative for HBV). Biochemical hepatitis was seen in 32 patients (23%) after transplantation and was thought to be related to HBV reactivation in 13 cases (9.5%). Hepatitis due to HBV reactivation was more common in HBsAg-positive patients than in HBsAg-negative patients (48% vs. 1.7%, $P = .023$) (hazard ratio, 33.3; 95% CI, 7.35 to 142.86; $P < .0001$). Among the HBsAg-positive patients, those with detectable serum HBV DNA (based on the Digene assay, which has a lower limit of detection of 10^5 copies/ml) before transplantation had a significantly higher risk of hepatitis due to HBV reactivation compared with those with no detectable serum HBV DNA.

Another study from the same group examined the risk of HBV reactivation in patients who have immunity against HBV at the time of transplantation.[8] In this study, 2 of 426 patients (0.5%) who were anti-HBs positive developed acute hepatitis B more than 2 years after BMT. In both cases, anti-HBs titers decreased to undetectable levels 6 months after BMT and both became HBsAg positive at the time of developing hepatitis.

Most studies on HBV reactivation have focused on the first 1 to 2 years after BMT. Hui and colleagues[9] examined the long-term serologic and liver-related outcomes of 803 consecutive patients who underwent allogeneic stem cell transplantation during a median follow-up of 83 months (range, 0.5 to 155 months). Late HBV-related hepatitis, defined as hepatitis occurring more than 12 months after BMT, was seen in 2 of 239 (0.8%) patients who were HBsAg negative at the time of transplantation compared with 16 of 82 (20%) HBsAg-positive recipients ($P < .001$) (**Fig. 39-2, A**). Eight of the 82 HBsAg-positive patients (9.8%) developed cirrhosis compared with none in the HBsAg-negative group ($P < .001$) (see **Fig. 39-2, B**).

Reverse seroconversion has been reported to occur several years after BMT. In a study by Knoll and colleagues, of six patients with a history of resolved hepatitis B who underwent allogeneic hematopoietic stem cell transplantation, three developed reverse seroconversion 12 to 22 months after transplantation.[10] Retrospective testing of stored blood samples found that serum HBV DNA was detected at increasing levels before HBsAg became positive. Two of these three patients were asymptomatic with normal aminotransferases, whereas the third patient developed an acute hepatitis, which was followed by HBsAg clearance.

Adoptive Transfer of Immunity

Reactivation of HBV replication and immune clearance of HBV infection have been reported after BMT.[11] Adoptive transfer of immunity against HBV leading to clearance of HBV infection has been documented in patients undergoing BMT who received bone marrow from donors who had recovered from prior HBV infection as well as donors who had been actively immunized against hepatitis B.[12,13]

Prevention and Treatment of HBV Reactivation

Lamivudine has been shown to be effective in preventing hepatitis associated with reactivation of HBV replication in

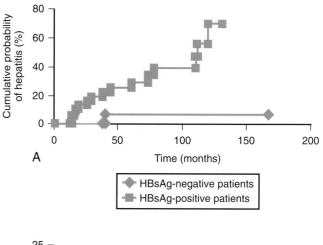

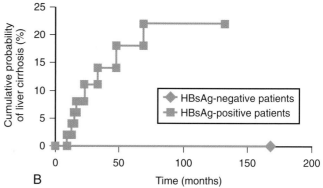

Fig. 39-2 **Cumulative probability of HBV-related hepatitis (A) and liver cirrhosis (B) in patients who were HBsAg positive and in those who were HBsAg negative before hematopoietic stem cell transplantation.** *(From Hui CK, et al. A long-term follow-up study on hepatitis B surface antigen-positive patients undergoing allogeneic hematopoietic stem cell transplantation. Blood 2005;106:464–469.)*

BMT recipients (**Fig. 39-3**).[14-16] Antiviral therapy is most effective when administered prophylactically at the onset of immunosuppressive therapy. In a study of early versus deferred preemptive lamivudine treatment for hepatitis B patients undergoing chemotherapy, Lau and colleagues[17] randomized 30 HBsAg-positive patients undergoing chemotherapy for lymphoma to either receive lamivudine 100 mg before chemotherapy or when there was evidence of HBV reactivation (defined as HBV DNA becoming positive from a previous negative state or a >1 log increase in HBV DNA from baseline value). None of the 15 patients who received lamivudine before chemotherapy had HBV reactivation compared with 8 of 15 patients (53%) who did not receive lamivudine ($P = .002$). Three patients who received lamivudine before chemotherapy developed biochemical hepatitis compared with 10 patients who did not receive lamivudine ($P = .02$). None of the 3 cases of hepatitis in the early treatment group were believed to be related to HBV reactivation, whereas 7 of the 10 patients in the deferred group were determined to be related to HBV reactivation. A systematic review of 14 studies, including 275 patients receiving cancer chemotherapy who received prophylactic lamivudine and 475 control patients, found that prophylactic lamivudine decreased

HBV reactivation, HBV-related hepatitis, HBV-related liver failure, and HBV-related death by 80% to 100%.[6]

The benefit of prophylactic antiviral therapy among HBsAg-positive patients undergoing BMT has been confirmed in several studies. In one study, 16 of 71 HBsAg-positive patients undergoing HSCT received prophylactic lamivudine.[14] Twenty-two patients (only 1 patient received prophylactic lamivudine) had hepatitis associated with HBV reactivation, 16 were icteric, and 7 had fulminant disease. In a multiple regression analysis, preemptive lamivudine therapy was the only significant factor associated with a decreased incidence of HBV-related hepatitis (hazard ratio, 0.122; 95% CI, 0.016 to 0.908; $P = .04$). It should be noted that lamivudine resistance mutations were detected in 10 of 16 (63%) patients after a median duration of treatment of 73 weeks (range, 19 to 153 weeks).

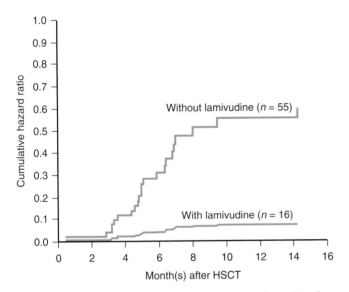

Fig. 39-3 **Cumulative hazards for HBV reactivation hepatitis after hematopoietic stem cell transplantation in HBsAg-positive patients who did or did not receive prophylactic lamivudine therapy.** *(From Hsiao LT, et al. Extended lamivudine therapy against hepatitis B virus infection in hematopoietic stem cell transplant recipients. Biol Blood Marrow Transplant 2006;12:84–94.)*

In another study, 32 patients with non-Hodgkin lymphoma who underwent chemotherapy and autologous HSCT were randomly assigned to either receive prophylactic lamivudine ($n = 20$) or no antiviral therapy ($n = 12$).[18] Patients who received lamivudine had a significantly lower incidence of HBV-reactivation hepatitis (10% vs. 50%, $P = .03$), severe hepatitis (0% vs. 25%, $P = .009$), and HBV-related mortality (0% vs. 25%, $P = .024$).

Prophylactic antiviral therapy must be continued for several months after completion of chemotherapy to prevent hepatitis flares and fatal decompensation as a result of a rebound in viremia upon withdrawal of antiviral therapy.[19] In a study by Hui and colleagues,[19] 46 patients who received prophylactic lamivudine were followed for a median period of 26 months (range, 5.7 to 75.7 months). Lamivudine was stopped a median of 3 months after chemotherapy was completed. Eleven patients (24%) developed hepatitis associated with viral relapse. Patients with higher levels of HBV DNA ($>10^4$ copies/ml) and those who were HBeAg positive before chemotherapy were more likely to have hepatitis associated with a relapse of viremia.

The need for antiviral prophylaxis in HBsAg-negative, anti-HBc–positive patients undergoing BMT is unclear. In a study of 244 HBsAg-negative patients undergoing chemotherapy for lymphoma, 7 of 152 anti-HBc–positive and 1 of 92 anti-HBc–negative patients had de novo HBV-related hepatitis.[20] The risk was higher in patients who received rituximab-containing regimens and highest in those who received rituximab plus steroid-containing regimens.

Based on available data, prophylactic antiviral therapy is recommended for all HBsAg-positive patients undergoing BMT regardless of baseline HBeAg or serum HBV DNA status (**Fig. 39-4**). If possible, treatment should be initiated before the start of immunosuppressive therapy. In patients with baseline low or undetectable serum HBV DNA, antiviral therapy should be continued for at least 4 to 6 months after discontinuation of immunosuppressive therapy; however, in patients with high baseline serum HBV DNA (more than 2000 IU/ml), antiviral therapy should be continued until the therapeutic endpoint for chronic hepatitis B is reached to prevent post-treatment hepatitis flares. For example, HBeAg-positive patients should continue treatment until the patient develops HBeAg seroconversion. Although hepatitis flares secondary to

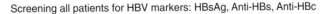

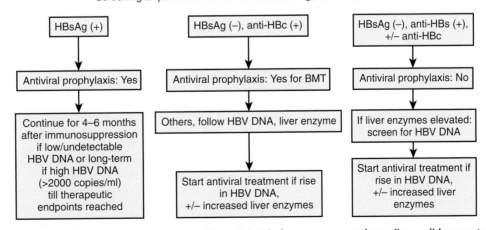

Fig. 39-4 **Recommended algorithm for the management of hepatitis B in bone marrow and non–liver solid organ transplant patients.**

reactivation of HBV replication are less common in HBsAg-negative, anti-HBc–positive patients, most experts would recommend prophylactic antiviral therapy in the setting of BMT because of the potential risks of severe and even fatal fulminant hepatitis and the safety of HBV antiviral therapy.

Most studies of prophylactic antiviral therapy in BMT patients have used lamivudine; however, long-term use of lamivudine is associated with a very high rate of antiviral drug resistance. Both entecavir and tenofovir have more potent antiviral activity and a much lower rate of drug resistance than lamivudine and are preferred even though these drugs have not been extensively studied in BMT patients.

Kidney Transplantation

Incidence and Risk Factors Associated with Reactivation of Hepatitis B

Morbidity and mortality from chronic liver disease is a common complication in patients who are HBsAg-positive at the time of kidney transplantation. The prevalence of HBsAg among hemodialysis patients has declined over the years in developed countries such as the United States from 7.8% in 1976 to less than 1% in 2002, secondary to implementation of HBV vaccination programs and universal precautions.[21] In countries where hepatitis B is endemic, the prevalence rates are much higher. HBsAg-positive patients who undergo kidney transplantation tend to have higher serum HBV DNA levels because of chronic immunosuppression, but not all patients have clinical hepatitis. The incidence of HBV reactivation, HBV-related biochemical hepatitis, and fatal hepatitis flare in kidney transplant recipients has not been well defined. Rates of HBV DNA reactivation of 50% to 94% have been reported in the absence of prophylactic antiviral therapy.[22,23] Not all patients with HBV reactivation have elevated aminotransferases but severe flares and liver failure had been reported in some patients. A rare but severe manifestation of hepatitis B, fibrosing cholestatic hepatitis (FCH), has been reported in kidney transplant patients.[24,25] FCH is associated with a rapid progression to liver failure.

Dusheiko and colleagues assessed the outcomes of 83 patients followed for up to 15 years after kidney transplantation.[26] Of these, 14 were HBsAg positive (4 were HBeAg positive). All four HBeAg-positive patients had persistently high levels of HBV replication posttransplant. Reactivation of hepatitis B was observed in eight patients of whom seven were HBsAg-positive and HBeAg-negative before transplantation, whereas the last patient was HBsAg negative, anti-HBc positive.

Reactivation of HBV replication has also been reported in HBsAg-negative, anti-HBs, and anti-HBc–positive patients, but the incidence is low (0.9% to 5%) and the majority of these patients are asymptomatic. Reverse seroconversion has been reported to occur as early as 8 weeks but may be as late as 15 years after kidney transplantation and appears to correlate with a fall in anti-HBs titers to less than 10 to 100 IU/ml. In the study by Berger and colleagues, 228 of 1512 patients had evidence of resolved HBV infection at the time of kidney transplantation.[27] Reverse seroconversion with the appearance of HBsAg was seen in two patients (0.9%) about 5 years after transplantation despite both patients being on low doses of immunosuppressive therapy. In another study, HBsAg reverse

seroconversion was observed in 2 of 49 patients (4%).[28] A third study on 23 patients who were HBsAg negative but anti-HBc positive (20 were anti-HBs positive before transplantation) found that 2 patients became HBsAg positive posttransplant. Two of 10 patients tested were also HBV DNA positive pretransplant compared with 10 of 23 who were positive posttransplant.[29] Occult HBV infection (HBsAg negative but HBV DNA detectable in serum or liver) has been reported in 3% to 36% of hemodialysis patients and in 1% to 2% of kidney transplant patients.[30]

Long-Term Outcomes

Several studies have shown that the long-term outcomes after kidney transplantation among HBsAg-positive patients is poor compared with those who are HBsAg negative.[31,32] The impaired outcomes in the HBsAg-positive patients are related to the accelerated progression of chronic hepatitis B to cirrhosis and hepatocellular carcinoma (HCC) and increased mortality, particularly liver-related mortality. It should be emphasized that most of these studies were conducted in an era before oral antiviral therapy was available for HBV.

In a case-control study of patients with and without evidence of hepatitis B or C, Mathurin and colleagues studied three groups of patients undergoing kidney transplantation: 128 HBsAg-positive, 216 anti-HCV–positive, and 490 without serologic markers of HBV or HCV infection.[33] HBsAg-positive patients and anti-HCV–positive patients had a significantly lower patient and graft survival compared with patients without serologic markers of HBV or HCV (**Fig. 39-5**). Among HBV- or HCV-infected patients with cirrhosis determined by a biopsy before transplant, the 10-year survival rate was only 26% ± 16% (HBV and HCV cases combined) compared with 69% ± 7% (P = .05). When HBV patients were compared with controls with no HBV or HCV infection, the presence of HBsAg and age at transplantation were independent factors for patient survival (P = .005 and P = .05, respectively), whereas only the presence of HBsAg was an independent predictor of graft survival (P < .001). The findings in this study suggest that the presence of chronic viral hepatitis adversely affects the outcome of kidney transplantation and histologic assessment should be considered in patients with chronic hepatitis B or C to improve the selection of patients undergoing kidney transplantation.

Fornairon and colleagues reported on the long-term virologic and histopathologic outcomes in 151 HBsAg-positive kidney transplant recipients followed for a median period of 125 months (range, 1 to 320).[34] Persistently high serum HBV DNA levels were found in 50% of patients, while reactivation of HBV was noted in 30% of patients. More importantly, histologic deterioration was observed in 85% of 101 patients who had follow-up liver biopsies after a mean interval of 66 months and 28% progressed to cirrhosis. HCC developed in 8 of 35 (23%) patients with underlying cirrhosis. Although the overall survival rate of the 151 HBsAg-positive patients was similar to the 1247 HBsAg-negative patients, liver disease was the leading cause of death in the HBsAg-positive group, especially among patients with cirrhosis.

In a recent study by that included three groups of patients (HBV-infected, HCV-infected, and patients with no HBV or HCV infection), HBV but not HCV infection was an independent predictor of patient survival (hazard ratio for death, 7.76;

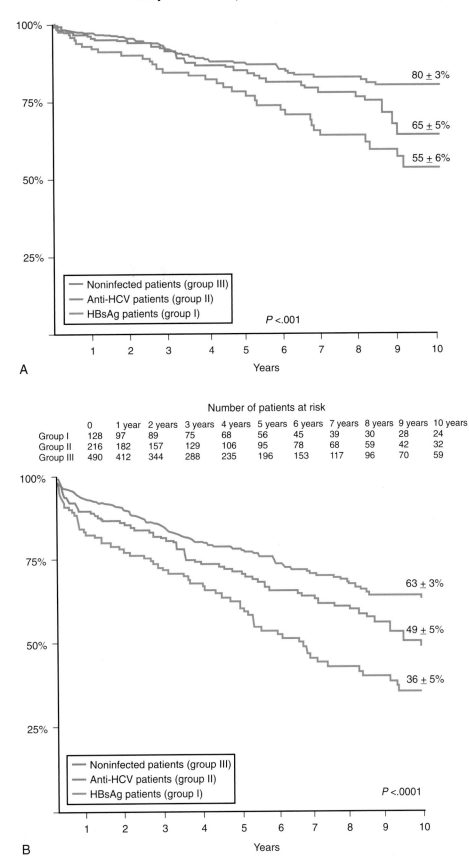

Fig. 39-5 **Patient (A) and graft (B) survival rates after kidney transplantation in HBsAg-positive patients, in anti-HCV–positive patients, and in patients not infected with HBV or HCV.** *(From Mathurin P, et al. Impact of hepatitis B and C virus on kidney transplantation outcome [see comments]. Hepatology 1999;29:257–263.)*

95% CI, 1.88 to 30.86; $P = .004$).[35] Both HBV and HCV groups had significantly higher rates of chronic allograft nephropathy compared with the group with no HBV or HCV infection.

In a recent meta-analysis of long-term outcomes after kidney transplantation, the presence of HBsAg was an independent predictor of poor outcome with a significantly higher rate of overall mortality (relative risk [RR], 2.49; 95% CI, 1.64 to 3.78) and also graft failure (RR, 1.4; 95% CI, 1.02 to 2.04).[36] Additionally, HBsAg-positive patients had a trend toward a higher risk of death because of complications of cirrhosis or HCC.

Recently, several studies have found no difference in graft function or liver enzymes among HBsAg-positive kidney transplant recipients compared with HBsAg-negative patients despite the occurrence of reactivation of HBV in the HBsAg-positive patients.[37-39] In these studies, the overall prevalence of hepatitis B was low and the mean duration of follow-up was about 5 years. Additionally, some patients received lamivudine therapy for HBV reactivation after transplantation,[38] which may have improved the outcome of the HBsAg-positive patients.

The American Society of Transplantation and the American Society of Transplant Surgeons (ASTP) Clinical Practice Guidelines for the care of kidney transplant recipients[40] recommend that all HBsAg-positive kidney transplant recipients receive antiviral prophylaxis, preferably with tenofovir or entecavir or lamivudine. Additionally the guidelines recommend that patients who have developed resistance to lamivudine should be treated with adefovir or tenofovir, and HBsAg-negative patients who have anti-HBs titer less than 10 mIU/ml should receive a booster vaccination to raise the titer to greater than 100 mIU/ml.

Transplantation of HBsAg-Positive Organs in Patients with Natural or Vaccine-Induced Immunity

Given the shortage of organs for transplantation, the possibility of transplanting HBsAg-positive donor organs in patients with protective anti-HBs titer from natural or vaccine-induced immunity has been raised. In one report of 41 patients undergoing kidney transplantation, 14 who were HBsAg-negative and anti-HBs positive received HBsAg-positive donor organs (group 1), whereas 27 who were HBsAg-positive received organs from HBsAg-negative donors (group 2).[41] Actuarial survival at 10 years was 92.8% and 62.5% in groups 1 and 2, respectively. None of the patients in group 1 received hepatitis B immune globulin or antiviral therapy and none became HBsAg positive. Only one death was seen in group 1 and was unrelated to hepatitis B, whereas 9 of 11 deaths in group 2 were related to hepatitis B complications. This study suggests that transplantation of HBsAg-positive donor kidneys into recipients who are anti-HBs positive appears to be safe, but these data should be confirmed before widespread use of kidneys from HBsAg-positive donors is implemented.

Prevention and Treatment of Reactivation of Hepatitis B

The introduction of nucleoside analogues for hepatitis B has made a significant impact on the prevention and treatment of reactivation of hepatitis B after kidney transplantation. Much of the available data is based on lamivudine.[22,42-44] Despite the high rate of drug-resistance mutations during long-term lamivudine therapy, outcomes are improved and prophylactic therapy appears to be better compared with initiating therapy after the onset of hepatic dysfunction.

In one of the earliest studies on antiviral therapy the effects of preemptive lamivudine on patient survival in HBsAg-positive kidney transplant recipients who were observed to have increasing serum HBV DNA with or without increasing ALT levels was reported.[43] A total of 26 HBsAg-positive patients met treatment criteria and received preemptive lamivudine for 32.6 ± 13.3 months. An additional 37 HBsAg-positive patients were transplanted before 1996. The outcomes of the HBsAg-positive patients transplanted after 1996, HBsAg-positive patients transplanted before 1996, and 442 HBsAg-negative patients were compared. Renal allograft survival was similar for all three groups. HBsAg-positive patients transplanted before 1996 had a decreased overall patient survival rate (RR, 9.4; 95% CI, 4.7 to 18.9); and increased liver-related mortality (RR, 68; 95% CI, 8.7 to 533.2) compared with HBsAg-negative controls. By contrast, HBsAg-positive patients transplanted after 1996 and who were eligible to receive preemptive lamivudine therapy had similar survival as the HBsAg-negative controls. These findings suggest that preemptive lamivudine in HBsAg-patients undergoing kidney transplantation who experienced an increase in serum HBV DNA with or without an increase in ALT levels may improve patient survival time and decrease liver-related mortality. Lamivudine has also been shown to reverse liver failure in patients with fibrosing cholestatic hepatitis (FCH).[45,46]

Long-term lamivudine use is associated with increasing rates of drug resistance, leading to virologic breakthrough and in some instances hepatitis flares. In a recent study, 14 of 20 HBsAg-positive patients who underwent kidney transplantation had reactivation of hepatitis B for a mean period of 16 months after transplantation. All 14 were treated with lamivudine and 13 had an initial response.[39] However, 7 of the 13 patients had virologic breakthrough after a mean of 9.2 ± 6.2 months of lamivudine therapy. Despite the high rate of drug resistance, the clinical outcome of HBsAg-positive kidney transplant recipients receiving lamivudine is improved compared with patients transplanted in the prelamivudine era. Ten-year patient and graft survival rates were significantly lower among 66 HBsAg-positive patients compared with 1988 HBsAg-negative patients (64% and 37% vs. 88% and 71%, respectively; $P < .0001$).[32] Among the 66 HBsAg-positive patients, the patient and graft survival rate was significantly higher in the group that received lamivudine ($n = 27$) compared with those that did not (85% and 59% vs. 50% and 23%, respectively; $P < .0001$) (**Fig. 39-6**). The cumulative incidence of virologic breakthrough was 53% at 5 years. All 3 patients with virologic breakthrough who were switched to adefovir responded with a decline in HBV DNA levels, while 3 of 10 patients who did not receive rescue therapy developed liver failure, with 2 who died and 1 who underwent a liver transplant. These findings highlight the importance of serum HBV DNA monitoring and prompt initiation of rescue therapy in patients with drug resistance.

The availability of newer oral antiviral agents, such as entecavir and tenofovir, that have more potent antiviral activity

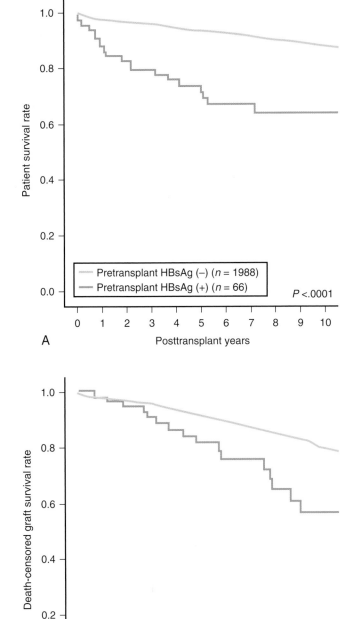

A

B

Fig. 39-6 **Patient survival (A) and graft survival rates (B) in patients who were HBsAg negative or HBsAg positive before transplantation.** *(From Ahn HJ, et al. Clinical outcome of renal transplantation in patients with positive pre-transplant hepatitis B surface antigen. J Med Virol 2007;79: 1655–1663.)*

and a lower rate of drug resistance is expected to further improve the outcomes of HBsAg-positive patients undergoing kidney transplantation. Despite the limited experience of these drugs in the kidney transplant setting, antiviral drugs with lower rates of drug resistance are preferred because of

the need for lifelong immunosuppression after kidney transplantation. Tenofovir has been reported to be associated with nephrotoxicity and renal tubular dysfunction, including Fanconi syndrome[47-49]; therefore entecavir is a better option in patients undergoing kidney transplantation. Although interferon is also approved for hepatitis B, it is not recommended in kidney transplant patients because of the high risk of interferon-induced graft rejection.[50]

Heart and Lung Transplantation

Incidence of HBV Reactivation and Outcomes

Limited information is currently available on the long-term outcomes of HBsAg-positive patients after thoracic organ (heart and lung) transplantation.[51] Available data suggest that the overall prevalence of HBV is low in these patients, but HBV reactivation and severe hepatitis flares have been reported. Cases of de novo HBV infection after transplantation have also been reported.

De novo infection (appearance of HBV DNA after transplantation among patients negative for serologic markers of HBV infection before transplantation) was seen in 4 of 781 patients (0.5%) undergoing heart or lung transplantation.[51] Additionally, one patient with isolated anti-HBc was noted to have detectable HBV DNA in serum in the posttransplant period. In this study, 20 patients who were HBsAg positive with undetectable HBV DNA in serum underwent heart or lung transplantation. Of these, reactivation of hepatitis B was seen in nine patients (45%) at a mean of 35.1 (range, 5.1 to 129.5) months after transplantation; two patients who had not received antiviral therapy died of decompensated hepatitis B following the HBV reactivation. The remaining seven patients were treated with lamivudine and did not have decompensation or death related to hepatitis B. In a second report, 69 of 874 patients (8%) undergoing heart transplantation acquired a new HBV infection (defined as the appearance of HBsAg in patients who were HBsAg negative before transplantation; anti-HBc status not reported), while an additional 11 patients acquired HBV and HCV co-infection.[52] The source of the new HBV infection was believed to be nosocomial transmission from patient to patient, most likely during endomyocardial biopsies. In another study, the prevalence of HBV infection after a heart transplant was 3.7% (11 of 297 patients 4 of whom were HBsAg positive and 7 who were negative for all serologic markers for HBV infection before transplantation) and nearly all patients developed chronic liver disease, with HBV-related mortality in 9% of patients.[53] In a more recent study, HBV reactivation was seen in seven of nine HBsAg-positive patients after heart transplantation (defined as elevated ALT and HBV DNA >200,000 copies/ml).[54] These seven patients were treated with lamivudine, and all responded. This study suggests that reactivation of underlying HBV infection is common after heart transplantation; and prophylactic antiviral therapy to prevent HBV reactivation should be administered in HBsAg-positive heart transplant patients.

HBV reactivation after lung transplantation has also been reported. Eleven patients (4 HBsAg-positive before transplantation and 7 who received organs from anti–HBc–positive donors) received prophylactic lamivudine therapy (all 11 patients had undetectable HBV DNA and normal ALT before therapy) for 12 months.[55] Reactivation of HBV with high HBV DNA levels and elevated ALT was seen in two patients, both of whom were HBsAg positive. This study also illustrated the safety of using anti-HBc–positive donors when prophylactic lamivudine was administered because none of the patients who received organs from anti-HBc–positive donors became HBsAg positive after transplantation during a median follow-up of 24 months. In another recent study of 456 lung transplant recipients, 29 received organs from anti-HBc–positive donors.[56] After a median follow-up of 24.5 months, patients who received lungs from anti-HBc–positive donors had similar 1-year survival compared with those who received lungs from anti-HBc–negative donors. In addition, none of the patients who received lungs from anti-HBc–positive donors developed clinical liver disease and all had undetectable serum HBV DNA during follow-up despite the fact that none of these patients received antiviral prophylaxis. It should be emphasized that all the patients in this study had received HBV vaccine before transplant.

Despite the limited data in thoracic organ transplantation, it is reasonable to consider similar recommendations that have been made for kidney transplant patients. It is advisable to initiate antiviral prophylaxis in HBsAg-negative recipients if they are receiving an organ from a donor who is HBsAg or anti-HBc positive. Although the optimal duration of antiviral prophylaxis has not been defined, it is reasonable to continue antiviral therapy until immunosuppressive therapy is tapered to a stable, minimal dose. Better studies are needed to clarify whether antiviral prophylaxis can be omitted in recipients with high titer anti-HBs and when antiviral prophylaxis can be discontinued. Among patients who are HBsAg positive before transplant, antiviral prophylaxis should be administered regardless of HBeAg or HBV DNA status and continued until HBeAg seroconversion in patients who are HBeAg positive before transplant and until HBV DNA becomes undetectable on a stable low-dose immunosuppression regimen in HBeAg-negative patients. Additionally, antiviral treatment should be initiated immediately in patients who are not on antiviral therapy but have developed reactivation of hepatitis B after transplantation.

Other Organs

A unique feature of transplanting avascular organs such as the cornea is that transmission of viral hepatitis (B or C) infection should be low or negligible, making it possible to transplant such organs even from donors who are HBsAg positive. However, there are at least two reported cases in the literature of acquired hepatitis B infection after corneal transplantation.[57] Both donors were HBsAg positive, whereas both recipients were seronegative for HBV infection at the time of surgery, and the donor corneal tissue was thought to be the only source of transmission of hepatitis B in both patients. In one study,[58] 17 HBsAg-positive cornea donors were tested for the presence of HBV DNA in both the serum and 29 corneal tissue specimens. HBV DNA was detected in the sera from 6 donors (35%), but not in the corneal tissue or the culture media in which the corneas were placed from the donors. These results suggest that despite the few reported cases, the risk of transmitting hepatitis B infection with corneal transplantation is very low even in HBsAg-positive donors.

Summary

In summary, HBV infection after hematopoietic and non-liver solid organ transplantation has a variable course with significant effects on both patient and graft survival rates in some patients. Recent studies have shown that the overall prevalence of HBV infection among transplant recipients has decreased; however, cases of de novo infection and reactivation of hepatitis B after transplantation are still being reported. Characterizing the serologic, virologic, and biochemical profile before transplantation and close monitoring of these parameters after transplantation are crucial. Antiviral prophylaxis is recommended for those who are at risk for reactivation of hepatitis B after transplantation. Monitoring of anti-HBs titers in patients who have immunity to HBV before transplantation and vaccinating those whose anti-HBs titers fall to low or below detectable levels may help prevent reactivation of hepatitis B in these patients. Studies using lamivudine both as prophylaxis to prevent reactivation of disease and as treatment of active infection have demonstrated a reduction in HBV-related hepatitis and an improvement in survival. The availability of antiviral drugs with lower risk of drug resistance will make the management of hepatitis B in transplant recipients much easier.

Hepatitis C

The prevalence of HCV infection among bone marrow or non-liver solid organ transplant recipients is higher than that in the general population. Screening of blood products for HCV and a decreased need for blood transfusions through the use of erythropoietin have decreased the prevalence of HCV infection in bone marrow and kidney transplant recipients in recent years. The outcome of patients with hepatitis C and bone marrow or non-liver solid organ transplantation is variable. Reactivation of HCV replication with resultant hepatitis flares appears to be less common than reactivation of hepatitis B. However, accelerated fibrosis progression and increased mortality from cirrhosis and HCC have been reported. In addition to HCV-related liver morbidity and mortality, patients with HCV infection have increased risk of posttransplant diabetes mellitus and renal disease compared with patients without HCV infection. The risk of sinusoidal obstruction syndrome after BMT is also higher.

Screening of bone marrow and solid organ donors for hepatitis C antibody (anti-HCV) has decreased the risk of transmission of HCV infection. However, there is an average window period of 68 days between the time of infection and the detection of anti-HCV. Whether application of nucleic acid testing can further decrease the risk of HCV transmission is being evaluated. In an attempt to relieve the shortage of donor organs, it has been proposed that the donor pool for non-liver solid organs be expanded to include anti-HCV–positive donors. Initial studies showed that there was no adverse effect on short-term patient or graft survival and the waiting time to transplant was shortened. Subsequent large cohort studies showed that kidney transplantation from HCV-positive donors was independently and significantly associated with diminished survival rates. Currently, it is recommended that organs from HCV-positive donors be used in HCV-positive recipients only.

Contrary to hepatitis B, oral antiviral agents that are well tolerated in transplant recipients are not available. Current treatment of hepatitis C involves a combination of pegylated interferon and ribavirin. Interferon is associated with many side effects, including bone marrow suppression and increased risk of rejection. The main side effect related to ribavirin is anemia. Ribavirin is renally excreted and contraindicated in patients with renal failure. Experience with antiviral therapy in bone marrow and non-liver solid organ transplant recipients is limited. Interferon therapy appears to result in a higher rate of sustained virologic response (SVR) in dialysis patients compared with patients with normal renal function and should be considered in selected kidney transplant candidates.

Bone Marrow Transplantation

Many patients who required BMT in the past were infected with HCV because they acquired HCV infection about the time of bone marrow transplantation from blood transfusions. Despite the screening of blood and marrow donors, a recent prospective study of the European Group for Blood and Marrow Transplantation, which included patients who received transfusions in the "postscreening" era, showed that 6% of stem cell transplant recipients were HCV RNA positive.[59] Therefore the long-term outcome of HCV-positive BMT recipients is an important concern.

Sinusoidal Obstruction Syndrome

Several studies have shown that HCV-positive BMT recipients have an increased incidence of sinusoidal obstruction syndrome (SOS) when compared with HCV-negative patients. In a study that included 62 HCV-positive and 292 HCV-negative BMT patients, severe SOS developed in 48% of HCV-positive and in 14% of HCV-negative patients (P <.0001).[60] Multivariable analysis found that pretransplant HCV infection and elevated serum aspartate aminotransferase (AST) levels in the weeks before the start of cytoreductive therapy was a predictor of severe SOS (RR, 9.6), while HCV infection alone or elevated AST alone was not. In another study, 5 of 6 (83%) patients with HCV infection before BMT died of SOS compared with 9 of 52 (17%) patients not infected with HCV (P <.005).[61] A more recent study found that activity and stage of underlying liver disease and components of the conditioning regimen and not HCV infection per se were risk factors for SOS.[62] This has led to the recommendation that a liver biopsy should be considered before the start of conditioning therapy if there is a clinical suspicion of cirrhosis or extensive fibrosis.[63]

Progression of Liver Disease

Systematic data on HCV replication, flares of hepatitis, and fibrosis progression after BMT are not available. In a study of BMT recipients followed for up to 10 years, HCV-positive patients had a greater frequency of AST elevation than HCV-negative patients at each time interval.[60] An acute flare in hepatitis (AST >10 times the upper limit of normal) was observed in 11 of 36 (31%) anti-HCV–positive and in only 6 of 115 (5%) anti-HCV–negative long-term survivors (P < .0001).

Of 96 HCV-positive BMT recipients who were followed for a median of 15.7 years after transplantation, 15 patients developed cirrhosis and 3 developed HCC, both determined by a biopsy.[64] The cumulative incidence of cirrhosis was 11% at 15 years and 24% at 20 years. The authors also compared the rate of progression to cirrhosis in these 96 patients with 158 HCV-infected patients who had a known date of infection, a liver biopsy, and had not undergone BMT. They found that the median time to development of cirrhosis in the BMT group was shorter, 18 years versus 40 years in the control group. It should be noted that the two groups differed in many respects such as age, alcohol consumption, HCV genotype, and hemosiderosis in the liver.

The incidence of cirrhosis in 3721 patients who survived 1 or more years after BMT was studied and 31 patients developed cirrhosis based on clinical (portal hypertension and/or liver failure) or histologic evidence.[65] The median time to development of cirrhosis after BMT was 10 years (range, 1.2 to 24.9) and HCV infection was the most common cause. Overall, the available data suggest that liver disease progression in adult HCV-positive BMT recipients may be accelerated compared with HCV-positive patients without BMT.

Limited studies suggest that the clinical course of hepatitis C in pediatric HCV-positive BMT recipients is not different compared with that seen in other children who acquired HCV infection at a young age and cirrhosis is uncommon after more than 10 years of follow-up. This may be related to a slow rate of progression of hepatitis C in children and young adults,[66] and a longer duration of follow-up will be necessary to determine the long-term outcomes of children who acquired HCV infection around the time of BMT.

Survival

A recent study compared 1-year survival rates in 31 HCV-positive BMT recipients and 31 HCV-negative BMT controls matched for age, diagnosis, disease stage, conditioning regimen, and donor type, and 1800 HCV-negative patients transplanted during the same period.[67] The overall 1-year survival for the three groups was 29%, 56%, and 56%, respectively and the 1-year nonrelapse mortality was 43%, 24%, and 23%, respectively. Multivariate analysis found that HCV infection was a significant predictor of mortality, with a hazard ratio of 3.1 (95% CI, 1.9 to 5.6; P <.001). Other studies have found that survival up to 10 years post-BMT is not decreased.[60,68] In a study of 355 BMT recipients, including 113 who were HCV RNA positive, the presence of HCV infection did not influence overall mortality up to 10 years after BMT.[60] However, these authors found that the cumulative incidence of cirrhosis among HCV-positive patients was 24% after 20 years of post-BMT follow-up. These data indicate that HCV-positive BMT recipients may have an impaired long-term (beyond 10 years) survival rate and that liver disease may be a major contributor to mortality.

Antiviral Treatment

There are very limited data on the experience of treating HCV infection in patients who underwent BMT. In one study, 22 patients were treated including 12 who had more than 1 course of treatment (a total of 41 courses).[69] Sustained virologic response (SVR) was achieved in 4 of 18 patients (22%) treated with a combination of pegylated interferon or standard interferon with ribavirin and in 2 of 20 (10%) patients who received interferon only. Hematologic side effects were more common in patients receiving combination therapy (39% vs. 5%), with the majority being anemia related to ribavirin therapy. Graft-versus-host disease was seen in three patients receiving standard interferon alone and in none of the patients receiving combination therapy. During long-term follow-up, all patients with an SVR were alive at the end of the study. In contrast 3 of 16 nonresponder patients (19%) and 7 of 14 untreated patients died during follow-up; nearly all (9 of 10) deaths were due to HCV-related complications. The results suggest that interferon is successful in some patients after BMT without a significant effect on graft function. However, treatment-related cytopenia remains a challenging issue in this patient population. It is recommended that HCV treatment be considered when the patient's immune response and bone marrow have recovered, immunosuppressive therapy has been stopped, and there is no evidence of graft-versus-host disease.

Kidney Transplantation

Hepatitis C is a common problem among kidney transplant patients. The prevalence of HCV infection among kidney transplant patients has been reported to be as high as 21%, whereas the prevalence among diseased donors ranged from 1% to 11.8% depending on the geographic location of the studies.[70] In a study by Abbott and colleagues,[71] of the 36,956 patients who underwent kidney transplantation in the United States between January 1, 1996 and May 31, 2001, 6.8% of the recipients and 2.4% of the donors were anti-HCV positive.

Reactivation of HCV replication after kidney transplantation has not been systematically studied. Available data suggest that an increase in HCV RNA levels may occur after kidney transplantation[72] but flares of hepatitis are uncommon. Studies on fibrosis progression in kidney transplant patients have yielded conflicting results, with some studies suggesting accelerated progression and others showing similar or even slower progression compared with nontransplant patients. Regardless, long-term follow-up studies showed that patient survival is worse in HCV-positive patients compared with HCV-negative patients. In addition, HCV-positive kidney transplant recipients have increased risk of new-onset diabetes, posttransplant glomerulonephritis, and sepsis. Ribavirin is contraindicated in patients with renal failure, but interferon monotherapy is well tolerated and appears to result in higher rates of SVR in dialysis patients compared with those with normal renal function. Available data suggest that interferon therapy in patients awaiting kidney transplantation might be safer and more effective than antiviral therapy after transplantation.

Liver Fibrosis

Cross-sectional studies found a high proportion of HCV-positive kidney transplant recipients had advanced fibrosis on liver biopsy, suggesting that immunosuppression associated with kidney transplantation may accelerate fibrosis progression in patients with hepatitis C; however, studies comparing paired biopsies from hepatitis C patients with and without kidney transplants found that fibrosis progression in kidney transplant recipients is similar or even slower.

In one study, 39 of 74 patients with hepatitis C underwent a liver biopsy after kidney transplantation.[73] Of the 13 patients with normal ALT, none had significant liver disease

while 12 of the 26 (46%) patients with abnormal ALT (30% of total) had bridging fibrosis. It should be noted that the interval between kidney transplantation and the performance of these biopsies was unclear. A study of 51 patients who had detectable serum HCV RNA at the time of kidney transplantation and had at least 2 liver biopsies (range, 2 to 4) found that fibrosis progressed in 21 patients (41%), remained stable in another 21 patients (41%), and regressed in 10 patients.[74]

Graft and Patient Survival

Chronic liver disease is a frequent complication after kidney transplantation, representing the fourth most common cause of death in some series.[75] A systematic review of eight studies of 6365 patients found that the presence of anti-HCV was an independent and significant risk factor for death and graft failure after kidney transplantation (RR, 1.79; 95% CI, 1.57 to 2.03).[76] In this study, cirrhosis and HCC were significantly more common in anti-HCV–positive patients compared with those who were anti-HCV negative.

Multicenter surveys and data bases have also confirmed increased mortality among kidney transplant recipient patients who are anti-HCV positive. Using the data from the Organ Procurement and Transplantation Network/Scientific Registry of Transplant Recipients in the United States ($N = $ 79,337: 3708 HCV-positive and 75,629 HCV-negative), Luan and associates found that a positive HCV serology conferred a significantly higher risk for patient death after kidney transplantation (hazard ratio [HR], 1.30; 95% CI, 1.20 to 1.41; $P = .0001$) compared with transplant recipients who were anti-HCV negative.[77] This effect was most pronounced in younger recipients. In contrast, an analysis of a total of 73,707 patients from the U.S. Renal Data System found that adjusted patient survival was superior for HCV-positive patients with overall incidence of death from all-cause mortality being 20% in anti-HCV–negative patients compared with 15.7% in those who were anti-HCV positive ($P = .02$).[78] These differences in survival time were seen during each of the initial 7 years after transplantation ($P = .01$); but at the end of year 8, overall survival time was similar (69%) between the two groups of patients. Although not directly comparable, the differences in patient survival rates in these two studies from the United States may be related to the differences in age and prevalence of diabetes between HCV-positive and HCV-negative recipients, which influence long-term outcomes after transplantation.

Historically, studies on the course of HCV-infected patients after kidney transplantation have reported lower rates of graft and patient survival rates with liver-related deaths and infections being a major problem, although death due to HCV-related kidney disease or graft dysfunction did not appear to influence overall patient survival time. Some recent studies, however, have reported similar patient survival rates compared with patients without hepatitis C[79-82] and one study from Taiwan even reported better survival.[83]

With regards to long-term graft and patient survival rates, several earlier studies have shown that the outcomes of HCV patients undergoing kidney transplantation may be inferior when compared with patients without HCV infection. One of the earlier studies that brought this issue to light found that compared with anti-HCV–negative patients, patients who were anti-HCV positive had a higher risk of death after kidney transplantation from all causes (RR, 1.41; 95% CI, 1.01 to 1.97), as well as liver disease or infection (RR, 2.39; 95% CI, 1.28 to 4.48).[84] In another recent study, anti-HCV–positive status was associated with both a decreased graft survival rate (56% vs. 75%, P = .0002) and a reduced overall patient survival rate at 13 years after transplantation (68% vs. 83%, P = .0028) when compared with patients who were anti-HCV negative.[85] In the meta-analysis of observational studies of patients undergoing kidney transplantation, anti-HCV–positive patients had a greater risk of overall mortality and renal graft failure compared with patients who were anti-HCV negative.[76] The presence of anti-HCV was an independent predictor of death (RR, 1.79; 95% CI, 1.57 to 2.03) and graft failure (RR, 1.56; 95% CI, 1.35 to 1.80) after kidney transplantation. In addition to studies showing a higher risk of overall mortality among anti-HCV–positive patients, liver-related morbidity and mortality due to complications of cirrhosis, including decompensation and development of HCC, has also been shown to be higher in anti-HCV–positive patients following kidney transplantation.

In a study from Taiwan,[83] anti-HCV–positive patients undergoing their first kidney transplantation had a higher incidence of chronic hepatitis and chronic allograft dysfunction, and also development of nephrotic syndrome or glomerulonephritis after transplantation. In this study of 299 patients (129 anti-HCV positive and 170 anti-HCV negative; all HBsAg negative), graft survival rate was decreased during long-term follow-up of up to 15 years in anti-HCV–positive patients. In contrast, overall patient survival time was better among patients with hepatitis C at 10 and 15 years compared with those without hepatitis C infection (86% and 71%, respectively, vs. 68% and 60%, P = .014). The reasons for better patient survival rates in the hepatitis C group was not clear, although these patients received less immunosuppression and no antilymphocyte induction therapy compared with patients who were anti-HCV negative.

More recently, in a study of 208 patients (144 HCV negative and 64 HCV positive) followed for up to 5 years after kidney transplantation, patient survival rates were similar between the HCV-positive and HCV-negative patients, especially in patients undergoing living-related kidney transplantation (71% vs. 75% at 5 years).[86]

A rare but a severe form of hepatitis C, fibrosing cholestatic hepatitis (FCH), has been described in HCV-positive patients undergoing kidney transplantation. In one study, 4 of 259 (1.5%) HCV-infected kidney transplant recipients developed FCH 2 to 36 months after transplantation.[87] Another manifestation of hepatitis C infection after kidney transplantation is de novo glomerulonephritis in renal allografts, which has been associated with graft loss especially in patients with membranoproliferative glomerulonephritis.

Diabetes After Kidney Transplantation

Several studies have shown that hepatitis C infection is an important factor in the development of diabetes after kidney transplantation. In one study, 427 nondiabetic patients who underwent kidney transplantation were retrospectively studied for the development of diabetes at 12 months after transplantation.[88] The incidence of posttransplant diabetes was more common in HCV-positive patients compared with HCV-negative patients (39% vs. 10%, P = .0005). In another

larger report,[89] 11,659 patients who received their first kidney transplant were studied. The overall incidence of diabetes increased with time after transplantation from 9% at 3 months to 24% at 36 months. Additionally, the presence of diabetes was independently associated with a significantly increased risk of graft failure (odds ratio [OR], 1.63; 95% CI, 1.46 to 1.84; P <.0001) and patient mortality (OR, 1.87; 95% CI, 1.60 to 2.18; P <.0001).

In a recent systematic review of 10 clinical studies involving a total of 2502 patients, the relationship between the presence of HCV infection after kidney transplantation (based on anti-HCV status) and development of diabetes was assessed.[90] The authors found a significant independent relationship between HCV status and diabetes after transplantation (summary estimate for adjusted OR of 3.97 (95% CI, 1.83 to 8.61; P <.05). The role of donor-recipient HCV status on the development of diabetes among a total of 28,942 patients undergoing kidney transplantation has been examined.[91] HCV-positive status in the donors was independently associated with a higher risk of developing posttransplant diabetes irrespective of the recipient status[91] (**Fig. 39-7**). This study also showed that posttransplant HCV infection and diabetes were independent risk factors for patient mortality on follow-up (adjusted HR, 3.36; 95% CI, 2.44 to 4.61; and adjusted HR, 1.81; 95% CI, 1.54 to 2.11, respectively).

The available studies to date suggest that hepatitis C infection after kidney transplantation is a risk for the development of diabetes, and the presence of diabetes may adversely affect both patient and graft survival in this population.

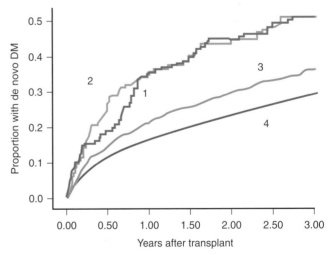

Time to de novo DM, by HCV seropairing

1 = D+/R–, 2 = D+/R+, 3 = D–/R+, 4 = D–/R–

D = donor, R = recipient serology for hepatitis C virus (ELISA)

Fig. 39-7 **Development of de novo diabetes mellitus in patients undergoing kidney transplantation, with outcomes based on donor-recipient HCV status.** Time to de novo posttransplantation diabetes was stratified by donor-recipient HCV status (limited to patients without known prevalent diabetes; N = 17,572). *(From Abbott KC, et al. Impact of diabetes and hepatitis after kidney transplantation on patients who are affected by hepatitis C virus. J Am Soc Nephrol 2004;15:3166–3174.)*

Treatment of Hepatitis C Before Transplantation

The rationale for treating patients pretransplant is to achieve viral clearance and hopefully prevent liver-related morbidity and mortality, and possibly even recurrent renal problems associated with HCV after transplantation. Also, interferon therapy has been shown to increase the risk of graft rejection after kidney transplantation, making treatment difficult in this setting. Although ribavirin is contraindicated in patients with renal failure, high rates of SVR have been reported in dialysis patients receiving interferon monotherapy possibly because of decreased renal clearance and increased drug exposure. Limited data suggest that hemodialysis patients who achieved SVR before kidney transplantation maintained this response posttransplant despite the institution of immunosuppressive therapy.

Interferon Monotherapy

Clinical trials of interferon (IFN) monotherapy with different dose regimens have reported SVR rates ranging between 14% and 78%, although the number of patients treated in each study is small and different studies used different durations of treatment[92] (**Table 39-1**).

Since the approval of pegylated interferon (PEG-IFN) therapy, several studies of PEG-IFN with a small number of patients in each trial have observed SVR rates ranging from 30% to 75% (**Fig. 39-8**). In a recent study of 12 patients with genotype 1 HCV infection on hemodialysis,[93] treatment with

Table 39-1 Clinical Trials of IFN Monotherapy in Hemodialysis Patients with Chronic Hepatitis C

STUDY	PATIENT POPULATION (n)	INTERFERON-ALPHA DOSE AND DURATION	COMPLETED TREATMENT	END OF TREATMENT RESPONSE	SVR	NO. OF PATIENTS DISCONTINUING TREATMENT BECAUSE OF SAE
Rocha et al.	Tx-naïve (46) G1: 86% RT: 20% Bridging fibrosis: 39%	3 MU 3×/wk for 12 months	29/46 (63%)	19/46 (41%)	10/46 (22%)	n = 11
Degos et al.*	Tx-naïve (37) G1: 78%	3 MU 3×/wk for 48 weeks	18/37 (49%)	12/37 (32.4%)	7/37 (19%)	n = 19
Chan et al.	No. pts (11) G1: 91%	1.5 MU 3×/wk for 2 weeks, then 3 MU 3×/wk for 24 weeks	11/11 (100%)	11 (100%)	3 (27%)	NR
Rivera et al.	No. pts (27)	3 MU, 2 to 3× week for 6 to 12 months (n = 20) or PEG-IFN alfa-2a (135 μg/ wk) for 12 months (n = 7)	NR	13/27 (48.1%) (IFN-α, 10/20; PEG-IFN-α, 3/7)	11/27 (40.7%)	n = 3
Grgurevic et al.	No. pts (15)	3 MU 3×/wk for 6 months or 5 MU 3×/wk for 3 months, then 5 MU/wk for 3 months	13/15 (86.7%)	9/15 (60%)	6/15 (40%)	n = 2
Uchihara et al.	No. pts (9)	3-6 MU/day for 2 weeks, then 3 MU 3×/wk for 24 weeks	6/9 (66.6%)	NR	3/9 (33.3%)	n = 3
Espinosa et al.	No. pts (13) G1: 40%	3 MU 3×/wk for 1 year	10/13 (76.9%)	8/13 (61.5%)	6/13 (46.2%)	n = 3
Mahmoud et al.	No. pts (18)	3 MU 3×/wk for 6 months	16/18 (88.9%)	NR	8[†]/18 (44.4%)	n = 2
Ozdemir et al.	No. pts (20)	6 MU 3×/wk for 6 months (n = 10) or 3 MU 3×/wk for 12 months (n = 10)	NR	15/20 (75%)	8/20 (40%)	NR

Adapted from Berenguer M. Treatment of chronic hepatitis C in hemodialysis patients. Hepatology 2008;48:1690–1699.

*Study interrupted because of frequency and severity of side effects.

[†]Two patients experienced relapses 6 and 9 months after transplantation.

G1, genotype 1; IFN, interferon; NR, not reported; RT, renal transplant; SAE, serious adverse event; SVR, sustained virologic response.

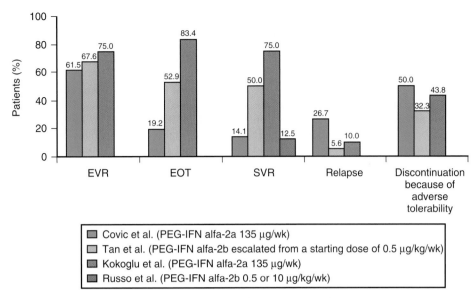

Fig. 39-8 Response to PEG-IFN-α monotherapy treatment of patients with chronic hepatitis C who were undergoing hemodialysis. EOT, end-of-treatment response (undetectable HCV RNA at week 48 of treatment); EVR, early virologic response (>2 log decrease in HCV RNA at week 12); PEG-IFN, pegylated interferon; SVR, sustained virologic response (undetectable HCV RNA 6 months after completion of therapy) *(From Berenguer M. Treatment of chronic hepatitis C in hemodialysis patients. Hepatology 2008;48:1690–1699.)*

pegylated interferon alfa-2a (PEG-IFN-α-2a) monotherapy at a lower dose (135 µg/wk) resulted in an SVR rate of 50% compared with 62% (29 of 47) of HCV-infected patients not on hemodialysis that were treated with the standard dose of PEG-IFN-α-2a (180 µg/week) in combination with ribavirin. A recent study of 14 patients with genotype 1 (*n* = 13) or 4 infection, patients treated with PEG-IFN-α-2a at a dose of 135 µg weekly for 48 weeks found that only 9 patients (64%) completed treatment and 5 patients (36%, all genotype 1) had SVR.[94]

These data suggest that SVR rates comparable with that achieved with standard doses of PEG-IFN and ribavirin in patients with normal renal function can be achieved with PEG-IFN monotherapy in hemodialysis patients, but it should be cautioned that the sample size in these studies was small and there may be publication bias. Despite the favorable response rates, withdrawal of treatment due to side effects was reported in 30% to 50% of patients.

Interferon and Ribavirin Combination Therapy

More recently, there have been several case series of combination therapy with standard IFN or PEG-IFN and ribavirin in patients with hepatitis C and end-stage renal disease. In these studies, SVR rates have ranged from 16% to 71% with standard IFN, and 29% to 97% with PEG-IFN.[95-98] One major concern with the use of ribavirin is hemolytic anemia. Ribavirin is excreted by the kidneys and is generally contraindicated in patients with end-stage renal disease. Recent studies suggested that ribavirin concentrations equivalent to that seen in patients with normal renal function receiving approved doses can be achieved in patients with end-stage renal disease using doses as low as 200 mg/day, and that combination therapy with PEG-IFN and ribavirin may lead to increased SVR rates; however, it is important to note that ribavirin levels

were closely monitored in these studies to maintain adequate levels and to guide dose adjustments.

Whether IFN is used alone or in combination with ribavirin, patients who achieved an SVR had improved outcomes after kidney transplantation. The outcomes of 69 anti-HCV–positive patients undergoing kidney transplantation using kidneys from anti-HCV–negative donors was assessed.[99] De novo glomerulonephritis after transplantation developed only among patients who were HCV RNA positive.

Recently two meta-analyses on the effect of interferon-based therapy in patients with hepatitis C on hemodialysis were reported. In one study that included 28 clinical trials (645 patients), of which 6 had a controlled design, the summary estimate for SVR was 39% (95% CI, 32% to 46%) for all patients and among patients with genotype 1 infection, SVR was 33% (95% CI, 19% to 47%).[92] When studies using PEG-IFN were analyzed, the overall summary estimate for SVR was 31% (95% CI, 7% to 55%). One group reported on a total of 25 studies with sample sizes of greater than 10 patients; 20 studies used standard IFN (total of 459 patients, all except one used IFN monotherapy, while one used low-dose ribavirin in combination); 3 used PEG-IFN (38 patients); and 2 used a PEG-IFN and ribavirin combination (49 patients).[100] The overall summary estimate of SVR was 41% for the standard IFN group (95% CI, 33% to 49%) and 37% for the PEG-IFN (PEG-IFN monotherapy only) group (95% CI, 9% to 77%). Treatment discontinuation rates were 25% (95% CI, 20% to 34%) and 28% (95% CI, 12% to 53%) in the groups that received IFN and PEG-IFN, respectively.

Transplantation of Kidneys from Anti-HCV–Positive Donors

The prevalence of anti-HCV in diseased kidney donors is higher compared with the general population, ranging between 1% and 12% in different countries.[70] A complete prohibition on the use of kidneys from anti-HCV–positive donors will result in an average rate of organ loss of 4%. Unlike hepatitis B, hyperimmune globulin and safe and well-tolerated antiviral therapy are not available to prevent HCV transmission when kidneys from HCV-positive donors are transplanted to HCV-negative recipients.

Transmission of HCV infection from anti-HCV–positive donors has been reported, although the rate of transmission is variable.[101-103] Factors associated with transmission include viral load in the donors, susceptibility of the recipients, and methods of organ preservation. One group showed that the highest rate of acquiring HCV infection after kidney transplantation occurred in the donor positive-recipient negative group (9.1%) followed by donor positive-recipient positive group (6.3%) and donor negative-recipient positive group (2.4%), whereas the lowest rate was in the donor negative-recipient negative group (0.2%).[91] The peak incidence of HCV infection was seen in the initial 6 months after kidney transplantation.

Outcomes

Studies with a short duration of follow-up found that transplantation of kidneys from HCV-positive donors was not associated with impaired patient or graft survival rates and waiting time was shortened for kidney transplantation.[104,105] However, studies with a long duration of follow-up showed that transplantation of kidneys from HCV-positive donors is associated with impaired patient survival, and a higher incidence of delayed allograft function as well as new-onset diabetes. There had also been case reports of fibrosing cholestatic hepatitis in kidney transplant patients who acquired HCV infection shortly before or after kidney transplantation.[106,107]

A retrospective review of 34 anti-HCV–positive (of whom 13 received kidneys from HCV-positive donors) and 111 anti-HCV–negative kidney transplant recipients was reported.[108] After a mean follow-up of about 36 months, no significant differences were observed between the HCV-positive and HCV-negative recipients with regard to patient survival, BK nephropathy, incidence of delayed allograft function, or new-onset diabetes. Graft survival rate was, however, lower in the HCV-positive group: 71% versus 84%, $P = .02$, and within the HCV-positive group, graft survival was lower in those who received kidneys from HCV-positive donors: 54% versus 81% ($P = .08$).

In another study, 259 HCV-positive recipients (60 received kidneys from HCV-positive donors and 199 from HCV-negative donors) and 506 HCV-negative recipients was examined and there was no difference in patient or graft survival among these three groups after a follow-up of 1 to 13 years.[109]

Studies of large databases have shown that the use of kidneys from HCV-positive donors is associated with a higher rate of patient mortality compared with transplantation of kidneys from HCV-negative donors. In one report, 17,697 adult patients undergoing kidney transplantation between 1994 and 1998 were studied.[110] Of 484 kidneys from anti-HCV–positive donors, 165 (34%) were given to anti-HCV–negative recipients. A positive donor HCV status was an independent predictor of patient mortality (HR, 1.46; 95% CI, 1.04 to 2.05; $P = .028$). In another study of 36,956 patients undergoing kidney transplantation between January 1996 and May 2001 were assessed.[71] A total of 2525 recipients (6.8%) and 873 (2.4%) donors were anti-HCV positive. The

kidneys from HCV-positive donors were transplanted into 280 HCV-negative and 593 HCV-positive recipients. The results showed that donor HCV-positive status was an independent predictor of increased mortality (adjusted HR, 2.12; 95% CI, 1.72 to 2.87; $P <.0001$). Among HCV-positive recipients, donor HCV-positive status was an independent predictor of increased mortality 2 years after transplantation (adjusted HR, 1.34; 95% CI, 1.04 to 1.74; $P = .026$). In a more recent study a total of 79,337 patients who underwent kidney transplantation (3708 HCV positive and 75,629 HCV negative) between January 1995 and December 2004 were studied.[77] Overall survival rate was reduced in HCV-positive compared with HCV-negative recipients.

Others have also shown that new-onset diabetes and posttransplant hepatitis C were independent predictors of increased risk of death (adjusted HR, 1.81; 95% CI, 1.54 to 2.11; and adjusted HR, 3.36; 95% CI, 2.44 to 4.61, respectively; $P <.001$ for both), and the presence of diabetes accounted for more years of life lost, especially among recipients of kidneys from HCV-positive donors.[91]

Despite the decrease in long-term survival rates compared with receipt of a kidney from HCV-negative donors, an analysis of 38,270 patients on the kidney transplant waiting list found that the survival rate was higher among patients receiving kidney transplants from HCV-positive donors compared with staying on the transplant waiting list.[111] It should be mentioned that 52% of the patients who received a kidney from an HCV-positive donor were also HCV positive and the outcomes in HCV-negative recipients may be different. These data suggest that transplantation of kidneys from HCV-positive donors to HCV-negative recipients should be avoided, but a net benefit may be attained for HCV-positive recipients compared with long-term dialysis.

One concern with transplanting kidneys from HCV-positive donors to HCV-positive recipients is the possibility of superinfection with another HCV genotype. There have been case reports of superinfection with an associated increase in aminotransferases but the frequency in which this occurs and the outcome has not been systematically studied. A large multicenter survey suggested that the type or number of HCV genotypes may not have a significant impact on survival rates among patients with end-stage renal disease.[112]

Treatment of Hepatitis C Posttransplantation

Treatment of hepatitis C infection after kidney transplantation is difficult because IFN can increase the risk of graft rejection. One small series in 14 kidney transplant recipients with chronic HCV infection was reported.[113] Eight patients received ribavirin alone, while the remaining six patients received IFN alone or in combination with ribavirin. While ribavirin therapy alone did improve or stabilize serum ALT levels in the majority of patients, only one of eight patients became HCV RNA negative. Of the six patients treated with IFN alone or in combination with ribavirin, SVR was seen in two (both receiving combination therapy). However, four of the six patients developed graft dysfunction, including one case of chronic allograft nephropathy, suggesting that IFN-related graft dysfunction may be irreversible in some patients.

A recent meta-analysis of 12 clinical trials of antiviral therapy for hepatitis C in kidney transplant patients showed that IFN-based therapy (IFN alone or in combination with ribavirin) is poorly tolerated.[114] The overall summary estimate for SVR was 18% (95% CI, 7% to 29%) and the drop-out rate was 35% (95% CI, 20% to 50%). The summary estimate for SVR among the nine studies using IFN alone was 12% (95% CIs 1% to 22%). Although a lower response rate was seen in patients with a genotype 1 infection, the difference compared with patients with genotype non-1 was not statistically significant. Graft dysfunction mostly due to acute rejection was common and was seen in 28 of 102 patients (27%), and it was frequently irreversible and steroid resistant.

There are some settings where IFN treatment should be considered despite the potential risk of renal graft loss; one such setting is the rare patient with fibrosing cholestatic hepatitis. Also among patients with evidence of renal graft failure, treatment for hepatitis C can be considered particularly if the patient is a candidate for retransplantation.

Heart and Lung Transplantation

Very limited information is currently available on the impact of HCV infection on the natural history of liver disease, as well as graft and patient survival rates in patients undergoing thoracic organ (heart and lung) transplantation. Available data at least in heart transplantation showed that donor HCV status might be associated with an increased risk of mortality, although overall experience has been limited. In one study, the authors reported that histologic progression of hepatitis C was slow and 5-year survival rates were unaffected by the patients' HCV status after heart transplantation.[52] However, in this study, all patients had acquired HCV infection at the time of transplantation and the follow-up may not have been long enough to influence the outcome of the liver disease in these patients. In another study of 499 patients undergoing heart transplantation over almost an 18-year period, 11 (2.2%) had evidence of chronic HCV infection.[115] In these 11 patients, aminotransferases remained stable after a mean duration of 32 months after transplantation. In a recent large study of 10,915 patients undergoing heart transplantation, 261 patients received an HCV-positive donor organ.[116] Mortality was significantly higher among the patients receiving an HCV-positive donor heart compared with HCV-negative donor hearts at 1, 5, and 10 years after transplantation. The receipt of an HCV-positive heart was an independent predictor of mortality (HR, 2.1; 95% CI, 1.60 to 2.75) and this association was independent of the recipients' HCV status or age. These findings suggest that the preferential allocation of HCV-positive donor hearts to patients with known HCV infection may not be beneficial with regards to patient survival after transplantation. Compared with patients who received an HCV-negative donor organ, patients receiving an HCV-positive heart were more likely to die of either liver disease or coronary artery disease. However, it is unknown how not transplanting these patients for the lack of a suitable organ influences survival rates relative to those who received HCV-positive organs.

In a study of 465 patients undergoing lung transplantation, 6 patients who had evidence of HCV infection before transplant were followed for up to 6 years after transplant.[117] Five of the six patients who had a liver biopsy pretransplant had no evidence of cirrhosis, and although follow-up liver biopsies were not done in any patient after their lung transplants, none had evidence of hepatic dysfunction. The overall graft and patient survival rate was similar to that seen in patients without HCV infection. It is important to note that the number of patients with HCV infection was small and the duration of follow-up may not be long enough to draw conclusions about the role of HCV infection on patient survival. In another report of three cases of acute HCV infection acquired after lung transplantation,[118] all three patients died 2 to 12 months after the diagnosis of hepatitis C. Two of the three patients died as a result of hepatic failure despite being initiated on treatment for hepatitis C, while the other patient died due to complications of fungal infection.

Summary

In summary, HCV infection after bone marrow transplantation and nonliver solid organ transplantation is associated with significant morbidity in some patients and a decrease in overall patient and graft survival rates after transplantation. Patients with HCV infection have increased risk of posttransplant diabetes, which in turn leads to an increased risk of patient mortality in patients undergoing kidney transplantation. Efforts should be made to treat patients with end-stage renal disease before transplantation if this is possible because eradication of HCV before kidney transplantation will improve the outcome after transplantation. Interferon-based treatment is associated with significant risk of graft dysfunction in kidney transplant recipients. Although direct antiviral agents for hepatitis C will likely be approved within the next 1 to 2 years, their safety and efficacy in transplant patients have not been determined and in the short term, these agents will have to be used in combination with PEG-IFN and ribavirin.

Key References

Abbott KC, et al. Hepatitis C and renal transplantation in the era of modern immunosuppression. J Am Soc Nephrol 2003;14:2908–2918. (Ref.71)

Abbott KC, et al. The impact of transplantation with deceased donor hepatitis C-positive kidneys on survival in wait-listed long-term dialysis patients. Am J Transplant 2004;4:2032–2037. (Ref.111)

Abbott KC, et al. Impact of diabetes and hepatitis after kidney transplantation on patients who are affected by hepatitis C virus. J Am Soc Nephrol 2004;15:3166–3174. (Ref.91)

Ahn HJ, et al. Clinical outcome of renal transplantation in patients with positive pre-transplant hepatitis B surface antigen. J Med Virol 2007;79:1655–1663. (Ref.32)

Akhan SC, Kalender B, Ruzgar M. The response to pegylated interferon alpha 2a in haemodialysis patients with hepatitis C virus infection. Infection 2008;36:341–344. (Ref.93)

Arango J, et al. Kidney graft survival in patients with hepatitis C: a single center experience. Clin Transplant 2008;22:16–19. (Ref.86)

Aroldi A, et al. Natural history of hepatitis B and C in renal allograft recipients. Transplantation 2005;79:1132–1136. (Ref.75)

Berger A, et al. HBV reactivation after kidney transplantation. J Clin Virol 2005;32:162–165. (Ref.27)

Bloom RD, et al. Association of hepatitis C with posttransplant diabetes in renal transplant patients on tacrolimus. J Am Soc Nephrol 2002;13:1374–1380. (Ref.88)

Brown KL, et al. Intermediate-term outcomes of hepatitis C-positive compared with hepatitis C-negative deceased-donor renal allograft recipients. Am J Surg 2008;195:298–302; discussion 303. (Ref.108)

Bruchfeld A, et al. Pegylated interferon and ribavirin treatment for hepatitis C in haemodialysis patients. J Viral Hepat 2006;13:316–321. (Ref.95)

Bucci JR, et al. Donor hepatitis C seropositivity: clinical correlates and effect on early graft and patient survival in adult cadaveric kidney transplantation. J Am Soc Nephrol 2002;13:2974–2982. (Ref.110)

Camarero C, et al. Hepatitis C virus infection acquired in childhood. Eur J Pediatr 2008;167:219–224. (Ref.66)

Cano O, et al. Course of patients with chronic hepatitis C virus infection undergoing heart transplantation. Transplant Proc 2007;39:2353–2354. (Ref.115)

Carreno MC, et al. Hepatitis C virus infection after lung transplantation: dim prognosis. J Heart Lung Transplant 2001;20:224. (Ref.118)

Carriero D, et al. Treatment of dialysis patients with chronic hepatitis C using pegylated interferon and low-dose ribavirin. Int J Artif Organs 2008;31:295–302. (Ref.97)

Challine D, Chevaliez S, Pawlotsky JM. Efficacy of serologic marker screening in identifying hepatitis B virus infection in organ, tissue, and cell donors. Gastroenterology 2008;135:1185–1191. (Ref.3)

Chan TM, et al. Preemptive lamivudine therapy based on HBV DNA level in HBsAg-positive kidney allograft recipients. Hepatology 2002;36:1246–1252. (Ref.43)

Chan TM, et al. Treatment of fibrosing cholestatic hepatitis with lamivudine. Gastroenterology 1998;115:177–181. (Ref.45)

Cruzado JM, et al. Pretransplant interferon prevents hepatitis C virus-associated glomerulonephritis in renal allografts by HCV-RNA clearance. Am J Transplant 2003;3:357–360. (Ref.99)

Delladetsima I, et al. The course of hepatitis C virus infection in pretransplantation anti-hepatitis C virus-negative renal transplant recipients: a retrospective follow-up study. Am J Kidney Dis 2006;47:309–316. (Ref.107)

Durlik M, et al. Long-term results of treatment of chronic hepatitis B, C and D with interferon-alpha in renal allograft recipients. Transpl Int 1998;11(Suppl 1):S135–S139. (Ref.50)

Dzekova P, et al. Long-term follow up of sustained viral response after treatment of hepatitis C with pegylated interferon alpha-2a in hemodialysis patients. Int J Artif Organs 2009;32:180–184. (Ref.94)

Fabrizi F, et al. Interferon monotherapy of chronic hepatitis C in dialysis patients: meta-analysis of clinical trials. J Viral Hepat 2008;15:79–88. (Ref.92)

Fabrizi F, et al. Meta-analysis: anti-viral therapy of hepatitis C virus-related liver disease in renal transplant patients. Aliment Pharmacol Ther 2006;24:1413–1422. (Ref.114)

Fabrizi F, et al. HBsAg seropositive status and survival after renal transplantation: meta-analysis of observational studies. Am J Transplant 2005;5:2913–2921. (Ref.36)

Fabrizi F, et al. Hepatitis C virus antibody status and survival after renal transplantation: meta-analysis of observational studies. Am J Transplant 2005;5:1452–1461. (Ref.76)

Fabrizi F, et al. Post-transplant diabetes mellitus and HCV seropositive status after renal transplantation: meta-analysis of clinical studies. Am J Transplant 2005;5:2433–2440. (Ref.90)

Fagiuoli S, et al. HBV and HCV infections in heart transplant recipients. J Heart Lung Transplant 2001;20:718–724. (Ref.53)

Finelli L, et al. National surveillance of dialysis-associated diseases in the United States, 2002. Semin Dial 2005;18:52–61. (Ref.21)

Gasink LB, et al. Hepatitis C virus seropositivity in organ donors and survival in heart transplant recipients. JAMA 2006;296:1843–1850. (Ref.116)

Ghafari A, Sanadgol H. Impact of hepatitis B and hepatitis C virus infections on patients and allograft outcomes in renal transplant recipients: a single center study. Transplant Proc 2008;40:196–198. (Ref.31)

Gordon CE, et al. Interferon treatment in hemodialysis patients with chronic hepatitis C virus infection: a systematic review of the literature and meta-analysis of treatment efficacy and harms. Am J Kidney Dis 2008;51:263–277. (Ref.100)

Grossi P, et al. Lamivudine treatment for HBV infection following thoracic organ transplantation. Transplant Proc 2001;33:1576–1578. (Ref.51)

Gupta SK. Tenofovir-associated Fanconi syndrome: review of the FDA adverse event reporting system. AIDS Patient Care STDS 2008;22:99–103. (Ref.49)

Han DJ, et al. Results on preemptive or prophylactic treatment of lamivudine in HBsAg (+) renal allograft recipients: comparison with salvage treatment after hepatic dysfunction with HBV recurrence. Transplantation 2001;71:387–394. (Ref.44)

Hartwig MG, et al. Hepatitis B core antibody positive donors as a safe and effective therapeutic option to increase available organs for lung transplantation. Transplantation 2005;80:320–325. (Ref.56)

Hassan AA, et al. Impact of hepatitis C on renal transplantation: a long-term study. Saudi J Kidney Dis Transpl 1999;10:487–492. (Ref.79)

Hogan WJ, et al. Hepatic injury after nonmyeloablative conditioning followed by allogeneic hematopoietic cell transplantation: a study of 193 patients. Blood 2004;103:78–84. (Ref.62)

Hoofnagle JH. Reactivation of hepatitis B. Hepatology 2009;49:S156–S165. (Ref.1)

Hsiao LT, et al. Extended lamivudine therapy against hepatitis B virus infection in hematopoietic stem cell transplant recipients. Biol Blood Marrow Transplant 2006;12:84–94. (Ref.14)

Huang H, et al. Lamivudine for the prevention of hepatitis B virus reactivation after high-dose chemotherapy and autologous hematopoietic stem cell transplantation for patients with advanced or relapsed non-Hodgkin's lymphoma single institution experience. Expert Opin Pharmacother 2009;10:2399–2406. (Ref.18)

Hui CK, et al. Hepatitis B reactivation after withdrawal of pre-emptive lamivudine in patients with haematological malignancy on completion of cytotoxic chemotherapy. Gut 2005;54:1597–1603. (Ref.19)

Hui CK, et al. Kinetics and risk of de novo hepatitis B infection in HBsAg-negative patients undergoing cytotoxic chemotherapy. Gastroenterology 2006;131:59–68. (Ref.20)

Hui CK, et al. A long-term follow-up study on hepatitis B surface antigen-positive patients undergoing allogeneic hematopoietic stem cell transplantation. Blood 2005;106:464–469. (Ref.9)

Hui CK, et al. Effectiveness of prophylactic anti-HBV therapy in allogeneic hematopoietic stem cell transplantation with HBsAg positive donors. Am J Transplant 2005;5:1437–1445. (Ref.15)

Hui CK, et al. Sexual transmission of hepatitis B infection despite the presence of hepatitis B virus immunity in recipients of allogeneic bone marrow transplantation. J Clin Virol 2005;32:173–178. (Ref.8)

Ingsathit A, et al. Different impacts of hepatitis B virus and hepatitis C virus on the outcome of kidney transplantation. Transplant Proc 2007;39:1424–1428. (Ref.35)

Izopet J, et al. Longitudinal analysis of hepatitis C virus replication and liver fibrosis progression in renal transplant recipients. J Infect Dis 2000;181:852–858. (Ref.72)

Jung S, et al. Four cases of hepatitis B virus-related fibrosing cholestatic hepatitis treated with lamivudine. J Gastroenterol Hepatol 2002;17:345–350. (Ref.46)

Kamar N, et al. Natural history of hepatitis C virus-related liver fibrosis after renal transplantation. Am J Transplant 2005;5:1704–1712. (Ref.74)

Kasiske BL, et al. Diabetes mellitus after kidney transplantation in the United States. Am J Transplant 2003;3:178–185. (Ref.89)

Kasprzyk T, et al. Long-term results of kidney transplantation from HCV-positive donors. Transplant Proc 2007;39:2701–2703. (Ref.109)

KDIGO clinical practice guideline for the care of kidney transplant recipients. Am J Transplant 2009;9(Suppl 3):S1–S155. (Ref.40)

Kempinska A, Kwak EJ, Angel JB. Reactivation of hepatitis B infection following allogeneic bone marrow transplantation in a hepatitis B-immune patient: case report and review of the literature. Clin Infect Dis 2005;41:1277–1282. (Ref.4)

Kliem V, et al. Relationship of hepatitis B or C virus prevalences, risk factors, and outcomes in renal transplant recipients: analysis of German data. Transplant Proc 2008;40:909–914. (Ref.37)

Knoll A, et al. Reactivation of resolved hepatitis B virus infection after allogeneic haematopoietic stem cell transplantation. Bone Marrow Transplant 2004;33:925–929. (Ref.10)

Knoll A, et al. Solid-organ transplantation in HBsAg-negative patients with antibodies to HBV core antigen: low risk of HBV reactivation. Transplantation 2005;79:1631–1633. (Ref.29)

Lau GK, et al. Preemptive use of lamivudine reduces hepatitis B exacerbation after allogeneic hematopoietic cell transplantation. Hepatology 2002;36:702–709. (Ref.16)

Lau GK, et al. High hepatitis B virus (HBV) DNA viral load as the most important risk factor for HBV reactivation in patients positive for HBV surface antigen undergoing autologous hematopoietic cell transplantation. Blood 2002;99:2324–2330. (Ref.7)

Lau GK, et al. Clearance of persistent hepatitis B virus infection in Chinese bone marrow transplant recipients whose donors were anti-hepatitis B core- and anti-hepatitis B surface antibody-positive. J Infect Dis 1998;178:1585–1591. (Ref.12)

Lau GK, et al. Resolution of chronic hepatitis B and anti-HBs seroconversion in humans by adoptive transfer of immunity to hepatitis B core antigen. Gastroenterology 2002;122:614–624. (Ref.13)

Lau GK, et al. Early is superior to deferred preemptive lamivudine therapy for hepatitis B patients undergoing chemotherapy. Gastroenterology 2003;125:1742–1749. (Ref.17)

Lin HH, et al. Impact of HCV infection on first cadaveric renal transplantation, a single center experience. Clin Transplant 2004;18:261–266. (Ref.83)

Liu CJ, et al. Lamivudine treatment for hepatitis B reactivation in HBsAg carriers after organ transplantation: a 4-year experience. J Gastroenterol Hepatol 2001;16:1001–1008. (Ref.23)

Locasciulli A, et al. The role of hepatitis C and B virus infections as risk factors for severe liver complications following allogeneic BMT: a prospective study by the infectious disease working party of the European blood and marrow transplantation group. Transplantation 1999;68:1486–1491. (Ref.59)

Loomba R, et al. Systematic review: the effect of preventive lamivudine on hepatitis B reactivation during chemotherapy. Ann Intern Med 2008;148: 519–528. (Ref.6)

Luan FL, et al. Impact of immunosuppressive regimen on survival of kidney transplant recipients with hepatitis C. Transplantation 2008;85:1601–1606. (Ref.77)

Lunel F, et al. Hepatitis virus infections in heart transplant recipients: epidemiology, natural history, characteristics, and impact on survival. Gastroenterology 2000;119:1064–1074. (Ref.52)

Mandal AK, et al. Shorter waiting times for hepatitis C virus seropositive recipients of cadaveric renal allografts from hepatitis C virus seropositive donors. Clin Transplant 2000;14:391–396. (Ref.105)

Manga Sahin G, et al. Impact of hepatitis C virus infection on patient and graft survival in kidney transplantation. Transplant Proc 2006;38:499–501. (Ref.80)

Mathurin P, et al. Impact of hepatitis B and C virus on kidney transplantation outcome (see comments). Hepatology 1999;29:257–263. (Ref.33)

Meier-Kriesche HU, et al. Hepatitis C antibody status and outcomes in renal transplant recipients. Transplantation 2001;72:241–244. (Ref.78)

Minz M, et al. Impact of anti-hepatitis C virus (HCV) antibody on outcomes in renal transplant recipients infected with HCV. Transplant Proc 2008;40: 2386–2388. (Ref.81)

Murakami R, et al. Reactivation of hepatitis and lamivudine therapy in 11 HBsAg-positive renal allograft recipients: a single centre experience. Clin Transplant 2006;20:351–358. (Ref.22)

Natov SN, et al. Hepatitis C virus genotype does not affect patient survival among renal transplant candidates. The New England Organ Bank hepatitis C study group. Kidney Int 1999;56:700–706. (Ref.112)

Natov SN. Transmission of viral hepatitis by kidney transplantation: donor evaluation and transplant policies (Part 1: hepatitis B virus). Transpl Infect Dis 2002;4:124–131. (Ref.70)

Park SK, et al. Outcome of renal transplantation in hepatitis B surface antigen-positive patients after introduction of lamivudine. Nephrol Dial Transplant 2001;16:2222–2228. (Ref.42)

Peffault de Latour R, et al. Treatment of chronic hepatitis C virus in allogeneic bone marrow transplant recipients. Bone Marrow Transplant 2005;36:709–713. (Ref.69)

Peffault de Latour R, et al. Long-term outcome of hepatitis C infection after bone marrow transplantation. Blood 2004;103:1618–1624. (Ref.64)

Peres AA, et al. Occult hepatitis B in renal transplant patients. Transpl Infect Dis 2005;7:51–56. (Ref.30)

Quimby D, Brito MO. Fanconi syndrome associated with use of tenofovir in HIV-infected patients: a case report and review of the literature. AIDS Read 2005;15:357–364. (Ref.48)

Ramos CA, et al. Impact of hepatitis C virus seropositivity on survival after allogeneic hematopoietic stem cell transplantation for hematologic malignancies. Haematologica 2009;94:249–257. (Ref.67)

Rendina M, et al. The treatment of chronic hepatitis C with peginterferon alfa-2a (40 kDa) plus ribavirin in haemodialysed patients awaiting renal transplant. J Hepatol 2007;46:768–774. (Ref.96)

Ridruejo E, et al. Hepatitis C virus infection and outcome of renal transplantation. Transplant Proc 2007;39:3127–3130. (Ref.85)

Romero E, et al. Hepatitis C virus infection after renal transplantation. Transplant Proc 2008;40:2933–2935. (Ref.82)

Sahi H, et al. Outcomes after lung transplantation in patients with chronic hepatitis C virus infection. J Heart Lung Transplant 2007;26:466–471. (Ref.117)

Santos L, et al. Impact of hepatitis B and C virus infections on kidney transplantation: a single center experience. Transplant Proc 2009; 41:880–882. (Ref.38)

Savas N, et al. Clinical course of hepatitis B virus infection in renal allograft recipients. Dig Dis Sci 2007;52:3440–3443. (Ref.39)

Sengler U, et al. Testing of corneoscleral discs and their culture media of seropositive donors for hepatitis B and C virus genomes. Graefes Arch Clin Exp Ophthalmol 2001;239:783–787. (Ref.58)

Sharma RK, et al. Chronic hepatitis C virus infection in renal transplant: treatment and outcome. Clin Transplant 2006;20:677–683. (Ref.113)

Shitrit AB, et al. Lamivudine prophylaxis for hepatitis B virus infection after lung transplantation. Ann Thorac Surg 2006;81:1851–1852. (Ref.55)

Socie G, de Latour RP, McDonald GB. Hepatitis C virus and allogeneic stem cell transplantation still matters! Haematologica 2009;94:170–172. (Ref.63)

Strasser SI, et al. Hepatitis C virus infection and bone marrow transplantation: a cohort study with 10-year follow-up. Hepatology 1999;29:1893–1899. (Ref.60)

Strasser SI, et al. Cirrhosis of the liver in long-term marrow transplant survivors. Blood 1999;93:3259–3266. (Ref.65)

Sumethkul V, Ingsathit A, Jirasiritham S. Ten-year follow-up of kidney transplantation from hepatitis B surface antigen-positive donors. Transplant Proc 2009;41:213–215. (Ref.41)

van Leusen R, et al. Pegylated interferon alfa-2a (40 kD) and ribavirin in haemodialysis patients with chronic hepatitis C. Nephrol Dial Transplant 2008;23:721–725. (Ref.98)

Weinbaum CM, et al. Recommendations for identification and public health management of persons with chronic hepatitis B virus infection. MMWR Recomm Rep 2008;57:1–20. (Ref.2)

Woodward CL, et al. Tenofovir-associated renal and bone toxicity. HIV Med 2009;10:482–487. (Ref.47)

Zampino R, et al. Heart transplantation in patients with chronic hepatitis B: clinical evolution, molecular analysis, and effect of treatment. Transplantation 2005;80:1340–1343. (Ref.54)

A complete list of references can be found at www.expertconsult.com.

Section VI

Immune Diseases of the Liver

Autoimmune Hepatitis

Christian P. Strassburg and Michael P. Manns

ABBREVIATIONS

AASLD American Association for the Study of Liver Diseases
AIH autoimmune hepatitis
AIRE autoimmune regulator
AMA antimitochondrial antibody
ANA antinuclear antibodies
ANCA antineutrophilic cytoplasmic antibody
APECED/APS1 autoimmune polyendocrinopathy–candidosis–ectodermal dystrophy
APS1 autoimmune polyendocrine syndrome type 1

ASGPR asialoglycoprotein receptor
cANCA cytoplasmic antineutrophilic cytoplasmic antibodies
FTCD formiminotransferase cyclodeaminase
HCC hepatocellular carcinoma
HCV hepatitis C virus
HDV hepatitis D virus
HLA human leukocyte antigen
HSP heat shock protein
HSV herpes simplex virus
IAIHG International Autoimmune Hepatitis Group
IgG immunoglobulin G

LC1 liver cytosolic type 1
LKM1 anti–liver-kidney microsomal type 1
MHC major histocompatibility complex
pANCA perinuclear antineutrophilic cytoplasmic antibody
PBC primary biliary cirrhosis
PSC primary sclerosing cholangitis
SLA/LP soluble liver antigen/liver pancreas
SMA anti–smooth muscle antibodies
TNF-α tumor necrosis factor-α
UDP uridine diphosphate
UGT UDP-glucuronosyltransferase

Introduction

Autoimmune hepatitis (AIH) is a chronic inflammatory disease in which loss of tolerance of hepatic tissue is presumed. Historically, AIH was first defined by Waldenström in 1950 when he described a form of chronic hepatitis in young women with jaundice, elevated γ-globulins, and amenorrhea, which eventually led to liver cirrhosis.[1] It was later recognized in combination with other extrahepatic autoimmune syndromes, and in particular, the presence of antinuclear antibodies (ANAs) led to the term lupoid hepatitis by Mackay and colleagues.[2] Systematic evaluation of the cellular and molecular immunopathology, clinical symptoms, and laboratory features has subsequently led to the establishment of AIH as a separate clinical entity that is serologically heterogeneous and treated with a specific therapeutic strategy.[3] A recently established and revised scoring system allows a reproducible and standardized approach to the diagnosis of AIH in a scientific context.[4-6] Use and interpretation of seroimmunologic and molecular biologic test results permit precise discrimination of AIH from other causes of chronic hepatitis, in particular, from chronic viral infection, the most common form of chronic hepatitis worldwide.[7,8]

Definition and Diagnosis of Autoimmune Hepatitis

Autoimmune hepatitis is usually present for more than 6 months before diagnosis. In 1992, an international panel met in Brighton, United Kingdom, to establish diagnostic criteria for AIH because it was recognized that several features, including histologic changes and clinical manifestation, are also prevalent in other chronic liver disorders.[9] In this and in a revised report the group noted that there is no single test specific for the diagnosis of AIH. In contrast, a set of diagnostic criteria were suggested in form of a diagnostic scoring system designed to classify patients as having probable or definite AIH (**Table 40-1**). According to this approach, diagnosis relies on a combination of specific features of AIH and exclusion of other causes of chronic liver disease (**Table 40-2**). AIH affects predominantly women in any age group and is characterized by marked elevation of serum globulins, in particular, γ-globulins, and circulating autoantibodies. The clinical manifestations range from an absence of symptoms to a severe or fulminant course, which responds to immunosuppressive treatment in most cases. An association

Table 40-1 International Diagnostic Criteria for the Diagnosis of Autoimmune Hepatitis

PARAMETER	SCORE
Sex	
Female	+2
Male	0
Serum biochemistry (ratio of elevation of serum alkaline phosphatase vs. aminotransferase)	
>3.0	−2
1.5-3	0
<1.5	+2
Total serum globulin, γ-globulin, or IgG (times upper limit of normal)	
>2.0	+3
1.5-2.0	+2
1.0-1.5	+1
<1.0	0
ANA, SMA, or LKM-1 autoantibodies in adults (titers by immunofluorescence on rodent tissues)	
>1:80	+3
1:80	+2
1:40	+1
<1:40	0
Antimitochondrial antibody	
Positive	−4
Negative	0
Hepatitis viral markers	
Negative	+3
Positive	−3
Other etiologic factors	
History of drug use	
Yes	−4
No	+1
Alcohol (average consumption)	
<25 g/day	+2
>60 g/day	−2
Genetic factors	
HLA-DR3 or HLA-DR4	+1
Other autoimmune diseases	+2
Response to therapy	
Complete	+2
Relapse	+3
Liver histology	
Interface hepatitis	+3
Predominant lymphoplasmacytic infiltrate	+1
Rosetting of liver cells	+1
None of the above	−5
Biliary changes	−3
Other changes	−3
Seropositivity for other defined autoantibodies	+2

From Alvarez F, et al. International Autoimmune Hepatitis Group Report: review of criteria for diagnosis of autoimmune hepatitis. J Hepatol 1999;31:929–938.

Interpretation of aggregate scores: definite autoimmune hepatitis (AIH), greater than 15 before treatment and greater than 17 after treatment; probable AIH, 10 to 15 before treatment and 12 to 17 after treatment.

ANA, antinuclear antibody; LKM, liver-kidney microsomal; SMA, smooth muscle antibody

Table 40-2 Differential Diagnosis of Autoimmune Hepatitis and Diagnostic Tests

SUSPECTED DIFFERENTIAL DIAGNOSIS	TEST PERFORMED FOR EXCLUSION
Hepatitis C virus (HCV) infection	Anti-HCV (HCV RNA)
Hepatitis B and D viruses (HBV, HDV)	HBsAg, anti-HBc (HBV DNA) Anti-HDV, HDV RNA only when HBsAg positive
Hepatitis A virus (HAV)	Antibodies, serology: IgG, IgM
Hepatitis E virus (HEV)	Only if suspected
Ebstein-Barr virus (EBV)	Only if suspected
Herpes simplex virus (HSV)	Only if suspected
Cytomegalovirus (CMV)	Only if suspected
Varicella-zoster virus (VZV)	Only if suspected
Drug-induced hepatitis	History; if applicable, withdrawal of drug LKM-2, LM autoantibody in selected cases
Primary biliary cirrhosis (PBC)	AMA Specificity of reactivity: PDH-E2, BCKD-E2 Liver histology: copper deposition in bile ducts Unresponsive to steroids
Primary sclerosing cholangitis (PSC)	Cholangiography
Wilson disease	Ceruloplasmin, urine copper, eye examination, quantitative copper in liver biopsy specimen
Hemochromatosis	Serum ferritin, serum iron, transferrin saturation Liver histology: iron staining, quantitative iron in biopsy specimen Genetic testing: C282Y, H63D mutation of HFE gene in Caucasian individuals
α_1-Antitrypsin deficiency	Phenotype testing: PiZZ/PiSS/PiMZ/PiSZ

AMA, antimitochondrial antibody; BCKD-E2, E2 subunit of branched-chain ketoacid dehydrogenase; HBc, hepatitis B core; HBsAg, hepatitis B surface antigen; LKM, liver-kidney microsomal; LM, liver microsomal; PDH-E2, E2 subunit of pyruvate dehydrogenase

with extrahepatic autoimmune diseases (**Table 40-3**), such as rheumatoid arthritis, autoimmune thyroiditis, ulcerative colitis, and diabetes mellitus, and a family history of autoimmune or allergic disorders has been reported.[10]

Autoantibodies are one of the distinguishing features of AIH. The discovery of autoantibodies directed against different cellular targets (**Table 40-4**), including endoplasmic reticulum membrane proteins, nuclear antigens, and cytosolic antigens, has led to a suggested subclassification of AIH based on the presence of three specific autoantibody profiles.

According to this approach, AIH type 1 is characterized by the presence of ANAs or anti–smooth muscle antibodies (SMAs) directed predominantly against smooth muscle actin. AIH type 2 is characterized by anti–liver-kidney microsomal type 1 (LKM1) autoantibodies directed against cytochrome P-450 (CYP) 2D6[11,12] and with lower frequency against uridine diphosphate (UDP)-glucuronosyltransferase (UGT).[13] AIH type 3[14,15] is characterized by autoantibodies against a soluble liver antigen/liver pancreas (SLA/LP) identified as the uridine, guanosine, and adenosine (UGA) suppressor serine tRNA-protein complex.[16-18]

Although the histologic appearance of AIH is characteristic, no specific histologic feature can be used to make the diagnosis.[19] Percutaneous liver biopsy should be performed for grading and staging, as well as for therapeutic monitoring. Histologic features usually include periportal hepatitis with lymphocytic infiltrates, plasma cells, and piecemeal necrosis. With advancing disease, bridging, panlobular, and multilobular necrosis may occur and can ultimately lead to cirrhosis. Lobular hepatitis can be present, but it is indicative of AIH only in the absence of copper deposits or biliary inflammation. In addition, granulomas and iron deposits argue against AIH.

Viral hepatitis should be excluded by the use of reliable, commercially available tests. Exclusion of ongoing infection with hepatitis A, B, and C viruses is sufficient in most cases. Exclusion of other hepatotropic viruses such as cytomegalovirus, Epstein-Barr virus, and herpes group viruses may be required only when such infections are suspected or if the diagnosis of AIH based on the aforementioned criteria remains inconclusive.

The probability of AIH decreases whenever signs of bile duct involvement are present, such as elevated alkaline

Table 40-3 Extrahepatic Associations of Autoimmune Hepatitis Are Present in 10% to 50% of Patients

Frequent

Autoimmune thyroid disease
Ulcerative colitis
Synovitis

Rare or Individual Reports

Rheumatoid arthritis
Lichen planus
Diabetes mellitus
CREST syndrome
Autoimmune thrombocytopenic purpura
Vitiligo
Nail dystrophy
Alopecia

CREST, calcinosis, Raynaud phenomenon, esophageal involvement, sclerodactyly, and telangiectasia

Table 40-4 Heterogeneity of Autoimmune Hepatitis Based on Serologic Findings: Molecular Definitions of the Most Important Autoantigens in Serologic Diagnostics

ANTIBODY	KD	TARGET ANTIGEN	DISEASE
Autoantigens of the Endoplasmic Reticulum (Microsomal Autoantigens)			
LKM1	50	Cytochrome P-450 2D6	Autoimmune hepatitis type 2 Hepatitis C
LKM2	50	Cytochrome P-450 2C9	Ticrynafen-induced hepatitis
LKM3	55	UGT1A	Hepatitis D–associated autoimmunity Autoimmune hepatitis type 2
LKM	50	Cytochrome P-450 2A6	APS1 Hepatitis C
LM	52	Cytochrome P-450 1A2	Dihydralazine-induced hepatitis Hepatitis with APS1
	57	Disulfidisomerase	Halothane hepatitis
	59	Carboxylesterase	Halothane hepatitis
	35	?	Autoimmune hepatitis
	59	?	Chronic hepatitis C
	64	?	Autoimmune hepatitis
	70	?	Chronic hepatitis C
Autoantigens of the Cytosol (Soluble Liver Proteins)			
LC1	58-62	Formiminotransferase cyclodeaminase	Autoimmune hepatitis type 2 Autoimmune hepatitis Hepatitis C?
SLA/LP	50	UGA repressor tRNA-associated protein	Autoimmune hepatitis (type 3)

APS1, autoimmune polyendocrine syndrome type 1; LC1, liver cytosolic type 1; LKM, liver-kidney microsomal; LM, liver microsomal; SLA/LP, soluble liver antigen/liver pancreas; UGA, uridine, guanosine, and adenosine; UGT1A, family 1 uridine diphosphate glucuronosyltransferase

phosphatase levels, histologic signs of cholangiopathy, and detection of antimitochondrial antibody (AMA). If one or more components of the scoring system are not evaluated, a score pointing to a probable diagnosis can be compiled (see **Table 40-1**).

Recently, a simplified scoring system that uses a limited number of generally available parameters has been presented by members of the International Autoimmune Hepatitis Group (IAIHG).[6]

Epidemiology of Autoimmune Hepatitis

Autoimmune hepatitis is a rare disorder. Based on limited epidemiologic data, the prevalence is estimated to range between 50 and 200 per 1 million Caucasian individuals in Western Europe and North America. The prevalence of AIH is similar to that of systemic lupus erythematosus, primary biliary cirrhosis (PBC), and myasthenia gravis, which also have an autoimmune etiology.[20,21] In the North American and western European Caucasian population, AIH accounts for about up to 20% of those with chronic hepatitis.[22] However, chronic viral hepatitis remains the major cause of chronic hepatitis in most Western societies. In countries in which viral hepatitis B and C are endemic, such as in Asia and Africa, the incidence of AIH appears to be significantly lower. Additional epidemiologic analyses are required to comprehensively elucidate the prevalence and geographic distribution of AIH.

Autoantibodies and Etiology of Autoimmune Hepatitis

There is no doubt that loss of self-tolerance is the pathophysiologic process that drives AIH and leads to the observed sequelae. A number of concepts have been pursued to elucidate the causative agents or mechanisms giving rise to AIH. Autoantibodies directed against the endoplasmic reticulum, in particular, autoantibodies against members of the CYP superfamily of proteins, also occur as markers of serologic autoimmunity in patients infected with hepatitis C virus (HCV) and hepatitis D virus (HDV),[23] as well as being frequent transient markers of drug-mediated allergic hepatic disease[24] and even in the context of genetically determined autoimmune disease such as autoimmune polyglandular syndrome type 1 (APS1).[25] The exact immunologic basis of AIH still remains unresolved despite awareness of its serologic features and considerable research effort invested in the autoantigen targets identified. When AIH is diagnosed, the disease is not usually in its early stages, and the initiating events are therefore not available for detailed analysis. The parallel serologic features of virus-associated autoimmunity and genuine AIH, however, have led to the hypothesis of an external trigger (infectious or chemical) for this disease. This suggests that inherent susceptibility in the host is a required co-factor. The epidemiology of AIH unfortunately offers very little information suggesting genetic susceptibility, mainly because familial risk has not been studied sufficiently. Apart from individual reports and in the absence of twin studies, AIH itself does not appear to segregate in families, but the prevalence of other autoimmune diseases, including autoimmune thyroid disease, celiac disease, ulcerative colitis, and others, is increased in relatives. Such findings are the basis for inclusion of first-degree relatives with autoimmune diseases in the revised international scoring system for AIH, a score that describes—for scientific purposes—the likelihood of the presence of AIH. The hypothesis of a trigger and genetic susceptibility is strengthened by a significant body of evidence linking major histocompatibility complex (MHC) genes with AIH.[26] MHC class I and II antigens are critical players in T-cell immunity because of their ability to present short antigenic peptides for recognition by antigen-specific T cells. Variants of MHC-encoded proteins therefore influence the precise interplay of T-cell receptor and human leukocyte antigens (HLAs), including the possibility of determining immunologic susceptibility and resistance. The study of autoantibodies and autoantigens, on the one hand, offers a window to identify the relevant antigenic determinants involved in the loss of tolerance, whereas the study of genetic associations,[27] on the other hand, leads to definition of the permissive genetic profile, and the combination represents the stage on which the pathophysiology of AIH unfolds.[28]

Autoantibodies in Autoimmune Hepatitis

Circulating autoantibodies are a hallmark of AIH. Autoantibodies are the single most important finding determining diagnosis, treatment, and discrimination of autoimmune disease from chronic viral infection. The identification, molecular cloning, and recombinant expression of hepatocellular autoantigens have enabled the implementation of precise testing systems and scientific evaluation of the humoral autoimmunity associated with AIH.[7,29] Autoantibodies with significance for AIH are ANAs, SMAs, LKM antibodies, SLA/LP antibodies, liver cytosolic type 1 (LC1) antibodies, and asialoglycoprotein receptor (ASGPR) antibodies.

ANAs are directed against functional and structural components of the cell nucleus and against nuclear membranes or DNA. The target antigens are a heterogeneous and incompletely defined group of cellular proteins.[30] To date, subtyping of the various ANAs offers no diagnostic or prognostic advantage. ANAs are also detected in patients with PBC, primary sclerosing cholangitis (PSC), viral hepatitis, drug-related hepatitis, and alcoholic liver disease, and investigations have been aimed at identifying target antigens that are specific for AIH. ANAs are determined by indirect immunofluorescence on cryostat sections of rat liver and on Hep.2 cell slides. Most commonly, a homogeneous (**Fig. 40-1**) or speckled immunofluorescence pattern is encountered. ANAs have been found to be reactive with centromeres, ribonucleoproteins, and cyclin A (**Fig. 40-2**).[31] They represent the most common autoantibody in AIH and occur in high titers that usually exceed 1:160.

SMAs are directed against components of the cytoskeleton such as actin, troponin, and tropomyosin.[32-34] They frequently occur in high titer in association with ANAs. However, SMA autoantibodies also occur in patients with advanced diseases of the liver of other cause, such as infectious diseases and rheumatic disorders. In these cases titers are often lower than 1:80. SMA autoantibodies are also determined by indirect immunofluorescence on cryostat sections of rat stomach

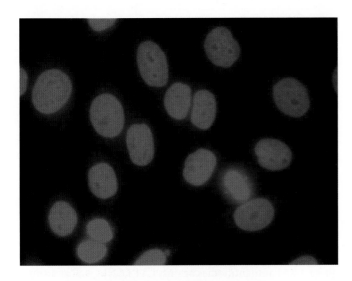

Fig. 40-1 **Indirect immunofluorescence micrograph of antinuclear antibodies detected on immobilized Hep.2 cells.** The typical aspect of homogeneous nuclear staining is found in a patient with type 1 autoimmune hepatitis at titers exceeding 1:160. These autoantibodies are frequently directed against double-stranded DNA and histones and are a typical finding in type 1 autoimmune hepatitis.

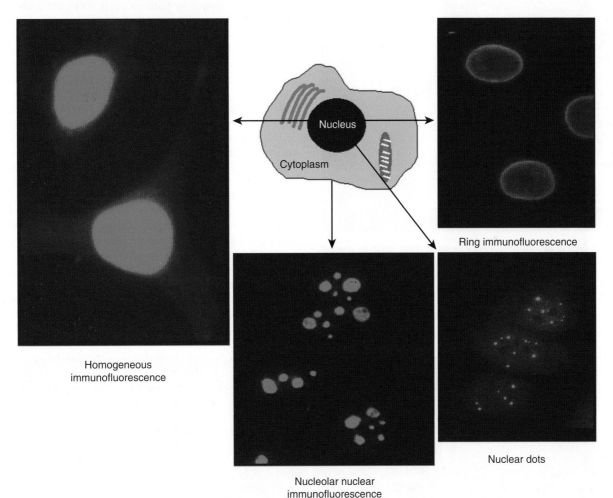

Fig. 40-2 **Indirect immunofluorescence micrographs of a variety of antinuclear antibodies (ANAs) found in autoimmune hepatitis and other autoimmune diseases and detected on immobilized Hep.2 cells.** An aspect of the nuclear membranous (rim) immunofluorescence pattern *(top right)* is found in a patient with autoimmune hepatitis type 1 at titers exceeding 1:160. In this pattern, autoantibodies are directed against lamins (lamin B, but also lamin A and C). Membranous immunofluorescence is not a frequent finding and can indicate the existence of mixed immune syndromes, including vasculitis and other features of systemic lupus erythematosus; it is clearly distinguished from a homogeneous pattern *(top left)*. The *middle panel* demonstrates a nucleolar ANA fluorescence pattern. This pattern is rarely seen in autoimmune hepatitis but is common in rheumatologic diseases such as scleroderma and polymyositis. If present in a patient with autoimmune hepatitis type 1, it can be indicative of overlap syndromes with rheumatologic disorders. The *lower right panel* shows *multiple nuclear dots*. This pattern is not typical of autoimmune hepatitis and is found mainly in about 20% of patients with primary biliary cirrhosis (PBC). Usually, antimitochondrial antibodies (AMAs) are present at the same time but can also be missing in cases of ANA-positive, AMA-negative PBC. These autoantibodies are directed against the sp100 nuclear antigen (100 kD).

(**Fig. 40-3**). SMAs are associated with the HLA-A1/B8/DR3 haplotype, and probably more as a reflection of this status, affected patients are reported to be younger at disease onset and have a poorer prognosis.

LKM autoantibodies are directed against proteins of the endoplasmic reticulum (microsomal protein). In 1973, Rizzetto and associates discovered autoantibodies reactive with the proximal renal tubules and hepatocellular cytoplasm by indirect immunofluorescence (**Fig. 40-4, *A* and *B***).[35] These autoantibodies, termed LKM1, were associated with a second form of AIH that is mostly ANA negative. Between 1988 and 1991, the 50-kD antigen of LKM1 autoantibodies was identified as CYP2D6. LKM1 autoantibodies recognize a major linear epitope between amino acids 263 and 270 of the CYP2D6 protein.[11,36-39] These autoantibodies inhibit

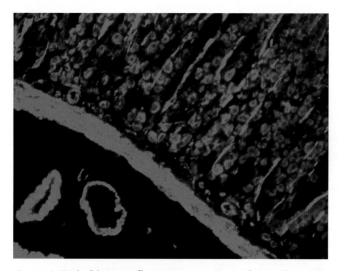

Fig. 40-3 **Typical immunofluorescence pattern of smooth muscle autoantibodies detected on rat stomach cryostat sections.** This serum shows immunoreactivity with the muscularis mucosae and propria mucosae layers of rat stomach. Note that the mucosa is excluded from reactivity. This autoantibody is often detected in conjunction with antinuclear antibodies in patients with autoimmune hepatitis type 1.

CYP2D6 activity in vitro and are capable of activating liver-infiltrating T lymphocytes. This indicates a combined humoral and cellular immune mechanism leading to the development of LKM autoantibodies. In addition to linear epitopes, LKM1 autoantibodies have also been shown to recognize conformation-dependent epitopes.[40] However, the recognition of epitopes located between amino acids 257 and 269 appears to be a specific autoimmune reaction of AIH and discriminates against LKM1 autoantibodies associated with chronic HCV infection (**Fig. 40-5**). The endoplasmic reticulum–based CYP2D6 has been found to be detectable on the hepatocellular surface, and its expression appears to be regulated by cytokines. Antibodies against microsomal proteins form a heterogeneous group spanning several immune-mediated diseases, including AIH, drug-induced hepatitis, autoimmune polyendocrinopathy–candidosis–ectodermal dystrophy (APECED/APS1), and chronic HCV and HDV infection (**Fig. 40-6**; also see **Table 40-4**). LKM autoantibodies against CYP1A2, as well as against CYP2A6, are found in patients with APECED and hepatic involvement. Anti-CYP2A6 autoantibodies also occur in HCV infection. Liver microsomal (LM) autoantibodies have an immunofluorescence pattern in which hepatocellular but not renal cell cytoplasm is stained selectively. LM autoantibodies have been found to be directed against CYP1A2, which is expressed only in the liver. These autoantibodies are also found in APECED syndrome with hepatic involvement and additionally occur in dihydralazine-induced hepatitis.[41] A second type of LKM autoantibodies, LKM2, are directed against CYP2C9 and are detectable in ticrynafen-associated hepatitis.[24,42] A third group of LKM autoantibodies, LKM3, were identified in 6% to 10% of patients with chronic HDV infection by Crivelli and co-workers in 1983.[43] These autoantibodies are directed against family 1 UDP-glucuronosyltransferases (UGT1A),[44] which are also a superfamily of drug-metabolizing proteins located in the endoplasmic reticulum membrane.[45] LKM3 autoantibodies have been identified in patients with HDV infection, as well as in those with AIH type 2.[13] They can also occur in patients with LKM1-negative and ANA-negative AIH. In addition, LKM-positive sera display reactivity with a number of thus far undefined antigens with molecular weights

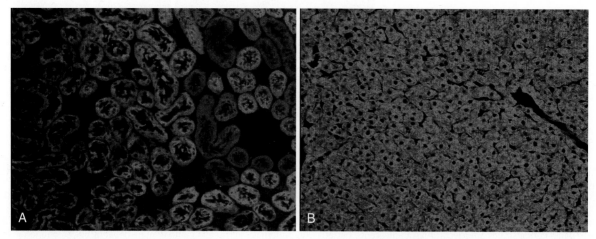

Fig. 40-4 **Indirect immunofluorescence showing liver-kidney microsomal type 1 (LKM1) autoantibodies on rat kidney and liver cryostat sections. A,** Typical indirect immunofluorescence pattern of LKM1 autoantibodies in the proximal (cortical) renal tubules but not in the distal tubules in the renal medulla, which corresponds to the tissue expression pattern of the autoantigen CYP2D6. **B,** Using rat hepatic cryostat sections, homogeneous cellular immunofluorescence staining is visualized, but not in hepatocellular nuclei (LKM1).

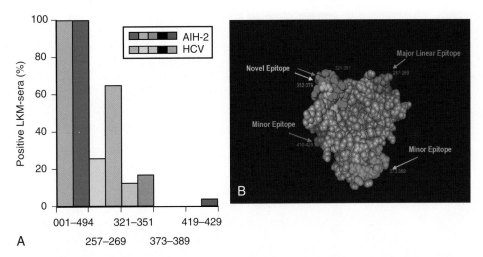

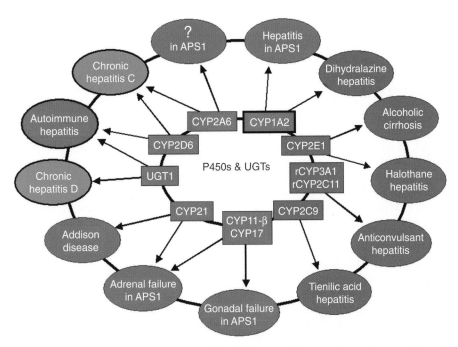

Fig. 40-5 **Liver-kidney microsomal type 1 (LKM1) autoantibodies directed against cytochrome P-450 (CYP) 2D6.** LKM1 autoantibodies display differences in autoepitope recognition in genuine autoimmune hepatitis type 2 (AIH2) and hepatitis C virus (HCV) infection. There are several epitope regions (**A**) targeted by LKM1 autoantibodies, and the greatest differences are seen in an epitope found between amino acids 257 and 269.[40] These epitopes, as well as a large conformation-dependent epitope between amino acids 321 and 379 (compare Table 40-6), are found at the surface of the three-dimensional structure of the CYP2D6 molecule (**B**).

Fig. 40-6 **Diversity of autoantibodies against endoplasmic reticulum (microsomal) targets in autoimmune hepatitis, drug-induced hepatitis, viral hepatitis, and genetic disease (autoimmune polyendocrinopathy–candidosis–ectodermal dystrophy/autoimmune polyglandular syndrome type 1 [APECED/APS1]).** CYP, cytochrome P-450; UGT, uridine diphosphate (UDP) glucuronosyltransferase

of 35, 57, 59, and 70 kD.[46] These autoantibodies are predominantly found in patients with AIH, HCV infection, and halothane-associated hepatitis (**Fig. 40-6**). LKM autoantibodies can be visualized by indirect immunofluorescence on rodent cryostat sections. Subclassification is achieved by enzyme-linked immunosorbent assay and Western blot, preferably using recombinant antigens.

Antibodies against SLA were detected in a patient with ANA-negative AIH.[14] It is now clear that LP antibodies recognize the same target protein structure, which has led to the designation SLA/LP autoantibodies.[15,18] Anti-SLA/LP was found to be highly specific for AIH and is detectable in about 10% to 30% of all patients with AIH. In 1992, Gelpi and colleagues identified specific autoantibodies present in patients with a severe form of autoimmune chronic hepatitis.[16] These antibodies precipitated a UGA suppressor serine tRNA-protein complex, which is probably involved in co-translational selenocysteine incorporation in human cells. Subsequently, SLA/LP antibodies have been identified as being directed against a UGA suppressor serine tRNA-protein complex and not against cytokeratin 8 or 18 or glutathione-*S*-transferases as previously suggested. The exact function and role of this

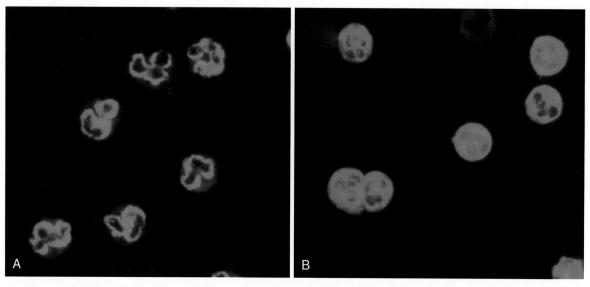

Fig. 40-7 Immunofluorescence study showing antineutrophil cytoplasmic antibodies (ANCAs) with a typical pANCA (A) and cANCA (B) distinction. These autoantibodies are found in up to 95% of patients with autoimmune hepatitis (AIH) type 1 (antinuclear antibody and smooth muscle antibody positive) but are not considered to be a specific diagnostic finding in AIH. When further analyzed, they frequently do not exhibit reactivity with myeloperoxidase (pANCA) or proteinase 3 (cANCA) in patients with AIH.

autoantigen in autoimmunity are thus far unclear. Regarding disease specificity, anti-SLA/LP may be linked to the pathogenesis of the autoimmune process.

Antibodies against LC1 were found in up to 50% of patients with AIH type 2.[47] Less frequently, anti-LC1 may be associated with SMAs and ANAs in sera from patients with AIH type 1 and chronic HCV infection. In addition, anti-LC1 proved to be the only serologic marker in 10% of patients with AIH. Anti-LC1 antibodies are visualized by indirect immunofluorescence; however, their characteristic staining may be masked by the more diffuse pattern of LKM1 antibodies. The antigen recognized by anti-LC1 was identified as formiminotransferase cyclodeaminase (FTCD). FTCD is a metabolic enzyme involved in the conversion of histidine to glutamic acid and is most highly expressed in the liver. It is bifunctional and composed of distinct FT and CD domains connected by a short linker. Anti-LC1 sera recognize distinct epitopes on FTCD preferentially localized to the FT domain.[48] Contrary to most other autoantibodies in AIH, anti-LC1 seems to correlate with disease activity and may be useful as a marker of residual hepatocellular inflammation in patients with AIH.

Antibodies against ASGPR were observed in up to 90% of all patients with AIH and can coexist with ANA, SMA and anti-LKM1.[49] However, they are not disease specific and can also be found in patients with viral hepatitis, drug-induced hepatitis, and PBC. Levels of anti-asialoglycoprotein antibodies correlate with inflammatory disease activity and might be used as an additional marker to monitor treatment efficacy. However, they are not part of the autoantibody spectrum routinely used as a diagnostic tool.

Perinuclear antineutrophilic cytoplasmic antibodies (pANCAs) were detected in 65% to 95% of sera from patients with AIH type 1 and additionally in sera from patients with PSC (**Fig. 40-7**). ANCAs are detected by immunofluorescence, which distinguishes two patterns: cANCA, which features diffuse cytoplasmic staining of neutrophils, and pANCA,

which exhibits rimlike staining of the perinuclear cytoplasm. In AIH, atypical pANCAs (also termed xANCAs) are usually found that display a pANCA immunofluorescence pattern but do not show reactivity with myeloperoxidase, one of the mayor autoantigens of classic ANCA. Discrimination of ANCAs is difficult because when using ethanol fixed for immunofluorescence staining, ANAs are frequently visible. The target antigen in AIH is unknown, but apart from myeloperoxidase, proteinase 3 and elastase have been ruled out as candidates. The role of ANCAs in AIH is unclear, but routine determination may be useful to identify patients formerly classified as having cryptogenic hepatitis.[4]

Etiology of Autoimmune Hepatitis

Conclusive evidence of a single cause of AIH has not yet emerged. Many findings have pointed toward a viral etiology, which has been investigated in numerous studies.[50,51] However, a viral cause of AIH remains a matter of controversy.[52]

A relationship of hepatitis A virus, hepatitis B virus, Epstein-Barr virus, and herpes simplex virus (HSV) with AIH has been implicated in anecdotal reports.[53-56] As a potential mechanism, molecular mimicry between viral and body proteins has been suggested. In this respect it was shown that the B-cell epitope of CYP2D6, which is targeted by LKM1 autoantibodies, displays homology with the immediate early antigen IE175 of HSV (**Fig. 40-8**). A case has been reported in which the only difference in HLA-identical twins with a discordant manifestation of AIH was HSV positivity.[51]

HCV infection is associated with a broad array of serologic markers of autoimmunity and immune-mediated syndromes. LKM autoantibodies are present in 3% to 5% of patients. However, this serologic autoimmunity differs with respect to recognition of antigen targets (CYP2D6 and CYP2A6), recognition of epitopes (AIH, mainly 257 to 269; HCV, more

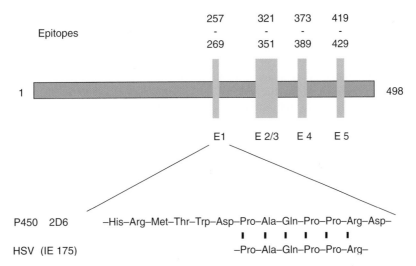

Epitopes

257 - 269   321 - 351   373 - 389   419 - 429

1   498

E1   E 2/3   E 4   E 5

P450 2D6   –His–Arg–Met–Thr–Trp–Asp–Pro–Ala–Gln–Pro–Pro–Arg–Asp–

HSV (IE 175)   –Pro–Ala–Gln–Pro–Pro–Arg–

Fig. 40-8 **Sequence homology between the herpes simplex virus (HSV) IE175 protein and cytochrome P-450 2D6 (CYP2D6), which is recognized by liver-kidney microsomal type 1 autoantibodies in patients with autoimmune hepatitis (AIH) type 2.** This has been suggested as a possible explanation for a virus-triggered onset of AIH by viral mimicry.[11]

Table 40-5 Differences Between Genuine Autoimmune Disease and Virus-Induced Serologic Autoimmunity

	AUTOIMMUNE HEPATITIS	VIRAL HEPATITIS
Autoantibody titer	↑↑↑	↑
Linear autoepitopes	+++	+
Conformational epitopes	+	++++
Inhibitory antibodies	++	++
Autoimmune response	Homogenous	Heterogeneous
Treatment	Immunosuppression	Antiviral

diverse and also more conformation-dependent epitopes) (see **Fig. 40-5**), and clinical manifestations (**Table 40-5**). From these considerations it is unlikely that HCV is etiologically responsible for AIH.[57]

Apart from viral agents, a genetic predisposition must be regarded as a mandatory prerequisite for the development of AIH. However, the genetic background of AIH does not follow a mendelian pattern, and a single genetic locus capable of explaining the etiology of AIH has not yet been conclusively identified. AIH is therefore considered a complex trait like most other human diseases, which means that there are one or more genes acting alone or in concert to reduce or increase the risk for that trait. The heritable component of AIH is currently regarded as small. However, absence of evidence does not mean evidence of absence, and these data have yet to be established.

The most conclusive association with AIH is related to the MHC alleles. Approximately 1000 HLA molecules have been identified to date. The MHC is encoded on a 4000–kilobase pair portion of chromosome 6p21.3. It is characterized by considerable genetic polymorphism and is divided into three regions: MHC class I and II encode HLA-A, HLA-B, HLA-Cw, HLA-DR, HLA-DQ, and HLA-DP, whereas the MHC class III

region encompasses several immune-reactive proteins, including the complement proteins C2, C4A, C4B, the heat shock protein (HSP-70) family, tumor necrosis factor-α (TNF-α) and TNF-β, and MHC class I chain-related proteins (MICA, MICB). Interest in HLA association in AIH stems from the fact that the molecular structure and variation of the MHC-peptide α-helical region at the floor of the peptide binding groove determine antigen presentation to the T-cell receptor and that most of the interindividual variability in HLA alleles is relevant to the amino acid sequence of this peptide binding groove. Patients with the HLA-A1/B8/DRB1*0301 haplotype were found to be younger at disease onset, relapse more often with immunosuppressive treatment, and more frequently require liver transplantation. Subsequent investigations of the encoding HLA alleles found that genetic susceptibility to AIH is related to the six–amino acid sequence LLEQKR at position 67 to 72 of the DRB1 polypeptide. Within these six amino acids the critical amino acid appears to be that found on position 71—namely, lysine or arginine on susceptibility alleles and alanine on resistance alleles. Polymorphisms within this region may affect the predisposition to autoimmune diseases by several mechanisms, including shaping of the T-cell repertoire, peptide selection and presentation, and peptide transport. Association of HLA-A1 and HLA-B8 with AIH had already been reported by Mackay and Morris in 1972.[58]

Genetic variability is not limited to the HLA I and II genes but equally affects TNF-α and TNF-β, complement genes, and MICA and MICB. Although the functional changes in TNF gene promoter polymorphisms are not clear, the role of the molecule in inflammation, cell death, apoptosis, and up-regulation of MHC expression make it an interesting candidate gene.

Association of HLA-A1, HLA-Cw7, HLA-B8, and HLA-DR3—which is inherited as a haplotype—and HLA-DR4 with AIH and other autoimmune diseases has been demonstrated conclusively in a number of studies.[59,60] In turn, an association with HLA-B, HLA-Cw, and TNF-α has been found not to be the major factor. Studies from Europe and the United States have identified DRB1*0301 and DRB1*0401 as susceptibility alleles and DRB1*1501 as a resistance allele (see **Table 40-2**).[61,62] However, these immunogenetic findings do not appear to apply universally, and it was noted that significant geographic differences exist. In Japan, DR2 (DRB1*1501) is a weak susceptibility rather than a resistance allele,[63] and in South American children, DRB1*1301 is a strong susceptibility allele[64] that has not been found in any of the other studies. Molecular comparison of amino acid residues at the α-helical binding groove region of the HLA molecule has suggested that risk for AIH appears to be conferred by histidine at position 13 in Japanese patients; by lysine at position 71 in U.S. and European patients, as well as in Japanese, Mexican, and Argentinian patients; and by valine at position 86 in South American children (see **Fig. 40-5**). These data illustrate that genetic association varies in study populations (**Table 40-6**). A number of explanations may account for this finding. An exogenous factor present in a distinct population may be necessary (molecular footprint), which is in line with the current hypothesis of an environmental trigger and genetic susceptibility, but the model may just be too simple altogether in its assumption of the relevance of differences in single amino acid residues. AIH is not likely to be a monogenetic or oligogenetic disease. It is obvious that a polygenetic profile of factors that remain to be elucidated will define predisposition for this disease.

Table 40-6 Heterogeneity of Autoimmune Hepatitis Based on Genetic Markers

	HLA-DR3	HLA-DR4
Genotype	DR B1*0301	DR B1*0401 (DR B1*0405 in Japanese)
Age at onset	<30	>40
Disease activity	+++	+
Treatment response	++	++++
Relapse after treatment	+++	+
Liver transplantation	+++	+
DR-β chain amino acid as risk factor	Lysine at amino acid 71	?

Non–Major Histocompatibility Complex Genes and Autoimmune Hepatitis

The CD152 (cytotoxic lymphocyte antigen-4, CTLA-4) molecule on immunoregulatory (CD25 positive) T cells interacts with CD80 and CD86 on the antigen-presenting cell with up to a 50-fold higher affinity than for CD28. Co-recognition of CD152 results in a reduction in the immune response. The CTLA-4 gene has been shown to exhibit more than 16 single nucleotide polymorphisms, and the CTLA-4 A+49G allele was found to be associated with diabetes, PBC, and autoimmune thyroiditis. An association with AIH makes biologic sense and is indeed the strongest non-MHC association yet.[65] Study of interleukin-1 and interleukin-10 did not reveal any associations. Variants of the vitamin D receptor, which is associated with a number of autoimmune diseases, as well as with the tyrosine phosphatase CD45, showed a weak association with AIH.[66,67]

Autoimmune Hepatitis in Autoimmune Polyendocrine Syndrome Type 1: A Model Disease?

APS1 syndrome is characterized by a number of autoimmune disorders involving endocrine and nonendocrine organs, including mucocutaneous candidiasis, hypoparathyroidism, and adrenal insufficiency (the diagnosis is established when two of the latter are present).[25] In 10% of patients, AIH is present. APS1 has greatly increased our understanding of autoimmune diseases because it has a monogenic association with mutations in the *AIRE* (autoimmune regulatory) gene. AIRE is expressed in medullary epithelial cells of the thymus and accounts for less than 0.1% of thymic cells.[68] The transcription factor encoded by the *AIRE* gene regulates the expression of a multitude of antigens required for the negative selection of autoreactive T cells in the thymus. In AIRE-deficient mice, less autoantigen is expressed in thymic medullary epithelial cells, thereby resulting in a higher number of more highly reactive T cells in the periphery, which contributes to the establishment of autoimmune disease.[69] AIH in APS1 syndrome leads to the formation of autoantibodies against CYP1A2 and CYP2A6. AIH may be the first clinically apparent component of this syndrome, particularly in children.[70] However, retrospective analysis of adult patients with AIH has not detected an increased frequency of variant *AIRE* alleles.[71]

Clinical Features

Systematically, AIH is part of the syndrome of chronic hepatitis, which is characterized by sustained hepatocellular inflammation of at least 6 months' duration and elevation of alanine and aspartate aminotransferase 1.5 times the upper limit of normal.[8] In about 49% of patients the onset of AIH is acute, and rare cases of fulminant AIH have been reported. In most cases, however, the clinical findings are not spectacular and include fatigue, right upper quadrant pain, jaundice, and occasionally, palmar erythema and spider nevi. In later stages, the consequences of portal hypertension dominate, including ascites, bleeding esophageal varices, and encephalopathy. A specific feature of AIH is the association of extrahepatic immune-mediated syndromes, including autoimmune thyroiditis, vitiligo, alopecia, nail dystrophy, ulcerative colitis, and rheumatoid arthritis, as well as diabetes mellitus and glomerulonephritis (see **Table 40-3**).

Subclassification

Immunserologic parameters assume a central role in the subclassification of AIH (see **Table 40-4**) and allow clinically differing groups of patients to be distinguished. The IAIHG has not recommended these subdivisions for other than research purposes because autoantibodies do not define distinct therapeutic groups. However, they noted that the distinction between AIH type 1 and type 2 has already been widely adopted in clinical practice.[72]

AIH type 1 is characterized by ANA and in most cases also SMA autoantibodies. In 97% of patients, hypergammaglobulinemia with elevated immunoglobulin G (IgG) is present. Representing 80% of cases of AIH, this form is the most prevalent subclass, which was historically first described as lupoid, classic, or idiopathic AIH. Seventy percent of patients are female, and it occurs at all ages.[73] However, 50% are older than 30 years.[73] An association with other immune syndromes is observed in 48%, with autoimmune thyroid disease, synovitis, and ulcerative colitis leading the list. The clinical course is often unspectacular and an acute onset is very rare. About 25% have cirrhosis at the time of diagnosis.

AIH type 2 is characterized by the presence of LKM1 autoantibodies against CYP2D6. In 10%, LKM3 autoantibodies against UDP-glucuronosyltransferases[74] are also present. In contrast to AIH type 1, additional organ-specific autoantibodies are present such as antithyroid, anti–parietal cell, and anti–Langerhans cell autoantibodies. The number of extrahepatic immune syndromes, such as diabetes, vitiligo, and autoimmune thyroid disease, is also more prevalent. Serum immunoglobulin levels are moderately elevated, with a reduction in IgA. AIH type 2 is a rare disorder that affects 20% of AIH patients in Europe but only 4% in the United States. There is a female preponderance. The age maximum is around 10 years, but AIH type 2 is also observed in adults, especially in Europe. AIH type 2 carries a higher risk for progression to cirrhosis and a fulminant course.

AIH type 3 is characterized by SLA/LP autoantibodies, but 74% also have other serologic markers of autoimmunity, including SMAs and AMAs. AIH type 3 has a lower prevalence than AIH type 2, affects female patients in 90% of cases, and has an age maximum between 20 and 40 years. This subclass of AIH is a matter of debate, and further evaluation is needed to determine whether it represents an entity in itself or is a variation of AIH type 1. However, it is important to diagnose anti-SLA/LP–positive AIH, which occurs in 10% of cases of AIH as the only serologic marker. This may therefore decrease the likelihood of misclassification.

Cryptogenic Hepatitis and Overlap Syndromes

Cryptogenic hepatitis is etiologically undefined chronic hepatitis. It is unclear how many of these patients in fact suffer from AIH without the presence of serum autoantibodies detectable with the available state-of-the-art techniques. In about 13% of these patients, who had initially been tested by

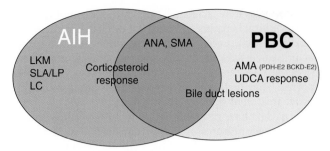

Fig. 40-9 **"Overlap syndrome" involving autoimmune hepatitis (AIH) and primary biliary cirrhosis (PBC).**[7] A true overlap is established by documentation of hepatitis and cholestasis biochemically, histology compatible with both diseases (presence of biliary lesions with otherwise typical features of AIH), and the presence of antimitochondrial autoantibodies (AMAs), as well as autoantibodies typical of AIH (i.e., antinuclear antibody [ANA]). For antibody nomenclature see Table 40-2. BCKD-E2, E2 subunit of branched-chain ketoacid dehydrogenase; LC, liver cytosolic; LKM, liver-kidney microsomal; PDH-E2, E2 subunit of pyruvate dehydrogenase; SLA/LP, soluble liver antigen/liver pancreas; UDCA, ursodeoxycholic acid.

indirect immunofluorescence for ANA, SMA, and LKM autoantibodies, it was possible to detect SLA autoantibodies, which contributed to diagnostic clarification. Clinically, this group of patients with cryptogenic hepatitis resembles those with AIH type 1 with respect to age and sex distribution, HLA types, inflammatory activity, and response to therapy.

Overlap syndromes are conditions in which there are leading symptoms of AIH but additional markers and symptoms point to other diseases in the differential diagnosis of AIH. Among these diseases are PBC in 8% with serum AMAs and histologic signs of cholangitis, PSC in 6% with typical changes noted on cholangiography, and autoimmune cholangitis in 10% with ANAs, SMAs, and histologic inflammation of the biliary system.[75] However, a concise and universally accepted definition of an overlap syndrome is currently lacking (**Fig. 40-9**). In addition, the frequency of this condition is a matter of controversy. The differences reported may reflect variations between serologic overlap and genuine clinical overlap of two autoimmune diseases. The latter appears to be very rare.[76]

A clinically significant association is virus-associated autoimmunity, which describes the coexistence of autoantibodies and virus infection.[10,23] The most important associations are HCV and HDV infection, in which LKM autoantibodies can be detected in 2% to 5% and 6% to 12% of patients, respectively. AIH type 2 and HCV infection with LKM autoantibodies are clinically distinct entities (see **Table 40-5**). LKM autoantibodies in patients with viral infection are present at lower titer and recognize more conformational and diverse epitopes than do those in patients with genuine AIH (see **Fig. 40-5**). This discrimination is relevant, as it forms the basis for mutually exclusive therapeutic strategies: immunosuppression for AIH and interferon for chronic virus hepatitis.[77]

Natural History and Prognosis

Data describing the natural history of AIH are scarce. The last placebo-controlled immunosuppressive treatment trial was published in 1980.[78] The value of these studies is limited since these patients were screened only for epidemiologic risk factors for viral hepatitis and were not evaluated by standardized diagnostic criteria. Nevertheless, these studies revealed that untreated AIH has a very poor prognosis, and 5- and 10-year survival rates of 50% and 10%, respectively, have been reported. They furthermore demonstrated that immunosuppressive treatment significantly improves survival.

Recent data have revealed that up to 30% of adult patients have histologic features of cirrhosis at diagnosis. In 17% of patients with periportal hepatitis, cirrhosis developed within 5 years, but cirrhosis develops in 82% when bridging necrosis or necrosis of multiple lobules is present. The frequency of remission (86%) and treatment failure (14%) is comparable in patients with and without cirrhosis at initial evaluation. Importantly, the presence of cirrhosis does not influence 10-year survival rates (90%), and these patients require a similarly aggressive treatment strategy.[79,80]

Almost half of children with AIH already have cirrhosis at the time of diagnosis. Long-term follow-up has revealed that only few children can completely stop all treatment and about 70% receive long-term treatment.[81,82] Most of these patients relapse when treatment is discontinued or if the dose of immunosuppressive drug is reduced. In about 15% of patients chronic liver failure develops, and they undergo transplantation before the age of 18 years.

In elderly patients, a more severe initial histologic grade has been reported, but the frequency of definite cirrhosis does not seem to differ from that in younger patients. At follow-up, cirrhosis is found in about 30% of patients. Response to immunosuppression is similar in older and younger patients, and up to 90% of older patients reach complete remission. However, in a study from the United Kingdom, 41% of the elderly patients with AIH received no immunosuppressive therapy and the prognosis did not appear to be worse than that in younger, usually treated patients.[83]

The risk for hepatocellular carcinoma (HCC) varies considerably in patients with PBC, PSC, and AIH. In particular, PSC can be complicated by cholangiocarcinoma, gallbladder carcinoma, and HCC. In contrast, the development of HCC in patients with AIH is a rare event and occurs only in those with long-standing cirrhosis.

Therapy

The indication for treatment of AIH is based on inflammatory activity and not so much on the presence of cirrhosis. In the absence of inflammatory activity, immunosuppressive treatment has only limited effects.

Independent of the clinically or immunoserologically defined type of AIH, treatment consists of prednisone or prednisolone alone or in combination with azathioprine. Both strategies are equally effective.[72] Prednisone and its metabolite prednisolone are also equally effective because chronic liver disease does not seem to have an effect on the synthesis of prednisolone from prednisone. However, exact differentiation between viral infection and AIH is important. Replicative viral hepatitis must not be treated with corticosteroids, and interferon must not be administered to patients with AIH, in whom it can lead to dramatic exacerbation of disease.

An indication for treatment is present when aminotransferases are elevated two-fold, γ-globulin levels are elevated two-fold, and histology shows moderate to severe periportal hepatitis. Symptoms of severe fatigue are also an indication for treatment. An absolute indication exists in patients with a ten-fold or higher elevation of aminotransferase levels, histologic signs of severe inflammation and necrosis, and progression of disease.[5]

The treatment regimen and suggested follow-up examinations are summarized in **Table 40-7**. Therapy is usually administered over the course of 2 years. The decision for monotherapy or combination therapy is guided by certain considerations. Long-term steroid therapy leads to cushingoid side effects, with the cosmetic side effects in particular decreasing patient

Table 40-7 Immunosuppressive Treatment Regimens for Adults with Autoimmune Hepatitis

	MONOTHERAPY WITH PREDNISONE ONLY* (mg/day)	COMBINATION THERAPY		
		Prednisone* (mg/day)	Azathioprine US (mg/day)	EU (mg/kg/day)
Week 1	60	30	50	1-2
Week 2	40	20	50	1-2
Week 3	30	15	50	1-2
Week 4	30	15	50	1-2
Maintenance until end point	20 and below	10	50	1-2
Reasons for preference	Cytopenia Thiopurine methyltransferase deficiency Pregnancy Malignancy Short course (≤6 mo)	Postmenopausal state Osteoporosis Brittle diabetes Obesity Acne Emotional lability Hypertension		

From Manns MP, et al. Diagnosis and management of autoimmune hepatitis. Hepatology 2010;51:2193–2213; adapted from Manns MP, Strassburg CP. Autoimmune hepatitis: clinical challenges. Gastroenterology 2001;120:1502–1517.

*Prednisolone can be used in place of prednisone at equivalent doses.

EU, European Union; US, United States.

Table 40-8 Typical Unwanted Drug Effects of Immunosuppressants

MEDICATIONS	SIDE EFFECTS
Prednisone and prednisolone	Acne Moon-shaped face Striae rubrae Dorsal hump Obesity Gain of weight Diabetes mellitus Cataract Hypertension
Azathioprine	Nausea Vomiting Abdominal discomfort Hepatotoxicity Rash Leukocytopenia Teratogenicity Oncogenicity

compliance considerably (**Table 40-8**). Serious complications such as steroid-induced diabetes, osteopenia, aseptic bone necrosis, psychiatric symptoms, hypertension, and cataract formation also have to be anticipated with long-term treatment. Side effects are present in 44% of patients after 12 months and in 80% after 24 months of treatment. However, prednisone or prednisolone monotherapy is possible in pregnant patients. Azathioprine, in contrast, leads to a decreased dose of prednisone. It has a theoretic risk for teratogenicity. In addition, abdominal discomfort, nausea, cholestatic hepatitis, rash, and leukopenia can be encountered. These side effects are seen in 10% of patients receiving a dose of 50 mg/day. From a general point of view, a postmenopausal woman with osteoporosis, hypertension, and elevated blood glucose would be a candidate for combination therapy. In young women, pregnant women, or patients with hematologic abnormalities, prednisone monotherapy may be the treatment of choice.

Treatment is initiated according to the regimen in **Table 40-7**. Ongoing administration is essential because most cases of relapse are the result of erratic changes in medication or dose (or both). Dose reduction is aimed at finding the maintenance dose. Because histologic findings lag 3 to 6 months behind normalization of serum parameters, therapy has to be continued beyond the normalization of aminotransferase levels. Usually, maintenance doses of prednisone range between 10 and 2.5 mg. After 12 to 24 months of therapy, prednisone or prednisolone can be tapered over the course of 4 to 6 weeks to test whether a sustained remission has been achieved. Tapering of regimens should be attempted with great caution and only after obtaining a liver biopsy specimen that demonstrates complete resolution of the inflammatory activity. Relapse of AIH and risk for progression to fibrosis are almost universal when immunosuppression is tapered in the presence of residual histologic inflammation.

Outcomes can be classified into four categories: remission, relapse, treatment failure, and stabilization.

Remission is complete normalization of all inflammatory parameters, including histology. This is achieved in 65% of patients after 24 months of treatment. The American Association for the Study of Liver Diseases (AASLD) 2010 practice guidelines for AIH have established normalization of aminotransferase levels as the definition of biochemical response.[5] Muratori and associates have shown in their single-center experience from Italy that only patients achieving normal aminotransferase levels with immunosuppressive therapy have a favorable long-term prognosis and that those in whom aminotransferase levels do not normalize progress.[84] These are the patients who need to be the focus of future drug development for AIH. This new definition of biochemical response as defined in the 2010 AASLD practice guidelines[5] differs from previous definitions in which less than twice the upper limit of normal was used. As a consequence, the percentage of patients achieving remission according to the 2010 AASLD practice guidelines is lower than that with the previous definition of less than twice the upper limit of normal.[85] Remission can be sustained with azathioprine monotherapy at 2 mg/kg body weight.[86] This prevents cushingoid side effects. However, side effects such as arthralgia (53%), myalgia (14%), lymphopenia (57%), and myelosuppression (6%) have been observed.

Relapse is characterized by a three-fold increase in aminotransferase levels and recurrence of clinical symptoms. Relapse occurs in 50% of patients within 6 months of treatment withdrawal and in 80% after 3 years. Relapse is associated with progression to cirrhosis in 38% and progression to liver failure in 14%. Occurrence of relapse calls for reinitiation of standard therapy and perhaps a long-term maintenance dose of prednisone/prednisolone or azathioprine monotherapy.

Treatment failure is characterized by progression of clinical, serologic, and histologic parameters during standard therapy. This is seen in about 10% of patients. In these cases the diagnosis of AIH has to be carefully reconsidered to exclude other causes of chronic hepatitis. Experimental regimens can be administered to these patients, or liver transplantation may ultimately become necessary.

Stabilization is achievement of partial remission. Because 90% of patients reach remission within 3 years, the benefit of standard therapy needs to be reevaluated in this subgroup of patients. Ultimately, liver transplantation provides a definitive treatment option.

If standard treatment fails or drug intolerance occurs, alternative therapies such as cyclosporine, tacrolimus, cyclophosphamide, mycophenolate mofetil, or rapamycin may be considered. The efficacy of these options has not yet been decided definitively.

Budesonide is a synthetic steroid with high first-pass metabolism in the liver, which should limit systemic side effects in comparison with conventional steroids. In a study in which 13 patients with AIH were treated with budesonide over a period of 9 months, the drug was well tolerated and aminotransferase levels normalized.[87] Our own initial experience has confirmed that budesonide is effective but does not offer an advantage over conventional steroids in patients with cirrhosis and portosystemic shunts.[88] In a more recent study, budesonide therapy was associated with a low frequency of remission and a high incidence of side effects.[89] However, these patients exhibited treatment failure, and it cannot be expected that such patients will benefit from topical steroids. In a recent study,[90] budesonide was shown to induce remission more effectively than prednisone, each being administered in combination with azathioprine. This controlled prospective study with more than noncirrhotic AIH 200 patients is the largest-ever prospective study on the treatment of AIH. It was performed in 30 centers from nine countries. It is also the most significant study on AIH after the discovery of HCV in 1989 in which the new definition of biochemical remission was used: normalization of aminotransferase levels. This study consisted of two phases. In the first 6 months, budesonide was compared with prednisone, each combined with azathioprine, for induction of remission. After 6 months in a second phase, patients receiving prednisone were switched to open-label budesonide to investigate whether a switch from prednisone to budesonide leads to a reduction in steroid-specific side effects. After 6 months there was a combined end point encompassing normalization of aminotransferase levels and lack of predefined steroid-specific side effects. The primary end point was achieved in 47% of budesonide-treated patients versus 19% of patients in the prednisone arm, each in combination with azathioprine. At 6 months, complete biochemical remission (normalization of aminotransferase levels) occurred in 60% of patients given budesonide as opposed to 39% of those given prednisone. Seventy-two percent of patients in the budesonide group did not have steroid-specifics side effects as compared with 47% in the prednisone arm. Among the 87 patients who were initially given prednisone and then received budesonide after 6 months, the incidence of steroid-specific side effects decreased from 45% to 26% at month 12. This was statistically significant. The main advantage of budesonide for the future treatment of AIH in noncirrhotic patients may be in replacing prednisone as long-term maintenance therapy to reduce the frequency of steroid-specific side effects.

Deflazacort has been proposed as an alternative corticosteroid for immunosuppression because it causes fewer side effects than conventional glucocorticoids do. In a recent study, deflazacort was used to treat 15 patients with AIH type 1 who had previously been treated with prednisone, with or without azathioprine, until biochemical remission was achieved. Remission was sustained during 2 years of follow-up. However, the long-term role of second-generation corticosteroids in sustaining remission in AIH patients with reduced treatment-related side effects requires further controlled studies.[91]

Cyclosporine is a lipophilic cyclic peptide of 11 residues produced by *Tolypocladium inflatum* that acts on calcium-dependent signaling and inhibits T-cell function via the interleukin-2 gene. Of all alternative agents, the greatest experience to date has been with cyclosporine. In these studies cyclosporine was used successfully for the treatment of AIH and was well tolerated.[92,93] The principal difficulty in advocating widespread use of the drug as first-line therapy relates to its toxicity profile, particularly with long-term use (increased risk for hypertension, renal insufficiency, hyperlipidemia, hirsutism, infection, and malignancy).[92-95]

Tacrolimus is a macrolide lactone compound with immunosuppressive capabilities that exceed those of cyclosporine. The mechanism of action is similar to that of cyclosporine, but it binds to a different immunophilin. Treatment of 21 patients with tacrolimus for 1 year led to an improvement in aminotransferase and bilirubin levels, with a minor increase in serum blood urea nitrogen and creatinine levels.[96] Although tacrolimus is a promising immunosuppressive candidate drug, larger randomized trials are required to assess its role in the treatment of AIH.

Mycophenolate has attracted attention as a transplant immunosuppressant with an important role as a steroid-free immunosuppressive therapy in patients who undergo transplantation for chronic HCV infection. Mycophenolate is a noncompetitive inhibitor of inosine monophosphate dehydrogenase, which blocks the rate-limiting enzymatic step in de novo purine synthesis. It has a selective action on lymphocyte activation, with a marked reduction in both T- and B-lymphocyte proliferation. In a recent pilot study, seven patients with AIH type 1 who either did not tolerate azathioprine or did not respond to standard therapy with complete normalization of aminotransferase levels were treated with mycophenolate in addition to steroids. In 5 of 7 patients, normalization of aminotransferase levels was achieved within 3 months. These preliminary data suggest that mycophenolate may be another promising strategy for treating AIH,[97] but these results were not confirmed in later retrospective studies.

Induction of remission with 1 to 1.5 mg/kg/day of cyclophosphamide in conjunction with steroids has been reported. However, the need for continued application of cyclophosphamide, with its potentially severe hematologic side effects, renders it a highly experimental treatment option.[98]

Ursodeoxycholic acid is a hydrophilic bile acid with putative immunomodulatory capabilities. It is presumed to alter HLA class I antigen expression on cellular surfaces and to suppress immunoglobulin production. Uncontrolled trials have shown a reduction in histologic abnormalities and clinical and biochemical improvement but no reduction in fibrosis in four patients with AIH type 1.[99-101] However, its role in AIH therapy or in combination with immunosuppressive therapy is still unclear.

Liver Transplantation

In approximately 10% of patients with AIH, liver transplantation remains the only lifesaving option. The indications for liver transplantation in patients with AIH are similar to those for other chronic liver diseases and include clinical deterioration, development of cirrhosis, bleeding esophageal varices, and coagulation abnormalities despite adequate immunosuppressive therapy.[102-107] There is no single indicator or predictor of the necessity for liver transplantation. Candidates for liver transplantation are usually patients who do not reach remission within 4 years of continuous therapy. Indicators of a high mortality associated with liver failure are histologic evidence of multilobular necrosis and progressive hyperbilirubinemia. In Europe, 4% of liver transplants are performed for AIH.[108] The long-term results of liver transplantation for AIH are excellent. The 5-year survival rate is up to 92%,[104,105,109] well within the range of other indications for liver transplantation.

The potential for AIH to recur after liver transplantation has been a matter of controversial debate. The first case of recurrent AIH after liver transplantation was reported in 1984 and was based on serum biochemistry, biopsy findings, and steroid reduction.[103] Studies published during the past years indicate that the rate of recurrence of AIH ranges between 10% and 35% and that the risk for recurrence of AIH is perhaps as high as 68% after 5 years of follow-up.[107,110-114] It is important, however, to consider the criteria on which the diagnosis of recurrent AIH is based.

When transaminitis is chosen as a practical selection parameter, many patients with mild histologic evidence of recurrent AIH may be missed. It is therefore suggested that all patients with suspected recurrence of AIH undergo liver biopsy, biochemical analysis of aminotransferases, and determination of immunoglobulins and autoantibody titers.[107] Significant risk factors for recurrence of AIH have not yet been identified, although it appears that the presence of fulminant hepatic failure before transplantation protects against the development of recurrent disease. An attractive risk factor for the development of recurrent AIH is the presence of specific HLA types that may predispose patients to more severe immunoreactivity. In two studies, recurrence of AIH appeared to occur more frequently in HLA-DR3–positive patients receiving HLA-DR3–negative grafts. However, this association was not confirmed in all studies. Interestingly, there have not been any conclusive data to support the hypothesis that a specific immunosuppressive regimen represents a risk factor for the development of recurrent AIH. Nonetheless, data indicate that 64% of patients who undergo liver transplantation for AIH require continuation of steroids versus 17% of patients receiving liver transplants for other conditions. Based on these results and other studies, it would appear that maintenance of steroid therapy in AIH patients is indicated to prevent not only cellular rejection but also graft-threatening recurrence of AIH.[107] Steroid withdrawal should therefore be performed with great caution. In addition to AIH recurrence, the development of de novo AIH after liver transplantation has been reported.[115]

Serum autoantibodies are an integral part of the diagnosis of AIH. Autoantibody prevalence and titers have been studied in patients undergoing liver transplantations for AIH and PBC. In general, autoantibody types persist in the majority of patients after transplantation. In patients with PBC, AMAs persisted, albeit at lower titer, in almost 100%, a finding confirmed by several groups.[116] In patients with AIH, autoantibodies of the specific subtype present before transplantation were detected at lower titer in 77% after transplantation in one study and were found in 82% of patients in whom recurrence of AIH did not develop. A recent study has suggested that an increase in titer exceeding levels detected before transplantation may be indicative of AIH recurrence. However, the majority of published data and our own experience presently do not support a prognostic role for autoantibodies in determining recurrence of AIH after liver transplantation.[107]

Key References

Agarwal K, et al. Cytotoxic T lymphocyte antigen-4 (CTLA-4) gene polymorphisms and susceptibility to type 1 autoimmune hepatitis. Hepatology 2000;31:49–53. (Ref.65)

Ahmed M, et al. Liver transplantation for autoimmune hepatitis: a 12-year experience. Transplant Proc 1997;29:496. (Ref.102)

Alvarez F, et al. International Autoimmune Hepatitis Group Report: review of criteria for diagnosis of autoimmune hepatitis. J Hepatol 1999;31:929–938. (Ref.4)

Alvarez F, et al. Short-term cyclosporine induces a remission of autoimmune hepatitis in children. J Hepatol 1999;30:222–227. (Ref.92)

Beaune PH, et al. Anti–cytochrome P450 autoantibodies in drug-induced disease. Eur J Haematol Suppl 1996;60:89–92. (Ref.24)

Bourdi M, et al. Anti–liver endoplasmic reticulum antibodies are directed against human cytochrome P-450IA2. A specific marker of dihydralazine hepatitis. J Clin Invest 1990;85:1967–1973. (Ref.41)

Calmus Y, et al. Hepatic expression of class I and class II major histocompatibility complex molecules in primary biliary cirrhosis: effect of ursodeoxycholic acid. Hepatology 1990;11:12–15. (Ref.99)

Cancado ELR, Porta G. Autoimmune hepatitis in South America. Boston: Kluwer, 2000. (Ref.22)

Czaja AJ. Frequency and nature of the variant syndromes of autoimmune liver disease. Hepatology 1998;28:360–365. (Ref.75)

Czaja AJ, Carpenter HA, Lindor KD. Ursodeoxycholic acid as adjunctive therapy for problematic type 1 autoimmune hepatitis: a randomized placebo-controlled treatment trial. Hepatology 1999;30:1381–1386. (Ref.100)

Czaja AJ, et al. Evidence against hepatitis viruses as important causes of severe autoimmune hepatitis in the United States. J Hepatol 1993;18:342–352. (Ref.57)

Czaja AJ, Lindor KD. Failure of budesonide in a pilot study of treatment-dependent autoimmune hepatitis. Gastroenterology 2000;119:1312–1316. (Ref.89)

Czaja AJ, Manns MP. Advances in the diagnosis, pathogenesis, and management of autoimmune hepatitis. Gastroenterology 2010;139:58–72, e54. (Ref.28)

Dalekos GN, et al. Epitope mapping of cytochrome P4502D6 autoantigen in patients with chronic hepatitis C during alpha-interferon treatment. J Hepatol 1999;30:366–375. (Ref.77)

Danielson A, Prytz H. Oral budesonide for treatment of autoimmune chronic hepatitis. Aliment Pharmacol Ther 1994;8:585–590. (Ref.87)

Debray D, et al. Efficacy of cyclosporin A in children with type 2 autoimmune hepatitis. J Pediatr 1999;135:111–114. (Ref.93)

Desmet VJ, et al. Classification of chronic hepatitis: diagnosis, grading and staging. Hepatology 1994;19:1513–1520. (Ref.8)

Devlin J, et al. Recurrence of autoimmune hepatitis following liver transplantation. Liver Transpl Surg 1995;1:162–165. (Ref.110)

Dienes HP, et al. Histologic features in autoimmune hepatitis. Z Gastroenterol 1989;27:327–330. (Ref.19)

Dighiero G, et al. Sera with high levels of anti–smooth muscle and anti-mitochondrial antibodies frequently bind to cytoskeleton proteins. Clin Exp Immunol 1990;82:52–56. (Ref.32)

Doherty DG, et al. Allelic sequence variation in the HLA class II genes and proteins on patients with autoimmune hepatitis. Hepatology 1994;19:609–615. (Ref.61)

Donaldson PT, Czaja AJ. Genetic effects on susceptibility, clinical expression, and treatment outcome of type 1 autoimmune hepatitis. Clin Liver Dis 2002;6:419–437. (Ref.26)

Donaldson PT, et al. Susceptibility to autoimmune chronic active hepatitis: human leukocyte antigens DR 4 and A1-B8-DR-3 are independent risk factors. Hepatology 1991;13:701–706. (Ref.59)

Durazzo M, et al. Heterogeneity of liver-kidney microsomal autoantibodies in chronic hepatitis C and D virus infection. Gastroenterology 1995;108:455–462. (Ref.46)

European Liver Transplant Registry. <http://www.eltr.org>; 1996.

Fernandez NF, et al. Cyclosporine therapy in patients with steroid resistant autoimmune hepatitis. Am J Gastroenterol 1999;94:241–248. (Ref.94)

Gelpi C, Sontheimer EJ, Rodriguez-Sanchez JL. Autoantibodies against a serine tRNA-protein complex implicated in cotranslational selenocysteine insertion. Proc Natl Acad Sci U S A 1992;89:9739–9743. (Ref.16)

Götz G, et al. Recurrence of autoimmune hepatitis after liver transplantation. Transplant Proc 1999;31:430–431. (Ref.114)

Gouw AS, et al. Is there recurrence of primary biliary cirrhosis after liver transplantation? A clinicopathologic study in long-term survivors. J Hepatol 1994;20:500–507. (Ref.116)

Gregorio GV, et al. Autoimmune hepatitis in childhood: a 20-year experience. Hepatology 1997;25:541–547. (Ref.81)

Guenguen M, et al. Identification of the main epitope on human cytochrome P450IID6 recognized by anti–liver kidney microsome antibody. J Autoimmun 1991;4:607–615. (Ref.36)

Guenguen M, et al. Anti–liver-kidney microsome antibody recognizes a cytochrome P450 from the IID subfamily. J Exp Med 1988;168:801. (Ref.37)

Heneghan MA, McFarlane IG. Current and novel immunosuppressive therapy for autoimmune hepatitis. Hepatology 2002;35:7–13. (Ref.95)

Hennes EM, et al. Simplified criteria for the diagnosis of autoimmune hepatitis. Hepatology 2008;48:169–176. (Ref.6)

Johnson PJ, McFarlane IG. Meeting report: International Autoimmune Hepatitis Group. Hepatology 1993;18:998–1005. (Ref.9)

Johnson PJ, McFarlane IG, Williams R. Azathioprine for long-term maintenance of remission in autoimmune hepatitis. N Engl J Med 1995;333:958–963. (Ref.86)

Kanzler S, et al. Cyclophosphamide as alternative immunosuppressive therapy for autoimmune hepatitis—report of three cases. Z Gastroenterol 1996;35:571–578. (Ref.98)

Kerkar N, et al. De-novo autoimmune hepatitis after liver transplantation. Lancet 1998;351:409–413. (Ref.115)

Lankisch TO, et al. Detection of autoimmune regulator gene mutations in children with type 2 autoimmune hepatitis and extrahepatic immune-mediated diseases. Autoimmune hepatitis. J Pediatr 2005; 146:839–842. (Ref.70)

Lenzi M, et al. Liver cytosolic 1 antigen-antibody system in type 2 autoimmune hepatitis and hepatitis C virus infection. Gut 1995;36:749–754. (Ref.50)

Manns M, et al. Characterisation of a new subgroup of autoimmune chronic active hepatitis by autoantibodies against a soluble liver antigen. Lancet 1987;1:292–294. (Ref.14)

Manns MP, et al. Diagnosis and management of autoimmune hepatitis. Hepatology 2010;51:2193–2213. (Ref.5)

Manns MP, et al. Correspondence: Reply to Muratori et al. Hepatology 2010; 52:1857–1858. (Ref.85)

Manns MP, et al. LKM-1 autoantibodies recognize a short linear sequence in P450IID6, a cytochrome P-450 monooxygenase. J Clin Invest 1991;88: 1370–1378. (Ref.11)

Manns MP, et al. Discordant manifestation of LKM-1 antibody positive autoimmune hepatitis in identical twins. Hepatology 1990;12:840. (Ref.51)

Manns MP, et al. Major antigen of liver kidney microsomal antibodies in idiopathic autoimmune hepatitis is cytochrome P450db1. J Clin Invest 1989;83:1066–1072. (Ref.12)

Manns MP, Kruger M. Immunogenetics of chronic liver diseases. Gastroenterology 1994;106:1676–1697. (Ref.27)

Manns MP, Strassburg CP. Autoimmune hepatitis: clinical challenges. Gastroenterology 2001;120:1502–1517. (Ref.72)

Manns MP, et al. Azathioprine with budesonide induces remission more effectively than with prednisone in patients with autoimmune hepatitis. Gastroenterology 2010;139:1198–1206. (Ref.90)

Milkiewicz P, et al. Recurrence of autoimmune hepatitis after liver transplantation. Transplantation 1999;68:253–256. (Ref.112)

Muratori L, et al. Detection of anti–liver cytosol antibody type 1 (anti-LC1) by immunodiffusion, counterimmunoelectrophoresis and immunoblotting: comparison of different techniques. J Immunol Methods 1995;187:259–264. (Ref.47)

Muratori L, et al. Distinct epitopes on formiminotransferase cyclodeaminase induce autoimmune liver cytosol antibody type 1. Hepatology 2001;34: 494–501. (Ref.48)

Muratori P, et al. Autoimmune hepatitis in Italy: the Bologna experience. J Hepatol 2009;50:1210–1218. (Ref.84)

Nakamura K, et al. Efficacy of ursodeoxycholic acid in Japanese patients with type 1 autoimmune hepatitis. J Gastroenterol Hepatol 1998;13:490–495. (Ref.101)

Newton JL, et al. Autoimmune hepatitis in older patients. Age Ageing 1997;26: 441–444. (Ref.83)

Nishioka M, et al. Frequency and significance of antibodies to P450IID6 protein in Japanese patients with chronic hepatiis C. J Hepatol 1997;26:992–1000. (Ref.20)

Nishioka M, Morshed SA, McFarlane IG. Geographical variation in the frequency and characteristics of autoimmune liver diseases. Amsterdam: Elsevier, 1998. (Ref.21)

Obermayer-Straub P, et al. Hepatic autoantigens in patients with autoimmune polyendocrinopathy–candidiasis–ectodermal dystrophy. Gastroenterology 2001;121:668–677. (Ref.25)

Ota M, et al. A possible association between basic amino acids of position 13 of DRB1 chains and autoimmune hepatitis. Immunogenetics 1992;36:40–55. (Ref.63)

Pando M, et al. Pediatric and adult forms of type I autoimmune hepatitis in Argentina: evidence for differential genetic predisposition. Hepatology 1999; 30:1374–1380. (Ref.64)

Philipp T, et al. Recognition of uridine diphosphate glucuronosyl transferases by LKM-3 antibodies in chronic hepatitis D. Lancet 1994;344:578–581. (Ref.44)

Pitkanen J, et al. Subcellular localization of the autoimmune regulator protein. Characterization of nuclear targeting and transcriptional activation domain. J Biol Chem 2001;276:19597–19602. (Ref.68)

Prados E, et al. Outcome of autoimmune hepatitis after liver transplantation. Transplantation 1998;66:1645–1650. (Ref.104)

Ramsey C, et al. Aire deficient mice develop multiple features of APECED phenotype and show altered immune response. Hum Mol Genet 2002;11: 397–409. (Ref.69)

Ratziu V, et al. Long-term follow-up after liver transplantation for autoimmune hepatitis: evidence of recurrence of primary disease. J Hepatol 1999;30: 131–141. (Ref.109)

Rebollo Bernardez J, et al. Deflazacort for long-term maintenance of remission in type I autoimmune hepatitis. Rev Esp Enferm Dig 1999;91:630–638. (Ref.91)

Richardson PD, James PD, Ryder SD. Mycophenolate mofetil for maintenance of remission in autoimmune hepatitis in patients resistant to or intolerant of azathioprine. J Hepatol 2000;33:371–375. (Ref.97)

Sanchez-Urdazpal L, Czaja AJ, Van Holk B. Prognostic features and role of liver transplantation in severe corticoid-treated autoimmune chronic active hepatitis. Hepatology 1991;15:215–221. (Ref.105)

Schüler A, Manns MP. Treatment of autoimmune hepatitis. In: Arroyo V, Bosch J, Rodés J, editors. Treatment in hepatology. Paris: Masson, 1995:375–383. (Ref.88)

Stechemesser E, Klein R, Berg PA. Characterization and clinical relevance of liver-pancreas antibodies in autoimmune hepatitis. Hepatology 1993;18:1–9. (Ref.15)

Strassburg CP, et al. Identification of cyclin A as a molecular target of antinuclear antibodies (ANA) in hepatic and non-hepatic autoimmune diseases. J Hepatol 1996;25:859–866. (Ref.31)

Strassburg CP, Kalthoff S, Ehmer U. Variability and function of family 1 uridine-5′-diphosphate glucuronosyltransferases (UGT1A). Crit Rev Clin Lab Sci 2008;45:485–530. (Ref.74)

Strassburg CP, Manns MP. Autoimmune hepatitis versus viral hepatitis C. Liver 1995;15:225–232. (Ref.10)

Strassburg CP, Manns MP. Autoimmune tests in primary biliary cirrhosis. Baillieres Best Pract Res Clin Gastroenterol 2000;14:585–599. (Ref.29)

Strassburg CP, Manns MP. Autoantibodies and autoantigens in autoimmune hepatitis. Semin Liver Dis 2002;22:339–352. (Ref.7)

Strassburg CP, Manns MP. [Primary biliary liver cirrhosis and overlap syndrome. Diagnosis and therapy.] Internist (Berl) 2004;45:16–26. (Ref.76)

Strassburg CP, Manns MP. Autoimmune hepatitis in the elderly: what is the difference? J Hepatol 2006;45:480–482. (Ref.73)

Strassburg CP, et al. Autoantibodies against glucuronosyltransferases differ between viral hepatitis and autoimmune hepatitis. Gastroenterology 1996; 111:1576–1586. (Ref.13)

Strassburg CP, Obermayer-Straub P, Manns MP. Autoimmunity in hepatitis C and D virus infection. J Viral Hepat 1996;3:49–59. (Ref.23)

Strassburg CP, Obermayer-Straub P, Manns MP. Autoimmunity in liver diseases. Clin Rev Allergy Immunol 2000;18:127–139. (Ref.3)

Strettell MD, et al. HLA-C genes and susceptibility to type 1 autoimmune hepatitis. Hepatology 1997;26:1023–1026. (Ref.62)

Sugimura T, et al. A major CYP2D6 autoepitope in autoimmune hepatitis type 2 and chronic hepatitis C is a three-dimensional structure homologous to other cytochrome P450 autoantigens. Autoimmunity 2002;35:501–513. (Ref.40)

Tan EM, et al. Antinuclear antibodies (ANAs): diagnostically specific immune markers and clues toward the understanding of systemic autoimmunity. Clin Immunol Immunopathol 1988;47:121–141. (Ref.30)

Tillmann HL, Jackel E, Manns MP. Liver transplantation in autoimmune liver disease—selection of patients. Hepatogastroenterology 1999;46:3053–3059. (Ref.106)

Treichel U, et al. Autoantibodies to human asialoglycoprotein receptor in autoimmune-type chronic hepatitis. Hepatology 1990;11:606–612. (Ref.49)

Tukey RH, Strassburg CP. Genetic multiplicity of the human UDP-glucuronosyltransferases and regulation in the gastrointestinal tract. Mol Pharmacol 2001;59:405–414. (Ref.45)

Van Thiel DH, et al. Tacrolimus: a potential new treatment for autoimmune chronic active hepatitis: results of an open-label preliminary trial. Am J Gastroenterol 1995;90:771–776. (Ref.96)

Vento S, et al. Autoimmune hepatitis type 1 after measles. Am J Gastroenterol 1996;91:2618–2620. (Ref.53)

Vento S, et al. Autoimmune hepatitis type 2 induced by HCV and persisting after viral clearance. Lancet 1997;350:1298–1299. (Ref.54)

Vento S, et al. Identification of hepatitis A virus as a trigger for autoimmune chronic hepatitis type 1 in susceptible individuals. Lancet 1991;337:1183–1187. (Ref.55)

Vento S, et al. Epstein-Barr virus as a trigger for autoimmune hepatitis in susceptible individuals. Lancet 1995;346:608–609. (Ref.56)

Vogel A, et al. Long-term outcome of liver transplantation for autoimmune hepatitis. Clin Transplant 2004;18:62–69. (Ref.107)

Vogel A, et al. Autoimmune regulator AIRE: evidence for genetic differences between autoimmune hepatitis and hepatitis as part of the autoimmune polyglandular syndrome type 1. Hepatology 2001;33:1047–1052. (Ref.71)

Vogel A, Manns MP, Strassburg CP. Autoimmunity and viruses. Clin Liver Dis 2002;6:451–465. (Ref.52)

Vogel A, Strassburg CP, Manns MP. Genetic association of vitamin D receptor polymorphisms with primary biliary cirrhosis and autoimmune hepatitis. Hepatology 2002;35:126–131. (Ref.66)

Vogel A, Strassburg CP, Manns MP. 77 C/G mutation in the tyrosine phosphatase CD45 and autoimmune hepatitis: evidence for a genetic link. Genes Immun 2003;4:79–81. (Ref.67)

Volkmann M, et al. Soluble liver antigen: isolation of a 35-kd recombinant protein (SLA-p35) specifically recognizing sera from patients with autoimmune hepatitis. Hepatology 2001;33:591–596. (Ref.17)

Wies I, et al. Identification of target antigen for SLA/LP autoantibodies in autoimmune hepatitis. Lancet 2000;355:1510–1515. (Ref.18)

Wright HL, et al. Disease recurrence and rejection following liver transplantation for autoimmune chronic active liver disease. Transplantation 1992;53:136–139. (Ref.113)

Zanger UM, et al. Antibodies against human cytochrome P-450db1 in autoimmune hepatitis type 2. Proc Natl Acad Sci U S A 1988;85:8256–8260. (Ref.39)

A complete list of references can be found at www.expertconsult.com.

Chapter **41**

Primary Biliary Cirrhosis

Keith D. Lindor and Cynthia Levy

ABBREVIATIONS

AIH autoimmune hepatitis	**FIS** Fatigue Impact Scale	**PDC** pyruvate dehydrogenase complex
ALT alanine aminotransferase	**GGT** γ-glutamyltransferase	**PPAR-α** peroxisome proliferator–activated
AMA antimitochondrial antibody	**HDL** high-density lipoprotein	receptor α
ANA antinuclear antibody	**HLA** human leukocyte antigen	**PSC** primary sclerosing cholangitis
APO E apolipoprotein E	**HRT** hormone replacement therapy	**SLC4A2** anion exchange family
AST aspartate aminotransferase	**IL-1** interleukin-1	**SLE** systemic lupus erythematosus
BMD bone mineral density	**LDL** low-density lipoprotein	**STAT-4** signal transducer and activator of
BSEP 4 bile salt export pump 4	**MELD** Model for End-Stage Liver Disease	transcription 4
CT computed tomography	**MHC** major histocompatibility complex	**TNF-α** tumor necrosis factor α
CTLA-4 cytotoxic T-lymphocyte	**MRCP** magnetic retrograde	**UDCA** ursodeoxycholic acid
antigen-4	cholangiopancreatography	**ULN** upper limit of normal
ELF enhanced liver fibrosis	**MRI** magnetic resonance imaging	**US** ultrasound
ELISA enzyme-linked immunosorbent	**2-OADC** 2-oxo acid dehydrogenase family	**UTI** urinary tract infection
assay	of multienzyme complexes	**VDR** vitamin D receptor
FXR farnesoid X receptor	**PBC** primary biliary cirrhosis	**VLDL** very-low-density lipoprotein

Epidemiology
Incidence and Prevalence

Descriptive studies from around the globe confirm that primary biliary cirrhosis (PBC) is an uncommon disease. Incidence and prevalence have been reported from multiple European countries, North America, Australia, Israel, India, and Japan. The annual incidence rates ranged from 0.7 to 49 cases per million, whereas point prevalence ranged from 6.7 to 402 cases per million, with higher prevalence rates seen in northern Europe and the United States.[1] Many of these studies provided time trends within long observation periods of the same specific geographic region, at times indicating an increase in incidence and/or prevalence of PBC over time. As an example, the annual incidence rate among residents of Sheffield, England, increased from 5.8 cases per million to 20.5 cases per million between 1977 and 1987. Between 1987 and 1999 no further increase was noticed in incidence rates. The prevalence, on the other hand, increased steadily from 54 cases per million in 1977, to 57 cases per million in 1987, to 136 cases per million in 1993, to 238 cases per million in 1996, possibly reflecting earlier diagnosis and/or prolonged survival. Similarly, the reported annual incidence in Finland increased by 3.5% between 1988 and 1999, whereas the prevalence increased by 5.1%.

Only two epidemiologic studies have been conducted in the United States. The first, in Olmsted County, Minnesota, identified 46 cases of PBC between 1975 and 1995, providing an annual incidence rate of 27 cases per million. The overall age-adjusted incidence in women was 45 per million. This number did not change over the 20-year study period. The age- and gender-adjusted prevalence rate in 1995 was 402 cases per million people, with much higher rates among females (654 cases per million) as compared with males (121 cases per million).[2] A second study performed in Alaska identified 18 cases of PBC between 1984 and 2000, implying a point prevalence of 160 cases per million.[3] When 5 cases of antimitochondrial antibody (AMA)-negative PBC and 6 cases of overlap with autoimmune hepatitis (AIH) were added, the estimated prevalence rose to 289 cases per million. Time trends were not offered in the study. Whether the increase in incidence and prevalence of PBC is real or apparent remains to be clarified: the use of more accurate laboratory tests and increased awareness among healthcare providers, as well as more widespread screening habits, may have led to earlier, more frequent diagnosis of PBC.

Race/Gender Variation

Historically, PBC is known to affect predominantly Caucasians, although it is reported in all races and ethnicities. The disease is far more common in women, with a female/male ratio near 10:1, and the mean age at diagnosis is 52 years.[2] Although extremely atypical, the disease has been diagnosed in teenagers. Disease presentation in males and females is similar; however, significant differences are seen between

Caucasian and non-Caucasian patients. Peters and colleagues reviewed clinical, demographic, and laboratory data on 535 patients who were screened for a multicenter clinical trial between 1989 and 1998 in 11 states in the United States.[4] As expected, more than 90% of patients were female, and the mean age at presentation was 52 years. The vast majority of patients were Caucasian (86.3%), although Hispanics (7.9%) and African Americans (3.9%) were also represented. After adjustment for age and body mass, non-Caucasians were found to have more severe disease by clinical and laboratory criteria; specifically, ascites, encephalopathy, and variceal bleeding were more common among non-Caucasians. Furthermore, non-Caucasians also had more severe pruritus and decreased activity level compared with Caucasian patients.

The manifestation of PBC among Asian patients is less understood given the infrequency of the disease in this population. In a recent report from Singapore, overall survival free of liver transplantation at 5 years was near 90%, which is significantly better than that quoted in European and North American studies.[5] However, a direct comparison among studies is not possible, and prior studies from Asian countries demonstrated 5-year survival rates near 70% to 80%, more consistent with the European experience.

Geographic Clustering

The incidence and prevalence of PBC vary considerably in different areas of the world, introducing the concept of geoepidemiology. To that extent, investigators have reported geographic clusters of PBC within specific subregions in Estonia, Sweden, and northern England,[6-8] pointing perhaps to a strong role of environmental factors in the development of PBC. In the United States clustering was observed near toxic waste sites in New York City and near areas with high levels of air pollution.[9] In addition, studies from Australia and Israel have demonstrated that the prevalence of PBC among European immigrants was much higher than the overall prevalence of PBC in these countries.[9] Together, these studies support the hypothesis that exposure to certain environmental factors contributes to the etiology of PBC.

Predisposing Factors

The strongest risk factor for PBC is family history of the disease, with a relative risk as high as 10.5 for an individual whose sibling has PBC.[10] In a study involving 16 pairs of twins, the concordance rate in identical twins was 63%, which is among the highest reported in autoimmune diseases. On the other hand, no concordant pair was found among dizygotic twins.[11] These findings support that a combination of genetic and environmental factors is required for the development of PBC.

Two case control studies conducted in the United States searched for factors that could trigger the disease in genetically predisposed individuals. The first study was based on questionnaires sent to 241 patients with PBC, 261 identified siblings, and 225 friends of patients with PBC.[12] This study found that compared with friends and relatives, patients diagnosed with PBC were more likely to develop several autoimmune conditions. Similarly, first-degree relatives of patients with PBC had a high prevalence of PBC. Other independent risk factors identified in this study were history of tonsillectomy,

urinary tract infection, vaginal infection, shingles, or cholecystectomy as well as a history of smoking. A second, larger study included 1032 patients with PBC and 1041 controls selected by random-digit dialing and was performed through phone interviews.[13] The study confirmed an increased familial occurrence, association with autoimmune diseases and smoking, and increased frequency of urinary tract infections; it also showed a new association with use of nail polish, and protection conferred by nulliparity. The strength of these risk factors is shown in **Table 41-1**. No associations were found with alcohol consumption, breast cancer, stressful life events, and pet ownership.

Etiopathogenesis

The current consensus is that PBC is an organ-specific autoimmune disease that occurs in genetically predisposed individuals. Most patients with PBC have antimitochondrial antibodies (AMAs) directed against the 2-oxo acid dehydrogenase family of multienzyme complexes (2-OADC), of which the main targets are the E2 and E3 subunits of the pyruvate dehydrogenase complex (PDC-E2 and PDC-E3). Interestingly, a key shared component of the B-cell auto-epitope within all these enzymes is a lipoic acid co-factor.

Although the 2-OADC is located in the inner mitochondrial membrane and is present in all nucleated cells, the immunologic response in PBC is primarily against biliary epithelial cells. In this population, PDC-E2 appears to be aberrantly expressed on the cell surface, especially in small bile duct biliary epithelial cells. Thus one of the most fascinating challenges in PBC is to explain the mechanisms leading to this localized breakdown in immune tolerance. In this regard, emerging data suggest a potentially crucial role of apoptosis in biliary epithelial cells as a mechanism for the tissue-specific autoimmune reactivity that is typical of PBC.[14]

Biliary epithelial cells, or cholangiocytes, can (1) regulate expression of adhesion molecules, major histocompatibility complex (MHC) classes I and II, tumor necrosis factor α (TNF-α), interferon γ (IFN-γ), and interleukin-1 (IL-1) in the setting of stimulation by specific proinflammatory cytokines and (2) act as antigen presenting cells. Furthermore, these cells are susceptible to apoptosis. Thus phagocytosis of apoptotic cells by biliary epithelial cells could lead to the expression of endogenous autoantigens, which in turn would lead to autoreactivity, progressive cholangiocyte destruction, and ductopenia, one of the hallmarks of PBC progression.[15]

Immunogenicity

The immunologic milieu of the liver in PBC is characterized by an infiltration with B- and T-cell lymphocytes, with a CD4[+]/CD8[+] ratio near 2.[16] The predominant cytokine profile follows a typical T_H1 response with high levels of expression of IFN-γ mRNA; nevertheless, IL-6 is also present in the bile ducts, indicating some contribution of a T_H2 response. A newly recognized regulatory T-cell subset, TH17, which is a major source of IL-17, was also found infiltrating liver tissues of patients with PBC.[17] These T cells react to the same epitopes recognized by the B-cell lymphocytes in PDC-E2.

CD8[+] T cells appear in greater numbers in the liver than in the peripheral blood of patients with PBC. In the peripheral

Table 41-1 Proposed Risk Factors and Associations for Primary Biliary Cirrhosis

VARIABLE	OR	95% CI	REFERENCE
Medical History			
Family history of PBC	10.74	4.23-27.27	13
Sjögren syndrome	5.81	1.28-26.44	13
SLE	2.23	1.26-3.96	13
Autoimmune diseases	4.92	2.38-10.18	12
UTI or vaginal infection	2.12	1.10-3.78	12
UTI	1.51	1.192-1.95	13
Shingles	2.73	1.12-6.67	12
Cholecystectomy	2.30	1.16-4.58	12
Tonsillectomy	1.86	1.02-3.39	12
Lifestyle			
Previous smoking	2.04	1.10-3.78	12
Ever smoked	1.57	1.29-1.91	13
Use of nail polish	1.002	1.00-1.003	13
Reproductive History			
Never pregnant	0.61	0.44-0.84	13
Ever used HRT	1.55	1.24-1.88	13

CI, confidence interval; HRT, hormone replacement therapy; OR, odds ratio; PBC, primary biliary cirrhosis; SLE, systemic lupus erythematosus; UTI, urinary tract infection

blood, precursors of CD8[+] T cells are found in greater numbers during early stage PBC as opposed to advanced disease, suggesting a role in the development of bile duct injury.[18] Also noticeable is a decrease in the reactivity of CD4[+]/CD25[+] regulatory T cells.[19] The innate response, on the other hand, is enhanced in PBC. As a result, more proinflammatory cytokines are released in response to a pathogen-associated stimulus. Consistent with that, a marked increase in number and activity of natural killer T cells is seen.

Although the predominant immunoglobulin subtypes of AMA have been identified as IgG1 and IgG3, the role of IgA-type AMA in the pathogenesis of PBC has recently resurfaced because the biliary epithelial cells can actively transfer IgA. In addition to the apical surface of biliary epithelial cells, these IgA-type AMAs are also detected in saliva, urine, and bile of individuals with PBC.

Several hypotheses exist to explain what exactly initiates the induction of autoimmunity in predisposed patients, including the spillage of autoantigens through apoptosis following cellular damage, and molecular mimicry, either through exposure to a bacterial or viral infection or by exposure to xenobiotics, leading to modification of the native PDC-E2.

Role of Infectious Agents and Xenobiotics

Escherichia coli, Chlamydia pneumoniae, Lactobacillus delbrueckii, Helicobacter pylori, Novosphingobium aromaticivorans, and others have all been proposed to lead to PBC through molecular mimicry. In addition to bacteria, a beta-retrovirus has also been identified in the liver and lymph nodes of patients

with PBC. Interestingly, culture of biliary epithelial cells exposed to such lymph nodes was shown to induce expression of PDC-E2–like antigens on the cell membrane.[20]

Xenobiotics are foreign compounds that can alter the molecular structure of self or non-self antigens enough to induce an immune response. This immune response would then recognize not only the altered self or non-self antigen but also the native forms. Furthermore, it has been shown that after being metabolized, certain chemicals can generate halogenated structures that are variants of the lipoic acid residue in the PDC, thus eliciting a specific immune response capable of AMA production.[21]

The PDC-E2 structure is highly conserved among many species, and the cross-reactivity of AMA against bacterial antigens is a well-recognized phenomenon. Thus it is proposed that a bacterial mimic of PDC-E2 or a chemically modified PDC-E2 would cause activation of antigen presenting cells. Alternatively, an integrating hypothesis states that a bacterial mimic containing lipoic acid would be an attractive target for xenobiotic-induced modifications, thus leading to activation of antigen presenting cells. These cells would in turn activate T- and B-cell lymphocytes, initiating a cascade of events that would culminate with biliary injury.[22] The deficiency in regulatory T cells and other unclear mechanisms would help perpetuate the damage.

Genetics

Several lines of evidence point to a strong role for genetics in the etiopathogenesis of PBC. First, the disease occurs much more frequently among relatives of patients with PBC, with a reported rate ranging between 1% and 7%.[23] Second, the concordance rate among identical twins is 63%, which is among the highest reported in autoimmune diseases.[11] Finally, the well-described female predominance and the increased frequency of X monosomy in women with PBC suggest a role for X chromosome defects in PBC.[24] The genetic background in PBC, however, is complex and cannot be explained by a single gene abnormality. Thus a "multi-hit" genetic model was conceived in which specific genes would predispose to a breach in immune tolerance, leading to disease onset, whereas others would determine disease progression. In addition to genetics, various other external factors are proposed to affect both disease onset and disease progression.

Given that specific MHC alleles have been found in association with other autoimmune diseases, their association with PBC has been explored as well. To date, the association with MHC class I genes is regarded as weak. The study of MHC class II alleles, on the other hand, provides important clues to the pathogenesis of PBC. In multiple studies from Germany, Spain, Sweden, and the United States, HLA-DR8 (DRB1*08) was found with higher frequency among Caucasian patients with PBC as compared with controls, suggesting that DR8 might be a risk factor for PBC. In Great Britain, the linkage of DQA1*0401 and DR8-DQB1*0402 was associated with disease progression, not onset. These findings have not been consistent throughout the rest of Europe and Japan, indicating perhaps that different alleles have different impact on the disease depending on the geographic location. Interestingly, although further characterization and unifying data are still needed, a recent large study from Canada and the United States strongly suggested that most of the risk of PBC derives from common variants across the HLA-DQB1, IL12A, and IL12RB2 loci.[25]

Results have also been conflicting with respect to associations with MHC class III genes, which encode for cytokines and other immunologic components, as well as with non-MHC genes. Polymorphisms of the genes encoding for TNF-α, cytotoxic T lymphocyte antigen-4 (CTLA-4), IL-1, IL-10, IL-12, 1,25-dihydroxyvitamin D receptor (VDR), and others have been inconsistently reported in PBC.[23] **Table 41-2** shows potential genetic associations with PBC.

Clinical Manifestations

PBC affects predominantly middle-age women, with mean age at presentation of 52 years. A minority of at most 10% of patients will be males. Up to 40% of patients will present at age greater than 65, with the clinical features of the disease in this population being identical to those observed in younger patients.

Asymptomatic Disease

The clinical presentation of patients with PBC has significantly changed since its original description in 1851. Currently, most patients are diagnosed while still asymptomatic. Unfortunately, the definitions of "asymptomatic disease" vary among the various published studies, but frequently indicate patients who do not have specific liver-related symptoms or complications. The most controversial symptom in this regard would be fatigue, which recently has been the focus of a large amount of research.

Table 41-2 Potential Genetic Associations with Susceptibility and/or Progression of Primary Biliary Cirrhosis

	SUSCEPTIBILITY	PROGRESSION
CTLA-4	Promote	
STAT4	Promote	
IL-10	Promote	
IL-12A and IL-12RB2	Promote	
VDR	Promote	
C4A-Q0	Promote	
HLA-DR8 (DRB1*08)	Promote	
HLA-DQB1	Promote	
HLA-DRB1*11 and *13	Suppress	
TNF	Suppress	Suppress
IL-1		Suppress
SLC4A2		Suppress
HLA-DQA1*0401 and DQB1*0402		Promote
APO E		Promote
BSEP4		Promote

APO E, apolipoprotein E; BSEP 4, bile salt export pump 4; CTLA-4, cytotoxic T lymphocyte antigen-4; HLA, human leukocyte antigen; IL, interleukin; SLC 4A2, anion exchange family; TNF-α, tumor necrosis factor-α; VDR, 1,25-dihydrodroxyvitamin D receptor

The proportion of patients presenting in the asymptomatic stage appears to be higher in Western countries and Japan, accounting for up to 85% of all patients. In these cases PBC is eventually diagnosed after patients are incidentally found to have abnormal liver biochemical values, usually during routine check-up visits. In India, Lithuania, Singapore, and Hong Kong the rate of asymptomatic disease at presentation ranges between 20% and 47%, perhaps indicating differences in their healthcare systems versus a true difference in the natural history of PBC.[26]

Symptomatic Disease

Fatigue and pruritus are by far the most common symptoms reported by patients with PBC. Jaundice, on the other hand, is a late event and is associated with a poor prognosis. Right upper quadrant abdominal pain is reported by approximately 10% of patients; symptoms related to portal hypertension and those attributed to extrahepatic complications are discussed later in this chapter.

Fatigue

In North America and Northern Europe, fatigue is reported in up to 85% of patients with PBC, and approximately 50% of these patients consider it their worst symptom. Even though this has been considered a subjective complaint, questionnaires assessing symptoms and health-related quality of life can provide some insight with respect to the impact of fatigue in patients with PBC. Using the Fatigue Impact Scale (FIS), investigators have shown that patients with higher fatigue scores may have increased mortality, mostly attributable to cardiovascular causes,[27] and excessive daytime somnolence.[28] Fatigue is known to impact family life and job performance,[29] and a Canadian study using the Fatigue Assessment Instrument (FAI) showed that individuals with PBC and fatigue had poor-quality sleep and were significantly more depressed.[30] In that study, fatigue did not correlate with severity of liver disease and was not alleviated by the use of ursodeoxycholic acid (UDCA), findings which were validated by other groups.[31-33] The association with depression was also noted in other studies, at variable rates.

Patients with PBC who are fatigued, both those with and those without cirrhosis, have lower heart rate variability and tend to be more hypotensive, all indicating autonomic dysfunction with sympathetic overactivity and impaired baroreflex sensitivity.[34] Furthermore, these patients have accelerated reduction in muscle function on repeated sustained activity that correlates with the severity of fatigue. Such peripheral muscle fatigability appears to be related to excess muscle acidosis after exercise and recent studies point to the possibility of mitochondrial dysfunction as a contributing factor.[35]

Thus a hypothesis to explain the pathophysiology of fatigue involves a central effect secondary to accumulation of toxic substances related to cholestasis, leading to primary disautonomy and secondary peripheral muscular dysfunction, attributable to a loss of blood pressure control and abnormal oxygen delivery to peripheral tissues. The fact that the degree of fatigue does not correlate with the degree of cholestasis or hepatocellular dysfunction challenges this hypothesis to some extent. However, the possibility of inflammatory cytokines (e.g., IL-6, IL-1, and TNF-α) or adipokines (e.g., leptin) serving as central mediators is now being explored. Other factors that may contribute to the development of fatigue include depression, sleep deprivation, medication side effects, anemia, and hypothyroidism.

Pruritus

Defined as an unpleasant sensation that triggers the need to scratch, pruritus is a common complaint among patients with PBC. It has been reported in up to 70% of patients, with more recent studies indicating a lower prevalence of around 20% to 30%. Prince and colleagues followed 770 patients with PBC for symptom progression and found that 18.9% reported pruritus at the time of diagnosis; the cumulative risk of having pruritus was 45% at 5 years and 57% at 10 years.[36] Later, the natural history of pruritus in PBC was evaluated in patients participating in clinical trials at the Mayo Clinic. The annual risk of developing pruritus among patients who did not have this complaint at entry and who were randomized to the placebo arm was 27%, whereas the annual risk of reporting resolution or improvement of pruritus was 23%.[37] Although this particular study indicated that the serum alkaline phosphatase level and the Mayo risk score were independent predictors of pruritus, this relationship has not been shown consistently. Indeed, it appears that there is no direct correlation between biochemical markers of cholestasis or disease stage with the presence of pruritus, except perhaps for an increased incidence of severe pruritus in patients with florid

duct lesions.[38] In addition, pruritus is known to improve or resolve once liver failure ensues in some patients.

Pruritus in PBC is often generalized and intermittent, although it can certainly be relentless, and the severity will more typically be mild to moderate. It leads to marked impact on quality of life because of impaired sleep and depression. Rarely, pruritus can be severe enough to be considered disabling, and there are reports of liver transplantation indicated on the basis of this symptom alone. Even though the pruritus in PBC is not secondary to skin lesions, the physical exam will often reveal evidence of chronic scratching, such as excoriations, hyperpigmentation, and prurigo nodularis.

Little is known with respect to the pathogenesis of pruritus in PBC. Early speculations that bile acid accumulation in the plasma and tissues of patients with PBC would cause pruritus remain largely unproven. The fact that pruritus may improve at the later stages of the disease, when serum concentrations of bile acids are the highest, does not support this hypothesis. Furthermore, studies do not support a role for histamine in cholestatic pruritus either. Instead, other endogenous pruritogenic substances and pathways are under scrutiny, including opioid peptides, serotonin, acetylcholine, endothelins, substance P, kallikreins, leukotrienes, and prostaglandins.

Several lines of evidence support a central role for an increased opioidergic tone in the pathogenesis of pruritus in PBC.[39] First, as opposed to healthy volunteers, patients with PBC develop withdrawal-like symptoms after taking an opioid antagonist. Second, central administration of opioids induces pruritus, which is then improved by an opioid antagonist. Third, patients with cholestatic liver disease have increased serum levels of the endogenous opioid peptides methionine-enkephalin and leucine-enkephalin, with down-regulation of μ-opioid receptors. Fourth, clinical trials show that opioid antagonists improve pruritus in the setting of cholestasis. Taken together, the data suggest that either there is increased central opioidergic neurotransmission leading to pruritus or the opioid antagonists can possibly inhibit the release of a pruritogen that has not yet been identified. As far as genetics, a single nucleotide polymorphism has been reported in exon 1 of opioid receptor μ-1, which possibly protects against the scratching behavior, and another in exon 25 of the multidrug resistance protein 2 gene, which was significantly associated with the presence of pruritus.

Portal Hypertension

Only a minority of patients with PBC will have signs and symptoms consistent with portal hypertension at the time of their diagnosis. In one of the largest population-based studies, 3% of patients had ascites, 1.3% had bleeding esophageal varices, and 1.4% had hepatic encephalopathy at presentation. It was estimated that 10 years later 20% would have ascites; 10%, bleeding esophageal varices; and 12.6%, hepatic encephalopathy.[36] Interestingly, cirrhosis does not need to be present to elicit portal hypertension in PBC. Approximately 10% to 20% of patients are considered to have precirrhotic portal hypertension, possibly through formation of nodular regenerative hyperplasia and presinusoidal portal hypertension. Clinical features of portal hypertension in PBC are similar to those in patients with other forms of chronic liver disease.

Extrahepatic Complications

Bone Disease

Osteoporosis is present in 20% to 40% of patients with PBC; in contrast, osteomalacia is only rarely seen in this patient population. Such increased prevalence of osteoporosis actually translates into a measurable two-fold increase in fracture risk.[40] Risk factors for osteoporosis include advanced age, low body mass index ($\leq 24\ kg/m^2$), and advanced histologic disease stage.[41] The severity of cholestasis, the PBC Mayo risk score, postmenopausal state, and intestinal calcium malabsorption have all been inconsistently reported as predictive of osteoporosis. Similarly, genetic polymorphisms have been considered to influence bone disease in PBC, but with conflicting results. Although the pathogenesis of hepatic osteodystrophy in PBC is still disputed, it appears to be characterized by a combination of decreased bone formation and increased bone resorption.

Fat-Soluble Vitamin Deficiency

As PBC progresses and cholestasis worsens, the lack of an available pool of bile salts required for absorption of fat-soluble vitamins may lead to malabsorption of vitamins A, D, E, and K. As such, data derived from a clinical trial involving 180 patients with PBC indicated that the proportion of patients with vitamin A, D, E, or K deficiency was 33.5%, 13.2%, 1.9%, or 7.8%, respectively.[42] In general, the risk of a fat-soluble vitamin deficiency is higher with more advanced disease and lower cholesterol or albumin levels.

Hyperlipidemia

Up to 85% of patients with PBC will have hyperlipidemia at presentation. Hypercholesterolemia is typical in early and intermediate stages, with marked elevation of high-density lipoproteins (HDLs) and modest elevations of low-density and very-low-density lipoproteins (LDLs and VLDLs, respectively).[43] As the disease advances, we observe that HDL levels decrease significantly, whereas LDL levels remain elevated because of a progressive decrease in LDL receptors in injured hepatocytes and subsequent decrease in LDL clearance. Also, the composition of LDL changes during this stage: the concentration of lipoprotein X, a particle of LDL that is believed to have antiatherogenic properties, is elevated as well.[44] Triglyceride levels are normal or mildly elevated in the advanced stages.

Xanthelasmas, yellowish subcutaneous cholesterol deposits found around the eyes, and xanthomas, cholesterol deposits around the tendons, bony prominences, and peripheral nerves, are commonly seen in patients with PBC. Xanthomas, but not xanthelasmas, directly correlate with the plasma cholesterol levels and are usually seen with cholesterol levels greater than 600 mg/dl. A clear correlation between hyperlipidemia and cardiovascular disease has not been demonstrated in patients with PBC and treatment decisions should be made based on the presence or absence of additional risk factors in each individual patient.[45,46]

Associated Autoimmune Diseases

A number of autoimmune diseases can be seen with increased frequency among patients with PBC (**Table 41-3**), including dry eyes/dry mouth syndrome (Sjögren's syndrome) (up to

Table 41-3 Differential Diagnosis of Primary Biliary Cirrhosis

Extrahepatic biliary tract obstruction
   Choledocholithiasis
   Strictures
   Malignancy
Primary sclerosing cholangitis
Drug-induced cholestasis (e.g., estrogens, phenothiazines)
Granulomatous hepatitis
Autoimmune hepatitis
Chronic hepatitis C
Alcoholic hepatitis
Sarcoidosis

70%), thyroiditis (15%), scleroderma/CREST syndrome (calcinosis, Raynaud phenomenon, esophageal involvement, sclerodactyly, and telangiectasia) (5% to 10%), rheumatoid arthritis (10%), celiac disease (6%), and systemic lupus erythematosus (2%). Other rarely reported associations include inflammatory bowel disease, sarcoidosis, idiopathic thrombocytopenic purpura, hemolytic anemia, polymyositis, pulmonary fibrosis, and pulmonary hypertension.

Malignancies

Earlier concerns of an increased incidence of breast cancer in patients with PBC have been dismissed. In turn, available data support an increased risk of hepatocellular carcinoma in patients with cirrhotic-stage PBC. The most consistent risk factor for hepatocellular carcinoma in PBC is advanced histologic stage, but older age, male gender, evidence of portal hypertension, and history of blood transfusion have also been implicated.[47-49]

Diagnosis

The diagnosis of PBC is frequently made based on a combination of laboratory findings— persistent elevation of serum alkaline phosphatase level for at least 6 months and presence of antimitochondrial antibodies (AMAs) at a titer of 1:40 or greater or a level greater than 0.1 unit. Demonstration of typical features on liver biopsy can further confirm the diagnosis. In AMA-positive patients, a liver biopsy is required when serum alkaline phosphatase level elevation is less than 1.5 times the upper limit of normal and/or the concentrations of serum transaminases are more than 5 times elevated.[50] Furthermore, all AMA-negative patients should undergo liver biopsy. The differential diagnosis of PBC is listed in **Table 41-4**.

Laboratory Findings

Although levels of serum transaminases can be elevated, features of cholestasis predominate, with more prominent elevation of serum alkaline phosphatase and γ-glutamyltransferase (GGT) levels. Typically, serum levels of immunoglobulin M will be elevated and variable degrees of hyperlipidemia will be present. Synthetic dysfunction with reduction of serum albumin level, elevation of total bilirubin level, and prolongation of prothrombin time can be evident in the setting of advanced liver disease.

Table 41-4 Systemic Conditions Associated with Primary Biliary Cirrhosis

FEATURE	PREVALENCE (%)
Sjögren syndrome	70
Renal tubular acidosis	50
Gallstones	30
Arthritis	20
Thyroid disease	20
Scleroderma	15
Raynaud syndrome	10
CREST syndrome	5
Celiac disease	4

CREST, calcinosis, Raynaud phenomenon, esophageal involvement, sclerodactyly, and telangiectasia

Antimitochondrial Antibodies

The diagnostic hallmark of PBC is the presence of AMAs, which has a specificity of 95% for PBC. However, this autoantibody can be absent in up to 10% of patients when indirect immunofluorescence is used. More recently, with the introduction of recombinant autoantigens and the use of immunoblotting, AMAs will be detected in up to 95% of patients with PBC. Before the diagnosis of AMA-negative PBC is made, a liver biopsy should definitely be obtained and reviewed by an expert pathologist.

Patients who lack AMA seropositivity have the same clinical, biochemical, and histologic features of those who are AMA positive.[51] Furthermore, they also have similar clinical outcomes and response to UDCA or liver transplantation.[52] Thus although the detection of AMAs in the serum is highly specific for PBC and aids in the process of making the diagnosis, their presence appears to be clinically irrelevant.

Asymptomatic patients in a rheumatology clinic with AMA titers of 1:40 or greater or AMA levels greater than 0.1 unit and normal liver biochemistry values have been followed for up to 30 years and the likelihood that these individuals will eventually develop clinically evident PBC is very high—at the end of follow-up, 80% of these patients will have definite PBC, and an additional 14% will have probable PBC.[53] Nevertheless, in the general population, in which up to 0.5% of individuals can test positive for AMA, PBC will actually develop in fewer than 10%.[54] Perhaps healthy individuals found to have AMA positivity should undergo annual evaluation of serum liver biochemistry values, although no specific guidelines currently exist.

Other Autoantibodies

Antinuclear antibodies (ANAs) are present in approximately half of all patients with PBC, and in up to 85% of those who are AMA negative. Different types of ANAs have been described in PBC and some are believed to have prognostic importance. Anticentromere antibodies, for instance, are associated with higher frequency of portal hypertension[55] whereas anti–nuclear envelope antibodies such as anti-gp210, which provides a perinuclear staining pattern, are associated with worse overall survival.[55,56] Other ANAs seen in PBC include

anti–multiple nuclear dots, with specificity against the sp100 soluble protein and the promyelocytic leukemia protein, and anti-dsDNA, frequently seen in the so-called overlap syndromes. Both the perinuclear/rimlike and the multiple nuclear dots staining patterns are considered PBC specific.[57]

In addition, in the presence of one of the above-mentioned associated autoimmune diseases, the corresponding autoantibody is likely to be detected as well: anti-SSA/Ro in sicca syndrome, anti-Scl70 in systemic scleroderma, and anticentromere antibody with CREST syndrome, for example.

Imaging Studies

Cross-sectional imaging of the liver can be obtained through ultrasound (US), computerized tomography (CT), or magnetic resonance imaging (MRI). Noninvasive and inexpensive, US is usually the first test performed to exclude extrahepatic biliary obstruction, which is part of the differential diagnosis of PBC. A more detailed exam with use of Doppler US, CT, or MRI can provide valuable information on the size and morphology of the liver and spleen, signs of hepatocellular carcinoma, degree of collateral circulation, presence of ascites, direction and velocity of portal vein flow, and presence of portal vein thrombosis and/or lymphadenopathy. Lymphadenopathy has been reported in 62% to 88% of all patients with PBC, mainly in the periportal region.[58] Frequently, portocaval, cardiophrenic, gastroduodenal, periaortic, and peripancreatic adenopathy is also reported. It appears that larger lymph nodes of up to 2 cm are more common with more advanced PBC. Although the risk of lymphoma is reportedly <1%, bulky lymphadenopathy may need further investigation to exclude malignancy.

Liver morphologic studies show that hepatic atrophy is not common, although hypertrophy of the left lobe or caudate is frequently seen. Investigators have reported a lacelike pattern of fibrosis, with thin or thick bands of low attenuation surrounding regenerating nodules, by T_2-weighted MRI and CT in advanced PBC.[59] This finding, however, is not specific for PBC. The "halo sign" by MRI—hypointense areas encircling small portal vein branches, which would represent areas of fibrous deposition around the portal triads—is thought to have some specificity to PBC.[58]

Finally, MRI with magnetic retrograde cholangiopancreatography (MRCP) can also be used to differentiate the pruning of small intrahepatic bile ducts seen with advanced-stage PBC from the typical beading pattern of stricturing and dilatations characteristic of primary sclerosing cholangitis (PSC).

Histology

With increased awareness of the disease among healthcare providers and improved sensitivity of newer-generation AMA tests, liver biopsy is no longer considered a requirement to make the diagnosis of PBC. Moreover, prognostic information can be obtained through well-validated mathematical models that do not require input regarding histologic results.

In PBC only bile ducts that are less than 100 μm in diameter are involved. Two staging systems have been used to describe the histologic progression of PBC—Ludwig's and Scheuer's systems, which are both similar. In *stage I* disease there is inflammation and nonsuppurative destruction of the bile ducts; the infiltrates contain lymphocytes, plasma cells,

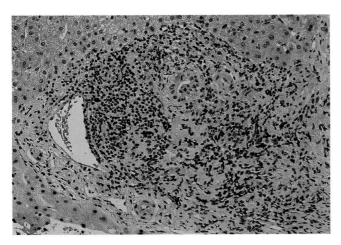

Fig. 41-1 **Florid duct lesion in stage I primary biliary cirrhosis.**

eosinophils, and mast cells, and the process is restricted to the portal tracts. Epithelioid noncaseating granulomas form very close to the injured bile duct, forming the so-called florid duct lesion (**Fig. 41-1**). They can occasionally be seen in the lobule as well. As the disease progresses, these damaged bile ducts disappear, causing ductopenia, a very important diagnostic hint. In *stage II* disease the inflammatory process extends to the interface with the hepatic parenchyma, and there may be ductal proliferation. Both stage I and stage II are considered "early." The presence of septal fibrosis indicates that the disease has progressed into *stage III*, and cirrhosis and regenerating nodules characterize *stage IV*.[60] Interestingly, features of all stages can overlap. For instance, a florid duct lesion can be seen in a biopsy specimen with septal fibrosis and interface hepatitis. These classification systems have been criticized for not allowing more detailed staging, especially with respect to the degree of fibrosis. **Figure 41-2** shows a schematic representation of the histologic stages of PBC.

Histologic progression does not necessarily occur at the same rate as clinical progression, and the presence of cirrhosis does not correlate with the presence of symptoms. Most untreated patients will progress histologically within 2 years.[61] Along with serum markers such as total bilirubin and albumin levels, the presence of piecemeal necrosis on liver biopsy appears to predict progression to cirrhosis.[62]

Natural History of Untreated Patients

Primary biliary cirrhosis (PBC) has a long protracted clinical course, and the following four distinct clinical phases are recognized: preclinical or silent, asymptomatic, symptomatic, and preterminal or liver failure. The rate of progression is highly variable and patients do not necessarily pass through all four phases (**Fig. 41-3**). They may first start at any of these phases and may skip phases as they progress.

The so-called silent phase is characterized by an incidentally found positive AMA, but with normal serum liver biochemistry measurements. Without treatment it can take up to 22 years for a patient to progress from an isolated positive AMA

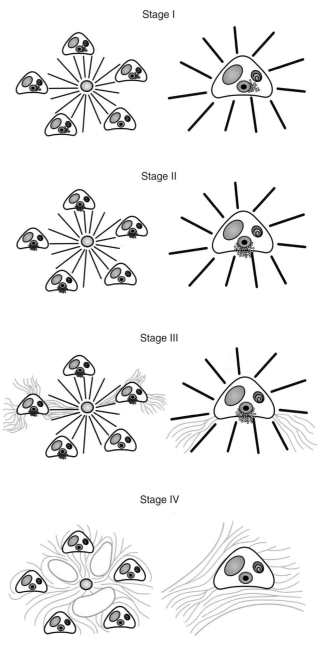

Stage I

Stage II

Stage III

Stage IV

Fig. 41-2 **Schematic representation of the staging system of primary biliary cirrhosis (Ludwig's classification).** Stage I is inflammation within the portal space, focused on the bile duct. Stage II occurs when the inflammation extends into the hepatic parenchyma (interface hepatitis or piecemeal necrosis). Stage III is fibrosis, and stage IV is cirrhosis with regenerative nodules.

to death. Metcalf and colleagues have been following a small cohort of 29 patients initially found to have an isolated positive AMA and normal liver chemistries. At diagnosis, most had liver biopsy findings that were at least consistent with PBC. After up to 18 years of follow-up, 76% developed symptoms and 83% proceeded to show abnormal liver tests in a cholestatic pattern characteristic of PBC.[63] More recently, an extended report with up to 30 years of follow-up suggested that perhaps patients who present this way have a more indolent course, because their overall survival was 12.8 years compared with

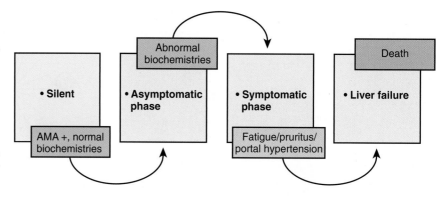

Fig. 41-3 **Schematic representation of the four phases in the natural history of primary biliary cirrhosis.**

9.6 years in an unselected group of 770 patients with PBC.[53] Median overall survival for PBC patients, symptomatic and asymptomatic combined, ranges between 6 and 10 years, with more recent studies showing longer survival times.

Most patients today present in the asymptomatic phase, which can last several years. Eventually, however, symptoms will develop; thus this phase is regarded as temporary only. In a study from England, half of 469 patients who were asymptomatic at presentation had developed symptoms at 5 years of follow-up, and it was estimated that only 5% remained asymptomatic after 20 years.[64] Liver-related mortality is decreased in asymptomatic patients compared with symptomatic patients, with median survival of 24.1 years versus 14.6 years, respectively. Unfortunately, it has been well demonstrated that even asymptomatic patients have a decreased survival compared with the general population. Those who remain asymptomatic over the years, however, appear to have similar survival as the age-and sex-matched population.[65]

As far as the impact of symptoms on survival, a high fatigue score appears to independently predict mortality after 4 years of follow-up, a finding that needs further validation.[27] More importantly, portal hypertension is known to predict a poor prognosis. Huet and colleagues confirmed this by demonstrating a clear correlation between higher hepatic vein gradients and worse survival among patients with PBC.[66] Liver failure is estimated to occur in 15% to 25% of patients after 5 years of follow-up.[36] Once fluid retention ensues, survival is significantly decreased, with approximately half of the patients deceased at 3 years.[67] Similarly, 3-year survival after the first episode of esophageal variceal bleeding is slightly below 50%.[68]

Treatment
Treatment of Primary Biliary Cirrhosis
Ursodeoxycholic Acid

Ursodeoxycholic acid (UDCA) is the only therapy approved by the U.S. Food and Drug Administration for the treatment of PBC. A dosage of 13 to 15 mg/kg/day is superior in terms of biochemical response and cost when compared with 5 to 7 mg/kg/day or 23 to 25 mg/kg/day dosages, and should be reinforced. Most studies using that dose have shown a decrease in serum total bilirubin, alkaline phosphatase, GGT,

Table 41-5 Observed Clinical Effects of Ursodeoxycholic Acid in Patients with Primary Biliary Cirrhosis

Laboratory Tests

Improves serum ALP, TB, GGT, AST, ALT, total cholesterol

Histology

Delays progression of fibrosis
Improves portal inflammation
Improves piecemeal necrosis

Symptoms

No clear effect on fatigue or pruritus

Complications of Primary Biliary Cirrhosis

Delays development of esophageal varices
Stabilizes or reduces portal vein gradient
Does not improve bone disease

Survival

Extends survival free of transplantation

ALP, alkaline phosphatase; ALT, alanine aminotransferase; AST, aspartate aminotransferase; GGT, γ-glutamyltransferase; TB, tuberculosis

cholesterol, and immunoglobulin M levels. Improvements in liver histologic results were also apparent: through mathematical modeling, investigators have shown a five-fold lower progression rate from early stage PBC to extensive fibrosis (7% per year with UDCA administration vs. 34% per year with placebo).[69] In addition to significantly delaying progression of fibrosis, UDCA reduces periportal necroinflammation and improves ductular proliferation. Likewise, one study suggested that UDCA can decrease the risk of developing esophageal varices in patients with PBC.[70] Unfortunately, UDCA has not demonstrated a consistent effect on the treatment of symptoms such as fatigue and pruritus, or on the management of bone disease associated with cholestasis. The proposed clinical effects of UDCA in PBC are shown in **Table 41-5.**

Many individual studies have been unable to show a survival benefit for patients receiving UDCA therapy. However, combined analyses of the largest trials lasting for a minimum of 2 years and using the endorsed dosage of 13 to 15 mg/kg/day clearly demonstrate an improved survival free of liver transplantation for UDCA users.[71] Even in this combined analysis, however, in which patients were treated for up to 4 years, a significant reduction in the likelihood of liver transplantation or death was only noticed for patients with moderate to severe disease. This is easy to explain, because PBC progresses very slowly and patients with early histologic disease at study entry were not likely to progress significantly over the 4-year study period. Thus it is not surprising that meta-analyses that included studies with shorter duration or lower dosages of UDCA failed to demonstrate improved survival in UDCA-treated patients.

More recently, an elegant Canadian study measured the portohepatic gradient in 132 patients with PBC at baseline and every 2 years thereafter. The investigators noticed that after 2 years of treatment with UDCA the gradient was either stabilized or decreased, and such response predicted better survival on multivariate analysis.[66] Another independent predictor was normalization of the serum aspartate aminotransferase (AST) level at 2 years. Patients who achieved both goals were considered "responders," and they had the same 15-year survival as the control population.

The definition of "response to therapy" has been the subject of debate, and defining who is a biochemical responder is important in identifying patients who could benefit from additional therapies. Pares and colleagues showed that patients with PBC who had normalization or at least a 40% decrease from baseline values toward the upper limit of normal (ULN) in the serum alkaline phosphatase level after 1 year of treatment with UDCA had similar survival times as the age- and gender-matched control population and significantly better outcomes than predicted by the Mayo risk score after up to 16 years of follow-up.[72] Interestingly, even patients without such biochemical response had some improvement in survival compared with that estimated by the Mayo risk score, albeit still substantially decreased compared with the control population. These predictors came to be known as the "Barcelona criteria."

In contrast, Corpechot and colleagues developed a new set of goals, known as the "Paris criteria," to define biochemical responders to UDCA. In this study involving 292 patients with PBC, investigators demonstrated that the combination of a serum bilirubin level of 1 mg/dl or lower, alkaline phosphatase level of three or less times the ULN, and AST level of two or less times the ULN after 1 year of therapy could accurately discriminate patients at lower risk of death or liver transplantation.[73] Indeed, patients who did not meet those criteria had a 2.5-fold increase in the risk of death or liver transplantation. Yet another conclusion of the study was that long-term treatment with UDCA over a 7-year period was associated with a 40% decrease in the risk of death or liver transplantation when compared with survival estimated by the Mayo risk score.

A subsequent Dutch study assessing the usefulness of serum albumin and bilirubin measurements in determining long-term prognosis was also able to validate the French criteria. The investigators reached the following conclusions: (1) patients with normal baseline values for serum albumin and bilirubin have survival similar to the general population; (2) normalization of serum albumin and/or bilirubin levels after 1 year of treatment with UDCA when one or both of these parameters was (were) abnormal at baseline is associated with increased survival free of liver transplantation, compared with patients who do not normalize these laboratory tests; and (3) the Paris criteria performed well in discriminating patients at

Table 41-6 Proposed Mechanisms of Action of Ursodeoxycholic Acid in Patients with Primary Biliary Cirrhosis

Hepatocytes
Stimulate biliary secretion of bile acids
Inhibit apoptosis
Activate glucocorticoid receptors
Reverse aberrant expression of HLA class I molecules

Cholangiocytes
Protect against cytotoxicity of hydrophobic bile acids
Possible antiapoptotic effect

Ileocytes
Inhibit bile acid carriers

Monocytes
Decrease cytokine secretion

higher mortality risk, but the Barcelona criteria only worked well for individuals with early stage disease (defined as normal baseline serum albumin and bilirubin concentrations).[74] Regardless of the stage of disease, all these studies show a long-term benefit of UDCA therapy in PBC in patients who have a biochemical response as defined by any of the previously mentioned criteria.

The mechanisms of action of UDCA in PBC are multiple[75,76] (**Table 41-6**). First, UDCA is a hydrophilic bile acid and, as such, lacks the cytotoxic effect on cell membranes that is so characteristic of more hydrophobic bile acids, such as lithocholic acid. Thus bile enrichment with UDCA protects the cholangiocytes against membrane damage. Second, UDCA has a known choleretic effect that has been demonstrated both in vitro and in vivo. This stimulation of biliary secretion is achieved mainly through up-regulation of synthesis, apical insertion, and activation of the bile salt export pump (Bsep) and the conjugate export pump (Mrp2); investigators also speculate about possible blockage of additional uptake of bile acids by UDCA through alterations in second messengers. Third, there is strong evidence that UDCA can stabilize the mitochondrial membrane and prevent its depolarization, thus reducing production of reactive oxygen species and preventing apoptosis. Hydrophobic bile acids, on the other hand, are known to increase mitochondrial permeability, leading to mitochondrial swelling and activation of caspase-9, thereby triggering a cascade of events that culminate with cell apoptosis. Finally, UDCA has immunomodulatory effects that have been demonstrated in patients with PBC. UDCA reverses aberrant expression of HLA class I molecules on hepatocytes and modulates secretion of cytokines by peripheral monocytes in vitro. It is possible that these effects are mediated through activation of the glucocorticoid receptor, which is currently being examined as a potential target for UDCA.

Other Drugs for Primary Biliary Cirrhosis

A variety of drugs have been tested without success in patients with PBC, including immunosuppressants (prednisolone, azathioprine, cyclosporine, chlorambucil, methotrexate, budesonide, and mycophenolate mofetil), antifibrotic agents (D-penicillamine and colchicine), malotilate, and thalidomide. As a result of the immune nature of PBC, corticosteroids and other immunosuppressants received early attention. However, despite a marginal effect noticed with some of these drugs given alone or in combination with UDCA, treatment-related irreversible side effects preclude their clinical use.

Methotrexate is still used by some experts for patients who fail to respond to UDCA. However, a large randomized control study of combination UDCA/methotrexate versus UDCA/placebo administration for a median follow-up time of 7.6 years did not demonstrate any additional benefit of methotrexate on progression of disease, development of esophageal varices, need for transplantation, or decreased mortality in comparison with the use of UDCA alone.[77] Aside from more bone marrow suppression in the methotrexate group, adverse events in this study were not different between treatment arms. This was different from prior trials showing more pulmonary toxicity, increased hair alopecia, and worsening fatigue among methotrexate-treated patients. A similar controversy exists with *colchicine*, an antifibrotic agent. A study comparing long-term use of methotrexate/UDCA versus colchicine/UDCA showed no difference between treatment arms, and estimated survival was as predicted by the Mayo risk score, indicating no change in the natural course of the disease.[78] Nevertheless, individual successful cases have encouraged its use by experts in special situations.

Budesonide is a newer glucocorticoid agent with greater than 90% first-pass metabolism that was used in combination with UDCA to treat patients with PBC. Benefits on histology and liver biochemistry analyses were noticed only in patients with early stage PBC, and further studies are warranted.[79] Of concern, development of portal vein thrombosis occurred in cirrhotic patients with portal hypertension while being treated with budesonide. Thus recent guidelines recommend against administering this drug to cirrhotic patients and consider its use among incomplete responders to UDCA who have early stage disease.[80]

A randomized controlled trial of the antiviral drug Combivir (lamivudine and zidovudine) versus placebo for 6 months was conducted in patients who failed UDCA in Canada and North America.[81] The only significant finding was a 50% reduction in serum AST level. Moreover, serious adverse events (variceal hemorrhage, fatigue, and alopecia) occurred in asymptomatic patients receiving Combivir, making its use unacceptable in that setting.

Lastly, combination trials of UDCA with other immunosuppressants—sulindac, silymarin, and atorvastatin—have also been unsuccessful.

Novel Agents

Small uncontrolled trials and case reports using the fibric acid derivatives *fenofibrate* or *bezafibrate* in the treatment of PBC with incomplete response to UDCA are available from Japan and the United Kingdom.[82-84] The proposed mechanism of action of these drugs is through activation of the peroxisome proliferator–activated receptor α (PPAR-α) pathway, with subsequent regulation of the immune response and cell proliferation. Such studies have consistently shown improvement in serum liver biochemistry and IgM measurements, and larger trials are warranted.

Pilot data on the use of rituximab, vitamin D3, and the farnesoid X receptor (FXR) ligand 6-ethylchenodeoxycholic acid appear encouraging but have only been presented in abstract form.[85-87]

Treatment of Associated Symptoms and Conditions

Pruritus

Cholestyramine is used as first-line therapy for pruritus based on its widespread use and safety. Starting dose is 4 g/day, which can be increased up to four times daily. Because this medication is a bile acid–binding resin, it should be administered at least 2 to 4 hours apart from UDCA and other medications to prevent loss of efficacy.

Rifampicin is a pregnane X receptor agonist and enzyme inducer, and has been used as a second-line agent to treat pruritus. Given a 10% to 15% risk of hepatitis, we recommend starting at only 150 mg/day and titrating up to a maximum of 300 mg twice a day.

Recent evidence of an increased opioidergic tone as a potential cause of pruritus in PBC led to studies using opioid antagonists such as naltrexone 25 to 50 mg/day as third-line therapy.[88] This has been dampened by adverse side effects including an opioid withdrawal–like reaction, pain, and confusion. Preloading the patient with escalating doses of intravenous naloxone has been advocated to prevent such a withdrawal-like syndrome. Nevertheless, results in clinical practice are not as encouraging. There are case reports of transdermal buprenorphine in the management of pruritus, which also requires further evaluation.

Finally, sertraline has been shown in small studies to improve pruritus in PBC and other cholestatic diseases and can be used instead of naltrexone as a third-line option.[89] The optimum dose is 75 to 100 mg/day, and is usually well tolerated.

Invasive approaches such as extracorporeal albumin dialysis, plasmapheresis, and bile duct drainage have been reported as rescue therapy for refractory cases. The use of vagal nerve stimulation remains experimental.

Fatigue

The first step in the management of fatigue is to exclude and/or treat conditions such as anemia, hypothyroidism, adrenal insufficiency, and depression, which could be contributing to the clinical presentation. Sleep disturbance should be addressed appropriately. Medications such as β-blockers and calcium channel blockers, which can exacerbate autonomic dysfunction, should be adjusted. For patients with excessive daytime somnolence and fatigue, use of modafinil 100 to 200 mg/day has been advocated through case series and small uncontrolled studies.[90] Otherwise, fluoxetine, ondansetron, and fluvoxamine have all failed to improve fatigue in patients with PBC.

Fat-Soluble Vitamin Deficiency

Patients with advanced-stage PBC should be tested annually for deficiencies of vitamins A, D, E, and K, and replacement should be prescribed as indicated, followed by a maintenance dose. The replacement and maintenance doses, respectively, are as follows: vitamin A, 50,000 and 10,000 U/day; vitamin

D, 1600 and 400 U/day; vitamin E, 10 U/kg/day and 30 U/day; vitamin K, 50 and 5 mg/day.

Hyperlipidemia

To date, no correlation has been found with respect to an increased risk of cardiovascular events in the setting of hyperlipidemia of PBC. Therefore treatment should be offered according to the patient's individual risk factors for cardiovascular disease. Statins have proven safe in small studies in this population.

Metabolic Bone Disease

The guidelines of the American Association for the Study of Liver Diseases (AASLD) recommend that a bone density study be obtained at baseline, when PBC is first diagnosed, and then every 2 to 3 years.[88] Supplementation with calcium 1000 to 1500 mg/day and vitamin D 800 to 1000 units/day is usually recommended for prevention of bone disease in this at-risk population. Vitamin D levels should be checked annually in those with advanced liver disease, and replacement with 50,000 units given two to three times per week in case of deficiency.

Only a few studies have been published on the management of bone disease in cholestatic patients. Hormone replacement therapy appears to be effective in increasing the bone mineral density (BMD) in patients with PBC, although cholestasis can worsen in some patients. The use of raloxifene, a selective estrogen receptor modulator, in a small study involving nine patients with PBC successfully increased BMD without apparent toxicity. Calcitonin, on the other hand, did not prove useful in this population. The best available data regarding PBC come from a randomized controlled trial of alendronate versus placebo involving 34 patients with PBC and osteopenia or osteoporosis. Alendronate 70 mg/week significantly improved BMD compared with placebo and was not associated with more adverse events.[91] Thus European clinical practice guidelines suggest the use of alendronate for those patients with a T-score less than −2.5 by DEXA scan or following pathologic fracture.[80] Its use in patients with T-scores less than −1.5 can be considered on an individual basis.

Liver Transplantation

Because it is the only definitive treatment for patients with advanced PBC, transplantation is performed for those who progress to liver failure despite available medical therapy. The indications to proceed with transplant are the same as for other etiologies of chronic liver disease. In this regard, the Model for End-Stage Liver Disease (MELD) score has been used for organ allocation since 2002. This model takes into account the serum bilirubin level, creatinine level, and international normalized ratio, as well as the need for dialysis. Refractory pruritus and excessive chronic fatigue have only rarely been used as indications for liver transplantation.

The greatest challenge is not to determine who will need a transplant, but to decide when the transplant will be needed. The ideal timing for liver transplant in patients with PBC is still a matter of debate. In 1998 a study using the Mayo risk score to evaluate patients undergoing liver transplantation in three large centers in the United States suggested that the risk of death after transplant, as well as resource utilization, is lower when transplant is performed for patients with Mayo risk scores of 7.8 or lower, although patients can certainly be transplanted with higher Mayo risk scores.[92] Alternatively, serum total bilirubin level can be used as a single indicator. Patients should be referred to a transplant center when the bilirubin concentration reaches 5.9 mg/dl, and transplant should be considered before the bilirubin level reaches 10 mg/dl.

The overall posttransplant survival is excellent, with a 5-year survival rate in the United States and Europe averaging 78% to 87%.[92] Quality of life is significantly improved, with posttransplant patients attesting to less fatigue, sleepiness, pruritus, and sick days. Likewise, they report better overall health and greater ability to carry on daily activities with minimal or no symptoms.

Recurrent Primary Biliary Cirrhosis

Primary biliary cirrhosis recurs in 11% to 34% of all patients who receive transplants for that indication.[93] Recurrent PBC is diagnosed mainly through histologic criteria, because AMA remains positive after transplant and serum alkaline phosphatase level may be elevated for multiple reasons. Thus the proportion of patients diagnosed with recurrence will vary according to the frequency with which liver biopsies are performed. In institutions where protocol biopsies are obtained at preestablished intervals the recurrence rate tends to be higher, whereas lower prevalence will be seen in institutions where biopsies are only obtained if clinically indicated. The median time to recurrence is 36 to 61 months.

Predictors of recurrence have been investigated in six studies to date. Interestingly, use of tacrolimus-based regimens was associated with increased recurrence rate in four of those studies.[92] Moreover, patients prescribed tacrolimus had earlier recurrence compared with those taking cyclosporin A. Two other independent variables linked to PBC recurrence were male sex and recipient age.

The effect of UDCA on recurrent PBC was evaluated in a retrospective study involving 154 patients undergoing transplantation for PBC. Of 52 (34%) patients with recurrent disease, 38 (73%) were treated with an average of 12 mg/kg/day of UDCA. Significantly more of the treated patients had normalization of the serum alkaline phosphatase level compared with untreated patients, but UDCA did not affect histologic progression over the 36 month-period.[94] Regardless, available data indicate that graft loss attributable to recurrent PBC is extremely rare.

Prognosis

Numerous predictors of prognosis have been evaluated in PBC, but only a few have been validated and are in use in clinical practice. The most commonly used are mathematical models, which will be discussed later, and several others are currently undergoing further investigation.

Laboratory Tests

Total bilirubin value is the best single laboratory test to independently predict survival; however, jaundice only occurs late in the disease. More recently, markers of fibrosis have been explored and exciting results were seen with the enhanced liver fibrosis (ELF) assay, which showed an area under the curve of 0.76 to predict advanced fibrosis and cirrhosis. Remarkably, by stratifying according to low, intermediate, and high values for the ELF assay, investigators were able to accurately predict clinical events. Each 1-point increase in ELF was associated with a three-fold increase in future clinical complications.[95] Other serologic tests that appear promising include the use of specific autoantibodies, such as the anti-gp210, which indicates increased risk of death by liver failure, and the anti-centromere, which appears to be associated with an increased risk of developing portal hypertension.[55] The use of certain genetic polymorphisms as a means to stratify patients according to likelihood of clinical/histologic progression may be a viable option in the future.

Histology

Although most investigators are performing fewer serial liver biopsies for prognostic purposes, histologic studies can provide helpful information and may be needed at times to identify patients who might need additional therapy. The presence of moderate to severe lymphocytic piecemeal necrosis indicates a higher risk of progression to cirrhosis.[62] Similarly, the presence of features that resemble overlap syndrome, such as severe interface hepatitis, is associated with worse overall survival.[96]

Elastography

Transient elastography (FibroScan) is an ultrasound exam that uses pulse-echo ultrasound acquisitions to measure liver stiffness in kilopascals (kPa). This technique allows for a noninvasive assessment of liver stiffness in a volume of liver that is approximately 100 times greater than that obtained from liver biopsy. Given that cirrhosis and portal hypertension are associated with poorer survival, it is worth identifying noninvasive methods to accurately predict the presence of fibrosis and portal hypertension. Corpechot and colleagues used FibroScan to assess for biliary fibrosis in patients with PBC and primary sclerosing cholangitis (PSC) and found a very significant correlation between the liver stiffness measurements and the histologic and fibrosis stages on biopsy.[97] The study could accurately predict the fibrosis stage in 69 of the 95 patients (72.6%). In a separate study from Spain involving 55 patients with PBC evaluated with liver biopsy and transient elastography, liver stiffness correlated well with histologic findings when the slides were examined by an independent blinded pathologist.[98] Recently, assessment of liver fibrosis in 45 patients with PBC was carried out with FibroScan, MRI, MR spectroscopy, and serum markers of fibrosis, and these results were compared with the findings obtained after liver biopsy. The investigators reported comparable results between MRI and FibroScan, with an accuracy of 80% to 83% in detecting fibrosis stages of II or greater.[99]

Elastography has not yet been shown to correlate with clinical outcomes in cholestatic liver diseases, but was found to correlate with portal pressure as measured by the hepatic vein pressure gradient mostly on hepatitis C virus (HCV)-induced liver disease.

Mathematic Models

Several mathematic models have been created and well validated, among which the Mayo risk score is the most widely used, at least in the United States. Indeed, a study conducted in Olmsted County, Minnesota, demonstrated not only that this prognostic index is reliable in predicting survival but also that it can be used in the community with the same accuracy.[2] Other models include the Oslo, Newcastle, European, and Barcelona risk scores. In all of these models, total bilirubin level is the most heavily weighted variable.

In the Mayo risk score, the patient's age, serum total bilirubin and albumin levels, prothrombin time, and presence or absence of edema and ascites as well as the use of diuretics are independent variables entered into a computer-generated model to generate a prediction. This is available at www.mayoclinic.org/gi-rst/mayomodel1.html. Histologic information is not required. The Mayo risk score has been shown to retain its accuracy in predicting survival for patients with PBC who are treated with UDCA.

Mayo risk score has also been used to optimize timing of liver transplantation[100] and to determine patients who are at higher risk for esophageal varices and who would benefit from a screening upper endoscopy.[70,101] Despite the accuracy of the Mayo risk score in predicting long-term survival without liver transplantation, the model tends to overestimate survival in patients with poor short-term outcomes; the mathematical models cannot yet replace good clinical judgment.

Special Populations
Antimitochondrial Antigen–Negative Primary Biliary Cirrhosis

The proportion of patients who are AMA negative is dependent on the population studied and also on the choice of test to detect the AMA. Immunofluorescence is insensitive; ELISA or immunoblotting will detect AMAs in up to 80% of patients considered to be AMA negative by immunofluorescence. Newer generations of ELISA directed against the PDC-E2 subunit may capture additional patients.

Frequently, AMA-negative patients will have detectable antinuclear or anti–smooth muscle antibodies. As previously mentioned, some antinuclear antibodies appear to be specific for PBC, including those targeted against gp210, nucleoporin p62, and nuclear pore complex, which generate a rimlike pattern on immunofluorescence, and those against sp100 or promyelocytic leukemia protein, which generate the multiple nuclear dots pattern. Therefore the presence of these autoantibodies does not indicate a diagnosis of AIH. Some investigators use the term "autoimmune cholangitis" to define AMA-negative PBC patients who do have detectable antinuclear or anti–smooth muscle antibodies. Whether this represents a distinct clinical entity is debatable.

An emerging body of literature indicates that patients who are AMA negative but with typical histologic findings have the same clinical and biochemical features of those who are AMA positive. Importantly, they also have similar outcomes with respect to response to therapy and survival without liver transplantation.

Overlap of Primary Biliary Cirrhosis and Autoimmune Hepatitis

The term "overlap syndrome" was coined to describe patients with AIH who also have typical features of PBC (overlap PBC-AIH) or of primary sclerosing cholangitis (overlap PSC-AIH). Although a precise and well-accepted definition is lacking, it is estimated that approximately 5% to 10% of patients initially diagnosed with AIH or with PBC actually have an overlap syndrome.

The diagnosis of overlap PBC-AIH requires that patients meet criteria for both diseases; the presence of ANAS in PBC patients is not enough to diagnose overlap, nor is the histologic finding of mild ductular changes in patients with AIH. Different case-finding methods have been described in this setting, with the easiest and yet more selective definition perhaps being the one used by Chazouilleres and colleagues.[102] These investigators proposed that overlap could be diagnosed in patients who met two out of three criteria for each disease, with at least moderate interface hepatitis being required in all cases. In this regard, at least two of the following three criteria were needed for the diagnosis of PBC: (1) AMA seropositivity; (2) serum alkaline phosphatase levels at least twice the upper limit of normal or serum γ-glutamyltransferase levels at least five times the upper limit of normal; and (3) bile duct lesions in the liver biopsy. For AIH at least two of the following criteria were required: (1) serum aminotransferase levels at least five times the upper limit of normal; (2) serum immunoglobulin G levels at least twice the upper limit of normal or positive anti–smooth muscle antibodies; and (3) a liver biopsy showing moderate or severe interface hepatitis.

More recently, double positivity for AMA and double-stranded DNA antibody (anti-dsDNA) was found in 47% of 15 patients with overlap PBC-AIH, whereas only 3% of 120 patients with PBC and 1% of 120 patients with AIH demonstrated the same pattern, suggesting perhaps that this double-positivity could serve as a serologic profile for overlap PBC-AIH.[103] Further studies are required to validate this hypothesis.

The pathophysiology of overlap syndromes is largely unknown. It has been proposed to represent a completely separate entity from AIH and PBC, or to represent a different manifestation of those diseases according to the genetic background. Because transition cases have clearly been demonstrated, with PBC patients developing well-defined AIH months to years after the original diagnosis and vice versa, some investigators have proposed that there is a continuum between PBC and AIH, with overlap being in the middle. However, this remains speculative.

Recognizing an overlap syndrome is important and may justify repeating liver biopsies in patients with incomplete response to UDCA or in patients who worsen after a long period of stability. It is possible that patients with overlap have a worse overall prognosis compared with patients with pure PBC, with more complications related to portal hypertension and more deaths.[96] Thus a more aggressive therapy with use of immunosuppressants is likely indicated in such cases and indeed has been shown to be effective in multiple small case series. According to European guidelines, the treating physician may decide whether to use corticosteroids and UDCA at the time of diagnosis of overlap or to start with UDCA and only add a corticosteroid if an appropriate response is not observed within 3 months.[80]

References

1. Lazaridis KN, Talwalkar JA. Clinical epidemiology of primary biliary cirrhosis: incidence, prevalence, and impact of therapy. J Clin Gastroenterol 2007;41:494–500.
2. Kim WR, et al. Epidemiology and natural history of primary biliary cirrhosis in a US community. Gastroenterology 2000;119:1631–1636.
3. Hurlburt KJ, et al. Prevalence of autoimmune liver disease in Alaska Natives. Am J Gastroenterol 2002;97:2402–2407.
4. Peters MG, et al. Differences between Caucasian, African American, and Hispanic patients with primary biliary cirrhosis in the United States. Hepatology 2007;46:769–775.
5. Wong RK, et al. Primary biliary cirrhosis in Singapore: evaluation of demography, prognostic factors and natural course in a multi-ethnic population. J Gastroenterol Hepatol 2008;23:599–605.
6. Danielsson A, Boqvist L, Uddenfeldt P. Epidemiology of primary biliary cirrhosis in a defined rural population in the northern part of Sweden. Hepatology 1990;11:458–464.
7. Prince MI, James OF. The epidemiology of primary biliary cirrhosis. Clin Liver Dis 2003;7:795–819.
8. Remmel T, et al. Primary biliary cirrhosis in Estonia. With special reference to incidence, prevalence, clinical features, and outcome. Scand J Gastroenterol 1995;30:367–371.
9. Gross RG, Odin JA. Recent advances in the epidemiology of primary biliary cirrhosis. Clin Liver Dis 2008;12:289–303; viii.
10. Jones DE, et al. Familial primary biliary cirrhosis reassessed: a geographically-based population study. J Hepatol 1999;30:402–407.
11. Selmi C, et al. Primary biliary cirrhosis in monozygotic and dizygotic twins: genetics, epigenetics, and environment. Gastroenterology 2004;127:485–492.
12. Parikh-Patel A, et al. Risk factors for primary biliary cirrhosis in a cohort of patients from the United States. Hepatology 2001;33:16–21.
13. Gershwin ME, et al. Risk factors and comorbidities in primary biliary cirrhosis: a controlled interview-based study of 1032 patients. Hepatology 2005;42:1194–1202.
14. Salunga TL, et al. Oxidative stress-induced apoptosis of bile duct cells in primary biliary cirrhosis. J Autoimmun 2007;29:78–86.
15. Allina J, et al. T cell targeting and phagocytosis of apoptotic biliary epithelial cells in primary biliary cirrhosis. J Autoimmun 2006;27:232–241.
16. Ishibashi H, et al. T cell immunity and primary biliary cirrhosis. Autoimmun Rev 2003;2:19–24.
17. Lan RY, et al. Hepatic IL-17 responses in human and murine primary biliary cirrhosis. J Autoimmun 2009;32:43–51.
18. Kita H, et al. Identification of HLA-A2-restricted CD8(+) cytotoxic T cell responses in primary biliary cirrhosis: T cell activation is augmented by immune complexes cross-presented by dendritic cells. J Exp Med 2002;195:113–123.
19. Lan RY, et al. Liver-targeted and peripheral blood alterations of regulatory T cells in primary biliary cirrhosis. Hepatology 2006;43:729–737.
20. Xu L, et al. Does a betaretrovirus infection trigger primary biliary cirrhosis? Proc Natl Acad Sci U S A 2003;100:8454–8459.
21. Leung PS, et al. Immunization with a xenobiotic 6-bromohexanoate bovine serum albumin conjugate induces antimitochondrial antibodies. J Immunol 2003;170:5326–5332.
22. Selmi C, Zuin M, Gershwin ME. The unfinished business of primary biliary cirrhosis. J Hepatol 2008;49:451–460.
23. Selmi C, et al. Genetics and geoepidemiology of primary biliary cirrhosis: following the footprints to disease etiology. Semin Liver Dis 2005;25:265–280.
24. Invernizzi P, et al. Frequency of monosomy X in women with primary biliary cirrhosis. Lancet 2004;363:533–535.
25. Hirschfield GM, et al. Primary biliary cirrhosis associated with HLA, IL12A, and IL12RB2 variants. New Engl J Med 2009;360:2544–2555.
26. Kumagi T, Onji M. Presentation and diagnosis of primary biliary cirrhosis in the 21st century. Clin Liver Dis 2008;12:243–259; vii.
27. Jones DE, et al. Four year follow up of fatigue in a geographically defined primary biliary cirrhosis patient cohort. Gut 2006;55:536–541.
28. Newton JL, et al. Fatigue in primary biliary cirrhosis is associated with excessive daytime somnolence. Hepatology 2006;44:91–98.

29. Witt-Sullivan H, et al. The demography of primary biliary cirrhosis in Ontario, Canada. Hepatology 1990;12:98–105.

30. Cauch-Dudek K, et al. Fatigue in primary biliary cirrhosis. Gut 1998;43: 705–710.

31. Goldblatt J, et al. The true impact of fatigue in primary biliary cirrhosis: a population study. Gastroenterology 2002;122:1235–1241.

32. Huet PM, et al. Impact of fatigue on the quality of life of patients with primary biliary cirrhosis. Am J Gastroenterol 2000;95:760–767.

33. Stanca CM, et al. Evaluation of fatigue in U.S. patients with primary biliary cirrhosis. Am J Gastroenterol 2005;100:1104–1109.

34. Newton JL, et al. Population prevalence and symptom associations of autonomic dysfunction in primary biliary cirrhosis. Hepatology 2007;45: 1496–1505.

35. Newton JL, et al. A predictive model for fatigue and its etiologic associations in primary biliary cirrhosis. Clin Gastroenterol Hepatol 2008; 6:228–233.

36. Prince M, et al. Survival and symptom progression in a geographically based cohort of patients with primary biliary cirrhosis: follow-up for up to 28 years. Gastroenterology 2002;123:1044–1051.

37. Talwalkar JA, et al. Natural history of pruritus in primary biliary cirrhosis. Clin Gastroenterol Hepatol 2003;1:297–302.

38. Poupon R, et al. Clinical and biochemical expression of the histopathological lesions of primary biliary cirrhosis. UDCA-PBC Group. J Hepatol 1999;30:408–412.

39. Bergasa NV. Pruritus in primary biliary cirrhosis: pathogenesis and therapy. Clin Liver Dis 2008;12:385–406, x.

40. Solaymani-Dodaran M, et al. Fracture risk in people with primary biliary cirrhosis: a population-based cohort study. Gastroenterology 2006;131: 1752–1757.

41. Menon K, et al. Bone disease in primary biliary cirrhosis: independent indicators and rate of progression. J Hepatol 2001;35:316–323.

42. Phillips J, et al. Fat-soluble vitamin levels in patients with primary biliary cirrhosis. Am J Gastroenterol 2001;96:2745–2750.

43. Crippin JS, et al. Hypercholesterolemia and atherosclerosis in primary biliary cirrhosis: what is the risk? Hepatology 1992;15:858–862.

44. Jahn CE, et al. Lipoprotein abnormalities in primary biliary cirrhosis. Association with hepatic lipase inhibition as well as altered cholesterol esterification. Gastroenterology 1985;89:1266–1278.

45. Solaymani-Dodaran M, et al. Risk of cardiovascular and cerebrovascular events in primary biliary cirrhosis: a population-based cohort study. Am J Gastroenterol 2008;103:2784–2788.

46. Sorokin A, Brown JL, Thompson PD. Primary biliary cirrhosis, hyperlipidemia, and atherosclerotic risk: a systematic review. Atherosclerosis 2007;194:293–299.

47. Suzuki A, et al. Clinical predictors for hepatocellular carcinoma in patients with primary biliary cirrhosis. Clin Gastroenterol Hepatol 2007;5:259–264.

48. Cavazza A, et al. Incidence, risk factors, and survival of hepatocellular carcinoma in primary biliary cirrhosis: comparative analysis from two centers. Hepatology 2009;50:1162–1168.

49. Deutsch M, et al. Risk of hepatocellular carcinoma and extrahepatic malignancies in primary biliary cirrhosis. Eur J Gastroenterol Hepatol 2008; 20:5–9.

50. Zein C, Angulo P, Lindor K. When is liver biopsy needed in the diagnosis of primary biliary cirrhosis? Clin Gastroenterol Hepatol 2003;1:89–95.

51. Invernizzi P, et al. Comparison of the clinical features and clinical course of antimitochondrial antibody–positive and –negative primary biliary cirrhosis. Hepatology 1997;25:1090–1095.

52. Kim WR, et al. Does antimitochondrial antibody status affect response to treatment in patients with primary biliary cirrhosis? Outcomes of ursodeoxycholic acid therapy and liver transplantation. Hepatology 1997; 26:22–26.

53. Swann RE, et al. Antimitochondrial antibody (AMA) positivity but normal LFTs—is this PBC as we know it? Hepatology 2008;48(4 (Suppl):601A.

54. Mattalia A, et al. Characterization of antimitochondrial antibodies in healthy adults. Hepatology 1998;27:656–661.

55. Nakamura M, et al. Anti-gp210 and anti-centromere antibodies are different risk factors for the progression of primary biliary cirrhosis. Hepatology 2007;45:118–127.

56. Invernizzi P, et al. Autoantibodies against nuclear pore complexes are associated with more active and severe liver disease in primary biliary cirrhosis. J Hepatol 2001;34:366–372.

57. Muratori L, et al. Antimitochondrial antibodies and other antibodies in primary biliary cirrhosis: diagnostic and prognostic value. Clin Liver Dis 2008;12:261–276, vii.

58. Wenzel JS, et al. Primary biliary cirrhosis: MR imaging findings and description of MR imaging periportal halo sign. AJR Am J Roentgenol 2001;176:885–889.

59. Haliloglu N, Erden A, Erden I. Primary biliary cirrhosis: evaluation with T2-weighted MR imaging and MR cholangiopancreatography. Eur J Radiol 2009;69:523–527.

60. Burt AD. Primary biliary cirrhosis and other ductopenic diseases. Clin Liver Dis 2002;6:363–380, vi.

61. Locke GR III, et al. Time course of histological progression in primary biliary cirrhosis. Hepatology 1996;23:52–56.

62. Corpechot C, et al. Biochemical markers of liver fibrosis and lymphocytic piecemeal necrosis in UDCA-treated patients with primary biliary cirrhosis. Liver Int 2004;24:187–193.

63. Metcalf JV, et al. Natural history of early primary biliary cirrhosis. Lancet 1996;348:1399–1402.

64. Prince MI, et al. Asymptomatic primary biliary cirrhosis: clinical features, prognosis, and symptom progression in a large population based cohort. Gut 2004;53:865–870.

65. Springer J, et al. Asymptomatic primary biliary cirrhosis: a study of its natural history and prognosis. Am J Gastroenterol 1999;94:47–53.

66. Huet PM, et al. Portal hypertension and primary biliary cirrhosis: effect of long-term ursodeoxycholic acid treatment. Gastroenterology 2008;135: 1552–1560.

67. Chan CW, et al. Survival following the development of ascites and/or peripheral oedema in primary biliary cirrhosis: a staged prognostic model. Scand J Gastroenterol 2005;40:1081–1089.

68. Gores GJ, et al. Prospective evaluation of esophageal varices in primary biliary cirrhosis: development, natural history, and influence on survival. Gastroenterology 1989;96:1552–1559.

69. Corpechot C, et al. The effect of ursodeoxycholic acid therapy on liver fibrosis progression in primary biliary cirrhosis. Hepatology 2000;32: 1196–1199.

70. Angulo P, et al. Utilization of the Mayo risk score in patients with primary biliary cirrhosis receiving ursodeoxycholic acid. Liver 1999;19:115–121.

71. Poupon R, et al. Combined analysis of randomized controlled trials of ursodeoxycholic acid in primary biliary cirrhosis. Gastroenterology 1997; 113:884–890.

72. Pares A, Caballeria L, Rodes J. Excellent long-term survival in patients with primary biliary cirrhosis and biochemical response to ursodeoxycholic acid. Gastroenterology 2006;130:715–720.

73. Corpechot C, et al. Biochemical response to ursodeoxycholic acid and long-term prognosis in primary biliary cirrhosis. Hepatology 2008;48: 871–877.

74. Kuiper EM, et al. Improved prognosis of patients with primary biliary cirrhosis that have a biochemical response to ursodeoxycholic acid. Gastroenterology 2009;136:1281–1287.

75. Paumgartner G, Beuers U. Ursodeoxycholic acid in cholestatic liver disease: mechanisms of action and therapeutic use revisited. Hepatology 2002;36: 525–531.

76. Beuers U. Drug insight: mechanisms and sites of action of ursodeoxycholic acid in cholestasis. Nat Clin Pract Gastroenterol Hepatol 2006;3: 318–328.

77. Combes B, et al. Methotrexate (MTX) plus ursodeoxycholic acid (UDCA) in the treatment of primary biliary cirrhosis. Hepatology 2005;42:1184–1193.

78. Kaplan MM, et al. A randomized controlled trial of colchicine plus ursodiol versus methotrexate plus ursodiol in primary biliary cirrhosis: ten-year results. Hepatology 2004;39:915–923.

79. Rautiainen H, et al. Budesonide combined with UDCA to improve liver histology in primary biliary cirrhosis: a three-year randomized trial. Hepatology 2005;41:747–752.

80. EASL Clinical Practice Guidelines: management of cholestatic liver diseases. J Hepatol 2009;51:237–267.

81. Mason AL, et al. Pilot studies of single and combination antiretroviral therapy in patients with primary biliary cirrhosis. Am J Gastroenterol 2004; 99:2348–2355.

82. Iwasaki S, et al. The efficacy of ursodeoxycholic acid and bezafibrate combination therapy for primary biliary cirrhosis: a prospective, multicenter study. Hepatol Res 2008;38:557–564.

83. Ohira H, et al. Fenofibrate treatment in patients with primary biliary cirrhosis. Am J Gastroenterol 2002;97:2147–2149.

84. Walker LJ, et al. Comment on biochemical response to ursodeoxycholic acid and long-term prognosis in primary biliary cirrhosis. Hepatology 2009;49:337–338; author reply 338.

85. Allina J, et al. High dose vitamin D3 treatment enhances macrophage phagocytosis of apoptotic cells and lowers bilirubin levels in PBC. Hepatology 2008;48(Suppl 4):611A.

86. Myers RP, et al. Rituximab for primary biliary cirrhosis (PBC) refractory to ursodeoxycholic acid (UDCA). Hepatology 2007;46(Suppl 1):550A.

87. Mason A, et al. Farnesoid X receptor agonists: a new class of drugs for the treatment of PBC? An international study evaluating the addition of INT-747 to ursodeoxycholic acid. J Hepatology 2010;52:S1–S2.

88. Lindor KD, et al. Primary biliary cirrhosis. Hepatology 2009;50:291–308.

89. Mayo MJ, et al. Sertraline as a first-line treatment for cholestatic pruritus. Hepatology 2007;45:666–674.

90. Jones DE, Newton JL. An open study of modafinil for the treatment of daytime somnolence and fatigue in primary biliary cirrhosis. Aliment Pharmacol Ther 2007;25:471–476.

91. Zein CO, et al. Alendronate improves bone mineral density in primary biliary cirrhosis: a randomized placebo-controlled trial. Hepatology 2005; 42:762–771.

92. Milkiewicz P. Liver transplantation in primary biliary cirrhosis. Clin Liver Dis 2008;12:461–472, xi.

93. Sylvestre PB, et al. Recurrence of primary biliary cirrhosis after liver transplantation: histologic estimate of incidence and natural history. Liver Transpl 2003;9:1086–1093.

94. Charatcharoenwitthaya P, et al. Long-term survival and impact of ursodeoxycholic acid treatment for recurrent primary biliary cirrhosis after liver transplantation. Liver Transpl 2007;13:1236–1245.

95. Mayo MJ, et al. Prediction of clinical outcomes in primary biliary cirrhosis by serum enhanced liver fibrosis assay. Hepatology 2008;48:1549–1557.

96. Silveira MG, et al. Overlap of autoimmune hepatitis and primary biliary cirrhosis: long-term outcomes. Am J Gastroenterol 2007;102: 1244–1250.

97. Corpechot C, et al. Assessment of biliary fibrosis by transient elastography in patients with PBC and PSC. Hepatology 2006;43:1118–1124.

98. Gomez-Dominguez E, et al. Transient elastography to assess hepatic fibrosis in primary biliary cirrhosis. Aliment Pharmacol Ther 2008;27:441–447.

99. Friedrich-Rust M, et al. Assessment of liver fibrosis and steatosis in PBC with FibroScan, MRI, MR-spectroscopy, and serum markers. J Clin Gastroenterol 2010;44:58–65.

100. Kim WR, et al. Optimal timing of liver transplantation for primary biliary cirrhosis. Hepatology 1998;28:33–38.

101. Levy C, et al. Prevalence and predictors of esophageal varices in patients with primary biliary cirrhosis. Clin Gastroenterol Hepatol 2007;5:803–808.

102. Chazouilleres O, et al. Primary biliary cirrhosis–autoimmune hepatitis overlap syndrome: clinical features and response to therapy. Hepatology 1998;28:296–301.

103. Muratori P, et al. The serological profile of the autoimmune hepatitis/ primary biliary cirrhosis overlap syndrome. Am J Gastroenterol 2009;104: 1420–1425.

VI

Chapter 42

Primary Sclerosing Cholangitis

Tom H. Karlsen, Kirsten Muri Boberg, and Erik Schrumpf

Introduction

Primary sclerosing cholangitis (PSC) is a chronic inflammatory condition of unknown origin that is characterized by strictures of the intrahepatic and extrahepatic bile ducts. Whereas PSC in most cases is a progressive condition leading to liver cirrhosis and the need for liver transplantation 10 to 15 years after onset, the disease course is highly variable among patients. In many ways, the heterogeneity of clinical features and severity in PSC can be considered a major characteristic of the disease, adding to other challenges in the management of these patients. The majority of patients (50% to 80%) have concurrent inflammatory bowel disease (IBD), mainly ulcerative colitis (UC), and there is also an increased frequency (25%) of other autoimmune conditions. PSC patients frequently (10% to 20%) develop cholangiocarcinoma, and patients with both PSC and UC exhibit a four-fold increased risk of colonic carcinoma as compared with patients with only UC. No medical treatment has been shown to influence disease progression in PSC, but symptomatic treatment and management of infections and dominant strictures of the bile ducts may benefit individual patients. PSC has become one of the leading indications for liver transplantation in northern Europe and the United States over the last decades. Although results are excellent, PSC may recur in the liver allograft, and the timing of liver transplantation with regard to the risk of cholangiocarcinoma remains a major challenge. Clearly, the treatment of PSC patients requires a multidisciplinary approach, and at some stage most patients will benefit from an evaluation at a tertiary referral center with dedicated expertise.

Epidemiology

While the first official case description of PSC occurred in the German literature in 1867 (Hoffman), it was not until 1924 that case reports started appearing in French and English journals. In the mid-1960s several case series were reviewed that established the link with UC and several other clinical characteristics of PSC. The introduction of endoscopic retrograde cholangiography (ERC) throughout the 1970s greatly facilitated diagnosis of PSC, and the definite clinical, radiologic, and histopathologic criteria still in practical use were stated by three articles in 1980 from the United States (Rochester, Minnesota), the United Kingdom (London), and Norway (Oslo).[1-3] Five years later, the association between PSC and cholangiocarcinoma was defined,[4] whereas an increased risk of colonic carcinoma among PSC patients with UC was not determined until 2002.[5] During the last 2 decades, increasing awareness of variant forms of PSC (small-duct PSC, overlap with autoimmune hepatitis [AIH] and immunoglobulin G4 [IgG4] associated sclerosing cholangitis) has further complicated the diagnosis and handling of patients, and emphasized the point that PSC is a heterogeneous disease.

Population-based data on PSC incidence and prevalence are scarce for several reasons. The primary obstacle is the lack of a simple and specific diagnostic test. Until the introduction of magnetic resonance cholangiography (MRC), the only means to establish the diagnosis was by ERC. An invasive technique with potential complications is not suitable for screening purposes, and it is thus likely that most of the ERC-based studies underestimate PSC frequency. Another important consideration is the insidious onset of PSC. Nearly half of patients are asymptomatic at diagnosis and the disease course is also typically fluctuating; therefore biochemical tests may intermittently be normal and the diagnosis overlooked. Finally, the lack of efficacious therapy raises ethical concerns regarding the value of diagnosis for epidemiologic purposes.

Epidemiology of Primary Sclerosing Cholangitis

In available population-based studies, the prevalence of PSC in northern European descendants is approximately 10 per 100,000. In southern Europe and Asia, the reported numbers are 10- to 100-fold lower. The annual incidence rate in northern European descendants is approximately 1 per 100,000. Although there are sporadic suggestions in the literature that PSC prevalence may be increasing, there is no definite evidence for this notion. Increased awareness of PSC and simplified diagnosis by MRC rather than ERC are likely explanations.

The first population-based epidemiologic study of PSC was published by Norwegian researchers in 1998.[6] Newly diagnosed cases of PSC within a population of 130,000 inhabitants in eastern Norway were prospectively registered during the period 1986 to 1995. A total of 17 cases of PSC were detected at a mean annual incidence rate of 1.3 per 100,000. The prevalence at the end of 1995 was calculated as 8.5 per 100,000. Two studies from Wales, conducted from 1984 to 2003 (prevalence 12.7/100,000; annual incidence rate, 0.91/100,000) and from Olmsted County, Minnesota, from 1976 to 2000 (prevalence of 13.6/100,000; annual incidence rate, 0.9/100,000) later reported similar results. Another study reported PSC frequency in southern Europe based on questionnaire-based reports retrieved by physicians at 23 Spanish hospitals from 1984 to 1988 (the total population covered was 19 million). The study design makes it likely that cases have been missed; however, the reported prevalence and annual incidence rates of 0.22 per 100,000 and 0.07 per 100,000, respectively, are still substantially lower than those observed in northern European descendants. From Asia, there is also only one population-based report on PSC frequency. In a Singaporean population of 750,000, 10 cases were retrospectively identified by review of medical records from 1989 to 1998 and a PSC prevalence of 1.3/100,000 was estimated. Although a study of approximately 100,000 Alaskan natives from 1984 to 2000 reported a PSC prevalence of zero, the limitations of the epidemiologic studies of PSC discussed previously make this result questionable.

Epidemiology of Primary Sclerosing Cholangitis in Patients with Inflammatory Bowel Disease

In patients with a verified diagnosis of IBD, the frequency of PSC is similar in different ethnicities. In ERC-based studies, prevalence rates of PSC in patients with UC are in the range of 2.3% to 4.6%. Prevalence rates of PSC in patients with Crohn disease range from 1.2% to 3.6%. Importantly, in Crohn disease, colitis is reported in all patients in whom PSC develops. Colonic involvement thus seems to be a prerequisite for the development of PSC in patients with IBD. With the exception of one study from Stockholm county in Sweden,[7]

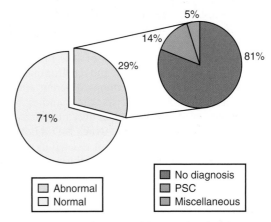

Fig. 42-1 **Prevalence of abnormal hepatic biochemistry measurements in patients with inflammatory bowel disease and distribution of chronic liver disease among patients with abnormal hepatic biochemistry measurements.** Miscellaneous causes included autoimmune hepatitis, hepatitis C, fatty liver, portal vein thrombosis, and metastatic cancer. *(Reprinted with permission from Mendes FD, et al. Abnormal hepatic biochemistries in patients with inflammatory bowel disease. Am J Gastroenterol 2007;102:344–350.)*

all reported studies are based on hospital series of IBD and PSC patients. It could thus be speculated that the frequency of PSC detected might be an overestimation of the true prevalence of PSC in IBD. However, two recent studies indicate that the opposite may actually be the case.

In a population of 544 patients with IBD seen at the Mayo Clinic in Rochester, Minnesota, in 2000,[8] abnormal hepatic biochemistry results were detected in 159 (29%) of the cases (**Fig. 42-1**). Among these 159 patients, a diagnosis of PSC preexisted in 23 (14%) cases. Together with the 2 PSC cases found among the 385 IBD patients without abnormal hepatic biochemistry results, the overall PSC prevalence in the study population was 4.6%. Support for the notion that subclinical and undiagnosed cases of PSC may exist among IBD patients has been reported in a small British study of 51 patients with IBD and normal hepatic biochemistry measurements.[9] Among the 51 patients, as many as 9 (18%) had biliary changes consistent with PSC on MRC. The clinical relevance of detecting these changes can only be clarified by further studies. From an epidemiologic point of view it is nevertheless clear that PSC and PSC-like changes at cholangiography may be more prevalent among patients with IBD than previously appreciated.

Epidemiology of Inflammatory Bowel Disease in Patients with Primary Sclerosing Cholangitis

The prevalence of IBD in PSC shows a significant geographic gradient. In northern European descendants the frequency of IBD in PSC is reported to range between 62% and 83% in series published after 1990, whereas in southern Europe the frequency is between 47% and 54%. In Asia the frequency of IBD in PSC is typically lower, ranging from 50% in India to 20% to 37% in Singapore and Japan. IBD in PSC typically runs a quiescent course,[10] and may be overlooked unless evaluation by total colonoscopy and histologic evaluation is performed. This is probably the reason why the prevalence of IBD in PSC in early case series in northern European descendants was reported as low as 25% to 30%, because direct assessment elsewhere does not suggest an increase of IBD in PSC.[7] The reason for the geographic differences of IBD in PSC is not known. The frequency of genetic and environmental risk factors for IBD in PSC may vary among different ethnicities and regions, and features noted in some studies of PSC without IBD (e.g., more females, older age) may also suggest that distinct subtypes of PSC exist in which IBD is not part of the pathology. It is, however, important to keep in mind that IBD in PSC may present after the onset of the liver disease and even after liver transplantation for PSC. This indicates that a precise distinction between groups of PSC patients with and without IBD is difficult.

According to standard clinical, endoscopic, and histologic criteria, the type of IBD in PSC in approximately 80% to 90% of the cases is compatible with UC whereas the remainder of the cases are diagnosed as Crohn disease or IBD unclassified. However, the distribution of IBD types among PSC patients varies between studies. One explanation for the problems in classifying IBD appears in two recent publications reporting on the frequencies of subcharacteristics of IBD in PSC; it was proposed that IBD in patients with PSC may represent a "third" IBD phenotype distinct from both UC and Crohn disease in several aspects.[11,12]

Epidemiology of Cancer in Patients with Primary Sclerosing Cholangitis

An increased frequency of cancer throughout the epithelial surfaces affected by the inflammation in PSC (liver, bile duct, and colonic mucosa) is the most severe and challenging component of PSC. With a relative risk in the range of 160 to 1560 as compared with the general population, cholangiocarcinoma is the most important cancer in PSC. There is also an approximately four-fold increased risk of colonic carcinoma in PSC patients with UC as compared with UC patients without PSC. An approximately 10-fold increase in the risk of gallbladder carcinoma and pancreatic cancer further supports the presence of a "field effect" in terms of neoplastic potential in PSC. The published prevalence rates of cholangiocarcinoma in PSC range from 4.8% to 36.4%. Population-based studies report lower frequencies (6.3% to 13%) than most transplant center series (12.2% to 36.4%). In parallel with the lower frequency of IBD, the frequency of cholangiocarcinoma in PSC is considerably lower in series of patients from southern Europe and Asia (3.3% to 5.7%). The frequency of colonic dysplasia and/or carcinoma among patients with PSC and UC is reported in the range of 20% to 31% at 20 years, as compared with approximately 5% in UC patients without PSC.[13] The overall frequency of gallbladder cancer in PSC has been reported within the range of 3.5% to 7.8%, and adenocarcinoma is found in approximately 60% of polyploid lesions of the gallbladder in PSC.[14] Hepatocellular carcinoma in PSC patients with cirrhosis has been reported from several centers, whereas single cases of Hodgkin and non-Hodgkin lymphoma in PSC may be incidental.

Unlike the association between hepatocellular carcinoma and cirrhosis, an advanced histologic stage is not a prerequisite for cholangiocarcinoma development in PSC. Very characteristically, up to 38% to 50% of the cholangiocarcinomas are diagnosed during the first year following the diagnosis of PSC. Probably the majority of these tumors were present before referral and detected because of the increased awareness imposed by a diagnosis of PSC. Following the initial peak, there is an annual incidence rate of 0.6% to 1.5%, and 10% of PSC patients develop cholangiocarcinoma more than 10 years after the diagnosis.[15] Whereas there is no definite evidence for an increased frequency of cholangiocarcinoma in PSC patients with IBD, a European multicenter study of 394 European PSC patients showed that the duration of IBD before diagnosis of PSC was significantly longer among the 48 patients who developed cholangiocarcinoma (median, 17.4 years) than among PSC patients without cholangiocarcinoma (median, 9.0 years).[15] Possibly the occurrence of cholangiocarcinoma in PSC is overrepresented in PSC patients with colonic dysplasia or colon cancer,[13] but the present literature does not allow for a definite conclusion.

The increased risk of colorectal cancer in UC was first reported in 1928 and is now well established. Cases of colorectal cancer in PSC have long been described, and in 1992 Broomé and colleagues proposed that PSC may serve as an independent risk factor for colonic dysplasia in UC.[16] Several subsequent studies disputed the clinical relevance of this initial report, and it was not until a meta-analysis of 564 cases of PSC with UC and 16,280 cases of UC without PSC in 2002 that the risk of colorectal dysplasia and cancer in PSC was established.[5] In this analysis, when dysplasia and cancer were considered together, the common odds ratio for patients with PSC developing colorectal neoplasia was 4.8 (95% confidence interval, 3.6 to 6.3). When adenocarcinoma only was considered, the common odds ratio was 4.1 (95% confidence interval, 2.9 to 5.8). The disparate results between the individual studies in the meta-analysis may have several explanations. Importantly, most study populations were too small to address the question because of the low prevalence of PSC. The mild course of UC in PSC also signifies that an increased neoplastic potential may simply reflect a longer duration of subclinical UC than in patients with UC without PSC.

Epidemiology of Primary Sclerosing Cholangitis Variants

Three PSC variants require particular consideration. Two of these, small-duct PSC and AIH-like PSC, show poor demarcation toward typical PSC and a continuum of intermediate cases exists. Both conditions may develop into typical PSC. A distinct form of sclerosing cholangitis characterized by elevated IgG4 levels (some authors have termed this IgG4-associated sclerosing cholangitis) was originally described within Japanese PSC populations, but was later shown to occur also in Western countries.

Small-duct PSC was introduced as a disease entity in 1985 by Ludwig, replacing the previous denomination "pericholangitis" for patients with typical clinical and histologic features of PSC, but without cholangiographic findings.[17] This group of patients was first identified during the 1960s, with cases detected both in Crohn disease and in UC. Although the presence of IBD was previously mandatory for the diagnosis, recent reports from Europe have included cases without IBD (see later). This must be considered when assessing studies of this subpopulation of PSC patients. The frequency of small-duct PSC has been reported in up to 20% of all PSC patients in the adult population, and is probably even higher in the pediatric population (36%). Whereas the overall frequency of IBD seems to be similar to that seen in large-duct PSC, there are several reports suggesting that the fraction of small-duct PSC is higher within the Crohn disease–associated PSC population that among those with UC.

The presence of biochemical, serologic, and histologic features of autoimmune hepatitis in a subset of PSC patients has long been recognized. The nomenclature for this group of patients is not clear. A similar phenomenon occurs in patients with primary biliary cirrhosis (PBC), and these subentities of PSC and PBC have traditionally been designated autoimmune hepatitis overlap syndromes. As will be discussed later, it may be more correct to consider these patients as typical PSC patients with autoreactive features in the pathogenesis. The frequency of this subgroup is dependent on the clinical definition used. In the application of traditional scoring criteria for autoimmune hepatitis, approximately 6% to 9% of adult PSC patients seem to have features of "probable" autoimmune hepatitis. However, using less strict criteria, up to 33% of the PSC patients may be scored as AIH.[18] Conversely, as many as 42% of the patients with autoimmune hepatitis and UC display abnormal cholangiographic results consistent with PSC, whereas the prevalence of cholangiographic abnormalities in the overall adult autoimmune hepatitis population is low (up to 10%). The frequency of a similar entity is considerably higher in pediatric patients with PSC, and some authors have denoted this condition autoimmune sclerosing cholangitis to emphasize the slight distinction of this childhood condition from adult PSC.[19]

Autoimmune pancreatitis was first reported from Japan in 1995, and was only recently recognized as a condition of worldwide relevance. Following these reports it has now been established that 7% to 23% of northern European descendants with PSC may actually exhibit features of this condition.[20] The disease is characterized by high levels of IgG4 and some authors refer to it as IgG4-associated sclerosing cholangitis. This PSC-like condition occurs as a subtype of autoimmune pancreatitis (syndromic autoimmune pancreatitis) and commonly affects other organ systems, resulting in inflammatory bowel disease, retroperitoneal fibrosis, and seronegative sialoadenitis.[21] The extent to which this condition helps explain the pancreatic involvement observed in a variable proportion of PSC patients (see later) is not clear. Whereas cholangiocarcinoma seems to be rare in IgG4-associated cholangitis, high carbohydrate antigen (CA) 19-9 levels may occur in IgG4-associated sclerosing cholangitis and can thus complicate the distinction from cholangiocarcinoma.

Epidemiology of Autoimmune Diseases in Patients with Primary Sclerosing Cholangitis

The association of IBD with autoimmune diseases of other organs has been consistently demonstrated. This needs to be taken into account when calculating the prevalence of other autoimmune conditions in PSC. By comparing 119 patients with both PSC and UC with 103 patients with UC alone, the prevalence of autoimmune diseases in patients with PSC

and ulcerative colitis was 24%, as compared with 8.3% in UC-only patients.[22] The most common conditions were type 1 diabetes, psoriasis, autoimmune thyroiditis, and rheumatoid arthritis. Case reports of a variety of other conditions have also been reported, and probably it should be considered likely that any chronic inflammatory condition would have the propensity to occur in conjunction with PSC. An important additional relationship is that between PSC and celiac disease. Given the therapeutic implications and overlapping, vague symptoms of weight loss and fatigue, awareness of this relationship is especially important. The reason for the association between PSC and other autoimmune disease is not known, but shared genetic susceptibility is likely to be important.

Pathogenesis

The etiology of PSC is not known. Any proposal needs to account for the heterogeneity of the patient population described earlier in this chapter (e.g., presence or absence of IBD, cholangiocarcinoma, other autoimmune conditions, and the PSC variants). Most consistently, genetic risk factors have been detected within the human leukocyte antigen (HLA) complex on chromosome 6p21 and at genetic loci known as precursors to inflammatory bowel disease,[23] but how these genetic variants effect the biliary changes has not yet been established. The earliest theories on PSC pathogenesis were based on the relationship with colonic inflammation, and it was proposed that PSC-like changes may be caused by bacteria or bacterial products activating macrophages and other immune cells in the liver (the "leaky gut" hypothesis). Based on immunologic observations in humans, it was later proposed that lymphocytes activated in the intestinal epithelium may be directed to the liver by endothelial cell features shared between the liver and the intestine (the "aberrant homing" hypothesis). Autoreactivity is definitely present in many PSC patients, as evident from the presence of autoantibodies against biliary epithelial cells. Studies in mice have shown that toxic constituents of bile, or defective protective systems against toxic effects from normal bile, may lead to PSC-like changes (the "toxic bile" hypothesis). Probably each of these hypotheses is at least partially correct. Moreover, because the biliary tract exhibits a very limited repertoire for reacting to any insult, the clinical syndrome that we today classify as PSC may actually represent a variety of conditions for which the underlying molecular pathogenesis differs.

Genetic Susceptibility

By the time diagnosis of PSC can be made by cholangiography, extensive scarring and strictures of the biliary tree have already occurred. The obstruction of bile flow leads to secondary inflammation and apoptosis, and it is thus impossible to determine whether observations at the cellular and molecular level are of primary importance in PSC pathogenesis or only secondary to the ongoing disease processes. The genetic constitution of an individual is not affected by these secondary phenomena, meaning that genetic risk factors may be the only readily available clues predicting PSC pathogenesis. In genetic terms, PSC is considered a complex phenotype, indicating that polymorphisms in several genes along with environmental factors are required for development of the disease. Studies of heritability have shown that siblings of PSC patients are 9 to 39 times more likely to develop PSC than the overall population. Siblings of PSC patients also have an approximately eight-fold increased risk of developing UC even without liver disease, signifying that shared genetic risk factors between PSC and UC are likely to exist. A major problem in the genetics of PSC is the scarcity of patients. Even for important disease genes the relative risk of genetic variants may be low, meaning that large study populations (thousands of patients and healthy controls) are required to detect them. Therefore a large fraction of the genetic risk in PSC cannot be accounted for by the genes identified at this time.

An HLA association in PSC was identified for HLA-B8 (i.e., HLA-B*08:01) and HLA-DR3 (i.e., DRB1*03:01) in 1982.[24] These two HLA variants are closely linked to other genes that were later shown to be associated with PSC (HLA-A1, HLA-C7 allele, the major histocompatibility complex class I chain–related A [MICA] *008/5.1 variant, and the tumor necrosis factor-α [TNF-α] 308 A variant). For unknown reasons, this string (haplotype) of genetic variants is associated with a wide range of autoimmune diseases, and possibly the increased frequency of other autoimmune conditions among patients with PSC arises because of this shared susceptibility. A cross-European study (Norway, Sweden, Great Britain, Italy, and Spain) concluded that consistent HLA associations also exist for a string of genes carrying DR6 (i.e., DRB1*13:01)[25] and in individuals negative for DR3 and DR6 an association with DR2 (i.e., DRB1*15:01) can be found. Protective HLA variants have also been detected, most importantly DR4 (no particular subtype) and DR7 (i.e., DRB1*07:01). Most importantly, the HLA associations in PSC and UC seem to differ, in contrast to PSC susceptibility genes outside this genetic region.[23]

An important question in HLA genetics is whether genetic associations are due to variation in the HLA class I or II genes, or to variation in neighboring genes. At this time, this cannot be concluded in PSC. Probably the HLA class II variants (e.g., DRB1*13:01) have a role in defining the specificity of the immune reaction, meaning that genetic associations arise because the patients are able to present particular antigens to the T-cell receptor. The antigens that are presented by the PSC-associated HLA variants have not been identified. A role for the HLA class I genes in autoimmune diseases is less clear, but may equally well be related to inhibitory signaling via so-called killer immunoglobulin-like receptors (KIRs) on natural killer cells and various T lymphocytes. In PSC it has been shown that HLA-B and HLA-C variants that provide particularly strong inhibitory signals to these cells may protect against PSC (HLA-Bw4 and HLA-C1, respectively).[26] Interestingly, the HLA-C1 variant has also been shown to protect against the development of biliary strictures and graft loss following liver transplantation.[27] Because more than one third of the 250 protein coding genes in the HLA complex have immunologic functions, it is possible that they may modify the risk imposed by the HLA class I and II molecules in HLA-associated conditions. Further studies are needed to clarify which of these genes may be particularly important in PSC.

Following the publishing of the human genome draft in 2000, it became possible to study genes with particularly interesting functions regarding PSC pathogenesis, so-called candidate gene studies. More than 20 such studies have been published over the last years, but none of the findings have been consistently reproduced. In most cases this is probably due to type I errors (false-positive findings) in the original reports, but it is not possible to exclude the presence of very weak statistical effects (which would not be detectable in small study populations) or the fact that important genetic variants may only be present in a few individuals (meaning they could not be detected using statistical association analysis at all). The cystic fibrosis transmembrane conductance regulator gene (CFTR) serves as a good example. The gene is of great interest because cystic fibrosis patients may indeed develop PSC-like changes. Furthermore, induction of colitis in mice lacking the cftr gene leads to bile duct injury. Whereas some studies have reported positive associations with CFTR variants, others have failed to confirm these results. There are hundreds of disease-causing variants of the CFTR gene, and therefore it cannot be excluded that the negative studies have failed to study the important ones or that the effects from these variants were too subtle to be detected.

So-called genome-wide association studies (GWAS) have now been performed in patients with PSC and UC. In these studies, hundreds of thousands of genetic markers distributed across all chromosomes are tested in patients and healthy controls. The studies aim to detect regions of the genome, or even single genes, where particular genetic variants are detected more or less frequently in the patients versus the healthy controls. Only rather small PSC populations have so far been studied, and three genes outside the HLA complex have been found at the time of the writing of this chapter.[23] Whereas these three genes also tend to show associations in IBD, no associations have been detected in PSC for most of the UC-associated genes. This corroborates the clinical observation that IBD in PSC may represent a distinct form of IBD (see later). The fact that a limited overlap exists, however, may explain why the IBD in a clinical setting has been classified as either UC or Crohn disease in most instances.

The function of the PSC-associated genes outside the HLA complex is poorly defined. The macrophage stimulating protein (MST1) encodes a circulating preprotein that is activated by various inflammatory stimuli and exerts negative feedback on macrophages to prevent excessive inflammation. Interestingly, the G-protein coupled bile acid receptor 1 (GPBAR1) also seems to mediate inhibition of macrophages, which could be useful in preventing excessive inflammation during cholestasis. GPBAR1 is activated by bile acids, and seems to be involved in the regulation of bile flow (inducing choleresis) and the amount of bicarbonate released via activation of chloride secretion by CFTR. The importance of these systems is also suggested by findings of reduced CFTR function in patients with PSC, even in the absence of mutations in the CFTR gene itself. The third genetic region found to be associated with PSC is as large as the HLA complex, but only contains two genes: glypican 5 (GPC5) and glypican 6 (GPC6). The function of the genes is not known, but silencing the GPC6 gene in cholangiocytes leads to an inflammatory response that could be important in disease pathogenesis.[23]

Immune-Mediated Bile Duct Injury

An unusual mixture of lymphocytes characterizes the normal liver. This may be related to the anatomic proximity of the portal and systemic circulations. Cells of the innate immune system are the most prominent feature, and up to 65% of normal liver lymphocytes are natural killer (NK) cells, γδ T lymphocytes, and natural killer T cells, as compared with the respective proportions in peripheral blood of 13%, 2%, and 2%. Similar to many autoimmune conditions, T lymphocytes constitute the majority of the mononuclear cells in the portal infiltrate in liver biopsies from patients with PSC. Even in early stage biopsies, most of these cells stain for markers typical of mature T lymphocytes, indicating that the inflammatory response has existed for some time when the diagnosis of PSC is made. Some studies report an increased frequency of NK cells in the portal infiltrate of patients with PSC when compared with other liver diseases, and also in the intestinal mucosa of patients with PSC when compared with UC patients without liver disease. γδ T lymphocytes are observed at increased frequencies in both adults and children with PSC. There is also an increase in Kupffer cells and perisinusoidal macrophages in PSC, but whether this is related to defective inflammatory inhibition for genetic reasons (e.g., lack of *MST1* or *GPBAR1* signaling) is not known.

The function of these various immune cells in PSC pathogenesis is not known. A series of studies from Birmingham, U.K., have investigated the possibility that lymphocytes activated in the gut may be responsible for biliary inflammation in PSC.[28] Following cell division and maturation in the regional lymph nodes, lymphocytes activated in mucosa-associated lymphoid tissues preferentially recirculate to the mucosal surfaces of antigen encounter. This phenomenon is called homing and is of particular interest because drugs that may block this process are currently being developed. Intestinal homing of T lymphocytes is ensured by the α$_4$β$_7$ integrin receptor on the lymphocytes and the corresponding mucosal addressin cellular adhesion molecule-1 (MAdCAM-1) ligand on intestinal endothelial cells. MAdCAM-1 is also expressed on portal vein and sinusoidal endothelium in inflammatory liver diseases. Intestinally activated T lymphocytes may thus influence hepatic inflammation in PSC. There is also evidence for an increased production of chemokine ligand 25 (CCL25) in PSC, along with an increased fraction of memory T lymphocytes expressing the corresponding chemokine receptor 9 (CCR9). The extent that expression of MAdCAM-1 and CCL25 is specific to PSC, or merely a general feature of inflammation in autoimmune liver disease, must still be established.

Antibodies against biliary as well as colonic epithelial cells have been reported in PSC.[29] Autoreactivity has also been demonstrated in animal models of PSC. The preferential usage of particular T-cell receptor gene segments of hepatic T cells and the presence of autoreactive T cells in peripheral blood from patients with PSC also suggest that tissue-specific antigens of relevance to PSC pathogenesis may exist. The nature of such antigens has not been defined, and the general pathogenetic importance of similar autoantigens in other autoimmune conditions is also not known. A variety of autoantibodies directed against nonspecific cellular components may be detected at low levels in PSC (e.g., antinuclear antibody [ANA], anti–smooth muscle antibody [SMA], anticardiolipin antibody, rheumatoid factor).[29] These probably also reflect the presence of autoimmune components in the disease process have no diagnostic value (see later). The most prevalent of these autoantibodies (up to 94% of the PSC patients) is a particular type of perinuclear antineutrophil cytoplasmic antibody (pANCA). This antibody is also observed in UC and type 1 autoimmune hepatitis, suggesting that common pathogenetic mechanisms for these conditions are likely to exist. Possibly, autoimmune mechanisms of bile duct injury may be particularly pronounced in AIH-like PSC.

Infectious Triggers

A series of studies in mice performed almost 20 years ago at the University of North Carolina suggested that innate immune responses to bacterial products of an inflamed gut may initiate the development of PSC-like changes.[30] Genetic background probably determines outcome in these models; for instance, Wistar and female Lewis rats are susceptible whereas Fischer and Buffalo rats are not. The findings warrant renewed interest for several reasons. Because the inflammation in these models was mediated by TNF-α, it is of interest to note increased levels of this cytokine also in human PSC as compared with healthy controls and patients with other chronic cholestatic liver diseases. Along with macrophages, both NK cells and T lymphocytes can produce TNF-α, which leads to the activation of inflammatory and apoptotic pathways. Because several of the genetic findings in PSC also implicate a role of innate immune responses, including the effector functions of macrophages and natural killer cells, the relationship between the genetic defects and translocation of bacterial components from the gut needs to be further explored. Interestingly, it has been shown that expression of Toll-like receptors 4 and 9 (TLR4 and TLR9) on biliary epithelial cells may be induced by antibodies against these cells.[31] These TLRs recognize bacterial products and viral DNA and activation may aggravate ongoing biliary inflammatory processes in conjunction with exacerbations of inflammatory bowel disease as well as systemic bacterial and viral infections.

Specific infectious agents have also been proposed. Bile-tolerant *Helicobacter* species have been detected in patients with PSC, but may also colonize the biliary tree in patients with other cholestatic liver diseases. Similarly, an increased frequency of α-hemolytic *Streptococci* has been detected, and possibly infectious processes following endoscopic procedures in PSC may play a role in disease progression.[32] An increased frequency of antibodies against the lipopolysaccharide component of an unspecified *Chlamydia* subtype among patients with PSC as compared with healthy controls has also been reported. Specific viral etiologies have also been discussed, but no causal relationship has yet been established. The presence of an infectious trigger or exacerbating factor in PSC is likely, but further studies are required to determine the nature and function of such a factor in PSC pathogenesis. It is possible that a diverse spectrum of infectious agents may cause breakdown of immunologic tolerance in the bile ducts in genetically susceptible individuals, leading to sustained immunologic reactions toward "self-antigens" even after the clearance of the infectious agent.

Bile Acid Toxicity and Liver Cirrhosis

The toxicity of bile has been a subject of interest since the days of Hippocrates. Exactly how bile acids and other constituents of bile exert their toxic effects in living human tissues is not known. The detergent effects of bile observed at high concentrations are probably less important than the activation of several apoptotic pathways. Regarding PSC-specific effects, it seems important to distinguish between toxic effects on bile duct tissue and on the liver itself.

A series of studies from the Netherlands and Austria have elaborated on the biliary effects of "toxic bile"; these studies were based on the findings of PSC-like changes in mice devoid of the phospholipid transporter multidrug resistance protein 2 (mdr2), called MDR3 in humans (**Fig. 42-2**). The most pronounced effect, from the regurgitation of bile acids from the disrupted biliary epithelium found in these mice, is the up-regulation of profibrotic pathways, which leads to

extensive scarring of bile ducts that mimicks human PSC. Cholangiocytes secrete a bicarbonate (HCO_3^-) rich fluid that constitutes about 25% of the daily bile formation.[33] This process is driven by the interactive effects of CFTR-mediated chloride secretion and a chloride/bicarbonate anion exchanger (AE2). Impaired CFTR or AE2 function (or both) thus leads to impaired hydration and alkalinization of bile, inspissated bile, and the bile duct injury observed in knockout animals for these genes. The relevance of bicarbonate secretion in the *mdr2* knockout mouse has been further demonstrated by the protective effect against bile duct injury induced by a bicarbonate-rich bile flow. Whereas defects in the human *MDR3* gene lead to progressive familial intrahepatic cholestasis type 3 (PFIC3), no associations between genetic variants

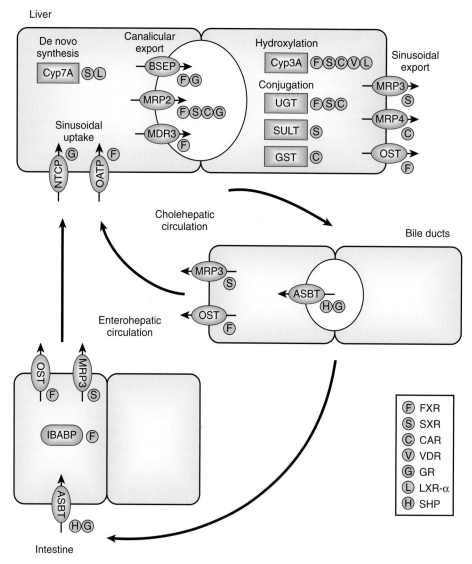

Fig. 42-2 Important transporter proteins *(ovals)* involved in the enterohepatic circulation of bile acids and micelle formation, along with key enzymes *(boxes)* of bile acid synthesis and detoxification. Nuclear receptors *(blue)* involved in the positive or negative regulation of respective genes are given adjacent to each individual protein. ASBT, apical sodium-dependent bile acid transporter; BSEP, bile salt export pump; CAR, constitutive androstane receptor; Cyp, cytochrome P-450; FXR, farnesoid X activated receptor; GR, glucocorticoid receptor; GST, glutathione *S*-transferase; IBABP, ileal bile acid–binding protein; LXR-α, liver X receptor α; MDR3, multidrug resistance protein 3; MRP2, MRP3, and MRP4, multidrug resistance-associated protein 2, 3, and 4, respectively; NTCP, Na$^+$-taurocholate co-transporting polypeptide; OATP, several organic anion transporting polypeptides; OST, organic solute transporter (OST-α-OST-β heterodimer); SHP, small heterodimer partner; SULT, sulfotransferase; SXR, steroid and xenobiotic receptor; UGT, uridine diphosphate glucuronosyltransferase; VDR, vitamin D receptor

of the *MDR3* gene and susceptibility to PSC have been reported. However, MDR3 may still serve as a "modifier gene," because particular genetic variants of the *MDR3* gene (also called *ABCB4*) have been associated with a more severe disease course. The role of bicarbonate-driven choleresis in human PSC remains to be established, but it has been speculated that ursodeoxycholic acid may exert parts of its beneficial effects via such mechanisms (see later).

During cholestasis, defense mechanisms aim at minimizing bile acid–induced liver damage. Bile acids are toxic to the hepatocytes, and are likely to contribute to the development of liver cirrhosis in PSC. The hepatocytes initiate adaptive responses during cholestasis, including the following: (1) down-regulation of bile acid synthesis and hepatocellular bile acid uptake; (2) increased hydroxylation and conjugation, making bile acids more water soluble; and (3) induction of bile acid efflux pumps on the sinusoidal membrane, leading to export of metabolized bile acids to the systemic circulation for renal elimination (see **Fig. 42-2**). Together with the constitutive androstane receptor (CAR) and farnesoid X activated receptor (FXR), the steroid and xenobiotic receptor (SXR) is a major determinant of the expression of the genes involved in this adaption. The observation that genetic variants of the SXR may lead to a more aggressive disease course in PSC is therefore in line with the importance of SXR in animal models of cholestasis.[34,35] Interestingly, the SXR ligand rifampicin has been used in the treatment of cholestatic pruritus, possibly stimulating 6-hydroxylation of bile acids via CYP3A4, followed by glucuronosyl conjugation and excretion in the urine. Whether SXR, CAR, or FXR stimulation may aid in slowing the development of liver cirrhosis in cholestatic liver disease is currently under study.

Pathogenesis of Cholangiocarcinoma in Patients with Primary Sclerosing Cholangitis

In cholestatic conditions, cholangiocytes probably actively interact with cells of the immune system. The "reactive" cholangiocyte is also involved in the proliferation of the small bile ducts, which can be observed on histologic examinations of biopsies from PSC patients (see later). Biliary dysplasia precedes the occurrence of cholangiocarcinoma in PSC,[36] meaning that, similar to colon cancer, cholangiocarcinoma develops via a dysplasia-adenocarcinoma sequence. Both persistent exposure to effector molecules of inflammatory pathways (e.g., interleukin-6 [IL-6]) and carcinogenic effects from accumulated bile acids during chronic cholestasis are probably important for the malignant transformation of cholangiocytes. The inflammatory and cholestatic environment functions as a "cancer ecosystem,"[37] and leads to a vicious circle of mutations and altered regulation of genes involved in DNA repair, cell proliferation/senescence and apoptosis, and vascular/invasive mechanisms (**Table 42-1**). Common cancer-associated mutations have been detected in patients with cholangiocarcinoma and PSC (e.g., *K-ra*, the tumor suppressor genes *p53* and *p16*). Chromosomal abnormalities have also been detected and may serve as a basis for diagnostic tests based on the binding of

Table 42-1 Molecular Pathology of Cholangiocarcinoma

MALIGNANT PHENOTYPE	DYSREGULATED GENES/PATHWAYS
Proliferation	IL-6, IL-6 receptor (gp130) HGF/Met ErbB-2 K-ras BRAF COX2
Apoptosis/evasion	Caspase-9 Mcl-1 Bcl-2 Bcl-XL COX2
Senescence/evasion	Telomerase
Cell cycle dysregulation	Cyclin D1 p21$^{waf1/cip1}$ p27^{kip1} pRb p53 mdm-2 DCP4/Smad4 p16^{INK4a}
Invasion/metastases	E-Cadherin αβ-Cadherin Aspartyl (asparaginyl) β-hydroxylase WISP1v Matrix metalloproteinases
Angiogenesis	VEGF TGF-β

Reprinted with permission from Blechacz B, Gores GJ. Cholangiocarcinoma: advances in pathogenesis, diagnosis, and treatment. Hepatology 2008;48:308–321.

fluorescently labeled DNA probes to chromosomes 3, 7, and 17 and chromosomal band 9p21 (fluorescent in situ hybridization [FISH]).[38]

Only parts of the molecular mechanisms of carcinogenesis in PSC have been described. Regarding carcinogenic effects from bile acids, they are at least in part mediated via DNA damage caused by reactive oxygen intermediates (oxidative stress). Defects of the DNA repair machinery have been detected in some patients with cholangiocarcinoma and may aggravate the effects of oxidative stress. A series of studies by Gores and colleagues have demonstrated the importance of autocrine effects from IL-6 on cholangiocarcinoma cell immortalization.[39] The effects from IL-6 are mediated via activation of the signal transducer and activator of transcription 3 (STAT3) protein, which leads to the up-regulation of several molecules involved in cancer cell apoptosis and proliferation. Interestingly, the IL-6–STAT3 signaling pathway has also been implicated in the pathogenesis of colorectal carcinoma in ulcerative colitis. Normally, the STAT3 activation is restricted via negative feedback by suppressor of cytokine signaling 3 (SOCS3). In cholangiocarcinoma, however, this negative feedback is defective because of inactivation of the promoter region of the *SOCS3* gene by methylation of the DNA. As reviewed elsewhere, similar mechanisms (called epigenetic alterations) may also be of more widespread importance in cholangiocarcinoma carcinogenesis.[40]

As part of the ongoing inflammation, and in response to the altered state of the dysplastic cholangiocytes, various immune cells play important roles in cholangiocarcinogenesis. Some of these cells may promote tumor growth and metastasis (e.g., macrophages), whereas others are probably trying to kill abnormal cholangiocytes (e.g., NK cells). The importance of this balance has been demonstrated by the finding of an association between genetic variants of the natural killer cell receptor NKG2D and cholangiocarcinoma.[41] Individuals who carried NKG2D variants that lead to less efficient killing by NK cells were more prone to develop cholangiocarcinoma than individuals with normal NK cell activity. The prevalence of cholangiocarcinoma among individuals with normal NKG2D variants was 4% to 8% as compared with 20% to 28% in individuals with a less effective NKG2D. Further studies of genetic risk factors for cholangiocarcinoma are warranted, particularly given the low risk in longstanding PSC, which suggests that a PSC patient is either likely or unlikely to develop cholangiocarcinoma.

Clinical Features

The diagnosis of PSC is made by cholangiography and exclusion of other causes of the typical presentation of multifocal biliary strictures and intervening dilatations. There are no specific symptoms, clinical findings, or biochemical tests to diagnose PSC. The patient may be jaundiced and experience pruritus, and other symptoms include pain in the upper abdomen as well as marked fatigue. For many patients the predominant symptoms are those of the associated conditions (e.g., diarrhea attributable to IBD). Biochemically, the typical finding is that of an increased alkaline phosphatase (ALP) level, whereas other findings vary markedly between patients and typically fluctuate with time. When the diagnosis is made late in the course of the disease, there may be signs of cirrhosis and liver failure. Unlike for primary biliary cirrhosis, there is no PSC-specific autoantibody test, and histologic findings are also nonspecific. The onset is typically insidious, but cases presenting with acute liver failure have been reported. In contrast to most autoimmune conditions, approximately two thirds of the PSC

patients are male. Most patients are also relatively young, with a median age at onset of 30 to 40 years, ranging from children younger than 10 years to elderly individuals 70 to 80 years old.

Symptoms and Signs

Because of increased awareness of PSC and early diagnosis, symptoms are currently reported at a lower frequency than seen in the early literature on PSC (**Table 42-2**). The symptoms of liver disease in PSC are vague, and to some extent related to the development of complications in terms of dominant strictures, bacterial cholangitis, liver cirrhosis, and cholangiocarcinoma.

More recent publications state that almost half of the patients (44%) are now asymptomatic at time of diagnosis. A series of 45 asymptomatic patients with PSC monitored for a median of 6.3 years at the Mayo Clinic in Rochester, Minnesota, during the period 1970 to 1987 was reported in 1991.[42] During follow-up, more than half of these patients (53%) developed symptoms of liver disease with or without associated physical signs. For the subgroup of 29 patients who had subsequent biopsies, 66% showed evidence for histologic progression. Follow-up studies showed that 18% of the patients died from liver failure and another 13% underwent orthotopic liver transplantation. Two patients developed cholangiocarcinoma and one patient adenocarcinoma of the pancreas. Whereas these results clearly demonstrate a progressive nature of asymptomatic PSC, other reports nevertheless emphasize that the disease course is less severe than in symptomatic patients. As discussed in detail later, it could be argued that asymptomatic patients have simply been diagnosed at an early disease stage and that progression is inevitable. However, it is also likely that heterogeneity regarding PSC severity exists, and that some patients, for genetic and other reasons, are less prone to develop symptomatic liver cirrhosis and cholangiocarcinoma.

A few particular suppositions can be presented with regard to abdominal pain, pruritus, and fatigue, because the cause of each of these symptoms in PSC is poorly understood. Abdominal pain could be speculated to arise from biliary obstruction arising at strictures. However, recent data from patients with small-duct PSC show that even in this group of patients, abdominal pain may occur at equal frequency (34%) as in

Table 42-2 Symptoms of Primary Sclerosing Cholangitis at Diagnosis						
SYMPTOM	**WARREN ET AL., 1967 (N = 42)**	**WIESNER ET AL., 1980 (N = 50)**	**CHAPMAN ET AL., 1980 (N = 29)**	**FARRANT ET AL., 1991 (N = 126)**	**BROOMÉ ET AL., 1996 (N = 305)**	**BOBERG ET AL., 2002 (N = 330)**
Abdominal pain	76%	50%	72%	51%	37%	22%
Jaundice	100%	68%	72%	54%	30%	28%
Pruritus	60%	62%	69%	48%	30%	25%
Fever	50%	28%	NA	NA	17%	8%
Weight loss	69%	28%	79%	29%	NA	14%
Fatigue	76%	NA	NA	65%	NA	23%

NA, not available

patients with large-duct biliary strictures. The genesis of abdominal pain in PSC is therefore unknown. The biologic basis of fatigue in PSC is also not known. It may in some cases be the dominant clinical feature, and can have serious implications for career building and family planning in young individuals. Importantly, there is no correlation with the severity of the liver disease, whereas a correlation with clinical depression has been noted. However, it can only be speculated whether fatigue leads to depression or whether depression is the leading force behind the fatigue. When it comes to pruritus, it is generally considered that pruritus in the presence of any cholestatic liver disease has the same pathogenesis. The cause is probably complex, because increased levels of endogenous opioids as well as hepatic and cutaneous effects from retained bile acids are not able to explain all cases. The pruritus may be intractable and debilitating, and in a few cases the primary indication for liver transplantation.

Clinical findings in PSC are caused by cholestasis (jaundice) and cirrhosis with portal hypertension. In two recent reports of a total of 603 European patients with PSC,[43,44] the frequency of hepatomegaly at diagnosis of PSC was 26% to 44%; splenomegaly, 9% to 29%; gastroesophageal varices, 7% to 10%; and ascites, 2% to 4%. Spider nevi have been reported in 10% of the cases.

Biochemistry and Immunologic Tests

The ALP level is typically markedly increased (more than three-fold the upper limit of normal) in the majority of patients with PSC. Alanine aminotransferase (ALT) and aspartate aminotransferase (AST) levels may be elevated, but usually less pronounced (2 to 3 times upper normal limits). Bilirubin level is not always elevated, and in patients with advanced liver disease there may be signs of liver failure as evident from an increased prothrombin time and decreased albumin levels.

In early series of PSC patients,[1-3] practically all patients (97% to 100%) were reported to have elevated levels of ALP. In a follow-up study at our center published in 1987,[45] it was noted that in one fourth of the patients with elevated ALP levels at diagnosis, there were no abnormalities registered at follow-up. This probably reflects the diagnostic setting of PSC, where biochemical abnormalities including elevated ALP level are among the motivators for cholangiography. Several reports later corroborated fluctuations in ALP levels in PSC, and also documented cases of cirrhotic-stage PSC with normal ALP levels. ALT and AST levels are often moderately elevated, but may be normal. As discussed later, the subgroup of PSC patients exhibiting features of autoimmune hepatitis is characterized by increased ALT and AST levels, and is important to identify because some of these patients may respond to corticosteroid treatment. In large series, bilirubin level is elevated in approximately 40% of the PSC cases. Like ALP, the elevation may be transiently caused by cholangitis, biliary calculi, or dominant strictures, and in a recent series[44] only 15% of the PSC patients showed persistent elevation of bilirubin level (>3 months). Bilirubin is a key component of most of the prognostic models in PSC (see later) and is also one of the parameters involved in the calculation of the Child-Pugh and Model for End-Stage Liver Disease (MELD) scores. Typically, the bilirubin level gradually increases toward the end of the disease course, reflecting advanced liver disease along with prolonged prothrombin time and low albumin levels. Intestinal malabsorption in the context of IBD may in some cases also contribute to low albumin levels. Notably, elevated amylase levels have been reported in 38% to 47% of patients with PSC, and are probably related to pancreatic duct abnormalities (see later). A few cases of PSC presenting with acute pancreatitis have been reported.

The main purpose of immunologic tests in PSC is to exclude other liver diseases (primary biliary cirrhosis and autoimmune hepatitis) or to confirm the presence of a therapeutically responsive PSC variant (IgG4-associated cholangitis and AIH-like PSC). A summary of the frequency of autoantibodies observed in PSC is provided in **Table 42-3**. The most prevalent autoantibody in PSC is atypical pANCA. However, this antibody is also observed in UC and type 1 autoimmune hepatitis, and the reported sensitivity and specificity (78% and 61%, respectively, for a cutoff titer of 1:40) for atypical pANCA are far too low to make the current indirect immunofluorescence assays valuable in the diagnostic workup of PSC patients.

Typical for PSC in terms of autoantibodies is the absence (<10%) of antimitochondrial antibodies (AMAs), and this aids in the differential diagnosis versus primary biliary cirrhosis. Detection of elevated levels of immunoglobulin G4 (IgG4) in 7% to 9% of the PSC patients is also clinically useful, because the subset of IgG4-associated sclerosing cholangitis typically responds remarkably well to corticosteroid treatment. When it comes to markers of autoimmune hepatitis, the situation is more complex. In a study of 114 PSC patients, elevated total IgG levels were found in 61% of the patients.[18] Markers of autoimmune hepatitis type 1 (ANAs and SMAs) were detected in 24% of the patients in this series. However, only a subset of these cases can be definitely classified as AIH-like PSC according to the revised scoring system for

Table 42-3 Autoantibodies Detected in Patients with Primary Sclerosing Cholangitis

ANTIBODY	PREVALENCE (%)
pANCA	26-94
AMA	0-9
Anti-LKM	0
Anti-SLA/LP	0
ANA	8-77
SMA	0-83
ASCA	44
Anticardiolipin	4-63
Rheumatoid factor	15
Anti-TPO	16
Anti-GBM	17

AMA, antimitochondrial antibody; ANA, antinuclear antibody; anti-GBM, antibodies against glomerular basement membrane; anti-LKM, liver-kidney microsomal antibodies; anti-SLA/LP, antibodies against soluble liver antigen/liver pancreas; anti-TPO, antibodies against thyroid peroxidase; ASCA, anti–*Saccharomyces cerevisiae* antibodies; pANCA, perinuclear antineutrophil cytoplasmic antibody; SMA, smooth muscle antibody

autoimmune hepatitis published in 1999,[46] which means that a consistent clinical correlate for these antibody observations in PSC does not exist. The typical markers of autoimmune hepatitis type 2, anti–liver-kidney-microsomal antibodies (anti-LKM), have not been reported in adult PSC. However, in a population of 27 children diagnosed with AIH-like PSC, Gregorio and colleagues found 1 anti-LKM–positive patient (4%), whereas the remainder of the patients had elevated ANA and SMA levels.[19] The overlap between PSC and autoimmune hepatitis is undefined and probably a continuum of shared pathogenetic factors exists, meaning that any immunologic observation in either of the conditions should be expected to occasionally occur in the other.

Cholangiographic Features

The typical cholangiographic finding in PSC is that of multiple strictures with intervening saccular dilatations of both the intrahepatic and the extrahepatic bile ducts (**Fig. 42-3**).

Typically, PSC affects both the intrahepatic and the extrahepatic bile ducts. Changes of the extrahepatic bile ducts only are rare, whereas isolated changes of the intrahepatic bile ducts have been reported in 20% to 28% of the cases. Dominant strictures, defined as strictures with a diameter of less than 1.5 mm of the common bile duct or less than 1.0 mm of a hepatic duct within 2 cm of the bifurcation, develop at an accumulated frequency of 36% to 57% throughout the disease course. Almost 90% of PSC patients have abnormal gallbladders,[47] and bile duct calculi are found in 8% to 26% of PSC patients. Pancreatic duct abnormalities may be observed, but there is no consensus in the literature regarding the frequency of such changes (from zero to 77%). In clinical practice there is a time lag of several years between the first biochemical abnormality consistent with PSC and the diagnostic cholangiography.[15]

The introduction of MRC in 1995 led to a still-ongoing discussion on the utility of MRC versus traditional ERC in the diagnosis of PSC. For both modalities, interobserver

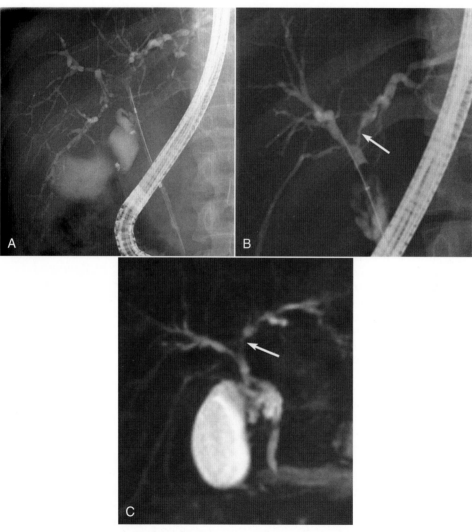

Fig. 42-3 **A,** Endoscopic retrograde cholangiography (ERC) showing bile duct caliber variation with multiple intrahepatic strictures and intervening dilatations ("beading"). In the extrahepatic bile ducts there is a uniform narrowing from the hilar region to the papilla of Vater. **B** and **C,** ERC and magnetic resonance cholangiography (MRC) from the same PSC patient showing nonmalignant stricture *(arrow)* with prestenotic dilatation. *(**B** and **C,** Reprinted with permission from Berstad AE, et al. Diagnostic accuracy of magnetic resonance and endoscopic retrograde cholangiography in primary sclerosing cholangitis. Clin Gastroenterol Hepatol 2006;4:514–520.)*

variability and the heterogeneous patient population make it difficult to precisely determine the specificity and sensitivity of each test. In a study in which 39 of 66 individuals had a confirmed diagnosis of PSC, comparable sensitivity and specificity for MRC (80% and 87%, respectively) and ERC (89% and 80%, respectively) have been reported.[48] Subtle intrahepatic changes may be missed at MRC, but there is no consensus on the extent of this problem. Some authors also claim that MRC is inferior to ERC in the detailed characterization of extrahepatic biliary changes, signifying that ERC should be performed for complete characterization of dominant strictures in PSC. In late-stage cirrhosis, false-positive results may be obtained by ERC as a result of distortion of the intrahepatic ducts. Keeping the limitations of either method in mind, MRC should be considered a cost-effective and accurate method for initial characterization of the liver and bile ducts in a patient where PSC is suspected.[49]

The main advantage of ERC over MRC is the opportunity to perform additional diagnostic (biliary brushings, cholangioscopy) or therapeutic (dilatations, stenting) procedures with ERC. Inherent to ERC and these associated procedures is also the risk of complications. The most common complications include pancreatitis, bacterial cholangitis, perforation, and papillotomy-related bleedings. In a recent review,[50] risk was mainly found to be related to ERCs that involved additional procedures (up to 15% to 30%) as compared with diagnostic ERC only (approximately 7% to 10%). The risk for complications is higher than in non-PSC patients (approximately 4%). In particular, cholangitis is a common complication despite the routine use of prophylactic antibiotics. Additional ERC procedures are performed in a significantly higher proportion of PSC versus non-PSC patients (73% versus 43%, respectively, in a series of 68 patients from the Mayo Clinic).[51] The role of cholangioscopy in patients with PSC has not yet been defined, but as discussed later, increased sensitivity and specificity in diagnosing cholangiocarcinoma as the cause of a dominant stricture in PSC have been noted.

Histopathologic Features

There are no specific histologic findings in PSC. Also, similar to the endoscopic changes, microscopic lesions are not uniformly distributed throughout the liver, leading to variability between different biopsies taken from the same patient. Microscopic findings suggestive of PSC are usually made in the portal tracts (**Fig. 42-4**), and the typical lesion is obliterative, nonsuppurative cholangitis with marked periductular fibrosis. This lesion, often referred to as "onion-skinning" of the small bile ducts because of the concentric layers of fibrous tissue, is observed in only 14% of the biopsies and can also be observed in ischemic cholangitis.[52] In many patients, the microscopic changes in PSC progress gradually toward cirrhosis, and in patients with biochemical and immunologic

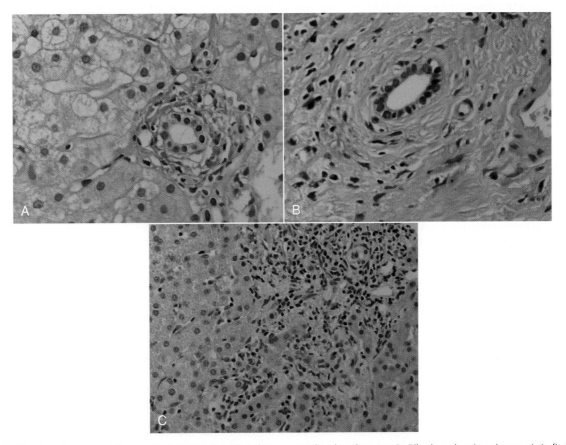

Fig. 42-4 **A,** Bile duct showing minimal epithelial changes with a few surrounding lymphocytes. **B,** Bile duct showing characteristic findings with more advanced epithelial changes and concentric fibrosis and scattered lymphocytes. **C,** AIH-like features with inflammatory interface activity and a small bile duct with epithelial changes *(upper right corner).*

findings compatible with AIH-like PSC, a biopsy may have therapeutic consequences. However, microscopic changes in PSC poorly reflect large-duct pathology, and the role of liver biopsies in the diagnosis and follow-up of typical cases of PSC can be questioned.

In a classic article from 1989, Ludwig defined four stages of the progressive nature of PSC.[53] In the early stages biopsy specimens may be normal,[3] or show only mild portal edema, inflammation, and proliferation of the small bile ducts and ductuli. Typically, these lesions may appear side by side with portal tracts where ducts are obliterated and replaced by fibrous tissue. In stage 2 the inflammation and fibrosis extend to involve the periportal tissue. In some cases piecemeal necrosis of hepatocytes can be observed and the portal tracts themselves are often enlarged. Fibrous septa stretching between neighboring portal tracts characterize stage 3, gradually progressing towards end-stage cirrhosis (stage 4) with regenerative noduli with ductular proliferation in the periphery. However, as will be described later, the timing of liver transplantation in PSC is dependent on a variety of factors, and in a revised prognostic model from the Mayo Clinic published in 2000 the requirement of a liver biopsy was omitted.[54] In a series of 79 PSC patients where liver biopsy was performed after completion of a diagnostic cholangiography, the biopsy resulted in a clinical consequence (e.g., corticosteroid administration) in only 3 cases of AIH-like PSC.[52]

The macroscopic appearance of the liver affected by PSC has been likened to a pruned tree. Fibrous cholangitis extends radially from the hilar region and is complicated by obliterated bile ducts and cholangiectases with biliary gravel and calculi and in some cases abscess formation.[55] Strictures are macroscopically defined by semicircular fibrous crests. Two types of cholangiectases have been reported. In some cases, the cholangiectasis is thin-walled and with excessive mucous exudation, but with little evidence of inflammation. In other cases, the cholangiectases have thick, fibrous walls lined with granulation tissue and inflammatory cells. The liver tissue itself may show any degree of biliary cirrhosis.

Lymphadenopathy in Patients with Primary Sclerosing Cholangitis

Enlarged abdominal lymph nodes have been reported in 65% to 100% of patients with PSC, particularly in the regions draining the liver. In some cases, even gross enlargement (>3 cm) can be found. In a study of 26 PSC patients with abdominal lymphadenopathy,[56] enlargement of the celiac nodes was found in 53%; of the paraaortic nodes in 23%; of the portal, pyloric, and left gastric nodes in 19% each; of the peripancreatic nodes in 15%; and of the superior mesenteric and aortocaval nodes in 12% each. Perihepatic lymphadenopathy is observed at high frequencies also in other autoimmune liver diseases (primary biliary cirrhosis and autoimmune hepatitis) as well as in chronic hepatitis C virus infection. The importance of lymphadenopathy in PSC is related to differential diagnostic considerations versus cholangiocarcinoma, lymphoma, IgG4-associated sclerosing cholangitis, and immunologic conditions with occasional PSC-like manifestations (e.g., Langerhans cell histiocytosis, sarcoidosis). Although the lymph nodes in PSC patients with metastatic cholangiocarcinoma may be more numerous and slightly larger and have a

reduced length/width ratio, lymphadenopathy in itself has limited predictive value with regard to the presence of malignancy in PSC. Unless cholangiocarcinoma or lymphoma is suspected otherwise, following up on incidentally observed lymphadenopathy in PSC (e.g., by endosonography-guided fine-needle aspiration) is therefore not advocated.

Clinical, Endoscopic, and Histologic Features of Inflammatory Bowel Disease in Patients with Primary Sclerosing Cholangitis

There is no temporal relationship between onset of PSC and onset of IBD in PSC. IBD in PSC presents at a younger age than in IBD patients without PSC,[12] and usually the diagnosis of PSC is made in patients with preexisting IBD. The typical PSC patient is a 30- to 40-year-old man with a diagnosis of UC or colonic Crohn disease and abnormal hepatic biochemistry results. However, in some cases the diagnosis of PSC precedes that of IBD by several years. IBD may even present after liver transplantation for PSC, and PSC may present in an IBD patient after colectomy. Paradoxically, the colitis is usually total but symptomatically mild, often with no rectal bleeding, and characterized by prolonged remissions. Inflammation is more pronounced in the right colon than in the left,[12] and colon cancer in IBD patients with PSC is also frequently right sided.

In a series of 71 PSC patients with IBD and 142 patients with UC, Loftus and colleagues found a frequency of pancolitis in PSC-IBD of 87% as compared with 54% in the UC control group.[11] The frequencies of rectal sparing (52% vs. 6%) and ileitis (51% vs. 7%) were also increased in the PSC-IBD group versus UC without PSC group. In colectomized patients, the frequency of pouchitis was 71% as compared with 30% in the UC group without PSC. In a subsequent series of 40 PSC patients with IBD and 40 patients with UC without PSC, the high frequency of pancolitis in PSC-IBD (85% vs. 45%) was verified.[12] In this study, only a modest increase in the frequency of ileitis (36% vs. 27%) and pouchitis (43% vs. 27%) was detected, and no increase in the frequency of rectal sparing (28% vs. 25%) was found. Backwash ileitis is defined histologically by mucosal inflammation involving a minimum of 3 cm of the terminal ileum in the absence of features of Crohn disease. The frequency of backwash ileitis in series of regular UC patients is in the range of 17% to 27% and predominantly seems to occur in patients with pancolitis. Notably, PSC cases are predominantly found in the subpopulation of UC patients with backwash ileitis. In conclusion, there is reason to believe that only the pancolitis-ileitis subtype of UC associates with PSC and that a substantial proportion of the patients with this form of IBD also exhibit rectal sparing (**Fig. 42-5**).

Full colonoscopy with biopsies is required to establish a diagnosis of either UC or Crohn disease in PSC. Whereas IBD in PSC clearly shows several features distinct from both UC and Crohn disease, the dichotomy of UC and Crohn disease has several practical implications for clinical handling. Because pathognomonic features of IBD in PSC do not exist, it is thus advisable that IBD in PSC is still categorized according to standard criteria. Crohn disease confined to the small intestine is not associated with PSC, but it has been suggested that PSC is equally common in extensive Crohn colitis as in extensive

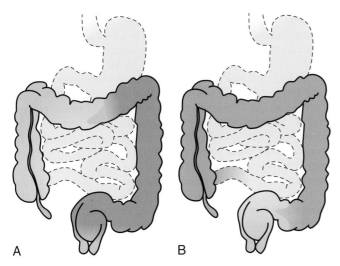

Fig. 42-5 Compared with regular UC (**A**), colitis in PSC (**B**) is usually mild with a right-sided predominance. Many of the patients have rectal sparing and backwash ileitis.

UC. The relative frequency of pancolitis in Crohn disease versus UC could thus explain the relative frequency of PSC in these two conditions. It has also been claimed that PSC severity may differ between UC and Crohn disease, based on the observation of a relatively high prevalence of Crohn disease among patients with small-duct PSC (17% to 21%).

The clinical severity of the colitis in PSC has two opposing facets—the relatively mild inflammation and the increased risk of colonic adenocarcinoma. In a report on 48 patients with UC and hepatobiliary disease by Schrumpf and associates in 1980,[3] IBD was classified as mild and moderate in 83% of the cases. In a follow-up study of 27 PSC patients from the same center,[45] further evaluation of the course of IBD showed that 44% had clinical disease activity only at onset of IBD, followed by quiescence. At follow-up colonoscopy, mild or inactive disease was found in 76% of the patients, moderate inflammation in 19%, and severe inflammation only in 5%. A detailed review of the histologic findings of IBD in PSC was only relatively recently given.[12] Whereas the pathologic findings were similar both in PSC patients with UC and in UC patients without PSC, the histologic inflammation grade was significantly lower in UC patients with PSC, and significantly less activity was detected in the left colon than in the right of these patients. The low activity of IBD in PSC is also reflected by a reduced need for surgery among these patients than in a matched UC population (28% vs. 46%, respectively).[11]

Clinical Features of Cholangiocarcinoma in Patients with Primary Sclerosing Cholangitis

Sudden deterioration of clinical (jaundice, fatigue, and weight loss) and biochemical (bilirubin and ALP levels in particular) parameters in a patient with preexisting PSC could be considered the obvious presentation of cholangiocarcinoma in PSC. However, similar symptoms may arise from benign strictures and during development of end-stage liver disease in PSC, and in many cases the clinical presentation of cholangiocarcinoma is far more insidious. Synchronous diagnosis of

cholangiocarcinoma and underlying PSC is made in 10% to 30% of the cases. Levels of the tumor marker carbohydrate antigen (CA) 19-9 may be grossly elevated (>100 U/ml), but this parameter is not specific and values may also be normal. In up to one third of the cholangiocarcinoma patients, no radiologic modality (ultrasound, computed tomography [CT], and ERC) is able to detect a tumor. Biliary brush cytology is a reliable means of establishing the diagnosis of biliary dysplasia and cancer, but the negative predictive value in an overall PSC population has been disputed. It has been reported that up to one third of the cases of cholangiocarcinoma are diagnosed during intended liver transplantation, in which the procedure is most often aborted and the liver allograft reallocated.

The difficulty in establishing the diagnosis of cholangiocarcinoma in PSC is underscored by the experiences from a U.S. series of 26 PSC patients with cholangiocarcinoma and 87 PSC patients without cholangiocarcinoma,[57] where the diagnosis was made by brush cytology in 15%, percutaneous biopsy in 23%, laparoscopy in 4%, laparotomy in 27% and during liver transplantation in 31% of the cases. In this series, there were no significant differences in symptoms, hepatic biochemistry measurements, liver disease severity, or IBD duration between patients with and without cholangiocarcinoma. The CA 19-9 values were significantly higher in cholangiocarcinoma patients (177 ± 89 U/ml) than in PSC patients without cholangiocarcinoma (61 ± 58 U/ml), but the range was wide and cholangiocarcinoma was found in patients with CA 19-9 levels less than 100 U/ml; conversely, CA 19-9 levels greater than 100 U/ml were found in patients without cholangiocarcinoma. In a large European series of 48 PSC patients with cholangiocarcinoma and 346 PSC patients without cholangiocarcinoma,[15] the frequency of jaundice and the levels of bilirubin were found to be higher among PSC patients with cholangiocarcinoma as compared with those without cholangiocarcinoma. The differences, however, did not remain significant when the patients diagnosed with cancer during the first year after diagnosis of PSC were excluded from the analysis. Most likely the cancer in many of the early cases is progressing at diagnosis of PSC and may even contribute to the PSC diagnosis reaching clinical attention. Also in this series, a high frequency of cholangiocarcinomas was not histologically confirmed until liver transplantation or autopsy (37%).

Although the American Joint Committee on Cancer TNM staging of cholangiocarcinoma is often applied, an important clinical distinction is that between intrahepatic and ductal cholangiocarcinoma. The clinical presentation of intrahepatic cholangiocarcinoma is that of a liver mass, and although the ALP level is usually elevated, the patients are rarely jaundiced. The clinical presentation of ductal cholangiocarcinoma is that of bile duct obstruction with silent jaundice and occasionally cholangitis. Hilar cholangiocarcinoma (also called Klatskin tumors) can be further classified according to Bismuth-Corlette, which is useful for selecting patients for surgery, but does not correlate with clinical presentation or patient survival. Relatively recently, an alternative staging system for ductal cholangiocarcinoma was proposed,[58] taking into account particular features of this form of cholangiocarcinoma. First, because of pronounced bile duct tropism, the ductal cholangiocarcinomas typically grow longitudinally before radial growth into a mass lesion. This means that they are difficult to visualize and often lack a measurable diameter. Second, the extensive perineural growth also often escapes imaging. Third, complicating vascular encasement in the portal tracts is the rule rather than the exception.

The exact prevalence of intrahepatic versus ductal cholangiocarcinoma in PSC is not known, but an impression of the distribution can be taken from the series of Ahrendt and colleagues,[59] who found 76% perihilar cancers, 16% intrahepatic cancers, and 8% cancers primarily involving the gallbladder in their population of 25 cholangiocarcinoma patients.[59] In 38 Nordic patients with biliary cancer detected in conjunction with intended liver transplantation, hilar or extrahepatic cancers were found in 58% of the cases, intrahepatic cancers in 16%, and gallbladder localization in 5%, whereas the exact origin was unknown in 21% of the cases. Metastatic disease has been reported at diagnosis in 52% to 63% of PSC patients with cholangiocarcinoma. In a series from the Mayo Clinic,[60] 47% of the patients with metastatic disease had intraabdominal metastases only, whereas 16% had both intraabdominal and extraabdominal metastases. The most common metastatic sites were regional lymph nodes (68%) and liver (37%), whereas some patients also had metastatic disease involving the lungs (10%), skin (10%), peritoneum (5%), and bone (5%). Skin metastasis in cholangiocarcinoma occurs as a complication of percutaneous biliary drainage procedures attributable to catheter seeding of tumor cells.

Diagnosis and Surveillance of Cholangiocarcinoma in Patients with Primary Sclerosing Cholangitis

An early diagnosis of cholangiocarcinoma in PSC is exceedingly difficult and often impossible to obtain. In clinical practice, tumor markers (CA 19-9 and carcinoembryonic antigen [CEA]) are often employed, but are not useful for detecting early disease. Biliary brushings may help distinguish between a malignant and a benign stenosis in PSC, but sensitivity is highly variable. Many diagnosticians consider MR imaging the most useful imaging modality, but is most often supplemented with CT, endoscopic ultrasound (EUS), and positron emission tomography (PET) scanning to elaborate on the possible presence of metastatic disease. Because tumor seeding is frequently reported after invasive procedures in cholangiocarcinoma, transcutaneous biopsy is normally discouraged if the patient is a candidate for resection or liver transplantation. Sensible application of each of these tests warrants further discussion of strengths and weaknesses.

The CA 19-9 antibody recognizes an epitope associated with the Lewis blood type antigen (which is not present in 5% of the population), and the normal range of test results may vary slightly. Even in PSC without cholangiocarcinoma and a variety of benign liver conditions, levels of CA 19-9 above the upper normal limit can be detected (alcoholic liver disease, primary biliary cirrhosis, chronic hepatitis B and C infection, and autoimmune hepatitis). Particularly high values can be observed in conjunction with acute cholangitis and choledocholithiasis. Among the many articles addressing the problems raised by this overlap, three deserve particular mentioning. Ramage and coworkers proposed that using a combination of CA 19-9 and CEA values with the formula CA 19-9 + (CEA × 40) and a cutoff value for this index of 400 would increase sensitivity (to 67%) and specificity (to 100%) compared with use of CA 19-9 alone (60% and 91%, respectively).[61] However,

retesting the performance of the Ramage score, Chalasani and colleagues found that a cutoff for CA 19-9 at 100 U/ml performed equally well (area under the curve, 0.78 for Ramage score >400; area under the curve, 0.76 for CA 19-9 >100 U/ml).[57] An important extension of these findings was made by Levy and colleagues,[62] who found that in serial measurements, the median CA 19-9 level change between two measurements in PSC patients without cholangiocarcinoma was 6.7 U/ml versus 664 U/ml in PSC patients with cholangiocarcinoma. By using a cutoff value of 63 U/ml for change in CA 19-9 level over time, a sensitivity of 90% and a specificity of 98% were obtained. With a cutoff value for the absolute value of CA 19-9 of 100 U/ml, sensitivity was 79% and specificity 97% in the same study population. By increasing the cutoff to 200 U/ml, sensitivity dropped to 71%, whereas specificity increased to 99%. A key problem is that by the time such levels are reached, most patients will have incurable disease, and reliance on CA 19-9 measurement as a "screening tool" for cholangiocarcinoma in PSC cannot be recommended.

Investigation of brush cytology specimens obtained by ERC in a region of a suspicious stricture has a specificity of close to 100% for cholangiocarcinoma in PSC in most published series. The problem with the method is the variable sensitivity (40% to 79%). Criteria for cytologic classification of biliary brush specimens are given in **Table 42-4** and histologic features of dysplasia and cholangiocarcinoma are shown in

Table 42-4 Criteria for Cytologic Classification of Bile Duct Epithelium

CATEGORY	CRITERIA
Insufficient material	Less than 60 normal epithelial cells
Normal epithelium and/or irregular nondysplastic changes	Sheets of cells in monolayer with even, relatively dense chromatin pattern and no nucleoli
Indefinite for dysplasia	Sheets with slight nuclear overlapping, slightly increased nuclear/cytoplasmic ratio, slight abnormality in chromatin structure
Low-grade dysplasia	Sheets and clusters of cells with nuclear overlapping, smooth nuclear shape, and moderately increased nuclear/cytoplasmic ratio. No dissociation of single cells. Nuclear chromatin shows mild clumping, and there are small, but clearly visible nucleoli
High-grade dysplasia/adenocarcinoma	Atypical cell clusters with marked increase in nuclear/cytoplasmic ratio, nuclear overlapping, and crowding. Nuclear membranes are irregular with signs of molding. Nuclei show coarse chromatin with distinct and prominent nucleoli

Reprinted with permission from Boberg KM, et al. Diagnostic benefit of biliary brush cytology in cholangiocarcinoma in primary sclerosing cholangitis. J Hepatol 2006;45:568–574.

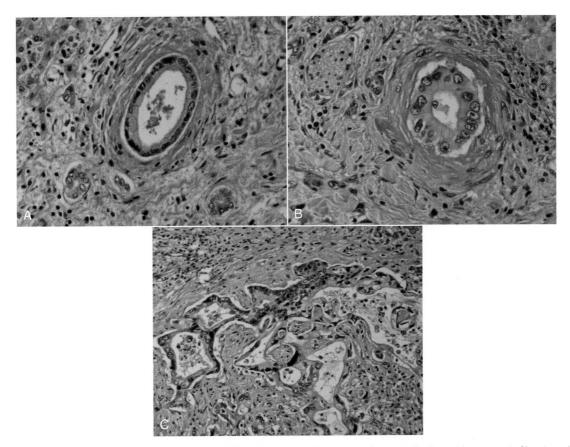

Fig. 42-6 Dysplasia and cholangiocarcinoma in the explanted liver from one PSC patient. A, Bile duct with concentric fibrosis and moderate dysplasia. **B,** Bile duct with concentric fibrosis and severe dysplasia. **C,** Intrahepatic cholangiocarcinoma with fibrosis.

Figure 42-6. Cytologist experience and differences in the definition criteria applied are likely to contribute to the variable sensitivity,[36] but intrinsic variability in the nature of ductal cholangiocarcinoma may also contribute. The technique of brushing is likely of importance but has not been studied systematically. High-quality samples have been obtained at our center by sampling nondilated strictures, using an over-the-wire brush. Brushing with the whole catheter, as opposed to moving the brush in and out of the catheter, may increase the yield, avoiding loss of material against the edge of the catheter. The brushings are retrieved by cutting the brush wire with pliers and then flushing the catheter into the same cytology conservation solution where the brush itself is contained.

In principle, all histopathologic variants of cholangiocarcinoma can occur in PSC and various histologic features may even be present in the same tumor. However, the most common appearance is that of a moderately to well-differentiated adenocarcinoma. Furthermore, cholangiocarcinoma in PSC is frequently "desmoplastic" and "scirrhous," referring to a picture of scarce chains of neoplastic cells with an excessive fibrotic response in the surrounding tissue (i.e., at least as many fibrous stroma as cancer cells). Important characteristics of scirrhous cholangiocarcinoma behavior (e.g., perineural growth) are often observed in cholangiocarcinoma in PSC. Another feature of cholangiocarcinoma in PSC is superficial distribution along the biliary mucosa

before invasive growth. Concepts such as "biliary tropism" of the cancer cells and "field cancerization" are used to describe this phenomenon, but further studies are needed to clarify the mechanism of this type of tumor growth in cholangiocarcinoma.

Several means of increasing sensitivity of brush cytology have been successfully applied. The first method is to repeat brushings, and it has been reported that three out of eight patients with cholangiocarcinoma and two negative brushings may yield a positive specimen on the third attempt. Another possibility is to include assessment of chromosomal aberrations by means of FISH. In a study of 131 patients being evaluated for possible malignant bile duct strictures, FISH increased sensitivity to 34% (from 15% to 21% by routine cytology in the same study).[38] Fluorescent probes hybridizing with centromeres of chromosomes 3, 7, and 17 as well as the 9p21 chromosomal band and a cutoff for malignancy of five or more polysomal cells were used. When only the PSC patients in this study were analyzed, the corresponding gain of sensitivity was from 29% to 41% by routine cytology to 50% by FISH. Digitized image analysis (DIA) allows for an objective assessment of chromatin distribution and nuclear morphology. In a population of 100 patients with biliary strictures of various etiologies, sensitivity for cholangiocarcinoma detection increased from 18% at routine cytology to 39% by DIA.[63] A slightly different approach was adopted by Boberg and associates,[64] who were concerned predominantly about the practical implication of a positive brush cytology report in terms of early liver transplantation in PSC. By jointly considering low-grade and high-grade dysplasias as suggestive of malignancy in PSC, a sensitivity of 100% was achieved at the cost of a reduced specificity (85%). When high-grade dysplasia only was considered, sensitivity was 73% and specificity 95%, values that are in line with most other series. It still needs to be decided if the gain in sensitivity of this strategy justifies liver transplantation in a few PSC patients with benign strictures. So far, mutational analysis (*p53* and *K-RAS*) has not been shown to improve performance of brush cytology investigations on suspected cholangiocarcinoma in PSC, but analysis of novel genetic and epigenetic alterations holds promise for improved accuracy in the future.

Imaging related to cholangiocarcinoma in PSC is associated with three principal challenges: (1) the similar appearance of benign strictures in PSC and ductal cholangiocarcinomas, (2) the high frequency of hilar lymphadenopathy in PSC without cholangiocarcinoma (see earlier), and (3) the staging of a verified malignancy to clarify whether the patient is a candidate for liver transplantation. A tumor identifiable by ultrasound has been reported in no more than 25% of cholangiocarcinoma cases, and in PSC a prestenotic dilatation of the bile ducts may be missing as a result of fibrosis. In a small study population of 45 PSC patients of whom 18 were diagnosed with cholangiocarcinoma, the sensitivity and specificity for detecting cholangiocarcinoma in PSC by CT were calculated as 82% and 80%, respectively.[65] In a recent study of 230 PSC patients of whom 23 were diagnosed with cholangiocarcinoma, the corresponding numbers for combined MR imaging and MRC were 89% and 75%, respectively.[66] Because of the inherent variability in PSC and cholangiocarcinoma behavior, these numbers are likely to vary depending on the manner in which the study population is recruited.

Based on clinical experience, contrast-enhanced (e.g., gadolinium) MR imaging with MRC is considered the imaging method of choice if cholangiocarcinoma is suspected in PSC. In case of pathologic findings, CT typically supplements with information on lymph node enlargement and the liver parenchyma (e.g., cirrhosis), and has been reported to be superior to MR imaging in terms of defining extrahepatic growth and vascular encasement. The role of EUS imaging in cholangiocarcinoma in PSC is limited to characterization of enlarged lymph nodes (including fine-needle aspiration) during staging. A similar role can be assigned to ^{18}F-deoxyglucose (FDG) positron emission tomography (PET) scanning, which is useful for detecting solid metastases, but unreliable for detecting biliary lesions not visible on MRI/CT or peritoneal carcinomatosis. In specialized centers, cholangioscopy, either alone or combined with intraductal ultrasound and lesion-directed biopsies, may supplement the other imaging modalities. Using cholangioscopy, a sensitivity of 92% and specificity of 93% in the diagnosis of malignant strictures in PSC have been reported,[67] as compared with 66% and 51% for ERC alone. The application of intraductal ultrasound correspondingly increased the sensitivity from 63% to 88% and specificity from 53% to 91%, respectively, when compared with ERC alone.[68] Further guidelines on the application of these latter two methods need to be established.

The probable diagnosis of cholangiocarcinoma in PSC is based on multiple tests of questionable sensitivity and specificity along with sound clinical judgment and experience. An extensive evaluation of CA 19-9 imaging and cytology-based techniques has been published from the Mayo Clinic.[66] Based on their data, an up-to-date algorithm for the screening and diagnosis of cholangiocarcinoma in PSC was proposed (**Fig. 42-7**). Although the usefulness of the algorithm requires confirmation in prospective series, the important conclusion from the authors is that almost two thirds of the cholangiocarcinomas were detected at an early stage during which potentially curative liver transplantation protocols were still applicable. In addition to the obvious benefits of an early diagnosis, it is evident that a definite diagnosis, either negative or positive, of malignancy status in PSC is of great practical concern and should be pursued by all means.

Differential Diagnosis and Primary Sclerosing Cholangitis Variants

Three groups of differential diagnoses exist in adult PSC: (1) secondary sclerosing cholangitis, (2) other distinct liver diseases that may have some clinical and biochemical similarities with PSC, and finally (3) PSC variants that are poorly defined entities with considerable similarities with regular PSC. In the pediatric population the situation is even more complex and a number of conditions may present with PSC-like features (**Table 42-5**). As alluded to repeatedly throughout this chapter, PSC is in many ways not a single disease, and as the origins of diseases that we today denominate "primary" are unraveled, the list of differential diagnoses is likely to grow.

As evident from **Table 42-6**, the spectrum of diagnoses constituting secondary sclerosing cholangitis is too diverse to allow for detailed elaboration and is reviewed elsewhere.[69] By definition, the cause of the secondary sclerosing cholangitis is always identified. In most cases this means considering the presence of trauma, gallstones, tumors, infections, and immunodeficiency and various systemic inflammatory conditions (e.g., sarcoidosis). However, rare causes need to be considered and may require careful reflection of patient history and associated conditions (e.g., Langerhans histiocytosis). In children particular attention needs to be directed to diagnoses of monogenic diseases (e.g., PFIC3 attributable to severe *MDR3* mutations) as opposed to congenital disorders (e.g., biliary atresia, congenital hepatic fibrosis, Caroli disease, choledochal cysts). Also, some findings should not immediately lead to the exclusion of a PSC diagnosis. The discovery of cholangiocarcinoma in young individuals should always raise the suspicion of underlying PSC and appropriate investigations should be

---

Table 42-5 Differential Diagnosis of Primary Sclerosing Cholangitis–Like Changes on Cholangiography in Children

Cystic fibrosis
Primary and secondary immunodeficiency
Langerhans cell histiocytosis
Neonatal sclerosing cholangitis
Biliary atresia
Ichthyosis with sclerosing cholangitis
Congenital bile duct abnormalities
Sickle cell disease
Progressive familial intrahepatic cholestasis type 3

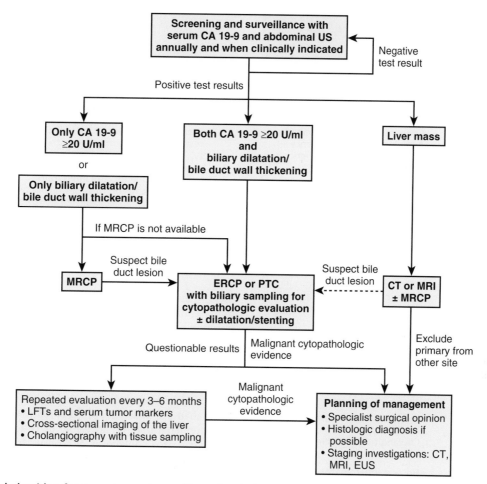

Fig. 42-7 **Proposed algorithm for screening and surveillance for cholangiocarcinoma in patients with PSC.** *(Reprinted with permission from Charatcharoenwitthaya P, et al. Utility of serum tumor markers, imaging, and biliary cytology for detecting cholangiocarcinoma in primary sclerosing cholangitis. Hepatology 2008;48:1106–1117.)*

initiated. Gallstones can be found in approximately 25% of PSC patients, and should in otherwise typical cases be considered part of the normal disease spectrum rather than an exclusion of the diagnosis.

In terms of other liver diseases, primary biliary cirrhosis can usually be excluded on the basis of AMA positivity (>90%) and histologic findings. However, PSC patients with elevated levels of AMAs have been reported.[18] Conversely, AMA negativity occurs in up to 10% of primary biliary cirrhosis patients. If other features are suggestive of PSC (e.g., presence of IBD), cholangiography should be performed. Viral hepatitis, alcoholic liver disease, and drug-induced reactions may also present with a cholestatic pattern of hepatic biochemistries and must be excluded on the basis of appropriate serologic tests and patient history.

It is important to remember that other causes of elevated hepatic biochemistry results in IBD may exist beside PSC (e.g., fatty liver).[8,10] However, it is probable that many previous notions of "non-specific abnormities" of hepatic biochemistries in patients with IBD may actually represent clinically quiescent forms of PSC.[9] The threshold for performing cholangiography to detect the presence of PSC in such patients should be low. To diagnose small-duct PSC, liver biopsy needs to be performed (**Table 42-7**), but liver biopsy interpretation relies on IBD status. In patients without IBD, typical changes suggestive of PSC should be required. In patients with concurrent IBD, the histologic changes should at least be compatible with PSC, but not necessarily typical or specific for the histologic pathology observed in large-duct PSC. Transition to large-duct PSC may occur, and cholangiography should be repeated when clinical deterioration is observed. Typically, however, small-duct PSC runs a quiescent course, and long-term survival is significantly better than that for large-duct PSC. Cholangiocarcinoma does not seem to occur in small-duct PSC patients unless transition into regular large-duct PSC has occurred. Other features of large-duct PSC, however, may be present in a subset of the patients (e.g., AIH-like features).

Compared with PSC and PBC, where cholangiography and AMA determination, respectively, may establish the diagnosis, autoimmune hepatitis is a more complex diagnosis. The diagnosis is based on criteria established by the International Autoimmune Hepatitis Group,[46,70] and includes measuring levels of autoantibodies and IgG, performing liver histologic studies, and determining viral hepatitis parameters for differential diagnostic purposes. For diagnosis of PSC with

Table 42-6 Secondary Sclerosing Cholangitis and Conditions Showing Primary Sclerosing Cholangitis–Like Changes on Cholangiography

Infection	Bacterial cholangitis Recurrent pyogenic cholangitis
Immunodeficiency related	Congenital immunodeficiency Acquired immunodeficiency Combined immunodeficiency Angioimmunoblastic lymphadenopathy
Congenital	Caroli disease Congenital hepatic fibrosis Cystic fibrosis Ductal plate abnormalities
Mechanic/toxic	Cholelithiasis/choledocholithiasis Intraarterial chemotherapy
Ischemic	Vascular trauma Hepatic allograft arterial occlusion Paroxysmal nocturnal hemoglobinuria
Pancreatic disease	Autoimmune pancreatitis Chronic pancreatitis
Infiltrative disorders	Amyloidosis Sarcoidosis Systemic mastocytosis Hypereosinophilic syndrome Hodgkin disease Cholangitis glandularis proliferans
Others	Hepatic inflammatory pseudotumor Neoplastic/metastatic disease Langerhans cell histiocytosis Hepatic allograft rejection Graft-versus-host disease

Partially reproduced from Abdalian R, Heathcote EJ. Sclerosing cholangitis: a focus on secondary causes. Hepatology 2006;44:1063–1074.

Table 42-7 Definition of Small-Duct Primary Sclerosing Cholangitis

1. Chronic cholestatic liver disease of at least 1 year of follow-up
2. Liver biopsy showing features of PSC:
   A. Patients without IBD should have typical changes suggestive of PSC
   B. Patients with concomitant IBD should have histologic results at least compatible with PSC but not necessarily typical or identical or specific to liver histologic results observed in large-duct PSC
3. Normal good-quality cholangiogram
4. Appropriate exclusion of other biliary and liver diseases

IBD, inflammatory bowel disease; PSC, primary sclerosing cholangitis

therapy, and patients do not seem to develop cholangiocarcinoma as frequently as PSC patients without features of autoimmune hepatitis.

Similar to autoimmune hepatitis, the diagnosis of autoimmune pancreatitis syndrome, including IgG4-associated sclerosing cholangitis, is based on multiple criteria.[21] Elevated levels of IgG4 (>135 mg/dl) are highly specific for IgG4-associated sclerosing cholangitis. However, sensitivity may be lower than previously reported (71% to 82%), and repeated measurements may be advisable in patients with suspected IgG4-associated cholangitis. If biopsies from diseased organs are available, staining for IgG4 may reveal the characteristic accumulation of IgG4-positive plasma cells, and moderate (11 to 30 cells/high-power field) to severe (>30 cells/high-power field) levels of these cells are considered diagnostic of IgG4-associated sclerosing cholangitis. In liver explant specimens from patients with PSC, positive IgG4 immunostaining for IgG4 has been reported in 23% of patients.[20] Some of the patients may also have inflammatory bowel disease, and there is also a male preponderance (8:1). On imaging, diffuse pancreatic enlargement in conjunction with pancreatic duct abnormalities is part of the diagnostic criteria.[20] Further studies are needed to elaborate on these observations. The discovery of IgG4-associated sclerosing cholangitis illustrates, however, that PSC most likely will divide into a heterogeneous group of diseases. Ultimately the definition of each of these disorders may indeed lead to successful therapy.

Natural History of Primary Sclerosing Cholangitis

Disease course in PSC is usually defined as the time from diagnosis to the combined end point of death or liver transplantation. The course of PSC following liver transplantation will be discussed separately (see later). Determination of the time point in which a patient becomes ill with PSC is not straightforward. One could use the patient's perspective, and state that it is the time when the first symptom attributable to PSC is reported. However, as we have discussed previously, symptoms are nonspecific and many patients only develop symptoms of PSC a long time after being diagnosed. One could also state that PSC begins at the time when the

AIH-like features, liver biopsy is the most important diagnostic modality. Typical findings include interface hepatitis, lymphocytic and lymphoplasmacytic infiltrates in the portal tracts and extending into the lobule, emperipolesis (active penetration by one cell into and through a larger cell), and finally hepatic rosette formation. Because initial versions of the scoring system led to as many as one third of PSC patients being classified as "probable" AIH,[18] a revised version reduced this proportion to 9% in the same PSC population.[71] Whereas suspicion of autoimmune features is easily raised in patients with PSC, diagnosis of PSC in a patient believed to present with autoimmune hepatitis is more easily missed. Typically, in the presence of IBD, an ALP/AST ratio higher than 3, and histologic evidence for periductal fibrosis, concurrent PSC should be suspected. In the pediatric population, where AIH-like features in PSC are common, ALP level cannot be used for diagnosis because of its inherent elevation associated with growing bones. There are reports that suggest a more benign disease course of AIH-like PSC, possibly related to effects from

first abnormal liver biochemistry test is seen. However, as discussed later, blood tests may be normal, and even when elevated they may become normal at a later stage, making it difficult to use blood tests to follow the disease course in PSC. It is therefore most common to assert that onset of PSC is the time when the first abnormal cholangiographic result is observed. Survival is then defined as the time from this abnormal cholangiography until death or liver transplantation.

During the late 1980s, it was generally established that the natural history of PSC is progressive. Sooner or later, most PSC patients are believed to develop liver cirrhosis with associated complications in terms of liver failure and portal hypertension with ascites, variceal bleeding, and hepatic encephalopathy. Median survival in published series ranges from 12 to 17 years. However, PSC patients show a remarkable variability in natural history, in contrast to other liver diseases such as primary biliary cirrhosis, which follows a relatively predictable prognostic course. Several studies have tried to define predictors of poor outcome. The most important of these is clearly cholangiocarcinoma (**Fig. 42-8**), which can occur at any time point (see earlier).[15] Also consistent in the majority of studies is the association between elevated bilirubin levels and poor outcome. Furthermore, patients with symptoms, particularly variceal bleeding, progress considerably faster to liver transplantation or death than asymptomatic patients. Evidently, it could be argued that asymptomatic patients with normal bilirubin levels have less liver and bile duct damage than those with symptoms and high bilirubin levels because the former have been diagnosed at an earlier stage. In most patients, the disease processes have been ongoing for years before the diagnosis is made, and probably the clinical parameters associated with poor outcome serve as indirect measures for underlying differences in these processes between patients (e.g., attributable to genetic variability, the so-called modifier genes).

Several attempts have been made to construct a PSC-specific prognostic model by which individual clinical parameters can be used to predict survival for any individual PSC patient. It has been argued that these models are more useful for predicting outcome in early stage PSC than other classifications such as the Child-Pugh score. Because biochemical parameters may change according to disease stage, it has also been argued that time-dependent models are more accurate than models that only consider parameters at one given point in time.[43] Most early models included histologic staging, but this requirement was later abandoned because of the invasive nature and inherent sampling variability of liver biopsies in PSC (see earlier).[54] Whereas the prognostic models are accurate in predicting outcome for groups of patients, they cannot be reliably used in clinical practice to predict outcome at the individual level. Furthermore, an important notion with regard to the relevance of present prognostic models came from studies on the effects of high-dose ursodeoxycholic acid discussed next. Whereas changes in prognostic indices suggested this treatment would be beneficial, direct observations later revealed adverse effects on outcome.[72] Evidently, there is more to disease course in PSC than can be captured by statistical modeling. New markers for disease activity and prognostic applications may hopefully be revealed in parallel with increasing understanding of the molecular pathogenesis of PSC. Given the long disease course, such markers will also prove useful in determining the efficacy of novel treatment regimens.

Treatment

With the introduction of liver transplantation as a treatment option for PSC in 1983, palliative surgical biliary drainage procedures were abandoned. The efficacy of these procedures had long been questioned, and previous biliary surgery negatively affects outcome following liver transplantation. The principal problem in treating PSC is the fact that by the time diagnosis by cholangiography is feasible, irreversible biliary fibrosis is already manifest. The main challenge is thus not to cure PSC, but to (1) prevent progression to end-stage liver disease and avoid the development of (2) complications and (3) cancer. No medical treatment has yet been shown to effectively achieve any of these three goals. Immunosuppressive therapy probably has a role in IgG4-associated sclerosing cholangitis and AIH-like PSC, but does not influence disease progression in regular PSC. Whereas an effect on need for liver transplantation and risk of death is questionable, there is clearly a place for endoscopic dilatation and stenting in reducing the risk of complications from dominant stenoses and the use of antibiotic for treating recurrent episodes of acute cholangitis. Survival following liver transplantation in PSC is excellent, but a major challenge is timing with regard to the risk of developing cholangiocarcinoma.

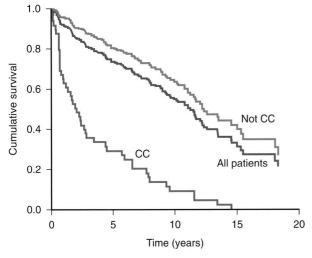

Fig. 42-8 Survival of the total group of PSC patients (*n* = 394) and the subgroups of patients with cholangiocarcinoma *(CC)* (*n* = 48) and without cholangiocarcinoma (*n* = 346). *(Reprinted with permission from Boberg KM, et al. Cholangiocarcinoma in primary sclerosing cholangitis: risk factors and clinical presentation. Scand J Gastroenterol 2002;37:1205–1211.)*

Ursodeoxycholic Acid in Patients with Primary Sclerosing Cholangitis

The physiologic effects of peroral ursodeoxycholic acid (UDCA) in healthy individuals and as treatment for various hepatobiliary conditions have been extensively studied. For more than 1000 years, the drug has been prescribed in traditional Chinese medicine for a variety of liver conditions in the form of dried bile ("Yutan") from black bears. In polar, black, and brown bears (Latin: *ursidae*) ursodeoxycholic acid constitutes 15% to 39% of biliary bile acids, but also occurs at low concentrations (1% to 3%) in humans. The beneficial effect of increasing biliary concentrations of the hydrophilic ursodeoxycholic acid in human cholestatic disease has been attributed to protection of hepatocyte and bile duct epithelial cells against hydrophobic bile acids, anti-apoptotic effects, immunomodulatory effects, and altered secretion of a variety of toxic and nontoxic biliary constituents. The relative importance of each of these mechanisms of action is not known. The cell membrane protection has been described to result from the incorporation of ursodeoxycholic acid and a cholesterol-like, stabilizing effect, but is more likely related to more favorable handling of hydrophobic bile acids by the mixed micelle compartment of bile. The antiapoptotic effects have been demonstrated for hepatocytes in several experimental settings, and for biliary epithelial cells during therapy for primary biliary cirrhosis. Proposed immunomodulatory effects are poorly understood and difficult to differentiate from secondary effects of other mechanisms of action. Finally, the most important changes in apical hepatobiliary transport systems induced by ursodeoxycholic acid are the increased expression of the Cl^-/HCO_3^- anion exchanger (AE2) MDR3 and the bile salt export pump (BSEP), leading to increased bile flow and phospholipid content. Basolaterally, an increased expression of MRP4 may facilitate the removal of retained bile acids from a cholestatic liver into the systemic circulation for elimination in the urine.

An understanding of the pharmacokinetics of ursodeoxycholic acid is required to comprehend the evolvement of treatment trials on this drug in PSC. After peroral administration, up to 30% to 60% of the administered dose of unconjugated ursodeoxycholic acid is transported throughout the small (80%) and large (20%) intestines. Because uptake is facilitated by the presence of biliary micelles, it is generally recommended that ursodeoxycholic acid be administered in conjunction with a meal.[33] First-pass uptake of ursodeoxycholic acid from the portal circulation amounts to approximately 60% of the administered dose, and is effectuated by broad specificity bile acid transporter molecules on the sinusoidal membrane of hepatocytes. Conjugation with glycine and taurine is subsequently performed, followed by biliary excretion and enterohepatic circulation. Ursodeoxycholic acid and corresponding conjugates that are not absorbed undergo bacterial conversion into hydrophobic lithocholic acid in the colon and are subsequently excreted in the feces.[33] With continuous treatment, ursodeoxycholic acid constitutes 40% to 60% of the bile acid pool in the enterohepatic circulation. However, inspiring the series of trials to be described next, there is an increasing enrichment of biliary ursodeoxycholic acid in patients with PSC from 43% to 47% at normal doses (10 to 17 mg/kg/day) to 56% to 59% at higher doses (18 to 32 mg/kg/day).[73]

The first randomized, double-blind, placebo-controlled trial of ursodeoxycholic acid for PSC was performed by Beuers and colleagues in 1992.[74] As confirmed in two subsequent studies, the investigators noted that both hepatic biochemistry values and histologic parameters of liver injury improved in the treatment group. None of the studies were able to demonstrate an improvement in transplant-free survival. The three largest studies to date were performed in the United States and Scandinavia and utilized different doses of ursodeoxycholic acid (13 to 15 mg/kg/day,[75] 17 to 23 mg/kg/day,[76] and 28 to 30 mg/kg/day[72]). Neither of these studies was able to demonstrate significant effects on risk of liver transplantation or death, as also confirmed in a recent meta-analysis of ursodeoxycholic acid treatment trials in PSC. Actually, contrary to suggestions made by pilot studies of high-dose ursodeoxycholic acid in PSC, the highest dose regimen (28 to 30 mg/kg/day) was significantly associated with a two-fold increased risk of liver transplantation or death as compared with placebo. The explanation for this is not clear, but speculations were made that higher doses may result in increased colonic conversion of unabsorbed ursodeoxycholic acid into the toxic metabolite lithocholic acid, or that the anti-apoptotic effects may actually also benefit cells involved in disease progression in PSC (e.g., stellate cells).[72] After consideration of all the trials, it can be concluded that ursodeoxycholic acid may be effective in reducing the activity of components in the disease process in PSC, possibly even at the histologic level, but these components do not seem to be important for the progression of the disease. General use of ursodeoxycholic acid in the treatment of PSC is therefore not recommended.[49]

The concept of "chemoprevention" by ursodeoxycholic acid in carcinogenesis in PSC is based on in vitro and animal data demonstrating reduced proliferation of cancer cells and tumors induced by several chemical carcinogens. In particular, it has been proposed that the reduced levels of fecal deoxycholic acid observed in ursodeoxycholic acid therapy may influence colonic carcinogenesis. In a 2001 cross-sectional study of 59 PSC patients with UC of whom 41 had received ursodeoxycholic acid therapy, a protective effect against the development of colonic dysplasia was shown.[77] A similar observation was made by retrospectively assessing the combined risk of colon cancer and dysplasia in 52 patients who had previously participated in a U.S. treatment trial with low-dose ursodeoxycholic acid (13 to 15 mg/kg/day).[78] In a small panel of IBD patients without PSC,[79] ursodeoxycholic acid was shown to prevent further progression of manifest low-grade colonic dysplasia. In cholangiocarcinoma, indirect evidence for a protective effect of ursodeoxycholic acid has been derived by retrospectively demonstrating a low prevalence of cholangiocarcinoma in PSC patients who received ursodeoxycholic acid. Because none of the large prospective high-dose ursodeoxycholic acid treatment trials have been able to confirm similar effects, general recommendations cannot presently be concluded. Possibly, low-dose ursodeoxycholic acid should be prescribed to PSC patients when additional risk factors are present (e.g., family history of colorectal cancer, previous colorectal neoplasia, longstanding extensive colitis).[49]

Immunosuppressive and Antibiotic Treatment in Patients with Primary Sclerosing Cholangitis

As reviewed by Cullen and Chapman,[80] a variety of immunosuppressive drugs ranging from corticosteroids to monoclonal antibodies against TNF-α have been tested in pilot studies as well as randomized, double-blind, placebo-controlled treatment trials in PSC. None of these agents have proven beneficial and should not be prescribed to the typical PSC patient.

Two exceptions should nevertheless be made: in AIH-like PSC and IgG4-associated cholangitis immunosuppressive therapy is indicated and may influence disease course and the cholangiographic changes in these subgroups.

The prognosis of AIH-like PSC is better than that of regular PSC, but significantly worse than that of autoimmune hepatitis. It could be speculated that this difference is due to a partial response to immunosuppressive therapy in this group of PSC patients. In principle, the AIH-like features of these patients have been addressed like autoimmune hepatitis without PSC, and in retrospective series treatment is associated with improved survival. The observation that progression to cirrhosis occurs in a majority of the patients despite immunosuppressive treatment indicates that some of the pathologic processes may be relatively inert to immunosuppression even in AIH-like PSC. In a series of 27 children with this condition,[19] parenchymal inflammatory damage was effectively reversed upon immunosuppression with corticosteroids and azathioprine, whereas none of the cholangiograms showed regression.

An immunosuppressive regimen for IgG4-associated sclerosing cholangitis has been proposed.[49,81] Prospective, randomized, placebo-controlled trials of immunosuppression in this condition are not likely to be performed. The reason for this is the excellent response to corticosteroid treatment in published series, along with notions of unfavorable outcome in patients not receiving corticosteroid treatment. Typically, pretreatment biliary dilatation and stenting is performed for quicker resolution of symptoms. A challenge in the handling of patients with IgG4-associated sclerosing cholangitis is the high rate of relapse, particularly in patients with proximal bile duct disease, following tapering of corticosteroids after the 3 recommended months of initial treatment.[81] Whereas most cases of relapse apparently can be handled with azathioprine, long-term corticosteroid treatment has been the preferred option at some centers.

Based on the frequent bacterial colonization of deranged bile ducts in PSC along with theories of chronic infectious processes possibly contributing to disease progression in PSC, antibiotic treatment in PSC may serve several important purposes. First, relapsing episodes of acute cholangitis may occur at any time point during PSC. Relevant bacterial species include those typically seen in acute cholangitis (e.g., *Escherichia coli*, *Klebsiella*, enterococci, *Pseudomonas*, and *Proteus* species), but antibiotic treatment should also consider peculiarities of the biliary colonization in PSC (e.g., α-hemolytic *Streptococci* and *Staphylococci*). Similar considerations should be made regarding prophylactic use of antibiotics in conjunction with ERC in patients with PSC, where typically a broader spectrum of bacteria are introduced than present in quiescent PSC. Finally, two studies have assessed the effects of long-term antibiotic treatment in PSC.[82,83] Whereas no significant influence on disease progression was observed in either of these studies, Färkkilä and associates observed a significantly larger decrease in ALP levels during metronidazole plus ursodeoxycholic acid treatment as compared with ursodeoxycholic acid alone. Although long-term antibiotics in some instances may be justified in PSC patients with dominant stenoses and recurrent attacks of acute cholangitis, prophylactic antibiotics should not be routinely prescribed to PSC patients. Rather, as will be discussed next, endoscopic therapy may be indicated.

Endoscopic Treatment of Primary Sclerosing Cholangitis

Endoscopic treatment is applicable to both long and short stenoses in the common bile duct as well as to short stenoses in the hepatic ducts within 2 cm of the bifurcation. In patients with extensive intrahepatic disease, endoscopic treatment is not effective and liver transplantation should be considered. The preferred endoscopic treatment option is balloon dilatation, and details of the procedure has been reviewed by Stiehl.[84] It remains to be clarified to what extent and in which patients short-term (<1 to 2 weeks) stenting is of additional value. Long-term stenting is not advisable because of the high frequency of stent occlusion and cholangitis, which seems to occur more frequently in patients with PSC than other forms of biliary stenoses (e.g., tumor). Biliary stones are frequently detected in conjunction with endoscopic therapy (50%) and should be extracted. Balloon dilatation and stenting in PSC patients with dominant stenoses effectively relieve pruritus and jaundice in 80% to 100% of the patients, but it can be noted that bilirubin level may transiently rise during the first days after intervention. In most cases, multiple treatments over the years are required to maintain the open bile ducts. In a series of 32 patients from the Netherlands, however, as many as 80% and 60% of the patients were free from additional endoscopic procedures 1 and 3 years, respectively, after the first dilation.[85]

The extent that endoscopic treatment may influence long-term outcome in patients with PSC and dominant stenoses is disputed. Some authors have claimed that predominantly the intrahepatic biliary changes are predictive of disease progression in PSC, and that intermittent cholestasis occurs in PSC patients regardless of the presence of dominant strictures. However, other studies have reported that the extent of extrahepatic biliary changes may be important, and a direct association between the presence of dominant strictures and poor outcome in PSC has been reported.[32] No randomized, prospective controlled trials have been performed to assess the efficacy of endoscopic treatment in PSC, and the application is presently performed at the discretion of the endoscopist based on careful assessment of each individual patient. Several retrospective studies have noted a significant increase in actual as compared with predicted 3- and 5-year survival rates (according to the Mayo risk score) following endoscopic treatment of dominant stenoses. Based on the sum of this experience, placebo-controlled studies of endoscopic treatment of PSC patients with dominant stenoses are not likely to be undertaken. Treatment seems justified for dominant stenoses with recurrent attacks of acute cholangitis and severe jaundice and pruritus. Further studies are needed on technical details of the procedure (e.g., stenting, extent of papillotomy) and long-term benefits, and the option of liver transplantation should continuously be considered in patients in whom multiple dilatations fail to achieve patency of the strictures.[49]

Liver Transplantation in Patients with Primary Sclerosing Cholangitis

The progressive nature of PSC means that for most patients the prospect of a future liver transplant is part of coping with the diagnosis. In the Nordic countries PSC is the most important indication for liver transplantation. In the United States

PSC is among the 5 leading indications, and even in low-prevalence countries such as Italy and Spain, PSC is among the 10 most common indications. Patient survival is excellent, with recent 1- and 5-year survival rates at most centers approaching 90% and 85%, respectively. However, liver transplantation in PSC poses several particular challenges. First, disease course is unpredictable, and some patients may require listing for liver transplantation before development of end-stage liver disease (e.g., because of uncontrollable and recurrent episodes of acute cholangitis). Second, the high risk of biliary and colonic malignancies indicates that thorough pretransplant evaluation regarding the presence of cancer must be performed. Finally, an increased risk of rejections (as compared with other indications), recurrence of PSC in the liver allograft in 20% to 30% of the cases, and risk of IBD exacerbation all pose particular challenges in the long-term handling of PSC patients after liver transplantation.[86]

Predicting transplant-free survival, as discussed earlier is virtually impossible at the level of an individual PSC patient. However, for patients with end-stage cirrhosis, timing of liver transplantation in PSC does not differ from that of other indications for liver transplantation. General considerations with regard to timing need to be made (e.g., MELD score, waiting time), taking into account the association between deaths of PSC patients on the waiting list and an advanced MELD score.[87] As pointed out in the previous edition of this book,[88] it seems advisable to refer PSC patients for liver transplantation early in the disease course. The argument is politically a difficult one, and some authors claim that early listing of patients with PSC based on intractable symptoms is not justifiable when MELD scores actually do predict long-term survival for this group of patients. Support for the latter notion is further given by PSC having among the lowest waiting list mortality of all diagnoses under the MELD system. The context of organ availability clearly needs to be taken into account, but in cases of severe recurrent cholangitis there is general consensus for liver transplantation to be considered even in noncirrhotic patients.[49]

The other problem of timing is related to the risk of cholangiocarcinoma. The problems of an early diagnosis of cholangiocarcinoma in PSC have been emphasized earlier in this chapter. Several comments to these problems can be made in the context of liver transplantation based on a study of 255 PSC patients listed for liver transplantation in the Nordic countries between 1990 and 2001.[89] Significant predictors of hepatobiliary malignancy in these patients were found to be short duration of PSC, absence of ursodeoxycholic acid treatment, previous diagnosis of colorectal carcinoma, and clinical suspicion of cancer. Given the high risk of cholangiocarcinoma during the first year following diagnosis of PSC, the risk factor is obvious. The next two risk factors in this study are related to the possible presence of a common denominator for biliary and colonic neoplasia in patients with PSC,[14] meaning that dysplasia in one of these locations should always raise suspicion about the condition of the other location. The final risk factor, clinical suspicion, is compound. Because a confirmed diagnosis of cholangiocarcinoma in many cases may not be possible before liver transplantation, a strong clinical suspicion should have two consequences: First, if clinical suspicion is substantiated by findings of dysplasia in biliary brushings, the patient should be considered for immediate listing and liver transplantation in the absence of solid tumors

on any imaging modality.[49] Second, if liver transplantation is otherwise indicated and malignancy cannot definitely be excluded, the patient should be listed and pretransplant explorative surgery performed.[86] In some cases this warrants interruption of the planned transplantation, indicating that a backup recipient should be available for organ reallocation and the original patient thoroughly informed on the possibility of this unfavorable outcome.[86]

An outline of the pretransplant evaluation of patients with PSC is given in **Figure 42-9**.[90] All the particular considerations pertain to the increased risk of malignancy, and general examinations (e.g., characterization of portal hypertension including the identification and eradication of esophageal varices) will not be discussed further in this text. Whereas suspected hepatocellular carcinoma in cirrhotic PSC patients can be managed according to standard guidelines based on the Milan criteria, the treatment of colorectal cancer and cholangiocarcinoma in the context of liver transplantation is less clearly defined. It seems reasonable that all PSC patients should undergo a full colonoscopy before liver transplantation. Based on the mild symptoms of IBD in PSC, the procedure should not be restricted to patients with a history of IBD. Pretransplant colectomy in PSC patients with colonic dysplasia and cirrhosis implicates a high risk of complications, and in some of these patients concomitant liver transplantation and colectomy may be justified. Regarding cholangiocarcinoma, the relatively high negative predictive value (89% to 100%) of brush cytology[64,66] warrants liberal application of this technique in PSC patients during pretransplant evaluation. Serum tumor markers (CA 19-9, CEA, and α-fetoprotein [AFP]) should be measured in conjunction with use of CT or MR with MRC, and, in suspected cases, also PET and EUS. As discussed earlier, the presence of perihepatic lymphadenopathy is not predictive of malignancy in patients with PSC. In suspicious cases, frozen section histologic studies of enlarged lymph nodes during pretransplant explorative surgery may be required to finally conclude on eligibility for transplantation. Inevitably, however, some PSC patients with undetectable cholangiocarcinoma will undergo transplantation and diagnosis made during pathologic examination of the explanted liver.

Also during posttransplant follow-up, PSC patients differ from other recipients in several important aspects. An increased risk of acute cellular rejection in PSC has been demonstrated in several series. Because high frequencies of acute cellular rejection have also been reported in recipients with underlying autoimmune hepatitis and primary biliary cirrhosis, it is not clear whether PSC patients are particularly at risk or whether the risk is generally related to autoimmune liver disease in the recipient. In a series of 150 PSC patients, Graziadei and colleagues found significantly more rejection episodes in patients with pretransplant IBD (1.16 episodes/patient) as compared with patients without IBD (0.67 episode/patient).[91] This notion is supported by others, and the risk of chronic rejection also seems to be higher in PSC patients with IBD. Based on these observations, some authorities recommend an intensified immunosuppressive regimen including life-long corticosteroids following liver transplantation for PSC,[86] whereas others cautiously prefer a regular regimen based on an association between aggressive immunosuppression and recurrent PSC (see later).[92]

The risks of hepatic artery thrombosis, non–skin malignancies, and biliary complications are all higher in patients with

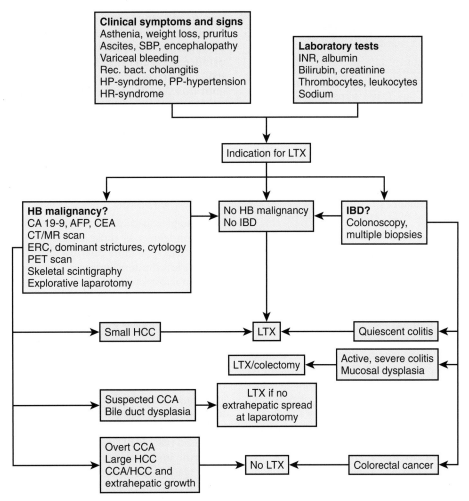

Fig. 42-9 **Pretransplant evaluation of patients with primary sclerosing cholangitis.** This schematic presentation illustrates common clinical problems and possible ways to address these problems. CCA, cholangiocarcinoma; HB malignancy, hepatobiliary malignancy; CT, computed tomography; HCC, hepatocellular carcinoma; HP-syndrome, hepatopulmonary syndrome; HR-syndrome, hepatorenal syndrome; IBD, inflammatory bowel disease; INR, international normalized ratio; LTX, liver transplant; MR, magnetic resonance; PET, positron emission tomography; PP-hypertension, portopulmonary hypertension; SBP, spontaneous bacterial peritonitis

PSC compared with other recipients. It is not known if the foundation for the increased risk of hepatic artery thrombosis in PSC patients (8.6% vs. 1.6% in non-PSC recipients[91]) is due to hematologic (e.g., the antiphospholipid antibodies frequently observed in PSC), vascular/surgical, or immunologic/infectious factors. In a recent series of 798 adult liver transplant recipients (of whom 127 were diagnosed with PSC),[93] PSC patients had the highest cumulative frequency of non–skin cancers of 6%, 10%, and 22% at 1, 5, and 10 years, respectively. Although PSC patients with IBD experienced a 3.5-fold increased risk for gastrointestinal cancers, other cancers were also increased. At 12 years follow-up, 19 of the 127 PSC patients had developed skin malignancies and 27 had developed non–skin malignancies (8 gastrointestinal, 6 hematologic, 3 lung, 3 breast, 2 kidney, and 2 other/metastatic). Yearly colonoscopy of transplanted PSC patients with IBD is recommended. Preemptive colectomy to bypass the risk of colorectal neoplasia is not yet advocated because posttransplant colectomy does not adversely affect outcome.

Assessing posttransplant biliary complications in patients with PSC is difficult. First, most of the patients will have a Roux-en-Y choledochojejunostomy rather than regular end-to-end anastomosis. This means that for imaging and intervention by ERC, access is only available via double-balloon endoscopy. For this reason, along with the desire to minimize surgery, some authors have advocated for a choledochoduodenostomy to be performed during liver transplantation in PSC, but studies are needed to assess long-term outcome by this approach. Second, distinguishing the many causes of biliary strictures (e.g., ischemia attributable to hepatic artery insufficiency, extended graft ischemic time and preservation injuries, ABO incompatibility, chronic rejection, live donor transplantation, ascending infections, PSC recurrence) is often challenging. Several of the causes may be present simultaneously; therefore determining the presence of recurrent PSC (rPSC) solely on the exclusion of other causes will lead to an underestimation of this important problem in post–liver transplantation follow-up in PSC, as first reported in 1998.

Depending to some extent on which diagnostic criteria are applied, the prevalence of rPSC following liver transplantation varies between 15% and 30%. The median time to diagnosis

Table 42-8 Definition of Recurrent Primary Sclerosing Cholangitis Following Liver Transplantation

1. Confirmed diagnosis of PSC before liver transplantation
2. Cholangiographic or histologic features compatible with recurrent PSC:
    A. Intrahepatic and/or extrahepatic biliary stricturing, beading, and irregularity >90 days following liver transplantation
    B. Fibrous cholangitis and/or fibroobliterative lesions with or without ductopenia, biliary fibrosis, or biliary cirrhosis
3. Appropriate exclusion of hepatic artery thrombosis/stenosis, established ductopenic rejection, anastomotic strictures alone, nonanastomotic strictures before posttransplant day 90, and ABO incompatibility between donor and recipient

Reprinted with permission from Graziadei IW, et al. Recurrence of primary sclerosing cholangitis following liver transplantation. Hepatology 1999;29: 1050–1056.

following liver transplantation for PSC is typically 3 to 5 years. Diagnostic criteria for rPSC were established in 1999 (**Table 42-8**).[94] Most often, relatively unspecific cholangiographic features similar to those of pretransplant PSC can be found. In terms of histologic features, posttransplant histologic findings of PSC patients have been compared with those of non-PSC patients both with and without Roux-en-Y biliary anastomoses.[95] Biliary obstruction was found in all patient groups, whereas fibrous cholangitis and fibroobliterative lesions were almost exclusively detected among patients with rPSC. A histologic distinction of rPSC versus chronic rejection was proposed by Demetris in 2006.[96] Whereas ductular reaction and ductular proliferation along with a mixed portal inflammatory infiltrate involving neutrophils, positive copper staining, and bile infarcts were often found in patients with rPSC, ductopenia along with perivenular lymphoplasmacytic inflammation, fibrosis, and often destruction of the peribiliary plexus were typical findings in patients with chronic rejection. However, because no features are diagnostic for rPSC, the diagnosis ultimately is that of a compound clinical decision.

A variety of different risk factors for the recurrence of PSC have been proposed, all of them only detected in one or a few studies each. The most consistent risk factor seems to be the presence of acute rejections, as also reflected by an association with the use of OKT3. However, prolonged corticosteroid administration does not seem to protect against rPSC.[92,94] Male sex and sex donor-recipient mismatch may also influence risk of rPSC. From a pathogenetic point of view, the association with an intact colon and use of maintenance steroids for UC following liver transplantation may allude to an influence from colonic inflammatory activity on the occurrence of rPSC.[97] The role of HLA matching and HLA genes is not defined. An association with the primary biliary cirrhosis associated HLA-DRB1*08 variant, which is not found in PSC alone, has been reported. Also, there is an increased frequency of biliary complications in patients undergoing liver transplantation homozygous for the PSC-associated HLA-C1 variant.[27] Importantly, HLA or other genetic factors may even prove detrimental, as suggested by recent studies proposing an increased risk of rPSC in living donor recipients, warranting further studies on this topic.[98] The role of ursodeoxycholic

acid in preventing or treating rPSC has not yet been established. Further studies are clearly needed. Indeed, recurrent PSC may prove an ideal setting to study early events of PSC pathogenesis and early treatment effects. The development of PSC-like changes in a genetically dissimilar and healthy liver graft over 3 to 5 years is astonishing, and further insight into the mechanisms behind these changes may in turn shed light on the development of PSC alone.

Treatment of Inflammatory Bowel Disease in Patients with Primary Sclerosing Cholangitis

In principle, medical treatment of IBD in PSC follows the same guidelines as those employed for IBD without PSC. However, despite more extensive disease, IBD in PSC generally requires less immunosuppression than regular IBD. Paradoxically, up to 50% to 60% of PSC patients with IBD experience an exacerbation after liver transplantation, and de novo IBD can occur at any time point following liver transplantation. Given the aggressive immunosuppression, these exacerbations are not easily explained in terms of immunologic mechanisms. A positive cytomegalovirus donor status and a negative recipient have been proposed to increase risk of IBD exacerbation, and cytomegalovirus infection should always be considered as a differential diagnosis in therapy-refractory colitis following liver transplantation. With regard to immunosuppressive regimens, tacrolimus seems to be associated with increased risk of IBD exacerbation, whereas cyclosporine, azathioprine, and corticosteroids seem to protect the patient from an increase in IBD severity.[99] Particularly, long-term continuation of corticosteroids may be advisable in patients with high pretransplant IBD activity, but no evidence-based recommendations can be given regarding the choice of immunosuppression following liver transplantation in patients with PSC and IBD. In refractory cases, proctocolectomy may be necessary.

Surgical treatment of IBD in PSC poses a particular challenge with regard to the risk of pouchitis following restorative proctocolectomy with ileal pouch-anal anastomosis (IPAA) versus the risk of stomal varices following ileostomy. Because IPAA avoids the risk of severe bleeding from stomal varices, it has been the surgical treatment of choice in patients with PSC and refractory IBD since the early 1990s. However, PSC patients undergoing IPAA seem to experience more perioperative complications (e.g., infections) than regular IBD patients. Furthermore, up to 43% to 79% of PSC patients with an IPAA develop chronic pouchitis as compared with 27% to 32% of IBD patients without PSC. For anatomic reasons it could be speculated that IPAA in PSC is related to the "backwash" ileitis found in many of the PSC patients with IBD (see earlier). Immunosuppressive therapy, however, is generally of limited value in controlling the pouchitis. The usefulness of antibiotic therapy (e.g., metronidazole) may point to the importance of intestinal bacteria, but other mechanisms have also been speculated (e.g., related to bile acid reabsorption).

It has been proposed that low-dose ursodeoxycholic acid helps reduce the risk of colorectal carcinoma in PSC patients with long-standing extensive colitis (see earlier). No protective effects from 5-aminosalicylic acid prescriptions have been reported in PSC. In the recent practice guidelines from the European Association for the Study of the Liver, yearly colonoscopies were recommended in all patients with PSC and IBD.[49] Adherence of patients to this program, however, is difficult.

Treatment of Cholangiocarcinoma in Patients with Primary Sclerosing Cholangitis

Only surgical therapy may lead to long-term recurrence-free survival in cholangiocarcinoma. The median survival for cholangiocarcinoma in PSC without surgery is less than 6 months. The main factors precluding surgery in cholangiocarcinoma in PSC are delayed diagnosis, presence of multiple neoplastic foci along the bile ducts of the same patient, and presence of cirrhosis. In addition, a biliary-enteric anastomosis may further increase the risk of cholangitis and de novo cholangiocarcinoma for which these patients are already predisposed.[37] Although resection should be considered in selected patients, the long-term results following resection of cholangiocarcinoma in PSC are dismal. In one of the largest series reported of only nine PSC patients with resected cholangiocarcinoma, the 1-, 3-, and 5-year survival rates were 56%, 28%, and 0%, respectively.[59] For comparison, the 5-year survival rate following resection of cholangiocarcinoma without PSC ranges from 11% to 44%.[37] For all these reasons patients with PSC and potentially resectable cholangiocarcinomas will in most cases benefit from an evaluation for liver transplantation.

Based on 5-year survival rates ranging from zero to 18%, liver transplantation for intrahepatic cholangiocarcinoma is not recommended.[37] In selected patients with hilar cholangiocarcinoma,[37] a protocol of aggressive pretransplant (neoadjuvant) radiation, chemotherapy, and brachytherapy has been established at the Mayo Clinic.[100] By 2009 a total of 76 PSC patients with hilar cholangiocarcinoma had been selected and undergone transplantation according to this protocol, with a 5-year survival rate of approximately 80%. In this series patients without PSC ($n = 43$) have a considerably worse outcome, with a 5-year survival rate of approximately 60%. Reasons for this may include the following: patients with PSC had been followed more closely than non-PSC patients; PSC patients were younger than non-PSC patients; and possibly the pathophysiologic characteristics of cholangiocarcinoma in PSC affect patient outcome. For comparison, in an unselected series of 36 PSC patients with cholangiocarcinoma undergoing liver transplantation, a 5-year survival rate of 35% was found.[89] The relative role of patient selection versus effects from neoadjuvant therapy needs to be further explored, but most likely liver transplantation for cholangiocarcinoma will become an increasingly important therapeutic option, particularly if diagnosis can be made at earlier stages.

Palliative endoscopic therapy plays an important role in cases where curative resection or liver transplantation is not possible. The goals of endoscopic therapy are relief of jaundice and pruritus, prevention of cholangitis, and avoidance of hepatic failure caused by progressive biliary obstruction. It seems that even unilateral drainage via plastic or metal stenting may suffice to accomplish these goals in patients with hilar cholangiocarcinoma. Endoscopic laser illumination following intravenous administration of a photosensitizer that accumulates in neoplastic tissue (a process called

photodynamic therapy) has been shown to significantly improve median survival, cholestasis, and quality of life in patients with cholangiocarcinoma. Importantly, marked effects were evident even in patients with inadequate response to biliary stenting alone, signifying that photodynamic therapy may prove a useful supplement to palliation by stenting.[37]

Concluding Remarks

Despite increased knowledge related to several aspects of PSC obtained during the last 3 decades, many important questions remain unanswered. Further studies of genetic susceptibility and the molecular pathogenesis of PSC are likely to yield an explanation for the heterogeneity of the patients and the close link with IBD. We anticipate that further exploration of disease mechanisms may lead to precise classification of different subtypes of PSC and possibly also to the design of therapeutic strategies for these subtypes. The development of tools for early diagnosis of PSC may prove crucial, because the stage at which the biliary pathology is now diagnosed may prove irreversible. Furthermore, sensitive and specific markers for the prediction and diagnosis of cholangiocarcinoma are urgently needed to allow for curative liver transplantation. While still awaiting effective medical therapy, further insight into the underlying mechanisms for the wide variability in disease severity between patients may simplify the prediction of prognosis and timing of liver transplantation in PSC. Given the young age of patients affected by this disease, the severity of the condition, and the risk of cancer, we believe that further research into all these topics should be considered a major challenge within hepatology.

References

1. Wiesner RH, LaRusso NF. Clinicopathologic features of the syndrome of primary sclerosing cholangitis. Gastroenterology 1980;79:200–206.
2. Chapman RW, et al. Primary sclerosing cholangitis: a review of its clinical features, cholangiography, and hepatic histology. Gut 1980;21:870–877.
3. Schrumpf E, et al. Sclerosing cholangitis in ulcerative colitis. Scand J Gastroenterol 1980;15:689–697.
4. Wee A, et al. Hepatobiliary carcinoma associated with primary sclerosing cholangitis and chronic ulcerative colitis. Hum Pathol 1985;16:719–726.
5. Soetikno RM, et al. Increased risk of colorectal neoplasia in patients with primary sclerosing cholangitis and ulcerative colitis: a meta-analysis. Gastrointest Endosc 2002;56:48–54.
6. Boberg KM, et al. Incidence and prevalence of primary biliary cirrhosis, primary sclerosing cholangitis, and autoimmune hepatitis in a Norwegian population. Scand J Gastroenterol 1998;33:99–103.
7. Broome U, et al. Liver disease in ulcerative colitis: an epidemiological and follow up study in the county of Stockholm. Gut 1994;35:84–89.
8. Mendes FD, et al. Abnormal hepatic biochemistries in patients with inflammatory bowel disease. Am J Gastroenterol 2007;102:344–350.
9. Bungay HK, et al. Prevalence and determinants of primary sclerosing cholangitis in a cohort of patients with inflammatory bowel disease and normal liver function tests. Gut 2008;57(Suppl 1):A107.
10. Schrumpf E, et al. Hepatobiliary complications of inflammatory bowel disease. Semin Liver Dis 1988;8:201–209.
11. Loftus EV Jr, et al. PSC-IBD: a unique form of inflammatory bowel disease associated with primary sclerosing cholangitis. Gut 2005;54:91–96.
12. Joo M, et al. Pathologic features of ulcerative colitis in patients with primary sclerosing cholangitis: a case-control study. Am J Surg Pathol 2009;33:854–862.
13. Broome U, et al. Primary sclerosing cholangitis and ulcerative colitis: evidence for increased neoplastic potential. Hepatology 1995;22:1404–1408.
14. Karlsen TH, Schrumpf E, Boberg KM. Gallbladder polyps in primary sclerosing cholangitis: not so benign. Curr Opin Gastroenterol 2008;24:395–399.

15. Boberg KM, et al. Cholangiocarcinoma in primary sclerosing cholangitis: risk factors and clinical presentation. Scand J Gastroenterol 2002;37: 1205–1211.

16. Broomé U, Lindberg G, Lofberg R. Primary sclerosing cholangitis in ulcerative colitis—a risk factor for the development of dysplasia and DNA aneuploidy? Gastroenterology 1992;102:1877–1880.

17. Ludwig J. Small-duct primary sclerosing cholangitis. Semin Liver Dis 1991;11:11–17.

18. Boberg KM, et al. Features of autoimmune hepatitis in primary sclerosing cholangitis: an evaluation of 114 primary sclerosing cholangitis patients according to a scoring system for the diagnosis of autoimmune hepatitis. Hepatology 1996;23:1369–1376.

19. Gregorio GV, et al. Autoimmune hepatitis/sclerosing cholangitis overlap syndrome in childhood: a 16-year prospective study. Hepatology 2001;33: 544–553.

20. Webster GJ, Pereira SP, Chapman RW. Autoimmune pancreatitis/IgG4-associated cholangitis and primary sclerosing cholangitis—overlapping or separate diseases? J Hepatol 2009;51:398–402.

21. Nishimori I, Otsuki M. Autoimmune pancreatitis and IgG4-associated sclerosing cholangitis. Best Pract Res Clin Gastroenterol 2009;23:11–23.

22. Saarinen S, Olerup O, Broome U. Increased frequency of autoimmune diseases in patients with primary sclerosing cholangitis. Am J Gastroenterol 2000;95:3195–3199.

23. Karlsen TH, et al. Genome-wide association analysis in primary sclerosing cholangitis. Gastroenterology 2010;138:1102–1111.

24. Schrumpf E, et al. HLA antigens and immunoregulatory T cells in ulcerative colitis associated with hepatobiliary disease. Scand J Gastroenterol 1982;17:187–191.

25. Spurkland A, et al. HLA class II haplotypes in primary sclerosing cholangitis patients from five European populations. Tissue Antigens 1999; 53:459–469.

26. Karlsen TH, et al. Particular genetic variants of ligands for natural killer cell receptors may contribute to the HLA associated risk of primary sclerosing cholangitis. J Hepatol 2007;46:899–906.

27. Hanvesakul R, et al. Donor HLA-C genotype has a profound impact on the clinical outcome following liver transplantation. Am J Transplant 2008;8:1931–1941.

28. Adams DH, Eksteen B. Aberrant homing of mucosal T cells and extra-intestinal manifestations of inflammatory bowel disease. Nat Rev Immunol 2006;6:244–251.

29. Hov JR, Boberg KM, Karlsen TH. Autoantibodies in primary sclerosing cholangitis. World J Gastroenterol 2008;14:3781–3791.

30. Lichtman SN, et al. Biliary tract disease in rats with experimental small bowel bacterial overgrowth. Hepatology 1991;13:766–772.

31. Karrar A, et al. Biliary epithelial cell antibodies link adaptive and innate immune responses in primary sclerosing cholangitis. Gastroenterology 2007;132:1504–1514.

32. Rudolph G, et al. Influence of dominant bile duct stenoses and biliary infections on outcome in primary sclerosing cholangitis. J Hepatol 2009;51: 149–155.

33. Beuers U. Drug insight: mechanisms and sites of action of ursodeoxycholic acid in cholestasis. Nat Clin Pract Gastroenterol Hepatol 2006;3:318–328.

34. Staudinger JL, et al. The nuclear receptor PXR is a lithocholic acid sensor that protects against liver toxicity. Proc Natl Acad Sci USA 2001;98: 3369–3374.

35. Karlsen TH, et al. Polymorphisms in the steroid and xenobiotic receptor gene influence survival in primary sclerosing cholangitis. Gastroenterology 2006;131:781–787.

36. Fleming KA, et al. Biliary dysplasia as a marker of cholangiocarcinoma in primary sclerosing cholangitis. J Hepatol 2001;34:360–365.

37. Blechacz B, Gores GJ. Cholangiocarcinoma: advances in pathogenesis, diagnosis, and treatment. Hepatology 2008;48:308–321.

38. Kipp BR, et al. A comparison of routine cytology and fluorescence in situ hybridization for the detection of malignant bile duct strictures. Am J Gastroenterol 2004;99:1675–1681.

39. Kobayashi S, et al. Interleukin-6 contributes to Mcl-1 up-regulation and TRAIL resistance via an Akt-signaling pathway in cholangiocarcinoma cells. Gastroenterology 2005;128:2054–2065.

40. Isomoto H. Epigenetic alterations associated with cholangiocarcinoma (review). Oncol Rep 2009;22:227–232.

41. Melum E, et al. Cholangiocarcinoma in primary sclerosing cholangitis is associated with NKG2D polymorphisms. Hepatology 2008;47:90–96.

42. Porayko MK, et al. Patients with asymptomatic primary sclerosing cholangitis frequently have progressive disease. Gastroenterology 1990;98: 1594–1602.

43. Boberg KM, et al. Time-dependent Cox regression model is superior in prediction of prognosis in primary sclerosing cholangitis. Hepatology 2002;35:652–657.

44. Tischendorf JJ, et al. Characterization, outcome, and prognosis in 273 patients with primary sclerosing cholangitis: a single center study. Am J Gastroenterol 2007;102:107–114.

45. Aadland E, et al. Primary sclerosing cholangitis: a long-term follow-up study. Scand J Gastroenterol 1987;22:655–664.

46. Alvarez F, et al. International Autoimmune Hepatitis Group Report: review of criteria for diagnosis of autoimmune hepatitis. J Hepatol 1999;3129–938.

47. Brandt DJ, et al. Gallbladder disease in patients with primary sclerosing cholangitis. AJR Am J Roentgenol 1988;150:571–574.

48. Berstad AE, et al. Diagnostic accuracy of magnetic resonance and endoscopic retrograde cholangiography in primary sclerosing cholangitis. Clin Gastroenterol Hepatol 2006;4:514–520.

49. EASL Clinical Practice Guidelines: management of cholestatic liver diseases. J Hepatol 2009;51:237–267.

50. Gluck M, et al. A twenty-year experience with endoscopic therapy for symptomatic primary sclerosing cholangitis. J Clin Gastroenterol 2008;42: 1032–1039.

51. Angulo P, et al. Magnetic resonance cholangiography in patients with biliary disease: its role in primary sclerosing cholangitis. J Hepatol 2000;33: 520–527.

52. Burak KW, Angulo P, Lindor KD. Is there a role for liver biopsy in primary sclerosing cholangitis? Am J Gastroenterol 2003;98:1155–1158.

53. Ludwig J. Surgical pathology of the syndrome of primary sclerosing cholangitis. Am J Surg Pathol 1989;13(Suppl 1):43–49.

54. Kim WR, et al. A revised natural history model for primary sclerosing cholangitis. Mayo Clin Proc 2000;75:688–694.

55. Ludwig J, et al. Intrahepatic cholangiectases and large-duct obliteration in primary sclerosing cholangitis. Hepatology 1986;6:560–568.

56. Johnson KJ, Olliff JF, Olliff SP. The presence and significance of lymphadenopathy detected by CT in primary sclerosing cholangitis. Br J Radiol 1998;71:1279–1282.

57. Chalasani N, et al. Cholangiocarcinoma in patients with primary sclerosing cholangitis: a multicenter case-control study. Hepatology 2000;31:7–11.

58. Blechacz BR, Sanchez W, Gores GJ. A conceptual proposal for staging ductal cholangiocarcinoma. Curr Opin Gastroenterol 2009;25:238–239.

59. Ahrendt SA, et al. Diagnosis and management of cholangiocarcinoma in primary sclerosing cholangitis. J Gastrointest Surg 1999;3:357–367; discussion 367–368.

60. Rosen CB, et al. Cholangiocarcinoma complicating primary sclerosing cholangitis. Ann Surg 1991;213:21–25.

61. Ramage JK, et al. Serum tumor markers for the diagnosis of cholangiocarcinoma in primary sclerosing cholangitis. Gastroenterology 1995;108:865–869.

62. Levy C, et al. The value of serum CA 19-9 in predicting cholangiocarcinomas in patients with primary sclerosing cholangitis. Dig Dis Sci 2005;50:1734–1740.

63. Baron TH, et al. A prospective comparison of digital image analysis and routine cytology for the identification of malignancy in biliary tract strictures. Clin Gastroenterol Hepatol 2004;2:214–219.

64. Boberg KM, et al. Diagnostic benefit of biliary brush cytology in cholangiocarcinoma in primary sclerosing cholangitis. J Hepatol 2006;45: 568–574.

65. Campbell WL, et al. Using CT and cholangiography to diagnose biliary tract carcinoma complicating primary sclerosing cholangitis. AJR Am J Roentgenol 2001;177:1095–1100.

66. Charatcharoenwitthaya P, et al. Utility of serum tumor markers, imaging, and biliary cytology for detecting cholangiocarcinoma in primary sclerosing cholangitis. Hepatology 2008;48:1106–1117.

67. Tischendorf JJ, et al. Cholangioscopic characterization of dominant bile duct stenoses in patients with primary sclerosing cholangitis. Endoscopy 2006;38:665–669.

68. Tischendorf JJ, et al. Transpapillary intraductal ultrasound in the evaluation of dominant bile duct stenoses in patients with primary sclerosing cholangitis. Scand J Gastroenterol 2007;42:1011–1017.

69. Abdalian R, Heathcote EJ. Sclerosing cholangitis: a focus on secondary causes. Hepatology 2006;44:1063–1074.

70. Hennes EM, et al. Simplified criteria for the diagnosis of autoimmune hepatitis. Hepatology 2008;48:169–176.

71. Kaya M, Angulo P, Lindor KD. Overlap of autoimmune hepatitis and primary sclerosing cholangitis: an evaluation of a modified scoring system. J Hepatol 2000;33:537–542.

72. Lindor KD, et al. High-dose ursodeoxycholic acid for the treatment of primary sclerosing cholangitis. Hepatology 2009;50:808–814.

73. Rost D, et al. Effect of high-dose ursodeoxycholic acid on its biliary enrichment in primary sclerosing cholangitis. Hepatology 2004;40:693–698.

74. Beuers U, et al. Ursodeoxycholic acid for treatment of primary sclerosing cholangitis: a placebo-controlled trial. Hepatology 1992;16:707–714.

75. Lindor KD. Ursodiol for primary sclerosing cholangitis. Mayo Primary Sclerosing Cholangitis–Ursodeoxycholic Acid Study Group. New Engl J Med 1997;336:691–695.

76. Olsson R, et al. High-dose ursodeoxycholic acid in primary sclerosing cholangitis: a 5-year multicenter, randomized, controlled study. Gastroenterology 2005;129:1464–1472.

77. Tung BY, et al. Ursodiol use is associated with lower prevalence of colonic neoplasia in patients with ulcerative colitis and primary sclerosing cholangitis. Ann Intern Med 2001;134:89–95.

78. Pardi DS, et al. Ursodeoxycholic acid as a chemopreventive agent in patients with ulcerative colitis and primary sclerosing cholangitis. Gastroenterology 2003;124:889–893.

79. Sjoqvist U, et al. Ursodeoxycholic acid treatment in IBD-patients with colorectal dysplasia and/or DNA-aneuploidy: a prospective, double-blind, randomized controlled pilot study. Anticancer Res 2004;24:3121–3127.

80. Cullen SN, Chapman RW. The medical management of primary sclerosing cholangitis. Semin Liver Dis 2006;26:52–61.

81. Ghazale A, et al. Immunoglobulin G4–associated cholangitis: clinical profile and response to therapy. Gastroenterology 2008;134:706–715.

82. Mistilis SP, Skyring AP, Goulston SJ. Effect of long-term tetracycline therapy, steroid therapy and colectomy in pericholangitis associated with ulcerative colitis. Australas Ann Med 1965;14:286–294.

83. Färkkilä M, et al. Metronidazole and ursodeoxycholic acid for primary sclerosing cholangitis: a randomized placebo-controlled trial. Hepatology 2004;40:1379–1386.

84. Stiehl A. Primary sclerosing cholangitis: the role of endoscopic therapy. Semin Liver Dis 2006;26:62–68.

85. Ponsioen CY, et al. Four years experience with short term stenting in primary sclerosing cholangitis. Am J Gastroenterol 1999;94:2403–2407.

86. Bjoro K, et al. Liver transplantation in primary sclerosing cholangitis. Semin Liver Dis 2006;26:69–79.

87. Brandsaeter B, et al. Liver transplantation for primary sclerosing cholangitis in the Nordic countries: outcome after acceptance to the waiting list. Liver Transpl 2003;961–969.

88. Broome U, Bergquist A. Primary sclerosing cholangitis. In: Boyer T, Manns M, Sanyal AJ, editors. Zakim & Boyer's hepatology: a textbook of liver disease, 5th ed. Philadelphia: Elsevier, 2006: 821–854.

89. Brandsaeter B, et al. Liver transplantation for primary sclerosing cholangitis; predictors and consequences of hepatobiliary malignancy. J Hepatol 2004;40:815–822.

90. Bjoro K, Schrumpf E. Liver transplantation for primary sclerosing cholangitis. J Hepatol 2004;40:570–577.

91. Graziadei IW, et al. Long-term results of patients undergoing liver transplantation for primary sclerosing cholangitis. Hepatology 1999;30: 1121–1127.

92. Kugelmas M, et al. Different immunosuppressive regimens and recurrence of primary sclerosing cholangitis after liver transplantation. Liver Transpl 2003;9:727–732.

93. Watt KD, et al. Long-term probability of and mortality from de-novo malignancy after liver transplantation. Gastroenterology 2009;137: 2010–2017.

94. Graziadei IW, et al. Recurrence of primary sclerosing cholangitis following liver transplantation. Hepatology 1999;29:1050–1056.

95. Harrison RF, et al. Fibrous and obliterative cholangitis in liver allografts: evidence of recurrent primary sclerosing cholangitis? Hepatology 1994;20: 356–361.

96. Demetris AJ. Distinguishing between recurrent primary sclerosing cholangitis and chronic rejection. Liver Transpl 2006;12(11 Suppl 2) :S68–72.

97. Alabraba E, et al. A re-evaluation of the risk factors for the recurrence of primary sclerosing cholangitis in liver allografts. Liver Transpl 2009;15: 330–340.

98. Tamura S, et al. The urgent need for evaluating recurrent primary sclerosing cholangitis in living donor liver transplantation. Liver Transpl 2009;15:1383–1384; author reply 1385.

99. Haagsma EB, et al. Inflammatory bowel disease after liver transplantation: the effect of different immunosuppressive regimens. Aliment Pharmacol Ther 2003;18:33–44.

100. Heimbach JK, et al. Liver transplantation for perihilar cholangiocarcinoma after aggressive neoadjuvant therapy: a new paradigm for liver and biliary malignancies? Surgery 2006;140:331–334.

Overlap Syndromes

G.M. Hirschfield and E.J. Heathcote

ABBREVIATIONS

AIH autoimmune hepatitis
ALP alkaline phosphatase
ALT alanine aminotransferase
AMA antimitochondrial antibody
ANA antinuclear antibody
ASC autoimmune sclerosing cholangitis
AST aspartate aminotransferase
PBC primary biliary cirrhosis
PSC primary sclerosing cholangitis
SMA smooth muscle antibody
UDCA ursodeoxycholic acid
ULN upper limit of normal

Introduction

Although combinations of clinical, biochemical, histologic, immunologic, and cholangiographic criteria do help to discriminate the major autoimmune liver diseases, individual components lack specificity. An intrinsic scope for overlap and "mistaken identity" is therefore present and there is frequently a temptation to apply the term overlap syndrome to patients with autoimmune liver disease. This term, however, should be applied sparingly and only when referring to the small number of patients who have clear features, predominantly histologic and radiologic as opposed to just serologic, either concurrently or sequentially of two autoimmune liver diseases. Lack of well-defined and accepted definitions, as well as prospectively followed cohorts, limits natural history studies, and debate remains as to whether these entities reflect simply the extremes of one disease or separate disease processes. Coincidental overlaps, most commonly viral hepatitis with autoimmune liver disease, are simply accidental, and their presence is largely related to the relative prevalence of viral liver disease in the population at risk.

The Dynamic Nature of Autoimmune Liver Disease

To fully appreciate the spectrum of autoimmune liver disease one must first remember that many patients are asymptomatic, and if symptomatic the symptoms need not necessarily be specific to liver disease. Second, liver biochemical measurements can be normal in the face of abnormal histologic or imaging studies, as well as fluctuate over time and/or be masked by treatment. Third, these diseases are more often chronic with very long clinical courses. Because autoimmune liver disease rarely has absolute diagnostic tests, any evaluation must be made by considering a composite of the history and physical examination in conjunction with biochemical, serologic/immunologic, and histologic features and reviewing the patient's response to therapy. This appraisal must be longitudinal and not just a single moment in time. Awareness of the challenges faced in interpreting histologic and radiologic data is essential, because it is an attempt to appreciate the limits of what is considered acceptable for a disease. Thus although bile duct destruction is generally not prominent in autoimmune hepatitis (AIH), approximately 10% of biopsies may show duct destruction, and an additional ≈10% show lymphocytic infiltration of bile duct epithelium without ductopenia.[1,2] Conversely, perhaps as many as 10% of patients with primary biliary cirrhosis (PBC) will appear at least clinically to have an AIH overlap.[3,4] Similarly, when dedicated liver magnetic resonance imaging (MRI) and liver histologic studies are evaluated in adults with AIH, as many as 12% may have detectable cholangiopathies according to one study.[5] In children the limits of disease appear to blur further, with upwards of half of those with clinical AIH having abnormal cholangiograms.[6]

Differential Diagnosis

In any patient with a chronic liver disease it is important to consider numerous possible explanations for disease etiology before entertaining an autoimmune foundation and especially before invoking the presence of an overlap. Because the presence of unexpected interface activity or the observation of biliary changes on biopsy is what commonly triggers the concern for overlap, recognition that drugs can cause such change is relevant, although this is rarely addressed in published case series. Potential agents may include prescribed medications (e.g., amoxicillin, clavulanic acid, "statins," ramipril) or herbal preparations.[7-9] In the case of cholestasis in AIH, one cause is the introduction of exogenous hormones such as the contraceptive pill, hormone replacement therapy, or testosterone. Treatment with hormones may induce symptomatic or asymptomatic cholestasis, but importantly without duct injury. Duct injury but not duct loss occasionally occurs in cases of otherwise typical AIH (however, once again without reported drug histories).[1] The temporal association between liver biochemical measurements and drug use must therefore always be carefully noted. In individuals with primary sclerosing cholangitis (PSC) it is not unusual to see fluctuating levels of serum aminotransferases. This may be related to common duct stones, the presence of sludge, or a resolving episode of bacterial cholangitis. Thus overlap with AIH should not be considered until the appropriate investigations have been performed and a longer-term perspective is available.

Autoantibodies in Serum of Patients with Liver Disease

When evaluating patients it should not be assumed that each facet of the investigation carries equal weight in reaching a diagnosis; for example, histologic and imaging studies are generally more important than biochemical and serologic evaluations. Serologic imprecision in liver disease is inevitable and reflects a combination of the component being evaluated by a specific autoantibody assay as well as the methodology applied.[10] Autoimmune serologic studies generally lack specificity for single diseases; in a patient with liver disease the temptation to associate the finding of autoantibodies in serum with the presence of autoimmune liver disease must be tempered by the fact that many individuals who have liver disease that is clearly not autoimmune in origin (e.g., alcoholic hepatitis) and chronic hepatitis C will test positive for the non–organ-specific and non–species-specific autoantibodies, including antinuclear antibody (ANA) or smooth muscle antibody (SMA).[11-13] These same autoantibodies may be detected in 2% to 14% of perfectly healthy individuals; the older the individual, the higher this value. Transient findings of so-called disease-specific antibodies can also be recognized (e.g., antimitochondrial antibody [AMA] in acute liver failure).[14] Thus their presence in the sera of individuals with liver disease does not necessarily indicate an autoimmune basis for the underlying disease. Furthermore, some patients may have classic features of one disease (autoimmune hepatitis on biopsy or sclerosing cholangitis on cholangiography) and yet have autoimmune serologic results that are more closely associated with alternative autoimmune liver disease. This alone is insufficient to justify the use of the term "overlap".

AMA-Positive Autoimmune Hepatitis

Patients with all the features of autoimmune hepatitis may be persistently AMA positive. The report by Kenny and colleagues[15] noted that AMAs, when detected in the sera of patients thought to have AIH, tended to be of low titer and sometimes were really microsomal antibodies rather than mitochondrial antibodies. This confusion arises because anti-LKM1 antibodies (markers of type 2 AIH) stain similarly by immunofluorescence and may therefore be confused with AMAs. Nevertheless, AMA is probably found in fewer than 10% of those with AIH. It is not synonymous with a PBC overlap, and in one long-term cohort single center study of AMA-positive patients with AIH, none had any histologic features suggestive of PBC.[16] These patients with overt AIH who test positive for AMAs at initial presentation and who were treated conventionally with steroids did not show clinical or histologic evidence of PBC despite the continued detection of AMAs over a long-term follow-up study.

AMA-Negative Primary Biliary Cirrhosis

In 1987 Brunner and Klinge[17] described three women who had clinical, histologic, and biochemical criteria for PBC but who all tested AMA negative and instead had high-titer ANAs. All were given treatment with immunosuppressive therapy, and at least in the short term an improvement was seen. They were given a diagnosis of immune cholangitis. Michielleti and colleagues[18] later described 17 patients referred for a randomized controlled trial of the efficacy of ursodeoxycholic acid (UDCA) for PBC treatment; these patients consistently tested negative for AMA by both immunofluorescence and immunoblotting, but otherwise had all the clinical, biochemical, and histologic features of PBC. These patients also all tested positive for ANA, generally in high titer. Subsequently, several other series of AMA-negative individuals, all of whom appeared to have PBC but tested positive in high titer for ANAs, were reported. These cases all had higher levels of IgG and lower levels of IgM, and somewhat higher serum aminotransferase levels than their AMA-positive counterparts; however, as a whole, liver histologic results showed the typical histologic features of PBC, and such patients are now recognized as having AMA-negative PBC. Subsequently, a study by Kim[19] reported that the response to UDCA in terms of changes in liver biochemistry was no different in AMA-negative PBC compared with AMA-positive PBC. The natural history of AMA-negative PBC is similar to that of AMA-positive PBC,[20] and to date one difference possibly appears to be their HLA associations. Whereas class II HLA DR8 is predominant in AMA-positive PBC, this was not the case in AMA-negative PBC.[21] The presence of ANA is very common in this setting, and specific ANA patterns on immunofluorescence are indeed characteristic. The immunofluorescence patterns for PBC-specific ANAs are described as either perinuclear/rimlike or multiple nuclear dot pattern.[22,23] The rimlike pattern results from autoantibodies directed against constituents of the nuclear envelope including gp210, a 210-kiladalton (kDa) transmembrane glycoprotein of the nuclear pore complex, lamin B receptor, and nucleoporin p62. The multiple nuclear dot pattern is caused by autoantibodies against two autoantigens that co-localize: sp100 and promyelocytic leukemia protein. ANAs reacting with gp210 occur in 10% to 40% of patients with AMA positivity and in up to 50% of patients with AMA-negative PBC, and are therefore an appropriate second-line investigation in this group of individuals. Thus although variations exist in the immunologic profiles of these patients, clinically there are no discernible differences of note, and although the diagnostic threshold is higher (i.e., liver biopsy is usually required), the treatment and prognosis mirror those of classic PBC. Previous terminology has therefore been abandoned in favor of the description AMA-negative primary biliary cirrhosis.

Primary Biliary Cirrhosis–Autoimmune Hepatitis Overlap Syndromes

There is rarely any confusion about making a diagnosis of PBC. Thus in the absence of any other extrinsic factor the combination of positive AMA and an elevated level of alkaline phosphatase (ALP) in a woman with or without symptoms of cholestasis is sufficient for the diagnosis of PBC. Liver histologic analysis confirms the diagnosis and assists with establishing a prognosis, but a liver biopsy is not considered essential to make a diagnosis of PBC.[24] The concept of AMA-positive PBC with overlapping features of AIH has arisen because some patients given a primary diagnosis of PBC have a greater elevation of serum transaminase levels than expected, usually arbitrarily defined as an aspartate aminotransferase/alanine aminotransferase (AST/ALT) ratio of greater than five times the upper limit of normal (ULN) (**Table 43-1**). This appreciation dates back many years. Before AMAs were identified as a hallmark for PBC, it had been recognized that certain individuals thought to have "postnecrotic cirrhosis" had additional features of cholestasis. Once endoscopic retrograde cholangiopancreatography (ERCP) became available, some of these individuals were found to have PSC. Others were found to test positive for AMA despite features of co-existent "hepatitis." In 1976 Geubel and colleagues[25] from the Mayo Clinic described 125 individuals given a diagnosis of severe chronic active hepatitis, 15 of whom had shown a poor response to immunosuppressive therapy. Other features that distinguished these poor responders were a high ALP/AST ratio, high IgM level, the presence of pruritus, and the presence of AMA in serum. In addition, the histologic analysis indicated that the patients who failed to respond to immunosuppressive therapy never had evidence of bridging necrosis. The degree of bile duct damage, cholestasis, or granulomas did not distinguish responders from non-responders, although the non-responders did have significantly fewer interlobular bile ducts

in the portal tracts than the responders. The poor responders to corticosteroids represented 12% of their population with postnecrotic cirrhosis, and such patients were thought to represent an overlap with PBC.

Chazouilleres and associates[4] examined 130 patients given an initial diagnosis of PBC and found that 12% had features of autoimmune hepatitis. The autoimmune features these authors chose were a composite of ALT levels (>5 times ULN), serum IgG levels (>2 times ULN), or positive SMA and a liver biopsy that showed moderate to severe periportal and periseptal lymphocytic piecemeal necrosis. Subsequently, Talwalkar[26] from the Mayo Clinic scrutinized a similar number of cases of PBC for features of AIH by applying the revised AIH scoring system.[27] He was unable to find any patients with PBC who scored in the definite range for AIH, though he did find that 19% of their PBC population scored in the probable range. It should of course be recognized that in developing the revised AIH scoring system, one goal was to ensure scores distinguished patients with biliary disease as distinct.

Lohse and co-authors[28] reported a series of 20 patients diagnosed with PBC, 20 patients diagnosed with autoimmune hepatitis, and 20 patients given a diagnosis of an overlap of PBC and AIH, and compared the biochemical, immunologic, and histologic features of the three groups. The designation of overlap was applied in 14 patients because they tested positive for AMA but had an ALT level more than twice the upper limit of normal, and in 6 patients because they tested strongly positive for AMA and their liver histologic results showed features of both AIH and PBC. In their 20 cases of overt AIH, 1 tested positive for AMA but repeat testing by enzyme-linked immunosorbent assay (ELISA) was negative, whereas 16 of the 20 overlaps consistently tested positive for AMA by both immunofluorescence and ELISA, and all 20 patients given a primary diagnosis of PBC were AMA positive. From this heterogeneous population the authors concluded that those with overlap in their series had more features in common with PBC, particularly in terms of elevation of serum alkaline phosphatase and serum IgM levels. However, they did note that the HLA pattern was more typical of that seen in patients with AIH, namely, more cases with HLA DR3 and/or DR4, and so concluded that these patients indeed had a PBC–AIH overlap. For this retrospective study the therapy given to each patient was not standardized. Patients thought to have predominant AIH responded well to immunosuppressive therapy. Of the 20 patients diagnosed with an overlap syndrome, 16 were also given immunosuppressive therapy for a minimum of 2 years. In follow-up studies, serum aminotransferase levels improved, as did the alkaline phosphatase levels in 12 of these 16 patients, but all were also given additional UDCA. Of the 20 individuals given a primary diagnosis of PBC, 4 received immunosuppressive therapy, 2 with some biochemical benefit. The rest of this group was treated with UDCA, seven of whom had liver biochemical tests that returned to normal. No data beyond 2 years were presented and the numbers under study were small. Thus it cannot be said whether these treatments were appropriate or effective in the long term; nor do we know the natural history of these so-called overlaps. Because both corticosteroid therapy and UDCA can be associated with an improvement in liver biochemical tests in almost all forms of liver disease, response to these therapies cannot be considered specific.

Table 43-1 AIH, PBC, AIH–PBC Overlap—Laboratory and Histologic Features

LABORATORY	AIH	PBC	AIH/PBC OVERLAP
ALP	+	+++	++
ALT	+++	+	++
AMA	−	+++	++
ANA	+++	+	++
SMA	++	+	+
IgG	+++	+	++
IgM	−	++	+/−
Liver Histology			
Piecemeal necrosis	+++	−	++
Bile duct loss	−	+++	++

AIH, autoimmune hepatitis; ALP, alkaline phosphatase; ALT, alanine aminotransferase; AMA, antimitochondrial antibody; ANA, antinuclear antibody; Ig, immunoglobulin; PBC, primary biliary cirrhosis; SMA, smooth muscle antibody

Silveira and colleagues[29] from the Mayo Clinic studied longer-term outcomes by reviewing 135 patients with PBC according to the revised AIH score and identifying 26 patients with features of PBC–AIH overlap. Over more than 5 years of follow-up studies, they found statistically higher rates of portal hypertension, esophageal varices, gastrointestinal bleeding, and ascites in overlap patients, as well as greater rates of death and/or orthotopic liver transplantation. If these data were to be robustly validated by others, then the increased risk for a poorer outcome would overcome the concerns regarding use of additional immunosuppressive therapy.

Sequential Primary Biliary Cirrhosis and Autoimmune Hepatitis

There are case reports of patients who were first given a diagnosis of AMA-positive PBC with typical biochemical and histologic features that responded to UDCA treatment, and who subsequently showed a complete change in their symptomatology, biochemistry, and histology, changing to autoimmune hepatitis, even with loss of AMA.[30,31] Only when treatment with immunosuppressive therapy was introduced were the features of the AIH adequately controlled. Poupon and co-workers[32] reported a series of 12 patients with consecutive occurrence of PBC and AIH (i.e., PBC followed by AIH). Among 282 PBC patients, 39 were identified who fulfilled criteria for probable or definitive AIH. AIH developed in 12 patients (4.3%). The baseline characteristics of the patients were similar to those of patients with classic PBC. The time elapsed between the diagnosis of PBC and the diagnosis of AIH varied from 6 months to 13 years. In contrast, Gossard and associates[33] described 8 patients (from 1476 with PBC) who developed AIH (on biochemical and histologic parameters) after the diagnosis of PBC was made. Muratori and colleagues[34] have recently suggested that concomitant AMA/anti-dsDNA seropositivity can be considered the serologic profile of AIH–PBC overlaps. It will be important to see if other groups can replicate this observation.

Interestingly, the finding of a sequential overlap from AIH to PBC is apparently very uncommon, based on the lack of any robust reports in the literature.

Management of Autoimmune Hepatitis–Primary Biliary Cirrhosis Overlaps

It has been known for 30 years that immunosuppressive therapy effectively improves survival in patients with severe AIH, although demonstrating the benefit of immunosuppressive therapy in all patients is difficult.[35] The current standard of care for PBC is UDCA 15 mg/kg/day. This treatment leads to slowed progression of fibrosis and liver failure. Most would argue that treatment with UDCA increases survival free of liver transplantation, especially for those achieving a biochemical response, but all acknowledge that this treatment does not cure PBC.[24] UDCA has also been used effectively—at

least in the short term—in patients with mild AIH, but it is not advised in the long term or for individuals with severe AIH. Thus there is much debate about the appropriate management of AIH with overlapping features of PBC, and vice versa, and no definitive answer. Corpechot and colleagues[36] have shown that in their patients with PBC outcome is worse in those who show lymphocytic piecemeal necrosis from liver histologic analysis. They have advocated additional treatment with corticosteroid therapy in this patient population, but this has not been evaluated in a prospective manner. In a long-term (7½ years) cohort study, the French group[37] presented data on 17 patients with simultaneous PBC and AIH. They described their observational data to suggest that combination therapy with UDCA and immunosuppression is the best treatment option. However, it should be noted that by using clinical trial data, in a retrospective study of patients with PBC and features of overlapping AIH, no difference in survival was observed in those patients with features of AIH, compared with those with PBC alone, when randomized to treatment with UDCA or placebo.[38]

Patients with PBC are at increased risk for osteoporosis, both because of their chronic cholestasis and because many are postmenopausal. Thus the major concern if steroid therapy is prescribed to those with PBC with or without overlapping features of AIH is that it may promote further osteoporosis. The same concern pertains to the treatment of AIH with features of PBC. For those patients in whom corticosteroid therapy is considered essential it is important to make an accurate assessment of bone fracture risk (including the following in addition to steroid use and recorded bone density: age, gender, smoking status, and history of prior fractures) and to subsequently utilize prophylaxis as appropriate with agents such as bisphosphonates.

Autoimmune Hepatitis and Primary Sclerosing Cholangitis Overlaps

Generally it seems that interface hepatitis is a common denominator in autoimmune liver disease. Thus although there are few convincing reports[39,40] of overlap between the small bile duct disease PBC and the large bile duct disease PSC, patients presenting with an overlap of PSC with AIH are both more common and more convincing. Even though a precise distinction has not been established for the conclusion of childhood disease and the commencement of adult disease, it seems that the frequency of overlapping presentation is related to the age of the patient. It also remains important that before employing the term "primary" for patients with a radiologic pattern of sclerosing cholangitis, appropriate efforts are made to exclude secondary etiologies. In particular, IgG₄-associated disease should be ruled out. This is not an overlap syndrome but a different disease, with a wide spectrum of presentation and a different natural history.[41]

Children

In 1995 Wilschanski and colleagues[42] described the clinical presentations and outcomes of 32 children with radiologic evidence of PSC in a retrospective review. Of these 32 children, 9 were originally diagnosed as having autoimmune hepatitis and the others had isolated features typical of AIH.

Intrahepatic biliary disease predominated, with only 3 of 32 having common bile duct involvement. Of the nine children with overt autoimmune hepatitis and PSC, five (55.6%) subsequently required a liver transplant. In contrast, only 5 of the 22 (22.7%) with PSC and only minor features of AIH progressed to liver transplant. Hence overt AIH and PSC appeared to carry a worse prognosis. Perhaps also relevant was the older age at presentation of the overt AIH–PSC group. It may be that their worse prognosis was related to the fact that their liver disease had been present but clinically silent for many years before diagnosis. No specific features reliably predicted which children had the AIH–PSC overlap at the time of initial presentation. Coexisting inflammatory bowel disease was just as common in those with PSC and mild isolated features of AIH as in those with overt overlap. In addition, despite the presence of biliary tract disease in all patients, half the children had normal levels of serum alkaline phosphatase. HLA typing did not show any consistent pattern, but the sample size was very small.

About 6 years later, Gregorio and colleagues[6] described a 16-year prospective study of children who at presentation were all given a primary diagnosis of autoimmune hepatitis. Between 1984 and 1997, 76 children were referred with clinical and/or biochemical evidence of liver disease associated with the presence of serum autoantibodies. Of these 76, 21 (27.6%) were considered too ill to undergo radiologic investigation of their biliary tree and were excluded from the study. The remaining 55 were evaluated and met the revised autoimmune hepatitis scoring system criteria for a diagnosis of AIH. In addition, they all underwent radiologic investigation of the biliary tree at the time of presentation (median time between diagnosis of AIH and ERCP, 1.1 months). Of these children, 23 (41.8%) were found to have abnormal cholangiography, but the typical stricturing and beading pattern well described in adults with PSC was only observed in 2 children (9%). The most common abnormality was mucosal irregularity of the common bile duct, which was present in 15 (65%) patients. An abnormal pancreatic duct was observed in three (13%), and stones were detected in the common duct/cystic duct/gallbladder in two (9%). The authors referred to those with AIH and an abnormal biliary tree as having autoimmune sclerosing cholangitis (ASC). Follow-up cholangiography was performed from 1 to 9 years later in 36 patients, 17 of whom had previously been diagnosed with ASC. Of these 17 patients, 9 (52.9%) were found to have static disease and 8 (47.1%) had progressive intra- or extrahepatic bile duct abnormalities. Of the 28 who did not have ASC at initial presentation, 17 (60.7%) underwent repeat cholangiography and all but 1 remained with a normal endoscopic retrograde cholangiopancreatography (ERCP) a median of 6 years later. The one child who was shown to change from having a normal duct to having advanced intra- and extrahepatic disease did so 8 years after her original presentation with AIH, ulcerative colitis, and urticaria pigmentosa.

All 55 children were alive at the time of publication, but 4 had required a liver transplant, 3 of whom had ASC and the fourth ductopenia on liver biopsy. Thus, just as in the retrospective study by Wilschanski and associates,[42] overlap of AIH with cholangitis appears to have a poorer prognosis than AIH alone.

In both these pediatric studies there were very few clinical features at presentation that distinguished those children with the overlap of AIH plus biliary tract disease from those with isolated AIH. Gregorio and colleagues[6] found that inflammatory bowel disease was more common in those with ASC (12 children [44%]) than in those with AIH alone (5 children [18%]), whereas a family history of autoimmune disease was found more commonly (20 [71%]) in children with AIH alone than in those with ASC (10 [37%]). Similarly, there were very few laboratory features that distinguished these groups of children. Although the presence of the antineutrophil cytoplasmic autoantibody (ANCA) was significantly more common in those with ASC (74%), ANCA was also positive in 33% of those with only AIH. In both groups the parenchymal lesions seen on liver biopsy responded to steroids, but half of the patients with ASC, also treated with 10 to 15 mg/kg UDCA, showed progression of their bile duct disease on follow-up ERCP. Of great practical relevance is that the height of neither the serum alkaline phosphatase level nor the γ-glutamyltransferase (GGT) level at presentation distinguished these children in either study. Thus co-existing biliary tract disease must be either confirmed or eliminated in all children given a diagnosis of AIH or PSC.

The experience of a separate center supports many of these points: Miloh and co-authors published their experience of childhood PSC[43] and reported 47 pediatric patients with biliary disease, most of whom had inflammatory bowel disease (59%) or autoimmune overlap (25%). Levels of serum liver enzymes normalized after therapy with UDCA, including patients with positive autoimmune markers without histologic features of autoimmune hepatitis. The nine children with established AIH–PSC overlap received immunosuppression as well. Liver transplantation was performed in nine patients (three with overlap syndrome and two with small-duct PSC) at a median time of 7 years after diagnosis.

Adults

The coexistence of AIH and PSC appears to be much less common in adults than in children. There have been case reports[44,45] describing patients who appear to have both AIH and PSC simultaneously (**Figs. 43-1 and 43-2**). A large study by Boberg and associates[46] reviewed cases of proven PSC and calculated their AIH score. The results suggested that features of AIH were indeed common in their population with PSC. However, although the AIH score may be helpful in confirming a case of AIH, it has not been validated in individuals with mixed forms of autoimmune liver disease. To rectify this confusion, this AIH score was revised. With the updated criteria[27] the Mayo Clinic found that only 1.4% and 6% of patients with proven PSC had scores qualifying for definite and probable AIH, respectively.[47] However, using the same revised scoring system, a group from the Netherlands in a somewhat younger cohort of patients with PSC found 8% with a definite AIH score.[48]

Abdo and co-authors[49] published a case series of six adults with AIH in whom PSC was first documented later (mean, 4.6 years) by ERCP. These patients had been reinvestigated because they had all become resistant to the treatment that in the past had controlled their AIH. Three of these individuals had undergone ERCP at the time of initial presentation, and in all three the biliary tree had appeared normal. None of the six had evidence of intrahepatic bile duct disease on histologic evaluation of their initial liver biopsy. In follow-up studies, all six were found to have changes typical of PSC on ERCP. Three of the six subsequently required a liver transplant.

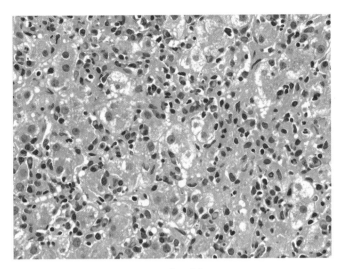

Fig. 43-1 **Liver biopsy.**

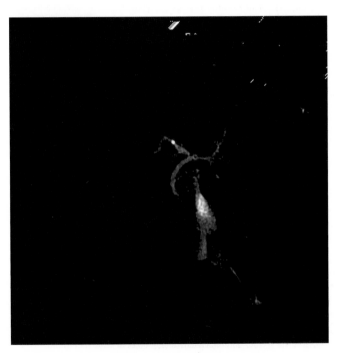

Fig. 43-2 **Magnetic resonance cholangiogram.**

overlap, retention of copper in the periportal hepatocytes can be a clue to suggest long-standing cholestasis.

There is debate regarding the significance of overlap in adult patients when identified solely by MR cholangiography. One study[5] evaluated 79 patients given a diagnosis of AIH (mean AIH score, 15.1 ± 3.4) with MR cholangiography for evidence of sclerosing cholangitis (SC). Results were reviewed by two radiologists. Clinical parameters were correlated with MRI findings. A histologic review of available liver biopsies (*n* = 29) was performed. Of the 79 patients surveyed, 8 (10%) had MRI findings consistent with cholangiopathy. Younger age at diagnosis (24.3 ± 11.9), higher baseline alkaline phosphatase level (186.4 ± 98.3), higher bilirubin level at time of MRI (45.8 ± 37.2), and greater lobular activity on initial liver biopsy were significantly associated with the detection of this overlap of SC with AIH, but not ALP/AST ratio, time between the initial diagnosis of AIH and the MRI, or the presence of cirrhosis on initial liver histologic analysis. Two cases with a normal MRI had histologic lesions typical of small-duct PSC. A limitation of MR cholangiography in patients with cirrhosis, however, is that it may demonstrate a biliary tree that simulates a sclerosing pattern, although this finding is usually limited to the periphery. A contrasting study from France[51] was not able to reproduce the initial Canadian finding suggesting a high prevalence of biliary overlap in AIH, indicating that overlap is much less common and specifically highlighting the concern that cirrhosis can affect cholangiographic evaluation. In the French study 59 consecutive patients with AIH diagnosed according to International Autoimmune Hepatitis Group score (women, 71%; mean age, 48 years; cirrhosis, 23%) underwent both MRI and percutaneous liver biopsy. A total of 27 patients with cirrhosis of nonbiliary or nonautoimmune cause served as controls. Fourteen AIH patients (24%) showed mild MRI abnormalities of intrahepatic bile ducts (IHBDs). None had abnormal common bile ducts or convincing evidence of sclerosing cholangitis on MRI or biopsy. A diagnosis of overlapping sclerosing cholangitis was nevertheless retained in one patient with MRI abnormalities who subsequently developed symptomatic cholestasis despite corticosteroid therapy. Fibrosis score was the only independent parameter associated with bile duct abnormalities on MRI; in this series the percentage of patients with IHBD MRI abnormalities was the same among AIH patients with advanced fibrosis (F3-F4, *n* = 24) as compared with cirrhotic controls (46% vs. 59%).

Management of Autoimmune Hepatitis–Primary Sclerosing Cholangitis Overlap

Specific Treatment

Once it has been recognized that a true overlap exists, each individual autoimmune liver disease requires the appropriate therapy. It is often the presence of a greater than 10-fold elevation in serum aminotransferase levels in the patient with PSC that prompts the clinician to consider overlapping autoimmune hepatitis. However, a transaminitis, at least in the early phases of acute cholestasis (as is seen with stones in the common bile duct), is not unusual in PSC. Thus in individuals who present with PSC it may be helpful to initiate treatment

Because the "gold standard" hallmark for PSC—namely, beading and stricturing of the intra- and/or extrahepatic biliary tree on cholangiography—is a late manifestation of the disease and may not be demonstrated even when histologic examination of the interlobular bile ducts suggests intrahepatic PSC, it is not possible to definitively state whether the overlap of AIH and PSC previously described was truly sequential. In this series of six adult cases (just as in the children with AIH and PSC) none of the usual laboratory markers for cholestasis—namely, the serum levels of GGT and alkaline phosphatase (ALP)–were indicative of biliary tract pathology. Improvements in immunohistochemistry during routine liver biopsy interpretation may aid the identification of early biliary disease (e.g., cytokeratin 7 staining),[50] and in the children with

that improves the biochemical cholestasis before the introduction of any immunosuppressive therapy. UDCA, although clearly not shown to improve survival in PSC, does improve the biochemical picture of cholestasis.[52-54] In those individuals who first present with features of autoimmune hepatitis and who are also shown to have PSC, it is probably optimal for immunosuppressive therapy to be the first line of treatment, particularly in patients who have florid symptoms and/or bridging necrosis on liver histologic analysis. UDCA may be added once the AIH has settled, although if this is chosen, the patient must be made aware that there are no convincing survival data for UDCA use in PSC.

Reports of the long-term follow-up of both pediatric studies of AIH–PSC (ASC) overlap indicate that the outcome was worse than in those patients with either AIH or PSC alone, and that those patients with the overlapping diseases frequently required liver transplantation. There are insufficient data to indicate whether this is also true for adults with AIH and PSC. Some retrospective studies do suggest this,[55] whereas others do not.[56]

Preventive Treatment

There are two significant nonhepatic complications of the AIH–PSC syndrome that may be adversely affected by the primary treatments for this disease.

Metabolic Bone Diseases

All forms of chronic cholestasis, particularly in the presence of jaundice, are complicated by the development of progressive osteopenia/osteoporosis. The need to administer corticosteroid therapy in those with an AIH–PSC overlap syndrome further increases the risk of thin bones in such individuals, who may also in addition have inflammatory bowel disease. Thus even in the young it is important that adequate calcium and vitamin D supplementation be provided. Studies in patients with PBC suggest that the bisphosphonate alendronate is effective in the prevention and management of osteoporosis in individuals with chronic cholestasis.[57] Prophylactic bisphosphonate therapy has also been shown to be beneficial in individuals who require long-term corticosteroids for any reason, although therapeutic decisions should be tailored to the individual.[58] In those with additional pancreatic involvement or celiac disease, osteomalacia caused by malabsorption of calcium and vitamin D may also be a feature of the complicating metabolic bone disease.

Sepsis

The requirement for corticosteroid therapy to control autoimmune hepatitis necessitates that all patients be well educated about the need for prompt treatment of any focus of infection; patient education to encourage prompt treatment of fever and/or chills is essential. In those individuals with additional sclerosing cholangitis it is particularly important to avoid procedures that could introduce infection into a poorly draining biliary system. Appropriate antibiotic coverage needs to be provided for invasive procedures.

Summary

With so many potential immunologic targets within the liver, it is not surprising that mixed presentations are observed when tolerance is overcome. Despite ongoing rigorous investigation into the pathogenesis of the autoimmune liver diseases, their etiology remains obscure. The pathogenesis is clearly multifactorial, with both exogenous influences and genetics playing a role. The presence of shared genetic risk factors across autoimmune disease highlights the complex pathophysiology[59] whereas the description of a single patient with features of PSC, AIH, and mitochondrial antibodies clinically epitomizes the underlying multifactorial processes in individuals.[60] The rarity and the heterogeneous nature of overlap syndromes unfortunately mean that there remain no clear diagnostic criteria, and at present it is unlikely that robust evidence will become available upon which to formally recommend appropriate management. Patient care should therefore remain based on a high level of clinical acumen.

References

1. Czaja AJ, Carpenter HA. Autoimmune hepatitis with incidental histologic features of bile duct injury. Hepatology 2001;34:659–665.
2. Czaja AJ, et al. Diagnostic and therapeutic implications of bile duct injury in autoimmune hepatitis. Liver Int 2004;24:322–329.
3. Czaja AJ. Frequency and nature of the variant syndromes of autoimmune liver disease. Hepatology 1998;28:360–365.
4. Chazouilleres O, et al. Primary biliary cirrhosis–autoimmune hepatitis overlap syndrome: clinical features and response to therapy. Hepatology 1998;28:296–301.
5. Abdalian R, et al. Prevalence of sclerosing cholangitis in adults with autoimmune hepatitis: evaluating the role of routine magnetic resonance imaging. Hepatology 2008;47:949–957.
6. Gregorio GV, et al. Autoimmune hepatitis/sclerosing cholangitis overlap syndrome in childhood: a 16-year prospective study. Hepatology 2001;33:544–553.
7. Yeung E, et al. Ramipril-associated hepatotoxicity. Arch Pathol Lab Med 2003;127:1493–1497.
8. Alla V, et al. Autoimmune hepatitis triggered by statins. J Clin Gastroenterol 2006;40:757–761.
9. Ramachandran R, Kakar S. Histological patterns in drug-induced liver disease. J Clin Pathol 2009;62:481–492.
10. Bogdanos DP, et al. Autoimmune liver serology: current diagnostic and clinical challenges. World J Gastroenterol 2008;14:3374–3387.
11. Lidman K. Clinical diagnosis in patients with smooth muscle antibodies. A study of a one-year material. Acta Med Scand 1976;200:403–407.
12. Lenzi M, et al. Prevalence of non–organ-specific autoantibodies and chronic liver disease in the general population: a nested case-control study of the Dionysos cohort. Gut 1999;45:435–441.
13. Kavanaugh A, et al. Guidelines for clinical use of the antinuclear antibody test and tests for specific autoantibodies to nuclear antigens. American College of Pathologists. Arch Pathol Lab Med 2000;124:71–81.
14. Leung PS, et al. Antimitochondrial antibodies in acute liver failure: implications for primary biliary cirrhosis. Hepatology 2007;46:1436–1442.
15. Kenny RP, et al. Frequency and significance of antimitochondrial antibodies in severe chronic active hepatitis. Dig Dis Sci 1986;31:705–711.
16. O'Brien C, et al. Long-term follow-up of antimitochondrial antibody–positive autoimmune hepatitis. Hepatology 2008;48:550–556.
17. Brunner G, Klinge O. A chronic destructive non-suppurative cholangitis-like disease picture with antinuclear antibodies (immunocholangitis). Dtsch Med Wochenschr 1987;112:1454–1458.
18. Michieletti P, et al. Antimitochondrial antibody negative primary biliary cirrhosis: a distinct syndrome of autoimmune cholangitis. Gut 1994;35:260–265.
19. Kim WR, et al. Does antimitochondrial antibody status affect response to treatment in patients with primary biliary cirrhosis? Outcomes of ursodeoxycholic acid therapy and liver transplantation. Hepatology 1997;26:22–26.
20. Invernizzi P, et al. Comparison of the clinical features and clinical course of antimitochondrial antibody-positive and -negative primary biliary cirrhosis. Hepatology 1997;25:1090–1095.
21. Stone J, et al. Human leukocyte antigen class II associations in serum antimitochondrial antibodies (AMA)-positive and AMA-negative primary biliary cirrhosis. J Hepatol 2002;36:8–13.

22. Muratori P, et al. Characterization and clinical impact of antinuclear antibodies in primary biliary cirrhosis. Am J Gastroenterol 2003;98: 431–437.
23. Rigopoulou EI, et al. Prevalence and clinical significance of isotype specific antinuclear antibodies in primary biliary cirrhosis. Gut 2005;54:528–532.
24. Lindor KD, et al. Primary biliary cirrhosis. Hepatology 2009;50:291–308.
25. Geubel AP, Baggenstoss AH, Summerskill WH. Responses to treatment can differentiate chronic active liver disease with cholangitic features from the primary biliary cirrhosis syndrome. Gastroenterology 1976;71:444–449.
26. Talwalkar JA, et al. Overlap of autoimmune hepatitis and primary biliary cirrhosis: an evaluation of a modified scoring system. Am J Gastroenterol 2002;97:1191–1197.
27. Alvarez F, et al. International Autoimmune Hepatitis Group Report: review of criteria for diagnosis of autoimmune hepatitis. J Hepatol 1999;31: 929–938.
28. Lohse AW, et al. Characterization of the overlap syndrome of primary biliary cirrhosis (PBC) and autoimmune hepatitis: evidence for it being a hepatitic form of PBC in genetically susceptible individuals. Hepatology 1999;29:1078–1084.
29. Silveira MG, et al. Overlap of autoimmune hepatitis and primary biliary cirrhosis: long-term outcomes. Am J Gastroenterol 2007;102:1244–1250.
30. Colombato LA, et al. Autoimmune cholangiopathy: the result of consecutive primary biliary cirrhosis and autoimmune hepatitis? Gastroenterology 1994;107:1839–1843.
31. Weyman RL, Voigt M. Consecutive occurrence of primary biliary cirrhosis and autoimmune hepatitis: a case report and review of the literature. Am J Gastroenterol 2001;96:585–587.
32. Poupon R, et al. Development of autoimmune hepatitis in patients with typical primary biliary cirrhosis. Hepatology 2006;44:85–90.
33. Gossard AA, Lindor KD. Development of autoimmune hepatitis in primary biliary cirrhosis. Liver Int 2007;27:1086–1090.
34. Muratori P, et al. The serological profile of the autoimmune hepatitis/ primary biliary cirrhosis overlap syndrome. Am J Gastroenterol 2009;104: 1420–1425.
35. Feld JJ, et al. Autoimmune hepatitis: effect of symptoms and cirrhosis on natural history and outcome. Hepatology 2005;42:53–62.
36. Corpechot C, et al. Primary biliary cirrhosis: incidence and predictive factors of cirrhosis development in ursodiol-treated patients. Gastroenterology 2002;122:652–658.
37. Chazouilleres O, et al. Long term outcome and response to therapy of primary biliary cirrhosis-autoimmune hepatitis overlap syndrome. J Hepatol 2006;44:400–406.
38. Joshi S, et al. Primary biliary cirrhosis with additional features of autoimmune hepatitis: response to therapy with ursodeoxycholic acid. Hepatology 2002;35:409–413.
39. Burak KW, Urbanski SJ, Swain MG. A case of coexisting primary biliary cirrhosis and primary sclerosing cholangitis: a new overlap of autoimmune liver diseases. Dig Dis Sci 2001;46:2043–2047.
40. Kingham JG, Abbasi A. Co-existence of primary biliary cirrhosis and primary sclerosing cholangitis: a rare overlap syndrome put in perspective. Eur J Gastroenterol Hepatol 2005;17:1077–1080.
41. Ghazale A, et al. Immunoglobulin G4-associated cholangitis: clinical profile and response to therapy. Gastroenterology 2008;134:706–715.
42. Wilschanski M, et al. Primary sclerosing cholangitis in 32 children: clinical, laboratory, and radiographic features, with survival analysis. Hepatology 1995;22:1415–1422.
43. Miloh T, et al. A retrospective single-center review of primary sclerosing cholangitis in children. Clin Gastroenterol Hepatol 2009;7:239–245.
44. Gohlke F, et al. Evidence for an overlap syndrome of autoimmune hepatitis and primary sclerosing cholangitis. J Hepatol 1996;24:699–705.
45. Luketic VA, et al. An atypical presentation for primary sclerosing cholangitis. Dig Dis Sci 1997;42:2009–2016.
46. Boberg KM, et al. Features of autoimmune hepatitis in primary sclerosing cholangitis: an evaluation of 114 primary sclerosing cholangitis patients according to a scoring system for the diagnosis of autoimmune hepatitis. Hepatology 1996;23:1369–1376.
47. Kaya M, Angulo P, Lindor KD. Overlap of autoimmune hepatitis and primary sclerosing cholangitis: an evaluation of a modified scoring system. J Hepatol 2000;33:537–542.
48. van Buuren HR, et al. High prevalence of autoimmune hepatitis among patients with primary sclerosing cholangitis. J Hepatol 2000;33:543–548.
49. Abdo AA, et al. Evolution of autoimmune hepatitis to primary sclerosing cholangitis: a sequential syndrome. Hepatology 2002;36:1393–1399.
50. Goldstein NS, Soman A, Gordon SC. Portal tract eosinophils and hepatocyte cytokeratin 7 immunoreactivity helps distinguish early-stage, mildly active primary biliary cirrhosis and autoimmune hepatitis. Am J Clin Pathol 2001;116:846–853.
51. Lewin M, et al. Prevalence of sclerosing cholangitis in adults with autoimmune hepatitis: a prospective magnetic resonance imaging and histological study. Hepatology 2009;50:528–537.
52. Mitchell SA, et al. A preliminary trial of high-dose ursodeoxycholic acid in primary sclerosing cholangitis. Gastroenterology 2001;121:900–907.
53. Olsson R, et al. High-dose ursodeoxycholic acid in primary sclerosing cholangitis: a 5-year multicenter, randomized, controlled study. Gastroenterology 2005;129:1464–1472.
54. Lindor KD, et al. High-dose ursodeoxycholic acid for the treatment of primary sclerosing cholangitis. Hepatology 2009;50:808–814.
55. Al-Chalabi T, et al. Autoimmune hepatitis overlap syndromes: an evaluation of treatment response, long-term outcome and survival. Aliment Pharmacol Ther 2008;28:209–220.
56. Floreani A, et al. Clinical course and outcome of autoimmune hepatitis/ primary sclerosing cholangitis overlap syndrome. Am J Gastroenterol 2005;100:1516–1522.
57. Guanabens N, et al. Alendronate is more effective than etidronate for increasing bone mass in osteopenic patients with primary biliary cirrhosis. Am J Gastroenterol 2003;98:2268–2274.
58. Saag KG, et al. Alendronate for the prevention and treatment of glucocorticoid-induced osteoporosis. Glucocorticoid-Induced Osteoporosis Intervention Study Group. New Engl J Med. 1998;339:292–299.
59. Hirschfield GM, et al. Primary biliary cirrhosis associated with HLA, IL12A, and IL12RB2 variants. New Engl J Med 2009;360:2544–2555.
60. Bhat M, et al. Transient development of anti-mitochondrial antibodies accompanies autoimmune hepatitis-sclerosing cholangitis overlap. Gut 2009;58(1):152–153.

Section VII

Vascular Diseases of the Liver

Budd-Chiari Syndrome and Sinusoidal Obstruction Syndrome (Hepatic Venoocclusive Disease)

Aurélie Plessier and Dominique Valla

ABBREVIATIONS

AFP α-fetoprotein	**IVC** inferior vena cava	**PNH** paroxysmal nocturnal hemoglobinuria
ALT alanine aminotcansferase	**JAK** Janus tyrosine kinase	
APLS antiphospholipid syndrome	**MELD** Model for End-Stage Liver Disease	**SOS** sinusoidal obstruction syndrome
BCS Budd-Chiari syndrome	**MPD** myeloproliferative disease	**TIPS** transjugular intrahepatic portosystemic shunt
FNH focal nodular hyperplasia	**PAI-1** plasminogen activator inhibitor-1	
HCC hepatocellular careinoma		**VOD** venoocclusive disease

Budd-Chiari syndrome (BCS) and sinusoidal obstruction syndrome (SOS) are two rare entities among vascular disorders of the liver. BCS is by consensus characterized by obstruction of the hepatic venous outflow tract, regardless of the mechanism and level of obstruction, but excluding cardiac and pericardial disease and SOS.[1,2] SOS is characterized by nonthrombotic obliteration of the sinusoids or central veins (or both), most often in the context of toxic exposure. Although the manifestations of these two vascular disorders may be similar, their epidemiology, cause, and therapy differ. Therefore they are discussed separately.

Budd-Chiari Syndrome

Epidemiology

Epidemiologic data on this rare disease are limited. In Denmark, search of a nationwide inpatient register for the years 1981 to 1985 resulted in an estimated incidence rate of 0.5 per million inhabitants per year. In Japan, a 1989 hospital questionnaire survey and autopsy register showed an estimated incidence rate of 0.2 per million per year and a prevalence rate of 2.4 per million inhabitants.[3] In France, a similar survey indicated an incidence of 0.4 per million per year.[4,5] Recently, in Sweden, using both inpatient and outpatient registers and covering a recent time period (1990 to 2001), mean age-standardized incidence and prevalence

rates were 0.8 per million per year and 1.4 per million inhabitants, respectively.[6]

The level of obstruction differs according to geographic region: pure or combined obstruction of the inferior vena cava (IVC) predominates in Asian countries, whereas pure obstruction of the hepatic veins appears to predominate in Western countries.[7] In Nepal, for reasons that may be linked to extreme poverty, IVC obstruction has accounted for an enormous proportion of the patients admitted for chronic liver disease (20%) and those undergoing liver biopsy (25%).[8]

Causes and Risk Factors

Budd-Chiari Syndrome is defined as secondary when the obstruction is due to compression or invasion by a lesion originating outside the vein (e.g., tumor, cyst), whereas BCS is regarded as primary when the obstruction is the result of an endoluminal venous lesion (e.g., thrombosis, stenosis).[1,2]

Secondary Budd-Chiari Syndrome

Hepatocellular carcinoma (HCC), renal and adrenal adenocarcinoma,[9,10] renal angiomyolipoma,[11] primary hepatic hemangiosarcoma,[12-14] epithelioid hemangioendothelioma, sarcoma of the IVC, right atrial myxoma,[15] intrahepatic cholangiocarcinoma,[16] and alveolar hydatid disease[17] have been reported to cause BCS by vascular invasion. Benign tumors (focal nodular hyperplasia [FNH])[18] and cysts developing in the central part of the liver may compress the hepatic veins.[19] Abscesses and parasitic and nonparasitic cysts of the liver may induce hepatic venous obstruction through combined compression and thrombosis. Compression or kinking of the hepatic veins may occur after liver transplantation or resection and cause secondary BCS.[20,21] Blunt abdominal trauma may induce BCS in several ways: compression of the veins by hematoma or by herniation of the liver through a ruptured diaphragm or thrombosis of the hepatic veins or IVC.[22-25]

Primary Budd-Chiari Syndrome

Congenital or acquired risk factors for thrombosis have been found in up to 70% of patients with primary BCS (**Table 44-1**).[26] In recent studies, 45% of patients had two or more risk factors for thrombosis. The major acquired risk factors include myeloproliferative disease (MPD), antiphospholipid syndrome (APLS), paroxysmal nocturnal hemoglobinuria (PNH), and Behçet disease. Oral contraceptive use and extreme poverty are major environmental risk factors. Factor V Leiden is the best-established inherited risk factor for BCS. Recognition of the underlying risk factors is important for appropriate prophylaxis of recurrent thrombosis.[27] The assistance of a hematologist with expertise in these diseases is invaluable.

MPDs are chronic clonal hematopoietic stem cell disorders characterized by proliferation of one or more of the myeloid lineages (i.e., granulocyte, erythroid, megakaryocyte). The incidence of thrombotic complications in large cohorts of

unselected patients with MPD has been estimated to be 11% to 20% for polycythemia vera and 11% to 40% for essential thrombocythemia or myelofibrosis.[28,29] BCS accounted for 5% to 30% of the thrombotic complications occurring in these patients.[29,30] A past history of thrombosis,[28] high leukocyte counts, and heightened activation of these cells interacting with platelets[31] are predictors of thrombosis. Transformation into acute leukemia at 100 months after diagnosis occurs in 10% to 20% of patients with polycythemia vera and in 4% to 15% of patients with essential thrombocythemia and myelofibrosis.[28,32]

In BCS patients, hemodilution and hypersplenism may mask the changes in peripheral blood cell counts that are considered essential for a diagnosis of MPD.[33] These mechanisms may account in part for the so-called atypical expression of MPD in peripheral blood in patients with BCS.[34] In fact, the combination of a platelet count higher than $200 \times 10^9/L$ and marked enlargement of the spleen (a spleen palpable beyond 5 cm under the 10th rib) is highly predictive of MPD in patients with BCS.[33] Recent advances have greatly facilitated the diagnosis of MPD in BCS patients. A specific acquired mutation (V617F) in the autoregulatory JH2 pseudokinase domain of the *JAK2* gene can be detected in approximately 90% of patients with polycythemia vera and 50% of patients with essential thrombocythemia or myelofibrosis.[35] This mutation confers constitutive kinase activity, which causes enhanced hematopoiesis independent of growth factors (e.g., erythropoietin). Indeed, the V617F mutation in *JAK2* has been found in the peripheral blood granulocytes of 39% to 58% of patients with BCS.[36-44] Hematologic data at diagnosis in a large retrospective study of 104 patients with BCS are presented in **Table 44-2**.[45] Interestingly, in this study the V617F *JAK2* mutation was found in 18% of the patients with normal or nonspecific bone marrow biopsy findings. However, a V617F mutation was not found in 14% of patients who had evidence of MPD at bone marrow biopsy, as shown by the presence of clusters of dystrophic megakaryocytes. Thus a

Table 44-1 Prevalence of Acquired and Inherited Risk Factors for Budd-Chiari Syndrome in Europe

ACQUIRED AND INHERITED DISORDER	N POSITIVE/N TESTED (%)[26]
Myeloproliferative disorders	56/143 (39)
JAK2+	35/121 (29)
Antiphospholipid syndrome	37/150 (25)
Paroxysmal nocturnal hemoglobinuria	15/77 (19)
Factor V Leiden mutation	18/47 (38)
Factor II mutation	5/143 (3)
Protein C deficiency	5/117 (4)
Protein S deficiency	3/108 (3)
Antithrombin deficiency	3/112 (3)
Hyperhomocysteinemia	28/129 (22)
Recent pregnancy	6/93 (6)
Recent oral contraceptive use	31/93 (33)
Systemic disease	37/163 (23)
Connective tissue disease	11
Inflammatory bowel disease	8
Behçet disease	4
Sarcoidosis	2
Dehydration	5
>1 risk factor	74/160 (46)

Table 44-2 Clinical and Biologic Characteristics of 47 Patients with the *JAK2* V617F Mutation Out of 104 Patients with Budd-Chiari Syndrome

	N = 47/104
JAK2+/BM+	27/35 (77%)
JAK2+/BM−	18/67 (27%)
BM+/JAK2−	8/57 (14%)
Platelets ($10^9/L$)	352 (284-456)
Spleen extending below the costal margin (cm)	1 (0-5)
Hemoglobin (g/dl)	15 (13-16)
Leukocytes ($10^9/L$)	10 (6-14)

Modified from Kiladjian JJ, et al. The impact of JAK2 and MPL mutations on diagnosis and prognosis of splanchnic vein thrombosis: a report on 241 cases. Blood 2008;111:4922–4929.

BM, absence of clusters of dystrophic megacaryocytes at bone marrow biopsy; BM+, presence of clusters of dystrophic megacaryocytes at bone marrow biopsy; JAK2−, absence of V617F JAK2 mutation; JAK2+, presence of V617F JAK2 mutation

search for the V617F *JAK2* mutation in peripheral blood granulocytes should constitute the first step in screening BCS patients for MPD. In patients testing negative, bone marrow biopsy should then be performed to ascertain the presence of MPD.

When combining the results of bone marrow biopsy and testing for the V617F *JAK2* mutation, MPD has been found in 40% to 50% of BCS patients.[43,45] Other MPD-associated mutations (*MPL* and *JAK2* exon 12 mutations) appear to play a minor role inasmuch as fewer than 10 patients with such mutations and BCS have thus far been reported.[41,46] A TET2 mutation was recently detected in 2 of 15 screened BCS patients, and the 46/1 haplotype was also detected in patients with BCS, as well as in family members of 1 BCS patient, with and without the *JAK2* V617F mutation, thus suggesting a predisposition to BCS independent of acquisition of the *JAK2* V617F mutation and a predisposition to latent MPD.[47]

The reasons why MPD is found in such a high proportion of patients with BCS remain unknown. By comparison, MPD is present in "only" 25% of patients with primary portal vein thrombosis and 1% to 5% of patients with cerebral vein thrombosis.[39] Recent observation of the V617F *JAK2* mutation in the hepatic venous endothelial cells of two BCS patients with MPD[48] and the finding of increased expression of circulating endothelial colony-forming cells in myelofibrosis patients with splanchnic vein thrombosis[49] suggest a role for MPD-specific abnormalities of endothelial cells in the splanchnic area. These interesting but preliminary findings need confirmation.

Treatment of MPD is currently based on hydroxyurea and low-dose aspirin.[50] Promising results have been reported with pegylated interferon alfa.[51] Peginterferon was shown to decrease the percentage of mutated *JAK2* alleles in 89% of treated patients.[51] New selective JAK1/JAK2 inhibitors are also very promising therapeutics, with clinical response obtained in 50% to 70% of patients with polycythemia vera and essential thrombocythemia.[52] In patients with BCS and portal hypertension, low-dose aspirin might be contraindicated because it increases the risk for gastrointestinal bleeding in those with cirrhosis.[53] Although patients with MPD appear to have more severe disease at initial evaluation, their short-term outcome does not seem to differ from that of patients with BCS of other causes.[41] The impact of specific treatment of MPD on overall outcome needs to be evaluated in patients with BCS.

APLS is characterized by arterial or venous thrombotic events (or both) or obstetric complications and a medium to high titer of antiphospholipid antibodies (lupus anticoagulant, anticardiolipin antibodies, or anti–β_2-glycoprotein 1 antibodies).[54,55] APLS is found in 20% to 25% of patients with BCS.[26,56-58] Among APLS patients with BCS, 40% have the secondary form of APLS, which is associated with systemic lupus erythematosus or other connective tissue diseases, and 60% have the primary form, in which connective tissue disease is not present. In patients with APLS, deep venous thrombosis, and no additional risk factors, the targeted international normalized ratio (INR) for anticoagulation therapy is 2.5 (INR range, 2 to 3). The recommended INR target is 3 (INR range, 2.5 to 3.5) in patients who have recurrent thromboembolic events while the INR is in the therapeutic target range and in those with other additional risk factors for thromboembolic events.[59] This issue needs to be evaluated in BCS patients.

PNH is a rare acquired clonal disorder of hematopoietic stem cells. The disease is often diagnosed in patients with hemolytic anemia, marrow failure, and episodes of venous thrombosis, mainly in the cerebral and splanchnic territories. PNH is related to a somatic mutation in the phosphatidylinositol glycan class A, X-linked gene, which is responsible for a deficiency in glycosylphosphatidylinositol-anchored proteins (GPI-APs).[60] Lack of one of the GPI-AP complement regulatory proteins (CD59) leads to hemolysis. Flow cytometry allows direct quantification of GPI-AP–deficient cells with the use of anti-CD59 and anti-CD55 antibodies. Thrombosis is the major prognostic factor in patients with PNH. Ten years after a diagnosis of PNH, the cumulative incidence of thrombosis is nearly 30%. Risk factors for thrombosis include older age, thrombosis at diagnosis, and transfusions. The propensity for thrombosis appears to be roughly proportional to the size of the PNH clone. New episodes or progression of thrombosis has been observed in patients with PNH despite the use of anticoagulants, antiplatelet agents, or both. The risk for fatal hemorrhage in patients with PNH is substantial and is mainly due to the frequent occurrence of thrombocytopenia.

The prevalence of BCS in large series of PNH cohorts is approximately 10% to 15%,[61-63] a considerable figure, whereas the prevalence of PNH in BCS patients is approximately 7%.[64] The short-term prognosis of patients with PNH and BCS does not seem to differ from that of patients with other causes of BCS. After a diagnosis of BCS, extension or recurrence of thrombosis occurred in 4 of 15 PNH patients (27%) despite anticoagulation therapy. Transjugular intrahepatic portosystemic shunt (TIPS) placement was successful in most patients in whom it was attempted.[64] Patients with BCS and PNH have been treated successfully with allogeneic stem cell transplantation.[65-68] Eculizumab is a humanized monoclonal antibody against terminal complement protein C5 that inhibits activation of the terminal complement. It has been shown to decrease hemolysis in PNH patients. Post hoc analyses have also shown a decreased incidence of thrombosis in patients receiving eculizumab.[69]

Behçet disease, an established cause of venous thrombophlebitis, accounts for less than 5% of cases of BCS in Western countries.[70] However, in countries in which Behçet disease is prevalent, such as Turkey, the corresponding figure is close to 40%.[71,72] Conversely, the incidence of BCS in patients with Behçet disease is 3% to 10%.[73,74] More than 80% of affected patients have IVC involvement with or without extension to the hepatic veins. Specific treatment of Behçet disease includes anticoagulation and immunosuppressive therapy for vasculitis.[73,75,76]

Celiac disease, particularly in North African populations,[77,78] and Crohn disease (ulcerative colitis) have been associated with BCS in small case series.[79-84] Epidemiologic or pathophysiologic data are lacking to explain these possible associations.

Isolated case reports have suggested an association of BCS with hypereosinophilic syndrome, whether idiopathic or related to 5q deletion syndrome.[85-87] Endothelial toxicity of eosinophil constituents has been incriminated.

Idiopathic granulomatous venulitis has been described in several case reports. The criteria for a diagnosis of sarcoidosis were fulfilled in some but not all cases. A good response to corticosteroid therapy has been recorded.[88-90]

Factor V Leiden and the prothrombin gene mutation are gain-of-function mutations that are cured by liver transplantation. The consequence of heterozygous or homozygous factor V Leiden mutation is resistance to activated protein C, which is found in about 25% of patients with BCS, whereas its prevalence is about 5% in the Caucasian population.[26,91,92] In patients with BCS, factor V Leiden is usually associated with another thrombotic risk factor. Certain subgroups of BCS patients seem to be particularly affected by factor V Leiden, namely, those with progressive IVC obstruction, those with acute BCS related to pregnancy, and oral contraceptive users. A diagnosis of factor V Leiden mutation is ruled out by a normal result on a test for activated protein C resistance. Confirmation of an abnormal test result is obtained by molecular biology.

The G20210A mutation in the prothrombin gene is responsible for increased plasma levels of prothrombin and a moderate increase in the risk for venous thrombosis. It is found in about 5% of BCS patients, whereas the background prevalence in Western countries is about 2%.[26,91,92] The diagnosis is made by molecular biology.

Antithrombin, protein C, and protein S are produced by the liver, and their plasma levels are nonspecifically decreased in many patients with BCS. Family studies are therefore necessary to establish a low plasma level as a primary deficiency. The high number of private mutations precludes direct molecular testing at present. Formulas taking into account the degree of liver insufficiency have yielded an estimated prevalence of about 25% for primary protein C deficiency in BCS patients.[26,91,92] However, these formulas require further validation. These three inherited thrombophilias are cured by transplantation of a liver from an unaffected donor.

Impaired fibrinolysis and increased plasma levels of factor VII, factor VIII, or homocysteine are established risk factors for venous thrombosis and may or may not be genetically determined.[93] Data on these factors in BCS patients are lacking, mainly because of the difficulties in interpreting plasma levels of these liver-derived substances in patients with liver disease. Genetic variations in the thrombin-activatable fibrinolysis inhibitor (TAFI) were shown to be associated with increased risk for hepatic or portal venous thrombosis, thus suggesting a possible role for TAFI in these diseases.[94] Hyperhomocysteinemia was more prevalent in patients with BCS than in controls (37% vs. 18%)[95] and was present in 22% of patients in a large BCS cohort.[26]

A case-control study has established oral contraceptives as a risk factor for BCS.[96] However, this study was performed in an era in which contraceptive pills had a high estrogen content. In a more recent study, the increased risk in oral contraceptive users fell short of statistical significance.[92] In both studies, oral contraceptive users generally had other risk factors for thrombosis. Therefore the role of current oral contraceptives should be reevaluated.

In 6% to 47% of women, BCS was diagnosed during or after pregnancy (hereafter referred to as BCS temporally related to pregnancy). However, data indicate that pregnancy is unlikely to cause BCS in the absence of other thrombotic risk factors.[97] In a recent study, the median number of risk factors for BCS (not including pregnancy) was two (range, zero to three) in women with BCS temporally related to pregnancy but only one (range, zero to five) in the 36 other women ($P = .30$). Furthermore, three of seven women with BCS temporally

related to pregnancy had a previous pregnancy uncomplicated by liver disease before the diagnosis of BCS.[97]

There is evidence from a large case-control study in Nepal that extreme poverty is a strong risk factor for the development of BCS related to obstruction of the IVC. The mechanisms that underlie this association are still unknown.[8,98]

Screening for Causes

According to recent recommendations, all patients with newly recognized BCS should undergo appropriate investigations, first to rule out a cause of secondary BCS, second to seek clinical evidence of systemic or gastrointestinal disease, and third to routinely check for risk factors for thrombosis as detailed in **Table 44-1**.[2]

Pathophysiology and Histopathology of Liver Damage

Former autopsy studies[99,100] and more recent analyses of explanted livers after transplantation[101,102] have allowed a detailed description of hepatic lesions at an advanced stage of the disease. Liver biopsy provides information on earlier stages of the disease,[103-105] but with considerable sampling variation because of inhomogeneous distribution of the lesions.[101,102]

Obstruction of a single main hepatic vein is clinically silent.[100] Obstruction of two or three main hepatic veins produces two types of hemodynamic change: increased sinusoidal blood pressure and reduced sinusoidal blood flow. Raised sinusoidal pressure is responsible for the liver enlargement, pain, and ascites via several mechanisms. (1) Sinusoidal dilation and congestion occur predominately in the central area of the hepatic lobules, where it is almost constant.[106] (2) The filtration of interstitial fluid increases, which leads to passage of this fluid through the liver capsule when the capacity for hepatic lymph drainage is exceeded. Usually, the filtrated fluid has a high protein content because of the high permeability of the sinusoidal wall to proteins. (3) Portal pressure increases.[107]

Changes in total hepatic blood flow have not been well characterized. Indirect evidence suggests that in the microcirculation of the areas with impaired outflow, perfusion with portal blood decreases whereas perfusion with arterial blood increases.[108,109] These alterations are unevenly distributed. Ischemic-type damage to liver cells is found in about 70% of cases.[100] Reperfusion injury may participate in the damage to liver cells, which would explain the rapid return of alanine transaminase (ALT) values in the majority of patients.[110] Centrilobular necrosis is probably potentiated by congestion.[111] When the hepatic and portal veins are both obstructed in the same region, confluent cell loss occurs in regions supplied by the preterminal and larger portal tracts.[102] Liver failure resulting from ischemic liver cell necrosis is rarely fulminant. Within a few weeks after obstruction of the hepatic veins, fibrosis develops and can predominate either in the centrilobular area (when there is pure hepatic vein obstruction) or in the periportal area (when there is associated obstruction of the portal veins).[102,106] Within a few months, nodular regeneration may take place, predominantly in the periportal area.[100-102,106] Cirrhosis can eventually develop but is found in only 10% to 20% of patients undergoing transplantation.[100-102]

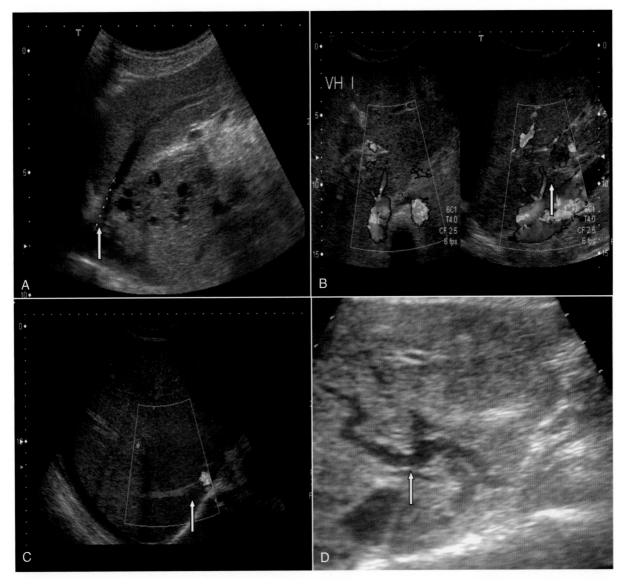

Fig. 44-1 **Doppler ultrasound images of Budd-Chiari syndrome. A,** Short stenosis of the left hepatic vein *(arrow).* **B,** Collateral circulation in the caudate lobe *(arrow).* **C,** Fibrous cord of the right hepatic vein *(arrow).* **D,** Venovenous collateral circulation *(arrow).*

Although there is evidence that increased sinusoidal pressure is a stable, permanent state, decreased hepatic perfusion appears to be inconstant. Indeed, centrilobular necrosis is lacking in 20% to 45% of patients.[105,112] Moreover, at the time of diagnosis, the ALT level is normal in more than half of patients and transient. Natural mechanisms that are able to compensate for the decreased perfusion may therefore be involved. Such mechanisms include (1) the development of venous collateral channels bypassing the obstructed veins (obvious in **Fig. 44-1**),[113,114] (2) redistribution of portal flow from areas where outflow is impaired toward areas where outflow is preserved,[108,109] (3) increased portal pressure, and (4) increased arterial flow.

Superimposed thrombosis of the intrahepatic portal veins appears to be common at an advanced stage, which can be explained by the combination of stagnant flow and an underlying thrombophilic state. Obstruction of the extrahepatic portal vein is present in 10% to 20% of patients.[57,115] Severe obliteration of the intrahepatic portal veins can be found in more than half of explanted livers at transplantation.[101,102] Areas where the portal and hepatic veins are simultaneously obstructed undergo infarction or parenchymal extinction.[101,102] Depending on whether only the hepatic veins or both the hepatic veins and portal vein are obstructed, bridging fibrosis can be found in a venovenous or in a portovenous or portoportal disposition, respectively.[101,102]

Because obstruction of the hepatic veins is usually asynchronous, atrophy of the liver areas affected early may coexist with congestive or hyperplastic enlargement of the areas affected late. In 80% of cases, the caudate lobe is hypertrophied and thereby causes IVC stenosis.[116,117] Enlargement of the caudate lobe is due to its veins draining directly into the IVC caudal to the ostia of the main hepatic veins; the veins are preserved for a considerable time from the thrombotic process affecting the main hepatic veins. Preservation of this drainage allows compensatory hypertrophy and also serves as an outflow for the intrahepatic venous collaterals. Conversely, obstruction of these veins usually causes severe liver disease.

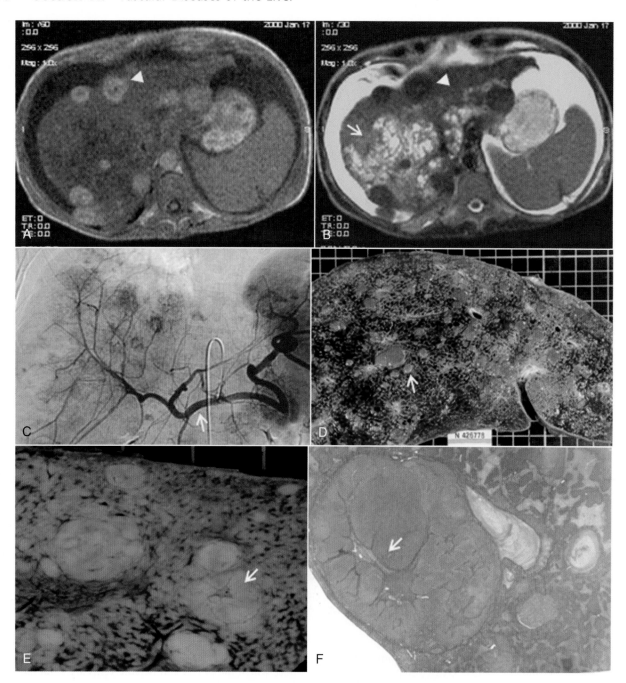

Fig. 44-2 Focal nodular regenerative hyperplasia–like lesions in a liver with Budd-Chiari syndrome. A, T1-weighed magnetic resonance imaging (MRI) showing multiple hyperintense nodules *(arrowhead)*. **B,** T2-weighed MRI showing that the nodules are hyperintense, some of them with a central scar *(arrowhead)*; the inhomogeneous area of hyperintensity is congestive *(arrow)*. **C,** Hepatic arteriography showing arterialization. The hepatic artery *(arrow)* is larger than the splenic artery, and there are multiple hypervascular areas. **D,** A sliced native liver at transplantation shows multiple nodules *(arrow)* in an otherwise congestive parenchyma. **E,** A fixed liver slice shows multiple pale nodules, some of them harboring a central scar *(arrow)*. **F,** Low-power view of a nodule showing the central scar devoid of the portal vein *(arrow)*; the neighboring liver parenchyma is congestive with two thrombosed hepatic veins.

A frequent feature of long-standing BCS is the development of multiple large regenerative nodules, some of them resembling FNH (**Fig. 44-2**).[101,102,118,119] These nodules can be viewed as a response to focal loss of portal perfusion and hyperarterialization in areas with preserved hepatic venous outflow.[101,102] There is no evidence at present that HCC results from the transformation of benign regenerative macronodules.[101,118] Distinction of benign FNH-like nodules from HCC may be difficult. Large, single, heterogeneous nodules are more likely

to be HCC.[120] A raised α-fetoprotein (AFP) level is specific for HCC in this population.[120] However, the data available are still too limited to conclude that stable, small FNH-like nodules will not transform into malignant nodules.[120] Indeed, there are several reports of HCC developing in patients with BCS.[120-125] In a recent study of 96 patients, the cumulative incidence of HCC during follow-up was 4%.[120] A strong association of HCC with cirrhosis and chronic IVC obstruction has been documented in most studies. HCC has also been associated with male sex (72.7% vs. 29.0%; $P = .007$) and with factor V Leiden (54.5% vs. 17.5%; $P = 0.01$).[120]

Although patients with BCS exhibit increased plasma volumes and activation of neurohumoral vasoactive systems, the cardiac index was significantly lower and systemic vascular resistance significantly higher in BCS patients than in cirrhotics. In fact, the cardiac index and systemic vascular resistance remained within the normal range in BCS patients.[126] These poorly understood changes might be related in part to the hematocrit being usually normal in BCS patients but decreased in cirrhotic patients.

Manifestations and Course

Patients with BCS are 39 years old on average, and most of them are females.[57] The cardinal features of BCS are ascites (80%), upper abdominal pain (60%), hepatic encephalopathy (10%), and less frequently, upper gastrointestinal bleeding (5%).[26] Ascites protein content higher than 3 g/dl (or a serum-ascites albumin gradient >1.1 g/dl) is suggestive of BCS in the absence of cardiac disease or SOS. Marked dilation of subcutaneous collaterals on the trunk is highly suggestive of vena cava obstruction.

The findings vary from a fulminant picture to an asymptomatic condition recognized fortuitously.[113] Several classifications into acute, acute-on-chronic, and chronic have been proposed because the prognosis and management would differ accordingly. An acute manifestation is characterized by a short illness, abdominal pain and fever, ascites, marked elevation in serum aminotransferases, and markedly decreased coagulation factors, whereas a chronic manifestation is characterized by the indolent development of ascites or portal hypertensive bleeding with normal or mildly increased serum aminotransferases (less than five times the upper limit of normal values) and moderately decreased plasma coagulation factors; jaundice is uncommon. The chronic manifestation and acute-on-chronic manifestation (an acute manifestation in patients with anatomic features of long-standing disease) are more frequent than an acute manifestation (patients seen acutely but without evidence of long-standing disease).[57] It has been shown that an acute-on-chronic manifestation is associated with a poorer outcome than is solely acute or chronic disease.[127]

The clinical findings appear to depend both on the extent and on the speed of the obstructive process.[100] Thus obstruction of only one major hepatic vein usually develops without symptoms; slow obstruction of two or three major veins produces a chronic course or, when accompanied by extensive collaterals, no symptoms at all.[113] According to this view, acute disease could result from abrupt occlusion of several veins simultaneously or from recent obstruction of a vein or a large collateral remaining patent while other veins have long been obstructed.

Diagnosis

A diagnosis of BCS should be suspected when ascites, liver enlargement, and upper abdominal pain are simultaneously present or when intractable ascites contrasts with moderate alterations in liver function test results, when liver disease occurs in a patient with known risk factors for thrombosis, or when the liver disease remains unexplained after other common or uncommon causes have been excluded. The diagnosis is often delayed: in a recent cohort study, a majority of patients had symptoms for more than 1 month before the diagnosis was made,[26] although evidence for the diagnosis could be found retrospectively at reexamination of the initial imaging data.

Hepatic Venous Outflow Tract Imaging

The diagnosis is made when hepatic venous outflow obstruction or collaterals of the hepatic veins or vena cava are seen. A strategy favoring minimally invasive diagnostic procedures by successively using ultrasonography and computed tomography (CT) or magnetic resonance imaging (MRI) has recently been recommended for the diagnosis of BCS. Venography is recommended only when the diagnosis remains uncertain or for planning interventional therapy. Liver biopsy is indicated only in patients in whom the large hepatic veins and IVC are shown to be clearly patent on all imaging procedures.[2]

Ultrasonography must combine color Doppler imaging and pulse Doppler analysis of hepatic vein waveforms (see **Fig. 44-1**). The examiner should be aware of the clinical suspicion of BCS and have sufficient experience to seek specific signs of obstruction. In this context, ultrasound has become the first choice for the noninvasive diagnosis of BCS. The following features can be considered specific for hepatic vein obstruction: (1) a large hepatic vein appearing to be void of flow signal or with reversed or turbulent flow; (2) large intrahepatic or subcapsular collaterals with continuous flow connecting the hepatic veins or the diaphragmatic or intercostal veins; (3) a spiderweb appearance, usually located in the vicinity of the hepatic vein ostia, together with the absence of a normal hepatic vein in the area; (4) an absent or flat hepatic vein waveform without fluttering; and (5) a hyperechoic cord replacing a normal vein.[109,128]

Absence of visualization or tortuosity of the hepatic veins on gray-scale real-time sonography, albeit with the presence of flow signals on Doppler imaging, is common but not specific in that it is also observed in patients with advanced cirrhosis of other origin. A distinctive feature, however, is the association with intrahepatic or subcapsular hepatic venous collaterals. This collateral circulation is the most sensitive feature for the diagnosis of BCS because it is found in more than 80% of patients.[109,128] Limits of this technique are the patient's body habitus and the examiner's awareness and experience.

MRI with spin-echo and gradient-echo sequences and intravenous gadolinium enhancement allows visualization of the obstructed hepatic veins and IVC, intrahepatic or subcapsular collaterals, and the spiderweb pattern.[108,109] MRI, however, is not as effective as sonography in demonstrating the intrahepatic collaterals, although it is sufficiently discriminatory to identify the caudate vein. It does not allow easy determination of flow direction.

On CT (**Figs. 44-3 and 44-4**), a striplike appearance or failure to visualize the hepatic veins suggests hepatic vein obstruction. However, false-positive and indeterminate results occur in approximately 50% of patients.[109] The accuracy of multiphasic helical CT for the diagnosis of BCS appears to be good, but it has not yet been fully evaluated.

Venography (**Fig. 44-5**; also see **Fig. 44-4**) is recommended when the diagnosis remains uncertain after the previously described imaging procedures or during a therapeutic procedure.[2] Three patterns of opacification are regarded as specific during retrograde catheterization: (1) a fine spiderweb

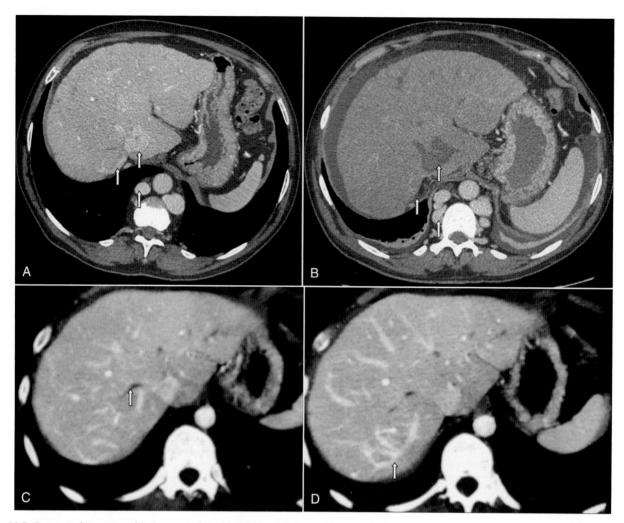

Fig. 44-3 Computed tomographic images of Budd-Chiari syndrome. A, Hepatic veins and paravertebral collaterals *(arrows)*. **B,** In the same patient 2 months later, thrombosis of the hepatic vein collaterals and the inferior vena cava *(arrows)* is apparent. Compensatory paravertebral circulation has developed, and ascites is visible. **C,** Diffuse distal hepatic vein thrombosis *(arrow)*. **D,** Venovenous collateral circulation *(arrow)*.

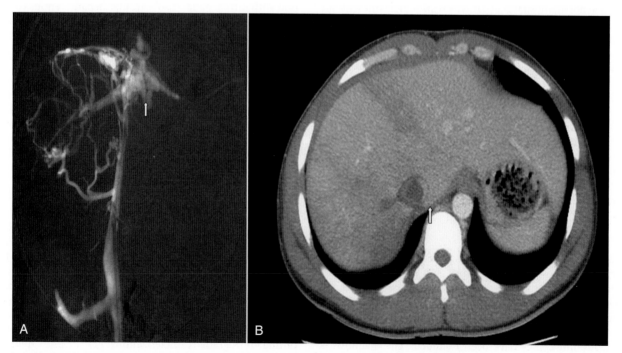

Fig. 44-4 Simultaneous hepatic and caval vein obstruction. A, Venography showing the hepatic vein and cavocaval collaterals *(arrow)*. **B,** Venous-phase computed tomography showing obstruction of the inferior vena cava *(arrow)* associated with thrombosis of the hepatic vein stump.

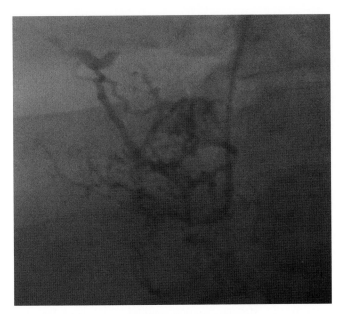

Fig. 44-5 **Spiderweb on venography.**

network pattern spreading out from the catheter tip wedged into a blocked vein without filling of venous radicals; (2) when there is incomplete occlusion of the hepatic veins, a coarse network of collateral veins that arch outward from the catheter tip and then come together again near the site of entry of the hepatic vein into the IVC; and (3) a patent vein upstream from a stricture. Diagnostic pitfalls include failure to cannulate the hepatic vein ostia and a distorted appearance of the hepatic veins. These two features are encountered in patients with cirrhosis of other origin. Direct percutaneous venography can show a localized obstruction in the vicinity of the ostia when the hepatic veins cannot be entered via retrograde cannulation. Inferior venacavography allows the demonstration of caval stenosis or occlusion. In many patients with pure hepatic vein thrombosis, the IVC appears to be narrowed at its intrahepatic portion with respect to the enlarged caudate lobe. An increased pressure gradient across the stenosis or the presence of a collateral cavacaval circulation is a better indication of the impact of intrahepatic stenosis on caval hemodynamics than is the apparent degree of stenosis.

Indirect Evidence for Budd-Chiari Syndrome at Liver Imaging or Liver Biopsy

Particular features can be highly suggestive of BCS. An enlarged caudate lobe is found in about 80% of patients.[117] This hypertrophy is explained by preservation of the multiple hepatic veins draining this lobe directly into the IVC. However, caudate lobe enlargement is also common in many cases of cirrhosis of other origin. Visibility and dilation (>3 mm in diameter) of the hepatic caudate veins on MRI or Doppler ultrasound may help differentiate BCS from cirrhosis.[129,130]

An altered parenchymal perfusion pattern is seen on CT or MRI after bolus intravenous injection of contrast material. The most characteristic pattern is early homogeneous central enhancement (particularly at the level of the caudate lobe), together with delayed patchy enhancement and prolonged retention of contrast medium in the periphery of the

liver.[109,131,132] This pattern is suggestive but neither sensitive nor specific, as it is observed in many other situations in which portal venous perfusion is compromised.[133] Among the latter conditions, constrictive pericarditis deserves special mention because clinically, it closely mimics hepatic venous obstruction and the diagnosis can be missed on echocardiography.[134]

Large regenerative hypervascular nodules are frequently seen in patients with BCS, as discussed earlier. They are usually multiple, with a typical diameter of 0.5 to 3 cm. On multiphasic helical CT, large regenerative nodules are markedly and homogeneously hyperattenuating on arterial phase images and remain slightly hyperattenuating on portal venous phase images. Large regenerative nodules are bright on T1-weighted MRI and show the same enhancement characteristics after intravenous bolus administration of gadolinium contrast material. They are predominantly isointense or hypointense relative to the liver on T2-weighted images. At present, there is no evidence yet that large regenerative nodules can become malignant, but a diagnosis of HCC may be difficult to make in this context. The combination of a hepatic nodule or nodules and a serum AFP level greater than 15 ng/ml is suggestive of malignancy, so in such a situation, biopsy of the largest nodule should be performed. When the serum AFP level is normal (<15 ng/ml), heterogeneous nodules with a diameter greater than 3 cm should be investigated further to rule out HCC.[120]

In view of the risk for bleeding in patients who are likely to receive anticoagulation or thrombolytic therapy, liver biopsy should be performed for a diagnosis of BCS only when an obstructed hepatic venous outflow tract has not been demonstrated on noninvasive imaging.[2] Liver specimens can be obtained by transcapsular needle puncture under sonographic guidance or during laparoscopy after having temporarily stopped the anticoagulation. The rare form of BCS that is due to involvement of the small hepatic veins with patent large veins is recognized only at liver biopsy.[135] Differentiation of this form from SOS is not always feasible solely on the basis of pathologic examination.[135,136] Liver biopsy specimens usually show the characteristic predominance of congestion, loss of liver cells, or fibrosis in the centrilobular area (see **Fig. 44-2, D**).[135] The differential diagnosis of congestion includes heart failure and constrictive pericarditis; for centrilobular liver cell loss with mild to marked congestion, circulatory failure, whatever its cause, and SOS should be eliminated. Isolated perivenular fibrosis is encountered in alcoholic or diabetic patients. Absence of congestion in the centrilobular area is a strong argument against the diagnosis of hepatic vein thrombosis. Surprisingly, small-vein thrombosis is relatively uncommon in biopsy specimens. At a late stage, differentiation of hepatic vein thrombosis complicated by cirrhosis from cardiac cirrhosis and from cirrhosis complicated by hepatic vein thrombosis may become difficult solely on pathologic grounds.[137]

Treatment

Treatment of the Cause

The recommended routine screening for all possible causes and risk factors presented earlier may enable one to identify conditions that require a specific therapy (as briefly discussed in the section Causes and Risk Factors) along with treatment of hepatic venous obstruction. In some patients, the disease appears to be adequately controlled just with treatment of the cause and anticoagulation therapy.[26,138] For example, immuno-suppressive therapy for Behçet disease[73] or hematopoietic stem cell transplantation for PNH[64] apparently sufficed to control the underlying disease and BCS. Oral contraceptive use should generally be stopped. In patients with known BCS that is well controlled, pregnancy should not be contraindicated because maternal outcome and fetal outcome beyond the 20th week of gestation are good.[139] Patients should be fully informed of the persistent risks associated with such pregnancies, mainly fetal loss, recurrent thrombosis, and bleeding at delivery, which occur in 30%, 8%, and 25% of pregnancies, respectively. Ideally, pregnant women with BCS would be managed by experienced clinicians in multidisciplinary centers.[139]

Anticoagulation Therapy

According to recent recommendations,[2] (1) anticoagulation therapy with low-molecular-weight heparin should be initiated immediately, with a target anti-Xa activity of 0.5 to 0.8 IU/ml, and be changed to an oral anticoagulation agent when clinically appropriate, with an INR target of between 2 and 3, and (2) anticoagulation therapy should be used long-term unless a major contraindication is present or a complication of anticoagulation therapy occurs. These recommendations have been based on the following circumstantial evidence: (1) an improved outcome since the introduction of systematic anticoagulation in nontransplant as well as in transplant patients,[105,140-142] (2) reports of recanalization of thrombosed hepatic veins and a thrombosed portal vein associated with thrombosed hepatic veins with just anticoagulation therapy,[143] (3) the efficacy of anticoagulation for recanalization of recent thrombosis of the portal vein or other deep veins,[144] and (4) reports of recurrent occlusion of the hepatic veins following angioplasty in patients not receiving anticoagulation.[145] In a recent multicenter prospective cohort study,[57] 86% of the patients received anticoagulation therapy with or without an invasive procedure, and 40% received only anticoagulation with or without diuretics and β-blockers. The 2-year survival rate was 82%. Variceal bleeding occurred in only 8% of patients receiving anticoagulation therapy.[26] However, a retro-spective cohort study involving 96 consecutive BCS patient treated with anticoagulation found a high incidence of major bleeding.[146] Bleeding contributed to death in 5 of the 96 patients.[146] Severe bleeding or death was more likely to occur in patients with the most severe BCS, in those who undergo invasive therapeutic procedures for BCS, or in patients with portal hypertension.[146] Low-molecular-weight heparins are generally preferred over unfractionated heparins because of a lower risk for heparin-induced thrombocytopenia and easier administration.[138] These recent data point to the need for improved anticoagulation with new agents or alternative protocols for periprocedural anticoagulation and bleeding prophylaxis (or both).[147]

Pharmacologic and Endoscopic Treatment of Portal Hypertension

The practice guidelines that have been proposed for the treatment of portal hypertension in patients with cirrhosis are considered to be applicable to BCS patients.[1] However, the tolerance and efficacy of β-adrenergic blocking agents should be monitored closely because baseline systemic hemodynamics differs in patients with BCS and those with cirrhosis, as discussed earlier.

Recanalization of the Hepatic Venous Outflow Tract by Thrombolysis, Angioplasty, or Stenting

Pharmacologic thrombolysis by local or systemic administration has been performed in patients with BCS, with or without recanalization procedures. Local administration appears to cause a similar rate of complications, but higher concentrations of agent are achieved at thrombosis sites, and it is more efficacious than systemic administration. A recent review of the limited data available concluded that thrombolysis appears to be effective only when the thrombus is relatively recent (hours to weeks), when thrombolysis is associated with angio-plasty of a stenosis, and when local infusion at the thrombosis site ensures a high concentration of the thrombolytic agent.[148] Patients with IVC obstruction may be better candidates for thrombolysis according to these criteria.[149] The potential benefits should be weighed against the expected risks before making a decision. Thrombolysis exposes patients to risk for hemorrhage (from variceal or intracranial sources or related to an invasive procedure), pulmonary embolism, and stroke. Recent reports highlighting the risk for dreadful complications with thrombolysis for acute portal vein thrombosis should make one cautious when considering thrombolytic therapy for BCS.

Percutaneous angioplasty with stenting aims to restore hepatic venous outflow by dilating an accessible, but obstructed vein; it has the advantage of restoring a physiologic hepatic circulation.[138,142,145,150-154] A short stenosis upstream from a patent segment is theoretically amenable to such treatment. Short stenoses have been seen in up to a third of BCS patients with pure hepatic vein obstruction and two thirds of those with IVC obstruction.[152,155,156] Attempts at recanalization have been made via the IVC or by combining a transhepatic-transvenous rendezvous approach for longer stenoses.[151,152] Combined angioplasty and stenting approaches and simultaneous recanalization of the hepatic veins and IVC have been reported.[151,152] Recanalization is reportedly achieved in 80% to 90% of selected patients, but reocclusion occurs frequently. Repeated assessment of patency and, when necessary, dilation improve secondary patency rates.[151,152] Anticoagulation appears to be helpful in preventing complete reocclusion.[151,152] Severe immediate complications are rare with the transvenous approach but more frequent with the transhepatic rendezvous technique.[151,152] Mortality seems to be low and not related to the procedure. However, data are too limited to allow proper assessment of long-term efficacy. Stent placement should not compromise future hepatic surgery or transplantation. The potential benefits of the procedure should be weighed against this risk and would be better discussed in a multidisciplinary context.

Portosystemic Shunting for Liver Decompression

The rationale for portosystemic shunting is to convert the portal vein into an outflow tract for the liver.[157] The drawback is that the liver is deprived of its portal inflow, which could be compensated by improved arterial perfusion. Several techniques have been used, depending on the patency of the veins (IVC, portal, and mesenteric) and on the size of the caudate lobe. Surgical mesocaval shunting with autologous jugular or prosthetic grafts and side-to-side portocaval shunting have been performed when the portal or mesenteric veins were patent. IVC obstruction precludes the use of these surgical shunts. A mesoatrial shunt or cavoatrial shunt followed by side-to-side portocaval shunts or IVC stenting has been proposed in this situation. The overall mortality rate has been 25% to 30%, and the rate of shunt thrombosis is 25%. Maintenance of shunt patency has a major impact on long-term survival.[158] However, of four large multivariate analyses evaluating the impact of surgical shunts on survival, only one found portosystemic shunting to have an overall favorable effect,[159] whereas in another study only a subgroup with an intermediate baseline prognosis would benefit.[112] These studies did not allow clarification of whether portosystemic shunting was not effective because of high operative mortality,

a high rate of secondary obstruction, or a deleterious influence on liver function. However, the absence of a beneficial effect on survival contrasted with the pathologic and clinical evidence of rapid and complete relief of hepatic congestion and control of ascites.

TIPS placement was first proposed for BCS patients in 1993.[160] The technique is more demanding in patients with BCS than in those with cirrhosis because the hepatic veins are obstructed, the caudate lobe is often markedly enlarged, the hepatic arteries are dilated, and the portal veins have a thickened wall and a smaller lumen. A learning curve effect is obvious.[138] In half of the patients it is possible to place the catheter in the remaining hepatic venous stump and, preferentially under ultrasonographic guidance, to direct the needle through the liver parenchyma toward the right intrahepatic branch of the portal vein. In the other half of patients, cannulation of the hepatic vein is not feasible, so direct puncture from the intrahepatic IVC toward the intrahepatic branch of the right portal vein is needed (**Fig. 44-6**).[38] In skilled hands,

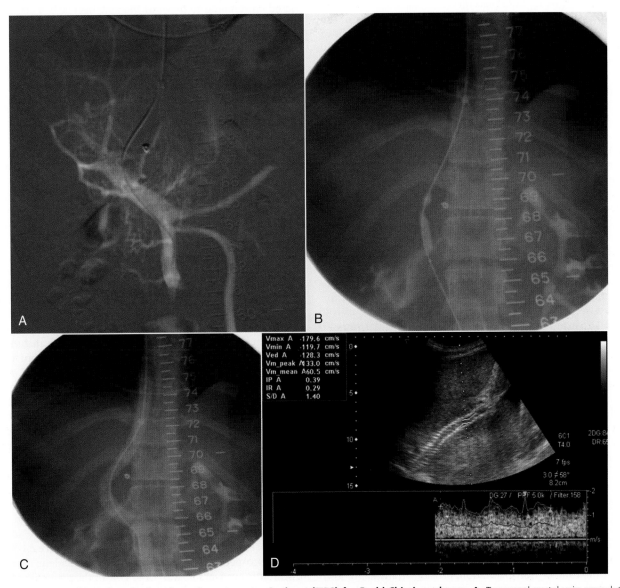

Fig. 44-6 Transcaval transjugular intrahepatic portosystemic shunt (TIPS) for Budd-Chiari syndrome. A, Transcaval portal vein cannulation. **B,** Balloon dilation of the portovenous tract. **C,** Expansion of the stent. **D,** Doppler ultrasound control of TIPS patency.

TIPS can be successfully placed in more than 90% of patients.[161,162] Several reports now confirm that even in high-risk patients, TIPS placement is effective in decreasing portal hypertension, improving liver function, and controlling ascites, thus suggesting that TIPS may improve survival.[138,161,163-168] In a large group of BCS patients treated with TIPS, recent data confirmed 1- and 5-year liver transplantation–free survival rates of 88% and 78%, respectively.[161] Factors associated with a poor prognosis following TIPS insertion were suggested to be age, high bilirubin, and high INR. Patients with the latter characteristics might benefit from directly undergoing liver transplantation, although this remains to be established.[161]

Resumption of anticoagulation therapy following TIPS insertion is a delicate issue given the risk for bleeding from intrahepatic or extrahepatic sources after this invasive procedure. Factors that could be taken into account are (1) the risk for early TIPS thrombosis, which might be related to an insufficient decrease in the portosystemic pressure gradient, and (2) the risk for procedure-related bleeding, which could be linked to the ease of TIPS placement.

TIPS dysfunction during follow-up is defined as any of the following: increase in the portal pressure gradient above 12 mm Hg, significant narrowing of the lumen on venography or ultrasound, or the appearance of reappearance of ascites or other complications of portal hypertension. It is recommended that clinical and biochemical parameters and ultrasound be used to monitor patients closely, initially at 1 month after TIPS, then at 3 months, and every 6 months thereafter. Hemodynamic evaluation has to be performed when clinical or ultrasound data suggest TIPS dysfunction.[161] The advent of polytetrafluoroethylene-covered stents for TIPS has proved to be most beneficial in preventing TIPS dysfunction in BCS patients.[161,162]

Liver Transplantation

Two large surveys have evaluated the use of orthotopic liver transplantation (OLT) in patients with BCS.[169,170] The European survey based on European Liver Transplantation Registry data included 248 patients who received transplants for BCS between 1988 and 1999. The overall actuarial survival rate was 76% at 1 year, 71% at 5 years, and 68% at 10 years.[169] Most of these patients were high-risk patients according to widely used prognostic indices. A proportion of them had previously received a TIPS that had either failed or been used as a bridge to liver transplantation. However, it is still difficult to evaluate what the outcome would have been with a strategy in which angioplasty or TIPS would have been put to more extensive use and considered definitive therapy. Retransplantation was performed in 15% of the patients. Most of the patients died within the first 3 months because of infection, multiorgan failure, graft failure, or hepatic artery thrombosis. Univariate analysis showed that renal failure, high bilirubin, and a previous surgical shunt or TIPS were associated with poor survival. In the American survey,[170] 510 transplants were performed in a 20-year period. Risk factors predicting graft loss or patient death included increased recipient age, hyperbilirubinemia, elevated creatinine, life support or hospitalization at the time of transplantation, previous transplantation, prior abdominal surgery, increased donor age, and prolonged cold ischemic time. Previous TIPS placement was not

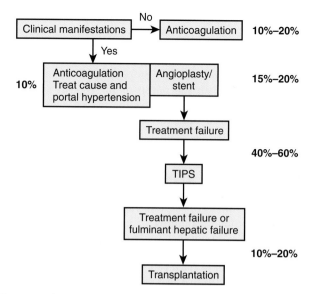

Fig. 44-7 Therapeutic strategy according to a graded approach based on response to previous therapy. The numbers on the *right* represent the approximate proportion of patients who can be permanently controlled at each step of the strategy. Data are based on recent cohort studies.[26,138,161]

associated with worse outcomes. Transplantation in the Model for End-Stage Liver Disease (MELD) era was associated with improved survival.[170]

Currently available percutaneous procedures have modified the indications for OLT. In a recent European prospective cohort, only 12% of patients underwent OLT.[26] Indications for OLT were mainly fulminant or rapidly progressive liver failure, absence of response or rescue treatment after failed previous interventions, and intractable variceal bleeding or ascites.[26]

Treatment Algorithm

Recent data support previous recommendations from expert panels for a graded approach based on response to previous therapy rather than on a time point or severity of the patient's condition.[1,171] According to this view, the therapies that should be successively implemented include the following (**Fig. 44-7**): (1) anticoagulation, treatment of the underlying condition, and symptomatic treatment of the complications of portal hypertension in all patients with primary BCS; (2) angioplasty/stenting of short venous stenoses in symptomatic patients; (3) TIPS placement in patients not suited for or unresponsive to angioplasty/stenting; and (4) liver transplantation in patients unresponsive to TIPS or with fulminant hepatic failure.

Recent clinical studies from specialized centers using this strategy indicate an overall probability of 5-year survival approaching 90% and, in patients with the most severe disease, a 5-year survival rate of 75% or higher.[138,161,172] The progressive improvement in survival with time according to the severity of disease in French cohorts is depicted in **Figure 44-8**. In a recent prospective international study of incident cases, the 24-month survival rate was 80%; 47% of the patients had been managed noninvasively, 40% had radiologic interventions, and only 12% underwent liver transplantation.[26]

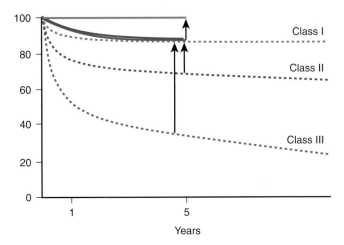

Fig. 44-8 Schematic representation of survival curves in two different periods in multicenter cohorts of European patients according to Rotterdam class at diagnosis. The *dotted lines* represent survival rates from Murad and colleagues[26] during a 17-year period before this therapeutic strategy was used, and the *solid blue line* represents survival rates from Plessier and colleagues[138] during an 8-year period from 1997 to 2005 when this therapeutic strategy was used. The strategy is depicted in Figure 44-7.

Current Outcome and Prognosis

In the last 4 decades the prognosis has improved, with current survival rates of 87% (95% confidence interval [CI], 82% to 93%) at 1 year and 82% (95% CI, 75% to 88%) at 2 years. Multivariate analyses have found ascites, male sex, and higher creatinine level to be associated with invasive interventions.[161] Serum albumin, bilirubin, prothrombin, ascites, and encephalopathy, or their combination as a Child-Pugh score, and serum creatinine were found to be independent prognostic factors for survival.[105,112,127,173] Several scores (Clichy, Rotterdam BCS index, New Clichy, and BCS-TIPS prognostic scores) based on a combination of these factors have been developed. These scores were recently compared with the Child-Pugh and MELD scores and found to be useful for stratification in clinical studies, but not accurate enough to be used for individual patients.[174] A recent study showed that, overall, high levels of ALT reflected acute, severe, but potentially reversible ischemic liver cell necrosis, but the subgroup with high ALT levels that decreased slowly had progressive liver disease and a poor outcome.[175] Although fibrosis, cirrhosis, and portal vein thrombosis have been associated with a poor prognosis in univariate analysis, no independent prognostic value of these conditions was shown in multivariate analysis once easily collected features of liver disease severity (Child-Pugh or MELD score components) are taken into account.

HCC developing in BCS patients[120] and polycythemia vera or essential thrombocythemic transformation in myelofibrosis or acute leukemia[33] are the current main concerns in patients with BCS once the initial manifestations of the disease have been recognized and treated.

Conclusion

Primary BVS is related to thrombosis of the hepatic veins or the IVC. In most patients the disease is caused by one or several blood disorders occurring in conjunction. MPDs,

factor V Leiden, and oral contraceptive use are the leading causes of primary BCS. At initial evaluation, these underlying disorders require routine testing with accurate laboratory tests, including testing for the V617F *JAK2* mutation for MPDs. The signs and symptoms are extremely variable from patient to patient and range from a fulminate manifestation to a completely asymptomatic condition, probably depending on the level, speed, and extent of the obstructive process. Treatment is based on successive implementation of anticoagulation and correction of the underlying disorders, percutaneous procedures for recanalization of the obstructed veins or TIPS, and liver transplantation. Currently, the disease can be fully controlled in most patients, and the survival rate is higher than 80% at 2 years, with half of these patients being treated conservatively. The long-term outcome might be jeopardized by malignant complications of liver disease (HCC) or by underlying blood disease.

Sinusoidal Obstruction Syndrome/Venoocclusive Disease

SOS (previously called venoocclusive disease [VOD]) is characterized by nonthrombotic obstruction of the sinusoids, which may extend to the central veins, in the absence of thrombosis or other underlying disorder of the hepatic veins.[2] SOS/VOD was first described as a clinical syndrome consisting of hepatomegaly, ascites, and jaundice in response to a toxic injury to the centrilobular zone of the liver. The first cases, reported in 1918 from South Africa, were related to the ingestion of plants containing pyrrolizidine alkaloids. Similar changes were reported later in patients receiving high-dose conditioning before hematopoietic stem cell transplantation. SOS/VOD has also been reported to occur after the ingestion of herbal teas containing pyrrolizidine alkaloid and has recently been described after adjuvant or neoadjuvant chemotherapies for solid cancer.

The initial lesion is a toxic injury to the sinusoids. Because central vein lesions are not required for recognition of the syndrome, the name has been changed from VOD to SOS. Indeed, 45% of patients with mild or moderate SOS and 25% of patients with severe SOS do not have occluded hepatic venules at autopsy.[176]

Pathogenesis

In vitro, sinusoidal cells are more sensitive to drug or toxin injury than hepatocytes are.[177] In the monocrotaline rat model of SOS, sinusoidal cells round up, and red cells penetrate into the space of Disse and dissect the sinusoidal lining. Kupffer cells, sinusoidal cells, and stellate cells will then embolize downstream and obstruct sinusoidal flow.[177] Depletion of glutathione by drugs or toxins, increased metalloproteinase activity, and depletion of nitric oxide (NO) play important roles in inducing experimental SOS/VOD.[178-180] Damage to hepatic sinusoidal endothelial cells initiates SOS, which is most commonly a consequence of myeloablative chemoirradiation or the ingestion of pyrrolizidine alkaloids such as monocrotaline. A recent study involving the monocrotaline rat model examined whether sinusoidal endothelial cells are of bone marrow origin, whether bone marrow injury and repair could be a determinant of the severity of liver injury, and whether treatment with bone marrow–derived progenitor cells could be beneficial. Bone marrow–derived progenitors replaced sinusoidal endothelial cells after injury, which suggested that toxicity to bone marrow progenitors impairs repair whereas timely infusion of bone marrow has therapeutic benefit.[181] Thus SOS/VOD might not be just a liver disease but a combined liver–bone marrow disease.

Causes

Pyrrolizidine Alkaloid–Containing Plants

It has been estimated that 3% of the flowering plants in the world contain pyrrolizidine alkaloids, and such plants are most often found in hot and dry climates. *Senecio, Crotalaria, Heliotropium,* and *Symphytum* (comfrey) are among the most commonly encountered plants containing pyrrolizidine alkaloids. An essential structural requirement for toxicity is the presence of an unsaturated pyrrolizidine ring structure. The alkaloids are metabolized to toxic pyrrole metabolites. Hepatotoxicity is related not only to the stability of the metabolites but also to the total dose ingested, route of exposure, and host susceptibility.[182] The first epidemic occurred in 1918 and was responsible for 80 cases in a 10-year period. It was caused by contamination of cereal grain with seeds of *Senecio;* the grain was insufficiently winnowed in old mills before being turned into bread.[183] This was accompanied by the fact that it occurred in poor populations during famine periods, with bread being the only food available in these populations. Similar epidemics in India, Afghanistan, and Tajikistan were reported later.[184-187]

Use of traditional remedies such as herbal or "bush teas," some of them widely sold in herbal or health food stores, accounts for the regular occurrence of cases, mostly described in Jamaica and the West Indies.[188] Recently, 10 cases of toxic hepatitis, including one clear SOS incident, that occurred after the consumption Herbalife products have been documented.[189] In adults, heavy or at least regular use seems to be needed to induce liver poisoning.[190,191] The severity of liver injury depends on host susceptibility and the quantity of toxin ingested. Children are more likely to be affected than adults, and in some, severe SOS/VOD has developed after acute exposure for less than 1 week.[192]

Chemotherapeutic Agents
Myeloablative Regimens Before Hematopoietic Stem Cell Transplantation

The incidence of SOS/VOD varies according to the toxicity of the conditioning regimens. In most studies the incidence approached 20% to 50%, with the most toxic regimens used including high-dose cyclophosphamide in combination with either busulfan, total-body irradiation, BCNU, carboplatin, or cytarabine.[193] In a recent review of 135 publications on SOS/VOD after myeloablative regimens for stem cell transplantation between 1979 and October 2007, the overall mean incidence was 13.7% (95% CI, 13.3% to 14.1%).[194] These variations in incidence may be due to modifications of doses and the type of conditioning regimens and better management of risk

factors. Among the latter, pharmacogenomics could play a great role. For example, cyclophosphamide requires bioactivation via cytochrome P-450 2B2. The endothelial toxicity is secondary to a cyclophosphamide metabolite, acrolein, formed simultaneously with phosphoramide mustard. Metabolism of cyclophosphamide is highly variable from person to person. When cyclophosphamide is coupled with other antineoplastic agents (busulfan or total-body irradiation), glutathione, which has a protective effect, is depleted.[193] Cyclophosphamide in conjunction with radiation doses higher than 13 Gy causes more severe and frequent liver injury.[193] Furthermore, it could be that busulfan predisposes patients to liver toxicity inasmuch as liver injury is more frequent when busulfan is given first than when it is given as a secondary drug.[195]

Finally, as discussed later, avoiding cyclophosphamide regimens, avoiding norethisterone (an estrogen that increases the risk for SOS/VOD), excluding patients with chronic hepatitis, and using lower doses of radiation have contributed to reducing the incidence of SOS/VOD after stem cell transplantation.

Other Agents in the Absence of Stem Cell Transplantation

Chemotherapy at conventional doses is associated with SOS/VOD in the absence of stem cell transplantation. Agents such as gemtuzumab ozogamicin, 6-thioguanine, urethane, 6-mercaptopurine, actinomycin D, dacarbazine, and azathioprine have been implicated.

Recently, SOS/VOD lesions have been described in patients receiving adjuvant chemotherapy, mainly with oxaliplatin, for colorectal liver metastases or pancreatic cancer.[196] Reports of clinically severe forms are extremely scarce despite an approximate 20% prevalence of such lesions[197] on routine examination of resected liver specimens.[198,199]

SOS/VOD has also been reported after lung, kidney, and liver transplantation.[200-203] Azathioprine and tacrolimus have both been implicated. Altered hepatic metabolism resulting in a prolonged half-life of their toxic metabolites has been incriminated.[200-203] The association with other risk factors has not been evaluated, and further studies are needed. The incidence of SOS/VOD after OLT was estimated to be 2% in a 9-year period.[204] SOS/VOD was associated with a high incidence of acute rejection, thus suggesting an immunologic alteration as a cause of the disease in this context.[204]

SOS/VOD has developed in patients with Crohn disease or APLS who were treated with azathioprine.[205,206] Here again, it is difficult to separate the role played by immunologic alterations from that played by azathioprine.

Radiotherapy

As a radiation-induced liver disease, SOS/VOD is seen in patients receiving 30 to 35 Gy.[195] There is interindividual variability in radiation-induced toxicity. Fractionated total-body irradiation possibly causes less sinusoidal toxicity and has the same efficacy as single-dose total-body irradiation.[207]

Alterations in Coagulation

An altered intrahepatic coagulation cascade secondary to sinusoidal endothelial cell damage has been suspected in patients with SOS/VOD. Indeed, low circulating levels of the anticoagulants protein C and antithrombin, high plasma levels of plasminogen activator inhibitor-1 (PAI-1) and transforming growth factor-β1, and reduced fibrinolysis have been found in patients with SOS/VOD. One small study found a higher incidence of factor II mutation than expected (13% vs. 1%), but no factor V Leiden mutation.[208] In another small study, there was an increased prevalence of the factor V Leiden mutation.[209] These discrepant findings need reevaluation. In the liver, immunohistology has demonstrated deposition of fibrinogen and factor VIII/von Willebrand factor in the perivenular zone.[179] Serum levels of endothelin-1, a mediator of hepatic sinusoidal constriction, are increased, whereas NO levels decrease in parallel with changes in sinusoidal flow.[179,210]

Manifestations and Course

Clinical and Laboratory Features

The clinical features in patients with SOS/VOD vary from an asymptomatic condition unexpectedly diagnosed on liver biopsy to severe disease leading to multiorgan failure and associated with a mortality rate of 84% (95% CI, 79.6% to 88.9%).[194,211] Symptomatic SOS/VOD has been described mainly after stem cell transplantation. In this setting, features regarded as typical for SOS include weight gain, ascites, right upper quadrant pain, hepatomegaly, and jaundice. Symptomatic SOS/VOD has been divided into three groups: mild SOS/VOD, in which the symptoms do not require specific treatment and the spontaneous course is favorable; moderate SOS/VOD, in which symptoms do require treatment (mainly diuretics or water balance) but resolve with treatment; and severe SOS, in which the symptoms require treatment but do not resolve before death or by day 100.[212]

In the context of myeloablative therapy, the onset of SOS/VOD is characterized by hepatomegaly, liver pain, and weight gain (related to fluid accumulation), beginning on day 1 after a cyclophosphamide-containing transplant regimen. Around day 20, hyperbilirubinemia develops. Later, SOS may develop with other conditioning regimens, such as busulfan-containing regimens, in which case SOS develops after day 30.[213] The Baltimore[214] and Seattle[212] classifications, shown in **Table 44-3**, have been elaborated and used mainly for research purposes.

Additional clinical and laboratory features that are also useful in individual patients include ALT elevation, isolated weight gain or jaundice, gallbladder wall edema, and pain. High serum bilirubin is a sensitive but not specific feature of SOS/VOD because it can be elevated in multiple other critical situations. Both classifications have a high positive predictive value for SOS/VOD in the absence of an alternative explanation for the liver anomalies.[212,214] However, SOS/VOD is a difficult clinical diagnosis to make because confounding factors are many, particularly in the setting of myeloablative therapy, and include viral hepatitis, toxicity of other drugs, graft-versus-host disease, and sepsis.

Imaging

Doppler ultrasound, MRI, and CT give no specific information for diagnosing SOS/VOD. These imaging procedures usually show hepatomegaly, ascites, and splenomegaly. They may allow diagnostic elimination of biliary obstruction, infiltrative tumors, or infectious lesions such as liver abscess and may detect hepatic or portal vein obstruction. When comparing SOS/VOD patients with a control group, the presence of splenomegaly, umbilical vein recanalization, gallbladder wall thickening, enlarged portal vein, slow or reversed portal flow, and increased resistive artery index were somewhat specific but late indicators of SOS/VOD.[215] Repeating Doppler ultrasound may help detect portal vein thrombosis, especially in patients with previously reversed flow.[215] On contrast-enhanced CT or MRI, periportal edema is visible and the gallbladder wall is seen to be hyperattenuated. A dysmorphic liver may develop late in the course. Indeed, the appearance of the liver changes with time.[216]

Liver Biopsy

When clinical and imaging information is not sufficient to make a diagnosis of SOS/VOD in patients with moderate or severe disease, liver biopsy is recommended.[2] A transjugular route is usually preferred in patients with a low platelet count or severe ascites. A hepatic venous gradient greater than 10 mm Hg is highly specific for SOS in the context of exposure to myeloablative therapy.[217] Lesions may have a heterogeneous distribution throughout the liver.[218] Findings on histology will become modified over time. As early as 6 days after myeloablative therapy, the subendothelial zone is widened and edematous and contains fragmented red cells and noncellular debris, the sinusoids are enlarged and congestive, red cells extravasate through the space of Disse, and perivenular hepatocyte necrosis occurs. Next, stellate cells are activated, and fibrosis of the sinusoids and venules increases. Later stages of fatal SOS are characterized by extensive collagenization of the sinusoids and venules. In a series of consecutive autopsies, clinically severe SOS/VOD was statistically correlated with several zone 3 acinar changes: hepatocyte necrosis and sinusoidal fibrosis, occluded hepatic venules (greater frequency and degree), eccentric luminal narrowing, and phlebosclerosis (**Fig. 44-9**).[219] Nodular regenerative hyperplasia is found in 2% to 30% of patients following bone marrow transplantation.[218,220] This architectural change may correspond to a nonspecific adaptation to heterogeneous hepatic blood flow.

Complications of liver biopsy in this population occur in 7% to 18% of patients and procedure-related death in 0% to 3%.[217]

Table 44-3 Clinical Criteria for the Diagnosis of Sinusoidal Obstruction Syndrome After Hematopoietic Cell Transplantation

SEATTLE CRITERIA	BALTIMORE CRITERIA
2 of 3 findings within 20 days of transplantation:	Hyperbilirubinemia plus ≥2 other criteria:
Bilirubin >34.2 μmol/L (2 mg/dl)	Bilirubin >34.2 μmol/L (2 mg/dl)
Hepatomegaly or right upper quadrant pain of liver origin	Hepatomegaly, usually painful
>2% weight gain attributable to fluid accumulation	≥5% weight gain
	Ascites

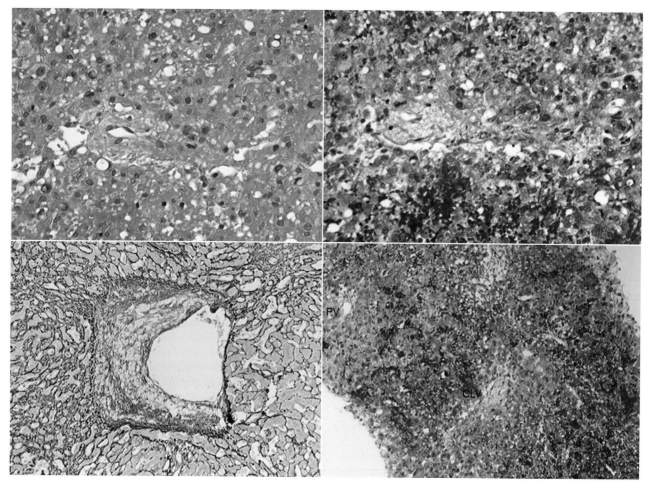

Fig. 44-9 **Histology of sinusoidal obstruction syndrome/venoocclusive disease.** A central vein is at the center of each panel. There is marked thickening of its wall with fibrosis and edema. Hepatocytes and sinusoidal endothelial cells have disappeared in the centrilobular area. The sinusoids are destroyed and congestion is apparent. *Upper left panel,* hematoxylin and eosin stain; *lower left panel,* reticulin stain; *right panels,* Masson trichrome stain.

Course and Prognosis

A model has been devised for predicting the development of severe SOS/VOD in patients conditioned with cyclophosphamide-containing regimens. This model, based on the slope of serum bilirubin and weight gain from day 1 through day 16, has not been validated with other regimens.[221] Other predictors of a poor outcome are higher serum ALT levels, higher hepatic venous pressure gradient, portal vein thrombosis, and multiorgan failure.[217,221-223] SOS/VOD is frequently associated with renal and cardiopulmonary failure. Criteria for systemic inflammatory response syndrome (SIRS) (persistent fever during cytoreductive therapy, falling oxygen saturation) are independent predictors of severe SOS/VOD and may play an independent role in the evolution of SOS/VOD.[212]

Prophylaxis

Adapting the Conditioning for Patients with High-Risk Factors

Patients at high risk for toxic liver injury should be identified before initiating myeloablative regimens to adapt the regimen.

Markers of high risk are preexisting extensive hepatic fibrosis, viral hepatitis, myelofibrosis with extramedullary hematopoiesis, nonalcoholic or alcoholic hepatitis, recent treatment with gemtuzumab ozogamicin, or a previous history of SOS/VOD.[224] Regimens that are less liver toxic include reduced-intensity regimens, regimens without cyclophosphamide, and regimens with lower doses of total-body irradiation (<12 Gy).[225] However, the advantages of preventing SOS/VOD in the short term should be weighed against an increased short- and long-term risk for graft-versus-host disease and an increased long-term risk for poor control of the underlying malignancy.

Once SOS/VOD has been recognized, markers of severity (e.g., renal or cardiorespiratory failure, SIRS) should be identified and their cause and consequences corrected when possible. In view of the frequency of associated renal failure, avoidance of nephrotoxic agents and maintenance of fluid and electrolyte balance appear to be most important.[224]

Medical Prophylaxis

Defibrotide is a single-stranded polydeoxyribonucleotide that has specific binding sites on vascular endothelium. Defibrotide up-regulates the release of prostaglandin E_2, thrombomodulin, NO, and tissue plasminogen activator and decreases thrombin generation, tissue factor expression, PAI-1, and endothelin activity.[226-229] Defibrotide has shown a benefit in preventing SOS/VOD and fatal SOS/VOD in a nonrandomized, historically controlled study.[230] In addition, 100-day event-free survival was significantly higher with defibrotide, and there was a trend for a better survival rate.[230] Randomized controlled trials are needed in this area.

In a meta-analysis, heparin was not found to be effective in preventing SOS/VOD.[231] However, methodologic weakness and heterogeneity between studies precluded a meaningful analysis. Two randomized trials showed that heparin was safe and effective in preventing mild to moderate SOS/VOD, but not severe fatal SOS/VOD. Therefore further studies are also needed in this area.

Prostaglandin E$_1$ reduced the overall incidence of SOS/VOD in one study, but no impact was shown on fatal SOS/VOD.[232] In conclusion, although several agents have been evaluated for prevention of SOS/VOD, no benefit in the prevention of fatal SOS/VOD has thus far been shown for any of them, so no recommendation can be made for their use.[233-237]

Treatment of Established Sinusoidal Obstruction Syndrome

In addition to nonspecific therapy for fluid retention, sepsis, and renal, respiratory, and circulatory failure, various specific treatments have been proposed once SOS/VOD is established.

Thrombolysis

Experience with thrombolysis using tissue plasminogen activator and heparin in nonrandomized studies has been reported. In two series of fewer than 50 patients, the survival rate was 30%.[238,239] Patients with multiorgan failure did not respond to thrombolytic therapy.[238] The risk for severe bleeding is high in these patients.[238,240] Therefore thrombolysis is not recommended.[2]

Defibrotide

Four uncontrolled trials are available. In patients with moderate to severe SOS, these trials showed complete resolution at day 100 in 36% to 50% of patients and survival at day 100 in 31% to 43%.[226,241-243] In the largest study, multiorgan failure was documented in 97% of patients, tracheal intubation was needed in 36%, and dialysis was necessary in 31%.[226] The mean duration of defibrotide therapy was 15 days, and mean doses were 20 to 40 mg/kg/day. Grade 1 and 2 toxicity, including nausea, fever, and vasomotor symptoms, was observed, but no grade 3 or 4 toxicity was recorded. Based on these inconclusive data, the American Association for the Study of Liver Diseases practice guidelines did not recommend using defibrotide as long as randomized controlled trials have not demonstrated efficacy.[2]

Transjugular Intrahepatic Portosystemic Shunt

Although TIPS placement was suggested to reduce ascites in isolated case reports,[244-246] no obvious effect on survival was shown in two larger series consisting of 6 to 10 patients.[247,248] In both series,[247,248] there was an immediate 50% mortality rate and a delayed mortality of 40% for other causes. Patients who survived exhibited resolution of SOS.[247,248] Special attention should be paid to heart and respiratory failure because acute respiratory distress syndrome has been reported following TIPS insertion in this setting.[249]

Liver Transplantation

There are anecdotal reports of successful OLT in patients with SOS/VOD.[250-253] However, three consecutive patients who underwent OLT were reported to die of hepatic failure, cerebral edema, and pneumonia.[254] Based on these limited data, it has been proposed that patients who undergo hematopoietic stem cell transplantation for a benign condition or in whom the underlying malignancy has a favorable prognosis after transplantation may be considered for OLT when severe SOS/VOD develops.[2]

Conclusion

SOS/VOD is a toxic injury to sinusoidal endothelial cells that produces portal hypertension and hepatic failure. An associated toxic effect on the bone marrow progenitors of sinusoidal endothelial cells is suggested and would satisfactorily explain the particular context in which SOS/VOD develops (myeloablative therapy, anticancer therapy, and myelotoxic pyrrolizidine alkaloids). There is little evidence that any form of therapy can prevent its development or limit its severity, apart from reducing the intensity of toxic interventions. Because defibrotide appears to have a favorable profile for side effects, it has been in extensive use despite a lack of definitive evidence for a beneficial effect.

Key References

Ansell J, et al. Pharmacology and management of the vitamin K antagonists: American College of Chest Physicians Evidence-Based Clinical Practice Guidelines (8th Edition). Chest 2008;133(6 Suppl):160S–198S. (Ref.59)

Arotcarena R, et al. Severe sinusoidal lesions: a serious and overlooked complication of oxaliplatin-containing chemotherapy? Gastroenterol Clin Biol 2006;30:1313–1316. (Ref.198)

Bachet JB, et al. Long-term portosystemic shunt patency as a determinant of outcome in Budd-Chiari syndrome. J Hepatol 2007;46:60–68. (Ref.158)

Bargallo X, et al. Sonography of the caudate vein: value in diagnosing Budd-Chiari syndrome. AJR Am J Roentgenol 2003;181:1641–1645. (Ref.129)

Barrault C, et al. [Non surgical treatment of Budd-Chiari syndrome: a review.] Gastroenterol Clin Biol 2004;28:40–49. (Ref.142)

Ben Ghorbel I, et al. Budd-Chiari syndrome associated with Behçet's disease. Gastroenterol Clin Biol 2008;32:316–320. (Ref.73)

Bresson-Hadni S, et al. [Alveolar echinococcosis: how to confirm the diagnosis?] Bull Acad Natl Med 2008;192:1141–1149; discussion 1150. (Ref.17)

Brinar M, et al. Chronic Budd-Chiari syndrome as a rare complication of Crohn's disease: a case report. Eur J Gastroenterol Hepatol 2010;22:761–764. (Ref.79)

Camera L, et al. Triphasic helical CT in Budd-Chiari syndrome: patterns of enhancement in acute, subacute and chronic disease. Clin Radiol 2006;61:331–337. (Ref.131)

Carnevale FC, et al. Long-term follow-up after successful transjugular intrahepatic portosystemic shunt placement in a pediatric patient with Budd-Chiari syndrome. Cardiovasc Intervent Radiol 2008;31:1244–1248. (Ref.168)

Carobbio A, et al. Leukocytosis is a risk factor for thrombosis in essential thrombocythemia: interaction with treatment, standard risk factors, and Jak2 mutation status. Blood 2007;109:2310–2313. (Ref.31)

Castro-Fernandez M, et al. [Influence of nonsteroidal antiinflammatory drugs in gastrointestinal bleeding due to gastroduodenal ulcers or erosions in patients with liver cirrhosis.] Gastroenterol Hepatol 2006;29:11–14. (Ref.53)

Cazals-Hatem D, et al. Arterial and portal circulation and parenchymal changes in Budd-Chiari syndrome: a study in 17 explanted livers. Hepatology 2003;37: 510–519. (Ref.101)

Chait Y, et al. Relevance of the criteria commonly used to diagnose myeloproliferative disorder in patients with splanchnic vein thrombosis. Br J Haematol 2005;129:553–560. (Ref.33)

Chalandon Y, et al. Prevention of veno-occlusive disease with defibrotide after allogeneic stem cell transplantation. Biol Blood Marrow Transplant 2004;10: 347–354. (Ref.230)

Colaizzo D, et al. New JAK2 gene mutation in patients with polycythemia vera and splanchnic vein thrombosis. Blood 2007;110:2768–2769. (Ref.36)

Colaizzo D, et al. Occurrence of the JAK2 V617F mutation in the Budd-Chiari syndrome. Blood Coagul Fibrinolysis 2008;19:459–462. (Ref.37)

Coppell JA, et al. Hepatic veno-occlusive disease following stem cell transplantation: incidence, clinical course and outcome. Biol Blood Marrow Transplant 2010;16:157–168. (Ref.194)

Corbacioglu S, et al. Defibrotide in the treatment of children with veno-occlusive disease (VOD): a retrospective multicentre study demonstrates therapeutic efficacy upon early intervention. Bone Marrow Transplant 2004;33:189–195. (Ref.242)

D'Amico EA, et al. Successful use of Arixtra in a patient with paroxysmal nocturnal hemoglobinuria, Budd-Chiari syndrome and heparin-induced thrombocytopenia. J Thromb Haemost 2003;1:2452–2453. (Ref.147)

Darwish Murad S, et al. Etiology, management, and outcome of the Budd-Chiari syndrome. Ann Intern Med 2009;151:167–175. (Ref.38)

de Bruijne EL, et al. Genetic variation in thrombin-activatable fibrinolysis inhibitor (TAFI) is associated with the risk of splanchnic vein thrombosis. Thromb Haemost 2007;97:181–185. (Ref.94)

de Franchis R. Evolving consensus in portal hypertension. Report of the Baveno IV consensus workshop on methodology of diagnosis and therapy in portal hypertension. J Hepatol 2005;43:167–176. (Ref.1)

de Latour RP, et al. Paroxysmal nocturnal hemoglobinuria: natural history of disease subcategories. Blood 2008;112:3099–3106. (Ref.61)

DeLeve LD, et al. Embolization by sinusoidal lining cells obstructs the microcirculation in rat sinusoidal obstruction syndrome. Am J Physiol Gastrointest Liver Physiol 2003;284:G1045–G1052. (Ref.177)

DeLeve LD, Valla DC, Garcia-Tsao G. Vascular disorders of the liver. Hepatology 2009;49:1729–1764. (Ref.2)

De Stefano V, et al. Incidence of the JAK2 V617F mutation among patients with splanchnic or cerebral venous thrombosis and without overt chronic myeloproliferative disorders. J Thromb Haemost 2007;5:708–714. (Ref.39)

De Stefano V, et al. Influence of the JAK2 V617F mutation and inherited thrombophilia on the thrombotic risk among patients with essential thrombocythemia. Haematologica 2009;94:733–737. (Ref.40)

Eapen CE, et al. Favourable medium term outcome following hepatic vein recanalisation and/or transjugular intrahepatic portosystemic shunt for Budd Chiari syndrome. Gut 2006;55:878–884. (Ref.172)

Elliott MA, Tefferi A. Thrombosis and haemorrhage in polycythaemia vera and essential thrombocythaemia. Br J Haematol 2005;128:275–290. (Ref.29)

Garcia-Pagan JC, et al. TIPS for Budd-Chiari syndrome: long-term results and prognostics factors in 124 patients. Gastroenterology 2008;135:808–815. (Ref.161)

Gelsi E, et al. [Association of Budd-Chiari syndrome with a coeliac disease in patient native from North Africa.] Gastroenterol Clin Biol 2004;28(10 Pt 1):903–905. (Ref.77)

Harb R, et al. Bone marrow progenitor cells repair rat hepatic sinusoidal endothelial cells after liver injury. Gastroenterology 2009;137:704–712. (Ref.181)

Havlioglu N, Brunt EM, Bacon BR. Budd-Chiari syndrome and hepatocellular carcinoma: a case report and review of the literature. Am J Gastroenterol 2003;98:201–204. (Ref.121)

Hernandez-Guerra M, et al. Systemic hemodynamics, vasoactive systems, and plasma volume in patients with severe Budd-Chiari syndrome. Hepatology 2006;43:27–33. (Ref.126)

Hernandez-Guerra M, et al. PTFE-covered stents improve TIPS patency in Budd-Chiari syndrome. Hepatology 2004;40:1197–1202. (Ref.166)

Hilliard NJ, Heslin MJ, Castro CY. Leiomyosarcoma of the inferior vena cava: three case reports and review of the literature. Ann Diagn Pathol 2005;9:259–266. (Ref.12)

Hillmen P, et al. Effect of the complement inhibitor eculizumab on thromboembolism in patients with paroxysmal nocturnal hemoglobinuria. Blood 2007;110:4123–4128. (Ref.69)

Hoekstra J, et al. Paroxysmal nocturnal hemoglobinuria in Budd-Chiari syndrome: findings from a cohort study. J Hepatol 2009;51:696–706. (Ref.64)

Ibarrola C, Castellano VM, Colina F. Focal hyperplastic hepatocellular nodules in hepatic venous outflow obstruction: a clinicopathological study of four patients and 24 nodules. Histopathology 2004;44:172–179. (Ref.119)

Imran H, et al. Use of prophylactic anticoagulation and the risk of hepatic veno-occlusive disease in patients undergoing hematopoietic stem cell transplantation: a systematic review and meta-analysis. Bone Marrow Transplant 2006;37:677–686. (Ref.231)

James C, et al. A unique clonal JAK2 mutation leading to constitutive signalling causes polycythaemia vera. Nature 2005;434:1144–1148. (Ref.35)

Jang JW, et al. Rapidly progressing Budd-Chiari syndrome complicated by hepatocellular carcinoma. Korean J Intern Med 2003;18:191–195. (Ref.122)

Janssen HL, et al. Budd-Chiari syndrome: a review by an expert panel. J Hepatol 2003;38:364–371. (Ref.171)

Kane S, Cohen SM, Hart J. Acute sinusoidal obstruction syndrome after 6-thioguanine therapy for Crohn's disease. Inflamm Bowel Dis 2004;10: 652–654. (Ref.205)

Kiladjian JJ, et al. High molecular response rate of polycythemia vera patients treated with pegylated interferon alpha-2a. Blood 2006;108:2037–2040.(Ref.51)

Kiladjian JJ, et al. The impact of JAK2 and MPL mutations on diagnosis and prognosis of splanchnic vein thrombosis: a report on 241 cases. Blood 2008;111:4922–4929. (Ref.41)

Korkmaz C. Is anticoagulation unnecessary in Behçet's disease with deep venous thrombosis? Clin Rheumatol 2008;27:405–406. (Ref.74)

Kuo GP, Brodsky RA, Kim HS. Catheter-directed thrombolysis and thrombectomy for the Budd-Chiari syndrome in paroxysmal nocturnal hemoglobinuria in three patient. J Vasc Interv Radiol 2006;17(2 Pt 1):383–387. (Ref.67)

Langlet P, et al. Clinicopathological forms and prognostic index in Budd-Chiari syndrome. J Hepatol 2003;39:496–501. (Ref.127)

Law JK, et al. Intrahepatic cholangiocarcinoma presenting as the Budd-Chiari syndrome: a case report and literature review. Can J Gastroenterol 2005;19:723–728. (Ref.16)

Lea NRL, et al. Prevalence of 46/1 JAK2 haplotype in patients with Budd-Chiari syndrome with and without JAK2V617F and TET2 mutations. Blood 2009;114:180. (Ref.47)

Mancuso A, et al. TIPS for acute and chronic Budd-Chiari syndrome: a single-centre experience. J Hepatol 2003;38:751–754. (Ref.164)

Martinez F, et al. Budd-Chiari syndrome caused by membranous obstruction of the inferior vena cava associated with coeliac disease. Dig Liver Dis 2004;36:157–162. (Ref.78)

McCabe JM, Mahadevan U, Vidyarthi A. An obscure harbinger. Difficult diagnosis of Crohn's disease. Am J Med 2009;122:516–518. (Ref.80)

McMullin MF, et al. Guidelines for the diagnosis, investigation and management of polycythaemia/erythrocytosis. Br J Haematol 2005;130:174–195. (Ref.50)

Mentha G, et al. Liver transplantation for Budd-Chiari syndrome: a European study on 248 patients from 51 centres. J Hepatol 2006;44:520–528. (Ref.169)

Mijnhout GS, et al. Sepsis and elevated liver enzymes in a patient with inflammatory bowel disease: think of portal vein thrombosis. Dig Liver Dis 2004;36:296–300. (Ref.81)

Mori T, et al. Altered metabolism of tacrolimus in hepatic veno-occlusive disease. Transpl Int 2005;18:1215–1217. (Ref.202)

Morris-Stiff G, Tan YM, Vauthey JN. Hepatic complications following preoperative chemotherapy with oxaliplatin or irinotecan for hepatic colorectal metastases. Eur J Surg Oncol 2008;34:609–614. (Ref.197)

Moucari R, et al. Hepatocellular carcinoma in Budd-Chiari syndrome: characteristics and risk factors. Gut 2008;57:828–835. (Ref.120)

Murad SD, et al. Etiology, management, and outcome of the Budd-Chiari syndrome. Ann Intern Med 2009;151:167–175. (Ref.26)

Murad SD, et al. Determinants of survival and the effect of portosystemic shunting in patients with Budd-Chiari syndrome. Hepatology 2004;39:500–508. (Ref.112)

Opitz T, et al. The transjugular intrahepatic portosystemic stent-shunt (TIPS) as rescue therapy for complete Budd-Chiari syndrome and portal vein thrombosis. Z Gastroenterol 2003;41:413–418. (Ref.167)

Patel RK, et al. Prevalence of the activating JAK2 tyrosine kinase mutation V617F in the Budd-Chiari syndrome. Gastroenterology 2006;130:2031–2038. (Ref.42)

Peffault de Latour R, Amoura Z, Socié G. [Paroxysmal nocturnal hemoglobinuria.] Rev Med Interne 2010;31:200–207. (Ref.62)

Plessier A, et al. Aiming at minimal invasiveness as a therapeutic strategy for Budd-Chiari syndrome. Hepatology 2006;44:1308–1316. (Ref.138)

Primignani M, et al. Role of the JAK2 mutation in the diagnosis of chronic myeloproliferative disorders in splanchnic vein thrombosis. Hepatology 2006;44:1528–1534. (Ref.43)

Quicios Dorado C, Allona Almagro A. [Renal angiomyolipoma causing inferior vena cava thrombus and secondary Budd-Chiari's syndrome.] Arch Esp Urol 2008;61:435–439. (Ref.11)

Rahhal RM, Pashankar DS, Bishop WP. Ulcerative colitis complicated by ischemic colitis and Budd Chiari syndrome. J Pediatr Gastroenterol Nutr 2005;40:94–97. (Ref.82)

Rajani R, et al. Budd-Chiari syndrome in Sweden: epidemiology, clinical characteristics and survival—an 18-year experience. Liver Int 2009;29: 253–259. (Ref.6)

Rautou L, et al. Bleeding in patients with Budd-Chiari syndrome (BCS). J Hepatol 2009;50(S1):S88. (Ref.146)

Rautou PE, et al. Pregnancy in women with known and treated Budd-Chiari syndrome: maternal and fetal outcomes. J Hepatol 2009;51:47–54. (Ref.139)

Rautou PE, et al. Levels and initial course of serum alanine aminotransferase can predict outcome of patients with Budd-Chiari syndrome. Clin Gastroenterol Hepatol 2009;7:1230–1235. (Ref.175)

Rautou PE, et al. Prognostic indices for Budd-Chiari syndrome: valid for clinical studies but insufficient for individual management. Am J Gastroenterol 2009; 104:1140–1146. (Ref.174)

Rautou PE, et al. Pregnancy: a risk factor for Budd-Chiari syndrome? Gut 2009; 58:606–608. (Ref.97)

Rosendaal FR. Venous thrombosis: the role of genes, environment, and behavior. Hematology Am Soc Hematol Educ Program 2005:1–12. (Ref.93)

Rosti V, et al. High frequency of circulating endothelial colony forming cells (ECFCs) in myeloproliferative neoplasms (MPNs) is associated with diagnosis of prefibrotic myelofibrosis, history of splanchnic vein thrombosis, and vascular splenomegaly. Blood 2009;114:131. (Ref.49)

Rubbia-Brandt L, et al. Severe hepatic sinusoidal obstruction associated with oxaliplatin-based chemotherapy in patients with metastatic colorectal cancer. Ann Oncol 2004;15:460–466. (Ref.196)

Rubbia-Brandt L, Mentha G, Terris B. Sinusoidal obstruction syndrome is a major feature of hepatic lesions associated with oxaliplatin neoadjuvant chemotherapy for liver colorectal metastases. J Am Coll Surg 2006;202: 199–200. (Ref.211)

Schoepfer AM, et al. Herbal does not mean innocuous: ten cases of severe hepatotoxicity associated with dietary supplements from Herbalife products. J Hepatol 2007;47:521–526. (Ref.189)

Schoppmeyer K, et al. TIPS for veno-occlusive disease following stem cell transplantation. Z Gastroenterol 2006;44:483–486. (Ref.244)

Segev DL, et al. Twenty years of liver transplantation for Budd-Chiari syndrome: a national registry analysis. Liver Transpl 2007;13:1285–1294. (Ref.170)

Seyahi E, et al. Infliximab in the treatment of hepatic vein thrombosis (Budd-Chiari syndrome) in three patients with Behçet's syndrome. Rheumatology (Oxford) 2007;46:1213–1214. (Ref.76)

Sharma S, et al. Pharmacological thrombolysis in Budd Chiari syndrome: a single centre experience and review of the literature. J Hepatol 2004;40: 172–180. (Ref.148)

Shin SH, et al. Characteristic clinical features of hepatocellular carcinoma associated with Budd-Chiari syndrome: evidence of different carcinogenic process from hepatitis B virus–associated hepatocellular carcinoma. Eur J Gastroenterol Hepatol 2004;16:319–324. (Ref.124)

Smalberg JH, et al. Myeloproliferative disease in the pathogenesis and survival of Budd-Chiari syndrome. Haematologica 2006;91:1712–1713. (Ref.44)

Socha P, et al. Hepatic vein thrombosis as a complication of ulcerative colitis in a 12-year-old patient. Dig Dis Sci 2007;52:1293–1298. (Ref.83)

Sozer S, et al. The presence of JAK2V617F mutation in the liver endothelial cells of patients with Budd-Chiari syndrome. Blood 2009;113:5246–5249. (Ref.48)

Takamura M, et al. Recurrence of hepatocellular carcinoma 102 months after successful eradication and removal of membranous obstruction of the inferior vena cava. J Gastroenterol 2004;39:681–684. (Ref.125)

Tang W, et al. Hepatic caudate vein in Budd-Chiari syndrome: depiction by using magnetic resonance imaging. Eur J Radiol 2011;77:143–148. (Ref.130)

Teofili L, et al. MPLSer505Asn induced hereditary thrombocytosis is associated with a high thrombotic risk, splenomegaly and progression to bone marrow fibrosis. Haematologica 2010;95:65–70. (Ref.46)

Tisman G, et al. Oxaliplatin toxicity masquerading as recurrent colon cancer. J Clin Oncol 2004;22:3202–3204. (Ref.199)

Valla D. Hepatic venous outflow tract obstruction etiopathogenesis: Asia versus the West. J Gastroenterol Hepatol 2004;19:204–211. (Ref.7)

Valla DC. Budd-Chiari syndrome and veno-occlusive disease/sinusoidal obstruction syndrome. Gut 2008;57:1469–1478. (Ref.5)

Vassiliadis T, et al. Late onset ulcerative colitis complicating a patient with Budd-Chiari syndrome: a case report and review of the literature. Eur J Gastroenterol Hepatol 2009;21:109–113. (Ref.84)

Vergniol J, et al. Paroxysmal nocturnal hemoglobinuria and Budd-Chiari syndrome: therapeutic challenge with bone marrow transplantation, transjugular intrahepatic portosystemic shunt, and vena cava stent. Eur J Gastroenterol Hepatol 2005;17:453–456. (Ref.68)

Verstovsek S, et al. A phase 2 study of INCB018424, an oral, selective JAK1/JAK2 inhibitor, in patients with advanced polycythemia vera (PV) and essential thrombocythemia (ET) refractory to hydroxyurea. Blood 2009;114:132. (Ref.52)

Wingard JR, Nichols WG, McDonald GB. Supportive care. Hematology Am Soc Hematol Educ Program 2004:372–389. (Ref.213)

A complete list of references can be found at www.expertconsult.com.

VII

Chapter 45

Portal and Splenic Vein Thrombosis

J.C. García-Pagán, S. Seijo, and Jaime Bosch

ABBREVIATIONS

BCS Budd-Chiari syndrome	**IPH** idiopathic portal hypertension	**PVT** portal vein thrombosis
CT computed tomography	**ISVT** isolated splenic vein thrombosis	**SMV** superior mesenteric vein
EBL endoscopic band ligation	**JAK2** Janus kinase-2	**TIPS** transjugular intrahepatic
ERCP endoscopic retrograde	**LMWH** low-molecular-weight heparin	portosystemic shunt
cholangiopancreatography	**MPD** myeloproliferative disease	**US** ultrasound
HCC hepatocellular carcinoma	**MRI** magnetic resonance imaging	
INR international normalized ratio	**OLT** orthotopic liver transplantation	

Introduction

Thrombosis can affect any of the different venous segments of the portal venous system (portal vein, splenic vein, superior mesenteric vein, and inferior mesenteric vein), either isolated or combined.[1-4] The underlying etiologic factors triggering thrombosis are independent of the venous segment involved, and for that reason they will be treated jointly in this chapter. Isolated splenic vein thrombosis and also portosplenomesenteric venous thrombosis occurring in children, in patients with cirrhosis, and in liver transplant recipients have distinctive clinical and management characteristics and will be considered separately. Portal thrombosis may present as two distinct clinical scenarios: acute or chronic portal vein thrombosis. These represent successive stages of the same disease and have similar causes but different management.

Physiology

Under normal circumstances the portal vein is responsible for approximately two thirds of the hepatic blood supply. After thrombosis of the portal venous system has occurred, two mechanisms develop to maintain the hepatic blood flow: an immediate hepatic arterial vasodilatation in response to decreased portal venous flow[2] and a very rapid development (within days) of a network of hepatopetal collateral veins (cavernous transformation of the portal vein) that bypass the thrombosed area.[4] However, these collaterals are not sufficient to carry all the portal blood flow, resulting in presinusoidal, prehepatic portal hypertension.

Epidemiology

In developed countries portal vein thrombosis (PVT) is present in approximately 1% of autopsies.[5] In Asia extrahepatic portal vein thrombosis is a common cause of portal hypertension, accounting for 30% of all cases of gastrointestinal variceal bleeding, and is the leading cause of bleeding in children.[6] In Western countries, however, most cases of PVT are related to cirrhosis or liver tumors, and only one third of cases are attributable to a noncirrhotic, nontumoral origin. Nonetheless, noncirrhotic, nontumoral PVT is the second leading cause of portal hypertension in the world (5% to 10%).[4]

Etiology

After an extensive workup is completed, a definite causal factor is identified in up to 70% of patients with noncirrhotic, nontumoral PVT (**Table 45-1**). In approximately 60% of these cases a systemic thrombophilic factor is documented, and in 30% to 40% predisposing local factors are documented.[4,7-10] In greater than 15% of patients multiple etiologic factors co-exist, supporting the view that portal vein thrombosis is a multifactorial disease[10,11]; therefore a complete etiologic study is required even after a thrombophilic or local factor has been identified. Nonetheless, PVT still remains idiopathic in up to 30% of patients.

Prothrombotic conditions can be acquired or inherited.

Acquired Prothrombotic Disorders

Chronic myeloproliferative diseases (MPDs) are the most frequent etiologic cause of PVT, found in up to 30% to 40% of cases.[1,4,9,12,13] The characteristic increase of blood cells observed in MPD is often masked by the presence of portal hypertension with its consequent expansion of plasma volume and hypersplenism.[7] Hence, all patients with PVT should be evaluated for MPD, even in the absence of polycythemia or thrombocytosis. The diagnosis of MPD has recently been facilitated by genetic testing of the V617F mutation of the Janus kinase 2 (*JAK2*) gene.[14] By testing for this mutation in the etiologic workup of patients with PVT, the probability of diagnosing an underlying MPD has increased from 27.5% to 35%.[15] However, the presence of this mutation does not define the phenotype of MPD. Hence, it is often necessary to perform additional hematologic studies, including bone marrow aspiration/biopsy, to specifically define the type of MPD.

Less common acquired diseases, such as antiphospholipid syndrome, paroxysmal nocturnal hemoglobinuria, or Behçet's syndrome, have also been associated with PVT.[12,16,17]

Pregnancy and the use of oral contraceptives are extremely rare causes of PVT but may trigger it if there are superimposed local or prothrombotic factors.[8,10,18,19]

Inherited Thrombophilic Disorders

Inherited prothrombotic disorders such as factor II or factor V Leiden mutations, and, less frequently, deficiencies of protein C, protein S, or antithrombin III, may cause PVT.[8,9] The diagnosis of these deficiencies (protein C, protein S, and antithrombin III) can be complicated in chronic causes because of impaired hepatic synthesis. Genetic testing of relatives and comparison of factor levels with the levels of other coagulative factors of hepatic synthesis can help to determine whether a specific deficit is primary or secondary.

Hyperhomocysteinemia is a relatively weak risk factor for thrombosis.[7] Moreover, homocysteine levels are highly influenced by diet and by vitamin B_{12} or folic acid deficiencies.[12] Recently, genetic variations in the gene inhibitor of thrombin-activated fibrinolysis (TAFI)[20] and methylenetetrahydrofolate reductase gene mutation have been described as candidate etiologic factors associated with both portal vein thrombosis (PVT) and Budd-Chiari syndrome (BCS).[20]

Local Factors

The presence of local factors (abdominal surgery, inflammation, or sepsis) does not exclude the concomitant presence of a thrombophilic condition, as both are frequently present in adult PVT (see **Table 45-1**). However, in children it is common to find a history of omphalitis or umbilical vein catheterization as the potential cause of PVT, not necessarily associated with the presence of a prothrombotic state.[21] Frequent intestinal infections and poor nutrition have also been implicated to explain the high incidence of PVT in children in Southeast Asia and the Indian subcontinent. Hepatic disorders such as cirrhosis, Budd-Chiari syndrome (BCS), and idiopathic portal hypertension (IPH) may also be complicated by the development of PVT.[22-24]

Clinical Findings

PVT may be manifested as an acute process characterized by abdominal pain and signs suggestive of acute intestinal venous ischemia. However, the acute episode is frequently

Table 45-1 Prevalence of Etiologic Factors in Noncirrhotic, Nontumoral Portal Vein Thrombosis

INHERITED CONDITIONS	PREVALENCE (%)	ACQUIRED CONDITIONS	PREVALENCE (%)
Systemic Factors			

Factor V Leiden mutation	3-8	Myeloproliferative diseases:
		  Polycythemia vera
		  Essential thrombocytopenia
		  Myelofibrosis
			17-35

Prothrombin gene *G20210A* mutation	9-22	Antiphospholipid syndrome	1-11
Protein C deficiency	1-9	Paroxysmal nocturnal hemoglobinuria (PNH)	0-3
Protein S deficiency	2-5	Hyperhomocysteinemia	11-22
C677T *MTHFR* gene mutations	11		

Antithrombin deficiency	0-2	External factors*:
		  Pregnancy
		  Oral contraceptives
			0-40
			7-44

Local Factors			

Inflammatory lesions:
  Omphalitis
  Pancreatitis
  Diverticulitis
  Cholecystitis
  Cholangitis
  Appendicitis
	7-34	Portal vein axis injury:
		  Splenectomy
		  Surgical portocaval shunt
		  Other intraabdominal
		    surgical procedures
			3-45

*See Plessier et al. (2009),[1] Janssen et al. (2000),[9] Primignani et al. (2005, 2006),[10,13] Turnes et al. (2008),[31] and Amitrano et al. (2007).[32]

asymptomatic or paucisymptomatic and portal vein thrombosis may be misdiagnosed until the development of manifestations of chronic portal hypertension.[25]

Acute Portal Vein Thrombosis
Clinical Manifestations

The presence and severity of symptoms in the acute episode are probably related to the velocity of development and the extent of acute venous thrombosis. Patients usually complain of abdominal or lumbar pain, nonspiking fever, and systemic inflammatory response.[26] In up to 80% of cases the abdominal pain is associated with nonspecific dyspeptic symptoms (nausea, postprandial fullness) and discomfort.[1] In many cases these manifestations overlap with those of the triggering factors, such as recent surgery or acute pancreatitis. In cases where thrombosis affects the small mesenteric arches or when diagnosis and treatment are delayed, features of intestinal ischemia may appear with continuous abdominal pain and ileus, which may lead to small-bowel infarction.[12] Ischemic bowel necrosis should be suspected when abdominal pain is accompanied by hematochezia, rebound tenderness at abdominal examination, accumulation of abdominal fluid, metabolic acidosis, and renal or respiratory failure.[4,27] Intestinal stenosis may be a late sequela of mesenteric venous ischemia. In earlier series, intestinal necrosis was a frequent and serious complication, associated with a high mortality rate between 20% and 50% even with surgical resection of the affected segment. Currently, this complication is less likely, probably as a consequence of an earlier diagnosis and immediate application of treatment. Indeed, in a recent prospective multicenter study including 101 patients with acute PVT, intestinal infarction developed in only 2 patients, with a good outcome after limited intestinal resection, and 2 patients died (one death attributable to a late malignancy and another resulting from sepsis).[1]

Isolated thrombosis of an intrahepatic portal vein branch (lobar or segmental) is a special situation, usually detected incidentally by conducting a routine imaging test after surgery, accompanied by a moderate transient increase in the levels of transaminases. The real impact of this alteration is not well known. Usually, in contrast to complete portal trunk thrombosis, it does not lead to development of chronic portal hypertension. However, if repermeabilization is not achieved, it may lead to extinction of the affected liver lobe with a compensatory hypertrophy of the rest of the parenchyma.

Diagnosis

Diagnosis of acute PVT should be suspected in any patient with recent-onset abdominal pain, especially if the patient is known to have an underlying prothrombotic disease or a local factor, including all patients with portal hypertension.

In most patients the diagnosis of acute PVT can be rapidly established using noninvasive imaging.[12] Doppler ultrasound performed by an experienced physician is the technique of choice because of its high sensitivity and lack of side effects. Sonography and Doppler ultrasound can demonstrate the presence of solid hyperechogenic material within the portal vein and turbulence, stasis, or absent or reversed flow. Contrast-enhanced ultrasound (US) has improved the visualization of the portal vein axis.[28] Computed tomography (CT) scanning and magnetic resonance angiography imaging (MRI) may provide additional information, especially regarding the extension of thrombosis and signs of bowel infarction. Lack of significant porto-portal collaterals, presence of a high luminal density in the thrombosed vessel on CT,[29] and lack of signs of chronic portal hypertension (gastrointestinal bleeding, portosystemic collateral circulation, or hypersplenism) are features that help to differentiate a recent thrombosis from the chronic form.[25] This is relevant because it has prognostic and therapeutic consequences (**Fig. 45-1, A**).

Furthermore, imaging techniques can identify the presence of local factors associated with PVT, such as abscesses, neoplasms, inflammatory bowel disease, and pancreatic or liver diseases.[30] In the acute phase, invasive diagnostic techniques such as angiography have almost been abandoned.

In some cases it may be difficult to differentiate between acute PVT and a rethrombotic episode in a patient with chronic PVT.

Treatment

The aims of treatment in acute PVT are to recanalize the occluded veins (to prevent the development of both intestinal

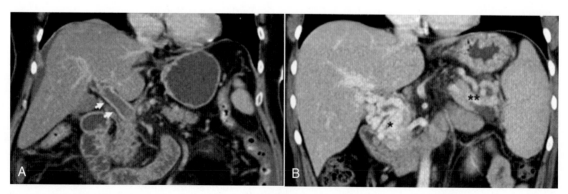

Fig. 45-1 **A,** Coronal CT showing the presence of high-density material within the portal vein trunk *(arrows)* that corresponds to a total thrombosis. Notice the lack of endoluminal enhancement of the portal vein that extends to the portosplenomesenteric confluence. The absence of collaterals suggests an acute episode of PVT. **B,** Coronal CT showing the presence of multiple tortuous collateral veins that bypass the thrombosed area: cavernous transformation of the portal vein *(asterisk)* and hepatopetal collateral veins in the perisplenic area *(double asterisks).*

infarction and portal hypertension) and to quickly correct causal local or systemic factors.[12]

Anticoagulation Therapy

Although no randomized controlled trials (RCTs) have been performed, after the diagnosis of acute PVT early initiation of anticoagulation therapy (within 30 days of the onset of symptoms) is recommended[6,25] based on the clinical observation that spontaneous recanalization is extremely infrequent.[1,26,31] In contrast, anticoagulation therapy allows partial or complete recanalization in a significant proportion of patients, approximately 40% according to recently published series.[1,26,31,32] It is important to initiate anticoagulation therapy as soon as possible. In a recent study the rate of recanalization, partial or complete, was 60% when anticoagulation therapy was started in the first week after the onset of symptoms but only 20% when it was started later (in the first 30 days).[31] Several factors—such as the extent of the initial thrombosis within the portal venous system, the presence of peritoneal fluid at diagnosis of acute PVT, and the presence of more than one prothrombotic disorder—have been identified in retrospective studies as negative predictive factors for recanalization.[26,31,32] A large European multicenter prospective study identified the presence of ascites (even when only detected by ultrasound) and extension of thrombosis to the splenic vein as the most important predictors of lack of recanalization despite early use of anticoagulation therapy.[1] These high-risk factors may be helpful for designing therapeutic studies for acute PVT.

Portal vein recanalization may be expected to occur up to 4 to 6 months after starting an anticoagulation regimen.[26,31] A recent study suggested that mesenteric and splenic veins may recanalize even later.[1] Therefore anticoagulation therapy is recommended for at least 6 months (or even for 12 months).[1,6,25] Although there are no specific studies, long-term anticoagulation administration seems rational in patients with identified prothrombotic disorders, recurrent thrombotic episodes, a personal history of intestinal ischemia, or a family history of deep venous thrombosis. In acute PVT, anticoagulation therapy should be initiated with heparin and maintained for 2 to 3 weeks. After this period, heparin can be changed to an oral vitamin K antagonist, targeting an international normalized ratio (INR) range of 2 to 3. Subcutaneous low-molecular-weight heparin (LMWH) is at least as effective and safe as intravenous heparin.[33] Moreover, LMWHs have a more predictable dose-response relationship, which makes monitoring unnecessary and confers a lower risk of bleeding and immune thrombocytopenia.

Major complications of anticoagulation therapy were reported in fewer than 5% of treated patients.[1,26,31] Anticoagulants should be introduced even in the presence of severe underlying diseases or thrombocytopenia.[1,31] Specific treatment for the underlying acquired prothrombotic disorder should also be initiated.

Other Treatments

Local thrombolytic therapy through a catheter introduced in the portal vein either through the skin (percutaneously) or by transjugular portal vein catheterization may be useful to achieve recanalization in the absence of contraindications.[34] However, this therapy carries a high rate of complications, and probably should be reserved for persistent or worsening symptoms despite systemic anticoagulation therapy.[35,36]

Insertion of a transjugular intrahepatic portosystemic shunt (TIPS) to maintain high portal blood flow velocity has also been proposed, particularly in patients with superimposed BCS.[23,37] There are no studies evaluating whether these invasive approaches offer advantages over early use of anticoagulation therapy.

Surgery is indicated when short-bowel damage is suspected.

Chronic Portal Vein Thrombosis: Portal Cavernoma

Clinical Manifestations

Frequently, the initial episode of PVT is asymptomatic and PVT is diagnosed at a late phase, either during the evaluation of a portal hypertension–related complication (thrombocytopenia, splenomegaly, variceal bleeding, and occasionally jaundice) or incidentally during a diagnostic imaging test performed for an unrelated issue.[25]

Portal hypertension–related complications are the main clinical manifestations of chronic PVT. Upper gastrointestinal endoscopy demonstrates varices in 20% to 55% of cases, mostly large in caliber.[26,31,32] Gastric varices are much more common in chronic PVT than in other causes of portal hypertension. Gastroesophageal varices can develop as early as 1 month after the acute PVT episode, but varices may develop later in those patients with a negative early endoscopy. Consequently, it is recommended that an early screening for varices (2 to 3 months after the diagnosis of acute PVT) be performed and then repeated 6 to 9 months later in the absence of varices or recanalization.[31] The best schedule for further follow-up screening endoscopies is unknown, but a 2- to 3-year interval may be adequate.[25] The presence of ectopic varices, most commonly in the duodenum, anorectal region, and gallbladder bed, is significantly more frequent than in patients with cirrhosis.[3,38] Portal hypertensive gastropathy is a rare feature of this condition.[3]

Variceal bleeding is a frequent manifestation of PVT.[6] Bleeding-related mortality in patients with PVT is much lower than that in cirrhotics, probably because of preserved liver function.[1,19,32,39,40]

Portal biliopathy is defined as abnormalities in the extrahepatic and intrahepatic bile ducts and gallbladder wall in patients with portal cavernoma.[3] It is attributed either to ischemic injury secondary to PVT or, more commonly, to biliary compression by the periportal collaterals composing the cavernoma.[41-43] Obstructive biliary signs, such as stenosis, dilatation, angulation, or irregularity of the bile ducts or choledochus, may be identified by cholangiography in more than 80% of patients after long-standing portal vein obstruction.[41,43] This is commonly associated with increased levels of serum alkaline phosphatase and γ-glutamyltransferase. Despite the high rate of biliary tract abnormalities, clinical manifestations are infrequent.[41] Severe and life-threatening complications (cholecystitis, cholangitis, obstructive jaundice) occur in 5%

to 35% of patients, depending on the severity of symptoms considered.[41,43,44]

Other symptoms such as early satiety, abdominal discomfort, and fullness may be related to massive splenomegaly.[45] Growth retardation attributed to reduced blood flow, resistance to growth hormone function, and reduced levels of insulin-like growth factor is common in childhood.[46]

Ascites is quite infrequent; it represents a late-phase manifestation and is usually associated with triggering events such as gastrointestinal bleeding or infection.[39] In our experience, the 2-year actuarial probability of developing ascites after acute PVT is 16%.[31] Ascites is usually easy to control by adherence to a low-sodium diet and use of diuretics.[47] If this is not the case, other causes for the ascites should be considered.

Overt encephalopathy is rare, but approximately half of the patients with noncirrhotic, nontumoral PVT may develop subclinical neurologic abnormalities compatible with minimal hepatic encephalopathy attributable to portosystemic shunting.[48,49] It is not well known whether these alterations may affect the quality of life and whether these complications are eliminated after blood flow restoration by surgical procedures, such as a mesenteric left portal vein bypass (Rex shunt) for children.[50]

A low prothrombin ratio, other abnormal coagulation parameters (including factor V, factor VII, protein C, protein S, and antithrombin), and a mild increase in the levels of transaminases occur commonly in association with PVT,[51] but the reason for these alterations is not well known. Restitution of the liver blood flow has been shown to revert abnormal coagulation parameters.[52] Furthermore, PVT causes changes in liver morphology, including nodular regenerative hyperplasia,[53] that may be related to hepatic apoptotic phenomena attributable to hypoperfusion despite compensatory arterial vasodilation.[54] The real impact of these abnormalities upon the clinical course or management remains unknown.

Morbidity is mainly related to variceal bleeding, recurrent thrombosis, symptomatic portal biliopathy, and hypersplenism.[25] Mortality among patients with PVT is low and is mainly related to associated diseases (e.g., myelofibrosis, acute leukemia transformation of MPD)[25] rather than to complications of portal hypertension.[55] In this last situation, half of deaths were due to gastrointestinal bleeding, and half due to extensive or recurrent thrombosis.[39] Predictors of survival have not been adequately studied.

Diagnosis

Diagnosis should be suspected in patients with signs of portal hypertension without a chronic liver disease, and confirmed by imaging techniques. Doppler US, CT, and MR angiography demonstrate splenomegaly, portosystemic collaterals, and the presence of portal cavernoma (see **Fig. 45-1, B**).[29,56] In this phase it is not uncommon to find an altered liver architecture (atrophy/hypertrophy complex) and even nodular images corresponding to areas of nodular regenerative hyperplasia in relation to altered hepatic perfusion. These nodules may be misdiagnosed as hepatocarcinoma. In some patients a large, prominent collateral vein at the porta hepatis can be erroneously considered as a normal portal vein. A liver biopsy can help to rule out chronic liver disease associated with PVT in patients with altered liver biochemistry measurements or an abnormal ultrasound. Liver morphologic CT studies of the

caudate lobe atrophy/hypertrophy complex could help to differentiate noncirrhotic PVT.[53] In addition, in our experience the finding of a normal or slightly elevated transient elastography value at FibroScan may also help to differentiate cirrhotic from noncirrhotic PVT.

To assess portal biliopathy, magnetic resonance cholangiography is the first choice technique.[43,57] Endoscopic retrograde cholangiopancreatography (ERCP) should be restricted to symptomatic cases requiring therapeutic intervention. Endoscopic ultrasonography may also show the characteristic lesions of portal biliopathy, but is rarely necessary.

Treatment

The goals of treatment in chronic PVT are (1) prevention and treatment of complications of portal hypertension, (2) prevention of recurrent thrombosis, and (3) treatment of portal biliopathy.

Anticoagulation Therapy

In patients with portal cavernoma anticoagulation therapy has been shown to prevent the progression and recurrence of thrombosis.[32,39] These beneficial effects have been observed without increasing the risk or severity of gastrointestinal bleeding provided that adequate prophylactic measures to prevent variceal bleeding or rebleeding are adopted before initiation of anticoagulation therapy.[39] Thus, although this should be decided on an individual basis, it is our policy to initiate long-term anticoagulation therapy in all patients with an underlying prothrombotic disorder or a history of previous thrombosis.[4] Oral contraceptives should be discontinued. If patients present any underlying acquired thrombophilic disorder, it should be treated.

Acute Bleeding Episode

The acute gastrointestinal bleeding episode should be managed by following the same protocol used in cirrhotic patients.[25] It is recommended that pharmacologic agents (terlipressin, somatostatin, or octreotide) be initiated as early as possible to control variceal bleeding and be maintained for 2 to 5 days.[40] Prophylactic antibiotics should also be instituted. After determination of the variceal origin of the bleeding by emergency endoscopy, appropriate endoscopic treatment should be instituted. Bleeding from isolated gastric varices may require endoscopic variceal obturation with tissue adhesives.[40]

Long-Term Therapy

Insufficient data are available resolving whether pharmacologic or endoscopic therapy is preferable for primary prophylaxis, although experts agree that prevention should always be recommended in patients with large varices.[25,58] Data are also scarce concerning the use of β-blockers with or without endoscopic therapy to prevent rebleeding.[39,40,59] Prospective randomized studies are needed before any firm recommendation can be made about this topic.[25] Endoscopic therapy has been shown to be effective in secondary prophylaxis.[40,60,61] Two studies have shown that, as in cirrhosis, variceal band ligation is superior to sclerotherapy for esophageal varices, with earlier variceal eradication and lower recurrent variceal bleeding and complications.[62] Preliminary data suggest that in the prevention of rebleeding, β-blockers and endoscopic band ligation are equally effective in terms of rebleeding and number and severity of side effects.[63]

Radiologic Treatments

Percutaneous stenting and TIPS in the setting of chronic portal vein thrombosis, although technically demanding, are sometimes possible in adults and children,[64,65] even with a challenging concomitant hepatic venous obstruction.[23,37]

Surgical Shunts

Decompressive surgery should be considered for patients in whom medical and endoscopic therapy is ineffective and who have patent splenic or mesenteric veins with a history of a major bleeding episode.[66,67] In our experience 37% of patients with PVT also had thrombosis of the splenic and superior mesenteric veins and therefore were not suitable for conventional derivative surgery. Other procedures, such as esophageal transection or splenectomy with variceal ligation, are less useful because of the high frequency of late rebleeding attributable to reappearance of the varices.

Novel shunting techniques, such as mesenteric vein bypass from the left portal branch (Rex shunt), show excellent results in children with symptomatic PVT. With this technique, resolution of symptoms, cessation of episodes of gastrointestinal bleeding, and normalization of splenic size, blood count, and coagulation parameters (including factors II, V, and VII) are achieved, and also the hepatic flow is preserved physiologically.[16,68-70] The experience with this technique in adults is still limited to a few case reports, but results are encouraging.[68,71]

Portal Biliopathy

No studies have prospectively evaluated the recommendations for the treatment of portal biliopathy, so these are based on personal experience and review of the scarce literature available.[43,72,73] Ursodeoxycholic acid (UDCA) has been empirically proposed for the treatment of patients with symptomatic portal biliopathy,[43] including those with abnormal cholestatic tests. This is based on the beneficial effects shown by UDCA in the treatment of other cholestatic disorders as well as the lack of adverse effects. Choledocholithiasis may complicate a bile duct stenosis. This necessitates ERCP with sphincterotomy, stone removal, and correction of the stenosis by stent placement.[74-76] When there is no evidence of common bile duct stones sphincterotomy may be ineffective and hazardous.[44,77] In some severe cases with recurrent cholangitis associated with biliary strictures, a portosystemic shunt is the best treatment because it abolishes the bleeding risk and decompresses collaterals.[78] Biliointestinal bypass, other than a second-line intervention (after previous portosystemic shunting), should be avoided because it has high morbidity and mortality.[43,79] Liver transplant has recently been reported to resolve biliary duct complications attributable to cavernoma.[80]

Outcome

The natural history of PVT remains elusive, because of the scarce data available and the heterogeneity of the patient population. The outcome has improved through early diagnosis, as a result of enhanced clinical awareness and improved diagnostic techniques, and probably also by the use of early anticoagulation[26] and antibiotic therapy,[81] which yield 5-year survival rates up to 85% and 81%, respectively, at 10 years.[16,19]

Special Situations
Portal Vein Thrombosis in Cirrhosis

Development of portal vein thrombosis is a significant event in the natural history of cirrhosis. It is usually associated with deterioration of liver function and occurrence of variceal bleeding, but it may be an incidental finding during routine ultrasonography. There are insufficient data to establish whether this association is causal or whether the development of PVT is only a further consequence of liver decompensation.[82] In addition, the natural history of PVT in cirrhosis and the way it may influence survival are not known. It is, however, clear that PVT increases morbidity and mortality associated with liver transplantation and that it may even contraindicate it, especially if the thrombus extends to the superior mesenteric vein.[83,84]

Among all cases of PVT, cirrhosis is the underlying cause in 22% to 32% of patients.[5,19,45] The prevalence of partial or total PVT in cirrhotic patients ranges from 0.6% to 26%.[83,85] It is approximately 11% when patients with hepatocellular carcinoma (HCC) are excluded and US is used for the diagnosis.[86] The prevalence increases with the severity of the disease (1% in compensated cirrhosis[86] and 8% to 25% in candidates for liver transplantation[87]). The incidence of de novo thrombosis has been estimated at 16% at 1-year follow-up in two small prospective studies.[22,85] Because of the widespread use of imaging techniques in patients with cirrhosis, it is highly likely that an increasing number of patients with PVT are being diagnosed.

PVT in liver cirrhosis is a multifactorial condition. The presence of factor V Leiden, prothrombin gene *G20210* mutation, and methylenetetrahydrofolate reductase gene *TT677* mutation is significantly increased in cirrhotic patients with PVT.[85,86] Other coagulation defects such as protein C, protein S, and antithrombin III deficiencies have also been described in patients with cirrhosis and PVT.[85,88] These potential hereditary procoagulative disorders have been suggested to be counterbalanced by impairment of the synthesis of procoagulant factors as a result of liver insufficiency in patients with cirrhosis. However, it is now evident that, in cirrhosis, the complex interactions among procoagulant and anticoagulant mechanisms do not always result in hypocoagulation and bleeding but even more frequently may predispose to a hypercoagulative state facilitating PVT.[89] As a local factor, a recent prospective study has suggested a major role for the reduced portal blood flow velocity, a consequence of portal hypertension, in the development of PVT in cirrhosis.[22] Other factors that have been statistically associated with increased risk of PVT in cross-sectional studies are male gender; previous abdominal surgery (especially splenectomy and portosystemic shunts); previous endoscopic treatment of portal hypertension; previous occurrence of variceal bleeding, encephalopathy, ascites, or low platelet count; and advanced liver failure.[22,83,84,87,90] The

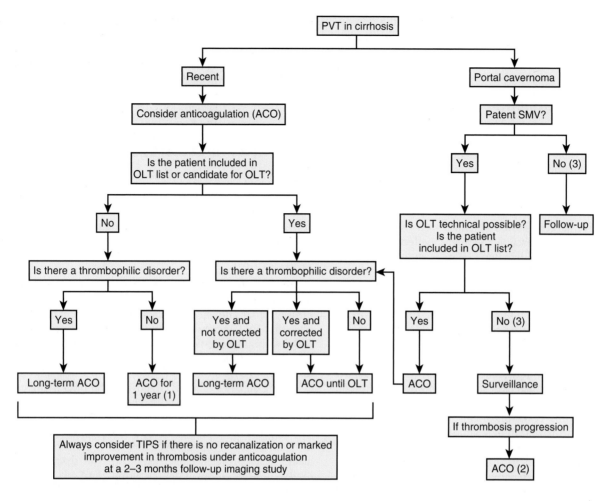

(1) If TIPS is not possible and there is no improvement of thrombosis at 6 months, consider stopping anticoagulation.

(2) If there is an underlying prothrombotic disease and it is not corrected by OLT, anticoagulation for life.

(3) Consider anticoagulation if there is an inherited or acquired thrombotic disorder.

OLT: Orthotopic liver transplantation
SMV: Superior mesenteric vein
TIPS: Transjugular intrahepatic portosystemic shunt

Fig. 45-2 **Algorithm of the proposed management of portal vein thrombosis (PVT) in patients with cirrhosis.**

extent that these factors are relevant in the development of PVT in cirrhosis needs further evaluation.

There are no current clinical guidelines regarding the management of PVT in cirrhosis; however, administering anticoagulation therapy, using transjugular portosystemic shunts, or refraining from intervention has been applied in case series. The aim of treatment should be to achieve recanalization or to prevent thrombosis progression. Therefore early detection of PVT is essential. This has been facilitated by the current approach of performing US every 6 months to screen for HCC provided the US operator is specifically advised to evaluate portal vein patency. However, very frequently patients are diagnosed when they already have a portal cavernoma. In this situation, if patients are candidates for orthotopic liver transplantation (OLT), the aim is to prevent the extension of thrombosis to the superior mesenteric vein, because this may preclude OLT. Anticoagulation therapy is the treatment option most frequently used, but there are limited data concerning its benefits. In a study of 29 cirrhotic patients listed for OLT,

partial or complete recanalization was significantly higher in those who received anticoagulation therapy than in those who did not; none of the patients developed severe anticoagulation-related complications.[87] Although more data are needed before a formal recommendation can be made, **Figure 45-2** summarizes our algorithm approach. TIPS may be considered when thrombosis extends despite anticoagulation therapy.

Portal Vein Thrombosis After Liver Transplantation

Portal vein thrombosis is a rare but serious complication after OLT, with a reported incidence of 1.16% to 2.7%.[12,91] PVT usually occurs at the anastomotic site in the early post-OLT period.[84] Post-OLT PVT can result in graft dysfunction, graft loss (associated with complete PVT in the early post-OLT), portal hypertension, and death. This risk of graft loss and mortality has been reduced as a result of systematic postoperative screening with Doppler-US and its multidisciplinary management.[12,91] Splenectomy during OLT, donor–recipient portal vein diameter mismatch, and modification of the standard portal vein anastomosis (mainly related to pre-OLT PVT) are the risk factors associated with PVT. Management includes angioplasty, systemic thrombolysis, surgical thrombectomy, retransplantation, splenorenal shunt, or wall-stent placement during laparotomy.[12,91]

Isolated Splenic Vein Thrombosis

Isolated splenic vein thrombosis (ISVT) usually results in left-side portal hypertension and isolated gastric fundal varices.[92] The most common cause of ISVT is chronic pancreatitis, with a reported incidence of up to 45%.[92] Occasionally splenic vein thrombosis has been described in relation to pancreatic pseudotumor, pancreatic pseudocyst, retroperitoneal abscess, renal neoplasms, perirenal abscess, and segmental splenic vein resection during removal of a pancreatic tumor (iatrogenic cause).

The triad of gastric varices with splenomegaly and normal liver function is highly suspicious of isolated splenic vein thrombosis.[93,94] Usually, splenic vein obstruction is diagnosed after a bleeding episode related to recurrent gastric varices.[92,94] The accuracy of US to diagnose ISVT may be limited[92] and other imaging techniques such as CT or MRI are often needed.

Because splenectomy eliminates venous collateral outflow and thereby decompresses surrounding varices, surgical treatment is clearly justified in patients presenting with variceal bleeding.[95] However, in patients without prior bleeding, a decision for splenectomy is questionable because of the low rate of variceal bleeding, the absence of mortality related to variceal hemorrhage, the lack of progression of varices on repeated follow-up endoscopy,[92,96] and the long-term care that will be required after splenectomy. This procedure should be avoided if possible, in cirrhotic patients, because the development of PVT following splenectomy may complicate or eliminate the chance of liver transplantation in the future. Splenic artery embolization is a second-line option for high operative risk patients or those in whom intervention is contraindicated.[97]

Portal Vein Thrombosis and Pregnancy

Management of PVT during pregnancy should consider (1) prevention of the progression of PVT as a result of the prothrombotic state characteristic of pregnancy, (2) treatment of the underlying prothrombotic disease, and (3) prevention and treatment of portal hypertension–related complications.

Anticoagulation therapy should be maintained during pregnancy if there is an underlying prothrombotic factor.[18] However, it remains unclear whether anticoagulation therapy should be started when no thrombophilia has been found.[18] Oral anticoagulants are associated with a high risk of miscarriage (14.6% to 56%) and congenital malformations (30%).[18] Therefore clinical practice guidelines recommend a pregnancy test as early as possible, and when pregnancy is confirmed heparin administration should be instituted in lieu of oral anticoagulants.[98] There are scarce data and no specific guidelines but, despite their risk of intrauterine growth retardation and fetal bradycardia, β-blockers should be considered as the first-line option for primary prophylaxis.[99] Variceal bleeding episodes complicated approximately 15% of pregnancies.[100] Despite these complications, maternal prognosis is good, with a less favorable prognosis for the fetus. The incidence of abortion, prematurity, small-for-gestational-age babies, and perinatal death is higher in these women.[6,18] The association of β-blockers and EBL may be a suitable alternative for secondary prophylaxis.

Pregnancy in these patients usually follows a normal course and vaginal delivery is recommended.[18] Cesarean section can be dangerous because of the possible presence of pelvic varices. If there is a specific underlying prothrombotic disease, its possible impact on pregnancy should be considered. All patients with PVT who wish to become pregnant should be properly informed and must be considered high-risk pregnancies.

Acknowledgments

We thank Drs. F. Cervantes, J.C. Reverter, R. Gilabert, M.A. García-Criado, J.G. Abraldes, and P. Tandon for their useful advice during the elaboration of this chapter. SSR was founded by "Río Hortega" Instituto de Salud Carlos III (CM08/00161). This work is supported in part by grants from Instituto de Salud Carlos III, Ministerio de Ciencia e innovación (FIS 06/0623, FIS 09/01261, and SAF 07/61298). Ciberehd Clínic Hospital, Barcelona, Spain, is funded by Instituto de Salud Carlos III.

References

1. Plessier A, et al. Acute portal vein thrombosis: a prospective multicenter follow-up study. Hepatology 2010;51:210–218.
2. Valla DC, Condat B. Portal vein thrombosis in adults: pathophysiology, pathogenesis and management. J Hepatol 2000;32:865–871.
3. Sarin SK, Agarwal SR. Extrahepatic portal vein obstruction. Semin Liver Dis 2002;22:43–58.
4. García-Pagán JC, Hernandez-Guerra M, Bosch J. Extrahepatic portal vein thrombosis. Semin Liver Dis 2008;28:282–292.
5. Ogren M, et al. Portal vein thrombosis: prevalence, patient characteristics and lifetime risk: a population study based on 23,796 consecutive autopsies. World J Gastroenterol 2006;12:2115–2119.
6. Sarin SK, et al. Consensus on extra-hepatic portal vein obstruction. Liver Int 2006;26:512–519.
7. Primignani M, Mannucci PM. The role of thrombophilia in splanchnic vein thrombosis. Semin Liver Dis 2008;28:293–301.
8. Denninger MH, et al. Cause of portal or hepatic venous thrombosis in adults: the role of multiple concurrent factors. Hepatology 2000;31: 587–591.
9. Janssen HL, et al. Factor V Leiden mutation, prothrombin gene mutation, and deficiencies in coagulation inhibitors associated with Budd-Chiari syndrome and portal vein thrombosis: results of a case-control study. Blood 2000;96:2364–2368.
10. Primignani M, et al. Risk factors for thrombophilia in extrahepatic portal vein obstruction. Hepatology 2005;41:603–608.
11. Rosendaal FR. Venous thrombosis: a multicausal disease. Lancet 1999;353: 1167–1173.
12. DeLeve LD, Valla DC, Garcia-Tsao G. Vascular disorders of the liver. Hepatology 2009;49:1729–1764.
13. Primignani M, et al. Role of the JAK2 mutation in the diagnosis of chronic myeloproliferative disorders in splanchnic vein thrombosis. Hepatology 2006;44:1528–1534.
14. Tefferi A, et al. Proposals and rationale for revision of the World Health Organization diagnostic criteria for polycythemia vera, essential thrombocythemia, and primary myelofibrosis: recommendations from an ad hoc international expert panel. Blood 2007; 110:1092–1097.
15. Kiladjian JJ, et al. The impact of JAK2 and MPL mutations on diagnosis and prognosis of splanchnic vein thrombosis: a report on 241 cases. Blood 2008;111:4922–4929.
16. Bittencourt PL, Couto CA, Ribeiro DD. Portal vein thrombosis and Budd-Chiari syndrome. Clin Liver Dis 2009;13:127–144.

17. Bayraktar Y, et al. Cavernous transformation of the portal vein: a common manifestation of Behcet's disease. Am J Gastroenterol 1995;90:1476–1479.
18. Perarnau JM, Bacq Y. Hepatic vascular involvement related to pregnancy, oral contraceptives, and estrogen replacement therapy. Semin Liver Dis 2008;28:315–327.
19. Janssen HL, et al. Extrahepatic portal vein thrombosis: aetiology and determinants of survival. Gut 2001;49:720–724.
20. de Bruijne EL, et al. Genetic variation in thrombin-activatable fibrinolysis inhibitor (TAFI) is associated with the risk of splanchnic vein thrombosis. Thromb Haemostasis 2007;97:181–185.
21. Pinto RB, et al. Portal vein thrombosis in children and adolescents: the low prevalence of hereditary thrombophilic disorders. J Pediatr Surg 2004;39:1356–1361.
22. Zocco MA, et al. Thrombotic risk factors in patients with liver cirrhosis: correlation with MELD scoring system and portal vein thrombosis development. J Hepatol 2009;51:682–689.
23. Darwish MS, et al. Pathogenesis and treatment of Budd-Chiari syndrome combined with portal vein thrombosis. Am J Gastroenterol 2006;101:83–90.
24. Chang PE, et al. Idiopathic portal hypertension in patients with HIV infection treated with highly active antiretroviral therapy. Am J Gastroenterol 2009;104:1707–1714.
25. De FR. Evolving consensus in portal hypertension. Report of the Baveno IV consensus workshop on methodology of diagnosis and therapy in portal hypertension. J Hepatol 2005;43:167–176.
26. Condat B, et al. Recent portal or mesenteric venous thrombosis: increased recognition and frequent recanalization on anticoagulant therapy. Hepatology 2000;32:466–470.
27. Kumar S, Sarr MG, Kamath PS. Mesenteric venous thrombosis. New Engl J Med 2001;345:1683–1688.
28. Rossi S, et al. Contrast-enhanced versus conventional and color Doppler sonography for the detection of thrombosis of the portal and hepatic venous systems. AJR Am J Roentgenol 2006;186:763–773.
29. Mathieu D, Vasile N, Grenier P. Portal thrombosis: dynamic CT features and course. Radiology 1985;154:737–741.
30. Lee HK, et al. Portal vein thrombosis: CT features. Abdom Imaging 2008;33:72–79.
31. Turnes J, et al. Portal hypertension-related complications after acute portal vein thrombosis: impact of early anticoagulation. Clin Gastroenterol Hepatol 2008;6:1412–1417.
32. Amitrano L, et al. Prognostic factors in noncirrhotic patients with splanchnic vein thromboses. Am J Gastroenterol 2007;102:2464–2470.
33. Dolovich LR, et al. A meta-analysis comparing low-molecular-weight heparins with unfractionated heparin in the treatment of venous thromboembolism: examining some unanswered questions regarding location of treatment, product type, and dosing frequency. Arch Intern Med 2000;160:181–188.
34. Lopera JE, et al. Percutaneous transhepatic treatment of symptomatic mesenteric venous thrombosis. J Vasc Surg 2002;36:1058–1061.
35. Hollingshead M, et al. Transcatheter thrombolytic therapy for acute mesenteric and portal vein thrombosis. J Vasc Interv Radiol 2005;16:651–661.
36. Smalberg JH, et al. Risks and benefits of transcatheter thrombolytic therapy in patients with splanchnic venous thrombosis. Thromb Haemostasis 2008;100:1084–1088.
37. Senzolo M, et al. Transjugular intrahepatic portosystemic shunt (TIPS), the preferred therapeutic option for Budd Chiari syndrome associated with portal vein thrombosis. Am J Gastroenterol 2006;101:2163–2164.
38. Chawla Y, Dilawari JB. Anorectal varices—their frequency in cirrhotic and non-cirrhotic portal hypertension. Gut 1991;32:309–311.
39. Condat B, et al. Current outcome of portal vein thrombosis in adults: risk and benefit of anticoagulant therapy. Gastroenterology 2001;120:490–497.
40. Spaander MC, et al. Endoscopic treatment of esophagogastric variceal bleeding in patients with noncirrhotic extrahepatic portal vein thrombosis: a long-term follow-up study. Gastrointest Endosc 2008;67:821–827.
41. Khuro MS, et al. Biliary abnormalities associated with extrahepatic portal venous obstruction. Hepatology 1993;17:807–813.
42. Dhiman RK, et al. Biliary changes in extrahepatic portal venous obstruction: compression by collaterals or ischemic? Gastrointest Endosc 1999;50:646–652.
43. Condat B, et al. Portal cavernoma-associated cholangiopathy: a clinical and MR cholangiography coupled with MR portography imaging study. Hepatology 2003;37:1302–1308.
44. Sezgin O, et al. Endoscopic management of biliary obstruction caused by cavernous transformation of the portal vein. Gastrointest Endosc 2003;58:602–608.
45. Cohen J, Edelman RR, Chopra S. Portal vein thrombosis: a review. Am J Med 1992;92:173–182.
46. Sarin SK, et al. Portal-vein obstruction in children leads to growth retardation. Hepatology 1992;15:229–233.
47. Rangari M, et al. Hepatic dysfunction in patients with extrahepatic portal venous obstruction. Liver Int 2003;23:434–439.
48. Minguez B, et al. Noncirrhotic portal vein thrombosis exhibits neuropsychological and MR changes consistent with minimal hepatic encephalopathy. Hepatology 2006;43:707–714.
49. Sharma P, et al. Minimal hepatic encephalopathy in patients with extrahepatic portal vein obstruction. Am J Gastroenterol 2008;103:1406–1412.
50. Mack CL, et al. Surgically restoring portal blood flow to the liver in children with primary extrahepatic portal vein thrombosis improves fluid neurocognitive ability. Pediatrics 2006;117:e405–e412.
51. Fisher NC, et al. Deficiency of natural anticoagulant proteins C, S, and antithrombin in portal vein thrombosis: a secondary phenomenon? Gut 2000;46:534–539.
52. Mack CL, Superina RA, Whitington PF. Surgical restoration of portal flow corrects procoagulant and anticoagulant deficiencies associated with extrahepatic portal vein thrombosis. J Pediatr 2003;142:197–199.
53. Vilgrain V, et al. Atrophy-hypertrophy complex in patients with cavernous transformation of the portal vein: CT evaluation. Radiology 2006;241:149–155.
54. Bilodeau M, et al. Evaluation of hepatocyte injury following partial ligation of the left portal vein. J Hepatol 1999;30:29–37.
55. Janssen HL. Role of coagulation in the natural history and treatment of portal vein thrombosis. J Gastroenterol Hepatol 2001;16:595–596.
56. Ueno N, et al. Color Doppler ultrasonography in the diagnosis of cavernous transformation of the portal vein. J Clin Ultrasound 1997;25:227–233.
57. Umphress JL, Pecha RE, Urayama S. Biliary stricture caused by portal biliopathy: diagnosis by EUS with Doppler US. Gastrointest Endosc 2004;60:1021–1024.
58. Condat B, Valla D. Nonmalignant portal vein thrombosis in adults. Nat Clin Pract Gastroenterol Hepatol 2006;3:505–515.
59. Orr DW, et al. Chronic mesenteric venous thrombosis: evaluation and determinants of survival during long-term follow-up. Clin Gastroenterol Hepatol 2007;5:80–86.
60. Sarin SK, Sachdev G, Nanda R. Follow-up of patients after variceal eradication. A comparison of patients with cirrhosis, noncirrhotic portal fibrosis, and extrahepatic obstruction. Ann Surg 1986;204:78–82.
61. Vleggaar FP, van Buuren HR, Schalm SW. Endoscopic sclerotherapy for bleeding oesophagogastric varices secondary to extrahepatic portal vein obstruction in an adult Caucasian population. Eur J Gastroenterol Hepatol 1998;10:81–85.
62. Zargar SA, et al. Endoscopic ligation vs. sclerotherapy in adults with extrahepatic portal venous obstruction: a prospective randomized study. Gastrointest Endosc 2005;61:58–66.
63. Gupta N, et al. Endoscopic variceal ligation and beta-blockers are equally effective in prevention of variceal rebleeding in patients with non cirrhotic portal hypertension: a randomized controlled trial. Hepatology 2009;50(4 Suppl):401A–402A.
64. Bilbao JI, et al. Transjugular intrahepatic portosystemic shunt (TIPS) in the treatment of venous symptomatic chronic portal thrombosis in non-cirrhotic patients. Cardiovasc Intervent Radiol 2004;27:474–480.
65. Senzolo M, et al. Transjugular intrahepatic portosystemic shunt for portal vein thrombosis with and without underlying cirrhosis. Cardiovasc Intervent Radiol 2007;30:545.
66. Warren WD, et al. Management of variceal bleeding in patients with noncirrhotic portal vein thrombosis. Ann Surg 1988;207:623–634.
67. Orloff MJ, et al. Bleeding esophagogastric varices from extrahepatic portal hypertension: 40 years' experience with portal-systemic shunt. J Am Coll Surg 2002;194:717–728.
68. de Ville de GJ, et al. Original extrahilar approach for hepatic portal revascularization and relief of extrahepatic portal hypertension related to later portal vein thrombosis after pediatric liver transplantation. Long term results. Transplantation 1996;62:71–75.
69. de Ville de GJ, et al. Direct bypassing of extrahepatic portal venous obstruction in children: a new technique for combined hepatic portal revascularization and treatment of extrahepatic portal hypertension. J Pediatr Surg 1998;33:597–601.
70. Superina R, et al. Correction of extrahepatic portal vein thrombosis by the mesenteric to left portal vein bypass. Ann Surg 2006;243:515–521.

71. Vanderlan WB, Bansal A, Abouljoud MS. Adult portal hypertension secondary to posttraumatic extrahepatic portal vein thrombosis treated with Rex shunt. J Trauma 2009;66:260–263.

72. Htun OY, et al. Symptomatic portal biliopathy: a single centre experience from the UK. Eur J Gastroenterol Hepatol 2009;21:206–213.

73. Dumortier J, et al. Diagnosis and treatment of biliary obstruction caused by portal cavernoma. Endoscopy 2003;35:446–450.

74. Thervet L, et al. Endoscopic management of obstructive jaundice due to portal cavernoma. Endoscopy 1993;25:423–425.

75. Bhatia V, Jain AK, Sarin SK. Choledocholithiasis associated with portal biliopathy in patients with extrahepatic portal vein obstruction: management with endoscopic sphincterotomy. Gastrointest Endosc 1995; 42:178–181.

76. Dhiman RK, et al. Portal hypertensive biliopathy. Gut 2007;56:1001–1008.

77. Mutignani M, et al. Endoscopic treatment of extrahepatic bile duct strictures in patients with portal biliopathy carries a high risk of haemobilia: report of 3 cases. Dig Liver Dis 2002;34:587–591.

78. Vibert E, et al. Therapeutic strategies in symptomatic portal biliopathy. Ann Surg 2007;246:97–104.

79. Chaudhary A, et al. Bile duct obstruction due to portal biliopathy in extrahepatic portal hypertension: surgical management. Br J Surg 1998;85:326–329.

80. Hajdu CH, et al. Intrahepatic portal cavernoma as an indication for liver transplantation. Liver Transpl 2007;13:1312–1316.

81. Plemmons RM, Dooley DP, Longfield RN. Septic thrombophlebitis of the portal vein (pylephlebitis): diagnosis and management in the modern era. Clin Infect Dis 1995;21:1114–1120.

82. García-Pagán JC, Valla DC. Portal vein thrombosis: a predictable milestone in cirrhosis? J Hepatol 2009;51:632–634.

83. Nonami T, et al. The incidence of portal vein thrombosis at liver transplantation. Hepatology 1992;16:1195–1198.

84. Yerdel MA, et al. Portal vein thrombosis in adults undergoing liver transplantation: risk factors, screening, management, and outcome. Transplantation 2000;69:1873–1881.

85. Amitrano L, et al. Inherited coagulation disorders in cirrhotic patients with portal vein thrombosis. Hepatology 2000;31:345–348.

86. Amitrano L, et al. Risk factors and clinical presentation of portal vein thrombosis in patients with liver cirrhosis. J Hepatol 2004;40:736–741.

87. Francoz C, et al. Splanchnic vein thrombosis in candidates for liver transplantation: usefulness of screening and anticoagulation. Gut 2005;54:691–697.

88. Martinelli I, et al. High levels of factor VIII and risk of extra-hepatic portal vein obstruction. J Hepatol 2009;50:916–922.

89. Northup PG. Hypercoagulation in liver disease. Clin Liver Dis 2009;13: 109–116.

90. Amitrano L, et al. Portal vein thrombosis after variceal endoscopic sclerotherapy in cirrhotic patients: role of genetic thrombophilia. Endoscopy 2002;34:535–538.

91. Cavallari A, et al. Treatment of vascular complications following liver transplantation: multidisciplinary approach. Hepatogastroenterology 2001;48:179–183.

92. Weber SM, Rikkers LF. Splenic vein thrombosis and gastrointestinal bleeding in chronic pancreatitis. World J Surg 2003;27:1271–1274.

93. Han DC, Feliciano DV. The clinical complexity of splenic vein thrombosis. Am J Surg 1998;64:558–561.

94. Goldberg S, et al. Isolated gastric varices due to spontaneous splenic vein thrombosis. Am J Gastroenterol 1984;79:304–307.

95. Sutton JP, Yarborough DY, Richards JT. Isolated splenic vein occlusion. Review of literature and report of an additional case. Arch Surg 1970;100: 623–626.

96. Heider TR, et al. The natural history of pancreatitis-induced splenic vein thrombosis. Ann Surg 2004;239:876–880.

97. Owman T, et al. Embolization of the spleen for treatment of splenomegaly and hypersplenism in patients with portal hypertension. Invest Radiol 1979;14:457–464.

98. Bates SM, et al. Venous thromboembolism, thrombophilia, antithrombotic therapy, and pregnancy: American College of Chest Physicians Evidence-Based Clinical Practice Guidelines (8th ed.). Chest 2008;133(6 Suppl): 844S–886S.

99. Mahadevan U, Kane S. American Gastroenterological Association Institute technical review on the use of gastrointestinal medications in pregnancy. Gastroenterology 2006;131:283–311.

100. Kochhar R, et al. Pregnancy and its outcome in patients with noncirrhotic portal hypertension. Dig Dis Sci 1999;44:1356–1361.

Chapter **46**

Liver Involvement in Osler-Weber-Rendu Disease (Hereditary Hemorrhagic Telangiectasia)

Martin Caselitz, Siegfried Wagner, and Michael P. Manns

ABBREVIATIONS

ACVRL1 activin receptor–like kinase-1
ALK1 activin receptor–like kinase-1
AVMs arteriovenous malformations
BMPs bone morphogenetic proteins

ENG endoglin
HCC hepatocellular carcinoma
HHT hereditary hemorrhagic telangiectasia
MRI magnetic resonance imaging

PAVMs pulmonary AVMs
TGF-β transforming growth factor-β
VEGF vascular endothial growth factor

General Aspects and Diagnostic Criteria

Hereditary hemorrhagic telangiectasia (HHT), or Osler-Weber-Rendu disease, is a rare hereditary autosomal dominant disorder of blood vessels. Mucocutaneous and visceral fibrovascular dysplasia leads to various arteriovenous malformations (AVMs) and telangiectasia in different organs. These manifestations predominantly involve the skin, mucosa, liver, gastrointestinal tract, lung, and brain (**Fig. 46-1**).

The following features are summarized in the classic triad of Osler disease:
1. Multiple mucocutaneous telangiectases (**Fig. 46-2**)
2. Epistaxis
3. Positive family history

The association of these features was described by Rendu in 1896 and independently by Osler in 1901 and Weber in 1907.[1-3] The names of these authors appear in various order in the common eponymous labels for this condition. In 1909, Hanes coined the term "hereditary hemorrhagic telangiectasia" in acknowledgment of the three features that by then defined the disorder.[4]

Initially, it was suspected that visceral involvement in HHT was a rare condition, but interpretation was based on the frequency of symptomatic patients seen by an astute physician. With the onset of modern imaging methods and asymptomatic screening programs, a much higher incidence of visceral involvement was seen.[4] Approximately a third of affected individuals have multiorgan involvement. Moreover, visceral involvement of HHT can be responsible for the high mortality rate of affected patients.[5,6] With regard to the importance of visceral involvement, an actual diagnostic score was developed based on the criteria described in **Table 46-1**.[5] These criteria permit a high level of clinical suspicion with limited diagnostic procedures.

Especially in young patients with a positive family history who do not fulfill the diagnostic clinical criteria for HHT, genetic testing for the two most common mutations (*endoglin*, activin receptor–like kinase-1 [*ALK1* or *ACVRL1*]) can be performed to assist in establishing a diagnosis of HHT. Genetic testing is complex because there are no "common mutations" or "hot spots" and not all genes that can cause HHT have been discovered. A clinical sensitivity/mutation detection rate of approximately 75% for sequence analysis of *endoglin* and *ACVRL1* has been reported (see later).[7]

Epidemiology

Hereditary hemorrhage telangiectasia occurs in many ethnic groups and has a wide geographic distribution, including Asia, Africa, and the Middle East.[8,9]

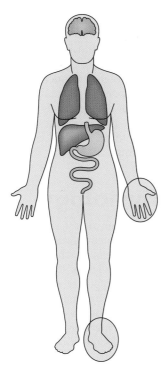

Fig. 46-1 **Distribution of organs affected in hereditary hemorrhagic telangiectasia.**

Table 46-1 Diagnostic Criteria (Curaçao Criteria) as Presented by Shovlin and Tarte
The diagnosis of hereditary hemorrhagic telangiectasia (HHT) is
• "Definite" if three or four criteria are present • "Possible" or "suspected" if two criteria are present • "Unlikely" if fewer than two criteria are present
Criteria

• Multiple telangiectases at characteristic sites:
  Lips (see Fig. 46.2)
  Oral cavity
  Fingers
  Nose
• Epistaxis: spontaneous, recurrent nosebleeds
• Family history: a first-degree relative with HHT according to these criteria
• Visceral manifestation
  Gastrointestinal telangiectases (with or without bleeding)
  Pulmonary arteriovenous malformations (AVMs)
  Hepatic AVMs
  Cerebral AVMs
  Spinal AVMs

Adapted from Shovlin CL, Letarte M. Hereditary haemorrhagic telangiectasia and pulmonary arteriovenous malformations: issues in clinical management and review of pathogenic mechanisms. Thorax 1999;54:714–729.

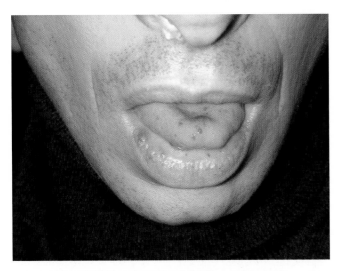

Fig. 46-2 **Telangiectasia of the lips and tongue.**

The prevalence of HHT ranges between 1 in 2000 and 1 in 40,000. There are considerable differences in the geographic distribution of HHT. HHT has been found to occur in 1 in 2351 persons in the French department of Ain, 1 in 3500 on the Danish island Fünen,[10] 1 in 5155 in the Leeward Islands (West Indies), 1 in 16,500 in the state of Vermont (United States),[11] and 1 in 39,000 in northern England.[12]

Genetic Background

Hereditary hemorrhagic telangiectasia is inherited in an autosomal dominant manner, with variable expression of clinical symptoms even among family members.[13] However, the penetrance of HHT is high (>95%), with an age-dependent phenotype that is nearly complete by the age of 40 to 45 years.[11,14] Up to 20% of patients lack a family history of HHT. The homozygous state appears to be lethal.[15]

Studies of families with HHT have identified five genes whose defects are believed to be responsible for the majority of cases of HHT.

The phenotype has thus been classified as HHT1 or HHT2, depending on the thus far well-described mutated genes *endoglin* and *ACVRL1*. Mutations in these two genes account for the majority of cases of HHT. Both genes code for two receptors of the transforming growth factor-β (TGF-β) superfamily.

TGF-β is a member of a supergene family of polypeptide growth factors that include activins, inhibins, and bone morphogenetic proteins (BMPs). TGF-β is produced by nearly every cell, and each cell expresses the corresponding receptors. This factor plays a significant role in the regulation of cell proliferation and differentiation, wound healing, angiogenesis, and embryonic development. In endothelium, TGF-β modulates endothelial cell functions (e.g., migration, proliferation, adhesion), interactions between endothelium and smooth muscle cell layers, and vascular tone.

HHT1 is caused by mutations of the *endoglin* gene on chromosome 9q3. Confirmation that *endoglin* (CD105, *ENG*) mutations are causative is provided by experiments in transgenic mice. Some mice carrying one normal and one mutated copy of the *endoglin* gene display features of HHT.[16] Endoglin is the most abundant TGF-β–binding protein found on endothelial cells. It consists of 658 amino acids and is an integral transmembrane protein that associates with TGF-β ligand–binding receptors and modulates cellular responses.

Endoglin interacts with and becomes a component of the TGF-β1 and TGF-β3 receptor complexes involved in endothelial cell signaling. More than 130 mutations have been identified to date, and disease severity has not been correlated with the type of mutation.

The mutant endoglin products seen in HHT1 are transient intracellular molecules that show no cell surface expression. Measurable levels of normal endoglin in HHT patients are thus reduced by 50%, even in "normal" vessels, thus suggesting that a single copy of the gene confers susceptibility to the disease but that a "second hit" or modifier genes probably contribute to the development of vascular abnormalities.[17]

HHT2—the second genetic defect—is mapped to chromosome 12q13. It results in a mutation in the *ALK1* or *ACVRL1* gene, which has similar affinity to the TGF-β complex as endoglin. Significant expression of this gene product occurs only in endothelium, but it may also be found in peripheral blood leukocytes. ACVRL1 is a type I cell surface receptor in the TGF-β superfamily. It modulates TGF-β signaling during regulation of angiogenesis and plays an important role in controlling blood vessel development and repair. ACVRL1 has the properties of a type I serine/threonine kinase receptor and binds to TGF-β1 only in association with TGF-β receptor type II in vitro; however, the ACVRL1 ligand in vivo remains unknown. More than 100 mutations have been identified so far.[18] Similar to endoglin, reduced levels of functional ACVRL1 are seen, thus suggesting a haploinsufficiency mechanism of disease.[19]

The presence of two disease loci provided the basis for genotype-phenotype studies of the disease.[20] Recently, a large questionnaire-based study led Berg and colleagues to the conclusion that the HHT1 phenotype is distinct from and more severe than the HHT2 phenotype.[21] In this study, an earlier onset of epistaxis and telangiectasia was seen in patients with HHT1. Additionally, pulmonary AVMs (PAVMs) were noted only in HHT1.[21] *ACVRL1* mutations were also identified in kindreds with pulmonary hypertension and HHT[22] (see later discussion).

In conclusion, mutations in both genes are associated with blood vessels with impaired wall integrity, which are more susceptible to dilation and remodeling during development and repair after injury.

Mutations in a third gene, *SMAD4*, have been reported in a subgroup of HHT individuals with or without signs of juvenile polyposis. Additional HHT genes have also recently been mapped to chromosomes 5 and 7.[23-25]

Genetic Background of Liver Involvement

Nikolopoulos and co-workers[26] and Piantanida and associates[27] described HHT families with an accumulation of liver involvement, which suggests a genotype-phenotype correlation of hepatic manifestation in HHT. These observations prompted another group to systematically screen for mutations in the *ENG* and *ACVRL1* genes in a group of HHT patients from Germany with and without liver involvement. The researchers found that hepatic manifestation in HHT patients is associated with mutations in the *ACVRL1* gene but is rarely also caused by *ENG* mutations.[28,29]

Recent analysis of the genotype-phenotype relationship revealed differences between HHT1 and HHT2 and within

HHT1 and HHT2 between men and women. Pulmonary and cerebral vascular malformations occur more often in HHT1, whereas hepatic vascular malformations are more frequent in HHT2 (40.6%) than in HHT1 (7.6%). Furthermore, in HHT1 and HHT2, there is a higher frequency of hepatic vascular malformations in women. Explanations for the sex-related differences have still not been precisely identified and include environmental factors, modifier genes, or hormonal differences. Additionally, within families there is a wide variety of expression of symptoms.[30]

Pathophysiology

In HHT the malformations consist of aberrant vascular development with multiple dilated vessels that are lined by a single layer of endothelium that is attached to a continuous basement membrane. The smallest of the hallmark telangiectases are focal dilations of postcapillary venules. In fully developed telangiectases, the venules are markedly dilated and convoluted with excessive layers of smooth muscle without elastic fibers. These venules often connect directly to dilated arterioles without intervening capillaries. This aberrant development is also associated with a perivascular mononuclear cell infiltrate. However, no single pathognomonic histologic characteristic for the telangiectasia in HHT exists.

Various explanations for the characteristic bleeding of these vessels include insufficient smooth muscle contractile elements, endothelial cell junction defects, perivascular connective tissue weakness, and endothelial cell degeneration.[15] Changes in the liver in HHT are described later.

Organ Manifestations

The diverse manifestations of HHT involve mostly vascular abnormalities of the nose, skin, lung, brain, and gastrointestinal tract. **Table 46-2** summarizes the most important organ manifestations of persons with HHT. However, angiodysplasia

Table 46-2 Clinical Manifestations of Hereditary Hemorrhagic Telangiectasia

AFFECTED ORGAN OR SYSTEM	TYPE OF LESION	FREQUENCY
Nose, skin, and oral cavity	Telangiectases	80%-100%
Lung	Arteriovenous malformations	15%-30%
Gastrointestinal tract	Telangiectases, angiodysplasia, arteriovenous malformations	11%-44%
Central nervous system (brain and spinal cord)	Telangiectases, arteriovenous malformations, arterial aneurysm, cavernous angioma	8%-31%
Liver	Arteriovenous malformations	Telangiectases in up to 78%

may occur in every organ. Cases of urogenital,[12,31,32] ophthalmologic,[33,34] and splenic[35] involvement in HHT have been reported in the literature. Furthermore, aneurysms of the coronary artery[36] and the aorta[37] are described.

Nose

Epistaxis caused by spontaneous bleeding from telangiectases of the nasal mucosa is the most common (95%) and earliest manifestation of HHT and occurs in the majority of affected persons, but not in all. The average age at onset of epistaxis is 12 years. It may be so severe that multiple transfusions and oral iron supplementation are required,[38] or it may be so mild that HHT is never suspected. Recurrent epistaxis begins by the age of 10 years in many patients and by the age of 21 years in most (>90%); it becomes more severe in the later decades in about two thirds of affected persons.

Skin

Telangiectases of the skin typically occur later in life than does epistaxis. By the age of 40, most affected persons (70%) have multiple telangiectases on the lips, tongue, palate, fingers, face, nail beds, or a combination of these sites[4,39] (Fig. 46-2). There may be bleeding from cutaneous telangiectases, but it is rarely clinically important. In these cases or for cosmetic concerns, laser ablation can be effective.

Lung

Pulmonary AVMs are thin-walled abnormal vessels that replace normal capillaries between the pulmonary arterial and venous circulations, and they often result in bulbous saclike structures.[5,40] They are frequently multiple and appear in both lungs, with a predilection for the lower lobes.[41] These "capillary-free" shunts give rise to three main clinical consequences[42]:
1. Pulmonary arterial blood cannot be oxygenated, thereby leading to hypoxemia.
2. The absence of a filtering capillary bed allows embolic particles to reach the systemic circulation, where they have an impact on other capillary beds (e.g., abscess in the central nervous system).
3. The fragile vessels may lead to hemorrhage into a bronchus or the pleural cavity.

Embolic cerebral events (cerebral abscess and embolic stroke) occur in patients regardless of the degree of respiratory symptoms and are still associated with significant morbidity and mortality.[5]

Complications of PAVMs can be limited if this condition is diagnosed and treated by transcatheter embolization, which offers the safest method of treatment. Recently published guidelines recommend screening all patients with possible or confirmed HHT for PAVMs. Initial screening should be performed with transthoracic contrast-enhanced echocardiography. The therapy of choice for PAVMs is transcatheter embolization.[43] Surgical management of PAVMs may be an alternative option in selected patients.[5] Long-term follow-up of treated patients is important because the growth of malformations may require further treatment. In addition, prophylactic antibiotics are recommended at the time of dental and surgical procedures to reduce the risk for brain abscess.

Central Nervous System

About 15% to 23% of patients with HHT may have cerebral involvement with telangiectases, AVMs, aneurysms, or cavernous angiomas.[5,44] Cerebral involvement can lead to migraine headache, seizures, ischemia of the surrounding tissue because of a steal effect, hemorrhage, and less commonly, paraparesis.[45] An important cause of neurologic complications is pulmonary embolism from PAVMs. It is estimated that in up to two thirds of those in whom neurologic symptoms develop, PAVMs are the source of the symptoms. In the remaining third, complications arise from cerebral AVMs. Screening of adult HHT patients for cerebral involvement by magnetic resonance imaging (MRI) with a protocol consisting of contrast-enhanced and non–contrast-enhanced images and sequences that detect blood products to maximize sensitivity is recommended.[43]

HHT patients with neurologic symptoms suggestive of cerebral involvement or pulmonary embolism deserve further assessment, as in the non-HHT population, by experienced neurointerventional centers.

Gastrointestinal Tract

The gastrointestinal tract is the second most common organ system involved in HHT after the respiratory system. Gastrointestinal manifestations of HHT can be found in every section of the gut.[39,46] Characteristically, gastrointestinal symptoms do not appear until the fifth or sixth decade of life.[4] Telangiectasia or AVM may occur in about 60% of patients with HHT (**Fig. 46-3**). Hemorrhage, the most common gastrointestinal manifestation, is seen in 10% to 45% of patients.[5,47] In a retrospective study, up to 40% of patients had an upper gastrointestinal source of bleeding, up to 10% had a lower gastrointestinal source, and 50% had an indeterminate bleeding site.[47] Thus far, no studies of capsular endoscopy are available in HHT patients. Transfusion of more than 100 units of blood because of gastrointestinal bleeding has been documented.[48] Hemobilia from hepatic telangiectasia has been proposed as a cause of gastrointestinal bleeding as well.[49]

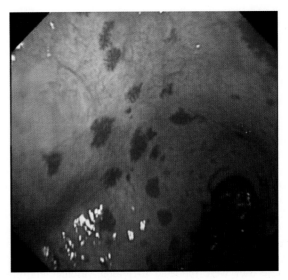

Fig. 46-3 **Angiodysplasia in the stomach.**

A recent consensus conference has recommended that all patients with HHT who are older than 35 years should have hemoglobin or hematocrit levels checked annually. If anemia disproportionate to epistaxis is found, the patient should undergo endoscopy to look for telangiectases. In those with the *SMAD4* mutation, screening for gastrointestinal polyps and malignancy should be performed.[43]

The basic principles for the management of acute gastrointestinal bleeding in patients with HHT are the same as for any other lesion. Early recognition of HHT is important for proper management. Endoscopy remains the most important tool for diagnosing and treating this condition. Endoscopic findings include AVMs or telangiectases similar to those seen in the oral or nasal mucosa.[50] Tagged red blood cell scans may be used to diagnose the origin of subacute bleeding but are of only limited use because of the often intermittent nature of the bleeding. In the setting of severe acute hemorrhage, angiography may demonstrate the origin of bleeding as well.[50]

Recurrent hemorrhage is most difficult to manage. Endoscopic treatment techniques include the use of laser and argon plasma coagulation; all methods have comparable results in the control of acutely bleeding telangiectases, with typical success rates exceeding 90%.[51,52] However, the long-term results of endoscopy have been disappointing because of the multifocal nature of the disease and recurrent episodes of bleeding from other sites in the gastrointestinal tract.

Asymptomatic, nonbleeding lesions should not be treated because of the risk of inducing acute or delayed bleeding (or both). Patients refractory to endoscopic treatment or those with lesions not amenable to endoscopic therapy may require angiography with arterial embolization or surgery after localization of the bleeding site. However, with the further development of endoscopic techniques, the need for surgical intervention has steadily decreased and it is now rarely required. Long-term treatment of hemorrhage in patients with HHT, regardless of the source, has been disappointing. In some small trials, hormonal treatment with estrogen-progestogen combinations (ethinylestradiol, 0.05 mg, and norethisterone, 1 mg daily, given orally) has been shown to decrease transfusion requirements in patients with gastrointestinal bleeding.[48] ε-Aminocaproic acid, a potent inhibitor of the fibrinolytic system, has been reported to decrease the frequency of bleeding episodes and the number of transfusions required.[50]

Danazol (Danocrine), 200 mg orally twice daily for 6 weeks and then continued in responders (200 mg daily), may be a beneficial alternative in men with fewer side effects. Another alternative is antifibrinolytic therapy with aminocaproic or tranexamic acid. Aminocaproic acid is usually started at 500 mg four times per day orally and increased to a maximum of 2500 mg four times daily (10 g/day). Tranexamic acid is usually started at 500 mg orally every 8 to 12 hours and increased to 1 to 1.5 g orally every 8 to 12 hours. Patients should be screened for pulmonary vascular malformations before initiating systemic therapies because of increased thrombogenic risk.[43]

A case report described regression of gastrointestinal telangiectases during immunosuppression with sirolimus after liver transplantation in a female patient with HHT. Sirolimus and aspirin were included in the posttransplant therapy because they were reported to inhibit vascular endothelial growth factor (VEGF).[53]

Hepatic Manifestations of Hereditary Hemorrhagic Telangiectasia

Historical Aspects and Epidemiology of Liver Involvement

Liver involvement in HHT was originally suspected by Osler in 1901. The first case report was published by van Bogaert in 1935.[54] Martini reviewed the literature in 1978 and grouped liver involvement into three histologic subtypes[55]:
1. Telangiectasia with fibrosis or cirrhosis
2. Cirrhosis without telangiectasia
3. Telangiectasia without fibrosis or cirrhosis

Patients in group 2 often had a superimposed disease present that caused the cirrhosis, such as posttransfusion hepatitis or iron overload. Vascular dilation and arteriovenous shunts with high-output cardiac failure were found in groups 1 and 3.[15]

Recent screening studies of HHT patients have reported a prevalence of hepatic vascular malformations of 32% to 72% with Doppler ultrasound and 67% to 78% with triphasic computed axial tomography. In none of these studies was a diagnostic gold standard (angiography) uniformly performed. However, these prevalences are all much higher than the symptomatic rate (8%), thus suggesting that these tests are sensitive. No screening studies have been performed in children.[43]

Histopathology and Pathophysiology of Hepatic Involvement

The liver has a unique vascular supply. Blood enters the liver from two sources, the portal vein and the hepatic artery; it merges at the level of the hepatic sinusoids and exits through the hepatic veins. Therefore the hepatic changes associated with HHT can be complex and multiple and include sinusoidal ectasia, arteriovenous shunts (direct communication between arterioles and sinusoids), arterioportal shunts (direct shunt between branches of the hepatic artery and the portal vein causing portal hypertension), and portovenous shunts (connections between portal veins and sinusoids).

Three forms of angiodysplasia have been identified:
1. Telangiectases are focal dilations that originate from capillaries and postcapillary venules (or sinusoids in the liver) (**Fig. 46-4**). These dilated vessels are lined by a single layer of endothelium attached to continuous basement membrane. The vessels are often surrounded by a mononuclear cell infiltrate.
2. AVMs are larger dilated tortuous vessels consisting of both arterial and venous elements with interrupted elastica lamina and variable thickness of the smooth muscle layers. AVMs are devoid of interlinking capillaries; therefore significant shunting occurs. In the liver, arteriovenous shunting, arterioportal shunting, and portovenous shunting may occur. The different types of shunts may explain the wide variety of clinical symptoms in HHT patients with hepatic involvement. The lesions are embedded in dense fibrous tissue. These fibrous bands may link, thereby entrapping

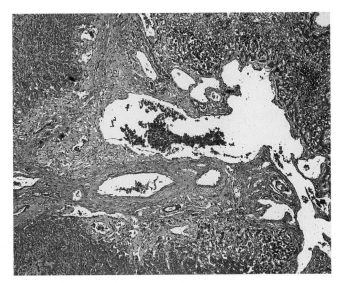

Fig. 46-4 **Microscopic aspect of hepatic involvement in hereditary hemorrhagic telangiectasia with dilated vessels.** (Hematoxylin-eosin stain, 100×.)

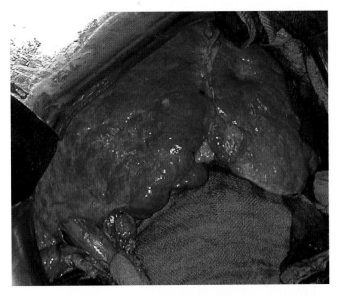

Fig. 46-5 **Nodular pattern of hepatic involvement in hereditary hemorrhagic telangiectasia (pseudocirrhosis).**

the hepatocytes and leading to a fine or coarse nodular appearance similar to cirrhosis (pseudocirrhosis) (**Fig. 46-5**). The hepatocellular architecture is preserved within these nodules, including central veins and portal areas. There may be little or no hepatocellular necrosis or inflammation. Reilly and Nostrant performed liver biopsy in 10 HHT patients with suspected liver involvement.[47] They found hepatic telangiectasia in 30%, iron overload in 50%, and periportal fibrosis in 80% of affected patients. However, no patient with fully developed cirrhosis, bridging necrosis, or chronic active hepatitis was found. These findings were confirmed by other authors.[56]

3. Aneurysms form large vessels secondary to fragmentation of the elastic lamina and loss of the vessel's muscularis.

Focal nodular hyperplasia (FNH)—independent of hormonal therapy—in patients with HHT is presumed to be

parenchymal hyperplasia secondary to hyperperfusion by large anomalous hepatic arteries.

Hepatomegaly (>15 cm at the midclavicular line), sometimes accompanied by splenomegaly, is found as a consequence of portal hypertension or intrahepatic AVMs in 44% of affected patients.[57]

Primary involvement of the liver must be distinguished from secondary hepatic complications occurring in patients with HHT. Viral hepatitis following transfusion for iron deficiency anemia may cause liver cirrhosis in older HHT patients. Patients with unexplained elevated liver enzyme levels for more than 6 months should undergo hepatitis B and C serologic evaluation and sonographic imaging (see later). HHT patients requiring blood transfusions should be vaccinated against hepatitis B. Hepatocellular carcinoma (HCC) has been described in a very few patients with hepatic manifestations of HHT.[58] However, HHT with liver involvement itself cannot be considered a risk factor for HCC, but the presence of viral hepatitis in affected patients may lead to HCC.

Furthermore, hepatic iron overload has been described as a complication of repetitive blood transfusions or iron supplementation in patients with HHT. Systemic AVMs may lead to high-output cardiac failure and congestion of the liver. The increased pressure in the sinusoids may induce fibrosis of the liver. Therefore cirrhosis in some HHT-affected patients may be caused by right-sided congestive heart failure (cardiac cirrhosis).

Up to 70% of HHT patients suffering from symptomatic liver involvement are female and in their fourth or fifth decade.[5,14,59,60] These findings have been confirmed by other authors when the initial problem was pulmonary[41,61] and cerebral[5,62] vascular malformations. The increasing magnitude of hepatic vascular malformations[37,63] and pulmonary arteriovenous fistulas during pregnancy indicates the potential role of hormones in the pathogenesis of vascular malformations.[64,65] This is supported by the observation that gastrointestinal bleeding may be treated successfully with estrogen-progestogen combinations,[48] and recurrent episodes of epistaxis are associated with menstruation.[5] However, thus far the exact mechanism of hormonal influence remains unclear.

Clinical Features

The manifestations of HHT are not generally present at birth, but telangiectases and malformations develop with increasing age. Therefore the clinical course can be divided into three periods:

1. An asymptomatic period during childhood
2. A hemorrhagic period with episodes of severe and recurrent epistaxis from puberty up to the third decade
3. A period of manifest organ involvement (e.g., pulmonary, hepatic) with clinical symptoms and secondary complications in some patients[66]

Liver involvement is generally asymptomatic. Symptoms appear around the age of 30 or later and occur predominantly in females. It appears that symptoms develop in only 8% of patients with HHT and hepatic vascular malformations.

Substantial morbidity and mortality occur in only a minority of patients with hepatic involvement. In the liver, arteriovenous shunting, arterioportal shunting, and portovenous shunting occur and explain the great variety of clinical symptoms. The three most common initial clinical manifestations are high-output heart failure, portal hypertension, and biliary ischemia (Garcia-Tsao types 1 to 3).[56]

Hepatic involvement in HHT can also be manifested clinically as abdominal angina secondary to arteriovenous shunting and as portosystemic encephalopathy secondary to portovenous shunts.[67]

Heart Failure

The most common finding is high-output heart failure caused by shunts between the hepatic artery and hepatic veins, and it occurs predominantly in middle-aged women. It is characterized by shortness of breath, dyspnea on exertion, ascites, or edema. A liver bruit has been reported to be present in half of affected patients. Laboratory testing reveals anicteric cholestasis (elevated γ-glutamyltransferase and alkaline phosphatase) in up to 73% of patients.[59]

Right heart catheterization is the gold standard for diagnosis, but an elevated cardiac output or cardiac index can be measured by echocardiography as well. Mean pulmonary pressure is only mildly elevated and correlates with pulmonary capillary wedge pressure. This is different from the primary pulmonary hypertension described in patients with HHT, in whom pulmonary arterial pressure is markedly elevated.[22]

Portal Hypertension

Shunting from the hepatic artery to the portal vein is the main cause of portal hypertension as a complication of liver involvement in patients with HHT. A second cause may be nodular regenerative hyperplasia in some patients. In contrast to high-output cardiac failure, portal hypertension is described in male and female patients equally. These patients exhibit ascites, varices, or variceal hemorrhage. Levels of bilirubin and alkaline phosphatase are elevated. Notably in HHT patients with portal hypertension, liver synthetic function and platelet counts are normal because these patients do not have cirrhosis and therefore liver insufficiency does not develop. In some patients, portal pressure measurements might be helpful to confirm the diagnosis (>5 mm Hg hepatic venous pressure gradient).

Biliary Ischemia

In contrast to the liver, the biliary system derives its blood supply solely from the hepatic artery. Shunting from the hepatic artery to the hepatic or portal vein may lead to biliary hypoperfusion. The subsequent biliary ischemia causes biliary strictures with or without cholangitis and biliary necrosis with cyst formation. This form of hepatic involvement occurs in women. Patients suffer from abdominal pain in the right upper quadrant and have clinical signs of cholestasis with or without cholangitis. Notably, the right upper quadrant pain observed in some patients is presumably due to thrombosis in telangiectasia independent of the biliary ischemia. Laboratory abnormalities include elevated levels of alkaline phosphatase and bilirubin.[67]

Portosystemic Encephalopathy

Portosystemic encephalopathy is a rare manifestation of hepatic involvement and occurs as a result of shunting from the portal to the hepatic vein. The development of encephalopathy depends on the magnitude of the shunt; if it is small,

encephalopathy is unusual. Recurrent hepatic encephalopathy is described in patients with liver failure, after gastrointestinal bleeding, and in patients with portovenous shunts.[68] Most HHT patients with portosystemic encephalopathy also have other clinical symptoms of hepatic vascular malformations.[67]

Abdominal Angina

In rare cases, abdominal AVMs may further induce a "steal syndrome," which may lead to symptoms of abdominal angina with consequent loss of weight.[59] The pathogenesis is related to shunting of blood away from the mesenteric circulation into the liver. The diagnosis is based on superior mesenteric angiographic findings.[43,67]

Diagnosis of Hepatic Involvement in Hereditary Hemorrhagic Telangiectasia

Screening for liver vascular malformations in patients with HHT who have no clinical evidence of liver involvement is not recommended because the prevalence is high and there is no effective treatment of asymptomatic vascular malformations. Diagnostic procedures for hepatic involvement might be helpful to clarify the diagnosis of HHT in patients with one or two Curaçao criteria (see **Table 46-1**) in whom genetic testing is inconclusive or not available.[67]

In contrast, in patients with accidentally diagnosed diffuse liver AVMs who do not fulfill the diagnostic clinical criteria for HHT (see **Table 46-1**), genetic testing for the two most common coding sequence mutations (*endoglin*, *ALK1*) can be performed to assist in establishing a diagnosis of HHT.

However, diagnosis of liver involvement is based on both clinical diagnostic criteria (as previously discussed) and imaging methods. Liver involvement is suspected by finding a thrill or bruit in the right upper quadrant of the abdomen.

Although anicteric cholestasis has been well described by several authors, laboratory tests are not appropriate to diagnose the hepatic manifestations of HHT. Percutaneous liver biopsy may reveal typical features such as telangiectasia, hepatic congestion, and periportal fibrosis.[47] Because of the considerable risk for bleeding following biopsy and the improvement in imaging methods, percutaneous liver biopsy should be avoided in patients with proven or suspected HHT. Transjugular biopsy may be an alternative to percutaneous biopsy in a very few selected patients.[43,67]

The diagnosis of hepatic vascular malformations is made by imaging procedures. Although a dilated hepatic artery (>7 mm) and intrahepatic hypervascularization are present in most HHT patients with liver involvement, the picture of hepatic involvement in HHT is highly variable. It may be confused with other comorbid conditions (**Table 46-3**) such as liver cirrhosis, FNH, and hepatic congestion. Angiography is the gold standard for the diagnosis of hepatic AVMs (**Fig. 46-6**). Characteristically, dilation and tortuosity of the hepatic artery and its branches are seen along with numerous telangiectatic lesions throughout the liver and early visualization of the hepatic veins, right heart chambers, or both. The angiographic appearance depends on the stage of development of the AVM. The differential diagnosis includes conditions of reduced portal venous blood flow, cavernous hemangiomas,

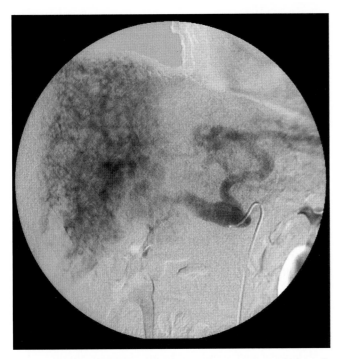

Fig. 46-6 **Angiographic findings of hepatic involvement in hereditary hemorrhagic telangiectasia.**

Table 46-3 **Differential Diagnosis of Sonographic Findings in Hepatic Involvement of Hereditary Hemorrhagic Telangiectasia**

Cirrhosis of the liver: irregular surface of the liver
Tumors of the liver (especially focal nodular hyperplasia): dilated and hypertrophic branches of the hepatic artery
Caroli syndrome, sclerosing cholangitis: dilated intrahepatic bile ducts (B-mode sonography)
Arteriovenous fistulas of other origin

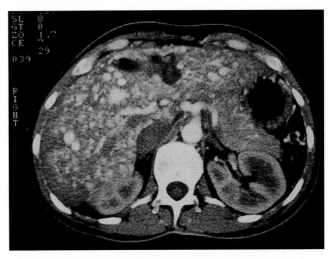

Fig. 46-7 **Computed tomographic scan showing intrahepatic vascular malformations.**

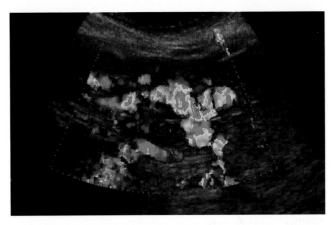

Fig. 46-8 **Intrahepatic hypervascularization caused by dilated branches of the hepatic artery.** (Color Doppler, 3.75-MHz convex transducer.)

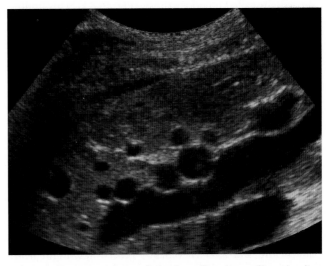

Fig. 46-9 **Tortuous course of the hepatic artery.** (B-mode ultrasound, 3.75-MHz convex transducer.)

highly vascularized liver tumors or metastatic neoplasms, cirrhosis, and hemangioendothelioma of infancy.[53,69,70]

One should, however, consider that selective angiography of the hepatic artery—the current gold standard—is expensive, invasive, and not readily available for repeated measurements. Doppler ultrasound, spiral and multidetector computed tomography (**Fig. 46-7**), and MRI are less invasive and have high sensitivity for establishing the diagnosis of liver involvement. Typical findings include hepatic artery dilation, disseminated telangiectasia, early filling of the hepatic vein, and a pseudonodular pattern in the liver. The aspects of the differential diagnosis are similar to those mentioned earlier.[51,71-73]

Ultrasound criteria were investigated in several studies. The characteristic sonographic picture of liver lesions in HHT consists of intrahepatic hypervascularization (**Fig. 46-8**) caused by a lack of normal tapering of arterial branches combined with a tortuous course of the dilated hepatic artery (>7 mm) (**Figs. 46-9 and 46-10**). Earlier stages of hepatic involvement include peripheral hypervascularization, increased flow velocity, or decreased resistance index of the hepatic artery.[67,74]

Another study demonstrated that one sonographic feature that appears to be linked to the more advanced stages of liver

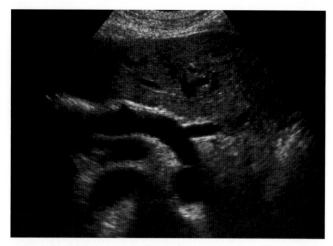

Fig. 46-10 **Dilated common hepatic artery.** (B-mode ultrasound, 3.75-MHz convex transducer.)

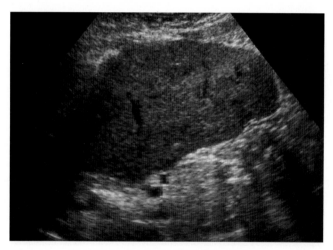

Fig. 46-11 **Sonographic aspect of the nodular pattern of hepatic involvement in hereditary hemorrhagic telangiectasia (pseudocirrhosis).** (B-mode ultrasound, 3.75-MHz convex transducer.)

involvement in HHT is an irregular, nodular surface of the liver, usually called pseudocirrhosis (**Fig. 46-11**). This finding needs to be distinguished from the regenerative nodules found in liver cirrhosis.[57]

A recent interobserver agreement study that involved three experienced investigators demonstrated very good agreement in determining the presence or absence of hepatic vascular malformations, but only moderate agreement in grading the severity of the AVMs.[75] Therefore ultrasound has been proposed as a noninvasive approach to investigate HHT patients and to diagnose and monitor hepatic HHT lesions.[8,54,69]

In addition to the criteria just mentioned, sonographic findings may reveal right heart failure, portal hypertension, and different types of focal liver lesions, such as hemangiomas and FNH.[54,69] The prevalence of FNH is much higher in HHT patients with liver involvement (2.9%) than in the general population (0.3%). Measurement of cardiac output is required to evaluate symptomatic patients with hepatic AVMs, especially before and after therapeutic procedures. Right heart catheterization with the use of thermodilution or noninvasive echocardiography can be used to calculate cardiac output.[59]

Abnormalities of the bile duct similar to those in Caroli disease or those in sclerosing cholangitis have been described in the literature.[49,56,76,77] Imaging methods such as computed tomography and sonography can show focal biliary dilation in the liver. In the event of inconsistent findings, biliary disease can be confirmed by magnetic resonance cholangiography. Diagnostic endoscopic retrograde cholangiography should be avoided because it significantly increases the risk for cholangitis.[67]

Therapy

No treatment is recommended for HHT patients with asymptomatic liver involvement. In those with symptomatic liver involvement, management depends on the clinical findings. Clinical complications of hepatic AVMs may be indications for therapeutic intervention. Such complications are grouped as follows[56]:

- Cardiac insufficiency induced by arteriovenous shunts
- Complications of portal hypertension
- Biliary ischemia
- Hepatic encephalopathy caused by portovenous shunts
- Abdominal angina induced by arteriovenous shunts

Because severe symptomatic hepatic involvement in HHT is quite rare and accompanied by multiple clinical features, a standard therapy cannot be recommended. Treatment of cardiac insufficiency and portal hypertension caused by increased cardiac output or arterioportal shunts should be conservative and based on pharmaceutical intervention. β-Blockers are the primary choice for these patients.[15] Further therapy includes correction of anemia, salt restriction, diuretics, antihypertensive agents, antiarrhythmic agents, and digoxin as clinically indicated. Complication of portal hypertension should be treated as recommend in patients with cirrhosis. Analgesics could be used in the case of abdominal complaints.

If medical treatment is insufficient, other therapeutic options must be considered. In general, there are three main options:

1. Liver transplantation
2. Surgical ligation or banding of the hepatic artery
3. Transcatheter embolization of the hepatic artery or appropriate branches

The different therapeutic options are based on different concepts and strategies. Liver transplantation should be considered only after failure of intensive medical therapy. After successful liver transplantation, recurrence of hepatic vascular malformations should not be expected, and this could be interpreted as a cure of HHT with regard to the liver. However, recent reports have described recurrence of vascular malformation after liver transplantation.[78]

Survival rates of up to 92% 5 years after liver transplantation and improving quality of life in 75% of HHT patients after liver transplantation have been reported.[79] Survival after liver transplantation in the subgroup of patients with portal hypertension appeared to be the worst, with an overall survival rate of 63% at a median follow-up period of 47 months.[78]

Surgical ligation or banding and embolization of the hepatic artery are performed to reduce the pathologic hepatic blood flow. Ligation of the hepatic artery has been reported in only very select cases in the past 25 years, as opposed to alternative methods of therapy.[80] Recently, Koscielny and co-workers reported a modified technique of flow-adapted hepatic artery banding as an alternative palliative procedure to hepatic artery ligation or embolization.[81]

The objective of transarterial embolization is to reduce arteriovenous or arterioportal shunting by embolizing branches of the hepatic artery. This method has been used by several investigators to treat vascular malformations in HHT. Amelioration or resolution of symptoms has been reported in most cases, but the procedure is associated with significant morbidity and mortality, mostly in form of biliary or hepatic necrosis, or both. Consequently, the clinical results after embolization differ considerably. Although some authors reported severe side effects or a fatal outcome,[56,80,82] others have described a successful outcome in up to 80% of treated patients.[59]

In recent guidelines and reviews, embolization of liver malformations is considered a temporizing and high-risk procedure and should be used only as a last resort in patients who are not candidates for liver transplantation.[43,67,83-86] In rare patients with symptomatic focal vascular malformations of the liver, resection of affected segments might be a therapeutic alternative as shown by an anecdotal report.[87] In HHT patients with portal hypertension caused by hepatic vascular malformations, a transjugular intrahepatic portosystemic shunt may be a alternative to liver transplantation.[88]

Bevacizumab is an antibody against VEGF. Administration of six courses of bevacizumab over a 12-week period at a dose of 5 mg/kg in a 47-year-old women with high-output cardiac failure because of hepatic vascular malformations led to a dramatic improvement in her clinical state. This improvement was confirmed by imaging of the liver (reduction of liver vascularity) and normalization of cardiac output. Further investigations are needed, however, before bevacizumab can be used as an alternative to liver transplantation or other therapeutic options.[89]

Comparison of the different therapeutic approaches is thus far based on case reports and small groups of patients. The literature was reviewed in several articles and has been summarized in guidelines and reviews.[43,67,83-86] In conclusion, treatment is not indicated in patients with asymptomatic liver involvement. In patients with symptoms, treatment depends on the clinical findings. Portal hypertension and heart failure are treated according to the standards of care. Biliary disease is treated with ursodeoxycholic acid and with analgetics for right upper quadrant pain. Liver transplantation is the only curative treatment and should be considered for acute biliary necrosis syndrome and intractable heart failure or intractable portal hypertension. Embolization can be considered in patients with intractable heart failure and hepatic artery steal syndrome who are not transplant candidates. It is contraindicated in patients with portosystemic shunting and biliary involvement. Finally, HHT patients with symptomatic liver involvement should be referred to specialized centers where interdisciplinary management by hepatologists, transplant surgeons, and interventional radiologists can be provided.

Summary

Also known as Osler-Weber-Rendu disease, HHT is an autosomal dominant disorder that results in fibrovascular dysplasia and the development of telangiectases and AVMs.

Telangiectases cause bleeding of the skin and mucosal membranes, whereas AVMs may lead to serious complications when they are located in the lungs, liver, and brain.

The clinical manifestations vary over time and are generally progressive. Classification of the phenotypes of HHT is based on the recently identified mutated genes *endoglin* (HHT1) and *ACVRL1* (HHT2). Both genes encode for two receptors of the TGF-β family. Other families with phenotypic HHT do not bear these mutations; therefore at least three other genes are involved.

Involvement of the liver with AVMs is associated with HHT2. Hepatic manifestations of HHT are reported in up to 78% of individuals affected by HHT, but only a minority of affected patients become symptomatic. Generally, hepatic involvement becomes clinically symptomatic predominantly in women during the fifth to sixth decade of life. Large hepatic AVMs can lead to significant complications, including high-output congestive heart failure, biliary ischemia, portal hypertension, hepatic encephalopathy, and abdominal ischemia.

Screening for hepatic involvement is not recommended in asymptomatic patients. In cases of suspected but not proven HHT or following the development of clinical symptoms, hepatic malformations can be diagnosed by imaging methods such as Doppler sonography, computed tomography, MRI, and angiography. Ultrasound is a method with high sensitivity and specificity in detecting hepatic involvement in HHT and is a low-cost, noninvasive bedside method that does not require the application of contrast media or radiation. Liver biopsy should be avoided.

Asymptomatic hepatic manifestations of HHT require no treatment. Symptomatic hepatic involvement should be treated according to the clinical symptoms, such as heart failure. In patients in whom medical treatment is insufficient, liver transplantation, which eradicates malformations, must be considered, especially in those with ischemic biliary necrosis, intractable heart failure, or intractable portal hypertension. Embolization of the hepatic artery is associated with significant morbidity and mortality and therefore an alternative option only for selected patients with intractable heart failure who are not transplant candidates.[43,67,83-86]

References

1. Rendu HJ. Epistaxis repetees chez un sujet porteur de petits angiomes cutanes et muqueux. Gaz Hop 1896;13:731–733.
2. Osler W. On a family form of recurrent epistaxis, associated with multiple telangiectases of the skin and mucous membranes. Bull Johns Hopkins Hosp 1901;12:333–337.
3. Weber FP. Multiple hereditary developmental angiomata (telangiectases) of the skin and mucous membranes associated with recurrent haemorrhages. Lancet 1907;2:160–162.
4. Guttmacher AE, Marchuk DA, White RIJ. Hereditary hemorrhagic telangiectasia. N Engl J Med 1995;333:918–924.
5. Shovlin CL, Letarte M. Hereditary haemorrhagic telangiectasia and pulmonary arteriovenous malformations: issues in clinical management and review of pathogenic mechanisms. Thorax 1999;54:714–729.
6. Kjeldsen AD, Vase P, Green A. Hereditary haemorrhagic telangiectasia: a population-based study of prevalence and mortality in Danish patients. J Intern Med 1999;245:31–39.
7. Prigoda NL, et al. Hereditary hemorrhagic telangiectasia: mutation detection, test sensitivity and novel mutations. J Med Genet 2006;43: 722–728.
8. Yamaguchi H, et al. A novel missense mutation in the endoglin gene in hereditary hemorrhagic telangiectasia. Thromb Haemost 1997;77:243–247.
9. El-Harith EA, et al. Hereditary hemorrhagic telangiectasia: a case report. Saudi Med J 1999;20:797–799.

10. Gallione CJ, et al. Two common endoglin mutations in families with hereditary hemorrhagic telangiectasia in the Netherland Antilles: evidence for a founder effect. Hum Genet 2000;107:40–44.

11. Guttmacher AE, McKinnon WC, Upton MD. Hereditary hemorrhagic telangiectasia: a disorder in search of the genetics community. Am J Med Genet 1994;52:252–253.

12. Porteous ME, Burn J, Proctor SJ. Hereditary haemorrhagic telangiectasia: a clinical analysis. J Med Genet 1992;29:527–530.

13. Shovlin CL. Molecular defects in rare bleeding disorders: hereditary haemorrhagic telangiectasia. Thromb Haemostat 1997;78:145–150.

14. Plauchu H, et al. Age-related clinical profile of hereditary hemorrhagic telangiectasia in an epidemiologically recruited population. Am J Med Genet 1989;32:291–297.

15. Larson AM. Liver disease in hereditary hemorrhagic telangiectasia. J Clin Gastroenterol 2003;36:149–158.

16. Bourdeau A, Dumont DJ, Letarte M. A murine model of hereditary hemorrhagic telangiectasia. J Clin Invest 1999;104:1343–1351.

17. Bourdeau A, et al. Potential role of modifier genes influencing transforming growth factor-beta1 levels in the development of vascular defects in endoglin heterozygous mice with hereditary hemorrhagic telangiectasia. Am J Pathol 2001;158:2011–2020.

18. Fernandez LA, et al. Hereditary hemorrhagic telangiectasia, a vascular dysplasia affecting the TGF-beta signaling pathway. Clin Med Res 2006;14:463–470.

19. Abdalla SA, et al. Analysis of ALK-1 and endoglin in newborns from families with hereditary hemorrhagic telangiectasia type 2. Hum Mol Genet 2000;9:1227–1237.

20. Johnson DW, et al. A second locus for hereditary hemorrhagic telangiectasia maps to chromosome 12. Genome Res 1995;5:21–28.

21. Berg J, et al. Hereditary haemorrhagic telangiectasia: a questionnaire based study to delineate the different phenotypes caused by endoglin and ALK1 mutations. J Med Genet 2003;40:585–590.

22. Trembath RC, et al. Clinical and molecular genetic features of pulmonary hypertension in patients with hereditary hemorrhagic telangiectasia. N Engl J Med 2001;345:325–334.

23. Gallione CJ, et al. SMAD4 mutations found in unselected HHT patients. J Med Genet 2006;43:793–797.

24. Cole SG, et al. A new locus for hereditary hemorrhagic telangiectasia (HHT3) maps to chromosome 5. J Med Genet 2005;42:577–582.

25. Bayrak-Toydemir P, et al. A fourth locus for hereditary hemorrhagic telangiectasia maps to chromosome 7. Am J Med Genet 2006;140:2155–2162.

26. Nikolopoulos N, Xynos E, Vassilakis JS. Familial occurrence of hyperdynamic circulation status due to intrahepatic fistulae in hereditary hemorrhagic telangiectasia. Hepatogastroenterology 1988;35:167–168.

27. Piantanida M, et al. Hereditary haemorrhagic telangiectasia with extensive liver involvement is not caused by either HHT1 or HHT2. J Med Genet 1996;33:441–443.

28. Kuehl HK, et al. Hepatic manifestation is associated with ALK1 in hereditary hemorrhagic telangiectasia: identification of five novel ALK1 and one novel ENG mutations. Hum Mutat 2005;25:320.

29. Brakensiek K, et al. Identification of eight novel mutations in German patients with hereditary hemorrhagic telangiectasia (HHT) and detection of a significant association between mutations in the ACVRL1 gene and hepatic involvement. Clin Genet 2008;74:171–177.

30. Letteboer TGW, et al. Genotype-phenotype relationship in hereditary hemorrhagic telangiectasia. J Med Genet 2006;43:371–377.

31. Hagspiel KD, Christ ER, Schopke W. Hereditary hemorrhagic telangiectasis (Osler-Rendu-Weber disease) with pulmonary, hepatic and renal disease pattern. Rofo 1995;163:190–192.

32. Cooke DA. Renal arteriovenous malformation demonstrated angiographically in hereditary haemorrhagic telangiectasia (Rendu-Osler-Weber disease). J R Soc Med 1986;79:744–746.

33. Brant AM, Schachat AP, White RI Jr. Ocular manifestations in hereditary hemorrhagic telangiectasia (Rendu-Osler-Weber disease). Am J Ophthalmol 1989;107:642–646.

34. Lepori JC, et al. Rendu-Osler familial hemorrhagic telangiectasia with retinal localization. Bull Soc Ophtalmol Fr 1981;81:641–644.

35. Secil M, et al. Splenic vascular malformations and portal hypertension in hereditary hemorrhagic telangiectasia: sonographic findings. J Clin Ultrasound 2001;29:56–59.

36. Kurnik PB, Heymann WR. Coronary artery ectasia associated with hereditary hemorrhagic telangiectasia. Arch Intern Med 1989;149:2357–2359.

37. Romer W, Burk M, Schneider W. Hereditary hemorrhagic telangiectasia (Osler's disease). Dtsch Med Wochenschr 1992;117:669–675.

38. Aassar OS, Friedmann CM, White RI Jr. The natural history of epistaxis in hereditary hemorrhagic telangiectasia. Laryngoscope 1991;101:977–980.

39. Haitjema T, et al. Hereditary hemorrhagic telangiectasia (Osler-Weber-Rendu disease): new insights in pathogenesis, complications, and treatment. Arch Intern Med 1996;156:714–719.

40. Kjeldsen AD, et al. Prevalence of pulmonary arteriovenous malformations (PAVMs) and occurrence of neurological symptoms in patients with hereditary haemorrhagic telangiectasia. J Intern Med 2000;248:255–262.

41. White RI Jr, et al. Pulmonary arteriovenous malformations: techniques and long-term outcome of embolotherapy. Radiology 1988;169:663–669.

42. Ference BA, et al. Life-threatening pulmonary hemorrhage with pulmonary arteriovenous malformations and hereditary hemorrhagic telangiectasia. Chest 1994;106:1387–1390.

43. Faughnan ME, et al. International guidelines for the diagnosis and management of hereditary hemorrhagic telangiectasia. J Med Genet 2011;48:73–87.

44. Fulbright RK, et al. MR of hereditary hemorrhagic telangiectasia: prevalence and spectrum of cerebrovascular malformations. AJNR Am J Neuroradiol 1998;19:477–484.

45. Roman G, et al. Neurological manifestations of hereditary hemorrhagic telangiectasia (Rendu-Osler-Weber disease): report of 2 cases and review of the literature. Ann Neurol 1978;4:130–144.

46. Vase P, Grove O. Gastrointestinal lesions in hereditary hemorrhagic telangiectasia. Gastroenterology 1986;91:1079–1083.

47. Reilly PJ, Nostrant TT. Clinical manifestations of hereditary hemorrhagic telangiectasia. Am J Gastroenterol 1984;79:363–367.

48. Van Cutsem E, Rutgeerts P, Vantrappen G. Treatment of bleeding gastrointestinal vascular malformations with oestrogen-progesterone. Lancet 1999;335:953–955.

49. Costa MT, et al. Hemobilia in hereditary hemorrhagic telangiectasia: an unusual complication of endoscopic retrograde cholangiopancreatography. Endoscopy 2003;35:531–533.

50. Sharma VK, Howden CW. Gastrointestinal and hepatic manifestations of hereditary hemorrhagic telangiectasia. Dig Dis 1998;16:169–174.

51. Longacre AV, et al. Diagnosis and management of gastrointestinal bleeding in patients with hereditary hemorrhagic telangiectasia. Am J Gastroenterol 2003;98:59–65.

52. Kitamura T, et al. Rendu-Osler-Weber disease successfully treated by argon plasma coagulation. Gastrointest Endosc 2001;54:525–527.

53. McAllister VC. Regression of cutaneous and gastrointestinal telangiectasia with sirolimus and aspirin in a patient with hereditary hemorrhagic telangiectasia. Ann Intern Med 2006;144:226–227.

54. Bernard G, et al. Hepatic involvement in hereditary hemorrhagic telangiectasia: clinical, radiological, and hemodynamic studies of 11 cases. Gastroenterology 1993;105:482–487.

55. Martini GA. The liver in hereditary haemorrhagic telangiectasia: an inborn error of vascular structure with multiple manifestations: a reappraisal. Gut 1978;19:531–537.

56. Garcia-Tsao G, et al. Liver disease in patients with hereditary hemorrhagic telangiectasia. N Engl J Med 2000;343:931–936.

57. Caselitz M, et al. Sonographic criteria for the diagnosis of hepatic involvement in hereditary hemorrhagic telangiectasia (HHT). Hepatology 2003;37:1139–1146.

58. Jameson CF. Primary hepatocellular carcinoma in hereditary haemorrhagic telangiectasia: a case report and literature review. Histopathology 1989;15:550–552.

59. Caselitz M, et al. Clinical outcome of transfemoral embolisation in patients with arteriovenous malformations of the liver in hereditary haemorrhagic telangiectasia (Weber-Rendu-Osler disease). Gut 1998;42:123–126.

60. Selmaier M, et al. Liver hemangiomatosis in Osler's disease. Dtsch Med Wochenschr 1993;118:1015–1019.

61. Shovlin CL, et al. Medical complications of pregnancy in hereditary haemorrhagic telangiectasia. Q J Med 1995;88:879–887.

62. Graf C, Perrett G, Torner J. Bleeding from cerebral arteriovenous malformations as part of their natural history. J Neurosurg 1983;58:331–337.

63. Bauer T, et al. Liver transplantation for hepatic arteriovenous malformation in hereditary haemorrhagic telangiectasia. J Hepatol 1995;22:586–590.

64. Gammon RB, Miksa AK, Keller FS. Osler-Weber-Rendu disease and pulmonary arteriovenous fistulas. Deterioration and embolotherapy during pregnancy. Chest 1990;98:1522–1524.

65. Livneh A, et al. Functionally reversible hepatic arteriovenous fistulas during pregnancy in patients with hereditary hemorrhagic telangiectasia. South Med J 1988;81:1047–1049.

66. Kirchner J, et al. Universal organ involvement in Rendu-Osler-Weber disease: interdisciplinary diagnosis and interventional therapy. Z Gastroenterol 1996;34:747–752.

67. Khalid SK, Garcia-Tsao G. Hepatic vascular malformations in hereditary hemorrhagic telangiectasia. Semin Liver Dis 2008;28:247–258.

68. Fagel WJ, Perlberger R, Kauffmann RH. Portosystemic encephalopathy in hereditary hemorrhagic telangiectasia. Am J Med 1988;85:858–860.

69. Buscarini E, et al. Hepatic vascular malformations in hereditary hemorrhagic telangiectasia: Doppler sonographic screening in a large family. J Hepatol 1997;26:111–118.

70. Hashimoto M, et al. Angiography of hepatic vascular malformations associated with hereditary hemorrhagic telangiectasia. Cardiovasc Intervent Radiol 2003;26:177–180.

71. Buscarini E, et al. Hepatic vascular malformations in hereditary hemorrhagic telangiectasia: imaging findings. AJR Am J Roentgenol 1994; 163:1105–1110.

72. Kakitsubata Y, et al. Intrahepatic portal-hepatic venous shunts demonstrated by US, CT, and MR imaging. Acta Radiol 1996;37:680–684.

73. Saxena R, et al. Coexistence of hereditary hemorrhagic telangiectasia and fibropolycystic liver disease. Am J Surg Pathol 1998;22:368–372.

74. Buscarini E, et al. Doppler ultrasound grading of hepatic vascular malformations in hereditary hemorrhagic telangiectasia—results of extensive screening. Ultraschall Med. 2004;25:348–355.

75. Buscarini E, et al. Interobserver agreement in diagnosing liver involvement in hereditary hemorrhagic telangiectasia by Doppler ultrasound. Ultrasound Med Biol 2008;34:718–725.

76. Hatzidakis AA, et al. Hepatic involvement in hereditary hemorrhagic telangiectasia (Rendu-Osler-Weber disease). Eur Radiol 2002;12(Suppl 4):S51–S55.

77. Hillert C, et al. Hepatic involvement in hereditary hemorrhagic telangiectasia: an unusual indication for liver transplantation. Liver Transpl 2001;7:266–268.

78. Lerut J, et al. Liver transplantation for hereditary hemorrhagic telangiectasia—report of the European liver transplant program. Ann Surg 2006;244:854–864.

79. Dupuis-Girod S, et al. Long-term outcome of patients with hereditary hemorrhagic telangiectasia and severe hepatic involvement after liver transplantation: a single center study. Liver Transpl 2010;16: 340–347.

80. Pfitzmann R, et al. Liver transplantation for treatment of intrahepatic Osler's disease: first experiences. Transplantation 2001;72:237–241.

81. Koscielny A, et al. Treatment of high output cardiac failure by flow-adapted hepatic artery banding (FHAB) in patients with hereditary hemorrhagic telangiectasia. J Gastrointest Surg 2008;12:872–876.

82. Whiting JH Jr, Korzenik JR, Miller FJ Jr. Fatal outcome after embolotherapy for hepatic arteriovenous malformations of the liver in two patients with hereditary hemorrhagic telangiectasia. J Vasc Interv Radiol 2000;11: 855–858.

83. Buscarini E, et al. Liver involvement in hereditary hemorrhagic telangiectasia: consensus recommendations. Liver Int 2006;26:1040–1046.

84. DeLeve LD, Valla DC, Garcia-Tsao G. AASLD guidelines: vascular disorders of the liver. Hepatology 2009;49:1729–1764.

85. Garcia-Tsao G. Liver involvement in hereditary hemorrhagic telangiectasia (HHT). J Hepatol 2007;46:499–507.

86. Sabba C, Pompili M. Review article: the hepatic manifestations of hereditary haemorrhagic telangiectasia. Aliment Pharmacol Ther 2008;28: 523–533.

87. Orlando G, et al. Non transplant surgical approach to liver based hereditary haemorrhagic telangiectasia: a first report. Liver Int 2008;28:574–577.

88. Cura MA, et al. Transjugular intrahepatic portosystemic shunt for variceal hemorrhage due to recurrent of hereditary hemorrhagic telangiectasia in a liver transplant. J Vasc Interv Radiol 2010;21:135–139.

89. Mitchell A, et al. Bevacizumab reverses need for liver transplantation in hereditary hemorrhagic telangiectasia. Liver Transpl 2008;14:210–213.

Section VIII

Liver Transplantation

Pretransplant Evaluation and Care

Scott W. Biggins

ABBREVIATIONS

AIDS acquired immunodeficiency syndrome
AMA antimitochondrial antibody
ANA antinuclear antibody
BMI body mass index
CT computed tomography
CTP Child-Turcotte-Pugh
DCD donation after cardiac death
DRI donor risk index
HAART highly active antiretroviral therapy
HAV hepatitis A virus

HBV hepatitis B virus
HCC hepatocellular carcinoma
HCV hepatitis C virus
HDV hepatitis D virus
HIV human immunodeficiency virus
INR international normalized ratio
MDRD modification of diet in renal disease equation
MELD Model for End-Stage Liver Disease
MELDNa Model for End-Stage Liver Disease with Sodium
MRI magnetic resonance imaging

NASH nonalcoholic steatohepatitis
NIDDK National Institute of Diabetes and Digestive and Kidney Diseases
OPTN Organ Procurement and Transplant Network
PBC primary biliary cirrhosis
PELD pediatric end-stage liver disease
PSC primary sclerosing cholangitis
UNOS United Network for Organ Sharing

Introduction

Liver transplantation has revolutionized the care of patients with end-stage liver disease. Since the first successful human liver transplant performed in 1967 by Dr. Thomas Starzl at the University of Colorado, advances in surgical technique, immunosuppression, and patient selection have made the procedure a standard life-saving treatment for patients with decompensated acute and chronic liver disease. Liver transplantation is available in most regions of the world, generally with excellent patient and graft survival rates. For example, in the United States, patient survival is 87%, 80%, and 73% at 1, 3, and 5 years after liver transplantation nationally, with single center reports of long-term survival rates as high as 68% and 64% at 10 and 15 years, respectively[1,2] (**Table 47-1, A and B**). The ubiquitous application of the procedure is limited by the scarcity of available donor liver grafts. Despite efforts to expand the donor pool and improve systems to triage liver grafts, death rates while waiting for liver transplantation remain high.[3] **Figure 47-1** shows the waiting list outcome for U.S. liver transplant candidates after 30, 60, and 90 days. Among the more than 15,900 patients active on the waiting list in the United States in 2009, there were 6320 who received a liver transplant and 1455 deaths in those who did not.[2] For patients with end-stage liver disease, the stakes are high. For their healthcare providers, knowledge of the appropriate pretransplant evaluation and management is paramount.

Pretransplant Evaluation

Appropriate evaluation of a patient for liver transplantation begins with recognition of a need for the procedure and a timely referral to a transplant center. At the initial evaluation, most transplant centers have a multidisciplinary approach that includes a detailed history and examination by a transplant hepatologist and transplant surgeon, an assessment by a mental health provider, a social worker, a transplant coordinator, and a financial counselor. The process can be quite stressful for the patient and accompanying care providers. For this reason, many centers offer counseling and educational sessions and the opportunity to meet with prior organ transplant recipients. Laboratory and imaging tests are performed to confirm the cause and severity of liver disease, estimate renal function, determine blood group, evaluate exposure and immunity to prior infections, screen for and assess the degree of comorbid medical conditions, and assess the technical feasibility of transplant surgery (**Table 47-2**). A thorough cardiopulmonary assessment is performed that typically includes an electrocardiogram, echocardiography, cardiac stress test, chest radiograph, and pulmonary function testing. Additionally, patients undergo specific screening for concurrent medical conditions that may warrant appeal for exceptional priority for liver transplant, such as hepatocellular carcinoma and hepatopulmonary syndrome (**Table 47-3**). The details of prior therapies for liver disease are collected. This is particularly

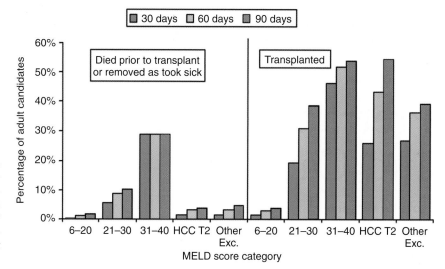

Fig. 47-1 U.S. liver transplant waiting list candidates events within 30, 60, and 90 days after snapshot (January 1, 2007) by MELD score, exceptional priority for stage 2 hepatocellular carcinoma (HCC T2) and other exceptional diagnosis (Other Exc). *(From Berg CL, et al. Liver and intestine transplantation in the United States 1998-2007. Am J Transplant 2009;9[4 Pt 2]:907–931. By permission.)*

Table 47-1A Unadjusted Patient Survival for Deceased Donor Liver Transplantation in the United States

PRIMARY DIAGNOSIS	3 mo*	1 yr*	5 yr†	10 yr‡
All	94	87	73	59
Noncholestatic liver disease/cirrhosis	94	87	72	56
Cholestatic liver disease/cirrhosis	96	91	81	69
Acute hepatic necrosis	90	85	71	61
Biliary atresia	94	92	90	84
Metabolic diseases	92	89	82	74
Malignant neoplasm	94	87	66	50
Other	91	84	76	65

From SRTR [online]. Cited April 4, 2010. Available from URL: www.srtr.org.

Based on data in the OPTN/SRTR as of May 1, 2008. Values are rounded to the nearest integer; the range of standard errors reported is 0.2% to 2.2%. Multiorgan transplants are excluded.

*A total of 10,522 patients during years 2005 and 2006.
†A total of 28,428 patients during years 2001 to 2006.
‡A total of 47,082 patients during years 1996 to 2006.

Table 47-1B Unadjusted Graft Survival for Deceased Donor Liver Transplantation in the United States

PRIMARY DIAGNOSIS	3 mo*	1 yr*	5 yr†	10 yr‡
All	90	82	68	53
Noncholestatic liver disease/cirrhosis	91	83	67	51
Cholestatic liver disease/cirrhosis	90	85	74	60
Acute hepatic necrosis	85	79	64	52
Biliary atresia	90	86	78	72
Metabolic diseases	87	82	74	66
Malignant neoplasm	92	83	62	45
Other	85	77	67	66

From SRTR [online]. Cited April 4, 2010. Available from URL: www.srtr.org.

Based on data in the OPTN/SRTR as of May 1, 2008. Values are rounded to the nearest integer; the range of standard errors reported is 0.3% to 2.1%. Multiorgan transplants are excluded.

*A total of 11,503 liver grafts during years 2005 and 2006.
†A total of 31,137 liver grafts during years 2001 to 2006.
‡A total of 51,910 liver grafts during years 1996 to 2006.

important for patients with HCV, HBV, and HIV where prior treatments may direct future treatment choices. Therapeutic options to control the patient's underlying liver disease are considered. Age- and gender-specific preventive healthcare, dental care, and cancer screening are generally requested. Patients should be committed to a healthy lifestyle including cessation of the use of tobacco products. Based on the initial evaluation, targeted specialist consultation is requested to evaluate and potentially intervene to mitigate the perioperative and postoperative surgical risk. For patients with severe renal insufficiency or failure, the assessment includes whether or not a combined liver-kidney transplantation may be indicated.[4,5]

The following fundamental questions of the pretransplant evaluation have been summarized in candidate selection guidelines[6]:
1. Is the patient in need of a liver transplant?
2. Can the patient survive the operation and immediate postoperative period?
3. Does the patient have other comorbid conditions that could so severely compromise graft or patient survival that transplantation would be futile and/or an inappropriate use of a scarce donor organ?
4. Can the patient be expected to comply with the complex medical regimen required after liver transplantation?

Table 47-2 Pretransplant Evaluation for Liver Transplantation

Standard Blood Tests

Complete blood count, liver chemistry, kidney profile, coagulation profile (PT, PTT)
ANA, smooth muscle antibody, AMA
Iron studies, ceruloplasmin, α_1-antitrypsin phenotype
CMV, EBV, HSV, VZV, HIV; syphilis; toxoplasmosis
HAV-HDV serology
α-Fetoprotein

Other Standard Tests

Abdominal ultrasound with Doppler, electrocardiogram, chest x-ray, pulmonary function tests, endoscopic evaluations
PPD skin tests

Standard Consultations

Dietary
Psychosocial
Women's health (Papanicolaou smear, mammogram in women older than 35)
Financial (insurance clearance must be obtained)
Overall assessment of patient (clinical judgment in addition to biochemical parameters)

Other Optional Tests

CT or MRI (to exclude HCC); angiography if needed to exclude vascular abnormalities
Carotid duplex scanning (for older or cardiovascular patients)
Contrast echocardiography (for suspected hepatopulmonary syndrome)
Cardiac catheterization (for suspected CAD)
Colonoscopy (history of IBD, PSC, polyps, family history of colon cancer, (+) FOBT
ERCP (in PSC)
Liver biopsy
Fungal serology (in areas endemic for dimorphic fungi)

Other Optional Measures

Pretransplant vaccines if needed (hepatitis A and B, pneumococcal vaccine, influenza vaccine, tetanus booster)

Adapted and reprinted with permission from Yu AS, Keeffe EB. Orthotopic liver transplantation. In: Boyer T, Zakim D, editors. Hepatology, 4th ed. Philadelphia: Harcourt Health Sciences. 2002: 1617–1656.

AMA, antimitochondrial antibody; ANA, antinuclear antibody; CAD, coronary artery disease; CMV, cytomegalovirus; CT, computed tomography; CTP, Child-Turcotte-Pugh; EBV, Epstein-Barr virus; ERCP, endoscopic retrograde cholangiopancreatography; ; FOBT, fecal occult blood test; HAV, hepatitis A virus; HDV, hepatitis D virus; HIV, human immunodeficiency virus; HSV, herpes simplex virus; IBD, inflammatory bowel disease; MRI, magnetic resonance imaging; PPD, purified protein derivative; PPT, partial prothrombin time; PSC, primary sclerosing cholangitis; PT, prothrombin time; VZV, varicella-zoster virus

Timing of Referral for Evaluation

Patients with decompensated liver disease, regardless of the cause, should be considered as potential candidates for liver transplantation. Assessing the urgency of a referral includes evaluating (1) the degree of liver disease, whether acute or chronic; (2) the availability of local expertise; and (3) the proximity of a transplant center. Several clinical tools exist to assist in assessing the degree of liver disease, both acute and chronic[7] (**Tables 47-4 and 47-5**). Nearly all transplant centers will provide triage assistance and emergent management advice at any time of day. When in doubt, an early referral is prudent.

When severe acute liver injury or acute liver failure occurs, urgent contact with a liver transplant center is indicated.

Patients with evidence of severe acute liver injury and signs of hepatocellular insufficiency (encephalopathy and/or coagulopathy with an international normalized ratio [INR] >1.5) should be admitted to the hospital and monitored closely for further deterioration. Acute liver failure, defined as acute hepatic deterioration without antecedent chronic liver disease, is characterized by the development of encephalopathy within 8 weeks of the onset of jaundice. If there are no clear contraindications to liver transplantation or to safe transportation of the patient, transfer to a liver transplant center should be considered. As rapid clinical deterioration is not uncommon, frequent assessment of the patient immediately before and during transfer is imperative. Attention to the patient's neurologic status and ability to protect his or her airway is necessary and a low threshold for intensive care level monitoring and endotracheal intubation is advised. Additionally, cause-specific therapies should be considered[8] (**Table 47-6**).

In acute liver failure, the interval from jaundice to encephalopathy is prognostic, with short intervals (<4 weeks) associated with a greater risk of brain edema and intracranial hypertension but an improved spontaneous survival rate. Longer intervals are associated with less brain edema but a lower spontaneous survival rate.[8] Coagulopathy, renal failure, and acidosis often occur in this setting, the degree to which is inversely correlated with transplant-free survival. Cause and early intervention can be predictive of the clinical course. Acetaminophen toxicity, the most common cause of acute liver failure in the United States and Europe, has the greatest spontaneous survival rate, whereas idiosyncratic drug-induced liver injury has one of the worst. Although many prognostic scores exist to predict low transplant-free recovery, the King's College criteria and Clichy criteria are the most used scores to identify the need for transplantation[9] (see **Table 47-4**). Although the King's College criteria provide a high accuracy in predicting death without liver transplantation (positive predictive value, 80% to 100%), they are less effective in predicting who will recover spontaneously (negative predictive value, 23% to 70%).[10,11] Therefore, although a patient with acute liver failure meeting the King's College criteria will likely require liver transplantation, not meeting these criteria does not accurately predict a lack of need for transplantation.

When chronic liver disease manifests with signs of decompensation, referral for liver transplantation should be considered. Such clinical signs include the presence of encephalopathy, portal hypertensive gastrointestinal bleeding, moderate ascites, spontaneous bacterial peritonitis, hepatorenal syndrome, or the development of hepatocellular carcinoma.[6] Each of these is associated with significantly increased mortality without liver transplantation when compared with compensated cirrhosis. Several general and disease specific prognostic tools exist to predict the natural history of liver disease.[7] Among these models, the Child-Turcotte-Pugh (CTP) score and the Model for End-Stage Liver Disease (MELD) score are most commonly used[12-14] (see **Table 47-5**). Recently, serum sodium, a long-known predictor of mortality in cirrhotics, has been incorporated along with the three MELD components (INR, total bilirubin, creatinine) as the MELDNa.[15] Guidelines from the American Association for the Study of Liver Disease recommend that patients with cirrhosis be referred for liver transplant evaluation when the CTP score reaches 7, the MELD score is 10, or the first major complication develops (ascites, variceal bleeding, encephalopathy, or

Table 47-3 Recognized Diagnosis and Criteria for Exceptional Priority for Liver Transplantation in the United States[41]

DIAGNOSIS	CRITERIA
Acute liver failure	Fulminant hepatic failure with onset of hepatic encephalopathy within 8 weeks of first symptoms of liver disease, the absence of pre-existing liver disease, and one of following three criteria: (1) ventilator dependence, (2) renal dialysis, or (3) INR >2.0 Primary nonfunction or hepatic artery thrombosis of transplanted liver graft within 7 days of transplant defined by AST ≥ 3000 and one of following: INR ≥2.5 or acidosis (arterial pH ≤7.30, venous pH ≤7.25, or lactate ≥4 mmol/L) Wilson disease with acute liver decompensation
Hepatocellular carcinoma	Contrast-enhanced cross-sectional imaging documenting hepatic lesion(s) with "vascular blush" and ≥2 cm in largest diameter but not exceeding 5 cm for a single lesion. For multiple lesions, no more than 3 lesions with the largest not exceeding 3 cm
Hepatoblastoma	Nonmetastatic disease
Cholangiocarcinoma	Neoadjuvant therapy protocol approved by UNOS committee Unresectable hilar cholangiocarcinoma of ≤3 cm in size documented by cross-sectional imaging and malignant appearing stricture on cholangiography and one of the following: carbohydrate antigen 19-9 ≥100 U/ml or biopsy or cytology results demonstrating malignancy or aneuploidy Intrahepatic and extrahepatic metastases should be excluded by cross-sectional imaging of chest and abdomen initially and every 3 months Exclusion of regional hepatic and peritoneal metastases by operative staging after neoadjuvant therapy and before liver transplantation Avoidance of transperitoneal aspiration or biopsy of primary tumor
Hepatopulmonary syndrome	Clinical evidence of portal hypertension, evidence of a right to left extracardiac shunt, PaO_2 <60 mm Hg, and no significant clinical evidence of underlying primary pulmonary disease
Portopulmonary syndrome	Previous MPAP >35 mm Hg and elevated transpulmonary gradient ≥12 mm Hg; presently controlled with MPAP <35 mm Hg and pulmonary vascular resistance <400 dynes/sec/cm⁵
Familial amyloid polyneuropathy	Documented amyloidosis, echocardiogram with an ejection fraction of >40%, ambulatory status, identification gene mutation, and amyloid proven by a biopsy
Primary hyperoxaluria	Documented primary hyperoxaluria, with AGT deficiency proven by liver biopsy, estimated GFR ≤25 ml/min/1.73 m² for 6 weeks or longer
Cystic fibrosis	Documented cystic fibrosis, signs of reduced pulmonary function, define by FEV_1 <40%

AGT, alanine–glyoxylate transaminase; AST, aspartate aminotransferase; FEV_1, forced expiratory volume in 1 second; GFR, glomerular filtration rate; MPAP, mean pulmonary artery pressure; INR, international normalized ratio; UNOS, United Network of Organ Sharing

type I hepatorenal syndrome).[6] Children with chronic liver disease are recommended to have a transplant evaluation when they deviate from the normal growth curve or develop evidence of hepatic dysfunction or portal hypertension.[6] The pediatric end-stage liver disease (PELD) score includes five factors (total bilirubin, albumin, INR, age less than 1, and growth failure) and, like MELD, has been shown to accurately predict waiting list short-term mortality in pediatric patients with chronic liver disease.[16]

Exploring Alternatives to Liver Transplantation

All efforts should be made to exhaust alternatives to liver transplantation before proceeding with the surgery.[6] Despite the success of liver transplantation as a treatment for acute and chronic liver disease, transplant surgery and posttransplant immunosuppression are associated with significant morbidity and mortality.[17,18] The challenge of assessing the risk/benefit ratio of liver transplantation is most evident in acute liver failure where the most gravely ill patient can, on occasion, have a dramatic and complete recovery without liver transplantation, and avoid lifelong immunosuppression and the associated morbidity. Patients with some chronic liver diseases, such as severe autoimmune hepatitis, chronic Wilson disease, and decompensated hepatitis B virus cirrhosis, may avert liver transplantation with timely and appropriate intervention (steroids, chelation therapy, or HBV antiviral agents, respectively). However, guidelines recommend concurrent pursuit of liver transplantation for critically ill patients with decompensated liver disease where the response to therapeutics is uncertain.[6]

Indications for Liver Transplantation

Liver transplantation is indicated for acute or chronic liver failure of any cause. Indications for liver transplantation can be categorized as noncholestatic, cholestatic, acute liver failure, metabolic disorders, vascular disorders, hepatic malignancy, and nonhepatic malignancy (**Table 47-7**). The leading indications for liver transplantation in the United States and Europe

Table 47-4 Criteria for Liver Transplantation in Patients with Acute Liver Failure

Criteria of King's College, London*

Patients taking acetaminophen
  pH <7.3, or
  Prothrombin time >6.5 (INR) and serum creatinine >3.4 mg/dl

Patients not taking acetaminophen
  Prothrombin time >6.5 (INR) or
  Any three of the following variables:
    Age <10 or >40 years
    Cause: non-A, non-B hepatitis; halothane hepatitis; idiosyncratic drug reaction
    Duration of jaundice before encephalopathy >7 days
    Prothrombin time >3.5 (INR)
    Serum bilirubin >17.5 mg/dl

Criteria of Hospital Paul-Brousse, Villejuif†

Hepatic encephalopathy, and factor V level:
  <20% in patient younger than 30 years or
  <30% in patient 30 years or older

Adapted and reprinted with permission from Yu AS, Ahmed A, Keeffe EB. Liver transplantation: evolving patient selection criteria. Can J Gastroenterol 2001;15:729–738.

*From O'Grady JG, Alexander GJ, Hayllar KM, Williams R. Early indicators of prognosis in fulminant hepatic failure. Gastroenterology 1989;97:439–445.

†From Bernuau J, et al. Criteria for emergency liver transplantation in patients with acute viral hepatitis and factor V below 50% of normal: a prospective study [abstract]. Hepatology 1991;14:49A.

INR, international normalized ratio

Table 47-5 Clinical Models to Assess the Degree of Liver Disease

MELD Score[13]

$MELD = 9.57 \times \log e \, (creatinine \, [mg/dl]) + 3.78 \times \log e \, (total \, bilirubin \, [mg/dl]) + 11.2 \times \log e \, (INR) + 6.43$
Laboratory values less than 1.0 are set to 1.0. The maximum serum creatinine considered is 4.0 mg/dl. For patients undergoing renal dialysis, creatinine is set to 4.0 mg/dl. An online calculator is available at www.mayoclinic.org/meld/mayomodel5.html

MELDNa Score[15]

$MELDNa = MELD - Na - [0.025 \times MELD \times (140 - Na)] + 140$
The MELD score is calculated as above. Serum sodium, Na, is in the unit mEq/L and is bounded by 125 to 140. An online calculator is available at www.mayoclinic.org/meld/mayomodel8.html

Child-Turcotte-Pugh Score

| | | POINTS | |
CRITERIA	1	2	3
Total bilirubin (mg/dl)	<2.0	2-3	>3	—
Albumin (g/dl)	>3.5	3.5-2.8	—	<2.8
INR	<1.7	1.7-2.2	—	>2.2
Ascites	—	Absent	Mild	Severe
Encephalopathy	Absent	—	Grade I-II	Grade III-IV

INR, international normalized ratio; MELD, Model for End-Stage Liver Disease

Table 47-6 Cause-Specific Treatment of Acute Liver Failure

CAUSE	TREATMENT
Acetaminophen	N-Acetylcysteine
Amanita	Penicillin G and N-acetylcysteine
Hepatitis B	Lamivudine
Autoimmune hepatitis	Methylprednisolone
Herpes simplex virus	Acyclovir
Acute fatty liver of pregnancy	Fetus delivery
HELLP syndrome	Fetus delivery

HELLP, hemolysis, elevated liver enzymes, and low platelet count

Table 47-7 Causes of Liver Disease in Patients Undergoing Liver Transplantation

Noncholestatic

Hepatitis C
Alcohol liver disease
Hepatitis B
Nonalcoholic steatohepatitis
Cryptogenic cirrhosis

Cholestatic

Primary biliary cirrhosis
Primary sclerosing cholangitis
Biliary atresia
Progressive familial intrahepatic cholestasis
Hyperalimentation induced

Acute Liver Failure

Drug or toxin
Hepatitis A or B or other viral
Cryptogenic
Wilson disease
Fatty liver of pregnancy
Primary nonfunction of liver graft after transplantation

Metabolic Disorders

Hereditary hemochromatosis
α_1-Antitrypsin deficiency
Wilson disease
Primary hyperoxaluria
Glycogen storage disease
Urea and branched-chain amino acid disorders

Vascular

Budd-Chari syndrome
Veno-occlusive disease

Hepatic Malignancy

Hepatocellular carcinoma
Hepatoblastoma
Cholangiocarcinoma
Hemangioendothelioma

Nonhepatic Malignancy

Neuroendocrine tumor

Other

Familial amyloidosis
Sarcoidosis
Cystic fibrosis
Adult polycystic disease
Nodular regenerative hyperplasia

Table 47-8A Liver Disease in Adult Transplant Recipients in the United States, 1987-2009, $N = 89,026$		
PRIMARY LIVER DISEASE	**NUMBER**	**%**
Hepatitis C	21,356	24
Alcoholic liver disease	11,924	13.4
Cryptogenic cirrhosis	7,924	8.9
Hepatocellular carcinoma	7,334	8.2
Primary sclerosing cholangitis	5,781	6.5
Acute liver failure	5,667	6.4
Hepatitis C and alcoholic	5,018	5.6
Primary biliary cirrhosis	4,968	5.6
Hepatitis B	3,164	3.6
Autoimmune hepatitis	3,049	3.4
Metabolic disease	2,693	3
Hepatitis C and B	567	0.6
Cholangiocarcinoma	356	0.4
Other	9,225	10.4
Total	89,026	100

Based on OPTN data as of April 16, 2010. Adults are defined as age 18 or older.

Table 47-8B Liver Disease of Pediatric Transplant Recipients in the United States, 1987-2009, $N = 12,079$		
PRIMARY LIVER DISEASE	**NUMBER**	**%**
Biliary atresia	4,923	40.8
Acute liver failure	1,433	11.9
Metabolic disease	1,354	11.2
Hyperalimentation induced	634	5.2
Cryptogenic	376	3.1
Hepatoblastoma	320	2.6
Autoimmune hepatitis	317	2.6
Primary sclerosing cholangitis	234	—
Secondary biliary cirrhosis	206	1.7
Other hepatic malignancy	99	0.8
Hepatitis C	86	0.7
Hepatocellular carcinoma	71	0.6
Benign neoplasm	34	0.3
Other	1,992	16.6
Total	12,079	100

Based on OPTN data as of April 16, 2010. Pediatric is defined as younger than 18 years.

are hepatic C infection and alcohol liver disease[2,19,20] (**Table 47-8, A and B**).

Acute Liver Failure

Acute liver failure has a dramatic presentation, yet fortunately is a relatively uncommon indication for liver transplantation, accounting for only 5.9% of transplants in the United States and 9% in Europe, annually.[20,21] Because of the rapidly evolving clinical course, patients with acute liver failure require urgent referral to and an expedited evaluation by the transplant center. Under most liver graft allocation systems, patients meeting criteria for acute liver failure are awarded the highest priority for available liver grafts. An emergent and thorough psychiatric and social assessment is required for suspected overdose or suicidal attempt. This is best performed before advanced encephalopathy. Even in the absence of a self-inflicted injury, the rapid onset of illness in often previously healthy individuals makes it challenging for both patients and family to fully grasp the enormity of the transplant evaluation, transplant surgery, and lifelong immunosuppression. Compared with transplantation for chronic liver disease, the graft survival rate is lower and rejection rates higher, likely at least in part due to medical compliance issues.[22]

Hepatitis C

There is a high burden of HCV disease in the United States and Europe, which has made HCV the leading cause of liver patients requiring liver transplantation.[19,20] In individuals with chronic HCV for 20 to 30 years, 10% to 20% will develop cirrhosis and 1% to 5% will develop hepatocellular

carcinoma.[23,24] Once decompensation occurs, the 5-year survival rate is less than 50% without liver transplantation.[25] When HCV viremia is present at the time of transplant, HCV infection of the liver graft is universal and has an accelerated natural history compared with nontransplant patients. By 5 years after transplantation, 10% to 30% will develop cirrhosis.[26] The development of an aggressive cholestatic variant recurrent HCV occurs in 2% to 5% of HCV-infected recipients and can lead to cirrhosis within the first few years after transplant.[26] In contrast to earlier studies, more recent large registry studies report reduced graft and patient survival time in HCV-infected recipients.[3,27] Patient survival at 3 years was 78% in more than 7400 HCV-seropositive recipients and 82% in more than 20,000 HCV-seronegative recipients.[27] Emerging data suggest that sustained viral response can be achieved with a combination of interferon and ribavirin therapy in compensated (Child class A and B) cirrhotics pretransplant, particularly those with HCV genotypes 2 and 3.[28] As tolerance of HCV treatment in this population is poor and complications common, efforts to eradicate HCV pretransplant should be carried out by experienced physicians at liver transplant centers.

Alcoholic Cirrhosis

Alcoholic liver disease is one of the leading causes of cirrhosis in the United States, accounting for 40% of all deaths from cirrhosis and 28% of all deaths from liver disease. It is the second leading indication for liver transplantation.[2,29] Alcohol abstinence is essential. Abstinence can allow for stabilization of decompensated cirrhosis that may be able to delay or even avert the need for liver transplantion.[30,31] Although an arbitrary pretransplant abstinence period of 6 months is often required, the duration of abstinence is only one component of the overall assessment.[30,32] The aim is to minimize risk of recidivist alcohol dependence and abuse that can have a dramatic negative effect on graft and patient survival.[33] Risk factors for recidivist alcohol use include age at the start of alcohol consumption, family history, and psychosocial stressors.[34] Graft survival rates for liver transplantation for alcohol cirrhosis appears to be similar to that of most other indications, yet higher rates of de novo posttransplant malignancies are reported, particularly oropharyngeal squamous cell carcinomas.[33]

Hepatitis B

Worldwide an estimated 350 million persons are infected with HBV.[35] Although the incidence of HBV in the United States has declined to an overall prevalence of 0.4%, it remains an important cause of acute and chronic liver disease, particularly in young adult Asian immigrants, in whom prevalence estimates are as high as 25%.[36] Patients with HBV can require liver transplant for a severe acute infection causing acute liver failure, an acute or chronic flare, decompensation of cirrhosis, or the development of hepatocellular carcinoma. Nucleoside antiviral therapy taken for several months may stabilize decompensated cirrhosis and occasionally avert the need for liver transplantation.[37] Interferon should be avoided in advanced or decompensated HBV. The risk of HBV recurrence after transplant is low with hepatitis B immunoglobulin and/or HBV antiviral agents.[38] Both the risk of recurrence and the choice of appropriate prophylactic regimen are informed by the degree of viremia at the time of transplantation. Long-term graft and patient survival rates are excellent.

Cholestatic Liver Diseases

Liver transplantation is the only effective therapy for end-stage liver disease resulting from primary biliary cirrhosis and primary sclerosing cholangitis and has excellent graft survival rates. In PBC patients without decompensated cirrhosis but with severe recalcitrant pruritus (associated sleep deprivation and emotional disturbance), liver transplantation can be indicated when medical treatment options have been exhausted.[6] Patients with PSC are at high risk for the development of cholangiocarcinoma, which is associated with a dramatically reduced survival time after transplantation because of high recurrence rates. Survival rates were only 74% and 38% at 1 and 5 years after transplant in a study of 280 patients transplanted with cholangiocarcinoma.[39] However, improved results have been reported in highly selected patients who undergo pretransplant neoadjuvant therapy. In patients with hilar cholangiocarcinoma, 3 cm or less in size, without nodal spread or metastasis and who undergo pretransplant neoadjuvant radiation and chemotherapy, patient survival at 1, 3, and 5 years is reported as 96%, 83%, and 72%, respectively.[40] Based on these results, patients with cholangiocarcinoma can receive higher priority for transplantation in the United States, if they meet the specified criteria, undergo an approved pretransplant neoadjuvant protocol, and have a negative pretransplant staging laparotomy[41] (see **Table 47-3**).

Biliary atresia is the most common indication for liver transplantation in children, accounting for more than 40% of all pediatric transplants. Other pediatric cholestatic indications include PSC, Alagille syndrome, nonsyndromic intrahepatic paucity of bile ducts, cystic fibrosis, and progressive familial intrahepatic cholestasis. Patient survival rates after liver transplantation for these indications are approximately 90% and 85% at 1 and 3 years, respectively.[42]

Hepatocellular Carcinoma

Hepatocellular carcinoma is the most frequent primary liver malignancy worldwide and is responsible for more than 600,000 deaths annually.[43] Patients with chronic hepatitis B infection with or without cirrhosis or cirrhosis from hepatitis C or hemochromatosis are at particularly increased risk. HCC is 3 to 4 times more common in men than women, and more common in Africans and Asians than in Caucasians.[44] In the appropriate clinical setting, dynamic cross-sectional imaging with computed tomography (CT) or magnetic resonance imaging (MRI) can establish the diagnosis without a liver biopsy. Recent consensus guidelines have established new imaging criteria for HCC.[45] These guidelines recommend the mandated use of dynamic contrast cross-sectional imaging with CT or MRI that includes late arterial, portal venous, and delayed phases.[45] Essential imaging characteristics of HCC include contrast enhancement in comparison with the background liver parenchyma on late arterial phase images, portal venous phase washout, late pseudocapsule enhancement, and documented interval growth on serial imaging[45] (**Tables 47-9 and 47-10**). When HCC is discovered, several surgical and nonsurgical treatments exist for HCC. The choice and response to treatment are influenced by tumor stage and liver function.[46-49]

Liver transplantation is considered the treatment of choice for patients with decompensated cirrhosis and HCC that is confined to the liver and not exceeding the Milan criteria or stage II on the tumor-node-metastasis classification.[48] This is defined as a single lesion 2 cm to 5 cm in size or no more than three lesions, with none greater than 3 cm in size and the absence of extrahepatic disease. Several centers have demonstrated that a modest expansion of the number and/or size of tumors can still result in satisfactory outcomes.[50] The expanded University of California San Francisco criteria (single tumor of 6.5 cm or two to three tumors with none >4.5 cm and with total tumor diameter of 8 cm) have had similar outcomes to the Milan criteria.[51] Further extensions beyond the Milan criteria in tumor size and/or number carry an increased risk of tumor recurrence, which as been conceptualized as a "metro ticket" by Llovet and colleagues; the greater the distance, the greater the cost[47] (**Figure 47-2**).

Surgical resection of hepatocellular carcinoma can be an alternative to liver transplantation in select patients. Solitary tumors less than 5 cm in size in noncirrhotic livers or well-compensated cirrhosis (Child A without portal hypertension defined as no varices, a platelet count >100,000/ μL, and a hepatic venous pressure gradient <10 mm Hg) may have a survival time that is only marginally less than transplant recipients.[45] Unfortunately, recurrent or de novo hepatocellular carcinoma after resection is not uncommon and the outcome of salvage transplant after resection appears to be inferior to a primary transplant strategy.[52]

Table 47-9 OPTN Classification System for Nodules on Imaging of Cirrhotic Livers

OPTN CLASS	DESCRIPTION	COMMENT
0	Incomplete or technically inadequate study	Repeat study is required for adequate assessment; automatic priority MELD points cannot be assigned on the basis of an OPTN class 0 classified imaging study
1	No evidence of HCC on good-quality, appropriate surveillance examination	Typically, surveillance would continue according to the routine practice at the respective transplant center
2	Benign lesion(s) or diffuse parenchymal abnormality with no dominant focal lesion	Typically, the need for any further imaging would be determined on a clinical basis according to the routine practice at the respective transplant center (MRI preferred over CT)
3	Abnormal findings on scan, indeterminate focal lesion(s), not currently meeting radiologic criteria for HCC	Typically, follow-up imaging would be performed in 6-12 months (MRI preferred over CT)
4	Abnormal findings on scan, indeterminate focal lesion(s), not currently meeting radiologic criteria for HCC	Consider short-term follow-up in 3 (maximum diameter of lesions ≥2 cm) to 6 months (maximum diameter of lesions <2 cm), with MRI preferred over CT or biopsy. Imaging follow-up should be considered if biopsy is negative or not possible
5	Meets radiologic criteria for HCC	Patient may be eligible for automatic priority MELD points on the basis of this imaging study. Please refer to definitions for class 5 criteria

Used with permission from Pomfret EA, et al. Report of a national conference on liver allocation in patients with hepatocellular carcinoma in the United States. Liver Transpl 2010;16:262–278.

CT, computed tomography; HCC, hepatocellular carcinoma; MELD, Model for End-Stage Liver Disease; MRI, magnetic resonance imaging; OPTN, Organ Procurement and Transplant Network

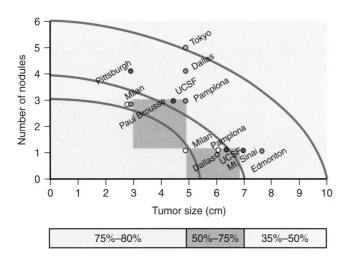

75%–80%	50%–75%	35%–50%

Expected 5-year survival

Fig. 47-2 The "metro ticket" concept: the greater the distance, the greater the cost. Expected 5-year survival rates after liver transplantation are shown for hepatocellular carcinoma by tumor size and number. *(From Yao FY. Liver transplantation for hepatocellular carcinoma: beyond the Milan criteria. Am J Transplant 2008;8:1982–1989. By permission.)*

Local regional therapy for hepatocellular carcinoma such as ablative and transarterial techniques is increasingly common and has the following aims (1) to prevent waitlist "drop out" (need for removal from the waitlist because of tumor progression to a stage associated with an unacceptable recurrence rate after transplantation); (2) to improve posttransplant survival; and/or (3) to downstage large tumors before liver transplantation.[45] Ablative treatment is generally used for tumors 3 cm in size and includes ethanol, cryoablation, and radiofrequency

modalities; it can be performed by percutaneous, laparoscopic, or laparotomy techniques.[53] Intraarterial therapy includes bland embolization, chemoembolization, and radioembolization (yttrium-90 microspheres) and is typically used for larger tumors (>3 cm).[54] Use of serial treatments is common. Although large randomized trials are lacking, use of a combination treatment modalities is common and may be superior to monotherapy.[55] Local regional therapy can decrease waitlist "drop out" for candidates with multifocal hepatocellular carcinoma or with a solitary tumor greater than 3 cm in size and who have waiting times of 3 to 6 months or greater.[45] Posttransplant survival rates in recipients with HCC treated with local regional therapy were equivalent to recipients without HCC in one single center report.[56] Protocols to use local regional therapy to "downstage" large tumors to a stage within the Milan criteria have been proposed.[45,50] A recent consensus meeting recommended the following as an investigative downstaging protocol: (1) The initial tumor should not exceed 8 cm in size or two to three tumors should not exceed 5 cm in size individually, with the total tumor burden not to exceed 8 cm and without vascular invasion; (2) α-fetoprotein level should be reduced to less than 500 ng/ml if the initial level was greater than 1000 ng/ml; and (3) successful downstaging is achieved to a tumor burden such that it meets, and is maintained, within the Milan criteria for at least 3 months before eligibility for active and priority listing for liver transplant.[45]

Other Primary Hepatic Malignancies

Several other malignancies of the liver occur, some in the absence of underlying liver disease. Fibrolamellar hepatocellular carcinoma has a better prognosis than HCC and when

Table 47-10 Imaging Criteria for OPTN Class 5 Lesion (Compatible with an Imaging Diagnosis of HCC)

OPTN CLASS	LESION SIZE	APPEARANCE	COMMENT
5A	Maximum diameter of lesion ≥1 cm and <2 cm, measured on later arterial or portal vein phase images	Increased contrast enhancement on late arterial phase (with respect to hepatic parenchyma) AND washout during later contrast phases AND peripheral rim enhancement (capsule/pseudocapsule) on delayed phase OR Increased contrast enhancement on late arterial phase (with respect to hepatic parenchyma) AND growth (maximum increase in diameter) of 50% or more documented on serial MRI or CT obtained ≤6 months apart. Growth criteria do not apply to ablated lesions	This category describes a T1-stage HCC that meets stringent qualitative imaging criteria diagnostic of HCC OR a rapidly growing T1-stage HCC with some qualitative imaging features diagnostic of HCC
5B	Maximum diameter of lesion ≥2 cm, measured on later arterial or portal vein phase images	Increased contrast enhancement on late hepatic arterial images (with respect to hepatic parenchyma)* AND washout on portal venous/delayed phase and/or late capsule or pseudocapsule enhancement OR Increased contrast enhancement on late hepatic arterial images (with respect to hepatic parenchyma)* AND growth (maximum increase in diameter) of 50% or more documented on serial MRI or CT obtained ≤6 months apart. Growth criteria do not apply to perviously ablated lesions	This category describes a T2-stage HCC that meets qualitative imaging criteria diagnostic of HCC OR a rapidly growing T2-stage HCC with some qualitative imaging features diagnostic of HCC. Class 5B lesions automatically qualify for automatic HCC exception MELD points
5T	Previous local/regional treatment of HCC	Past local/regional treatment of HCC (OPTN class 4 or biopsy proven before ablation) AND evidence of persistent/recurrent HCC such as nodular or crescentic extrazonal or intrazonal enhancing tissue on later arterial imaging (with respect to hepatic parenchyma)	This category describes residual or recurrent HCC after previous local ablative therapy

Used with permission from Pomfret EA, Washburn K, Wald C, et al. Report of a national conference on liver allocation in patients with hepatocellular carcinoma in the United States. Liver Transpl 2010;16:262–278.

*Isovascular and hypovascular HCC may occur that does not exhibit this feature; consider biopsy if this is suspected.

CT, computed tomography; HCC, hepatocellular carcinoma; MELD, Model for End-Stage Liver Disease; MRI, magnetic resonance imaging; OPTN, Organ Procurement and Transplant Network

limited to the liver, responds well to liver transplantation.[6,44] Hemangioendothelioma is a rare vascular endothelial tumor that can be treated successfully with chemotherapy and liver transplantation despite the extrahepatic spread that often exists at presentation.[57] In children, hepatoblastoma is the most common primary hepatic malignancy. The prognosis is generally better than hepatocellular carcinoma, and liver transplantation, with neoadjuvant chemotherapy, should be considered when the tumor is confined to the liver and not amenable to resection.[6,58]

Retransplantation: Recurrent Disease and Graft Failure

Repeat liver transplant is a relatively uncommon procedure, yet accounted for 7% to 9% of all liver transplant procedures annually in the United States during the years 2000 to 2008 and 458 (7.2 %) of the 6320 liver transplants in 2009.[2] The vast majority of liver retransplants are performed early in the posttransplant period (<90 days) for primary graft nonfunction, hepatic artery thrombosis, or technical reasons related to the first procedure.[3] Retransplantations performed later are generally for ischemic-type biliary lesions, chronic rejection, or recurrent disease.[3] Nearly all diseases that prompted the first liver transplant can occur in the liver graft. The procedure is a more technically challenging surgery and the patients are generally older and sicker than those presenting for first transplant. Survival after retransplantation is approximately 15% to 20% lower than first transplant recipients at most time points but can be much worse, particularly those with early aggressive recurrent hepatitis C.[3] Several models exist to assist with candidate selection by predicting survival rates; most models identified that increasing recipient age, bilirubin, creatinine, and time to retransplantation were associated with worse outcome.[59]

Contraindications for Liver Transplantation: Absolute and Relative

The goal of liver transplantation is to improve a patient's survival time and quality of life. Assessing whether liver transplantation can achieve these goals is fundamental to the pretransplant evaluation and is individualized within a transplant center. Medical, psychosocial, and technical issues, individually or in summation, may establish that liver transplant is contraindicated (**Table 47-11**).

Medical Issues

Patients who are not expected to survive liver transplant surgery or have a meaningful neurologic or functional recovery should not undergo the procedure. This assessment can be complicated and may require the expertise of consultants.

Cardiovascular Disease

Cardiac contraindications for liver transplantation include symptomatic ischemic heart disease, advanced cardiomyopathy, severe ventricular dysfunction, severe pulmonary

Table 47-11 Absolute Contraindications to Liver Transplantation

CATEGORY	EXAMPLE
Medical	
Unstable, active cardiopulmonary disease	Symptomatic CAD
	Severe pulmonary HTN
Incurable, active extrahepatic malignancy	Metastatic HCC
	CCA with adjacent tissue spread
Uncontrolled, active sepsis	Endocarditis, fungemia
Uncontrolled, active HIV or AIDS	HIV unresponsive to HAART
Severe, irreversible neurologic disease	Uncal herniation
Psychosocial	
Active substance abuse	Active alcohol or illicit drug use
Inadequate social support	No or unreliable support person
Uncontrolled psychiatric disorder	Active, uncontrollable psychosis
Severe psychosocial dysfunction	Interferes with medial compliance
Surgical	
Extensive vascular thrombosis	No viable splanchnic venous inflow

AIDS, acquired immunodeficiency syndrome; CAD, coronary artery disease; CCA, cholangiocarcinoma; HAART, highly active antiretroviral therapy; HCC, hepatocellular carcinoma; HIV, human immunodeficiency syndrome; HTN, hypertension

hypertension, and aortic stenosis with significant pressure gradient and poor ventricular function. Cardiovascular complications are one of the leading causes of non–graft-related death after liver transplantation.

Much like the general population, the coronary artery disease risk profile is worsening in patients presenting as liver transplant candidates. At the time of presentation, liver transplant candidates are increasingly older, more obese, and enriched for atherosclerotic disease because of the rising proportion of nonalcoholic steatohepatitis (NASH)-induced cirrhosis.[60] Estimates of asymptomatic significant coronary artery disease in liver transplant candidates vary from 2.9% to 28%.[61,62] The perioperative assessment for liver transplantation, as in guidelines for noncardiac surgery preoperative assessment, is based on risk factor profiling (age >50, cigarette smoking, diabetes, personal and family history) followed by noninvasive functional testing to identify those who may benefit from invasive angiography and revascularization (**Fig. 47-3**). Low-risk patients undergo noninvasive screening. For this purpose, direct inotropic stimulation with dobutamine stress echocardiography may be preferable to vasodilator provocation with adenosine or dipyridamole. Yet the use of β-blockers can limit the utility of dobutamine stress echocardiography, and β-blockers may need to be temporarily stopped to optimize the test's performance. In predicting significant intraoperative cardiac events, dobutamine stress echocardiography has negative and positive predictive value of 78% and 30%, respectively.[61] Patients with positive or nondiagnostic noninvasive screening should be considered for coronary angiogram. For candidates at intermediate or high risk for coronary events based on their risk factor assessment, proceeding directly to a coronary angiogram may be preferable. Percutaneous coronary revascularization can be attempted before liver transplantation. The degree of coagulopathy, the risk of gastrointestinal bleeding, and especially the time to a potential transplant influence the choice of balloon angioplasty, bare metal stent, or drug eluting stent.[63] Surgical revascularization before transplant has been reported in small cohort studies yet is associated with significant mortality—17% to 30% in cirrhotics.[61] Medical therapy with perioperative β-blockers, if tolerated, may reduce risk of cardiovascular mortality associated with liver transplantation.[64]

Increasingly, nonischemic cardiac disease has been implicated in cardiovascular complications following liver transplantation, including myocarditis with fibrosis caused by hepatitis C or hemochromatosis, cirrhotic cardiomyopathy, and cardiac chronotropic incompetence. Dobutamine echocardiography, with less than 82% of maximal heart rate or peak rate-pressure product of less than 16,333, may identify patients at higher risk for perioperative cardiac events.[62,65]

Pulmonary Disease

Pulmonary contraindications to liver transplantation include advanced pulmonary fibrosis, severe chronic obstructive pulmonary disease, and severe pulmonary hypertension. Patients with chronic liver disease are at risk for two distinct pulmonary vascular disorders: portopulmonary syndrome and hepatopulmonary syndrome.

Portopulmonary syndrome occurs in 2% to 4% of patients with cirrhosis and is characterized by elevated mean pulmonary artery pressure (>25 mm Hg), increased pulmonary

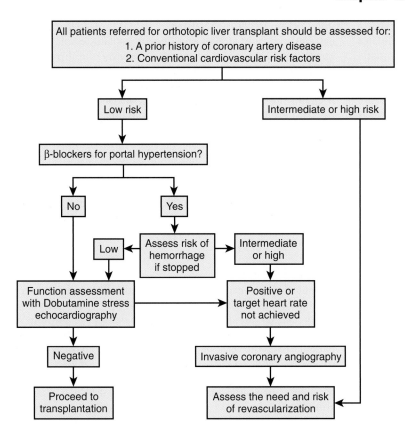

Fig. 47-3 **Coronary artery disease screening algorithm for liver transplant candidates.** *(From Ehtisham J, et al. Coronary artery disease in orthotopic liver transplantation: pretransplant assessment and management. Liver Transpl 2010;16:550–557. By permission.)*

vascular resistance (>240 dynes/cm⁵), and either low pulmonary artery occlusion pressure (<15 mm Hg) or elevated transpulmonary gradient (>12 mm Hg) in chronic liver disease.[66] The diagnosis can be suspected based on echocardiogram, yet confirmation with direct pressure measurement is required. Severe uncontrolled pulmonary hypertension (>60 mm Hg) has a prohibitively high mortality with liver transplantation, with only rare reports of long-term survival. Yet when the pulmonary pressure is less than 35 mm Hg, obtained with or without pharmacologic intervention, post-transplantation survival rates are satisfactory.[66-68] Pulmonary hypertension resolves or improves in some but certainly not all recipients after liver transplantation. Long-term treatment may be required, but many new pharmacologic therapies are available in injectable, inhaled, and oral formulations.[69]

Hepatopulmonary syndrome occurs in 5% to 29% of patients with cirrhosis and is characterized by intrapulmonary vascular dilation, with right to left extracardiac shunting and arterial hypoxemia (A-a [alveolar-arterial] gradient of less than 15 mm Hg) in portal hypertension. Pulse oximetry can be used for screening, yet arterial blood gas is more appropriate to use for establishing the diagnosis. Delayed shunting on contrast echocardiography or abnormal brain uptake (>6%) on a ⁹⁹ᵐTc-macroaggregated albumin lung perfusion scan can be confirmatory.[70] The latter is particular useful in the presence of current asthma, lung fibrosis, chronic obstructive lung disease, or hepatic hydrothorax. The degree of hypoxemia correlates with the degree of portal hypertension and the mortality risk without liver transplant. Oxygen supplementation can ameliorate symptoms, yet liver transplantation is the treatment of choice. Although severe hepatopulmonary syndrome may be associated with prolonged recovery and oxygen

requirement, it generally is not considered a contraindication to liver transplantation.

Renal Failure

Renal failure is common with or because of end-stage liver disease. Impaired renal function or failure is associated with higher rates of death without liver transplant and increased morbidity and mortality after liver transplantation, but is not a contraindication to the procedure.[5] Although creatinine based measures (MDRD, Cockcroft-Gault) of the glomerular filtration rate are used most commonly, they overestimate renal function in cirrhotics.[71] Renal insufficiency with liver disease can be related to the liver disease (hepatorenal syndrome, hepatitis C membranoproliferative glomerulonephritis, hepatitis B membranous nephropathy), to intrinsic renal disease (diabetic or nondiabetic glomerulosclerosis, ischemic nephropathy), or a mixture of both. Complete renal recovery from hepatorenal syndrome after liver transplant is common, yet the time to recovery is dependent on its duration and severity before transplantation and the presence of other concomitant renal disease.

Determining the presence and degree of irreversible kidney disease is a deciding factor on whether a combined liver-kidney transplant should be pursued. Although a combined transplant can improve survival time for the liver-kidney recipient, it also decreases the availability of a kidney graft that could improve the survival rate for a patient on the kidney transplant waiting list. The expertise of a transplant nephrologist is often sought and information generated from two consensus meetings can guide this evaluation and decision-making process.[4,5] In an effort to optimize the utility of available kidney grafts, these guidelines suggest the following criteria for simultaneous liver-kidney transplantation in candidates with end-stage renal disease, cirrhosis, and symptomatic portal hypertension: (1) chronic kidney disease with a glomerular filtration rate of 30 ml/min or less, (2) acute kidney insufficiency or hepatorenal syndrome with a creatinine more than 2.0 mg/dl and dialysis for 8 weeks or longer, or (3) chronic kidney disease and a kidney biopsy showing greater than 30% glomerulosclerosis or fibrosis.[5]

Infection

Patients with end-stage liver disease are immunosuppressed and prone to infection. Uncontrolled sepsis is an absolute contraindication to liver transplantation. Other infections should be treated aggressively before the procedure. Patients with evidence of latent tuberculosis should undergo treatment before transplant when possible, yet caution is advised given the potential toxicity of isoniazid. Rifampin may be considered as an alternative to isoniazid when liver dysfunction is severe.

Human immunodeficiency virus (HIV) infection is no longer an absolute contraindication to liver transplantation. With the advent of highly active antiretroviral therapy (HAART), liver disease has become a leading cause of death in people with HIV and has inspired a growing worldwide experience in liver transplantation in this population.[72] Causes of liver disease in HIV-infected persons include co-infection (with HCV or HBV), hepatotoxicity (HAART, alcohol), hepatocellular carcinoma related to HBV or HCV, NASH, and immune reconstitution inflammatory syndrome.[72] Proper candidate selection and care by an experienced multidisciplinary team are paramount to the success of liver transplantation in the HIV-infected patient. Available data suggest that compared with non–HIV-infected liver transplant recipients, recipients with HIV and HBV or HIV infection alone had similar survival rates.[72,73] However, most studies report a significantly reduced posttransplant survival time in patients with HCV and HIV co-infection, with a 5-year survival rate of 50% or lower.[72] Data-driven exclusion criteria are still emerging but include: CD4 count under 100 cells per milliliter, HIV that is predicted to be unresponsive to available HAART, untreatable opportunistic infections (progressive multifocal leukoencephalopathy, chronic cryptosporidiosis, multidrug resistant HIV, systemic fungal infection), and HIV-associated lymphoma.[72] Patient selection is particularly important in the HCV and HIV co-infected candidates because subsets of this group have been shown to have better survival rates; favorable candidate characteristics include low MELD score (<20), higher body mass index (BMI) (>18), non–African American race, and absence of renal insufficiency.[72]

Extrahepatic Malignancy

Active extrahepatic malignancy, with rare exception, is a contraindication to liver transplantation. Exceptions include nonmelanoma skin cancer, neuroendocrine tumors (carcinoid gastrinoma, insulinoma, somatostatinoma), and hemangioendothelioma. Previous nonhepatic malignancy is not an absolute contraindication, although these patients are likely at higher risk for recurrence because of posttransplant immunosuppression. Recurrence risk estimates have been extrapolated from studies of kidney transplant recipients and appear to be dependent on the type of cancer and the interval before transplant. Low-risk (<10 %) prior malignancies are incidental renal tumors, lymphomas, thyroid cancer, carcinoma of the testis, uterus, and cervix; intermediate risk (11% to 25%) are uterine body carcinoma, Wilms tumor, and carcinoma of the prostate and breast; high risk (>25%) are bladder carcinoma, sarcoma, malignant melanoma, symptomatic renal carcinoma, and nonmelanoma skin cancer and myeloma.[74] There is no consensus on the optimal tumor free duration. At least a 2-year observation period following curative cancer treatment is generally recommended and longer periods of up to 5 years are advised for malignant melanomas, and breast and colon carcinomas.

Advanced Age

Advanced age, by itself, is not a contraindication to liver transplantation but is an independent risk factor for coronary artery disease, vascular disease, and malignancy.[6,61,75] Although several centers report short-term survival rates in selected patients over the ages of 60 and 70 are similar to younger recipients, older recipients have a diminished long-term survival rate.[75-77] In a review of more than 5600 U.S. transplant recipients, 10-year posttransplant patient survival was 42% and 60% for those over age 65 and for those 65 or younger.[76] A thorough evaluation for co-morbid conditions should be performed during the transplant evaluation with an understanding of the synergistic negative effect of advanced age.

Obesity

Based on World Health Organization estimates, there are 400 million obese (BMI >30) adults worldwide. In the United States, approximately two thirds of adults are overweight (BMI >25) or obese (BMI >30) and the proportion of obese patients undergoing liver transplant increased from 15% in the 1990s to more than 25% by 2003.[78] The obese, particular those with fatty liver, are at increased risk for cardiovascular disease and diabetes, but the data on the association with a reduced posttransplant survival rate are mixed. A study of the UNOS database, not correcting for ascites, found that the class II (BMI >35) and class III (BMI >40) obese had significantly lower posttransplant survival rates at 1 month, 1 year, 3 years, and 5 years after transplant.[79] However, a subsequent study of the NIDDK database, corrected for ascites at the time of transplant, found no difference in survival at the same time points after transplant across a BMI range from 18.5 to greater than 40.[78] Therefore current data suggest that obesity alone should not preclude liver transplantation, yet in combination with other negative risk factors it may.

Active Alcohol or Substance Abuse

Liver transplantation is contraindicated with alcohol or substance abuse yet may proceed once sincere recovery is established. Addiction is common in patients with end-stage liver disease and recidivism is common in addiction. Formal evaluation and management by an addiction specialist can aid in risk stratification and mitigation. Common substances of abuse include alcohol, tobacco, prescription medications such as narcotics and benzodiazepines, and recreational and illicit drugs. Documentation of ongoing participation in a formal recovery plan is generally mandated by transplant centers and third-party payers, and often includes random drug screening.

Psychosocial Issues

Psychosocial challenges to a patient's candidacy for liver transplantation are common. Lack of ability to comply with medical recommendations or lack of adequate social support is a contraindication to transplant. Cirrhotic patients have both poor quality of life and low perceived well-being. Depression and isolation can impair medical compliance. Significant psychiatric disorders should be under the care of a mental health provider and under excellent control. Addiction of any form should be addressed before liver transplantation. Tobacco product cessation should be mandated because it can improve operative outcomes.[80]

Technical Issues

Advances in surgical technique and preoperative imaging have trimmed the list of technical contraindications for liver transplantation. Portal vein thrombosis is not an absolute contraindication yet does pose a greater technical challenge, particularly if the entirety of the portal venous system is occluded or atrophied.[81] However, more extensive thrombosis occluding the entire portomesenteric system can be prohibitive.

Monitoring and Management

Once the patient is selected as a candidate and registered on the wait list, ongoing, well-coordinated monitoring and management is critical. The importance of an excellent primary care provider and system cannot be overstated. Timely and clear communication among the transplant center, the primary care provider, and the patient and patient's home support team improves delivery of the often complicated care plans.

Patients with end-stage liver disease have complex medical care and are at high risk for the development of complications. Regular updating of laboratory tests is required to evaluate the progression of liver disease and update the patient's priority status on the waiting list. The frequency of this requirement increases as priority increases. Failure to provide timely results can result in a temporary loss of priority status. Where appropriate, documentation of compliance with a substance abuse recovery plan is requested. Routine health maintenance includes age-specific cancer screening and vaccinations. Vaccinations for hepatitis A and B, when appropriate, are of value as well as annual influenza and pneumococcal vaccines every 5 years. Early detection of hepatocellular carcinoma is possible with routine screening by imaging, such as ultrasound, CT, and MRI.[82] Identification of HCC, depending on the stage, may give the patient an opportunity for additional transplant priority in the United States. This is also true for hepatopulmonary syndrome and controlled portopulmonary syndrome.[41] Patients and their families should be aware that

uncontrolled and even minimal encephalopathy may increase the risk of motor vehicle accidents, so alternative transportation plans should be considered.[83] Generally, cirrhotic patients should not restrict protein given the significant risks of cachexia, yet sodium restriction (<2 g/day) is warranted when portal hypertensive fluid retention is present. Regular exercise, as tolerated, should be encouraged to minimize debilitation.

Allocation and Distribution Systems

Allocation refers to how patients on a waiting list are ranked or prioritized for available donor organs. Candidates for liver transplantation are most commonly prioritized using an urgency-based system where candidates with the highest likelihood of dying or becoming too sick for transplant receive the greatest priority. In the United States and several countries worldwide, the MELD and PELD scores are used to assess the risk of death and hence priority for transplantation.[84] Up until February 2002, the U.S. allocation system used the Child-Turcotte-Pugh score for this purpose. Since then, the MELD score has been used. The MELD score has been shown to have several advantages as an allocation tool, including improved accuracy and reproducibility because of the avoidance of subjective predictors such as ascites and encephalopathy.[84-86] MELD can accurately predict short-term waitlist mortality for the vast majority (83% to 87%) of liver transplant candidates.[86] Yet for the minority of patients with acute liver failure or liver disease in which the prognosis is not predicted by derangements in the MELD score, an alternative priority system is required. Under the MELD-based allocation system in the United States, patients meeting specific criteria are eligible for additional priority or MELD exception score (see **Table 47-3**). Hepatocellular carcinoma is the most common reason for such additional priority and has been the topic of new consensus guidelines for establishing the diagnosis of HCC and revising the priority schema[3,45] (see **Tables 47-9 and 47-10**).

Distribution of available donor organs to a waiting list is typically defined by geographic areas but in some countries it is defined by a transplant center's assigned donor area. In patient-based distribution, as in the United States, donor organ offers go first to the highest priority patient nearest the organ donor in the local area known as a designated service area, then to a larger regional area, then nationally. An exception to this schema is made for patients with an estimated survival time of less than 7 days without liver transplantation and listed as "status 1." Under these conditions, donor organs are drawn from the entire region. The United States is divided into 58 donor service areas that contain one to several transplant centers and 11 regions that contain one to several donor service areas. Under center-based distribution, such as in the United Kingdom, donor organs are offered to transplant centers, who then allocate the organ to the most appropriate and highest priority candidate at that center.[87]

Donor Liver Choices

Donor livers for transplantation are a scarce, life-saving resource. Given this scarcity, efforts have been made to expand the donor options available to patients in need of liver transplantation. Unfortunately, the ideal donor liver is often not available. Therefore the patient, in consultation with the transplant team, should decide on which less-than-ideal donor liver he or she would consider. This important risk–benefit discussion is typically an ongoing and dynamic process. It begins at the time of initial evaluation in the hypothetical and culminates at the time of a viable offer with the specific risks associated with the characteristics of that donor organ.[88,89] Issues to consider in this decision include the transplant candidates underlying liver disease, the disease-specific risk for becoming too sick for transplantation, the risk of posttransplant complications and graft failure, and the local expertise of the transplant team. An analysis of the U.S. transplant experience showed that with an increasing severity of illness, as measured by MELD, there is an increasing benefit of transplantation with less-than-ideal liver grafts as measured by the donor risk index (DRI).[90] Available donor options include a whole or split graft from a standard deceased donor who had a brain death, a donor who had a cardiac death, a live donor, an older age donor, and a donor at higher than average risk for transmitting disease.

The availability and type of donor liver is determined by the cultural, religious, and demographic makeup of the surrounding population. For example, deceased donor organ donation is less common in much of Asia, making live donor organ procurement the most common donor source. This experience has allowed the advancement of adult-to-child and adult-to-adult live donor liver donation using either the left or right liver lobes as a liver graft. At experienced centers, patient and graft survival after live-donor liver transplantation are similar to deceased donor transplantation, yet the rates of biliary complications and hospitalizations are higher.[91,92] The safety of the person being considered as a live donor is imperative because this individual does not otherwise require a surgical procedure nor the associated risks.[93,94] In Europe and Northern America, deceased organ donation is much more accepted and accounts for the vast majority of available donor livers. The demographics of these donors reflect the general population. Deceased donors are increasingly older and with metabolic syndrome risk factors that are associated hepatic steatosis, both of which can have detrimental effects on early and late graft survival.[95,96] The effect of these risk factors can vary widely based on the potential recipients underlying disease, particularly in recipients with HCV infection.[3,97] For example in a study using the UNOS database, compared with younger donors aged 21 to 30, the risk of graft failure with older donors aged 41 to 50 years and over 60 was 22% and 89% higher in recipients without viral hepatitis and 67% and 121% higher in recipients with HCV, respectively.[97]

Several other donor options exist. Deceased donor livers are typically procured after brain death, yet organ donation after cardiac death, known as DCD, is uncommon but increasing. Use of DCD livers in the United States increased from 0.9% to 5% between 2000 and 2006 in the United States and accounted for 307 liver transplants in 2007.[2,3] Because of a 10% to 15% lower graft survival compared with livers from brain-dead donors, practice guidelines exist to select appropriate recipients for this valuable donor option.[19,98] Good-quality deceased donor livers can be split to provide grafts for two recipients, generally one pediatric and one adult patient. When split liver grafts are from younger donors (<30 years old) and lack other poor prognostic factors, outcomes can be comparable with whole liver grafts.[99] Rates of transmission of infections via the donor in liver transplantation can

be predicted with only fair accuracy based on reported donor risk factors, so rapid testing of all donors is routine. Although rapid testing cannot exclude the risk of transmission of HIV, when modern testing is negative, the absolute risk of transmission is low with an estimated probability from standard- and high-risk donors of 2.4 and 46 in 100,000 transplants, respectively.[89] HCV-infected donors without evidence of significant hepatic fibrosis have been used successfully in HCV-infected recipients. HCV recipient infection is universal and use of HCV-positive organs should be avoided if the recipient has a more treatment-responsive HCV genotype. HBV core positive donors without evidence of significant hepatic fibrosis are associated with comparable graft survival rates to other liver donors but must receive antiviral drugs following transplantation.[100]

Conclusion

For patients whose lives depend on liver transplantation, timely and appropriate evaluation for liver transplantation is of paramount importance. When assessing indications and contraindications to liver transplantation, the concepts of beneficence, nonmaleficence, and futility are considered. Patients with well-compensated or reversible liver disease may benefit from avoiding transplant whereas other patients who may have hastened progression of a malignancy, may have no meaningful neurologic function or may not survive the procedure or perioperative period. In this case, two individuals may be harmed; that is, the recipient and the other potential recipient who was not allocated that donor liver. Patients with relative contraindications should be considered for a preliminary discussion with the liver transplant selection committee before embarking on a time-consuming and costly evaluation. Once a patient is selected as a candidate and registered on the transplant waiting list, well-coordinated care between the transplant center and the patient's primary care team provide the patient with the greatest chance of surviving until an appropriate donor liver is available. As the urgency for transplant grows, serious consideration of alternative donor sources by the patient and transplant team is warranted.

References

1. Busuttil RW, et al. Analysis of long-term outcomes of 3200 liver transplantations over two decades: a single-center experience. Ann Surg 2005;241:905–916; discussion 916–918.
2. OPTN [online]. Cited April 4, 2010. Available from URL: http://optn.transplant.hrsa.gov.
3. Thuluvath PJ, et al. Liver transplantation in the United States, 1999-2008. Am J Transplant 2010;10:1003–1019.
4. Davis CL, et al. Simultaneous liver-kidney transplantation: evaluation to decision making. Am J Transplant 2007;7:1702–1709.
5. Eason JD, et al. Proceedings of Consensus Conference on Simultaneous Liver Kidney Transplantation (SLK). Am J Transplant 2008;8:2243–2251.
6. Murray KF, Carithers RL Jr. AASLD practice guidelines: evaluation of the patient for liver transplantation. Hepatology 2005;41:1407–1432.
7. Durand F, Valla D. Assessment of prognosis of cirrhosis. Semin Liver Dis 2008;28:110–122.
8. Stravitz RT, et al. Intensive care of patients with acute liver failure: recommendations of the U.S. acute liver failure study group. Crit Care Med 2007;35:2498–2508.
9. O'Grady JG, et al. Early indicators of prognosis in fulminant hepatic failure. Gastroenterology 1989;97:439–445.
10. Shakil AO, et al. Acute liver failure: clinical features, outcome analysis, and applicability of prognostic criteria. Liver Transpl 2000;6:163–169.

11. Yantorno SE, et al. MELD is superior to King's College and Clichy's criteria to assess prognosis in fulminant hepatic failure. Liver Transpl 2007;13: 822–828.

12. Malinchoc M, et al. A model to predict poor survival in patients undergoing transjugular intrahepatic portosystemic shunts. Hepatology 2000;31:864–871.

13. Kamath PS, et al. A model to predict survival in patients with end-stage liver disease. Hepatology 2001;33:464–470.

14. Kamath PS, Kim WR. The Model for End-Stage Liver Disease (MELD). Hepatology 2007;45:797–805.

15. Kim WR, et al. Hyponatremia and mortality among patients on the liver-transplant waiting list. N Engl J Med 2008;359:1018–1026.

16. McDiarmid SV, Anand R, Lindblad AS. Development of a pediatric end-stage liver disease score to predict poor outcome in children awaiting liver transplantation. Transplantation 2002;74:173–181.

17. Laryea M, et al. Metabolic syndrome in liver transplant recipients: prevalence and association with major vascular events. Liver Transpl 2007; 13:1109–1114.

18. Ojo AO, et al. Chronic renal failure after transplantation of a nonrenal organ. N Engl J Med 2003;349:931–940.

19. Berg CL, et al. Liver and intestine transplantation in the United States 1998-2007. Am J Transplant 2009;9(4 Pt 2):907–931.

20. ELTR [online]. Cited April 4, 2010. Available from URL: http://www.eltr.org.

21. SRTR [online]. Cited April 4, 2010. Available from URL: www.srtr.org.

22. Liou IW, Larson AM. Role of liver transplantation in acute liver failure. Semin Liver Dis 2008;28:201–209.

23. Davis GL, et al. Projecting future complications of chronic hepatitis C in the United States. Liver Transpl 2003;9:331–338.

24. Burroughs A, McNamara D. Liver disease in Europe. Aliment Pharmacol Ther 2003;18(Suppl 3):54–59.

25. Fattovich G, et al. Morbidity and mortality in compensated cirrhosis type C: a retrospective follow-up study of 384 patients. Gastroenterology 1997; 112:463–472.

26. Gane EJ. The natural history of recurrent hepatitis C and what influences this. Liver Transpl 2008;14(Suppl 2):S36–S44.

27. Forman LM, et al. The association between hepatitis C infection and survival after orthotopic liver transplantation. Gastroenterology 2002;122: 889–896.

28. Everson GT, et al. Treatment of advanced hepatitis C with a low accelerating dosage regimen of antiviral therapy. Hepatology 2005;42: 255–262.

29. Kim WR, et al. Burden of liver disease in the United States: summary of a workshop. Hepatology 2002;36:227–242.

30. Veldt BJ, et al. Indication of liver transplantation in severe alcoholic liver cirrhosis: quantitative evaluation and optimal timing. J Hepatol 2002;36: 93–98.

31. Vanlemmens C, et al. Immediate listing for liver transplantation versus standard care for Child-Pugh stage B alcoholic cirrhosis: a randomized trial. Ann Intern Med 2009;150:153–161.

32. Everhart JE, Beresford TP. Liver transplantation for alcoholic liver disease: a survey of transplantation programs in the United States. Liver Transpl Surg 1997;3:220–226.

33. Cuadrado A, et al. Alcohol recidivism impairs long-term patient survival after orthotopic liver transplantation for alcoholic liver disease. Liver Transpl 2005;11:420–426.

34. Consensus Conference: Indications for Liver Transplantation, Jan 19-20, 2005, Lyon-Palais Des Congres: text of recommendations (long version). Liver Transpl 2006;12:998–1011.

35. Lavanchy D. Hepatitis B virus epidemiology, disease burden, treatment, and current and emerging prevention and control measures. J Viral Hepat 2004; 11:97–107.

36. Kim WR, et al. Trends in waiting list registration for liver transplantation for viral hepatitis in the United States. Gastroenterology 2009;137: 1680–1686.

37. Yao FY, Bass NM. Lamivudine treatment in patients with severely decompensated cirrhosis due to replicating hepatitis B infection. J Hepatol 2000;33:301–307.

38. Lok AS. Prevention of recurrent hepatitis B post-liver transplantation. Liver Transpl 2002;8(10 Suppl 1):S67–S73.

39. Becker NS, et al. Outcomes analysis for 280 patients with cholangiocarcinoma treated with liver transplantation over an 18-year period. J Gastrointest Surg 2008;12:117–122.

40. Rea DJ, et al. Transplantation for cholangiocarcinoma: when and for whom? Surg Oncol Clin N Am 2009;18:325–337, ix.

41. UNOS [online]. Cited April 4, 2010. Available from URL: www.unos.org.

42. Roberts MS, et al. Survival after liver transplantation in the United States: a disease-specific analysis of the UNOS database. Liver Transpl 2004;10:886–897.

43. Schutte K, Bornschein J, Malfertheiner P. Hepatocellular carcinoma: epidemiological trends and risk factors. Dig Dis 2009;27:80–92.

44. El-Serag HB. Hepatocellular carcinoma: recent trends in the United States. Gastroenterology 2004;127(5 Suppl 1):S27–S34.

45. Pomfret EA, et al. Report of a national conference on liver allocation in patients with hepatocellular carcinoma in the United States. Liver Transpl 2010;16:262–278.

46. Llovet JM, et al. Sorafenib in advanced hepatocellular carcinoma. N Engl J Med 2008;359:378–390.

47. Llovet JM, Schwartz M, Mazzaferro V. Resection and liver transplantation for hepatocellular carcinoma. Semin Liver Dis 2005;25:181–200.

48. Mazzaferro V, et al. Liver transplantation for the treatment of small hepatocellular carcinomas in patients with cirrhosis. N Engl J Med 1996; 334:693–699.

49. Bruix J, Sherman M. Management of hepatocellular carcinoma. Hepatology 2005;42:1208–1236.

50. Yao FY. Liver transplantation for hepatocellular carcinoma: beyond the Milan criteria. Am J Transplant 2008;8:1982–1989.

51. Yao FY, et al. Liver transplantation for hepatocellular carcinoma: validation of the UCSF-expanded criteria based on preoperative imaging. Am J Transplant 2007;7:2587–2596.

52. Adam R, et al. Liver resection as a bridge to transplantation for hepatocellular carcinoma on cirrhosis: a reasonable strategy? Ann Surg 2003;238:508–518; discussion 518–519.

53. Lin SM, et al. Randomised controlled trial comparing percutaneous radiofrequency thermal ablation, percutaneous ethanol injection, and percutaneous acetic acid injection to treat hepatocellular carcinoma of 3 cm or less. Gut 2005;54:1151–1156.

54. Liapi E, Geschwind JF. Intra-arterial therapies for hepatocellular carcinoma: where do we stand? Ann Surg Oncol 2010;17:1234–1246.

55. Wang W, Shi J, Xie WF. Transarterial chemoembolization in combination with percutaneous ablation therapy in unresectable hepatocellular carcinoma: a meta-analysis. Liver Int 2010;30:741–749.

56. Lu DS, et al. Percutaneous radiofrequency ablation of hepatocellular carcinoma as a bridge to liver transplantation. Hepatology 2005;41: 1130–1137.

57. Kayler LK, et al. Epithelioid hemangioendothelioma of the liver disseminated to the peritoneum treated with liver transplantation and interferon alpha-2B. Transplantation 2002;74:128–130.

58. Faraj W, et al. Liver transplantation for hepatoblastoma. Liver Transpl 2008;14:1614–1619.

59. Biggins SW, et al. Retransplantation for hepatic allograft failure: prognostic modeling and ethical considerations. Liver Transpl 2002;8:313–322.

60. Kadayifci A, et al. Clinical and pathologic risk factors for atherosclerosis in cirrhosis: a comparison between NASH-related cirrhosis and cirrhosis due to other aetiologies. J Hepatol 2008;49:595–599.

61. Ehtisham J, et al. Coronary artery disease in orthotopic liver transplantation: pretransplant assessment and management. Liver Transpl 2010;16:550–557.

62. Findlay JY, Wen D, Mandell MS. Cardiac risk evaluation for abdominal transplantation. Curr Opin Organ Transplant Mar 2010;15:363–367.

63. Brilakis ES, Banerjee S, Berger PB. Perioperative management of patients with coronary stents. J Am Coll Cardiol 2007;49:2145–2150.

64. Safadi A, et al. Perioperative risk predictors of cardiac outcomes in patients undergoing liver transplantation surgery. Circulation 2009;120: 1189–1194.

65. Umphrey LG, et al. Preoperative dobutamine stress echocardiographic findings and subsequent short-term adverse cardiac events after orthotopic liver transplantation. Liver Transpl 2008;14:886–892.

66. Swanson KL, et al. Survival in portopulmonary hypertension: Mayo Clinic experience categorized by treatment subgroups. Am J Transplant 2008;8: 2445–2453.

67. Fix OK, et al. Long-term follow-up of portopulmonary hypertension: effect of treatment with epoprostenol. Liver Transpl 2007;13:875–885.

68. Krowka MJ, et al. Pulmonary hemodynamics and perioperative cardiopulmonary-related mortality in patients with portopulmonary hypertension undergoing liver transplantation. Liver Transpl 2000;6: 443–450.

69. Mucke HA. Pulmonary arterial hypertension: on the way to a manageable disease. Curr Opin Investig Drugs 2008;9:957–962.

70. Krowka MJ. Hepatopulmonary syndrome and portopulmonary hypertension: implications for liver transplantation. Clin Chest Med 2005; 26:587–597, vi.

71. Bambha KM, Biggins SW. Inequities of the Model for End-Stage Liver Disease: an examination of current components and future additions. Curr Opin Organ Transplant 2008;13:227–233.

72. Samuel D, et al. Are HIV-infected patients candidates for liver transplantation? J Hepatol 2008;48:697–707.

73. Mindikoglu AL, Regev A, Magder LS. Impact of human immunodeficiency virus on survival after liver transplantation: analysis of United Network for Organ Sharing database. Transplantation 2008;85:359–368.

74. Penn I. The effect of immunosuppression on pre-existing cancers. Transplantation 1993;55:742–747.

75. Lipshutz GS, et al. Outcome of liver transplantation in septuagenarians: a single-center experience. Arch Surg 2007;142:775–781; discussion 781–784.

76. Kemmer N, et al. Liver transplantation trends for older recipients: regional and ethnic variations. Transplantation 2008;86:104–107.

77. Keswani RN, Ahmed A, Keeffe EB. Older age and liver transplantation: a review. Liver Transpl 2004;10:957–967.

78. Leonard J, et al. The impact of obesity on long-term outcomes in liver transplant recipients: results of the NIDDK liver transplant database. Am J Transplant 2008;8:667–672.

79. Nair S, Verma S, Thuluvath PJ. Obesity and its effect on survival in patients undergoing orthotopic liver transplantation in the United States. Hepatology 2002;35:105–109.

80. Lindstrom D, et al. Effects of a perioperative smoking cessation intervention on postoperative complications: a randomized trial. Ann Surg 2008;248:739–745.

81. Manzanet G, et al. Liver transplantation in patients with portal vein thrombosis. Liver Transpl 2001;7:125–131.

82. Cabibbo G, Craxi A. Hepatocellular cancer: optimal strategies for screening and surveillance. Dig Dis 2009;27:142–147.

83. Bajaj JS, et al. Minimal hepatic encephalopathy is associated with motor vehicle crashes: the reality beyond the driving test. Hepatology 2009;50:1175–1183.

84. Freeman RB Jr. The model for end-stage liver disease comes of age. Clin Liver Dis 2007;11:249–263.

85. Wiesner R, et al. Model for End-Stage Liver Disease (MELD) and allocation of donor livers. Gastroenterology 2003;124:91–96.

86. Biggins SW, Bambha K. MELD-based liver allocation: who is underserved? Semin Liver Dis 2006;26:211–220.

87. Freeman RB, et al. Who should get a liver graft? J Hepatol 2009;50:664–673.

88. Halpern SD, et al. Informing candidates for solid-organ transplantation about donor risk factors. N Engl J Med 2008;358:2832–2837.

89. Freeman RB, Cohen JT. Transplantation risks and the real world: what does "high risk" really mean? Am J Transplant 2009;9:23–30.

90. Schaubel DE, et al. The survival benefit of deceased donor liver transplantation as a function of candidate disease severity and donor quality. Am J Transplant 2008;8:419–425.

91. Merion RM, et al. Hospitalization rates before and after adult-to-adult living donor or deceased donor liver transplantation. Ann Surg 2010;251:542–549.

92. Freise CE, et al. Recipient morbidity after living and deceased donor liver transplantation: findings from the A2ALL retrospective cohort study. Am J Transplant 2008;8:2569–2579.

93. Rhee J, et al. Organ donation. Semin Liver Dis 2009;29:19–39.

94. Iida T, et al. Surgery-related morbidity in living donors for liver transplantation. Transplantation 2010;89:1276–1282.

95. Briceno J, et al. Impact of donor graft steatosis on overall outcome and viral recurrence after liver transplantation for hepatitis C virus cirrhosis. Liver Transpl 2009;15:37–48.

96. McCormack L, et al. Hepatic steatosis is a risk factor for postoperative complications after major hepatectomy: a matched case-control study. Ann Surg 2007;245:923–930.

97. Lake JR, et al. Differential effects of donor age in liver transplant recipients infected with hepatitis B, hepatitis C and without viral hepatitis. Am J Transplant 2005;5:549–557.

98. Reich DJ, et al. ASTS recommended practice guidelines for controlled donation after cardiac death organ procurement and transplantation. Am J Transplant 2009;9:2004–2011.

99. Lee KW, et al. Factors affecting graft survival after adult/child split-liver transplantation: analysis of the UNOS/OPTN data base. Am J Transplant 2008;8:1186–1196.

100. Yu L, et al. Survival after orthotopic liver transplantation: the impact of antibody against hepatitis B core antigen in the donor. Liver Transpl 2009;15:1343–1350.

Transplantation of the Liver

Parsia A. Vagefi and Sandy Feng

Brief History of Liver Transplantation

"... liver, brain, and heart, these sovereign thrones"
(William Shakespeare, *Twelfth Night*, Act 1, Scene 1)

The history of modern liver transplantation began in 1955 in the laboratories of Stuart Welch at Albany Medical College and Jack Cannon at the University of California, Los Angeles. Welch was the first to demonstrate the technique of auxiliary liver transplantation, experiments that he performed in dogs in which the native liver was left undisturbed and the transplanted liver was placed in a heterotopic position.[1,2] It was Cannon who first demonstrated the technique of orthotopic liver transplantation in which the native liver was removed, and a graft put in its place.[3] Unfortunately, none of the dogs survived. Finally, in 1958, Francis Moore in Boston and Thomas Starzl in Denver demonstrated technical success, achieving recipient survival in canine models of orthotopic liver transplantation. However, the success was short-lived because rejection led to graft and recipient demise within the first weeks after transplantation.[4,5] Following the technical success in canine models, Starzl attempted the first liver transplant in a human in 1963. The recipient was a 3 year old with biliary atresia, who succumbed in the operating room because of hemorrhage before the completion of the transplant. Over

the ensuing year there would be six more attempts at liver transplantation in Denver, Paris, and Boston, all of which resulted in recipient mortality within 23 days of transplantation. Given the dismal results, a moratorium was imposed in 1964, which lasted for just over 3 years. In 1967, Starzl performed the first successful liver transplantation in an 18-month-old child with hepatoblastoma. She survived for 400 days before succumbing to disseminated malignancy. Although this initial success spawned more clinical activity, the 1-year survival rate following liver transplantation remained below 50%[5] because two major hurdles stood in the way of successful liver transplantation: rejection and optimization of organ preservation.

Initial efforts at organ preservation were simplistic, with the use of chilled normal saline or lactated Ringer solution, which achieved organ preservation for a maximum of 6 hours. Gradually, it was realized that preservation solutions should contain an impermeant and/or a colloid to prevent cellular edema, strong buffering capacity to combat acidosis, an electrolyte composition to simulate either the intracellular or the extracellular milieu, and finally antioxidants to scavenge free radicals. In 1987, a University of Wisconsin solution emerged as the leading preservation solution and allowed for cold static liver preservation for up to 18 to 24 hours.[6]

Concomitant with efforts to optimize organ preservation were efforts to understand transplant rejection. In 1944, Peter Medawar demonstrated that allograft rejection was an immune-mediated phenomenon.[7] More than a decade later, Sir Roy Calne demonstrated that 6-mercaptopurine, and subsequently azathioprine, prolonged the life of kidney allografts.[8] In 1967, the concept of induction immunosuppression—administration of an agent for a short course at the time of transplantation—emerged with the introduction of antilymphocyte globulin used in conjunction with maintenance therapy consisting of azathioprine and prednisone. This comprised the first triple drug immunosuppression regimen.[9] It was, however, the discovery of cyclosporine in 1969 by Jean-Francois Borel that truly revolutionized organ transplantation. Derived from a fungus sample cultured from soil, it was first used with success by Sir Roy Calne in rodent models of heart transplantation.[10] Cyclosporine was first used in humans in 1978, and U.S. Food and Drug Administration approval came in 1983. Cyclosporine achieved 1-year liver transplant survival rates of 70% and was rapidly accepted as the gold standard of maintenance immunosuppression.[11] Six years later, tacrolimus, isolated from the culture broth of a soil sample from the Tsukuba area of northern Japan,[12] was introduced. Its superiority to cyclosporine was quickly demonstrated such that it supplanted cyclosporine as the mainstay of maintenance regimens, a position it retains to this day.

Indications and Contraindications to Liver Transplantation

Indications

Transplantation has become the procedure of choice for a wide range of liver diseases in both adult and pediatric patients. These conditions range from acute or chronic liver disease to metabolic/congenital conditions and hepatic malignancy. **Table 48-1** summarizes the indications for liver transplantation in adult and pediatric patients. Despite the varying causes of these diseases, the onset of decompensated liver disease is often the common final pathway that leads to liver transplantation.

Noncholestatic liver disease remains the most common indication for transplantation overall, accounting for 57% and 39% of deceased and living donor liver transplants, respectively.[13] In adults, noncholestatic liver disease is dominated by hepatitis C cirrhosis, the most common indication for liver transplantation. However, it is anticipated that over the next 1 to 2 decades hepatitis C will substantially diminish, while nonalcoholic steatohepatitis will correspondingly escalate as an indication for liver transplantation. Among children, biliary atresia remains the most common indication, accounting for nearly two thirds of liver transplants. **Table 48-2** demonstrates the diagnoses for adult and pediatric recipients of donor livers from deceased individuals from 1998 to 2007, and **Table 48-3** demonstrates the diagnoses for adult and pediatric recipients of livers from living donors from 1998 to 2007.

Contraindications

Table 48-4 lists the absolute and relative contraindications to liver transplantation. Among the relative contraindications to liver transplantation, special note should be made of human

Table 48-1 Indications for Hepatic Transplantation

Acute Liver Injury

Viral hepatitis
Toxic injury (acetaminophen [paracetamol], halothane, mushroom, others)
Fulminant Wilson disease
Fulminant tyrosinemia

Chronic Liver Injury

Cholestatic disease (primary biliary cirrhosis, primary sclerosing cholangitis, biliary atresia, familial cholestatic syndromes)
Hepatocellular disease (viral hepatitis, alcoholic cirrhosis, autoimmune hepatitis)
Vascular disease (Budd-Chiari, veno-occlusive disease)
Massive steatosis

Mass-Occupying Lesions

Hepatocellular carcinoma
Hepatoblastoma
Hemangioendothelioma
Metastatic neuroendocrine tumor
Polycystic liver disease
Multiple adenomatosis

Metabolic Diseases

α_1-Antitrypsin deficiency
Wilson disease
Tyrosinemia
Hemochromatosis
Glycogen storage disease types I and IV
Cystic fibrosis
Erythropoietic protoporphyria
Crigler-Najjar syndrome
Oxalosis
Urea cycle enzyme deficiency
Protein C deficiency
Hemophilia A

Graft Failure

Rejection (acute, chronic)
Primary graft failure
Technical failure

immunodeficiency virus (HIV) infection. The advent of highly active antiretroviral therapy (HAART) has dramatically improved the prognosis for people with HIV infection. At the University of California, San Francisco (UCSF), criteria for inclusion of HIV-positive recipients for liver transplants are those predicted to achieve viral load suppression after transplantation it unable to tolerate HAART before transplant, have a CD4[+] T-cell count of more than 100 cells per microliter for 6 months, and have no history of opportunistic infections nor HIV-related neoplasms.[14] In a prospective series of liver transplant recipients infected with HIV, 1- and 3-year survival rates were 91% and 64%, respectively. In addition, 1- and 3-year liver graft survival rates were 82% and 64%, respectively.[15] These results suggest that liver transplantation remains an option for a select group of HIV-infected patients.

Obesity is another relative contraindication that deserves special mention, particularly because its prevalence is greatly increasing in the United States. Many transplant centers have body mass index (BMI) limitations to qualify for transplantation, although there is certainly no uniformity in

Table 48-2 **Liver Deceased Donor Transplant Recipients by Diagnosis, 1998-2007**

	1998	1999	2000	2001	2002	2003	2004	2005	2006	2007
Noncholestatic cirrhosis (%)	63	64	64	64	62	59	60	61	59	57
Hepatitis C (%)	24	26	28	28	29	27	27	24	23	22
Alcoholic cirrhosis (%)	13	13	12	11	11	12	11	12	11	11
Both hepatitis C and alcoholic (%)	8	8	7	8	5	5	6	8	7	7
Autoimmune hepatitis (%)	4	3	4	3	3	3	2	3	2	2
Hepatitis B only (%)	4	4	3	4	4	3	3	2	2	2
Cryptogenic, idiopathic, NASH (%)	9	9	9	8	7	7	7	7	6	6
Other noncholestatic (%)	1	1	1	1	1	1	2	3	2	2
Cholestatic liver disease (%)	13	11	10	10	10	10	9	8	9	9
Acute hepatic necrosis (%)	8	9	9	8	7	7	7	7	6	6
Biliary atresia	5	4	4	4	3	3	3	3	2	3
Metabolic disorders (%)	4	3	4	4	3	3	3	3	3	3
Malignant neoplasms (%)	2	2	2	3	7	7	8	10	12	13
Other (%)	6	6	7	8	7	11	9	8	9	10

From 2008 OPTN/SRTR Annual Report 1998-2007.
Recipients with both hepatitis B and hepatitis C are counted in the hepatitis C category.
NASH, nonalcoholic steatohepatitis

Table 48-3 **Liver Living Donor Transplant Recipients by Diagnosis, 1998-2007**

	1998	1999	2000	2001	2002	2003	2004	2005	2006	2007
Noncholestatic cirrhosis (%)	22	38	44	56	52	46	50	46	39	39
Hepatitis C (%)	9	21	24	37	28	23	22	20	15	17
Alcoholic cirrhosis (%)	3	4	6	8	8	8	9	9	6	5
Both hepatitis C and alcoholic (%)	1	3	2	4	4	2	3	4	3	2
Autoimmune hepatitis (%)	5	4	2	4	3	2	4	2	2	3
Hepatitis B only (%)	1	3	1	3	3	2	1	2	2	2
Cryptogenic, idiopathic, NASH (%)	2	5	8	7	6	9	11	8	11	9
Other noncholestatic (%)	0	0	0	1	1	1	0	1	0	1
Cholestatic liver disease (%)	7	11	18	16	21	21	23	21	23	18
Acute hepatic necrosis (%)	7	10	6	5	4	7	3	4	6	3
Biliary atresia	42	20	14	9	9	12	7	8	13	12
Metabolic disorders (%)	5	5	4	3	2	2	3	3	2	4
Malignant neoplasms (%)	2	9	8	6	5	3	7	8	9	12
Other (%)	15	7	7	6	6	8	8	10	8	12

From 2008 OPTN/SRTR Annual Report 1998-2007.
Recipients with both hepatitis B and hepatitis C are counted in the hepatitis C category.
NASH, nonalcoholic steatohepatitis

practice. Obese recipients pose a substantial technical challenge that is reflected in the increased frequency of postoperative complications. Although it has been reported that severe obesity (BMI >40 kg/m^2) is a significant predictor of death following liver transplantation,[16] correction of the BMI to account for the extent of ascites volume has demonstrated that an adjusted BMI did not independently predict patient or graft survival.[17] Indeed, in selected obese patients, satisfactory outcomes, similar to that obtained in nonobese recipients, can be achieved.[17] One proposed approach for the management of pretransplant obesity has been the use of laparoscopic bariatric procedures.[18] The latter approach remains investigational; however, preliminary evidence has demonstrated that bariatric surgery is not only safe and well tolerated, but can improve the candidacy of patients awaiting transplantation. Larger studies will be needed to assess the safety, feasibility, and efficacy of bariatric surgery in morbidly obese patients with cirrhosis awaiting transplantation.

Candidate Evaluation and Listing

Evaluation

Patients with end-stage liver disease who are referred for liver transplantation undergo evaluation either as an outpatient or

Table 48-4 Contraindications to Hepatic Transplantation

Absolute

Patient unable to understand and comply with immunosuppression
Active extrabiliary sepsis
Metastatic hepatocellular carcinoma
Advanced cardiopulmonary disease
Active alcoholism and drug addiction
Acquired immunodeficiency syndrome (AIDS)
Documented anatomic anomalies precluding transplantation
Recent history of extrahepatic cancer

Relative

Age older than 75 years
Active sepsis of hepatobiliary origin
Active infection of extrahepatic organs
Retransplantation for recurrence of hepatitis C
Cholangiocarcinoma
Severe malnutrition
Diabetes mellitus with coronary artery disease
Multiple organ failure requiring cardiopulmonary support
Patients in coma stage IV
Human immunodeficiency virus (HIV) infection
Morbid obesity

an inpatient. The latter is often associated with the onset of acute hepatic decompensation, or severe, life-threatening complications of end-stage liver disease (i.e., bleeding, encephalopathy, infection) that necessitate expedited assessment. Evaluation begins with standard blood tests and serologic profiles. Radiologic studies should include, at a minimum, a chest x-ray and an ultrasound with Doppler examination of the abdomen, with particular focus on the liver and kidneys. In patients with hepatocellular carcinoma, a computed tomography (CT) scan of the abdomen is obtained. Further diagnostic studies include upper endoscopy to assess for esophageal and/or gastric varices, portal hypertensive gastropathy, and peptic ulcer disease. Cardiovascular evaluation is tailored to the candidate's demographics and cardiac risk factors. Typically, an electrocardiogram, transthoracic echocardiogram, and a noninvasive stress test are standard. Right and/or left heart catheterization, CT coronary angiography, and cardiac magnetic resonance imaging (MRI) are reserved for specific indications. Up-to-date routine health maintenance studies such as colonoscopy, mammography, Papanicolaou smear, and testing for prostate-specific antigen is typically required.

In addition to the battery of laboratory, radiographic, and procedural assessments, candidates seeking transplantation undergo thorough evaluation by a hepatologist, a transplant surgeon, a social worker, a financial counselor, and, if needed, a substance abuse expert and/or a psychiatrist to determine their suitability for transplantation. Following completion of the pretransplant evaluation process, each candidate is presented and discussed by a multidisciplinary team and his or her candidacy is thus determined.

Assessment of Disease Severity and Waiting List Stratification

In 1964 C. Garner Child and Jeremiah Turcotte of the University of Michigan proposed a scoring system that stratified the degree of end-stage liver disease. Their scoring system, the first of its kind, relied on five clinical parameters: total bilirubin, serum albumin, nutritional status, extent of ascites, and degree of hepatic encephalopathy.[19] The Child-Turcotte scoring system was developed to preoperatively standardize the severity of chronic liver disease using a reliable set of clinical criteria, which allowed for the prediction of postoperative outcome. The scoring system was modified by Pugh in 1972 to allow for consideration of the bleeding tendency in patients with portal hypertension. The Child-Turcotte-Pugh (CTP) score replaced the criterion of nutritional status with the prothrombin time.[20] Lacking any other standardized method, the CTP score, combined with waiting time on the transplant list, was used to stratify liver transplant candidates for organ allocation. However, the CTP score required the subjective assessment of ascites and severity of encephalopathy. Dissatisfaction with the subjective components of the CTP score helped prompt the development of a completely objective scoring system for organ allocation.

The Model for End-Stage Liver Disease (MELD) score was originally developed as a method to predict 3-month survival rates in patients undergoing transjugular intrahepatic portosystemic shunts (TIPS).[21] Based on the patient's total serum bilirubin, serum creatinine, and the international normalized ratio (INR), the MELD score did not rely on the subjective assessments of ascites and encephalopathy severity inherent to the CTP score. The MELD score also proved to be superior to the CTP score in predicting transplant waitlist survival. In February 2002 the United Network of Organ Sharing (UNOS) adopted the MELD allocation system, and in doing so gave priority to the sickest patients based upon objective parameters and deemphasized the importance of waitlist time. A pediatric scoring system entitled the pediatric end-stage liver disease (PELD) score based on four clinical parameters, total bilirubin, INR, albumin, and extent of growth failure,[22] was adopted for patients younger than 12 years.

Candidates with Hepatocellular Carcinoma

Early results for the treatment of hepatocellular cancer (HCC) by liver transplantation were unfavorable, consisting of poor survival rates and a high incidence of posttransplantation recurrence.[23] In 1996, Mazzaferro and colleagues reported results that have led to the codification of the Milan criteria, thereby defining the subset of patients with unresectable HCC for whom liver transplantation is the appropriate treatment.[24] Transplantation within the Milan criteria (single tumor of 5 cm in diameter, or two to three tumors of 3 cm in diameter) resulted in overall and recurrence-free survival rates of 85% and 92%, respectively, at 4 years. Therefore HCC with tumor burden within the Milan criteria gained wide acceptance as a legitimate indication for liver transplantation.

As patients with HCC often have preserved hepatic function, their calculated MELD score predicted a low risk of death from their liver disease alone. To provide HCC candidates access to liver transplantation before HCC progression beyond the Milan criteria, MELD exception points were awarded to this subset of liver transplant candidates. Under the initial HCC-adjusted MELD scheme of organ allocation, patients with stage 1 HCC (1 lesion <2 cm) were given a MELD score of 24, corresponding to an expected 15% 3-month dropout rate because of tumor progression beyond the Milan criteria.

Those with stage 2 HCC (one lesion 2 to 5 cm, two to three nodules all 3 cm) were assigned a MELD score of 29, which reflected an expected 30%, 3-month dropout rate. For every 3 months on the waiting list, HCC candidates who remained within the Milan criteria were awarded additional exception points equivalent to a 10% increase in mortality risk. Since its inception, there has been a growing body of evidence that HCC was overvalued in the original MELD allocation, prompting two subsequent adjustments in the attribution of MELD points for HCC patients in April 2003 and January 2004.[23] Currently, stage 1 HCC candidates no longer receive any MELD exception points, and stage 2 HCC candidates are now awarded a MELD score of 22.

The application of Milan criteria in the selection of liver transplant candidates in patients with HCC has led to excellent posttransplant survival rates (61% at 5 years), thus demonstrating that liver transplantation is the treatment of choice in patients with advanced cirrhosis and HCC.[25] The excellent results obtained has prompted further investigation into whether the Milan criteria could be expanded to include patients with a larger HCC tumor burden. In 2001, Yao and colleagues at UCSF proposed expansion of the Milan criteria for HCC liver transplant candidates.[26] Termed the UCSF criteria, these patients with HCC had a single tumor 6.5 cm in diameter, or two or three tumors, none exceeding 4.5 cm in diameter and whose sum of tumor diameters did not exceed 8 cm. For this cohort, liver transplantation allowed for 1- and 5-year survival rates of 90% and 75%, respectively, thus demonstrating equivalent rates of long-term survival when compared with the Milan criteria.

Locoregional therapy has been proposed as an effective strategy to not only retard HCC progression and prevent dropout from the transplant waitlist, but also as a means of downstaging patients to within the Milan criteria, and thus achieve eligibility for transplantation.[27] There remains a wide array of locoregional therapies for the management of HCC in candidates awaiting liver transplantation. These therapies range from surgical resection, percutaneous or laparoscopic radiofrequency ablation, percutaneous ethanol injection, and transarterial chemoembolization. Locoregional therapy may not only prevent dropout from the waitlist, it may also improve survival rates following liver transplantation for HCC.[28]

Liver Transplantation: Deceased and Living Donors

Historical Perspectives

The world's first human-to-human transplant of a solid organ was performed in April 1933 by the Russian surgeon Yu Yu Voronoy.[29] The recipient of the kidney allograft was a 26-year-old woman who had succumbed to acute renal failure after ingesting 4 g of mercuric chloride in an apparent suicide attempt. The donor kidney was obtained from an ABO incompatible 60-year-old gentleman who had died from a head injury 6 hours prior. The renal allograft did not function, and the recipient succumbed 2 days later. This event, however,

marked the first procurement of an organ from a deceased (non–heart beating) donor for transplantation. It would not be until December 23, 1954, that Boston surgeon Joseph Murray would perform the first living donor transplant. He transplanted a kidney procured from 23-year-old Ronald Herrick for his twin brother Richard Herrick, who suffered from advanced glomerulonephritis.[30] The transplant was a success, and Richard Herrick went on to live for 9 years after transplantation before succumbing to a heart attack.

Deceased Donors—Brain Death versus Cardiac Death

The concept of a brain dead donor was formalized in 1968 by an ad hoc committee at Harvard Medical School. They suggested revising the definition of death such that a subset of patients with a devastating neurologic injury would be suitable for organ donation under the dead donor rule.[31] The definition of brain death requires the complete and irreversible loss of all brain function including brainstem function, and is a clinically measurable condition. In donation after cardiac death (DCD or non–heart beating donors), patients with severe brain injuries, but who do not meet the clinical definition of brain death, can serve as organ donors at the bequest of their family after they sustain cardiac death. The potential DCD donor undergoes withdrawal of life-sustaining therapy and is subsequently pronounced dead by his or her physician.[32] To avoid obvious conflicts of interest, neither the surgeon who recovers the organs, nor any other personnel involved in transplantation, can participate in end-of-life care or the declaration of death for a DCD donor.[33] As autoresuscitation (spontaneous return of circulation) has not been reported to occur after 65 seconds of asystole, the Institute of Medicine recommends a 5-minute interval between pronouncement of death and the start of organ procurement.[34,35] DCD donors accounted for 5% of the 5625 deceased donors in 2007 and are expected to further increase.[13]

Expanded-Criteria Donors

The organ shortage has driven many transplant centers to accept expanded-criteria donors (ECD). This term, however, connotes a wide range of increased risk, including donors who pose a risk of transmitting malignancy or infection to the recipient. Increased infection risk refers to donors with evidence of hepatitis B, hepatitis C, human T-cell lymphotrophic virus I/II, human immunodeficiency virus (HIV), or donors with Centers for Disease Control and Prevention (CDC) high-risk social behavior. ECD also refers to donors whose liver poses a risk for poor function above the standard donor. The exact definition of what constitutes a functional ECD liver donor remains elusive. While many studies offer a definition,[36,37] a recognition that donor quality extends across a wide spectrum has led to the development of a donor risk index (DRI)—a continuous and quantitative assessment of the risk of graft failure for a specific donor liver compared with an ideal donor.[38] The donor and graft characteristics significantly associated with liver allograft failure include increasing donor age, African American race (compared with Caucasian donors), decreased donor height, nontraumatic causes of donor death, DCD donors, and split or partial grafts. The DRI allows for stratification of potential donors based upon the quality of the allograft. This not only facilitates the transplant team's decision regarding organ acceptance, but also allows for a quantitative consideration of donor-recipient pairing, using the DRI to describe donor quality and the MELD score to describe the potential recipient's disease severity.[39]

Organ Procurement Operation

Once a potential organ donor is identified and declared brain dead, the local organ procurement organization (OPO) begins to assists in the donor's management. OPO personnel thoroughly assess and document the donor's history of present illness and hospitalization along with his or her past medical and social history. Serological testing to determine blood and HLA type, and previous exposure to specific viruses and pathogens (cytomegalovirus, Epstein-Barr virus, HIV, hepatitis B and C virus, and syphilis) is obtained. Subsequent nucleic acid amplification testing for HIV and hepatitis C can be considered, too. For the donor liver, a list of potential recipients in rank order of disease severity is generated by UNOS. The donor liver is then offered to the highest-priority candidate by notifying the relevant transplant center. The transplant team then accepts or refuses the organ based on an assessment of the donor, the recipient, and the suitability of the match between the two. By policy, the transplant team has only 1 hour to make its decision. If the liver allograft is not accepted, the OPO staff then offers it to the transplant center of the next listed candidate until it is placed. During the organ allocation period, the OPO staff continues to actively manage the donor with the aim of optimizing organ quality. It is important to remember that brain dead donors are often hemodynamically unstable, with a high potential for metabolic and electrolyte abnormalities secondary to the devastating brain injury.

Once all of the organs appropriate for transplantation are allocated, a time is set for the organ procurement. Separate procurement teams may be deployed for each placed organ necessitating a coordinated effort to ensure a smooth donor operation. Techniques for liver procurement can vary among procurement teams and depends on the donor type. For brain dead donors, many surgeons perform some dissection before cardiopulmonary arrest and infusion of cold preservation, whereas others excise the abdominal organs en bloc and separate them on the back table. For DCD donors, it is critical to remember that organ ischemia begins as soon as the donor becomes hypotensive and/or hypoxic after the withdrawal of life support. Therefore, when a DCD procurement begins following the pronouncement of death and the obligatory period to ensure the absence of auto-resuscitation, the first goal is to expeditiously establish vascular access for flushing of organs with preservation solution, followed by placing ice slush in the abdomen for topical cooling. Organs can then be removed individually or en bloc. For DCD or brain dead donors, the donor's iliac artery and vein are procured because they may be used as vascular conduits during graft implantation.

Once organs, from either brain dead or cardiac death donors are excised, they are brought to the back table where additional flush and/or dissection can be done. In addition to arterial and portal venous flushing, the billary tree of the liver allograft is flushed via the common bile duct. The liver is then packaged with three barrier layers, placed on ice, and transported to the recipient's hospital. Although modern preservation

solutions have extended liver preservation for up to 24 hours, most surgeons prefer to limit the cold ischemic time to less than 12 hours because the incidence of biliary strictures and graft dysfunction increase exponentially thereafter.

Reduced-Sized and Split Livers

The size discrepancy between the typical pediatric liver transplant recipient, an infant or toddler, and the adult donor, necessitated a series of technical innovations over the past 3 decades that exploited the segmental anatomy of the liver and its regenerative capacity (**Fig. 48-1**). In reduced-sized liver transplantation, the liver is procured whole. Reduction hepatectomy to achieve a graft of appropriate size, typically a left lateral segment (segments 2 and 3) or a left lobe (segments 2 to 4) is then performed ex vivo (on the back table) and the residual liver is discarded. The first use of a partial liver graft was reported in 1979, albeit in the heterotopic position.[40] Five years later came the first report of a reduced-sized liver graft transplanted in the orthotopic position.[41] Reduced liver transplantation increased the transplant options for children but at the expense of the adult waiting list because it did not increase the overall number of available organs. The technical advance of split liver transplantation whereby one liver could be divided into two partial grafts for successful transplantation into two recipients—a child and an adult—emerged in 1988[42] (**Fig. 48-2**). The liver of a 23-year-old man was split ex vivo

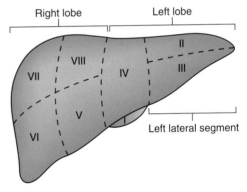

Fig. 48-1 Anatomic segments of the liver based upon its blood supply. The segmental blood supply to the liver, along with its regenerative capacity, allows partial, split, and living donor liver transplantation.

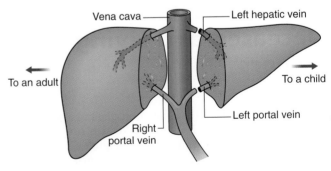

Fig. 48-2 Split liver transplantation, performed either in situ or ex vivo, allows for the creation of two functional allografts. The size of the left lateral segment is suitable for a pediatric recipient, whereas the right lobe allograft is suitable for adult recipients. (Hepatic artery and bile duct are not shown, but course alongside the portal branches.)

following a deceased donation, yielding an extended right lobe graft (segments 1 and 4 to 8), which was transplanted into a 63-year-old woman with primary biliary cirrhosis; the left lateral segment graft (segments 2 and 3) was transplanted into a 2-year-old pediatric recipient with congenital biliary atresia.

Although partial liver transplantation from deceased donors was the foundation that supported the development of living donor transplantation (see Living Donor section), living donor liver transplantation in turn refined split liver transplantation through the concept of in situ splitting.[43] Dissection of the vascular structures and division of the liver parenchyma in the donor while the liver is perfused facilitates identification of critical structures, eliminates the incremental cold ischemia time incurred with ex vivo splitting, and mitigates the problem of reperfusion hemorrhage from the cut edge.[44] Recent data has shown that 54% of split grafts are performed ex vivo, with the remaining 46% performed in situ.[45] Given the infrequency with which splitting is performed, direct comparisons of the in situ and ex vivo techniques are limited. However, in situ split liver transplantation may provide superior results by limiting the prolonged cold ischemia times encountered with the ex vivo technique.[46,47]

Living Donor: Historical Perspectives

The scarcity of organs that fueled surgical innovation leading to reduced and split deceased donor liver transplantation (DDLT) similarly motivated the development of living donor liver transplantation (LDLT). The first living donor liver transplant was done in 1988 by a Brazilian team.[48] The donor was a 23-year-old mother who donated her left lateral segment to her 4-year-old daughter with biliary atresia. The donor was discharged home on postoperative day four. The recipient developed a hemolytic reaction following a blood transfusion, resulting in renal failure. The recipient subsequently died on the sixth postoperative day during a hemodialysis session. The following year marked the first successful living donor transplant when a 15-month-old child with biliary atresia received his mother's left lateral segment.[49] Four years later, living donor transplantation was reported using right lobe grafts, thus ushering in the modern era of adult-to-adult living donor liver transplantation (A2ALL).[50] Indeed the advantages of living donation include its elective nature, the ability to control the timing of transplantation relative to the recipient's disease severity, and minimization of cold ischemia time for the allograft.

Living Donor: Preoperative Evaluation and Planning

The inherent risk associated with major hepatic surgery in the setting of a healthy donor poses a formidable challenge even in the most experienced of hands. Once blood type compatibility is ascertained, the potential living donor undergoes a battery of tests to determine medical, psychosocial, and anatomic suitability. Formal consultation with the surgeon to better understand liver donation, as well as the attendant risks and benefits, is undertaken, and a donor advocate is appointed. Donors who choose to proceed undergo radiological imaging to assess their suitability for donation. Once the potential donor is deemed suitable based upon evaluation of his or her liver anatomy, the

next steps are a thorough medical and psychosocial evaluation. The complete donor evaluation is then subjected to multidisciplinary review before proceeding to transplant.[51-53]

Although some centers begin with an ultrasound with Doppler examination as an initial screening modality, the organ-specific evaluation for liver donation is largely based upon either a helical multiphase CT examination or MRI, both of which delineate parenchymal quality and vascular anatomy. The configuration of the biliary tree is typically visualized by either CT or MR cholangiography. Calculation of graft and whole liver volume is done to ensure appropriate donor graft and remnant liver volumes.[54-56] Transplant centers differ in their requirement for routine versus selective predonation liver biopsy. It has been shown that the procedure can be performed with minimal morbidity.[57] As an example, one set of criteria for a selective approach requires a biopsy for any potential donor with a body mass index (BMI) greater than 28, a history of substance abuse, a family history of immune-mediated liver disease, or any abnormal liver test or imaging study.[57] These criteria necessitated a biopsy for 22% of potential donors and, the authors would contend, allowed for a zero incidence of preventable aborted donor hepatectomies.[57]

For A2ALL, the right liver lobe (segments 5 to 8) is most often procured, accounting for approximately 60% of the donor's liver volume. For an adult-to-child liver transplant, the left lateral segment (segments 2 and 3) is most often procured, accounting for 20% of the donor's liver (see **Fig. 48-2**). Historically, the left lobe (segments 1 to 4), accounting for 35% to 40% of the donor's liver, has been used to achieve transplantation for older children. There is, however, a concerted effort to increase the use and the success of left lobes for adult living donor transplantation because the left lobe, compared with right lobe donor hepatectomy, is associated with lower morbidity for the donor. The size of a liver graft is estimated as a volume, but measured by weight. Functionally meaningful assessment of graft size takes the recipient into account, as exemplified by graft-to-recipient body weight ratio (GBWR) or graft volume to standard liver volume (GV/SV) ratio. The minimum acceptable GBWR is 0.8%, which corresponds to a GV/SV of 40%. Thus the canonical 70-kg recipient should receive a 560-g donor liver graft. The minimum graft size guidelines have been established to minimize the risk of small-for-size syndrome (SFSS).[58] SFSS is defined as a graft size smaller than the liver volume required for the intended recipient, and is manifested as graft dysfunction or nonfunction during the first postoperative week that is not attributable to other causes (i.e., rejection, infection, vascular complications).[59] Following reperfusion of a SFS graft, a state of hyperperfusion of the liver allograft ensues, which leads to paradoxical ischemic changes within the allograft. The hyperdynamic portal flow, and resultant liver injury, is clinically manifested usually within the first week following transplantation, along with encephalopathy and/or ascites and a laboratory profile of persistent coagulopathy and worsening hyperbilirubinemia. Liver biopsies demonstrate periportal sinusoidal endothelial denudation with focal hemorrhage into the portal tract and periportal hepatic parenchyma, as well as areas of ischemic cholangitis and parenchymal infarction.[60] It is, however, becoming clearer that while smaller grafts may be more vulnerable to SFSS, many recipient and transplant factors interplay to determine the graft outcome. Current strategies aimed at mitigating SFSS focus on reducing portal pressures through creation of portosystemic shunts, with or without splenectomy, at the time of liver transplantation.[61]

Final preparations for donor hepatectomy includes preoperative donation of autologous blood to minimize the small risk of infection associated with allogeneic blood transfusion. Intraoperatively, blood salvage and acute isovolemic hemodilution are routinely used. Hemodilution is achieved by removing two to four units of whole blood after the induction of anesthetic, preserving the blood in citrate phosphate dextrose storage bags, and using crystalloid and colloid infusions for replacement of the intravascular volume. Acute isovolemic hemodilution has been demonstrated to be safe and effective in limiting the use of banked blood in living donor right hepatectomies.[62]

Living Donor: Hepatectomy

Although a left lateral segmentectomy allograft can be procured through an upper midline incision, a right hepatic lobectomy requires either a unilateral or bilateral subcostal incision with a midline extension. The portion of the liver to be procured is freed of its ligamentous attachments. Dissection of the suprahepatic inferior vena cava (IVC) is performed to isolate the graft's hepatic venous outflow. A cholecystectomy is typically performed, followed by an intraoperative cholangiogram via the cystic duct to visualize the biliary anatomy. Hilar dissection is performed to identify and isolate the hepatic artery, portal vein, and bile duct for the planned donor graft. Temporary occlusion of the isolated hepatic artery and portal vein can be done to delineate the appropriate plane of parenchymal transection. To minimize blood loss and optimize hemostasis, parenchymal transection is often performed under reduced central venous pressures and with transient interruption of blood flow as needed. Intraoperative ultrasound can serve as a useful adjunct during the parenchymal transection to identify large tributaries of the portal and hepatic venous system. Complete parenchymal transection leaves the graft attached only by its biliary and vascular structures (**Figs. 48-3 and 48-4**). The bile duct to the graft is sharply divided and the resulting stump is oversewn with extreme care to prevent narrowing the donor's common hepatic duct. Intravenous heparin is administered, vascular clamps are applied, vessels are sequentially divided (hepatic artery, then portal vein, then hepatic vein), and the graft is immediately flushed with several liters of preservation solution to remove donor blood and to achieve rapid cooling. To minimize ischemia time, coordination between the donor and recipient teams helps to ensure that the recipient hepatectomy is completed by the time the donor liver graft is available for transplantation. For the living donor, the immediate postdonation time period is focused on ensuring hemodynamic stability, lack of hemorrhage, and preservation of normal liver function. Transient rises in INR or bilirubin are often seen in the postoperative period, and should be followed until they return to normal. Due to the rapid regeneration of liver volume, aggressive phosphate repletion is of paramount importance in the living donor.[63]

The safety of the living donor remains of utmost importance. The worldwide donor death rate has been estimated to range from 0.15% to 0.20%. In a 2006 report, 13 of the 19 donor deaths (as well as 1 donor left in a chronic vegetative state) were directly attributed to the donors' surgery. Two deaths were considered possibly related to the donors' surgery, and four were considered unlikely to have resulted from the

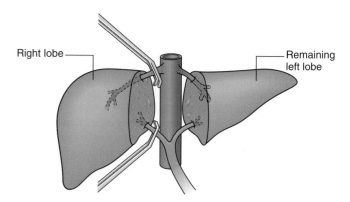

Fig. 48-3 The segmental anatomy that allows for split or partial liver transplantation, also allows for living donor liver transplantation. A right hepatectomy is depicted in the figure. In a living donation, parenchymal transection proceeds before the division of the vascular structures to minimize ischemia in the allograft.

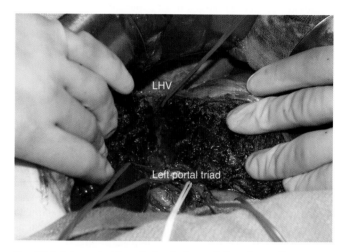

Fig. 48-4 **Intraoperative photo during a living donor liver transplant.** The left hepatic vein *(LHV)* and the left-sided portal structures have been isolated, but not yet divided. The liver parenchyma has been divided in anticipation of procurement of the left lateral segment for donation.

donors' surgery. Twelve patients involved right lobe donation, two involved left lateral segment donation, and six involved donation of an unknown lobe.[64] Morbidity following liver donation can be significant, especially for right lobe donors. As many as two thirds of right lobe donors suffer complications.[51,65] Results from the nine A2ALL centers demonstrated an overall complication rate of 38% for the study period of 1998-2003.[66] Of the 393 patients who underwent donation at the A2ALL centers, 148 suffered 220 complications. Twelve donors experienced an aborted hepatectomy based on intraoperative findings. Among successful donors, 82 (21%) experienced a single complication, 40 (10.2%) experienced two complications, 16 (4.1%) experienced three complications, and 10 (2.6%) experienced four to seven complications. All complications were graded according to the Clavien classification,[67] in which grade I complications are considered minor with complete recovery, grade II complications are potentially life threatening but do not have any lasting disability, grade III complications have lasting functional disability, and grade IV complications result in the need for transplantation or death. Of the 220 complications in the A2ALL experience, 48% were classified as grade I, 47% were grade II, 4% were grade III, and 1% were grade IV. The most common postoperative complications were infections (12.5%), biliary leak (persistent leak beyond postoperative day 7) (9.2%), and incisional hernia (5.6%). Additional complications included pleural effusion requiring intervention (5%), neurapraxia (4%), reexploration (3%), wound infections (3%), and intraabdominal abscess (2%). Of the donors who experienced grade IV complications, one patient died from a biliary leak that led to pancreatitis and multisystem organ failure during the initial hospitalization, whereas the other two donors died from drug overdose and suicide more than a year after donation. The average length of hospital stay following donation surgery was 7 days; however, 13% of donors required hospital readmission, and 4% required two to five readmissions.

Given the morbidity associated with the open operation for a living liver donor, there have been recent reports of laparoscopic-assisted donor hepatectomies.[68-70] Procurement of the left lateral lobe can be performed with a discrete suprapubic incision made for removal of the donor allograft. The larger right lobe can be mobilized laparoscopically; however, subsequent parenchymal, biliary, and vessel transection is often performed through a small upper midline incision, which also serves as the site of donor allograft removal.

Living Donor: Impact on the Waiting List

Based on Organ Procurement and Transplantation Network (OPTN) data, 1541 wait-listed candidates died without the benefit of liver transplantation in 2008. Of the 6319 adult and pediatric liver transplants performed in 2008, only 249 (4%) were from living donors. At the peak of living donor liver transplantation in 2001, before the publicized report of a donor death,[71] 524 living donor transplants were performed. Living donation combined with the use of split liver transplantation currently falls short in supplying the increased demands of the adult end-stage liver disease population.

Liver Transplantation: The Recipient Operation

Once a suitable organ has been accepted for a candidate, he or she is brought into the hospital, unless already hospitalized. The liver procurement team directly communicates with the accepting surgeon regarding the suitability of the liver allograft and the anticipated time of organ availability to optimally schedule the recipient transplant procedure, and thereby minimize cold ischemic time. The candidate is brought to the operating room and general anesthesia is induced. Coagulopathy, if severe, is corrected before placement of invasive monitoring and resuscitation lines. Intravenous antibiotics are then administered in preparation for the surgical incision, followed by induction immunosuppression.

Recipient Hepatectomy

Although varying incisions can be employed for entry into the abdominal cavity depending on the recipient's body habitus, the most common is a bilateral subcostal incision with a midline extension to the xiphoid process (**Fig. 48-5**). Ascites, if present, is removed, and inspection to rule out surgical contraindications to transplantation, such as extrahepatic malignancy or infection, is performed. The recipient hepatectomy is then begun by division of the falciform ligament and subsequently mobilization of the suspensory ligaments of the liver. The suprahepatic and infrahepatic IVC are circumferentially exposed. The common bile duct is identified and divided, as are the left and right hepatic arteries, and finally the portal vein is exposed. There are two common methods of recipient hepatectomy that then determine the reconstruction strategy. The liver can be removed with the intrahepatic segment of the recipient's vena cava necessitating subsequent use of the donor intrahepatic IVC (caval interposition technique), or alternatively the recipient vena cava can be left in situ and the donor liver placed onto the recipient IVC (piggyback technique).[72-74]

There are clearly pros and cons for each caval reconstruction technique. For the caval interposition technique, once the liver has been fully mobilized, clamps are placed on the portal

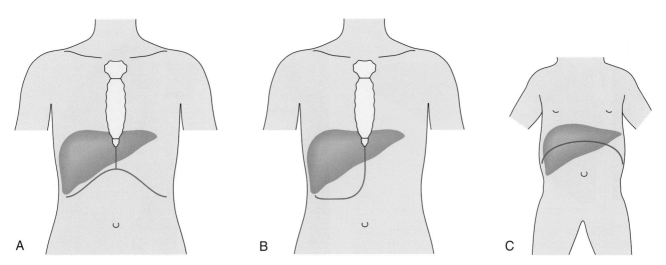

Fig. 48-5 Various incisions can be employed for liver transplantation. **A,** Bilateral subcostal incision with a midline extension to the xiphoid process; **B,** right subcostal incision; and **C,** bilateral subcostal incision (commonly used in pediatric recipients).

vein and the suprahepatic and infrahepatic IVC. These structures are divided and the liver explanted (**Fig. 48-6**). The caval interposition technique requires less dissection than the piggyback technique, and thus expedites the hepatectomy. However, clamping of the IVC results in major fluid and hemodynamic shifts, and necessitates massive volume loading in preparation for the precipitous loss of systemic venous return from below the diaphragm. In the piggyback technique, which is always used for living donor liver transplantation, the numerous small and fragile retrohepatic tributaries between the IVC and the caudate and right lobes of the liver must be meticulously divided and the hepatic veins isolated. A clamp is placed on the portal vein, as well as the hepatic veins as they enter the vena cava to allow for uninterrupted systemic vena caval venous return (**Fig. 48-7**). These vessels are divided and the liver is explanted (**Fig. 48-8**).

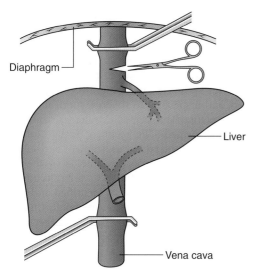

Fig. 48-6 Caval interposition technique of liver transplantation requires removal of the recipient IVC during recipient hepatectomy via incision of the suprahepatic and infrahepatic IVC. This results in subsequent loss of systemic subdiaphragmatic venous return during the anhepatic phase.

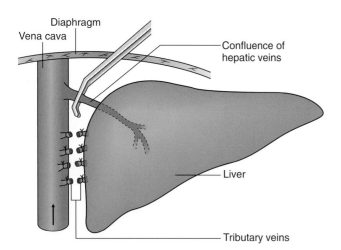

Fig. 48-7 Piggyback technique of liver transplantation allows for continued subdiaphragmatic systemic venous return by preservation of the recipient IVC. This technique is more time-consuming because it requires a meticulous dissection of the right lobe of the liver off of the IVC. The liver is separated from the IVC at the confluence of the hepatic veins.

For those patients undergoing the caval interposition technique, venovenous bypass (VVB) remains an option to improve intraoperative hemodynamics by allowing for continuation of systemic venous return, with or without continuation of portal venous return as well. For VVB, cannulation of the femoral and/or portal vein is performed, with flow of the systemic and/or splanchnic venous circulation through a third return cannula placed in the axillary, subclavian, or jugular vein (**Fig. 48-9**). The femoral cannula and the return cannula can be placed under direct visualization or percutaneously. Ultrasound guidance should be employed to limit the morbidity associated with percutaneous placement.[75] The VVB technique avoids the portal venous congestion associated with clamping and can help maintain hemodynamic stability during the anhepatic phase. However, VVB lengthens operative time and incurs complications, including: embolism, hemorrhage, hematoma/lymphocele formation, injury to arteries and nerves during cannulation, and fibrinolysis.[75,76] VVB has been demonstrated to maintain renal perfusion pressure during the anhepatic phase, avoiding the venous hypertension within the native kidneys that occurs with caval clamping.[77] However, it remains to be determined whether the use of VVB alters the course of postoperative renal dysfunction often seen following liver transplantation.[78]

Venous, Arterial, and Biliary Anastomoses

Following the recipient hepatectomy, the preservation solution within the donor allograft is flushed out, and the donor liver is brought to the operative field for implantation. Caval reconstruction is done first. The caval interposition technique requires two end-to-end anastomoses between the donor and recipient suprahepatic and infrahepatic cava (**Fig. 48-10**). The piggyback technique requires only a single anastomosis between the donor's suprahepatic cava and the confluence of recipient's hepatic veins. In this technique, to ensure a widely patent anastomosis, the recipient's confluence of hepatic veins is often enlarged by incising onto the anterior wall of the IVC.

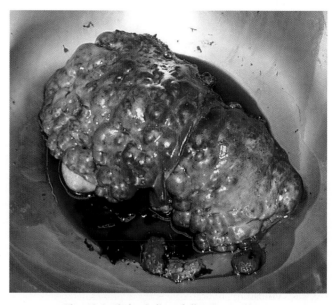

Fig. 48-8 Cirrhotic liver following explant.

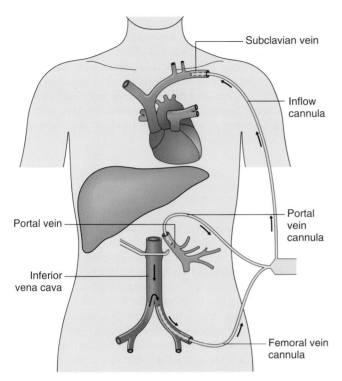

Fig. 48-9 Depiction of complete venovenous bypass during the anhepatic phase of liver transplantation. Systemic venous return via the femoral vein, and splanchnic venous return via the portal vein, are bypassed to the subclavian, axillary, or internal jugular vein. Partial bypass includes return of systemic venous blood alone (not shown).

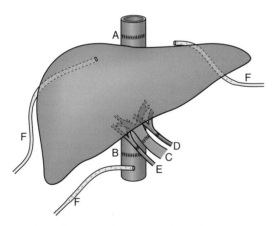

Fig. 48-10 Completion of liver transplantation using the caval interposition technique. The donor suprahepatic IVC *(A)* infrahepatic IVC, *(B)* portal vein, *(C)* hepatic artery, *(D)*, and bile duct *(E)* are anastomosed to the respective recipient counterpart. Drains are left in the subdiaphragmatic space and adjacent to the biliary anastomosis *(F)*.

The donor's infrahepatic vena cava is then stapled or oversewn. For a living donor allograft, the donor hepatic vein is sewn to the recipient's hepatic vein, or directly onto the vena cava. Once the caval anastomosis is complete, the donor and recipient portal veins are connected, and the liver is reperfused with venous blood. Preoperative portal vein thrombosis occurs commonly in patients with end-stage liver disease. Eversion thromboendovenectomy is frequently used to restore

adequate inflow for standard recipient-to-donor portal venous anastomosis. If adequate thromboendovenectomy cannot be achieved, a bypass graft can be constructed from the mesenteric circulation to the donor portal vein, most frequently using the donor iliac vein. In the event of extensive thrombosis of the portal system involving the portal, splenic, and mesenteric veins, the liver allograft's portal inflow can be constructed from the systemic circulation.[79,80]

After venous reperfusion, attention is then turned toward arterial reconstruction where the donor hepatic artery is anastomosed to the recipient's hepatic artery. Severe disease within the recipient's native arterial system may require implantation of the donor hepatic artery into an alternative site, such as the supraceliac or infrarenal aorta, to achieve sufficient arterial inflow. Variations in donor anatomy, particularly an accessory or replaced right hepatic artery emanating from the superior mesenteric artery, may necessitate back table reconstruction to enable a single in situ anastomosis.

A cholecystectomy is performed and then biliary reconstruction is typically done using one of two methods. The first is a direct anastomosis between the donor and recipient common bile ducts (choledochocholedochostomy), with or without a T-tube. The alternative is to directly implant the donor bile duct into a loop of jejunum (choledochojejunostomy), with or without a stent. Choledochojejunostomy is the preferred reconstruction method for recipients with large duct disease, such as primary sclerosing cholangitis or Caroli disease.[81] Often during biliary reconstruction, one can observe production of bile by the functioning allograft. In preparation for closing the abdomen, hemostasis is ensured, the abdomen is irrigated with antibiotic-containing solution, and closed suction drains are placed.

Post-Reperfusion Syndrome

Post-reperfusion syndrome of the liver is characterized by hemodynamic instability of variable magnitude following venous reperfusion. The delivery of oxygenated blood to a liver that has undergone cold preservation generates the massive release of free radicals, endotoxin, and inflammatory cytokines, which precipitously reduces systemic vascular resistance resulting in hypotension. Moreover, the influx of lactic acid following the unclamping of the portal circulation further contributes to hemodynamic instability. Post-reperfusion syndrome was initially defined as a decrease in the mean arterial pressure to less than 70% of the baseline value for at least 1 minute, and occurring within 5 minutes of reperfusion. By this definition, this syndrome was noted to occur in up to 30% of liver transplant recipients; however, all patients exhibited some degree of hemodynamic instability intraoperatively.[82] Further studies have led to a stratification of the varying degrees of post-reperfusion syndrome, and thus classification of a mild and a significant form.[83] Again, all patients demonstrated some degree of instability. The mild form was characterized by a decrease in blood pressure and/or heart rate less than 30% of the anhepatic levels and of short-lived duration (5 minutes). The mild form also responded to calcium chloride (1 g intravenously) and/or epinephrine intravenous boluses (100 µg) without requiring the continuous infusion of vasopressor agents. The significant form of post-reperfusion syndrome was defined as persistent hypotension (a decrease >30% of the anhepatic level), asystole, or hemodynamically significant arrhythmias. Recipients who required vasopressor infusion during the intraoperative period, or who had prolonged or recurrent fibrinolysis requiring antifibrinolytic agents, were considered to have significant post-reperfusion syndrome as well. Although there was no significant difference between the two groups in survival rates at 3 years, those with significant post-reperfusion syndrome (55% of the cohort) had a higher incidence of primary graft nonfunction requiring retransplantation, and had longer hospital and ICU stays, as well as a longer duration of mechanical ventilation. Supportive care is the mainstay of therapy for post-reperfusion syndrome because investigation into pharmacologic preconditioning regimens and variations on surgical reperfusion techniques to limit ischemia/reperfusion injury have yet to demonstrate efficacy.

Postoperative Complications of Liver Transplantation

Assessment of Early Allograft Function

Primary nonfunction (PNF) is an uncommon occurrence following liver transplantation, occurring in 2% to 6% of transplants.[84] The actual causes of immediate graft failure are incompletely understood. However, the common final pathway of massive hepatocyte injury and decreased regenerative activity create immediate danger in the early posttransplant period. Risk factors associated with PNF are predominantly related to the donor and include increased donor age, prolonged length of stay in the intensive care unit, uncorrected hypernatremia, hepatic steatosis, DCD status, and prolonged cold preservation times.[85-89]

PNF is manifested clinically by elevated liver enzymes, coagulopathy, unremitting acidosis, encephalopathy, hemodynamic instability, and multiorgan system failure. Retransplantation is the procedure of choice for this surgical emergency. Although retransplantation for PNF is traditionally thought to have lower rates of patient survival,[90] more recent data has demonstrated that retransplantation for PNF resulted in patient survival rates of 66% at 1 year, 60% at 5 years, and 48% at 10 years after transplantation. These outcomes were similar to those observed in recipients retransplanted for causes other than PNF.[84]

Postoperative Bleeding

The postoperative liver transplant recipient is at high risk for bleeding for multiple reasons. First, the cirrhotic enters the operating room with portal hypertension, coagulopathy, and thrombocytopenia. Next, he or she undergoes an extensive dissection of the upper abdomen and retroperitoneum to explant the native liver, leaving a sizable area of raw surfaces. The transplant necessitates multiple vascular anastomoses, and on full reperfusion the ischemia/reperfusion injury activates fibrinolysis. Adequate function of the new allograft, along with appropriate correction of acidosis, coagulopathy, thrombocytopenia, and avoidance of hypothermia, optimizes medical hemostasis. Following transplantation, evidence of brisk blood loss, hemodynamic instability, and/or abdominal

compartment syndrome are indications for an emergent return to the operating room for reexploration. In addition, a steady and persistent need for red cell transfusions, particularly after correction of coagulation parameters, should also prompt consideration of reexploration. The goals of reexploration are a thorough reinspection for surgically correctable sources of bleeding, and evacuation of clot that can provide an ongoing stimulus for fibrinolysis and serve as a nidus for future infection.

Technical Complications: Vascular

Although complications can involve any of the vascular anastomoses, hepatic artery thrombosis (HAT) and portal vein thrombosis (PVT) remain the most common vascular complications following liver transplantation.[91] Whereas PVT complicates 3% to 7% of liver transplants, HAT is reported to complicate 4% to 15% of liver transplants. The latter is more frequent following pediatric liver transplantation, a direct consequence of the smaller diameter of the involved vessels. Other risk factors predisposing to HAT include inadequate inflow secondary to proximal stenosis, use of bypass grafts, arterial intima trauma or injury, and anomalous anatomy necessitating complex back table arterial reconstruction procedures.

The presentation of HAT is extremely varied. At one extreme, HAT may have dramatic elevations of aminotransferases indicating fulminant acute allograft ischemia and/or infarction, particularly if it occurs in the early posttransplantation period. At the other extreme, HAT may be clinically silent and an incidental finding on radiographic assessment of the allograft, particularly if it occurs late (more than 6 months) after transplantation. Both the early and late form of HAT often result in ischemia of the biliary tree. In the early form of HAT, this can manifest as necrosis with an associated biliary leak and/or intrahepatic abscess formation. In the late form of HAT, biliary ischemia often results in diffuse stricturing and dilation of the biliary tree with or without intrahepatic abscess formation. Diagnosis of HAT is suggested when duplex ultrasound cannot identify flow in the hepatic artery, and should be confirmed by visceral angiography. The definitive and most common treatment for early HAT is retransplantation. Additional therapies for early HAT include surgical exploration with thrombectomy or revision of the hepatic artery anastomosis, and catheter-based thrombolysis or systemic anticoagulation. Intervention for late presentations of HAT include retransplantation, arterial stent placement, hepatic resection of affected segments, or nonoperative management with biliary drainage.[92]

Factors predisposing to PVT include pretransplant PVT, small portal vein size, portal vein redundancy, prior splenectomy, and reconstructions involving a graft or conduit. PVT can have elevated aminotransferases with or without acute allograft dysfunction, or with clinical symptoms of portal hypertension, such as gastrointestinal bleeding or new-onset ascites. Diagnosis of PVT is typically suggested by duplex ultrasound examination and confirmed on CT or magnetic resonance venography. Treatment of portal vein thrombosis includes open surgical thrombectomy with or without anastomotic revision, systemic anticoagulation, catheter-directed thrombolysis, portosystemic shunt creation, or retransplantation.

In a large single center study review from UCLA, which included 4234 liver transplants from 1984 to 2007, HAT occurred in 5% of cases. HAT reduced overall patient and graft survival rates in this study; however, the former did not reach statistical significance.[91] In the same study, PVT occurred less often than HAT, affecting 2% or fewer of deceased donor liver transplants.[91] However, PVT significantly reduced both graft and patient survival rates.[91]

Hepatic vein stenosis is rare, with a reported frequency of 2%. There is an increased incidence following the piggyback technique compared with the caval replacement technique.[93] Although the outflow obstruction can be caused by a technical error during reconstruction, in living transplant recipients the rapid hypertrophy of the partial liver graft may cause twisting or external compression of the hepatic vein, resulting in outflow obstruction.[94] Patients commonly present months after transplantation with symptoms ranging from new-onset ascites, with or without lower extremity edema, variceal bleeding, renal insufficiency, or rising liver test values. Diagnosis can be suggested by conventional imaging modalities, including US with Doppler, CT scan, or MRI. However, venography with pressure measurements is considered the gold standard and should be done as a confirmatory test. A gradient greater than 10 mm Hg between the hepatic vein and the right atrium is commonly used to determine significance and necessity for intervention.[95,96] Percutaneous intervention consisting of balloon angioplasty, with or without stent placement, offers an 80% success rate,[96] although repetitive intervention may be required for long-term success. Surgical intervention or retransplantation should be reserved for cases refractory to percutaneous intervention.

Technical Complications: Biliary

Biliary complications occur more commonly than vascular complications following liver transplantation, occurring in 10% to 30% of whole-organ liver recipients, and can be classified as either leaks or strictures.[97] Partial liver transplants, such as reduced, split, or living donor grafts, are associated with an increased risk of biliary complications with a reported incidence of 10% to 60%. The majority of biliary complications occur within the first 6 months following transplantation. The signs and symptoms are often nonspecific but can include abdominal pain or elevated liver test results. Ultrasonography is the first-line investigation of choice. Because of the frequent association of biliary complications with the presence of hepatic artery thrombosis or stenosis, concomitant Doppler examination is recommended.

Biliary leaks occur less frequently than biliary strictures, accounting for a third of all biliary complications, and typically occur early in the posttransplant period. In recipients of DDLT, leaks most often occur at the site of biliary anastomosis and can be related to technical errors in reconstruction, or ischemic necrosis of the donor common bile duct because of disruption of the ductal blood supply. In recipients of living donor allografts, or deceased donor split liver transplants, bile can leak from the cut surface of the hepatic parenchyma, in addition to the anastomotic site. Diagnosis can be suggested by radiographic imaging, although demonstration of the leak through endoscopic retrograde cholangiopancreatography (ERCP), or percutaneous transhepatic cholangiogram (PTC) in the setting of choledochojejunostomy, is essential. These diagnostic studies can frequently be combined with a therapeutic intervention, including sphincterotomy

and/or stent placement, to allow for decompression of the biliary system and spontaneous closure of the biliary fistula. Any biliomas resulting from the bile leak should be managed with drainage. Large biliary fistulas in the early postoperative period may require operative intervention with revision of the biliary anastomosis. Healing of a nonoperatively managed biliary fistula may result in late stricture formation and thus may necessitate future surgical biliary revision.

Biliary strictures account for two thirds of biliary complications following liver transplantation, often with elevated liver values and/or abdominal pain. Biliary obstruction with ascending cholangitis or intrahepatic abscess formation remains a serious complication. Whereas early anastomotic stricture is usually related to errors in the surgical technique, late biliary stricture formation is often at the level of the anastomosis and secondary to ischemia. Ultrasound examination in liver transplant recipients has a low sensitivity (50%) in establishing a diagnosis of biliary stricture given the frequent lack of ductal dilation.[98] Liver allograft biopsies often provide the first clue if histologic findings of biliary obstruction and/or chronic cholangitis are present.[97] ERCP, or PTC in the case of choledochojejunostomy, is again essential to diagnose and treat a biliary stricture. The endoscopic approach has yielded success rates of 62% for deceased donor recipients, and 75% for living donor recipients.[99] Frequently, more than one endoscopic procedure is required for resolution of the biliary obstruction. Recipients with anastomotic reconstruction using choledochojejunostomy require percutaneous transhepatic biliary drainage to accomplish biliary decompression, followed by transhepatic dilation and stent placement (**Fig. 48-11**). Rare but serious complications associated with the transhepatic route include hemobilia, hepatic artery pseudoaneurysm formation, arterio-portal fistula creation, and portal vein thrombosis.[100] Failure of nonsurgical therapies necessitates operative intervention, which is more common for late compared with early anastomotic strictures. Operative intervention entails surgical excision of the stricture, with conversion of the choledochocholedochostomy to a choledochojejunostomy. In cases of a preexisting choledochojejunostomy, revision is undertaken.

Although anastomotic strictures are the most frequent type of biliary stricture in the liver transplant recipient, diffuse intrahepatic strictures are far more problematic. Generalized ischemia of the entire biliary tree is believed to be the etiologic agent leading to the diffuse stricture disease. The latter occurs in hepatic artery thrombosis, prolonged cold preservation times, or DCD allografts. Diffuse intrahepatic strictures are associated with microscopic or macroscopic abscesses, and commonly recurrent biliary sepsis.[101] Diffuse strictures are generally not amenable to conventional endoscopic or percutaneous therapy.[102] Hepatic resection is occasionally curative, although retransplantation is typically the only true definitive treatment.

DDLT is associated with a 15% to 25% biliary stricture rate,[103] whereas LDLT has a significantly higher incidence of biliary complications (30%).[104] It remains debatable as to whether the type of biliary reconstruction is an independent predictor of subsequent stricture. Retrospective reviews have demonstrated a lower stricture rate in patients undergoing choledochojejunostomy (8.3% for Roux-en-Y choledochojejunostomy vs. 26.6% for duct-to-duct choledochocholedochostomy reconstruction). However, the duct-to-duct

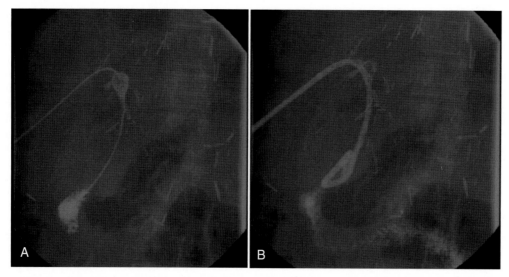

Fig. 48-11 Percutaneous transhepatic management of a choledochojejunostomy anastomotic stricture in a recipient of a living donor liver transplant. A transhepatic wire is placed into the biliary tree under fluoroscopic guidance across the stricture, with contrast opacification of the jejunum confirming passage across the anastomotic stricture (**A**). A transhepatic drain is left in the biliary tree across the stricture, with the tip of the drain in the jejunal roux limb (**B**).

anastomosis was shown to have a significantly lower incidence of leakage (4.7% for choledochocholedochostomy vs. 12.4% for choledochojejunostomy).[105] Additional studies, however, have shown no difference in the stricture rate between the two reconstruction approaches.[99]

Current Outcomes of Liver Transplantation

In 2007 the median time to liver transplantation was 361 days, with 6489 liver transplants performed: 96% from deceased donors and 4% from living donors. Of the liver transplants performed, 7.8% were retransplants. At the end of 2007, 12,213 patients remained on the liver transplant waitlist.[13] UNOS data continue to demonstrate excellent patient and graft survival rates. Adjusted patient survival rates for DDLT were 87%, 73%, and 59% at 1, 5, and 10 years, respectively. Adjusted patient survival rates for LDLT demonstrated improved results when compared with DDLT, with 92%, 78%, and 71% survival rates at 1, 5, and 10 years, respectively. Graft survival rates for DDLT were 82%, 68%, and 53% at 1, 5, and 10 years, respectively, whereas LDLT graft survival rates were 85%, 71%, and 62% at 1, 5, and 10 years, respectively.[13] The improved results seen in recipients of LDLT has been attributed to the shorter duration of time spent on the waiting list, and transplantation at a lower MELD score, when compared with DDLT recipients.[106]

Age exerts a substantial effect on posttransplant outcomes. At the extremes, the infant (<1 year of age) and elderly (>65 years of age) recipients suffer the lowest adjusted 1-year patient survival rates following DDLT. Older adults (>50 years of age) demonstrated decreased survival rates when compared with younger adults. Compared to female recipients, males enjoyed a significant, albeit small, improvement in survival rates at 1 year posttransplantation (88% for men vs. 86% for women), but this advantage did not persist over time after

transplantation. Although short-term posttransplant survival did not differ significantly according to recipient race, African American recipients demonstrated the lowest 5-year patient survival rates at 66%, compared with 77% for Asians and 75% for Hispanics, a difference that persisted for 10 years after transplantation. Finally, graft origin and type exert a sizable impact on posttransplant outcomes. Livers procured from DCD compared with brain dead donors, and partial grafts compared with whole grafts, are extremely potent negative risk factors for patient and graft survival.[13]

Conclusion

With advances in surgical technique, immunosuppression, and critical care, liver transplantation has become the management of choice for patients with acute and chronic liver failure, metabolic diseases with their primary defect residing in the liver, and unresectable primary liver tumors without evidence of extrahepatic spread. Advances in immunosuppression regimens have improved both graft and patient survival rates. However, side effects associated with chronic immunosuppression continue to cause substantial long-term morbidity and mortality. Innovative techniques such as split-liver and living donor liver transplantation, as well as donor pool expansion with DCD and extended-criteria donors, have been pursued in response to the severe shortage of donor organs. Indeed, it is the shortage of donor organs and the need for chronic immunosuppression that represent the remaining formidable obstacles to the greater application and long-term success of liver transplantation.

Key References

A definition of irreversible coma: report of the ad hoc committee of the Harvard Medical School to examine the definition of brain death. JAMA 1968;205:337–340. (Ref.31)

Abt PL, et al. Survival following liver transplantation from non-heart-beating donors. Ann Surg 2004;239:87–92. (Ref.37)

Aggarwal S, et al. Postreperfusion syndrome: hypotension after reperfusion of the transplanted liver. J Crit Care 1993;8:154–160. (Ref.82)

Arcari M, et al. An investigation into the risk of air embolus during veno-venous bypass in orthotopic liver transplantation. Transplantation 1999;68:150–152. (Ref.76)

Baker T, et al. Laparoscopy-assisted and open living donor right hepatectomy: a comparative study of outcomes. Surgery 2009;146:817–825. (Ref.70)

Barr ML, et al. A report of the Vancouver forum on the care of the live organ donor: lung, liver, pancreas, and intestine data and medical guidelines. Transplantation 2006;81:1373–1385. (Ref.52)

Belghiti J, et al. A new technique of side to side caval anastomosis during orthotopic hepatic transplantation without inferior vena caval occlusion. Surg Gynecol Obstet 1992;175:270–272. (Ref.73)

Berg CL, et al. Improvement in survival associated with adult-to-adult living donor liver transplantation. Gastroenterology 2007;133:1806–1813. (Ref.106)

Berg CL, et al. Liver and intestine transplantation in the United States 1998-2007. Am J Transplant 2009;9(4 Pt 2):907–931. (Ref.13)

Bernat JL. Are organ donors after cardiac death really dead? J Clin Ethics 2006; 17:122–132. (Ref.32)

Bernat JL. The boundaries of organ donation after circulatory death. N Engl J Med 2008;359:669–671. (Ref.34)

Bharat A, et al. Pre-liver transplantation locoregional adjuvant therapy for hepatocellular carcinoma as a strategy to improve longterm survival. J Am Coll Surg 2006;203:411–420. (Ref.28)

Bismuth H, Houssin D. Reduced-sized orthotopic liver graft in hepatic transplantation in children. Surgery 1984;95:367–370. (Ref.41)

Budd JM, et al. Morbidity and mortality associated with large-bore percutaneous venovenous bypass cannulation for 312 orthotopic liver transplantations. Liver Transpl 2001;7:359–362. (Ref.75)

Buell JF, et al. Long-term venous complications after full-size and segmental pediatric liver transplantation. Ann Surg 2002;236:658–666. (Ref.96)

Busuttil RW, et al. Analysis of long-term outcomes of 3200 liver transplantations over two decades: a single-center experience. Ann Surg 2005;241:905–916. (Ref.103)

Calne R. Recollections from the laboratory to the clinic. In: Terasaki PI, editor. History of transplantation: thirty-five recollections. Los Angeles: UCLA Tissue Typing Laboratory, 1991: 227–243. (Ref.10)

Caruso S, et al. Imaging in liver transplantation. World J Gastroenterol 2009;15: 675–683. (Ref.56)

Chan SC, et al. Resurgence of biliary cast syndrome. Liver Transpl 2005;11: 242–243. (Ref.101)

Cherqui D, et al. Liver transplantation with preservation of portacaval flow: comparison with the conventional technique. Ann Chir 1994;48:980–985. (Ref.74)

Cherqui D, et al. Laparoscopic living donor hepatectomy for liver transplantation in children. Lancet 2002;359:392–396. (Ref.68)

Child CG, Turcotte JG. Surgery and portal hypertension. In: Child CG, editor. The liver and portal hypertension. Philadelphia: WB Saunders, 1964: 50–64. (Ref.19)

Cholongitas E, et al. Risk factors for recurrence of primary sclerosing cholangitis after liver transplantation. Liver Transpl 2008;14:138–143. (Ref.81)

Clavien PA, et al. Definition and classification of negative outcomes in solid organ transplantation: application in liver transplantation. Ann Surg 1994;220: 109–120. (Ref.67)

Concejero A, et al. Donor graft outflow venoplasty in living donor liver transplantation. Liver Transpl 2006;12:264–268. (Ref.93)

Dahm F, Georgiev P, Clavien PA. Small-for-size syndrome after partial liver transplantation: definition, mechanisms of disease and clinical implications. Am J Transplant 2005;5:2605–2610. (Ref.59)

Demetris AJ, et al. Pathophysiologic observations and histopathologic recognition of the portal hyperperfusion or small-for-size syndrome. Am J Surg Pathol 2006;30:986–993. (Ref.60)

Detre KM, et al. Influence of donor age on graft survival after liver transplantation—United Network for Organ Sharing Registry. Liver Transpl Surg 1995;1:311–319. (Ref.87)

Dick AA, et al. Liver transplantation at the extremes of the body mass index. Liver Transpl 2009;15:968–977. (Ref.16)

Duffy JP, et al. Vascular complications of orthotopic liver transplantation: experience in more than 4,200 patients. J Am Coll Surg 2009;208:896–903. (Ref.91)

Emond JC, et al. Functional analysis of grafts from living donors. Implications for the treatment of older recipients. Ann Surg 1996;224:544–552. (Ref.58)

Fan ST, et al. Biliary reconstruction and complications of right lobe live donor liver transplantation. Ann Surg 2002;236:676–683. (Ref.100)

Feng S, et al. Characteristics associated with liver graft failure: the concept of a donor risk index. Am J Transplant 2006;6:783–790. (Ref.38)

Fortner JG, et al. The case for and technique of heterotopic liver grafting. Transplant Proc 1979;11:269–275. (Ref.40)

Ghobrial RM, et al. A2ALL study group. Donor morbidity after living donation for liver transplantation. Gastroenterology 2008;135:468–476. (Ref.66)

Goss JA, et al. In situ splitting of the cadaveric liver for transplantation. Transplantation 1997;64:871–877. (Ref.46)

Grande L, et al. Effect of venovenous bypass on perioperative renal function in liver transplantation: results of a randomized, controlled trial. Hepatology 1996;23:1418–1428. (Ref.78)

Gunsar F, et al. Late hepatic artery thrombosis after orthotopic liver transplantation. Liver Transpl 2003;9:605–611. (Ref.92)

Hamilton DNH, Reid WA. Yu Yu Voronoy and the first human kidney allograft. Surg Gynecol Obstet 1984;159:289–294. (Ref.29)

Hilmi I, et al. The impact of postreperfusion syndrome on short-term patient and liver allograft outcome in patients undergoing orthotopic liver transplantation. Liver Transpl 2008;14:504–508. (Ref.83)

Ikegami T, et al. Current concept of small-for-size grafts in living donor liver transplantation. Surg Today 2008;38:971–982. (Ref.61)

Institute of Medicine, National Academy of Sciences. Non-heartbeating organ transplantation: practice and protocols. Washington, DC: National Academy Press, 2000. (Ref.35)

Kalayoglu M, et al. Extended preservation of the liver for clinical transplantation. Lancet 1988;19:617–619. (Ref.6)

Kasahara M, et al. Biliary reconstruction in right lobe living-donor liver transplantation: comparison of different techniques in 321 recipients. Ann Surg 2006;243:559–566. (Ref.105)

Kino T, et al. FFK506, a novel immunosuppressant isolated from a Streptomyces. I. Fermentation, isolation, and physico-chemical and biological characteristics. J Antibiot (Tokyo) 1987;40:1249–1255. (Ref.12)

Ko GY, et al. Endovascular treatment of hepatic venous outflow obstruction after living-donor liver transplantation. J Vasc Interv Radiol 2002;13:591–599. (Ref.95)

Koffron AJ, et al. Laparoscopic-assisted right lobe donor hepatectomy. Am J Transplant 2006;6:2522–2525. (Ref.69)

Lee HW, et al. Classification and prognosis of intrahepatic biliary stricture after liver transplantation. Liver Transpl 2007;13:1736–1742. (Ref.102)

Leonard J, et al. The impact of obesity on long-term outcomes in liver transplant recipients: results of the NIDDK liver transplant database. Am J Transplant 2008;8:667–672. (Ref.17)

Liu XL, et al. Treatment of hepatic venous outflow stenosis after living donor liver transplantation by insertion of an expandable metallic stent. Hepatobiliary Pancreat Dis Int 2009;8:424–427. (Ref.94)

Malinchoc M, et al. A model to predict poor survival in patients undergoing transjugular intrahepatic portosystemic shunts. Hepatology 2000;31:864–871. (Ref.21)

Marino IR, et al. Effect of donor age and sex on the outcome of liver transplantation. Hepatology 1995;22:1754–1762. (Ref.88)

Mazzaferro V, et al. Liver transplantation for the treatment of small hepatocellular carcinomas in patients with cirrhosis. N Engl J Med 1996;334:693–699. (Ref.24)

McDiarmid SV, Anand R, Lindblad AS, Principal Investigators and Institutions of the Studies of Pediatric Liver Transplantation (SPLIT) Research Group. Development of a pediatric end-stage liver disease score to predict poor outcome in children awaiting liver transplantation. Transplantation 2002;74: 173–181. (Ref.22)

Miller C, et al. Fulminant and fatal gas gangrene of the stomach in a healthy live liver donor. Liver Transpl 2004;10:1315–1319. (Ref.71)

Paskonis M, et al. Surgical strategies for liver transplantation in the case of portal vein thrombosis: current role of cavoportal hemitransposition and renoportal anastomosis. Clin Transplant 2006;20:551–562. (Ref.80)

Pichlmayr R, et al. Transplantation of a donor liver to 2 recipients (splitting transplantation): a new method in the further development of segmental liver transplantation. Langenbecks Arch Chir 1988;373:127–130. (Ref.42)

Pomfret EA, Feng S. Striving for perfection: evaluation of the right lobe live liver donor. Am J Transplant 2006;6:1755–1756. (Ref.53)

Pomfret EA, et al. Live donor adult liver transplantation using right lobe grafts: donor evaluation and surgical outcome. Arch Surg 2001;136:425–433. (Ref.51)

Pomposelli JJ, et al. Life-threatening hypophosphatemia after right hepatic lobectomy for live donor adult liver transplantation. Liver Transpl 2001;7: 637–642. (Ref.63)

Pugh RN, et al. Transection of the oesophagus for bleeding oesophageal varices. Br J Surg 1973;60:646–649. (Ref.20)

Radtke A, et al. Preoperative volume prediction in adult living donor liver transplantation: how much can we rely on it? Am J Transplant 2007;7: 672–679. (Ref.55)

Raia S, Nery JR, Mies S. Liver transplantation from live donors. Lancet 1989;2: 497. (Ref.48)

Renz JF, et al. Split-liver transplantation in the United States: outcomes of a national survey. Ann Surg 2004;239:172–181. (Ref.45)

Renz JF, et al. Utilization of extended donor criteria liver allografts maximizes donor use and patient access to liver transplantation. Ann Surg 2005;242: 556–563. (Ref.36)

Reyes J, et al. Split-liver transplantation: a comparison of ex vivo and in situ techniques. J Pediatr Surg 2000;35:283–289. (Ref.47)

Rhim CH, et al. Intra-operative acute isovolemic hemodilution is safe and effective in eliminating allogeneic blood transfusions during right hepatic lobectomy: comparison of living donor versus non-donors. HPB (Oxford) 2005;7:201–203. (Ref.62)

Roayaie K, Feng S. Allocation policy for hepatocellular carcinoma in the MELD era: room for improvement? Liver Transpl 2007;13(11 Suppl 2):S36–S43. (Ref.23)

Rogiers X, et al. In situ splitting of cadaveric livers. The ultimate expansion of a limited donor pool. Ann Surg 1996;224:331–339. (Ref.43)

Roland ME, et al. HIV-infected liver and kidney transplant recipients: 1- and 3-year outcomes. Am J Transplant 2008;8:355–365. (Ref.15)

Schaubel DE, Sima CS, Goodrich NP. The survival benefit of deceased donor liver transplantation as a function of candidate disease severity and donor quality. Am J Transplant 2008;8:419–425. (Ref.39)

Shah SA, et al. Biliary strictures in 130 consecutive right lobe living donor liver transplant recipients: results of a Western center. Am J Transplant 2007;7:161–167. (Ref.99)

Simpson MA, et al. Successful algorithm for selective liver biopsy in the right hepatic lobe live donor (RHLD). Am J Transplant 2008;8:832–838. (Ref.57)

Soejima Y, et al. Biliary strictures in living donor liver transplantation: incidence, management, and technical evolution. Liver Transpl 2006;12:979–986. (Ref.104)

Starzl TE. History of liver and other splanchnic organ transplantation. In: Busutill RW, Klintmalm GB, editors. Transplantation of the liver. Philadelphia: WB Saunders, 1996: 3–22. (Ref.5)

Starzl TE, et al. Liver transplantation with use of cyclosporin A and prednisone. N Engl J Med 1981;305:266–269. (Ref.11)

Starzl TE, et al. The use of heterologous antilymphoid agents in canine renal and liver homotransplantation and in human renal homotransplantation. Surg Gynecol Obstet 1967;124:301–308. (Ref.9)

Steinbrook R. Organ donation after cardiac death. N Engl J Med 2007;357: 209–213. (Ref.33)

Stock PG, et al. Kidney and liver transplantation in human immunodeficiency virus-infected patients: a pilot safety and efficacy study. Transplantation 2003;76:370–375. (Ref.14)

Strasberg SM, et al. Selecting the donor liver: risk factors for poor function after orthotopic liver transplantation. Hepatology 1994;20(4 Pt 1):829–838. (Ref.85)

Strong RW, et al. Successful liver transplantation from a living donor to her son. N Engl J Med 1990;322:1505–1507. (Ref.49)

Takata MC, et al. Laparoscopic bariatric surgery improves candidacy in morbidly obese patients awaiting transplantation. Surg Obes Relat Dis 2008;4:159–164. (Ref.18)

Taketomi A, et al. Donor risk in adult-to-adult living donor liver transplantation: impact of left lobe graft. Transplantation 2009;87:445–450. (Ref.65)

Totsuka E, et al. Influence of high donor serum sodium levels on early postoperative graft function in human liver transplantation: effect of correction of donor hypernatremia. Liver Transpl Surg 1999;5:421–428. (Ref.86)

Trotter JF, et al. Documented deaths of hepatic lobe donors for living donor liver transplantation. Liver Transpl 2006;12:1485–1488. (Ref.64)

Tzakis A, Todo S, Starzl TE. Orthotopic liver transplantation with preservation of the inferior vena cava. Ann Surg 1989;210:649–652. (Ref.72)

Tzakis AG, et al. Liver transplantation with cavoportal hemitransposition in the presence of diffuse portal vein thrombosis. Transplantation 1998;65:619–623. (Ref.79)

Uemura T, et al. Liver retransplantation for primary nonfunction: analysis of a 20-year single-center experience. Liver Transpl 2007;13:227–233. (Ref.84)

Veroli P, el Hage C, Ecoffey C. Does adult liver transplantation without venovenous bypass result in renal failure? Anesth Analg 1992;75:489–494. (Ref.77)

Wang ZJ, et al. Living donor candidates for right hepatic lobe transplantation: evaluation at CT cholangiography: initial experience. Radiology 2005;235: 899–904. (Ref.54)

Wojcicki M, Milkiewicz P, Silva M. Biliary tract complications after liver transplantation: a review. Dig Surg 2008;25:245–257. (Ref.97)

Yamaoka Y, et al. Liver transplantation using a right lobe graft from a living related donor. Transplantation 1994;57:1127–1130. (Ref.50)

Yao FY, et al. Liver transplantation for hepatocellular carcinoma: expansion of the tumor size limits does not adversely impact survival. Hepatology 2001;6:1394–1403. (Ref.26)

Yao FY, et al. A prospective study on downstaging of hepatocellular carcinoma prior to liver transplantation. Liver Transpl 2005;11:1505–1514. (Ref.27)

Yersiz H, et al. Split liver transplantation. Transplant Proc 2006;38:602–603. (Ref.44)

Yersiz H, et al. Correlation between donor age and the pattern of liver graft recovery after transplantation. Transplantation 1995;60:790–794. (Ref.89)

Yoo HY, Maheshwari A, Thuluvath PJ. Retransplantation of liver: primary graft nonfunction and hepatitis C virus are associated with worse outcome. Liver Transpl 2003;9:897–904. (Ref.90)

Yoo HY, et al. The outcome of liver transplantation in patients with hepatocellular carcinoma in the United States between 1988 and 2001: 5-year survival has improved significantly with time. J Clin Oncol 2003;21: 4329–4335. (Ref.25)

Zoepf T, et al. Diagnosis of biliary strictures after liver transplantation: which is the best tool? World J Gastroenterol 2005;11:2945–2948. (Ref.98)

A complete list of references can be found at www.expertconsult.com.

Post–Liver Transplantation Management

Douglas Hunt and Sammy Saab

ABBREVIATIONS

ACE angiostensin-converting enzyme
ACR acute cellular rejection
ALG antilymphocyte globulins
AS anastomotic biliary stricture
ATG antithymocyte globulins
AZA azathioprine
BMI body mass index
CIT cold ischemia time
CMV cytomegalovirus
CNI calcineurin inhibitor
CYA cyclosporine
DBD donation after brain death
DCD donation after cardiac death
DD deceased donor
DDLT deceased donor liver transplantation

EBV Epstein-Barr virus
EGD early graft dysfunction
HAT hepatic artery thrombosis
HCC hepatocellular carcinoma
HCV hepatitis C virus
HMC CoA 3-hydroxy-3-methylglutaryl coenzyme A
ICU intensive care unit
IFN-γ interferon-γ
IL-1 interleukin-1
IV intravenous
LDL low-density lipoprotein
LDLT living donor liver transplantation
MELD Model for End-Stage Liver Disease
MMF mycophenolate mofetil

MRSA methicillin-resistant *Staphylococcus aureus*
mTOR mammalian target of rapamycin
NAS nonanastomotic biliary stricture
OKT3 muromonab-CD3
PCP *Pneumocystis carinii* pneumonia
PNF primary nonfunction
PTLD posttransplantation lymphoproliferative disease
PVT portal vein thrombosis
TAC tacrolimus
TNF-α tumor necrosis factor-α
UNOS United Network for Organ Sharing

Introduction

Liver transplantation is the standard of care for the treatment of patients with decompensated liver disease. There has been a steady increase in the number of transplants performed since liver transplantation became an acceptable treatment modality in the mid 1980s.[1] However, the number of patients needing a liver transplantation as a lifesaving modality has unfortunately outpaced the number of organs available.

Improvements in medical care, operative techniques, and immunosuppressive therapies have led to improvements in posttransplant patient and graft survival rates. Three-year patient and graft survival rates in liver transplant recipients are currently 79% and 74%, respectively.[1] As a result, there are an increasing number of recipients living, and living longer. There are an estimated 40,000 to 50,000 liver transplant recipients currently being managed posttransplant. Thus there is increasing interest in long-term management issues in liver transplantation recipients, such as quality of life, complications related to extended immunosuppressants, natural development of co-morbidities, and recurrent disease.

This chapter will focus on management of liver transplant recipients. We will identify posttransplant prognostic factors, review available immunosuppressive medications, and detail the short- and long-term complications that occur posttransplant, elucidating strategies for diagnosing, managing, and preventing these complications.

Posttransplantation Prognostic Factors

Background

An understanding of the specific post–liver transplantation complications and their management would be incomplete without a discussion of the factors that have been shown to negatively affect graft survival in liver transplant patients. These factors can be stratified into donor factors, graft factors, and recipient factors (**Fig. 49-1**).

Donor Factors

A number of donor factors have been demonstrated to negatively affect graft survival in liver transplant recipients. Donor age is the most extensively studied risk factor for graft failure. Results are conflicting, especially among small single institution studies, but most of the largest studies incorporating data from liver transplant registries have confirmed advanced donor age to be a risk factor for graft failure.[2-4] Evidence in patients transplanted for hepatitis C virus (HCV) is even more striking, with most studies showing a significant decrement in graft and patient survival rates for those with HCV who receive grafts from older donors.[5,6] Indeed, it has been demonstrated that the progression of fibrosis and the development of cirrhosis is more advanced in HCV-infected

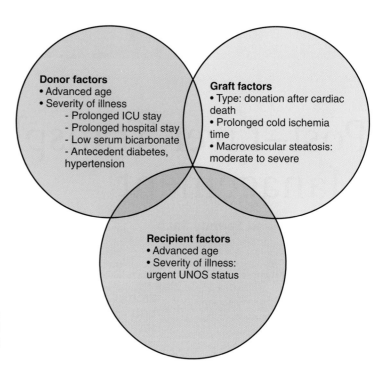

Donor factors
• Advanced age
• Severity of illness
 - Prolonged ICU stay
 - Prolonged hospital stay
 - Low serum bicarbonate
 - Antecedent diabetes, hypertension

Graft factors
• Type: donation after cardiac death
• Prolonged cold ischemia time
• Macrovesicular steatosis: moderate to severe

Recipient factors
• Advanced age
• Severity of illness: urgent UNOS status

Fig. 49-1 **Donor, graft, and recipient factors that have been shown to adversely affect posttransplant patient survival rates.** ICU, intensive care unit; UNOS, United Network for Organ Sharing.

patients receiving grafts from older donors.[7] Despite evidence of generally poorer outcomes with grafts from donors of advanced age, use of these grafts has increased from 2.5% of all deceased donors in 1988 to 34.7% in 2008.[8] This increase results from the large-scale shortage of available organs for transplantation; grafts from older donors have been identified as possibly the most important type of extended criteria donor to counter this shortage. There is evidence that if recipients are chosen carefully, grafts from older donors can be used with survival rates comparable with normal populations. For instance, first-time liver recipients over the age of 45 with body mass index (BMI) less than 35, non–status 1 United Network for Organ Sharing (UNOS) registration, cold ischemia time (CIT) less than 8 hours, and either hepatocellular carcinoma (HCC) or an indication for transplantation other than HCV who receive grafts from donors with advanced age have been shown to have similar 3-year patient survival rates compared with patients without grafts from donors of advanced age.[3]

Severity of the donor's illness has been demonstrated to predict poorer outcomes in some large studies. Prolonged intensive care unit (ICU) stay has been shown to increase histologically proven liver preservation injury,[9] to be a significant predictor of donor infection,[10] and to predict poorer graft survival rates.[11] Similarly, in a large single-center study involving 3200 liver transplantations, donor length of hospital stay greater than 6 days reduced recipient survival rates. Low bicarbonate level and antecedent hypertension and diabetes mellitus have also been demonstrated to predict poorer graft survival rates.[2,11]

Graft Factors

Graft type is an important determinant of the prognosis of liver transplantation recipients. The majority of transplants use allografts from deceased donors (DD). Deceased donor grafts can be defined as either a donation after brain death

(DBD) or a donation after cardiac death (DCD). Donation after brain death enables a period of donor resuscitation and graft evaluation before procurement. Donation after cardiac death occurs in situations where criteria for brain death are not met. In these cases procurement is deferred until after cardiopulmonary death, followed by a period of observation to exclude spontaneous resuscitation. Donation after cardiac death represents another strategy for expanding the available pool of organs for transplantation. It is not surprising that DCD organs—by definition exposed to ischemia during cardiopulmonary death and deprived of directed resuscitation before procurement—have been shown to have worse outcomes, including inferior graft survival rates, compared with DBD organs.[2,12-14] A number of studies have documented a significant increase in biliary complications in DCD transplants,[13,15] as well as an increased rate of retransplantation.[12] Similar to other risk factors, however, careful donor-recipient matching using DCD grafts to minimize additional risk factors can yield survival rates similar to DBD graft recipients, specifically avoiding a donor age greater than 60 years, warm ischemia time greater than 30 minutes, cold ischemia time greater than 10 hours, its use for retransplantation, and recipient cardiopulmonary support.[13]

Prolonged cold ischemia time has been consistently shown to worsen posttransplant outcomes. Analysis of 34,664 patients in the European Liver Transplant Registry revealed that CIT greater than 13 hours increased 3- and 12-month mortality.[4] In a large single center study, CIT greater than 10 hours predicted an elevated risk of death.[16] The combination of advanced donor age and prolonged CIT leads to significantly worsened survival rates. Indeed, when grafts are obtained from donors 45 years of age or older and with a CIT of 12 hours or more, an additional 1 of 16 grafts will fail when compared with grafts without these negative prognostic factors.[17,18] Though the precise threshold for prolonged CIT is not known, efforts for its minimization should be undertaken, especially in the setting of other risk factors for poor outcomes.

Graft steatosis is believed by many to compromise post-transplant outcomes. Steatosis is present in up to 30% of donors, and given the increasing prevalence of diabetes and obesity may be expected to become more prevalent in the future.[19] Graft steatosis can be histologically classified as microvesicular or macrovesicular. Microvesicular steatosis is defined histologically by diffuse cytoplasmic small droplet vacuolization. Macrovesicular steatosis classically demonstrates a single large vacuolar deposit with displacement of the nucleus.[20] Macrovesicular steatosis can be classified based on the percentage of hepatocytes involved: mild (<30%), moderate (30% to 60%), or severe (>60%).[21] Data on the effect of steatosis on posttransplant outcomes are at first glance contradictory. Upon closer review, however, the effects of steatosis are consistent when evaluated by type and severity of steatosis. Microvesicular steatosis of any severity, as well as mild macrovesicular steatosis, has been shown not to significantly affect outcomes.[19,22] Most studies have shown that use of grafts with severe macrovesicular steatosis significantly worsens outcomes,[5] and as a result most transplant surgeons discard grafts with severe macrovesicular steatosis. Use of grafts with moderate macrovesicular steatosis is controversial. They are considered marginal grafts and can worsen outcomes, especially if coupled with other risk factors.[9] Of note, many grafts demonstrate mixed patterns of microvesicular and macrovesicular stenosis, complicating the ability to prognosticate outcomes for recipients of these grafts.[23]

Recipient Factors

Recipient age has been shown in a number of studies to worsen posttransplant prognosis.[4] Despite this, the number of liver transplant recipients in the United States over the age of 65 has increased approximately 2.5-fold. Interestingly, in a study that stratified older recipients between ages 65 and 75 versus greater than 75, no difference in 10-year survival rates were noted.[24] Of note, there is some evidence that recipients over 65 years experience less graft rejection,[25] which could be accounted for by immune system senescence. Currently, no consensus on an age limit for undergoing liver transplantation exists, and these patients are evaluated on an individual basis.

Severity of recipient disease pretransplant is believed by many to portend poorer posttransplant prognosis. Indeed, a number of studies have shown that urgent UNOS status at transplant leads to poorer survival rates posttransplant.[4,16,18] Data for the impact of the Model for End-Stage Liver Disease (MELD) score on posttransplant outcomes are conflicting. Some studies, including a large study involving 15,878 patients from the UNOS database, have shown poorer outcomes with elevated MELD score.[3] Other studies, however, have shown no effect of MELD score on posttransplant outcomes.[26]

Immunosuppressive Medications

Background

Immunosuppressive management after liver transplantation is a cornerstone of posttransplant care. Refinements in immunosuppressive strategies have greatly improved posttransplant

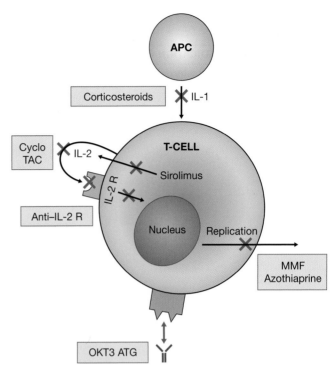

Fig. 49-2 Mechanisms of action of commonly used immunosuppressive therapies. APC, antigen-presenting cells; ATG, antithymocyte globulins; IL-1, interleukin-1; MMF, mycophenolate mofetil; OKT3, muromonab-CD3; TAC, tacrolimus.

outcomes. The goal of immunosuppressive therapy is to prevent allograft rejection, optimize graft function, and maximize patient survival rates and quality of life while concomitantly maintaining immunologic control over infection and neoplasia, and minimizing side effects and their sequelae. Knowledge of the available options for immunosuppressive therapy, along with an understanding of their mechanisms of action, side effects, and drug–drug interactions is critical for optimal posttransplant immunosuppressive management. **Table 49-1** details the most commonly used immunosuppressive agents, their mechanisms, and associated side effects. Their mechanisms are also illustrated in **Figure 49-2**. In general, immunosuppressive therapy can be divided into two phases. Induction therapy is usually initiated immediately posttransplant and continued for 1 to 2 weeks. Two or three drugs are used in the induction phase, most commonly a calcineurin inhibitor, an antimetabolite, and a glucocorticoid. Maintenance therapy begins after the induction phase, the cornerstone of which is a calcineurin inhibitor, most commonly tacrolimus.

Corticosteroids

Corticosteroids have been used in the transplant setting since the earliest days of liver transplantation in the 1960s. Steroids are used for induction, maintenance, and treatment of allograft rejection. They have both antiinflammatory and immunomodulatory effects. They suppress prostaglandin and leukotriene release, and stabilize lysosomal membranes.[27] In addition, they alter antigen presentation by dendritic cells, reduce circulating CD4$^+$ T cells, diminish monocyte and macrophage effectiveness, and inhibit lymphocyte activation via

Table 49-1 Summary of Immunosuppressive Agents

AGENT	MEDICATION CLASS	MECHANISM	ADVERSE EFFECTS
Prednisone	Corticosteroid	Suppresses prostaglandin/leukotriene release, stabilizes lysosomal membranes, alters antigen presentation by dendritic cell, reduces CD4+ T-cell levels, inhibits lymphocyte activation	Hypertension, dyslipidemia, glucose intolerance, peptic ulcer disease, psychiatric disturbance, obesity, cushingoid features, osteoporosis, avascular necrosis, impaired wound healing, adrenal suppression, cataracts
Azathioprine (AZA)	Antiproliferative, purine analogue	Inhibits DNA and RNA synthesis in T and B cells, inhibits CD28 co-stimulation	Bone marrow toxicity, hepatotoxicity, pancreatitis
Mycophenolate mofetil (MMF)	Antiproliferative	Inhibits DNA synthesis by targeting inosine monophosphate dehydrogenase to block synthesis of guanosine nucleotides	Bone marrow toxicity, nausea, vomiting, diarrhea, abdominal pain
Cyclosporine (CYA)	Calcineurin inhibitor (CNI)	Reduces phosphatase activity of calcineurin, which leads to decreased transcription of IL-2 and resultant inhibition of T-cell activation	Acute/chronic renal failure, neurotoxic effects, obesity, hypertension, hyperlipidemia, hirsutism, gingival hyperplasia
Tacrolimus (TAC)	CNI	Reduces phosphatase activity of calcineurin, which leads to decreased transcription of IL-2 and resultant inhibition of T-cell activation	Acute/chronic renal failure, neurotoxic effects, insulin resistance, diarrhea, alopecia, electrolyte disturbances, thrombotic microangiopathy
Antithymocyte globulins (ATG)	Polyclonal T cell–depleting agents	Deplete lymphocytes via complement-mediated cell lysis	Fever, allergic reaction, serum sickness, thrombocytopenia
Antilymphocyte globulins (ALG)	Polyclonal T cell–depleting agents	Deplete lymphocytes via complement-mediated cell lysis	Fever, allergic reaction, serum sickness, thrombocytopenia
Muromonal-CD3 (OKT3)	Monoclonal T cell–depleting agent	Depletes lymphocytes via T-cell CD3 targeting, which results in complement-mediated cell lysis	Cytokine release syndrome (fever, diarrhea, nausea, vomiting, headaches, myalgias, and/or shortness of breath)
Alemtuzumab	Monoclonal T cell–depleting agent	Depletes lymphocytes via T-cell CD52 targeting, which results in complement-mediated cell lysis	Infectious complications
Daclizumab	IL-2 receptor blocker	Antagonizes IL-2 receptor with resultant inhibition of IL-2–mediated T-cell activation	Infection, gastrointestinal upset, pulmonary edema/bronchospasm
Basiliximab	IL-2 receptor blocker	Antagonizes IL-2 receptor with resultant inhibition of IL-2–mediated T-cell activation	Infection, gastrointestinal upset, pulmonary edema/bronchospasm
Sirolimus	mTOR inhibitor	Inhibits mammalian target of rapamycin, which results in diminished intracellular signaling distal to IL-2 receptor and arrested T-cell replication	Leukopenia, thrombocytopenia, hyperlipidemia, oral ulcers, proteinuria, acne, peripheral edema, interstitial pneumonitis
Everolimus	mTOR inhibitor	Inhibits mammalian target of rapamycin, which results in diminished intracellular signaling distal to IL-2 receptor and arrested T-cell replication	Leukopenia, thrombocytopenia, hyperlipidemia, oral ulcers, proteinuria, acne, peripheral edema, interstitial pneumonitis

IL-2, interleukin-2; mTOR, mammalian target of rapamycin

reduction in interleukin-1 (IL-1), IL-2, IL-6, interferon-γ (IFN-γ), and tumor necrosis factor-α (TNF-α) transcription.[28,29] These immunosuppressive effects are unfortunately accompanied by a number of well-recognized side effects. These include hypertension, dyslipidemia, glucose intolerance, peptic ulcers, psychiatric disturbances, obesity, cushingoid features, osteoporosis, avascular necrosis, poor wound healing, adrenal suppression, and cataract development. In addition, there is some evidence that high-dose pulsed corticosteroids can worsen the severity of HCV recurrence.[30] An immunosuppressive strategy that avoids abrupt reductions in steroid doses, however, has been shown to mitigate this intensification of HCV recurrence.[31]

Due to the myriad adverse effects of corticosteroids, efforts have been made to remove them from immunosuppressive regimens altogether. Two meta-analyses evaluating corticosteroid-free immunosuppression showed no differences in mortality or graft survival rates, and demonstrated reduced cholesterol levels, de novo diabetes mellitus, and cytomegalovirus (CMV) infection. Both meta-analyses also demonstrated lower rates of HCV recurrence with steroid-free regimens. Overall rates of rejection were increased in individual studies in which steroids were not substituted with other immunosuppressives; however, when steroids were replaced, rejection rates were not elevated.[32,33] As a result of these data, many transplant centers endeavor to rapidly taper or even completely avoid steroids in the setting of liver transplantation. Indeed, the rate of corticosteroid avoidance among transplant centers has increased from 8% in 1999 to 20% in 2004.[34] Patients undergoing liver transplantation for immunologic liver diseases, such as autoimmune hepatitis, primary biliary cirrhosis, and sclerosing cholangitis, may have less chance of long-term success with a steroid-sparing strategy.[35]

Antiproliferative Agents

Azathioprine (AZA) and mycophenolate mofetil (MMF) comprise the class of antiproliferative immunosuppressive agents. AZA was part of the immunosuppressive regimen used for the first successful liver transplantation in 1967.[36] MMF came into use for liver transplantation in the 1990s.[37] AZA and MMF reduce immune-mediated graft injury by reducing the expansion of activated T and B cells. AZA is a purine analogue that inhibits DNA and RNA synthesis in rapidly proliferating T and B cells, and also inhibits CD-28 co-stimulation of T lymphocytes. MMF is more selective than AZA. It is converted in the liver to mycophenolic acid, which targets inosine monophosphate dehydrogenase, ultimately inhibiting DNA synthesis by blocking synthesis of guanosine nucleotides.[29] Use of AZA and MMF can be limited by bone marrow toxicity. AZA has also been shown to cause hepatotoxicity and pancreatitis. MMF is most commonly associated with gastrointestinal side effects, with nausea, vomiting, diarrhea, or abdominal pain occurring in as many as 25% of patients.[38] The specificity of action of MMF is believed to result in fewer serious side effects than AZA, while maintaining superior efficacy with regards to prevention of rejection when used in conjunction with calcineurin inhibitors (CNIs) and corticosteroids.[39,40] As a result of these data, MMF has largely replaced AZA in immunosuppressive regimens during the last decade.[41] The majority of transplant centers use MMF in conjunction with CNIs and corticosteroids for maintenance therapy during the first 6 months posttransplant. The antiproliferative agents, particularly MMF, have also been used to minimize or eliminate CNIs in patients with CNI-induced renal insufficiency. Replacement of CNIs with MMF has been consistently shown to result in renal improvement, as well as improvement in hypertension in these patients,[42,43] though this strategy may be somewhat limited by side effects and rejection, particularly when CNIs are discontinued rather than reduced.[44,45]

Calcineurin Inhibitors

Calcineurin inhibitors have been a mainstay of immunosuppressive regimens for liver transplantation since the introduction of cyclosporine and its resultant dramatic improvements in post–liver transplant survival rates in the early 1980s.[46] As of 2004, 97% of patients were discharged home after liver transplantation with an immunosuppressive regimen incorporating a calcineurin inhibitor.[34] Cyclosporin (CYA) and tacrolimus (TAC) inhibit T-cell activation by binding specific intracellular proteins to form a drug–protein complex, which reduces the phosphatase activity of calcineurin, resulting in decreased transcription of IL-2.[29] Calcineurin inhibitors have several major side effects, including acute and chronic renal failure, and neurotoxic effects. In addition to these effects, CYA and TAC carry distinct side effect profiles. CYA manifests in higher rates of obesity, hypertension, hyperlipidemia,

hirsutism, and gingival hyperplasia, while TAC results in higher rates of insulin resistance, diarrhea, alopecia, electrolyte disturbances, and thrombotic microangiopathy.[47] Many of these side effects are dose dependent. These agents are metabolized by the cytochrome P-450 system, and as a result are prone to drug–drug interactions. Another concerning feature of calcineurin inhibitors is their association with malignancy. Both CYA and TAC have been shown to be independent risk factors for recurrence of HCC posttransplant,[48,49] and therefore CNI exposure should be minimized in patients transplanted for HCC. Overall, TAC has largely replaced CYA in clinical use based on evidence of its superior efficacy. Indeed, a Cochrane review in 2006 demonstrated that treating 100 patients with TAC in place of CYA would result in 9 fewer cases of acute rejection, 7 fewer cases of steroid-resistant rejection, 5 fewer cases of graft failure, and 2 fewer deaths.[47]

T Cell–Depleting Agents

Polyclonal antibodies can be used for induction or for treatment of rejection, and include antithymocyte globulins (ATG) and antilymphocyte globulins (ALG). Antilymphocyte globulins were a component of the first successful immunosuppressive regimens in the 1960s. Polyclonal antibodies deplete lymphocytes via complement-mediated cell lysis, resulting in uptake of opsonized T cells by the reticuloendothelial system.[29] These agents are used for induction in approximately 20% of transplant centers, and they have been shown in preliminary studies to have acceptable levels of efficacy in CNI-minimizing immunosuppressive regimens.[50] Moreover, their use in treatment of steroid-resistant rejection has modestly increased in recent years to a rate of 38% in 2004.[34] The overall use of polyclonal antibodies has been curbed by significant side effects, which occur in approximately 80% of patients. These side effects include fever, allergic reactions, serum sickness, and thrombocytopenia.

During the 1970s, in response to the frequent side effects associated with polyclonal antibodies, monoclonal antibodies were designed using hybridoma technology in an effort to achieve more targeted antibody-mediated immunosuppression.[51] Muromonab-CD3 (OKT3) is a monoclonal antibody directed against CD3, a cell surface antigen found on all T lymphocytes. Its use results in rapid T-cell depletion, which can result in a cytokine release syndrome characterized by fever, diarrhea, nausea, vomiting, headaches, myalgias, and/or shortness of breath. A number of older studies demonstrated acceptable outcomes with the use of OKT3 induction therapy in regimens designed to delay initiation of CYA.[52,53] Current use of OKT3 has been reduced to only a small percentage of inductions and 28% of cases of steroid-resistant rejection.[34] Alemtuzumab is a newer monoclonal antibody that targets CD52, a prominent antigen on all lymphocytes and monocytes. It has been shown to enact profound and long-lasting T-cell depletion, but unfortunately has also been associated with a high risk of infectious complications, and currently is only rarely used in liver transplantation.[28]

Interleukin-2 Receptor Blockers

Daclizumab and basiliximab are monoclonal antibodies that antagonize the IL-2 receptor, with resultant inhibition of IL-2–mediated T-cell activation. These medications were developed in the 1990s and due to their selective action, they have minimal side effects and are generally well tolerated. Side effects include infections, gastrointestinal upset, and in rare cases pulmonary edema/bronchospasm. Both agents have been demonstrated in prospective, randomized controlled trials to effectively suppress rejection without significant side effects or infectious complications when combined with other CNIs and/or corticosteroids during induction.[54,55] Their low incidence of side effects has led to their increasing usage in steroid-sparing[56,57] and CNI-minimizing regimens, particularly in patients with underlying renal insufficiency.[54]

mTOR Inhibitors

Sirolimus and its derivative everolimus enact their immunosuppressive effects by inhibiting the mammalian target of rapamycin (mTOR), arresting cell replication, diminishing intracellular signaling distal to the IL-2 receptor, and preventing T-cell replication. Side effects include leukopenia, thrombocytopenia, hyperlipidemia, oral ulcers, proteinuria, acne, peripheral edema, and interstitial pneumonitis.[27] Stemming from sparse data from early trials, which showed increased rates of wound infections and hepatic artery thrombosis with use of high-dose sirolimus—including the temporary discontinuation of a trial using sirolimus due to development of hepatic artery thrombosis (HAT) in five patients—use of sirolimus has been tempered, particularly as primary immunosuppression after liver transplantation. More recent studies, however, have not borne out the earlier findings of increased wound infections and HAT.[58]

Sirolimus has been most commonly studied in the setting of CNI-induced renal failure, with overall mixed results. Many small, retrospective single-center trial results showed improvement in renal function with acceptable side effects and rejection prevention. However, the results of two prospective, randomized, single-center trials did not demonstrate significant improvement in long-term renal function compared with a low-dose CNI strategy, and also showed high rates of side effects.[59,60] Currently, sirolimus is used for maintenance immunosuppression in approximately 14% of liver transplant patients, most commonly for the prevention of, or mitigation of, the effects of CNI-induced renal failure.[61] Multicenter, randomized controlled trials are needed. An intriguing aspect of mTOR inhibitors is their anticancer effect. They have been shown in vitro to inhibit angiogenesis and to have a direct intracellular signaling effect that can regulate cancer cell growth. Sirolimus has been shown to inhibit HCC tumor growth in mice,[62] but its effect on minimizing tumor proliferation and preventing de novo malignancy in humans has not been clearly demonstrated to date and requires further study.[63]

Posttransplantation Complications
Background

Posttransplant outcomes have gradually improved during the last 4 decades, and 1-year graft survival rates now exceed 80%.[2] The spectrum of posttransplant complications and causes of mortality has changed with time as management challenges have been overcome, often giving way

Table 49-2 Early and Late Complications Following Liver Transplantation

EARLY COMPLICATIONS	LATE COMPLICATIONS
Hepatic	
Postsurgical	Immunologic
Primary nonfunction	Chronic rejection
Early graft dysfunction	Disease recurrence
Vascular	Hepatocellular carcinoma
Hepatic artery thrombosis	Viral hepatitis
Portal vein thrombosis	Autoimmune disease
Hepatic vein thrombosis	Alcoholic liver disease
Biliary	Nonalcoholic fatty liver
Bile leak	disease
Biliary stricture	
Immunologic	
Acute cellular rejection	
Nonhepatic	
Infectious	Metabolic/cardiovascular
Bacterial infection	Hypertension
Fungal infection	Dyslipidemia
Cytomegalovirus infection	Diabetes mellitus
	Obesity
	Renal failure
	Atherosclerotic
	cardiovascular disease
	Neoplastic
	Cutaneous malignancy
	Posttransplant
	lymphoproliferative
	disease
	Solid organ malignancy
	Infectious
	Late-onset cytomegalovirus
	infection

to new challenges as patients survive longer. Posttransplant complications can be loosely divided between early and late complications (**Table 49-2**), and a number of these early and late complications have been demonstrated to worsen graft and/or patient survival rates (**Table 49-3**). It should be noted, however, that there is considerable variation in the timing of all posttransplant complications.

Early Complications

Primary Nonfunction and Early Graft Dysfunction

Though definitions of primary nonfunction (PNF) vary, it is generally defined as primary graft failure resulting in death or retransplantation shortly after transplant in the absence of recurrent disease, graft-versus-host disease, rejection, or vascular thrombosis. The incidence of PNF varies with the specific definition used, from 1.4% to 14%.[64] Primary nonfunction manifests clinically with rapidly rising transaminitis and severe coagulopathy, high lactate level, absence of bile production, and hemodynamic instability. Pathologically, allograft biopsy shows coagulative necrosis. Though the cause is unknown, female donors, advanced donor age, donor days in the ICU, retransplantation, prolonged CIT, and prolonged operating room time have been suggested to increase risk for PNF.[65] Early retransplantation is the only proven therapy for PNF. In situations where a liver is not immediately available

Table 49-3 Complications that Have Been Shown to Adversely Affect Patient and/or Graft Survival Rates

EARLY COMPLICATIONS	LATE COMPLICATIONS
Hepatic	
Postsurgical	Immunologic
Primary nonfunction	Chronic rejection
Vascular	Disease recurrence
Hepatic artery thrombosis	Hepatocellular carcinoma
Portal vein thrombosis	Viral hepatitis
Nonhepatic	
Infectious	Metabolic/cardiovascular
Fungal infection	Diabetes mellitus
(*Aspergillus*)	Chronic renal failure
Cytomegalovirus infection	Neoplastic
	Posttransplant
	lymphoproliferative
	disease
	Solid organ malignancy
	Infectious
	Late-onset cytomegalovirus
	infection

and severe cardiopulmonary instability is present, rescue hepatectomy can result in immediate, short-term clinical improvement.[66] Short- and long-term patient survival rates are diminished in patients with PNF.

Similar to PNF, the definition of early graft dysfunction (EGD) is not well defined. It is generally characterized by posttransplant transaminitis and cholestasis in the absence of encephalopathy, coagulopathy, renal failure, or severe hemodynamic instability. Unlike PNF, EGD is largely reversible, and does not mandate retransplantation.

Hepatic Artery Thrombosis

Hepatic artery thrombosis is the most common and most devastating post–liver transplantation vascular complication, occurring with an incidence of 2% to 9% of adult recipients.[67] Early HAT occurs within days of transplantation, and usually presents with abnormal liver function tests, often progressing rapidly to acute graft failure. Late HAT generally has a more subtle manifestation, often with biliary and infectious complications (chronic cholangitis, hepatic abscesses, and biliary sepsis) likely because the hepatic artery provides the sole vascular supply to the biliary epithelium.[67] Hepatic artery thrombosis can be asymptomatic—in as many as 37% of patients in one series. As a result, many transplant centers employ screening Doppler ultrasound in the first few days posttransplant to screen for HAT.[68] Doppler sonography is the primary modality for diagnosis, which is generally followed by contrast-enhanced ultrasound, Computed tomography (CT) angiography, magnetic resonance (MR) angiography, or catheter angiography for confirmation. Sensitivity of ultrasound for early HAT has been reported to be as high as 100%, but declines when performed later after transplant. The lower sensitivity with a late manifestation is probably due to establishment of blood flow through collateral vessels.[69] Risk factors for HAT include pediatric recipient, transarterial chemoembolization, HCC, aberrant arterial anatomy requiring complex reconstruction, prolonged CIT, ABO incompatibility, acute rejection, cytomegalovirus

mismatch, retransplantation, prolonged operative time, low recipient weight, and low-volume transplantation center.[70,71] Early HAT requires urgent management because mortality rates without revascularization or retransplantation in these patients have been reported to be greater than 80%.[72] Therapeutic options include catheter-based therapy, surgical thrombectomy or revascularization, or retransplantation. Patient and graft survival rates for patients whose liver transplantation is complicated by HAT are diminished compared with the general posttransplant population.[70,71]

Portal Vein and Hepatic Vein Thrombosis

Portal vein thrombosis (PVT) occurs after approximately 1% of liver transplants, and is more common among pediatric transplant recipients.[70] Hepatic vein thrombosis is uncommon, occurring in less than 1% of transplants.[73] Symptoms result from portal hypertension, in the form of esophageal variceal bleeding, massive ascites, or hepatic encephalopathy. Diagnosis is made with ultrasonography, which can be confirmed with CT, MR venography, or portography. Commonly used management options include anticoagulation, catheter-based therapy, surgical thrombectomy or shunt placement, or retransplantation. Patient and graft survival are significantly compromised by the occurrence of PVT.[70]

Biliary Complications

For decades biliary complications have been considered the "Achilles' heel" of liver transplantation because they are a leading cause of posttransplant morbidity, resulting in increased need for hospitalizations and invasive procedures.[74] Biliary complications occur with an incidence rate of 11% to 25%,[75] and include bile leaks, biliary strictures, bile duct stones, bile casts, and sphincter of Oddi dysfunction. Bile leaks and biliary strictures are the most common posttransplant biliary complications, and these complications are more common after living donor liver transplantation (LDLT) than deceased donor liver transplantation (DDLT).[76] Bile leak is the most common complication in the first few weeks posttransplant. Patients with bile leak may be asymptomatic or have signs and symptoms of peritonitis. Bile leaks commonly occur at sites of biliary anastomosis, or at the T-tube exit site, particularly after tube removal.[77] Management options include endoscopic, percutaneous, and surgical strategies, though some bile leaks can be managed conservatively. Bile leak has been consistently shown to be a risk factor for biliary strictures.[78]

Biliary strictures can be classified as anastomotic (AS) or nonanastomotic (NAS). Anastomotic strictures most commonly arise because of technical factors related to the transplant surgery. Nonanastomotic strictures are often a result of ischemic injury, and because the hepatic artery is the lone blood supply to the biliary tree, urgent evaluation of the patency of the hepatic artery is imperative in these cases. Less common causes of NAS include rejection, prolonged ischemia time, infection, recurrent autoimmune disease, and external compression due to posttransplant lymphoproliferative disease (PTLD). Cholangiography, whether endoscopic or percutaneous, is the gold standard for evaluation of biliary strictures, and though relatively easy to perform in patients with T-tubes, is associated with procedure-related complications. Though ultrasound is often employed as an initial diagnostic test to assess for hepatic artery flow, MRCP has been shown to be the noninvasive diagnostic modality of choice for evaluating the biliary anatomy, with a sensitivity approaching 90%.[79] Management of posttransplant strictures has shifted significantly toward endoscopic strategies during the last decade. In DDLT, endoscopic management is now considered first-line therapy.[80] Endoscopic therapy for post-LDLT strictures is less well established because the limited available evidence demonstrates diminished efficacy, particularly with NAS.[76] Surgery is reserved for cases not amenable to endoscopic management.

Acute Cellular Rejection

Acute cellular rejection (ACR) is a common complication in the early posttransplant period, occurring in approximately 15% to 57% of transplants.[81,82] The human liver is an immunologically advantaged organ, with lower rates of allograft rejection compared with other transplanted organs. Indeed, some patients are able to achieve "operational tolerance" because immunosuppression can eventually be completely withdrawn with stable rejection-free graft function.[83] Clinically evident ACR occurs most commonly within the first month after transplantation. ACR is at times asymptomatic in mild cases, and sometimes occurs with fever, abdominal tenderness, reduced bile flow, and liver function test abnormalities. Diagnosis is based on histology because clinical presentation is variable and laboratory findings are not sensitive or specific. Histologic findings include mixed but mostly mononuclear portal inflammation, bile duct inflammation and damage, and subendothelial inflammation in portal veins or hepatic venules. At least two of these features must be found to confirm the diagnosis of ACR. Acute cellular rejection is graded histologically based on the Banff criteria.[84]

The majority of cases of ACR are mild, result in no long-term detriment to the graft, and are effectively managed with optimization of baseline immunosuppression and intravenous (IV) methylprednisolone.[82,85] ACR uncommonly progresses to graft failure.[86] Histologic evidence of ACR without evidence of graft dysfunction is often encountered when protocol biopsies are performed posttransplant. Only 14% of these patients develop clinically significant graft dysfunction; therefore it has been suggested that withholding adjuvant therapy with close monitoring of graft function in these patients is safe and reasonable.[87] Approximately 18% of cases of ACR are steroid resistant, and management options for these patients include T cell–depleting agents and IL-2 receptor blockers.[34]

Bacterial Infections

Liver transplant patients are prone to postoperative infectious complications because of risks associated with the presence of end-stage liver disease, poor nutrition, major surgery, frequent need for invasive diagnostic procedures after transplantation, and immunosuppressive therapy. In general, infections in transplant patients are more difficult to detect because of muted inflammatory responses as a result of immunosuppression. Infectious complications occur in greater than one third of patients in the first month posttransplant, and the majority of infections occurring in the first weeks after the transplant are attributed to common nosocomial bacterial infections.[88] These primarily include surgical site infections, catheter-related blood stream infections, pneumonias, urinary tract infections, and colitis due to *Clostridium difficile*. Liver transplant recipients have been demonstrated to have a greater risk of respiratory tract infections than pancreatic or renal transplant recipients, and severe pneumonia has been shown to result in 37% mortality in liver transplant recipients.[89] Unfortunately, multidrug-resistant pathogens are commonly implicated in posttransplant infections, including methicillin-resistant *Staphylococcus aureus* (MRSA), vancomycin-resistant *Enterococcus*, *C. difficile* colitis, and resistant gram-negative rods, with relative rates varying with prevalence of prophylaxis regimens and center-specific microbial patterns.[90] Many centers give prophylactic antibiotics for the first 1 to 2 days after transplantation, which are targeted to cover skin flora, gastrointestinal flora including biliary *Enterococcus* species, and, if there is high risk or known colonization, multidrug resistant organisms. Routine antimicrobial prophylaxis for *Pneumocystis carinii* pneumonia (PCP) using trimethoprim-sulfamethoxazole has largely eliminated PCP pneumonia in transplant patients; this provides the additional benefit of antimicrobial coverage against some gram negatives, some community-acquired MRSA, *Nocardia*, and *Toxoplasma gondii*.

Fungal Infections

Candida and *Aspergillus* species account for most invasive fungal infections in liver transplant recipients, and commonly occur within the first month after transplant. Prominent risk factors for invasive fungal infections in liver transplant patients include reoperation after transplant, retransplantation, and renal failure requiring renal replacement therapy.[91] Indeed renal failure requiring hemodialysis is associated with a 15-fold to 21-fold risk for invasive fungal infections in liver transplant recipients.[92] Common manifestations of post–liver transplant invasive candidiasis infections are intraabdominal abscesses, peritonitis, wound infections, and fungemia.[93] Invasive *Aspergillus* most commonly manifests with pulmonary involvement. Central nervous system lesions due to *Aspergillus* are also well documented. Though less common than candidal infections, invasive *Aspergillus* infections carry a high rate of mortality (40% to 100%). Early diagnosis and initiation of appropriate therapy is a prerequisite to providing a chance for survival.[94] Fortunately the incidence of invasive fungal infections has decreased in the past decade because of improved surgical techniques, improvements in immunosuppressive regimens, and institution of antifungal prophylaxis.[95]

Antifungal prophylaxis in transplant patients is controversial, though frequently used in clinical practice. Two meta-analyses have recently explored this issue in liver transplant recipients. Overall they demonstrated a reduction in invasive fungal infections, particularly invasive candidiasis, without a benefit in the overall mortality, and with some evidence for an increased incidence of infections with non-*albicans Candida* among those receiving prophylaxis. In addition to potential selection for these often triazole-resistant candidal strains, the downside of antifungal prophylaxis is unnecessary antifungal exposure, with its attendant costs, drug interactions, and drug-associated toxicities.[96,97] At some transplant centers, antifungal prophylaxis is universally administered after transplantation, whereas other centers only offer prophylaxis to high-risk patients. Of note, a recent multicenter prospective observational study showed a low rate of invasive fungal infections in patients who were not given prophylaxis based on estimated low risk because of minimal risk factors,[98] lending evidence to the theory that patients can be effectively risk stratified for receiving, or not receiving, fungal prophylaxis. Overall, in light of available evidence, targeting prophylaxis only to high-risk patients is likely a more efficient and cost-effective strategy. When used, prophylaxis duration should be limited to 6 weeks or less.[99]

Cytomegalovirus Infection

Cytomegalovirus is a member of the human herpesvirus group, and is an important viral infection in liver transplant recipients. In the absence of preventive antiviral therapy, CMV disease commonly occurs in the early posttransplant period.[100] Cytomegalovirus involvement can be classified as either CMV infection or tissue-invasive CMV disease. CMV infection can be asymptomatic or symptomatic, and is defined using assays for CMV antigenemia (pp65) or DNA PCR to demonstrate CMV in any tissue specimen. Tissue-invasive disease is defined as the presence of end-organ symptoms, as well as histologic evidence of invasive CMV. An allograft biopsy is sometimes needed to differentiate CMV hepatitis from acute allograft rejection.[101] Symptoms of tissue-invasive disease most often involve fever and neutropenia. Gastrointestinal disease, hepatitis, lymphadenopathy, thrombocytopenia, pneumonitis, pancreatitis, chorioretinitis, and meningoencephalitis can also occur.[102] Donor and recipient serologic CMV status are the most important contributors to determining risk of CMV infection. The highest risk occurs with the combination of a seropositive donor (D^+) and seronegative recipient (R^-). Polyclonal antibody T cell–depleting immunosuppressives also increase the risk for CMV disease.[103]

Treatment of CMV disease classically entails administration of IV ganciclovir in concert with minimization of immunosuppression. Because of its poor bioavailability, oral ganciclovir should not be used for active CMV disease. Valganciclovir is a prodrug of ganciclovir, and has been recently shown to have similar short- and long-term outcomes when compared with IV ganciclovir in a randomized controlled noninferiority trial for treatment of active CMV disease in transplant patients with non–life-threatening CMV disease.[104] Although only a small percentage of patients in this study were liver transplant recipients, these results may lead to more widespread usage of oral valganciclovir in the treatment of selected liver transplant patients with CMV disease. Cases of ganciclovir-resistant CMV disease, though rare, have been identified in liver transplant patients, and this issue merits careful monitoring and an effort to minimize further resistance.

Two strategies have been extensively used for prevention of CMV infection. Universal prophylaxis involves administration of antiviral therapy to all patients shortly after transplantation, usually for a duration of 3 months. Preemptive therapy, on the other hand, entails close monitoring of transplant recipients for evidence of viral replication. Treatment is initiated when there is evidence of CMV infection in an effort to prevent progression to clinical disease.[105] The optimal preventive strategy continues to be debated, but antiviral preventive therapy has clearly demonstrated excellent results, lending to

a 72% to 80% lower likelihood of developing CMV invasive disease and resulting in lower rates of allograft rejection[106] and death.[107] Despite the success in minimizing early-onset CMV, late-onset CMV disease has emerged as a prominent challenge, particularly in patients who have received antiviral prophylaxis. Late-onset CMV has been associated with increased mortality in liver transplant recipients.[108] Strategies such as extending the duration of prophylaxis and aggressively minimizing immunosuppression are currently being explored as possibilities for preventing late-onset CMV.[109]

Late Complications

Background

Hepatic, as well as nonhepatic factors, contribute to late posttransplant mortality (see **Table 49-3**). Chronic rejection and recurrence of the primary hepatic disease, which led to transplantation, are important hepatic factors. Chronic rejection will be discussed later, and recurrent disease will be explored in detail in Chapter 50. Nonhepatic factors play an increasing role in patient mortality as time passes posttransplant, and beyond 3 years posttransplant 58% of deaths are related to nonhepatic causes, largely due to cardiovascular disease and malignancy.[110] The incidence of a number of prominent cardiovascular disease risk factors increase after liver transplantation, and identifying and managing these risk factors is a critical component of posttransplant management.

Hypertension

Hypertension is the most common cardiovascular complication after liver transplantation. The prevalence of de novo arterial hypertension is as high as 77% posttransplant.[111] A number of mechanisms have been identified that contribute to this phenomenon. First of all, preexisting masked hypertension can be exposed with liver transplantation when pretransplant portal hypertension–mediated systemic vasodilation is reversed.[112] More importantly, immunosuppressive medications play a significant role in causing posttransplant hypertension. Calcineurin inhibitors, particularly CYA, have been clearly demonstrated to cause arterial hypertension via stimulation of renin release, up-regulation of angiotensin II receptors,[113] increased thromboxane release, and impairment of prostacyclin and nitric oxide-mediated vasodilation.[114] They have also been shown to cause sympathetic activation.[115] The sum of these effects is systemic vasoconstriction, resulting in hypertension. Corticosteroids have also been reported to contribute to hypertension via renin-angiotensin system activation,[116] increased sympathetic responsiveness, reduction of vasodepressor systems,[117] and direct activation of vascular smooth muscle glucocorticoid receptors.[118]

In addition to lifestyle modification involving weight loss, dietary sodium restriction, smoking cessation, regular exercise, and avoidance of excessive alcohol intake, many liver transplant patients require pharmacologic management of hypertension. Calcium channel blockers are generally considered first-line agents due to their proposed ability to counteract CNI-induced vasoconstriction.[111] Dihydropyridine calcium channel blockers are preferred agents due to interactions of nondihydropyridine calcium channel blockers with CNI metabolism. β-Blockers have also been used with success in liver transplant patients. Indeed, a recent controlled clinical trial demonstrated that monotherapy with carvedilol was as effective, and was better tolerated than nifedipine.[119] Circulating renin levels are low during the first year after liver transplantation, then steadily increase after the first posttransplant year, suggesting that the use of angiotensin-converting enzyme (ACE) inhibitors for treatment of hypertension may be ineffective in the first transplant year, but possibly efficacious afterward.[111] Combined therapy with nifedipine and ramipril has been shown to be more effective than combination carvedilol and ramipril.[119] ACE inhibitors must be used with particular caution, however, due to the prevalence of renal failure posttransplant. Modification of immunosuppressive regimens has also been shown to improve hypertension in liver transplant patients. Strategies involving replacement of CYA with TAC, as well as elimination of CNIs altogether, with or without substitution with MMF, have been shown to improve hypertension.[120-122] Corticosteroid withdrawal late after transplant improves hypertension.[123]

Dyslipidemia

Hypercholesterolemia is present in approximately 62% of liver transplant patients[111] and has been shown to be an independent risk factor for cardiovascular events in these patients.[124] Risk factors for posttransplant hyperlipidemia include pretransplant hyperlipidemia, as well as posttransplant renal dysfunction.[125] Genetics, obesity, and diabetes mellitus are also likely to contribute, but immunosuppressive agents are the most important contributors to posttransplant hyperlipidemia. Calcineurin inhibitors, particularly CYA, as well as sirolimus and corticosteroids have been shown to cause hyperlipidemia. CYA increases low-density lipoprotein (LDL) levels by inhibiting their catabolism via an effect on LDL receptor synthesis,[126] and also inhibits sterol 27-hydroxylase, an important enzyme for bile acid biosynthesis.[127] Sirolimus causes mixed hyperlipidemia, inducing hypertriglyceridemia via alterations in the insulin signaling pathway.[128] The lipid-altering effects of sirolimus are significantly more when used with CYA compared with TAC.[129] Corticosteroids increase total cholesterol, very-low-density lipoprotein, and triglycerides, and reduce high-density lipoprotein via activation of acetyl-CoA carboxylase, free fatty acid synthetase, and 3-hydroxy-3-methul glutaryl coenzyme A (HMG-CoA) reductase.[130]

Given the high prevalence of hyperlipidemia in liver transplant patients, screening for this complication should occur at least annually.[130] In addition to lifestyle modifications, many patients require lipid-lowering medications. HMG-CoA reductase inhibitors are first-line agents for treatment of hypercholesterolemia, and the efficacy of pravastatin and atorvastatin has been demonstrated in liver transplant patients.[131,132] To avoid toxicity, these medications should be started at low dosages, and titrated up slowly with close monitoring for side effects and drug interactions. Interestingly, some evidence suggests that HMG-CoA reductase inhibitors may have antimicrobial and immunosuppressive effects, which could expand their benefit in transplant patients.[133,134] When lipid-lowering pharmacologic therapies are unsuccessful for management of hyperlipidemia, changes in immunosuppression can be considered. Reduction of CNI dose,[121] conversion from CYA to TAC,[135] and withdrawal of corticosteroids[123] have been shown in small studies to improve hyperlipidemia.

Diabetes Mellitus

As many as 36.5% of liver transplant recipients develop new-onset diabetes mellitus in the post–liver transplant setting, and this complication has been clearly associated with diminished patient and graft survival rates.[136] Risk factors vary among studies, but older age, ethnic background (African American and Hispanic), family history, HCV virus status, and, most important, immunosuppressive therapies are the most clearly identified risk factors for new-onset diabetes mellitus after transplant.[137] Glucocorticoids increase the risk of diabetes mellitus by increasing gluconeogenesis and inducing insulin resistance.[138] CNIs directly damage pancreatic islet cells,[139] and the diabetogenic effects of TAC are enhanced in patients with HCV infection.[140] Unlike most other metabolic complications, new-onset diabetes mellitus occurs more frequently with TAC than with CYA.[47]

Based on published consensus guidelines, all posttransplant patients should be screened for diabetes; at least once a week for the first 4 weeks after transplantation, at 3, 6, and 12 months posttransplant; and then annually after the first year. New-onset diabetes mellitus posttransplant is treated in a manner similar to type 2 diabetes in the general population.[141] Insulin is often needed for management of early postoperative hyperglycemia, a condition that is often reversible. In persistent new-onset diabetes posttransplant, when dietary and lifestyle modifications fail to improve glucose control, an oral hypoglycemic agent is often used. Because many oral diabetic drugs are metabolized by the liver, however, these agents should not be initiated in the setting of unstable graft function.[142] Evidence regarding the safety and efficacy of specific agents is largely lacking. Rosiglitazone and pioglitazone, both thiazolidinedione insulin sensitizers, have been demonstrated to be safe and effective in treatment of posttransplant patients in single-center, noncontrolled trials. Sulfonylureas, metformin, meglitinide analogs, and α-glucosidase inhibitors have been used in transplant patients, though they have not been formally studied. Randomized controlled trials using oral agents and/or insulin in the posttransplant setting are needed before clear conclusions can be drawn. In the meantime, oral agents should be administered based on individual patient characteristics, as well as medication safety and side effect profiles. Steroid withdrawal has been shown in a meta-analysis to minimize de novo diabetes mellitus development.[33] Conversion from TAC to CYA is generally well tolerated and results in improvement of diabetes,[143] but often at the expense of worsened hypertension and dyslipidemia. Conversion from CNIs to MMF can improve diabetes control, but may increase the risk of rejection.[44]

Obesity

The prevalence of obesity, defined as a BMI greater than $30 \text{mm}^2/\text{kg}$, has been steadily increasing in the United States. Liver transplant recipients are no exception. The mean weight of liver transplant recipients has increased by approximately 1 kg/year from 1990 to 2006. Currently, approximately 25% of patients undergoing liver transplantation are obese.[144] The incidence of new-onset obesity posttransplant is also high.[145]

Studies of the effect of obesity on overall patient and graft survival rates have revealed conflicting results. A number of studies, including a study that involved 23,000 patients using the Scientific Registry of Transplant Recipients database, reported a decrement in survival rates in obese patients.[146] These studies, however, generally did not correct BMI for ascites volume, which could alter the results. The largest study to date that corrected BMI for ascites volume, involving 704 patients, did not find an effect of BMI on survival rates.[144] Reasons for development of obesity posttransplant include increased dietary intake due to improved health, genetic factors,[147] and immunosuppressive medications, namely corticosteroids and CYA.

Not surprisingly, the cornerstone of management of posttransplant obesity involves dietary and lifestyle modifications. Also, minimization of steroids and conversion from CYA to TAC have been shown to result in weight reduction in transplant patients.[120] For patients who are unresponsive to these interventions, pharmacotherapy and bariatric surgery are emerging options. A 6-month course of orlistat has been shown to be well tolerated and decreased waist circumference in liver transplant patients, though no change in BMI was noted.[148] Laparoscopic Roux-en-Y gastric bypass surgery after liver transplantation, as well as gastric band placement during liver transplantation surgery, have been performed successfully, but are not widely practiced at this time.[149,150]

Renal Disease

The incidence of post–liver transplant renal failure (glomerular filtration rate less than 30 ml/min/1.73 m^2) is 18% at 5 years,[151] and the incidence of end-stage renal disease in liver transplant patients is between 4.5% and 9.5% at 5 years.[152] Chronic renal failure posttransplant significantly increases posttransplant mortality. Renal failure in the early postoperative period is common, though largely reversible, and is often related to drug toxicities, acute tubular necrosis, or hypovolemia. Risk factors for persistent posttransplant renal failure vary among studies, but include pretransplant renal disease, older age at transplant, hypertension, diabetes mellitus, HCV, and use of CNIs. Chronic renal failure occurs more commonly with CYA than TAC,[151] and the pathogenesis of CNI-induced renal failure is related to compromise of the glomerular filtration rate due to reduced renal blood flow and reduction of the glomerular capillary ultrafiltration coefficient. Calcineurin inhibitors also cause renal interstitial fibrosis.[153]

Identification and aggressive management of risk factors for renal failure is important in liver transplant patients. Hypertension and diabetes should be aggressively controlled. Nephrotoxic agents should be avoided. Patients should be counseled to avoid salicylates and nonsteroidal antiinflammatory drugs because of their propensity for causing renal failure.[154] Calcineurin inhibitor-induced nephrotoxicity can often be managed by lowering the CNI dose or by substituting MMF or sirolimus for the CNI.[155,156] Liver transplant patients requiring renal replacement therapy should be considered for renal transplantation because recipients of renal transplants, despite a transient increase in mortality during the first month posttransplant, have a lower long-term risk of death than patients who are not transplanted.[151]

Atherosclerotic Cardiovascular Disease

Given the propensity of the above risk factors in liver transplant recipients, it is not surprising that the risk of cardiac ischemic events and death due to cardiovascular causes in these patients is higher than age- and sex-matched nontransplant populations.[157] Studies have confirmed that familiar cardiovascular risk factors, namely advanced age, gender, hypertension, diabetes, body weight, and dyslipidemia, also portend cardiovascular risk in liver transplant patients.[158] Indeed, cardiovascular events account for 21% of deaths in liver transplant recipients who survive more than 3 years posttransplant.[110] This elevated rate of cardiovascular risk is even more striking when considering that pretransplant patients with known symptomatic coronary artery disease are routinely excluded from transplantation at many centers, therefore the posttransplant population may be starting with a lower overall cardiovascular risk burden than the general population.[159] Diligent screening for, and aggressive management of, the previously stated reversible risk factors are integral components of posttransplant management. Also, careful management of immunosuppressive agents in an effort to strike a balance between minimization of cardiovascular side effects and suppression of rejection is also of paramount importance in the transplant setting.

Chronic Rejection

Chronic rejection causes approximately 16% of deaths in liver transplant recipients surviving more than 3 years.[110] Chronic rejection is often asymptomatic, with gradual worsening results in liver function tests—predominantly elevation of alkaline phosphatase and mild transaminitis. Graft biopsy is required to differentiate chronic rejection from disease recurrence, biliary complications, and other diseases. The Banff criteria for histologic diagnosis of chronic rejection include the presence of diffuse biliary epithelial senescence changes with or without bile duct loss, foam cell obliterative arteriopathy, or bile duct loss affecting greater than 50% of the portal tracts.[160] Obliterative arteriopathy, when present, causes changes that can also be noted on angiography. Chronic rejection classically occurs within the first 12 months after transplant, but exceptions exist. A reduction from previously measured rates has occurred during the last 2 decades due to advances in immunosuppressive therapies and increased histopathologic sophistication. The incidence of chronic rejection is currently less than 4% in liver transplant recipients.[86] Episodes of acute rejection often precede the onset of chronic rejection. Unlike acute rejection, however, chronic rejection is often irreversible, carries a poor prognosis, and often leads to graft failure. Indeed, chronic rejection accounts for approximately 14% of liver retransplantations.[161] When diagnosed early, however, alterations of the immunosuppressive regimen can sometimes salvage the graft.

Malignancy

The incidence of cancer is significantly higher among transplant patients than in the general population. The incidence of de novo nonmelanomatous skin cancer is increased threefold in liver transplant recipients. Not unexpectedly, the prognosis for transplant patients with de novo malignancy is worse than that for transplant patients without cancer.[162] Indeed, in some studies, de novo malignancy is the most common cause of posttransplant death in patients surviving more than 3 years after transplantation.[110] Loss of immunologic surveillance because of immunosuppressive medications, effects of cancer-promoting viruses, and direct oncogenic effects of immunosuppressive medications contribute to the increased risk of malignancy in posttransplant patients. Type and quantity of immunosuppressive therapy received appears to alter the risk of malignancy. Alcohol abuse, tobacco use, and advanced age also increase the rate of posttransplant malignancy.[163,164]

Cutaneous Malignancy

Skin cancer is the most common type of post–liver transplant cancer, occurring at higher rates than in the general population, and comprising approximately 54% of posttransplant malignancies.[163] Squamous and basal cell carcinomas are more common than melanomas,[165] and there is evidence that squamous cell carcinomas are more aggressive in transplant patients than in age- and sex-matched nontransplant populations.[166] Given the increased frequency and more aggressive nature of posttransplant cutaneous malignancies, many transplant centers recommend annual dermatologic evaluations for all patients. This strategy should be strongly considered for patients with additional risk factors for skin cancer, such as fair skin, previous skin cancer, and residence in an area where sun exposure is common.

Posttransplantation Lymphoproliferative Disease

Posttransplantation lymphoproliferative disease (PTLD) is defined as a lymphoid proliferation or lymphoma that develops as a consequence of pharmacologic immunosuppression following transplantation.[167] It is commonly of B-cell origin and is strongly associated with the Epstein-Barr virus (EBV) infection, a nearly ubiquitous latent infection in immunocompetent hosts that in immunocompromised patients is able to proliferate because of diminished T-cell immunity. Recipient EBV seronegativity is a prominent risk factor for development of PTLD. Clinical presentation is variable, ranging from lymphadenopathy to mononucleosis-like syndrome to systemic disease. Similarly, the spectrum of pathologic findings is wide, ranging from benign lymphoid hyperplasia to high-grade invasive lymphoma.[168] PTLD occurs with an incidence rate of less than 4% in adult liver transplant recipients, with approximately one half of cases occurring within 1 year of transplantation.[168,169] Diagnosis is made based on a biopsy taken from affected tissue and/or lymph nodes. Management options, none of which have been sufficiently evaluated with large, prospective randomized controlled trials, include reduction of immunosuppression to enhance immune function, anti–B-cell monoclonal antibodies and/or cytoxic chemotherapy to destroy lymphoma cells, and antiviral therapy to eliminate EBV. In patients without aggressive forms of PTLD, reduction of immunosuppression is generally considered first-line therapy if the risk of rejection is not considered to be prohibitive. Rituximab, a chimeric anti-CD20 IgG monoclonal antibody, is considered by many to be the first-line pharmacologic agent for patients who do not respond to initial immunosuppression reduction.[167] In patients with particularly high-grade histologic variants of PTLD, or those who do not respond to rituximab, cytotoxic chemotherapy is often used.[170] Overall, the mortality rate for PTLD is high.

Solid Organ Tumors

Noncutaneous, nonhematologic malignancies represent approximately 35% of posttransplant de novo malignancies. They have been shown to significantly worsen survival rates in transplant patients. One recently published large multicenter study demonstrated the 10-year probability of developing a gastrointestinal, lung, female genitourinary, or oropharyngeal cancer to be 3.6%, 2.0%, 1.8%, and 1.1%, respectively.[163] Oropharyngeal squamous cell carcinomas and lung cancers are suggested to be as much as 7.6 and 3.7 times more common, respectively, in liver transplant patients than in the general population, and are particularly common among those transplanted for alcoholic liver disease.[164,171] Prognosis with colorectal adenocarcinoma and lung cancer is worse in transplant recipients than in the general population.[171,172] Of note, there is some evidence that the incidence of breast and gynecologic cancers is lower in the posttransplant population,[173] possibly due to widespread screening programs for these malignancies before transplantation. Unfortunately, the majority of posttransplant noncutaneous cancers are diagnosed at late stages where treatment options are limited.[164] Routine cancer screening is an integral component of posttransplant management. At minimum, screening guidelines for specific cancers in the general population should be strictly followed in liver transplant patients, if not exceeded in particularly high-risk patients. For example, patients transplanted for primary sclerosing cholangitis with inflammatory bowel disease have a very high risk of de novo colon cancer posttransplant and should undergo annual colonic surveillance.[174]

Summary

Clearly management of liver transplant recipients is an important, diverse, and ever-evolving endeavor. Advances in posttransplantation management have led to improved long-term outcomes in liver transplant recipients. In the transplant setting, awareness of factors that determine posttransplant survival rates allows for optimal balancing of donor and recipient risk factors such as advanced donor and recipient age, donor and recipient severity of illness, and graft factors such as steatosis and CIT, enabling long-term posttransplant success without prohibitively restricting the number of organs available for transplantation. Understanding the efficacies and mechanisms, as well as the adverse effects and interactions of immunosuppressive medications, allows for informed administration of these medications in a manner that can strike a balance between suppression of rejection and minimization of side effects. Minimization, as well as comprehensive management, of early and late posttransplant vascular, biliary, immunologic, infectious, metabolic, cardiovascular, and neoplastic complications can sustain patient and graft survival rates and optimize patient quality of life.

Key References

Asberg A, et al. Long-term outcomes of CMV disease treatment with valganciclovir versus IV ganciclovir in solid organ transplant recipients. Am J Transplant 2009;9:1205–1213. (Ref.104)

Baccarani U, et al. De novo tumors are a major cause of late mortality after orthotopic liver transplantation. Transplant Proc 2009;41:1303–1305. (Ref.162)

Bekker J, Ploem S, de Jong KP. Early hepatic artery thrombosis after liver transplantation: a systematic review of the incidence, outcome and risk factors. Am J Transplant 2009;9:746–757. (Ref.71)

Berenguer M, et al. Significant improvement in the outcome of HCV-infected transplant recipients by avoiding rapid steroid tapering and potent induction immunosuppression. J Hepatol 2006;44:717–722. (Ref.30)

Burroughs AK, et al. 3-Month and 12-month mortality after first liver transplant in adults in Europe: predictive models for outcome. Lancet 2006;367:225–232. (Ref.4)

Burroughs SG, Busuttil RW. Optimal utilization of extended hepatic grafts. Surg Today 2009;39:746–751. (Ref.15)

Busuttil RW, et al. Analysis of long-term outcomes of 3200 liver transplantations over two decades. Ann Surg 2005;241:905–918. (Ref.16)

Campsen J, et al. Adjustable gastric banding in a morbidly obese patient during liver transplantation. Obes Surg 2008;18:1625–1627. (Ref.150)

Cassiman D, et al. Orlistat treatment is safe in overweight and obese liver transplant recipients: a prospective, open label trial. Transpl Int 2006;19:1000–1005. (Ref.148)

Cerutti E, et al. Bacterial- and fungal-positive cultures in organ donors: clinical impact in liver transplantation. Liver Transpl 2006;12:1253–1259. (Ref.10)

Chan EY, et al. Ischemic cholangiopathy following liver transplantation from donation after cardiac death donors. Liver Transpl 2008;14:604–610. (Ref.74)

Cicinnati VR, et al. Clinical trial: switch to combined mycophenolate mofetil and minimal dose calcineurin inhibitor in stable liver transplant patients: assessment of renal and allograft function, cardiovascular risk factors and immune monitoring. Aliment Pharmacol Ther 2007;26:1195–1208. (Ref.42)

Creput C, et al. Long-term effects of calcineurin inhibitor conversion to mycophenolate mofetil on renal function after liver transplantation. Liver Transpl 2007;13:1004–1010. (Ref.156)

Cross TJ, et al. Liver transplantation in patients over 60 and 65 years: an evaluation of long-term outcomes and survival. Liver Transpl 2007;13:1382–1388. (Ref.25)

Cruciani M, et al. Antifungal prophylaxis in liver transplant patients: a systematic review and meta-analysis. Liver Transpl 2006;12:850–858. (Ref.96)

Cuende N, et al. Donor characteristics associated with liver graft survival. Transplantation 2005;79:1445–1452. (Ref.11)

de Boccardo G, et al. The burden of chronic kidney disease in long-term liver transplant recipients. Transplant Proc 2008;40:1498–1503. (Ref.152)

Demetris AJ, et al. Liver biopsy interpretation for causes of late liver allograft dysfunction. Hepatology 2006;44:489–501. (Ref.160)

de Vera ME, et al. Liver transplantation using donation after cardiac death donors: long-term follow-up from a single center. Am J Transplant 2009;9:773–781. (Ref.13)

Duffy JP, et al. Vascular complications of orthotopic liver transplantation: experience in more than 4,200 patients. J Am Coll Surg 2009;208:896–905. (Ref.70)

Dumortier J, et al. Conversion from tacrolimus to cyclosporine in liver transplanted patients with diabetes mellitus. Liver Transpl 2006;12:659–664. (Ref.143)

Eschenauer GA, Lam SW, Carver PL. Antifungal prophylaxis in liver transplant recipients. Liver Transpl 2009;15:842–858. (Ref.99)

Ferraz-Neto BH, et al. Analysis of liver transplantation outcome in patients with MELD score > or = 30. Transplant Proc 2008;40:797–799. (Ref.26)

Fishman JA. Infection in solid-organ transplant recipients. N Engl J Med 2007;357:2601–2614. (Ref.102)

Freeman RB, et al. Liver and intestine transplantation in the United States, 1997-2006. Am J Transplant 2008;8:958–976. (Ref.1)

Galioto A, et al. Nifedipine versus carvedilol in the treatment of de novo arterial hypertension after liver transplantation: results of a controlled clinical trial. Liver Transpl 2008;14:1020–1028. (Ref.119)

Gastaca M. Extended criteria donors in liver transplantation: adapting donor quality and recipient. Transplant Proc 2009;41:975–979. (Ref.21)

Geissler EK. The impact of mTOR inhibitors on the development of malignancy. Transplant Proc 2008;40:S32–S35. (Ref.63)

Geissler EK, Schlitt HJ. Immunosuppression for liver transplantation. Gut 2009;58:452–463. (Ref.28)

Gluckelberger O, et al. Validation of cardiovascular risk scores in a liver transplant population. Liver Transpl 2006;12:394–401. (Ref.124)

Gomez CM, et al. Endoscopic management of biliary complications after adult living-donor versus deceased-donor liver transplantation. Transplantation 2009;88:1280–1285. (Ref.76)

Goodwin JE, Zhang J, Geller DS. A critical role for vascular smooth muscle in acute glucocorticoid-induced hypertension. J Am Soc Nephrol 2008;19:1291–1299. (Ref.118)

Gornicka B, et al. Pathomorphological features of acute rejection in patients after orthotopic liver transplantation: own experience. Transplant Proc 2006;38:221–225. (Ref.82)

Grinyo JM, Cruzado JM. Mycophenolate mofetil and calcineurin-inhibitor reduction: recent progress. Am J Transplant 2009;9:2447–2452. (Ref.41)

Groth CG. Forty years of liver transplantation: personal recollections. Transplant Proc 2008;40:1127–1129. (Ref.36)

Guckelberger O, et al. Coronary event rates in liver transplant recipients reflect the increased prevalence of cardiovascular risk-factors. Transpl Int 2005;18:967–974. (Ref.158)

Haddad E, et al. Cyclosporin versus tacrolimus for liver transplanted patients. Cochrane Database Syst Rev 2006;4:CD005161. (Ref.47)

Hellinger WC, et al. Risk stratification and targeted antifungal prophylaxis for prevention of aspergillosis and other invasive mold infections after liver transplantation. Liver Transpl 2005;11:656–662. (Ref.91)

Hodson EM, et al. Antiviral medications for preventing cytomegalovirus disease in solid organ transplant recipients. Cochrane Database Syst Rev 2008;2:CD003774. (Ref.107)

Hodson EM, et al. Antiviral medications to prevent cytomegalovirus disease and early death in recipients of solid-organ transplants: a systematic review of randomized controlled trials. Lancet 2005;365:2105–2115. (Ref.100)

Horrow MM, et al. Sonographic diagnosis and outcome of hepatic artery thrombosis after orthotopic liver transplantation in adults. AJR Am J Roentgenol 2007;189:346–352. (Ref.69)

Jensen GS, Wiseman A, Trotter JF. Sirolimus conversion for renal preservation in liver transplantation: not so fast. Liver Transpl 2008;14:601–603. (Ref.61)

Johnson EE, et al. A 30-year analysis of colorectal adenocarcinoma in transplant recipients and proposal for altered screening. J Gastrointest Surg 2007;11:272–279. (Ref.172)

Ju MK, et al. Invasive pulmonary aspergillosis after solid organ transplantation: diagnosis and treatment based on 28 years of transplantation experience. Transplant Proc 2009;41:375–378. (Ref.94)

Kalil AC, et al. Meta-analysis: the efficacy of strategies to prevent organ disease by cytomegalovirus in solid organ transplant recipients. Ann Intern Med 2005;143:870–880. (Ref.106)

Karie-Guiges S, et al. Long-term function in liver transplant recipients and impact of immunosuppressive regimens (calcineurin inhibitors alone or in combination with mycophenolate mofetil): the TRY study. Liver Transpl 2009;15:1083–1091. (Ref.155)

Kawecki D, et al. Etiological agents of bacteremia in the early period after liver transplantation. Transplant Proc 2007;39:2816–2821. (Ref.90)

Kemmer N, et al. Liver transplantation trends for older recipients: regional and ethnic variations. Transplantation 2008;86:104–107. (Ref.24)

Kitazono MT, et al. Magnetic resonance cholangiography of biliary strictures after liver transplantation: a prospective double-blind study. J Magn Reson Imaging 2007;25:1168–1173. (Ref.79)

Klintmalm GB, et al. Corticosteroid-free immunosuppression with daclizumab in HCV + liver transplant recipients: 1-year interim results of the HCV-3 study. Liver Transpl 2007;13:1521–1531. (Ref.56)

Kuene S, Blair J. Viral and fungal infections after liver transplantation: part II. Liver Transpl 2006;12:2–11. (Ref.103)

Leonard J, et al. The impact of obesity on long-term outcomes in liver transplant recipients: results of the NIDDK liver transplant database. Am J Transplant 2008;8:667–672. (Ref.144)

Lerut J, Sanchez-Fueyo A. An appraisal of tolerance in liver transplantation. Am J Transplant 2006;6:1774–1780. (Ref.83)

Limaye AP, et al. Impact of cytomegalovirus in organ transplant recipients in the era of antiviral prophylaxis. Transplantation 2006;81:1645–1652. (Ref.108)

Lupo L, et al. Basiliximab versus steroids in double therapy immunosuppression in liver transplantation: a prospective randomized clinical trial. Transplantation 2008;86:925–931. (Ref.57)

Marchetti P. New-onset diabetes after liver transplantation: from pathogenesis to management. Liver Transpl 2005;11:612–620. (Ref.142)

Mateo R, et al. Risk factors for graft survival after liver transplantation from donation after cardiac death donors: an analysis of OPTN/UNOS data. Am J Transplant 2006;6:791–796. (Ref.14)

Matinlauri IH, et al. Changes in liver graft rejections over time. Transplant Proc 2006;38:2663–2666. (Ref.86)

Meier-Kriesche HU, et al. Immunosuppression: evolution in practice and trends, 1994-2004. Am J Transplant 2006;6:1111–1131. (Ref.34)

Mells G, Neuberger J. Reducing the risks of cardiovascular disease in liver allograft recipients. Transplantation 2007;83:1141–1150. (Ref.130)

Moon JI, et al. Negative impact of new-onset diabetes mellitus on patient and graft survival after liver transplantation: long-term follow up. Transplantation 2006;82:1625–1628. (Ref.136)

Moore DE, et al. Impact of donor, technical, and recipient risk factors on survival and quality of life after liver transplantation. Arch Surg 2005;140: 273–277. (Ref.18)

Neuberger JM, et al. Delayed introduction of reduced-dose tacrolimus, and renal function in liver transplantation: the "ReSpECT" study. Am J Transplant 2009;9:327–336. (Ref.54)

Nickkholgh A, et al. Utilization of extended donor criteria in liver transplantation: a comprehensive review of the literature. Nephrol Dial Transplant 2007;22:S29–S36. (Ref.20)

Noujaim HM, et al. Expanding postmortem donor pool using steatotic liver grafts: a new look. Transplantation 2009;87:919–925. (Ref.23)

Pappas PG, et al. Invasive fungal infections in low-risk liver transplant recipients: a multi-center prospective observational study. Am J Transplant 2006;6: 386–391. (Ref.98)

Perez-Daga JA, et al. Impact of donor age on the results of liver transplantation in hepatitis C virus-positive recipients. Transplant Proc 2008;40:2959–2961. (Ref.5)

Piselli P, et al. Incidence and timing of infections after liver transplant in Italy. Transplant Proc 2007;39:1950–1952. (Ref.88)

Pons JA, et al. Immunosuppression withdrawal improves long-term metabolic parameters, cardiovascular risk factors and renal function in liver transplant patients. Clin Transpl 2009;23:329–336. (Ref.121)

Razonable RR. Cytomegalovirus infection after liver transplantation: current concepts and challenges. World J Gastroenterol 2008;14:4849–4860. (Ref.109)

Reese PP, et al. Donor age and cold ischemia interact to produce inferior 90-day liver allograft survival. Transplantation 2008;85:1737–1744. (Ref.17)

Roy A, et al. Tacrolimus as intervention in the treatment of hyperlipidemia after liver transplant. Transplantation 2006;82:494–500. (Ref.135)

Sanchez-Perez B, et al. Influence of immunosuppression and effect of hepatitis C virus on new onset diabetes mellitus in liver transplant recipients. Transplant Proc 2008;40:2994–2996. (Ref.140)

Segev DL, et al. Minimizing risk associated with elderly liver donors by matching to preferred recipients. Hepatology 2007;46:1907–1918. (Ref.3)

Segev DL, et al. Steroid avoidance in liver transplantation: meta-analysis and meta-regression of randomized trials. Liver Transpl 2008;14:512–525. (Ref.32)

Selck FW, et al. Utilization, outcomes, and retransplantation of liver allografts from donation after cardiac death. Ann Surg 2008;248:599–606. (Ref.12)

Selzner M, et al. Recipient age affects long-term outcome and hepatitis C recurrence in old donor livers following transplantation. Liver Transpl 2009; 15:1288–1295. (Ref.6)

Sgourakis G, et al. Corticosteroid-free immunosuppression in liver transplantation: a meta-analysis and meta-regression of outcomes. Transpl Int 2009;22:892–905. (Ref.33)

Sharma S, Gurakar A, Jabbour N. Biliary strictures following liver transplantation: past, present and preventive strategies. Liver Transpl 2008;14: 759–769. (Ref.75)

Shenoy S, et al. Sirolimus conversion in liver transplant recipients with renal dysfunction: a prospective, randomized, single-center trial. Transplantation 2007;83:1389–1392. (Ref.59)

Short KR, Bigelow ML, Nair KS. Short-term prednisone use antagonizes insulin's anabolic effect on muscle protein and glucose metabolism in young healthy people. Am J Physiol Endocrinol Metab 2009;297:1260–1268. (Ref.138)

Sun HY, Singh N. Antimicrobial and immunomodulatory attributes of statins: relevance in sold-organ transplant recipients. Clin Infect Dis 2009;48:745–755. (Ref.133)

Svoboda J, Kotloff R, Tsai DE. Management of patients with post-transplant lymphoproliferative disorder: the role of rituximab. Transpl Int 2006;19: 259–269. (Ref.167)

Taner CB, Bathala V, Nguyen JH. Primary nonfunction in liver transplantation: a single-center experience. Transplant Proc 2008;40:3566–3568. (Ref.64)

Taylor AL, et al. Anthracycline-based chemotherapy as first-line treatment in adults with malignant posttransplant lymphoproliferative disorder after solid organ transplantation. Transplantation 2006;82:375–381. (Ref.170)

Taylor AL, Watson CJ, Bradley JA. Immunosuppressive agents in solid organ transplantation: mechanisms of action and therapeutic efficacy. Crit Rev Oncol Hematol 2005;56:23–46. (Ref.29)

Tichansky DS, Madan AK. Laparoscopic Roux-en-Y gastric bypass is safe and feasible after orthotopic liver transplantation. Obes Surg 2005;15:1481–1486. (Ref.149)

Toniutto P, et al. Weight gain after liver transplantation and the insertion/ deletion polymorphism of the angiotensin-converting enzyme gene. Transplantation 2005;79:1338–1343. (Ref.147)

Uemura T, et al. Liver retransplantation for primary nonfunction: analysis of a 20-year single-center experience. Liver Transpl 2007;13:227–233. (Ref.65)

United Network for Organ Sharing. Transplants [Online]. Cited Jan 16, 2010. Available from URL: www.unos.org. (Ref.8)

Vivarelli M, et al. Influence of steroids on HCV recurrence after liver transplantation: a prospective study. J Hepatol 2007;47:793–798. (Ref.31)

Vivarelli M, et al. Liver transplantation for hepatocellular carcinoma under calcineurin inhibitors. Ann Surg 2008;248:857–862. (Ref.48)

Vivarelli M, et al. Analysis of risk factors for tumor recurrence after liver transplantation for hepatocellular carcinoma: key role of immunosuppression. Liver Transpl 2005;11:497–503. (Ref.49)

Waki K. UNOS Liver Registry: ten year survivals. Clin Transpl 2006:29–39. (Ref.2)

Watson CJ, et al. A randomized controlled trial of late conversion from calcineurin inhibitor-based to sirolimus-based immunosuppression in liver transplant recipients with impaired renal function. Liver Transpl 2007;13: 1694–1702. (Ref.60)

Watt KD, et al. Long-term probability of and mortality from de novo malignancy after liver transplantation. Gastroenterology 2009;137:2010–2017. (Ref.163)

Welling TH, et al. Biliary complications following liver transplantation in the model for end-stage liver disease era: effect of donor, recipient, and technical factors. Liver Transpl 2008;14:73–80. (Ref.78)

Xia D, et al. Postoperative severe pneumonia in adult liver transplant recipients. Transplant Proc 2006;38:2974–2978. (Ref.89)

Zanus G, et al. Alcohol abuse and de novo tumors in liver transplantation. Transplant Proc 2009;41:1310–1312. (Ref.164)

Zhang J, et al. Effects of sirolimus on the growth of transplanted hepatocellular carcinoma. Chin J Hepatol 2009;17:413–416. (Ref.62)

A complete list of references can be found at www.expertconsult.com.

Recurrent Viral Diseases after Liver Transplantation

Jennifer C. Lai and Norah A. Terrault

ABBREVIATIONS

ACR acute cellular rejection
AR acute rejection
ATG antithymocyte globulin
CI confidence interval
CMV cytomegalovirus
CTL cytotoxic T lymphocyte
DDLT deceased donor liver transplant
DRI donor risk index
HBcAg hepatitis B core antigen
HBeAg hepatitis B e antigen
HBIG hepatitis B immune globulin
HBsAg hepatitis B surface antigen
HBV hepatitis B virus

HCC hepatocellular carcinoma
HCIG hepatitis C immune globulin
HCV hepatitis C virus
HDV hepatitis D virus
HIV human immunodeficiency virus
HLA human leukocyte antigen
HR hazard ratio
HVPG hepatic venous pressure gradient
IL interleukin
IL-2RA IL-2 receptor antagonist
KIR killer immunoglobulin–like receptor
LDLT living donor liver transplant
MELD Model for End-Stage Liver Disease

MHC major histocompatibility class
MMF mycophenolate mofetil
NA nucleotide analogue
NK natural killer cell
NKT natural killer T cell
PD1 programmed cell death-1
RR relative risk
SCID severe combined immunodeficiency
SVR sustained virologic response
Treg regulatory T lymphocyte
UNOS United Network for Organ Sharing

Hepatitis B and Liver Transplantation

Among transplant programs in North America and western Europe, hepatitis B virus (HBV) disease accounts for 5% to 10% of the total transplants performed. In other areas of the world where HBV is endemic, it is the leading indication for liver transplantation. Over the last 2 decades there has been a significant decline in decompensated cirrhosis as an indication for liver transplantation in HBV-infected patients in the United States, probably because of the benefits of antiviral therapy in preventing and treating HBV-related cirrhosis.[1] Concurrently, there has been an upward trend in the proportion of patients undergoing liver transplantation for HBV-associated hepatocellular carcinoma (HCC), most likely because of the increasing use of liver transplantation for the treatment of small HCCs and the prioritization of patients with HCC for transplantation (**Fig. 50-1**).[1]

Natural History after Transplantation

The early experience with liver transplantation in HBV-infected patients revealed a high rate of reinfection and accelerated progression of disease after transplantation, which resulted in 5-year survival rates of less than 50%.[2,3] The availability of prophylactic therapies—first, hepatitis B immune globulin (HBIG), and later, oral antivirals such as lamivudine—transformed the outcomes of patients with HBV infection undergoing liver transplantation. In a retrospective study of HBV-infected adults undergoing primary liver transplantation in the United States between 1987 and 2002, the 1-year survival probability improved from 71% in 1987 to 1991 to 87% in 1997 to 2002, and the 5-year survival rate increased from 53% in 1987 to 1991 to 76% in 1997 to 2002 (**Fig. 50-2**).[4] The progressive improvement in survival rates parallels the availability of therapeutic interventions to prevent and treat HBV disease in transplant recipients.[4] The current experience with liver transplantation in HBV-infected patients is demonstrated in a contemporary U.S. multicenter cohort of 170 HBV-infected patients who underwent transplantation between 2001 and 2007 in which the 5-year survival rate was 85% or greater, with minimal variation by racial subgroup.[5]

Natural history studies from the era before the use of prophylactic therapies showed that the level of HBV DNA at the time of transplantation was the principal factor affecting the posttransplant risk for recurrent infection. In a landmark paper by Samuel and colleagues in which 372 European hepatitis B surface antigen (HBsAg)-positive patients underwent

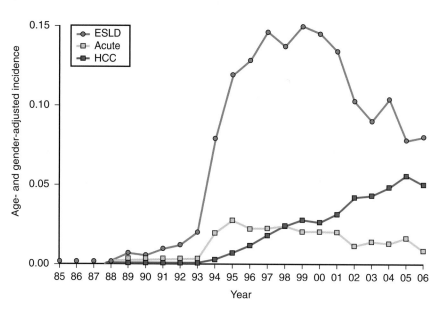

Fig. 50-1 **Incidence rates of end-stage liver disease (ESLD) cirrhosis and hepatocellular carcinoma among waiting list registrants for transplantation for HBV-related liver disease.** Over the last 2 decades there has been a significant decline in decompensated cirrhosis as an indication for liver transplantation in HBV-infected patients in the United States, which probably reflects the benefits of antiviral therapy on prevention and treatment of HBV-related cirrhosis. HCC, hepatocellular carcinoma. *(From Kim WR, et al. Trends in waiting list registration for liver transplantation for viral hepatitis in the United States. Gastroenterology 2009;137:1680–1686.)*

liver transplantation from 1977 to 1990 (the majority without prophylaxis), the 3-year actuarial risk for HBV recurrence was highest (83%) in those with HBV-related cirrhosis and an HBV DNA content of 10^5 copies/ml or greater at time of transplantation, intermediate in those without detectable HBV DNA or Hepatitis B e antigen (HBeAg) (58%), and lowest in those with hepatitis D virus (HDV) co-infection (32%) or fulminant HBV infection (17%) (**Fig. 50-3**).[6]

Similarly, in the current era of routine use of prophylactic therapies to prevent HBV recurrence, failure of prophylactic therapy with the development of recurrent HBV infection is most consistently associated with levels of HBV DNA before transplantation,[7,8] although the overall frequency of recurrent HBV infection with current combination prophylactic regimens is very low.[9,10] Other factors identified as being of potential importance are recurrence of HCC,[11] with HBV replication in tumor cells possibly serving as a source for recurrence of HBV infection, and the presence of drug-resistant HBV strains before transplantation,[9,10,12] with preexistence of mutations making such patients less likely to be protected by single-agent prophylactic regimens.

Pathology of Hepatitis B after Transplantation

In general, the histopathologic findings of recurrent HBV infection in a liver allograft are similar to those in a non-transplanted liver with HBV.[13,14] Acute and chronic pathologic features may be seen, as well as a unique variant form of severe recurrent HBV termed the fibrosing cholestatic variant. The latter, first described in liver transplant recipients,[15] has also been identified in renal and bone marrow transplant recipients,[16,17] and there is one case report of a patient with chronic HBV infection treated with immunosuppressive therapy.[18]

In the absence of prophylactic therapy, the earliest manifestations of recurrent HBV infection include cytoplasmic and nuclear expression of hepatitis B core antigen (HBcAg) in hepatocytes by immunostaining 2 to 5 weeks after transplantation, typically in the absence of hepatocyte necrosis or inflammation.[2] Acute hepatitis, which develops on average 8 to 10 weeks after transplantation, is manifested histologically as diffuse hepatocyte ballooning and lobular disarray with spotty hepatocyte necrosis.[13,14] A portal-based mononuclear infiltrate of varying severity is seen. There is a gradual increase in the percentage of hepatocytes containing both nuclear and cytoplasmic HBcAg, especially during the evolution of acute to chronic disease.[14] Ground glass cells are infrequently seen during the acute and early phase of infection.[13] There is no significant bile duct damage or endothelial injury, thus making the distinction between early recurrent HBV infection and acute cellular rejection quite straightforward. In a small percentage of patients, a more severe hepatitis with bridging and submassive necrosis is seen and is typically associated with rapid progression to cirrhosis or graft loss.[14]

Over time, the changes associated with acute hepatitis evolve into those of chronic hepatitis, with portal-based inflammation and fibrosis and the presence of piecemeal necrosis and ground glass cells, typically in inverse proportion to the necroinflammatory activity.[13] The inflammatory infiltrates are predominantly of the plasma lymphocytic type (**Fig. 50-4, A**). Immunohistochemical studies reveal HBcAg in the cytoplasm and nucleus of a large number of hepatocytes (see **Fig. 50-4, B**). Overall, the histologic features in the chronic phase of infection are the same as those in nontransplant patients except for the rapidity of progression over time. Evolution to recurrent cirrhosis can occur within 2 years in the absence of antiviral therapy.[19]

As mentioned earlier, fibrosing cholestatic HBV is an infrequent form of HBV disease that is seen only in immunosuppressed patient populations. Unique histologic features include extensive hepatocyte ballooning, marked ductular reaction and cholestasis, pericellular and portal fibrosis, and a paucity of inflammatory infiltrates (**Fig. 50-5, A**).[15,20] High levels of viral replication are present as evidenced by high levels of expression of HBcAg and HBsAg in the liver (see **Fig. 50-5, B**),[21,22] thus lending support to the concept of a direct

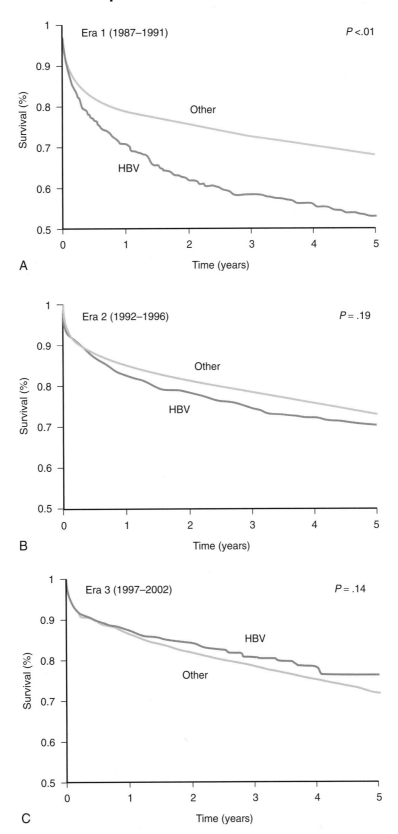

Fig. 50-2 Comparison of survival after liver transplantation between recipients with HBV and those with other diagnoses. A, 1987 to 1991; B, 1992 to 1996; C, 1997 to 2002. The 1-year survival probability in patients undergoing liver transplantation for HBV infection improved from 71% in 1987 to 1991 to 87% in 1997 to 2002, and the 5-year survival probability increased from 53% in 1987 to 1991 to 76% in 1997 to 2002. *(From Kim WR, et al. Outcome of liver transplantation for hepatitis B in the United States. Liver Transpl 2004;10:968–974.)*

cytopathic form of liver injury. Biochemical features include markedly abnormal serum bilirubin levels and prothrombin times, but only modest increases in serum aminotransferase levels and signs of progressive liver failure. In the absence of antiviral therapy, the outcome is rapidly fatal.[23]

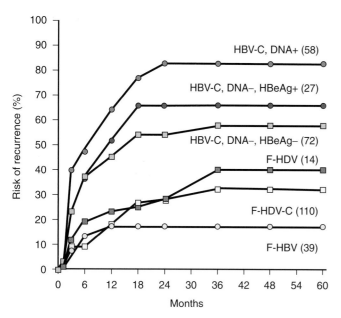

Fig. 50-3 **Actuarial risk for recurrence of HBV infection as indicated by the reappearance of hepatitis B surface antigen (HBsAg) according to initial liver disease and pretransplant viral replication status.** Among 372 European HBsAg-positive patients who underwent liver transplantation from 1997 to 1990 (the majority without prophylaxis), the 3-year actuarial risk for HBV recurrence was highest (83%) in those with HBV-associated cirrhosis (HBV-C) and an HBV DNA content of 10^5 copies/ml or greater at time of transplantation, intermediate in those without HBV DNA detectable or HBeAg present (58%), and lowest in those with HDV co-infection (HDV-C) (32%) and fulminant HBV infection (F-HBV) (17%). HBeAg, hepatitis B e antigen. *(From Samuel D, et al. Liver transplantation in European patients with the hepatitis B surface antigen. N Engl J Med 1993;329:1842–1847.)*

Pathogenesis of Posttransplantation HBV Disease

The mechanism of liver injury in liver transplant recipients with recurrent HBV disease is incompletely understood.[24] Levels of HBV DNA increase significantly after transplantation, presumably related to the administration of immunosuppressive drugs. Although HBV is known to have a corticosteroid-responsive promoter region within its genome that activates HBV replication,[25] the exact mechanisms by which other immunosuppressive drugs affect HBV replication are less certain. In early in vitro studies, prednisolone and azathioprine were associated with approximately twofold and four-fold increases, respectively, in intracellular viral DNA and RNA levels, whereas cyclosporine had no significant effect on viral RNA or DNA levels.[26] However, the combination of all three immunosuppressive agents increased the level of intracellular viral DNA eight-fold, indicative of an additive effect.[26] Major changes in immunosuppression, such as occurs in the treatment of acute rejection (AR), may be particularly important in promoting HBV replication and liver injury.

High viral replication is associated with the production of viral proteins in large quantities, and the clinicopathologic entity of fibrosing cholestatic hepatitis is hypothesized to represent a variant of injury that is primarily cytotoxic and related to the accumulation of viral proteins.[21] Pre-S mutants and precore mutants have been linked with severe recurrence, including fibrosing cholestatic hepatitis.[27-29] Mutants with deletions in the pre-S1 region that are capable of replication but exhibit defective secretion of viral particles, including surface protein, may lead to the cellular accumulation of viral replicative intermediates.[27] With available prophylaxis, this pathologic entity is rare but has been described with the emergence of drug-resistant HBV after transplantation.[30,31]

In most transplant recipients, immune-mediated liver injury is the primary mechanism of progressive fibrosis and graft loss. The immunologic events that determine the outcome of recurrent infection are only partially understood. In immunocompetent patients with self-limited HBV infection, a vigorous, polyclonal, and multispecific CD4+ (T helper

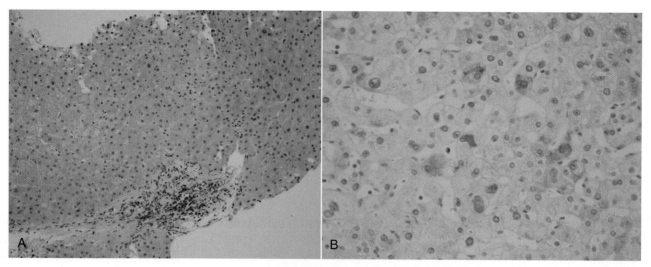

Fig. 50-4 **Histopathologic features of chronic recurrent HBV infection. A,** The inflammatory infiltrates are predominantly of the plasma lymphocytic type. **B,** Immunohistochemical studies reveal that HBcAg is detectable in the cytoplasm and nucleus of a large number of hepatocytes. *(Photomicrographs courtesy of Linda Ferrell, University of California, San Francisco.)*

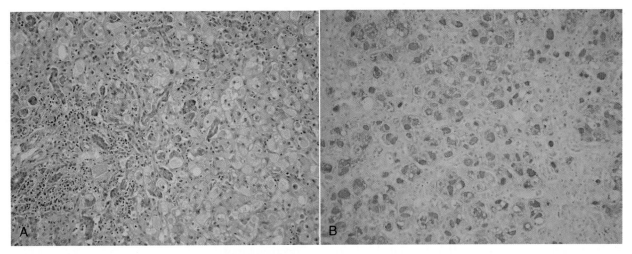

Fig. 50-5 **Histopathologic features of fibrosing cholestatic HBV infection. A,** Unique histologic features include extensive hepatocyte ballooning, marked ductular reaction and cholestasis, pericellular and portal fibrosis, and a paucity of inflammatory infiltrates. **B,** High levels of viral replication are present as evidenced by high levels of expression of HBcAg and HBsAg in the liver. *(Photomicrographs courtesy of Linda Ferrell, University of California, San Francisco.)*

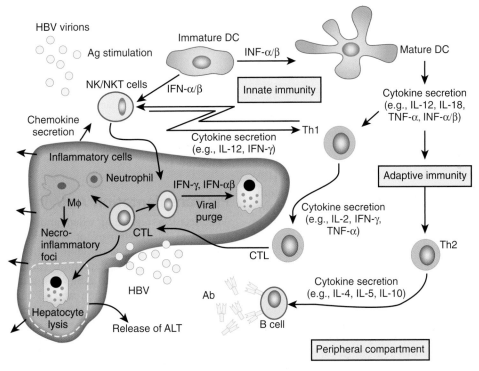

Fig. 50-6 **Innate and adaptive immune responses to HBV infection.** In immunocompetent patients with self-limited HBV infection, a vigorous, polyclonal, and multispecific CD4+ (Th1 profile predominant) and cytotoxic T-lymphocyte (CTL) response are seen. Additionally, the innate immune response to HBV plays an important role in determining the outcome of acute infection. Ab, antibody; Ag, antigen; ALT, alanine transaminase; DC, dendritic cell; IFN, interferon; IL-12, interleukin-12; Mø, macrophage; NK, natural killer cell; NKT, natural killer T cell; TNF-α, tumor necrosis factor-α. *(From Lee JY, Locarnini S. Hepatitis B virus: pathogenesis, viral intermediates, and viral replication. Clin Liver Dis 2004;8:301–320.)*

1 [Th1] profile predominant) and cytotoxic T-lymphocyte (CTL) response is seen (**Fig. 50-6**).[32] HBV peptides presented by HLA class I molecules on hepatocytes targeted by CTLs expressing the same HLA antigen provide the major effector mechanism for the control of HBV replication.[33] In the liver transplant setting, where HLA matching is not typically present (because it is not required for transplantation), this primary mechanism of HBV immune control is likely to be altered. Studies evaluating whether the degree of HLA matching influences the risk and severity of HBV recurrence have yielded inconsistent results.[34-37] Some of this inconsistency may be methodologic (e.g., HLA antigens are determined by phenotype rather than genotype), whereas the number and quality of the matches may be another explanation. Moreover,

with the low rates of recurrence of HBV infection seen with current prophylactic protocols, the ability to discern an independent contribution of HLA matching to graft recurrence rates is quite limited. In a recent European cohort of 85 liver transplant recipients with HBV, matching of HLA-A and HLA-B was associated with lower rates of HBV recurrence and better graft survival than were zero matches.[35]

An alternative, class I–independent pathway of immune-mediated viral clearance has been demonstrated and is probably relevant in the transplant setting.[38] Following transplantation, the new liver graft is repopulated by antigen-presenting cells and mononuclear cells from the recipient.[39] Studies have shown that intrahepatic infiltrates in HBV-reinfected allografts are predominantly composed of CD4+ T lymphocytes. It is proposed that viral antigens on newly infected hepatocytes are presented to recipient T helper cells in association with antigen-specific HLA class II molecules on recipient Kupffer cells and macrophages that repopulate the liver after engraftment. This interaction triggers expansion and activation of antigen-specific CD4+ T cells and the subsequent production of proinflammatory cytokines, especially tumor necrosis factor, which leads to further amplification of the inflammatory response and injury to virally infected hepatocytes.[24,40] Additionally, as shown in immunocompetent patients, the innate immune response to HBV plays an important role in determining the outcome of acute infection[41] (see **Fig. 50-6**), but studies in liver transplant recipients are lacking.

As prophylactic therapies have become more effective and recurrent infection a less frequent and less devastating complication, emphasis has shifted toward studying the immune response under the effects of prophylactic therapies to better understand factors contributing to the failure of prophylaxis.[40,42] In a study of transplant recipients treated with prophylactic antivirals without HBIG, the frequency and magnitude of peripheral CD4+ T-cell responses against HBV envelope and nucleocapsid antigens were found to be significantly lower in patients who were HBV negative with prophylaxis than in pretransplant patients with chronic HBV and in posttransplant patients with recurrence.[40] In another study of liver transplant recipients given only HBIG as prophylaxis, peripheral CD4+ T-cell responses were not detected, but CD8+ T-cell responses, especially against nucleocapsid antigens, were present, although the responses were fewer and stronger than in patients with chronic hepatitis.[42] In this study, patients receiving HBIG prophylaxis had a cellular immune profile most similar to subjects with chronic HBV infection with suppressed HBV DNA.[42] Differences in prophylaxis, patient characteristics, and methods of measuring HBV responses (e.g., defined mostly by HLA-A2–restricted epitopes vs. overlapping peptides of nucleocapsid and envelope proteins) may partially explain the differences in results. Additional studies of immune responses in transplant recipients undergoing different prophylactic regimens may help identify correlates of immune protection that would allow more individualized prophylactic treatment.

Prevention of Recurrent HBV Disease

The most effective strategy to prevent recurrent HBV disease consists of pretransplant HBV viral suppression

Table 50-1 Prophylactic Therapies for HBV-Infected Transplantation Recipients

RISK FOR RECURRENT HBV	PROPHYLACTIC TREATMENT OPTIONS
Low Risk	
No known drug resistance Undetectable HBV DNA levels at transplantation	Short-term HBIG + indefinite antivirals or combination oral antiviral drugs[50-52]
Higher Risk	
Preexisting drug resistance HBV DNA positive at transplantation HIV co-infected HDV co-infected Retransplantation Noncompliance	Long-term HBIG + combination oral antiviral drugs[53-59]

HBIG, hepatitis B immune globulin; HBV, hepatitis B virus; HDV, hepatitis D virus; HIV, human immunodeficiency virus

with oral nucleoside/nucleotide analogues (NAs), followed by posttransplant combined prophylactic therapy with HBIG and NAs. Posttransplant combination HBIG/NA regimens vary with respect to dose, duration, and method of administration of HBIG, but this combined approach is highly effective and reduces HBV recurrence rates to less than 10%.[10,43-49] In recent years, with the availability of potent antiviral drugs with low rates of drug resistance, alternative protocols have been used, including short-term or low-dose HBIG (or both) combined with long-term NA therapy (**Table 50-1**).[50-59]

Pretransplantation Antiviral Treatment

The decision regarding when and what oral antiviral to initiate in the pretransplant setting is determined by the patient's replication status (level of HBV DNA) and the anticipated time until transplantation. The goals of pretransplant antiviral treatment are to achieve an undetectable HBV DNA level before transplantation and to minimize the risk for emergence of resistant viral strains. Although the largest published experience of pretransplant antiviral therapy is with lamivudine and adefovir, alternative antivirals with lower rates of resistance, such as tenofovir and entecavir, are the preferred drugs for wait-listed patients.[53] However, in resource-constrained situations, lamivudine—when given for a limited duration of treatment before transplantation to minimize the risk for pretransplant resistance—may be an acceptable low-cost option.[60]

Lamivudine, a nucleoside analogue, has been shown to be safe and effective in patients awaiting liver transplantation, including those with decompensated cirrhosis.[61-63] Monotherapy with lamivudine in the pretransplant setting has been associated with loss of HBV DNA in 80% to 100% of patients within 2 to 6 months of therapy and an excellent safety profile.[61-67] In a trial of 23 patients with decompensated cirrhosis secondary to chronic HBV infection, pretransplant treatment with lamivudine monotherapy resulted in a statistically significant survival advantage in comparison with a historical cohort of untreated controls.[61] However, the major limitation of pretransplant use of lamivudine has been development of the rtM204V/I mutation in the HBV DNA polymerase gene in 8% to 27% of treated patients after 9 to 18 months of therapy, which is associated with a risk for hepatic decompensation as a result of virologic breakthrough.[61-64,67]

For patients with lamivudine-resistant HBV infection, the use of adefovir results in viral suppression and a low rate of resistance after 1 to 2 years of treatment.[68] In a multicenter, open-label study of 128 patients awaiting liver transplantation—98% of whom had lamivudine-resistant HBV—81% had undetectable HBV DNA levels by polymerase chain reaction after 48 weeks of treatment with a mean change in serum HBV DNA of −3.5 $\log_{10}$ copies/ml.[54,68] As expected, patients with lower baseline HBV DNA levels, defined as 5 $\log_{10}$ copies/ml or less, were more likely to experience viral suppression by 48 weeks than were patients with baseline HBV DNA levels of 5 $\log_{10}$ copies/ml or greater (100% vs. 60%).[68] The adefovir resistance mutation rtN236T was identified in only 2 of 114 (2%) patients at the end of 96 weeks of follow-up, and discontinuation of the drug secondary to treatment-related adverse events occurred in only 4% of the pretransplant study cohort.[54]

Newer-generation NAs, including entecavir, telbivudine, and tenofovir, have been approved for the treatment of chronic HBV infection. When compared with lamivudine or adefovir, these drugs have been shown to have greater antiviral potency and to result in a more rapid decline in HBV DNA levels in both HBeAg-positive and HBeAg-negative noncirrhotic patients.[69-72] Fewer studies, however, have been performed in patients with advanced liver disease and in the pretransplant setting. In a study that included 120 patients with advanced fibrosis, treatment with entecavir resulted in undetectable HBV DNA levels in 91% of HBeAg-positive patients and 96% of HBeAg-negative patients versus 57% and 61% treated with lamivudine, respectively.[73] In none of these patients did resistance to entecavir develop after 48 weeks of treatment.[73] In 70 treatment-naïve decompensated cirrhotics in a separate study, 75% of HBeAg-positive and 98% of HBeAg-negative patients achieved HBV DNA suppression.[74] Telbivudine has been found to be more effective than lamivudine for HBV DNA suppression, but resistance rates are higher than seen with entecavir, with 1- and 2-year resistance rates of 4% and 22% to 25% for HBeAg-positive patients and 3% and 9% to 11% for HBeAg-negative patients.[72,75] Therefore caution is advised with the use of telbivudine monotherapy in the pretransplant setting. Data on the use of tenofovir disoproxil in decompensated cirrhotics are limited to case reports,[76,77] but data on noncirrhotic patients indicate a favorable profile with high antiviral potency and the absence of resistance with treatment periods of up to 3 years.[78]

Prophylactic Therapy
Combination Hepatitis B Immune Globulin and Nucleoside/Nucleotide Analogues after Liver Transplantation

Earlier studies using HBIG monotherapy for prevention of graft reinfection after liver transplantation demonstrated HBV recurrence-free rates of 81% to 86% at 2 years when high-dose HBIG was used to maintain trough anti-HBs titers higher than 500 IU/L.[7,79] More recently, combination HBIG

and NA therapy has proved to be more effective at minimizing graft reinfection and has thus become the standard of care for HBV-infected liver transplant recipients in the majority of transplant centers. This combination approach has reduced HBV recurrence rates to approximately 7% (**Table 50-2**).[10,43-49,80] Three recent metaanalyses have clearly demonstrated the superiority of combination HBIG plus lamivudine over HBIG alone, with a reduction in posttransplant HBV recurrence by 62% to 81% with the combination regimen.[81-83] One meta-analysis reported a significant reduction in the development of YMDD (rtM204V) mutants with HBIG plus lamivudine versus lamivudine monotherapy (relative risk [RR] = 0.4; 95% confidence interval [CI], 0.23 to 0.72).[82] Only one study has evaluated the efficacy of combination HBIG and entecavir versus HBIG plus lamivudine.[84] The rate of HBV DNA recurrence was 0% in the HBIG/entecavir group versus 11% in the HBIG/lamivudine group ($P < .05$), but there was no difference in overall survival between the two groups.[84] No studies have yet reported the results of the combined use of HBIG and tenofovir, and although tenofovir-induced nephrotoxicity is a potential concern, the efficacy of such a regimen would be expected to be at least comparable with that of HBIG/lamivudine or HBIG/entecavir regimens.

Alternatives to Long-Term Combination HBIG plus Antiviral Therapy

To date, no consensus exists on the optimal dosing, duration, and route of HBIG therapy. Alternatives to high-dose, long-term intravenous HBIG therapy have been sought because of the high cost and inconvenience of this treatment.

INTRAMUSCULAR HBIG

Two large studies of 261 HBV-infected transplant recipients evaluating the use of lamivudine plus intramuscular HBIG, administered at doses of 400 to 800 IU daily for the first week, then monthly thereafter, demonstrated an actuarial risk for HBV recurrence of 1% at 1 year and 4% at 5 years in one study[10] and 14% at 1 year and 15% at 2 years in the other study.[43] In both studies, the most important predictor of HBV recurrence was an HBV DNA level of greater than 10⁶ copies/ ml at the time of transplantation.[10,43] Given the significantly lower cost and comparable efficacy of low-dose intramuscular and higher-dose intravenous HBIG,[85] intramuscular HBIG in combination with lamivudine may be viewed as the optimal strategy for the prevention of HBV recurrence, especially for patients with low HBV DNA levels at the time of transplantation. However, there may still be a role for higher-dose intravenous HBIG in patients at greatest risk for recurrence (e.g., those with HBV DNA >10⁵ copies/ml before transplantation) (see **Table 50-1**).

DISCONTINUATION OF HBIG

An alternative strategy to the use of long-term HBIG therapy is to transition from combination HBIG/NA to NA therapy alone after a defined period. In a trial of 29 patients—all of whom had undetectable HBV DNA at the time of transplantation—who were randomized after 1 month of intravenous HBIG therapy to receive combination lamivudine/HBIG (15 patients) versus lamivudine monotherapy (14 patients), 29 of 29 (100%) patients remained HBsAg negative at the end of the 18-month follow-up

Table 50-2 Prevention of HBV Recurrence after Liver Transplantation with Lamivudine and HBIG

AUTHORS	PATIENTS (N)	PRETREATMENT VIROLOGIC STATUS OF TRANSPLANT PATIENTS		HBV DNA⁺ AT OLT	TRANSPLANTED (N)	PREVENTION OF HBV RECURRENCE		HBV RECURRENCE, N (%)	FOLLOW-UP, MONTHS, MEDIAN (RANGE)
		HBV DNA⁺	HBeAg⁺			Pre-OLT Duration, Months, Median (Range)	Post-OLT		
Markowitz et al.[44]	14	5	1	1	14	LAM, 3 (0.7-7.8)	LAM + HBIG IV	0 (0%)	13 (NA)
Rosenau et al.[45]	21	11	3	5	21	LAM, 4.6 (0.06-14.1)	LAM + HBIG IV	2 (9.5%)	21 (2-49)
Marzano et al.[46]	33	26	7	0	26	LAM, 4.6 (0.6-14.1)	LAM + HBIG IV	1 (4%)	30 (NA)
Han et al.[47]	59	NA	NA	NA	59	LAM, NA	LAM + HBIG IV	0 (0%)	15 (1-61.8)
Roche et al.[48]	15	15	5	4	15	LAM, 4.6 (0.3-13)	LAM + HBIG IV	1 (6.6%)	15 (3-36)
Seehofer et al.[49]	17	17	9	5	17	LAM, 10.6 (1-28)	LAM + HBIG IV	3 (18%)	25 (9-49)
Zheng et al.[43]	114	NA	NA	NA	114	LAM, NA	LAM + HBIG IM	16 (14%)	16 (8-36)
Gane et al.[10]	147	121	46	121	147	LAM, 3 (0-59)	LAM + HBIG IM	7 (4.7%)	62 (1-125)
Total	420				413			30 (7.3%)	19

Adapted from Terrault N, Roche B, Samuel D. Management of the hepatitis B virus in the liver transplantation setting: a European and an American perspective. Liver Transpl 2005;11:716–732.

HBeAg, hepatitis B e antigen; HBIG, hepatitis B immune globulin; HBV, hepatitis B virus; IV, intravenous; LAM, lamivudine; NA, not available; OLT, orthotopic liver transplantation

period.[50] The YMDD mutation was detected in 3 of 29 (10%) patients who were HBV DNA–positive by polymerase chain reaction only.[50] Given the low genetic barrier to resistance with lamivudine monotherapy, a strategy involving combinations of oral antivirals after HBIG discontinuation is predicted to be more efficacious. A small retrospective review of 10 patients who received combination HBIG/lamivudine therapy for 6 months followed by combination lamivudine/adefovir revealed a 0% HBV recurrence rate at a mean follow-up of 21 months (range, 16 to 25 months),[51] but it is important to note that all patients were HBV DNA negative at the time of transplantation and were therefore at low risk for HBV recurrence. In an Australasian trial of patients who had shown no evidence of HBV recurrence after 12 months of combination HBIG/lamivudine therapy—16 of whom were randomized to receive lamivudine/adefovir and 18 to continue HBIG/lamivudine—there were no documented cases of HBV recurrence in either arm after a median follow-up of 21 months.[52] A comparison of costs of the two arms revealed a 40% annual cost savings in the lamivudine/adefovir arm over the HBIG/lamivudine arm.[52] Based on the available data, discontinuation of HBIG in favor of NAs (either as monotherapy or as combination NA therapy) is an effective alternative to long-term HBIG therapy, at least in patients with low HBV viral loads at the time of

transplantation and with adequate adherence to NA therapy (see **Table 50-1**).

VACCINATION AFTER DISCONTINUATION OF HBIG

Although earlier studies reported successful prevention of HBV recurrence with use of the recombinant HBV vaccine followed by discontinuation of HBIG,[86,87] more recent studies have raised doubt regarding the efficacy of this strategy.[88-93] Even though these more recent studies were heterogeneous in the timing of HBV vaccination and NA use after discontinuation of HBIG, the overall response rate to HBV vaccination was low, with HBsAg titers greater than 100 IU/L developing in only 8 of 126 (6%) patients in the studies.[88-93] Until larger studies with longer follow-up are conducted to evaluate which patients are most appropriate for this strategy, HBV vaccination in lieu of HBIG cannot be recommended.

Viral Detection in Patients Receiving Prophylaxis

Despite overall low rates of recurrent HBV disease with current prophylaxis regimens, some studies have demonstrated that low-level HBV DNA can be detected in the serum, liver, and peripheral blood mononuclear cells of patients without serologic evidence of HBV recurrence.[46,94,95] Of 25 patients who received combination HBIG and lamivudine continuously after transplantation and remained HBsAg negative, HBcAg was found in 4 (16%) by immunochemical staining of liver biopsy specimens.[46] In two recent studies that included 66 patients without evidence of HBV recurrence, 23 of 66 (35%) had total HBV DNA and 11 of 66 (17%) had covalently closed circular (ccc) HBV DNA detected in posttransplant liver biopsy specimens.[88,89] In contrast, in a study that included 24 patients who received long-term HBIG immunoprophylaxis and had undetectable HBV DNA after transplantation, none had HBcAg detected in the liver or HBV DNA detected in peripheral blood mononuclear cells.[48] Although there may be a subset of patients in whom HBV infection is completely eradicated after transplantation or whose own immune system can control the infection,[95a] thus far the clinically applicable diagnostic tools to identify this group of patients are lacking. The presence of HBV DNA in liver and peripheral blood mononuclear cells provides the rationale for lifelong HBV prophylaxis to prevent recurrent HBV disease.

Treatment of Recurrent HBV Disease

Given the safety, tolerability, and efficacy of current prophylactic therapies for the prevention of HBV reinfection, recurrence of HBV after transplantation, as defined by the reappearance of serum HBsAg, is uncommon. In patients in whom recurrence develops despite optimal prophylaxis,

long-term treatment with antivirals is required to prevent progressive fibrosis and graft loss. Lifelong antiviral therapy prolongs graft survival, and with current antiviral options, graft loss from recurrent HBV disease is infrequent. Given the need for long-term therapy, a drug or drug combination with a low likelihood of virologic breakthrough is desirable, and monitoring of response to treatment by checking HBV DNA levels at regular intervals is needed.

The limitations of suboptimal antiviral therapy after transplantation are highlighted by the previous experience with lamivudine. As in the nontransplant setting, high rates of lamivudine resistance approaching 40% after 1 to 5 years of follow-up were seen with posttransplant lamivudine monotherapy.[96-100] Among 16 patients in whom YMDD mutations developed in the setting of posttransplant lamivudine monotherapy, severe clinical hepatitis developed in 3 of 16 (19%), and 2 of 16 (13%) died of hepatic failure.[97,98,100]

For transplant recipients with lamivudine resistance, there is cross-resistance with the nucleoside analogues telbivudine and emtricitabine and reduced efficacy of entecavir. Thus, for patients with resistance to lamivudine or any of the nucleoside analogues, the only treatment options are the nucleotide analogues adefovir and tenofovir (**Table 50-3**).* Combination therapy is recommended once drug resistance is documented to minimize the risk for subsequent treatment failure and the development of multidrug-resistant HBV.[53] The largest study

---

*References 54, 55, 58, 68, 84, 101, and 102.

Table 50-3 Treatment Options for Liver Transplantation Recipients with Recurrent HBV Infection and Drug Resistance*

RESISTANCE PROFILE[†]	DRUG OPTIONS	PERCENTAGE WITH UNDETECTABLE HBV DNA	COMMENTS
Nucleotide resistance Lamivudine Telbivudine Entecavir	(1) Add adefovir[54,68,101]	34%-64% at week 48 65% at week 96 78% at week 144	25% with elevated creatinine 4% discontinuation rate
	(2) Add tenofovir[55,102]	80%-88% at 64-76 weeks	Limited safety data after transplantation Monitor for nephrotoxicity
	(3) Change to tenofovir-emtricitabine[58]	38% at a median of 42 months[‡]	Limited safety data after transplantation Monitor for nephrotoxicity
Nucleoside resistance Adefovir Tenofovir[‡]	(1) Add lamivudine[54,68,101]	34%-64% at week 48 65% at week 96 78% at week 144	25% with elevated creatinine 4% discontinuation rate
	(2) Add entecavir	No data available	Entecavir monotherapy shown to be safe and effective after transplantation[84]
	(3) Add telbivudine	No data available	Reports of myositis
	(4) Change to tenofovir-emtricitabine[58]	38% at median of 42 months[‡]	Limited safety data after transplantation Monitor for nephrotoxicity

*Combination therapy is recommended to minimize the risk for subsequent treatment failure.
[†]Resistance testing recommended to further guide antiviral choices.
[‡]Data from HBV-HIV co-infected liver transplant recipients.
HBV, hepatitis B virus; HIV, human immunodeficiency virus.

to date of combination NA therapy involved the use of adefovir plus lamivudine in 241 posttransplant patients with lamivudine-resistant recurrent HBV and found undetectable serum HBV DNA in 65% of patients at week 96 and in 78% at week 144.[54] It is important to note that 46% of these patients experienced treatment-related adverse events—25% of whom had elevated creatinine levels—but adverse events of any kind resulted in discontinuation of treatment in only 4% of patients.[54] Moreover, the study was uncontrolled, thus limiting interpretation of the creatinine abnormalities in a posttransplant population. Studies evaluating the addition of tenofovir are limited, but one study that included eight lamivudine-resistant patients who received tenofovir reported that 7 (88%) of the patients had undetectable HBV DNA levels after a median follow-up of 19.3 months (range, 14 to 26 months).[55] Given its high potency against HBV in the nontransplant setting, tenofovir is likely to emerge as the antiviral of choice for posttransplant nucleotide-resistant HBV (see **Table 50-3**).

Several reports have demonstrated the emergence of multidrug-resistant HBV strains in both the pretransplant and posttransplant settings.[103,104] Preexisting viral variants, as well as the selection of mutations during exposure to sequential antiviral therapies and HBIG, contribute to the emergence of complex multidrug-resistant HBV.[104]

Management of Hepatitis B in Special Populations

HIV Co-Infected Patients

As our experience in managing HBV/human immunodeficiency virus (HIV) co-infection grows, liver transplantation in these patients has been gaining wider acceptance. Two retrospective studies that included a total of eight HBV/HIV co-infected patients who underwent liver transplantation reported no patient or graft loss after a follow-up range of 1.5 to 7 years.[56,57] The median CD4[+] T-cell count before transplantation was 229×10^6/L (range, 104 to 439), and all patients had undetectable HBV DNA levels at the time of transplantation.[56,57] A recent prospective cohort study of 22 co-infected patients confirmed these favorable survival rates—when compared with an HBV mono-infected cohort, patient and graft survival were similar (85% for co-infected vs. 100% for mono-infected patients; $P = .08$ log rank) at a median follow-up of 4 years.[58] All patients were maintained on combination HBIG/nucleotide analogue (NA) therapy after transplantation, and no patients had evidence of HBV recurrence.[58] However, 7 of 16 (44%) had detectable HBV DNA in serum by sensitive detection methods, thus suggesting that these patients need to maintain lifelong HBV prophylaxis. Overall, these data support the efficacy of liver transplantation for the treatment of end-stage liver disease in HBV/HIV co-infected patients.

HDV Co-Infected Patients

Although earlier studies evaluating posttransplant outcomes in HDV co-infected patients revealed HDV reinfection rates of 80% to 100%,[105,106] the universal use of prophylactic HBV therapy has greatly reduced the burden of HDV recurrence. Long-term administration of HBIG monotherapy in 68 HDV co-infected patients resulted in a 5-year actuarial survival rate of 88%.[107] Although liver HDV antigen or serum HDV RNA was detected in 88% of patients within the first year, active HBV and HDV replication and clinical hepatitis developed in only 7 of 68 (10%) patients.[107] A more recent study that included 25 HBV/HDV co-infected patients who received combination HBIG/lamivudine immunoprophylaxis reported a 0% HBV and HDV recurrence rate after a mean follow-up of 40 (range, 13 to 74) months.[59]

Recipients of Anti–HBc-Positive Donors

To increase the total number of grafts available in the donor pool, transplant centers have increasingly used extended-criteria donors, including anti-HBc–positive donors. Approximately 4% of the donor liver grafts used in the United States are anti-HBc positive and HBsAg negative.[108] Transplantation of these organs is accompanied by an increased risk for de novo HBV infection. Among 133 consecutive anti-HBc-positive donors, only 8.2% of the liver grafts showed evidence of HBV DNA on biopsy.[109] One recent systematic review involving 903 recipients of anti-HBc–positive liver grafts in 39 studies reported that 5-year graft survival rates were similar between HBsAg-positive patients receiving anti-HBc–positive grafts (67%) and HBsAg-positive patients receiving anti-HBc–negative grafts (68%).[110] De novo infection developed in 149 of 788 (19%) of HBV naive patients at a median of 24 (5 to 54) months after transplantation, but only 30 (8%) de novo infections occurred in patients receiving HBV prophylaxis ($n = 366$) versus 119 (28%) in patients not receiving prophylaxis ($n = 422$, $P < .001$).[110] In addition, HBV-naïve recipients experienced increased rates of de novo HBV infection in comparison with anti-HBc/anti-HBs–positive recipients (48% vs. 15%, respectively; $P < .001$).[110] In a separate systematic review of 13 studies of anti-HBc–positive graft recipients, there was no significant difference in the rates of de novo infection among the 73 patients who received lamivudine monotherapy versus the 110 patients who received combination lamivudine/HBIG (2.7% vs. 3.7%, respectively; $P = .74$).[111] These data suggest that with the routine administration of prophylactic therapy, transplantation of anti-HBc–positive grafts is a safe and effective means of increasing the availability of donor livers. In addition, lamivudine monotherapy in HBsAg-negative recipients of anti-HBc–positive liver grafts is highly effective, low in cost, and, therefore, may be the preferred therapy.[111]

Retransplantation

With the widespread use of prophylactic therapies, retransplantation for recurrence of HBV disease is an infrequent event. For the rare patients in whom drug-resistant HBV disease develops that is not controlled with antivirals, retransplantation can still be considered with the knowledge that high-dose HBIG combined with antivirals is likely to be effective. This was demonstrated during the early experience with lamivudine-resistant recurrent disease.[112] In this scenario, high-dose HBIG and maintenance of anti-HBs titers of 500 IU/L or greater may be critical,[112] and HBIG in combination with NAs should be continued in the long term to prevent HBV recurrence in the second graft.[112,113]

Hepatitis C and Liver Transplantation

Chronic infection with hepatitis C virus (HCV) is the leading indication for liver transplantation in the Western world. In the United States, more than 50% of all liver transplants from 1985 to 2006 were performed for complications of HCV disease.[1] Over the past 2 decades, the number of transplants for HCV-associated decompensated cirrhosis has plateaued, whereas the number of transplants for HCV-related HCC has increased dramatically (**Fig. 50-7**).[1,114] The latter reflects introduction of the Model for End-Stage Liver Disease (MELD) score prioritization for HCC, as well as an increased incidence of HCC in HCV-infected persons.[1] Projections of the number of patients needing liver transplantation suggest an increasing disease burden over the next 5 to 10 years and then a decline related to a lower prevalence of HCV in the population, as well as the beneficial effects of successful HCV treatment.[1]

Natural History after Transplantation

Viral recurrence after liver transplantation is universal in patients who are viremic before transplantation.[115,116] Alanine or aspartate aminotransferase levels are elevated persistently or intermittently in the majority of transplant recipients, but up to 30% of patients have persistently normal levels despite the presence of histologic damage on biopsy specimens.[117] Thus serum aminotransferase levels are not a reliable marker of recurrent HCV, and protocol liver biopsies are useful to assess the severity and progression of liver disease. Approximately 60% to 80% of recipients show evidence of recurrent histologic disease at 1 year following transplantation.[116,118] Delayed, spontaneous clearance of HCV infection has been reported after liver transplantation but is rare.[119-123]

Hepatitis C disease progression is accelerated in liver transplant recipients in comparison with immunocompetent patients with HCV.[124,125] The rate of HCV-associated progression of fibrosis is nonlinear and highly variable (**Fig. 50-8**).[116,118,124,126] The median time to cirrhosis is 9 years, but in up to 30% of patients cirrhosis develops within the first 5 years.[124,125,126] Once cirrhosis is established, patients have a 30% to 42% annual risk for decompensation—a rate that is markedly elevated relative to immunocompetent patients with HCV-associated cirrhosis.[124,128,129]

Overall survival is reduced in HCV-infected patients in comparison with HCV-negative patients, with 5-year patient and graft survival rates of 64% to 70% and 57% to 76%, and 10-year patient and graft survival rates of 51% to 69% and 57% to 63%, respectively.[125,130-134] In a large retrospective study using data from 11,000 transplants (4400 were HCV positive) available through the United Network for Organ Sharing (UNOS) registry, patients who received transplants for HCV-related liver disease had a 23% increased risk for death and a 30% increased risk for graft loss at 5 years when compared with patients who received transplants for non–HCV-related causes (**Fig. 50-9**).[125] The major causes of death and graft loss in HCV-infected transplant recipients are complications related to recurrent HCV-associated cirrhosis.[116,130,135]

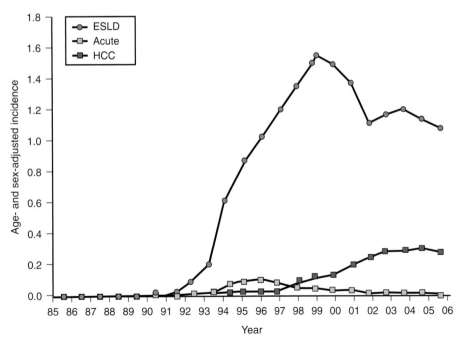

Fig. 50-7 **Incidence rates of decompensated cirrhosis and hepatocellular carcinoma (HCC) in waiting list registrants for transplantation for HCV-related liver disease.** Over the last 2 decades, the number of transplants for HCV-associated end-stage liver disease (ESLD) has plateaued, whereas the number of transplants for HCV-related HCC has increased dramatically. Incidence rates per year for waiting list registrants infected with HCV, adjusted for age and sex, are shown. *(From Kim WR, et al. Trends in waiting list registration for liver transplantation for viral hepatitis in the United States. Gastroenterology 2009;137:1680–1686.)*

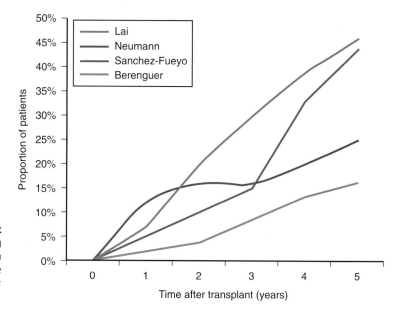

Fig. 50-8 Rates of advanced fibrosis in HCV transplant recipients. The reported proportions of patients with bridging fibrosis or cirrhosis at each year after transplantation from different transplant centers in the United States and Europe are shown. (*Data from Lai et al.,[126] 2009; Neumann et al.,[116] 2004; Sanchez-Fueyo et al.,[118] 2002; and Berenguer et al.,[124] 2000.*)

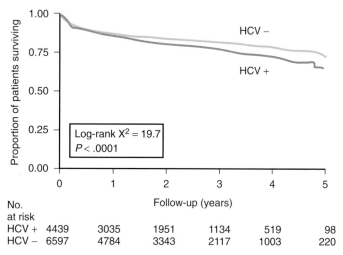

Log-rank $X^2 = 19.7$
$P < .0001$

No. at risk						
HCV +	4439	3035	1951	1134	519	98
HCV −	6597	4784	3343	2117	1003	220

Fig. 50-9 Survival of U.S. adult liver transplant recipients with and without HCV infection. Kaplan-Meier estimates of posttransplant patient survival according to hepatitis C status show that patients who received transplants because of HCV-related liver disease had a 23% increased risk for death and a 30% increased risk for graft loss at 5 years when compared with patients who received transplants for non-HCV causes. The number of patients in each group at each time point is indicated. (*From Forman LM, et al. The association between hepatitis C infection and survival after orthotopic liver transplantation. Gastroenterology 2002;122: 889–896.*)

Assessment of Hepatic Fibrosis in Liver Transplantation Recipients

Although liver biopsy is currently the favored method for assessing disease severity, this procedure is cumbersome as a repeat measure of fibrosis, is associated with some risk, and may understage the severity of fibrosis, especially with smaller specimens and those stained with hematoxylin and eosin alone (without trichrome).[136-138] Given these limitations of liver biopsy, alternative methods for staging disease

have been examined (**Table 50-4**).[139-144] Transient elastography measures the velocity of a low-frequency shear wave across the hepatic parenchyma and correlates impedance with the severity of fibrosis. In two studies of liver transplant recipients with HCV, an elastography score cutoff of 8.5 kPa had 90% sensitivity and 81% specificity, and a cutoff of 10.1 kPa had 94% sensitivity and 89% specificity in distinguishing stage 0 to 1 from stage 2 to 4 disease (on a 4-point scale).[139,140] Recent data have suggested that the slope of liver stiffness measured every 3 months in the first year after liver transplantation may identify patients at risk for rapid versus slow progression of fibrosis (slope of 0.42 vs. 0.05, respectively; $P < .0001$).[145] Measurement of the hepatic venous pressure gradient (HVPG) has also been evaluated as a predictor of disease severity and graft survival.[141,142] Two studies have found a significant correlation between fibrosis stage and HVPG.[141,142] The disadvantage of HVPG as a predictive test is its invasive nature and the need for specialized expertise. Elastography, in contrast, is noninvasive and technically less demanding.

Serum fibrosis markers have also been studied as an alternative method of staging recurrent disease (see **Table 50-4**). In a study of 133 recipients, a composite score of 2 or greater derived from three serum fibrosis markers—serum hyaluronic acid, amino-terminal propeptide of type III procollagen, and tissue inhibitor of matrix metalloproteinase type 1—accurately identified 12 of 20 (60%) patients with bridging fibrosis or cirrhosis and 15 of 17 (88%) patients with clinically significant portal hypertension (defined as an HVPG ≥10).[144] In a small study of 49 HCV-infected recipients, a serum hyaluronic acid level of 90 μg/L or greater had a sensitivity and specificity of 80%, and a YKL-40 level of 200 μg/L or greater had a sensitivity and specificity of 87% and 100%, respectively, for identifying recipients with rapid progression of fibrosis as defined by an increase in fibrosis score by 2 or more points (on a 6-point Ishak fibrosis scale) within a mean of 39 ± 6 months (range, 29 to 49 months).[143] Pending further multicenter confirmatory studies of the accuracy and feasibility of these methods in posttransplant patients, liver biopsy remains

Table 50-4 Alternative Methods for Detection of Advanced Recurrent HCV Disease in Liver Transplantation Recipients

TEST	CUTOFF VALUE	OUTCOME	SENSITIVITY (%)	SPECIFICITY (%)	POSITIVE PREDICTIVE VALUE (%)	NEGATIVE PREDICTIVE VALUE (%)
Transient elastography[139]	8.5 kPa	Bridging fibrosis/cirrhosis	90	81	79	92
Transient elastography[140]	10.1 kPa	Bridging fibrosis/cirrhosis	94	89	81	94
Hepatic venous pressure gradient[141,142]	≥6	Bridging fibrosis/cirrhosis	72	89	72	89
Hyaluronic acid[143]	≥90 µg/L	Rapid progression of fibrosis*	80	80	67	89
YKL-40[143]	≥200 µg/L		87	100	100	87
Composite score (serum HA, PIIINP, TIMP-1)[144]	≥2	Bridging fibrosis/Cirrhosis	65	94	83	84

*2 of 6 points from first biopsy (5 ± 2 months post-LT) to second biopsy (39 ± 6 months post-LT).

HCV, hepatitis C virus; kPa, kilopascal; PIIINP, amino-terminal propeptide of type III procollagen; TIMP-1, tissue inhibitor of matrix metalloproteinase type 1

the gold standard for assessing both disease severity and progression.

Pathology of Hepatitis C after Transplantation

Although findings may vary, early histopathologic features of recurrent HCV infection include lobular inflammation and focal apoptotic hepatocyte necrosis (**Fig. 50-10, A**). Steatosis is a nonspecific finding of early HCV recurrence,[146] and portal inflammation—mainly with mononuclear cells often as lymphoid aggregates—may be found as the disease progresses. Any bile duct injury, if present, is typically mild.[147] Severe necroinflammation lesions, including focal necrosis, interface hepatitis, and confluent necrosis, may be seen and are highly associated with the early development of cirrhosis.[148] Over time, the histology of recurrent chronic HCV infection is indistinguishable from that seen in the nontransplant setting (see **Fig. 50-10, B**).

An aggressive variant of recurrent HCV infection has been recognized and called cholestatic hepatitis C; it occurs in 2% to 8% of transplants for HCV-related liver disease.[135,149-152] Initially labeled fibrosing cholestatic hepatitis based on similarities to fibrosing cholestatic hepatitis in transplant recipients with recurrent hepatitis B, cholestatic hepatitis C is characterized clinically by severe hyperbilirubinemia (mean rise in serum bilirubin of 24.7 mg/dl) in the setting of high HCV RNA levels, typically occurring within the first 2 years after transplantation.[149] Examination of biopsy specimens reveals lobular inflammation, bile duct proliferation, and cholestasis; areas of bridging and confluent necrosis can be rapidly replaced by fibrosis (see **Fig. 50-10, C**).[149,152] In the absence of treatment, cholestatic hepatitis can lead to early graft loss.

Another variant of recurrent hepatitis C is plasma cell or autoimmune-like hepatitis.[153-156] This has been described in the context of antiviral therapy and has unique histologic findings. Some cases are associated with elevated levels of autoantibodies (antinuclear antibody, anti–smooth muscle antibody, and anti–liver-kidney-microsomal antibody) and elevated immunoglobulin levels.[155,156] The key histologic features include severe interface inflammatory activity consisting predominantly of plasma cells and perivenular necroinflammation (see **Fig. 50-10, D**).[155,156] In a recent study of 40 patients in whom plasma cell hepatitis developed after transplantation for HCV-related liver disease, graft failure occurred in 19 of 40 (48%) patients and cirrhosis developed in an additional 7 of 40 (18%) after a median follow-up of 67 months.[154] Clinical and histologic responses to treatment with corticosteroids and amplification of baseline immunosuppression have been reported and are associated with good outcomes.[153,156]

Acute Rejection in Patients with Hepatitis C

Histopathologically, AR may be difficult to differentiate from recurrent HCV, with some[157] but not all[158] studies reporting low interobserver and intraobserver agreement in the diagnosis. Because recurrent HCV disease occurs universally after liver transplantation, most biopsy samples will have evidence of the presence of HCV, and the features of ACR are superimposed on that background. Features that are characteristically associated with acute cellular rejection (ACR)—and not recurrent HCV—include bile duct injury and necrosis with overlapping nuclei, endotheliitis, and inflammatory infiltrates around the portal tracts consisting of eosinophils, lymphocytes, and occasional neutrophils.[159,160]

New tools to improve the accuracy of diagnosis of ACR in the setting of HCV infection are highly desired. MxA protein, a marker for type I interferon production that is strongly expressed by hepatocytes in the presence of HCV, has yielded mixed results.[161,162] In a retrospective study of 54 HCV-infected patients with or without ACR, the Cylex immune function assay, which measures levels of adenosine triphosphate

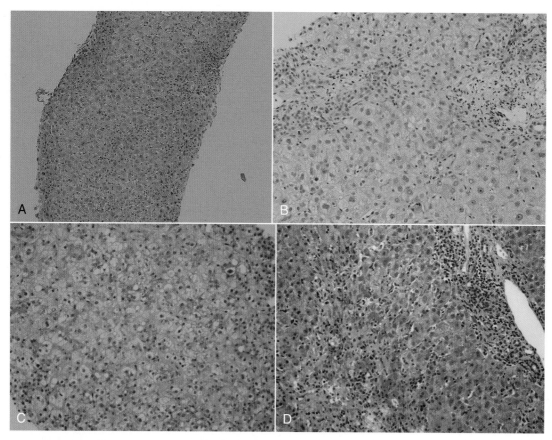

Fig. 50-10 Histopathologic features of recurrent HCV infection. A, Early, acute recurrent HCV infection is characterized by multiple apoptotic bodies in the hepatic lobule and minimal inflammatory infiltrates. **B,** Chronic recurrent HCV infection is characterized by expansion of portal tracts with lymphocytic inflammation and varying degrees of interface activity, lobular inflammation, and lobular necrosis (Councilman bodies) with intact bile ducts. Early fibrosis is present surrounding the portal tracts. **C,** Cholestatic hepatitis is characterized by swelling of hepatocytes *(left)* and accumulation of bile in tissue (cholestasis). Other features of cholestatic hepatitis include minimal portal and lobular inflammation and periportal ductular reaction. **D,** Plasma cell hepatitis is characterized by expanded portal tract showing clusters of plasma cells and in the area of bridging necrosis. *(B, Courtesy of Raga Ramachandran, M.D., University of California, San Francisco; C, courtesy of Vivian Tan, M.D., University of California, San Francisco; D, courtesy of Swan Thung, M.D., Mount Sinai Hospital, New York.)*

released from CD4[+] T cells, found that a cutoff of 220 ng/ml had 88.5% sensitivity and 90.9% specificity for identifying ACR.[163] Finally, various immunohistochemical stains, including those for lymphocyte expression of minichromosome maintenance protein-2 (Mcm-2), C4d, and IG222 monoclonal antibody against HCV-E2 glycoprotein, in addition to CD28 expression on peripheral blood mononuclear cells, have shown promise in small single-center studies.[164-167] At the present time, none of these biomarkers are ready for routine clinical use, and liver biopsy remains the gold standard for diagnosis of AR.

Pathogenesis of Posttransplantation HCV Infection

The mechanism of liver injury following liver transplantation probably involves both viral and immune-mediated mechanisms (**Table 50-5**).[168-180] Although much is known about the mechanisms of injury in HCV-infected immunocompetent patients, study of the mechanisms of liver injury in HCV-infected liver transplant recipients is made more complex by the HLA mismatch between the recipient and allograft, the altered hepatocyte milieu as a result of ischemia-reperfusion injury early after transplantation, the viral inoculum size (larger than a needlestick), the preexisting HCV-specific adaptive immune response (dysfunctional T cells and ineffective neutralizing antibodies), and the concomitant use of immunosuppressive drugs (**Fig. 50-11**).[181] The ultimate consequence of chronic infection, with its associated immune-mediated injury, is fibrosis, with activated hepatic stellate cells playing a central role. The posttransplant setting is unique in that several cofactors, in addition to chronic HCV infection, may act synergistically to activate and perpetuate stellate cell activation, including ischemia-reperfusion damage, cholestasis, allograft rejection, and infection with other viruses such as cytomegalovirus (CMV), and thereby accelerate progression of fibrosis.

Viral Kinetics and Quasispecies Evolution

Serum HCV RNA levels decline rapidly during the reperfusion phase of the operation and then gradually increase to peak in the first few weeks to months after transplantation.[182,183] The intrahepatic events that correlate with the changes in serum viral load presumably reflect the liver's binding and removal

Table 50-5 Putative Protective and Adverse Immunologic Mechanisms in HCV Recurrence

Protective

HCV-specific CD4+ T cells early after infection[169,170]
HCV-specific CD8+ T cells in the setting of antiviral therapy[169,171]
Pretransplant level of CD56+ lymphocytes[171,172]

Adverse

Decreased CD56+ lymphocytes before transplantation[172]
T-cell depletion treatments[173,174]
Mismatching of KIR–HLA-C ligands between donor-recipient pairs and presence of KIR2DL3 in the recipient[175]
Cytokine gene polymorphisms[176,177]
Impaired innate interferon signaling within hepatocytes (unknown)
Allograft-restricted T-cell responses[178,179]
Relative allograft expression of CD81 and other HCV receptors with immune properties (unknown)[180]

Data from Hughes MG Jr, Rosen HR. Human liver transplantation as a model to study hepatitis C virus pathogenesis. Liver Transpl 2009;15:1395–1411.
HCV, hepatitis C virus; HLA, human leukocyte antigen; KIR, killer cell immunoglobulin–like receptor

of the virus from the circulation and the extrahepatic clearance of virus. Kinetic modeling studies indicate that the majority of the virus infecting the new liver during the first 24 to 48 hours after perfusion is derived from the circulation, with only a small proportion from extrahepatic sources (<5%).[184,185] Donor liver factors, including the age of the donor, and the early immunologic milieu related to ischemia-reperfusion and regeneration may influence the efficacy of viral binding to receptors, internalization, and establishment of the viral replication machinery. Prolonged warm ischemia time and the presence of preservation injury have been linked with subsequent disease severity, but whether and how early graft "health" influences initial viral and immunologic events are unknown. More rapid uptake of HCV during reperfusion and a more rapid rise in HCV viral load to pretransplant levels are seen in living donor recipients than in deceased donor recipients,[185] which supports the concept that better early graft function may facilitate viral entry and replication. Alternatively, the regenerating living donor graft may be more susceptible to these early viral replicative events. Recent studies have shown that only a portion of the HCV quasispecies population that are present in the recipient before transplantation gain entry into new hepatocytes and establish infection and that selection of this viral species occurs early, probably from the time of reperfusion.[180,186] Moreover, postperfusion viral species were more closely related to each other than to the

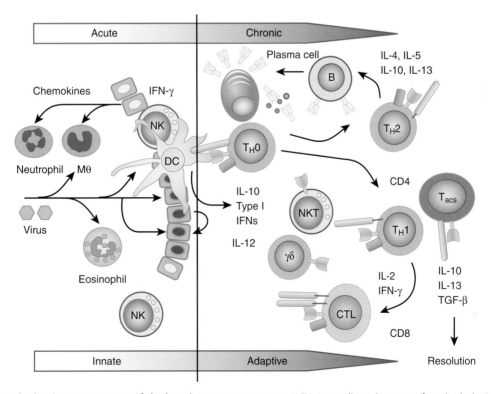

Fig. 50-11 Innate and adaptive components of the host immune response to HCV. A coordinated response from both the innate and adaptive arms of the host immune system is required for a successful HCV immune response. Natural killer *(NK)* cells are the primary innate antiviral effector population and provide the earliest and most rapid response. Activated dendritic cells *(DCs)* prime naive CD4+ T cells *(T_H0)*, thereby inducing a predominantly inflammatory *(T_H1)* and cytotoxic CD8+ T-cell response. Natural killer T cells *(NKTs)* and γδ T-cell responses may also be invoked, as well as the production of antibody by B cells activated to differentiate into plasma cells. Constitutive and induced regulatory T cells modulate the inflammatory response. IFN, interferon; IL-4, interleukin-4; TGF-β, transforming growth factor-β. *(From Golden-Mason L, Rosen HR. Natural killer cells: primary target for hepatitis C virus immune evasion strategies? Liver Transpl 2006;12:363–372.)*

pretransplant HCV viral population, thus suggesting that the selection process may occur at the level of cell attachment and entry.[180] Once infection is established, HCV quasispecies diversity and complexity evolve, but studies evaluating the relationship between HCV quasispecies and the severity of HCV recurrence have yielded conflicting results.[186-189]

Innate Immune Responses

The innate immune response is the first line of defense in the liver following HCV infection. The key cellular components of this response are natural killer (NK) and natural killer T (NKT) cells, with which the liver is enriched. These immune cells eliminate virally infected cells through cytolytic mechanisms, produce cytokines that inhibit viral replication (e.g., interferon), and recruit and activate other immune cells, including dendritic cells and T cells. NK cell activity is controlled by multiple activating and inhibitory cell surface receptors that interact with major histocompatibility class (MHC) I and MHC class I–like molecules.[190] Studies in nontransplant patients suggest that HCV evades the initial NK response by several different mechanisms,[181] but studies in liver transplant patients are limited. One small study evaluating pretransplant NK and NKT cell frequencies as a predictor of posttransplant disease severity showed that low frequencies of CD56[+] NK/NKT cells before liver transplantation were associated with more severe posttransplantation.[172] Another study of circulating NK and NKT cells before and after transplantation found that the proportions declined during the first week after transplantation and that lower HCV RNA levels correlated with a lower proportion of circulating NK cells.[191] This may be interpreted as showing that viral replication is linked with NK compartmentalization.[192] The importance of NK cells in early control of HCV infection was demonstrated in a study of adoptive transfer of donor liver lymphocytes pretreated with interleukin-2 (IL-2)/OKT3 into transplant recipients with HCV; reduced HCV RNA levels and a delay in HCV recurrence by months were achieved, effects that may be, at least partially, due to enhanced production of interferon by NK and NKT cells.[192] Indeed, the innate immune response, though not HCV specific, does result in killing of infected hepatocytes and, as a result of their ability to produce Th1 cytokines, may be a significant contributor to liver disease.

One of the key NK receptor families recognized is the killer immunoglobulin–like (KIR) receptor. Genetic polymorphisms in these activating and inhibitory receptors have been associated with disease outcomes in HCV infection.[193-195] A small study of liver transplant recipients found that a significantly higher percentage of NKT cells in those with recurrence expressed the inhibitory receptor NKG2A relative to HCV-negative nontransplant controls with liver disease.[172] Another study of 151 transplant recipients found that the presence of the KIR2DL3 receptor in the recipient correlated with a higher rate of progression to liver fibrosis and that mismatching of KIR–HLA-C ligands between donor-recipient pairs of HLA-KIR ligands favored the progression of recurrent hepatitis to fibrosis in the presence of KIR2DL3.[175] These early studies suggested an important role of the innate immune response in the outcome of HCV disease after transplantation, but larger-scale studies are needed to address the complex interactions among NK cells, their ligands, and posttransplant outcomes.

Humoral Response to HCV

The relevance of the neutralizing antibody response in acute HCV infection remains controversial because HCV can be cleared in hypogammaglobulinemic patients without an antibody response[196] whereas HCV has been shown to persist in the face of cross-neutralizing antibodies in some but not all studies.[197-200] Additionally, a neutralizing antibody response may be rendered ineffective because of viral escape mutations.[201] The HCV surface glycoproteins E1 and E2 are believed to mediate viral entry into hepatocytes via interactions with cell surface receptors and co-receptors, including CD81, claudin-1, scavenger receptor class B type I, occludin, low-density lipoprotein, and others.[167] Antibodies directed against either the E2 glycoprotein or the cell surface receptors of HCV may offer unique methods to prevent reinfection of the liver allograft. In a chimpanzee model of acute infection, hepatitis C immune globulin (HCIG) was shown to delay or prevent the development of acute infection.[202] However, in two clinical studies of hepatitis C antibody therapy in liver transplant recipients, no difference in HCV recurrence rates was evident with the use of this therapy.[203,204] The first study used a polyclonal HCIG product derived from blood donors,[203] and the second used a humanized monoclonal antibody directed against the E2 region.[204] In the latter study, a modest decline in HCV RNA levels was seen in the highest-dose cohort (≈1.5 log greater than controls), but the effect was lost when antibody was administered less frequently at 7 days after transplantation.[204] More recent studies of humanized monoclonal antibodies targeting the E2 region of HCV and the hepatocyte cell surface receptor cluster of differentiation 81 CD81 have been shown to prevent HCV infection.[205,206] In an in vivo model, human liver–uPA–severe combined immunodeficiency (SCID) mice that received prophylactic treatment with anti-CD81 antibodies were completely protected from subsequent challenge with HCV.[206] Antibodies to claudin-1 have been also shown to inhibit HCV infection in vitro.[207] These studies suggest a potential future role for a combination of antibodies to prevent allograft reinfection.

Cellular Adaptive Immune Responses

Both CD4[+] and CD8[+] T-cell responses are important in HCV pathogenesis. Priming of naïve T cells by dendritic cells expressing HCV peptides in the context of MHC molecules is critical for the induction of adaptive responses. In comparing the liver and peripheral compartments, HCV-specific CD4[+] T cells were found more frequently in the liver than in blood (47% vs. 23%) and were more frequently detectable within the first 6 months after transplantation than later (78% vs. 49%).[171] Strong, multispecific CD4[+] T-cell responses early after transplantation were associated with milder histologic injury at 1 year after transplantation in one study[168] and are more frequently detectable against nonstructural proteins.[169,171] Overall, the magnitude of activated CD4[+] T-cell expansion was significantly lower in liver transplant patients with HCV infection than in those without HCV infection.[208] Of interest, improvement in the activated CD4[+] T-cell population in posttransplant patients achieving sustained suppression of HCV viremia with antiviral therapy is well documented, with response levels comparable with those of liver transplant recipients not infected with HCV.[208,209] Regarding T-cell helper subtypes, a small study reported that Th1 cytokine profiles (tumor necrosis factor-α, interferon-γ, and IL-2) are similar in liver transplant recipients with HCV and nontransplant patients with chronic HCV but that the Th2 cytokines (interleukin-10 and interleukin-4) are increased in HCV transplant recipients with cholestatic hepatitis compared with those with chronic HCV. This finding suggests that up-regulation of Th2 cytokines favors this more severe presentation of recurrent HCV.[210]

The peripheral CTLs present after transplantation were clonotypically identical to those present within the recipient liver explant, defined at the level of the T-cell receptor β chain.[169] There is evidence of CD8+ HCV-specific T-cell responses as early as 6 weeks to 3 months after transplantation,[169,171] but proliferation of CD8+ T cells is significantly impaired in comparison with non–HCV-infected liver transplant recipients.[169,211,212] The impairment of CD8+ T cells in posttransplant patients is probably multifactorial and appears to be reversible. Transplant recipients achieving a sustained virologic response (SVR) exhibit a significant and multispecific increase in the CD8+ T-cell response that is long lasting, though found mainly in peripheral blood.[212] T-cell exhaustion, defined as functional impairment related to chronic stimulation by antigen, may be important. Programmed cell death 1 (PD1), a marker of such functionally exhausted T cells,[213] has been studied in patients with chronic HCV infection and found to correlate with loss of effector function, with more severe dysfunction being evident in the liver than in the periphery.[214] Studies in HCV-infected transplant recipients are lacking, but studies of PD1 expression in liver transplant recipients are of interest in that the PD1/PD ligand pathway is also important for induction for allograft tolerance.[215]

Regulatory T lymphocytes (Tregs) are important modulators of the adaptive immune response to chronic infection and prevent overly vigorous T-cell activation, which would lead to excessive inflammatory responses and liver injury. In a study of Tregs in subsets of liver transplant recipients 1 and 5 years after transplantation, circulating Treg cells were overexpressed in all HCV-infected recipients compared with non–HCV-infected recipients, but the Tr1 markers (indicative of CD4+ T cells secreting IL-10) were overexpressed only in patients with severe HCV recurrence.[216] In another study of recipients at a mean of 5.6 years after transplantation, Tregs were shown to be significantly decreased in all transplant recipients (relative to HCV-infected and healthy controls), but with significantly higher levels of Tregs in HCV-infected (n = 29) than in HCV-negative liver transplant recipients (n = 24).[208] Collectively, studies of Tregs remain challenging since most Treg markers also induce activated T cells and Treg expansion may be influenced by a number of different factors (e.g., rapamycin, transforming growth factor-β).[217] Nonetheless, these studies suggest a modulating effect of Tregs on HCV infection in the posttransplant setting.

Factors Associated with Disease Progression and Graft Loss

Several viral-, recipient-, donor-, and transplant-related factors influence the rate of progression of HCV disease and the risk for graft loss (**Table 50-6**). Recipient factors most consistently associated with worse posttransplant outcomes include older age and African-American race. Older donor age

Table 50-6 Strength of Association of Risk Factors for HCV Disease Severity or Graft Loss

FACTOR	STRENGTH OF ASSOCIATION	
	Disease Severity	*Graft Loss*
Recipient Related		
Older age	No association	++
African American race	+	+++
HIV co-infection	+	+
Female sex	+	+
Donor Related		
Older donor age	+++	+++
HCV-positive donor	No association	No association
Steatosis	±	±
Cold ischemia time	+	+
Living donor	No association	No association
Virus Related		
Genotype 1b (vs. others)	±	No association
High pretransplant viral load	±	±
Early posttransplant viral load	++	±
Transplant Related		
Warm ischemia time	±	±
Episodes of treated acute cellular rejection	+++	++
Cytomegalovirus infection	+++	++
Insulin resistance/diabetes	++	±

is the most important donor factor associated with risk for recurrent cirrhosis. Viral factors have not been consistently linked with risk for recurrent disease or survival. Posttransplant factors of importance include a history of treated AR, diabetes, and CMV infection. Immunosuppressive therapy is likely to be of some importance, but there are a very limited number of randomized controlled studies evaluating the effect of specific immunosuppressive drugs on the outcome of HCV disease. At present, no specific immunosuppressive regimen has established itself to be superior to others.

Recipient Factors
Recipient Age

Older recipient age has been shown to be associated with patient mortality and graft loss,[218-221] but not disease progression.[222] A single-center study of 500 transplants over the course of a decade reported that age older than 52 years was associated with a 1.8-fold increased risk for death in comparison with recipients 52 years or younger (P <.01).[218] A UNOS registry–based study found a more modest, but statistically significant effect, with patients older than 60 years experiencing a 5-year survival rate of 66.5% versus 70.3% for recipients 60 years or younger (P <.01).[219]

Recipient Race

African American race has also been recognized to be a predictor of death and graft loss.[126,219,223] In a study evaluating nearly 3500 HCV-related transplants from the Scientific Registry of Transplant Recipients, African American race was associated with a statistically significant hazard ratio (HR) of 1.28 for graft loss and 1.30 for death in comparison with Caucasian transplant recipients.[222] Although studies linking race with recurrent HCV severity are more limited, an association between African American race and increased rate of progression of fibrosis has been shown.[124,224]

HIV Co-Infection

Studies evaluating the outcomes of liver transplant recipients co-infected with HIV and HCV have shown decreased graft survival and higher rates of recurrent HCV cirrhosis compared with HCV-infected liver transplant recipients without HIV (**Fig. 50-12**). Graft survival rates vary among studies but range from 78% to 94% at 1 year, 29% to 80% at 2 years, and 29% to 51% at 5 years; however, the studies are limited because of small numbers of patients.[57,225-228] In a study of 35 co-infected recipients, fibrosis scores were significantly higher in the co-infected group than in the mono-infected group at 2 years after transplantation (1.4 ± 1.1 versus 2.4 ± 1.3, P = .01), and death was more common in the patients in whom the aggressive variant of recurrent HCV, cholestatic hepatitis, developed.[226] In a U.S. multicenter study of 81 HIV-HCV co-infected patients, treated AR occurred at a two-fold higher rate in co-infected than in mono-infected recipients (35% vs. 18%, respectively) and was associated with a three-fold increase (HR = 2.9; 95% CI, 1.2 to 7.0; P = .02) in graft loss.[229]

Recipient Sex

Limited studies have shown recipient female sex to be associated with increased graft loss[124,126,229a] and recurrent HCV disease progression.[126,230] However, this finding has not been replicated in other studies[116,135,150,219,231] and therefore remains controversial as a predictor of disease progression and graft loss.

Donor- and Peritransplantation-Related Factors

Older Donor Age

The single most important risk factor for both graft loss and disease progression in HCV-infected transplant recipients is older donor age. Using donors younger than 40 years as a reference group, a UNOS registry–based study of HCV-infected transplant recipients from 1995 through 2001 found an increasing risk for graft loss with donors between the ages of 41 and 50 years (HR = 1.67; 95% CI, 1.34 to 2.09), donors between 51 and 60 years of age (HR = 1.86; 95% CI, 1.48 to 2.34), and donors older than 60 years (HR = 2.21; 95% CI, 1.73 to 2.81).[223] Although increasing donor age has also been associated with increased mortality in HCV-negative recipients, a stronger effect has been shown in HCV-positive recipients (**Fig. 50-13**).[223,232] Several other single-center studies have supported this finding.[231,233,234] Older donor age has also been associated with a significantly increased risk for early recurrent disease and progression to cirrhosis.[116,231,233,235] One single-center study of 183 HCV-positive recipients reported that an organ from a donor older than 33 years increased the risk for the development of any fibrosis within the first year after transplantation by 3.3-fold (95% CI, 1.7 to 6.5; P = .001).[116]

Donor Risk Index and Cold Ischemia Time

The donor risk index (DRI),[236] an algorithm consisting of seven donor and graft characteristics, including donor age, predicts the risk of graft failure associated with a particular donor liver. In a UNOS registry–based cohort of HCV-positive recipients, in the RR of patient and graft loss was significantly higher in patients with higher DRI.[237] When compared with a DRI of 1, a DRI of 2 was associated with a two-fold increase in graft failure (RR = 2.03; 95% CI, 1.85 to 2.23), and a DRI of 3 was associated with a four-fold increase (RR = 4.12; 95% CI, 3.41 to 4.97).[237] Prolonged cold ischemia time (>10 to 12

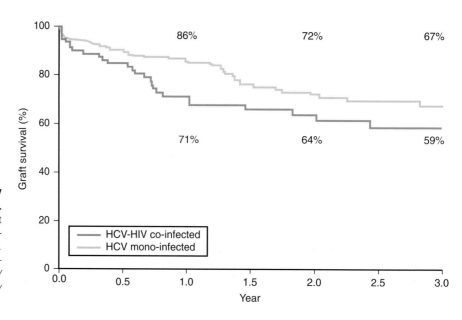

Fig. 50-12 Graft survival in HCV-HIV co-infected liver transplant recipients. Kaplan-Meier estimates of posttransplant graft survival are lower in co-infected than in mono-infected patients (P = .01). *(From Terrault NA, et al. Survival and risk of severe HCV recurrent in liver transplant recipients coinfected with HIV and HCV. [The HIV in Solid Organ Multi-Site Transplant (HIVTR) Study Group] Hepatology 2009;50 Suppl:A195.)*

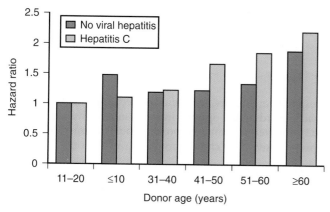

Fig. 50-13 Risk for recipient death by donor age in U.S. adult liver transplant recipients with and without HCV. In patients who underwent transplantation for HCV-related liver disease, there was an increasing risk for graft loss with donors between the ages of 41 and 50 years (hazard ratio [HR] = 1.67; 95% confidence interval [CI], 1.34 to 2.09), donors between 51 and 60 years (HR = 1.86; 95% CI, 1.48 to 2.34), and donors older than 60 years (HR = 2.21; 95% CI, 1.73 to 2.81). *(From Lake JR, et al. Differential effects of donor age in liver transplant recipients infected with hepatitis B, hepatitis C and without viral hepatitis. Am J Transplant 2005;5: 549–557.)*

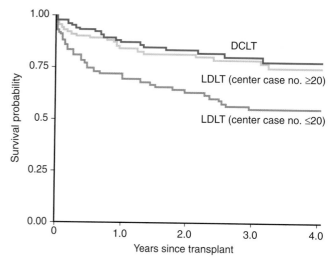

Fig. 50-14 Graft survival in living donor liver transplant (LDLT) recipients versus deceased donor liver transplant (DDLT) recipients. Graft survival after DDLT *(red line)*, LDLT ≤20 *(blue line;* first 20 cases at each center), and LDLT >20 *(yellow line;* cases beyond the first 20 at each center). Graft survival was significantly lower in LDLT ≤20 than in LDLT >20 (*P* = .0023) and DDLT (*P* = .0007). However, there was no significant difference in graft survival between LDLT >20 and DDLT (*P* = .66, log-rank test). *(From Terrault NA, et al. Outcomes in hepatitis C virus–infected recipients of living donor vs. deceased donor liver transplantation. Liver Transpl 2007;13:122–129.)*

hours), one of the seven factors included in the DRI, was found to be an independent predictor of progression of fibrosis in some[238] but not all studies.[218,219]

HCV-Positive Donors

The use of HCV-positive donors for patients with HCV disease has gained broad acceptance in the liver transplant community. The studies available have shown that overall graft survival in recipients of livers from anti–HCV-positive donors was similar to that in recipients of livers from anti–HCV-negative donors.[239-241] A single-center study suggested an interaction between donor HCV status and donor age, with recipients of anti–HCV-positive allografts from donors 50 years or older experiencing higher rates of graft failure (HR = 2.74; 95% CI, 1.34 to 5.61) and advanced fibrosis than seen with the use of matched donor HCV-negative allografts.[241]

Donor Macrosteatosis

Several single-center studies have examined the association between donor macrosteatosis and recurrence of HCV disease.[238,242-244] The majority found that mild to moderate donor steatosis (5% to 45%) was not associated with more severe HCV disease recurrence or a higher risk for graft loss. However, the studies were of limited sample size and underpowered to control for the multiple confounding donor and recipient factors influencing HCV-associated outcomes.

Live Donors

A number of studies have reported worse outcomes for living donor liver transplant (LDLT) recipients than for deceased donor liver transplant (DDLT) recipients.[245-251] In a study evaluating 764 HCV-infected LDLT recipients matched with 1470 HCV-infected DDLT recipients in the UNOS registry from 1998 to 2001, LDLT recipients experienced an increased risk for graft failure in comparison with DDLT recipients (HR = 1.6; 95% CI, 1.1 to 2.5).[245] Other studies, however, have

shown no difference in mortality between the types of transplants.[248-251] The Adult-to-Adult Living Donor Transplantation Cohort Study (A2ALL), a consortium of nine experienced liver transplant centers in the United States, compared the outcomes of 181 LDLT and 94 DDLT recipients and found that overall 3-year unadjusted graft and patient survival rates were 68% and 74% for LDLT versus 80% and 82% for DDLT (*P* = .04), respectively, but when the analysis was restricted to only LDLTs after the first 20 cases at each center, graft and patient survival rates were not significantly different (79% and 84% for LDLTs vs. 80% and 82% for DDLTs, *P* = .74) (**Fig. 50-14**).[252] In other words, survival of LDLT recipients was not different from that of DDLT recipients once centers had sufficient experience with LDLTs. Similarly, although initial studies found a higher rate of severe HCV recurrence in LDLT than in DDLT recipients, subsequent studies have not confirmed this finding.[246,247,253]

Ischemia-Reperfusion Injury

Preservation and ischemia-reperfusion injuries have been predictive of graft survival and HCV disease severity in some studies, but the associations have not been consistent. Warm ischemia time of 30, 60, or 90 minutes was correlated with rates of severe disease recurrence of 19%, 40%, and 65%, respectively, 1 year after transplantation (*P* = .04).[254] A separate study found a 2.3% increase in risk for graft failure for every minute increase in warm ischemia time (HR = 1.02; 95% CI, 1.01 to 1.04; *P* <.01).[218] A small study suggested that when compared with HCV-positive patients without evidence of histologic preservation injury, HCV-positive patients with evidence of histologic preservation injury had increased rates of advanced progression of fibrosis (43% vs. 9%, *P* = .02) and decreased 3-year survival rates (59% vs. 88%, *P* <.01).[255]

Viral Factors
Genotype and High Pretransplant Viral Load

There are conflicting results from studies evaluating the association between HCV genotype 1b and recurrent HCV disease severity.[116,150,218,222,256,257] High pretransplant viral load has not been linked with greater risk for severe histologic disease and higher graft loss in most,[124,221,258] but not all studies.[116] However, high HCV RNA levels in the early posttransplant period (first 7 days to 12 weeks) appear to be predictive of more severe histologic disease at 1 year than in those who have milder histologic disease.[258-260] Prospective studies to define the viral load "cutoff" that best predicts the risk for rapidly progressive disease have not been performed.

Transplantation-Related Factors
Treated Acute Rejection

Treatment of AR with either steroid boluses or antilymphocyte therapies is associated with an increased risk for severe recurrent HCV disease[116,124,127,222] and mortality.[133,261] A large single-center prospective study showed that advanced fibrosis developed in 47% of patients who required treatment for at least one episode of AR as compared with 22% of recipients without an episode of AR (P < .01).[222] In a prospective, multicenter study of patients enrolled in the National Institute of Diabetes and Digestive and Kidney Diseases Liver Transplantation Database, patients treated for AR had an 2.9-fold increase in mortality (P = .03) in comparison with those not treated for AR.[221]

Cytomegalovirus Infection

Independent of the number of episodes of AR, CMV infection has also been identified as a risk factor for graft loss[234] and recurrent disease progression.[262] A greater proportion of patients with CMV infection after liver transplantation progressed to cirrhosis at 5 years than did patients without CMV viremia (37.5% vs. 11%),[263] and CMV infection was associated with an increased risk for graft failure (RR = 2.62; 95% CI, 1.21 to 5.67).[234]

Metabolic Syndrome

Recent studies have convincingly shown that diabetes, insulin resistance, and metabolic syndrome are important risk factors for graft failure[219] and disease progression.[264-266] Moreover, HCV infection per se is an important risk factor for the development of de novo diabetes after transplantation.[267,268] In a study of UNOS transplant registrants, HCV-infected liver transplant recipients with diabetes were found to have a 61.8% 5-year survival rate versus 71.8% for nondiabetics (P <.01), although is it important to note that this effect was also seen in HCV-negative recipients (77.7% vs. 81.5%, P = .03), but to a lesser degree.[219] In a Mayo Clinic study of 160 HCV-infected transplant recipients, the Homeostasis Model Assessment of Insulin Resistance was associated with a two-fold increased risk for the development of advanced fibrosis (HR = 2.07; 95% CI, 1.10 to 3.91; P = .02), but glycosylated hemoglobin levels (HR = 0.94; 95% CI, 0.77 to 1.15; P = .56) and steatosis (HR = 0.88; 95% CI, 0.42 to 1.86; P = .73) were not.[264] In another study, metabolic syndrome, defined by the Adult Treatment Panel III criteria, was an independent predictor of progression of fibrosis after the first year after transplantation—and was a better predictor than obesity or diabetes.[266]

Immunosuppression and Acute Rejection

Despite many studies, few definitive recommendations can be made regarding the optimal immunosuppressive regimen for HCV-infected patients. Proposed benefits of specific immunosuppressive drug choices are shown in **Table 50-7**.

Corticosteroids

Although corticosteroid boluses for the treatment of AR are associated with a risk for advanced fibrosis, the effect of corticosteroids in standard immunosuppressive regimens remains a controversial issue. Multiple randomized trials have evaluated the effect of corticosteroid-containing versus corticosteroid-avoiding regimens and found no clear effect on progression of fibrosis,[269-271] mortality,[270-272] or graft survival.[270,271,273-276] A recent metaanalysis of 19 randomized trials before 2007 demonstrated a significant reduction in disease recurrence (RR = 0.90; 95% CI, 0.82 to 0.99; P = .03), but interpretation of these results was limited by the heterogeneity among the trials, especially with respect to the immunosuppressive "potency" of the comparator arms.[277] Of note,

Table 50-7 Theoretic Benefits of Specific Immunosuppressive Drugs in Patients with Hepatitis C

IMMUNOSUPPRESSIVE DRUG	THEORETIC BENEFITS
Induction Therapy	
Induction antibody therapy	Associated with decreased rates of acute rejection; Often used in conjunction with steroid-sparing regimens
Maintenance Corticosteroids	
Corticosteroid avoidance	May slow HCV recurrence; Associated with a lower risk for de novo diabetes
Calcineurin Inhibitors	
Cyclosporine	Inhibits HCV replication in vitro; May improve sustained virologic response rates to antiviral therapy
Tacrolimus	Lower risk for acute rejection
Antiproliferative Drugs	
Azathioprine	Shares antiviral properties with ribavirin; May decrease severity of HCV recurrence
Mycophenolate mofetil	Shares antiviral properties with ribavirin; Associated with decreased risk for graft loss in comparison with azathioprine
Rapamycin Inhibitors	
Sirolimus	Has antiproliferative and antifibrotic effects in vitro

studies reveal no detrimental effects of corticosteroid-free immunosuppressive regimens on HCV outcomes. In addition, corticosteroid avoidance has been shown to reduce metabolic complications, including de novo diabetes,[269,271,273] and this, in turn, may be important in minimizing the risk for progression of HCV disease.

Another area of controversy is whether the rate of corticosteroid tapering after transplantation affects HCV-related outcomes.[278-281] Retrospective and small prospective studies found an increased risk for progression of rapid fibrosis in patients who received a rapid corticosteroid taper as opposed to either a slow corticosteroid taper or an indefinite posttransplant corticosteroid course.[279-281] Although the factors underlying this increased risk for progressive disease are unclear, in vitro data suggest that it may be due to vigorous immune reconstitution after a previous period of intensive immunosuppression.[282]

Calcineurin Inhibitors

Cyclosporine has been shown to inhibit HCV replication in vitro,[283,284] but there are no convincing data that cyclosporine-based versus tacrolimus-based immunosuppression influences the progression of HCV disease. A recent metaanalysis that included five randomized controlled trials found no differences in mortality, graft survival, biopsy-proven AR, or progression to advanced fibrosis.[285] Interestingly, several retrospective studies evaluating predictors of SVR to peginterferon and ribavirin therapy have found that use of a cyclosporine- versus tacrolimus-based immunosuppressive regimen is associated with up to a doubling of overall rates of SVR.[283,286,287]

Antiproliferative Drugs

Mycophenolate mofetil (MMF) and azathioprine, both antiproliferative drugs, are used as part of immunosuppressive regimens in combination with calcineurin inhibitors and corticosteroids, but MMF is most commonly used.[288] Both inhibit inosine monophosphate dehydrogenase and share some antiviral actions with ribavirin,[289] thus leading to speculation that these drugs have some specific benefits in HCV-infected liver transplant recipients. In a systematic review evaluating the effects of MMF versus azathioprine on HCV-associated outcomes, the authors found that more studies reported a benefit of azathioprine (5 of 9) than a benefit of MMF (2 of 17), but the majority of studies were retrospective and observational.[290] Additionally, because azathioprine was used more before 2000 and MMF used more since 2000, the observed effects on HCV outcomes may reflect other transplant-related changes (i.e., donor and recipient factors) rather than the choice of antiproliferative agent. A large study of 3463 HCV-positive recipients from the Scientific Registry of Transplant Recipients found that when compared with tacrolimus plus corticosteroids alone, a regimen consisting of MMF, tacrolimus, and corticosteroids was associated with a reduced risk for overall graft loss (HR = 0.83, P = .01) but no difference in HCV-associated graft or patient loss (HR = 1.03, P = .84).[291] Prospective studies comparing azathioprine and MMF are few in number and limited by either small sample size[292,293] or lack of histologic follow-up.[294]

Rapamycin Inhibitors

The rapamycin inhibitors sirolimus and everolimus are not approved for use in liver transplant recipients but have been used in patients intolerant of calcineurin inhibitors, particularly those with nephrotoxicity.[295-297] Additionally, sirolimus has antiproliferative and antifibrotic effects in vitro, which has led to speculation of potential benefits against recurrent HCV disease.[298] However, no clinical studies have evaluated HCV-specific benefits. Moreover, de novo use in liver transplant recipients is not recommended given the black-box warning of higher risk for hepatic artery thrombosis and mortality in the posttransplant setting with the use of sirolimus in combination with tacrolimus or cyclosporine. Additionally, a numerically but not statistically significant increase in mortality in liver transplant recipients converted from calcineurin inhibitor–based therapy to sirolimus was evident in a multicenter study and prompted the Food and Drug Administration to issue an alert regarding the use of sirolimus in this clinical setting.[299]

Induction Antibody Therapy

Induction antibody therapy, including antithymocyte globulin (ATG) and IL-2 receptor antagonists (IL-2RAs), has been used in corticosteroid-sparing and calcineurin inhibitor minimization strategies.[270,300-304] A study evaluating the efficacy of ATG induction (versus no ATG or corticosteroids) reported lower rates of AR and similar overall and HCV-associated graft survival.[300] Randomized controlled studies have examined the effect of the IL-2RAs daclizumab and basiliximab and found no significant adverse effect on graft survival or HCV disease progression in the short term.[270,301] In the HCV3 study, which compared transplant recipients with HCV who received tacrolimus/MMF/corticosteroids with recipients of daclizumab/tacrolimus/MMF, there were no significant differences in rates or severity of HCV recurrence after 2 years of follow-up.[302] In contrast to the results with daclizumab and basiliximab, the limited data on alemtuzumab induction in HCV-infected liver transplant recipients suggest significantly higher rates of severe HCV disease and graft failure than with conventional treatment.[303]

Treatment of Acute Rejection

As AR requiring treatment with corticosteroid boluses and lymphocyte-depleting drugs is associated with higher risk for severe posttransplant HCV disease,[116,124,127,222] the goal of immunosuppression is to provide sufficient immunosuppression to avoid the need to treat AR without contributing to accelerated HCV disease progression. Additionally, abrupt changes in the amount of immunosuppression may be associated with increased risk for immune-mediated liver injury, as suggested by studies using rapid corticosteroid tapering[279-281] and lymphocyte-depleting therapies,[303,304] and should therefore be avoided. In the management of AR, experts recommend against the treatment of mild AR, in part because of the difficulty in identifying this entity on a background of recurrent HCV infection.[305] For mild to moderate AR, amplification of baseline immunosuppression is generally used, with corticosteroids being reserved for nonresponders to this measure. Corticosteroid boluses and the use of lymphocyte-depleting

Table 50-8 Treatment Strategies for HCV-Infected Liver Transplantation Recipients

TREATMENT STRATEGY	TIMING OF TREATMENT	TARGET POPULATION	OUTCOMES ACHIEVED IN STUDIES TO DATE
Before transplantation	Initiated before transplantation with the goal of achieving an undetectable viral load before transplantation	Best results in patients with mildly to moderately decompensated cirrhosis	Prevents recurrence of HCV infection
Prophylactic	Initiated at the time of transplantation and continued after transplantation with the goal of preventing recurrent infection	Unknown	Does not prevent infection of new graft
Preemptive	Initiated early in the posttransplant period (typically within the first 8 weeks) before the onset of biochemical and histologic evidence of disease	Best tolerated by LDLT recipients and patients with lower MELD scores. Absence of current or recent rejection	Viral eradication in a proportion of treated patients. Possibly milder histologic disease, even in virologic nonresponders
After transplantation	Initiated only after biochemical and histologic evidence of recurrent (and typically progressive) disease	Any stage eligible Given the high risk for decompensation once cirrhosis occurs, treatment should be initiated at an early stage of fibrosis (1-2 on a scale of 4). Absence of rejection	Viral eradication in a proportion of treated patients. Histologic improvements in the majority of responders. Whether earlier treatment is more likely to yield SVR is unknown

From Terrault NA, Berenguer M. Treating hepatitis C infection in liver transplant recipients. Liver Transpl 2006;12:1192–1204.
HCV, hepatitis C virus; LDLT, living donor liver transplant; MELD, Model for End-Stage Liver Disease; SVR, sustained virologic response

drugs are reserved for those with moderate to severe rejection.

Prevention and Treatment of Recurrent Disease

Management of HCV infection to prevent or treat recurrent disease can be considered (1) before transplantation, (2) in the perioperative and early posttransplant phase, or (3) in delayed fashion when there is evidence of histologic recurrence after transplantation (**Table 50-8**).[306] Prevention of recurrent infection is best achieved by obtaining SVR before transplantation. Additionally, a significant proportion of patients who have an undetectable HCV RNA level on treatment at the time of transplantation will be free of HCV after transplantation. Prophylactic antibody therapy, given intraoperatively and for variable periods in the posttransplant setting, has been tested but found to be ineffective in preventing HCV recurrence. For those who have detectable HCV RNA at the time of transplantation, recurrent infection develops after transplantation, and antiviral therapy can be considered early after transplantation or delayed until there is evidence of progressive histologic disease.

Pretransplantation Antiviral Therapy

Pretransplant antiviral treatment is reserved for patients who are able to tolerate peginterferon and ribavirin. Studies confirm that achievement of SVR before transplantation confers protection against recurrent HCV.[307-311] In studies treating patients to achieve SVR, rates ranged from 7% to 30% for genotypes 1 or 4 and 44% to 50% for genotypes 2 or 3.[308,310,311] Moreover, an important additional observation from these studies was that some patients who are HCV RNA

negative as a result of treatment and underwent transplantation before completing a full course remained HCV free after transplantation. This provided the impetus to treat patients on the waiting list with the primary goal of achieving an undetectable level of HCV RNA before transplantation. Studies with a mean of 8 to 12 weeks of pretransplant antiviral therapy reported on-treatment virologic response rates ranging from 18% to 56% in recipients with genotypes 1 or 4 and 82% to 100% in those with genotypes 2 or 3.[307,309-313] Of the studies that reported posttransplant follow-up, rates of SVR after transplantation ranged from 33% to 87%, with the lower rates reported for genotype 1 patients (33% to 50%) (see **Table 50-6**).[296-298,300] Interim analysis of a randomized trial of 79 patients registered in the Adult-to-Adult Liver Transplantation Cohort Study demonstrated that 41% of patients with genotypes 1, 4, 5, or 6 and 53% of patients with genotypes 2 or 3 achieved an on-treatment response by week 12 and that 18% of genotype 1, 4, 5, or 6 recipients and 39% of genotype 2 or 3 recipients remained HCV free after transplantation (**Table 50-9**).[307,308,310-312,314,315]

The tolerability of peginterferon and ribavirin is reduced in the posttransplant as opposed to the nontransplant setting. Even though some studies used a graduated dosing regimen, growth factors, and transfusions to manage anemia and nentropenia, serious adverse events were still frequent[308,314] and occurred at a higher rate than in untreated patients.[315] Patients with more advanced liver disease had the lowest response rates and poorest tolerabilty.[312,313,314] Deaths have been reported but do not appear to be higher than in untreated controls with similar severity of disease.[310,315] In patients with MELD scores lower than 20 at the start of treatment, wait list mortality in treated patients was 14% versus 15% in untreated controls (P = nonsignificant).[315] Based on evidence to date, experts recommend considering pretransplant treatment in patients with a MELD score of 18 to 20 or lower.[305,316] Patients

Table 50-9 Studies of Patients Receiving Pretransplant Antiviral Therapy with Combination Interferon and Ribavirin

AUTHOR	N	IFN TYPE	ON-TREATMENT RESPONSE		HCV-RNA NEGATIVE AFTER LIVER TRANSPLANTATION		DISCONTINUATION RATE
			Genotype 1/4	Genotype 2/3	Genotype 1/4	Genotype 2/3	
Crippin et al.,[312] 2002	6	IFN-α-2b	1/6 (17%)	Not available	0/6 (0%)	Not available	4/6 (67%)
Forns et al.,[307] 2004	30	IFN-α-2b	6/25 (24%)	3/5 (60%)	3/6 (50%)	3/3 (100%)	10/30 (33%)
Everson,[308] 2005	124	IFN-α-2b or PEG-IFN-α-2b (graduated ascending dose)	26/86 (30%) (G1 only)	31/38 (82%) (non-G1)	11/86 (13%) (G1 only)	19/38 (50%) (non-G1)	16/124 (13%)
Iacobellis et al.,[310] 2007	66	PEG-IFN-α-2b	13/44 (30%)	18/22 (83%)	3/44 (7%)	10/22 (41%)	13/66 (20%)
Tekin et al.,[311] 2008	20	PEG-IFN-α-2a (graduated ascending dose)	9/20 (45%)	Not available	6/20 (30%)	Not available	8/20 (40%)
Massoumi et al.,[314] 2009	90	PEG-IFN-α-2a (graduated ascending dose)	40/69 (58%)	17/19 (89%)	7/69 (10%)	6/19 (32%)	30/90 (33%)
Everson et al.,[315] 2009	59	PEG-IFN-α-2b (graduated ascending dose)	9/22 (41%)	9/18 (53%)	4/22 (18%)	7/18 (39%)	8/59 (15%)
Total (median %)	395		30%	82%	13%	46%	23%

G, genotype; IFN, interferon; PEG-IFN, pegylated interferon (peginterferon)

listed as having HCC as their primary indication for transplantation and patients with living donors with lower MELD scores may be ideal candidates for such therapy. In addition, the risk/benefit ratio of pretransplant antiviral therapy favors use in patients with the best chance of achieving an on-treatment response, such as previous relapsers, patients with genotypes 2 or 3, and treatment-naïve genotype 1 patients with low viral loads.

Prophylactic Antibody Therapy

Although HBIG can successfully prevent recurrent hepatitis B, human HCIG has not been shown to be effective in preventing recurrent HCV. In a randomized, double-blind, multicenter phase I clinical trial of HCIG, there was no suppression of HCV RNA levels with either a low dose (75 mg/kg) or high dose (200 mg/kg), and dose reductions occurred in 75% of patients because of symptomatic adverse effects.[202] HCV-Ab[XTL]68, a neutralizing, high-affinity, fully human monoclonal antibody that binds E2 glycoprotein, was associated with a modest and transient decrease in HCV RNA levels at the highest doses used (240 mg), but recurrent HCV infection occurred in all patients.[204] Based on these limited studies, there is no current indication for HCIG, which has orphan drug status in some countries, nor are there any effective prophylactic therapies available for patients undergoing liver transplantation for HCV disease.

Preemptive and Early Post–Liver Transplantation Antiviral Therapy

Preemptive treatment is typically initiated within the first 8 weeks following transplantation. The rationale for early treatment rests on the knowledge that histologic disease is minimal and HCV burden may be lower than at later times after transplantation, both features that offer the theoretic advantage of increased efficacy. These potential advantages, however, are countered by the presence of posttransplant complications, including AR, and a greater frequency of cytopenia related to immunosuppression in the early posttransplant period. In one prospective study of preemptive antiviral therapy, only 40% of transplant recipients were clinically suitable for initiation of therapy within 4 to 8 weeks of transplantation.[317] In three separate studies that included an aggregate total of 128 patients, preemptive therapy with combination interferon and ribavirin resulted in SVR rates between 9% and 39%.[317-319] Adverse events requiring dose reduction or discontinuation of therapy occurred in 31% to 85% of patients, thus reinforcing the fact that this strategy may be limited only to the most clinically stable recipients. In one study, preemptive therapy was associated with a trend toward a reduced risk for subsequent advanced fibrosis (HR = 0.52; 95% CI, 0.24 to 1.12; P = .09).[320]

Early antiviral therapy initiated beyond the first 8 weeks but within the first 6 months of transplantation targets patients with early histologic disease. This approach focuses on patients better able to tolerate therapy inasmuch as they are more fully recovered from transplant-related events but yet are likely to have mild disease and be more responsive to antiviral therapy as a consequence. In the largest controlled trial evaluating early antiviral treatment, 115 U.S. patients were randomized to peginterferon alfa-2a and ribavirin 10 to 26 weeks after liver transplantation or observation for 48 weeks.[321] Clinically apparent HCV recurrence was less frequent in treated patients than in untreated controls (16% vs. 41%).[321] However, 44% of patients in the early treatment arm discontinued therapy, and only 22% of patients achieved SVR. In contrast, a smaller study of 24 patients with genotype 1 from Spain reported that 58% of patients achieved an end-of-treatment response, with 35% achieving SVR.[322] Based on these mixed results, it is unclear whether early treatment offers any specific benefits over delayed initiation of treatment. However, most experts recommend consideration of early antiviral therapy in patients with risk factors for progressive disease, such as those with early severe hepatitis or patients who have undergone retransplantation for recurrent HCV.

Treatment of Recurrent Disease

Given the limited applicability and modest response rates of pretransplant and preemptive anti-HCV therapy, most clinicians initiate antiviral therapy only if there is histologic evidence of recurrent disease, namely, fibrosis stage ≥ 2 (on a 4-point scale) on a biopsy specimen or cholestatic hepatitis.[305] Over 20 studies, including more than 700 patients, have evaluated the efficacy of combination therapy with peginterferon and ribavirin.[286,323-342] The majority of studies used peginterferon alfa-2b and ribavirin doses ranging from 600 to 800 mg/day. Overall SVR rates ranged from 21% to 48%, with genotypes 1 or 4 patients experiencing lower rates (13% to 40%) than those with non-1/4 genotype (33% to 100%). Although at least 70% of the studies allowed the use of growth factors for the management of cytopenia, dose reductions were common and occurred in 21% to 88% of patients, and treatment discontinuation occurred in 22% to 43% of patients.* Predictors of SVR are listed in **Table 50-10**.† Histologic

responses were difficult to assess in the studies given the variability in follow-up times and fibrosis measures used. However, benefit was generally limited to patients who achieved SVR,[338,343] and two studies showed a significantly increased 5-year survival rate in those who were treated and achieved SVR versus those who were not (66% to 69%).[335,345] In a recent Cochrane Collaboration systematic review of the randomized trials of antiviral therapy to treat recurrent HCV disease, there was no difference in mortality, graft rejection, or retransplantation in treated versus untreated patients.[346] However, this review was limited by significant heterogeneity in the studies included.

Treatment of recurrent HCV disease is limited by increased rates of adverse effects, decreased tolerability, and additional concerns regarding graft rejection. Studies evaluating posttransplant treatment with combination peginterferon and ribavirin have reported that cytopenia is the most common adverse effect requiring dose reduction (32% to 74%) or discontinuation of treatment (21% to 43%).* Use of growth factors for anemia (25% to 38%) and leukopenia (15%% to 44%) was common.[326,331,334] Rates of AR were highly variable, with studies reporting rates of 0% to 22%,† but the two randomized studies that reported rates of rejection showed no significant difference between treated and untreated groups.[328,343]

Treatment of Recurrent Disease in Special Populations

Cholestatic Hepatitis

Though associated with a high rate of graft failure if untreated, cholestatic hepatitis has been shown to be responsive to interferon-based therapy.[333,347-349] Rates of biochemical response to combination interferon (pegylated and nonpegylated forms) and ribavirin are reported to be 57% to 70%, but 20% or fewer patients achieved SVR.[333,348] Although recipients with cholestatic hepatitis who were nonresponders or relapsers were at risk for the development of severe recurrent cholestatic hepatitis, most responded to reinitiation and long-term continuation of antiviral therapy.[333,348,349]

HIV Co-Infected Patients

Similar to the nontransplant population, progression of HCV disease occurs more rapidly in HIV co-infected patients than in mono-infected patients after liver transplantation. Severe cholestatic hepatitis developed in a median of 23% (range, 9% to 60%) of co-infected recipients, a rate that was elevated relative to the mono-infected population.[226,227,350,351] Limited data are available on treatment outcomes in co-infected transplant recipients. Of the 43 patients in these studies who received combination pegylated or standard interferon plus ribavirin treatment, a median of 47% (range, 21% to 100%) achieved on-treatment virologic response, with 20% (range, 16% to 27%) achieving SVR.[226,227,350-352] As in HCV mono-infected liver transplant recipients, tolerability of full-dose interferon

---

*References 330, 331, 333, 334, 338, 339, and 341 to 343.

†References 286, 330, 331, 333, 334, 338, 339, 341, and 342.

Table 50-10 Predictors of Sustained Virologic Response with Antiviral Treatment of Recurrent Hepatitis C

Baseline Characteristics
Non–genotype 1
Low pretreatment viral load
Donor age <60 years
Use of cyclosporine-based immunosuppression
Milder histologic recurrent disease
IL-28B genotype
On-Treatment Factors
Early virologic response
Absence of drug interruptions or dose reductions
Use of growth factors

---

*References 319, 324, 325, 327, 330, 333, 334, and 343.

†References 319, 325, 326, 330, 331, 334, and 343.

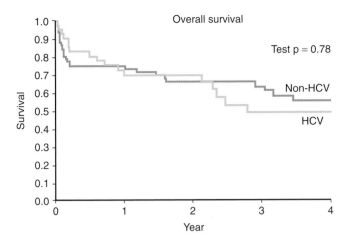

Fig. 50-15 Overall survival after liver retransplantation for HCV-related versus non–HCV-related disease. Patients undergoing retransplantation for HCV-related disease experienced similar survival rates as patients undergoing retransplantation for non–HCV-related liver disease, with 1- and 3-year survival rates of 69% and 49% versus 73% and 55%, respectively ($P = .78$). (From McCashland T, et al. Retransplantation for hepatitis C: results of a U.S. multicenter retransplant study. Liver Transpl 2007;13:1246–1253.)

and ribavirin was limited and use of growth factors during treatment was frequent.[227]

Retransplantation

Despite efforts to prevent or slow disease progression with antiviral therapy, recurrent HCV disease remains the most common cause of graft failure requiring retransplantation in patients receiving transplants for HCV-related liver disease.[124,127] Although survival rates after retransplantation are lower than those after primary liver transplantation for any cause, several single-center studies have reported significantly shorter overall survival rates for HCV-related retransplants than for non–HCV-related retransplants.[353-355] When evaluated in a multicenter study of 43 HCV-related and 73 non–HCV-related retransplants, 1-year (69% vs. 73%) and 3-year (49% vs. 55%) survival rates for the HCV-positive cohort were decreased, but not significantly ($P = .74$), relative to the HCV-negative cohort (**Fig. 50-15**).[356]

Worse outcomes have been associated with older donor age,[353,355,357] elevated prothrombin time,[353] elevated serum creatinine,[355,358] elevated serum bilirubin,[358] and MELD score of 16 or higher.[356,359] The International Liver Transplantation Society Expert Panel indicated that the following were the key variables associated with a worse outcome after retransplantation:[305]

- Bilirubin level of 10 mg/dl or greater
- Creatinine level of 2.0 mg/dl or greater (or creatinine clearance of less than 40 ml/min)
- Recipient age older than 55 years
- Donor age older than 40 years
- Early HCV recurrence (cirrhosis less than 1 year after liver transplantation)

Currently, guidelines recommend that listing for retransplantation be considered only if the expected 1-year survival rate after retransplantation is greater than 60%, which is the lowest acceptable target survival rate for primary liver

transplantation. Of 156 patients included in the multicenter study of retransplantation, common reasons for not listing patients for retransplantation include recurrent hepatitis C within 6 months of transplantation (22%), fibrosing cholestatic hepatitis C (19%), advanced renal insufficiency (18%), and other reasons (28%) such as older age and patient request.[356]

Based on the current data, optimal retransplantation outcomes for HCV-infected recipients would be anticipated with the use of organs from young donors offered early in the recurrent cirrhosis course, when patients still have good synthetic function and renal function. However, such a strategy is difficult given the current MELD-based organ allocation system. Therefore retransplantation for recurrent HCV disease remains a controversial issue, and policies regarding relisting vary among transplant centers.

Key References

Angus PW, et al. A randomized study of adefovir dipivoxil in place of HBIG in combination with lamivudine as post–liver transplantation hepatitis B prophylaxis. Hepatology 2008;48:1460–1466. (Ref.52)

Berenguer M, et al. Clinical benefits of antiviral therapy in patients with recurrent hepatitis C following liver transplantation. Am J Transplant 2008;8: 679–687. (Ref.345)

Bihl F, et al. [What's new in the treatment of hepatitis B infection?] Rev Med Suisse 2009;5:1720–1722, 1724. (Ref.42)

Borgogna C, et al. Expression of the interferon-inducible proteins MxA and IFI16 in liver allografts. Histopathology 2009;54:837–846. (Ref.161)

Briceno J, et al. Impact of donor graft steatosis on overall outcome and viral recurrence after liver transplantation for hepatitis C virus cirrhosis. Liver Transpl 2009;15:37–48. (Ref.232)

Broering TJ, et al. Identification and characterization of broadly neutralizing human monoclonal antibodies directed against the E2 envelope glycoprotein of hepatitis C virus. J Virol 2009;83:12473–12482. (Ref.205)

Burra P, et al. Donor livers with steatosis are safe to use in hepatitis C virus–positive recipients. Liver Transpl 2009;15:619–628. (Ref.243)

Bzwej N, et al. Liver transplantation outcomes among Caucasians, Asian Americans, and African Americans with hepatitis B. Liver Transpl 2009;15: 1010–1020. (Ref.5)

Bzwej N, et al. PHOENIX: A randomized controlled trial of peginterferon alfa-2a plus ribavirin as a prophylactic treatment after liver transplantation for hepatitis C virus. Liver Transpl 2011;17:528-538. (Ref. 321)

Caccamo L, et al. Role of lamivudine in the posttransplant prophylaxis of chronic hepatitis B virus and hepatitis delta virus coinfection. Transplantation 2007;83:1341–1344. (Ref.59)

Carambia A, Herkel J. CD4 T cells in hepatic immune tolerance. J Autoimmun 2010;34:23–28. (Ref.215)

Carpenter A, et al. Increased expression of regulatory Tr1 cells in recurrent hepatitis C after liver transplantation. Am J Transplant 2009;9:2102–2112. (Ref.216)

Carrión JA, et al. Serum fibrosis markers identify patients with mild and progressive hepatitis C recurrence after liver transplantation. Gastroenterology 2010;138:147–141. (Ref.144)

Carrión JA, et al. Liver stiffness identifies two different patterns of fibrosis progression in patients with hepatitis C virus recurrence after liver transplantation. Hepatology 2010;51:147–158. (Ref.145)

Cescon M, et al. Predictors of sustained virological response after antiviral treatment for hepatitis C recurrence following liver transplantation. Liver Transpl 2009;15:782–789. (Ref.286)

Cholongitas E, Papatheodoridis GV, Burroughs AK. Liver grafts from anti–hepatitis B core positive donors: a systematic review. J Hepatol 2010;52: 272–279. (Ref.110)

Ciuffreda D, et al. Hepatitis C virus infection after liver transplantation is associated with lower levels of activated CD4(+)CD25(+)CD45RO(+) IL-7ralpha(high) T cells. Liver Transpl 2010;16:49–55. (Ref.208)

Ciuffreda D, et al. Polyfunctional HCV-specific T-cell responses are associated with effective control of HCV replication. Eur J Immunol 2008;38: 2665–2677. (Ref.211)

Coffin CS, et al. Virologic and clinical outcomes of hepatitis B virus infection in HIV-HBV coinfected transplant recipients. Am J Transplant 2010;10: 1268–1275. (Ref.58)

Corradi F, et al. Assessment of liver fibrosis in transplant recipients with recurrent HCV infection: usefulness of transient elastography. Dig Liver Dis 2009;41:217–225. (Ref.139)

Dale CH, et al. Spontaneous clearance of hepatitis C after liver and renal transplantation. Can J Gastroenterol 2009;23:265–267. (Ref.120)

de Arias AE, et al. Killer cell immunoglobulin–like receptor genotype and killer cell immunoglobulin–like receptor–human leukocyte antigen C ligand compatibility affect the severity of hepatitis C virus recurrence after liver transplantation. Liver Transpl 2009;15:390–399. (Ref.175)

Degertekin B, et al. Impact of virologic breakthrough and HBIG regimen on hepatitis B recurrence after liver transplantation. Am J Transplant 2010;10: 1823–1833. (Ref.9)

D'Errico-Grigioni A, et al. Tissue hepatitis C virus RNA quantification and protein expression help identify early hepatitis C virus recurrence after liver transplantation. Liver Transpl 2008;14:313–320. (Ref.117)

De Simone P, et al. Conversion from a calcineurin inhibitor to everolimus therapy in maintenance liver transplant recipients: a prospective, randomized, multicenter trial. Liver Transpl 2009;15:1262–1269. (Ref.295)

Duclos-Vallee JC, et al. Survival and recurrence of hepatitis C after liver transplantation in patients coinfected with human immunodeficiency virus and hepatitis C virus. Hepatology 2008;47:407–417. (Ref.226)

Everson GT, et al. Interim analysis of a controlled trial of pre-transplant peginterferon alfa-2b/ribavirin (PEG/RBV) to prevent recurrent hepatitis C virus (HCV) infection after liver transplantation (LT) in the Adult-to-Adult Liver Transplantation (A2ALL) Study. Hepatol 2009;50. (Ref.315)

Faria LC, et al. Hepatocellular carcinoma is associated with an increased risk of hepatitis B virus recurrence after liver transplantation. Gastroenterology 2008;134:1890–1899; quiz 2155. (Ref.11)

Fiel MI, Schiano T. Acute cellular rejection and its sequelae developing in a 42-year-old man after liver transplantation. Hepatology 2009;50:650–651. (Ref.160)

Firpi RJ, et al. The natural history of hepatitis C cirrhosis after liver transplantation. Liver Transpl 2009;15:1063–1071. (Ref.128)

Gane EJ, et al. Lamivudine plus low-dose hepatitis B immunoglobulin to prevent recurrent hepatitis B following liver transplantation. Gastroenterology 2007;132:931–937. (Ref.10)

Gedaly R, et al. Prevalent immunosuppressive strategies in liver transplantation for hepatitis C: results of a multi-center international survey. Transpl Int 2008;21:867–872. (Ref.288)

Germani G, et al. Azathioprine in liver transplantation: a reevaluation of its use and a comparison with mycophenolate mofetil. Am J Transplant 2009;9: 1725–1731. (Ref.290)

Guo L, et al. Living donor liver transplantation for hepatitis C–related cirrhosis: no difference in histological recurrence when compared to deceased donor liver transplantation is attributable to the difference in donor age. Liver Transpl 2008;14:1778–1786. (Ref.251)

Gurusamy KS, et al. Antiviral therapy for recurrent liver graft infection with hepatitis C virus. Cochrane Database Syst Rev 2009;(1):CD006803. (Ref.346)

Hanouneh IA, et al. The significance of metabolic syndrome in the setting of recurrent hepatitis C after liver transplantation. Liver Transpl 2008;14: 1287–1293. (Ref.266)

Hashimoto K, et al. Measurement of CD4$^+$ T-cell function in predicting allograft rejection and recurrent hepatitis C after liver transplantation. Clin Transplant 2010;24:701–708. (Ref.163)

http://www.fda.gov/Drugs/DrugSafety/PostmarketDrugSafetyInformationfor PatientsandProviders/DrugSafetyInformationforHeathcareProfessionals/ ucm165015.htm. 6/11/2009. (Ref.299)

Hughes MG Jr, Rosen HR. Human liver transplantation as a model to study hepatitis C virus pathogenesis. Liver Transpl 2009;15:1395–1411. (Ref.168)

Hussain M, et al. Presence of intrahepatic (total and ccc) HBV DNA is not predictive of HBV recurrence after liver transplantation. Liver Transpl 2007;13:1137–1144. (Ref.95)

Katz LH, et al. Prevention of recurrent hepatitis B virus infection after liver transplantation: hepatitis B immunoglobulin, antiviral drugs, or both? Systematic review and meta-analysis. Transpl Infect Dis 2010;12:292–308. (Ref.83)

Kawamoto K, et al. Transforming growth factor beta 1 (TGF-beta1) and rapamycin synergize to effectively suppress human T cell responses via upregulation of FoxP3$^+$ Tregs. Transpl Immunol 2010;23:28–33. (Ref.217)

Kim WR, et al. Trends in waiting list registration for liver transplantation for viral hepatitis in the United States. Gastroenterology 2009;137:1680–1686. (Ref.1)

Klintmalm GB, et al. Hepatitis C (HCV)-3 study: does immunosuppression affect HCV recurrence progression after liver transplantation? [abstract] Transplantation 2008;86:97. (Ref.302)

Knapp S, et al. Consistent beneficial effects of killer cell immunoglobulin–like receptor 2DL3 and group 1 human leukocyte antigen-C following exposure to hepatitis C virus. Hepatology 2010;51:1168–1175. (Ref.193)

Krieger SE, et al. Inhibition of hepatitis C virus infection by anti–claudin-1 antibodies is mediated by neutralization of E2-CD81-claudin-1 associations. Hepatology 2010;51:1144–1157. (Ref.207)

Kuo A, et al. Long-term histological effects of preemptive antiviral therapy in liver transplant recipients with hepatitis C virus infection. Liver Transpl 2008;14:1491–1497. (Ref.320)

Lai CL, et al. Telbivudine versus lamivudine in patients with chronic hepatitis B. N Engl J Med 2007;357:2576–2588. (Ref.72)

Lai JC, et al. Hepatitis C virus infected females are at higher risk of graft loss after liver transplantation: a multicenter cohort study. Gastroenterol Hepatol (N Y) 2010;6:226–228. (Ref.126)

Lanier LL. Evolutionary struggles between NK cells and viruses. Nat Rev Immunol 2008;8:259–268. (Ref.189)

Lenci I, et al. Total and covalently closed circular DNA detection in liver tissue of long-term survivors transplanted for HBV-related cirrhosis. Dig Liver Dis 2010;42:578–584. (Ref.94)

Lenci I, et al. Safety of complete and sustained prophylaxis withdrawal in patients liver transplanted for HBV-related cirrhosis at low risk of HBV recurrence. J Hepatol 2011 [epub ahead of print]. (Ref.95a)

Liaw YF, et al. 2-Year GLOBE trial results: telbivudine is superior to lamivudine in patients with chronic hepatitis B. Gastroenterology 2009;136:486–495. (Ref.75)

Llado L, et al. Impact of immunosuppression without steroids on rejection and hepatitis C virus evolution after liver transplantation: results of a prospective randomized study. Liver Transpl 2008;14:1752–1760. (Ref.271)

Lok AS, McMahon BJ. Chronic hepatitis B: update 2009. Hepatology 2009;50: 661–662. (Ref.53)

Loomba R, et al. Hepatitis B immunoglobulin and lamivudine improve hepatitis B–related outcomes after liver transplantation: meta-analysis. Clin Gastroenterol Hepatol 2008;6:696–700. (Ref.81)

Luo Y, et al. Hepatitis B virus–specific CD4 T cell immunity after liver transplantation for chronic hepatitis B. Liver Transpl 2009;15:292–299. (Ref.40)

Macquillan GC, et al. Hepatocellular MxA protein expression supports the differentiation of recurrent hepatitis C disease from acute cellular rejection after liver transplantation. Clin Transplant 2010;24:252–258. (Ref.162)

Maluf DG, et al. Impact of the donor risk index on the outcome of hepatitis C virus–positive liver transplant recipients. Liver Transpl 2009;15:592–599. (Ref.237)

Manousou P, et al. Outcome of recurrent hepatitis C virus after liver transplantation in a randomized trial of tacrolimus monotherapy versus triple therapy. Liver Transpl 2009;15:1783–1791. (Ref.272)

Marcellin P, et al. Tenofovir disoproxil fumarate versus adefovir dipivoxil for chronic hepatitis B. N Engl J Med 2008;359:2442–2455. (Ref.71)

Massoumi H, et al. An escalating dose regimen of pegylated interferon and ribavirin in HCV cirrhotic patients referred for liver transplant. Transplantation 2009;88:729–735. (Ref.304)

Meuleman P, et al. Anti-CD81 antibodies can prevent a hepatitis C virus infection in vivo. Hepatology 2008;48:1761–1768. (Ref.205)

Mondelli MU, Varchetta S, Oliviero B. Natural killer cells in viral hepatitis: facts and controversies. Eur J Clin Invest 2010;40:851–863. (Ref.41)

Nakamoto N, et al. Functional restoration of HCV-specific CD8 T cells by PD-1 blockade is defined by PD-1 expression and compartmentalization. Gastroenterology 2008;134:1927–1937, 1937 e1-e2. (Ref.214)

Neff GW, et al. Combination therapy in liver transplant recipients with hepatitis B virus without hepatitis B immune globulin. Dig Dis Sci 2007;52:2497–2500. (Ref.51)

Ohira M, et al. Adoptive immunotherapy with liver allograft–derived lymphocytes induces anti-HCV activity after liver transplantation in humans and humanized mice. J Clin Invest 2009;119:3226–3235. (Ref.191)

Pang PS, et al. The effect of donor race on the survival of Black Americans undergoing liver transplantation for chronic hepatitis C. Liver Transpl 2009;15:1126-1132. (Ref.224)

Pungpapong S, et al. Serum fibrosis markers can predict rapid fibrosis progression after liver transplantation for hepatitis C. Liver Transpl 2008;14: 1294–1302. (Ref.142)

Rao W, Wu X, Xiu D. Lamivudine or lamivudine combined with hepatitis B immunoglobulin in prophylaxis of hepatitis B recurrence after liver transplantation: a meta-analysis. Transpl Int 2009;22:387–394. (Ref.82)

Rehermann B. Hepatitis C virus versus innate and adaptive immune responses: a tale of coevolution and coexistence. J Clin Invest 2009;119:1745–1754. (Ref.197)

Roche B, et al. Hepatitis C virus therapy in liver transplant recipients: response predictors, effect on fibrosis progression, and importance of the initial stage of fibrosis. Liver Transpl 2008;14:1766–1777. (Ref.341)

Roland ME, et al. HIV-infected liver and kidney transplant recipients: 1- and 3-year outcomes. Am J Transplant 2008;8:355–365. (Ref.228)

Rosen HR. Transplantation immunology: what the clinician needs to know for immunotherapy. Gastroenterology 2008;134:1789–1801. (Ref.177)

Rosen HR, et al. Pretransplantation CD56(+) innate lymphocyte populations associated with severity of hepatitis C virus recurrence. Liver Transpl 2008;14:31–40. (Ref.171)

Rosenau J, et al. Failure of hepatitis B vaccination with conventional HBsAg vaccine in patients with continuous HBIG prophylaxis after liver transplantation. Liver Transpl 2007;13:367–373. (Ref.92)

Saab S, et al. Decision analysis model for hepatitis B prophylaxis one year after liver transplantation. Liver Transpl 2009;15:413–420. (Ref.60)

Saab S, et al. Comparison of different immunoprophylaxis regimens after liver transplantation with hepatitis B core antibody–positive donors: a systematic review. Liver Transpl 2010;16:300–307. (Ref.111)

Sadamori H, et al. Immunohistochemical staining of liver grafts with a monoclonal antibody against HCV-Envelope 2 for recurrent hepatitis C after living donor liver transplantation. J Gastroenterol Hepatol 2009;24:574–580. (Ref.164)

Schiff E, et al. Adefovir dipivoxil for wait-listed and post–liver transplantation patients with lamivudine-resistant hepatitis B: final long-term results. Liver Transpl 2007;13:349–360. (Ref.54)

Schiff E, et al. Efficacy and safety of entecavir in patients with chronic hepatitis B and advanced hepatic fibrosis or cirrhosis. Am J Gastroenterol 2008;103:2776–2783. (Ref.73)

Segev DL, et al. Steroid avoidance in liver transplantation: meta-analysis and meta-regression of randomized trials. Liver Transpl 2008;14:512–525. (Ref.277)

Selzner N, et al. Antiviral treatment of recurrent hepatitis C after liver transplantation: predictors of response and long-term outcome. Transplantation 2009;88:1214–1221. (Ref.287)

Shackel NA, et al. Early high peak hepatitis C viral load levels independently predict hepatitis C–related liver failure post–liver transplantation. Liver Transpl 2009;15:709–718. (Ref.260)

Shim JH, et al. Efficacy of entecavir in treatment-naive patients with hepatitis B virus–related decompensated cirrhosis. J Hepatol 2010;52:176–182. (Ref.74)

Tekin F, et al. Safety, tolerability, and efficacy of pegylated-interferon alfa-2a plus ribavirin in HCV-related decompensated cirrhotics. Aliment Pharmacol Ther 2008;27:1081–1085. (Ref.311)

Terrault NA. Hepatitis C therapy before and after liver transplantation. Liver Transpl 2008;14(Suppl 2):S58–S66. (Ref.316)

Terrault NA, et al. Survival and risk of severe HCV recurrent in liver transplant recipients coinfected with HIV and HCV. (The HIV in Solid Organ Multi-Site Transplant [HIVTR] Study Group) Hepatology 2009;50 Suppl:A195. (Ref.229)

Thuluvath PJ, et al. Survival after liver transplantation for hepatocellular carcinoma in the Model for End-Stage Liver Disease and pre–Model for End-Stage Liver Disease eras and the independent impact of hepatitis C virus. Liver Transpl 2009;15:754–762. (Ref.133)

Tretheway D, et al. Should trichrome stain be used on all post–liver transplant biopsies with hepatitis C virus infection to estimate the fibrosis score? Liver Transpl 2008;14:695–700. (Ref.137)

Unitt E, et al. Minichromosome maintenance protein-2–positive portal tract lymphocytes distinguish acute cellular rejection from hepatitis C virus recurrence after liver transplantation. Liver Transpl 2009;15:306–312. (Ref.163)

Varchetta S, et al. Prospective study of natural killer cell phenotype in recurrent hepatitis C virus infection following liver transplantation. J Hepatol 2009;50:314–322. (Ref.190)

Veldt BJ, et al. Impact of pegylated interferon and ribavirin treatment on graft survival in liver transplant patients with recurrent hepatitis C infection. Am J Transplant 2008;8:2426–2433. (Ref.342)

Veldt BJ, et al. Insulin resistance, serum adipokines and risk of fibrosis progression in patients transplanted for hepatitis C. Am J Transplant 2009;9:1406–1413. (Ref.264)

Ward SC, et al. Plasma cell hepatitis in hepatitis C virus patients post–liver transplantation: case-control study showing poor outcome and predictive features in the liver explant. Liver Transpl 2009;15:1826–1833. (Ref.153)

Weber NK, Trotter JF. Spontaneous clearance of hepatitis C virus after liver transplantation. Transplantation 2009;87:1102–1103. (Ref.123)

Xi ZF, et al. The role of entecavir in preventing hepatitis B recurrence after liver transplantation. J Dig Dis 2009;10:321–327. (Ref.84)

Yu L, et al. Survival after orthotopic liver transplantation: the impact of antibody against hepatitis B core antigen in the donor. Liver Transpl 2009;15:1343–1350. (Ref.108)

Yuefeng M, et al. Long-term outcome of patients with lamivudine after early cessation of hepatitis B immunoglobulin for prevention of recurrent hepatitis B following liver transplantation. Clin Transplant 2010 Jun 15 [Epub ahead of print]. (Ref.12)

Zhao H, et al. Impact of human leukocyte antigen matching on hepatitis B virus recurrence after liver transplantation. Hepatobiliary Pancreat Dis Int 2010;9:139–143. (Ref.36)

A complete list of references can be found at www.expertconsult.com.

Treatment of Recurrent Nonviral Disease

James Neuberger

Introduction

Many diseases recur after liver transplantation; prompt recognition and diagnosis and appropriate treatment are necessary to prevent unnecessary complications and maintain good graft function (**Table 51-1**).

Primary Biliary Cirrhosis

The reported incidence of recurrent primary biliary cirrhosis (rPBC) has been uncertain, with a recent systematic review of 16 studies suggesting a recurrence rate of 18% with a range between 4% and 33%.[1] This wide variation of reported recurrence rates reflects largely the heterogeneity of the studies, which is partly attributable to the differences in criteria used to define recurrence and the variations in protocol biopsies, sample sizes, and follow-up intervals. In the majority of cases, the impact of recurrence of PBC on graft function and survival is minimal for the first decade after transplantation, with end-stage disease affecting fewer than 5%.

Diagnosis

The diagnostic criteria for PBC in the native liver are based on clinical history, abnormal cholestatic liver tests, elevations of immunoglobulins (especially IgM), and positive antimitochondrial antibodies (AMAs) (**Table 51-2**). Liver histologic studies may be normal but usually show the characteristic noncaseating granulomatous cholangitis. The interpretation of these tests in the posttransplant setting is more complicated because features of recurrence may be modified by immunosuppression and the graft is subject to other causes of damage, including immunologic, ischemic, and toxic factors.

Symptoms of PBC such as lethargy and pruritus are not specific for PBC and so are not diagnostic of disease recurrence. Similarly, liver function tests are of limited value in the diagnosis of recurrent PBC because of their lack of specificity. Histologic evidence of rPBC can be seen within the background of normal liver function tests.[2] The presence of AMAs represents a high sensitivity and specificity for the disease in the native liver; however, AMAs may be present even in the absence of histologic evidence of recurrence and therefore may not be diagnostic of disease in the allograft.[2]

Histologic studies remain the primary tool for the diagnosis of recurrent PBC. The main finding is florid duct lesions on liver biopsy, including mononuclear inflammatory infiltrates, formation of lymphoid aggregates, epithelioid granulomas, and bile duct damage.[3] The differential diagnosis includes cytomegalovirus (CMV) infection, hepatitis C infection, graft-versus-host disease, and acute and chronic rejection.[4] Hence it is important but relatively easy to exclude other causes before the diagnosis of recurrent PBC is made.

Outcome

The effects of recurrent disease on graft function and patient survival are usually minor, with only a small number of cases reporting progression from recurrent disease to graft failure and retransplantation.[5] However, as more long-term data emerge, the reported incidence may increase.

Risk Factors and Management

The association of specific immunosuppressive agents with rPBC is controversial. Individual studies have suggested that use of tacrolimus is associated with earlier and more

Table 51-1 Nonviral Diseases that Recur after Transplantation

Presumed autoimmune
    Primary biliary cirrhosis
    Primary sclerosing cholangitis
Metabolic
    Budd-Chiari syndrome (some causes)
    Nonalcoholic fatty liver disease
Alcohol

Table 51-2 Features of Recurrent Primary Biliary Cirrhosis

Frequency and Outcome

Recurrence: 18% rate
Graft loss: less than 5% rate at 5 years

Diagnosis

Specific
    Liver histology
Nonspecific
    Persistence of antimitochondrial antibodies
    Liver tests
    Recurrence of symptoms

Liver Biopsy Finding Suggestive of Primary Biliary Cirrhosis

Florid duct lesions that include mononuclear inflammatory
    infiltrates, formation of lymphoid aggregates, epithelioid
    granulomas, and bile duct damage

Risk Factors

Tacrolimus may be associated with more aggressive and
    earlier recurrent disease when compared with cyclosporine

Treatment

Ursodeoxycholic acid
    Improves liver test values
    May delay progression

Table 51-3 Features of Recurrent Primary Sclerosing Cholangitis

Frequency and Outcome

Recurrence: 50% rate
Graft loss: up to 25% rate at 5 years

Diagnosis

Specific
    Demonstration of multiple nonanastomotic biliary strictures
    Exclusion of other causes
    Liver histology (diagnostic lesions uncommon)
Nonspecific
    Liver tests
    Recurrence of symptoms

Risk Factors

Controversial but may include:
    Male gender
    Rejection acute/multiple episodes
    Cytomegalovirus infection
    Intact colon after surgery

Treatment

Ursodeoxycholic acid
    Improves liver test values
    May delay progression

According to the current but limited evidence, it seems reasonable to offer ursodeoxycholic acid at a daily dose of 10 to 15 mg/kg to patients with evidence of rPBC (although the drug is not licensed for use in this indication). There is no evidence, to date, that preemptive treatment with UDCA, substitution of tacrolimus with cyclosporine, or addition of corticosteroids will affect either the risk of recurrence or the rate of progression.

Primary Sclerosing Cholangitis

Primary sclerosing cholangitis (PSC) is a chronic progressive condition that involves inflammation and fibrosis of both intrahepatic and extrahepatic bile ducts, resulting in progressive chronic liver disease; it is commonly associated with inflammatory bowel disease. Similar to PBC, the reported prevalence of recurrent PSC differs widely among studies.

Evidence for recurrent PSC was based originally on a comparison of allograft liver histologic and imaging studies of the biliary tree between patients grafted for PSC and patients transplanted for non-PSC conditions but with biliary reconstruction. Nonanastomotic biliary strictures and characteristic biliary histologic findings were significantly more common in the PSC group.[14] Other studies have since confirmed such findings.[15,16] Recurrent PSC is seen in up to 50% of patients at 5 years and may lead to graft loss in up to 25% at 5 years.

Diagnosis

As with PSC in the native liver, the diagnosis of rPSC is based on a combination of biochemical, radiologic, and histologic findings and exclusion of other causes (**Table 51-3**). Histologic changes suggestive of rPSC include biliary fibrosis, fibrous cholangitis, and fibroobliterative lesions; however, these findings are used more commonly as criteria that support the

aggressive recurrence of PBC, compared with cyclosporine.[6,7] Cyclosporine has been shown to be effective in the treatment of PBC in the native liver.[8] Some researchers have suggested that lack of corticosteroids may increase the risk of recurrence whereas other studies have suggested that withdrawal of immunosuppression may increase the probability of recurrent disease.[9,10] The heterogeneity of published studies, both in diagnostic criteria and in follow-up interval, makes interpretation of these findings difficult.

Good evidence exists on the use of ursodeoxycholic acid (UDCA) in the treatment of PBC in the native liver but the mechanism of action remains uncertain; many, but not all, studies have demonstrated improvement in liver function tests, delay in histologic progression, and improvement in survival in patients with PBC.[11] The promising result seen with the use of UDCA in the native liver may translate into the posttransplant setting. Studies on the use of UDCA in recurrent PBC have so far demonstrated improvement in liver function tests.[12,13] Currently there is no evidence to suggest any benefit on patient and/or graft survival; however, with further studies using larger sample sizes and longer follow-up periods, any effect can be established.

diagnosis, mostly because of patchy involvement and consequent sample variability as well as the relative lack of specificity of the findings. Findings that are suggestive of rPSC can also be seen in other pathologic conditions, including ischemia, recurrent biliary sepsis, and reperfusion injuries.[17] Ductopenic rejection shares some features, making it difficult to distinguish between the two, but it is unusual for chronic rejection to cause multiple nonanastomotic strictures, increased deposition of copper-binding protein is not characteristic of chronic rejection, and the prognosis is said to be poor compared with recurrent PSC.

The gold standard for the diagnosis of PSC, both in the native liver and in the graft (with the exception of small duct disease variant), is demonstration of abnormal intrahepatic and extrahepatic ducts on imaging and exclusion of causes of secondary cholangitis. Other diseases can also give a similar picture of bile duct injury, including hepatic artery thrombosis/stenosis, drug toxicity, established ductopenia rejection, reperfusion injury, biliary sepsis, anastomotic strictures, and the consequences of donor/recipient ABO incompatibility.[17] Hence the diagnosis of rPSC is one of exclusion. Endoscopic retrograde cholangiopancreatography (ERCP) has largely been replaced by the use of magnetic resonance cholangiography (MRC). Percutaneous cholangiography may also be used. There are limited data on the use of MRC for the diagnosis of recurrent PSC, but early evidence suggests it offers a reliable and noninvasive test for the identification of biliary pathology seen in recurrent PSC.[18]

Risk factors for the development of recurrent PSC include male gender,[19] an intact colon before or during transplantation,[19] steroid-resistant rejection,[18] active colitis posttransplantation,[20] use of OKT3 for the treatment of cellular rejection,[21] gender mismatch between donor,[22] cytomegalovirus infection,[23] recurrent acute cellular rejection,[15] and the presence of specific HLA haplotypes (e.g., HLA-DRB1*08).[24] However, there is little consistency between series.

Early studies with short follow-up intervals that compared patient survival have demonstrated no difference between patients with or without recurrent PSC.[25] However, longer-term data suggest recurrent disease can lead to graft loss.[26]

Treatment

Ursodeoxycholic acid has been advocated for the treatment of PSC in the native liver: studies have demonstrated improvement in biochemical parameters, symptoms, disease progression, and survival time although higher doses may be toxic. Currently there are no robust data on the use of UDCA in the posttransplant setting for recurrent PSC. However, UDCA may be beneficial not only in avoidance of the possible development and/or progression of rPSC but also in prevention of colon cancer in patients who have associated colitis.[27] Those with both PSC and ulcerative colitis have a greater risk of such complications after liver transplantation.[28] Although colectomy, before or during transplantation, may protect against recurrent disease, there is no indication for prophylactic colectomy merely to prevent recurrence of PSC.

Autoimmune Hepatitis

As with PBC and PSC, autoimmune hepatitis (AIH) can recur following transplantation. The reported rates of recurrence

Table 51-4 Features of Recurrent Autoimmune Hepatitis

Frequency and Outcome
Recurrence: up to 25% rate Graft loss: approximately 25% rate at 5 years
Diagnosis

Specific
   Immunology (increase in titer or de novo autoantibodies)
   Liver histology
Nonspecific
   Liver tests
   Recurrence of symptoms

Liver Biopsy Finding Suggestive of Autoimmune Hepatitis
Interface hepatitis
Risk Factors
Certain HLA matches/mismatches Reduction in corticosteroids
Treatment

Corticosteroid reintroduction or increased dose
Switch to tacrolimus or sirolimus
   Improves liver test values
   May delay progression

differ widely.[29] The diagnosis of AIH in the native liver incorporates a combination of clinical, biochemical, immunologic, and histologic findings; a response to immunosuppression; and the exclusion of other possible diagnoses (**Table 51-4**). The scoring system developed by the International Autoimmune Hepatitis Group[30] has not been validated for use in recurrent AIH and many aspects included in this scoring system cannot be simply and uncritically translated into the posttransplant setting.

Studies using protocol liver biopsies have shown that recurrent AIH can also occur in the presence of normal liver function; therefore the use of abnormal transaminase level as a marker of possible recurrent disease is limited in the diagnosis of recurrent AIH.[31] High-titer autoantibodies and hypergammaglobulinemia are useful screening tools in the diagnosis of suspected AIH in the native liver and, as with PBC, such markers can remain detectable posttransplantation and in other causes of graft damage.[32,33] An increase in the titer of autoantibodies after liver transplantation may indicate recurrent disease, but evidence is limited and titers may be affected by immunosuppression.[34] Thus liver histologic analysis is essential to establish the diagnosis of recurrent disease and evaluate disease severity. Histologic findings consistent with recurrent disease include mononuclear inflammatory infiltrates, abundant plasma cells, and interface hepatitis (piecemeal necrosis). However, such findings are not unique to recurrent AIH, and can be seen in viral hepatitis and cellular rejection.[35]

The reported outcome of recurrent disease varies.[29,36] Risk factors for rAIH are uncertain: recipient HLA DR3 positivity and donor HLA DR3 negativity may be correlated with an increased risk of recurrent disease. Both chronic ductopenic and acute cellular rejection are more common in patients with recurrent disease, possibly reflecting an increase in autoimmune responsiveness of the recipient.[37]

Treatment

Immunosuppression plays an important role both in the treatment and in the prevention of recurrent AIH. The reduction of immunosuppression, in particular corticosteroids, increases the risk of recurrence; therefore administration of long-term, low-dose corticosteroids (e.g., prednisolone 5 to 7.5 mg/day) has been suggested in patients who have received liver transplants for AIH.[38,39] In those who are not maintained with a treatment regimen of corticosteroids, regular monitoring of immunoglobulin levels, titers of autoantibodies, and use of protocol biopsies will be required to detect recurrence and allow early intervention. Small studies have suggested that treatment with tacrolimus and sirolimus are effective in the management of recurrent disease.[40,41]

Nonalcoholic Fatty Liver Disease

The extent and consequences of recurrent nonalcoholic fatty liver disease (NAFLD) in the allograft are uncertain: it is believed that many cases labeled as cryptogenic cirrhosis are "burnt out" NAFLD; therefore distinguishing de novo from recurrent NAFLD in the graft may be difficult. The diagnosis of NAFLD in the native liver involves the combination of clinical history and identifying component of the metabolic syndrome, abnormal liver function tests, exclusions of other liver disease, and identification of fatty liver using radiologic imaging or histologic studies, and often liver biopsy. Newer diagnostic tools, including blood tests and imaging (e.g., FibroScan), are of some value in both diagnosis and staging of NAFLD in the native liver.[42]

The diagnosis of recurrent NAFLD is similar to that in the native liver. Liver tests are not specific and radiologic findings of a fatty liver are suggestive of NAFLD but cannot differentiate NAFLD from other causes of fatty liver (e.g., diabetes mellitus, some infections, alcohol and other toxins); liver histologic studies may be needed to confirm the diagnosis, establish the extent of disease, and exclude other causes. Histologic evidence of NAFLD can be seen in patients with normal liver function.[43]

Factors associated with recurrence are related to the metabolic syndrome, and include high triglyceride level, hypertension, increased body mass index, and the presence of diabetes before or following liver transplantation.[44,45] Immunosuppression can further exacerbate and/or trigger such risk factors: corticosteroids, calcineurin inhibitors, and sirolimus can be associated with hypertension, increase in insulin resistance, obesity, and hypertension.[46]

Treatment

Currently there is no definitive treatment for NAFLD and no study has yet looked at treatments for recurrent posttransplant NAFLD. The main focus of treatment for NAFLD is modification of components associated with the metabolic syndrome. Treatment of the metabolic syndrome may not only prevent recurrent NAFLD in the liver graft but also reduce the cardiovascular risk. Treatment includes weight reduction in the form of diet, exercise, and, in selected patients, bariatric surgery.

Bariatric surgery is often high risk in the liver allograft recipient because of the consequences of the previous surgery and adhesions; therefore laparoscopic techniques are often not appropriate. Newer antiobesity drugs such as cannabinoid receptor antagonists, lipase inhibitors, and serotonin and glucagon-like protein-1 receptor agonists have all provided early promising results in the treatment of NAFLD in the native liver.[47-49] Thiazolidinediones and metformin have shown some benefit.[48-53] Control of hypertension using agents that block the angiotensin system and treatment for dyslipidemia with lipid-lowering medications, such as statins and gemfibrozil, have also been suggested to improve NAFLD.[54-56] As yet, there is little evidence for the benefit of each treatment in the allograft recipient and few agents have a license for use in this indication.

Alcoholic Liver Disease

The reported rate of relapse following transplantation for alcoholic liver disease (ALD) is highly variable, in part because of lack of standardization for the definition of recidivism. Many different strategies have been suggested in the detection of recidivism. Self-reporting is most common, and the success rate may be increased if the patient is interviewed by someone outside the transplant team. The use of reporting by family members, friends, and caregivers may further improve the sensitivity.

Biochemical tests including blood and urine alcohol levels, carbohydrate-deficient transferrin (CDT) level, alanine transaminase (ALT) to aspartate aminotransferase (AST) ratio, mitochondrial AST (mAST) level, γ-glutamyltransferase (GGT) level, and mean corpuscular volume (MCV) have all been well studied in the detection of alcohol abuse in the general population.[59] Other tests have also been developed (e.g., sialic acid, sialic acid index of apolipoprotein J, β-hexosaminidase, acetaldehyde adducts, the urinary ratio of serotonin metabolites, 5-hydroxytryptophol, and 5-hydroxyindoleacetic acid) but are used less often and their role in this context is not fully tested. Measurement of blood, breath, or urine alcohol concentration is a well-recognized tool in identifying patients with recent alcohol consumption, and it has been used in a number of studies in the posttransplant setting. However, its value is limited by the relatively short detectable half-life of alcohol. The use of CDT measurement may overcome this shortfall, because of its longer half-life of between 14 and 17 days. An increase in CDT level correlates with alcohol consumption exceeding 50 to 80 g/day for 2 to 3 weeks; although CDT measurement is considered to be unaffected by liver disease, its use in the posttransplant setting has still provided mixed results.[58-61]

With evidence pointing towards the different outcomes between harmful drinking and slips, the main aim in the prevention and treatment of recurrent disease should be total abstinence. Limited data exist on the treatment of recidivism in the posttransplant setting. Medications that are commonly used for the treatment of alcohol dependence include acamprosate, naltrexone, and disulfiram.[62] However, the effectiveness and safety of these agents have not been fully evaluated in the posttransplant setting. There is a concern regarding the possible interaction between these medications and immunosuppression therapy. Psychotherapeutic interventions, such as the use of motivational enhancement therapy (MET), have been shown to be useful in the nontransplant setting in the treatment of alcohol abuse, and a few studies in the posttransplant setting have demonstrated promising results, but further research is needed.[63,64]

Budd-Chiari Syndrome

In Western countries the most common causes of Budd-Chiari syndrome (BCS) are hematologic or thrombotic conditions. Budd-Chiari syndrome may also be the early herald of a myeloproliferative disorder. In some cases, where the thrombotic defect arises in the liver (e.g., factor V Leiden mutation; protein C, protein S, antithrombin III deficiency), liver transplantation will correct the predisposing defect.

The incidence of recurrent disease ranges from between 0% and 10% and complications from other thrombotic events are not uncommon.[65] Because of the risk of recurrent disease relating to hypercoagulable conditions from some causes, most patients begin anticoagulation therapy following liver transplantation. Thus the need for anticoagulation medication will depend on the indication.

However, despite the use of anticoagulation therapy, patients can still develop recurrent disease, leading to graft failure and 71&Q death.[66-68] In many such cases, subtherapeutic anticoagulation levels can be identified as a factor to recurrent disease and this may reflect in difficulties in the dosage of warfarin attributable to its narrow therapeutic window and need for long-term monitoring. If recurrence does occur, management includes medical treatment of complications from portal hypertension, surgical shunt, transjugular intrahepatic portosystemic shunt (TIPS), and retransplantation.[68] Once again, because of the small number of cases, recommendation on the best treatment cannot be made and should be determined on an individual basis.

Metabolic Diseases

Liver transplantation is curative for those metabolic diseases where the metabolic defect lies within the liver (e.g., Wilson disease, α_1-antitrypsin deficiency, tyrosinemia, Crigler-Najjar syndrome, some urea cycle defects and glycogen storage diseases). It remains uncertain whether liver replacement "cures" hemochromatosis; however, most evidence suggests that, at least in the medium term, iron accumulation does not occur. The defects in most lipid storage disorders are not confined to the liver, so liver transplantation alone is not curative and these diseases persist.

References

1. Gautam M, Cheruvattath R, Balan V. Recurrence of autoimmune liver disease after liver transplantation: a systematic review. Liver Transpl 2006; 12:1813–1824.
2. Klein R, et al. Antimitochondrial antibody profiles in patients with primary biliary cirrhosis before orthotopic liver transplantation and titres of antimitochondrial antibody-subtypes after transplantation. J Hepatol 1994; 20:181–189.
3. Hubscher S, et al. Primary biliary cirrhosis. Histological evidence of disease recurrence after liver transplantation. J Hepatol 1993;18:173–184.
4. Neuberger JM. Recurrent primary biliary cirrhosis. Liver Transpl 2003;9: 539–546.
5. Garcia R, et al. Transplantation for primary biliary cirrhosis: retrospective analysis of 400 patients in a single center. Hepatology 2001;33:22–27.
6. Wong PY, et al. Recurrence of primary biliary cirrhosis after liver transplantation following FK506-based immunosuppression. J Hepatol 1993;17:284–287.
7. Neuberger J, et al. Immunosuppression affects the rate of recurrent primary biliary cirrhosis after liver transplantation. Liver Transpl 2004;10:488–491.
8. Lombard M, et al. Cyclosporin A treatment in primary biliary cirrhosis: results of a long-term placebo controlled trial. Gastroenterology 1993;104: 519–526.
9. Mazariegos GV, et al. Weaning of immunosuppression in liver transplant recipients. Transplantation 1997;63:243–249.
10. Yoshida EM, et al. Late recurrent post-transplant primary biliary cirrhosis in British Columbia. Can J Gastroenterol 1997;11:229–233.
11. Angulo P, et al. Long-term ursodeoxycholic acid delays histological progression in primary biliary cirrhosis. Hepatology 1999;29:644–647.
12. Guy JE, et al. Recurrent primary biliary cirrhosis: peritransplant factors and ursodeoxycholic acid treatment post-liver transplant. Liver Transpl 2005;11: 1252–1257.
13. Charatcharoenwitthaya P, et al. Long-term survival and impact of ursodeoxycholic acid treatment for recurrent primary biliary cirrhosis after liver transplantation. Liver Transpl 2007;1:1236–1245.
14. Sheng R, et al. Cholangiographic features of biliary strictures after liver transplantation for primary sclerosing cholangitis: evidence of recurrent disease. Am J Roentgenol 1996;166:1109–1113.
15. Harrison RF, et al. Fibrous and obliterative cholangitis in liver allografts: evidence of recurrent primary sclerosing cholangitis? Hepatology 1994;20: 356–361.
16. Sheng R, et al. Cholangiographic features of biliary strictures after liver transplantation for primary sclerosing cholangitis: evidence of recurrent disease. Am J Roentgenol 1996;166:1109–1113.
17. Graziadei IW. Recurrence of primary sclerosing cholangitis after liver transplantation. Liver Transpl 2002;8:575–581.
18. Brandsaeter B, et al. Recurrent primary sclerosing cholangitis after liver transplantation: a magnetic resonance cholangiography study with analyses of predictive factors. Liver Transpl 2005;11:1361–1369.
19. Vera A, et al. Risk factors for recurrence of primary sclerosing cholangitis of liver allograft. Lancet 2002;360:1943–1944.
20. Cholongitas E, et al. Risk factors for recurrence of primary sclerosing cholangitis after liver transplantation. Liver Transpl 2008;14:138–143.
21. Kugelmas M, et al. Different immunosuppressive regimens and recurrence of primary sclerosing cholangitis after liver transplantation. Liver Transpl 2003;9:727–732.
22. Khettry U, et al. Liver transplantation for primary sclerosing cholangitis: a long-term clinicopathologic study. Hum Pathol 2003;34:1127–1136.
23. Jeyarajah DR, et al. Recurrent primary sclerosing cholangitis after orthotopic liver transplantation: is chronic rejection part of the disease process? Transplantation 1998;66:1300–1306.
24. Alexander J, et al. Risk factors for recurrence of primary sclerosing cholangitis after liver transplantation. Liver Transpl 2008;14:245–251.
25. Faust TW. Recurrent primary biliary cirrhosis, primary sclerosing cholangitis, and autoimmune hepatitis after transplantation. Liver Transpl 2001;7:S99–S108.
26. Rowe IA, et al. The impact of disease recurrence on graft survival following liver transplantation: a single centre experience. Transpl Int 2008;21: 459–465.
27. Pardi DS, et al. Ursodeoxycholic acid as a chemopreventive agent in patients with ulcerative colitis and primary sclerosing cholangitis. Gastroenterology 2003;124:889–893.
28. Loftus EV Jr, et al. Risk of colorectal neoplasia in patients with primary sclerosing cholangitis and ulcerative colitis following orthotopic liver transplantation. Hepatology 1998;27:685–690.
29. Gautam M, Cheruvattath R, Balan V. Recurrence of autoimmune liver disease after liver transplantation: a systematic review. Liver Transpl 2006;12:1813–1824.
30. Alvarez F, et al. International Autoimmune Hepatitis Group report: review of criteria for diagnosis of autoimmune hepatitis. J Hepatol 1993;31: 929–938.
31. Ahmed M, et al. Liver transplantation for autoimmune hepatitis; a 12-year experience. Transplant Proc 1997;29:496.
32. Götz G, et al. Recurrence of autoimmune hepatitis after liver transplantation. Transplant Proc 1999;31:430–431.
33. Ratziu V, et al. Long-term follow-up after liver transplantation for autoimmune hepatitis: evidence of recurrence of primary disease. J Hepatol 1999;30:131–141.
34. González-Koch A, et al. Recurrent autoimmune hepatitis after orthotopic liver transplantation. Liver Transpl 2001;7:302–310.
35. Hubscher SG. Recurrent autoimmune hepatitis after liver transplantation: diagnostic criteria, risk factors, and outcome. Liver Transpl 2001;7:285–291.
36. Milkiewicz P, et al. Recurrence of autoimmune hepatitis after liver transplantation. Transplantation 1999;68:253.
37. Ayata G, et al. Liver transplantation for autoimmune hepatitis: a long-term pathologic study. Hepatology 2000;32:185–192.

38. Neuberger J, et al. Recurrence of autoimmune chronic active hepatitis following orthotopic liver grafting. Transplantation 1984;37:363–365.
39. González-Koch A, et al. Recurrent autoimmune hepatitis after orthotopic liver transplantation. Liver Transpl 2001;7:302–310.
40. Rumbo C, et al. Rapamycin successfully treats post-transplant autoimmune hepatitis. Am J Transplant 2005;5:1085–1089.
41. Hurtova M, et al. Successful tacrolimus therapy for a severe recurrence of type 1 autoimmune hepatitis in a liver graft recipient. Liver Transpl 2001;7:556–558.
42. Beckebaum S, et al. Assessment of allograft fibrosis by transient elastography and noninvasive biomarker scoring systems in liver transplant patients. Transplantation 2010;89:983–993.
43. Contos MJ, et al. Development of nonalcoholic fatty liver disease after orthotopic liver transplantation for cryptogenic cirrhosis. Liver Transpl 2001;7:363–373.
44. Cauble MS, et al. Lipoatrophic diabetes and end-stage liver disease secondary to nonalcoholic steatohepatitis with recurrence after liver transplantation. Transplantation 2001;71:892–895.
45. Ong J, et al. Cryptogenic cirrhosis and posttransplantation nonalcoholic fatty liver disease. Liver Transpl 2001;7:797–801.
46. Benten D, Staufer K, Sterneck M. Orthotopic liver transplantation and what to do during follow-up: recommendations for the practitioner. Nat Clin Pract Gastroenterol Hepatol 2009;6:23–36.
47. Gary-Bobo M, et al. Rimonabant reduces obesity-associated hepatic steatosis and features of metabolic syndrome in obese zucker fa/fa rats. Hepatology 2007;46:122–129.
48. Assy N, Hussein O, Abassi Z. Weight loss induced by orlistat reverses fatty infiltration and improves hepatic fibrosis in obese patients with non-alcoholic steatohepatitis. Gut 2007;56:443–444.
49. Tushuizen ME, et al. Incretin mimetics as a novel therapeutic option for hepatic steatosis. Liver Int 2006;26:1015–1017.
50. Aithal GP, et al. Randomized, placebo-controlled trial of pioglitazone in nondiabetic subjects with nonalcoholic steatohepatitis. Gastroenterology 2008;135:1176–1184.
51. Sanyal AJ, et al. A pilot study of vitamin E versus vitamin E and pioglitazone for the treatment of non-alcoholic steatohepatitis. Clin Gastroenterol Hepatol 2004;2:1107–1115.
52. Belfort R, et al. A placebo controlled trial of pioglitazone in subjects with nonalcoholic steatohepatitis. New Engl J Med 2006;355:15–25.
53. Nair S, et al. Metformin in the treatment of non-alcoholic steatohepatitis: a pilot open label trial. Aliment Pharmacol Ther 2004;20:23–28.
54. Yokohama S, et al. Inhibitory effect of angiotensin II receptor antagonist on hepatic stellate activation in non-alcoholic steatohepatitis. World J Gastroenterol 2006;12:322–326.
55. Gómez-Domínguez E, et al. A pilot study of atorvastatin treatment in dyslipidemidic, non-alcoholic fatty liver patients. Aliment Pharmacol Ther 2006;23:1643–1647.
56. Basaranoglu M, Acbay O, Sonsuz A. A controlled trial of gemfibrozil in the treatment of patients with non-alcoholic steatohepatitis. J Hepatol 1999;31:384.
57. Niemelä O. Biomarkers in alcoholism. Clin Chim Acta 2007;377:39–49.
58. DiMartini A, et al. Alcohol use following liver transplantation: a comparison of follow-up methods. Psychosomatics 2001;42:55–62.
59. Schmitt VM, et al. Carbohydrate-deficient transferrin is not a useful marker for the detection of chronic alcohol abuse. Eur J Clin Invest 1998;28:615–621.
60. Heinemann A, et al. Carbohydrate-deficient transferrin: diagnostic efficiency among patients with end-stage liver disease before and after liver transplantation. Alcohol Clin Exp Res 1998;22:1806–1812.
61. Berlakovich GA, et al. Carbohydrate-deficient transferrin for detection of alcohol relapse after orthotopic liver transplantation for alcoholic cirrhosis. Transplantation 1999;67:1231–1235.
62. Mann K. Pharmacotherapy of alcohol dependence: a review of the clinical data. CNS Drugs 2004;18:485–504.
63. Georgiou G, et al. First report of a psychosocial intervention for patients with alcohol-related liver disease undergoing liver transplantation. Liver Transpl 2003;9:772–775.
64. Björnsson E, et al. Long-term follow-up of patients with alcoholic liver disease after liver transplantation in Sweden: impact of structured management on recidivism. Scand J Gastroenterol 2005;40:206–216.
65. Cruz E, et al. High incidence of recurrence and hematologic events following liver transplantation for Budd-Chiari syndrome. Clin Transplant 2005;19:501–506.
66. Jamieson NV, Williams R, Calne RY. Liver transplantation for Budd–Chiari syndrome. Ann Chir 1991;45:362.
67. Halff G, et al. Liver transplantation for the Budd–Chiari syndrome. Ann Surg 1990;211:43.
68. Srinivasan P, et al. Liver transplantation for Budd–Chiari syndrome. Transplantation 2002;73:973.

Section IX

Liver Affected by Other Organs or Conditions (Diseases)

The Liver in Pregnancy

Ghassan M. Hammoud and Jamal A. Ibdah

ABBREVIATIONS

ABC ATP-binding cassette
AFLP acute fatty liver of pregnancy
AIH autoimmune hepatitis
ALT alanine aminotransferase
APAP acetaminophen
AST aspartate aminotransferase
BCS Budd-Chiari syndrome
BSEP bile-salt export pump
BSP sulfobromophthalein
CoA coenzyme A
CT computed tomography
DIC disseminated intravascular coagulopathy
EIA enzyme immunoassay
ERCP endoscopic retrograde cholangiopancreatography
GGT γ-glutamyltransferase
HAV hepatitis A virus

HBIG hepatitis B immunoglobulin
HBV hepatitis B virus
HCC hepatocellular carcinoma
HCV hepatitis C virus
HDL high-density lipoprotein
HELLP hemolysis, elevated liver enzymes, and low platelet count
HEV hepatitis E virus
HG hyperemesis gravidarum
HIV human immunodeficiency virus
ICP intrahepatic cholestasis of pregnancy
LCHAD long-chain 3-hydroxyacyl-CoA dehydrogenase
LDH lactate dehydrogenase
LDL low-density lipoprotein
LMWH low-molecular-weight heparin
MRI magnetic resonance imaging

MRP2 multidrug resistance–associated protein-2
MTP mitochondrial trifunctional protein
NAC N-acetylcysteine
NTCP Na⁺/taurocholate co-transporting polypeptide
NVP nausea and vomiting of pregnancy
PFIC progressive familial intrahepatic cholestasis
PHT portal hypertension
PT prothrombin time
PVT portal vein thrombosis
SAMe S-adenosyl-L-methionine
TIPS transjugular intrahepatic portosystemic shunt
UDCA ursodeoxycholic acid
UGT uridine glucuronosyltransferase

Introduction

Physiologic and anatomic alterations arise in many organs during the course of pregnancy. These physiologic changes tend to occur in the early stages of pregnancy in preparation for the incoming fetus. Examples include alterations in blood volume, blood constituents, cardiac output, and levels of sex hormones and plasma lipids. The liver is influenced by the physiologic state of pregnancy and thus abnormalities that may usually signify hepatic dysfunction may not represent actual liver damage and should be interpreted with caution. In addition, the anatomic location of the liver is changed because it is shifted superiorly as pregnancy progresses secondary to the enlarging gravid uterus. Therefore liver that is palpable below the right subcostal margin during pregnancy usually indicates an ongoing pathologic hepatic process. Liver disease in pregnancy is uncommon and in the majority of cases there is no need for a change in management of a liver disorder until pregnancy ends. However, special consideration must always be given to both mother and baby during pregnancy, delivery, and the postpartum period. In general, most liver abnormalities that occur in pregnancy are secondary to conditions not specific to pregnancy and therefore such conditions should be considered along with those specific to pregnancy when evaluating liver dysfunction.

Liver diseases unique to pregnancy can be classified according to their association with preeclampsia (**Table 52-1**) or their time of onset during pregnancy (**Table 52-2**). These disorders and their period of onset include the following:

1. Hyperemesis gravidarum (HG)—Usually occurs in the first trimester of pregnancy and is not associated with preeclampsia.
2. The syndrome of hemolysis, elevated liver enzymes, and low platelets (HELLP)—Usually occurs in the third trimester and is associated with preeclampsia.
3. Intrahepatic cholestasis of pregnancy (ICP)—Can occur at any time during pregnancy and is not associated with preeclampsia.
4. Acute fatty liver disease of pregnancy (AFLP)—Usually occurs in the third trimester and is associated with preeclampsia.

The aspects of liver function and liver disease during pregnancy that are discussed in this chapter include (1) normal anatomic, physiologic, and biochemical changes in hepatic function and metabolism during pregnancy; (2) liver diseases not specific to pregnancy; and (3) liver diseases unique to

Table 52-1 Classification of Liver Diseases Unique to Pregnancy According to Their Association with Preeclampsia/Eclampsia

ASSOCIATED WITH PREECLAMPSIA/ECLAMPSIA	NOT ASSOCIATED WITH PREECLAMPSIA/ECLAMPSIA
HELLP syndrome	Hyperemesis gravidarum
Acute fatty liver disease of pregnancy	Intrahepatic cholestasis of pregnancy

HELLP, hemolysis, elevated liver enzymes, and low platelet count

Table 52-2 Classification of Liver Diseases Unique to Pregnancy According to Their Onset during Pregnancy

FIRST TRIMESTER	SECOND TRIMESTER	THIRD TRIMESTER
Hyperemesis gravidarum		HELLP syndrome
		Acute fatty liver of pregnancy
	Intrahepatic cholestasis of pregnancy	

HELLP, hemolysis, elevated liver enzymes, and low platelet count

pregnancy. The reader is encouraged to refer to detailed discussions of liver diseases not specific to pregnancy in other chapters of this book.

Changes in Liver Anatomy and Function during Normal Pregnancy

Liver Anatomy and Histology

Anatomically, the gross appearance of the liver does not change during pregnancy. In the third trimester, the gravid uterus displaces the liver upward towards the chest and a palpable liver is considered abnormal. Histologically, subtle changes may be seen but are not specific. These changes include (1) increased variability in hepatocyte size and shape; (2) enhanced granularity of hepatocyte cytoplasm; (3) increased numbers of cytoplasmic fat vacuoles in centrilobular hepatocytes; and (4) hypertrophied Kupffer cells. Hepatocytes in women during normal pregnancy also exhibit proliferation of the smooth and rough endoplasmic reticula; enlarged, rod-shaped, and giant mitochondria with paracrystalline inclusions; and increased numbers of peroxisomes. Many of these changes are also observed in women taking oral contraceptives.

Hemodynamics and Hepatic Blood Flow

Pregnancy is characterized by an increase in extracellular and plasma volume of 50% to 70%. This progressive increase in blood volume starts at 6 to 8 weeks of gestation and reaches its maximum level by 32 to 34 weeks. Red blood cell mass also increases, but the increase is moderate (20% to 30%) and delayed. As the total blood volume increases, hemodilution occurs as a consequence. Plasma volume and red blood cell mass decrease rapidly after delivery. This phenomenon of hemodilution should be considered during interpretation of all serum concentrations during pregnancy. Cardiac output increases to a similar degree as the blood volume until the second trimester, and then decreases and normalizes near term. Absolute hepatic blood flow remains unchanged, but the percentage of cardiac output to the liver decreases.

Changes in Liver Function

Drug Metabolism

Medication use during pregnancy is common and includes prescription, over-the-counter, and herbal products. A study of U.S. and Canadian women found that, on average, 2.3 drugs were used during pregnancy; however, 28% reported using more than 4 medications.[1] The liver plays a major role in drug metabolism and detoxification. Various hemodynamic changes during pregnancy, such as the increase in blood volume, cardiac output, and glomerular filtration rate, may contribute to altered drug metabolism, disposition, and clearance.[2] Gastrointestinal absorption or bioavailability of drugs may vary because of changes in gastric secretion and motility. Drug properties such as lipid solubility, protein-binding characteristics, and ionization constant influence the placental passage of drugs. Moreover, changes in the activity of maternal and fetal drug-metabolizing enzymes may affect maternal drug distribution and clearance.

Pregnancy alters the ability of a drug to be distributed within the body, in part by causing reduced concentrations of both albumin and α_1-acid glycoprotein. Moreover, the increase in body weight in late pregnancy results in a decrease in dose per kilogram. Caffeine metabolism is reduced during pregnancy because of decreased activity of CYP1A2. The activity of P-450 2A6 is increased and drugs such as nicotine exhibit substantially lower serum concentrations. Likewise, the activity of CYP3A4 is increased and drugs such as nifedipine, carbamazepine, midazolam, indinavir, lopinavir, and ritonavir have an increased clearance. Drugs such as metoprolol, fluoxetine, citalopram, and nortriptyline may exhibit increased clearance.[3] The dose of selective serotonin reuptake inhibitors (SSRIs) must be increased to maintain efficacy in pregnancy. Furthermore, glomerular filtration rate is increased in pregnancy because of an increase in cardiac output; therefore drugs that are eliminated by renal mechanisms have increased clearance rates, such as ampicillin, cefuroxime, ceftazidime, cephradine, cefazolin, piperacillin, atenolol, sotalol, digoxin, and lithium. Both estrogen intake and pregnancy impair hepatic activity of glucuronosyltransferase (UGT), and progestational agents induce hepatic mixed-function oxidase activity in animals. Acetaminophen (APAP) metabolism is unchanged in pregnancy. Acetaminophen crosses the placenta and is detected in the neonatal serum after birth. Glucuronidation, the main metabolic pathway that safely metabolizes acetaminophen in adults, is markedly reduced in the neonate, leaving sulfation as the major pathway for acetaminophen metabolism. APAP toxicity in pregnancy is not rare and can

Table 52-3 FDA Category by Class in Pregnancy for Common Drug Therapy in Liver Disease

FDA CATEGORY B	FDA CATEGORY C	FDA CATEGORY D	FDA CATEGORY X
Ursodeoxycholic acid	Interferon alfa	Azathioprine	Ribavirin
Octreotide	Prednisone	D-Penicillamine	Vasopressin
Acyclovir	Lamivudine		Warfarin
	Adefovir		
	Entecavir		
	Telbivudine		
	Tenofovir		
	Mycophenolate mofetil		
	Tacrolimus		
	Sirolimus		
	Trientine		
	Zinc sulfate		
	Cyclosporine		
	Propranolol (in first trimester)	Propranolol (in second/third trimester)	
	Nadolol (in first trimester)	Nadolol (in second/third trimester)	
	Heparin		

FDA, Food and Drug Administration

result in significant morbidity and mortality in both the mother and the fetus. *N*-Acetylcysteine (NAC) can be safely administered during pregnancy and should be given early after APAP overdose. Clinicians must vigilantly monitor both the dose of drugs and the patient's response during pregnancy. **Table 52-3** lists the categories by class of the Food and Drug Administration (FDA) during pregnancy for common drug therapy used in pregnant patients with liver disease.

Serum Proteins and Lipids

Normally, up to 10 g of albumin is produced and secreted by the liver daily. Serum albumin concentrations decrease during the second trimester and continue to decline throughout pregnancy, reaching concentrations approximately 70% to 80% of normal values at the time of delivery secondary to hemodilution. In pregnancy the intravascular mass of albumin does not change and the rates of albumin synthesis and catabolism are not affected. By contrast, there is an increase in serum concentration of some proteins such as α_2-macroglobulin, α_1-antitrypsin, and ceruloplasmin.

Levels of fibrinogen and most coagulation factors (II, VIII, IX, and XII) increase, protein S levels decrease, and fibrinolysis is inhibited. These physiologic changes in hemostasis limit bleeding during delivery but are associated with an increased risk of thromboembolism during pregnancy and the postpartum period. Prothrombin time (PT) reflects the extrinsic clotting pathway involving factors II, V, VII, and X and is used to assess hepatic synthetic function. PT is considered a universal indicator of liver failure and is prolonged in acute liver failure. PT is generally not affected by pregnancy and any change in the prothrombin time during pregnancy should be considered pathologic and warrants further investigation. Serum albumin has a long half-life of 20 days and is not a good indicator of

hepatic synthetic function in acute liver disease. However, the half-lives of blood clotting factors are quite short (about 1 day) and are useful indicators of liver injury.

Serum cholesterol, triglyceride, and phospholipid concentrations increase in late pregnancy. Levels of total serum cholesterol, high-density lipoprotein (HDL) cholesterol, and low-density lipoprotein (LDL) cholesterol increase 25% to 50%, whereas concentrations of serum triglycerides increase twice to four times their nonpregnancy levels. This hyperlipidemia is a result of the metabolic adaptation to the pregnancy state. Consequently, measurement of serum lipid concentrations is rarely useful during pregnancy, an exception being the pregnant woman suffering from acute pancreatitis. Serum concentrations of α- and β-globulins are increased whereas levels of γ-globulins are decreased. **Table 52-4** lists changes in laboratory profiles during normal pregnancy.

Bilirubin

Bilirubin is formed through the degradation of heme by heme oxygenase, which results in the formation of carbon monoxide, iron, and biliverdin as end products. Biliverdin is then converted to unconjugated bilirubin by biliverdin reductase. Normal serum bilirubin values represent a balance between the production of bilirubin as a result of heme degradation (unconjugated bilirubin) and the hepatic elimination of bilirubin (conjugated bilirubin). In the liver, uridine diphosphate glucuronosyltransferases (UGTs) conjugate the water-insoluble bilirubin to glucuronic acid, and conjugated bilirubin is then excreted into the bile. Defects in UGT activity result in indirect hyperbilirubinemia and impaired biliary excretion results in direct hyperbilirubinemia. The normal value for serum total bilirubin level is 1 mg/dl, of which 70% is unconjugated bilirubin.

Table 52-4 Changes in Laboratory Profile during Normal Pregnancy

TEST	CHANGE
WBCs	Increased
Hemoglobin	Decreased
Platelets	—
Albumin	Decreased
Aminotransferases	—
Alkaline phosphatase	Increased
GGT	—
Bilirubin	—/Decreased
Prothrombin time	—
Fibrinogen	Increased
Globulins	Increased in α- and β-globulins; decreased in γ-globulin
Glucose	—
Creatinine	—
Uric acid	—
Bile acids	—
Cholesterol	Increased
Triglycerides	Increased
α-Fetoprotein	Increased
Ceruloplasmin	Increased
Ferritin	Increased

GGT, γ-glutamyltransferase; WBC, white blood cell

In pregnant women the total and free bilirubin concentrations are significantly lower during all three trimesters as are concentrations of conjugated bilirubin during the second and third trimesters. Hemodilution could at least be partly responsible for the decrease in bilirubin concentration because albumin is the protein that transports bilirubin. Gilbert syndrome is characterized by mild unconjugated nonhemolytic hyperbilirubinemia. Gilbert syndrome generally affects 7% to 10% of the average population. In 80% to 100% of patients diagnosed with Gilbert syndrome, the (TA)-insertion in the promoter-region of the gene is present in homozygous (TA)7/(TA)7 form, and leads to a decrease in the amount of functionally active enzyme. This will result in mild indirect hyperbilirubinemia with serum total bilirubin levels of 5 mg/dl or less. The disease is not associated with cholestasis or pruritus and serum bile acid level is normal. HELLP syndrome has been associated with postpartum indirect hyperbilirubinemia and should be differentiated from Gilbert syndrome. There is no association between HELLP syndrome and Gilbert syndrome.[4] The management of patients with Gilbert syndrome is the same for both pregnant and nonpregnant patients. Conservative management and reassurance should be provided.

Patients with Crigler-Najjar type 1 (CN1) disorder have an unconjugated hyperbilirubinemia attributable to the complete absence of uridine diphosphate glucuronosyltransferase activity, a bilirubin-conjugating enzyme. In pregnant women with CN1, the fetus is at high risk of being adversely affected by the bilirubin, because unconjugated bilirubin can cross the placenta and may cause kernicterus, a potentially neurotoxic condition. Successful pregnancy in patients with Crigler-Najjar syndrome has been reported with the use of phenobarbital and phototherapy.[5-7]

Dubin-Johnson syndrome (DJS) is a rare benign chronic disorder of bilirubin metabolism, characterized by conjugated hyperbilirubinemia, darkly pigmented liver, and the presence of abnormal pigment in hepatic parenchymal cells. Pregnancy and use of oral contraceptives in women with Dubin-Johnson syndrome cause a reversible increase in serum conjugated bilirubin level. Placental concentrations of bile acids remain normal. Affected women may be deeply jaundiced during pregnancy, but pruritus and signs of generalized cholestasis are absent.

Bile Acids

Increases in serum concentrations of certain bile acids have been reported during pregnancy, and it has been suggested that pregnancy could be associated with subclinical cholestasis. Organic anion transport, including bilirubin and sulfobromophthalein (BSP), is impaired during pregnancy. These changes are likely caused primarily by estrogen/pregnancy-induced decreases in the canalicular organic anion–transporting pump multidrug resistance-associated protein-2 (MRP2: ABC C2).[8] The changes in concentrations of serum bile acids in pregnancy are in fact minimal and observed mainly in the postprandial state. Concentrations of bile salts in blood are within the normal range in most pregnant women, but levels of glycocholate, taurocholate, and chenodeoxycholate may rise progressively until term and exceed levels measured early in pregnancy by two- to three-fold. Pregnancy- or estrogen-induced decreases in bile-salt transport are likely attributable to reductions in both sinusoidal (Na⁺/taurocholate co-transporting polypeptide [NTCP]) and canalicular (bile-salt export pump [BSEP], ATP-binding cassette [ABC] B11) bile-salt transporters. In clinical practice, when a woman experiences pruritus during pregnancy, the measurement of serum bile acid concentration may be useful for the diagnosis of cholestasis, especially when routine liver function tests are still within normal limits.

Changes in Liver Function Test Values

Close monitoring of serum liver function test values is essential in the management of liver diseases in both pregnant and nonpregnant patients. Routine liver function tests usually include measurement of levels of total and conjugated bilirubin, aminotransferases, and alkaline phosphatase as well as determination of prothrombin time. In addition, γ-glutamyltransferase (GGT) or 5′-nucleotidase activity may be used to confirm the hepatobiliary origin of increased levels of alkaline phosphatase. Measurement of serum bile acid concentrations may be useful for the management of cholestasis, especially during pregnancy. Awareness of the physiologic changes in liver function tests is indispensable for the interpretation of these test values during pregnancy (see **Table 52-4**).

Measurement of serum alanine aminotransferase (ALT) and aspartate aminotransferase (AST) activity levels is the most useful test for the routine diagnosis of liver diseases. The effects of pregnancy on serum ALT and AST activity levels are somewhat controversial. In a few studies, a slight increase in ALT and/or AST activity has been found during the third trimester. However, in the majority of published studies, serum ALT and AST activity levels remain within the normal limits established in nonpregnant women. Thus it should be emphasized that serum AST or ALT activity values above the upper limit of normal values before labor should be considered pathologic and should lead to further investigations. Serum alkaline phosphatase activity levels increase in late pregnancy, mainly during the third trimester. By contrast, serum alkaline phosphatase levels have been found to be lower in oral contraceptive users. This increase during pregnancy is not due to an increase in the hepatic isoenzyme but rather largely attributable to the production of the placental isoenzyme. During the third trimester, there is also an increase in the production of the bone isoenzyme as documented by an increase in its serum level up to 6 weeks after delivery. These findings document that the measurement of serum alkaline phosphatase activity is not a suitable test for the diagnosis of cholestasis during late pregnancy and in the postpartum period.

Liver-Related Symptoms and Physical Examination in Pregnancy

Nausea and vomiting are common symptoms of early pregnancy and occur in more than half of all pregnant women. Although this condition was traditionally named morning sickness, the symptoms frequently persist throughout the day. By contrast, hyperemesis gravidarum, usually defined by severe vomiting beginning in early pregnancy and often requiring hospitalization, is much less frequent. Nausea or vomiting occurring during the second or third trimester should be considered pathologic and prompt investigation, including measurement of serum aminotransferases activity. It should be noted that jaundice and generalized pruritus are never considered normal features in pregnancy. Vascular spiders and palmar erythema are commonly associated with chronic liver disease and pregnancy. Vascular spiders were found in 14% of Caucasian women by the second month of pregnancy and in 66% by the ninth month of pregnancy. The frequency of these vascular spiders was noted to be lower in African American women, with 8% occurring in the fourth month of pregnancy and 14% in the ninth month. In this study,[9] the vascular spiders were no longer visible in approximately 75% of the women by the seventh week after delivery. In the same study, palmar erythema was observed in 63% of the Caucasian women and in 35% of the African American women. By the time of the postpartum consultation, palmar erythema had faded in all but 9% of the women. During pregnancy, these cutaneous vascular changes are not usually associated with hepatic dysfunction but may be related to sex steroids circulating in the blood. Physical examination of the liver is normal although it is difficult in late pregnancy because of the expanding uterus. In the postpartum period, after normal delivery, the liver and spleen may be palpable.

Hepatobiliary Ultrasonography in Pregnancy

Ultrasonography of the liver and biliary tract is widely used in the management of liver diseases outside pregnancy and is safe during pregnancy. In normal pregnancy, ultrasonographic examination reveals no dilatation of the biliary tract, but fasting gallbladder volume and residual volume after contraction are increased. The lithogenic or cholesterol saturation index of bile increases during pregnancy. Indeed, biliary sludge frequently occurs during pregnancy but is generally asymptomatic and often disappears spontaneously after delivery. Gallstones are much less common (2% in an Italian study, 12% in a Chilean study)[10,11] and may be associated with biliary pain. In the absence of suggestive symptoms, systematic ultrasound (US) examination of the gallbladder as an extension of the routine pelvic US is not justified because silent stones in pregnant women need no treatment.

Liver Disease Not Specific to Pregnancy

Abnormal liver function tests in pregnancy are mainly caused by conditions that are not related to the pregnancy itself and have no deleterious effect on pregnancy. However, sometimes liver disease unique to pregnancy may result in abnormal liver function test values. Therefore it is important to emphasize that conditions not specific to pregnancy should be considered along with those unique to pregnancy when evaluating liver dysfunction during pregnancy. Liver diseases not specific to pregnancy can be either preexisting or coincidental to pregnancy. It should also be emphasized that pregnancy in patients with chronic liver disease is uncommon. Generally, fertility is reduced with the onset of chronic liver disease. Hepatocellular dysfunction alters sex hormone metabolism and leads to amenorrhea and anovulation. However, with the improvement in the management of chronic liver disease, menstruation may occur as well as ovulation and pregnancy may ensue. Pregnant women with chronic liver disease are at risk for worsening liver disease including an increase in portal pressure, hepatic variceal bleeding, portosystemic encephalopathy, ascites, and liver failure. Indeed, the impact is also significant to the developing fetus. Premature labor, stillbirth, and low birth weight are major risks. The impact of chronic liver disease on pregnancy is also affected by the underlying condition. Alcoholic liver disease and autoimmune hepatitis may improve during pregnancy but pregnancy in chronic liver injury secondary to viral hepatitis carries a poor outcome. Here we discuss the major causes of liver disease not specific to pregnancy. The reader is encouraged to seek detailed discussion of these diseases in other chapters of this book.

Viral Hepatitis

Viral hepatitis—caused by hepatitides A, B, C, D, or E; herpes simplex; cytomegalovirus; and Epstein-Barr virus—accounts for 40% of jaundice in pregnant women in the United States.[12] Hepatitides A, B, and C have the same frequency in the pregnant and nonpregnant populations and during each of the three trimesters of pregnancy. The clinical and serologic

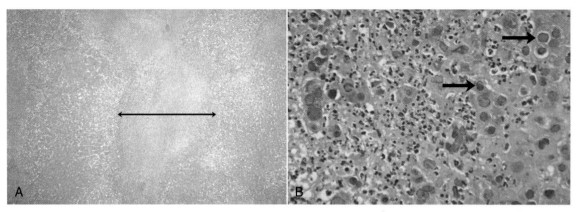

Fig. 52-1 **Herpes simplex hepatitis during pregnancy. A,** Large area of confluent hepatocellular necrosis *(double-headed arrow).* **B,** Infected hepatocytes with intranuclear eosinophilic Cowdry type A inclusions *(arrows).* (Hematoxylin and eosin stain)

Table 52-5 Summary of Mode of Transmission, Effect on Pregnancy, and Management of Viral Hepatitides A, B, C, and E in Pregnancy

TYPE OF VIRUS	MODE OF TRANSMISSION	EFFECT ON PREGNANCY	MANAGEMENT
Hepatitis A	Fecal–oral	Perinatal transmission rare Acute infection associated with preterm labor and maternal complications	Supportive care Safety of vaccination not determined Postexposure immunoglobulin safe Breastfeeding not contraindicated
Hepatitis B	Perinatal, sexual, and parenteral	Acute infection can cause fetal and neonatal hepatitis	Supportive care Active and passive immunization recommended Lamivudine, given during second and third trimesters, decreases risk of transmission Breastfeeding not contraindicated
Hepatitis C	Perinatal, sexual, and parenteral	No effects on pregnancy and fetal outcome	Supportive care Breastfeeding appears to be safe
Hepatitis E	Similar to hepatitis A	Preterm labor and increased maternal mortality in third trimester	Supportive care Breastfeeding appears to be safe No therapy to prevent transmission

course of acute hepatitis in the Western world is generally the same as that observed in the nonpregnant patient. Moreover, viral hepatitis does not appear to affect the pregnant state adversely; an exception to this is hepatitis E, which in the third trimester of pregnancy may lead to fulminant liver failure and may carry a high mortality (up to 31.1%).[13] Herpes simplex hepatitis is rare in previously healthy adults. The disease tends to be severe and the death rate is about 40%. More often, patients with herpes hepatitis present with severe or fulminant "anicteric" hepatitis in the third trimester. Hepatitis is characterized by markedly elevated levels of serum aminotransferases (>1000 units) and coagulopathy but low bilirubin levels. Transjugular liver biopsy is preferable to percutaneous transthoracic puncture because of the presence of coagulopathy. If liver biopsy is performed, histologic analysis demonstrates the presence of confluent coagulative necrosis, scant amounts of inflammatory infiltrate, and "ground-glass" nuclear inclusions or Cowdry type A inclusions at the periphery of areas of necrosis that are positive on immunohistochemical stain as

shown in **Figure 52-1.** Early treatment with antiviral therapy such as acyclovir or vidarabine is life-saving. In general, the management of the pregnant patient with acute viral hepatitis is supportive, and viral hepatitis is not an indication for termination of pregnancy, performance of a cesarean section, or discouragement for breastfeeding.[12] **Table 52-5** summarizes mode of transmission, effect on pregnancy, and management of common viral hepatitis causes.

Hepatitis A

Hepatitis A virus (HAV) is a small (27 nm) RNA virus that causes either symptomatic or asymptomatic infection in humans. The average incubation period is 28 days (range, 15 to 50 days). HAV replicates within the liver and is excreted in bile, with the highest viral concentrations in the stool late in the incubation period. This represents the window of greatest infectivity. Person-to-person transmission is the primary means of HAV infection in the United States. Serious complications of HAV infection are uncommon; the overall case/fatality ratio among reported cases is less than 1% and does not lead to chronic infection, although 10% to 15% of symptomatic individuals can have a prolonged or relapsing disease lasting up to 6 months.

If a pregnant woman becomes infected with hepatitis A, generally the baby is not affected. Intrauterine transmission of hepatitis A virus is very rare; however, perinatal transmission could occur. A recent study evaluating the impact of acute hepatitis A on pregnancy reported that acute HAV infection during pregnancy was associated with high risk of maternal complications and preterm labor.[14] The management of acute HAV in pregnancy does not differ from that used in nonpregnant patients. Maternal immunization embraces the concepts that vaccines given to pregnant women enhance their resistance to vaccine-preventable diseases, and passive antibodies that cross the placenta protect the neonate for the first 3 to 6 months of life.[15]

The safety of hepatitis A vaccination during pregnancy has not been determined; however, because hepatitis A vaccine is produced from an inactivated hepatitis A virus, the theoretical risk to the developing fetus is expected to be low. The risk associated with vaccination should be weighed against the risk for infection with hepatitis A in women who may be at high risk for exposure to hepatitis A virus. It was observed that passively acquired maternal anti-HAV resulted in a significantly lower antibody response when infants were administered hepatitis A vaccine. This is possibly due to interference between maternal antibodies and hepatitis A vaccination in young infants. It is proposed that all pregnant women should be screened at delivery for anti-HAV antibodies and children born to anti-HAV–negative mothers should be vaccinated early during the first year of life, whereas vaccination may be postponed in children born to anti-HAV–positive mothers if necessary. Mothers infected with hepatitis A virus are encouraged to breastfeed and HAV infection is not a contraindication for breastfeeding.[16]

Hepatitis B

Hepatitis B virus (HBV) is a hepatotropic double-stranded DNA (dsDNA) virus and a member of the Hepadnaviridae family. An estimated 350 million people worldwide are chronically infected with HBV, including 1.25 million in the United States.[17] Virtually 100% of hepatocytes are affected once infection is established. Carriers with chronic HBV are at risk for the development of liver cirrhosis, hepatic decompensation, and hepatocellular carcinoma (HCC). HBV is generally noncytolytic but liver injury is attributed to host immune response. In rare cases, acute liver failure ensues. In contrast to hepatitis C virus (HCV) that replicates in the cytoplasm of the hepatocyte, HBV (dsDNA) enters into the nucleus and is converted to a covalently closed circular form known as cccDNA. This is a remarkably stable species from which all viral mRNAs are transcribed and is resistant to antiviral therapy. HBV is transmitted mainly by perinatal, sexual, and parenteral exposure. Perinatal transmission represents the most common route in China and East Asia and sexual transmission is common in Europe and North America.

Hepatitis B virus has a high rate of vertical transmission, causing fetal and neonatal hepatitis. Because it is highly pathogenic and infectious, perinatal transmission of HBV infection represents the single largest cause of chronically infected individuals worldwide. Approximately 10% to 20% of women who are seropositive for hepatitis B surface antigen (HBsAg) alone transmit the virus to their neonates in the absence of neonatal immunoprophylaxis. However, if the mother is seropositive for both HBsAg and hepatitis B e-antigen (HBeAg), the frequency of vertical transmission increases to approximately 90% without neonatal prophylaxis. Therefore the American Congress of Obstetricians and Gynecologists and the Centers for Disease Control and Prevention recommend universal screening for HBsAg in all pregnant women during the third trimester.

The diagnosis of HBV infection is established by the detection of HBsAg in serum by enzyme immunoassays (EIAs). The presence of anti-HB surface antibody (HBsAb) confers lifelong protective immunity. Testing for the hepatitis B virus is generally a standard test performed on all pregnant women at or before their first prenatal visit (usually before 12 to 14 weeks of gestation). Pregnant women who are directly exposed to hepatitis B virus should receive a hepatitis B immunoglobulin (HBIG) injection ideally within 72 hours of exposure and then a hepatitis B vaccine within 7 days of exposure. HBV vaccine is then administered two more times—at 1 month and 6 months after the first vaccination. It is recommended that every infant receive three doses of HBV vaccines. The current vaccines contain noninfectious HBsAg and should cause no potential risk to the fetus. Hepatitis B vaccine administration to pregnant women is relatively safe and its benefits outweigh its risks. Sporadic cases of Guillain-Barré syndrome (GBS) have been reported in association with HBV vaccine although heated debate in the United States and Europe still exists on the actual causality.[18,19] Hepatitis B vaccination can be delayed more than 24 hours after the baby's birth but should be given within the first week of delivery. The combination of passive and active immunization is very effective in reducing the frequency of perinatal transmission of hepatitis B virus (85% to 95% efficacy). Several antiviral therapies are currently available for HBV. The current (2009) FDA-approved therapy for HBV includes subcutaneous injection of interferon/pegylated interferon-alfa and orally administered nucleoside/nucleotide analogues such as lamivudine, adefovir, entecavir, telbivudine, and tenofovir. Interferon is considered an FDA Category C drug in pregnancy and is not recommended. Lamivudine, an oral nucleoside analogue that is classified as an FDA Category C drug in terms of safety (see **Table 52-3**), is given to mothers with high HBV DNA during the second and third trimesters to reduce the risk of transmission at the time of delivery.[20,21] It is generally not recommended for use against HBV in the first trimester of pregnancy. However, potential benefits may justify the potential risk.[22] Data describing the safety of adefovir, entecavir, telbivudine, and tenofovir use in pregnancy are limited.[23]

Hepatitis C

Hepatitis C virus is a hepatotropic positive single-stranded RNA virus of the Hepacivirus genus and a member of the Flaviviridae family. It replicates primarily in hepatocytes using both host and viral enzymes. HCV is the most common cause of chronic blood-borne infection in the United States. Chronic HCV infection is estimated to affect 170 million people worldwide, including 2 to 3 million Americans (1.8%

of the general population). There are six HCV genotypes (1, 2, 3, 4, 5, and 6) and a large number of subtypes (e.g., 1a, 1b, 1c) have been identified. The major risk factor for HCV transmission is injection drug use. Other risk factors include exposure to clotting factor therapy before 1987, blood transfusion before 1992, contaminated therapeutic equipment, occupational needlestick, and sexual and perinatal transmission. The most remarkable feature of hepatitis C virus is its ability to establish chronic infection in 55% to 85% of acute cases. Approximately 20% of chronically infected patients eventually develop cirrhosis, hepatic decompensation, and hepatocellular carcinoma after 20 to 30 years of infection. The risk of hepatocellular carcinoma in HCV-infected patients with cirrhosis is 2% to 3.5% per year. The incidence of acute hepatitis C has declined markedly since 1990. Therefore data about vertical HCV transmission are based on chronic hepatitis C. Vertical HCV transmission rates range from 2% to 8%, with maternal viremia defined as detectable HCV RNA in blood, an almost uniform prerequisite for transmission. In pregnancies among HCV-infected mothers who were HCV RNA negative, vertical transmission was rare. Maternal co-infection with human immunodeficiency virus (HIV) significantly increases the risk of vertical HCV transmission to as much as 44%.[24,25] In a recent cohort study, risk factors associated with increased rate of vertical HCV transmission were higher maternal HCV viral titer, prolonged membrane rupture during labor (6 hours or longer), and use of internal fetal monitoring during labor.[26] The risk of transmission through amniocentesis appears to be low for women who are chronically infected, although the number of cases studied in the literature is small.

Serologic confirmation of exposure to HCV is performed by detecting serum or plasma HCV antibodies by third-generation enzyme immunoassays (EIAs). Confirmation of viremia is established through testing for HCV RNA by a sensitive assay with a lower limit of detection of 50 units/ml or less. Currently, unlike HBV there are no preventable measures available to lower the risk of vertical HCV transmission. Routine prenatal HCV screening is not recommended; however, women with significant risk factors for infection should be offered antibody screening. The treatment for chronic HCV infection in nonpregnant women is combination therapy of pegylated interferon-alfa and ribavirin. Ribavirin is an FDA Pregnancy Category X product (Table 52-3), indicating that its use is contraindicated in women who are pregnant. However, interferon has been used safely for the treatment of T-cell leukemias during pregnancy and its potential role as an anti-HCV therapy for both maternal and fetal/neonatal benefit warrants further studies. Both HCV antibodies and HCV RNA have been detected in colostrum; however, breastfeeding appears to be safe.

Hepatitis E

The epidemiologic features of hepatitis E virus (HEV) are similar to those of hepatitis A. The disease has been reported rarely in the United States, and the highest rates of infection occur in regions of the developing world or among immigrants or travelers from endemic countries. Hepatitis E is primarily a water-borne disease; epidemics have been reported in areas where fecal contamination of drinking water is common. In general, HEV produces a self-limited viral infection followed by recovery; the incubation period is 3 to 8

weeks, with a mean of 40 days. HEV infection is known to cause severe hepatitis, fulminant liver failure, preterm labor, and increased mortality in pregnant women, especially in their third trimester with reported maternal death rates as high as 20% to 31.1%.[13,27] The mechanism of fulminant hepatitis E in pregnancy is not clear but is thought to be attributable to induction of type 2 (T_H2) cytokines.[28] Maternal–fetal transmission of hepatitis E virus has been reported. In two prospective studies conducted in India, mother-to-child transmission of hepatitis E virus infection ranged between 33.3% and 50%.[29,30] There is no current evidence regarding the transmissibility of HEV through breast milk. At the present time, it appears that it would be especially important to continue breastfeeding during epidemics of HEV in underdeveloped and endemic areas to prevent a greater risk of infant mortality from other infectious diseases.

Autoimmune Hepatitis

Autoimmune hepatitis (AIH) is a disease of interest to hepatologists, endocrinologists, and obstetricians because it predominantly affects younger women. AIH is a syndrome of progressive hepatitis characterized by loss of tolerance to hepatic autoantigens. This results in hepatocellular necroinflammation characterized by elevated levels of serum aminotransferases, hypergammaglobulinemia, and detection of serum autoantibodies.[31] The histologic features of AIH are characterized by portal tract inflammation with moderate to marked infiltration by lymphocytes, and numerous plasma cells, with periportal interface inflammatory activity (piecemeal necrosis/interface hepatitis).[32] The disease frequently responds to immunosuppressive medication, which is considered part of its diagnostic requirement. AIH occurs predominantly among women, particularly in their younger years. In the United States AIH affects 100,000 to 200,000 patients with an incidence of 1.9 per 100,000 per year and a point incidence of 16.9 per 100,000 persons per year.[33] If untreated, severe active disease eventually leads to cirrhosis and carries a high mortality.

Pregnant women with AIH have a reduced fertility rate secondary to amenorrhea and anovulation, which might be related to hypothalamic-pituitary dysfunction. However, AIH has been reported to occur de novo during pregnancy or the postpartum period.[34] Because of improved management of AIH patients and reduced hepatocellular injury from use of immunosuppression therapy, menstruation may ensue and more women with AIH are able to conceive. Previous reports described increased incidence of obstetric complications among pregnant patients with AIH. In a retrospective study[35] the rate of serious maternal complications was 9% and a high rate (52%) of postpartum exacerbation was noted. The rate of adverse pregnancy outcome was 26%, which was highly associated with the presence of antibodies to SLA/LP and Ro/SSA. A review of the literature from February 1966 to January 2004[36] revealed that in the 101 pregnancies documented with AIH, there were 47 flare-ups, 5 clinical improvements, and 45 stabilizations of the disease during pregnancy. The perinatal mortality was 4%; 19 fetal deaths and 2 maternal deaths were also reported. In an earlier study of 35 pregnancies with autoimmune hepatitis in which more than one third had a diagnosis of cirrhosis before conception, there were 31 live births. Exacerbations in disease activity were seen in four women during pregnancy and in another four women within 3 months postpartum.[34] These data and others illustrate that pregnancy can ameliorate autoimmune hepatitis,[37,38] whereas delivery can exacerbate it.[39,40]

The diagnosis of AIH requires exclusions of other causes of liver injury. Patients with AIH have a diverse clinical presentation that ranges from asymptomatic to an acute presentation with liver failure.[41] Asymptomatic presentation represents 34% of the cases,[42] whereas acute hepatitis is noted in up to 30% of patients. Nonspecific symptoms such as malaise, fatigability, anorexia, nausea, and mild upper abdominal discomfort are also noted.

Immunosuppressive therapy with azathioprine (AZA) and corticosteroids is the principal treatment regimen used in AIH. Corticosteroid therapy induces clinical, laboratory, and histologic improvements in 80% of patients with autoimmune hepatitis,[43] but most women with AIH require maintenance immunosuppression therapy. At this time successful completion of pregnancy is a realistic expectation for patients with well-controlled AIH.[44] Corticosteroids and azathioprine are generally safe during pregnancy but birth defects have been described.[34] The placenta forms a relative barrier to AZA and its metabolites. 6-Thioguanine nucleotides (6-TGNs) can be detected in the red blood cells (RBCs) of the infant; however, 6-methylmercaptopurine (6-MMP) was not.[45] Pregnant women with AIH need careful monitoring during pregnancy and for several months postpartum.

Wilson Disease

Wilson disease is a rare autosomal recessive disorder of hepatic copper transport leading to inhibition of biliary copper excretion. This causes an increase in copper deposition in vital organs such as liver, kidney, brain, and eyes. Two copper-transporting ATPases, Menkes (ATP7A; MNK) and Wilson (ATP7B; WND), are expressed in the placenta and both are involved in placental copper transport.[46] Pregnancy does not seem to have an adverse effect on the clinical course of Wilson disease although recurrent abortions are common in untreated patients, which can be seen in 26% of cases.[47] Indeed, untreated symptomatic women with Wilson disease tend to suffer amenorrhea, oligomenorrhea, irregular menses, and multiple miscarriages. However, pregnancy in women with Wilson disease is safe and successful when treatment with a chelating drug is continued uninterrupted. With the current available copper chelators such as D-penicillamine, trientine, and zinc, fertile women are able to conceive. Penicillamine and trientine have teratogenic effects in animals, and penicillamine has known teratogenic effects in humans as well. D-Penicillamine probably inhibits thyroperoxidase activity in utero. Infants born to mothers with Wilson disease may develop transient goitrous hypothyroidism.[48] In a retrospective analysis of 16 fertile women with Wilson disease who had conceived at least once, 16 patients had conceived on 59 occasions, resulting in 30 successful pregnancies, 24 spontaneous abortions, 2 medical terminations of pregnancy, and 3 stillbirths.[49] In this study of 102 patients, teratogenicity was not observed with low-dose penicillamine and zinc sulfate. In a study from the National Center for the Study of Wilson Disease[50] that included 43 women with this disorder, 71 pregnancies occurred, yielding 69 normal neonates and 2 abortions. Zinc appears to be safe during pregnancy and can maintain a low serum copper level by inducing metallothionein, which sequesters copper in hepatocytes and enterocytes. Zinc intake at a dose of 25 to 50 mg three times daily in pregnancy appears to be safe with very minimal teratogenicity.[50] It is important that treatment of Wilson disease with anticopper agents continues during pregnancy without interruption. Both mother and baby should be monitored while on chelation therapy.

Portal Vein Thrombosis

Portal vein thrombosis (PVT) is a rare occurrence during pregnancy. PVT is caused by a combination of local and systemic risk factors. Local factors are more frequently recognized during the acute stage of PVT and are responsible for 30% to 40% of PVT cases. Malignant tumors, cirrhosis, and other causes of intraabdominal inflammation (e.g., pancreatitis, appendicitis, cholecystitis, duodenal ulcer, inflammatory bowel disease) are the leading local risk factors.[51] Additionally, systemic prothrombotic risk factors such as myeloproliferative disorders; antiphospholipid syndrome; protein C, protein S, and antithrombin deficiency; and factor V Leiden, factor II, and methylenetetrahydrofolate reductase gene mutations are other potential risk factors for PVT and are responsible for 60% to 70% of cases.[52,53]

Clinical Manifestations

Acute PVT usually presents with abdominal or lumbar pain that either is sudden in onset or progresses over a few days. Abdominal guarding is generally absent unless an inflammatory focus is the source or PVT is complicated with intestinal infarction. Partial thrombosis of the portal vein is associated with fewer symptoms. Rapid and complete obstruction of the portal or mesenteric veins, without involvement of mesenteric venous arches, induces intestinal congestion that is manifested by severe and continuous colicky abdominal pain with occasional nonbloody diarrhea. Acute septic PVT referred to as acute pyelophlebitis is characterized by infected thrombus. The presentation is spiking fever and chills, a tender liver, and occasionally shock. Persistence of severe pain beyond 5 to 7 days, bloody diarrhea, and ascites along with features of acidosis and renal or respiratory dysfunction are suggestive of intestinal infarction. In the absence of treatment, intestinal perforation, peritonitis, shock, and death from multiorgan failure ensue.[51] The manifestations of chronic PVT are variable and include biliary symptoms related to compression of large bile ducts, which could result in portal cholangiopathy and portal hypertension.[54]

Laboratory and Imaging Features

Liver function is preserved in both acute and chronic PVT because increased hepatic arterial blood flow compensates for the decreased portal inflow. Rapid formation of collateral circulation develops from preexisting veins in the porta hepatis. The diagnosis of acute or chronic PVT can be rapidly established using cross-sectional imaging of the abdomen. Abdominal US with Doppler studies of the portal veins reveals absent or sluggish flow, establishing the diagnosis. Persistent pain, presence of ascites, or development of multiorgan failure indicates that intestinal infarction is likely and surgical exploration should be considered. A tumor-like cavernoma, a rare form of chronic PVT, is characterized by tiny collateral channels forming a mass that encases the main bile duct and can be confused with carcinoma of the main bile duct.[54]

Treatment

Management differs in acute and chronic PVT in pregnancy. The goal of treatment in acute PVT is to recanalize the obstructed veins, which may prevent intestinal infarction and subsequent portal hypertension. Correction of the causal factors should be achieved as soon as possible. In the presence of pyelophlebitis, antibiotics should be administered. Anticoagulation therapy in acute PVT is logical but still not firmly validated. There have been no controlled studies of anticoagulation therapy in patients with acute PVT. The optimal duration of anticoagulation therapy for acute PVT has not been determined. A panel of international experts has recommended that in patients with acute PVT, anticoagulation medication should be administered for at least 3 months and permanent anticoagulation therapy should be considered for patients with prothrombotic conditions.[55] Other treatment modalities such as surgical thrombectomy, systemic or in situ thrombolysis, and transjugular intrahepatic portosystemic shunt (TIPS) are extremely limited and some are associated with development of major procedure-related complications.[56] Emergency laparotomy is reserved for patients with intestinal infarction.

Pregnant patients with chronic PVT should be offered screening for gastroesophageal varices. In pregnant patients with gastroesophageal varices, anticoagulation therapy should not be initiated until after adequate prophylaxis for variceal bleeding. Additionally, long-term anticoagulation therapy should be considered only in patients with chronic PVT, without cirrhosis, and with a permanent risk factor for venous thrombosis that cannot be corrected otherwise, provided that there is no major contraindication.

Budd-Chiari Syndrome

Budd-Chiari syndrome (BCS), also known as hepatic venous outflow tract obstruction, is characterized by occlusion of the hepatic venous outflow tract at various levels from small hepatic veins to the inferior vena cava (IVC), resulting from thrombosis or its fibrous sequelae.[55,57] Primary BCS is associated with an increased risk of a hypercoagulable state because of myeloproliferative disorders; protein C, protein S, antithrombin III, or factor V Leiden mutations; prothrombin gene mutation; hyperhomocysteinemia; and oral contraceptive use. Pregnancy is associated with an increase in the serum level of estrogen and a decrease in the serum level of antithrombin III, leading to increased risk of hypercoagulable state.[58-59]

Clinical and Laboratory Features

In most cases, the underlying disorders causing thrombosis of the hepatic venous outflow tract are unrecognized at presentation. Presentation can range from complete absence of symptoms to fulminant hepatic failure. This syndrome usually presents in the last trimester or the puerperium. The characteristic clinical triad of acute BCS is right upper quadrant pain, hepatomegaly, and ascites.[58,59] Chronic thrombosis typically evolves slowly with dull abdominal pain. Other signs and symptoms include lower extremity edema, gastrointestinal

bleeding, and hepatic encephalopathy; these symptoms may be absent in patients with overt BCS.[60] Jaundice is relatively uncommon. Marked dilation of subcutaneous veins on the trunk has a high specificity but a low sensitivity for IVC obstruction. Levels of serum aminotransferases and alkaline phosphatase can be normal or increased. Levels of serum albumin, serum bilirubin, and prothrombin can be normal or abnormal, and in some patients are markedly abnormal. The protein level in ascitic fluid varies from patient to patient. Ascites protein content is greater than 3.0 g/dl, and a serum-ascites albumin gradient (SAAG) greater than 1.1 is generally suggestive of portal hypertension.

Imaging Features

Diagnostic modalities including right upper quadrant abdominal US with Doppler studies of the hepatic veins have the advantages of being noninvasive or minimally invasive. The examiner's experience and awareness of a clinical suspicion of BCS appear to be key factors for a high diagnostic yield at Doppler sonography. A distinctive feature for BCS is the association with intrahepatic or subcapsular hepatic venous collaterals, which is found in more than 80% of the cases. In the patient presenting with acute or chronic liver disease, Doppler sonography by an experienced operator has sufficed to establish or rule out BCS in most patients when the operator was aware of the diagnostic suspicion. MRI allows better delineation of the vascular anatomy of splanchnic vessels without use of contrast agents and is also able to better differentiate acute from chronic BCS. MRI with gadolinium-based contrast agents can be performed in pregnancy, as suggested by the European Society of Radiology guidelines. In contrast, the American College of Radiology has a more cautious attitude and recommends a case-by-case risk/benefit analysis before using gadolinium chelates.[61,62]

Treatment

In clinical practice, a woman with an identified history of BCS who wishes to become pregnant should be screened for portal hypertension by upper endoscopy and, when indicated, prophylaxis of varices should be initiated. Most patients begin long-term warfarin therapy if nonpregnant, and if pregnant, patients are also administered low-molecular-weight heparin (LMWH) as soon as possible, preferably before conception. Because glomerular filtration rate (GFR) and distribution volume are increased during pregnancy, and because of the presence of placental heparinase, anti–factor Xa activity should be monitored once a month. Preference should be given to twice-daily dosing of LMWH because of the short half-life of once-daily dosing. Delivery should be scheduled 24 hours after the last therapeutic dose and restarted 12 hours after vaginal delivery or 24 hours after cesarean section either with LMWH or with warfarin.

When BCS is diagnosed during pregnancy, Doppler US should be used as the first modality. Treatment of BCS patients presenting during pregnancy is no different from treatment used for nonpregnant BCS patients, except for the contraindication of warfarin (FDA category X). LMWH at a curative dose should be started as soon as the diagnosis is established.

Pharmacologic and endoscopic therapy for portal hypertension can be applied as previously discussed (see Portal

Vein Thrombosis). Angioplasty and TIPS insertion have been reported for refractory variceal bleeding, although TIPS should be used with caution because of fetal irradiation.

Hereditary Hemorrhagic Telangiectasia

Hereditary hemorrhagic telangiectasia (HHT), or Rendu-Osler-Weber syndrome, is a rare genetic disease with an autosomal dominant inheritance pattern; it is characterized by widespread cutaneous, mucosal, and visceral arteriovenous malformations that can involve the lung, brain, and/or liver. Liver vascular malformations are widespread and include both microscopic and macroscopic malformations of variable size, ranging from tiny telangiectasias to discrete arteriovenous malformations. The majority of cases are asymptomatic. The three most common initial clinical presentations of HHT are high-output heart failure, portal hypertension, and biliary ischemia.[63,64] High-output heart failure is the most severe presentation and is characterized by shortness of breath, dyspnea on exertion, ascites, and/or edema. Portal hypertension is generally present with ascites, but also with varices and possible variceal hemorrhage. The diagnosis of HHT can be readily established using less invasive methods such as Doppler US. Treatment is not indicated in patients with HHT who have asymptomatic liver involvement. In patients with symptomatic HHT, treatment is directed toward the clinical manifestation of heart failure and portal hypertension.

Cirrhosis and Portal Hypertension

Pregnancy in the setting of cirrhosis is an uncommon condition possibly secondary to hepatocellular damage and altered metabolism of sex hormones by the liver. The incidence of cirrhosis in pregnancy is estimated to be approximately 1 in 5950 pregnancies.[65] The co-existence of pregnancy in patients with cirrhosis represents a complex clinical dilemma for the clinician. In patients with portal hypertension (PHT) splanchnic blood flow and intrahepatic sinusoidal pressure increase, resulting in deviation of the blood to the azygos venous system and formation of collaterals. During pregnancy a hypervolemic state develops, leading to an increase in portal flow and elevation of portal pressure transmitted to the collateral veins with increased risk of variceal bleeding.[66] PHT occurs during the last stages of the second trimester of pregnancy and is associated with increased risk of variceal bleeding in the later stages of pregnancy. Esophageal variceal bleeding has been reported in 18% to 32% of pregnant women with cirrhosis and in up to 50% of those with known portal hypertension. Of those with preexisting varices, 78% will have gastrointestinal bleeding during pregnancy, with a mortality of 18% to 50%.[67] Pregnant patients with cirrhosis face unique risks. These include higher rates of spontaneous abortion, prematurity, pulmonary hypertension, splenic artery aneurysm rupture, and postpartum hemorrhage, and a potential for life-threatening variceal hemorrhage and hepatic decompensation.[67-69] Although cirrhosis is the most common cause of portal hypertension in the United States, noncirrhotic portal hypertension (NCPH) represents an important contributing factor in developing countries, but with favorable outcome to pregnant women and their babies.[70] Variceal bleeding is the most common complication in pregnancies with NCPH, occurring in 34% of cases, but the majority (88.2%) of patients respond to endoscopic sclerotherapy.[71] Pregnancy outcome may be influenced by the underlying cause of liver disease.[67] Pregnant cirrhotic patients with an underlying diagnosis of autoimmune hepatitis and alcoholic liver disease tend to have a favorable outcome in comparison with those with viral hepatitis. The management of a parturient with esophageal varices and thrombocytopenia requires multidisciplinary care. Endoscopic surveillance and banding of esophageal varices is recommended during pregnancy. Upper endoscopy in general appears to be safe during pregnancy, with the main risk being fetal hypoxia from sedative drugs or procedure positioning. No cases of premature labor or fetal malformations have been reported in patients who have undergone endoscopy during pregnancy.[72] On the basis of the endoscopic findings, primary prophylaxis with nonselective β-blockers such as propranolol and/or nadolol (designated by the FDA as Pregnancy Category C) is recommended. The risks of nonselective β-blockers include fetal bradycardia, hypotension, hypoglycemia, and intrauterine growth retardation.[73] Endoscopic banding ligation seems to be a safe procedure in pregnancy.[74] When bleeding is not arrested endoscopically, an emergency TIPS procedure should be considered, but data in pregnant cirrhotic women are scarce.[75,76] Ascites rarely occurs in pregnant women with cirrhosis and the mainstay of treatment is sodium restriction and the use of diuretics. Hepatic encephalopathy in pregnancy may be related to a wide variety of acute and chronic liver diseases, including acute viral hepatitis, acute fatty liver of pregnancy, and preeclampsia-related liver injury. In the setting of cirrhosis, pregnant women can develop portosystemic hepatic encephalopathy secondary to medications, sepsis, hypoxia, gastrointestinal bleeding, and hypotension. Treatment with lactulose and antibiotics is effective. Postpartum uterine hemorrhage occurs in 7% to 10% of pregnancies in patients with cirrhosis and represents a potential source of maternal morbidity and mortality. Vaginal delivery is usually safe and early assistance with forceps delivery or vacuum extraction should be considered to prevent further rise in portal pressure secondary to prolonged straining during labor. Termination of pregnancy is warranted in the presence of progressive hepatic decompensation.

Gallstones and Biliary Tract Disease

There are several changes that occur during the course of pregnancy that lead to the formation of biliary sludge and gallstones. Among these changes is a decline in the contractility of the gallbladder that results in stasis of bile with an increase in residual volume. It appears that this is most likely caused by hormonal changes during pregnancy, with progesterone having the greatest effect. In addition to changes in gallbladder emptying, there is also an alteration in the content of bile. Compared with bile acids and phospholipids, cholesterol secretion increases in the second and third trimesters, leading to supersaturated bile that is more lithogenic. The formation of biliary sludge and stones is strongly associated with frequency and number of pregnancies. Up to 10% of patients develop stones or sludge over the course of pregnancy, with obesity and high serum leptin levels being risk factors.[77] Despite their prevalence in 5% to 12% of pregnant women, symptomatic gallstones occur in only 0.1% to 0.3% of pregnancies. The most typical clinical presentations are biliary pain and gallstone pancreatitis, and the least common manifestation is acute cholecystitis. The clinical features of biliary disease and pancreatitis are the same as those in the nonpregnant patient, which can occur at any time of gestation, and may recur during future pregnancy and into the postpartum period.

Management of symptomatic uncomplicated biliary tract disease is usually conservative. A more aggressive approach may be required in cases of severe disease such as cholecystitis, choledocholithiasis, cholangitis, and/or gallstone pancreatitis. Recent data show that cholecystectomy during pregnancy is not associated with a high rate of fetal demise.[78] Likewise, recent reports indicate that a laparoscopic cholecystectomy is probably a safe option.[79-80] Irrespective of the surgical approach, surgery is considered to be safest if performed during the second trimester of pregnancy. Endoscopic management of biliary tract disease using endoscopic retrograde cholangiopancreatography (ERCP) is also a viable option. Two recent retrospective studies provide further evidence to support the safety of ERCP during pregnancy, provided that all possible measures are taken to minimize fetal radiation exposure and that the clinical situation warrants intervention.[81,82]

Liver Disease Unique to Pregnancy

Four unique disorders of liver dysfunction have been recognized during pregnancy. These include (1) hepatic involvement in HG, (2) ICP, (3) HELLP syndrome, and (4) AFLP.

Hepatic Involvement in Hyperemesis Gravidarum

Nausea and vomiting of pregnancy (NVP) are common symptoms and affect up to 70% to 80% of pregnant women.[83] Although NVP is very common, it is usually mild and resolves spontaneously with no serious complications. HG is a severe and persistent form of NVP that predominantly affects pregnant women in their first trimester and is characterized by intractable vomiting that leads to loss of 5% or more of prepregnant body weight and dehydration. In a large cohort study, hyperemesis occurred in 473 of 100,000 live births.[84] The prevalence is directly related to socioeconomic status and geographic region. For example, women born in western Europe had the lowest prevalence of HG (0.8%), whereas those born in India and Sri Lanka had the highest (3.2%).[85] HG is one of the leading causes for hospitalization in pregnant women in early gestation[86] and can be associated with dehydration, imbalanced electrolyte levels, ketonuria, abnormal levels of liver enzymes, low birth weight, avitaminosis, and Wernicke's encephalopathy; rarely, it can be fatal.[87-89] Moreover, it can be associated with a substantial increase in cost and economic burden.[90]

Etiology and Pathophysiology

The underlying mechanism of maternal liver disease associated with hyperemesis gravidarum is not clear. Women with previous history of hyperemesis gravidarum, previous molar pregnancy, preexisting diabetes, gastrointestinal disorders, asthma, singleton female pregnancies, pregnancies with multiple male fetuses, multiple gestations, hyperthyroid disorders, psychiatric illness, and low prepregnancy body weight are at increased risk.[91] On the other hand, woman who have a history of smoking and a maternal age older than 30[92] as well as working women and women who lived with a partner[93] appear to have a decreased risk. The relationship between infection with *Helicobacter pylori* and HG is not clear. Few studies reported an association,[94,95] whereas others were contradictory.[94,96,97] The pathogenesis of liver injury in HG is not clear. Intense vomiting leads to dehydration, ketonuria, starvation, and malnutrition. This may result in depletion of glycogen stores and an increase in mitochondrial injury caused by oxidative stress. HG is also associated with an increase in levels of maternal estrogen and human chorionic gonadotropin (β-hCG).[98] This may contribute to the elevation in concentrations of liver transaminases as well.[99] Impaired mitochondrial fatty acid oxidation has also been attributed to play a role in HG-induced liver injury.[100]

Diagnosis

Intense nausea and vomiting in the first trimester associated with a 5% or greater weight loss, dehydration, ketonuria, electrolyte imbalance, and metabolic alkalosis is highly suggestive of hyperemesis gravidarum. The presence of fever, abdominal pain, headache, elevation in white blood cell count, anemia, thrombocytopenia, and coagulopathy should elude to nausea and vomiting of other causes. The most common hepatic abnormality associated with hyperemesis gravidarum is mild elevation of levels of liver transaminases (usually <300 U/L). Jaundice is uncommon and the total bilirubin level is generally less than 4 mg/dl. These liver abnormalities are seen only in 20% to 30% of patients. Other laboratory abnormalities include elevation of free thyroxine level and/or suppressed thyroid-stimulating hormone (TSH) activity, and mild increases in amylase and lipase concentrations. The differential diagnosis should include biliary pancreatitis, acute cholecystitis, choledocholithiasis, preeclampsia, and acute viral hepatitis. Liver biopsy is generally not indicated unless necessary to rule out other causes; if biopsy is performed, it may show no abnormalities or bland cholestasis.

Management

Fewer than 1% of patients with hyperemesis gravidarum require admission to the hospital.[92] In one retrospective analysis, elevated liver function tests had a negative predictive value for readmission to the hospital.[101] Nutritional support, hydration, and control of emesis are the mainstay of therapy. Ginger has been shown to be effective in reducing nausea and vomiting in several well-controlled, double-blinded, randomized clinical studies.[102-105] Metoclopramide and vitamin B_6 appear to be safe and effective.[106,107] Thiamine supplementation for women with prolonged vomiting is recommended to prevent Wernicke-Korsakoff syndrome. Nerve stimulation therapy is effective in reducing nausea and vomiting and in promoting weight gain in symptomatic women in the first trimester of pregnancy.[108] Treatment with antidepressants before and during early pregnancy does not appear to affect the incidence of NVP.[109] Low-dose prednisolone has been shown to have a similar effect as promethazine in reducing nausea and vomiting with fewer side effects.[110] The addition of parenteral and oral corticosteroids to treatment of women with hyperemesis gravidarum did not reduce the need for rehospitalization later in pregnancy.[111] Ondansetron does not appear to be associated with an increased risk for major malformations but demonstrated no benefit over promethazine.[112,113] Adverse infant outcomes associated with hyperemesis are a consequence of, and mostly limited to, women with poor maternal weight gain.[114] Women with poor maternal weight gain have a poor predictive fetal outcome.[114]

Intrahepatic Cholestasis of Pregnancy

Also known as obstetric cholestasis, ICP is a unique liver disorder in pregnancy that is most commonly seen in the third trimester. ICP is characterized by a generalized distressing pruritus and elevated levels of maternal serum bile acids in the absence of dermatologic causes of pruritus. Although most affected pregnant women have a mild form of the disease, the disease can be associated with meconium staining in 45%, spontaneous preterm labor in 44%, and intrapartum fetal distress in 22% of pregnancies,[115-117] as well as low birth weight.[118]

Epidemiology

Intrahepatic cholestasis of pregnancy is a rare, recurrent, and reversible disease of pregnancy. It is the second most common cause of jaundice in pregnant women after viral hepatitis. The incidence of ICP varies based on demographics and geographic region. In the United States the incidence is estimated to be around 1 in 1000 to 10,000 pregnancies. Latino Americans have higher incidence rates (5.6%).[119] The overall incidence in Europe is 0.7%.[120] The highest incidence is seen among the Araucanian (27.6%) and Aymara (11.8%) Indians of Chile.[121] It has been suggested that winter months are associated with a higher incidence of this disease in Chile secondary to lower levels of serum selenium.[122] Twin pregnancies have a higher incidence than single pregnancies (20.9% vs. 4.7%, respectively).[123]

Etiology

The etiology of ICP is still unknown. Genetic, hormonal, environmental, and dietary factors have been suggested. The genetic basis of the disease has been attributed secondary to its occurrence within familial clustering and endemic ethnic groups.[124] Heterozygous nonsense mutation of the multidrug resistance–associated protein-3 (*MDR3*) gene has been implicated in familial intrahepatic cholestasis of pregnancy.[125] Estrogen is known to induce cholestasis in animal models.[126,127] High levels of maternal sex hormones in a susceptible patient may lead to ICP. Hypersensitivity to estrogen and estrogen-sulfated metabolites is considered to be the main precipitant. The disease is most common in the third trimester—when maternal estrogen concentration is at its peak. Moreover, ovarian hyperstimulation has been reported.[128] It has been suggested that women with previous symptoms of pruritus associated with intake of oral contraceptives are at risk.

Selenium deficiency and low selenium concentration have also been shown to play a role.

Pathophysiology

Cholestasis is an abnormal physiologic state characterized by impairment of bile flow. Bile acid secretion is an energy-dependent process and its secretion into the biliary canaliculi is based on multiple protein transporters such as the canalicular bile-salt export pump (BSEP), familial intrahepatic cholestasis-1 (FIC1), PFIC2, PFIC3, MDR3, MDR1, and others.[129] The exact gene defect in bile acid secretion has not been defined. Low serum selenium concentration[130] and lower levels of serum placental protein 10 (PP10) have also been noted in ICP patients.[131]

Diagnosis

The diagnosis is established by the presence of a typical history of generalized intractable pruritus in the second or third trimester of pregnancy with elevated levels of maternal serum bile acids in the absence of radiologic evidence of biliary obstruction. Pruritus is severe and tends to follow an ascending pattern of distribution. Initially it involves the palms of the hands and the soles of the feet and subsequently the arms, legs, and trunk are involved. Pruritus tends to abate after resolution of gestation but to occur in subsequent pregnancies. Elevated levels of maternal serum bile acids are the hallmark of cholestasis and are usually 10 μmol/L or greater. A cutoff level of serum bile acids of 40 μmol/L or greater is associated with impaired fetal outcome.[132] Serum aminotransferase levels are usually elevated but less than 1000 U/L. Levels of cholestatic enzymes, such as alkaline phosphatase, are also elevated; however, use of alkaline phosphatase level as a single indicator of the disease is not recommended because it is produced by both placenta and bone. Serum γ-glutamyltranspeptidase (GGT) level is normal or slightly elevated. Bilirubin level is increased but usually less than 5 mg/dl. Liver biopsy is generally not required but if performed demonstrates cholestasis with no inflammation or bile duct injury, as shown in **Figure 52-2**.[133]

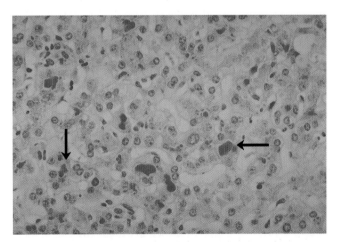

Fig. 52-2 **Intrahepatic cholestasis of pregnancy showing canalicular bile plugs (*arrows*) with well-preserved hepatocytes containing yellow pigment.** (Hematoxylin and eosin [H & E] stain)

Management

In addition to the symptomatic relief of pruritus, strict fetal monitoring must be carried out, especially during the last few weeks of pregnancy when rates of fetal morbidity and mortality are increased. Cholestasis and pruritus are reversible once pregnancy ceases. Ursodeoxycholic acid (UDCA), a tertiary bile acid available in minute amounts in the body, is the primary medication used to alleviate pruritus and cholestasis. In a randomized, double-blinded, placebo-controlled clinical trial, UDCA was safe and effective in attenuating pruritus and improving levels of liver transaminases as well as serum bilirubin in pregnant ICP patients.[134,135] Moreover, UDCA reduces fetal bile acid concentration by preventing its passage from the maternal serum to the fetus.[136] The recommended dose is 15 mg/kg/day in divided doses. A 3-week treatment regimen of UDCA improves levels of liver transaminases, lowers levels of serum bile acids, and relieves pruritus.[137] UDCA treatment in ICP decreased urinary excretion of disulfated progesterone metabolites, suggesting that amelioration of pruritus is connected to stimulation of hepatobiliary excretion of progesterone disulfates.[138] Of interest, women who have transient pruritus with normal bile salts and liver biochemistry measurements appear to have higher intrapartum and postpartum complications and require increased vigilance.[139] Other therapy for pruritus, such as hydroxyzine, ondansetron, and S-adenosyl-L-methionine (SAMe), has shown to be of some benefit.[140] On the other hand, dexamethasone was determined to be noneffective in one randomized clinical trial.[137] Pregnant patients with ICP should be counseled on future recurrence of this disorder if further pregnancies are anticipated.

Syndrome of Hemolysis, Elevated Liver Enzymes, and Low Platelet Count

The diagnostic criteria for preeclampsia are defined as the presence of edema, proteinuria, and hypertension with a blood pressure greater than 140/90 mm Hg in a previously normotensive patient or worsening hypertension in a patient with preexisting vascular hypertension in the second or third trimester of pregnancy. The exact cause remains unknown and the definitive treatment is still delivery.[141] The liver involvement in preeclampsia may manifest as HELLP syndrome. HELLP syndrome has been described in the literature both with and without symptoms of preeclampsia and is currently considered a variant of preeclampsia.[142,143] The incidence of HELLP syndrome is approximately 0.6% of pregnancies and 3.1% to 12% of patients with preeclampsia.[144] HELLP syndrome can be life-threatening to both the mother and the fetus. The associated liver disease may progress to the point that liver transplantation may become necessary. HELLP syndrome occurs in the antepartum period in 70% to 92% of cases and during the postpartum period in 8% to 30% of patients.

Pathogenesis

Many theories have been proposed to explain the pathophysiology of HELLP syndrome. One theory emphasizes structural and functional changes in the systemic vasculature as a major role in the development of HELLP syndrome. In one prospective study of total hepatic blood flow in patients with severe preeclampsia, the authors observed that decreased hepatic blood flow was predictive of the subsequent development of HELLP syndrome in these patients.[145] Another theory is that placenta-derived proteins mediate apoptosis of liver cells. In animal models interaction of placenta-derived CD95 (APO-1, Fas) with its ligand, CD95L (FasL), induces apoptosis in hepatic cells. A new therapeutic agent (LY498919) that blocks CD95-induced apoptosis is under investigation.[146]

Clinical Findings

Patients are typically seen in the early third trimester with nonspecific symptoms including right upper quadrant pain, malaise, nausea, and vomiting. Concomitant signs and symptoms of preeclampsia (hypertension, proteinuria, and edema) may or may not be present. Jaundice and bleeding attributable to thrombocytopenia are a very uncommon mode of presentation. Severe right upper quadrant abdominal pain that is radiated to the neck or shoulder may herald impending hepatic rupture or the presence of hepatic hematoma.

Diagnosis

Two major diagnostic classification systems are currently used for the classification of HELLP syndrome (**Table 52-6**). In the Tennessee classification system,[142] a diagnosis of the complete form of HELLP syndrome requires the presence of all three major components, whereas partial or incomplete HELLP syndrome consists of only one or two elements of the triad.[147,148] The presence of an abnormal peripheral smear (e.g., microangioplastic anemia with schistocytosis), thrombocytopenia, and elevated levels of AST, ALT, bilirubin, and lactate dehydrogenase (LDH) is diagnostic.[141] The Mississippi classification system (see **Table 52-6**) has been proposed for

Table 52-6 Main Diagnostic Criteria of HELLP Syndrome

TENNESSEE CLASSIFICATION*	MISSISSIPPI CLASSIFICATION†
Complete syndrome: Platelets ≤100 × 10⁹/L AST ≥70 units/L LDH ≥600 units/L	Class 1: platelets ≤50 × 10⁹/L AST or ALT ≥70 units/L LDH ≥600 units/L
Incomplete syndrome: Any one or two of the above	Class 2: platelets ≤100 × 10⁹/L ≥50 × 10⁹/ AST or ALT ≥70 units/L LDH ≥600 units/L
	Class 3: platelets ≤150 × 10⁹/L ≥100 × 10⁹/L AST or ALT ≥40 units/L LDH ≥600 units/L

*Modified from Audibert F, et al. Clinical utility of strict diagnostic criteria for the HELLP (hemolysis, elevated liver enzymes, and low platelets) syndrome. Am J Obstet Gynecol 1996;175:460–464.

†Adopted from Martin JN Jr, et al. The spectrum of severe preeclampsia: comparative analysis by HELLP (hemolysis, elevated liver enzyme levels, and low platelet count) syndrome classification. Am J Obstet Gynecol 1999;180(6 Pt 1):1373–1384.

ALT, alanine aminotransferase; AST, aspartate aminotransferase; HELLP, hemolysis, elevated liver enzymes, and low platelet count; LDH, lactate dehydrogenase

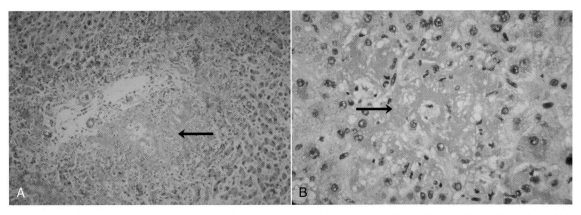

Fig. 52-3 **Liver in HELLP syndrome. A,** Periportal patchy hemorrhage and necrosis *(arrow)*. **B,** Sinusoidal deposition of fibrin *(arrow)*. (H & E stain)

assessment of the severity of the pathologic process, with class 1 HELLP syndrome having a worse prognosis and longer hospital stay than either class 2 or class 3. This classification system is based on the degree of thrombocytopenia and the extent of elevation in transaminase and LDH levels, as shown in **Table 52-6.** The platelet count and serum LDH levels are found not only to be moderately predictive of the severity of the disease but also to indicate the speed of recovery.

Because of an initial nonspecific presentation, HELLP syndrome can be confused with acute viral hepatitis, hemolytic uremic syndrome (HUS), thrombotic thrombocytopenic purpura (TTP), antiphospholipid syndrome, and acute fatty liver of pregnancy (AFLP). Both HELLP syndrome and acute fatty liver of pregnancy occur in the third trimester and have similar presentations, but liver dysfunction is usually more pronounced in the latter and is more frequently associated with coagulopathy, hypoglycemia, and renal failure. The coagulopathy of AFLP is due to liver failure, whereas in HELLP syndrome coagulopathy develops as a part of disseminated intravascular coagulation (DIC) syndrome.

The histologic features of HELLP syndrome include diffuse deposition of fibrin along the sinusoids and periportal patchy necrosis and hemorrhage, as shown in **Figure 52-3.**

Management

Because of significant morbidity and mortality, HELLP syndrome is considered an indication for immediate delivery.[149,150] Although controversial, expectant management may be recommended in rare cases when the patient is stable and the term of gestation is unfavorable for fetal survival.[141,151]

After initial stabilization, decision should be made about time and method of delivery with prompt delivery if the term of gestation is greater than 34 weeks, fetal testing results are nonreassuring, or any of the following conditions are present: maternal multiorgan dysfunction, DIC, liver infarction or hematoma, renal failure, or abruptio placentae. In addition to prompt delivery, seizure prophylaxis with magnesium sulfate and blood pressure control is also required.[141]

If both mother and fetus are stable before 34 weeks of gestation, corticosteroids should be administered to promote fetal lung maturity.[141] Delivery is then usually performed within 48 hours. Few studies have suggested beneficial effects of corticosteroids for both mother and fetus in the setting of HELLP

syndrome; however, the greatest benefit was demonstrated in class 1 HELLP syndrome.[152] However, only a few randomized studies have been reported that demonstrated an improvement of maternal laboratory values and renal output but with no difference in serious maternal morbidity. Platelet transfusion is recommended in the case of bleeding or severe thrombocytopenia (platelet count $<20 \times 10^9/L$).[153] After delivery, initial worsening of laboratory values with subsequent spontaneous recovery is observed. The speed of recovery depends upon the severity of the initial presentation and the presence of complications.

Complications of HELLP Syndrome

Serious maternal complications are common, including DIC, abruptio placentae, acute renal failure, eclampsia, pulmonary edema, acute respiratory distress syndrome, ascites, subcapsular hematoma, hepatic failure, and wound hematomas.[141,151,154,155] Indications to proceed with liver transplantation include persistent bleeding from a hematoma or hepatic rupture or liver failure from extensive necrosis.[156] Hepatic hemorrhage without rupture in a hemodynamically stable patient is managed conservatively with close hemodynamic monitoring in an intensive care unit. Exogenous trauma in the form of deep abdominal palpation, convulsions, emesis, and unnecessary transportation should be avoided.

Liver rupture is a rare, life-threatening complication of HELLP syndrome that carries a very high maternal mortality. It is usually preceded by an intraparenchymal hemorrhage progressing to a contained subcapsular hematoma in the right hepatic lobe in patients with severe thrombocytopenia. Hepatic rupture usually requires immediate laparotomy and evacuation of the hematoma with pressure packing and drainage, followed by consideration of hepatic artery embolization or ligation, partial hepatectomy, or oversewing of the laceration. In the rare hemodynamically stable patient, angiographic embolization may be considered. Abdominal CT scans (**Fig. 52-4**) may be the most sensitive and specific way to detect hepatic hemorrhage and/or rupture.

Recurrence of HELLP Syndrome

HELLP syndrome can recur in subsequent pregnancies. Subsequent pregnancies in patients with HELLP syndrome carry

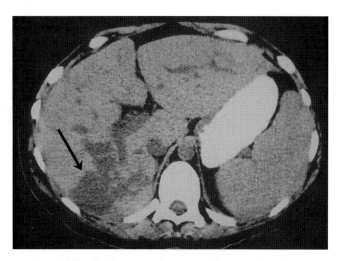

Fig. 52-4 Abdominal computed tomography scan showing a subcapsular hematoma *(arrow)* in the right lobe in a woman with HELLP syndrome.

a high risk of complications such as preeclampsia, recurrent HELLP, prematurity, intrauterine growth retardation, abruptio placentae, and perinatal mortality.

Acute Fatty Liver of Pregnancy

Acute fatty liver of pregnancy is a rare clinical entity unique to pregnancy that occurs during the third trimester. Although it is a rare condition, it carries significant perinatal and maternal mortality. AFLP was first described in 1934 by Stander as "yellow acute atrophy of the liver" and in 1940 a specific clinical entity was described by Sheehan. The reported incidence of AFLP is 1 in 7270 to 13,000 deliveries.[157] There is no ethnic or regional variability in the disease. Clinical findings in AFLP vary and its diagnosis is complicated by a significant overlap in clinical and biochemical features with HELLP syndrome. AFLP is more common in primiparous women and generally occurs between 30 and 38 weeks of gestation. Multiple gestations and gestations with male fetuses result in generally higher prevalence of AFLP when compared with the average population. The disease tends to recur in future pregnancies.

Pathogenesis

Until recently the pathogenesis of AFLP was unknown and still has not been fully elucidated. Recent molecular advances suggest that AFLP may result from mitochondrial dysfunction. Several reports have documented a strong association between AFLP and a deficiency of the enzyme long-chain 3-hydroxyacyl-CoA dehydrogenase (LCHAD) in the fetus, a disorder of mitochondrial fatty acid β-oxidation.

Mitochondrial Fatty Acid Oxidation Defects

Mitochondrial β-oxidation of fatty acids is a complex process that consists of multiple transport steps and four enzymatic reactions resulting in the sequential removal of two-carbon, acetyl-coenzyme A units (**Fig. 52-5**).[157] The first step in the spiral, as shown in **Figure 52-6**,[157] is an acyl-CoA dehydrogenase reaction, catalyzed by very long–chain

acyl-CoA dehydrogenase (VLCAD) and its homologous enzymes: long-chain acyl-CoA dehydrogenase (LCAD), medium-chain acyl-CoA dehydrogenase (MCAD), or short-chain acyl-CoA dehydrogenase (SCAD). The second step in the pathway is catalyzed by either a long-chain 2,3-enoyl-CoA hydratase (LCEH) or a short-chain 2,3-enoyl-CoA hydratase (SCEH). The third step is catalyzed by a long-chain 3-hydroxyacyl-CoA dehydrogenase (LCHAD) or a short-chain 3-hydroxyacyl-CoA dehydrogenase (SCHAD). The fourth and last step in the spiral is mediated by a long-chain 3-ketoacyl-CoA thiolase (LKAT), medium-chain 3-ketoacyl-CoA thiolase (MKAT), or short-chain 3-ketoacyl-CoA thiolase (SKAT). For long chain–length fatty acids, the last three steps are mediated by an enzyme complex called mitochondrial trifunctional protein (MTP), which is associated with the inner mitochondrial membrane trifunctional protein.[158] MTP is a hetero-octamer of four α-subunits and four β-subunits. The α-subunit amino-terminal domain contains the long-chain 3-enoyl-CoA hydratase enzymatic activity whereas the LCHAD enzymatic activity resides in the carboxy-terminal domain. The β-subunit has the long-chain 3-ketoacyl-CoA thiolase enzymatic activity. Both subunit genes, *HADHA* and *HADHB*, have been localized to chromosome 2p23.[159] Both genes have been found to be arranged in a head-to-head manner and share a promoter that is bidirectional.[160] MTP defects have emerged as an important group of errors of metabolism because of their clinical implications. Human defects in the MTP complex are recessively inherited and cause either isolated LCHAD deficiency, with normal or partially reduced thiolase and hydratase activity, or complete MTP deficiency, with markedly reduced activity of all three enzymes. Patients have been described with either an isolated LCHAD deficiency or an MTP deficiency. In the literature, the majority of patients reported have been described as having isolated LCHAD deficiency.[161] A few hours or several months after birth, children with these recessively inherited disorders present with nonketotic hypoglycemia and hepatic encephalopathy, which may progress to coma and death if untreated.[162] They can also present with cardiomyopathy, slowly progressing peripheral neuropathy, skeletal myopathy, or sudden, unexpected death.[163,164] Two teams, independent of each other, delineated the G1528C mutation in exon 15 of the α-subunit, which changes amino acid 474 from glutamic acid to glutamine (E474Q).[165,166] In a subsequent study, Ibdah and colleagues reported the α-subunit molecular defects and phenotypes in 24 patients with documented isolated LCHAD deficiency or complete MTP deficiency.[161] Of the 24 patients, 19 were diagnosed with isolated LCHAD deficiency and presented with the hepatic phenotype and 5 were diagnosed with complete trifunctional protein deficiency, of which 3 displayed the cardiac phenotype and the other 2 presented with the neuromuscular phenotype. Patients with isolated LCHAD deficiency presented predominantly with a Reye-like syndrome of liver dysfunction and carried the prevalent G1528C missense mutation on one or both alleles.

Fetal Mitochondrial Trifunctional Protein Defects and Acute Fatty Liver of Pregnancy

Several studies in the literature have documented strong and somewhat unique causative association between fetal

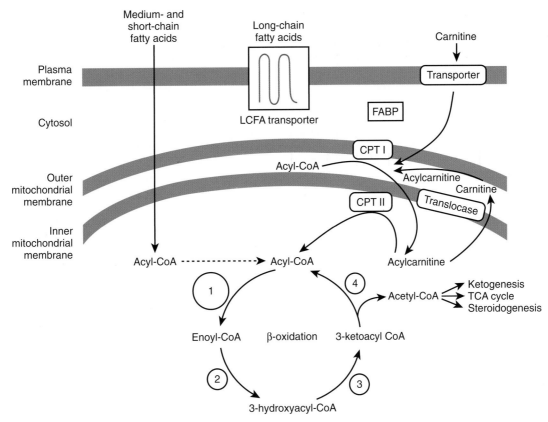

Fig. 52-5 Fatty acid import into the mitochondria and fatty acid β-oxidation. Long-chain fatty acids (*LCFA*) are actively transported across the plasma membrane, esterified to coenzyme A, carried by fatty acid–binding proteins (*FABP*) through the cytoplasm to the mitochondria, and translocated across the mitochondrial membranes by the carnitine shuttle into the mitochondrial matrix. The fatty acid is subsequently cleaved two carbons shorter by the β-oxidation spiral. CPT, carnitine palmitoyltransfease. *(Modified from Ibdali JA. Acute fatty liver of pregnancy: an update on pathogenesis and clinical implications. World J Gastroenterol 2006;12:7397–7404.)*

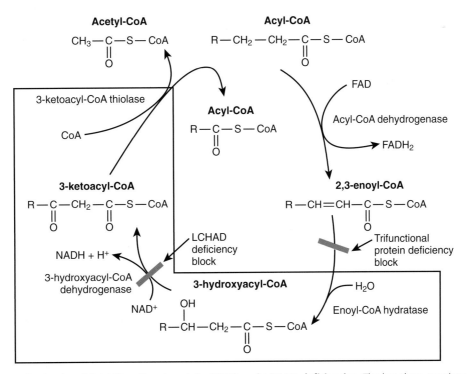

Fig. 52-6 Biochemistry of mitochondrial trifunctional protein (MTP) and LCHAD deficiencies. The last three reactions of the mitochondrial fatty acid β-oxidation spiral where the trifunctional protein catalyzes long-chain fatty acid substrates. In isolated LCHAD deficiency, the pathway is blocked after the enoyl Co-A hydratase reaction and before the 3-hydroxyacyl Co-A dehydrogenase reaction, causing the accumulation of medium- and long-chain 3-hydroxy fatty acids and their metabolites. In complete MTP deficiency, the pathway is blocked after the acyl Co-A dehydrogenase reaction and before the enoyl Co-A dehydrogenase reaction, causing the accumulation of straight-chain fatty acids and their metabolites. *(Modified from Ibdali JA. Acute fatty liver of pregnancy: an update on pathogenesis and clinical implications. World J Gastroenterol 2006;12:7397–7404.)*

mitochondrial trifunctional protein (MTP) defects and AFLP. Schoeman and colleagues were first to note an association between recurrent maternal acute fatty liver of pregnancy and a fetal fatty acid oxidation disorder in their study of two affected siblings who both died at 6 months of age.[167] Other case reports in the early 1990s have also associated affected infants with LCHAD deficiency to the occurrence of severe preeclampsia, HELLP syndrome, or AFLP in the infant's mother during pregnancy.[165,168,169] In a study in which Ibdah and colleagues examined the association between MTP defects in children and liver disease in their mothers during pregnancy,[161] maternal liver disease was diagnosed in 15 of 24 women (62%) during their pregnancies, whereas 9 of the 24 women had normal pregnancies. In five of the normal pregnancies, the affected infant did not have the G1528C mutation, but rather other MTP mutations. The remaining four normal pregnancies were associated with fetal LCHAD deficiency. Thus 15 of 19 pregnancies associated with fetal LCHAD deficiency were complicated by maternal liver disease and none of the pregnancies associated with complete MTP deficiency were complicated by maternal liver disease. The results in this study suggest that when carrying an LCHAD-deficient fetus, there is a 79% chance that the pregnancy will be complicated by AFLP.

In a subsequent study, Ibdah and colleagues evaluated fetal genotypes and pregnancy outcomes in 83 pregnancies in 35 families with documented pediatric MTP defects; 24 pregnancies were complicated by AFLP, HELLP syndrome, or severe preeclampsia.[170] Of the 24 pregnancies, 20 were complicated by AFLP, 2 by HELLP syndrome, and 2 by preeclampsia; in all 24 pregnancies, the LCHAD-deficient fetus carried the G1528C mutation on one or both alleles. Five pregnancies had fetuses with complete MTP deficiency (none of the mutations were G1528C); however, there were no associated maternal complications in those pregnancies. These studies provide strong evidence that carrying a fetus with LCHAD deficiency is associated with a high risk for developing AFLP during pregnancy. With the growing evidence suggesting that carrying an LCHAD-deficient fetus is associated with AFLP, it is recommended that neonates born to pregnancies complicated by AFLP be tested for the common G1528C mutation. When this genetic testing is performed early after birth, it can be life-saving because it identifies LCHAD-deficient children before they manifest the disease, allowing early dietary intervention by institution of a diet low in fat and high in carbohydrates and by substitution of long-chain fatty acids with medium-chain fatty acids.

To further assess the significance of the association between maternal AFLP and fetal LCHAD deficiency, Yang and colleagues prospectively screened for MTP mutations in mothers who developed AFLP (27 pregnancies) or HELLP syndrome (81 pregnancies) and in their newborn infants.[170] The molecular screening was based solely on the maternal history. Of the 27 women who developed AFLP, 5 carried fetuses with MTP mutations. Three were homozygous for the G1528C mutation and two were compound heterozygotes with one mutant allele carrying the common G1528C and the other mutant allele carrying a novel mutation. Only one woman diagnosed with HELLP syndrome was heterozygous for a G1528C mutation that was not detected in her infant. None of the children born to the 81 women diagnosed with HELLP syndrome carried MTP mutations. This study documents that in approximately one of five pregnancies complicated by AFLP, the fetus is LCHAD deficient. This strong association between AFLP and the common G1528C mutation in the fetus is significant. Therefore screening the progeny of women who develop AFLP at birth for this mutation can be life-saving.

In addition, identification of MTP mutations in the progeny of pregnancies complicated by AFLP allows genetic counseling for the mothers. Prenatal diagnosis can be performed in subsequent pregnancies to identify pregnancies at risk for development of AFLP.[171] The precise mechanism by which an LCHAD-deficient fetus causes AFLP in a heterozygote mother is still unclear. However, several factors appear to contribute to this fetal–maternal interaction as illustrated in **Figure 52-7**.[157] First, the heterozygosity of the mother for an MTP defect reduces her capacity to oxidize long-chain fatty acids, resulting in the buildup of toxic metabolites. Second, the metabolic stress present in the third trimester of pregnancy concomitant with its changes in metabolism (e.g., increased lipolysis, decreased β-oxidation) permit the accumulation of toxic metabolites and the development of liver disease. Third, environmental stress in the presence of the G1528C mutation may lead to the accumulation of potentially hepatotoxic

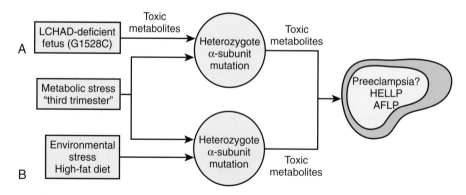

Fig. 52-7 Hypothesis illustrating the possible role of fetal and maternal MTP mutations in developing AFLP. A, Carrying an LCHAD-deficient fetus is the major determining factor in the development of maternal illness. Hepatotoxic metabolites produced by the fetus and/or placenta may cause liver disease in the obligate heterozygous mother when combined with the metabolic stress of the third trimester. **B,** Environmental stress may lead to the further accumulation of toxic metabolites in the genetically susceptible mother, causing maternal liver disease. *(Modified from Ibdali JA. Acute fatty liver of pregnancy: an update on pathogenesis and clinical implications. World J Gastroenterol 2006;12:7397–7404.)*

long-chain 3-hydroxyacyl fatty acid metabolites in the maternal circulation.

The role of other fatty acid oxidation (FAO) defects in the development of AFLP is not clear and remains controversial. Only a small number of case reports describe possible association between maternal liver disease and fetal FAO defects other than those in MTP. There are few reports of the involvement of fetal hepatic carnitine palmitoyltransferase (CPT I) deficiency and maternal medium-chain acyl-CoA dehydrogenase (MCAD) deficiency in AFLP.[172,173] CPT I deficiency usually presents as a Reye's-like syndrome in children ages 8 to 18 months. There is one case report of recurrent AFLP and hyperemesis gravidarum in two successive pregnancies in a patient whose offspring were diagnosed with CPT I deficiency.[174] Undiagnosed MCAD deficiency in AFLP was also reported in a woman who delivered a baby without enzyme abnormalities.[173] One study that looked at the incidence of maternal liver disease in pregnancies with fetal FAO defects suggested that fetal long-chain defects are 50 times more likely to develop a liver disease in pregnancy when compared with healthy controls; and short- and medium-chain FAO defects are 12 times more likely to develop liver disease.[172]

Clinical Findings

Acute fatty liver of pregnancy usually occurs in the late term of pregnancy, most commonly in the third trimester with a few case reports in the second trimester. Initial presentation is very nonspecific with malaise, nausea, vomiting, and headache and can be easily misdiagnosed. Right upper quadrant pain and epigastric abdominal pain are common (50% to 80% of cases).[157] Fever, headache, diarrhea, back pain suggestive of acute pancreatitis, and myalgias are occasionally seen in the initial presentation. Rarely patients may present with frank liver failure and bleeding attributable to liver failure–induced coagulopathy, but generally these symptoms are seen 1 to 2 weeks later. Preeclampsia co-exists in >50% of patients with AFLP. Occasionally, the patient may present with signs and symptoms of eclampsia (agitation, increased thirst, premature labor, seizures). Hypertension is mild or may be absent because of a decrease in peripheral vascular resistance associated with hepatic failure. Rarely AFLP may present as asymptomatic elevation of transaminase levels. Jaundice is seen on initial presentation in severe cases.[175] Physical findings are often minimal. Early in the disease, right upper quadrant tenderness may be the only abnormality found. The liver is usually nonpalpable. As the disease progresses, jaundice, altered mental status, ascites, and edema arise.

Complications

Early complications include acute renal failure, acute pancreatitis, hypoglycemia, and infection. Hepatic encephalopathy is generally a late complication and heralds the onset of acute liver failure. Any combination of these complications may lead to significant maternal and fetal mortality. Delivery is often complicated with severe postpartum bleeding. Diabetes insipidus may also complicate AFLP.[175]

AFLP is mainly diagnosed clinically. A moderate elevation in the levels of transaminases is usually seen, ranging from just slightly above normal to a value more than 1000 U/L above normal. The degree of elevation of liver transaminases

does not accurately reflect the severity of liver dysfunction. Normocytic anemia and leukocytosis are seen. Thrombocytopenia is common when DIC is present; otherwise, it is unusual in AFLP. Coagulation studies show a pattern of DIC in many cases. The peripheral smear contains nucleated red blood cells and, in cases with DIC, fragmented erythrocytes and burr cells. Elevation of blood urea nitrogen (BUN) and creatinine values is observed. As liver function progressively worsens, encephalopathy, hypoglycemia, and elevated ammonia concentration develop. Although liver biopsy is a gold standard for diagnosis of AFLP, it is not routinely done because of the urgency of the clinical situation and risk of hemorrhage. Liver biopsy is especially helpful early in the disease or in mild cases of AFLP, when the diagnosis is not clear. Liver biopsy shows cytoplasmic vacuolization predominantly in the perivenular and midzonal regions with microvesicular fatty infiltration as shown in **Figure 52-8**. In severe cases lobular disarray is seen with cell dropout and fatty change may be diffuse and involve all zones.[176] Portal inflammatory changes can be seen as well, suggestive of cholangitis; therefore histopathologic studies should be interpreted with the consideration of clinical presentation. Imaging studies are of little value in the diagnosis of AFLP.[157] They are mainly useful for excluding other pathologic processes in the liver (e.g., hepatic ischemia, hepatic infarct, Budd-Chiari syndrome, or hepatic hematoma/rupture). Liver US and CT were inconsistent in detecting fatty infiltration of the liver in patients with AFLP; the role of MRI and spectroscopy in particular requires further investigation.

Differential Diagnosis

The distinguishing features of liver diseases unique to pregnancy are shown in **Table 52-7**. Clinical and laboratory features of AFLP have significant overlap with those of HELLP syndrome (see **Table 52-7**). Both conditions present late in pregnancy and both can be associated or complicated with preeclampsia. The presence of hypoglycemia and/or prolongation of prothrombin time is suggestive of AFLP.[157] Moreover, patients with preeclampsia-associated liver disease and HELLP have more profound hematologic abnormalities. AFLP can be confused with fulminant liver failure attributable to acute viral hepatitis. A history of exposure and viral serologic testing are the key in making the diagnosis. The degree of elevation of liver transaminase levels is much higher in patients with acute viral hepatitis than in AFLP and DIC is generally uncommon. Additionally, the histopathology is also different in these pathologic processes. The histologic feature of HELLP syndrome is virtually nonexistent in AFLP. Extensive hepatocellular necrosis, a common histologic feature of HELLP syndrome, is absent in AFLP, and microvesicular fatty infiltration, the predominant feature of AFLP, is generally absent in HELLP syndrome.[157]

Management

Prompt diagnosis is the key to a successful outcome. Patients are usually very ill and require hospitalization in the intensive care unit. If AFLP is suspected, patients should be admitted for further evaluation and management. Timely delivery after initial patient stabilization will cure the patient, similar to most pregnancy-associated liver diseases.[175,177] Depending on the presence of complications, complete recovery from AFLP

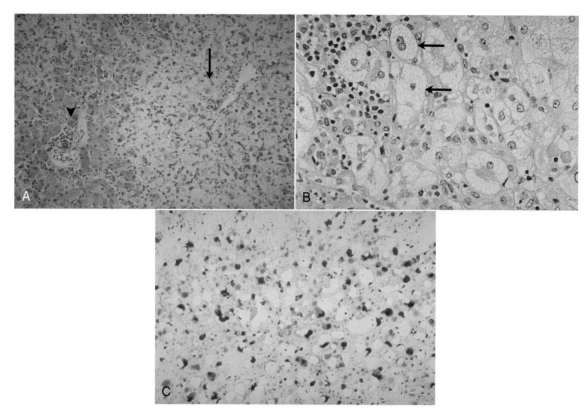

Fig. 52-8 **Acute fatty liver of pregnancy. A,** Fat accumulation is greater in pericentral hepatocytes *(arrow)* compared with periportal hepatocytes *(arrowhead).* (H & E stain.) **B,** The small (microvesicular) fat droplets surround but do not displace hepatocyte nuclei *(arrows).* (H & E stain.) **C,** Fat is readily appreciated with oil-red O stain on frozen liver tissue.

Table 52-7 Distinguishing Features of Liver Diseases Unique to Pregnancy

DISEASE/FEATURES	HG	ICP	HELLP	AFLP
Incidence in pregnancy	0.3%-2%	0.1%-0.01% (US)	0.2%-0.6%	0.005%-0.01%
Onset during pregnancy	First trimester	Third trimester, but can occur in second trimester	Third trimester or postpartum	Third trimester or postpartum
Presence of preeclampsia	No	No	Yes	>50%
Clinical features	Intense nausea and vomiting, dehydration, electrolyte abnormality	Generalized pruritus, elevated maternal serum bile acids	Hemolysis, thrombocytopenia	Liver failure with coagulopathy, encephalopathy, hypoglycemia, and DIC
Aminotransferases	Usually <300 units/L	Mild to 20-fold increase	Typically >500 units/L	Typically 300-500 units/L
Bilirubin	Usually <4 mg/dl	<5 mg/dl	<5 mg/dl	<5 mg/dl
Imaging	Normal	Normal	May show hepatic rupture or infarction	May show fatty infiltrate
Histology	Normal or bland cholestasis	Cholestasis	Patchy/extensive necrosis and hemorrhage	Microvesicular steatosis in zone 3
Perinatal/fetal outcomes	Preterm and low birth weight	Preterm and low birth weight, meconium staining	Perinatal mortality, prematurity	Fetal mortality 9%-23%

AFLP, acute fatty liver disease of pregnancy; HELLP, hemolysis, elevated liver enzymes, and low platelet count; HG, hyperemesis gravidarum; ICP, intrahepatic cholestasis of pregnancy

may take anywhere from days to weeks. Because clotting factors have short half-lives, prothrombin time improvement is the first sign of hepatic recovery. Patients may require supportive management including dialysis, multiple transfusions, mechanical ventilation, or glucose infusions. In general, if the patient recovers from complications, there are no hepatic sequelae postpartum after AFLP. Rarely, liver transplantation is needed for management of severe acute hepatic failure in the setting of AFLP.

Key References

Anger GJ, Piquette-Miller M. Pharmacokinetic studies in pregnant women. Clin Pharmacol Ther 2008;83:184–187. (Ref.1)

Araujo AC, et al. Characteristics and treatment of hepatic rupture caused by HELLP syndrome. Am J Obstet Gynecol 2006;195:129–133. (Ref.144)

Arora N, Choudhary S. Pregnancy with Crigler-Najjar syndrome type II. J Obstet Gynaecol 2009;2942–244. (Ref.5)

Arrese M, Reyes H. Intrahepatic cholestasis of pregnancy: a past and present riddle. Ann Hepatol 2006;5:202–205. (Ref.116)

Arrese M, et al. Molecular pathogenesis of intrahepatic cholestasis of pregnancy. Expert Rev Mol Med 2008;10:e9. (Ref.124)

Aytac S, et al. *Helicobacter pylori* stool antigen assay in hyperemesis gravidarum: a risk factor for hyperemesis gravidarum or not? Dig Dis Sci 2007;52:2840–2843. (Ref.96)

Bailit JL, Bailit JL. Hyperemesis gravidarum: epidemiologic findings from a large cohort. Am J Obstet Gynecol 2005;193(3 Pt 1):811–814. (Ref.84)

Barton JR, Sibai BM. Diagnosis and management of hemolysis, elevated liver enzymes, and low platelets syndrome. Clin Perinatol 2004;31:807–833, vii. (Ref.155)

Baxter JK, Weinstein L. HELLP syndrome: the state of the art. Obstet Gynecol Surg 2004;59:838–845. (Ref.154)

Bittencourt PL, Couto CA, Ribeiro DD. Portal vein thrombosis and Budd-Chiari syndrome. Clin Liver Dis 2009;13:127–144. (Ref.53)

Boccia D, et al. High mortality associated with an outbreak of hepatitis E among displaced persons in Darfur, Sudan. Clin Infect Dis 2006;42:1679–1684. (Ref.13)

Bozzo P, et al. The incidence of nausea and vomiting of pregnancy (NVP): a comparison between depressed women treated with antidepressants and non-depressed women. Clin Invest Med 2006;29:347–350. (Ref.109)

Browning MF, et al. Fetal fatty acid oxidation defects and maternal liver disease in pregnancy. Obstet Gynecol 2006;107:115–120. (Ref.172)

Bryer E, Bryer E. A literature review of the effectiveness of ginger in alleviating mild-to-moderate nausea and vomiting of pregnancy. J Midwifery Womens Health 2005;50:e1–e3. (Ref.102)

Candia L, Marquez J, Espinoza LR. Autoimmune hepatitis and pregnancy: a rheumatologist's dilemma. Semin Arthritis Rheum 2005;35:49–56. (Ref.36)

Cissoko H, et al. Neonatal outcome after exposure to beta adrenergic blockers late in pregnancy. Arch Pediatr 2005;12:543–547. (Ref.73)

Condat B, et al. Portal cavernoma-associated cholangiopathy: a clinical and MR cholangiography coupled with MR portography imaging study. Hepatology 2003;37:1302–1308. (Ref.54)

Cooper GS, Stroehla BC. The epidemiology of autoimmune diseases. Autoimmun Rev 2003;2:119–125. (Ref.33)

Czaja AJ. Autoimmune liver disease. Curr Opin Gastroenterol 2004;20:231–240. (Ref.41)

Czaja AJ. Diverse manifestations and evolving treatments of autoimmune hepatitis. Minerva Gastroenterol Dietol 2005;51:313–333. (Ref.42)

Czaja AJ. Current and future treatments of autoimmune hepatitis. Expert Rev Gastroenterol Hepatol 2009;3:269–291. (Ref.43)

Darwish Murad S, et al. Determinants of survival and the effect of portosystemic shunting in patients with Budd-Chiari syndrome. Hepatology 2004;39:500–508. (Ref.60)

de Boer NK, et al. Azathioprine use during pregnancy: intrauterine exposure to metabolites. Am J Gastroenterol 2006;101:1390–1392. (Ref.45)

de Franchis R. Evolving consensus in portal hypertension. Report of the Baveno IV consensus workshop on methodology of diagnosis and therapy in portal hypertension. J Hepatol 2005;43:167–176. (Ref.55)

Dodds L, et al. Outcomes of pregnancies complicated by hyperemesis gravidarum. Obstet Gynecol 2006;107(2 Pt 1):285–292. (Ref.114)

Einarson A, et al. The safety of ondansetron for nausea and vomiting of pregnancy: a prospective comparative study. Br J Obstet Gynaecol 2004;111:940–943. (Ref.112)

Elinav E, et al. Acute hepatitis A infection in pregnancy is associated with high rates of gestational complications and preterm labor. Gastroenterology 2006;130:1129–1134. (Ref.14)

Fell DB, et al. Risk factors for hyperemesis gravidarum requiring hospital admission during pregnancy. Obstet Gynecol 2006;107(2 Pt 1):277–284. (Ref.92)

Ferrero S, et al. Prospective study of mother-to-infant transmission of hepatitis C virus: a 10-year survey (1990-2000). Acta Obstet Gynecol Scand 2003;82:229–234. (Ref.24)

Fonseca JE, et al. Dexamethasone treatment does not improve the outcome of women with HELLP syndrome: a double-blind, placebo-controlled, randomized clinical trial. Am J Obstet Gynecol 2005;193:1591–1598. (Ref.153)

Fontana RJ. Side effects of long-term oral antiviral therapy for hepatitis B. Hepatology 2009;49(5 Suppl):S185–S195. (Ref.23)

Fontana RJ. Hepatitis B: a "GLOBAL" health challenge. Gastroenterology 2009;136:389–392. (Ref.17)

Gajdos V, et al. Successful pregnancy in a Crigler-Najjar type I patient treated by phototherapy and semimonthly albumin infusions. Gastroenterology 2006;131:921–924. (Ref.6)

Gall SA. Maternal immunization. Obstet Gynecol Clin North Am 2003;30:623–636. (Ref.15)

Garcia-Tsao G. Liver involvement in hereditary hemorrhagic telangiectasia (HHT). J Hepatol 2007;46:499–507. (Ref.64)

Ghidirim G, et al. Prophylactic endoscopic band ligation of esophageal varices during pregnancy. J Gastrointest Liver Dis 2008;17:236–237. (Ref.74)

Glantz A, et al. Intrahepatic cholestasis of pregnancy: a randomized controlled trial comparing dexamethasone and ursodeoxycholic acid. Hepatology 2005;42:1399–1405. (Ref.137)

Glantz A, Hanns-Ulrich M, Lars-Ake M. Intrahepatic cholestasis of pregnancy: Relationships between bile acid levels and fetal complication rates. Hepatology 2004;40:467–474. (Ref.132)

Glantz A, et al. Intrahepatic cholestasis of pregnancy: amelioration of pruritus by UDCA is associated with decreased progesterone disulphates in urine. Hepatology 2008;47:544–551. (Ref.138)

Golberg D, et al. Hyperemesis gravidarum and *Helicobacter pylori* infection: a systematic review. Obstet Gynecol 2007;110:695–703. (Ref.94)

Hanukoglu A, et al. Hypothyroidism and dyshormonogenesis induced by D-penicillamine in children with Wilson's disease and healthy infants born to a mother with Wilson's disease. J Pediatr 2008;153:864–866. (Ref.48)

Haram K, Svendsen E, Abildgaard U. The HELLP syndrome: clinical issues and management. A review. BMC Pregnancy Childbirth 2009;9:8. (Ref.147)

Hardman B, et al. Hormonal regulation of the Menkes and Wilson copper-transporting ATPases in human placental Jeg-3 cells. Biochem J 2007;402:241–250. (Ref.46)

Hay JE. Liver disease in pregnancy. Hepatology 2008;47:1067–1076. (Ref.12)

Hollingshead M, et al. Transcatheter thrombolytic therapy for acute mesenteric and portal vein thrombosis. J Vasc Interv Radiol 2005;16:651–661. (Ref.56)

Holstein A, et al. Successful photo- and phenobarbital therapy during pregnancy in a woman with Crigler-Najjar syndrome type II. Scand J Gastroenterol 2005;40:1124–1126. (Ref.7)

Hutchins GF, John LG. Recent developments in the pathophysiology of cholestasis. Clin Liver Dis 2004;8:i–v. (Ref.129)

Ibdah JA. Acute fatty liver of pregnancy: an update on pathogenesis and clinical implications. World J Gastroenterol 2006;12:7397–7404. (Ref.157)

Janssen HL, et al. Budd-Chiari syndrome: a review by an expert panel. J Hepatol 2003;38:364–371. (Ref.57)

Jelin EB, et al. Management of biliary tract disease during pregnancy: a decision analysis. Surg Endosc 2008;22:54–60. (Ref.80)

Kahaleh M, et al. Safety and efficacy of ERCP in pregnancy. Gastrointest Endosc 2004;60:287–292. (Ref.81)

Karaca C, et al. Is lower socio-economic status a risk factor for *Helicobacter pylori* infection in pregnant women with hyperemesis gravidarum? Turk J Gastroenterol 2004;15:86–89. (Ref.97)

Kawabata I, Nakai A, Takeshita T. Prediction of HELLP syndrome with assessment of maternal dual hepatic blood supply by using Doppler ultrasound. Arch Gynecol Obstet 2006;274:303–309. (Ref.145)

Ko CW, et al. Incidence, natural history, and risk factors for biliary sludge and stones during pregnancy. Hepatology 2005;41:359–365. (Ref.77)

Ko H, Yoshida EM. Acute fatty liver of pregnancy. Can J Gastroenterol 2006;20:25–30. (Ref.177)

Kumar A, et al. Hepatitis E in pregnancy. Int J Gynaecol Obstet 2004;85:240–244. (Ref.29)

Lee RH, et al. The prevalence of intrahepatic cholestasis of pregnancy in a primarily Latina Los Angeles population. J Perinatol 2006;26:527–532. (Ref.119)

Letson GW, et al. Effect of maternal antibody on immunogenicity of hepatitis A vaccine in infants. J Pediatr 2004;144:327–332. (Ref.16)

Liaw YF, et al. Asian-Pacific consensus statement on the management of chronic hepatitis B: a 2005 update. Liver Int 2005;25:472–489. (Ref.22)

Lin SP, Brown JJ. MR contrast agents: physical and pharmacologic basics. J Magn Reson Imaging 2007;2584–2899. (Ref.62)

Lodato F, et al. Transjugular intrahepatic portosystemic shunt: a case report of rescue management of unrestrainable variceal bleeding in a pregnant woman. Dig Liver Dis 2008;40:387–390. (Ref.75)

Lopez-Mendez E, Avila-Escobedo L. Pregnancy and portal hypertension: a pathology view of physiologic changes. Ann Hepatol 2006;5:219–223. (Ref.66)

Louik C, et al. Nausea and vomiting in pregnancy: maternal characteristics and risk factors. Paediatr Perinat Epidemiol 2006;20:270–278. (Ref.83)

Markl GE, et al. The association of psychosocial factors with nausea and vomiting during pregnancy. J Psychosom Obstet Gynecol 2008;29:17–22. (Ref.93)

Martin JN Jr, Rose CH, Briery CM. Understanding and managing HELLP syndrome: the integral role of aggressive glucocorticoids for mother and child. Am J Obstet Gynecol 2006;195:914–934. (Ref.152)

Mast EE, et al. Risk factors for perinatal transmission of hepatitis C virus (HCV) and the natural history of HCV infection acquired in infancy. J Infect Dis 2005;192:1880–1889. (Ref.26)

Matsuo K, et al. Hyperemesis gravidarum in Eastern Asian population. Gynecol Obstet Invest 2007;64:213–216. (Ref.91)

Mattison D, Zajicek A. Gaps in knowledge in treating pregnant women. Gend Med 2006;3:169–182. (Ref.3)

Mjahed K, et al. Acute fatty liver of pregnancy. Arch Gynecol Obstet 2006;274:349–353. (Ref.175)

O'Mahony S. Endoscopy in pregnancy. Best Pract Res Clin Gastroenterol 2007;21:893–899. (Ref.72)

Outlaw WM, Ibdah JA. Impaired fatty acid oxidation as a cause of liver disease associated with hyperemesis gravidarum. Med Hypotheses 2005;65:1150–1153. (Ref.100)

Pal R, et al. Immunological alterations in pregnant women with acute hepatitis E. J Gastroenterol Hepatol 2005;20:1094–1101. (Ref.28)

Pavek P, Ceckova M, Staud F. Variation of drug kinetics in pregnancy. Curr Drug Metab 2009;10:520–529. (Ref.2)

Piwko C, et al. The weekly cost of nausea and vomiting of pregnancy for women calling the Toronto Motherisk Program. Curr Med Res Opin 2007;23:833–840. (Ref.90)

Pongrojpaw D, et al. A randomized comparison of ginger and dimenhydrinate in the treatment of nausea and vomiting in pregnancy. J Med Assoc Thai 2007;90:1703–1709. (Ref.103)

Safioleas MC, Moulakakis KG. A rare cause of intra-abdominal haemorrhage: spontaneous rupture of the splenic vein. Acta Chir Belg 2006;106:237–239. (Ref.69)

Santos L, et al. Acute liver failure in pregnancy associated with maternal MCAD deficiency. J Inherit Metab Dis 2007;30:103. (Ref.173)

Savage C, et al. Transjugular intrahepatic portosystemic shunt creation for recurrent gastrointestinal bleeding during pregnancy. J Vasc Interv Radiol 2007;18:902–904. (Ref.76)

Schramm C, et al. Pregnancy in autoimmune hepatitis: outcome and risk factors. Am J Gastroenterol 2006;101:556–560. (Ref.35)

Shames BD, et al. Liver transplantation for HELLP syndrome. Liver Transpl 2005;11:224–228. (Ref.156)

Sibai BM. Diagnosis, controversies, and management of the syndrome of hemolysis, elevated liver enzymes, and low platelet count. Obstet Gynecol 2004;103(5 Pt 1):981–991. (Ref.141)

Sibai BM. Diagnosis, prevention, and management of eclampsia. Obstet Gynecol 2005;105:402–410. (Ref.151)

Sigel CS, Harper TC, Thorne LB. Postpartum sudden death from pulmonary hypertension in the setting of portal hypertension. Obstet Gynecol 2007;110(2 Pt 2):501–503. (Ref.68)

Singh S, et al. Mother-to-child transmission of hepatitis E virus infection. Indian J Pediatr 2003;70:37–39. (Ref.30)

Sinha S, et al. Successful pregnancies and abortions in symptomatic and asymptomatic Wilson's disease. J Neurol Sci 2004;217:37–40. (Ref.49)

Smith C, et al. A randomized controlled trial of ginger to treat nausea and vomiting in pregnancy. Obstet Gynecol 2004;103:639–645. (Ref.104)

Strand S, et al. Placenta-derived CD95 ligand causes liver damage in hemolysis, elevated liver enzymes, and low platelet count syndrome. Gastroenterology 2004;126:849–858. (Ref.146)

Sumana G, et al. Non-cirrhotic portal hypertension and pregnancy outcome. J Obstet Gynaecol Res 2008;34:801–804. (Ref.70)

Tan J, Surti B, Saab S. Pregnancy and cirrhosis. Liver Transpl 2008;14:1081–1091. (Ref.67)

Tan PC, et al. Readmission risk and metabolic, biochemical, haematological and clinical indicators of severity in hyperemesis gravidarum. Aust N Z J Obstet Gynaecol 2006;46:446–450. (Ref.101)

Terrabuio DR, et al. Follow-up of pregnant women with autoimmune hepatitis: the disease behavior along with maternal and fetal outcomes. J Clin Gastroenterol 2009;43:350–356. (Ref.44)

van Zonneveld M, et al. Lamivudine treatment during pregnancy to prevent perinatal transmission of hepatitis B virus infection. J Viral Hepat 2003;10:294–297. (Ref.21)

Vikanes A, et al. Variations in prevalence of hyperemesis gravidarum by country of birth: a study of 900,074 pregnancies in Norway, 1967-2005. Scand J Public Health 2008;36:135–142. (Ref.85)

Webb JA, Thomsen HS, Morcos SK. The use of iodinated and gadolinium contrast media during pregnancy and lactation. Eur Radiol 2005;15:1234–1240. (Ref.61)

Wong LFA, Shallow H, Connell MPO. Comparative study on the outcome of obstetric cholestasis. J Matern Fetal Neonatal Med 2008;21:327–330. (Ref.118)

Xu WM, et al. Lamivudine in late pregnancy to prevent perinatal transmission of hepatitis B virus infection: a multicentre, randomized, double-blind, placebo-controlled study. J Viral Hepat 2009;16:94–103. (Ref.20)

Yoong W, et al. Pregnancy outcomes of women with pruritus, normal bile salts and liver enzymes: a case control study. Acta Obstet Gynecol Scand 2008;87:419–422. (Ref.139)

Zamah AM, Yasser YE-S, Amin AM. Two cases of cholestasis in the first trimester of pregnancy after ovarian hyperstimulation. Fertil Steril 2008;90:1202.e7–1202.e10. (Ref.128)

Zapata R, et al. Ursodeoxycholic acid in the treatment of intrahepatic cholestasis of pregnancy. A 12-year experience. Liver Int 2005;25:548–554. (Ref.135)

Ziaei S, et al. The efficacy low dose of prednisolone in the treatment of hyperemesis gravidarum. Acta Obstet Gynecol Scand 2004;83:272–275. (Ref.110)

A complete list of references can be found at www.expertconsult.com.

Nonalcoholic Fatty Liver Disease

Puneet Puri and Arun J. Sanyal

ABBREVIATIONS

ABCA1 ATP-binding cassette lipid transporter-1
ALT alanine aminotransferase
AMPK adenosine-5′-monophosphate–activated protein kinase
AP1 activator protein-1
AST aspartate aminotransferase
ATP adenosine triphosphate
BCL2 B-cell lymphoma-2
BMI body mass index
CB1 cannabinoid receptor
CCL2 C-C motif chemokine ligand-2
ChREBP carbohydrate response element–binding protein
CI confidence interval
CoA acyl-coenzyme A
CRN Clinical Research Network
CT computed tomography
DNL de novo lipogenesis
EMT epithelial-mesenchymal transition
ER endoplasmic reticulum
ERAD ER-associated degradation
FABP fatty acid–binding protein
FFA free fatty acid
FOXa2 forkhead box protein-a2
GGT γ-glutamyltransferase

GLUT4 glucose transporter-4
HDL high-density lipoprotein
HR hazard ratio
HSC hepatic stellate cell
HIV human immunodeficiency virus
IKK-β inhibitor kappa beta kinase-β
IL-6 interleukin-6
iNOS inducible nitric oxide synthetase
IR insulin resistance
JNK Jun N-terminal kinase
KLF6 Kruppel-like factor-6
LXR liver X receptor
Mlx maxlike protein X
MDB Mallory-Denk bodies
MRI magnetic resonance imaging
MTP microsomal transfer protein
NAFL nonalcoholic fatty liver
NAFLD nonalcoholic fatty liver disease
NAS NAFLD activity score
NASH nonalcoholic steatohepatitis
NF-κB nuclear factor-κB
NHANES III National Health and Nutrition Examination Survey III
NIH National Institutes of Health
OSA obstructive sleep apnea

PAI-1 plasminogen activator inhibitor-1
PPAR peroxisome proliferator–activated receptor
PPARGC1 PPAR-α and PPAR-γ coactivator-1
PUFA polyunsaturated fatty acids
RBP4 retinol-binding protein 4
RNS reactive nitrogen species
ROS reactive oxygen species
RXR retinoid X receptor
SOCS suppressors of cytokine signaling
SREBP sterol regulatory element–binding protein
sXBP spliced X box–binding protein
TF tissue factor
TGF-β transforming growth factor-β
TIMP tissue inhibitor of metalloproteinase
TNF-α tumor necrosis factor-α
TLR Toll-like receptors
TRAIL TNF-α–related apoptosis-inducing ligand
UDCA ursodeoxycholate acid
UPR unfolded protein response
VLDL very-low-density lipoprotein

Introduction

Nonalcoholic fatty liver disease (NAFLD) is the most common cause of persistent abnormalities in liver enzyme test results in North America.[1] The rising prevalence of NAFLD is related to the epidemic of obesity. Although the histologic picture resembles that of alcohol-induced liver injury, NAFLD occurs in patients who do not abuse alcohol. The histologic hallmark of NAFLD is predominantly macrovesicular steatosis.[2] NAFLD is now increasingly being recognized as a cause of end-stage liver disease and is associated with increased rates of hepatocellular carcinoma, liver transplantation, and death.[3,4] The terminology, histopathology, epidemiology, pathogenesis, clinical evaluation, and management of NAFLD are discussed in this chapter.

Terminology

Historically, abnormal liver chemistry in patients with obesity and diabetes has been referred to by different names, including idiopathic steatohepatitis, pseudoalcoholic liver disease, fatty liver hepatitis, and alcohol-like liver disease.[5] NAFLD is the currently accepted term, which by definition requires exclusion of alcohol as a cause. Other commonly used terminologies are used variably in the published literature and are described

Table 53-1 Terminology for Nonalcoholic Fatty Liver Disease

TERM	DESCRIPTION
NAFLD	Indicates the presence of fatty infiltration of the liver Defined as fat >5%-10% of liver weight Hepatic steatosis >5% in biopsy specimens
Simple steatosis	Fatty infiltration with no or minimal inflammation and no fibrosis
NASH	Hepatic steatosis with inflammation, ballooned hepatocytes, and/or fibrosis, which may progress to cirrhosis
"Primary" NAFLD	Occasionally used in the literature but not uniformly accepted Indicates typical disease associated with features of metabolic syndrome but without a specific, additional cause
"Secondary" NAFLD	NAFLD associated with a specific cause Implies the absence of insulin resistance May represent exacerbation of underlying primary NAFLD Distinction not very useful
"Presumed" NAFLD	Presumptive diagnosis of NAFLD Used in epidemiologic and pediatric studies
Basis	Abnormal liver enzyme levels Negative results of viral studies Exclusion of other common causes of liver disease Echogenic or bright liver on imaging, often on abdominal ultrasound consistent with fatty infiltration
Types of NAFLD (Matteoni et al.)	Type 1: Simple steatosis (no inflammation or fibrosis) Type 2: Steatosis with lobular inflammation but absent fibrosis or balloon cells Type 3: Steatosis, inflammation, and fibrosis of varying degrees (NASH) Type 4: Steatosis, inflammation, ballooned cells, and Mallory hyaline or fibrosis (NASH)

NAFLD, nonalcoholic fatty liver disease; NASH, nonalcoholic steatohepatitis

in **Table 53-1**. The spectrum of NAFLD is defined on the basis of liver histology, which encompasses nonalcoholic fatty liver (NAFL) and nonalcoholic steatohepatitis (NASH).

Histopathology of Nonalcoholic Fatty Liver Disease

The characteristic histopathologic features of adult NAFLD include mainly zone 3 macrovesicular steatosis; lobular inflammation; cellular injury, represented by cytologic ballooning, Mallory-Denk bodies (MDBs), or both; and pericellular fibrosis. Based on these characteristics, NAFLD has two broad histologic patterns: hepatic steatosis, or NAFL, and steatohepatitis (NASH). Contrary to its literal meaning, steatohepatitis does not simply represent the presence of steatosis and inflammation. Steatohepatitis is defined by the presence of hepatic steatosis with varying degrees of inflammation along with evidence of cell injury, usually in the form of cytologic ballooning (**Fig. 53-1**).[6] Fibrosis is not required for the diagnosis of steatohepatitis. These changes are typically most marked in the centrilobular regions. The inflammation associated with steatohepatitis is generally modest and mainly lobular in distribution. Portal inflammation exists to varying degree in individual subjects. The inflammation is often neutrophilic in nature,[7] but a mixed inflammatory infiltrate may also be seen.[8] A dense lymphocytic infiltrate in the portal areas is not typical of NAFLD, and an alternative cause of such an infiltrate, such as hepatitis C, should be sought when it is present. Portal fibrosis may be associated with NAFLD, particularly in pediatric subjects and in those who are morbidly obese.[9,10]

Grading and Staging

The grade of steatohepatitis reflects the necroinflammatory activity and the degree of cell injury that is present. The stage of the disease reflects the degree of fibrosis or how far an individual has progressed toward cirrhosis. An optimal system for grading and staging should be easy to use, be highly reproducible, relate to long-term outcomes, show sensitivity to change, and capture the entire spectrum of disease. Unfortunately, such an ideal system for grading and staging of NAFLD remains to be defined.

A fundamental requirement of any scoring system is a high degree of reproducibility. To assess reproducibility, 19 individual parameters grouped under steatosis, hepatocyte injury, inflammation, and fibrosis were examined in a blinded manner by four pathologists and twice by two pathologists.[11] Substantial concordance was observed with respect to assessment of the extent of steatosis, sinusoidal location of the steatosis, perivenular fibrosis, stage of fibrosis, ballooning degeneration, and glycogen nuclei. There was, however, considerable interobserver variation in the assessment of inflammation. These findings have been corroborated by the National Institutes of Health (NIH)-sponsored NASH Clinical Research Network (CRN).[12]

Several systems for grading and staging NAFLD have been proposed, but only two systems have been validated to any degree. A landmark study by Brunt and colleagues examined 10 separate histologic parameters.[13] Based on these parameters, a three-grade, four-stage system of classifying NAFLD was developed. Significant histologic lesions included steatosis, ballooning, and inflammation. The necroinflammatory grade correlated with alanine aminotransferase (ALT) activity. The staging score reflected both location and the extent of fibrosis.

More recently, using the Brunt classification as a starting point, the NIH-sponsored NASH CRN proposed and validated a scoring system.[12] Although 14 separate parameters were evaluated, 4 were scored semiquantitatively, including steatosis (0 to 3), cytologic ballooning (0 to 2), lobular

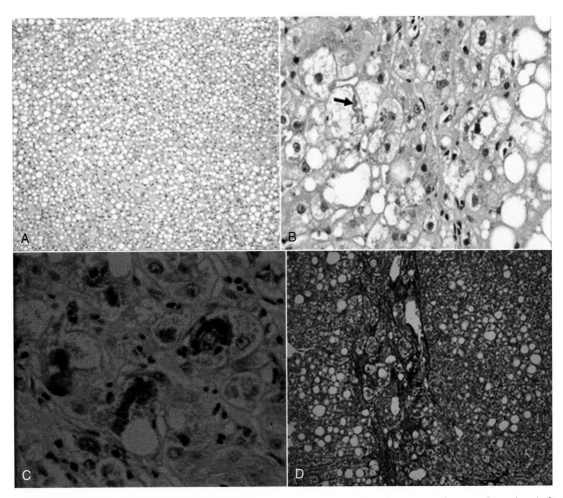

Fig. 53-1 Histologic features of nonalcoholic steatohepatitis. A, Macrovesicular steatosis. (Low power, hematoxylin and eosin [H & E] stain.) **B,** Cytologic ballooning with eosinophilic Mallory-Denk bodies *(arrow).* **C,** "Ropy" Mallory-Denk bodies stained with antibodies to ubiquitin. **D,** Pericellular fibrosis in centrilobular location. (Masson trichrome stain.)

inflammation (0 to 2), and fibrosis (0 to 4). A NAFLD activity score (NAS) was then developed that included the unweighted scores for steatosis, inflammation, and cytologic ballooning (**Table 53-2**). The NAS correlated well with the presence of steatohepatitis during a blinded validation process and was typically associated with a score of 5 or higher. Those with a score of 3 or less were not usually found to have steatohepatitis, whereas a score of 4 was associated with some divergence of opinion (**Fig. 53-2**). It is, however, important to note that the NAS cannot be used to diagnose the presence of steatohepatitis, which is identified by the presence of steatosis, inflammation, and cytologic ballooning in a typical pattern. The NASH CRN staging system divides stage 1 into several subsets (**Table 53-3**), thereby improving its sensitivity to change in earlier stages of the disease. This system is highly valuable as a research tool for the design and analysis of clinical trials related to NASH. However, its role in routine clinical practice remains to be established.

A major limitation of any histologic scoring system is sampling variability. In one study, two biopsy specimens were obtained from the same site at the same time.[14] About 20% of subjects had at least a one-stage variability between specimens, whereas 12% had a two-stage variation. Similar data have been obtained from studies in which biopsy specimens from the left and right lobes were compared.[15] This limitation may be overcome by using samples of adequate length and diameter. Although a 4-cm core is ideal,[16] a minimum biopsy core length of 2 cm obtained with a 15- to 16-gauge needle is generally recommended.

Distinguishing Nonalcoholic Steatohepatitis from Alcoholic Steatohepatitis

Although features such as steatosis and mild steatohepatitis may occur in either group, several histologic findings can suggest the presence of alcohol-related liver disease, including canalicular cholestasis, extensive deposition of dense perisinusoidal collagen, and cholangiolitis. Large, dense MDBs are also more common in alcoholic hepatitis than in NASH. In addition, noncirrhotic alcoholic hepatitis may actually exist without steatosis; this is not true of noncirrhotic NASH.[17,18]

Table 53-2 NASH Clinical Research Network Scoring System: NAFLD Activity Score

STEATOSIS GRADE		LOBULAR INFLAMMATION		HEPATOCELLULAR BALLOONING	
Degree	Description	Degree	Description	Degree	Description
0	<5%	0	None	0	None
1	5%-33%	1	<2 foci/20× optical field	1	Mild; few
2	34%-66%	2	2-4 foci/20× optical field	2	Moderate to marked; many
3	>66%	3	>4 foci/20× optical field		

NAFLD, nonalcoholic fatty liver disease; NASH, nonalcoholic steatohepatitis

Table 53-3 NASH Clinical Research Network Scoring System: Fibrosis Score

DEGREE	DESCRIPTION
0	None
1a	Mild (delicate) zone 3 perisinusoidal fibrosis
1b	Moderate (dense) zone 3 perisinusoidal fibrosis
1c	Portal/periportal fibrosis only
2	Zone 3 perisinusoidal fibrosis with portal/periportal fibrosis
3	Bridging fibrosis
4	Cirrhosis

NAFLD, nonalcoholic fatty liver disease; NASH, nonalcoholic steatohepatitis

Table 53-4 ATP III Clinical Identification of Metabolic Syndrome

RISK FACTOR	DEFINING LEVEL
Abdominal obesity (waist circumference) Men Women	>102 cm (>40 in) >88 cm (>35 in)
Triglycerides	>150 mg/dl
HDL cholesterol Men Women	<40 mg/dl <50 mg/dl
Blood pressure	≥130/≥85 mm Hg
Fasting glucose	≥110 mg/dl

ATP III, Adult Treatment Panel III; HDL, high-density lipoprotein

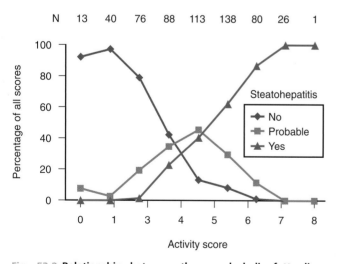

Fig. 53-2 **Relationship between the nonalcoholic fatty liver disease activity score (NAS) and the probability of having steatohepatitis.** A group of experienced pathologists diagnosed steatohepatitis to be present, absent, or probable and also independently scored the same biopsy specimens while unaware of their own interpretation to determine the NAS. A score higher than 4 was associated with a high probability of being considered to have steatohepatitis. *(Adapted from Kleiner DE, et al. Design and validation of a histological scoring system for nonalcoholic fatty liver disease. Hepatology 2005;41:1313–1321.)*

Epidemiology and Conditions Associated with Nonalcoholic Fatty Liver Disease

Nonalcoholic fatty liver disease represents the hepatic manifestation of metabolic syndrome.[19] Metabolic syndrome is characterized by obesity, diabetes, hypertension, hypertriglyceridemia, and low high-density lipoprotein (HDL) cholesterol (**Table 53-4**).[20] It is estimated that about 47 million U.S. individuals are afflicted with metabolic syndrome and more than 80% of such subjects have NAFLD.[21,22] On the other hand, more than 90% of subjects with NAFLD have some features of metabolic syndrome.[23] The prevalence of NAFLD increases as the severity and number of metabolic syndrome parameters increase.

About 66% of adults in the United States are overweight, and half of those are obese as reported by the Centers for Disease Control and Prevention. Obesity is projected to increase to 45% by 2025 in the United States.[24] Similarly, the projected percent increase in type 2 diabetes mellitus by 2030 is 32% in Europe, 72% in the United States, and 150% or greater in sub-Saharan Africa, India, and the Middle East.[24]

These are important risk factors for NAFLD and make it likely that the prevalence of NAFLD will rise to epidemic proportions globally.

The presence of underlying insulin resistance (IR) is the common link between the disorders that define metabolic syndrome.[25] Although several systems for defining metabolic syndrome have been proposed,[20,26,27] they do not capture the presence of the underlying IR with optimal sensitivity. Indeed, many individuals in the general population have biochemical evidence of IR, even in the absence of features of metabolic syndrome.[28,29] It may be argued that the development of metabolic syndrome is analogous to the development of end-organ disease. Thus, even though it is important to identify those with end-organ disease for treatment, it may be even more important to identify those at risk (i.e., those with IR before metabolic syndrome develops). This would appear to be a rational approach given the impact of IR-related disorders on overall morbidity and mortality in the general population.[30]

The prevalence of NAFLD in the general population is estimated to range from 2.8% to 46%, depending on the methodology, the study population, and the type of screening test used.[31] Although hospital-based studies are flawed because of ascertainment bias, population-based studies use noninvasive imaging studies (e.g., sonography) to define the presence of NAFLD.[32] Unfortunately, sonography has poor specificity for the diagnosis of NAFLD.[33] Recently, magnetic resonance imaging has been used to define and quantify the amount of hepatic steatosis.[34-36] This technique has been validated and used to define the prevalence of hepatic steatosis in the general population. Based on this technique, it is estimated that 31% of the U.S. population has hepatic steatosis.[37]

In contrast, depending on the definition used, between 2.8% and 24% of U.S. adults have NAFLD according to a comprehensive National Health and Nutrition Examination Survey III (NHANES III) data set–based analysis.[38] The prevalence of NAFLD in the Dionysos study[38a] was noted to be 94% in obese patients (body mass index [BMI] of 30 kg/m² or higher), 67% in overweight patients (BMI of 25 kg/m² or higher), and 25% in patients with normal weight.[39] Assessment of NAFLD is further confounded by the fact that approximately 70% to 80% of subjects with NAFLD have normal ALT loevels.[40] These data are in keeping with the observation that 7.9% of the U.S. population has persistently elevated ALT values and that most individuals with such elevations have underlying NAFLD.[41] Among type 2 diabetics, 40% to 70% have associated NAFLD.[42] In a recent ¹H-magnetic resonance spectroscopy–based case-control study, patients with type 2 diabetes had up to 200% more fat in their liver than did matched controls.[43]

In an autopsy series in which liver histology was used to define the presence of a fatty liver,[44] hepatic steatosis was found in approximately 2.7% of lean individuals and 18.5% of obese individuals. Similar data have been reported from autopsies of air crash victims.[45] A relationship between BMI and the presence of a fatty liver has also been established in otherwise apparently healthy individuals being considered as donors for living donor liver transplantation.[46] Clearly, no single marker or test has sufficient positive or negative predictive power for diagnosing NAFLD.

Regardless of the methodology used, several aspects of the epidemiology of NAFLD are consistently observed. Fatty liver, as well as NASH, occurs in all age groups, including children.[47]

Although studies published before 1990 emphasized that NASH occurs mostly in women (53% to 85% of all patients),[2,48] more recent studies have shown that NASH occurs with equal frequency in males (≈50%).[8,49] The prevalence of NAFLD is directly related to BMI, with more than 80% of subjects with a BMI higher than 35 kg/m² having steatosis.[19,50] Waist circumference may be an even better predictor of underlying IR and NAFLD than the BMI is.[51]

Other factors that influence the prevalence are discussed in the following sections.

Ethnicity

In Hispanic subjects, the prevalence of NAFLD reaches 45%, whereas African Americans have a lower prevalence (24%). An apparent paradox in African Americans of high IR but decreased visceral adiposity and hepatic steatosis has been documented in a large population study by imaging techniques for quantitating steatosis and determining body fat distribution.[37]

Familial and Genetic Factors

The phenotype of this complex condition is highly likely to reflect complex interactions between environmental and lifestyle-related factors and genetic predisposition. Obesity and diabetes often cluster within families.[52,53] The causes of such familial clustering include both genetic and environmental factors.[54] In a study of eight families, a total of 18 members with NAFLD, including NASH with cirrhosis, were described.[55] A clear-cut pattern of inheritance of risk for NAFLD was not identified. Another recent small study showed a trend toward familial clustering and maternal linkage for IR in patients with NAFLD.[56]

Several studies have now identified a specific polymorphism in the promoter of the *PNPLA3* gene to be specifically related to the presence of NAFLD. Recently, Kruppel-like factor 6 (KLF6) has been linked with NASH, as well as hepatic stellate cell (HSC) activation in response to inflammation and hepatocyte growth. NAFLD subjects with a certain KLF6 polymorphism had advanced NASH, and a protective functional polymorphism was also identified.[57] An in-depth review of current published work in genetics and NAFLD is covered elsewhere.[58]

Impact of Recent and Past Consumption of Alcohol on NAFLD

An important and controversial factor that may affect the severity and progression of NAFLD is previous alcohol use and ongoing social consumption of modest amounts of alcohol. The precise levels of alcohol consumption that separate those with alcoholic liver disease from NAFLD have not been clearly defined. It is widely accepted that ingestion of less than 10 g/day for women and less than 20 g/day for men is considered insignificant alcohol consumption. It is certainly feasible that subjects with risk factors for NAFLD may be at higher risk for hepatic steatosis if they consume alcohol in any quantity. Indeed, it has been found that obese individuals who regularly consume alcohol have the highest prevalence of hepatic steatosis.[59]

Other Conditions Associated with NAFLD

Several other conditions have also been associated with NAFLD (**Table 53-5**), including abetalipoproteinemia and some rare syndromes characterized by severe IR, such as lipoatrophic diabetes and Mauriac syndrome.[60-62] The liver disease in both abetalipoproteinemia and lipodystrophy can progress to advanced fibrosis and cirrhosis.[63] NAFLD has also been associated with the use of several drugs, such as amiodarone, tamoxifen, and diltiazem. The mechanisms involved in the development of steatosis are somewhat variable across these conditions, and ideally they should be considered separately from the fatty liver disease associated with metabolic syndrome.

Hepatic steatosis can also be present in those infected with hepatitis C virus or human immunodeficiency virus (HIV).[64,65] Hepatic steatosis is a risk factor for increased hepatic fibrosis in subjects with hepatitis C[66] and is associated with the presence of underlying metabolic syndrome in most subjects with genotype 1 infection.[67] It is also associated with a higher chance of failing to respond to antiviral therapy.[68] The development of steatosis in those with HIV infection has been linked to the use of highly active antiretroviral therapy and the presence of lipodystrophy, dyslipidemia, and IR.[69,70] A detailed description of these conditions is beyond the scope of this chapter, and readers are referred to recent reviews for more information on the subject.[71]

Table 53-5 Conditions Associated with Nonalcoholic Fatty Liver Disease

Insulin resistance
Obesity
  Sedentary lifestyle
  Type 2 diabetes
  Hypertriglyceridemia
  Hypertension
Drugs
  Tamoxifen
  Corticosteroids
  Amiodarone
  Estrogens
  Calcium channel blockers (case reports, true association uncertain)
Toxins
  Extensive exposure to volatile hydrocarbons
Dietary abnormalities
  Carbohydrate excess (e.g., dietary, total parenteral nutrition)
  Protein deficiency
  Rapid weight loss
  Vitamin B_{12} deficiency
  Choline deficiency (?)
Altered small bowel anatomy
  Obesity surgery with a blind loop of the small bowel
  Small bowel diverticula
  Short gut
Metabolic diseases (resulting in NASH-like histology)
  Hypobetalipoproteinemia
  Abetalipoproteinemia
  Wilson disease
  Lipodystrophies
  Andersen disease
  Weber-Christian syndrome
  Mauriac syndrome
Infections
  Chronic hepatitis C (usually genotype 3)
  AIDS
  Bacillus cereus infection (?)

AIDS, acquired immunodeficiency syndrome; NASH, nonalcoholic steatohepatitis

Pathogenesis of Nonalcoholic Fatty Liver Disease

Fatty liver and steatohepatitis constitute the spectrum of NAFLD. The common notion is that the fatty liver phenotype is a result of the ability of the liver to adapt to the development of hepatic steatosis whereas an inadequate adaptive response would lead to steatohepatitis. This formed the basis for the two-hit hypothesis in which development of a fatty liver was the first hit and an additional hit was required to cause steatohepatitis.[72] It is now thought that multiple mechanisms are concurrently operative to produce the phenotype of steatohepatitis. A generally accepted construct is that NAFLD reflects disordered energy homeostasis. To appreciate how disordered energy homeostasis leads to steatosis and steatohepatitis, one must first understand the normal physiology of energy homeostasis.

Normal Energy Homeostasis

Normal energy homeostasis is a complex balance of multiple processes in which the metabolic and neurohormonal compartments are integrated. Obesity is a fundamental problem of energy balance. In simple terms, energy intake in excess of energy expenditure is reflected by an increase in fat stores. Although the overall principle of energy imbalance seems logical and simple, factors influencing this imbalance are complex in nature and are discussed in this section.

Adipose tissue plays a critical role in normal energy homeostasis. It serves as an "energy bank" in which excess energy is stored and then released to meet the energy needs of the body. During periods of caloric excess, the extra "energy" is stored as triglyceride, which is the most efficient "currency" because oxidation of free fatty acids (FFAs) yields more energy than does oxidation of proteins or carbohydrates. When diet-derived calories are not available or are inadequate to meet the "energy" requirements of the body, adipose tissue triglycerides undergo lipolysis to release FFAs and glycerol into the circulation, where they can be taken up by the liver. This is regulated by the adipokine profile at a given adipose tissue location (**Table 53-6**) and several hormones.

Mechanisms by Which Metabolic Pathways Are Regulated in Adipose Tissue and the Liver

Adipose tissue, in addition to being an "energy bank," is also a metabolically active organ with endocrine and inflammatory functions. This is especially true of visceral fat, which is an important source of a variety of cytokines, collectively referred

Table 53-6 Adipocytokines and Their Known Effects on Inflammation and Insulin Actions

ADIPOCYTOKINE	EFFECT ON INFLAMMATION	EFFECT ON INSULIN ACTIONS
TNF-α	↑ ICAM1, VCAM1, MCP1 ↑ E selectin ↑ EC apoptosis ↑ NF-κB	↓ Insulin signaling ↑ Lipolysis
Leptin	↑ NO and ET1 ↑ EC and VSMC proliferation ↑ Macrophage survival/ proliferation ↑ Angiogenesis	↑ Glucose transport ↑ Sympathetic tone Corrects insulin resistance in lipodystrophy
IL-6	↑ ICAM1, VCAM1, MCP1 ↑ Acute phase reactants	↑ Insulin resistance ↑ Preadipocyte differentiation
Ang II	↑ ICAM1, VCAM1, MCP1 ↓ NO and ↑ NF-κB ↑ Fibrosis	
Resistin	↑ ET1 release ↑ ICAM1, VCAM1, MCP1 ↓ TRAF3	↓ Glucose clearance in muscle ↑ Hepatic insulin resistance
PAI-1	↑ Fibrinolysis	?
Adipsin	Complement activation	?
Adiponectin	↓ ICAM1, VCAM1, selectins ↓ NF-κB	↑ Lipid oxidation ↑ Insulin sensitivity
Visfatin	↑ Susceptibility to endotoxin- mediated EC injury in lungs	↑ Insulin signaling

Ang II, angiotensin II; EC, endothelial cell; ET1, endothelin-1; ICAM1, intercellular adhesion molecule-1; IL-6, interleukin-6; MCP1, monocyte chemotactic protein-1; NF-κB, nuclear factor κB; NO, nitric oxide; PAI-1, plasminogen activator inhibitor-1; TNF-α, tumor necrosis factor-α; TRAF3, TNFR-associated factor-3; VCAM1, vascular cell adhesion molecule-1; VSMC, vascular smooth muscle cell

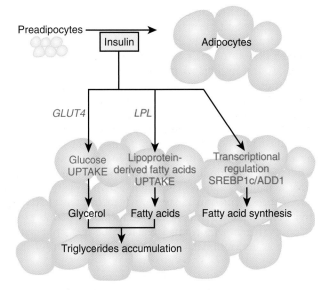

Fig. 53-3 Actions and effects of insulin on adipocytes. Insulin stimulates the differentiation of preadipocytes to adipocytes. In mature adipocytes, insulin promotes lipogenesis by stimulating the uptake of glucose and lipoprotein-derived fatty acid. Insulin also participates in transcriptional regulation by inducing sterol regulatory element–binding protein-1c *(SREBP1c)*/adipocyte determination and differentiation-dependent factor-1 *(ADD1)*, which regulate genes promoting fatty acid synthesis and lipogenesis. FFA, free fatty acid; GLUT4, glucose transporter-4; LPL, lipoprotein lipase.

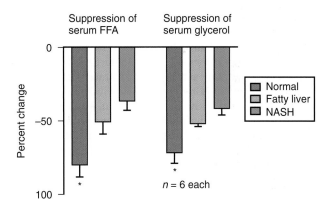

Fig. 53-4 Effects of insulin infusion on serum free fatty acid *(FFA)* and glycerol concentrations. There was a stepwise decrease in insulin-mediated suppression of FFA and glycerol concentrations from normal individuals to those with fatty liver and then nonalcoholic steatohepatitis *(NASH)*, thus confirming that there is increased peripheral lipolysis in those with nonalcoholic fatty liver disease. *Asterisk*, statistical significance. *(Adapted from Sanyal AJ, et al. Nonalcoholic steatohepatitis: association of insulin resistance and mitochondrial abnormalities. Gastroenterology 2001;120:1183–1192.)*

to as adipocytokines or adipokines. This is one of the mechanisms by which visceral adiposity contributes to NAFLD.

Hormones

Insulin is crucial in maintaining energy homeostasis because it regulates the fat depot by coordinating the actions in adipose tissue, liver, and muscle. Insulin is a critical regulator of most aspects of adipocyte biology and promotes lipogenesis (**Fig. 53-3**) while inhibiting lipolysis (**Fig. 53-4**). Furthermore, adipocytes are one of the most highly insulin-responsive cell types. The actions of insulin are balanced by counterregulatory hormones, such as growth hormone and glucagon. In addition to endocrine, paracrine, and autocrine regulation of adipose tissue, β_3-adrenergic neurons innervating adipose tissue add another layer of regulatory influence on the balance between lipogenesis and lipolysis.[73]

Insulin promotes glucose uptake and utilization by either glycogen synthesis or glycolysis. It also promotes lipogenesis, and under conditions of long-term energy excess, glucose is converted to triglycerides for storage. These are important mechanisms for the postprandial control of metabolism and for utilization of the calories that are consumed. In the interdigestive phase, the glucose supply for tissues that are critically dependent on it is provided by glycogenolysis and gluconeogenesis. Similarly, during periods of food deprivation or during periods of increased energy requirements, such as growth, wound healing, or inflammation, there is increased mobilization of FFAs from adipose stores and their use as a source of fuel to feed the energy-requiring processes. These are provided by increased levels of counterregulatory hormones that antagonize the effects of insulin, such as glucagon. The immediate effects of insulin and its counterregulatory hormones are mediated by alterations in signal transduction cascades following binding of the hormones to their receptors. These signaling pathways alter the activity of regulatory kinases, such as protein kinase A, which in turn affect the activity of specific enzymes in various metabolic pathways. In the long term, these hormones regulate the metabolic pathways by transcriptional up- or down-regulation of key enzymes.

Adipokines

Adipocytes produce polypeptides, including leptin, adiponectin, resistin, and plasminogen activator inhibitor-1 (PAI-1), and many cytokines, such as tumor necrosis factor-α (TNF-α) and interleukin-6 (IL-6).[74] These adipocyte products have potent autocrine, paracrine, and endocrine functions. Of these products, TNF-α, IL-6, and PAI-1 have been implicated in promoting inflammation and the atherothrombotic predilection in subjects with obesity and metabolic syndrome.[75] On the other hand, a low adiponectin level has been associated with IR and NAFLD.[76]

TNF-α is a proinflammatory cytokine that is secreted by adipose tissue and macrophages.[77] It regulates inflammation, cell viability, metabolism, and other cytokines and plays a central role in the response to endotoxin by generating both inflammation and apoptosis. TNF-α interferes with insulin signaling through the activation of intracellular signaling pathways such as Jun N-terminal kinase (JNK) and inhibitor kappa beta kinase-β (IKK-β).[78] In addition, it inhibits adiponectin, which has many important actions with respect to insulin sensitivity and lipid metabolism.[79] Thus the high levels of TNF-α seen in the setting of low adiponectin contribute to the development of disordered lipid metabolism, severe IR, and a proinflammatory state.[80] TNF-α levels increase in a stepwise manner from obesity to simple steatosis to NASH.[81] NAFLD has been associated with promoter polymorphisms in the TNF receptor, as well as increased expression of TNF-α in both adipose tissue and the liver.[82]

Adiponectin is another adipokine that bears similarity to complement.[83] It increases fatty acid β-oxidation in muscle and liver.[84] It also improves hepatic insulin sensitivity and thereby results in improved insulin-mediated suppression of hepatic glucose output.[85] It acts upstream of adenosine-5′-monophosphate–activated protein kinase (AMPK), an allosteric inhibitor of acyl-coenzyme A (CoA) carboxylase, the rate-limiting step in lipogenesis.[86] AMPK also promotes fatty acid oxidation in the mitochondria. By decreasing lipogenesis and increasing FFA oxidation, adiponectin decreases hepatic steatosis. Low levels of adiponectin have been associated with NAFLD[87] and been shown to have a negative correlation with hepatic steatosis.[88] In murine models of NAFLD, recombinant adiponectin inhibits TNF-α and improves insulin sensitivity and hepatic steatosis.[89] Thus an imbalance in the TNF-α/

adiponectin ratio may be important for the development NASH.

Resistin is a proinflammatory cytokine that is also associated with impairment of insulin action.[81] In contrast to adiponectin, increased resistin levels have been correlated with the severity of NAFLD and development of NASH.[90]

IL-6 is secreted largely by visceral fat and is associated with NALFD and obesity.[91] Increased systemic IL-6 is associated with increased inflammation and fibrosis in patients with NAFLD.[92] In a transgenic mouse model, increased IL-6 levels resulted in IR, presumably through the steatosis-induced IKK-β and nuclear factor-κB (NF-κB) pathway, and IR improved significantly with the administration of anti–IL-6 antibody.[93]

Transcriptional Factors that Mediate the Effects of Cytokines and Hormones

Several transcriptional factors play an important role in metabolic homeostasis and mediate the effects of insulin and its counterregulatory hormones (**Table 53-7**). The sterol regulatory element–binding protein (SREBP) group of basic helix-loop-helix-leucine zipper transcription factors are important transcriptional regulators of lipogenesis. They are synthesized as inactive precursors bound to the endoplasmic reticulum (ER). Activation of them requires cleavage and transport to the Golgi apparatus, where they undergo further cleavage to release the NH_2 terminal of the protein, which translocates to the nucleus and binds to sterol response elements in the promoters of their target genes. Three isoforms of SREBP are known: SREBP1a, SREBP1c, and SREBP2. Of these, SREBP1c plays a major role in mediating insulin-directed lipogenic activity. SREBP1c increases de novo lipogenesis (DNL) by transcriptionally increasing the expression of several key lipogenic enzymes (**Fig. 53-5**). It also increases the expression of acetyl-CoA synthetase, which increases the production of acetyl CoA, the starting point for lipogenesis.[94] SREBP1c further contributes to a positive triglyceride balance by inhibiting expression of microsomal transfer protein (MTP), which results in decreased formation of very-low-density lipoprotein (VLDL).[95]

The cellular abundance of SREBP is affected by dietary nutrients, metabolites, hormones, and cytokines. Whereas glucose, saturated fats, and sterols increase SREBP abundance, polyunsaturated fats decrease SREBP and thus decrease lipogenesis.[96] Insulin mediates its signature "lipogenic activation" profile via liver X receptor (LXR)-mediated activation of SREBP1c.[97]

LXR is another important transcriptional regulator of metabolism. LXR binds its response elements (LXRE) in the DNA promoters of its target genes along with its heteromeric partner retinoid X receptor (RXR).[98] On ligand binding, co-repressor proteins are inactivated and co-activation proteins are recruited, which results in gene transcription.[99] LXR-α is present in liver and adipose tissue and is activated by oxysterols and insulin. LXR increases lipogenesis by increasing SREBP1c transcription.[97] It also promotes cholesterol utilization by increasing primary bile acid synthesis.[100] LXR activates adenosine triphosphate (ATP)-binding cassette lipid transporter-1 (ABCA1) and promotes cholesterol efflux.[101]

The carbohydrate response element–binding protein (ChREBP) is another important transcriptional regulator of

Table 53-7 Transcription Factors Involved in Fatty Acid and Cholesterol Synthesis

TRANSCRIPTION FACTOR	TARGET GENES	LOCATION	FUNCTION
SREBP1c	ACC, FAS, ACS ATP citrate lyase	1. Liver 2. Adipose tissue	↑ Lipogenesis
SREBP2	HMG-CoA reductase LDL receptor	1. Liver 2. Constitutive	↑ Cholesterol synthesis
ChREBP	Pyruvate kinase FAS ACC	1. Liver 2. Adipose tissue	↑ Lipogenesis (in carbohydrate excess states)
PPAR-α	ACS FATP1, CPT1 ABCA1	1. Liver 2. Muscle	1. ↑ FA catabolism 2. ↑ Cholesterol efflux
PPAR-γ	LPL FATP ACS	1. Adipose tissue 2. Intestines	1. ↑ TG synthesis/storage 2. Adipocyte differentiation
LXR	CYP7A1 ABCG1, ABCA1 SREBP1c LPL, CETP, Apo E	1. Liver 2. Intestines 3. Adipose tissue	1. FA synthesis, BA synthesis 2. XOL/PL absorption and synthesis 3. Lipoprotein metabolism

Modified from Sanyal AJ. Mechanisms of disease: pathogenesis of nonalcoholic fatty liver disease. Nat Clin Pract Gastroenterol Hepatol. 2005;2(1):46–53.
ABCA, ATP-binding cassette genes; ACC, acyl-CoA carboxylase; ACS, acyl-CoA synthetase; ATP, adenosine triphosphate; BA, bile acid; CETP, cholesterol ester transporter protein; ChREBP, carbohydrate response element–binding protein; CoA, coenzyme A; CPT1, carnitine palmitoyltransferase; FA, fatty acid; FAS, fatty acid synthetase; FATP1, fatty acid transporter protein-1; LPL, lipoprotein lipase; HMG CoA, 3-hydroxy-3-methylglutaryl CoA; LXR, liver X receptor; PL, phospholipid; PPAR, peroxisome proliferator–activated receptor; SREBP, sterol regulatory element–binding protein; TG, triglyceride; XOL, cholesterol

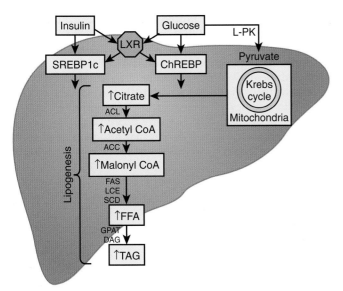

Fig. 53-5 Transcriptional regulation of lipogenesis in the liver. Hyperinsulinemia and hyperglycemia regulate sterol regulatory element–binding protein 1c *(SREBP1c)* and carbohydrate response element–binding protein *(ChREBP)* expression through the liver X receptor *(LXR)*, which leads to the transcriptional activation of lipogenic genes. Simultaneously, ChREBP transcriptionally activates liver X pyruvate kinase *(LPK)*. The synergistic actions of SREBP1c and ChREBP coordinately regulate the conversion of excess glucose to fatty acids. Thus, in the setting of insulin resistance, free fatty acids *(FFAs)* entering the liver from the periphery, as well as those derived from de novo lipogenesis, will be preferentially esterified to triglycerides. ACC, acyl-CoA carboxylase; ACL, ATP citrate lyase; DAG, diacylglycerol; FAS, fatty acid synthase; GPAT, glycerol-3-phosphate acyltransferase; LCE, long-chain fatty acyl elongase; SCD, stearoyl-CoA desaturase; TAG, triacylglycerol

metabolism. In periods of carbohydrate overload, it promotes the conversion of carbohydrates to lipids by a transcriptional increase in expression of the enzymes involved in lipogenesis.[102] It is activated by glucose and, along with its heteromeric partner maxlike protein X (Mlx), binds to carbohydrate response elements of the pyruvate kinase, acetyl-CoA carboxylase, and fatty acid synthetase genes, thereby increasing their transcription.[103]

Carbohydrate feeding affects energy balance and lipid homeostasis by increasing carbohydrate oxidation and lipogenesis as a result of increased SREBP and ChREBP activity. Interestingly, ChREBP was recently identified as direct target for LXR,[104] thus establishing LXR as the master lipogenic transcription factor that enhances hepatic fatty acid synthesis (see **Fig. 53-5**). As shown for oxysterols, glucose may effectively bind and activate LXR.[105] The integration of glucose sensing and control of lipogenesis in a single protein may provide an explanation for the observation that a low-fat, high-carbohydrate diet induces hypertriglyceridemia; LXR can thus sense surplus glucose, induce fatty acid synthesis, and promote hepatic export of VLDL.

The peroxisome proliferator–activated receptors (PPARs) play a major role as metabolic regulators as well. Three isoforms have been identified: PPAR-α, PPAR-β/δ, and PPAR-γ. PPAR-α is expressed in organs where fatty acid oxidation is an important source of energy utilization, such as the liver, heart, and kidney, whereas PPAR-γ is preferentially expressed in adipose tissue and the intestine.[106] Long-chain fatty acids and oxidized phospholipids activate PPAR-α, which increases FFA uptake, activation to acyl-CoA esters, and β-oxidation of mitochondrial FFAs.[107] PPAR-α agonists increase fatty acid utilization and limit the availability of FFAs for lipogenesis.[108]

In the small intestine, PPAR-β/δ increases fatty acid–binding protein (FABP) and may play a role in the intestinal adaptation to changes in dietary lipid content.[109] PPAR-γ promotes adipocyte differentiation and lipoprotein lipase activity, thereby making triglyceride-derived fatty acids available for uptake. It also induces fatty acid transport protein and acyl-CoA synthetase, which increases adipose tissue lipogenesis. PPAR-γ induces adiponectin, an important insulin-sensitizing cytokine.[110] PPARs and LXRs increase the expression of each other.[111] PPAR-γ also antagonizes NF-κB and thus has anti-inflammatory effects.[112]

When hepatic fatty acid levels increase, PPAR-α and PPAR-γ coactivator-1 (PPARGC1) are activated and promote fatty acid oxidation and the production of VLDL, the net effect being catabolism and clearance of fatty acids.[113] PPAR-α also directly interacts with PPARGC1. This interaction, in conjunction with forkhead box protein-a2 (FOXa2), also known as hepatic nuclear factor 3a, cooperatively stimulates fatty acid oxidation and VLDL production.[113] Because IR results in disrupted phosphorylation of FOXa2 and dissociation from PPARGC1,[114] this pathway may contribute to the development of NAFLD. Moreover, PPARGC1 increases SREBP1 and LXR-dependent transcriptional activity, thereby coupling lipid synthesis and lipoprotein secretion.[115]

AMPK decreases gluconeogenesis and fatty acid synthesis while increasing fatty acid oxidation. The mechanisms involved include suppression of SREBP1 and ChREBP, respectively,[116,117] and inhibition of acetyl-CoA carboxylase, which in turn increases fatty acid oxidation via decreased malonyl CoA.[118]

During weight gain and visceral fat accumulation, increased secretion of retinol-binding protein 4 (RBP4) directly impairs insulin signaling in adipocytes and induces hepatic expression of phosphoenolpyruvate carboxykinase, thereby reducing insulin's action in suppressing glucose production.[119] Increased serum levels of RBP4 have been found in patients with NAFLD[120] and in subjects with subclinically increased liver fat.[121] The close inverse association between RBP4 and adiponectin in patients with NAFLD further favors the concept that the degree of insulin sensitivity depends on the balance between TNF-α, IL-6, and RBP4 on one hand and adiponectin on the other.

Endocannabinoids

The endocannabinoids are endogenous lipid mediators that participate in controlling energy intake and regulation and produce effects similar to those of marijuana.[122] The actions of endogenous endocannabinoids are mediated via cannabinoid (CB1) receptors, which are mainly expressed in the central nervous system but are also found on adipocytes and hepatocytes. Stimulation of CB1 receptors can induce increased lipogenesis, decreased adiponectin, increased leptin and IR, and decreased fatty acid oxidation. CB1 blockade improves increased adiposity and hepatic steatosis in rat models. In a 2-year randomized, placebo-controlled human trial, the CB1 antagonizer rimonabant resulted in significant weight loss, improved waist circumference, and enhanced plasma triglyceride and insulin sensitivity.[123] Unfortunately, because this drug can induce severe depression, its development has been halted.

Integration of Systemic and Local Mechanisms of Regulation of Intermediary Metabolism

The ability of the body to respond to different substrate concentrations and varying energy requirements depends on closely integrated regulation of carbohydrate and lipid metabolism (Fig. 53-6). From a physiologic perspective, the formation of acetyl CoA is a key step that connects the glycolytic pathway to the Krebs cycle, as well as to the lipogenic pathway. Even though these pathways exist in all cells, there is organ-specific differentiation of the various limbs of these pathways. The rapid uptake of glucose by striated muscle and liver tissue allows clearance of the postprandial glucose load. This is stored mainly as glycogen in the short term and as triglyceride within adipocytes, muscle, and liver tissue in the long term.

Thus, during periods of caloric abundance, excess carbohydrate-derived energy can be diverted via acetyl CoA to lipid synthesis via the lipogenesis pathway under the control of insulin and several transcriptional factors noted earlier, such as LXR and ChREBP. Similarly, excess dietary fat can be stored as triglycerides. Acetyl CoA may also be derived from FFA oxidation and serve as a substrate for FFA synthesis again if required.

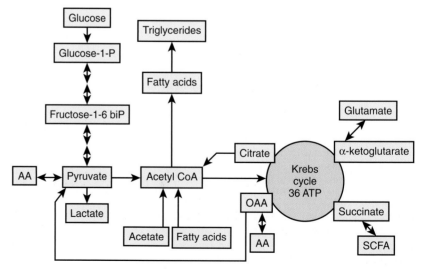

Fig. 53-6 **Integrated view of intermediary metabolism.** Glycolysis leads to the formation of pyruvate. Under anaerobic condition, lactate formation is used for the generation of adenosine triphosphate (*ATP*) (Embden-Meyerhof pathway). Under aerobic conditions, pyruvate enters the Krebs cycle, which yields 36 ATP molecules. During periods of caloric excess, extra calories are shunted into acetyl CoA, which is used to form triglycerides and cholesterol. During periods of starvation, oxaloacetic acid (*OSS*) can lead to phosphoenolpyruvate and reverse synthesis of glucose (gluconeogenesis). Under conditions of severe starvation, amino acids (*AAs*) can be transaminated to yield metabolic intermediates that can be used in the Krebs cycle. Short-chain fatty acids (*SCFAs*) can also be converted to succinate, an intermediate in the Krebs cycle.

Yet another source of acetyl CoA is citrate via citrate lyase, another insulin-sensitive enzyme. This pathway assumes importance when the Krebs cycle slows down because of an altered reduced nicotinamide adenine dinucleotide phosphate/nicotinamide adenine dinucleotide (NADPH/NAD) ratio, and citrate accumulates in the cell.[124,125] In addition, when energy is required, proteins may be deaminated to keto acids or to intermediates in the Krebs cycle, thereby providing a source of acetyl CoA and energy. This pathway is particularly important for the response to starvation or severe caloric deficiency. FFAs derived from lipolysis may be oxidized to release acetyl CoA, which can be used for the Krebs cycle. FFAs interfere with hepatic insulin signaling and are associated with an increase in local and systemic lipolytic cytokines, such as TNF-α.[126]

There is increasing evidence that FFAs themselves may play an important role as the integrator of lipid and carbohydrate metabolism. FFAs, the major metabolic product of adipocytes, have direct effects on intermediary metabolism and also specifically affect insulin signal transduction pathways.[127] FFAs, particularly those derived from visceral adipose tissue, impair insulin signaling and promote gluconeogenesis.[128] Thus insulin regulates lipolysis and therefore the availability of FFA, whereas FFA regulates the function of insulin.

Insulin Resistance and Its Effects on Energy Homeostasis

Insulin resistance is linked to the pathogenesis of NAFLD. The original clinical descriptions of NAFLD noted a relationship between obesity and diabetes, the two conditions best known to be associated with IR.[2] Patients with NASH have lower IR and higher insulin secretion rates than do age- and gender-matched normal controls. IR, as measured by the homeostatic model (IR$_{HOMA}$), is nearly universal in subjects with NASH (65/66), as opposed to those with metabolic syndrome (55/66).[23] IR was present in lean as well as obese individuals. Finally, the presence of IR has been confirmed via euglycemic, hyperinsulinemic clamping in nondiabetic, precirrhotic individuals with fatty liver, as well as NASH.[25]

The development of IR is multifactorial and involves both genetic and environmental factors. Inherited disorders of IR are extremely rare and include leprechaunism, Rabson-Mendenhall syndrome, and type A IR syndrome. The genetics of IR and the phenotypic variations that may be observed as a consequence of isolated gene defects have been studied in detail in single-gene knockout mouse models. Although these models are excellent tools for understanding the specific mechanisms of IR, they do not reflect the genomic alterations associated with the actual disease process in the body. The reason for this difficulty is due to the polygenic nature of IR and the polymorphism of different genes involved in the process of pancreatic insulin secretion and their action on specific target organs.

Recent studies have shed light on the early events in the genesis of IR.[129] With increasing adipose mass, especially visceral adipose mass, the adipose tissue is infiltrated by macrophages. Relative hypoxia with release of hypoxia-inducible factor, specific dietary constituents, hormones (e.g., leptin), and gut flora–derived products have all been implicated in this process.[130] The interactions between these activated macrophages and adipocytes cause release of adipokines with a net proinflammatory profile, which produce a chronic inflammatory state within this tissue.[131] They also have metabolic effects that cause IR. These cytokines further affect the liver and lead to an acute phase reaction. The net effect is a net systemic proinflammatory and fibrogenic state along with metabolic IR.

Recently, suppressors of cytokine signaling (SOCS) have emerged as important regulators of insulin signaling. SOCS3 inhibits signaling by Janus kinase–signal transducers and activators of transcription (JAK-STAT) and activates JNK signaling, which further worsens insulin signaling and activates inflammatory signaling pathways. SOCS3 is virtually absent in basal conditions, but it is rapidly and robustly induced in response to cytokines and appears to promote the development of fatty liver, probably as a consequence of IR-mediated activation of SREBP1.[132]

Metabolic Consequences of Insulin Resistance

Insulin sensitivity and IR are defined by the ability of insulin to clear glucose from blood.[28] Importantly, sensitivity to insulin is measured on a continuous rather than a categoric scale. Thus insulin sensitivity and resistance vary along a continuous scale, and there is no threshold insulin cutoff value that marks the onset of IR in a given individual. The fundamental physiologic abnormality in the insulin-resistant state is an impairment in the insulin-mediated suppression of lipolysis (see **Fig. 53-4**). Visceral adipose tissue is less sensitive than subcutaneous adipose tissue to insulin-mediated suppression of lipolysis. This is probably due to increased expression of 11β-hydroxysteroid dehydrogenase, which is the rate-limiting enzyme for steroid synthesis. Thus increased FFA release from visceral adipose tissue affects hepatocytes, where they interfere with insulin signaling and cause increased gluconeogenesis and impaired glucose utilization. In striated muscle, FFAs impair glucose uptake by impairment of insulin signaling and decreased translocation of glucose transporter-4 (GLUT4) to the cell surface.[133] Increased FFA levels and glucose load because of impaired clearance result in pancreatic compensation and hyperinsulinemia. Thus insulin levels for a given plasma glucose concentration are elevated; this is the biochemical hallmark of the insulin-resistant state.

It is possible that different organs and metabolic pathways may have differential sensitivity to insulin. Consequently, even though IR exists almost universally in subjects with NAFLD, it is important to delineate the specific metabolic pathways that are affected. Thus, although there is considerable resistance to the effects of insulin on lipolysis, its effects on lipogenesis are maintained and rates of lipogenesis are increased.[134,135] This may be due to the effects of hyperinsulinemia on SREBP and lipogenic enzyme expression and activity.

Insulin Resistance and the Pathogenesis of Hepatic Steatosis

Nonalcoholic fatty liver disease is characterized by lipid accumulation in the liver, mainly in the form of triglycerides. Triglycerides accumulate in the liver from an imbalance between production and turnover. Triglycerides are formed by

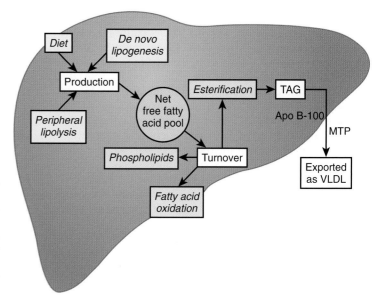

Fig. 53-7   Genesis of hepatic steatosis. Hepatic steatosis is due to either increased production or impaired output/oxidation (or both) of triacylglycerol *(TAG)*. TAG is formed from either de novo lipogenesis or reesterification of free fatty acids *(FFAs)* taken up from circulation. The availability of FFAs for TAG synthesis is further affected by their utilization for phospholipid synthesis or fatty acid oxidation. TAG is packaged into very-low-density lipoproteins *(VLDLs)* by the addition of apolipoprotein B-100 *(Apo B-100)* in a step requiring microsomal transfer protein *(MTP)*.

the esterification of a glycerol moiety with three fatty acid molecules. Triglyceride synthesis in the liver is linked to the genesis of hepatic steatosis (**Fig. 53-7**): The net pool of FFAs available for triglyceride synthesis depends on the balance between the formation and utilization of fatty acids. There are two major sources of FFA in the liver: FFAs that are taken up from the circulation and FFAs that are formed in the hepatocyte itself. The availability of FFA for triglyceride synthesis also depends on its utilization for phospholipid synthesis and for oxidation.

The two main sources of FFA in the circulation are diet and peripheral lipolysis. There are limited data on the dietary intake of subjects with NAFLD and its contribution to circulating FFA levels. A high saturated fat level, high concentration of refined sugars, and low fiber content in diet have all been associated with the development of IR.[136] There are, however, no data comparing subjects with NAFLD and those with obesity but without NAFLD to see whether there are any specific excesses or deficiencies in their diet. Although increased fat intake correlated with increased steatosis, increased carbohydrate intake correlated with the presence of inflammation in the liver.[137] IR is associated with increased peripheral lipolysis and higher levels of fasting FFA concentrations.[138] NAFLD is associated with higher fasting FFA concentrations than in age-, gender-, and race-matched controls.[25] Moreover, fatty liver and steatohepatitis are associated with progressive resistance to insulin-mediated suppression of lipolysis as determined by the rates of appearance of glycerol during euglycemic hyperinsulinemic clamping.[25] DNL also contributes to the hepatic pool of FFAs. Under physiologic circumstances, DNL contributes to only 5% to 8% of the triglycerides synthesized in the liver.[139] The physiologic relevance of DNL is not currently well understood. The substrates for DNL include acetate, carbohydrate-derived acetyl CoA, and acetyl CoA derived from lipid oxidation. NAFLD is associated with increased DNL.[140] As noted earlier, the enzymes of DNL are under the control of SREBP1c, which is an insulin-sensitive transcriptional factor.[141] NAFLD is associated with hyperinsulinemia.[25] It appears that despite the resistance to insulin's

effects on lipolysis in peripheral adipose tissue, its effects on DNL in the liver are maintained in NAFLD. It is likely that this is facilitated by low adiponectin levels, which would decrease AMPK activity and thus disinhibit acyl-CoA carboxylase, the rate-limiting enzyme in DNL.[142] Low levels of polyunsaturated fatty acids (PUFAs) in the liver may also promote maturation of SREBP1c from the ER-Golgi system.[143] This forms the rationale for the use of PUFAs in subjects with NAFLD. DNL is also increased by the intake of fructose, especially high-fructose corn syrup, a common additive to many foods and beverages.[144] Fructose bypasses the regulated steps in carbohydrate metabolism and forms glycerol-3-phosphate and acetyl CoA, which can both serve as precursors for DNL. The national consumption of total fructose has been increasing and correlates well with the increasing prevalence of obesity in the United States.

It is well known that acetyl CoA can be used either for the formation of malonyl CoA or for the formation of mevalonate. The former leads to FFA synthesis and is under the control of SREBP1c, whereas the latter leads to cholesterol synthesis and is regulated by SREBP2.[145] The two pathways are known to be coordinately regulated. If so, up-regulation of DNL should be accompanied by increased cholesterol synthesis. However, the principal features of the dyslipidemia associated with metabolic syndrome and NAFLD are hypertriglyceridemia and low HDL cholesterol. LXR affects ABCA1 and modulates the export of cholesterol to HDL cholesterol.[146] In addition, steroyl-CoA desaturase, a SREBP1c-sensitive enzyme that forms monounsaturated fatty acids, destabilizes ABCA1 function.[147] This can possibly cause the low HDL cholesterol levels in subjects with NAFLD.

The availability of FFAs for triglyceride synthesis is also affected by their utilization for oxidation and phospholipid synthesis. There are no systemic defects in the incorporation of FFAs into phospholipids in subjects with NAFLD.[25] The availability of FFAs for triglyceride synthesis is also affected by their utilization for oxidation. FFAs can undergo β-oxidation in the mitochondria or peroxisomes. They may also be oxidized by the microsomal enzyme or cytochrome P-450 system. NAFLD is associated with increased β-hydroxybutyrate levels and higher lipid oxidation rates than in matched controls.[25] Moreover, during euglycemic clamping, normal individuals suppress β-hydroxybutyrate levels, which indicates that mitochondrial fatty acid oxidation is normally suppressed by insulin. In contrast, fatty liver and NASH are associated with impairment in the insulin-mediated suppression of serum β-hydroxybutyrate levels, thus confirming that these conditions are associated with resistance to the effects of insulin on fatty acid oxidation. These data are compatible with the known effects of increased FFA delivery on mitochondrial fatty acid oxidation. At a molecular level, FFAs may directly interfere with insulin signaling and inhibit insulin-mediated suppression of ketogenesis.[148,149] In addition, increased activity of SOCS1 has been associated with impairment of insulin signaling pathways.[132,150] Peroxisomal proliferation has been reported in those with NAFLD, although there are no definite human data on peroxisomal fatty acid oxidation in subjects with NASH.[151]

Triglyceride Export from the Liver and the Genesis of Hepatic Steatosis

There are no accurate quantitative flux rates for the amounts of triglyceride synthesized via DNL versus reesterification of circulating FFA versus transport from the liver in subjects with NAFLD. Triglycerides are packaged into VLDLs in the liver by a process requiring MTP and apolipoprotein B-100. Defects in MTP or in VLDL assembly can result in rare syndromes of NAFLD.[152,153]

Hepatic steatosis is thus the net result of either or both increased synthesis and decreased export from the liver. IR contributes to hepatic steatosis in multiple ways by increasing FFAs for reesterification, increasing DNL, and providing the substrates for DNL.

In summary, overall integration of the metabolic pathways is closely regulated to maintain homeostasis (**Fig. 53-8**). An imbalance in hepatic lipid metabolism (synthesis and import versus metabolic utilization and export) causes accumulation of fat in hepatocytes. Imbalances in these processes, which are controlled by transcriptional factors such as SREBP, result from dysregulated transcriptional control, which in turn is influenced by the abnormal endocrine and paracrine milieu associated with IR. All of these layers of complexity are further modulated by many factors such as genetic makeup, diet, and lifestyle. Metabolism thus represents a complex biologic state, which explains why simple paradigms focused on a single mechanism fail in one or more clinical scenarios.

Pathogenesis of Steatohepatitis

Steatohepatitis is characterized by the presence of inflammation, increased cell injury, apoptosis, and the development of fibrosis. As originally proposed, an additional hit in the presence of IR that produces hepatic steatosis is required for the development of steatohepatitis.[72] In recent years it has become apparent that the situation is more complex in that some pathophysiologic mechanisms of cell injury are present in both fatty liver and NASH. IR has been shown to directly or indirectly promote hepatic steatosis, hepatocyte injury, inflammation, and fibrosis. Moreover, the pathways involved in each of these processes affect the pathogenesis of all of the other end points that produce the phenotype of steatohepatitis.

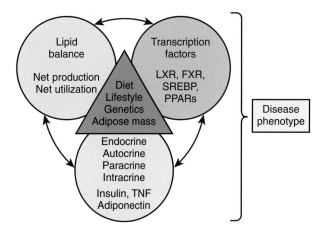

Fig. 53-8 The disease phenotype is a result of a complex interaction modulated by a variety of factors to produce an accumulation of lipid in the liver. Dysregulation of lipid balance, which involves net production (synthesis and import) and net utilization (oxidation and export), can lead to accumulation of lipid. These processes are normally closely regulated by a number of transcriptional factors, which are in turn influenced by cytokines, hormones, and other substances. Diet, lifestyle, genetic background, and adipocyte mass/distribution can affect all of these steps, thus creating a complex biologic system. FXR, farnesoid X receptor; LXR, liver X receptor; PPARs, peroxisome proliferator–activated receptors; SREBP, sterol regulatory element–binding protein; TNF, tumor necrosis factor.

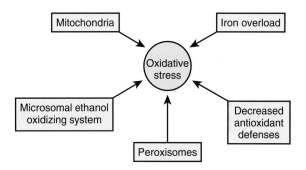

Fig. 53-9 Potential sources of oxidative stress in nonalcoholic fatty liver disease.

Role of Oxidative Stress

Oxidative stress is a key mechanism in the genesis of steatohepatitis. Oxidative stress has been observed in both animal models and human NAFLD.[25,154] In human NAFLD, increased levels of lipid peroxide are seen with both hepatic steatosis and NASH. However, subjects with NAFL have lower levels than do those with NASH.[25]

Oxidative stress is a result of an imbalance between prooxidant and antioxidant species. This could be due to either increased production of prooxidants (reactive oxygen species [ROS] or reactive nitrogen species [RNS]) or decreased antioxidant defenses. Potential sources of ROS in the liver include the mitochondria, the peroxisomes, the microsomal oxidative system, and iron overload (**Fig. 53-9**).

The structure of mitochondria in NASH hepatocytes is markedly abnormal with loss of cristae and a ballooned appearance (**Fig. 53-10**).[25,155] This is accompanied by the formation of paracrystalline intramitochondrial inclusions.

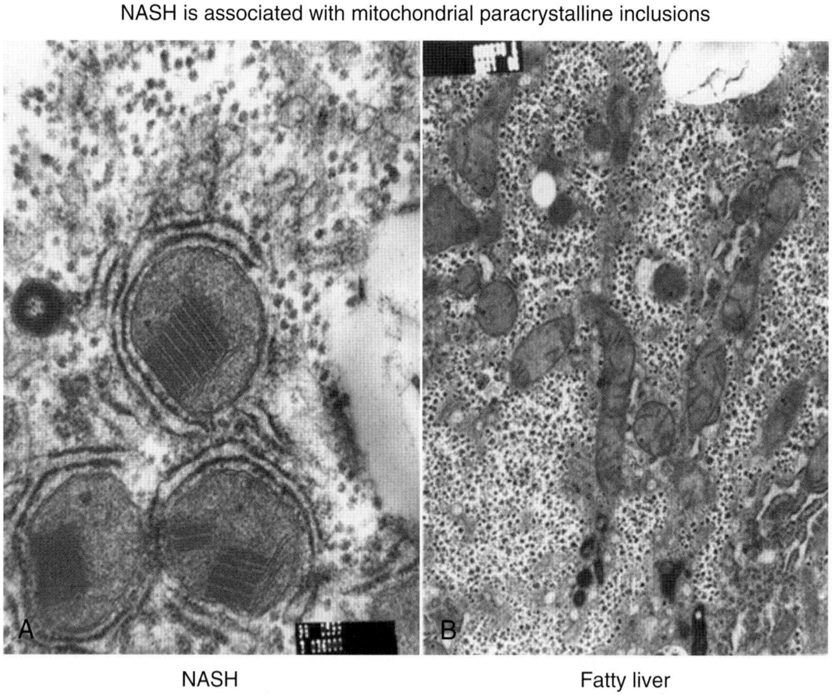

NASH is associated with mitochondrial paracrystalline inclusions

Fig. 53-10 **Mitochondrial morphology in nonalcoholic steatohepatitis (NASH).** Although hepatocyte mitochondria in a fatty liver are generally normal (right panel), the mitochondria in NASH are often ballooned with loss of cristae and the development of paracrystalline inclusions (left panel). (Adapted from Sanyal AJ, et al. Nonalcoholic steatohepatitis: association of insulin resistance and mitochondrial abnormalities. Gastroenterology 2001;120:1183–1192.)

NASH   Fatty liver

These changes are relatively specific for NASH and are not commonly seen in NAFL. Ten percent to 40% of mitochondria within each hepatocyte demonstrate these abnormalities. These mitochondrial structural defects in NASH are associated with impaired mitochondrial respiratory chain activity, thereby producing a state of uncoupled oxidation and phosphorylation that leads to ROS production and enhanced oxidative stress.[156,157] This concept is further supported by evidence of decreased ATP formation in the liver of subjects with NASH.[158]

Another source of oxidative stress is the cytochrome P-450 system. This system, particularly CYP2E1, is overexpressed in subjects with NAFLD.[159] Hepatic cytochrome P4502E1 activity in nondiabetic patients is also increased in those with NASH.[160] CYP2E1 can be induced by the insulin-resistant state, as well as by FFAs.[161] The impaired insulin signaling induced by CYP2E1 overexpression in NASH is most likely secondary to posttranslational enzyme stabilization, although more direct transcriptional control may also have a role in this process. It is believed that overexpression of this enzyme is associated with futile cycling of the enzyme that generates ROS. CYP2E1 induction is seen in subjects with NAFL, and additional mechanisms must be required to produce steatohepatitis. CYP2E1 can also be induced in subjects with metabolic syndrome in the absence of fatty liver.[162]

Peroxisomes also oxidize long-chain fatty acids but do not generate ATP. As a consequence, peroxisomal fatty acid oxidation causes ROS formation. An increased number of peroxisomes is seen in subjects with alcoholic as well as nonalcoholic fatty livers.[151] Iron overload has been associated with increased oxidative stress.[163] Even though some studies have shown an association between NASH and iron overload,[164] others have failed to find such an association.[165]

The antioxidant pathways in the liver of subjects with NASH have not been well described. Antioxidant paraoxonase-1

activity is decreased in those with metabolic syndrome.[166] Promoter polymorphisms in Mn-superoxide dismutase may affect the progression of NASH. Levels of superoxide dismutase, a key antioxidant, are increased by dehydroepiandrosterone.[167] Low circulating dehydroepiandrosterone levels can thus explain the reduced expression of superoxide dismutase in NASH patients.[168] Moreover, the mitochondrial free cholesterol content appears to be critical in precipitating steatohepatitis by sensitizing hepatocytes to TNF-α and Fas through depletion of mitochondrial glutathione.[169]

Oxidative stress produces its biologic effects through several mechanisms, including direct lipid peroxidation of the membranes of organelles, oxidative changes in DNA, mitochondrial DNA depletion, and alterations in the expression of redox-sensitive genes.[170] These changes in gene expression have far-reaching effects on a multitude of cellular functions and can lead to adaptive changes or cell death. For an in-depth appraisal of this subject, readers are referred to other reviews.[171,172]

Mechanisms of Cell Injury and Death

The phenotype of steatohepatitis is due to the presence of cytologic ballooning and Mallory hyaline, forms of cell injury associated with apoptosis, inflammation, and pericellular fibrosis (**Figs. 53-11 and 53-12**).[173]

Cell Injury in Steatohepatitis

The pathogenesis of cytologic ballooning is not well known. A priori, one would expect a defect in the maintenance of normal cell volume regulation because an increase in cell volume is the hallmark of cytologic ballooning.

Cell volume is regulated by a number of complex processes, including osmotic receptors and the intracellular actin

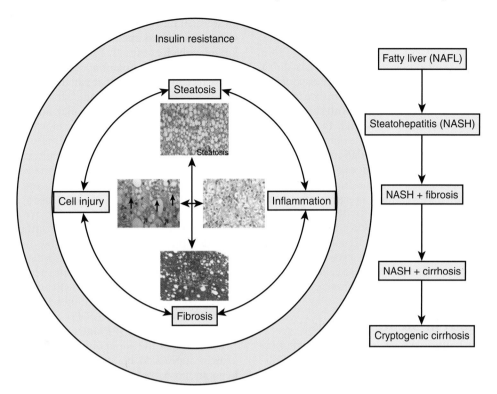

Fig. 53-11 **Role of insulin resistance in the pathogenesis of nonalcoholic steatohepatitis (NASH).** Insulin resistance promotes steatosis, cell injury, inflammation, and fibrosis. Each of these factors further promotes each other and eventually causes cell injury, inflammation, and fibrosis—hallmarks that distinguish steatohepatitis from steatosis alone. Depending on these factors, increasing fibrosis and eventually cirrhosis can develop in up to 15% to 20% patients with NASH. Following the development of cirrhosis, the hepatic steatosis and the other features of NASH may disappear and lead to the appearance of cryptogenic cirrhosis. NAFL, nonalcoholic fatty liver

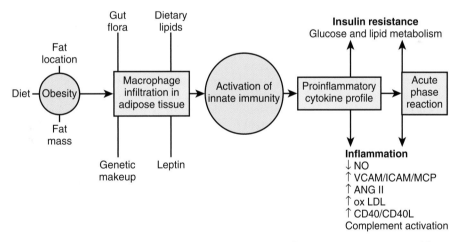

Fig. 53-12 **Pathophysiologic events in the development of insulin resistance.** As fat mass increases, a variety of factors, including relative ischemia, dietary components, cytokines (e.g., leptin), and gut flora, lead to chemotaxis of macrophages into adipose tissue. This is most prominent in visceral adipose tissue. The cell–cell interactions between macrophages and adipocytes lead to the activation of macrophages (part of the innate immune system) and production of proinflammatory cytokines. These substances have metabolic effects that promote insulin resistance. They also promote inflammation. These cytokines further stimulate the liver to produce additional cytokines that are part of the acute phase reaction often accompanying the insulin-resistant state. ANG II, angiotensin II; ICAM, intercellular adhesion molecule; MCP, monocyte chemotactic protein; NO, nitric oxide; VCAM, vascular cell adhesion molecule

network, which tethers the cell membranes.[174] Their large cell volume may be related to increased fluid in the cytosol.[18] It can also result from microtubular disruption and from alterations in the intermediate filament cytoskeleton in severe cell injury preceding lytic necrosis.[175] Displacement of cytoskeletal filaments K8/18 to the periphery has been observed on immunohistochemistry.[176] It is also unclear why occasional cells undergo cytologic ballooning whereas other adjacent cells do not.

Recently renamed Mallory-Denk bodies, MDBs are composed of heat shock proteins that are ubiquitinated but fail to undergo proteosomal degradation.[177] MDBs, which are perinuclear, "ropy" eosinophilic aggregates, are composed of misfolded, ubiquitinated K8/18 filaments together with stress-induced and ubiquitin-binding protein p62, heat shock proteins 70 and 25, and αβ-crystallin.[178] Heat shock proteins are a family of proteins that are produced in response to a variety of cellular stress, including oxidative stress, a direct function of IR and uncoupling of oxidation and phosphorylation in mitochondria. It is likely that these proteins are induced in response to the oxidative stress in subjects with either NAFL or NASH. However, in subjects with NASH, there may be defects in protein trafficking to proteosomes or in proteosomal function itself, which leads to accumulation of these proteins within intermediate filaments. It is speculated that MDBs may actually be hepatoprotective by sequestering abnormal, possibly deleterious proteins given the association of p62 (an immediate early response gene product) with ubiquitinated keratins and the protective role played by K8/18 filaments in guarding hepatocytes from apoptosis. Of note, MDBs are almost always seen within ballooned hepatocytes. The mechanistic relationship between altered cytologic ballooning and the development of MDBs also remains unknown.

Hepatocyte Death in Steatohepatitis

Nonalcoholic steatohepatitis is also characterized by extensive apoptotic activity.[179] Apoptosis is a highly regulated, metabolically active form of cell death. There are extrinsic and intrinsic pathways for apoptosis that converge on the final effector caspases to mediate cell death. The extrinsic pathway is activated by death ligands and their receptors, such as Fas and FasL, and by TNF-α–related apoptosis-inducing ligand (TRAIL); the intrinsic pathway is activated by mechanisms of cell and membrane stress (lysosomal, ER, and mitochondrial injury).[180]

Several mechanisms have been invoked to explain the proapoptotic state in NASH. Triglyceride accumulation itself increases apoptosis by the interaction of unoxidized palmitoyl CoA with serine to form dihydrosphingosine, a precursor of ceramide.[181] Ceramide is a potent inducer of apoptosis via an inducible nitric oxide synthetase (iNOS)-mediated pathway that requires the transcriptional factor NF-κB.[182] It has also been shown that increased FFA delivery to hepatocytes, secondary to increased peripheral lipolysis in the insulin-resistant state, may produce lipotoxicity and induce apoptosis.[126] FFAs induce translocation of Bax to lysosomes, where it causes the release of cathepsin. Cathepsin, acting via NF-κB, induces TNF-α and activation of TNF receptor–associated death pathways.

Recently, the potential role of ER stress in the development of cell injury in NASH has gained interest. The ER is the principal site for synthetic activity within cells. Such activity requires not only appropriate synthesis but also local mechanisms to ensure that the proteins are correctly folded because this is essential for their recognition by appropriate receptors and trafficking to their final destination. Under conditions in which there is increased protein or lipid synthetic activity in the ER, depletion of ATP, depletion of calcium, or altered glucose homeostasis, the regulatory function of the ER in maintaining normal synthetic function is disrupted. This leads to the activation of an intracellular program called the unfolded protein response (UPR).[183] Activation of the UPR initially leads to an adaptive response in which protein synthesis decreases and allows restoration of normal ER function. Simultaneously, proteosomal degradation of unfolded proteins is increased (ER-associated degradation [ERAD]).

However, if the initiating factors are not corrected, alarm pathways are activated, including activation of a number of stress kinases, which eventually results in activation of homologous protein (CHOP), a potent apoptosis-inducing factor.

We recently observed that patients with NAFLD have a variable degree of UPR activation.[184] Inositol requiring enzyme-1 (IRE-1) activation appears to play an important role in the genesis of cell injury in NASH via activation of JNK phosphorylation. Interestingly, there seems to be a close association of IRE-1 activation with the histologic activity of the disease. Failure to generate ER degradation-enhancing α-mannosidase-like protein (EDEM) in response to spliced X box–binding protein (sXBP) in some subjects raises the possibility that patients with the lowest EDEM levels are at particular risk of progressing to cirrhosis because of insufficient degradation of unfolded proteins, thus perpetuating the ER stress. Despite increased phosphorylated eIF-2a, patients with NASH are apparently unable to up-regulate activating transcription factor 4 (ATF4), CHOP, and growth arrest and DNA damage-34 (GADD34), which contributes to the failure to recover from ER stress.[184] Thus NASH is specifically associated with failure to generate sXBP1 and activation of JNK.[184]

Interestingly, the antiapoptotic B-cell lymphoma-2 (BCL2) protein appears to be strongly expressed in human steatohepatitis, probably representing an adaptive response.[185] Thus, on the basis of the recognized significance of hepatocyte apoptosis in the pathogenesis of NAFLD, it has been proposed that the development of progressive NAFLD in some patients but not in others may be the result of increased susceptibility of steatotic hepatocytes to apoptosis arising from abnormal regulation of BCL2 proteins, alteration in JNK activation, or preferential activation of ER stress.[180,186]

Mechanisms of Inflammation

Nonalcoholic steatohepatitis is characterized by a scattered, predominantly lobular, mixed inflammatory infiltrate. The precise mechanisms of inflammation in NASH have not been defined. It is generally presumed that the products of cell death and release of inflammatory cytokines within the liver cause changes in blood flow and endothelial function that promote inflammation. At a cellular level, activation of proinflammatory pathways is associated with activation of the stress kinase JNK (**Fig. 53-13**). JNK can be activated by ER stress, oxidative stress, and inflammatory cytokines such as TNF-α.[187-189] JNK may also be activated by TNF-independent pathways.[190] Activation of JNK can lead to activation of the transcriptional factors NF-κB and activator protein-1 (AP1), which cause transcriptional induction of inflammatory cytokines such as TNF-α.[191]

Role of the Innate Immune System

The role of the innate immune system in the initiation and maintenance of inflammation within the liver is currently under active investigation. The innate immune system is an important factor in the promotion and progression of inflammation in the liver in subjects with NASH. A key consequence of the expansion of adipose tissue, as well as an early event in the development of IR, is the infiltration of adipose tissue by macrophages,[129] especially visceral adipose tissue. Relative tissue hypoxemia, induction of hypoxia-inducible factor-1, increased expression of the C-C motif chemokine ligand-2

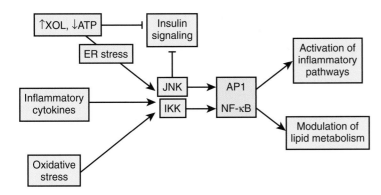

Fig. 53-13 Cellular pathways involved in steatohepatitis. Endoplasmic reticulum stress *(ER stress)*, inflammatory cytokines, and oxidative stress all lead to activation of c-Jun terminal kinase *(JNK)* and inhibitor κB kinase *(IKK)*, which results in activation of the transcriptional factors activator protein-1 *(AP1)* and nuclear factor κB *(NF-κB)*. These factors increase expression of genes regulating proinflammatory cytokines and also further impair metabolic homeostasis and cause both glucose intolerance and hepatic steatosis. ATP, adenosine triphosphate; XOL, cholesterol

(CCL2) within adipose tissue, and several dietary constituents have been implicated in this process. These macrophages produce a number of proinflammatory cytokines that further induce the production of additional cytokines from adjacent adipocytes.[75,192] These cytokines antagonize insulin-mediated suppression of lipolysis and also produce a proinflammatory milieu within the adipose tissue.[74] In addition, they enter the circulation and induce an acute phase reaction by the liver. IL-6 plays a key role in this process.[193] These cytokines and the secondary cytokines produced in the liver alter endothelial function and promote vascular dysfunction and leukocyte adherence and migration.

Fatty acids can directly activate inflammatory signaling and hepatic IR as ligands for Toll-like receptors (TLRs) with downstream, intracellular activation of JNK and IKK. All resident cells of the liver express TLRs, and TLR2 and TLR4 in particular have been demonstrated to play a role in animal models of NASH. Furthermore, inhibitors of TLRs have been shown to decrease inflammation and fibrosis in dietary animal models.

Role of Gut Microbiota

Endotoxin, one of the components of the outer wall of gram-negative bacteria, is released by the microbiota in the gut and is directly introduced into the liver via portal blood. Endotoxin is considered to play an important role in the promotion of inflammation in NAFLD. Endotoxin stimulates an inflammatory response via TLR4, including increasing levels of TNF-α. Kupffer cells, the first line of defense, are activated by endotoxin.[194] Marked activation of Kupffer cells has been observed in human NASH. In a study of 40 morbidly obese patients with NAFLD, the circulating lipopolysaccharide-binding protein (a surrogate marker of endotoxin) level was elevated in NASH.[195] Similarly, plasma endotoxin was elevated in NAFLD patients in comparison to healthy controls,[196] as well as increased small bowel bacterial overgrowth. Metabolic alterations related to loss of diversity of the gut microbiota as a result of energy use and storage in obesity have been demonstrated in twin studies in humans.[197]

Mechanisms of Fibrosis

Pericellular fibrosis in the hepatic sinusoids is a histologic hallmark of NASH. It results from activation of quiescent HSCs, which then produce a collagenous matrix. Over time, the fibrosis extends to form central-to-central and central-to-portal bridges, which then evolve into cirrhosis. Several factors have been implicated in the activation of HSCs, including a variety of cytokines, of which transforming growth factor-β

(TGF-β) is the most well known.[198] Both hyperinsulinemia and increased leptin levels increase collagen synthesis by activated HSCs.[199] It is also conceivable that if HSC apoptosis is inhibited, the total fibrotic process may be enhanced. Recent studies have focused on the role of N-cadherin, tissue inhibitor of metalloproteinase (TIMP), and endocannabinoids in this process.[200,201] The mechanisms involved in activation and perpetuation of the fibrotic process constitute an area of active investigation. Importantly, after improvement of IR, hepatic fibrosis can regress.[202,203]

NASH is characterized by perisinusoidal deposition of a collagenous matrix by activated HSCs. In NASH, HSC activation correlates with portal and lobular inflammation, but not with steatosis alone, thus suggesting that the mechanisms implicated in fibrogenesis are probably related to signals that not only lead to hepatic fat deposition but are also proinflammatory and profibrotic in their own right. One such signal could be adiponectin, known to inhibit HSC proliferation and migration and expression of the classic fibrogenic cytokine TGF-β, respectively.[204] Adiponectin-mediated activation of HSCs may occur via activation of AMPK,[205] NF-κB,[206] or Kruppel-like factors.[57] It has also been shown that insulin and glucose are capable of inducing the synthesis of connective tissue growth factor by HSCs.[207] Endocannabinoids have recently emerged as a potent mediator of hepatic steatosis, HSC activation, and fibrosis.[208] CB1 is expressed at low density on hepatocytes, quiescent HSCs, and endothelial cells, and its expression is strongly induced in subjects with fibrosis and cirrhosis.[209,210] Although CB1 receptors on hepatocytes promote lipogenesis, expression on HSCs accelerates a fibrogenic response associated with chronic liver injury, independently of the offending agent.[211]

An emerging area of active investigation is the process of epithelial-mesenchymal transition (EMT), by which local factors induce mature epithelial cells to differentiate into cells with mesenchymal phenotypic markers and functions. Its role has been demonstrated in a variety of inflammatory conditions of solid organs and organs with endocrine or exocrine function (or both), as well as in cancers of solid organs. EMT has recently been shown to occur in diseases of the biliary system,[212] but the role of EMT in the fibrosis associated with NAFLD/NASH is currently under active investigation.

Progression of NASH to Cirrhosis

The progression of NASH to cirrhosis reflects a balance between cell injury versus repair and regeneration (**Fig. 53-14**).

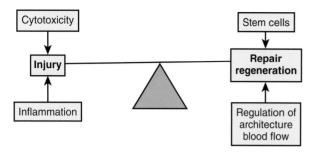

Fig. 53-14 Progression of nonalcoholic steatohepatitis to cirrhosis is a function of cell injury and death versus repair and regeneration. Cell injury can result from the metabolic disturbances caused by insulin resistance or from the proinflammatory milieu within the liver. Cell repair and regeneration are still not well understood but presumably involve stem cells derived from the circulation, as well as the liver, and changes in regulation of the hepatic architecture and microcirculation.

Cell injury results from both the metabolic disturbances related to IR and the inflammatory state in the liver. The latter is associated with the presence of proinflammatory cytokines (e.g., TNF-α) and products of inflammation (e.g., leukotrienes). In contrast, tissue repair involves both repair of cells that have sublethal injury and removal and replacement of dead hepatocytes with either new hepatocytes derived from stem cells or scar tissue. Very little is currently understood about the mechanisms of hepatic tissue repair and pathologic wound healing in disease states. Specifically, the mechanisms by which the hepatic architecture is disrupted with progression to cirrhosis remain poorly understood.

Clinical Features of Nonalcoholic Fatty Liver Disease

Most subjects with NAFLD are asymptomatic. The diagnosis is often made incidentally in these individuals because of either abnormal liver enzyme levels or features of a fatty liver on an imaging study when such tests are performed for unrelated reasons. In others, NAFLD may be diagnosed either as a result of an unusual appearance of the liver during abdominal surgery or because of persistent hepatomegaly. It is important to recognize that in only a minority of subjects has NAFLD been diagnosed and that it currently remains undiagnosed in the great majority of afflicted individuals.

Symptoms and Signs

Most patients have vague complaints of fatigue or malaise and a sensation of fullness or discomfort on the right side of the upper part of the abdomen without signs of chronic liver disease at the time of diagnosis. Such symptoms often antedate the diagnosis of NAFLD in a third of patients.[213]

Abdominal obesity and hepatomegaly are the most common physical findings. Obesity is present in 50% to 90% of subjects.[19] About two thirds of subjects with NAFLD also have other features of metabolic syndrome. We recently confirmed abdominal obesity as a marker of both steatosis and grade of

the disease. In addition, we demonstrated that about 28% of subjects had increased dorsocervical fat, which correlated strongly with histologic severity.[214] Acanthosis nigricans may be found in individuals with NAFLD and is suggestive of an underlying insulin-resistant state.

Hepatomegaly is the most common liver-related physical finding in subjects with NAFLD.[8] A minority of people have stigmata of chronic liver disease such as spider angiomas or palmar erythema. Jaundice and features of portal hypertension, such as ascites and variceal hemorrhage, are the initial findings in a small minority of subjects with advanced liver disease.[215]

Other Clinical Conditions Commonly Encountered in Patients with NAFLD

The association of NAFLD with obesity, diabetes, hypertriglyceridemia, and hypertension is well known. Other associations include cardiovascular morbidity and mortality, sleep abnormalities, psychiatric illness, chronic fatigue and pain syndrome, and abnormalities of the coagulation cascade.

Cardiovascular Morbidity and Mortality

Recent studies have highlighted the importance of a fatty liver as an independent risk factor for a variety of end points related to metabolic syndrome. In a 5-year follow-up study of 633 subjects, those with abnormal liver enzyme levels had a 2.2- to 2.8-fold increase in risk for the development of full-blown metabolic syndrome, which outperformed C-reactive protein as a risk factor.[216] Similarly, other studies have shown that those with abnormal liver enzymes have a higher risk for the development of hypertension and diabetes.[217,218] The presence of NAFLD (either NAFL or NASH) is also independently associated with endothelial dysfunction, abnormal vascular reactivity, increased carotid intimal thickness, and the number of plaques in the carotids.[219] These data indicate that although the presence of a fatty liver may not have many clinical consequences for the liver, it may have many deleterious effects on health in general.

Sleep Abnormalities

Patients with NAFLD often complain of increased sleepiness during the day. This is associated with disturbed sleep patterns, and patients often wake up feeling tired. Many subjects have associated sleep disorders and, on direct questioning, will acknowledge that they snore. In addition, obstructive sleep apnea (OSA) has been associated with NAFLD. In a recent prospective series of adults seen in a sleep clinic, a three-fold increase in the likelihood of elevated liver enzyme levels was found in subjects with newly diagnosed severe OSA.[220] Liver biopsy, performed only on subjects with abnormal liver enzymes in this same study, identified NASH in the vast majority of subjects with severe OSA, whereas just a minority of subjects with mild or no OSA had biopsy-proven NASH. The presence of NASH was related to the apnea-hypopnea index, independent of age and BMI. Subjects with severe OSA, however, had more pronounced IR. Thus it is not clear whether OSA or the increased IR in these subjects contributed to the development of NASH.

It has recently been recognized that the IR syndrome is not simply a function of diet and lifestyle but is also markedly affected by abnormal sleep patterns.[221] Thus abnormal sleep leads to IR, and the IR syndrome is associated with abnormal sleep patterns.[222] The relationship of other abnormalities in patients with sleep disorders and IR remains poorly defined.

Association with Psychiatric Illness

We performed a detailed inventory of associated symptoms and conditions in a cohort of 61 subjects with NAFLD. In addition to confirming the classic associations with NAFLD, we found that 25% suffered from chronic depression, 10% had an anxiety disorder, and more than 50% of subjects were taking a psychotropic drug at the time of diagnosis. On detailed questioning, the onset of weight gain often corresponded with a life event that was also associated with depression or anxiety, such as divorce, an accident, or childbirth. In some of these cases, the onset of weight gain is often temporally related to development of the behavioral disorder and the use of an antidepressant drug. Given the propensity of several antidepressant drugs to cause weight gain, the potential role of such drugs in the weight gain and subsequent development of IR is an important and yet unexplored question.

The relationship of depression and anxiety disorders to NAFLD is not clear and merits further evaluation. Moreover, the prevalence of NAFLD in the general population of subjects with chronic pain or fatigue is unknown. One should, however, be aware that NAFLD may also be present in subjects with chronic fatigue, fibromyalgia, and depression.

Chronic Fatigue and Pain Syndrome

Fatigue is often present in patients with NAFLD and is frequently the most debilitating aspect of the condition for the individual subject. In the experience of these authors, fatigue is the most common symptom in this patient population. Several clinical variations of fatigue syndrome can be recognized. Most commonly, subjects complain of chronic malaise and severe lethargy. Some patients have mixed patterns of fatigue, which are often difficult to evaluate and manage. Approximately 25% of subjects with NAFLD also have chronic fatigue syndrome. Some patients complain of aching soreness in their muscles along with fatigue, and about 20% of all subjects suffer from a chronic pain disorder.[223] At our institution, 27% of the subjects in whom NAFLD was diagnosed were taking analgesics, including narcotics (7%), at the time of diagnosis.

Abnormalities of the Coagulation Cascade

Coagulation abnormalities are associated with IR and metabolic syndrome, which are present in more than 75% and 90% of subjects with NAFLD, respectively.[23] Metabolic syndrome predisposes to a prothrombotic state with increased concentrations of circulating tissue factor (TF) and factor VII.[224] The severity of IR (i.e., hyperinsulinemia) and adipose tissue mass both determine the levels of TF and factor VII.[225-227] TF forms a complex with factor VII. This complex activates factor X, which together with factor V converts prothrombin to thrombin. This step is further amplified by activation of factor IX

by the TF–factor VII complex, as well as thrombin itself, along with recruitment of cofactors V and VIII. Thrombin converts fibrinogen to fibrin to form a clot. Metabolic syndrome has also been associated with high factor VIII and fibrinogen levels, which further promotes the procoagulant state in this condition.[228]

The tendency to form clots is counteracted by inhibitors of the clotting pathways and by fibrinolysis, which is initiated by plasminogen activators. The impact of IR on inhibitors of coagulation (e.g., protein C, protein S, and TF pathway inhibitor) has not been fully defined. PAI-1 is the principal physiologic inhibitor of fibrinolysis. IR is associated with increased PAI-1 levels as a result of increased production and release by adipose tissue and adipose tissue–associated stromal cells.[229] PAI-1 expression is increased by TNF-α, TGF-β, insulin, hyperglycemia, increased FFAs, and triglycerides.[230,231]

In summary, in those with risk factors for NAFLD, the presence of right upper quadrant discomfort, hepatomegaly or elevated liver enzymes should trigger an evaluation for NAFLD. Other subjects with persistently elevated liver enzymes (e.g., ALT) who do not have viral hepatitis, hemochromatosis, or other liver diseases, including autoimmune hepatitis and metabolic disorders such as Wilson disease, should likewise be evaluated for NAFLD. It is also important to remember that there are no symptoms or signs that distinguish those with NAFL from those with NASH.

Laboratory Abnormalities

Suspicion for NAFLD is triggered by abnormal results on liver chemistry tests that are usually performed for non–liver-related reasons. Approximately 7.9% of the U.S. population has persistently abnormal liver enzymes with negative tests for viral hepatitis and other common causes of liver diseases.[41] The majority of these subjects could have NAFLD if they have risk factors associated with NAFLD, such as the presence of features of metabolic syndrome. It is also important to note that a large number of subjects with NAFLD have persistently normal liver enzyme levels, and the entire histologic spectrum of NAFLD can be seen in such individuals.

Mild to moderate elevation in serum aminotransferases (ALT and aspartate aminotransferase [AST]) is the most common and often the only laboratory abnormality found in patients with NAFLD. When these values exceed 300 IU/L, alternative causes of liver disease should be sought carefully. The AST/ALT ratio is usually less than 1 but can be reversed in those with advanced fibrosis or cirrhosis. A mild to modest increase in serum alkaline phosphatase and γ-glutamyltransferase (GGT) can be seen in patients with NAFLD, but the degree of elevation is less than that seen in those with alcoholic hepatitis, as is the case with an increased AST/ALT ratio.

Findings of chronic liver disease together with the presence of hypoalbuminemia, coagulopathy, hyperbilirubinemia, and thrombocytopenia suggest advanced liver disease with probable cirrhosis. Serum albumin and the prothrombin time become abnormal before bilirubin becomes elevated. In diabetic subjects, isolated hypoalbuminemia can result from diabetic nephropathy. Hematologic parameters are usually normal unless cirrhosis and portal hypertension lead to hypersplenism. In fact, a large proportion of patients with cryptogenic cirrhosis share many of the clinical and demographic features of patients with NAFLD, thus suggesting that cryptogenic cirrhosis is unrecognized NAFLD in an advanced stage.

About 30% to 50% of subjects with NAFLD have elevated blood glucose and about 60% also have associated hypertriglyceridemia, low HDL cholesterol, or both.[23] An elevated ferritin level is also often seen in subjects with NAFLD.[164] It is, however, not associated with iron overload in most cases and usually reflects an acute phase response.[8]

From a practical point of view, the laboratory evaluation of a subject with suspected NAFLD involves excluding alternative causes of liver enzyme abnormalities, documenting hepatic steatosis, making the distinction between hepatic steatosis and steatohepatitis, assessing the stage of the disease, and evaluating for the presence and severity of IR and other complications of metabolic syndrome. Each of these factors must be considered carefully when making a decision about the aggressiveness with which the answer to each of these is sought. It is important to remember that liver enzymes are notably poor predictors of steatosis and significant fibrosis. Therefore liver biopsy remains the gold standard for diagnosing steatohepatitis and for staging the liver disease, unless clinically evident cirrhosis is present.

Diagnostic Approach to Nonalcoholic Fatty Liver Disease

Complete evaluation of a patient with NAFLD includes confirmation of the diagnosis, assessment of the cause, and delineation of the grade and stage of the disease. The diagnosis of NAFLD requires two steps: establishment of the presence of fatty liver disease and confirmation of the "nonalcoholic"

nature of the condition. In addition, several other forms of chronic liver disease are extremely prevalent in the general population (e.g., hepatitis C) and can often coexist with NAFLD.[67] It is therefore imperative that the initial evaluation include appropriate laboratory studies to exclude other common causes of liver disease.

The gold standard for the diagnosis of fatty liver disease is liver biopsy. However, given the invasive nature, cost, and risks associated with liver biopsy, there is considerable interest in trying to make the diagnosis with noninvasive methods.

Noninvasive Methods for the Diagnosis of NAFLD

Two-dimensional sonography, computed tomography (CT), and magnetic resonance imaging (MRI) are the most studied methods that are also available at most medical centers. The sonographic features of NAFLD include increased hepatic parenchymal echotexture and vascular blurring (**Fig. 53-15, A**). These findings are, however, also seen in those with any form of chronic liver disease, and though sensitive (85% to 95%), they are nonspecific (positive predictive value of 62%).[8] Moreover, the ability to detect fatty liver by sonography drops off markedly once the degree of hepatic steatosis decreases to 30% or less.[33]

CT of the liver provides a more specific method for the noninvasive diagnosis of NAFLD (see **Fig. 53-15, B**). Hepatic steatosis decreases the CT attenuation of the liver. When hepatic parenchymal attenuation is 10 or more Hounsfield units lower than that of the spleen on a non–contrast-enhanced scan, a diagnosis of hepatic steatosis can be made. When intravenous contrast material is administered, hepatic enhancement lags behind enhancement of the spleen, and the liver-to-spleen attenuation differential exceeds 20 Hounsfield units.[232] Even though these features allow hepatic steatosis to

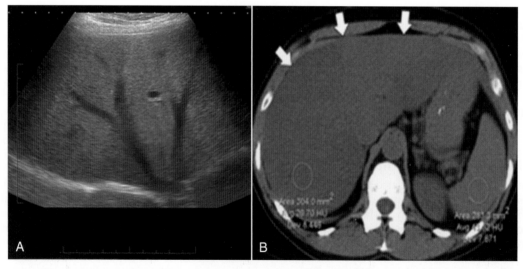

Fig. 53-15 **A,** Ultrasound image of hepatic steatosis. The parenchyma is hyperechogenic. In addition, the edges of the blood vessels are blurred. **B,** Computed tomographic images of hepatic steatosis. In non–contrast-enhanced scans, the decreased liver attenuation results in prominence of the blood vessels. Moreover, the liver is darker than the spleen. When intravenous contrast material is administered, liver attenuation increases, but to a lesser degree than in the spleen. When the difference exceeds 20 Hounsfield units, hepatic steatosis can be diagnosed with relative specificity.

be defined with a 76% positive predictive value,[33] they do not permit distinction between fatty liver and steatohepatitis. In addition, the diagnostic sensitivity of the test depends on the severity of the steatosis and decreases when the steatosis is mild. CT also does not provide any information on the stage of fibrosis in the liver unless features of portal hypertension are present. This occurs only in the presence of cirrhosis of the liver. Finally, it is worth remembering that CT is substantially more expensive than sonography.

MRI is even more sensitive than CT for the assessment of hepatic steatosis. Recently, MRI techniques have been refined to provide a highly reproducible and validated measure of hepatic triglyceride content.[36] Unfortunately, MRI also has many of the same limitations of CT just noted. It is even more expensive than CT and is not universally available. In clinical practice, a hepatic sonogram is the most commonly used modality for evaluation of the presence of steatosis. However, it is important to note that none of these methods can diagnose steatohepatitis or accurately assess the stage of the disease.

Role of Liver Biopsy in the Diagnosis of NAFLD

Liver biopsy is the gold standard for the diagnosis of NAFLD because it can distinguish those with a fatty liver alone from those with steatohepatitis and can be used to assess the stage of hepatic fibrosis. Unfortunately, it is invasive, uncomfortable, and expensive and occasionally causes severe morbidity and mortality. There is now some hope for patients with steatohepatitis as specific pharmacologic treatment of NASH becomes available in the near future. Establishing a diagnosis of NASH versus NAFL may therefore allow the use of specific treatment interventions in routine clinical practice.

To make intelligent decisions regarding whom to perform biopsy on and when to perform it, one must consider the information to be obtained and how it will affect the individual undergoing liver biopsy. The key information provided by liver biopsy includes the following:

1. A diagnosis of persistently abnormal liver chemistry can be established after excluding other common causes.
2. Hepatic steatosis and steatohepatitis (NASH) can be distinguished only on the basis of the histologic features described earlier.
3. Liver biopsy is the best way to assess the degree of fibrosis in the liver and stage the disease.
4. It may also be useful in determining the effect of medical treatment.

Thus liver biopsy can establish the presence of NASH, which can progress to cirrhosis in up to 15% to 20% of patients. Additionally, liver biopsy can help identify those with bridging fibrosis or cirrhosis even in the presence of normal ALT levels inasmuch as up to a third of these patients can have an advanced stage of liver disease. Also, weight loss surgery has been shown to improve NASH. In cases in which NASH is found on liver biopsy, this option may be considered if the BMI exceeds 35 kg/m². However, once cirrhosis develops, the amount of steatosis and cytologic ballooning may decrease or they may disappear completely and thus make NASH difficult to diagnosis. Such cases are labeled as cryptogenic cirrhosis or "burned-out" NASH. In these settings, the diagnosis can be suspected only from the clinical profile of the patient and the presence of risk factors for NAFLD. In some circumstances, the presence of bridging fibrosis may direct management. For example, in a morbidly obese subject who is likely to be turned down for liver transplant listing because of obesity, the presence of bridging fibrosis may lead the treating physician to consider aggressive weight loss measures. These possibilities should be discussed with the patient together with the fact that once the diagnosis and stage of the disease are established, physicians can intervene aggressively in a multidisciplinary manner, including pharmacologic and surgical weight loss, which may have its own set of challenges.

In a decision analysis study to determine the benefits of early liver biopsy for the diagnosis and early treatment of NASH, an initial liver biopsy strategy was projected to lead to lower mortality than in the group with no initial liver biopsy and result in fewer transplant-listed patients after 5 years.[233] With early biopsy and early intervention, the relative return of preventing advanced liver disease per liver biopsy was high. This decision tree model provides a context for balancing the risks and benefits of liver biopsy in patients with NAFLD. In addition, the risk of having advanced fibrosis (i.e., bridging fibrosis or cirrhosis) increases with increasing age and BMI and the presence of diabetes.[234] These criteria may be used to identify those who are most likely to benefit from biopsy. It is important to remember, however, that the gold standard of liver biopsy is subject to sampling error, differences in histopathologic interpretation, and selection and ascertainment bias.

Natural History of Nonalcoholic Fatty Liver Disease: Nonalcoholic Steatohepatitis, Cirrhosis, and Hepatocellular Carcinoma

Only limited data are available on the natural history of NAFLD. Most studies are cross-sectional in nature and have focused on highly selected patient populations. In such studies, the majority of subjects have NAFL. It is generally believed that NAFL rarely progresses to more advanced liver disease. However, there are several reported cases of the development of steatohepatitis in subjects with NAFL, particularly after rapid weight loss following bariatric surgery.[235] This occurred more frequently after jejunoileal bypass and only rarely after proximal gastric bypass or vertical banded gastroplasty.[236,237]

The long-term natural history of subjects with NAFLD is affected by the presence of underlying metabolic syndrome, and these patients are at risk from the morbidity related to diabetes and cardiovascular disease. A recent study found that cardiovascular mortality was higher in subjects with cirrhosis secondary to NASH than in those with hepatitis C.[238] Subjects with metabolic syndrome are also at risk for the development of gallstones. Although gallstones are well known to occur in subjects with obesity, the specific prevalence of gallstones in subjects with NAFLD is unknown.

A recent study evaluated the natural history of NAFLD by chart review of subjects in whom NAFLD was diagnosed in the last 20 years in Olmstead County.[239] The overall survival of subjects with NAFLD was lower than that of a matched population in Minnesota. Higher mortality was associated with increased age (hazard ratio [HR] per decade = 2.2; 95% confidence interval [CI], 1.003 to 1.76), impaired blood glucose control (HR = 2.6; 95% CI, 1.3 to 5.2), and cirrhosis (HR = 3.1; 95% CI, 1.2 to 7.8). Liver disease was the third leading cause of death in this population, whereas it was the thirteenth cause of death in Minnesota. These data confirm previous studies in which the presence of cirrhosis and steatohepatitis was shown to be associated with increased mortality.[240]

Only limited data are available on the progression of NASH to cirrhosis. Most studies are retrospective and methodologically flawed. However, based on the limited data available, the risk for progression to cirrhosis is estimated to be about 20%.[241] In a study of 103 subjects who underwent multiple liver biopsies over a median duration of 3.2 years, 37% showed progression of fibrosis and 29% showed regression.[242] It is, however, unclear whether these findings reflect sampling variability. It has been reported that a biopsy specimen about 4 cm long is required to obviate such variability,[16] but this length is rarely obtained in routine clinical practice. In cross-sectional studies, increasing age, diabetes, and high BMI have been associated with advanced fibrosis.[234] In other studies, severely

obese individuals with a combination of hypertension, abnormal ALT, and IR_{HOMA} have been found to have a higher probability of having advanced fibrosis.[50] Evaluation of the existing literature suggests that older subjects with additional features of metabolic syndrome (e.g., diabetes, hypertension) are more likely to have advanced disease.

Once cirrhosis develops, the natural history of NASH is characterized by an approximately 4% annual rate of decompensation.[238] In a 10-year follow-up of 150 subjects with cirrhosis secondary to NASH, the rate of decompensation was found to be slightly but significantly lower than in a matched population of subjects with hepatitis C and cirrhosis. These differences were mainly due to lower rates of development of ascites and synthetic failure (**Fig. 53-16**). Although some studies have suggested that hepatocellular cancer occurs frequently in patients with NASH, these studies have not evaluated the population at risk (i.e., the denominator).[243,244] It has recently been found that hepatocellular cancer developed in 10 of 149 subjects with cirrhosis secondary to NASH over a 10-year time frame as compared with 25 of 147 subjects with hepatitis C (**Fig. 53-17**).[238]

Another aspect of NASH is that hepatic steatosis and other features of steatohepatitis decrease after cirrhosis develops.[215] In some patients these findings disappear completely, and

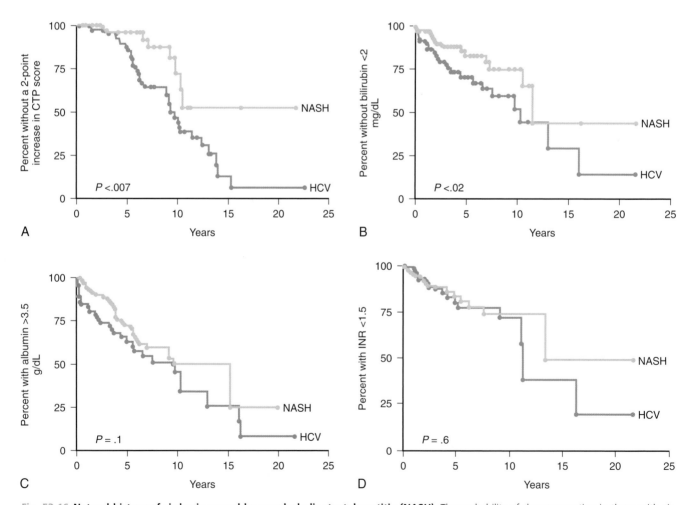

Fig. 53-16 **Natural history of cirrhosis caused by nonalcoholic steatohepatitis (NASH).** The probability of decompensation in those with cirrhosis secondary to NASH is less than that seen in subjects with cirrhosis secondary to hepatitis C virus (HCV). Similar observation is made for other laboratory parameters. CTP, Child-Turcotte-Pugh; INR, international normalized ratio.

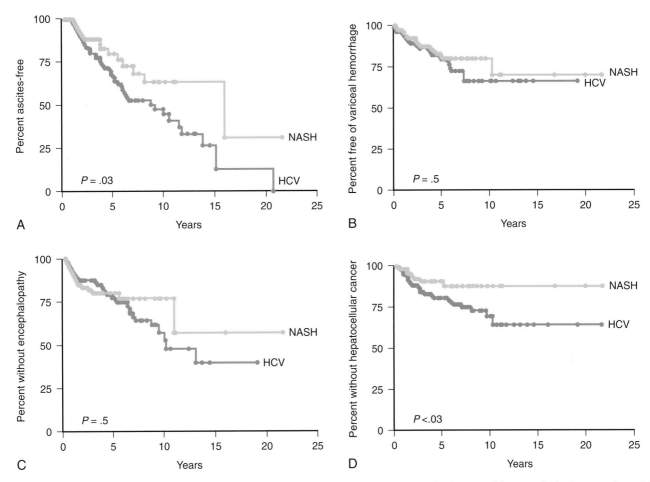

Fig. 53-17 Long-term risk of complications of cirrhosis developing in patients with cirrhosis caused by nonalcoholic steatohepatitis (NASH) or hepatitis C virus (HCV). The hazard of ascites (**A**), variceal hemorrhage (**B**), encephalopathy (**C**), and hepatocellular carcinoma (**D**) developing is shown as time to failure via the Kaplan-Meier method. Across-group differences were analyzed with the log-rank test. Patients with cirrhosis secondary to NASH had a significantly lower risk of ascites and hepatocellular carcinoma developing than did those with cirrhosis secondary to hepatitis C.

such cases are manifested as cryptogenic cirrhosis. In fact, most subjects with cryptogenic cirrhosis have underlying fatty liver disease. Currently, about 7% to 14% of subjects referred for liver transplantation have cryptogenic cirrhosis.[3,245] Hepatic steatosis develops universally in subjects with cryptogenic cirrhosis after liver transplantation, as opposed to 20% of those with hepatitis B, primary biliary cirrhosis, and alcoholic liver disease.[246] Steatohepatitis develops at a later time, and most such subjects have recurrence of disease between 2 and 5 years after transplantation. However, graft function is maintained over the first 5 to 10 years after transplantation, and there is no evidence of a higher rate of graft loss than in subjects undergoing transplantation for other indications.

Treatment of Nonalcoholic Fatty Liver Disease

At present there are no established treatment guidelines and no single approved therapy for the treatment of NAFLD. Based on our current understanding of the natural history of

this disease, one may propose to treat only patients with NASH or those at risk for the development of liver cirrhosis. This approach may change as our understanding of disease pathophysiology improves and potential targets of therapy evolve. The focus of management remains treatment of the risk factors for NASH (i.e., IR, obesity), with the objective of preventing disease progression or regression of already established fatty liver or NASH.

Dietary modification and lifestyle changes are the principal methods used for weight management. Although several drugs have been used for either weight control or treatment of IR, their role remains experimental.

Weight Management

The goal of weight management is to bring the weight as close to ideal body weight as possible (**Fig. 53-18**). However, it is not essential for the weight to normalize to improve the metabolic status of overweight or obese individuals. Even modest weight loss can be accompanied by substantial improvement in IR.[247] There have been a large number of studies on various dietary and lifestyle interventions to improve body weight in

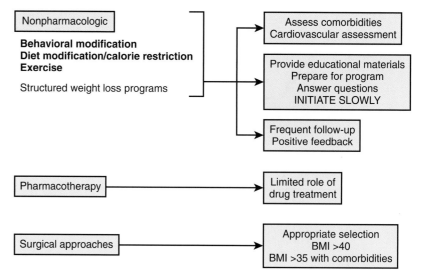

Fig. 53-18 Approach to weight management in patients with nonalcoholic fatty liver disease. A nonpharmacologic approach is the cornerstone of therapy either alone or in combination with other modalities as depicted by the large arrow. Pharmacotherapy is least likely to result in long-term weight loss, whereas weight loss surgery is increasingly being considered for appropriate candidates with improvement in metabolic profile and liver disease. BMI, body mass index.

subjects with obesity. The results are somewhat heterogeneous but still allow certain conclusions to be made.

First, most diets work in the short term. However, long-term weight loss with diet alone is difficult to accomplish. Similarly, lifestyle interventions often appear to be effective in the short term but are difficult to sustain. Combined approaches using intense diet and exercise interventions have also been limited because of the very high recidivism rate after discontinuation of the studies. The data underscore the need for diet and lifestyle changes that are palatable to the patient and easy to accomplish and maintain in the context of the socioeconomic, family, and cultural milieu in which a given patient lives. This further indicates that it is unlikely that a single magic solution will work for all subjects. Using a transtheoretic model to analyze the behavioral status of patients with NASH, a preliminary report indicated that most subjects are in the precontemplation phase.[248] This indicates that most subjects with NASH do not perceive in their mind that they have a weight-related problem; these data provide a clue about why most patients with NASH do not achieve long-term benefits from lifestyle interventions.

It is the practice of these authors to provide as much education to the patient before embarking on a diet and exercise program. In addition, in those with long-standing diabetes or other cardiovascular risk factors, it is prudent to perform a basic cardiac, vascular, ophthalmic, and neurologic evaluation before starting an exercise program. In subjects who are overweight or obese, the National Heart, Lung, and Blood Institute guidelines for weight management are the best evidence-based treatment guidelines.[249] It is generally recommended that the diet should be planned to achieve a daily caloric deficit of 500 to 1000 calories. Furthermore, an increase in everyday activities should be encouraged. For diabetic individuals, the American Diabetes Association guidelines for diet should be followed.[250] Subjects with a BMI higher than 30 kg/m^2 or with a BMI higher than 27 along with other comorbid conditions (e.g., sleep apnea), pharmacologic weight management with orlistat or sibutramine may be considered.[249] The latter is a serotonin reuptake antagonist and is contraindicated in subjects with heart disease. Orlistat causes fat malabsorption, and a recent nonrandomized trial suggested that this agent could produce a beneficial effect on NAFLD.[251]

Both proximal gastric bypass and vertical banded gastroplasty have been shown to be safe in subjects with NASH (**Fig. 53-19**). In the first few months following these procedures, the steatosis decreases while the inflammation may worsen.[235] However, in the long term, the severity of hepatic steatosis, cell injury, and fibrosis all regress once the weight stabilizes following these operations.[235,252] In subjects with a BMI higher than 35 kg/m^2, these operations are a viable treatment option provided that the operative risks are within an acceptable range.

Pharmacologic Treatment of NASH

Several drug therapies have been tried in both research and clinical setting, yet no agent has been approved by the Food and Drug Administration for the treatment of NAFLD (**Fig. 53-20**). The results of the most recent pioglitazone versus vitamin E versus placebo for the treatment of nondiabetic patients with nonalcoholic steatohepatitis (PIVENS) trial may guide future therapeutic options.

Insulin Sensitizers

Two classes of drugs have been shown to correct IR: biguanides (e.g., metformin) and thiazolidinediones (e.g., rosiglitazone, pioglitazone). The former works by a mechanism not well defined and can modulate AMPK activity. The roles of all of the pharmacologic agents discussed in the following sections are experimental at this time.

Metformin

In an animal model of steatohepatitis, metformin treatment improved hepatic steatosis and inflammation. However, in human studies, although ALT improved and liver size decreased, metformin was not consistently found to improve liver histology.[253] In a recent open-label randomized trial, metformin (2 g/day given orally) improved ALT more often than did vitamin E (800 IU/day) (odds ratio = 3.1, P <.001).[254] However, only limited histologic data are available from this study. The role of metformin remains experimental, and a large-scale clinical trial is currently in progress to define the utility of metformin for NASH.

Parameter	RYGBP	BPD-DS	VBG	LAGB
	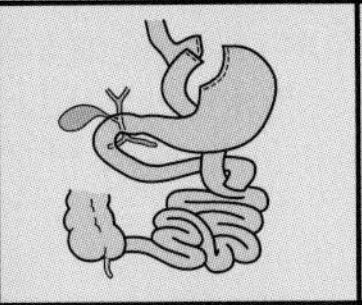	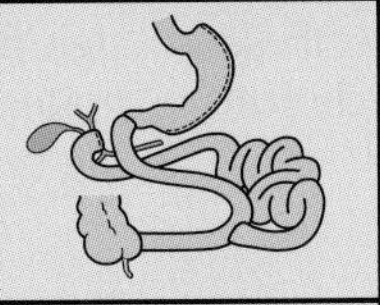	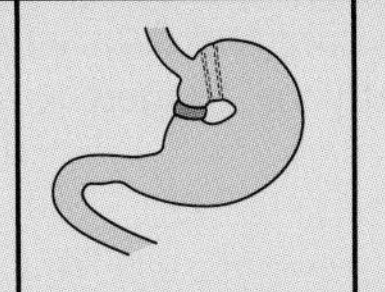	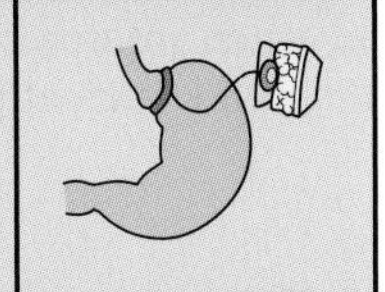
Weight loss % EBW % BMI	65–70 35	~70 ~35	50–60 25–30	50 25
NAFLD	SI	SI	SI except fibrosis, may get worse	SI
Diabetes	SI or R 65–95%	SI or R 65–95%	SI or R	I or R 40–65%
Operative Mortality Morbidity Complication	0.5–1% 5% Stomach dilation, ventral hernia	1% 5% Malabsorption Increased AST/ALT, resolve after 6 mos	0.1% 5% Food/pill impaction Outlet obstruction	0.1% 5% Gastric prolapse, stomal obstruction, pouch dilation
Type	Restrictive/malabsorptive	Malabsorptive/restrictive	Restrictive	Restrictive
Use in the United States	87%	2%	1.4%	9%

Fig. 53-19 Surgical weight loss. Some of the different types of weight loss surgeries, their benefit in patients with nonalcoholic fatty liver disease *(NAFLD)* and diabetes, and associated risks and complications are summarized. As shown, the most common type of procedure in the United States is RYGBP. ALT, alanine transaminase; AST, aspartate transaminase; BMI, body mass index; BPD-DS, biliopancreatic diversion with duodenal switch; EBW, excess body weight; I, improvement; LAGB, laparoscopic adjustable gastric banding; R, resolved; RYGBP, Roux-en-Y gastric bypass; SI, significant improvement; VBG, vertical band gastroplasty

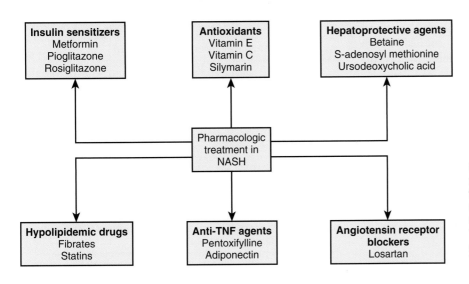

Insulin sensitizers
Metformin
Pioglitazone
Rosiglitazone

Antioxidants
Vitamin E
Vitamin C
Silymarin

Hepatoprotective agents
Betaine
S-adenosyl methionine
Ursodeoxycholic acid

Pharmacologic treatment in NASH

Hypolipidemic drugs
Fibrates
Statins

Anti-TNF agents
Pentoxifylline
Adiponectin

Angiotensin receptor blockers
Losartan

Fig. 53-20 Pharmacologic approach to the management of nonalcoholic steatohepatitis *(NASH).* Several drugs under different categories have been investigated for the treatment of NASH, with some encouraging results. Theses agents remain experimental until approved by the Food and Drug Administration. TNF, tumor necrosis factor

Thiazolidinediones

This class of drugs acts via PPAR-γ and improves insulin sensitivity.[202,203,255-258] A small nonrandomized trial of troglitazone demonstrated an improvement in ALT in 9 of 10 subjects and improvement in inflammatory scores in 5 subjects. Troglitazone has also been shown to be beneficial in those with NAFLD associated with lipodystrophy. Recent pilot trials support the use of thiazolidinediones for NASH. These are the basis for a large ongoing NIH-sponsored clinical trial. Caution should be exercised when interpreting these data because of the small number of subjects. In a recent trial, the greatest benefit of rosiglitazone was seen on hepatic steatosis, whereas the effects on cytologic ballooning and inflammation were less impressive. Thiazolidinediones also cause weight gain that is not lost when use of the drugs is discontinued. In addition, on discontinuation, liver histology returns to baseline. Given the potential risk for hepatotoxicity with these drugs, one must exercise caution when interpreting the data with these drugs, and their use should currently be limited to clinical trials only.

Lipid-Lowering Agents

In one controlled trial, clofibrate had no beneficial effects on liver function or hepatic histology, whereas in another small controlled trial, gemfibrozil improved liver chemistry.[259] However, no histologic data are available from the latter study. Thus, in general, such agents are not used for the treatment of NASH.

Vitamin E

In one published series of 11 pediatric patients with NASH who received vitamin E (*d*-α-tocopherol), 400 to 1200 IU, ALT improved.[202,260,261] However, no follow-up liver histologic evaluation was available from this study, which limits knowledge about whether this was a cosmetic effect or whether the hepatic histology was indeed improved. In a recent study we found that 400 IU of *d*-α-tocopherol improved hepatic steatosis significantly but only produced a trend toward improvement in other histologic parameters. In a single pilot study, a combination of vitamin E and C (1000 IU of vitamin E and 1000 mg/day of vitamin C) improved hepatic fibrosis but did not affect inflammation.

Ursodeoxycholate

Ursodeoxycholate (UDCA) is a hydrophilic bile acid that is associated with hepatoprotective properties. In one study, UDCA produced improvement in liver enzymes and a decrease in hepatic steatosis.[262] The long-term benefits of UDCA and the optimal dose of UDCA remain to be established. A 1996 randomized clinical trial was unable to establish the benefits of UDCA for NASH.[263]

Taurine

Taurine is believed to function as a lipotropic factor and to improve the mobilization of hepatic fat. In another single uncontrolled series, 10 children treated with taurine supplements orally had radiologic resolution of their fatty liver.[264] Radiologic improvement was accompanied by a decrease in glycine/taurine-conjugated bile acids.

Betaine

Betaine is a precursor of *S*-adenosylmethionine, a hepatoprotective factor. In one study, 10 subjects received anhydrous betaine for 12 months in two daily divided doses. Seven of 10 subjects completed 1 year of treatment. In this group, an improvement in aminotransferase activity, as well as liver histology, was noted.[265,266] Similar data were reported in another study in which betaine was administered along with diethanolamine glucuronate and nicotinamide ascorbate.[267] In a recent randomized placebo-control study, 55 patients with biopsy-proven NASH received oral betaine (20 g daily).

Patients randomized to betaine had a decrease in steatosis grade without a significant change in intragroup or intergroup differences in NAS or fibrosis stage. Moreover, there was no significant change in adiponectin, insulin, glucose, proinflammatory cytokines, and oxidant stress in NASH patients receiving betaine therapy.[266]

Pentoxifylline

Pentoxifylline antagonizes TNF-α and is orally available for long-term use. In two small pilot studies,[268,269] ALT improved after several months of treatment at a dose of 400 mg three times a day. However, histologic data are not available. In addition, although the drug was well tolerated in one study, 9 of 20 subjects in the other study dropped out because of side effects, especially nausea. Several trials are currently under way to confirm these initial findings.

Losartan

Angiotensin II has been implicated in HSC activation and matrix production.[270] In a small pilot study of an angiotensin receptor blocker, losartan, an improvement in ALT was noted.[271] These data also require validation in large-scale studies before any recommendations can be made.

Key References

Abdelmalek MF, et al. Familial aggregation of insulin resistance in first-degree relatives of patients with nonalcoholic fatty liver disease. Clin Gastroenterol Hepatol 2006;4:1162–1169. (Ref.56)

Abdelmalek MF, et al. Betaine for nonalcoholic fatty liver disease: results of a randomized placebo-controlled trial. Hepatology 2009;50:1818–1826. (Ref.266)

Abrams GA, et al. Portal fibrosis and hepatic steatosis in morbidly obese subjects: a spectrum of nonalcoholic fatty liver disease. Hepatology 2004;40:475–483. (Ref.9)

Adachi M, Brenner DA. High molecular weight adiponectin inhibits proliferation of hepatic stellate cells via activation of adenosine monophosphate–activated protein kinase. Hepatology 2008;47:677–685. (Ref.205)

Adams LA, et al. The natural history of nonalcoholic fatty liver disease: a population-based cohort study. Gastroenterology 2005;129:113–121. (Ref.239)

Adams LA, et al. The histological course of nonalcoholic fatty liver disease: a longitudinal study of 103 patients with sequential liver biopsies. J Hepatol 2005;42:132–138. (Ref.242)

Aller R, et al. Influence of insulin resistance and adipokines in the grade of steatosis of nonalcoholic fatty liver disease. Dig Dis Sci 2008;53:1088–1092. (Ref.88)

Alvarez Cosmea A, et al. [Differences in the prevalence of metabolic syndrome according to the ATP-III and WHO definitions.] Med Clin (Barc) 2005;124:368–370. (Ref.27)

Balasubramanyam A, et al. Pathophysiology of dyslipidemia and increased cardiovascular risk in HIV lipodystrophy: a model of "systemic steatosis." Curr Opin Lipidol 2004;15:59–67. (Ref.65)

Baldan A, et al. ATP-binding cassette transporter G1 and lipid homeostasis. Curr Opin Lipidol 2006;17:227–232. (Ref.101)

Belfort R, et al. A placebo-controlled trial of pioglitazone in subjects with nonalcoholic steatohepatitis. N Engl J Med 2006;355:2297–2307. (Ref.257)

Belfort R, et al. Dose-response effect of elevated plasma free fatty acid on insulin signaling. Diabetes 2005;54:1640–1648. (Ref.148)

Bellentani S, et al. The epidemiology of fatty liver. Eur J Gastroenterol Hepatol 2004;16:1087–1093. (Ref.39)

Bilzer M, Roggel F, Gerbes AL. Role of Kupffer cells in host defense and liver disease. Liver Int 2006;26:1175–1186. (Ref.194)

Browning JD, et al. Prevalence of hepatic steatosis in an urban population in the United States: impact of ethnicity. Hepatology 2004;40:1387–1395. (Ref.37)

Bugianesi E, et al. A randomized controlled trial of metformin versus vitamin E or prescriptive diet in nonalcoholic fatty liver disease. Am J Gastroenterol 2005;100:1082–1090. (Ref.254)

Bugianesi E, et al. Plasma adiponectin in nonalcoholic fatty liver is related to hepatic insulin resistance and hepatic fat content, not to liver disease severity. J Clin Endocrinol Metab 2005;90:3498–3504. (Ref.76)

Burns MP, et al. The effects of ABCA1 on cholesterol efflux and Abeta levels in vitro and in vivo. J Neurochem 2006;98:792–800. (Ref.146)

Cai D, et al. Local and systemic insulin resistance resulting from hepatic activation of IKK-beta and NF-kappaB. Nat Med 2005;11:183–190. (Ref.93)

Caligiuri A, et al. Adenosine monophosphate–activated protein kinase modulates the activated phenotype of hepatic stellate cells. Hepatology 2008;47:668–676. (Ref.206)

Cha JY, Repa JJ. The liver X receptor (LXR) and hepatic lipogenesis. The carbohydrate-response element–binding protein is a target gene of LXR. J Biol Chem 2007;282:743–751. (Ref.104)

Charlton M, et al. Low circulating levels of dehydroepiandrosterone in histologically advanced nonalcoholic fatty liver disease. Hepatology 2008;47:484–492. (Ref.168)

Cheung O, et al. The impact of fat distribution on the severity of nonalcoholic fatty liver disease and metabolic syndrome. Hepatology 2007;46:1091–1100. (Ref.214)

Clark JM. The epidemiology of nonalcoholic fatty liver disease in adults. J Clin Gastroenterol 2006;40(Suppl 1):S5–S10. (Ref.38)

Conti A, et al. Expression of the tumor necrosis factor receptor–associated factors 1 and 2 and regulation of the nuclear factor-kappaB antiapoptotic activity in human gliomas. J Neurosurg 2005;103:873–881. (Ref.78)

Dey D, et al. Involvement of novel PKC isoforms in FFA induced defects in insulin signaling. Mol Cell Endocrinol 2006;246:60–64. (Ref.149)

Diehl AM. Lessons from animal models of NASH. Hepatol Res 2005;33:138–144. (Ref.79)

Donnelly KL, et al. Sources of fatty acids stored in liver and secreted via lipoproteins in patients with nonalcoholic fatty liver disease. J Clin Invest 2005;115:1343–1351. (Ref.140)

Evans JL, Maddux BA, Goldfine ID. The molecular basis for oxidative stress–induced insulin resistance. Antioxid Redox Signal 2005;7:1040–1052. (Ref.172)

Fantuzzi G. Adipose tissue, adipokines, and inflammation. J Allergy Clin Immunol 2005;115:911–919; quiz 920. (Ref.75)

Fishbein M, et al. Hepatic MRI for fat quantitation: its relationship to fat morphology, diagnosis, and ultrasound. J Clin Gastroenterol 2005;39:619–625. (Ref.35)

Fontana L, et al. Visceral fat adipokine secretion is associated with systemic inflammation in obese humans. Diabetes 2007;56:1010–1013. (Ref.91)

Gaidos JK, Hillner BE, Sanyal AJ. A decision analysis study of the value of a liver biopsy in nonalcoholic steatohepatitis. Liver Int 2008;28:650–658. (Ref.233)

Gastaldelli A, et al. Importance of changes in adipose tissue insulin resistance to histological response during thiazolidinedione treatment of patients with nonalcoholic steatohepatitis. Hepatology 2009;50:1087–1093. (Ref.258)

Handschin C, Meyer UA. Regulatory network of lipid-sensing nuclear receptors: roles for CAR, PXR, LXR, and FXR. Arch Biochem Biophys 2005;433:387–396. (Ref.100)

Hanley AJ, et al. Liver markers and development of the metabolic syndrome: the insulin resistance atherosclerosis study. Diabetes 2005;54:3140–3147. (Ref.216)

Harada K, et al. Epithelial-mesenchymal transition induced by biliary innate immunity contributes to the sclerosing cholangiopathy of biliary atresia. J Pathol 2009;217:654–664. (Ref.212)

Harrison SA, et al. Orlistat for overweight subjects with nonalcoholic steatohepatitis: A randomized, prospective trial. Hepatology 2009;49:80–86. (Ref.251)

Harsch IA, Hahn EG, Konturek PC. Insulin resistance and other metabolic aspects of the obstructive sleep apnea syndrome. Med Sci Monit 2005;11:RA70–RA75. (Ref.222)

Hossain P, Kawar B, El Nahas M. Obesity and diabetes in the developing world—a growing challenge. N Engl J Med 2007;356:213–215. (Ref.24)

Hunt KJ, et al. National Cholesterol Education Program versus World Health Organization metabolic syndrome in relation to all-cause and cardiovascular mortality in the San Antonio Heart Study. Circulation 2004;110:1251–1257. (Ref.30)

Hurwitz BE, et al. HIV, metabolic syndrome X, inflammation, oxidative stress, and coronary heart disease risk: role of protease inhibitor exposure. Cardiovasc Toxicol 2004;4:303–316. (Ref.69)

Jarrar MH, et al. Adipokines and cytokines in non-alcoholic fatty liver disease. Aliment Pharmacol Ther 2008;27:412–421. (Ref.81)

Kabir M, et al. Molecular evidence supporting the portal theory: a causative link between visceral adiposity and hepatic insulin resistance. Am J Physiol Endocrinol Metab 2005;288:E454–E461. (Ref.128)

Kleiner DE, et al. Design and validation of a histological scoring system for nonalcoholic fatty liver disease. Hepatology 2005;41:1313–1321. (Ref.12)

Kola B, et al. Expanding role of AMPK in endocrinology. Trends Endocrinol Metab 2006;17:205–215. (Ref.142)

Kotronen A, et al. Liver fat is increased in type 2 diabetic patients and underestimated by serum alanine aminotransferase compared with equally obese nondiabetic subjects. Diabetes Care 2008;31:165–169. (Ref.43)

Kunde SS, et al. Spectrum of NAFLD and diagnostic implications of the proposed new normal range for serum ALT in obese women. Hepatology 2005;42:650–656. (Ref.40)

Lackner C, et al. Ballooned hepatocytes in steatohepatitis: the value of keratin immunohistochemistry for diagnosis. J Hepatol 2008;48:821–828. (Ref.176)

Lazo M, Clark JM. The epidemiology of nonalcoholic fatty liver disease: a global perspective. Semin Liver Dis 2008;28:339–350. (Ref.31)

Lefkowitch JH. Morphology of alcoholic liver disease. Clin Liver Dis 2005;9:37–53. (Ref.17)

Lin J, et al. Hyperlipidemic effects of dietary saturated fats mediated through PGC-1beta coactivation of SREBP. Cell 2005;120:261–273. (Ref.115)

Ma L, Robinson LN, Towle HC. ChREBP*Mlx is the principal mediator of glucose-induced gene expression in the liver. J Biol Chem 2006;281:28721–28730. (Ref.103)

Malhi H, Gores GJ. Molecular mechanisms of lipotoxicity in nonalcoholic fatty liver disease. Semin Liver Dis 2008;28:360–369. (Ref.180)

Malhi H, Gores GJ, Lemasters JJ. Apoptosis and necrosis in the liver: a tale of two deaths? Hepatology 2006;43:S31–S44. (Ref.186)

Marchesini G, et al. WHO and ATPIII proposals for the definition of the metabolic syndrome in patients with type 2 diabetes. Diabet Med 2004;21:383–387. (Ref.26)

Mari M, et al. Mitochondrial free cholesterol loading sensitizes to TNF- and Fas-mediated steatohepatitis. Cell Metab 2006;4:185–198. (Ref.169)

Miele L, et al. The Kruppel-like factor 6 genotype is associated with fibrosis in nonalcoholic fatty liver disease. Gastroenterology 2008;135:282–291, e1. (Ref.57)

Mitro N, et al. The nuclear receptor LXR is a glucose sensor. Nature 2007;445:219–223. (Ref.105)

Nguyen MT, et al. JNK and tumor necrosis factor-alpha mediate free fatty acid–induced insulin resistance in 3T3-L1 adipocytes. J Biol Chem 2005;280:35361–35371. (Ref.190)

Nieuwdorp M, et al. Hypercoagulability in the metabolic syndrome. Curr Opin Pharmacol 2005;5:155–159. (Ref.224)

Nomura K, et al. Efficacy and effectiveness of liver screening program to detect fatty liver in the periodic health check-ups. J Occup Health 2004;46:423–428. (Ref.32)

Ong JP, et al. Predictors of nonalcoholic steatohepatitis and advanced fibrosis in morbidly obese patients. Obes Surg 2005;15:310–315. (Ref.51)

Osei-Hyiaman D, et al. Endocannabinoid activation at hepatic CB1 receptors stimulates fatty acid synthesis and contributes to diet-induced obesity. J Clin Invest 2005;115:1298–1305. (Ref.211)

Pacher P, et al. Modulation of the endocannabinoid system in cardiovascular disease: therapeutic potential and limitations. Hypertension 2008;52:601–607. (Ref.122)

Pagano C, et al. Increased serum resistin in nonalcoholic fatty liver disease is related to liver disease severity and not to insulin resistance. J Clin Endocrinol Metab 2006;91:1081–1086. (Ref.90)

Parfieniuk A, Flisiak R. Role of cannabinoids in chronic liver diseases. World J Gastroenterol 2008;14:6109–6114. (Ref.208)

Patton HM, et al. The impact of steatosis on disease progression and early and sustained treatment response in chronic hepatitis C patients. J Hepatol 2004;40:484–490. (Ref.68)

Puri P, et al. Activation and dysregulation of the unfolded protein response in nonalcoholic fatty liver disease. Gastroenterology 2008;134:568–576. (Ref.184)

Ramalho RM, et al. Apoptosis and Bcl-2 expression in the livers of patients with steatohepatitis. Eur J Gastroenterol Hepatol 2006;18:21–29. (Ref.185)

Ramesh S, Sanyal AJ. Evaluation and management of non-alcoholic steatohepatitis. J Hepatol 2005;42(Suppl):S2–S12. (Ref.223)

Ratziu V, et al. Sampling variability of liver biopsy in nonalcoholic fatty liver disease. Gastroenterology 2005;128:1898–1906. (Ref.14)

Ruiz AG, et al. Lipopolysaccharide-binding protein plasma levels and liver TNF-alpha gene expression in obese patients: evidence for the potential role of endotoxin in the pathogenesis of non-alcoholic steatohepatitis. Obes Surg 2007;17:1374–1380. (Ref.195)

Sampath H, Ntambi JM. Polyunsaturated fatty acid regulation of genes of lipid metabolism. Annu Rev Nutr 2005;25:317–340. (Ref.143)

Sanyal AJ, et al. Similarities and differences in outcomes of cirrhosis due to nonalcoholic steatohepatitis and hepatitis C. Hepatology 2006;43:682–689. (Ref.238)

Schwimmer JB, et al. Histopathology of pediatric nonalcoholic fatty liver disease. Hepatology 2005;42:641–649. (Ref.10)

Siegmund SV, et al. Anandamide induces necrosis in primary hepatic stellate cells. Hepatology 2005;41:1085–1095. (Ref.201)

Stefan N, et al. High circulating retinol-binding protein 4 is associated with elevated liver fat but not with total, subcutaneous, visceral, or intramyocellular fat in humans. Diabetes Care 2007;30:1173–1178. (Ref.121)

Sterling RK, et al. Impact of highly active antiretroviral therapy on the spectrum of liver disease in HCV-HIV coinfection. Clin Gastroenterol Hepatol 2004; 2:432–439. (Ref.70)

Stranges S, et al. Body fat distribution, liver enzymes, and risk of hypertension: evidence from the Western New York Study. Hypertension 2005;46:1186–1193. (Ref.218)

Tanne F, et al. Chronic liver injury during obstructive sleep apnea. Hepatology 2005;41:1290–1296. (Ref.220)

Targher G, et al. Nonalcoholic fatty liver disease is independently associated with an increased incidence of cardiovascular events in type 2 diabetic patients. Diabetes Care 2007;30:2119–2121. (Ref.219)

Teixeira-Clerc F, et al. CB1 cannabinoid receptor antagonism: a new strategy for the treatment of liver fibrosis. Nat Med 2006;12:671–676. (Ref.209)

Thomas EL, et al. Hepatic triglyceride content and its relation to body adiposity: a magnetic resonance imaging and proton magnetic resonance spectroscopy study. Gut 2005;54:122–127. (Ref.36)

Thuy S, et al. Nonalcoholic fatty liver disease in humans is associated with increased plasma endotoxin and plasminogen activator inhibitor 1 concentrations and with fructose intake. J Nutr 2008;138:1452–1455. (Ref.196)

Timlin MT, Parks EJ. Temporal pattern of de novo lipogenesis in the postprandial state in healthy men. Am J Clin Nutr 2005;81:35–42. (Ref.139)

Tolman KG, et al. Narrative review: hepatobiliary disease in type 2 diabetes mellitus. Ann Intern Med 2004;141:946–956. (Ref.42)

Trayhurn P, Bing C, Wood IS. Adipose tissue and adipokines—energy regulation from the human perspective. J Nutr 2006;136:1935S–1939S. (Ref.85)

Turnbaugh PJ, et al. A core gut microbiome in obese and lean twins. Nature 2009;457:480–484. (Ref.197)

Ueki K, Kadowaki T, Kahn CR. Role of suppressors of cytokine signaling SOCS-1 and SOCS-3 in hepatic steatosis and the metabolic syndrome. Hepatol Res 2005;33:185–192. (Ref.150)

van der Poorten D, et al. Visceral fat: a key mediator of steatohepatitis in metabolic liver disease. Hepatology 2008;48:449–457. (Ref.92)

Van Gaal LF, et al. Long-term effect of CB1 blockade with rimonabant on cardiometabolic risk factors: two year results from the RIO-Europe Study. Eur Heart J 2008;29:1761–1771. (Ref.123)

Wilfred de Alwis NM, Day CP. Genes and nonalcoholic fatty liver disease. Curr Diab Rep 2008;8:156–163. (Ref.58)

Wolfrum C, Stoffel M. Coactivation of Foxa2 through Pgc-1beta promotes liver fatty acid oxidation and triglyceride/VLDL secretion. Cell Metab 2006;3:99–110. (Ref.113)

Wu H, et al. Serum retinol binding protein 4 and nonalcoholic fatty liver disease in patients with type 2 diabetes mellitus. Diabetes Res Clin Pract 2008;79:185–190. (Ref.120)

Yaggi HK, Araujo AB, McKinlay JB. Sleep duration as a risk factor for the development of type 2 diabetes. Diabetes Care 2006;29:657–661. (Ref.221)

Yang Q, et al. Serum retinol binding protein 4 contributes to insulin resistance in obesity and type 2 diabetes. Nature 2005;436:356–362. (Ref.119)

Yip WW, Burt AD. Alcoholic liver disease. Semin Diagn Pathol 2006;23:149–160. (Ref.18)

Zatloukal K, et al. From Mallory to Mallory-Denk bodies: what, how and why? Exp Cell Res 2007;313:2033–2049. (Ref.178)

Zhang K, Kaufman RJ. The unfolded protein response: a stress signaling pathway critical for health and disease. Neurology 2006;66:S102–S109. (Ref.183)

A complete list of references can be found at www.expertconsult.com.

The Liver in Systemic Illness

Jayant A. Talwalkar

Introduction

A number of systemic conditions affecting other organs can produce signs and symptoms that are indistinguishable from primary liver disease. The hepatic manifestations in these disorders may range from mild enzyme abnormalities to significant liver injury and liver failure. In this chapter, we will review liver involvement in selected systemic disorders originating from the cardiovascular, connective tissue, hematologic, gastrointestinal, endocrine, and oncologic systems. Other systemic disorders with hepatic involvement, such as granulomatous systemic diseases including sarcoidosis and sepsis, are covered elsewhere in this textbook.

Cardiovascular Disease

Liver involvement occurs in patients with both acute and chronic heart disease and its spectrum ranges from asymptomatic increases in liver biochemical values to fulminant liver failure. The liver receives a significant portion of the cardiac output. In turn, conditions that reduce cardiac output will lead to a decrease in hepatic perfusion. The liver compensates for changes in hepatic blood flow via vasoactive mechanisms and by increasing oxygen extraction during periods of hepatic hypoperfusion.[1] However, when critical levels of left or right heart failure are reached, hepatic injury may occur.

Congestive Hepatopathy

The effects of congestive heart failure on the liver result from three pathogenic factors: decreased hepatic blood flow, increased hepatic venous pressure, and decreased arterial oxygen saturation. Elevated central venous pressure is transmitted by the hepatic veins to the small hepatic venules that drain hepatic acini. This results in atrophy of zone 3 hepatocytes.[2] Elevated hepatic venous pressure also results in sinusoidal congestion and enlargement of the sinusoidal fenestrae, allowing protein-rich fluid to move into the space of Disse. The resulting perisinusoidal edema may impair diffusion of oxygen and nutrients to hepatocytes.[2,3] Excess fluid in the space of Disse can be drained into hepatic lymphatics, but exudes from the surface of the liver into the peritoneal cavity when the lymphatic system is overwhelmed. This exudation may result in the high-protein ascites seen among patients with congestive hepatopathy.[3] Sustained passive congestion can result in zone 3 liver fibrosis, and the degree of fibrosis is variable throughout the parenchyma.[4] As cardiac output declines further, compensatory mechanisms become inadequate, and hypoxia ensues.

Clinical Manifestations

In a large study of 175 patients with both acute and chronic right heart failure,[5] physical examination showed hepatomegaly in more than 90% and splenomegaly in 20% of these patients. Other findings of right heart failure, such as peripheral edema, pleural effusion, and ascites, were also frequently present. Ascites is more prominent in patients with chronic right heart failure than in those with acute right heart failure (**Table 54-1**).

Several signs and symptoms of congestive heart failure (e.g., ascites, pedal edema, mild hyperbilirubinemia) may be difficult to distinguish from patients with decompensated hepatic cirrhosis. In a prospective study of 13 patients with cardiac ascites, the serum ascites albumin concentration gradient was

Table 54-1 Symptoms and Signs of Congested Livers in 175 Patients with Right-Side Heart Failure

SYMPTOM/SIGN	ACUTE HEART FAILURE (%)	CHRONIC HEART FAILURE (%)
Hepatomegaly	99	95
Peripheral edema	77	71
Pleural effusion	25	17
Splenomegaly	20	22
Ascites	7	20

Adapted from Richman SM, Delman AJ, Grob D. Alterations in indices of liver function in congestive heart failure with particular reference to serum enzymes. Am J Med 1961;30:211.

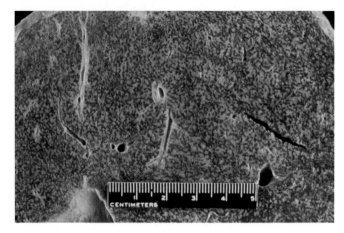

Fig. 54-1 **"Nutmeg" liver.** In chronic passive congestion of the liver, red cells pool and distend the sinuses around the central vein. These regions develop a darker red-violet color, in contrast to the surrounding tan liver parenchyma. This color stippling is reminiscent of the cut surface of a nutmeg.

1.1 g/dl and the total protein concentration was 2.5 g/dl.[6] Additionally, the ascitic fluid associated with cardiac ascites had significantly higher red blood cell counts and higher levels of lactate dehydrogenase. The degree of liver damage and the ensuing changes in related hemodynamic parameters do not seem to correlate with the amount of ascites in congestive heart failure.[5] Physical examination may reveal a pulsatile liver in patients with tricuspid valve disease. Loss of hepatic pulsatility in patients with long-standing congestive hepatopathy suggests progression to cardiac cirrhosis. The congested liver is usually enlarged and firm, often associated with slight enlargement of the spleen.

Congestive hepatopathy is often associated with serum liver test abnormalities. Modest elevations in levels of aspartate aminotransferase (AST), alanine aminotransferase (ALT), lactate dehydrogenase (LDH), γ-glutamyltransferase (GGT), and alkaline phosphatase are often noticed in patients with congestive hepatopathy.[7,8] Serum liver test elevations appear most commonly when the cardiac index less than 1.5 L/min/m^2.

Hyperbilirubinema occurs in more than 20% of patients.[5] The elevation is usually less than 3 mg/dl and composed predominantly of unconjugated bilirubin.[9] Jaundice increases with prolonged and repeated bouts of congestive heart failure.[7,8] When jaundice is accompanied by significantly elevated levels of serum aminotransferase in patients with acute cardiac decompensation, the clinical presentation may simulate that of acute viral hepatitis.[10,11] Multiple factors—including hepatocellular dysfunction, hemolysis, pulmonary infarction, canalicular obstruction with bile thrombi, and medications—are often associated with hyperbilirubinemia. Serum albumin levels are decreased in more than 30% of patients with values rarely less than 2.5 g/dl. The degree of hypoalbuminemia does not correlate with the degree of histologic liver damage. Serum prothrombin time values are usually normal.

Liver histologic specimens from patients with congestive hepatopathy exhibit several unique features when compared with histologic specimens of patients with primary liver diseases. On gross inspection, the congested liver will be enlarged with blunt edges.[6] The liver is often described as having a "nutmeg" appearance caused by alternating areas of normal-appearing parenchyma contrasting with congested, hemorrhagic areas (**Fig. 54-1**). Microscopic examination of the liver

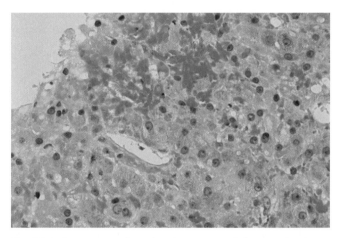

Fig. 54-2 **Liver congestion.** The sinuses around the central vein are distended by normal red cells. As the severity of this lesion increases, the adjacent hepatocytes become atrophic (Hematoxylin and eosin [H & E] stain).

may reveal sinusoidal engorgement, degeneration, and variable degrees of hemorrhagic necrosis in zone 3 (**Fig. 54-2**).

Additional features include steatosis and cholestasis with bile thrombi in the canaliculi (see **Fig. 54-2**). As the damage progresses with chronic or recurrent episodes of heart failure, there is collapse of the central vein reticulin network and degeneration of zone 3 hepatocytes. This creates the deposition of collagen in fibrotic bands that radiates outward from the central vein. Extension of these bands toward central veins and portal regions culminates in the development of cardiac cirrhosis (see Treatment and Prognosis).[7] The degree of cardiac decompensation or its duration is not strongly associated with the degree of hepatic fibrosis. Clinical manifestations, such as jaundice, splenomegaly, and ascites, also do not correlate with histologic results.[7,12]

Treatment and Prognosis

Treatment of the underlying heart disease may improve congestive hepatopathy. Jaundice, hepatic congestion, and ascites

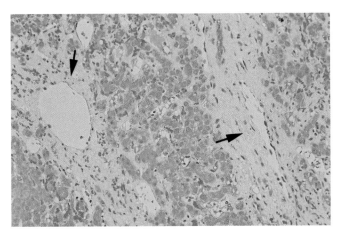

Fig. 54-3 **Cardiac cirrhosis.** Dense fibrous bands emanate from the central veins *(arrows)* to surround a nodule of regenerating hepatocytes (Trichrome stain).

may respond dramatically to diuretic therapy. In patients with severely impaired cardiac output, excessive diuresis may reduce hepatic perfusion and precipitate further necrosis in zone 3 hepatocytes. The treatment of refractory ascites in cardiac cirrhosis involves large-volume paracentesis with albumin replacement. Peritoneovenous shunts should not be offered as an alternative for treatment, and transjugular intrahepatic portosystemic shunt (TIPS) placement is generally contraindicated because shunting of portal venous blood to the right heart may increase pulmonary arterial pressure and precipitate heart failure. Other complications of portal hypertension are managed according to recommendations for noncardiac etiologies of cirrhosis.[12]

The prognosis of patients with congestive hepatopathy is related to the degree of underlying cardiac dysfunction. Effective medical management of heart failure may also resolve early histologic changes of passive hepatic congestion. Prolonged hepatic congestion may result in cardiac cirrhosis. The major causes of cardiac cirrhosis are ischemic heart disease (31%), cardiomyopathy (23%), valvular heart disease (23%), restrictive lung disease (15%), and pericardial disease (8%).[8] Cardiac cirrhosis itself does not confer a poor prognosis because jaundice and hepatic synthetic function can be similar in patients with cardiac cirrhosis or simple passive congestion (**Fig. 54-3**). [7,12] Several cases of fulminant hepatic failure with coma have been reported to occur secondary to congestive heart failure.[12,13] Most, but not all, of these cases occurred in the setting of superimposed shock, and all cases seem to have been caused by hepatic ischemia rather than passive congestion alone.

Ischemic Hepatitis

Ischemic hepatitis can be defined as hepatocellular necrosis associated with a decrease in hepatic perfusion.[14-16] This condition affects all age groups, although it is most frequently reported in older adults.[17] The most commonly reported risk factor for the development of ischemic hepatitis is cardiogenic shock from myocardial infarction, arrhythmia, or cardiac tamponade. Episodes of hypotension resulting in ischemic hepatitis are usually brief when documented. Although diminished hepatic perfusion from systemic hypotension appears to

be essential, a recent study suggested that systemic hypotension or shock alone is insufficient to cause ischemic hepatitis.[18] Furthermore, there may be different mechanisms responsible for hypoxic hepatitis based on noncardiac etiologies, such as respiratory failure and sepsis, that may also be responsible for ischemic hepatitis. In a recent study a shock state was observed in only about 50% of documented cases.[18] Other causes of ischemic hepatitis include hypovolemic shock from hemorrhage, dehydration, and heat stroke.[19-21]

The pathophysiology of ischemic hepatitis is determined by the relationship between hepatic blood flow and liver oxygen status. Of the total hepatic blood flow 70% is derived from the portal venous system, whereas the remaining 30% is delivered by the hepatic artery.[8] Hepatic oxygen delivery is dependent on total hepatic blood flow. As hepatic blood flow declines in proportion to a reduction in cardiac output, the liver compensates by increasing the extraction of oxygen. This process usually maintains oxygenation of hepatocytes in zones 1 and 2 but not in zone 3.[16] This remarkable compensatory mechanism most likely accounts for the low incidence of liver damage in shock states. In contrast, the presence of congestive hepatopathy from heart failure appears to render the liver susceptible to acute ischemic injury. Reduced cardiac output in patients with this condition leads to an approximate threefold decrease in total hepatic blood flow.[1] In a recent clinical study, all patients with a clinical diagnosis of ischemic hepatitis were found to have clinically significant cardiac disease (94% had right-side heart failure) as compared with a group of patients with trauma and documented hypotension (**Table 54-2**).[18]

Clinical Manifestations

The clinical presentation of ischemic hepatitis is often masked by the overall disease state in which it occurs. Fluctuations in serum liver enzyme levels are commonly observed. Serum AST and ALT levels rise rapidly after an ischemic episode and peak within 1 to 3 days. Serum ALT and AST activities are strikingly elevated and may exceed 200 times the upper limits of normal (**Fig. 54-4**). With treatment of the underlying illness, levels of serum aminotransferases usually return to nearly normal within 7 to 10 days of the initial insult. In many cases, a 30% to 50% reduction in serum aminotransferase levels every 24 to 48 hours is highly indicative of uncomplicated ischemic hepatitis. Persistent elevation of serum aminotransferase levels beyond this period implies a poor prognosis because of continued hepatic hypoperfusion. Less marked elevations (<500 U/L) have also been reported in biopsyproven ischemic hepatitis. Serum LDH activity is also markedly elevated and parallels serum aminotransferase activity. Marked elevations of alkaline phosphatase level or serum bilirubin level are unusual in ischemic hepatitis.[18,22]

The pathologic hallmark of ischemic hepatitis is centrilobular (zone 3) necrosis in the absence of significant inflammation.[18,23] With prolonged ischemia, central hepatocyte necrosis can extend to the midzonal hepatocytes.[24] Gibson and Dudley studied 17 patients with these characteristic histologic findings and concluded that a diagnosis of ischemic hepatitis could be made without a liver biopsy in the appropriate clinical setting (i.e., patients who had a potential cause for a drop in cardiac output and a rapid rise in serum aminotransferase levels).[22]

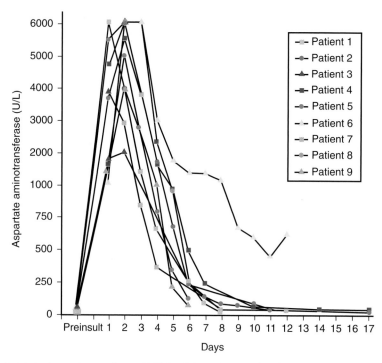

Fig. 54-4 Ischemic hepatitis. Serial alanine aminotransferase (ALT) levels in patients with ischemic hepatitis. *(Adapted from Gitlin N, Serio KM. Ischemic hepatitis: widening horizons. Am J Gastroenterol 1992;87:831, with permission.)*

Table 54-2 Liver Tests of 175 Patients with Right-Side Heart Failure

LIVER TESTS	ACUTE HEART FAILURE		CHRONIC HEART FAILURE	
	N	*Abnormal (%)*	*N*	*Abnormal (%)*
Bilirubin	86	37	57	21
BSP retention	71	87	55	71
Alkaline phosphatase	80	10	55	9
Aspartate aminotransferase	67	48	37	5
Alanine aminotransferase	53	15	29	3
Globulins	100	60	67	37
Prothrombin time	68	84	43	74
Albumin	100	32	67	27
Cholesterol	87	49	60	42

Adapted from Richman SM, Delman AJ, Grob D. Alterations in indices of liver function in congestive heart failure with particular reference to serum enzymes. Am J Med 1961;30:211.
BSP, bromosulfophthalein

Treatment and Prognosis

The treatment of ischemic hepatitis is directed at the underlying illness. Pharmacologic and interventional therapies to improve cardiac output may also improve hepatic perfusion with variable effects on ischemic hepatitis. Similarly, volume resuscitation for patients with hemorrhagic shock and appropriate treatment for septic shock will indirectly improve cardiac output and hepatic perfusion. Limited data suggest that intravenous dopamine leads to preservation of hepatic blood flow. However, it has not been demonstrated that dopamine improves serum liver enzyme values.[25] There are no data

to support the use of vitamin C, vitamin E, glutathione, and allopurinol.[12] Ischemic hepatitis is often a benign and self-limited condition. Hepatic synthetic function is often maintained. In some cases, the prothrombin time rarely is prolonged by more than 3 seconds. Although the peak serum aminotransferase levels do not seem to have any prognostic significance, the persistence of AST level elevation appears more common in patients who die in the setting of ischemic hepatitis.[14] The severity of the liver injury correlates with the duration and extent of the hemodynamic compromise, but the overall prognosis remains associated with the underlying systemic disease.[22] One-month death rates of 50% have been reported in patients with ischemic hepatitis.[26] Of note, fulminant hepatic failure also may result in patients with ischemic hepatitis that complicates cirrhosis, which is associated with death rates ranging from 60% to 100%.[27]

Constrictive Pericarditis and Restrictive Cardiomyopathy

Constrictive pericarditis is characterized by a thick, noncompliant pericardium. This results in decreased diastolic filling of the heart and the ensuing clinical syndrome of right heart failure. Common etiologies are viral pericarditis, previous cardiac surgery or radiation exposure, chronic inflammatory disease (systemic lupus erythematosus, rheumatoid arthritis), uremia, and malignancy.[28]

Restrictive cardiomyopathy involves reduced diastolic volumes of either or both ventricles with normal or near-normal systolic function.[29] Common causes include amyloidosis, sarcoidosis, hemochromatosis, scleroderma, endomyocardial fibrosis, hypereosinophilic syndrome, carcinoid syndrome, radiation exposure, malignancy, anthracycline toxicity, and idiopathic factors.[28]

Clinical Manifestations

In both conditions, symptoms may develop weeks to decades after an episode of pericarditis or cardiac trauma. Constrictive pericarditis can present with peripheral edema, abdominal swelling, and hepatomegaly. Physical examination may disclose pulsus paradoxus, pericardial knock, pulsatile hepatomegaly, splenomegaly, and ascites.[28] Of 231 cases from 4 studies during the 1950s,[30-33] an elevated jugular venous pulse (JVP) was identified in 96% and ascites in 57% of patients. It has been noted that ascites is more prominent than pedal edema.[28]

Using two-dimensional echocardiography, small ventricles with intact systolic function are seen in constrictive pericarditis, whereas restrictive cardiomyopathy is characterized by increased wall thickness of both ventricles.[28] With computed tomography (CT) and magnetic resonance (MR) imaging, a pericardial thickness of 4 mm (normal, <2 mm) or more is highly suggestive of constrictive pericarditis. Pericardial thickening may also be localized rather than diffuse.[34] CT imaging additionally detects pericardial calcification when present.[35] Invasive hemodynamic evaluation generally cannot distinguish between constrictive pericarditis and restrictive cardiomyopathy.[28]

The most distinctive feature that differentiates constrictive pericarditis from restrictive cardiomyopathy is pericardial thickening. However, the presence of a thickened pericardium does not always imply constriction because physiologic constriction may occur with a normal-appearing pericardium on imaging. Therefore hemodynamic documentation of constrictive/restrictive physiology by echocardiography is required as a first step to differentiate between the two disorders.[1] Note that in patients with clinical and hemodynamic features of restrictive cardiomyopathy, the presence of constrictive pericarditis must still be excluded.[28]

Although rarely performed once a diagnosis is made, liver biopsy in patients with either disorder reveals nonspecific histologic features including diffuse centrilobular congestion, necrosis, and fibrosis. Occasionally, there can be prominent sinusoidal dilation and hemorrhagic necrosis that can mimic histologic findings associated with Budd-Chiari syndrome.[36,37]

Treatment and Prognosis

Pericardiectomy (cardiac decortication) represents the treatment of choice for patients with constrictive pericarditis. The in-hospital death rate has been reported to vary between 0% and 10%,[38-40] with a 7-year survival rate after surgery approaching 87%. Pericardiectomy for radiation-related constriction has a higher complication rate and is an independent predictor of postoperative death.[41] In contrast, patients with established restrictive cardiomyopathy have a poor prognosis. Treatment is usually based on palliative care.[28]

Connective Tissue Diseases
Systemic Lupus Erythematosus

Systemic lupus erythematosus (SLE) is an autoimmune disorder involving the skin, kidneys, cardiovascular system, and central nervous system. Strict criteria reflecting multiorgan involvement have been established by the American College of Rheumatology, yet the presence of liver injury is not one of the criteria.[42]

Clinical Manifestations

Serum liver enzyme tests may be abnormal in 25% to 50% of patients at some time during the course of their illness.[43] From a study including more than 200 patients with SLE,[44] 21% of patients had abnormal liver enzyme levels that could not be attributed to other nonhepatic etiologies or conditions. In 20% of patients, the first elevations in liver enzyme levels were noted during an exacerbation of SLE. Elevations of serum aminotransferase and alkaline phosphatase levels were less than four-fold the upper limits of normal. However, approximately 25% of the patients developed jaundice with three patients dying from liver failure. In Rothfield's series of 365 SLE patients, abnormal measurements of serum liver enzymes were present at the time of diagnosis in 30% of cases.[45] Jaundice occurred in 25% of patients with SLE, hepatomegaly was found in 20% to 39%, splenomegaly in 6%, and ascites in 11% over the course of their lifetimes. In contrast, a review of Japanese autopsy registry data for 1468 patients with SLE found that evidence for chronic liver disease occurred in <5% of cases.[46] It should also be noted that these results are potentially confounded by several issues, such as the possibility of co-existent drug-induced liver injury and occult chronic hepatitis C infection.

Serum autoantibodies to ribosomal P proteins have been linked to patients with SLE and lupoid hepatitis.[43] However, a retrospective study by Fox and colleagues determined that unexplained deranged liver function tests were uncommon in their cohort of 200 patients with SLE (2.5%). They concluded these abnormalities were rarely of clinical significance and there was no association with ribosomal P antibodies.[47]

Table 54-3 Liver Disease Associated with Adult and Juvenile Rheumatoid Arthritis	
ADULT RHEUMATOID ARTHRITIS	**JUVENILE RHEUMATOID ARTHRITIS**
Hepatic steatosis	Acute hepatitis
Primary biliary cirrhosis	Chronic nonspecific hepatitis
Autoimmune hepatitis	Massive liver enlargement
Nodular regenerative hyperplasia	Drug toxicity
Amyloidosis	Salicylate or methotrexate hepatotoxicity

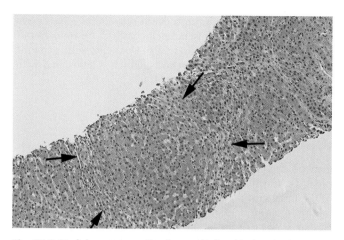

Fig. 54-5 **Nodular regenerative hyperplasia.** Thin bands of atrophic hepatocytes *(arrows)* outline a central focus of hepatocyte regeneration, producing a nodular appearance throughout the liver. The reticulin in the atrophic areas is condensed but there is no fibrosis (H & E stain).

Liver histologic findings in SLE are variable. Lobular inflammation with a paucity of lymphoid infiltrates has been described. When inflammatory cells are present, they are predominantly lymphocytes. Round cell infiltration of portal tracts, periportal hepatitis, and piecemeal necrosis have also been documented in SLE.[48,49] In an autopsy study of 52 patients with SLE,[46] an estimated 21% of patients had histologic evidence of arteritis.

The management of hepatitis related to SLE is based on treating the other manifestations of the disease. Increased immunosuppression with prednisone may be beneficial in reducing SLE-related ascites, once other causes have been carefully excluded.[50]

Rheumatoid Arthritis

Elevated concentrations of serum liver enzymes may occur in up to 6% of patients with rheumatoid arthritis (RA).[51,52] Specific increases in alkaline phosphatase and serum γ-glutamyltransferase levels, rather than serum aminotransferase levels, have also been described.[51] In studies of alkaline phosphatase fractionation tests, almost one third of patients with RA had elevated levels of hepatobiliary alkaline phosphatase, suggesting liver involvement. Other investigators have demonstrated that the degree of total alkaline phosphatase elevation varies with the number of joints involved[53] and changes over time.[54] As with SLE, drug-induced liver injury from salicylates, gold therapy, methotrexate, and other immunosuppressive/biologic agents may play a role in the liver abnormalities associated with RA (**Table 54-3**).[55]

Liver histologic studies in patients with RA and elevated levels of serum liver enzymes are usually nonspecific and include the findings of Kupffer cell hyperplasia, fatty cell infiltration, and infiltration of periportal areas with mononuclear cells.[56] Among 117 unselected patients with RA, an estimated 65% of cases had reactive hepatitis (43%) or fatty infiltration (22%) on biopsy even when normal serum enzyme levels were present.[52] Ruderman and associates[57] published an autopsy study of hepatic histology in 182 patients with RA. The most common finding was hepatic congestion, although it is likely that this lesion was a result of the terminal event. As in SLE, hepatic steatosis was common (23%), whereas 11% of patients had fibrosis, 5% showed evidence of amyloidosis, and 3% exhibited cirrhosis.

Felty syndrome (defined by the combination of RA, splenomegaly, and neutropenia) rarely involves the liver. Blendis and colleagues reported that 5 of 12 patients in their series exhibited hepatomegaly and increased serum alkaline phosphatase levels.[58] Liver histologic studies in eight patients showed diffuse sinusoidal lymphocytic infiltration with Kupffer cell hyperplasia. Three patients had periportal fibrosis with lymphocytic infiltration and one had macronodular cirrhosis. There was no correlation between abnormal liver chemistry and the histologic findings. From an independent series, hepatomegaly was found in 68% and elevated serum liver enzymes were noted in 25% of cases.[59] Portal hypertension with esophageal varices and gastrointestinal bleeding may be a major complication in Felty syndrome.[60] Nodular regenerative hyperplasia of the liver has also been noted in Felty syndrome (**Fig. 54-5**). The pathogenesis of nodular regenerative hyperplasia is not known, although some authors have suggested it is related to drug toxicity or underlying portal venous thromboses.[46,61]

Antiphospholipid Syndrome

Antiphospholipid syndrome (APS) is characterized by the presence of antiphospholipid antibodies (anticardiolipin antibodies and/or lupus anticoagulant) in association with venous/arterial thromboses, recurrent fetal loss, and thrombocytopenia. Although APS can be a primary disorder, it is frequently seen in patients with SLE and other connective tissue disorders. The most commonly described hepatic manifestation of APS is Budd-Chiari syndrome.[62-64] Several other liver disorders have been reported in patients with APS and these are summarized in **Table 54-4**.[62,64-67]

Scleroderma

Scleroderma is a multisystem autoimmune rheumatic disorder characterized by fibrogenesis within multiple organs including the skin. Although hepatic involvement is thought to be rare, as many as 50% of patients may have elevated serum liver enzyme values.[68] In contrast, a review of 727 patients with scleroderma demonstrated that only 8 (1.1%) cases had evidence for hepatic involvement.[43]

The liver disease most often associated with scleroderma is primary biliary cirrhosis (PBC). Reynolds and colleagues[69]

Table 54-4 Liver Complications in Antiphospholipid Syndrome

Budd-Chiari syndrome
Hepatic venoocclusive disease
Nodular regenerative hyperplasia
Transient elevation of hepatic enzymes becaue of multiple
   fibrin thrombi
Infarction of liver
Autoimmune hepatitis
HELLP syndrome

HELLP, hemolysis, elevated liver enzymes, and low platelet count

described six patients with typical PBC and varying features of scleroderma and CREST syndrome (calcinosis, Raynaud phenomenon, esophageal dysmotility, sclerodactyly, and telangiectasia). Since then, the association between these two autoimmune disorders has been well established and demonstrated by the finding of positive serum antimitochondrial antibodies in patients with scleroderma and serum anticentromere antibody in patients with PBC. Although the prevalence of PBC in patients with scleroderma is not clear, about 15% of patients with PBC have been reported to have scleroderma, with approximately 4% of patients having the variant of limited scleroderma while testing positive for serum anticentromere antibody.

Sjögren Syndrome

Primary Sjögren syndrome (SS) is a chronic inflammatory autoimmune disorder that mainly affects exocrine glands and usually presents as xerostomia and keratoconjunctivitis sicca. A limited number of studies have examined liver involvement in primary SS, with prevalence rates between 6% and 22%.[70,71] In 1 study, 300 patients with primary SS were investigated for liver disease using clinical, biochemical, immunologic, and histologic data. Seven percent of patients showed evidence of liver disease, either subclinical (2%) or asymptomatic (5%) with raised levels of serum liver enzymes.[72] Furthermore, the liver disease in patients with primary SS did not lead to cirrhosis. Subsequent investigations have essentially supported these observations.[43]

An overlap between PBC and primary SS is well known.[73] The exact prevalence of PBC in primary SS is unknown, but has been estimated at 6%.[43] Recently, a number of investigations have explored the relationship between chronic hepatitis C virus (HCV) and SS. The reported prevalence of HCV in patients with SS depends on the methods of detection, the population studied, and the criteria for diagnosing primary SS. In European patients, the prevalence ranges between 14% and 19% by third-generation enzyme-linked immunosorbent assay (ELISA) and between 5% and 19% by the second-generation immunoblot (RIBA2) method, whereas HCV prevalence by RIBA2 was only as high as 1% in American patients.[74,75] Based on the current evidence, HCV seems to be a rare cause of primary SS except in patients with liver involvement or cryoglobulinemia.[75] Furthermore, HCV is a sialotropic virus and morphologic evidence of sialadenitis is found in a significant proportion of patients with chronic HCV infection.[76,77] In HCV-related sialadenitis, the lymphocytic infiltrate is predominantly pericapillary (unlike periductal, in primary SS) and clinical symptoms of dryness are infrequent.

Adult-Onset Still Disease

Adult-onset Still disease is a rare systemic inflammatory disorder of unknown etiology. This disease is characterized by quotidian or double-quotidian spiking fevers, an evanescent rash, arthritis, and multiorgan involvement. Adult-onset Still disease occurs worldwide and affects women slightly more often than men. An estimated 75% of patients are diagnosed between 16 and 35 years of age.[78-81] However, an epidemiologic survey from Japan reported that 67% of the cases presented after the age of 35.[82]

The etiology of adult-onset Still disease remains unknown. A genetic component has been suggested, linking the disease with a number of human leukocyte antigens (HLAs)[83] and viruses such as rubella, mumps, echovirus 7, cytomegalovirus, Epstein-Barr virus, parainfluenza, coxsackievirus B4, adenovirus, influenza A, human herpes/virus 6, parvovirus B19, hepatitis B, and hepatitis C.[84,85] More recently, it has been suggested that alterations in cytokine production have an important pathophysiologic role in adult-onset Still disease.[86]

Clinical Manifestations

Adult-onset Still disease typically manifests as a triad of symptoms that include high-spiking fevers, a characteristic rash, and arthritis/arthralgias. Fever generally exceeds 39° C and is transient, lasting typically less than 4 hours with the highest temperatures seen in the late afternoon or early evening.[78] The rash is a salmon-pink, maculopapular lesion involving the proximal limbs and trunk. The most common joints affected are the knees, wrists, and ankles.[11,23] Less common manifestations include pleuritis (26%), pericarditis (24%), and splenomegaly (44%).[87]

Hepatomegaly and elevated levels of serum liver enzymes are present in approximately 50% to 75% of patients, and frequently occur concomitantly with fever and exacerbations of arthritis.[78] Serum ferritin levels in adult-onset Still disease are usually higher than those found in patients with other autoimmune or inflammatory diseases. In most studies a threshold for serum ferritin levels of 1000 ng/ml has been used to suggest adult-onset Still disease.[88] However, levels ranging from 4000 to 30,000 ng/ml are not uncommon.[89] Adult-onset Still disease can also present with jaundice and hepatic failure requiring liver transplantation, yet this is exceedingly rare.[90,91] Liver biopsy typically shows mild periportal inflammation with monocyte infiltration.[83]

Treatment and Prognosis

The treatment of adult-onset Still disease has been empiric, mainly consisting of nonsteroidal antiinflammatory agents, corticosteroids, and antirheumatic agents to control systemic symptoms. Most patients are treated with corticosteroids at some point in their disease course, with responses ranging from 76% to 95%.[92,93] Intravenous γ-globulin (IVIG) and anti–tumor necrosis factor blocking agents have also been employed in uncontrolled studies.[94-96] Serious complications from hepatic disease that affect prognosis are rare.[84]

Henoch-Schönlein Purpura

Henoch-Schönlein purpura (HSP) is the most common systemic vasculitis in childhood. The annual incidence of HSP is 10 to 22 cases per 100,000, with a peak at age 5 to 7 years.[97-100] It occurs particularly in the autumn and winter. The diagnostic criteria for HSP include palpable purpura (a mandatory criterion) in the presence of at least one of the following: (1) diffuse abdominal pain; (2) biopsy showing predominant IgA deposition; (3) arthritis or arthralgia; and (4) renal involvement (hematuria and/or proteinuria).[101]

HSP is mediated by immune deposits (typically with IgA) that cause necrosis of the walls of small- and medium-sized arteries, resulting in features consistent with leukocytoclastic vasculitis (LCV). Note that IgA deposition in capillary walls is characteristic of HSP.[101]

HSP is associated with infections, medications, vaccines, and tumors, although a cause-and-effect relationship is not always proven. Upper respiratory tract infections occur in 35% to 52% of patients. Group A hemolytic streptococcus and parvovirus B19 have been implicated as common etiologies but evidence remains controversial.[102] Adults may have malignancies associated with HSP, with specific reference to non–small-cell lung cancer followed by prostate cancer and Hodgkin and non-Hodgkin lymphoma.[103] HSP has also been associated with campylobacteriosis, shigellosis, salmonellosis (both typhi and nontyphi), amebiasis, and cytomegalovirus.[101]

Clinical Manifestations

Palpable purpura is noted in 55% to 70% of patients. Skin biopsy is often consistent with LCV. Joint involvement occurs in 4% to 8% of patients with HSP as a symmetric oligoarthritis involving the ankles, feet, or knees. Renal involvement occurs in 30% to 55% of patients with HSP, usually manifesting as hematuria. Gastrointestinal (GI) tract features of HSP include abdominal pain, nausea, vomiting, or bleeding in 50% to 75% of patients.[99,101] In children intussusception is the most common complication of HSP requiring surgical intervention, but is uncommon in adults and children younger than 3 years. Other complications of HSP include obstruction and stricture formation of the duodenum or ileum.[104] Mesenteric vasculitis is uncommon in HSP.[101]

Hepatobiliary manifestations of HSP include LCV involving the gallbladder, which can result in acute acalculous cholecystitis.[105,106] Hydrops of the gallbladder has been described with spontaneous resolution.[107] Vasculitis of the peribiliary vessels may cause ischemic necrosis and stenosis of the bile ducts and, ultimately, obstructive biliary cirrhosis.[107] Nine percent of patients with HSP may develop right upper quadrant pain, hepatomegaly, and nausea associated with elevated levels of serum ALT. These findings resolve within 3 to 7 days of beginning corticosteroid treatment.[108] Other rare manifestations of HSP are hemorrhagic ascites with serositis[109] and chylous ascites.[110]

Treatment and Prognosis

Analgesics are useful for joint pain and fever. Nonsteroidal antiinflammatory drugs can be used to treat major arthritis, but should be avoided in patients with GI and renal manifestations. The efficacy of corticosteroids to prevent severe complications or relapses is controversial, and should be reserved for patients who have a high risk of renal involvement. Signs and symptoms of liver involvement, including elevated concentrations of serum liver enzymes, are noted to resolve within 3 to 7 days of initiation of corticosteroid treatment. Plasma exchange, IVIG, and dapsone have also been empirically used as treatment with success in anecdotal cases.[101-103]

More than 80% of patients recover within 2 weeks following treatment initiation. About 30% of patients have one or more recurrences of symptoms with more than 90% of these recurrences occurring within 4 months.[101] HSP in adults, unlike that in children, is associated with more frequent and severe kidney disease.[111]

Hematologic Disease
Primary and Secondary Amyloidosis

Amyloid is currently classified by placing an "A" in front of the abbreviation for the precursor protein (**Table 54-5**). There are at least 16 different variants. Many of these occur only focally in aged or tumorous organs and do not directly involve the liver.

Primary or AL amyloidosis is related to the deposition of immunoglobulin light-chain or heavy-chain protein.[112,113] Immunoglobulin is a normal component of the humoral immune system and is typically found in the serum in a kappa/lambda 2:1 ratio. In lymphoplasmocytic disorders such as multiple myeloma or Waldenström macroglobulinemia, there is an overproduction of portions of the immunoglobulin molecule, generally the light chain. The light-chain protein itself or its breakdown products then precipitate out of the serum to form amyloid. Most patients with amyloidosis have precipitated lambda light chains, suggesting that this form is more likely to produce a beta-pleated-sheet arrangement.

Secondary or AA amyloidosis is associated with chronic infections such as osteomyelitis or tuberculosis. Cytokines associated with the inflammation, such as IL-1, IL-6, and tumor necrosis factor, stimulate the liver to produce serum amyloid A.[114,115] The normal human AA protein is continuously produced during chronic infections.[116] Although most individuals cleave amyloid A into small peptides, some patients can only cleave it into larger sizes consistent with the amyloid subunit.

Mutations in the transthyretin gene are associated with familial amyloidotic polyneuropathy (FAP). This is the most common type of heritable amyloidosis. The transthyretin gene product is a normal serum protein largely produced by the liver and it carries serum thyroxine and retinal-binding protein. The protein is a tetramer of identical subunits that is encoded by a single gene on chromosome 18. At least 78 different amino acid substitutions occurring at 51 different sites in the transthyretin gene have been reported.[117] Most of these mutations are amyloidogenic. Although inherited as an autosomal dominant disorder, symptoms generally do not arise until the third to fourth decade of life. The disorder has been seen in Portugal, Sweden, Japan, and the United States. The U.S. kindreds usually exhibit the defects associated with their country of origin. The clinical onset can be quite variable

Table 54-5 Different Types of Amyloidosis

VARIANT	PRECURSOR PROTEIN	SITES INVOLVED	DISEASE	MUTATION
AL	Immunoglobulin light chain	Systemic	Myeloma	
ATTR	Transthyretin	Systemic	Hereditary	Chromosome 18; Val30Met most common
AA	(Apo)serum AA	Systemic	Chronic infection	AA gene on 11p; FMF 16p
Aβ_2M	β_2-Microglobulin	Systemic	Chronic hemodialysis	
AApoAI	Apoprotein AI	Nerves, kidney, liver	Hereditary	Chromosome 11; Gly26Arg most common
ALys	Lysozyme variants	Kidney	Hereditary	
AGel	Gelsolin	Cornea, nerves, skin	Hereditary	
AFib	Fibrinogen a-chain	Kidney	Hereditary	
ACys	Cystatin C	Cerebral blood vessels	Hereditary	
Aβ	Aβ-Protein precursor	Brain	Alzheimer's disease	Chromosome 21
APrPsc	Prion protein	Nervous system	Spongiform encephalopathy	PRNP gene chromosome 20
ACal	(Pro)calcitonin	Thyroid	Medullary carcinoma	
AIAPP	Islet amyloid protein	Islet of Langerhans		
AANF	Atrial natriuretic factor	Heart		
APro	Prolactin	Aging pituitary	Prolactinoma	

among these ethnic groups, even in those patients with the same mutation. The patients usually have a lower limb neuropathy that progresses to the upper limbs. Autonomic nervous system involvement is also usually extensive, often resulting in diarrhea and weight loss. Rarely, the heart and corneas can be involved.

Patients undergoing chronic hemodialysis develop amyloid secondary to precipitation of the β_2-microglobulin protein.[118] β_2-Microglobulin is a normal serum protein. The hemodialysis itself is thought to produce localized excess concentrations of this precursor, resulting in the deposition of amyloid. Generally, the musculoskeletal system and the kidneys are involved.

Table 54-6 Manifestations of Hepatic Amyloidosis

Hepatosplenomegaly
Splenomegaly
Ascites
Prolongation of prothrombin time because of acquired factor X deficiency
Cholestasis
Jaundice
Acute liver failure
Spontaneous rupture

Clinical Manifestations

Amyloidosis can present with symptoms related to renal failure, heart failure secondary to cardiomyopathy, peripheral neuropathy, rash, and blood dyscrasias.[119] The most common finding related to the liver is hepatomegaly.[113] Several other forms of presentation of hepatic amyloidosis are summarized in **Table 54-6**. Jaundice and cholestasis can be two of the initial manifestations of hepatic amyloidosis.[120,121] When present, they are an ominous finding and suggest an increased short-term mortality risk. Ascites attributable to sinusoidal occlusion can also be a presenting symptom.[122] Serum aminotransferase levels are minimally elevated, and jaundice is rare. Imaging studies may show an infiltrative process but are generally not helpful in gauging the extent of disease.

The demonstration of amyloid deposition within affected tissues is generally required to make the diagnosis. Fat pad aspirations are the easiest and most common approach to diagnose amyloidosis. When fat pad aspiration is negative,

rectal or skin biopsies are obtained with biopsies of affected organs performed if the diagnosis of amyloid remains in doubt. Amyloid deposition in the liver occurs in three basic patterns. The most common pattern is protein deposition in the spaces of Disse (**Fig. 54-6**). As the material accumulates, it encroaches on the hepatocytes, causing extensive atrophy. Remarkably, the amyloid deposition rarely causes portal hypertension. Use of Congo red stain remains a mainstay in detecting tissue-based amyloid. The staining properties with Congo red are related to the beta-pleated-sheet arrangement of the proteins. Generally, all types of amyloid stain with Congo red dye. However, in some patients with AL amyloid, it may be very difficult to obtain a satisfactory staining reaction. In these cases, it may be useful to implement other stains, such as thioflavins T and S, crystal violet, and methyl violet.[123]

Therapy is generally directed at treating the underlying condition.[124,125] In the case of primary amyloid, therapy directed

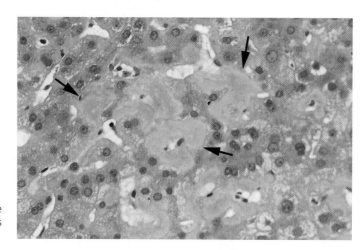

Fig. 54-6 Liver in amyloidosis. Amyloid is usually deposited in the space of Disse (arrows). As the deposits increase, the hepatocytes become sunken ribbons (H & E stain).

against the underlying lymphoplasmocytic neoplasm can sometimes improve survival.[126] Liver transplantation has been performed in this disorder and short-term survivors have been noted.[127] Stem cell transplantation has also been employed, with mixed results.[128] However, fatal complications from cardiac or renal failure eventually ensue. In the cases of amyloidosis attributable to chronic infections, eradication of underlying infection should be attempted. Orthotopic liver transplantation has been very successful in patients with FAP.[129] Most centers recommend transplantation in patients with FAP as soon as symptoms occur, because liver with or without heart transplantation has been shown to diminish the disease progression. In general, there is little improvement in the autonomic dysfunction when it is already established. Patients with advanced disease, including both upper and lower motor neuron symptoms, generally do poorly.[130]

Sickle Cell Anemia

Patients with sickle cell anemia may have a variety of hepatic abnormalities involving both the hepatic parenchyma and the biliary tract. These abnormalities may be present during the asymptomatic phase of sickle cell disease as well as during episodes of sickle cell crisis. The incidence of hepatic involvement is very difficult to estimate because of the confounding effects of chronic hemolysis, which may elevate serum bilirubin aminotransferase levels.[131]

Hepatic Crisis

Hepatic crisis is characterized by right upper quadrant abdominal pain, jaundice, hepatomegaly, and fever. This constellation of findings is also suggestive of acute cholecystitis or cholangitis, which can occur in this population as well. It has been estimated that 7% to 10% of hospitalizations for sickle cell anemia were complicated by hepatic crises.[132]

The most marked serum biochemical abnormality is elevation of serum total bilirubin level. Total bilirubin values are usually less than 15 mg/dl. This marked hyperbilirubinemia may not necessarily be associated with a worse prognosis.[132,133] A large component of this bilirubin is the direct fraction, which may be as much as 50% of the total bilirubin in many cases. Levels of serum aminotransferases are usually less than

10 times the upper limits of normal. Elevation of serum LDH level is also common based on hemolysis associated with sickle cell crisis. Deaths related to fulminant hepatic failure in the absence of other identifiable etiologies have been reported.[131] Recent data suggest that acute hepatopathy attributable to sickle cell anemia should be considered a contraindication to percutaneous liver biopsy because serious bleeding or death has been reported.[134]

Biliary Tract Disease

Pigment gallstones develop in 40% to 80% of patients with sickle cell anemia.[131,135] Choledocholithiasis was found in 18% of 65 patients undergoing cholecystectomy.[131] In contrast to hepatic crisis, the occurrence of cholecystitis and cholangitis will ultimately require endoscopic and/or surgical intervention. Schubert reviewed published reports on 97 patients who underwent cholecystectomy and found 15% of patients had complications that were deemed serious, including pneumonia, seizures, and sickle cell crisis. Thus cholecystectomy should be reserved for those patients with documented symptomatic gallstones or for those in whom hepatic crisis and biliary tract disease cannot be adequately differentiated.[131]

Viral Hepatitis

As expected from the large numbers of transfusions required by many patients with sickle cell anemia, viral hepatitis has been reported to occur, although from published reports, the incidence is difficult to determine. In patients with liver test abnormalities, the incidence of hepatitis B virus (HBV) or histologic changes of chronic hepatitis has ranged from 5% to 47%.[136,137] The reported prevalence of hepatitis C in patients with sickle cell anemia is 10% to 35%.[138] Not surprisingly, the risk of hepatitis C was directly related to the number of transfusions received. The impact of hepatitis C infection on the natural history of patients with sickle cell anemia is currently unknown.

Hepatic Histology

A wide variety of liver histopathologic features occur in patients with sickle cell disease.[139] Hepatic sinusoidal distention, erythrocyte sickling, and erythrophagocytosis are

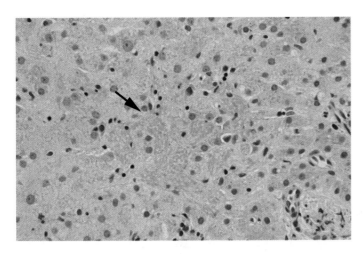

Fig. 54-7 **Liver in sickle cell anemia.** Numerous sickled red blood cells distend the sinuses of the liver *(arrow)* (H & E stain).

observed in nearly all patients affected by hepatic crisis (**Fig. 54-7**). Massive iron deposition is frequently identified by routine iron stains in the majority of patients. Also, there can be changes consistent with acute or chronic viral hepatitis.[137] Cirrhosis has been reported to occur in 15% to 20% of patients with sickle cell anemia and may be due to hypoxic injury from sickling and intrasinusoidal sludging of erythrocytes, chronic viral hepatitis, or massive hemosiderosis.[137,140]

Hemophagocytic Syndrome

Hemophagocytic syndrome, also known as hemophagocytic lymphohistiocytosis (HLH), is characterized by the proliferation of benign macrophages that participate in phagocytosis of blood cells in hematopoietic organs, including bone marrow, spleen, or lymph nodes. This syndrome, which was first described in patients with several viral infections, occurs in association with various conditions of altered immunity (lymphoproliferative disorder), severe bacterial infections, acquired immunodeficiency syndrome, systemic lupus erythematosus, immunosuppressive therapy, or neoplastic diseases.[141]

The pathophysiology of hemophagocytic syndrome is not well understood. Upon triggering of the immune system, histiocytes (macrophages and dendritic cells), natural killer (NK) cells, and cytotoxic lymphocytes are activated and mutually stimulate each other. This concerted action leads to killing of the infected cell, removal of antigen, and termination of the immune response. Defective cytotoxic activity impairs not only the elimination of cellular targets that express antigens but also the down-regulation of the immune response. Sustained immune activation with persistently high cytokine levels then leads to the clinical presentation of hemophagocytic syndrome.[142]

Clinical Manifestations

The diagnostic criteria for hemophagocytic syndrome[143] include (1) the presence of familial disease/known genetic defect and/or (2) the presence of at least five of the following criteria: fever; splenomegaly; cytopenia in two cell lines with the hemoglobin content less than 9 g/dl, platelet count less than 100×10^9/L, and neutrophil count less than 1×10^9/L; hypertriglyceridemia and/or hypofibrinogenemia; ferritin level greater than 500 µg/L; sCD25 greater than 2400 U/ml; decreased or absent NK-cell activity; and hemophagocytosis in bone marrow, cerebro spinal fluid (CSF), or lymph nodes. Supportive evidence includes elevated serum aminotransferase values, hyperbilirubinemia, and increased LDH activity. Patients suspected of having hemophagocytic syndrome should undergo bone marrow examination and a lumbar puncture at an experienced center. Marrow with normal or increased cellularity is typical. Unfortunately, hemophagocytosis is often absent initially but may be found by a repeat examination.

Hepatomegaly, cholestasis, and fulminant hepatic failure have been reported in association with hemophagocytic syndrome.[141] It has been suggested that liver changes are caused by the underlying disease[144] or secondary to an increased number of histiocytes with or without hemophagocytosis in hepatic sinusoids, or as a result of focal hepatocellular necrosis.[144,145] In a recent retrospective study of 30 patients with hemophagocytic syndrome and liver involvement,[144] the association of fever, jaundice, and hepatomegaly or splenomegaly was present in 50% of cases, with 24 patients exhibiting hepatomegaly; 19, splenomegaly; 18, jaundice; 7, ascites; and 3, hepatic encephalopathy. Fifteen patients presented with the combination of persistent fever, fatigue, jaundice, and hepatomegaly or splenomegaly. In 19 patients, hepatic manifestations were the reasons for hospitalization. An underlying condition predisposing to hemophagocytic syndrome was identified in 29 patients.

Serum ALT values were five times the upper limit of normal, and serum alkaline phosphatase activity was two to three times the upper limit of normal. Average total bilirubin values were approximately 8 mg/dl. Serum ferritin and triglyceride levels were increased in all patients. There was no correlation between the magnitude of liver biochemical test changes and the magnitude of serum ferritin or serum triglyceride elevation, or with liver histologic findings.[144]

In selected patients who underwent liver biopsy, sinusoidal dilatation with hemophagocytic histiocytosis was found in the biopsy specimen in all patients. Liver biopsy was diagnostic for the underlying condition in 15 patients (including 8 cases with nonspecific bone marrow biopsy findings). All specimens showed sinusoidal dilatation, congestion, and hyperplasia of Kupffer cells. These cells were markedly increased both in size and in number. Hemophagocytosis was seen in all patients, with only erythrophagocytosis in 16 cases. In the 14 other patients, erythrophagocytosis was associated with intracytoplasmic accumulation of pigment. Hemophagocytosis was not present in portal tracts. In this study, liver biopsy was obtained before bone marrow biopsy in 15 patients because of predominant liver manifestations. In 8 of these 15 cases, liver biopsy identified a condition not seen at bone marrow biopsy. Among the 22 patients in whom lymphoma or leukemia was diagnosed, 14 presented with isolated hepatic manifestations. However, liver histologic studies may not be as helpful when interpreted as chronic hepatitis because hemophagocytosing macrophages may be absent in the periportal infiltrate.[144]

Severe manifestations can be treated by corticosteroids, which are cytotoxic for lymphocytes and inhibit expression of cytokines and differentiation of dendritic cells. Because dexamethasone crosses the blood–brain barrier more easily than prednisolone, it is the preferred drug in pediatric protocols. High-dose prednisolone (30 mg/kg × 3days) is often used with good response.[146] Cyclosporine has proved to be effective for maintaining remission in genetic HLH.[147] Etoposide, which was introduced to the treatment of HLH in 1980, is highly active in monocytic and histiocytic diseases.[148] In genetic HLH, stem cell transplantation as the only curative method is the ultimate aim.[149]

In the study of 30 patients with predominant hepatic manifestations, there were 12 deaths mainly attributable to multiorgan failure or generalized sepsis. Among the 21 patients in whom an underlying disease was identified and appropriately treated, cure of hemophagocytic syndrome and complete remission of the underlying disease were obtained in 15. In 15 patients treated using systemic combination chemotherapy for malignancy, 11 survived. Among the four patients treated by intravenous acyclovir for viral infection, three survived. One patient who received antituberculous chemotherapy for disseminated infection survived. The remaining patient who was treated by antibiotics alone died. Of the nine patients in whom no underlying disease was identified before death, six received no treatment and five died. High serum bilirubin level, elevated serum alkaline phosphatase activity, low factor V level, and lack of treatment for the underlying disease were associated with a poor prognosis.[144]

Mastocytosis

Mastocytosis is a systemic disorder that can involve the liver.[150] When seen in adults, it often presents with fever, hepatosplenomegaly, diarrhea, and weight loss. Levels of serum liver enzymes are usually minimally abnormal with jaundice being uncommon. Liver histologic analysis demonstrates irregular areas of fibrosis containing numerous eosinophils and a background of lymphocytes and other mononuclear cells (**Fig. 54-8**).[151] These mononuclear cells are mast cells that may be recognized by a number of methods including toluidine blue and chloroacetate esterase staining. These fibrotic clusters may be located either in the portal tracts or in the parenchyma. When the lesions abut the central veins, they may be responsible for the rare cases of portal hypertension associated with the disease.[152]

Hypereosinophilic Syndromes

Hypereosinophilic syndromes are a rare group of hematologic diseases characterized by unexplained blood and tissue

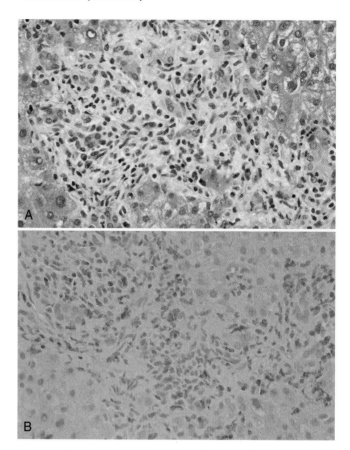

Fig. 54-8 **A,** Hepatic mastocytosis (H & E stain). It may involve the portal tracts or lobule, or both. The lesion is a stellate region of fibrosis occupied by lymphocytes, eosinophils, and cells with larger pale nuclei—the mast cell. **B,** Hepatic mastocytosis (Leder stain). In this section of the liver the numerous mast cells *(red)* of systemic mastocytosis stand out against the background counterstain. (Chloroacetate esterase [Leder] stain).

eosinophilia. In 1975 Chusid and colleagues established four diagnostic criteria for hypereosinophilic syndromes including (1) eosinophilia greater than 1.5×10^9/L; (2) eosinophilia lasting longer than 6 months; (3) exclusion of other known causes of eosinophilia; and (4) evidence of organ dysfunction directly attributable to eosinophils.[153]

Two main mechanisms responsible for eosinophilia have been identified in HES patients to date. First, eosinophilia can be induced by genetic abnormalities leading to a clonal and uncontrolled expansion of the myeloid linage, including the eosinophil lineage. Second, eosinophilia can also follow an overproduction of eosinophilopoietic cytokines (mainly IL-5) by abnormal circulating T-cell subsets.[154]

Clinical Manifestations

The clinical manifestations of hypereosinophilic syndrome usually involve the heart, skin, lung, nervous system, and/or gastrointestinal tract (**Table 54-7**). Depending on the study, the frequency of each organ involvement is as high as 50%.[155] Cardiac involvement represents the major complication and cause of death of patients with hypereosinophilic syndromes. Digestive tract involvement can manifest as abdominal pain and/or diarrhea, and is usually demonstrated by intestine biopsies. Ascites develops when eosinophils infiltrate the

Table 54-7 Clinical Manifestations of Hypereosinophilic Syndromes

Cardiovascular	Myocarditis, endocardial thrombi, endomyocardial fibrosis
Integumentary	Angioedema, erythematous and/or urticarial lesions, purpura, pruritus, Raynaud phenomenon, nail-fold splint hemorrhages, mucosal ulcerations
Neurologic	Confusion, encephalopathy, stroke, peripheral neuropathies
Gastrointestinal	Abdominal pain, diarrhea, ascites, colitis and enteritis, pancreatitis, cholangitis
Respiratory	Cough, bronchial hyperreactivity, pulmonary infiltrates
Hematologic	Hepatomegaly, splenomegaly, anemia, thrombocytopenia, arterial or venous thrombosis

deeper layers of the intestinal wall. Hepatomegaly and splenomegaly are common as well.[155,156]

Treatment and Prognosis

The major indication for specific treatment is the demonstration of eosinophil-mediated tissue injury. This approach signifies that truly asymptomatic patients with chronic eosinophilia could potentially be left untreated if a complete evaluation failed to reveal evidence of target organ involvement. Corticosteroids and tyrosine kinase inhibitors such as imatinib are considered first-line agents. Salvage therapies include administration of medications such as hydroxyurea and interferon alfa, mepolizumab, and alemtuzumab as well as bone marrow transplantation.[155]

Gastrointestinal Disease
Celiac Disease

Celiac disease has been recognized as a multisystem disorder that may affect other organs, such as the nervous system, bones, skin, heart, and liver.[157]

The prevalence of abnormal levels of serum liver enzymes ranges between 40% and 55% of cases with a concurrent atypical presentation of celiac disease.[158] Celiac disease has also been associated with an eight-fold increased risk of death from liver cirrhosis.[159]

The mechanism by which celiac disease affects the liver is poorly understood. Intestinal permeability is increased in celiac disease from inflammation of the intestine,[160] and patients with a significant increase in intestinal permeability have elevated levels of serum liver enzymes. The permeability may encourage translocation of toxins, antigens, and inflammatory substances to the portal circulation, and these mediators may have a role in the liver involvement seen in patients with celiac disease.[161] Serum autoantibodies including tissue transglutaminase are present in the liver and other extraintestinal tissues, which raises the possibility of a pathogenic role for the humoral-mediated immune responses in the liver injury.[162]

Clinical Manifestations

Most patients are asymptomatic or complain of vague symptoms such as fatigue and myalgias. Physical examination is normal in most patients,[161] yet palmar erythema, jaundice, finger clubbing, spider angiomata, ascites, hepatomegaly, and splenomegaly have been described when patients with celiac disease have cirrhosis.[163]

Mild to moderate elevations in serum AST and/or ALT levels (less than five times the upper limit of normal) are highly common. The isolated elevation of alkaline phosphatase level (4% to 20%) is less common and may reflect secondary hyperparathyroidism.[158,161] Hypoalbuminemia, a prolonged prothrombin time, and hyperbilirubinemia suggest that cirrhosis may have already developed.[163]

Liver histologic examination in celiac disease is generally mild and nonspecific. Features include periportal inflammation, bile duct obstruction, mononuclear infiltration in the parenchyma, steatosis, and mild fibrosis. Extensive fibrosis and cirrhosis have also been reported.[164]

Treatment

Utilization of a gluten-free diet can lead to normalization of levels of serum aminotransferases in 75% to 95% of cases within 1 year.[158] Treatment responses have also been observed in patients with advanced fibrosis and cirrhosis.[163] Note that an alternative cause for liver injury should be explored with persistently abnormal levels of serum liver enzymes despite use of a gluten-free diet.[161]

Endocrine Disease
Hyperthyroidism

Despite an increase in cardiac output, hepatic blood flow is not increased in hyperthyroidism. Thus a reduced oxygen supply to centrilobular hepatocytes may occur, resulting in the tissue hypoxia that is likely responsible for the hepatic dysfunction seen in most cases of hyperthyroidism.[165]

Clinical Manifestations

Increases in serum AST and ALT levels occur in 30% and 40% of cases, respectively. Mild elevation of alkaline phosphatase level is encountered in up to 65% of patients with hyperthyroidism. This elevation is not specific to the liver because a high turnover in bones may contribute. Elevations of γ-glutamyltransferase and bilirubin concentrations usually do not exceed 20% of normal values. Jaundice primarily occurs in the setting of infection or heart failure.[165,166] Thus, in a patient with uncomplicated mild hyperthyroidism, the presence of jaundice is more likely from co-existent hepatobiliary disease or a hemolytic disorder.[167]

Mild histologic changes are common, but cases of fulminant hepatic failure with centrizonal necrosis have been described. Long-term untreated hyperthyroidism can ultimately lead to cirrhosis.[165]

Thyrotoxic crisis or storm occurs more commonly in untreated or inadequately treated patients, and is usually precipitated by surgery or complicating illness (usually sepsis). Extreme irritability, delirium or coma, fever, tachycardia, restlessness, hypotension, vomiting, and diarrhea characterize the syndrome. Significant liver injury is frequently observed in thyroid crisis, and may present as acute or fulminant liver failure.[168]

Pharmacologic therapies have also been associated with liver injury in patients with hyperthyroidism. Treatment with methimazole or carbimazole can be a rare cause of reversible cholestasis. Propylthiouracil (PTU) most commonly causes a mild transient asymptomatic elevation in serum AST and ALT levels; however, severe cases of PTU-induced liver injury have been reported. Although PTU generally can be continued in patients who have mild elevations of serum aminotransferase levels, these patients must be followed closely with frequent laboratory testing, especially during the early treatment period. In rare severe cases of PTU-induced liver injury, the drug must be discontinued. Corticosteroid therapy may be helpful, but there are no controlled trials that establish the benefit of this therapy.[169,170]

Hypothyroidism

The mechanisms of liver injury with hypothyroidism also relate to decreased hepatic oxygen consumption, bile acid production, bile flow, and bile salt excretion.[165]

Serum liver enzyme values are mildly disturbed in almost 50% of patients with hypothyroidism despite normal histologic findings. Occasionally, in severe cases of myxedema, marked elevations in serum aminotransferase and bilirubin levels attributable to congestive heart failure and hepatomegaly can be observed. Myxedema ascites in hypothyroidism is rare and may be a long-standing overlooked and/or isolated sign of the disease. The serum-to-ascites albumin gradient is usually greater than 1.1 g/dl with a high protein content. Although considered to be the result of hypothyroidism-related chronic right heart failure, it is mainly attributed to increased permeability of vascular endothelium.[165,171] Primary biliary cirrhosis is not uncommonly associated with primary autoimmune diseases of the thyroid.[172]

Histologically, hypothyroidism produces a specific central congestive fibrosis of the liver, which occurs predominantly in patients with co-existent myxedema ascites.[173] Accurate diagnosis and treatment with thyroid replacement therapy should lead to a reversal of all these symptoms.

Oncologic Disease
Stauffer Syndrome

Stauffer syndrome is a paraneoplastic syndrome of liver test abnormalities in patients with renal cell carcinoma.[174] The prevalence of this condition is between 4% and 40% according to data gathered from previous studies.[175,176] Strickland and Schenker reviewed 29 published cases of nephrogenic hepatic dysfunction in which sufficient data were available to apply strict criteria for the diagnosis.[176] Fever and weight loss were the most common symptoms. Hepatomegaly was present in two thirds of patients. Elevation of alkaline phosphatase level was the most common biochemical abnormality, occurring in 90% of reported cases, whereas abnormalities in levels of serum aminotransferases and serum bilirubin were much less common. Histologic examination of the liver in patients with

nephrogenic hepatic dysfunction has shown only nonspecific changes. Steatosis, mild focal hepatocyte necrosis, portal lymphocytic infiltration, and Kupffer cell hyperplasia have all been reported.[176] Recent evidence suggests that interleukin-6 (IL-6) is responsible for causing various paraneoplastic syndromes seen in renal cell carcinoma.[177] Abnormalities of hepatic function usually resolve within 1 to 2 months after the primary tumor has been resected.[176] With recurrence of renal cell carcinoma, clinical and biochemical characteristics of liver injury may again become evident.[178]

Hodgkin Lymphoma

Hepatic involvement in Hodgkin lymphoma has been reported to occur in 5% of patients at the time of diagnosis, with as many as 50% of cases diagnosed at the time of autopsy.[179]

Elevated serum alkaline phosphatase levels are noted in up to 40% of patients with the majority of cases having stage III or stage IV disease. Increased alkaline phosphatase levels may also be seen in the absence of hepatic involvement when fever as a systemic manifestation of Hodgkin disease is present. Jaundice occurs infrequently in Hodgkin lymphoma, except in the late stages of the illness. The most common cause of jaundice is intrahepatic infiltration by the tumor, which was seen in 45% of jaundiced patients at the time of autopsy.[179,180] Extrahepatic biliary tract obstruction occurs much less frequently and accounts for only 5% to 10% of jaundiced patients.[180] A small number of patients with Hodgkin lymphoma have been described who have evidence of severe intrahepatic cholestasis with dramatic elevations in serum bilirubin and alkaline phosphatase levels in the absence of tumor infiltration or bile duct obstruction.[179] The cause of this syndrome is not known but one report suggested that it could be related to vanishing bile duct syndrome.[181] Acute liver failure with encephalopathy, jaundice, and coagulopathy has also been reported in patients with Hodgkin and non-Hodgkin lymphoma either attributable to direct hepatic involvement[182] or caused by a paraneoplastic syndrome.[183]

A diagnosis of hepatic involvement in Hodgkin disease requires observation of Reed-Sternberg cells (**Fig. 54-9**).

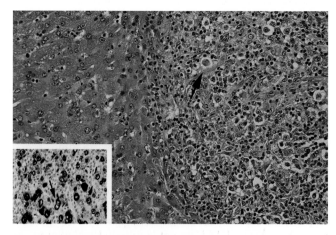

Fig. 54-9 **Liver in Hodgkin lymphoma.** Classic Reed-Sternberg cell (*arrow*) is seen in a polymorphous background of lymphocytes, plasma cell, and eosinophils, which greatly expands a portal tract. (H & E stain.) The *inset* shows the Reed-Sternberg cells marked with anti-CD-30. (Modified immunoperoxidase method.)

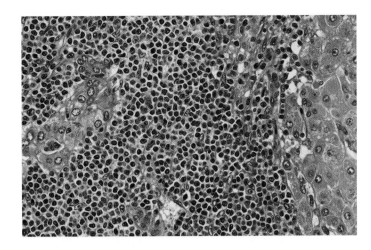

Fig. 54-10 Hepatic B-cell lymphoma. Sheets of small lymphocytes surround a regenerative liver nodule. The portal tract also appears to be involved. The B-cell nature of the infiltrate can be confirmed by immunohistochemistry or flow cytometry (H & E stain).

Nonspecific inflammatory infiltrates are seen in 50% of cases and by itself they do not constitute grounds for diagnosing hepatic involvement. Noncaseating epithelioid granulomas may be seen in 25% of patients.[184]

Non-Hodgkin Lymphoma

Hepatic involvement in non-Hodgkin lymphomas occurs very frequently, with estimates ranging between 24% and 43%.[185] The hepatic infiltrate usually involves the portal triads and has a nodular appearance (**Fig. 54-10**). Epithelioid granulomas may also be seen in the liver of these patients. Immunophenotyping using monoclonal antibodies may be performed on snap-frozen liver biopsy tissues to characterize the infiltrates.[186] Rarely, primary hepatic lymphoma in the absence of systemic lymphoma has been reported.[187]

The clinical manifestations of hepatic infiltration with non-Hodgkin lymphoma are similar to those seen with Hodgkin disease. Patients may remain asymptomatic despite extensive hepatic infiltration or present with fulminant hepatic failure. Mild to moderate elevations in serum alkaline phosphatase levels and moderate to marked elevations of LDH activities may be present. In contrast to Hodgkin disease, non-Hodgkin lymphomas are more likely to produce jaundice as a result of extrahepatic obstruction, usually at the porta hepatis, rather than by direct hepatic infiltration.[185,187] Although some reports have suggested that HCV may have a role in the development of non-Hodgkin lymphoma, other reports have failed to confirm such an association.[188]

Patients with lymphoma and severe liver dysfunction (due to either lymphoma involvement or co-existing liver problem) pose a significant therapeutic problem because of their inability to tolerate conventional chemotherapeutic agents. Ghobrial and colleagues summarized their experience with 41 such patients seen at the Mayo Clinic over a 5-year period. The authors found that mechlorethamine, high-dose corticosteroids, and rituximab are safe and effective in this patient population.[189]

Multiple Myeloma

Direct plasma cell infiltration of the liver may occur in up to 30% of patients with multiple myeloma. The patients generally present with hepatomegaly or ascites.[190] It is important to distinguish myeloma involvement from autoimmune hepatitis in patients with evidence of clinical liver injury. In myeloma, the plasma cell infiltrate predominantly involves the sinusoids, with relative sparing of the portal tracts. This is distinct from autoimmune hepatitis, where the infiltrate is predominantly in the portal area. Another pattern of liver injury in myeloma patients is nodular regenerative hyperplasia.[191]

Waldenström macroglobulinemia is a neoplastic disorder of B-lymphocytes and plasma cells that may co-exist with multiple myeloma.[192] The neoplastic cells secrete immunoglobulin heavy chain, which has rarely been associated with the development of amyloidosis. The lymphoplasmocytic tumor can directly involve the liver. Clinical liver disease in these patients is often mild, with minimal elevation in levels of transaminases and alkaline phosphatase. Their symptoms are usually referred to the extrahepatic problems associated with the disease. Histologically, the infiltrate shows expanded portal tracts with lymphocytes and plasma cells, and larger atypical cells with occasional mitotic figures.

Key References

Abraham S, Begum S, Isenberg D. Hepatic manifestations of autoimmune rheumatic diseases. Ann Rheum Dis 2004;63:123. (Ref.43)

Akritidis N, Giannakakis I, Giouglis T. Ferritin levels and response to treatment in patients with adult Still's disease. J Rheumatol 1996;23:201. (Ref.89)

Bacon BR, Joshi SN, Granger DN. Ischemia, congestive heart failure, Budd–Chiari syndrome, and veno-occlusive disease. In: Kaplowitz N, editor. Liver and biliary diseases, 2nd ed. Philadelphia: Williams & Wilkins, 1996: 421. (Ref.16)

Bardella MT, et al. Prevalence of hypertransaminasemia in adult celiac patients and effect of gluten-free diet. Hepatology 1995;22:833. (Ref.158)

Blanco R, et al. Henoch-Schonlein purpura in adulthood and childhood: two different expressions of the same syndrome. Arthritis Rheum 1997;40: 859. (Ref.97)

Bull RK, Edwards PD, Dixon AK. CT dimensions of the normal pericardium. Br J Radiol 1998;71:923. (Ref.35)

Calvino MC, et al. Henoch-Schonlein purpura in children from northwestern Spain. A 20-year epidemiologic and clinical study. Medicine (Baltimore) 2001;80:279. (Ref.99)

Cavagna L, et al. Infliximab in the treatment of adult Still's disease refractory to conventional therapy. Clin Exp Rheumatol 2001;19:329. (Ref.96)

Chang WL, et al. Gastrointestinal manifestations in Henoch-Schonlein purpura: a review of 261 patients. Acta Pediatr 2004;93:1427. (Ref.98)

Chao HC, Kong MS, Lin SJ. Hepatobiliary involvement of Henoch-Schonlein purpura in children. Acta Paediatr Taiwan 2000;41:63. (Ref.108)

Chen DY, et al. Predominance of Th1 cytokine in peripheral blood and pathological tissues of patients with active untreated adult onset Still's disease. Ann Rheum Dis 2004;63:1300. (Ref.86)

Chinnaiyan KM, Leff CB, Marsalese DL. Constrictive pericarditis versus restrictive cardiomyopathy: challenges in diagnosis and management. Cardiol Rev 2004;12:314. (Ref.28)

Chung DJ, et al. Radiologic findings of gastrointestinal complications in an adult patient with Henoch-Schonlein purpura. Am J Roentgenol 2006;187:396. (Ref.104)

Clemente MG, et al. Early effects of gliadin on enterocyte intracellular signaling involved in intestinal barrier function. Gut 2003;52:218. (Ref.160)

Comenzo RL. Hematopoietic cell transplantation for primary systemic amyloidosis: what have we learned? Leuk Lymph 2000;37:245. (Ref.128)

Comenzo RL, et al. Dose-intensive melphalan with blood stem-cell support for the treatment of AL (amyloid light-chain) amyloidosis: survival and responses in 25 patients. Blood 1998;91:3662. (Ref.126)

de Kerguenec C, et al. Hepatic manifestations of hemophagocytic syndrome: a study of 30 cases. Am J Gastroenterol 2001;96:852. (Ref.144)

Dillmann WH. Thyroid storm. Curr Ther Endocrinol Metab 1997;6:81. (Ref.168)

Dimopoulos MA, Galani E, Matsouka C. Waldenström's macroglobulinemia. Hematol Oncol Clin North Am 1999;13:1351. (Ref.192)

Dino OPG, et al. Fulminant hepatic failure in adult onset Still's disease. J Rheumatol 1996;23:784. (Ref.91)

Dolezal MV, et al. Virus-associated hemophagocytic syndrome characterized by clonal Epstein-Barr virus genome. Am J Clin Pathol 1995;103:188. (Ref.145)

Dourakis SP, et al. Fulminant hepatic failure as a presenting paraneoplastic manifestation of Hodgkin's disease. Eur J Gastroenterol Hepatol 1999;11:1055. (Ref.183)

Drueke TB. Beta2-microglobulin and amyloidosis. Nephrol Dial Transpl 2000;15:17. (Ref.118)

Ebert EC. Gastrointestinal manifestations of Henoch-Schonlein purpura. Dig Dis Sci 2008;53:2011. (Ref.101)

Efthimiou P, Paik PK, Bielory L. Diagnosis and management of adult onset Still's disease. Ann Rheum Dis 2006;65:564. (Ref.87)

Escudero FJ, et al. Rubella infection in adult onset Still's disease. Ann Rheum Dis 2000;59:493. (Ref.85)

Farrell GC. Drug-induced liver disease. London: Churchill Livingstone, 1994: 388. (Ref.55)

Fautrel B. Ferritin levels in adult Still's disease: any sugar? Joint Bone Spine 2002;69:355. (Ref.88)

Fox RA, et al. Liver function test abnormalities in systemic lupus erythematosus [abstract]. Br J Rheumatol 1997;36(Suppl):S10. (Ref.47)

Fuchs S, et al. Ischemic hepatitis. Clinical and laboratory observations of 34 patients. J Clin Gastroenterol 1998;26:183. (Ref.15)

Garcia-Porrua C, et al. Henoch-Schonlein purpura in children and adults: clinical differences in a defined population. Semin Arthritis Rheum 2002;32:149. (Ref.111)

Gardner-Medwin JMM, et al. Incidence of Henoch-Schonlein purpura, Kawasaki disease, and rare vasculitides in children of different ethnic origins. Lancet 2002;360:1197. (Ref.100)

Gertz MA, Kyle RA. Amyloidosis: prognosis and treatment. Semin Arthritis Rheum 1994;24:124. (Ref.124)

Gertz MA, Kyle RA. Hepatic amyloidosis: clinical appraisal in 77 patients. Hepatology 1997;25:118. (Ref.119)

Gertz MA, Lacy MQ, Dispenzieri A. Amyloidosis. Hematol Oncol Clin North Am 1999;13:1211. (Ref.112)

Ghobrial IM, et al. Therapeutic options in patients with lymphoma and severe liver dysfunction. Mayo Clinic Proc 2004;79:169. (Ref.189)

Giallourakis CC, Rosenberg PM, Friedman LS. The liver in heart failure. Clin Liver Dis 2002;6:947. (Ref.12)

Gillmore JD, Lovat LB, Hawkins PN. Amyloidosis and the liver. J Hepatol 1999;30:117. (Ref.113)

Haram K, et al. Severe syndrome of hemolysis, elevated liver enzymes and low platelets (HELLP) in the 18th week of pregnancy associated with antiphospholipid-antibody syndrome. Acta Obstet Gynaecol Scand 2003; 82:679. (Ref.66)

Hassan M, et al. Hepatitis C virus in sickle cell disease. J Nat Med Assoc 2003; 95:939. (Ref.138)

Henrion J, et al. Hypoxic hepatitis. Clinical and hemodynamic study in 142 consecutive cases. Medicine (Baltimore) 2003;82:392. (Ref.26)

Henter JI, et al. HLH-2004: diagnostic and therapeutic guidelines for hemophagocytic lymphohistiocytosis. Pediatr Blood Cancer 2007;166:124. (Ref.143)

Hogan SP, et al. Eosinophils: biological properties and role in health and disease. Clin Exp Allergy 2008;38:709. (Ref.154)

Horne A, et al. Haematopoietic stem cell transplantation in haemophagocytic lymphohistiocytosis. Br J Haematol 2005;129:622. (Ref.149)

Horny H-P, et al. Systemic mast cell disease (mastocytosis). General aspects and histopathological diagnosis. Histol Histopathol 1997;12:1081. (Ref.151)

Huang MJ, Liaw YF. Clinical association between thyroid and liver diseases. J Gastroenterol Hepatol 1995;10:344. (Ref.166)

Husni ME, et al. Etanercept in the treatment of adult patients with Still's disease. Arthritis Rheum 2002;46:1171. (Ref.95)

Imashuku S, et al. Requirement for etoposide in the treatment of Epstein-Barr virus-associated hemophagocytic lymphohistiocytosis. J Clin Oncol 2001;19:2665. (Ref.148)

Janka GE. Hemophagocytic syndromes. Blood Rev 2007;21:245. (Ref.141)

Kahn JE, Blétry O, Guillevin L. Hypereosinophilic syndromes. Best Pract Res Clin Rheumatol 2008;22:863. (Ref.155)

Kaukinen K, et al. Celiac disease in patients with severe liver disease: gluten-free diet may reverse hepatic failure. Gastroenterology 2002;122:881. (Ref.163)

Kim HJ, et al. The incidence and clinical characteristics of symptomatic propylthiouracil-induced hepatic injury in patients with hyperthyroidism: a single-center retrospective study. Am J Gasteronterol 2001;96:165. (Ref.170)

Korponay-Szabo IR, et al. In vivo targeting of intestinal and extraintestinal transglutaminase 2 by celiac autoantibodies. Gut 2004;53:641. (Ref.162)

Lee TH, et al. Concurrent occurrence of chylothorax and chylous ascites in a patient with Henoch-Schonlein purpura. Scand J Rheumatol 2003;32:378. (Ref.110)

Loechelt BJ, et al. Immunosuppression: preliminary results of alternative maintenance therapy for familial hemophagocytic lymphohistiocytosis (FHL). Med Pediatr Oncol 1994;22:325. (Ref.147)

Loustaud-Ratti V, et al. Prevalence and characteristics of Sjogren's syndrome or Sicca syndrome in chronic hepatitis C virus infection: a prospective study. J Rheumatol 2001;28:2245. (Ref.77)

Magadur-Joly G, et al. Epidemiology of adult Still's disease. J Epidemiol 1997;7:221. (Ref.81)

Mahmud T, Hughes GR. Intravenous immunoglobulin in the treatment of refractory adult Still's disease. J Rheumatol 1999;26:2067. (Ref.94)

McFadden PM, et al. Pericardiectomy for pericardial constriction. Am J Surg 1996;62:304. (Ref.39)

McFarlane M, Harth M, Wall WJ. Liver transplant in adult Still's disease. J Rheumatol 1997;24:2038. (Ref.90)

Memeo L, et al. Primary non-Hodgkin's lymphoma of the liver. Acta Oncol 1999;38:655. (Ref.185)

Mohr A, et al. Hepatomegaly and cholestasis as primary clinical manifestations of an AL-kappa amyloidosis. Eur J Gastroenterol Hepatol 1999;11:921. (Ref.120)

Monteiro E, Freire A, Barroso E. Familial amyloid polyneuropathy and liver transplantation. J Hepatol 2004;41:188. (Ref.129)

Murakami T, Uchino M, Ando M. Genetic abnormalities and pathogenesis of familial amyloidotic polyneuropathy. Pathol Int 1995;45:1. (Ref.117)

Naschitz JE, et al. Heart diseases affecting the liver and liver diseases affecting the heart. Am Heart J 2000;140:111. (Ref.8)

Nowak G, et al. Liver transplantation as rescue treatment in a patient with primary AL kappa amyloidosis. Transpl Int 2000;13:92. (Ref.127)

Pauls JD, et al. Mastocytosis: diverse presentations and outcomes. Arch Intern Med 1999;15:9401. (Ref.150)

Pawlotsky JM, et al. Extrahepatic immunologic manifestations in chronic hepatitis C virus serotypes. Ann Intern Med 1995;122:169. (Ref.76)

Pelletier S, et al. Antiphospholipid syndrome as the second cause of non-tumorous Budd–Chiari syndrome. J Hepatol 1994;21:76. (Ref.64)

Peters RA, et al. Primary amyloidosis and severe intrahepatic cholestatic jaundice. Gut 1994;35:1322. (Ref.121)

Peters U, et al. Causes of death in patients with celiac disease in a population-based Swedish cohort. Arch Intern Med 2003;163:1566. (Ref.159)

Pioltelli P, et al. Hepatitis C virus in non-Hodgkin's lymphoma. A reappraisal after a prospective case-control study of 300 patients. Am J Hematol 2000;64: 95. (Ref.188)

Pollock DJ. The liver in celiac disease. Histopathology 1997;1:421. (Ref.164)

Ramanan A, Laxer R, Schneider R. Secondary hemophagocytic syndromes associated with rheumatic diseases. In: Weitzman S, Egeler RM, editors. Histiocytic disorders of children and adults, Cambridge University Press: Cambridge, 2005: 380. (Ref.146)

Ramos-Casals M, et al. Sjögren's syndrome and hepatitis C virus. Clin Rheumatol 1999;18:93. (Ref.75)

Roberts G, et al. Acute renal failure complicating HELLP syndrome, SLE and antiphospholipid-antibody syndrome: successful outcome using plasma exchange therapy. Lupus 2003;12:251. (Ref.67)

Rostom A, Murray JA, Kagnoff MF. American Gastroenterological Association (AGA) Institute technical review on the diagnosis and management of celiac disease. Gastroenterology 2006;131:1981. (Ref.157)

Rubio-Tapia A, Murray JA. The liver in celiac disease. Hepatology 2007;46: 1650. (Ref.161)

Ruderman EM, et al. Histologic liver abnormalities in an autopsy series of patients rheumatoid arthritis. Br J Rheum 1997;36:210. (Ref.57)

Santiago J, et al. Henoch-Schonlein purpura with hemorrhagic ascites and intestinal serositis. Gastrointest Endosc 1996;44:624. (Ref.109)

Seeto R, Fenn B, Rockey DC. Ischemic hepatitis: clinical presentation and pathogenesis. Am J Med 2000;109:109. (Ref.18)

Skopouli FN, Barbatis C, Moutsopoulos HM. Liver involvement in primary Sjögren's syndrome. Br J Rheumatol 1994;33:745. (Ref.72)

Stinchcombe J, Bossi G, Griffiths GM. Linking albinism and immunity: the secrets of secretory lysosomes. Science 2004;305:55. (Ref.142)

Suhr OB, et al. Liver transplantation for hereditary transthyretin amyloidosis. Liver Transplant 2000;6:263. (Ref.130)

Tan SY, Pepys MB, Hawkins PN. Treatment of amyloidosis. Am J Kidney Dis 1995;26:267. (Ref.125)

Tsutsumi A, Koike T. Hepatic manifestations of the antiphospholipid syndrome. Intern Med 2000;39:6. (Ref.62)

Urieli-Shoval S, Linke RP, Matzner Y. Expression and function of serum amyloid A, a major acute-phase protein, in normal and disease states. Curr Opin Hematol 2000;7:64. (Ref.116)

Viola S, et al. Ischemic necrosis of bile ducts complicating Schonlein-Henoch purpura. Gastroenterology 1999;117:211. (Ref.107)

Wakai K, et al. Estimated prevalence and incidence of adult Still's disease: findings by a nationwide epidemiological survey in Japan. J Epidemiol 1997;7:221. (Ref.82)

Walther MM, et al. Serum interleukin-6 levels in metastatic renal cell carcinoma before treatment with interleukin-6 correlates with paraneoplastic syndromes but not patient survival. J Urol 1998;159:718. (Ref.177)

Wang ZJ, et al. CT and MR imaging of pericardial disease. RadioGraphics 2003;23:S167. (Ref.34)

Wanless IR, Liu JJ, Butany J. Role of thrombosis in the pathogenesis of congestive hepatic fibrosis. Hepatology 1995;21:1232. (Ref.4)

Weller PF, Bubley GJ. The idiopathic hypereosinophilic syndrome. Blood 1994;83:2759. (Ref.156)

Woolf GM, et al. Acute liver failure due to lymphoma: a diagnostic concern when considering liver transplantation. Dig Dis Sci 1994;39:1351. (Ref.182).

Youssef WI, Mullen KD. The liver in other (nondiabetic) endocrine disorders. Clin Liver Dis 2002;6:879. (Ref.165)

Zakaria N, et al. Acute sickle cell hepatopathy represents a potential contraindication for percutaneous liver biopsy. Blood 2003;101:101. (Ref.134)

Zurada JM, Ward KM, Grossman ME. Henoch-Schonlein purpura associated with malignancy in adults. J Am Acad Dermatol 2006;55(5 Suppl):S65. (Ref.103)

A complete list of references can be found at www.expertconsult.com.

The Liver and Parenteral Nutrition

Khalid M. Khan, Navaneeth C. Kumar, and Rainer W. Gruessner

ABBREVIATIONS

BSEP bile-salt export pump
CCK cholecystokinin
FXR farnesoid X receptor
GGT γ-glutamyltranspeptidase
GLP glucagon-like peptide
HBD hepatobiliary disorder
Ig immunoglobulin

IL interleukin
PN parenteral nutrition
PNAC PN-associated cholestasis
PUFA polyunsaturated fatty acid
PXR pregnane X receptor
SAMe S-adenosylmethionine
SBS short bowel syndrome

SGA small for gestational age
SIBO small intestinal bacterial overgrowth
STEP serial transverse enteroplasty
TNF-α tumor necrosis factor-α
UDCA ursodeoxycholic acid
VLDL very-low-density lipoprotein

Introduction

Nutrition administered intravenously, also termed parenteral nutrition (PN), can be used to supplement an inadequate enteral intake or it can be formulated to provide the majority of the nutritional requirements of the body. PN is life-saving for patients without remaining options for enteral nutrition and has been used in routine clinical practice for more than 5 decades for adults and children, including premature neonates. Complications of PN include those related to the safety and adequacy of its content and administration. Liver-related issues, the main focus of this chapter, range from biochemical abnormalities in asymptomatic individuals to biliary disease, steatosis, severe cholestasis, and end-stage liver disease. An awareness of the natural history and underlying contributing factors to PN-related liver disease will allow the clinician to make appropriate adjustments to circumvent or reduce the potential for the most serious complications and consider therapies such as intestinal transplantation for those patients with a poor prognosis with medical therapy alone.

Indications

In the inpatient setting PN is used for ill patients with limited ability or inability to use the enteral route, often in a catabolic state. Long-term PN is used in patients with structural and/or functional intestinal failure, a major malabsorptive state, or an inaccessible intestine. In cases not involving intestinal loss, the situation typically develops in adults with chronic illness or malignancy whereas in children it is most often related to congenital intestinal problems and prematurity (**Table 55-1**).

The characteristics of the underlying disease state may also determine the way PN is used, even in the long term. For instance, in widespread malignant disease involving the abdomen, PN may be necessary despite the presence of an intact small intestine because of symptoms related to enteral feeding.

Complications

Whether PN is necessary for a short or long time, complications related to venous access can be expected to occur. PN diluted for administration through a peripheral vein may lead to venous thrombophlebitis, and extravasation of PN into surrounding soft tissues can also occur. Such complications are also possible with central venous catheters. In addition, problems arising from central line placement or displacement are more likely with longer duration of PN. The impending loss of suitable venous access sites is an indicator for intestinal transplantation.[1]

Bacterial and fungal organisms both introduced and colonized through the central venous catheter can result in life-threatening sepsis. In turn, septicemia is a risk factor for loss of venous access and end-organ damage from cardiovascular collapse, hematologic compromise, and embolic phenomena. Bacterial sepsis is specifically related to hepatobiliary complications associated with PN (discussed later).

The preexisting nutritional status and nutritional requirements of the patient and the characteristics of the infusate have a key impact on complications in the initial days after PN is commenced. Early complications include fluid,

Table 55-1 Common Causes of Intestinal Failure*

Adults

Crohn disease
Midgut volvulus and small bowel incarceration
Small intestinal mesenteric thromboembolism
Trauma and surgical resection
Abdominal malignancy (including radiation)
Pseudoobstruction

Infants

Necrotizing enterocolitis
Gastroschisis
Malrotation and volvulus
Intestinal atresia
Pseudoobstruction
Aganglionosis
Congenital or immune enteropathy

*The list represents the most common underlying conditions in patients who need long-term parenteral nutrition. Intestinal failure may occur from a combination of a short small intestine, dysmotility, mucosal loss, ischemia, scarring, and infiltration.

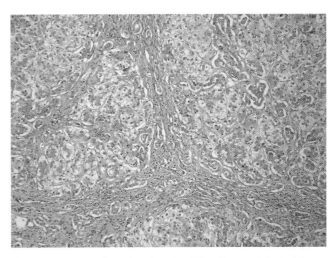

Fig. 55-1 Hematoxylin and eosin stain of liver from an infant with parenteral nutrition–related cholestatic liver showing portal inflammation, cholestasis with hepatocellular rosette formation, bile duct proliferation, and severe fibrosis.

Table 55-2 Hepatobiliary Pathology Associated with Parenteral Nutrition*

Acalculous cholecystitis
Biliary sludge
Cholestasis (predominant; infants)
Cholelithiasis and its complications
Fibrosis
Micronodular cirrhosis
Steatosis (predominant; adults)
Steatohepatitis

*More than one pathologic finding is typically present in patients receiving long-term parenteral nutrition. Hemosiderosis is also common in histologic liver specimens.

acid-base, and electrolyte abnormalities.[2] Some of these issues arise from refeeding and can be anticipated. Longer-term complications are less predictable and may be exacerbated by the presence of preexisting co-morbidities and underlying disorders, variability in nutritional requirements, inadequate composition of PN solution, or failure to monitor PN adequately. Potential complications include the whole gamut of nutritional deficiencies, in particular protein, essential fatty acid, trace mineral, and vitamin deficiencies; metabolic bone disease; and hepatobiliary disorders (HBDs).

Hepatobiliary Complications

Incidence and Pathology

Hepatic and biliary complications of PN are encountered in pediatric and adult patients (**Table 55-2**). The overall frequency of PN-associated liver complications is reported to range from 7.4% to 84%[3]; the wide variation in the reported frequency is the result of the heterogeneity in the population studied, the duration and composition of PN, and the liver complications reported in the studies.[4] For infants the incidence of PN-induced liver disease associated with intestinal failure is about 40% to 60%.[5] However, reported incidences vary from center to center and for different time periods.[6,7] In a survey conducted over 3 decades by Kubota and colleagues, the incidence of PN in infants appeared to have dropped from 57% in the 1970s to 25% in the 1990s.[8] The authors postulated that improvements in PN composition and advancements in sepsis control were the reasons for the progress. The most common and severe manifestation in infancy of PN-induced hepatobiliary disease is *cholestasis,* which may progress to potentially life-threatening liver dysfunction.[1,5] The pathology of the liver appears to transition through a number of stages in infants. In a histologic study steatosis (with portal eosinophilia and extramedullary hematopoiesis) was seen during the first 5 days of PN, canalicular cholestasis was observed in 84.2% of infants after 10 days of PN, and bile duct proliferation was found in 63.6% of infants after 3 weeks of PN.[9] Moderate to severe portal fibrosis was noted after 90 days, and one infant developed micronodular cirrhosis after 5 months. In a report of 24 infant autopsies, about 80% of specimens showed inflammation, cholestasis, bile duct proliferation, and extramedullary hematopoiesis.[10] Steatosis was common and more than 70% of the specimens showed fibrosis. **Figure 55-1** illustrates the histologic characteristics of PN-related liver disease from an infant who subsequently underwent liver transplantation.

In the adult population, including patients receiving home PN, the reported incidence of liver disease also varies widely. The severity ranges from minimal and transient increases in the levels of liver enzymes to cirrhosis and liver failure. In adults the typical presentation includes abnormal levels of liver enzymes and steatosis reported in 40% to 55% of cases.[5,11] In one report, however, the majority of adult patients administered PN for longer than 90 days exhibited steatosis.[12] PN-induced hepatic steatosis is characterized by centrilobular, microvesicular, and macrovesicular patterns. Steatosis may progress to steatohepatitis and fibrosis.[3] Steatohepatitis is characterized by the presence of mixed inflammatory infiltrates and focal necrosis.[1] End-stage liver disease occurs in 15% to 20% of adults administered PN.[13] In one report of adults with intestinal failure, cholestasis developed in 72% after 6 years of PN, and microsteatosis was present in 53% of biopsy samples.[14] In a European multicenter survey, up to 40% of patients reported fatty liver, and cirrhosis was observed in up to 25% of cases.[15] Other hepatocellular features reported in adults include hemosiderosis[16] and phospholipidosis.[1]

Sludging of bile is common in both adults and children administered long-term PN.[17] Sludge was reported in 50% of patients after 4 to 6 weeks of beginning PN[18] and 23% had gallstones. Gallstone formation occurs in almost half of the patients with shortened small bowel from resection.[19]

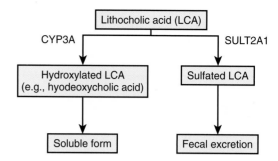

Fig. 55-2 Cytochrome P-450 3A (CYP3A) converts lithocholic acid (LCA) to more soluble nontoxic bile acids. Sulfation by hydroxysteroid sulfotransferase 2A1 (SULT2A1) reduces the ability to reabsorb LCA.

Pathogenesis

Pathogenesis is discussed here under the broad categories of cholestasis, steatosis, and biliary disorders. Evidence points to a number of risk factors for each of these PN-associated liver disorders; some factors are ubiquitous whereas others are unique to a specific liver disorder.

Cholestasis

PN-associated cholestasis (PNAC) is often defined as an increase in the concentration of serum-conjugated bilirubin to 2 mg/dl or greater.[20] It is typically accompanied by an increase in the levels of transaminases, alkaline phosphatase, or γ-glutamyltranspeptidase (GGT). Cholestasis is the most commonly noted liver disease associated with PN in infants.[1,5] It may develop within 2 weeks after beginning PN, but usually takes longer.[21] As noted earlier in this chapter, steatosis is also commonly present concurrently; fibrosis, cirrhosis, and, eventually, liver failure may occur.[10,22]

The duration of PN is a risk factor for PNAC. The severity of histopathologic changes progresses in relation to the duration of PN administration.[9] Children administered PN for less than 2 weeks were observed to have almost no fibrosis, whereas those with more than 6 weeks of PN developed moderate to severe fibrosis.[10] Similar results have been observed for cholestasis and bile duct proliferation. In a study involving 172 infants administered PN for at least 1 week (including 32 infants receiving PN for at least 7 weeks), increased severity of cholestatic jaundice directly correlated with duration of PN.[23] Low birth weight is an important risk factor for PNAC; Beale and colleagues, almost 3 decades ago, found a 50% incidence of cholestatic liver disease in infants weighing less than 1000 g.[6] Infants with a birth weight over 1500 g had only a 7% incidence. Being small for gestational age (SGA) is an independent risk factor for PNAC.[24] Low-birth-weight infants who were SGA and administered PN for more than 7 days, despite being more mature than appropriate-for-gestational-age infants, had an increased predilection for PNAC and developed it earlier in life.[25] There is a body of evidence showing a greater prevalence and an increased severity of PNAC with greater degrees of prematurity.[5,19,26]

Hepatic Maturation

The increased incidence of PNAC in premature infants indicates that its development is related to immaturity of the neonatal liver.[27] Particularly in premature infants, the total bile salt pool is reduced. Hepatic uptake and synthesis of bile salts is diminished, and enterohepatic circulation is decreased, in comparison with full-term infants or adults.[3,28] The canalicular bile-salt export pump (BSEP) is the major transporter of bile acids and therefore bile flow. BSEP and other bile-salt pumps in the ileum and canaliculi are under the control of nuclear transcription factors, most notably farnesoid X receptor (FXR), which controls the expression of BSEP.[29] Both classes of proteins are expressed at low levels in neonates; this may account for the propensity for cholestasis, especially in less mature infants.[30]

Bile Acid Toxicity

The ability to remove detergent bile acids by rendering them soluble depends on the bile acid transporter mechanism. In particular, chenodeoxycholate is dehydroxylated to the secondary bile acid lithocholate, a toxic derivative that is lethal to some species of animal even in small amounts. In increased amounts, lithocholic acid promotes a reduction in bile flow with subsequent cholestasis, gallstone formation, and bile duct proliferation.[31] In animal models it has been shown to cause bile duct injury.[32] The normal processing of lithocholate is facilitated by enzymes controlled by a nuclear transcription factor pregnane X receptor (PXR). In humans the presence of lithocholate is sensed by the PXR, which can activate the genes required for effective conversion and elimination of lithocholate.[33] These include cytochrome P450 3A, which hydroxylates it to a more soluble form, and sulfotransferase (SULT2A1); sulfation enhances its fecal excretion (**Fig. 55-2**).[34] PXR also up-regulates expression of the membrane transporters that excrete lithocholate metabolites.[33] Low enzyme levels of PXR, as seen in fetuses and neonates, contribute to lithocholate toxicity.[30] Other detoxifying processes may also be deficient in early life because of similar ontogeny. As discussed later, increased availability and reabsorption of lithocholate also play a role in cholestasis related to PN in children and adults with small intestine disease.

Bile Acid Conjugation and Antioxidant Depletion

Prematurity and the newborn period are characterized by low levels of cystathionase activity, with a reduction in the ability to convert methionine to cysteine and therefore taurine and

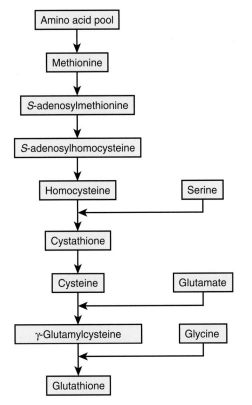

Fig. 55-3 Glutathione is necessary to counter cellular oxidant injury. It is synthesized from glutamate, cysteine, and glycine. Cysteine is derived from methionine via the hepatic transsulfuration pathway.

glutathione (**Fig. 55-3**).[35] Taurine is a part of the conjugation process of bile acids and reduced levels may therefore affect bile flow.[36] Involving the same pathway, the ability to adequately synthesize S-adenosylmethionine (SAMe), a methyl donor derived from methionine and ATP, is deficient in prematurity and the newborn period.[37] The deficiency of glutathione and SAMe, both antioxidants, potentially increases the risk of liver damage from free radicals, especially during oxidative stress such as hypoxia and hypoperfusion[38]; glutathione also conjugates bile acids. In rodents SAMe has been shown to facilitate bile flow by maintaining normal plasma membrane Na^+,K^+-ATPase activity.[39]

Composition of Infusate

Cholestasis can be related to PN composition as a result of a deficiency state, an excess or accumulation of a potential toxin, and an imbalance of nutrients.[40] The best-documented contaminants in pediatric PN are phytosterols, derived from soy and noted to be present in commercial lipid preparations. Sterols are difficult to metabolize and displace cholesterol in cell membranes, affecting membrane-related function including bile acid transporters.[41] Sterols were also shown to directly antagonize FXR.[42] Proteins (amino acids) are a necessary part of PN; however, in rodent studies infusion of amino acids has been shown to cause reduced bile flow; methionine infusion resulted in cholestasis and an elevation of homocysteine levels.[43] A study that examined the amount of protein in PN showed that with high protein concentrations cholestasis develops at a relatively earlier stage.[44] Conversely, methionine, which is an essential amino acid, is necessary for cellular antioxidant function and bile flow (see previous section).[45] Carbohydrate in the form of dextrose is the main nonprotein caloric source in PN. In a rodent model hyperglycemia was shown to reduce bile flow by a mechanism independent of bile flow.[46] An observational study of adult patients administered PN found that cholestatic individuals received higher caloric (fat and protein) intakes compared with noncholestatic individuals.[47] A reduction in PN in cholestatic individuals was associated with reversal of jaundice and improvement in liver biochemistry and histologic results. Lipids are routinely added to PN to provide a portion of the nonprotein calories. To avoid deficiency of essential fatty acids and fat-soluble vitamins, infusion of small amounts of lipid (0.5 g/kg/day) is necessary.[40] Lipid infusion has been shown to be related to cholestasis in both adults and children[40,48,49] and in particular at a rate greater than 1 g/kg/day.[14,40]

ω3 and ω6 Polyunsaturated Fatty Acids

The standard lipid emulsions for parenteral use in the United States contain soy or safflower oil. Of these long-chain fatty acids, ω-polyunsaturated fatty acids (PUFAs) are the most abundant; they result in plasma-free fatty acids, such as arachidonic acid, and do not reflect the balance with ω3 in cell membranes. Of note, ω6 PUFAs have been shown to cause monocyte proinflammatory cytokine release and monocyte–endothelium interaction.[50] Furthermore, infused lipids interfere with cholesterol metabolism, macrophage function, clearance of endotoxin, and lipid peroxidation.[48]

Fish oil–based lipid emulsions are primarily composed of ω3 PUFAs. In a mouse model such emulsions protected against liver injury; the same investigators found them to be safe and have some efficacy in children with PN-related cholestatic liver disease.[51] Similarly, in a sepsis model addition of ω3 lipid emulsions significantly increased the ω3/ω6 fatty acid ratios in the plasma-free fatty acid fraction and in the monocyte membrane lipid pool, markedly suppressing monocyte generation of tumor necrosis factor-alpha (TNF-α) and interleukin-1 (IL-1), IL-6, and IL-8 in response to endotoxin.[52] In addition, ω3 lipid emulsions significantly inhibited both monocyte–endothelium adhesion and migration.[52] The role of endotoxin and cytokines in causing cholestasis is discussed in the next section.

Altered Intestinal Physiology and Absence of Enteral Feeding

The combination of lack of enteral intake, altered anatomy (especially with a very short bowel and/or absent ileocecal valve), and severe dysmotility can lead to severe cholestasis and end-stage liver disease in infants. This is also the case for adults or older children who undergo massive small intestine loss. Andorsky and colleagues examined children with short bowel syndrome (SBS) administered PN for at least 3 months and found that shorter small intestine length, longer time with a stoma, more frequent episodes of sepsis, and fewer days of enteral feeding correlated with higher peak bilirubin levels.[53]

Intraluminal nutrients stimulate cholecystokinin (CCK) release.[1] In the absence of CCK release gallbladder emptying is reduced, leading to biliary stasis and depletion of the enterohepatic circulation. Levels of other gut hormones and growth factors necessary for enterocyte development and consequent function are also reduced in the absence of stimulation by enteral intake, resulting in hypoplasia of the enterocyte mass.[54] Gut immunity is impaired in the absence of enteral feeding in individuals receiving PN; immunoglobulin A (IgA) secretion, gut-associated lymphoid tissue, and lymphocyte populations are reduced.[55,56] Intestinal hypoplasia and a reduced level of gut immunity will likely alter the balance between intestinal bacteria and translocation of bacteria to the systemic circulation. This effect is further compounded by decreased small intestinal motility.[57] Translocation of bacteria activates inflammatory pathways through an increase in portal endotoxin levels. The lipopolysaccharide in endotoxin is known to stimulate macrophages/Kupffer cells to release cytokines and has a role in steatosis and cholestasis.[58] Cholestasis occurs from a number of mechanisms; the most direct involves reduction of uptake and secretion of bile acids into canaliculi by the action of endotoxin on the bile acid pumps and the multispecific organic ion transporter (Mrp2) present on the hepatocyte canalicular membrane.[59] Endotoxin also acts directly on stellate cells, further compounding inflammation and fibrosis. Even a small amount of enteral intake has a significant impact on reducing hepatobiliary complications.[60]

Short bowel syndrome is a malabsorptive state resulting from anatomic or functional loss of small intestine. The ability to secrete ileal hormones (e.g., enteroglucagon, glucagon-like peptides [GLPs] 1 and 2, peptide YY, neurotensin) may be lost in patients with SBS and the adaptive process may cause small intestinal dilation. Patients with any of the following conditions will develop small intestinal bacterial overgrowth (SIBO): untreatable intestinal disorders (e.g., intestinal pseudoobstruction); very short remaining small bowel segments; loss of the ileocecal valve; or small bowel strictures with stasis.[5,21] Bacterial overgrowth may result in increased lithocholate formation by deconjugation. Furthermore, bacteria translocate to extraintestinal sites that include the liver.[61] In patients with intestinal failure being administered PN, central venous catheter infection is the most prevalent infectious complication[62] and may be from enteric organisms or skin commensals.[63] As noted earlier in this chapter, release of bacterial endotoxin from all these sources triggers a cytokine cascade that contributes to cholestasis.

Steatosis

Although steatosis (either microvesicular or macrovesicular) is a common complication of PN in adults, steatohepatitis is less common.[64] Steatosis is known to occur in specific situations including metabolic diseases, diabetes, malnutrition and starvation, refeeding obesity, and toxin exposure,[19] and mechanisms responsible for steatosis in these disorders may contribute to PN-induced steatosis.

Composition of Infusate

An imbalance of nonprotein macronutrients, particularly carbohydrate and fat, in PN solutions is the most basic cause for steatosis. Steatosis results from infusion of venous glucose outside of the portal system, particularly in the absence of lipid.[64] Lipogenesis results from excess glucose that cannot be oxidized, from increased plasma insulin levels, and from an altered insulin/glucagon level balance; fatty acid synthesis and esterification are stimulated, whereas fatty acid oxidation is depressed.[65,66] In adults the glucose infusion rate for optimal glucose oxidation is approximately 5 mg/kg/min and lipogenesis may be expected at higher rates.[67] Newborn and particularly premature infants are able to tolerate higher rates of glucose infusion; this may account for steatosis not being a dominant feature in PN-related liver disease in infants. An imbalance between carbohydrate and nitrogen levels can also cause steatosis.[21] As discussed earlier, intravenous lipid in PN induces an inflammatory cascade that alters fatty acid metabolism and therefore contributes to steatosis as well as cholestasis. Excessive infused lipid itself is scavenged and therefore ends up in Kupffer cells, rather than entering the hepatocytes.[68]

Choline is necessary to synthesize very-low-density lipoprotein (VLDL); without transport out of the hepatocyte, triglyceride accumulates in the liver, resulting in steatosis. In a rat model a choline-free regimen was shown to cause steatosis[69] and low levels of choline are documented in cirrhotic patients.[70] In PN a small amount of choline is provided in the form of phosphatidylcholine; however, low serum levels of choline have been documented with PN regimens and shown to correlate with the degree of steatosis.[71,72] In both adults and children with elevated levels of aminotransferases, steatosis has been noted to improve when they receive choline.[71,72] Low choline levels may also be from reduced synthesis attributable to immaturity or depletion of the transsulfuration pathway (see next section).

Carnitine is essential for fat metabolism, transporting long-chain fats across the mitochondrial membrane. Methionine is a precursor for carnitine synthesis; therefore impairment in hepatic transsulfuration may diminish carnitine levels as well as levels of other sulfa-containing products (e.g., choline, lecithin, taurine, glutathione) (see **Fig. 55-3**). Peripherally metabolized intravenous (rather than enteral) methionine may not be available for hepatic consumption.[73] In practice monitoring long-term PN in adults and children has not revealed deficiency states.[74,75] On the other hand, adding carnitine to PN enhances ketogenesis and fat metabolism in premature infants.[76,77]

Infection, Inflammation, and Antioxidants

Steatosis is common in individuals with chronic infection and receiving PN; this is mediated through endotoxin release. An increase in free fatty acids released from triglycerides, an increase in hepatic uptake of triglycerides, and increased hepatic synthesis have been shown to occur in animals after the infusion of endotoxin.[78] Moreover, these changes are partially reversed by the administration of antibiotics or TNF-α antibodies in animals.[79,80] The effect of SIBO is similarly mediated.[81]

Hepatic oxidant injury and glutathione depletion have been reported to occur with PN.[73] Oxidative stress impairs glucose uptake and adversely affects lipid metabolism. Although infants are particularly at risk because of the immaturity of the glutathione synthesis pathway, it has been argued that hepatic steatosis is largely due to infused oxidants and/or to decreased antioxidant capacity.[1,21] In a liver model, exposure of PN solutions to light has been linked to alterations in hepatobiliary function and histology[82]; such alterations have been demonstrated in vivo.[83] Exposing multivitamins in PN solution to light results in photooxidation, leading to peroxide formation (mainly hydrogen peroxide). Parenteral fat formulations contain lipid peroxides that undergo further peroxidation when exposed to light.[84-86] Peroxides are associated with hepatic steatosis and fibrosis as well as cholestasis (discussed earlier).[87] In parenterally fed premature infants, protecting the intravenous line from light decreased the load of infused peroxides.[88] Photooxidized products of amino acids are also implicated in steatosis.[89] In an experimental model a decrease in hepatic nitric oxide synthesis has been shown to induce severe hepatic steatosis, which can be reversed with arginine.[90]

Biliary Disorders

Bile becomes primed for stone formation by reduced gallbladder contractility combined with abnormal and excessive bile saturation. With sludging of bile, the amounts of mucin glycoproteins, unconjugated bilirubin, and cholesterol monohydrate crystals increase.[91] Biliary sludge will eventually result in gallstones.[92]

Risk Factors for Biliary Disease

The composition of bile is altered in patients receiving PN because gallbladder emptying is reduced and bile flow is impaired by PN administration.[93,94] The major risk for biliary problems in individuals receiving PN is the absence of enteric nutrition to stimulate bile flow. The gallbladder motor function is impaired, potentially resulting in gallbladder dilatation, biliary sludge, gallstones, and acalculous cholecystitis. Pigment (calcium bilirubinate) stones typically develop from biliary sludging during long-term PN use (approximately 4 months).[1,21,95] Disruption of the enterohepatic circulation leads to a relative increase in cholesterol saturation because of the loss of bile salts.[96] Not surprisingly, gallstones are common after ileal disease and after ileal resection.[97] In patients with SBS, treatment of massive stoma output with octreotide (a long-acting somatostatin analogue), opiates, and anticholinergics reduces gallbladder contractility and increases the risk of cholelithiasis[98]; it also promotes SIBO and thereby creates more lithogenic bile.

Treatment

The definitive treatment for patients with HBDs is to discontinue PN and thereby reestablish enteral nutrition. This maneuver has to be effected in a timely manner to prevent the development of major health issues (e.g., sepsis-related morbidity and mortality, loss of venous access sites, end-stage liver disease). Biliary disease and nutritional deficiency states can be managed; however, quality of life may not be normal if PN therapy is a known lifelong prospect. Medical and surgical therapies may be able to reduce the impact of PN on the liver; however, for those with no prospect of discontinuing PN, intestinal transplantation is the only real option.

Formulation and Administration of Parenteral Nutrition and Monitoring of Patients

Nutritional requirements need to be calculated accurately for patients receiving PN. Overfeeding of macronutrients can be

an issue with PN, especially in infants; potential growth failure is always a concern. Optimizing the proportions of macromolecules by adding a suitable amount of lipid as a nonprotein calorie source (30% in adults) and keeping the glucose infusion rate at or less than 5 mg/kg/min may reduce conversion of excessive carbohydrate to fat and weaken the stimulus for insulin secretion.[47,99] In rats the addition of glucagon to PN has been shown to reduce hepatic lipid level, portal insulin/glucagon ratio, and periportal fatty infiltration[100] as well as to reverse hepatic steatosis.[101] Thus glucagon may be useful in established hepatic steatosis. Cycling the PN infusion allows the levels of insulin and of counter-regulatory hormones to normalize. In infants and adults it was shown to improve cholestasis.[102,103] High-dose lipid infusion should be considered a risk factor and the infusion rate should be reduced to 1 g/kg/day or less if cholestasis is beginning to be a concern.[14,104] The amounts of ω6 PUFAs, phospholipids, and phytosterols infused with the lipid emulsions can be reduced by using a mixture of long-chain and medium-chain triglycerides; a reduction in the incidence of liver enzyme abnormality has been reported.[105] Currently, ω3 PUFAs are not added routinely to PN. As noted earlier there are early data to support their use in PN; however, clinical experience is limited in using fish oil–based regimens (the primary source of ω3 PUFAs) in comparison with conventional regimens.[106] More data are needed addressing the possibility of complications such as essential fatty acid deficiency and the true potential of ω3 PUFAs in cholestatic liver disease.[107]

Taurine is an important consideration in neonates and premature infants; it is necessary for conjugation of bile acids.[36,108] There is, however, no clear evidence that supplementation has any role in PN-related liver disease in children or adults.

Checking plasma free choline levels and supplementing low levels should be considered. Low levels are reported in adults and children administered long-term PN and reversal of steatosis in adults with choline supplementation has been demonstrated.[72,109]

Intravenous carnitine, especially in patients with a deficiency, stimulates fatty acid oxidation and thereby helps reduce steatosis and cholestasis.[110] Supplementation was observed to improve cholestasis, hypoglycemia, and muscle weakness in a carnitine-deficient patient.[111]

Effective monitoring of patients' nutritional and fluid status is necessary to adjust the composition of PN. Regulation of the levels of fat-soluble and essential fatty acids and assessment of the development of micronutrient deficiencies are important in the management of PN-related liver disease (**Table 55-3, Fig. 55-4**). Biliary excretion is the major elimination pathway for manganese (and copper) and therefore manganese may accumulate in cholestasis. In children with cholestatic liver disease, basal ganglia changes were seen with high manganese levels.[112]

Biliary Function, Enteral Feeding, and Intestinal Hormones

Screening for gallbladder problems and removing the gallbladder should be considered in patients using long-term PN, because of the potential for dysfunction and eventual sepsis and gallstone formation.[113] In particular, patients with a very short small intestine appear to lose the normal gallbladder

Table 55-3 Practical Considerations in the Management of Parenteral Nutrition–Associated Liver Disease*

MANAGEMENT	WHEN TO CONSIDER
Assessment of macromolecule and fluid needs and adjustment of PN (including anthropometry and calorimetry)	Periodically while on long-term PN
Assessment of micronutrient needs	Periodically while on long-term PN
PN Administration	
Central line care	Review if repeated line infections
Cycling of PN	As soon as convenient
Monitor maximum infusion rate of glucose	Especially when cycling PN
PN Composition	
Lipids	With liver disease consider reducing to <1 g/kg/day and supplementing ω3 in infants
Fat-soluble vitamins	Monitor
Amino acids (carnitine, choline)	Monitor and supplement
Ursodeoxycholic acid	Evidence of PN-associated liver disease
Cholecystokinin	Gallbladder distention, no enteral intake, progressive cholestasis
Enteral feeding	Whenever possible
Glutamine	Small intestinal mucosal disease and short bowel syndrome
Glucagon	Steatosis
Antibiotics and probiotics	Sepsis, bacterial overgrowth
Antioxidants (including shielding PN solutions from light and arginine)	As listed above, other antioxidants† may be considered for progressive liver disease related to PN

*The common therapies currently used for liver disease related to PN are listed here. Some therapeutic options such as glucagon-like peptide 2 have future potential.

†Antioxidant regimens specifically for PN-related liver disease are yet to be defined. Although there is good evidence for use of proinflammatory cytokines, the potential for overwhelming sepsis precludes their routine use.

PN, parenteral nutrition

contraction response to CCK.[114] With a functioning gallbladder, intake of even a small amount of long-chain triglycerides or a small amount of protein stimulates the secretion of CCK and gallbladder contraction. The effect has been demonstrated with rapid intravenous infusions of amino acids (mimicking the effect of an enteral meal)[115] and prokinetics (e.g., the macrolide antibiotics erythromycin, cisapride, and indomethacin).[116] Administration of intravenous CCK improves bile flow and reduces the serum bilirubin concentration; however, no clear benefit on outcome has been demonstrated and side effects may occur.[117-119]

Enteral nutrition has a major protective role in PN-related HBDs. It reverses mucosal atrophy in patients who have previously been unable to feed, and it improves motility, thus reducing the potential for bacterial translocation. Bile flow is enhanced by stimulation of the enterohepatic circulation, and stores of precursors of glutathione are increased, thereby reducing oxidative damage to hepatocytes.[120]

Ursodeoxycholic acid (UDCA), a hydrophilic bile acid, reduces cholesterol crystallization. A choleretic agent, UDCA replaces bile acids that are toxic to the liver.[121] It has been shown to inhibit apoptosis by preventing mitochondrial membrane permeability and therefore antagonizes production of reactive oxygen species.[122] UCDA has been shown to be clinically effective in reducing or preventing PN-related intrahepatic cholestasis and is now routinely used in the management of patients with intestinal failure who are receiving PN.[123,124]

Antimicrobial, Antiinflammatory, and Antioxidant Therapies

Control of SIBO has a role in reducing cholestasis. Antibiotic treatment is largely empiric, given the difficulty of isolating specific bacteria from the small intestine, although a duodenal aspirate may reveal a dominant species. Metronidazole and gentamicin administered during PN have been shown to have a liver protective effect.[125,126] There is good evidence for treating chronic sepsis and/or interrupting the downstream cytokine release to circumvent PN-related liver disease.[78-81] Although there are animal data to suggest that antibodies to TNF-α would be effective in this role,[126] there is potential risk of bacterial sepsis. Probiotics also have a role in the reduction of SIBO.[126]

Glucagon-like polypeptide 2 is an enteroendocrine hormone that plays a significant role in the enhancement of intestinal function and growth, especially in SBS patients. It aids small intestine adaptation and improves the integrity of the small intestinal mucosa, potentially improving enteral intake and reducing bacterial translocation.[127,128]

L-Glutamine, a nonessential amino acid, accounts for one third of all the amino acid nitrogen in the plasma. It is the primary energy source for enterocytes. When added to rodent PN, it reduced PN-associated mucosal atrophy and bacterial translocation.[129] Furthermore, it has a protective effect against intestinal reperfusion injury after ischemia and bacterial translocation, improves immunoglobulin and T-lymphocyte populations, and enhances nitrogen balance.[130] In patients receiving PN, glutamine supplementation may be an indirect way of enhancing host defenses and decreasing infectious morbidity. Glutamine is also involved in glutathione production, and could help reduce oxidant-related hepatocyte damage.

Increasing evidence suggests that oxidation has a role in disease states ranging from cancer to ischemic cardiovascular and neurovascular disorders. In terms of the liver, cellular glutathione in its reduced form neutralizes reactive hydroxyl free radicals as well as oxygen-centered free radicals. Depletion of cellular glutathione results in cell death. Exogenous glutathione does not significantly affect the intracellular levels, but treatment with *N*-acetylcysteine replenishes stores by providing cysteine. Other repletion strategies have included α-lipoic

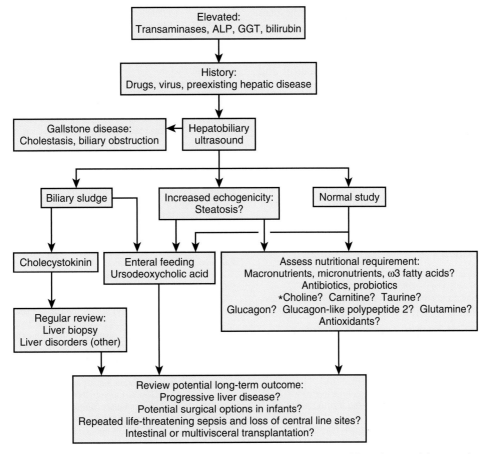

Fig. 55-4 The algorithm as followed by the author. Progression of PN-related liver disease is variable and no guidelines can be offered for timing of specific interventions. Asterisk, Data on cellular repletion and antioxidant therapies for application to PN-related liver disease are limited.

acid, ascorbic acid, and taurine. Not all glutathione precursors have shown potential for improving glutathione stores, yet animal data suggest that SAMe may prevent and treat cholestasis without discontinuation of PN.[131] Newer antioxidants with potential to attenuate oxidative liver damage in certain circumstances are being examined,[1] including curcumin.[132] In a rat model β-carotene was shown to reduce apoptosis of hepatocytes by blocking the production of reactive oxygen species generated by hydrophobic bile acids.[133] Selenium is an integral component of glutathione peroxidase, and acts synergistically with vitamin E in its action against lipid peroxidation, which is responsible for some of the destructive effects of free radicals on cell membranes. Data on these antioxidants having an impact on PN-associated liver disease are lacking. In a report on adults with chronic cholestatic liver disease, plasma levels of a panel of antioxidants appeared to be normal.[134]

Surgical Options

An infant with SBS who has a dysmotile, dilated, poorly functioning remnant and who is receiving PN is at great risk for developing cholestasis that will progress to end-stage liver disease. Removing strictures, tapering dilated areas of intestine, and performing intestinal lengthening procedures (Bianchi and serial transverse enteroplasty [STEP]) may help in reestablishing enteral nutrition and reducing SIBO. The recently created STEP Registry reported an increase of 116% in enteral tolerance in 38 patients; nearly half discontinued PN after a median follow-up time of about 1 year.[135]

Liver and Intestinal Transplantation

Patients with end-stage liver disease should be referred for a combined liver-intestine transplant. In light of the death rate of intestinal transplant candidates on the waiting list, early referral is preferred.[136] In patients with no effective enteral intake despite corrective surgery, or from pseudoobstruction or congenital enteropathy, an isolated small intestine transplant should be considered—before liver disease significantly progresses. An isolated liver transplant can be effective in infants with SBS where the lack of subsequent adaptation can be predicted.[137]

Prognosis and Conclusion

The prognosis for adults receiving PN for malignancy-related complications is determined by the primary problem. Of those receiving PN for nonmalignant causes, one study found that 11% of deaths were from PN-related complications and the 5-year survival rate was 62%.[138] In another series of adults using home PN, 15% developed cirrhosis.[13] Infants, including those that are premature, will recover—unless they have a primary intestinal disease such as pseudoobstruction or lose a large part or all of the small intestine. Persistent cholestasis remains a poor prognostic indicator in children; in a cohort study of 93 children with mainly SBS, the death rate was 58% in those with a persistently elevated bilirubin level.[124] Furthermore, this group was also least responsive to medical and surgical rehabilitation. Progressive hyperbilirubinemia is a poor prognostic indicator in children with intestinal failure and should prompt referral for intestinal transplantation.[139] Patients with decompensated cirrhosis should also be referred for liver transplantation. Greater focus on the PN formulation (particularly the role of antioxidants), further developments in small intestinal surgery, and improved outcomes of intestinal transplantation will help to reduce the need for long-term PN and the more severe consequences of PN-related liver disease.

Key References

Adamkin DH. Total parenteral nutrition-associated cholestasis: prematurity or amino acids? J Perinatol 2003;23:437–438. (Ref.27)

Andorsky DJ, et al. Nutritional and other postoperative management of neonates with short bowel syndrome correlates with clinical outcomes. J Pediatr 2001;139:27–33. (Ref.53)

Angelico M, Della Guardia P. Hepatobiliary complications associated with total parenteral nutrition. Alim Pharmacol Ther 2000;2:54–57. (Ref.17)

Balasubramaniyan N, et al. Multiple mechanisms of ontogenic regulation of nuclear receptors during rat liver development. Am J Physiol Gastrointest Liver Physiol 2005;288:G251–G260. (Ref.30)

Bao W, et al. Curcumin alleviates ethanol-induced hepatocytes oxidative damage involving heme oxygenase-1 induction. J Ethnopharmacol 2010;128:549–553. (Ref.132)

Baserga MC, Sola A. Intrauterine growth restriction impacts tolerance to total parenteral nutrition in extremely low birth weight infants. J Perinatol 2004;24:476–481. (Ref.25)

Belli DC, et al. S-Adenosylmethionine prevents total parenteral nutrition-induced cholestasis in the rat. J Hepatol 1994;31:18–23. (Ref.39)

Berg RD. Bacterial translocation from the gastrointestinal tract. Adv Exp Med Biol 1999;473:11–30. (Ref.61)

Bhatia J, et al. Total parenteral nutrition-associated alterations in hepatobiliary function and histology in rats: is light exposure a clue? Pediatr Res 1993;33:487–492. (Ref.83)

Bonner CM, et al. Effects of L-carnitine supplementation on fat metabolism and nutrition in premature infants. J Pediatr 1995;126:287–292. (Ref.77)

Btaiche IF, Khalidi N. Parenteral nutrition-associated liver complications in children. Pharmacotherapy 2002;22:188–211. (Ref.4)

Btaiche IF, Khalidi N. Metabolic complications of parenteral nutrition in adults, Part 2. Am J Health Syst Pharm 2004;61:2050–2057; quiz 2058–2059. (Ref.20)

Buchman AL, et al. Choline deficiency causes reversible hepatic abnormalities in patients receiving parenteral nutrition: proof of a human choline requirement: a placebo-controlled trial. JPEN J Parenter Enteral Nutr 2001;25:260–268. (Ref.72)

Buchman AL, et al. Choline deficiency: a cause of hepatic steatosis during parenteral nutrition that can be reversed with intravenous choline supplementation. Hepatology 1995;22:1399–1403. (Ref.71)

Buchman AL, Scolapio J, Fryer J. AGA technical review on short bowel syndrome and intestinal transplantation. Gastroenterology 2003;124:1111–1134. (Ref.136)

Bueno J, et al. Factors impacting the survival of children with intestinal failure referred for intestinal transplantation. J Pediatr Surg 1999;34:27–32. (Ref.139)

Carter BA, et al. Stigmasterol, a soy lipid-derived phytosterol, is an antagonist of the bile acid nuclear receptor FXR. Pediatr Res 2007;62:301–306. (Ref.42)

Catton JA, Dobbins BM, Wood JM. The routine microbial screening of central venous catheters in home parenteral nutrition patients. Clin Nutr 2004;23:171–175. (Ref.63)

Cavicchi M, et al. Prevalence of liver disease and contributing factors in patients receiving home parenteral nutrition for permanent intestinal failure. Ann Intern Med 2000;132:525–532. (Ref.14)

Chan S, et al. Incidence, prognosis, and etiology of end-stage liver disease in patients receiving home parenteral nutrition. Surgery 1999;126:28–34. (Ref.13)

Chesney RW, et al. The role of taurine in infant nutrition. Adv Exp Med Biol 1998;442:463–476. (Ref.36)

Chessex P, et al. Photooxidation of parenteral multivitamins induces hepatic steatosis in a neonatal guinea pig model of intravenous nutrition. Pediatr Res 2002;52:958–963. (Ref.87)

Colomb V, et al. Role of lipid emulsions in cholestasis associated with long-term parenteral nutrition in children. JPEN J Parenter Enteral Nutr 2000;24:345–350. (Ref.48)

Cowles RA, et al. Reversal of intestinal failure-associated liver disease in infants and children on parenteral nutrition: experience with 93 patients at a referral center for intestinal rehabilitation. J Pediatr Surg 2010;45:84–87. (Ref.124)

de Meijer VE, et al. Fish oil–based lipid emulsions prevent and reverse parenteral nutrition–associated liver disease: the Boston experience. JPEN J Parenter Enteral Nutr 2009;33:541–547. (Ref.51)

Dilger K, et al. No relevant effect of ursodeoxycholic acid on cytochrome P450 3A metabolism in primary biliary cirrhosis. Hepatology 2005;41:595–602. (Ref.34)

Ding LA, Li JS. Effects of glutamine on intestinal permeability and bacterial translocation in TPN-rats with endotoxemia. World J Gastroenterol 2003;9:1327–1332. (Ref.129)

Dzakovic A, et al. Trophic enteral nutrition increases hepatic glutathione and protects against peroxidative damage after exposure to endotoxin. J Pediatr Surg 2003;38:844–847. (Ref.120)

Enotomo E, et al. Role of Kupffer cells and gut-derived endotoxins in alcoholic liver injury. J Gastroenterol Hepatol 2000;15:D20–D25. (Ref.58)

Fell JM, et al. Manganese toxicity in children receiving long-term parenteral nutrition. Lancet 1996;347:1218–1221. (Ref.112)

Fickert P, et al. Lithocholic acid feeding induces segmental bile duct obstruction and destructive cholangitis in mice. Am J Pathol 2006;168:410–422. (Ref.32)

Floreani A, et al. Plasma antioxidant levels in chronic cholestatic liver diseases. Aliment Pharmacol Ther 2000;14:353–358. (Ref.134)

Fuchs M, Sanyal AJ. Sepsis and cholestasis. Clin Liver Dis 2008;12:151–172. (Ref.59)

Grattagliano I, et al. Starvation impairs antioxidant defence in fatty livers of rats fed a choline-deficient diet. J Nutr 2000;130:2131–2136. (Ref.69)

Guglielmi FW, et al. Hepatobiliary complications of long-term home parenteral nutrition. Clin Nutr 2001;20:51–55. (Ref.16)

Guglielmi FW, et al. Cholestasis induced by total parenteral nutrition. Clin Liver Dis 2008;12:97–110. (Ref.21)

Gumpricht E, et al. Beta-carotene prevents bile acid–induced cytotoxicity in the rat hepatocyte: evidence for an antioxidant and anti-apoptotic role of beta-carotene in vitro. Pediatr Res 2004;55:814–821. (Ref.133)

Heird WC. Amino acids in pediatric and neonatal nutrition. Curr Opin Clin Nutr Metab Care 1998;1:73–78. (Ref.45)

Hwang TL, Lue MC, Chen LL. Early use of cyclic TPN prevents further deterioration of liver functions for the TPN patients with impaired liver function. Hepatogastroenterology 2000;47:1347–1350. (Ref.103)

Iyer KR, Spitz L, Clayton P. New insight into mechanisms of parenteral nutrition associated cholestasis: role of plant sterols. J Pediatr Surg 1998;33:1–6. (Ref.41)

Jensen AR, et al. The association of cyclic parenteral nutrition and decreased incidence of cholestatic liver disease in patients with gastroschisis. J Pediatr Surg 2009;44:183–189. (Ref.102)

Kakkos SK, Yarmenitis SD, Kalfarentzos F. Gallbladder contraction induced by intravenous erythromycin administration. Relation to body mass index. Hepatogastroenterology 1996;43:1540–1543. (Ref.116)

Kelly DA. Liver complications of pediatric parenteral nutrition—epidemiology. Nutrition 1998;14:153–157. (Ref.3)

Kelly DA. Intestinal failure-associated liver disease: what do we know today? Gastroenterology 2006;130:S70–S77. (Ref.5)

Khashu M, et al. Impact of shielding parenteral nutrition from light on routine monitoring of blood glucose and triglyceride levels in preterm neonates. Arch Dis Child Fetal Neonatal Ed 2009;94:F111–F115. (Ref.88)

Koletzko B, Goulet O. Fish oil containing intravenous lipid emulsions in parenteral nutrition–associated cholestatic liver disease. Curr Opin Clin Nutr Metab Care 2010;13:321–326. (Ref.107)

Kubota A, et al. Total parenteral nutrition–associated intrahepatic cholestasis in infants: 25 years' experience. J Pediatr Surg 2000;35:1049–1051. (Ref.8)

Kudsk KA, Renegar KB, Li J. Loss of upper respiratory tract immunity with parenteral feeding. Ann Surg 1996;223:629–638. (Ref.56)

Kumar D, Tandon RK. Use of ursodeoxycholic acid in liver diseases. J Gastroenterol Hepatol 2001;16:3–14. (Ref.121)

Laborie S, Lavoie JC, Chessex P. Paradoxical role of ascorbic acid and riboflavin in solutions of total parenteral nutrition: implications in photo-induced peroxide generation. Pediatr Res 1998;43:601–606. (Ref.85)

Lavoie JC, et al. Admixture of a multivitamin preparation to parenteral nutrition: the major contributor to in vitro generation of peroxides. Pediatrics 1997;99:E61–E70. (Ref.84)

Li J, et al. Effects of parenteral nutrition on gut-associated lymphoid tissue. J Trauma 1995;39:44–52. (Ref.55)

Li N, et al. S-Adenosylmethionine in treatment of cholestasis after total parenteral nutrition, laboratory investigation and clinical application. Hepatobiliary Pancreat Dis Int 2002;1:96–100. (Ref.131)

Li Z, et al. Probiotics and antibodies to TNF inhibit inflammatory activity and improve nonalcoholic fatty liver disease. Hepatology 2003;37:343–350. (Ref.127)

Ling PR, et al. Cholecystokinin (CCK) secretion in patients with severe short bowel syndrome (SSBS). Dig Dis Sci 2001;46:859–864. (Ref.114)

Luman W, Shaffer JL. Prevalence, outcome and associated factors of deranged liver function tests in patients on home parenteral nutrition. Clin Nutr 2002; 21:337–343. (Ref.11)

Mayer K, et al. Parenteral nutrition with fish oil modulates cytokine response in patients with sepsis. Am J Respir Crit Care Med 2003;167:1321–1328. (Ref.52)

Mayer K, et al. Short-time infusion of fish oil-based lipid emulsions, approved for parenteral nutrition, reduces monocyte proinflammatory cytokine generation and adhesive interaction with endothelium in humans. J Immunol 2003;171:4837–4843. (Ref.50)

Messing B. Guidelines for management of home parenteral support in adult chronic intestinal failure patients. Gastroenterology 2006;130:S43–S51. (Ref.104)

Messing B, et al. Prognosis of patients with nonmalignant chronic intestinal failure receiving long-term home parenteral nutrition. Gastroenterology 1995;108:1005–1010. (Ref.138)

Misra S, et al. Plasma choline concentrations in children requiring long-term home parenteral nutrition: a case control study. JPEN J Parenter Enteral Nutr 1999;23:305–308. (Ref.109)

Modi BP, et al. First report of the International Serial Transverse Enteroplasty Data Registry: indications, efficacy, and complications. J Am Coll Surg 2007;204:365–371. (Ref.135)

Moss RL, Amii LA. New approaches to understanding the etiology and treatment of total parenteral nutrition–associated cholestasis. Semin Pediatr Surg 1999; 8:140–147. (Ref.38)

Moss RL, et al. Methionine infusion reproduces liver injury of parenteral nutrition cholestasis. Pediatr Res 1999;45:664–668. (Ref.43)

Mullady DK, O'Keefe SJ. Treatment of intestinal failure: home parenteral nutrition. Nat Clin Pract Gastroenterol Hepatol 2006;3:492–504. (Ref.64)

Murphy MS. Growth factors and the gastrointestinal tract. Nutrition 1998;14: 771–774. (Ref.54)

Neuzil J, et al. Oxidation of parenteral lipid emulsion by ambient and phototherapy lights: potential toxicity of routine parenteral feeding. J Pediatr 1995;126:785–790. (Ref.86)

Nightingale JM. Hepatobiliary, renal and bone complications of intestinal failure. Best Pract Res Clin Gastroenterol 2003;17:907–929. (Ref.95)

Nightingale JMD, Kamm MA, van der Sijp JR. Gastrointestinal hormones in SBSPeptide YY may be the colonic brake to gastric emptying. Gut 1996;39:267. (Ref.57)

Oshita M, et al. Significance of administration of fat emulsion: hepatic changes in infant rats receiving total parenteral nutrition with and without fat. Clin Nutr 2004;23:1060–1068. (Ref.65)

Pappo I, et al. Antitumor necrosis factor antibodies reduce hepatic steatosis during total parenteral nutrition and bowel rest in rat. JPEN J Parenter Enteral Nutr 1995;19:80–82. (Ref.80)

Parente F, et al. Incidence and risk factors for gallstones in patients with inflammatory bowel disease: a large case-control study. Hepatology 2007;45: 1267–1274. (Ref.97)

Pereira SP, et al. Bile composition in inflammatory bowel disease: ileal disease and colectomy, but not colitis, induce lithogenic bile. Aliment Pharmacol Ther 2003;17:923–933. (Ref.96)

Piper SN, et al. Hepatocellular integrity after parenteral nutrition: comparison of a fish-oil–containing lipid emulsion with an olive-soybean oil–based lipid emulsion. Eur J Anaesthesiol 2009;26:1076–1082. (Ref.106)

Raman M, Allard JP. Parenteral nutrition related hepato-biliary disease in adults. Appl Physiol Nutr Metab 2007;32:646–654. (Ref.1)

Reimund JM, et al. Catheter-related infection in patients on home parenteral nutrition: results of a prospective survey. Clin Nutr 2002;21:33–38. (Ref.62)

Richards CE, et al. Effect of different chloride infusion rates on plasma base excess during neonatal parenteral nutrition. Acta Paediatr 1993;82:678–682. (Ref.2)

Rintala RJ, Lindahl H, Pohjavuori M. Total parenteral nutrition–associated cholestasis in surgical neonates may be reversed by intravenous cholecystokinin: a preliminary report. J Paediatr Surg 1995;30:827–830. (Ref.118)

Robinson DT, Ehrenkranz RA. Parenteral nutrition–associated cholestasis in small for gestational age infants. J Pediatr 2008;152:59–62. (Ref.24)

Rodrigues CM, et al. A novel role for ursodeoxycholic acid in inhibiting apoptosis by modulating mitochondrial membrane perturbation. J Clin Invest 1998;101:2790–2799. (Ref.122)

Roth B, et al. Lipid deposition in Kupffer cells after parenteral fat nutrition in rats: a biochemical and ultrastructural study. Intensive Care Med 1996;22: 1224–1231. (Ref.68)

Rubin M, et al. Structured triacylglycerol emulsion, containing both medium and long chain fatty acids, in long-term home parenteral nutrition: a double blind randomized cross-over study. Nutrition 2000;16:95–100. (Ref.105)

Sandhu IS, Jarvis C, Everson GT. Total parenteral nutrition and cholestasis. Clin Liver Dis 1999;3:489–508. (Ref.12)

Shaffer JL, ESPEN-HAN Group. A European survey on management of metabolic complications in home parenteral nutrition. Clin Nutr 1997;16:79. (Ref.15)

Shattuck KE, et al. The effect of light exposure on the in vitro hepatic response to an amino acid–vitamin solution. JPEN J Parenter Enteral Nutr 1995;19:398–402. (Ref.82)

Sigalet DL, et al. Glucagon-like peptide-2 induces a specific pattern of adaptation in remnant jejunum. Dig Dis Sci 2006;51:1557–1566. (Ref.128)

Sokol RJ, et al. Hepatic oxidant injury and glutathione depletion during total parenteral nutrition in weanling rats. Am J Physiol 1996;270:G691–G700. (Ref.73)

Spagnuolo MI, et al. Ursodeoxycholic acid for treatment of cholestasis in children on long-term total parenteral nutrition: a pilot study. Gastroenterology 1996;111:716–719. (Ref.123)

Spagnuolo MI, Ruberto E, Guarino A. Isolated liver transplantation for treatment of liver failure secondary to intestinal failure. Ital J Pediatr 2009;35:28. (Ref.137)

Staudinger JL, et al. The nuclear receptor PXR is a lithocholic acid sensor that protects against liver toxicity. Proc Natl Acad Sci U S A 2001;98:3369–3374. (Ref.33)

Suchy FJ, Ananthanarayanan M. Bile salt excretory pump: biology and pathobiology. JPEN J Pediatr Gastroenterol Nutr 2006;43:S10–S16. (Ref.29)

Teitelbaum DH, et al. Use of cholecystokinin to prevent the development of parenteral nutrition–associated cholestasis. JPEN J Parenter Enteral Nutr 1997;21:100–103. (Ref.119)

Thompson JS. The role of prophylactic cholecystectomy in the short-bowel syndrome. Arch Surg 1996;131:556–560. (Ref.113)

Wigg AJ, et al. The role of small intestinal overgrowth, intestinal permeability, endotoxemia, and TNF alpha in the pathogenesis of non-alcoholic steatohepatitis. Gut 2001;48:206–211. (Ref.81)

Wu GH, et al. Glutamine supplemented parenteral nutrition prevents intestinal ischemia-reperfusion injury in rats. World J Gastroenterol 2004;10:2592–2594. (Ref.130)

Zambrano E, et al. Total parenteral nutrition induced liver pathology: an autopsy series of 24 newborn cases. Pediatr Dev Pathol 2004;7:425–432. (Ref.10)

Zheng JF, Wang HD, Liang LJ. Protective effects of nitric oxide on hepatic steatosis induced by total parenteral nutrition in rats. Acta Pharmacol Sin 2002;23:824–828. (Ref.90)

A complete list of references can be found at www.expertconsult.com.

IX

Chapter **56**

Preoperative and Postoperative Hepatic Dysfunctions

Thomas D. Boyer

Introduction

It is estimated that up to 10% of cirrhotic patients will undergo surgery in the final 2 years of their lives.[1,2] This leads to the need for a careful review of preoperative and postoperative liver dysfunction in this group of patients. In this chapter, we will review many aspects of what is known with regard to how the normal and diseased liver reacts to operative procedures.

The liver is the major site for the metabolism of many drugs and is responsible for the synthesis of most serum proteins and the removal of endogenous and exogenous toxins. Therefore postoperative liver dysfunction may slow the recovery of a patient who has undergone surgery. Because of the liver's role in drug metabolism, it is susceptible to injury by a variety of xenobiotics. Alterations in hepatic blood flow may also affect liver function, especially in the patient with underlying chronic liver disease. Therefore it is not unexpected that abnormalities of liver tests are noted frequently in patients after surgery.[2] However, clinical jaundice is rare (<1%) in patients with normal livers, and its development should prompt a thorough evaluation of its cause. Before reviewing the causes of postoperative liver dysfunction, there will be a brief discussion of the evaluation of the patient with abnormal liver test results found during preoperative testing. If the surgery is critical to the patient, the presence of preoperative liver dysfunction should have no effect on the decision to operate. However, if the surgery is elective, the finding of abnormal liver test results preoperatively should prompt an evaluation as to their cause, and an estimate of liver function and reserve should be made.

Preoperative Liver Dysfunction

The frequency of unsuspected liver disease is approximately 1 in 700 of otherwise healthy surgical candidates, making this a common clinical problem.[3,4] Of most concern to surgeons and anesthesiologists are elevations of the serum aspartate aminotransferase (AST), alanine aminotransferase (ALT), bilirubin, and disorders of coagulation. Elevations of alkaline phosphatase or γ-glutamyltranspeptidase are of little clinical significance and should not prompt an evaluation unless associated with other clinical findings (see Chapter 14). The significance of a low serum albumin alone is difficult to interpret because of the multiple causes of a fall in the concentration of this protein (see Chapter 14). It is useful to combine patients with preoperative liver dysfunction into three groups: (1) asymptomatic with normal physical examination; (2) symptomatic; and (3) physical and biochemical findings of chronic liver disease.

Asymptomatic patients with a normal physical examination and abnormal liver test results (increased AST/ALT) are encountered frequently (9.8% of adults in the United States),[5] raising concerns that they have underlying liver disease that may increase the risk of surgery. The abnormal liver test results most likely reflect a subacute or chronic form of liver injury, resulting from viral hepatitis, drugs, and/or alcohol, or especially fatty liver.[6] We lack information whether this group of patients is at any increased risk from surgery, but it is the authors' opinion that if the serum bilirubin, albumin, and clotting tests are normal and the increase in aminotransferases is mild (two-fold to five-fold), there is little, if any, increase in surgical risk. Deciding to perform surgery and ensuring its successful completion in this type of patient should not be an end to the evaluation of the liver disease. After surgery the liver tests need to be monitored; if persistently abnormal, a thorough evaluation should be performed.

Greater increases in aminotransferases are more problematic only because they suggest more significant hepatic injury. Anesthetic agents may adversely affect hepatic function because of decreases in splanchnic blood flow and thereby oxygen delivery to the liver.[7,8] Early studies suggested that this may be a real clinical concern when an increase in operative mortality was observed in patients with acute hepatitis.[9-11]

However, in other studies no increase in mortality has been found when surgery was performed in patients with coincidental acute viral hepatitis.[12-14] All of these studies suffer from being anecdotal and reporting on small numbers of patients. In addition many patients were jaundiced, suggesting the presence of significant liver injury. Despite these uncertainties, if the surgery is elective, a delay in the operation is the most conservative approach. Liver tests should be performed 2 to 3 weeks later, and if the abnormalities persist for several months, the patient should be evaluated completely. If it is decided to perform an elective operation when AST/ALT is elevated more than five-fold but a normal albumin, prothrombin time, and bilirubin levels are noted, the risk to the patient probably remains small. However, if the liver test results worsen postoperatively, defining whether the surgery or the initial illness is at fault will be difficult. Because there is no evidence that the presence of liver disease increases the risk of developing anesthetic-induced hepatitis[15] (see Chapter 25), there is no need to alter the choice of anesthetic agent used for the surgery.

Isolated elevations in the serum bilirubin are usually due to Gilbert syndrome (see Chapter 62); this syndrome does not increase the risk of surgery. If the elevations of bilirubin are seen in association with elevations of AST/ALT or alkaline phosphatase, the cause of the liver injury needs to be determined before any elective surgery is performed. Isolated prolongation of the prothrombin time is an unusual manifestation of liver disease but suggests the presence of cirrhosis or a severe acute or subacute injury.

The symptomatic patient with elevated liver test results is of greater concern when elective surgery is planned. The presence of symptoms (nausea, vomiting) in association with elevated liver test results suggests that the patient is developing an acute illness that may worsen before it improves. Therefore if the patient is subjected to surgery and the test results worsen, it will be very difficult to determine whether the patient is suffering from a preexisting condition or a complication of surgery (i.e., anesthetic-induced hepatitis). In addition, there is uncertainty as to whether or not acute viral hepatitis increases the risk of surgery[10-14]; therefore, elective surgery should be postponed until the hepatitis has resolved.

A special subset of the symptomatic patient is represented by patients with markedly elevated transaminases. This group is varied as to cause of these elevations: causes range from ischemic hepatitis or cardiac dysfunction, drugs, liver trauma, cancer metastases to the liver, to rhabdomyolysis. A review demonstrated that the overall mortality of patients with serum AST greater than 3000 IU/L was 55% and that ischemic hepatitis patients had a 75% mortality compared with 33% for all other causes. This group should clearly be excluded from consideration for any elective surgery.[16]

The presence of clinical (i.e., splenomegaly, spiders, palmar erythema, ascites) and biochemical (i.e., low albumin, prolonged prothrombin time) evidence of chronic liver disease is of greatest concern when planning elective surgery. The risk of the surgery is determined by how well the liver is functioning[17] and the presence or absence of symptoms. For example, patients with chronic hepatitis appear to have an increased surgical risk if they are symptomatic.[17,18] Elective surgeries in patients with evidence of chronic liver disease should be delayed until the cause of the liver disease is determined and the severity of the injury is fully assessed.

The most common cause of chronic liver disease in the Western world is alcoholism. Alcoholic liver disease can manifest as fatty liver, alcoholic hepatitis, cirrhosis, or a combination of these conditions (see Chapter 28). The risk associates with surgery in patients with fatty liver appears to be small.[17] Surgical studies would suggest that it is not uncommon to find unsuspected cirrhosis in obese patients at the time of bariatric surgery. A report of 125 patients with cirrhosis detected at surgery, the authors were able to proceed with their planned bariatric surgery in 74% of patients; the result was no intraoperative deaths and only a 4% mortality rate.[19] Alcoholic hepatitis can be present as an asymptomatic illness or may be associated with jaundice and liver failure. Elective surgery in a patient with decompensated liver disease resulting from any cause is ill advised. Even in patients with better-preserved liver function, elective surgery in patients with acute symptomatic alcoholic hepatitis is associated with increased morbidity and mortality and should not be performed.[17,20] The effect of asymptomatic alcoholic hepatitis on surgical mortality has been studied best in patients undergoing portosystemic shunt surgery.[21-24] The presence of large amounts of alcoholic hyaline in a liver biopsy specimen indicated a high likelihood of mortality in some series.[25,26] In another series, the 1-year survival rate of patients after the insertion of a portosystemic shunt was 70% to 74% in the absence of alcoholic hyaline and only 10% in those with alcoholic hyaline in a liver biopsy. In contrast, other investigators have found no correlation between the presence of alcoholic hyaline and survival rates.[22-24] Despite these uncertainties, performance of elective surgery in a patient with alcoholic hepatitis should be avoided. It is very difficult, however, to determine whether an alcoholic patient has a fatty liver or a more serious lesion (i.e., alcoholic hepatitis) based on liver test results alone. Therefore the most conservative approach in a chronic alcoholic patient who requires elective surgery and who has abnormal liver test results is either to perform a liver biopsy to define the nature of the liver injury or a period of abstinence (2 to 3 months) to allow the acute injury to resolve preceding surgery.

There is little question that the presence of cirrhosis increases the risk of performing surgery, especially if it is an intraabdominal operation.[27-30] Published mortality rates vary from 0% to 100% depending on the type of surgery and the severity of liver disease.[17] These differences in survival rates reflect the variability in the clinical state of the patients reported in the different studies. The risk of performing surgery is defined best by the clinical severity of the cirrhosis (i.e., Child classification, Model for End-Stage Liver Disease [MELD] score).[17,27-29] Patients with good hepatic function, no ascites, and a good nutritional state (Child class A) do well with surgery, whereas those with jaundice, low serum albumin, ascites, and muscle-wasting have a high operative mortality and postoperative morbidity. **Figure 56-1** shows the relationship between the MELD score and postoperative mortality at 30 and 90 days.[29] Although there is no clear inflection point, when the MELD score exceeds 10 the expected mortality exceeds 10%, a meaningful number when one is discussing elective surgery. At MELD scores of greater than 20, the expected mortality exceeds 50%. A single-point increase in the MELD score was associated with a 14% to 15% increase in mortality risk at 30 and 90 days, respectively.[29] Elective surgery can be performed in patients with decompensated liver disease but the surgeon must have experience in the

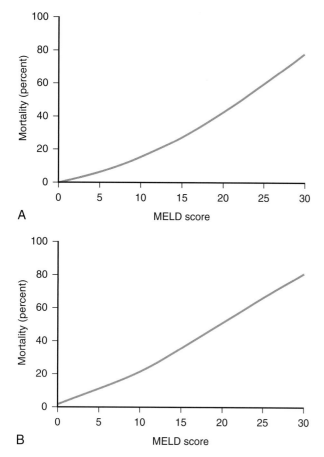

Fig. 56-1 **Relationship between Model for End-Stage Liver Disease (MELD) score and postoperative survival rates. A,** Thirty-day mortality. **B,** Ninety-day mortality. *(Reproduced with permission from Teh SH, et al. Risk factors for mortality after surgery in patients with cirrhosis. Gastroenterology 2007;132:1261–1269.)*

management of this type of patient to minimize the risks of surgery. Emergent surgery appears to carry a high risk of in-hospital mortality for certain procedures as compared with elective operations. The presence of portal hypertension also appeared to increase the surgical risk.[30]

A difficult problem that many surgeons face is performing a cholecystectomy in a patient with cirrhosis. Mortality rates of 7.5% to 25.5% and morbidity rates of 4.8% to 25% have been reported.[27,31-38] In addition, many patients require transfusions, especially if they have decompensated liver disease.[31] A subtotal cholecystectomy used to be suggested for patients with cirrhosis and portal hypertension.[32] Previously, open cholecystectomy had been recommended for patients with cirrhosis, but recent studies suggest that in Child class A and B patients, elective laparoscopic cholecystectomy is preferred because there is less bleeding, fewer wound infections, and less time in the hospital compared with open cholecystectomy.[17,33-38] The complication rates after urgent cholecystectomy are significantly higher (36%) compared with elective laparoscopic cholecystectomy in cirrhotics (16%), suggesting that, if possible, stabilization of the patient with medical management followed by elective surgery would be preferable.[37] Given the high rates of mortality and morbidity in patients with advanced cirrhosis undergoing cholecystectomy and the increased difficulty associated with liver transplantation in patients with a previous cholecystectomy, we believe that the

presence of recurrent cholecystitis in a patient with advanced liver disease should be considered an indication for liver transplantation while conservative management is being performed. This may require filing an appeal with the United Network for Organ Sharing for U.S. patients to allow them to have a higher-priority MELD score. In the acutely ill patient, percutaneous cholecystostomy tubes may be attempted but may be difficult to perform in patients with significant ascites.

Complication rates are also quite high for cirrhotics with abdominal surgeries other than just cholecystectomy. The overall mortality rate for urgent abdominal surgery has been reported to be 45% to 57% versus 10% to 18% with elective surgeries. Important predictive factors associated with mortality in some studies include the presence of ascites ($P = .006$), encephalopathy ($P = .002$), and coagulopathy ($P = .021$).[27,39-41] The mortality rates by the Child classification likewise demonstrate a progressive increased risk as liver disease worsens and are reported at 10% for class A, 30% to 31% for class B, and 76% to 82% for class C cirrhotics. The causes of the death from gastrointestinal surgeries in a series by Mansour and colleagues were coagulopathy or sepsis in 81% of cases.[39] A prior report classified 87% of deaths as being due to multisystem organ failure.[27] These data suggest that the surgery should be converted from an emergent procedure to an elective one, wherever possible, but this may depend on the situation. It remains to be seen if the new MELD scores will be more predictive of operative morality for these procedures than is the Child classification. Given that coagulopathy plays a major role in postoperative abdominal surgery complications seen in cirrhotics, it is interesting to speculate what the future role of recombinant factor VIIa (rFVIIa) may be for these patients. Data on the use of rFVIIa have been increasingly seen in the literature, and there are scattered reports of use of this medication for limited abdominal procedures, such as diagnostic laparoscopy and some other radiologic and surgical procedures.[42-44] It is unclear whether this effect is transient in nature, and if surgery is performed what impact this would have on overall postoperative bleeding complications and patient survival rates. Use of rFVIIa has been shown to be ineffective in controlling variceal bleeding and its use during intraabdominal operations clearly has not been of any benefit.[45]

Cardiac surgery in more advanced cirrhotic patients likewise has a reported high complication rate.[46,47] Little mortality was noted in Child class A patients who underwent cardiac surgery but mortality was reported to be 42% to 50% in Child class B patients for similar surgeries and 100% in Child class C cirrhotics. Higher MELD scores were also predictive of a worse outcome following cardiac surgery.[29] Probable contributors to the increased mortality include liver perfusion injuries related to cardiopulmonary bypass, as well as bypass aggravation of the coagulopathy, which may be already be present in these patients. New advances in the use of cardiac stents and valvuloplasty techniques may help these patients avoid thoracotomy.

Postoperative Liver Dysfunction

Table 56-1 lists the most common causes of liver dysfunction and jaundice in postoperative patients. In a review of surgical complications in cirrhotics, the 30-day mortality rate was

Table 56-1 **Causes of Postoperative Liver Dysfunction**
Hepatitis-Like
Drugs
Anesthetic needs
Ischemia
Cardiac
Shock (noncardiac)
Iatrogenic (ligation hepatic artery)
Viral hepatitis
Cholestasis
Benign postoperative cholestasis
Sepsis drugs
Antibiotics, antiemetics
Bile duct injury
Choledocholithiasis/pancreatitis
Cholecystitis

reported to be 11.6%, with a 30.1% perioperative complication rate.[34] The causes of this mortality rate are separated into two large groups but many patients have a mixed picture, which increases the difficulty in making a correct cause-to-outcome association.

Anesthetic-Induced Liver Injury

Anesthetic-induced hepatitis is of most concern because of a high incidence of hepatic failure; it is discussed in detail in Chapter 25. Liver injury resulting from any of the currently used anesthetics is rare.[48,49] By 1985 more than 500 cases of halothane hepatitis had been reported; however, the estimated frequency of hepatitis resulting from halothane is 1 in 10,000 operations.[15,49] The putative toxin is a metabolic product of halothane; therefore other halogenated anesthetic agents that are less extensively metabolized than halothane have an even lower incidence of hepatotoxicity.[15,49] Published mortality rates vary from 10% to 80%, with rates of 10% to 30% being most representative.[49]

The development of symptoms (fever or jaundice) is seen 7 to 14 days after a single exposure and 5 to 7 days after multiple exposures to halothane. Patients at greatest risk are obese females, but adverse reactions have been seen in all types of patients. Fever is the most common symptom of halothane-induced hepatitis and may be present in the absence of jaundice. Laboratory test results show a marked increase (greater than ten-fold above normal) in serum levels of aminotransferases. Patients with severe injury may have a rise in serum bilirubin and prolongation of the prothrombin time. Many patients, however, have only a rise in aminotransferase levels without clinical icterus, and therefore the injury may be missed unless laboratory tests are obtained in patients with postoperative fever.[47-51] Eosinophilia and renal insufficiency may also be present.[49-51] The other halogenated anesthetics also cause a hepatitis-like injury with clinical features that are similar to those seen with halothane hepatitis.

Separately, the use of anesthetics is known to reduce the hepatic arterial blood flow and oxygen uptake by hepatocytes.[7,8,51-53] In healthy volunteers, this reduction averaged 35% and was seen in the first 30 minutes of induction but returns to baseline during the procedure. It is possible that this fall in oxygen delivery may adversely affect the cirrhotic liver.

Ischemic Hepatitis

Surgery is commonly performed in patients with cardiac disease, and, if they develop congestive heart failure, they may develop ischemic hepatitis. Ischemic hepatitis is marked by a rapid rise in serum levels of AST, ALT, and lactate dehydrogenase (LDH). The levels are frequently greater than tenfold above normal and in severe cases may be associated with jaundice and prolongation of the prothrombin time.[54,55] In contrast to halothane hepatitis, elevated liver enzyme values can be seen any time after surgery and is not associated with fever or eosinophilia. In addition, the liver test results tend to return rapidly to normal (elevations last 3 to 11 days).[54] Noncardiogenic shock liver is seen in association with hypotensive episodes (resulting from bleeding or sepsis) and also is marked by a rapid rise and fall in serum levels of AST and ALT. When comparing all causes of massive elevations of AST (more than 3000 IU/L), ischemic hepatitis is associated with a mortality rate of 75% versus 33% for all other causes combined.[56] Accidental or deliberate ligation of the hepatic artery or its branches may result in hepatic ischemia and necrosis associated with a rise in serum levels of AST and ALT.[57] When accidental ligation of the hepatic artery occurs, it is usually during cholecystectomy, and should be suspected in a patient who develops a rise in serum levels of AST and ALT after that operation.

Acute Viral Hepatitis

The development of acute viral hepatitis in the postoperative period is rare if patients are shown to have normal liver test results preceding the surgery. If the patient does develop acute viral hepatitis, a gradual rise in the serum levels of AST and ALT will be observed with or without other systemic symptoms. Of note, the serum levels of LDH are only slightly increased relative to the degree of elevation of the AST and ALT; hence, measurement of the serum LDH is a useful test for separating ischemic and drug-induced hepatitis from viral hepatitis. The appropriate tests for the diagnosis of acute viral hepatitis are discussed in Chapters 29 to 34.

Drug-Induced Hepatitis

There are a large number of drugs that may cause an acute hepatitis-like injury and these are discussed in detail in Chapter 25. Acetaminophen is a direct hepatotoxin and is commonly used in the postoperative patient. Toxicity from acetaminophen is generally observed when more than 7.5 g is ingested as a single dose.[58] However, it has become apparent that therapeutic doses of acetaminophen ingested by alcoholics may be associated with significant hepatic injury.[58,59] In addition, the toxic metabolite of acetaminophen is formed by P-450 2E1; this enzyme is susceptible to induction by a number of drugs, including alcohol.[58] The co-administration of an inducing agent may increase the generation of the toxic metabolite of acetaminophen and cause toxicity with ingestion of therapeutic doses (3 to 4 g/day) of the drug. Therefore, if a patient develops an increase in serum levels of AST/ALT postoperatively, the amount of acetaminophen taken by the patient should be determined. Most hepatitis-like drug reactions are idiosyncratic and can be due to a variety of agents, as discussed in Chapter 25. An important fact in the differential diagnosis of postoperative liver dysfunction is that most idiosyncratic drug reactions develop after at least 2 weeks of therapy. Therefore the development of abnormal liver test results within 2 weeks of surgery is unlikely to be due to drugs started after the operation. In addition, drugs taken for more than 12 months preceding the surgery are unlikely causes of postoperative liver dysfunction.

Benign Postoperative Cholestasis

The development of jaundice postoperatively is observed in fewer than 1% of patients undergoing major surgery. Patients with preexisting liver or cardiovascular disease and who suffer trauma have a significantly higher incidence of postoperative jaundice.[2] The cause of the jaundice is multifactorial and includes anesthetic-induced reduction in liver function because of decreased hepatic blood flow, increased pigment load from hematomas and transfused blood, and impaired bile formation secondary to bacterial sepsis.[2,60-63] The breakdown of 50 ml of blood yields 250 mg of bilirubin, which can be easily handled by the normal liver but leads to a rapid rise in serum bilirubin in patients with impaired liver function.[2] A fall in liver blood flow is observed with almost all general anesthetics, which may lead to a decline in liver function, especially in patients with underlying liver disease.[7,8,17] If the patient has suffered an episode of hypotension, it will affect hepatocyte function and predispose the patient to the development of cholestasis.[2] Finally, endotoxemia reduces bile flow, and intraabdominal sepsis is frequently associated with abnormal liver test results and jaundice.[60,63]

Benign postoperative cholestasis develops most commonly within the first 10 days after surgery. Cholestasis is observed most frequently in patients with sepsis, after cardiovascular surgery, and after prolonged operations during which and after the patient received multiple transfusions.[60-64] Although an increase in serum bilirubin is common and may reach levels of 40 mg/dl, it is not universal. Serum levels of alkaline phosphatase are frequently elevated, whereas AST and ALT levels are normal or only mildly elevated (less than five-fold). Serum albumin levels may be normal or slightly reduced, and the prothrombin time is usually normal. Cholestasis and variable degrees of fat are seen in a liver biopsy.[2,62]

The condition is referred to as benign because, if the patient recovers from the surgery and any associated complications, the cholestasis resolves. However, patients developing postoperative cholestasis have a significant mortality. Patients with serum bilirubin levels of greater than 6 mg/dl have a 46% mortality if they have suffered abdominal trauma and an 86% mortality if they have intraabdominal sepsis.[64] These latter groups of patients frequently die, with the syndrome termed multiple organ system failure, and worsening liver function is seen in association with renal failure and acute respiratory distress syndrome.[36,65] The liver plays a passive role in multiple organ system failure in that acute liver failure (encephalopathy with a coagulopathy) is not the cause of death.

Bile Duct Obstruction

A common concern is the development of extrahepatic bile duct obstruction in the postoperative patient who becomes icteric. Coincidental choledocholithiasis after surgery is rare. A far more common occurrence is bile duct injury after biliary tract or gastric surgery. Bile duct injury after laparoscopic cholecystectomy is an increasingly common problem and frequently goes unrecognized during the cholecystectomy.[66,67] The patient develops clinical jaundice with or without signs of cholangitis days to weeks after the initial surgery. Diagnosis is made by endoscopic retrograde cholangiopancreatography or transhepatic cholangiography (see Chapter 61). Postoperative pancreatitis may also cause bile duct obstruction because of edema in the head of the pancreas. The diagnosis is made by finding an elevated serum level of amylase and through a computed tomography scan of the abdomen showing edema of the pancreas and bile duct dilation. The jaundice resolves as the patient recovers from the pancreatitis.[68] In the postoperative jaundiced patient who has not undergone biliary or gastric surgery and who does not have evidence of pancreatitis, biliary tract disease is uncommon and other causes of jaundice should be considered initially. Acute cholecystitis (calculous or acalculous) may occur postoperatively and can be associated with abnormal liver test results and jaundice.[69] The presence of right upper quadrant abdominal pain and fever suggests the diagnosis: ultrasound findings of pericholecystic fluid, thickening of the gallbladder wall, and perhaps stones supporting the clinical suspicion.[70] Gangrene, perforation, and empyema of the gallbladder are common in the postoperative patient and associated with high mortality.[68]

Abnormal liver test results are frequently observed in patients receiving total parenteral nutrition, which is discussed in detail in Chapter 55. Fatty liver with mild elevations of the serum aminotransferases and alkaline phosphatase is commonly observed.[70] Less common, but of greater concern, especially in children, is the development of jaundice. The abnormal liver test results develop days to weeks after the institution of therapy.[71] The liver biopsy findings are nonspecific and the diagnosis is one of excluding the other causes of postoperative hepatic dysfunction. The cause of the disorder remains poorly understood.

Evaluation of Patients with Postoperative Liver Dysfunction

If the patient is within the first 2 weeks of surgery and has a hepatitis-like injury, anesthetic-related hepatitis or ischemic hepatitis is of major concern (**Table 56-2**). Injury by a direct hepatotoxin such as acetaminophen should also be considered. The development of cholestasis in the immediate postoperative period in a patient who has undergone biliary or gastric surgery suggests bile duct injury. If the patient has undergone major cardiac or abdominal surgery and is infected or has received multiple blood transfusions, benign postoperative cholestasis should be the initial diagnosis. If the abnormal liver test results develop more than 2 weeks after surgery, drug or total parenteral nutrition-induced liver injury should

Table 56-2 Differential Diagnosis of Postoperative Liver Dysfunction

DISORDER	TYPE OF SURGERY	FEVER	ONSET POSTOPERATIVELY	ALT (U/L)	AP
Halothane hepatitis	No relationship	Common	2-15 days	>500	Slight ↑
Viral hepatitis	No relationship	Uncommon	>3 weeks	>500	Slight ↑
Benign postoperative jaundice	Major surgery with sepsis	Common	<7 days	Slight ↑	↑↑
Shock	No relationship (cardiac disease)	Uncommon	1-4 days	>500	Slight ↑(LDH)
Bile duct injury	Biliary tract and stomach	Common	Days to weeks	200–300	↑↑

ALT, alanine aminotransferase; AP, alkaline phosphatase; LDH, lactate dehydrogenase; ↑, increase; ↑↑, greater increase

be considered, as should bile duct injury if gallbladder surgery had been performed. Postoperative cholecystitis is associated with abdominal pain and fever, which are unusual features of the other types of injury; abdominal ultrasonography should be performed in this situation. Hepatitis C should be considered in the transfused patient who develops elevated AST/ALT levels more than 3 weeks after exposure to blood products but is very rare unless the donor was incubating the virus when the blood was donated. Antibody test results may be negative during the acute illness and identification of viral ribonucleic acid in the serum by polymerase chain reaction may be required (see Chapter 31). Tests for acute hepatitis A and B are not usually necessary because they rarely cause posttransfusion hepatitis.

References

1. Jackson FC, Christophersen EB, Peternel WW. Preoperative management of patients with liver disease. Surg Clin North Am 1968;48:907–930.
2. LaMont JT. Postoperative jaundice. Surg Clin North Am 1974;54:637–645.
3. Schemel WH. Unexpected hepatic dysfunction found by multiple laboratory screening. Anesth Analg 1976;55:810–812.
4. Watanecyawech M, Kelly KA Jr. Hepatic diseases unsuspected before surgery. N Y State J Med 1975;75:1278–1281.
5. Ioannou GN, Boyko EJ, Lee SP. The prevalence and predictors of elevated serum aminotransferase activity in the United States in 1999-2002. Am J Gastroenterol 2006;101:76–82.
6. Ioannou GN, et al. Elevated serum alanine aminotransferase activity and calculated risk of coronary heart disease in the United States. Hepatology 2006;43:1145–1151.
7. Ngai SH. Effects of anesthetics on various organs. N Engl J Med 1980;302:564–566.
8. Cooperman LH. Effects of anesthesia on the splanchnic circulation. Br J Anaesth 1972;44:967–970.
9. Harville DD, Summerskill WHJ. Surgery in acute hepatitis. Causes and effects. JAMA 1963;184:257–261.
10. Powell-Jackson P, Greenway B, Williams R. Adverse effects of exploratory laparotomy in patients with unsuspected liver disease. Br J Surg 1982;69:449–451.
11. Shaldon S, Sherlock S. Virus hepatitis with features of prolonged bile retention. Br Med J 1957;2:734–738.
12. Hardy KJ, Hughes ESR. Laparotomy in viral hepatitis. Med J Aust 1968;1:710–712.
13. Strauss AA, et al. Decompression by drainage of the common bile duct in subacute and chronic jaundice: a report of 73 cases with hepatitis or concomitant biliary duct infection as cause. Am J Surg 1959;97:137–140.
14. Bourke JB, Cannon P, Ritchie HD. Laparotomy for jaundice. Lancet 1967;2:521–523.
15. Farrell GC. Postoperative hepatic dysfunction. In: Zakim D, Boyer TD, editors. Hepatology: a textbook of liver disease, 2nd ed. Philadelphia: WB Saunders, 1990: 869–890.
16. Johnson RD, O'Connor ML, Kerr RM. Extreme serum elevations of aspartate aminotransferase. Am J Gastroenterol 1995;90:1244–1245.
17. O'Leary JG, Yachimski P, Friedman LS. Surgery in the patient with liver disease. Clin Liver Dis 2009;13:211–231.
18. Hargrove MD. Chronic active hepatitis: possible adverse effect of exploratory laparotomy. Surgery 1971;68:771–773.
19. Brolin RE, Bradley LJ, Taliwal RV. Unsuspected cirrhosis discovered during elective obesity operations. Arch Surg 1998;133:84–88.
20. Greenwood SM, Leffler CT, Minkowitz S. The increased mortality rate of open liver biopsy in alcoholic hepatitis. Surg Gynecol Obstet 1972;134:600–604.
21. Eckhauser F, et al. Hepatic pathology as a determinant of prognosis after portal decompression. Am J Surg 1980;139:105–112.
22. Kanel GC, et al. Survival in patients with post necrotic cirrhosis and Laennec's cirrhosis undergoing therapeutic portacaval shunt. Gastroenterology 1977;73:679–683.
23. Bell RH, Miyai K, Orloff MJ. Outcomes in cirrhotic patients with acute alcoholic hepatitis after emergency portacaval shunt for bleeding esophageal varices. Am J Surg 1984;147:78–84.
24. Reichle FA, Fahmy W, Golsorkhi M. Prospective comparative clinical trial with distal splenorenal and mesocaval shunts. Am J Surg 1979;137:13–21.
25. Mikkelsen W. Therapeutic portacaval shunt. Preliminary data on controlled trial. Arch Surg 1974;108:302–305.
26. Pande N, et al. Cirrhotic portal hypertension. Morbidity of continued alcoholism. Gastroenterology 1978;74:64–69.
27. Garrison RN, et al. Clarification of risk factors for abdominal operations in patients with hepatic cirrhosis. Ann Surg 1984;199:648–655.
28. Klemperer JD, et al. Cardiac operations in patients with cirrhosis. Ann Thorac Surg 1998;65:85–87.
29. Teh SH, et al. Risk factors for mortality after surgery in patients with cirrhosis. Gastroenterology 2007;132:1261–1269.
30. Nguyen GC, Correia AJ, Thuluvath PJ. The impact of cirrhosis and portal hypertension on mortality following colorectal surgery: a nationwide, population-based study. Dis Colon Rectum 2009;52:1367–1374.
31. Bloch RS, Allaben RD, Wait AJ. Cholecystectomy in patients with cirrhosis: a surgical challenge. Arch Surg 1985;120:669–672.
32. Bornman PC, Terblanche I. Subtotal cholecystectomy: for the difficult gallbladder in portal hypertension and cholecystitis. Surgery 1985;98:1–6.
33. Yerdel MA, et al. Laparoscopic cholecystectomy cirrhotic patients: expanding indications. Surg Laparosc Endosc 1993;3:180–183.
34. Yerdel MA, et al. Laparoscopic cholecystectomy in cirrhotic patients: a prospective study. Surg Laparosc Endosc 1997;7:483–486.
35. Sleeman D, et al. Laparoscopic cholecystectomy in cirrhotic patients. J Am Coll Surg 1998;187:400–403.
36. D'Alburquerque LA, et al. Laparoscopic cholecystectomy in cirrhotic patients. Surg Laparosc Endosc 1995;5:272–276.
37. Friel CM. Laparoscopic cholecystectomy in patients with hepatic cirrhosis: a five-year experience. J Gastrointest Surg 1999;3:286–290.
38. Curro G, et al. Laparoscopic cholecystectomy in patients with mild cirrhosis and symptomatic cholelithiasis. Transplant Proc 2007;39:1471–1473.

39. Mansour A, et al. Abdominal operations in patients with cirrhosis: still a major surgical challenge. Surgery 1997;122:730–735.
40. Doberneck RC, Sterling WA, Allison DC. Morbidity and mortality after operation in nonbleeding cirrhotics. Am J Surg 1983;146:306–309.
41. Aranha GV, Greenlee HB. Intra-abdominal surgery in patients with advanced cirrhosis. Arch Surg 1986;121:275–277.
42. Bernstein DE. Recombinant factor VIIa corrects prothrombin time in cirrhotic patients: a preliminary study. Gastroenterology 1997;113:1930–1937.
43. Berstein DE. Effectiveness of the recombinant factor VIIa in patients with the coagulopathy of advanced Child's B and C cirrhosis. Semin Thromb Hemost 2000;26:437–438.
44. Jeffers L, et al. Safety and efficacy of recombinant factor VIIa in patients with liver disease undergoing laparoscopic liver biopsy. Gastroenterology 2002;123:118–126.
45. Shah NL, Caldwell SH, Berg CL. The role of anti-fibrinolytics, rFVIIa and other pro-coagulants: prophylactic versus rescue? Clin Liver Dis 2009;13:87–93.
46. Morris JJ, et al. Three patients requiring both coronary artery bypass surgery and orthotopic liver transplantation. J Cardiothorac Vasc Anesth 1995;9:322–332.
47. Pollard RJ, Sidi A, Gibby GL. Aortic stenosis with end stage liver disease: prioritizing surgical and anesthetic therapies. J Clin Anesth 1998;10:253–257.
48. Kenna JG. Mechanism, pathology, and clinical presentation of hepatotoxicity of anesthetic agents. In: Kaplowitz N, DeLeve LD, editors. Drug-induced liver disease, 2nd ed. New York: Informa Healthcare, 2007: 465–484.
49. Benjamin SB, et al. The morphologic spectrum of halothane-induced hepatic injury: analysis of 77 cases. Hepatology 1985;5:1163–1171.
50. Cousins MJ, Plummer JL, Hau PM. Risk factors for halothane hepatitis. Aust N Z J Surg 1989;59:5–14.
51. Friedman LS. The risk of surgery in patients with liver disease. Hepatology 1999;29:1617–1623.
52. Strunin L. Anesthetic management of patients with liver disease. In: Millward-Sadler GH, Wright R, Arthur MJP, editors. Wright's liver and biliary disease. London: WB Saunders, 1992: 1381.
53. Cowan RE, et al. Effects of anesthetics and abdominal surgery on the liver blood flow. Hepatology 1991;14:1161–1166.
54. Gibson PR, Dudley FJ. Ischemic hepatitis: clinical features, diagnosis and prognosis. Aust N Z J Med 1984;14:822–825.
55. Seeto RK, Fenn B, Rockey DC. Ischemic hepatitis: clinical presentation and pathogenesis. Am J Med 2000;109:109–113.
56. Johnson RD, O'Connor ML, Kerr RM. Extreme serum elevations of aspartate aminotransferase. Am J Gastroenterol 1995;90:1244–1245.
57. Brittain RS, et al. Accidental hepatic artery ligation in humans. Am J Surg 1964;107:822–832.
58. Lee WM, Ostapowicz G. Acetaminophen: pathology and clinical presentation of hepatotoxicity. In: Kaplowitz N, DeLeve LD, editors. Drug-induced liver disease, 2nd ed. New York: Informa Healthcare, 2007: 389–405.
59. Kumar S, Rex DK. Failure of physicians to recognize acetaminophen hepatotoxicity in chronic alcoholics. Ann Intern Med 1991;151:1189–1191.
60. Gottlieb JE, Menashe PI, Cruz E. Gastrointestinal complications in critically ill patients: the intensivists' overview. Am J Gastroenterol 1986;81:227–238.
61. LaMont JT, Isselhacher KJ. Postoperative jaundice. N Engl J Med 1973;288:305–307.
62. Schmid M, et al. Benign postoperative intrahepatic cholestasis. N Engl J Med 1965;272:545–550.
63. Kantrowitz PA, et al. Severe postoperative hyperbilirubinemia simulating obstructive jaundice. N Engl J Med 1967;276:591–598.
64. Boekhorst T, et al. Etiologic factors of jaundice in severely ill patients. A retrospective study in patients admitted to intensive care unit with severe trauma or with septic intraabdominal complications following surgery and without evidence of bile duct obstruction. J Hepatol 1988;7:111–117.
65. Waxman K. Postoperative multiple organ failure. Crit Care Clin 1987;3:429–440.
66. Moossa AR, et al. Laparoscopic injuries to the bile duct. A cause for concern. Ann Surg 1992;215:203–208.
67. Davidoff AM, et al. Mechanisms of major biliary injury during laparoscopic cholecystectomy. Ann Surg 1992;215:196–202.
68. Thompson JS, et al. Postoperative pancreatitis. Surg Gynecol Obstet 1988;167:377–380.
69. Frazee RC, Nagorney UM, Mucha P. Acute acalculous cholecystitis. Mayo Clin Proc 1989;64:163–167.
70. Becker CD, Burckhardt B, Terrier F. Ultrasound in postoperative acalculous cholecystitis. Gastrointest Radiol 1986;11:47–50.
71. Ukleja A, Romano MM. Complications of parenteral nutrition. Gastroenterol Clin North Am 2007;36:23–46.

Section X

Tumors of the Liver and Gallstones

Hepatocellular Carcinoma

Jorge A. Marrero

ABBREVIATIONS

AFB aflatoxin B	**HBV** hepatitis B virus	**PcG** polycomb gene group
AFP α-fetoprotein	**HCC** hepatocellular carcinoma	**PDGF** platelet-derived growth factor
BMI body mass index	**HCV** hepatitis C virus	**PEI** percutaneous ethanol injection
CBP CREB-binding protein	**H-DN** high-grade dysplastic nodule	**PIP$_3$** phosphatidilinositol triphosphate
CREB cAMP response element binding protein	**HGF** hepatocyte growth factor	**PI3K** phosphatidylinositol-3′-kinase
	HIF1 hypoxia inducible factor-1	**PKB** protein kinase B
CT computed tomography	**HSP70** heat shock protein 70	**RECIST** Response Evaluation Criteria in Solid Tumors
DCP des-gamma carboxyprothrombin	**IGF2** insulin-like growth factor-2	
EGF epidermal growth factor	**LDLT** living donor liver transplantation	**RFA** radiofrequency ablation
FGF fibroblast growth factor	**L-DN** low-grade dysplastic nodule	**TACE** transarterial chemoembolization
GPC3 glypican-3	**MAPK** mitogen-activated protein kinase	**TNF-α** tumor necrosis factor-α
GS glutamine synthetase	**MRI** magnetic resonance imaging	**TNM** tumor-node-metastasis
HALT-C Hepatitis C Antiviral Long-Term Treatment Against Cirrhosis	**mTOR** mammalian target of rapamycin	**US** ultrasound
	NF-κB nuclear factor kappa B	**VEFG** vascular endothelial growth factor
HBeAg hepatitis B e antigen	**OLT** orthotopic liver transplantation	**WHO** World Health Organization

Introduction

Hepatocellular carcinoma (HCC), the most common primary liver tumor, was once thought as an uncommon cancer in the Western world. Now it is one of the solid tumors with a fast-rising incidence rate and the leading cause of death among patients with cirrhosis. The risk factors are well known and with surveillance, a significant number of patients are diagnosed at early stages, allowing for curative therapy. This chapter summarizes the current state regarding the epidemiology, pathogenesis, diagnosis, and treatment of this neoplasm.

Epidemiology

Hepatocellular carcinoma is a common cancer worldwide and accounts for approximately 5.6% of all cancers. It is the fifth most common cancer in the world and the third most common cause of cancer death.[1] There is considerable geographic variation in the incidence of HCC. The largest concentration of HCC cases in the world is in Asia, followed by Africa, Europe, and North and South America as shown in **Figure 57-1**.[2] China alone accounts for more than 50% of the world's cases.[3] Other high-rate (>20/100,000) areas include Senegal (male, 28.47/100,000; female, 12.2/100,000), Gambia (male, 39.67/100,000; female, 14.6/100,000), and South Korea (male,

48.8/100,000; female, 11.6/100,000). The incidence of HCC varies among ethnic groups, with increasing incidence rates found in Japanese (5.5/100,000 in men and 4.3/100,000 in women), African American (7.1/100,000 in men and 2.1/100,000 in women), Hispanics (9.8/100,000 in men and 3.5/100,000 in women), and Chinese (16.2/100,000 in men and 5/100,000 in women) populations.[4] The worldwide prevalence of HCC is seen in **Figure 57-2**.

Liver cancer incidence increased in Japan and many Western countries during the last several decades. More recent data indicates that the HCC rates may be stabilizing or falling. Fluctuations in HCC incidence are largely a cohort effect. For instance, as the cohort of people with hepatitis C (HCV) infected between the end of World War II and approximately 1970 in Europe and North America, the incidence of HCV-related HCC increases 20 to 30 years later.[5,6] In Japan the epidemic of HCV occurred right at the time of World War II and seems to have fallen over the last decade.[7] Immigration to Europe and North America from countries where chronic viral infections are endemic has also contributed to the incidence of HCC. Immigrants to Western countries tend to have higher HCC rates than the native-born population. For example, in the United States the age-adjusted HCC incidence is highest in Korean immigrants, followed by Chinese and Philipino.[8] This is probably related to the varying prevalence of underlying liver disease in these populations. In Korean men in the United States, the age-adjusted incidence ratio is

PREVALENCE PER 100,000 PERSONS

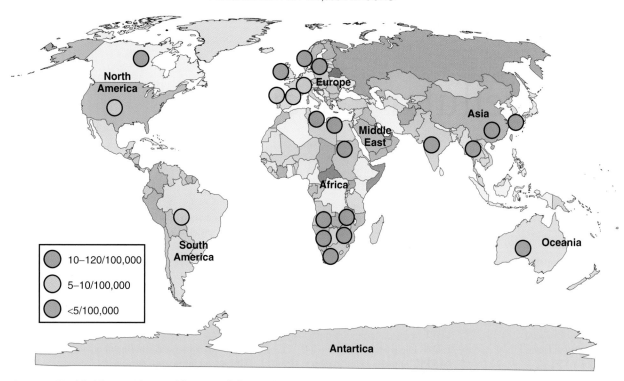

Fig. 57-1 Worldwide prevalence of hepatocellular carcinoma. *(Adapted from Bosch FX, et al. Primary liver cancer: worldwide incidence and trends. Gastroenterology 2004;127[5 Suppl 1]:S5–S16.)*

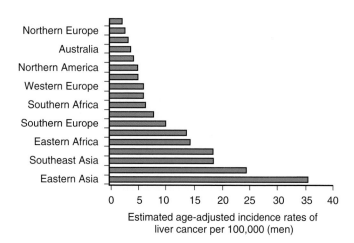

Fig. 57-2 Worldwide incidence of hepatocellular carcinoma. *(Adapted from Parkin DM, et al. Global cancer statistics in the year 2000. Lancet Oncol 2001;2:533–543.)*

20.71 compared with 3.81 for Caucasian men. In Korea, the age-adjusted incidence ratio in chronic hepatitis B virus (HBV) carriers is in excess of 98.8. Thus, in Western countries the increase in HCC incidence is also fed by importation of immigrants who bring with them the high prevalence of chronic viral hepatitis from their home countries. Interestingly, the second-generation immigrants have a lower incidence of HCC than do their parents. This has been documented in the United States and in Australia.[8,9] Although the prevalence of the underlying risk factors has not been studied, it is likely that this decrease in HCC incidence reflects a fall in the prevalence of chronic viral hepatitis in the second-generation immigrants.

HCC is the fastest-growing cause of cancer-related death in men in the United States. Age-adjusted HCC incidence rates increased more than two-fold between 1985 and 2002, with the trend being patients with HCC being diagnosed at an earlier age compared with previous decades.[10,11] The average annual, age-adjusted rates of HCC verified by histology or cytology increased from 1.3 per 100,000 during 1978 to 1980 to 3.3 per 100,000 during 1999 to 2001.[12] At all ages and in all racial/ethnic groups in the United States, HCC is three to four times more common in men than women. Higher levels of testosterone, higher body mass index, and higher rates of liver disease are possible explanations for the higher risk in men. Rates of HCC are two times higher in Asians than African Americans, which are two times higher than those in Caucasians (**Fig. 57-3**).The increase in HCC started in the mid-1980s, with the greatest proportional increases occurring during the late 1990s. The largest proportional increases occurred among whites (Hispanics and non-Hispanics), whereas the lowest proportional increases occurred among Asians. The mean age at diagnosis is approximately 65 years, 74% of cases occur in men, and the racial distribution is 48% Caucasian, 15% Hispanic, 13% African American, and 24% other race/ethnicity (predominantly Asian). During recent years as incidence rates increased, the age distribution of HCC patients has shifted toward relatively younger ages, with the greatest proportional increases between ages 45 and 60.

In almost all populations, males have higher liver cancer rates than females, with male/female ratios usually averaging between 2:1 and 4:1.[13] At present, the largest discrepancies in rates (>4:1) are found in medium-risk European populations.

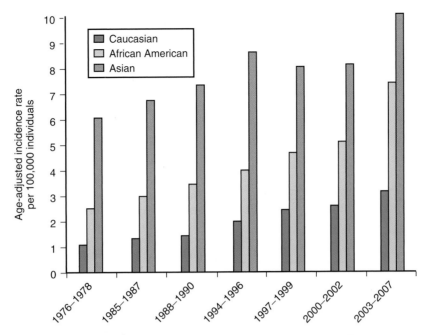

Fig. 57-3 **Age-adjusted incidence rates of hepatocellular carcinoma in the United States according to race.** (*Adapted from El-Serag HB. Hepatocellular carcinoma: recent trends in the United States. Gastroenterology 2004;127:S27–S34.*)

Typical among these ratios are those reported from Geneva, Switzerland (4.1:1), and Varese, Italy (5.1:1).[14] Among 10 French registries listed in Volume VIII of *Cancer in Five Continents,* 9 report male/female ratios of greater than 5:1. In contrast, typical ratios currently seen in high-risk populations are those of Qidong, China (3.2:1); Osaka, Japan (3.7:1); Gambia (2.8:1); and Harare, Zimbabwe (2.4:1).[8]

The overall survival rates of HCC is improving. Overall, survival rates increased for short-, intermediate-, and longer-term follow-up intervals over the time period of study, with a doubling of 2- to 4-year cause-specific survival rates according to population data in the United States.[15] Increases in survival rates occurred as more patients were diagnosed with localized stage HCC (28% in 1992 to 1993, 44% in 2003 to 2004) and 1-year survival rates for patients with localized HCC increased from 41% to 67%. Among patients with localized HCC with reported therapy, 1-year survival rates increased from 65% in 1992 to 1993 to 83% in 2003 to 2004. One-year survival rates for patients with localized HCC who received surgery increased from 81% to 91% between 1992 to 1993 and 2003 to 2004. Survival rates also increased among patients with regional HCC who reported therapy. Although changes in survival rates for cases with distant HCC were less pronounced, patients reporting treatment had higher survival rates. This is likely a reflection of understanding the risk factors that lead to this tumor, and these are shown in **Table 57-1.**

Risk Factors

Hepatocellular carcinoma has well-known important risk factors, especially the hepatotropic viruses. Chronic HCV and HBV infections are classified by the World Health Organization (WHO) as carcinogens. Significant risk factors known to be attributed to HCC that vary geographically are shown in **Table 57-2.** The most important risk factors will be discussed in more detail.

Hepatitis B

Chronic HBV infection is the most important risk factor for HCC worldwide. In Asia and Africa, more than 80% of patients with HCC have an underlying chronic HBV infection.[16] Chronic HBV infection is the most common underlying cause of HCC in the world.[17] The increased HCC risk associated with HBV infection particularly applies to areas where HBV is endemic. In these areas, it usually is transmitted from mother to newborn (vertical transmission) and up to 90% of infected persons follow a chronic course. This pattern is different in areas with low HCC incidence rates where HBV is acquired in adulthood through sexual and parenteral routes (horizontal transmission), with more than 90% of acute infections resolving spontaneously. The annual HCC incidence in chronic HBV carriers in Asia ranges between 0.4% and 0.6%.[18] This figure is lower in Alaskan natives (0.26%/year), and is lowest in Caucasian HBV carriers.[19] Several other factors have been reported to increase HCC risk among HBV carriers, including male sex; older age (or longer duration of infection); Asian or African race; cirrhosis; family history of HCC; exposure to aflatoxin, alcohol, or tobacco; or co-infection with HCV.[3] HCC risk also is increased in patients with higher levels of HBV replication, as indicated by the presence of hepatitis B e antigen (HBeAg) and high HBV DNA levels.[20,21] The same authors also showed that HBV carriers with low viral loads have a five-fold increased risk of HCC compared with controls (patients with chronic liver disease not attributable to viral hepatitis).[22] Therefore viral replication seems to be an important risk factor for HCC among these patients. In addition, it has been suggested in Asian studies that genotype C is associated with more severe liver disease than genotype B,[23] but genotypes do not affect treatment of the disease or clinical practice. One study estimated by mathematical modeling that for the year 2000, there were 620,000 persons who died worldwide from HBV-related causes, with 580,000 (94%) from chronic infection–related cirrhosis and HCC.[24] In the

Table 57-1 Common Factors Affecting the Progression to Hepatocellular Carcinoma in Patients with Cirrhosis

Host Related

Age
Gender
Liver disease severity
Iron overload
Diabetes
Obesity

Viral Related

Duration of infection
Viral replication (HBV)
Genotype (HBV, HCV, HIV)
Co-infection (HBV, HCV, HIV)

External

Smoking
Alcohol
Aflatoxin

HBV, hepatitis B; HCV, hepatitis C; HIV, human immunodeficiency virus

Table 57-2 Major Risk Factors for Primary Liver Cancer and Estimates of Attributable Fractions

RISK FACTORS	EUROPE AND UNITED STATES (%)	JAPAN (%)	AFRICA AND ASIA (%)
Hepatitis B virus	22 (4-58)*	20 (18-44)	60 (40-90)
Hepatitis C virus	60 (12-72)	63 (48-94)	20 (9-56)
Alcohol	45 (8-57)	20 (15-33)	10 (6-41)
Tobacco	10 (5-29)	14 (8-47)	13 (9-34)
Aflatoxin	Limited exposure	Limited exposure	Important exposure

Adapted from Bosch FX, et al. Primary liver cancer: worldwide incidence and trends. Gastroenterology 2004;127(5 Suppl 1):S5–S16.
*Estimate (range).

surviving birth cohort for the year 2000, the model estimated that without vaccination, 64.8 million would become infected with HBV and 1.4 million would die from HBV-related disease. Routine infant hepatitis B vaccination, with 90% coverage and the first dose administered at birth, would prevent 84% of global HBV-related deaths. HBV infection continues to be a significant healthcare problem and an important risk factor for HCC worldwide.

Hepatitis C

The causal agents leading to HCC have been largely established. In Japan, Europe, and America about 60% of the patients with HCC are attributed to chronic HCV infection, whereas about 20% are attributed to chronic HBV infection and about 20% between cryptogenic and alcoholic liver

disease.[8] Chronic HCV infection is found in a variable proportion of HCC cases in different populations, accounting for 75% to 90% of cases in Japan, 31% to 47% in the United States, 44% to 76% in Italy, and 60% to 75% of HCC cases in Spain.[15] A higher but undefined proportion of HCC patients might have had HCV detected by polymerase chain reaction testing of liver tissue and/or serum, even if antibody to HCV (anti-HCV) was nondetectable. In a meta-analysis of 21 case-control studies in which second-generation enzyme immunoassay tests for anti-HCV were used, HCC risk was increased 17-fold in HCV-infected patients compared with HCV-negative controls (95% confidence interval [CI], 14 to 22).[25] The likelihood of development of HCC among HCV-infected persons is difficult to determine because of the paucity of adequate long-term cohort studies; however, the best estimate is 2% to 3% after 30 years.[26] A recent multicenter prospective study in the United States of 1005 patients (41% with cirrhosis) showed that the 3-year cumulative incidence rate for HCC was 2%, which increases to 5% at 5 years.[27] In this study the rate of development of HCC was significantly higher in cirrhotics compared with those without cirrhosis but with advanced fibrosis (7.0% vs. 4.1%). HCV increases HCC risk by promoting fibrosis and eventually cirrhosis. Once HCV-related cirrhosis is established, HCC develops at an annual rate of 1% to 4%, although rates of up to 7% have been reported in Japan.[28-30] In HCV-infected patients, host and environmental factors appear to be more important than viral factors in determining progression to cirrhosis. In a population-based study of 12,008 men, being anti-HCV positive conferred a 20-fold increased risk of HCC compared with anti-HCV–negative subjects.[31] Other important factors included older age, older age at the time of acquisition of infection, male sex, heavy alcohol intake (>50 g/day), diabetes, obesity, and co-infection with human immunodeficiency virus (HIV) or HBV.[31] There is no strong evidence that HCV viral factors such as genotype, load, or quasispecies are important in determining the risk of progression to cirrhosis or HCC.

Cirrhosis

Cirrhosis is the most important risk factor for the development of HCC, regardless of the cause.[30] The risk of HCC in persons with HBV-related cirrhosis is 2.2 to 4.3 per 100 person-years, whereas it is less than 1 per 100 person-years in noncirrhotic patients.[18] It is estimated that about 20% of patients with HBV-related HCC present without cirrhosis, indicating that other factors are important in hepatocarcinogenesis.[32] The risk of HCC among patients with chronic HCV infection also occurs in the setting of patients with cirrhosis.[18] A more recent study in the United States showed that for patients with chronic HCV infection, the incidence of HCC was higher in cirrhotics than in noncirrhotics.[27] Alcoholic cirrhosis is another well-established major etiologic risk factor for the development of HCC.[33-35] An association between nonalcoholic liver disease and HCC has been made,[36] but prospective cohort studies evaluating the natural history of nonalcoholic fatty liver disease are needed. Other causes of chronic liver disease, such as hemochromatosis, primary biliary cirrhosis, autoimmune hepatitis, and α_1-antitrypsin deficiency are less common causes of chronic liver disease, with prevalence rates in patients with HCC between 1% and 8%.[37-40] Furthermore, improvements in the survival rates of patients with cirrhosis because of better specialty care may further increase the number of individuals at risk for developing HCC.[41]

Alcohol and Tobacco

Heavy alcohol intake is a well-established HCC risk factor. Although heavy intake is associated strongly with the development of cirrhosis, there is little evidence of a direct carcinogenic effect of alcohol otherwise. However, there is evidence that the risk of HCC increases with a daily alcohol intake of 40 to 60 g/day.[42,43] There is evidence for a synergistic effect of heavy alcohol ingestion and viral hepatitis. An Italian study investigated the dose-effect relation between alcohol drinking and HCC considering HBV and HCV virus infections.[44] They enrolled 464 subjects (380 men) with a first diagnosis of HCC as cases and 824 subjects (686 men) unaffected by hepatic diseases as controls, of whom 24% of HCC had HBV infection. There was a steady linear increase in the odds ratio (OR) for HCC with an increase in alcohol intake starting at a value of greater than 60 g of ethanol per day, with no substantial differences between men and women. A synergism between alcohol drinking and viral infection was found, with approximately a two-fold increase in the OR for each hepatitis virus infection for drinkers of greater than 60 g/day. A Greek case-control study of 333 incident HCC cases and 360 controls investigated the role of tobacco in HCC.[45] The authors found a significant dose-response, positive association between smoking and HCC risk (more than two packs per day; OR = 2.5). This association was stronger in individuals without chronic infection with either HBV or HCV (≥2 packs per day; OR = 2.8). Interestingly, the authors also found evidence of a super-multiplicative effect of heavy smoking and heavy drinking in the development of HCC (OR for both exposures = 9.6). This interaction was particularly evident among individuals with viral infection (OR for both exposures = 10.9). A large Korean study of 1,283,112 men and women free of cancer at baseline were followed prospectively for 10 years, and 3807 died from liver cancer during follow-up.[46] Current smoking was associated with increased risk of mortality from HCC in men (relative risk [RR] = 1.4; 95% CI, 1.3 to 1.6) but not in women. Heavy alcohol drinking was associated with hepatocellular carcinoma mortality risk in the subgroup of men who also had HBV infection (RR = 1.5; 95% CI, 1.2 to 2.0). All patients with chronic viral hepatitis should be completely abstinent from alcohol and tobacco to reduce the risk of developing HCC.

Aflatoxin

Aflatoxin B (AFB) is a mycotoxin produced by the *Aspergillus* fungus. This fungus grows readily on foodstuffs, such as corn and peanuts, stored in warm, damp conditions. In most areas where AFB exposure is a problem, chronic HBV infection also is highly prevalent. A p53 mutation has been observed in 30% to 60% of HCC tumors in AFB-endemic areas.[47] There was a 60-fold increased risk of HCC in individuals with excreted AFB metabolites who were HBV carriers.[48] A recent study concluded that about 25,200 to 155,000 cases per year of HCC may be attributable to AFB exposure.[49] Most cases occur in sub-Saharan Africa, Southeast Asia, and China, where populations suffer from both high HBV prevalence and largely uncontrolled aflatoxin exposure in food. AFB-infected food

sources are still a significant healthcare problem in Africa and efforts are ongoing to combat this exposure.[50] In addition to HBV vaccination as the major preventive tactic, persons already chronically infected could benefit by eliminating AFB exposure. Such practice is being promoted in high-rate countries and has lead to excellent results in some areas.[51]

Obesity

Evidence indicating that obesity is an important risk factor for liver cancer came from a prospectively followed adult cohort in the United States. In a study of more than 900,000 individuals, obesity was associated with increased death rates for multiple solid tumors; the greatest impact of obesity was on liver cancer.[52] The relative risk of death from liver cancer among adults with a body mass index (BMI) greater than 35 was 5.2 compared with those with a BMI less than 30; the risk may be higher if weights before diagnosis of HCC were available. Two other population-based cohort studies also showed increased risk of HCC among obese individuals.[53,54] The mechanism by which obesity leads to cancer is unclear; insulin resistance and its subsequent inflammatory cascade and insulin growth factor (IGF)-1 have been implicated.[55] A case-control study done in the United States showed a synergistic interaction among heavy alcohol consumption, heavy tobacco smoking, and obesity regarding the risk of HCC.[56] Although the evidence linking obesity to HCC is relatively scant, even small increases in risk related to obesity could translate into a large number of HCC cases.

Diabetes Mellitus

Diabetes has been shown to be a risk factor for the development of HCC. There have been 10 case-control and 5 prior cohort studies from 7 countries since 1986 that reported a relationship between diabetes and HCC, all of which show a significant association (mean RR = 2.4 with a range of 1.27 to 4.88).[57] These studies concluded that diabetes is an important and consistent risk factor for HCC. However, the current studies have not established that diabetes precedes HCC or considered the possibility that both HCC and diabetes might be the product of other factors, particularly chronic liver disease. The only study performed in a HBV-endemic area followed a prospective cohort of 54,979 subjects enrolled in a population-based study of disease surveillance.[58] A total of 138 confirmed HCC cases, in which diabetes preceded the development of these tumors, were identified either through a two-stage liver cancer screening or linkage with the National Cancer Registry. After controlling for age, sex, HBV infection, HCV infection, smoking, and alcohol consumption, the association of diabetes and HCC was statistically significant (adjusted hazard ratio [HR] = 2.08, 95% CI, 1.03 to 4.18), especially in HCV-negative individuals. An American study cohort of 173,643 patients with diabetes and 650,620 patients without diabetes showed that the incidence for HCC was 2.39 versus 0.87 per 10,000 person-years, respectively ($P < .0001$).[59] Diabetes was associated with a relative risk of 2.16 (1.86 to 2.52) for HCC. HCC and diabetes have repeatedly been shown to occur together too consistently among diverse studies to be due to chance or bias alone. Further studies are needed to make the observation that diabetes precedes HCC and to determine whether diabetes (abnormal glucose and insulin metabolism) precedes liver disease that leads to HCC or whether liver disease precedes the diabetes.

Prevention

Cancer prevention is an important aspect in the care of patients. Because viral hepatitis is the predominant cause of HCC, the prevention data center on vaccines and antiviral medications. For the other risk factors of HCC, such as tobacco, alcohol, diabetes, and obesity, there are no prospective studies to determine whether eliminating these risks will decrease HCC. Most of the data come from retrospective studies. A study from Japan reported that increased smoking in the 5 years before development of HCC increases the risk for developing this tumor three-fold.[60] To date, despite its undoubted importance as a risk factor, there is limited evidence to support the effectiveness of alcohol reduction interventions in reducing the incidence of HCC. While lifestyle modifications that include dietary restriction and exercise to achieve judicious weight loss is recommended to treat nonalcoholic fatty liver disease, diabetes, and obesity,[61] they have not been shown to reduce the risk of HCC. However, it is prudent to counsel patients with chronic liver disease in regard to smoking and alcohol cessation and weight loss, which can lead to healthier lifestyles.

Regardless of the mechanisms for the occurrence of hepatocarcinogenesis in patients with viral hepatitis, eliminating the virus is of utmost importance in decreasing the risk of HCC. The HBV vaccine is the first vaccine shown to prevent cancer. A study of Taiwanese children found that the average annual incidence of liver cancer decreased from 0.70 per 100,000 between 1981 and 1986 to 0.57 per 100,000 between 1986 and 1990 and to 0.36 per 100,000 between 1990 and 1994 (P <.0001).[62] It is anticipated that the implementation of global vaccination of all newborns will ultimately lead to a worldwide reduction in incidence of HBV-related HCC, although it may take a few decades for the impact to be observed among adults.

For the 350 million persons estimated to have chronic HBV infection worldwide, HBV vaccination would not be effective in preventing HCC. The best strategy for prevention is eliminating the modifiable risk factors, such as alcohol and tobacco, and to treat with agents aimed at eliminating viral replication. A meta-analysis of seven studies that evaluated the use of interferon alfa showed that treatment reduced the risk of HCC by 6.4%.[63] The recent development of newer antivirals such as lamivudine, adefovir, and entecavir may increase the potential to prevent HCC further. There has been one randomized controlled trial that aimed to determine whether treatment with lamivudine can prevent HCC.[64] The authors randomly assigned 651 patients who were HBeAg positive and/or had detectable HBV DNA (98% Asian and 85% male) to receive lamivudine or a placebo. HCC occurred in 3.9% ($n = 17$) of those in the lamivudine group and 7.4% ($n = 17$) of those in the placebo group (HR = 0.49; P = .047). Even though this trial was very well done and provided some insights, there are still questions remaining about whether treatment should be directed toward those with a high viral load and whether treatment is effective for those with lower HBV DNA levels. Questions also remain about the appropriate length of treatment, resistance to

medications, and end points. The development of newer and more powerful antivirals raises the possibility for improved prevention of HCC among those with chronic HBV infection.

Cirrhosis is by far the single most important risk factor for the development of HCC in patients with chronic HCV infection. It is also known that male gender, older age, co-infection with HBV, alcohol, tobacco, obesity, and diabetes are important risk factors for HCC. As with HBV, only alcohol, tobacco, and obesity are modifiable but no studies have been performed to evaluate whether these factors can prevent HCC. There are three randomized controlled trials that focused on prevention of HCC as an outcome.[65-67] The largest trial from Japan randomized 90 patients based on whether they received treatment. HCC developed in 33 of the untreated patients and in only 12 of the treated patients according to a follow-up study conducted 8.2 years later (P <.001). The other studies suffer from lack of an adequate sample size, long-term follow-up, and small overall effect. The largest trial to date for secondary prevention of HCC is a multicenter trial in the United States that randomized nonresponders with advanced fibrosis to chronic pegylated interferon alfa for 3 years versus no treatment.[68] The results showed that chronic interferon therapy did not reduce the risk of HCC or hepatic decompensation when compared with the best supportive care for those with advanced fibrosis that are nonresponders to previous antiviral therapy. As better antivirals are developed, the potential ability to prevent HCC development in patients with viral hepatitis will improve as the ability to develop sustained virologic responses improves.

Pathogenesis

In the last several years there have been important gains in the understanding of the pathogenesis of HCC and the appreciation of the critical oncogenic and tumor suppressor pathways involved in hepatocarcinogenesis. Perhaps most important is the growing appreciation of the critical role of unrestricted cellular proliferation in the process of carcinogenesis. Currently, the dominant paradigm suggests that carcinogenesis occurs through a multistep process resulting in the progression of normal cells through preneoplastic states into invasive cancers.[69] The key phenotypic characteristics of cancer cells are self-sufficiency in growth signals, insensitivity to growth-inhibitory signals, evasion of apoptosis, limitless replicative potential, sustained angiogenesis, and tissue invasion and metastasis. It has been proposed that the acquisition of each of these phenotypic characteristics is necessary for the eventual development of the full neoplastic phenotype.[70] Although there is substantial evidence to support this view, it is also becoming increasingly clear that the predominant cellular event necessary for the development of cancer is unconstrained cell proliferation. This "cancer platform" concept suggests that the key event driving carcinogenesis is the simultaneous development of deregulated proliferation and reduced cell death; the subsequent development of the additional phenotypes of invasion, angiogenesis, metastasis, and immune evasion are secondary to the development of unrestricted proliferation.[71] Because of the presence of a complex network of molecules within both the oncogenic and antiapoptotic programs, genetic or epigenetic alterations may affect different molecules but have similar results on the overall cellular

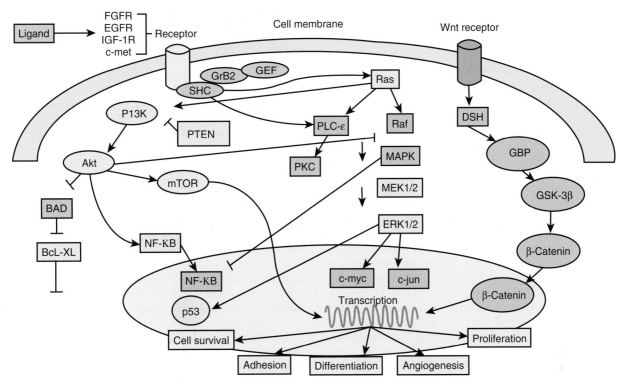

Fig. 57-4 **Major cellular pathways in hepatocellular carcinoma that ultimately lead to cell survival, adhesion, differentiation, angiogenesis, and proliferation.** *(Adapted from Thorgiersson SS, Grisham JW. Molecular pathogenesis of human hepatocellular carcinoma. Nat Genet 2002;31:339–346.)*

phenotype. A typical example of the interaction between pathogenic mechanisms in the development of HCC is illustrated by the synergism between dietary aflatoxin intake and chronic HBV infection in carcinogenesis. Aflatoxin exposure results in *p53* mutations, most commonly at codon 249. Wild-type *p53* promotes apoptosis and is induced by many oncogenes in a negative feedback loop to limit proliferation. Inactivation of *p53* by mutation severely compromises oncogene-induced apoptosis and also leads to defects in DNA damage checkpoints and to gross aneuploidy.[72] The majority of HCCs develop in patients with chronic inflammation related to chronic hepatitis B or C virus infection, chronic alcohol abuse, or other causes. Evidence from the Mdr2 knockout mouse model of hepatitis-induced carcinogenesis suggests that infiltrating endothelial and inflammatory cells release tumor necrosis factor-α (TNF-α), which acts on nearby hepatocytes by activating nuclear factor κB (NF-κB).[73]

We will now discuss the major cellular signaling mechanisms known to play a role in hepatocarcinogenesis for which targeted agents are currently under development or in clinical trials for modulation of these pathways in the treatment of cancer. These major pathways ultimately lead to cell survival, adhesion, differentiation, angiogenesis, and proliferation as shown in **Figure 57-4**.

Receptor Tyrosine Kinase Pathways

The Ras mitogen-activated protein kinase (MAPK) and phosphatidylinositol-3′-kinase (PI3K)-Akt kinase signaling pathways are activated by ligand binding and phosphorylation of several growth factor tyrosine kinase receptors, including the vascular endothelial growth factor (VEFG) receptor,

epidermal growth factor (EGF) receptor, platelet-derived growth factor (PDGF) receptor, fibroblast growth factor (FGF) receptor, the hepatocyte growth factor (HGF) receptor c-met, and the stem cell growth factor receptor (c-kit).[74] The downstream consequences of activation of these receptors are multiple and include activation of the Grb2/Shc/SOS adapter molecule complex and downstream activation of the Ras/MAPK pathway, which results in activation of transcriptional activators c-fos and c-jun and consequent induction of transcription of genes that drive cell proliferation. Sorafenib is an example of an agent that blocks this pathway and has been used in clinical medicine.[75]

Wnt/β-Catenin Pathway

Wnts are secreted cysteine-rich glycoprotein ligands that act as ligands for the Frizzled family of cell surface receptors and activate receptor-mediated signaling pathways; the best-studied Wnt pathway activates β-catenin.[76] Activation of the Wnt pathway occurs in approximately 30% to 40% of HCCs and is due to mutations in the β-catenin gene in 12% to 26% of human HCCs and to mutations in AXIN1 or AXIN2 in 8% to 13% of human HCC.[77] Wnts are involved in regulation of liver regeneration and in the maintenance and self-renewal of pluripotent stem cells and progenitor cells; hence, they may play a role in the maintenance of the cancer stem cell compartment and may be ideal targets for cancer therapy.[78] Agents under development for targeting the Wnt pathway in cancer include small molecule inhibitors that block interaction of β-catenin with TCF, such as the fungal derivatives PKF115-854 and CGP049090[79] or interaction of β-catenin with cAMP response element binding protein (CREB), such as the small molecule ICG-001,[80] and therapeutic monoclonal antibodies against Wnts.[81]

PI3K/AKT/mTOR Pathway

Multiple cellular growth factors, including insulin and insulin-like growth factors and cytokines such as interleukin-2, activate the PI3K family of enzymes, which produce the lipid second messenger phosphatidylinositol triphosphate (PIP_3) and related second messengers. PIP_3 in turn activates Akt/protein kinase B (PKB). Activated Akt phosphorylates several cellular target proteins, including the proapoptotic protein BAD, which is inactivated by phosphorylation, and also the mammalian target of the rapamycin (mTOR) subfamily of proteins.[82] mTOR proteins in turn regulate the phosphorylation of p70 S6 kinase, a serine-threonine kinase, and the translational repressor protein PHAS-1/4E-BP. These proteins regulate translation of cell cycle regulatory proteins and promote cell cycle progression.[83] In a recently reported study, overexpression of phospho-mTOR was found in 15% of HCCs and mTOR phosphorylation was associated with increased expression of total p70 S6 kinase, which was found in 45% of HCCs. In vitro experiments showed that rapamycin reduced p70 S6K phosphorylation and markedly inhibited proliferation of both HepG2 and Hep3B HCC cell lines.[84] Rapamycin and other mTOR kinase inhibitors show significant activity against cancers with activated PI3K/Akt pathways,[85,86] and are currently under investigation in clinical trials.

Angiogenic Pathways

Substances produced by cancer cells in response to local hypoxia or the interaction of the proliferating mass of cells with surrounding stromal tissue stimulate the growth of new blood vessels from the surrounding parenchyma into the tumor. Signaling pathways critical to the angiogenic process include growth factor–mediated pathways such as VEGF and FGF receptor signaling, as well as the nitric oxide signaling pathway. Hypoxia induces expression of hypoxia inducible factor 1 (HIF1) and insulin-like growth factor 2 (IGF2), both of which stimulate expression of VEGF and other growth factors.[87] HCCs are highly vascular and presumably dependent on active neoangiogenesis for their growth. These factors presumably have both antiproliferative and antiangiogenic effects. In parallel with the increase in angiogenic stimuli, it has been shown that the expression of collagen XVIII, the precursor of the antiangiogenic molecule endostatin, is decreased in larger and more vascular HCCs.[88] Angiogenesis is a critical process in HCC and forms the basis for the majority of treatments.

Telomerase

Telomeres are specialized protein-DNA structures at the ends of chromosomes that contain long stretches of TTAGGG hexameric repeats. Telomeres prevent degradation of chromosome ends and end-to-end fusion with other chromosomes. Aging of somatic cells is associated with reduction in telomere length because of the inability of traditional DNA polymerases to replicate completely the end of the chromosomal DNA. In contrast, germ line and neoplastic cells express telomerase,

an enzyme that restores telomere length. There is progressive shortening of telomeres during progression from chronic hepatitis to cirrhosis and eventually to HCC.[89,90] Hepatocarcinogenesis is characterized by the evolution of clones of hepatocytes with increased telomerase expression and an immortalized phenotype. Therefore almost all HCCs show reactivation of telomerase activity.[91,92] Telomerase is an attractive target for anticancer drug development. Because it is usually not expressed in normal cells, it is likely that there will be no serious side effects from treatments that abrogate telomerase activity.

Stem Cells

Recently, applying the principles of stem cells to understand tumor development and progression has emerged because they share similar characteristics. The acquisition of stem cell–like properties in various tumors has been indicated to regulate cellular self-renewal potential and promote cell proliferation.[93] A signaling pathway that connects this "stemness" feature in tumorigenesis is Bmi-1. Bmi-1 belongs to the Polycomb gene group (PcG) involved in maintaining target genes in their transcriptional state. The ability of Bmi-1 to immortalize cells by inducing telomerase activity and promote tumorigenesis through repression of the p16[INK4a] and p19[ARF] expression indicates the involvement of the Bmi-1 "stemness" function in neoplastic proliferation.[94] Bmi-1 overexpression may cause hepatocyte immortalization through the suppression of p16 and the activation of human telomerase. However, the exact mechanistic role of Bmi-1 in tumorigenesis is not yet clear. This is an area of rapid growth that may lead to important clinical implications.

Early Detection

The overall goal of screening or surveillance is to reduce morbidity and mortality from cancer. Screening is the use of a relatively simple, inexpensive test in a large number of individuals to determine whether they are likely or unlikely to have the cancer for which they are being screened.[95] Screening can be further defined as the one-time application of a test that allows detection of a disease before the symptoms appear and at a stage where curative intervention may improve the goal of reducing morbidity and mortality. Surveillance is the continuous monitoring of disease occurrence (using the screening test) within a population to achieve the same goals of screening. Criteria have been developed, first promoted by the WHO, to ensure the benefits of screening or surveillance for a specific disease[96]: (1) the disease in question should be an important health problem; its significance may be defined by disease burden, including morbidity and mortality; (2) there should be an identifiable target population; (3) treatment of occult disease (i.e., disease diagnosed before the symptoms appear) should offer advantages compared with the treatment of symptomatic disease; (4) a screening test should be affordable and provide benefits justifying its cost; (5) the test must be acceptable to the target population and to healthcare professionals; (6) there must be standardized recall procedures; and (7) screening tests must achieve an acceptable level of accuracy in the population undergoing screening. HCC meets all of these criteria for establishing a surveillance program. Before starting a surveillance program, it is critical

Table 57-3 Risk for Development of Hepatocellular Carcinoma Is Greater Than 1.5% Per Year for the Following Patients Who Would Benefit from Surveillance

Hepatitis B Carriers

Asian men >40 years
Asian women >50 years
Cirrhosis
First-degree relative with HCC
Africans >20 years

Non–Hepatitis B Cirrhosis

Hepatitis C
Alcohol
Genetic hemochromatosis
Primary biliary cirrhosis
Nonalcoholic fatty liver disease

Adapted from Bruix J, et al. Management of hepatocellular carcinoma. Hepatology 2005;42:1208–1236.

to decide what level of risk for HCC is significant enough to warrant initiation of surveillance, what screening tests are to be applied and at what frequency, and how to handle abnormal results from screening tests (diagnosis or recall).

To decide what level of risk of a disease is significant to warrant the start of a surveillance program, most investigators use the incidence rates of the disease in an at-risk population to determine the risk, as well as whether intervention increases longevity. An intervention is considered effective if it provides an increase in longevity of about 100 days, (i.e., about 3 months).[97] Although the levels were set years ago, and may not be appropriate today, interventions that can be achieved at a cost of less than about $50,000 per year of life gained are considered cost effective.[98] There are several decision analysis models that have shown that the surveillance of HCC is a cost effective strategy.[99-101] These studies showed that an incidence rate of HCC of at least 1.5% per year should trigger surveillance, that there is an increase survival rate with surveillance, and that the surveillance strategy was cost effective. The patients at risk for HCC should be divided among those with chronic HBV infection and those without HBV given the different natural histories and disease progression.[30] **Table 57-3** shows the patients in which the risk of developing HCC is greater than 1.5% per year and that warrant surveillance.

Hepatitis B

The seminal work of Beasley showed for the first time that patients with chronic HBV infection are at risk for HCC.[102,103] He showed that the overall incidence of HCC was 0.5% per year but increased to 1% in older patients (>70 years old) and increased further to 2.5% per year in patients with cirrhosis. In North America, the incidence of HCC among these patients varies widely, up to 0.46%.[104-106] In Europe, the patients who develop HCC are mostly patients with cirrhosis.[107-108] Non-Asian patients with no evidence of viral replication and who do not have cirrhosis seem to be at a very low risk for developing HCC.[109-111] However, Asian patients that do not have cirrhosis are at risk for HCC if they have persistent viral replication.[20,112,113] Prospective studies have shown that the

annual incidence rate for patients is 2.2% to 4.3% in patients with HBV cirrhosis, 0.1% to 1% in patients with chronic hepatitis, and 0.02% to 0.2% in inactive carriers.[18] Men older than 40 years of age have a significant risk factor for HCC.[103] In the presence of a first-degree relative, HCC surveillance should start at the age of 40 years.[114] Natives of Africa seem to develop HCC at younger ages when compared with other ethnicities with chronic HBV infection, and therefore should start surveillance for HCC at the age of 20 years.[115,116]

Hepatitis C

The risk of HCC among those with chronic HCV infection is mainly limited to those with cirrhosis, and the reported incidence rate is between 2% and 8% per year.[26-31] Patients without cirrhosis are at a low risk for developing HCC.[117] None of the viral factors such as replication status, genotype, or age have been shown to increase the risk of HCC further.

Cirrhosis Resulting from Nonviral Causes

The incidence of HCC among patients without viral hepatitis is not accurately known. Alcoholic cirrhosis has a significant risk for HCC of greater than 2% per year.[118] Alcoholic cirrhosis also accounts for about a third of patients with HCC.[119,120] Nonalcoholic fatty liver disease has been associated with HCC.[36] However, the incidence among patients with nonalcoholic steatohepatitis is unknown. It has been shown that up to 40% of patients with HCC have cryptogenic liver disease.[121] Therefore the evidence indicates that patients with cryptogenic cirrhosis, most of these related to nonalcoholic fatty liver disease, are at risk for developing HCC and therefore should undergo surveillance. Patients with genetic hemochromatosis and primary biliary cirrhosis that have progressed to cirrhosis are also at risk for developing HCC and should undergo surveillance.[122-124]

Surveillance Tests and Efficacy

The most commonly used surveillance tests for HCC is α-fetoprotein (AFP) and hepatic ultrasound (US). The studies on surveillance should be evaluated separately in those with chronic HBV (studies from Asian countries) and those with cirrhosis in Western countries given the differences in populations studied.

For patients with chronic HBV infection, the surveillance strategy of AFP plus US was recently evaluated in two randomized trials. In both trials, surveillance was conducted every 6 months and compared with patients who did not receive any routine screening. The first study evaluated 17,920 carriers of the HBV virus who were randomized to surveillance ($n = 8109$) or no surveillance ($n = 9711$) and followed for an average of 14.4 months.[125] Of the patients randomized to the surveillance group, 38 patients developed HCC, of whom 29 (76.3%) were detected at early stages, whereas 18 patients developed HCC in the no-surveillance group, of whom none were detected at an early stage ($P <.01$). A higher proportion of patients in the surveillance group met criteria for surgical therapy, with 24 patients having surgical resection in the surveillance group compared with zero patients in the no-screening group. Accordingly, the 1-year and 2-year survival rates for the surveillance group were 88.1% and 77.5%, respectively, compared with a 0% survival rate at 1 year for the no-screening group. The authors concluded that surveillance would reduce HCC-associated mortality rates. The second randomized controlled trial evaluated 19,200 HBV carriers who were randomized to surveillance ($n = 9757$) and no surveillance ($n = 9443$).[126] A total of 86 patients developed HCC in the surveillance group, of which 45% were early stage compared with 67 patients with HCC in the no-surveillance group, of whom none were early stage. The mortality rate of patients undergoing surveillance was significantly lower than the control group (83.2 vs. 131.5 per 100,000, $P < .01$), with an HR of 0.63 (95% CI, 41 to 98). These results demonstrate that the strategy of surveillance with AFP and US among patients with chronic HBV infection reduces overall mortality.

There are no randomized trials of surveillance in patients with non-HBV infection (mostly HCV infection), which mostly involved patients with cirrhosis in Western countries. AFP and US have been the most used surveillance tests. It has been shown in a study of patients with HCC (60% having advanced HCC) that the optimal balance of sensitivity and specificity for AFP is achieved by a cutoff level of 20 ng/ml.[127] However, this cutoff leads to sensitivities between 41% and 60% and specificities between 80% and 94%.[128-130] A major problem with the data is that these studies were heterogenous in nature with regard to sample size and length of follow-up, were performed before better diagnostic tests were developed, and, importantly, did not follow the guidelines set forth for the evaluation of surveillance tests.[131] A large recent multi-center case-controlled study of 417 cirrhotics without HCC and 419 HCC cases, of whom 208 (49.6%) had early-stage HCC, was performed to evaluate the true performance of AFP in the large number of patients with early-stage HCC.[132] AFP had a sensitivity of 66% for early-stage HCC. In a large prospective cohort study of 1145 patients with chronic HCV infection, called the HALT-C (Hepatitis C Antiviral Long-Term Treatment Against Cirrhosis) trial, a total of at least 48 patients developed HCC.[27] A nested case-control study involving 39 patients that developed HCC and 77 matched controls without HCC who were part of the HALT-C trial evaluated the performance of AFP and US.[133] The results showed that at the time of HCC, AFP had a sensitivity of 61% that decreased to 57% 6 months before the diagnosis. Although AFP is not specific for HCC,[134] the evidence shows that it can lead to detection of early-stage HCC with or without US and it is also a marker of prognosis of HCC.[135]

The other commonly used surveillance test for HCC is US. As the goal of screening is to reduce mortality by detecting patients with occult disease, the performance characteristics of a test used for diagnosis and/or staging (e.g., computed tomography [CT], magnetic resonance imaging [MRI]) cannot be assumed to be the same when used in a surveillance/screening situation. The sensitivity and specificity of US has been shown to be between 58% and 78% and 93% and 98%, respectively.[136-138] A recent meta-analysis evaluated prospective studies in cirrhotics to determine the sensitivity of US to detect early-stage HCC.[139] The authors showed that surveillance US had a sensitivity of 63% to detect early-stage HCC, whereas AFP provided no additional benefit to US, and meta-regression analysis demonstrated a significantly higher sensitivity for early HCC with US every 6 months versus annual surveillance. Importantly, the authors showed that there was

significant heterogeneity with these current studies with significant limitations, such as verification bias, varying sample size, and poor overall power, and the lack of reproducibility testing for US. When verification bias was evaluated, the overall sensitivity of US decreased to 33%. In the nested case-control study of the HALT-C trial, 24 patients had early-stage HCC, detected by US in 14 patients (60%), doubling of AFP in 5 patients (20%), and a combination of AFP and US (20%).[133] When US is done in a best-case scenario, for the planning of RFA for tumors less than 2 cm in patients with cirrhosis, the sensitivity of US was 71% (in 77 out of 248 planning US for RFA, the tumors were not seen on CT or MRI).[140] The experience of the operator is also an important aspect of the performance of US in HCC, especially occurring in a liver that is cirrhotic or that has chronic liver disease.[141] These results show that US is the best surveillance test for HCC in cirrhosis, although the problems of operator dependency and the visualization in cirrhotic patients are important limitations. AFP does contribute to the early detection of HCC by being complementary to US, and has been shown to be a cost-effective strategy in patients with cirrhosis.[99-101] Both AFP and US are the best current surveillance tests for patients with non-HBV cirrhosis.

There is a need for new biomarkers for the detection of early HCC. One of these tests is des-gamma carboxyprothrombin (DCP). DCP is an abnormal prothrombin protein that is generated as a result of an acquired defect in the post-translational carboxylation of the prothrombin precursor in malignant hepatic cells.[142] A single-center case-controlled study showed that DCP was more sensitive and specific than total AFP.[143] Several prospective cohort studies in patients with cirrhosis without HCC have been performed to determine the performance of DCP.[144-146] The sensitivities for detecting HCC ranged from 23% to 57% compared with 14% to 71% for AFP. A multicenter case-control study in the United States showed that AFP had a better performance than DCP for the diagnosis of early-stage HCC.[132] However, the prospective nested case-control study of the HALT-C trial showed that DCP had a sensitivity of 74% at the time of diagnosis, which decreased to 63% 6 months before the diagnosis of HCC.[133] The combination of DCP and AFP increased the sensitivity to 86% 6 months before the diagnosis of HCC. DCP does indeed show promise as a biomarker, and future studies should evaluate if DCP is complementary to US for the early detection of HCC.

Several variants of AFP with differences in lectin affinities have been identified. One variant, the fucosylated variant, has a high affinity of the sugar chain to *Lens culinaris* (or lectin-bound AFP). Lectin-bound AFP or AFP-L3 has been shown to be more specific for HCC in patients with chronic HBV infection.[147] Prospective studies in patients with cirrhosis have shown sensitivities for AFP-L3 ranging from 55% to 75% and specificities from 68% to 90%.[148-150] However, two studies included only HCC patients with elevated total AFP at baseline, making it impossible to compare the accuracy of AFP-L3 with total AFP. A prospective study evaluated the clinical utility of AFP-L3 in a North American multicenter cohort.[151] The authors evaluated 332 patients with HCV cirrhosis and 34 developed HCC. The sensitivity, specificity, positive predictive value (PPV), and negative predictive value (NPV) for AFP (cutoff >20 ng/mL) was 61%, 71%, 34%, and 88%, respectively, whereas for AFP-L3 (cutoff 10%) it was 36%, 91%, 51%, and 85%, respectively. In a recent large case-control study that included a large number of patients with early-stage HCC, AFP-L3 was shown to have a poor sensitivity.[132] At this time there is no evidence of AFP-L3's efficacy in the surveillance of patients with cirrhosis or that these are better than AFP and ultrasound in this capacity.

Glypican-3 (GPC3) is a member of the glypican family of cell-surface heparan sulfate proteoglycans, recently found to be up-regulated in early-stage HCC compared with normal hepatic tissue.[152] Evaluation of GPC3 as a serum marker for HCC has been reported.[153] In this study, GPC3 expression in liver was detected using immunohistochemistry in none of 22 cirrhotics without dysplasia or HCC, 1 of 5 cirrhotics with high-grade dysplasia, and 21 of 29 with HCC. For tumors less than 3 cm, GPC3 expression was detected in 11 of 11 and AFP in only 2 of cirrhotics without cancer. Using enzyme-linked immunoassay (ELISA), GPC3 was detected in the serum from 18 of 34 (53%) patients with HCC and only 1 of 20 (5%) patients with cirrhosis, ($P = .0049$). More recently, it was found that GPC3 expression was an independent histologic marker for differentiating early HCC from cirrhosis.[154] Further studies are needed to determine if the sensitivities can be improved in the serum in order for GPC3 to be used in the surveillance for HCC.

GP73 is a resident Golgi protein that is up-regulated in virus-infected hepatocytes.[155] Using Western blot assay, GP73 has been detected in serum with significantly higher levels among cirrhotics and patients with HCC than in normal subjects and patients with chronic hepatitis. In a phase II biomarker study, a total of 352 patients (152 cirrhosis controls and 144 HCC cases) were studied.[156] Serum GP73 levels were significantly higher in patients with HCC compared with those with cirrhosis ($P <.001$). GP73 had a sensitivity of 69% and a specificity of 75% at the optimal cutoff point of 10 relative units, with an area under the receiver operating curve of 0.79 versus 0.61 for AFP ($P = .001$). GP73 levels had significantly higher sensitivity (62%) than AFP (25%) for diagnosing early HCC ($P <.0001$). Moreover, GP73 levels were elevated in the serum of 57% (32 of 56) individuals with HCC who had serum AFP levels less than 20 ng/ml. GP73 should be tested in a larger sample set to determine the performance characteristics for the diagnosis of early-stage HCC.

Other markers such as squamous cell carcinoma antigen,[157] human hepatocyte growth factor,[158] insulin growth factor-1,[159] and osteopontin[160] are being evaluated, but the data are preliminary. The field of proteomics may provide the tools to determine novel serum biomarkers in HCC.[161] However, none of these have been externally validated nor are they ready for clinical use.

The recommended surveillance test for patients with chronic HBV infection is US and AFP with the highest level of evidence (**Table 57-4**). For non-HBV cirrhotic patients, the data indicates that US and AFP appear to be complementary in detecting early stage HCC at a lower level of evidence (see **Table 57-4**). Better-quality studies are needed to determine if biomarkers such as DCP add to US and AFP.

Diagnosis

Once an abnormal screening test is obtained in a cirrhotic patient, it is necessary to perform the diagnostic evaluation to determine the presence of HCC. Pathologic examination and

Table 57-4 Recommended Surveillance Tests for Heaptocellular Carcinoma and Level of Evidence

SURVEILLANCE TEST	LEVEL OF EVIDENCE
Hepatitis B Carriers	
α-Fetoprotein	I
Ultrasound	I
Nonhepatitis B Cirrhosis	
Ultrasound	II-2
α-Fetoprotein	II-2

Based on Practice Guidelines Committee of the American Association for the Study of Liver Disease.[30]

radiology are the main tools to make the diagnosis of HCC. We will discuss these in more detail.

Pathology

Low-grade dysplastic nodules (L-DNs) can be nodular because of the presence of a peripheral fibrous scar. L-DNs show a mild increase in cell density with a monotonous pattern and have no cytologic atypia.[162] Architectural changes beyond clearly regenerative features are not present; these lesions do not contain pseudoglands or markedly thickened trabeculae. Unpaired arteries are sometimes present in small numbers.[163] Nodule-in-nodule lesions are not present in L-DNs. L-DNs may have diffuse siderosis or diffusely increased copper retention. The distinction between these regenerative nodule and L-DNs cannot be made confidently by morphology alone and remain a task for the future.[164] Fortunately, this distinction does not appear to have significant practical consequence at present.

High-grade dysplastic nodules (H-DNs) may be distinctly or vaguely nodular in the background of cirrhosis and are more likely to show a vaguely nodular pattern than LDNs. An HDN is defined as having architectural and/or cytologic atypia, but the atypia is insufficient for a diagnosis of HCC. These lesions most often show increased cell density, sometimes more than two times higher than the surrounding nontumoral liver, often with an irregular trabecular pattern.[165] Small cell change (also known as small cell dysplasia) is the most frequently seen form of cytologic atypia in HDNs.[166] A nodule-in-nodule appearance is occasionally found in H-DNs, and subnodules often have a higher labeling index of Ki-67 or proliferating cell nuclear antigen than that of H-DN parenchyma. When a nodule with largely HDN features contains a subnodule (i.e., nodule-in-nodule) of HCC, the subnodule of HCC is usually well-differentiated with a well-defined margin. The diagnostic discrepancy between HDNs and early HCC has improved because of the recognition of stromal invasion as a diagnostic criterion for the differentiation of HDN from early HCC.[164] If areas of questionable invasion are present, immunostaining for keratins 7 or 19 may be useful; if such staining demonstrates a ductular reaction, the focus is considered a pseudoinvasion and does not warrant a diagnosis of HCC.[167]

Early HCC can be characterized by major histologic features. This includes (1) increased cell density more than two

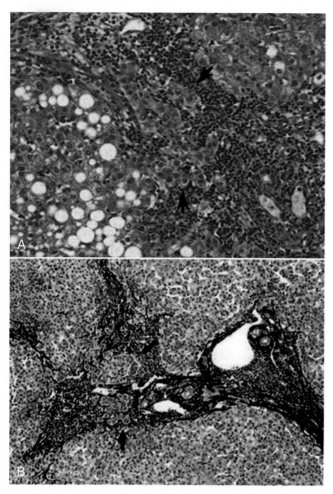

Fig. 57-5 Stromal invasion in hepatocellular carcinoma. The *arrows* in panel **A** indicate a low power view of stromal invasion of hepatocellular carcinoma. Panel **B** indicates a high-power field view of the trabecular pattern of the stromal invasion in well-differentiated HCC as shown by the *arrow.*

times that of the surrounding tissue, with an increased nuclear/cytoplasm ratio and an irregular, thin trabecular pattern; (2) varying numbers of portal tracts within the nodule (intratumoral portal tracts); (3) pseudoglandular pattern; (4) diffuse fatty change; and (5) varying numbers of unpaired arteries.[164,168-170] Any of these listed features may be diffuse throughout the lesion or may be restricted to an expansile subnodule (nodule-in-nodule). Most importantly, because all of these features may also be found in HDNs, it is important to note that stromal invasion remains most helpful in differentiating early HCC from H-DNs as shown in **Figure 57-5.** Stromal invasion is defined at tumor cell invasion into the portal tracts or fibrous septa within vaguely nodular lesions.[164]

Various novel biomarkers have also been shown to be able to distinguish HCC from HDNs or regenerative nodules. GPC3, a cell-surface heparan sulfate proteoglycan that is secreted into the plasma, has recently become established as a tissue marker for HCC. GPC3 immunoreactivity has a reported sensitivity of 77% and a specificity of 96% in the diagnosis of small HCC; therefore GPC3 positivity is a strong indicator of malignancy.[153] Another biomarker is heat shock

protein 70 (HSP70), which belongs to a class of heat shock proteins implicated in the regulation of cell cycle progression, in apoptosis, and in tumorigenesis.[171] HSP70 immunoreactivity was recently reported in the majority of HCCs, including early and well-differentiated forms, but not in nonmalignant nodules, which suggests its use as a marker of malignancy.[172] Glutamine synthetase (GS) catalyzes the synthesis of glutamine from glutamate and ammonia in the mammalian liver.[173] There is a stepwise increase in GS immunoreactivity from precancerous lesions to early HCC to progressed HCC.[174] When applying a panel of these three markers (GPC3, HSP70, and GS) to resected small lesions, the finding of any two positive markers had a sensitivity of 72% and a specificity of 100% to detect malignancy.[175] The diagnostic accuracy of this panel of markers in liver biopsies of hepatocellular nodules has not been yet tested in a prospective manner but holds promise.

Radiology

Radiologic imaging is the most important aspect in the diagnostic evaluation of patients with HCC because the imaging characteristics can be diagnostic of HCC, and it provides the true determination of the overall tumor burden. The development of varying degrees of cellular and architectural atypia suggests that nodular lesions in the liver represent a pathway of carcinogenesis, which involves neoangiogenesis, leading to a gradual change in blood supply from portal to arterial, as a dysplastic nodule becomes hepatocellular carcinoma.[176,177] Studies based on findings at CT during arterial portography and CT during hepatic arteriography with pathologic correlation have shown that as the grade of malignancy within the nodules evolves, there is a gradual reduction of the normal hepatic arterial and portal venous supply to the nodule followed by an increase in the abnormal arterial supply via newly formed abnormal arteries, a process known as neoangiogenesis.[178] Histopathologically, this corresponds to a diminution in the portal tracts (portal vein and hepatic artery), which are virtually absent in HCC.[177] Moreover, unpaired arteries and sinusoidal capillarization are most common in HCC, less common in dysplastic nodules, and rare in regenerative nodules.[179] This process of neoangiogenesis or arterial recruitment forms the basis for the most important imaging feature of HCC, which is arterial enhancement. Arterial enhancement (hypervascularity) is considered an essential radiologic characteristic of HCC.[180-182] Arterial enhancement of HCC relative to surrounding parenchyma is often moderate in comparison with the enhancement of other hypervascular lesions, such as hemangioma and focal nodular hyperplasia. Enhancement is heterogeneous in large lesions and is homogeneous in small lesions.[183] As noted previously, other hepatic lesions also have arterial enhancement and therefore this is not specific of HCC.[184] The value of venous washout of an arterially enhancing lesion has been recognized and shown in **Figure 57-6.**[185] This is due to lack of arterial contrast in the portal venous delayed phases that leads to a hypointense characteristic of the HCC relative to the adjacent hepatic parenchyma. The reported overall sensitivity and specificity of venous washout was 89% and 96%, respectively.[186] Therefore the most important radiologic characteristic for HCC is dynamic imaging showing enhancement in the arterial phase followed by washout in the venous phases.

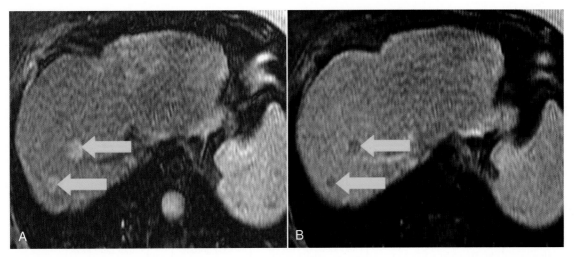

Fig. 57-6 **Washout in hepatocellular carcinoma. A,** Enhancement of two nodules in the arterial phase *(arrows).* **B,** The same nodules in the portal venous phase indicating no enhancement *(arrows).*

Both dynamic triple-phase CT and dynamic contrast-enhanced MRI are the most important diagnostic modalities in HCC. Recent studies have compared both modalities in cirrhotic patients, with liver transplantation as the gold standard.[187-191] MRI was more sensitive and specific compared with CT scans. The sensitivity of dynamic MRI ranges from 61% to 95% compared with 51% to 86% for triple-phase CT in these studies. In one study MRI was able to detect more lesions, especially smaller lesions (<2 cm), compared with CT, but the overall sensitivity was similar between the two modalities.[192] Ultrasound is used more as a surveillance test and its performance as a diagnostic test has been poor.[193] Positron emission tomography has shown poor performance in the diagnosis of HCC.[194]

For lesions in cirrhotic patients that are greater than 2 cm in diameter that enhance in the arterial phase and have washout, the positive predictive value is 95% and these should be treated as HCC.[195,196] If the imaging characteristics are not classic for HCC (i.e., no enhancement in the arterial phase, no washout), then a liver biopsy is recommended.[30,197] Recent studies have evaluated contrast-enhanced US as a modality that can be useful to evaluate lesions in cirrhotics.[198,199] However, these are small studies and it is not clear that it would add more information than CT or MRI.

Lesions between 1 and 2 cm in diameter, are harder to evaluate. From a radiologic standpoint, the typical imaging characteristics of HCC (enhancement in the arterial phase followed by washout in the venous phase) are less commonly seen and posed a significant challenge to diagnose. The majority of these lesions are not malignant.[200] However, some of these small lesions can have aggressive behavior leading to vascular invasion and poor prognosis.[201-203] The American Association for the Study of Liver Disease guidelines for the diagnosis of lesions in cirrhotics that are greater than 2 cm indicated that two imaging techniques with typical radiologic characteristics (enhancement in the arterial phase followed by washout in the venous phase) were needed to make the diagnosis of HCC without liver biopsy (see **Fig. 57-6**).[30] However, a recent study showed that for HCCs between 1 and 2 cm, one technique (CT or MRI) showing typical HCC characteristics was the best strategy, with a sensitivity of 65% and a specificity of 100%.[204]

If these small lesions show atypical characteristics on imaging, then a liver biopsy should be performed. There are concerns with conducting a liver biopsy, such as bleeding and obtaining an insufficient tissue sample; however, it seems that tumor seeding along the needle track does not appear to be a major concern.[205] As discussed in the pathology section, there are now criteria in place that can determine the difference between HDN and well-differentiated HCC more accurately. Patients in whom biopsy was negative for malignancy should undergo further follow-up with enhanced imaging and/or repeat biopsy. This strategy of performing a biopsy of atypical lesions and continued follow-up if the initial biopsy is negative has been validated.[206] In this study, the first biopsy was positive in 42 of 60 (70%) patients with HCC, and subsequent follow-up and biopsies (up to three biopsies performed in 17%) lead to the diagnosis. Therefore the imaging characteristics for patients with these small lesions will be critical for determining whether the patient has HCC or whether a liver biopsy is needed. If the workup for these small lesions is negative, it is important to continue follow-up because these patients may in fact have HCC.

Lesions less than 1 cm have a low likelihood of being HCC,[207] even if these lesions are seen on CT or MRI.[208] Therefore these lesions should be followed about every 3 to 6 months to determine if there has been growth or a change in their imaging characteristics.[209]

Table 57-5 shows the radiologic-pathologic characteristics of early-stage HCC. The most important feature from a pathologic standpoint is the presence of stromal invasion, whereas arterial hypervascularity is the most important radiologic finding in early stage HCC (though it can be isovascular or hypovascular in nature). If a nodule in the liver of a patient at risk for HCC has atypical features, a biopsy will be important for the evaluation. **Figure 57-7** shows the algorithm used for a mass found in someone at risk for developing HCC.

There are novel imaging techniques that may improve our ability to diagnose HCC. One of the improvements is the development of novel contrast agents for MRI, and one such agent is gadoxetate disodium (Eovist). This agent is selectively taken up by hepatocytes, which will increase the signal intensity of normal liver parenchyma on T1-weighted images.[210]

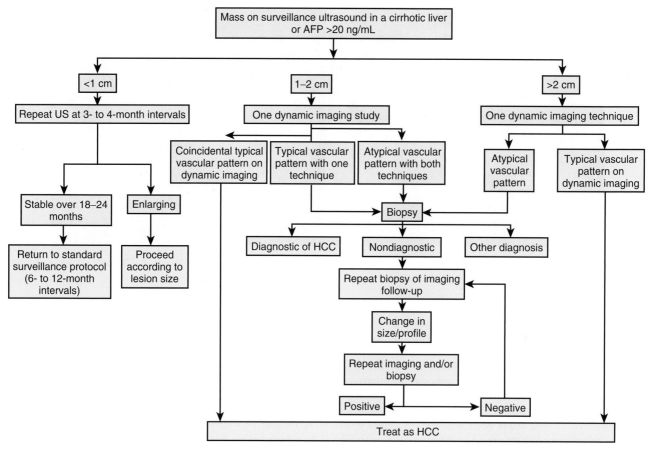

Fig. 57-7 **Evaluation of a nodule found during surveillance in patients with cirrhosis on dynamic imaging.** HCC, hepatocellular carcinoma. *(Adapted from Bruix J, et al. Management of hepatocellular carcinoma. Hepatology 2005;42:1208–1236.)*

Table 57-5 Clinicopathologic Features of Early-Stage Hepatocellular Carcinoma

	L-DN	H-DN	WD-HCC	MD-HCC
Pathologic Features				
Gross appearance			Vaguely nodular	Nodular
Stromal invasion	No	No	Yes	Yes
Radiologic Features				
Arterial supply	Iso/hypo	Iso/hypo	Iso/hypo (rarely hyper)	Hyper
Portal vein supply	Yes	Yes	Yes	No
Classification	Premalignant	Premalignant	Early HCC	Progressed HCC

HCC, hepatocellular carcinoma; H-DN, high-grade dysplastic nodule; hypo, hypovascular; hyper, hypervascular; iso, isovascular; L-DN, low-grade dysplastic nodule; MD-HCC, moderately differentiated hepatocellular carcinoma; WD-HCC, well-differentiated hepatocellular carcinoma

This results in improved lesion-to-liver contrast because malignant tumors either do not contain hepatocytes or their functioning is hampered, leading them to be seen as a hypointense lesion. This contrast agent can provide arterial, portal venous, delayed, and hepatobiliary phases. **Figure 57-8** shows an example of a typical HCC lesion with gadoxetate disodium. Importantly, this contrast agent may be helpful in the diagnosis of patients with HCC between 1 and 2 cm as seen in **Figure 57-9**. More studies are needed to better determine the role of this contrast agent.

Another important aspect of radiology in HCC is to evaluate response to local therapy. Tumor response was initially measured according to the WHO criteria,[211] and afterward according to the Response Evaluation Criteria in Solid Tumors (RECIST) guidelines.[212] Both methods offer simple approaches to determining anatomic size and lesion changes during treatment as an indicator of response. Target lesions are measured using either the bilinear product approach (WHO) or single linear summation (RECIST). The WHO criteria and RECIST were designed primarily for the evaluation of cytotoxic agents.

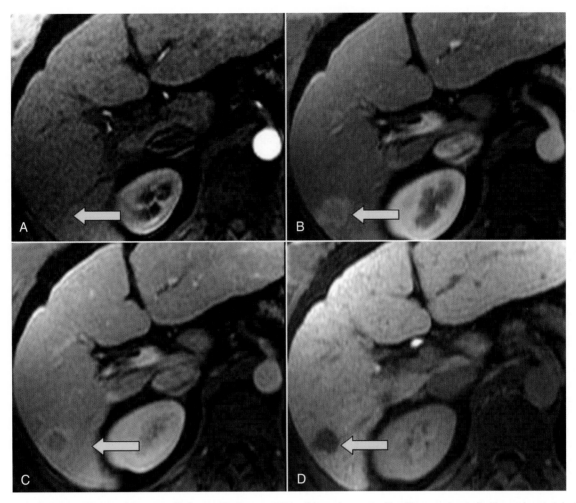

Fig. 57-8 **Typical characteristics of hepatocellular carcinoma on MRI with gadoxetate disodium contrast. A,** The early arterial phase with no enhancement of the lesion. **B,** The late arterial phase with homogenous enhancement. **C,** The lesion with central washout but rim enhancement. **D,** A hypoenhancing lesion in the hepatobiliary phase. *Arrows* point to the lesions.

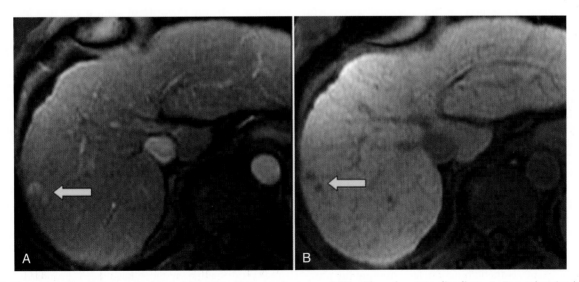

Fig. 57-9 **Characteristics of very early (<2 cm) hepatocellular carcinoma on MRI with gadoxetate disodium. A,** Two enhancing lesions on arterial phase. **B,** The same lesions in the hepatobiliary phase. *Arrows* point to the lesions.

They do not address measures of antitumor activity other than tumor shrinkage. As acknowledged in the original RECIST publication, assessments based solely on changes in tumor size can be misleading when applied to other anticancer drugs, such as molecular-targeted therapies, or other therapeutic interventions. In the case of HCC, there is poor correlation between the clinical benefit provided by new agents such as molecular targeted therapy or by locoregional interventional therapies and conventional methods of response assessment.[213] The modified RECIST (mRECIST) criteria were created specifically for HCC.[214]

The first step is to standardize the response assessment with regard to image acquisition, image interpretation, and assessment of tumor lesions at baseline. Patients can be followed with either contrast-enhanced spiral CT—preferably with use of multislice scanners—or contrast-enhanced dynamic MRI. The administration of intravenous contrast is recommended for all CT or MRI studies if not medically contraindicated. In contrast-enhanced studies, it is mandatory to obtain a dual-phase imaging of the liver. Every effort should be made to time the contrast administration so that high-quality arterial-phase imaging is obtained throughout the liver on the first run, and high-quality portal venous–phase imaging is obtained throughout the liver on the second run. To use the mRECIST criteria, an HCC lesion should meet all the following criteria: the lesion can be classified as a RECIST measurable lesion (i.e., the lesion can be accurately measured in at least one dimension as 1 cm or more), the lesion is suitable for repeat measurement, and the lesion shows intratumoral arterial enhancement on contrast-enhanced CT or MRI.

The second aspect is the definition of response and tumor progression by mRECIST criteria as shown on **Table 57-6**. The definition of a complete response is the disappearance of any intratumoral arterial enhancement, which is quite different from the standard RECIST criteria. These new criteria need to be further examined as have other, previously used methods. First, a one–time point pathologic correlation with tumor measurements will be required. Second, the effect of specific antiangiogenic agents changing the tumor inflow of blood might also have an impact in the response assessment. However, these criteria provide a guide to determine response to therapy that is unique to HCC.

Staging

The natural history of HCC is now well known. Recently, a meta-analysis of survival rates of untreated HCC that were randomized to a nontreatment arm was performed.[215] The pooled estimates of the survival rates were 17.5% at 1 year and 7.3% at 2 years. Significant heterogeneity among studies was highly significant both for 1-year and 2-year survival rates, and persisted when randomized trials were stratified according to all patient and study features. Through meta-regression, impaired performance status, Child-Pugh B-C class, and presence of portal vein thrombosis were all independently associated with shorter survival rates. HCC leads to different natural history based on certain tumor-related factors, performance status and hepatic synthetic function. Determining the prognosis of patients with HCC is important to account for these factors.

When determining the prognosis of patients with solid tumors, tumor staging and tumor grading are important

Table 57-6 Assessment of Target Lesions in Hepatocellular Carcinoma

RECIST	mRECIST FOR HCC
CR = disappearance of all target lesions	CR = disappearance of any intratumoral arterial enhancement in all target lesions
PR = at least a 30% decrease in the sum of diameters of target lesions, taking as reference the baseline sum of the diameters of target lesions	PR = at least a 30% decrease in the sum of diameters of viable (enhancement in the arterial phase) target lesions, taking as reference the baseline sum of the diameters of target lesions
SD = any cases that do not qualify for either partial response or progressive disease	SD = any cases that do not qualify for either partial response or progressive disease
PD = an increase of at least 20% in the sum of the diameters of target lesions, taking as reference the smallest sum of the diameters of target lesions recorded since treatment started	PD = An increase of at least 20% in the sum of the diameters of viable (enhancing) target lesions, taking as reference the smallest sum of the diameters of viable (enhancing) target lesions recorded since treatment started

Adapted from Lencioni R, Llovet JM. Modified RECIST (mRECIST) assessment for hepatocellular carcinoma. Semin Liver Dis 2010;30:52–60.
HCC, hepatocellular carcinoma; RECIST, Response Evaluation Criteria in Solid Tumors; mRECIST, Modified Response Evaluation Criteria in Solid Tumors

factors to take into account. Tumor staging describes the extent of an individual's tumor burden in the original primary organ and spread throughout the body. Staging is important because it helps plan treatment, it can be used to estimate the person's prognosis, and it provides a standardized platform to evaluate new treatment and to compare the results of different studies.[216] In the majority of solid organ tumors, staging is determined at the time of surgery and by pathologic examination of the resected specimen leading to the tumor-node-metastasis (TNM) classification, as in HCC.[217] The main downside of the TNM system in HCC is that it only takes into account pathology and not other important parameters such as hepatic synthetic function. The presence of underlying liver cirrhosis in patients with HCC adds an important dimension that cannot be ignored when discussing prognosis and treatment for these patients, and it is what differentiates HCC from other solid tumors. The majority of patients with HCC have underlying cirrhosis, and the degree of hepatic dysfunction is an independent prognostic factor and frequently determines if therapy can be used for HCC.[218] Another important independent risk factor in the prognosis of patients with HCC is performance status.[218,219] Therefore the prognosis of patients with HCC will rely on tumor burden, hepatic function, and performance status.

Several staging systems have been proposed for HCC, including the TNM (tumor node metastasis),[220] Okuda,[221] BCLC (Barcelona Clinic Liver Cancer),[222] CLIP (Cancer of Liver Italian Program),[223] French (Groupe d'Etude de Traitement du Carcinoma Hepatocellulaire),[224] CUPI (Chinese

Table 57-7 Composition of the Various Staging Systems that Have Been Proposed for Hepatocellular Carcinoma

STAGING SYSTEM	HEPATIC FUNCTION	α-FETOPROTEIN	PERFORMANCE STATUS	TUMOR STAGING
TNM[220]	No	No	No	Number of nodules, tumor size, presence of PVT, and presence of metastasis
Okuda[221]	Ascites, albumin, bilirubin	No	No	Tumor > or <50% of cross-sectional area of liver
BCLC[222]	CTP	No	Yes	Tumor size, number of nodules, and PVT
CLIP[223]	CTP	< or ≥400 ng/ml	No	Number of nodules, tumor > or <50% area of liver, and PVT
GETCH[224]	Bilirubin, alkaline phosphatase	< or ≥35 μg/L	Yes	PVT
CUPI[225]	Bilirubin, ascites, alkaline phosphatase	< or ≥500 ng/ml	Presence of symptoms	TNM
JIS[226]	CTP	No	No	TNM

BCLC, Barcelona Clinic Liver Cancer; CLIP, Cancer of Liver Italian Program; CTP, Child-Turcotte-Pugh; CUPI, Chinese University Prognostic Index; GETCH, Groupe d'Etude de Traitement du Carcinoma Hepatocellulaire; JIS, Japan Integrated System; PVT, portal vein thrombosis; TNM, tumor-node-metastasis.

University Prognostic Index),[225] and JIS (Japanese Integrated System)[226] classifications as shown on **Table 57-7.** The TNM is limited in that it only evaluates tumor burden and does not take into account hepatic function and performance status, and it also is limited because pathologic information can only be obtained in the minority of patients undergoing surgical therapy. The CLIP, GRETCH, and CUPI systems were each determined based on the results of a multivariate analysis for survival factors in a cohort of patients with HCC. This leads to several problems limiting their value: applicable only to the population studied (leading to lack of transportability), validation in an independent cohort is critical at the development of such a system and not performed; not all factors that determine tumor burden, hepatic function, or performance status were included; and lack of a link to treatment. Okuda realized that tumor burden and hepatic function were the most important factors that determine prognosis in HCC. However, assessment of tumor burden was crude and applicable only to advanced stages of HCC: tumor occupying more or less than 50% of the liver, and measures of hepatic function included only ascites, albumin, and bilirubin.

Several studies have shown that CLIP has limited value in determining prognosis of patients with HCC.[227,228] A number of limitations of the CLIP scoring system have been reported.[229] First, the tumor morphology categories used may be too general to be globally applicable, particularly in countries such as Japan where more patients are diagnosed with very small solitary tumors largely because of the established screening programs in place. Second, although patient populations with a CLIP score appear to be well discriminated from one another, there is no clear difference among patient populations with a CLIP score of 4 to 6. Indeed, in the prospective validation of this scoring system performed by the founding group,[223] patients with a CLIP score of 4 to 6 were placed into one group. The CLIP score also includes AFP, which is sensitive in

about 60% of patients,[132] and therefore not reliable in patients with HCC. Finally, all studies evaluating the CLIP score reported to date show that a high proportion of patients are categorized as CLIP score 0 to 2, suggesting poor stratification ability with this system.

The BCLC system was developed in Spain[222] and has been validated in Italy,[230] the United States,[218] and Taiwan.[231] This system has also been compared with the other common systems and has been shown to be the most effective at determining prognosis.[232] One of the most important observations for the development of the BCLC staging system came from the follow-up of patients with nonresectable and nontransplantable HCC who were randomized to a placebo in three different trials.[219] In this study, the multivariate study identified performance status, constitutional syndrome, vascular invasion, and extrahepatic spread as independent predictors for mortality. The authors show that the 1-, 2-, and 3-year survival rates for the 48 patients without adverse factors (BCLC intermediate stage) were 80%, 65%, and 50%, respectively, and 29%, 16%, and 8% in the 54 patients with at least one adverse parameter (BCLC advanced stage). The overall BCLC staging system is shown in **Figure 57-10.** The main advantage of the BCLC system is that it links staging based on prognosis and survival rates to an evidence-based treatment algorithm. It identifies those with early-stage HCC who may benefit from curative therapies and those at intermediate or advanced stages who may benefit from palliative therapies. At the present time the evidence points toward the BCLC as the staging system that provides the best prognostic information and linkage to an evidence-based treatment algorithm. It has been externally validated in several populations when all systems are included. However, as in all areas of medicine, as our ability to diagnose and treat HCC improves, the validity of BCLC and other tumor staging systems need to be reevaluated. This staging system has been endorsed by several associations.[30,197]

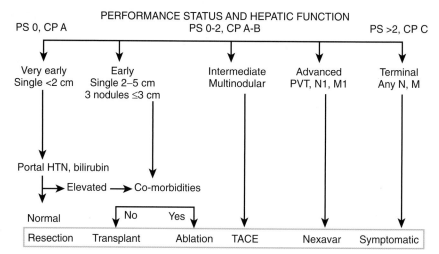

PERFORMANCE STATUS AND HEPATIC FUNCTION

Fig. 57-10 Barcelona staging classification. CP, Child-Pugh class; M, metastasis; N, node; PS, performance status; PVT, portal vein thrombosis (tumor thrombus); TACE, transarterial chemoembolization. *(Adapted from Bruix J, et al. Management of hepatocellular carcinoma. Hepatology 2005;42:1208–1236.)*

The recent advances in molecular biology may change our ability to further define the prognosis of patients with HCC; at the moment we rely on for clinical parameters as discussed in the previous paragraphs. The attempts to classify HCC have relied on whole-genome approaches.[233] Unsupervised clustering of microarray data obtained from human HCC samples identified diverse groups of patients according to their similarities in gene expression. Integrative analysis with other genomic parameters (i.e., changes in DNA copy number, point mutations, activation of signaling pathways) outlined at least two clear-cut groups of HCCs characterized by either activation of the WNT signaling pathway or overexpression of genes implicated in cell cycling and proliferation.[234] The fact that different research teams identified both classes, using different genomic platforms and after studying a wide clinical range of human HCCs, guaranteed their robustness.[235,236] A pioneering study of global gene expression patterns in 91 human HCCs to define the molecular characteristics of the tumors and to test the prognostic value of the expression profiles.[237] Tumors from the low-survival subclass have strong cell proliferation and anti-apoptosis gene expression signatures. In addition, the low-survival subclass displayed higher expression of genes involved in ubiquitination and histone modification, suggesting an etiologic involvement of these processes in accelerating the progression of HCC. Genome-wide expression data obtained from adjacent nontumoral liver tissue have also proved extremely useful for patient classification. In a seminal study, HCV-related early HCC patients treated with surgical resection were evaluated and a gene signature was identified that predicted overall survival rates.[238] Therefore the prognosis prediction in HCC rests on three pillars: (1) clinical parameters, as described in the BCLC algorithm; (2) genomic data obtained from the tumor; and (3) genomic data obtained from the adjacent nontumoral tissue. At the current time we rely on clinical parameters, but genomic data are emerging rapidly and may alter how we stage patients with HCC. Validation studies of these gene signatures will be critical to make progress in this aspect.

Treatment

Significant advances have been made with regard to the treatment of HCC over the last 10 years. Treatment can be divided into radical (curative) or palliative interventions. Radical therapies include tumor resection, orthotopic liver transplantation (OLT), and ablative techniques such as radiofrequency ablation (RFA), all of which offer the hope of achieving a long-term response and thereby improving survival rates. Palliative therapies are those that aim to prolong survival for patients with advanced HCC and include transarterial chemoembolization (TACE), intraarterial radioembolization, and systemic chemotherapy. **Figure 57-8** shows the Barcelona staging system that is linked to an evidence-based treatment strategy.

Hepatic Resection

Hepatic resection is the treatment of choice for patients with HCC without cirrhosis, who represent about 5% of patients in the West in contrast to up to 40% in Asia.[239] Resection of HCC in cirrhotic patients requires a thorough selection of the candidates—meaning adequate knowledge of the stage of the disease and the risk factors for postoperative morbidity and mortality, recurrence, and survival—and adequate skills in the performance of the surgical procedure. Advancements in the knowledge of both have increased the efficacy of treatment. Today, the selection of candidates for resection has been refined and the surgical technique (e.g., ultrasonic dissector, Pringle maneuver) and the immediate postoperative management have been optimized. In addition, the implementation of anatomic resections according to Couinaud criteria has ensured a surgical approach based on sound oncologic principles.[240] The degree of hepatic function clearly affects survival following resection as evaluated by MELD or Child-Pugh scores. Patients who are Child class B or C have decreased overall survival rates when compared with Child A patients.[241-243] In addition, patients with MELD scores of greater than 9 have relatively high mortality rates following resection (29%), making other therapies more attractive in these patients.[244] Clinically significant portal hypertension (platelet count <100,000/mm^3 or hepatic vein pressure gradient >10 mm Hg) have been used to assess surgical risk and remain a relative exclusion to surgical therapy in most centers.[245] A study showed that a normal bilirubin and no portal hypertension leads to excellent 5-year survival rates as shown in **Figure 57-11**.[246] Case series have established that a planned small future liver remnant of less than 40% of total liver volume contributes to mortality in patients with chronic

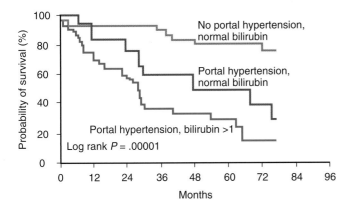

Fig. 57-11 Survival rates after surgical resection for early-stage hepatocellular carcinoma. The *blue lines* indicate survival rates for those with normal bilirubin and no portal hypertension. The *purple line* indicates those with normal bilirubin but with portal hypertension. The *red line* shows those with elevated bilirubin and portal hypertension. (*Adapted from Llovet JM, Fuster J, Bruix J. Intention-to-treat analysis of surgical treatment for early heaptocellular carcinoma: resection versus transplantation. Hepatology 1999;30:1434–1440.*)

liver disease.[247] These same authors showed that candidates with decreased planned liver remnant are eligible for preoperative portal vein embolization to the portion planned for resection to allow compensatory hypertrophy of the unaffected side allowing an increase in the planned future liver remnant. Therefore, assessment of hepatic synthetic function, portal hypertension, and planned future liver remnant are critical to determining candidates eligible for resection.

When patients are properly selected without significant portal hypertension and normal bilirubin levels, the overall 5-year survival rates are greater than 50%.[248-250] However, applying these criteria, the resectability rate is only 5% to 10% of patients with HCC. In the largest experience of resection in the world (>12,000 patients), the best results were in patients with single tumors less than 2 cm with a 5-year survival rate of 66%.[251] In the largest experience in the United States (788 patients) with early-stage HCC (<5 cm in diameter), the 5-year survival rate was 39%.[252] Other reports of hepatic resection for very early HCC (HCC <2 cm) have shown 5-year survival rates between 54% and 93%.[253-255] The 5-year survival rate after operations for patients with HCC between 2 and 5 cm in diameter have been shown to be between 38% and 53%,[252,256] while the 5-year survival rate worsens to less than 39% in patients with tumors greater than 5 cm.[257] Perioperative mortality rates are generally on the order of 4.0% to 4.7% for resections for HCC[257] and reflects the underlying chronic liver disease among patients with HCC. Therefore the best results with hepatic resection are those with normal liver function, no clinically significant portal hypertension, and tumors less than 5 cm in diameter. Laparoscopic liver resection is gaining favor at a variety of centers as surgical technologies continue to evolve. The best report at the present time is a matched case series with reported reductions in length of stay, decreased blood loss, and decreased complications in select cases.[258] Similar to other fields where laparoscopy has been used, additional benefits for a laparoscopic approach will likely be described in the near future.

The success of surgical therapy has been linked to tumor characteristics as well. Tumor size, tumor number, and the presence of macrovascular or microvascular invasion have been the most important factors and correlate with a reduction of survival rates postresection.[259] The most important factor is vascular invasion with a reduction from 41% to 57% in the 5-year survival rate down to 10%.[260] Other variables have been evaluated to provide prognostic information on the success of surgical therapy, the most important of which is AFP level. AFP levels have been shown to directly correlate with the presence of vascular invasion, with AFP levels above 1000 ng/mL in one study[261] and above 200 ng/ml in another[262] being shown to have vascular invasion in 61% of patients. Attention to these criteria is important and will lead to better outcomes.

One of the major downsides to hepatic resection is the recurrence rate, which can be up to 70% over 5 years, reflecting either intrahepatic metastases (true recurrences) or the development of de novo tumors.[263-266] Interferon has shown positive results in four randomized control trials in patients with hepatitis C infection, but the efficacy is limited to developing a sustained virologic response.[267-270] Interestingly, HCC has developed in patients with cirrhosis who have developed a sustained virologic response to antiviral therapy, and therefore these patients should continue to undergo surveillance for HCC. Unfortunately, these trials lacked an adequate sample size to provide robust conclusions, and a meta-analysis would be underpowered (overall sample of 150 patients) and is not clinically sound because of the heterogeneity of treatments and end points, namely recurrence or survival. However, the development of novel antivirals may affect the outcome of recurrences and de novo tumors. Clinical trials assessing adjuvant therapies after resection are urgently needed, and this should constitute a priority area of investigation. Molecular targeted therapies offer great potential as adjuvant therapies to prevent recurrence.

Liver Transplantation

Orthotopic liver transplantation offers the unique ability not only to treat the HCC but also the underlying cirrhosis. In a landmark study in Milan, Italy, the authors showed that a 75%, 4-year survival rate was achieved when adhering to the pretransplant tumor assessment of single tumors less than or equal to 5.0 cm or 2 to 3 tumors, with the largest being less than or equal to 3.0 cm in the absence of portal vein involvement and extrahepatic metastasis (called the Milan criteria).[271] This survival rate improved to 85% when the explant examination also met these criteria, and the recurrence rate in this study was 10%. Following this pivotal study, organ allocation systems worldwide have adopted the Milan criteria for transplanting patients with HCC. The results of applying the Milan criteria to transplants for HCC have been recently examined in Europe and the United States using official national data. The overall reported 5-year patient survival rate of 8273 OLT for HCC in Europe between 1988 and 2008 is 60%.[272] The data from the United States included 4482 patients with HCC transplanted between 1998 and 2006, after the Milan criteria were applied, and showed a 5-year patient survival rate of 65% when meeting the Milan criteria as shown in **Figure 57-12**.[273] These results show that adherence to the Milan criteria yields excellent posttransplant outcomes for HCC and is the best treatment for HCC.

Besides the overall influence of tumor size, tumor number, and absence of portal vein involvement and/or extrahepatic

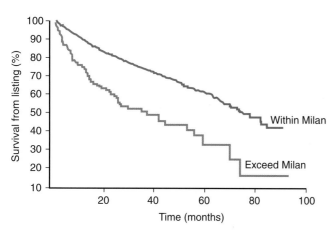

Fig. 57-12 **Survival since listing for hepatocellular carcinoma.** The *red line* indicates those who meet the Milan criteria and the *blue line* indicates those that exceed the Milan criteria. *(Adapted with permission from Pelletier SJ, et al. An intention-to-treat analysis of liver transplantation for hepatocellular carcinoma using organ procurement transplant network data. Liver Transpl 2009;15:859–868.)*

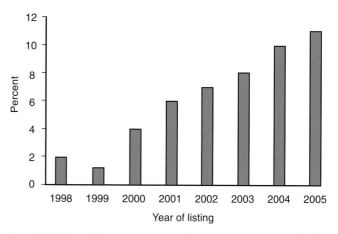

Fig. 57-13 **The rising percentage of patients who exceed the Milan criteria.** *(Adapted with permission from Pelletier SJ, et al. An intention-to-treat analysis of liver transplantation for hepatocellular carcinoma using organ procurement transplant network data. Liver Transpl 2009;15:859–868.)*

metastasis, other prognostic factors have been evaluated for their effects on outcomes of transplantation for HCC. In particular, multivariate single-center analyses have shown that the presence of macrovascular and microvascular invasion and AFP greater than 300 ng/ml were negative prognostic factors.[274,275] Therefore attention to these factors is important when selecting patients for liver transplantation.

The role of "bridging therapy" or neoadjuvant therapy remains controversial before liver transplantation. TACE has been the treatment most commonly used for those waiting for liver transplantation.[276] However, a recent report from the United Network of Organ Sharing showed that patients who have undergone liver transplantation for HCC showed a minimally improved 3-year survival rate of 79% versus 75% (*P* = .03) when compared with HCC patients who were not treated.[277] It has been discussed that pretransplant therapy benefits those in whom the waiting times are expected to be more than 6 months and responses to therapy can be used as measures of tumor biology, which can help determine candidacy for some patients.[278] Certainly, randomized trials are required to firmly determine the role and application of "bridging therapy" but until these data are available, it seems that pretransplant therapy does improve outcomes.

Over the past 10 years, adult living donor liver transplantation (LDLT) has developed as an alternative to deceased donor transplantation because of the scarcity of donor livers. Despite the number of procedures performed, enthusiasm for LDLT has waned because of the need for a highly skilled group of senior liver surgeons, the increased surgery-related morbidity, and the risk of donor mortality.[279] There are three large case series that supported LDLT for HCC. The first study from Japan reported an overall 3-year survival rate of 54%, whereas a study from the United States showed a 3-year survival rate of 86% in patients within the Milan criteria and 42% for patients with expanded criteria.[280,281] In Japan, a survey including 316 patients reported better 3-year survival and lower recurrence rates for patients within versus outside the Milan limits (79% vs. 60% and 1.4% vs. 22.2%, respectively).[282] The authors indicated that LDLT for HCC outside of Milan should be considered given the 3-year survival rate found in this study.

However, it has been argued that this approach is unethical due to worse outcomes in these patients and the risk undertaken by a healthy donor.[283] The Adult-to-Adult Living Donor Liver Transplantation study group in the United States evaluated 106 consecutive transplant candidates with cirrhosis and HCC who had a potential living donor evaluated between January 1998 and February 2003 at the nine participating centers.[284] A total of 58 underwent LDLT, and 34 deceased donor liver transplants were performed. Relative to deceased-donor transplant recipients, LDLT recipients had a shorter time from listing to transplant (mean, 160 vs. 469 days) and a higher rate of HCC recurrence within 3 years than deceased-donor recipients (29% vs. 0%), but there was no difference in mortality. The waiting time in deceased-donor transplant likely serves as a measure of tumor biology by selecting out those that ultimately will have better outcomes. The enthusiasm for LDLT for the treatment of HCC has dampened somewhat and should be performed in highly selected individuals.

In recent years, several groups from different countries have challenged the Milan criteria for OLT for HCC as too strict. The number of patients who exceed the Milan criteria are rising in the United States based on a recent report, as shown in **Figure 57-13**.[273] There are reports that support the idea of expanding the criteria. The criteria that have gained notoriety and have been validated prospectively are the University of California–San Francisco (UCSF) criteria. The criteria include 1 lesion of 6.5 cm in diameter, or 2 to 3 lesions each of 4.5 cm with a total tumor diameter of 8 cm,[285] which was then validated in another cohort of patients by the same group of investigators.[285,286] Other reports have shown that expansion of the criteria can lead to 5-year survival rates between 30% and 50%.[287-291] However, a recent model showed that expanding the criteria to transplant beyond the Milan criteria will increase the mortality among those listed without HCC.[292] The criteria should expand only in those regions that have patients with lower MELD scores (<20). Expansion of the Milan criteria is reasonable and can lead to excellent long-term results in some individuals. However, because transplantation relies on a scarce resource, it is better to maximize the efficacy of transplant for HCC. Because the number of deceased donors has not increased, the current recommendation from the United Network of Organ Sharing is not to expand the Milan criteria.[293]

Ablative Therapies

Of the ablative therapies for patients with early-stage HCC, RFA has emerged as the treatment of choice. The goal of RFA is to induce thermal injury to the tissue through electromagnetic energy deposition. An alternating electric field is created within the tissue of the patient. There is high electrical resistance of tissue in comparison with metal electrodes and marked agitation of ions present in the target tissue that surrounds the electrodes. The discrepancy between the small surface area of the needle electrode and the large area of the ground pads causes the generated heat to be focused and concentrated around the needle electrode.[294] Ideally, temperatures between 60° C and 100° C in the area of ablation induces immediate coagulation necrosis, leading to a 360-degree, 0.5- to 1-cm-thick ablative margin around the tumor. The other commonly used ablative technique is percutaneous ethanol injection (PEI). Ethanol induces coagulation necrosis of the lesion as a result of cellular dehydration, protein denaturation, and chemical occlusion of small tumor vessels.[295]

RFA has been compared with PEI in several randomized control trials in early-stage HCC as shown in **Table 57-8**.[296-300] These investigations consistently show that RFA has a higher anticancer effect than PEI, leading to better local tumor control. The overall survival rate was improved in the three Asian studies while there was no difference in the two European studies. In patients with early-stage HCC treated with percutaneous ablation, the long-term survival rate is influenced by multiple interventions, given that close to 80% of the patients will develop recurrent intrahepatic HCC nodules within 5 years of initial treatment.[301] Three independent meta-analyses of ablative techniques have confirmed that RFA offers a survival benefit compared with PEI, particularly for tumors greater than 2 cm in diameter, establishing RFA as the standard percutaneous technique.[302-304]

Recent reports on long-term outcomes of RFA-treated patients have shown that in patients who are Child class A with tumors less than 2 cm, 5-year survival rates between 51% and 64% have been shown, and may reach 76% in those who would have been eligible for hepatic resection.[305-308] Therefore there is the possibility that RFA may be a first-line treatment for solitary, very early HCC instead of hepatic resection. In fact, a randomized controlled trial evaluating RFA versus

hepatic resection in patients with Child class A and early-stage HCC showed equivalent results (4-year survival rate of 64% with RFA vs. 67.9% with resection; $P > .5$) with an overall reduction in morbidity in the RFA group when compared with the resection group.[309] There are questions about the power and end point of the study (neither overall survival nor disease-free survival were the main end points), but it appears that both surgical resection and RFA may be similar in terms of overall survival rate. The decrease in morbidity with an excellent 5-year survival rate indicates that RFA may be the treatment of choice for small HCC.

One of the problems with RFA is that it is limited by the location of the tumor. Tumors located near large vessels (>3 mm) result in a drop of greater than 50% of complete response because of heat loss caused by perfusion-mediated tissue cooling within the ablated area.[310] In addition, subcapsular tumors and those adjacent to the gallbladder are also associated with incomplete ablation and may result in complications.[311-314] The choice of surgical resection or RFA will be determined by the tumor location, liver function, degree of portal hypertension, and tumor size (<3 cm for RFA).

Other local ablative techniques such as microwave ablation have been studied as an alternative to RFA. One randomized control trial compared RFA and microwave ablation.[315] There were no differences in survival rate and efficacy of response, but there was a tendency favoring RFA in terms of lower recurrences and complication rates. Newer devices for microwave ablation may lead to trials that challenge RFA. Cryoablation is a technique in which a liquid nitrogen cooled cryoprobe is directly placed into the tumor and an ice ball is created in the target. This technique has not been shown to be efficacious in HCC.[316] In addition, the complication rate is not negligible because of the risk of cryoshock. There are no randomized trials that support its use in HCC.

Transarterial Tumor Therapy

Hepatocellular carcinoma exhibits intense neoangiogenic activity during its progression, and therefore TACE performed via intraarterial infusion of chemotherapy (mostly doxorubicin and cisplatin) followed by embolization of the blood vessel leads to a strong cytotoxic effect combined with ischemia. TACE is the mainstay of treatment and has been evaluated in several randomized controlled studies for patients who have nontransplantable or nonresectable disease (i.e., Barcelona stage B).[317-323] A meta-analysis of these trials showed an improved 2-year survival rate with an OR of 0.53 (95% CI,

Table 57-8 Randomized Studies Comparing Radiofrequency Ablation with Percutaneous Ethanol Ablation

AUTHOR	N	TUMOR SIZE	CR (%) WITH PEI RFA	NO. SESSIONS PEI RFA	SURVIVAL DIFFERENCE
Lencioni[296]	102	Milan	82 (91)	5.4 (1.1)	No
Lin[297]	157	<4 cm	88 (96)	6.5 (1.6)	Yes
Shiina[298]	232	Milan	NA	6.4 (2.1)	Yes
Lin[299]	187	<3 cm	88 (96)	4.9 (1.3)	Yes
Brunello[300]	139	Milan	66 (96)	4.3 (1.2)	No

CR, complete response; Milan, Milan criteria; NA, not available; PEI, percutaneous ethanol ablation; RFA, radiofrequency ablation

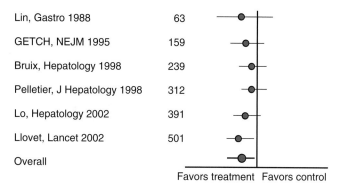

Lin, Gastro 1988	63	
GETCH, NEJM 1995	159	
Bruix, Hepatology 1998	239	
Pelletier, J Hepatology 1998	312	
Lo, Hepatology 2002	391	
Llovet, Lancet 2002	501	
Overall		

Favors treatment   Favors control

Fig. 57-14 **Meta-analysis of randomized controlled trials of trans-arterial chemoembolization for hepatocellular carcinoma.** (*Adapted from Llovet JM, et al. Arterial embolisation or chemoembolisation versus symptomatic treatment in patients with unresectable hepatocellular carcinoma: a randomised controlled trial. Lancet 2002;359:1734–1739.*)

0.32 to 0.89; $P = .17$) when TACE was compared with best supportive care for patients not suitable for resection, transplant, or RFA as shown in **Figure 57-14**.[324] Sensitivity analysis showed that there is no benefit for embolization alone or in patients with portal vein invasion. The outcome of TACE appears to be dependent on careful patient selection. In one of the randomized studies that recruited patients with compensated cirrhosis (70% Child class A), absence of cancer-related symptoms (81% with performance status of 0) and large or multinodular tumors with neither vascular involvement nor extrahepatic spread, the 2-year survival rate reached 63% compared with 27% of the untreated arm ($P = .0009$).[323] TACE is the standard of care for patients with multinodular tumors, relatively preserved hepatic function, absence of cancer-related symptoms, and no vascular involvement or extrahepatic spread (intermediate tumors based on the Barcelona staging).

The tolerability of conventional TACE seems to be affected by the type of regimen and the frequency of treatment. A French study evaluated a schedule of TACE with cisplatin every 2 months in patients with unresectable HCC without severe liver disease.[319] This schedule was associated with hepatic decompensation in 30 of 50 patients treated. Conversely, the study from Spain evaluated a schedule of TACE treatment with doxorubicin at baseline, 2 months, 6 months, and every 6 months thereafter, with only 2 of 40 developing hepatic decompensation.[323] This is important to take into account when performing this procedure.

The ideal TACE procedure should allow maximal and sustained concentration of chemotherapeutic drug within the tumor with minimal systemic exposure combined with calibrated tumor vessel embolization. Conventional TACE does not allow for this ideal scenario. A strategy is the introduction of embolic microspheres that have the ability to actively sequester chemotherapeutic drugs, such as doxorubicin, via drug-eluting beads and release them in a controlled and sustained fashion. This strategy has been shown to substantially diminish the amount of chemotherapy that reaches the systemic circulation compared with traditional regimens, thus significantly increasing the local concentration of drug and the antitumoral efficacy.[325] In a multicenter phase II randomized study of 201 patients with Barcelona stage B disease,

doxorubicin-eluting beads TACE resulted in a marked and statistically significant reduction in liver toxicity and drug-related adverse events compared with conventional TACE.[326] Importantly, patients randomized to the doxorubicin-eluting beads TACE had higher rates of objective responses and disease control rates compared with conventional TACE. The added value of chemotherapeutic agent over the bland embolic bead TACE has been evaluated in a randomized control trial.[327] The authors showed that the overall response and the delay in tumor progression were better in the doxorubicin-eluting bead arm compared with the bland embolization arm. At this time, it appears that drug-eluting beads may lead to better tumor control with a better adverse event profile than conventional TACE.

There does appear to be a role for downstaging of tumors that exceed the Milan criteria. Downstaging is possible with the use of TACE in as many as 70% of patients, with a 2-year posttransplant survival rate of 81% after performance of the downstaging therapy.[328] One caveat for this study is that the authors waiting at least 3 months with a tumor response before listing and the median time from listing to transplantation was 9 months. Therefore it appears that for downstaging to be effective there has to be complete response and a significant amount of time of at least 6 months before listing leads to better outcomes. Prospective studies are needed in this area.

Radioembolization is an infusion of radioactive substances into the hepatic artery. The rationale is that conventional external-beam radiation therapy in HCC has been limited by low tolerance of the cirrhotic liver leading to hepatoxicity or radiation-induced hepatitis.[329] The most popular form of radioembolization is the use of yttrium-90 (Y90), a β-emitting isotope. Y90 radioembolization is delivered in glass microspheres of 20 to 30 micrometers that are minimally embolic. Given the hypervascularity of HCC, intraarterially injected microspheres will be preferentially delivered to the tumor-bearing area and selectively emit high-energy, low-penetration radiation to the tumor. The safety of Y90 radioembolization has been documented in several phase I and II studies.[330-332] There are two absolute contraindications for Y90 microsphere radioembolization. The first includes a pretreatment technetium-99m–labeled macroaggregated albumin scan demonstrating significant hepatopulmonary shunting that would result in greater than 30 Gy being delivered to the lungs with a single infusion. The second includes the inability to prevent deposition of microspheres to the gastrointestinal tract. Therefore, before performing this procedure, a microaggregated albumin scan is performed to evaluate for pulmonary shunting and a selective angiogram is done to determine the hepatic blood flow. However, because of the minimal embolic effects of Y90 microsphere radioembolization, treatment can be safely applied to patients with portal vein thrombosis.[333] The largest experience evaluated 291 patients with HCC in a single-center cohort study.[334] Toxicities included fatigue (57%), pain (23%), and nausea/vomiting (20%), and 19% exhibited elevations of total bilirubin. Those with Child class A did better than those with Child class B, and the study included patients at the BCLC intermediate stage and advanced stages, both of which have different natural history. Therefore, it is hard to determine its true efficacy. There are no randomized control studies comparing TACE with Y90 radioembolization for those at the intermediate stage of HCC or in advanced HCC, but radioembolization may be an option in certain conditions in which TACE cannot be performed.

Systemic Therapy

The importance of developing effective systemic therapy in this disease has been well appreciated for decades as a result of the dismal prognosis for patients with advanced disease and the high recurrence rate after definitive surgical resection. Unfortunately, systemic therapy with various classes of agents, including hormone and cytotoxic agents, has provided no or marginal benefits. Several agents have been investigated as systemic therapy for advanced HCC. These agents have shown essentially no effect against HCC when compared with control and include: tamoxifen,[335] doxorubicin,[336] combination cisplatin/interferon alfa-2b/doxorubicin/fluorouracil,[337] seocalcitol,[338] nolatrexed,[339] and thalidomide.[340] Doxorubicin has been the most used agent in HCC. Doxorubicin has been the most used systemic cytotoxic therapy in advanced HCC. In a large study assessing doxorubicin in advanced HCC, no responses were noted among 109 patients.[341] Among 475 patients who received doxorubicin in various studies, a 16% response rate was documented, with a median survival rate of 3 to 4 months.[337] None of these systemic agents have efficacy in HCC.

Increasing knowledge of carcinogenic pathways in HCC has lead to the development of targeted molecular therapies as shown in **Table 57-9**. One of these agents, sorafenib, has activity against tyrosine kinases, such as the VEGF receptor 2, PDGF receptor, and c-kit receptors and also has activity against serine/threonine kinases (b-Raf/Ras/MAPKK pathway).[342,343] Thus cell proliferation and angiogenesis are inhibited by sorafenib. In a phase II study of 137 patients with advanced HCC, sorafenib provided orally at 400 mg twice daily induced a partial response in 2.2% of patients, a minor response in 5.8%, and stable disease lasting 4 months in 34%.[344] Median time to progression (TTP) was 4.2 months, and the median overall survival rate was 9.2 months. In a randomized phase III clinical trial of patients with advanced

HCC, a total of 602 patients were randomized to sorafenib (n = 299 patients) or to a placebo (n = 303).[345] More than 95% had Child class A compensated cirrhosis. There was a significant increase in median survival rate from 7.9 months to 10.7 months (HR = 0.58; 95% CI, 0.45 to 0.74) in those treated with sorafenib compared with a placebo as shown in **Figure 57-15**. Sorafenib also delayed the time to progression from 2.8 months in the placebo group to 5.5 months (P = .0000007). Overall this therapy was well tolerated with the majority of side effects being mild to moderate; however, grade III diarrhea, hand and foot skin reaction, and fatigue were observed; only 8% of patients suffered grade III toxicities (diarrhea or hand and foot skin reaction). Another randomized trial was performed in Asia in advanced HCC, the majority being patients with chronic HBV infection.[346] **Figure 57-16** shows the efficacy results for the Western study (North American and Europe) and the Asian study of sorafenib for advanced HCC. These results show that sorafenib risk reduction in mortality and time to progression is the same in both studies

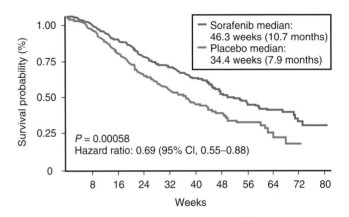

Fig. 57-15 **Survival rate of patients treated with sorafenib *(red line)* and placebo *(blue line)* in a randomized trial of advanced hepatocellular carcinoma.** *(Adapted from Llovet JM, et al. Sorafenib in advanced hepatocellular carcinoma. N Engl J Med 2008;359:378–390.)*

Table 57-9 **Most Promising Single-Agent Molecular Targeted Therapies in Trials for Advanced Hepatocellular Carcinoma**

AGENT	TARGET INHIBITION	STUDY PHASE	TTP (mo)	PFS (mo)	MEDIAN SURVIVAL (mo)
Sorafenib[345]	VEGFR, PDGFR	III	5.5	NR	10.7
Bevacizumab[351]	VEGF	II	NR	6.9	12.4
Sunitinib[355]	VEGFR, PDGFR	II	NR	3.9	9.8
Erlotinib[359]	EGFR	II	3.1	4.1	13
Gefinitib[361]	EGFR	II	NR	2.8	6.5
Lapatinib[362]	EGFR, HER2	II	NR	2.3	6.2
Cetuximab[363]	EGFR	II	NR	1.4	9.6
Brivanib[365]	VEGFR, FGFR	II	2.8	NR	10
AZD6244[366]	MEK, ERK	II	2	NR	NR

EGFR, epidermal growth factor receptor; ERK, extracellular signal-regulated protein kinase; FGFR, fibroblast growth factor receptor; HER2, human EGFR–related-2 receptor; PDGFR, platelet derived growth factor receptor; VEGF, vascular endothelial growth factor; VEGFR, vascular endothelial growth factor receptor

End point	Asia-Pacific[347]		Europe-N. America[346]	
	Hazard ratio (95% CI)	P value	Hazard ratio (95% CI)	P value
Overall survival	0.68 (0.50–0.93)	.014	0.69 (0.55–0.87)	<.001
Time to progression	0.57 (0.42–0.79)	<.001	0.58 (0.45–0.74)	<.001

Fig. 57-16 Risk reduction in overall survival rate and time to progression of sorafenib for advanced hepatocellular carcinoma in two randomized clinical trials.

and represents the first-line therapy for patients with advanced HCC.

HCC are vascular tumors, and increased levels of VEGF and microvessel density have been observed.[347,348] High VEGF expression has been associated with worse survival rates.[349,350] Therefore inhibition of angiogenesis represents a potential therapeutic target in HCC, and several antiangiogenic agents have entered clinical studies in HCC. Bevacizumab is a recombinant humanized monoclonal antibody that targets VEGF. A phase II study was completed in HCC.[351] Two dosages of bevacizumab, 5 and 10 mg/kg administered intravenously once every 2 weeks, were tested in patients with HCC with no overt extrahepatic metastases or invasion of major blood vessels. Of the 46 patients with data available for efficacy, 6 had objective responses (13%; 95% CI, 3 to 23), and 65% were progression free at 6 months. Median progression-free survival (PFS) time was 6.9 months (95% CI, 6.5 to 9.1), and the median survival rate was 12.4 months (95% CI, 9.4 to 19.9). Bevacizumab has been combined with cytotoxic agents and in one study it was combined with gemcitabine and oxaliplatin in advanced HCC.[352] This regimen had moderate antitumor activity in HCC with an overall response rate of 20% in evaluable patients. An additional 27% of patients had stable disease with a median duration of 9 months (range, 4.5 to 13.7 months). The median overall survival rate was 9.6 months and the median PFS was 5.3 months. A combination of bevacizumab and erlotinib (EGF receptor inhibitor) was given.[353] Bevacizumab was provided at 10 mg/kg intravenously once every 14 days and erlotinib at 150 mg orally daily. Of the 40 patients with efficacy data available, a 25% response rate was observed. The median PFS was 9 months and overall survival rate was 15 months. These studies demonstrated early evidence of antitumor activity of bevacizumab in HCC. Despite the overall good tolerability profiles, the risk of bleeding, hypertension, and thromboembolic events remain to be further characterized and limit its general use at the current time. Moreover, as a result of the nonrandomized nature, small sample size, and patient selection bias inherent in single-arm studies, the relative contributions, if any, from any chemotherapy regimens remain unknown and warrant further investigations.

Sunitinib is an oral multikinase inhibitor that targets receptor tyrosine kinases, including VEGF receptor-1, PDGF receptor, c-kit, and RET kinases.[354] A phase II study in patients with advanced HCC used sunitinib at 37.5 mg orally once daily on a standard 4-weeks-on, 2-weeks-off regimen (6 weeks per cycle).[355] The primary end point of the study was PFS. Of the 34 patients enrolled, 1 had a partial response of 20 months'

duration, and an additional 10 patients (38.5%) had stable disease of at least 12 weeks' duration. The median PFS was 3.9 months and overall survival rate was 9.8 months. In another phase II study, sunitinib was administered at 50 mg daily for 4 weeks every 6 weeks to patients with unresectable HCC.[356] The primary end point of the study was overall response rate. Of the 37 patients enrolled, one patient (2.7%) experienced a partial response, and 13 patients (35%) had stable disease as their best response. The median overall survival rate was 8.0 months and PFS was 3.7 months. In terms of toxicity, the studies that used the lower dose (37.5 mg) reported acceptable safety profiles. The most common adverse events included hematologic toxicities, fatigue, and an increase in transaminases. A phase III study comparing sunitinib with sorafenib is ongoing.

Increasing evidence has highlighted the importance of EGF receptor, (human EGFR related) HER1 and its ligands EGF and transforming growth factor-alpha (TGF-α), in hepatocarcinogenesis. The expression of several EGF family members, specifically EGF, TGF-α, and heparin-binding epidermal growth factor, as well as EGF receptor, has been described in several HCC cell lines and tissues.[357,358] One of the agents that blocks EGF receptor tyrosine kinase is erlotinib. In a phase II study of erlotinib in advanced HCC, 3 (9%) of 38 patients experienced partial response, and 12 patients (32%) were free of progression of disease at 6 months.[359] Median overall survival rate for this cohort was 13 months. In another phase II study of erlotinib in advanced HCC, 17 (43%) of 40 patients achieved PFS at 16 weeks, and the PFS rate at 24 weeks was 28%.[360] No partial or complete responses were observed in this study. The median time to failure, defined as either disease progression or death, was 13.3 weeks. The median time of overall survival rate was 25.0 weeks (95% CI, 17.9 to 42.3) from the date of erlotinib therapy initiation. Gefitinib, another EGF receptor tyrosine kinase inhibitor, was also studied in advanced HCC.[361] The 250-mg daily dose was examined in a single-arm phase II study. A two-stage design was used, and 31 patients were accrued in the first stage. One patient had a partial response and seven patients had stable disease. The median PFS was 2.8 months (95% CI, 1.5 to 3.9) and the median overall survival rate was 6.5 months (95% CI, 4.4 to 8.9). The criterion for second-stage accrual was not met, and the authors concluded that gefitinib as a single agent was not active in advanced HCC. Lapatinib, a selective dual inhibitor of both EGF receptor and HER2 tyrosine kinases, also demonstrated modest activity in HCC.[362] Among the 40 patients with advanced HCC, the response rate was 5%, PFS 2.3 (95% CI, 1.7 to 5.6) months, and overall survival rate of 6.2 (95% CI, 5.1 to infinity) months. Cetuximab, a chimeric monoclonal antibody against EGF receptor, was tested in a phase II study in patients with advanced HCC.[363] A total of 30 patients with advanced HCC were enrolled. The initial dose of cetuximab was 400 mg/m² provided intravenously, followed by weekly intravenous infusions at 250 mg/m². No responses were seen. Five patients had stable disease (median time, 4.2 months; range, 2.8 to 4.2 months). The median overall survival rate was 9.6 months (95% CI, 4.3 to 12.1) and the median PFS was 1.4 months (95% CI, 1.2 to 2.6). Cetuximab trough concentrations were not notably altered in patients with Child-Turcotte-Pugh A and B cirrhosis. Combinations of cetuximab with cytotoxic or other targeted therapies are being planned.

Brivanib alaninate is a dual inhibitor of VEGF receptor and FGF receptor signaling pathways that can induce tumor growth inhibition in the mouse HCC xenograft model.[364] A phase II study was conducted to assess the efficacy and safety of brivanib in patients with unresectable locally advanced or metastatic HCC who had received either no prior systemic therapy (cohort A) or one prior regimen of angiogenesis inhibitor (cohort B).[365] The treatment schedule consisted of continuous daily dosing of brivanib at 800 mg. Of the 96 patients enrolled, 55 patients were in cohort A and 41 in cohort B, including 38 whose disease failed to respond to sorafenib. In cohort A, the median overall survival rate was 10 months and time to progression was 2.8 months (95% CI, 1.4 to 3.9). Partial response was seen in 5% of patients, and disease control rate was 47%. Interestingly, a greater than 50% decrease in serum AFP from baseline was seen in more than 40% of patients in both cohorts A and B. Most frequently observed grade 3 or 4 adverse events included fatigue (16%), high levels of transaminases (19%), and hyponatremia (41%) in cohort A and hypertension (7.3%), diarrhea (4.9%), and headache (4.9%) in cohort B. Brivanib is undergoing additional evaluation in phase III studies in both the first-line setting in comparison with sorafenib and in the sorafenib-refractory setting in comparison with best supportive care in advanced HCC.

HCC is characterized by frequent mitogen-induced extracellular kinase (MEK)/extracellular signal-regulated protein kinase (ERK) activation in the absence of RAS or RAF mutation. A multicenter, single-arm phase II study with a two-stage design was conducted with AZD6244, a specific inhibitor of MEK, in advanced HCC.[366] AZD6244 was administered orally at a dose of 100 mg twice a day. Of the 19 patients enrolled, 16 had response data available. Despite the good tolerability of AZD6244, it showed minimal activity in advanced HCC. No response was observed, and stable disease was observed in 37.5% of the patients. The median TTP was only 8 weeks (95% CI, 6.6 to 11.1). These data need to be further tested in other cohorts.

mTOR functions to regulate protein translation, angiogenesis, and cell-cycle progression in many cancers, including HCC.[367] Preclinical data have demonstrated that mTOR inhibitors were effective in inhibiting cell growth and tumor vascularity in HCC cell lines and HCC tumor models. A number of mTOR inhibitors (sirolimus, temsirolimus, and everolimus) are available clinically. Retrospective studies in patients who underwent liver transplantation for HCC have shown that patients who received sirolimus for immunosuppression had a much lower rate of tumor recurrence than those who received calcineurin inhibitors.[368] Clinical studies with mTOR inhibitors alone and in combination with either targeted agents or chemotherapeutic agents in advanced HCC are at an early stage of clinical development. A recent randomized phase I pharmacokinetic study of everolimus in advanced HCC was reported.[369] Two different schedules were tested: continuous daily dosing and once-weekly dosing. A total of 36 patients were enrolled. Dose-limiting toxicities observed included hyperbilirubinemia, high levels of alanine aminotransferase, thrombocytopenia, infection, diarrhea, and cardiac ischemia. The maximum tolerated dose for weekly and daily dosing schedules was determined to be 70 and 7.5 mg, respectively. Interestingly, reactivation of hepatitis B and C virus was observed in four patients and one patient,

respectively. The disease control rate of 31 evaluable patients was 61% (10 of 16) and 46.7% (7 of 15, including one case of PR) of patients receiving daily and weekly treatment, respectively. Phase II and III studies are expected for advanced HCC in the next few years.

The identification of the molecular pathways in HCC has led to a new era in the treatment of this tumor. At the moment most of the studies are targeting patients with advanced HCC. However, these new therapies can change the treatment paradigm in HCC by combining molecular therapies with local therapies, such as surgical resection, RFA, and transarterial therapies. Ongoing studies are evaluating these combinations, which may further improve the treatments for patients with HCC.

Key References

Altekruse SF, McGlynn KA, Reichman ME. Hepatocellular carcinoma incidence, mortality, and survival trends in the United States from 1975 to 2005. J Clin Oncol 2009;27:1485–1491. (Ref.15)

Bandyopadhyay R, Kumar M, Leslie JF. Relative severity of aflatoxin contamination of cereal crops in West Africa. Food Addit Contam 2007;24:1109–1114. (Ref.50)

Beasley RP. Diabetes and hepatocellular carcinoma. Hepatology 2006;44:1 408–1410. (Ref.57)

Belli G, et al. Laparoscopic versus open liver resection for hepatocellular carcinoma in patients with histologically proven cirrhosis: short- and middle-term results. Surg Endosc 2007;21:2004–2011. (Ref.258)

Bosetti C, et al. Trends in mortality from hepatocellular carcinoma in Europe: 1980-2004. Hepatology 2008;48:137–145. (Ref.14)

Boyault S, et al. Transcriptome classification of HCC is related to gene alterations and to new therapeutic targets. Hepatology 2007;45:42–52. (Ref.235)

Brown DB, et al. Image-guided tumor ablation: standardization of terminology and reporting criteria. J Vasc Interv Radiol 2009;20:S377–S390. (Ref.295)

Brunello F, et al. Radiofrequency ablation versus ethanol injection for early hepatocellular carcinoma: a randomized controlled trial. Scand J Gastroenterol 2008;43:727–735. (Ref.300)

Cabibbo G, et al. A meta-analysis of survival rates of untreated patients in randomized clinical trials of hepatocellular carcinoma. Hepatology 2010;51:1274–1283. (Ref.215)

Chan HL, et al. High viral load and hepatitis B virus subgenotype ce are associated with increased risk of hepatocellular carcinoma. J Clin Oncol 2008;26:177–182. (Ref.23)

Chen CJ, et al. Risk of hepatocellular carcinoma across a biological gradient of serum hepatitis B virus DNA level. JAMA 2006;295:65–73. (Ref.21)

Chen JD, et al. Carriers of inactive hepatitis B virus are still at risk for hepatocellular carcinoma and liver-related death. Gastroenterology 2010;138:1747–1754. (Ref.22)

Chen L, et al. Randomized, phase I, and pharmacokinetic (PK) study of RAD001, an mTOR inhibitor, in patients (pts) with advanced hepatocellular carcinoma (HCC). J Clin Oncol 2009;27(Suppl):4587. (Ref.369)

Chen MS, et al. A prospective randomized trial comparing percutaneous local ablative therapy and partial hepatectomy for small hepatocellular carcinoma. Ann Surg 2006;243:321–328. (Ref.309)

Cheng AL, et al. Efficacy and safety of sorafenib in patients in the Asia-Pacific region with advanced hepatocellular carcinoma: a phase III randomised, double-blind, placebo-controlled trial. Lancet Oncol 2009;10:25–34. (Ref.346)

Chiang DY, et al. Focal gains of VEGFA and molecular classification of hepatocellular carcinoma. Cancer Res 2008;68:6779–6788. (Ref.236)

Cho YK, et al. Systematic review of randomized trials for hepatocellular carcinoma treated with percutaneous ablation therapies. Hepatology 2009;49:453–459. (Ref.303)

Choi D, et al. Percutaneous radiofrequency ablation for early-stage hepatocellular carcinoma as a first-line treatment: long-term results and prognostic factors in a large single-institution series. Eur Radiol 2007;17:684–692. (Ref.306)

Cillo U, et al. Prospective validation of the Barcelona Clinic Liver Cancer staging system. J Hepatol 2006;44:723–731. (Ref.230)

Di Bisceglie AM, et al. Prolonged therapy of advanced chronic hepatitis C with low-dose peginterferon. N Engl J Med 2008;359:2429–2441. (Ref.68)

Di Tommaso L, et al. Diagnostic value of HSP70, glypican 3, and glutamine synthetase in hepatocellular nodules in cirrhosis. Hepatology 2007;45:725–734. (Ref.178)

Duffy JP, et al. Liver transplantation criteria for hepatocellular carcinoma should be expanded: a 22-year experience with 467 patients at UCLA. Ann Surg 2007;246:502–511. (Ref.287)

Dutkowski P, et al. Current and future trends in liver transplantation in Europe. Gastroenterology 2010;138:802–809. (Ref.272)

El-Serag HB, Rudolph KL. Hepatocellular carcinoma: epidemiology and molecular carcinogénesis. Gastroenterology 2007;132:2557–2576. (Ref.3)

Faivre S, et al. Safety and efficacy of sunitinib in patients with advanced hepatocellular carcinoma: an open-label, multicentre, phase II study. Lancet Oncol 2009;10:794–800. (Ref.356)

Fisher RA, et al. Hepatocellular carcinoma recurrence and death following living and deceased donor liver transplantation. Am J Transplant 2007;7:1601–1608. (Ref.284)

Forner A, et al. Diagnosis of hepatic nodules 20 mm or smaller in cirrhosis: prospective validation of the noninvasive diagnostic criteria for hepatocellular carcinoma. Hepatology 2008;47:97–104. (Ref.206)

Forner A, et al. Evaluation of tumor response after locoregional therapies in hepatocellular carcinoma: are response evaluation criteria in solid tumors reliable? Cancer 2009;115:616–623. (Ref.213)

Germani G, et al. Clinical outcomes of radiofrequency ablation, percutaneous alcohol and acetic acid injection for hepatocelullar carcinoma: a meta-analysis. J Hepatol 2010;52:380–388. (Ref.304)

Gianelli G, et al. Clinical validation of combined serological biomarkers for improved hepatocellular carcinoma diagnosis in 961 patients. Clin Chim Acta 2007;383:147–152. (Ref.160)

Gish RG, et al. Phase III randomized controlled trial comparing the survival of patients with unresectable hepatocellular carcinoma treated with nolatrexed or doxorubicin. J Clin Oncol 2007;25:3069–3075. (Ref.339)

Guglielmi A, et al. Comparison of seven staging systems in cirrhotic patients with hepatocellular carcinoma in a cohort of patients who underwent radiofrequency ablation with complete response. Am J Gastroenterol 2008;103:597–604. (Ref.232)

Hara M, Tanaka K, Sakamoto T. Case-control study on cigarette smoking and the risk of hepatocellular carcinoma among Japanese. Cancer Sci 2008;99:93–97. (Ref.60)

Hoshida Y, et al. Gene expression in fixed tissues and outcome in hepatocellular carcinoma. N Engl J Med 2008;359:1995–2004. (Ref.238)

Huynh H, et al. Bevacizumab and rapamycin induce growth suppression in mouse models of hepatocellular carcinoma. J Hepatol 2008;49:52–60. (Ref.364)

Hytiroglou P, et al. Hepatic precancerous lesions and small hepatocellular carcinoma. Gastroenterol Clin North Am 2007;36:867–887. (Ref.173)

Ibrahim SM, et al. Radioembolization for the treatment of unresectable hepatocellular carcinoma: a clinical review. World J Gastroenterol 2008;14:1664–1669. (Ref.330)

International Consensus Group for Hepatocellular Neoplasia. Pathologic diagnosis of early hepatocellular carcinoma: a report of the international consensus group for hepatocellular neoplasia. Hepatology 2009;49:658–664. (Ref.164)

Kim MJ, et al. Sonography guided percutaneous radiofrequency ablation of hepatocellular carcinoma: effect of cooperative training on the pretreatment assessment of the operation's feasibility. Korean J Radiol 2008;9:29–37. (Ref.141)

Kim SW, et al. Percutaneous radiofrequency ablation of hepatocellular carcinomas adjacent to the gallbladder with internally cooled electrodes: assessment of safety and therapeutic efficacy. Korean J Radiol 2009;10:366–376. (Ref.312)

Kojiro M, et al. Pathology of hepatocellular carcinoma. Oxford, UK: Blackwell, 2006. (Ref.172)

Kulik LM, et al. Safety and efficacy of 90Y radiotherapy for hepatocellular carcinoma with and without portal vein thrombosis. Hepatology 2008;47:71–78. (Ref.333)

Lai MS, et al. Type 2 diabetes and hepatocellular carcinoma: a cohort study in high prevalence area of hepatitis virus infection. Hepatology 2006;43:1295–1302. (Ref.58)

Lammer J, et al. Prospective randomized study of doxorubicin-eluting-bead embolization in the treatment of hepatocellular carcinoma: results of the PRECISION V study. Cardiovasc Intervent Radiol 2010;33:41–52. (Ref.326)

Lencioni R, et al. Radiofrequency ablation of liver cancer. Tech Vasc Interv Radiol 2007;10:38–46. (Ref.294)

Lencioni R, Llovet JM. Modified RECIST (mRECIST) assessment for hepatocellular carcinoma. Semin Liver Dis 2010;30:52–60. (Ref.214)

Libbrecht L, et al. Glypican-3 expression distinguishes small hepatocellular carcinomas from cirrhosis, dysplastic nodules, and focal nodular hyperplasia-like nodules. Am J Surg Pathol 2006;30:1405–1411. (Ref.177)

Liu L, et al. Sorafenib blocks the RAF/MEK/ERK pathway, inhibits tumor angiogenesis, and induces tumor cell apoptosis in hepatocellular carcinoma model PLC/PRF/5. Cancer Res 2006;66:11851–11858. (Ref.343)

Liu Y, Wu F. Global burden of aflatoxin-induced hepatocellular carcinoma: a risk assessment. Environ Health Perspect 2010;118:818–824. (Ref.49)

Livraghi T, et al. Sustained complete response and complications rates after radiofrequency ablation of very early hepatocellular carcinoma in cirrhosis: is resection still the treatment of choice? Hepatology 2008;47:82–89. (Ref.308)

Llovet JM, et al. A molecular signature to discriminate dysplastic nodules from early hepatocellular carcinoma in HCV cirrhosis. Gastroenterology 2006;131:1758–1767. (Ref.154)

Llovet JM, et al. Sorafenib in advanced hepatocellular carcinoma. N Engl J Med 2008;359:378–390. (Ref.345)

Lok AS, et al. Des-gamma-carboxy prothrombin and alpha-fetoprotein as biomarkers for the early detection of hepatocellular carcinoma. Gastroenterology 2010;138:493–502. (Ref.133)

Lok AS, et al. Incidence of hepatocellular carcinoma and associated risk factors in hepatitis C-related advanced liver disease. Gastroenterology 2009;136:138–148. (Ref.27)

Malagari K, et al. Prospective randomized comparison of chemoembolization with doxorubicin-eluting beads and bland embolization with BeadBlock for hepatocellular carcinoma. Cardiovasc Intervent Radiol 2010;33:541–551. (Ref.327)

Marrero JA, et al. Alpha-fetoprotein, des-gamma carboxyprothrombin, and lectin-bound alpha-fetoprotein in early hepatocellular carcinoma. Gastroenterology 2009;137:110–118. (Ref.132)

Maturen K, et al. Lack of tumor seeding of hepatocellular carcinoma after percutaneous needle biopsy using coaxial cutting needle technique. AJR Am J Roentgenol 2006;187:1184–1187. (Ref.205)

Mendel DB, et al. In vivo antitumor activity of SU11248, a novel tyrosine kinase inhibitor targeting vascular endothelial growth factor and platelet-derived growth factor receptors: determination of a pharmacokinetic/pharmacodynamic relationship. Clin Cancer Res 2003;9:327–337. (Ref.354)

N'Kontchou G, et al. Radiofrequency ablation of hepatocellular carcinoma: long-term results and prognostic factors in 235 Western patients with cirrhosis. Hepatology 2009;50:1475–1483. (Ref.307)

Nathan H, et al. Predictors of survival after resection of early hepatocellular carcinoma. Ann Surg 2009;249:799–805. (Ref.252)

O'Neill BH, et al. A phase II study of AZD6244 in advanced or metastatic hepatocellular carcinoma. J Clin Oncol 2009;27(15s):A15574. (Ref.366)

Onaca N, et al. Expanded criteria for liver transplantation in patients with hepatocellular carcinoma: a report from the International Registry of Hepatic Tumors in Liver Transplantation. Liver Transpl 2007;13:391–399. (Ref.291)

Orlacchio A, et al. Percutaneous cryoablation of small hepatocellular carcinoma with US guidance and CT monitoring: initial experience. Cardiovasc Intervent Radiol 2008;31:587–594. (Ref.315)

Orlando A, et al. Radiofrequency thermal ablation vs. percutaneous ethanol injection for small hepatocellular carcinoma in cirrhosis: meta-analysis of randomized controlled trials. Am J Gastroenterol 2009;104:514–524. (Ref.302)

Park YN, et al. Ductular reaction is helpful in defining early stromal invasion, small hepatocellular carcinomas, and dysplastic nodules. Cancer 2007;109:915–923. (Ref.170)

Pelletier SJ, et al. An intention-to-treat analysis of liver transplantation for hepatocellular carcinoma using organ procurement network data. Liver Transpl 2009;15:859–868. (Ref.273)

Pomfret EA, et al. Report of a national conference on liver allocation in patients with hepatocellular carcinoma in the United States. Liver Transpl 2010;16:262–278. (Ref.293)

Ramanathan RK, et al. A phase II study of lapatinib in patients with advanced biliary tree and hepatocellular cancer. Cancer Chemother Pharmacol 2009;64:777–783. (Ref.362)

Raoul JL, et al. An open-label phase II study of first- and second-line treatment with brivanib in patients with hepatocellular carcinoma (HCC). J Clin Oncol 2009;27(15s):A4577. (Ref.365)

Rhim H, et al. Planning sonography to assess the feasibility of percutaneous radiofrequency ablation of hepatocellular carcinomas. AJR Am J Roentgenol 2008;190:1324–1330. (Ref.140)

Salem R, et al. Radioembolization for hepatocellular carcinoma using Yytrium-90 microspheres: a comprehensive report of long-term outcomes. Gastroenterology 2010;138:52–64. (Ref.334)

Sakata J, et al. Preoperative predictors of vascular invasion in hepatocellular carcinoma. Eur J Surg Oncol 2008;34:900–905. (Ref.261)

Sangiovanni A, et al. The diagnostic and economic impact of contrast imaging techniques in the diagnosis of small hepatocellular carcinoma in cirrhosis. Gut 2010;59:638–644. (Ref.204)

Sherman M. Hepatocellular carcinoma: epidemiology, surveillance and diagnosis. Semin Liver Dis 2010;30:3–16. (Ref.2)

Shimizu T, et al. Outcome of MR-guided percutaneous cryoablation for hepatocellular carcinoma. J Hepatobiliary Pancreat Surg 2009;16:816–823. (Ref.316)

Siegel AB, et al. Phase II trial evaluating the clinical and biologic effects of bevacizumab in unresectable hepatocellular carcinoma. J Clin Oncol 2008;26:2992–2998. (Ref.351)

Singal AG, et al. Meta-analysis: surveillance with ultrasound for early-stage hepatocellular carcinoma in patients with cirrhosis. Aliment Pharmacol Ther 2009;30:37–47. (Ref.139)

Starley BQ, Calcagno CJ, Harrison SA. Nonalcoholic fatty liver disease and hepatocellular carcinoma: a weighty connection. Hepatology 2010;51:1820–1832. (Ref.55)

Sterling RK, et al. Clinical utility of AFP-L3% measurement in North American patients with HCV-related cirrhosis. Am J Gastroenterol 2007;102:2196–2205. (Ref.151)

Tanaka S, et al. Integral role of transcription factor 8 in the negative regulation of tumor angiogenesis. Cancer Res 2009;69:1678–1684. (Ref.83)

Thomas MB, et al. Phase 2 study of erlotinib in patients with unresectable hepatocellular carcinoma. Cancer 2007;110:1059–1067. (Ref.360)

Thomas MB, et al. Phase II trial of the combination of bevacizumab and erlotinib in patients who have advanced hepatocellular carcinoma. J Clin Oncol 2009;27:843–850. (Ref.353)

Thuluvath P, et al. Liver transplantation in the United States, 1999-2008. Am J Transplant 2010;10:1003–1019. (Ref.277)

Torres DM, Harrison SA. Diagnosis and treatment of nonalcoholic steatohepatitis. Gastroenterology 2008;134:1682–1698. (Ref.61)

Toso C, et al. Sirolimus-based immunosuppression is associated with increased survival after liver transplantation for hepatocellular carcinoma. Hepatology 2010;51:1237–1243. (Ref.368)

Umemura T, et al. Epidemiology of hepatocellular carcinoma in Japan. J Gastroenterol 2009;44(Suppl 19):102–107. (Ref.7)

Varela M, et al. Chemoembolization of hepatocellular carcinoma with drug eluting beads: efficacy and doxorubicin pharmacokinetics. J Hepatol 2007;46:474–481. (Ref.325)

Vecchia CL. Alcohol and liver cancer. Eur J Cancer Prev 2007;16:495–497. (Ref.42)

Vibert E, et al. Progression of alphafetoprotein before liver transplantation for hepatocellular carcinoma in cirrhotic patients: a critical factor. Am J Transplant 2010;10:129–137. (Ref.135)

Villanueva A, et al. Hepatocellular carcinoma: novel molecular approaches for diagnosis, prognosis, and therapy. Annu Rev Med 2010;61:317–328. (Ref.233)

Villanueva A, et al. Pivotal role of mTOR signaling in hepatocellular carcinoma. Gastroenterology 2008;135:1972–1983. (Ref.367)

Villanueva A, Toffanin S, Llovet JM. Linking molecular classification of hepatocellular carcinoma and personalized medicine: preliminary steps. Curr Opin Oncol 2008;20:444–453. (Ref.234)

Volk ML, et al. A novel model measuring the harm of transplanting hepatocellular carcinoma exceeding Milan criteria. Am J Transplant 2008;8:839–846. (Ref.292)

Volk ML, et al. Who decides? Living donor liver transplantation for advanced hepatocellular carcinoma. Transplantation 2006;82:1136–1139. (Ref.283)

Wang JH, et al. The efficacy of treatment schedules according to Barcelona Clinic Liver Cancer staging for hepatocellular carcinoma: survival analysis of 3892 patients. Eur J Cancer 2008;44:1000–1006. (Ref.231)

Willat J, et al. MR Imaging of hepatocellular carcinoma in the cirrhotic liver: challenges and controversies. Radiology 2008;247:311–330. (Ref.185)

Yao FY, et al. Liver transplantation for hepatocellular carcinoma: validation of the UCSF-expanded criteria based on preoperative imaging. Am J Transplant 2007;7:2587–2596. (Ref.285)

Yao FY, et al. Excellent outcome following down-staging of hepatocellular carcinoma prior to liver transplantation: an intention-to-treat analysis. Hepatology 2008;48:819–827. (Ref.328)

Zhu AX, et al. Phase 2 study of cetuximab in patients with advanced hepatocellular carcinoma. Cancer 2007;110:581–589. (Ref.363)

A complete list of references can be found at www.expertconsult.com.

Chapter 58

X

Cholangiocarcinoma

Konstantinos N. Lazaridis and Gregory J. Gores

ABBREVIATIONS

CC cholangiocarcinoma
CDK cell division kinase
COX2 cyclooxygenase-2
DAPI 4′,6-Diamidino-2-phenylindole
DIA digitized image analysis
EBRT external beam radiation therapy
EGF epidermal growth factor
EGFR epidermal growth factor receptor
ERCP endoscopic retrograde cholangiopancreatography
EUS endoscopic ultrasound
FISH fluorescence in situ hybridization
FLIP flice-inhibitory protein

HAAH human aspartyl β-hydroxylase
HCV hepatitis C virus
HGF hepatocyte growth factor
HIV human immunodeficiency virus
hMLH1 human Mut L homologue-1
hTERT human telomerase reverse transcriptase
IL-6 interleukin-6
MAPK mitogen-activated protein kinase
Mcl-1 myeloid cell leukemia-1
MMP matrix metalloproteinase
MRCP magnetic resonance cholangiopancreatography

MRI magnetic resonance imaging
NO nitric oxide
PDT photodynamic therapy
PSC primary sclerosing cholangitis
PTC percutaneous transhepatic cholangiography
STAT signal transducer and activator of transcription
TNF tumor necrosis factor
TNM tumor-node-metastasis
WISP1v WNT1-inducible signaling pathway protein-1

Introduction

Cholangiocarcinoma (CC) is a malignancy of the bile ducts with rising incidence. CC is caused by malignant transformation of the cholangiocyte—the epithelial cell that lines the bile ducts—and/or possibly biliary stem cells.[1] CC accounts for 10% to 20% of all hepatobiliary neoplasms.[2] Anatomically, CC is divided into two types (intrahepatic and extrahepatic) based on its location along the biliary tree, each having discrete epidemiologic and clinical features, and probably independent etiopathogenetic origins.[1] Despite progress, we need a better understanding of the biology of CC. More knowledge will likely improve early detection and hopefully treatment of CC.[3]

Epidemiology and Risk Factors
Epidemiology

Over past decades the incidence of CC has increased.[4,5] Approximately 5000 new cases of CC are diagnosed every year in the United States.[6,7-9] Of those, about two thirds involve the extrahepatic bile ducts and the remaining one third affect the intrahepatic biliary tree. However, it should be noted that in several registries, hilar CCs, which involve the right and left hepatic ducts and their confluence, are classified as intrahepatic CCs. We believe this is erroneous and consider hilar CCs to be extrahepatic given their clinical and biologic characteristics.[10]

The epidemiology of intrahepatic as opposed to extrahepatic CC is different. Possible misclassification between these two kinds of CC may affect reported epidemiologic parameters. In the United States, based on the Surveillance Epidemiology and End Results registries, the age-adjusted incidence rate of intrahepatic CC increased from 0.32 per 100,000 in 1975 to 1979 to 0.85 per 100,000 in 1995 to 1999.[4] In contrast, the incidence of extrahepatic CC decreased slightly from 1.08 per 100,000 in 1979 to 0.82 per 100,000 in 1998.[4] Because of the epidemiologic disparity, we discuss independently the epidemiology of intrahepatic versus extrahepatic CC.

The incidence of intrahepatic CC varies across the world.[11] It is highest in northeast Thailand (96/100,000 in men and 38/100,000 in women), probably because of the high prevalence of liver-fluke infestations. In the past, the average age of diagnosis of intrahepatic CC was the mid-50s, with recent age shift toward the mid-60s. This observation might relate to: (1) development of CC in the context of ever-increasing chronic liver disease in the aging population; and (2) improved follow-up and treatment of risk factors (i.e., primary sclerosing cholangitis [PSC], choledochal cysts) in younger individuals. Caucasians and African Americans have a comparable age-adjusted incidence of intrahepatic CC. In contrast, the incidence among Asians is twice as high as that of Caucasians. However, Caucasians are the only ethnic group in which there is a reported gradual increase in the age-adjusted incidence of intrahepatic CC.

The mortality related to intrahepatic CC is also increasing worldwide.[11] In fact, intrahepatic CC mortality increased by a greater percentage than that observed for hepatocellular carcinoma. In the United States, the age-adjusted mortality rate for intrahepatic CC increased from 0.07 per 100,000 in 1973 to 0.69 per 100,000 in 1997.[12] Overall, the 5-year survival rate of patients with intrahepatic CC remains disappointingly low and practically unchanged over the last 2 decades.[7-9] This lack of progress occurs despite earlier detection and employment of aggressive surgical approaches (i.e., hepatectomy.).

The incidence of extrahepatic CC also differs across the globe. In the United States, the age-adjusted incidence of extrahepatic CC has been reported to be 1.2 per 100,000 for men and 0.8 per 100,000 for women. As mentioned previously, the overall incidence of extrahepatic CC is slightly decreasing. The age-adjusted mortality rates of extrahepatic CC are declining in Western world,[11] with the exception of Italy and Japan. In the United States, age-adjusted mortality rates declined from 0.6 per 100,000 in 1979 to 0.3 per 100,000 in 1998.[12] Indeed, there is evidence of minor improvements in 5-year survival rates of extrahepatic CC from 11.7% in 1973 to 1977 to 15.1% in 1983 to 1987.[13] Nevertheless, the small decline in extrahepatic CC in the United States is followed by a true increase of intrahepatic CC, which determines the overall rising incidence of CC.[4]

Risk Factors

Most patients in whom is CC diagnosed do not have or have not been exposed to known risk factor(s) associated with the disease (**Table 58-1**).[5] Primary sclerosing cholangitis (PSC) is a definite risk factor for CC. The risk for developing CC in a patient with PSC is approximately 1.5% per year after diagnosis of the cholestatic liver disease.[14] Of interest, among the PSC patients who develop CC, about 30% will be found to have malignancy of the bile duct[11] within 2½ years of the diagnosis of PSC.[15,16]

Liver flukes, namely, *Opisthorchis viverrini* and *Clonorchis sinensis*, are strongly associated with CC. These liver worms inhabit the bile ducts and sporadically the gallbladder. Individuals become infected with these parasites by eating undercooked fish. In patients with choledochal cysts (i.e., congenital

cystic dilation of bile ducts), the lifetime risk of developing CC is about 10% to 15%, and the median age of diagnosis is 34 years.[17] Intrahepatic biliary stones (i.e., hepatolithiasis) are found frequently in Asia but are rare in Western countries. Studies have reported the association of hepatolithiasis with peripherally located intrahepatic CC.[18] Thorotrast is a colloidal suspension of $^{232}ThO_2$, which mainly emits α-particles and was used as a contrast agent in radiology from the 1930s to 1950s. Exposure to Thorotrast has been linked to the development of CC. Thorotrast causes microsatellite instability and subsequently CC, probably via clonal expansion of cholangiocytes and inactivation of human Mut L homologue-1 (hMLH1) by hypermethylation.[19] In addition, toxins such as dioxin and polyvinyl chloride have been postulated to contribute to development of CC. Recently, chronic viral hepatitis, obesity, and human immunodeficiency virus (HIV) have been added to the list of risk factors for development of CC.[5,20,21]

Common features among several of the risk factors of CC include chronic inflammation of the bile ducts and cholestasis. As discussed later, both these events likely contribute to the malignant transformation of biliary epithelia.

Molecular Pathogenesis

Since the mid-1990s, there has been considerable progress in understanding the pathogenesis of CC. It is widely accepted that malignant transformation of cholangiocytes takes place amid a milieu of chronic inflammation of the bile ducts along with persistent cholestasis. This environment causes increased production of cytokines and reactive oxygen species, resulting in protracted cellular (i.e., cholangiocyte) stresses and accrual of irreversible DNA damage.[1] Subsequently, cholangiocytes undergo malignant transformation; namely, they undergo molecular changes and develop cellular and subcellular characteristics that are otherwise lacking in normal conditions. The molecular alteration of cholangiocytes, which leads to carcinogenesis, is a multifaceted process of interrelated events. **Table 58-2** shows the proposed contributing pathways. The described molecular mechanisms of cholangiocarcinogenesis are mainly derived from experimental studies of intrahepatic CC because of the easy access to tissue. It remains uncertain, however, whether these pathogenetic pathways are pertinent to extrahepatic CC. For example, hilar CCs are highly desmoplastic and therefore obtaining adequate cells for studies is challenging.

Under normal conditions, cholangiocytes retain tissue homeostasis despite exposure to proliferation signals. However, chronic biliary inflammation causes local interleukin 6 (IL-6) and hepatocyte growth factor (HGF) production, which are initially derived from periductal stromal cells (i.e., stellate cells). IL-6 is a powerful mitogen involved in cholangiocyte proliferation, as reported in both animal and human studies.[22-25] IL-6 binds to its plasma membrane receptor, forming the active heterodimer gp80/gp130, which in turn stimulates cellular transcription through the mitogen-activated protein kinase (MAPK)/signal transducer and activator of transcription (STAT) pathway.[26] Of interest, malignant, but not normal, cholangiocytes also produce high levels of IL-6[27] and overexpress the gp80/gp130 heterodimer. HGF also promotes cholangiocyte growth via its plasma membrane receptor, c-met.[22,28] In addition, CC cells achieve an endogenous capacity to produce HGF and up-regulate

Table 58-1 Risk Factors for Cholangiocarcinoma

Age (>65 years old)
Primary sclerosing cholangitis (PSC)
Liver fluke infestation
   Opisthorchis viverrini
   Clonorchis sinensis
Caroli disease
Choledochal cysts
Bile duct adenoma and biliary papillomatosis
Chronic intraductal stones (i.e., hepatolithiasis)
Liver cirrhosis
Chronic viral hepatitis
Human immunodeficiency virus
Thorotrast
Surgical biliary-enteric drainage procedures
Toxins (dioxin, polyvinyl chloride)
Obesity

Table 58-2 Molecular Alterations of Cholangiocyte Malignant Transformation

CONTRIBUTION IN CARCINOGENESIS	MOLECULAR MECHANISMS	REFERENCES
Autologous proliferation signaling	IL-6, gp80/gp130 up-regulation	Sugawara et al.[27]
	HGF/c-*met* up-regulation	Yokomuro et al.,[24] Lai et al.[29]
	EGF/c-*erb*B-2	Ito et al.,[32] Kiguchi et al.[34]
	COX2 up-regulation	Chariyalertsak et al.,[36] Endo et al.,[37] Yoon et al.[43]
	K-*ras* mutations	Kang et al.,[39] Tannapfel et al.[40]
Loss of antigrowth signaling	*p53* mutations	Kang et al.[39]
	p21/WAF mutations	Furubo et al.[104]
	Mdm-2 up-regulation	Furubo et al.[104]
	p16^{INK4} mutation	Tannapfel et al.,[40] Ahrendt et al.[48]
Evasion of apoptosis	FLIP up-regulation	Que et al.[50]
	NO inhibition of caspases	Torok et al.[51]
	Bcl2 up-regulation	Harnois et al.[105]
	Bcl-X_L up-regulation	Okaro et al.[106]
	Mcl-1 up-regulation	Yoon et al.[43]
	COX2 up-regulation	Nzeako et al.[52]
Unlimited replicative potential	Telomerase expressed	Itoi et al.[55,56]
Angiogenesis	VEGF expressed	Benckert et al.[57]
Tissue invasiveness and metastasis	E-cadherin decreased	Ashida et al.[107]
	α-Catenin and β-catenin decreased	Ashida et al.[107]
	Matrix metalloproteinase (MMP) up-regulation	Terada et al.[59]
	Human aspartyl (asparaginyl)	Lavaissiere et al.,[60] Ince et al.,[61] Maeda et al.[62]
	β-Hydroxylase expression	Tanaka et al.[63]
	WISP1v expression	

Modified from Berthiaume EP, Wands J. Molecular pathogenesis of cholangiocarcinoma. Semin Liver Dis 2004;24:127–137.

COX-2, cyclooxygenase-2; EGF, epidermal growth factor; FLIP, flice-inhibitory protein; HGF, hepatocyte growth factor; IL-6, interleukin-6; NO, nitric oxide; VEGF, vascular endothelial growth factor; WAF, wild-type p53 activated fragment-1; WISP1v, WNT1-inducible signaling pathway protein-1

its c-met receptor.[24,29,30] Hence, through the IL-6 and HGF pathways, malignant cholangiocytes maintain autologous proliferating mechanisms.

Another mechanism that contributes to cholangiocarcinogenesis is the epidermal growth factor (EGF) and its receptor (EGFR).[31,32] Interaction of EGF with EGFR leads to activation of the MAPK pathway.[33] The c-erb-B2 protein, a homolog of the EGFR, is a tyrosine kinase, which is activated in CC.[30] Indeed, constitutive expression of c-erb-B2 in gallbladder epithelium leads to adenocarcinoma.[34]

Cyclooxygenase-2 (COX2), an isoform that catalyzes the formation of prostaglandins from arachidonic acid, is induced by mitogens and cytokines[35] and is involved in the pathogenesis of CC. COX2 is overexpressed in malignant, but not normal, cholangiocytes.[36,37] The complex and interrelated processes of carcinogenesis in bile ducts is indicated by the fact that IL-6, HGF, and EGF stimulate COX2 expression in cholangiocytes.[34,38] Nonetheless, the exact mechanism by which COX2 causes CC is uncertain, but it likely involves inhibition of apoptotic pathways.

K-*ras* is an oncogene that plays an important role in mitogenic cellular signals. Mutations of this gene have been detected in 20% to 100% of CC proven by a biopsy.[39,40] K-*ras* mutations have also been associated with hilar CC and periductal tumor extension.[39,41]

In addition to biliary inflammation as a precipitant of cholangiocarcinogenesis, CC demonstrates an inherent tropism for bile. For example, bile acids have been reported to transactivate the EGFR and to promote the expression of COX-2 in cholangiocytes.[42,43]

Critical pathways that inhibit cell proliferation are usually lost in the development of cholangiocarcinogenesis. For instance, loss of heterozygosity for the tumor suppressor gene *p53* is frequent in CC.[44] The *p53* gene directs the cellular machinery of cell cycle and apoptosis. Regarding the cell cycle, *p53* regulates the p21/WAF1 (wild-type *p53* activated fragment-1) protein, which binds to the cell division kinase (CDK) 4-cyclin D complex. Thus *p53* causes negative feedback of the CDK4–cyclin D complex, therefore averting phosphorylation of Rb and, as a result, release of the E2F transcription factor (**Fig. 58-1**). Subsequently, the E2F molecule controls the transcription of multiple cellular proteins important in the S phase of the cell cycle.[45,46] Moreover, *p53* can induce apoptosis by promoting Bax insertion in the mitochondrial membrane and stimulating mitochondrial depolarization and subsequently apoptosis (see **Fig. 58-1**). Inactivation of the p14/mdm/*p53* pathway and the *p16* (a tumor suppressor gene) via a variety of molecular mechanisms has been described in CC and in PSC-associated CC.[47,48] As shown in **Table 58-2**, *p53*, *p21/WAF1*, and *p16* mutations are involved in the loss of critical cell signaling, which may allow the development of CC.

Apoptosis is an important cellular mechanism that controls tissue homeostasis. Disarrangement of apoptosis may lead to aberrant cell proliferation and subsequently to carcinogenesis. Ligand activation of the Fas/TRAIL (tumor

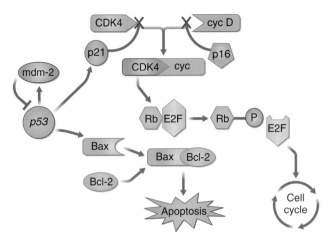

Fig. 58-1 *p53* regulates both cholangiocyte cell cycle and apoptosis. *p53* controls the cell division kinase (CDK) 4-cyclin D complex via the p21/ WAF1 protein, which binds to the latter. As a result, *p53* causes negative feedback of the CDK4–cyclin D complex, therefore averting phosphorylation of Rb and leading to release of the E2F transcription factor. Subsequently, E2F regulates the transcription of multiple proteins in the S-phase of the cell cycle. *p53* can also induce apoptosis by promoting Bax insertion into the mitochondrial membrane, stimulating mitochondrial depolarization and resulting in apoptosis. The p16 protein also inhibits the CDK4–cyclin D complex. *(Modified from Berthiaume EP, Wands J. Molecular pathogenesis of cholangiocarcinoma. Semin Liver Dis 2004;24: 127–137.)*

necrosis factor [TNF]-related apoptosis-inducing ligand)/ TNF-receptor family or release of cytochrome c by mitochondria causes activation of caspases, resulting in DNA fragmentation and cell destruction.[49] As mentioned previously, both chronic biliary inflammation and chronic cholestasis cause persistent cholangiocyte stress and DNA damage. Thus apoptosis serves as a scavenger for cells that develop malignant transformation. As a result, loss of the protective function of apoptosis in cholangiocytes may result in development of CC.

Cholangiocytes express the Fas receptor on plasma membrane[38] and respond to FAS ligand stimulation with apoptosis. Nevertheless, in a CC cell line there was diminished responsiveness of the Fas/FAS ligand because of alteration of the flice-inhibitory protein (FLIP).[38] FLIP inhibits activation of procaspase-8, causing diminished signaling of the Fas/FAS ligand pathway.[50] Moreover, cholangiocytes under the effect of nitric oxide (NO) display inhibition of both caspase-3 and -9, likely via nitrosylation, and become relatively resistant to apoptosis.[51] Overall, it is the balance of proapoptotic and antiapoptotic signals in the cholangiocyte that guides the depolarization of the mitochondrial membrane, releasing cytochrome c into the cytosol and then the activation of caspases.

COX2 induced by inflammation is antiapoptotic. Up-regulation of COX2 inhibits Fas/FAS ligand-induced apoptosis by increasing expression of the inhibitory protein myeloid cell leukemia-1 (Mcl-1).[52] Of interest, bile acids, which are elevated in CC, have a positive effect on the expression of Mcl-1 protein via inhibition of proteosome degradation.[42] Besides bile acids, inflammatory mediators could up-regulate Mcl-1. As a result, potential malignant cholangiocytes are averted from apoptosis.

CCs are able to grow perpetually. In contrast, normal cholangiocytes, like other types of cells, undergo a defined number of cellular divisions before undergoing senescence. Key to this process is progressive telomere shortening. Telomeres are long stretches of repeat sequences present at the end of chromosomes that are involved in DNA synthesis. After multiple cell cycles, telomere shortening causes chromosomal instability and renders cells unable to divide.[53] Preservation of telomere shortening via overexpression of the human telomerase reverse transcriptase (hTERT) allows cancers, including CCs, to sustain chromosomal replication and therefore to maintain eternal proliferation.[54] In fact, detectable hTERT activity and increased expression of hTERT mRNA have been reported in intrahepatic CC.[55,56]

Angiogenesis is promoted by many malignancies to ensure the adequate blood supply of oxygen and nutrients to constantly dividing tumor cells. CCs have a high vascular supply and intrahepatic CCs express vascular endothelial growth factor (VEGF).[57] Moreover, in a CC cell line, increased expression of VEGF was dependent on transforming growth factor-β stimulation.[57]

A feature of neoplasia is invasiveness of the surrounding tissue and metastasis. E-cadherin, a cell surface protein, is involved in cellular adhesion. Mutations or deletions of the gene cause diminished cell adhesiveness, facilitating tissue invasion and metastasis. Intrahepatic CCs have reduced expression of E-cadherin associated with advanced tumor histologic stage.[58] Matrix metalloproteinases (MMP) have been reported to be up-regulated in CC, an event which was associated with clinical invasiveness.[59] Moreover, the human aspartyl β-hydroxylase (HAAH), a protein involved in tumor invasion, is expressed in hepatocellular carcinoma and CC.[60] HAAH involves posttranscriptional hydroxylation of β-carbons on specific residues present in EGF-like domains of proteins that participate in cell migration and motility.[60] Expression of HAAH in transfected cell lines was associated with anchorage-independent growth and tumor development in nude mice.[61] CC cell lines have been reported to overexpress HAAH.[62] Another protein associated with the connective tissue growth factor family, termed WISP1v (WNT1-inducible signaling pathway protein-1), is also overexpressed in CC.[63] Overexpression of WISP1v was linked with lymphatic and perineural CC invasion.[63]

Pathology and Classification

Both intrahepatic and extrahepatic CCs are adenocarcinomas by histopathology. They usually are well- to moderately differentiated tubular adenocarcinomas within a dense, desmoplastic stroma. Other histologic variants of CC include papillary adenocarcinoma, signet ring carcinoma, squamous cell or mucoepidermoid carcinoma, and a lymphoepithelioma-like form.

CC is classified into intrahepatic and extrahepatic (**Fig. 58-2**). The extrahepatic variety constitutes about two thirds of all CCs and is subdivided into: (1) hilar or Klatskin tumor; (2) middle; and (3) distal tumors. Hilar tumors represent approximately 60% of extrahepatic CC. The Bismuth-Corlette classification of hilar CC is shown in **Figure 58-3**. Based on growth patterns, extrahepatic CC is grouped into sclerosing, nodular, and papillary. The sclerosing type is the most common and causes annular thickening of the bile ducts because of

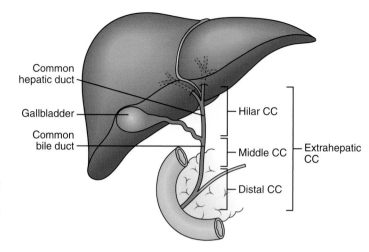

Fig. 58-2 The term *cholangiocarcinoma (CC)* refers to tumors involving the entire (i.e., intrahepatic and extrahepatic) biliary tree. Intrahepatic CC denotes malignancies affecting the bile ducts inside the liver. Extrahepatic CCs are divided into hilar or Klatskin tumor, middle, and distal tumors.

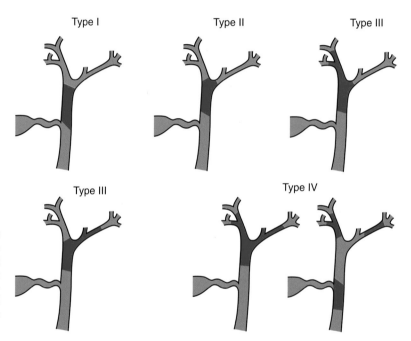

Fig. 58-3 Type I cholangiocarcinoma (CC) affects the common hepatic duct; type II CC involves the common hepatic duct and the confluence of the right and left hepatic ducts; type IIIa and IIIb CC includes the common hepatic duct and either the right or left hepatic duct, respectively; and type IV CC involves the biliary confluence and extends to both right and left hepatic ducts or refers to multifocal bile duct tumors.

infiltration and fibrosis. Intrahepatic CC grows as a mass lesion, accounts for about one third of bile duct tumors, and can be confused with hepatocellular carcinoma. Intrahepatic CC could be solitary or multinodular. It might also be well demarcated as a mass lesion or as a diffuse, infiltrating neoplasm growing along the intrahepatic bile ducts.

Clinical Findings and Diagnosis

Extrahepatic CC

Patients with extrahepatic CC have symptoms, signs, and biochemical laboratory tests of obstructive cholestasis. They often complain of jaundice, dark urine, pale stools, pruritus, malaise, and weight loss. Laboratory tests reveal an increased alkaline phosphatase and bilirubin. The serum level of CA 19-9 can be elevated. CA 19-9 detects circulating high-molecular-weight mucin glycoproteins coated with sialylated blood group epitopes (i.e., sialyl Lewis).[64] Therefore CA 19-9 blood levels depend on the Lewis phenotype.[65] Approximately 7% of the population are Lewis negative, and thus these individuals have an undetectable CA 19-9 in the presence of malignancy.[66] In addition, CA 19-9 is not specific for CC. Pancreatic, gastric, colorectal, and gynecologic cancers, as well as bacterial cholangitis and smoking, can cause elevation of CA 19-9.

In extrahepatic CC, imaging studies demonstrate dilation of the biliary tree and often localize the level of biliary obstruction. Unilobular bile duct obstruction usually causes atrophy of the affected lobe along with hypertrophy of the nonaffected lobe, a phenomenon known as the atrophy–hypertrophy complex.[67] Endoscopic retrograde cholangiopancreatography (ERCP) and magnetic resonance cholangiopancreatography (MRCP) are common procedures to define the position and extent of CC along the biliary tree. Brush cytology and endoscopic biopsies of the bile ducts can be obtained during ERCP for histopathologic diagnosis. An

ERCP of a patient with a hilar CC is shown in **Figure 58-4**. Nevertheless, tissue-proven diagnosis can be challenging because CC is a highly desmoplastic tumor consisting of excessive fibrous tissue with few aggregations of malignant cholangiocytes. This desmoplastic reaction surrounds the bile ducts and extends into the submucosal tissue, and the diagnosis of CC based on biliary cytology findings is seen in only in approximately 30% of cases.[3]

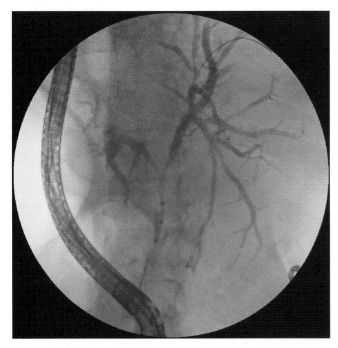

Fig. 58-4 **Endoscopic retrograde cholangiopancreatography demonstrating a hilar cholangiocarcinoma causing obstruction of the biliary bifurcation.**

Fluorescence in situ hybridization (FISH) is a promising method to assess cellular aneuploidy and chromosomal duplication in CC. FISH uses fluorescently labeled DNA probes to detect cholangiocytes with chromosomal alterations (**Fig. 58-5**). The presence of significant populations of cells with chromosomal gains indicates the possibility of biliary malignancy. A positive test is defined when 5 or more cells display gains of two or more chromosomes, or 10 or more cells demonstrate a gain of a single chromosome. Nevertheless, a positive biliary FISH study does not identify the position or type of bile duct malignancy. To perform a FISH study, bile duct brushings are collected at the time of ERCP and cells are fixed on a slide. Then four fluorescently labeled DNA probes hybridize to the centromere of chromosomes 3, 7, and 17 and the *p16* gene on chromosome 9 (9p21). After hybridization, the slide is stained with the nuclear counterstain 4′,6-diamidino-2-phenylindole (DAPI) and fluorescence microscopy is used to scan the slide for atypical cells (i.e., gains of chromosomes 3, 7, 9, and 17) (see **Fig. 58-5**). If the number of cells with chromosomal gains (i.e., polysomy, trisomy) observed is adequate to declare the test positive, then the percentage of abnormal cells is calculated. In a large study of 498 consecutive patients undergoing ERCP for pancreatobiliary strictures, polysomy of FISH had high sensitivity (42.9%) compared with routine cytology (20.1%), and both tests displayed identical specificity.[68,69]

Endoscopic ultrasound (EUS) has applicability in determining the nature of biliary strictures. EUS-guided fine-needle aspiration biopsy of suspected CC has a specificity, sensitivity, and a positive predictive value of 86%, 100%, and 100%, respectively.[70] EUS with fine-needle aspiration was reported to have a positive effect on the clinical management of 84% of patients with CC.[70] The contribution of magnetic resonance imaging (MRI) in the management of CC is to aid the diagnosis and to evaluate tumor resectability. In hilar CC, MRCP images may show moderately irregular thickening of

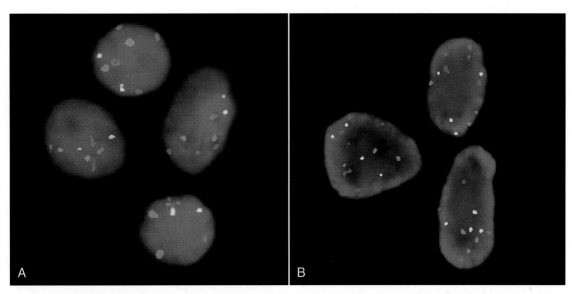

Fig. 58-5 **Fluorescently labeled DNA probes decorating genomic loci on four separate chromosomes.** *Red* indicates chromosome 3, *green* specifies chromosome 7, *gold* points to chromosome 9, and *aqua* identifies chromosome 17. Normal cholangiocytes (**A**) have two duplicates of each probe, as expected for normal diploid cells. Malignant cholangiocytes (**B**) reveal gains of chromosomal probes, suggesting polysomy.

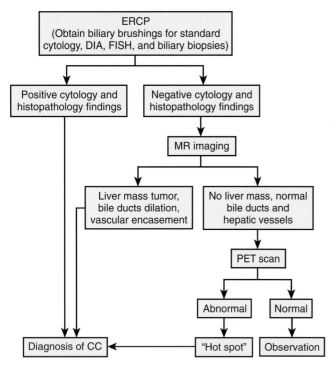

Fig. 58-6 Algorithm for the management of a primary sclerosing cholangitis patient having a dominant biliary stricture. CC, cholangiocarcinoma; DIA, digitized image analysis; ERCP, endoscopic retrograde cholangiopancreatography; FISH, fluorescence in situ hybridization; MR, magnetic resonance; OLT, orthotopic liver transplantation; PET, positron emission tomography.

the bile duct wall associated with proximal biliary dilation.[71] In clinical practice, it is not uncommon to make the diagnosis of extrahepatic CC based solely on clinical, laboratory, and imaging findings in the absence of a tissue-proven diagnosis. Perhaps the greatest challenge is to diagnose CC in patients with PSC. The patient may have a dominant biliary stricture, which makes it difficult to differentiate between a benign lesion and CC. In a patient with PSC, sudden and unexpected clinical deterioration, coupled with progressive elevation of alkaline phosphatase and serum CA 19-9 values greater than 100 U/ml, in the absence of bacterial cholangitis, strongly indicates the development of CC. **Figure 58-6** provides an algorithm for evaluation of these patients.

Intrahepatic CC

Intrahepatic CC has nonspecific symptoms, such as abdominal pain, anorexia, weight loss, malaise, and night sweats, as well as signs of a liver mass lesion. An incidental abdominal mass during physical examination or imaging study may be the sole finding in asymptomatic patients. Laboratory test results reveal an elevated alkaline phosphatase with a normal bilirubin; CA 19-9 is likely increased.[3] The diagnosis of intrahepatic CC is commonly made by the exclusion of other primary or metastatic hepatic mass lesions, which on many occasions could imitate the former. Using cross-sectional MR, intrahepatic CC appears hypointense and hyperintense on T1- and T2-weighted images, respectively. Positron emission tomography (PET) is emerging as a diagnostic study of

intrahepatic CC.[72] At times, a liver biopsy of the mass lesion is the definitive approach to make the correct diagnosis.

Staging

Clinical staging of CC is necessary to identify potential candidates for surgical resection. **Tables 58-3 and 58-4** describe the tumor-node-metastasis (TNM) classification for intrahepatic and extrahepatic CC, respectively. Nevertheless, the value of the TNM categorization system for extrahepatic CC is limited. This is because the TNM system relates to histopathology but not to clinical extension of the disease, and the latter is more important in making decisions for surgical resection of the tumor (**Table 58-5**). During clinical staging of extrahepatic CC, the proximal and distal margins of the tumor should be clearly identified. Obtaining high-quality imaging studies of the bile ducts and liver can attain this aim. ERCP, MRCP, and percutaneous transhepatic cholangiography (PTC) can be used, at times in combination, to map the tumor boundaries. It is also crucial to rule out vascular encasement of the contralateral (i.e., nonaffected) liver lobe by the CC before committing to partial hepatectomy, as well as to verify the patency of the portal vein and hepatic artery. Regional metastases should be excluded. To this end, EUS is superior compared with conventional cross-sectional abdominal imaging (i.e., computed tomography, MRI) to exclude metastatic disease. This is particularly important for doubtful-appearing regional lymph nodes, where biopsy can be taken during EUS to rule out metastatic disease. Indeed, 15% to 20% of CC patients with unremarkable abdominal imaging studies have metastatic lymph node involvement based on EUS evaluation.[73] Nevertheless, the current TNM system (see **Tables 58-3 and 58-4**) is based on surgical acquisition of tissue, which limits the clinical assessment of patients with CC. An ideal classification system should include information about disease extent without subjecting the affected patients to surgical resection. Such staging systems for intrahepatic and extrahepatic CC have been proposed and may facilitate the evaluation of nonsurgical therapies.[74,75]

Table 58-3 Tumor-Node-Metastasis (TNM) Pathologic Classification of Intrahepatic Cholangiocarcinoma

STAGE	TUMOR	NODE	METASTASIS
I	T1	N0	M0
II	T2	N0	M0
III	T3	N0	M0
IVA	T4 or any T	N1	M0
IVB	Any T	Any N	M1

From Sobin LH, Gospodarowicz MK, Wittekind CH, editors. International Union Against Cancer (UICC): TNM classification of malignant tumors, 7th ed. Oxford, UK: Wiley-Blackwell, 2009.

M0, no distant metastasis; M1, distant metastasis; N0, no regional lymph node metastasis; N1, regional lymph node metastases; T1, solitary tumor without vascular invasion; T2a, solitary tumor with vascular invasion; T2b, multiple tumors with vascular invasion; T3, tumor perforating the visceral peritoneum or involving the local extrahepatic structures by direct invasion; T4, tumor(s) with direct invasion of adjacent organs other than gallbladder or with perforation of visceral peritoneum

Table 58-4 Tumor-Node-Metastasis (TNM) Pathologic Classification of Proximal and Distal Extrahepatic Cholangiocarcinoma

PROXIMAL EXTRAHEPATIC BILE DUCT (RIGHT, LEFT, AND COMMON HEPATIC DUCTS)

Stage	Tumor	Node	Metastasis
I	T1	N0	M0
II	T2a-b	N0	M0
III A	T3	N0	M0
III B	T1-T3	N1	M0
IV A	T4	Any N	M0
IV B	Any T	Any N	M1

M0, no distant metastasis; M1, distant metastasis; N1, regional lymph node metastasis; T1, ductal wall; T2a, beyond ductal wall; T2b, adjacent hepatic parenchyma; T3, unilateral portal vein or hepatic artery branches; T4, main portal vein or branches bilaterally

DISTAL EXTRAHEPATIC BILE DUCTS (FROM CYSTIC DUCT INSERTION INTO COMMON HEPATIC DUCT)

Stage	Tumor	Node	Metastasis
I A	T1	N0	M0
I B	T2	N0	M0
II A	T3	N0	M0
II B	T1-T3	N1	M0
III	T4	Any N	M0
IV	Any T	Any N	M1

From Sobin LH, Gospodarowicz MK, Wittekind CH, editors. International Union Against Cancer (UICC): TNM classification of malignant tumors, 7th ed. Oxford, UK: Wiley-Blackwell, 2009.

M0, no distant metastasis; M1, distant metastasis; N1, regional; T1, ductal wall; T2a, beyond ductal wall; T3, adjacent organs; T4, celiac axis or superior mesenteric artery

Table 58-5 Proposed, Preoperative T-Stage Criteria for Hilar Cholangiocarcinoma

STAGE	CRITERIA
T1	Tumor involving biliary confluence ± unilateral extension to second-order biliary radicles
T2	Tumor involving biliary confluence ± unilateral extension to second-order biliary radicles *and* ipsilateral portal vein involvement ± ipsilateral hepatic lobar atrophy
T3	Tumor involving biliary confluence ± bilateral extension to second-order biliary radicles; *or* unilateral extension to second-order biliary radicles with contralateral portal vein involvement; *or* unilateral extension to second-order biliary radicles with contralateral hepatic lobar atrophy; *or* main or bilateral portal vein involvement

Modified from Jarnagin WR, et al. Staging, resectability, and outcome in 225 patients with hilar cholangiocarcinoma. Ann Surg 2001;234:507–517; discussion 517–519.

Therapy

Surgical resection is a potentially curative treatment for both intrahepatic and extrahepatic CC. For all intrahepatic and most extrahepatic CCs, complete surgical removal of the malignancy necessitates a major hepatectomy. To this end, many patients do not qualify for surgery because of other comorbidities. Unfortunately, more than half of CC patients have advanced unresectable disease. In such cases, palliative therapies (i.e., biliary stenting, PDT) provide symptom relief and may have a positive effect on survival rates.

To date, chemotherapy and/or radiation therapy for CC have not been evaluated in randomized controlled trials, including adjuvant treatment after surgical resection to diminish the risk of recurrence.[3,76] A very small fraction of selected patients with CC may undergo orthotopic liver transplantation (OLT) with curative intent at selected liver transplant centers. **Figure 58-7** provides an algorithm for the management of CC.

Surgical Therapy

Extrahepatic CC

Most extrahepatic CCs involve the biliary bifurcation (i.e., hilar tumors). CC implicating the distal bile ducts usually requires pancreaticoduodenectomy. In this section, we discuss surgical therapy for hilar tumors. Clinical staging of patients with extrahepatic CC is key before considering surgical resection. Jarnagin and colleagues have proposed staging criteria for hilar CC (see **Table 58-5**). These criteria do correlate with tumor resectability (i.e., 60% in stage T1 and 0% in stage T3) and patient survival rates.[77] The evaluation for resectability of extrahepatic CC demands appropriate patient selection and careful assessment of imaging studies. During this assessment process, about one third of patients will be deemed unresectable. Yet 25% to 30% of those who had been considered good candidates for surgical resection will be found to have an unresectable tumor during laparotomy.[78] To this extent, laparoscopy before resection of extrahepatic CC has become the standard surgical approach.

In general, patients with resectable extrahepatic CC require partial hepatic resection to have tumor-free margins. Patients with tumor-free margins have a 20% to 40% 5-year survival rate.[77,79] Other independent prognostic factors for long-term survival rates include lymph node status and the differentiation grade of the tumor.[80] Therefore the primary aim of surgical resection is negative margins proven by a biopsy and local lymph node resection. To achieve this goal for extrahepatic CC, resection of the tumor/extrahepatic bile ducts and subhilar lymphadenopathy is usually needed.[79] Indeed, concurrent en bloc partial hepatectomy is associated with a higher degree of negative resection margins.[77] In a recent study, survival rates of patients with node-negative CC was higher in those with more than seven lymph nodes harvested.[81] Moreover, patients with R1 resection (i.e., positive resection margins) had better survival rates than did unresected patients.[81] Of note, extrahepatic CC involving the biliary confluence almost always engages the main caudate duct and demands caudate lobe removal. Regional lymph node metastases are associated with reduced 3- and 5-year survival rates.[82] However, it is not

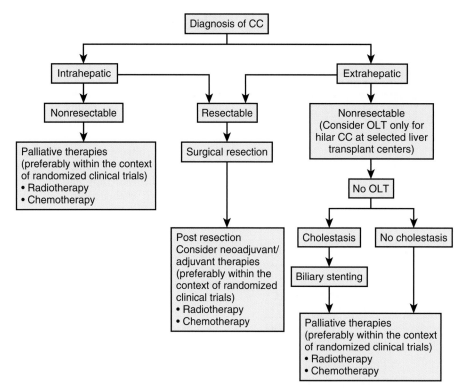

Fig. 58-7 **Overview for the clinical management of cholangiocarcinoma (CC).** OLT, orthotopic liver transplantation.

clear whether extended lymph node resection improves patient survival rates.

Resection of extrahepatic CC is major surgery, with 5% to 10% mortality and notable morbidity, even at medical centers with significant expertise.[79] Preoperative biliary drainage of the liver remnant is recommended if the remnant is less than 30% of the initial organ volume.[83] Postoperative mortality is dominated by infective complications.[77] In addition to curative intent, surgery can be used to palliate obstructive jaundice in extrahepatic CC. This goal can be achieved by choledochojejunostomy or hepaticojejunostomy. Nonetheless, improvements of current endoscopic modalities (i.e., biliary stenting, PDT, brachytherapy), as well as the high cost and morbidity of surgical approaches, have rendered the endoscopic approach a good choice for palliation of jaundice.

Intrahepatic CC

Surgery is also the best option for treatment of intrahepatic CC. In general, intrahepatic CCs are large tumors at the time of diagnosis and patients need major liver resections. Prognostic factors indicating poor outcome after surgical resection of intrahepatic CC are shown in **Table 58-6**. Although tumor metastasis to regional lymph nodes predicts survival, the effect of surgical node dissection on survival rates is unclear. Following surgical resection of intrahepatic CC with negative margins proven by a biopsy, the 1- and 5-year survival rate is 72.4% and 30.4%, respectively.[84]

Palliative Therapeutic Approaches

Many patients with intrahepatic or extrahepatic CC have unresectable disease. Because CC usually affects the elderly,

Table 58-6 Prognostic Factors Associated with Unfavorable Outcome after Surgical Treatment of Intrahepatic Cholangiocarcinoma

Preoperative CA 19-9 levels >1000 U/ml
Multifocal disease
Liver capsule invasion
Lack of cancer-free surgical margins
Regional lymph node metastases
Mass-forming or periductal infiltrating-type CC growth
Expression of mucin 1 (MUC1) by CC cells

CC, cholangiocarcinoma

a notable proportion of surgical candidates have other co-morbidities, which preclude surgical resection of the tumor. Surgical bypass approaches designed to offer palliation of jaundice have been successful but have high operative mortality, morbidity, and cost. Palliative therapy focuses on relieving of obstructive jaundice and/or reducing the tumor bulk, which improves patient symptoms but is less likely to prolong survival time. Although nonsurgical approaches to treat obstructive jaundice can be performed endoscopically or percutaneously, next we discuss endoscopy-based therapies.

Biliary Stents

Amelioration of obstructive jaundice in CC improves patient symptoms and quality of life but not survival rates. Biliary stents are an effective modality in relieving malignant bile duct obstruction with subsequent decline of jaundice. Studies have shown that biliary drainage of only 25% to 30% of the hepatic parenchyma is required to accomplish adequate palliation of obstructive jaundice. In patients with CC, there are several issues to consider before palliative therapy of obstructive jaundice with endoscopic biliary stents.[85] Host parameters (i.e., patient life expectancy, position and degree of biliary obstruction, hepatic lobe atrophy) and the appropriate selection of the type and number of biliary stents (i.e., plastic vs. metallic; single vs. double drainage) are important considerations in optimizing treatment.[85] For example, a jaundiced patient with Bismuth type I hilar CC can be successfully palliated with a single biliary stent. However, there is a lack of consensus among experts for biliary stenting of hilar CC Bismuth types II, III, and IV. In a prospective, randomized controlled trial of patients with hilar CC, it was concluded that unilateral drainage was adequate to alleviate biliary obstruction; moreover, efforts to place a second biliary stent may result in complications (i.e., bacterial cholangitis) without survival rate benefits.[86]

In current clinical practice, MRCP is used to assist with the disease diagnosis and the endoscopic placement of biliary stents to relieve jaundice. Obtaining an MRCP before ERCP helps the endoscopist in choosing the optimal bile ducts for stenting and in avoiding atrophied hepatic segments, thus minimizing the risk of postprocedure cholangitis.[87] Both plastic and metallic biliary stents have been used to alleviate obstruction of extrahepatic CC. Plastic stents are of smaller diameter and become occluded more easily compared with self-expandable metal stents.[85] The latter are also cost effective in patients with CC who are expected to survive for more than 6 months after diagnosis of the malignancy.

Photodynamic Therapy

Photodynamic therapy (PDT) is more suitable for palliation of extrahepatic CC. This therapy is an ablative procedure that involves systemic preadministration of a nontoxic, photosensitizer drug, which accumulates principally within the CC. Subsequently, the patient undergoes ERCP to activate the photosensitizer via direct nonthermal laser application on the tumor. During activation, the drug reaches an excited reactive state (triplet state) and subsequently, energy is transferred from the triplet state of the photosensitizer to molecular oxygen. This event creates singlet molecular oxygen ($^1O_2$), which results in direct or indirect photodamage of the targeted tissue. The photosensitizer agent localizes to mitochondria and induces apoptosis of malignant bile duct cells and other supporting tissues, resulting in tumor regression.

There are several types of photosensitizers. The most commonly used are derivatives of hematoporphyrin, such as porfimer sodium (Photofrin), HpD, and Photosan II. Sodium porfimer is given intravenously at 2 mg/kg. Studies have shown that porfimer enrichment in CC is adequate for employing PDT between days 1 and 4 following intravenous administration. Intraluminal photoactivation is achieved by laser light (wavelength, 630 nm; light dose, 180 J/cm²). The tumoricidal depth penetration of PDT with porfimer is about 4 to 6 mm. A plethora of parameters determine the depth and extent of tissue damage, including the kind and quantity of photosensitizer used, the oxygen concentration in the affected tissue, and the intensity, absorption, and distribution of

Table 58-7 Indications and Contraindications of Photodynamic Therapy for Hilar Cholangiocarcinoma

Indications
Preliminary indication: nonresectable hilar CC with unrelieved cholestasis
Relative indications (i.e., within clinical trials)
Nonresectable hilar CC with successful biliary drainage
Inoperable co-morbid patient with resectable hilar CC
Borderline resectability of hilar CC (neoadjuvant photodynamic therapy for purging of intrahepatic ducts from tumor cells beyond the tumor margins)

Contraindications
Porphyria (all genetic types)
Recent use of photosensitizing or dermatotoxic drugs (e.g., bleomycin)
Insertion of a coated metal stent
Severe hepatic or renal failure
Relative contraindications
Peritoneal carcinomatosis (cholestasis palliated)
Karnofsky performance status <30%
Biliary empyema or liver abscess

Modified from Berr F. Photodynamic therapy for cholangiocarcinoma. Semin Liver Dis 2004;24:177–187.

activating laser light. Indications and contraindications of PDT are shown in **Table 58-7**.

Following injection of porfimer, patients can tolerate artificial room light; however, they must keep out of bright direct or indirect sunlight to prevent phototoxicity of the skin. PDT can produce mild to moderate epigastric pain for up to 3 days after the ERCP. A temporary elevation of aspartate aminotransferase and leukocytosis is expected 2 to 3 days after PDT. Complications of PDT include biloma and hemobilia. Biliary perforations have not been reported and the rate of cholangitis is not increased following PDT compared with placement of biliary stents alone.

Patients should follow specific instructions to "bleach out" the accumulated porfimer in the skin. This goal can be achieved with step-by-step short exposures (5 to 10 minutes) of the skin after day 4 to mild evening sunlight before sunset. If this exposure is endured without skin sunburn, then slow progression of reexposure is suggested until bright sunlight can be tolerated.

Pilot nonrandomized studies of PDT for unresectable CC have demonstrated promising results on: (1) prompt improvement of cholestasis; (2) stabilization of the Karnofsky performance status at almost normal or moderately diminished rates; and (3) improvement or preservation of quality of life.[88] A multicenter prospective randomized trial from Europe evaluated the effect of biliary stenting followed by PDT (group A) compared with biliary stenting alone (group B) in patients with unresectable CC.[89] Patients in group A demonstrated prolonged survival (n = 20; median survival, 493 days; 95% confidence interval [CI], 276 to 710) compared with patients in group B (n = 19; median survival, 98 days; 95% CI, 87 to 107) (P <.0001).[89] Of interest, this study failed to improve biliary obstruction and jaundice in the second group (sole bile duct stenting), as expected. Thus it is likely that the survival rate benefit reported in the first group (biliary stenting and PDT) relates to amelioration of cholestasis rather than tumor burden.[90] In a recent retrospective study from the United States, there was a significant increase in the survival rate in the PDT group (16.2 + 2.4 months) compared with the biliary stent group (7.4 ± 1.6 months). Nevertheless, more prospective randomized trials on PDT for unresectable extrahepatic CC, including patients with concurrent PSC, are needed to further assess the utility of this promising approach.

Intraluminal Brachytherapy

The assumption is that this intraluminal approach permits focal, higher, and more effective doses of radiation compared with external beam radiation therapy (EBRT). In the course of intraluminal brachytherapy (IB), premounted iridium-192 seeds are deployed within a catheter and placed across the neoplastic biliary stricture(s) during ERCP or PTC.[91,92] IB should extend the palliation of obstructive jaundice and avoid unnecessary radiation damage of the surrounding tissues and organs. To date, the therapeutic effects of IB on CC are unclear.[92,93] Additional studies are necessary to evaluate this palliative approach.

Other Palliative Therapies

To reduce the tumor bulk and to improve symptoms, systemic chemotherapy with gemcitabine-based regimens[94] and radioembolization with yttrium-90 microspheres[95] have been used. Indeed, gemcitabine alone or in combination with cisplatin is associated with improved control of advanced or metastatic CC.[94] The response rate to these therapies are not well studied. More therapeutic trials are needed to address the effectiveness of these palliative treatments.

Liver Transplantation for Unresectable CC

Former experience with OLT for CC was disappointing.[96] Recurrence of the malignancy was very common and the 5-year survival rates were only 5% to 15%. As a result, most liver transplant centers considered CC a contraindication for OLT. Nevertheless, a selected group of patients who underwent OLT and had negative surgical resection margins and negative regional lymph nodes demonstrated long-term survival.[97] Moreover, in a small number of patients treated with radiation and brachytherapy plus 5-fluorouracil, the observed 5-year survival rate was 22%.[98] Because of these favorable observations, in 1993 we developed an experimental liver transplant protocol for therapy of selected patients with early-stage unresectable hilar CC or CC arising in the background of PSC. For patients to be enrolled into the protocol, they have to be diagnosed with CC based on either biopsy, biliary brush cytology, or aneuploidy of biliary epithelia. If the malignancy forms a mass lesion, the diameter had to be less than 3 cm on cross-sectional imaging studies. Furthermore, the CC has to be deemed unresectable surgically after evaluation by an experienced hepatobiliary team. Tumor vascular encasement causing absence of blood flow without evidence of vessel invasion is not a contraindication to enrollment.

Enrolled patients have to be suitable for radiation therapy, chemotherapy, and liver transplantation, as determined by the interdisciplinary team. Patients who meet eligible criteria receive neoadjuvant chemotherapy and radiation therapy.

EBRT (at a total dose of 4500 cGy in 30 sessions) is completed in 3 weeks. 5-fluorouracil is given intravenously at 500 mg/m^2 daily as bolus for 3 consecutive days in the beginning of EBRT. ERBT can cause nausea, vomiting, leukopenia, cholangitis, gastrointestinal ulceration, and liver abscess. Following completion of ERBT, patients receive brachytherapy of the tumor using a transcatheter loaded with ^{192}iridium seeds (total dose, 2000 to 3000 cGy). In the course of brachytherapy, they are also treated with 5-fluorouracil at 225 mg/m^2 daily. Subsequently, patients continue to receive the above dose of 5-fluorouracil or capecitabine (2000 mg/m^2 daily) for 2 of 3 weeks until liver transplantation is performed. Once neoadjuvant chemoradiation therapy is finished, patients undergo staging laparotomy, which includes biopsy of regional lymph nodes. Patients with negative staging proceed with OLT. Cadaveric livers or living donor right liver grafts can be used. Transplanted patients receive standard immunosuppression therapy.

Between 1993 and 2008, 148 patients with CC were enrolled in this protocol at the Mayo Clinic in Rochester, Minn. Thirty-nine patients were removed from the protocol because of disease progression or death.[99] Ninety patients have undergone OLT, of whom 19 died following OLT and 71 are currently alive. The patient survival rate following liver transplantation was 90% at 1 year and 71% at 5 years.[99] The outcome of patients on our liver transplant protocol for CC exceeds the outcome of surgical resection with curative intent, which is considered the standard therapy for CC. Liver transplant protocols for CC have been developed at other medical centers.[100,101] A recent study suggests that negative ^{18}F-fluorodeoxyglucose (FDG) PET predicts recurrence-free survival after OLT without the need for chemo-radiation before transplant.[102]

Future Therapeutic Directions

Given the increasing incidence of intrahepatic CC, progress has to be made to improve the survival rate of patients afflicted with this devastating disease. Currently, no survival benefit has been attained in patients with CC treated with chemotherapy and/or radiation therapy.[3,103] Better staging systems and randomized, controlled clinical trials are needed to evaluate the usefulness of novel therapeutic agents and/or radiation therapy.[75] As our understanding of the pathogenesis of CC improves, we expect that better pharmacologic inhibitors will be available in treating these tumors, alone or in combination with chemotherapeutic agents.

Key References

Ahrendt SA, et al. Chromosome 9p21 loss and p16 inactivation in primary sclerosing cholangitis-associated cholangiocarcinoma. J Surg Res 1999;84: 88–93. (Ref.48)

Aishima SI, et al. C-erbB-2 and c-Met expression relates to cholangiocarcinogenesis and progression of intrahepatic cholangiocarcinoma. Histopathology 2002;40:269–278. (Ref.30)

Ashida K, Terada T, Kitamura Y. Expression of E-cadherin, alpha-catenin, beta-catenin, and CD44 (standard and variant isoforms) in human cholangiocarcinoma: an immunohistochemical study. Hepatology 1998;27:974–982. (Ref.107)

Benckert C, et al. Transforming growth factor beta 1 stimulates vascular endothelial growth factor gene transcription in human cholangiocellular carcinoma cells. Cancer Res 2003;63:1083–1092. (Ref.57)

Bergquist A, Broome U. Hepatobiliary and extra-hepatic malignancies in primary sclerosing cholangitis. Best Pract Res Clin Gastroenterol 2001;15: 643–656. (Ref.14)

Berr F. Photodynamic therapy for cholangiocarcinoma. Semin Liver Dis 2004;24:177–187. (Ref.88)

Blechacz B, Gores GJ. Cholangiocarcinoma: advances in pathogenesis, diagnosis, and treatment. Hepatology 2008;48:308–321. (Ref.1)

Blechacz BR, Sanchez W, Gores GJ. A conceptual proposal for staging ductal cholangiocarcinoma. Curr Opin Gastroenterol 2009;25:238–239. (Ref.75)

Boccaccio C, et al. Hepatocyte growth factor (HGF) receptor expression is inducible and is part of the delayed-early response to HGF. J Biol Chem 1994;269:12846–12851. (Ref.28)

Breitenstein S, Apestegui C, Clavien PA. Positron emission tomography (PET) for cholangiocarcinoma. HPB (Oxford) 2008;10:120–121. (Ref.72)

Broome U, et al. Natural history and prognostic factors in 305 Swedish patients with primary sclerosing cholangitis. Gut 1996;38:610–615. (Ref.15)

Bruha R, et al. Intraluminal brachytherapy and self-expandable stents in nonresectable biliary malignancies: the question of long-term palliation. Hepatogastroenterology 2001;48:631–637. (Ref.92)

Buys CH. Telomeres, telomerase, and cancer. N Engl J Med 2000;342:1282–1283. (Ref.53)

Carriaga MT, Henson DE. Liver, gallbladder, extrahepatic bile ducts, and pancreas. Cancer 1995;75:171–190. (Ref.13)

Chariyalertsak S, et al. Aberrant cyclooxygenase isozyme expression in human intrahepatic cholangiocarcinoma. Gut 2001;48:80–86. (Ref.36)

Cong WM, et al. Multiple genetic alterations involved in the tumorigenesis of human cholangiocarcinoma: a molecular genetic and clinicopathological study. J Cancer Res Clin Oncol 2001;127:187–192. (Ref.47)

De Palma GD, et al. Unilateral versus bilateral endoscopic hepatic duct drainage in patients with malignant hilar biliary obstruction: results of a prospective, randomized, and controlled study. Gastrointest Endosc 2001;53:547–553. (Ref.86)

De Palma GD, et al. Unilateral placement of metallic stents for malignant hilar obstruction: a prospective study. Gastrointest Endosc 2003;58:50–53. (Ref.87)

Eloubeidi MA, et al. Endoscopic ultrasound-guided fine needle aspiration biopsy of suspected cholangiocarcinoma. Clin Gastroenterol Hepatol 2004;2:209–213. (Ref.70)

Endo K, et al. E-cadherin gene mutations in human intrahepatic cholangiocarcinoma. J Pathol 2001;193:310–317. (Ref.58)

Endo K, et al. ERBB-2 overexpression and cyclooxygenase-2 up-regulation in human cholangiocarcinoma and risk conditions. Hepatology 2002;36:439–450. (Ref.37)

Evan GI, Vousden KH. Proliferation, cell cycle and apoptosis in cancer. Nature 2001;411:342–348. (Ref.45)

Everhart JE, Ruhl CE. Burden of digestive diseases in the United States part I: overall and upper gastrointestinal diseases. Gastroenterology 2009;136: 376–386. (Ref.7)

Everhart JE, Ruhl CE. Burden of digestive diseases in the United States part II: lower gastrointestinal diseases. Gastroenterology 2009;136:741–754. (Ref.8)

Everhart JE, Ruhl CE. Burden of digestive diseases in the United States part III: liver, biliary tract, and pancreas. Gastroenterology 2009;136:1134–1144. (Ref.9)

Foo ML, Gunderson LL, Bender CE, External radiation therapy and transcatheter iridium in the treatment of extrahepatic bile duct carcinoma. Int J Radiat Oncol Biol Phys 1997;39:929–935. (Ref.98)

Fritcher EG, et al. A multivariable model using advanced cytologic methods for the evaluation of indeterminate pancreatobiliary strictures. Gastroenterology 2009;136:2180–2186. (Ref.68)

Fuks D, et al. Biliary drainage, photodynamic therapy and chemotherapy for unresectable cholangiocarcinoma with jaundice. J Gastroenterol Hepatol 2009;24:1745–1752. (Ref.76)

Furubo S, et al. Protein expression and genetic alterations of p53 and ras in intrahepatic cholangiocarcinoma. Histopathology 1999;35:230–240. (Ref.104)

Gerhards MF, et al. Results of postoperative radiotherapy for resectable hilar cholangiocarcinoma. World J Surg 2003;27:173–179. (Ref.93)

Gores GJ. A spotlight on cholangiocarcinoma. Gastroenterology 2003;125: 1536–1538. (Ref.90)

Gores GJ. Cholangiocarcinoma: current concepts and insights. Hepatology 2003;37:961–969. (Ref.103)

Gores GJ. Early detection and treatment of cholangiocarcinoma. Liver Transpl 2000;6:S30–S34. (Ref.73)

Harada K, Terada T, Nakanuma Y. Detection of transforming growth factor-alpha protein and messenger RNA in hepatobiliary diseases by immunohistochemical and in situ hybridization techniques. Hum Pathol 1996;27:787–792. (Ref.31)

Harnois DM, et al. Bcl-2 is overexpressed and alters the threshold for apoptosis in a cholangiocarcinoma cell line. Hepatology 1997;26:884–890. (Ref.105)

Heinrich PC, et al. Principles of interleukin (IL)-6-type cytokine signalling and its regulation. Biochem J 2003;374:1–20. (Ref.26)

Hengartner MO. The biochemistry of apoptosis. Nature 2000;407:770–776. (Ref.49)

Ibrahim SM, et al. Treatment of unresectable cholangiocarcinoma using yttrium-90 microspheres: results from a pilot study. Cancer 2008;113: 2119–2128. (Ref.95)

Ince N, et al. Overexpression of human aspartyl (asparaginyl) beta-hydroxylase is associated with malignant transformation. Cancer Res 2000;60:1261–1266. (Ref.61)

Isa T, et al. Analysis of microsatellite instability, K-ras gene mutation and p53 protein overexpression in intrahepatic cholangiocarcinoma. Hepatogastroenterology 2002;49:604–608. (Ref.44)

Ito Y, et al. Expression and clinical significance of the erbB family in intrahepatic cholangiocellular carcinoma. Pathol Res Pract 2001;197:95–100. (Ref.32)

Itoi T, et al. Detection of telomerase reverse transcriptase mRNA in biopsy specimens and bile for diagnosis of biliary tract cancers. Int J Mol Med 2001;7:281–287. (Ref.56)

Itoi T, et al. Detection of telomerase activity in biopsy specimens for diagnosis of biliary tract cancers. Gastrointest Endosc 2000;52:380–386. (Ref.55)

Jarnagin WR, et al. Staging, resectability, and outcome in 225 patients with hilar cholangiocarcinoma. Ann Surg 2001;234:507–517; discussion 517–519. (Ref.77)

Jemal A, et al. Cancer statistics, 2003. CA Cancer J Clin 2003;53:5–26. (Ref.6)

Jonas S, et al. Extended liver resection for intrahepatic cholangiocarcinoma: a comparison of the prognostic accuracy of the fifth and sixth editions of the TNM classification. Ann Surg 2009;249:303–309. (Ref.84)

Kaiser GM, et al. Liver transplantation for hilar cholangiocarcinoma: a German survey. Transplant Proc 2008;40:3191–3193. (Ref.101)

Kang YK, et al. Mutation of p53 and K-ras, and loss of heterozygosity of APC in intrahepatic cholangiocarcinoma. Lab Invest 1999;79:477–483. (Ref.39)

Kennedy TJ, et al. Role of preoperative biliary drainage of liver remnant prior to extended liver resection for hilar cholangiocarcinoma. HPB (Oxford) 2009;11:445–451. (Ref.83)

Khan SA, et al. Guidelines for the diagnosis and treatment of cholangiocarcinoma: consensus document. Gut 2002;51(Suppl 6):vi1–vi9. (Ref.3)

Khan SA, et al. Changing international trends in mortality rates for liver, biliary and pancreatic tumours. J Hepatol 2002;37:806–813. (Ref.11)

Khan SA, Toledano MB, Taylor-Robinson SD. Epidemiology, risk factors, and pathogenesis of cholangiocarcinoma. HPB (Oxford) 2008;10:77–82. (Ref.5)

Kiguchi K, et al. Constitutive expression of ErbB-2 in gallbladder epithelium results in development of adenocarcinoma. Cancer Res 2001;61:6971–6976. (Ref.34)

Kitagawa Y, et al. Lymph node metastasis from hilar cholangiocarcinoma: audit of 110 patients who underwent regional and paraaortic node dissection. Ann Surg 2001;233:385–392. (Ref.82)

Kloek JJ, et al. Surgery for extrahepatic cholangiocarcinoma: predictors of survival. HPB (Oxford) 2008;10:190–195. (Ref.80)

Kornberg A, et al. Recurrence-free long-term survival after liver transplantation in patients with 18F-FDG non-avid hilar cholangiocarcinoma on PET. Am J Transplant 2009;9:2631–2636. (Ref.102)

Lai GH, et al. Unique epithelial cell production of hepatocyte growth factor/ scatter factor by putative precancerous intestinal metaplasias and associated "intestinal-type" biliary cancer chemically induced in rat liver. Hepatology 2000;31:1257–1265. (Ref.29)

Lavaissiere L, et al. Overexpression of human aspartyl(asparaginyl)beta-hydroxylase in hepatocellular carcinoma and cholangiocarcinoma. J Clin Invest 1996;98:1313–1323. (Ref.60)

Lee CH, et al. Viral hepatitis-associated intrahepatic cholangiocarcinoma shares common disease processes with hepatocellular carcinoma. Br J Cancer 2009;100:1765–1770. (Ref.21)

Levine AJ. p53, the cellular gatekeeper for growth and division. Cell 1997;88:323–331. (Ref.46)

Levy MJ, et al. Palliation of malignant extrahepatic biliary obstruction with plastic versus expandable metal stents: an evidence-based approach. Clin Gastroenterol Hepatol 2004;2:273–285. (Ref.85)

Liu D, et al. Microsatellite instability in Thorotrast-induced human intrahepatic cholangiocarcinoma. Int J Cancer 2002;102:366–371. (Ref.19)

Maeda T, et al. Antisense oligodeoxynucleotides directed against aspartyl (asparaginyl) beta-hydroxylase suppress migration of cholangiocarcinoma cells. J Hepatol 2003;38:615–622. (Ref.62)

Manfredi R, et al. Magnetic resonance imaging of cholangiocarcinoma. Semin Liver Dis 2004;24:155–164. (Ref.71)

Matsumoto K, et al. Human biliary epithelial cells secrete and respond to cytokines and hepatocyte growth factors in vitro: interleukin-6, hepatocyte growth factor and epidermal growth factor promote DNA synthesis in vitro. Hepatology 1994;20:376–382. (Ref.22)

Meyer CG, Penn I, James L. Liver transplantation for cholangiocarcinoma: results in 207 patients. Transplantation 2000;69:1633–1637. (Ref.96)

Montemaggi P, et al. Intraluminal brachytherapy in the treatment of pancreas and bile duct carcinoma. Int J Radiat Oncol Biol Phys 1995;32:437–443. (Ref.91)

Moreno Luna LE, et al. Advanced cytologic techniques for the detection of malignant pancreatobiliary strictures. Gastroenterology 2006;131:1064–1072. (Ref.69)

Nathan H, et al. A proposed staging system for intrahepatic cholangiocarcinoma. Ann Surg Oncol 2009;16:14–22. (Ref.74)

Nzeako UC, et al. COX-2 inhibits Fas-mediated apoptosis in cholangiocarcinoma cells. Hepatology 2002;35:552–559. (Ref.52)

Okaro AC, et al. The expression of antiapoptotic proteins Bcl-2, Bcl-X(L), and Mcl-1 in benign, dysplastic, and malignant biliary epithelium. J Clin Pathol 2001;54:927–932. (Ref.106)

Ortner ME, et al. Successful photodynamic therapy for nonresectable cholangiocarcinoma: a randomized prospective study. Gastroenterology 2003;125:1355–1363. (Ref.89)

Park J, et al. Inhibition of interleukin 6-mediated mitogen-activated protein kinase activation attenuates growth of a cholangiocarcinoma cell line. Hepatology 1999;30:1128–1133. (Ref.23)

Patel T. Increasing incidence and mortality of primary intrahepatic cholangiocarcinoma in the United States. Hepatology 2001;33:1353–1357. (Ref.12)

Que FG, et al. Cholangiocarcinomas express Fas ligand and disable the Fas receptor. Hepatology 1999;30:1398–1404. (Ref.50)

Rea DJ, et al. Major hepatic resection for hilar cholangiocarcinoma: analysis of 46 patients. Arch Surg 2004;139:514–523; discussion 523–525. (Ref.79)

Rocha FG, et al. Hilar cholangiocarcinoma: the Memorial Sloan-Kettering Cancer Center experience. J Hepatobiliary Pancreat Surg 2010;17:490–496. (Ref.81)

Rosen CB, Heimbach JK, Gores GJ. Surgery for cholangiocarcinoma: the role of liver transplantation. HPB (Oxford) 2008;10:186–189. (Ref.99)

Schlessinger J. Ligand-induced, receptor-mediated dimerization and activation of EGF receptor. Cell 2002;110:669–672. (Ref.33)

Shaib Y, El-Serag HB. The epidemiology of cholangiocarcinoma. Semin Liver Dis 2004;24:115–125. (Ref.2)

Shaib YH, et al. Rising incidence of intrahepatic cholangiocarcinoma in the United States: a true increase? J Hepatol 2004;40:472–477. (Ref.4)

Shaib YH, et al. Risk factors of intrahepatic cholangiocarcinoma in the United States: a case-control study. Gastroenterology 2005;128:620–626. (Ref.20)

Shay JW, Bacchetti S. A survey of telomerase activity in human cancer. Eur J Cancer 1997;33:787–791. (Ref.54)

Shimoda M, et al. Liver transplantation for cholangiocellular carcinoma: analysis of a single-center experience and review of the literature. Liver Transpl 2001;7:1023–1033. (Ref.97)

Shimonishi T, et al. Up-regulation of Fas ligand at early stages and down-regulation of Fas at progressed stages of intrahepatic cholangiocarcinoma

reflect evasion from immune surveillance. Hepatology 2000;32:761–769. (Ref.38)

Simeone D. Gallbladder and biliary tree: anatomy and structural anomalies. In: Yamada T, editor. Textbook of gastroenterology. Philadelphia: Lippincott, 1999: 2244–2257. (Ref.17)

Sudan D, et al. Radiochemotherapy and transplantation allow long-term survival for nonresectable hilar cholangiocarcinoma. Am J Transplant 2002;2:774–779. (Ref.100)

Sugawara H, et al. Relationship between interleukin-6 and proliferation and differentiation in cholangiocarcinoma. Histopathology 1998;33:145–153. (Ref.27)

Tanaka S, et al. Human WISP1v, a member of the CCN family, is associated with invasive cholangiocarcinoma. Hepatology 2003;37:1122–1129. (Ref.63)

Tannapfel A, et al. Frequency of p16(INK4A) alterations and K-ras mutations in intrahepatic cholangiocarcinoma of the liver. Gut 2000;47:721–727. (Ref.40)

Terada T, Okada Y, Nakanuma Y. Expression of immunoreactive matrix metalloproteinases and tissue inhibitors of matrix metalloproteinases in human normal livers and primary liver tumors. Hepatology 1996;23: 1341–1344. (Ref.59)

Torok NJ, et al. Nitric oxide inhibits apoptosis downstream of cytochrome C release by nitrosylating caspase 9. Cancer Res 2002;62:1648–1653. (Ref.51)

Valle JW, et al. Gemcitabine alone or in combination with cisplatin in patients with advanced or metastatic cholangiocarcinomas or other biliary tract tumours: a multicentre randomised phase II study—the UK ABC-01 study. Br J Cancer 2009;101:621–627. (Ref.94)

Vestergaard EM, et al. Reference values and biological variation for tumor marker CA 19-9 in serum for different Lewis and secretor genotypes and evaluation of secretor and Lewis genotyping in a Caucasian population. Clin Chem 1999;45:54–61. (Ref.65)

Weber SM, et al. Staging laparoscopy in patients with extrahepatic biliary carcinoma. Analysis of 100 patients. Ann Surg 2002;235:392–399. (Ref.78)

Welzel TM, et al. Impact of classification of hilar cholangiocarcinomas (Klatskin tumors) on the incidence of intra- and extrahepatic cholangiocarcinoma in the United States. J Natl Cancer Inst 2006;98:873–875. (Ref.10)

Yokomuro S, et al. The effect of interleukin-6 (IL-6)/gp130 signalling on biliary epithelial cell growth, in vitro. Cytokine 2000;12:727–730. (Ref.25)

Yokomuro S, et al. Growth control of human biliary epithelial cells by interleukin 6, hepatocyte growth factor, transforming growth factor beta1, and activin A: comparison of a cholangiocarcinoma cell line with primary cultures of non-neoplastic biliary epithelial cells. Hepatology 2000;32:26–35. (Ref.24)

Yoon JH, et al. Bile acids induce cyclooxygenase-2 expression via the epidermal growth factor receptor in a human cholangiocarcinoma cell line. Gastroenterology 2002;122:985–993. (Ref.43)

Yoon JH, et al. Bile acids inhibit Mcl-1 protein turnover via an epidermal growth factor receptor/Raf-1-dependent mechanism. Cancer Res 2002;62:6500–6505. (Ref.42)

A complete list of references can be found at www.expertconsult.com.

Benign Liver Tumors

Massimo Colombo, Massimo Iavarone, and Riccardo Lencioni

ABBREVIATIONS

AFP α-fetoprotein	**GGT** γ-glutamyl transpeptidase	**IL-6** interleukin-6
APC adenomatous polyposis coli	**HA** hepatocellular adenoma	**MRI** magnetic resonance imaging
CEA carcinoembryonic antigen	**HCC** hepatocellular carcinoma	**NRH** nodular regenerative hyperplasia
CRP C-reactive protein	**HNF-1α** hepatocyte nuclear factor-1α	**RES** reticuloendothelial system
CT computed tomography	**HUMARA** human androgen receptor assay	**SAA** serum amyloid protein
FNH focal nodular hyperplasia		**SPECT** single-photon emission CT

Introduction

Benign liver tumors are a heterogeneous group of nodular lesions that originate from different cell lines. Such tumors include hemangiomas, which are the most common benign nodes found in the liver, and hepatocellular neoplasms, which are clinically more relevant lesions (**Table 59-1**). For hepatocellular lesions, a descriptive nomenclature was set forward by an international panel of experts sponsored by the World Congress of Gastroenterology in 1994.[1] This chapter focuses on hemangioma, focal nodular hyperplasia (FNH), hepatocellular adenoma (HA), and nodular regenerative hyperplasia (NRH). These lesions have gained increased recognition following the widespread use of imaging tests, which has led to the identification of an increased number of affected patients. As far as HA is concerned, a molecular classification has recently been proposed that has changed our understanding of this condition, particularly with respect to diagnosis and prognosis.

Hepatic Hemangioma

Hepatic hemangiomas are benign vascular tumors of the liver and the second most common liver mass after metastatic cancer.

Epidemiology

Hemangiomas affect 1% to 2% of the general population and are typically discovered incidentally during evaluation for nonspecific abdominal complaints.[2,3] The reported female/male gender ratios range from 1.6:1 to 6:1. The prevalence of hemangioma has been overestimated in autopsy series (from 2% to as high as 20%) because of overrepresentation of elderly patients with co-morbid illnesses[4-7] (**Table 59-2**). The majority of hemangiomas are small (<4 cm). Liver nodes larger than 4 cm in size are defined as cavernous hemangiomas.

Pathogenesis

The pathogenesis of hemangioma is unknown, but congenital hamartoma is a likely candidate. A pathogenic role of sex hormones has been postulated because of consistent predominance of larger tumors in females, tumor enlargement/recurrence in hysterectomized women undergoing estrogen replacement therapy, and development of tumors in women with long-term use of oral contraceptives.[8] Cavernous hemangiomas may exhibit accelerated growth during pregnancy and often display estrogen receptors. However, tumor growth was also induced or influenced by such drugs as metaclopramide.[9]

Pathology

Macroscopically, hepatic hemangiomas are ovoid, soft, reddish-purple or blue masses separated from the surrounding parenchyma by a fibrous pseudocapsule. Varying degrees of fibrosis, hyalinization, calcification, thrombosis, and shrinking are seen. Extensive fibrosis and hyalinization with narrowing or obliteration of vessels are typical of sclerosed hemangiomas. Microscopically, hemangiomas are vascular abnormalities characterized by multiple blood-filled sinusoidal spaces and vascular lakes lined by endothelial cells. Vascular channels are separated by fibrous tissue. They are fed by branches of the hepatic artery, and their internal circulation is slow. Blood vessels and arteriovenous shunting may be seen in large septa. The tumors seem to grow by ectasia rather than by hyperplasia or hypertrophy.[8]

Clinical Features

Characteristically, hemangioma is an incidental finding on hepatic imaging (**Table 59-3**), and the majority of patients have a single tumor node (**Table 59-4**). However, a few patients may have isolated diffuse hemangiomatosis, and this condition may occur in association with Rendu-Osler-Weber disease or skeletal hemangiomatosis.[8] Cavernous hemangiomas are typically silent, clinically benign, and rarely expanding or symptomatic tumors. The few patients with symptoms complain of one of the following: abdominal swelling, abdominal pain, early satiety, anorexia, abdominal mass, and hepatomegaly. The presence of symptoms correlated with the size of hemangiomas in one study[13] but not in another.[5] In addition, there seems to be no correlation between symptoms and the number of tumors. Atypical hemangiomas exist and form arteriovenous shunts that may cause severe symptoms, including heart failure.[14] Other unusual clinical manifestations of hepatic hemangioma include hemobilia, inflammatory pseudotumor caused by recurrent intranodal thrombosis, caval thrombosis, portal hypertension, and torsion of a pedunculated tumor.

Table 59-1 Classification of Benign Nodular Lesions of the Liver

Hepatocellular	Regenerative lesions: 　Monoacinar regenerative nodule 　Diffuse nodular hyperplasia without 　　fibrous septa (nodular regenerative 　　hyperplasia) 　Diffuse nodular hyperplasia with fibrous 　　septa or in cirrhosis 　Multiacinar regenerative nodule 　Lobar or segmental hyperplasia 　Focal nodular hyperplasia Dysplastic or neoplastic lesions: 　Hepatocellular adenoma 　Dysplastic focus 　Dysplastic nodule
Biliary	Bile duct adenoma Biliary hamartoma Biliary cystoadenoma Biliary papillomatosis
Vascular	Hemangioma Infantile hemangioendothelioma Hereditary hemorrhagic telangiectasia Lymphangiomatosis
Mesenchymal	Leiomyoma Lipoma Myelolymphoma Angiomyolipoma Pseudolymphoma Fibrous mesothelioma Hamartoma Benign teratoma

Table 59-3 Clinical Findings Leading to Diagnosis in Patients with a Liver Hemangioma

CLUES TO DIAGNOSIS	TERKIVATAN ET AL.,[10] 2001 (N = 103)	WEIMANN ET AL.,[11] 1997 (N = 238)	FARGES ET AL.,[12] 1995 (N = 163)
Incidental	64 (62%)	114 (48%)	38 (23%)
Abdominal pain	24 (23%)	99 (42%)	87 (53%)
Suspected metastases	4 (4%)	7 (3%)	25 (15%)
Palpable mass	2 (2%)	5 (2%)	0
Nonspecific complaints	9 (9%)	13 (5%)	13 (8%)

Table 59-4 Clinical Features and Characteristics of Hemangiomas Detected in 123 Patients Undergoing Screening with Abdominal Ultrasound

No. of males	41 (33%)
Patients age (yr)	56 (20-79)

NO. OF TUMORS	TUMOR SIZE (cm)
1	93 (75%)
2	26 (21%)
>2	4 (4%)
<2	75 (61%)
2-5	31 (25%)
>5	17 (14%)

From Gandolfi L, et al. Natural history of hepatic haemangiomas: clinical and ultrasound study. Gut 1991;32:677–680.

Table 59-2 Prevalence of Hemangiomas in Population-Based Screening Programs with Abdominal Ultrasound and Autopsy Series

TYPE OF STUDY	AUTHOR	NO. OF PATIENTS	PREVALENCE OF HEMANGIOMA (%)
Population studies	Lu et al.,[2] 1990	923	1.4
	Gandolfi et al.,[3] 1991	21,280	1.4
Autopsy series	Karhunen,[4] 1986	95	20.0
	Reddy and Schiff,[5] 1993	256	6.1
	Rubin and Mitchell,[6] 1996	284	5.2
	Dodd et al.,[7] 1999	508	1.7

Diagnosis

Liver function test results are typically normal in patients with hemangiomas. A few patients with cavernous hemangiomas may have coagulopathy (i.e., thrombocytopenia, hypofibrinogenemia).[15] Fine-needle aspiration biopsy is considered reasonably safe in patients with hepatic hemangiomas, as long as the aspiration route is through a layer of normal liver tissue, but it lacks sensitivity. The aspirate consists mainly of blood with only a few noncharacteristic spindle cells of benign appearance. In 36 consecutive fine-needle aspiration biopsies of liver hemangiomas in Helsinki, a cytologic diagnosis of hemangioma was obtained in 21 (58%). One patient (3%) had uneventful intraperitoneal bleeding after the aspiration.[16] The sensitivity of percutaneous biopsy (microhistology) for the diagnosis of hemangioma is higher (75% to 91%), with a specificity of 100%.[17]

Imaging Findings
Ultrasound and Contrast-Enhanced Ultrasound

The most common ultrasound appearance of hemangioma is a sharply demarcated lesion with uniformly increased echogenicity relative to normal liver tissue (**Fig. 59-1**). This pattern is observed in about 70% of hemangiomas detected by ultrasound. The remaining cases show atypical ultrasound patterns and appear either as hypoechoic lesions with a hyperechoic border or as lesions with heterogeneous internal structure.[18] Heterogeneity is commonly observed in large hemangiomas.

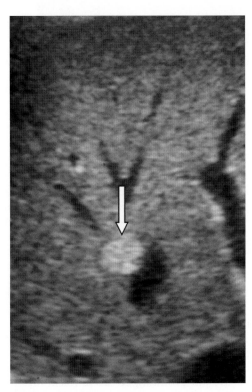

Fig. 59-1 Hemangioma, ultrasound appearance. The lesion shows typical features and appears as a round, well-defined, hyperechoic nodule (arrow).

Although no vascular patterns can be used to reliably diagnose hemangioma on conventional color or power Doppler ultrasound, early clinical experience with ultrasound contrast agents has suggested that contrast-enhanced ultrasound can provide useful information.[19,20] Most liver hemangiomas (78% to 93%) show peripheral nodular enhancement during the early phase of the contrast-enhanced study, with progressive centripetal fill-in.[21] Diffuse contrast enhancement with homogeneous fill-in or a persistent hypoechoic appearance because of absent contrast enhancement can be observed in small, high-flow hemangiomas or thrombosed hemangiomas, respectively.[21]

Computed Tomography

The standard spiral computed tomography (CT) protocol for suspected hemangioma includes baseline and contrast-enhanced scans in the arterial, portal venous, and delayed phases. Most hemangiomas appear hypoattenuating on baseline scans, show peripheral nodular enhancement or vascular attenuation on arterial and portal phase imaging, and are hyperattenuating with possible central hypoattenuation or isoattenuation relative to vascular spaces in the delayed phase. This pattern has a sensitivity of 67% to 86% and a specificity of 99% to 100% for the diagnosis of hemangioma.[22,23] Atypical features on CT are observed in hemangiomas with either high flow or very slow flow. High-flow hemangiomas show rapid filling after the administration of contrast material, which results in homogeneous enhancement during the hepatic arterial or portal venous phase.[23] This feature is relatively common in small hemangiomas. Differentiation of high-flow hemangiomas from hypervascular malignant tumors may be difficult and relies on attenuation equivalent to that of the aorta during all phases of CT, including the delayed phase. Very slow-flow hemangiomas appear either as nonenhancing lesions or as lesions with weak peripheral enhancement without centripetal progression. These features may be related to thrombosis or abundant fibrosis and mimic a hypovascular malignant tumor.

Magnetic Resonance Imaging

The magnetic resonance imaging (MRI) protocol for characterizing suspected hemangiomas includes gradient-echo T1-weighted sequences, fast-spin-echo T2-weighted sequences with short and long (>200 ms) echo times, and serial dynamic gadolinium-enhanced gradient-echo T1-weighted sequences. Hemangiomas appear as homogeneous focal lesions with smooth, well-defined margins. The lesion is hypointense with respect to liver parenchyma on T1-weighted images and strongly hyperintense relative to liver parenchyma on T2-weighted images. The high signal intensity on heavily T2-weighted (long echo time) MRI gives hemangiomas a consistent "light bulb" pattern with 100% sensitivity and 92% diagnostic specificity.[24] Dynamic contrast-enhanced MRI shows quite a typical perfusion pattern in hemangiomas: peripheral nodular enhancement in the early phase with centripetal progression to uniform or almost uniform enhancement during the portal venous and delayed phases (**Fig. 59-2**). Such a characteristic enhancement pattern has a sensitivity of 77% to 91% and a specificity of 100% for the diagnosis of hemangioma.[25,26] However, very small (<1.5 cm), high-flow hemangiomas frequently exhibit a hypervascular pattern with uniform enhancement in the arterial phase that may persist

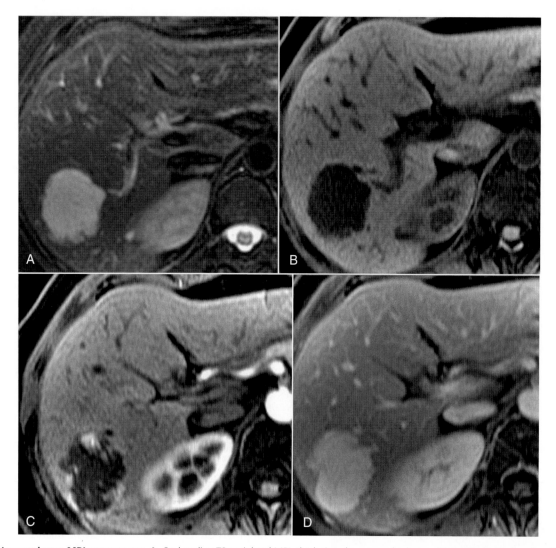

Fig. 59-2 **Hemangioma, MRI appearance. A,** On baseline T2-weighted MRI, the lesion shows very high signal intensity. **B,** On baseline T1-weighted MRI, the hemangioma is hypointense in relation to surrounding liver parenchyma. **C,** During the arterial phase of the contrast-enhanced dynamic study, the lesion shows peripheral globular enhancement. **D,** In the delayed phase, complete homogeneous enhancement is observed within the lesion.

into the portal venous and delayed phases (**Fig. 59-3**).[26] In these cases, diagnostic assessment may be difficult and requires careful analysis of baseline and contrast-enhanced images. Hemangiomas show a peculiar feature after the injection of MRI agents that target the reticuloendothelial system (RES): hyperintensity on T1-weighted, contrast-enhanced images. This is due to the T1 effect of superparamagnetic iron oxide particles trapped within the slow-flow vascular channels of the lesion.[27]

99mTc-Labeled Red Blood Cell Scintigraphy

99mTc-pertechnetate–labeled red blood cell scintigraphy is a relatively specific examination for characterizing hemangioma. With this method, there is decreased activity on early dynamic images and increased activity on delayed blood pool images. Comparison between 99mTc-pertechnetate–labeled red blood cell single-photon emission CT (SPECT) and MRI has shown that MRI has higher sensitivity and specificity than SPECT, especially for lesions smaller than 2 cm in diameter.[28]

Diagnostic Workup

The recommended diagnostic workup for suspected hemangioma is dependent on the clinical scenario. If a hemangioma with typical ultrasound features is incidentally detected in a patient with neither a history of malignancy nor chronic liver disease, no additional investigation may be required. It has been shown that in this clinical setting the risk of misinterpreting a malignant tumor for hemangioma is negligible (0.5%). Conversely, in patients with incidentally detected lesions with ultrasound features atypical of hepatic hemangioma, further diagnostic workup is recommended. Additional investigation is also mandatory—regardless of the ultrasound features—for any lesion detected in a patient at increased risk for malignancy. MRI is currently the most accurate technique for diagnostic confirmation of suspected hemangioma.[29] Despite promising results in recent investigations, contrast-enhanced ultrasound is at an early stage of clinical application.[30] On the other hand, spiral CT has limitations in achieving a reliable diagnosis of small lesions, especially in the

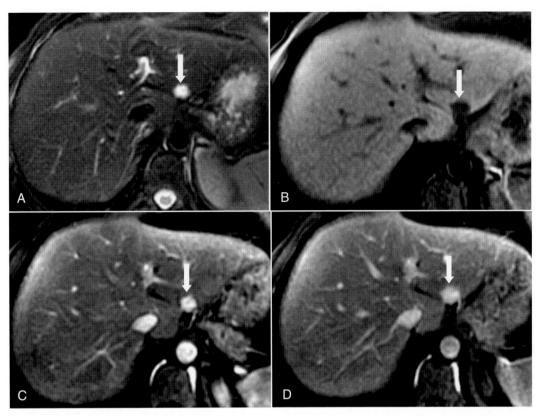

Fig. 59-3 Hemangioma, MRI appearance. A, On baseline T2-weighted MRI, a tiny lesion is detected as a hyperintense nodule *(arrow)*. **B,** On baseline T1-weighted MRI, the hemangioma is hypointense relative to the liver *(arrow)*. **C,** In the arterial phase of the contrast-enhanced dynamic MRI study, the small lesion shows uniform enhancement *(arrow)*. **D,** In the delayed phase, the lesion remains hyperintense because of persistent enhancement *(arrow)*.

setting of cirrhosis.[23,31] Indeed, high-flow hemangiomas that enhance homogeneously in the arterial phase of CT may not be confidently distinguished from small hypervascular hepatocellular carcinoma (HCC).[23] Because MRI has greater sensitivity to small differences in contrast enhancement and because several fast MRI sequences can be used to track the passage of a small, tight bolus of contrast material, MRI may show the characteristic enhancement patterns of hemangioma and HCC better than CT does.[31] In addition, besides the information provided by the dynamic gadolinium-enhanced study, MRI can offer an improved capability of characterizing lesions through analysis of lesion signal intensity on baseline sequences, especially heavily T2-weighted sequences.[29] In the setting of cirrhosis, diagnosis of hemangioma should meet strict CT or MRI criteria, whereas percutaneous biopsy can be used to solve uncertain diagnosis.

Treatment

Treatment is not indicated for asymptomatic tumors less than 5 cm in size. Current indications for surgical management of these benign liver masses include uncertain diagnosis with a suspicion of malignancy, severe or progressive symptoms because of size, and less commonly, risk for hemorrhage or rupture.[13] Indeed, elective surgical resection has been advocated in selected young patients with asymptomatic hemangiomas larger than 10 cm to eliminate the risk for hemorrhage, thrombosis, and rupture. Enlarging tumors and those that become symptomatic have been treated successfully by resection, with relief of symptoms in 90% of cases.[13] Patients with multiple hemangiomas and those with extensive hilar involvement may be considered for either angiographic embolization or liver transplantation. The former treatment is indicated for patients with one or few tumors that have favorable vascular anatomy, as debulking therapy before surgery, to reduce blood loss at the time of surgery, or to treat atypical tumors with arteriovenous shunts. When local ethanol injection therapy was delivered to 37 patients with symptomatic hemangiomas (41% with multiple nodes, 60% with cavernous tumors), the tumors shrunk in 27 (73%) of the patients, and pain disappeared in 10 (35%) of the 29 patients with symptoms.[14]

Liver transplantation may be indicated for large, unresectable tumors; for extensive multiple tumors; or when surgical resection is not feasible. Hepatic resection and transcatheter hepatic embolization are effective treatment modalities for Kasabach-Merritt syndrome, although in a few instances unresectable cavernous hemangiomas with this complication may be an indication for liver transplantation.[32] There is little evidence of the efficacy of radiotherapy, which carries a risk for radiation-induced hepatitis. In a PubMed MEDLINE search,[33] 32 patients with spontaneously ruptured hemangiomas (range, 6 to 25 cm in diameter) were identified. Thirteen (41%) underwent hepatic resection, 5 (16%) were treated by suturing, and 4 (13%) underwent tamponade. Three of the 13 resected patients, 2 of 5 suture patients, and 3 of 4 patients who underwent tamponade died.

Table 59-5 Longitudinal Studies Assessing Changes in Volume of Hemangiomas During Follow-Up

| AUTHOR | NO. OF PATIENTS | MONTHS OF FOLLOW-UP* | TUMOR SIZE | |
			Decreased	Increased
Gandolfi et al.,[3] 1991	123	22 (12-60)	0	1 (1%)
Farges et al.,[12] 1995	78	92	0	1 (1%)
Weimann et al.,[11] 1997	104	32 (7-123)	7 (7%)	11 (11%)
Terkivatan et al.,[10] 2001	78	45 (24-72)	0	1 (1%)
Okano et al.,[34] 2001	64	19 (6-58)	1 (2%)	0

*Median (range).

Prognosis and Natural History

The risk that abdominal pain will develop in a patient with an asymptomatic hemangioma is negligible.[11,13] In a series of patients with abdominal pain, the pain disappeared in most either after treatment of co-morbid conditions or without specific treatment. Interestingly, the pain persisted in two thirds of patients who underwent treatment of hemangioma by hepatic resection, embolization, or arterial ligation.[12] The mechanism of the development of symptoms or pain is unclear but may include expansion of tumor size with pressure effects on adjacent hepatic parenchyma or the capsule of Glisson. In a few cases, the symptoms are related to intralesional hemorrhage, localized thrombosis, or torsion of a pedunculated hemangioma. Patients with Kasabach-Merritt syndrome—disseminated intravascular coagulation in the setting of a cavernous hemangioma of the liver and cutaneous hemangiomas—have abdominal pain and signs of bleeding. During a follow-up of 3 to 180 months, a tiny (10%) minority of patients with hemangioma showed a decrease in tumor size, whereas in a similar percentage of patients the tumor grew in size[12] (**Table 59-5**).

The risk for rupture of hepatic hemangiomas is negligible, the only reports involving patients with cavernous hemangiomas and trauma-induced or spontaneous rupture. Rupture is associated with a sudden onset of severe abdominal pain, abdominal distention, hypotension or shock, and increased serum transaminase levels and prothrombin time. A PubMed MEDLINE search has identified up to 32 cases of spontaneous rupture of hepatic hemangioma (mostly cavernous hemangiomas) in adults without a history of trauma.[35]

Focal Nodular Hyperplasia

Focal nodular hyperplasia of the liver is a rare, completely benign lesion characterized by nodular hyperplasia of the hepatic parenchyma around a central scar containing an anomalous artery; it usually occurs in a normal liver and is frequently multinodular.

Epidemiology

Focal nodular hyperplasia is the second most common benign tumor of the liver, with an estimated prevalence of 0.4% to 0.8% in unselected autopsy series.[35] The tumor has a female/male ratio of between 2:1 and 26:1, and the average age at diagnosis is between 35 and 50 years.

Pathogenesis

Focal nodular hyperplasia appears to be the result of a hyperplastic response of the hepatic parenchyma to an arterial lesion or portal venous ischemia (or both). A congenital vascular malformation is suggested by the presence of a central fibrous scar containing abundant arteries with spiderlike malformations and its association with other vascular abnormalities, such as hepatic hemangioma and hereditary hemorrhagic telangiectasia[36-38] (Rendu-Osler-Weber disease) or congenital absence of the portal vein. The finding of an unbalanced expression of angiopoietin-1 and angiopoietin-2 genes coupled with expression of the angiopoietin-1 protein by the endothelial cells of dystrophic vessels suggests a role of angiopoietin genes in FNH.[39] Clonality studies and overexpression of important genes involved in cell homeostasis, such as Bcl-2 and transforming growth factor-α, support the important role of hepatocellular proliferation in FNH.[40] Conversely, the role of oral contraceptives in FNH is disputed. A hospital-based case-control study in women with histologically proven FNH showed a quantitatively proportional increase in the risk for FNH in patients who ever used oral contraceptives.[41] Their use has been associated with increase in size and vascularity of FNH nodes, and tumor regression was observed after drug withdrawal.[36] However, the association among pregnancy, estrogen, and FNH was negated by a 8-year study involving 216 women in Paris.[42]

Pathology

Macroscopically, the vast majority of patients have pale tan to light brown lesions that give rise a central scar radiating into the liver tissue. The majority of solitary tumors are located in the right lobe. In a pathologic study of 305 lesions in Paris (mostly symptomatic), 21% of the patients had 2 to 5 nodules in the liver and 3% had 15 to 30 nodular lesions.[43] The size of the lesions ranged from 1 mm to 19 cm (median, 3 cm), and occasionally, the lesions were either pedunculated or encapsulated. A large vascular pedicle was observed in a tiny minority (6%) of the patients. The previously classified atypical or telangiectatic FNH is now recognized as a subtype of HA in the new molecular classification. Eighty percent of patients have the classic form, which is characterized by abnormal nodular architecture, malformed-appearing vessels, and bile duct proliferation. The majority of classic forms contain one to three macroscopic scars. Microscopically, classic FNH lesions show nodular hyperplastic parenchyma, with the nodules being completely or incompletely surrounded by fibrous septa. The central scar contains malformed vessels of various caliber, mostly large and tortuous arteries showing intimal or muscular fibrous hyperplasia. However, apart from the dystrophic vessels in the scar, the morphology of the vessels in the lobular parenchyma confirms that FNH retains the overall organization of normal liver tissue.[44] Dense bile duct hilar proliferation accompanies the vascular structures both in the central scars and in the radiating septa with histologic cholestasis. A mild degree of macrovascular steatosis is often present. Multiple FNH syndrome is the presence of at least two FNH lesions and one or more of the following: liver hemangioma, central nervous system vascular malformation, meningioma, and astrocytoma.[1]

Molecular Features Associated with Focal Nodular Hyperplasia

Clonal analysis using the human androgen receptor assay (HUMARA) demonstrated the reactive polyclonal nature of liver cells in 50% to 100% of FNH lesions.[44-46] Although genetic analysis failed to identify somatic mutations in the genes for β-catenin, TP53, adenomatous polyposis coli (APC), or hepatocyte nuclear factor-1α (HNF-1α),[46-48] recent studies have shown modification of the mRNA expression levels of the angiopoietin genes (*ANGPT1* and *ANGPT2*) involved in vessel maturation, with an increased ANGPT1/ANGPT2 ratio being noted in all FNH samples analyzed.[45,49]

Clinical Features

Focal nodular hyperplasia is usually an incidental finding, but a few patients may have symptoms such as a palpable mass or hepatomegaly (**Table 59-6**).

Diagnosis

Liver chemistry is usually unaltered. In a few patients, FNH may cause slight elevations in serum γ-glutamyl transpeptidase (GGT) levels. The serum tumor markers α-fetoprotein (AFP), CA 19.9, and carcinoembryonic antigen (CEA) are invariably negative. Lesions lacking a central scar and smaller lesions with indeterminate vascular characteristics may be diagnosed by ultrasound-guided thin biopsy.[50]

Imaging Findings
Ultrasound and Contrast-Enhanced Ultrasound

FNH may have variable ultrasound features. It usually appears as a round mass that is slightly hypoechoic or slightly hyperechoic in comparison with liver parenchyma. Some lesions may be isoechoic with the liver and be detected only because of vascular displacement. The lesion is frequently homogeneous. In fact, detection of the central scar on baseline ultrasound is uncommon. Typical findings on color or power Doppler ultrasound include the presence of a central feeding artery with a stellate or spoke-wheel pattern caused by vessels running into radiating fibrous septa originating from the central scar. Doppler spectral analysis can show an intralesional pulsatile waveform with high diastolic flow and a low resistive index.[51] The specificity of ultrasound for the diagnosis of FNH has improved following the introduction of ultrasound contrast agents. On contrast-enhanced ultrasound, FNH shows a central vascular supply with centrifugal filling in the early arterial phase, followed by homogeneous enhancement in the late arterial phase. In the portal phase the lesion remains hyperechoic relative to normal liver tissue and becomes isoechoic in the late phase.[19,20] This pattern has been observed in 85% to 100% of patients with FNH.[52] The central scar becomes detectable as a hypoechoic area in the portal phase of the contrast-enhanced study.

Computed Tomography

Focal nodular hyperplasia is usually isoattenuating or slightly hypoattenuating relative to surrounding liver tissue on baseline CT. The detection rate of the central scar—which appears as a hypoattenuating structure—is related to the size of the lesion. It may be identified in 35% of lesions smaller than 3 cm in diameter and in 65% of those exceeding 3 cm.[53] FNH shows strong homogeneous enhancement during the arterial phase of contrast-enhanced CT. The central scar is typically hypoattenuating during the arterial phase. In the portal venous and delayed phases, FNH becomes isoattenuating in relation to hepatic parenchyma. On delayed images, the central scar may become hyperattenuating because of distribution of contrast material within its fibrous stroma. Features evident on CT may enable correct characterization of FNH in 78% of cases.

Magnetic Resonance Imaging

Magnetic resonance imaging is the most accurate imaging method for characterizing FNH. Because of the affinity of its cells with normal hepatocytes, FNH is usually slightly hypointense or isointense with respect to normal liver parenchyma on T1-weighted images and slightly hyperintense or isointense on T2-weighted images.[54] The hallmark of the lesion, the central stellate scar, is usually depicted because of its hypointensity on T1-weighted images and hyperintensity on T2-weighted images, thus reflecting its pathologic substratum of vascularized connective tissue.[54] On baseline MRI, however, the aforementioned typical features—homogeneous structure, isointensity with respect to liver, and presence of the central scar—are observed in only 22% of patients.[55]

Table 59-6 Clinical Findings Leading to Diagnosis in Patients with Focal Nodular Hyperplasia		
CLUES TO DIAGNOSIS	**WEIMANN ET AL.,[11] 1997 (N = 150)**	**NGUYEN ET AL.,[43] 1999 (N = 130)**
Incidental finding	66 (44%)	46 (35%)
Abdominal pain	49 (37%)	75 (58%)
Palpable mass	3 (2%)	5 (4%)
Abnormal liver function test results	18 (12%)	17 (13%)

Diagnostic confirmation requires contrast-enhanced MRI. This is usually performed by serial dynamic imaging following the administration of a gadolinium chelate.[56] FNH shows strong, homogeneous enhancement in the arterial phase with sparing of the central scar, whereas it becomes isointense relative to liver parenchyma in the portal venous and delayed phases (**Fig. 59-4**). The central scar may show uptake of contrast medium in the delayed phase because of the interstitial distribution of the contrast agent. These features have a specificity of greater than 95% for the diagnosis of FNH.[56] However, even with the administration of gadolinium chelates, the central scar may not be detectable in as many as 22% of FNH lesions, including 80% of those smaller than 3 cm.[56] A liver-specific MRI contrast agent provides an alternative strategy for diagnosing FNH. Because of the affinity of its cells with hepatocytes, FNH takes up hepatocyte-targeted agents, similar to normal parenchyma. These agents are then trapped within the lesion because FNH is unable to effectively eliminate the compound via biliary excretion. Hence, it appears hyperintense relative to normal parenchyma on T1-weighted images.[57] In addition, the central scar—which does not take up the hepatocyte-targeted agent—becomes well delineated in up to 90% of patients (**Fig. 59-5**).[58] This approach may enable diagnosis of 90% of FNH lesions with atypical features on baseline and conventional contrast-enhanced dynamic studies.[56] The diagnosis of FNH has also been achieved with the use of RES-targeted agents. Because of its rich Kupffer cell population, FNH takes up iron oxide particles and shows a marked decrease in signal intensity on T2-weighted images. The central scar is usually well delineated on contrast-enhanced images because it does not contain RES cells and therefore maintains high signal intensity.[55]

Technetium ^{99m}Tc Sulphur Colloid Scintigraphy

Technetium ^{99m}Tc sulphur colloid scintigraphy has long been used to characterize FNH. In fact, up to 80% of these lesions show uptake because of their Kupffer cell population.[59] Unfortunately, the uptake of sulphur colloid is not highly specific. In a series of 20 lesions, sulphur colloid studies were diagnostic in only 16% of FNH lesions larger than 3.5 cm and in 14% of lesions smaller than 3.5 cm.[60]

Diagnostic Workup

Focal nodular hyperplasia is usually detected incidentally. Diagnostic confirmation can rely solely on imaging findings,

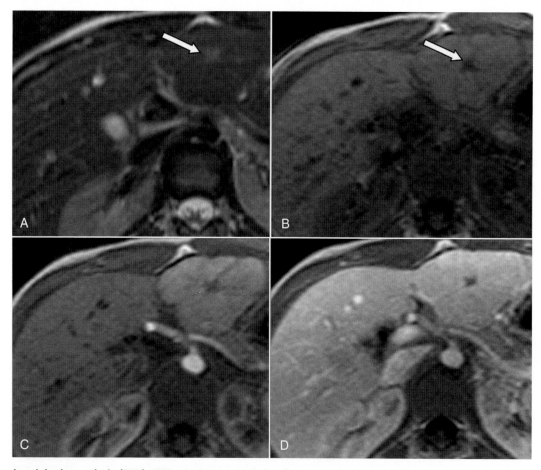

Fig. 59-4 **Focal nodular hyperplasia (FNH), MRI appearance. A,** On baseline T2-weighted MRI, the lesion is determined to be FNH and appears isointense relative to surrounding liver parenchyma (i.e., undetectable); the central scar is detected as an hyperintense area *(arrow)*. **B,** On baseline T1-weighted MRI, the lesion is isointense relative to the liver, and the scar is detected as a hypointense zone *(arrow)*. **C,** In the arterial phase of the contrast-enhanced dynamic MRI study, rapid homogeneous enhancement sparing the central scar is observed. **D,** In the delayed phase, the lesion becomes isointense with respect to surrounding parenchyma.

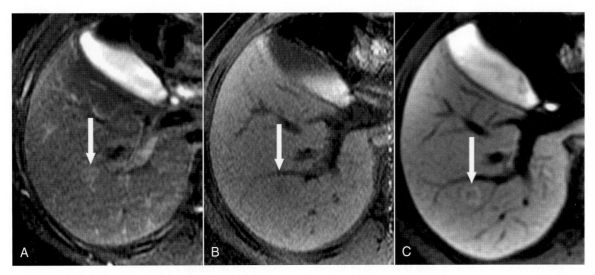

Fig. 59-5 Focal nodular hyperplasia, MRI appearance. A, On baseline T2-weighted MRI, the lesions is slightly hyperintense relative to the liver *(arrow).* **B,** On baseline T1-weighted MRI, the lesion is hypointense with respect to surrounding parenchyma *(arrow).* **C,** After the administration of a hepatobiliary contrast agent (manganese dipyridoxyldiphosphate [MnDPDP]), the lesion appears hyperintense relative to normal parenchyma on the T1-weighted image *(arrow),* and the central scar is detected as a hypointense area.

provided that typical features are shown in the proper clinical setting. CT can be used to characterize lesions of medium to large size but has limitations in the diagnosis of small lesions.[23,61] Although promising results have recently been reported with the use of contrast-enhanced ultrasound, MRI is the most accurate technique for diagnosing FNH.[29] MRI—besides the information provided by baseline and dynamic gadolinium-enhanced studies—can offer improved capability in characterizing lesions through the use of liver-specific agents, especially with small lesions.[29] The use of percutaneous biopsy should be restricted to patients with questionable findings.[61]

Associated Conditions

The syndrome of multiple FNH consists of the presence of FNH, HAs, and disorders of the central nervous system such as meningioma, astrocytoma, and arterial malformations. This syndrome has been described in association with Klippel-Trénaunay-Weber syndrome, a nonhereditary congenital condition characterized by capillary malformations, hemihypertrophy, and venous stasis.[36] The association between FNH and fibrolamellar carcinoma is disputed.

Treatment

Treatment is rarely indicated. FNH lesions do usually not bleed or undergo malignant transformation. Hemorrhage, clinically important symptoms, and uncertain diagnosis are indications for surgical resection. Treatment of FNH should also be reserved for patients with a lesion that demonstrates growth on sequential imaging. In a series of 150 patients with FNH in Hannover, Germany, 5 (3%) underwent hepatic resection because of the onset of symptoms. Recurrence or persistence of symptoms following resection may occur in excess of 20% of patients.[10]

Prognosis and Natural History

Focal nodular hyperplasia is a completely benign condition that has the potential to change in size. In one study,[11] 4% of the lesions decreased in size, whereas they increased in size in 3% of 136 patients who were monitored for 9 years. In recent reports, the size of the lesions did not increase during oral contraceptive treatment and pregnancy,[42] nor did it expand in patients receiving immunosuppressive therapy.[62] The risk for bleeding of FNH lesions seems remote,[5,63] and neoplastic transformation has never been reported. In a few patients, FNH has been reported to progress to the development of clinically important symptoms.[63] In a series of 53 patients observed in Hannover for 3 years, upper abdominal symptoms developed in 21 (40%) and were severe in 2 (4%).[11]

Hepatocellular Adenoma

Hepatocellular adenoma is a rare, frequently capsulated nodular lesion of the liver characterized by benign monoclonal proliferation of liver cells. HA can be divided into three groups according to histologic features and into four subgroups according to genotype and phenotypic features.

Epidemiology

Hepatocellular adenoma is by far a less frequent disease than FNH. In a series of patients collected between 1989 and 1992, the adenoma/FNH ratio was 1:10.[64] HA occurs more commonly in women of reproductive age who use oral contraceptives. In one study,[65] the relative risk for HA was 25 for women who used oral contraceptives for more than 109 months in comparison with those who used contraceptives for less than 12 months. Although the female/male ratio is 4:1,[11] the incidence of HA appears to have increased in males because the use of anabolic drugs has become widespread in sports.[66] The tumor may also be associated with underlying metabolic diseases, including type 1 glycogen storage disease and iron overload related to β-thalassemia or hemochromatosis.[67-69] In a few patients, the tumor may be manifested as 10 or more adenomas in an otherwise normal liver (liver adenomatosis) with a male/female distribution of approximately 3 : 1 and an increased risk for complications.[70]

Pathogenesis

Hepatocellular adenomas are monoclonal tumors[40,46] that may have different molecular signatures. One group of HAs is characterized by mutations in the transcription factor 1 (*TCF1*) gene. This gene encodes HNF-1α, which has been identified as a human tumor suppressor factor involved in hepatic carcinogenesis.[71] HAs harboring HNF-1α mutations show inhibition of gluconeogenesis coordinated with activation of the glycolysis citrate shuttle and fatty acid synthesis, which may lead to high rates of lipogenesis. These changes are accompanied by silencing of liver fatty acid binding protein (L-FABP), which encodes a liver fatty acid bridging protein, thus suggesting that impaired fatty acid traffic may also contribute to the fatty phenotype of HA.[72]

A few HAs harbor mutation of the wnt/β-catenin pathway,[47,73,74] which pathogenetically links these adenomas with a subgroup of HCCs characterized by mutations in β-catenin.[75] In a series of patients with HA, those with β-catenin activation were in fact shown to be at risk for malignant transformation.[73] The fact that no case of HA with both β-catenin and biallelic inactivation of HNF-1α was identified suggests that these two signaling pathways are mutually exclusive.

A third type of HA is characterized by increased expression of members of the acute-phase inflammatory response, such as serum amyloid protein (SAA), C-reactive protein (CRP),[74] and the interleukin-6 (IL-6) signaling pathway.[76] The fact that most inflammatory HAs harbor small in-frame deletions that target the bridging site of gp130 for IL-6 probably accounts for the activation of the acute inflammatory phase signals observed in tumor hepatocytes.[76]

Based on these three molecular pathways of activation, a new classification has been proposed for HA, and a panel of four specific antibodies has been identified.

Group 1: HNF-1α Mutations

Biallelic-inactivating mutations of the *TCF1* gene leading to inactivation of HNF-1α are detected in more than a third of all HAs. Most mutations are somatic and occur in a histologically homogeneous group of tumors characterized by marked steatosis in the absence of cytologic abnormalities, inflammatory infiltrates, and tumor expression of L-FABP. Patients with the germline HNF-1α mutation are younger, frequently have a history of liver adenomatosis, and do not express L-FABP.[73,74]

Group 2: β-Catenin Mutations

In a series of HAs, a fifth harbored an activating β-catenin gene mutation, with preference for HA with cytologic abnormalities and an acinar pattern.[73] β-Catenin mutations were rarely detected in patients with steatosis and those with inflammatory changes in the liver. Most HAs with mutated β-catenin are borderline lesions between adenoma and HCC and are more frequently associated with the development of HCC than are other HA subtypes.[73,74,77] Risk factors include exposure to male hormones, glycogenesis, and familial polyposis. Glutamine synthetase overexpression and β-catenin are frequently found in both the cytoplasm and nucleus.

Group 3: Inflammatory Features

A third of HAs are characterized by overexpression of SAA and CRP and, histologically, by inflammatory infiltrates, sinusoidal dilation, dystrophic vessels, and bile duct proliferation.[46,78] In fact, these HAs correspond to a variant previously defined as telangiectatic FNH.[79] A tiny minority (10%) of adenomas with inflammatory features have mutations in the β-catenin gene as well. The risk for HCC transformation is lower than in group 2.

Group 4: None of the Aforementioned Alterations

This group represents less than 5% to 10% of all cases of HA.

Pathology

Hepatic adenomas are soft, yellow lesions, often with a highly vascularized surface and capsule and focal areas of hemorrhage in the parenchyma. The histologic features are two-cell (or more) -thick sheets of hepatocytes without cellular atypia (to differentiate from adenocarcinoma), portal tracts (to differentiate from liver cell regeneration), and biliary ductules and fibrosis (to differentiate from FNH). Recently, a classification of HA according to typical histologic features has been proposed and validated[80,81]: steatotic HAs (overlapping with the HNF-1α mutation subgroup of the molecular classification), telangiectatic HAs (overlapping with the inflammatory subgroup of the molecular classification), and unclassified HAs. Steatotic HA is characterized by prominent steatosis (>60%) without other specific features. Telangiectatic HA is characterized by the presence of portal tract remnants associated with vascular changes, inflammatory infiltrates, or both. When no specific histologic features are present, HAs are considered unclassified. Foci of malignant transformation have been described that may escape detection in small specimens obtained by thin-needle liver biopsy.

Clinical Features

Hepatocellular adenomas are usually solitary. Approximately 30% of patients have multiple nodules, and the presence of 10 or more adenomas defines liver adenomatosis[82]; somatic HNF-1α mutations are frequently found in these patients.[10] In approximately half of the patients with adenoma, they have been detected incidentally, whereas the remaining have had such symptoms as pain or an abdominal mass (**Table 59-7**). In the literature, 10 patients (26%) with liver adenomatosis became symptomatic because of intraperitoneal bleeding, and 9 of these patients were taking oral contraceptives.[82] Patients with HA have a higher prevalence of symptoms at initial evaluation than do patients with hemangioma or FNH, probably because of the high rate of intratumoral or intraabdominal

Table 59-7 Clinical Findings Leading to Diagnosis of Hepatocellular Adenoma

CLUES TO DIAGNOSIS	WEIMANN ET AL.,[11] 1997 (N = 44)	HERMAN ET AL.,[83] 2000 (N = 10)	TERKIVATAN ET AL.,[10] 2001 (N = 33)
Incidental finding	12 (27%)	2 (20%)	10 (30%)
Abdominal pain	19 (43%)	8 (80%)	10 (30%)
Elevated γ-glutamyl transpeptidase	3 (7%)	4 (40%)	0
Bleeding	6 (13%)	NA	12 (36%)

NA, not available

hemorrhage.[10,84] The risk for hemorrhage does not appear to relate to the number of HAs but to its pathologic characteristics, with a lower risk in patients with steatotic HA. The diagnosis of liver adenomatosis is made by the presence of complications of adenomas (intraperitoneal bleeding, intratumoral hemorrhage, or necrosis-producing acute pain), by the presence of hepatomegaly with or without symptoms, or as an incidental finding. Even though the massive form of liver adenomatosis is rare and can be unilobular, most patients have multifocal liver adenomatosis distributed in both lobes.[82]

Diagnosis

Laboratory tests are not helpful during the diagnostic workup. However, negative tests for serum AFP and hepatitis B and C corroborate the exclusion of malignant disease. Percutaneous liver biopsy has been considered to be of little value because of the possible lack of specific features in a small specimen and the risk of needle-induced bleeding in hypervascular nodes. However, recent data have raised the possibility of using liver biopsy specimens for identification of the various HA subtypes. In liver adenomatosis, a two-fold or three-fold increase in alkaline phosphatase or GGT levels has been described[82]; in particular, inflammatory HAs are more often associated with an increased level of GGT and occur more frequently in overweight patients.[10,85] A diagnosis of liver adenomatosis is better obtained by exploration of the liver via laparoscopy or laparotomy, which allows the operator to obtain biopsy specimens of several different lesions without the risk of hemorrhage.[82]

Imaging Findings
Ultrasound and Contrast-Enhanced Ultrasound

Hepatocellular adenoma has variable sonographic appearances. The lesion may appear as slightly hypoechoic, isoechoic, or hyperechoic. When necrotic or hemorrhagic changes occur, adenoma appears as a complex mass with a large cystic component. On color or power Doppler, the arterial hypervascularity is well demonstrated by arterial vessels running along the border of the lesion in a "basket" pattern.[86,87] On contrast-enhanced ultrasound, adenoma shows intense enhancement during the arterial phase. During the portal venous and equilibrium phases, adenomas may appear as an isoechoic or slightly hyperechoic mass.[88] None of these features, unfortunately, is specific enough for diagnosis.

Computed Tomography

Baseline CT can easily detect the presence of fat or recent hemorrhage within the lesion, features that can suggest the diagnosis of adenoma. During dynamic contrast-enhanced CT, noncomplicated adenomas may enhance rapidly and appear homogeneously hyperdense in comparison with the liver. The enhancement does not usually persist in adenomas because of arteriovenous shunting within the lesion. Larger or complicated adenomas may be highly heterogeneous as a result of necrotic phenomena or intralesional hemorrhage (**Fig. 59-6**).

Magnetic Resonance Imaging

Magnetic resonance imaging is considered the most comprehensive and noninvasive imaging technique for evaluating HA.[89-92] MRI findings include fatty, necrotic, and hemorrhagic components, but a homogeneous hypervascular appearance may also be observed. These characteristics overlap with those of other hypervascular hepatic tumors. Laumonier and colleagues recently demonstrated a correlation between specific MRI features and the two most frequently identified subtypes of HA: HNF-1α–inactivated and inflammatory HA.[93] This study showed that HNF-1α–inactivated HA can be confidently recognized on MRI if a homogeneous fat distribution is observed because of the known marked steatosis typical of this subgroup of HA associated with the activation of liponeogenesis.

Patients with inflammatory HA also displayed specific MRI features: markedly hyperintense signal on T2-weighted images and strong arterial enhancement that persists in the delayed phases. The combination of these features was found to be sensitive (85%) and specific (88%) for the radiologic diagnosis of inflammatory HA in this population of 50 patients with HA.

Finally, the only two cases of HA with β-catenin activation displayed strong arterial enhancement with marked wash-out at the portal venous phase, which is the typical pattern of HCC.

Diagnostic Workup

Radiologic diagnosis of adenoma is very difficult, and more data are needed to confirm the new findings on MRI. The only finding that may suggest the diagnosis is detection of intratumoral hemorrhage. The role of liver biopsy should be reevaluated because of the new molecular classification of HA.

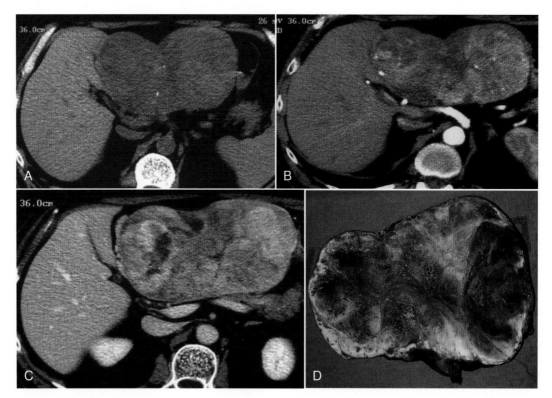

Fig. 59-6 Hepatocellular adenoma, appearance on CT. A, Baseline CT showing a large, heterogeneous mass in the left liver lobe. **B,** In the arterial phase of the contrast-enhanced CT study, rapid, inhomogeneous enhancement of the lesion is detected. **C,** In the portal venous phase, the lesion shows heterogeneous features with hypoattenuating and hyperattenuating areas. **D,** Resected specimen showing hepatocellular adenoma with intralesional hemorrhage and necrosis.

Associated Conditions

Adenoma has been associated with glycogen storage disease, anabolic drug use, and diabetes.[82]

Treatment

Management of patients with adenoma is evolving. In principle, patients should not be managed according to the number of HAs, but according to the risk for complications, which is related to the subtype and the size of the HA. For patients taking oral contraceptives with incidentally discovered adenomas smaller than 4 cm, the best option would be withdrawal of the contraceptives and close monitoring with sequential ultrasound examinations of the abdomen. Although patients with adenoma regression may escape or delay surgical treatment or locoregional ablation, those with larger, symptomatic adenomas unresponsive to withdrawal of contraceptives should be considered for surgical treatment. Any nodule larger than 4 cm should be removed to avoid the risk for hemorrhage (frequent) and HCC (rare). In a retrospective analysis of 122 patients with single and multiple HAs at Beaujon Hospital in Clichy, France, patients with HAs larger than 5 cm, those with telangiectatic or unclassified subtypes, and men were shown to have an increased risk for complications and were therefore identified as having an indication for hepatic resection.[80] Tumor ablation should be also considered for patients who for medical reasons cannot stop oral contraceptive use or for those who plan to become pregnant.[11] With any

HA discovered in a pregnant woman, close follow-up with frequent ultrasound imaging seems reasonable. Treatment of patients with ruptured adenoma requires stabilization with selective arterial embolization before resection.[10] Management of liver adenomatosis is problematic. The unilobular, massive form can be treated by hepatic resection. For patients with liver adenomatosis, surgery on the largest or complicated adenomas is an option. Because it is often impossible to resect all tumors in patients with multiple HAs, liver transplantation has been proposed, especially in those with more than 10 HAs.[94-96]

Prognosis and Natural History

The potential for adenomas to increase in size is not well established for women taking oral contraceptives, whereas regression of the lesion has been documented on cessation of oral contraceptive use.[8] The potential for β-catenin–mutated HA to progress to cancer is certainly a strong argument for removing it; however, more studies on carcinogenesis are warranted before this becomes a universal recommendation. The other clinical concern associated with adenoma, bleeding, involves approximately a quarter of all patients. In 12 patients with HA over a 10-year period in Taiwan, 4 had pathologic findings of intratumor hemorrhage on resection, and 1 patient in fact had had hemoperitoneum from rupture of the adenoma. In another series of 33 patients in Rotterdam, 14 were managed by observation, and 1 of them had a ruptured adenoma.[10] Spontaneous bleeding occurred in 20% of 122 patients with HA treated in Clichy, France, from 1990 to 2004 and was almost exclusively confined to patients with tumors larger than 5 cm.[80] In the same series of patients, malignant transformation of HA was present in 10% of patients, as previously reported by others.[94,97]

Nodular Regenerative Hyperplasia

Nodular regenerative hyperplasia of the liver is a condition in which nodules of proliferating hepatocytes develop in a liver with preserved architecture without fibrous septa. The lesion is commonly seen at the hepatic hilum or around large portal tracts and may be associated with features of portal hypertension and subclinical cholestasis.[98]

Epidemiology

Nodular regenerative hyperplasia occurs in both males and females. Two autopsy series including approximately 3000 subjects demonstrated NRH in approximately 2.5%,[99,100] with a female/male ratio of approximately 1:1 to 2:1. The disease affects predominantly patients older than 60 years and those with portal hypertension or portal vein thrombosis.[99] However, NRH has been reported in children as young as 7 months, as well as in young adults.

Pathogenesis

The pathogenesis of NRH is still unknown, but two theories have been proposed to explain the pathogenesis of this disease. The basic pathologic lesion leading to NRH may be obliteration or thrombosis of the portal vein system causing ischemic atrophy in the central zones of the hepatic acinus,[101] the centrolobular atrophy being compensated for by a proliferation of liver cells from the periportal areas that form regenerative nodules. This sequence of events is accounted for by several portal venous abnormalities, such as venous thrombi and phlebosclerosis.[99,100] NRH could also be a generalized proliferative disorder of the liver with the potential to progress to HCC,[102] an interpretation that is corroborated by the frequent occurrence of liver cell dysplasia in patients with NRH.

Pathology

Nodular regenerative hyperplasia has been defined as a secondary and nonspecific tissue adaptation to the heterogeneous distribution of blood flow that occurs as part of a spectrum of architectural changes known as nodular transformation.[100] Nodular transformation is recognized by the presence of regions of atrophy of liver tissue juxtaposed to normal or hyperplastic areas with a curved contour and no interviewing fibrous septa. Diffuse nodular hyperplasia may also be associated with fibrous septa or be superimposed on a previously cirrhotic liver.[1]

Macroscopically, the liver is normal in size and shows nodules 1 to 10 mm in diameter that are centered on a larger portal tract, and it may mimic micronodular cirrhosis. Partial nodular transformation of the liver is no longer used to define

the NRH that forms confluent masses in association with high-grade obstruction of the medium-sized or larger portal veins. Microscopically, the nodes show liver cell plates that are one or two cells thick, whereas the sinusoids are narrow. In the intranodular regions the cell plates are one cell thick, hepatocytes may be atrophic, and the sinusoids are usually dilated. NRH differs from a multiacinar regenerative nodule, which contains more than one portal tract located in a cirrhotic liver, or from severe disease of the portal veins, hepatic veins, or sinusoids.[1]

Clinical Features

The clinical manifestations of NRH are heterogeneous and may range from asymptomatic to end-stage liver disease. Hepatomegaly and splenomegaly occur in fewer than half of the patients with NRH.[99] NRH is often an incidental finding in patients with features of hepatic disease or lymphoproliferative disorders. In patients with a clinical history of vasculitis, hepatic artery fibrosis is found. Portal hypertension is present in half of the patients with NRH but only in a minority of patients as an initial feature.[100] Life-threatening bleeding and death are uncommon. In a few patients, liver failure requiring liver transplantation was the initial feature.[103]

Diagnosis

The typical manifestation of NRH is bleeding from esophageal varices because of portal hypertension. However, most patients with NRH have no specific signs or symptoms related to their hepatic disease. Liver function test results are normal in most patients. Alkaline phosphatase is elevated to more than 1.5 times the upper limit of normal in a third of patients.[99] Liver biopsy may allow a diagnosis of NRH. However, because NRH, incomplete cirrhosis, and complete cirrhosis may occur in different regions of the same liver, large quantities of liver tissue have to be examined for a complete diagnosis.[100] Deterioration of portal pressure is an additional key to the diagnosis of NRH. The procedure of transjugular liver biopsy allows both histopathologic diagnosis and hepatic venography and hepatic vein pressure measurement to be performed in parallel. The differential diagnosis of NRH includes Budd-Chiari syndrome.

Imaging Findings

Sonography may show multiple isoechoic or hyperechoic nodules. They may become hypoechoic or anechoic as a result of intratumoral hemorrhage.[104] Findings on color or power Doppler ultrasound include the presence of intratumoral vessels and sometimes the presence of a central feeding artery.[105] On baseline CT, the lesions are usually isodense relative to liver tissue. Subcapsular lesions may distort the surface of the liver. During the dynamic study, both hypervascular lesions and nodules with the same attenuation as normal parenchyma are visible.[106] The lesions are frequently isointense with respect to normal liver tissue on T1- and T2-weighted images. However, some nodules may show high signal intensity on T1-weighted images, probably because of copper deposits[100,107,108] (**Fig. 59-7**). Following the administration of hepatobiliary contrast agents, nodules become hyperintense relative to the liver because they contain normal

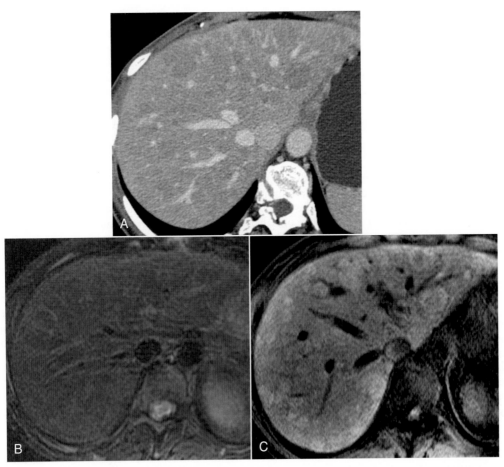

Fig. 59-7 Nodular regenerative hyperplasia, appearance on CT and MRI. A, CT shows inhomogeneous liver tissue with subtle hypoattenuating nodules. **B,** On T2-weighted MRI, no focal abnormality is detected. **C,** On T1-weighted MRI, multiple small hyperintense nodules are detected throughout the liver parenchyma.

hepatocytes and a dysfunctional biliary system. As a result of their Kupffer cell population, nodules take up iron oxide particles and show a decrease in signal intensity on T2-weighted images, similar to normal parenchyma.[109] Unfortunately, the imaging findings of NRH are nonspecific. The diffuse nature of involvement, the associated portal hypertension, and the clinical history are all features that may allow characterization of this entity.

Associated Conditions

Nodular regenerative hyperplasia is associated with lymphoproliferative, rheumatologic, vascular, and storage diseases. The condition has been seen in patients receiving anabolic steroids, chemotherapeutic agents, and azathioprine.[8]

Disease Complications

Portal hypertension with symptoms of variceal bleeding and ascites may develop in 5% to 13% of patients.[100] Compression of the intrahepatic portal radicles by the regenerating nodules and thrombosis of the portal vein/venules are probably pathogenetic mechanisms. Hepatic failure occurs rarely.

Treatment

In most patients, NRH is a slowly evolving, asymptomatic condition that requires no treatment. The few patients with symptomatic portal hypertension and variceal bleeding have been treated with repeated endoscopic therapy or a portocaval shunt.[8] Three patients with progressive liver failure from NRH underwent orthotopic liver transplantation, and in at least one of these patients NRH has recurred after transplantation.[103]

Prognosis and Natural History

Nodular Regenerative Hyperplasia tends to run an indolent course. The few patients in whom clinical decompensation develops will exhibit slow progression to end-stage liver disease. A rare complication reported in the literature is exacerbation of disease in patients receiving chemotherapy for associated myeloproliferative disease or hemoperitoneum because of rupture of a regenerative nodule.[110]

Conclusion

Benign liver tumors are usually identified by imaging and only in a few instances require treatment. Single or multiple imaging methods may be used to achieve acceptable diagnostic specificity. Lesions failing to fulfill specific diagnostic criteria on radiologic imaging require either biopsy or surgical resection. In patients suspected of having cavernous hemangioma, asymptomatic tumors require surveillance with sequential imaging, and if stable, no further testing is required. Conversely, treatment is advisable for patients with a typical symptomatic hemangioma or one larger than 15 cm in diameter. Patients with an atypical hemangioma require enhanced follow-up or biopsy. If the tumor enlarges, resection should be considered. Patients with FNH require imaging follow-up whenever CT, MRI, or technetium ^{99m}Tc sulphur colloid scintigraphy demonstrates a central scar. Biopsy or resection is advocated in patients with expanding large masses or those with atypical features. Masses with the typical features of HA are often recommended for surgical resection or ablation because of concern for bleeding and progression to HCC. Biopsy is also required to distinguish NRH from cirrhosis, which in the majority of the patients requires no treatment.

Key References

Albrecht T, et al, for the EFSUMB Study Group. Guidelines for the use of contrast agents in ultrasound. January 2004. Ultraschall Med 2004;25: 249–256. (Ref.30)

Al-Mukhaizeem KA, Rosenberg A, Sherker AH. Nodular regenerative hyperplasia of the liver: an under-recognized cause of portal hypertension in haematological disorders. Am J Hepatol 2004;75:225–230. (Ref.110)

Bartolozzi C, et al. Focal liver lesions: MR imaging–pathologic correlation. Eur Radiol 2001;11:1374–1388. (Ref.54)

Bartolozzi C, et al. Differentiation of hepatocellular adenoma and focal nodular hyperplasia of the liver: comparison of power Doppler imaging and conventional color Doppler sonography. Eur Radiol 1997;7:1410–1415. (Ref.86)

Ba-Ssalamah A, et al. Atypical focal nodular hyperplasia of the liver: imaging features of nonspecific and liver-specific MR contrast agents. AJR Am J Roentgenol 2002;179:1447–1456. (Ref.55)

Bioulac-Sage P, Balabaud C, Wanless IR. Diagnosis of focal nodular hyperplasia not so easy. Am J Surg Pathol 2001;25:1322–1325. (Ref.49)

Bioulac-Sage P, et al. Hepatocellular adenoma management and phenotypic classification: the Bordeaux experience. Hepatology 2009;50:481–489. (Ref.81)

Bioulac-Sage P, et al. Hepatocellular adenomas. Liver Int 2009;29:142. (Ref.50)

Bioulac-Sage P, et al. Clinical, morphologic, and molecular features defining so-called telangiectatic focal nodular hyperplasias of the liver. Gastroenterology 2005;128:1211–1218. (Ref.46)

Bioulac-Sage P, et al. Hepatocellular adenomas subtype classification using molecular markers and immunohistochemistry. Hepatology 2007;46:740–748. (Ref.74)

Birnbaum BA, Weinreb JC, Megibow AJ. Definitive diagnosis of hepatic hemangiomas: MR vs Tc-99m labeled red blood cell SPECT. Radiology 1990;176:95–105. (Ref.28)

Bläker H, et al. Analysis of somatic APC mutations in rare extracolonic tumors of patients with familial adenomatous polyposis coli. Genes Chromosomes Cancer 2004;41:93–98. (Ref.48)

Bluteau O, et al. Bi-allelic inactivation of TCF1 in hepatic adenomas. Nat Genet 2002;32:312–315. (Ref.71)

Brancatelli G, et al. Hemangioma in the cirrhotic liver: diagnosis and natural history. Radiology 2001;219:69–74. (Ref.31)

Brancatelli G, et al. Focal nodular hyperplasia: CT findings with emphasis on multiphasic helical CT in 78 patients. Radiology 2001;219:61–68. (Ref.53)

Brancatelli G, et al. Large regenerative nodules in Budd-Chiari syndrome and other vascular disorders of the liver: CT and MR imaging findings with clinicopathologic correlation. AJR Am J Roentgenol 2002;178:877–883. (Ref.106)

Brancatelli G, et al. CT and MR imaging evaluation of hepatic adenoma. J Comput Assist Tomogr 2006;30:745–750. (Ref.92)

Broglia L, et al. Computerized tomography, magnetic resonance, and nuclear medicine in the non-invasive diagnosis of focal nodular hyperplasia of the liver. Radiol Med 1998;96:218–225. (Ref.60)

Buscarini E, et al. High prevalence of hepatic focal nodular hyperplasia in subjects with hereditary hemorrhagic telangiectasia. Ultrasound Med Biol 2004;30:1089–1097. (Ref.38)

Charny CK, et al. Management of 155 patients with benign liver tumours. Br J Surg 2001;88:808–813. (Ref.13)

Chen PJ. Genetic mutation in hepatic adenoma: seeing is believing. J Hepatol 2006;45:767–769. (Ref.77)

Chen YW, et al. P53 gene and Wnt signaling in benign neoplasms: beta-catenin mutations in hepatic adenoma but not in focal nodular hyperplasia. Hepatology 2002;36:927–935. (Ref.47)

Cherqui D, et al. Management of focal nodular hyperplasia and hepatocellular adenoma in young women: a series of 41 patients with clinical, radiological, and pathological correlations. Hepatology 1995;22:1674–1681. (Ref.64)

Chiche L, et al. Liver adenomatosis: reappraisal, diagnosis, and surgical management: eight new cases and review of the literature. Ann Surg 2000;231:74–81. (Ref.82)

Cho SW, et al. Surgical management of hepatocellular adenoma: take it or leave it? Ann Surg Oncol 2008;15:2795–2803. (Ref.97)

Choi CS, Freeny PC. Triphasic helical CT of hepatic focal nodular hyperplasia: incidence of atypical findings. AJR Am J Roentgenol 1998;170:391–395. (Ref.61)

Chung KY, et al. Hepatocellular adenoma: MR imaging features with pathologic correlation. AJR Am J Roentgenol 1995;165:303–308. (Ref.89)

Corigliano N, et al. Hemoperitoneum from a spontaneous rupture of a giant hemangioma of the liver: report of a case. Surg Today 2003;33:459–463. (Ref.33)

de La Coste A, et al. Somatic mutations of the beta-catenin gene are frequent in mouse and human hepatocellular carcinoma. Proc Natl Acad Sci U S A 1998;95:8847–8851. (Ref.75)

Dodd GD 3rd, et al. Spectrum of imaging findings of the liver in end-stage cirrhosis: part II, focal abnormalities. AJR Am J Roentgenol 1999;173: 1185–1192. (Ref.7)

Dokmak S, et al. A single-center surgical experience of 122 patients with single and multiple hepatocellular adenomas. Gastroenterology 2009;137:1698–1705. (Ref.80)

Farges O, Daradkeh S, Bismuth H. Cavernous hemangiomas of the liver: are there any indications for resection? World J Surg 1995;19:19–24. (Ref.12)

Feurle GE. Arteriovenous shunting and cholestasis in hepatic hemangiomatosis associated with metoclopramide. Gastroenterology 1990;99:258–262. (Ref.9)

Fujita S, et al. Liver-occupying focal nodular hyperplasia and adenomatosis associated with intrahepatic portal vein agenesis requiring orthotopic liver transplantation. Transplantation 2006;81:490–492. (Ref.95)

Gaffey MJ, Iezzoni JC, Weiss LM. Clonal analysis of focal nodular hyperplasia of the liver. Am J Pathol 1996;4:1089–1096. (Ref.40)

Gaiani S, et al. Hemodynamics in focal nodular hyperplasia. J Hepatol 1999; 31:576. (Ref.51)

Gandolfi L, et al. Natural history of hepatic haemangiomas: clinical and ultrasound study. Gut 1991;32:677–680. (Ref.3)

Golli M, et al. Hepatocellular adenoma: color Doppler US and pathologic correlation. Radiology 1994;190:741–744. (Ref.87)

Grazioli L, et al. Liver adenomatosis: clinical, histopathologic, and imaging findings in 15 patients. Radiology 2000;216:395–402. (Ref.90)

Grazioli L, et al. Focal nodular hyperplasia: morphologic and functional information from MR imaging with gadobenate dimeglumine. Radiology 2001;221:731–739. (Ref.56)

Haber M, et al. Multiple focal nodular hyperplasia of the liver associated with hemihypertrophy and vascular malformations. Gastroenterology 1995;108:1256–1262. (Ref.36)

Heilo A, Stenwig AE. Liver hemangioma: US-guided 18-gauge core-needle biopsy. Radiology 1997;204:719–722. (Ref.17)

Herman P, et al. Hepatic adenoma and focal nodular hyperplasia: differential diagnosis and treatment. World J Surg 2000;24:372–376. (Ref.83)

Hoso M, Terada T, Nakanuma Y. Partial nodular transformation of liver developing around intrahepatic portal venous emboli of hepatocellular carcinoma. Histopathology 1996;29:580–582. (Ref.98)

Hussain SM, et al. Hepatocellular adenoma: findings at state-of-the-art magnetic resonance imaging, ultrasound, computed tomography and pathologic analysis. Eur Radiol 2006;16:1873–1886. (Ref.91)

International Working Party. Terminology of nodular hepatocellular lesions. Hepatology 1995;22:983–993. (Ref.1)

Kim MJ, et al. Evaluation of hepatic focal nodular hyperplasia with contrast-enhanced gray scale harmonic sonography: initial experience. J Ultrasound Med 2004;23:297–305. (Ref.52)

Kim T, et al. Discrimination of small hepatic hemangiomas from hypervascular malignant tumors smaller than 3 cm with three-phase helical CT. Radiology 2001;219:699–706. (Ref.23)

Laumonier H, et al. Hepatocellular adenomas: magnetic resonance imaging features as a function of molecular pathological classification. Hepatology 2008;48:808–818. (Ref.93)

Lencioni R, et al. Magnetic resonance imaging of liver tumors. J Hepatol 2004; 40:162–171. (Ref.29)

Loinaz C, et al. Orthotopic liver transplantation in 4 patients with portal hypertension and non-cirrhotic nodular liver. Hepatogastroenterology 1998; 45:1787–1794. (Ref.103)

Longeville JH, et al. Treatment of a giant haemangioma of the liver with Kasabach-Merritt syndrome by orthotopic liver transplant: a case report. HPB Surg 1997;10:159–162. (Ref.32)

Mathieu D, et al. Oral contraceptive use and focal nodular hyperplasia of the liver. Gastroenterology 2000;118:560–564. (Ref.42)

Mathieu D, et al. Association of focal nodular hyperplasia and hepatic hemangioma. Gastroenterology 1989;97:154–157. (Ref.37)

McEntee MF, et al. Non cirrhotic portal hypertension and nodular regenerative hyperplasia of the liver in dogs with mucopolysaccharidosis type I. Hepatology 1998;28:385–390. (Ref.101)

McFarland EG, et al. Hepatic hemangiomas and malignant tumors: improved differentiation with heavily T2-weighted conventional spin-echo MR imaging. Radiology 1994;193:43–47. (Ref.24)

Montet X, et al. Specificity of SPIO particles for characterization of liver hemangiomas using MRI. Abdom Imaging 2004;29:60–70. (Ref.21)

Moody AR, Wilson SR. Atypical hepatic hemangioma: a suggestive sonographic morphology. Radiology 1993;188:413–417. (Ref.18)

Nakanuma Y. Nodular regenerative hyperplasia of the liver: retrospective survey in autopsy series. J Clin Gastroenterol 1990;12:46–50. (Ref.99)

Nguyen BN, et al. Focal nodular hyperplasia of the liver: a comprehensive pathologic study of 305 lesions and recognition of new histologic forms. Am J Surg Pathol 1999;23:1441–1454. (Ref.43)

Nicolau C, Bru C. Focal liver lesions: evaluation with contrast-enhanced ultrasonography. Abdom Imaging 2004;29:348–359. (Ref.88)

Nino-Murcia M, et al. Focal liver lesions: pattern-based classification scheme for enhancement at arterial phase CT. Radiology 2000;215:746–751. (Ref.22)

Nzeako UC, Goodman ZD, Ishak KG. Hepatocellular carcinoma and nodular regenerative hyperplasia: possible pathogenetic relationship. Am J Gastroenterol 1996;91:879–884. (Ref.102)

Okano H, et al. Natural course of cavernous hepatic hemangioma. Oncol Rep 2001;8:411–414. (Ref.34)

Ozenne V, et al. Liver tumours in patients with Fanconi anaemia: a report of three cases. Eur J Gastroenterol Hepatol 2008;20:1036–1039. (Ref.69)

Paradis V, et al. Telangiectatic focal nodular hyperplasia: a variant of hepatocellular carcinoma. Gastroenterology 2004;126:1323–1329. (Ref.78)

Paradis V, et al. A quantitative gene expression study suggests a role for angiopoietins in focal nodular hyperplasia. Gastroenterology 2003;124: 651–659. (Ref.39)

Paradis V, et al. Telangiectatic adenoma: an entity associated with increased body mass index and inflammation. Hepatology 2007;46:140–146. (Ref.85)

Paradis V, et al. Evidence for the polyclonal nature of focal nodular hyperplasia of the liver by the study of X-chromosome inactivation. Hepatology 1997;26:891–895. (Ref.45)

Quaia E, et al. Characterization of focal liver lesions with contrast-specific US modes and a sulfur hexafluoride–filled microbubble contrast agent: diagnostic performance and confidence. Radiology 2004;232:420–430. (Ref.21)

Rebouissou S, et al. Frequent in-frame somatic deletions activate gp130 in inflammatory hepatocellular tumours. Nature 2009;457:200–204. (Ref.76)

Rebouissou S, et al. HNF1alpha inactivation promotes lipogenesis in human hepatocellular adenoma independently of SREBP-1 and carbohydrate-response element-binding protein (ChREBP) activation. J Biol Chem 2007;282:14437–14346. (Ref.72)

Reddy KR, Schiff ER. Approach to a liver mass. Semin Liver Dis 1993;13:423–435. (Ref.5)

Reddy SK, et al. Resection of hepatocellular adenoma in patients with glycogen storage disease type 1a. J Hepatol 2007;47:658–663. (Ref.68)

Reimer P, Balzer T. Ferucarbotran (Resovist): a new clinically approved RES-specific contrast agent for contrast-enhanced MRI of the liver: properties, clinical development, and applications. Eur Radiol 2003;13:1266–1276. (Ref.109)

Rubin RA, Mitchell DG. Evaluation of the solid hepatic mass. Med Clin North Am 1996;80:907–928. (Ref.6)

Sadowski DC, et al. Progressive type of focal nodular hyperplasia characterized by multiple tumors and recurrence. Hepatology 1995;61:210–214. (Ref.63)

Savellano DH, et al. Assessment of sequential enhancement patterns of focal nodular hyperplasia and hepatocellular carcinoma on mangafodipir trisodium enhanced MR imaging. Invest Radiol 2004;39:305–312. (Ref.58)

Scalori A, et al. Oral contraceptives and the risk of focal nodular hyperplasia of the liver: a case-control study. Am J Obstet Gynecol 2002;186:195–197. (Ref.41)

Scoazec JY, et al. Focal nodular hyperplasia of the liver: composition of the extracellular matrix and expression of cell-cell and cell-matrix adhesion molecules. Hum Pathol 1995;26:1114–1125. (Ref.44)

Semelka RC, et al. Hepatic hemangiomas: a multi-institutional study of appearance on T2-weighted and serial gadolinium-enhanced gradient-echo MR images. Radiology 1994;192:401–406. (Ref.26)

Siegelman ES, et al. MR imaging of hepatic nodular regenerative hyperplasia. J Magn Reson Imaging 1995;5:730–732. (Ref.108)

Soler R, et al. Benign regenerative nodules with copper accumulation in a case of chronic Budd-Chiari syndrome: CT and MR findings. Abdom Imaging 2000;25:486–489. (Ref.107)

Strobel D, et al. Tumor-specific vascularization pattern of liver metastasis, hepatocellular carcinoma, hemangioma and focal nodular hyperplasia in the differential diagnosis of 1,349 liver lesions in contrast-enhanced ultrasound. Ultraschall Med 2009;30:376–382. (Ref.19)

Suzuki H, et al. Preoperative transcatheter arterial embolization for giant cavernous hemangioma of the liver with consumption coagulopathy. Am J Gastroenterol 1997;92:688–691. (Ref.15)

Taavitsainen M, et al. Fine-needle aspiration biopsy of liver hemangioma. Acta Radiol 1990;31:69–71. (Ref.16)

Tan M, et al. Successful outcome after transplantation of a donor liver with focal nodular hyperplasia. Liver Transpl 2001;7:652–655. (Ref.62)

Tanaka A, et al. Atypical liver hemangioma with shunt: long-term follow-up. J Hepatobiliary Pancreat Surg 2002;9:750–754. (Ref.14)

Terkivatan T, et al. Indications and long-term outcome of treatment for benign hepatic tumors: a critical appraisal. Arch Surg 2001;136:1033–1038. (Ref.10)

Toso C, et al. Hepatocellular adenoma and polycystic ovary syndrome. Liver Int 2003;23:35–37. (Ref.67)

Trillaud H, et al. Characterization of focal liver lesions with SonoVue-enhanced sonography: international multicenter-study in comparison to CT and MRI. World J Gastroenterol 2009;15:3748–3756. (Ref.20)

Trotter JF, Everson GT. Benign focal lesions of the liver. Clin Liver Dis 2001;5:17–42. (Ref.8)

Wanless IR. Micronodular transformation (nodular regenerative hyperplasia) of the liver: a report of 64 cases among 2500 autopsies and a new classification of benign hepatocellular nodules. Hepatology 1990;11:787–797. (Ref.100)

Wanless IR, et al. Multiple focal nodular hyperplasia of the liver associated with vascular malformations of various organs and neoplasia of the brain: a new syndrome. Mod Pathol 1989;2:456–462. (Ref.35)

Weimann A, et al. Benign liver tumors: differential diagnosis and indication for surgery. World J Surg 1997;21:983–990. (Ref.11)

Weimann A, et al. Critical issues in the diagnosis and treatment of hepatocellular adenoma. HPB 2000;2:25–32. (Ref.94)

Whitney WS, et al. Dynamic breath-hold multiplanar spoiled gradient-recalled MR imaging with gadolinium enhancement for differentiating hepatic hemangiomas from malignancies at 1.5 T. Radiology 1993;189:863–870. (Ref.25)

Zech CJ, et al. Diagnostic performance and description of morphological features of focal nodular hyperplasia in Gd-EOB-DTPA–enhanced liver magnetic resonance imaging: results of a multicenter trial. Invest Radiol 2008;43:504–511. (Ref.57)

Zucman-Rossi J, et al. Genotype-phenotype correlation in hepatocellular adenoma. New classification and relationship with HCC. Hepatology 2006;43:515–524. (Ref.73)

A complete list of references can be found at www.expertconsult.com.

Surgery for Liver Tumors

Réal Lapointe and Henri Bismuth

Introduction

As of 1950, major progress had been made in liver tumor surgery. Today, imaging is still improving and enormous strides have been made to better understand liver disease. Increasing experience and new surgical techniques have allowed a widespread acceptance of liver resection for benign and malignant tumors because of two factors: (1) the reduction in operative mortality and morbidity; and (2) the proven impact on prognosis.[1-4] For example, over the past decade many large series on resection of colorectal liver metastases (CRLM) and hepatocellular carcinoma (HCC) have shown better results, with operative mortality rates between 0% and 3% in high-volume centers (**Table 60-1**). Nowadays, the surgery of either benign or malignant liver tumors can be performed on normal or cirrhotic livers with acceptable morbidity and mortality rates in specialized hepatobiliary centers. The operative technique should be compared with an "à la carte" menu; that is, the surgical approach is adapted to each patient's liver tumors according to its performance status, the underlying liver disease, and complete tumor removal with margin of hepatic transection clear of the tumor.

General Principles

Liver resection for benign tumors should be done only for symptomatic patients, in the presence of a questionable diagnosis, or for tumors with known malignant potential. A minimal amount of liver parenchyma should be then removed. The principle of complete tumor removal also applies to malignant primary and secondary liver tumors, but a microscopic negative margin (R0 resection) is mandatory. However, even if it is still better to have a margin of at least of 1 cm, inability to get this wide margin should not restrain the surgeon from performing a liver resection for malignant tumors.

Criteria of resectability in metastatic disease are not based on either the number, the size, or distribution of tumors, but must guarantee complete R0 resection and preserve a sufficient volume of functioning liver parenchyma. In cirrhotic patients, liver resection is much more demanding and poses a risk of postoperative complications and mortality. Consequently, liver resection should be reserved only for patients with good liver function; the surgical technique should be limited to minimal mobilization and transection of cirrhotic liver with complete removal of tumor as long as preservation of maximal residual liver is ensured to minimize postoperative hepatic failure and susceptibility to infections.

A major concern during parenchymal transection is bleeding mainly from the hepatic veins and the inferior vena cava or in the presence of portal hypertension. The use of inflow with or without outflow vascular occlusion of the liver has limited morbidity and mortality related to intraoperative blood loss. Furthermore, knowledge of the segmental anatomy of the liver is essential for a safe performance of liver resection.

Anatomy and Classification

Safe and effective liver surgery cannot be performed without a perfect knowledge of the anatomy of the liver, including the blood vessels and bile ducts.[11,12] The liver is divided in two hemilivers, each divided into segments supplied by branches of the portal triads and drained by the hepatic veins (**Fig. 60-1**). The current nomenclature is based on the anatomic descriptions of Couinaud in 1957[13] and then by Bismuth in 1982.[11] This functional vascular anatomy was reviewed by the terminology committee of the International Hepato-Pancreato-Biliary Association in 2000 in order to standardize the nomenclature worldwide.[14] In general, a major liver resection is defined as the resection of three or more hepatic

Table 60-1 Large Series of Resection of Liver Tumors

STUDY (REF NO.)	YEAR	TYPE OF LIVER TUMORS	NO. OF PATIENTS	PERIOPERATIVE MORTALITY (%)	5-YEAR SURVIVAL RATE (%)	10-YEAR SURVIVAL RATE (%)
Fong (5)	1999	CRLM	1001	2.8	36	22
Fan (6)	1999	HCC	110	0	—	—
Minagawa (7)	2000	CRLM	235	0	38	26
Choti (2)	2002	CRLM	226	1	40	26
Kato (8)	2003	CRLM	585	—	33	—
Imamura (9)	2003	HCC	445	0	—	—
Wei (3)	2006	CRLM	423	1.6	47	28
Shah (10)	2007	CRLM	841	3	43	—
Rees (4)	2008	CRLM	929	1.5	36	23

CRLM, colorectal liver metastases; HCC, hepatocellular carcinoma

Table 60-2 Nomenclature of Major Hepatic Resections

SEGMENTS	COUINARD (1999)	BRISBANE (2000)
5, 6, 7, 8	Right hepatectomy	Right hemihepatectomy*
4, 5, 6, 7, 8	Right lobectomy	Right trisectionectomy or extended right hepatectomy or extended right hemihepatectomy*
2, 3	Left lobectomy	Left lateral sectionectomy or bisegmentectomy 2,3
2, 3, 4	Left hepatectomy	Left hepatectomy or left hemihepatectomy
2, 3, 4, 5, 8	Extended left hepatectomy	Left trisectionectomy or extended left hepatectomy or extended left hemihepatectomy*

*Stipulate with or without segment 1.

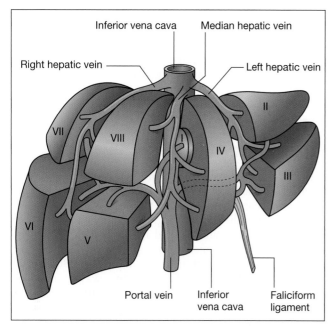

Fig. 60-1 **Schematic illustration of the anatomy of the liver.**

segments (hemihepatectomy and extended hepatectomy); a minor resection is defined as the resection of fewer than three segments, including wedge resections (**Table 60-2**).

Techniques for Liver Parenchymal Transection

The open approach was the only one used for performing liver resection until recently when the laparoscopic approach was proposed as an alternative in selected patients with either benign or malignant liver tumors. Pain, reduced mobility, a longer hospital stay, and more time off work are more frequent outcomes with open compared with laparoscopic surgery. The development of the laparoscopic approach has been directly related to technological refinements in laparoscopic instruments and the hepatic surgeon's learning curve. The main experience of laparoscopic liver resection is still limited to highly specialized centers worldwide.[15-18]

Various techniques of liver resection have been described to control bleeding during the parenchymal transection. The most commonly used method is the clamp crushing technique, first described by Bismuth.[11] The liver also may be cut with new devices, such as the ultrasonic dissector,[19] the hydrojet,[20,21] and the radiofrequency dissection sealer (RFDS).[20,22-24] Recently, alternative devices have been developed: the vessel sealing system (LigaSure)[25,26] and the ultrasonic activated device (Harmonic Scalpel).[27,28] In the last decade, other devices based on new energy sources (radiofrequency, microwave) have been produced.[29,30] The main purpose of these technical innovations is to decrease the bleeding during transection of hepatic parenchyma because excessive blood loss and blood transfusion have been associated with increased risk of both postoperative morbidity and mortality.[31-33]

A recently published meta-analysis of randomized controlled trials on different techniques for liver parenchymal transection has shown the clamp crushing technique is more rapid and is associated with lower rates of blood loss and otherwise similar outcomes (mortality, morbidity, liver dysfunction, or intensive therapy unit and hospital stay) when compared with other methods of parenchymal transection. It represents the reference standard against which new methods may be compared.[34] Two other randomized controlled trials[20,26] also concluded that the clamp crushing technique is the most efficient and the most cost-effective device.[20] However, the use of alternative devices that coagulate and/or dissect hepatic parenchyma is mandatory for laparoscopic liver surgery.[27,35,36]

Vascular Occlusion Techniques

Prevention of intraoperative blood loss is of prime concern in any type of liver resection. Intraoperative blood loss has been shown to influence adversely the short-term prognosis and may be associated with an increased risk of recurrence in patients undergoing surgery for a hepatobiliary malignancy because of impairment of the patient's immune response.[31-33] Although liver resections may be safely performed without vascular clamping, the basic principle in liver surgery is to minimize blood loss through control of major vascular structures. This may be achieved in several ways that range from segmental portal control to total hepatic vascular occlusion (**Fig. 60-2**).[37] However, the common drawback of any vascular occlusion technique is ischemic injury to remnant liver parenchyma. The type of hepatic vascular clamping is usually selected according to the site of the tumor, the presence of underlying liver disease, and the patient's cardiovascular status.

Inflow Vascular Control

The hemihepatic vascular clamping using the extrahepatic approach was first described by Lortat-Jacob in 1952. It consists of individually dissecting, ligating, and dividing the component portal inflow structures at the hepatic hilum and the hepatic vein before transecting the liver parenchyma. This technique has two advantages: (1) the primary vascular control permits demarcation between the two livers by the darkening of the ipsilateral liver; and (2) good vascular control results in a decrease in intraoperative bleeding. However, the technique has two disadvantages: (1) the risk of causing an injury to the hepatic vein; and (2) the risk of devitalizing the remaining liver by an erroneous ligation of an element of the porta hepatis, a risk which is increased by the frequency of anatomic abnormalities. An alternative technique is the intrahepatic anterior or posterior approach in which the whole sheath of the

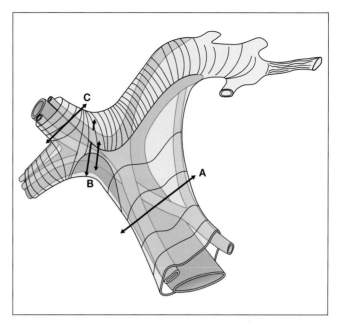

Fig. 60-2 **Modalities of vascular clamping. A,** Inflow exclusion or Pringle maneuver. **B,** Selective hemihepatic clamping (extrafascial or intrafascial). **C,** Suprahilar clamping.

portal pedicle is isolated within the substance of the liver during parenchymal transection and secured using a ligature or vascular stapling device.[11,38-40] The potential advantages include its avoidance of time-consuming and risky extrahepatic dissection, as well as the ligation of vessels of hepatic hilum by mistake because of anatomic abnormalities. However, the main drawback is the persistence of intraoperative bleeding in the resection plane from the nonoccluded liver. To overcome this drawback, a technique called the liver hanging maneuver has been described lately in which the liver is lifted by tape passed between the anterior surface of the vena cava and the liver, thereby providing effective vascular control.[41,42]

To decrease blood loss during the liver transection, the Pringle maneuver of total occlusion of the hepatic pedicle has been popularized in the late 1980s. Intermittent clamping is the preferred method over continuous clamping because it minimizes the ischemic injury during liver surgery.[43] However, notwithstanding the effectiveness of this procedure in reducing blood loss, it may still cause ischemic damage to the remaining liver, with risk of a poor postoperative outcome; therefore it is undesirable for use in circumstances such as in a small liver remnant, underlying liver disease, advanced age, steatosis, preoperative jaundice, and prolonged chemotherapy.[44,45] An alternative to intermittent clamping is ischemic preconditioning, in which a brief period of ischemia and reperfusion is applied before the prolonged ischemic insult (10 minutes of ischemia and 10 minutes of reperfusion).[46,47] It reduces reperfusion injury after warm ischemia, particularly in steatotic patients.

Hepatic Vascular Exclusion

Hepatic vascular exclusion (HVE) combines inflow and outflow vascular occlusion of the liver. The procedure completely isolates the liver from the systemic circulation and aims to prevent bleeding and air embolism from injuries to major

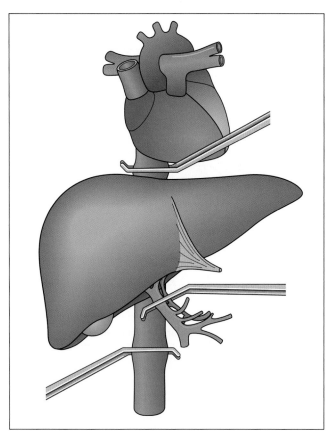

Fig. 60-3 **Total vascular exclusion.**

hepatic veins and/or the inferior vena cava (IVC). In this technique the liver has to be totally mobilized and the IVC dissected above and below the liver. HVE can be performed in different ways with total or selective hepatic vascular exclusion representing the most commonly applied techniques. Total hepatic vascular exclusion (THVE) combines portal triad clamping with suprahepatic and infrahepatic clamping of the IVC (**Fig. 60-3**). This technique allows a blood-free transection of the liver parenchyma.[48] Main indications are major resections for lesions involving the main hepatic veins or cavohepatic junction and when there is intolerance to lower central venous pressure. The main limit of this procedure is the low tolerance rate to clamping because of the inability of the myocardium to maintain an adequate cardiac output.

However, it is possible to overcome these hemodynamic drawbacks by using a selective hepatic vascular exclusion (SHVE), also known as hepatic vascular exclusion, with the preservation of caval flow.[49] This alternative technique consists of portal triad clamping plus transient occlusion of the hepatic veins without IVC clamping.

Even if a recent systematic review and meta-analysis study revealed that HVE does not offer any benefit regarding outcome of patients undergoing hepatic resection compared with portal triad clamping alone,[50] the HVE or SHVE technique should be considered very useful when there is invasion of the remnant hepatic vein or the IVC.

Value of Intraoperative Ultrasound

The inspection and palpation of the liver remain suboptimal to evaluate the deep hepatic tumors and/or discover other unrecognized hepatic tumors by preoperative imaging modalities. This is mainly due to the texture and thickness of the liver. Therefore the routine use of intraoperative ultrasound (IOUS) ensures the detection of all tumoral disease.[51] A systematic anatomic study of the liver should be performed in all cases, beginning with the three hepatic veins, the portal bifurcation, and its branches. Only when the segmental architecture has been understood are the known lesions examined, including paying attention to their location and relationship to the intrahepatic vascular structures. Scanning of the remaining parenchyma for occult lesions ends the examination of the liver. Today IOUS is mandatory for the planning of an adapted surgical procedure. It shows the relationship between a lesion and the neighboring vascular structures and may demonstrate that no clear margin is available without sacrificing a vessel to achieve a R0 resection. Despite the advances in preoperative imaging modalities, the frequency of unrecognized liver tumors found during IOUS and its use for surgical guidance has not changed significantly. Currently, routine use of IOUS modifies the operative strategy in about 20%.[52]

Because intraoperative ultrasound is the only method to see the intrahepatic vascular architecture of the liver, this has led to the evolution of segment-based resection, which is preferable from an oncologic standpoint, avoiding the need of extensive "blind" resections, thus sparing the maximal amount of nontumoral parenchyma, especially in patients with underlying liver disease with reduced hepatic reserve.[53,54]

Evolving Concept of Resectability

The concept of what constitutes "resectable" disease continues to evolve.[55] Lesions that would previously be deemed unresectable may now be considered resectable. However, despite significant improvement in techniques and outcomes of liver resection, only 20% to 30% of patients who have colorectal liver metastases have resectable disease and this remains a major limiting factor.[56-58] Lessons learned from living donor liver transplantation and the development of innovative surgical techniques have increased the possibility of operating on liver tumors previously deemed unresectable. Unresectability of liver lesions can be related to technical considerations such as: (1) large or ill-located tumors; (2) multiple bilateral lesions; and (3) when resection of a large area, although necessary, cannot be performed because the amount of the remnant liver is likely to result in liver failure.

It is usually accepted that a noncirrhotic healthy liver may tolerate a resection of up to 70% to 80% of its total volume. The enormous regenerative capacity enables functional compensation within a few weeks and regeneration of up to 75% of the preoperative liver volume within 1 year.[59,60] Computed tomography (CT) scans provide an accurate and reproducible method for preoperative liver volume calculation using three-dimensional CT volumetry. As there is some variability in liver volume calculation, it is suggested that the safe limit of resection should leave between 20% and 30% of functional normal liver parenchyma intact. Complications associated with technical aspects of liver surgery have shifted toward those related on the basis of liver remnant volume after major hepatic resection. Acceptable outcomes have been reported with living donor and partial liver transplantation by use of graft-volume to standard-liver-volume ratios of 30%.[61,62] Similarly, extended resections of up to 80% of the functional hepatic parenchyma can be performed with acceptable morbidity rates in patients with primary and metastatic disease.[63-65] Other studies revealed that future liver remnants of less than 25% of total liver volume were associated with an increased incidence of postoperative dysfunction in patients with normal liver.[66] The lessons learned from transplant volumetry and their application in liver surgery have widened the indications for extended hepatectomy for primary and secondary liver malignancies.[64,65] Recent studies have even reported combined resection of the liver and IVC with primary reconstruction of IVC or with synthetic or autogenous grafts.[67,68]

Portal Vein Embolization

One of the prerequisites for hepatic resection is that there is sufficient remaining parenchyma to prevent postoperative liver failure. Preoperative portal embolization (PVE) is a technique that induces an atrophy of the liver to be resected, leading to a compensatory hypertrophy of the remnant liver.[69,70] The portal system is most commonly accessed percutaneously through an ipsilateral or contralateral transhepatic approach under ultrasound guidance (**Fig. 60-4**). The choice of approach is at the discretion of the radiologist and the decision may be based on multiple factors that include the extent of the embolization and surgery, the preference of a specific agent, the tumor burden within the liver, and the experience of the radiologist with one technique more than another. The main advantage of the ipsilateral approach is that it avoids puncturing through healthy future remnant liver (FRL) parenchyma. Furthermore, it allows straightforward catheterization of segment IV branches in cases of planned extended right hepatectomy. On the other hand, the contralateral approach is performed through the future remnant liver with the

advantage of antegrade catheterization of right portal branches without the sharp angulation seen with the ipsilateral approach. The ratio of the volumes of the embolized and nonembolized parts of the liver is monitored by CT scans with three-dimensional reconstruction taken before and after embolization. The most important information obtained through volumetry is the ratio of the FRL to the total liver volume (TLV). Most surgical teams consider patients with a normal liver and with a ratio below 20% to 30% (depending on each center) to be candidates for preoperative PVE based on the FRL/TLV ratio. In cases of cirrhotic liver, some centers recommend PVE in all patients before a right-side hepatectomy to reduce postoperative complications such as liver failure.[71]

A period of 4 to 5 weeks is usually necessary for obtaining an FRL/TLV ratio sufficient enough to allow liver resection. In livers with impaired function this time interval can be increased up to 8 weeks. In the experience of French multicenter study, in 188 PVE procedures, the complication rate was 6%, but only in 1% of cases was planned liver surgery precluded. Transient liver insufficiency, with a bilirubin level exceeding two-fold the baseline value, occurred significantly more often in cirrhotic patients than in noncirrhotic patients.[72] PVE is a safe, modern, minimally invasive technique that may not only increase the pool of patients who are candidates for liver resection but may also increase the safety of resection.[63,69,73,74]

Two-Stage Hepatectomy

The ability of the liver to regenerate may also be used in situations where multiple bilobar disease would have previously precluded surgery. Staged resections can be performed without

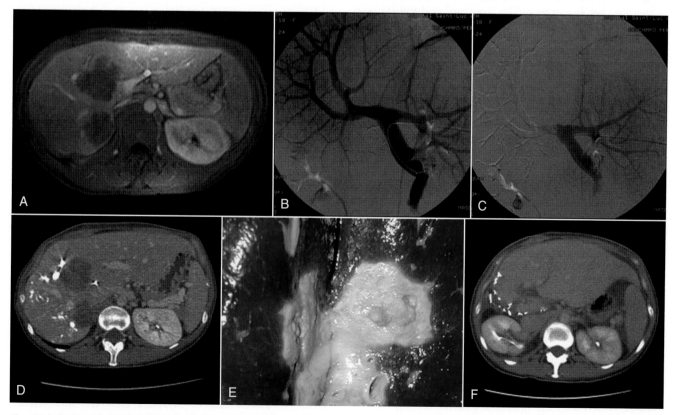

Fig. 60-4 **A,** Preembolization CT scan. **B,** Preportal embolization portography. **C,** Postportal embolization portography. **D,** One-month postportal embolization CT scan. **E,** Macroscopic pattern of portal pedicle fibrosis. **F,** Two-month postoperative CT scan.

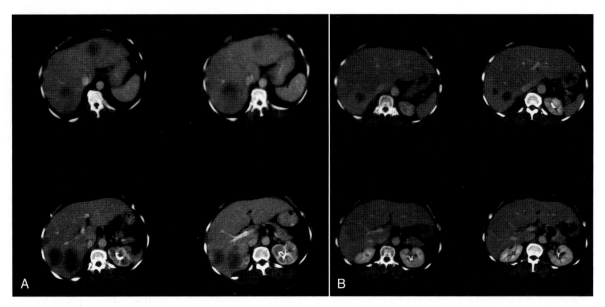

Fig. 60-5 **Downstaging by neoadjuvant chemotherapy.** Metastatic deposit in the liver before (**A**) and after (**B**) systematic neoadjuvant chemotherapy with fluorouracil and oxaliplatin.

inducing liver insufficiency by resecting large amounts of liver parenchyma in two separate sessions, thus allowing the liver time to regenerate between resections. This two-stage hepatectomy procedure is planned at the first liver resection and re-resection is usually performed within 3 to 6 months. During this time interval patients received chemotherapy, starting 3 weeks after the first hepatectomy to prevent interference with initial liver regeneration, and normally the same drug protocol is used as before surgery. This systemic chemotherapy is administered to limit the growth and spread of the remaining tumors.[75-79] As part of a multidisciplinary approach, this strategy can achieve long-term outcome in up to 70% of patients with a 5-year survival rate of 42%, which is not different from patients that undergo a single curative hepatectomy.[79]

Neoadjuvant Chemotherapy

Since it was recognized that neoadjuvant therapy could aid initially unresectable colorectal liver metastases, the use of neoadjuvant chemotherapy has expanded rapidly. However, there are no randomized trials of such neoadjuvant treatment to date, but several groups have reported evidence of improved survival rate after different chemotherapeutic regimens.[58,80] Also, some authors have noted that response to preoperative chemotherapy may be a surrogate marker of resection success and of response to postoperative chemotherapy, as well as 5-year survival rate.[81] Using this aggressive approach, liver resection has been routinely reconsidered in all cases of objective response to the treatment, permitting the tumor resectability rate to be increased from 20% to 30% (**Fig. 60-5**). The overall 5-year patient survival rate is 34%.[82] These results emphasize the importance of reconsidering liver resection in patients who were not candidates for primary surgery at first, but who responded well to chemotherapy. Independent of the type of chemotherapy used, the main point is that this approach offers a chance of cure to patients initially thought to have unresectable disease.[83]

PROS AND CONS OF PREOPERATIVE CHEMOTHERAPY

Pros
    Decrease size
    Control micrometastatic disease
    Assessment of activity of chemotherapy
    Better chemotherapy tolerance
    Surrogate marker for success of lives surgery

Cons
    Liver toxicity
        Steatosis
        Sinusoidal dilation
        Steatohepatitis
    Risk for progression or growth of new sites
    Complete response may make surgery more difficult
    Secondary splenomegaly
    Selection of resistant clones

Fig. 60-6 **Pros and cons of preoperative chemotherapy.** *(From Kemeny N. Presurgical chemotherapy in patients being considered for liver resection. Oncologist 2007;12:825–839.)*

Although surgical resection alone is regarded as the standard of care in initially resectable patients, patients are increasingly receiving preoperative chemotherapy as well.[84] No guidelines currently exist to guide this decision, and until recently, no randomized prospective trials have adequately investigated the risks and benefits. Proponents of preoperative chemotherapy in initially resectable patients mainly argue that this approach decreases tumor size, thereby potentially reducing resection volumes, while also offering earlier control of micrometastatic disease.[85] Opponents of preoperative chemotherapy contend that chemotherapy regimens are generally hepatotoxic, which may increase surgical complications, and that reducing tumor size is not necessarily a good thing, especially if tumors achieve complete response and become undetectable.[86-88] **Figure 60-6** summarizes the potential risks and benefits associated with preoperative chemotherapy in initially and potentially resectable patients.

Repeat Hepatectomy

The long-term outcome achieved after liver resection for malignant disease is often compromised by tumor recurrence. About 60% of patients develop recurrence after hepatectomy for colorectal metastases in the first two postoperative years and approximately a third of them have isolated liver recurrence.[89-92] Treatment of recurrent cancer after liver resection is usually palliative, and includes chemotherapy, with disappointing results.[90] However, with the improvement of surgical techniques and with increased range of sophisticated nonoperative modalities, it is possible to have a more radical approach. Therefore repeat resection has been more frequently performed in patients with isolated liver recurrence. This is due to recent advances in the early detection of recurrences, the efficacy of chemotherapy, and improvements in liver surgery. Patients submitted to a repeat resection for liver recurrence can achieve similar results to those of initial liver resection, with a reported survival benefit of 30% to 40% at 5 years and without additional perioperative mortality.[91,92]

Nonsurgical Treatment of Liver Tumors

Nonoperative ablative modalities such as radiofrequency ablations (RFAs) may be very useful in selected patients with primary or secondary liver malignancies.[93-95] RFA allows localized thermal treatment designed to produce tumor destruction by heating tumor tissue to temperatures that exceed 60° C. It can be performed percutaneously, laparoscopically, or with open surgery. Each technique has its own set of advantages and disadvantages; however, open surgery is the most effective and permits the greatest flexibility. Ideally, a zone of 1 cm width around the tumor should be destroyed to ensure a rim of nonmalignant tissue. RFA should not be applied to tumors near the hilum because it can damage the large bile ducts in the area, resulting in bile duct strictures. It also should not be applied to tumors in subcapsular locations, as it is associated with a high risk of neoplastic seeding. RFA should not be considered as a replacement for resection of colorectal liver tumors, but rather as an extension of treatment in unresectable patients. Combining hepatic resection with ablation expands the number of patients who may be candidates for liver surgery with a perioperative morbidity and mortality comparable with those seen after resection alone.[96-98] Patients with tumors larger than 3 cm have high local recurrence rates with RFA and are not optimal candidates for this procedure.[99] In patients with hepatocellular carcinoma (HCC), RFA should be considered when patients are not candidates for liver transplantation or are awaiting transplantation. The benefit of RFA relative to surgical resection for potentially resectable HCC remains controversial. Few retrospective series report long-term outcomes after RFA,[100,101] but the results are comparable with those of resection but with lower complication rates. In a Chinese randomized trial comparing partial hepatectomy with percutaneous local ablative therapy for solitary HCCs 5 cm or smaller, overall and disease-free survival rates were comparable in the two groups at 1, 2, 3, and 4 years.[102] Despite these data, the choice of treatment between RFA and surgical resection will depend on different clinical and radiologic

criteria: degree of liver failure (Child-Pugh class A, B, or C), intrahepatic location, solitary or multiple lesions, tumor size, presence or absence of vascular invasion and negative margin.

Microwave therapy has emerged as a new imaging-guided local thermal ablation within the past decade, mainly as a minimally invasive management technique for the treatment of HCC.[103,104] One advantage of microwave ablation (MWA) over radiofrequency ablation is the possibility of doing multiple ablations simultaneously. Even if MWA is reported as a safe and effective method for treating unresectable liver tumors with a low rate of local recurrence, the technique has not been widely available until now.

Conclusion

Despite the evolution of nonsurgical treatment in recent years, the surgical approach, whenever possible, remains the most favorable choice of treatment for benign and malignant hepatic tumors. The postoperative morbidity and mortality rates are low and very extensive resections can be carried out safely. Recent advances in medical technology and surgical techniques, better knowledge of segmental liver anatomy, improved imaging modalities for identifying liver tumors, and improved critical care management have allowed most patients to undergo liver resections with minimal morbidity and virtually no mortality. However, these patients are best managed in specialized centers where a multidisciplinary team with a medical, surgical, and oncologic expertise in treatment of liver tumors can take charge of these patients. As part of this dedicated team, the surgeons must be familiar with all aspects of both complex hepatobiliary surgery and liver transplantation.

Key References

Abdalla EK, et al. Improved resectability of hepatic colorectal metastases: expert consensus statement. Ann Surg Oncol 2006;13:1271–1280. (Ref.99)

Abdalla EK, et al. Extended hepatectomy in patients with hepatobiliary malignancies with and without preoperative portal vein embolization. Arch Surg 2002;137:675–680. (Ref.63)

Abdalla EK, et al. Total and segmental liver volume variations: implications for liver surgery. Surgery 2004;135:404–409. (Ref.60)

Abdalla EK, et al. Recurrence and outcomes following hepatic resection, radiofrequency ablation, and combined resection/ablation for colorectal liver metastases. Ann Surg 2004;239:818–827. (Ref.98)

Abulkhir A, et al. Preoperative portal vein embolization for major liver resection. A meta-analysis. Ann Surg 2008;247:49–57. (Ref.74)

Adam R, et al. Five-year survival following hepatic resection after neoadjuvant therapy for nonresectable colorectal liver metastases. Ann Oncol 2001;8: 347–353. (Ref.82)

Adam R, et al. Rescue surgery for unresectable colorectal liver metastases downstaged by chemotherapy: a model to predict long-term survival. Ann Surg 2004;240:644–657. (Ref.58)

Adam R, et al. Two-stage hepatectomy: a planned strategy to treat irresectable liver tumors. Ann Surg 2000;232:777–785. (Ref.75)

Adam R, et al. Two-stage hepatectomy approach for initially unresectable colorectal hepatic metastases. Surg Oncol Clin N Am 2007;16:525–536. (Ref.76)

Adam R, et al. Tumor progression while on chemotherapy: a contraindication to liver resection for multiple colorectal metastases? Ann Surg 2004;240: 1052–1061. (Ref.81)

Adam R, et al. Patients with initially unresectable colorectal liver metastases: is there a possibility of cure? J Clin Oncol 2009;27:1829–1835. (Ref.83)

Adams RB. Intraoperative ultrasound of the liver: techniques for liver resection and transplantation. In: Blumgart LH, et al, editors. Surgery of the liver, biliary tract, and pancreas, 4th ed. Philadelphia: WB Saunders, 2007: 1484–1524. (Ref.51)

Aldrighetti L, et al. Ultrasonic-mediated laparoscopic liver transection. Am J Surg 2008;195:270–272. (Ref.27)

Allen PJ, et al. Importance of response to neoadjuvant chemotherapy in patients undergoing resection of synchronous colorectal liver metastases. J Gastrointest Surg 2003;7:109–117. (Ref.80)

Arita J, et al. Randomized clinical trial of the effect of a saline-linked radiofrequency coagulator on blood loss during hepatic resection. Br J Surg 2005;92:954–959. (Ref.22)

Belghiti J, et al. Liver hanging manoeuvre: a safe approach to right hepatectomy without liver mobilization. J Am Coll Surg 2001;193:109–111. (Ref.41)

Belli G, et al. Ultrasonically activated device for parenchymal division during open hepatectomy. HPB (Oxford) 2008;10:234–238. (Ref.28)

Benoist S, et al. Complete response of colorectal liver metastases after chemotherapy: does it mean cure? J Clin Oncol 2006;24:3939–3945. (Ref.88)

Bleicher RJ, et al. Radiofrequency ablation in 447 complex unresectable liver tumors: lessons learned. Ann Surg Oncol 2003;10:52–58. (Ref.94)

Bryant R, et al. Laparoscopic liver resection—understanding its role in current practice. The Henri Mondor Hospital experience. Ann Surg 2009;250:103–111. (Ref.16)

Buell JF, et al. The international position on laparoscopic liver surgery. The Louisville statement, 2008. Ann Surg 2009;250:825–830. (Ref.18)

Chen MS, et al. A prospective randomized trial comparing percutaneous local ablative therapy and partial hepatectomy for small hepatocellular carcinoma. Ann Surg 2006;243:321–328. (Ref.102)

Cherqui D, et al. Laparoscopic liver resections: a feasibility study in 30 patients. Ann Surg 2000;232:753–762. (Ref.15)

Choti MA, et al. Trends in long-term survival following liver resection for hepatic colorectal metastases. Ann Surg 2002;235:759–766. (Ref.2)

Chouker A, et al. Effects of Pringle manoeuvre and ischaemic preconditioning on haemodynamic stability in patients undergoing elective hepatectomy: a randomized trial. Br J Anaesth 2004;93:204–211. (Ref.47)

Chun YS, et al. Management of chemotherapy-associated hepatotoxicity in colorectal liver metastases. Lancet Oncol 2009;10:278–286. (Ref.87)

Clavien PA, et al. A prospective randomized study in 100 consecutive patients undergoing major liver resection with versus without ischemic preconditioning. Ann Surg 2003;238:843–850. (Ref.46)

Couinaud C. Liver anatomy: portal (and suprahepatic) or biliary segmentation. Dig Surg 1999;16:449–467. (Ref.12)

Covey AM, et al. Combined portal vein embolization and neoadjuvant chemotherapy as a treatment strategy for resectable hepatic colorectal metastases. Ann Surg 2008;247:451–455. (Ref.73)

Cresswell AB, et al. Evaluation of intrahepatic, extra-Glissonian stapling of the right porta hepatis vs classical extrahepatic dissection during right hepatectomy. HPB (Oxford) 2009;11:493–498. (Ref.39)

Cunningham SC, Choti MA, Pawlik TM. Two-stage hepatectomy for colorectal cancer hepatic metastases. Curr Colorectal Cancer Rep 2008;4:93–99. (Ref.77)

de Baere T, Denys A, Madoff DC. Preoperative portal vein embolization: indications and technical considerations. Tech Vasc Interv Radiol 2007;10:67–78. (Ref.70)

de Jong MC, et al. Repeat curative intent liver surgery is safe and effective for recurrent colorectal liver metastasis: results from an international multi-institutional analysis. J Gastrointest Surg 2009;13:2141–2151. (Ref.91)

de Jong MC, et al. Rates and patterns of recurrence following curative intent surgery for colorectal liver metastasis: an international multi-institutional analysis of 1669 patients. Ann Surg 2009;250:440–448. (Ref.89)

De Matteo RP, et al. Anatomical segmental hepatic resection is superior to wedge resection as an oncologic operation for colorectal liver metastases. J Gastrointest Surg 2000;4:178–184. (Ref.53)

Delis S, et al. Clamp-crush technique vs radiofrequency-assisted liver resection for primary and metastatic liver neoplasms. HPB (Oxford) 2009;11:339–344. (Ref.24)

Delis SG, Madariaga J, Ciancio G. Combined liver and inferior vena cava resection for hepatic malignancy. J Surg Oncol 2007;96:258–264. (Ref.67)

Di Stefano DR, et al. Preoperative percutaneous portal vein embolization: evaluation of adverse events in 188 patients. Radiology 2005;234:625–630. (Ref.72)

Dionigi G, et al. Effect of perioperative blood transfusion on clinical outcomes in hepatic surgery for cancer. World J Gastroenterol 2009;15:3976–3983. (Ref.31)

Ellsmere J, et al. Intraoperative ultrasonography during planned liver resections: Why are we still performing it? Surg Endosc 2007;21:1280–1283. (Ref.52)

Fan ST, et al. Hepatectomy for hepatocellular carcinoma: toward zero hospital deaths. Ann Surg 1999;229:322–330. (Ref.6)

Fan ST, et al. Safety of donors in live donor liver transplantation using right lobe grafts. Arch Surg 2000;135:336–340. (Ref.61)

Farges O, et al. Portal vein embolization before right hepatectomy: prospective clinical trial. Ann Surg 2003;237:208–217. (Ref.71)

Fong Y, et al. Clinical score for predicting the recurrence after hepatic resection for metastatic colorectal cancer. Analysis of 1001 consecutive cases. Ann Surg 1999;230:309–321. (Ref.5)

Gumbs A, Gayet B, Gagner M. Laparoscopic liver resection: when to use the laparoscopic stapler device. HPB (Oxford) 2008;10:296–303. (Ref.36)

Hemming AW, et al. Combined resection of the liver and inferior vena cava for hepatic malignancy. Ann Surg 2004;239:712–721. (Ref.68)

Hilal MA, Lodge JPA. Pushing back the frontiers of resectability in liver cancer surgery. Eur J Surg Oncol 2008;34:272–280. (Ref.55)

Ikeda M, et al. The vessel sealing system (LigaSure) in hepatic resection. A randomized controlled trial. Ann Surg 2009;250:199–203. (Ref.26)

Imamura H, et al. One thousand fifty-six hepatectomies without mortality in 8 years. Arch Surg 2003;138:1198–1206. (Ref.9)

Jaeck D, et al. A two-stage hepatectomy procedure combined with portal vein embolization to achieve curative resection for initially unresectable multiple and bilobar colorectal liver metastases. Ann Surg 2004;240:1037–1051. (Ref.78)

Jarnagin WR, et al. Improvement in perioperative outcome after hepatic resection: analysis of 1,803 consecutive cases over the past decade. Ann Surg 2002;236:397–406. (Ref.1)

Kato T, et al. Therapeutic results for hepatic metastasis of colorectal cancer with special reference to effectiveness of hepatectomy: analysis of prognostic factors for 763 cases recorded at 18 institutions. Dis Colon Rectum 2003;46:S22–S31. (Ref.8)

Kemeny N. Presurgical chemotherapy in patients being considered for liver resection. Oncologist 2007;12:825–839. (Ref.85)

Kishi Y, et al. Three hundred and one consecutive extended right hepatectomies. Evaluation of outcome based on systematic liver volumetry. Ann Surg 2009;250:540–548. (Ref.65)

Kooby DA, et al. Influence of transfusions on perioperative and long-term outcome in patients following hepatic resection for colorectal metastases. Ann Surg 2003;237:860–869. (Ref.33)

Kornprat P, et al. Role of intraoperative thermoablation combined with resection in the treatment of hepatic metastasis from colorectal cancer. Arch Surg 2007;142:1087–1092. (Ref.96)

Kwon AH, Matsui Y, Kamiyama Y. Perioperative blood transfusion in hepatocellular carcinoma: influence of immunologic profile and recurrence free survival. Cancer 2001;91:771–778. (Ref.32)

Launois B, Tay KH, Meunier B. The posterior intrahepatic approach to liver resection. Hepatopancreatobiliary Surg 1999;1:209–214. (Ref.40)

Leelaudomlipi S, et al. Volumetric analysis of liver segments in 155 living donors. Liver Transpl 2002;8:612–614. (Ref.62)

Lesurtel M, Belghiti J. Open hepatic parenchymal transection using ultrasonic dissection and bipolar coagulation. HPB (Oxford) 2008;10:265–270. (Ref.19)

Lesurtel M, et al. Clamping techniques and protecting strategies in liver surgery. HPB (Oxford) 2009;11:290–295. (Ref.43)

Lesurtel M, et al. How should transection of the liver be performed? A prospective randomized study in 100 consecutive patients: comparing four different transection strategies. Ann Surg 2005;242:814–823. (Ref.20)

Liang P, et al. Prognostic factors for survival in patients with hepatocellular carcinoma after percutaneous microwave ablation. Radiology 2005;235:299–307. (Ref.104)

Liddo G, et al. The liver hanging manoeuvre. HPB (Oxford) 2009;11:296–305. (Ref.42)

Livraghi T, et al. Sustained complete response and complication rates after radiofrequency ablation of very early hepatocellular carcinoma in cirrhosis: Is resection still the treatment of choice? Hepatology 2008;47:82–89. (Ref.100)

Lupo L, et al. Randomized clinical trial of radiofrequency-assisted vs clamp-crushing liver resection. Br J Surg 2007;94:287–291. (Ref.23)

Martin RC, Scoggins CR, McMasters KM. Safety and efficacy of microwave ablation of hepatic tumors: a prospective review of a 5-year experience. Ann Surg Oncol 2010;17:171–178. (Ref.103)

Minagawa M, et al. Extension of the frontiers of surgical indications in the treatment of liver metastases from colorectal cancer: long-term results. Ann Surg 2000;231:487–499. (Ref.7)

N'Kontchou G, et al. Radiofrequency ablation of hepatocellular carcinoma: long-term results and prognostic factors in 235 Western patients with cirrhosis. Hepatology 2009;50:1475–1483. (Ref.101)

Nguyen KT, Gamblin TC, Geller DA. World review of laparoscopic liver resection—2,804 patients. Ann Surg 2009;250:831–841. (Ref.17)

Nicholl MB, Bilchik AJ. Thermal ablation of hepatic malignancy: useful but still not optimal. Eur J Surg Oncol 2008;34:318–323. (Ref.95)

Nordlinger B, et al. Perioperative chemotherapy with FOLFOX4 and surgery versus surgery alone for resectable liver metastases from colorectal cancer

(EORTC Intergroup trial 40983): a randomized controlled trial. Lancet 2008;371:1007–1016. (Ref.84)

Nordlinger B, et al. Combination of surgery and chemotherapy and the role of targeted agents in the treatment of patients with colorectal liver metastases: recommendations from an expert panel. Ann Oncol 2009;20:985–992. (Ref.57)

Pai M, et al. Liver resection with bipolar radiofrequency device: Habib™4X. HPB (Oxford) 2008;10:256–260. (Ref.29)

Pamecha V, et al. Techniques for liver parenchymal transection: a meta-analysis of randomized controlled trials. HPB (Oxford) 2009;11:275–281. (Ref.34)

Pawlik TM, Choti MA. Surgical therapy for colorectal metastases to the liver. J Gastrointest Surg 2007;11:1057–1077. (Ref.97)

Pawlik TM, Schulick RD, Choti MA. Expanding criteria for resectability of colorectal liver metastases. Oncologist 2008;13:51–64. (Ref.56)

Petrowsky H, et al. Second liver resections are safe and effective treatment for recurrent hepatic metastases from colorectal cancer. A bi-institutional study. Ann Surg 2002;235:863–871. (Ref.92)

Rahbari NN, et al. Portal triad clamping versus vascular exclusion for vascular control during hepatic resection: a systematic review and meta-analysis. J Gastrointest Surg 2009;13:558–568. (Ref.50)

Rau HG, Duessel AP, Wurzbacher S. The use of water-jet dissection in open and laparoscopic liver resection. HPB (Oxford) 2008;10:275–280. (Ref.21)

Rees M, et al. Evaluation of long-term survival after hepatic resection for metastatic colorectal cancer: a multifactorial model of 929 patients. Ann Surg 2008;247:125–135. (Ref.4)

Ribero D, et al. Portal vein embolization before major hepatectomy and its effects on regeneration, resectability and outcome. Br J Surg 2007;94: 1386–1394. (Ref.69)

Saiura A, et al. Liver transection using the LigaSure sealing system. HPB (Oxford) 2008;10:239–243. (Ref.25)

Satoi S, et al. Long-term outcome of hepatocellular carcinoma patients who underwent liver resection using microwave tissue coagulation. HPB (Oxford) 2008;10:289–295. (Ref.30)

Serracino-Ingnotti F, Habbib NA, Mathie RT. Hepatic ischaemia-reperfusion injury. Am J Surg 2001;58:160–166. (Ref.45)

Shah SA, et al. Survival after liver resection for metastatic colorectal carcinoma in a large population. J Am Coll Surg 2007;205:676–683. (Ref.10)

Shoup M, et al. Volumetric analysis predicts hepatic dysfunction in patients undergoing major liver resection. J Gastrointest Surg 2003;7:325–330. (Ref.66)

Slakey D. Laparoscopic liver resection using a bipolar vessel-sealing device: LigaSure®. HPB (Oxford) 2008;10:253–255. (Ref.35)

Strasberg SM, Drebin JA, Lineban D. Use of a bipolar vessel-sealing device for parenchymal transection during liver surgery. J Gastrointest Surg 2002;6: 569–574. (Ref.44)

Sutherland LM, et al. Radiofrequency ablation of liver tumors. A systematic review. Arch Surg 2006;141:181–190. (Ref.93)

Tanaka K, et al. Role of neoadjuvant chemotherapy in treatment of multiple colorectal metastases to the liver. Br J Surg 2003;90:963–969. (Ref.90)

Terminology Committee of the International Hepato-Pancreato-Biliary Association IHPBA. Brisbane 2000 terminology of liver anatomy & resections. HPB (Oxford) 2000;2:333–339. (Ref.14)

Torzilli G, et al. Anatomical segmental and subsegmental resection of the liver for hepatocellular carcinoma: a new approach by means of ultrasound-guided vessel compression. Ann Surg 2010;251:229–235. (Ref.54)

Vauthey JN, et al. Is extended hepatectomy for hepatobiliary malignancy justified? Ann Surg 2004;239:722–730. (Ref.64)

Wei AC, et al. Survival after hepatic resection for colorectal metastases: a 10-year experience. Ann Surg Oncol 2006;13:668–676. (Ref.3)

Wicherts DA, et al. Long-term results of two-stage hepatectomy for irresectable colorectal cancer liver metastases. Ann Surg 2008;248:994–1005. (Ref.79)

Zografos GN, et al. Total vascular exclusion for liver resections: pros and cons. J Surg Oncol 1999;72:50–55. (Ref.48)

Zorzi D, et al. Chemotherapy-associated hepatotoxicity and surgery for colorectal liver metastases. Br J Surg 2007;94:274–286. (Ref.86)

A complete list of references can be found at www.expertconsult.com.

Chapter **61**

Management of Gallstones

J. Kettelle and Priti Sud

ABBREVIATIONS

BMI body mass index
CT computed tomography
ERCP endoscopic retrograde
  cholangiopancreatography

ES endoscopic sphincterotomy
EUS endoscopic ultrasound
GERD gastroesophageal reflux disease
MELD Model of End-Stage Liver Disease

MRCP magnetic resonance
  cholangiopancreatography
NOTES natural-orifice transluminal
  endoscopic surgery

Introduction

Gallstones are increasingly prevalent; among digestive diseases they are second in cost only to gastroesophageal reflux disease (GERD). Treating patients with gallstones exceeds the expense of treating patients with colorectal cancer or peptic ulcer disease.[1]

The causes of gallbladder disease are multifactorial. In developed countries it is most commonly due to the formation of cholesterol-type gallstones. Risk factors for cholesterol gallstone formation include pregnancy, obesity, older age, type 2 diabetes mellitus, hypertriglyceridemia, insulin resistance, ethnic background, and family history. Dietary factors including high total calorie intake, high carbohydrate intake, and lack of fiber consumption also predispose to gallbladder disease.[2] A Swedish twin study confirmed the association between increasing body mass index (BMI) and gallbladder disease. That same study demonstrated a negative effect of increased alcohol consumption on gallbladder disease.[3] Obesity and female gender appear to be risk factors for gallbladder disease even in children and adolescents.[4] The dramatically elevated risk of gallstones in one Native American population has been well described.[5] German researchers found that cholesterol-type gallstones were strongly linked to a common variant of the gene encoding the hepatocanalicular cholesterol transporter protein ABCG5/G8.[6]

Cholesterol, mixed, and pigment are the three most common types of stones. Cholesterol gallstones occur when bile that is supersaturated with cholesterol begins to precipitate cholesterol crystals, which then become the nidus for stone formation. Mixed gallstones are a combination of cholesterol and pigment gallstones but have less than 70% cholesterol by weight. Pigment gallstones contain the calcium salts of bilirubin and other anions. Pigment stones are associated with bile duct obstruction, biliary stasis, and hemolysis. Pigment gallstones are further subclassified into brown and black subtypes: brown pigment gallstones are associated with biliary infections and are seen most commonly in Asia; black pigment stones are common in the Western population.

The treatment for pigment gallstones is equivalent to the treatment for cholesterol and mixed gallstones, except that pigment gallstone response to medical therapy is worse.[7] This chapter emphasizes endoscopic and surgical management of gallstones, as medical therapy is now seldom used.

Cholecystectomy is the most common general surgical operation performed. In 2006, according to the U.S. Centers for Disease Control and Prevention (CDC), 414,000 cholecystectomies were performed as inpatient procedures[8] and 503,000 as outpatient procedures.[9] The overall number of outpatient surgical procedures has increased markedly over the last decade; laparoscopic cholecystectomy has followed this trend.

With the litany of advances in endoscopic techniques, endoscopic retrograde cholangiopancreatography (ERCP) has become a successful approach for gallstone removal. For the first 30 years of its use, ERCP served as the only effective diagnostic and therapeutic entity for patients with pancreaticobiliary diseases, but is now primarily a therapeutic tool for such patients; its use dramatically increased from 1988 to 1996. With the advent of noninvasive diagnostic techniques such as endoscopic ultrasound (EUS) and magnetic resonance cholangiopancreatography (MRCP), the use of ERCP for diagnosis has steadily declined since 1996. From 1988 to 1996, the age-adjusted rate of diagnostic ERCP use increased nearly three-fold, from 25 per 100,000 up to nearly 75 per 100,000, but then began to decline, dropping to 59 per 100,000 by the year 2002. The age-adjusted rate of therapeutic ERCP use, however, continued to rise from approximately 14 per 100,000 in 1988, up to about 40 per 100,000 by 2002.[10]

Laparoscopic Cholecystectomy

The French surgeon Phillipe Mouret is credited with performing the first human laparoscopic cholecystectomy in 1987. Reddick and Olsen published the first reports of laparoscopic cholecystectomy and developed laparoscopic cholangiography.[11]

Laparoscopic cholecystectomy begins with creation of a pneumoperitoneum by carbon dioxide insufflation. Gas-tight trocars are then inserted into the peritoneal cavity. Traditionally, three or four trocars are inserted. A forward-viewing or angled laparoscope is inserted through one port; retraction and dissection are carried out through the other ports. The cystic duct and cystic artery are circumferentially dissected. Lateral retraction of the gallbladder is essential in order to identify the triangle of Calot (**Fig. 61-1**). Once completely dissected, the cystic duct and cystic artery are secured with surgical clips and divided. The gallbladder is then dissected off the gallbladder fossa and removed through a trocar.

A number of innovative approaches to laparoscopic cholecystectomy have now been developed, with the goal of reducing or eliminating abdominal wall incisions. Single-incision laparoscopic surgery (SILS) involves placing multiple trocars in close proximity to one another, or using a specially designed multiple-port trocar through a single small incision typically placed at the umbilicus.[12] Articulating laparoscopic instruments have been designed to facilitate this approach. Natural-orifice transluminal endoscopic surgery (NOTES) uses flexible endoscopes and endoscopic instrumentation through a natural orifice to perform intraabdominal operations. NOTES cholecystectomy has now been performed in humans via transvaginal and transgastric routes (**Fig. 61-2**).[13-15]

Endoscopic Procedures

In 1968 the first ERCP was reported in the United States; in 1974 the first endoscopic sphincterotomy (ES) was performed in Japan.[16-18] Subsequently a number of new techniques have been introduced, but controversy still exists in several clinical areas. For example, no clear consensus has been reached regarding performing a cholecystectomy after ERCP and ES in patients who have common bile duct stones but are otherwise asymptomatic.

Retained or recurrent common bile duct stones are found in about 5% of patients who have undergone cholecystectomy.[19] The possibility of de novo synthesis of stones in the common bile duct may favor leaving the gallbladder in situ following a sphincterotomy. A study by Saito showed a relatively favorable long-term outcome for patients with choledocholithiasis and cholecystolithiasis who underwent endoscopic papillotomy. The authors concluded that cholecystectomy after endoscopic papillotomy was not always necessary in the management of cholecystolithiasis.[20]

Subsequent studies have shown a higher incidence of recurrent biliary events in those in whom the gallbladder was not removed. Boerma and colleagues studied 120 patients over a period of 2 years. Recurrent biliary events were observed significantly more often in the group randomized to watchful waiting (47%) than in the group randomized to early cholecystectomy (2%). At the end of the study, 37% of the patients originally assigned to watchful waiting required cholecystectomy; in addition, the conversion rate to open cholecystectomy was higher in that group.[21] Similar results were found in a meta-analysis of five randomized trials published in the Cochrane Database.[22]

Those studies supported the trend to offer cholecystectomy to healthy patients after ERCP but to implement a wait-and-watch policy for older patients or those with a high operative risk. However, a recent study in China involving patients older than 60 showed that cholecystectomy after endoscopic treatment of bile duct stones reduced recurrent biliary events and should be recommended, even in older patients.[23] Similar studies must be conducted in the United States before the data can be extrapolated.

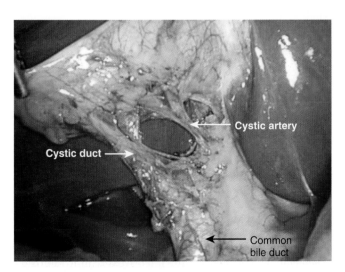

Fig. 61-1 **Triangle of Calot's.**

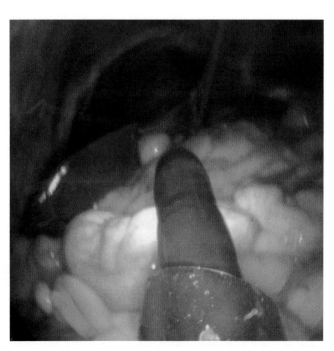

Fig. 61-2 **Transvaginal cholecystectomy.**

Symptomatic Cholelithiasis

The overall prevalence of gallstone disease in the United States is 15% to 20% of the adult population. Of these adults, 80% are asymptomatic. Symptoms of gallbladder disease include epigastric or right upper quadrant abdominal pain, dyspepsia, bloating, jaundice, fatty food intolerance, and flatulence. Recurrent episodes of cystic duct obstruction over time cause inflammation and scarring of the gallbladder. Surgery remains the mainstay of treatment for symptomatic gallstone disease. The presence of related symptoms, if gallstones are documented by imaging, is an indication for cholecystectomy in patients with acceptable medical risks.

Laparoscopic cholecystectomy significantly improves the quality of life in patients with either symptomatic or asymptomatic gallstones.[24] Prolonged waiting time for the treatment of gallstones has been shown to increase overall morbidity.[25]

Intraoperative diagnosis of choledocholithiasis may be made by cholangiography or laparoscopic ultrasound. Detected common bile duct stones may then be managed by laparoscopic common bile duct exploration, intraoperative ERCP, or open common bile duct exploration; most commonly, however, stones are deferred for postoperative ERCP.[26]

Acute Cholecystitis

Acute cholecystitis occurs secondary to obstruction of the cystic duct, resulting in bile stasis, with inflammation and edema of the gallbladder wall. Cholelithiasis, the most common cause of cystic duct obstruction, accounts for 95% of acute cholecystitis cases. Secondary infection of the bile with gut organisms may occur. *Escherichia coli* and *Bacteroides* are the most commonly isolated species.[27] Early laparoscopic cholecystectomy for patients with acute cholecystitis has been shown to be safe, with no significant increase in postoperative complications or in the conversion rate to an open procedure. Patients who undergo early cholecystectomy have a shorter hospital length of stay.[28] Acute acalculous cholecystitis is much less common, accounting for only 5% of acute cholecystitis cases; it tends to occur in critically ill patients. Gallbladder stasis and ischemia have been postulated as causative factors.

Choledocholithiasis

Choledocholithiasis occurs in 3% to 10% of patients undergoing cholecystectomy.[29] Common clinical presentations include bile duct obstruction, pancreatitis, and cholangitis. Common bile duct stones may be discovered preoperatively, intraoperatively, or postoperatively. Elevated serum bilirubin, alkaline phosphatase, and γ-glutamyltransferase levels may indicate common bile duct stones.[30] Transabdominal ultrasound, computed tomography (CT), EUS, and MRCP may aid in preoperative diagnosis. As previously discussed, ERCP was the gold standard for preoperative diagnosis of common bile duct stones but is now primarily used therapeutically. MRCP and EUS offer the opportunity to accurately visualize the biliary system while avoiding the risks of pancreatitis, cholangitis, and radiation exposure.[31] Gallstones can be documented within the common bile duct by EUS with an accuracy similar to that of ERCP.[31-35] MRCP documents gallstones with a somewhat lower accuracy. Intraoperative cholangiography has been shown to be less sensitive than both MRCP and EUS.[36-41]

A recent meta-analysis found that by first performing EUS, ERCP may be safely avoided in two thirds of patients suspected to have common bile duct stones. Use of EUS to select patients for therapeutic ERCP significantly reduces complications.[42]

Postoperative ERCP is commonly used when bile duct stones are found at the time of surgery.[26] ERCP complicated by difficult duodenal anatomy, prior gastric surgery, or other technical factors may necessitate laparoscopic or open common bile duct exploration. Percutaneous transhepatic stone extraction or lithotripsy may also be used. Endoscopic sphincterotomy during ERCP has been an essential technique in the removal of common bile duct stones. However, endoscopic sphincterotomy and attempted stone extraction by Dormia basket are unsuccessful in 10% to 15% of patients.[43] In the vast majority of such patients, the two main problems are large stone size (>15 mm in diameter) and tapering of the distal common bile duct.

Stones that are difficult to remove can be extracted by such methods as mechanical lithotripsy, intraductal shock wave lithotripsy, extracorporeal shock wave lithotripsy, biliary stenting, and chemical dissolution. Balloon sphincteroplasty is another method used to enlarge the biliary sphincter opening; although popular in Asia, this method is not widely used in the United States because of the associated risk of pancreatitis.[44-46] A modified technique, involving large-diameter balloon dilation after a limited endoscopic sphincterotomy, has recently been shown to be safe and easy to perform.[47,48] Direct, peroral cholangioscopy with intubation of the biliary orifice allows for electrohydraulic lithotripsy;[43] perforation of the bile duct has been reported with this technique, but is uncommon.[49] With the use of the previously listed methods, endoscopic stone extraction is successful in 98% of cases.[50,51]

Endoscopic removal of common bile duct stones has a low rate of morbidity and mortality. The most common complication is pancreatitis, which occurs in 1% to 7% of patients. Less common complications include hemorrhage, perforation, cholangitis, cholecystitis, and cardiopulmonary events (fewer than 1% of patients). The mortality is low (an estimated 0.2% to 0.4%).[52-54] The complication rate is highest when ERCP is performed for suspected sphincter of Oddi dysfunction (21.7%) and lowest for removal of stones within 30 days after laparoscopic cholecystectomy (4.9%).[53]

Cholangitis

Acute cholangitis is an ascending bacterial infection of the biliary tract that occurs with some degree of ductal obstruction. The most common cause of obstruction is gallstones. The most frequent organisms cultured from bile in patients with cholangitis are *E. coli* and *Klebsiella, Enterococcus,* and *Bacteroides* species.[55] Cholangitis may manifest as a relatively mild infection with fever and jaundice or as severe septic shock. The clinical triad of jaundice, fever, and right upper quadrant abdominal pain was described by Jean-Martin Charcot in 1877.[56] Hypotension and mental status changes were added by B.M. Reynolds in 1959 to form the eponymous pentad.[57]

Initial treatment requires antibiotics and fluid resuscitation. Severely ill patients may require intensive care unit admission and pressor support. Emergency decompression of the bile ducts may be necessary, which can be accomplished by endoscopic or percutaneous drainage. Surgical treatment with bile duct exploration and T-tube drainage is reserved for situations where endoscopic or percutaneous treatment is not possible.

Mirizzi Syndrome

Mirizzi syndrome, or functional hepatic syndrome, was first described in 1948. This rare and late symptom of gallbladder disease was described as biliary obstruction with jaundice secondary to severe inflammation in the triangle of Calot caused by gallstone impaction in the cystic duct or gallbladder.[58] A classification system for Mirizzi syndrome is developed based on the degree of bile duct involvement. This system grades the cholecystobiliary involvement from type I (external compression of the bile duct) to type IV (complete destruction of the bile duct).[59] Mirizzi syndrome has also been associated with cholecystoenteric fistula formation. Beltran and colleagues proposed a new classification system that included cholecystoenteric fistula formation.[60]

Laparoscopic treatment of patients with Mirizzi syndrome is feasible, particularly for type I disease.[61] Careful preoperative workup is essential to prevent injury to the bile duct. Yet laparoscopic treatment presents a formidable challenge. A recent review showed a conversion rate of 41%, a complication rate of 20%, and a reoperation rate of 6%.[62] Interestingly, gallbladder carcinoma has been described as mimicking Mirizzi syndrome; conversely, Mirizzi syndrome has been noted to mimic gallbladder carcinoma.[63,64]

Gallstone Pancreatitis

An estimated 237,000 people per year are hospitalized for acute pancreatitis.[8] Although most cases are mild, 10% to 20% of patients will have moderate or severe forms of pancreatitis, graded by various scoring systems such as Ranson's criteria, Acute Physiology and Chronic Health Evaluation (APACHE) II, and the 1992 Atlanta Symposium guidelines.[65-67] Gallstones and alcohol use remain the chief causes of pancreatitis, each accounting for about 40% of all cases. Gallstones are suspected as the cause of acute pancreatitis when gallstones are visualized, when common bile duct dilation is detected by ultrasound or CT, or when elevations in measurements of liver function tests are found.[67]

Up to two thirds of patients whose acute pancreatitis is caused by gallstones will develop recurrent symptoms unless the gallstones are eliminated. Patients with resolving mild pancreatitis should undergo laparoscopic cholecystectomy with intraoperative cholangiography. Some evidence shows that cholecystectomy should be carried out during the index hospital admission in most patients, but it may have to be delayed until laboratory indices of inflammation or malnutrition have returned to normal.[68,69] Patients with mild to moderate acute gallstone pancreatitis who undergo selective postoperative ERCP (as compared with routine preoperative ERCP) and common bile duct stone extraction have shorter hospital stays, incur less cost, and experience no increase in combined treatment failure rates.[70] ERCP is reserved for patients with evidence of retained gallstones after cholecystectomy or poor surgical candidates.[71] A study involving 238 patients with mild pancreatitis and a serum bilirubin concentration lower than

5 mg/dl found no difference in survival between the early ERCP group and the delayed selective ERCP group. The early ERCP group also had more severe complications.[72]

Urgent ERCP is performed in patients with severe pancreatitis or accompanying cholangitis.[71] In a randomized multicenter trial, 153 patients with predicted severe gallstone pancreatitis without cholangitis were prospectively followed. The trial compared conservative treatment versus early ERCP within 72 hours after symptom onset (at the discretion of the treating physician) for complications and mortality. Early ERCP was associated with fewer complications in patients with severe gallstone pancreatitis if cholestasis (defined by a bilirubin concentration >2.3 mg/dl) was present.[73] EUS or MRCP may be useful in determining the need for ERCP in patients with a complicated clinical course, including those not improving in a timely manner, pregnant women, patients for whom ERCP is a difficult or high-risk procedure, and patients whose pancreatitis may not have a biliary cause.[74,75]

Despite the advances in our understanding of gallstone pancreatitis the overall mortality remains approximately 15%. Only half of the patients hospitalized for gallstone pancreatitis throughout the United States undergo cholecystectomy before discharge, suggesting suboptimal adherence on the part of clinicians to national guidelines.[76]

Gallstone Ileus

Gallstone ileus is a mechanical obstruction of the gastrointestinal tract secondary to gallstone impaction. It most commonly occurs in conjunction with a cholecystoenteric fistula. The phenomenon has also been described after ERCP with stone extraction.[77] Bouveret syndrome is obstruction of the duodenum with an impacted gallstone. Gallstone ileus typically involves obstruction of the terminal ileum but it has been described in numerous locations, from the stomach to the sigmoid colon. Treatment usually requires surgery with enterolithotomy and retrieval of the obstructing stone. Controversy exists regarding the benefit of a single-stage operation with enterolithotomy alone (leaving the fistula in place) versus enterolithotomy with fistula closure.[78] Both procedures have been performed laparoscopically.[79-82] Fistula closure adds significant time to the operation. Leaving the fistula in place appears to add little postoperative morbidity.[83] Gallstone ileus has also been treated endoscopically, with stone retrieval or fragmentation from the duodenum, the proximal jejunum, and the terminal ileum. Endoscopic lithotripsy and extracorporeal lithotripsy have also been used to successfully treat gallstone ileus.[84,85]

Cholecystectomy in Pregnancy

Pregnancy is an important factor in the pathogenesis of gallstones. Changes in the enterohepatic circulation and hormonal influences on cholesterol concentration in bile have been linked to gallstone formation. In the animal model, gallstone formation has been observed after prolonged administration of progesterone and estradiol.[86]

Gallbladder volume is increased and the percentage of gallbladder emptying is decreased during pregnancy. The large retained volume after gallbladder emptying in pregnancy may result in retention of cholesterol crystals with subsequent gallstone formation.[87]

Table 61-1 **SAGES Guidelines for Laparoscopic Surgery in Pregnancy 2007**	
Ultrasonographic imaging during pregnancy is safe and useful in identifying the etiology of acute abdominal pain in the pregnant patient. Expeditious and accurate diagnosis should take precedence over concerns for ionizing radiation. Radiation dosage should be limited to 5-10 rad in the first 25 weeks of pregnancy. Contemporary multidetector CT protocols deliver a radiation dose to the fetus below detrimental levels and may be considered as an appropriate test during pregnancy, depending on the clinical situation. Magnetic resonance imaging can be performed at any stage of pregnancy without the use of intravenous gadolinium. Nuclear medicine administration of radionucleotides can generally be accomplished at fetal radiation levels of exposure that are well below any known detrimental levels. Intraoperative and endoscopic cholangiography exposes the mother and fetus to minimal radiation and may be used selectively during pregnancy. The lower abdomen should be shielded when performing cholangiography during pregnancy to decrease the radiation exposure to the fetus. Diagnostic laparoscopy is safe and effective when used selectively in the workup and treatment of acute abdominal processes in pregnancy. Laparoscopic treatment of acute abdominal processes has the same indications in pregnant and nonpregnant patients. Laparoscopy can be safely performed during any trimester of pregnancy. Gravid patients should be placed in the left lateral recumbent position to minimize compression of the vena cava and the aorta.	Initial access can be safely accomplished with open (Hassan), Veress needle, or optical trocar technique if the location is adjusted according to fundal height, previous incisions, and experience of the surgeon. CO_2 insufflation of 10-15 mm Hg can be safely used for laparoscopy in the pregnant patient. Intraabdominal pressure should be sufficient to allow for adequate visualization. Intraoperative CO_2 monitoring by capnography should be used during laparoscopy in the pregnant patient. Intraoperative and postoperative pneumatic compression devices and early postoperative ambulation are recommended prophylaxis for deep venous thrombosis in the gravid patient. Laparoscopic cholecystectomy is the treatment of choice in the pregnant patient with gallbladder disease regardless of trimester. Choledocholithiasis during pregnancy may be managed with preoperative endoscopic retrograde cholangiopancreatography (ERCP) with sphincterotomy followed by laparoscopic cholecystectomy, intraoperative laparoscopic transcystic or choledochotomy common bile duct exploration, or postoperative ERCP depending on local resources and clinical scenario. Fetal heart monitoring should occur pre- and postoperatively in the setting of urgent abdominal surgery during pregnancy. Obstetric consultation can be obtained pre- and/or postoperatively based on the acuteness of the patient's disease, gestational age, and availability of the consultant. Tocolytics should not be used prophylactically, but should be considered perioperatively in coordination with obstetric consultation when signs of preterm labor are present.

Adapted from Yumi H. Guidelines for diagnosis, treatment, and use of laparoscopy for surgical problems during pregnancy: this statement was reviewed and approved by the Board of Governors of the Society of American Gastrointestinal and Endoscopic Surgeons (SAGES), Sept 2007. It was prepared by the SAGES Guidelines Committee. Surg Endosc 2008;22:849–861.

In a large study gallstones were detected in 12.2% of women screened within 48 hours postpartum versus 1.3% of an age-matched nulliparous control group. One third of the postpartum women with documented gallstones were also found to have been symptomatic with biliary colic during the pregnancy.[88] Biliary sludge is also frequently found in pregnancy; it is generally asymptomatic and, in a high percentage of patients, is believed to resolve after pregnancy.[89]

Laparoscopic cholecystectomy has been safely performed in all trimesters of pregnancy and has for some time been the preferred treatment for gallbladder disease during the second trimester.[90] Other minimally invasive techniques including percutaneous aspiration or cholecystostomy, as well as ERCP, have also been used successfully in all trimesters.[91] A more recent analysis based on quality pregnancy weeks found laparoscopic cholecystectomy to be superior to nonoperative management in both the first and second trimesters.[92] The guidelines of the Society of American Gastrointestinal and Endoscopic Surgeons (SAGES) were updated in 2008 to reflect that laparoscopic cholecystectomy is now the treatment of choice for gallbladder disease in pregnancy, regardless of trimester[93] (**Table 61-1**).

Cholecystectomy in Cirrhosis

Cholelithiasis is common in patients with cirrhosis because of intravascular hemolysis and functional changes of the gallbladder.[94]

Open cholecystectomy in patients with cirrhosis has been described as a formidable operation, with an 83% mortality. Deaths have been related to hepatic encephalopathy, ascites, sepsis, and hemorrhage.[95] In 1992 the U.S. National Institutes of Health (NIH) Consensus Development Conference on Gallstones and Laparoscopic Cholecystectomy declared cirrhosis with portal hypertension as a relative contraindication to laparoscopic cholecystectomy.[96] Since then, multiple studies have shown the feasibility of laparoscopic cholecystectomy in patients with compensated Child-Pugh class A and B cirrhosis. A meta-analysis of 400 patients with cirrhosis who underwent laparoscopic (as compared with open) cholecystectomy showed less operative blood loss, shorter operative times, and shorter length of hospital stay.

However, the aforementioned meta-analysis and other studies have failed to draw conclusions regarding Child-Pugh class C cirrhosis, given the small number of patients in that category.[97,98] A single-institution experience that included four patients with Child-Pugh class C cirrhosis who underwent laparoscopic cholecystectomy showed 50% mortality and 75% morbidity.[99-101] A retrospective review involving 55 patients with cirrhosis who underwent laparoscopic cholecystectomy did not find the Model for End-Stage Liver Disease (MELD) score to be useful in predicting morbidity.[102] Percutaneous gallbladder aspiration and percutaneous cholecystostomy with deployment of a pigtail catheter have both been shown to be effective alternatives to laparoscopic cholecystectomy in patients with Child-Pugh class C cirrhosis.[103] Subtotal laparoscopic cholecystectomy has also been described as an alternative to complete laparoscopic cholecystectomy in patients with cirrhosis; the posterior wall of the gallbladder is left in place, while the anterior surface of the gallbladder and its luminal contents are removed.[104]

Key References

Allen JW, et al. Totally laparoscopic management of gallstone ileus. Surg Endosc 2003;17:352. (Ref.81)

Amouyal P, et al. Diagnosis of choledocholithiasis by endoscopic ultrasonography. Gastroenterology 1994;106:1062–1067. (Ref.35)

Antoniou SA, Antoniou GA, Makridis C. Laparoscopic treatment of Mirizzi syndrome: a systematic review. Surg Endosc 2010;24:33-39. (Ref.62)

Aranha GV, Sontag SJ, Greenlee HB. Cholecystectomy in cirrhotic patients: a formidable operation. Am J Surg 1982;143:55–60. (Ref.95)

Arnold JC, et al. Endoscopic papillary balloon dilation vs sphincterotomy for removal of common bile duct stones: a prospective randomized pilot study. Endoscopy 2001;33:563–567. (Ref.46)

Auyang ED, et al. Human NOTES cholecystectomy: transgastric hybrid technique. J Gastrointest Surg 2009;13:1149–1150. (Ref.15)

Balan G, et al. Retrograde cholangiopancreatography (ERCP) and endoscopic sphincteropapillotomy (ES) in the diagnosis and treatment of common bile duct (CBD) lithiasis. Rev Med Chir Soc Med Nat Iasi 1995;99:56–62. (Ref.54)

Bang S, et al. Endoscopic papillary balloon dilation with large balloon after limited sphincterotomy for retrieval of choledocholithiasis. Yonsei Med J 2006;47:805–810. (Ref.48)

Banks PA, Freeman ML. Practice guidelines in acute pancreatitis. Am J Gastroenterol 2006;101:2379–2400. (Ref.67)

Baron TH, Harewood GC. Endoscopic balloon dilation of the biliary sphincter compared to endoscopic biliary sphincterotomy for removal of common bile duct stones during ERCP: a metaanalysis of randomized, controlled trials. Am J Gastroenterol 2004;99:1455–1460. (Ref.45)

Beltran MA, Csendes A, Cruces KS. The relationship of Mirizzi syndrome and cholecystoenteric fistula: validation of a modified classification. World J Surg 2008;32:2237–2243. (Ref.60)

Benchellal ZA, et al. Mirizzi syndrome mimicking a gallbladder carcinoma. Presse Med 2009;38:1191–1193. (Ref.64)

Bingener J, et al. Can the MELD score predict perioperative morbidity for patients with liver cirrhosis undergoing laparoscopic cholecystectomy? Am Surg 2008;74:156–159. (Ref.102)

Binmoeller KF, et al. Treatment of difficult bile duct stones using mechanical, electrohydraulic and extracorporeal shock wave lithotripsy. Endoscopy 1993;25:201–206. (Ref.43)

Boerma D, et al. Wait-and-see policy or laparoscopic cholecystectomy after endoscopic sphincterotomy for bile-duct stones: a randomised trial. Lancet 2002;360:761–765. (Ref.21)

Braverman DZ, Johnson ML, Kern F Jr. Effects of pregnancy and contraceptive steroids on gallbladder function. N Engl J Med 1980;302:362–364. (Ref.87)

Burtin P, et al. Diagnostic strategies for extrahepatic cholestasis of indefinite origin: endoscopic ultrasonography or retrograde cholangiography? Results of a prospective study. Endoscopy 1997;29:349–355. (Ref.34)

Cappell MS. Acute pancreatitis: etiology, clinical presentation, diagnosis, and therapy. Med Clin North Am 2008;92:889–923, ix–x. (Ref.74)

Cappellani A, et al. Retrospective survey on laparoscopic cholecystectomy in the cirrhotic patient. Eur Rev Med Pharmacol Sci 2008;12:257–260. (Ref.98)

Chamberlain RS, Sakpal SV. A comprehensive review of single-incision laparoscopic surgery (SILS) and natural orifice transluminal endoscopic surgery (NOTES) techniques for cholecystectomy. J Gastrointest Surg 2009;13:1733–1740. (Ref.12)

Chang L, et al. Preoperative versus postoperative endoscopic retrograde cholangiopancreatography in mild to moderate gallstone pancreatitis: a prospective randomized trial. Ann Surg 2000;231:82–87. (Ref.70)

Chang WH, et al. Outcome of simple use of mechanical lithotripsy of difficult common bile duct stones. World J Gastroenterol 2005;11(4):593–596. (Ref.51)

Chiappetta Porras LT, et al. Minimally invasive management of acute biliary tract disease during pregnancy. HPB Surg 2009;2009:829020. (Ref.91)

Csendes A, et al. Mirizzi syndrome and cholecystobiliary fistula: a unifying classification. Br J Surg 1989;76:1139–1143. (Ref.59)

Cullen KA, Hall MJ, Golosinskiy A. Ambulatory surgery in the United States, 2006. Natl Health Stat Report 2009;(11):1–25. (Ref.9)

Curro G, et al. Laparoscopic cholecystectomy in patients with mild cirrhosis and symptomatic cholelithiasis. Transplant Proc 2007;39:1471–1473. (Ref.100)

Curro G, Cucinotta E. Percutaneous gall bladder aspiration as an alternative to laparoscopic cholecystectomy in Child-Pugh C cirrhotic patients with acute cholecystitis. Gut 2006;55:898–899. (Ref.103)

Curro G, et al. Laparoscopic cholecystectomy in Child-Pugh class C cirrhotic patients. JSLS 2005;9:311–315. (Ref.101)

Date RS, Kaushal M, Ramesh A. A review of the management of gallstone disease and its complications in pregnancy. Am J Surg 2008;196:599–608. (Ref.90)

DeFrances CJ, Cullen KA, Kozak LJ. National Hospital Discharge Survey: 2005 annual summary with detailed diagnosis and procedure data. Vital Health Stat 2007;(165):1–209. (Ref.8)

Doko M, et al. Comparison of surgical treatments of gallstone ileus: preliminary report. World J Surg 2003;27:400–404. (Ref.78)

Elewaut A, Afschrift M, Barbier F. Gallstone ileus treated with extracorporeal shock wave lithotripsy. J Clin Ultrasound 1993;21:343–345. (Ref.85)

Eshghi F, Abdi R. Routine magnetic resonance cholangiography compared to intra-operative cholangiography in patients with suspected common bile duct stones. Hepatobiliary Pancreat Dis Int 2008;7:525–528. (Ref.41)

Espinel J, Pinedo E. Large balloon dilation for removal of bile duct stones. Rev Esp Enferm Dig 2008;100:632–636. (Ref.47)

Folsch UR, et al. Early ERCP and papillotomy compared with conservative treatment for acute biliary pancreatitis. The German Study Group on Acute Biliary Pancreatitis. N Engl J Med 1997;336:237–242. (Ref.72)

Freeman ML, et al. Complications of endoscopic biliary sphincterotomy. N Engl J Med 1996;335:909–918. (Ref.53)

Grunhage F, et al. Increased gallstone risk in humans conferred by common variant of hepatic ATP-binding cassette transporter for cholesterol. Hepatology 2007;46:793–801. (Ref.6)

Hekimoglu K, et al. MRCP vs ERCP in the evaluation of biliary pathologies: review of current literature. J Dig Dis 2008;9:162–169. (Ref.33)

Hermann RE. The spectrum of biliary stone disease. Am J Surg 1989;158:171–173. (Ref.19)

Horio T, et al. Cholecystic adenosquamous carcinoma mimicking Mirizzi syndrome. Can J Surg 2009;52:E71–E72. (Ref.63)

Jelin EB, et al. Management of biliary tract disease during pregnancy: a decision analysis. Surg Endosc 2008;22:54–60. (Ref.92)

Kaechele V, et al. Prevalence of gallbladder stone disease in obese children and adolescents: influence of the degree of obesity, sex, and pubertal development. J Pediatr Gastroenterol Nutr 2006;42:66–70. (Ref.4)

Katsika D, et al. Body mass index, alcohol, tobacco and symptomatic gallstone disease: a Swedish twin study. J Intern Med 2007;262:581–587. (Ref.3)

Kawai K, et al. Endoscopic sphincterotomy of the ampulla of Vater. Gastrointest Endosc 1974;20:148–151. (Ref.18)

Knaus WA, et al. APACHE II: a severity of disease classification system. Crit Care Med 1985;13:818–829. (Ref.66)

Kozarek RA. Balloon dilation of the sphincter of Oddi. Endoscopy 1988;20(Suppl 1):207–210. (Ref.44)

Lau JY, et al. Cholecystectomy or gallbladder in situ after endoscopic sphincterotomy and bile duct stone removal in Chinese patients. Gastroenterology 2006;130:96–103. (Ref.23)

Lawrentschuk N, Hewitt PM, Pritchard MG. Elective laparoscopic cholecystectomy: implications of prolonged waiting times for surgery. ANZ J Surg 2003;73:890–893. (Ref.25)

Leandros E, et al. Laparoscopic cholecystectomy in cirrhotic patients with symptomatic gallstone disease. ANZ J Surg 2008;78:363–365. (Ref.99)

Lichten JB, Tehrani K, Sekons D. Laparoscopically assisted enterolithotomy for a gallstone ileus in an atypical location. Surg Endosc 2003;17:1496–1497. (Ref.80)

Lipsett PA, Pitt HA. Acute cholangitis. Front Biosci 2003;8:s1229–s1239. (Ref.55)

Liu CL, et al. Comparison of early endoscopic ultrasonography and endoscopic retrograde cholangiopancreatography in the management of acute biliary pancreatitis: a prospective randomized study. Clin Gastroenterol Hepatol 2005;3:1238–1244. (Ref.75)

Liu CL, et al. Detection of choledocholithiasis by EUS in acute pancreatitis: a prospective evaluation in 100 consecutive patients. Gastrointest Endosc 2001;54:325–330. (Ref.32)

Loperfido S, et al. Major early complications from diagnostic and therapeutic ERCP: a prospective multicenter study. Gastrointest Endosc 1998;48:1–10. (Ref.52)

Makary MA, et al. The role of magnetic resonance cholangiography in the management of patients with gallstone pancreatitis. Ann Surg 2005;241:119–124. (Ref.40)

Maringhini A, et al. Biliary sludge and gallstones in pregnancy: incidence, risk factors, and natural history. Ann Intern Med 1993;119:116–120. (Ref.89)

Mayer AD, et al. Operations upon the biliary tract in patients with acute pancreatitis: aims, indications and timing. Ann R Coll Surg Engl 1984;66:179–183. (Ref.68)

Mazen Jamal M, et al. Trends in the utilization of endoscopic retrograde cholangiopancreatography (ERCP) in the United States. Am J Gastroenterol 2007;102:966–975. (Ref.10)

McAlister VC, Davenport E, Renouf E. Cholecystectomy deferral in patients with endoscopic sphincterotomy. Cochrane Database Syst Rev 2007;4:CD006233. (Ref.22)

McCune WS, Shorb PE, Moscovitz H. Endoscopic cannulation of the ampulla of Vater: a preliminary report. Ann Surg 1968;167:752–756. (Ref.17)

Mendez-Sanchez N, et al. Role of diet in cholesterol gallstone formation. Clin Chim Acta 2007;376:1–8. (Ref.2)

Mentes BB, et al. Gastrointestinal quality of life in patients with symptomatic or asymptomatic cholelithiasis before and after laparoscopic cholecystectomy. Surg Endosc 2001;15:1267–1272. (Ref.24)

Moberg AC, Montgomery A. Laparoscopically assisted or open enterolithotomy for gallstone ileus. Br J Surg 2007;94:53–57. (Ref.79)

Nathanson LK, et al. Postoperative ERCP versus laparoscopic choledochotomy for clearance of selected bile duct calculi: a randomized trial. Ann Surg 2005;242:188–192. (Ref.26)

Nguyen GC, Tuskey A, Jagannath SB. Racial disparities in cholecystectomy rates during hospitalizations for acute gallstone pancreatitis: a national survey. Am J Gastroenterol 2008;103:2301–2307. (Ref.76)

Norton SA, Alderson D. Prospective comparison of endoscopic ultrasonography and endoscopic retrograde cholangiopancreatography in the detection of bile duct stones. Br J Surg 1997;84:1366–1369. (Ref.31)

Palanivelu C, et al. Laparoscopic cholecystectomy in cirrhotic patients: the role of subtotal cholecystectomy and its variants. J Am Coll Surg 2006;203:145–151. (Ref.104)

Peng WK, et al. Role of liver function tests in predicting common bile duct stones in acute calculous cholecystitis. Br J Surg 2005;92:1241–1247. (Ref.30)

Pertkiewicz J, et al. Interventional radiological and endoscopical techniques in biliary tract obstruction. Med Sci Monit 2001;7(Suppl 1):72–75. (Ref.16)

Petrov MS, Savides TJ. Systematic review of endoscopic ultrasonography versus endoscopic retrograde cholangiopancreatography for suspected choledocholithiasis. Br J Surg 2009;96:967–974. (Ref.42)

Proceedings of the NIH Consensus Development Conference on Gallstones and Laparoscopic Cholecystectomy, Bethesda, MD, Sept 14-16, 1992. Am J Surg 1993;165:387–548. (Ref.96)

Puggioni A, Wong LL. A metaanalysis of laparoscopic cholecystectomy in patients with cirrhosis. J Am Coll Surg 2003;197:921–926. (Ref.97)

Ramos AC, et al. NOTES transvaginal video-assisted cholecystectomy: first series. Endoscopy 2008;40:572–575. (Ref.14)

Ranson JH, et al. Prognostic signs and the role of operative management in acute pancreatitis. Surg Gynecol Obstet 1974;139:69–81. (Ref.65)

Reddick EJ, Olsen DO. Laparoscopic laser cholecystectomy. A comparison with mini-lap cholecystectomy. Surg Endosc 1989;3:131–133. (Ref.11)

Romagnuolo J, et al. Magnetic resonance cholangiopancreatography: a meta-analysis of test performance in suspected biliary disease. Ann Intern Med 2003;139:547–557. (Ref.39)

Sackmann M, et al. Gallstone ileus successfully treated by shock-wave lithotripsy. Dig Dis Sci 1991;36:1794–1795. (Ref.84)

Saito M, et al. Long-term outcome of endoscopic papillotomy for choledocholithiasis with cholecystolithiasis. Gastrointest Endosc 2000;51:540–545. (Ref.20)

Sampliner RE, et al. Gallbladder disease in Pima Indians. Demonstration of high prevalence and early onset by cholecystography. N Engl J Med 1970;283:1358–1364. (Ref.5)

Sandler RS, et al. The burden of selected digestive diseases in the United States. Gastroenterology 2002;122:1500–1511. (Ref.1)

Sandzen B, et al. Cholecystectomy and sphincterotomy in patients with mild acute biliary pancreatitis in Sweden 1988-2003: a nationwide register study. BMC Gastroenterol 2009;9:80. (Ref.69)

Schirmer BD, Winters KL, Edlich RF. Cholelithiasis and cholecystitis. J Long Term Eff Med Implants 2005;15:329–338. (Ref.29)

Sharma VK, Howden CW. Metaanalysis of randomized controlled trials of endoscopic retrograde cholangiography and endoscopic sphincterotomy for the treatment of acute biliary pancreatitis. Am J Gastroenterol 1999;94:3211–3214. (Ref.71)

Siegel JH, Kasmin FE. Biliary tract diseases in the elderly: management and outcomes. Gut 1997;41:433–435. (Ref.50)

Silva MA, Wong T. Gallstones in chronic liver disease. J Gastrointest Surg 2005;9:739–746. (Ref.94)

Snow LL, et al. Evaluation of operative cholangiography in 2043 patients undergoing laparoscopic cholecystectomy: a case for the selective operative cholangiogram. Surg Endosc 2001;15:14–20. (Ref.38)

Soloway RD, Trotman BW, Ostrow JD. Pigment gallstones. Gastroenterology 1977;72:167–182. (Ref.7)

Soto DJ, Evan SJ, Kavic MS. Laparoscopic management of gallstone ileus. JSLS 2001;5:279–285. (Ref.82)

Swahn F, et al. Ten years of Swedish experience with intraductal electrohydraulic lithotripsy and laser lithotripsy for the treatment of difficult bile duct stones: an effective and safe option for octogenarians. Surg Endosc 2010;24:1011-1016. (Ref.49)

Tan YM, Wong WK, Ooi LL. A comparison of two surgical strategies for the emergency treatment of gallstone ileus. Singapore Med J 2004;45:69–72. (Ref.83)

Uchiyama K, et al. Timing of laparoscopic cholecystectomy for acute cholecystitis with cholecystolithiasis. Hepatogastroenterology 2004;51:346–348. (Ref.28)

Valdivieso V, et al. Pregnancy and cholelithiasis: pathogenesis and natural course of gallstones diagnosed in early puerperium. Hepatology 1993;17:1–4. (Ref.88)

van Santvoort HC, et al. Early endoscopic retrograde cholangiopancreatography in predicted severe acute biliary pancreatitis: a prospective multicenter study. Ann Surg 2009;250:68–75. (Ref.73)

Videhult P, Sandblom G, Rasmussen IC. How reliable is intraoperative cholangiography as a method for detecting common bile duct stones? A prospective population-based study on 1171 patients. Surg Endosc 2009;23:304–312. (Ref.37)

Williams IM, et al. Gall stone ileus following multiple endoscopic retrograde cholangiopancreatographies. J R Coll Surg Edinburgh 1997;42:423. (Ref.77)

Yeh CN, Jan YY, Chen MF. Laparoscopic treatment for Mirizzi syndrome. Surg Endosc 2003;17:1573–1578. (Ref.61)

Yumi H. Guidelines for diagnosis, treatment, and use of laparoscopy for surgical problems during pregnancy: this statement was reviewed and approved by the Board of Governors of the Society of American Gastrointestinal and Endoscopic Surgeons (SAGES), Sept 2007. It was prepared by the SAGES Guidelines Committee. Surg Endosc 2008;22:849–861. (Ref.93)

Zanlungo S, Nervi F. The ACAT2 gene encodes a gatekeeper of intestinal cholesterol absorption that regulates cholesterolemia and gallstone disease. Hepatology 2001;33:760–761. (Ref.27)

Zidi SH, et al. Use of magnetic resonance cholangiography in the diagnosis of choledocholithiasis: prospective comparison with a reference imaging method. Gut 1999;44:118–122. (Ref.36)

Zorron R, et al. NOTES. Transvaginal cholecystectomy: report of the first case. Surg Innov 2007;14:279–283. (Ref.13)

A complete list of references can be found at www.expertconsult.com.

Section XI

Inherited and Pediatric Liver Diseases

Bilirubin Metabolism and Its Disorders

Jayanta Roy-Chowdhury and Namita Roy-Chowdhury

ABBREVIATIONS

ABC ATP-binding cassette
ATF2 activating transcription factor-2
BSEP bile-salt export pump
BSP bromosulfophthalein
CAR constitutive androstane receptor
CO carbon monoxide
DBSP dibromosulfophthalein
DDT dichlorodiphenyltrichloroethane
ELB "early-labeled peak" of bilirubin
ER endoplasmic reticulum
GST glutathione-S-transferase
HO heme oxygenase

HPLC high-pressure liquid chromatography
ICG indocyanine green
IL interleukin
MRP2 multidrug resistance–associated protein-2
NADPH reduced form of nicotinamide adenine dinucleotide phosphate
NHANES III Third National Health and Nutrition Examination Survey

NTCp N⁺/taurocholate co-transporting polypeptide
SHP gene short heterodimer partner
TCDD tetrachlorodibenzo-p-dioxin
UGT uridinediphosphoglucuronate glucuronosyltransferase
UGT1A1 uridinediphosphoglucuronate glucuronosyltransferase 1A1 (also called bilirubin-uridinediphosphoglucuronate glucuronosyltransferase)

Introduction

Bilirubin is the degradation product of heme, and the bulk of bilirubin is derived from hemoglobin of senescent erythrocytes and hepatic hemoproteins. Bilirubin is potentially toxic, but is normally rendered harmless by binding to plasma albumin and by efficient hepatic clearance. In some disease states, severe unconjugated hyperbilirubinemia can result in encephalopathy (kernicterus).

Perhaps because of its distinctive color, bilirubin has attracted the attention of physicians since antiquity. Hippocrates considered it one of the four important humors of the body: blood, phlegm, black bile, and yellow bile.[1] *Ayurveda*, the ancient Indian book of medicine, also included it among its three principal factors—gases, bile, and phlegm—the proper balance of which was considered critical for health. During the last 3 centuries, the chemistry, metabolism, and disposal of bilirubin have been investigated meticulously by generations of chemists, biologists, and clinical investigators. Excretion of bilirubin by the liver has also been studied as a model for hepatic disposal of other biologically important organic anions of limited aqueous solubility. Several inherited disorders of bilirubin metabolism and excretion have been described in humans and animals. Investigation of these inborn errors has provided important information regarding its metabolic pathways. Definitive treatment of some of these disorders continues to be a therapeutic challenge and an

impetus for further research. Although bilirubin has interested physiologists mainly as a toxic metabolic product, as an antioxidant it may serve as a defense mechanism against oxidative damage.

Jaundice as an Indicator of Hepatic Dysfunction

Jaundice is a sensitive indicator of liver dysfunction. As a sign and symptom, jaundice and hyperbilirubinemia are among the frequently used liver function tests. In acute hepatitis, jaundice is common and usually transient. In contrast, in other hepatocellular diseases such as alcoholic hepatitis and alcoholic or nonalcoholic liver cirrhosis and drug-induced hepatitis, jaundice has a dismal prognosis. In the intensive care unit, in septic or multitrauma patients, jaundice is associated with a high mortality rate. In primary biliary cirrhosis, jaundice is a major indicator of poor prognosis and serial serum bilirubin measurement is one of the tests used for determining the appropriate timing of liver transplantation. Impairment of bile flow caused by obstruction of the intrahepatic or extrahepatic biliary tract leads to jaundice. Because this is a postconjugation event, conjugated bilirubin accumulates in the blood. After relief of obstruction of the bile duct, jaundice usually resolves within 1 week, although elevated plasma bilirubin levels may linger because of the covalent binding of conjugated bilirubin to albumin. Acquired causes of hyperbilirubinemia, which include hemolysis, liver disease, or biliary obstruction, need to be differentiated from inborn errors of bilirubin metabolism.

Although jaundice is a common symptom, its clinical significance varies according to the underlying disease. In some cases, a simple bilirubin level determination has more clinical predictive power than a battery of expensive diagnostic tests, including invasive techniques. However, a sound knowledge of the pathophysiology of bilirubin metabolism is required for interpretation of this simple and valuable liver function test.

Formation of Bilirubin

Breakdown of heme results in the daily production of 250 to 400 mg of bilirubin in humans. Normally, about 80% of bilirubin originates from the hemoglobin of senescent erythrocytes,[2] and the remainder is derived from heme-containing enzymes (e.g., tissue cytochromes, catalase, peroxidase, tryptophan pyrrolase) and from myoglobin. A fraction of bilirubin is also derived from free heme. After the heme precursors glycine and δ-aminolevulinic acid are radiolabeled and injected into humans or rats, radioactivity is incorporated into bile pigments in two phases.[2-4] The "early-labeled peak" of bilirubin (ELB) contains 20% of the radiolabel and is excreted in bile within 3 days. The initial "fast" component of ELB comprises two thirds of the peak in humans and is largely derived from hepatic hemoproteins, such as cytochromes, catalase, peroxidase, and tryptophan pyrrolase,[4] and from a rapidly conveying pool of free heme in the cytosol of hepatocytes, a fraction of which may be degraded without incorporation into heme proteins.[5] Induction of hepatic cytochrome P-450 increases the ELB.[6] Because δ-aminolevulinic acid is preferentially incorporated into hepatic hemoproteins, when labeled δ-aminolevulinic acid is used as a precursor, only the initial component of the ELB incorporates radioactivity. The relatively "slower" phase of the ELB, which normally comprises one third of the peak, is derived from both erythroid and nonerythroid sources. This slower phase is enhanced in conditions associated with "ineffective erythropoiesis," such as congenital dyserythropoietic anemias, megaloblastic anemias, iron-deficiency anemia, lead poisoning, and erythropoietic porphyria.[4] This phase is also increased during accelerated erythropoiesis, probably because of intramedullary breakdown of normoblasts, destruction of reticulocytes in the peripheral circulation,[7] and trimming of reticulocytes during maturation.[8] The "late-labeled peak," normally comprising 80% of the radiolabel, is derived from the hemoglobin of senescent erythrocytes and is associated with the life span of erythrocytes (approximately 50 days in rats and 110 days in humans). When the erythrocyte life span is reduced, as in hemolytic syndromes or intravascular or extravascular hemolysis, the "late-labeled peak" appears earlier.

Opening of the Heme Ring by Heme Oxygenase

Heme (ferroprotoporphyrin IX) is a ring of four tetrapyrroles connected by methene bridges (**Fig. 62-1**). The ring is opened by cleavage of the α-methene bridge, catalyzed by microsomal heme oxygenase (HO). Initially, an electrophilic attack at Fe(II) by a reducing agent, such as the reduced form of nicotinamide adenine dinucleotide phosphate (NADPH), and oxygen results in the formation of α-oxyheme (see **Fig. 62-1**).[9] Subsequently, the α-methene bridge carbon is eliminated as carbon monoxide (CO) and the porphyrin ring carbons that flank the α-methene bridge are oxidized using two additional oxygen molecules, resulting in the two lactam oxygens of biliverdin and bilirubin.[10] Iron is released from the open

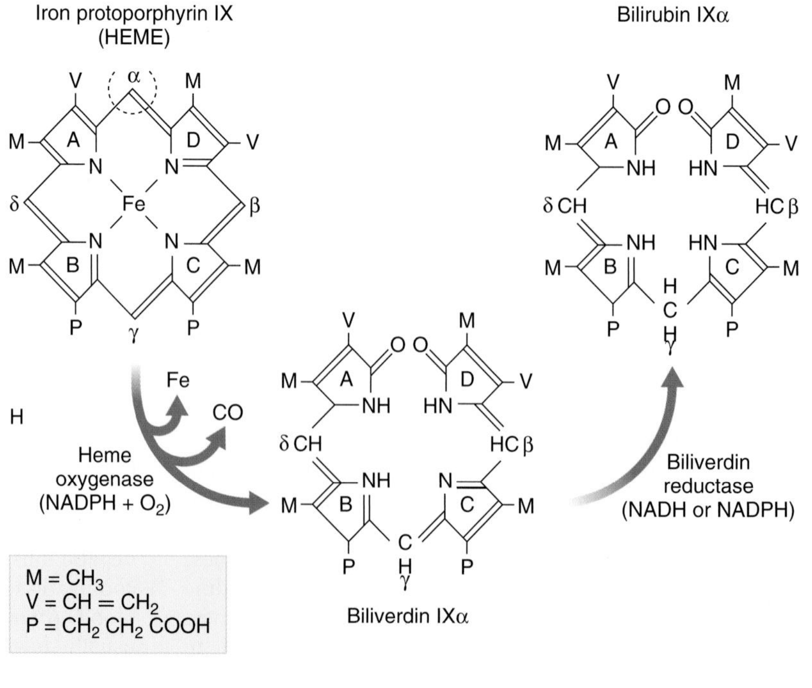

Fig. 62-1 **Mechanism of heme ring opening and subsequent reduction of biliverdin to bilirubin.** The α-carbon bridge, marked with an interrupted arc, is the site of cleavage catalyzed by heme oxygenase.

$M = CH_3$
$V = CH = CH_2$
$P = CH_2\ CH_2\ COOH$

tetrapyrrole after addition of electrons, suggesting that conversion of ferric to ferrous iron is required.[11] Only a minute fraction of heme is opened at the β, γ, or δ bridges, resulting in the excretion of traces of bilirubin IXβ, IXγ, or IXδ, respectively, in bile.

HO catalyzes physiologic heme degradation. It consists of three structurally related isozymes: HO-1, HO-2, and HO-3. HO-1 is the inducible form, HO-2 is a constitutive isoform, and HO-3 is a minor isoform present in spleen, liver, thymus, heart, kidney, brain, and testis.[12] HO-2 is the isoform in hepatocytes and spleen responsible for biliverdin and CO production under normal physiologic conditions. High levels of HO-2 activity are present in cells involved in the breakdown of hemoproteins, such as cells in the spleen, where senescent erythrocytes are sequestered. In the liver both hepatocytes and Kupffer cells have HO activity; the activity in the Kupffer cells is as high as that in the spleen.[13] Apart from breakdown of heme from circulating hemoglobin, constitutive HO-2 is important for cellular hemoprotein homeostasis. HO-2 also appears to function as an oxygen sensor in the lungs. HO-2–deficient mice are severely hypoxic and data suggest that HO-2 is responsible for matching the ventilation to perfusion. HO-1 is a 32-kilodalton (kDa) protein that is induced by lipopolysaccharides, cytokines, heavy metals, reactive oxygen species, protoheme IX, oxidized low-density lipoprotein, hypoxia, and probably also by shear stress in endothelial cells in the cirrhotic liver.[14,15] NF-κB and p38 MAPK signaling pathways mediate the lipopolysaccharide-dependent induction of HO-1 gene expression via DNA sequences in the proximal promoter region. HO-1 acts as a stress-response protein and, by converting prooxidant heme to antioxidant biliverdin and bilirubin, it plays a role in the cellular defense against oxidative injury. A prerequisite for this antioxidant action is that toxic ferrous iron that is released upon cleavage of the porphyrin ring is efficiently scavenged by ferritin. HO-1 deficiency in humans is associated with growth retardation, hyperlipidemia, endothelial cell damage with consumption coagulopathy, and microangiopathic hemolytic anemia. Inducible HO-1 is particularly important for cytoprotection in vascular endothelium and renal tubular epithelium. HO-1–deficient mice show early atherosclerosis, in particular when they are also hypercholesterolemic.

In addition to these cellular effects, it should be realized that the products of the HO reaction, CO and bilirubin, may have more distant effects. CO is a signaling molecule with vasodilatory effects[16] and effects on intestinal motility and sphincters.[17] Moreover, a possible negative correlation between circulating bilirubin levels and coronary heart disease has been reported. Whether this protective effect of bilirubin also holds for patients with Gilbert syndrome is unclear.

Binding of heme to HO requires the propionic acid substituents in the C-6 and C-7 positions and a metal, such as iron, tin, or zinc. Oxygen binds to ferrous heme and undergoes reductive activation. Non-iron metalloprotoporphyrins, such as tin- and zinc-protoporphyrins, bind HO with even greater affinity, but do not activate oxygen and are therefore not degraded by HO. These metalloporphyrins are dead-end inhibitors of heme degradation.[18] Tin- and zinc-protoporphyrins also disrupt the integrity of HO-2, but not of HO-1. The loss of integrity of HO-2, the more abundant form of HO, may partly account for the suppression of bilirubin formation by tin-protoporphyrin.

Conversion of Biliverdin to Bilirubin

The immediate product of HO-mediated ring opening is the green pigment biliverdin, which is the major bile pigment in many amphibian, avian, and fish species. In most mammals, biliverdin is converted to the orange pigment bilirubin. Being less polar, bilirubin crosses placental membranes more readily than does biliverdin,[19,20] although some placentate animals, such as nutria and rabbits, excrete biliverdin as the main bile pigment.[21] Conversely, bilirubin formation has been found in early vertebrates, such as teleost and elasmobranch fish,[21,22] that precede the evolution of the placenta.

Reduction of biliverdin to bilirubin is catalyzed by biliverdin reductase (see **Fig. 62-1**), a family of cytosolic enzymes that use the reduced form of nicotinamide adenine dinucleotide (NADH) at pH 6.7 and NADPH at pH 8.5 as co-factors. Guinea pig liver biliverdin reductase is a 70-kDa protein.[23] Several interconverting forms of biliverdin reductase found in rat liver and spleen are produced by tissue-specific posttranslational modification of a single gene product.[24] Recently biliverdin reductase was shown to induce activating transcription factor-2 (ATF2). ATF2 controls the transcription of the *HO-1* gene. This thus provides for a regulatory loop in which HO-1 and biliverdin reductase expression are interdependent.

Potential Beneficial Effects of Products of Heme Breakdown

Both biliverdin and bilirubin are strong antioxidants, which may be particularly important in the newborn period, when the levels of other natural antioxidants are low. Biliverdin appears to attenuate graft rejection in both cardiac and small intestine transplant models.[25,26] Bilirubin is also a strong antioxidant and has been reported to have cytoprotective activity, although at higher concentrations it is neurotoxic. The evolutionary development and conservation of the energetically expensive mechanisms of bilirubin production and elimination suggest a physiologic benefit for bilirubin. In a large cohort of insurance applicants, the relative mortality rate was higher in individuals who had serum bilirubin levels lower than those in the middle 50% of the population.[27] An inverse relationship between serum bilirubin levels and risk of coronary artery disease supports this hypothesis.[28] Analysis of more than 176 million individuals in the Third National Health and Nutrition Examination Survey (NHANES III) in the United States showed a significant inverse relationship between serum bilirubin concentrations and history of colorectal cancer.[29] The odds ratios for colorectal cancer per 1 mg/dl increase in serum bilirubin levels for men and women were 0.295 (confidence interval [CI], 0.291 to 0.299) and 0.186 (CI, 0.183 to 0.189), respectively. This observation is consistent with another large study showing an inverse relationship between serum bilirubin levels and cancer mortality in a Belgian population.[30] However, despite the impressive difference in odds ratios, such database analyses do not establish firmly a cause-and-effect relationship, because of the possible existence of known and unknown confounding variables. Overweight children developing nonalcoholic fatty liver disease were reported to have lower mean serum bilirubin levels than those who did not develop fatty liver.[31] Notably, heme oxygenase and biliverdin reductase, the two enzymes involved in bilirubin production, may also exert beneficial effects directly. For example, cell surface biliverdin reductase has been implicated in biliverdin-induced antiinflammatory effects via phosphatidylinositol 3-kinase and Akt signaling.[32]

Measurement of Bilirubin Production

At steady state, bilirubin production equals the synthesis and breakdown of biologically important hemoproteins. Because bilirubin is almost quantitatively excreted in bile, bilirubin production can be measured by determining its biliary excretion in bile duct–cannulated experimental animals. A portion of the unconjugated bilirubin excreted in bile may undergo enterohepatic cycling. This may become important in patients with terminal ileum dysfunction, such as in Crohn disease, where unabsorbed bile acids may spill over into the cecum, solubilizing deconjugated bilirubin and increasing its reabsorption.[33,34] In humans, and in animals with an intact enterohepatic circulation, bilirubin production can be estimated by quantification of fecal and urinary urobilinogen and stercobilinogen levels, the bacterial degradation products of bilirubin.[35]

A more convenient method utilizes the turnover of radioisotopically labeled bilirubin. Following intravenous injection of radiolabeled albumin-bound bilirubin, plasma bilirubin concentration and radioactivity are measured at frequent intervals.[36] Plasma bilirubin clearance (the fraction of plasma from which bilirubin is irreversibly extracted) is calculated from the area under the radiobilirubin disappearance curve.[37] Bilirubin removal is measured as the product of plasma bilirubin concentration and clearance. At steady-state levels of plasma bilirubin, the removal rate of bilirubin equals the rate of its synthesis. This method does not take into account a small portion of bilirubin that is produced in the liver and excreted directly into bile without appearing in the circulation and therefore slightly underestimates bilirubin production.

Because heme oxygenase–mediated oxidation of the α-carbon bridge of heme is the main source of endogenous CO, bilirubin formation can also be quantified by measuring CO production. The subject breaths into a closed rebreathing system. In the absence of anoxia, the body CO stores equilibrate rapidly with the CO in the rebreathed air. CO production is calculated from the CO concentration in the breathing chamber or from an increment in blood carboxyhemoglobin saturation.[38] A fraction of CO in expired air may be derived from non-heme sources (e.g., halogenated methane and polyphenolic compounds, including catecholamines).[39] In addition, intestinal bacteria contribute a small fraction of the CO.[40] Therefore CO production exceeds plasma bilirubin turnover by 12% to 18%.

Chemistry of Bilirubin

The systemic name of bilirubin IXα is 1′,8′-dioxo-1,3,6,7-tetramethyl-2,8-divinylbiladiene-*a,c*-dipropionic acid.[41] The planar chemical structure of bilirubin, as determined by Fischer and Plieninger,[42] was confirmed by x-ray diffraction analysis.[43] The carbon bridges between pyrrolenone rings *A* and *B* (C-4) and rings *C* and *D* (C-15) are in *trans* or *Z*

configuration. The oxygen attached to the outer pyrrolenone ring is in a lactam rather than lactim configuration. Titration of bilirubin in aqueous solutions suggests a p*K* value of 7 to 8.[44] However, as bilirubin forms insoluble aggregates below pH 8.0, titration of aqueous solutions of bilirubin can yield misleading p*K* values.[44] [13]C nuclear magnetic resonance spectra and potentiometric and spectrophotometric titrations in aqueous solutions indicate that the p*K* value of the two carboxyl groups is 4.4 and that of the two lactam groups is 13.0.[45]

Physical Conformation and Solubility of Bilirubin IXα

Precise determination of the solubility of bilirubin IXα is difficult because the pigment is unstable in aqueous solutions and tends to form dimers, colloids, or surface films.[44] Crystallized bilirubin IXα-*Z*, with two protonated carboxyl groups, is virtually insoluble in water, but is readily soluble in polar solvents, provided the intramolecular hydrogen bonds can be disrupted.[46] Bilirubin and polar ligands, such as sulfonamides, share a binding site in the polar region of albumin[45] with other polar substances, such as sulfonamides.[47] Therefore, despite its insolubility in water at physiologic pH, bilirubin should be considered a relatively polar substance, the mechanism of toxicity of which may differ from that of truly lipophilic toxins, such as dichlorodiphenyltrichloroethane (DDT).[47]

Despite the presence of two propionic acid side chains, four amino groups, and two lactam oxygens, bilirubin IX is insoluble in water at physiologic pH. Fog and Jellum[48] and Kuenzle and colleagues[49,50] proposed that bilirubin IXα may be internally stabilized by hydrogen bonding between the carboxyl and the two external pyrrolenone rings (**Fig. 62-2**). X-ray diffraction studies of crystalline bilirubin confirmed hydrogen bonding between each propionic acid side chain and the pyrrolic and lactam sites in the opposite half of the molecule.[43] These hydrogen bonds constrain the molecule into a "ridgetile" conformation (see **Fig. 62-2**). Because both carboxylic groups, all NH groups, and the two lactam oxygens are engaged by hydrogen bonding, the molecule is insoluble in water. The integrity of the hydrogen-bonded structure requires the interpyrrolic bridges at the 4- and 15-positions of bilirubin to be in *trans* or *Z* configuration.[51] Addition of methanol, ethanol, or 6 mol/L urea interferes with the hydrogen-bonded structure and makes bilirubin more labile,[50] water soluble, and rapidly reactive with diazo reagents. In the body, bilirubin IXα requires conversion to a polar molecule before excretion. Conjugation of the propionic acid carboxyls with sugar moieties disrupts the hydrogen bonds, resulting in the formation of water-soluble conjugates that are readily excreted in bile. Resonance Raman spectroscopic studies of bilirubin-sphingomyelin complexes suggest that the intramolecular hydrogen bonds are disrupted in such complexes, and the propionic acid carboxyls form ion pairs with the quaternary ammonium ion of the choline moiety of sphingomyelin.[52]

Absorption Spectra and Circular Dichroism

Bilirubin IXα has a main absorption band at 450 to 474 nm in most organic solvents with an extinction coefficient of 48.0

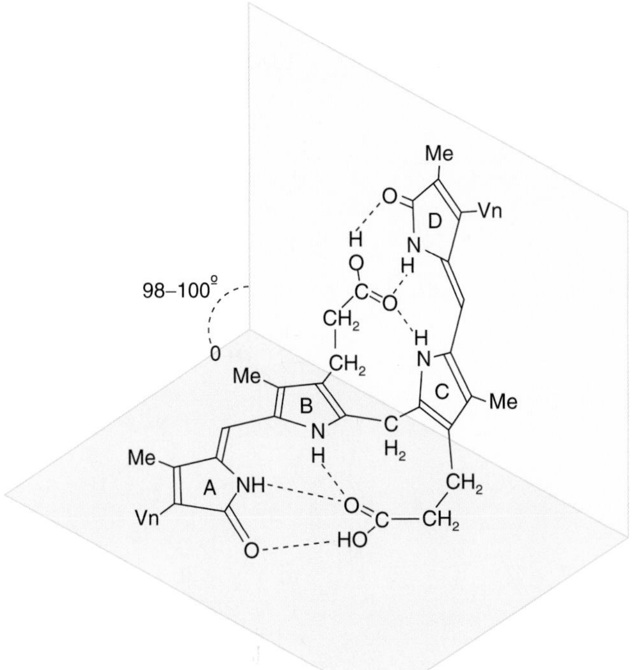

Fig. 62-2 **The x-ray crystallographic structure of bilirubin.** The linear structure shown in Figure 62-1 is contorted into a ridge-tile–like configuration caused by internal hydrogen bonding *(dashed line)* of the propionic acid carboxyls to the amino groups and the lactam oxygen of the pyrrolenone rings of the opposite half of the molecule. The carbon bridges connecting pyrrolenone rings *A* and *B* (C-4) and rings *C* and *D* (C-15) are in the *Z* (*trans*) configuration. Because the polar groups, the propionic acid carboxyls, and the amino and lactam groups are all engaged by hydrogen bonding, bilirubin is very sparsely soluble in water. The hydrogen bonding bends the molecule along the central carbon bridge (C-10) and buries the central bridge deep within the molecule, thereby restricting the access of diazo reagents to the central bridge. Therefore bilirubin reacts very slowly with diazo reagents, unless the hydrogen bonds are opened by adding "accelerator" reagents ("indirect diazo reaction," discussed later in the text).

to 63.4 mmol/L at its absorption maximum at 1-cm path length.[53] Circular dichroism spectroscopy shows that biliverdin preferentially adopts a minus-helicity conformation when bound to human serum albumin, whereas bilirubin IXα prefers a plus-helicity conformation. Reduction of human serum albumin-bound biliverdin to bilirubin results in a conformational inversion from minus to plus helicity.[54] Such sign inversion also occurs on addition of halothane, chloroform, or other volatile anesthetics to the albumin–bilirubin complex, suggesting that the volatile anesthetics alter the internal topography of receptor sites, influencing the stereoselectivity of ligand binding.[55]

Photochemistry of Bilirubin

Conformational Isomerization and Cyclization

Exposure of circulating bilirubin to light changes the configuration of one or both of the interpyrrolic bridges at positions

5 and 15 from *Z* (*trans*) to *E* (*cis*) (**Fig. 62-3**). The resulting 4*Z*,15*E* or 4*E*,15*Z* isomers lack hydrogen bonds in one half of the molecule, whereas bilirubin IXα-*EE* lacks hydrogen bonds in both halves of the molecule. Of these conformations, the 4*Z*,15*E* isomer is more abundant.[56] Blue light is more efficient in mediating the conformational changes. The conversion of the *E* forms back to the *Z* forms may be reduced in serum albumin-bound bilirubin by competitive internal conversion processes.[57] Following absorption of two photons,[56] the vinyl substituent at position C-3 of bilirubin IXα-4*E*,15*Z* is cyclized with the methyl substituent on the internal pyrrole ring, forming the structural isomer *E*-cyclobilirubin, or lumirubin.[58,59] Although cyclization of bilirubin occurs at a slower rate than formation of configurational isomers, because of the relative stability of cyclobilirubin, this form may be quantitatively more important in phototherapy of neonatal jaundice.[58] The conformational isomers are more polar than is bilirubin IXα-*ZZ* and can be excreted in bile without conjugation.[60]

Fluorescence

Although pure bilirubin does not fluoresce, when dissolved in detergents, albumin, or alkaline methanol it exhibits intense fluorescence at 510 to 530 nm,[61] which has been used for quantification of blood bilirubin concentrations and the unsaturated bilirubin-binding capacity of albumin.

Photooxidation and Degradation

In the presence of light and oxygen, bilirubin undergoes a self-sensitized reaction involving singlet oxygen, resulting in the formation of colorless fragments, chiefly maleimides and propentdyopent adducts.[62] A small amount of biliverdin is also formed.

Dismutation

When bilirubin IXα is irradiated in deoxygenated aqueous solution, free radical disproportionation results in the formation of the symmetric molecules bilirubin IIIα and bilirubin XIIIα, which are nonphysiologic isomers of bilirubin.[63] The reaction is enhanced in the presence of acid and oxygen and is inhibited by ascorbate.

Bilirubin Toxicity

The cerebral toxicity of bilirubin in neonatal jaundice has been known for at least 5 centuries. Degeneration of brain tissues associated with yellow pigmentation was reported in 1949.[64] The association of kernicterus, or bilirubin-induced encephalopathy with severe unconjugated hyperbilirubinemia, was subsequently established.[65] The study of mutant rats (Gunn strain) that lack hepatic bilirubin glucuronidating activity has contributed greatly to the current knowledge of bilirubin toxicity. Although the cerebral toxicity of bilirubin has been studied in detail, other organ systems are also affected. Bilirubin neurotoxicity is related to the free (non–protein-bound) fraction of unconjugated bilirubin, which exists predominantly as a protonated diacid that can diffuse across cell membranes. At the cellular level, moderately

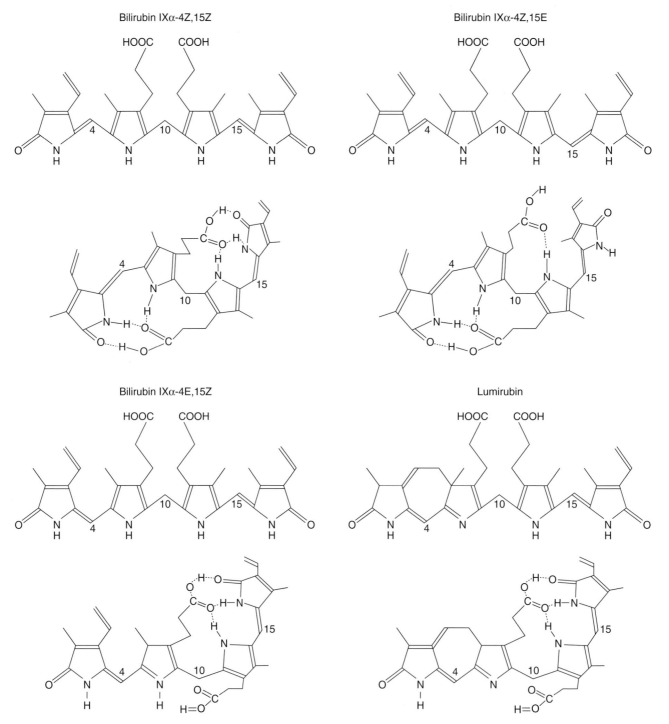

Fig. 62-3 Photoisomerization of bilirubin IXα. The linear *(upper row)* and hydrogen-bonded structures of bilirubin IXα and its photoisomers are shown. Bilirubin IXα-4Z,15Z is the preferred configuration of unconjugated bilirubin, in which carbon bridges at both the 4 and the 15 position are in Z or *trans* configuration, allowing hydrogen bonding on both halves of the molecule. Upon exposure to light, configurational isomers, 4Z,15E and 4E,15Z, are formed. As shown in the figure, there is disruption of hydrogen bonds in the dipyrrolic half of the molecule that bears an E configuration. The 4E,15Z isomer becomes cyclized to produce the stable structural isomer lumirubin, which, because of its stability, is quantitatively the most important photoisomer of bilirubin formed during phototherapy.

increased intracellular bilirubin levels affect astrocytes and neurons, causing mitochondrial damage, which impairs energy metabolism and may induce apoptosis. Cell membrane perturbation can also inhibit the transport of neurotransmitters. Protective mechanisms against bilirubin encephalopathy include active export of bilirubin from cells to plasma by

adenosine triphosphate (ATP)-consuming pumps in the brain capillary endothelium and the choroid plexus epithelium. Binding to cytosolic proteins lowers the intracellular free bilirubin concentration, thereby reducing its toxicity. Because bilirubin cytotoxicity is modified by multiple pathophysiologic factors, the incidence and extent of bilirubin encephalopathy cannot be predicted simply on the basis of plasma bilirubin and albumin concentrations.

Bilirubin Encephalopathy in Gunn Rats

Bilirubin deposition at specific areas of the brain accompanied by structural damage is termed kernicterus. The Gunn rat is the only animal model in which spontaneous bilirubin-induced brain damage has been observed. Normally, albumin binding inhibits bilirubin deposition in the brain. Displacement of bilirubin from albumin-binding sites by drugs such as salicylates or sulfonamides increases bilirubin accumulation in the brain and may precipitate kernicterus.[66] Gunn rats that are rendered genetically analbuminemic by cross-breeding with Nagase analbuminemic rats have serum bilirubin levels that are only 25% that of other Gunn rats, whereas their cerebral bilirubin content is 1.2- to 2.7-fold higher.[67] Such hybrid rats die within 3 weeks of birth. Therefore, for clinical purposes, it is important to calculate the molar ratio between plasma albumin and bilirubin. However, the plasma free bilirubin level does not correlate well with brain bilirubin concentration[68] and it is not certain whether unbound bilirubin is the only toxic species of the pigment.

Abnormalities of the cochlear nuclei, associated with various degrees of hearing deficiency, commonly occur as a complication of neonatal hyperbilirubinemia. Brainstem auditory evoked potential studies in Gunn rats indicate functional abnormalities of the central auditory pathways at and rostral to the cochlear nuclei[69] beginning at 17 days of age. Similar changes are found in human neonates with severe hyperbilirubinemia.

Sulfonamides displace bilirubin from albumin binding, thereby promoting the net transfer of bilirubin into neural tissues. Administration of sulfonamides results in reversible brainstem auditory evoked potential abnormalities in Gunn rats.[70] Under these conditions, focal bilirubin staining occurs in Purkinje cells of the cerebellum, hippocampus, and basal ganglia. Similar changes occur in human infants with fully developed kernicterus. A large number of Purkinje cells are affected in the cerebellum of Gunn rats at the age of 7 days; most of these cells degenerate and disappear between days 12 and 30, resulting in cerebellar hypoplasia.[71] The remaining Purkinje cells recover and persist into adult life. However, synapse formation among these Purkinje cells or with other neural cells may be abnormal. Cerebellar mitochondria are enlarged and distorted in Gunn rats.[72] Increased activities of the lysosomal enzymes arylsulfatase and cathepsin occur in the cerebellum of Gunn rats by the eighth day of life.[73] Cerebellar cyclic guanosine monophosphate (cGMP) concentrations decrease progressively from day 15 to day 30, but cyclic adenosine monophosphate (cAMP) levels remain normal.[74]

Clinical Features of Bilirubin Encephalopathy

Except in patients with inherited deficiency of bilirubin glucuronidation (discussed later in this chapter), the occurrence of kernicterus is usually limited to the neonatal period and the first few months of life. Bilirubin encephalopathy may present with a broad spectrum of neurologic features. In the most severe cases, overt kernicterus presents between the third and sixth days of life. The normal Moro reflex is lost, the muscles become hypotonic, the cry is high-pitched, athetoid movements appear, and reflex opisthotonos occurs in response to a startling stimulus. This may progress to lethargy, atonia, and death. Occasionally, in some children with Crigler-Najjar syndrome type 1, bilirubin encephalopathy may present late with cerebellar symptoms as the presenting feature.[75] Those who survive acute kernicterus may develop chronic hearing abnormalities, athetoid movements, paralysis of upward gaze, and mental retardation, in various combinations. The cochlear nucleus is commonly affected by hyperbilirubinemia. Cells of the auditory system that receive synaptic input from end-bulbs or calyces appear to be early targets.[76] In Gunn rat pups, these morphologic changes correlate with abnormalities of brainstem auditory evoked potentials.[77] Sensitivity of auditory evoked potential testing can be increased by recording binaural difference waves obtained by subtracting the sum of two monaural brainstem auditory evoked potentials from a binaural brainstem auditory evoked potential.[78]

Bilirubin staining of the hippocampus, basal ganglia, and nuclei of the cerebellum and brainstem occurs in infants dying in the acute phase of bilirubin encephalopathy[79]; however, such staining is not found in children dying in the chronic stage of the disorder. Clinical manifestations precede histologic evidence of brain damage by approximately 72 hours.[80] Focal necrosis of neurons and glial cells occurs later. Gliosis of the affected areas is seen in chronic cases.[80] Because these histologic lesions are not present from the onset of clinical kernicterus, these may not be the initiating pathophysiologic events in bilirubin-induced brain damage. Nonspecific signs of encephalopathy in the neonate may result from other causes, such as cerebral hemorrhage,[81] and therefore kernicterus cannot always be diagnosed without pathologic documentation. Conversely, focal bilirubin staining of the brain may occur in other forms of brain injury. Thus, in the absence of neuronal degeneration, bilirubin staining alone does not establish the diagnosis of classic kernicterus.[82]

Peak serum bilirubin levels of up to 10 to 12 mg/dl are usually considered safe. The prognostic significance of a moderate degree of hyperbilirubinemia is not entirely clear. Serum bilirubin levels that are not high enough to cause kernicterus have been reported to result in an increased incidence of neurologic abnormalities or decreased intellectual performance later in life.[83]

The Blood–Brain Barrier and Cerebral Bilirubin Clearance

The equilibration of hydrophilic water-soluble substances and proteins between the blood and the brain is restricted by a functional blood–brain barrier.[84] Tight junctions between capillary endothelial cells and foot processes of astroglial cells represent the structural component of this barrier.[84] Specific transport mechanisms that are involved in the translocation of ions, water, and nutrients from plasma to brain may provide the functional counterpart of the blood–brain barrier. Conventionally, immaturity of the blood–brain barrier in neonates has been implicated in the high incidence of kernicterus in this age group. However, it has been difficult to confirm a more rapid passage of labeled markers[85] or lipophilic substances[86] into the immature brain. Therefore there is no firm evidence to support the concept of an immature blood–brain barrier in the neonate.

The efficiency of cerebral bilirubin clearance may be inversely related to the cerebral toxicity of bilirubin. Experimentally, the blood–brain barrier can be unilaterally and reversibly opened without causing brain damage by infusion of hypertonic urea[87] or arabinose.[84] The hyperosmolarity-associated shrinkage of the capillary endothelial cells results in temporary opening of the tight junctions. When the blood–brain barrier is opened in newborn rats by this technique, intravenously administered albumin-bound bilirubin rapidly enters the brain. Following the reversal of the blood–brain barrier, bilirubin is rapidly cleared from the brain. The clearance of bilirubin from brain parallels its clearance from serum, suggesting that bilirubin is cleared by diffusion or actively transported back into the general circulation.[88] Damaged brain, which may be edematous, may bind bilirubin[89] to such an extent that it is unable to clear bilirubin rapidly. The damaged brain therefore may be more vulnerable to bilirubin toxicity.

Endothelial cells of cerebral microvessels and the choroid plexus together form the blood–brain barrier and cerebrospinal fluid–blood barrier. Recent studies show that these endothelial cells are richly supplied with ATP-dependent transporters belonging to the ATP-binding cassette (ABC) superfamily of transporting proteins. Notably, MDR1 (multidrug resistance protein-1, a P-glycoprotein) and the multidrug resistance–associated proteins MRP1, MRP4, MRP5, and, to a lesser extent, MRP6 are expressed in these tissues.[90-93] The MRPs located in the microvascular endothelial cells and the basolateral membranes of the choroid plexus epithelial cells act as efflux pumps, stimulating the efflux of drugs from the brain and the cerebrospinal fluid to the blood.[91-93] MRP1 is preferentially expressed in the astroglial component of the blood–brain barrier. Recent evidence indicates that bilirubin is a substrate for MRP1 (ABCC1). According to these concepts the blood–brain barrier is not merely a passive anatomic structure, but is an active tissue that can pump bilirubin and other metabolites and drugs out of the brain, thus reducing their intracellular concentrations. Substrate competition at the level of these pumps may be another way by which drug exposure can modulate bilirubin brain toxicity.

Biochemical Basis of Bilirubin Toxicity

Bilirubin has a broad range of toxicity on organs, cells, subcellular organelles, and cellular functions. It is not clear which of these toxic effects are relevant in bilirubin encephalopathy. In rat neuronal primary cultures, bilirubin increases protein and lipid peroxidation, lowers the reduced glutathione concentration, and increases cell death, indicating a role of oxidative stress in bilirubin cytotoxicity.[94] Interestingly, inhibition of cell division and enhancement of cellular apoptosis by bilirubin have been linked to the induction of a tumor suppressor protein, phosphatase, and tensin homolog (PTEN).[95] In the human neuroblastoma cell line SH-SY5Y, exposure to

bilirubin resulted in reactive oxygen species–mediated DNA damage as shown by the formation of 8-hydroxyguanine and the increase in the number of abasic sites in chromosomal DNA.[96] Proteomic studies showed differential expression of proteins involved in cell proliferation, intracellular trafficking, protein degradation, and oxidative stress response after exposure to bilirubin. Notably, the redox-sensitive chaperone protein DJ-1 was up-regulated. Bilirubin toxicity in this cell line was decreased by up-regulation of DJ-1 and increased by down-regulation of this neuroprotective protein. Bilirubin uncouples oxidative phosphorlyation and inhibits ATPase activity of brain mitochondria.[97] Bilirubin reduces local cerebral metabolic rates for glucose in immature rats.[98] All areas of the brain are affected, but decreased glucose utilization is particularly pronounced in auditory, visual, hypothalamic, and thalamic regions. The findings of large glycogen vacuoles in neonatal Gunn rat brains,[69] reduced brain pyruvate concentration, and decreased activity of glycolytic enzymes[99] suggest an inhibition of glycogenolysis by bilirubin. Decreased choline acetyltransferase activity has been observed in substantia nigra and amygdala of Gunn rat brain, whereas the enzyme activity was increased in the olfactory bulb.[100] Bilirubin has been shown to inhibit cAMP-dependent protein kinase activity in vitro[101] and non–cAMP-dependent protein kinase activity in vivo.[102]

In a cell-free system, bilirubin irreversibly inhibits calcium-activated, phospholipid-dependent protein kinase C activity and cAMP-dependent protein kinase activity.[103] Because protein phosphorylation is the final common pathway of neuronal signal transmission, inhibition of protein kinase C by bilirubin may play a role in bilirubin encephalopathy in the newborn.

Bilirubin Nephrotoxicity

Renal medullary deposition of unconjugated bilirubin results in medullary necrosis and formation of bilirubin crystals on the renal papillae[104] in Gunn rats and in hyperbilirubinemic infants.[105] In adult Gunn rats, abnormality of the ascending loop of Henle[104] leads to an impairment of urinary concentration, which is ameliorated by reduction of serum bilirubin levels.[106] The urinary concentration defect has not been found in mature neonates with hyperbilirubinemia[107] or in patients with Crigler-Najjar syndrome type 1 who survive to adult age.[108]

Disposition of Bilirubin

Bilirubin is transported in the circulation bound to plasma proteins, predominantly to albumin. In the hepatic sinusoids the albumin–bilirubin complex dissociates and bilirubin is internalized. Bilirubin is stored in the hepatocytes bound to cytosolic proteins. Bilirubin uridinediphosphoglucuronate glucuronosyltransferase (UGT1A1), located in the endoplasmic reticulum (ER), mediates the conjugation of bilirubin with glucuronic acid. Conjugated bilirubin first needs to cross the endoplamic reticulum membrane to be transported across the bile canalicular membrane into the bile. This multistep process is summarized in **Figure 62-4**. Many of these steps are shared by other organic anions and cholephilic

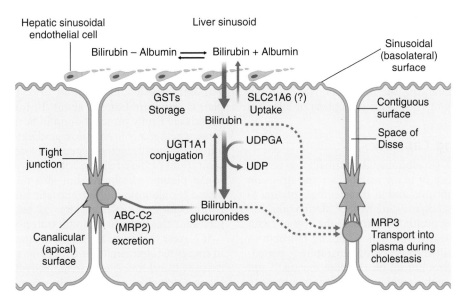

Fig. 62-4 **A schematic diagram summarizing bilirubin metabolism by hepatocytes.** During its carriage in plasma, bilirubin is strongly, but reversibly, bound to albumin. In hepatic sinusoids, this complex comes in direct contact with the basolateral domain of the hepatocyte plasma membrane through fenestrae of the specialized hepatic endothelial cells. At the hepatocyte surface, dissociation of the albumin–bilirubin complex occurs, and bilirubin enters hepatocytes by a specific uptake mechanism(s). A fraction of the bilirubin is also derived from catabolism of hepatocellular heme proteins. Storage within the hepatocyte is accomplished by binding of bilirubin to a group of cytosolic proteins, glutathione-*S*-transferases (GSTs) (also termed ligandin or Y-protein). Binding to these proteins keeps bilirubin in solution and inhibits its efflux from the cell, thereby increasing the net uptake. Conjugation of bilirubin in the endoplasmic reticulum is catalyzed by bilirubin-uridinediphosphoglucuronate glucuronosyltransferase (UGT1A1), forming bilirubin monoglucuronide and diglucuronide. Both conjugates may bind to GSTs in the cytosol. Conjugation is obligatory for efficient transport across the bile canaliculus. Bilirubin glucuronides are secreted across the bile canaliculus by an energy-consuming process mediated by MRP2 (previously termed cMOAT). This process is normally rate-limiting in bilirubin throughput, and is shared by other organic anions, but not bile salts.

metabolites. These processes are briefly discussed in the following paragraphs.

The Role of Albumin

Bilirubin is carried in the circulation bound to plasma albumin. As discussed previously, unconjugated bilirubin is only sparingly soluble in water at physiologic pH. Binding to albumin prevents its precipitation and deposition in tissues, thereby facilitating the transport of bilirubin from its site of production to its organ of elimination—the liver. Albumin binding prevents bilirubin from entering the brain. The reserve binding capacity of albumin acts as a buffer by accommodating for sudden rises in serum bilirubin concentrations (e.g., during acute hemolysis). The endothelial lining of the hepatic sinusoids is fenestrated and the albumin–bilirubin complex entering the liver through the portal circulation passes through the fenestrae to reach the space of Disse, where bilirubin has direct contact with the sinusoidal and basolateral plasma membrane domains of the hepatocyte (see **Fig. 62-4**). Albumin enables bilirubin to be transported across the so-called unstirred water layer, a thin layer of water that surrounds the hepatocytes. By gradually releasing ligands to hepatocytes along the acinus, albumin distributes the ligands to all zones of the acinus, thereby establishing a considerable metabolic reserve. Bilirubin, but not albumin, passes into the hepatocyte, indicating that bilirubin dissociates from albumin close to or at the hepatocyte surface. It is unclear whether or

not an albumin receptor at the hepatocyte surface facilitates this dissociation.

Bilirubin Binding Sites and Competition by Other Ligands
Binding Sites

There is a primary and a secondary binding site on albumin for bilirubin.[109] Affinity labeling studies indicate that the primary binding site of bilirubin is located at residues 124 to 297 and, to a lesser extent, at residues 446 to 547.[110] Lysine 240 in human albumin and lysine 238 in bovine serum albumin appear to be the sites of bilirubin binding.[111]

Binding Capacity and Effect of Competitive Substrates

Albumin inhibits the neurotoxic effects of unconjugated bilirubin following intravenous injection in puppies.[112] The role of albumin in preventing bilirubin toxicity is clearly shown in analbuminemic-Gunn hybrid rats, which die of bilirubin encephalopathy shortly after birth. Binding of other ligands to albumin affects its bilirubin binding capacity. The other ligand may bind at the same site as does bilirubin, resulting in competitive displacement, or bind at a different site, causing noncompetitive displacement of bilirubin. Noncompetitive binding may not affect bilirubin binding or may produce conformational changes that enhance (cooperative binding) or diminish (anticooperative) bilirubin binding. Sulfonamides, antiinflammatory drugs, and contrast media used for cholangiography displace bilirubin competitively from albumin.[113] Prophylactic use of sulfonamides in newborns enhances bilirubin encephalopathy,[114] probably by enhancing the dissociation of bilirubin from albumin, thereby increasing the net uptake of bilirubin into neural tissues.[115]

"Reserve" Binding Capacity

Binding of bilirubin to albumin is normally reversible. Because of the influence of many metabolites and drugs on albumin binding of bilirubin and its transfer from plasma to the central nervous system, measurement of plasma bilirubin concentration does not accurately estimate the risk of brain damage from unconjugated bilirubin. Unbound bilirubin in serum has been quantified by gel chromatography,[116] peroxidase treatment,[117] electrophoresis on cellulose acetate,[118] and fluorometry of serum with or without detergent treatment.[119] Free bilirubin concentration may be roughly estimated as the product of serum bilirubin concentration, the concentration of reserve bilirubin binding sites on albumin, and the association constant for bilirubin.[120] Competitive binding by a ^{14}C-labeled ligand, monoacetyl-4,4'-diaminodiphenylsulfone, or by a spin-labeled ligand, 1-*N*-(2,2,6,6-tetramethyl-1-oxy-4-piperidinyl)-5-*N*-(1-aspartate)-2,4-dinitrobenzene,[121] has been used to determine reserve binding capacity.

Irreversible Binding of Bilirubin to Albumin

During prolonged conjugated hyperbilirubinemia, bilirubin becomes covalently bound to albumin.[122] This fraction of bile pigments is not cleared by the liver or kidney and persists for a long time in the circulation, reflecting the long half-life of serum albumin.

Bilirubin Metabolism in Genetic Analbuminemia

In view of this discussion it is interesting to note that analbuminemia is compatible with life and that elimination of amphipathic compounds such as bilirubin and bromosulfophthalein (BSP) is disturbed to a relatively minor degree in analbuminemic rats.[123,124] For example, elimination of a tracer dose of bilirubin was entirely normal, although the biliary recovery after a loading dose was decreased.[124] Other plasma proteins, such as high-density lipoproteins, can assume some of the assigned roles of albumin.

Hepatic Bilirubin Uptake

For efficient liver uptake, bilirubin needs to be delivered to hepatocytes via the sinusoidal blood. In the presence of portosystemic collaterals that develop in patients with portal hypertension, or surgically produced portosystemic shunts, bilirubin generated in the spleen is diverted to the systemic circulation. In these circumstances, first-pass clearance of bilirubin by the liver does not occur, resulting in mild hyperbilirubinemia. Similarly, an open ductus venosus in the newborn may intensify and prolong the "physiologic" jaundice in premature infants. Hepatic uptake of amphiphilic organic anions is carrier mediated. Recent studies have elucidated various aspects of this transport process. A brief discussion of these mechanisms follows.

Energy Requirements

The intrahepatic concentration of a ligand can exceed the plasma concentration by about 10-fold. However, because ligands are firmly protein bound in both plasma and hepatocytes, whether a concentration gradient exists with respect to a free (unbound) ligand depends not only on respective concentrations of the ligand on both sides of the hepatocyte sinusoidal plasma membrane, but also on the affinities of the ligand for albumin and intrahepatic binding proteins. These considerations are relevant for a discussion about the driving forces for this potentially uphill transport.

It is clear that there are multiple uptake systems that differ in energy requirement.[125] In any uptake system, organic anions must be translocated against an inside negative plasma membrane potential of approximately -35 mV that is generated by Na^+/K^+-ATPase. Electrical neutrality must be maintained by intracellular association with counterions, by co-transport with cations such as H^+, or by countertransport with anions such as OH^- or Cl^-.

Transporters

The basolateral hepatocyte membrane contains various transporter proteins that function as carriers for the uptake of a multitude of endogenous and exogenous substances. The uptake carriers in human hepatocytes are listed in **Table 62-1**. NTCP (SLC10A1) in humans (ntcp, Slc10a1 in rodents) has a narrow range of substrate specificity and is a specialized carrier for the Na^+-dependent hepatic uptake of bile salts.[126] BSP and its glutathione conjugate are widely used model substrates in transport studies and indeed are substrates for a number of uptake transporters. Also the thyroid hormones, thyroxine and triiodothyronine, are transported by a number of uptake carriers. Organic cations are transported by members of the OCT/oct family. These are particularly active in the kidney. Hepatic uptake of unconjugated bilirubin has been investigated in numerous classic studies using membrane fractions of various degrees of purity, isolated hepatocytes, isolated perfused rat livers, or whole animals. Concentrative bilirubin uptake in the liver can partly be explained by sinusoidal dissociation from albumin and binding to intrahepatocellular proteins. Before bilirubin binds to intracellular proteins, it must cross the sinusoidal domain of the hepatocyte plasma membrane. Bilirubin's polarity is sufficiently low that it can cross membranes without the aid of transporter proteins. Zucker and Goessling have proposed a non–carrier-mediated transmembrane diffusion of unconjugated bilirubin, in which dissociation from albumin is rate-limiting.[127] However, because concentrative bilirubin uptake is a liver-specific function, a hepatocyte-specific carrier protein is thought to be involved. OATP2 (also termed OATP-C or SLC21A6) in human liver and Oatp4 (Slc21a10) in rat liver are high-affinity transporters of organic anions, such as BSP, taurocholate, estradiol-17β-glucuronide, LTC4, estrone-3-sulfate, estrone-1-sulfate, dehydroepiandrosterone sulfate, triiodothyronine, and thyroxine.[128,129] OATP-C has also been reported to transport unconjugated bilirubin,[128] but other studies did not confirm this conclusion.[130] Thus the

Table 62-1 Organic Anion Uptake Transporters in the Basolateral Membrane of Human Hepatocytes

	NTCP SLC10A1	OATP-A SLC21A3 OATP1 OATP	OATP-B SLC21A9	OATP-C SLC21A6 LST-1 OATP2	OATP8 SLC21A8	PGT SLC21A2
Bilirubin				+	−	
Bromosulfophthalein	++	+	−	+	+/−	
Taurocholate		+	+	+	+/−	
Estrone-3-sulfate	−	+		+	+	
Estradiol	−	++	+	+	+	
17β-Glucuronide	−	+	−	−	+	
Dehydroepiandrosterone sulfate	−	−		−	+	
Ouabain				+		
Digoxin	−	+++	−	−	−	
Pravastatin		−		+	+	
N-Methylquinine	−	+	−	+	−	++
Leukotriene C$_4$	−	−	−	−	−	
Prostaglandin E$_2$						
Tissue distribution	H	B	H, B	H	H	W
References	125, 128	128	128	127, 139	127	124, 125

B, brain; H, hepatocytes; M, muscle; W, wide tissue distribution

transport mechanism of bilirubin across the sinusoidal surface membrane of the hepatocytes remains to be conclusively identified.

Acquired and Genetic Abnormalities of Hepatic Uptake

The expression of hepatic uptake carrier proteins is regulated at both transcriptional and posttranscriptional levels. For instance, cellular swelling in the isolated perfused rat liver causes a cAMP-mediated translocation of ntcp from intracellular storage sites to the basolateral plasma membrane.[131] Delivery and insertion of ntcp into the plasma membrane require microtubules and microfilaments.[132] Prolactin induces ntcp by Stat-5–regulated enhancement of transcription.[133] The transcriptional and posttranscriptional regulation of uptake transporters has been studied. Endotoxin, tumor necrosis factor-α, interleukin-1β) (IL-1β), and IL-6 reduce bile salt and organic anion uptake. These cytokines downregulate expression of ntcp and Oatp4.[134,135] They mediate their effect most probably via the nuclear hormone receptors retinoid X receptor (RXR) and retinoic acid receptor (RAR).[136] They bind to the RXR-RAR heterodimer response elements within the promoter region of the *ntcp* and *oatp4* genes. High intracellular bile salt concentrations decrease ntcp expression. The mechanism of this down-regulation has been elucidated. Bile salts bind to the farnesoid X-receptor (FXR), a cytosolic nuclear hormone receptor. Upon binding bile salts, this receptor associates with RXR and the heterodimer then translocates to the nucleus. Here it binds to an FXR-RXR response element that is present in a number of genes, including the

SHP gene (short heterodimer partner). Thus high bile salt concentration activates SHP expression and the up-regulated SHP protein interferes with RAR-RXR binding to the *ntcp* gene, inhibiting transcription. Also OATP-C expression in humans and Oatp4 expression in rats are down-regulated in cholestasis. OATP-C is under transcriptional control of hepatocyte nuclear factor-1α (HNF-1α) and HNF-1α expression is controlled by HNF-4α. SHP inhibits HNF-4α–mediated transactivation of the HNF-1α promoter in co-transfection assays. In addition, the human HNF-4α gene promoter is repressed by CDCA through an SHP-independent mechanism. This explains why, in addition to NTCP, OATP-C is also down-regulated in cholestatic liver disease. Because in most liver diseases conjugated bilirubin rather than unconjugated bilirubin is the dominant bile pigment in serum, it is likely that down-regulation of bilirubin transport is a postconjugation event affecting canalicular transport. As discussed later in this chapter, an elegant explanation for the accumulation of conjugated bilirubin in plasma in cholestatic conditions is now available. MRP2, the biliary export pump for conjugated bilirubin, is down-regulated during cholestasis,[137-139] whereas MRP3, a transporter with affinity for conjugated bilirubin, is up-regulated in the basolateral membrane. Via this transporter, conjugated bilirubin is pumped from the hepatocyte into blood.[140,141] Subsequent clearance of bilirubin conjugates by the kidneys in cholestasis is helped by the up-regulation of renal mrp2 expression.

From this discussion it is clear that bile acid and bilirubin are incorporated into the hepatocyte partly via separate mechanisms. This explains the discrepancy between the extent of elevation of plasma bile acid and bilirubin levels in some clinical situations. For example, early in the course of primary biliary cirrhosis, bile acid levels are elevated, but bilirubin levels may still be normal.[142,143] Reduced hepatic bilirubin uptake has been observed in some cases of Gilbert syndrome (discussed later).

Storage of Bilirubin within the Hepatocyte

Within the hepatocyte bilirubin is kept in solution predominantly by binding to cytosolic proteins. Gel permeation chromatography of hepatic cytosol containing ^{3}H-bilirubin revealed that radioactivity is associated with two protein fractions, which were originally named Y and Z.[144] Tracer quantities of anions bind almost exclusively to the Y fraction, whereas in the presence of higher concentrations, binding to the Z fraction becomes apparent, suggesting that components of the Y fraction are the predominant proteins to which organic anions bind within hepatocytes.[144] The Y proteins bind many compounds, including drugs, hormones, and organic anions. This led to the designation of a Y protein as a "ligandin." Later, ligandin was found to be a family of proteins, identical to the α class of glutathione-S-transferases (GSTs).[145] Studies of bilirubin transport in isolated perfused rat liver showed that hepatic ligandin concentration did not affect the influx rate of bilirubin, but increased the net uptake by reducing the efflux rate.[146]

Conjugation of Bilirubin

Biliary excretion of bilirubin requires its conversion to polar derivatives by enzyme-catalyzed conjugation of the propionic acid carboxyls with sugar moieties, which disrupts the internal hydrogen bonds (**Fig. 62-5**). Glucuronic acid is the predominant conjugating sugar in vertebrate bile; glucuronidation of one or both propionic acid carboxyls results in the formation of bilirubin monoglucuronide or bilirubin diglucuronide, respectively, both of which are efficiently excreted in bile.[147] In normal bile from humans and most other mammals, bilirubin diglucuronide is the predominant conjugate.[148,149] In addition, small amounts of glucosyl and xylosyl conjugates have been described in mammalian bile.[150]

Enzyme-Catalyzed Glucuronidation of Bilirubin

Glucuronidation of bilirubin is catalyzed by a specific isoform of a family of enzymes termed uridinediphosphoglucuronate glucuronosyltransferase (UDP-glucuronosyltransferase, EC 2.4.1.17, recommended abbreviation: UGT). UGTs are concentrated in the ER and nuclear envelope of a variety of cells.[151] These enzymes catalyze the transfer of the glucuronosyl moiety of UDP-glucuronate to a wide spectrum of aglycons, forming ether, ester, thiol, and N-glucuronides.[152] Substrates of UGT include hormones (e.g., steroid hormones, thyroid hormones, catecholamines), endogenous metabolites (e.g., bile salts, bilirubin), numerous drugs and their intermediate metabolites, toxins (e.g., carcinogens), and laboratory xenobiotics.[152] Glucuronidation renders the aglycon substrates more polar and, in general, less biologically active. Thus UGTs

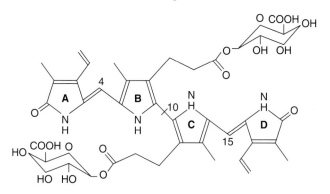

Fig. 62-5 **Effect of sugar conjugation on the structure of bilirubin.** The fully hydrogen-bonded structure of bilirubin IXα-Z,Z is shown in the *top panel*. In bilirubin glucuronides *(bottom panel)*, glucuronidation of the propionic acid carboxyls disrupts the hydrogen bonds. This makes the molecule water-soluble and rapidly excretable in the bile. Disruption of the hydrogen bonds exposes the central carbon bridge (C-10) to diazo reagents, resulting in direct diazo reaction.

constitute one of the most important detoxification mechanisms of the body.

Latency of UGTs

UGTs are integral membrane proteins that require specific membrane lipids for function.[153] UGT activity in microsomal vesicles is partially latent. Membrane perturbation by physical,[154,155] enzymatic,[156] or detergent treatment[155] removes the latency, making the enzyme fully active. Two mechanisms have been proposed to explain the latency and activation of UGT in microsomal membranes. In the compartmental model, the catalytic site of the enzymes is envisioned to be located inside the lumen of the ER. Analysis of their amino acid sequences reveals a putative transmembrane domain near the carboxy-terminal end, leaving only a small segment of the proteins on the cytosolic side of the ER. This cytosolic tail is believed to contain the ER-localizing signal.[157] In view of the hydrophilic nature of UDP-glucuronic acid, the presence of a transporter protein to mediate the movement of UDP-glucuronic acid from the cytosol to the ER lumen is likely. Mechanisms of transport of UDP-glucuronic acid into the ER cisternae are being investigated, but the putative transporters have not been fully characterized or cloned.[158-160] UDP-N-acetylglucosamine activates hepatic microsomal UGT activity at low concentrations and has been postulated to be a physiologic activator of the transferase. Two alternatives have been proposed to explain this. UDP-*N*-acetylglucosamine could increase the access of UDP-glucuronate either by activating a putative transporter or by physically increasing the permeability of the lipid membranes to UDP-glucuronic acid.[161] An alternative hypothesis proposes that the UGT activity is "constrained" by the membrane. Physical or chemical activators, such as UDP-*N*-acetylglucosamine, may act by releasing the enzyme from such constraints.[162] In this model, UDP-*N*-acetylglucosamine is envisioned as an allosteric activator of UGTs. The two models may not be mutually exclusive and neither has been reliably excluded by firm experimental evidence.

Multiple Forms of UGT

The UGT system consists of a family of structurally related enzymes that are functionally heterogeneous. The isoforms differ from each other in ontogenic development[163] and their response to enzyme-inducing agents.[164,165] Several laboratories have isolated multiple UGT isoforms from solubilized liver microsomes.[166] Cloning of cDNAs and genomic DNA has provided a large amount of information on the structure and evolutionary divergence of UGTs. This topic has been reviewed.[167] Based on the degree of structural homology among the various UGT cDNAs, UGTs may be separated into two major families.[167] One family (UGT1) contains the bilirubin conjugating form in human and rat liver, and at least two phenol conjugating UGTs. The second family (UGT2) includes

a number of UGT isoforms that mediate the conjugation of steroids and other endogenous and exogenous substrates. One of these isoforms is inducible by phenobarbital. The UGT2 subfamily also includes two UGT isoforms located in the olfactory tissues that are thought to be responsible for the cessation of chemical olfactory signals.[168]

Organization of the UGT1A Gene Locus

Members of the UGT1A family, including the form that accepts bilirubin as a substrate (UGT1A1) and two phenol-UGT isoforms (UGT1A6 and UGT1A7), are expressed from a locus, termed *UGT1A*.[169] This locus, shown schematically in **Figure 62-6**, is located on human chromosome 2 at region 2q37.[170] The 3′ domain of this gene contains four consecutive exons (exons 2 through 5) that are shared by all UGT isoforms expressed from the UGT1A locus and encode their identical carboxy-terminal domains. This "common region" is highly conserved in evolution and is responsible for UDP-glucuronate binding.[171] Upstream to these exons are a series of at least 12 exons (exons 1A1 through 1A12), each encoding the variable NH₂-terminal region of a different UGT1A isoform. Each variable region exon is preceded by a separate promoter sequence. Depending on promoter selection during transcription, transcripts of various lengths are produced. During processing of the transcript to mRNA, the exon (which is located at the 5′ end of the transcript) is always spliced to exon 2 (the

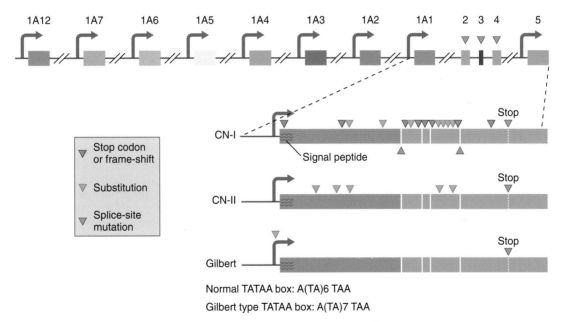

Normal TATAA box: A(TA)6 TAA
Gilbert type TATAA box: A(TA)7 TAA

Fig. 62-6 **A schematic representation of the human *UGT1A* locus at human chromosome 2q37 that comprises several genes encoding the UGT1A family of isoforms.** At the 3′ end of the locus there are 4 exons (exons 2, 3, 4, and 5, shown as *solid bars*), which are used in all UGT1A isoforms (UGT1A1 through UGT1A12) expressed from this locus. Upstream to these common region exons there is a series of variable region exons, designated 1A1 through 1A12, only one of which is used in a given UGT isoform. Each of these exons encodes the variable NH₂-terminal region of one UGT isoform. Each variable region exon has an upstream promoter element, and is differentially regulated. Depending on which promoter is used, transcripts of various lengths are produced. In each transcript, the exon located at the 5′ end of the transcript is spliced to exon 2; the intervening stretch of RNA is spliced out. The genes are named according to their unique region exons. For example, when the transcription starts at exon 1A1, the processed mRNA will consist of exons 1A1, -2, -3, -4, and -5. This gene is termed *UGT1A1*. If the transcription starts at exon 1A6, the mRNA will consist of exons 1A6, -2, -3, -4, and -5 and the gene is termed *UGT1A6*. *UGT1A1* expresses the only UGT isoform that significantly contributes to bilirubin glucuronidation. Genetic nonsense *(red triangle)* or missense *(orange triangle)* mutations of any of the five exons of UGT1A1 can abolish or reduce UGT1A1 activity, causing CN-1. In the case of CN-2 all mutations are of the missense type *(orange triangle)*. Genetic lesions of exon 1A1 only affect bilirubin glucuronidation, whereas those of exons 2, 3, 4, or 5 affect all isoforms of the UGT1A subfamily. Mutations within introns at splice sites can also give rise to CN-1 *(blue triangles)*. Gilbert syndrome is associated with the insertion of a TA dinucleotide within the TATAA element upstream to exon 1A1.

first of the four common region exons), the whole intervening sequence being spliced out. The amino-terminal domain of a given UGT1A isoform encoded by a unique exon confers the aglycon substrate specificity to that isoform.[172] The genes for the various UGT1A isoforms are named according to the unique exon used in that mRNA. For example, exon 1A1 encodes the amino-terminal domain of UGT1A1 (bilirubin-UGT) and this gene is termed *UGT1A1*. UGT1A1 is the only isoform that significantly contributes to the conjugation of bilirubin.[173] Two other genes, *UGT1A6* and *UGT1A7*, encode isoforms that conjugate phenols.[167]

The presence of a separate regulatory *cis* element upstream to each unique exon permits UGT1A isoforms to be independently regulated, explaining their different organ distribution and expression during ontogeny, enzyme induction, or carcinogenesis. Enzyme activity toward 4-nitrophenol and other simple phenolic substrates develops in late fetal life in rats, whereas activity toward bilirubin develops after birth.[163] UGT1A6, a 3-methylcholanthrene–inducible isoform, is permanently overexpressed in carcinogen-induced preneoplastic nodules in rat liver.[174] Triiodothyronine treatment results in a three-fold increase in rat liver phenol-UGT activity, whereas bilirubin glucuronidation is reduced by 80%.[165]

Bile Canalicular Secretion of Bilirubin Conjugates and Related Organic Anions

Excretion across the canalicular membrane is rate limiting in overall disposition of many cholephilic compounds and represents the most important concentrative step. Indeed, for all classes of organic compounds, including cations, anions, and bile acids, this step creates a larger concentration gradient than that observed across the sinusoidal/basolateral membrane. For example, for organic anions such as dibromosulfophthalein (DBSP), a liver to bile concentration ratio of 1:1000 can be reached.[175] These concentration gradients are too large to be accounted for by the membrane potential difference over the canalicular membrane. For most classes of compounds, active, energy-consuming transport systems have been demonstrated.

ATP-Dependent Organic Anion Transport

ATP-dependent transporters are important in the canalicular excretion of bilirubin glucuronides. ABCC2/MRP2 is a canalicular efflux pump for organic anions. This protein is also expressed in intestine and kidneys.[176-178] In the liver ABCC2 functions as the efflux pump for many organic anions, most of which are products of phase II drug metabolism. Bilirubin monoglucuronide and bilirubin diglucuronide are among its substrates.[179] Genetic deficiency of ABCC2 in humans leads to Dubin-Johnson syndrome, characterized by hyperbilirubinemia.[180,181] The TR⁻ rat is an animal model with conjugated bilirubinemia caused by a single nucleotide deletion in the *MRP2/ABCC2* gene.[182] MRP1 (mrp1 in rodents) is expressed during liver regeneration and endotoxin-mediated cholestasis.[138,183] MRP3 (mrp3 in rodents) is expressed at very low levels in normal liver, but is greatly induced during cholestasis and hyperbilirubinemia.[140,184,185] Both mrp1 and mrp3 are located in the basolateral membrane of hepatocytes. Mrp1 and

mrp3 are mainly pumps for glucuronides, including bilirubin glucuronides,[186,187] whereas mrp1 pumps glutathione-*S*-conjugates[141] and, as has recently been reported, unconjugated bilirubin. Mrp3 expression is strongly enhanced during cholestasis, in the liver of mrp2-deficient Eisai hyperbilirubinemic rats (EHBR) rats, and in UGT1A1-deficient Gunn rats.[187,188] Thus MRP3/mrp3 functions as a reverse transporter, which pumps substrates back to the blood when biliary excretion of glucuronides is reduced because of an inherited deficiency of ABCC2/MRP2 or its down-regulation in cholestatic conditions.

CAR, the constitutive androstane receptor, is the dominant transcriptional regulator of MRP3. Phenobarbital is the prototypical substrate of CAR. MRP3 expression is enhanced in patients with Dubin-Johnson syndrome and in Eisai hyperbilirubinemic rats, suggesting that conjugated bilirubin may also be a CAR substrate. The bilirubin conjugate transporter MRP2/ABCC2 is a multispecific pump that contributes to bile formation by transporting glutathione, a major driving force for bile salt–independent bile flow. In addition, ABCC2/MRP2 also has a role in canalicular anionic phase II conjugate transport. ABCC2/MRP2 expression in rat liver responds to inducing agents and is down-regulated by endotoxin, cytokines, and bile duct ligation. A dose- and time-dependent induction of *abcc2* expression was observed in isolated rat hepatocytes cultured in the presence of xenobiotics, including vincristine, tamoxifen, or the pregnane x receptor (PXR)-ligand rifampicin,[189] indicating that *abcc2* gene transcription may respond to substrates of ABCC2 itself. The promoter regions of human *ABCC2/MRP2* and rat *abcc2/mrp2* genes have been isolated.[187,190] Sequence analysis of the human *ABCC2/MRP2* promoter showed a number of putative consensus binding sites for both ubiquitous and liver-enriched transcription factors, including activating protein-1 (AP1), specificity protein 1 (SP1), hepatocyte nuclear factor-1 (HNF1), and HNF-3β[190,191] as well as CAR, PXR, and FXR. An unusual sequence was identified 440 base pairs (bp) upstream of the *MRP2* transcription initiation site that binds with high-affinity to PXR, CAR, and FXR as heterodimers with RXR. Human and rodent hepatocytes reacted with a robust induction of ABCC2/MRP2 mRNA levels on exposure to the PXR, CAR, and FXR agonists—rifampicin, dexamethasone, pregnenolone 16α-carbonitrile, and spironolactone (PXR); phenobarbital (CAR); and chenodeoxycholic acid (FXR). *Ugt1A1* in rodents has also been reported to be a PXR target gene. Like *ABCC2/MRP2*, *UGT1A1* contains a multicomponent enhancer element in its promoter region with CAR, PXR, and AhR motifs. In addition, both glucuronidation and secretion are induced by PXR and CAR agonists. Thus PXR and CAR are major regulators of bilirubin uptake, glucuronidation, and secretion. The various secretion transporters and the substances that they handle are listed in **Table 62-2**.

Transport of Bile Acids and Non–Bile Acid Organic Anions

Human MDR1 (ABCB1), MDR3 (ABCB4), ATP8B1, and BSEP (ABCB11)—and their rat orthologues Mdr1a and Mdr1b, Mdr2, Atp8b1, and Bsep, respectively—are P-glycoproteins that are constitutively expressed in the canalicular membrane of the hepatocyte. MDR3/Mdr2 and

Table 62-2 Organic Anion Secretion Transporters in Human Liver

	MRP1 (ABCC1)	MRP2(ABCC2 OR CMOAT)	MRP3(ABCC3)	MRP6(ABCC6)
Glutathione (GSH)	+	+		
Glutathione disulfide (GSSG)	+	+		
Leukotriene C_4	+	+		
Gluthatione-S-conjugates	+	+		
Bilirubin monoglucuronide	+	+	*	
Bilirubin diglucuronide	+	+	*	
Estradiol 17β-D-glucuronide	+	+	+	
Taurocholate			+	
Glycocholate			+	
3α-Sulfotaurochenodeoxy cholate			+	
6α-Glucuronosyl hyodeoxycholate	+			
3α-Sulfotaurolithocholate	+		+	
Ochratoxin A		+		
Methotrexate	+	+	+	
BQ-123				+
Regulation	LPS↑[29] PH↑[46]	LPS↓[30]↑[29] BDL↓dexamethasone ↑[125,126]	BDL[127,128] EHBR rats↑[126] Gunn rats↑[127] Phenobarbital↑[51]	
Polarity	Basolateral	Canalicular	Basolateral	Basolateral Canalicular
Tissue distribution	H, E, B	H, I, K	H, C	H
References	140, 193	184, 185, 188-190	144, 191-195	

Alternative names are given in parentheses.
*, Probable.
B, brain; BDL, bile duct ligation; C, cholangiocytes; E, erythrocytes; H, hepatocytes; K, kidney; LPS, lipopolysaccharide; PH, partial hepatectomy

BSEP/Bsep are expressed in the liver only, whereas MDR1 and ATP8B1 are also expressed in various nonhepatic secretory epithelia. The canalicular bile-salt export pump (BSEP/ABCB11) is of paramount importance for bile formation and liver function. BSEP/ABCB11 appears to be the principal driving force in the enterohepatic circulation of bile salts. Also the bile-salt–dependent fraction of bile flow depends on BSEP/ABCB11. Bile salts are the major, if not the only, substrates of BSEP/ABCB11. Rat, mouse, and human *BSEP/ABCB11* genes have been cloned.[191-195] Inherited deficiency of ATP8B1 and BSEP/ABCB11 leads to progressive familial intrahepatic cholestasis types I and II, respectively. Both these conditions lead to severe life-threatening cholestatic liver disease, associated with both conjugated and unconjugated hyperbilirubinemia. Surprisingly, some mutations of ATP8B1 and BSEP/ABCB11 also cause forms of benign intrahepatic cholestasis.[196,197] MDR3/ABCB4 in humans (mdr2 in mice) is involved in the biliary secretion of phosphatidylcholine, the only phospholipid in bile. Mice with a knockout mutation of the *mdr2* gene produce bile in which phospholipids are absent.[198] These mice and humans with a similar defect develop severe liver disease characterized by bile duct proliferation, portal fibrosis, and eventually cirrhosis.[199,200] Heterozygosity for MDR3/ABCB4 deficiency is also in part responsible for intrahepatic cholestasis of pregnancy as well as for intrahepatic and gallbladder cholesterol stone formation. Approximately a third of adult patients presenting with unexplained cholestasis have mutations in the coding region of at least one ABCB4 allele.[196] ABCB4 mutations also cause acute recurrent biliary pancreatitis, biliary cirrhosis, and fibrosing cholestatic liver disease in adults with or without biliary symptoms.[196,197]

Role of Nuclear Receptors in the Orchestration of Various Steps Involved in Bilirubin Throughput

The capacity of the various steps involved in bilirubin throughput appears to be matched in vivo. Thus reduction of any of the following can lead to hyperbilirubinemia: transport, storage, conjugation, or excretion. On the other hand, enhanced excretion of bilirubin, for example, in response to an increased bilirubin load, would require a coordinated increase in the capacity of each step involved in the uptake and elimination process. It has been proposed that the nuclear receptor CAR serves as the coordinating mechanism for physiologic modulation of each of these steps.[201,202]

Fate of Bilirubin in the Gastrointestinal Tract

Conjugated bilirubin reaching the intestinal tract is not substantially absorbed.[203] Absorption of unconjugated bilirubin from the intestine may be enhanced in the presence of maternal milk and may contribute to neonatal hyperbilirubinemia.[204] A small amount of bilirubin may be reabsorbed from the gallbladder in animals.[205] Bilirubin glucuronides are deconjugated by intestinal bacteria[206] and degraded to a series of urobilinogens and related products.[207] Urobilinogens are not glucuronidated; it is not known whether deconjugation precedes or follows bilirubin degradation. After absorption from the intestine, urobilinogen is excreted in the bile and, to a lesser extent, in the urine. Variability of reabsorption of urobilinogen by renal tubules and instability of the pigment in acid urine make the measurement of urinary urobilinogen concentration an unreliable indicator of metabolism. However, the absence of urobilinogen in stool and urine indicates complete obstruction of the bile duct or severe cholestasis, as seen in the early presentation of acute hepatitis. In most liver diseases and in states of increased bilirubin production, urinary urobilinogen excretion is increased. Urobilinogen is colorless. Its oxidation product, urobilin, is yellow and contributes to the color of normal urine and stool.

Extrahepatic Handling of Bilirubin

Renal Handling of Bilirubin

Only 3% of labeled unconjugated bilirubin is excreted by the kidney after intravenous administration. Even in the presence of high bilirubin levels, bile remains the main route of bilirubin excretion. Renal excretion of conjugated bilirubin depends on the glomerular filtration of a small, non–protein-bound fraction of conjugated bilirubin.[208] Unconjugated bilirubin, which is tightly bound to albumin, is not filtered to a significant extent by normal renal glomeruli and does not appear in the urine. There is evidence for tubular reabsorption but not tubular secretion of bilirubin.[209] Because, normally, less than 5% of total bilirubin in plasma is conjugated, bilirubin is not present in urine in the absence of albuminuria.

During cholestasis, the kidney assumes a major role in bilirubin disposal. Upon infusion of radiolabeled bilirubin into plasma of animals with experimental bile duct ligation[210,211] and in children with biliary atresia,[212] 50% to 90% of injected radioactivity is excreted in urine. Urinary excretion becomes the major excretory pathway for bilirubin in the presence of complete biliary obstruction.[208]

Intestinal Bilirubin Metabolism

Intestinal mucosal epithelia, particularly cells of the proximal small intestinal villi, have bilirubin-UGT activity.[151] The relative contribution of small intestinal glucuronidation in the overall disposition of bilirubin is not clearly known.

Alternative Pathways of Bilirubin Elimination

Photoisomerization

Configurational and cyclic isomers of bilirubin formed in the presence of ambient light or during phototherapy (discussed previously in this chapter; see Photochemistry of Bilirubin) are excreted in bile in unconjugated form.[213,214] A significant amount of bilirubin is degraded to polar diazo-negative compounds that are excreted in bile and urine.[215]

Enzyme-Catalyzed Oxidation

Oxidation of bilirubin may be mediated by mixed-function oxidases in liver and other organs. Inducers of the mixed-function oxidase cytochrome P-450c, such as 2,3,7,8-tetra-chlorodibenzo-p-dioxin (TCDD) or 3-methylcholanthrene, reduce plasma bilirubin levels in bilirubin-UGT–deficient Gunn rats.[216] Induction of cytochrome P-450c by chlorpromazine resulted in the reduction of serum bilirubin levels in one patient with Crigler-Najjar syndrome type 1.[217] Degradation of bilirubin in vitro by cytochrome P-450-1A1 supports the concept that bilirubin oxidation in the liver may be a functional alternative pathway of bilirubin disposal. Induction of this enzyme system by substances such as indole-3-carbinol may convert bilirubin to colorless metabolites.[218] The relative contribution of microsomal oxidation to the overall turnover of bilirubin in vivo is not clear, but this pathway may play a significant role in bilirubin disposition in cases where the normal pathways are deficient; for example, in patients with Crigler-Najjar syndrome type 1 or in Gunn rats.[219]

Quantification of Bilirubin

Serum bilirubin is an important marker of liver function. In the newborn period, the total serum bilirubin concentration and the fractional concentration of free (non–protein-bound) bilirubin need to be monitored to determine the need to institute therapy to reduce serum bilirubin level. Clinically, serum bilirubin is usually measured after conversion to stable azo derivatives. Quantification of the various species of bilirubin as intact tetrapyrroles is more accurate and of value mainly for research purposes. Currently available methods of bilirubin analysis have been reviewed.[220]

Conversion of Bilirubin to Azo Derivatives

Quantification of bilirubin is facilitated by derivatization with diazo reagents that transform it to stable dipyrrolic derivatives. Electrophilic attack by a diazonium ion at the carbons flanking the central carbon bridge (C-9 and C-11 positions of bilirubin)[221] converts the tetrapyrrole to two diazotized azodipyrroles, the central bridge carbon being eliminated as formaldehyde. Unconjugated bilirubin yields two unconjugated dipyrroles: bilirubin diconjugates form two conjugated azodipyrroles, and bilirubin monoconjugates form one conjugated and one unconjugated azodipyrrole. In 1916 van den Bergh and Muller described that one species of serum bilirubin reacts with the sulfanilic acid diazo reagent within minutes ("direct"-reacting fraction), whereas another species only reacts rapidly when accelerator substances, such as methanol or caffeine, are present ("indirect"-reacting fraction).[222] Later, it was understood that indirect-reacting bilirubin represents unconjugated bilirubin, whereas the direct-reacting fraction roughly corresponds to conjugated bilirubin.[223] Variations of the van den Bergh reaction are currently used for the clinical determination of bilirubin conjugates.

The direct diazo reacting fraction of bilirubin overestimates the levels of conjugated bilirubin, because solutions of unconjugated bilirubin may show as much as 10% to 15% of the total pigment as direct-reacting. Usually, a direct-reacting bilirubin concentration of less than 15% of total is considered normal. The diazo reaction does not differentiate between noncovalently albumin-bound conjugated bilirubin and the fraction of bilirubin that becomes irreversibly bound to serum proteins, particularly albumin, during conjugated hyperbilirubinemia,[224] because both fractions give direct diazo reaction. The irreversibly protein-bound bilirubin is slowly cleared from serum after reversal of biliary obstruction. Therefore finding direct-reacting bilirubin during this period may give a false impression of continued biliary obstruction. Certain metabolites, such as indican, which accumulate in serum during renal failure, may interfere with the diazo reaction.[225] In circumstances in which it is critical to know whether conjugated bilirubin is present in the plasma, it is necessary to perform chromatographic analysis of bile pigments.

Chromatographic Analysis of Bilirubin Species as Intact Tetrapyrroles

Thin-Layer and High-Pressure Liquid Chromatography

Bilirubin and its conjugates can be separated by thin-layer chromatography.[226] High-resolution analysis of bilirubin and its conjugates is possible using high-pressure liquid chromatography (HPLC). Methyl esters formed by alkaline methanolysis of bilirubin mono- and diconjugates are easy to extract from serum and analyze by HPLC.[227] However, as the conjugating sugars are replaced by methyl groups, this method does not identify the type of sugar conjugate. Methods for separation and quantification of intact bilirubin tetrapyrrole conjugates by HPLC have been developed[228,229] and offer accurate and sensitive means to identify and quantify bilirubin conjugates in body fluids and in vitro.

Measurement of the Irreversibly Protein-Bound Fraction

Most chromatographic methods require extraction of serum bile pigments into organic solvents, whereby the irreversibly protein-bound fraction of bilirubin (also known as δ-bilirubin) is lost. To measure this fraction, along with other fractions of unconjugated and conjugated bilirubin, reverse-phase HPLC is performed on incompletely deproteinated serum.[224] Investigations utilizing this method

indicate that the irreversibly protein-bound serum bilirubin fraction is formed in conditions associated with conjugated hyperbilirubinemia.

Slide Tests

A convenient slide test measures conjugated, unconjugated, and irreversibly protein-bound bilirubin. The Ektachem TIBL slide is used to quantify total bilirubin by a diazo technique.[230] Another slide is specially coated to allow only the free and reversibly protein-bound forms of bilirubins to react with the diazo reagent.[231] Irreversibly protein-bound bilirubin can be estimated from the difference between measurements of total bilirubin and the sum of conjugated and unconjugated bilirubin, as estimated by the second slide. Corroboration with chromatographic methods indicates that results obtained by the Ektachem slide tests are consistent and reliable.[230,231]

Transcutaneous Bilirubinometry

Determination of the rate of increase of serum bilirubin levels during the first 24 to 48 hours of life by repeated measurement of serum bilirubin levels can be helpful in predicting peak serum bilirubin level during the neonatal period. Such measurements can be performed painlessly and at low expense by the measurement of the yellow color of the skin by analysis of reflected light.[232] On-board computers in these analyzers are programmed to measure the yellow color without interference by underlying skin pigmentation or erythema. Transcutaneous bilirubinometry in 900 term and premature infants of different races provided estimated serum bilirubin concentrations that correlated well with values obtained by a standard diazo method using serum samples.[233-235]

The Nature and Significance of Bilirubin in Body Fluids

Bilirubin in Plasma

When measured by accurate chromatographic techniques, unconjugated bilirubin is normally the predominant plasma bile pigment: only up to 4% of the pigments are conjugated. When there is an overproduction of bilirubin, the proportion of the unconjugated and conjugated fractions remains unchanged despite the increase in total bilirubin levels. In contrast, when the serum level increases because of a deficiency of bilirubin glucuronidation, the absolute concentration of conjugated bilirubin may remain normal or may be reduced, resulting in a reduced proportion of conjugated bilirubin.

During biliary obstruction, intrahepatic cholestasis, or hepatocellular diseases, both conjugated bilirubin and unconjugated bilirubin accumulate in plasma, and the proportion of conjugated bilirubin increases. As discussed previously, during cholestasis MRP2 is down-regulated, reducing biliary excretion of conjugated bilirubin. Bile pigments accumulating in hepatocytes may be pumped into plasma by MRP3, which is up-regulated in basolateral membranes during cholestasis. When there is a prolonged accumulation of conjugated bilirubin, a fraction of the pigment becomes irreversibly bound to albumin. This fraction, termed δ-bilirubin, has a direct diazo reaction and can be identified by chromatographic analysis. After successful surgical correction of biliary obstruction, the reversibly protein-bound fraction of serum bilirubin is rapidly excreted in bile, resulting in an increase in the proportion of the irreversibly protein-bound fraction of serum bilirubin. If biliary obstruction persists, both reversibly protein-bound and irreversibly protein-bound fractions are retained; therefore the proportion of the irreversibly bound fraction does not show a marked increase.[122]

Bilirubin in Urine

Because unconjugated bilirubin is tightly bound to albumin, it is not normally filtered in renal glomeruli. Conjugated bilirubin is less strongly bound to albumin and therefore appears in urine. In the absence of proteinuria, excretion of bilirubin in the urine indicates the presence of conjugated bilirubin in the plasma. Covalently protein-bound bile pigment (δ-bilirubin) is not excreted in urine.

Bilirubin in Bile

More than 80% of bilirubin in normal hepatic bile is the diglucuronide form. Unconjugated bilirubin accounts for only 4% of biliary pigments. In the presence of complete deficiency of bilirubin-UGT activity, as in the case of Crigler-Najjar syndrome type 1, little or no bilirubin glucuronides are excreted in bile. When bilirubin glucuronidation is partially deficient, as in Crigler-Najjar syndrome type 2 or Gilbert syndrome, the proportion of bilirubin monoglucuronide and unconjugated bilirubin increases in bile. The presence of a significant amount of conjugated bilirubin in bile reliably differentiates Crigler-Najjar syndrome type 1 from Crigler-Najjar syndrome type 2 (see Crigler-Najjar Syndrome Type 2: Laboratory Tests).

Bilirubin in Tissue Fluids

Tissue fluids with high protein content contain albumin-bound bilirubin. Therefore a comparison of the serum bilirubin concentration with the concentration of bilirubin in body fluids can help to differentiate between exudates and transudates. A pleural fluid/serum bilirubin ratio of 0.6 or higher is strongly indicative of an exudate.[234] Bilirubin is excreted in sweat, semen, and breast milk in hyperbilirubinemic patients. Bilirubin is present in synovial and ocular fluids. However, xanthopsia is extremely rare in jaundice. Interestingly, paralyzed limbs are less deeply jaundiced than other parts of the body.

Bilirubin in Cerebrospinal Fluid

Because of the low protein concentration of the cerebrospinal fluid, bilirubin concentration in cerebrospinal fluid is much lower than that in the serum. When an increase in the cerebrospinal fluid protein concentration co-exists with jaundice (e.g., in leptospirosis) the cerebrospinal fluid may contain bilirubin.

Bilirubin in Skin and Sclera

Bilirubin binds avidly to the elastic tissue of skin and sclera. Therefore scleral icterus is a sensitive clinical feature of hyperbilirubinemia. Scleral icterus often outlasts hyperbilirubinemia. Yellow discoloration of skin and mucous membranes is more intense in conjugated hyperbilirubinemia, probably because of better penetration of the water-soluble conjugates into body fluids. During prolonged conjugated hyperbilirubinemia, oxidation of bilirubin to biliverdin may produce a greenish pigmentation of the skin.

Disorders of Bilirubin Metabolism

Increased bilirubin production and abnormalities in any of the four distinct but interactive steps of hepatic bilirubin throughput—namely, uptake from the circulation, intracellular binding or storage, conjugation, and biliary excretion—may result in hyperbilirubinemia. Many clinical disorders, such as hepatitis or cirrhosis, affect multiple steps of this process. In contrast, in several inherited disorders, a specific step of bilirubin throughput may be involved. From the viewpoint of bilirubin metabolism, these disorders may be classified into those that cause predominantly unconjugated hyperbilirubinemia and those that are characterized by elevation in levels of both conjugated and unconjugated bilirubin in plasma.

Disorders Associated with Unconjugated Hyperbilirubinemia

Neonatal Hyperbilirubinemia

When compared with healthy adults, all newborns have higher serum bilirubin concentrations. Clinically obvious jaundice occurs in about 50% of neonates during the first 5 days of life. In normal, full-term babies, serum bilirubin levels increase from 1 to 2 to 5 to 6 mg/dl in approximately 72 hours and subsequently decrease to below 1 mg/dl in 7 to 10 days.[235] In this "physiologic jaundice," serum bilirubin is predominantly unconjugated. Exaggeration of physiologic jaundice may expose infants to the risk of kernicterus. In approximately 16% of newborns, maximum serum bilirubin concentrations reach or exceed 10 mg/dl; in 5% the level exceeds 15 mg/dl.[236] Physiologic jaundice of the newborn may result from a combination of increased bilirubin production and a lower than adult level of the capability of the liver to dispose of bilirubin. Exaggeration of one or more of the normal restrictions characteristic of the newborn period and/or superimposition of additional mechanisms may result in a pathologic level of neonatal hyperbilirubinemia. A brief discussion of these mechanisms follows.

Increased Bilirubin Load

Premature breakdown of erythrocytes or ineffective erythropoiesis causes hyperbilirubinemia despite normal liver function. Increased bilirubin production in the newborn period is evidenced by increased endogenous carbon monoxide production,[237] early-labeled peak of bilirubin from erythroid and nonerythroid sources, and decreased erythrocyte half-life.[238] In the past hemolytic diseases of the fetus, such as rhesus incompatibility between mother and fetus, were a common cause of severe neonatal jaundice. Today this condition is managed by treatment of the mother with anti-rhesus immunoglobulins.[239] However, ABO blood group incompatibility remains a common cause of exaggerated neonatal hyperbilirubinemia.[240] Inherited disorders, such as sickle cell disease and hereditary spherocytosis, and toxic or idiosyncratic drug reactions are common causes of hemolytic jaundice in the newborn period. Ineffective erythropoiesis occurs in thalassemia, vitamin B_{12} deficiency, and congenital dyserythropoietic anemias. In the presence of normal liver function, serum bilirubin levels rarely exceed 4 mg/dl. In some cases, the high bilirubin throughput may result in the accumulation of some conjugated bilirubin in serum in addition to the predominantly unconjugated fraction.

Immaturity of Hepatic Bilirubin Uptake

Hepatic bilirubin uptake capacity is low at birth compared with adult levels, and may remain so for the first few days of life. Maturation of the net hepatic bilirubin uptake may correlate with the expression of hepatic GSTs[241] that bind bilirubin, thereby reducing its efflux from the liver. When the closure of the ductus venosus is delayed, portal blood bypasses the liver, thereby reducing hepatic uptake.[242] Reduced caloric intake may contribute to hyperbilirubinemia by reducing hepatic bilirubin clearance.

Bilirubin Conjugation

Hepatic UGT1A1 activity is very low in mammalian fetuses and is only 1% of normal adult levels at birth in humans.[243] Regardless of gestational age at birth, bilirubin glucuronidating activity rapidly increases to adult levels by the fourteenth week of life.[244] Reduced hepatic levels of UGT1A1 may linger in some cases because of an inherited inhibitory factor or factors in maternal milk or serum as described in the following paragraphs.

Maternal Milk Jaundice

Breastfed infants have higher serum bilirubin levels than do formula-fed babies.[245] Occasionally, serum bilirubin levels may increase to 15 to 24 mg/dl within 10 to 19 days of life. This transient nonhemolytic unconjugated hyperbilirubinemia may take up to 4 weeks to disappear, but promptly resolves upon discontinuation of breastfeeding. Kernicterus is rare, but has been reported.[246] The presence of an inhibitor of bilirubin glucuronidation in maternal milk[247,248] is responsible for this syndrome. A progestational steroid, $3',20\beta$-pregnanediol, isolated from the milk of mothers of infants with this syndrome, was reported to inhibit o-aminophenol glucuronidation by guinea pig, rat, and rabbit livers,[244,248] but not by human liver. The free fatty acid concentration in maternal milk correlates positively with its inhibitory effect on human UGT1A1 activity. The inhibition is more pronounced with polyunsaturated free fatty acids.[249] The presence of a lipolytic enzyme in specific maternal milk

samples has been reported by some investigators, who have suggested that lipolysis may be responsible for the increased free fatty acid concentrations in the milk. The inhibitory effect of maternal milk on bilirubin glucuronidation increases on storage and is destroyed by heating at 56° C.[249]

Maternal Serum Jaundice

In this condition, termed Lucey-Driscoll syndrome,[250,251] jaundice occurs within the first 4 days of life. Peak serum bilirubin concentrations of 8.9 to 65 mg/dl are reached within 7 days. An unidentified inhibitor of UGT1A1 is present in the serum of mothers of these infants. Jaundice begins earlier than in maternal milk jaundice, is more severe, and can be associated with kernicterus.

Canalicular Bilirubin Excretion

During the late newborn period, uptake and conjugation of bilirubin mature to adult levels, but the bilirubin load continues to be high. During this period of life, canalicular excretion becomes rate-limiting in hepatic disposition of bilirubin. In cases where the bilirubin load is further increased, conjugated bilirubin accumulates in serum.[252] However, as discussed previously, a small amount of conjugated bilirubin may accumulate in plasma even when the bilirubin load does not exceed the maximum canalicular excretory capacity.

Increased Intestinal Reabsorption

Hydrolysis of conjugated bilirubin by intestinal β-glucuronidase releases unconjugated bilirubin in the intestine.[253] Because the intestinal flora is not yet established in the newborn, there is a reduced level of bacterial degradation of bilirubin, resulting in an increased absorption of unconjugated bilirubin.[253] Maternal milk may also increase intestinal absorption of unconjugated bilirubin.

Hyperbilirubinemia Caused by Bilirubin Overproduction

Except in the presence of abnormal liver function, overproduction of bilirubin rarely causes serum bilirubin to reach levels greater than 3 to 4 mg/dl. Common causes of hemolytic jaundice include sickle cell anemia, hereditary spherocytosis, and toxic or idiosyncratic drug reactions in susceptible individuals. In hemolytic jaundice, a small amount of conjugated bilirubin produced in the liver may appear in the circulation[254]; however, the unconjugated/conjugated bilirubin ratio remains normal. Ineffective erythropoiesis that occurs in thalassemia and other hematologic disorders is often associated with hyperbilirubinemia.[255] Hereditary dyserythropoietic anemias are a group of rare disorders characterized by ineffective erythropoiesis, intramedullary normoblastic hyperplasia, secondary hemochromatosis, and unconjugated hyperbilirubinemia.[256]

Inherited Disorders of Bilirubin Glucuronidation

Three grades of inherited deficiency of UGT1A1 activity have been described in humans. A virtual absence of UGT1A1 activity results in the most severe of these disorders, Crigler-Najjar

Table 62-3 Features of Inherited Disorders Resulting in Unconjugated Hyperbilirubinemia

	CRIGLER-NAJJAR SYNDROME TYPE 1	CRIGLER-NAJJAR SYNDROME TYPE 2	GILBERT SYNDROME
Serum bilirubin levels	340-850 μmol/L	<340 μmol/L	Usually <50 μmol/L
Routine liver function tests	Normal	Normal	Normal
Serum bile acid levels	Normal	Normal	Normal
Oral cholecystography	Normal	Normal	Normal
Liver histology	Normal	Normal	Normal
Bile conjugates	Usually pale: contains small amounts of unconjugated bilirubin	Increased proportion of bilirubin monoglucuronide	Increased proportion of bilirubin monoglucuronide
Hepatic UGT1A1 activity	None	10% of normal or less	25%-40% of normal
Effect of phenobarbital on serum bilirubin levels	None	Reduction by 25% or more	Reduction
Mode of inheritance	Autosomal recessive	Autosomal recessive	Autosomal recessive
Prevalence	Rare	Uncommon	Common, ≈5% in general population
Prognosis	Kernicterus is the rule	Usually benign; kernicterus is rare	Benign
Animal model	Gunn rat	—	Bolivian squirrel monkey ? Mutant Southdown sheep

UGT1A1, bilirubin-uridinediphosphoglucuronate glucuronosyltransferase

syndrome type 1. Severe but incomplete deficiencies of the transferase activity lead to Crigler-Najjar syndrome type 2, also known as Arias syndrome. A mild reduction of UGT1A1 activity is found in the common, mostly innocuous disorder, termed Gilbert syndrome. **Table 62-3** summarizes the clinical and diagnostic features of these disorders.

Crigler-Najjar Syndrome Type 1

This rare disorder was described by Crigler and Najjar in 1952 in six infants from three unrelated families.[257] Subsequently, the disease was found to result from an absence of bilirubin-UGT activity.[258] Severe indirect hyperbilirubinemia in the absence of hemolysis was observed in all cases within the first few days of life, and persisted life long. Five of the six infants in the initial series died of kernicterus by the age of 15 months. The single survivor was free of neurologic disease until 15 years of age, but then developed kernicterus and died 6 months later. In a related patient neurologic symptoms developed at 18 years of age; she died at the age of 24.[259] These early cases suggested the heterogeneity of Crigler-Najjar syndrome, which became clearly established when Arias and associates subsequently described a milder variant of the condition, termed Crigler-Najjar syndrome type 2.[260] Several other recessively inherited traits, such as Morquio syndrome, homocystinuria, metachromatic leukodystrophy, and bird-headed dwarfism, were found in some families, but were subsequently not found to be associated with Crigler-Najjar syndrome. Since the initial report, several hundred patients with Crigler-Najjar syndrome type 1 have been described.[261] The syndrome occurs in all races and is transmitted as an autosomal recessive trait.[257,258] The incidence appears to be approximately one in a million live births, although the precise frequency of this disease in various populations is not known. As in all rare autosomal recessive disorders, a high incidence of consanguinity among the parents has been observed. Physical examination is normal except for jaundice, and sometimes, evidence of neurological damage. The institution of routine use of phototherapy and intermittent application of exchange transfusion for clinical emergencies has extended the life expectancy beyond adolescence. However, around puberty phototherapy becomes less effective and the bilirubin load increases. Therefore patients always are at risk for kernicterus[261] and liver transplantation remains the only definitive treatment.

Laboratory Tests

Serum biochemical tests are normal in Crigler-Najjar syndrome type 1, except for a high serum bilirubin level, which usually ranges from 18 to 30 mg/dl, but may be as high as 50 mg/dl.[261] Because all the serum bilirubin is present in the unconjugated form, bilirubin is not present in the urine. Plasma bilirubin concentrations fluctuate according to the level of exposure to the sun or other light, and increase during intercurrent illness.[258,261] The bile lacks bilirubin glucuronides and may contain only small amounts of unconjugated bilirubin. Although fecal urobilinogen excretion is reduced, stool color remains normal.[257] Bilirubin production rate is normal[257,262] and there is no evidence of hemolysis.[257,260] Intact bile canalicular excretion mechanisms are evidenced by normal plasma disappearance of BSP[259] and indocyanine green,[257] and radiologic visualization of the biliary tree by cholecystographic agents.

Liver biopsy reveals normal histologic results, except for bilirubin plugs in bile canaliculi and bile ducts,[257,261] probably resulting from biliary excretion of unconjugated bilirubin or its photoisomers. A high incidence of pigment gallstones, often requiring cholecystectomy, is seen in patients with Crigler-Najjar syndrome. Electron microscopy of the liver shows no specific pathologic change.[263]

Abnormalities of Hepatic UGTs and Their Molecular Mechanisms

All Crigler-Najjar syndrome type 1 patients lack hepatic UGT activity toward bilirubin, but some have additional abnormalities of phenol glucuronidation.[264] The mechanism of the abnormality of single or multiple isoforms of hepatic UGTs in Crigler-Najjar syndrome type 1 was clarified when the molecular basis of this disorder was determined in 1992.[265-267] The structure of the UGT1A locus dictates that genetic lesions located in any of the four common region exons (exons 2 to 5) should cause a defect of all isoforms expressed from the UGT1A locus (see **Fig. 62-6**), whereas sequence abnormalities within the unique exon 1A1 should affect only bilirubin glucuronidation, which is mediated by UGT1A1.

Since these initial reports, more than 50 genetic lesions have been identified in more than 100 Crigler-Najjar syndrome patients and in many of their immediate relatives. Huang and colleagues reviewed and tabulated these studies. Analysis of this cumulative experience shows that genetic lesions, such as point mutations, deletions, or insertions, within any of the five exons constituting UGT1A1 mRNA, can inactivate the enzyme. Effects of single amino acid substitutions are being studied by site-directed mutagenesis of expression vectors, followed by transfection into COS cells. Furthermore, in three cases, intronic mutations at the splice donor or splice acceptor sites have been found to cause abnormal splicing at cryptic splice sites within exons, leading to frameshift and truncation of the enzyme.[268,269]

The molecular genetic studies confirm the autosomal recessive inheritance pattern of Crigler-Najjar syndrome type 1. A high incidence of consanguinity in the families is reflected by the observation that, in the majority of patients, both alleles contain the same genetic lesion. However, in some cases no history of consanguinity exists and the patients are compound heterozygotes; that is, a different genetic lesion is present in each allele. Although in a great majority of cases the genetic lesion is inherited from both parents, recently an instance of uniparental isodisomy has been reported in which both mutant alleles were inherited from the father.[270] The mother's UGT1A1 genotype was normal. This case underscores the need for analyzing the genotype of both parents in order to ascertain the mode of inheritance of inherited jaundice.

The availability of modern molecular biologic techniques has made it feasible to identify sequence abnormalities of the UGT1A1 gene from genomic DNA extracted from any nucleated cell (e.g., blood leukocytes, buccal smear). This should assist genetic counseling by the identification of heterozygous carriers and the establishment of a prenatal diagnosis based on genomic DNA analysis of cultured chorionic villous cells.

The Gunn Rat, an Animal Model of Crigler-Najjar Syndrome Type 1

In 1938 Gunn described a mutant strain of Wistar rats that exhibited lifelong hyperbilirubinemia, inherited as an autosomal recessive characteristic.[271] Although the mechanism of the nonhemolytic unconjugated hyperbilirubinemia was not known at that time, William E. Castle maintained the mutants for more than 15 years, until the deficiency of bilirubin glucuronidation was shown to be the mechanism of jaundice in this strain.[272] The Gunn rat is both a metabolic and a molecular model of Crigler-Najjar syndrome type 1.[273] Studies using this animal model have led to major advances in understanding bilirubin throughput and toxicity. As in Crigler-Najjar syndrome type 1, Gunn rats have high concentrations of serum bilirubin, all in the unconjugated form. The bile contains no conjugated bilirubin and liver histologic studies are normal.[273-275]

The Gunn rat is the only animal model that develops bilirubin encephalopathy spontaneously.[274] Much of the present information on bilirubin encephalopathy was derived from studies conducted using the Gunn rat (see the previous section on bilirubin toxicity). Studies performed in the Gunn rat also helped in developing new treatment modalities for hyperbilirubinemia, including cell transplantation and gene therapies.

Enzyme and molecular abnormalities in Gunn rats include the lack of UGT activity toward bilirubin found in Gunn rat livers.[272] Canalicular transport of exogenously administered conjugated bilirubin is normal.[275] In addition to lacking hepatic bilirubin-UGT activity, Gunn rat livers lack UGT activity toward digitoxigenin monodigitoxoside[276] and the methylcholanthrene-inducible phenol-UGT activity.[277,278] Abnormality of multiple isoforms of the UGT1A family is explained by the genetic lesion in Gunn rats, which consists of deletion of a single guanosine residue from exon 4 of the *ugt1a1* gene. This genetic lesion results in a premature stop codon, leading to the truncation of 150 amino acids at the carboxy-terminal end of the UGTs and the inactivation of their catalytic function.[279] Because this deletion is in one of the common region exons, all isoforms of the UGT1A subfamily are affected. UGT isoforms expressed from other genes are normal. Several UGT isoforms with normal catalytic activity have been isolated from the liver of Gunn rats.[277]

Treatment of Crigler-Najjar Syndrome Type 1

Conventional treatment aims at reducing serum bilirubin levels. Unlike the results in patients with Crigler-Najjar syndrome type 2 and Gilbert syndrome, serum bilirubin levels in Crigler-Najjar syndrome type 1 are not significantly reduced by phenobarbital administration.[260]

PHOTOTHERAPY

Phototherapy is the mainstay of medical therapy for severe unconjugated hyperbilirubinemia.[280] Banks of fluorescent lamps with devices for shielding the eyes or "light blankets" effectively lower serum bilirubin levels by mechanisms that have been discussed in the section Chemistry of Bilirubin: Photochemistry of Bilirubin. About the time of puberty, phototherapy becomes progressively less effective because of thickening of the skin, increased skin pigmentation, and decreased surface area in relation to body mass.[261]

PLASMAPHERESIS

In neurologic emergencies, plasmapheresis is an efficient method for reducing serum bilirubin concentration acutely.[259,261] Because bilirubin is tightly bound to plasma albumin, removal of albumin results in the withdrawal of equimolar amounts of bilirubin. This is followed by mobilization of tissue bilirubin stores to the plasma. Attempts to remove plasma bilirubin by affinity chromatography on albumin-conjugated agarose gel columns were successful in Gunn rats,[281] but were limited by the additional removal of formed elements of simian or human blood.[282]

ORTHOTOPIC LIVER TRANSPLANTATION

Because, at present, there is no other definitive long-term treatment for patients with this condition, orthotopic liver transplantation has become a standard treatment of Crigler-Najjar syndrome type 1. Although this procedure is not without risk, it has been curative in several patients and has dramatically changed the prognosis of Crigler-Najjar syndrome type 1 patients.[283]

Experimental Methods Aimed at Reduction of Serum Bilirubin Levels

Inhibition of Heme Oxygenase

Administration of non–iron-metalloporphyrins for inhibition of microsomal HO activity[19] has resulted in the suppression of neonatal hyperbilirubinemia in rats[284] and rhesus monkeys.[285] Administration of tin-mesoporphyrin, 0.5 μmol/kg three times a week for 13 to 23 weeks, to two 17-year-old boys with Crigler-Najjar syndrome type 1 resulted in only a modest and variable degree of reduction in serum bilirubin levels.[286] Although the place of this agent in the treatment of Crigler-Najjar syndrome type 1 is not fully clarified, these agents may have a role in reducing serum bilirubin levels during acute emergencies.

Bilirubin Degradation by Bilirubin Oxidase

Bilirubin oxidase from *Myrothecium verrucaria*[287] catalyzes the oxidation of bilirubin to a colorless product. Bilirubin oxidase, linked to polyethylene glycol for increasing its half-life in circulation, has been administered intravenously,[288] and resulted in substantial reduction of serum bilirubin levels in Gunn rats for 3 hours.

Induction of P-450c

As discussed earlier, the induction of P-450c causes increased oxidative degradation of serum bilirubin in Gunn rat liver, resulting in the reduction of serum bilirubin levels. Several naturally occurring indoles extracted from cruciferous vegetables, such as cabbage, cauliflower, and brussels sprouts, induce the P-450 isoforms CYP1A1 and CYP1A2 in rat liver and intestine.[289] Indole-3-carbinol, an inducer of CYP1A2, has been reported to reduce serum bilirubin levels temporarily in patients with Crigler-Najjar syndrome type 1.[290]

Methods Aimed at Replacing Hepatic UGT1A1 Activity

Because UGT1A1 activity is present in excess in normal liver, partial replacement of the enzyme should ameliorate hyperbilirubinemia in Crigler-Najjar syndrome type 1. As rat kidney contains a low but significant level of UGT1A1 activity, transplantation of a normal Wistar rat kidney into homozygous Gunn rat results in the excretion of bilirubin glucuronides in bile and reduction of serum bilirubin concentrations.[291] However, human kidney lacks bilirubin-UGT activity and therefore renal transplantation cannot be used for the treatment of Crigler-Najjar syndrome type 1.

Hepatocyte Transplantation

Transplantation of hepatocytes is technically easier than liver transplantation and, because the host liver is retained, the consequence of graft loss is minimized. For these reasons, liver cell transplantation is being evaluated as a potential treatment for Crigler-Najjar syndrome type 1. Based on experience in rodent and murine models,[292,293] hepatocytes were transplanted into a 10-year-old girl with Crigler-Najjar syndrome type 1.[294] Transplantation of 7.5 billion hepatocytes resulted in partial amelioration of jaundice, and permitted reduction of the daily duration of phototherapy. Two and a half years later, bilirubin glucuronide excretion in bile continued, but the serum bilirubin level gradually increased, probably as a result of increased bilirubin production or reduced effectiveness of phototherapy. The patient received an auxiliary liver transplantation, which has kept her serum bilirubin level within normal limits (J. Roy-Chowdhury, personal communication). Experience in this case, as well as worldwide experience with hepatocyte transplantation, indicates that the number of adult hepatocytes that can be transplanted at a single procedure is not likely to be sufficient for a complete cure of inherited metabolic diseases of the liver.[295,296] Moreover, the shortage of good-quality donor livers for hepatocyte isolation has limited more general application of hepatocyte transplantation.[295,297] Preparative irradiation and other manipulations of the host liver are being explored for inducing preferential proliferation of the engrafted hepatocytes.[298,299]

Gene Therapy

Because the metabolic defect in Gunn rats and in Crigler-Najjar syndrome type 1 results from lesions of a single gene, supplementation with a normal bilirubin-UGT gene would be an attractive potential therapeutic modality. Methods for gene introduction into the liver using recombinant viruses or ligands that mediate receptor-directed endocytosis are being evaluated for this purpose. In the ex-vivo approach, liver cells harvested from a mutant subject or animal by partial hepatectomy are established in primary culture, transduced with normal (therapeutic) genes, and transplanted back into the donor.[300] In the in-vivo approach, genes are introduced into the organ of live organisms using recombinant viruses or nonviral vectors.[301] Recombinant adenoviral vectors are highly efficient in transferring therapeutic genes into the liver. However, because adenoviruses are episomal, the effect is not permanent. Moreover, the host immune response toward adenoviral proteins can cause toxicity and precludes repeated injection of the vector. Adenoviral vectors have been developed that do not evoke an immune response, because of the co-expression of an immunosuppressive gene product.[302] However, the safety of abrogating host immunity toward adenoviruses, which are potential human pathogens, remains doubtful. A T-antigen–deleted recombinant simian virus 40 has been used successfully in gene therapy in Gunn rats.[303] These vectors integrate into the host genome and are not immunogenic.[304] Site-directed gene repair by triggering the cells' gene repair enzymes using RNA-DNA hybrid oligonucleotides has been used to replace the deleted G residue in Gunn rats, resulting in expression of normal UGT1A1 and partial amelioration of jaundice.[305] This last approach, although highly interesting, has not yet provided enough efficiency for application in clinical gene therapy. These approaches, and other approaches that are currently being investigated, raise the hope that hepatocyte transplantation, gene therapy, or the combination of the two should eventually result in curative medical therapy for Crigler-Najjar syndrome and other inherited metabolic liver diseases.[306]

Crigler-Najjar Syndrome Type 2 (Arias Syndrome)

Clinical Features

In 1962 Arias showed that some patients with chronic unconjugated hyperbilirubinemia differ from patients with classic Crigler-Najjar syndrome type 1 in that they have somewhat lower serum bilirubin concentrations. The serum bilirubin levels of these patients are reduced by at least 25% following phenobarbital treatment and, in general, this patient population has a better prognosis.[260,307] In most patients jaundice is noted before the age of 1 year, but occasionally it can elude detection until the patient is an adult. Serum bilirubin concentrations usually range from 8 to 18 mg/dl, and are mostly indirect reacting. Hepatic bilirubin-UGT activities are markedly reduced. As in Crigler-Najjar syndrome type 1, red cell survival is normal and there is no other clinical abnormality.

Kernicterus is uncommon in Crigler-Najjar syndrome type 2, but can occur under stressful situations. Serum bilirubin concentration may rise to very high levels following general anesthesia and surgery, with precipitation of encephalopathy. In a female patient who developed signs of bilirubin encephalopathy at the age of 43 years and died at the age of 44, autopsy disclosed a small brain.[260] There was no bilirubin staining, but histologic features typical of kernicterus were seen. Several additional cases were reported of patients with Crigler-Najjar syndrome type 2 who developed neurologic lesions.[308,309]

Laboratory Tests

As in Crigler-Najjar syndrome type 1, laboratory examination reveals normal values except for serum bilirubin concentrations of 8 to 18 mg/ml. Serum bilirubin levels may increase to as high as 40 mg/dl during fasting[307] or intercurrent illness.[310] By diazo analysis, serum bilirubin is mostly indirect reacting. In contrast to Crigler-Najjar syndrome type 1, the bile contains significant amounts of bilirubin glucuronides, although less than 50% of estimated daily bilirubin production is excreted into bile.[260,309] The proportion of bilirubin monoglucuronide in bile exceeds 30% of total conjugated bilirubin,[310,311] reflecting the reduced UGT1A1 activity in the liver. Liver histologic analysis is normal. Hepatic UGT1A1 activity is markedly reduced, but is detectable using sensitive techniques.[309,310]

Molecular Mechanism and Inheritance

As in Crigler-Najjar syndrome type 1, this syndrome is caused by genetic lesions within the various exons that constitute the coding region of *UGT1A1*.[311] However, in Crigler-Najjar syndrome type 2, the genetic lesions always consist of single amino acid substitutions that reduce, but do not completely abolish, UGT1A1 activity. In some cases, the residual enzyme activity is enough to result in only a minor elevation of serum bilirubin levels, compatible with the diagnosis of Gilbert syndrome. Mutations of the coding region of *UGT1A1* that are known to partially reduce the enzyme activity have been

reviewed and tabulated, as shown in the work of Kadakol and colleagues.[268]

Both autosomal dominant transmission with incomplete penetrance[260] and autosomal recessive transmission[312] had been suggested for Crigler-Najjar syndrome type 2. Molecular genetic studies have confirmed autosomal recessive inheritance. Part of the confusion about the mode of inheritance arose from the observation that some family members of patients with Crigler-Najjar syndrome types 1 and 2 have intermediate levels of hyperbilirubinemia. A molecular explanation for this phenomenon is now available. In heterozygous carriers of Crigler-Najjar syndrome, if the allele with the normal coding region carries a variant promoter ("Gilbert-type" TATAA element; see The Genetic Basis of Gilbert Syndrome), expression of the only normal allele is reduced. Because Gilbert syndrome is very common in the general population, this type of compound heterozygosity is a more common cause of intermediate levels of hyperbilirubinemia than is homozygosity for a coding region mutation.[313]

Gilbert Syndrome

A common disorder characterized by mild, chronic, fluctuating increase of serum unconjugated bilirubin levels was described by Gilbert and Lereboullet in 1901.[314] Although various investigators have used other names for this disorder, such as constitutional hepatic dysfunction, hereditary hemolytic bilirubinemia, and familial nonhemolytic jaundice, Gilbert syndrome is the most commonly used name for this condition.

Clinical Features

Gilbert syndrome is usually diagnosed in young adults who are found to have mild, predominantly unconjugated hyperbilirubinemia. Diagnosis is often made inadvertently when blood tests are being performed for other reasons, such as for preemployment or preinsurance screening or because of intercurrent illness. In most cases, bilirubin levels are less than 3 mg/dl, but fluctuate with time, and increase during intercurrent illness, stress, or menstrual periods.[315] Jaundice is the only positive finding on physical examination. The vague constitutional symptoms, such as fatigue and abdominal discomfort, experienced by some patients[315] may be manifestations of anxiety. Routine laboratory tests are normal, except for the predominantly unconjugated hyperbilirubinemia. Oral cholecystography allows visualization of the gallbladder. Liver biopsy is not routinely indicated, but when performed shows normal histologic results. Hepatic UGT1A1 activity is reduced to approximately 30% of normal.[316] Gilbert syndrome is diagnosed with much more frequency in males than in females,[317] probably reflecting higher rates of bilirubin production in males.[29] Gilbert syndrome is often diagnosed around puberty, which may be related to increased hemoglobin turnover and possibly the inhibition of bilirubin glucuronidation by endogenous steroid hormones.[318]

The Genetic Basis of Gilbert Syndrome

The molecular background of reduced UGT activity in patients with Gilbert syndrome has been unraveled. The promoter region of the *UGT1A1* gene contains a TATAA element with a common A(TA)$_6$TAA motif. Caucasian patients with Gilbert syndrome are homozygous for a longer TATAA element, A(TA)$_7$TAA.[319] The *UGT1A1* gene with this variant TATAA element has been termed *UGT1A1*28*. The frequency of the variant promoter is approximately 30% among Caucasian and African American populations,[319,320] resulting in homozygosity in about 9%. Although homozygosity for the Gilbert-type promoter is required for Gilbert syndrome in these populations, all subjects who are homozygous for this polymorphism do not manifest the full clinical phenotype of Gilbert syndrome. For example, Gilbert syndrome is diagnosed infrequently in women. Additional factors, such as increased bilirubin production, may be required for manifestation of the Gilbert phenotype. In some, but not all, subjects with Gilbert syndrome, a defect of hepatic bilirubin uptake has been observed. However, the relationship between the uptake defect and reduced bilirubin glucuronidation is unclear. Promoter-reporter studies show that an increased TATAA box length reduces *UGT1A1* expression.[319] Patients with the Gilbert genotype have been shown to have lower hepatic microsomal UGT1A1 activity.[321]

In people of African origin, a small percentage of the population have an even longer TATAA element, A(TA)$_8$TAA. Others have a shorter than usual TATAA element, A(TA)$_5$TAA. There appears to be an inverse relationship between TATA box length and gene expression: TATA boxes with seven and eight repeats are associated with a decreased expression and five TA repeats with an increased expression.[322]

The A(TA)$_7$TAA variant is less frequent among Japanese populations. In Japanese, Korean, and Chinese people heterozygosity for missense mutations in the *UGT1A1* coding region has been reported to be a more common cause of Gilbert syndrome.[323-325] Compound heterozygotes for the common structural G71R mutation and the variant TATAA element have also been described. So far, these mutations have only been found in races originating in the Far East.

Gilbert syndrome genotypes have been reported to be associated with accelerated or prolonged neonatal jaundice.[326-328] In children with a combination of glucose-6-phosphate dehydrogenase deficiency and the Gilbert-type TATAA element, neonatal serum bilirubin concentrations can rise to dangerously high levels.[329] In patients with splenomegaly (P.L.M. Jansen, unpublished observation) and in liver transplant recipients, the Gilbert-type promoter can cause prolonged spontaneous unconjugated hyperbilirubinemia.[330,331] Gilbert syndrome is also correlated with early development of gallstones in patients with hereditary spherocytosis.[332] Oxidative acetaminophen metabolism is associated with drug toxicity. Conflicting evidence has been obtained for a possibly increased oxidative metabolism and a decreased acetaminophen glucuronidation in patients with Gilbert syndrome.[333-335] Gilbert syndrome is associated with a high incidence of diarrhea in patients treated with the anticancer drug irinotecan.[336]

Organic Anion Transport

Although all subjects with Gilbert syndrome have reduced bilirubin-UGT activity, some patients exhibit additional abnormalities of organic anion transport. Clearance of intravenously administered bilirubin is reduced in patients with Gilbert syndrome.[337] Goresky and associates found normal initial uptake in Gilbert syndrome, suggesting that the reduced

clearance is due to decreased glucuronidation.[338] However, multicompartmental analysis suggests that the reduction of plasma clearance may also be related to decreased hepatic bilirubin uptake.[339] Subsequent studies have shown that subjects with Gilbert syndrome may be heterogeneous in terms of organic anion transport. In two subsets, bromosulfophthalein (BSP)[340] and indocyanine green (ICG),[341] plasma disappearance is abnormal. In one group, reduced plasma clearance of BSP and ICG appears to be due to decreased hepatic uptake. In the other group compartmental analysis showed a defect in BSP transport at a later stage in the transport process. Because the excretion of BSP and ICG into bile is normal in Crigler-Najjar syndrome type 1 and Gunn rats, decreased clearance of these organic anions in Gilbert syndrome cannot be attributed to reduced UGT1A1 activity. At this time, no mechanism for the association of decreased UGT1A1 activity and reduced organic anion uptake is known, and the presence of the two apparently unrelated abnormalities in subsets of subjects with Gilbert syndrome appears be coincidental, perhaps owing to the high prevalence of Gilbert syndrome in the general population.

Effect of Fasting

A two-fold to three-fold increase in serum bilirubin levels occurs in patients with Gilbert syndrome upon reduction of daily caloric intake to 400 kcal for 48 hours.[342] Because fasting also increases serum bilirubin levels in normal individuals[343,344] and in individuals with other hepatobiliary disorders,[344] the fasting test is of limited use in the differential diagnosis of Gilbert syndrome.

Fasting-induced hyperbilirubinemia in normal individuals probably results from multiple physiologic factors. Clearly, reduction of bilirubin glucuronidation cannot be the sole reason, because fasting also exacerbates hyperbilirubinemia in homozygous Gunn rats.[345] Increased heme catabolism during fasting has been reported.[333,335,344,346] Decreased intestinal motility during fasting may contribute to the bilirubin load by increasing bilirubin reabsorption from the gut.[347] However, earlier kinetic studies had indicated that reduced hepatic clearance of bilirubin from plasma was a more important contributor to fasting hyperbilirubinemia than increased bilirubin load.[348] Reduced hepatic uptake of bilirubin attributable to down-regulation of organic anion transport[349] or competition with serum free fatty acids may explain these observations.[350,351] Although increased bilirubin load and reduced hepatic uptake appear to contribute to fasting hyperbilirubinemia, an inverse relationship between hepatic UGT1A1 activity and the increase of serum bilirubin concentration during caloric restriction has been demonstrated.[352] In normal subjects, homozygous for a normal UGT1A1 TATA element sequence [A(TA)$_7$TAA], the mean increase in serum bilirubin levels after caloric restriction was 9.6 and 4.1 mmol/L in males and females, respectively. In subjects who were homozygous for the Gilbert-type promoter [A(TA)$_8$TAA], the increment was significantly greater (20.5 ± 7.2 mmol/L), but in these subjects there was no significant sex difference. Interestingly, the mean increment in serum bilirubin levels was also slightly, but significantly, increased in heterozygotes for the promoter [A(TA)$_7$TAA/ A(TA)$_8$TAA], suggesting a rate-liming role of UGT1A1 in serum bilirubin clearance, particularly during fasting. It has suggested that a reduction of hepatic UDP-glucuronic acid content during fasting may result in a reduction of UGT1A1 activity in vivo.[353]

Effect of Nicotinic Acid Administration

Intravenous nicotinic acid administration increases unconjugated hyperbilirubinemia, probably by increasing erythrocyte fragility, splenic HO activity, and splenic bilirubin formation.[354] Consistent with this, splenectomy prevents nicotinic acid–induced unconjugated hyperbilirubinemia.[355] Although nicotinic acid administration has also been proposed as a provocative test for the diagnosis of Gilbert syndrome,[355,356] like fasting, it does not clearly separate patients with Gilbert syndrome from normal subjects or those with hepatobiliary disease.[356]

Bilirubin Conjugates in Bile

Similar to Crigler-Najjar syndrome type 2, an increased proportion of bilirubin glucuronides excreted in bile in Gilbert syndrome is bilirubin monoglucuronide.[310] The alteration of the bilirubin diglucuronide/monoglucuronide ratio may reflect reduced hepatic bilirubin-UGT activity in these syndromes.

Diagnosis

Gilbert syndrome is conventionally diagnosed in individuals with mild unconjugated hyperbilirubinemia without evidence of hemolysis or structural liver disease. Hemolysis is not a feature of Gilbert syndrome; however, co-existent compensated hemolysis is found in many patients with Gilbert syndrome because increased bilirubin production makes the hyperbilirubinemia more clinically apparent.[356] A presumptive diagnosis of Gilbert syndrome is made when mild unconjugated hyperbilirubinemia is noted on several occasions, and serum levels of glutamic-oxaloacetic/pyruvic transaminase, alkaline phosphatase, γ-glutamyltranspeptidase, and fasting and postprandial bile acids are normal. If confirmation of diagnosis is essential, chromatographic determination of the relative contents of bilirubin monoglucuronide and bilirubin diglucuronide in bile is of potential use in the diagnosis of Gilbert syndrome. Genetic analysis has greatly facilitated the diagnosis of Gilbert syndrome.

Animal Model

Bolivian squirrel monkeys have higher serum unconjugated bilirubin concentration than do the closely related Brazilian squirrel monkeys.[357] The difference in bilirubin levels becomes exaggerated in the fasting state. Compared with the Brazilian population, Bolivian monkeys have slower plasma clearance of intravenously administered bilirubin, a lower level of hepatic bilirubin-UGT activity, and a higher bilirubin monoglucuronide/diglucuronide ratio in bile. The two populations of squirrel monkeys have comparable erythrocyte life span and hepatic GST activity. In these respects, the Bolivian squirrel monkeys are a model of human Gilbert syndrome. Fasting hyperbilirubinemia is rapidly reversed by oral or intravenous administration of carbohydrates, but not by lipid administration.[358]

Disorders Resulting in Predominantly Conjugated Hyperbilirubinemia

Conjugated bilirubin may accumulate in the serum because of leakage of bilirubin glucuronides from hepatocytes, reverse transport from hepatocyte to the plasma, or regurgitation from bile. When the accumulation of conjugated bilirubin in plasma is due to inflammatory diseases of the hepatocyte, intrahepatic cholestasis, or biliary obstruction, plasma concentrations of bile salts and various hepatocellular proteins are also expected to increase. However, in specific disorders of organic anion storage or transport (e.g., Rotor or Dubin-Johnson syndrome, respectively), plasma bile acid concentrations and liver enzyme levels remain normal, and hyperbilirubinemia is the predominant biochemical abnormality. Because of partial hydrolysis by hepatic β-glucuronidase and reversibility of the UGT1A1-catalyzed reaction, conjugated hyperbilirubinemia is always associated with various degrees of unconjugated hyperbilirubinemia.

Acquired Defects of Hepatobiliary Transport

Cholestasis is the result of impaired hepatobiliary transport. Hepatobiliary transport starts at the level of the basolateral membrane of hepatocytes and includes transcellular and canalicular transport; cholestasis may result from disturbances in either of these transport mechanisms. In addition, bile flow in the intrahepatic or extrahepatic part of the biliary tree may be impaired.

Clinical cholestasis mainly results from disturbances of bile flow through inflammation or obstruction of the intrahepatic or extrahepatic biliary tree. Common cholestatic diseases include primary biliary cirrhosis, primary sclerosing cholangitis, cholangiocarcinoma, gallstone disease, and papillary or pancreatic tumors. In addition, inflammation of the liver parenchyma, as occurs in hepatitis, usually causes some degree of cholestasis. Some drugs are well-known for cholestatic reactions.[359]

Experimental cholestasis can result from impaired hepatic uptake, reduced Na$^+$/K$^+$-ATPase activity, increased permeability of tight junctions, disturbed function of microtubules or microfilaments, reduced ATP generation, impaired canalicular transport, or the formation of precipitates within the bile canaliculi. **Table 62-2** reviews the canalicular transporters and their substrates. Ethinylestradiol is one of the best-studied cholestatic agents, and results obtained from using this drug have led to major insights into the pathophysiology of bile secretion. Ethinylestradiol alters the membrane fluidity and decreases Na$^+$/K$^+$-ATPase activity in the basolateral membrane. It inhibits the hepatic uptake and the canalicular secretion of bile acids and, to a lesser extent, that of conjugated bilirubin.[360,361] In rodents, estrogen administration reduces the expression and/or activity of several transporters, including ABC, *bsep*,[362] *mdr1a/1b*, two MDR1 isoforms,[363] and the multidrug resistance–associated protein-2 (mrp2).[364] In addition, estrogen-induced cholestasis is associated with a reduced activity of the Na$^+$/taurocholate co-transporting polypeptide (ntcp)[363,365] and a reduction of endogenous bile acid synthesis.[365] Most known physiologic actions of estrogens are mediated by binding of the estrogen receptor to an estrogen response element in the *cis*-regulatory elements in genes. In addition, estrogens increase the hepatic expression of the short heterodimer partner, an atypical nuclear receptor that does not have a DNA-binding domain, represses the activity of several nuclear hormone receptors in vitro, and is a target for FXR ligands.[366] 6-Ethylchenodeoxycholic acid, an FXR ligand, protects against estrogen-induced cholestasis.[367]

Cholestasis is characterized by the accumulation of both bilirubin and bile acid conjugates in the blood. Under normal physiologic conditions the basolateral membrane of the hepatocyte contains efflux carriers that mediate the secretion of metabolites from liver to blood. Physiologically these transporters may transport compounds that are metabolized in the liver to the blood for subsequent excretion by the kidney. In experimental cholestasis, as occurs during ethinylestradiol administration, bile duct ligation, or endotoxin administration, a reorientation of ABC transporters takes place, resulting in a loss of polarity of hepatocytes. Under these conditions, ATP-dependent transporters such as mrp3 and mrp1, which are expressed at very low levels in normal liver, are induced and localize to the basolateral membrane of hepatocytes.[187] Canalicular mrp2 and, to a lesser extent, bsep are down-regulated during cholestasis.[138,368] Mrp3 and mrp1 mediate the active transport of glucuronides, glutathione-conjugates, and bile salts.[141,369] The basolateral expression of these ABC transporters may help to remove metabolites that could otherwise inhibit hepatic metabolism. Down-regulation of the Na$^+$-dependent taurocholate co-transporter may also serve to protect the hepatocyte in cholestatic conditions.[370] Common cholestatic agents, such as chlorpromazine and cyclosporine, inhibit hepatic transport at multiple levels.

Cyclosporine therapy is frequently associated with jaundice. Cyclosporine inhibits the hepatic uptake of both bile acids and non–bile acid organic anions.[371] It is a competitive inhibitor of taurocholate uptake in both basolateral and canalicular membrane vesicles but not of Na$^+$-dependent alanine uptake.[372] In addition to canalicular ATP-dependent transport of taurocholate, the drug also strongly inhibits the ATP-dependent transport of leukotriene C$_4$ (an mrp2 substrate) and of daunorubicin (a P-glycoprotein substrate).[372] In the rat cyclosporine impairs both the bile acid–dependent and the bile acid–independent components of bile flow. As with ethinylestradiol, administration of cyclosporine to rats increases serum bile acid levels.[372] With these drugs, serum bile acid levels are more sensitive indicators of cholestasis than are serum bilirubin levels.

Inherited Disorders of Excretion of Conjugated Bilirubin

Dubin-Johnson Syndrome

In 1954, Dubin and Johnson[373] and Sprinz and Nelson[374] described a syndrome with chronic nonhemolytic jaundice characterized by accumulation of conjugated bilirubin in serum and grossly pigmented, but otherwise histologically normal, livers.

Clinical Findings

Except for mild icterus, physical examination results are within normal limits. Patients are usually asymptomatic, although an occasional patient complains of weakness and vague abdominal pain, and, rarely, hepatosplenomegaly is observed.[375,376] Because serum total bile acid levels are normal,[377] pruritus is absent. Hyperbilirubinemia is increased by intercurrent illness, oral contraceptives, and pregnancy.[377] The diagnosis is often made after puberty, although some patients have been diagnosed during the neonatal period.[376,378] Sometimes the disorder is noted for the first time when a woman becomes pregnant or receives oral contraceptives, which increase the hyperbilirubinemia to a clinically detectable level.[377]

Laboratory Tests

Complete blood count, prothrombin time, and serum levels of bile acids, transaminases, alkaline phosphatase, and albumin are normal.[376,377] Serum bilirubin concentration is usually between 2 and 5 mg/dL but can be as high as 20 to 25 mg/dL. More than 50% of total serum bilirubin is direct-reacting. Serum bilirubin levels fluctuate and individual measurements may yield normal results. Because of the general abnormality of canalicular transport of non–bile acid organic anions, oral cholecystography, even using a "double dose" of contrast material, usually does not visualize the gallbladder. However, visualization may occur 4 hours after administration of intravenous contrast medium.[379] The liver is grossly black and light microscopy reveals a dense pigment (**Fig. 62-7**), which on electron microscopy appears to be contained within lysosomes.[380] Histochemical staining and physicochemical properties of the pigment suggest that the pigment is related to

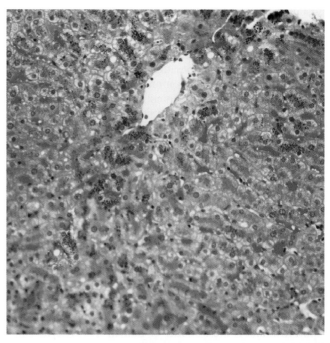

Fig. 62-7 **Pigmentation of the liver in Dubin-Johnson syndrome.** Hematoxylin and eosin–stained section of the liver shows deep brown pigments in hepatocytes, particularly in the perivenous zone (zone 3).

melanin.[381] Following infusion of [³H]epinephrine into mutant Corriedale sheep (an animal model for Dubin-Johnson syndrome), the isotope is incorporated into the hepatic pigment,[382] supporting the concept that the pigment is a melanin-like derivative. However, electron spin resonance spectroscopy shows that the pigment differs from authentic melanin.[383] It may be composed of polymers of epinephrine metabolites.[384,385] Interestingly, following liver disease, such as acute viral hepatitis, the pigment is cleared from the liver.[386] Following recovery, the pigment reaccumulates slowly, starting from the centrizonal region.

Organic Anion Transport

The hepatic secretion of bilirubin glucuronides and the glutathione conjugate of BSP is disturbed in these patients.[275,387] The hepatic secretion of negatively charged iopanoic acid is disturbed whereas the secretion of neutral iopamide is normal. The bile acid secretion is unaffected.[387] Pharmacokinetic analysis of plasma disappearance of bilirubin, BSP, and ICG revealed normal hepatic storage but impaired secretion.[275,387,388] Impaired canalicular secretion of non–bile acid organic anions represents the basic defect of this syndrome. After intravenous injection of BSP, plasma BSP concentration decreases at near-normal rate for 45 minutes. However, in 90% of patients, plasma BSP concentration increases after this time, such that the concentration at 90 minutes is greater than that at 45 minutes.[363] This secondary rise results from reflux of glutathione-conjugated BSP from hepatocytes into the circulation. A similar secondary rise occurs after intravenous administration of bilirubin.[387] The secondary rise of plasma BSP level has been observed in other hepatobiliary disorders,[388] and is therefore not diagnostic of Dubin-Johnson syndrome.

The Genetic Background of Dubin-Johnson Syndrome

Dubin-Johnson syndrome is caused by mutations of the *MRP2* gene causing a deficiency of canalicular MRP2 expression.[180-182] More than a dozen genetic lesions, including nucleotide transition of a single-nucleotide deletion, resulting in amino acid substitutions, premature truncation, or exon skipping, have been reported to cause Dubin-Johnson syndrome.[389] Some of the reported mutations may lead to impaired glycosylation of the MRP2 protein, impaired sorting to the canalicular membrane, and premature proteasome-dependent degradation.[390] As in TR⁻ rats and EHBR rats, the absence of MRP2 (mrp2 in rats) in the canalicular membrane causes severe impairment of canalicular secretion of bilirubin conjugates, the leukotriene LTC₄, reduced and oxidized glutathione, and numerous glucuronide and glutathione conjugates.[391] As a consequence, these patients and animals have a mild conjugated hyperbilirubinemia. Experiments with the animal models provided firm evidence for the existence of different pathways for the canalicular secretion of bilirubin conjugates and bile acids.[392] In contrast to bile acids with a free 3-hydroxyl, 3-hydroxyl-conjugated bile acids are transported by mrp2, rather than bsep, as evidenced by impaired secretion of bile acid conjugates in TR⁻ and EHBR rats.[393] On feeding TR⁻ rats a diet enriched with tryptophan, tyrosine, and phenylalanine, intravenous injection of metanephrine results in the accumulation of a black lysosomal pigment in hepatocytes, identical to that seen in patients with Dubin-Johnson

syndrome.[394] Despite the absence of MRP2, the serum bilirubin levels are only mildly elevated in Dubin-Johnson syndrome and in the two rat models of the disease, suggesting alternative canalicular secretion pathways for bilirubin conjugates.[395] Members of the mrp family, other than Mrp2, have been described in the rat bile canaliculi.[396,397] Whether these mrps accept bilirubin glucuronides as substrates needs to be studied. MRP3 is expressed in the basolateral domain of the hepatocyte plasma membrane in patients with Dubin-Johnson syndrome. The activity of this transporter contributes to the conjugated hyperbilirubinemia by actively pumping bilirubin conjugates from liver to blood in these patients.[140] Thus the accumulation of conjugated bilirubin in the plasma of Dubin-Johnson syndrome patients may not be caused by passive "leakage" only, but also by active transport of bilirubin conjugates out of the hepatocytes.

Inheritance

Dubin-Johnson syndrome is rare, but occurs in both sexes and in virtually all races. The syndrome occurs frequently (1 : 1300) in Persian Jews,[376] in whom it is associated with clotting factor VII deficiency.[398,399] It had been difficult to ascertain the inheritance pattern from clinical analysis,[377] but with respect to urinary coproporphyrin excretion (see the following paragraph), Dubin-Johnson syndrome is inherited as an autosomal recessive characteristic.[400,401]

Urinary Coproporphyrin Excretion

Urinary coproporphyrin I excretion is increased in patients with Dubin-Johnson syndrome to a greater degree than in patients with other hepatobiliary disorders.[401] Of the two isomers of coproporphyrin, isomers I and III, coproporphyrin III is a precursor of heme, whereas other porphyrin isomers are metabolic byproducts of unknown significance and are excreted in urine and bile.[400] Normally, approximately 75% of total urinary coproporphyrin is coproporphyrin isomer III. In Dubin-Johnson syndrome, total urinary coproporphyrin excretion is normal, but more than 80% is coproporphyrin I (**Fig. 62-8**).[401,402] Although neonates normally have elevated urinary content of coproporphyrin I as compared with adults, levels are not as high as those seen in Dubin-Johnson syndrome.[403] In obligate heterozygotes (e.g., unaffected parents, children of subjects with Dubin-Johnson syndrome), total urinary coproporphyrin excretion was reduced by 40% of normal.[401,403] The mechanism of the abnormal urinary porphyrin excretion and its relationship to the organic anion transport defect are not known. When the history and physical examination are consistent, the urinary coproporphyrin excretion pattern is diagnostic of Dubin-Johnson syndrome. However, the overlap of results in carriers with those in controls[401] makes identification of heterozygotes difficult.

Animal Models
MUTANT CORRIEDALE SHEEP

This mutant strain has an inherited defect that closely resembles the Dubin-Johnson syndrome. Biliary excretion of conjugated bilirubin, glutathione-conjugated BSP, iopanoic acid, and ICG is decreased, whereas taurocholate transport is normal.[403,404] The secretion of the organic cation procainamide ethobromide is unaffected[406] and, interestingly, the

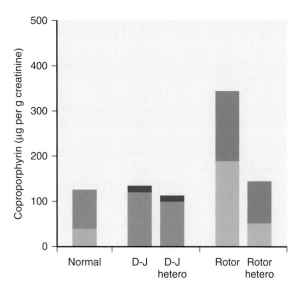

Fig. 62-8 Urinary coproporphyrin excretion in normal subjects and in patients with Dubin-Johnson (D-J) syndrome and Rotor's syndrome. The bars represent total urinary coproporphyrin excretion, normalized to creatinine excretion. Coproporphyrin I *(light orange, light blue, and light cyan)* excretion and coproporphyrin III *(deep orange, deep blue, and deep cyan)* excretion are also shown. In D-J syndrome the total urinary coproporphyrin excretion is normal, but the proportion of coproporphyrin I is markedly elevated (>80%). In contrast, both total urinary coproporphyrin and the proportion of coproporphyrin I are increased in Rotor's syndrome. *(Data from Wolkoff AW, et al. Rotor's syndrome: a distinct inheritable pathophysiologic entity. Am J Med 1976;60:173.)*

secretion of unconjugated BSP is unimpaired.[405] These sheep have a mild hyperbilirubinemia, with 60% of the bilirubin being conjugated. The liver is pigmented as in Dubin-Johnson syndrome,[406] but the histologic results are otherwise normal. Total urinary coproporphyrin excretion is normal with increased excretion of coproporphyrin isomer I and decreased isomer III excretion.

TR⁻ RATS AND EHBR RATS

These rats have a hepatic excretory abnormality that strongly resembles that of the mutant Corriedale sheep and patients with Dubin-Johnson syndrome. The biliary excretion of conjugated bilirubin and many other organic anions is impaired.[407-409] As in Dubin-Johnson syndrome, coproporphyrin I constitutes a major fraction of the total urinary coproporphyrins.[407] As explained previously, the *Mrp2* gene defect of TR⁻ and EHBR rats has been characterized. Different single-nucleotide deletions cause an absence of canalicular Mrp2 expression in these two animal models.[182,410]

Rotor Syndrome
Clinical Findings

In 1948 Rotor and colleagues described several individuals from two families who had chronic predominantly conjugated hyperbilirubinemia.[411] As in Dubin-Johnson syndrome, routine hematologic tests and routine blood biochemistries are normal, except for conjugated hyperbilirubinemia.[411,412] There is no evidence of hemolysis. Histomorphologic analysis of the liver is normal and, in contrast to the findings in

Dubin-Johnson syndrome, the liver is not pigmented.[413] Rotor syndrome is rare, but has been described in several races. Although Rotor syndrome shares many clinical features with Dubin-Johnson syndrome, the basic abnormalities of these disorders are different.[412]

Organic Anion Excretion

In contrast to the findings in Dubin-Johnson syndrome, more than 25% of injected BSP is retained in serum at 45 minutes after intravenous administration of 5 mg/kg BSP.[414] There is no secondary rise of plasma BSP level in Rotor syndrome and conjugated BSP is not found in plasma.[413] Following intravenous administration, there is also marked plasma retention of unconjugated bilirubin[414] and ICG.[415] Phenotypically normal obligate heterozygotes for Rotor syndrome have mildly abnormal BSP retention at 45 minutes, which is intermediate between results in affected patients and normal controls.[414] Oral cholecystographic agents usually do not visualize the gallbladder in Dubin-Johnson syndrome, whereas roentgenographic visualization is usually possible in Rotor syndrome.[413]

The hepatic storage capacity and the transport maximum of BSP have been determined by a constant infusion technique.[414,415] In Dubin-Johnson syndrome the transport is severely abnormal, whereas the hepatic storage capacity is normal. In contrast, in Rotor syndrome, the storage capacity was reduced by 75% to 90%, whereas the transport maximum was reduced by only 50%.[414,416] The findings in Rotor syndrome are similar to those in hepatic storage disease, a familial disorder manifested by predominantly conjugated hyperbilirubinemia and normal liver histologic results.[417,418] These two disorders may represent a single pathophysiologic entity.

Urinary Coproporphyrin Excretion

In contrast to the findings in Dubin-Johnson syndrome, total urinary coproporphyrin is increased by 250% to 500% over normal in Rotor syndrome, and the proportion of coproporphyrin I in urine is approximately 65% of the total (**Fig. 62-8**).[412] In one report, however, two brothers with clinical Rotor syndrome had more than 80% of urinary coproporphyrins as isomer I.[419] These results are similar to those seen in many other hepatobiliary disorders.[420] Obligate heterozygotes have a coproporphyrin excretory pattern that is intermediate between that of control subjects and patients with Rotor syndrome. With respect to urinary coproporphyrin excretion, Rotor syndrome is inherited as an autosomal recessive characteristic.[412] The urinary coproporphyrin abnormality in Rotor syndrome is most likely caused by reduced biliary excretion of coproporphyrins, with a concomitant increase in renal excretion. The nature of the organic anion transport defect in Rotor syndrome is unknown. Similar and differential features of Dubin-Johnson syndrome and Rotor syndrome are listed in **Table 62-4**.

Acknowledgment

This work was partly supported by the following grants: NYSTEM Grant CO24346 (to J.R.-C.); National Institutes of Health Grants RO1-DK 39137 (to N.R.-C.), RO1-DK 46057 (to J.R.-C.), and P30-DK 41296 (to Liver Research Center).

Table 62-4 Inherited Disorders Associated with Elevation of Conjugated Bilirubin

	DUBIN-JOHNSON SYNDROME	ROTOR SYNDROME
Serum bilirubin pattern and concentrations	Predominantly conjugated Usually 50-85 µmol/L; can be as high as 340 µmol/L	Predominantly conjugated Usually 50-100 µmol/L; occasionally as high as 340 µmol/L
Routine liver function tests	Normal except for hyperbilirubinemia	Normal except for hyperbilirubinemia
Serum bile salt levels	Normal	Normal
Plasma BSP retention	Normal at 45 minutes; secondary rise at 90 minutes	Elevated; no secondary rise at 90 minutes
BSP infusion studies	T_m very low; storage normal	T_m and storage both reduced
Oral cholecystography	Usually does not visualize gallbladder	Usually visualizes gallbladder
Urinary coproporphyrin excretion pattern	Total: normal; >80% as coproporphyrin I	Total: elevated; ≈50%-75% coproporphyrin I
Appearance of liver	Grossly black	Normal
Histology of liver	Dark pigments, predominantly in centrilobular areas; otherwise normal	Normal, no increase in pigmentation
Mode of inheritance	Autosomal recessive	Autosomal recessive
Prevalence	Rare (1:1300 in Persian Jews)	Rare
Prognosis	Benign	Benign
Animal model	Mutant TR⁻ rats/mutant Corriedale sheep/golden lion tamarin monkey	None

BSP, bromosulfophthalein

Key References

Akaba K, et al. Neonatal hyperbilirubinemia and a common mutation of the bilirubin uridine diphosphate-glucuronosyltransferase gene in Japanese. J Hum Genet 1999;44:22. (Ref.326)

Bancroft JD, Kreamer B, Gourley GR. Gilbert syndrome accelerates development of neonatal jaundice. J Pediatr 1998;132:656. (Ref.327)

Battaglia E, Radominska-Pandya A. A functional role for histidyl residues of the UDP-glucuronic acid carrier in rat liver endoplasmic reticulum membranes. Biochemistry 1998;37:258. (Ref.159)

Beigneux AP, et al. The acute phase response is associated with retinoid X receptor repression in rodent liver. J Biol Chem 2000;275:16390. (Ref.136)

Beutler E, Gelbart T, Demina A. Racial variability in the UDP-glucuronosyltransferase 1 (UGT1A1) promoter: a balanced polymorphism for regulation of bilirubin metabolism? Proc Natl Acad Sci U S A 1998;95:8170. (Ref.322)

Bohan A, Boyer JL. Mechanisms of hepatic transport of drugs: implications for cholestatic drug reactions. Semin Liver Dis 2002;22:123. (Ref.391)

Borst P, et al. The multidrug resistance protein family. Biochim Biophys Acta 1999;1461:347. (Ref.396)

Brink MA, et al. Enterohepatic cycling of bilirubin: a putative mechanism for pigment gallstone formation in ileal Crohn's disease [see comments]. Gastroenterology 1999;116:1420. (Ref.33)

Brito MA, et al. Bilirubin injury to neurons: contribution of oxidative stress and rescue by glycoursodeoxycholic acid. Neurotoxicology 2008;29:259. (Ref.94)

Cesaratto L, et al. Bilirubin-induced cell toxicity involves PTEN activation through an APE1/Ref-1-dependent pathway. J Mol Med 2007;85:1099. (Ref.95)

Cui Y, et al. Hepatic uptake of bilirubin and its conjugates by the human organic anion-transporting polypeptide 2 (symbol SLC21A6). J Biol Chem 2000;276:9626. (Ref.128)

de Vree JM, et al. Mutations in the MDR3 gene cause progressive familial intrahepatic cholestasis. Proc Natl Acad Sci U S A 1998;95:282. (Ref.199)

Deganuto M, et al. A proteomic approach to the bilirubin-induced toxicity in neuronal cells reveals a protective function of DJ-1 protein. Proteomics 2010;10:1645. (Ref.96)

del Giudice EM, et al. Coinheritance of Gilbert syndrome increases the risk for developing gallstones in patients with hereditary spherocytosis. Blood 1999;94:2259. (Ref.332)

Denson LA, et al. Interleukin-1α suppresses retinoid transactivation of two hepatic transporter genes involved in bile formation. J Biol Chem 2000;275:8835. (Ref.134)

Dhawan A, et al. Human hepatocyte transplantation: current experience and future challenges. Nat Rev Gastroenterol Hepatol 2010;7:288. (Ref.296)

Dranoff JA, et al. Short-term regulation of bile acid uptake by microfilament-dependent translocation of rat ntcp to the plasma membrane. Hepatology 1999;30:223. (Ref.132)

Fernandez M, Bonkovsky HL. Increased heme oxygenase-1 gene expression in liver cells and splanchnic organs from portal hypertensive rats. Hepatology 1999;29:1672. (Ref.15)

Fiorucci S, et al. Protective effects of 6-ethyl chenodeoxycholic acid, a farnesoid X receptor ligand, in estrogen induced cholestasis. J Pharmacol Exp Ther 2005;313:604. (Ref.367)

Fox IJ, et al. Treatment of Crigler-Najjar syndrome type I with hepatocyte transplantation. N Engl J Med 1998;333:1422. (Ref.294)

Fox IJ, Roy-Chowdhury J. Hepatocyte transplantation. J Hepatol 2004;40:878. (Ref.295)

Fulks M, Stout RL, Dolan VF. Mortality associated with bilirubin levels in insurance applicants. J Insur Med 2009;41:49. (Ref.27)

Ganguly TC, et al. Regulation of the rat liver sodium-dependent bile acid cotransporter gene by prolactin. Mediation of transcriptional activation by Stat5. J Clin Invest 1997;99:2906. (Ref.133)

Gantla S, et al. Splice site mutations: a novel genetic mechanism of Crigler-Najjar syndrome type 1. Am J Hum Gen 1998;62:585. (Ref.269)

Gerloff T, et al. The sister of P-glycoprotein represents the canalicular bile salt export pump of mammalian liver. J Biol Chem 1998;273:10046. (Ref.192)

Ghosh SS, et al. Liver-directed gene therapy: promises, problems and prospects at the turn of the century. J Hepatol 2000;32(Suppl 1):238–252. (Ref.306)

Green RM, Hoda F, Ward KL. Molecular cloning and characterization of the murine bile salt export pump. Gene 2000;241:117. (Ref.195)

Guha C, et al. Long-term normalization of serum bilirubin levels by massive repopulation of Gunn rat liver by normal hepatocytes, transplanted after preparative hepatic irradiation and partial hepatectomy. Hepatology 2002;36:354. (Ref.298)

Hirohashi T, et al. Hepatic expression of multidrug resistance-associated protein-like proteins maintained in Eisai hyperbilirubinemic rats. Mol Pharmacol 1998;53:1068. (Ref.184)

Hirohashi T, Suzuki H, Sugiyama Y. Characterization of the transport properties of cloned rat multidrug resistance-associated protein 3 (MRP3). J Biol Chem 1999;274:15181. (Ref.141)

Hirohashi T, et al. ATP-dependent transport of bile salts by rat multidrug resistance-associated protein 3 (mrp3). J Biol Chem 2000;275:2905. (Ref.369)

Huang L, et al. MRP2 is essential for estradiol-17 beta (beta-d-glucuronide)-induced cholestasis in rats. Hepatology 2000;32:66. (Ref.364)

Huang W, et al. Induction of bilirubin clearance by the constitutive androstane receptor. Proc Natl Acad Sci U S A 2003;100:4156. (Ref.201)

Ishihara T, et al. Role of UGT1A1 mutation in fasting hyperbilirubinemia. J Gastroenterol Hepatol 2001;16:678. (Ref.352)

Iyer L, et al. Genetic predisposition to the metabolism of irinotecan (CPT-11). Role of uridine diphosphate glucuronosyltransferase isoform 1A1 in the glucuronidation of its active metabolite (SN-38) in human liver microsomes. J Clin Invest 1998;101:847. (Ref.336)

Jedlitschky G, et al. ATP-dependent transport of bilirubin glucuronides by the multidrug resistance protein MRP1 and its hepatocyte canalicular isoform MRP2. Biochem J 1997;327:305. (Ref.137)

Kadakol A, et al. Genetic lesions of bilirubin uridinediphosphoglucuronate glucuronosyltransferase causing Crigler-Najjar and Gilbert's syndromes: correlation of genotype to phenotype. Hum Mutat 2000;16:297. (Ref.268)

Kadakol A, et al. Interaction of coding region mutations and the Gilbert-type promoter abnormality of the UGT1A1 gene causes moderate degrees of unconjugated hyperbilirubinemia and may lead to neonatal kernicterus. J Med Genet 2001;38:244. (Ref.313)

Kamisako T, et al. Transport of monoglucuronosyl and bisglucuronosyl bilirubin by recombinant human and rat multidrug resistance protein 2. Hepatology 1999;30:485. (Ref.179)

Kauffman HM, et al. Influence of redox-active compounds and PXR-activators on human MRP1 and MRP2 gene expression. Toxicology 2002;171:137. (Ref.189)

Kauffmann HM, Schrenk D. Sequence analysis and functional characterization of the 5′-flanking region of the rat multidrug resistance protein 2 (mrp2) gene. Biochem Biophys Res Commun 1998;245:325. (Ref.191)

Keitel V, et al. Impaired protein maturation of the conjugate export pump multidrug resistance protein 2 as a consequence of a deletion mutation in Dubin-Johnson syndrome. Hepatology 2000;32:1317. (Ref.390)

Keppler D, Konig J. Hepatic secretion of conjugated drugs and endogenous substances. Semin Liver Dis 2000;20:265. (Ref.186)

Konig J, et al. Characterization of the human multidrug resistance protein isoform MRP3 localized to the basolateral hepatocyte membrane. Hepatology 1999;29:1156. (Ref.140)

Kool M, et al. Expression of human MRP6, a homologue of the multidrug resistance protein gene MRP1, in tissues and cancer cells. Cancer Res 1999; 59:175. (Ref.397)

Kouzuki H, et al. Contribution of sodium taurocholate co-transporting polypeptide to the uptake of its possible substrates into rat hepatocytes. J Pharmacol Exp Ther 1998;286:1043. (Ref.126)

Kren B, et al. Correction of the UDP-glucuronosyltransferase gene defect in the Gunn rat model of Crigler-Najjar syndrome type I. Proc Natl Acad Sci USA 1999;96:10349. (Ref.305)

Kren B, et al. Gene therapy as an alternative for liver transplantation. Liver Transplant 2002;8:1089. (Ref.301)

Kubitz R, et al. Benign recurrent intrahepatic cholestasis associated with mutations of the bile salt export pump. J Clin Gastroenterol 2006;40:171. (Ref.197)

Lai K, Harnish DC, Evans MJ. Estrogen receptor α regulates expression of the orphan receptor small heterodimer partner. J Biol Chem 2003;278: 36418–36429. (Ref.366)

Lecureur V, et al. Cloning and expression of murine sister of P-glycoprotein reveals a more discriminating transporter than MDR1/P-glycoprotein. Mol Pharmacol 2000;57:24. (Ref.194)

Lee JM, et al. Expression of the bile salt export pump is maintained after chronic cholestasis in the rat. Gastroenterology 2000;118:163. (Ref.368)

Lin Y-C, et al. Variants in the UGT1A1 gene and the risk of pediatric nonalcoholic fatty liver disease. Peditrics 2009;124:e1221. (Ref.31)

Machida I, et al. Mutation analysis of the multidrug resistance protein 2 (MRP2) gene in a Japanese patient with Dubin-Johnson syndrome. Hepatol Res 2004; 30:86. (Ref.389)

Makino N, et al. Altered expression of heme oxygenase-1 in the livers of patients with portal hypertensive diseases. Hepatology 2001;33:32. (Ref.14)

Maruo Y, et al. Gilbert syndrome caused by a homozygous missense mutation (Tyr486Asp) of bilirubin UDP-glucuronosyltransferase gene. J Pediatr 1998; 132:1045. (Ref.323)

Mills CO, et al. Different pathways of canalicular secretion of sulfated and non-sulfated fluorescent bile acids: a study in isolated hepatocyte couplets and TR⁻ rats. J Hepatol 1999;31:678. (Ref.393)

Nakao A, et al. Biliverdin protects the functional integrity of a transplanted syngeneic small bowel. Gastroenterology 2004;127:595. (Ref.25)

Nishikawa Y, et al. In vivo role of heme oxygenase in ischemic coronary vasodilation. Am J Physiol Heart Circ Physiol 2004;286:H2296. (Ref.16)

Ogawa K, et al. Characterization of inducible nature of MRP3 in rat liver. Am J Physiol Gastrointest Liver Physiol 2000;278:G438. (Ref.185)

Petit FM, et al. Parental isodisomy for chromosome 2 as the cause of Crigler-Najjar syndrome type I syndrome. Eur J Hum Genet 2005;13:278. (Ref.270)

Raijmakers MT, et al. Association of human liver bilirubin UDP-glucuronyltransferase activity with a polymorphism in the promoter region of the UGT1A1. J Hepatol 2000;33:348. (Ref.321)

Rao VV, et al. Choroid plexus epithelial expression of MDR1 P glycoprotein and multidrug resistance-associated protein contribute to the blood–cerebrospinal fluid–drug permeability barrier. Proc Natl Acad Sci U S A 1999;96:3900. (Ref.91)

Rattan S, Al Haj R, De Godoy MA. Mechanism of internal anal sphincter relaxation by CORM-1, authentic CO, and NANC nerve stimulation. Am J Physiol Gastrointest Liver Physiol 2004;287:G605. (Ref.17)

Roy-Chowdhury J, Locker J, Roy-Chowdhury N. Nuclear receptors orchestrate detoxification pathways. Dev Cell 2003;4:607. (Ref.202)

Roy-Chowdhury J, et al. Hepatocyte transplantation in humans: gene therapy and more. Pediatrics 1998;102:647. (Ref.297)

Roy-Chowdhury N, et al. Presence of the genetic marker for Gilbert syndrome is associated with increased level and duration of neonatal jaundice. Acta Paediatr 2002;91:100. (Ref.328)

Sauter BV, et al. Gene transfer to the liver using a replication-deficient recombinant SV40 vector results in long-term amelioration of jaundice in Gunn rats. Gastroenterology 2000;119:1348. (Ref.303)

Schauer R, et al. Treatment of Crigler-Najjar type 1 disease: relevance of early liver transplantation. J Pediatr Surg 2003;38:1227. (Ref.283)

Stieger B, et al. Drug- and estrogen-induced cholestasis through inhibition of the hepatocellular bile salt export pump (bsep) of rat liver. Gastroenterology 2000; 118:422. (Ref.362)

Stockel B, et al. Characterization of the 5′-flanking region of the human multidrug resistance protein 2 (MRP2) gene and its regulation in comparison with the multidrug resistance protein 3 (MRP3) gene. Eur J Biochem 2000; 267:1347. (Ref.187)

Strautnieks SS, et al. A gene encoding a liver-specific ABC transporter is mutated in progressive familial intrahepatic cholestasis. Nat Genet 1998;20:233. (Ref.193)

Strayer DS, et al. Durability of transgene expression and vector integration: recombinant SV40-derived gene therapy vectors. Mol Ther 2002;6:227. (Ref.304)

Suzuki H, Sugiyama Y. Transport of drugs across the hepatic sinusoidal membrane: sinusoidal drug influx and efflux in the liver. Semin Liver Dis 2000;20:251. (Ref.129)

Takahashi M, et al. A novel strategy for in vivo expansion of transplanted hepatocytes using preparative hepatic irradiation and FasL-induced hepatocellular apoptosis. Gene Ther 2003;10:304. (Ref.299)

Tanaka T, et al. The human multidrug resistance protein 2 gene: functional characterization of the 5′-flanking region and expression in hepatic cells. Hepatology 1999;30:1507. (Ref.190)

Tanaka Y, et al. Increased renal expression of bilivubin glucronide transporters in a rat model of obstructive jaundice. Am J Physiol Gastrointest Liver Physiol 2002;282:G656. (Ref.210)

Tayba R, et al. Non-invasive estimation of serum bilirubin. Pediatrics 1998; 102:28. (Ref.235)

Temme EHM, et al. Serum bilirubin and 10-year mortality risk in a Belgian population. Cancer Causes Control 2001;12:887. (Ref.30)

Thummala NR, et al. A non-immunogenic adenoviral vector, coexpressing CTLA4Ig and bilirubin-uridinediphosphoglucuronateglucuronosyltransferase permits long-term, repeatable transgene expression in the Gunn rat model of Crigler-Najjar syndrome. Gene Ther 2002;9:981. (Ref.302)

Trauner M, et al. Endotoxin downregulates rat hepatic ntcp gene expression via decreased activity of critical transcription factors. J Clin Invest 1998;101:2092. (Ref.135)

Trauner M, et al. The rat canalicular conjugate export pump (mrp2) is down-regulated in intrahepatic and obstructive cholestasis. Gastroenterology 1997;113:255. (Ref.139)

Vajro P, et al. Unusual early presentation of Gilbert syndrome in pediatric recipients of liver. J Pediatr Gastroenterol Nutr 2000;31:238. (Ref.331)

Van Aubel RA, et al. Expression and immunolocalization of multidrug resistance protein 2 in rabbit small intestine. Eur J Pharmacol 2000;400:195. (Ref.178)

Van Aubel RA, et al. Multidrug resistance protein Mrp2 mediates ATP-dependent transport of classic renal organic anion p-aminohippurate. Am J Physiol Renal Physiol 2000;279:F713. (Ref.177)

Van Mil SW, et al. Benign recurrent intrahepatic cholestasis type 2 is caused by mutations in ABCB11. Gastroenterology 2004;127:379. (Ref.196)

Vos TA, et al. Up-regulation of the multidrug resistance genes, mrp1 and mdr1b, and down-regulation of the organic anion transporter, mrp2, and the bile salt transporter, spgp, in endotoxemic rat liver. Hepatology 1998;28:1637. (Ref.138)

Vos TA, et al. Regulation of hepatic transport systems involved in bile secretion during liver regeneration in rats. Hepatology 1999;29:1833. (Ref.183)

Wang P, et al. The human organic anion transport protein SLC21A6 (OATP2) is not sufficient for bilirubin transport. J Biol Chem 2003;278:20695. (Ref.130)

Webster CR, et al. Cell swelling-induced translocation of rat liver Na$^+$/taurocholate cotransport polypeptide is mediated via the phosphoinositide 3-kinase signaling pathway. J Biol Chem 2000;275:29754. (Ref.131)

Wegiel B, et al. Cell surface biliverdin reductase mediates biliverdin-induced anti-inflammatory effects via phosphatidylinositol 3-kinase and Akt. J Biol Chem 2009;284:21369. (Ref.32)

Wells PG, et al. Glucuronidation and the UDP-glucuronosyltransferases in health and disease. Drug Metab Dispos 2004;32:281. (Ref.335)

Wijnholds J, et al. Multidrug resistance protein 1 protects the choroid plexus epithelium and contributes to the blood–cerebrospinal fluid barrier. J Clin Invest 2000;105:279. (Ref.92)

Yamashita K, et al. Biliverdin, a natural product of heme catabolism, induces tolerance to cardiac allografts. FASEB J 2004;18:765. (Ref.26)

Zhang Y, et al. Expression of various multidrug resistance-associated protein (MRP) homologues in brain microvessel endothelial cells. Brain Res 2000;876:148. (Ref.93)

Zimmerman HJ. Drug-induced liver disease. Clin Liver Dis 2000;4:73–96. (Ref.359)

Zucker SD, Goessling W. Mechanism of hepatocellular uptake of albumin-bound bilirubin. Biochim Biophys Acta 2000;1463:197. (Ref.127)

Zucker SD, Horn PS, Serman KE. Serum bilirubin levels in the US population: gender effect and inverse correlation with colorectal cancer. Hepatology 2004;40:827. (Ref.29)

A complete list of references can be found at www.expertconsult.com.

Wilson Disease

Eve A. Roberts and Diane W. Cox

ABBREVIATIONS

ATPase adenosine triphosphatase	**MRI** magnetic resonance imaging	**XIAP** X-linked inhibitor of apoptosis
DMT1 divalent cation transporter	**NF-κB** nuclear factor kappa B	
IgG immunoglobulin G	**SOD1** superoxide dismutase	

Copper Disorders

Copper is essential for biologic processes in plants, bacteria, yeast, and complex organisms. Copper can exist in two oxidation states (Cu^+ or Cu^{+2}). This characteristic makes it a versatile co-factor for numerous enzymes and permits it to participate in reactions that produce activated oxygen species. Although mammals absolutely require copper for normal cellular functions, they use trace amounts—far lower than what is absorbed from the diet. Excess copper is highly toxic in tissues, and the disposition of copper is tightly controlled. Copper-associated diseases occur when this control is disturbed. There are two human diseases involving copper transport that are due to defective metal-transporting P-type adenosine triphosphatases (ATPases). Menkes disease is an X-linked defect in transport of copper from the intestine that results in copper deprivation in many organs. Wilson disease, an autosomal recessive disorder, leads to copper overload in the liver and other organs. Two other human diseases characterized by hepatic copper overload have been described—Indian childhood cirrhosis and Tyrolean cirrhosis—but their possible genetic basis and disease mechanisms have not been determined and may not be identical. No human counterpart to the Bedlington terrier hereditary hepatic copper toxicosis associated with mutations in the *COMMD1* gene has yet been identified. Exogenous copper intoxication occurs rarely, and hepatic accumulation of copper is a well-known consequence of severe chronic cholestasis, but neither of these conditions will be discussed further.

Wilson Disease: History

Wilson disease presents a prototype of 20th-century biomedical progress through research in clinical and basic science. Kinnear Wilson, an American neurologist working in England, first described Wilson disease in 1912 as a familial disorder characterized by progressive, lethal neurologic disease along with chronic liver disease[1] and a corneal abnormality known as the Kayser-Fleischer ring, which had been reported approximately 10 years earlier. Although numerous observations over the next few decades pointed to copper overload as being important in Wilson disease, the etiologic role of copper was not firmly established until 1948.[2] The importance of low concentrations of plasma ceruloplasmin, the major serum protein containing copper, was recognized in 1952. By the mid-1950s the main diagnostic criteria for Wilson disease were clear, and in 1956, oral chelation therapy with penicillamine, a sulfhydryl-containing metabolite of penicillin, was first used. This treatment radically changed the outlook for the disease because many, if not most patients could be restored to good health Although Wilson disease could be treated successfully, knowledge of its pathobiology remained incomplete. A defect in biliary excretion of copper appeared to be the most likely mechanism of disease, but this remained unproven. An autosomal recessive pattern of inheritance was confirmed in 1960. In 1985 the gene was localized to chromosome 13, and in 1993, the abnormal gene in Wilson disease was identified.[3,4] The gene *ATP7B* encodes the metal-transporting P-type ATPase ATP7B (Wilson ATPase), which has six copper-binding motifs. The N-terminal of the Wilson ATPase, including all the copper-binding domains, was expressed in 1997, and the copper-binding action of this domain was characterized.[5] The structure of the Wilson ATPase was first demonstrated by homology modeling in 2002.[6] Subsequent studies provided a basis for predicting the functional effects of mutations. Since identification of the abnormal gene in Wilson disease more than 15 years ago, approximately 500 mutations have been described worldwide. Several animal models have been identified: the Long-Evans cinnamon rat, the Rauch toxic milk mouse (C57/Bl6 strain), the Jackson toxic milk mouse (C3H strain), and a knockout mouse with the entire gene disrupted.

Copper Pathway

The average diet includes ample amounts of copper, and ordinary daily intake of copper ranges from 1 to 10 mg/day, usually around 2 to 5 mg/day, depending on the mix of meat, legumes, shellfish, and chocolate. The recommended daily intake is 0.9 mg/day. Most (85%) of the dietary copper is excreted, with only 15% being retained in body tissues (**Fig. 63-1**). The predominant route for excretion of dietary copper is hepatobiliary. There is no enterohepatic recirculation of copper. Typically, the kidneys account for less than 5% of copper excretion, unless renal tubular reabsorption capacity is exceeded, as occurs in Wilson disease. Thus, in a normal individual, close regulation of excretion of copper in bile is critically important for whole-body copper homeostasis.

Dietary copper, as well as copper found in bile, salivary and gastric secretions, and pancreatic juice, is absorbed in the small intestine, mainly in the duodenum and proximal jejunum. Absorption is probably via human CTR1 expressed on enterocytes, although the divalent cation transporter (DMT1), which is mainly involved in iron uptake, may play a small role. Once absorbed, copper binds reversibly to serum albumin and to various amino acids, of which histidine is the most important. Copper–albumin and copper–histidine complexes distribute copper to various tissues, mainly to the liver. Copper loosely bound to amino acids is filtered in the kidneys and reabsorbed in the tubules. Copper is essential for many cellular processes.[7] Trace amounts of copper are required for the action of essential enzymes such as lysyl oxidase, which is involved in connective tissue production and elastin cross-linking. Cu/Zn superoxide dismutase (SOD1), a cytoplasmic free radical scavenger; cytochrome-c oxidase, which is integral to mitochondrial electron transfer; tyrosinase, which is required for pigment production; dopamine β-monooxygenase, an enzyme involved in neurotransmission; and peptidyl α-aminating monooxygenase, which plays a role in processing neurotransmitters, all require copper.

Molecular copper does not exist freely within cells. In hepatocytes and other cells it is always bound to low-molecular-weight proteins called metallochaperones, each of which delivers copper to different specific target molecules within the cell for use in cellular processes or further protein synthesis.[8] In hepatocytes, copper is incorporated into the ferroxidase ceruloplasmin, an α_2-glycoprotein with a molecular weight of 132 kD that contains six molecules of copper. As a ferroxidase, ceruloplasmin oxidizes iron for transport from ferritin to transferrin. Ceruloplasmin lacking copper (apoceruloplasmin) is devoid of ferroxidase activity; its half-life within the plasma compartment is comparatively brief, on the order of 24 hours. When copper is inserted into apoceruloplasmin, the resulting protein is ceruloplasmin (technically known as holoceruloplasmin), which is enzymatically active. The Wilson

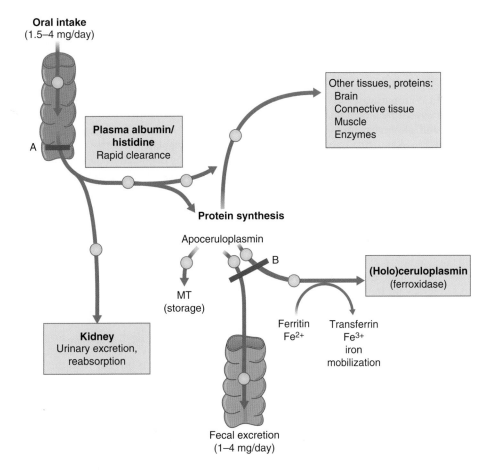

Oral intake
(1.5–4 mg/day)

A

Plasma albumin/ histidine
Rapid clearance

Other tissues, proteins:
Brain
Connective tissue
Muscle
Enzymes

Protein synthesis

Apoceruloplasmin

B

MT
(storage)

(Holo)ceruloplasmin
(ferroxidase)

Ferritin
Fe^{2+}

Transferrin
Fe^{3+}
iron
mobilization

Kidney
Urinary excretion,
reabsorption

Fecal excretion
(1–4 mg/day)

Fig. 63-1 Simplified overview of the pathways for copper ion transport, with excretion predominantly via bile. MT, metallothionein (copper storage), represents copper. Two sites of transport disorders are shown: A, Menkes disease (*ATP7A* gene); B, Wilson disease (*ATP7B* gene).

ATPase appears to be essential for synthesizing ceruloplasmin. Approximately 95% of the copper in plasma is contained within ceruloplasmin, and therefore this copper is not exchangeable. Both enterocytes and hepatocytes contain metallothioneins, a class of low-molecular-weight cysteine-rich proteins that are inducible and can sequester copper in a nontoxic form. Copper can also form complexes with intracellular glutathione.

Epidemiology

Incidence and Geographic Distribution

Wilson disease is found worldwide. It occurs on average in 30 individuals per million (i.e., 1 per 30,000) population, with a corresponding carrier frequency of approximately 1 in 90. In some populations it is quite rare, on the order of 1 per 100,000 population. In other populations, such as Sardinians and Chinese, the frequency is higher than average. Wilson disease is relatively infrequent in populations of African origin.

Pathogenesis

Basic Defect

Cloning of the genes for the two known human metal-transporting P-type ATPases provided the first key insights into the basic cellular defects in Wilson disease. *ATP7A*, the gene abnormal in Menkes disease, an X-linked disorder, was cloned by using a chromosomal breakpoint in an affected female. It was found to be related to bacterial copper resistance genes. The abnormal gene in Wilson disease (*ATP7B*) is found on chromosome 13. It was cloned by a combination of conventional linkage analysis and physical mapping of the relevant region of chromosome 13q14 and, finally, by capitalizing on its extensive homology with the Menkes disease gene.[3,4] The coding region of *ATP7B* is 4.1 kilobases in length, with mRNA of approximately 8 kilobases. It consists of 21 exons, and its 5′ untranslated region has also been defined. All functionally important regions of *ATP7B* are conserved as compared with bacteria and yeasts. Although *ATP7A* is expressed in many tissues, including muscle, kidney, heart, and intestine, *ATP7B* has a different and to some extent complementary pattern of tissue expression. *ATP7B* is expressed predominantly in the liver and kidneys, with minor expression in the brain, lungs, and placenta.

The product, known as the Wilson ATPase, is an intracellular membrane-spanning P-type ATPase consisting of 1411 amino acid residues with a molecular mass of approximately 165 kD. P-type ATPases are functionally diverse, but all have a cation channel and phosphorylation domains with a highly conserved aspartate-containing motif, DKTGT, in which the aspartate residue is transiently phosphorylated during the transport cycle. The Wilson ATPase retains this feature and also a highly characteristic CPC motif in a transmembrane segment. The Wilson ATPase is notable for having six tandemly arranged Copper-binding domains, each including the motif CXXC, in addition to eight transmembrane segments that form a pore and an ATPase loop region.[9] Its structure was originally determined by homology mapping using SERCA1, the sarcoplasmic Ca^{2+} P-type ATPase, as a model.[6] More recently, extensive crystallographic structural analyses are becoming available. The Wilson ATPase N-terminal Copper-binding region binds copper with the stoichiometry of one copper molecule per metal-binding domain through a cooperative mechanism.[5] Bound copper is in the +1 oxidation state and is coordinated by two cysteines in a distorted linear geometry, and the N-terminal region undergoes secondary and tertiary conformational changes in response to binding of copper. Conformational changes may influence the function of the Wilson ATPase, depending on the copper concentration, in which case the N-terminal region would exert a regulatory role.

Copper Transport and Homeostasis in Hepatocytes

Copper loosely bound to albumin or histidine is available for uptake into hepatocytes across the sinusoidal plasma membrane (**Fig. 63-2**). Because copper associated with these transporters is in the cupric form (+2 valence state), it must be reduced to the cuprous form (+1 valence state) before hepatocellular uptake. After the available copper is reduced by a reductase presumed to be located on the outer surface of the hepatocyte membrane or possibly by dietary reductants, it is taken up into hepatocytes via the transmembrane transporter CTR1 (a member of the solute ligand carrier superfamily), which is encoded by the gene *SLC31A1*. Human CTR1 is a membrane-spanning protein that appears to exist as a trimer to form a channel in the hepatocellular plasma membrane. Somewhat analogous to the Wilson ATPase, human CTR1 has a copper-binding domain near the N-terminal, but these domains consist of a different motif: a methionine cluster (MXXM), as opposed to a cysteine cluster (CXXC). Copper uptake may be linked to potassium transport. Although CTR1 is not the regulatory control point for copper homeostasis, it appears to be degraded in the presence of high concentrations of copper. A second copper transporter, known as human CTR2, mediates low-affinity copper uptake. The role of DMT1 in hepatocellular copper uptake, apart from that mediated by CTR1, is controversial.

Once inside the hepatocyte, small proteins called metallochaperones or copper chaperones coordinate the movement of copper to specific sites in the cell.[10] CCS1 guides copper to SOD1. Cox17 supplies copper to cytochrome-*c* oxidase in mitochondria. Sco1 and Sco2 mediate the transfer of copper to subunit II of cytochrome-*c* oxidase, and other metallochaperones might be involved. The chaperone ATOX1 transports copper to the Wilson ATPase, located in the trans-Golgi network region. ATOX1 has a single CXXC copper-binding domain; it interacts directly with the Wilson ATPase to transfer copper, possibly through specific copper-binding domains; all details of the interaction between the Wilson ATPase and ATOX1 remain to be established.[11]

The intracellular action of the Wilson ATPase is two-fold: it has a role both in incorporating copper into ceruloplasmin and in facilitating excretion of copper into bile. In vitro studies using various continuous cell lines have shown that the intracellular location of the Wilson ATPase changes with increased intracellular copper concentration. When the

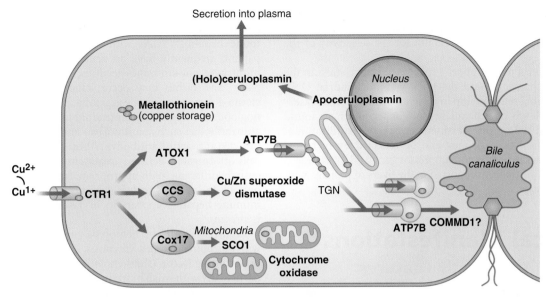

Fig. 63-2 Proposed model of the intracellular pathways of copper trafficking within the hepatocyte, with the major proteins involved shown. Low-molecular-weight copper "chaperones" (ATOX1, SCO1/Cox17, and CCS) each deliver copper to a specific target protein (ATP7B, cytochrome oxidase, and superoxide dismutase, respectively). SCO1 transports copper across the mitochondrial membrane. ATP7B (shown as a channel) traffics from the trans-Golgi network (TGN) to cytoplasmic vesicles that deliver copper to the bile canaliculus. COMMD1 is proposed to be involved in excretion of copper from the cell but may have other functions in the intracellular disposition of copper.

intracellular copper concentration is elevated, the Wilson ATPase redistributes from the trans-Golgi network to vesicles in the apical region of the hepatocyte; that is, to the vicinity of the bile canalicular membrane.[10,12,13] The sixth copper-binding domain appears to be essential for normal intracellular trafficking. Interaction of the Wilson ATPase and the dynactin subunit p62 may be part of the mechanism of this intracellular redistribution.[14] Many details of the cellular mechanism of biliary excretion of copper remain unknown. There may be more than one mechanism, one being direct exocytosis from cytoplasmic vesicles in the endosome–lysosome spectrum. Whether the Wilson ATPase actually resides transiently in the bile canalicular membrane to transport copper into bile remains unclear.[9] A paracellular pathway has also been suggested.[15]

Discoveries regarding the inherited copper toxicosis in Bedlington terriers have identified a possible new component of the copper transport system. This hepatic copper toxicosis is inherited recessively. Clinical expression is variable, with death occurring at 2 to 3 years of age or a long chronic course. The abnormal gene in this disorder was identified in a region equivalent to human chromosome 2 and not on chromosome 13, where the Wilson disease gene is located. The causative gene for this condition was proposed to be *COMMD1*, originally known as *MURR1*, in which one of the three coding exons was found to be completely deleted in affected dogs.[16] However, some affected dogs lack the deletion.[17] This raises the question of whether *COMMD1* is truly the defective gene responsible for canine copper toxicosis. *COMMD1* has various functions. In addition to interacting with the copper-binding region of Wilson ATPase,[18] it interacts with the X-linked inhibitor of apoptosis (XIAP)[19] and inhibits nuclear factor nuclear factor kappa beta (NF-κB), a transcription factor affecting immune responses and cell cycle regulation, by affecting the association of NF-κB with chromatin in the nucleus. Because its effect on cellular copper distribution is modest, *COMMD1* cannot yet be regarded as having a proven major role in copper transport. A family of related genes has now been identified, named *COMMD* genes, that contain the copper metabolism gene *MURR1* domain.[20]

Some aspects of cellular metal transport are not specific. Platinum (including organic platinum compounds used as chemotherapy for neoplasia) appears to use all of the hepatocellular machinery evolved for the disposition of copper.[21] Resistance to the chemotherapeutic effect of cisplatin in some types of neoplasia has been related to function of the Wilson ATPase.[22] By contrast, zinc has its own family of transporters.[23]

Consequences of Copper Storage

Because copper is a prooxidant, liver damage in patients with Wilson disease is attributed to oxidative stress. Accumulated copper is probably a source of activated oxygen species (e.g., superoxide $O_2^{\cdot}$, hydrogen peroxide, hydroxyl radicals) through a Fenton-type reaction. Generation of peroxides and hydroxyl radicals leads to nuclear DNA damage. Studies using primary cultures of rat hepatocytes have shown that copper generates more activated oxygen species and causes more lipid peroxidation than cadmium does.[24] Incubation of Hep G2 cells with increasing concentrations of copper led to the generation of activated oxygen species in a dose-responsive pattern, whereas incubation with zinc did not have this effect.[25]

Copper toxicity in the brain also appears to involve oxidative stress. The amyloid precursor protein may regulate copper action in the brain, but it is not clear whether it functions as a metallochaperone. Increased concentrations of copper in the milieu surrounding neurons or altered activities of key copper-containing enzymes in the brain may contribute to the neuronal damage and possibly account for the selectivity of the damage.

Some clinical data support a role for oxidative stress in the disease mechanism. Focal deletions in mitochondrial DNA typical of aging may develop in patients with Wilson disease.[26] Subnormal levels of antioxidants such as vitamin E are found in untreated Wilson disease, thus suggesting overutilization.[27] Oxygen radical damage may also be reflected by increased mutations in the p53 tumor suppressor gene and by increased nitric oxide synthase, as reported in the livers of patients with Wilson disease.

Clinical Manifestations
Clinical Diagnostic Features

The clinical findings in patients with Wilson disease are extremely variable. Age at the onset of symptoms is usually from 6 years old to about 45 years old. Patients outside these age limits continue to be reported and pose important diagnostic challenges. Wilson disease with hepatic involvement has been identified in patients younger than 5 years old[28] and in patients older than 50 years old; that is, in their 70s.[29] Wilson disease may be manifested clinically as chronic or fulminant liver disease, as a progressive neurologic disorder without evident hepatic dysfunction, or as rather nondescript psychiatric illness.[30-32] Some patients have one or more episodes of isolated, self-limited acute hemolysis. This degree of clinical variability frequently makes confirmation of the diagnosis very difficult. A diagnostic algorithm has been proposed[33] but requires further validation. Currently, validation has been performed only for Wilson disease in childhood.[34]

Hepatic Involvement

Wilson disease is manifested as liver disease more commonly in children[35,36] but should be considered as the cause of any acute or chronic liver disease in adults. Wilson disease should be considered as a possible diagnosis in any child, whether symptomatic or not, who has hepatomegaly, persistently elevated serum aminotransferases, or evidence of fatty liver. Symptoms may be vague and nonspecific: fatigue, anorexia, or abdominal pain. Occasionally, patients of any age are found to have a self-limited clinical illness resembling acute hepatitis, with malaise, anorexia and nausea, jaundice, elevated serum aminotransferases, and abnormal coagulation test results. Frequently, this hepatic disorder resembles acute autoimmune hepatitis. Some patients have a history of self-limited jaundice, apparently caused by unexplained hemolysis. Patients with hepatic Wilson disease may have severe, established chronic liver disease as shown by hepatosplenomegaly, ascites, congestive splenomegaly, low serum albumin, and persistently abnormal coagulation. Many of these findings relate more to portal hypertension as a consequence of Wilson disease than to the metabolic disorder itself. A few patients have been encountered with isolated splenomegaly, without hepatomegaly, or indeed without any evidence of hepatic dysfunction. Initial manifestation as splenic rupture has been reported.

Wilson disease may be manifested in children and young adults as clinical liver disease that looks exactly like autoimmune hepatitis.[37,38] As with actual autoimmune hepatitis, patients frequently have an acute onset. In Wilson disease mimicking autoimmune hepatitis, fatigue, malaise, arthropathy, and rashes may occur; laboratory findings include elevated aminotransferases, greatly increased serum immunoglobulin G (IgG) concentration, and positive nonspecific autoantibodies such as antinuclear antibody and anti–smooth muscle (anti-actin) antibody. Wilson disease must be specifically investigated because treatment of the two diseases is entirely different. With appropriate treatment, the long-term outlook for patients with Wilson disease manifested as autoimmune hepatitis appears to be favorable even if cirrhosis is present.

Recurrent bouts of hemolysis may lead to cholelithiasis with bilirubinate stones. Cirrhosis, if present, may be a further predisposing factor. Children with unexplained cholelithiasis, particularly with small bilirubinate stones, should be tested for Wilson disease. Hepatocellular carcinoma is rare in patients with Wilson disease, as opposed to other chronic liver diseases, but recent reports suggest that it is not as rare as generally thought.[39] Reported age at diagnosis of hepatocellular carcinoma in patients with Wilson disease includes all decades from the teens to the 60s, including the youngest, a 12-year-old boy with clinically unsuspected hepatocellular carcinoma.[40] Cholangiocarcinoma may also occur.

Neurologic Involvement

Neurologic Wilson disease tends to occur in the second and third decades or later, but it has been reported in children as young as 6 to 10 years old. If Kayser-Fleischer rings and prominent cupriuria are not present or if the neuropsychiatric syndrome is either atypical or nonspecific, diagnosis can be difficult.[31,32,41] Most, but not all, patients with the neurologic form have hepatic involvement; however, the hepatic disease may be entirely asymptomatic. Approximately 40% of patients with a neurologic manifestation of Wilson disease have cirrhosis. Neurologic Wilson disease follows two main patterns: (1) increased or abnormal movement disorder, which may be characterized by tremor or dystonia, or (2) a relative loss of movement that resembles parkinsonian rigidity. Movement disorders tend to occur earlier and include tremors, poor coordination, and loss of fine motor control. The earliest symptoms may be subtle and attributed to other factors; for example, familial tremor has erroneously been implicated in some patients. Dystonia involves a sustained focal movement disorder, and patients may also have a facial grimace. The disorders with reduced movement and rigidity generally develop later. These disorders strongly resemble a parkinsonian phenotype, with masklike facies, gait disturbance, and pseudobulbar involvement, such as dysarthria, drooling, and difficulty swallowing. The features suggesting pseudobulbar involvement may, however, occur in any patient with neurologic Wilson disease. Various speech disorders may occur with any of these neurologic manifestations: speech abnormalities include slurred or scanned speech, garbled speech described as difficulty getting the words out, and hypophonia, a soft whispery voice. Epilepsy, including status epilepticus, can occur in patients with Wilson disease. Generally, intellect is not impaired.

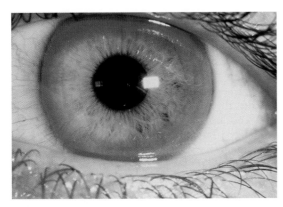

Fig. 63-3 **Kayser-Fleischer ring, a golden-brown deposit seen at the outer rim of the cornea, in the membrane of Desçemet.** Kayser-Fleischer rings are present in 50% to 95% of patients, depending on the type of onset. *(Courtesy of the late Professor Dame Sheila Sherlock, London.)*

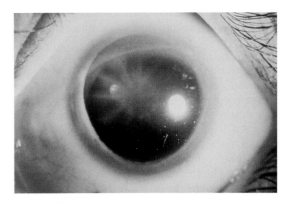

Fig. 63-4 **Sunflower cataract, an infrequent ocular manifestation, caused by copper deposits in the lens.** *(Courtesy of the late Dr. Irmin Sternlieb, New York.)*

In patients who have predominantly hepatic disease, neurologic involvement is often subtle. Direct questioning may be required to determine whether the patient has significant mood disturbance, recent deterioration in academic or occupational performance, clumsiness, and disorganized or cramped handwriting.

Psychiatric Aspects

As many as 20% of patients may have purely psychiatric symptoms.[42-44] These symptoms are highly variable, although depression is common. Neurotic behavior such as phobias or compulsive behavior has been reported; aggressive or antisocial behavior may also occur, as well as psychosis. In some younger patients the psychiatric disorder seems disproportionately severe for age. In most patients with purely psychiatric features of Wilson disease, the diagnosis is delayed to older age.

Ocular Features

The classic Kayser-Fleischer ring is caused by deposition of copper in the membrane of Desçemet (**Fig. 63-3**). Although copper is distributed throughout the cornea, fluid streaming favors accumulation of copper here, especially at the superior and inferior poles and eventually circumferentially around the iris. Kayser-Fleischer rings are visible on direct inspection only when the iris is lightly pigmented and copper deposition is heavy. A careful slit-lamp examination is mandatory. Kayser-Fleischer rings may be absent in approximately 50% of patients with exclusively hepatic involvement and in presymptomatic patients. They are less commonly found in children. Most patients with neurologic features of Wilson disease have Kayser-Fleischer rings; however, approximately 5% do not. Kayser-Fleischer rings are not specific for Wilson disease. They may be found in patients with other types of chronic liver disease, usually with a prominent cholestatic component, such as primary biliary cirrhosis. With effective chelation, the Kayser-Fleischer rings disappear; the lateral edges are resorbed first and the superior and inferior poles last. Disappearance of Kayser-Fleischer rings with treatment should not be

interpreted as casting doubt on the original diagnosis of Wilson disease.

Copper can be deposited in the lens and lead to the so-called sunflower cataract (**Fig. 63-4**), which does not interfere with vision. Like Kayser-Fleischer rings, they disappear with effective chelation therapy.

Involvement of Other Systems

Wilson disease can be accompanied by various extrahepatic disorders, apart from neurologic disease. Episodes of hemolytic anemia can result from sporadic release of copper into blood. Renal disease, mainly Fanconi syndrome, may be prominent. Abnormalities include microscopic hematuria, aminoaciduria, phosphaturia, and defective acidification of urine, and nephrolithiasis has been reported. Arthritis, affecting mainly the large joints, may occur as a result of synovial copper accumulation. Other musculoskeletal problems include osteoporosis and osteochondritis dissecans. Vitamin D–resistant rickets may develop as a result of the renal damage. Copper deposition in the heart can lead to cardiomyopathy or cardiac arrhythmias.[45] Sudden death in patients with Wilson disease has been attributed to cardiac involvement, but this is rare. Copper deposition in skeletal muscle can cause rhabdomyolysis. Pancreatitis, possibly caused by deposition of copper in the pancreas, may also occur.

Endocrine disorders can occur. Hypoparathyroidism has been attributed to copper deposition. Amenorrhea and testicular problems appear to be due to Wilson disease itself, not as a consequence of cirrhosis. Infertility or repeated spontaneous abortions occur with untreated Wilson disease.[46]

Biochemical Diagnostic Features

The two main disturbances in hepatocellular copper disposition in Wilson disease are absent or decreased incorporation of copper into ceruloplasmin and greatly decreased biliary excretion of copper. Abnormalities in clinical biochemistry revolve around the serum ceruloplasmin concentration. The normal serum concentration of ceruloplasmin in adults is 200 to 600 mg/L.[47] In the neonatal period, serum ceruloplasmin levels are low (50 to 260 mg/L), and in the first few years of life, levels run in the high end of the normal range (300 to

500 mg/L), with adult serum concentrations being reached by adolescence. Ceruloplasmin is an acute-phase protein whose serum levels are increased by inflammatory hepatic disease, pregnancy, or estrogen supplements. The serum ceruloplasmin concentration is typically decreased in patients with Wilson disease, and therefore serum copper is also decreased. A serum ceruloplasmin level lower than 50 mg/L is a significant diagnostic finding. It is now recognized that many patients with hepatic Wilson disease, up to 30% to 40% depending on the reported series, have a normal or nearly normal serum ceruloplasmin concentration. This is in part methodologic. The immunologic methods routinely used in most clinical laboratories measure both apoceruloplasmin and holoceruloplasmin; these methods overestimate the true amount of ceruloplasmin in plasma. With an immunologic type of assay, a serum ceruloplasmin level lower than 140 mg/L may be an informative finding for Wilson disease.[48] Enzymatic assays, which measure the ferroxidase activity of ceruloplasmin, the routine method of the 1960s, are to be preferred. They provide a more reliable measure of ceruloplasmin for the diagnosis of Wilson disease by measuring ceruloplasmin that is enzymatically active by virtue of containing copper.[49] The enzymatic assay permits a reliable, reasonably accurate estimate of non–ceruloplasmin-bound copper and may indicate early copper deficiency when oxidized activity is completely absent.[50] In some patients with hepatic Wilson disease, hepatic inflammation may be sufficient to increase serum ceruloplasmin levels to the normal range. In very young children the level may appear normal but is actually low for age.

Serum ceruloplasmin by itself is not a sufficient diagnostic test for Wilson disease because protein synthesis may be decreased in other types of severe chronic liver disease. Protein loss from intestinal malabsorption, nephrotic syndrome, or severe malnutrition can cause a reduction in concentration. Furthermore, subnormal serum ceruloplasmin concentrations are found in at least 10% of heterozygotes for Wilson disease. Near-absence of ceruloplasmin is found in hereditary aceruloplasminemia, a rare autosomal recessive disease caused by mutations in the structural gene for ceruloplasmin on chromosome 3. Aceruloplasminemia is associated with neurologic, retinal, and pancreatic degeneration as a result of iron accumulation in the brain, retina, and pancreas.[51] Anemia with increased serum ferritin is found. Excessive hepatic iron storage occurs, as in hereditary hemochromatosis. Study of patients with hereditary aceruloplasminemia has indicated the critical function of ceruloplasmin as a ferroxidase, and targeted disruption of the ceruloplasmin gene in a mouse model has confirmed its key role in transporting iron out of cells. Theoretically, patients with Wilson disease who are undergoing prolonged, aggressive chelation therapy could show similar effects if copper deprivation reduces the ferroxidase activity of ceruloplasmin to undetectable levels. This has been found in a few patients after prolonged treatment and in those with particularly low ceruloplasmin levels.[52]

Typically, the serum copper concentration parallels the serum ceruloplasmin level. In severe or untreated Wilson disease, the non–ceruloplasmin-bound copper concentration is elevated. This concentration can be estimated by subtracting the amount of copper associated with ceruloplasmin from the total serum copper content. The arithmetic method is performed by multiplying the serum ceruloplasmin concentration (in milligrams per liter) by 3.15 (the amount of copper,

in micrograms, per milligram ceruloplasmin) to determine the amount of copper (in micrograms per liter) associated with ceruloplasmin. If total serum copper is reported in micromoles per liter, it must be converted to micrograms per liter by multiplying that value by 63.5, the molecular weight of copper. The ceruloplasmin-bound copper is then subtracted from the total serum copper. In normal individuals, the non–ceruloplasmin-bound copper concentration is approximately 50 to 100 µg/L. In Wilson disease, the concentration is higher than 200 µg/L, or even 10 times higher in the presence of fulminant hepatic failure and intravascular hemolysis. The usefulness of this calculation is highly dependent on the accuracy of the copper and ceruloplasmin measurements. Serum ceruloplasmin measured immunologically may be misleading in this calculation. A direct method for measuring non–ceruloplasmin-bound copper has recently become available.[53] Neither the estimated version nor this direct measurement has been validated as a diagnostic criterion.

Studies of urinary copper excretion, preferably with three separate 24-hour collections, prove useful for diagnosis. It is critically important to ensure that collection is complete and precautions are taken against contamination with copper in the collection process; in general, problems with urine collection are not sufficient to invalidate the usefulness of testing. "Spot" urine samples are not suitable as a basis for diagnosis. The volume and urine creatinine concentration should be measured to show completeness of the 24-hour collection. The conventional cutoff for diagnosing Wilson disease has been greater than 100 µg/24 h (>1.6 µmol/24 h) in symptomatic patients. Recent studies suggest that this threshold for diagnosis is too high in that basal 24-hour urinary copper excretion may be less than 100 µg/24 h in up to a quarter of patients. Using 40 µg/24 h (equivalent to 0.6 µmol/24 h) appears to be a better diagnostic cutoff for Wilson disease.[32,54,55] Reference values for normal urinary copper excretion may vary from laboratory to laboratory. Heterozygotes usually have normal 24-hour urinary copper excretion, although occasionally it is borderline abnormal.

A provocative test of urinary copper excretion, in which D-penicillamine (500 mg orally every 12 hours) is given while a 24-hour urinary collection is obtained, sometimes provides useful information.[56] Although a normal person may excrete as much as 20 times the baseline level after D-penicillamine administration, a patient with Wilson disease will excrete considerably more. Urinary copper excretion of 25 µmol or greater of copper per 24 hours (≥1600 µg/24 h) is taken as being diagnostic of Wilson disease. This provocative test has been suggested to be more reliable than measurement of the hepatic tissue content of copper.[56] Though well-validated in children, this test has not been validated in adults. Some patients with Wilson disease do not reach the 25-µmol threshold, and therefore the sensitivity of this test is not as great as initially thought.[57] From a practical point of view, it is worthwhile carrying out this test on 3 successive days and making three separate 24-hour urine collections during D-penicillamine administration.

Serum uric acid and phosphate concentrations may be low because of the renal tubular dysfunction associated with untreated Wilson disease, but these findings are not specific for Wilson disease nor particularly sensitive. Urinalysis may show microscopic hematuria; if possible, aminoaciduria, phosphaturia, and proteinuria should be quantified.

The hepatic tissue copper concentration, usually measured by neutron activation analysis or atomic absorption spectrometry, may provide important diagnostic information. Hepatic copper content higher than 250 µg/g dry weight is considered diagnostic of Wilson disease. Conversely, hepatic parenchymal copper concentrations less than 40 µg/g dry weight are taken as strong evidence against the diagnosis of Wilson disease. A recent study placed the upper limit of normal for hepatic parenchymal copper at 55 µg/g dry weight.[58] Liver biopsy samples must be collected without extraneous copper contamination, but disposable liver biopsy needles can be used. In early stages of Wilson disease, when copper is distributed diffusely in the liver cell cytoplasm and therefore not detected by histochemical stains, this measurement may clearly indicate hepatic copper overload. In later stages of hepatic Wilson disease, measurement of hepatic copper is less reliable because copper is distributed unequally in the liver. However, liver biopsy may not be safe in some patients because of coagulopathy or ascites. The use of transjugular liver biopsy may circumvent this contraindication to percutaneous biopsy. Some patients with Wilson disease have a hepatic tissue copper concentration intermediate between normal and definitely elevated (between 55 and 250 µg/g dry weight). Because the 250-µg/g dry weight threshold may be too high, a cutoff of 70 µg/g dry weight has been suggested.[59] If the hepatic parenchymal copper concentration is in the 70- to 250-µg/g dry weight range, further diagnostic testing (particularly genetic) is warranted, especially if other clinical features are present. Parenchymal copper measurement is also highly susceptible to sampling problems. An adequate core of the liver biopsy specimen, at least 1 cm in length, should be analyzed. Paraffin-embedded tissue can be used for retrospective analysis. An elevated hepatic copper concentration is not specific; patients with chronic cholestasis or diseases such as Indian childhood cirrhosis may have elevated hepatic copper levels. Some heterozygotes have similar moderate elevations of liver tissue copper.

Because impaired production of ceruloplasmin is an important aspect of the hepatocellular pathology of Wilson disease, measurement of the incorporation of copper into apoceruloplasmin has been used as a diagnostic test. Radioactive isotopes (^{64}Cu, ^{67}Cu) or, preferably, a stable (^{65}Cu) copper isotope can be used. Following oral or intravenous administration of copper isotope, patients with Wilson disease show little or no incorporation of labeled copper into plasma ceruloplasmin. Unfortunately, heterozygotes cannot always be differentiated from presymptomatic homozygous patients. This test is obsolete and rarely used.

Imaging Studies

Sonography of the liver may reveal features associated with fatty infiltration of the liver or advanced chronic liver disease with portal hypertension and splenomegaly. Magnetic resonance imaging (MRI) of the brain may be highly informative in the neurologic form of Wilson disease[60-62] and should also be performed in any patient with hepatic Wilson disease.

Histopathology

Wilson disease can exhibit a broad range of histologic findings on liver biopsy specimens, many of which are nonspecific.[63,64]

In the earliest stages the features are nonspecific and include steatosis, focal necrosis, glycogenated nuclei in hepatocytes, and occasional apoptotic bodies. Mallory-Denk hyaline has been reported sometimes. As the parenchymal damage progresses, possibly by repeated episodes of lobular necrosis, periportal fibrosis develops. The cirrhosis is usually macronodular but may be micronodular. With treatment the cirrhosis may regress.

Early in the disease, hepatocellular copper is bound mainly to metallothionein and distributed diffusely in the cytoplasm of hepatocytes. Histochemical stains for copper are negative. With disease progression, hepatocellular copper exceeds the storage capacity of available metallothionein and is deposited in lysosomes. Staining techniques for copper or copper-binding protein (e.g., rubeanic acid, orcein) detect these lysosomal aggregates of copper. Copper is usually distributed throughout the lobule or nodule, but in a cirrhotic liver, some nodules may have no stainable copper.

If the clinical features resemble autoimmune hepatitis, findings on liver biopsy may also suggest an autoimmune process. Inflammation is sometimes severe, with classic piecemeal necrosis. Features not typical of autoimmune hepatitis may be found, such as Mallory-Denk hyaline and hepatocellular copper aggregates. When Wilson disease is manifested as fulminant hepatic failure, histologic findings confirm the pre-existing liver disease. Cirrhosis is found, but parenchymal copper is deposited mainly in Kupffer cells rather than in hepatocytes.

Changes in hepatocellular mitochondria, identified by electron microscopy, are an important feature in Wilson disease.[65] The mitochondria vary in size; dense bodies in mitochondria may be increased in number. The most striking change is dilation of the tips of the mitochondrial cristae as a result of separation of the inner and outer membranes of the cristae. The intercristal space is widened such that it looks bulbous or, if more extreme, has an irregular cystic shape. This finding, though not absolutely specific, can be helpful diagnostically, even in quite young and minimally affected patients. Not all hepatocytes in a given lobule are affected, and some lobules may be more severely affected than others. The mitochondrial changes are probably a consequence of oxidative damage from excessive copper in the liver.[66]

Diagnosis by Mutation Analysis

Characteristic clinical features, accompanied by typical biochemical parameters, can provide a diagnosis of Wilson disease in some cases. However, gene mutation analysis has highlighted that many of these traditional parameters can often be misleading because of overlap with other liver diseases or borderline biochemical results. Diagnosis by DNA mutation analysis plays an important role in providing a reliable diagnosis. DNA diagnosis is possible from liver biopsy samples or blood. Mutation analysis is valuable in any case in which the biochemical and clinical features are atypical, in early stages of the disease when biochemistry may be borderline, and in patients undergoing liver transplantation because of fulminant hepatic failure. In the latter case, DNA analysis will not alter treatment but is essential for appropriate follow-up of siblings. Even when the original patient is deceased, accurate diagnosis is important for other family members.

More than 500 mutations in the *ATP7B* gene have been reported from a variety of populations worldwide and are listed in the Wilson disease database maintained at the University of Alberta (available at www.uofa-medical-genetics.org/wilson/index.php), along with all relevant references.[67] Although *ATP7B* is a large gene with 21 exons and a coding region of 4.1 kilobases, modern technologies make DNA diagnosis feasible. High-throughput analytic methods include direct sequencing, denaturing high-performance liquid chromatography,[68] and automated single-strand conformation polymorphism analysis. New methods involving microarray techniques may expedite genetic diagnosis in some populations.[69] Certain mutations in a limited number of exons are often characteristic of specific populations, and thus feasible methods for mutation analysis can be devised to improve cost-effectiveness. Most patients are compound heterozygotes; namely, they carry two different mutations of *ATP7B*. This is helpful for DNA diagnosis in that one mutation may be sufficient to confirm the diagnosis when the patient has the typical clinical signs and at least one biochemical assay indicating increased copper storage. Identification of only one mutation is not adequate when copper assays are borderline and the clinical features are ambiguous (e.g., psychiatric features, slight abnormalities in liver function). Mutation identification is very likely to become the diagnostic aid of choice when clinical and biochemical features arouse suspicion for Wilson disease. Nevertheless, genetic data are not always simple to interpret.[70,71]

Specific mutations are typical of certain ethnic origins of patients. Different populations may have a typical spectrum of mutations. The most common mutation, histidine1069glutamine (His1069Gln or H1069Q), is present as at least one of the two mutations in 35% to 75% of affected patients of European origin, particularly those from eastern Europe.[72,73] This mutation is not found in Chinese and related populations, in whom arginine778leucine (Arg778Leu, R778L) is common.[74,75] Patients from most populations have a large number of mutations, with none in a particularly high frequency. One of the exceptions is the island of Sardinia, where the majority of patients have a 15–base pair deletion in the promoter region.[76] This is the only population in which a promoter mutation has been identified to date. In some populations, feasible mutation identification schemes can be developed for rapid mutation assessment in 90% of patients, as in Sardinia[77] and eastern Germany.[78] Examples of other populations with a characteristic limited spectrum of mutations include those in Iceland, Korea, Japan, and the Canary Islands.[55] Of interest, the spectrum of mutations in Brazil is similar to that in the Canary Islands.[79]

Mutations have been identified throughout the gene and in the promoter region. Most mutations identified to date in *ATP7B*, as recorded in the mutation database, are missense mutations (57%), small deletions and insertions (28%), nonsense mutations (7%), and splice site mutations (8%). The mutation spectrum for *ATP7A*, abnormal in Menkes disease, differs from that for *ATP7B*.[80] Large gene deletions, found in approximately 20% of patients with Menkes disease, are apparently rare. Missense mutations tend to lie predominantly within functional domains, but their functional effects are difficult to predict. In contrast, deletions, duplications, and nonsense mutations can be predicted to affect production of the Wilson ATPase severely.

Given the large number of missense mutations, an important challenge is to ensure that mutations identified within *ATP7B* are actually responsible for the defective function causing Wilson disease. When only one mutation is used to support the diagnosis, that one mutation must be definitely established as causing disease. Prediction of disruption of the molecule, conservation of the specific residue between species, and absence in at least 50 controls are among the features examined in attempts to identify which mutations are causing disease. Changes in size, shape, and hydrophobicity are compared. Examination of mutation location by using a model of *ATP7B* based on the crystallized calcium transporter SERCA1 can assist in assessing which mutations lie in critical regions of the protein.[6,81] Examination of sequence homology can also be used to predict whether a change in an amino acid will affect overall protein function.[82] Functional assays are useful, although carried out for a limited number of mutations. The components of the copper transport system are completely conserved between yeast and humans. Therefore a yeast assay is useful to determine whether the mutant Wilson ATPase is capable of transporting copper, a requirement for its normal function.[83,84] Cell culture assays in Chinese hamster ovary or hepatoma cell lines can indicate whether *ATP7B* is distributed normally[85,86] and can traffic within the cell from the trans-Golgi network to cytoplasmic vesicles in response to elevated copper concentrations.[87] With certain mutations, such trafficking, required for biliary excretion of copper, does not occur.

Specific Mutations and Clinical Features

Because most patients have two different mutations of the *ATP7B* gene, correlation of clinical features with specific mutations is difficult. Data from a number of laboratories indicate that there is not a high correlation between clinical disease (phenotype) and a specific mutation (genotype).[88] However, in general, the more severe mutations that interfere with production of intact Wilson ATPase result in an earlier age at onset and tend to be associated with a hepatic manifestation of disease.[28,89,90] For the most common His1069Gln mutation, age at onset in homozygous patients ranges from approximately 10 to 50 years (mean age, approximately 20 years), somewhat more frequently in those with neurologic onset.[73] In addition to functional defects in the Wilson ATPase because of specific mutations in the patient, disease severity and clinical features are probably influenced by numerous other modifying factors that could be genetic or environmental. Monozygotic twins with different clinical forms of Wilson disease have been reported.[91,92] Apolipoprotein E polymorphisms may affect the severity of Wilson disease.[93]

Diagnosis of Presymptomatic Siblings

Because Wilson disease is a recessive condition, brothers and sisters of a patient have a 25% chance of also being affected and a 50% risk of being heterozygotes. Reliable diagnosis is essential for presymptomatic individuals before embarking on lifetime treatment. Because of the variability of biochemical tests, diagnosis in the presymptomatic stage can be difficult. However, initiation of treatment before tissue damage occurs

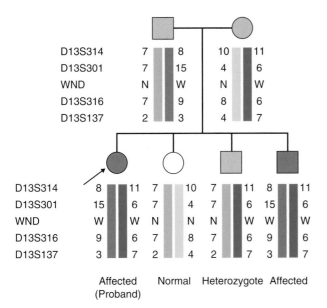

D13S314	7	8	10	11
D13S301	7	15	4	6
WND	N	W	N	W
D13S316	7	9	8	6
D13S137	2	3	4	7

D13S314	8	11	7	10	7	11	8	11
D13S301	15	6	7	4	7	6	15	6
WND	W	W	N	N	N	W	W	W
D13S316	9	6	7	8	7	6	9	6
D13S137	3	7	2	4	2	7	3	7

Affected   Normal   Heterozygote   Affected
(Proband)

Fig. 63-5 Polymorphic DNA microsatellite markers, which can be used to reliably diagnose the status of siblings of a confirmed patient. One or preferably two informative markers should flank the gene on each side. DNA markers are listed in centromeric to telomeric order. Numbers represent the alleles of each marker listed. The proband *(arrow)* and presymptomatic siblings, confirmed as affected, are shown as a *filled circle* or *square*. Markers indicate the genotype of each sibling. The specific chromosome segment can be followed through the family. Mutation identification is not necessary when the patient has a firm diagnosis of Wilson disease.

offers the best outlook for a normal span and quality of life. Genetic diagnosis performed expertly offers the only secure diagnosis. If both *ATP7B* mutations have been identified in the patient, sibling diagnosis can be carried out directly by mutation analysis. In cases in which the diagnosis of Wilson disease is secure in the proband by clinical and biochemical criteria but DNA analysis has not been undertaken or when only one mutation has been identified, DNA marker analysis can be used without knowledge of the specific mutations present in the initial patient. Preferred markers are variable regions in the DNA within the gene or in regions closely flanking the gene. The specific markers allow tracking of the disease gene, along with its accompanying markers, from each parental chromosome (**Fig. 63-5**). When using this approach, the flanking markers must be appropriate and informative on both sides of the gene to avoid possible error because of a recombination event. Many single nucleotide polymorphisms have been identified throughout the genome, and these can also be used for marker analysis. The importance of DNA analysis for sibling diagnosis has been demonstrated by the occurrence of occasional heterozygotes with borderline normal results in copper parameters such as ceruloplasmin, urinary copper, and even liver copper.

When sibling diagnosis by haplotype is carried out without mutation analysis, the initial patient must have an unequivocal diagnosis of Wilson disease. This analysis assumes that there is no other similar disease of copper storage, and such is the case, given our present knowledge. Very rare patients with an uncharacterized congenital glycosylation disorder who have isolated liver disease (hepatic steatosis with

abnormal serum aminotransferases and subnormal ceruloplasmin but entirely normal basal 24-hour urinary copper excretion) have been described.[94] An important issue is whether mutations in *COMMD1* could cause copper storage in humans. No mutations of *COMMD1* were identified in a series of patients with early-onset childhood cirrhosis or in 24 patients with some features of copper storage.[95] These findings were confirmed in a larger study from Italy.[96] In another study, a polymorphic codon alteration that resulted in no change in amino acid appeared to influence age at onset.[97] There is still no rigorous evidence that mutations in *COMMD1* cause a human hereditary copper toxicosis.

In the absence of marker analysis or until these results are available, screening should include physical examination, liver function tests, serum copper and ceruloplasmin, 24-hour urinary copper measurement, and a careful slit-lamp examination of the eyes. Children 6 years old or younger who appear to be unaffected should be rechecked at annual intervals over the next 5 to 10 years. Genetic screening with the use of flanking markers or by direct mutation analysis remains the most reliable way of identifying affected siblings when the patient's DNA is available. For deceased patients, tissue from autopsy or biopsy can be used.

Thus far, clinical Wilson disease has not developed in any known heterozygotes, and liver tissue from a heterozygote is approved for living donor liver transplantation. Confirmation of genotype is highly recommended before treatment is initiated because a heterozygote should not unnecessarily be consigned to lifelong treatment with the inherent risk for adverse side effects. Then again, some mutations may be functionally more severe than others. Reassessment of heterozygotes for hepatic copper accumulation at approximately 50 years of age may have merit. Surveillance should include liver function tests, serum copper and ceruloplasmin, basal 24-hour urinary copper excretion, and a liver sonogram. If total body copper overload is detected, treatment with zinc might be considered, although no clinical studies are currently available to determine whether treatment is ever warranted. Heterozygotes should be counseled to maintain good liver health by avoiding abdominal obesity and excessive use of alcohol.

Diagnosis by Population Screening

Mass screening of infants or very young children is an emerging diagnostic intervention related to Wilson disease. Various methods have been proposed and investigated.[98-100] The rationale for such testing is that early diagnosis with institution of treatment affords the best prognosis for patients with Wilson disease. Various technical issues require further refinement. Mass screening may not identify all affected individuals. It potentially avoids the difficulties associated with confirming the diagnosis of Wilson disease in patients who have atypical clinical findings. Importantly, what still remains uncertain is the optimal age for starting treatment and the best treatment to use in patients identified by very early mass screening.

Treatment

Medical treatment of Wilson disease involves either chelation or induction of metallothioneins (**Table 63-1**). Treatment options appear limited[38,101]; however, effective pharmacologic

Table 63-1 Treatment of Wilson Disease

DRUG	DOSE	ASSESSMENT OF EFFICACY	MONITORING OF SIDE EFFECTS
D-Penicillamine*	Initial: 1-1.5 g/day (adult) or 20 mg/kg/day (child), divided into 2 or 3 equal oral doses	24-h urinary copper: 200-500 µg (3-8 µmol)/day as a target	Complete blood count, urinalysis, skin examination
	Maintenance: 0.75-1 g/day (in 2 doses) orally to maintain cupruresis		
Trientine	Initial: 1-1.5 g/day (adult) or approximately 20 mg/kg/day (child), divided into 2 or 3 equal doses orally	24-h urinary copper: 200-500 µg (3-8 µmol)/day as a target	Complete blood count, urinalysis, serum iron and iron-binding capacity
	Maintenance: same		
Zinc	Initial: 50 mg elemental zinc/day (adult) or 25 mg elemental zinc/day (child 5-12 years old), 3 times/day orally, ≥1 h away from meals if possible	24-h urinary copper: <75 µg (1.2 µmol)/ day as a target[†]	Serum creatinine, urinalysis, serum zinc (also to monitor compliance), serum AST and ALT
	Maintenance: titrate the dose as required to achieve indicators of efficacy		

*Plus pyridoxine, 25-50 mg daily by mouth.

[†]Urinary copper excretion in 24 hours generally reflects the total body copper load and can be used to monitor zinc treatment, even though zinc does not cause cupruresis; alternatively, an estimated serum non–ceruloplasmin-bound copper of less than 150 µg/L can be used.

ALT, alanine aminotransferase; ASP, aspartate aminotransferase

therapy can be found for most patients. Based on extensive clinical experience with chronic chelator treatment, it is evident that most patients live normal, healthy lives with effective treatment. There are two generally accepted oral chelating agents: D-penicillamine and trientine. The potent chelator tetrathiomolybdate is relatively new and remains an experimental treatment modality. Zinc interferes with copper uptake from the intestinal contents and stabilizes hepatic copper by inducing metallothioneins. Early institution of treatment is critical to the overall success of treatment. The outcome is best for patients who begin treatment when their disease is diagnosed before the onset of symptoms ("presymptomatic"). The role of adjunctive treatments such as antioxidants has not been formally established, and the potential utility of gene transfer therapy is currently undetermined. New treatments based on improving the intracellular function of misfolded mutant versions of the Wilson ATPase are being developed.[102]

Chelation

Penicillamine was introduced in 1956 by Walshe, has been the first-line treatment of Wilson disease for decades, and is effective in most patients. Penicillamine is the sulfhydryl-containing amino acid cysteine substituted with two methyl groups (β,β-dimethylcysteine). D-Penicillamine is in clinical use. It can be administered orally and is rapidly absorbed with bioavailability on the order of 50%. D-Penicillamine greatly increases urinary excretion of copper. Studies in the Long-Evans cinnamon rat model of Wilson disease indicate that penicillamine inhibits the accumulation of copper in hepatocellular lysosomes and, once accumulated, solubilizes copper for mobilization from these particles, but not from cytoplasmic metallothionein.[103] The action of D-penicillamine involves reductive chelation in which copper bound to proteins as Cu^{+2} is reduced to Cu^+, thus diminishing the affinity of the protein for copper and permitting chelation to D-penicillamine.[104] Copper is incompletely removed from the liver by D-penicillamine. In addition to its chelating action, D-penicillamine inhibits collagen crosslinking and acts as an immunosuppressant.

D-Penicillamine is effective, but it can have serious adverse side effects. In some patients a febrile reaction with rash and proteinuria develops within the first 7 to 10 days after beginning treatment. Although D-penicillamine can be restarted slowly, along with corticosteroids, changing to an alternative chelator may be safer and has become the customary management. The neurologic status of patients with neurologic Wilson disease may deteriorate initially after D-penicillamine treatment is started; the reported frequency of this effect varies widely, with the typical incidence being in the 10% to 22% range. Structural changes in the central nervous system have been reported. Most, but certainly not all, patients recover despite continued use of D-penicillamine. Recent evidence supports discontinuing D-penicillamine and substituting an alternative treatment, usually zinc.[105] Use of D-penicillamine as a first-line drug for the treatment of neurologic Wilson disease is currently being reevaluated.

A host of other adverse side effects can occur at any time during chronic treatment. Some side effects are minor (loss of taste, gastrointestinal upset, and arthralgias), whereas others are severe (proteinuria, leukopenia, or thrombocytopenia). Aplastic anemia occurs rarely and does not always reverse when use of D-penicillamine is stopped. Nephrotic syndrome, Goodpasture syndrome, myasthenia syndrome, and a systemic disease resembling lupus erythematosus have all been reported. All these severe side effects require immediate discontinuation of D-penicillamine and use of a different chelator. A severe-enough adverse effect of D-penicillamine that change in treatment is required develops in up to 30% of patients with Wilson disease.[106] Hepatotoxicity of D-penicillamine itself has occasionally been suspected. Adverse reactions involving the skin include an assortment of rashes but, more importantly, pemphigus and elastosis perforans serpiginosa. D-Penicillamine is intrinsically less toxic than L-penicillamine, which is why the racemic mixture is not used. Some chronic toxicities such as optic neuritis may be due to pyridoxine insufficiency, and accordingly, pyridoxine supplementation (25 to 50 mg by mouth daily) is routine with D-penicillamine use.

The overall safety of lifelong treatment with D-penicillamine is unknown. Quality of life in patients with Wilson disease may be compromised by drug toxicity. Patients who have taken D-penicillamine may have chronic skin changes with loss of elastic tissue or other significant skin lesions.[107] Whether the antifibrotic effect weakens vascular connective tissues is not known. Anecdotal observations suggest that damage to collagen may accrue over decades in patients maintained indefinitely on D-penicillamine, but this risk has not been adequately assessed. Chronic depletion of copper can occur, as shown by complete absence of enzymatically active ceruloplasmin[50] or very low 24-hour urinary copper excretion, but it seems to be a rare consequence of long-term treatment at appropriate maintenance doses. Patients taking D-penicillamine long-term should be maintained on the lowest effective dose, preferably taken before meals.

Trientine, or triethylene tetramine dihydrochloride (2,2,2-tetramine; official short name, trien), introduced by Walshe in the early 1980s, is the usual second-line treatment for patients intolerant of D-penicillamine. A major logistic problem with its clinical use is that it remains an orphan drug, neither universally available nor absolutely ensured to remain in pharmaceutical production. Trientine differs chemically from D-penicillamine; as a polyamine chelator, it has a different structure and lacks sulfhydryl groups. Copper is chelated by forming a stable complex with the four constituent nitrogens in a planar ring. Trientine increases urinary copper excretion and may interfere with intestinal absorption of copper.[108,109] Trientine is a less potent chelator than D-penicillamine, but this difference is not clinically important.

Trientine is relatively nontoxic, apart from causing occasional gastritis and inducing iron deficiency, apparently by chelating dietary iron. Bone marrow suppression may occur but is rare. Sideroblastic anemia has rarely been reported. Neurologic worsening after beginning treatment with trientine may occur. Most importantly, the adverse effects of D-penicillamine resolve and do not recur when patients intolerant of D-penicillamine are converted to treatment with trientine. Trientine appears to be an attractive first-line treatment, but sufficient clinical data are lacking to permit this recommendation as a routine. It is well tolerated in adults[110] and children.[111] Its use in pregnancy is based on favorable, but extremely limited, experience. Apart from use in patients with Wilson disease, trientine is being investigated for treatment of

cardiovascular and renal disease in diabetics because of its antioxidant effects.

Ammonium tetrathiomolybdate may be especially suitable for the treatment of severe neurologic Wilson disease because unlike D-penicillamine, it is not associated with early neurologic deterioration.[112,113] Tetrathiomolybdate interferes with copper absorption from the intestine and binds to plasma copper with high affinity. Studies in Long-Evans cinnamon rats indicate that unlike D-penicillamine, tetrathiomolybdate removes copper from metallothionein at low doses; at higher doses, an insoluble copper complex is deposited in the liver.[114] Even though tetrathiomolybdate is regarded as nontoxic, bone marrow suppression is an important and potentially serious adverse side effect, although it may be due to copper deficiency.[115] Serum aminotransferase elevations may occur with treatment. Little is known about where the mobilized copper, as well as molybdate, might be deposited. Cerebral deposition of molybdate is associated with an organic brain syndrome. The dose and length of treatment, in addition to long-term side effects, must still be determined, but short-term use for acute neurologic involvement may be the role for this drug. Systemic copper deficiency might be associated with prolonged use of this potent copper-binding drug. Tetrathiomolybdate also has antiangiogenic action.[116] Its use is investigational.

Induction of Metallothioneins and Interference with Absorption

Zinc, used in Europe since the late 1960s, has been extensively developed as a treatment modality in North America in the past 20 years. Its mechanism of action differs from that of chelators. In pharmacologic doses, zinc interferes with absorption of copper from the gastrointestinal tract and increases copper excretion in stool. Induction of metallothionein in enterocytes is the principal mechanism of action. This metallothionein has greater affinity for copper than for zinc and preferentially binds copper from the intestinal contents. Once bound, the copper is not absorbed but is lost in feces as enterocytes are shed in normal turnover. Because some non–ceruloplasmin-bound copper is secreted into the intestinal contents through gastric and pancreatic secretions and bile, chronic treatment can lead to an overall decrement in total body copper stores. Although copper induces hepatic metallothionein, it is possible that zinc also has this effect because the hepatic parenchymal copper concentration does not decrease during chronic treatment with zinc.

Zinc treatment appears to be effective, with few adverse side effects.[117,118] Recent studies in children support these observations.[119] In a randomized controlled trial comparing D-penicillamine and zinc sulfate, both were equally effective in stabilizing the clinical disease, but adverse side effects were more numerous with D-penicillamine. Gastritis is the most common side effect with zinc. Use of salts other than sulfate may minimize the gastritis, but any zinc salt is equally acceptable for the treatment of Wilson disease. Food interferes with effectiveness, and some authors recommend taking no food for 1 hour before or after the zinc dose. This tends to increase the severity of gastritis and may be sufficiently inconvenient to compromise compliance, such as in adolescents. An alternative approach is to be less strict about taking zinc away from mealtimes but to titrate the dose against the estimated serum non–ceruloplasmin-bound copper concentration.

Rare patients experience deterioration in hepatic Wilson disease when zinc therapy is started. Zinc may have immuno-suppressant effects and may reduce leukocyte chemotaxis. Studies in rats suggest possible interference with bone formation. Zinc excess is associated with increased serum cholesterol, but in the doses used for Wilson disease, the adverse effects on blood lipids appear to be very modest. Zinc interferes with the absorption of quinolone antibiotics. The long-term effectiveness and adverse side effects of zinc are currently being assessed. Although the data available indicate that chronic zinc therapy is effective and comparatively non-toxic,[101,118] outcomes may vary. Comparison of long-term outcomes with zinc monotherapy in patients with Wilson disease have indicated that hepatic Wilson disease may not be as well treated with zinc as neurologic Wilson disease.[120] Problems with adherence seem to be the main contributor to clinical deterioration. In one recent study, comparison of cerebral MRI showed progressive structural deterioration with zinc monotherapy as compared with D-penicillamine treatment, although no functional deterioration was found in the zinc-treated patients.[121] Patients with Wilson disease treated long-term with zinc monotherapy require regular detailed follow-up for changes in serum aminotransferase and neurologic status.

The combination of zinc with a conventional chelator (D-penicillamine or trientine) has become a popular treatment strategy despite a lack of laboratory studies to provide a rationale or systematic clinical evidence as validation. If zinc and a chelator are used together, the two types of treatment must be temporally dispersed through the day, with at least 4 to 5 hours between administration of either drug, or else they may neutralize each other. In general, the routine is to alternate the drugs through the day at 6-hour intervals such that zinc, 50 mg elemental, is given as the first and third doses and D-penicillamine or trientine (250 or 500 mg) given as the second and fourth doses. The regimen thus involves taking some medication four times a day. This intensive treatment may thus be best suited to patients with very severe hepatic or neurologic disease, in whom it has mainly been used.[122,123] It is fundamentally an induction regimen, suitable for a treatment duration of approximately 3 to 6 months; patients who respond and stabilize clinically can then be transitioned to a simpler standard regimen, either full-dose zinc or full-dose chelator monotherapy. The limited clinical data available suggest that of the two chelators in clinical use, trientine is preferable for this therapeutic strategy, but further data are required before the strategy can be recommended confidently. Prompt diagnosis and early institution of pharmacologic treatment in patients with severe hepatic decompensation but without encephalopathy may be critical.[28,124]

Conversion to zinc monotherapy in patients initially treated with a chelator is an important, relatively new aspect of the clinical management of Wilson disease. A patient eligible for this change in treatment should be clinically well, with normal serum aminotransferase levels and good hepatic synthetic function. In general, the change to zinc from chelator is not made until the patient has been satisfactorily treated with chelator for 1 to 5 years; laboratory test results reflecting copper status should be normal or stable.[38] Limited clinical data about such treatment conversion are currently available. Patients should be aware that zinc therapy may be less convenient

than the twice-daily dosing schedule for a chelator. Adherence to drug treatment remains the key issue. No patient should be permitted to discontinue treatment indefinitely (unless, of course, the patient has received a liver transplant).

Antioxidants

Antioxidants such as α-tocopherol may be an important adjunctive treatment of Wilson disease, either to prevent or to reverse progressive liver damage, but its value remains theoretical. The clinical importance of low serum levels of vitamin E in patients with Wilson disease is unclear.[27] Anecdotal evidence favors the use of α-tocopherol in patients with severe hepatic decompensation; however, rigorous clinical data related to this strategy are not available. Conventional pharmacologic doses (400 IU by mouth daily) might be considered as an adjunct to definitive treatment. Likewise, the role of N-acetylcysteine as treatment of severe hepatic Wilson disease has not yet been investigated systematically. Selenium appears to be sufficient in Wilson disease.

Dietary Management

Most patients should eliminate copper-rich foods from their diet, especially during the first year of treatment. Although detailed dietary management can be designed, the main foods to be avoided are organ meats, shellfish, nuts, chocolate, and mushrooms. In the North American diet, the main problem is eliminating chocolate. Vegetarians require specific dietary counseling. If there is reason to believe that the drinking water is high in copper, the water should be analyzed and a copper-removing device possibly installed in the plumbing system. Dietary management alone is not sufficient to establish control of the disease. Attention to adequacy of the nutritional components supporting good bone health (as well as pertinent lifestyle habits) should be part of the management plan for patients with Wilson disease.

Liver Transplantation

The role of liver transplantation for Wilson disease is limited, but it can be lifesaving. Fulminant hepatic failure in patients with Wilson disease necessitates liver transplantation for recovery. Some patients with severe liver disease that is unresponsive to drug therapy may also proceed to early transplantation. The potential for rescue by combination therapy with temporally dispersed trientine plus zinc, used along with vitamin E and other antioxidants, has not been well explored. It has not been established that liver transplantation improves severe neurologic disease. Favorable[125] and unfavorable[92,126] results have been reported, but experience is limited and subject to subtle bias. On balance, this intervention cannot be recommended, especially since its rationale is not apparent. Therefore liver transplantation should be reserved for patients with severe, decompensated liver disease unresponsive to therapy or for those with fulminant failure. Living related transplants, in which the graft may be from a heterozygote, have been found to function adequately, albeit with minor defects in copper disposition, as encountered in heterozygotes.

Survival rates after liver transplantation for Wilson disease are highly favorable, on the order of 70% to 88% or greater in early studies[127,128] and recent smaller studies[129,130] and also in those with exclusively living related donors.[131,132] The renal failure that often accompanies the fulminant liver failure in patients with Wilson disease generally resolves in the post-transplant period. Kayser-Fleischer rings resorb after liver transplantation. Pediatric patients with Wilson disease may be more prone than other children undergoing liver transplantation to neurologic complications after liver transplantation.[133] Patients with neuropsychiatric features of Wilson disease may have poorer outcomes after liver transplantation, in part because of difficulties adhering to the medical regimen.[134]

Gene Therapy

Liver cell transplantation has shown promising results in various animal models.[135,136] The practicality of gene transfer therapy requires further investigation, although good outcomes have been reported in experimental models.[137-139] After further refinement, these could be effective curative strategies in the future.[140]

Special Situations

Pregnancy

Treatment must be continued throughout pregnancy. There is a risk for postpartum hepatic decompensation if treatment is stopped altogether. Many successful pregnancies have been carried out during D-penicillamine treatment,[141-143] although D-penicillamine is regarded as carrying a 5% risk for fetotoxicity. The severe collagen defects reported occasionally in the offspring could in part be due to copper deficiency from prolonged aggressive treatment, as well as from the teratogenic effects of D-penicillamine.[144] Zinc treatment may pose less risk for adverse effects on developing collagen in the fetus.[145] Trientine has also been used as treatment during pregnancy.[146,147] Judicious reduction of the dose of D-penicillamine or trientine, by approximately 25% of the prepregnancy dose, is advisable in the third trimester, especially if delivery by cesarean section is anticipated.[38,148] Meticulous attention to diet, iron sufficiency, and folic acid supplementation is important in pregnant women with Wilson disease. The absence of enzymatically active ceruloplasmin may be a possible early sign of copper depletion, a problem of uncertain significance for the fetus.

Women with undiagnosed and thus untreated Wilson disease may have difficulty conceiving and maintaining pregnancy if they do conceive.[143,149] Wilson disease should be part of the differential diagnosis of recurrent spontaneous abortion. Copper accumulates in the placenta in untreated Wilson disease. Both the Wilson and Menkes ATPases play important roles in copper, as well as possibly iron, homeostasis in the maternal-fetal unit.[150] Parous women with Wilson disease require counseling regarding contraception because some contraceptive drugs are not tolerated well with chronic liver disease. They should not use copper-containing intrauterine devices.

No firm consensus exists whether a mother who has Wilson disease should breastfeed her infant. The disease itself does not appear to impose a contraindication. D-Penicillamine can enter breast milk and is potentially toxic to the infant. Therefore taking D-penicillamine, even in relatively low doses, is regarded as a contraindication to breastfeeding. The safety of trientine is not known, and it is not clear whether trientine is secreted into breast milk. Zinc is secreted into breast milk, and although its safety is uncertain, breastfeeding seems to be acceptable. The currently available data are too limited to make any firm recommendations. Caution should be exercised.

Fulminant Liver Failure

With at least 80 cases reported and additional cases in liver transplantation databases, this form of Wilson disease is more common than was initially supposed.[151,152] It accounts for approximately one third of all patients with Wilson disease undergoing liver transplantation. Although chronic liver disease (usually cirrhosis) is present, the diagnosis is not initially suspected. Wilsonian fulminant hepatic failure occurs predominantly in females. Most patients are in the 10- to 30-year-old age bracket, but a few very young children have been reported with Wilsonian fulminant liver failure. The fulminant liver failure form of Wilson disease has clinical and biochemical features that, when considered together, distinguish it from acute liver failure associated with acute viral infection or drug hepatotoxicity. Coombs-negative acute intravascular hemolysis occurs. Renal failure is often present and progresses rapidly. If the patient has not been suspected of having underlying liver disease, fulminant viral hepatitis is usually the working diagnosis. Unlike fulminant viral hepatitis, fulminant Wilson disease is usually characterized by serum aminotransferases that are disproportionately low (usually <2000 U/L) for the severity of the liver failure from the onset of clinically apparent disease. Serum alkaline phosphatase levels are strikingly reduced—in the normal range or even low for age,[153] although the mechanism of this distinctive finding remains obscure. Serum bilirubin levels may be very high because of hemolysis. Urinary copper excretion is greatly elevated, as is the estimated non–ceruloplasmin-bound copper concentration; however, these results may not be available soon enough to be diagnostically useful. Slit-lamp examination, if it can be performed, may reveal Kayser-Fleischer rings.

Simple biochemical indices for the diagnosis or prognostication of Wilsonian fulminant hepatic failure have been formulated. In some patients, the level of aspartate aminotransferases (AST) is higher than that of alanine aminotransferases (ALT), thus suggesting a primary mitochondrial lesion, but this is not a reliable feature of the disorder. The most recent iteration of a simple biochemical index is a combination of the ratio of alkaline phosphatase to total bilirubin of less than 4 and a aminotransferases ratio (AST/ALT) of less than 2.2; this combination, calculated in American units, appears to be more helpful for the diagnosis of Wilsonian fulminant hepatic failure in adults than is serum ceruloplasmin.[154] In children with Wilsonian fulminant hepatic failure, this ratio, in international units per micromole, was less than 2, and it distinguished patients with Wilson disease from those with fulminant hepatic failure of other cause.[155] An index based on serum AST, total serum bilirubin, and prolongation of the prothrombin time identifies cases of Wilsonian fulminant hepatic failure with fair accuracy but fails to prognosticate cases of decompensated chronic hepatic Wilson disease.[156] A recent revision of this index, consisting of total serum bilirubin, white blood count, international normalized ratio (INR), serum albumin, and serum AST, showed excellent predictive value, with the threshold for a bad prognosis being a score of 11.[35] These indices may be helpful in difficult cases.

Very rarely, patients with Wilson disease have acute liver failure because of intercurrent viral hepatitis. The clinical and biochemical features may then be those typical of viral hepatitis. Concurrent chronic hepatitis C in a patient with Wilson disease has also been reported.

Liver biopsy findings in Wilsonian fulminant hepatic failure usually reveal cirrhosis with intracellular copper detectable in both hepatocytes and Kupffer cells.[157] Extensive hepatocellular apoptosis may account for this disease pattern.[158]

Patients with typical Wilsonian fulminant hepatic failure require liver transplantation urgently. Referral to a transplant center should not be delayed. They do not respond to chelation treatment, although this may be instituted. Plasmapheresis and exchange transfusion,[159] hemofiltration,[160] or hemodialysis can be used to minimize renal injury before liver transplantation. Albumin dialysis[161,162] and related techniques, including the molecular adsorbent recycling system,[163] may serve as valuable temporizing measures until liver transplantation can be performed. In general, these measures delay, but do not eliminate, the need for liver transplantation in patients with established Wilsonian fulminant hepatic failure; a single exception to this experience has been reported.[164]

With Wilson disease, variations in the clinical pattern of ostensibly acute liver failure need to be recognized. If the contemporary, more inclusive definition of acute liver failure is used—namely, new-onset liver disease with coagulopathy (INR >1.5) and any grade of hepatic encephalopathy—some patients with Wilson disease in whom decompensated chronic liver disease with some degree of lethargy is present initially may be classified as having Wilsonian fulminant hepatic failure. Such patients do not necessarily end up requiring liver transplantation.[165] Intensive treatment with trientine plus zinc, as described previously, may be effective. Very early institution of albumin dialysis may interrupt the downward course.[166-168] In some patients with Wilson disease and rapidly progressive liver failure, intractable liver disease has developed because of failure to adhere to the treatment regimen. Whether the same intensive clinical management can salvage such patients without liver transplantation has not been established. Nevertheless, with any patient who has Wilson disease and is in liver failure, arrangement for liver transplantation as a possible intervention is recommended.

Disease Complications

Patients who stop taking all treatment have a very poor prognosis. New neurologic abnormalities, such as dysarthria, may develop. Rapidly progressive hepatic decompensation has been observed; it occurs on average within 3 years but has been reported as early as 8 months after stopping treatment. This reactivated liver damage is usually refractory to reinstitution of chelator therapy. These patients typically require liver transplantation.

Consideration of Risk for Copper Deficiency

Deficiencies in trace metals may develop with the use of any chelator, although it is not yet clear whether these deficiencies are clinically important. Abnormal iron metabolism leading to hepatic iron overload and anemia, as in hereditary aceruloplasminemia, can be predicted if ceruloplasmin oxidase activity is reduced to zero.[50] Likewise, this activity is very low or not measurable in patients with severe copper deficiency because of overly aggressive chelation therapy.

Prognosis and Natural History

Patients with Wilson disease are generally regarded as having a good prognosis if the disease is diagnosed promptly and treated consistently. Presymptomatic siblings, with the condition diagnosed on biochemical or genetic grounds before any sign of clinical impairment, have the best long-term outlook with prompt institution of treatment. The best time to begin treatment in very young asymptomatic children has not been established. Treatment of infants and very young children must be evaluated carefully in view of the risk associated with copper depletion during a critical period of growth. Patients with early hepatic disease have a generally favorable prognosis as long as treatment is consistent and well tolerated. Severe neurologic disease may not resolve entirely with treatment. Adequate adherence to an effective drug regimen may be the most important prognosticator apart from early diagnosis.

Conclusion

Wilson disease is an uncommon disorder of copper disposition that affects mainly the liver and brain. The pattern of inheritance is autosomal recessive. Its distribution is worldwide, with an average incidence of 30 affected individuals per million population; the incidence is higher in some more isolated populations. Numerous mutations have been identified since the gene was first cloned in 1993. Compound heterozygotes predominate. This may account in part for the clinical heterogeneity and has certainly made it more difficult to find correlations between genotype and phenotype. Treatment is usually very effective, but these patients require regular follow-up to monitor clinical well-being, compliance, and the possible development of adverse effects of long-term drug treatment.

Key References

Aagaard NK, et al. A 15-year-old girl with severe hemolytic Wilson's crisis recovered without transplantation after extracorporeal circulation with the Prometheus system. Blood Purif 2009;28:102–107. (Ref.164)

Ala A, et al. Wilson disease in septuagenarian siblings: raising the bar for diagnosis. Hepatology 2005;41:668–670. (Ref.29)

Allen KJ, et al. Liver cell transplantation leads to repopulation and functional correction in a mouse model of Wilson's disease. J Gastroenterol Hepatol 2004;19:1283–1290. (Ref.136)

Arnon R, et al. Wilson disease in children: serum aminotransferases and urinary copper on triethylene tetramine dihydrochloride (trientine) treatment. J Pediatr Gastroenterol Nutr 2007;44:596–602. (Ref.111)

Asfaha S, et al. Plasmapheresis for hemolytic crisis and impending acute liver failure in Wilson disease. J Clin Apher 2007;22:295–298. (Ref.166)

Askari FK, et al. Treatment of Wilson's disease with zinc. XVIII. Initial treatment of the hepatic decompensation presentation with trientine and zinc. J Lab Clin Med 2003;142:385–390. (Ref.122)

Bartee MY, Lutsenko S. Hepatic copper-transporting ATPase ATP7B: function and inactivation at the molecular and cellular level. Biometals 2007;20: 627–637. (Ref.9)

Becuwe C, et al. Elastosis perforans serpiginosa associated with pseudo-pseudoxanthoma elasticum during treatment of Wilson's disease with penicillamine. Dermatology 2005;210:60–63. (Ref.107)

Brewer GJ. Tetrathiomolybdate anticopper therapy for Wilson's disease inhibits angiogenesis, fibrosis and inflammation. J Cell Mol Med 2003;7:11–20. (Ref.116)

Brewer GJ. Neurologically presenting Wilson's disease: epidemiology, pathophysiology and treatment. CNS Drugs 2005;19:185–192. (Ref.41)

Brewer GJ, et al. Treatment of Wilson disease with ammonium tetrathiomolybdate: IV. Comparison of tetrathiomolybdate and trientine in a double-blind study of treatment of the neurologic presentation of Wilson disease. Arch Neurol 2006;63:521–527. (Ref.113)

Brewer GJ, et al. Treatment of Wilson disease with ammonium tetrathiomolybdate: III. Initial therapy in a total of 55 neurologically affected patients and follow-up with zinc therapy. Arch Neurol 2003;60:379–385. (Ref.112)

Burstein E, et al. A novel role for XIAP in copper homeostasis through regulation of MURR1. EMBO J 2004;23:244–254. (Ref.19)

Burstein E, et al. COMMD proteins: a novel family of structural and functional homologs of MURR1. J Biol Chem 2005;280:22222–22232. (Ref.20)

Cater MA, et al. ATP7B mediates vesicular sequestration of copper: insight into biliary copper excretion. Gastroenterology 2005;130:493–506. (Ref.13)

Chiu A, Tsoi NS, Fan ST. Use of the molecular adsorbents recirculating system as a treatment for acute decompensated Wilson disease. Liver Transpl 2008;14: 1512–1516. (Ref.167)

Collins KL, et al. Single pass albumin dialysis (SPAD) in fulminant Wilsonian liver failure: a case report. Pediatr Nephrol 2008;23:1013–1016. (Ref.162)

Coronado VA, et al. COMMD1 (MURR1) as a candidate in patients with copper storage disease of undefined etiology. Clin Genet 2005;68:548–551. (Ref.95)

Coronado VA, et al. New haplotypes in the Bedlington terrier indicate complexity in copper toxicosis. Mamm Genome 2003;14:483–491. (Ref.17)

Czlonkowska A, Gromadzka G, Chabik G. Monozygotic female twins discordant for phenotype of Wilson's disease. Mov Disord 2009;24:1066–1069. (Ref.91)

Davies LP, Macintyre G, Cox DW. New mutations in the Wilson disease gene, ATP7B: implications for molecular testing. Genet Test 2008;12:139–145. (Ref.70)

de Bie P, et al. Molecular pathogenesis of Wilson and Menkes disease: correlation of mutations with molecular defects and disease phenotypes. J Med Genet 2007;44:673–688. (Ref.88)

Deguti MM, et al. Wilson disease: novel mutations in the ATP7B gene and clinical correlation in Brazilian patients. Hum Mutat 2004;23:398. (Ref.79)

deWilde A, et al. Tryptic peptide analysis of ceruloplasmin in dried blood spots using liquid chromatography–tandem mass spectrometry: application to newborn screening. Clin Chem 2008;54:1961–1968. (Ref.100)

Dhawan A, et al. Wilson's disease in children: 37-year experience and revised King's score for liver transplantation. Liver Transpl 2005;11:441–448. (Ref.35)

Dolgova NV, et al. The soluble metal-binding domain of the copper transporter ATP7B binds and detoxifies cisplatin. Biochem J 2009;419:51–56, 3 p following 56. (Ref.22)

Dufner-Beattie J, et al. Structure, function, and regulation of a subfamily of mouse zinc transporter genes. J Biol Chem 2003;278:50142–50150. (Ref.23)

Efremov RG, et al. Molecular modelling of the nucleotide-binding domain of Wilson's disease protein: location of the ATP-binding site, domain dynamics and potential effects of the major disease mutations. Biochem J 2004;382: 293–305. (Ref.81)

Eisenach C, et al. Diagnostic criteria for acute liver failure due to Wilson disease. World J Gastroenterol 2007;13:1711–1714. (Ref.165)

Erol I, et al. Neurological complications of liver transplantation in pediatric patients: a single center experience. Pediatr Transplant 2007;11:152–159. (Ref.133)

Ferenci P, et al. Diagnosis and phenotypic classification of Wilson disease. Liver Int 2003;23:139–142. (Ref.33)

Ferenci P, et al. Diagnostic value of quantitative hepatic copper determination in patients with Wilson's disease. Clin Gastroenterol Hepatol 2005;3:811–818. (Ref.59)

Gojova L, et al. Genotyping microarray as a novel approach for the detection of ATP7B gene mutations in patients with Wilson disease. Clin Genet 2008;73: 441–452. (Ref.69)

Gu YH, et al. Mutation spectrum and polymorphisms in ATP7B identified on direct sequencing of all exons in Chinese Han and Hui ethnic patients with Wilson's disease. Clin Genet 2003;64:479–484. (Ref.75)

Hardman B, et al. Distinct functional roles for the Menkes and Wilson copper translocating P-type ATPases in human placental cells. Cell Physiol Biochem 2007;20:1073–1084. (Ref.150)

Hernandez S, et al. ATP7B copper-regulated traffic and association with the tight junctions: copper excretion into the bile. Gastroenterology 2008;134: 1215–1223. (Ref.15)

Hsi G, Cox DW. A comparison of the mutation spectra of Menkes disease and Wilson disease. Hum Genet 2004;114:165–172. (Ref.80)

Hsi G, et al. Sequence variation in the ATP-binding domain of the Wilson disease transporter, ATP7B, affects copper transport in a yeast model system. Hum Mutat 2008;29:491-501. (Ref.84)

Huster D, et al. Defective cellular localization of mutant ATP7B in Wilson's disease patients and hepatoma cell lines. Gastroenterology 2003;124:335–345. (Ref.85)

Huster D, et al. Rapid detection of mutations in Wilson disease gene ATP7B by DNA strip technology. Clin Chem Lab Med 2004;42:507–510. (Ref.78)

Kenney SM, Cox DW. Sequence variation database for the Wilson disease copper transporter, ATP7B. Hum Mutat 2007;28:1171-1177. (Ref.67)

Koppikar S, Dhawan A. Evaluation of the scoring system for the diagnosis of Wilson's disease in children. Liver Int 2005;25:680–681. (Ref.34)

Korman JD, et al. Screening for Wilson disease in acute liver failure: a comparison of currently available diagnostic tests. Hepatology 2008;48: 1167–1174. (Ref.154)

Kozic D, et al. MR imaging of the brain in patients with hepatic form of Wilson's disease. Eur J Neurol 2003;10:587–592. (Ref.61)

Kroll CA, et al. Retrospective determination of ceruloplasmin in newborn screening blood spots of patients with Wilson disease. Mol Genet Metab 2006;89:134–138. (Ref.98)

La Fontaine S, Mercer JF. Trafficking of the copper-ATPases, ATP7A and ATP7B: role in copper homeostasis. Arch Biochem Biophys 2007;463:149–167. (Ref.10)

Leiros da Costa M, et al. Wilson's disease: two treatment modalities. Correlations to pretreatment and posttreatment brain MRI. Neuroradiology 2009;51: 627–633. (Ref.121)

Lim CM, et al. Copper-dependent interaction of dynactin subunit p62 with the N terminus of ATP7B but not ATP7A. J Biol Chem 2006;281:14006–14014. (Ref.14)

Linn FH, et al. Long-term exclusive zinc monotherapy in symptomatic Wilson disease: experience in 17 patients. Hepatology 2009;50:1442–1452. (Ref.120)

Lovicu M, et al. The canine copper toxicosis gene MURR1 is not implicated in the pathogenesis of Wilson disease. J Gastroenterol 2006;41:582–587. (Ref.96)

Lovicu M, et al. Efficient strategy for molecular diagnosis of Wilson disease in the Sardinian population. Clin Chem 2003;49:496–498. (Ref.77)

Lovicu M, et al. RNA analysis of consensus sequence splicing mutations: implications for the diagnosis of Wilson disease. Genet Test Mol Biomarkers 2009;13:185–191. (Ref.71)

Lu J, et al. Triethylenetetramine and metabolites: levels in relation to copper and zinc excretion in urine of healthy volunteers and type 2 diabetic patients. Drug Metab Dispos 2007;35:221–227. (Ref.109)

Luoma LM, et al. Functional analysis of mutations in the ATP loop of the Wilson disease copper transporter, ATP7B. Hum Mutat 2010;31:569-577. (Ref.86)

Macintyre G, et al. Value of an enzymatic assay for the determination of serum ceruloplasmin. J Lab Clin Med 2004;144:294–301. (Ref.50)

Mak CM, Lam CW, Tam S. Diagnostic accuracy of serum ceruloplasmin in Wilson disease: determination of sensitivity and specificity by ROC curve analysis among ATP7B-genotyped subjects. Clin Chem 2008;54:1356–1362. (Ref.48)

Mandato C, et al. Cryptogenic liver disease in four children: a novel congenital disorder of glycosylation. Pediatr Res 2006;59:293–298. (Ref.94)

Manolaki N, et al. Wilson disease in children: analysis of 57 cases. J Pediatr Gastroenterol Nutr 2009;48:72–77. (Ref.36)

Marcellini M, et al. Treatment of Wilson's disease with zinc from the time of diagnosis in pediatric patients: a single-hospital, 10-year follow-up study. J Lab Clin Med 2005;145:139–143. (Ref.119)

Markiewicz-Kijewska M, et al. Liver transplantation for fulminant Wilson's disease in children. Ann Transplant 2008;13:28–31. (Ref.168)

Martin AP, et al. A single-center experience with liver transplantation for Wilson's disease. Clin Transplant 2008;22:216–221. (Ref.129)

McMillin GA, Travis JJ, Hunt JW. Direct measurement of free copper in serum or plasma ultrafiltrate. Am J Clin Pathol 2009;131:160–165. (Ref.53)

Medici V, et al. Liver transplantation for Wilson's disease: the burden of neurological and psychiatric disorder. Liver Transpl 2005;11:1056–1063. (Ref.134)

Medici V, et al. Diagnosis and management of Wilson's disease: results of a single center experience. J Clin Gastroenterol 2006;40:936–941. (Ref.30)

Meng Y, et al. Restoration of copper metabolism and rescue of hepatic abnormalities in LEC rats, an animal model of Wilson disease, by expression of human ATP7B gene. Biochim Biophys Acta 2004;1690:208–219. (Ref.139)

Merle U, et al. Serum ceruloplasmin oxidase activity is a sensitive and highly specific diagnostic marker for Wilson's disease. J Hepatol 2009;51:925–930. (Ref.49)

Merle U, et al. Clinical presentation, diagnosis and long-term outcome of Wilson's disease: a cohort study. Gut 2007;56:115–120. (Ref.32)

Merle U, et al. Truncating mutations in the Wilson disease gene ATP7B are associated with very low serum ceruloplasmin oxidase activity and an early onset of Wilson disease. BMC Gastroenterol 2010;10:8. (Ref.90)

Muller T, et al. Re-evaluation of the penicillamine challenge test in the diagnosis of Wilson's disease in children. J Hepatol 2007;47:270–276. (Ref.57)

Nagata Y, et al. Bridging use of plasma exchange and continuous hemodiafiltration before living donor liver transplantation in fulminant Wilson's disease. Intern Med 2003;42:967–970. (Ref.160)

Nakayama K, et al. Early and presymptomatic detection of Wilson's disease at the mandatory 3-year-old medical health care examination in Hokkaido Prefecture with the use of a novel automated urinary ceruloplasmin assay. Mol Genet Metab 2008;94:363–367. (Ref.99)

Ng PC, Henikoff S. SIFT: predicting amino acid changes that affect protein function. Nucleic Acids Res 2003;31:3812–3814. (Ref.82)

Nuttall KL, Palaty J, Lockitch G. Reference limits for copper and iron in liver biopsies. Ann Clin Lab Sci 2003;33:443–450. (Ref.58)

Pabon V, et al. Long-term results of liver transplantation for Wilson's disease. Gastroenterol Clin Biol 2008;32:378–381. (Ref.130)

Panagiotakaki E, et al. Genotype-phenotype correlations for a wide spectrum of mutations in the Wilson disease gene (ATP7B). Am J Med Genet A 2004;131A:168–173. (Ref.89)

Piga M, et al. Brain MRI and SPECT in the diagnosis of early neurological involvement in Wilson's disease. Eur J Nucl Med Mol Imaging 2008;35:716–724. (Ref.62)

Pinter R, Hogge WA, McPherson E. Infant with severe penicillamine embryopathy born to a woman with Wilson disease. Am J Med Genet A 2004;128:294–298. (Ref.144)

Roberts EA, et al. Diagnosis and outcome of Wilson disease in a paediatric cohort [abstract]. J Pediatr Gastroenterol Nutr 2004;39(Suppl 1):A128. (Ref.54)

Roberts EA, Robinson BH, Yang S. Mitochondrial structure and function in the untreated Jackson toxic milk (tx-j) mouse, a model for Wilson disease. Mol Genet Metab 2008;93:54–65. (Ref.66)

Roberts EA, Schilsky ML. Diagnosis and treatment of Wilson disease: an update. Hepatology 2008;47:2089–2111. (Ref.38)

Rodriguez-Granillo A, Crespo A, Wittung-Stafshede P. Conformational dynamics of metal-binding domains in Wilson disease protein: molecular insights into selective copper transfer. Biochemistry 2009;48:5849–5863. (Ref.11)

Safaei R, et al. The role of copper transporters in the development of resistance to Pt drugs. J Inorg Biochem 2004;98:1607–1613. (Ref.21)

Savas N, et al. Hepatocellular carcinoma in Wilson's disease: a rare association in childhood. Pediatr Transplant 2006;10:639–643. (Ref.40)

Schilsky ML. Wilson disease: current status and the future. Biochimie 2009;91:1278–1281. (Ref.140)

Senzolo M, et al. Different neurological outcome of liver transplantation for Wilson's disease in two homozygotic twins. Clin Neurol Neurosurg 2007;109:71–75. (Ref.92)

Seth R, et al. In vitro assessment of copper-induced toxicity in the human hepatoma line, Hep G2. Toxicol In Vitro 2004;18:501–509. (Ref.25)

Sinha S, et al. Successful pregnancies and abortions in symptomatic and asymptomatic Wilson's disease. J Neurol Sci 2004;217:37–40. (Ref.143)

Stapelbroek JM, et al. The H1069Q mutation in ATP7B is associated with late and neurologic presentation in Wilson disease: results of a meta-analysis. J Hepatol 2004;41:758–763. (Ref.73)

Stuehler B, et al. Analysis of the human homologue of the canine copper toxicosis gene MURR1 in Wilson disease patients. J Mol Med 2004;82:629–634. (Ref.97)

Sutcliffe RP, et al. Liver transplantation for Wilson's disease: long-term results and quality-of-life assessment. Transplantation 2003;75:1003–1006. (Ref.128)

Taly AB, et al. Wilson disease: description of 282 patients evaluated over 3 decades. Medicine (Baltimore) 2007;86:112–121. (Ref.31)

Tao TY, et al. The copper toxicosis gene product Murr1 directly interacts with the Wilson disease protein. J Biol Chem 2003;278:41593–41596. (Ref.18)

Tissieres P, et al. Fulminant Wilson's disease in children: appraisal of a critical diagnosis. Pediatr Crit Care Med 2003;4:338–343. (Ref.155)

Turski ML, Thiele DJ. New roles for copper metabolism in cell proliferation, signaling, and disease. J Biol Chem 2009;284:717–721. (Ref.7)

Valbonesi M, et al. Role of intensive PEX in a patient with fulminant hepatic failure due to Wilson's disease (WD) in preparation for orthotopic liver transplantation (OLT). Int J Artif Organs 2003;26:965–966. (Ref.159)

van den Berghe PV, et al. Reduced expression of ATP7B affected by Wilson disease–causing mutations is rescued by pharmacological folding chaperones 4-phenylbutyrate and curcumin. Hepatology 2009;50:1783–1795. (Ref.102)

Walshe JM. The conquest of Wilson's disease. Brain 2009;132:2289–2295. (Ref.2)

Walshe JM, et al. Abdominal malignancies in patients with Wilson's disease. QJM 2003;96:657–662. (Ref.39)

Wiggelinkhuizen M, et al. Systematic review: clinical efficacy of chelator agents and zinc in the initial treatment of Wilson disease, Aliment Pharmacol Ther 2009;29:947–958. (Ref.101)

Yoshitoshi EY, et al. Long-term outcomes for 32 cases of Wilson's disease after living-donor liver transplantation. Transplantation 2009;87:261–267. (Ref.132)

A complete list of references can be found at www.expertconsult.com.

Hemochromatosis

Paul C. Adams

ABBREVIATIONS

ALT alanine aminotransferase
AST aspartate aminotransferase
Dcytb duodenal cytochrome *b*
DMT1 divalent metal transport protein-1

ESR erythrocyte sedimentation rate
HFE hemochromatosis gene
HIV human immunodeficiency virus
HJV juvenile hemochromatosis gene

HLA human leukocyte antigen
LDL low-density lipoprotein
MHC major histocompatibility complex
MRI magnetic resonance imaging

Introduction

Hemochromatosis is the most common genetic disease in populations of European ancestry. Despite estimates based on genetic testing that hemochromatosis is present in 1 of every 200 Caucasians, many physicians consider hemochromatosis to be a rare disease. The diagnosis can be elusive because of the nonspecific nature of the symptoms. The discovery of the hemochromatosis gene (*HFE*) in 1996[1] has provided new insights into the pathogenesis of the disease and innovative diagnostic strategies.[2]

A fundamental issue that has arisen since the discovery of the *HFE* gene is whether the disease "hemochromatosis" should be defined strictly on the basis of phenotype, such as the degree of iron overload (as measured by transferrin saturation, ferritin level, liver biopsy results, hepatic iron concentration, iron removed by venesection therapy), or be defined on the basis of genotype, because it is a familial disease in Europeans most commonly associated with C282Y mutation of the *HFE* gene and varying degrees of iron overload. It is important to realize that there are many causes of iron overload other than hemochromatosis (**Table 64-1**) and there are a growing number of new non-*HFE* genetic mutations that can be associated with iron overload.[3]

History of Hemochromatosis

In 1865 Trousseau described an association between cirrhosis of the liver, diabetes, pancreatic disease, and pigmentation of the skin. These clinical features are associated with advanced stages of the disease and are now rarely seen by clinicians. The term hemochromatosis was used by Von Recklinghausen in 1889 because he suspected that the increased pigment originated from the blood. Many variations in the nomenclature have been suggested (e.g., *HFE*-linked hemochromatosis,

hereditary hemochromatosis, iron overload disease). In 1935 Sheldon published his classic monograph, summarizing his results from 311 cases.[4] The relative roles of genes and alcoholism were debated for many years but the familial aspects of the disease were clearly elucidated in pedigree studies by Simon in Brittany, France, in 1977, including a close linkage of the disease to the human leukocyte antigen (HLA) complex on chromosome 6. Genetic studies concentrated on this region of the chromosome but informative genetic recombinations were rarely found. The hemochromatosis gene (*HFE*) was finally discovered a long distance from the HLA complex by Mercator Genetics in 1996.[1] This discovery led to the development of a simple genetic blood test that has demonstrated that more than 90% of typical hemochromatosis patients are homozygous for the C282Y mutation of the *HFE* gene.

Most patients with hemochromatosis can trace their ancestry to northern Europe. Because of the high prevalence of hemochromatosis in Brittany, it has been hypothesized that the original couple with hemochromatosis were born in Brittany around 800 AD. Many people from Brittany crossed the English Channel during the Norman Conquest in 1066 and resettled in the United Kingdom, and currently residents of Wales and Ireland share traditional language and music with Brittany.

Because the Vikings were exploring Brittany extensively during those years, it is possible that some of the original genes were of Nordic ancestry. Further evidence for this hypothesis can be ascertained from the high prevalence of the *HFE* gene in Iceland, which was explored by the Vikings but not by French explorers. However, Irish women may have been absconded by the Vikings to Iceland. Furthermore, there has been evidence presented that the gene originated much earlier in mainland Europe before 4000 BC.[5] The hemochromatosis gene can be used as a genetic marker to study the migration of Europeans to North and South America, South Africa, and Australia. Most studies have linked *HFE*-related hemochromatosis to northern Europe but there is also a high prevalence of this condition in Portugal.[6]

Table 64-1 Differential Diagnosis of Iron Overload

HFE-Related Hemochromatosis

C282Y homozygotes (95%)
C282Y/H63D compound heterozygotes (4%)
H63D homozygotes (1%)

Non–HFE-Related Hemochromatosis

Ferroportin disease
Transferrin receptor 2 mutation
Juvenile hemochromatosis (young adults with cardiac and
  endocrine dysfunction)

Miscellaneous Iron Overload

African American iron overload
African iron overload
Transfusional iron overload
Insulin resistance–related iron overload
Aceruloplasminemia
Alcoholic siderosis
Iron overload secondary to end-stage cirrhosis
Porphyria cutanea tarda
Post-portacaval shunt

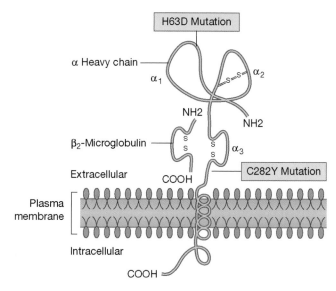

Fig. 64-1 Schematic representation of the *HFE* protein, with the location of the common mutations for hemochromatosis illustrated.

Epidemiology

The typical genetic pattern (C282Y homozygote) is found in approximately 1 in 227 Caucasians.[7] However, the clinical symptoms of hemochromatosis are much less common and many of the symptoms are nonspecific. The regions with the highest prevalence of hemochromatosis are Ireland, northern Portugal, western France, and regions where migration from these countries has occurred (Australia, Canada, United States, South Africa).[6] Iron overload can occur from a variety of genetic and environmental factors and the geographic distribution of iron overload is much broader than that for *HFE*-linked hemochromatosis.

Pathogenesis of Hemochromatosis

In healthy people, most dietary iron is absorbed from the proximal duodenum. Both ionic iron and heme iron are absorbed across the enterocyte at the tip of the intestinal villi. The mechanisms involved in the absorption of heme iron have not been established. In regard to non-heme iron absorption, it is becoming more apparent that there is a cascade of iron-related proteins involved in normal and abnormal iron absorption. This concept is similar to the cascade of events that occurs with blood coagulation or complement activation. In hemochromatosis, increased iron absorption from the intestine and inappropriate iron absorption in the presence of total body iron overload occur. There is a disruption of the regulation of iron absorption and whether this occurs at the level of the intestinal enterocyte or at a more distant site is a subject of current research. Iron proteins at the brush border include divalent metal transport protein-1 (DMT1) and duodenal cytochrome *b* (Dcytb), a ferrireductase. Iron transport within the enterocyte has not been well-defined but a number of iron-related proteins including transferrin, transferrin

receptor, ferritin, iron regulatory peptide, and hepcidin have been described. The transfer of iron from the enterocyte into the portal circulation involves another series of transport proteins including hephaestin and ferroportin (IREG1) (**Fig. 64-1**).[3,8]

The *HFE* gene produces a major histocompatibility complex (MHC) class 1 protein (see **Fig. 64-1**) that is expressed in many cells but has a high concentration in the duodenal crypts. It interacts with transferrin receptor to facilitate iron uptake into cells. In hemochromatosis, patients have a mutated *HFE* protein, resulting in a conformational change in the protein that alters the interaction between the *HFE* protein and transferrin receptor. The C282Y mutation has a more pronounced effect on *HFE* protein function than the H63D mutation. Because the *HFE* protein is not abundant at the intestinal villus where iron absorption occurs, it has been necessary to implicate other iron proteins in the pathogenesis of hemochromatosis.[9]

Hepcidin is a hepatic peptide that may be the key regulator of iron metabolism. Hepcidin deficiency in knockout mice results in severe iron overload.[10] Hepcidin may also have a direct effect on the uptake of iron by intestinal epithelia.[11] Conversely, a relative deficiency of hepcidin can result in increased iron efflux from macrophages. This is consistent with the paradoxical observation in *HFE*-related hemochromatosis of relative iron deficiency in the spleen and within macrophages. Hepcidin expression in liver tissue, serum, and urine has suggested a relative deficiency in *HFE*-linked hemochromatosis.[12] However, at the present time it is unclear whether the defect in hepcidin is the primary abnormality in hemochromatosis, or a downstream effect of abnormalities in the *HFE* protein. The control of hepcidin may be related to a cellular iron-sensing mechanism that includes bone morphogenetic protein-6 (BMP6), transferrin receptors 1 and 2, *HFE* protein, hemojuvelin, and Smad proteins (**Fig. 64-2**).[13-16] It is intriguing to speculate whether alterations in non-*HFE* iron proteins could explain the wide range of clinical expression seen in hemochromatosis. The concept is that the most severe

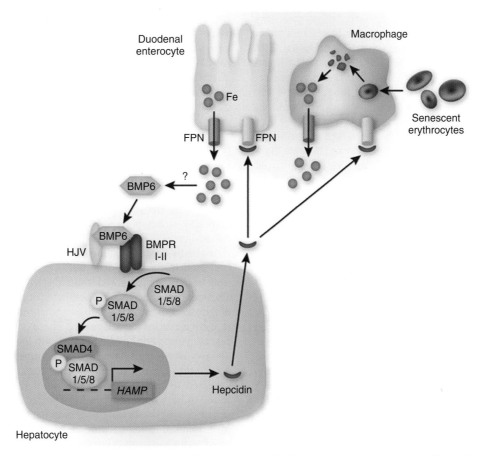

Fig. 64-2 Schematic representation of the *HFE* protein, a class 1 MHC protein that is involved in iron metabolism with a cascade of other iron proteins. Typical hemochromatosis patients are homozygous for the C282Y mutation of *HFE,* which cause conformational changes in the protein that impair intracellular trafficking. BMP, bone morphogenetic protein; Fe, iron; HJV, juvenile hemochromatosis gene

cases of *HFE*-related hemochromatosis may be heterozygotes for a mutation in another iron-related protein. These mutations would need to be very common to fit this hypothesis. A tantalizing theory has been suggested that the hemochromatosis gene has not been found yet and that the *HFE* gene is only a modifying gene.[17]

Clinical Features of Hemochromatosis

A major problem has been the attribution of clinical symptoms in hemochromatosis to iron overload. Earlier studies did not use control populations and recent population screening studies have drawn increasing attention to the nonspecific nature of the clinical symptoms, such as arthralgias, fatigue, and even diabetes. It has been assumed that the symptoms of hemochromatosis are related to iron overload causing tissue injury. However, iron depletion does not reverse many of the symptoms of hemochromatosis. Of all the putative symptoms of hemochromatosis, liver disease is the most consistent. A prospective study of C282Y homozygotes in Australia suggested that 28% of men and only 1% of women have iron-related symptoms.[18] Although the disease was originally called "bronze diabetes," several studies have now suggested that the prevalence of diabetes is similar between

C282Y homozygotes and a control population.[19,20] The study of the possible symptoms in C282Y homozygotes without biochemical iron overload may provide more information on the relationship of symptoms to the degree of iron overload. Another unresolved issue is whether early iron depletion in an asymptomatic C282Y homozygote will prevent the development of symptoms.

Liver Disease

Although hemochromatosis is often classified as a liver disease, it should be emphasized that it is a systemic genetic disease with multisystem involvement. The liver has a great capacity to accumulate iron within hepatocytes initially without any obvious sequelae in terms of both clinical symptoms and abnormal liver biochemistry results. Because hepatic iron presumably accumulates from birth in this genetic disease, a relationship between iron level and age is predictable. However, this may only apply serially within an individual patient because the correlation coefficient between age and hepatic iron concentration was not significant in 410 homozygotes ($r = 0.07$; $P = .12$).[21] Hepatomegaly remains one of the more common physical signs in hemochromatosis but may not be present in the young asymptomatic homozygote. In older studies in which patients presented with clinical features of chronic liver disease in the fifth or sixth decade, cirrhosis was invariably present. Because patients are detected as young adults through pedigree studies or population screening studies, the prevalence of cirrhosis is much lower. In a study of 410 referred homozygotes from Canada and France, 22% had cirrhosis of the liver at the time of diagnosis. The mean aspartate aminotransferase (AST) and alanine aminotransferase (ALT) values were within the normal range in these 410 patients. Cirrhotic patients and patients with concomitant alcohol abuse were more likely to have abnormal levels of liver enzymes.[22] A clinical presentation with marked elevations in liver enzymes and iron levels should suggest an alternate diagnosis such as alcoholic liver disease, chronic viral hepatitis, or nonalcoholic steatohepatitis. A study of the critical hepatic iron concentration associated with cirrhosis in C282Y homozygotes using receiver operating characteristic curve analysis suggested that the critical iron concentration was greater than 283 μmol/g (normal, 0 to 35 μmol/g).[23] However, there were many patients with much higher liver iron concentrations who did not have cirrhosis. Liver damage at lower iron concentrations was usually associated with other risk factors such as alcohol abuse or chronic viral hepatitis. Therefore it seems likely that factors other than iron overload contribute to the development of cirrhosis in hemochromatosis.[24] It should also be emphasized that women can have significant liver involvement in hemochromatosis. In a study of 176 women matched with males for year of birth, there was no difference in the hepatic iron concentration.[22] Many of these studies are subject to referral bias with only the sickest patients being sent for medical evaluation. Population screening studies have rarely identified patients with cirrhosis.[25-27]

Hepatocellular carcinoma has been described in 18.5% of cirrhotic patients with hemochromatosis.[28] It has rarely been described in noncirrhotic hemochromatosis patients. The relative risk is approximately 200-fold, which is similar to that for cirrhotic patients with chronic viral hepatitis. Screening for hepatocellular carcinoma remains a controversial topic because of the expense of the screening program, the shortage of organs available for liver transplantation, and the small number of candidates who are cured by surgical resection. In the case of the hemochromatosis patient with cirrhosis, screening could be considered but this is not an evidence-based recommendation.

Diabetes in Hemochromatosis

Many patients with cirrhosis of any origin have glucose intolerance or diabetes and this is true for hemochromatosis patients as well. The presence of diabetes in hemochromatosis is usually related to the presence of liver disease and glucose intolerance; diabetes has been found in 85% of hemochromatosis patients with cirrhosis.[29] There has also been a higher prevalence of diabetes found in family members of hemochromatosis patients with diabetes. Earlier morphologic studies of iron deposition in the pancreas suggested pancreatic damage as the cause of diabetes. However, subsequent studies have demonstrated that the presence of high circulating insulin levels (insulin resistance secondary to liver disease) is more common than low circulating insulin levels[30] related to islet cell damage. Metabolic studies of insulin and glucose have not clearly demonstrated a reversal of these changes with iron depletion.[31,32] This is consistent with the clinical observation that diabetes rarely resolves with therapy. Insulin resistance in obese patients has also been associated with iron overload in

patients without the typical genetic profile for hemochromatosis.[33] Most of these cases have a moderate elevation in serum ferritin level with a normal transferrin saturation. However, most obese patients with elevated ferritin concentrations have normal liver iron concentrations and likely manifest a mild elevation in serum ferritin level (<1000 μg/L) secondary to steatohepatitis.

Cardiac Disease in Hemochromatosis

Cardiac disease in hemochromatosis includes both cardiomyopathy and arrhythmias. In a series of 410 patients, cardiac disease was only present in 10% of probands and 3% of discovered cases.[21] Dyspnea is the most common symptom associated with dilated cardiomyopathy. Echocardiography is the preferred initial diagnostic test. The cardiac iron concentration is significantly lower than the liver iron concentration. Transvenous cardiac biopsies have occasionally missed the diagnosis of hemochromatosis and should not be considered to have excluded the diagnosis. There have been uncommon cases of young adults who present with life-threatening cardiac disease. These cases have been called juvenile hemochromatosis and the gene for juvenile hemochromatosis (*HJV*) has been localized to chromosome 1. Some of these cases have been found to have mutations in the hepcidin gene.[34] These patients can also have life-threatening ventricular arrhythmias requiring implantable defibrillators or potentially hepatotoxic medications such as amiodarone. Cardiac dysfunction is more common in secondary iron overload conditions such as thalassemia and is a common cause of death. C282Y homozygotes have been demonstrated to have lower levels of total cholesterol and low-density lipoprotein (LDL) cholesterol than in a control population.[35,36]

Arthropathy of Hemochromatosis

Arthralgias are perhaps the most common symptom of hemochromatosis. Pain is typically reported in the proximal interphalangeal joints of the hands, but the wrists, shoulders, knees, and feet are commonly affected. The features of the arthropathy are more similar to osteoarthritis and less commonly chondrocalcinosis. Radiologic features are often nonspecific but on occasion the diagnosis is suggested by an astute radiologist. Subchondral cyst formation, osteopenia, squaring of the metacarpophalangeal joint heads, and chondrocalcinosis have all been described in patients with hemochromatosis. Joint complaints are particularly common in women. Arthritis has been demonstrated to be the major factor affecting quality of life in hemochromatosis.[37] Because arthritis is common in the general population, it has been difficult to attribute the arthritis in an aging population to hemochromatosis.

Endocrine Abnormalities

The most common symptom of endocrine dysfunction is impotence in men with hemochromatosis. This has been estimated to be present in 40% of cases and is almost universal in male cirrhotic patients. Most cases will have low levels of luteinizing and follicle-stimulating hormones and low levels of testosterone. Amenorrhea and infertility can be seen in women. Hypothyroidism is a less common endocrine manifestation of hemochromatosis. Hemochromatosis patients are predisposed to osteoporosis. This is likely related to the low testosterone level and an independent effect of cirrhosis. Many patients will receive testosterone supplementation without a major effect on their impotence but possibly an improvement in bone density. The effect of androgens potentially increasing the risk of hepatocellular carcinoma in a cirrhotic hemochromatosis patient is another consideration in the clinical management.

Pigmentation of the Skin

The characteristic pigmentation of hemochromatosis is caused by melanin, not iron. In the late stages of hemochromatosis, iron can be seen in the sweat glands and in the basal layers of the epidermis. The prevalence of pigmentation depends to an extent on the age of the patient and the severity of the iron overload. It was estimated to be present in 47% of proband cases and 18% of discovered cases[37] but, like all signs and symptoms of hemochromatosis, is observed less frequently because of earlier diagnosis.

Infections

Yersinia infections have been described in cases of hemochromatosis and secondary iron overload. Other infections have included *Pasteurella pseudotuberculosis, Vibrio vulnificus,* and *Listeria monocytogenes.* It has been implied that the bacterial iron metabolism of these species encourages their growth in an iron-rich environment.

Fatigue

Although a nonspecific symptom, fatigue is one of the most common reported symptoms of hemochromatosis. The presence of fatigue often leads to biochemical iron studies and the physician who was expecting a low value is surprised to find iron overload. Because more than half of patients attending a general medical clinic complain of fatigue, this has been one of the most difficult symptoms to attribute to hemochromatosis. Screening projects within chronic fatigue syndrome clinics have not demonstrated an enhanced case detection for hemochromatosis.

Diagnosis of Hemochromatosis

A paradox of genetic hemochromatosis is the observation that the disease is underdiagnosed in the general population and overdiagnosed in patients with secondary iron overload. A case definition that appeals to all experts has been elusive.[38] Minimum criteria for the diagnosis of hemochromatosis are increased iron stores in the absence of a cause for secondary iron overload. Genetic testing for *HFE* mutations (C282Y and H63D) has been a major advance, with a single mutation explaining most typical cases; however, there are a growing number of new genetic mutations in other genes that make an *HFE*-specific case definition unsatisfactory. The original descriptions of 311 cases of iron overload described by

Sheldon in 1935[4] were likely C282Y related, and many experts continue to use the presence of homozygosity for the C282Y mutation of the *HFE* gene as the cornerstone for the diagnosis of hemochromatosis. A more broad case definition dependent on the degree of iron overload in the liver or the existence of iron mobilized by phlebotomy allows for the consideration of an expanding number of newer genetic mutations that may result in iron overload. An increasing awareness that iron overload can be a sequelae of a wide range of chronic liver diseases has led to many previous cases of "hemochromatosis" being reclassified as iron overload secondary to cirrhosis. From a practical perspective, the clinician should not get too immersed in the debate about whether an individual patient has "hemochromatosis" because this is largely a semantic debate. The focus should be on identifying treatable causes of iron overload and initiating the appropriate diagnostic tests and therapies in the patient and other affected family members.

Underdiagnosis of Hemochromatosis

Many physicians consider hemochromatosis to be a rare disease. This belief is due to a lack of penetrance of the gene (nonexpressing homozygote) and failure of physicians to consider the diagnosis. It is likely that both of these factors are contributory. A major problem in the diagnosis of hemochromatosis is the lack of symptoms and the nonspecific nature of symptoms. An elderly patient who presents with joint symptoms and diabetes is rarely considered to have genetic hemochromatosis. Many patients assume that the routine blood tests done frequently at ambulatory clinics would have tested their iron status; however, unless iron deficiency is suspected, measurement of iron level is not in the usual panel of blood tests. The presenting features vary depending on age and gender but fatigue is the most common complaint. Women are more likely to have fatigue, arthralgia, and pigmentation rather than liver disease.[22]

Diagnostic Tests for Hemochromatosis

A number of diagnostic algorithms based on laboratory tests have been proposed for the diagnosis of hemochromatosis (**Fig. 64-3**). These should be used as guidelines for the clinician and do not replace clinical judgment based on history and physical examination, imaging studies, pathologic findings, and pedigree studies.

Transferrin Saturation

Transferrin saturation is often elevated in patients with *HFE*-linked hemochromatosis (**Fig. 64-4**). A two-step test that is widely available is used for its determination. Transferrin saturation can be calculated by using the serum iron concentration and one of the following: total iron binding capacity, unsaturated iron binding capacity, or transferrin level. The serum iron concentration, although often elevated in hemochromatosis, has been a less reliable test than the transferrin saturation. The transferrin saturation has been reported to have a sensitivity of greater than 90% for hemochromatosis.

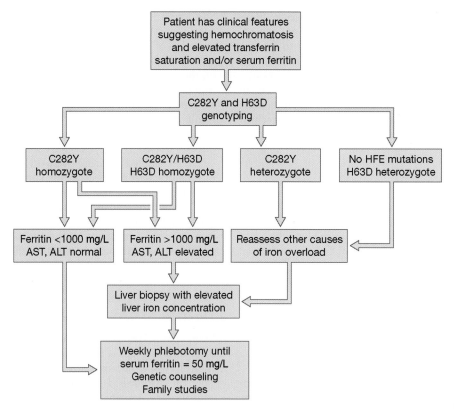

Fig. 64-3 Proposed diagnostic algorithm for patients with suspected hemochromatosis.

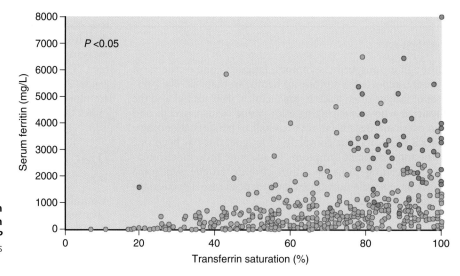

Fig. 64-4 **Relationship between transferrin saturation and serum ferritin concentration in C282Y homozygotes (*n* = 411, *r* = 0.37, *P* < .0001).** The *solid circles* represent patients with cirrhosis.

The sensitivity and specificity of transferrin saturation have usually been established at referral centers where most of the patients have *HFE*-linked hemochromatosis. The sensitivity of transferrin saturation is lower in population screening studies designed to detect C282Y homozygotes and was only 52% (threshold >50%) in a large screening study from San Diego that included a significant number of cases with normal serum ferritin levels.[19] The transferrin saturation continues to have a high sensitivity for the detection of an iron-loaded hemochromatosis patient. Transferrin saturation is often elevated in young adults with hemochromatosis before the development of iron overload or a rise in ferritin concentration. The

threshold to pursue further diagnostic studies has varied from 45% to 62% in previous studies. A lower threshold identifies more patients with hemochromatosis but also leads to more investigations in patients without hemochromatosis. A common threshold used in screening studies is >45% in women and >50% in men. A higher threshold leads to fewer investigations overall with a greater possibility of missing some patients. An elevated transferrin saturation in the presence of a normal serum ferritin level rarely indicates significant iron overload but may be a marker that iron overload may develop over time in that patient. There appears to be a wide biologic variability in transferrin saturation that also

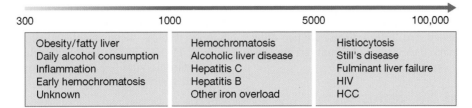

Fig. 64-5 Differential diagnosis of an elevated serum ferritin level differs according to the degree of elevation. Reference range: men, 15 to 200 μg/L; women, 30 to 300 μg/L. HCC, hepatocellular carcinoma; HIV, human immunodeficiency virus

limits its use as a screening test. There is no advantage to using fasting samples versus random samples for the detection of C282Y homozygotes.[39]

Newer genetic mutations may not share this typical pattern of an elevated transferrin saturation and elevated ferritin level. A marked elevation (>1000 μg/L) in the presence of a normal transferrin saturation may still represent significant iron overload and further investigations may be indicated to differentiate iron overload from an inflammatory elevation of ferritin level.

Serum Ferritin Level

The relationship between serum ferritin level and total body iron stores has been clearly established by strong correlations with hepatic iron concentration and amount of iron removed by venesection.[40] However, ferritin level can be elevated secondary to obesity, chronic alcohol consumption, steatohepatitis, chronic inflammation including viral hepatitis, and histiocytic neoplasms. A major diagnostic dilemma in the past was deciding whether the serum ferritin level was related to hemochromatosis or to another underlying liver disease such as alcoholic liver disease, chronic viral hepatitis, or nonalcoholic steatohepatitis (with or without insulin resistance).[41] It is likely that some of these difficult cases will now be resolved by genetic testing. As the ferritin concentration increases, the risk of significant liver disease also increases. The investigation of hyperferritinemia can be challenging. It may be helpful to classify the most common causes of an elevated ferritin level according to the degree of ferritin elevation (**Fig. 64-5**). Extreme elevations of serum ferritin level (>50,000 μg/L) are usually not related to hemochromatosis. Because serum ferritin is a glycosylated protein secreted by macrophages, neoplasms of macrophages, such as histiocytosis, can produce extreme elevations in ferritin level. These diseases can cause elevations in levels of liver enzymes associated with infiltration of the liver, and a variant called histiocytic medullary reticulocytosis can present with acute liver failure.

Elevations of serum ferritin level in the range of 1000 to 5000 μg/L can be associated with clinical hemochromatosis but a careful investigation for hepatitis B and C, alcoholic liver disease, and nonalcoholic steatohepatitis should be considered. If another liver disease is the predominant clinical diagnosis, it is more likely that the ferritin level elevation is secondary to that disease rather than the concomitant presence of genetic hemochromatosis. In this range of serum ferritin concentrations, liver biopsy is often recommended and review of liver pathologic studies, iron staining results, and liver iron concentration measurements is often diagnostic.

Table 64-2 A Clinical Approach to Elevated Serum Ferritin Level

Is this a new or chronic observation?
Is the ferritin level rising?
Is the transferrin saturation elevated?
Is obesity present?
Is daily alcohol consumption present?
Is inflammation present?
Is there a family history of iron overload?

The most common problem is the assessment of mild elevations in serum ferritin level in the range of 300 to 1000 μg/L. The prevalence of an increased serum ferritin level is so common in men that the origin and appropriateness of a reference range of up to 300 μg/L have been questioned. Genetic testing can be useful to detect early hemochromatosis but most cases will have normal *HFE* testing, and heterozygosity for an *HFE* mutation is an unlikely explanation for an elevated ferritin level.[42] Although it had been considered that heterozygotes could have mild iron overload, since genetic testing has become available it has become apparent that most of these apparent heterozygotes with mild iron overload were actually compound heterozygotes (C282Y/H63D).[43] The epidemic of obesity has likely contributed to this high prevalence of ferritin level elevations because fatty liver may be the most common cause of an elevated serum ferritin level. This is assumed to be related in most cases to inflammation secondary to steatohepatitis and not to iron overload.[44] However, many liver biopsies do not show large amounts of inflammatory cells and correlations with inflammatory markers such as C-reactive protein or erythrocyte sedimentation rate (ESR) have been inconsistent. A clinical approach to the assessment of these patients is shown in **Table 64-2**. A liver biopsy is often unappealing to the physician and the patient in the setting of a mild elevation in ferritin concentration. Serial monitoring is often done and a ferritin level exceeding 1000 μg/L is an indication for more investigations or empirical phlebotomy therapy. Noninvasive investigations such as magnetic resonance imaging (MRI) may be most useful in this clinical setting. Phlebotomy therapy can be considered; however, because the ferritin level is more likely to be an inflammatory indicator rather than an indicator of iron overload, the patient will likely become anemic after several phlebotomies without a marked decrease in the serum ferritin level. Voluntary blood donation may also be an alternative in healthy patients.

There are patients with marked elevations in serum ferritin concentration without iron overload. The presence of cataracts at a young age is a clue to the diagnosis of the hyperferritinemia-cataract syndrome.[45] Still disease and human immunodeficiency virus (HIV) disease are two other conditions in which marked elevations of serum ferritin level without iron overload can occur.

Iron Removed by Venesection as Diagnostic Criterion

Because hemochromatosis was usually diagnosed when symptoms developed in the fifth or sixth decade, patients typically had significant iron overload at the time of diagnosis. The weekly removal of 500 ml of blood (0.25 g of iron) was well tolerated often for years without the development of significant anemia. If a patient became anemic (hemoglobin <10 g/dl) after only six venesections, it suggested mild iron overload incompatible with the diagnosis of hereditary hemochromatosis. These guidelines may no longer apply as population and pedigree studies uncover hemochromatosis patients in the second and third decades of life. This is another historic diagnostic criterion for hemochromatosis that will no longer be as relevant in the era of genetic testing. Furthermore, these guidelines were established in C282Y-linked hemochromatosis and patients with other types of iron overload such as aceruloplasminemia and ferroportin mutations commonly become anemic with phlebotomy without achieving iron depletion.

Liver Biopsy

Liver biopsy has previously been the gold standard test for diagnosing hemochromatosis. Liver biopsy has shifted from a major diagnostic tool to a method of estimating prognosis and concomitant disease. The need for liver biopsy seems less clear now in the young asymptomatic C282Y homozygote where there is a low clinical suspicion of cirrhosis based on history, physical examination, and liver biochemistry results. A large study conducted in France and Canada suggested that C282Y homozygotes with a serum ferritin level of less than 1000 µg/L, a normal aspartate aminotransferase (AST) level, and the absence of hepatomegaly have a very low risk of cirrhosis.[46] C282Y homozygotes with a ferritin level higher than1000 µg/L, an elevated AST level, and a platelet count lower than 2.0×10^9/L had a 77% to 81% chance of having cirrhosis.[33] Serum hyaluronic acid has also been used as a noninvasive test to predict cirrhosis in hemochromatosis.[47] Hepatic elastography is another tool being used to assess the presence of fibrosis in hemochromatosis patients.[48]

Liver biopsy has not been widely accepted by hematologists, public health physicians, geneticists, and some hemochromatosis patients, and should always be considered optional. Liver biopsy is considered in typical C282Y homozygotes with liver dysfunction; however, it is most useful in the patient without *HFE* mutations because it may demonstrate that iron overload is not present and therefore phlebotomy therapy is not required. The distribution of iron within the liver can still provide clues to the cause of the iron overload. Typical C282Y-linked hemochromatosis patients have a portal to central vein gradient of iron distribution within hepatocytes. A predominance of iron within macrophages in the absence of transfusions may suggest a ferroportin mutation. If the liver biopsy suggests another diagnosis such as alcoholic hepatitis

or chronic viral hepatitis with patchy iron distribution in macrophages, the iron is likely secondary to the primary disease. Simple C282Y heterozygotes, compound heterozygotes (C282Y/H63D), and patients with other risk factors (alcohol abuse, chronic viral hepatitis) with moderate to severe iron overload (ferritin >1000 µg/L) may be considered for liver biopsy.

Hepatic Iron Concentration and Hepatic Iron Index

The traditional method of assessing iron status by liver biopsy uses the semiquantitative staining method of Perls. This is adequate when there is no iron staining or massive parenchymal iron overload. However, when moderate iron overload is present, the degree of iron overload can be difficult to interpret. There have been more comprehensive methods developed to analyze liver iron staining and distribution but these are not widely utilized. Hepatic iron concentration can be measured using atomic absorption spectrophotometry. This can be done on a piece of paraffin-embedded tissue; therefore special preparation is not required at the time of the biopsy. An advantage of cutting the tissue from the block is that one is more certain that the tissue assayed is the same as the tissue examined under the microscope. For example, a piece of tissue set aside for iron analysis at the time of the biopsy may represent intercostal muscle rather than liver tissue. The normal reference range for hepatic iron concentration is 0 to 35 µmol/g dry weight (<2000 µg/g). The hepatic iron concentration (µmol/g) divided by age (years) is the hepatic iron index. This was demonstrated to be a useful test in differentiating the patient with genetic hemochromatosis from the patient with alcoholic siderosis. The index remains a useful test in this clinical application. A threshold of 1.9 for the hepatic iron index had a 91% sensitivity for hemochromatosis, and the area under the receiver operating characteristic curve was 0.94 (0.9 to 0.99, 95% confidence interval).[49] Early diagnoses in population screening and pedigree studies have demonstrated many homozygotes with a hepatic iron index lower than 1.9. Increasing awareness of the concept of moderate iron overload in cirrhosis of any cause has demonstrated many patients without hemochromatosis but with a hepatic iron index higher than 1.9. The hepatic iron index has become less useful with the advent of genetic testing. Liver biopsy reports should not include statements confirming a diagnosis of genetic hemochromatosis on the basis of a hepatic iron index >1.9. It will remain a tool to aid clinicians with their clinical judgment concerning an individual case. It may be most useful in the unusual hemochromatosis patient who is negative by conventional genetic testing but clinically seems to have genetic hemochromatosis. There are patients with 1 to 2+ iron staining on liver biopsy who have a normal liver iron concentration and the liver iron concentration can be used to assess the need for phlebotomy therapy.

Imaging Studies of the Liver

Magnetic resonance imaging can demonstrate moderate to severe iron overload of the liver. Proponents of MRI have emphasized the noninvasive nature of this test as an advantage over liver biopsy.[50] In a study of 174 patients, Gandon and colleagues demonstrated that a simple MRI protocol could detect hepatic iron overload greater than 60 μmol/g (normal range, 0 to 36 μmol/g) with a sensitivity of 89%.[51] A modification of this protocol was used by a second group in a study of 112 patients in which a correlation coefficient of 0.94 was demonstrated between liver iron concentration and MRI estimation of liver iron concentration.[52] These techniques are improving and may be ideally suited to exclude iron overload in a patient in whom an inflammatory condition may be responsible for the elevations in iron test values, such as severe alcoholic hepatitis. MRI can also demonstrate the clinical features of cirrhosis such as nodularity of the liver, ascites, portal hypertension, and splenomegaly as well as hepatocellular carcinoma, but these features can be more readily assessed by abdominal ultrasound at a lower cost. Magnetic susceptibility has been studied using a superconducting quantum interference device (SQUID) to estimate liver iron concentration but the technology is not widely available.[53]

Genetic Testing for Hemochromatosis

A major advance that stems from the discovery of the hemochromatosis gene (*HFE*) is the use of a diagnostic genetic test. Clinical studies in well-defined hemochromatosis pedigrees reported that 90% to 100% of typical hemochromatosis patients were homozygous for the C282Y mutation of the *HFE* gene. The presence of a single mutation in most patients is in marked contrast to other genetic diseases in which multiple mutations were discovered (cystic fibrosis, Wilson disease, α_1-antitrypsin deficiency). A second minor mutation, H63D, was also described in the original report. This mutation does not cause the same intracellular trafficking defect of the *HFE* protein. Compound heterozygotes (C282Y/H63D) and less commonly H63D homozygotes[54] may resemble C282Y homozygotes with mild to moderate iron overload.[55] These genotypes are much more common than C282Y homozygotes in the general population yet are not commonly reported in large series of typical hemochromatosis patients. Large population studies have demonstrated that most patients with C282Y/H63D or H63D/H63D mutations have normal iron studies.[7,55] A polymorphism on intron 4 of the *HFE* gene (5569A) was independently reported by several laboratories to lead to false-positive genetic testing in which a C282Y heterozygote appears to be a homozygote.[56,57] This should be considered during the evaluation of a "non-expressing" C282Y homozygote. The correct diagnosis can be confirmed by direct DNA sequencing. Other hemochromatosis *HFE* mutations have not been clearly established in large studies to explain iron overload in non-C282Y homozygotes. It is likely that more mutations will be found but they will only be relevant to a minority of patients. The interpretation of the test in several settings is shown in **Table 64-3**.

Genetic discrimination has been a major concern with the widespread use of genetic testing.[58] A positive genetic test even without iron overload could disqualify a patient for health or life insurance. In the largest population screening study (Hemochromatosis and Iron Overload Screening [HEIRS] Study), there was no evidence of genetic discrimination at 1

Table 64-3 Interpretation of Genetic Testing for Hemochromatosis

C282Y Homozygote

This is the classic genetic pattern that is seen in >90% of typical cases. Expression of disease ranges from no evidence of iron overload to massive iron overload with organ dysfunction. Siblings have a 1 in 4 chance of being affected and should have genetic testing. For children to be affected the other parent must be at least a heterozygote. If iron studies are normal, false-positive genetic testing or a nonexpressing homozygote should be considered.

C282Y/H63D Compound Heterozygote

This patient carries one copy of the major mutation and one copy of the minor mutation. Most patients with this genetic pattern have normal iron studies. A small percentage of compound heterozygotes have been found to have mild to moderate iron overload. Severe iron overload is usually seen in the setting of another concomitant risk factor (alcoholism, viral hepatitis).

C282Y Heterozygote

This patient carries one copy of the major mutation. This pattern is seen in about 10% of the Caucasian population and is usually associated with normal iron studies. In rare cases the iron studies are high in the range expected in a homozygote rather than a heterozygote. These cases may carry an unknown hemochromatosis mutation and liver biopsy is helpful to determine the need for venesection therapy.

H63D Homozygote

This patient carries two copies of the minor mutation. Most patients with this genetic pattern have normal iron studies. A small percentage of these cases have been found to have mild to moderate iron overload. Severe iron overload is usually seen in the setting of another concomitant risk factor (alcoholism, viral hepatitis).

H63D Heterozygote

This patient carries one copy of the minor mutation. This pattern is seen in about 20% of the Caucasian population and is usually associated with normal iron studies. This pattern is so common in the general population that the presence of iron overload may be related to another risk factor. Liver biopsy may be required to determine the cause of the iron overload and the need for treatment in these cases.

No HFE Mutations

There are other iron overload diseases associated with mutations in other iron-related genes (transferrin receptor 2, ferroportin, HJV). Genetic testing is not widely available for these conditions. There will likely be other hemochromatosis mutations discovered in the future. If iron overload is present without any *HFE* mutations, a careful history for other risk factors must be reviewed and liver biopsy may be useful to determine the cause of the iron overload and the need for treatment. Most of these cases are isolated, nonfamilial cases.

From Gurrin LC, et al. HFE C282Y/H63D compound heterozygotes are at low risk of hemochromatosis-related morbidity. Hepatology 2009;50:94–101.

year.[59] In the case of hemochromatosis, the advantages of early diagnosis in young adulthood of a treatable disease outweigh the disadvantages of genetic discrimination.

The widespread use of genetic testing for hemochromatosis has also led to misinterpretation of the test results by both the

Table 64-4 Genetic Diseases of Iron Metabolism

CLINICAL FEATURE	*HFE*-LINKED HEMOCHROMATOSIS	FERROPORTIN DISEASE	JUVENILE HEMOCHROMATOSIS	TRANSFERRIN RECEPTOR 2	ACERULOPLASMINEMIA
Gene location	6p21.3	2q32	1q21 (*HJV*), 19q13.1 (hepcidin)	7q22	3q25
Inheritance pattern	Autosomal recessive	Autosomal dominant	Autosomal recessive	Autosomal recessive	Autosomal recessive
Organs involved	Liver, endocrine, heart	Liver, spleen	Heart, endocrine, liver	Liver, endocrine, heart	Retina, basal ganglia, pancreas, liver
Hepatic iron distribution	Hepatocytes	Macrophages	Hepatocytes	Hepatocytes	Hepatocytes
Anemia	No	Yes	No	No	Yes
Response to phlebotomy	Excellent	Anemia	Excellent	Excellent	Anemia

patient and the physician. For example, a H63D heterozygote, which is seen in 1 of 5 Caucasians, may be interpreted as evidence of hemochromatosis. This can occur because of the complexity of the genetic test report, and is also commonly seen when the patient would prefer to attribute their lifestyle-induced liver disease to a genetic problem. In this setting, the patient often accredits every symptom to this genetic test result and may be seeking disability benefits. This is clearly an adverse effect of genetic testing. Genetic testing is not recommended for children because organ damage is not typically seen in childhood and early detection may lead to insurance discrimination, labeling, or stigmatization.

Most cases of familial iron overload are C282Y homozygotes but there are a growing number of less common genetic mutations that may result in iron overload (**Table 64-4**). Some of these conditions have been labeled *HFE2*, *HFE3*, and *HFE4*; however, because they do not refer to mutations in the *HFE* gene, this nomenclature is not recommended. In an isolated case with hepatic iron overload, consideration should first be given to a secondary cause of iron overload. The identification of an iron-loaded family member is a powerful clinical clue to the presence of a genetic disorder in iron metabolism. Siblings have the highest yield in an autosomal recessive disease. Pedigree studies have become difficult in some countries because of geographic separation, differences in healthcare providers, and new privacy legislation.

Ferroportin Disease

Ferroportin-associated iron overload is an autosomal dominant disorder in iron metabolism resulting from a mutation of the *SLC40A1* gene on chromosome 2q32.[60] The ferroportin protein is normally involved in iron transport out of macrophages; consequently, ferroportin mutation results in an accumulation of iron in hepatic macrophages. The typical clinical findings include a progressive elevation in serum ferritin level and mild hypochromic anemia. Transferrin saturation may be normal or rise as the iron overload increases. In an original report from the Netherlands, several cases were described of severe hepatic iron overload with normal transferrin saturation and normal ferritin levels.[61] Liver disease can include

hepatic fibrosis but this is usually less severe than *HFE*-linked hemochromatosis. MRI scanning can demonstrate iron overload in the liver and spleen, in contrast to *HFE*-linked hemochromatosis in which there is a relative paucity of iron in the spleen. Ferroportin mutations have been described in a wide range of ethnic groups and countries including Caucasians, African Americans, and Asians. A ferroportin mutation has been found in a patient from the Solomon Islands, suggesting that the previously described Polynesian iron overload may be related to a ferroportin mutation.[62] Treatment is by a slow phlebotomy protocol (500 ml, once per month) because anemia develops with weekly phlebotomy.

Aceruloplasminemia

The original description of this genetic mutation on chromosome 3q25 was of progressive retinal and basal ganglia degeneration, diabetes, and ataxia. Hepatic iron overload has been demonstrated and serum ceruloplasmin is either absent or present at very low levels. Treatment of this condition has been problematic because of the development of anemia with phlebotomy.[63]

Juvenile Hemochromatosis

The typical clinical profile of a patient with juvenile hemochromatosis was a male in the second or third decade presenting with severe congestive heart failure, ventricular arrhythmias, and hypogonadism. The disease was often fatal and severe iron overload was demonstrated in the liver, heart, and endocrine organs. Although considered to be a single disease, recent advances in the genetics of juvenile hemochromatosis suggest that this is genetically heterogeneous. A gene on chromosome 1 (*HJV*) produces hemojuvelin.[34] This iron protein appears to interact with BMP6 to regulate hepcidin. A growing number of genetic mutations have been described in the *HJV* gene. Mutations in the hepcidin gene on chromosome 19 also produce a clinical presentation similar to that of juvenile hemochromatosis. Treatment of juvenile hemochromatosis may require twice-weekly phlebotomy and careful cardiac supportive care. Phlebotomy can

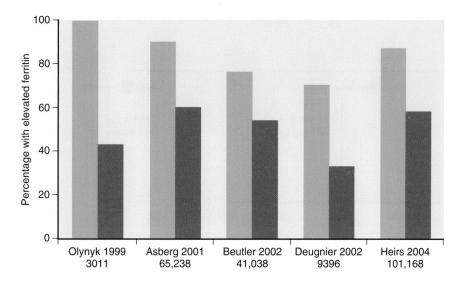

Fig. 64-6 Percentage of C282Y homozygotes (men *[blue]*, women *[green]*) in population screening studies with an elevated serum ferritin level at the time of discovery.

lead to a marked improvement in symptoms and cardiac function. Arrhythmia management can be challenging because chronic amiodarone therapy can be hepatotoxic and many patients have cirrhosis at the time of diagnosis. Pacemakers and implantable defibrillators have been used to manage arrhythmias. Testosterone replacement therapy is often required.

Transferrin Receptor-2 Mutation

Several European family studies have identified mutations in the transferrin receptor-2 gene (chromosome 7q22) associated with hepatic iron overload. The liver findings were similar to those for *HFE*-linked hemochromatosis with a predominance of iron in the hepatocytes. This is an autosomal recessive condition and can be treated by phlebotomy.[64]

Genetic Testing for Non–*HFE* Iron Overload

The genetic tests for mutations in ferroportin, hepcidin, hemojuvelin, and transferrin receptor-2 are not likely to become widely available commercially because of the low prevalence of these mutations. Research centers are more likely to be interested in a pedigree of iron overload before initiating newer genetic tests, which can be expensive and often are uninformative. As more polymorphisms are described, the genotypic–phenotypic correlations have been difficult to establish and it is important to ascertain the prevalence of these new polymorphisms in larger populations of affected and unaffected cases. Newer advances in microarrays and gene chips may allow for the simultaneous identification of multiple iron genes.[65]

Nonexpressing Homozygotes

As genetic testing has become more available, an increasing number of persons have been found who have the hemochromatosis gene but do not have iron overload. This includes siblings within well-defined hemochromatosis pedigrees.[66] Pooled estimates from 14 studies have suggested that 50% of

C282Y homozygotes may not have iron overload.[67] The prevalence of an elevated ferritin level in C282Y homozygotes from screening studies is shown in **Figure 64-6**. The term nonexpressing homozygote has been used for C282Y homozygotes with normal values for ferritin concentration and transferrin saturation or with normal transferrin saturation and elevated ferritin level; in addition, this term can be used for asymptomatic homozygotes with elevated iron tests. Patients who are homozygous for the C282Y mutation should be considered at risk of developing iron overload; however, if there are no abnormalities in transferrin saturation or ferritin concentration in adulthood, it seems more likely that these patients are nonexpressing homozygotes rather than patients in whom iron overload will develop later in life. The risk for development of a serum ferritin level higher than 1000 μg/L has been estimated based on the presenting transferrin saturation, ferritin level, age, and gender from a population study in Melbourne.[68] The follow-up of adult C282Y homozygotes with a normal serum ferritin level has not demonstrated a marked increase in serum ferritin concentration.[69] At the present time it seems appropriate to repeat the serum ferritin and transferrin saturation measurements every 5 years in non–iron-loaded C282Y homozygotes to understand more about their natural history. The study of the nonexpressing homozygote may provide additional information about new modifying genes that counteract the effect of the hemochromatosis gene.

Family Studies in Hemochromatosis

Once the proband case is identified and confirmed with the genetic test for the C282Y mutation, family testing is strongly recommended.[70,71] Siblings have the highest chance of carrying the gene and should be screened with genetic testing (C282Y and H63D mutations) and measurement of transferrin saturation and serum ferritin level (**Fig. 64-7**). Phenotypic expression can vary widely among siblings, suggesting that environmental factors are contributory.[71,72] Patients are

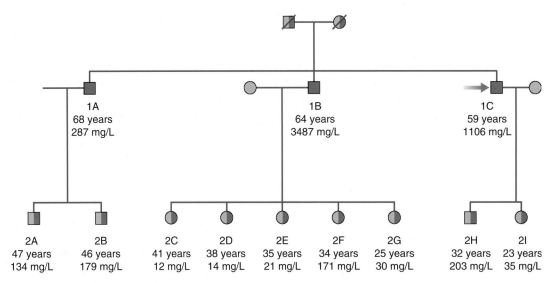

Fig. 64-7 Pedigree in a hemochromatosis family carrying the C282Y mutation. Homozygotes are the single-color symbols and heterozygotes are the dual-colored symbols. Age and serum ferritin concentration are displayed. Note the presence of a nonexpressing 68-year-old C282Y homozygous male with a normal serum ferritin level (1A) with two expressing younger siblings (1B and 1C).

usually very concerned about their children and may have difficulty with the concept of autosomal recessive transmission. The risk to a child is dependent on the prevalence of heterozygotes in the community and is probably greater than 1 in 20 and much lower if the spouse is non-Caucasian.[73] A cost-effective strategy is to test the spouse for the C282Y mutation to assess the risk in the children.[74] If the spouse is not a C282Y heterozygote or homozygote, the children will be obligate heterozygotes. This assumes paternity and excludes another gene or mutation causing hemochromatosis. This strategy is particularly advantageous for situations in which the children are geographically separated or insured by different healthcare systems.

If an isolated heterozygote is detected by genetic testing, it is recommended to test siblings. Extended family studies are less revealing than a family study with a homozygote; however, extended family studies are more likely to uncover a homozygote than random population screening. The risk to family members is illustrated in **Table 64-5**. The impact of the H63D mutation is far less than that of the C282Y mutation.

Genetic counseling for an autosomal recessive disease such as *HFE*-linked hemochromatosis has been within the realm of practice of the gastroenterologist or hepatologist. However, as additional mutations are discovered, new polymorphisms are identified that may contribute to iron overload, and multiple genes are tested simultaneously, genetic counseling becomes far more complex and may require additional support from medical geneticists.

Diagnosis of Non-*HFE* Hemochromatosis and Secondary Iron Overload

It is important to remember that there will be patients who will be negative for the C282Y mutation but who have a clinical presentation indistinguishable from that for genetic hemochromatosis. In non-Caucasians iron overload is not commonly associated with *HFE* mutations.[60] Therefore screening for *HFE* mutations in African Americans and Asians has not been clinically useful. Many Asians have been found to have elevations in serum ferritin level and transferrin saturation, although documented cases of iron overload remain rare.[75] Hispanic populations have been found to have *HFE* mutations, which is likely related to their Spanish heritage. Iron overload and ferroportin mutations have been described in African Americans[75] but many of these cases had other risk factors for iron overload and pedigree studies have not been commonly reported. The iron overload described in sub-Saharan Africans may be related to another iron loading gene,[76] and a linkage to iron overload in African Americans is an intriguing hypothesis that awaits the identification of the responsible gene.

A negative C282Y test should alert the physician to question the diagnosis of genetic hemochromatosis and reconsider secondary iron overload related to cirrhosis, alcohol abuse, viral hepatitis, or iron-loading anemias. If no other risk factors are found, the patient should begin venesection treatment similar to any other hemochromatosis patient. The decision to classify this group of patients as non-*HFE* hemochromatosis or idiopathic iron overload is a matter of semantics and ideology surrounding case definition. Quantification of iron burden by hepatic iron concentration or quantitative phlebotomy will be important to further characterize this group of patients.

In most cases of iron overload secondary to blood diseases, the patient has anemia with iron overload from increased iron absorption and/or multiple transfusions. These patients will not tolerate venesections and will require chelation therapy. A liver biopsy and echocardiogram may be helpful to determine if the secondary iron overload is causing organ damage. Because parenteral deferoxamine therapy has chronic side effects, clinical judgment is required in each case to assess whether the benefits outweigh the toxicity of chelation therapy. Oral iron chelators such as deferasirox and deferiprone have been used in these patients.

Table 64-5 Predicting Risk to Family Members with Hemochromatosis

A. Risks for Iron Overload in Relatives of C282Y/C282Y Proband*

	CHANCE OF					
RISK TO	**C282Y/ C282Y (%)**	**C282Y/C282Y WITH IRON OVERLOAD (%)**	**C282Y/ H63D (%)**	**C282Y/H63D WITH IRON OVERLOAD (%)**	**H63D/ H63D (%)**	**H63D/H63D WITH IRON OVERLOAD (%)**
Father	5.6	5.0	28.5	0.6	Does not occur	0.0
Mother	5.6	2.8	28.5	0.3	Does not occur	0.0
Brother	26.4	23.8	7.9	0.2	0.0	0.0
Sister	26.4	13.2	7.9	0.1	0.0	0.0
Son	5.5	4.9	15.0	0.3	Does not occur	0.0
Daughter	5.5	2.7	15.0	0.2	Does not occur	0.0

B. Risks for Iron Overload in Relatives of C282Y/H63D Proband

	CHANCE OF					
RISK TO	**C282Y/ C282Y (%)**	**C282Y/C282Y WITH IRON OVERLOAD (%)**	**C282Y/ H63D (%)**	**C282Y/H63D WITH IRON OVERLOAD (%)**	**H63D/ H63D (%)**	**H63D/H63D WITH IRON OVERLOAD (%)**
Father	2.8	2.5	20.1	0.4	8.1	0.1
Mother	2.8	1.4	20.1	0.2	8.1	0.0
Brother	1.4	1.3	27.9	0.6	3.8	0.0
Sister	1.4	0.7	27.9	0.3	3.8	0.0
Son	2.7	2.5	10.2	0.2	7.5	0.1
Daughter	2.7	1.4	10.2	0.1	7.5	0.0

Adapted from Adams P, Acton R, Walker A. A primer for predicting risk of disease in HFE-linked hemochromatosis. Genet Testing 2001;5:311–316.

*The risks to family members are based on Hardy-Weinberg equilibrium. It assumes that a Caucasian marries another Caucasian and that there are no paternity issues. The risk to a sibling of a C282Y homozygote is slightly higher than 1 in 4 (25%) at 26.4% because the parents have a rare chance of being C282Y homozygotes or compound heterozygotes. Allele frequency: C282Y = 0.05, H63D = 0.15. Risk of iron overload was based on available estimates from population screening studies and assumes that 90% of male and 50% of female C282Y homozygotes will have elevated iron tests. Risks of iron overload in C282Y/H63D and H63D/H63D homozygotes are much lower because most participants with these genotypes have normal iron studies.

Treatment of *HFE*-Linked Hemochromatosis

Treatment of hemochromatosis continues to be the medieval therapy of periodic bleeding (i.e., phlebotomy). The goal of therapy is to remove excess iron to prevent any further tissue damage. Phlebotomy therapy has never been subjected to a randomized clinical trial and this has hindered our understanding of the natural history of untreated disease. Although most experts believe that iron depletion can stabilize liver disease, improve cardiac function and dyspnea, and reduce skin pigmentation, there are still skeptics who have suggested there is no evidence to support phlebotomy therapy.[17] At our center, patients attend an ambulatory care facility and the venesections are performed by a nurse using a kit containing a 16-gauge straight needle and collection bag (Blood Pack MR6102, Baxter, Deerfield, IL). Blood is removed over 15 to 30 minutes with the patient in the reclining position. A hemoglobin measurement is done at the time of each venesection. If the hemoglobin level decreases to less than 10 g/dl the venesection schedule is modified to 500 ml every other week. The concomitant administration of a salt-containing sports beverage (e.g., Gatorade) is a simple method of maintaining plasma volume during the venesection. Maintenance venesections after iron depletion of three to four venesections per year are done in most patients although the rate of iron reaccumulation is highly variable.[77] The transferrin saturation will remain elevated in many treated patients and will not normalize unless the patient becomes iron deficient. In some cases, a component of the elevation in serum ferritin level is related to inflammation rather than iron overload; therefore the ferritin level does not decrease with treatment as the patient becomes anemic. In these cases, a careful review of the liver biopsy including hepatic iron concentration may be helpful in deciding whether to discontinue treatment or to decrease the frequency of phlebotomies. There are different ways to follow the progress of phlebotomy therapy. At our center, patients are treated until the serum ferritin concentration is approximately 50 µg/L. This is at the low end of the normal range and allows some room for iron reaccumulation into the normal range. Patient support groups have advocated for more intensive phlebotomy therapy but fatigue begins to intervene as iron deficiency is approached. The transferrin saturation may not decrease until the patient is on the brink of iron deficiency, and therefore we discontinue phlebotomy therapy in some patients with a low ferritin level but an elevated transferrin saturation (**Fig. 64-8**). Other approaches to monitoring

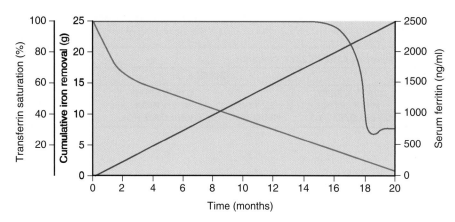

Fig. 64-8 **Response of indirect markers of iron overload to phlebotomy therapy.** This figure illustrates the reciprocal relationship between the serum ferritin level *(green line)* and the degree of removal of excess iron stores *(blue line)*. The *red line* represents transferrin saturation.

phlebotomy therapy include continuing weekly phlebotomy until anemia develops (hemoglobin <10 g/dl) or monitoring the mean corpuscular volume (MCV) during therapy. Many patients enjoy the concept of maintenance therapy particularly if they can be voluntary blood donors.[78] The evidence supporting the need for maintenance therapy is lacking[77] and it may be useful to repeat a serum ferritin level measurement in 6 months following cessation of therapy to estimate the risk of iron reaccumulation. Repeat liver biopsy is rarely done and is not recommended.

Chelation therapy with deferoxamine is not recommended for hemochromatosis. The therapy is expensive, inefficient, cumbersome, and potentially toxic. Oral chelators such as deferasirox are under investigation as a treatment for hemochromatosis but side effects and cost are less appealing than phlebotomy therapy. Erythrocytapheresis has been used but is more expensive than simple phlebotomy therapy.

Patients are advised to avoid oral iron therapy and alcohol abuse but there are no proven dietary restrictions. Patient support groups are discouraged because of the practice of iron fortification of foods, but much of this iron is in an inexpensive form with poor bioavailability. Iron fortification has been removed from food in Sweden and a decrease in the mean serum ferritin level has been demonstrated in the healthy population.[79] Tea consumption has been shown to decrease intestinal iron absorption. Many patient support groups recommend avoidance of shellfish because of the increased risk of *Vibrio* infections from iron overload.

Liver Transplantation for Hemochromatosis

In a patient with decompensated cirrhosis from hemochromatosis, liver transplantation can be performed. Despite the high prevalence of hemochromatosis, it remains an uncommon indication for liver transplant, and many cases that we labeled as hemochromatosis are more likely to have had iron overload secondary to cirrhosis from other causes. Pretransplant phlebotomy may improve cardiac function and is recommended if tolerated. Chelating agents have been suggested in several case reports. Recurrence of iron overload after liver transplantation has been infrequent.[80,81] Transplantation of iron-loaded livers from C282Y homozygotes into recipients

has usually resulted in the mobilization of hepatic iron over time, and the transplantation of a small intestine and liver into a recipient resulted in the development of iron overload in the recipient.[82] A liver transplant from an iron-loaded C282Y homozygote into a recipient was associated with an elevated serum hepcidin level.[83] These transplant experiments have been fertile ground for speculation on the pathogenesis of hemochromatosis.[83]

Population Screening for Hemochromatosis

Identification of persons at risk of developing the sequelae of hemochromatosis is preferred. The plan is to screen a population of asymptomatic individuals with no personal or family history to suggest that they are at higher risk for the disease than the rest of the population. The screening program aims to detect disease in presymptomatic individuals in order to provide more effective treatment in the early stages of disease. Because screening programs are initially associated with increased healthcare costs, it is imperative that before implementation of screening protocols, all the risks and benefits as well as the diagnostic strategy relevant to the disease are considered. Population screening for hemochromatosis meets most of the criteria established by the World Health Organization for screening for medical disease. However, the area of greatest concern is the uncertainty about the natural history of untreated hemochromatosis. An important aspect of a screening project is the demonstration of a difference between screened and unscreened cases. If unscreened cases would never develop significant morbidity the utility of population screening is greatly decreased. If most C282Y homozygotes are asymptomatic and are not progressing to cirrhosis or diabetes, then the early identification and treatment of patients may not be as cost effective as initially had been projected.[36,84]

Sporadic screening studies have been performed to establish the utility of various tests and the prevalence of hemochromatosis in a target population before the use of genetic testing. Target populations have included blood donors; hospital inpatients, outpatients, and employees; diabetic patients; and military recruits. Initial testing and test thresholds also varied and have included serum iron, unsaturated iron-binding capacity (UIBC), transferrin saturation, ferritin, and combinations of these tests. Since the advent of genetic testing in 1996, many studies have used an iron test (transferrin saturation, ferritin, UIBC) as the initial screening test with follow-up genetic testing in those with elevated iron test results. This strategy minimizes the potential for genetic discrimination in C282Y homozygotes with normal iron tests and it also has the potential to detect non-*HFE* iron overload.

An example of this approach is a study of 65,238 Norwegians attending a health appraisal clinic.[46] Genetic testing was only done in cases with an elevated transferrin saturation. In this study, there were liver biopsies performed in 149 patients and cirrhosis of the liver was detected in 3.7% of men and none of the women. The symptoms in the C282Y homozygotes did not significantly differ from those of the control population.[77] The screening of 41,038 primary care patients in San Diego detected 152 C282Y homozygotes. In an analysis of clinical symptoms only, liver disease was significantly more common in C282Y homozygotes compared with participants without *HFE* mutations. There was no difference in diabetes, arthritis, impotence, or pigmentation between these two groups.[15] The Hemochromatosis and Iron Overload Screening (HEIRS) Study screened 101,168 participants in North America. Iron overload was found predominantly in Caucasian male C282Y homozygotes. Elevations in iron tests were common and genetic testing was well accepted.[85] A large prospective study in Melbourne demonstrated iron-related disease in 28% of the male and 1% of the female C282Y homozygotes.[18,86]

In general, the screening studies to date have demonstrated a high prevalence of *HFE* mutations in Caucasian populations but low morbidity. If a study is designed to screen healthy people, many symptomatic and treated patients will not be represented in the studies. These studies have also highlighted the nonspecific nature of the symptoms that have been historically attributed to hemochromatosis. The observation that there is significant disease in referred cases and much less disease in screened cases is not unique to hemochromatosis and occurs in most screening studies. Another example of this phenomenon can be seen in the study of hepatitis C. The unresolved issue is whether these asymptomatic C282Y homozygotes would develop cirrhosis or diabetes if untreated. There have been population studies for other diseases in which genetic testing for hemochromatosis was done many years into the study. This has led to observations on the natural history of untreated disease in C282Y homozygotes who were unaware of the diagnosis. The serum ferritin level in these cases is not always rising, so progressive iron overload is not inevitable without treatment.[68,87] A clinical trial randomizing C282Y homozygotes to treatment or nontreatment seems unlikely to be conducted because of ethical concerns of withholding treatment.

Screening in diabetes and arthritis clinics has also been studied. Unfortunately, by the time diabetes is present, organ damage is also evident. Arthritis is a common cause of an elevation in serum ferritin level that will increase the number of false-positive patients who will then have invasive testing. The use of genetic testing within an arthritis clinic would likely improve the screening algorithm but several studies in diabetes and arthritis clinics have not shown an increased prevalence of *HFE* mutations.[88]

At the present time, it seems likely that mass population screening studies will not be recommended.[85,89] Targeted screening in young males could be considered in countries with a homogeneous Caucasian population.

End-Stage Cirrhosis

It is well recognized that iron overload can complicate many forms of end-stage liver disease.[90] The most common liver diseases associated with secondary iron overload are alcoholic liver disease, hepatitis B or C, and nonalcoholic steatohepatitis (NASH). Iron overload is much less common in chronic cholestatic liver diseases. It is important to recognize that most patients with these liver diseases have elevations in serum ferritin level and/or transferrin saturation without iron overload. This is a source of diagnostic confusion, and performing a liver biopsy and measuring liver iron concentration are often helpful in this clinical setting. The role of *HFE* mutations (C282Y heterozygotes, compound heterozygotes C282Y/H63D, H63D homozygotes and heterozygotes) in the pathogenesis of mild iron overload in these other liver diseases has been controversial but a study of liver explants for patients without hemochromatosis demonstrated no increase in prevalence of *HFE* mutations compared to a screened population.[91] Alcoholic siderosis is an uncommon manifestation of alcoholic liver disease and historical reports of an increase in alcoholism in hemochromatosis patients are likely attributable to patients with alcoholic liver disease being misdiagnosed as hemochromatosis patients.[92] Hepatitis C has also been typically associated with elevated iron tests but atypically associated with significant elevations in liver iron concentrations. Phlebotomy therapy has been shown to decrease levels of liver enzymes but without a consistent effect on hepatitis C virus RNA in controlled trials studying the effects of phlebotomy and antiviral therapy. The role of *HFE* mutations and their contribution to fibrogenesis remains controversial in hepatitis C but theories have invoked non–iron-related mechanisms because many cases have normal liver iron concentrations.[93-95] The prevalence of *HFE* mutations has also been studied in NASH patients with conflicting results.[96] Insulin resistance has been associated with mild to moderate iron overload in NASH independent of *HFE* mutations.[33] A typical NASH patient is obese, with an elevated ferritin level and normal transferrin saturation.

Porphyria cutanea tarda (PCT) is a cutaneous complication of chronic liver disease including hepatitis C, alcoholic liver disease, and hemochromatosis. *HFE* mutations have been found to be more common in PCT patients in many studies.[97] Phlebotomy therapy is useful in these cases and leads to improvement in the skin rash.

The presence of anemia should immediately suggest that *HFE*-linked hemochromatosis is not the correct diagnosis. Mild anemia has been seen in other iron overload genetic diseases such as ferroportin mutations and aceruloplasminemia.[98] The initial investigations include review of the peripheral blood smear, which may provide clues towards the diagnosis of spherocytosis, sickle cell disease, or thalassemia. Further investigations may include hemoglobin electrophoresis and bone marrow examination. Hepatic iron overload can occur even in the absence of blood transfusions, and the liver biopsy in an untransfused thalassemia patient can be indistinguishable from that of an *HFE*-linked hemochromatosis patient. Transfusional iron overload is characterized by iron deposits in the macrophages in the liver.

Prognosis of Patients with Hemochromatosis

The major factor affecting the long-term outcome in hemochromatosis is the presence of cirrhosis. Cirrhotic patients have a 5.5-fold increased relative risk of death compared with noncirrhotic patients. Diabetes is also a risk factor affecting long-term prognosis but most diabetic patients with hemochromatosis also have cirrhosis. Cirrhotic patients are also at risk of hepatocellular carcinoma, which is a common cause of death. The long-term survival rate in cirrhotic hemochromatosis patients compared with noncirrhotic patients is shown in **Figure 64-9**. These findings are the major stimulus for screening programs that attempt to identify and treat hemochromatosis patients at a precirrhotic stage of the disease. However, there is likely a large group of hemochromatosis patients who despite the absence of phlebotomy therapy never progress to cirrhosis or diabetes. We currently lack the ability to distinguish those patients who do not need phlebotomy until iron overload has occurred.

Conclusion

The clinical profile of a typical hemochromatosis patient has not changed significantly since the scholarly descriptions of Sheldon in 1935. However, the inclusion of control patients in population-based studies has resulted in uncertainty about the attribution of many of the symptoms of hemochromatosis to iron overload. Of all the symptoms, liver disease has the most consistent relationship to hemochromatosis and the prognosis of hemochromatosis is most closely linked to the degree of iron overload. The discovery of the *HFE* gene in 1996 was a major advancement in the field, and most Caucasian patients with typical hemochromatosis can be diagnosed with a commercially available genetic test. However, a growing number of new iron-related genes have been discovered and linked to other iron overload syndromes. These newer tests will prove useful in the future as we better understand the pathophysiology of the iron-overloaded state.

References

1. Feder JN, et al. A novel MHC class I-like gene is mutated in patients with hereditary hemochromatosis. Nat Genet 1996;13:399–408.
2. Adams PC. The natural history of untreated HFE-related hemochromatosis. Acta Haematol 2009;122:134–139.
3. Pietrangelo A. Hereditary hemochromatosis: a new look at an old disease. N Engl J Med 2004;350:2383–2397.
4. Sheldon JH. Haemochromatosis. Oxford, England: Oxford Medical Publications, 1935: 164–340.
5. Distante S, et al. The origin and spread of the HFE-C282Y haemochromatosis mutation. Hum Genet 2004;115:269–279.
6. Lucotte G, Dieterlen F. A European allele map of the C282Y mutation of hemochromatosis: Celtic versus Viking origin of the mutation? Blood Cells Mol Dis 2003;31:262–267.
7. Adams PC, et al. Hemochromatosis and iron-overload screening in a racially diverse population. N Engl J Med 2005;352:1769–1778.
8. Andrews NC, Schmidt PJ. Iron homeostasis. Annu Rev Physiol 2007;69:69–85.
9. Muckenthaler M, et al. HFE acts in hepatocytes to prevent hemochromatosis. Cell Metab 2008;7:173–178.
10. Muckenthaler M, et al. Regulatory defects in liver and intestine implicate abnormal hepcidin and Cybrd1 in mouse hemochromatosis. Nat Genet 2003;34:102–106.
11. Yamaji S, et al. Inhibition of iron transport across human intestinal epithelial cells by hepcidin. Blood 2004;104:2178–2180.
12. Bridle K, et al. Disrupted hepcidin regulation in HFE-associated haemochromatosis and the liver as a regulator of body iron homeostasis. Lancet 2003;361:661–673.
13. Camaschella C. BMP6 orchestrates iron metabolism. Nat Genet 2009;41: 387–389.
14. Ganz T. Iron homeostasis: fitting the puzzle pieces together. Cell Metab 2008; 7:288–290.
15. Andriopoulos B Jr, et al. BMP6 is a key endogenous regulator of hepcidin expression and iron metabolism. Nat Genet 2009;41:482–487.
16. Meynard D, et al. Lack of the bone morphogenetic protein BMP6 induces massive iron overload. Nat Genet 2009;41:478–481.
17. Beutler E. Natural history of hemochromatosis. Mayo Clin Proc 2004;79: 305–306.
18. Allen KJ, et al. Iron-overload-related disease in HFE hereditary hemochromatosis. N Engl J Med 2008;358:221–230.
19. Beutler E, et al. Penetrance of the 845G to A (C282Y) HFE hereditary haemochromatosis mutation in the USA. Lancet 2002;359:211–218.
20. McLaren GD, et al. Clinical manifestations of hemochromatosis in *HFE* homozygotes identified by screening. Can J Gastroenterol 2008;22:923–930.
21. Adams PC, et al. The relationship between iron overload, clinical symptoms and age in 410 patients with genetic hemochromatosis. Hepatology 1997; 25:162–166.
22. Moirand R, et al. Clinical features of genetic hemochromatosis in women compared to men. Ann Intern Med 1997;127:105–110.
23. Adams PC. Is there a critical threshold for hepatic iron concentration causing cirrhosis in hemochromatosis? Am J Gastroenterol 2001;96:567–569.
24. Fletcher L, et al. Excess alcohol greatly increases the prevalence of cirrhosis in hereditary hemochromatosis. Gastroenterology 2002;122:563–565.
25. Asberg A, et al. Screening for hemochromatosis—high prevalence and low morbidity in an unselected population of 65,238 persons. Scand J Gastroenterol 2001;36:1108–1115.
26. Powell LW, et al. Screening for hemochromatosis in asymptomatic subjects with or without a family history. Arch Int Med 2006;166:294–301.
27. Adams PC, et al. Liver diseases in the Hemochromatosis and Iron Overload Screening Study. Clin Gastroenterol Hepatol 2006;4:918–923.
28. Adams PC. Hepatocellular carcinoma in hereditary hemochromatosis. Can J Gastroenterol 1993;7:37–41.
29. Niederau C, et al. Long-term survival in patients with hereditary hemochromatosis. Gastroenterology 1996;110:1107–1119.
30. McClain D, et al. High prevalence of abnormal glucose homeostasis secondary to decreased insulin secretion in individuals with hereditary haemochromatosis. Diabetologia 2006;49:1661–1669.

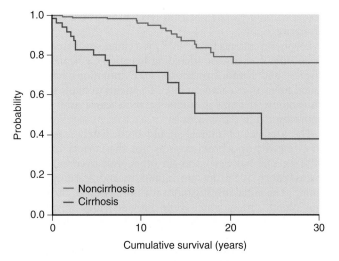

Fig. 64-9 Long-term survival in C282Y homozygotes. Cirrhotic patients had a significantly decreased survival compared with noncirrhotic patients (*n* = 392, *P* <.0001, log-rank test).

31. Niederau C, et al. Hyperinsulinaemia in non-cirrhotic haemochromatosis: impaired hepatic insulin degradation. Diabetologia 1984;26:441–444.

32. Hramiak I, Finegood D, Adams PC. Factors affecting glucose tolerance in hereditary hemochromatosis. Clin Invest Med 1997;20:110–118.

33. Mendler MH, et al. Insulin resistance-associated hepatic iron overload. Gastroenterology 1999;117:1155–1163.

34. Papanikolaou G, et al. Mutations in HFE2 cause iron overload in chromosome 1q-linked juvenile hemochromatosis. Nat Genet 2004;36:77–82.

35. Adams PC, et al. *HFE* C282Y homozygosity is associated with lower total and LDL cholesterol: the Hemochromatosis and Iron Overload Screening (HEIRS) Study. Circ Cardiovasc Genet 2009;2:34–37.

36. Pankow JS, et al. HFE C282Y homozygotes have reduced low-density lipoprotein cholesterol: the Atherosclerosis Risk in Communities (ARIC) Study. Translat Res 2008;152:3–10.

37. Adams PC, Speechley M. The effect of arthritis on the quality of life in hereditary hemochromatosis. J Rheumatol 1996;23:707–710.

38. Adams PC. Hemochromatosis case definition—out of focus? Nat Clin Gastroenterol Hepatol 2006;3:178–179.

39. Adams PC, et al. Biological variability of transferrin saturation and unsaturated iron binding capacity. Am J Med 2007;120:999,e1–999,e7.

40. Brissot P, et al. Assessment of liver iron content in 271 patients: a reevaluation of direct and indirect methods. Gastroenterology 1981;80:557–565.

41. Wong K, Adams PC. The diversity of liver diseases associated with an elevated serum ferritin. Can J Gastroenterol 2007;20:467–470.

42. Moirand R, et al. Phenotypic expression of HFE mutations: a French study of 1110 unrelated iron-overloaded patients and relatives. Gastroenterology 1999;116:372–377.

43. Lim EM, et al. Hepatic iron loading in patients with compound heterozygous HFE mutations. Liver Int 2004;24:631–636.

44. Yoneda M, et al. Serum ferritin is a clinical biomarker in Japanese patients with nonalcoholic steatohepatitis (NASH) independent of HFE gene mutation. Dig Dis Sci 2010;55:808–814.

45. Roetto A, et al. Pathogenesis of hyperferritinemia cataract syndrome. Blood Cell Mol Dis 2002;29:532–535.

46. Guyader D, et al. Non-invasive prediction of fibrosis in C282Y homozygous hemochromatosis. Gastroenterology 1998;115:929–936.

47. Crawford DH, et al. Serum hyaluronic acid with serum ferritin accurately predicts cirrhosis and reduces the need for liver biopsy in C282Y hemochromatosis. Hepatology 2009;49:418–425.

48. Adhoute X, et al. Diagnosis of liver fibrosis using FibroScan and other noninvasive methods in patients with hemochromatosis: a prospective study. Gastroenterol Clin Biol 2008;32:180–187.

49. Adams PC, Bradley C, Henderson AR. Evaluation of the hepatic iron index as a diagnostic criterion in hereditary hemochromatosis. J Lab Clin Med 1997;130:509–514.

50. St Pierre T, et al. Noninvasive measurement and imaging of liver iron concentrations using proton magnetic resonance. Blood 2005;105:855–861.

51. Gandon Y, et al. Non-invasive assessment of hepatic iron stores by MRI. Lancet 2004;363:357–360.

52. Alustiza J, et al. MR Quantification of hepatic iron concentration. Radiology 2004;230:479–484.

53. Nielsen P, et al. Non-invasive liver iron quantification by SQUID-biosusceptometry and serum ferritin iron as new diagnostic parameters in hereditary hemochromatosis. Blood Cells Mol Dis 2002;29:451–458.

54. Aguilar-Martinez P, et al. Variable phenotypic presentation of iron overload in H63D homozygotes: are gene modifiers the cause? Gut 2001;6:836–842.

55. Gurrin LC, et al. HFE C282Y/H63D compound heterozygotes are at low risk of hemochromatosis-related morbidity. Hepatology 2009;50:94–101.

56. Jeffrey G, et al. Polymorphism in intron 4 of HFE may cause overestimation of C282Y homozygote prevalence in haemochromatosis. Nat Genet 1999;22:325–326.

57. Somerville M, et al. An HFE intronic variant promotes misdiagnosis of hereditary hemochromatosis. Am J Hum Genet 1999;65:924–926.

58. Shaheen N, et al. Insurance, employment, and psychosocial consequences of a diagnosis of hereditary hemochromatosis in subjects without end-organ damage. Am J Gastroenterol 2003;98:1175–1180.

59. Hall MA, et al. Genetic screening for iron overload: no evidence of discrimination at one year. J Fam Pract 2007;56:829–833.

60. Pietrangelo A. Non-HFE hemochromatosis. Hepatology 2004;39:21–29.

61. Njajou O, et al. Dominant hemochromatosis due to N144H mutation of SLC11A3: clinical and biological characteristics. Blood Cell Mol Dis 2002;29:439–443.

62. Wallace D, et al. Novel mutation in ferroportin 1 is associated with autosomal dominant hemochromatosis. Blood 2002;100:692–694.

63. Hellman N, et al. Hepatic iron overload in aceruloplasminemia. Gut 2003;47:858–860.

64. Camaschella C, et al. The gene TFR2 is mutated in a new type of haemochromatosis mapping to 7q22. Nat Genet 2000;25:14–15.

65. Kotze M, et al. Molecular diagnosis of hereditary hemochromatosis: application of a newly-developed reverse-hybridization assay in the South African population. Clin Genet 2004;65:317–321.

66. Adams PC, Chakrabarti S. Genotypic/phenotypic correlations in genetic hemochromatosis: evolution of diagnostic criteria. Gastroenterology 1998;114:319–323.

67. Bacon BR. Hemochromatosis: diagnosis and management. Gastroenterology 2001;120:718–725.

68. Gurrin LC, et al. The natural history of serum iron indices for HFE C282Y homozygosity associated with hereditary hemochromatosis. Gastroenterology 2008;135:1945–1952.

69. Yamashita C, Adams PC. Natural history of the C282Y homozygote of the hemochromatosis gene (HFE) with a normal serum ferritin level. Clin Gastroenterol Hepatol 2003;1:388–391.

70. Gleeson F, et al. Clinical expression of haemochromatosis in Irish C282Y homozygotes identified through family screening. Eur J Gastroenterol Hepatol 2004;16:859–863.

71. Jacobs EM, et al. Severity of iron overload of proband determines serum ferritin levels in families with HFE-related hemochromatosis: the HEmochromatosis FAmily Study. J Hepatol 2009;50:174–183.

72. Lazarescu A, Snively B, Adams PC. Phenotype variation in C282Y homozygotes for the hemochromatosis gene. Clin Gastroenterol Hepatol 2005;3:1043–1046.

73. Adams PC, Walker AP, Acton RT. A primer for predicting risk of disease in HFE-linked hemochromatosis. Genet Testing 2001;5:311–316.

74. Adams PC. Implications of genotyping of spouses to limit investigation of children in genetic hemochromatosis. Clin Genet 1998;53:176–178.

75. Harris EL, et al. Serum ferritin and transferrin saturation in Asians and Pacific Islanders. Arch Intern Med 2007;167:722–726.

76. Gordeuk V, et al. Iron overload in Africa. Interaction between a gene and dietary iron content. N Engl J Med 1992;326:95–100.

77. Adams PC, Kertesz AE, Valberg LS. Rate of iron reaccumulation following iron depletion in hereditary hemochromatosis. Implications for venesection therapy. J Clin Gastroenterol 1993;16:207–210.

78. Levstik M, Adams PC. Eligibility and exclusion of hemochromatosis patients from voluntary blood donation. Can J Gastroenterol 1998;12:61–63.

79. Olsson K, et al. The effect of withdrawal of food iron fortification in Sweden as studied with phlebotomy in subjects with genetic hemochromatosis. Eur J Clin Nutr 1998;51:782–786.

80. Crawford DH, et al. Patient and graft survival after liver transplantation for hereditary hemochromatosis: implications for pathogenesis. Hepatology 2004;39:1655–1662.

81. Kowdley K, et al. Survival after liver transplantation in patients with hepatic iron overload: the National Hemochromatosis Transplant Registry. Gastroenterology 2005;129:494–503.

82. Adams PC, et al. Transplantation of haemochromatosis liver and intestine into a normal recipient. Gut 1999;45:783.

83. Adams PC, et al. Is serum hepcidin causative in hemochromatosis? Novel analysis from a liver transplant with hemochromatosis. Can J Gastroenterol 2008;22:851–853.

84. Adams PC. Population screening for haemochromatosis. Gut 2000;46:301–303.

85. Adams PC, et al. Screening for iron overload: lessons from the Hemochromatosis and Iron Overload Screening (HEIRS) study. Can J Gastroenterol 2009;23:769–772.

86. Allen K, et al. The HealthIron Study: a longitudinal study of the natural history and burden of disease of hereditary hemochromatosis. Hepatology 2006;44:221A.

87. Andersen RV, et al. Hemochromatosis mutations in the general population: iron overload progression rate. Blood 2004;103:2914–2919.

88. DuBois S, Kowdley K. Targeted screening for hereditary haemochromatosis in high-risk groups. Alimen Pharm Ther 2004;20:1–14.

89. Whitlock E, et al. Screening for hereditary hemochromatosis: a systematic review for the U.S. Preventative Services Task Force. Ann Intern Med 2006;145:209–223.

90. Ludwig J, et al. Hemosiderosis in cirrhosis: a study of 447 native livers. Gastroenterology 1997;112:882–888.

91. Alanen K, et al. Prevalence of the C282Y mutation of the hemochromatosis gene in liver transplant recipients and donors. Hepatology 1999;30:665–669.

92. Adams PC, Agnew S. Alcoholism in hereditary hemochromatosis revisited: prevalence and clinical consequences among homozygous siblings. Hepatology 1996;23:724–727.

93. Fontana RJ, et al. Iron reduction before and during interferon therapy of chronic hepatitis C: results of a multicenter, randomized, controlled trial. Hepatology 2000;31:730–736.

94. Bonkovsky HL, et al. Roles of iron and HFE mutations on severity and response to therapy during retreatment of advanced chronic hepatitis C. Gastroenterology 2006;131:1440–1451.

95. Price L, Kowdley K. The role of iron in the pathophysiology and treatment of chronic hepatitis C. Can J Gastroenterol 2009;23:822–828.

96. Bataller R, North K, Brenner D. Genetic polymorphisms and the progression of liver fibrosis: a critical appraisal. Hepatology 2003;37:493–503.

97. Bonkovsky HL, et al. Porphyria cutanea tarda, hepatitis C, and HFE gene mutations in North America. Hepatology 1998;27:1661–1669.

98. Xu X, et al. Aceruloplasminemia: an inherited neurodegenerative disease with impairment of iron homeostasis. Ann N Y Acad Sci 2004;1012:299–305.

α₁-Antitrypsin Deficiency

David Perlmutter

ABBREVIATIONS

α₁AT α₁-antitrypsin
ER endoplasmic reticulum
IL interleukin

MPT mitochondrial permeability transition
PBA 4-phenylbutyric acid

SERPIN serine protease inhibitor
SNP single nucleotide polymorphism

Introduction

α₁-Antitrypsin (α₁AT) deficiency is an autosomal co-dominant disorder associated with premature development of pulmonary emphysema, chronic liver disease, and hepatocellular carcinoma. A point mutation results in a protein that is retained in the endoplasmic reticulum (ER) of liver cells rather than secreted into the blood and body fluids. The mutant protein is prone to polymerization within the ER. Loss of function permits uninhibited proteolytic destruction of the connective tissue matrix of the lung, ultimately leading to emphysema. Cigarette smoking exacerbates the development of emphysema because residual α₁AT molecules are functionally inactivated by the increased load of active oxygen intermediates that are produced by smokers' alveolar macrophages. In contrast, liver disease results from a gain-of-toxic function mechanism whereby the retention of mutant α₁AT in liver cells somehow triggers a series of events that lead to liver injury and a predilection for hepatocellular carcinoma. Although it is the most common genetic cause of liver disease in children, clinically significant liver disease develops in only approximately 10% of affected homozygotes, an observation that has provided the basis for the notion that genetic modifiers and environmental factors play a role in susceptibility to and/or protection from liver disease in α₁AT deficiency. Even though there are several attractive new concepts for chemoprophylaxis and treatment of liver disease in this deficiency, the only effective treatment currently available is liver transplantation.

Epidemiology

The incidence of α₁AT deficiency is 1 in 1800 to 1 in 2000 live births in most populations that have been carefully studied.[1] Most of the studies of lung and liver disease in this population have been biased in ascertainment because they involve patients referred to specialty clinics. The only unbiased study comes from nationwide screening of all newborns in Sweden in the 1970s.[2,3] More than 200,000 newborns were screened and 127 homozygotes for the α₁AT Z alleles were identified; most of these individuals have now been followed for almost 30 years. The results show that only 14 of these individuals (11%) had prolonged obstructive jaundice in infancy and only 9 (7%) have developed clinically significant liver disease. Of the remaining α₁AT-deficient population, 85% have shown persistently normal transaminase levels as they have aged. Liver biopsies have not been done in this study and therefore it is not known whether some of these seemingly unaffected individuals have subclinical histologic abnormalities and will develop clinical signs of liver disease as they reach the fourth and fifth decades of life. Although it is widely believed that lung disease affects a higher percentage of homozygotes,[4] a valid determination of incidence will not be possible until the Swedish prospective cohort reaches the peak age range for emphysema, 40 to 60 years of age.

Pathogenesis

As the archetype of the serine protease inhibitor (SERPIN) family, α₁AT mainly functions as a blood-borne inhibitor of destructive neutrophil proteases, including elastase, cathepsin G, and proteinase 3. α₁AT is predominantly derived from parenchymal liver cells, constituting the most abundant glycoprotein secreted by the liver. α₁AT is also considered a positive acute-phase reactant because its plasma concentration increases during the host response to inflammation/tissue injury.

The classic deficiency mutant α₁ATZ is characterized by a point mutation that results in the substitution of lysine for glutamate 342 and by itself accounts for defective secretion. The mutant α₁ATZ molecule is retained in the ER of liver cells (**Fig. 65-1**). Studies by Carrell and Lomas have shown that this substitution reduces the stability of α₁ATZ as a monomer and increases the formation of polymers by a "loop-sheet" insertion mechanism.[5] Although polymers have been detected by electron microscopy in hepatocytes of a liver biopsy specimen

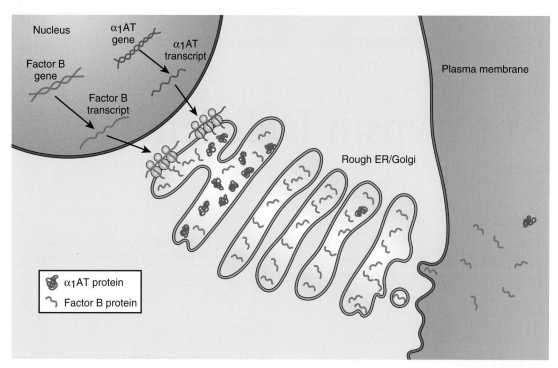

Fig. 65-1   Secretory defect in α₁AT deficiency. The mutant α₁AT protein is retained in the endoplasmic reticulum, whereas another hepatic secretory protein, complement factor B, is distributed throughout the secretory pathway and is efficiently secreted. *(Reproduced from Perlmutter DH. Alpha-1-antitrypsin deficiency. In: Walker WA, et al, editors. Pediatric gastrointestinal disease. Philadelphia: BC Decker, 1991:979, with permission.)*

from an α₁AT-deficient individual[6] and by sucrose density gradient centrifugation in transfected cell lines that express mutant α₁ATZ,[7,8] it is still not clear whether polymerization is responsible for ER retention of mutant α₁ATZ. The strongest evidence supporting this theory is derived from studies showing partial correction of the secretory defect by insertion of a second mutation into α₁ATZ that suppresses polymerization.[9-11] However, those studies do not exclude the possibility that there is an abnormality in folding that is distinct from the tendency to polymerize and that is also partially corrected by the second, experimentally introduced mutation. More recent studies cast some doubt on the concept that polymerization is the cause of ER retention. First, naturally occurring variants of α₁AT with truncated carboxyl-terminal tails are retained in the ER of liver cells even though they do not form polymers.[7,8] Second, only a minor proportion (≈15%) of the intracellular pool of α₁ATZ at steady state in model cell lines is in the form of polymers.[7,8] Third, new structural information implies that alteration in folding of α₁ATZ precedes polymerization.[12] Thus most of what we know suggests that polymerization is not the cause of α₁ATZ retention in the ER but rather is the result of its retention. As it accumulates in the ER of liver cells polymers of α₁ATZ form and become insoluble. Even though it might not cause the retention and accumulation, the formation of polymers in that intracellular compartment appears to have a specific impact on how the liver cell responds and, moreover, to dictate the pathobiology of liver inflammation, fibrosis, and carcinogenesis, as explained later in this section.

There is relatively limited information available describing how ER retention of mutant α₁ATZ causes liver injury by a gain-of-toxic function mechanism. Recent studies have shown that liver from α₁AT-deficient patients is characterized by significant mitochondrial injury and mitochondrial autophagy as well as activation of caspase-3 and caspase-9.[13,14] These mitochondrial changes and caspase activation were also seen in transfected cell lines and transgenic model systems. Indeed, treatment of one transgenic mouse model with cyclosporin A, which inhibits the mitochondrial permeability transition (MPT) pore, resulted in diminished hepatic mitochondrial injury and caspase activation and improved survival.[13] This may mean that ER retention of α₁ATZ causes mitochondrial injury by a direct interaction between the distended ER and adjacent mitochondria. In fact, recent studies in model cell lines with inducible expression have shown that ER retention of α₁ATZ activates BAP31,[15] an ER protein that mediates direct interactions between ER and mitochondria that are pro-apoptotic.[16] It is also possible that mitochondria are injured as innocent bystanders of an overexuberant autophagic response that is activated by ER retention of α₁ATZ. Autophagy is a ubiquitous, highly conserved cellular mechanism by which senescent and/or denatured constituents in the cytoplasm and intracellular organelles or whole organelles are sequestered from the rest of the cytoplasm within newly formed vacuoles that then fuse with lysosomes for degradation (**Fig. 65-2**). It is believed to be a mechanism for turnover of cellular constituents during nutritional deprivation, stress states, morphogenesis, differentiation, and aging. Our previous studies have shown that ER retention of α₁ATZ is a powerful stimulus for the autophagic response.[13,17,18] A marked increase in autophagosomes has been observed in several different model cell lines genetically engineered to express α₁ATZ, including human

Normal liver cell

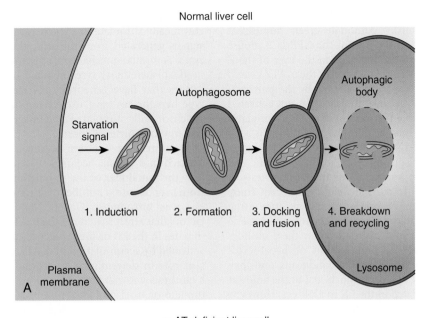

α₁AT-deficient liver cell

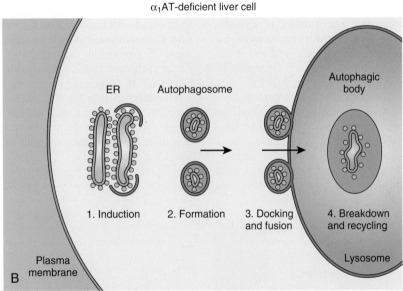

Fig. 65-2 **Autophagosomes in (A) normal and (B) α₁AT-deficient liver cells.** In the normal liver cell, stress, such as starvation, leads to induction of vacuolar membranes, formation of an autophagosome that envelops cytoplasm and organelles, docking and fusion of the autophagosome with lysosome, and breakdown of its contents within the lysosome. In the α₁AT-deficient cell, accumulation of mutant α₁ATZ in the endoplasmic reticulum *(ER)* leads to induction of vacuolar membranes and pinching-off of ER to form autophagosomes. *(Adapted from Klionsky DJ, Emr SD. Autophagy as a regulated pathway of cellular degradation. Science 2000;290:1717–1721, with permission.)*

fibroblasts, murine hepatoma, and rat hepatoma cell lines.[17] Moreover, in a HeLa cell line engineered for inducible expression of α₁ATZ, autophagosomes appear as a specific response to the expression of α₁ATZ and its retention in the ER. There is a marked increase in autophagosomes in hepatocytes in transgenic mouse models of α₁AT deficiency and a disease-specific increase in autophagosomes in liver biopsies from patients with the deficiency.[17] Autophagy clearly plays a major role in disposal of the mutant α₁ATZ molecule, as demonstrated in autophagy-deficient mammalian cell lines[19] and yeast strains.[20] Indeed, in yeast it appears that the autophagic pathway is specialized for disposal of the insoluble forms of α₁ATZ that accumulate at higher levels of expression.[20] Kruse

and colleagues have discovered that a mutant subunit of fibrinogen that aggregates in the ER of liver cells in a rare inherited form of fibrinogen deficiency depends on autophagy for disposal.[21] Interestingly, this type of fibrinogen deficiency is associated with a chronic liver disease, providing evidence both for the concept that the accumulation of aggregation-prone protein in the ER is hepatotoxic and for the notion that autophagy is particularly specialized for disposal of insoluble mutant proteins. The autophagic pathway is also specifically and selectively activated by accumulation of α₁ATZ in the ER. This has been definitively determined by breeding the Z mouse model, which has hepatocyte-specific inducible expression of α₁ATZ, with the GFP-LC3 mouse, which renders autophagosomes fluorescent (LC3 is an autophagosomal membrane-specific protein).[19] Although green fluorescent autophagosomes are seen in the liver of the GFP-LC3 mouse only after starvation, they were observed in the liver of the Z ×GFP-LC3 simply by inducing expression of the α_1ATZ gene.[19] This effect appears to be specifically elicited by the polymerizing properties of α_1ATZ because autophagy is not activated when the nonpolymerogenic Saar variant of α_1AT accumulates in the ER of liver cells. Thus the autophagic pathway is activated when insoluble α_1ATZ accumulates in the ER and then it plays a critical role in disposing of the insoluble α_1ATZ.

There is also very little known about the pathogenesis of hepatocellular carcinoma in α_1AT deficiency. A recent study by Rudnick and colleagues[14] has suggested an interesting hypothesis. Using bromodeoxyuridine labeling in the PiZ transgenic mouse model of α_1AT deficiency, these authors demonstrated an increase in proliferation of hepatocytes in the liver of these mice under resting conditions, and they hypothesized that this increase is proportional to the amount of α_1AT that has accumulated in the ER in globules. However, the cells that proliferate are the ones that do not have the globules. Previous studies of transgenic mouse models of α_1AT deficiency have shown that the number of globule-devoid hepatocytes and the area of the liver occupied by globule-devoid hepatocytes increase with age and this is the area where adenomas and carcinomas arise.[22] Interestingly, autophagosomes are predominantly found in liver cells that contain globules in the PiZ mouse.[17] Several studies have shown that autophagic activity inhibits tumorigenesis in vivo.[23] Taken together, these observations suggest that hepatocytes that have accumulated significant α_1AT and have formed globules are sick but not dead, that globule-devoid hepatocytes therefore have a selective proliferative advantage and, most importantly, that adenomas and eventually carcinomas

evolve in the globule-devoid hepatocytes because they are chronically stimulated to regenerate in an "injury milieu" by signals generated from the sick, globule-containing hepatocytes. A similar mechanism appears to occur in the mouse model of hereditary tyrosinemia.[24] In the latter model, hepatocytes that have genetically reverted or transplanted wild-type hepatocytes have a selective proliferative advantage and are chronically stimulated by damaged cells that are unable to undergo complete cell death.

To address the question of how a subpopulation of α_1AT-deficient individuals becomes susceptible to liver disease and how the remainder of the population is apparently protected from liver disease, a number of years ago the following hypothesis was introduced: Genetic modifiers or environmental factors that affect the fate of the α_1ATZ molecule once it accumulates in the ER or the protective cellular response pathways activated by accumulation of α_1ATZ in the ER play an important role in determining susceptibility to liver disease. This hypothesis was validated by a series of experiments in which the fate of α_1ATZ in skin fibroblast cell lines from deficient individuals with liver disease (susceptible hosts) was compared with its fate in skin fibroblast cell lines from deficient individuals without liver disease (protected hosts) after expression was established in each by stable gene transduction techniques.[25] The results showed that α_1ATZ was retained in the ER in each case, but it was degraded more efficiently in cell lines from the protected hosts (**Fig. 65-3**).

The mechanisms for the degradation of mutant α_1ATZ once it has accumulated in the ER are very complex. There appear to be ubiquitin-dependent proteasomal[26] and ubiquitin-independent proteasomal[27] as well as nonproteasomal pathways involved. The proteasome is part of a pathway for degradation that has been termed ERAD (ER-associated degradation) and involves a mechanism by which proteins

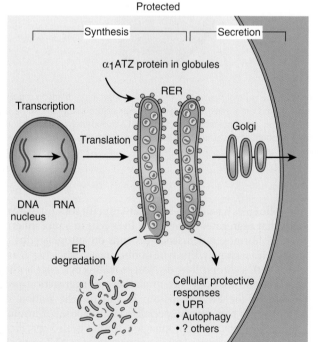
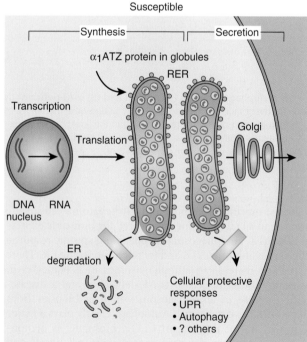

Fig. 65-3 Fate of mutant α_1ATZ in liver cells from protected and susceptible hosts. In the susceptible hosts, there is a subtle block in endoplasmic reticulum *(ER)* degradation of α_1ATZ or cellular protective responses to α_1ATZ. RER, rough endoplasmic reticulum; UPR, unfolded protein response

that are destined for disposal are translocated retrograde from the ER to the cytoplasm. At least two nonproteasomal pathways, a tyrosine phosphatase–dependent pathway[28] and autophagy,[19] have already been implicated. The studies of Kruse and colleagues[20] have suggested that there is another pathway for disposal of α₁ATZ in yeast that involves transit to the *trans*-Golgi and then targeting to the vacuole. A comparable pathway for degradation of α₁ATZ in mammalian cells has not yet been described. Genetic modifiers that affect the function of any of these pathways would theoretically increase susceptibility to liver disease. Indeed, a single nucleotide polymorphism (SNP) in the downstream flanking region of the gene for ER mannosidase I has been implicated in early-onset liver disease among α₁AT-deficient individuals.[29] Because ER mannosidase I plays a role in the ERAD pathway, a polymorphism that affects its function would be a prime candidate for a genetic modifier of liver disease in α₁AT deficiency according to our hypothetical paradigm. However, further epidemiologic studies are needed to determine if this SNP is truly affecting liver disease susceptibility, and further cellular studies are needed to identify how it later affects α₁ATZ accumulation in the ER. In another study a SNP in the upstream flanking region of the α₁AT gene itself has been implicated in liver disease susceptibility.[30] However, this study could have led to an entirely different conclusion with a legitimate alternate way of classifying one of the patient groups.

The protective cellular response pathways that are activated by ER retention of mutant α₁ATZ could also be the target of genetic modifiers. The autophagic response is certainly one of these.[19] It now appears that the signally pathway associated with the transcription factor NF-κB is another specific response pathway activated by accumulation of α₁ATZ in the ER.[31] Interestingly, gene expression profile studies demonstrate that a distinct subgroup of the known target genes of the NF-κB signaling pathways is altered in expression when α₁ATZ accumulates in the ER,[32] suggesting that NF-κB is activated in a very specific way. Again, genetic modifiers that affect these response pathways could theoretically increase or even decrease susceptibility to liver disease. Chemical or genetic manipulation of these cellular responses could also constitute strategies for chemoprophylaxis or treatment for liver disease in α₁AT deficiency.

Indomethacin could represent an environmental modifier of liver disease in α₁AT deficiency. In one study, indomethacin administration to the PiZ mouse model resulted in increased hepatic α₁ATZ accumulation and hepatocyte injury.[33] The effect of indomethacin appeared to involve increased expression of α₁AT at the transcriptional level via interleukin-6 (IL-6) signaling.

Clinical Features

In many cases this liver disease first becomes apparent at 4 to 8 weeks of age because of persistent jaundice (**Table 65-1**). Conjugated bilirubin and transaminase levels in the blood are mildly to moderately elevated. The liver may be enlarged, but symptoms, signs, or laboratory abnormalities that suggest significant liver injury are rarely present. It is very difficult to clinically differentiate these infants from infants affected by many other causes of neonatal liver disease, including infections, metabolic diseases, and even the destructive

Table 65-1 α₁-Antitrypsin Deficiency–Associated Liver Disease

Clinical Manifestations	
Infancy	Prolonged obstructive jaundice Elevated transaminases Symptoms of cholestasis
Early childhood	Elevated transaminases Asymptomatic hepatomegaly Severe liver dysfunction
Late childhood/adolescence	Chronic active hepatitis Cryptogenic cirrhosis Portal hypertension Hepatocellular carcinoma
Diagnostic Features	
Diminished serum levels of ATZ (10%-15% of normal levels) Abnormal mobility of antitrypsin in isoelectric focusing (PIZ) Periodic acid–Schiff-positive, diastase-resistant globules in liver cells	

hepatobiliary lesions of biliary atresia; therefore α₁AT deficiency is usually considered one of the causes of a broad diagnostic category termed neonatal hepatitis syndrome. Occasionally the diagnosis will be discovered in a newborn with bleeding symptoms such as hematemesis, melena, bleeding from the umbilical stump, or bruising.[34] In some cases there may be cholestatic manifestations including icterus, pruritus, and laboratory abnormalities such as hypercholesterolemia. Indeed, this subgroup of α₁AT-deficient infants may have severe biliary epithelial cell damage and even paucity of the intrahepatic bile ducts detected in their liver biopsies.[35] α₁AT deficiency rarely manifests with severe progressive liver disease in the first year of life.[36]

The liver disease of α₁AT deficiency may also be diagnosed later in childhood because of asymptomatic hepatomegaly, elevated levels of transaminases detected incidentally, or jaundice that develops during an intercurrent illness. Finally, this disease can first present in childhood, adolescence, or adult life with complications of portal hypertension, including splenomegaly, hypersplenism, gastrointestinal bleeding from varices, ascites, and/or hepatic encephalopathy (see **Table 65-1**). It should be part of the differential diagnosis in any adult patient with chronic liver disease, cryptogenic cirrhosis, or hepatocellular carcinoma. An autopsy study done in Sweden suggested that as many as 25% of α₁AT-deficient men who die between the ages of 40 and 60 have evidence of liver inflammation, necrosis, and/or carcinoma.[37]

The natural history of liver disease in α₁AT deficiency is quite variable. Most infants who present with prolonged jaundice are asymptomatic by the time they reach 1 year of age. In the majority of these cases there is no further evidence of liver disease for many years. Because this diagnosis has only existed for approximately 35 years, it is not yet clear what proportion of these individuals progress to develop liver disease and/or hepatocellular carcinoma. The only prospective data on the course of α₁AT deficiency are available from the Swedish nationwide screening study started by Sveger in the early 1970s.[2] In that study, 200,000 newborn infants were screened, and 127 were found to have the classical form of α₁AT deficiency. Of the 127 affected patients, 14 had prolonged obstructive jaundice and 9 of these 14 had clinically significant liver disease. Another 8 of the 127 had hepatomegaly with or without elevated bilirubin or transaminase levels. Approximately 50% of the remaining population had elevated transaminase levels alone. The long-term outcome for these infants was last published when their mean age was 18 years,[3] but unpublished observations by Sveger indicate that little has changed for the population well into their third decade of life. There has been no evidence for the development of clinically significant liver disease in any of the patients since the first year of life. This indicates that only 8% of the population have encountered clinically significant liver disease to date. Of the remaining population of α_1AT-deficient children identified in this cohort, 85% showed persistently normal transaminase levels as they aged. Liver biopsies have not been conducted in this study and therefore it is not known whether some of these seemingly unaffected individuals have subclinical histologic abnormalities and will develop clinical signs as they reach the fourth and fifth decades of life.

Even patients with severe liver disease caused by α_1AT deficiency may have a stable or relatively slowly progressing course. In one retrospective review of a pediatric hepatology service, 9 of 17 patients with α_1AT deficiency and cirrhosis or portal hypertension, or both, had a prolonged, relatively uneventful disease course for at least 4 years after the diagnosis of cirrhosis or portal hypertension was made.[38] Two of these patients eventually underwent liver transplantation but seven were leading relatively healthy lives for as long as 23 years while carrying a diagnosis of severe α_1AT deficiency–associated liver disease.

It has not yet been possible to identify specific clinical and/or laboratory signs that can be used to predict a poor prognosis for liver involvement in α_1AT deficiency. Results of one early study suggested that persistence of hyperbilirubinemia, development of hard hepatomegaly or splenomegaly, and progressive prolongation of the prothrombin time were indicators of poor prognosis.[39] In another study, elevated transaminase levels, prolonged prothrombin time, and lower trypsin inhibitory capacity correlated with a worse prognosis.[40] In my experience the first definitive evidence of poor prognosis is typically a complication that affects the overall life functioning of the patient.

It is still unclear whether heterozygotes for the classical form of α_1AT deficiency are predisposed to liver disease. Early studies of liver biopsy collections suggested that there was a relationship between heterozygosity and the development of liver disease.[41] This has been confirmed by later studies of liver biopsy collections. In particular, the liver biopsies from patients who have undergone liver transplantation show a higher-than-expected prevalence of heterozygosity for the classic form of α_1AT deficiency without another diagnostic explanation for severe liver disease.[42] However, these studies and others like them have an inherent bias in ascertainment. In a cross-sectional study of patients with α_1AT deficiency in a referral-based Austrian university hospital, who were reexamined with recently developed, more sensitive and sophisticated diagnostic assays, results suggested that liver disease in heterozygotes could be accounted for, to a large extent, by infections with hepatitis C virus or by autoimmune disease.[43] Unfortunately neither type of study has provided convincing evidence supporting or refuting a predisposition to liver disease in PiMZ individuals. Nevertheless, my experience with numerous PiMZ individuals with severe liver disease and no other plausible explanation leads me to believe that the predisposition does exist.

Liver disease has been described for several other allelic variants of α_1AT. Children with compound heterozygosity for the S and Z alleles are affected by liver disease in a manner similar to PIZZ children.[2,3] Interestingly, α_1AT S forms heteropolymers with α_1ATZ[44] and this compound heterozygous state is probably associated with retention of the mutant protein in a polymeric form within the ER of liver cells.[45] There have been several reports of liver disease in the α_1AT deficiency PiM Malton.[46,47] This is an interesting association, because the abnormal α_1AT Malton molecule has been shown to undergo polymerization and retention in the ER.[46] Because it has only been reported in single patients with other allelic variants of α_1AT,[48] it is not clear whether liver disease is causally related to those variants.

Destructive lung disease/emphysema caused by α_1AT deficiency probably does not clinically manifest until late in the third decade. Although there are a few reports of younger individuals with lung disease, the diagnosis of α_1AT deficiency in these cases was not convincing.[49]

There is still limited information available about the incidence of liver disease in α_1AT-deficient individuals with established emphysema. In a study of 22 PIZZ patients with emphysema, there were elevated transaminase levels in 10 patients and cholestasis in 1 patient.[50] Because liver biopsies were not done in this study, the extent and incidence of liver disease in adults with emphysema as their predominant clinical problem may be underestimated.

Diagnosis

α_1-Antitrypsin deficiency should be considered in anyone with elevated levels of transaminases or conjugated bilirubin, asymptomatic hepatomegaly, signs or symptoms of portal hypertension or cholestasis, or bleeding/bruising with a prolonged prothrombin time. It should be considered in adults with chronic idiopathic hepatitis, cryptogenic cirrhosis, and hepatocellular carcinoma.

The diagnosis is established by means of serum α_1AT phenotype (PI type) determination using isoelectric focusing electrophoresis or agarose gel electrophoresis at acid pH (**Fig. 65-4**). Serum concentrations can be used for screening with follow-up PI typing of any values below normal (85 to 215 mg/dl). A retrospective study of all pediatric patients who had both serum concentrations and PI typing done at one center indicated that the serum concentration determination had a positive predictive value of 94% and a negative predictive value of 100% for homozygous PIZZ α_1AT deficiency[51]; however, because of the inherent limitations of retrospectively defining a patient population for the analysis, the results of the study are not necessarily applicable to each diagnostic situation that might be encountered. In my experience it is wise to both measure the serum concentration and perform PI typing when seriously considering this diagnosis. Serum concentrations increase during the host response to inflammation and therein may reach normal levels in heterozygotes and near-normal levels in homozygotes. Both the serum concentrations and the PI type will be needed to confirm the homozygous and compound heterozygous as well as the heterozygous

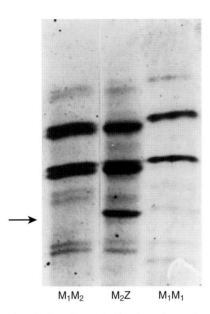

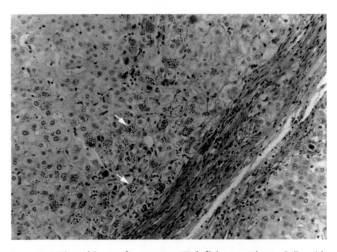

Fig. 65-5 **Liver biopsy from an α₁AT-deficient patient.** Cells with periodic acid–Schiff-positive, diastase-resistant globules are shown with *arrows. (Reproduced from Perlmutter DH. Alpha-1-antitrypsin deficiency. In: Snape WJ, editor. Consultations in gastroenterology. Philadelphia: WB Saunders, 1996:793, with permission.)*

Fig. 65-4 **Isoelectric focusing gel.** Blood specimens from three individuals are shown: normal with M₁ and M₂ alleles; heterozygote with M₂ and Z alleles *(arrow)*; normal with two M₁ alleles. *(Reproduced from Perlmutter DH. Alpha-1-antitrypsin deficiency. In: Snape WJ, editor. Consultations in gastroenterology. Philadelphia: WB Saunders, 1996:791–801, with permission.)*

states that can be present at the α₁AT locus. In some cases, phenotype determinations of parents and other relatives are necessary to confirm the diagnosis if there is any discrepancy and to ensure the distinction between the ZZ and SZ allotypes, for which isoelectric focusing may not be straightforward. This distinction and the others will be important for genetic counseling.

The PI type is particularly important in the neonatal period because it may be very difficult to distinguish patients with α₁AT deficiency from those with biliary atresia. Moreover, it is not uncommon for neonates with a PIZZ phenotype to have no biliary excretion on scintigraphic studies.[52] There is one report of α₁AT deficiency and biliary atresia in a single patient.[53] I have seen several patients with homozygous PIZZ α₁AT deficiency and cholestasis for whom there was no biliary excretion of technetium-labeled mebrofenin, but with more prolonged observation, in each of these cases, cholestasis remitted such that it was then obvious that the patients did not have biliary atresia.

The distinctive histologic feature of homozygous PIZZ α₁AT deficiency—periodic acid–Schiff-positive, diastase-resistant globules in the ER of hepatocytes—substantiates the diagnosis (**Fig. 65-5**). According to some observers, these globules are not as easy to detect in the first few months of life.[54] The presence of these inclusions should not be interpreted as diagnostic of α₁AT deficiency. Similar structures are occasionally present in other liver diseases.[55] The inclusions are eosinophilic, round to oval, and 1 to 40 μm in diameter. They are most prominent in periportal hepatocytes but may also be seen in Kupffer cells and biliary epithelial cells.[56] The liver biopsy may also be characterized by variable degrees of hepatocellular necrosis, inflammatory cell infiltration, periportal fibrosis, and/or cirrhosis. There is often evidence of biliary epithelial cell destruction. Recent studies have also shown evidence for autophagosomes and mitochondrial injury[17] (**Fig. 65-6**).

Treatment

There is no specific therapy for α₁AT deficiency–associated liver disease; therefore clinical care involves avoidance of cigarette smoking to prevent exacerbation of destructive lung disease/emphysema, supportive management of symptoms caused by liver dysfunction, and prevention of complications of liver disease. Cigarette smoking markedly accelerates the lung disease associated with α₁AT deficiency, reduces quality of life, and significantly shortens the longevity of these patients.[57]

Progressive liver dysfunction and failure in children with α₁AT deficiency has been managed successfully with liver transplantation, with survival rates well over 92% for 5 years.[58] Nevertheless, a number of homozygotes with severe liver disease, even cirrhosis or portal hypertension, may have a relatively low rate of disease progression and lead a relatively normal life for extended periods. With the availability of living related donor transplantation techniques it may be possible to observe these patients for some time before transplantation becomes necessary.

Patients with α₁AT deficiency and emphysema have been treated with purified plasma or recombinant α₁AT administered intravenously or by means of aerosol as replacement therapy.[59] This therapy is associated with improvement both in α₁AT concentrations in serum and bronchoalveolar lavage fluid and in neutrophil elastase inhibitory capacity in lavage fluid without significant side effects. Although results of initial studies have suggested that there is a slower decline in forced expiratory volume in patients undergoing replacement therapy, this only occurred in a subgroup of patients and the study was not randomized.[60] This therapy is designed for established and progressive emphysema. Protein replacement therapy is not being considered for patients with liver disease because there is no evidence that deficient

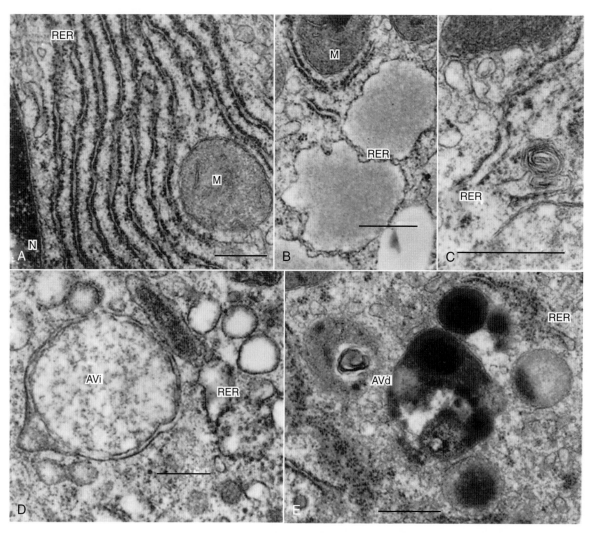

Fig. 65-6 **Electron micrographs of liver biopsy from an α₁AT-deficient patient. A,** Rough endoplasmic reticulum *(RER)* from a normal liver cell. **B,** RER distended with proteinaceous material. **C,** Autophagic vacuole pinching-off RER. **D,** Early autophagosomes *(AVi)* adjacent to RER. **E,** Degradative autophagosomes *(AVd)* adjacent to RER. Black bans = 100nm. M, mitochondrion *(Reproduced from Teckman JH, Perlmutter DH. Retention of the mutant secretory protein α1-antitrypsin Z in the endoplasmic reticulum induces autophagy. Am J Physiol 2000;279:G961–G974, with permission.)*

serum levels of α₁AT play a role in the development of liver injury.

A number of patients with severe emphysema from α₁AT deficiency are being treated with lung transplantation. Over a 13-year experience, 86 patients with α₁AT deficiency underwent lung transplantation in St. Louis with an approximately 60% 5-year survival rate.[61]

A number of novel strategies for chemoprophylaxis and treatment of α₁AT deficiency have been proposed recently. Because treatment of the PiZ mouse with cyclosporin A resulted in reduced hepatic mitochondrial damage, absent hepatic caspase-3 activation, and improved tolerance of starvation,[14] cyclosporin A and other drugs that prevent the mitochondrial permeability transition appear to be candidates for treatment of α₁AT deficiency–associated liver disease. This strategy is particularly attractive because it involves a mechanism of action at a distal step in the pathway of liver damage that is still effective, even though the primary pathologic phenomenon, mutant α₁ATZ, continues to accumulate in the ER.

Several studies have shown that a class of compounds called chemical chaperones can reverse the cellular mislocalization or misfolding of mutant plasma membrane, lysosomal, nuclear, and cytoplasmic proteins including CFTRαF508, prion proteins, mutant aquaporin molecules associated with nephrogenic diabetes insipidus, and mutant galactosidase A associated with Fabry disease.[62] These compounds include nonspecific chaperones such as glycerol, trimethylamine oxide, deuterated water, and 4-phenylbutyric acid (PBA) as well as specific chaperones that have antagonistic or agonistic pharmacologic bases. Burrows and colleagues determined that glycerol and PBA mediate a marked increase in the secretion of α₁ATZ in a model cell line.[63] Moreover, oral administration of PBA was well tolerated by the PiZ mouse and consistently mediated an increase in blood levels of human α₁AT, reaching 20% to 50% of the levels present in PiM mice and normal humans. PBA did not affect the synthesis or intracellular degradation of α₁ATZ. The α₁ATZ secreted in the presence of PBA was functionally active, in that it could form an inhibitory complex with neutrophil elastase. Because PBA has been used safely as an oral drug in children with urea cycle disorders, it was considered an excellent candidate for chemoprophylaxis of α₁AT deficiency. However, PBA did not mediate an increase in blood levels of α₁AT in a recent pilot human trial.[64] The explanation for the discrepancy between the mouse model and humans is not apparent but one prominent possibility is that humans are unable to tolerate the doses required for its salutary effect in mice. Studies of other candidate chemical chaperones will be important because the approach has the potential to prevent liver damage both by reducing the burden of α₁ATZ that accumulates in the cell and by increasing the secretion of α₁AT and therein the amount of α₁AT that reaches the lung to inhibit elastases.

Alternative strategies for at least partial correction of α₁AT deficiency may result from further studies of the fate of α₁ATZ in the ER. For instance, small molecules that prevent polymerization by inserting into specific conformationally important sites within the structure of α₁ATZ have been proposed. Indeed, a drug has been identified using this strategy that mediates an increase in degradation of α₁ATZ in a cell line model.[65] Another potential strategy involves drugs that enhance autophagy. Several FDA-approved drugs have been shown to enhance autophagic disposal of other aggregation-prone mutant proteins.[66,67] Replacement of α₁AT by means of somatic gene therapy has been discussed in the literature for a number of years.[68] This strategy is potentially less expensive than replacement therapy with purified protein and may avert the need for weekly or even monthly medication administration. As a form of replacement therapy, however, this strategy will only be useful for lung disease in α₁AT deficiency. There are still significant issues that need to be addressed before gene therapy becomes a realistic alternative. The most important prerequisite will be demonstration that replacement therapy with purified plasma α₁AT is truly associated with an ameliorative effect. Several novel types of gene therapy—such as repair of mRNA by trans-splicing ribozymes,[69,70] chimeric RNA/DNA oligonucleotides,[71-73] triplex-forming oligonucleotides,[74] small fragment homologous replacement,[75] or RNA silencing[76,77]—are theoretically attractive alternative strategies for the prevention of liver disease associated with α₁AT deficiency because they would prevent the synthesis of mutant α₁ATZ and accumulation in the ER. However, there has been limited progress in development of strategies to deliver these molecules in vivo.

Other studies have shown that transplanted hepatocytes can repopulate the diseased liver in several mouse models,[78,79] including a mouse model of the childhood metabolic liver disease hereditary tyrosinemia. Replication of transplanted hepatocytes only occurs when there is injury and/or regeneration in the liver. The results provide evidence that it may be possible to use hepatocyte transplantation techniques to treat hereditary tyrosinemia and, perhaps, other metabolic liver diseases in which the underlying defect is cell autonomous. For instance, α₁AT deficiency involves a cell-autonomous defect and would be an excellent candidate for this strategy.

References

1. de Serres FJ, Blanco I, Fernandez-Bustillo E. Genetic epidemiology of alpha-1 antitrypsin deficiency in North America and Australia/New Zealand: Australia, Canada, New Zealand and the United States of America. Clin Genet 2003;64:382–397.
2. Sveger T. Liver disease in α₁-antitrypsin deficiency detected by screening of 200 000 infants. N Engl J Med 1976;294:1316–1321.
3. Piitulainen E, et al. Alpha1-antitrypsin deficiency in 26-year-old subjects: lung, liver and protease/protease inhibitor studies. Chest 2005;128:2076–2081.
4. DeMeo DL, Silverman EK. Alpha₁-antitrypsin deficiency. 2: genetic aspects of alpha(1)-antitrypsin deficiency: phenotypes and genetic modifiers of emphysema risk. Thorax 2004;59:259–264.
5. Carrell RW, Lomas DA. Conformational disease. Lancet 1997;350:134–138.
6. Lomas DA, et al. The mechanism of Z α₁-antitrypsin accumulation in the liver. Nature 1992;357:605–607.
7. Lin L, et al. A naturally occurring non-polymerogenic mutant of α₁-antitrypsin characterized by prolonged retention in the endoplasmic reticulum. J Biol Chem 2001;276:33893–33898.
8. Schmidt B, Perlmutter DH. GRP78, GRP94 and GRP170 interact with α₁AT mutants that are retained in the endoplasmic reticulum. Am J Physiol 2005;289:6444–6455.
9. Kim J, et al. A thermostable mutation located at the hydrophobic core of α₁-antitrypsin suppresses the folding defect of the Z-type variant. J Biol Chem 1995;270:8597–8601.
10. Sidhar SK, et al. Mutations which impede loop-sheet polymerization enhance the secretion of human α₁-antitrypsin deficiency variants. J Biol Chem 1995;270:8393–8396.
11. Kang HA, Lee KN, Yu M-H. Folding and stability of the Z and Siiyama genetic variants of human α₁-antitrypsin. J Biol Chem 1997;272:510–516.
12. Yamasaki M, et al. Crystal structure of a stable dimer reveals the molecular basis of serpin polymerization. Nature 2008;455:1255–1259.
13. Teckman JH, et al. Mitochondrial autophagy and injury in the liver in alpha 1-antitrypsin deficiency. Am J Physiol Gastrointest Liver Physiol 2004;286:G851–G862.
14. Rudnick DA, et al. Analyses of hepatocellular proliferation in a mouse model of alpha-1-antitrypsin deficiency. Hepatology 2004;39:1048–1055.
15. Hidvegi T, et al. Accumulation of mutant α₁ATZ in the ER activates caspases-4 and -12, NFκB and BAP31 but not the unfolded protein response. J Biol Chem 2005;280:39002–39015.
16. Wang B, et al. Uncleaved BAP31 in association with A4 protein at the endoplasmic reticulum is an inhibitor of fas-initiated release of cytochrome c from mitochondria. J Biol Chem 2002;278:14461–14468.
17. Teckman JH, Perlmutter DH. Retention of the mutant secretory protein α₁-antitrypsin Z in the endoplasmic reticulum induces autophagy. Am J Physiol 2000;279:G961–G974.
18. Teckman JH, et al. Effect of fasting on liver in a mouse model of α₁-antitrypsin deficiency: constitutive activation of the autophagic response. Am J Physiol 2003;283:G1117–G1124.
19. Kamimoto T, et al. Intracellular inclusions containing mutant α₁-antitrypsin Z are propagated in the absence of autophagic activity. J Biol Chem 2006;281:4467–4476.
20. Kruse KB, Brodsky JL, McCracken AA. Characterization of an ERAD gene as VPS30/ATG6 reveals two alternative and functionally distinct protein quality control pathways: one for soluble A1PiZ and another for aggregates of A1PiZ. Mol Biol Cell 2006;17:203–212.
21. Kruse KB, et al. Mutant fibrinogen cleared from the endoplasmic reticulum via endoplasmic reticulum-associated protein degradation and autophagy: an explanation for liver disease. Am J Pathol 2006;168:1300–1308.
22. Geller SA, et al. Hepatocarcinogenesis is the sequel to hepatitis in Z#2 α₁-antitrypsin transgenic mice: histopathological and DNA ploidy studies. Hepatology 1994;9:389–397.
23. Liang X, et al. Induction of autophagy and inhibition of tumorigenesis by beclin 1. Nature 1999;402:672–676.
24. Vogel A, et al. Chronic liver disease in murine hereditary tyrosinemia type 1 induces resistance to cell death. Hepatology 2004;39:433–443.
25. Wu T, et al. A lag in intracellular degradation of mutant α₁-antitrypsin correlates with the liver disease phenotype in homozygous PiZZ α₁-antitrypsin deficiency. Proc Natl Acad Sci U S A 1994;91:9014–9018.
26. Qu D, et al. Degradation of mutant secretory protein, α₁-antitrypsin Z, in the endoplasmic reticulum requires proteasome activity. J Biol Chem 1996;271:22791–22795.
27. Teckman JH, Gilmore R, Perlmutter DH. The role of ubiquitin in proteasomal degradation of mutant α₁-antitrypsin Z in the endoplasmic reticulum. Am J Physiol 2000;278:G39–G48.
28. Cabral CM, et al. Organizational diversity among distinct glycoprotein endoplasmic reticulum-associated degradation programs. Mol Biol Cell 2002;13:2639–2650.
29. Pan S, et al. Single nucleotide polymorphism–mediated translational suppression of endoplasmic reticulum mannosidase I modifies the onset of end-stage liver disease in alpha1-antitrypsin deficiency. Hepatology 2009;50:275–281.

30. Chappell S, et al. A polymorphism of the alpha1-antitrypsin gene represents a risk factor for liver disease. Hepatology 2008;47:127–132.

31. Hidvegi T, et al. Accumulation of mutant alpha-1-antitrypsin Z in the ER activates caspases-4 and -12, NFκB and BAP31 but not the unfolded protein response. J Biol Chem 2005;280:39002–39015.

32. Hidvegi T, et al. Regulator of G signaling 16 is a marker for the distinct endoplasmic reticulum stress state associated with aggregated mutant α1-antitrypsin Z in the classical form of α1-antitrypsin deficiency. J Biol Chem 2007;282:27769–27780.

33. Rudnick DA, et al. Indomethacin increases liver damage in a murine model of liver injury from alpha-1-antitrypsin deficiency. Hepatology 2006;44: 976–982.

34. Hope PL, et al. Alpha-1-antitrypsin deficiency presenting as a bleeding diathesis in the newborn. Arch Dis Child 1982;57:68–70.

35. Hadchouel M, Gautier M. Histopathologic study of the liver in the early cholestatic phase of alpha-1-antitrypsin deficiency. J Pediatr 1976;89: 211–215.

36. Grishan FR, Gray GF, Green HL. α1-antitrypsin deficiency presenting with ascites and cirrhosis in the neonatal period. Gastroenterology 1983;85: 435–438.

37. Eriksson S, Carlson J, Velez R. Risk of cirrhosis and primary liver cancer in α1-antitrypsin deficiency. N Engl J Med 1986;314:736–739.

38. Volpert D, Molleston JP, Perlmutter DH. α1-antitrypsin deficiency–associated liver disease may progress slowly in some children. J Pediatr Gastroenterol Nutr 2001;32:265–269.

39. Nebbia G, et al. Early assessment of evolution of liver disease associated with α1-antitrypsin deficiency in childhood. J Pediatr 1983;102:661–665.

40. Ibarguen E, et al. Liver disease in α1-antitrypsin deficiency: prognostic indicators. J Pediatr 1990;117:864–870.

41. Hodges JR, et al. Heterozygous MZ α1-antitrypsin deficiency in adults with chronic active hepatitis and cryptogenic cirrhosis. N Engl J Med 1981;304: 357–360.

42. Gradziadei IW, et al. Increased risk of chronic liver failure in adults with heterozygous α1-antitrypsin deficiency. Hepatology 1998;28:1058–1063.

43. Propst T, et al. High prevalence of viral infection in adults with homozygous and heterozygous α1-antitrypsin deficiency and chronic liver disease. Ann Intern Med 1992;117:641–645.

44. Mahadeva R, et al. Heteropolymerization of S, I, and Z α1-antitrypsin and liver cirrhosis. J Clin Invest 1999;103:999–1006.

45. Teckman JH, Perlmutter DH. The endoplasmic reticulum degradation pathway for mutant secretory proteins α1-antitrypsin Z and S is distinct from that for an unassembled membrane protein. J Biol Chem 1996;271: 13215–13220.

46. Curiel DT, et al. Molecular basis of the liver and lung disease associated with the α1-antitrypsin deficiency allele M$_{malton}$. J Biol Chem 1989;264: 13938–13945.

47. Reid CL, et al. Diffuse hepatocellular dysplasia and carcinoma associated with the M$_{malton}$ variant of α1-antitrypsin. Gastroenterology 1987;93:181–187.

48. Lomas DA, et al. α1-antitrypsin M$_{malton}$ (Phe^{52} deleted) forms loop-sheet polymers in vivo: evidence for the C-sheet mechanism of polymerization. J Biol Chem 1995;270:16864–16870.

49. Perlmutter DH. Alpha-1-antitrypsin deficiency. In: Schiff ER, Sorrell MF, Maddrey WD, editors. Schiff's disease of liver, Vol. 2, 9th ed. Philadelphia: Lippincott-Raven, 2002: 1206–1229.

50. von Schonfeld J, et al. Liver function in patients with pulmonary emphysema due to severe alpha-1-antitrypsin deficiency (PIZZ). Digestion 1996;57: 165–169.

51. Steiner SJ, et al. Serum levels of α1-antitrypsin predict phenotypic expression of the α1-antitrypsin gene. Dig Dis Sci 2003;48:1793–1796.

52. Johnson K, Alton HM, Chapman S. Evaluation of mebrofenin hepatoscintigraphy in neonatal-onset jaundice. Pediatr Radiol 1998;28: 937–941.

53. Nord KS, et al. Concurrence of α1-antitrypsin deficiency and biliary atresia. J Pediatr 1987;111:416–418.

54. Mowat AP. Hepatitis and cholestasis in infancy: intrahepatic disorders. In: Mowat AP, editor. Liver disorders in children. London: Butterworth, 1982: 50.

55. Qizibash A, Yong-Pong O. Alpha-1-antitrypsin liver disease: differential diagnosis of PAS-positive diastase-resistant globules in liver cells. Am J Clin Pathol 1983;79:697–702.

56. Yunis EJ, Agostini RM, Glew RH. Fine structural observations of the liver in α1-antitrypsin deficiency. Am J Pathol 1976;82:265–286.

57. Wilson-Cox D. Alpha-1-antitrypsin deficiency. In: Scriver CB, et al, editors. The metabolic basis of inherited disease. New York: McGraw-Hill, 1989: 2409–2437.

58. Kemmer N, et al. Alpha-1-antitrypsin deficiency: Outcomes after liver transplantation. Transplant Proc 2008;40:1492–1494.

59. Wewers MD, et al. Replacement therapy for alpha 1-antitrypsin deficiency associated with emphysema. N Engl J Med 1987;316:1055–1062.

60. The Alpha-1-Antitrypsin Deficiency Registry Study Group. Survival and FEV$_1$ decline in individuals with severe deficiency of α1-antitrypsin. Am J Respir Crit Care Med 1998;158:49–59.

61. Cassivi SD, et al. Thirteen-year experience in lung transplantation for emphysema. Ann Thorac Surg 2002;74:1663–1670.

62. Perlmutter DH. Chemical chaperones: a pharmacological strategy for disorders of protein folding and trafficking. Pediatr Res 2002;52:832–836.

63. Burrows JA, Willis LK, Perlmutter DH. Chemical chaperones mediate increased secretion of mutant alpha 1-antitrypsin (α1-AT) Z: a potential pharmacological strategy for prevention of liver injury and emphysema in α1-AT deficiency. Proc Natl Acad Sci U S A 2000;97:1796–1801.

64. Teckman JH. Lack of effect of oral 4-phenylbutyrate on serum alpha-1-antitrypsin in patients with α1-antitrypsin deficiency: a preliminary study. J Pediatr Gastroenterol Nutr 2004;39:34–37.

65. Maliya M, et al. Small molecules block the polymerization of Z alpha-1-antitrypsin and increase the clearance of intracellular aggregates. J Biol Chem 2007;50:5357–5363.

66. Sarkar S, et al. Small molecules enhance autophagy and reduce toxicity in Huntington's disease models. Nat Chem Biol 2007;3:331–338.

67. Zhang L, et al. Small molecule regulators of autophagy identified by an image-based high-throughput screen. Proc Natl Acad Sci U S A 2007;104: 19023–19028.

68. Crystal RG. Alpha-1-antitrypsin deficiency, emphysema and liver disease: genetic basis and strategies for therapy. J Clin Invest 1990;95:1343–1352.

69. Long MB, et al. Ribozyme-mediated revision of RNA and DNA. J Clin Invest 2003;112:312–318.

70. Garcia-Blanco MA. Messenger RNA reprogramming by spliceosome-mediated RNA trans-splicing. J Clin Invest 2003;112:474–480.

71. Kren BT, Bandyopadhyay P, Steer CJ. In vivo site-directed mutagenesis of the factor IX gene by chimeric RNA/DNA oligonucleotides. Natl Med 1998;4:285–290.

72. Metz R, et al. Mode of action of RNA/DNA oligonucleotides. Chest 2002; 121:915–925.

73. Kmiec EB. Targeted gene repair—in the arena. J Clin Invest 2003;112: 632–636.

74. Seidman MM, Glazer PM. The potential for gene repair via triple helix formation. J Clin Invest 2003;114:487–494.

75. Gruenert DC, et al. Sequence-specific modification of genomic DNA by small DNA fragments. J Clin Invest 2003;112:637–641.

76. Davidson BL. Hepatic diseases—hitting the target with inhibitor RNAs. N Engl J Med 2003;349:2357–2359.

77. Rubinson DA, et al. A lentivirus-based system to functionally silence genes in primary mammalian cells, stem cells and transgenic mice by RNA interference. Nat Gen 2003;33:401–406.

78. Rhim JA, et al. Replacement of diseased mouse liver by hepatic cell transplantation. Science 1994;263:1149–1152.

79. Overturf K, et al. Hepatocytes corrected by gene therapy are selected in vivo in a murine mouse model of hereditary tyrosinemia type I. Nat Genet 1996; 12:226–273.

Inborn Errors of Metabolism that Lead to Permanent Liver Injury

Fayez K. Ghishan

ABBREVIATIONS

ADP adenosine diphosphate
ALT alanine aminotransferase
AMP adenosine monophosphate
AST aspartate aminotransferase
ATP adenosine triphosphate
BSEP bile-salt export pump
BSP sulfobromophthalein
CFTR cystic fibrosis transmembrane regulator
CoA coenzyme A
DHCA 3α,7α-dihydroxy-5β-cholestan-26-oic acid

DHA docosahexaenoic acid
FAH fumarylacetoacetate hydrolase
FDPase fructose-1,6-diphosphatase
GBE glycogen branching enzyme
GGTP γ-glutamyl transpeptidase
GSD glycogen storage disease
H&E hematoxylin and eosin
HFI hereditary fructose intolerance
MDR3 multidrug-resistant-3
NADH nicotinamide-adenine dinucleotide
NADPH nicotinamide-adenine dinucleotide phosphate

NTBC2 (2-nitro-4-trifluoro-methylbenzoyl)-1,3-cyclohexanedione
PAF1 peroxisome assembly factor-1
PAS periodic acid–Schiff
PFIC progressive familial intrahepatic cholestasis
P$_i$ inorganic phosphate
PRPP phosphoribosyl pyrophosphate
TPN total parenteral nutrition
UDP uridine diphosphate

Introduction

The liver is often affected by inborn errors of metabolism, but only a few of these injure the liver severely enough to cause permanent damage. Percutaneous liver biopsy has proved safe in infants and children, and this has allowed for the histologic, biochemical, and genetic evaluation of liver specimens from living patients, permitting rapid progress in the study of metabolic diseases during the past few years. Advances in molecular genetics promise greater advances in diagnosis and treatment of metabolic illnesses as our understanding of the pathophysiology of such disorders improves. **Table 66-1** lists the major metabolic diseases that involve the liver. Those marked with asterisks may lead to progressive disease and are discussed here or elsewhere in this book.

Evaluation of Hepatic Metabolic Disorders

The clinical history and physical examination are the first essentials in evaluating infants and children with metabolic

liver disorders. Of particular importance is a family history of any metabolic liver disease. Symptoms that may be associated with metabolic liver disorders are usually nonspecific and include vomiting, diarrhea, jaundice, seizures, and abnormal urinary odor. Clinical findings include hepatosplenomegaly, hypotonicity or hypertonicity, coarse facial features, and respiratory distress. In general, storage diseases usually cause marked hepatomegaly. By contrast, disorders resulting in hepatocellular damage cause only modest hepatomegaly. The physical examination should include adequate ophthalmologic examination by slit lamp for corneal, lenticular, and retinal alterations. Psychomotor evaluation to detect developmental delays is important in identifying those diseases that may involve the central nervous system. Initial laboratory screening tests such as analysis of the urine for reducing substances may help in early diagnosis of galactosemia. The peripheral blood smear may reveal vacuolation of the lymphocytic cytoplasm, which signifies deposition of storage material. Skeletal radiographs may reveal changes consistent with certain storage diseases, as in the case of mucopolysaccharidosis. Confirmatory tests depend on assays of appropriate enzymes in tissues such as leukocytes, skin fibroblasts, intestine, and liver, and

Table 66-1 Inborn Errors of Metabolism Resulting in Injury to the Liver

Inborn Errors of Carbohydrate Metabolism

Glycogen storage disease, types I-XII[a]
Galactosemia*
   Fructose-1-phosphate aldolase deficiency
   Fructose-1,6-diphosphatase deficiency

Inborn Errors of Protein Metabolism

Tyrosinemia*
Urea cycle enzymic defects

Inborn Errors of Lipid Metabolism

Gaucher disease
Niemann-Pick disease
Gangliosidosis
Acid cholesterol ester hydrolase deficiency*
   Wolman disease
   Cholesterol ester storage disease
Lipodystrophy

Inborn Errors of Mucopolysaccharide Metabolism

Inborn Errors of Porphyrin Metabolism

Protoporphyria*

Inborn Errors of Bile Acid Metabolism

Progressive familial intrahepatic cholestasis*
   Type I (Byler disease)*
   Type II (Byler syndrome)*
   Type III*
Hereditary lymphedema with recurrent cholestasis (Aagenaes syndrome)

Disorders of Peroxisome Biogenesis

Zellweger syndrome*
Alagille syndrome (arteriohepatic dysplasia)*

Inborn Errors of Copper Metabolism

Wilson disease (discussed in Chapter 63)*

Unclassified

α_1-Antitrypsin deficiency*
Cystic fibrosis*

*Diseases that lead to progressive disease and are discussed in this chapter or other sections of this book.
THCA, 3α,7α,12α-trihydroxy-5β-cholestan-26-oic acid

DNA analysis for mutations in those disorders with known genetic defects.

Disorders of Carbohydrate Metabolism

Three inborn errors in carbohydrate metabolism that may result in permanent liver damage are: (1) disorders of fructose metabolism; (2) disorders of galactose metabolism; and (3) certain glycogen storage diseases (GSDs) (**Fig. 66-1**). These three abnormalities are discussed separately.

Inborn errors resulting from the abnormal metabolism of lipids are mostly untreatable at present, and most of the errors in protein metabolism that respond to treatment require relatively stringent dietary restrictions. In contrast, most errors in carbohydrate metabolism that respond favorably to treatment

do so with relatively modest dietary restrictions. Liver diseases that occur in untreated patients with inborn errors of carbohydrate metabolism, such as fructose intolerance and galactosemia, are usually preventable. Although these particular conditions are relatively rare (about 1 in 30,000 live births for fructose intolerance and 1 in 20,000 live births for galactosemia), their combined incidence is similar to that of phenylketonuria (about 1 in 14,000 births in the United States). Considering the outcome in untreated patients and the simplicity of either measuring urinary reducing sugar or assaying the blood sample that is obtained to screen for phenylketonuria, it seems reasonable to implement the practice of routine screening of all newborn infants for both galactosemia and fructose intolerance.

Disorders of Fructose Metabolism

Fructose Phosphate Aldolase Deficiency (Hereditary Fructose Intolerance) and Fructose-1,6-Diphosphatase Deficiency

Until the mid-1950s, the only identified defect in fructose metabolism was the benign disorder essential fructosuria.[1] It was recognized in some patients in 1956 that ingestion of fructose was followed by vomiting, severe hypoglycemia, and liver disease.[2] A year later, this illness was characterized and named hereditary fructose intolerance (HFI).[3] A third disorder of fructose metabolism was identified in 1970. It was associated with fasting-induced and diet-induced hypoglycemia, but more strikingly, both fasting and dietary fructose caused lactic acidosis.[4] Each of these three disorders is distinct from the others both clinically and biochemically. Essential fructosuria is due to deficient activity of hepatic fructokinase; HFI is due to deficiency of fructose-1-phosphate aldolase; and the third condition results from deficiency of fructose-1,6-diphosphatase (FDPase). Essential fructosuria does not cause liver injury. Patients with FDPase deficiency may show transient fatty infiltration of the liver. In contrast, liver injury may be a significant feature of HFI.

Hereditary Fructose Intolerance

In 1957, Froesch and colleagues described the typical syndrome of HFI in two siblings and two relatives.[3] They recognized that the disorder, like essential fructosuria, was inherited and was associated with urinary excretion of fructose. They also realized that it was due to a different enzymatic defect and had different prognostic implications.

MOLECULAR BASIS OF HEREDITARY FRUCTOSE INTOLERANCE

Hereditary fructose intolerance occurs with a frequency of 1 in 20,000 individuals. It has a recessive mode of inheritance, and is caused by a deficiency of fructose-1-phosphate aldolase (aldolase B), which is normally present in the liver, kidneys, and small intestine. The enzymatic activities of the two other aldolase isoenzymes, aldolase A in muscle and aldolase C in the brain, are normal. The three isoenzymes are related and are derived from a single ancestral gene.

The aldolase B gene has been sequenced and is mapped to human chromosome 9q13→q32.[5] The gene has nine exons encoding 364 amino acids.[5,6] The gene consists of 14,500 base

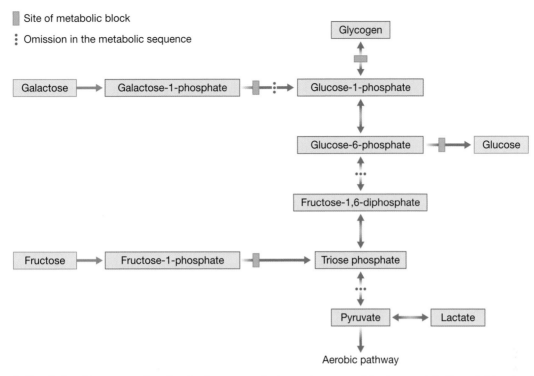

■ Site of metabolic block

⋮ Omission in the metabolic sequence

Fig. 66-1 **Metabolic relationship among disorders in glycogen, galactose, glucose, and fructose metabolism.** *Solid rectangle* indicates site of metabolic block; *red dots* indicate omission in the metabolic sequence.

pairs. The first mutation described was a G→C transversion in exon 5, which resulted in an amino acid substitution (alanine→proline) at position 149 of the protein within a region critical for substrate binding (A149P). The G→C transversion created a new recognition site for the restriction enzyme Aha II.[7] The alanine at position 149 is a conserved amino acid because it is present in the aldolase B gene of humans, rats, and chickens.[8] The substitution of proline is likely to disrupt the spatial configuration of juxtaposed residues in aldolase B and adversely affects its catalytic activity. The mutation alanine→proline was found in 67% of 50 HFI patients studied by Cross and colleagues.[9] This mutation is encountered more frequently in patients from northern than from southern Europe. Several other mutations have been described, such as alanine 174→aspartic acid (A174D) and asparagine 334→lysine (N334K).[10] Tolan and Brooks characterized the molecular defects in the aldolase B gene in 31 North Americans with HFI. Fifty-nine percent of mutant North American alleles were alanine 149→proline. Alanine 174→aspartic acid and asparagine 334→lysine represented 11% and 2% of North American alleles, respectively. Nine subjects (32%) had HFI alleles that were not these common, missense mutations.[11] Thus far, 25 mutations have been reported. The missense mutations could be classified into two groups: catalytic mutants with retained tetrameric structure but altered kinetic properties (W147R, R303W, and A337V) and structural mutations in which heterotetramers dissociate into subunits with impaired enzymatic activity (A149P, A174D, N334K).[12]

CLINICAL FEATURES

Patients with HFI may be extremely ill and may die after continuous exposure to fructose. However, affected patients are generally healthy and symptom-free so long as they do not ingest fructose or fructose-containing foods.[13,14] For this reason, symptoms do not arise until breast milk or cow's milk formulas are supplemented with fructose-containing foods. In fortunate cases, fructose is not introduced until after an affected infant is 5 to 6 months of age. By this time, the child is likely to associate nausea, vomiting, and symptoms of hypoglycemia with sweet-tasting food. In such cases, aversion to sweets is probably life-saving, and the diagnosis may go undetected until adulthood.[15] When this occurs, the diagnosis may be suspected on the basis of a careful history that recognizes the extreme aversion to dietary "sweets."

The largest single collection of patients consists of 55 patients diagnosed between 1961 and 1977 as having HFI.[16] Fifty of the patients had become symptomatic because of dietary fructose, and five were diagnosed shortly after birth because an older sibling of each infant was known to have HFI. Fourteen patients received fructose in their first feedings, and symptoms usually appeared within a few days. The remaining patients received a fructose-free diet (breast milk or cow's milk formula). Their symptoms began immediately after introduction of dietary fructose or sucrose. Thirty-two (64%) were diagnosed as having HFI at less than 6 months of age, 12 (24%) between 6 and 12 months of age, and 6 (12%) after 1 year of age. The younger patients were usually admitted to the hospital on an emergency basis with acute liver impairment, sepsis, bleeding diathesis, shock, or dehydration. Patients less than 6 months old developed a triad of jaundice, edema, and a tendency to bleed. Older patients were admitted more often because of liver enlargement, ascites, or both. Vomiting and hepatomegaly were observed in all patients, and about half had anorexia, weight retardation, and a tendency to bleed. About a third had jaundice, diarrhea, edema or ascites or both, and growth retardation. Thirteen of the 50 had developed an aversion to sweet foods. This aversion had developed as early as 3 months of age and in two patients had resulted in continued breastfeeding until 9 months of age. Vomiting and diarrhea in young children were sometimes severe enough to cause dehydration.

The laboratory findings were variable, but liver tests were severely deranged in the younger patients in this series.[16] Deficiency of clotting factors and elevated alanine aminotransferase (ALT) were present in all but one of the patients less than 6 months old. Two patients also had serum albumin levels of 2.8 g/dl. Fifteen patients had aminoaciduria; the predominant amino acids were tyrosine and methionine in 3 of the 15. All patients showed complete resolution of laboratory abnormalities in response to removal of fructose from the diet during a succeeding 2-week period.

Histologic abnormalities were found in the livers of all patients. Fibrosis without inflammation was present in either periportal or intralobular areas in most; all but three patients had some steatosis. These three patients were older and had voluntarily restricted themselves to diets with small amounts of fructose.[16]

Treatment of the symptomatic patients consisted of immediate cessation of fructose intake. Those with normal liver test results were given fructose-free diets normal in protein content. Infants who had acute liver dysfunction were given a glucose-electrolyte mixture intravenously and were given exchange transfusion when they had a serious bleeding tendency. Thereafter a fructose-free, low-protein diet was fed; when the liver dysfunction had been corrected, a diet with normal protein levels began. Clinical and biochemical improvement was dramatic after exchange transfusion. Vomiting ceased immediately. The bleeding tendency disappeared in less than 24 hours, and renal tubular dysfunction disappeared within 3 days. All patients showed resolution of symptoms and normalization of laboratory findings within 2 weeks. Catch-up growth occurred within 2 to 3 years. The only persistent abnormality was hepatomegaly with steatosis, which was present from birth in the five patients with restricted dietary fructose.[16] Although there were no deaths in the series reported by Odievre and co-workers,[16] the continuous intake of fructose may cause death because of hypoglycemic seizures or progressive liver failure and inanition. The second child of such a family may profit from experience with the first child by more rapid recognition of the illness.

With greater awareness, more cases of HFI in children are being diagnosed, and the condition is arrested by feeding fructose-restricted diets. One cautionary note is that a number of proprietary milks, primarily the soy-based formulas, contain sucrose as a significant source of the carbohydrate calories. The remaining carbohydrate is usually a glucose oligosaccharide. Hypoglycemia and seizures may not be a problem in affected infants fed these formulas because the remaining carbohydrate is glucose. The liver disease caused by fructose ingestion may be progressive, however, and infants fed these formulas may simply fail to thrive, have hepatomegaly and vomiting, or progress to chronic liver failure and death. Acute liver failure because of fructose intolerance is exceedingly unusual, and the absence of hepatomegaly in an infant who has severe liver disease and has reducing sugar in the urine should make one doubt the diagnosis of HFI. Follow-up studies of infants and recognition of older patients

with HFI indicate a normal life expectancy. Patients retain their sensitivity to dietary fructose as adults, but the hypoglycemic response to fructose may be somewhat more delayed in adults than in infants (45 to 60 minutes in infants; 60 to 90 minutes in adults).[14] The sensitivity to fructose may be life-threatening for adult patients. For example, patients with known HFI have been given sorbitol intravenously after surgery. Because sorbitol is metabolized to fructose, the patients died of complications from the sorbitol infusion.[17,18]

BIOCHEMICAL CHARACTERISTICS

The clinical and biochemical abnormalities seen in patients with HFI result from decreased activity of hepatic fructose-1-phosphate aldolase (aldolase B). This enzyme is normally present in the liver, renal tubular cells, and intestinal mucosa.[19] It catalyzes the conversion of fructose-1-phosphate to D-glyceraldehyde and dihydroxyacetone phosphate (reaction 1). The metabolic consequences of this enzymatic deficiency are the accumulation of large amounts of fructose-1-phosphate in the liver and depletion of inorganic phosphate (P_i) and adenosine triphosphate (ATP). The inability to metabolize fructose-1-phosphate in cells of affected patients leads to sequestration of large amounts of P_i. One of the many effects secondary to this sequestration of P_i is an inability to regenerate ATP, a process that depends on the presence of P_i. The clinical and laboratory features of HFI can be understood on the basis of this simple scheme (**Fig. 66-2**).

Patients with HFI have been shown to have levels of activity of fructose-1-phosphate aldolase ranging from 0% to 12% of normal.[14,20,21] In addition, most patients have reduced levels of activity of hepatic fructose-1,6-diphosphate aldolase ranging from 25% to 85% of normal.[20,22] The differential between the activities of the two aldolase enzymes suggests that they are separate protein moieties. However, Gurtler and Leuthardt have crystallized human liver aldolase and have shown that both enzymatic activities are attributable to a single liver aldolase.[23] In addition, slight alterations of the aldolase molecule, such as splitting off an end-terminal residue, may change the ratio of its affinity for fructose-1-phosphate or fructose-1,6-diphosphate.[24,25]

Patients with HFI produce a protein that has the immunologic properties of fructose-1-phosphate aldolase but is biologically inactive.[26] On the basis of these findings, it seems probable that a mutation of the structural gene is responsible for the enzyme defect in HFI. More recent studies suggest that the mutation in HFI affects aldolase B function by decreasing substrate affinity, maximal velocity, and/or enzyme activity.[27]

Accumulation of fructose-1-phosphate apparently causes the major manifestations of the disease through inhibition of other enzymatic reactions. Two metabolic pathways studied most extensively are gluconeogenesis and glycogenolysis. Their inhibition by fructose-1-phosphate explains fructose-induced hypoglycemia. Concentrations of fructose-1-phosphate in excess of 10 mmol/l completely inhibit fructose-1,6-diphosphate aldolase activity in vitro.[28] This finding suggests that fructose-1-phosphate inhibits gluconeogenesis at this enzymatic step. Inhibition at this site is further supported by the finding that fructose-induced hypoglycemia is not prevented by simultaneous infusions of gluconeogenic precursors, such as dihydroxyacetone or glycerol. In addition, liver

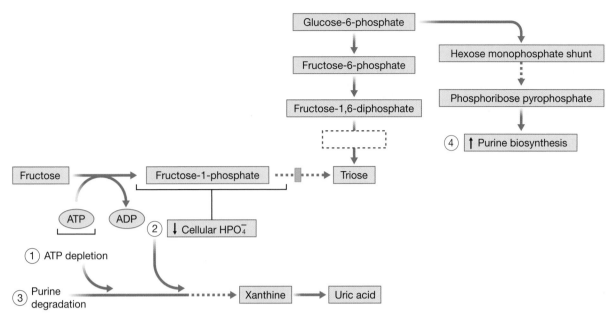

Fig. 66-2 Mechanism of hyperuricemia and hypophosphatemia in hereditary fructose intolerance. After fructose intake, there is rapid phosphorylation to fructose-1-phosphate, causing adenosine triphosphate (ATP) depletion *(1)* because of the aldolase block. The accumulated fructose-1-phosphate inhibits the aldolase step, preventing ATP generation from anaerobic glycolysis. Phosphate (HOP$_4^-$) is not released from the sugar, causing depletion of intracellular phosphate *(2)*. Low ATP and HOP$_4^-$ levels favor degradation of preformed purines to uric acid *(3)*. There is a compensatory increase in purine biosynthesis *(4)*. *Solid rectangle* indicates site of metabolic block. ADP, adenosine diphosphate

specimens from patients with HFI do not form glucose from ^{14}C-glycerol when fructose is present, whereas oxidation of ^{14}C-glycerol is apparently unaffected by fructose (reaction 2).[29]

Patients with HFI apparently also have inhibition of glycogenolysis after fructose intake. This inhibition occurs above the level of phosphoglucomutase. In support of this idea was the finding that when galactose is administered together with fructose, hypoglycemia is less pronounced and does not last as long as when fructose is given alone (reaction 3).[13] Thus a defect in the phosphorylation of glycogen to glucose-1-phosphate is incriminated. Several studies of normal liver indicate that depletion of P_i and accumulation of fructose-1-phosphate may contribute to an almost complete failure of glycogen mobilization.[30-32] In addition, depletion of intracellular ATP levels may contribute to the lack of glycogen degradation to glucose-1-phosphate.[32-34]

A variant of fructose intolerance has been described in which the red cell galactose-1-phosphate uridyl transferase activity was normal but galactose and fructose caused hypoglycemia.[35] The nature of this finding is unclear because a reevaluation of these patients 12 years later showed normal blood glucose responses to fructose and galactose.[36]

Results of studies by Schwartz and colleagues suggest that newborn infants delivered at term have less capacity for fructose metabolism in the first few days of life compared with later in life.[37] This is believed to be caused by the immaturity of the enzymes for handling fructose. In their studies, a rapid infusion of fructose caused a prompt but transient decrease in blood glucose and suppressed the glucagon-induced elevation of blood glucose. Although hepatic aldolase was not measured, the findings suggest that until further studies are completed, the use of fructose or sorbitol as a calorie source (as in total parenteral nutrition [TPN]) for term infants in the first few days of life may not be justified. Enzymatic

maturation may take longer in premature infants, although definitive studies have not been reported.

LABORATORY FEATURES

The primary laboratory features of HFI are fructose-induced hypoglycemia and hypophosphatemia and/or chronic liver disease. In addition, serum and urinary urate levels may be increased.

Hypoglycemia

Hypoglycemia induced by dietary or intravenous fructose is a characteristic of the illness. The hypoglycemia is not due to excess circulating insulin.[28,38] Sorbitol provokes hypoglycemia before substantial amounts of fructose are released into the circulation and is evidence against a direct effect of fructose on blood glucose levels.[14] More likely, the adverse effects of fructose result from intracellular accumulation of a fructose metabolite, such as fructose-1-phosphate.[28,39] This metabolite impairs both gluconeogenesis and glycogenolysis (reactions 2 and 3). Studies with ^{14}C-glucose indicate a complete cessation of hepatic glucose release after fructose infusion.[38] Also, glucagon does not increase blood glucose after fructose-induced hypoglycemia, even in the presence of normal to slightly elevated hepatic glycogen content.[40]

Hypophosphatemia

This is the second prominent feature of fructose-induced hypoglycemia. The reduction of inorganic phosphorus precedes that of glucose and may be the only abnormal finding when a small dose of fructose is administered.[14] Hypophosphatemia appears to be a consequence of binding and sequestration of phosphorus in the form of fructose-1-phosphate within the hepatocytes.[39,41] The first step in fructose metabolism is phosphorylation of the sugar by ATP. With large doses of fructose, ATP is depleted rapidly. With deficient activity of aldolase, as occurs in HFI, P_i is not released back into the cell. To compensate, phosphate from the serum is sequestered by the liver, with a resulting reduction in available circulating phosphate levels.[14] Phosphorylation of fructose decreases intracellular phosphate in normal individuals, but the phosphate sequestered in normal liver is made available by further metabolism of fructose-1-phosphate. Thus changes in serum levels of phosphate are extremely transient in a normal individual and depend on the amount of fructose ingested.

Hepatic Enzyme Elevation

This appears to be the direct effect of increased hepatic fructose-1-phosphate levels. Within $1\frac{1}{2}$ hours of a large dose of fructose, aminotransferase levels may increase more than two-fold.[34] The mechanism of liver cell damage is not clear, but it may result from a combination of depletion of ATP and a direct toxic effect of elevated levels of the phosphorylated hexose.

Hyperuricemia and Increased Urate Excretion

These conditions appear to result from depletion of intracellular ATP and P_i. This depletion of ATP and P_i increases the rate of purine degradation to uric acid (see **Fig. 66-2**).[32,33]

Other laboratory findings are less consistent. Some patients show substantial decreases in serum potassium and increases in serum magnesium after fructose intake.[14,40] Some have increases in serum lactate and pyruvate levels.[13,14,20] These changes appear to be related to the extent of liver damage and the severity of hypoglycemia. Granulocytosis may be noted with chronic fructose ingestion. A galactose infusion may relieve the hypoglycemia, but this is also an inconsistent finding. As blood glucose declines after fructose ingestion, insulin and insulin-like activity decrease and levels of glucagon, epinephrine, and growth hormone increase. In response to these hormonal changes, the nonesterified fatty acids in plasma increase more than two-fold, a response not observed in normal subjects.[13,20,42,43]

Renal tubular acidosis and a Fanconi-like syndrome with renal tubular reabsorptive defects have been reported.[16,44,45] The renal tubular acidosis is normalized in most patients as soon as fructose intake ceases.[46,47] Fructose-1-phosphate aldolase is normally present in the renal tubules but it is absent in patients with HFI. Hence, the transient renal disturbance in affected patients may be due to accumulation of fructose-1-phosphate in renal tubular cells after fructose intake.[19]

Pathology

Within $1\frac{1}{2}$ to 2 hours of a single dose of fructose, "glycogen-associated membrane arrays" and cytolysosomes in various stages of development are seen in the liver. The latter may represent lysosomes ingesting the accumulated fructose-1-phosphate in an attempt to get rid of it by acid hydrolysis. With chronic ingestion of fructose, the primary histologic changes are lipid accumulation, varying stages of hepatocellular necrosis, and bile duct proliferation. Liver disease may progress to cirrhosis with impairment of liver-dependent coagulation factors.[48] Despite extremely severe hepatic disease, the liver shows a remarkable ability to regenerate once dietary fructose is excluded. For example, a 3-month-old child who had cirrhosis, hypoalbuminemia, hypoprothrombinemia, and ascites had normal liver function and disappearance of ascites

after 3 weeks of a fructose-free diet. Except for slight fibrosis, the hepatic architecture was normal 3 years later.[40]

The pathogenesis of acute and chronic liver cell injury following fructose intake has not been studied in detail. By analogy with galactosemia, a six-carbon sugar phosphorylated at carbon 1 may have a direct cytotoxic effect, whereas phosphorylation of the carbon-6 position apparently has no obvious hepatic toxicity. In addition, the severe alterations in energy metabolism seen in patients with HFI may have a role in derangement of liver cell function and may thereby result in the pathologic changes observed after ingestion of dietary fructose. The reason for lipid accumulation is also unclear, but it may represent general cellular dysfunction seen in a number of unrelated conditions.[13,20,42,43]

Although renal function may be severely impaired, little histologic change occurs in the kidneys other than some increase in medullary lipid. The teeth of patients who have HFI are unusually free of caries. This has been taken to indicate that fructose and sucrose are important cariogenic substrates.[49] Despite the recurrent episodes of hypoglycemia and seizures that are common in undiagnosed cases, the brain is remarkably free of abnormalities. In contrast to patients with galactosemia, who commonly show psychomotor retardation, HFI patients surviving even the most severe forms of liver disease appear to have normal intelligence after being given fructose-free diets.

Genetics

The genetic findings are compatible with an autosomal recessive trait. Levels of hepatic fructose-1-phosphate aldolase activity in five parents of patients with HFI were normal.[50] In addition, carriers usually metabolize substantial fructose loads without difficulty. This is in contradistinction to carriers of galactosemia, who metabolize galactose at slower rates than normal and who may develop lenticular opacification with chronic galactose ingestion.

As already mentioned, the molecular basis of HFI is missense mutations in the gene. Testing for these mutations in amplified DNAs by the polymerase chain reaction with a limited panel of allele-specific oligonucleotides identifies more than 95% of patients. A reverse dot blot method is available as a screening tool, and can detect the two most common mutations (A149P and A174D).[51]

Differential Diagnosis

During infancy, various conditions may be associated with hypoglycemia,[52,53] but most of them are associated with fasting. Hypoglycemia after eating should be a clue to the possibility of HFI, particularly in the presence of urinary reducing sugar. Other diseases that are associated with hypoglycemia following ingestion of food include deficiency of fructose diphosphatase, galactosemia, and leucine intolerance. In addition, premature infants may have transient fructose intolerance because of immaturity of hepatic aldolase activity.[37] Some patients with Tay-Sachs disease have deficient levels of fructose-1-phosphate aldolase.[54,55] Three such patients were given fructose loads but did not develop hypoglycemia, hypophosphatemia, or hypermagnesemia. The relationship of the decreased enzymatic activity to the pathogenesis of Tay-Sachs disease is unknown, although measurement of fructose-1-phosphate aldolase activity has been used as a marker to detect the carrier state of Tay-Sachs disease.[55,56]

The diagnosis of HFI can be made by an intravenous fructose tolerance test. The smallest dose that produces the typical symptoms without causing nausea and vomiting is 0.25 g/kg body weight.[14] A dose of 0.25 g/kg body weight or 3 g/m^2 surface area is given as a single rapid injection. Marked, prolonged reductions of blood glucose and phosphate levels occur regularly with this dose. However, at least one infant with notable hepatomegaly and severely deranged hepatic function did not have the typical changes in blood glucose and phosphate until the intravenous dose was doubled. Thus with severe liver disease, blood and urinary levels of fructose are inconsistently elevated with the lesser fructose load. The lower dose of fructose may be a valuable aid as an initial screen for HFI, but a negative result, as described earlier, should not be used to rule out the diagnosis of HFI. Because the fructose load may cause symptomatic hypoglycemia, vomiting, and derangement of liver function, measurement of intestinal aldolase activity may be preferable in patients strongly suspected of having HFI.[57] The presumptive diagnosis made from tolerance tests should be confirmed by assay of enzyme activity in percutaneous liver biopsy specimens.

Treatment

A diet containing no fructose alleviates all the symptoms and liver dysfunction associated with HFI.[3,11-15] It is important that children and their parents receive detailed dietary counseling about which foods contain fructose. Older children commonly may associate discomfort with specific foods and regularly avoid them. However, infants are completely dependent on dietary selections made by their parents.

The common practice of adding small amounts of sugar to processed foods demands almost constant attention to avoid substantial fructose intake. One patient with HFI who continued to consume small amounts of fructose had chronic slight elevations in aspartate aminotransferase (AST) levels and hepatic fat accumulation. Because pharmacologic doses of folate are known to cause nonspecific increases in both aldolase activities, the patient was treated with 5 mg of folate daily, with a resultant 53% increase in hepatic fructose-1-phosphate aldolase activity. With no change in dietary intake, there were decreases in AST levels and hepatic lipid content. Tolerance tests, however, showed that folate treatment did not increase this patient's ability to handle a large dietary intake of fructose.[57]

Prognosis

Patients maintained on fructose-free diets have developed entirely normally, with normal life spans, although most continue to have slight hepatomegaly with hepatic steatosis.[16] Even infants with severely deranged liver function and substantial hepatic fibrosis can achieve remarkable recoveries once fructose is removed from their diets.

Fructose Diphosphatase Deficiency

In 1970, Baker and Winegrad described a patient who had a third type of genetic defect in fructose metabolism.[4] The predominant clinical findings were hepatomegaly and fasting-induced hypoglycemia with lactic acidosis. The patient was shown later to have deficient hepatic FDPase activity. Other cases with similar clinical and laboratory findings have subsequently been reported.[58] The primary difference between

patients with FDPase deficiency and patients with HFI is that fasting and dietary fructose induces symptoms in patients with deficiencies of FDPase. As a result, an occasional patient with FDPase deficiency has been incorrectly diagnosed as having type IB GSD. Several patients have been found to have "partial" FDPase deficiencies. These patients do not have lactic acidosis but develop hypoglycemia during fasting or secondary to dietary intake of fructose or glycerol. One such patient had many of the characteristics of the syndrome ketotic hypoglycemia.[59] Others have been erroneously diagnosed during infancy as having acute tyrosinosis. The deficiency of FDPase is inherited as an autosomal recessive trait. The diagnosis can be made by measurement of FDPase in cultured lymphocytes[60] and confirmed by detections of mutations in the FDPase gene.[61]

Disorders of Galactose Metabolism

In 1935, Mason and Turner provided the first detailed description of a patient intolerant of galactose.[62] Since then, numerous case reports have described the constellation of nutritional failure, liver disease, cataracts, and mental retardation that results from a deficiency of hepatic galactose-1-phosphate uridyl transferase activity.[63-65] The defect in galactosemia was initially thought to be a lack of synthesis of the transferase protein.[66] Advances in molecular cloning have shown, however, that there are missense mutations in the gene coding for the transferase enzyme in the majority of patients with galactosemia (discussed later). Subsequently, Gitzelmann described the case of a 44-year-old patient with galactosuria and early-onset cataracts.[67] Later reports indicated that this patient represented a second defect in galactose metabolism, which was a deficiency of galactokinase.[68,69] The latter defect apparently does not result in progressive liver disease and mental retardation. In 1972, Gitzelmann discovered a third type of galactosemia caused by uridine diphosphate (UDP): galactose-4-epimerase deficiency.[70] This condition has been considered benign to the extent that the deficiency is limited to leukocytes and erythrocytes, and affected individuals show no other laboratory or clinical abnormalities.[71] More recently, generalized epimerase deficiency has been described.[72-75] These patients show signs and symptoms identical to those of transferase-deficiency galactosemia. Because each of these conditions results in milk-induced galactosemia but represents three distinct biochemical entities, it has been suggested that the term galactosemia be supplemented by the specific enzymatic defect; that is, transferase-deficiency galactosemia, galactokinase-deficiency galactosemia, and epimerase-deficiency galactosemia.

Transferase-Deficiency Galactosemia

Human beings are capable of metabolizing large quantities of galactose, as demonstrated by the rapid elimination of galactose from blood.[76,77] Elevation of the level of plasma glucose occurs shortly after galactose infusion as a result of conversion of galactose to glucose. Tracer studies indicate that as much as 50% of galactose may be found in body glucose pools within 30 minutes of injection.[77] Under normal circumstances, plasma galactose is removed so rapidly by the liver that the rate of galactose clearance has been used as an index of hepatic blood flow[78] and liver function.[79] The removal mechanism is saturated at plasma levels of about 50 mg/dl, a level corresponding to the limits of the ability of galactokinase to phosphorylate the sugar. With a load of galactose that increases blood levels by 30 to 40 mg/dl, urinary losses may be substantial because the kidney threshold is at plasma levels of 10 to 20 mg/dl.[80]

Almost half of the calorie source in most mammalian milks is from hydrolysis of lactose to its two monosaccharides: glucose and galactose. Consequently, the series of enzymatic steps involved in conversion of galactose to glucose are most stressed during infancy. As a consequence, enzymatic defects of this pathway are most likely to produce clinical signs and symptoms, as well as marked elevations of blood and urinary galactose levels during this crucial period of development.

The first described defect resulting in galactosemia comes from deficient activity of the enzyme required for the second of four steps in galactose metabolism (**Fig. 66-3**). The consequences of this defect are much more severe than are those of the other defects in galactose metabolism, galactokinase deficiency, and UDP-galactose-4-epimerase deficiency.

MOLECULAR BASIS OF TRANSFERASE-DEFICIENCY GALACTOSEMIA

Transferase deficiency is an autosomal recessive disorder. The sequence of the homologous protein from *Escherichia coli*,[81] from *Saccharomyces cerevisiae*,[82] and from humans shows overall sequence identity of 35%. The cDNA coding for the human transferase enzyme is 1295 nucleotide bases in length and predicts a 43-kDa protein.[83] The gene has been mapped to chromosome 9p18 and spans 4 kb with 11 exons. The amino acids histidine (164)-proline-histidine (166) form an active site sequence that is essential for activity of the enzyme.[84] Southern, Northern, and Western blotting experiments suggest that the majority of galactosemia mutations are missense mutations that result in low or undetectable enzyme activity. The two most commonly characterized mutations are glutamine 188→arginine (Q188R) and lysine 285→asparagine (K285N), which account for 75% of all mutations in Caucasian and Hispanic populations.[85] Arginine 333→tryptophan mutation occurs at a highly conserved domain in the homologous enzymes from *E. coli*, yeast, and humans. Several other mutations have been described, such as valine 44→methionine (M) and methionine 142→lysine (K). Mutation S135L involving leucine substitution by serine occurs mostly in African Americans. Mutation N314D involves an asparagine to aspartate change as the basis for the Duarte variant. This variant is benign as the transferase expresses diminished but adequate enzyme activity.[86] These other mutations result in low or total loss of activity of the transferase. Therefore it appears that transferase-deficiency galactosemia results from missense mutations that tend to occur in regions that are highly conserved throughout evolution.[87] So far more than 219 mutations have been described.[88]

CLINICAL FEATURES

Since transferase-deficiency galactosemia was first described in 1935, numerous patients with the disorder have been monitored for long periods. In 1970, Komrower and Lee reported the results of long-term follow-up of the 60 known cases of galactosemia in the United Kingdom.[89] Long-term follow-up studies from 47 families have been reported from Los Angeles as well.[90] The disease varies in severity. Some patients may have an acute, fulminant illness after the first milk feedings or more commonly as a subacute illness with gastrointestinal symptoms (i.e., jaundice, failure to thrive). In milder cases, moderate intestinal upset after galactose ingestion may be the only manifestation. In severe cases, anorexia, abdominal distention, diarrhea, vomiting, and hypoglycemic attacks may occur shortly after birth. The most common initial symptoms are failure to thrive and vomiting, usually starting within the first few days of milk ingestion. **Table 66-2** lists the more common findings in 43 symptomatic patients.[74] Within the first week of life, hepatomegaly and jaundice are usually noted.

Table 66-2 Common Clinical Findings in 43 Symptomatic Galactosemic Patients

	NUMBER OF PATIENTS	INCIDENCE (%)
Anorexia and weight loss	23	53
Hepatomegaly	39	91
Jaundice	34	79
Ascites and/or edema	7	16
Vomiting	17	40
Abdominal distention	9	21
Cataracts	21	49
Infection	10	23
Sepsis	5	12

Reproduced from Koch R, et al. Galactosemia. In: Kelley VC, editor. Practice of pediatrics. Hagerstown, Md: Harper & Row, 1979:14, with permission.

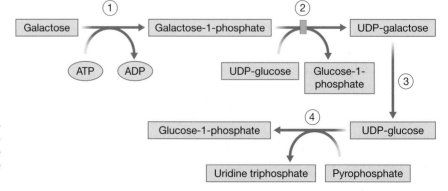

Fig. 66-3 Reactions in the conversion of galactose to glucose. *1,* Galactokinase; *2,* galactose-1-phosphate uridyltransferase; *3,* uridine diphosphate (UDP) galactose-4-epimerase; *4,* UDP glucose pyrophosphorylase

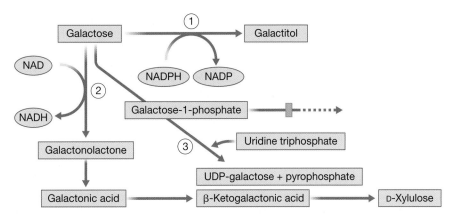

Fig. 66-4 **Alternative pathways of galactose metabolism.** *1,* Aldose reductase or L-hexonate dehydrogenase; *2,* galactose dehydrogenase; *3,* uridine diphosphate galactose pyrophosphorylase

In fact, prolonged obstructive jaundice in a neonate is a common presenting feature, and examination of urine for reducing sugar should be done in all infants with clinical jaundice. The jaundice from intrinsic liver disease may be accentuated in some infants with galactosemia by severe hemolysis and erythroblastosis. With continued galactose ingestion, ascites may develop as early as 2 to 5 weeks after birth. Cataracts may be seen within a few days after birth, or, if the mother has consumed large amounts of milk late during gestation, they may be present at delivery. The cataracts, consisting of punctate lesions in the nucleus of the fetal lens, may be so small that they can only be seen with slit-lamp examination. Retardation of mental development may be apparent after the first several months. A few patients homozygous for the disorder have been entirely asymptomatic while ingesting milk. These patients, who are usually black, may be capable of metabolizing moderate amounts of galactose.[75,91]

Since milk-substitute formulas have become easily accessible, infants who have recurrent vomiting and poor weight gain during the first few weeks of life are often given trials of one of the lactose-free formulas. An occasional infant with galactosemia may be unwittingly changed to such a formula, with resulting improvement without any awareness of the child's underlying defect. In such instances, the patient may have the disease undetected until months or years later, when he or she may have motor retardation, hepatomegaly, and cataracts.[92]

An important clinical observation about galactosemia is that of Levy and associates, who showed the strong association between galactosemia and *E. coli* sepsis.[93] In routine screening of more than 700,000 infants during a 12-year period, 8 infants were identified with classic transferase-deficiency galactosemia. Four of these infants had septicemia at the time galactosemia was detected (second week of life), and three of the four died. A review of results from eight other states that routinely screen newborns for galactosemia indicates that in screening more than 2.5 million newborns, 35 such patients were identified. Of the 35 patients, 10 are known to have had systemic infection, and 9 of the 10 died of bacteremia despite therapy. Infections usually develop at the end of the first week or during the second week of life, and their incidence appears to correlate directly with continued intake of galactose. These findings suggest that infants with *E. coli* sepsis should be considered possibly galactosemic and that infants recently diagnosed as galactosemic should be considered possibly infected with *E. coli.*

With initiation of a galactose elimination diet, all acute manifestations of the disease usually improve within 72 hours, and hepatic dysfunction begins to normalize by 1 week. During the first year of life, small amounts of dietary galactose may cause symptoms; however, around puberty, most patients show an improved tolerance to dietary galactose. To account for this improved tolerance, an alternative metabolic pathway for galactose has been postulated to develop about the time of puberty. This pathway is thought to bypass the deficient transferase step by forming UDP-galactose from the interaction of galactose-1-phosphate and uridine triphosphate (**Fig. 66-4**).[94] This reaction in the liver and brain would reduce the concentration of galactose-1-phosphate to normal levels and would thus protect against the effects of the defective pathway. Although this hypothesis represents an attractive explanation for the increased ability to tolerate galactose later in life, tracer studies do not support an increased rate of galactose metabolism. A third pathway, involving the formation of xylulose, is unimportant in normal humans but may permit survival of some patients who continue to ingest galactose (see **Fig. 66-4**).

LABORATORY FINDINGS

Routine laboratory findings may be varied but include elevated blood and urinary levels of galactose, hyperchloremic acidosis, albuminuria, aminoaciduria, hypoglycemia, and blood changes reflecting deranged liver function. Occasionally, infants may have severe and prolonged hypoglycemia. The galactosuria may be intermittent because of poor food intake or may disappear within 3 or 4 days of intravenous feeding. Thus, if the urine is not tested for reducing sugar during a period of galactosuria, the diagnosis may not be suspected. The finding of a urinary reducing substance that does not react with the glucose oxidase test should alert one to the possibility of galactosemia. This finding does not establish the diagnosis because several other conditions such as fructosuria, lactosuria (from deficient intestinal lactase), and severe liver disease of any origin may impair the clearance of blood galactose and result in the presence of urinary reducing sugar that is not glucose.[92]

BIOCHEMICAL CHARACTERISTICS AND PATHOGENESIS OF GALACTOSE TOXICITY

The hepatic manifestations of transferase-deficiency galactosemia are entirely due to the abnormal metabolism of galactose. Toxicity apparently results from accumulation of the metabolic products of galactose rather than from galactose itself. The two compounds that have been studied most extensively are galactose-1-phosphate and galactitol, the product of an alternate pathway (see **Fig. 66-4**). The biochemical causes of toxicity in individual organs may differ, depending on the metabolic patterns and functions of the involved organs. For example, cataracts are apparently caused by galactitol accumulation, whereas this compound appears to have little, if any, relation to the renal abnormalities or hepatic dysfunction.

Hypoglycemia

Hypoglycemia that may occur after galactose ingestion is apparently caused by inhibition of glucose release from glycogen. The mechanism responsible is postulated to be high levels of galactose-1-phosphate that interfere with phosphoglucomutase, the enzyme that catalyzes the conversion of glucose-1-phosphate to glucose-6-phosphate.[95] In addition, there is an inhibition of glucose formation through gluconeogenesis.[96] The galactose-1-phosphate may be toxic in other ways as well, although investigations aimed at answering this question depended primarily on changes induced in normal animals fed high-galactose diets and do not necessarily reflect the changes that occur in patients who have deficiencies of enzymatic activity.

Lenticular Changes

Changes in the lens appear to result primarily from accumulation of galactitol. Van Heyningen showed galactitol accumulation, and Kinoshita and associates showed that an increase in galactitol concentration caused a concomitant increase in water content secondary to the oncotic pressure from the galactitol.[97-99] The poor diffusion of the alcohol from the lens makes this organ particularly susceptible. Reversing the osmotic effect of the galactitol accumulation with an osmotically balanced incubation medium prevents the lenticular opacification.[98] Many biochemical alterations occur concurrently in the lens as it undergoes cataract formation. These include decreases in amino acid transport, protein synthesis, several enzymatic activities, and alteration of ion fluxes.[99-104] Glycolysis and respiration of the lens are reduced by about 30% after about 2 days of galactose feeding and remain at this level until cataracts develop.[103] It is not surprising then that nutrient supplements can alter the rate of cataract formation in galactose-fed animals.[105] Thus nutrient imbalances and alterations in lenticular water content from galactitol formation together are prime initiators of lenticular opacification. The causes of cellular damage in other organs are less clear.

Liver

The concentration of both galactose-1-phosphate and galactitol in the liver is elevated in patients fed galactose.[106,107] However, the liver damage seen in patients with transferase deficiencies does not occur in normal animals fed high-galactose diets despite high hepatic levels of galactose-1-phosphate and high hepatic galactitol levels.[108,109] In addition, patients with galactokinase deficiencies form large amounts of galactitol but show no liver damage. This suggests that some other metabolite or metabolites accumulate to act singly or in concert to cause cellular toxicity. In this respect,

galactosamine, which was increased in the liver of one patient, is known to induce hepatocellular changes in animals.[109]

Kidneys

Kidneys of transferase-deficient patients develop renal tubular dysfunction after galactose ingestion. They accumulate both galactose-1-phosphate and galactitol.[106,107] However, accumulation of galactitol alone does not appear toxic because patients with galactokinase deficiencies do not develop renal dysfunction but do excrete large amounts of galactitol. This suggests that the alcohol is not the primary renal insult in patients with transferase deficiency. Aminoaciduria can be induced in both normal humans and rats by large amounts of galactose.[110,111] This could be because of an accumulation of galactose-1-phosphate that secondarily impairs amino acid accumulation by the tubules.[112] If analogous to that in the human intestine, the inhibition is noncompetitive.[113]

Brain

Changes in the brains of patients with transferase-deficiency galactosemia may not be entirely reversible after galactose restriction. For this reason, substantial efforts have been made to delineate the pathogenesis of galactose-induced brain damage. Galactitol accumulates in higher concentrations in the brains of patients and those of rats fed galactose than in any other tissue except the lens.[108,114] This observation suggests that galactitol accumulation may be important in the pathogenesis of brain abnormality. However, in patients with galactokinase deficiencies, galactitol accumulation does not appear to damage tissues other than the lens.

Studies in chick brain showed that galactose administration diminished ATP, reduced brain glucose and glycolytic intermediates, redistributed hexokinase, enhanced fragility of neural lysosomes, and decreased fast axoplasmic transport.[115-119] The effects could be temporarily reversed by glucose.[120] Changes in the chick brain appear to be related to several factors such as hyperosmolality,[119] alterations in energy metabolism,[116] abnormal serotonin levels,[121] and interference with active uptake of glucose into the neurons. It remains to be determined whether these changes in chicks are similar to galactose-induced abnormalities in patients with transferase deficiencies.

Although intestinal epithelium of patients with galactosemia is also deficient in transferase activity, this deficiency does not appear to alter intestinal transport of galactose. Many infants develop intestinal symptoms of vomiting and diarrhea after galactose ingestion, but it is unclear whether this is a direct effect on the intestine or secondary to the effects of galactose on the central nervous system.

Gonads

Ninety percent of galactosemic females have ovarian failure, which is present shortly after birth. Biochemically, follicle-stimulating hormone (FSH) is high whereas antimüllerian hormone (AMH) is low compared with controls (hypergonadotropic hypogonadism).[122] Males with galactosemia have normal testicular function. The mechanism underlying ovarian failure in galactosemic women is not known, although galactose toxicity has been implicated. It is interesting to note that tissues with the highest transferase activity are target organs for the dysfunction and are affected to the greatest extent in galactosemia. In this regard, the ovary has five times more transferase activity and transferase mRNA than the testis.[123]

Pathology

Early hepatic lesions, present in the first weeks of life, consist of cholestasis and diffuse fatty vacuolation with little or no inflammatory reaction. The fatty changes are extensive and generalized throughout the lobule. Later, disorganization of the liver cells with pseudoductular and pseudoglandular formation occurs. This tendency toward pseudoglandular orientation of cells has been described as characteristic of galactosemia but is relatively nonspecific. As the disease progresses, delicate fibrosis appears, first in the periportal regions, eventually extending to bridge adjacent portal tracts. Regenerating nodules and hepatic fibrosis are late features that, with continued galactose ingestion, progress to cirrhosis that is similar in many respects to the cirrhosis of ethanol abuse. Death usually occurs in the first year of life unless galactose intake is decreased or curtailed. Frank cellular necrosis is unusual but may occur with large amounts of dietary galactose. Despite the severity of the hepatic lesion, there is a remarkable lack of infiltration by inflammatory cells.[124]

Except for cataract formation in the lens, other tissues show only minor changes. Kidneys show dilation of tubules at the corticomedullary junction. The spleen enlarges as a result of portal hypertension. Lesions in the brain are subtle, with minor loss of nerve cells and gliosis in the dentate nucleus and in the cerebral cortex and gray matter.[125]

Genetics

Investigations of red blood cell and leukocytic transferase activities in family members indicate that the disorder is transmitted as an autosomal recessive trait.[126] Heterozygotes have about 50% of normal activity, and genotype detection is more accurate when the transferase/galactokinase ratio is determined.[127] Population studies indicate that the incidence of heterozygosity for galactosemia is between 0.9% and 1.25% and that between 8% and 13% carry the Duarte gene.[128] Incidences of transferase-deficiency galactosemia derived from large-scale screening in neonatal nurseries have been between 1 in 10,000 and 1 in 70,000 live births.[129,130] At least one patient with transferase-deficiency galactosemia has delivered a normal heterozygous infant.[90]

Diagnostic Screening for Galactosemia

The rationale for genetic screening is three-fold: (1) to detect disease at its incipient stage and thereby offset harmful expression of the mutant gene through appropriate medical treatment; (2) to identify a variant genotype for which reproductive options (family planning) may be provided; and (3) to identify gene frequency or biologic significance and natural history of variant phenotypes.

Various screening methods have been used for galactosemia.[131] The original Guthrie test used filter paper blood samples from which a microbiologic assay detected elevated galactose levels. The newer Beutler test assays the erythrocyte transferase activity directly from dried filter paper, and the Paigen assay is an improved bacteriologic method that includes detection of elevated levels of galactose and galactose-1-phosphate. Measurements of elevated galactose require that the infant receive sufficient dietary galactose or a false-negative

test will result. Conversely, the normal enzyme may become inactive in a hot or humid climate, and a false-positive (negative enzyme activity) may be reported.

The relatively common inaccuracies of the screening tests for galactosemia and the low prevalence of the illness, coupled with the observation that infants born into families without a known history of galactosemia may be affected at birth, have prompted some screening centers not to screen for galactosemia. For example, in Quèbec, the spaces on the blood sample filter paper assigned to galactosemia were given over to screening for congenital hypothyroidism, with a striking increase in cost effectiveness.

In utero assay for galactosemia is indicated in pregnant women with a family history of galactosemia. Cultured fibroblasts from amniotic fluid can be assayed for transferase activity. Additionally, the technique of chorionic villus sampling has been used to detect galactosemia during the tenth week of gestation.[132] Cloning of the cDNA encoding for the transferase enzyme and the finding that the majority of galactosemic patients have missense mutations have allowed for rapid molecular approaches using the polymerase chain reaction to detect common mutations.

Diagnosis

The presumptive diagnosis of galactosemia in an infant with vomiting and failure to thrive on milk feedings may be made by identification of a urinary reducing sugar that does not react with glucose oxidase reagents. It should be remembered that lactose, fructose, and pentose may give similar results, but if the formula is milk based and there is no other dietary sugar, galactosemia is the presumed diagnosis, and restriction of dietary galactose should be initiated immediately. Identification of the sugar can be made by paper or gas-liquid chromatography. Paper impregnated with galactose oxidase makes screening for galactosuria easier. Normal premature and some normal term infants may excrete as much as 60 mg/dl urinary galactose during the first week or two of life.

Unlike suspected fructose intolerance, which may be diagnosed by use of a fructose tolerance test, demonstration of galactosuria or galactosemia by a galactose tolerance test should never be used. Although not clearly documented, it has been suggested that a single large exposure to galactose may result in severe and prolonged hypoglycemia, with resulting brain damage. For this reason, the definitive diagnosis should be made on the basis of direct measurement of transferase activity and not by a tolerance test.[75,76]

The red cell UDP-glucose consumption test has been used extensively as a screening test for the past decade.[92,129,130,133] It is based on the assay of UDP-glucose before and after incubation of galactose-1-phosphate with red cell hemolysate as the source of transferase. Conversion of UDP-glucose to UDP-glucuronic acid by UDP-glucose dehydrogenase forms NAD from nicotinamide-adenine dinucleotide (NADH), which is measured spectrophotometrically. With this procedure, a complete absence of red cell transferase activity is found in homozygous patients, and intermediate levels are found in heterozygous carriers. Infants identified as having 50% of normal activity should have further tests to rule out other variants that may be homozygous and provide 50% of enzymatic activity (see later discussion).

With the advent of screening for galactosemia, multiple variants of this disease have become apparent, the variants being more prevalent than classic transferase-deficiency galactosemia.[134] There are three homozygotic types:

1. "Classic" galactosemia is autosomal recessive, and there is no transferase activity in erythrocytes, fibroblasts, liver, and presumably in any other tissue. In heterozygotic, unaffected carriers, activity is 50% of normal.

2. The Duarte variant is the most common form of galactosemia and is only detected by enzyme screening because these infants are asymptomatic. Red cell activity is 50% of normal, and the enzyme migrates faster than normal on starch gel electrophoresis. Red cells of patients who have this variant produce two distinct bands rather than the single normal transferase band. In addition, red cells of a parent of a Duarte-homozygous patient have three bands for the variant enzyme. Homozygotic Duarte erythrocytes have 50% of normal enzyme activity; heterozygous Duarte erythrocytes have 75% of normal activity. Ten percent to 15% of the population may have Duarte-variant galactosemia. The Duarte gene is apparently allelic with the normal and galactosemic genes because the most frequently detected abnormality on neonatal screening tests is the compound heterozygous state, consisting of classic galactosemia with the Duarte variant. Two protein bands are present on protein electrophoresis, and erythrocyte transferase activity is 25% of control. Although some of these infants appear asymptomatic at birth and remain so during infancy, others have systemic symptoms with metabolic manifestations of galactosemia.

3. In the "Negro" variant, erythrocytic transferase activity is absent, but 10% of normal activity is present in the liver and intestine. The Duarte and the Negro variants may be asymptomatic despite galactose ingestion, although patients with the variant may develop a galactose toxicity syndrome in the neonatal period.

In addition to the homozygotic variants, several heterozygotic variants have been identified:

1. An Indiana variant in which erythrocytic transferase activity is approximately 35% of normal and is highly unstable (mobility on starch gel electrophoresis is slower than normal).

2. A Rennes variant, which has about 7% to 10% of normal transferase activity (this variant also travels more slowly than normal by electrophoresis).

3. The Los Angeles variant, which has erythrocytic transferase activity higher than normal (about 140%); this has been detected in six families. Electrophoretic mobility of this variant of the enzyme is similar to that of the Duarte variant. West German and Chicago variants have also been identified by screening procedures.

Treatment

Although the cause of the entire toxicity syndrome in transferase deficiency is uncertain, there is no disagreement that elimination of galactose intake reverses the biochemical manifestations of transferase-deficiency galactosemia. Some patients seem to have increasing tolerance to galactose with advancing age; however, studies using ^{14}C-galactose do not support the clinical impression that alternate pathways of galactose metabolism develop at puberty,[90-92] nor is there any indication that any drug will increase galactose oxidation, although some patients with variant forms of transferase deficiencies can oxidize limited amounts of galactose.

The only acceptable treatment at present is elimination of dietary galactose. Permissible diets are described in at least two publications.[77,90] Preparations used in treating infants are Pregestimil, Nutramigen, and the soybean milk preparations. Both Pregestimil and Nutramigen are prepared from casein and may contain small amounts of lactose, but this amount of lactose does not appear to be sufficient to impair therapeutic efficacy. The soybean formulas contain small amounts of galactose in raffinose and stachyose, and other dietary constituents contain small amounts of galactosides, but these carbohydrates are not digested by human intestinal enzymes and should not affect the efficacy of treatment.[90] Because of the frequent addition of milk to a number of proprietary food items, strict attention must be given to the diet during and after weaning. Concern has been raised regarding the presence of galactose in grains, fruits, and vegetables.[135] These foods contain significant amounts of soluble galactose, although newer information related to substantial endogenous production of galactose has minimized this concern.[136]

It is important to be aware that asymptomatic heterozygotic mothers may have elevated serum galactose levels after ingestion of diets high in milk. Infants delivered of such mothers may have the galactosemic syndrome at birth. For this reason, restriction of galactose during the pregnancies of women who have previously borne children with galactosemia is recommended.[90-92] The use of uridine and aldose reductase inhibitors in galactosemic patients has not been shown to be effective despite their theoretical advantage.[137,138]

Prognosis

When untreated, galactosemia results in early deaths of many affected children and is attended by the prospect of mental retardation of those who survive. In a series of 43 galactosemic patients described by Koch and colleagues, there were 13 neonatal deaths.[90] The deaths occurred at an average age of 6 weeks and were usually attributed to infection. Levy and co-workers noted that 9 of 35 patients died of *E. coli* infections and strongly recommended early cultures and institution of antibiotics effective against *E. coli* in any infant with galactosemia who appears ill.[93]

Treatment of galactosemic patients with a galactose-free diet results in survival with reversal of the acute symptoms, normal growth, and complete recovery of liver function; however, the long-term outcome (particularly for intellectual development) is not entirely certain. Experience gained in the long-term follow-up of 59 patients in the Los Angeles area indicates that many patients have developed very well and have attained college-level educations.[90] Others who were equally well treated with galactose restriction have had various intellectual deficiencies, including verbal dyspraxia, reduced intelligence, learning disabilities, and neurologic deficits.[139] The causes of the variability in the responses to treatment need further exploration.

Hypergonadotropic hypogonadism is another long-term disorder observed in galactosemic women.[140,141] Although successful pregnancy is possible, 90% of galactosemic women develop ovarian failure with atrophic gonads. The mechanism is believed to be related to excess galactose exposure during fetal and childhood development[142] or to galactose restriction and a specific galactose need during ovarian development. The male gonads, however, appear more resistant to the effects of galactosemia.[143]

Osteoporosis is a frequent complication among females with galactosemia. The mechanisms underlying this complication may relate to low calcium intake, lack of sex hormones associated with ovarian failure, and an independent defect in collagen synthesis resulting in disturbances in bone mineralization.[144,145] Renner and co-workers have shown that treatment with hormone replacement and vitamin D therapy (1000 IU/day) resulted in the onset of menarche and increased bone density in two 28-year-old galactosemic twins when treatment was started at 25 years of age.[145]

Although genetic and social factors may influence results of intelligence tests, such factors do not explain all the differences observed. The association of thyroid dysfunction with galactosemia may have some role in the outcome.[146,147] A factor that definitely affects outcome is the age of the patient at diagnosis. Evidence supports the previous impression that a more favorable outcome can be expected when a patient is treated at an early age. For example, the mean IQ of 16 patients treated before 7 days of age was 99.5, whereas that of patients treated between 4 and 6 months of age was 62. It is generally desirable to institute treatment at the earliest possible age, and neonatal screening is an important step in this direction. Although diagnosis and treatment at birth are desirable objectives, it is also possible that homozygotic galactosemic infants may have experienced unfavorable intrauterine exposure to galactose or its metabolites. Even with maternal dietary restriction of lactose during pregnancy, levels of erythrocytic galactose-1-phosphate in samples of cord blood from 12 homozygotic infants still averaged 11.3 mg/dl. Thus it appears that the intrauterine environment is not ideal for a homozygotic galactosemic fetus.[90]

Galactokinase-Deficiency Galactosemia

Galactokinase deficiency is less common than classic transferase deficiency, with an incidence of about 1 in 10,000.[148] It does not result in progressive liver disease and mental retardation, but galactose exposure may result in cataract formation.[67-69] It is appropriate to compare this entity with transferase deficiency because it affects the first reaction (kinase) and the transferase, the second reaction of the galactose pathway (see **Fig. 66-3**). Comparison of patients with these two defects and the defect involving the third reaction (epimerase) has helped to define some of the mechanisms of toxicity in several organs, including the development of cataracts. With galactokinase deficiency, there is no accumulation of galactose-1-phosphate, no systemic manifestations, and no mental retardation. Cataract formation is related to synthesis of galactitol in the lens and osmotic disruption of lens fiber architecture, as discussed in the previous section. Maternal galactokinase deficiency may result in fetal cataract formation.[148] Because of the potential for cataract formation, lifelong elimination of galactose is suggested. The gene has been mapped to chromosome 17q24, and 20 mutations have been described in galactokinase gene, resulting in loss of the activity of the enzyme.[149]

Uridine Diphosphate Galactose-4-Epimerase-Deficiency Galactosemia

Galactose epimerase catalyzes the third reaction of galactose metabolism (see **Fig. 66-3**). Epimerase deficiency was discovered incidentally while screening for galactosemia and has an incidence of about 1 in 46,000 in Switzerland. Patients have normal erythrocyte transferase activity but elevated levels of galactose-1-phosphate.[70,71] One form of this condition is apparently caused by a decreased stability of the epimerase and leads to enzyme deficiency in those cells in which its turnover is slow or absent, such as erythrocytes.[150] It is therefore considered to be a benign illness in as much as the enzyme deficiency is limited to leukocytes and red blood cells. Affected persons with the form limited to leukocytes and red blood cells have no symptoms but patients with generalized epimerase deficiency have been described.[72,74] The latter patients have signs and symptoms identical to transferase-deficiency galactosemia.

By contrast with transferase deficiency, in which uridine diphosphogalactose can be formed from uridine diphosphoglucose, one patient with generalized epimerase deficiency was unable to synthesize the galactose precursor necessary for synthesis of glycoproteins and glycolipids. These glycosylated compounds are necessary for cell membrane integrity, especially in the central nervous system. Thus, in contrast to patients with transferase deficiency, the rare patient with systemic epimerase deficiency may require small quantities of galactose for normal growth and development. One patient with epimerase deficiency continued to show slightly elevated levels of galactose-1-phosphate in red cells even with dietary restriction of galactose. Appropriate treatment of this disorder therefore requires frequent monitoring of erythrocyte galactose-1-phosphate levels to best determine the optimal dietary level of galactose.

Glycogen Storage Diseases

Clinical and pathologic recognition of GSD affecting the liver and kidneys was described by von Gierke in 1929.[151] Three years later, Pompe recognized another type of GSD that involved not only the liver and kidneys but most other organs as well.[152] In 1952, Cori and Cori showed that hepatic glucose-6-phosphatase activity was deficient in patients with von Gierke disease.[153] This marked the beginning of a classification of glycogenoses by the types of enzymatic defects and the primary organs of involvement. In most types of GSD, the glycogen content of liver or muscle or both is excessive. In unusual cases, the glycogen content may be less than normal, the molecular structure of glycogen may be abnormal, or both may occur. Despite differences in the specific enzymatic defects, most of the syndromes are not readily distinguishable on clinical grounds alone, and tissue analyses for glycogen content and enzymatic activity are necessary to confirm the diagnoses.[154,155] Deficiencies of enzymes involving almost every step of glycogen synthesis and degradation have been identified. Their locations in the sequence of glycogen synthesis and degradation are illustrated in **Figure 66-5**.

Most enzymatic defects giving rise to hepatic glycogenosis involve degradation of glycogen to glucose-6-phosphate or, in rare instances, the synthesis of glycogen from glucose-6-phosphate.[154-157,163] On the other hand, patients with von Gierke disease are deficient in the activity of glucose-6-phosphatase, a gluconeogenic enzyme. As a consequence of this enzymatic difference, many of the clinical and chemical features of von Gierke disease, or type I GSD (GSD-I), are unique among the

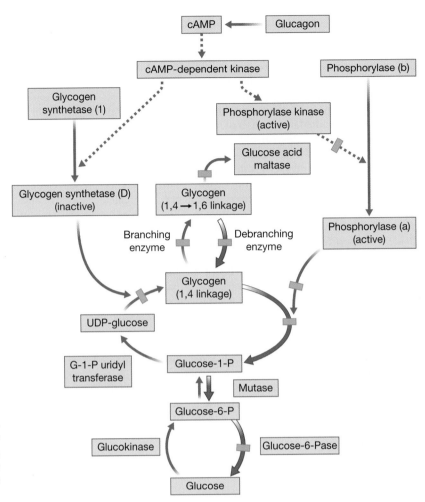

Fig. 66-5 Pathway for glycogen synthesis and degradation to glucose. *Broken lines* indicate enzymatic activation after glucagon stimulation; *thick arrows* indicate glycogen degradation from glucagon infusion; and *hatched boxes* indicate points in the metabolic sequence where enzymatic defects have been identified.

GSDs. For example, the tetrad of a bleeding tendency from thrombasthenia, urate stones from hyperuricemia, hyperlipidemia, and lactic acidosis accompanies GSD-I and is not part of the aberrations seen with other glycogenoses.

Despite the number of enzymatic deficiencies leading to the glycogenoses, only types 0 (glycogen synthetase deficiency) and IV (α-1,4-glucan: α-1,4-glucan 6-glycosyl transferase deficiency) invariably lead to cirrhosis and liver failure. Patients who have type I (glucose-6-phosphatase deficiency) may develop benign hepatic adenomas and hepatic adenocarcinomas, and patients with type III (amylo-1,6-glucosidase deficiency; debrancher enzyme deficiency) may develop hepatic fibrosis or cirrhosis. Because only a few patients have been reported with type 0 GSD, only types I, III, and IV are discussed in detail in this chapter.

Type I Glycogenosis (Glucose-6-Phosphatase Deficiency)

Classification of Type I Glycogenesis

Glycogen storage disease type I (GSD-I) represents a defect in glycogenosis. Originally, GSD-I was thought to represent four subtypes. GSD-IA is a deficiency in glucose-6-phosphatase (G6Pase), GSD-IB is a deficiency in glucose-6-phosphate transporter (G6PT), GSD-IC is a deficiency in the Pi

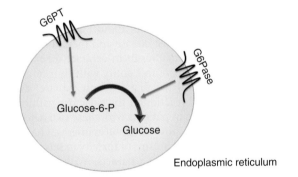

Defect in G6Pase leads to GSD type1a.
Defect in G6PT leads to GSD type1b.

Fig. 66-6 Schematic model of hepatic microsomal glucose-6-phosphatase. Glucose-6-phosphate entry into the endoplasmic reticulum is via a transport protein (G6PT). Hydrolysis occurs by the catalytic subunit of the glucose-6-phosphatase.

transporter, and GSD-ID is a deficiency in the glucose transporter.[158-162] Recent studies confirmed the molecular identity of GSD-IA and -IB; however, the identity of GSD-IC and -ID has not been defined and indeed they may represent a mutation in G6PT, suggesting that G6PT may be also a G6P and Pi transporter.[163] **Figure 66-6** represents schematically the different GSD subtypes.

Molecular Basis of Glycogen Storage Disease Type I

The cDNA encoding the murine glucose-6-phosphatase enzyme was cloned by screening a mouse liver cDNA library differentially with mRNA populations representing the normal and the albino deletion mouse known to express a markedly reduced level of glucose 6-phosphatase enzyme.[164] This discovery allowed the cloning of the human glucose-6-phosphatase cDNA by homology screening. The human gene spans 12 kb, is composed of five exons, and encodes for a 357 amino acid protein.[165-167] The gene has been localized to chromosome 17q21. The glucose-6-phosphatase mRNA is expressed in the liver, kidney, and intestine; however, it is not expressed in human neutrophils/monocytes.[165] To date, more than 84 mutations have been identified in the glucose-6-phosphatase gene of patients with type Ia.[167-173] The two most common mutations are R83C and Q347X, which account for more than 70% of mutations in Caucasian populations.[174] The common mutation Q347X causes a protein truncation of the last 10 carboxy-terminal amino acids that contain the signal for retention of the enzyme in the endoplasmic reticulum.

Clinical Characteristics

Type Ia is the most commonly diagnosed type and represents about a fourth of all cases diagnosed. A general discussion of type IA (designated GSD-I) is presented, followed by a brief discussion of type IB. The clinical picture is one of severe hepatomegaly, which may be apparent within the first 2 weeks of life. Profound hypoglycemia may develop shortly after birth or may not be prominent for several weeks, depending on the frequency of feeding, the presence of intercurrent infection, and the severity of the disease. Because glucose-6-phosphatase activity is also deficient in the kidneys, patients have a substantial enlargement of the kidneys. Serum transaminase levels may be slightly elevated but become normal with effective treatment that maintains blood glucose between 75 and 110 mg/dl at all times. Neither the liver nor the kidneys show functional abnormalities other than the inability to release free glucose into the circulation. In this regard, patients who receive a renal transplant remain unable to maintain normal fasting blood glucose levels.[175] Consanguinity of parents is common, and the disease is transmitted as an autosomal recessive. During the past decade, major improvements in therapy have been documented.[176-179] The study of mechanisms whereby deficiencies of glucose-6-phosphatase activity can cause striking abnormalities in lipid, purine, and carbohydrate metabolism has been instrumental in these therapeutic advances. To place GSD-I in metabolic perspective, the mechanisms by which this single enzyme deficiency can have such profound effects on other metabolic pathways are reviewed.

Biochemical Characteristics

BLOOD GLUCOSE CHANGES

The most consistent and life-threatening feature of GSD-I is the low blood glucose levels that result from relatively short periods of fasting. Fasting for as short a time as 2 to 4 hours is almost always associated with decreases in blood glucose to less than 70 mg/dl, and it is not uncommon to observe levels of 5 to 10 mg/dl after 6 to 8 hours of fasting. In normal individuals, blood glucose levels are maintained within a relatively narrow range by hepatotropic agents such as glucagon, which releases glucose either from stored glycogen or by gluconeogenesis.[180] In GSD-I, degradation of glycogen can occur, or lactate or other gluconeogenic precursors can be converted to glucose-6-phosphate, but in the absence of glucose-6-phosphatase, glucose is not released, and blood glucose levels continue to decline. Blood hormone measurements indicate that during periods of hypoglycemia, insulin levels are appropriately low and glucagon levels are high. After a glucose load, there is a substantial although somewhat delayed insulin release, with concomitant decreases in glucagon and alanine levels.[155,176,181] Thus the hormonal response to changes in blood glucose concentrations appears appropriate.

LACTIC ACID CHANGES

Under normal circumstances, most circulating lactate is generated by muscle glycolysis during exercise. Removal and metabolism of this lactate are efficiently performed by the liver.[180] On the other hand, much of the circulating lactate in patients with GSD-I is generated by hepatic glycolysis.[182] This phenomenon is apparently the result of hepatic stimulation to release glucose from glycogen in combination with inefficient gluconeogenesis. Excess glucose-6-phosphate formed during glycogenolysis cannot be hydrolyzed to free glucose because of the lack of glucose-6-phosphatase activity. Instead, glucose-6-phosphate is diverted through the glycolytic pathway. This metabolic diversion appears to be the basis for enhancement of lactate formation, as illustrated in **Figure 66-7**.

HYPERLIPIDEMIA

Elevation of plasma lipids is a consistent and striking abnormality.[183,184] Levels of triglyceride may reach 6000 mg/dl, with associated cholesterol levels of 400 to 600 mg/dl. Free fatty acid levels are also usually elevated. Near puberty, xanthomas can appear over extensor surfaces, but they may also appear in childhood, with involvement of the nasal septum. Those located on the septum may contribute to the frequency of prolonged nosebleeds seen in some patients.

As with lacticemia, elevated levels of triglyceride and cholesterol appear to be a consequence of increased rates of glycogenolysis and glycolysis. Observations by Sadeghi-Nejad and co-workers suggest that excess hepatic glycolysis increases hepatic levels of NADH, nicotinamide-adenine dinucleotide phosphate (NADPH), and acetyl coenzyme A (CoA), three compounds important in fatty acid and cholesterol synthesis.[182] Thus increases in glycerol-3-phosphate and acetyl CoA generated by the glycolytic pathway, together with high levels of reduced co-factors, could sustain an increased rate of triglyceride and cholesterol synthesis.[185,186] In addition to this apparent increased rate of lipid synthesis, an event concomitant with hypoglycemia is lipolysis from peripheral lipid stores. This further augments the tendency for hyperlipidemia and hepatic steatosis to occur by increasing circulating free fatty acids.[183-187]

Hyperuricemia

Although blood levels of uric acid and the tendency to develop gouty arthritis and nephropathy vary among patients, those who survive puberty often have gouty complications.[188,189] Hyperuricemia was originally attributed to the increased

Type I glycogen storage disease

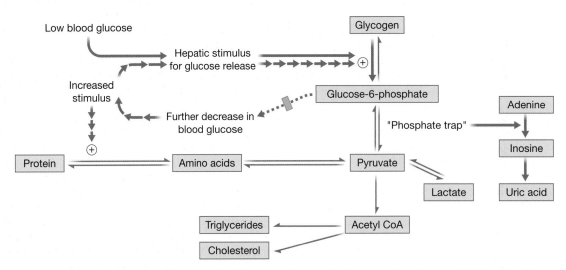

Fig. 66-7 Biochemical basis for the primary laboratory findings in patients with glucose-6-phosphatase deficiency *(solid rectangles).* The increased production of glucose-6-phosphate that results from continuous stimulation of glycogen breakdown apparently increases glycolysis, which in turn results in a net increase *(dark arrows)* in the production of lactate, triglyceride, cholesterol, and uric acid. Both glycogenolysis and gluconeogenesis are involved in the overproduction of substrate.

levels of serum lactate and lipid, which competitively inhibit urate excretion.[184] However, the high level of urate excretion, together with the rate of incorporation of ^{14}C-L-glycine into plasma and urinary urate, indicates that an increased rate of purine synthesis de novo is probably more important in the genesis of hyperuricemia than is a decrease in urate excretion.[190,191] The rate of purine synthesis can be influenced by at least two mechanisms: (1) alteration of the substrate (precursor) concentration (i.e., phosphoribosyl pyrophosphate (PRPP) and glutamine levels); and (2) alteration of the end product, or purine concentration (i.e., low intracellular purine levels increase purine synthesis).[192-194] In support of the former, two substrates, PRPP and glutamine, are necessary for the first committed reaction. This reaction transfers the amine from L-glutamine to PRPP to form 5-phosphoribosyl-1-amine and is apparently rate limiting for the entire sequence of purine synthesis (reaction 4). Although tissue glutamate and glutamine levels have not been measured, blood levels of the two substrates obtained from hyperuricemic patients with GSD I are three-fold to eight-fold higher than are values obtained after urate is normalized by glucose infusion.[186] In addition to the possibility of increased availability of glutamine, the high levels of glucose-6-phosphate produced during periods of hypoglycemia and excessive glycogenolysis may increase synthesis of the second important substrate in purine synthesis, ribose-5-phosphate.[184,188,195] These findings suggest that an apparent increased availability of purine precursors, glutamine, and ribose-5-phosphate may cause a secondary increase in PRPP and thus increase the rate of purine synthesis. Studies using human leukocytes indicate, however, that an increase in availability of glutamine and ribose-5-phosphate alone will not increase the generation of PRPP.[196] Assuming this is true in the liver, the second mechanism, alteration of end-product concentration, should be more important in modulating the increased rate of purine synthesis in patients with GSD-I.

In support of the second mechanism for hyperuricemia, a decreased concentration of purine ribonucleotides would favor an increase in the rate of purine biosynthesis by releasing the glutamine pyrophosphate-ribose-phosphate amidotransferase from end-product inhibition.[197] Although hepatic nucleotide levels during hypoglycemic episodes have not been determined directly, indirect evidence suggests that in patients with GSD-I, hypoglycemia can reduce adenyl ribonucleotide levels. Such a conclusion is based on measured values of hepatic ATP before and after simulating the effects of hypoglycemia with intravenous glucagon administration.[198] Seven patients had a three-fold decrease in hepatic ATP levels with concomitant 1.3-fold decreases in adenosine diphosphate (ADP). Such a reduction in ATP has been shown to favor the rapid degradation of adenyl or guanyl ribonucleotides to xanthine and uric acid. The latter set of reactions is also favored by low intracellular phosphate levels, which apparently occur through phosphate trapping of the phosphorylated sugar. Normally, this accumulation of glucose-6-phosphate is prevented by the action of glucose-6-phosphatase.[199,200]

These observations suggest that the increase in urate production is secondary to recurrent episodes of hypoglycemia (reaction 5), which result in compensatory glucagon release. This hepatotropic agent stimulates glycogen degradation to glucose-6-phosphate. The absence of phosphatase activity results in a phosphate-trapping effect and lowering of ATP levels, which in turn promotes degradation of preformed purines to uric acid (reaction 5).[25,200,201] Finally, the decrease in end-product (purine) concentration promotes a high rate of purine biosynthesis (reaction 5).

HYPOPHOSPHATEMIA

Low serum phosphate levels are not an invariable finding but are more likely to be present during periods of hypoglycemia and acidosis. It has been noted that a glucagon injection is followed by an acute decrease in serum phosphate that spontaneously reverts to the preinjection level within 3 hours. This suggests that cellular (P_i) levels are rapidly depleted by the glucagon effects and that there is a compensatory shift of phosphate out of the circulating pool. A well-demonstrated corollary occurs after fructose ingestion in patients with HFI. This has been shown to result from phosphate trapping on the fructose moiety because of blockage of the aldolase step.[14,25,200,201] As a result of the inability to release P_i from sugar, the liver cell must take up phosphorus from serum (reaction 6). For example, when 6.6 mmol of fructose is administered to an 8.8-kg infant, the fructose load exceeds the amount of P_i mole per mole in the entire extracellular fluid.[14]

A phenomenon analogous to that in HFI apparently occurs because of the phosphate trap created as a result of glucose-6-phosphatase deficiency. A relative metabolic block at the aldolase step would also be expected because of the progressive increase in NADH formed during the initial phase of the reaction cascade from glucose-6-phosphate to pyruvate. The demonstrated decrease in hepatic glycogen content by a mean of 2.3% after a glucagon injection provides a large amount of glucose-6-phosphate that cannot be hydrolyzed to release the bound P_i (reaction 7).[198] The series of reactions (reaction 7) reflects the phosphate trapping by the accumulated sugars of the anaerobic pathway, thus causing an acute shift of circulating phosphate to the intracellular pool. As the phosphate is lost from the sugars, there will be a compensatory shift of phosphate back into the circulation.

RECURRENT FEVER

A few patients have recurrent fever in association with acidosis and hypoglycemia. In these patients, the fever can be reproduced by intravenous injection of glucagon if the patient is already slightly hypoglycemic (blood glucose, 35 to 55 mg/dl) and acidotic (arterial blood pH, 7.28 to 7.36). The febrile response begins 8 to 12 minutes after glucagon injection (0.1 mg/kg given over 3 minutes), and usually peaks 12 to 16 minutes later. If the low blood glucose level is corrected by intravenous administration of glucose and the acidosis is corrected by sodium bicarbonate, the temperature usually returns to normal within 45 minutes of glucagon infusion.

If the explanation for hypophosphatemia just postulated is correct, the febrile response may represent an uncoupling of oxidative phosphorylation secondary to a lack of P_i. For example, glucagon results in the excessive formation of glucose-6-phosphate from glycogen. Because of the glucose-6-phosphatase deficiency, a burst of glycolysis results in excess production of reduced co-factors, which normally produce high-energy phosphates. Because of low intracellular phosphate levels, oxidative phosphorylation—were it to occur—would have to be uncoupled, leading to production of heat rather than chemical energy in the form of ATP (reaction 8).

PLATELET DYSFUNCTION

Patients with GSD-I usually have prolonged bleeding times secondary to abnormal platelet aggregation. Corby and co-workers examined platelet function in 13 patients, each with deficient hepatic activity of one of the following enzymes: glucose-6-phosphatase, debrancher enzyme, phosphorylase, or phosphorylase kinase.[201] Only the seven patients with glucose-6-phosphatase deficiencies had abnormal platelet aggregation, and four of these also had abnormal platelet adhesiveness. The defect appears to be intrinsic because crossover and resuspension studies using patients' platelets in normal plasma and normal platelets in patients' plasma did not alter in vitro platelet function. Two such patients had the ADP content of affected platelets measured, and in both instances it was normal. Nevertheless, the release of ADP from platelets in response to added collagen and epinephrine was markedly impaired. These observations suggest that the functional defect is an impairment of the ability of the platelet membrane to release ADP. Cooper has shown a similar defect in ADP release from platelets with elevated cholesterol content.[202] The elevated cholesterol content impaired the fluidity of the membrane, causing secondary impairment of ADP and epinephrine-induced aggregation. Although platelet cholesterol levels of patients with GSD-I have not been measured, the elevated serum cholesterol content might reflect elevated platelet cholesterol content and therefore may contribute to the abnormality of platelet function in patients with GSD-I. If this postulate is correct, then treatment that lowers blood and platelet cholesterol levels should also normalize platelet function. One of the author's patients was found to have abnormal platelet function but had normal serum cholesterol and triglyceride levels. This finding does not support the hypothesis.

GROWTH IMPAIRMENT

Children who have GSD-I are of short stature but without disproportionate head sizes or limb or trunk lengths. The abdomen is usually massively enlarged as a result of hepatomegaly. Bones may be osteoporotic, and some patients have delayed bone age. The mechanism leading to these changes is not clear. Growth hormone and thyroid hormone levels are normal or increased.[155,176] Measurements of calorie-protein intake in three patients for 2 weeks indicated adequate caloric consumption. Observations suggest that chronic lactic acidosis and concomitant reversal of the insulin/glucagon ratio may be more important factors in preventing normal growth.

Hepatic Adenomas and Carcinomas

Most patients with GSD-I who are more than 15 years old are now found to develop adenomas. This is at variance with the previously held view that they occur only infrequently. Adenomas develop in most patients during the second decade of life, but they may be found in 3-year-old children. The nodules, which are best demonstrated by ultrasonography and radioisotopic scanning, show increased echodensity and decreased isotope uptake. During a laparotomy, they appear as discrete, pale nodules that range in number from one to many and in size from 1 to 5 cm. A number of patients have been found to have solitary hepatocellular adenocarcinomas in individual nodules.[203-206] The mechanism causing the adenomas or their malignant degeneration is unknown, but treatment with portacaval shunting does not prevent their development. The author now has two patients who had adenomas before nocturnal feedings, but after 3 years of treatment, nodules were no longer detectable by scanning (**Fig. 66-8**). Another older patient (age 16 years) developed adenomas during treatment with nocturnal feedings; the feedings were later found to be inadequate to maintain blood glucose above 75 mg/dl. After readjustment of therapy, the nodules decreased in size but did not show complete resolution. This suggests that chronic stimulation of the liver by hepatotropic agents (glucagon and

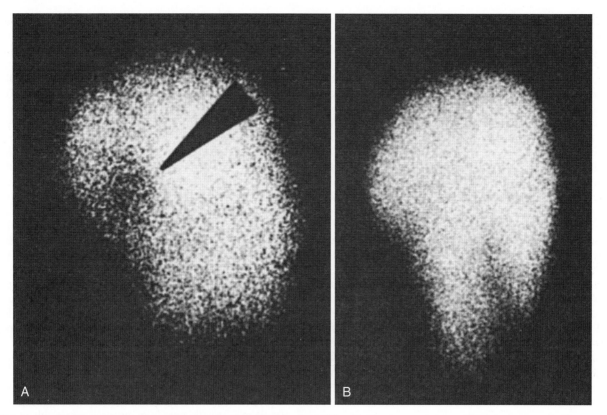

Fig. 66-8 **Technetium scan of the liver, showing regression of hepatic filling defect in response to dietary therapy. A,** The *arrowhead* indicates a hepatic adenoma before therapy. **B,** Disappearance of the adenoma and reduction in the size of the liver after 4 years of dietary therapy.

others) that increase blood glucose levels may be important in the genesis of the adenomas.

The tendency for adenoma formation and malignant transformation is highest in young adult patients and appears to be a consequence of supportive therapy, which currently ensures survival into childhood and young adulthood. The mechanism leading to hepatic malignancy is unknown. A similar progression has been observed in experimental hepatocarcinogenesis from exposure to *N*-nitrosomorpholine. The progression from normal hepatocytes to malignancy appears to be as follows. First, multifocal areas of cells containing excessive glycogen develop. The cells in these areas also show decreased glucose-6-phosphatase activity. Second, the focal cluster of cells develops a gradual reduction in glycogen content and a concomitant increase in ribosomes, reflected as basophilia by hematoxylin and eosin (H&E) staining. Finally, the foci enlarge and acquire the phenotypic markers of hepatocellular carcinoma. These experimental observations, coupled with the findings in patients with GSD-I, have led Bannasch and associates to postulate that the metabolic disturbance leading to hepatocellular glycogenesis is fixed at the genetic level in both the experimental animals and the patients and is causally related to the neoplastic transformation.[207]

Severity of Illness

Despite the fact that there is no difference in activities of the phosphatase enzyme between patients, the expression of symptoms and of chemical anomalies varies substantially from one patient to another without detectable differences in management. Some patients may have only moderate abnormalities in blood chemistry and slightly decreased growth rates, whereas others may have marked alterations in blood lipids, require frequent hospitalizations for fever and lactic acidosis, or even die in infancy or early childhood. In addition, hypoglycemia seems to abate somewhat after patients have reached adulthood. In fact, a few patients who had moderately severe symptoms during childhood improved so dramatically during adulthood that they were able to have successful pregnancies.[208,209]

Glucose Production

In 1969, Havel and colleagues reported that two adult patients with GSD I showed near-normal basal rates of glucose production using ^{14}C-glucose as a marker.[210] This observation has been confirmed in patients of all ages by several investigators who used dideuteroglucose as the isotopic marker.[211-214] These studies defined several features of the illness that have important therapeutic implications:

1. Patients with GSD I can release glucose into the circulation at close to normal basal rates.
2. Patients cannot increase glucose release during hypoglycemia or after a pharmacologic dose of glucagon; therefore, their basal rates of glucose production are also their maximal rates of production.
3. Maximal glucose production is variable between patients but is not related to residual activity of hepatic glucose-6-phosphatase. However, the tendency for fasting-induced hypoglycemia and severity of the clinical illness is directly related to maximal rates of glucose production.

4. Endogenous glucose production is not inhibited unless an exogenous source of glucose is provided at a rate of 8 mg/kg per minute, an amount that maintains blood glucose levels at about 90 mg/dl.

5. The improvement in ability to fast for a longer time after the second decade of life appears to result from a decrease in glucose use rather than an increase in glucose production.

Diagnosis

Characteristically, these patients have no increase in blood glucose levels after administration of glucagon or epinephrine, and usually they show substantial decreases in blood glucose within 20 minutes of the intravenous administration of glucagon. As mentioned in the previous section, a major product of glycogenolysis is lactate rather than glucose. In some patients who are already slightly acidotic, glucagon stimulation may cause severe acidosis. Aside from the glucagon tolerance test, other tolerance tests have been used as an aid in diagnosing the type of glycogenosis. For example, neither galactose nor fructose is converted to free glucose in patients with GSD-I, and a tolerance test with either of these sugars results in a flat blood glucose curve. These tolerance tests have the advantage of avoiding a liver biopsy. On the other hand, a substantial volume of blood is required to complete all the tolerance testing, and not infrequently the results are inconclusive. For example, the author has had several patients referred with erroneous diagnoses based on tolerance tests. Thus, for accurate diagnosis, the author believes that measurement of hepatic enzyme activity is necessary. To provide a basis for some selectivity in the enzymatic analyses of biopsy specimens, the author's practice is to determine serial blood glucose and lactate measurements during a 4- to 6-hour fast, followed by the maximum glucose response to glucagon before a liver biopsy. For example, a rise in glucose of more than 30 mg/dl generally indicates a defect in phosphorylase kinase, which is not routinely measured from needle biopsy material.

Before an effective form of treatment was available, the need for accurate diagnosis was less important than it is today. Because of the effectiveness of treatment of patients with glucose-6-phosphatase deficiency, the suspected diagnosis of GSD should be confirmed by enzymatic assay of hepatic tissue. A diagnosis can be confirmed by examination of needle biopsy material, which avoids potential complications of surgery and general anesthesia.[215] Recent identification of gene mutations has allowed accurate diagnosis using DNA from blood samples.

Pathology

In GSD-I, the liver cells are distended with glycogen and often contain medium-sized to large lipid vacuoles. The lipid content in the liver of an untreated patient is substantially greater than that in the liver of a patient who has been treated, but in either instance, hepatic steatosis is a prominent morphologic feature. The liver cells are pale staining and have prominent plasma membranes. Three notable features differentiate GSD-I from other glycogenoses: (1) the presence of substantial steatosis; (2) a lack of associated fibrosis; and (3) nuclear hyperglycogenosis. Nuclear glycogenosis is commonly noted in hepatocytes of normal children, but in GSD-I (and GSD-III), the nuclei are grotesquely enlarged; that is, hyperglycogenosis is present.

It is not possible to distinguish between normal and elevated levels of cytoplasmic glycogen in the liver in any of the forms of glycogenosis through the use of periodic acid–Schiff (PAS) stain.[216] Thus, to make a diagnosis of excessive glycogen content, a quantitative determination is necessary. It is also important to note that the livers of normal individuals and those of patients with glucose-6-phosphatase deficiencies can degrade glycogen. Thus postmortem analyses of surgical specimens that are not frozen promptly may give inappropriately low (e.g., "normal") levels.

Treatment

Patients with some glycogenoses—for example, those who have deficiencies of hepatic phosphorylase kinase activity—and some patients with GSD-III (debrancher deficiency) have an excellent prognosis without specific treatment. In fact, with the exception of those who have defects in glycogen synthesis (i.e., generalized glycogenosis [acid maltase deficiency; GSD-II; Pompe disease]) or glucose-6-phosphatase deficiencies, most patients who have hepatic glycogenoses have favorable prognoses and are successfully treated with attention to frequencies of food intake. This, however, has not been true of most patients who have GSD-I.

Current recommendations for treatment of GSD-I stem primarily from the studies by Folkman and associates,[217] who first illustrated the reversal of most biochemical abnormalities after TPN. Their observation that both TPN and portacaval shunting[218,219] delivered nutrients primarily into the systemic circulation suggested that hepatic exposure to nutrients was important in the pathogenesis of many of the biochemical abnormalities. Nevertheless, it was later demonstrated that the same beneficial effect seen with TPN or portacaval shunting could be achieved with an intragastric infusion of a nutrient solution similar in content to that used for TPN.[220] This suggested that bypassing the liver with nutrients was not the most important factor in reversing the abnormalities. The similarity in the three types of treatment (i.e., portacaval shunting, TPN, continuous intragastric infusion of glucose) was that a hormonal stimulus to the liver to produce glucose was decreased or averted. Specifically, both TPN and continuous intragastric feeding prevented an hepatic stimulus for glucose release by maintaining blood glucose levels in the range of 90 to 150 mg/dl, whereas the portacaval shunt prevented such a stimulus by diverting pancreatic and enteric blood into systemic circulation. On this basis, the hypothesis for treatment illustrated in **Figure 66-9** was formulated.

The hypothesis states that, as blood glucose falls below a critical level, compensatory mechanisms cause glycogen degradation to glucose-6-phosphate. In the absence of glucose-6-phosphatase, glucose-6-phosphate is not hydrolyzed to release free glucose, and the hepatic stimulus for glycogenolysis results in formation of other intermediates such as lactate, triglycerides, and cholesterol. To interrupt the stimulus, treatment with an exogenous source of glucose inhibits the release of hepatotropic stimuli and thus the excess glycogenolysis. If this postulate is correct, any method of treatment that maintains blood glucose above a critical level should also prevent, or at least alleviate, biochemical manifestations of the illness. In addition, the hypothesis suggests that diversion of portal vein blood flow should dilute hepatotropic agents in the systemic

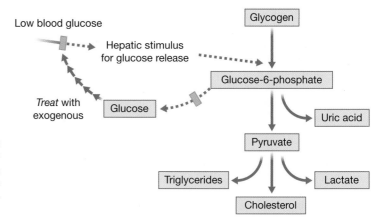

Fig. 66-9 A biochemical basis for management of patients with glucose-6-phosphatase deficiency (*solid rectangles*). By preventing the decrease in blood glucose with an exogenous supply of glucose, excessive glycolysis and gluconeogenesis are prevented. This results in a net decrease in production of circulating triglyceride, cholesterol, lactate, and uric acid.

circulation. This dilution should result in less stimulation of glycogenolysis.

Theoretically, either portacaval shunting or continuous infusion of a high-glucose diet should be effective in reversing most manifestations of the illness, with the exception that portacaval shunting should have little or no beneficial effect on hypoglycemia. Thus portacaval shunting is not recommended as the sole form of treatment for those patients who are expected to have frequent episodes of very low blood glucose levels or for small children, in whom shunts may be more likely to close spontaneously.

Although TPN and continuous intragastric infusion of glucose are effective treatment modalities for GSD-I, they are impractical on a long-term basis. A more practical method was devised to maintain blood glucose at physiologic concentrations or at levels that would prevent stimulation of excess glycogenolysis and glycolysis. This treatment consisted of a high-glucose diet given to simulate TPN. Thus it was given enterally either by nasogastric tube or by gastrostomy during nighttime sleep, along with a high-starch diet, which was consumed at frequent intervals while the patient was awake. Such a regimen has successfully maintained a large number of patients relatively symptom-free for more than 10 years and has provided normal or near-normal growth and development.[221,222]

Chen and colleagues found that a number of patients can maintain normal blood glucose levels by taking cold, uncooked cornstarch (2 g/kg) at 6-hour intervals.[223] This regimen has been used by a number of patients to avoid the continuous nocturnal feedings. A number of the younger children have not been able to maintain normal glucose and lactate levels with the cornstarch regimen as well as they had with the continuous nocturnal feeding regimen.[224,225] In the author's experience, growth rates were less with the raw starch regimen than with continuous feedings, and one patient consumed such large quantities of cornstarch that protein intake was insufficient to maintain normal secretory proteins (albumin, transferrin, and retinol-binding protein). Thus, although the cornstarch feedings can be beneficial as a time-release form of glucose in some patients, a dose response to the starch preparation and careful monitoring of blood glucose levels should be carried out to ensure that treatment is appropriate for individual patients. The author believes that many patients require an intensive feeding regimen at least until they have stopped growing. This consists of high starch feedings at 2- to 3-hour intervals during the day, continuous nocturnal feeding of a complete, low lipid–containing (<5% calories) formula,

and periodic monitoring to ensure normal blood glucose and lactate levels throughout the day and night. As patients become fully grown and have a relatively lower requirement for glucose, the uncooked cornstarch regimen may allow discontinuation of the nighttime nasogastric feedings. Recently, using modified corn starch has shown benefit in ameliorating the metabolic complications.[226]

Prognosis

Until the use of nocturnal feedings, the first few years of life were usually marked by frequent hospitalizations for treatment of hypoglycemia and acidosis, with a high rate of death or permanent central nervous system impairment from recurrent and prolonged episodes of hypoglycemia. Patients who survived puberty appeared to have fewer problems than they had when younger. Patients with persistent hyperuricemia had gouty complications during the second and third decades of life, and many patients had complications of hyperlipemia, with xanthomas, and with higher rates of cardiovascular disease and pancreatitis than those in the general population.[154-156,180,227] Recognition of hepatic adenomas has been relatively recent, and the incidence of complications from benign hepatic adenomas is unclear, although several patients have developed hepatomas.[203,205]

Long-term follow-up of the results of portacaval shunting or nocturnal feedings is not complete. Ten-year follow-up of patients treated with nocturnal feedings indicates that infants thus treated have many fewer problems than they had before treatment and that some patients with hepatic adenomas may show resolution after a few years of treatment. Too few patients have been monitored into the third decade of life to permit conclusions, but early observations indicate that, for optimal treatment, the nocturnal feedings are necessary for most young patients, whereas raw cornstarch administration may suffice for older patients. On the other hand, patients generally have less tendency to hypoglycemia after the age of 20. A 22-year-old patient, severely affected at the age of 15 years, had been treated with nocturnal feedings for $6\frac{1}{2}$ years, with complete resolution of all chemical manifestations of the illness except hypoglycemia (blood glucose, 62 mg/dl) and lactate elevation (7 mmol/L) after a 9-hour fast. She was weaned off nocturnal feedings by gradually decreasing the hourly feeding over a period of a month. After $2\frac{1}{2}$ years of no nocturnal feedings, she continues to have completely normal blood chemistry results after an 8-hour fast. There is still no hepatic glucose-6-phosphatase activity, however. As long as blood glucose is consistently maintained between 70 and 120 mg/dl, most children appear to lead fairly normal, healthy lives, with normal growth and development, although in at least one patient the disease has been unresponsive to this type of management.[228]

Chen and colleagues observed that older patients (>18 years) with suboptimal treatment have a high incidence of progressive renal disease. The affected individuals show progressive glomerular sclerosis with proteinuria as an early manifestation.[229] Renal involvement appears initially with microalbuminuria and hyperfiltration progressing to frank proteinuria and hypertension.[230] Although the cause of the lesion is unclear, it appears that the incidence is lowered by good control of blood glucose and other blood abnormalities because none of the author's nine patients aged 25 to 34 show renal abnormalities.

Glycogen Storage Disease Type IB

In 1968, Senior and Loridan described a patient with clinical and laboratory features identical to GSD-I, except that no enzyme defect was identified from frozen liver.[231] Subsequently, a number of similar patients have been identified.[232-240] In addition to the hepatic abnormality, patients have repeated infections because of neutropenia and abnormal leukocyte migration,[235-239] and some show decreased neutrophil phagocytosis-stimulated oxygen consumption, decreased nitroblue tetrazolium reduction,[238] defective bactericidal activity, defective hexose monophosphate shunt activity, and increased incidence of inflammatory bowel disease.[239,241] These patients have been diagnosed as having GSD-IB. There has been little mention of a familial occurrence in the reports of GSD-IB. This is curious because a number of patients with GSD-I have affected siblings. One of the authors' patients with GSD-IB has seven unaffected siblings. The number of reported cases is small, however; and the mode of inheritance is presumed to be autosomal recessive.

The reason for the discrepancy between the in vitro and in vivo activity of glucose-6-phosphatase in patients with GSD-IB is not known. Steady-state kinetic measurements led Arion and associates to conclude that the normal microsomal glucose-6-phosphatase enzyme is a two-compartment system consisting of a specific glucose-6-phosphate carrier on the outer bilayer of the membrane of the endoplasmic reticulum and a catalytic phosphorylase component located on the inner half of the membrane.[239] Because disruption of isolated microsomes in patients with GSD-IB with cholate or freeze-thawing results in a marked increase in activity, the general assumption has been that the defect in GSD-IB is a deficiency of the translocase or carrier portion of the enzyme system,[232-234,240] although the putative translocase has never been identified in microsomes from a normal liver. Zakim and Edmonson, using methods to measure pre–steady-state kinetics,[242] have shown that the limiting step in the reaction is not glucose release from the enzyme but the release of phosphate. These findings in normal liver microsomes are similar in the liver of a patient with GSD-IB, although the pre–steady-state kinetics are blunted. These findings question the general concept of a translocase and suggest that patients with GSD-IB may have a configurational abnormality in the enzyme membrane interaction that can be overcome by alteration of the membrane lipid rather than by an opening of the microsomal vesicle.[242,243]

Molecular Basis of Glycogen Storage Disease Type IB

GSD type IB is caused by mutation in the gene encoding microsomal glucose-6-phosphate transporter.[244] The gene has been mapped to chromosome 11q23 and is composed of nine exons spanning a genomic region of 4 kb. The gene is expressed in the liver, kidney, and leukocytes.[245] More than 69 mutations have been described in the gene, resulting in functional deficiency of glucose-6-phosphate transporter, which explains the neutropenia and neutrophil-monocyte dysfunction characteristic of GSD type IB.[244,246] No genotype–phenotype correlations have been described for type IA or IB disorders.[247]

Treatment of GSD-IB is identical to that of GSD-IA, with the possible exception that prophylactic antibiotics may lessen the tendency for frequent infection.[235-239,248] Improvement in neutrophil function with treatment has been reported by some investigators.[238,239] However, the authors' experience was that the neutropenia and abnormal migration persisted even after 3 months of management that normalized all parameters of disease in the blood, and even after subsequent portacaval shunting.[248,249] The lack of improvement in neutrophil function in some of the well-treated patients suggests that the defect in GSD-IB is intrinsic to both the liver and leukocytes. The functional impairment in neutrophils is related to impaired glucose production by neutrophils, resulting in endoplasmic stress and increased apoptosis.[250] Improvement of neutropenia and neutrophil dysfunction occurs in response to granulocyte colony-stimulating factor.[251]

Type III Glycogen Storage Disease (GSD-III) Amylo-1,6-Glucosidase (Debrancher) Deficiency

This glycogenosis accumulates a polysaccharide that has a structure similar to limit Dextrin produced by degradation of glycogen with phosphorylase and oligo-1,4-1,4 glucan-transferase but no debrancher activity (reaction 9).[252] As depicted, the terminal α-1,4-glucosyl units are hydrolyzed by the combined activity of oligo-1,4-1,4-glucanotransferase and phosphorylase, but the inner branch points of α-1,6 linkages (MG) are not hydrolyzed by the debranching enzyme. Thus the glycogen molecule is abnormal, with an excessive number of branch points (1,6 linkages). The debrancher enzyme contains two catalytic subunits on a single polypeptide chain. The two activities are oligo-1,4-1,4-glucantransferase and amylo-1,6-glucosidase.

Molecular Basis of Type III Glycogen Storage Disease

The human gene encoding for glycogen debranching enzyme is 85 kb in length and consists of 35 exons.[253] The gene has been localized to chromosome 1p21.[254] The cDNA includes a 4545-bp encoding region and 2371-bp 3′-untranslated region. The predicted protein is approximately 172 kDa, consistent with the estimated size of the purified protein.[255] Six mRNA isoforms have been identified.[256] Isoform 1 is expressed in the liver; isoforms 2, 3, and 4 are muscle specific. Isoforms 5 and 6 are minor isoforms. Mutations in the glycogen debranching gene have been described in patients with type IIIA and IIIB. These mutations include missense, nonsense, splicing, and deletion insertion defects.[257] Specific mutations in exon 3 such as 17delAG and Q6x are only seen in type IIIB.[258] The splice mutation IVS32-12A→G was found to cause mild clinical symptoms, whereas mutations 3965delT and 4529insA are associated with a severe phenotype and early onset of clinical symptoms.[259]

Depending on the tissue(s) involved and enzymatic characteristics, subtypes of GSD-III have been described (i.e., GSD-IIIA, GSD-IIIB, and so on). Type IIIA describes patients who exhibit complete absence of debrancher enzyme activity in hepatic and muscle tissue, whereas type IIIB describes patients with liver involvement only.

Clinical Characteristics

By physical examination alone, these patients cannot be readily distinguished from patients who have type I glycogenosis (GSD-I). Early in life, hepatomegaly and growth failure may be striking. However, a few patients may develop splenomegaly at 4 to 6 years of age.[260] These patients usually have evidence of hepatic fibrosis but do not necessarily develop cirrhosis and liver failure.

In addition to hepatic involvement, a number of patients with GSD-III have muscle weakness. Rapid walking and climbing result in increased weakness without cramps.[261] Some patients may have a progressive myopathy. Glycogen may also accumulate in the heart, and moderate cardiomegaly with nonspecific electrocardiographic changes is sometimes present.[222] However, congestive heart failure and cardiac arrhythmias are not reported. There is no renal enlargement in GSD III, in contradistinction to GSD-I.

The clinical course in GSD-III is generally much milder than that of GSD-I in that severe hypoglycemia is not a problem except with prolonged fasting. Some patients have shown relative decreases in liver size around puberty,[252,262] but rare patients have shown evidence of progressive fibrosis and liver failure.[154,263,264] The latter patients may have an additional phosphorylase or phosphorylase kinase deficiency.[154] In a study of 41 patients with type III GSD, 31 patients had involvement of the liver and muscle (type IIIA), 4 patients had liver involvement only (type IIIB), 3 patients had unknown muscle status, and 3 patients had isolated deficiency of transferase activity with retention of glucosidase activity.[265]

Biochemical Characteristics and Laboratory Findings

Lipid levels in plasma are variably elevated and to some extent appear to be related to the individual tendency toward fasting-induced hypoglycemia.[262] That is, the patients who develop lower glucose levels with 6- to 8-hour fasts tend to have higher blood lipid levels. However, none of the patients approach the severe elevations of 4000 to 6000 mg/dl seen with GSD I. Uric acid levels are generally normal, but rare patients reportedly have slight elevations. Serum transaminase levels are consistently moderately elevated (300 to 600 IU; normal <40 IU),[64] although some patients show elevations of 900 to 2000 IU.

Galactose and fructose are readily converted to glucose by these patients; similarly, protein and amino acid mixtures induce small and prolonged increases in blood glucose levels.[181,262] Both glucagon and epinephrine increase blood

glucose when given between 1½ and 3 hours after a meal but elicit little response after a 14-hour fast (double glucagon tolerance test).[266] This result is interpreted to indicate available 1,4 glucosyl linkages that can be degraded by phosphorylase shortly after a meal. The glycogen in this case is degraded only until 1,6 linkages are encountered. Access to 1,4 linkages is blocked by terminal 1,6 glycosyl linkages that would be present after a prolonged fast, and these would prevent glucose increase after glucagon administration. Unfortunately, the glucose response to the double glucagon tolerance test is not a consistent finding, and it should not be used as a definitive diagnostic test. Because glucagon also stimulates gluconeogenesis, the inconsistency of the test results is possibly due to glucose formation via this pathway.

The liver content of glycogen is often markedly increased (to as much as 17.4 g/100 g tissue) in GSD-III.[252] By various techniques, the glycogen is found to have abnormally short outer branch points. Many patients also show some depression of glucose-6-phosphatase activity. Hug has found several patients with combined defects in phosphorylase and phosphorylase kinase. These patients are generally more severely affected and tend to develop cirrhosis.[154]

A series of techniques is available for measuring debrancher activity: (1) liberation of glucose from phosphorylase-treated limit dextrin; (2) incorporation of ^{14}C-glucose into glycogen; (3) 1,4→1,4 transfer of an oligoglucan (glucan transferase activity); and (4) hydrolysis of singly branched oligosaccharides. Using these various techniques, Hers and associates have identified a series of biochemical subtypes of GSD-III. These subtypes are also divided according to types of muscle glycogen.[252,267,268]

Pathology

The liver in GSD-III is very similar in appearance to that in GSD-I, with two notable exceptions: (1) the presence of fibrous septa or frank cirrhosis; and (2) the paucity of fat (**Fig. 66-10**). Progression of the fibrosis to cirrhosis has been demonstrated. Hug reports that progression to cirrhosis is more likely to occur in patients who have combined enzymatic defects.[154,266] The ultrastructural appearance of the liver is not distinguishable from that in GSD-I, except that in GSD-III lipid vacuoles are small and are less common.[268]

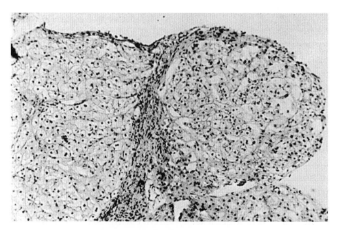

Fig. 66-10 **Percutaneous liver biopsy specimen from a patient with glycogen storage disease type III, showing increased fibrosis.** The hepatocytes do not contain fat deposition. (×80.)

If muscle is affected, excessive glycogen is readily demonstrable in ethanol-fixed specimens by the PAS method. Glycogen accumulates between intact myofibrils and in the subsarcolemmal position, locations in which glycogen usually occurs but not in abundance. The diagnosis depends on demonstration of deficient activity of amylo-1,6-glucosidase (debrancher enzyme).[216]

Treatment

Treatment of this disorder remains investigative. Treatment should be restricted to patients who have obvious muscle involvement, progressive fibrotic changes in the liver, or both. An accurate correlation between the type of glycogen accumulation and the progression of liver disease, such that a clear-cut prognosis could be assigned to each patient, would be helpful in showing a positive therapeutic response.

Present investigative efforts combine the technique of nocturnal feedings with the known responses to protein and amino acids.[181,262,269] Slonim and co-workers have shown improved growth and increased muscle strength in a patient given a high-protein diet during the day and continuous nocturnal intragastric feedings of a high-protein liquid formula (Sustacal) at night.[270] Borowitz and Greene[271] have found that growth and transaminase and blood glucose levels were more positively influenced by a high-starch diet with a standard (recommended dietary allowance) protein intake. This therapy is therefore virtually identical to that for GSD-I. This outcome is encouraging, but more extensive follow-up evaluation over a longer period of treatment is needed.

Type IV Glycogenosis (α-1,4 Glucan-6-Glycosyl Transferase Deficiency; GSD-IV)

Type IV GSD, a rare form of glycogenosis, was first described clinically and pathologically in 1952 by Anderson.[272] Illingsworth and Cori showed that the glycogen possessed abnormally long outer and inner chains of glucose units.[273] More than 10 years later, Brown and Brown demonstrated the absence of branching enzyme activity in this disorder.[274] The few descriptions of the disorder (about 20 documented cases) have illustrated its unusual clinical, biochemical, and pathologic aspects.[275-281]

Clinical Characteristics

Infants are normal at birth and for some months thereafter. The onset of symptoms during the first year of life is insidious. Symptoms may manifest as early as 3 months or as late as 15 months of age. The disorder is usually diagnosed because of hepatosplenomegaly, abdominal distention, signs and symptoms referable to hepatic dysfunction, nonspecific gastrointestinal symptoms, and failure to thrive. Muscle hypotonia and wasting may be present. Superficial veins over the distended abdomen are prominent as the disease progresses. Patients who live beyond infancy develop cirrhosis with accompanying portal hypertension, ascites, and esophageal varices. The terminal course is usually due to chronic hepatic failure and jaundice with bleeding esophageal varices. Variants include a cardiopathic form of childhood in which patients develop cardiac failure, apparently from myofibrillar damage caused by polysaccharide deposits within myocardial

cells. Intercurrent infection is a common terminal complication. The duration of survival after diagnosis is usually 2 to 37 months, although an occasional patient may survive 3 to 4 years.

A neuromuscular variant has been reported that may involve the skeletal muscles, peripheral nervous system, and central nervous system. The level and extent of the neuromuscular lesions appear to vary from patient to patient, and at least one patient showed signs of involvement of muscles and nervous system simultaneously.[281]

A 59-year-old man with GSD-IV had deficient branching enzyme in skeletal muscle with normal muscle glycogen and low normal enzyme activity in leukocytes.[282] The man had a 30-year history of progressive, asymmetric limb-girdle weakness and a vacuolar myopathy. The vacuoles contained glycogen, which was partially resistant to diastase. Ultrastructural changes resembled the amylopectin polysaccharide deposits encountered in childhood GSD-IV. Three other adult patients have been reported with an amylopectin-like storage myopathy; two of these later developed involvement of the heart and brain, but none showed hepatic involvement.[283-285]

Approximately 50% of infants with GSD-IV have signs suggestive of involvement of the neuromuscular system and abnormal deposits of polysaccharide in skeletal muscle.[279,281,286,287] The pathologic changes can occur in the absence of clinical changes.[279] Because the majority of these patients have not had comparative measurements of branching enzyme activity in fibroblasts, liver, muscle, and leukocytes, it is not possible to correlate apparent clinical and pathologic findings with enzymatic changes. It has been suggested that two branching enzymes may be acting at different sites[274,275] and that the clinical expression of this disease depends on deficiency of organ-specific brancher isoenzymes.

The author has had experience in managing two unusual patients with deficient branching enzyme measured in both the liver and skin fibroblasts (by Dr. Barbara Brown, St. Louis). The first patient, a male, showed the usual progression to cirrhosis and liver failure by 18 months of age.[288] At 2 years of age, he underwent liver transplantation and standard treatment with immunosuppressants. Six years after transplantation the patient had normal liver function and shows no evidence of nerve, muscle, or cardiac abnormalities. Thus, despite the generalized nature of the defect, transplantation of a normal liver has not been associated with obvious progression in other organs. The second patient, a 6-year-old boy, was noted at 3 years of age to have hepatomegaly and chronically elevated serum aminotransferases.[289] An open liver biopsy showed moderate, generalized micronodular fibrosis and typical PAS-positive, diastase-resistant deposits in about 25% of the hepatocytes. Electron microscopy showed accumulation of Drochman fibrils characteristic of GSD-IV, but these fibrils were not present in all cells. During the succeeding 3 years, the boy showed normal growth and development with spontaneous normalization of liver test results. A liver biopsy at the age of 6 years showed minimal periportal fibrosis with no PAS-positive, diastase-resistant deposits present in any hepatocytes and normal-appearing glycogen using electron microscopic analysis. Assays of hepatocytes and skin fibroblasts showed no detectable branching enzyme activity. These two patients plus previous reports of GSD-IV indicate that branching enzyme deficiency may present in various ways, the classic infantile variety primarily affecting the liver. As more patients have the opportunity for transplantation, it is anticipated that a more accurate classification system can be found for the various subgroups of this unusual disorder.

Laboratory Findings

Blood electrolytes are usually within normal limits except in patients with renal tubular defects, who have low bicarbonate concentrations. Serum transaminase and alkaline phosphatase levels are usually elevated to three to six times normal. Except with malnutrition, late in the disease, serum cholesterol is often slightly elevated. Until liver failure develops, serum albumin, globulin, bilirubin, and ammonia are normal. All liver test results become abnormal as liver failure becomes severe. Glucagon and epinephrine tolerance tests cause a positive glucose response, with increases in levels of 15 to 23 mg/dl and the maximum response occurring about 30 minutes after hormone injection and 2 hours after a meal.[276] Both hormones may allow detection of urinary ketone bodies. Hypoglycemia is not a characteristic feature of the illness until terminal liver failure occurs. Chronic and severe acidosis may occur secondary to a renal tubular defect in hydrogen ion excretion.[277-279] Oral glucose and fructose tolerance test results show no abnormality, and serum lactate and pyruvate levels are normal.[276]

Biochemical Characteristics

The stored polysaccharide in GSD-IV is a glucose polymer whose properties differ from those of normal mammalian glycogen. The normal level of liver glycogen in a child in the fed state is roughly 6% of the hepatic wet weight.[290,291] Normal glycogen has the following characteristics: (1) at least 36% of the glucose units are susceptible to phosphorylase-catalyzed degradation; (2) chain lengths are 8 to 12 glycosyl units; (3) branch points (1,6 linkages) make up 8%; and (4) the $KI:I_2$ absorption band is at 460 nm.[21]

Patients with GSD-IV usually have hepatic glycogen levels slightly lower than normal (3.5% to 5%), although one patient had a level of 10.7%. Hepatic glycogen in these patients is unusually susceptible to phosphorylase-induced hydrolysis (>40% phosphorylase degradation), suggesting that it has longer outer chain lengths and fewer branch points (about 6%) than does normal glycogen. The polysaccharide is highly chromogenic, with a maximal $KI:I_2$ absorption band at about 525 nm.[292] About half the extracted polysaccharide may be insoluble and poorly characterized. Muscle glycogen appears normal; leukocytic glycogen is abnormal, as is brancher enzyme activity in these cells.

Although the deficiency of branching enzyme explains the formation of an amylopectin-like polysaccharide, it does not account for the presence of an appreciable proportion of branch points in the abnormal glycogen. Brown and Brown suggest that normal liver contains two enzymes with branching activities of different specificities, only one of which is measured by the methods used.[274] Another possibility is that the mutant gene in this disorder has produced a protein with substantially modified enzymatic specificity such that branching occurs mainly with long outer chains.[275] The liver glycosyl deposits and myocardial deposits are believed to be biochemically the same because they appear similar histochemically and are both resistant to digestion by α-amylase. This resistance to digestion by amylase is difficult to explain because there is no other evidence for the existence of an α-amylase-resistant glycogen.

Pathology

Examination of the liver shows a uniform micronodular cirrhosis with broad bands of fibrous tissue extending around and into the lobules. Portal veins, lymphatic channels, and hepatic arteries are normal with slight portal biliary duct proliferation. Liver cell plates are distorted, and, as the disease progresses, the lobules develop prominent sinusoidal channels with fibrous walls coursing between thick liver plates.

Pale amphophilic or basophilic deposits occur in liver cells, cardiac and skeletal muscle, and brain.[275,278,281] The deposits in cardiac muscle resemble cardiac colloid, and those in brain resemble Lafora bodies.[218,221] Liver cell nuclei are frequently eccentric in position. They appear (with H&E stain) to be displaced by pale, slightly eosinophilic or colorless inclusions deposited in the cytoplasm. This is the most striking and characteristic finding and is generally limited to the periphery of the lobule. The inclusions vary from hyaline to reticulate and are usually sharply demarcated from normal cytoplasm. Clear halos may surround the contents of the inclusions. In the late stages of the disease, nodular accumulations of a slightly different hyaline, fibrillar material are scattered throughout the hepatic lobules. This material is birefringent, appearing in polarized light as sheaths of crystals that cannot be easily distinguished from deposits that typify α_1-antitrypsin deficiency, except perhaps on the basis of their greater frequency and larger size in GSD-IV. In both conditions, the peripheral lobular deposits are PAS positive and diastase resistant.[290]

Examination of myocardial tissue shows hypertrophied muscle fibers with large rectangular nuclei. Within the fibers, colorless discrete deposits similar to those in the liver are found. These deposits are uniformly distributed, with only a slight predilection for subendocardial regions. The epicardium and vessels are normal, without significant myocardial fibrosis, endocardial sclerosis, necrosis, or calcification.

PAS-positive material may be present within foamy macrophages of the spleen and lymph nodes, smooth muscle of the gastrointestinal tract and large blood vessels, and skeletal muscle around the larynx, diaphragm, tongue, and esophagus. Peripheral skeletal muscle is usually free of any abnormality except for scant amounts of abnormal polysaccharide.

Central nervous system abnormalities have been found in only 6 of 20 reported cases. In these instances, discrete, spherical PAS-positive globules were widely scattered throughout the neuraxis. They were usually most prominent in white matter and in subependymal and subapical regions but were also numerous in gray matter. Peripheral nerves also contain PAS-positive globules in the endoneurium. The PAS-positive deposits in neuronal tissue are also resistant to amylase digestion.[281]

Electron microscopic studies show a decrease in cytoplasmic organelles. The organelles are found in tongues of cytoplasm extending between large, irregular aggregates of low electron density. The contents of these aggregates are variable, and they contain two or three components: glycogen rosettes or the alpha particles of Drochman fibrils and granular material. The fibrils are straight or curved and are about 65 nm wide.[280] Some areas, which contain primarily glycogen, frequently fail to stain well despite the use of lead citrate.

Myocardial fibers are distended by zones of material with low electron density, similar to those seen in the liver. Unlike liver cells, cardiac cells rarely contain material thought to be glycogen. Electron microscopic examination of skeletal muscle reveals granulofibrillar deposits similar to those in the viscera but less conspicuous; beta glycogen is more prominent in these deposits. Ultrastructural studies of the central nervous system tissue show the presence of large numbers of globules with a granulofibrillar appearance and of medium electron density. In some deposits, the fibrils are oriented radially, and in others, they assume a whorled appearance. The material is mostly restricted to astrocytic processes. It is not found within neuronal perikarya or processes.[276,281]

Histochemical stains of the liver deposits indicate that the material is an abnormal glycogen with fewer branch points than usual. The deposits also have properties that are unusual for a glucose polymer: a positive colloidal iron stain and resistance to α-amylase digestion of conventional duration. Only pectinase was able to reduce the PAS and colloidal iron reactions significantly.

Molecular Basis of Type IV Glycogen Storage Disease

Type IV GSD is a rare autosomal recessive disorder caused by deficiency of the glycogen branching enzyme (GBE), leading to accumulation of amylopectin-like compounds in various tissues. The human GBE cDNA is 3 kb in length, and encodes a 702 amino acid protein. The GBE gene is located on chromosome 3p14 and has 16 exons. Mutations in GBE have been reported.[291]

Treatment

Three types of treatment, without decided improvement, were used for one patient.[292] First, a high-protein, low-carbohydrate diet with corn oil added to the milk fat caused no change in weight gain or in the progression of cirrhosis. Second, with progression of the disease, treatment with purified α-glucosidase from *Aspergillus niger* was given for 6 days. This treatment resulted in a striking decrease in hepatic glycogen content, from 10% to 2%. Although no unfavorable reaction occurred, liver size did not decrease. Glycogen content was maintained at 3% by a third treatment, intramuscular injection of zinc-glucagon, 1 mg three times a day for 24 days. Any positive effect of these treatments remains doubtful. On the other hand, the poor clinical results following the treatments might have been related to the advanced state of cirrhosis before their initiation.

Other than supportive nutritional management[288] for terminal cirrhosis, no specific treatment appears to be beneficial. The finding that the *Aspergillus* extract caused a striking decrease in hepatic glycogen suggests that, if the accumulation of abnormal glycogen is in some way hepatotoxic, this form of treatment might be studied in patients before the onset of severe cirrhosis.

A study by Starzl's group suggests that liver transplantation in GSD-IV results in resorption of extrahepatic deposits of amylopectin, possibly by systemic microchimerism (i.e., cells of the host organs became mixed with cells with the donor genomes that had migrated from the allograft into the recipient tissues and presumably serve as enzyme carriers).[293]

Inborn Errors of Amino Acid Metabolism

Hereditary tyrosinemia is the only inborn error of amino acid metabolism that results in permanent liver injury. This section summarizes the normal metabolic pathway of tyrosine, and then discusses the disorders associated with abnormal tyrosine metabolism.

Tyrosine Metabolism

The principal hepatic pathway for degradation of tyrosine is shown in **Figure 66-11**. These reactions normally catabolize 99% of tyrosine. The steady-state plasma concentration of tyrosine is determined by two primary factors: (1) gastrointestinal uptake, which is regulated by an active transport system; and (2) the rate of production of tyrosine from phenylalanine and its subsequent catabolism to carbon dioxide and water. Most of the ingested phenylalanine is catabolized via tyrosine. The rate-limiting reaction in the tyrosine oxidation pathway is that catabolized by tyrosine aminotransferase (see **Fig. 66-11**, reaction 1).[294,295] Pyridoxal phosphate is the coenzyme. Tyrosine aminotransferase is mainly found in the cytosol of the liver and its activity shows a circadian rhythm. Also, the activity of tyrosine aminotransferase is induced by various compounds, including corticosteroids.[296-298]

p-Hydroxyphenylpyruvic hydroxylase is the second enzyme involved in tyrosine catabolism. This enzyme is found in the cytosol of the human liver and kidney.[299,300] It catalyzes the conversion of *p*-hydroxyphenylpyruvic acid to homogentisic acid (see **Fig. 66-11**, reaction 2) and converts phenylpyruvic acid to *p*-hydroxyphenylacetic acid.[301] The enzyme requires a reducing agent and ascorbic acid can serve both in vivo and in vitro in this capacity.[302] *p*-Hydroxyphenylpyruvic acid is not normally found in urine. When its normal catabolism to homogentisic acid is blocked, the levels of both the α-keto acid and tyrosine in the plasma may be increased. At the same time, *p*-hydroxyphenyl lactic acid is formed through the action of lactic dehydrogenase. *p*-Hydroxyphenylacetic acid can also be formed from decarboxylation of *p*-hydroxyphenylpyruvic acid. Homogentisic acid oxidase catalyzes the conversion of homogentisic acid to maleylacetoacetic acid. This reaction also requires vitamin C for maximal activity in vivo. Fumarylacetoacetase acts on maleylacetoacetic acid to yield fumaric acid and acetoacetic acid.

Disorders of Tyrosine Metabolism

Several conditions associated with abnormalities in tyrosine metabolism have been described; however, only hereditary tyrosinemia (hepatorenal type) is associated with permanent injury to the liver. Other abnormalities in tyrosine metabolism, summarized in **Table 66-3**, are discussed briefly.

Tyrosinosis

The first known case of abnormal excretion of a tyrosine metabolite was described by Medes and colleagues in 1927.[303] The patient, a 49-year-old Russian Jew who had myasthenia gravis, was found to have an unusual reducing substance in

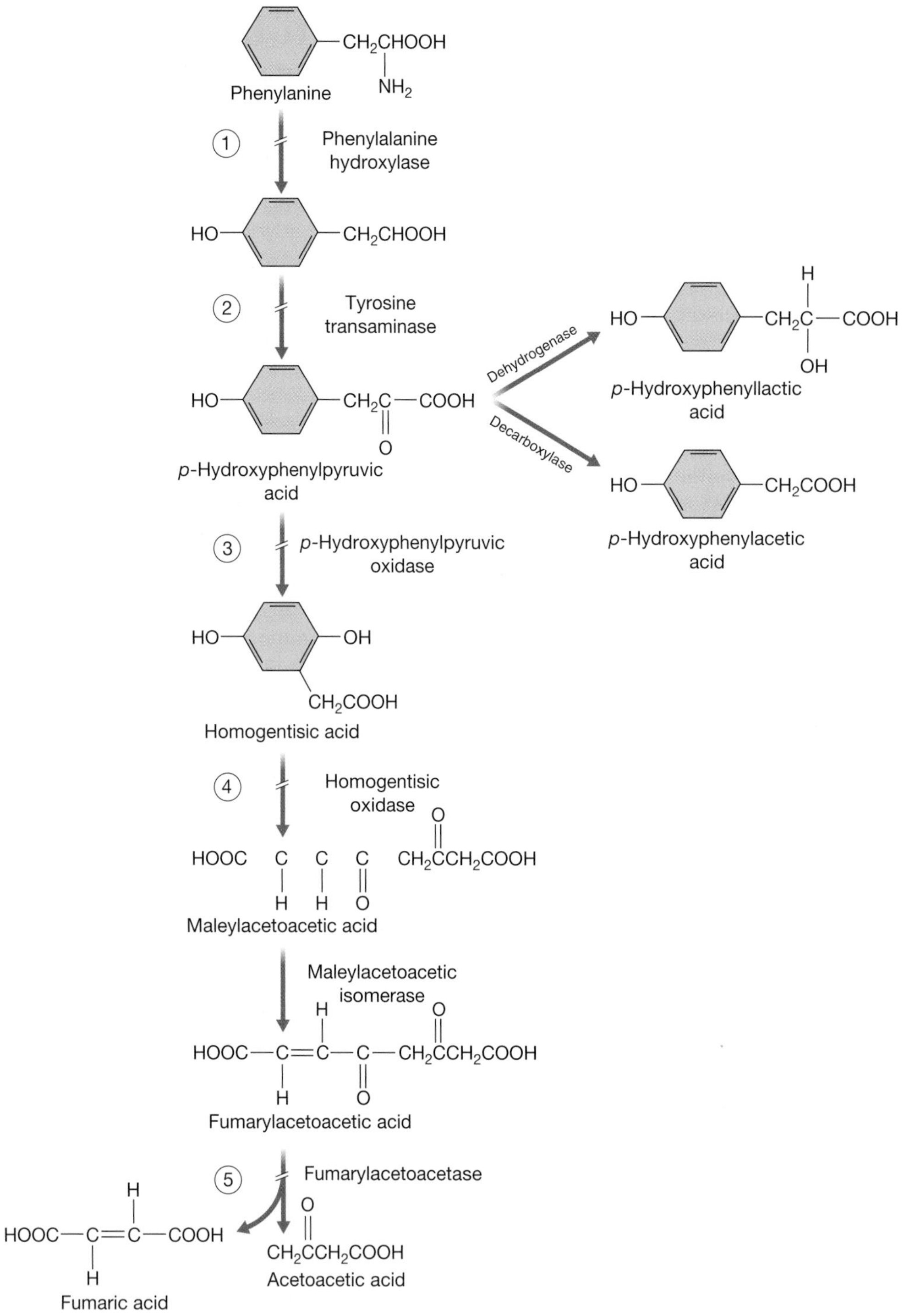

Fig. 66-11 **Metabolic pathway of phenylalanine and tyrosine.** *Double lines,* Block in the metabolic pathway; *1,* block in phenylketonuria; *2,* block in persistent hypertyrosinemia; *3,* block in Medes tyrosinemia patient; *4,* block in alkaptonuria; *5,* block in hereditary tyrosinemia

the urine. The reducing compound was later isolated and identified as *p*-hydroxyphenylpyruvic acid, the α-keto acid of tyrosine. Medes named this condition tyrosinosis.[304] When the patient was fasting, the urine contained 1.6 g *p*-hydroxyphenylpyruvic acid in a 24-hour period. This quantity was considered to represent endogenous production from the catabolism of endogenous protein. When the patient was fed a regular diet, the amount of urinary

p-hydroxyphenylpyruvic acid doubled, and tyrosine could also be isolated from his urine. One of the interesting findings was that feeding large amounts of tyrosine also led to the excretion of 3,4-dihydroxyphenylalanine (dopa), a product of the minor pathway of tyrosine metabolism. Medes postulated a defect in the conversion of *p*-hydroxyphenylpyruvic acid to homogentisic acid. No other case of tyrosinosis has been described.

Table 66-3 Conditions Associated with Hypertyrosinemia

	ENZYME DEFICIENCY	CLINICAL FEATURES
Transitory tyrosinemia of the newborn	p-Hydroxyphenylpyruvic acid oxidase	None
Tyrosinosis (Medes' patient)	p-Hydroxyphenylpyruvic acid oxidase	Mental retardation Skin and eye lesions
Persistent tyrosinemia	Cytosol tyrosine transaminase in one case	No hepatic or renal disease
Hereditary tyrosinemia (hepatorenal type)	Fumarylacetoacetase	Cirrhosis, hepatomas Renal tubular defects
Hypertyrosinemia secondary to liver disease	Generalized partial defects of tyrosine transaminase, p-hydroxyphenylpyruvic acid oxidase, and homogentisic acid oxidase	

Transitory Tyrosinemia of the Newborn

This condition affects approximately 30% of premature infants and as many as 10% of full-term infants.[305-307] It is assumed that the hepatic enzymes catalyzing the early steps of tyrosine metabolism are not well developed in these infants.[308,309] Administration of vitamin C, which is known to protect p-hydroxyphenylpyruvate oxidase from unphysiologic levels of its own substrate, usually corrects the transitory tyrosinemia.[310] The transitory tyrosinemia in infants usually disappears within a few weeks but occasionally persists for several months. A reduction in protein intake to 1.5 to 2 g/kg/day with administration of vitamin C should correct the condition. Although it is generally assumed that transitory tyrosinemia is harmless, this may not be true, because persistent hypertyrosinemia (see later discussion) is regularly associated with mental retardation. There is a definite need for prospective studies of infants, specifically premature infants with transitory hypertyrosinemia.

Persistent Hypertyrosinemia (Tyrosinemia II, Richner-Hanhart Syndrome)

Several patients with persistent tyrosinemia without associated hepatic or renal disease have been described.[311-316] The patients were reported to have cataracts, corneal ulcers, keratotic skin lesions, and neuropsychiatric abnormalities. Enzymatic studies were carried out in four patients. A total deficiency of cytosolic tyrosine transaminase was found in two[313]; however, the activity was only reduced in two others.[317] The keratotic lesions abated in response to low-phenylalanine, low-tyrosine diets in two cases.[315,318] Large doses of vitamin C had no effect on the tyrosinemia in those patients.

Hypertyrosinemia Secondary to Liver Disease

Patients with hepatic cirrhosis have a reduced capacity to metabolize tyrosine and other amino acids.[319] Cirrhotic patients have significantly increased fasting levels of plasma tyrosine and basal levels of p-hydroxyphenylpyruvic acid. They have impaired tolerance to oral loading doses of tyrosine, p-hydroxyphenylpyruvic acid, and homogentisic acid.[320] These findings suggest generalized partial defects in tyrosine transaminase, p-hydroxyphenylpyruvate oxidase, and homogentisic acid oxidase enzymes in patients with cirrhosis. Levels of tyrosine are also slightly elevated in other diseases, including cystic fibrosis (CF),[321] hypoxia with respiratory failure,[322] and rheumatoid arthritis.[323]

Hereditary Tyrosinemia (Hepatorenal Tyrosinemia)

In 1956, Baber reported the case of a 9-month-old infant with failure to thrive, abdominal distention, and diarrhea. The child was found to have cirrhosis of the liver, a renal tubular defect with gross aminoaciduria of a distinct type, and vitamin D–resistant rickets.[324] In 1957 to 1959, Sakai and co-workers reported the case of another patient with a similar clinical picture and marked p-hydroxyphenyllactic aciduria. They drew attention to the abnormal metabolism of tyrosine in this patient and named the condition atypical tyrosinosis.[325-327] Since then, many cases have been reported from Norway,[328] Canada,[329,330] Sweden,[331] and the United States.[332,333] Although many names have been given to the disorder in these cases, hereditary tyrosinemia is generally accepted.

Clinical Features

Hereditary tyrosinemia may be either acute or chronic.[329,334] Symptoms appear in the first month with acute disease, and the patient usually dies with hepatic failure within the first 3 to 9 months.[329] In the chronic form of the disease, the symptoms appear later. The life spans of these patients are longer than those of patients who have the acute form.[329-334] Both forms can occur within the same family. The main symptoms are failure to thrive, vomiting, diarrhea, anorexia, hepatosplenomegaly, ascites, edema, jaundice, bruising, and rickets.[328] Some patients have slight mental deficiencies.

In the chronic form of the disease, hepatoma may develop. A review of the literature by Weinberg and colleagues in 1976 disclosed 16 cases of hepatoma in 43 patients surviving beyond 2 years of age. This incidence is higher than that in adults with macronodular cirrhosis.[335]

Laboratory Findings

Elevated serum levels of AST and ALT are common, and total and direct bilirubin were elevated in 19 of 20 patients thus tested.[328] However, total serum bilirubin levels were usually less than 10 mg/dl until the appearance of signs of liver failure, at which time they became markedly elevated. Synthetic function of the liver is also disturbed, as evidenced by low levels of serum albumin and vitamin K–dependent clotting factors. Hematologic studies show mild anemia, elevated reticulocyte counts, and normal serum iron levels. Bone marrow aspirates show erythroid hyperplasia. These findings suggest a hemolytic anemia, which may be related to an intracorpuscular defect secondary to abnormal accumulation of tyrosine metabolites.[336] In the chronic form of the disease, anemia, leukopenia, and thrombocytopenia are present secondary to hypersplenism.

A tendency to develop hypoglycemia has been found in association with hereditary tyrosinemia.[336,337] Marked hyperplasia of the islets of Langerhans is a rather constant finding, but insulin levels are reported to be normal. The responses to epinephrine and glucagon of two patients thus examined showed flat curves.[336] These findings suggest a disturbance in the release of glucose from glycogen; however, hepatic glycogen content and structure and glycogenolytic enzymes are normal and the glycolytic enzymes are also normal.

The laboratory findings related to the renal tubular defects include hyperphosphaturia, glucosuria, proteinuria, and gross aminoaciduria. Biochemical evidence of rickets secondary to hypophosphatemia is seen in almost all cases.[329] The urinary excretion of amino acids follows a distinctive pattern.[338] The aminoaciduria is more pronounced in the acute disease. The pattern of urinary excretion of tyrosine and phenolic acids (p-hydroxyphenyllactic, p-hydroxyphenylpyruvic, and p-hydroxyphenylacetic acids) by tyrosinemic patients is similar to that described for premature infants with transitory tyrosinemia.[339]

Chromatography of the serum amino acids reveals slight hypertyrosinemia and, frequently, hypermethioninemia. Other amino acids, including phenylalanine, are occasionally slightly elevated. Some of these results must be interpreted with caution because liver damage may cause modest elevations of these amino acids.

In six patients with hereditary tyrosinemia, urinary δ-aminolevulinic acid levels were elevated to as much as 100-fold above control values. In two of these cases, attacks of abdominal pain and paresis of a peripheral type (resembling acute intermittent porphyria) prompted investigation for porphyria. The amounts of porphobilinogen and porphyrins excreted were normal or slightly elevated, but δ-aminolevulinic acid levels were markedly elevated.[340] Similarly, an abnormal pyrrole metabolism was found by Kang and Gerald in a patient with hereditary tyrosinemia. δ-Aminolevulinic acid synthetase activity in liver tissue was increased[333] and it was believed that the abnormality of pyrrole metabolism is a secondary process related to induction of δ-aminolevulinic acid synthetase activity by one of the accumulated metabolites of tyrosine. However, Lindblad and colleagues[341] and Melancon and associates[342] have shown that accumulation of succinyl acetoacetate inhibits porphobilinogen synthetase (δ-aminolevulinic acid dehydratase), leading to increased excretion of δ-aminolevulinic acid. This observation has been confirmed by others and thus the cause of the high levels of δ-aminolevulinic acid is unclear.[343]

Biochemical Features

Patients with hereditary tyrosinemia are reported to lack or to have markedly reduced activity of p-hydroxyphenylpyruvic acid oxidase in their liver and kidneys.[344,345] There is reason to question whether deficiency of this enzyme can account for the clinical manifestations in patients with hereditary tyrosinemia. Thus activity of p-hydroxyphenylpyruvic acid oxidase is reduced in 30% of premature infants, 10% of full-term infants, and patients with persistent hypertyrosinemia (but these patients have no derangement of function of the liver or kidneys). Perry and colleagues induced experimental hypertyrosinemia in vitamin C–deficient newborn guinea pigs fed diets containing large amounts of tyrosine. There was no evidence of a liver or kidney disturbance.[346] Gaull and associates therefore proposed that deficiency of p-hydroxyphenylpyruvic acid oxidase is not the primary defect in patients with hereditary tyrosinemia. These researchers believe that there are deficiencies in the methionine-activating enzyme and cystathionine synthetase in affected patients and that the signs and symptoms of the disease reflect these deficiencies.[347,348]

Feeding large amounts of methionine to guinea pigs in fact produced a syndrome similar to that in infants with hereditary tyrosinemia. The animals showed hypertyrosinemia, hypermethioninemia, generalized aminoaciduria, hypoglycemia, and pancreatic islet cell degeneration.[346] Hence, some metabolite of methionine may be the toxic factor responsible for the pathologic and biochemical changes in hereditary tyrosinemia. Some findings, however, do not support this idea:

1. Hypertyrosinemia usually precedes hypermethioninemia in infants with hereditary tyrosinemia.
2. Transient neonatal hypermethioninemia is an apparently benign condition unassociated with tyrosinemia.
3. Weaning rats fed high-methionine diets have increases of methionine, taurine, and alanine, but not tyrosine, in the serum.[349]

An apparently identical clinical and biochemical picture resembling hereditary tyrosinemia has occasionally been found in patients with hereditary fructosemia[350-352] but not in galactosemia, although severe liver damage is noted in both conditions. Plasma levels of tyrosine and methionine and the excretion of phenolic acid decreased markedly with the exclusion of fructose from the diets of patients with hereditary fructosemia.[351]

Lindblad and associates[341] reported increased excretion of succinyl acetone and succinyl acetoacetate in the urine of patients with hereditary tyrosinemia. These compounds presumably originate from maleylacetoacetate or fumarylacetoacetate or both. Their accumulation indicates a block in metabolism of tyrosine at the fumarylacetoacetase reaction (see Fig. 66-11). These observations have been confirmed by others.[342] Since then, several groups have confirmed the defect in fumarylacetoacetase in liver tissues from patients with hereditary tyrosinemia.[353-357] Additionally, the activity of fumarylacetoacetase was found to be greatly decreased in patients with the acute form of hereditary tyrosinemia. It is reasonable to conclude that severe liver and kidney damage in hereditary tyrosinemia is secondary to accumulation of succinyl acetone and succinyl acetoacetate, which can bind to the SH group of proteins, thereby destroying their function. The liver and kidneys would be the organs principally affected by these metabolites because these tissues are the only ones with p-hydroxyphenylpyruvate hydroxylase activity; that is, metabolism of tyrosine to potentially toxic metabolites depends on the presence of this enzyme. Of interest in this regard are the findings of Lindblad indicating that patients with the more benign form of hereditary tyrosinemia have lower levels of activity of *p*-hydroxyphenylpyruvate hydroxylase in their livers than do patients who have more serious forms of the illness. The cause of the low activity of *p*-hydroxyphenylpyruvic hydroxylase in hereditary tyrosinemia remains to be determined. The possibility of a defect in a regulatory gene common to *p*-hydroxyphenylpyruvic hydroxylase and fumarylacetoacetase can be considered. Continued search for other possible biochemical defects that may be responsible for all the clinical and biochemical features is needed.

Molecular Basis of Hereditary Tyrosinemia

The gene responsible for hereditary tyrosinemia fumarylacetoacetate hydrolase (FAH) has been cloned and mapped to chromosome 15q23-25. The cDNA encodes for a 419 amino acid cytosolic homodimer protein, which is present in the liver, kidney, lymphocytes, erythrocytes, fibroblast, and chorionic villi.[358] Several mutations in the FAH have been described. The IVS12+5G→A allele accounts for more than 95% of mutant FAH allele in the Saguenay-Lac St-Jean area of Québec.[359,360] Certain populations have specific mutations, including W262x in Finns[361,362] and Q64H in Pakistanis.[363]

Pathology

The major pathologic findings are in the liver and kidneys.[364-366] Macroscopically, the liver is enlarged, firm, and nodular. The kidneys are enlarged, with poor architectural demarcations. Microscopically, the architecture of the liver is distorted by extensive fibrosis and infiltration of the portal areas by lymphocytes and plasma cells. The liver cell cords have a pseudoglandular appearance. The hepatocytes show fatty metamorphosis, and some may undergo acidophilic degeneration and, occasionally, giant-cell transformation. Glycogen is either lacking or notably decreased.[364-366]

Genetics

Tyrosinemia has been found with increased frequency in French Canadians. Inheritance is autosomal recessive. The carrier rate in northeastern Québec is 1:14, for an estimated frequency of 14.6 cases per 10,000 population.[367] An automated fluorometric test for hypertyrosinemia has been described,[368] and in the province of Québec, a neonatal screening program has been developed. The association of increased serum levels of alpha fetoprotein with hypertyrosinemia distinguishes patients with hereditary tyrosinemia from patients with transient hypertyrosinemia of the newborn.[369] Prenatal diagnosis has been accomplished by measurement of fumarylacetoacetase in cultured amniotic fluid cells.[370]

Treatment

A diet low in phenylalanine and tyrosine has been used in management of the acute and chronic forms of the disease by several groups of investigators.[328,332,371-373] This diet decreases serum tyrosine levels. It increases serum phosphorus secondary to enhanced renal tubular reabsorption of phosphorus.[328] Similar beneficial effects on renal function are reflected by reductions of glycosuria, hyperaminoaciduria, and proteinuria. The effect of diet on hepatic dysfunction is uncertain. In only one acute case of tyrosinemia were reductions of fibrosis

and infiltration of the liver by inflammatory cells found.[374] Other patients did not respond to the diet in this manner.[330,373,375] The available evidence suggests that a diet low in phenylalanine and tyrosine should be given to patients with the acute and chronic forms of the disease. Signs of deficiency of phenylalanine and tyrosine should be monitored in patients receiving this diet. The amounts of phenylalanine and tyrosine used in such diets are approximately 25 mg/kg/day of each; however, there is some variation in the optimal minimum requirements for individual patients.

In one case, dietary treatment returned the elevated levels of phenylalanine and tyrosine to normal in the serum of a patient with hereditary tyrosinemia. However, the patient continued to have hypermethioninemia and clinical evidence of liver disease. Strict control of his dietary intake of methionine, as well as phenylalanine and tyrosine, returned all serum amino acid levels to normal and eliminated the hepatic abnormalities.[376] Large doses of vitamin D (10,000 to 15000 U/day), together with dietary restrictions of phenylalanine and tyrosine, are necessary to correct the rickets seen in patients with hereditary tyrosinemia.

Other recent treatment modalities pioneered by the Québec investigators include use of 2-(2-nitro-4-trifluoromethylbenzoyl)-1,3-cyclohexanedione (NTBC). NTBC appears to block the conversion of 4-hydroxyphenylpyruvate to homogentisate and to maleylacetoacetate. The treatment protocol includes maintenance of a plasma tyrosine level below 400 μmol/L by dietary phenylalanine and tyrosine restriction. NTBC is given at a starting dose of 1 mg/kg/day in two divided doses, and adjusted to achieve plasma NTBC concentration of greater than 50 μmol/L and no detectable urinary and blood succinylacetone. In asymptomatic patients diagnosed by neonatal screening, none developed hepatic nodules and no acute liver crises have been seen when treated with this regimen. However, in patients who have liver disease, progression to cirrhosis was noted, requiring transplantation.[377] The major complication of NTBC treatment has been thrombocytopenia, leucopenia, cutaneous disorder, corneal crystals, photophobia, and ocular inflammation. Hepatocellular carcinoma has developed in FAH-deficient mice despite NTBC treatment.[378]

Liver transplantation has been carried out in four patients with chronic hereditary tyrosinemia and hepatoma. All were reported to be alive and well 3 months to 3 years after transplantation. Therefore this modality of therapy needs to be considered in patients who develop hepatoma as a complication of their chronic hereditary tyrosinemia.[379] A follow-up of 10 patients who underwent liver transplantation for tyrosinemia suggests the feasibility of this therapy.[380] The indications for liver transplantation were hepatoma in three, acute liver failure in two, and progressive chronic liver disease in five. One patient died during surgery. Of the remaining nine, seven patients are alive 6 months to 6½ years after transplantation. Two died of complications.

Prognosis

Patients who have acute hereditary tyrosinemia die in the first few months of life. Unfortunately, this is the most common form of the disease.[329,334] In patients with the chronic form, the disease progresses slowly, with the eventual development of cirrhosis. Hepatoma has been reported to occur in 37% of patients with chronic hereditary tyrosinemia.[335]

Inborn Errors of Lipid Metabolism
Intracellular Metabolism of Cholesterol

Metabolism of cholesterol and cholesterol esters has been studied primarily in cultured human fibroblasts. Study of patients with inborn errors of lipid metabolism has provided information that tends to support most of the general hypotheses developed from growing fibroblasts in cultures. A brief discussion of the origin, transport, and degradation of free cholesterol and cholesterol esters is included to provide a basis for understanding the metabolic consequences of a deficiency of lysosomal acid lipase.

Peripheral cells can synthesize free cholesterol and cholesterol esters, but they derive most cholesterol from exogenous sterols circulating in the serum as low-density lipoproteins. Intracellular levels of cholesterol are the primary regulators of the rate of synthesis of cholesterol and of uptake from low-density lipoproteins. The metabolism of cholesterol esters is illustrated schematically in **Figure 66-12**.

The initial event in the intracellular metabolism of low-density lipoproteins (i.e., particles enriched in cholesterol esters) is binding to receptors on the cell surface. Low-density lipoprotein receptors bind only those human plasma lipoproteins that contain apolipoproteins B and E (e.g., low-density lipoprotein and very-low-density lipoprotein). After low-density lipoprotein is bound to its specific receptor site, the lipoprotein remains metabolically inactive until the endosomes fuse with lysosomes. At this point, the protein component is hydrolyzed by lysosomal enzymes to products that mostly consist of free amino acids and small peptides (molecular mass <1000). The cholesterol ester component of low-density lipoprotein is hydrolyzed by a lysosomal acid lipase. The liberated cholesterol is then available for metabolic use by the cell.[381] A consequence of the uptake and storage of low-density lipoprotein cholesterol is that the synthesis of cholesterol in nonhepatic tissues is maintained at a low level.

Patients with isolated deficiencies of acid hydrolase activity (Wolman disease) should develop predictable changes in tissue lipids. For example, cholesterol ester as cholesterol linoleate should accumulate in lysosomes of affected individuals. This has been shown to occur.[312,313] Because of a reduced rate of generation of free cholesterol within cells, there should also be decreased suppression of the activity of 3-hydroxy-3-methylglutaryl CoA reductase and reduced activation of endogenous cholesterol acyltransferase. These two events result in increased cholesterol synthesis by the cell and decreased cholesterol esterified with oleic acid, respectively. These abnormalities have been shown to occur in patients with cholesterol ester storage disease.[382,383] However, patients with Wolman disease have additional abnormalities such as accumulation of oxygenated steryl esters, which are difficult to explain solely on the basis of an isolated deficiency of acid hydrolase.[384] Similarly, patients with Wolman disease have unexplained steatorrhea, which may be secondary to defects in the metabolism of bile acids.

Molecular Basis of Lysosomal Acid Lipase Disorders (Wolman Disease and Cholesterol Ester Storage Disease)

Deficiency of lysosomal acid lipase leads to either Wolman disease or the more benign cholesterol ester storage disease. Both disorders are inherited as autosomal recessive diseases and are associated with reduced activity and genetic defects of lysosomal acid lipase. The gene for lysosomal acid lipase (LIPA) has been cloned and mapped to chromosome 10q23.2-q23.3. The gene is expressed in most tissues with high expression in the hepatocytes, splenic and thymic cells, small intestinal villus cells, and adrenal cortex.[385] Homozygotes for the exon-8 splice junction mutation, resulting in incomplete exon skipping, has been described in many Wolman disease patients.[386] Cholesterol ester storage disease is distinct from Wolman disease in that at least one mutant allele has the potential to produce some residual enzymatic activity to ameliorate the phenotype. Thus, in the majority of cholesterol ester storage disease cases, a single splicing mutation occurs in one allele.[387] A knockout mouse model of Wolman disease has been produced by targeted disruption of the lysosomal acid lipase gene.[388]

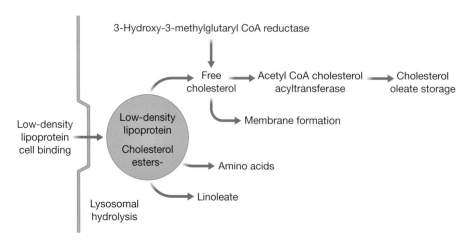

Fig. 66-12 **Metabolism of cholesterol esters.**

Wolman Disease

Enzymatic Abnormalities

In 1956 Abramov and colleagues reported an infant who died at 2 months of age after a short illness characterized by abdominal distention, severe vomiting, diarrhea, hepatosplenomegaly, and radiographic evidence of calcification of the adrenal glands.[389] Wolman and co-workers reported in 1961 on the cases of two siblings of their first patient who were found to have the same illness.[390] Accumulations of cholesterol esters and triglycerides were found in the liver, spleen, lymph nodes, and adrenal glands. The disorder was reported under the title generalized xanthomatosis with calcified adrenals.[390] In 1965 Crocker and associates described three patients with this disorder as having Wolman disease; since then, the latter term has been widely accepted.[391] Patrick and Lake confirmed in 1969 that the accumulated cholesterol was esterified and demonstrated an acid hydrolase deficiency in the livers and spleens of those patients.[392] The activity of acid hydrolase was also deficient in cultured fibroblasts of patients with Wolman disease.[393]

Deficiency of acid hydrolase or acid esterase manifests in two phenotypic forms. Wolman disease represents the clinically acute and severe form. Affected patients die in the first year of life. Cholesterol ester storage disease represents a chronic form of deficiency of acid hydrolase. Patients who have this latter disorder do not have adrenal calcifications, and they live to adulthood.[382] Forty patients with Wolman disease and more than 20 patients with cholesterol ester storage disease have been described so far.

Clinical Features

The majority of patients have similar clinical courses: projectile vomiting, diarrhea, abdominal distention, and failure to thrive, with the first noticeable symptoms appearing in about the second week of life.[389,390] Some patients are jaundiced.[391,394] Neurologic development of these infants is not normal. A decrease in activity may be noticed in the second month of life. It is not clear whether these symptoms are related to severe malnutrition or reflect neurologic defects. Konno and associates reported the case of an infant who had exaggerated tendon reflexes, ankle clonus, and opisthotonos.[394] Electroencephalography was reported to show no abnormality in this patient or several others.[383,395] On physical examination, a patient is usually slightly feverish, irritable, and wasted. Nonspecific skin eruptions may be observed. Abdominal distention with hepatosplenomegaly is noted in all patients; lymphadenopathy is detected in some. Subsequently progressive hepatosplenomegaly and abdominal distention, fever, and vomiting and diarrhea occur, persisting until the death of the patient, usually in the first 6 months of life.[389,390]

Laboratory Findings

Anemia usually appears early in the course of the disease, and hemoglobin levels progressively decrease to as low as 5 g/dl. Peripheral blood lymphocytes show intracytoplasmic and intranuclear vacuolation.[391,394,395] Acanthocytosis was found in a Japanese infant.[394] Lipid-laden histiocytes or foam cells are seen in bone marrow aspirates and in the peripheral blood.[389]

Total serum bilirubin and the conjugated fraction are elevated in some patients.[390,391,394] Some have elevated serum levels of AST and ALT.[391,394] Steatorrhea is present, evidenced by a high fecal fat content[391,394,395] and an abnormal [163]I-triolein absorption test.[395] The most consistent diagnostic finding, present in all reported cases of Wolman disease, is calcification of the adrenal glands. The adrenal glands are symmetrically enlarged and show extensive punctate calcifications (**Fig. 66-13**).[389,390] This is the only disease that causes such calcification of the adrenal glands. In all other conditions, the calcifications are scattered. In most patients, the responses of the adrenal glands to adrenocorticotropic hormone stimulation are depressed. Plasma cholesterol and triglycerides are usually normal in patients with Wolman

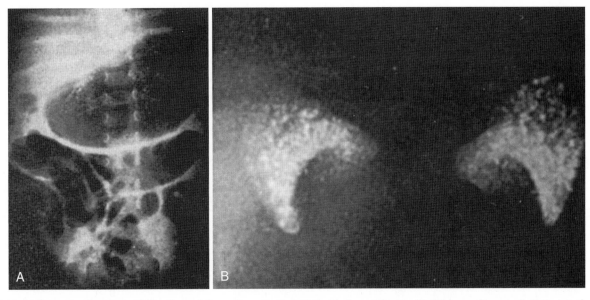

Fig. 66-13 **Radiograms showing calcification of the enlarged adrenal glands in a patient with Wolman disease. A,** Patient in the supine position; **B,** the adrenals after removal at autopsy. *(Reproduced from Crocker AC, et al. Wolman's disease: three new patients with a recently described lipidosis. Pediatrics 1965;35:627–640, with permission.)*

disease.[390,391,395-397] Triglycerides and very-low-density lipoproteins were elevated in two patients.[396] It is expected that low-density lipoprotein levels should be high because the acid hydrolase deficiency decreases cellular metabolism of low-density lipoproteins. Some patients, however, had hypolipoproteinemia.[395] The severe inanition and reduced production of lipoproteins by the liver probably offset the tendency toward hyperlipoproteinemia.

Biochemical Characteristics

Most of the enzymes that hydrolyze fatty acid esters are active at neutral or alkaline pH. An ester hydrolase active at acidic pH (4.0 to 5.6) has been found in lysosomes and cell membranes.[392] This enzyme requires no co-factors and uses triglycerides and cholesterol ester as substrates. Lysosomal acid lipase/cholesteryl ester hydrolase has been purified,[398] and the cDNA encoding the human enzyme has been cloned and expressed.[399] Accumulation of cholesterol esters apparently results from the deficiency of cholesterol ester hydrolase activity.[400] Accumulations of triglycerides and other lipid products in large quantities are more difficult to explain. These biochemical abnormalities are discussed in more detail in Cholesterol Ester Storage Disease. **Table 66-4** shows the results of analyses of lipids in various tissues in Wolman disease.

The triglyceride content is several-fold greater in the liver and as much as 100-fold greater in the spleen of a patient with Wolman disease than in comparable tissues of controls.[392] The total cholesterol in liver and spleen is elevated in every case of Wolman disease. The majority of the increase is in the cholesterol ester fraction. Similar accumulations of triglycerides and cholesterol esters have been found in bone marrow, the thymus, and lymph nodes. Slight increases were also detected in the lungs and kidneys.[396] Cholesterol and triglyceride contents of the brain were reported to be elevated in some patients[391,396]; however, they were normal in others.[394]

That severe malabsorption is seen in Wolman disease but not in cholesterol ester storage disease could be explained by the differences in bile acid metabolism in these two diseases. Total serum bile acid levels were either normal or increased in patients with cholesterol ester storage disease.[383] Assmann and colleagues found oxygenated steryl esters in Wolman disease but not in cholesterol ester storage disease. The accumulation of these oxygenated esters would suggest a defect in bile acid synthesis in Wolman disease.[384] Boyd suggested that cholesterol linoleate may be the precursor in 7α-hydroxycholesterol formation.[401] If the pathway from 7α-hydroxycholesterol to

bile acids were blocked, an accumulation of oxygenated steryl esters would occur. These speculations await confirmation by the study of bile acid metabolism in Wolman disease, and the finding of such a defect in bile acid synthesis in Wolman disease would explain the steatorrhea.

Pathology

LIVER

Enlargement of the liver is a constant finding. The liver is firm and appears yellow on gross examination. The hepatic architecture is usually distorted. The hepatic parenchymal cells show marked steatosis. Sinusoids are plugged by swollen histiocytes with foamy, vacuolated cytoplasm. Kupffer cells are distended and vacuolated. The portal areas are enlarged, with increased fibrosis that extends to the periportal areas. The fibrosis may be extensive, and a classic picture of hepatic cirrhosis may be seen.[389,390,396,397]

Electron microscopic examination of the liver shows that parenchymal organelles are distorted by the accumulation of large osmiophilic lipid droplets, which are neutral lipids. These droplets are seen mostly in the lysosomes. The smooth endoplasmic reticulum and rough endoplasmic reticulum appear distended but are usually empty. The Kupffer cells are so distended that they almost obstruct the sinusoids.[397]

SPLEEN AND LYMPH NODES

The spleen is greatly enlarged, is firm, and appears mottled with yellowish flecks. Microscopic section shows that the reticular cells are transformed into large foam cells. The lymphatic follicles are atrophied and compressed. The lymph nodes are enlarged, firm, and yellowish. Microscopically, the lymph nodes are similar to the spleen. The same changes are also seen in the bone marrow and thymus.[391,396]

INTESTINES

The small intestine is usually thickened and has a yellowish serosal surface. The mucosa is greasy, yellowish, and granular. Microscopic sections show thick, flattened villi with numerous foamy, lipid-filled histiocytes in the lamina propria. Some of the foam cells extend into the muscularis mucosa. These changes are most evident in the proximal intestine or occasionally in the colon.[391,396]

ADRENAL GLANDS

Both glands are symmetrically enlarged, firm, and difficult to cut. The cortex on cut sections is yellowish, whereas medially,

Table 66-4 Tissue Lipid Analysis in Patients with Wolman Disease

	TRIGLYCERIDE	TOTAL CHOLESTEROL	FREE	ESTERIFIED
Liver, wet weight (mg/g)	137	97	38	59
	61	170	9	161
	44	32	14	18
Upper limit of normal	20	5	4	1
Spleen, weight (mg/g)	8	26	10	16
	99	35	8	27
	29	8	4	4
Upper limit of normal	1	5	4	<1

the tissue is whitish. Microscopic sections of the glands show preservation of the architecture of the cortex. Many of the cells are swollen and vacuolated and contain sudanophilic lipid. Some of the foam cells are necrotic and appear as lipid cysts. Most of the calcium deposition occurs in a finely granular pattern; however, in some regions it may be condensed to form crystalline bumps.[396] Extensive fibrosis is found in the inner cortical areas. The medullary cells are normal.

Electron microscopic sections show that the innermost part of the adrenal cortex is necrotic, with calcification. The histiocytes are filled with large amounts of both crystalline and droplet lipid. Histochemical analysis of the lipid indicates the presence of cholesterol esters and triglycerides.[396,397]

OTHER ORGANS

The vascular endothelium shows lipid deposition, but frank atherosclerosis is not seen. Foam cells have been observed in the intestinal tissue and in the lungs, thyroid, testes, ovaries, leptomeninges, Purkinje cells, Auerbach plexus, and Meissner plexus.

Genetics

Wolman disease is inherited as an autosomal recessive trait. Seven of the patients reported so far have been Jews of Iraqi or Iranian origin. The other patients have been from Japan, western Europe, and North America. Young and Patrick reported that the enzyme acid hydrolase in the leukocytes of the parents and a sibling of one patient had half the normal activity.[400] Kyriakides and associates reported similar findings in skin fibroblasts from the parents of a patient.[393] A prenatal diagnosis using cultured amniotic fluid cells has been described.[402]

Differential Diagnosis

Calcifications of the adrenal glands, invariably present in Wolman disease, can be seen in conditions such as Addison disease, adrenal hemorrhage, neuroblastoma, ganglioneuroma, adrenal cysts, pheochromocytoma, cortical carcinoma, and adrenal teratoma.[389,403] However, the calcifications in Wolman disease characteristically outline the shape of the adrenal gland. Niemann-Pick disease may result in gastrointestinal symptoms, hepatosplenomegaly, and failure to thrive in early infancy, but adrenal calcifications are absent. The definitive diagnosis of Wolman disease depends on the clinical picture and assay of acid hydrolase in cultured leukocytes or skin fibroblasts, using *p*-nitrophenyl laurate as a substrate.[404] Acid hydrolase activity that is less than 5% of normal confirms the diagnosis.

Treatment and Prognosis

Several therapeutic approaches have been tried, including TPN[405] and bone marrow transplantation.[406] A diet free of hydrophobic esters in which cholesterol and the essential fatty acids are bound to protein has been proposed by Wolman.[407]

Cholesterol Ester Storage Disease

Clinical Picture

In 1963 Fredrickson reported the first known case of hepatic cholesterol ester storage disease. The patient was a child with hepatomegaly and hyperlipidemia.[408] In 1967 Lageron and co-workers reported the case of a French adult with the same disease.[409,410] Schiff and associates reported in 1968 the cases of a brother and sister with the disease. Mild cirrhosis was evident in liver biopsy specimens, along with notable increases in fat content. Four of five younger siblings were found to have hepatomegaly. Liver biopsy specimens from three of the siblings showed vacuoles in their hepatocytes similar to those seen in the hepatocytes of the original patients.[383] Partin and Schubert found deposits of cholesterol esters in the lamina propria and mucosal smooth muscle and vascular pericytes[411] in jejunal tissue from two of the severely affected children in the family described by Schiff.

The majority of patients come to medical attention early in childhood, but one patient sought treatment at the age of 23 years. Hepatomegaly has been present in all patients reported.[382,383,408-415] In one patient hepatomegaly was present at birth. Hepatomegaly is progressive; eventually, hepatic fibrosis develops. Splenomegaly was found in 54% of patients, and esophageal varices secondary to portal hypertension were present in 27%. One patient had recurrent episodes of abdominal pain without a known cause.[410,412] Two of the patients were reported to have had delays in sexual maturation.[409,411]

Laboratory Findings

The results of liver tests are usually normal. Jaundice has not been found, except in two patients who may have developed hepatitis with lethal complications.[400,413] Schiff and colleagues studied the serum bile acid profiles of two patients and those of five siblings, both parents, an uncle, and a grandfather of these patients. Total serum bile acids were markedly elevated in one patient and in all but three relatives. The ratio of cholic acid to chenodeoxycholic acid was decreased in duodenal bile obtained from one of the two patients.[383] Plasma lipoprotein patterns show hypercholesterolemia and some hypertriglyceridemia. The majority of the patients have increased levels of low-density lipoprotein. Two patients had low levels of high-density lipoprotein.

Biochemical Characteristics

Results of lipid analyses of liver tissue obtained from three patients with cholesterol ester storage disease are shown in **Table 66-5**. The major abnormality was the marked increase

Table 66-5 **Lipid Concentrations in Liver Tissue of Patients with Cholesterol Ester Storage Disease**

	TOTAL LIPIDS	TRIGLYCERIDES	TOTAL	FREE CHOLESTEROL	ESTERIFIED
Lipids, wet weight (mg/g)	280	64	121	9	187
	244	36	112	11	174
Upper limit of normal		19	4	3	1

in cholesterol esters. The fatty acid composition of the cholesterol esters showed a predominance of oleic and linoleic acids.[383,389] The stored esters contained less than the expected amount of cholesterol linoleate.

Increased levels of low-density lipoproteins in serum are routinely found in cholesterol ester storage disease. The presence of atherosclerosis in two patients with cholesterol ester storage disease is of interest because current speculation about the role of acid hydrolase in arterial intima predicts that accelerated atherosclerosis will be a consequence of the enzymatic deficiency.

The reason for the different clinical courses of Wolman disease and cholesterol ester storage disease is unclear. It may be that there is a small but critical difference between the levels of residual acid hydrolase in the two groups of patients. A slightly greater deficiency of acid hydrolase in tissues has been recorded for patients with Wolman disease.[382] Another possibility is that the two diseases are different at the levels of the enzymatic defects. For example, liver tissue from a patient with Wolman disease did not hydrolyze DL-hexadecanyl-1,2-dioleate, whereas liver tissue from a patient with cholesterol ester storage disease hydrolyzed this substrate at a normal rate.[416] There could be isoforms of acid hydrolase with deficiency of different isoenzymes in Wolman disease and cholesterol ester storage disease. Alternatively, it may be that the nature of the defect in a single type of acid hydrolase differs in these disorders.

Burton and co-workers reported that the intracellular acid hydrolase activity in cultured cells from Wolman's patients was 10% to 20% of control hydrolytic activity, whereas cholesterol ester storage disease cells exhibited 30% to 45% of control activity. These differences were only found when intracellular rather than cell lysate activity of the enzyme was measured.[417]

Pathology

The pathologic changes are secondary to the intralysosomal deposition of cholesterol esters and triglycerides.

LIVER

Macroscopically, the liver is greatly enlarged and appears orange. On microscopic examination, the hepatic parenchymal cells and Kupffer cells show deposition of lipid droplets (**Fig. 66-14**). In frozen sections, the lipid droplets in the hepatocytes are birefringent but not autofluorescent. Those in Kupffer cells are not birefringent but show yellow autofluorescence. The differences are thought to be due to peroxidation of the fatty acids of cholesterol esters in macrophages but not in parenchymal cells. Electron microscopic studies show the lipid deposits to be limited by a

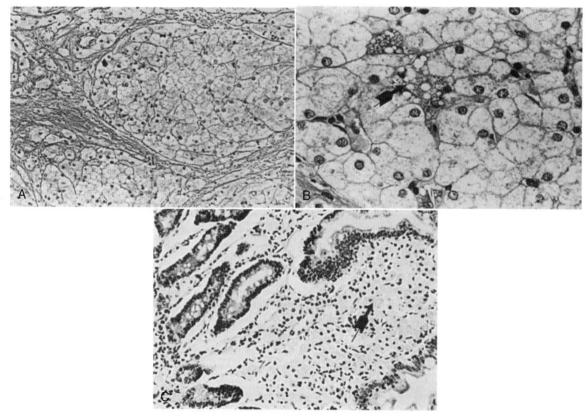

Fig. 66-14 Biopsy specimens from a patient with cholesterol ester storage disease. A, Liver showing dense bands of connective tissue extending through the liver and forming nodules. (Wilder reticulum stain, ×200.) **B,** The individual foam vacuoles of different sizes plus acinar clefts interpreted as cholesterol, indicated by the *arrow*. (Gomori's trichrome, ×500.) **C,** The lamina propria of the small intestine, containing foam cells, indicated by the *arrow*, in dense nodules distorting the involved villus. (Gomori's trichrome, ×200.) *(Reproduced from Beaudet AL, et al. Cholesterol ester storage disease: clinical, biochemical, and pathological studies. J Pediatr 1977;90:910–914, with permission.)*

single trilaminar membrane. The deposits in the hepatocytes are electron lucent; however, those in the Kupffer cells are interspersed with electron-dense material. In the majority of patients, dense bands of fibrous tissue extend through the liver, forming lobules of different sizes. Fibrosis may progress in some patients to give a classic picture of cirrhosis, with the development of portal hypertension and esophageal varices.[413]

OTHER TISSUES

Partin and Schubert[411] studied small intestinal biopsy specimens from two patients. The biopsy specimens had an orange tinge. In contradistinction to Tangier disease, which features storage of cholesterol esters, abnormal coloration of the colonic mucosa or the tonsils has not been found in cholesterol ester storage disease. Histologic sections of the small bowel show that the epithelial cells are normal; however, foam cells were found in the lacteal area and were especially abundant in the villus tips. Free droplets of fat were present in the extracellular spaces of the lamina propria.[382]

Electron microscopic studies of the small intestine show foam cells in clusters beneath the basement membrane of the epithelial cells surrounding the lacteals. The cytoplasm of the lacteal endothelium is distended by numerous large osmiophilic lipid vacuoles. Smooth muscle fiber cells, vascular pericytes, fibrocytes, and Schwann cells of nerve fibers contain lucent lipid droplets. Deposits of lipids, similar to those seen in Wolman disease, were found in other tissues. Although clinically there was no evidence of atherosclerosis in patients with cholesterol ester storage disease, two of three patients examined by necropsy had atherosclerosis.[413]

Genetics

Cholesterol ester storage disease is inherited as an autosomal recessive trait.[382] There is a preponderance of females among the patients reported. It is possible to detect heterozygotes by quantitation of acid hydrolase activity in leukocytes or cultured fibroblasts. Heterozygotes have 40% to 50% of the reported normal enzymatic activity.[413] Prenatal diagnosis can be established using cultured amniotic fluid cells. Different mutations in the lyosomal acid lipase can explain the level of the residual enzyme activity. Therefore the genotype can predict the severity of the phenotype.[418]

Treatment and Prognosis

Cholesterol ester storage disease is relatively benign although death in childhood from hepatic complications has been reported.[413] Two patients died at 43 years of age.[409,419]

Two reports suggested the utility of inhibitors of 3-hydroxy-3-methylglutaryl-coenzyme A reductase as a safe and effective treatment for children with acid lipase deficiency. A significant decrease in hepatomegaly and the levels of cholesterol and triglycerides was observed in the treated patients.[420,421]

Inborn Errors of Bile Acid Metabolism (see Chapter 5)

Inborn errors of bile acid metabolism include disorders involving molecular defects in the genes encoding canalicular transport proteins, peroxisomal disorders, and a heterogeneous group of disorders, including Alagille syndrome with mutations in the Jagged-1 gene and CF with mutations in the cystic fibrosis transmembrane regulator (CFTR).

PROGRESSIVE FAMILIAL INTRAHEPATIC CHOLESTASIS

Progressive familial intrahepatic cholestasis (PFIC) is a heterogeneous group of autosomal recessive disorders in which hepatocellular cholestasis often presents in the neonatal period or the first year of life, leading to death from liver failure during the childhood to adolescent periods. The clinical, biochemical, and histologic features and the advances in the understanding of the canalicular membrane transport proteins in the liver have provided evidence for the heterogeneity of this clinical entity and suggested defects in bile secretion and/or bile acid metabolism without anatomic obstruction. Three types of PFIC have been described based on the recent molecular and genetic studies that allowed identification of the molecular basis of these three types.

Progressive Familial Intrahepatic Cholestasis Type 1 (Byler Disease)

The first type is called PFIC1, also known as Byler disease and originally described in 1965 by Clayton and associates. They described a syndrome of progressive intrahepatic cholestasis in an extensive study of Amish descendants from Jacob Byler, who was born in the United States in 1799. Six members of four interrelated, inbred Amish sibships were described in Clayton's original abstract.[422] The disease was characterized by onset of pruritus, jaundice, steatorrhea, and hepatosplenomegaly early in infancy. Four of the six patients died between 17 months and 8 years of age. Similar cases have been reported from France and Japan.[423-425] Biochemically, all of Clayton's patients had conjugated hyperbilirubinemia and elevated serum alkaline phosphatase with normal serum cholesterol levels. Subsequently, Byler disease patients are characterized as having low serum γ-glutamyltransferase concentrations, high serum bile salt concentrations, and low biliary chenodeoxycholic bile salt concentrations. This form of progressive familial intrahepatic cholestasis has been mapped by positional cloning to chromosome 18q21-22.[426,427]

Clinical Features

Progressive intrahepatic cholestasis usually manifests between the ages of 1 and 10 months.[426,428] In four of the reported cases, onset of the disease occurred in the first week of life.[426] Pruritus and jaundice are the earliest symptoms. In infants, pruritus may be severe enough to interfere with sleep. The jaundice is usually accompanied by dark urine and pale stools that may become totally acholic. The stools are loose, foul smelling, and greasy because of steatorrhea.[426,429] Some patients may have watery diarrhea that continues even after liver transplantation.[430,431] The level of jaundice usually fluctuates. Recurrent cholestatic episodes alternate with periods of remission. The cholestatic episodes have been reported to be triggered by upper respiratory tract infections.[426] After several months, remissions are less frequent. Rickets is seen in some patients, most of whom have growth retardation; developmental retardation was found in 30% of the reported patients.[426,432]

Bleeding episodes secondary to hypoprothrombinemia have been reported for approximately half the patients. Some patients have clubbing of the fingers.[433] Xanthomatosis of the skin does not occur. Hepatomegaly has been present in all patients reported so far, but splenomegaly has been found in only half. Liver enlargement persists during remissions, and with the progression of disease, the liver becomes hard, irregular, and nodular. Extraintestinal manifestations include pancreatitis and hearing impairment.[434,435] The majority of patients die between the ages of 2 and 15 years, but occasionally a patient has survived until the age of 25 years.[425] Dahms reported the cases of twin brothers with Byler disease, both of whom developed hepatocellular carcinomas. The two brothers died of liver failure at 13 and 17 years of age.[436]

Laboratory Findings

All reported patients have had elevations of total serum bilirubin. Levels of 40 to 50 mg/dl are not unusual during the cholestatic episodes.[429] The direct fraction is usually half of the total bilirubin.[423-425] The serum AST and ALT levels are elevated. Serum cholesterol is usually normal or low.[423] Serum γ-glutamyl transpeptidase (GGTP) levels are normal despite the elevation of serum alkaline phosphatase levels.[437] Levels of GGTP in the liver are reported to be elevated.[438] Serum GGTP could be used as a marker for Byler disease because normal values were found in 22 of 28 patients with the disease.[439] Prothrombin time and thromboplastin time are increased secondary to malabsorption of vitamin K. Malabsorption studies reveal severe steatorrhea and excretion of fat amounting to 50% to 80% of intake.[424] Both T_m and storage capacity for sulfobromophthalein (BSP) are markedly reduced. A parent heterozygotic for the trait is clinically normal but may have an abnormally decreased BSP T_m.[423] Sweat chloride levels are elevated in PFIC1.

Total serum bile acids have been elevated in the patients studied. Total bile acids in duodenal aspirates of one patient studied by Linarelli and associates were 0.07 to 0.5 mmol/L, which is below the critical micellar concentration of 2 mmol/L.[440,441] The clearance of labeled cholic acid and chenodeoxycholic acid was normal at 20 minutes and slightly impaired at 60 minutes. The half-life of the labeled bile acid was prolonged. The major loss of the isotopes was in urine rather than feces. Serum lithocholic acid was reported to be high in Linarelli's patient. Radiographic examination of the biliary tree by operative cholangiography showed patency of the biliary tree in the patients studied. In the series reported from France, cholelithiasis and intrapancreatic calcification were found in some patients.[425]

The biochemical findings suggest a defect in the excretion of bile acids across the canalicular membrane of the liver cell. The gene for PFIC1 is called FIC1, which encodes for a P-type ATPase that is predominantly expressed in the small intestine and the liver and likely to be important in the transfer of amino phospholipids from the outer to the inner leaflet of the plasma membrane bilayer (aminophospholipid flippase).[427] Mutations in this transporter, ATP8B1, are responsible for PFIC1.[442-444] Another entity known as benign recurrent intrahepatic cholestasis (BRIC type 1) appear to represent a mild disease characterized by episodes of cholestasis. Missense mutation in ATP8B$_1$ are associated with BRIC type 1. Therefore the current concept is that both BRIC and PFIC1 represent a continuum of a single entity.

Pathology

Light microscopy of liver biopsy specimens early in the disease shows normal hepatic architecture. Hepatocellular and canalicular cholestasis with pseudoacinar transformation is commonly seen. Bile duct damage leading to ductal paucity is seen in 70% of older patients. The striking feature of all liver biopsy specimens is the marked cholestasis in the parenchymal cells and in canaliculi. As the disease progresses, the classic picture of biliary cirrhosis develops.[445,446] Electron microscopic studies show markedly abnormal biliary duct canaliculi. The pericanalicular ectoplasm is greatly thickened, and the microvilli are swollen, fused, or blunted. The canalicular lumina are filled with coarsely particulate and amorphous granular material.[446] In contrast, in biopsies from livers with other causes of cholestasis, the canalicular membrane lumen contains amorphous bile.

Prognosis

Death usually occurs between the ages of 17 months and 8 years from hepatic complications, such as liver failure, bleeding, and malnutrition. An occasional patient has survived to 25 years of age.

Therapy

Oral ursodeoxycholic acid appears effective in all types of progressive familial intrahepatic cholestasis for improving the clinical status of some children.[446] Alagille and Odievre reported rapid relief of cholestasis in four patients in whom cholecystojejunostomy was performed; however, the long-term benefit from such a major surgical procedure is unknown.[425] Similarly, Whitington and Whitington have shown improvement in cholestasis with external biliary drainage.[447] The researchers' experience suggests heterogeneity in the response to biliary diversion. Some patients improved greatly; others showed no improvement. The latter patients had liver transplantation, and favorable experience with liver transplantation in patients with Byler disease has been reported.[448]

Progressive Familial Intrahepatic Cholestasis Type 2

Patients with initial typical findings of familial progressive intrahepatic cholestasis type 1, and unrelated to the Byler family, have Byler syndrome. Cases have been described in isolated populations, the Middle East, Greenland, and Sweden.[449-452] Homozygosity mapping and linkage analysis in six consanguineous patients of Middle Eastern origin have resulted in identification of a gene location on chromosome on 2q24.[452] Patients with type 2 familial progressive intrahepatic cholestasis have severe pruritus, low serum γ-glutamyltransferase activity and cholesterol levels, high concentration of serum primary bile acids, and low biliary primary bile acid concentrations. Clinically these patients have more severe and permanent jaundice with the onset of rapid liver failure. Liver histology shows an absence of ductular proliferation with canalicular cholestasis and periportal biliary metaplasia of hepatocytes.[436,446] However, the liver architecture is more severely altered with lobular and portal fibrosis and inflammation and giant cell proliferation compared with PFIC1. More recent studies suggest that the defect may reside in the canalicular bile salt export pump (BSEP). At least 10 BSEP mutations have been determined in PFIC2 patients from several different populations.[453] Moreover, the human BSEP gene has been mapped to the 2q24 locus, which is the gene locus for the PFIC2. The findings of mutations in BSEP are consistent with the decreased canalicular excretion of bile acids described in these patients. Indeed, patients with PFIC2 were found to have a close correlation between BSEP gene mutations and canalicular BSEP expression, resulting in a decrease in the concentration of biliary bile acids in these deficient patients.[454] The BSEP transporter is now known as ABCB11.[455] Another entity known as BRIC2 has been described with mutations in ABCB11. These patients have gallstones.

Progressive Familial Intrahepatic Cholestasis Type 3

Patients with PFIC3 usually have cholestasis and the potential for development of biliary cirrhosis and liver failure at a later age. These patients can be distinguished from the other types of progressive intrahepatic cholestasis by the finding of very high serum γ-glutamyltransferase activity and a liver histology that shows portal fibrosis with bile duct proliferation and inflammatory infiltrate in the early stages, despite the fact that their intrahepatic and extrahepatic bile ducts are patent.[432] The genetic basis of PFIC3 has been shown to be related to mutations in ABCB4 (multidrug-resistant-3 [MDR3] P-glycoprotein), which transports phospholipids into the biliary system.[456,457] The finding of mutation on MDR3 was based on the finding that analysis of bile in these patients shows very low concentration of phospholipid and the phenotype of the analogous MDR2 knockout mouse.[458] MDR3 belongs to the family of ABC transporters and is expressed in the canalicular membrane of the hepatocytes. Immunohistochemistry revealed the lack of canalicular staining for MDR3 in the liver tissue of patients with PFIC3. Mutations in the MDR3 gene have been described in patients with PFIC3. Some of these mutations lead to a truncated MDR3 protein, which lacks at least one ABC motif. Additional nonsense mutations and missense mutations associated with low biliary phospholipid levels have been identified in patients with PFIC3. The liver pathology may be related to the toxic effects of bile acids on bile canaliculi and the biliary epithelium in the absence of phospholipids. Recent studies have also suggested that the heterozygous state for a MDR3 gene defect may represent a genetic predisposition in families with cholestasis, noted during pregnancy.[459,460] The MDR3 gene has been mapped to 7q21-36. One study has identified 16 different mutations in 17 different patients. These mutations include frameshift, nonsense, and missense. Gallstones or episodes of cholestasis of pregnancy were found in patients or parents. Children with missense mutations had a less severe disease and more often a beneficial effect of ursodeoxycholic acid therapy was noted in this group of patients.[458]

Hereditary Lymphedema with Recurrent Cholestasis (Norwegian Cholestasis; Aagenaes Syndrome)

In 1968 Aagenaes and associates reported the cases of 16 patients from Norway in whom hereditary recurrent intrahepatic cholestasis appeared during the neonatal period.[461] In 1971 Sharp and Krivit reported two sisters of Norwegian extraction with a similar syndrome.[462] Consanguinity was present in six of the seven parental couples in the series reported by Aagenaes and co-workers, suggesting an autosomal recessive inheritance. In 1974 Aagenaes described two additional families with a similar syndrome.[463] All patients had early onset of intrahepatic cholestasis with elevated levels of total and direct serum bilirubin. Lymphedema of the lower extremities appeared late in childhood in all of Aagenaes' patients. Lymphedema appeared early and at the onset of cholestatic jaundice in the patients of Sharp and Krivit.

Clinical Features

All reported patients became jaundiced during the first month of life.[462-464] The jaundice lasted about 1 to 6 years, and during this period, the patients had severe pruritus. Growth retardation with complications of malabsorption, such as rickets, anemia, and a bleeding tendency, was evident during the period of cholestasis. When the cholestasis resolved, catch-up growth occurred, such that the patients' adult heights were normal. One or more further episodes of cholestasis have occurred in all adult patients. Lymphedema, once present, persists throughout life.

Laboratory Findings

Total serum bilirubin is elevated, with the direct fraction accounting for 50% to 80% of the total. Serum AST and ALT levels are increased, especially during periods of cholestasis and in the first year of life.[462-465] Serum alkaline phosphatase levels are always increased. Results of the BSP excretion test are abnormal, with retention of 25% to 40% at 45 minutes. Serum cholesterol and triglyceride levels are elevated. Lipoprotein electrophoresis shows increases in pre-β and β-lipoproteins. Protein electrophoresis shows elevation of the α_2-globulin fraction with low serum albumin. Prothrombin time and thromboplastin time are elevated secondary to malabsorption of vitamin K. Fecal fat measurements show excretion of about 30% to 50% of ingested fat. Fecal nitrogen excretion is normal.

Lymphangiography with visualization of the deep lymphatics was attempted in only one case. The lymphatics were found to be abnormally tortuous. Injection of blue dye into the interdigital spaces in another patient resulted in a chicken-wire pattern, indicative of an absence of deep lymphatics.[463]

Pathology

Examination of liver biopsy specimens reveals intact architecture with marked bile stasis, giant cell transformation, and minimal hepatic cell necrosis. The portal areas show a slight increase in fibrosis, and in most instances, biliary ducts are difficult to find. In one patient, repeat liver biopsies at 10 years of age showed progression to cirrhosis.

Biochemical Characteristics

The elevated total serum bile acids and retention of BSP suggest a defect in the excretory function of the liver. However, the nature of the defect is not known. The association of lymphedema of both lower extremities and cholestasis raises the possibility of abnormal lymphatic drainage from the liver. Aagenaes and colleagues injected colloidal gold into the liver capsule of one of their patients. Instead of normal excretion by lymphatic vessels, there was puddling of the isotope in the liver, which suggests a defect in the hepatic lymphatic system.[464] The close functional relationship between lymphatic and biliary drainage systems of the liver was shown experimentally in animals. After experimental obstruction of the common bile duct, bilirubin and bile acids rapidly appeared in the lymphatic system before their elevation in the serum.[465-468] Conversely, an increased biliary flow with increased excretion of bilirubin and bile acids occurred after interruption of the hepatic lymphatics in cats.[464] Thus it is possible that abnormalities of the lymphatics of the liver contribute to the pathogenesis of this entity. The locus for Aagenaes syndrome has been mapped to a 6.6-cm interval on chromosome 15q.[469]

Prognosis

Initially, the syndrome was thought to carry a favorable prognosis[462]; however, a subsequent report indicated that one of the earlier reported patients had died of liver failure. As previously mentioned, in another patient, a repeat liver biopsy at 10 years of age showed evidence of cirrhosis.[463]

Therapy

No effective therapy is available. Cholestyramine has been used to alleviate pruritus during the cholestatic episodes. Because of the cholestasis, fat-soluble vitamins and fats in the form of medium-chain triglycerides should be given.

Alagille Syndrome (Arteriohepatic Dysplasia)

Although reports of biliary duct hypoplasia and chronic liver disease appeared in the early 1950s,[470-472] it was not until 1973 that Watson and Miller described the cases of nine patients who had neonatal liver disease and familial pulmonary dysplasia.[473] A full description of the syndrome was provided by Alagille and co-workers. These investigators emphasized the characteristic facial appearance and vertebral and cardiovascular anomalies.[474] The syndrome is not rare, as investigators were able to report large groups of patients.[474-478] The recent identification of Jagged-1 gene mutations in patients with Alagille syndrome made it possible to understand the mechanism of the disease and explain the various clinical manifestations.[479,480]

Clinical Features

The major features of this syndrome are chronic liver disease, characteristic facies, cardiovascular and vertebral anomalies, and ophthalmologic abnormalities. Minor features include central nervous system, renal, endocrine, pancreas, gut, systemic vascular system, ear, lung, and larynx abnormalities. **Table 66-6** summarizes the major and minor abnormalities.

Chronic Liver Disease

The syndrome is associated with cholestasis, which may develop during the neonatal period and usually becomes apparent in the first 2 years of life.[481-483] Pruritus develops early in infancy and persists despite the disappearance of jaundice. The liver is usually enlarged, firm, smooth, and not tender. The spleen may be enlarged even in the absence of portal hypertension. The stools may be clay colored and the urine

Table 66-6 Clinical Features of Alagille Syndrome

Major Features	
Liver	Paucity of intrahepatic ducts
Heart	Peripheral pulmonary stenosis
Eye	Posterior embryotoxon
Facies	Prominent forehead, deep-set eyes, mild hypertelorism, small pointed chin
Vertebra	Butterfly vertebrae
Minor Features	
Congenital heart disease	Coarctation of the aorta, tetralogy of Fallot, ventricular and atrial septal defects, patent ductus arteriosus, truncus arteriosus, abnormal venous return, right ventricular hypoplasia
Systemic vascular malformations	Arterial hypoplasia, renal artery stenosis, carotid artery aneurysm, intracranial hemorrhage
Skeletal anomalies	Spina bifida, short distal phalanges and metacarpal bones, clinodactyly, short distal ulna and radius
Eye abnormalities	Retinal pigmentation, iris strands, cataract myopia, strabismus, glaucoma
Renal abnormalities	Cystic disease, renal agenesis, horseshoe kidney, renal hypoplasia, mesangiolipidosis, tubular dysfunction
Pancreas abnormalities	Exocrine pancreatic dysfunction, diabetes mellitus
Lung abnormalities	Tracheal and bronchial stenosis
Ear abnormalities	Deafness, chronic otitis media
Gut abnormalities	Small bowel atresia

dark yellow. Xanthomas may be seen on the extensor surfaces of the fingers and in creases of the palms, anal folds, and popliteal and vaginal areas. These xanthomas are due to long-standing severe intrahepatic cholestasis. With the progression of the disease about the beginning of the second year of life, jaundice may subside or disappear, but cholestasis persists. The long-term outlook for the liver disease is variable, with 10% to 50% of the patients developing cirrhosis and portal hypertension. In one study, only 3 of 36 patients monitored by the Alagille group developed hepatic cirrhosis.[425]

Characteristic Facies

The face is small, with a prominent, broad forehead. The eyes are set widely and deeply (hypertelorism). The mandible is small and pointed, giving the appearance of a triangular face.[481-483] The peculiar facies become more prominent with increasing age.

Cardiovascular Abnormalities

All patients have cardiac murmurs as infants. Most have peripheral pulmonary stenosis, which is usually mild and does not necessitate surgery.[482] Other cardiac lesions, including ventricular septal defects, coarctation of the aorta, and cyanotic heart disease, have also been reported (see **Table 66-6**).

Osseous Abnormalities

The hands show various degrees of shortening of the distal phalanges, stiffening, swelling, and limitation of motion at the proximal interphalangeal joints. Radiographs of the spine show either frank or incomplete butterfly vertebrae and decreased interpediculate distances in the lumbar spine.[475]

Ocular Findings

Posterior embryotoxon (prominent Schwalbe ring), visible to the unaided eye by slit-lamp examination, or on gonioscopy, is the most important ocular abnormality and occurs in 56% to 95% of patients. In addition, retinal pigmentary changes are usually found. Nischal and co-workers reported ultrasound evidence of optic disk drusen in a large percentage of Alagille's patients.[484] Other abnormalities include microcornea, keratoconus, exotropia, iris hypoplasia, and abnormalities of the optic disk.[485-488]

Central Nervous System Findings

Gross motor delays and mental retardation were reported in a small number of patients.[477] Intracranial bleeding is the most significant neurologic complication and occurs in approximately 15% of patients[476,485] and in 30% to 50% the bleeding is fatal. It is of note that many of the patients with bleeding did not have coagulopathy, raising the issue of cerebral vascular malformation.[476] A recent study supported these observations by documenting the spectrum of vascular anomalies, including intracranial aneurysms and internal carotid artery anomalies in these patients.[489] Moyamoya disease (progressive arterial occlusion of the distal intracranial carotids) has been reported in patients with Alagille syndrome.[490,491] In support of the involvement of the central nervous system is the observation that the autosomal dominant cerebral arteriopathy with subcortical infarct and leukoencephalopathy is also caused by a mutation in Notch 3.[492]

Pancreatic Abnormalities

Chong and his associates described pancreatic insufficiency in some patients with Alagille syndrome.[493] Other investigators have shown that 41% of their patients had pancreatic insufficiency; some of this group also developed diabetes mellitus.[494] Indeed, tissue-specific knockout Jagged-1 in mice results in malformed pancreas, acinar cell death, fibrosis, and pancreatic insufficiency.[495]

Other Abnormalities

Growth retardation, which decreased with age, was documented in the majority of cases of children. Slight to moderate mental retardation has also been documented in some of these cases. Renal function is impaired, with hyperuricemia and decreased creatinine clearance in some patients. Hypogonadism was suspected to be present in six male patients reported by Alagille and colleagues. Testicular biopsy showed no abnormality in two; in two others, fibrous tissue proliferation was present. In the other two, spermatogenic cells were almost completely lacking.[474] Bleeding tendency has been reported to occur spontaneously or following surgical procedures.[496]

Laboratory Findings

Total serum bilirubin is elevated during infancy, with levels between 4 and 14 mg/dl. The direct fraction is 30% to 50% of the total. Serum bilirubin usually returns to normal after the second year of life.[474] Some patients remain deeply jaundiced, with bilirubin levels greater than 20 mg/dl. Serum cholesterol levels may be as high as 2000 mg/dl. Serum triglyceride levels range from 500 to 1000 mg/dl. Serum alkaline phosphatase and glutamyl transferase levels are very high. Serum AST and ALT are slightly elevated. Despite the return of serum bilirubin to normal, biochemical evidence of severe cholestasis is usually found. Total serum bile acids have been markedly elevated in the patients thus studied, with increases in both cholic acid and chenodeoxycholic acid. No major unidentified chromatographic peak was present in the serum or duodenal bile of the patients who were investigated.[481]

Retention of BSP at 45 minutes is abnormal; however, storage capacity for BSP is normal. Prothrombin time and partial thromboplastin time are abnormal secondary to malabsorption of fats. Both values return to normal in response to intramuscular administration of vitamin K.

Pathology

Exploratory laparotomy of a patient who has arteriohepatic dysplasia shows uniformly patent extrahepatic biliary ducts. In the neonatal period, liver biopsy shows intact hepatic architecture, with marked cholestasis. The hepatocytes may be swollen, with balloon degeneration and minimal giant cell transformation. The most dramatic changes are in the portal areas, where a decrease in the number of biliary ducts is observed, with a slight increase in connective tissue. However, Ghishan and colleagues reported finding biliary duct proliferation in two patients with arteriohepatic dysplasia whose livers were sampled when they were 5 and 49 days old, respectively. Subsequent liver biopsies, when the patients were 2 and 27 months old, respectively,[497] showed a paucity of biliary ducts in the portal areas. Biopsies of the livers of adult patients with arteriohepatic dysplasia have shown no biliary ducts in the portal areas with variable progression to biliary cirrhosis. Indeed, 3 of 26 patients followed by the Alagille group developed hepatic cirrhosis. Other investigators reported the finding of cirrhosis in as many as 50% of patients.[476,477]

Genetics

Alagille syndrome is inherited as an autosomal dominant trait with reduced penetrance and variable expression when both parents are clinically normal; the percentage of sporadic cases is 45% to 50%. Byrne and colleagues first noted deletions of the short arm of chromosome 20.[498] Since then, several investigators mapped the gene for Alagille syndrome to chromosome 20p12.[499-503] The gene was eventually identified as the Jagged-1 gene (*JAG1*) by physical, genetic, and gene mapping covering the 20p12 region.[504,505] Mutations in the *JAG1* gene have been demonstrated in 60% to 75% of patients with Alagille syndrome. Analysis of 233 cases revealed that 72% of the reported mutations lead to frameshifts that cause a premature termination codon.[506] The spectrum of mutations identified is consistent with haploinsufficiency for *JAG1* being a mechanism for Alagille syndrome. The *JAG1* gene encodes a protein, which belongs to the family of Notch ligands. The Notch signaling pathway is important for control of cell fate during embryogenesis. *JAG1* is expressed ubiquitously in tissues of humans, including liver biliary epithelia as well as the heart, kidney, eye, and brain.[507] The role of *JAG1* in remodeling embryonic vasculature has been delineated by a null mouse model. Mice homozygous for *JAG1* mutations die from bleeding during early embryogenesis. Heterozygotic mice show eye malformations.

Biochemical Characteristics

The majority of the patients with Alagille syndrome have elevated conjugated hyperbilirubinemia. Serum bile acids and γ-glutamyltransferase levels are elevated as well. Liver aminotransferase levels are modestly elevated.

Therapy

Phenobarbital and cholestyramine have not been shown to be effective in the treatment of Alagille syndrome; however, Alagille and colleagues reported alleviation of pruritus and reductions of serum cholesterol, triglyceride, and bilirubin levels in response to very high doses of cholestyramine—12 to 15 g/day.[425] Antihistamines, rifampin, and naltrexone have been used to relieve pruritus.[508] Some patients were subjected to biliary drainage.[509] Improved nutrition via gastrostomy with supplements of fat-soluble vitamins has been used. Pancreatic enzyme replacement for patients with pancreatic insufficiency is indicated.

Prognosis

Data from early studies suggest that the long-term prognosis is good. Cirrhosis developed in 3 of Alagille's 26 patients,[425] but recent reports suggest that liver cirrhosis and portal hypertension develop in 10% to 50% of patients. Hepatocellular carcinoma has been reported. Liver transplantation is eventually necessary in 21% to 31% of patients.[477,478] Hoffenberg and colleagues have estimated that 50% of patients will eventually require liver transplants.[476]

Inborn Errors of Peroxisome Biogenesis

Zellweger Syndrome (Cerebrohepatorenal Syndrome)

In 1964 Bowen and associates described an autosomal recessive disease occurring in two siblings. It was characterized by severe hypotonia, growth and mental retardation, renal cortical cysts, and hepatic dysfunction. Both patients died before the age of 5 months.[510] Patients with a similar clinical syndrome were described by Smith and co-workers[511] and by Passarge and McAdams.[512] In 1969 Opitz and colleagues described four new patients and identified iron deposition in the liver. Because the original two patients were Hans Zellweger's patients, his name was used by Opitz's group as an eponymic designation for this condition.[513] Goldfischer and co-workers in 1973 described mitochondrial abnormalities and the lack of peroxisomes in electron microscopic studies of liver biopsy specimens from patients with Zellweger syndrome.[514] In 1975 Danks and associates reported finding pipecolic acid in the urine of four patients.[515] In 1979 Hanson and colleagues described a defect in bile acid synthesis found in three patients with Zellweger syndrome.[516]

Studies conducted in the 1980s confirmed that Zellweger syndrome belongs to a group of disorders of peroxisome biogenesis.[517] The group of peroxisomal disorders now includes 17 different diseases, such as neonatal adrenoleukodystrophy, infantile Refsum disease, and hyperpipecolic acidemia. Affected patients have reduced or absent peroxisomes with multiple enzyme defects that are normally present within peroxisomes. The peroxisomal functions include β-oxidation of long-chain fatty acids, ether-phospholipid biosynthesis, glyoxylate metabolism, degradation of pipecolic acid, and oxidation of phytanic acid.

Clinical Features

Severe hypotonia with simian creases is common, together with camptodactyly, which may involve several fingers. There may be some ulnar deviation of hands and fingers. Partial flexion of the knees with various degrees of equinovarus deformities of the feet is often seen. All patients have high foreheads with shallow supraorbital ridges and flat facies. External ear deformities and redundant skin folds in the neck are commonly seen. Sucking and swallowing difficulties, generalized seizures, and delays in psychomotor developmental maturation are common. Patent ductus arteriosus and septal defects are present in approximately 40% of patients. Hepatomegaly is common; splenomegaly is occasionally found. Jaundice is evident in 30% to 50% of patients.[515]

Laboratory Findings

Hematologic investigations have shown elevated serum iron and nearly total saturation of the serum iron-binding protein in more than half the cases reported.[518] The true incidences of these abnormalities may be higher because iron status has not been determined in many cases. Tissue concentrations of iron in the liver, spleen, kidneys, and lungs are increased. In one reported case, tissue iron in the liver was 50 mg/100 g wet weight (normal values for the same age group range from 7 to 21 mg/100 g). Ferrokinetic studies in this case demonstrated a rapid disappearance of iron and a markedly increased plasma iron turnover.[518] Iron incorporation into circulating red cells was significantly impaired, with abnormal accumulation of the radiolabeled iron in the liver. Intestinal absorption of iron was normal. Desferrioxamine induced a marked increase in urinary iron excretion. However, ferrokinetic studies of a second patient done by the same investigator showed no abnormality.[518]

Prothrombin time and thromboplastin time are usually prolonged, secondary to hepatic dysfunction. Serum AST and ALT levels are moderately elevated. Conjugated hyperbilirubinemia may be detected. Aminoaciduria was present in four cases. Urinary excretion of pipecolic acid, a minor breakdown product of lysine, was found to be notably increased in four infants in whom adequate qualitative tests were made.[515] Hanson and colleagues showed that three infants excreted excessive 3α,7α-dihydroxy-5β-cholestan-26-oic acid (DHCA), 3α,7α,12α-trihydroxy-5β-cholestan-26-oic acid (THCA), and 3α,7α,12α,24-tetrahydroxy-5β-cholestan-26-oic acid (varanic acid). These compounds are precursors of chenodeoxycholic acid and cholic acid that have undergone only partial side chain oxidation.[516] These findings were confirmed in two other cases of Zellweger syndrome.[519] Increased accumulation of very-long-chain fatty acids in tissues, blood cells, and plasma is present in these patients secondary to defective β-oxidation of long-chain fatty acids.[520] Accumulation of phytanic acid and pristanic acid also occurs secondary to defective oxidation.[521] Tissue levels of plasmalogens are reduced secondary to defective synthesis.[522] These abnormalities reflect defective peroxisomal function.[523] Deficient docosahexaenoic acid (DHA) in erythrocytes and plasma has been documented.[524]

Radiographic studies of patients with Zellweger syndrome reveal certain characteristic findings, mainly the presence of patches of calcification in cartilage. These have a dense cortex and a reticular central region and characteristically are present in the triradiate cartilage in the acetabulum, the patellae, the sternum, and the scapulae.[525]

Pathology

LIVER

Macroscopically, the liver appears unremarkable. Histologic sections of biopsy and autopsy specimens of the liver show changes that may vary from minimal to severe diffuse fibrosis with cirrhosis.[515] The original patients were described as having biliary dysgenesis; however, recent reports show normal biliary ducts in the portal areas, with various degrees of portal fibrosis. The hepatic lobules may contain foci of liver cell necrosis and loss. Prussian blue staining for iron shows a marked increase in iron deposition, mainly in the reticuloendothelial cells.[513] Some patients have minimal or no deposition of iron.[515,526] There is no correlation between the extent of liver damage and iron deposition.[515] Electron microscopic studies show swollen hepatocytes filled with glycogen. The mitochondria are often extremely dense and reduced in number; their cristae are twisted and irregular, with dilation of the intracristate spaces. Typical arrays of rough endoplasmic reticulum are sparse. No peroxisomes can be found in the hepatocytes.[514]

KIDNEYS

Macroscopically, the surface is studded with small (<3 mmol/L in diameter) fluid-filled cysts. Microscopically, the cysts contain dysplastic glomerular and tubular elements and are lined by cuboidal or flattened epithelium. Cysts of glomerular origin and others that appear to be dilated tubular structures are also present. Ultrastructural studies demonstrate a lack of peroxisomes in the proximal tubules.[513,514]

Central Nervous System

Severe cerebral gliosis, subependymal cyst formation, macrogyria, and polymicrogyria were noted. Myelinization was incomplete or lacking.[513] Prussian blue staining shows deposition of iron. Ultrastructurally, the mitochondria of the cortical astrocytes are abnormally dense and often appear degenerate.[514]

Biochemical Features

The mitochondria in the livers, kidneys, and brains of patients with Zellweger syndrome are structurally abnormal. Functionally, oxygen consumption of mitochondrial fractions prepared from the livers and brains of two patients was diminished by 70%. Addition of ADP to the mitochondrial fractions failed to stimulate respiration, although this response was elicited in the control mitochondria.[514]

In vitro studies suggest that the formation of C24 bile acids (chenodeoxycholic acid and cholic acid) from cholesterol is defective in affected patients. It seems that mitochondrial defects are the cause of the abnormalities in bile acid synthesis (see Chapter 5). Because cholic acid and chenodeoxycholic acid are present in these patients, the defect in synthesis is not a complete one. It is possible that, in Zellweger syndrome, chenodeoxycholic and cholic acids are synthesized via an alternate pathway requiring only microsomal enzymes.[527,528]

Molecular Basis of Zellweger Syndrome

The primary defect in Zellweger syndrome is impaired assembly of peroxisomes.[529] A rat cDNA encoding the peroxisome assembly factor-1 (PAF1) was cloned.[530] This cDNA encodes for a 35-kDa protein that restores the assembly of peroxisomes in the peroxisome-deficient Chinese hamster ovary cell.[531] A human cDNA has been cloned that complements the disease symptoms, including defective peroxisome assembly in fibroblasts from a patient with Zellweger syndrome.[530] A point mutation in the cDNA of a patient with Zellweger syndrome resulted in premature termination of PAF1.[532] These observations were extended to show that at least 23 proteins are required for proper peroxisome assembly.[530-535] Complementation analysis indicated that 12 different complementation groups are defective in patients with peroxisomal disorder. The genes involved in protein assembly of peroxisomes (peroxins) are termed PEX genes. Mutations in 10 different PEX genes have been described.[535-545]

Zellweger syndrome is caused by mutations in any of several different genes involved in peroxisome biogenesis, including *PEX1*, *PEX2*, *PEX5*, *PEX6*, *PEX10*, *PEX12*, *PEX13*, *PEX16*, and *PEX19*.[530] The gene affected in complementation group 1 is *PEX1*. Approximately 65% of patients with peroxisomal biogenesis disorders harbor mutations in *PEX1*. A complete lack of PEX1 protein was found to be associated with Zellweger syndrome; however, residual amounts of PEX1 protein were found in a milder phenotype (neonatal adrenoleukodystrophy and infantile Refsum disease). The most common mutation described is G843D. This missense mutation results in a misfolded protein.[546]

Prognosis

Patients who have Zellweger syndrome die in the first year of life of malnutrition, liver failure, and intercurrent infections.[513,515] Desferrioxamine enhances urinary excretion of iron but unfortunately does not influence the ultimate outcome.

Genetics

An autosomal recessive inheritance is suggested by family studies. A prenatal diagnosis based on detection of elevated levels of a very-long-chain fatty acid, hexacosanoic acid (C26:0), in cultured amniotic fluid cells has been described.[547] The impaired oxidation of very-long-chain fatty acids is secondary to the absence of the peroxisomes seen in Zellweger patients. Determination of mutations in *PEX* genes will eventually replace the biochemical analysis of urine in these patients.

Cystic Fibrosis

Cystic fibrosis (CF) is the most common cause of chronic obstructive pulmonary disease and of pancreatic insufficiency in the first 3 decades of life in the United States. Today, as more patients with CF reach reproductive age, the hepatic complications of CF are encountered with increasing frequency. In her first review of cystic fibrosis of the pancreas, Anderson found three CF patients with hepatic cirrhosis already reported and added one of her own.[548] Farber provided an excellent description of an unfamiliar type of cirrhosis with gross lobulation of the liver, which he found in a few of his 87 patients with CF. Early histologic changes in the liver included enlargement of the portal areas with biliary duct proliferation and accumulation of eosinophilic material within the lumens of the biliary ducts. The cirrhotic change was attributed to obstruction of the biliary ductules by inspissated secretions.[549] Bodian described focal cirrhotic lesions in one fourth of 62 patients with CF examined at necropsy. These findings were present in virtually all patients older than 1 year. Bodian proposed the descriptive term focal biliary cirrhosis. This lesion had been asymptomatic in all of Bodian's patients.[550] Craig and associates found 7 patients with cirrhosis of the liver among 150 patients with CF examined at necropsy. Microscopically, the investigators found obstruction of biliary ductules by eosinophilic amorphous material surrounded by areas marked by fibrosis and biliary duct proliferation. The focal character of the extensive hepatic damage was emphasized.[551]

Blanc and di Sant'Agnese described CF and multilobular hepatic cirrhosis in seven patients 4 to 10 years old. To establish the evolution of the hepatic lesions, Blanc and di Sant'Agnese reviewed the autopsy material of 116 patients with CF. Of 25 patients who had cirrhotic lesions, 16 had single or multiple lesions of focal biliary cirrhosis. The changes were more extensive in nine. A multilobular biliary cirrhosis was found in six of these. Younger patients had focal biliary cirrhosis; older patients had multilobular cirrhosis.[552]

Clinical Features

LIVER DISEASE IN INFANCY

Cystic fibrosis may be manifested in the newborn period as obstructive jaundice.[553-559] In all of 10 such infants, the onset of jaundice was before 3 weeks of age, and it occurred before 10 days of age in 8.[549] Jaundice persisted from 20 days to 6 months. Meconium ileus with or without small intestinal atresia or combined with volvulus was found in approximately half of these patients. In three patients subjected to laparotomy, accumulation of thick, viscid bile was thought to have caused extrahepatic obstruction.[557-560] Bile duct proliferation without plugging by inspissated material was detected in the livers of five of nine patients with meconium ileus and intestinal atresia whose livers were examined. However, the authors do not rule out that the obstruction might have occurred in more central ducts.[554] Neonatal hepatitis with marked giant cell transformation of the hepatocytes was documented in a 2-month-old patient with CF and obstructive jaundice.[560] Some infants may make a complete recovery, and some may die of liver failure and other complications of CF. The diagnosis is suspected on the basis of a history of meconium ileus. Steatosis may be seen secondary to malnutrition and nutrient deficiencies.

LIVER DISEASE IN CHILDHOOD AND ADOLESCENCE

Symptomatic liver disease was noted in 2.2%[561,562] to 16%[559] of patients with CF in two series. In the largest reported series

(from Boston), portal hypertension developed in 48 of 2500 patients with CF. The incidence of portal hypertension increases more than ten-fold for patients who are adolescents or older.[563,564] Interestingly, several members of the same family developed cirrhosis and its complications. A similar observation was reported by Stern and colleagues. Initial symptoms of hepatic complications begin between 9 and 19 years of age. Of 693 patients with CF observed during a period of 18 years, clinical hepatic disease developed in 15, an incidence of 2.2%. In 13 of these 15 patients, all symptoms were related to portal hypertension, such as gastrointestinal bleeding or hypersplenism. Hepatocellular dysfunction was the principal feature in one of the remaining two cases, and massive hepatomegaly and failure to thrive were dominant in the other.[561] A similar experience was reported from Switzerland. Of 204 unselected patients with CF, 7 were found to have hepatic cirrhosis, an incidence of 3.4%. Two of the 7 patients came to medical attention because of hematemesis. The hepatic abnormality in the others was detected because of hepatosplenomegaly and failure to thrive.[565] In two further studies, 24% of 233 U.K. adults with CF had abnormal results of liver tests.[566] Similarly, 35% of 31 Swedish teenagers with CF had hepatosplenomegaly.[567] A subset (approximately 3% to 5%) of patients with CF developed severe liver disease with portal hypertension. It has been reported recently that the α_1-antitrypsin deficiency (*SERPINA1*) Z allele is a risk factor for liver disease in CF. Patients who carry the Z allele are at greater risk (odds ratio, approximately 5) of developing severe liver disease with portal hypertension.[568]

To assess the evolution of liver disease in CF patients, Ling and co-workers prospectively followed 124 children with CF for 4 years. At the initial assessment, 42% had hepatic biochemical abnormalities, 35% ultrasound abnormalities, and 6% had clinical abnormalities of the liver. In cross-sectional analysis, abnormal biochemistry was present in 40% of children with ultrasound and clinical abnormalities. Sixty-eight percent of the children showed ultrasound or clinical evidence of liver abnormality at some point during the 4-year follow-up. However, no association between liver disease and nutritional status was found.[569]

Documentation of mild hepatic involvement is often difficult because clinical manifestations, including jaundice, may be lacking. Results of liver tests may be normal. The BSP excretion test may be of help in detecting early hepatic involvement.[570] The best early indication of hepatic involvement is an elevated level of the hepatic isoenzyme of alkaline phosphatase.[571,572] Total serum alkaline phosphatase activity is not reliable in the evaluation of hepatic involvement in children with CF because age-related normal values for alkaline phosphatase are hard to establish. Also, puberty is often delayed in patients with CF; hence, total alkaline phosphatase may appear to be normal in the presence of liver disease.[565] γ-Glutamyltransferase levels are usually elevated.

It is important to emphasize that hepatic disease, including portal hypertension, may be present in patients with CF even when results of liver tests are normal or only slightly abnormal. In fact, the first manifestation of CF may be portal hypertension in a previously asymptomatic patient. Thus children and young adults with unexplained portal hypertension or other hepatic abnormalities should be tested by pilocarpine iontophoresis and by chemical determination of the chloride level in sweat.

Gallbladder Disease

Clinical symptoms of cholelithiasis and cholecystitis have been found in some patients with CF. Microgallbladder has been reported to be present in approximately 15% of cases and poor or nonvisualization of the gallbladder in another 25%.[573] Gallbladder stones are found in as many as 8% of patients.[574] The gallbladder disease in these patients may be related to occlusion of the cystic duct by precipitation of abnormal secretions and to abnormal biliary lipid composition.[575]

The pathogenesis of the increased incidence of gallbladder stones in CF was investigated by analysis of biliary lipid in 26 patients with CF, 7 children with cholelithiasis without CF, and 13 controls. For 14 patients with CF who had stopped taking pancreatic enzymes a week earlier, the molar percentage of lipid composition accounted for by cholesterol (mean $\pm$ SE, 16.3 ± 2.9) and the saturation index (2.0 ± 0.3) were comparable with values obtained for the group with cholelithiasis but no CF. For 12 patients with CF taking pancreatic enzymes, the molar percentage of cholesterol (8.6 ± 1.7) and the saturation index (1.0 ± 0.1) did not differ from those of controls. Bile salt analysis revealed a striking preponderance of cholic acid over chenodeoxycholic acid, and the glycine/taurine ratio of conjugated bile acids was lower in enzyme-treated patients with CF than in those not currently receiving treatment. The high ratio of cholic acid to chenodeoxycholic acid is a well-known response to malabsorption of bile acids. The decrease of this ratio and the concomitant normalization of biliary lipids during treatment of patients with CF with pancreatic enzymes suggest that the lithogenic bile in CF is secondary to bile acid malabsorption.[575]

Biochemical Characteristics

Cystic fibrosis is related to an abnormality in secretions of the exocrine glands. These secretions contain high concentrations of sodium chloride, and defective chloride secretion is the hallmark of the disease.[576-578] The biochemical characteristics of the liver disorder are not well understood. Intrahepatic obstruction by eosinophilic concentrations of mucus occurs early in the disease and has been proposed as the cause of cirrhosis. Shwachman found that cirrhosis did not develop in patients with CF who had pulmonary involvement without pancreatic involvement. Thus defects in digestion and absorption appear to be prerequisites for liver disease, except possibly during the neonatal period.[579] Patients with CF and pancreatic insufficiency have markedly elevated fecal bile acid excretion compared with age-matched controls.[580] Bile acid kinetics were investigated by double-isotope dilution technique in six children with previously untreated CF. All six children had pancreatic insufficiency. The bile acid pool sizes were small and turned over rapidly in untreated patients. When fat excretion was reduced by therapy, the turnover rate of the pool decreased, with two-fold enlargement of the pool size. These findings suggest an interruption of enterohepatic circulation.[581] The pathophysiologic mechanism of the interruption of the enterohepatic circulation and its relation to hepatobiliary disease has not been defined.

Molecular Basis

The CF gene has been cloned and mapped to chromosome 7.[582] The gene spans 250,000 base pairs and encodes a membrane protein of 1480 amino acids termed cystic fibrosis transmembrane conductance regulator (CFTR).[583] CFTR is believed to be a cyclic adenosine monophosphate (cAMP)-regulated chloride channel.[584] CFTR is predicted to have five domains: two membrane-spanning domains, two nucleotide-binding domains, and a unique regulatory (R) domain. The membrane-spanning domains appear to contribute to the organization of the chloride channel because mutations of specific amino acid residues within the first membrane-spanning domain alter the anion selectivity of the channel. Phosphorylation of the (R) domain, generally by cAMP-dependent protein kinase, is essential for opening of the channel.[585] More than 1500 mutations within the CF gene have been reported.[586] The most common mutation is a 3-bapa deletion removing a phenylalanine residue at amino acid position 508 (Δ508). The 508 mutation accounts for approximately 70% of CF cases in the United States.[587] There are four mechanisms by which mutations disrupt the function of CFTR (**Fig. 66-15**).[585] Class I mutations (defective protein products) result in production of little or no full-length protein, with loss of CFTR chloride channel function. These mutations produce premature termination signals because of frameshifts as a result of insertions, deletions, or nonsense mutations.[588] Class II mutations (defective protein processing) result in failure to direct the CFTR to the correct cellular location.[589] This class includes the most common mutation (ΔF508). Class III mutations (defective regulation) result from mutations in the nucleotide-binding proteins.[589] Class IV mutations lead to defective chloride conduction. Several mutations in the first membrane-spanning domain affect arginine residues located in putative membrane-spanning sequences. These mutations result in markedly reduced rates of ion flow through single open channels in inside-out membrane patches. The development of liver disease in patients with CF was not found to be related to specific mutations in the gene; other environmental or gene modifiers may influence the development of liver disease. In this regard a recent study showed that the presence of liver cirrhosis in CF patients is significantly associated with the presence of mutated mannose-binding lectin variants.[590] Mannose lectin binding is an important protein of the immune system and has been shown to be a modulating protein in the respiratory involvement of CF.

Laboratory Findings

Sweat chloride levels are elevated in all patients with CF. Total pancreatic exocrine dysfunction is found in 80% to 85% of the patients. Five percent to 10% of patients have partial insufficiency. The remainder have normal exocrine function. Steatorrhea and azotorrhea are the major consequences of the pancreatic insufficiency. Malabsorption of fat-soluble vitamins A, D, E, and K is the result of pancreatic insufficiency and the use of antibiotics to treat the pulmonary infections also alters the bacterial flora of the intestinal tract. Vitamin K deficiency may occur in the first year of life and produce overt hemorrhage.[591] Vitamin A levels are low in the serum but normal or elevated in the liver. A defect in the transport of vitamin A out of the liver is probable. Night blindness and benign increases in intracranial pressure secondary to low vitamin A levels in blood have been reported.[592,593] Vitamin D is poorly absorbed; however, overt rickets is rare. Serum levels of 25-OH vitamin D are reported to be similar to values obtained for normal controls.[594] Low serum levels of 25-OH

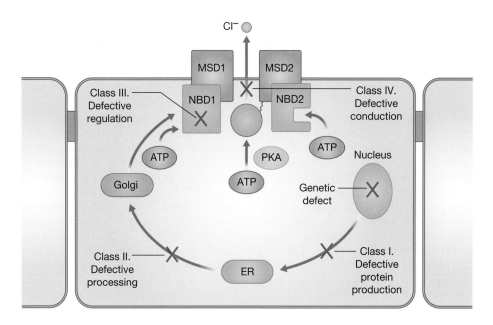

Fig. 66-15 Biosynthesis and function of cystic fibrosis transmembrane regulator (CFTR). ATP, adenosine triphosphate; ER, endoplasmic reticulum; MSD, membrane-spanning domain; NBD, nuclear-binding domain *(Adapted from Welsh MJ, Smith AE. Molecular mechanisms of CFTR chloride channel dysfunction in cystic fibrosis. Cell 1993;73:1251–1254, with permission.)*

vitamin D in 4 of 17 patients have been demonstrated in one series[595] and in all 21 patients in another.[596] Differences in serum levels reflect different assays and the times of the year during which the patients were studied because 85% of circulating 25-OH vitamin D is of endogenous origin.[594] When patients were studied in winter and early spring, values of serum 25-OH vitamin D were low[595]; however, the other studies were conducted in the summer and early fall.[594,596] These observations suggest a subtle deficiency of vitamin D in patients who have CF and are deprived of sunlight and endogenous vitamin D production.

Liver test results usually show no abnormality. Conjugated hyperbilirubinemia and elevations of serum AST, ALT, GGT, and alkaline phosphatase are noted in neonates with obstructive jaundice secondary to CF. Some infants with CF have hypoproteinemia and edema as a result of protein malabsorption, particularly infants who have been breastfed or fed soybean-based formulas. Breast milk contains only 1.1% protein; although adequate for normal infants, it is suboptimal for those who have CF. Soybean-based formula contains small amounts of antitryptic activity, which may potentiate the existing malabsorption.

Detecting mild liver involvement in CF is often difficult. The best early indication is elevated alkaline phosphatase of hepatic origin. Measurement of total serum alkaline phosphatase is not helpful due to active bone formation in children. The kinetics of BSP excretion show a decrease in hepatic removal rate and biliary secretion and an increase in hepatic-to-plasma reflux as liver disease progresses.[570] In patients with CF and biliary cirrhosis, abnormal liver function and hematologic abnormalities or hypersplenism are usually detected.

Pathology

Focal biliary cirrhosis is found in approximately 25% of patients with CF examined by necropsy.[552] Progression to a multilobular cirrhosis occurs in about 5% of surviving children and adolescents. Three histologic types of lesions were identified by Oppenheimer and Esterly[597] in young infants with CF:

1. Focal biliary cirrhosis, characterized by bile duct proliferation, inspissated granular eosinophilic material filling the biliary ducts, infiltration of the liver with chronic inflammatory cells, and variable degrees of fibrosis, is most common. The lesions are focal in distribution and vary in number and severity. The incidence of focal biliary cirrhosis increases with age.

2. Excess mucus in biliary duct radicles or in the linings of epithelial cells with periportal changes may be present. The distribution of the biliary mucus is variable and focal, but it is found most often in the large intrahepatic ducts. Biliary duct proliferation and, less commonly, metaplasia of the ductal epithelium are observed. The periportal changes include edema and an inflammatory cell infiltrate. This type of lesion is commonly seen in infants younger than 1 year.

3. Periportal changes without biliary mucus may be seen on biopsy. These changes are common in infants younger than 3 months but are not observed in older children.

It appears that the periportal changes are nonspecific and transitory. The accumulation of biliary mucus appears to be related to CF, and because its frequency decreases with age, this indicates that biliary mucus is only one factor in the pathogenesis of focal biliary cirrhosis. Why multilobular biliary cirrhosis develops in such a small percentage of the patients (5%) remains uncertain. Shwachman noted a familial tendency for the development of hepatic complications.[579] Nutritional deficiencies and intercurrent infection do not explain the progression to multilobular cirrhosis. The relationship in CF between the abnormalities in bile salt metabolism and hepatobiliary disease awaits further investigation.

Hemosiderosis and fatty infiltration of the liver are two other pathologic features of the liver in CF. The increased intestinal absorption of iron that occurs in untreated patients with pancreatic insufficiency may produce hepatic hemosiderosis. The early institution of supplemental pancreatic enzymes reduces the increased absorption of iron.[598] Hepatic infiltration with fat secondary to chronic malnutrition is frequently observed with CF.[579]

Genetics

Cystic fibrosis is inherited as an autosomal recessive trait.[599] The highest reported incidence of CF is in Caucasians, primarily those of European origin. The incidence in the Caucasian population in the United States is approximately 1 : 2000.[600] The disease is less frequent in blacks and Asians.[601] No good incidence figures are available for nonwhites, with the exception of Hawaiians, for whom the incidence has been reported to be 1 : 90,000.[602] Prenatal diagnosis can be accomplished by a number of techniques, including reverse dot blots, amplification refractory, mutation detection systems, oligonucleotide ligation assays, the invader assay, and nanochip systems.[603,604]

Therapy

Hepatic complications of CF that need treatment include those of newborns with obstructive jaundice and those of patients first seen for treatment as adolescents with multilobular biliary cirrhosis and portal hypertension. Jaundiced neonates may escape severe hepatic involvement later in their lives. Drugs that stimulate bile flow are not helpful. Flushing of the extrahepatic biliary tree with normal saline has been successful in two cases.[557,559] In some cases, spontaneous relief of the jaundice has occurred without treatment.[559] The hydrophilic bile acid, ursodeoxycholic acid, has been recommended by the U.S. Cystic Fibrosis Foundation Hepatobiliary Disease Consensus Group[605] for parents with established liver disease. However, the Cochrane collaboration concluded that there was insufficient evidence to justify the use of ursodeoxycholic acid.[606] Vitamin supplementation with ADEK preparation appears to reduce the incidence of vitamin K deficiency.[607] More recently, Nathanson and co-workers showed that ursodeoxycholic acid stimulates ATP secretion by isolated hepatocytes, thus promoting bile flow.[608] The decision to perform portosystemic shunting in an older patient with portal hypertension depends largely on the pulmonary status of the patient. Patients who have severe pulmonary disease are poor candidates for surgery. The long-term survival rates of these patients is poor, and the complication rate for such a major operation is very high. Those patients who have had single episodes of hemorrhaging or have esophageal varices with good pulmonary function are considered candidates for the shunting procedure.[563,564] Liver, lung, and heart transplantation has been performed in a number of patients with CF.

Key References

Anderson RA, Bryson GM, Parks JS. Lysosomal acid lipase mutations that determine phenotype in Wolman and cholesterol ester storage disease. Mol Genet Metab 1999;68:333–345. (Ref.387)

Annabi B, et al. The gene for glycogen-storage disease type 1b maps to chromosome 11q23. Am J Hum Genet 1998;62:400–405. (Ref.245)

Arnell H, et al. Progressive familial intrahepatic cholestasis (PFIC): evidence for genetic heterogeneity by exclusion of linkage to chromosome 18q21-q22. Hum Genet 1997;100:378–381. (Ref.449)

Bahttacharya K, et al. A novel starch for the treatment of glycogen storage disease. J Inherit Metab Dis 2007;30:350–357. (Ref.226)

Bao Y, Dawson TL Jr, Chen YT. Human glycogen debranching enzyme gene (AGL): complete structural organization and characterization of the 5′ flanking region. Genomics 1996;38:155–165. (Ref.253)

Bao Y, et al. Isolation and nucleotide sequence of human liver glycogen debranching enzyme mRNA: identification of multiple tissue-specific isoforms. Gene 1997;197:389–398. (Ref.256)

Bartlett JR, et al. Genetic modifiers of liver disease in cystic fibrosis. JAMA 2009;302:1076–1083. (Ref.568)

Berrocal T, et al. Syndrome of Alagille: radiological and sonographic findings. A review of 37 cases. Eur Radiol 1997;7:115–118. (Ref.475)

Braverman N, et al. Human PEX7 encodes the peroxisomal PTS2 receptor and is responsible for rhizomelic chondrodysplasia punctata. Nat Genet 1997;15:369–376. (Ref.538)

Bull L, et al. Clinical and biochemical features of FIC1 (ATP8B1) and BSEP (ABCB11) disease. Hepatology 2002;36:310a. (Ref.434)

Bull LN, et al. Genetic and morphological findings in progressive familial intrahepatic cholestasis (Byler disease [PFIC-1] and Byler syndrome): evidence for heterogeneity. Hepatology 1997;26:155–164. (Ref.451)

Bull LN, et al. Mapping of the locus for cholestasis-lymphedema syndrome (Aagenaes syndrome) to a 6.6-cM interval on chromosome 15q. Am J Hum Genet 2000;67:994–999. (Ref.469)

Bull LN, et al. A gene encoding a P-type ATPase mutated in two forms of hereditary cholestasis. Nat Genet 1998;18:219–224. (Ref.427)

Calderon FR, et al. Mutation database for the galactose-1-phosphate uridyltoursferase. (GALT) gene. Hum Mutat 2007;28:939–943. (Ref.88)

Chang CC, et al. Isolation of the human PEX12 gene, mutated in group 3 of the peroxisome biogenesis disorders. Nat Genet 1997;15:385–388. (Ref.542)

Chen LY, et al. Structure-function analysis of the glucose-6-phosphate transporter deficient in glycogen storage disease type Ib. Hum Mol Genet 2002;11:3199–3207. (Ref.246)

Chen SY, et al. The glucose-6-phosphate transporter is a phosphate-linked antiporter deficient in glycogen storage disease type Ib and Ic. FASEB J 2008;22:2206–2213. (Ref.163)

Cheng K, Ashby D, Smyth R. Ursodeoxycholic acid for cystic fibrosis-related liver disease. Cochrane Database Syst Rev 2000;2:CD000222. (Ref.606)

Cheung YY, et al. Impaired neutrophil activity and increased susceptibility to bacterial infection in mice lacking glucose-6-phosphate-beta. J Clin Invest 2007;117:784–793. (Ref.250)

Chou JY, Masfield B. Mutations in the glucose-6-phosphate (G6PC) gene that cause type 1a glycogen storage disease. Hum Mutat 2008;29:921–930. (Ref.173)

Chou JY, et al. Type I glycogen storage diseases: disorders of the glucose-6-phosphatase complex. Curr Mol Med 2002;2:121–143. (Ref.158)

de Vree JM, et al. Mutations in the MDR3 gene cause progressive familial intrahepatic cholestasis. Proc Natl Acad Sci U S A 1998;95:282–287. (Ref.456)

Dixon PH, et al. Heterozygous MDR3 missense mutation associated with intrahepatic cholestasis of pregnancy: evidence for a defect in protein trafficking. Hum Mol Genet 2000;9:1209–1217. (Ref.460)

Du H, et al. Targeted disruption of the mouse lysosomal acid lipase gene: long-term survival with massive cholesteryl ester and triglyceride storage. Hum Mol Genet 1998;7:1347–1354. (Ref.388)

Egawa H, et al. Intractable diarrhea after liver transplantation for Byler's disease: successful treatment with bile adsorptive resin. Liver Transpl 2002;8:714–716. (Ref.431)

Elpeleg ON. The molecular background of glycogen metabolism disorders. J Pediatr Endocrinol Metab 1999;12:363–379. (Ref.247)

Emerick KM, et al. Features of Alagille syndrome in 92 patients: frequency and relation to prognosis. Hepatology 1999;29:822–829. (Ref.477)

Eppens EF, et al. FIC1, the protein affected in two forms of hereditary cholestasis, is localized in the cholangiocyte and the canalicular membrane of the hepatocyte. J Hepatol 2001;35:436–443. (Ref.443)

Esposito G, et al. Structural and functional analysis of aldolase B mutants related to hereditary fructose intolerance. FEBS Lett 2002;531:152–156. (Ref.27)

Gabolde M, et al. The mannose binding lectin gene influences the severity of chronic liver disease in cystic fibrosis. J Med Genet 2001;38:310–311. (Ref.590)

Gauderer MW, Boyle JT. Cholecystoappendicostomy in a child with Alagille syndrome. J Pediatr Surg 1997;32:166–167. (Ref.509)

Golson ML, et al. Ductal malformation and pancreatitis in mice caused by conditional Jag 1 deletion. Gastroenterology 2009;136:1761–1771. (Ref.495)

Hemrika W, Wever RA. New model for the membrane topology of glucose-6-phosphatase: the enzyme involved in von Gierke disease. FEBS Lett 1997;409:317–319. (Ref.168)

Hingorani M, et al. Ocular abnormalities in Alagille syndrome. Ophthalmology 1999;106:330–337. (Ref.485)

Hiraiwa H, et al. Inactivation of the glucose 6-phosphate transporter causes glycogen storage disease type 1b. J Biol Chem 1999;274:5532–5536. (Ref.244)

Jacquemin E, et al. Heterozygous non-sense mutation of the MDR3 gene in familial intrahepatic cholestasis of pregnancy. Lancet 1999;353:210–211. (Ref.459)

Jacquemin E, et al. The wide spectrum of multidrug resistance 3 deficiency: from neonatal cholestasis to cirrhosis of adulthood. Gastroenterology 2001;120: 1448–1458. (Ref.457)

Jacquemin E, et al. Ursodeoxycholic acid therapy in pediatric patients with progressive familial intrahepatic cholestasis. Hepatology 1997;25:519–523. (Ref.446)

Jansen PL, et al. Hepatocanalicular bile salt export pump deficiency in patients with progressive familial intrahepatic cholestasis. Gastroenterology 1999;117: 1370–1379. (Ref.454)

John HA, et al. A study of pancreatic function in 17 children with Alagille syndrome. Gastroenterology 1998;114:A885. (Ref.494)

Kamath BM, et al. Vascular anomalies in Alagille syndrome: a significant cause of morbidity and mortality. Circulation 2004;109:1354–1358. (Ref.489)

Kikawa Y, et al. Identification of genetic mutations in Japanese patients with fructose-1,6-bisphosphatase deficiency. Am J Hum Genet 1997;61:852–861. (Ref.61)

Kikawa Y, et al. Diagnosis of fructose-1,6-bisphosphatase deficiency using cultured lymphocyte fraction: a secure and noninvasive alternative to liver biopsy. J Inherit Metab Dis 2002;25:41–46. (Ref.60)

Klomp LW, et al. A missense mutation in FIC1 is associated with Greenland familial cholestasis. Hepatology 2000;32:1337–1341. (Ref.442)

Klomp LW, et al. Characterization of mutations in ATP8B1 associated with hereditary cholestasis. Hepatology 2004;40:27–38. (Ref.444)

Krause C, Rosewichtl, Gartner J. Rational diagnostic strategy for Zellweger syndrome spectrum patients. Eur J Hum Genet 2009;17:741–748. (Ref.521)

Lau J, Tolan DR. Screening for hereditary fructose intolerance mutations by reverse dot-blot. Mol Cell Probes 1999;13:35–40. (Ref.51)

Li L, et al. Alagille syndrome is caused by mutations in human Jagged1, which encodes a ligand for Notch1. Nat Genet 1997;16:243–251. (Ref.480)

Ling SC, et al. The evolution of liver disease in cystic fibrosis. Arch Dis Child 1999;81:129–132. (Ref.569)

Lohse P, et al. Compound heterozygosity for a Wolman mutation is frequent among patients with cholesteryl ester storage disease. J Lipid Res 2000;41: 23–31. (Ref.386)

Louis AA, et al. Hepatic jagged1 expression studies. Hepatology 1999;30: 1269–1275. (Ref.507)

Lykavieris P, et al. Bleeding tendency in children with Alagille syndrome. Pediatrics 2003;111:167–170. (Ref.496)

Lykavieris P, et al. Progressive familial intrahepatic cholestasis type 1 and extrahepatic features: no catch-up of stature growth, exacerbation of diarrhea, and appearance of liver steatosis after liver transplantation. J Hepatol 2003;39: 447–452. (Ref.430)

Manis FR, et al. A longitudinal study of cognitive functioning in patients with classical galactosaemia, including a cohort treated with oral uridine. J Inherit Metab Dis 1997;20:549–555. (Ref.137)

Matsuzono Y, et al. Human PEX19: cDNA cloning by functional complementation, mutation analysis in a patient with Zellweger syndrome, and potential role in peroxisomal membrane assembly. Proc Natl Acad Sci U S A 1999;96:2116–2121. (Ref.545)

Mitchell GA, et al. Tyrosinemia. In: Suchy FJ, Sokol RJ, Balistreri WF, editors. Liver disease in children, 2nd ed. Philadelphia: Lippincott Williams & Wilkins, 2001: 667–685. (Ref.377)

Moser HW. Genotype-phenotype correlations in disorders of peroxisome biogenesis. Mol Genet Metab 1999;68:316–327. (Ref.534)

Moses SW, Parvari R. The variable presentations of glycogen storage disease type IV: a review of clinical, enzymatic and molecular studies. Curr Mol Med 2002;2:177–188. (Ref.291)

Motley AM, et al. Rhizomelic chondrodysplasia punctata is a peroxisomal protein targeting disease caused by a non-functional PTS2 receptor. Nat Genet 1997;15:377–380. (Ref.539)

Muntau AC, et al. Defective peroxisome membrane synthesis due to mutations in human PEX3 causes Zellweger syndrome, complementation group G. Am J Hum Genet 2000;67:967–975. (Ref.533)

Nathanson MH, et al. Stimulation of ATP secretion in the liver by therapeutic bile acids. Biochem J 2001;358:1–5. (Ref.608)

Nischal KK, et al. Ocular ultrasound in Alagille syndrome: a new sign. Ophthalmology 1997;104:79–85. (Ref.484)

Oda T, et al. Identification and cloning of the human homolog (JAG1) of the rat Jagged1 gene from the Alagille syndrome critical region at 20p12. Genomics 1997;43:376–379. (Ref.504)

Oda T, et al. Mutations in the human Jagged1 gene are responsible for Alagille syndrome. Nat Genet 1997;16:235–242. (Ref.479)

Okubo M, et al. Glycogen storage disease type IIIa: first report of a causative missense mutation (G1448R) of the glycogen debranching enzyme gene found in a homozygous patient. Hum Mutat 1999;14:542–543. (Ref.257)

Okumoto K, et al. Mutations in PEX10 is the cause of Zellweger peroxisome deficiency syndrome of complementation group B. Hum Mol Genet 1998;7: 1399–1405. (Ref.543)

Pagani F, et al. New lysosomal acid lipase gene mutants explain the phenotype of Wolman disease and cholesteryl ester storage disease. J Lipid Res 1998;39: 1382–1388. (Ref.418)

Pan CJ, et al. Transmembrane topology of glucose-6-phosphatase. J Biol Chem 1998;273:6144–6148. (Ref.169)

Parvari R, et al. Glycogen storage disease type 1a in Israel: biochemical, clinical, and mutational studies. Am J Med Genet 1997;72:286–290. (Ref.171)

Pollet N, et al. Construction of an integrated physical and gene map of human chromosome 20p12 providing candidate genes for Alagille syndrome. Genomics 1997;42:489–498. (Ref.505)

Portsteffen H, et al. Human PEX1 is mutated in complementation group 1 of the peroxisome biogenesis disorders. Nat Genet 1997;17:449–452. (Ref.537)

Purdue PE, et al. Rhizomelic chondrodysplasia punctata is caused by deficiency of human PEX7, a homologue of the yeast PTS2 receptor. Nat Genet 1997;15: 381–384. (Ref.540)

Quiros-Tejeira RE, et al. Variable morbidity in Alagille syndrome: a review of 43 cases. J Pediatr Gastroenterol Nutr 1999;29:431–437. (Ref.478)

Rellos P, Sygusch J, Cox TM. Expression, purification, and characterization of natural mutants of human aldolase B. Role of quaternary structure in catalysis. J Biol Chem 2000;275:1145–1151. (Ref.12)

Renner C, et al. Hormone replacement therapy in galactosaemic twins with ovarian failure and severe osteoporosis. J Inherit Metab Dis 1999;22:194–195. (Ref.145)

Reuber BE, et al. Mutations in PEX1 are the most common cause of peroxisome biogenesis disorders. Nat Genet 1997;17:445–448. (Ref.536)

Richards CS, Grody WW. Prenatal screening for cystic fibrosis: past, present and future. Expert Rev Mol Diagn 2004;4:49–62. (Ref.603)

Richards CS, Haddow JE. Prenatal screening for cystic fibrosis. Clin Lab Med 2003;23:503–530, x–xi. (Ref.604)

Sanders RD, et al. Biomarkers of ovarian function in girls and women with classic galactosemia. Fertil Steril 2009;92:344–351. (Ref.122)

Sangiuolo F, et al. Biochemical characterization of two GALK1 mutations in patients with galactokinase deficiency. Hum Mutat 2004;23:396. (Ref.149)

Shen JJ, Chen YT. Molecular characterization of glycogen storage disease type III. Curr Mol Med 2002;2:167–175. (Ref.259)

Sokol RJ, Durie PR. Recommendations for management of liver and biliary tract disease in cystic fibrosis. Cystic Fibrosis Foundation hepatobiliary disease consensus group. J Pediatr Gastroenterol Nutr 1999;28(Suppl 1):S1–S13. (Ref.605)

South ST, Gould SJ. Peroxisome synthesis in the absence of preexisting peroxisomes. J Cell Biol 1999;144:255–266. (Ref.544)

Spinner NB, et al. Jagged1 mutations in Alagille syndrome. Hum Mutat 2001;17: 18–33. (Ref.506)

Strautnieks SS, et al. A gene encoding a liver-specific ABC transporter is mutated in progressive familial intrahepatic cholestasis. Nat Genet 1998;20:233–238. (Ref.453)

Strautnieks SS, et al. Identification of a locus for progressive familial intrahepatic cholestasis PFIC2 on chromosome 2q24. Am J Hum Genet 1997;61:630–633. (Ref.452)

Stroppiano M, et al. Mutations in the glucose-6-phosphatase gene of 53 Italian patients with glycogen storage disease type Ia. J Inherit Metab Dis 1999;22: 43–49. (Ref.174)

Tyfield L, et al. Classical galactosemia and mutations at the galactose-1-phosphate uridyl transferase (GALT) gene. Hum Mutat 1999;13:417–430. (Ref.85)

Tygstrup N, et al. Recurrent familial intrahepatic cholestasis in the Faeroe Islands. Phenotypic heterogeneity but genetic homogeneity. Hepatology 1999;29:506–508. (Ref.435)

van Mil SW, et al. Benign recurrent intrahepatic cholestasis type 2 is caused by mutations in ABCB11. Gastroenterology 2004;127:379–384. (Ref.455)

Visser G, et al. Neutropenia, neutrophil dysfunction, and inflammatory bowel disease in glycogen storage disease type Ib: results of the European study on glycogen storage disease type I. J Pediatr 2000;137:187–191. (Ref.241)

Walter C, et al. Disorders of peroxisome biogenesis due to mutations in PEX1: phenotypes and PEX1 protein levels. Am J Hum Genet 2001;69:35–48. (Ref.546)

Walter JH, Collins JE, Leonard JV. Recommendations for the management of galactosaemia. UK galactosaemia steering group. Arch Dis Child 1999;80: 93–96. (Ref.136)

Wanders RJ. Metabolic and molecular basis of peroxisomal disorders: a review. Am J Med Genet 2004;126A:355–375. (Ref.524)

Wanders RJ. Peroxisomal disorders: clinical, biochemical, and molecular aspects. Neurochem Res 1999;24:565–580. (Ref.535)

Wang BB, et al. Molecular and biochemical basis of galactosemia. Mol Genet Metab 1998;63:263–269. (Ref.86)

Wilson DC, et al. Treatment of vitamin K deficiency in cystic fibrosis: effectiveness of a daily fat-soluble vitamin combination. J Pediatr 2001;138: 851–855. (Ref.607)

Woolfenden AR, et al. Moyamoya syndrome in children with Alagille syndrome: additional evidence of a vasculopathy. Pediatrics 1999;103:505–508. (Ref.491)

Yerushalmi B, et al. Use of rifampin for severe pruritus in children with chronic cholestasis. J Pediatr Gastroenterol Nutr 1999;29:442–447. (Ref.508)

Zielenski J. Genotype and phenotype in cystic fibrosis. Respiration 2000;67: 117–133. (Ref.586)

A complete list of references can be found at www.expertconsult.com.

Fibrocystic Diseases of the Liver

R. Brian Doctor, Maxwell L. Smith, Brett E. Fortune, Steve M. Helmke, and Gregory T. Everson

---

ABBREVIATIONS

ADPKD autosomal dominant polycystic kidney disease
AP1 activating protein 1
ARPKD autosomal recessive polycystic kidney disease
CA 19-9 carbohydrate antigen 19-9
CEA carcinoembryonic antigen
CT computed tomography
CXCR2 human chemokine receptor-2
ENA-78 epithelial neutrophil activating peptide

ER endoplasmic reticulum
ERCP endoscopic retrograde cholangiopancreatography
LDL low-density lipoprotein
IL-8 interleukin-8
MRCP magnetic resonance cholangiopancreatography
PC1 polycystin-1
PC2 polycystin-2
PCLD polycystic liver disease

PKC protein kinase C
PRKCSH protein kinase C substrate 80K-H gene
PTC percutaneous transhepatic cholangiography
STAT signal transducer and activator of transcription
TIPS transjugular intrahepatic portosystemic shunt
VEGF vascular endothelial growth factor

Introduction

Fibrocystic liver diseases constitute a group of congenitally acquired conditions that target bile ducts and surrounding portal tracts within the liver and biliary tree. These diseases include autosomal dominant polycystic kidney disease (ADPKD), polycystic liver disease (PCLD), congenital hepatic fibrosis, autosomal recessive polycystic kidney disease (ARPKD), Caroli disease, choledochal cysts, and solitary hepatic cysts (**Table 67-1**). Although these diseases are distinct from one another, they share common features including proliferation of biliary ductular epithelium, biliary ectasia, cyst formation, and periductular fibrosis. The last decade has witnessed enormous advances in understanding the genetic, molecular, and cellular events that underlie fibrocystic liver diseases. These advances will be highlighted in the first section of the chapter, Biology of Fibrocystic Liver Diseases. In Histopathology of Fibrocystic Liver Diseases, the gross anatomic and histopathologic features of these disorders are presented. In Section 3, Clinical Manifestations and Treatments of Fibrocystic Liver Diseases, the clinical features and therapies are described for each form of fibrocystic liver disease. Since the previous edition of this chapter, mechanism-based therapies have been initiated and are showing clinical potential. It is hoped that continued advances in the laboratory will translate into improved medical therapies for patients afflicted with fibrocystic liver diseases.

Biology of Fibrocystic Liver Diseases

Ductal Plate Malformation Hypothesis

Formation of the biliary tree begins during the first trimester of fetal life, when precursor cells lying in contact with the mesenchymal tissue of the portal tracts differentiate into a glandular morphology and give rise to the ductal plate.[1,2] This intermediary biliary structure consists of a double-layered tube of biliary epithelial cells surrounding the periphery of the future portal tracts and its formation proceeds from the central portion of the liver toward progressively smaller and more peripheral branches of the biliary tree (**Fig. 67-1**). During the beginning of the second trimester of fetal life, remodeling of the ductal plate normally begins with one portion, which is destined to become the functional bile duct, becoming embedded within the connective tissue of the portal tract, while other sections of the circumferential ductal plate gradually degenerate and disappear. This process is completed following birth, and a discontinuous vestige of the ductal plate can be identified by cytokeratin staining in newborns.[3]

Histopathologic examination of livers from patients with fibrocystic liver diseases commonly shows abnormal biliary structures that are reminiscent of the ductal plate stage of fetal

Table 67-1 Fibrocystic Diseases of the Liver

	ADPKD	PCLD	CONGENITAL HEPATIC FIBROSIS	CHOLEDOCHAL CYSTS	CAROLI DISEASE	SOLITARY HEPATIC CYST
Affected gene	*PKD1* (85%-90%) Chromosome 16 p13.3-p13.12; 230 distinct mutations in *PKD1* have been described	*PKD2* (10-15%) Chromosome 4 q21-q23; 60 mutations have been described	Protein kinase C substrate 80K-H (PRKCSH); chromosome 19p13	*sec63*	Given its association with ARPKD, thought to be related to mutations in *PKHD1* (chromosome 6p)	Unknown	Associated with mutations in *PKHD1* and possibly *PKD1*, or some other site	Unknown
Affected protein	Polycystin-1 (~460 kDa)	Polycystin-2 (110 kDa)	Hepatocystin (59 kDa)	SEC63p (63 kDa)	Possibly fibrocystin (447 kDa)	Unknown	Possibly fibrocystin	Unknown
Anatomic features	Development of multiple large cysts in kidneys and liver		Development of multiple large cysts in liver only	Extensive fibrosis and malformations of the interlobular bile ducts	Cystic dilations or diverticula of the extrahepatic bile ducts	Cystic dilation of the intrahepatic bile ducts that communicate with the extrahepatic biliary tree	Intrahepatic cyst formation that does not communicate with the biliary tree
Hepatic histopathologic features	Macrocystic disease; cysts lined by simple flattened to columnar epithelium; immunohistochemical profile similar to biliary epithelium		Macrocystic disease; cysts lined by simple flattened to columnar epithelium; immunohistochemical profile similar to biliary epithelium	Ductal plate malformations of the interlobular bile ducts, associated with extensive fibrosis	Biliary or intestinalized epithelium; often with extensive denudation; inflammation and reactive epithelial changes	Dilation of large bile ducts with marked periductal inflammation; bridges, and soft tissue protrusions into dilated ducts	Simple epithelium; rounded contour
Clinical presentation of liver cysts	Hepatomegaly and abdominal pain; incidence of hepatic cysts increases with age and gender; disease related to *PKD2* mutations typically has later onset and associated with greater life expectancy		Similar to the hepatic presentation of ADPKD, PCLD typically presents with hepatomegaly and abdominal pain	Portal hypertension, recurrent cholangitis; typically diagnosed early in childhood; incidence of 1:20,000-1:40,000	Chronic intermittent abdominal pain, jaundice, and recurrent cholangitis; can be congenital or acquired	Typically presents with recurrent cholangitis or complications of portal hypertension	Typically asymptomatic and discovered incidentally, although right upper quadrant pain can occur when cysts exceed 5 cm in diameter
Radiographic findings	CT, US, and MRI scanning shows multiple, large noncommunicating cysts within the hepatic and renal parenchyma		CT, US, and MRI scanning shows multiple, large noncommunicating cysts within the hepatic parenchyma only	Large multilobulated liver with rare cysts	Cholangiography shows cystic dilation of bile duct without overt obstruction; dilations can also be seen on CT, MRCP, or EUS	Cholangiography shows nonobstructing cystic dilations that communicate with the biliary tree	Ultrasound can distinguish simple hepatic cysts from other cystic lesions
Treatment options	Radiographic cyst aspiration and sclerosis; surgical fenestration; liver resection; liver transplantation		Radiographic cyst aspiration and sclerosis; surgical fenestration; liver resection; liver transplantation	Management focused on treatment of complications of cholangitis and portal hypertension	Given increased risk of cholangiocarcinoma, surgical resection is indicated	Adequate biliary drainage is mainstay; often requires lobectomy or liver transplant	Conservative management usually appropriate, if symptomatic radiographic aspiration and sclerosis

ADPKD, autosomal dominant polycystic kidney disease; CT, computed tomography; EUS, endoscopic ultrasound; MRCP, magnetic resonance cholangiopancreatography; MRI, magnetic resonance imaging; PCLD, polycystic liver disease; US, ultrasound

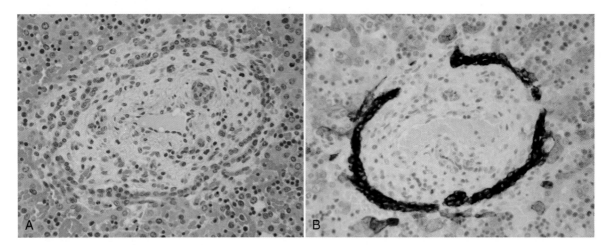

Fig. 67-1 Morphology of portal tracts during development at approximately 20 weeks' gestation. A, Evidence of residual ductal plate structures can be seen in the fetal liver at the periphery of portal area. **B,** Residual biliary structures are highlighted with cytokeratin 19. (H & E, ×400; anticytokeratin 19 immunostain, ×400.)

Fig. 67-2 "Two-hit" hypothesis of cyst formation in ADPKD. The germline mutation predisposes biliary epithelium to cystic transformation, but a second somatic mutation is required to initiate cystogenesis within a single cell. Clonal expansion of this single biliary epithelial cell stimulates budding and subsequent detachment from the biliary ductule. Cyst expansion and growth ensues under regulation of a number of factors defined within the text.

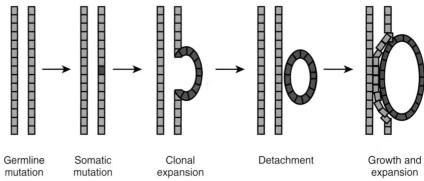

Germline mutation → Somatic mutation → Clonal expansion → Detachment → Growth and expansion

development. This similarity was first noted by Jorgensen who termed the lesion ductal plate malformation.[4] Isolated lesions are often referred to as biliary microhamartoma or von Meyenburg complexes and may be observed in normal livers. Desmet expanded on the observations of Jorgensen to hypothesize that many cystic liver diseases represent malformations of biliary development.[2,5] Although studies have not yet completely validated this hypothesis, the concept is useful to explain the similarities in the histologic findings in patients with various fibrocystic diseases. Immunohistochemical characterization of the epithelia within ductal plate malformations in a variety of fibrocystic diseases demonstrates similarity to the phenotype of normal embryonic ductal plates after 20 weeks of gestational age.[6] Anomalous ductal plate morphology is also observed in the hepatic conditions associated with renal polycystic disease and a number of other genetic syndromes, including Meckel syndrome.[5,7]

The "Two-Hit" Hypothesis of Cyst Development in ADPKD and PCLD

Although the pattern of expression of ADPKD and PCLD within families is consistent with these diseases being autosomal dominant in nature, ADPKD and PCLD are likely "molecular recessive" diseases. In this case, affected individuals have a germline mutation in one copy of the responsible gene (i.e., first hit) and acquire a mutation in the second copy of the responsible gene within individual bile duct epithelial cells during the individual's lifetime (i.e., second hit) (**Fig. 67-2**). The developmental pattern of liver cysts in ADPKD and PCLD is consistent with this two-hit hypothesis. Unlike the early and pervasive involvement of bile ducts in ARPKD/Caroli disease, liver cysts in ADPKD and PCLD develop focally along the bile duct during the lifetime of the individual. Genetic screening of *PKD1* and *PKD2* of cyst lining epithelial cells indicates these cells have undergone a loss of heterozygosity or other somatic mutations.[8,9] Genetic mouse models of ADPKD also support the two-hit hypothesis. Homozygous knockout models of ADPKD generally die in the late embryonic stages. In contrast, *pkd2(WS25/−)* mice develop kidney and liver cysts in a post-puberty pattern that mirrors the human condition.[10] Importantly, these mice have one true knockout in the *pkd2* gene (homolog of one of the two genes linked to ADPKD in humans; approximating first hit) and a recombinant sensitive allele (i.e., *WS25*) in the second copy of the *pkd2* gene. Appropriate recombination of the *WS25* allele results in a loss of its function (approximately second hit) and initiation of cyst development.

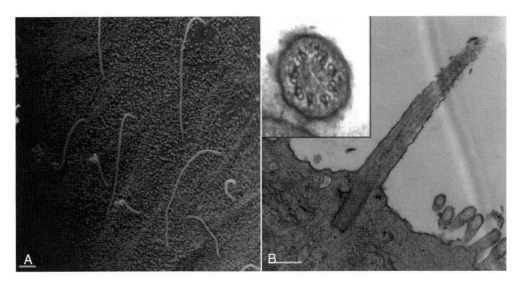

Fig. 67-3 Primary cilia extend from the apical surface of cholangiocytes, detect flow of fluid over the surface of the cell, and transduce flow information into the cell interior. **A,** Scanning electron micrograph of primary cilia extending from the apical surface of rat intrahepatic bile duct epithelial cells (cholangiocytes). **B,** Transmission electron micrograph showing the ultrastructure at the base of a primary cilium, including the basal body at the base of the primary cilium and the primary cilium extending into the lumen. *Inset* shows a cross-section of a primary cilium and the ring of microtubules that form the core of the primary cilium.

Primary Cilia Contribute to Cystogenesis

Epithelial cells, including bile duct epithelial cell, have a single primary cilium that extends from their luminal surface[11] (**Fig. 67-3**). Research over the last decade has led to a wealth of information regarding the molecular, structural and functional aspects of primary cilia. Primary cilia are a non-motile, microtubule-based organelle that arise from the basal body and can extend several microns in length into the lumen of the duct. The primary cilia serve to sense and transduce information about the luminal fluid osmolarity, composition and flow rate.[11-13] As the proteins that contribute to the structure and function of the primary cilium have been discovered, it has become apparent that a variety of genetic syndromes and diseases are associated with the dysfunction of primary cilia. These diseases, coined celiopathies, have a number of shared features and often include the development of cysts.[14,15] In the liver, polycystin-1 (PC1)/(PC2) and polycystin-2, the proteins linked to ADPKD, and fibrocystin, the protein linked to ARPKD, congenital hepatic fibrosis, and Caroli disease, localize to the primary cilium of biliary epithelial cells. The specific functions of these three proteins and their mechanistic contributions to cystogenesis will be covered in greater detail in the following sections. Parenthetically, the proteins linked to PCLD, hepatocystin, and sec63p are among the few "cystogenic" proteins that have not yet been found to distribute to or moderate the function of the primary cilium or basal body.

Genes and Proteins of Fibrocystic Liver Diseases

The last decade has witnessed the discovery and characterization of the genes and proteins responsible for different forms of cystic diseases. The following section will describe the genes, proteins, and functions linked to human ADPKD,

PCLD, and ARPKD/Caroli disease. For more comprehensive descriptions of the responsible genes and proteins, there are a number of excellent reviews.[16-18]

Autosomal Dominant Polycystic Kidney Disease

The most common form of autosomal dominant polycystic liver disease coexists with renal cystic disease (ADPKD) and is linked to mutations in either *PKD1* or *PKD2*.[19-23] Mutations in *PKD1* occur in approximately 85% of ADPKD patients; mutations in *PKD2* account for approximately 15% of the disease.[24] The phenotypic characteristics stemming from mutations in *PKD1* and *PKD2* are quite similar, but patients with mutations in *PKD2* have a later onset of disease and approximately 16 years of increased life expectancy compared with patients with mutations in *PKD1*.[25]

PKD1 *and Polycystin-1*

In 1957 Dalgaard demonstrated autosomal dominant inheritance in more than 90% of cases of polycystic renal disease.[26] In 1985 linkage techniques localized the first gene for ADPKD, coined *PKD1*, to the short arm of chromosome 16 p13.3-p13.12.[27] The *PKD1* gene was subsequently cloned, sequenced, and the resultant protein characterized.[28] *PKD1* encodes a 14.1-kb message that translates into a 4304 amino acid protein, polycystin-1.[29,30] Additional copies of exons 1 to 34 lie adjacent to the active *PKD1* locus. These duplicated copies are probably nonfunctional and fail to express protein, but their presence has hampered the development of molecular genetic testing.

There are more than 230 distinct mutations identified within the *PKD1* gene.[31] Evenly dispersed without evidence for clustering, the majority of mutations are missense or nonsense mutations but splicing mutations and gene rearrangements have also been reported. Approximately 60% of all mutations introduce premature stop codons that result in truncated proteins. Specific mutations and their locations have been associated with intracranial aneurysms and more severe polycystic disease within individual ADPKD families.[32,33] For example, mutations in the 5′ end of *PKD1* are predictive of a more rapid development and greater severity of end-stage renal disease.[34] The effect of mutational type or location on hepatic cystic disease has not been specifically analyzed.

PKD1 encodes for polycystin-1 (PC1), a 460-kDa integral membrane protein with a large extracellular NH_2-terminal domain, 11 transmembrane domains, and a comparatively small intracellular COOH-terminal domain. Although its function remains to be clarified, PC1 is predicted to help transduce extracellular signals from the cell surface to the cell interior. Constituting two thirds of the protein, the NH_2-terminus of the protein contains a number of domains that are consistent with initiating signaling through protein–protein and protein–carbohydrate interactions. The extracellular NH_2-terminus contains a region of leucine-rich repeats, a segment with C-type lectin characteristics, a segment with low-density lipoprotein (LDL)-like features, 12 immunoglobulin-like *PKD* repeats, an REJ domain, and a G protein–coupled receptor site.[35-37] The *PKD* repeat domains permit direct PC1/PC1 interaction. In other proteins, REJ domains moderate fluxes in ion channel complexes. Its presence supports the hypothesis that PC1 serves, in part, to regulate Ca^{2+} signaling. Specific protein–protein interactions of the intracellular COOH-terminal domain with other proteins, including heterotrimeric G-proteins, JAK2 kinase, and polycystin-2 (PC2)[38] further the notion that PC1 serves to transduce extracellular cues into intracellular signals. PC1 also has cleavage-sensitive sites: one within its extracellular G protein–coupled receptor site and two within its intracellular tail. All three sites are anticipated to have physiologic significance and contribute to cyst formation in pathologic states. Regarding its localization and site of activity, PC1 was originally described to reside along the basolateral membrane of epithelial cells where it could participate in cell–cell and cell–matrix interactions. The more recent localization of PC1, along with PC2, within the membrane of primary cilia has focused investigative efforts into understanding the function and relationship of these two proteins within this organelle.

PKD2 *and Polycystin-2*

In 1993 a second genetic locus linked to ADPKD was discovered on chromosome 4 q21-q23[22,23] and 3 years later the *PKD2* gene was identified, sequenced, and cloned.[39] *PKD2* produces a 5.3-kb message that codes for the 968 amino acid polycystin-2 protein. There are more than 60 identified mutations of the *PKD2* gene and, like the mutations of *PKD1*, the mutations of *PKD2* are evenly dispersed throughout the gene without clustering at any particular position.[40] Relationships of the mutations of *PKD2* to phenotypic expression of polycystic disease are under study but no clear-cut relationships have been reproducibly defined.[41]

Polycystin-2 (PC2; also referred to as TRPP2) is a 110-kDa integral membrane protein with six transmembrane domains and intracellular NH_2 and COOH tails. Sequence homology and functional characteristics place PC2 within the transient receptor potential (TRP) superfamily of ion channels. PC2 can form homotetramers and function as a cation channel.[42-45] The PC2-dependent Ca^{2+} transients may be further amplified by hetero-multimerizing with other transient receptor

potential channels.[46] Initially found along the lateral membranes and endoplasmic reticulum of epithelial cells, PC2 was subsequently discovered within the primary cilium as well. A wide variety of distinct proteins have been shown to bind with PC2,[17] supporting the prediction that PC2 participates in organizing an extracellular signal transduction complex.

PC1 and PC2 Form a Mechanosensory Complex

The discovery of PC1 and PC2 interactions through coiled-coil domains in their respective COOH-tails and co-distribution of the two proteins within primary cilia led to studies investigating the functions of the PC1/PC2 complex.[38,47] In cultured embryonic renal epithelial cells, flow of fluid across the cell bends the primary cilium and triggers calcium influx into the cell. This normal response is blocked by pretreatment of embryonic renal epithelial cells with channel-blocking antibodies directed against PC2 or genetic mutations that impair PC1 synthesis.[48] In these cases, fluid flow across the epithelial surface fails to elicit an increase in Ca^{2+}_i. This co-dependency of PC1 and PC2 for transducing flow information into an intracellular Ca^{2+}_i signal was confirmed in vitro by studies demonstrating PC1 modified the ion channel gating of PC2. Consistent with an impairment of calcium influx in ADPKD cells, the calcium levels in cyst-derived cells were significantly lower when compared with NHK cells.[49] In addition to flow-dependent Ca^{2+}_i signaling, the PC1/PC2 complex is integrated into additional signaling pathways. For example, PC1 constitutively activates heterotrimeric G-proteins to initiate downstream effects[50,51] and PC2 antagonizes this constitutive activity.[51] Significant research efforts are currently being invested to understand how these PC1/PC2 transduction pathways result in cystogenesis and cyst growth.

Mechanisms for PC1/PC2 Complexes to Influence Cell Proliferation

Increased cell proliferation is considered a cornerstone of cyst growth and the loss of functional PC1/PC2 complex activity is predicted to induce cell proliferation. Cystic epithelial cells can overexpress proto-oncogenes and growth factor receptors, suggesting a role for PC1 and PC2 in nuclear regulation. Distinct lines of investigation have implicated the PC1/PC2 complex in moderating cell cycle progression through the AP1 nuclear transcription factor, the JAK-STAT signaling pathway, the ERK signaling pathway, and mammalian target of rapamycin (mTOR) signaling (**Fig. 67-4**). First, PC1 and PC2 can independently or coordinately mediate the activity of the AP1 nuclear transcription factor complex through pathways involving small G proteins, PKC, p38, and JNK.[52,53] In cells overexpressing PC1, the carboxy-terminus of PC1 can be cleaved from the intact protein, translocate into the nucleus, and directly activate AP1.[54] Co-expression of PC2 blunts the effect of cleaving of the carboxy-terminus of PC1, suggesting that PC2 can modulate the AP1 signal by buffering the concentration of the PC1 carboxy-terminus available for nuclear signaling. Second, PC1 can bind and activate JAK2 in a PC2-dependent manner, resulting in the phosphorylation and activation of at least two STAT transcription factors, including STAT1.[55] Phosphorylated STAT (STAT-P) can then enter the nucleus and arrest cell cycle progression. Loss of either PC1 or PC2 would

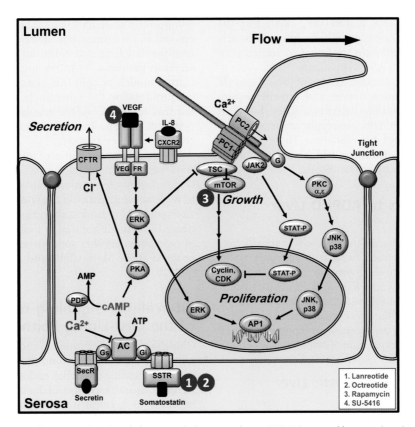

Fig. 67-4 Polycystin signaling pathways and rational therapeutic interventions. ADPKD is caused by mutations in the genes *PKD1* and *PKD2*, which code for the proteins polycystin-1 (PC1) and polycystin-2 (PC2). PC1 and PC2 have been implicated in many different signaling pathways that affect epithelial secretion, growth, and proliferation (ADPKD down-regulated pathways in *red*, up-regulated in *green*). PC1 and PC2 interact as part of a complex found in the primary cilium, which acts as a flow-regulated Ca^{2+} channel. Defects in any of the proteins reduce Ca^{2+} influx and lead to low intracellular concentrations. Ca^{2+} inhibits adenyl cyclase (AC) and activates phosphodiesterase (PDE), and thus low intracellular Ca^{2+} results in increased levels of cAMP and the activation of PKA. PKA acts on CFTR to increase Cl^- secretion into the cyst lumen. This process is also stimulated by secretin binding to the secretin receptor (SecR) signaling through Gs. AC is normally inhibited by somatostatin acting through its receptor SSTR and Gi. Therefore, to lower the abnormally high cAMP levels in ADPKD, long-acting somatostatin analogs, such as lanreotide and octreotide, are being tested in clinical trials. Low Ca^{2+} also allows PKA to activate the ERK pathway, which can increase proliferation. The PC1/PC2 complex binds and activates JAK2, which phosphorylates STAT. STAT normally inhibits the cyclin/CDK pathways so its down-regulation in ADPKD would increase epithelial proliferation. PC1 and PC2 signal via G proteins and distinct PKC isoforms to activate JNK and p38, which in turn stimulate AP1. PC1 binds tuberin, a component of the tuberous sclerosis complex (TSC), which normally inhibits mTOR, a central regulator of growth and proliferation. Loss of this regulation in ADPKD leads to greatly increased mTOR activity, stimulating cell growth and the cyclin/CDK pathway. Activated mTOR is a promising target for therapeutic intervention, and transplant recipients receiving the mTOR inhibitor rapamycin for immunosuppression exhibited a reduction in liver cyst volume. VEGF, whose production is increased by mTOR, is secreted both basolaterally and apically into the cyst lumen where it can bind back to apically localized VEGFR and activate ERK. Another cyst fluid component, IL-8, can bind to the CXCR2 and enhance the VEGFR signaling to ERK. ERK can inhibit tuberin and thus further activate mTOR, creating a feedback loop that leads to increased proliferation. The VEGFR antagonist SU-5416 can block this signaling and blunt the growth of liver cysts in a mouse model of PKD.

be predicted to diminish activated STAT levels and allow cells to reenter the cell cycle and promote cell proliferation. Third, although cAMP tends to inhibit ERK signaling in normal epithelial cells, calcium restriction allows cAMP in cystic epithelial cells to activate ERK.[56] Increased levels of cAMP itself observed in a murine PKD model[57] could also be the result of calcium restriction because calcium can inhibit adenyl cyclase (AC) and activate cAMP phosphodiesterase (PDE). Activated ERK can promote an increase in cell proliferation both by entering the nucleus and initiating a transcriptional cascade and by moderating the tuberous sclerosis complex (TSC) activity, which leads to an increase in mTOR activity. The JAK/STAT and mTOR pathways include activating specific cyclin-dependent kinases (CDK) to drive the progression in the cell cycle. In nonorthologous cystic animal models, treatment with roscovitine, a potent CDK inhibitor, significantly blunted kidney cyst growth.[58] Similarly, moderating CDK activity by decreasing miRNA15A abundance reduces the disease severity in rodent models of ARPKD.[59] The effects of CDK inhibition on ADPKD liver cyst growth will be of great interest.

Additional lines of evidence point to the potential significance of the mTOR pathway in driving errant proliferation of cystic epithelial cells. PC1 can directly bind the tuberin component of the TSC, which normally inhibits the activity of mTOR. Loss of this regulation would account for the inappropriate activation of mTOR observed in ADPKD cyst epithelial cells.[60] Described in greater detail later, liver cyst epithelial cells are likely to be tonically stimulated by vascular endothelial growth factor (VEGF). VEGF also can promote cell proliferation through ERK and mTOR.[61] Reflecting the efficacy in treating renal cyst growth in animal models with mTOR inhibitors, rapamycin treatment correlated with diminished liver volumes in ADPKD patients.[62]

Many of the details and interrelationships of these disparate pathways for regulating transcription and growth require additional investigation. It is important to recognize, however, the emerging evidence for PC1/PC2 in regulation or coordination of cell proliferation and differentiation. These pathways can now be investigated to determine which pathways, when disrupted, give rise to fibrocystic liver disease.

Contributing Events to ADPKD Liver Cyst Disease

In ADPKD, the clinical course of the disease is markedly heterogeneous even among identical twins. Although part of this heterogeneity is likely due to differences in the specific germline and somatic mutations in *PKD1* and *PKD2* that occur within individual subjects, additional factors likely contribute to promoting the growth of the liver cysts. Potential contributing factors include modifier genes, estrogen exposure, luminal fluid secretion, and altered expression of cytokines and growth factors.

Modifier Genes Influence Cystic Liver Disease Severity

Modifier genes, genes that are not directly linked to a genetic disease but influence the disease expression and severity, influence a number of genetic diseases. In ADPKD, modifier genes have been directly implicated and identified.[63,64] A comprehensive list of genes that specifically modify the development of cystic liver diseases has not yet been compiled but is likely to be forthcoming and will provide insight into the cellular mechanisms that moderate the disease severity.

Estrogen Has an Impact on Cystic Liver Disease Severity

ADPKD liver cyst severity is much greater in women than in men. Studies showing a positive correlation between liver cyst volumes and numbers of pregnancies, estrogen-based birth control, and postmenopausal estrogen therapy indicate that estrogen promotes liver cyst growth and is responsible for the sexual dimorphism observed in ADPKD liver cyst disease.[19,65] At the cellular level, cholangiocytes express α- and β-estrogen receptors, estrogen induces cholangiocyte proliferation, and estrogen receptor inhibition blocks the proliferative response to serum and liver cyst fluid.[66-68]

Fluid Secretion by Cyst-Lining Epithelial Cells May Contribute to Cyst Growth

In the normal liver, cholangiocytes have a robust capacity to secrete a bicarbonate-rich fluid into the ductular lumen.[69] This secretion is regulated in large part through the levels of specific gut hormones. For example, secretin binding activates adenylyl cyclase and drives cAMP-dependent secretion of Cl^-, HCO_3^-, and water while somatostatin binding inhibits the secretin response to block ductular secretion. Human liver cysts retain this regulated secretory capacity, generate a positive intraluminal cyst pressure under basal conditions, and have increased rates of fluid secretion following intravenous administration of secretin.[70,71] Studies on isolated liver cyst epithelial cells from genetic mouse models of ADPKD further confirm that liver cyst epithelial cells retain these regulated secretory pathways.[72,73] Increasing intraluminal pressure in cell culture models of epithelial cysts increases rates of epithelial cell proliferation.[74,75] Accordingly, increased epithelial stretching that follows from the regulated secretion into enclosed cysts will likely promote proliferation of the lining epithelial cells and drive cyst growth.

The therapeutic potential of inhibiting these secretory pathways has been highlighted in a recent clinical trial.[76] In this 6-month study, liver volumes in untreated patients continued to increase while patients receiving lanreotide, a somatostatin analogue, had a modest decrease in liver volumes. A similar phase II to III clinical trial to evaluate the therapeutic benefit of octreotide, another somatostatin analogue, is currently in progress at the Mayo Clinic and anticipated to be completed in 2010.

Intercellular Signaling for Proliferation of the Cyst-Lining Epithelium

Cholangiocytes use cytokines and growth factors to communicate information regarding the local environmental status with surrounding epithelial, endothelial, and immune cells. In ADPKD, apical secretion of factors would be confined and expected to accumulate. Analysis of liver cyst fluid from human ADPKD subjects showed that levels of IL-8, ENA-78, VEGF, and IL-6 are specifically elevated to physiologically relevant levels.[77] CXCR2, a receptor for both IL-8 and ENA-78, and receptors for VEGF are expressed on the apical domain of human liver cyst epithelial cells.[77,78] Interestingly, CXCR2 and VEGFR2 signaling pathways can act synergistically to drive cellular proliferation.[79] In vitro studies treating isolated mouse liver cyst epithelial cells with CXCR2 and VEGFR2 agonists similarly resulted in a robust increase in cellular proliferation. Thus an autocrine/paracrine loop is established in the cyst lumen where these factors can be released, accumulate, and drive proliferation of the cyst-lining epithelium. As part of the intracellular signaling pathways that drive the VEGF-induced increases in cell proliferation, VEGFR2 activates the MAPK-ERK signaling pathway (see **Fig. 67-4**).[80]

Angiogenesis and Vascularization of the Liver Cyst Wall

In monolayers of liver cyst epithelial cells, cytokines and growth factors were also secreted across the basolateral membrane.[77] Basolateral secretion of potent angiogenic factors, such as VEGF and IL-8, would position these factors to initiate angiogenesis. Treatment of cultured human endothelial cells with human liver cyst fluid induced both cellular proliferation and angiogenic differentiation.[81-83] Liver cyst walls are vascularized and angiogenic factors, such as VEGF and IL-8, likely promote angiogenesis within the cyst wall. The potential of the cyst wall vasculature to serve as a therapeutic target is highlighted by both mouse and human studies. Long-term treatment of *pkd2(WS25/−)* mice with SU-5416, a VEGFR2 inhibitor, markedly inhibited liver cyst growth.[81] Subsequent studies suggest the VEGF signaling effect in ADPKD may be more robust in mice with defective polycystin-2 versus polycystin-1.[61] Implicating the therapeutic potential of inhibiting angiogenesis and vascular maintenance in humans, embolization of the liver cyst wall vasculature in ADPKD patients resulted in a significant decrease in liver cyst volumes.[84,85]

Polycystic Liver Disease

In contrast to the concurrent renal and liver cystic disease characteristic of ADPKD, PCLD gives rise to polycystic livers with no discernible renal manifestations. This phenotypic distinction is paralleled by disparate genetic linkages. To date, PCLD has been definitively linked to two genes, *PRKCSH* and *Sec63*. Early analysis suggests these two genes account for a minority of PCLD cases, indicating there are one or more genetic loci to be linked to PCLD.

PRKCSH and Hepatocystin

The first demonstration that PCLD was genetically distinct from *PDK1* and *PKD2* was from phenotypic and genetic studies of a family affected by polycystic liver disease without renal cystic disease in three generations.[86] PCLD was initially linked to mutations in protein kinase C substrate 80K-H gene (*PRKCSH*) on chromosome 19p13.2-13.1.[87-89] *PRKCSH* encodes for a 527 amino acid protein of 59 kDa, termed hepatocystin, that is expressed in a number of different tissues.[88] The protein contains a membrane translocation signal sequence for the endoplasmic reticulum (ER) at its amino end, an LDL-α domain, two EF-hand domains, a glutamic acid–rich region, and an ER retrieval sequence at its carboxyl end. There have been several reported functions for hepatocystin, but the weight of evidence indicates its primary role is being the noncatalytic subunit of the glucosidase II protein complex.[89,90] Glucosidase II is localized in the endoplasmic reticulum where it modifies protein glycosylation and contributes to posttranslational processing of newly synthesized glycoproteins. Mutations that truncate or alter mRNA splicing of hepatocystin have been reported in PCLD families. Initial studies suggest there may be a correlation between the site of the mutation and the severity of the disease but this awaits confirmation in studies with a larger population base.

Sec63 and *Sec63p*

The association of PCLD with the ER and protein processing was bolstered by the linkage of a second gene, *Sec63*, to PCLD. In humans, the *Sec63* gene is on chromosome 6q21, and mutations are distributed throughout the gene.[91,92] The protein product of the *Sec63* gene is designated as Sec63p, an integral membrane protein within the ER that functions as a component of the protein translocation complex. This protein processing step is upstream of the glycosylation modification step that is performed by glycosidase II. Interestingly, despite the apparent liver specificity of PCLD that is initiated by *Sec63* mutations, *Sec63* is broadly expressed in a number of tissues including the kidney.

Comparative Mechanisms of PCLD and ADPKD

The developmental characteristics of liver cysts in ADPKD and PCLD are markedly similar. In both diseases, liver cysts develop after puberty, clinical manifestations generally appear around the fourth decade of life, and disease expression is sexually dimorphic with women having a greater degree of cyst progression. The striking difference between these two diseases is that ADPKD affects the kidneys, vasculature, and liver whereas expression of PCLD is largely limited to the liver. As described previously, the proteins linked to ADPKD form a mechanosensory signal transduction complex within the primary cilia. In contrast, proteins linked to PCLD participate in the translocation, processing, and quality control of ER proteins. Understanding how the loss of function of the disparate proteins associated with ADPKD versus PCLD results in the phenotypic emergence of liver cysts may reveal the pivotal steps that underlie liver cystogenesis. Clinically, PCLD patients have more and larger liver cysts than ADPKD patients but have a more benign clinical course.[93]

Autosomal Recessive Polycystic Kidney Disease (Caroli Disease)

ARPKD is a rare genetic disorder, occurring in approximately 1 in 20,000 live births, with a high degree of morbidity and mortality.[94,95] Key gross features of livers in ARPKD patients include malformation of the bile ducts with biliary ectasia and fibrosis of the portal tracts. Over 99% of ARPKD cases are linked to the *PKHD1* (polycystic kidney and hepatic disease 1) gene.

PKHD1 and Fibrocystin

PKHD1 is a large, alternatively spliced gene located on chromosome 6p12. More than 100 mutations in the *PKHD1* gene have been cataloged. The majority of affected individuals are compound heterozygotes. The presence of two truncation mutations is correlated with a severe phenotype and high mortality rates in the perinatal and neonatal period. *PKHD1* encodes for a 4074 amino acid, 447-kDa integral membrane protein termed fibrocystin. Fibrocystin has a large extracellular NH$_2$-terminal domain, a single transmembrane domain, and a small COOH-terminal domain. Little is definitively known about the molecular functions of fibrocystin. The dozen immunoglobulin-like motifs in the NH$_2$-terminal extracellular domain suggest fibrocystin may serve as a surface receptor.[16] The COOH-terminal domain contains a nuclear localization signal that can be liberated from the protein through proteolysis.[96,97] This has led to speculation that fibrocystin can participate in nuclear signaling and transcriptional regulation. Finally, several lines of evidence indicate that fibrocystin can bind and modify polycystin-2 activity.[98-100] This fibrocystin/polycystin-2 interaction is of specific interest because it implicates a common molecular pathway for cystogenesis in these two related diseases.

As anticipated by its interaction with polycystin-2, fibrocystin localizes to the primary cilium in rat intrahepatic bile duct epithelial cells.[101,102] In cell culture and animal models where bile duct epithelial cells lacked fibrocystin, the primary cilia are shorter and more bulbous.[102,103] Tomography of the biliary tree showed that loss of fibrocystin is paralleled by marked distortions of the biliary tree, including ductular dilation and focal budding.[104] More recent studies are identifying distinct molecular pathways that are modified in fibrocystin-compromised cells and establishing hypotheses on how these modifications produce the fibrocystic phenotype.[105-108] Early efforts to affect the liver disease progression in *cpk* rats, an orthologous ARPKD model, through mechanism-based therapies have yielded promising results.[109]

Histopathology of Fibrocystic Liver Diseases

Autosomal Dominant Polycystic Liver Disease

The histopathologic features of liver cysts in ADPKD and PCLD are indistinguishable. Gross anatomic examination shows varying degrees of enlargement because of the expansion of multiple fluid-filled cysts (**Fig. 67-5**). Involvement can be either diffuse or segmental within the liver, although diffuse disease is more common. In segmental disease, the left lobe is preferentially affected. Cysts appear to cluster along the track of major vascular/portal structures within the liver, but mature cysts do not communicate with the biliary tree.[110] The presence of cysts is commonly associated with the presence of biliary microhamartomas, and these structures have been proposed as cyst precursors.[19,22,23]

The lining of the cysts is composed of a simple epithelium of cuboidal to columnar-type cells that overlie a dense band of fibrous connective tissue (**Figs. 67-6 and 67-7**). Inflammation is generally not found around cysts except in the cases where they show evidence of infection with predominantly acute inflammatory cells. The cytologic features of the cyst lining cells resemble the epithelia of interlobular bile ducts, and immunohistochemically both structures express a particular subset of cytokeratin proteins (so-called biliary types CK7 and CK19).[71] Cyst-lining cells show only weak reaction, with antibodies recognizing tumor markers such as CA 19-9 and carcinoembryonic antigen (CEA).[111] MUC1 is an oncofetal mucin antigen that is expressed in the epithelial cells lining many types of hepatic cysts, including those of ADPKD. Interestingly, only interlobular bile ducts in patients with

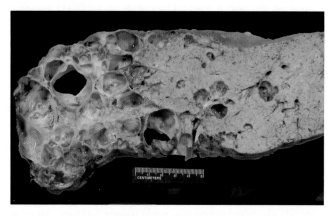

Fig. 67-5 Autosomal dominant polycystic liver disease. In a macroscopic view of segmental polycystic disease, less involved hepatic parenchyma is present on the *right side* of the slide where isolated cystic structures are seen in proximity to large portal tracts.

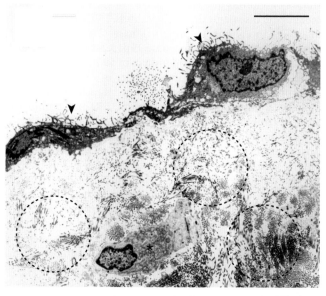

Fig. 67-7 Autosomal dominant polycystic liver. Electron microscopy demonstrates the thickened fibrotic matrix underlying cystic epithelial cells.

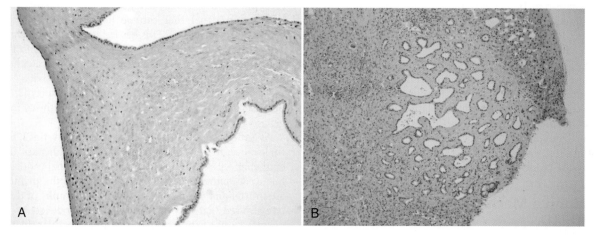

Fig. 67-6 Autosomal dominant polycystic liver. A, Epithelial variation within cysts ranges from flattened cells *(left vertical surface)* to cuboidal *(top horizontal surface)* to columnar *(lower right side)*. (H & E, ×100.) **B,** Biliary microhamartomas (von Meyenburg complexes) are often seen in association with ADPLD. In this figure, dilated and irregularly shaped bile duct structures are seen embedded in a dense fibrotic stroma. (H & E, ×100.)

ADPKD showed abnormal MUC1 expression in contrast to interlobular bile ducts in normal livers or livers with solitary cysts.[112] Development of cholangiocarcinoma, while rare, is a recognized complication of ADPKD that may arise following a dysplasia-carcinoma sequence in the epithelium of peribiliary cysts.[113]

Congenital Hepatic Fibrosis and Autosomal Recessive Polycystic Kidney Disease

Congenital hepatic fibrosis (**Figs. 67-8 and 67-9**) demonstrates one of two histopathologic broad patterns: either focal or diffuse.[2,5] In focal disease, there is enlargement of individual portal tracts associated with the presence of many abnormal biliary structures suggestive of maldevelopment of fetal ductal plates, but without bridging fibrosis of the type seen in the diffuse form. The diffuse form of the disease shows similar abnormal biliary structures; however, these are embedded within prominent irregular bands of fibrosis that connect portal tracts to other portal tracts and occasionally to hepatic venules. Inflammation is generally nonexistent to minimal. As yet, prospective studies have not shown that specific histologic patterns affect patient prognosis. Although many patients have portal hypertension in early childhood, patients without coincident renal disease may remain asymptomatic or have portal hypertension as adults.[114,115] Some cases demonstrate decreased numbers or a decreased size of portal vein branches that may represent a presinusoidal contribution to the portal hypertension in these patients.[110] Typically, cystic lesions are rarely identified in patients with congenital hepatic fibrosis by gross inspection of the liver after explantation or at the time of postmortem examination. However, some patients with congenital hepatic fibrosis also manifest biliary cysts.[2,5,110] In these cases, biliary cystic dilations may be prominent.

Caroli Disease

This disease is defined by the presence of congenitally dilatated intrahepatic bile ducts in the absence of obstruction, and the disease may be superimposed on congenital hepatic fibrosis (ARPKD) or polycystic disease (ADPKD)[116,117] (**Figs. 67-10 and 67-11**). Several studies have correlated radiologic and pathologic findings in patients with Caroli disease or syndrome.[118,119] By macroscopic examination, bridges and protrusions of soft tissue are seen within the lumens of the large, ectatic bile ducts. Brown pigmented stones, composed of inspissated bile, may also be present within the ducts. Upon microscopic examination, some protrusions contain hepatic arteries and portal vein branches, suggesting that the biliary dilation is related to maldevelopment of fetal ductal plates at the level of the central biliary branches. Inflammation is usually prominent around the areas showing cystic change. In

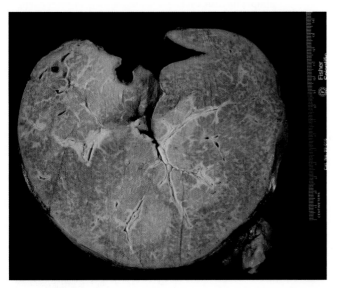

Fig. 67-8 **Congenital hepatic fibrosis.** A macroscopic view of congenital hepatic fibrosis shows a markedly enlarged liver with a reticular pattern of fibrosis.

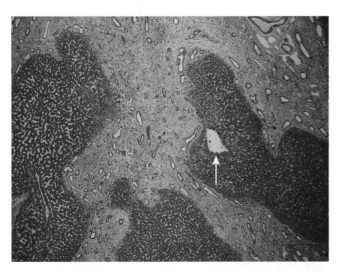

Fig. 67-9 **Congenital hepatic fibrosis showing a jigsaw puzzle pattern of fibrosis (blue) with preservation of the central veins (arrow).** Embedded within the fibrosis are numerous bile ducts, some of which are dilated. (Trichrome stain, ×40.)

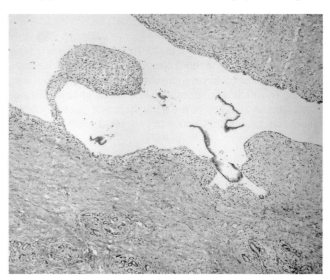

Fig. 67-10 **Caroli disease.** Ectatic bile ducts in the hilum of the liver show papillary protrusions into duct lumen. (H & E, ×100.)

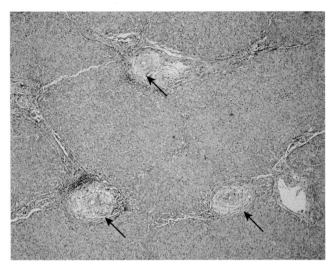

Fig. 67-11 **Caroli disease.** Other ducts show marked periductal chronic inflammation (H & E, ×100). The peripheral bile ducts do not show evidence of ductal plate malformation, although this case shows periductal fibrosis indicating secondary biliary sclerosis. (H & E, ×50.)

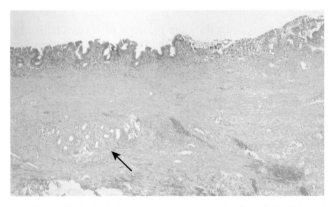

Fig. 67-12 **Choledochal cyst.** Low-power examination of the lining of a choledochal cyst shows peribiliary glands within the cyst wall *(arrow)* with epithelial denudation *(right side)* adjacent to an island of preserved epithelium *(left side)*. (H & E, ×50.)

some cases, small peripheral portal tracts may show relatively normal morphology without abnormal ductal plate elements, although periductal fibrosis suggestive of secondary sclerosing cholangitis can be seen. In other cases, ductal plate malformation occurs at all levels of the biliary tree and microhamartomatous structures can be seen in peripheral portal tracts.

Choledochal Cysts

These lesions represent one end of a spectrum that includes Caroli disease, because considerable overlap in histologic findings exists. Classification is usually based on the radiographic appearance. Choledochal cysts typically show extensive denudation of the epithelial lining[120] (**Fig. 67-12**). When the lining is present, there is most commonly a simple epithelium with reactive cytologic and architectural features. Whereas some authors report a predominance of intestinal-type epithelium in younger patients with evolution to a nondescript columnar or biliary epithelium in older patients,[121] others suggest that the likelihood of finding intestinalized epithelium increases

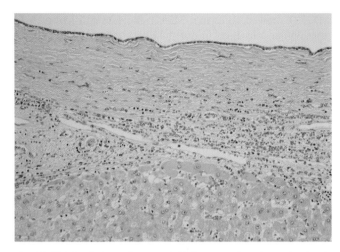

Fig. 67-13 **Simple hepatic cysts.** A high-power view shows the simple low cuboidal epithelial lining and a variably thickened fibrotic capsule seen in simple hepatic cysts. (H & E, ×200.)

with patient age.[122] Subepithelial inflammation is usually present and of variable density with a mixture of inflammatory cell types represented. Inflammatory infiltration is probably related to epithelial disruption and bacterial overgrowth associated with bile stasis that may also predispose cysts to metaplastic and dysplastic changes.[123] The risk of carcinoma is increased five-fold to 35-fold in patients with choledochal cysts, and risk appears to increase with the patient's age.[124]

Simple (Nonneoplastic, Nonparasitic, Noncommunicating) Hepatic Cysts

This common lesion (affecting roughly 1% to 2% of the general population) is generally referred to as solitary hepatic cyst although as many as 40% of patients may have multiple lesions.[125,126] The size of these lesions is generally small, although giant lesions as large as 27 cm in diameter have been reported.[127] Histologically, the epithelial lining of these hepatic cysts is a single layer of low cuboidal to columnar epithelium (**Fig. 67-13**). Epithelial cells may show mucinous features but without goblet cell formation. Immunohistochemical features of cytokeratin and mucin expression are similar to cysts arising in ADPKD.[111,112] Cyst-lining cells show only weak immunohistochemical expression of tumor markers such as CA 19-9 and CEA despite elevated levels of these markers in cyst fluid.[111,128]

Clinical Manifestations and Treatment of Fibrocystic Liver Diseases

Polycystic Liver Disease

Natural History

The natural history of autosomal dominant forms of polycystic liver disease is strikingly similar, regardless of etiologic mutation (*PKD1, PKD2, PRKSCH, Sec63*). The prevalence and

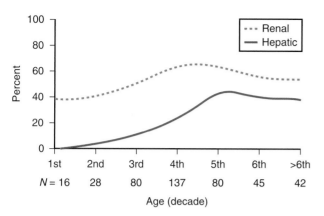

Fig. 67-14 **Prevalence of hepatic and renal cysts in ADPKD.** The frequency of renal and hepatic cysts is displayed by age in at-risk members of kindreds known to be affected by autosomal dominant polycystic kidney disease. Cysts were detected by real-time ultrasonography. The population at risk included 239 patients with ADPKD and 189 unaffected family members. Hepatic cysts are rarely detected before puberty, but by the fifth decade of life, approximately 80% of patients with renal cysts have liver cysts.

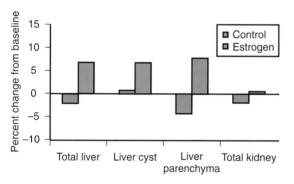

Fig. 67-15 **Postmenopausal estrogen selectively increases liver volume.** Percentage of volume change in liver and kidney following 1 year of postmenopausal estrogen treatment is shown. Estrogen-treated patients are depicted by *black bars* and nontreated controls as *hatched bars.* Estrogen treatment increases hepatic volume and hepatic cystic disease but does not influence renal cystic disease.

number of hepatic cysts in patients with ADPKD increase with increasing age (**Fig. 67-14**), female gender, severity of renal cystic disease, and severity of renal dysfunction. By age 60 nearly 80% of ADPKD patients have hepatic cysts.[19,21-23,129,130] Men and women have an equal lifetime risk for developing hepatic cysts but women experience greater numbers and larger sizes of hepatic cysts. Severe hepatic cystic disease correlates with both pregnancy and use of exogenous female steroid hormones. One longitudinal study of anovulatory women with ADPKD treated with hormone replacement suggested that estrogens selectively increase severity of hepatic cystic disease (**Fig. 67-15**).[131] Female tendency to develop massive hepatic cystic disease is also characteristic of isolated PCLD.[86]

Molecular Diagnostics

The molecular diagnostic approaches to ADPKD have advanced considerably with the availability of direct gene sequencing. Using commercially available methods,

pathologic mutations are detected in up to 90% of families with mutations of *PKD1* and *PKD2*.*

Molecular genetic testing is relatively new and consensus guidelines are lacking. Ultrasonography is a reasonable screening tool in adults. In young (age <30 years), presymptomatic individuals at risk for ADPKD, molecular genetic testing may offer a number of advantages over other approaches. In this group ultrasonography may lack sensitivity and linkage analysis is impractical. The identification of a *PKD1* or *PKD2* mutation could affect family planning or choice of future diagnostic studies. Discovery of ADPKD mutations may also encourage regular blood pressure monitoring and screening for associated conditions, such as cerebral aneurysm or mitral valve prolapse. Genetic testing may also have a role in the evaluation of young family members being considered as living donors for renal transplantation to another family member with renal failure from ADPKD. Clarifying the mutation status as negative in such potential donors would reduce future risks to both the donor and the recipient.

Clinical genetic testing for PCLD is also available and includes genetic sequencing of *PRKCSH* and *SEC63*.[134] Because the sensitivity of ultrasonography in PCLD is undefined, use of *PRKCSH* and *SEC63* testing to identify presymptomatic patients at risk of the disease may have even more relevance than in ADPKD. Although genetic testing results may not immediately alter the management of a PCLD-affected patient, the ability to screen other asymptomatic at-risk family members (and potential transplant donors) for mutations is important for patient care. As patients are frequently concerned about the risks to their offspring, formal genetic counseling is recommended even when the mutation status is unknown. An algorithm for use of genetic tests is presented in **Figure 67-16**.[135,136]

Clinical Features

Patients with small (<2 cm) or few hepatic cysts tend to be clinically asymptomatic. In contrast, patients who develop massive hepatic cystic disease, based upon a definition for massive of a total liver cyst/parenchyma volume ratio greater than 1, become symptomatic with abdominal pain or discomfort, early postprandial fullness, or shortness of breath (**Table 67-2**).[129,131] Consequences of progressive ADPKD include renal failure, requirement for hemodialysis, and renal transplantation. Dialysis, in particular, is thought to increase risk for hepatic complications. A single center reported that 21% of polycystic patients on dialysis experienced hepatic complications, mainly hepatic cyst infection, hemorrhage, or cyst carcinoma,[137] a finding that was not confirmed in a subsequent report by a different center.[138]

Typically, liver parenchymal volume is preserved despite extensive hepatic cystic disease and extraordinary distortion of hepatic architecture.[139] The only blood test abnormality is modest elevation of GGT, which correlates with hepatic cyst burden. The diagnosis of polycystic liver is readily established by its characteristic appearance on CT scan (**Figs. 67-17 and 67-18**). Quantitative tests of liver function indicate impairment of metabolic capacity and increased portal-systemic shunt in patients with massive polycystic disease

---

*References 31, 34, 40, 91, 92, 132, and 13.

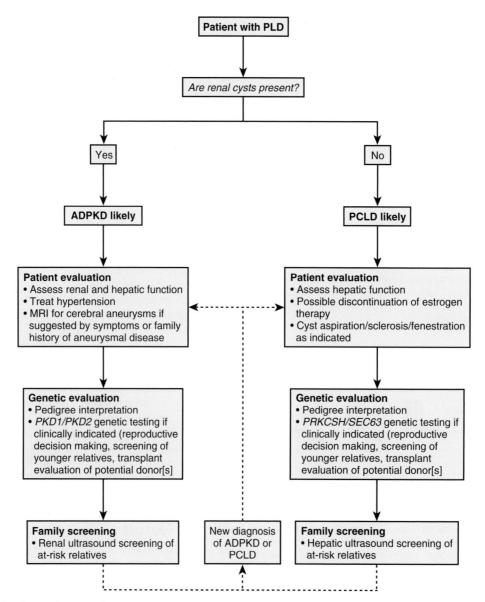

Fig. 67-16 Algorithm for evaluation of patients with known or suspected polycystic liver, (PCLD). ADPKD, autosomal dominant polycystic kidney disease; MRI, magnetic resonance imaging

in the absence of any obvious clinical manifestations.[21] Rarely, a patient with polycystic liver disease will experience hepatic decompensation and variceal hemorrhage, ascites, or encephalopathy.

The most common, clinically relevant complications arising in hepatic cysts are intracystic hemorrhage,[140] infection, or posttraumatic rupture (**Table 67-3**). Cyst adenocarcinoma, biliary obstruction, Budd-Chiari syndrome,[141,142] or hepatic failure are rarely reported. Associated conditions include mitral valve prolapse, diverticulosis, inguinal hernia, and cerebral aneurysm.[143]

Therapy

Medical Treatments

There are no definitive medical therapies for polycystic liver disease. Initial studies with somatostatin analogues, which block secretin effects, failed to demonstrate any significant benefit on hepatic cyst growth or size.[144] A recent double-blinded, placebo-controlled randomized trial evaluated the effects of a somatostatin analogue, lanreotide, on liver volume. The total liver volume of patients with ADPKD or PCLD (N = 54) decreased slightly but significantly (2.9% decrease in lanreotide vs. 1.6% increase in the placebo group; $P <.01$) after 6 months of treatment.[76] Longer follow-up of this same group is currently in progress to determine whether there is long-term reduction in liver volume.

Another modality under study includes the inhibition of cyst epithelial growth by blocking mTOR, which may regulate cyst epithelial proliferation. Sirolimus, an inhibitor of mTOR, could have a potential effect on cyst volume reduction by inhibiting the growth of cystic epithelium. Qian and colleagues examined seven kidney transplant patients with ADPKD who also had hepatic cysts. Patients treated with sirolimus-based therapy experienced reduction in liver volume when compared with patients receiving tacrolimus-based therapy without sirolimus ($P <.05$).[62]

Table 67-2 Gastrointestinal Symptoms in Patients with Polycystic Liver Disease

	PLD VS. CONTROL	PLD$_{min}$ VS. PLD$_{mass}$
Esophageal		
Belching	0.055	NS
Dysphagia	NS	NS
Odynophagia	NS	NS
Regurgitation	NS	NS
Heartburn	NS	NS
Hematemesis	NS	NS
Upper Gastrointestinal Tract		
Postprandial fullness	0.010	0.015
Bloating	0.0005	0.014
Pain	0.003	0.0005
Melena	NS	NS
Nausea	NS	NS
Vomiting	NS	NS
Lower Gastrointestinal Symptoms		
Diarrhea	NS	NS
Nocturnal diarrhea	NS	NS
Constipation	0.079	NS
Liver Specific Symptoms		
Jaundice	NS	NS
Bilirubinuria	NS	NS
Acholic stools	NS	NS
Pruritus	NS	NS

The significance of differences in the frequency of symptoms was assessed by the chi-square test.

NS, not significant; PLD, patients with polycystic liver disease; PLD$_{mass}$, patients with PLD and a liver cyst/parenchymal volume ratio of greater than 1; PLD$_{min}$, patients with PLD and a liver cyst/parenchymal volume ratio of less than 1

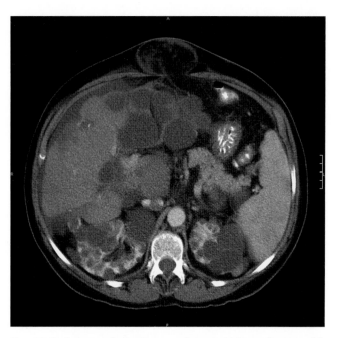

Fig. 67-17 Autosomal dominant polycystic kidney disease with liver cysts. CT demonstrates numerous cysts in liver and both kidneys. This patient also demonstrates a large umbilical hernia, which may complicate massive polycystic disease.

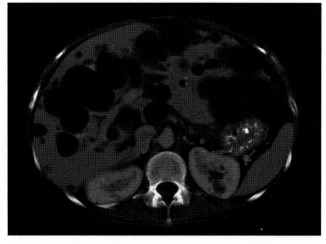

Fig. 67-18 Polycystic liver with minimal renal involvement in a patient from ADPKD cohort. CT demonstrates numerous hepatic cysts with uninvolved kidneys.

Some observations suggest a role for estrogen in stimulating hepatic cystic disease. Hepatic cystic disease, but not renal cystic disease, worsens under the influence of female gender or pregnancy. One study of anovulation in women demonstrated that use of hormone replacement therapy increased hepatic but not renal cysts.[131] These observations suggest that women with polycystic liver disease should avoid estrogen replacement therapy. However, proof that avoidance of estrogen effectively alters the course of hepatic cystic disease is lacking. The clinician must individualize hormonal replacement therapy in polycystic patients by weighing the potentially deleterious effect on hepatic cystic disease against other potential benefits and risks.

Radiologic Cyst Aspiration and Sclerosis

Symptomatic patients with one or few dominant cysts may be considered for cyst aspiration and sclerosis. Cyst aspiration and sclerotherapy requires ultrasonographic or CT-guided percutaneous puncture of the targeted cyst and placement of an intracystic drainage catheter. Success in obliterating individual cysts in polycystic patients is approximately 70% to 90%.[145-147] However, most patients with polycystic disease have too many cysts or cysts are of insufficient size to warrant this approach.

Cyst Fenestration

Cyst fenestration is a common surgical treatment in the management of symptomatic massive hepatic cystic disease.[148-151] Two approaches have been used: laparoscopy and (now less commonly) open laparotomy. Several series of open

Table 67-3 Complications of Polycystic Liver Disease

CLASSIFICATION	SPECIFIC TYPE	DIAGNOSTIC TESTS	TREATMENT
Arising within a Cyst			
	Infection	MRI, indium WBC scan	Fluoroquinolones
			Drainage
	Hemorrhage	CT or MRI	Pain control
			Drainage (rare)
	Carcinoma	CT or MRI	Surgery
			Aspiration cytology
Compression by a Cyst			
	Biliary obstruction	ERCP	Stent placement
			Cyst decompression
	Venous obstruction	Hepatic venography	Cyst decompression
	Hepatic	Resection	Transplantation
	Portal	MRI/MRA	Cyst decompression
		Mesenteric angiography	Resection
			Transplantation
Hepatic Dysfunction			
	Portal hypertension	Endoscopy (varices)	Band ligation
		US/CT/MRI	Cyst decompression
			Resection
			Transplantation
	Hepatic failure	Exceedingly rare	Transplantation
		Look for other cause	

CT, computed tomography; ERCP, endoscopic retrograde cholangiopancreatography; MRA, magnetic resonance angiography; MRI, magnetic resonance imaging; US, ultrasound; WBC, white blood cell

Table 67-4 Outcome after Laparoscopic Cyst Decompression

	SERIES 1	SERIES 2	SERIES 3	SERIES 4	TOTALS
Recurrent symptoms	62%	57%	33%	72%	58%
Conversion to open	0%	29%	11%	9%	10%
Complications	46%	57%	33%	10%	35%
Number of patients	13	7	9	11	40

Data from references 147 to 150.

laparotomy, encompassing large numbers of patients, indicate that this approach results in satisfactory resolution of symptoms. However, open laparotomy is associated with prolonged hospitalization, morbidity (bleeding, infection, bile leak, ascites) of major abdominal surgery (0% to 50%), and even mortality (<1%).[152] Because of its less invasive nature, laparoscopic cyst fenestration is gaining increasing acceptance as an alternative surgical technique. Advantages of laparoscopic surgery include: less morbidity, reduced hospital stay, and the potential for outpatient surgical management. One review,[151] totaling 40 cases, indicated that symptoms recurred in about half, necessitating repeat laparoscopic cyst fenestration. Although there were no deaths, surgical conversion to open cyst fenestration occurred in 10% of cases and 35% of patients suffered complications (**Table 67-4**).[148-151] Recurrence of large symptomatic cysts in appropriately selected patients remains low (10% to 11%).[152]

Liver Resection

One center reported their experience with partial liver resection in the management of 31 patients with highly symptomatic, massive hepatic polycystic disease.[153] Their ages ranged from 34 to 69, the sex ratio (M : F) was 3 : 28, and renal function varied from normal to dialysis dependency. Nearly all patients experienced significant relief from symptoms and long-term sustained reduction in symptoms was common (>95%). However, more than 50% experienced significant

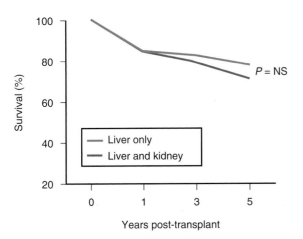

Fig. 67-19 **Patient survival rates after liver transplantation for polycystic liver disease.*** Results for combined liver–kidney and isolated liver transplantation are shown. Immediate survival is adversely affected by hemorrhage related to extensive dissection, infection, and complications related to renal dysfunction. The difference at 5 years, between the two types of transplants, is not statistically significant.

perioperative morbidity and there was one perioperative death (due to rupture of an intracranial aneurysm). Most surgeons reserve hepatic resection for those cases that are refractory to cyst decompression.

Liver Transplantation

Polycystic liver patients with symptoms refractory to other treatments or symptomatic hepatic cystic disease with end-stage renal cystic disease may be considered for liver or combined liver–kidney transplantation.[154-159] Rarer indications for hepatic transplantation include variceal hemorrhage, ascites, obstruction of hepatic venous outflow (Budd-Chiari equivalent), or biliary tract obstruction by extensive cystic disease not amenable to other interventions. One-, three-, and five-year survival rates for patients undergoing isolated hepatic transplantation ($n = 198$ between 2002 and 2008) are 84.8%, 78.5%, and 71.1%, respectively. One-, three-, and five-year survival rates for patients undergoing combined liver–kidney transplantation (n = 179 between 2002 and 2008) are 84.9%, 82.2%, and 77.9%, respectively (**Fig. 67-19**). The genetic basis of polycystic liver disease warrants caution with respect to living donor liver transplantation.

Congenital Hepatic Fibrosis

Characteristics

Congenital hepatic fibrosis is a rare, inherited, autosomal-recessive disorder that is most often associated with ARPKD. Other clinical associations of congenital hepatic fibrosis include renal dysplasia, nephronophthisis, Meckel-Gruber syndrome, Ivemark syndrome, Jeune syndrome, vaginal atresia, and tuberous sclerosis. Congenital hepatic fibrosis can co-exist with other fibrocystic liver diseases, such as Caroli disease and choledochal cyst.[160-162]

---

*Analyses provided by the U.S. Scientific Registry of Transplant Recipients, March 4, 2010.

Clinical Features

Congenital hepatic fibrosis presents in three clinical forms: portal hypertension, recurrent cholangitis, and asymptomatic or latent disease.[160] The first two forms are usually diagnosed in early childhood in patients who have variceal hemorrhage or unexplained biliary sepsis. In contrast, some patients will be detected later, during their adult years, when they are evaluated for unexplained hepatomegaly or portal hypertension. Rarely, patients have evidence of both portal hypertension and cholestasis, the latter because of either associated biliary anomalies (Caroli disease) or intrinsic destructive cholangiopathy. In general, hepatic function is well preserved, despite portal hypertension or bouts of cholangitis, although some patients experience progressive hepatic failure in long-term follow-up.

Treatment

The first-line treatment of variceal hemorrhage is endoscopic variceal eradication with ligation. If intolerant to endoscopic therapy, one could consider institution of β-adrenergic blockade. In most cases, varices may be successfully obliterated by the endoscopic approach, thereby controlling this potentially life-threatening complication. Surgical shunts or transjugular intrahepatic portosystemic shunt (TIPS) are reserved for patients who fail endoscopic therapy, bleed from gastric varices, or who have portal hypertensive gastropathy. Occasionally patients will experience progressive hepatic fibrosis and hepatic dysfunction after long-standing portosystemic shunt surgery, and development of this complication may necessitate consideration for liver transplantation.

In patients with cholangitis, radiologic imaging (ultrasonography, biliary radioscintigraphy, CT, or MRI) may be required to determine whether the patient with congenital hepatic fibrosis has concomitant biliary cystic disease. If the latter is present, the treatment of cholangitis is centered around the provision of adequate biliary drainage, relief of obstruction (papillotomy with stone extraction or stricture dilation), and control of infection with antibiotics. In the absence of biliary cystic disease or cholangiocarcinoma (6% of cases of congenital hepatic fibrosis), cholestasis may be related to idiopathic inflammatory destructive cholangiopathy and responds to UDCA therapy. Indications for hepatic transplantation include variceal hemorrhage or hemorrhage from portal hypertensive gastropathy that is not responsive to endoscopic treatment or amenable to portosystemic shunt surgery or TIPS, recurrent cholangitis that is not amenable to medical, endoscopic, radiologic, or surgical therapy; and hepatic failure (development of coagulopathy, biochemical deterioration, ascites, or portosystemic encephalopathy).

Caroli Disease

Characteristics

In 1973 Caroli described a syndrome of congenital ductal plate malformations of intrahepatic bile ducts characterized by segmental cystic dilation of the intrahepatic ducts, increased incidence of biliary lithiasis, cholangitis and liver abscesses, absence of cirrhosis and portal hypertension, and association of renal cystic disease.[116] Subsequent to Caroli initial reports, two distinct forms of the disease have been recognized: the simple type, which is associated with medullary sponge kidney in 60% to 80% of cases; and the periportal fibrosis variant, which is associated with congenital hepatic fibrosis, cirrhosis, portal hypertension, and esophageal varices.[163]

Clinical Features

The most common initial symptoms of Caroli disease are recurrent episodes of fever, chills, and abdominal pain caused by cholangitis, with peak incidence in early adult life. Males and females are equally affected, in contrast to the female predominance of massive polycystic liver disease, simple hepatic cysts, and choledochal cysts. More than 80% have symptoms before the age of 30 years. Rarely, the disease presents later in life with evidence of portal hypertension and its complications, most commonly bleeding esophageal varices. The lifetime risk of development of cholangiocarcinoma in Caroli disease is about 7%. Biliary lithiasis is found in one third of cases and predisposes patients to recurrent episodes of cholangitis because of obstruction and ascending infections. Occasionally patients also experience multiple liver abscesses.

The molecular pathogenesis of Caroli disease is not fully understood. Caroli disease has been associated with mutations in *PKHD1* (polycystic kidney and hepatic disease 1), the gene responsible for autosomal recessive polycystic kidney disease (ARPKD).[164] In rarer instances, it has been described in the setting of *PKD1* mutations, one of the two genes implicated in autosomal dominant polycystic kidney disease (ADPKD).[165] Other chromosomal mutations may be involved in inherited forms of Caroli disease not associated with renal cystic disease.[166]

Diagnosis

Caroli disease is typically discovered by imaging modalities performed during evaluation of biliary obstruction or cholangitis.[167] These studies typically demonstrate bile duct ectasia and nonobstructive saccular or fusiform dilation of the intrahepatic bile ducts. Communication of the intrahepatic cysts with the biliary tree and an otherwise normal common bile duct is the key feature of the diagnosis and is usually confirmed by ultrasonography, scintigraphy, CT scan after biliary contrast, magnetic resonance cholangiopancreatography (MRCP), endoscopic retrograde cholangiopancreatography (ERCP), or percutaneous transhepatic cholangiography (PTC). PTC and ERCP provide detailed examination of the biliary tree and may aid in therapy (**Fig. 67-20**). Magnetic resonance cholangiography with a dynamic contrast-enhanced study is an excellent screening tool for Caroli disease and allows for the diagnosis to be made without invasive imaging of the biliary tree.[168]

Treatment

Adequate biliary drainage is the primary approach in the management of Caroli disease. Endoscopic therapy with ERCP is effective in removing sludge or stones from the CBD but is of limited utility in providing adequate drainage of intrahepatic cysts. In contrast, PTC is more effective in draining these cysts and avoids recurrent episodes of cholangitis, especially if patients comply with periodic flushing and changing of drainage catheters. During episodes of acute cholangitis, patients may require courses of antibiotics and use ursodeoxycholic acid for severe cholestasis.[169] Rarely the cystic disease is confined to one hepatic lobe, and in this circumstance hepatic lobectomy may be curative. Although some have advocated

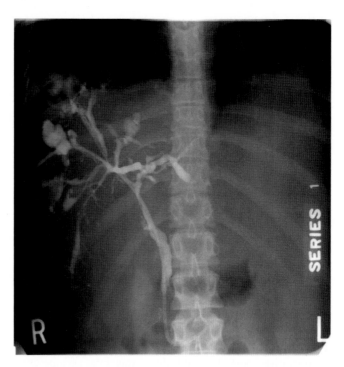

Fig. 67-20 Caroli disease. A cholangiogram demonstrates ectatic biliary ducts and saccular dilations of both intrahepatic and extrahepatic ducts.

hepaticojejunostomy after partial hepatectomy as the primary therapy, the long-term efficacy of this procedure is uncertain, and the extensive surgery could compromise the outcome from hepatic transplantation. There are three indications for hepatic transplantation in Caroli disease: hepatic decompensation, recurrent cholangitis that is unresponsive to endoscopic or radiologic interventions, and development of focal adenocarcinoma.[170]

Choledochal Cysts

Characteristics

Choledochal cysts are usually diagnosed in childhood but may remain silent and undetected until adulthood in up to 50% of patients.[171-173] Choledochal cysts are cystic dilations that may occur throughout the macroscopic intrahepatic and extrahepatic biliary tree. Although the term choledochal cyst has been used for any cystic dilation of the biliary tree, isolated choledochal cysts are usually restricted to only the common hepatic or bile duct. Despite the uncommon occurrence of choledochal cysts, there are hundreds of reports in the literature encompassing more than 3000 cases. Choledochal cyst is a rare condition in the Western hemisphere, but it is relatively more common among Japanese and other Asian populations. Several classifications of choledochal cysts have been proposed but the most commonly cited in the medical literature is by Todani (**Fig. 67-21**).[174] In this system, the most common is type I cyst, representing more than 80% of cases. The pattern of inheritance is unclear.

Clinical Features

The most common clinical presentation of choledochal cyst is a relatively young patient (child or adolescent) with pain, mass in the right upper quadrant or epigastrium, and jaundice. In

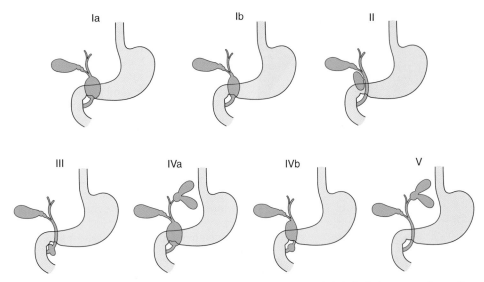

Fig. 67-21 Anatomic classification of choledochal cysts. The various anatomic types of choledochal cysts are shown. Type *Ia*, choledochal cyst; type *Ib*, segmental choledochal dilation; type *Ic*, diffuse or cylindric duct dilation (not shown); type *II*, extrahepatic duct diverticulum; type *III*, choledochocele; type *IVa*, multiple intrahepatic and extrahepatic duct cyst; type *IVb*, multiple extrahepatic duct cyst; type *V*, intrahepatic duct cyst (Caroli disease).

one series of 740 cases, jaundice was the most common and consistent presenting feature. In infants, jaundice is often the only sign and the disorder may be difficult to distinguish from biliary atresia. In the majority of the patients choledochal cysts have been diagnosed before the age of 30 years, and the male/female ratio in most series is about 1:4.

Reported complications include spontaneous and traumatic rupture. Rupture and increased levels of secondary bile acids may contribute to cyst metaplasia and carcinoma. The tumors may originate in different parts of the pancreatobiliary system, including liver, gallbladder, intrahepatic ducts, pancreatic ducts, and pancreas.

Diagnosis

The diagnosis of a choledochal cyst should be suspected when a patient has recurrent abdominal pain, jaundice, raised serum amylase, and cystic mass on imaging. Initial imaging of the biliary tree by ultrasonography or radioscintigraphy (HIDA scans) is usually diagnostic. Confirmation and anatomic definition may require CT, ERCP, or PTC (**Figs. 67-22 and 67-23**). Patients with extrahepatic choledochal cysts have an increased incidence of anomalous pancreaticobiliary junction, which requires ERCP when planning for excision of the cyst. In recent years, MRCP has shown to be equivalent to ERCP in detecting and defining not only choledochal cysts but also the presence of an anomalous union of the pancreatic and bile ducts. MRCP can also define the length of extrahepatic bile duct involved by the cyst, which is important when planning a surgical approach. Particularly in the pediatric population, MRCP offers an attractive noninvasive diagnostic alternative with the lack of ionizing radiation. Endoscopic ultrasonography has also been a useful imaging method for patients with suspected anomalous pancreaticobiliary junction. Prenatal ultrasonography can detect choledochal cysts in utero, which may help antenatal counseling because early neonatal cyst excision and duct revision may be required.

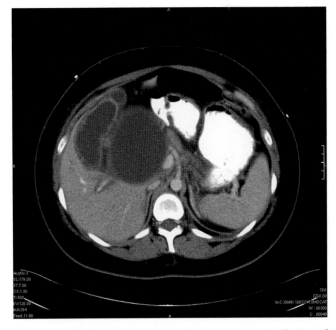

Fig. 67-22 Choledochal cyst. CT demonstrates cystic dilation of common hepatic duct near the gallbladder fossae.

Treatment

It is generally agreed that choledochal cysts require surgical treatment given their potential malignant risk. The preferred surgical treatment is complete cyst excision with Roux-en-Y hepaticojejunostomy.[171-176] This eliminates any opportunity for stasis, infection, stone formation, and possible development of cholangiocarcinoma. The procedure provides excellent long-term results with low morbidity and mortality,

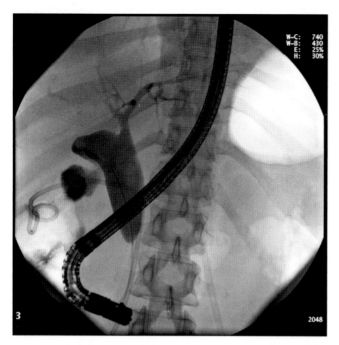

Fig. 67-23 **Choledochal cyst.** ERCP demonstrates a Todani type I choledochal cyst.

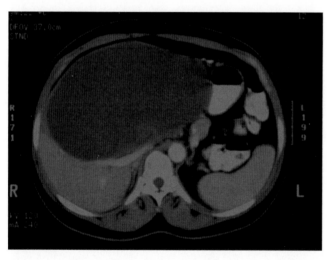

Fig. 67-24 **Solitary hepatic cyst.** CT demonstrates large solitary cyst in left lobe of liver.

but lifelong follow-up may be necessary to avoid potential problems, such as biliary cirrhosis. Internal cyst drainage procedures (cystoduodenostomy, cystojejunostomy) have often been unsatisfactory with a complication rate as high as 50%; this procedure may make transplantation difficult.

Solitary Hepatic Cyst

Characteristics

Solitary hepatic cysts are relatively common, usually asymptomatic, and most often discovered incidentally during the evaluation of abdominal symptoms or disorders (**Fig. 67-24**).[177] Exact prevalence of solitary hepatic cysts for the U.S.

population is unknown, but the female/male ratio is approximately 4:1. In a European study of 26,000 patients undergoing diagnostic ultrasonography, the prevalence of solitary hepatic cyst was 2.8%.[178] A Taiwanese study used ultrasonography in a large-scale screening program for simple hepatic cysts to explore age- and gender-specific prevalence.[179] A total of 3600 subjects underwent screening ultrasonography, and 156 simple hepatic cysts in 132 study subjects were detected. The overall prevalence was 3.6%. Prevalence increased with age, ranging from 0.83% below age 40 to 7.81% in subjects older than 60 years. The sizes of 219 hepatic cysts in 167 hospitalized patients were measured; 53% had diameters between 1 and 3 cm, and only 7% were larger than 5 cm. Cysts occurred more commonly in the right lobe and were twice as prevalent in women. All of these cysts were asymptomatic and none of the patients suffered clinical consequences.

Treatment

Asymptomatic solitary hepatic cysts are best managed conservatively. The preferred treatment of symptomatic cysts is ultrasound- or CT-guided percutaneous cyst aspiration followed by sclerotherapy.[146,177,180-182] This approach is more than 90% effective in controlling symptoms and ablating the cyst cavity. The recurrence rate after successful ablation is only 5% to 15%. If the radiologically guided, percutaneous approach is ineffective or unavailable, treatment may include either laparoscopic or open surgical cyst fenestration. The laparoscopic approach is increasingly used for anatomically accessible cysts and greater than 90% efficacy has been reported.

Key References

Alvaro D, et al. Alfa and beta estrogen receptors and the biliary tree. Mol Cell Endocrinol 2002;193:105–108. (Ref.66)

Alvaro D, et al. Estrogens and the pathophysiology of the biliary tree. World J Gastroenterol 2006;12:3537–3545. (Ref.67)

Alvaro D, et al. Morphological and functional features of hepatic cyst epithelium in autosomal dominant polycystic kidney disease. Am J Pathol 2008;172: 321–332. (Ref.68)

Ammori BJ, et al. Surgical strategy for cystic diseases of the liver in a western hepatobiliary center. World J Surg 2002;26:462–469. (Ref.181)

Amura CR, et al. CXCR2 agonists in APKD liver cyst fluids promote cell proliferation. Am J Physiol 2008;294:C786–C796. (Ref.82)

Amura CR, et al. VEGF receptor inhibition blocks liver cyst growth in pkd2(ws25/-) mice. Am J Physiol Cell Physiol 2007;293:C419–C428. (Ref.81)

Ananthakrishnan AN, Saeian K. Caroli's disease: identification and treatment strategy. Curr Gastroenterol Rep 2007;9:151–155. (Ref.169)

Awasthi A, et al. Morphological and immunohistochemical analysis of ductal plate malformation: correlation with fetal liver. Histopathology 2004;45: 260–267. (Ref.6)

Banales JM, et al. Hepatic cystogenesis is associated with abnormal expression and location of ion transporters and water channels in an animal model of autosomal recessive polycystic kidney disease. Am J Pathol 2008;173: 1637–1646. (Ref.105)

Banales JM, et al. The cAMP effectors Epac and protein kinase a (PKA) are involved in the hepatic cystogenesis of an animal model of autosomal recessive polycystic kidney disease (ARPKD). Hepatology 2009;49:160–174. (Ref.108)

Bhunia AK, et al. PKD1 induces p21(waf1) and regulation of the cell cycle via direct activation of the JAK-STAT signaling pathway in a process requiring PKD2. Cell 2002;109:157–168. (Ref.55)

Bogert PT, LaRusso NF. Cholangiocyte biology. Curr Opin Gastroenterol 2007; 23:299–305. (Ref.69)

Brodsky KS, et al. Liver cyst cytokines promote endothelial cell proliferation and development. Exp Biol Med (Maywood) 2009;234:1155–1165. (Ref.83)

Cantiello HF. Regulation of calcium signaling by polycystin-2. Am J Physiol 2004;286:F1012–F1029. (Ref.46)

Chauvet V, et al. Mechanical stimuli induce cleavage and nuclear translocation of the polycystin-1 c terminus. J Clin Invest 2004;114:1433–1443. (Ref.54)

Davila S, et al. Mutations in SEC63 cause autosomal dominant polycystic liver disease. Nat Genet 2004;36:575–577. (Ref.91)

Delmas P, et al. Constitutive activation of g-proteins by polycystin-1 is antagonized by polycystin-2. J Biol Chem 2002;277:11276–11283. (Ref.51)

Deltas CC. Mutations of the human polycystic kidney disease 2 (PKD2) gene. Hum Mutat 2001;18:13–24. (Ref.40)

Devuyst O, Persu A, Vo-Cong MT. Autosomal dominant polycystic kidney disease: modifier genes and endothelial dysfunction. Nephrol Dial Transplant 2003;18:2211–2215. (Ref.63)

Doctor RB, et al. Regulated ion transport in mouse liver cyst epithelial cells. Biochim Biophys Acta 2007;1772:345–354. (Ref.72)

Drenth JPH, et al. Germline mutations in PRKCSH are associated with autosomal dominant polycystic liver disease. Nat Genet 2003;33:345–347. (Ref.89)

Drenth JP, et al. Abnormal hepatocystin caused by truncating PRKCSH mutations leads to autosomal dominant polycystic liver disease. Hepatology 2004;39:924–931. (Ref.90)

Eriguchi N, et al. Treatments of non-parasitic giant hepatic cysts. Kurume Med J 2001;48:193–195. (Ref.127)

Everson GT, Taylor MR. Management of polycystic liver disease. Curr Gastroenterol Rep 2005;7:19–25. (Ref.136)

Everson GT, Taylor MR, Doctor RB. Polycystic disease of the liver. Hepatology 2004;40:774–782. (Ref.135)

Fabris L, et al. Effects of angiogenic factor overexpression by human and rodent cholangiocytes in polycystic liver diseases. Hepatology 2006;43:1001–1012. (Ref.78)

Fain PR, et al. Modifier genes play a significant role in the phenotypic expression of PKD1. Kidney Int 2005;67:1256–1267. (Ref.64)

Fliegauf M, Benzing T, Omran H. When cilia go bad: cilia defects and ciliopathies. Nat Rev Mol Cell Biol 2007;8:880–893. (Ref.14)

Gonzales-Perrett S, et al. Voltage dependence and pH regulation of human polycystin-2-mediated cation channel activity. J Biol Chem 2002;277:24959–24966. (Ref.43)

Gonzales-Perrett S, et al. Polycystin-2, the protein mutated in APKD, is a Ca^{2+}-permeable nonselective cation channel. Proc Natl Acad Sci U S A 2001;98:1182–1187. (Ref.42)

Gustafsson BI, et al. Liver transplantation for polycystic liver disease—indications and outcomes. Transplant Proc 2003;35:813–814. (Ref.159)

Guy F, et al. Caroli's disease: magnetic resonance imaging features. Eur Radiol 2002;12:2730–2736. (Ref.168)

Harris PC, Torres VE. Polycystic kidney disease. Annu Rev Med 2009;60:321–337. (Ref.16)

Hateboer N, et al. Location of mutations within the PKD2 gene influences clinical outcome. Kidney Int 2000;57:1444–1451. (Ref.41)

Hiesberger T, et al. Proteolytic cleavage and nuclear translocation of fibrocystin is regulated by intracellular Ca^{2+} and activation of protein kinase C. J Biol Chem 2006;281:34357–34364. (Ref.96)

Hoevenaren IA, et al. Polycystic liver: clinical characteristics of patients with isolated polycystic liver disease compared with patients with polycystic liver and autosomal dominant polycystic kidney disease. Liver Int 2008;28:264–270. (Ref.93)

Ibraghimov-Beskrovnaya O, et al. Strong homophilic interactions of the Ig-like domains of polycystin-1, the protein product of an APKD gene, PKD1. Hum Mol Genet 2000;9:1641–1649. (Ref.37)

Jordan PH Jr, et al. Some considerations for management of choledochal cysts. Am J Surg 2004;187:790–795. (Ref.171)

Kaimori JY, et al. Polyductin undergoes notch-like processing and regulated release from primary cilia. Hum Mol Genet 2007;16:942–956. (Ref.97)

Kim I, et al. Fibrocystin/polyductin modulates renal tubular formation by regulating polycystin-2 expression and function. J Am Soc Nephrol 2008;19:455–468. (Ref.100)

Koulen P, et al. Polycystin-2 is an intracellular calcium release channel. Nat Cell Biol 2002;4:191–197. (Ref.45)

Kuehn EW, Walz G. Prime time for polycystic kidney disease: does one shot of roscovitine bring the cure? Nephrol Dial Transplant 2007;22:2133–2135. (Ref.58)

Lee KF, Lai EC, Lai PB. Adult choledochal cyst. Asian J Surg 2005;28:29–33. (Ref.173)

Lee SO, et al. MicroRNA15a modulates expression of the cell-cycle regulator Cdc25a and affects hepatic cystogenesis in a rat model of polycystic kidney disease. J Clin Invest 2008;118:3714–3724. (Ref.59)

Levy AD, et al. Caroli's disease: radiologic spectrum with pathologic correlation. AJR Am J Roentgenol 2002;179:1053–1057. (Ref.119)

Li A, et al. Mutations in PRKCSH cause isolated autosomal dominant polycystic liver disease. Am J Hum Genet 2003;72:691–703. (Ref.88)

Malhas AN, Abuknesha RA, Price RG. Interaction of the leucine-rich repeats of polycystin-1 with extracellular matrix proteins: possible role in cell proliferation. J Am Soc Nephrol 2002;13:19–26. (Ref.36)

Masyuk AI, et al. Cholangiocyte primary cilia are chemosensory organelles that detect biliary nucleotides via p2y12 purinergic receptors. Am J Physiol Gastrointest Liver Physiol 2008;295:G725–G734. (Ref.13)

Masyuk AI, et al. Cholangiocyte cilia detect changes in luminal fluid flow and transmit them into intracellular Ca^{2+} and camp signaling. Gastroenterology 2006;131:911–920. (Ref.11)

Masyuk T, Masyuk A, LaRusso N. Cholangiociliopathies: genetics, molecular mechanisms and potential therapies. Curr Opin Gastroenterol 2009;25:265–271. (Ref.15)

Masyuk TV, et al. Biliary dysgenesis in the PCK rat, an orthologous model of autosomal recessive polycystic kidney disease. Am J Pathol 2004;165:1719–1730. (Ref.104)

Masyuk TV, et al. Defects in cholangiocyte fibrocystin expression and ciliary structure in the PCK rat. Gastroenterology 2003;125:1303–1310. (Ref.102)

Masyuk TV, et al. Octreotide inhibits hepatic cystogenesis in a rodent model of polycystic liver disease by reducing cholangiocyte adenosine 3',5'-cyclic monophosphate. Gastroenterology 2007;132:1104–1116. (Ref.109)

Muchatuta MN, et al. Structural and functional analyses of liver cysts from the BALB/c-cpk mouse model of polycystic kidney disease. Exp Biol Med (Maywood) 2009;234:17–27. (Ref.73)

Nardello O, et al. Dysplastic cysts of the liver: our experience. Minerva Chir 2004;59:351–362. (Ref.126)

Nauli SM, et al. Polycystins 1 and 2 mediate mechanosensation in the primary cilium of kidney. Nat Genet 2003;3:129–137. (Ref.48)

Nichols MT, et al. Secretion of cytokines and growth factors into autosomal dominant polycystic kidney disease liver cyst fluid. Hepatology 2004;40:836–846. (Ref.77)

Olsson AK, et al. VEGF receptor signalling—in control of vascular function. Nat Rev Mol Cell Biol 2006;7:359–371. (Ref.80)

Onuchic LF, et al. PKHD1, the polycystic kidney and hepatic disease 1 gene, encodes a novel large protein containing multiple immunoglobulin-like plexin-transcription-factor domains and parallel beta-helix 1 repeats. Am J Hum Genet 2002;70:1305–1317. (Ref.162)

Park F, et al. Chronic blockade of 20-HETE synthesis reduces polycystic kidney disease in an orthologous rat model of ARPKD. Am J Physiol Renal Physiol 2009;296:F575–F582. (Ref.106)

Perrone RD, Ruthazer R, Terrin NC. Survival after end-stage renal disease in autosomal dominant polycystic kidney disease: contribution of extrarenal complications to mortality. Am J Kidney Dis 2001;38:777–784. (Ref.138)

Petreaca ML, et al. Transactivation of vascular endothelial growth factor receptor-2 by interleukin-8 (IL-8/CXCL8) is required for IL-8/CXCL8-induced endothelial permeability. Mol Biol Cell 2007;8:5014–5023. (Ref.79)

Pirenne J, et al. Liver transplantation for polycystic liver disease. Liver Transpl 2001;7:238–245. (Ref.158)

Plata-Munoz JJ, et al. Complete resection of choledochal cyst with Roux-en-Y derivation vs. cyst-enterostomy as standard treatment of cystic disease of the biliary tract in the adult patient. Hepatogastroenterology 2005;52:13–16. (Ref.176)

Pozniczek M, et al. Sclerosant therapy as first-line treatment for solitary liver cysts. Dig Surg 2004;21:452–454. (Ref.180)

Praetorius HA, Spring KR. The renal cell primary cilium functions as a flow sensor. Curr Opin Nephrol Hypertens 2003;12:517–520. (Ref.12)

Qian Q, et al. Sirolimus reduces polycystic liver volume in APKD patients. J Am Soc Nephrol 2008;19:631–638. (Ref.62)

Robinson TN, Stiegmann GV, Everson GT. Laparoscopic palliation of polycystic liver disease. Surg Endosc 2005;19:130–132. (Ref.151)

Rossetti S, et al. The position of the polycystic kidney disease 1 (PKD1) gene mutation correlates with the severity of renal disease. J Am Soc Nephrol 2002;13:1230–1237. (Ref.34)

Rossetti S, et al. Association of mutation position in polycystic kidney disease 1 (PKD1) gene and development of a vascular phenotype. Lancet 2003;361:2196–2201. (Ref.33)

Rossetti S, et al. Comprehensive molecular diagnostics in autosomal dominant polycystic kidney disease. J Am Soc Nephrol 2007;18:2143–2160. (Ref.133)

Rossetti S, et al. Mutation analysis of the entire PKD1 gene: genetic and diagnostic implications. Am J Hum Genet 2001;68:46–63. (Ref.31)

Russell RT, Pinson CW. Surgical management of polycystic liver disease. World J Gastroenterol 2007;13:5052–5059. (Ref.152)

Sasaki M, et al. Intrahepatic cholangiocarcinoma arising in autosomal dominant polycystic kidney disease. Virchows Arch 2002;441:98–100. (Ref.113)

Sergi C, et al. Study of the malformation of ductal plate of the liver in Meckel syndrome and review of other syndromes presenting with this anomaly. Pediatr Dev Pathol 2000;3:568–583. (Ref.7)

Sgro M, et al. Caroli's disease: prenatal diagnosis, postnatal outcome and genetic analysis. Ultrasound Obstet Gynecol 2004;23:73–76. (Ref.164)

Shillingford JM, et al. The motor pathway is regulated by polycystin-1, and its inhibition reverses renal cystogenesis in polycystic kidney disease. Proc Natl Acad Sci U S A 2006;103:5466–5471. (Ref.60)

Spirli C, et al. Erk1/2-dependent vascular endothelial growth factor signaling sustains cyst growth in polycystin-2 defective mice. Gastroenterology 2010; 138:360–371, e367. (Ref.61)

Tagaya N, Nemoto T, Kubota K. Long-term results of laparoscopic unroofing of symptomatic solitary nonparasitic hepatic cysts. Surg Laparosc Endosc Percutan Tech 2003;13:76–79. (Ref.182)

Tahvanainen P, et al. Polycystic liver disease is genetically heterogeneous: clinical and linkage studies in eight Finnish families. J Hepatol 2003;38:39–43. (Ref.92)

Takei R, et al. Percutaneous transcatheter hepatic artery embolization for liver cysts in APKD. Am J Kidney Dis 2007;49:744–752. (Ref.85)

Tsiokas L. Function and regulation of TRPP2 at the plasma membrane. Am J Physiol Renal Physiol 2009;297:F1–F9. (Ref.18)

Ubara Y. New therapeutic option for autosomal dominant polycystic kidney disease patients with enlarged kidney and liver. Ther Apher Dial 2006;10: 333–341. (Ref.84)

van Keimpema L, Hockerstedt K. Treatment of polycystic liver disease. Br J Surg 2009;96:1379–1380. (Ref.147)

van Keimpema L, et al. Lanreotide reduces the volume of polycystic liver: a randomized, double-blind, placebo-controlled trial. Gastroenterology 2009; 137:1661–1668, e1661–e1662. (Ref.76)

Vassilev PM, et al. Polycystin-2 is a novel cation channel implicated in defective intracellular Ca²⁺ homeostasis in polycystic kidney disease. Biochem Biophys Res Comm 2001;282:341–350. (Ref.44)

Visser BC, et al. Congenital choledochal cysts in adults. Arch Surg 2004;139:855–860; discussion 860–862. (Ref.172)

Waanders E, et al. Secondary and tertiary structure modeling reveals effects of novel mutations in polycystic liver disease genes PRKCSH and SEC63. Clin Genet 2010;78:47–56. (Ref.134)

Waechter FL, et al. The role of liver transplantation in patients with Caroli's disease. Hepatogastroenterology 2001;48:672–674. (Ref.170)

Wang S, et al. Fibrocystin/polyductin, found in the same protein complex with polycystin-2, regulates calcium responses in kidney epithelia. Mol Cell Biol 2007;27:3241–3252. (Ref.99)

Ward CJ, et al. Cellular and subcellular localization of the ARPKD protein; fibrocystin is expressed on primary cilia. Hum Mol Genet 2003;12:2703–2710. (Ref.101)

Weston BS, Malhas AN, Price RG. Structure-function relationships of the extracellular domain of the APKD-associated protein, polycystin-1. FEBS Lett 2003;538:8–13. (Ref.35)

Woollard JR, et al. A mouse model of autosomal recessive polycystic kidney disease with biliary duct and proximal tubule dilatation. Kidney Int 2007;72:328–336. (Ref.103)

Wu Y, et al. Kinesin-2 mediates physical and functional interactions between polycystin-2 and fibrocystin. Hum Mol Genet 2006;15:3280–3292. (Ref.98)

Yamaguchi T, et al. Calcium restores a normal proliferation phenotype in human polycystic kidney disease epithelial cells. J Am Soc Nephrol 2006;17:178–187. (Ref.49)

Yamaguchi T, et al. Calcium restriction allows camp activation of the B-Raf/ERK pathway, switching cells to a cAMP-dependent growth-stimulated phenotype. J Biol Chem 2004;279:40419–40430. (Ref.56)

Yasoshima M, et al. Matrix proteins of basement membrane of intrahepatic bile ducts are degraded in congenital hepatic fibrosis and Caroli's disease. J Pathol 2009;217:442–451. (Ref.107)

Yoder BK, Hou X, Guay-Woodford LM. The polycystic kidney disease proteins, polycystin-2, polaris and cystin are co-localized in renal cilia. J Am Soc Nephrol 2002;13:2508–2516. (Ref.47)

Zeitoun D, et al. Congenital hepatic fibrosis: CT findings in 18 adults. Radiology 2004;231:109–116. (Ref.115)

Zhou J. Polycystins and primary cilia: primers for cell cycle progression. Annu Rev Physiol 2009;71:83–113. (Ref.17)

A complete list of references can be found at www.expertconsult.com.

Pediatric Cholestatic Syndromes

Deirdre Kelly

ABBREVIATIONS

α₁AT α₁-antitrypsin
ABC ATP-binding cassette
AGS Alagille syndrome
ASBT apical sodium-dependent bile acid transporter
ATP adenosine triphosphate
ATPase adenosine triphosphatase
BCAA branched-chain amino acid
BEC biliary epithelial cell
BRIC benign recurrent intrahepatic cholestasis
CMV cytomegalovirus
EHBA extrahepatic biliary atresia

ERCP endoscopic retrograde cholangiopancreatography
FIC1 familial intrahepatic cholestasis-1 protein
HDN hemorrhagic disease of the newborn
HLA human leukocyte antigen
ICAM1 intercellular adhesion molecule-1
JAG1 jagged-1 gene
MARS molecular absorbent recirculating system
MCT medium-chain triglyceride
MDR3 multidrug resistance-3 gene
MMR measles, mumps, and rubella

MRP2 multidrug resistance–associated protein-2
NCAM neural cell adhesion molecule
NSC neonatal sclerosing cholangitis
PCR polymerase chain reaction
PFIC progressive familial intrahepatic cholestasis
PN parenteral nutrition
PTC percutaneous transhepatic cholangiography
PUFA polyunsaturated fatty acid
VDRL Venereal Disease Research Laboratory

Introduction

Neonatal jaundice is common and transient in most normal infants. In the majority it is related to the immaturity of glucuronosyltransferase or to breastfeeding.[1] Conjugated hyperbilirubinemia, in contrast, is always significant and due to one of several underlying disorders. The most important of these disorders is extrahepatic biliary atresia (EHBA), the leading cause of morbidity and mortality of all the childhood liver diseases.[2] However, there are several other important causes of cholestasis in neonates that also benefit from early diagnosis. It is therefore important to distinguish between jaundice attributable to normal variation and that caused by disease. All infants with jaundice that occurs or persists after the age of 14 days require evaluation so that cholestasis can be recognized and appropriate investigations and management instituted promptly when necessary. This is especially pertinent for EHBA, for which early surgical treatment is vital.

Recent advances have been made in our understanding of the etiology and pathogenesis of many causes of cholestasis. These advances, together with improved investigative techniques and management strategies, have improved not only the accuracy of diagnosis but also the outcome for many children. This is of major importance because a number of cholestatic syndromes that occur in infancy can lead to significant childhood illness and, in some cases, to end-stage liver disease.

These conditions can be divided into disorders of a primarily extrahepatic or intrahepatic nature (**Table 68-1**). Extrahepatic disorders include EHBA, choledochal cyst, spontaneous perforation of the bile duct, bile or mucous plugs, or indeed, a mass compressing the extrahepatic biliary tree. Intrahepatic ones include bile duct paucity syndromes, progressive familial intrahepatic cholestasis (PFIC), inborn errors of bile metabolism, anatomic disorders such as Caroli disease, and certain metabolic disorders, including α₁-antitrypsin (α₁AT) deficiency and cystic fibrosis. The most common intrahepatic disorders come under the heading of neonatal hepatitis, for which many causes, often infectious, have now been elucidated. In this chapter the more common causes of cholestatic syndromes are discussed.

Clinical Manifestations

Cholestasis occurring in early infancy may be due to any of several causes. Diagnosis is usually not possible on clinical grounds alone, although the history and physical examination are important in differentiating among major types of disorders (see **Table 68-1**).

The most pressing need is to distinguish EHBA from other causes of cholestasis, most often from neonatal hepatitis. In

Table 68-1 Causes of Infantile Cholestatic Syndromes

I. Extrahepatic abnormalities
  A. Extrahepatic biliary atresia (EHBA)
  B. Choledochal cyst
  C. Caroli disease
  D. Neonatal sclerosing cholangitis
  E. Spontaneous perforation of the bile duct
  F. Bile plug syndrome/inspissated bile syndrome
  G. Agenesis of the extrahepatic bile ducts
  H. Bile duct stenosis
  I. Duplication of the biliary tree
  J. Bile duct tumors
  K. Agenesis of the extrahepatic bile ducts
  L. Gallstones
  M. Extramural compression of the common bile duct
II. Intrahepatic disorders
  A. Neonatal hepatitis syndrome
    1. Intrauterine infection
      a. Toxoplasmosis
      b. Rubella
      c. Cytomegalovirus
      d. Herpes simplex
      e. Varicella-zoster
      f. Syphilis
      g. Parvovirus B19
      h. Paramyxovirus
      i. Coxsackievirus
      j. Reovirus type 3
      k. Echovirus
      l. Adenovirus
      m. Human immunodeficiency virus
      n. Human herpesvirus-6
      o. Hepatitis B virus
      p. Listeriosis
      q. Tuberculosis
    2. Endocrine
      a. Hypopituitarism
      b. Hypothyroidism
    3. Chromosomal
      a. Trisomy 18
      b. Trisomy 13

    c. Trisomy 21
    d. Cat's eye syndrome
    4. Idiopathic
  B. Syndromic
    1. Alagille syndrome
    2. Arthrogryphosis renal dysfunction cholestasis (ARC) (VPS33B)
    3. Hereditary cholestasis with lymphedema (Aagenaes syndrome)
  C. Progressive familial intrahepatic cholestasis (PFIC)
    1. PFIC1
    2. Benign recurrent intrahepatic cholestasis (BRIC)
    3. PFIC2
    4. PFIC3
  D. Inborn errors of bile acid metabolism
    1. 3β-Δ^5-C27-hydroxysteroid oxoreductase deficiency
    2. Δ^4-3-Oxosteroid-5β-reductase deficiency
    3. 3β-Hydroxy-Δ^5-steroid dehydrogenase isomerase deficiency
    4. Zellweger syndrome (cerebrohepatorenal syndrome) and other peroxisomal disorders
    5. Microfilament dysfunction
  E. Metabolic disorders
    1. Disorders of lipid metabolism
      a. Wolman disease
      b. Niemann-Pick C disease
      c. Gaucher disease
    2. Disorders of carbohydrate metabolism
      a. Galactosemia
      b. Fructosemia
      c. Glycogenosis III/IV
    3. Metabolic disease (other)
      a. α_1-Antitrypsin (α_1AT) deficiency
      b. Cystic fibrosis
      c. Familial erythrophagocytic lymphohistiocytosis
  F. Intestinal failure–associated liver disease

EHBA, the baby is most often born at term with normal birth weight, whereas a child with neonatal hepatitis or α_1AT deficiency often has low birth weight and may be premature. Jaundice may be present soon after birth and certainly by 4 weeks of age and is associated with the development of completely acholic (clay-colored) stools. In some babies, associated situs inversus or cardiac or renal abnormalities may also alert the clinician to the possibility of EHBA, whereas the abnormal facies associated with Alagille syndrome (AGS) may be present in both infants and parents. A family history of cardiac or renal problems points to AGS as opposed to EHBA. Other dysmorphic features are suggestive of neonatal hepatitis.

Timing of the onset of jaundice, whether present from birth or late in onset, is important. Intermittent jaundice is seen in those with familial intrahepatic cholestasis and choledochal cysts.

A detailed antenatal and birth history revealing an infectious episode or fever during pregnancy is sometimes noted in infants with neonatal hepatitis. A family history, including consanguinity and previous neonatal or in utero deaths, is more indicative of a possible metabolic disorder. Cardiac or renal problems in family members may indicate AGS.

Examination often reveals pale stools and dark urine. Completely acholic stools indicate EHBA, although occasionally

those with AGS have very similar findings, and thus careful investigation is required to distinguish the two to avoid unnecessary laparotomy.

Hepatosplenomegaly is seen in late manifestations of EHBA but earlier with neonatal hepatitis, especially when there is an infectious cause. An intraabdominal mass may be present in those with a choledochal cyst.

Investigations

Because the clinical manifestations of many of these disorders are similar, investigation needs to exclude both serious and common causes of cholestasis (see **Table 68-1**).

Extrahepatic Disorders
Extrahepatic Biliary Atresia

Incidence
The incidence of EHBA in 1963 was reported to be 1 in 25,000. In recent reviews the incidence has been reported to be 1 in 20,000 in metropolitan France,[3] 1 in 16,700 in England,[4] 1 in

3500 live births in French Polynesia,[3] and between 1 in 2500 and 1 in 8000 in Soweto.[5] EHBA occurs more frequently in girls than in boys.[6]

Etiology

Extrahepatic biliary atresia is defined as an idiopathic, localized, complete obliteration or discontinuity of the hepatic or common bile ducts at any point in the extrahepatic biliary tract from the porta hepatis to the duodenum, and it results in complete obstruction to bile flow.[6]

The etiology remains obscure. It is unlikely to be an inherited disorder, except perhaps in a very small minority of cases.[7] There is little evidence of classic genetic inheritance of biliary atresia (BA). Thus it rarely occurs within families, and in twins it is rarely concordant.[8] Exceptional cases have been reported, including one North American Indian family with affected dizygotic twins and another sibling[9] and apparent vertical inheritance in which a mother with corrected type 3 BA gave birth to a baby with type 1 BA.[10]

Human leukocyte antigen (HLA)-identical twins are seen who are discordant for EHBA.[11] A single study reported an increase in HLA-B12 in individuals with BA that was three times that of controls in a European population, but these findings have not been replicated. Associations with HLACw4/7[12] and, in Japan, with A33, B44, and DR6[13] have been reported. However, two further studies did not detect any HLA association. The most recent study reported a significant increase in HLA-B8 and HLA-DR3 in 18 Egyptian children with EHBA.[14] This is of particular interest inasmuch as both these HLA subtypes are associated with primary sclerosing cholangitis and inflammatory bowel disease.

Initially, a seasonal variation was reported,[15] but the actual results are conflicting, with one recent large study of 119 Japanese infants with BA failing to show any evidence of seasonal clustering.[16]

No association was found among smoking, maternal age, education, alcohol use, folic acid, gravidity, parity, income, infant sex, preterm birth, infant birth weight, and plurality.[15]

Environmental toxins have produced a picture similar to EHBA in sheep, but no such evidence has been found in humans.[17]

Several studies looking for the presence of viral agents have been carried out. Viruses that may be etiologically implicated in EHBA include reovirus and rotavirus C, and they have been suggested to provoke an immune reaction with an inflammatory response.

In a mouse model, 2-day-old mice were injected with rotavirus RRV and SA11-FM strains, and jaundice with hepatic histology similar to EHBA developed.[18,19] Similar findings have been found with reovirus and cytomegalovirus (CMV) inoculation in mice. Serologic studies have also suggested an increased incidence of reovirus in patients with BA,[20] but this finding was not confirmed by polymerase chain reaction (PCR) techniques in liver tissue.[21]

Rotavirus C is also of the Reoviridae family. Reverse transcriptase–PCR for rotavirus C in hepatobiliary tissues showed positivity in 50% of livers with EHBA and none in control livers,[22] and a mouse model of EHBA induced by rotavirus infection has also been developed,[23] thus further supporting the idea that viral infection plays a role in the etiopathogenesis of this condition.

Although it is unlikely that EHBA is directly caused by viruses, it is possible that viral infection may have been the trigger for an inflammatory reaction in which viruses such as reovirus induce the expression of tumor necrosis factor (TNF)-related apoptosis–inducing ligand (TRAIL) in human biliary epithelial cells (BECs). This innate immune response is activated by the virus and leads to cell apoptosis and death.[24]

Clinically, CMV infection in infants with BA has a more severe clinical course and may represent a second hit in a liver already susceptible to damage through genetic or immunologic dysregulation.[25]

About 20% of patients with EHBA have associated anomalies or malformations.[26] These are divided into three groups: one (29%) with anomalies within the laterality sequence, including polysplenia or asplenia, cardiovascular defects, abdominal situs inversus, intestinal malrotation, and anomalies of the portal vein and hepatic artery; the second (59%) with single or dual anomalies involving the cardiac, gastrointestinal, and urinary systems not following a recognizable pattern; and a third, smaller group (12%) with intestinal malrotation and some similarity to the laterality sequence group. This last group may represent a more limited phenotypic result of faulty situs determination.[26] Davenport and colleagues studied the splenic malformation syndrome by analyzing the case records of 308 infants with EHBA for extrahepatic anomalies.[27] Twenty-three (7.5%) had polysplenia and four had other splenic malformations (two with a double spleen and two with asplenia). The presence of other anomalies such as situs inversus and portal vein anomalies suggested that they formed part of a larger association, for which they proposed the term biliary atresia splenic malformation syndrome as a distinct subgroup of patients with EHBA who tended to have a worse prognosis and required special attention to vascular anatomy at transplantation.

Other reported extrahepatic anomalies in EHBA include intestinal malrotation with partial abdominal heterotaxia and craniofacial anomalies; esophageal, duodenal, and pancreatic atresia; anorectal and esophageal atresia; and Kabuki syndrome.

EHBA with abnormalities in laterality might prove a suitable candidate for a major gene mutation, but the data thus far are limited. A mutation in the inversin (inv) gene in the mouse leads to anomalous development of the hepatobiliary system.[28] The human inv gene has recently been mapped, but no consistent mutations were found in 64 patients with heterotaxia, and specifically there were no mutations in 7 patients with EHBA and various congenital laterality defects.[29] Mutations in the CFC1 gene encoding for the human CRYPTIC protein have also been examined. The precise function of CRYPTIC is unknown, but it appears to be a co-factor in the Nodal pathway, which determines left-right axis development. Bamford and associates studied 144 patients with laterality defects.[30] Of nine with heterozygous mutations in the CRYPTIC gene, one had EHBA and polysplenia syndrome. Jacquemin and co-workers further identified two brothers with laterality defects, one with EHBA who had heterozygous gene mutations in CFC1.[31] However, although these findings are interesting, they do not represent the major underlying cause of EHBA, and teratogenic, infectious, and polygenic multifactorial causes may play a more significant role in EHBA associated with "nonsyndromic" organ system anomalies.

Morphologic abnormalities as a result of defective development of the biliary tree have also been suggested to play a role in the development of EHBA. The occurrence of ductal plate malformation of the intrahepatic bile ducts has been reported in up to 38% of patients with EHBA.[32] Early severe forms of EHBA suggest an antenatal onset of the disease process. Developmental anomalies of the intrahepatic bile ducts in EHBA include a report of EHBA in association with Caroli disease and the combination of common hepatic duct stricture (possibly a forme fruste of EHBA) and histologic congenital hepatic fibrosis. It has been proposed that EHBA may be caused by failure of remodeling of the ductal plate at the liver hilum, with the persistence of fetal bile ducts poorly supported by mesenchyme.[33] Bile leakage from these abnormal ducts may trigger an inflammatory reaction with subsequent obliteration of the biliary tree. Hepatic innervation is also abnormal in individuals with EHBA: neural cell adhesion molecule (NCAM)-positive and S100-positive nerve fibers were found to be increased near branches of the hepatic artery and portal vein, whereas no nerve fibers were observed around the bile ducts and periportal ductules that themselves became NCAM positive.[34] The possibility of cell signaling proteins and transcription factors involved in bile duct development being altered in EHBA has also begun to be explored. Jagged1, a ligand for the Notch signaling pathway that is involved in cell fate decisions and regulates cellular differentiation and proliferation, is known to be mutated in patients with AGS. Recent studies suggest that it may also play a role as a modifying factor in EHBA.[35,36] This may be via its effect on Hes1. Hes1 is a basic helix-loop-helix protein encoded by the gene *Hes1* whose expression is controlled by the Notch pathway. Hes1 is expressed in extrahepatic biliary epithelium throughout development. A recent study has demonstrated that Hes1-deficient mice have gallbladder agenesis and severe hypoplasia of the extrahepatic bile ducts.[37] Another basic helix-loop-helix protein regulated by Notch is Hex, which is important in the regulation of liver development in the zebrafish. Murine knockouts of hnf6, a transcription factor also important in early liver development, cause a ductal plate malformation associated with abnormalities of the hepatic artery, thus highlighting a link in vascular and biliary development.[38] Newly formed bile ducts in utero are in very close proximity to branches of the hepatic artery, and it has been suggested that a vasculopathy related to insufficient vascularization of the biliary tree may be the primary lesion in patients with EHBA. In support of this proposal, experimental atresia of bile ducts can be induced in fetal rabbits and sheep by ligation of the hepatic artery or its branches. Definite proof of an ischemic origin in human EHBA, however, is lacking.

In several cholestatic liver diseases there is marked formation of abnormal ductular reactive cells. In EHBA this is especially prominent with an increase in cells similar to those seen in formation of the ductal plate in utero.[6] Cytokeratin studies have been performed to determine the nature of bile duct formation and compared with patterns of cytokeratin expression in EHBA. These studies have demonstrated that the ductular reactive cells in EHBA have an immature phenotype, are flattened and smaller than mature BECs, and stain not only for cytokeratins 8, 18, and 19 but also for cytokeratin 7, which is normally present only on developing BECs from 20 weeks' gestation until shortly after birth.[39] The ductular reactive cells occurring in persons with cholestasis also display certain neuroendocrine features, including the presence of NCAM, not seen on normal BECs but also associated with a more primitive phenotype.[40] This finding further highlights the possibility of abnormalities in ductal plate formation in EHBA.

Progression of disease in patients with EHBA seems to involve an immunologically mediated mechanism of recruitment and activation of various immune factors, including T-lymphocyte and macrophage activation, which may have a role in the continued inflammation. Both CD4[+] lymphocytes and CD56[+] natural killer (NK) cells are increased in the livers of patients with EHBA.[41] Increased macrophage infiltration may also be associated with a poorer outcome.[41]

A characteristic histologic feature is an inflammatory response within both the liver and the systemic circulation. This response is seen as a periductal infiltrate of mononuclear cells with expression of HLA-DR on vascular and biliary epithelium and expression of a variety of intracellular adhesion molecules (e.g., ICAM-1, E-selectin).[41] In the latter there are elevated levels of soluble inflammatory adhesion molecules and cytokines (e.g., interleukin-2 [IL-2], IL-18, and TNF-α) that persist despite apparently successful surgery.[42] Lymphocyte-mediated biliary inflammation may be the mechanism for the bile duct damage in BA, although the trigger remains unknown.

Gene expression microarrays of RNA from extrahepatic biliary tissue and gallbladders from rotavirus-induced murine models of BA and from humans have demonstrated up-regulation of many genes regulating immunity.[43,44] Specifically, the interferon (IFN) inducer *Irf7* and *Irf9* genes were identified in the early stages of disease, with IFN-γ and IFN-γ–activated genes being more obvious at the time of bile duct obstruction. These findings suggest that up-regulation of proinflammatory genes may play a regulatory role in the pathogenesis of BA.[43] Microarray gene expression analysis of human BA samples has also shown overexpression of immune regulatory genes, specifically the transcription factor binding sites of the nuclear factor-κB (NF-κB)/c-Rel family of genes.[45]

Bile duct damage may be secondary to apoptosis from the synergistic role of IFN-γ and TNF-α.[46] Inflammatory cytokines such as IL-2, IL-12 IFN-γ, and TNF-α are up-regulated in patients with BA,[47] as are Kupffer cells, NK cells, CD3[+] and CD8[+] T cells, and lymphocyte chemokine receptor CXCR3[+] cells.[48] Oligoclonal expansion of CD4[+] and CD8[+] T cells within the liver and extrahepatic bile ducts suggests that there may be a response to specific antigenic stimulation.[47]

In the rotavirus mouse model, EHBA was more likely to develop when the type I IFN receptor was inactivated, thus implying that immune deregulation may play a role.[49]

It has also been suggested that an alloimmune process similar to graft-versus-host disease (GVHD) may occur with maternal microchimerism following the discovery of increased maternal chimeric CD8[+] T cells in EHBA liver cells.[50,51]

In conclusion, EHBA probably represents a common phenotype induced by diverse triggering and pathogenetic mechanisms. These mechanisms are presumably multifactorial in most instances. The resulting obliteration of variable segments of the biliary tree leads to cholestasis, which involves retention of potentially toxic hydrophobic bile salts and proliferation of reactive ductules producing several cytokines.[6] Retention of chenodeoxycholic acid (or other toxic bile acids) induces hepatocyte apoptosis and necrosis. Bile acids appear to have an impact on mitochondrial function (with altered oxidative metabolism and release of oxygen free radicals). It has been proposed that the sequence of mitochondrial injury, oxidant stress, adenosine triphosphate (ATP) depletion, increased cytosolic free calcium, and activation of degradative hydrolases leads to bile salt–induced hepatocellular injury.[6] Hepatocytes, in turn, may release additional factors that stimulate fibrosis. The fibrotic process is enhanced by profibrogenic cytokines released from proliferating ductules. The evolving processes of parenchymal injury and regeneration in a fibrosing environment finally result in secondary biliary cirrhosis.

Pathogenesis

Two theories of disease progression in EHBA have been proposed. It has been considered a congenital anomaly because of failure of recanalization of the bile duct, thought to be occluded by proliferating epithelial cells early in fetal life. Alternatively, it is thought to be due to progressive destruction of developed extrahepatic and even intrahepatic bile ducts by an inflammatory process of unspecified nature.[6] The latter is now taken to be the most likely. This has led to a change in emphasis to EHBA being an acquired disorder. Landing proposed the concept of infantile obstructive cholangiopathy based on the histologic similarity of liver lesions in patients with neonatal hepatitis, EHBA, and choledochal cyst.[52] This suggests that EHBA may be the result of a cholangiopathic process that starts in postnatal life in most cases because of an inflammatory process that destroys liver parenchymal cells and bile duct epithelium with subsequent obliteration of bile duct lumina. This concept has had a great impact on subsequent literature on the subject, but it is still a hypothesis. Its main merit is in stimulating thought about EHBA as an acquired progressive and destructive process. However, when considering EHBA as a postnatally acquired disorder, the subgroup of patients with associated malformations and the minority of patients with a familial aspect must be taken into account. Thus it may be that there are two types of EHBA, a fetal-embryonic form and a perinatally or postnatally acquired form of the disease.[6] The fetal-embryonic form is characterized clinically by an early onset of jaundice and no jaundice-free interval, with physiologic jaundice in the newborn changing into a pathologic, conjugated hyperbilirubinuria in the second or third week of life. This has been taken as evidence that atresia of the bile ducts commences in the embryonic or fetal period in this subgroup of patients. These patients have a poorer prognosis.[6]

The more common perinatal or postnatal form of EHBA is characterized clinically by a jaundice-free period after birth. This often lasts only a few days, but in some cases it may be as long as several weeks. Bile duct remnants may be demonstrated in this group as segments with epithelium-lined lumina or epithelial clusters. Other malformations are not seen. At present, the distinction between two clinical forms of EHBA is generally accepted.[6]

Pathology of the Extrahepatic Biliary Tree
Macroscopic

There are several anatomic variants of EHBA. These variants range from total absence of the system at one extreme to complete normality at the other, with presence or absence and stenosis or patency of all or any parts in between.

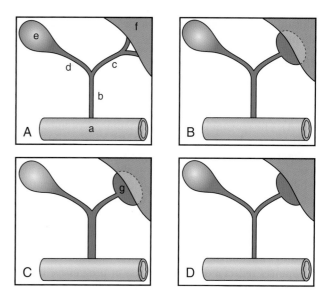

Fig. 68-1 Three main anatomic types of extrahepatic biliary atresia (EHBA). A, Type I. The common bile duct is partially or completely occluded or is reduced to a fibrous cord, with the more proximal extrahepatic bile duct segments left intact. **B,** Type IIa. The common hepatic duct is obliterated. There may also be atresia of its main branches. The common bile duct and cystic duct are patent, and the gallbladder is intact. Bile ducts at the porta hepatis are dilated. **C,** Type IIb. The common bile duct and hepatic and cystic ducts are obliterated. The gallbladder is not involved. The bile ducts at the porta hepatis are dilated. **D,** Type III. The common, hepatic, and cystic ducts are obliterated. There are no ducts that can be anastomosed at the porta hepatis. A prehilar fibrous cone is present. Types I, IIa, and IIb represent approximately 10% of cases of EHBA. The majority are type III. *a,* duodenum; *b,* common bile duct; *c,* common hepatic duct; *d,* cystic duct; *e,* gallbladder; *f,* liver; *g,* cystically dilated ducts at the porta hepatis *(Modified from Schweizer P, Müller G. Cholestase-syndrome im Neugeborenen und Säuglingsalter. Stuttgart: Hippokrates Verlag, 1984.)*

Kasai proposed a classification of the numerous observed anatomic variants that features three main types[53] (**Fig. 68-1**); the classification distinguishes between correctable forms (in which only part of the extrahepatic tree is involved and anastomosis of the remaining bile ducts is possible) and uncorrectable ones. Type I corresponds to atresia of the common bile duct, whereas the more proximal extrahepatic bile duct segments are intact. Type IIa represents obliteration of the common hepatic duct with or without atresia of its main branches; the common bile duct, cystic duct, and gallbladder are normal. Reanastomosis in this type of EHBA is performed through cystically dilated ducts near the porta hepatis. Type IIb also belongs to the correctable category, although all main branches of the extrahepatic system of bile ducts (common duct, hepatic ducts, and cystic ducts) are obliterated or missing. Reanastomosis with the duodenum is possible through cystically dilated ducts in the hilum, but the value of this type of corrective surgery has been questioned. Unfortunately, the correctable types I, IIa, and IIb are found in fewer than 10% of all patients with EHBA, with 90% or more patients belonging to type III, which represents noncorrectable BA (i.e., lack of or atresia of the common, hepatic, and cystic ducts). There are no cystically dilated hilar ducts that can be used for anastomosis in patients with type III. Frequently, a peculiar prehilar fibrous cone is present. The gallbladder is involved in the atretic process in about 80% of patients.

Microscopic

The diagnosis of EHBA is confirmed by identifying complete fibrous obliteration of at least part of the extrahepatic biliary tree. Usually, only a segment is reduced to a fibrous cord (**Fig. 68-2, A**). The remaining parts reveal remnants of lumina and inflammatory changes (see **Fig. 68-2, B**). The variable histologic appearances have been categorized into three or four types,[54] depending on the presence or absence of a lumen lined by biliary epithelium and the presence or absence of inflammatory infiltration (see **Fig. 68-2, C and D**). In a proportion of specimens the lumen is filled either with cellular debris and macrophages containing bile or with a biliary concrement. In other instances the lumen appears free but narrowed by surrounding inflammatory tissue. These variable histologic appearances reflect a dynamic process of progressive inflammatory destruction of the extrahepatic bile ducts, with the degree of fibrous obliteration increasing with increasing age of the patient, in parallel with increasing fibrosis in the liver.

The earliest stage corresponds to periductal inflammation with necrosis and sloughing of the epithelial lining, followed by progressive periductal fibrosis and narrowing of the lumen. The end stage is a complete fibrous scar of a destroyed epithelium-lined tube that remains identifiable as a fibrous cord in which the collagen texture is denser than the surrounding connective tissue. The most advanced stage of complete obliteration is frequently seen at the distal end of the common hepatic duct,[54] whereas the more proximal segments and the prehepatic fibrous cone often show the early stages of inflammatory destruction. This has led to the hypothesis that the lesion represents an ascending progressive inflammatory process.[54]

Clinical Features

The clinical course of EHBA is that of an unremitting, progressive jaundice. The patient is usually born at term with a normal birth weight. Jaundice is typically present from shortly after birth, often continuous with physiologic jaundice. There may be some variability in intensity; however, jaundice can readily be identified in affected infants by 4 weeks of age. Yellow or dark urine with increasingly pale stools, which eventually become acholic, is noted, although initially there may be variation in stool color, which may be confusing.

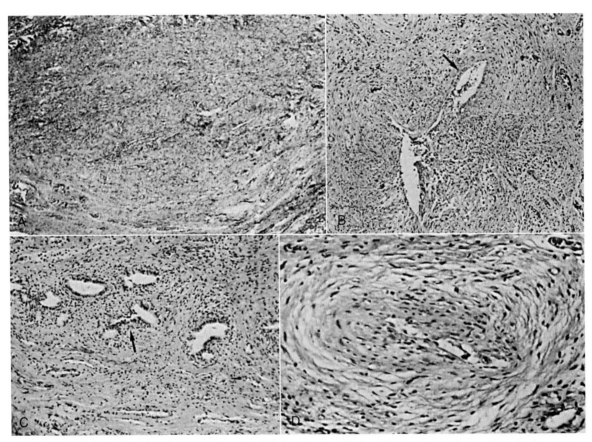

Fig. 68-2 **The four histologic types of fibrous remnant of the extrahepatic bile duct seen in extrahepatic biliary atresia. A,** No remaining extrahepatic bile duct. Instead, the bile duct is replaced by dense fibrous connective tissue. (Hematoxylin and eosin stain [H & E stain], ×64.) **B,** A cluster of small epithelium-lined tubes lies embedded in connective tissue, which shows inflammatory cell infiltration and the beginnings of fibrosis. Note the degenerative changes (e.g., nuclear pyknosis) *(arrow)* in part of the lining epithelial cells. (H & E stain, ×128.) **C,** Most of the lining bile duct epithelium is destroyed; some segments remain *(arrow)*. A lumen can still be recognized, but it is surrounded by granulation-like tissue rich in fibroblasts and inflammatory cells. (H & E stain, ×160.) **D,** The epithelial lining of the duct has virtually disappeared. A slitlike lumen surrounded by concentric fibrosis is still discernible. Collapse of the lumen and further fibrosis would lead to the formation of a fibrous cord. (H & E stain, ×40.)

Table 68-2 Differentiating Features of Neonatal Cholestatic Liver Disorders

INITIAL FEATURES	DIFFERENTIAL DIAGNOSIS
Intrauterine growth retardation, prematurity	α_1-Antitrypsin deficiency Neonatal hepatitis Alagille syndrome
Intermittent jaundice	PFIC Choledochal cyst
Cardiovascular abnormalities	"Syndromic" EHBA Alagille syndrome
Renal abnormalities	Alagille syndrome "Syndromic" EHBA
Microcephaly	Hypopituitarism Neonatal hepatitis
Hypoglycemia	Hypopituitarism Metabolic liver disease
Abnormal facies	Alagille syndrome Hypopituitarism Chromosomal disorders (e.g., Down syndrome)

EHBA, extrahepatic biliary atresia; PFIC, progressive familial intrahepatic cholestasis

Atypical findings may be seen. Prematurity has been reported as a more frequent feature in a recent epidemiologic study from New York.[55]

It is important to differentiate EHBA from other causes of neonatal cholestasis to prevent unnecessary surgery (**Table 68-2**). Neonatal hepatitis, α_1AT deficiency, and AGS in particular often have similar findings as EHBA. There are, however, features that may distinguish them from EHBA (see **Table 68-1**).

Findings on examination of patients with EHBA include hepatomegaly with a firm liver. Splenomegaly is a late sign. Failure to thrive despite adequate feeding is due to the high nutritional requirements and fat malabsorption in such infants.

Around 30% have associated cardiovascular anomalies (ventricular or atrial septal defects). Polysplenia syndrome, including a preduodenal portal vein, situs inversus, absence of the inferior vena cava, and malrotation, is also well recognized. Vitamin K–responsive coagulopathy is more common in breastfed infants who did not receive vitamin K at birth. Ascites and pruritus are late complications indicating progression to cirrhosis.

Late diagnosis is still a problem because of neonatal jaundice being wrongly ascribed to physiologic or breast milk jaundice. In an attempt to reduce this problem there have been several awareness campaigns, including the yellow-baby alert in the United Kingdom and pilot schemes using color charts to detect acholic stools.

Specific Investigations

The aim of investigations is to establish atresia of the extrahepatic ducts and at the same time to exclude alternative diagnoses (see **Tables 68-1 and 68-2**). Prompt investigation is vital so that if possible, surgery can be carried out before the age of 8 weeks.

Liver Function

1. Serum conjugated bilirubin at initial evaluation ranges from 40 to 200 μmol/L (normal range, <15 μmol/L).
2. Serum aminotransferases are always abnormal; concentrations of aspartate aminotransferase (AST) and alanine aminotransferase (ALT) are typically in the range of 80 to 200 U/L (normal range, <50 U/L).
3. Serum alkaline phosphatase is usually elevated to higher than 1000 U/L (normal range, 150 to 700 U/L) because of biliary damage or rickets.
4. γ-Glutamyltransferase (GGT) is usually elevated (10× normal).
5. Serum albumin is generally normal.
6. Cholesterol may be elevated but triglycerides are normal.
7. The prothrombin time is normal, although 5% to 10% of patients have vitamin K–responsive coagulopathy.
8. Blood glucose is typically normal.

Ultrasound Scan of the Abdomen

Abdominal ultrasonography is performed after a 4-hour fast and may not demonstrate a gallbladder or only a contracted gallbladder. Rarely, a dilated extrahepatic biliary tree is seen, consistent with distal, correctable atresia; dilated intrahepatic bile ducts are uncommonly found. Polysplenia with situs inversus and any renal abnormalities can be seen, as well as abnormal vascular anatomy consistent with polysplenia syndrome.

Recently, newer ultrasound techniques have been developed and two novel findings have been reported that may be of more diagnostic significance. Choi and co-authors reported the triangular cord sign as being specific for EHBA.[56] This is a unique triangular or tubular echogenic density representing the fibrous cone of a bile duct remnant at the porta hepatis. Overall results show 98% specificity and 80% sensitivity. A further study using a higher-frequency transducer (13 MHz as opposed to 7 MHz) identified abnormalities in gallbladder shape, wall thickness, and morphology that are characteristic of EHBA.[57]

Hepatobiliary Scanning Using DISIDA or TBIDA

Hepatobiliary scintigraphy with DISIDA (diisopropyliminodiacetic acid) or TBIDA (trimethylbromoiminoacetic acid) excludes the diagnosis of EHBA when biliary excretion of isotope into the intestine is demonstrated. If it fails to demonstrate passage of the radiolabeled substance into the intestinal tract over a 24-hour period, EHBA is likely. However, though about 95% sensitive, the results are not 100% specific and patients with cystic fibrosis, severe neonatal hepatitis, and bile duct paucity syndromes may fail to excrete isotope into the intestine. Phenobarbital induction, with at least 3 days' pretreatment (5 mg/kg/day for 3 to 5 days), is now used to promote excretion of isotope and thus increase the specificity of the test.

Percutaneous Liver Biopsy

Biopsy is essential and has high diagnostic specificity. Features of bile duct obstruction, such as proliferation of bile ductules, bile plugs in small bile ducts, and portal tract edema, are usually obvious, along with variable fibrosis and some giant cell transformation (**Fig. 68-3**). The earlier the liver biopsy is

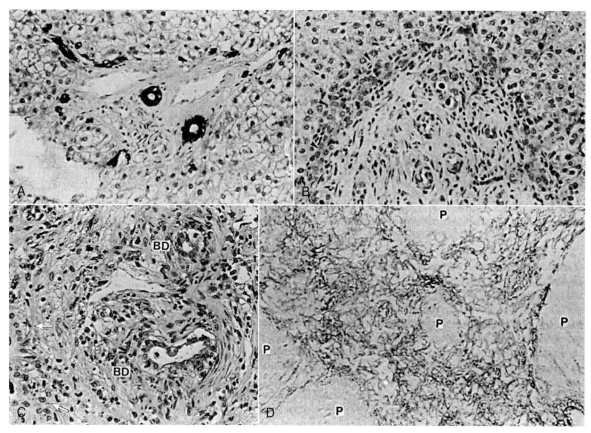

Fig. 68-3 **Histology of the portal tract in normal liver and in extrahepatic biliary atresia. A,** Normal adult liver. Bile ducts are present in the portal tract together with small ductules at the portal–parenchymal interphase, as stained with immunoperoxidase polyclonal anticytokeratin (immunoperoxidase stain with polyclonal rabbit antikeratin, wide-spectrum screening [Dako Corporation, Santa Barbara, CA], and counterstained with hematoxylin, ×400.) **B,** Extrahepatic biliary atresia in an infant age 43 days. The portal tract shows mild mononuclear cell infiltration. The bile duct contains bile concrements. Immediately surrounding the bile duct are ductular reactive cells at any early stage. (H & E stain, ×400.) **C,** Extrahepatic biliary atresia in an infant aged 8 weeks. A portal tract with two bile ducts (BD) shows swelling, vacuolization, attenuation, and sloughing of their lining epithelial cells. A mild inflammatory infiltrate is present. Ductular reactive cells are demonstrable at the margins of the portal tract (arrows). (H & E stain, ×400.) **D,** Extrahepatic biliary atresia in an infant aged 10 months with biliary cirrhosis. There is extensive fibrosis and an increase in ductular reactive cells between the nodular parenchymal areas (P). (Shikata orcein stain, ×160.)

performed, the more difficult it may be to interpret because of the overlap with giant cell hepatitis.

In recent years the diagnostic accuracy of liver biopsy is up to 90% to 95% with specimens of sufficient size that include five to seven portal tracts.[6]

CLASSIC EXTRAHEPATIC BILIARY ATRESIA

The histologic features of classic EHBA represent a dynamic process and change in the course of the disease (see **Fig. 68-3**). The timing of these stages is only approximate. In the early stage (from about 1 to 4 weeks), nonspecific features of bilirubin stasis predominate. Granules of bile pigment are seen in hepatocytes, along with intercellular bile plugs. A few hepatocytes may show degeneration and necrosis, but no inflammatory infiltration is present.

From about 4 to 7 weeks the portal tracts show characteristic changes consisting of rounding of the portal tract, edema, dilation of lymph vessels, and ductular proliferation (see **Fig. 68-3, B**). The increase in ductules typically occurs at the periphery of the portal tracts, so-called marginal bile duct proliferation, and is associated with an inflammatory infiltrate

of both lymphocytes and polymorphonuclear leukocytes and destruction of bile ducts. Periportal fibrosis is noted. This stage is considered diagnostic of EHBA and explains the recommendation by some to postpone diagnostic liver biopsy until the sixth week of life.

Later biopsy specimens (after 7 to 8 weeks) show progressive portal and periportal fibrosis, together with extension of the ductular reaction, but a decrease in inflammatory infiltration and the number of intact bile ducts (see **Fig. 68-3, C**). Periportal fibrosis eventually leads to biliary fibrosis and subsequent biliary cirrhosis (see **Fig. 68-3, D**), which is characterized by nodular regeneration of the parenchyma and perinodular septal fibrosis.

SEVERE EARLY FORM OF EXTRAHEPATIC BILIARY ATRESIA

The basic lesion of the intrahepatic bile ducts in the severe early form of EHBA corresponds to a lack of resorption and remodeling of the fetal ductal plate, termed ductal plate malformation. Bile ducts here differ in appearance from those in classic EHBA in that they are hyperplastic. Ductal plate

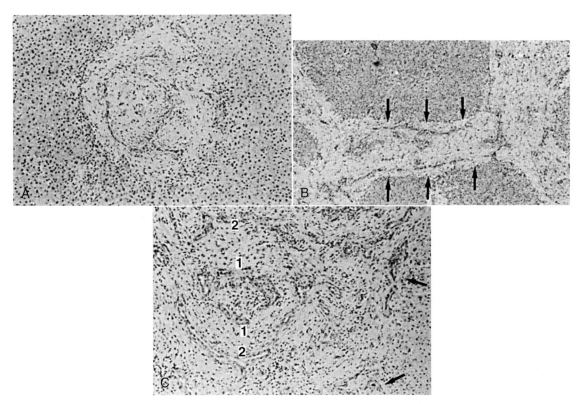

Fig. 68-4 **Histology of the portal tract in extrahepatic biliary atresia with ductal plate malformation. A,** Portal tract in an infant aged 43 days with extrahepatic biliary atresia. Bile ducts are seen in a ductal plate configuration. Some segments of the ductal plate show epithelial irregularities and involution. A mild ductular reaction occurs at the interphase between the portal tract and parenchyma. Note the prominent arteries and poorly developed portal vein in the portal tract. (H & E stain, ×160.) **B,** Extrahepatic biliary atresia in an infant aged 30 days. There is disturbed liver architecture with bridging between large portal areas. The portal tracts contain several bile ducts. Some of them appear in a ductal plate configuration *(arrows)*. This degree of fibrosis at the age of 30 days represents early, severe extrahepatic biliary atresia. Note the resemblance to congenital hepatic fibrosis. (H & E stain, ×64.) **C,** Extrahepatic biliary atresia in an infant aged 48 days. An enlarged portal tract with moderately dense inflammatory infiltration is shown. Two concentric rings of bile ducts in a ductal plate configuration can be recognized *(1, 2)*. Ductular reactive cells occur at the portal–parenchymal interface *(arrows)*. (H & E stain, ×160.)

malformation is the basic lesion of several disorders, including congenital hepatic fibrosis, infantile polycystic disease, von Meyenburg complexes, Ivemark syndrome, Meckel syndrome, Caroli disease, and some other rare disorders. However, it may also be associated with EHBA (**Fig. 68-4**). This histologic feature is combined with the typical features of classic EHBA.

Duodenal Intubation for Bilirubin Content

This investigation is performed by visually examining a 24-hour collection of duodenal fluid or by examining bile flow under direct endoscopic visualization following the intravenous injection of cholecystokinin. A positive result excludes EHBA. A negative result is not diagnostic because intrahepatic cholestasis may also cause complete lack of bile flow into the intestine. This test is not routinely used now.

Cholangiography

Cholangiography is performed to identify patency of the bile ducts and is necessary if the diagnosis is uncertain. Usually, an intraoperative cholangiogram is performed so that if EHBA is diagnosed, it is possible to proceed to hepatoportoenterostomy. Endoscopic retrograde cholangiopancreatography (ERCP) and magnetic resonance cholangiography are possible

alternatives. Percutaneous transhepatic cholangiography (PTC) is not generally helpful because the intrahepatic bile ducts are rarely dilated.

ERCP can be performed successfully and without complication in patients with EHBA following the development of instruments designed specifically for pediatric use. Considerable skill and expertise on the part of the endoscopist are required because the diagnostic result depends on failure to visualize the biliary tree. However, some experienced centers do not think that ERCP adds considerable value to the evaluation of infants with EHBA because the procedure is costly, requires substantial endoscopic skill, and is not without potential complications. False-positive results may be seen in children with AGS.

Magnetic resonance cholangiopancreatography was thought to have a role in diagnosis, but more recent evidence indicates that differentiation of severe intrahepatic cholestasis from EHBA may be difficult because of low bile flow.

Treatment and Prognosis

Optimal therapy for EHBA remains the Kasai procedure, or portoenterostomy, which should be carried out as soon as possible after diagnosis. General management strategies must be put in place as soon a child is known to have a cholestatic liver disease, including optimization of nutrition and fat-soluble vitamin intake (see later in General Management of Cholestatic Liver Disease). This is of particular importance in EHBA because resting energy expenditure is increased and long-term outcome is improved with optimal nutrition. Appropriate counseling of parents is vital, and psychological support is necessary for many families (see later in General Management of Cholestatic Liver Disease).

Surgical Management
Historical Perspective

Surgical treatment of EHBA was first discussed by Holmes in 1916, with successful surgery first reported in 1928 by Ladd. However, only limited success was reported between 1927 and 1970. The progress in understanding the varying forms of neonatal cholestasis led to a variety of approaches over the next few decades because it appeared that surgery could be harmful in infants with neonatal hepatitis. It was therefore recommended that surgery be postponed until the patient was 4 months old because the diagnosis of EHBA versus neonatal hepatitis could not be established in most infants during the early months of life. This was obviously not of benefit to those with EHBA.

It was not until the 1950s that a reliable surgical procedure was developed in Japan. In 1957, Dr. Morio Kasai performed exploratory surgery on an infant and found no patent extrahepatic ducts. He made a shallow exploration into the porta hepatis, just anterior to the portal vein, and found a small amount of bile seepage. A segment of small bowel was anastomosed to the liver capsule around this opening into the liver. Good flow of bile developed subsequently, and the patient remained healthy for more than 17 years. An account of this surgical approach—hepatoportoenterostomy, or the Kasai operation—was originally published in Japanese in 1959 but not in the English literature until 1968.[58] It was met with skepticism initially, and these two factors combined led to a delay in wider implementation of this surgical technique. It is now recognized that hepatoportoenterostomy and its subsequent modifications are the treatment of choice for EHBA. The work of Kasai demonstrated that the intrahepatic bile ducts were patent from the interlobular ducts of the liver to the porta hepatis in nearly all patients during the first 2 or 3 months after birth. The interlobular bile ducts appeared to be destroyed rapidly and their number decreased progressively after 2 months of age. This explained why surgery was most effective in patients younger than 10 weeks, which made early and rapid investigation mandatory. Increased experience worldwide with hepatoportoenterostomy has revealed that the intrahepatic component of duct inflammation and destruction is of great importance in determining the prognosis, even in patients with good bile flow soon after surgery.

The rationale for performing hepatoportoenterostomy lies in establishing continuity between the bile ducts near the porta hepatis and the intestinal lumen. Theoretically, successful restoration of bile flow is expected in patients with patent biliary structures near the porta hepatis. Postoperative bile flow would be expected to be greatest in patients with biliary structures having the largest diameters or in patients with the greatest numbers of such structures, or both. Investigations by Kasai indicated that satisfactory postoperative flow of bile is achieved only when the diameter of the patent ducts near the porta hepatis is at least 200 μm.[53] Subsequent studies have suggested that duct lumina 100 μm in diameter are sufficient for ensuring adequate bile flow. Some authors recommend intraoperative frozen section confirmation of the presence of microscopically patent ducts at the level of the anastomosis in portoenterostomy. However, there is not always a correlation between the presence of patent ducts and postoperative flow of bile in these studies. Furthermore, others have reported no correlation between postoperative drainage of bile and the number or size of bile ducts at the porta hepatis. Gautier and Eliot found, for example, that 6 of 13 patients with no demonstrable bile ducts at the porta hepatis had adequate bile flow postoperatively.[54]

Although refinement in recognition and measurement of bile ducts draining at the porta hepatis might help ensure a better predictive value of operative intervention, this still does not explain the occurrence of adequate bile flow in patients without recognizable epithelial structures. These puzzling cases raise the question of how bile is drained when there is no duct continuity and point to alternative pathways such as lymphatic drainage of bile constituents. The concept of lymphatic drainage forms the basis for some modifications of the Kasai procedure (omentopexy).

Surgical Prognostic Factors

The prognosis of patients with EHBA is dependent on several factors. The age at diagnosis and age at subsequent surgery are critical determinants of both short-term and long-term outcome. If portoenterostomy is performed within the first 60 days of life by an experienced surgeon, bile drainage should occur in at least 70% to 80% of patients.[59] If performed between 60 and 90 days of age, 40% to 50% show bile drainage, and after 90 days, in only up to 25% will bile drainage be present.[3] These figures have recently been updated following a European survey.[60] However, age at surgery is not the only factor. Two recent studies have examined the extremes of age for portoenterostomy. Volpert and associates found that outcome was worse in terms of the need for transplantation if surgery was performed before 30 days.[61] This may be due to a different phenotype occurring earlier, because these infants did not have a jaundice-free interval. At the other end of the spectrum, there is no strict upper age limit for portoenterostomy because the time of onset of disease, its rate of progression, and its severity vary.[62] In fact, concerns regarding late performance of portoenterostomy, after 100 days, have recently been challenged by Davenport and colleagues.[63] Of a total of 422 patients in whom EHBA was diagnosed, 35 were 100 days of age or older, 34 of whom underwent surgery. Of the 35 infants, 5- and 10-year survival rates with native liver were 45% and 40%, respectively.[62]

The expertise of the surgeon is also important as shown by a prospective study from the United Kingdom in which it was demonstrated that greater experience in performing the portoenterostomy, with more than five such procedures being performed annually, is associated with improved survival with native liver.[4,59,63] In this study there was an 80% 10-year survival rate with native liver for children who underwent a successful operation.[64] Thus it appears that with improving surgical techniques and better preoperative and postoperative care, portoenterostomy should be considered unless there are signs of decompensating liver disease.

Other prognostic factors include the anatomic pattern of atresia (with complete extrahepatic atresia being associated with a worse outcome), the presence of polysplenia, and the degree of fibrosis. When disease is already advanced at diagnosis, portoenterostomy is less likely to be successful.

Postoperative Care

Protocols for the management of EHBA postoperatively include ursodeoxycholic acid, which is often used to stimulate bile flow,[65] and prophylactic antibiotics, which are given to protect against ascending cholangitis.[66] Nutritional and fat-soluble vitamin supplementation is often necessary.

The role of corticosteroids in improving biliary drainage postoperatively is controversial. Steroids may stimulate bile salt–independent flow[67] or act as antiinflammatory and immunomodulatory agents in reducing the development of bile duct injury and fibrosis. A number of small retrospective studies have suggested a beneficial effect,[68,69] but this was not confirmed in a prospective randomized placebo-controlled study.[70] A recent systematic review (20 studies) of 1175 infants who received steroids and 645 who had no steroid treatment after Kasai portoenterostomy showed an improvement in clearance of jaundice and survival with the use of steroids.[71] A large prospective placebo-controlled trial is currently recruiting in the United States through the Biliary Atresia Research Consortium.[72]

Complications
Ascending Cholangitis

Cholangitis is the most important complication and has a significant bearing on long-term outcome and potential need for early liver transplantation. It is very common in children with EHBA after portoenterostomy—occurring in 40% to 60% of patients. It must be treated early because infection may encourage progressive biliary cirrhosis and lead to the early development of liver failure. The organisms responsible are mainly enteric ones, although fungal infection may occur. The use of prophylactic antibiotics decreases the incidence of recurrence,[66] and varying regimens have been used. Much consideration has been given to corticosteroid use after portoenterostomy to theoretically reduce ongoing bile duct injury and fibrosis. However, there are as yet no published randomized controlled trials of effectiveness. Many centers have used short-term (1- to 2-week) courses postoperatively, and one study found that an 8- to 10-week course after portoenterostomy improved outcome when compared with historical controls.

Pruritus and Nutrition

Treatment of pruritus and management of nutrition are as detailed at the end of the chapter.

Intrahepatic Biliary Cysts

The development of intrahepatic biliary cysts following portoenterostomy was first reported in 1980 and occurs in up to 21% of patients.[73] It is thought to be due to progressive inflammation and cirrhosis in the intrahepatic lobular spaces and subsequent intrahepatic biliary obstruction and cyst formation.[73] Treatment with antibiotics may not be effective,

percutaneous transhepatic cholangiography with drainage is not always effective, and patients may require liver transplantation.

Cirrhosis and Portal Hypertension

Cirrhosis and portal hypertension develop in the majority of patients. Progressive splenomegaly and a decrease in size of the liver with a firm texture and variceal bleeding are early signs. They may eventually progress to decompensated liver disease, with ascites, hypoalbuminemia, encephalopathy, or hepatopulmonary syndrome. Management of these complications is the same as for any other cause of portal hypertension or liver decompensation. The presence of variceal bleeding alone, without a rise in bilirubin, is not an indication for urgent transplantation[74,75] unless medical and endoscopic therapy has failed.

Medium-Term Outcome

In the medium term, prevention of cholangitis is the main aim. Recurrent cholangitis leads to progression of fibrosis and earlier decompensation. Thus, to avoid transplantation, use of prophylactic antibiotics in high-risk children and prompt treatment of any suspected episodes of cholangitis are vital.

It is important to maintain good nutrition to ensure adequate growth and development. All infants need to be monitored to detect signs of decompensating liver disease and the development of portal hypertension.[63]

Long-Term Outcome

Successful portoenterostomy is defined as one in which bile drainage is achieved, as documented by normalization of serum bilirubin at 3 months postoperatively. Although at least two thirds of patients have a successful outcome of surgery, cure is not possible for the majority. Long-term results after 10 and 20 years of follow-up indicate that only a minority appear to be cured following hepatic portoenterostomy.[59,76] Even those with normal liver function test results 10 years after portoenterostomy are found to have fibrosis or cirrhosis on liver biopsy.[77]

In approximately a third of patients, bile flow after portoenterostomy is inadequate and progressive fibrosis and cirrhosis develop, which leads to death by the age of 2 years without liver transplantation. In other children, cirrhosis develops at a slower rate despite bile drainage, and transplantation is required later in childhood. In France, a 10-year study of 472 patients with EHBA found that the actuarial survival rate with native liver was 29% at 10 years, with a 5-year survival rate after liver transplantation of 71%.[59]

Indications for Transplantation

Extrahepatic biliary atresia is the most common indication for liver transplantation in childhood, with two thirds of patients requiring transplantation following portoenterostomy. Technical advances, including the use of cut-down and split livers and living related donation, have addressed issues of donor availability and extended transplantation to infants. The age of the child is no longer a contraindication to transplantation, and 1-year survival rates following transplantation are approaching 90% for all ages.

Indications for liver transplantation in patients with EHBA are decompensating liver function, intractable portal hypertension with recurrent variceal bleeding or severe malnutrition and fat-soluble vitamin deficiency, and metabolic bone disease resulting in pathologic fractures. Elective transplantation is associated with better short-term survival than is transplantation for acute liver failure.[78] A number of risk factors have been established by Rodeck and co-authors, one or more of which indicate the need for urgent transplantation: bilirubin greater than 340 µmol/L, albumin lower than 33 g/L, and standard deviation score for weight of less than −2.2.[79] In comparing posttransplantation survival in these groups, there is a statistically significant difference at 1 year (57% vs. 90.5%) and 4 years (49% vs. 90.5%) after transplantation ($P = .0001$, log-rank test). More recently, a Pediatric End-Stage Liver Disease (PELD) score has been developed from data accumulated by the Studies for Pediatric Liver Transplantation Research Group.[80] PELD uses five variables to predict 3-month survival of children listed for liver transplantation: serum bilirubin, international normalized ratio, albumin, growth failure (height or weight z score of less than −2), and age younger than 1 year. This may assist in early referral and listing but does not appear to affect outcome.

Overall survival rates for elective BA repair are up to 95% at 1 year and 89% at 5 years.[81]

Choledochal Cyst

Choledochal cysts were first described in 1959. They are a group of congenital malformations of the pancreatobiliary system that involve the intrahepatic or extrahepatic bile ducts (or both). They are frequently accompanied by pancreatobiliary malunion.[57] Choledochal cysts have been classified into six types.[82] They are unusual in Western countries but common in Asia. There is a female preponderance (female/male ratio, 5:1).

Clinical Features and Diagnosis

Choledochal cysts may occur at any age. The classical manifestation is a triad of symptoms consisting of jaundice, abdominal mass, and pain, but this is unusual in the neonatal period. Most affected infants have jaundice, an abdominal mass or distention, and acholic stools,[83] and differentiation from BA or choledocholithiasis is important. Later development is associated with biliary colic, acute cholangitis, or gallstone pancreatitis.

The diagnosis is made by identifying the choledochal cyst on ultrasound examination of the liver. The diagnosis can also be made antenatally in the fetus by prenatal sonography.[83,84] Cholangiography, either percutaneous or endoscopic, is used to confirm the diagnosis. Hepatobiliary scanning has limited utility for diagnosis. Liver function test results are compatible with biliary obstruction.

Treatment and Outcome

Treatment is aimed at surgical removal. Excision of the cyst with hepaticoenterostomy offers the best outcome.[85] Complications occur less frequently with early surgical intervention and specific modifications of the hepaticojejunostomy.[86] Surgery should be performed promptly in infants with conjugated hyperbilirubinemia in whom choledochal cysts are diagnosed prenatally. If the infant remains free of jaundice, elective surgical resection of the choledochal cyst may be postponed until the infant is 1 month old, but it should not be delayed to any great extent. Although approximately 50% of infants with prenatally identified bile duct dilation have hepatic fibrosis and a few have cirrhosis, most of these infants do well. In older patients in whom the cirrhosis is advanced, transplantation may be necessary. A minority of infants may have correctable BA, and close follow-up is warranted. Pancreatitis may also occur. In the longer term, there is a risk for malignancy, but this is low in childhood (<1% in children younger than 10 years); however, it rises with age such that the risk is greater than 10% by the third decade.[86]

Caroli Disease

Caroli disease (also known as type V choledochal cyst) is characterized by congenital segmental saccular dilation of the intrahepatic bile ducts but without hepatic fibrosis or portal hypertension. It more commonly affects boys and is often associated with autosomal recessive polycystic kidney disease.[87] It is now thought to be a disorder of primary cilia.[88-90] Caroli disease is rarely evident in infancy. The main initial feature is jaundice as a result of acute cholangitis, which may be complicated by intrahepatic calculi and hepatic abscess formation.[87] Some newborn infants with severe autosomal recessive polycystic kidney disease have extensive cystic bile duct changes, but renal insufficiency dominates the clinical picture. Ultrasound of the liver is often adequate for diagnosing Caroli disease; cholangiography is confirmatory. The outcome is related to the severity of the renal disease or the development of cholangitis, intrahepatic gallstones, or portal hypertension.

Caroli syndrome is considered to be present if there is congenital hepatic fibrosis, which occurs in infancy and is characterized by hepatomegaly and either autosomal recessive polycystic kidney disease or systemic hypertension. Jaundice and abnormal serum aminotransferase levels are uncommon. Treatment depends on the clinical features. If disease is localized to one hepatic lobe, hepatectomy relieves the symptoms and possibly also the risk for malignancy. The outcome is variable and depends on progression of the hepatic and renal disease, as noted previously. Malignancy may complicate Caroli disease in approximately 7% of cases.[87]

Neonatal Sclerosing Cholangitis

Neonatal sclerosing cholangitis (NSC) was first reported in 1987 with a few subsequent reports.[91,92] It is characterized by irregular narrowing of the extrahepatic or intrahepatic bile ducts. The cause of this condition is unknown but it may have a genetic basis. The genetic basis of one form of NSC has been identified. Infants with NSC and ichthyosis (NISCH syndrome) have mutations in the claudin-1 gene severe enough to interfere with the production of claudin-1 protein and thus render tight junctions leaky. Cutaneous findings include decreased scalp hair, scarring alopecia, and ichthyosis.[93] As only a few such patients have been identified, NSC must be a heterogeneous disease with more than one disease mechanism. NSC is distinguished from childhood primary sclerosing cholangitis by its manifestation in early infancy as conjugated hyperbilirubinemia, which then resolves within 3 to 6 months.[94] Recurrent hyperbilirubinemia develops 1 to 2 years later or in midchildhood (8 to 10 years old). This is distinct from childhood primary sclerosing cholangitis developing in infancy, in which there is no early cholestatic jaundice. Other features include hepatosplenomegaly, biliary cirrhosis, and portal hypertension.

Investigations reveal obstructive biliary disease with elevated serum alkaline phosphatase and GGT. Endoscopic or percutaneous cholangiography demonstrates beaded irregularity of medium to large intrahepatic bile ducts in all patients and the extrahepatic ducts in 80%. Liver histology shows portal fibrosis with ductal proliferation developing into biliary cirrhosis. Surgical treatment with Kasai portoenterostomy is not indicated, and nutritional and supportive management is required. The disease is progressive, with liver transplantation being required at some stage.

Spontaneous Perforation of the Common Bile Duct

Spontaneous perforation of the common bile duct is a highly specific clinical entity in infancy and should always be considered in an infant in whom jaundice develops after an anicteric period of good health. It is a rare condition: some 60 cases have been reported since 1932.[94] Its cause is unknown.

In the majority of patients the perforation occurs at the union of the cystic and common ducts. This suggests a developmental weakness at this site, but a viral infection has also been suggested as a cause of this disease. Some cases are associated with distal obstruction resulting from sludge or EHBA.

Clinical signs of the disease are commonly noted between 1 week and 2 months after birth, although instances of later onset have been reported. A single case was diagnosed before birth.[95] The clinical findings may be those of an intraabdominal catastrophe. Usually, however, fluctuating jaundice, acholic stools, and dark urine develop slowly. Symptoms may be so mild that the development of an inguinal or umbilical hernia secondary to ascites may be the first sign of illness. In some cases, general symptoms of weight loss, irritability, and vomiting may be noted before jaundice.

On clinical examination there is abdominal distention from bile ascites and sometimes bile staining of the umbilicus or scrotum caused by bile tracking along patent hernial sacs. Signs of peritonitis and pyrexia are usually lacking. Laboratory investigation reveals a moderate rise in serum levels of bilirubin and normal hepatic aminotransferase levels, which differentiates this condition from EHBA. Definitive preoperative diagnosis can be made by abdominal paracentesis, which yields fluid with a high concentration of bilirubin. Intravenous cholangiography demonstrates a leak in the extrahepatic bile ducts.

Operative treatment depends on the findings at the time of surgery.

Bile Plug Syndrome and Inspissated Bile Syndrome

The terms bile plug syndrome and inspissated bile syndrome are often used interchangeably, although Bernstein and co-workers stated explicitly that obstruction of the common duct by a plug of secretions and bile is to be differentiated from the so-called inspissated bile syndrome.[96]

The majority of infants have massive hemolysis-induced jaundice caused by rhesus and ABO blood group incompatibility. The histologic feature of bile plugs in the parenchyma is the result rather than the cause of the cholestasis and is caused by bilirubin overload of the liver and by dehydration. Hemolytic disease of the newborn caused by blood group incompatibility is now partially preventable with maternal anti-D treatment, can be treated by exchange transfusion, and thus has become more infrequent.

Clinically, bile plug syndrome cannot be differentiated from EHBA. Ultrasonography is diagnostic and the findings confirmed at exploratory laparotomy. The inspissated material is removed by irrigation of the biliary tree or with the use of a mucolytic agent. On occasion, inspissation may proceed to the production of stones, which necessitates manual removal of the calculi, or it may resolve spontaneously. Choledochal cyst formation may develop after inspissated bile syndrome.

Bile Duct Stenosis

Localized narrowing of the distal part of the common bile duct is a rare cause of extrahepatic obstruction in children beyond the neonatal age. Fewer than 15 cases have been reported. In three such cases the proximal segments of the duct were dilated and contained small biliary concrements that had accumulated near the narrowed part of the bile duct. The condition was cured by simple choledochotomy and cleaning of the duct.

Two cases of posttraumatic stricture of the common bile duct have been reported, possibly caused by previous blunt abdominal trauma, and two cases of partial stenosis of the confluence of the hepatic ducts without evidence of antecedent trauma. Further abnormalities have recently been reported in association with bile duct stenosis, including ductal plate malformation, eosinophilia, and pancreatitis.[97]

Duplication of the Biliary Tree

Duplication of the biliary tree is a condition of exceptional rarity. The cause is identical to that of intestinal duplication. Clinical symptoms include abdominal pain and recurring intestinal obstruction with or without cholestasis. A hard mass of variable size is palpated in the right hypochondrium. The diagnosis is made during surgical intervention for presumed cholangitis or choledochal cyst.

Agenesis of Extrahepatic Bile Ducts

Schwartz and co-authors described five neonates with obstructive jaundice in whom exploration revealed absence of the proximal extrahepatic biliary ducts (four cases) or total absence of the extrahepatic ducts and gallbladder (one case).[98] Jaundice was diagnosed from birth to 3 weeks of age. Surgery revealed absence of bile duct remnants, lack of inflammation, and a fibrous mass at the porta hepatis. Liver biopsy specimens showed histologic evidence of cholestasis, minimal bile duct proliferation and fibrosis, and nearly complete absence of inflammation. The authors concluded that this group of patients represents true agenesis of the extrahepatic bile ducts rather than EHBA and that liver transplantation is the primary mode of treatment of this rare entity.

Gallstones

Cholelithiasis is being reported with increasing frequency in infants and neonates because of the widespread use of ultrasonography. The pigmentary nature of cholelithiasis has been established in most cases, but the pathogenesis of stone formation remains unclear.[99] Gallstone formation can occur in the fetus and in premature infants treated with parenteral nutrition (PN) and furosemide. Intrahepatic bile stone formation has been ascribed to *Ascaris lumbricoides* infestation. Other possible causes include chronic hemolytic disease, mucoviscidosis, bile duct malformations, and septicemia.

In contrast to adult gallstone disease, there is no female preponderance. Reviews of the clinical features, diagnostic procedures, and therapy have been published.[99]

Bile Duct Tumors

Tumors of the extrahepatic bile ducts are extremely rare in children. The tumors correspond to embryonal rhabdomyosarcoma and exceptionally to liposarcoma.[100,101] Clinical symptoms are those of complete cholestasis with a progressive onset; an abdominal mass may be palpable. Operative cholangiography reveals the obstruction, which is often located near the ampullary region. Treatment consists of surgical excision. The prognosis is poor.

Extramural Compression of the Common Bile Duct

Occasionally, extrahepatic cholestasis is secondary to extrinsic compression of the common bile duct. A case of bile duct obstruction by peritoneal bands has been reported, and cure was achieved by simple division of the constricting bands. Other causes include malignant tumors of lymph nodes near the porta hepatis (Hodgkin and non-Hodgkin lymphomas) and benign lesions such as chronic pancreatitis and posttraumatic cyst of the pancreas. Both benign and malignant tumors of the pancreas or duodenum may cause obstructive jaundice in infants (duodenal fibrosarcoma and carcinoma and hemangioendothelioma of the pancreas).

Intrahepatic Disorders
Neonatal Hepatitis Syndrome

Etiology and Pathogenesis

Neonatal hepatitis was first described in 1952 by Craig and Landing, who reported a "form of hepatitis in the neonatal period simulating biliary atresia." The disease appears clinically as obstructive jaundice indistinguishable from EHBA and is histologically characterized by parenchymal giant cell transformation. The biliary tree is found to be patent on abdominal exploration or postmortem examination. The histologic picture was initially interpreted as "active hepatitis having the characteristics of viral hepatitis," but a viral cause remained unproven.

Failure to identify a specific viral infection in the majority of cases and the clinical similarity to EHBA have led to terms such as neonatal hepatitis syndrome and infantile obstructive cholangiopathy. Many causes of prolonged, conjugated neonatal hyperbilirubinuria have now been identified (see **Table 68-1**). Early detection of specific infectious diseases, toxins, and disorders of amino acid, lipid, and carbohydrate metabolism is important because in many instances cholestasis attributable to these factors is treatable and reversible. A similar clinical picture of obstructive jaundice may be seen in patients with homozygous $\alpha_1 AT$ deficiency and in those with cystic fibrosis. Endocrine disorders (hypopituitarism and hypothyroidism) may also be associated with cholestasis. There remains a subgroup with unclear etiology and for whom the term idiopathic neonatal hepatitis remains.

In neonatal hepatitis, the disease process is thought to focus on the hepatocyte and not, or only secondarily, on intrahepatic and extrahepatic segments of the biliary tree. Intralobular cholestasis may be due to infectious, metabolic, toxic, and unknown causes. Neonatal hepatitis syndrome thus represents a continuously evolving spectrum of problems.

It is important to distinguish neonatal hepatitis from EHBA and to avoid exploratory laparotomy, which may have a harmful effect on the prognosis of patients with neonatal hepatitis. In a follow-up study from France it was noted that progression to cirrhosis was more likely in patients who had undergone surgery, but this may also have been related to advanced liver disease at the time of surgery. A poor prognosis has been observed in patients with neonatal hepatitis mimicking EHBA; that is, severe forms with complete cholestasis.

Intrauterine Infection

This is the largest subgroup of disorders that result in giant cell hepatitis. Most are due to in utero viral infections (see **Table 68-1**).

Toxoplasmosis, Rubella, Cytomegalovirus, Herpes Simplex (TORCH) Infections

Congenital infections grouped under the acronym TORCH often have very similar clinical features: hepatosplenomegaly, jaundice, pneumonitis, petechial or purpuric rash, and a tendency to prematurity or poor intrauterine growth. Fulminant hepatic failure in the newborn period is common with herpes simplex infection. Whenever possible, direct identification of viral infection or measurement of specific immunoglobulin M antibodies should be sought for rapid diagnosis; relying on conventional TORCH titers is less preferable.

TOXOPLASMOSIS

Congenital toxoplasmosis is comparatively rare. Infection is acquired through maternal ingestion of raw or undercooked meat or food, especially fruit or vegetables, contaminated with infected cat feces. Rates of transmission to the fetus via transplacental infection are up to 40%[102] and vary with gestational age at the time of infection. Maternal infection in the third trimester is more likely to cause fetal infection than that earlier in pregnancy. Neonatal hepatitis is an important feature but may be less obvious than central nervous system involvement with chorioretinitis (with large pigmented scars), hydrocephaly, or microcephaly. Intracranial calcification is usually prominent and leads to convulsions, nystagmus, and evidence of increased intracranial pressure. Liver biopsy may demonstrate a nonspecific hepatitis or portal fibrosis with biliary ductule proliferation. Spiramycin or pyrimethamine therapy may prevent progression of the ocular, central nervous system, and liver disease.[102] The prognosis depends on the extent of neurologic or optic disease.

RUBELLA

Congenital infection with rubella was first identified in 1941 by Gregg. The virus is now rare because of immunization in the Western world. However, with recent controversies over the measles, mumps, and rubella (MMR) vaccine, immunization has fallen and congenital infection could conceivably become a problem. Transplacental transmission of the virus occurs during the first trimester of pregnancy, with severity increasing the earlier during pregnancy that the infection occurs. Risk is low after 17 weeks' gestation. Teratogenicity leads to intrauterine growth retardation, anemia/thrombocytopenia, congenital heart disease (patent ductus arteriosus or pulmonary artery stenosis), cataracts, chorioretinitis ("salt and pepper" appearance), mental retardation, and sensorineural deafness. Hepatosplenomegaly is usual. Liver histology shows typical giant cell hepatitis. The disease may be self-limited or progress to cirrhosis.

CYTOMEGALOVIRUS

Cytomegalovirus is the most common cause of congenital infection, with 0.15% to 2% of newborns being affected, almost 90% of whom are asymptomatic at birth.[103] It is thought to be more likely in association with maternal primary infection in the second and third trimester, but recent studies examining the severity of congenital CMV infection after recurrent infection have demonstrated equivalent severity.[103] Those with evident disease may have intrauterine growth retardation or be premature. Fetal ascites may occur, but CMV rarely causes acute liver failure in the newborn.

The most common initial features include jaundice, petechiae, and hepatosplenomegaly. Clinical findings include petechial rash, hepatosplenomegaly, and jaundice in 60% to 80%. CMV infection often affects the central nervous system and gives rise to microcephaly, intracranial calcification, and chorioretinitis; progressive sensorineural deafness or cerebral palsy may develop later in childhood.

Liver biopsy demonstrates giant cell hepatitis; the classic inclusion bodies are rarely seen in neonatal infection. In a study of liver tissue in infants with neonatal hepatitis or EHBA, Chang and colleagues found CMV DNA in 23 of 50 infants with neonatal hepatitis by PCR, in only 2 of 26 with EHBA, and in none of control specimens.[104] Although differentiation from BA is usually easy, CMV may be associated with EHBA. In one report of fraternal twins, both had congenital CMV infection: one had hepatitis only and the other had late-pattern EHBA. In addition, 25% of infants with EHBA have been found to have CMV infection and were referred later than those without CMV infection.[105] CMV is a candidate virus for causing late-appearing EHBA because it can infect bile duct epithelial cells directly and increase the expression of major histocompatibility class II antigens.[106] Infants with congenital CMV infection and persisting conjugated hyperbilirubinemia should have EHBA excluded.

Conclusive diagnosis requires culture of CMV from the infant within the first 4 weeks of life. Serologic studies and clinical features provide support for the presence of CMV infection but do not distinguish congenital from early postnatal infection. Treatment with ganciclovir has been suggested; it appears to improve the outcome with regard to hearing loss. However, neutropenia was a significant side effect in two thirds of those receiving intravenous ganciclovir for 6 weeks, and no report was made regarding other parameters. Ganciclovir and the oral version valganciclovir may also improve congenital CMV-associated liver disease.

In most children CMV hepatitis is mild and resolves completely. Hepatic fibrosis or noncirrhotic portal hypertension develops in a few children. Intrahepatic calcification has been reported. Cirrhosis with chronic cholestasis necessitated liver transplantation in one child. Persisting neurodevelopmental abnormalities become the main problem in the majority of patients.[103]

HERPES SIMPLEX VIRUS

Both type 1 and type 2 herpesviruses can lead to perinatal infection and cause a severe multisystem disorder consisting of encephalitis, severe hepatitis, or acute liver failure. Type 2 virus shed from genital herpes at birth is the most common route of transmission with the greatest risk if maternal infection involves the cervix. A true congenital infection from in utero viral infection is less common but may be associated with extensive hepatic calcifications.[107] Liver biopsy shows areas of necrosis with viral inclusions in intact hepatocytes; however, profound coagulopathy may preclude biopsy. Scrapings from vesicular skin lesions reveal herpes simplex virus, but these typical herpetic skin, mouth, or eye lesions may not be present in neonates. Antiviral treatment with acyclovir should be administered to avert the otherwise high mortality, although the outcome is more severe if disseminated disease or encephalitis is present.

Other Viral Infections

VARICELLA

Infection with varicella may occur following maternal infection. Infection in early pregnancy is associated with complications in 0.4% to 2% of infants[108]; complications are more likely if the infection occurs within 14 days of delivery, but disease is mild in term infants after 10 days of age. Early manifestation or protracted disease in an infant of any gestational age may lead to a fatal outcome. Jaundice and multisystem involvement occur, especially pneumonia, and infection is usually but not always associated with skin lesions. In fatal cases hepatic parenchymal involvement can be demonstrated. Prompt administration of zoster immune globulin to infants born of mothers with chickenpox and treatment of infection with acyclovir may ameliorate the symptoms.

Syphilis

Congenital syphilis is now rare in the developed world, but its incidence is rising in eastern Europe, the former Soviet Union, and the United Kingdom,[109] and it is common in sub-Saharan Africa. It causes a multisystem illness that may include intrauterine growth retardation and subsequent failure to thrive, severe anemia and thrombocytopenia, nephrotic syndrome, periosteal reaction and metaphyseal dystrophy, nasal discharge, rash with symmetric superficial desquamation of the hands and feet, diffuse lymphadenopathy, and hepatosplenomegaly. Infants may be born with hydrops fetalis, or jaundice may develop within 24 hours of birth or following treatment. Cholestasis has been reported in premature infants. Central nervous system involvement occurs in up to 30% of infants.

Liver histology in untreated congenital syphilis may reveal numerous treponemes in hepatic tissue, but after treatment with penicillin, giant cell hepatitis without detectable treponemes is the usual finding. Diagnosis involves serologic testing, including the Venereal Disease Research Laboratory (VDRL) test and confirmatory testing for specific antitreponemal antibodies. Radiographs of long bones may show typical bone abnormalities in the first 24 hours of life and aid in rapid diagnosis.

Other Viruses Associated with Neonatal Hepatitis

Several other viruses may cause neonatal hepatitis syndrome (see **Table 68-1**). Such viruses include parvovirus B19, which may lead to hydrops fetalis and death in utero, and paramyxovirus, which may cause a severe syncytial giant cell hepatitis that progresses to cirrhosis and usually requires liver transplantation.

Bacterial Infections Associated with Neonatal Hepatitis

Both generalized sepsis and localized infections may lead to cholestasis in neonates. Galactosemia must be excluded in all jaundiced infants with gram-negative septicemia because infection is a common initial feature. More unusual infections that may result in cholestasis include congenital listeriosis, in which infants may have hepatosplenomegaly and occasionally jaundice, as well as meningitis and tuberculosis. Hepatosplenomegaly is common in infants with congenital tuberculosis, but jaundice is rare and indicates severe disease.

Endocrine
Hypopituitarism

Pituitary-adrenal dysfunction is associated with neonatal hepatitis syndrome in 30% to 70% of patients. The cause of the hypopituitarism is variable, and it may be due to hypothalamic dysfunction or deficiency of anterior or posterior pituitary function (or both). Adrenal insensitivity to adrenocorticotropin has also been described. Clinical features include conjugated hyperbilirubinemia, hypoglycemia, and septooptic dysplasia. The hypoglycemia commences perinatally and is usually symptomatic and persistent. Septooptic dysplasia is a neurooptic malformation with a defect in ventral midline development (absence of the septum pellucidum or corpus callosum) and hypoplasia of one or both optic nerves in association with hypopituitarism. There may also be midline facial abnormalities, nystagmus, and in boys, microgenitalia.[110]

The diagnosis is confirmed by detecting an extremely low random or 9.00 AM cortisol level in association with low thyroid-stimulating hormone and thyroxine levels.[110,111] Liver biopsy usually reveals typical giant cell hepatitis, but severe cholestasis may be present with dilated bile canaliculi and hepatocellular necrosis. Delayed excretion may be seen on radioisotope scanning. Treatment with hormone replacement is essential, including thyroxine, corticosteroids, and growth hormone when appropriate. Progression of the disease to cirrhosis and portal hypertension has been reported when there was delay in hormone replacement.[110] There is also a report of association of septooptic dysplasia with congenital hepatic fibrosis.[111]

Hypothyroidism, usually associated with unconjugated hyperbilirubinemia, may be found in those with neonatal hepatitis syndrome and should be excluded in every patient.

Chromosomal Disorders

Trisomy 18 has been reported as being associated with both giant cell hepatitis and EHBA. Other cytogenetic abnormalities, including trisomy 13, deletion of the short arm of chromosome 18, and 49XXXXY, have also been reported in association with EHBA. Trisomy 21 has been reported in association with neonatal cholestasis and EHBA, but this is rare. Severe hepatic fibrosis associated with transient myeloproliferative disorder has likewise been reported with trisomy 21, thus raising the possibility that hepatic fibrogenesis may be due to high concentrations of growth factors derived from megakaryocytes.

Cat's eye syndrome is a rare developmental disorder in humans that is associated with the presence of three or four copies of a segment of chromosome 22q11.2, usually in the form of a bisatellite, isodicentric supernumerary chromosome.[112] It is characterized by a variety of congenital defects, including ocular coloboma, anal atresia, preauricular tags/pits, heart and kidney defects, dysmorphic facial features, and mental retardation. It is also reported to be associated with EHBA.

Idiopathic Neonatal Hepatitis

Recent advances in molecular biology and genetics have significantly reduced the frequency of diagnosis of idiopathic neonatal hepatitis,[113] and unresolved cases are likely to represent an as yet undefined genetic or infectious cause. Nevertheless, idiopathic neonatal hepatitis is found in preterm babies, particularly since many more infants are resuscitated and survive. They may have cholestasis because of immaturity of the biliary tree, have difficulty feeding, or need to be maintained on PN. It is important to differentiate this condition from other known causes of neonatal hepatitis, PN-associated liver disease, and EHBA, which may have an atypical manifestation in this gestational age group and occur at the corrected age for term. Examination of stool for pigment and a fasting ultrasound examination to determine gallbladder size are useful investigations to exclude BA. Liver biopsy is indicated only if there is persistent elevation of conjugated bilirubin, abnormal liver biochemistry, or both. The prognosis is good.[114]

Clinical Features

Conjugated hyperbilirubinemia may occur at any time after birth. If detected in the first 24 hours of life, infection is usually the cause. Most causes of neonatal hepatitis syndrome have similar findings: jaundice, which may not be obvious at first, together with dark urine and pale yellow stools.

Abnormal stool color, though suggestive of liver disease, is neither a specific nor reliable feature. Infants may be small for gestational age, especially those with AGS, metabolic liver disease, and intrauterine infection. Failure to thrive or poor feeding may also be a feature. Dysmorphic features should be sought and are present in those with trisomy 18, trisomy 21, AGS, Zellweger syndrome, and certain congenital infections. Hypoglycemia may suggest metabolic liver disease, hypopituitarism, or severe liver disease. Hepatomegaly and splenomegaly may be present. Ascites is rarely evident except in metabolic liver disease. Cardiac murmurs or neurologic abnormalities are associated with specific congenital syndromes. Bleeding from vitamin K deficiency or thrombocytopenia may occur.

Distinguishing neonatal hepatitis from EHBA may be difficult. Hepatomegaly is often obvious in the first or second week in neonatal hepatitis, whereas liver enlargement usually becomes detectable in the third or fourth week of life in those with EHBA. In EHBA, conjugated hyperbilirubinemia rises more progressively than in neonatal hepatitis. Hepatic aminotransferases are not helpful in discrimination. In the first 3 months of life neonatal hepatitis may cause higher elevations in AST and ALT, whereas GGT levels are more abnormal in patients with EHBA.[115]

Different scoring systems based on clinical and laboratory data have been developed in attempts to better differentiate EHBA from neonatal hepatitis. According to Alagille,[116] clinical features and laboratory data allow differentiation between EHBA and neonatal hepatitis in 83% of infants before the age of 3 months. The following characteristics occurred more frequently in infants with neonatal hepatitis than in those with EHBA: male gender (66% vs. 45%), low birth weight (mean, 2680 vs. 3230 g), other congenital anomalies (32% vs. 17%), onset of jaundice (mean, 23 vs. 11 days of age), onset of acholic stools (mean, 30 vs. 16 days), white stools during the first 10 days after admission (26% vs. 79%), and enlarged liver with a firm or hard consistency (53% vs. 87%).[116]

Histology

The histologic abnormalities in infants with idiopathic neonatal cholestasis are more prominent in the parenchyma than in the portal tracts. There is more extensive parenchymal giant cell transformation than in EHBA; giant cells are larger, appear more hydropic or ballooned, and often show degenerative features (**Fig. 68-5**). Necrosis of parenchymal giant cells may be associated with infiltration by neutrophils; this may require differentiation from so-called surgical necrosis in surgically resected wedge biopsy specimens. There is also a peculiar large type of cell with strongly eosinophilic cytoplasm and a bizarrely shaped, homogeneously staining nucleus. It is difficult to differentiate these cells from megakaryocytes, and their nature remains unclear. Foci of extramedullary hematopoiesis are found more often in neonatal hepatitis than in EHBA. Hemosiderin deposition in parenchymal cells and Kupffer cells is more conspicuous in neonatal hepatitis than in EHBA. Intralobular inflammation and Kupffer cell hyperplasia are usually more striking in neonatal hepatitis, whereas portal and periportal inflammation predominates in EHBA. Cholestasis is variable but may be marked, with pigmented granules present in parenchymal cells and Kupffer cells, as well as intercellular bile plugs. Ductular proliferation at the periphery of portal tracts may be observed in some cases, but not to the extent found in EHBA. Intralobular fibrosis is common in

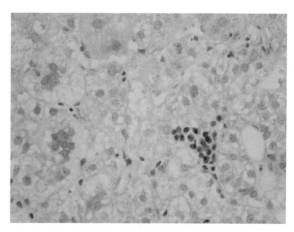

Fig. 68-5 **Liver histology of neonatal hepatitis in an infant age 47 days.** There is expansion of the portal tract with prominent giant cells. (H & E stain, ×160.)

neonatal hepatitis, in contrast to the periportal predominance of fibrosis in EHBA.

The reason for formation of parenchymal giant cells is unknown. It has been suggested that they represent a morphologic marker of infantile obstructive cholangiopathy.[52] However, parenchymal giant cells occur in virtually all liver disorders of early infancy and may represent a nonspecific reaction to various types of injury. It is more age specific than disease specific. Nonetheless, parenchymal giant cells have also been observed in adults, in patients with viral hepatitis, and in those with drug-induced liver disease. Parenchymal giant cells may be the result of faulty development of hepatocytes with aplasia of intercellular canaliculi, possibly on a hereditary basis. Alternatively, these multinucleated cells may arise by nuclear multiplication not followed by cell division, thereby resulting in multinucleated plasmodial cells. They may represent syncytial masses formed by the fusion of several mononuclear hepatocytes. The spontaneous disappearance of giant cells is similarly unresolved. Serial biopsy specimens from infants with giant cell transformation suggest that giant cells have a limited life span of only around up to 6 months. Their disappearance parallels recovery from cholestasis. The bile ducts in idiopathic neonatal hepatitis appear normal. A few infants with severe inflammation may have a paucity of small bile ducts.

Management and Treatment

The specific management of neonatal hepatitis is dependent on its cause (see earlier). Nevertheless, all require nutritional support and promotion of bile excretion, as for EHBA (see General Management of Cholestatic Liver Disease). Follow-up is indicated until the liver disease resolves.

Prognosis

The outcome of infants with neonatal hepatitis is highly variable and depends on the etiology, but is usually good. It is better in sporadic cases without known associated factors, whereas the prognosis is poor in genetic cases. Other predictors of a poor prognosis include prolonged severe jaundice (beyond 6 months of age), acholic stools, persistent hepatomegaly, and severe inflammation on biopsy. The peak bilirubin level is not necessarily predictive of outcome, and the prognostic importance of ductopenia has not been rigorously investigated. Septic complications may lead to decompensation. Overall mortality is 13% to 25%. The long-term outlook for infants surviving the first year of life with little evidence of chronic liver disease is very good.

Bile Duct Paucity

Alagille Syndrome

Also known as arteriohepatic dysplasia, AGS is a complex inherited disorder characterized by cholestatic liver disease and a paucity of intralobular bile ducts.[117,118] It was originally noted by Daniel Alagille in 1969 and was formally described in 1975[93] in a subgroup of children with cholestatic liver disease, idiopathic bile duct paucity, and complex congenital heart disease, most often peripheral pulmonary artery stenosis. The incidence of AGS is at least 1 in 70,000, although this figure may be an underestimate that reflects only those with disease severe enough to be recognized clinically. Inheritance is autosomal dominant with variable penetrance. The phenotype has considerable variability and can appear from the neonatal period through adult life, depending on the severity of disease. It affects the sexes equally.

Etiology and Pathogenesis

The underlying cause of AGS is now well known.[119] Some patients have been found to have deletions of chromosome 20p11-12. In 1997 the gene for Jagged1 was mapped to chromosome 20p12. It was tested as a candidate gene for AGS, and coding mutations in Jagged1 were shown to be present in four families with AGS.[120] A number of frameshift and splice donor mutations were also found at this time in the gene for Jagged1 in individuals with AGS.[121] Further studies in greater numbers of patients with AGS have confirmed that there are a considerable number of different mutations in the Jagged1 gene (*JAG1*) identified in up to 70% of patients with AGS. Very few are total gene deletions (6%), a few are missense mutations (12%), and the majority (82%) are protein-truncating mutations.[122,123] There is a high frequency of sporadic cases, up to 70%,[124] whereas fewer than 1% have mutations in the *Notch2* gene.[125]

Jagged1 is a ligand for the Notch receptor, part of a highly conserved and fundamental signaling pathway in the normal development of many organs. In humans there are at least five ligands for the Notch receptor. These are designated Jagged1 and Jagged2 and Delta1, Delta3, and Delta4. There are also four known members of the Notch receptor family in humans, Notch1 to Notch4, known to be essential for normal development in other organs, such as in hematopoiesis and formation of the pancreas,[126] as well as in blood vessel formation.

Notch signaling is vital for development and function of the cardiovascular system in both humans and mouse models, and mutations in either *JAGGED* or *NOTCH* may cause congenital heart disease. Recent data from a mouse model indicate that abnormal Notch-Jagged signaling within second heart field progenitors may cause some forms of congenital heart disease, which has direct relevance to AGS.[127]

Both ligand and receptor are transmembrane and contain epidermal growth factor–like motifs. Mutations in *JAG1* are thought to lead to protein haploinsufficiency and depleted numbers of BECs.[124] Alternatively, there could be a dominant negative effect of a resulting truncated Jagged1 protein produced from genetic mutations in *JAG1* such that the abnormal protein antagonizes the activity of remaining wild-type protein, thus inhibiting the normal function of the protein.[124]

In mouse models, *JAG1* knockouts die in utero of vascular defects, with heterozygous mutations leading to very limited ocular defects.[128] When mice are doubly heterozygous for a *JAG1* null allele and a *Notch2* hypomorphic allele, more clinical features of AGS become manifested, including bile duct, cardiac, ocular, and renal abnormalities.[129] It is likely that the *Notch2* gene may act as a genetic modifier to interact with a *JAG1* mutation, possibly as a digenic disorder but most likely to be in the form of polymorphisms in Notch2, which may influence the severity of AGS.[129] It is clear that *JAG1* plays an important role inasmuch as immunohistochemical studies indicate that Jagged1 is present in human fetal liver on the portal vein,[130] on the ductal plate,[36,131,132] and on BECs in normal pediatric[36,132] and adult liver. Notch receptor expression has been described in fetal, pediatric,[36] and adult liver. There appears to be up-regulation of Notch2 and Notch3 in AGS,[39] whereas data from *Notch2* and *Jag1* mouse knockouts have demonstrated the crucial role of this pathway, in particular with respect to gene dosage, in biliary morphogenesis.[133] Overall, there is poor genotype-phenotype correlation with *JAG1* mutations in AGS. Even in families with a single mutation, expression of the disorder ranges from mild to severe.[120]

Fringe genes encode glycosyltransferases, which modify Notch and alter ligand-receptor affinity. A recent study has suggested that they may be potential genetic modifiers of the Notch-mediated hepatic phenotype. In this study, double heterozygous mouse models were created that were haploinsufficient for both *Jag1* and one of three paralogous Fringe genes: Lunatic (*Lfng*), Radical (*Rfng*), and Manic (*Mfng*). Mice heterozygous for mutations in *Jag1* and the Fringe genes demonstrated bile duct proliferation, which was not apparent in the newborn mice. It is possible that the Fringe genes regulate postnatal bile duct growth and remodeling and therefore could be modifiers of the hepatic phenotype in AGS.[134]

Discordant phenotype has also been reported in monozygotic twins. One study demonstrated that in four sporadic cases, in which *JAG1* mutations occurred in the domain of the gene encoding for the binding region of Jagged1 to the Notch receptor (the DSL region), which led to total deletion of the DSL domain, outcome was poor, with progressive liver failure requiring transplantation at an early age.[135] There is also a single family with isolated heart disease in 11 individuals who have is a mutation in exon 6 of *JAG1*. This is a missense mutation in a region necessary for ligand-receptor interaction.[136]

Clinical Features

Alagille syndrome was originally defined as a paucity of intralobular bile ducts in association with at least three of five other main clinical features: (1) cholestasis, (2) cardiac disease with pulmonary artery stenosis, (3) skeletal abnormalities seen as abnormally shaped butterfly vertebrae, (4) ocular abnormalities with posterior embryotoxon, and (5) characteristic facies[117,118] (**Fig. 68-6**). Since then, a wide range of further abnormalities have also been noted in this group of patients, including renal abnormalities, pancreatic insufficiency, growth and developmental delay, and increased risk for intracranial hemorrhage.[137,138]

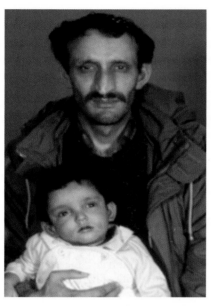

Fig. 68-6 **Father and son demonstrating the characteristic triangular facies, high forehead, and deep-set eyes.** The father is normal, but the baby has severe intrahepatic cholestasis.

In the majority, AGS is fairly benign. Most patients with clinically important AGS have conjugated hyperbilirubinemia in the neonatal period.[137] The liver disease in AGS most commonly becomes evident in the neonatal period, with cholestatic jaundice developing in a similar manner to EHBA or later in childhood with pruritus as a predominant feature. Earlier disease manifestation correlates with a poorer outcome.[139] The cholestasis may be sufficiently severe to produce acholic stools and dark urine, and it may be confused with EHBA. In the past some children with AGS have mistakenly undergone portoenterostomy. Chronic cholestasis with pruritus and fat malabsorption is occasionally exacerbated by exocrine pancreatic insufficiency. The other major features are as follows.

CARDIAC DISEASE

Cardiac lesions are present in more than 95% of patients with AGS. They are mainly right sided, the most common being peripheral pulmonary artery stenosis and severe hypoplasia of the pulmonary artery branches. Other abnormalities include pulmonary atresia, tetralogy of Fallot, pulmonary valve stenosis, aortic stenosis, ventricular septal defect, atrial septal defect, truncus arteriosus, and anomalous pulmonary venous return. The severity of cardiac disease varies among patients, and careful assessment is required, particularly if liver transplantation is being contemplated.

SKELETAL ABNORMALITIES

Skeletal abnormalities, including butterfly vertebrae because of failure of fusion of the anterior arch of the vertebral body, are found in the thoracic spine in approximately two thirds of patients.[140] Multiple vertebral anomalies may be seen in individual patients, including a decreased interpedicular distance in the lumbar spine, spina bifida occulta, and fusion of adjacent vertebrae.[140] Absent 12th rib, shortened distal ulna and radius, shortened phalanges, and fifth finger clinodactyly may also occur.

OCULAR ABNORMALITIES

Ocular abnormalities in patients with AGS may be very diverse.[141] The most common is posterior embryotoxon, an abnormal prominence of the Schwalbe line (junction of the Descemet membrane with the uvea at the angle of the anterior chamber), seen in up to 95% of patients.[141] It requires slit-lamp examination for detection. It is not pathognomonic for AGS because it occurs in 8% to 15% of the normal population. Optic disc drusen, or calcific deposits in the extracellular space of the optic nerve head, are also common in AGS and are not seen in other cholestatic conditions. They are detected by ocular ultrasound examination. Abnormal retinal pigmentation without evidence of functional retinal degeneration may occur. Strabismus, iris abnormalities, ectopic pupil, microcornea, and hypotrophic optic discs with or without abnormal retinal vessels have been reported. The development of benign intracranial hypertension, which may lead to optic atrophy and blindness, has been reported both before and after transplantation.[142] Regular funduscopy is essential to diagnose this treatable cause of blindness.

CHARACTERISTIC FACIES

Patients typically have a broad forehead, deep-set eyes, mild hypertelorism, a straight nose, and a small pointed chin. The facies may not be evident in the first months of life, and the classic childhood appearance differs from the adult form, in which the face becomes elongated.[143] This is a fairly "soft" feature and even experienced pediatricians may have difficulty detecting it accurately.[143]

In addition, failure to thrive in association with intrauterine retardation is common, with severe malnutrition being present in up to half of patients. This may be part of the syndrome or secondary to fat malabsorption or gastroesophageal reflux.

MINOR FEATURES

A number of other features may be present in children with AGS. Renal disease may be present, including renal tubular acidosis, nephrolithiasis, or structural abnormalities such as small kidneys, congenital single kidney, or renal cystic disease.[144] Histologic examination may reveal a membranous nephropathy or lipid accumulation in the kidney (mesangiolipidosis). Renal artery stenosis has also been documented, and therefore monitoring children with AGS for hypertension is important.

Noncardiac vascular anomalies have been reported in 9% of patients with AGS.[145] Such anomalies include decreased intrahepatic portal vein radicals, coarctation of the aorta, aortic aneurysm, intracranial vessel abnormalities leading to cerebrovascular accident, and moyamoya disease.[146] The most significant is intracranial bleeding, which occurs in up to 15% of patients.[137] In 30% to 50%, the bleeding is fatal.

Hypercholesterolemia is common. Associated xanthomas can be disfiguring. Other documented associations include delayed puberty or hypogonadism; abnormal cry or voice; mental retardation, learning difficulties, or antisocial behavior; hypothyroidism and pancreatic insufficiency; recurrent otitis media; recurrent chest infections, perhaps secondary to gastrointestinal reflux and aspiration pneumonia; supernumerary digital flexion creases; and craniosynostosis. Neurologic abnormalities, such as peripheral neuropathy, may be related to vitamin E deficiency from severe chronic cholestasis.

Diagnosis

The diagnosis of AGS is based on the aforementioned characteristic clinical features together with characteristic liver histologic findings.

LIVER FUNCTION TESTS

Neonates have conjugated hyperbilirubinemia, which may improve with age. AST and alkaline phosphatase concentrations are usually elevated by around 10 times above normal values. The GGT concentration can be elevated 3 to 20 times above normal. Serum cholesterol and triglyceride may be raised to values three times or more the upper limit of normal. Serum albumin and the prothrombin time are usually normal unless there is decompensated liver disease.

IMAGING

Abdominal ultrasound may show normal findings or a small contracted gallbladder.

Radioisotope scanning may show delayed or no excretion if the intrahepatic cholestasis is severe. This has led to confusion with EHBA in the past and even to portoenterostomy, especially if the liver biopsy specimen does not show the classic bile duct paucity.

LIVER BIOPSY

Histology shows that atresia of the intrahepatic bile ducts is not usually complete but consists of a reduced ratio of the number of interlobular bile ducts to the number of portal tracts (**Fig. 68-7**). An adequate biopsy specimen is therefore required to evaluate the number of bile ducts effectively. Alagille and colleagues recommended surgical liver biopsy to obtain sufficient numbers of portal tracts,[117] although this is not a universal opinion. For optimal evaluation, between 6 and 20 portal tracts should be present. Hypoplasia of the intrahepatic bile ducts is present if the ratio of interlobular bile ducts to the number of portal areas is less than 0.5 (normal, 0.9 to 1.8). It may be lower in premature infants. The portal areas without bile ducts usually appear hypoplastic as a whole. The total number of portal tracts per square millimeter of tissue is also reduced.

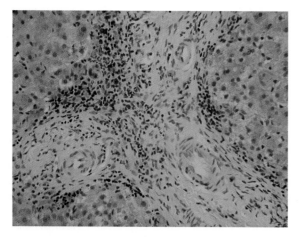

Fig. 68-7 **Liver histology in an infant aged 69 days with Alagille syndrome.** There are prominent arteries but no bile ducts visible. (H & E stain, ×160.)

Diagnostic confusion can arise when there is both EHBA and hypoplasia of the interlobular bile ducts, and care must be taken in differentiating the two conditions. This is especially important because interlobular bile duct paucity is not always present on the initial biopsy specimen in AGS, particularly in young infants. During the first few weeks of life, interlobular bile ducts can be demonstrated in the portal areas of liver biopsy specimens from patients with AGS, but their number gradually diminishes over time,[147] perhaps because of destructive inflammation. Some patients have an almost complete lack of interlobular ducts during the first 4 weeks of life, whereas in others paucity develops later.[147] Ductular proliferation may also be seen during the phase of inflammatory destruction. Hence, paucity of interlobular bile ducts may be diagnostically unreliable in the earlier stages of AGS.[147]

The bile ducts are infiltrated with mononuclear leukocytes, and the epithelial lining cells of the bile ducts show desquamation and necrobiosis. Gradually, the lumen is obliterated by connective tissue, with fading of the inflammatory component.

Periportal or centrilobular fibrosis is usually absent in infancy, but progressive disease with biliary cirrhosis develops in 15% to 20% of patients.

If there are problems in confirming the diagnosis histologically, exploratory laparotomy may be necessary to confirm patency of the extrahepatic ducts, although the presence of extrahepatic manifestations (characteristic facies, vertebral abnormalities, heart murmur, and posterior embryotoxon) is helpful.

GENETIC TESTING

Genetic testing is not yet widespread and is currently most often used as a research tool to investigate the types and number of *JAG1* mutations present in a given population. However, in some families it may be important. Kamath and colleagues have shown that in 34 patients with AGS and known *JAG1* mutations, when 53 family members were studied, 11 (21%) of mutation-positive relatives had features diagnostic of AGS, and another 17 (32%) had mild features suggestive of AGS.[148] This obviously has important implications for genetic counseling and certainly implies that a detailed history and examination are necessary to exclude AGS in the first-degree relatives of patients with newly diagnosed AGS.

Management

Management depends on the severity of associated extrahepatic disease and cholestasis. Cholestasis requires supportive management (see later).

Cardiac anomalies may require corrective surgery, with balloon dilation or surgical correction of pulmonary valve or pulmonary artery stenosis. Detailed discussion of the varying management strategies is beyond the scope of this book. Close liaison with an experienced cardiologist may be necessary, especially when transplantation is being considered. The outcome after transplantation in general, even with elevated right ventricular pressure, appears to be good.

NUTRITION AND GROWTH

Nutritional support is vital. Children with AGS often have poor growth.[149] Rovner and co-workers recently demonstrated that in a group of 26 prepubertal children with AGS, more than half were less than the 5th percentile for height or weight (or both) and 20% had inadequate calorie and fat-soluble vitamin intake contributing to this finding despite being recommended a high-calorie, high-fat diet by their physicians.[149] In particular, poor calcium intake correlated with lower height-age z scores. This highlights the ongoing need to optimize nutritional intake. Feeding via a nasogastric tube may be necessary in an attempt to achieve optimal growth. Additional fat-soluble vitamins are required.

Hypercholesterolemia is related to the severity of hyperbilirubinemia and is difficult to treat but may respond partially to a modified fat diet and bile salt resins in some children, although not all respond. In severe cases associated with disabling pruritus, partial external biliary drainage may lead to the resolution of xanthomas and decrease cholesterol levels significantly.[150] The use of statins is not recommended in young children, and it is not yet known whether they will effectively decrease any cholesterol-related cardiac complications in older patients. Pruritus is frequently far more severe than in other pediatric cholestatic disease and is ongoing in up to 80% of patients.[139]

Renal disease, including renal tubular acidosis, nephrolithiasis, and structural abnormalities, requires specific management as indicated.

LIVER TRANSPLANTATION

Indications for liver transplantation include the development of cirrhosis and chronic liver failure, marked deterioration in quality of life such as intense refractory pruritus, or malnutrition with recurrent bone fractures despite optimal nutrition.[139] Occasionally, early liver transplantation is indicated before the development of severe pulmonary hypertension.

Children with AGS are prone to bleeding episodes without definite abnormalities in coagulation. Special caution must be exercised with respect to head trauma.

Prognosis

Most estimates put overall mortality at 20% to 30% as a result of cardiac disease, intercurrent infection, or progressive liver disease,[137,139] the outcome depending on disease severity. The largest study of outcome showed that in 163 children with AGS and liver involvement, 44 (33%) required liver transplantation, with manifestation as neonatal cholestasis more likely to result in a worse outcome.[139] Actuarial survival rates with native liver were 51% and 38% at 10 and 20 years, respectively, and overall survival rates were 68% and 62%, respectively. Liver transplantation should be reserved for patients with hepatic failure, intolerable pruritus unresponsive to medical treatment, and severe growth failure. Catch-up growth after transplantation may occur, but not in all cases.

Nonsyndromic Paucity of Bile Ducts

Paucity of bile ducts is seen in a number of conditions other than AGS. These disorders fall into the broad categories of infection, genetic (with chromosomal abnormalities), and metabolic diseases. When idiopathic neonatal hepatitis is clinically severe, bile duct paucity may also be present.

Among congenital infections, CMV is the most important cause. Chromosomal abnormalities associated with duct paucity include trisomy 18 and 21. Metabolic disorders associated with duct paucity in infants are diverse and include α_1AT deficiency (which usually indicates more severe liver disease and a poor prognosis), PFIC, and rarely, cystic fibrosis or Zellweger syndrome. Duct paucity may also develop in the late stages of EHBA following Kasai portoenterostomy or in those with primary sclerosing cholangitis.

When no specific associated condition can be found, isolated nonsyndromic bile duct paucity can be diagnosed. These children are reported to have a less favorable outlook than children with AGS, with persistent severe cholestasis and progressive liver damage. The relationship of childhood nonsyndromic duct paucity to idiopathic adult ductopenia, which has recently been described and may be familial, remains uncertain.

Hereditary Cholestasis with Lymphedema (Aagenaes Syndrome)

Aagenaes syndrome is a very rare disorder characterized by cholestasis and lower limb edema. It was initially reported in a Norwegian kindred but has also been described in children of Norwegian descent and in other ethnic groups. Neonatal hepatitis evolves to a chronic cholestatic condition with pruritus and fat-soluble vitamin deficiencies requiring treatment. While the initial cholestasis resolves in early childhood, recurrent bouts of cholestasis, similar to benign recurrent cholestasis, and lymphedema become a prominent problem in adulthood. Chronic liver disease with portal hypertension has not been reported.[151] Abnormal development of hepatic lymphatics has been postulated as being part of the pathogenesis of this condition.

The lymphatic disorder may be due to abnormal development of hepatic lymphatics and can be manifested later than the cholestasis as localized lower limb lymphedema despite normal serum albumin or as hemangioma or lymphangioma (or both).

The genetic basis of this familial cholestatic disorder remains unknown, but the genetic locus has been mapped to chromosome 15q.[152]

Progressive Familial Intrahepatic Cholestasis

Progressive familial intrahepatic cholestasis consists of a group of autosomal recessive disorders with characteristic clinical, biochemical, and histologic features. Much recent progress has been made in understanding the genetic basis of some of these disorders, as well as reclassification into specific subgroups with inborn errors of bile acid biosynthesis and bile acid transport.

Control of bile salt metabolism is complex. Bile formation at the level of the canalicular membrane is driven by ATP-dependent transporters (**Fig. 68-8**). These transporters include the ATP-binding cassette (ABC) proteins MDR1 and MDR3 and multidrug resistance–associated protein-2 (MRP2). The main bile salt export pump is BSEP, which mediates mainly secretion of conjugated cholic acids and other hydrophobic bile acids. It has been proposed that familial intrahepatic cholestasis-1 (FIC1) protein may mediate transport of the more hydrophilic bile acids. Other genes involved in bile salt metabolism include the apical sodium-dependent bile acid transporter (ASBT) and the farsenoid X-receptor (FXR), a bile

BILE SALT TRANSPORT PROTEINS

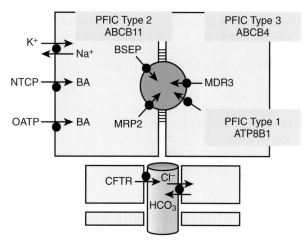

Fig. 68-8 Bile salt transport protein. BA, bile acid; BSEP, bile salt export protein; CFTR, cystic fibrosis transmembrane conductance regulator; MDR, multidrug resistance–associated protein; NTCP, sodium taurocholate co-transport protein; OATP, organic anion transporting polypeptide; PFIC, progressive familial intrahepatic cholestasis

acid–activated transcription factor that mediates transcriptional repression of genes important in bile acid and cholesterol homeostasis.[153]

This section deals with the three types of PFIC associated with specific gene defects in one of the members of the ABC superfamily: (1) PFIC1 (known originally as Byler disease) and benign recurrent intrahepatic cholestasis (BRIC), caused by mutations in the *FIC1* gene; (2) PFIC2, now renamed BSEP deficiency because of mutations in the *BSEP* gene and previously known as Byler syndrome; and (3) PFIC3, with abnormalities in the *MDR3* gene.

Progressive Familial Intrahepatic Cholestasis Type 1

Genetics

Type 1 PFIC was first described in the Amish population. It was originally known as Byler disease because the patients were all descendants of Jacob and Nancy Byler.[154]

Recently, PFIC1 was discovered to be due to mutations of the coding sequence of the *FIC1* gene (ATP8B1). This is located on chromosome 18q21. Roughly 50% of all mutations described to date are missense mutations, with point mutations often affecting conserved amino acid residues. The *FIC1* gene encodes the FIC1 protein,[155] which is expressed in many tissues, including the liver, pancreas, and small intestine.[155] In the liver, FIC1 is localized to the canalicular membrane of hepatocytes and cholangiocytes.

ATP8B1 DISEASE (PFIC1, BRIC1)

The role of ATP8B1 disease in cholestasis is now emerging.[155,156] ATP8B1 translocates aminophospholipids such as phosphatidylserine (PS) from the outer to the inner leaflet of the plasma membrane bilayer. In animal models of mice homozygous for an *Atp8b1* missense substitution mutation (mimicking PFIC1 mutation), PS, cholesterol, and certain enzymes were lost from canalicular membranes during increased bile acid secretion.[155] Membrane instability may impair bile salt transport and decrease hepatocyte resistance to bile salts. ATP8B1 may also, via FXR, up-regulate transcription of ABCB11.[157] Thus the defect in ATP8B1 reduces transport of bile acids in the liver and the gut, which results in cholestasis and watery diarrhea.

Mutations in the *ATP8B1* gene also give rise to BRIC and Greenland familial cholestasis.

Clinical Features

Type 1 PFIC is often manifested as recurrent episodes of intrahepatic cholestasis without anatomic obstruction in the first 6 months of life and leads to permanent cholestasis, intractable pruritus, fibrosis, and eventually, liver failure in the first decade.[157] Other features include short stature, diarrhea, and occasionally, hearing loss. The diarrhea and growth failure persist after liver transplantation, presumably because of the defective transporter in the ileum. In some cases it may become intractable when bile salt secretion is restored.

Investigation

Investigation of familial intrahepatic cholestasis is as described earlier and can differentiate between PFIC3 and either PFIC1 or PFIC2 (**Table 68-3**). Specific immunohistochemistry may also differentiate between the variants but is not widely available. Genetic testing is the only reliable method of distinguishing between PFIC1 and PFIC2 and may become more widespread in the future.

In all types of familial intrahepatic cholestasis, serum bile salt concentrations are high and cholesterol is normal.

Ultrasound should be performed to exclude any anatomic obstruction.

Liver Biopsy

Patients from the original Byler kindred were found to have minimal giant cell transformation, no bile duct paucity or ductular reaction, and bland intracanalicular cholestasis.[158] Initial biopsy often shows mild abnormalities, unremarkable canalicular cholestasis, and minimal hepatocyte degeneration, bile duct proliferation, or fibrosis. Later, the liver architecture may be distorted, with giant cell transformation and some inflammation.

Fibrosis and subsequent cirrhosis develop with increasing age, without ductular proliferation.

On electron microscopy there is a paucity of canalicular microvilli and a thickened canalicular network of microfilaments and coarse granular bile called Byler bile.

Management

Treatment is unsatisfactory. Ursodeoxycholic acid may decrease the cholestasis, but its effect on disease progression is unknown. Cholestyramine or rifampicin may be effective for pruritus.

Partial biliary diversion may be efficacious in some patients and results in a significant decrease in symptoms. If performed early enough, it may even delay or interrupt hepatic injury. There may be long-term amelioration of pruritus with this treatment and even catch-up growth. Histologic changes may also show some improvement.

Table 68-3 Investigation of a Cholestatic Infant

Blood

Liver function tests	Total and unconjugated bilirubin, AST, ALT, albumin, total protein, ALP, GGT
Electrolytes	Sodium, potassium, urea, creatinine, calcium, phosphate, magnesium, bicarbonate, glucose
Metabolic investigations	Fasting blood for cortisol, glucose, lactate, 3-hydroxybutyrate, free fatty acids and amino acids, cholesterol and triglycerides
Specific metabolic tests	Galactosemia and tyrosinemia screen; thyroid function tests, parathyroid hormone; chitotriosidase; immunoreactive trypsin; α_1-antitrypsin level and phenotype
Vitamin levels	Vitamins A and E
Hematology	Full blood count with differential and reticulocyte count; clotting screen, including fibrinogen; blood group and Coombs test
Serology	*Toxoplasma* antibodies, CMV IgM, adenovirus antibody; consider herpes simplex PCR, hepatitis B/C serology, syphilis

Urine

General	Urine pH, glucose, ketones, and protein. Protein/creatinine ratio if protein is present
Clinical chemistry	Amino acids and organic acids, reducing substances, bile acids (if possible), tubular reabsorption of phosphate
Virology	CMV culture
Microbiology	Urine microscopy and culture

Stool

Sample should be inspected for pigment

Radiology

Abdominal ultrasound (after a 4-h fast)

TBIDA scan if acholic stools

Liver Biopsy

Histology, electron microscopy, and snap-frozen and stored metabolic disorder suspected

INVESTIGATION	PFIC1	BRIC	PFIC2	PFIC3
GGT	Low/normal	Low/normal	Low/normal	High (>10× normal)
Aminotransferases	<10× normal	<3× normal	<10× normal	5× normal
Liver biopsy Histology	Minimal giant cell transformation, intracanalicular cholestasis, no ductular proliferation, minimal inflammation, fibrosis late	Normal or cholestasis; no ductular proliferation; minimal inflammation; fibrosis rare	Giant cell transformation, intracanalicular cholestasis, no ductular proliferation, moderate inflammation, fibrosis	Giant cell transformation, intracanalicular cholestasis, ductular proliferation, moderate inflammation, marked fibrosis
Electron microscopy	Coarsely granular bile within the colliculus	—	Amorphous/filamentous bile within the colliculus	—
Immunohistochemistry			Absent canalicular BSEP staining	Absent canalicular MDR3 staining
Genetics	Mutations in *FIC1* on chromosome 18q21	Mutations in *FIC1* on chromosome 18q21	Mutations in *BSEP* on chromosome 2q4n	Mutations in *MDR3* on chromosome 7q21

ALP, alkaline phosphatase; ALT, alanine aminotransferase; AST, aspartate aminotransferase; BSEP, bile salt export pump; CMV, cytomegalovirus; GGT, γ-glutamyltransferase; IgM, immunoglobulin M; PCR, polymerase chain reaction; TBIDA, trimethylbromoiminodiacetic acid

Although liver transplantation is successful in treating the pruritus and liver failure, there may not be any catch-up growth, liver steatosis has been described, and there may be worsening of the diarrhea with poor quality of life.[159] Pancreatitis may occur for the first time following transplantation. A recent report of the development of hepatobiliary tumors requires that annual monitoring be performed.[160]

Benign Recurrent Intrahepatic Cholestasis
Genetics

Benign recurrent intrahepatic cholestasis is also due to mutations in the *ATP8B1* gene. One missense mutation is common in BRIC patients in western Europe, with considerable variation in phenotype, but the phenotype is very different from that of PFIC1. Other mutations are rare. However, there is evidence that there may be locus heterogeneity in BRIC inasmuch as families have been described in whom it did not map to chromosome 18q21. The alternative loci are as yet undefined.

Initial Features

This disorder can appear with the first episode of cholestasis at any age, from 2 months to middle age. Patients tend to have pruritus, although a subgroup of up to 15% may not have pruritus and sometimes, but not always, jaundice.

Attacks are associated with pregnancy and oral contraceptive pills. The number of attacks and frequency also vary considerably, from annually to less than one attack per decade. Each attack may last weeks to months and be severely debilitating.[161]

During attacks there is severe jaundice, pruritus, steatorrhea, and weight loss. Between attacks patients are completely asymptomatic. The frequency of episodes may decrease with age.

There is a small subgroup in whom progressive disease may eventually develop similar to PFIC1, thus suggesting that there is a continuum rather than strict separation of the two disorders.[162]

Investigation

See **Table 68-3**.

Liver Biopsy

Findings on biopsy may be entirely normal. Alternatively, biopsy may show signs of cholestasis with minimal or no inflammation. There is usually no progression to chronic liver disease. Fibrosis is rare.

Management

Ursodeoxycholic acid does not prevent attacks in patients with BRIC, although it may reduce their duration.[163] Partial external biliary diversion or nasobiliary drainage may be helpful.[164] In extreme cases of BRIC, liver transplantation for severe pruritus may be necessary.

Progressive Familial Intrahepatic Cholestasis Type 2
Genetics

PFIC Type 2 is due to mutations in the *BSEP* or *ABCB11* gene on chromosome 2q24.[165] This gene encodes the canalicular BSEP, a P-glycoprotein belonging to the ABC transporter superfamily.[166] This protein is liver specific and is located in the canalicular domain of the hepatocyte plasma membrane. There are many mutations in the *BSEP* gene that give rise to cholestasis[167] and heterogeneous abnormalities in BSEP protein.[168] Two mutations are common: E297G and D482G, found in 25 and 16 families of European descent, respectively. Affected individuals may be homozygotes or compound heterozygotes, which implies that most patients have sporadic disease. A defective BSEP is expressed that leads to impaired bile salt secretion, accumulation of bile salts in hepatocytes, and subsequent hepatocellular injury, apoptosis, or necrosis. Genotype–phenotype correlation in a large cohort of patients with *PFIC* and *ABCB11* mutations found less severe disease when missense mutations were present, thus suggesting that truncating mutations confer an increased risk for hepatobiliary malignancy.[169]

Clinical Features

It is not always easy to differentiate between PFIC1 and PFIC2 by clinical findings. The clinical features and progression of disease may be more severe in PFIC2 than in PFIC1. In patients with PFIC2, jaundice is usually continuous from the outset, and the disease is associated with nonspecific giant cell hepatitis. Progression to decompensated liver disease is often rapid, with liver transplantation being required in the first few years of life. Other clinical features are similar to those of PFIC1 and consist of severe pruritus, growth failure, and cholelithiasis.[167] Diarrhea is not a prominent feature.

Investigation

The results of investigation in this disorder are similar to those for PFIC1 (see **Table 68-3**).

Liver Biopsy

Findings on biopsy may be similar to those of PFIC1. However, the liver architecture is more disturbed. The initial biopsy may show nonspecific giant cell hepatitis, similar to idiopathic neonatal hepatitis. Canalicular cholestasis is demonstrable, but with no real ductular proliferation. There is periportal metaplasia of hepatocytes. This progresses to more inflammatory activity, giant cell transformation, and lobular and portal fibrosis than seen with PFIC1. In the early stages bile duct loss occurs, and hepatocellular carcinoma can develop later.

The bile in patients with PFIC2 is amorphous or filamentous on electron microscopy.

In the majority of patients, immunohistochemical staining for canalicular BSEP is negative.

Management

Patients with PFIC2 do not respond to ursodeoxycholic acid and may have an increase in symptoms or a rise in bile acids without any increase in biliary bile acid secretion.

Partial external biliary diversion may be useful, and in the majority it produces a significant improvement in symptoms. If performed early enough, it may even delay or interrupt the hepatic injury. There may be long-term amelioration of pruritus with this treatment, as well as catch-up growth. Histologic changes may also show some improvement.

Liver transplantation is successful in this group of patients,[167] but recurrence after transplantation has been reported.[170]

Progressive Familial Intrahepatic Cholestasis Type 3
Genetics

Patients with PFIC3 have a defect in ABCB4, the multidrug resistance-3 gene (*MDR3*) on chromosome 7q21.[171] MDR3 is a class III multidrug resistance P-glycoprotein. It is an ABC transporter, acts as phospholipid translocator involved in biliary phospholipid (phosphatidylcholine [PC]) excretion, and is expressed mainly in the hepatocyte canalicular membrane.[172]

ABCB4 abnormalities result in impaired excretion of PC into bile.[155] PC in bile is a major component of the mixed micelles into which salts of bile acids are emulsified. Functional deficiency of ABCB4 permits bile acids to damage hepatocytes and cholangiocytes.[172]

Mutations in *MDR3* were initially suspected to be responsible for PFIC3 because the histologic features are similar to those of mice with a homozygous disruption in mdr2 (the murine equivalent of MDR3), the mdr2$^{-/-}$ mouse. Several different types of mutation have been discovered; it appears that those with missense mutations may have a milder form, more likely to respond to ursodeoxycholic acid and less likely to require liver transplantation. Those in whom the resulting protein is truncated are more likely to require early transplantation.[172] This may be of use in the future when genetic testing is more widely available to monitor patients more effectively and determine the most appropriate treatment.

Genetic defects in *MRD3* are also responsible for intrahepatic cholestasis of pregnancy and probably cholesterol gallstone formation as well.[172,173]

Initial Features

Patients usually have jaundice, pale stools, hepatosplenomegaly, or pruritus. However, short stature and pruritus may be less noticeable than in patients with PFIC1 or PFIC2. Age at onset varies from infancy to adulthood. In a recent review of 31 patients, clinical features of cholestasis were noted within the first year of life in 12, although only in 2 in the neonatal period.[172] Older patients are more likely to have signs of portal hypertension such as variceal bleeding. Progression is usual, with chronic cholestasis and liver failure developing.

Investigation

The investigative features of PFIC3 are very different from those of PFIC1 and PFIC2 (see **Table 68-3**).

Liver Biopsy

Portal fibrosis with a mixed inflammatory infiltrate is present, together with giant cell transformation of hepatocytes. Inflammatory changes are demonstrable from the early stages despite patency of the intrahepatic and extrahepatic bile ducts and normal cholangiographic findings. Cholestasis may be present in the lobules, and there is extensive ductular proliferation in the portal tract.[171,172] Portal and periportal fibrosis is often present. Older patients have more extensive fibrosis and biliary cirrhosis.

Management

Ursodeoxycholic acid is useful in around half of affected patients, with either normalization or improvement in liver function test results.[172] Children with a missense mutation in *MDR3* appear to have less severe disease than do those with a mutation leading to a truncated protein. This seems to have a later onset and is more likely to respond to ursodeoxycholic acid. It may be due to residual transport activity of MDR3 where there is a missense mutation.

When ursodeoxycholic acid fails, liver transplantation may be necessary. In a study of 31 patients, liver transplantation was performed in 18 for liver failure, persistent cholestatic jaundice, or severe portal hypertension at a mean age of 7.5 years.[172]

Inborn Errors of Bile Acid Synthesis

Deficiencies of enzymes involved in primary bile acid synthesis cause some instances of neonatal hepatitis in which serum GGT values do not rise despite conjugated hyperbilirubinemia (see **Table 68-1**). Disorders in bile acid synthesis can be diagnosed by identification of changes in bile acid composition within serum and urine (lack of primary bile acid, high concentrations of intermediary metabolites). Such disorders are important to recognize because many can easily be treated by supplementing the diet with primary bile acids, which can be lifesaving. The fed bile acids stimulate the nuclear receptor FXR and thereby down-regulate bile acid synthesis; fewer toxic precursor species are generated.[174]

Defects in bile acid synthesis are manifested as neonatal cholestasis with low GGT and resemble PFIC2. Because there are 16 enzymes in the breakdown of cholesterol into primary bile acids, disorders of primary bile acid synthesis are common.[174]

A defect in 3β-Δ^5-C27-hydroxysterol oxoreductase has been described as a cause of giant cell hepatitis. Other deficiencies leading to neonatal hepatitis and cholestasis involve Δ4-3-oxosteroid-5β reductase and 3β-hydroxy-Δ^5-steroid dehydrogenase isomerase. The diagnosis is made by detecting the abnormal metabolites in bile or urine.[175]

Other genetic forms of cholestasis also exist and may be due to disorders in hepatic transport. These include Zellweger syndrome and microfilament dysfunction.

Metabolic Disorders Manifested as Cholestasis

A number of metabolic disorders may give rise to a cholestatic picture in the neonatal period (see **Table 68-1**). Of the disorders of lipid metabolism, Niemann-Pick type C in particular must be excluded if hepatosplenomegaly is present. Gaucher and Wolman diseases should also be considered.

Of the disorders of carbohydrate metabolism, galactosemia must be considered, especially where septicemia is present, because although the jaundice is most often unconjugated, cholestasis may occur. Galactose-free milk should be used until the diagnosis is excluded. Rarer disorders of carbohydrate metabolism include fructosemia and glycogenosis III/IV.

Other rare disorders include lymphohistiocytosis. The more common disorders to consider, however, include α$_1$-AT deficiency (see the next section) and cystic fibrosis. Both of these disorders must be excluded because they may coexist with other conditions.

α$_1$-Antitrypsin Deficiency

For a detailed description of this disorder, see Chapter 65. However, it is worth mentioning in the context of infant cholestasis.

Clinical Features

α$_1$-Antitrypsin is manifested as conjugated hyperbilirubinemia in infancy in 10% of PiZZ patients. It is the most common genetic cause of liver disease in children and the most frequent genetic diagnosis leading to liver transplantation.

The most frequent finding is jaundice progressing from physiologic jaundice. Jaundice may, however, commence at any time within the first 4 months of life and usually lasts around 3 months but occasionally up to 1 year. Stools may be pale and urine dark. Most of these babies are small for gestational age and may show poor weight gain. Hepatomegaly is usually present with splenomegaly in around 50%. There may be pruritus.

Differentiation from EHBA is important because the histology may be similar. Features in favor of α_1AT deficiency over EHBA include low birth weight and stools that are incompletely acholic (see **Table 68-1**).

In approximately 5% of cases occurring in infancy, α_1AT deficiency is tragically manifested as late hemorrhagic disease of the newborn (HDN). Bleeding occurs between 2 and 6 weeks of age. Minor bleeding may have been overlooked initially and the child may suffer intracranial bleeding, with its long-term consequences. Vitamin K is traditionally administered at birth in an attempt to prevent such bleeding. This is particularly important for breastfed babies because there is little vitamin K in breast milk and any fat malabsorption secondary to cholestasis may leave them vulnerable to clotting abnormalities.[176] Since the controversy surrounding the use of intramuscular vitamin K, oral vitamin K regimens have been introduced. These vary in dosage, frequency, and type of vitamin K preparation administered. In many units four doses of oral vitamin K are given (2 mg at birth and at 2, 4, and 6 weeks of age), but late HDN is still seen, with an incidence of 2 in 30 breastfed infants with α_1AT deficiency.[177] In Denmark, vitamin K is given orally on a weekly basis until children are 3 months old if they are mainly breastfed (2 mg at birth and then 1 mg weekly). This has resulted in no cases of HDN because of vitamin K deficiency from 1992 to 2000.[178] The vitamin K deficiency seen in infants with cholestasis is rapidly correctable with parenteral vitamin K.

The reasons for very early findings in only a subgroup of patients with α_1AT deficiency are not clear. It has been suggested that there may be an association with intrauterine infection because these babies tend to be small for gestational age. However, such an association has not been substantiated. As mentioned earlier, breastfed babies are more likely to suffer the effects of deranged clotting because of vitamin K deficiency and may be affected earlier than their bottle-fed counterparts.

An alternative theory is that genetic differences in the rate of polymer degradation occur and may account for the variability in clinical findings, with those affected early and having more significant liver dysfunction exhibiting far slower degradation rates of the abnormal Z phenotype.[177]

Patients with α_1AT deficiency in whom neonatal cholestasis develops are more likely to have more severe abnormalities than those in whom liver dysfunction develops later in childhood. Although some recover completely, cirrhosis develops in others, and end-stage liver disease develops in up to a third in childhood.[179] Progressive liver disease in childhood is associated with more prolonged infantile jaundice (>6 weeks), more severe derangement of liver aminotransferases, and the presence of fibrosis or even cirrhosis on the initial liver biopsy specimen. Both clinical findings and liver histology may mimic EHBA, with marked ductular reaction in the portal tracts.

Investigation

LIVER FUNCTION TESTS

Conjugated hyperbilirubinemia is present but may improve with age. AST and alkaline phosphatase concentrations are usually elevated up to around 10 times normal values. The GGT concentration can be elevated up to five times normal.

α_1AT SERUM LEVEL

The serum level of α_1AT in patients with the PiZZ phenotype is often reduced to less than 0.6 g/L (normal range, 0.8 to 1.8 g/L). However, because α_1AT is an acute-phase reactant and may therefore be artificially elevated in patients with liver inflammation, these levels cannot be relied on and phenotype must be determined in all patients with cholestasis.[177]

α_1AT PROTEASE INHIBITOR (Pi) PHENOTYPE

This is assessed by isoelectric focusing on polyacrylamide gels. The normal phenotype is PiMM, and the most common homozygous form leading to α_1AT deficiency is PiZZ. Other forms may also result in liver disease, including the PiSZ phenotype. Note that it is essential that the test be performed in an experienced laboratory. CMV infection may cause a spurious Z band.

Genotype

Genotyping is available only in reference laboratories and is not a commonly used diagnostic tool. There are PCR primers available for the M, Z, and S alleles.

Liver Biopsy

An acute hepatitis of varying severity occurs in early infancy. This may resemble idiopathic neonatal hepatitis, but giant cells are rarely prominent. Liver histology may also mimic EHBA, with marked ductular reaction in the portal tracts. Fatty infiltration may be seen around the portal tracts. There is hepatocellular necrosis and inflammatory cell infiltrate. Fibrosis may be present, with or without portal bridging. Cirrhosis has been described as early as 8 weeks of age.

Periodic acid–Schiff–positive diastase-resistant granules may be seen in hepatocytes. These granules are 2 to 20 nm in diameter and correspond to amorphous material within the endoplasmic reticulum, as seen on electron microscopy. However, they may not be prominent in early biopsy samples and become marked only after 3 months of age.

With increasing age, the cholestasis, inflammation, and hepatocellular necrosis begin to settle. By 1 to 2 years of age, the inflammation becomes limited to expanded portal tracts and adjacent hepatocytes. In children in whom the cholestatic features and fibrosis have been prominent, cirrhosis may develop. However, if there is little early fibrosis or a paucity of interlobular bile ducts on the initial biopsy specimen, cirrhosis is less likely to develop.

Management

Management of neonates with α_1AT deficiency includes the general management for cholestatic liver disease (see later). Nutritional support and fat-soluble vitamin supplementation are important. Close follow-up throughout childhood at a specialist center is mandatory to detect signs of progressive liver disease and the possible need for transplantation.

It is important to counsel the family because this is a recessive disorder. All siblings should be screened and parents informed of the risks in future pregnancies.

Indications for Transplantation

Overall, α_1AT deficiency is the second most common indication for liver transplantation in childhood. Francavilla and associates documented that of 26 children with end-stage liver disease because of α_1AT deficiency, 21 had a neonatal onset of disease at a median age of 2.1 months.[179] Eighteen of the 21 affected as neonates had jaundice for more than 6 weeks. However, some children with early onset of liver disease are stable and exhibit only slow progression of liver disease. Thus transplantation should be avoided unless there is evidence of liver decompensation; hence the need for close follow-up.

Intestinal Failure–Associated Liver Disease

For a detailed description of this disorder, see Chapter 57. Intestinal failure–associated liver disease (IFALD) is more common in infants than in adults or older children and is the most frequent indication worldwide for combined liver and intestinal transplantation.

Survival of infants with intestinal failure has improved greatly in recent years because of improvements in both neonatal intensive care and PN.[180] Parenteral solutions are now safer to use, and improvements in catheter design and placement techniques have reduced septic complications. Hepatobiliary dysfunction remains a significant life-threatening complication and is an important indication for combined liver and small bowel transplantation.

The underlying causes of intestinal failure in infants include anatomic abnormalities and surgical excision of the bowel because of complications of prematurity, gastroschisis, intestinal volvulus, or dysmotility as a result of primary or secondary intestinal pseudoobstruction. The spectrum of IFALD differs in adults and children. Cholestasis occurs in 40% to 60% of infants, steatosis occurs in 40% to 55% of adults, and biliary sludge and cholelithiasis are seen in both adults and children. The cause is multifactorial and the incidence varies according to the population.

Etiology of Cholestasis

In infants, the development of cholestasis is associated with prematurity, sepsis, and possibly lack of enteral feeding.[181] In adults, it is related to the length of the bowel (<50 cm) and the concentration of lipid infusions.

Many studies have noted a close relationship among the development of IFALD, prematurity, and low birth weight.[181,182] Because many infants requiring PN are likely to be premature with low birth weight, it is difficult to ascertain whether these are independent risk factors. However, when Beale and colleagues reviewed 62 premature infants maintained on PN, the overall incidence of cholestasis was 23%, but infants receiving therapy for more than 60 days had an incidence of 80%, which increased to 90% in those treated for more than 3 months.[182] The incidence of cholestasis was 50% in infants with a birth weight of less than 1000 g but fell to 7% if the birth weight was greater 1500 g. This has been confirmed by Beath and co-workers,[181] who found the highest incidence in infants younger than 34 weeks' gestation and who weighed less than 2 kg. The increased incidence of IFALD in premature babies suggests that development of disease may be related to immaturity of the neonatal liver. It is known that the total bile salt pool in premature infants is reduced. There is both diminished hepatic uptake and synthesis of bile salts and reduced enterohepatic circulation as

compared with full-term infants or adults. It is possible that other essential components of bile secretion such as glutathione may be reduced in newborns because hepatic glutathione depletion has been demonstrated in young animals given PN.

Sulfation, an important step in the solubilization of toxic bile salts such as lithocholic acid, is also deficient in the fetus and neonate. It is therefore likely that the liver and biliary system of premature infants is more susceptible to toxic damage of any kind.

IFALD is more common in neonates who have recurrent episodes of sepsis, regardless of whether this is related to central line infections or bacterial translocation from bacterial overgrowth.[181] Bacterial overgrowth from intestinal stasis has been related to the development of IFALD, possibly because of the combination of a reduction in bile flow, production of secondary bile salts, and sepsis from bacterial translocation. Hepatic failure also appears to be closely related to septic episodes or peritonitis (or both). The mechanism by which early bacterial or fungal infection develops is also important. Sondheimer and colleagues reviewed 42 patients who underwent intestinal resection in the neonatal period and subsequently became dependent on PN.[183] Cholestasis developed in 67%, and 25% of these patients progressed to liver failure. The overall number of septic episodes was similar in all patients, even those without cholestasis, but the development of liver failure was associated with significantly younger age at first infection.

An inability to establish enteral feeding is common in children requiring PN and is one of the important indications for intravenous feeding. Nevertheless, IFALD is more likely to develop in children who are unable to tolerate any enteral feeding than in those with partial enteral feeding, although not all studies concur.[181] Experimental studies have shown that short-term fasting has several metabolic and endocrine consequences on intestinal and liver function. Levels of gastrointestinal hormones in patients maintained on total PN are reduced, which may lead not only to intestinal stasis but also to reduced gallbladder contractility. Intestinal stasis may result in bacterial overgrowth, bacterial translocation, and sepsis, which may increase cholestasis,[181] and in the production of lithocholic acid, which has been shown to be toxic to the liver. The reduction in release of cholecystokinin may influence gallbladder size and contractility and cause the development of biliary sludge. Fasting may reduce the size of the bile salt pool and bile formation, thereby compounding the difficulties with gallbladder contractility and the formation of sludge.

Components of PN itself may be detrimental to the liver. It has long been suggested that IFALD may be associated with bacterial or chemical toxins in PN solutions. Both animal and clinical studies have suggested a direct effect of amino acid infusions on the hepatocyte canalicular membrane in the production of cholestasis, but this is unlikely to be a significant problem with modern solutions. Alternatively, the hepatotoxicity may be related to deficiency of an essential amino acid (e.g., tyrosine, cysteine). In older infants and adults, cysteine and taurine are synthesized from methionine, but their production is diminished in premature infants. Not only is taurine one of the main bile acid conjugates in the neonate, but it has also been shown to increase bile flow and protect against lithocholate toxicity. Nonetheless, the benefits of taurine supplementation are unproven. One recent suggestion is that choline deficiency may exacerbate hepatic steatosis in adults and children. In a pilot study the addition of 2 g of choline reduced steatosis in adults, as demonstrated by normalization of hepatic aminotransferases and findings on computed tomography.[184]

There are also potentially toxic components in PN. Historically, degradation of tryptophan in feeding solutions contaminated by sodium bisulfate was thought to produce cholestatic metabolites, but this is not relevant to modern solutions. Although aluminum toxicity is well recognized in patients receiving PN and may lead to bone disease, there is no evidence that it is implicated in IFALD. Chromium toxicity has been reported in animals. Both serum and urine chromium levels are higher in children undergoing long-term PN than in controls, although no correlation with liver disease has been detected.

Manganese toxicity, in contrast, is important in the development of IFALD. A number of studies have reported the effects of manganese toxicity in children receiving long-term parenteral nutrition. Fell and associates studied 57 children undergoing long-term PN, including the multi–trace element solutions of Pedel or Addamel.[185] Forty-five children (79%) had whole blood manganese concentrations above the reference range. Children with impaired liver function had the highest manganese levels, and there was a significant correlation between whole blood manganese levels, AST ($r = .63$, $P \leq .001$), and total plasma bilirubin ($r = 0.64$, $P \leq .001$). Eleven children had both hypermagnesemia and cholestasis, and four of them died. In the seven survivors, whole blood manganese declined when manganese supplements were reduced or withdrawn,[185] and both the brain and liver disease resolved.[186] Because manganese is excreted in bile, the toxic effect may be secondary to cholestasis, and thus monitoring of manganese levels is important in patients with IFALD cholestasis.

There is now some evidence that lipid emulsions induce cholestasis, as well as steatosis. It has been accepted that excess lipid calories may lead to hepatic steatosis, hyperlipidemia, and thrombocytopenia and that close monitoring of triglyceride levels is necessary to monitor for lipemia, particularly in neonates with hepatic dysfunction. More recently, Colomb and co-authors correlated episodes of cholestasis in 23 infants with altered lipid concentrations,[187] and Cavicchi and colleagues demonstrated that cholestasis in adults was related to the use of more than 1 g/kg of lipid.[187a] It has been suggested that the mechanism may be due to a direct effect of lipid on hepatocytes, accumulation of phytosterols, or the production of inflammatory cytokines.

Acalculous cholecystitis, biliary sludge, gallbladder distention, and gallstones have all been reported in adults and children maintained long-term on PN.[180] The incidence of biliary sludge increases with the duration of PN, from 6% at 3 weeks to 100% at 6 to 13 weeks,[188] as does the incidence of gallstone formation, particularly in children who have had ileal resection or disease. The increase in gallbladder size noted in parenterally fed infants as opposed to enterally fed infants is related to the reduction in cholecystokinin production and other gut hormones. Gallbladder stasis may be prevented by the administration of cholecystokinin, by stimulating the endogenous release of cholecystokinin through pulsed infusions of large volumes of amino acids, or by the introduction of small amounts of enteral nutrition.

Clinical Features

The earliest clinical sign of cholestasis is a rise in conjugated bilirubin, particularly during episodes of intercurrent sepsis.[181] Persistent elevation of serum bilirubin (>200 μmol/L) has an adverse prognosis.[181,189] In 22 children evaluated for combined liver and small bowel transplantation, a raised plasma bilirubin concentration (>200 μmol/L) predicted death from liver failure within 6 months in the 11 children who subsequently died of liver failure.

Even in children without obvious cholestasis, hepatic dysfunction with portal fibrosis and splenomegaly may be present. In 37 children referred for small bowel and liver transplantation, splenomegaly was a constant feature in 75% of this group irrespective of cholestasis. Despite extensive hepatic fibrosis and splenomegaly, esophageal varices are infrequent in these children.[189]

Investigation
Liver Function Tests

There is a rise in conjugated bilirubin, particularly during episodes of intercurrent sepsis, associated with an increase in alkaline phosphatase, aminotransferases, and GGT.

Liver Biopsy

The histopathologic changes associated with IFALD include centrilobular cholestasis, portal inflammation, and necrosis with or without fatty infiltration (**Fig. 68-9**). As the liver disease advances, portal fibrosis, pericellular fibrosis, and bile ductule proliferation are seen, together with pigmented Kupffer cells and eventually cirrhosis. Cholestasis is not always present. Biliary cirrhosis is a late development that may be associated with death within 6 months.[189]

Management

Intestinal failure–associated liver disease is potentially reversible if the PN can be discontinued before the development of severe fibrosis or cirrhosis. In many children and adults this is not possible, and prevention or treatment of IFALD includes a number of approaches. The most important strategy is prevention of sepsis, especially early in life.[183] There is a marked difference between the incidence and the age at development of liver disease in children whose central line catheter care is managed by units with nutritional care teams that have experience in PN than in those without.[181] Strict catheter care and reduction of central line infections are important methods to prevent the development of IFALD.

The introduction of some enteral feeding will encourage normal biliary dynamics, decrease gallbladder size, improve bile flow, and reduce intestinal stasis and bacterial overgrowth, as well as potentially decrease episodes of bacterial translocation and sepsis. If enteral feeding is impossible, reducing the duration of daily PN or using cyclic infusions may be helpful. If the cholestasis is severe, restriction of lipid intake and control of manganese and copper levels are important.

To improve bile flow and reduce the formation of biliary sludge, oral ursodeoxycholic acid may be advantageous. Spagnuolo and co-authors reported biochemical resolution with ursodeoxycholic acid in seven children maintained long-term

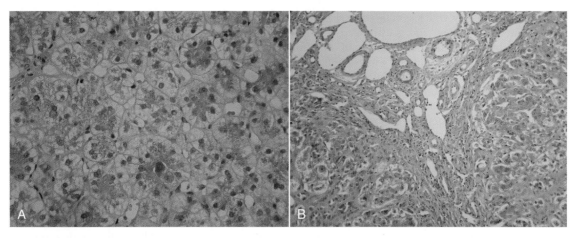

Fig. 68-9 Liver histology in intestinal failure–associated liver disease (IFALD). A, Cholestasis in an infant aged 79 days. There are prominent bile plugs with a mild inflammatory infiltrate. No fibrosis is present. (H & E stain, ×160.) **B,** Advanced IFALD in an infant aged 5 months. There is prominent fibrosis with parenchymal nodular formation. Some inflammatory cell infiltrate and prominent bile plugs are seen in the parenchyma. (H & E stain, ×64.)

on PN,[190] but another study in infants given ursodeoxycholic acid prophylactically found no benefit.[191]

Other strategies to prevent bacterial overgrowth include the addition of fiber to enteral feeding if tolerated because this reduces bacterial translocation. Addition of glutamine to PN solutions may be beneficial in that glutamine reverses the inhibition of mitochondrial metabolism observed in endotoxemia while also improving intestinal adaptation. *Saccharomyces boulardii*, a nonpathogenic yeast, may also have a trophic effect on the gut and reduce bacterial translocation.

It is possible that the presence of liver dysfunction and portal hypertension may prevent adequate intestinal adaptation. Weber and Keller demonstrated that survival and time to the development of feeding tolerance were related to the severity of liver dysfunction,[192] and a number of authors have drawn attention to the improvement in feeding intolerance after isolated liver transplantation in children with severe IFALD.[193]

If prevention of liver failure is not possible, combined liver and small bowel transplantation is a successful option with a 5-year survival rate of greater than 50%.[194] Therefore this must be considered as a therapeutic option in children with intestinal failure. Current results suggest that isolated small bowel transplantation has more favorable long-term results than does combined small bowel and liver transplantation, and this has important implications for children with intestinal failure, but the benefits of isolated liver transplantation in children with severe liver disease and potentially salvageable intestines should be considered.[195]

General Management of Cholestatic Liver Disease

Whatever the underlying diagnosis, a number of general measures should be taken in the management of infantile cholestasis.

Table 68-4 Pathophysiology of Malnutrition in Liver Disease

ABNORMALITY	ETIOLOGY
Decreased calorie intake	Anorexia Fat malabsorption Unpalatable food Use of bile salt resins Portal hypertension
Increased metabolic needs	Energy expenditure Calorie requirements
Inappropriate substrate utilization	Abnormal nitrogen metabolism Negative protein balance Reduction in glycogen stores
Hormonal dysregulation	GH/IGFI Insulin resistance

GH, growth hormone, IGF-1, insulin-like growth factor-1

Nutritional Support

Malnutrition is present in 50% to 80% of children with chronic liver disease. The pathophysiology is complex and multifactorial (**Table 68-4**). Infants with chronic cholestatic liver disease are particularly vulnerable to the effects of malnutrition because of their high energy and growth requirements.

Anorexia is common in children with chronic liver disease, who often take less than the recommended requirements or less than appropriate for their energy consumption because of increased energy expenditure. Energy requirements may be increased up to 140%. Mechanisms implicated include portosystemic shunting and ascites, abnormal intermediate metabolism, and the energy demands of specific complications such as sepsis and variceal hemorrhage.

Fat malnutrition develops first with loss of fat stores. Protein malnutrition is a late development and is associated with a reduction in muscle bulk, stunting, and significant motor developmental delay. In time, children with significant malnutrition will have impaired growth and psychosocial development,[196] and thus malnutrition is not only an important indication for liver transplantation but also one of the most important prognostic factors for survival after liver transplantation.

Nutritional Assessment

Accurate nutritional assessment is essential for the management of children with cholestatic liver disease. It is important to start with a comprehensive clinical and feeding history and a careful physical examination. Serial anthropometric examination is critical and may identify early malnutrition. Standard weight and height ratios are of little value in children with liver disease because of misinterpretation as a result of fluid overload, ascites, and visceromegaly. Many researchers, using sophisticated methods such as whole-body potassium and dual-energy x-ray absorptiometry, have demonstrated that body weight underestimates the incidence of malnutrition by 50% in both adults and children, and for this reason, simple methods of measuring body composition such as body impedance analysis are not reliable in children with liver disease.

Thus assessment of malnutrition should be performed with a number of parameters such as triceps or subscapular skinfold, midarm circumference, and arm muscle measurements (midarm muscle area). Triceps skinfold and midarm circumference are useful indicators of body fat and protein, and serial recording demonstrates early loss of fat stores before changes in weight and height become obvious. Although linear growth is a sensitive parameter, it is a late sign of growth failure in infancy in that stunting (or negative height velocity) may not be apparent until 1 year of age.

Growth data are best expressed as standard deviation scores (or z scores) related to the median value for the child's age and sex, with a z score of 0 equaling the 50th percentile. This is particularly useful in comparisons among centers and for evaluation of new feeding regimens.

Biochemical evaluation of vitamin deficiency is a useful adjunct to nutritional assessment (see **Table 68-3**). Plasma vitamin A levels can be measured but may not reflect hepatic stores. Plasma β-carotene or the ratio of plasma retinol to retinol-binding protein may be helpful. Vitamin E deficiency is monitored by determining serum vitamin E levels or the ratio of vitamin E to total lipid. Vitamin D deficiency is evaluated by measuring serum levels of calcium, phosphate, and alkaline phosphatase, whereas the diagnosis of rickets is confirmed by x-ray examination of the wrist or knee. In some centers it is possible to measure 25-hydroxyvitamin D levels. Vitamin K deficiency is identified by measuring coagulation times and monitoring the response to parenteral vitamin K.

Indications for Nutritional Therapy

The aim of nutritional therapy is to prevent or treat malnutrition by providing adequate calories for energy and sufficient nitrogen for protein synthesis to restore plasma amino acid imbalance, prevent vitamin and trace element deficiency, and achieve normal growth and activity. The need for nutritional support is often underestimated, particularly in infants with liver disease, who may have an increased appetite in the first few months of life.

Strategies for Nutritional Support
(Table 68-5)

Increased Energy Intake

As the resting energy requirements are increased, it is important to increase the energy intake to 140% to 200% of estimated average requirements. This can be achieved by using concentrated formulas (the formula is concentrated 13% to 15%, which increases kilocalories from 67 to 80 kcal/100 ml) or by supplementing milk feeding with extra carbohydrate and fat to produce a feed with an energy density of 4.18 kJ/ml (1 kcal/ml or greater). Because such feeding may have high

Table 68-5 Investigation and Management of Nutritional Deficiencies in Patients with Cholestatic Liver Disease

NUTRITIONAL DEFICIT	INVESTIGATION	MANAGEMENT
Protein	Plasma proteins (albumin)	Ensure adequate protein (3-4 g/kg/day)
	BCAA/AAA ratio	BCAA-enriched protein (32%)
	Protein stores: muscle mass	Albumin infusion if serum albumin <25 g/L
Fat	Triceps skinfold thickness	Change fat intake to 50:50
	Body composition	MCT/LCT
	EFA deficiency	Provide saturated fats high in EFA
	Plasma lipid profile	? Supplement DHA
Energy/carbohydrate	Calorie intake	Increased calorie intake to 130%-150% EAR
	Energy expenditure	Overnight enteral feeding
Fat-soluble vitamins	Vitamin D: plasma 25-OH-vitamin D, skeletal radiography, DEXA	Exposure to light Vitamin D$_{1\alpha}$ (50 ng/kg)
	Vitamin E and A: plasma levels	Vitamin E (50-400 IU/day) (as TPGS) Vitamin A (5000-10,000 IU/day)
Water-soluble vitamins	Specific levels Full blood count	Supplement as required
Trace elements	Specific levels Cardiac evaluation	Supplement as required

AAA, aromatic amino acid; BCAA, branched-chain amino acid; DEXA, dual-energy x-ray absorptiometry; DHA, docosahexanoic acid; EAR, estimated average requirement; EFA, essential fatty acid; LCT, long-chain triglyceride; MCT, medium-chain triglyceride; TBK, total body potassium; TBN, total body nitrogen; TPGS, tocopherol polyethyleneglycol-1000 succinate

osmolality (500 to 800 mmol/L), it should be introduced gradually to establish intestinal tolerance. Calorie supplementation added to drinks may be effective for older children. If there is no response to an increase in energy intake alone, nocturnal enteral feeding by nasogastric tube may be required. An alternative is placement of a gastrostomy tube if nasogastric tubes are poorly tolerated, but this should be avoided in children with severe portal hypertension because of the development of stomal varices.

Medium-Chain Triglycerides

Hydrolyzed protein infant formulas that contain 50% medium-chain triglycerides (MCTs) will maximize fat absorption and improve steatorrhea. Formulas with more than 80% MCTs may lead to essential fatty acid deficiency. In older children, MCT oil may be added to meals and should be balanced by fats with a high polyunsaturated fatty acid (PUFA) content.

Long-Chain Polyunsaturated Fatty Acids

It is important to ensure adequate intake of PUFAs. The minimal intake of linoleic acid recommended for infants is 1% to 2% of energy in a ratio of linoleic to linolenic acid of 5 : 15.1. The diet can be supplemented by the addition of soy bean or rape seed oil or dietary products such as egg yolk (which is rich in essential amino acids) or fish oil (which is rich in docosahexaenoic acid). Alternatively, infants may be given conventional PUFA-supplemented formula feedings, which are available commercially.

Structured Lipids

Recently, chemically defined structured lipids have been developed to increase the absorption of both medium- and long-chain fat and essential fatty acids. These lipids combine pure MCTs with long-chain triglycerides, which results in a triglyceride that contains combinations of short-, medium-, and long-chain fatty acids on a single glycerol backbone that should be absorbed like MCTs. To date, clinical studies in adults have evaluated structured lipids in postoperative patients receiving PN and demonstrated that they are safe and effective in comparison with PUFA emulsion. Although clinical studies of these modified lipids in children are currently in the preliminary stages, animal studies in rats have demonstrated improved fat absorption and reversal of essential fatty acid deficiency in vitro in caco-2 cells.[197] If successful, there might be considerable benefit for cholestatic infants.

Carbohydrate

Carbohydrate is a major source of energy and is particularly useful for increasing calorie intake. It can be given as a monomer, short-chain polymer, or starch, but complex carbohydrates such as maltodextrin or glucose polymer restrict the osmolality of the feed while maintaining a high energy density of greater than 1 kcal/ml, thereby allowing fluid restriction if necessary while providing up to 20 g/kg/day of carbohydrate. In infants, glucose polymers are best added to milk feedings, whereas in older children they may be provided as supplemental drinks.

Protein

The historical advice of restricting protein in patients with advanced end-stage liver disease is now considered inappropriate in both children and adults. Children with end-stage liver disease require a minimal protein intake of around 2 to 3 g/kg/day but will tolerate up to 4 g/kg/day without the development of encephalopathy or a significant increase in plasma amino acid abnormalities. Severe protein restriction below 2 g/kg/day may be required for acute severe encephalopathy but should be avoided in the long term because it may lead to endogenous muscle protein consumption. There is no necessity to use semielemental diets or protein hydrolysates because there is no evidence of protein malabsorption.

In view of the abnormal ratio of essential amino acids to branched-chain amino acids (BCAAs), there has been considerable interest in the use of modified amino acid formulations designed to improve this imbalance. BCAA-enriched formulas may have significant nutritional benefit in children. A study that compared a formula containing 32% BCAAs with standard feeding demonstrated improved lean body mass in children awaiting liver transplantation but no improvement in amino acid levels.[198] In another study, the effect of a modified amino acid feeding containing 50% BCAAs was compared with an isonitrogenous formula containing 22% BCAAs in infants with liver disease by measuring whole-body protein turnover. The BCAA-supplemented feeding improved protein retention when compared with the standard formula by suppressing endogenous protein catabolism and normalizing the plasma amino acid profile. Formulas rich in BCAAs complete with MCTs and vitamin and mineral supplements have been developed for use in infants (Generaid or Generaid Plus), and oral supplements rich in BCAAs are available for older children, but both are particularly unpalatable.

Fat-soluble vitamins are required in all children with prolonged or cholestatic liver disease. Most children will be maintained adequately with oral administration of fat-soluble vitamins, but monthly intramuscular administration is occasionally required for children with severe cholestasis.

Growth Hormone Therapy

In view of the disruption of the growth hormone–insulin-like growth factor-1 axis, it is tempting to prescribe growth hormone therapy for children with significant growth failure, but this has not proved beneficial to date.

Parenteral Nutrition

Parenteral nutrition should be considered only in children with chronic liver disease if they cannot be enterally fed because of feeding intolerance or complications such as recurrent variceal bleeding or abdominal sepsis. Standard amino acid and lipid solutions are well tolerated in stable patients, and lipids may be particularly beneficial in achieving adequate calorie intake. If encephalopathy develops, the amino acid content of the feeding could be reduced to 1 to 2 g/kg/day, but lipid administration requires careful monitoring in children with severe liver dysfunction, hepatic encephalopathy, and sepsis.

In general, the use of PN in children with established liver disease is for short-term purposes only, and thus biliary sludge and gallstones are unlikely to develop from the prescription

First-line therapy
Ursodeoxycholic acid: 5–7 mg/kg tds (maximum 45 mg/kg/day) Rifampicin: 3–10 mg/kg/day Cholestyramine: Under 6 years 2 g/day; over 6 years 4 g/day in divided doses Phenobarbitone: 3–5 mg/kg/day

Central action
Ondansetron: Ages under 12 years 2–4 mg bd; over 12 years 4–8 mg bd Naltrioxone: 6–20 mg/day Trimeprazine: Ages 6–12 months 250 g/kg qds; ages 1–2 years 2.5 mg qds; ages 2–12 years 5 mg qds; ages 12–18 years 10 mg tds MARS therapy (see text)

The above can be used singly or in combination. However, it is recommended that single agents be tried in the order given above, to assess effectiveness. Cholestyramine may be poorly tolerated; phenobarbitone should be administered at night to avoid daytime drowsiness.

Fig. 68-10 **Therapy for pruritus.** MARS, molecular absorbent recirculating system

of PN alone, although prescription of ursodeoxycholic acid, 15 to 20 mg/kg, may be of value.

Management of Pruritus

In recent years many advances have been made in the treatment of intractable pruritus. In many units it is standard practice to commence ursodeoxycholic acid in all cholestatic children, with the addition of other agents as required either singly or in combination (**Fig. 68-10**). Cholestyramine is very effective but unfortunately unpalatable to many children, thus leading to the more common use of other agents. The use of a pruritus score (1 to 10) may help in objective assessment and management.

Biliary Diversion

Partial external biliary diversion may be a very effective tool for the treatment of cholestasis. This procedure involves diversion of bile from the gallbladder through a loop of jejunum connecting the dome of the gallbladder to the skin of the abdomen. It therefore interrupts the enterohepatic circulation of bile salts. Biliary diversion can be a useful long-term treatment to relieve the symptoms of cholestasis and allow normalization of liver function test results.[164,199]

A new alternative treatment of intractable pruritus is the molecular absorbent recirculating system (MARS) or the Prometheus system. Both are forms of extracorporeal albumin dialysis. It was originally developed for patients with acute liver failure. The resulting decrease in bilirubin levels led it to be tried in patients with severe pruritus. Such management appears to reduce pruritus successfully for 6 to 12 months, but more research in this area is needed to determine the

frequency and duration of therapy and possible longer-term benefits and side effects.

Cholangitis

When surgical management is necessary, especially for EHBA, cholangitis is a risk. Prophylaxis regimens vary in the duration of rotating antibiotics and overall duration of prophylaxis. Current regimens involve rotating prophylactic cephalosporins, trimethoprim, and amoxicillin. Aggressive management is vital, with intravenous antibiotics being administered for at least 2 weeks when cholangitis is proven and there is a high index of suspicion. If the symptoms do not settle completely, changing to second-line antibiotics is essential.

Psychological Support

Psychological support is important, especially in families with the diagnosis of a lifelong, life-threatening, or inherited disorder. A multidisciplinary team that provides accurate and timely information and support is invaluable as part of the ongoing management of the child. Such support includes dietetic, social, and psychological input, as well as that of a dedicated nurse specialist to explain the diagnosis, ongoing treatment, and likelihood of outcomes.

Liver Transplantation

As discussed earlier, for many of these conditions liver transplantation may be the only option for some children in whom the disease is life-threatening or severely impairs quality of life. Survival is now greatly improved, with up to a 95% 1-year survival rate and 80% to 90% 5-year survival rate in some cases. It is important to not postpone transplantation until too late because the outcome is better when the procedure is elective than performed for acute liver failure.

Summary

There are many causes of neonatal cholestasis, and early diagnosis is beneficial for an improved outcome, particularly in infants with EHBA. With modern molecular and genetic developments, the diagnosis of many conditions is now possible. There have been significant advances in treatment, especially in liver transplantation and intensive care, as well as improved nutrition and antipruritic agents, which have dramatically changed the outcome for children with persistent cholestasis.

Improvements are likely to continue with the development of new therapies such as MARS, further understanding of the genetic and developmental components of many disorders, and increasing experience of many centers in managing rare conditions. Many children with neonatal cholestasis now have the prospect of a childhood spent achieving normal educational and recreational goals and survival with minimal morbidity into adulthood.

Key References

Allen SR, et al. Effect of rotavirus strains on the murine model of biliary atresia. J Virol 2007;81:1671–1679. (Ref.19)

Balistreri WF, Bezerra JA. Whatever happened to "neonatal hepatitis"? Clin Liver Dis 2006;10:27–53. (Ref.113)

Benjamin IS. Biliary cystic disease: the risk of cancer. J Hepatobiliary Pancreat Surg 2004;10:335–339. (Ref.87)

Bezerra JA, et al. Genetic induction of proinflammatory immunity in children with biliary atresia. Lancet 2002;360:1653–1659. (Ref.44)

Bu LN, et al. Prophylactic oral antibiotics in prevention of recurrent cholangitis after the Kasai portoenterostomy. J Pediatr Surg 2003;38:590–593. (Ref.66)

Carvalho E, et al. Analysis of the biliary transcriptome in experimental biliary atresia. Gastroenterology 2005;129:713–717. (Ref.43)

Caton AR, Druschel CM, McNutt LA. The epidemiology of extrahepatic biliary atresia in New York State, 1983-98. Pediatr Perinat Epidemiol 2004;18:97–105. (Ref.55)

Chardot C. Treatment for biliary atresia in 2003. J Pediatr Gastroenterol Nutr 2003;37:407–408. (Ref.2)

Clotman F, et al. The onecut transcription factor HNF6 is required for normal development of the biliary tract. Development 2002;129:1819–1828. (Ref.38)

Colliton RP, et al. Mutation analysis of Jagged1 (JAG1) in Alagille syndrome patients. Hum Mutat 2001;17:151–152. (Ref.122)

Crosnier C, et al. Fifteen novel mutations in the JAGGED1 gene of patients with Alagille syndrome. Hum Mutat 2001;17:72–73. (Ref.123)

Davenport M, et al. Seamless management of biliary atresia in England and Wales (1999-2002). Lancet 2004;363:1354–1357. (Ref.63)

Davenport M, et al. Immunohistochemistry of the liver and biliary tree in extrahepatic biliary atresia. J Pediatr Surg 2001;36:1017–1025. (Ref.41)

Davenport M, et al. The outcome of the older (> or =100 days) infant with biliary atresia. J Pediatr Surg 2004;39:575–581. (Ref.62)

Davenport M, et al. Randomized, double-blind, placebo-controlled trial of corticosteroids after Kasai portoenterostomy for biliary atresia. Hepatology 2007;46:1821–1827. (Ref.70)

Dell Olio D, et al. Immunosuppression in infants with short bowel syndrome undergoing isolated liver transplantation. Pediatr Transplant 2006;10:677–681. (Ref.195)

Deutsch GH, et al. Proliferation to paucity: evolution of bile duct abnormalities in a case of Alagille syndrome. Pediatr Dev Pathol 2001;4:559–563. (Ref.147)

Dillon PW, et al. Immunosuppression as adjuvant therapy for biliary atresia. J Pediatr Surg 2001;36:80–85. (Ref.68)

Drivdal M, et al. Prognosis, with evaluation of general biochemistry, of liver disease in lymphoedema cholestasis syndrome 1 (LCS1/Aagenaes syndrome). Scand J Gastroenterol 2006;41:465–471. (Ref.151)

Eldadah ZA, et al. Familial tetralogy of Fallot caused by mutation in the jagged1 gene. Hum Mol Genet 2001;10:163–169. (Ref.136)

Emerick KM, et al. Bile composition in Alagille syndrome and PFIC patients having partial external biliary diversion. BMC Gastroenterol 2008;8:47. (Ref.150)

Erickson N, et al. Temporal-spatial activation of apoptosis and epithelial injury in murine experimental biliary atresia. Hepatology 2008;47:1567–1577. (Ref.46)

Escobar MA, et al. Effect of corticosteroid therapy on outcomes in biliary atresia after Kasai portoenterostomy. J Pediatr Surg 2006;41:99–103. (Ref.69)

Farrant P, et al. Improved diagnosis of extrahepatic biliary atresia by high frequency ultrasound of the gallbladder. Br J Radiol 2001;74:952–954. (Ref.57)

Flynn DM, et al. Notch receptor expression in human fetal and pediatric liver: role in bile duct development and disease. J Pathol 2004;204:55–64. (Ref.36)

Frankenberg T, et al. The membrane protein ATPase class I type 8B member 1 signals through protein kinase C zeta to activate the farnesoid X receptor. Hepatology 2008;48:1896–1905. (Ref.156)

Golson ML, et al. Jagged1 is a competitive inhibitor of Notch signaling in the embryonic pancreas. Mech Dev 2009;126:687–699. (Ref.126)

Gyorffy A, et al. Promoter analysis suggests the implication of NFkappaB/C-Rel transcription factors in biliary atresia. Hepatogastroenterology 2008;55:1189–1192. (Ref.45)

Hadj-Rabia S, et al. Claudin-1 gene mutations in neonatal sclerosing cholangitis associated with ichthyosis: a tight junction disease. Gastroenterology 2004;127:1386–1390. (Ref.93)

Hadzic N, et al. Long-term survival following Kasai portoenterostomy: is chronic liver disease inevitable? J Pediatr Gastroenterol Nutr 2003;37:430–433. (Ref.77)

Hansen KN, Minousis M, Ebbesen F. Weekly oral vitamin K prophylaxis in Denmark. Acta Paediatr 2003;92:802–805. (Ref.178)

Harada K, et al. Innate immune response to double-stranded RNA in biliary epithelial cells is associated with the pathogenesis of biliary atresia. Hepatology 2007;46:1146–1154. (Ref.24)

Harger JH, et al. Frequency of congenital varicella syndrome in a prospective cohort of 347 pregnant women. Obstet Gynecol 2002;100:260-265. (Ref.108)

Hayashida M, et al. The evidence of maternal microchimerism in biliary atresia using fluorescent in situ hybridization. J Pediatr Surg 2007;42:2097–2101. (Ref.51)

Heubi JE, et al. Tauroursodeoxycholic acid (TUDCA) in the prevention of total parenteral nutrition–associated liver disease. J Pediatr 2002;141:237–242. (Ref.191)

High FA, et al. Murine Jagged1/Notch signaling in the second heart field orchestrates Fgf8 expression and tissue-tissue interactions during outflow tract development. J Clin Invest 2009;119:1986–1996. (Ref.127)

Jacquemin E, et al. FCI gene mutation and biliary atresia with polysplenia syndrome. J Pediatr Gastroenterol Nutr 2002;34:326–327. (Ref.31)

Jara P, et al. Recurrence of bile salt export pump deficiency after liver transplantation. N Engl J Med 2009;361:1359–1267. (Ref.170)

Kader HH, et al. HLA in Egyptian children with biliary atresia. J Pediatr 2002;141:432–433. (Ref.14)

Kamath BM, et al. Consequences of JAG1 mutations. J Med Genet 2003;40:891–895. (Ref.148)

Kamath BM, et al. Facial features in Alagille syndrome: specific or cholestasis facies? Am J Med Genet 2002;112:163–170. (Ref.143)

Kamath BM, et al. Vascular anomalies in Alagille syndrome: a significant cause of morbidity and mortality. Circulation 2004;109:1354–1358. (Ref.146)

Knisely AS, et al. Hepatocellular carcinoma in ten children under five years of age with bile salt export pump deficiency. Hepatology 2006;44:478–486. (Ref.160)

Kobayashi K, et al. Mother-to-daughter occurrence of biliary atresia: a case report. J Pediatr Surg 2008;43:1566–1568. (Ref.10)

Kohsaka T, et al. The significance of human Jagged 1 mutations detected in severe cases of extrahepatic biliary atresia. Hepatology 2002;36:904–912. (Ref.35)

Kuebler JF, et al. Type-I but not type-II interferon receptor knockout mice are susceptible to biliary atresia. Pediatr Res 2006;59:790–794. (Ref.49)

Kurbegov AC, et al. Biliary diversion for progressive familial intrahepatic cholestasis: improved liver morphology and bile acid profile. Gastroenterology 2003;125:1227–1234. (Ref.164)

Leung AK, Sauve RS, Davies HD. Congenital cytomegalovirus infection. J Natl Med Assoc 2003;95:213–218. (Ref.103)

Libbrecht L, et al. Expression of neural cell adhesion molecule in human liver development and in congenital and acquired liver diseases. Histochem Cell Biol 2001;116:233–239. (Ref.34)

Lina Y, Satlinb LM. Polycystic kidney disease: the cilium as a common pathway in cystogenesis. Curr Opin Pediatr 2004;16:171–176. (Ref.89)

Loomes KM, et al. Bile duct proliferation in liver-specific Jag1 conditional knockout mice: effects of gene dosage. Hepatology 2007;45:323–330. (Ref.133)

Loomes KM, et al. Characterization of Notch receptor expression in the developing mammalian heart and liver. Am J Med Genet 2002;112:181–189. (Ref.131)

Low Y, Vijayan V, Tan CE. The prognostic value of ductal plate malformation and other histologic parameters in biliary atresia: an immunohistochemical study. J Pediatr 2001;139:320–322. (Ref.32)

Luketic VA, Shiffman ML. Benign recurrent intrahepatic cholestasis. Clin Liver Dis 2004;8:133–149, vii. (Ref.161)

Lykavieris P, et al. Outcome of liver disease in children with Alagille syndrome: a study of 163 patients. Gut 2001;49:431–435. (Ref.139)

Lykavieris P, et al. Progressive familial intrahepatic cholestasis type 1 and extrahepatic features: no catch-up of stature growth, exacerbation of diarrhea, and appearance of liver steatosis after liver transplantation. J Hepatol 2003;39:447–452. (Ref.159)

Mack CL, et al. Oligoclonal expansions of CD4+ and CD8+ T-cells in the target organ of patients with biliary atresia. Gastroenterology 2007;133:278–287. (Ref.47)

Marchetti D, Iascone MR, Pezzoli L. Novel human pathological mutations. Gene symbol: JAG1 disease: Alagille syndrome. Hum Genet 2009;126:349–350. (Ref.119)

Martin S. Congenital toxoplasmosis. Neonatal Netw 2001;20:23–30. (Ref.102)

Mazariegos GV. Intestinal transplantation: current outcomes and opportunities. Curr Opin Organ Transplant 2009;14:515–521. (Ref.194)

McCright B, Lozier J, Gridley T. A mouse model of Alagille syndrome: Notch2 as a genetic modifier of Jag1 haploinsufficiency. Development 2002;129:1075–1082. (Ref.129)

McDaniell R, et al. NOTCH2 mutations cause Alagille syndrome, a heterogeneous disorder of the notch signaling pathway. Am J Hum Genet 2006;79:169–173. (Ref.125)

McDiarmid SV, Anand R, Lindblad AS. Development of a Pediatric End-Stage Liver Disease score to predict poor outcome in children awaiting liver transplantation. Transplantation 2002;74:173–181. (Ref.80)

McKiernan PJ, et al. British paediatric surveillance unit study of biliary atresia: outcome at 13 years. J Pediatr Gastroenterol Nutr 2009;48:78–81. (Ref.64)

Miga D, et al. Survival after first esophageal variceal hemorrhage in patients with biliary atresia. J Pediatr 2001;139:291–296. (Ref.74)

Minami K, et al. Septo-optic dysplasia with congenital hepatic fibrosis. Pediatr Neurol 2003;29:157–159. (Ref.111)

Muraji T, et al. Maternal microchimerism in underlying pathogenesis of biliary atresia: quantification and phenotypes of maternal cells in the liver. Pediatrics 2008;121:517–521. (Ref.50)

Narayanaswamy B, et al. Serial circulating markers of inflammation in biliary atresia—evolution of the post-operative inflammatory process. Hepatology 2007;46:180–187. (Ref.42)

Narula P, et al. Visual loss and idiopathic intracranial hypertension in children with Alagille syndrome. J Pediatr Gastroenterol Nutr 2006;43:348–352. (Ref.142)

Neimark E, Shneider B. Novel surgical and pharmacological approaches to chronic cholestasis in children: partial external biliary diversion for intractable pruritus and xanthomas in Alagille syndrome. J Pediatr Gastroenterol Nutr 2003;36:296–297. (Ref.199)

Nicolas I, et al. [Ursodeoxycholic acid treatment shortens the course of cholestasis in two patients with benign recurrent intrahepatic cholestasis.] Gastroenterol Hepatol 2003;26:421–423. (Ref.163)

Paulusma CC, et al. Atp8b1 deficiency in mice reduces resistance of the canalicular membrane to hydrophobic bile salts and impairs bile salt transport. Hepatology 2006;44:195–204. (Ref.155)

Petersen C, et al. European biliary atresia registries: summary of a symposium. Eur J Pediatr Surg 2008;18:111–116. (Ref.60)

Roberts E. The jaundiced baby. In: Diseases of the liver and biliary system in children, 3rd ed. New York: Blackwell/Wiley, 2008:57–105. (Ref.114)

Rosmorduc O, Poupon R. Low phospholipid associated cholelithiasis: association with mutation in the MDR3/ABCB4 gene. Orphanet J Rare Dis 2007;2:29. (Ref.173)

Rovner AJ, et al. Rethinking growth failure in Alagille syndrome: the role of dietary intake and steatorrhea. J Pediatr Gastroenterol Nutr 2002;35:495–502. (Ref.149)

Russell DW. The enzymes, regulation, and genetics of bile acid synthesis. Annu Rev Biochem 2003;72:137–174. (Ref.174)

Ryan MJ, et al. Bile duct proliferation in Jag1/fringe heterozygous mice identifies candidate modifiers of the Alagille syndrome hepatic phenotype. Hepatology 2008;48:1989–1997. (Ref.134)

Saito T, et al. Lack of evidence for reovirus infection in tissues from patients with biliary atresia and congenital dilatation of the bile duct. J Hepatol 2004;40:203–211. (Ref.21)

Sanderson E, et al. Vertebral anomalies in children with Alagille syndrome: an analysis of 50 consecutive patients. Pediatr Radiol 2002;32:114–119. (Ref.140)

Schon P, et al. Identification, genomic organization, chromosomal mapping and mutation analysis of the human INV gene, the ortholog of a murine gene implicated in left-right axis development and biliary atresia. Hum Genet 2002;110:157–165. (Ref.29)

Setchell KD, et al. Liver disease caused by failure to racemize trihydroxycholestanoic acid: gene mutation and effect of bile acid therapy. Gastroenterology 2003;124:217–232. (Ref.175)

Shen C, et al. Relationship between prognosis of biliary atresia and infection of cytomegalovirus. World J Pediatr 2008;4:123–126. (Ref.25)

Shinkai M, et al. Increased CXCR3 expression associated with CD3-positive lymphocytes in the liver and biliary remnant in biliary atresia. J Pediatr Surg 2006;41:950–954. (Ref.48)

Sokol RJ. New North American research network focuses on biliary atresia and neonatal liver disease. J Pediatr Gastroenterol Nutr 2003;36:1. (Ref.72)

Strautnieks SS, et al. Severe bile salt export pump deficiency: 82 different ABCB11 mutations in 109 families. Gastroenterology 2008;134:1203–1214. (Ref.169)

Sumazaki R, et al. Conversion of biliary system to pancreatic tissue in Hes1-deficient mice. Nat Genet 2004;36:83–87. (Ref.37)

The NS, et al. Risk factors for isolated biliary atresia, National Birth Defects Prevention Study, 1997-2002. Am J Med Genet A 2007;143A:2274–2284. (Ref.15)

Todani T, et al. Classification of congenital biliary cystic disease: special reference to type Ic and IVA cysts with primary ductal stricture. J Hepatobiliary Pancreat Surg 2003;10:340–344. (Ref.82)

van Hasselt PM, et al. Vitamin K deficiency bleeding in cholestatic infants with alpha-1-antitrypsin deficiency. Arch Dis Child Fetal Neonatal Ed 2009;94:F456–F460. (Ref.176)

van Heurn LW, Saing H, Tam PK. Portoenterostomy for biliary atresia: long-term survival and prognosis after esophageal variceal bleeding. J Pediatr Surg 2004;39:6–9. (Ref.75)

van Ooteghem NA, et al. Benign recurrent intrahepatic cholestasis progressing to progressive familial intrahepatic cholestasis: low GGT cholestasis is a clinical continuum. J Hepatol 2002;36:439–443. (Ref.162)

Volpert D, et al. Outcome of early hepatic portoenterostomy for biliary atresia. J Pediatr Gastroenterol Nutr 2001;32:265–269. (Ref.61)

Wada H, et al. Insignificant seasonal and geographical variation in incidence of biliary atresia in Japan: a regional survey of over 20 years. J Pediatr Surg 2007;42:2090–2092. (Ref.16)

Wang L, Soroka CJ, Boyer JL. The role of bile salt export pump mutations in progressive familial intrahepatic cholestasis type II. J Clin Invest 2002;110:965–972. (Ref.168)

Weber TR, Keller MS. Adverse effects of liver dysfunction and portal hypertension on intestinal adaptation in short bowel syndrome in children. Am J Surg 2002;184:582–586. (Ref.192)

Yamataka A, et al. Recommendations for preventing complications related to Roux-en-Y hepatico-jejunostomy performed during excision of choledochal cyst in children. J Pediatr Surg 2003;38:1830–1832. (Ref.86)

Yang H, et al. Steroids should be administered after Kasai porto-enterostomy for biliary atresia: a systematic review and meta-analysis. Vienna: United European Gastroenterology Federation, 2008:136, poster 0645. (Ref.71)

Yarlagadda S, et al. A syphilis outbreak: recent trends in infectious syphilis in Birmingham, UK, in 2005 and control strategies. Int J STD AIDS 2007;18:41041–41042. (Ref.109)

Yuan ZR, et al. The DSL domain in mutant JAG1 ligand is essential for the severity of the liver defect in Alagille syndrome. Clin Genet 2001;59:330–337. (Ref.135)

A complete list of references can be found at www.expertconsult.com.

Viral Hepatitis in Children

Scott A. Elisofon and Maureen M.F. Jonas

ABBREVIATIONS

AAP American Academy of Pediatrics
ACIP Advisory Committee on Immunization Practices
ALT alanine aminotransferase
CDC Centers for Disease Control and Prevention
CMV cytomegalovirus
EBV Epstein-Barr virus
ELISA enzyme-linked immunosorbent assay
ELU ELISA-linked units

HAI histologic activity index
HAV hepatitis A virus
HBeAg hepatitis B e antigen
HBsAg hepatitis B surface antigen
HBV hepatitis B virus
HCC hepatocellular carcinoma
HCV hepatitis C virus
HDV hepatitis D virus
HEV hepatitis E virus
HHV6 human herpesvirus-6
HIV human immunodeficiency virus

IFN-α interferon-alfa
Ig immunoglobulin
IgM immunoglobulin M
LKM1 liver-kidney microsomal antibody type 1
PCR polymerase chain reaction
SPLIT Studies of Pediatric Liver Transplantation
VCA viral capsid antigen

Introduction

Viral hepatitis is a systemic infection with predominant involvement in the liver. Agents include hepatitis A, B, C, D, and E viruses. These infections lead to a wide array of clinical entities, including asymptomatic infection, acute icteric hepatitis, fulminant hepatitis, and chronic hepatitis. It is important to recognize that the epidemiology, natural history, clinical features, and treatment options are different in children compared with adults, and differ among age groups in children. This recognition has led to specific prophylaxis regimens and treatment protocols for children and adolescents.

In addition to the hepatotropic viruses, other viruses contribute to the viral hepatitis seen in children. These viruses are more age specific, including herpes simplex virus, enteroviruses, and adenovirus in infants, as well as parvovirus B19, Epstein-Barr virus (EBV), and others in children and adolescents. Beside viral causes, the differential diagnosis for acute hepatitis in children is different from that in adults, and should be considered during evaluation (**Table 69-1**).

Hepatitis A in Children

Infection with hepatitis A virus (HAV) continues to be a reported disease in the United States, but the incidence continues to reported decrease with the implementation of vaccination for more individuals. This is important because of the greater risk of serious disease in adults older than 50 years and patients with underlying liver disease. Although children are responsible for many cases and much of the transmission of hepatitis A, they are less ill and use fewer medical dollars for their care. Seven percent of children under 15 years of age with acute hepatitis A infection are hospitalized, in comparison with 27% of adults older than 45 years.[1]

Epidemiology

Hepatitis A virus is primarily acquired by the fecal–oral route. The virus is found in the stool and blood of an infected individual for up to 2 to 3 weeks before clinical symptoms, and it can persist in stool from 1 to 2 weeks after symptom onset. HAV may be transmitted by personal contact or water/food ingestion. Transfusion-acquired HAV from viremic donors is rare because this phase of the infection is very brief. Of 431 children younger than 15 years with acute infection in 2007, 31.1% acquired HAV from international travel, 23.3% from household or sexual contacts, 15.1% from day care, and 6.6% from contact with a day care attendee or worker. Other sources of infection were unknown (41.5%), contact with hepatitis A patient (18%), food- or water-borne outbreak (6.7%), homosexual activity, and intravenous drug use.[2]

Hepatitis A is reported in all age groups. In 1997 the highest incidence remained in children 5 to 14 years of age, at a reported rate of 15 to 20 per 100,000 population. Children under 5 years were infected at a rate of 10 per 100,000 population.[3] The incidence decreased in 2006 to 1.4 cases per 100,000 population for children 5 to 14, and 0.7 cases per 100,000 population in children under 5 years.[3] These numbers are considered underestimates because many young children have asymptomatic infections or show only nonspecific

Table 69-1 Differential Diagnosis of Acute Hepatitis in Infants and Children	
NEONATE AND INFANTS <6 MO	**CHILDREN >6 MO**
Viral	Viral
Hepatitis B	Hepatitis A
Herpes simplex virus	Hepatitis B
Adenovirus	Hepatitis C
Enteroviruses	Hepatitis E
Human herpesvirus-6	Epstein-Barr virus
Metabolic disorders	Parvovirus B19
Neonatal hemochromatosis	Other viruses
Tyrosinemia	Hemophagocytic syndrome
Galactosemia	Hepatotoxicity
Fatty acid oxidation defects	Medications
Other metabolic disorders	Toxins/herbs
Hemophagocytic syndrome	Autoimmune hepatitis
	Metabolic disorders
	Fatty acid oxidation defects
	Mitochondrial disorders
	Other metabolic disorders

clinical features. Nonetheless, the decrease is dramatic, and is attributed to more routine immunization practices. As a result, adolescents are no longer the most affected cohort, and there is equal distribution among all age groups.[3,4]

Before 2006, the incidence of hepatitis A in the United States varied with race, socioeconomic status, and location, but by 2006, rates by region, age, race, and sex were equal, with ethnicity being the only difference. Although Hispanics had a dramatically lower incidence of infection since more widespread vaccination was introduced, it was still two to four times that of non-Hispanics.[3] With continued widespread vaccination, the most recent data from 2007 show no ethnic disparity in new hepatitis A infections.[2]

Pathogenesis

The pathogenesis of HAV infection is still not completely known, although it is thought to be immune-mediated hepatic injury. This hypothesis has been supported by active replication of HAV in cell cultures without cell death,[5] lack of complement-dependent antibody-mediated cytolytic activity in sera,[6] and evidence of HAV-specific cytotoxic T-lymphocytes in the liver.[7] Pathogenesis is probably the same in children as in adults, although children typically have milder disease.

Clinical Features

Infections in infants and young children may be completely asymptomatic, or children may have gastroenteritis symptoms. Jaundice is rare in this age group, which makes the diagnosis of acute HAV infection difficult. Older children and adolescents, like adults, may have a prodrome of fever, headache, and malaise for several days. These symptoms are followed by jaundice, abdominal pain, nausea, vomiting, and anorexia. In cases of acute hepatitis A reported to the Centers for Disease Control and Prevention (CDC) in 2007, 78% of children aged 5 to 14 had jaundice.[2] As with adults, hyperbilirubinemia typically resolves within 4 weeks.

On physical examination, the older child may be dehydrated and jaundiced and have a mildly enlarged, tender liver. Splenomegaly is rare. Aminotransferases are usually elevated at the time of jaundice and can range from 20 to 100 times the upper limit of normal. They usually improve significantly within 2 to 3 weeks.

Atypical manifestations of HAV seem to be infrequent in children. Cholestatic hepatitis, with jaundice and significant pruritus lasting more than 12 weeks, and biphasic or relapsing hepatitis are uncommon in children, but have been reported.[8,9] Extrahepatic manifestations such as cutaneous vasculitis,[10] arthritis, and cryoglobulinemia are also rare in children.[11] Pancreatitis has been reported during acute HAV infection.[12,13]

Diagnosis

The diagnosis of HAV infection in children is made as in adults, with detection of immunoglobulin M (IgM) to HAV (IgM anti-HAV). This antibody is present in serum approximately 5 to 10 days before the onset of symptoms and can remain for up to 6 months. Immunoglobulin G to HAV (IgG anti-HAV) appears early and will remain for the individual's lifetime, conferring long-term immunity.

Differential Diagnosis

In infants and children with acute HAV, because clinical symptoms of viral gastroenteritis are common, differential diagnosis includes viral infections such as rotavirus or other enteroviruses, and bacterial or parasitic enteritis. Aminotransferases and bilirubin are not usually measured in children with these symptoms.

In older children with acute hepatitis symptoms, other viral etiologies, such as EBV, acute hepatitis B, and acute hepatitis C, must be considered. Other possible infections include herpes simplex virus and cytomegalovirus (CMV) in immunocompromised patients, as well as non–A-E hepatitis, which frequently leads to fulminant hepatic failure. Causes such as parvovirus B19 infection, autoimmune hepatitis, and medication or toxin hepatotoxicity must be considered in the appropriate clinical settings.

Prognosis and Natural History

Acute HAV infection resolves spontaneously and fully in most cases. Few children have the atypical manifestations, as described previously. The most significant complication is fulminant hepatic failure causing death or requiring transplantation. In the United States, fewer than 1% of fulminant hepatic failure cases in children are attributed to hepatitis A.[14] This is in contrast to Latin America, where more than 40% of pediatric fulminant liver failure is caused by HAV.[15] The risk of hepatic failure is higher in children less than 5 years old[16] and patients with chronic hepatitis C infection.[17] In 2006 there were five reported deaths in the United States because of acute hepatitis A infection; none of these were in children.[3] According to the Studies of Pediatric Liver Transplantation (SPLIT) registry, which collects data from 37 North American pediatric liver transplant centers, only 2 (0.1%) of the 2291 pediatric transplants between 1995 and June 2006 were for fulminant hepatitis A.[18]

Treatment

Treatment of acute hepatitis A infection is purely supportive. For young children with vomiting or diarrhea, close monitoring of hydration is important. Any evidence of altered mental status or bleeding indicates that the child must be followed for development of fulminant hepatic failure.

Immunoprophylaxis

Prophylaxis for hepatitis A can be given actively with vaccine or passively with immunoglobulin (Ig). This decision depends on multiple factors. For travel to endemic areas, children under 1 year requiring preexposure prophylaxis should receive immune globulin intramuscularly (0.02 ml/kg) because a vaccine is not yet approved for this age group. This confers protection for 3 months. If longer protection (3 to 5 months) is required, a dose of 0.06 ml/kg is recommended. If the child is at least 1 year old, vaccination is appropriate if provided more than 2 to 4 weeks before travel.

For postexposure prophylaxis, children less than 1 year should be given 0.02 ml/kg Ig intramuscularly within 2 weeks.[19,20] Testing for anti-HAV is not needed for these children before the Ig. The Advisory Committee of Immunization Practices (ACIP) now recommends that healthy, unvaccinated children or adolescents with HAV exposure receive only hepatitis A vaccine at the age-appropriate dose.[20] This is based on a randomized, double-blind noninferiority trial comparing the efficacy of hepatitis A vaccine versus Ig after exposure to HAV.[21] Children who are less than 1 year, immunocompromised, or affected by chronic liver disease should still receive Ig for postexposure prophylaxis.

Effective vaccines for HAV have been available since 1995. In 1999, after reviewing data from 1987 to 1997, the CDC suggested routine vaccination for children living in areas of the United States that had HAV incidence rates of at least 20 per 100,000 (Alaska, Arizona, California, Idaho, Nevada, New Mexico, Oklahoma, Oregon, South Dakota, Utah, and Washington) and consideration of vaccination in states (Arkansas, Colorado, Missouri, Montana, Texas, Wyoming) and counties with more than 10 per 100,000 during that time period.[22] When these recommendations were implemented, the incidence in these states became comparable with those in northeastern states. The number of reported hepatitis A infections was lower in 2001 than ever before, with the greatest decline in children aged 5 to 14 years.[23] Subsequently, routine administration of HAV was recommended for all children 1 to 18 years.[19] As mentioned previously, the HAV vaccine is approved for use in children 1 year of age and older. Children aged 1 to 17 should receive two doses (an initial dose and one 6 to 12 months later) of either Havrix (SmithKline Beecham Biologicals) 720 ELISA-linked units (ELU) or Vaqta (Merck) 25 units.

Studies have demonstrated good immunogenicity and safety with HAV vaccination in children with chronic liver disease.[24,25]

Daily Activities

Children with acute hepatitis A should be excluded from activities, day care, or school for at least 1 week after the onset of clinical symptoms. Attention to personal hygiene is important to prevent secondary cases.

Conclusion

Hepatitis A is an acute hepatitis that is frequently asymptomatic or well tolerated in the pediatric population. Although most children recover from this illness, vaccinations can prevent sequelae such as fulminant hepatitis or hepatitis in adult contacts. Currently, universal vaccination is recommended for children 1 year and older.

Hepatitis B

Hepatitis B virus (HBV) infection is a worldwide health issue for all populations, but the epidemiology, modes of transmission, clinical features, and natural progression of the disease are different in children. Because of these differences, monitoring and treatment decisions are not the same for children and adults.

Epidemiology

The prevalence of HBV and its modes of transmission differ significantly in populations around the world. High-prevalence areas of HBV include densely populated areas of Africa and Asia. Vertical transmission from mother to infant, either in utero or around the time of delivery, is a dominant mode of HBV acquisition in these areas. Vertical transmission accounts for 40% to 50% of the transmission in Asia, and chronic HBV infections in these endemic populations are established before 2 years of age.[26] The risk of a newborn becoming infected by a hepatitis B surface antigen (HBsAg)-positive, hepatitis B e antigen (HBeAg)-positive mother is 85% to 90%.[26a] Vertical transmission carries the highest risk of chronic HBV and the lowest risk of acute symptomatic hepatitis. Vertical transmission must be addressed in hepatitis B prevention programs because the likelihood of chronic infection is inversely proportional to the age at acquisition.[27]

Horizontal transmission, from child to child, is the main mode of transmission for children in the United States because perinatal transmission is prevented with neonatal hepatitis B immune globulin (HBIg) administration and vaccination. Children at risk for horizontal transmission include those living in households with chronically infected individuals and children living in communities in which HBV is highly endemic. Adolescents at risk for infection are those who engage in high-risk behavior, including unprotected sexual activity and intravenous drug use. Most children with chronic hepatitis B infection in this country are immigrant or adopted children from HBV-endemic regions of the world.

Data collected by the CDC over the last 20 years have shown the declining incidence of hepatitis B infection in the United States, secondary to routine screening of pregnant women, wide use of the HBV vaccines, and changing practices among intravenous drug users. Before 1982, when the first vaccine became widely available, at least 20,000 U.S. children were infected annually.[28] From 1986 to 2000, the rate of acute hepatitis B infection in children aged 1 to 9 years declined by more than 80%, from 0.9 to 0.13 per 100,000 children aged 1 to 9 years.[29] Between 1990 and 2006, acute hepatitis B had declined by 98% among young people up to age 15 years.[3] Although these data demonstrate a decline in acute HBV cases in children, they do not reflect all new pediatric cases because of immigration of already-infected children, and chronic asymptomatic infections that are due to perinatal or early childhood infections in high-risk groups.

Pathogenesis

The primary difference in pathogenesis of HBV infection between adults and children is reflected in the percentage of children who become chronically infected. Most infants who acquire the virus perinatally have immune tolerance that permits chronic infection with high rates of viral replication and minimal immune response. These children usually have minimal hepatic inflammation or mild hepatitis. Immune tolerance may be induced by transplacental exposure to HBeAg in utero. This has been substantiated by the absence of T-cell responses to HBcAg (hepatitis B core antigen) in children born to HBsAg-positive, HBeAg-positive mothers, but an active response of T cells to HBcAg in infants with acute hepatitis B born to HBeAg-negative mothers.[30]

Clinical Features

There is a wide spectrum of clinical manifestations of acute and chronic hepatitis B infection in children. Manifestations are different for neonates compared with older children.

Vertically infected neonates are usually asymptomatic, with normal aminotransferases. However, fulminant hepatitis B, albeit rare in the United States, has been reported and is more common in endemic areas such as Taiwan, and in infants born to HBeAg-negative mothers.[31-33] Children with fulminant hepatitis B have jaundice and abnormal aminotransferases by 2 to 3 months of age. The mortality of this condition is very high.[34]

Young children and adolescents may also have asymptomatic infections, with the diagnosis discovered through routine laboratory tests. When symptoms do occur, they may include a prodrome consisting of fatigue, malaise, nausea, low-grade fever, or a serum sickness-like reaction. Within a week or two of the prodrome, children may develop icteric hepatitis. During this icteric phase, children may experience nausea, vomiting, or pruritus. Physical findings may include tender hepatomegaly or splenomegaly.

In addition to constitutional symptoms, children with acute HBV infections will occasionally exhibit extrahepatic manifestations. Most of these are attributed to immune complexes. As stated earlier, children may exhibit a serum sickness-like illness, consisting of arthralgia or arthritis, urticaria or angioedema, and a maculopapular rash. These symptoms usually improve with the onset of jaundice. Young children will rarely develop Gianotti-Crosti syndrome, which includes papular acrodermatitis of the face, extremities, and trunk, with lymphadenopathy. This may be the only clinical sign of hepatitis B infection, but can be seen with other viral infections as well.[35]

Chronic hepatitis B infection in children is usually asymptomatic. The children usually grow well and are clinically healthy. Children with chronic hepatitis B infection occasionally develop membranoproliferative glomerulonephritis or nephrotic syndrome,[36-38] but other extrahepatic manifestations are rare. HBV-associated glomerular disease in children has been shown to improve with antiviral therapy.[39-41] Chronic HBV infection in children may not be manifest until symptoms of cirrhosis or hepatocellular carcinoma (HCC) develop.

Diagnosis

The diagnosis of acute HBV infection in children is made as it is in adults, by detection of HBsAg and IgM antibody to hepatitis B core (anti-HBc). Chronic HBV infection is defined by the presence of HBsAg in serum for more than 6 months.

Chronic infections are further characterized as with or without active viral replication, depending on the detection of HBeAg or HBV DNA in serum (see Chapter 30). Most chronic HBV infections in children are associated with high levels of viral replication, leading to very high levels of viremia. ALT values may either be normal, reflecting lack of significant immune response, or elevated, indicating immune-mediated hepatocellular injury.

Differential Diagnosis

Acute Hepatitis

Acute hepatitis B in neonates is rare. Neonatal hepatitis is more commonly seen with herpes simplex virus,[42] echoviruses,[43] and adenoviruses[44] (see **Table 69-1**). These neonates are usually quite ill, with coagulopathy and other evidence of fulminant hepatic failure. The differential diagnosis of acute hepatitis in toddlers, children, and adolescents includes infection with hepatitis A, hepatitis C, EBV, and parvovirus B19,[45] as well as noninfectious disorders (see **Table 69-1**). Acute hepatitis because of superinfection of children with chronic HBV infection by hepatitis D virus (HDV) is uncommon.

Chronic Hepatitis

In addition to chronic HBV, chronic aminotransferase elevations in childhood may be due to hepatitis C, α_1-antitrypsin deficiency, Wilson disease, autoimmune hepatitis, and medication hepatotoxicity. Other causes include tyrosinemia, cystic fibrosis, or other metabolic disorders, such as carbohydrate metabolism defects or fatty acid oxidation defects (**Table 69-2**).

Associated Conditions and Infections

In addition to the clinical features discussed earlier, co-infection with HDV, human immunodeficiency virus (HIV), or hepatitis C virus (HCV) is rare, but does occur. A 1985 report from Italy, an endemic region for HDV, indicated that 13 of 102 (12.7%) HBV-infected Italian children had HDV co-infection.[46] However, HDV is seen with decreasing frequency, even in endemic areas. Recent data regarding prevalence of HDV infection in children are not available.

Disease Complications Pertinent to Infection Acquired in Childhood

As discussed earlier, extrahepatic manifestations in children are uncommon, with glomerular disease being the only

Table 69-2 Differential Diagnosis of Chronic Hepatitis in Children

Viral
  Hepatitis B
  Hepatitis C
  Hepatitis D
Autoimmune hepatitis
Nonalcoholic fatty liver disease
Primary sclerosing cholangitis
Hepatotoxicity because of medications or toxins
α_1-Antitrypsin deficiency
Wilson disease
Hereditary hemochromatosis
Celiac disease
Cystic fibrosis
Metabolic disorders
  Fatty acid oxidation defects
  Mitochondrial disorders
  Tyrosinemia
  Carbohydrate metabolism
  Amino acid metabolism
  Bile acid synthesis disorders
  Others

condition reported.[36-38] One center in Turkey reported 14 children with HBV-related glomerulonephritis over 20 years.[38]

Of greatest concern in infants with perinatally acquired disease is severe hepatitis with fulminant hepatic failure. Since implementation of universal HBV vaccination programs, the incidence of fulminant hepatitis B in children that had a mortality rate as high as 61% to 77% had decreased.[34] In Taiwan the infant mortality rate from HBV infection of 5.36 per 100,000 in the years 1975 to 1984 (before immunization) declined to 1.71 per 100,000 in years 1985 to 1998 after programs of mass vaccination.[47] Over the last several years, there have been no reported deaths from acute hepatitis B in U.S. children younger than 15 years old.[2] It has been shown in the United States, Taiwan, and Japan that HBV-associated fulminant hepatic failure is more common in infants born to HBeAg-negative or anti-HBe–positive mothers.[31,32]

Prognosis and Natural History

Age at infection is the most important factor in determining the risk of chronic hepatitis B.[27] Approximately 90% of infants infected during the perinatal period will develop chronic infection. This compares with 25% to 50% of children infected between ages 1 and 5 years, and 6% to 10% of older children.[48]

In Asia, infants with perinatally acquired HBV will have high levels of HBV DNA and continue to be HBeAg-positive into late childhood. These children usually have minimal liver disease and normal alanine aminotransferase (ALT).[49] Spontaneous seroconversion from HBeAg to anti-HBe occurs in fewer than 2% per year of children under 3 years, and 4% to 5% per year of children over 3 years.[50]

In contrast to the Asian population, long-term studies conducted in Italy and Spain demonstrate outcomes of chronic hepatitis B in Caucasian children. In one series of 76 Italian children followed longitudinally for 1 to 12 years (mean, 5 years) HBeAg-positive children seroconverted to anti-HBe and lost HBV DNA at a mean annual rate of 16%.[51] This represents an overall 70% rate of seroconversion and loss of HBV DNA during the observation period. Those patients who lost HBeAg had higher ALT values, indicating more active liver disease. Five of the 76 children cleared HBsAg.[51]

Another outcome study from Italy and Spain included 185 children with chronic hepatitis B and no other underlying chronic disorders. Ninety-one percent of these children were HBeAg-positive.[52] The mean age of these children was 5 years, and only 14% were known to have contracted hepatitis B perinatally. Five children (3%) had cirrhosis at entrance to the study. In a follow-up that averaged 13 years, more than 80% of the HBeAg-positive children developed anti-HBe seroconversion and normal ALT before adulthood. Of the children who originally had anti-HBe, 88% achieved sustained normalization of ALT.[52] Children with natural seroconversion have subsequently been followed long term.[53] With a mean follow-up of 14 years, only 4 of 85 (4.7%) HBeAg-negative children had reactivation, 3 of whom developed HBeAg-negative chronic hepatitis. There were no deaths in 20 years of follow-up.

The differences in the rate of early seroconversion between Asian and Western children are most likely because of the age of infection. Later infection is associated with a significantly better immune response.

Liver histology in HBeAg-positive children usually shows mild inflammation and fibrosis. This inflammation is usually milder than in adults.[54] Cirrhosis is an uncommon finding during childhood, but if present, usually develops early and is often noted on the initial biopsy.[52]

Of greatest concern for longstanding hepatitis B infection is the risk of hepatocellular carcinoma (HCC) and its poor prognosis, with fewer than 30% of children surviving 5 years.[55,56] HCC is a rare cancer in children without chronic HBV, or an inborn error of metabolism known to be associated with HCC. Pediatric HCC associated with chronic HBV has been described in both Asian and Western populations.[57,58] Although HCC is usually thought to occur after decades of chronic infection, studies have shown a significant incidence of childhood HCC in HBV-endemic areas.[59] Before hepatitis B vaccine was available, the annual incidence of HCC was 0.7 per 100,000 children aged 6 to 14 in Taiwan,[59] and 0.05 for Caucasians and 0.02 for Afican American per 100,000 children under 15 years in the United States.[60] Subsequent studies from Taiwan have demonstrated a significant decrease in HCC incidence: from 0.70 per 100,000 children from 1981 to 1986, 0.57 from 1986 to 1990, and 0.36 from 1990 to 1994.[59] A recent 20 year follow-up of vaccinated children has confirmed these data.[61]

Early seroconversion or the presence of anti-HBe in patients with HCC has been shown in other studies in both Asian and Western populations. Many of these children have had rapid development of cirrhosis.[62,63] These data suggest that early HBeAg seroconversion, especially in the presence of early cirrhosis, is an important risk factor for HCC in childhood.

No specific recommendations for HCC screening in children have been made, but many practitioners will obtain annual α-fetoprotein levels and, beginning in later childhood or adolescence, periodic hepatic ultrasounds in children with chronic HBV.

Treatment

Acute hepatitis B has no proven treatment, and care is purely supportive. There has been no proven role for antiviral medications during acute or fulminant infection in children but this has been studied in adults with limited success.[64]

As discussed previously, children are frequently immune tolerant and most often do not have significant liver disease in childhood. The natural history and factors associated with liver disease progression are different in children and adults. Because of this, therapeutic strategies for adults cannot be extrapolated to infants and children. The treating physician must take into consideration the patient's age, age at acquisition, and level of immune reactivity. General principles of management of these patients are listed in **Table 69-3**.

Although in adults the therapeutic benefit of reducing viremia has been established, this is controversial in children. Treatment during the immune-tolerant stage, with normal ALT, has not been proven of benefit, even though viral levels are quite high. In addition, the available agents are not effective at inducing HBeAg seroconversion at this stage. Once aminotransferases are documented as persistently greater than 1.5 to 2 times the upper limit of normal for at least 3 to 6 months, treatment can be considered. Treatment candidates should have evidence for active HBV replication, such as positive HBeAg or HBV DNA of at least 4 log (measured by quantitative polymerase chain reaction [PCR] assays) in serum. It is crucial to ensure that elevated aminotransferases are not indicative of active seroconversion because in this case treatment is not indicated or necessary. This is done by following the ALT values and HBeAg for at least 4 to 6 months before initiating therapy. Before any treatment, a liver biopsy should be considered to confirm that hepatitis B is the only cause of the hepatitis, and to quantify the degree of inflammation and fibrosis. Genotype evaluation before therapy has not been fully studied in children, but data from both children and adults show certain genotypes to be more likely to respond to interferon treatment.[65-67]

Currently, three medications are approved by the U.S. Food and Drug Administration for the treatment of chronic hepatitis B in children. Interferon-alfa (IFN-α) and lamivudine are approved for children aged 2 to 17 years. Adefovir dipivoxil is approved for children 12 to 17 years of age.

Interferon-Alfa

Interferon-alfa has been evaluated in individual populations and in large, multinational studies. It is tolerated well in children, with a good safety profile. Data from Western countries show loss of HBV DNA or HBeAg seroconversion to be 20% to 58% in IFN-treated children compared with 8% to 17% in controls.[68-70] These data differed from that from Chinese populations, with responses ranging from 3% to 17% HBeAg seroconversion or loss of HBV DNA.[71-73] Originally, these differences were thought to be secondary to the early age of infection in the Chinese population, as well as genetic and immunologic factors. More recently, these differences have been attributed to the inclusion of large numbers of children with normal or nearly normal ALT values in these studies.

A multinational, randomized, controlled trial included 144 children with chronic hepatitis B and ALT values averaging greater than twice the upper limit of normal.[70] Twenty-six percent of children who received IFN-α at 6 MU/m^2 three times a week for 24 weeks lost HBeAg and HBV DNA compared with 11% of controls. HBsAg became negative in 10% of treated patients and 1% of controls. In contrast to previous studies, there was no significant difference in response rates between Asians (22%) and non-Asians (26%). Response rates appeared to be higher in patients under 13 years, females, and those with low levels of HBV DNA. Responses to IFN-α can be delayed up to 1 year after the end of therapy. Factors that have been shown to be associated with response to IFN-α in children are listed in **Table 69-4**. IFN-α appears to be more successful in inducing HBeAg seroconversion in patients with HBV genotypes A and B.[65-67]

Early side effects of IFN-α in children include flulike symptoms of fever, myalgia, headache, arthralgia, and anorexia. Bone marrow suppression, specifically neutropenia, has been shown as frequently as 39% during the first month of treatment. Some children require dose adjustments, but most do not require discontinuation.[74] Children may have personality changes, irritability, and temper tantrums.[70,74] Weight gain and growth velocity may be compromised in children during therapy.[75,76] Data from a multinational study indicated that children undergoing treatment have temporary delays in both growth and weight gain in comparison with control children with chronic hepatitis B. Growth velocity and weight gain improved in the 6 months after treatment, becoming similar to those of untreated patients with chronic hepatitis B.[75]

IFN-α is effective for the treatment of hepatitis B in children with immune activation demonstrated by high ALT values. In addition to inducing HBeAg seroconversion, there is a higher rate of loss of HBsAg, and the treatment duration is finite as opposed to long term. Given that IFN-α therapy has more favorable outcomes with certain genotypes, treatment may be influenced by this factor, but this strategy has not yet been rigorously tested in children.

Table 69-3 Management of Chronic Hepatitis B in Children[172]

1. Prove chronic infection by at least two HBsAg-positive samples 6 months apart or anti-HBc, not IgM
2. Measure ALT every 6 months in children older than 2 years
3. Yearly HBeAg and anti-HBe in patients with normal ALT to detect spontaneous seroconversion
4. Liver biopsy, and consider treatment for children older than 2 years with ALT >1.5-2× upper limit of normal for more than 3 to 6 months and no evidence of seroconversion
5. Regular physical examinations for evidence of chronic liver disease
6. Immunize all household contacts and test for immunity
7. Immunize all hepatitis B patients with hepatitis A vaccine
8. Yearly serum α-fetoprotein and liver ultrasound*

Adapted from Broderick A, Jonas MM. Management of hepatitis B in children. In: Tran TT, Martin P, editors. Clinics in liver disease. Philadelphia: WB Saunders, 2004:387–401.

*No data to support optimal age to begin liver ultrasound surveillance and optimal interval between ultrasound scans.

ALT, alanine aminotransferase; anti-HBc, IgM antibody to hepatitis B core; anti-HBe, antibody to hepatitis B e antigen; HBeAg, hepatitis B e antigen; HBsAg, hepatitis B surface antigen; IgM, immunoglobulin M.

Table 69-4 Variables Associated with Virologic Response to Interferon alfa,[70,173-177] Lamivudine[79,80] and Adefovir Dipivoxil[83] in Children with Chronic Hepatitis B

Interferon Alfa

Associated with higher likelihood of response:
ALT ≥2× the upper limit of normal
Female sex
Low level of hepatitis B virus DNA
Age less than 13 years, if ALT ≥2 × upper limit of normal
Genotype A
Active inflammation on liver biopsy*
No association with likelihood of response:
Ethnicity
Body surface area

Lamivudine

Associated with higher likelihood of response:
Elevated baseline ALT
High baseline histologic activity index score
No association with likelihood of response:
Baseline hepatitis B virus DNA level
Race/ethnicity
Age
Gender
Previous interferon therapy
Baseline weight
Baseline body mass index

Adefovir Dipivoxil

Associated with higher likelihood of response:
Age 12 to 17 years
Elevated baseline ALT
Lower hepatitis B virus DNA level
No association with likelihood of response:
Age <12 years

*Shown to be associated with higher response in adults, and presumed to be similar in children.
ALT, alanine aminotransferase

Peginterferon has not been studied in randomized trials in children as it has in adults.[77]

Lamivudine

Lamivudine is an orally administered nucleoside analog, making it an attractive option in children. The pharmacokinetics and safety of this drug were originally studied in 53 European children with chronic hepatitis B infection.[78] Proper dosing was determined to be 3 mg/kg up to the adult maximum of 100 mg/day.

A randomized, double-blind, placebo-controlled multicenter trial of lamivudine for 52 weeks was reported in 2002.[79] In this study of children aged 2 to 17 years, 191 were assigned to receive lamivudine and 97 were given a placebo. All children had been HBsAg positive for at least 6 months, were positive for HBeAg, anti-HBe negative, and had detectable HBV DNA and an ALT greater than 1.3 times the upper limit of normal but less than 500 IU/L. Twenty-three percent of children who received lamivudine became HBeAg negative and had undetectable HBV DNA after 52 weeks in comparison with 13% of those who had received the placebo. This response rate was

35% in children whose ALT was at least twice the normal. Sustained normalization of ALT level was achieved in 55% of patients treated with lamivudine and 12% of children treated with the placebo. Logistic regression analyses showed that higher ALT values and higher histologic activity index (HAI) scores were associated with a greater likelihood of response.[80] In addition, there was no difference in virologic response between patients who had previously failed interferon and those who did not. Virologic response was not influenced by age, gender, or ethnic origin (see **Table 69-4**). In this study, 31 of 166 (19%) treated children developed the mutation conferring lamivudine resistance after 52 weeks of treatment. Of these, only one had HBeAg seroconversion. Results of prolonged treatment with lamivudine in children indicate that additional virologic responses can be achieved, and that seroconversions are durable in 88% of the treated children.[81] The frequency of viral resistance continues to increase, as in adults, with a frequency of 64% after 3 years of treatment.[81]

The safety profile of lamivudine appears to be quite good in children, and it is well tolerated in liquid or tablet form. Serious side effects were not reported in up to 3 years of therapy.[82] In comparison with treatment with IFN-α, decreased height velocity and weight loss were not observed.

Although this medication is well tolerated and was the first effective nucleoside analog in children, concerns regarding resistance should prompt reservation of this product for special circumstances. For example, lamivudine may be of value to inhibit viral replication during chemotherapy, stem cell transplantation, or organ transplantation when children or their donors have a remote or current hepatitis B infection.

Adefovir Dipivoxil

A randomized, double-blind, placebo-controlled multicenter pediatric trial of adefovir dipivoxil for 48 weeks was conducted in 2008.[83] In this study, 173 treatment-naïve or -experienced children with HBeAg-positive chronic hepatitis B were studied. Randomization was stratified by age and prior treatment. All children had been HBsAg positive for at least 6 months, were positive for HBeAg and anti-HBe negative, and had detectable HBV DNA, and ALT was greater than 1.5 times the upper limit of normal. Approximately half of these patients had received prior therapy, but not within the previous 6 months.

Only patients age 12 to 17 years significantly achieved the primary efficacy endpoint of HBV DNA of less than 1000 copies/ml and normal ALT in comparison with the placebo (23% vs. 0%). There was no statistical difference in outcomes in children ages 2 to 11 who were on either the study drug or the placebo, despite comparable plasma concentrations of adefovir in all age groups. Overall, there was more HBeAg seroconversion (15.9%) in adefovir patients than in placebo patients (5.3%). No resistance mutations were detected after 48 weeks. Side effect profiles were similar to those in adults. Given these findings, the U.S. Food and Drug Administration approved the use of adefovir dipivoxil in children 12 to 17 years of age.

Other Treatment Options

Peginterferon, entecavir, telbivudine, and tenofovir are options for adults with chronic hepatitis B infection. Although entecavir is approved for adolescents age 16 and older, the other agents are not approved for children younger than 18 years, although some are currently being tested in this population.

Immunoprophylaxis

There has been substantial progress in prevention of hepatitis B over the last 20 years. Vaccine recommendations regarding infants, children, and adolescents have evolved since the 1991 ACIP of the CDC made five major recommendations, but these are still the mainstays of the prevention strategy:

1. Screening all pregnant women for HBsAg
2. Immunizing and implementing HBIg and HBV vaccine within 12 hours for babies born to HBsAg-seropositive mothers
3. Vaccine administration within 12 hours of birth to infants of untested mothers
4. Universal immunization for all babies born to HBsAg-negative mothers
5. Vaccination of high-risk adolescents and adults

Since that time, the fifth recommendation has been broadened to include vaccination of all children aged up to 18 years.[84]

Currently, the recommendation is to start the HBV vaccine series at birth, while the infant is in the nursery. In 1999 there was some concern regarding mercury exposure from thimerosal, a preservative used in the vaccine. By 2000, this compound was eliminated from HBV vaccines, but not all pediatricians have resumed HBV vaccination at birth for all infants.[85] In addition, during the period of postponement of HBV vaccination at birth, one study demonstrated a six-fold increase in the number of hospitals not vaccinating all high-risk infants,[86] even though there have been no documented cases of injury from thimerosal.

Significant progress has been made toward decreasing transmission, acute infection, and chronic hepatitis in the pediatric population. After introduction of universal hepatitis B vaccination in Taiwan, fulminant neonatal hepatitis B mortality decreased from 5.36 to 1.71 per 100,000.[47] In 1994 the chronic HBV prevalence rate was zero in Alaskan native children under 10 years of age who had been vaccinated at birth, in comparison with 16% of those aged 11 to 30 years who had not.[87]

The current recommendation is three intramuscular doses starting in infancy. If administered according to the recommended schedule, the vaccine will promote a protective response in 95% of infants, children, and adolescents. For those children born to hepatitis B-infected mothers, anti-HBs and HBsAg should be checked after 12 months to determine the success of the HBV vaccines and HBIg. Anti-HBs should also be checked in patients co-infected with HIV, those with other immunodeficiencies, hemodialysis patients, and those living with chronically infected individuals. It is not necessary in other healthy children. Studies from Hong Kong have shown that more than 80% of children immunized with three doses had anti-HBs greater than 10 mIU/ml 12 years later, and that additional booster doses were not required.[88]

Daily Activities

Chronically infected children should not be allowed to share toothbrushes, razors, or any other items that may be contaminated with blood. Children with chronic HBV infection should be allowed to participate in all activities without restrictions because universal precautions are recommended for all children in schools, sports, or day care situations. Although HBV has been detected in breast milk, mothers who are HBV-infected may continue to breastfeed if the infants are appropriately immunized.[48]

Conclusion

Hepatitis B infection acquired during childhood is similar in some respects to that acquired by adults, but there are important differences in epidemiology, clinical features, natural history, and treatment. Chronic hepatitis B infection in children confers risks of cirrhosis and HCC. Other important considerations are patient selection for treatment and the timing of optimal treatment, which, according to recent studies, appears to be when there is evidence of active hepatitis as determined by abnormal ALT values and high HAI scores.[70,79,80] Currently in the United States, IFN-α and lamivudine are available for children aged 2 to 17 years with chronic hepatitis B, and adefovir dipivoxil in children ages 12 to 18. Testing of the newer agents is important because viral resistance limits the potential usefulness of first generation nucleoside or nucleotide analogs. Prevention remains a primary goal because safe and effective vaccines are available.

Hepatitis C

Children are only a small proportion of the HCV-infected population, but there are a significant number of children with chronic HCV. Chronic infection may not have clinical findings during childhood, but can lead to significant morbidity and mortality, such as cirrhosis and HCC, later in life. Understanding that HCV in children has different modes of acquisition, complications, and natural history will influence management and treatment decisions.

Epidemiology

The seroprevalence of antibody to HCV in the United States is approximately 1.8%, which is close to 4 million people. Data from the CDC have shown the seroprevalence to be 0.2% for children 6 to 11 years, and 0.4% for those aged 12 to 19 years.[89] Other studies in the United States have shown prevalence in urban adolescents to be 0.1% in Boston and Cambridge, Massachusetts,[90] and 0.1% in children under 12 years of age in a large cohort from Baltimore, Maryland.[91] Prevalence rates in European countries are similar, such as that in Italy (0.4%),[92] with a higher prevalence of 0.5% to 10% in countries of northern Africa.[93,94]

Exposures to hepatitis C such as intravenous drug use, needle sticks, and sexual contact are more common in adults than children. Before 1992, the primary route of HCV transmission in children was from transfusion of blood or blood products, including antihemophilic factor, factor IX concentrates, and immune globulin. The risk of infection appeared to correlate with the amount of transfusion exposure. After 1992 and universal testing of blood products, vertical transmission has become the leading source of infection for children.[95] Vertical transmission is much less common than that for hepatitis B, averaging about 5% in most studies.[96-102] The likelihood of HCV transmission to newborns increases to 14% (range, 5% to 36%) if mothers are infected with both HCV and untreated HIV.[98,101-105] Most HCV/HIV co-infected women have higher levels of HCV viremia, which contributes to transmission.[96,106] Rupture of membranes for 6 hours and internal fetal scalp monitoring have been associated with a higher risk of vertical transmission.[102]

Infected household contacts may pose a small risk to children, although this has not been clearly documented. Seroprevalence rates in household contacts have ranged from zero in developed countries to 6.5% in less developed countries. There may be increasing risk with age and/or duration of exposure for sexual and nonsexual contacts.[107,108] The mechanism of nonsexual, nonperinatal infection in children is not known. Child-to-child transmission is extremely rare, and the American Academy of Pediatrics (AAP) has advised that there is no need to restrict school or day care attendance. This includes full contact sports and other routine activities.[109]

Pathogenesis

Acute hepatitis C is often not clinically recognized, so limited information is available. The mechanism for hepatocellular injury is thought to be both direct cytopathic effect and immune-mediated injury. Children have a propensity to develop chronic infection, although perhaps less frequently than adults.[110,111] One hypothesis regarding the mechanism for viral persistence implicates a weak HCV-specific immune response that may occur through insufficient induction of a primary response or inability to maintain the response.[112] Another hypothesis involves viral evasion of the immune responses, secondary to development of quasispecies, mutations, and different genotypes. Immune responsiveness to HCV has not been compared between adults and children.

Clinical Features

The incubation period of hepatitis C infection averages 6 to 7 weeks, with a range of 2 weeks to 6 months. Most children are asymptomatic. However, when symptomatic with acute infection, the presentation is usually mild, with fewer than 25% of patients developing jaundice. Rarely, children may have associated anorexia, malaise, or abdominal pain. Occasionally, more severe acute hepatitis is seen.[113]

Most children with chronic hepatitis C are asymptomatic. Children have normal to mild elevation of aminotransferases. End-stage liver disease is extremely uncommon during the childhood years.[114]

Diagnosis

Because hepatitis C is uncommon in children, many pediatricians are unsure of which children should be tested for this infection. Universal screening is not cost effective or useful in children. The AAP Committee on Infectious Disease has made recommendations for the risk factors that should prompt testing for HCV (**Table 69-5**).

The diagnostic strategy for HCV infection is the same for children and adults. The first test is anti-HCV antibody. If this is positive, most clinicians will look for HCV RNA by a

Table 69-5 Indications for Testing for Hepatitis C in Children and Adolescents

Infants born to hepatitis C virus–infected mothers
Receipt of blood or blood products before 1992
Hemodialysis
History of injection drug use
Receipt of intravenous immunoglobulin April 1993 to March 1994
Acute or chronic hepatitis with negative workup for hepatitis B and other disorders
International adoptee

PCR-based assay to distinguish active infection from previous exposure to the virus or a false-positive antibody. Care must be taken in patients with suspected acute hepatitis C because anti-HCV may not appear until 5 to 6 weeks after symptoms of acute hepatitis. In this situation, testing for HCV RNA may be required. In immunocompromised children, or those receiving chemotherapy, anti-HCV may not develop, and testing directly for HCV RNA may be necessary.

Infants born to anti-HCV–positive mothers will most likely have anti-HCV at birth because of transplacental transfer of maternal antibody. The duration of this anti-HCV in the infant's serum in the absence of true infection depends on the titer, but is usually less than 12 to 15 months.[102] To evaluate for perinatal viral transmission early in infancy, PCR has been used. Several studies have confirmed the best time for testing of HCV RNA to be the third or fourth month of life.[115] However, even in some of these infants with HCV, the infection will resolve spontaneously in the first 2 to 3 years.

Children and adolescents with positive anti-HCV should have a qualitative PCR for HCV RNA to confirm infection. Once infection is confirmed, HCV genotype may be ascertained. Quantitative HCV RNA testing is reserved for assessment of response to treatment.

Differential Diagnosis

Acute Hepatitis

Acute hepatitis C in the pediatric population is uncommon, but some children do have mild to moderate elevation of aminotransferases during infancy and childhood. The differential diagnosis has been discussed (see **Table 69-1**). In most instances of acute hepatitis, liver biopsy is not indicated. Histologic features are usually suggestive of a viral process, but occasionally may be confused with those of autoimmune hepatitis.

Chronic Hepatitis

As discussed earlier, children may have chronic hepatitis secondary to α_1-antitrypsin deficiency, hepatitis B, Wilson disease, autoimmune hepatitis, medication or toxin injury, as well as other metabolic diseases and cystic fibrosis (see **Table 69-2**). Of note, liver biopsy specimens from children and adolescents with chronic hepatitis C may demonstrate steatosis, suggestive of metabolic disorders such as nonalcoholic fatty liver disease, fatty acid oxidation defects, or Wilson disease.

Associated Conditions

Extrahepatic manifestations, including cryoglobulinemia,[116] vasculitis,[117] and membranoproliferative glomerulonephritis[118] have not been reported in children. Children may be co-infected with HBV or HIV, especially if infected by perinatal transmission.

Non–organ-specific autoantibodies are commonly reported in children with hepatitis C, most commonly liver-kidney microsomal antibody type 1 (LKM1).[119,120] This antibody, usually associated with type 2 autoimmune hepatitis, has been demonstrated in approximately 10% of HCV-infected children in European studies. Antinuclear antibody and anti-smooth muscle antibodies have also been identified in this patient population. A multicenter study indicated that LKM1-positive children with hepatitis C had higher fibrosis scores on liver biopsies, more severe liver disease, poorer response to interferon and, in some cases, required corticosteroid therapy for presumed autoimmune hepatitis.[121]

Prognosis and Natural History Pertinent to Infection Acquired in Childhood

Although more data are being collected regarding the natural history of HCV infection in children, the frequency with which complications develop from infection acquired during childhood has not been fully elucidated. Studies have shown the importance of age at infection as a predictor of chronic viremia.

The first long-term studies in children involved mostly transfusion-acquired infections. A large study of more than 400 children who had blood transfusions during cardiac surgery before 1991 demonstrated a 14.6% acquisition rate of hepatitis C as evidenced by anti-HCV. Of these infected children, 55% developed chronic hepatitis, and were PCR positive after a mean follow-up of 17 years (range, 12 to 27 years).[110] Most of these patients did not have clinical or biochemical signs of liver disease and 1 of 17 patients who underwent liver biopsy had cirrhosis.

In the United States, a large cohort of HCV-infected cancer survivors who had been transfused before 1992 has been followed at St. Jude's Children's Research Hospital (Memphis, Tenn.). In 1995, 81% of anti-HCV-seropositive patients were PCR positive, after a median time from diagnosis of malignancy of 15.9 years. ALT abnormalities were seen in 30% of these PCR-positive patients and biopsies showed mild to moderate fibrosis in 64%, and cirrhosis in 13%.[122] A previous report from this cohort had described one patient who died of liver failure 9 years after onset of HCV, and two others who died of HCC after 25 and 27 years.[123]

Since the screening of blood products, perinatal transmission has been the focus of pediatric HCV natural history and prognosis studies. Vertical transmission is associated with a high incidence of viremia and abnormal aminotransferases during the first 12 months. Of 70 prospectively followed infants in five European centers from 1990 to 1999, 93% had abnormal ALT during the first 12 months, and only 19% cleared HCV RNA and normalized ALT by 30 months of age.[124] Clearance of viremia was independent of sex and maternal HIV co-infection. Peak ALT greater than five times

normal during the first 18 months and genotype 3 were more common in the patients in whom viremia eventually resolved spontaneously.

A European study with a cohort of 200 HCV-infected children was reported on in 2003.[125] The majority had genotype 1b, 45% from vertical transmission and 39% from transfusion. Fifteen percent of these patients had normal ALT, and none had jaundice or extrahepatic manifestations. After follow-up of 1 to 17.5 years (mean, 6.2), only 6% achieved sustained virologic clearance and normalization of ALT. Liver biopsies were performed in 118 patients at various times during follow-up; the majority (76%) had mild hepatitis and low fibrosis scores. One patient (1%) had cirrhosis and 1 (1%) had severe hepatitis. Greater degrees of fibrosis were seen in children older than 15 years, suggesting progressive effects of chronic HCV infection.

Expounding on this European study, results from a cohort of 504 consecutive Italian children with chronic hepatitis C, followed retrospectively and prospectively from 1990 to 2005 in an Italian national observatory, have been reported.[114] The aims of the study were to evaluate the natural history of chronic HCV and the rates of spontaneous HCV RNA clearance in untreated children. In this cohort, vertical transmission had occurred in 56%, and parenteral transmission in 31%. Of the 389 infections genotyped, the majority were genotype 1 (62%). The mean follow up was 10.6 ± 6 years from the putative time of exposure. Of the 359 HCV RNA positive children who were not treated with interferon, only 8% had spontaneous viral clearance. Six of the children with continued viremia (1.8%), and mean duration of HCV exposure of 9.87 ± 5.9 years, progressed to decompensated cirrhosis.

The histopathology of the liver in children with chronic hepatitis C has been studied in four large series. All have shown that findings such as sinusoidal lymphocytosis, steatosis, portal lymphoid aggregates, and bile duct epithelial damage occur in relatively the same frequency in children as in adults.[126-129] The first large study from Japan evaluated 109 liver specimens. The majority of these patients were infected via transfusion; biopsies were from patients with a mean duration of infection of 2.6 years, and genotypes were unknown. Ninety-seven percent of the specimens had no fibrosis or periportal fibrosis with intact architecture. Three percent had septal fibrosis with architectural distortion, and no patients had cirrhosis.[127] In contrast, a study from the United States demonstrated portal fibrosis in 78% of 40 liver biopsies.[126] Fibrosis was mild in 26%, moderate in 22%, and severe in 22%, with cirrhosis in 8%. Two of the children with cirrhosis were young adolescents who had acquired HCV perinatally. In comparison with the Japanese study, the mean duration of infection before biopsy was longer (6.8 years). Genotype 1a was present in 60% of this population, and 1b in 32%. A third series was a collection of 80 children from Italy and Spain, mostly infected with genotype 1, with a mean duration of infection of 3.5 years.[128] Necroinflammatory scores were low in this population, and the frequency and severity of bile duct damage and lymphoid follicles increased with patient age. Fibrosis was seen in 72.5% of the biopsies, and increased with age and duration of disease, as in the American series. Only one child had cirrhosis. The most recent publication of 121 children with chronic hepatitis C, predominantly genotype 1 (82%), and perinatally acquired (78%) demonstrated a similar finding.[129] Fibrosis was absent in 14%, portal/periportal in

80%, and bridging in 4%, and cirrhosis was found in 2%. Necrosis and inflammation were again mild. This study also demonstrated an association with obesity and more severe fibrosis. These four series have shown that, although necrosis and inflammation are usually mild, fibrosis is seen and worsens with age or duration.

Another complicating factor in children is the co-existence of autoantibodies, such as LKM1, as previously discussed.[120,121] Although they include only small numbers of patients, these studies have shown higher fibrosis scores and more significant hepatic flares during interferon therapy. Of the three anti-LKM-positive patients in a European study who received interferon, treatment needed to be discontinued in all secondary to persistent viremia and ALT abnormalities.[121]

Potential long-term sequelae of chronic HCV infection in children are cirrhosis and HCC. HCC secondary to hepatitis C is extremely rare during childhood, and there have been only a few case reports.[130-132]

Liver transplantation for complications of chronic hepatitis C during childhood is uncommon. According to the SPLIT registry that collects data from 37 North American pediatric centers, chronic hepatitis C with cirrhosis or "subacute hepatitis C" was the reason for transplant in 13 of 2291 children (0.6%) from 1995 through June 2006.[18]

Despite some complications that arise in childhood, HCV infection is benign during the first 2 decades in most cases. Severe liver disease and decompensated cirrhosis are rare during childhood. The greatest concern to the pediatric hepatologist regarding children with chronic HCV is the development of complications during adulthood.

Treatment

In 2003 the FDA approved the combination of interferon and ribavirin for the treatment of chronic HCV in children aged 3 to 17 years. In 2009 combination therapy with peginterferon alfa-2b and ribavirin was approved for the same age group. However, deciding to treat a child with hepatitis C may not be straightforward because physicians must consider the natural history and treatment efficacy in children. Safety profiles must be recognized and appropriate monitoring instituted because some children have comorbidities that may complicate therapy (**Table 69-6**).

Interferon

Interferon monotherapy was studied in children in small clinical trials, but it has not been tested in a large multicenter trial. Sustained virologic response rates were significantly better than in large trials in adults. A systematic analysis of multiple studies included 270 treated patients and 37 control subjects. The overall sustained virologic response in the treated children was 35%. There was a difference in response by genotype: 26% for genotype 1 and 70% for the other genotypes.[133]

Interferon-Alfa and Ribavirin

In a study conducted from 1998 to 2001, 118 children aged 3 to 17 years with chronic hepatitis C were given IFN alfa-2b, 3 MU per meter squared of body surface area three times a week, and 15 mg/kg of ribavirin daily for 24 weeks.[134] Therapy

Table 69-6 Special Considerations Regarding Hepatitis C Therapy in Children[178]
Differences in natural history
Mode of acquisition: perinatal
Shorter duration of infection
Fewer co-infections and co-morbid diseases
Longer anticipated life expectancy
Differences in liver disease
Milder grades of necroinflammation
Less frequent severe fibrosis or cirrhosis
Response to interferons with or without ribavirin
Similar frequency of response, similar predictive factors
Better compliance
Fewer drug discontinuations because of side effects
Unknown long-term side effects
No cost-benefit data

Adapted from Jonas MM. Treatment of chronic hepatitis C in pediatric patients. In: Keeffe EB, editor. Clinics in liver disease. Vol. 4. Philadelphia: WB Saunders, 1999:855–867, with permission.

was continued for an additional 24 weeks if they demonstrated undetectable HCV RNA or greater than a 2 log decrease in viremia. Most patients were infected via vertical transmission (54%) and were infected with genotype 1 (78%). Overall, 46% had a sustained virologic response (HCV RNA <100 copies/ml) 24 weeks after completion of therapy. Factors associated with the likelihood of sustained virologic response were age less than 12 years, genotypes 2 and 3, and fewer than 2 million copies/ml of HCV RNA in those children with genotype 1 infection. Variables not associated with sustained virologic response were ethnicity, gender, mode of acquisition, duration of infection, baseline ALT, and ribavirin preparation (tablet versus liquid) (**Table 69-7**). The side effects of combination therapy were similar to those seen in adults, but less severe. Adverse events led to dosage modifications in 31% and discontinuation in 7% of the treated children.

Peginterferon and Ribavirin

Several studies have evaluated combination therapy with peginterferon and ribavirin for children with chronic hepatitis C. Given previous pediatric data suggesting interferon monotherapy may be equal to combination therapy, a multicenter randomized trial compared the efficacy and safety of peginterferon alfa-2a alone ($1.80 \mu g/1.73 m^2$/wk) to peginterferon with ribavirin (15 mg/kg/day) as treatment for children ages 5 to 17 years.[135] Treatment groups were similar for age, gender, racial background, ALT, histologic activity and score, as well as genotype. Among the 114 children participating, SVR was significantly higher in children receiving combination therapy (53% vs. 21%). Sustained virologic response was attained in 47% of genotype 1, and 80% of non–genotype 1 patients using combination therapy. These SVR rates are similar to those in adults and have shown ribavirin to be critical in treatment of children with chronic hepatitis C.

A recent open label study of 107 children used peginterferon alfa-2b ($60 \mu g/m^2$/wk) and ribavirin (15 mg/kg/day) for 24 weeks for genotype 2 and low viral load genotype 3 (<600,000 IU/ml), and 48 weeks for genotypes 1 and 4 and high viral load genotype 3 (>600,000 IU/ml).[136] The majority

Table 69-7 Variables Associated with Sustained Virologic Response to Interferon-Alfa/Ribavirin[134] or Peginterferon/Ribavirin[135,136,179] in Children with Chronic Hepatitis C

INTERFERON AND RIBAVIRIN		PEGINTERFERON AND RIBAVIRIN	
Association	*No Association*	*Association*	*No Association*
≤12 years of age	Baseline ALT	Genotype 2 and 3[135,136,179]	Baseline ALT[136,179]
Genotype 2 and 3	Gender		Age[136]
If genotype 1, hepatitis C virus RNA ≤2 million copies/ml	Mode of acquisition		Mode of acquisition[179]
Receiving at least 80% of the medication doses and completing ≥38 weeks of treatment	Estimated duration of infection		
	Ethnicity		

ALT, alanine aminotransferase

of patients were between ages 3 and 11 (63%), had acquired HCV by vertical transmission (70%), and had genotype 1 (67%). Overall, 65% of treated children attained SVR: 53% with genotype 1, 93% with genotype 2 or 3, and 80% with genotype 4. SVR rates were independent of age and baseline ALT (see **Table 69-7**).

Given these data, combination therapy for children using peginterferon and ribavirin appears as safe as interferon/ribavirin therapy. Some studies demonstrate a slightly higher SVR rate with peginterferon. It is now the standard treatment for children ages 3 to 17 years. Therapy is indicated for the child with advanced fibrosis on liver biopsy. Other patients should have treatment plans on an individual basis, taking into account age, genotype, and other co-morbidities.

Daily Activities

Chronically infected children should not be allowed to share toothbrushes, razors, or any other items that may be contaminated with blood. Teenagers, if sexually active, must also be advised regarding the unlikely—but not impossible—risk of sexual transmission to their partners. Mothers who are HCV-infected may continue to breastfeed according to recommendations of the CDC, but should probably abstain if their nipples are cracked or bleeding.[109] Universal precautions are recommended for all children in school, sports, or day care situations, regardless of HCV status. Children with chronic hepatitis C should not be restricted in activities or school settings.

Conclusion

Hepatitis C infection continues to be a healthcare burden in children despite its changing epidemiology from transfusion acquired to vertical transmission. At this point, there are no proven methods to prevent perinatal transmission, so chronic HCV will continue to be seen by pediatricians. Further research is needed to delineate the factors that predict progression of disease and fibrosis in children. Randomized, prospective trials are required to determine optimal type and timing

of the treatment, as well as to study newer agents in this population.

Hepatitis in Children Caused by Other Viral Agents

As in adults, hepatitis A, hepatitis B, and hepatitis C are the predominant hepatitis viruses in children. Other hepatotropic viruses and other viral agents should be considered in the appropriate clinical settings and age groups.

Hepatitis D

Hepatitis D virus is an uncommon infection in children. It is not usually transmitted perinatally because most mothers with HDV are usually anti-HBe positive, with low levels of HBV DNA viremia.[137] It appears that most pediatric cases are due to horizontal spread. The most common regions for HDV infection in children are southern Italy, parts of eastern Europe, South America, Africa, and the Middle East. HDV infection is rare in the Far East, so it will be uncommon in children adopted from or emigrated from Asia. The clinical course appears to be similar to that in adults, in that HBV-infected children with HDV have more advanced liver disease.[137] Treatment of HDV infection in children with IFN-α had some short-term effects on HDV RNA, but did not appear to cause significant long-term virologic response or histologic change in European trials.[138,139] Universal immunization of infants for HBV will decrease the risk of HDV infection.

Hepatitis E

In the United States, hepatitis E virus (HEV) is a rare cause of hepatitis in children and is only slightly more common in the adult population. It is seen in individuals who have recently traveled from endemic areas, which include parts of India, areas of central and Southeast Asia, northwest China, and parts of Africa. Multiple studies of sporadic acute hepatitis in parts of Africa have shown HEV to be a significant contributor.[140,141] There have also been reports that children in endemic areas who are co-infected with HEV and HAV may have a more severe course than with either infection alone.[142] Diagnosis is made by HEV IgM antibody in serum. There is no therapy, and most children recover uneventfully.

Enteroviruses

The nonpolio enteroviruses (coxsackieviruses, echoviruses, and others) are those most commonly associated with severe hepatitis in neonates.[43] Transmission may be prenatal, intrapartum, or perinatal. Mothers of these infants usually have a history of a viral syndrome, with fever or diarrhea approximately 1 week before delivery. Most affected infants have a mild course, but severe neonatal hepatitis can occur within the first week, with jaundice, coagulopathy, and ascites. Echovirus 11 appears to be the most common, but Coxsackie B virus has been implicated as well.[43,143-145] Diagnosis can now be made by PCR in serum or urine. There has been a report of clinical improvement in infants with severe hepatitis using pleconaril, an agent that inhibits viral uncoating and blocks viral attachment to host cell receptors.[144] Currently, pleconaril is available only in research protocols.

Herpes Simplex Viruses

Herpes simplex virus may cause severe hepatitis in the neonatal period.[42] This is usually in conjunction with disseminated infection, and most commonly presents in the first week of life. Associated clinical symptoms include the typical cutaneous vesicular lesions, hepatosplenomegaly, fever, and coagulopathy. The treatment for these children is acyclovir, which must be instituted promptly. Occasionally, liver transplantation is necessary, with continued acyclovir after transplantation.[146]

In addition to infection in neonates, herpes simplex virus may cause hepatitis in immunocompromised children and adolescents, such as bone marrow and solid organ transplant recipients.[147,148]

Adenovirus

Adenovirus is a common neonatal infection, usually of the respiratory tract. Neonatal hepatitis because of adenovirus usually presents within the first week of life. This may be associated with overwhelming, potentially fatal, multisystem infection. Clinical findings are hepatomegaly, hepatitis, and bleeding secondary to thrombocytopenia and coagulopathy. Other symptoms include lethargy, pneumonia, and fever or hypothermia.[44]

Adenovirus may cause hepatitis in immunocompromised individuals as well.[149,150] Cidofovir, a monophosphate nucleotide analogue of cytosine that inhibits viral DNA polymerases, is available for treatment of significant adenovirus infection in both stem cell and solid organ transplant patients.[151,152] Side effects, such as nephrotoxicity need to be monitored closely in these patients, but the drug is usually well tolerated.[153]

Cytomegalovirus

Congenital CMV infection is often asymptomatic, but a minority of infected newborns will develop hepatitis, hepatosplenomegaly, conjugated hyperbilirubinemia, and/or thrombocytopenia. The diagnosis of CMV infection may be made by liver biopsy, urine CMV culture, or IgM antibody to CMV. CMV does not cause chronic infection in immunocompetent children.[154]

Acute CMV hepatitis is usually not a disorder of healthy children or adolescents, but is a common disease in immunocompromised hosts.[155,156] Treatment with ganciclovir or valganciclovir is indicated.

Parvovirus B19

Parvovirus B19 is the virus associated with erythema infectiosum (fifth disease). Typical clinical features are fever, a lacy maculopapular rash, and erythematous "slapped" cheeks. Occasionally, children will develop acute hepatitis and, rarely, fulminant hepatitis. It has been suggested that fulminant hepatitis because of parvovirus B19 has a better prognosis than that caused by other viral infections.[157] Associated with fulminant hepatic failure, some children develop aplastic anemia.[158] Diagnosis of acute infection is confirmed by parvovirus B19 IgM antibody or PCR. There is no treatment for this infection.

Epstein-Barr Virus

Clinical symptoms of infectious mononucleosis because of the Epstein-Barr virus (EBV) infection include fever, pharyngitis, lymphadenopathy, splenomegaly, and hepatitis with jaundice.[159] Abnormal aminotransferases are present in up to 80% of patients, although only a small percentage develop jaundice.[160] Fulminant hepatitis and EBV-associated hemophagocytic syndrome are rare complications.[161,162] Diagnosis may be made with a monospot or heterophile antibody, but there are frequent false-negative results for this test in children younger than 4 years, and false positives in older children with other viral infections or medical conditions. Serum IgM to the EB viral capsid antigen (VCA) is both more sensitive and specific, and has usually developed by the time of clinical presentation. Hepatitis associated with infectious mononucleosis usually resolves spontaneously and fully over 2 to 3 weeks.

Human Herpesvirus-6

Human herpesvirus-6 (HHV6) is the etiologic agent of roseola infantum in children. The typical presentation is high fever for several days, followed by rapid defervescence and the development of an erythematous maculopapular rash. Several studies have documented HHV6 in the livers of infants and adults with acute liver failure.[163-165] However, whether HHV6 is the actual etiologic agent causing the liver disease is controversial because almost all children are seropositive for the virus by 2 years of age, and the virus may persist and reactivate.[166,167] This claim was further substantiated by reports that HHV6 was detected in serum or bone marrow by PCR in hospitalized children with other chronic medical problems[168] and has been detected via PCR in the livers of 36 of 48 children (75%) with various liver diseases.[169]

HHV6 may reactivate in immunocompromised children, especially those with stem cell or solid organ transplants.[170,171] No established therapy is available, but some of these patients have received either ganciclovir or foscarnet.[171]

Summary

Although adults and children may develop hepatitis from the same viruses, the epidemiology, clinical findings, and natural history of these infections may be quite different. Identifying and recognizing these differences are important in terms of understanding pathogenesis, prevention, and treatment. Etiologic agents of hepatitis may be different in neonates and infants. Children may have substantial morbidity later in life from chronic hepatitis, such as cirrhosis or HCC. Determination of optimal treatment regimens for chronic HBV and HCV infections in children requires further research through large trials with new medications or combinations of medications. Prevention is still the most important mechanism for avoiding these sequelae. Broadening HAV and HBV vaccine usage, and development of other vaccines, as well as prevention of perinatal transmission of hepatitis C, will decrease the numbers of children with acute and chronic viral hepatitis in the future.

Key References

Advisory Committee on Immunization Practices (ACIP), Centers for Disease Control (CDC). Update: prevention of hepatitis A after exposure to hepatitis A virus and in international travelers. Updated recommendations from the Advisory Committee on Immunization Practices (ACIP). MMWR Morb Mortal Wkly Rep 2007;56:1080–1084. (Ref.20)

Advisory Committee on Immunization Practices (ACIP), et al. Prevention of hepatitis A through active or passive immunization: recommendations of the Advisory Committee on Immunization Practices (ACIP). MMWR Recomm Rep 2006;55:1–23. (Ref.19)

Agarwal K, et al. Acute pancreatitis with cholestatic hepatitis: an unusual manifestation of hepatitis A. Ann Trop Paediatr 1999;19:391–394. (Ref.12)

American Academy of Pediatrics. Hepatitis B. In: Pickering L, editor. 2000 Red book: report of the committee on infectious diseases. Elk Grove Village, Ill: American Academy of Pediatrics, 2000: 289–301. (Ref.48)

American Academy of Pediatrics. Hepatitis C. In: Pickering LK. Red book: report of the committee on infectious diseases. Elk Grove Village, IL: American Academy of Pediatrics, 2003: 336–340. (Ref.109)

American Academy of Pediatrics. Human herpesvirus 6 (including roseola) and 7. In: Pickering L, editor. 2000 Red book: report of the committee on infectious diseases. Elk Grove Village, IL: American Academy of Pediatrics, 2000: 322–324. (Ref.166)

Aradottir E, Alonso EM, Shulman ST. Severe neonatal enteroviral hepatitis treated with pleconaril. Pediatr Infect Dis J 2001;20:457–459. (Ref.144)

Armstrong GL, et al. Childhood hepatitis B virus infections in the United States before hepatitis B immunization. Pediatrics 2001;108:1123–1128. (Ref.28)

Arslan S, et al. Relapsing hepatitis A in children: report of two cases. Acta Paediatr Taiwan 2002;43:358–360. (Ref.9)

Badizadegan K, et al. Histopathology of the liver in children with chronic hepatitis C viral infection. Hepatology 1998;28:1416–1423. (Ref.126)

Bell BP, et al. The diverse patterns of hepatitis A epidemiology in the United States: implications for vaccination strategies. J Infect Dis 1998;178:1579–1584. (Ref.1)

Bhadri VA, Lee-Horn L, Shaw PJ. Safety and tolerability of cidofovir in high-risk pediatric patients. Transpl Infect Dis 2009;11:373–379. (Ref.153)

Bortolotti F, et al. Chronic hepatitis B in children after e antigen seroclearance: final report of a 29-year longitudinal study. Hepatology 2006;43:556–562. (Ref.53)

Bortolotti F, et al. Outcome of chronic hepatitis B in Caucasian children during a 20-year observation period. J Hepatol 1998;29:184–190. (Ref.52)

Bortolotti F, et al. Hepatitis C virus infection associated with liver-kidney microsomal antibody type 1 (LKM1) autoantibodies in children. J Pediatr 2003;142:185–190. (Ref.121)

Bortolotti F, et al. Changing epidemiologic pattern of chronic hepatitis C virus infection in Italian children. J Pediatr 1998;133:378–381. (Ref.95)

Bortolotti F, et al. Long-term course of chronic hepatitis C in children: from viral clearance to end-stage liver disease. Gastroenterology 2008;134:1900–1907. (Ref.114)

Broderick AL, Jonas MM. Management of hepatitis B in children. In: Tran TT, Martin P, editors. Clinics in liver disease. Vol. 8. Philadelphia: WB Saunders, 2004: 387–401. (Ref.172)

Carter BA, et al. Intravenous cidofovir therapy for disseminated adenovirus in a pediatric liver transplant recipient. Transplantation 2002;74:1050–1052. (Ref.151)

Castellino S, et al. The epidemiology of chronic hepatitis C infection in survivors of childhood cancer: an update of the St Jude Children's Research Hospital hepatitis C seropositive cohort. Blood 2004;103:2460–2466. (Ref.122)

Centers for Disease Control (CDC). Update: recommendations to prevent hepatitis B virus transmission—United States. MMWR Morb Mortal Wkly Rep 1999;48:33–34. (Ref.84)

Centers for Disease Control and Prevention (CDC). Hepatitis B vaccination—United States, 1982-2002. MMWR Morb Mortal Wkly Rep 2002;51:549–552, 563. (Ref.29)

Centers for Disease Control and Prevention (CDC). Hepatitis surveillance report 58. Atlanta: US Department of Health and Human Services, Public Health Service, CDC, 2003. (Ref.23)

Chang MH, et al. Decreased incidence of hepatocellular carcinoma in hepatitis B vaccinees: a 20-year follow-up study. J Natl Cancer Inst 2009;101:1348–1355. (Ref.61)

Chen HL, et al. Pediatric fulminant hepatic failure in endemic areas of hepatitis B infection: 15 years after universal hepatitis B vaccination. Hepatology 2004;39:58–63. (Ref.33)

Cheng LL, et al. Probable intrafamilial transmission of coxsackievirus B3 with vertical transmission, severe early-onset neonatal hepatitis, and prolonged viral RNA shedding. Pediatrics 2006;118:e929–e933. (Ref.145)

Cheung T, Teich S. Cytomegalovirus infection in patients with HIV infection. Mt Sinai J Med 1999;66:113–124. (Ref.156)

Chevret L, et al. Human herpesvirus-6 infection: a prospective study evaluating HHV-6 DNA levels in liver from children with acute liver failure. J Med Virol 2008;80:1051–1057. (Ref.165)

Ciocca M, et al. Hepatitis A as an etiologic agent of acute liver failure in Latin America. Pediatr Infect Dis J 2007;26:711–715. (Ref.15)

Clark S, et al. Hepatitis B vaccination practices in hospital newborn nurseries before and after changes in vaccination recommendations. Arch Pediatr Adolesc Med 2001;155:915–920. (Ref.86)

Comanor L, et al. Impact of chronic hepatitis B and interferon-alfa therapy on growth of children. J Viral Hepat 2001;8:139–147. (Ref.75)

Comanor L, et al. Statistical models for predicting response to interferon-alfa and spontaneous seroconversion in children with chronic hepatitis B. J Viral Hepat 2000;7:144–152. (Ref.177)

Committee on Infectious Diseases, American Academy of Pediatrics. Hepatitis C virus infection. Pediatrics 1998;101:481–485. (Ref.89)

Connor F, et al. HBV associated nephrotic syndrome: resolution with oral lamivudine. Arch Dis Child 2003;88:446–449. (Ref.40)

Conte D, et al. Prevalence and clinical course of chronic hepatitis C virus (HCV) infection and rate of HCV vertical transmission in a cohort of 15,250 pregnant women. Hepatology 2000;31:751–755. (Ref.115)

Czauderna P, et al. Hepatocellular carcinoma in children: results of the first prospective study of the International Society of Pediatric Oncology group. J Clin Oncol 2002;20:2798–2804. (Ref.55)

Dalekos G, et al. Interferon-alpha treatment of children with chronic hepatitis D virus infection: the Greek experience. Hepatogastroenterology 2000;47:1072–1076. (Ref.139)

Daniels D, et al. Surveillance for acute viral hepatitis—United States, 2007. MMWR Surveill Summ 2009;58:1–27. (Ref.2)

El-Kamary SS, et al. Prevalence of hepatitis C virus infection in urban children. J Pediatr 2003;143:54–59. (Ref.91)

Ertekin V, Selimoglu M, Orbak Z. An unusual combination of relapsing and cholestatic hepatitis A in childhood. Yonsei Med J 2003;44:939–942. (Ref.8)

Ferreira C, et al. Immunogenicity and safety of hepatitis A vaccine in children with chronic liver disease. J Pediatr Gastroenterol Nutr 2003;37:258–261. (Ref.24)

Ferrero S, et al. Prospective study of mother-to-infant transmission of hepatitis C virus: a 10-year survey (1990-2000). Acta Obstet Gynecol Scand 2003;82:229–234. (Ref.106)

Filler G, et al. Another case of HBV associated membranous glomerulonephritis resolving on lamivudine. Arch Dis Child 2003;88:460. (Ref.39)

Gonzalez-Peralta RP, et al. Interferon alfa-2b in combination with ribavirin for the treatment of chronic hepatitis C in children: efficacy, safety, and pharmacokinetics. Hepatology 2005;42:1010–1018. (Ref.134)

Gonzalez-Peralta RP, et al. Hepatocellular carcinoma in 2 young adolescents with chronic hepatitis C. J Pediatr Gastroenterol Nutr 2009;48:630–635. (Ref.132)

Goodman ZD, et al. Pathology of chronic hepatitis C in children: liver biopsy findings in the Peds-C trial. Hepatology 2008;47:836–843. (Ref.129)

Gregorio G, et al. Autoantibody prevalence in children with liver disease due to chronic hepatitis C virus (HCV) infection. Clin Exp Immunol 1998;112: 471–476. (Ref.120)

Guido M, et al. Chronic hepatitis C in children: the pathological and clinical spectrum. Gastroenterology 1998;115:1525–1529. (Ref.128)

Harma M, Hockerstedt K, Lautenschlager I. Human herpesvirus-6 and acute liver failure. Transplantation 2003;76:536–539. (Ref.163)

Harpaz R, et al. Elimination of new chronic hepatitis B virus infections: results of the Alaska immunization program. J Infect Dis 2000;181:413–418. (Ref.87)

Hom X, et al. Predictors of virologic response to lamivudine treatment in children with chronic hepatitis B infection. Pediatr Infect Dis J 2004;23: 441–445. (Ref.80)

Hou J, et al. Genetic characteristics of hepatitis B virus genotypes as a factor for interferon-induced HBeAg clearance. J Med Virol 2007;79:1055–1063. (Ref.67)

Hsiao CC, et al. Patterns of hepatoblastoma and hepatocellular carcinoma in children after universal hepatitis B vaccination in Taiwan: a report from a single institution in southern Taiwan. J Pediatr Hematol Oncol 2009;31:91–96. (Ref.56)

Hsu HY, et al. Changes of hepatitis B surface antigen variants in carrier children before and after universal vaccination in Taiwan. Hepatology 1999;30: 1312–1317. (Ref.26)

Ichai P, et al. Herpes simplex virus–associated acute liver failure: a difficult diagnosis with a poor prognosis. Liver Transpl 2005;11:1550–1555. (Ref.148)

Jacobson KR, et al. An analysis of published trials of interferon monotherapy in children with chronic hepatitis C. J Pediatr Gastroenterol Nutr 2002;34:52–58. (Ref.133)

Jara P, et al. Chronic hepatitis C virus infection in childhood: clinical patterns and evolution in 224 white children. Clin Infect Dis 2003;36:275–280. (Ref.125)

Jonas MM. Treatment of chronic hepatitis C in pediatric patients. In: Keeffe EB, editor. Treatment of chronic hepatitis C. Vol. 3. Philadelphia: WB Saunders, 1999: 855–867. (Ref.178)

Jonas MM, et al. Clinical trial of lamivudine in children with chronic hepatitis B. N Engl J Med 2002;346:1706–1713. (Ref.79)

Jonas MM, et al. Safety, efficacy, and pharmacokinetics of adefovir dipivoxil in children and adolescents (age 2 to <18 years) with chronic hepatitis B. Hepatology 2008;47:1863–1871. (Ref.83)

Jonas MM, Little NR, Gardner SD. Long-term lamivudine treatment of children with chronic hepatitis B: durability of therapeutic responses and safety. J Viral Hepat 2008;15:20–27. (Ref.82)

Kao J, et al. Universal hepatitis B vaccination and the decreased mortality from fulminant hepatitis in infants in Taiwan. J Pediatr 2001;139:349–352. (Ref.47)

Kao JH, et al. Hepatitis B genotypes and the response to interferon therapy. J Hepatol 2000;33:998–1002. (Ref.66)

Khetsuriani N, et al. Neonatal enterovirus infections reported to the national enterovirus surveillance system in the United States, 1983-2003. Pediatr Infect Dis J 2006;25:889–893. (Ref.143)

Kumar M, et al. A randomized controlled trial of lamivudine to treat acute hepatitis B. Hepatology 2007;45:97–101. (Ref.64)

Lau GK, et al. Peginterferon alfa-2a, lamivudine, and the combination for HBeAg-positive chronic hepatitis B. N Engl J Med 2005;352:2682–2695. (Ref.77)

Li DY, Boitnott J, Schwarz K. Human herpes virus 6 (HHV-6): a cause for fulminant hepatic failure or an innocent bystander? J Pediatr Gastroenterol Nutr 2003;37:95. (Ref.168)

Ljungman P, Singh N. Human herpesvirus-6 infection in solid organ and stem cell transplant recipients. J Clin Virol 2006;37(Suppl 1):S87–S91. (Ref.171)

Luman E, et al. Impact of thimerosal-related changes in hepatitis B vaccine birth-dose recommendations on childhood vaccination coverage. JAMA 2004;291:2351–2358. (Ref.85)

Majda-Stanislawska E, Bednarek M, Kuydowicz J. Immunogenicity of inactivated hepatitis A vaccine in children with chronic liver disease. Pediatr Infect Dis J 2004;23:571–574. (Ref.25)

Mast EE, et al. Risk factors for perinatal transmission of hepatitis C virus (HCV) and the natural history of HCV infection acquired in infancy. J Infect Dis 2005;192:1880–1889. (Ref.102)

Miras A, Morris K, Soper C. Hepatitis C virus prevalence in children in a highly endemic region of Egypt. Pediatr Infect Dis J 2002;21:987. (Ref.93)

Ozaki Y, et al. Frequent detection of the human herpesvirus 6–specific genomes in the livers of children with various liver diseases. J Clin Microbiol 2001;39: 2173–2177. (Ref.169)

Ozdamar S, Gucer S, Tinaztepe K. Hepatitis-B virus associated nephropathies: a clinicopathological study in 14 children. Pediatr Nephrol 2003;18:23–28. (Ref.38)

Prevention of hepatitis A through active or passive immunization: recommendations of the Advisory Committee on Immunization Practices (ACIP). MMWR Recomm Rep 1999;48:1–37. (Ref.22)

Rehermann B. Immunopathogenesis of hepatitis C. In: Liang T, Hoofnagle J, editors. Hepatitis C. San Diego: Academic Press, 2000: 147–166. (Ref.112)

Resti M, et al. Mother to child transmission of hepatitis C virus: prospective study of risk factors and timing of infection in children born to women seronegative for HIV-1. BMJ 1998;317:437–441. (Ref.100)

Resti M, et al. Clinical features and progression of perinatally acquired hepatitis C virus infection. J Med Virol 2003;70:373–377. (Ref.124)

Schooley R. Epstein-Barr virus (infectious mononucleosis). In: Mandell GL, Bennett JE, Dolin R, editors. Principles and practice of infectious diseases, Philadelphia: Churchill Livingstone, 2000: 1599–1613. (Ref.160)

Schwarz KB, et al. Peginterferon with or without ribavirin for chronic hepatitis C in children and adolescents: final results of the PEDS-C trial [abstract]. Hepatology 2008;48(4 Suppl):418A. (Ref.135)

Sokal EM, et al. Interferon alfa therapy for chronic hepatitis B in children: a multinational randomized controlled trial. Gastroenterology 1998;114:988–995. (Ref.70)

Sokal EM, et al. Long-term lamivudine therapy for children with HBeAg-positive chronic hepatitis B. Hepatology 2006;43:225–232. (Ref.81)

Sokal EM, et al. A dose ranging study of the pharmacokinetics, safety, and preliminary efficacy of lamivudine in children and adolescents with chronic hepatitis B. Antimicrob Agents Chemother 2000;44:590–597. (Ref.78)

Squires RH Jr, et al. Acute liver failure in children: the first 348 patients in the pediatric acute liver failure study group. J Pediatr 2006;148:652–658. (Ref.14)

Strickland D, Jenkins J, Hudson M. Hepatitis C infection and hepatocellular carcinoma after treatment of childhood cancer. J Pediatr Hematol Oncol 2001; 23:527–529. (Ref.131)

Strickland DK, et al. Hepatitis C infection among survivors of childhood cancer. Blood 2000;95:3065–3070. (Ref.123)

Studies of pediatric liver transplantation: 2006 annual report. 2006. (Ref.18)

Symeonidis N, et al. Invasive adenoviral infections in T-cell–depleted allogeneic hematopoietic stem cell transplantation: high mortality in the era of cidofovir. Transpl Infect Dis 2007;9:108–113. (Ref.150)

Vento S, et al. Fulminant hepatitis associated with hepatitis A virus superinfection in patients with chronic hepatitis C. N Engl J Med 1998;338: 286–290. (Ref.17)

Victor JC, et al. Hepatitis A vaccine versus immune globulin for postexposure prophylaxis. N Engl J Med 2007;357:1685–1694. (Ref.21)

Vogt M, et al. Prevalence and clinical outcome of hepatitis C infection in children who underwent cardiac surgery before the implementation of blood-donor screening. N Engl J Med 1999;341:866–870. (Ref.110)

Wai CT, et al. HBV genotype B is associated with better response to interferon therapy in HBeAg(+) chronic hepatitis than genotype C. Hepatology 2002;36:1425–1430. (Ref.65)

Wasley A, et al. Surveillance for acute viral hepatitis—United States, 2006. MMWR Surveill Summ 2008;57(2):1–24. (Ref.3)

Wasley A, Samandari T, Bell BP. Incidence of hepatitis A in the United States in the era of vaccination. JAMA 2005;294:194–201. (Ref.4)

Wen W, et al. The development of hepatocellular carcinoma among prospectively followed children with chronic hepatitis B virus infection. J Pediatr 2004;144: 397–399. (Ref.63)

Wirth S, et al. Peginterferon alfa-2b plus ribavirin treatment in children and adolescents with chronic hepatitis C. Hepatology 2005;41:1013–1018. (Ref.179)

Wirth S, et al. Children with HCV infection show high sustained virologic response rates on peginterferon alfa-2b plus ribavirin treatment [abstract]. Hepatology 2008;48(4 Suppl):392A. (Ref.136)

Yoshikawa T. Human herpesvirus-6 and -7 infections in transplantation. Pediatr Transplant 2003;7:11–17. (Ref.170)

Yuen MF, et al. Twelve-year follow-up of a prospective randomized trial of hepatitis B recombinant DNA yeast vaccine versus plasma-derived vaccine without booster doses in children. Hepatology 1999;29:924–927. (Ref.88)

Yusuf U, et al. Cidofovir for the treatment of adenoviral infection in pediatric hematopoietic stem cell transplant patients. Transplantation 2006;81: 1398–1404. (Ref.152)

A complete list of references can be found at www.expertconsult.com.

Index

Note: Page numbers followed by "b" indicate boxes; those followed by "f" indicate figures; those followed by "t" indicate tables.